Second Edition

DERMATOLOGY

Commissioning Editor: Thu Nguyen
Development Editor: Sven Pinczewski
Editorial Assistant: Kirsten Lowson
Project Manager: Glenys Norquay
Designer: Jayne Jones
Illustration Manager: Bruce Hogarth
Illustrator: Richard Tibbitts
Marketing Manager(s) (UK/USA): Clara Toombs/Todd Liebel

Second Edition

DERMATOLOGY

EDITED BY

Jean L Bolognia MD
Professor of Dermatology
Department of Dermatology
Yale Medical School
New Haven, CT, USA

Joseph L Jorizzo MD
Professor and Former (Founding) Chair
Department of Dermatology
Wake Forest University School of Medicine
Winston-Salem, NC, USA

Ronald P Rapini MD
Professor and Chair
Department of Dermatology
University of Texas Medical School
and MD Anderson Cancer Center
Houston, TX, USA

ASSOCIATE AND ARTWORK EDITOR

Julie V Schaffer MD
Assistant Professor of Dermatology and Pediatrics
Director of Pediatric Dermatology
Department of Dermatology
New York University School of Medicine
New York, NY, USA

SECTION EDITORS

Jeffrey P Callen MD FACP
Professor of Medicine (Dermatology)
Chief, Division of Dermatology
University of Louisville
Louisville, KY, USA

Stuart J Salasche MD
Clinical Professor
University of Arizona Health Sciences Center
Research Scientist
University of Arizona Cancer Center
Tucson, AZ, USA

Mary Seabury Stone MD
Professor of Dermatology and Pathology
Department of Dermatology
University of Iowa
Roy J. and Lucille A. Carver College of Medicine
Iowa City, IA , USA

Thomas D Horn MD MBA
CarisCohenDX
Newton, MA, USA
Consultant Dermatologist
Lahey Clinic
Burlington, MA, USA

Thomas Schwarz MD
Professor and Chairman
Department of Dermatology and Allergology
University Hospital Schleswig-Holstein
Kiel, Germany

Anthony J Mancini MD
Associate Professor of Pediatrics and Dermatology
Northwestern University Feinberg School of Medicine
Head, Division of Pediatric Dermatology
Children's Memorial Hospital
Chicago, IL, USA

Georg Stingl MD
Professor and Chairman
Department of Dermatology
Division of Immunology,
Allergy and Infectious Diseases (DIAID)
University of Vienna Medical School
Vienna, Austria

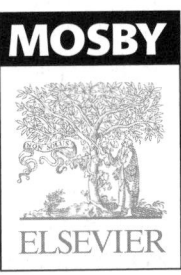

MOSBY

ELSEVIER

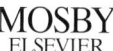

MOSBY
ELSEVIER

An imprint of Elsevier Limited

First published 2003
Reprinted 2003 (twice)
Reprinted 2004
Second edition 2008
Reprinted 2008, 2009

ISBN: 9781416029991
ISBN (E-dition): 9781416032694

British Library Cataloguing in Publication Data
A catalogue record for this book is available from the British Library

Library of Congress Cataloging in Publication Data
A catalog record for this book is available from the Library of Congress

Notice
Medical knowledge is constantly changing. Standard safety precautions must be followed, but as new research and clinical experience broaden our knowledge, changes in treatment and drug therapy may become necessary or appropriate. Readers are advised to check the most current product information provided by the manufacturer of each drug to be administered to verify the recommended dose, the method and duration of administration, and contraindications. It is the responsibility of the practitioner, relying on experience and knowledge of the patient, to determine dosages and the best treatment for each individual patient. Neither the Publisher nor the authors assume any liability for any injury and/or damage to persons or property arising from this publication.

The Publisher

Printed in Spain
Last digit is the print number: 9 8 7 6 5 4 3

Contents

Preface

The practice of dermatology is based upon a visual approach to clinical disease, with the development of an appreciation of recurrent patterns and images. The entire spectrum of our discipline, from the generation of clinicopathologic differential diagnoses to the orientation of rotational flaps, relies upon imagery. As a result, visualization also plays a critical role in how we integrate new information into pre-existing frameworks that serve as the hard drives of our medical memory.

In the textbook *Dermatology* there is a strong emphasis on visual learning. This commitment is reflected in the use of schematic diagrams to convey the principles of skin biology as well as cutaneous surgery, and the inclusion of algorithms, which provide a logical as well as practical approach to commonly encountered clinical problems. The majority of the basic science is integrated throughout the book and appears as introductory chapters to the various sections. All illustrations and graphics are in color and photomicrographs demonstrating key histologic findings are found interspersed within the clinical chapters. These chapters also contain tables that attempt to provide weighted differential diagnoses and a 'ladder' approach to therapeutic interventions. Lastly, color-coding of sections allows easy and rapid access to required information.

The ultimate goal of *Dermatology* is for it to never make its way to the bookshelf because it is being used on a weekly, or perhaps even daily, basis. Hopefully, this book will function as a colleague, albeit a non-verbal one, who is easily approachable and possesses the necessary expertise to provide succinct, up-to-date information that is both precise and practical. Realizing this goal required the time and energy of our contributors who have unselfishly shared their knowledge and experience with literally thousands of patients from around the world, and we thank them.

JB, JJ and RR
2008

List of Contributors

MA Abdallah MD
Professor of Dermatology and
Sexually Transmitted Diseases
Faculty of Medicine
Ayn Shams University
Cairo, Egypt

Sandra Albert MBBS MD DNB
Visiting Fellow
St John's Institute of Dermatology
St Thomas' Hospital
London, United Kingdom

**Macrene R Alexiades-Armenakas
MD PhD PC**
Director
Dermatology and Laser Surgery
New York, NY, USA

Carl M Allen MD
Associate Professor of Pathology
Section of Oral and Maxillofacial
Surgery and Pathology
College of Dentistry
The Ohio State University
Columbus, OH, USA

David M Allen MD
Assistant Clinical Professor
Department of Dermatology
University of Utah
Ogden, UT, USA

Masayuki Amagai MD PhD
Professor and Chair
Department of Dermatology
Keio University School of Medicine
Tokyo, Japan

R Rox Anderson MD
Professor of Dermatology
Harvard Medical School
Wellman Center for Photomedicine
Massachusetts General Hospital
Boston, MA, USA

Richard Antaya MD
Director, Pediatric Dermatology
Department of Dermatology
Yale University School of Medicine
New Haven, CT, USA

Zsolt B Argenyi MD
Director of Dermatopathology
Professor of Dermatology and
Pathology
Department of Pathology
University of Washington Medical
Center
Seattle, WA, USA

Meral J Arin MD
Assistant Professor
Department of Dermatology
University of Cologne
Cologne, Germany

Kenneth A Arndt MD
Clinical Professor of Dermatology
Yale University School of Medicine
SkinCare Physicians of Chestnut Hill
Chestnut Hill, MA, USA

Anna Asplund PhD
Doctor of Pathology
Department of Genetics and
Pathology
Uppsala University Hospital
Uppsala, Sweden

Chalid Assaf MD
Associate Professor of Dermatology
Department of Dermatology and
Allergy
Berlin-Charité – Universitätsmedizin
Berlin
Berlin, Germany

Alison Sharpe Avram MD
Clinical Instructor
Harvard Medical School
Department of Dermatology
Massachusetts General Hospital
Boston, MA, USA

Mathew Avram MD JD
Director
Massachusetts General Hospital
Dermatology
Laser and Cosmetic Center
Department of Dermatology
Massachusetts General Hospital
Boston, MA, USA

Christopher Baker MBBS FACD
Clinical Associate Professor of
Dermatology
Department of Dermatology
University of Melbourne
St Vincent's Hospital Melbourne
Fitzroy, VIC, Australia

Raymond L Barnhill MD
Clinical Professor of Dermatology
and Pathology
University of Miami
Coral Gables, FL, USA

Terry L Barrett MD
Clinical Professor of Pathology and
Dermatology
University of Texas Southwestern
Medical Center
Dallas, TX, USA

Susan J Bayliss MD
Professor of Internal Medicine
(Dermatology) and Pediatrics
St Louis Children's Hospital
St Louis, MO, USA

Paul R Bergstresser MD
Professor and Chair
Department of Dermatology
UT Southwestern Medical Center at
Dallas
Dallas, TX, USA

Philippe Bernard MD
Professor
Department of Dermatology
Hospital Robert Debre
Reims, France

Jeffrey D Bernhard MD
Professor of Medicine
University of Massachusetts
Medical School
Worcester, MA, USA

Sachin S Bhardwaj MD
University of Minnesota
Minneapolis, MN, USA

Anne Kobza Black MD FRCP
The St John's Dermatology Center
St Thomas' Hospital
London, United Kingdom

Martin M Black MD FRCP FRCPath
Emeritus Professor of
Dermatological Immunopathology
and Honorary Consultant
Dermatologist
St John's Institute of Dermatology
St Thomas Hospital
London, United Kingdom

Jean L Bolognia MD
Professor of Dermatology
Department of Dermatology
Yale Medical School
New Haven, CT, USA

Luca Borradori MD
Associate Professor
Head of the Outpatient Unit
Dermatology Clinic
University Hospital
Geneva, Switzerland

Julie Brantley MD
Resident
Department of Dermatology
University of Texas Medical Branch
Galveston, TX, USA

David G Brodland MD
Private Practice
Assistant Clinical Professor
Departments of Dermatology and
Otolaryngology
University of Pittsburgh
Clairton, PA, USA

Leena Bruckner-Tuderman MD
Professor of Dermatology
Department of Dermatology
University Medical Center
University of Freiburg
Freiburg, Germany

Craig G Burkhart MD MPH
Clinical Professor
University of Toledo College of
Medicine
Toledo, OH, USA

Craig N Burkhart MD MSBS
Pediatric Dermatologist
Department of Dermatology
Northwestern University
Chicago, IL, USA

Barbara K Burton MD
Professor of Pediatrics
Northwestern University Medical
School
Division of Genetics
Children's Memorial Hospital
Chicago, IL, USA

Claude S Burton MD
Associate Professor of Medicine
Duke University Medical Center
Durham, NC, USA

Jeffrey P Callen MD FACP
Professor of Medicine
(Dermatology)
Chief, Division of Dermatology
University of Louisville School of
Medicine
Louisville, KY, USA

**Francisco M Camacho-Martínez
MD PhD**
Head Professor of Dermatology
Department of Dermatology
School of Medicine
University of Seville
Seville, Spain

Charles Camisa MD
Affiliate Associate Professor
Department of Dermatology and
Cutaneous Surgery
University of South Florida, Tampa
Senior Staff Dermatologist
Department of Dermatology
Cleveland Clinic Foundation
Naples, FL, USA

Daniel Carrasco MD
Postdoctoral Fellow
Departments of Dermatology,
Microbiology, Immunology and
Internal Medicine
University of Texas Medical Branch
at Galveston
Galveston, TX, USA

Christie L Carroll MD
Department of Dermatology
Wake Forest University
Winston-Salem, NC, USA

Alastair Carruthers FRCPC
Clinical Professor
Department of Dermatology and
Skin Science
University of British Columbia
Vancouver, BC, Canada

**Jean Carruthers MD FRCSC
FRC(Ophth) FASOPRS**
Clinical Professor
Department of Ophthalmology and
Visual Sciences
University of British Columbia
Vancouver, BC, Canada

John Carucci MD
Assistant Professor and Chief
Mohs Micrographic and
Dermatologic Surgery
Weill Medical College of Cornell
University
New York, NY, USA

Lorenzo Cerroni MD
Associate Professor of
Dermatology
Department of Dermatology
Medical University of Graz
Graz, Austria

Mary Wu Chang MD
Associate Clinical Professor
Dermatology and Pediatrics
University of Connecticut School
of Medicine
Farmington, CT, USA

Mark A Chastain MD
Clinical Assistant Professor
Department of Dermatology
Emory University
Clinical Assistant Professor
Department of Dermatology
Tulane University School of
Medicine
Atlanta, GA, USA

Suephy Chen MD
Assistant Professor
Department of Dermatology
Emory University
Department of HRS+D
Division of Dermatology
Atlanta, GA, USA

T Minsue Chen MD
Mohs Research in Advanced
Dermatologic Surgery Education
Fellow
Department of Dermatology
University of Texas – MD Anderson
Cancer Center
Houston, TX, USA

Angela M Christiano PhD
Associate Professor
Departments of Dermatology/
Genetics & Development
Columbia University
College of Physicians & Surgeons
New York, NY, USA

David H Chu MD PhD
Visiting Fellow
The Rockefeller University
New York, NY, USA

Lorinda S Chung MD
Department of Medicine –
Immunology and Rheumatology
and Center for Clinical
Immunology
Stanford School of Medicine
Stanford, CA, USA

Anna S Clayton MD
Assistant Professor
Division of Dermatology and
Cutaneous Surgery
University of Texas Health Science
Center at San Antonio
San Antonio, TX, USA

Clay J Cockerell MD
Clinical Professor
Department of Dermatology and
Pathology
University of Texas Southwestern
Medical Center
Cockerell and Associates
Dallas, TX, USA

Bernard A Cohen MD
Department of Pediatric
Dermatology
Johns Hopkins University School of
Medicine
Baltimore, MD, USA

David E Cohen MD
Assistant Professor of Dermatology
New York University
Hewlett, NY, USA

William P Coleman III MD
Clinical Professor of Dermatology
Adjunct Professor of Surgery
(Plastic Surgery)
Tulane University Health Sciences
Center
New Orleans, LA, USA

M Kari Connolly MD
Professor of Dermatology and
Medicine
Department of Dermatology
University of California San Francisco
San Francisco, CA, USA

Susan M Cooper MD MRCP
Consultant Dermatologist
Department of Dermatology
Churchill Hospital
Oxford, United Kingdom

Kevin D Cooper MD
Professor and Chair
Department of Dermatology
Director
Skin Diseases Research Center
University Hospitals of Cleveland
and Case Western Reserve
University
Cleveland, OH, USA

Melissa I Costner MD
Assistant Professor
Dermatology
University of Texas Southwestern
Medical Center at Dallas
Dallas, TX, USA

Thomas N Darling MD PhD
Associate Professor of Dermatology
Department of Dermatology
Uniformed Services University of
the Health Sciences
Bethesda, MD, USA

Marc Darst MD
Resident
Division of Dermatology
Wright State University School of
Medicine
Dayton, OH, USA

Daniel Davis MD
Assistant Professor of Dermatology
and Pathology
Department of Dermatology
University of Arkansas for the
Medical Sciences
Little Rock, AR, USA

Mark DP Davis MD
Professor of Dermatology
Department of Dermatology
Mayo Clinic
Rochester, MN, USA

Aerlyn G Dawn MD
Research Fellow
Department of Dermatology
Wake Forest University School of
Medicine
Winston-Salem, NC, USA

Vincent A Deleo MD
Chairman
Department of Dermatology
St Luke's Roosevelt Hospital Center
and Beth Israel Medical Center
New York, NY, USA

Michael Detmar MD
Professor of Pharmacogenomics
Institute of Pharmaceutical Sciences
Zurich, Switzerland

Thomas L Diepgen MD
Professor
Department of Social Medicine,
Occupational and Environmental
Dermatology
University of Heidelberg
Heidelberg, Germany

A Cigdem Atahan Dogramaci MD
Assistant Professor
Department of Dermatology
Mustafa Kemal University Faculty of
Medicine
Hatay, Turkey

Jeffrey S Dover MD FRCPC
Associate Professor of Clinical
Dermatology
Yale University School of Medicine
Adjunct Professor of Medicine
(Dermatology)
Dartmouth Medical School
SkinCare Physicians of Chestnut Hill
Chestnut Hill, MA, USA

Zoe Diana Draelos MD
Dermatology Consulting Services
High Point, NC, USA

Raymond G Dufresne Jr MD
Associate Professor of Dermatology
University Dermatology, Inc.
Rhode Island Hospital
Providence, RI, USA

Boni E Elewski MD
Professor of Dermatology
Department of Dermatology
University of Alabama at
Birmingham
Birmingham, AL, USA

George Elgart MD
Dermatologist
Department of Dermatology
University of Miami School of
Medicine
Miami, FL, USA

Peter M Elias MD
Senate Emeritus
S/M Dermatology Service
University of California San
Francisco
Veteran Affairs Medical Center
San Francisco, CA, USA

Dirk M Elston MD
Chairman
Department of Dermatology
Geisinger Medical Center
Danville, PA, USA

Odile Enjolras MD
Director
Multidisciplinary Clinics for
Pediatric Vascular Anomalies
Department of Maxillo-facial and
Plastic Surgery
Armand-Trousseau Children's
Hospital
Paris, France

Vaishali Escaravage MD
Clinical Research Fellow
Wound Management Institute
Duke University Medical Center
Durham, NC, USA

Augustin España MD
Professor of Dermatology
Department of Dermatology
University Clinic of Navarra
School of Medicine
Pamplona, Spain

Janet A Fairley MD
Professor and Head of Dermatology
Department of Dermatology
University of Iowa Hospitals and
Clinics
Iowa City, IA, USA

Kenneth R Feingold MD
Department of Dermatology and
Medicine
University of California San
Francisco
Dermatology and Medical
(Metabolism) Services
Veterans Affairs Medical Center
San Francisco, CA, USA

Jo-David Fine MD MPH FRCP
Professor of Medicine
(Dermatology) and Pediatrics
Vanderbilt University School of
Medicine
Head, National Epidermolysis
Bullosa Registry
Nashville, TN, USA

David F Fiorentino MD PhD
Professor of Dermatology
Assistant Professor of Medicine
(Rheumatology)
Department of Dermatology
Stanford University School of
Medicine
Palo Alto, CA, USA

Alan B Fleischer Jr MD
Professor, Chair
Director of the General
Dermatology Clinic
Wake Forest University School of
Medicine
Winston-Salem, NC, USA

Franklin P Flowers MD
Professor of Dermatology
Division of Dermatology &
Cutaneous Surgery
University of Florida College of
Medicine
Gainesville, FL, USA

xi

Timothy Corcoran Flynn MD
Clinical Professor
Department of Dermatology
Cary Skin Center
Cary, NC, USA

Jorge Frank MD
Professor of Dermatology
Department of Dermatology
Academic Hospital Maastricht
Maastricht, The Netherlands

Ingolf Franke MD
Department of Dermatology and
Venerology
Otto-von-Guericke University
Magdeburg, Germany

Thomas J Franz MD
Executive Medical Director
PRACS Institute, Ltd
Portland, OR, USA

Lars E French MD
Professor of Dermatology,
Chairman
Department of Dermatology
Zurich University Hospital
Zurich, Switzerland

Ilona J Frieden MD
Professor of Clinical Dermatology
and Pediatrics
Department of Dermatology
University of California San
Francisco
San Francisco, CA, USA

Peter S Friedmann MD
Professor of Dermatology
University of Southampton
Dermatopharmacology Unit
Southampton General Hospital
Southampton, United Kingdom

Peter O Fritsch MD
Chairman, Professor of
Dermatology
Department of Dermatology
Innsbruck Medical University
Innsbruck, Austria

Maria C Garzon MD
Associate Professor of Clinical
Dermatology and Clinical
Pediatrics
Department of Dermatology
Columbia University
New York, NY, USA

Amy Geng MD
University Dermatology, Inc.
Rhode Island Hospital
Providence, RI, USA

Kamran Ghoreschi MD
Senior Fellow
Department of Dermatology
Eberhard Karls University of
Tübingen
Tübingen, Germany

Amy E Gilliam MD
Assistant Professor of Dermatology
and Pediatrics
Department of Dermatology
University of California at San
Francisco
San Francisco, CA, USA

Richard G Glogau MD
Clinical Professor
Department of Dermatology
University of California, San
Francisco
San Francisco, CA, USA

Glenn Goldman MD
Associate Professor of Medicine
and Dermatology
Director of Dermatologic Surgery
Division of Dermatology
The University of Vermont
Fletcher Allen Health Care
Burlington, VT, USA

Mitchel P Goldman MD
Volunteer Clinical Professor of
Dermatology/Medicine
University of California, San Diego
Medical Director
La Jolla Spa MD
La Jolla, CA, USA

Harald Gollnick MD
Department of Dermatology and
Venerology
Otto-von-Guericke University
Magdeburg, Germany

Warren T Goodman MD
HealthPartners Medical Group
Departments of Dermatology and
Pathology
Assistant Professor of Laboratory
Medicine and Pathology
University of Minnesota
St Paul, MN, USA

Clive E H Grattan MA MD FRCP
Consultant Dermatologist
Dermatology Centre
Norfolk and Norwich University
Hospital
Norwich, United Kingdom

Malcolm W Greaves MD PhD FRCP
Emeritus Professor of Dermatology
St Johns Institute of Dermatology
St Thomas' Hospital
London Allergy Centre
London, United Kingdom

Daniela Guzman Sanchez MD
Research Fellow
Department of Dermatology
Wake Forest University Baptist
Medical Center
Winston Salem, NC, USA

Allan C Halpern MD MS
Chief, Dermatology Service
Member, Department of Medicine
Memorial Sloan-Kettering Cancer
Center
New York, NY, USA

Analisa Vincent Halpern MD
Assistant Professor of Medicine
Division of Dermatology
Cooper University Hospital
UMDNJ Robert Wood Johnson
Cooper Hospital
Camden, NJ, USA

John LM Hawk BSc MD FRCP
Head of Medicine and Pediatrics
Division of Dermatology
UMDNJ-Robert Wood Johnson
Marlton, NJ, USA

Warren R Heymann MD
Clinical Associate Professor
UPenn School of Medicine
Professor of Medicine
Head, Division of Dermatology
University of Medicine and
Dentistry of New Jersey
Marlton, NJ, USA

Satoshi Hirakawa MD PhD
Assistant Professor of Dermatology
Department of Dermatology
Ehime University Graduate School
of Medicine
Toon-shi, Ehime, Japan

Ranella J Hirsch MD FAAD
Director
Skincare Doctors
Cambridge, MA, USA

Herbert Hönigsmann MD
Professor of Dermatology
Division of Special & Environmental
Dermatology
University of Vienna Medical
School
Vienna, Austria

Daniel Hohl MD
Professor of Medicine
CHUV Department of Dermatology
Beaumont Hospital
Lausanne, Switzerland

Walter M Holleran MD
Department of Dermatology and
Medicine
University of California San
Francisco
Dermatology and Medical
(Metabolism) Services
Veterans Affairs Medical Center
San Francisco, CA, USA

Thomas D Horn MD MBA
CarisCohenDX
Newton, MA, USA

Amy Howard MD
Assistant Professor of Dermatology
and Pathology
Emory University School of
Medicine
Atlanta, GA, USA

George J Hruza MD
Clinical Associate Professor of
Dermatology and Otolaryngology
St Louis University
Director, Laser and Dermatologic
Surgery Center
St Louis, MO, USA

Christopher M Hull MD
Assistant Professor of
Dermatology
Department of Dermatology
University of Utah Health Sciences
Center
Salt Lake City, UT, USA

Harry J Hurley Jr MD
Clinical Professor of Dermatology
University of Pennsylvania School
of Medicine
Upper Darby, PA, USA

Heidi T Jacobe MD
Chief Resident
Department of Dermatology
The University of Texas
Southwestern Medical Center
Dallas, TX, USA

Joseph L Jorizzo MD
Professor and Former (Founding)
Chair
Department of Dermatology
Wake Forest University School of
Medicine
Winston-Salem, NC, USA

Jacqueline M Junkins-Hopkins MD
Associate Professor of
Dermatology
Department of Dermatology
University of Pennsylvania
Philadelphia, PA, USA

Hideko Kamino MD
Director of Dermatopathology
Dermatopathology Section
New York University School of
Medicine
New York, NY, USA

Kefei Kang MD
Associate Professor
Department of Dermatology
University Hospitals of Cleveland
Case Western Reserve University
Cleveland, OH, USA

Yoko Kano MD
Associate Professor
Department of Dermatology
Kyorin University School of Medicine
Tokyo, Japan

Bory Kea BS BA
Medical Student
School of Medicine
Stanford University
Stanford, CA, USA

Paul Kelly MD
Professor and Chief
Division of Dermatology
King/Drew Medical Center
Los Angeles, CA, USA

Robert Kelly MBBS FACD
Consultant Dermatologist
St Vincent's Hospital
Melbourne, VIC, Australia

Jay Kincannon MD
Department of Dermatology
University of Arkansas for Medical
Sciences, Child Study Center
Little Rock, AR, USA

Reinhard Kirnbauer MD
Professor of Dermatology
Division of Immunology, Allergy and
Infectious Disease (DIAID)
Department of Dermatology
Medical University of Vienna
Vienna, Austria

Robert S Kirsner MD
Associate Professor
Department of Dermatology and
Cutaneous Surgery
Department of Epidemiology and
Public Health
University of Miami School of
Medicine
Miami, FL, USA

Sandra R Knowles BScPhm
Lecturer, Faculty of Pharmacy
Sunnybrook Health Sciences Centre
University of Toronto
Toronto, ON, Canada

Peter J Koch PhD
Associate Professor of
Dermatology
Department of Dermatology
University of Colorado at Denver
and Health Sciences Center
Aurora, CO, USA

Sabine Kohler MD
Professor of Pathology and
Dermatology
Director of Dermatopathology
Department of Pathology
Stanford University School of
Medicine
Stanford, CA, USA

John Koo MD
Professor and Vice Chairman
Department of Dermatology
Director, UCSF Psoriasis Treatment
Center
University of California San
Francisco Medical Center
San Francisco, CA, USA

Tamara Koss MD
Instructor in Clinical Dermatology
Columbia University
New York, NY, USA

Maranke I Koster PhD
Assistant Professor of Dermatology
Department of Dermatology
University of Colorado at Denver
and Health Sciences Center
Aurora, CO, USA

Alfons L Krol MD FRCPC
Professor of Dermatology &
Pediatrics
Oregon Health and Sciences
University
Portland, OR, USA

Stéphane Kuenzli MD
Consultant Dermatologist
Department of Dermatology
Geneva University Hospital
Fribourg, Switzerland

Emanuel G Kuflik MD
Clinical Professor of Dermatology
UMDNJ – New Jersey Medical
School
Newark, NJ, USA

Fiona Larsen MD FRACP
Dermatopathology Fellow
Department of Dermatology
University of Texas Southwestern
Medical Center
Dallas, TX, USA

Mark Lebwohl MD
Professor and Chairman
Department of Dermatology
The Mount Sinai School of
Medicine
New York, NY, USA

Lela A Lee MD
Professor of Dermatology and
Medicine
University of Colorado School of
Medicine
Chief of Dermatology
Denver Health Medical Center
Denver, CO, USA

Chai Sue Lee MD MS
Assistant Professor of Dermatology
Department of Dermatology
University of California Davis
School of Medicine
Sacramento, CA, USA

Kristin M Leiferman MD
Professor of Dermatology
Department of Dermatology
University of Utah School of
Medicine
Salt Lake City, UT, USA

Petra Lenz MD
Clinical Fellow
Laboratory of Pathology
NIH National Cancer Institute
Bethesda, MD, USA

Jack Lesher MD
Professor and Chief
Division of Dermatology
Medical College of Georgia
Augusta, GA, USA

Henry W Lim MD
Chairman and C. S. Livingood Chair
Department of Dermatology
Henry Ford Medical Center
Detroit, MI, USA

Cynthia A Loomis MD PhD
Assistant Professor of Dermatology
and Cell Biology
New York University School of
Medicine
Department of Pathology
New York, NY, USA

Joakim Lundeberg PhD
Professor of Molecular Biology
Royal Institute of Technology
Department of Gene Technology
AlbaNova University Center
Stockholm, Sweden

Omar Lupi MD Msc PhD
Adjunct Professor of Dermatology
Federal University of Rio de Janeiro
Professor of Dermatology
Postgraduate Course of
Dermatology
Institute of Dermatology Prof.
Azulay/SCMRJ, PGRJ and UFRJ
Rio de Janeiro, Brazil

Catherine Maari MD
Fellow
Department of Dermatology
Children's Hospital and Health
Center
San Diego, CA, USA

Vandana Madkan MD
Clinical Research Fellow
Center for Clinical Studies, Texas
Houston, TX, USA

Anthony J Mancini MD
Associate Professor of Pediatrics &
Dermatology
Head, Division of Pediatric
Dermatology
Northwestern University Feinberg
School of Medicine
Children's Memorial Hospital
Chicago, IL, USA

James G Marks Jr MD
Professor of Medicine
Department of Dermatology
Milton S Hershey Medical Center
Hershey, PA, USA

Amalia Martínez-Mir PhD
Research Scientist
Department of Medical
Biochemistry and Molecular
Biology
Faculty of Medicine
University of Seville
Seville, Spain

José M Mascaró Jr MD MS
Associate Professor
Department of Dermatology
Hospital Clinic and Barcelona
University Medical School
Barcelona, Spain

W Trent Massengale MD
Assistant Clinical Professor
Department of Dermatology
Louisiana State University
Baton Rouge, LA, USA

Seth L Matarasso MD
Clinical Professor of Dermatology
University College School of
Medicine
San Francisco, CA, USA

Theodora Mauro MD
Associate Professor of Dermatology
University of California San
Francisco
Chief, Dermatology Service
San Francisco Veterans' Hospital
San Francisco, CA, USA

Timothy H McCalmont MD
Professor of Clinical Pathology
Co-Director
UCSF Dermatopathology Service
Departments of Pathology and
Dermatology
Mount Zion Medical Center
University of California at San
Francisco
San Francisco, CA, USA

Thomas W McGovern MD
Private Practice of Dermatology
and Mohs Surgery
Fort Wayne Dermatology
Fort Wayne, IN, USA

Amy McMichael MD
Associate Professor of Dermatology
Department of Dermatology
Wake Forest University School of
Medicine
Winston-Salem, NC, USA

Shane Meehan MD
Associate Director of
Dermatopathology
Assistant Professor of Dermatology
& Pathology
Dermatopathology Section
New York University School of
Medicine
New York, NY, USA

Stephanie Mehlis MD
Director, Clinical Research
Evanston Northwestern Healthcare
Division of Dermatology
Skokie, IL, USA

Terri L Meinking PhD
President
Global Health Associates of Miami
Miami, FL, USA

Gregg M Menaker MD
Assistant Professor of Dermatology
Northwestern University Feinberg
School of Medicine
Director, Dermatologic Surgery
Evanston Northwestern Healthcare
Skokie, IL, USA

Natalia Mendoza MD Msc
Assistant Professor
Department of Dermatology
El Bosque University
Bogotá, Columbia
Center for Clinical Studies
Houston, TX, USA

Gopinathan K Menon PhD
Senior Research Fellow
Head, Skin Biology Research
Global Research & Development
Department
Avon Products, Inc.
Suffern, NY, USA

Jami L Miller MD
Assistant Professor
Division of Dermatology
Vanderbilt University Medical
Center
Nashville, TN, USA

Gary D Monheit MD
Associate Professor
Department of Dermatology
University of Alabama at
Birmingham Medical Center
Birmingham, AL, USA

Samuel L Moschella MD
Clinical Professor Harvard Medical
School
Senior Consultant
Lahey Clinic Foundation
Burlington, MA, USA

Celia Moss DM FRCP MRCPCH
Consultant Dermatologist
Department of Dermatology
Birmingham Children's Hospital
Birmingham, United Kingdom

Christen M Mowad MD
Associate Professor
Department of Dermatology
Geisinger Medical Center
Danville, PA, USA

xiii

Susan T Nedorost MD
Assistant Professor of Dermatology
Lakeside Department of
Dermatology
Case Western Reserve University
Cleveland, OH, USA

Lee T Nesbitt Jr MD
Henry Jolly Professor and Head of
Dermatology
Department of Dermatology
Louisiana State University Health
Sciences Center
New Orleans, LA, USA

Frank O Nestle MD
Mary Dunhill Chair of Cutaneous
Medicine and Immunotherapy
St John's Institute of Dermatology
Division of Genetics and Molecular
Medicine
King's College London School of
Medicine at Guy's
King's College & St Thomas'
Hospitals
London, United Kingdom

Paula E North MD PhD
Professor and Chief of Pediatric
Pathology
Department of Dermatology
Medical College of Wisconsin
Milwaukee, WI, USA

Carlos H Nousari MD
Director
Institute for Immunofluorescence
Dermpath Diagnostics
Weston, FL, USA

Julia R Nunley MD
Professor
Department of Dermatology
Virginia Commonwealth University
Richmond, VA, USA

Martin M Okun MD PhD
Associate Medical Director
Abbott Immunology
Dean Medical Center
Abbott Park, IL, USA

Suzanne Olbricht MD
Associate Professor of Dermatology
Harvard Medical School
Chair, Department of Dermatology
Lahey Clinic
Burlington, MA, USA

Seth J Orlow MD PhD
Professor of Dermatology, Cell
Biology and Pediatrics
Department of Dermatology
New York University Medical Center
New York, NY, USA

Luz Orozco-Covarrubias MD
Associate Professor of Pediatric
Dermatology
Department of Dermatology
National Institute of Pediatrics
Mexico City, Mexico

Jean-Paul Ortonne MD
Professor and Chairman
Department of Dermatology
Hôpital l'Archet
Nice, France

Clark C Otley MD
Associate Professor of Dermatology
Mayo Clinic and Mayo Medical
School
Chair, Division of Dermatologic
Surgery
Mayo Clinic
Rochester, MN, USA

Amy S Paller MD
Professor and Chair
Department of Dermatology
Children's Memorial Hospital
Chicago, IL, USA

James W Patterson MD
Professor and Director of
Dermatopathology
University of Virginia Medical
Center
Charlottesville, VA, USA

Michèle Pauporté MD
Dermatologist
University of California San
Francisco
San Francisco, CA, USA

Ralf Paus MD
Department of Dermatology
University Hospital Schleswig-
Holstein
Campus Lübeck
University of Lübeck
Lübeck, Germany

Stefan Peker MD
Department of Dermatology
University Hospital Schleswig-
Holstein
Campus Lübeck
University of Lübeck
Lübeck, Germany

Donna Pellowski MD
Assistant Professor of Dermatology
and Internal Medicine
Department of Dermatology
University of Arkansas for the
Medical Sciences
Little Rock, AR, USA

David Pharis MD
Private Practice
Georgia Dermatology Surgery
Center
Atlanta, GA, USA

Tania Phillips MD FRCPC
Professor of Dermatology
Dermatology Department
Boston University School of
Medicine
Boston, MA, USA

Warren Piette MD
Department of Dermatology
John H Stroger Hospital of Cook
County
Chicago, IL, USA

Bianca Maria Piraccini MD PhD
PhD in Dermatology
Department of Dermatology
University of Bologna
Bologna, Italy

Gerd Plewig MD
Chairman and Professor of
Dermatology
Clinic and Policlinic for
Dermatology and Allergology
Munich, Germany

Pamela Poblete-Gutiérrez MD
Dermatologist
Madrid, Spain

Sheldon V Pollack MD
Associate Professor of Medicine
(Dermatology)
Faculty of Medicine
University of Toronto
Toronto, ON, Canada

Amy M Polster MD
Associate Staff
Department of Dermatology
Cleveland Clinic
Cleveland, OH, USA

Fredrik Pontén MD
Associate Professor of Pathology
Department of Genetics and
Pathology
Uppsala University Hospital
Uppsala, Sweden

Julie Powell MD FRCPC ABD
Clinical Associate Professor of
Pediatrics / Dermatology
Department of Dermatology
Sainte-Justine Hospital
Montreal, QC, Canada

Christa Prins MD
Department of Dermatology
Geneva University Hospital
Geneva, Switzerland

John Pui MD
Dermatopathology
New York University Medical
Center
New York, NY, USA

Harold Rabinovitz MD
Plantation, FL, USA

Ben G Raimer MD
Professor of Pediatrics
University of Texas Medical Branch
Galveston, TX, USA

Sharon S Raimer MD
Professor and Chair of
Dermatology
Department of Dermatology
University of Texas Medical Branch
Galveston, TX, USA

Marcia Ramos-e-Silva MD PhD
Associate Professor and Head of
Dermatology
Clemente Fraga Filho University
Hospital
Federal University of Rio de Janeiro
Rio de Janeiro, Brazil

Ronald P Rapini MD
Professor and Chair
Department of Dermatology
University of Texas Medical School
and MD Anderson Cancer Center
Houston, TX, USA

Désirée Ratner MD
George Henry Fox Associate Clinical
Professor of Dermatology
Director of Dermatologic Surgery
Department of Dermatology
Columbia University Medical
Center
New York, NY, USA

Alfredo Rebora MD
Professor and Chairman
Dermatology Clinic
University of Genoa
Genoa, Italy

Norbert Reider MD
Professor of Dermatology
Department of Dermatology
University of Innsbruck
Innsbruck, Austria

George T Reizner MD
Professor of Dermatology
Department of Dermatology
University of Wisconsin
Madison, WI, USA

Adrienne Rencic MD PhD
Division of Immunodermatology
Johns Hopkins Medical Institutions
Baltimore, MD, USA

Jean Revuz MD
Professor of Dermatology
Chairman, Department of
Dermatology
Hospital Henri Mondor
University of Paris XII
Creteil, France

**Maria Cristina Ribeiro de Castro
MD MS**
Dermatologist
Sector of Dermatology and Post
Graduation Course
Federal University of Rio de Janeiro
Rio de Janeiro, Brazil

Phoebe Rich MD
Associate Professor of
Dermatology
University of Oregon
Portland, OR, USA

Gabriele Richard MD
Associate Clinical Director
GeneDx
Adjunct Associate Professor of
Dermatology
Thomas Jefferson University
Philadelphia
Gaithersburg, MD, USA

Shawn Richards MD
Consultant Dermatologist
Skin and Cancer Foundation
Westmead, NSW, Australia

Darrell S Rigel MD
Clinical Professor of Dermatology
New York University Medical Center
Rigel Dermatology
New York, NY, USA

Armin Rieger MD
University Clinic for Dermatology
Medical University Vienna
Vienna, Austria

Franziska Ringpfeil MD
Assistant Professor of Dermatology
Department of Dermatology
Jefferson Medical College
Jefferson University
Philadelphia, PA, USA

Martin Röcken MD
Professor and Chairman
Department of Dermatology
Eberhard Karls University of
Tübingen
Tübingen, Germany

Randall K Roenigk MD
Professor and Chair
Department of Dermatology
Mayo Clinic
Rochester, MN, USA

Franco Rongioletti MD
Associate Professor of Dermatology
Dermatology Clinic
University of Genoa
Genoa, Italy

Dennis R Roop PhD
Professor of Dermatology
Department of Dermatology
Director of Degenerative Medicine
and Stem Cell Biology
University of Colorado Denver and
Health Sciences Center
Aurora, CO, USA

Ramón Ruiz-Maldonado MD
Professor of Dermatology and
Pediatric Dermatology
Department of Dermatology
National Institute of Pediatrics
Mexico City, Mexico

Thomas M Rünger MD PhD
Professor of Dermatology,
Pathology and Laboratory Medicine
Department of Dermatology
Boston University School of
Medicine
Boston, MA, USA

Neil S Sadick MD FACP FAACS
Clinical Professor of Dermatology
Cornell University Medical College
New York, NY, USA

Miguel Sanchez MD
Associate Professor of Clinical
Dermatology
Department of Dermatology
New York University Medical Center
New York, NY, USA

Omar P Sangueza MD
Professor of Dermatology and
Pathology
Department of Pathology
Wake Forest University School of
Medicine
Winston-Salem, NC, USA

Jean-Hilaire Saurat MD
Professor of Medicine, Dermatology
University Hospitals of Geneva
Geneva, Switzerland

Julie V Schaffer MD
Associate Professor of Dermatology
Department of Dermatology
New York University
New York, NY, USA

Joost Schalkwijk MD
Professor of Experimental
Dermatology
Nijmegen, The Netherlands

Martin Schaller MD PhD
Professor of Dermatology
Assistant Medical Director of
Dermatology
Department of Dermatology
University of Tübingen
Tübingen, Germany

Thomas Schwarz MD
Professor and Chairman
Department of Dermatology and
Allergology
University Hospital Schleswig
Holstein
Kiel, Germany

**David Julian Seager MD MBBS
ABHRS**
Director
Seager Hair Transplant Center
The Court at Centenary Hospital
Toronto, ON, Canada

Ayelet Shani-Adir MD
Pediatric Dermatologist
Department of Dermatology
Haemek Medical Center
Afula, Israel

Lori E Shapiro MD FRCPC
Assistant Professor of Dermatology
Sunnybrook Dermatology
University of Toronto
Toronto, ON, Canada

Neil H Shear MD FRCP FACP
Professor and Chief of
Dermatology
Sunnybrook Dermatology
University of Toronto
Toronto, ON, Canada

Tetsuo Shiohara MD PhD
Professor and Chairman
Department of Dermatology
Kyorin University School of
Medicine
Tokyo, Japan

Jeff K Shornick MD MHA
Private Practice
Groton, CT, USA

Michael L Smith MD
Division of Dermatology
Vanderbilt Medical Center
Nashville, TN, USA

Bruce R Smoller MD
Professor and Chair
Department of Pathology
University of Arkansas Medical
Sciences
Little Rock, AR, USA

Jenny O Sobera MD
Department of Dermatology
University of Alabama at
Birmingham
Eye Foundation Hospital
Birmingham, AL, USA

Richard D Sontheimer MD
Professor & Vice-Chairman
Department of Dermatology
Richard and Adeline Fleischaker
Chair in Research
University of Oklahoma Health
Sciences Center
Oklahoma City, OK, USA

Leonard C Sperling MD
Professor of Dermatology and
Pathology
Department of Dermatology
Uniformed Services University
Bethesda, MD, USA

Karan Sra MD
Dermatology Resident
Department of Dermatology
University of Texas, Medical Branch
Galveston, TX, USA

Angelika Stary MD PhD
University Professor
Medical Director
Outpatients' Centre for
Venerodermatological Infectious
Diseases
Vienna, Austria

Thomas Stasko MD
Associate Professor of Medicine
Division of Dermatology
Vanderbilt University Medical
Center
Nashville, TN, USA

Wolfram Sterry MD
Professor of Dermatology
Department of Dermatology and
Allergy
Charité-Universitätsmedizin Berlin
Berlin, Germany

Cloyce L Stetson MD
Associate Professor and Chairman
Department of Dermatology
Texas Tech University
Lubbock, TX, USA

Seth R Stevens MD
Medical Director
Inflammation
Amgen
Thousand Oaks, CA, USA

Georg Stingl MD
Professor and Chairman
Division of Immunology, Allergy
and Infectious Diseases (DIAID)
Department of Dermatology
University of Vienna Medical
School
Vienna, Austria

Mary Seabury Stone MD
Professor of Dermatology and
Pathology
Department of Dermatology
University of Iowa Carver College of
Medicine
Iowa City, IA, USA

Dow B Stough MD
Clinical Assistant Professor of
Dermatology
The Stough Clinic
Hot Springs, AR, USA

John P Sundberg MD
The Jackson Laboratory
Bar Harbor, ME, USA

Virginia P Sybert MD
Staff Dermatologist
Group Health Cooperative
Clinical Professor
Division of Medical Genetics
University of Washington School of
Medicine
Seattle, WA, USA

Michael D Tharp MD
The Clark W Finnerud MD Professor
and Chair
Department of Dermatology
Rush University Medical Center
Chicago, IL, USA

Diane M Thiboutot MD
Associate Professor of Dermatology
Department of Dermatology
The Pennsylvania State University
College of Medicine
Milton S Hershey Medical Center
Hershey, PA, USA

Whitney D Tope MPhil MD
Dermatologist and Dermatologic
Surgeon
Advancements in Dermatology
Edina, MN, USA

Antonella Tosti MD
Professor of Dermatology
Department of Dermatology
University of Bologna
Bologna, Italy

Jui-Chen Tsai PhD
Department of Clinical Pharmacy
College of Medicine
National Cheng Kung University
Tainan, Taiwan

Hensin Tsao MD PhD
Associate Professor
Harvard Medical School
Department of Dermatology
Massachusetts General Hospital
Boston, MA, USA

Stephen K Tyring MD PhD MBA
Professor
Department of Dermatology
Microbiology/Molecular Genetics
and Internal Medicine
University of Texas Health Science
Center
Houston, TX, USA

Jouni Uitto MD PhD
Professor and Chair
Department of Dermatology and
Cutaneous Biology
Jefferson Medical College
Jefferson University
Philadelphia, PA, USA

Edward Upjohn MD
Dermatology Registrar
St John's Institute of Dermatology
St Thomas' Hospital
London, United Kingdom

Annemarie Uliasz MD
Department of Dermatology
Mount Sinai School of Medicine
New York, NY, USA

Laurence Valeyrie-Allanore MD
Assistant
Department of Dermatology
Hospital Henri Mondor
University of Paris XII
Creteil, France

Peter CM van de Kerkhof MD
Professor and Chairman
Department of Dermatology
University Medical Center
Nijmegen
Nijmegen, The Netherlands

Michael Veness MBBS MMed
FRANZCR
Senior Radiation Oncologist
Clinical Senior Lecturer
Department of Radiation Oncology
Westmead Hospital
Sydney University
Westmead, NSW, Australia

Jonathan Vogel MD
Senior Investigator
National Institutes of Health
Dermatology Branch
Bethesda, MD, USA

David H Walker MD
Professor and Chairman
Department of Pathology
University of Texas Medical Branch
Director, WHO Collaborating Center
for Tropical Diseases
Galveston, TX, USA

Tomi L Wall MD
Clinical Instructor
Department of Dermatology
Harvard Medical School
Massachusetts General Hospital
Boston, MA, USA

Guy F Webster MD PhD
Professor
Department of Dermatology
Thomas Jefferson University
Medical College
Philadelphia, PA, USA

Robert A Weiss MD
Associate Professor of Dermatology
Johns Hopkins University School of
Medicine
Maryland Laser, Skin & Vein Institute
Hunt Valley, MD, USA

Elke Weisshaar MD
Consultant Dermatologist
Department of Social Medicine,
Occupational and Environmental
Dermatology
University Hospital of Heidelberg
Heidelberg, Germany

James Wharton MD
Springdale Dermatology Clinic
Springdale, AR, USA

Clifton R White Jr MD
Professor of Dermatology and
Pathology
Department of Dermatology
Oregon Health and Science
University
Portland, OR, USA

Jeffrey M Whitworth MD FAAD
Assistant Clinical Professor
Department of Dermatology
The New Jersey Medical School
Newark, NJ, USA

Mark Wilkinson MD FRCP
Consultant Dermatologist
Department of Dermatology
Leeds Teaching Hospitals NHS Trust
The General Infirmary
Leeds, United Kingdom

Rein Willemze MD
Professor and Chairman
Department of Dermatology
Leiden University Medical Centre
Leiden, The Netherlands

Harry L Winfield MD
Cleveland Skin Pathology
Laboratory, Inc.
Beachwood OH, USA

Fenella Wojnarowska FRCP DM
Professor of Dermatology
Department of Dermatology
Churchill Hospital
Oxford, United Kingdom

Stephen Wolverton MD
Professor of Clinical Dermatology
Vice Chair of Clinical Affairs
Department of Dermatology
Indiana University School of
Medicine
Indianapolis, IN, USA

Gary S Wood MD
Johnson Professor and Chairman
Department of Dermatology
University of Wisconsin
Madison, WI, USA

Carol McConnell Woody MD
Private Practice Dermatologist
Greensboro, NC, USA

Kim B Yancey MD
Professor and Chair
Department of Dermatology
University of Texas Southwestern
Medical Center
Dallas, TX, USA

Carole L Yee BS
Research Biologist
National Institutes of Health
Dermatology Branch
Bethesda, MD, USA

Gil Yosipovitch MD
Associate Professor
Department of Dermatology &
Neuroscience
Wake Forest University School of
Medicine
Winston-Salem, NC, USA

Andrea L Zaenglein MD
Associate Professor of Dermatology
and Pediatrics
Department of Dermatology
Penn State Milton S Hershey
Medical Center
Hershey, PA, USA

Jennifer C Zampogna MD
Department of Otolaryngology
University of Florida College of
Medicine
Gainesville, FL, USA

Jonathan Zonana MD
Professor
Department of Molecular and
Medical Genetics
Oregon Health Science University
Portland, OR, USA

John J Zone MD
Professor and Chair
Department of Dermatology
University of Utah
Salt Lake City, UT, USA

User Guide

VOLUMES, SECTIONS AND COLOR CODING

Dermatology is divided into two volumes. The book is divided into 22 sections, which are color-coded as follows for reference:

VOLUME ONE

SECTION 1	– Overview of basic science
SECTION 2	– Pruritus
SECTION 3	– Papulosquamous and eczematous dermatoses
SECTION 4	– Urticarias, erythemas and purpuras
SECTION 5	– Vesiculobullous diseases
SECTION 6	– Adnexal diseases
SECTION 7	– Rheumatologic diseases
SECTION 8	– Metabolic and systemic diseases
SECTION 9	– Genodermatoses
SECTION 10	– Pigmentary diseases
SECTION 11	– Hair, nails and mucous membranes
SECTION 12	– Infections, infestations and bites

VOLUME TWO

SECTION 13	– Disorders due to physical agents
SECTION 14	– Disorders of Langerhans cells and macrophages
SECTION 15	– Atrophies and disorders of dermal connective tissue
SECTION 16	– Disorders of subcutaneous fat
SECTION 17	– Vascular disorders
SECTION 18	– Neoplasms of the skin
SECTION 19	– Medical therapy
SECTION 20	– Physical treatment modalities
SECTION 21	– Surgery
SECTION 22	– Cosmetic surgery

BASIC SCIENCE CHAPTERS

Basic science chapters in the book are highlighted on the upper corner of each page with the following skin biology symbol:

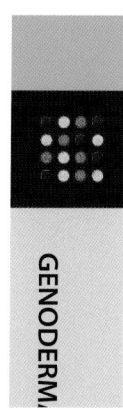

GENODERM.

THERAPEUTIC LADDERS

Therapeutic ladders have been standardized for measuring levels of evidence.

KEY TO EVIDENCE-BASED SUPPORT:

(1) prospective controlled trial
(2) retrospective study or large case series
(3) small case series or individual case reports.

Dermatology Website

The supporting website for the book, which includes all of the book's content in searchable format, can be found at **http://www.dermtext.com**

Dedication

This book is dedicated to our families, in particular Dennis Cooper MD, who endured our work on this project and who unwittingly were part of the team, and to all the rest of the team at Elsevier who made it all happen, especially Sven Pinczewski.

Acknowledgments

We are grateful to the authors for sharing their expertise and putting forth their best efforts to bring up-to-date educational material to the readers. In addition, we wish to acknowledge the contributions of the London team, led by Karen Bowler, and the Edinburgh team, led by Glenys Norquay.

We would also like to thank the following people for their help during this project: Donna Carroll, Russell Gabbedy, Misty Godwin, Kenneth Greer MD, Robert Hartman MD, Amor Khachemoune MD, Julie Karen MD, José Mascaró MD, Annette Myers, and Kalman Watsky MD.

The following figures were sourced from the **Yale Residents' Slide Collection**:
I.13, I.19, 2.9, 9.1, 9.4, 9.6A, 9.7, 9.8, 9.9, 9.10, 9.11, 9.13, 9.15, 9.16, 9.17, 9.18, 10.3A,B, 10.5, 10.7A, 10.8, 10.13, 10.14, 10.15, 11.1, 12.6, 12.7, 12.8, 12.9B, 12.9C, 12.10, 12.12, 12.13, 12.15, 12.16, 12.18A, 12.19, 12.23, 12.24A, 12.27A, 13.3, 13.4, 13.5, 13.6, 13.8, 13.9, 13.14, 13.15, 14.2B, 14.4, 15.4B, 15.6, 15.7, 15.9, 15.15D, 15.19, 18.12D, 19.1A,B, 19.2, 19.12, 20.1, 20.2, 20.6, 21.1B,C,E, 21.2, 21.6B, 21.7, 21.8A, 21.10, 21.12B, 22.1, 22.2, 22.3, 22.4, 22.6B, 22.6D, 22.7, 22.10A, 22.10B, 22.11, 22.15A, 22.18, 23.1C, 23.5A, 24.9, 25.1C, 25.1D, 25.1E, 25.4A,B, 25.5B, 25.6, 25.10, 25.12B, 25.12C, 26.4, 27.2, 27.8B, 27.9, 27.10, 28.3, 28.4, 28.7, 31.2, 31.5C, 31.13, 31.15, 31.18, 32.2A, 32.3, 32.11, 33.2, 33.3, 33.7, 33.8, 35.2A, 35.3, 35.5, 35.6, 35.7, 35.10, 35.11, 35.12, 35.13, 35.14, 37.5, 37.6, 37.7, 37.8A, 37.11, 38.3B, 38.4, 38.5, 38.6, 38.8, 38.10, 38.12B, 38.13A, 39.1, 39.2, 39.3, 39.4, 39.5, 39.14, 39.15, 40.7, 40.8, 40.14A, 40.15, 42.3A,B,E,F,G, 42.7B, 42.10, 42.11, 42.12, 42.13, 42.15, 44.2, 44.4, 44.5A, 44.6, 46.2, 46.11, 46.13A, 46.13B, 47.7, 47.8B, 47.9, 48.1, 49.3A, 49.5, 49.7, 50.7, 51.8, 51.9B, 51.10, 51.11, 52.21, 52.22, 56.4A, 56.7, 56.16, 57.3, 57.6B, 57.9, 57.11, 57.13, 57.14, 57.15, 58.2B, 58.11, 59.4B, 60.2, 60.6, 60.7, 60.14, 60.15, 60.16, 60.17, 60.18, 60.19, 60.20, 60.21, 61.5A,B, 61.6, 61.7, 61.10, 61.11, 61.13, 62.2, 62.12A,B, 62.14C, 62.15C, 62.17, 63.4, 63.14C, 63.16, 63.19, 65.15, 65.16, 65.18A,D,E,F, 65.19, 65.20, 65.21, 65.22, 65.26, 65.28, 66.3, 66.18B, 68.7A,D, 68.16H,I, 68.18B, 69.5, 70.9, 70.11, 70.13, 72.13A, 72.15A, 73.1B, 73.3, 73.6, 73.12, 73.15, 73.18, 73.24, 73.25, 74.16B, 74.17, 74.18, 74.19, 74.21, 74.23, 75.5, 75.6, 76.3B, 76.4, 76.5, 76.6, 76.10, 76.13C, 76.18, 76.22A, 76.29B,C, 77.4, 77.5, 77.7A, 77.9, 77.10, 77.13A,B,C, 78.7A, 79.9, 79.13C, 79.15, 79.16, 79.17, 79.21, 80.4, 80.5, 80.7, 80.10B, 80.13B, 80.14A, 81.5C, 81.7, 81.8, 81.9A,C, 81.13, 81.21, 82.4B, 82.10, 83.4A,D, 83.5, 83.10, 84.1, 84.2, 84.12, 86.22A,C,D, 87.3A, 87.9B, 89.7, 89.9, 90.1A,C, 91.2, 91.11, 91.12, 92.2A, 92.6, 92.7, 92.14, 93.1, 93.4B, 95.4, 95.6, 96.5, 96.8, 96.13B, 97.2D, 97.4A,B,D, 97.8B, 98.2, 98.3, 98.4, 98.5, 98.6, 98.8B, 98.11, 100.13, 103.4, 103.6, 103.7C, 103.8, 104.3A, 104.10, 104.14, 104.15, 104.17, 105.7, 105.8A, 105.9, 105.10, 105.11, 105.14, 105.15, 106.10, 108.5D, 108.6, 108.7, 108.8, 108.9, 108.11A,B,C, 108.16B, 108.17A, 108.20, 109.10D, 110.2, 110.22, 111.1, 111.3, 111.4, 111.10, 111.13, 111.19, 111.22A, 111.24, 111.28, 111.32, 111.34, 111.35, 111.38, 112.1, 112.6, 112.8, 112.9, 112.10 (inset), 112.14A, 112.27B, 113.6, 113.7A, 113.10B, 113.11A, 113.14, 114.6, 114.13, 116.22, 116.26, 117.2, 117.9, 118.7, 118.8, 121.1, 121.4A, 121.7, 122.2, 122.3, 122.5, 122.6, 125.7, 125.9, 130.1, 130.3, 134.6, 139.7E

The following figures were sourced from the **NYU Slide Collection**:
10.2B, 10.7B, 11.5, 11.6, 11.7, 12.9A, 12.13, 12.18B, 17.6, 19.13, 23.6, 25.1B, 25.5A, 26.6, 30.7B,C, 31.6A, 39.8, 48.4, 63.15A, 66.1A,B, 66.2, 68.10B, 68.17, 69.11, 71.4, 72.6B, 72.18B, 73.1A, 73.10B,C, 73.13, 73.19, 75.7, 77.7B, 80.9A, 80.10A, 81.11, 86.2, 86.3B, 92.12, 96.4, 96.9A, 98.10, 101.13B, 130.4, 133.3

The following figures were sourced from the **USC Residents' Slide Collection**:
7.6, 12.24B, 15.4A, 46.8, 58.18, 60.19, 61.4B, 61.5A,C, 66.10, 66.11, 68.16C, 73.23, 74.13, 76.20A,B, 76.21, 76.23A,B, 76.25A,B, 81.9B, 83.4B,C, 87.9B, 96.15, 99.5A, 101.6, 104.9, 111.27A, 114.4, 116.33, 121.9

The following figures were sourced from the **SUNY Stony Brook Residents' Slide Collection**:
65.18C, 96.12B

Ultraviolet Light

85

Thomas M Rünger

Key features

- Exposure of the skin to UV light has acute, short-term effects and chronic, long-term effects, both of which are wavelength-dependent. Profound effects also occur with non-erythemogenic doses of UV light

- UV light affects the skin's immune system, exerting both pro- and anti-inflammatory responses

- UV light induces several different types of DNA damage in a wavelength-dependent manner, such as pyrimidine dimers and oxidative guanine base modifications

- Several DNA repair pathways are involved in the processing of UV light-induced DNA damage, including nucleotide excision repair, base excision repair, translesional DNA synthesis, and recombination repair

- UV light-induced mutations, which play a pivotal role in photocarcinogenesis, are different from those induced by other mutagens. Some base substitution mutations (e.g. C→T, CC→TT) are so typical for UV light that they have been termed 'signature mutations'

- Disorders with an increased frequency of UV-induced skin cancers are characterized by an impaired cellular or host response to the effects of UV light

INTRODUCTION

Dermatologists are confronted daily with the effects of UV light on the skin, and often deal with them in a seemingly contradictory way. On the one hand, they have the responsibility of warning their patients against the deleterious effects of sunlight, such as sunburn, photoaging and sun-induced skin cancers, and on the other hand, they use UV radiation to treat skin disease. As with all medical interventions, dermatologists are only weighing the risks versus the benefits when they use UV light for therapeutic purposes. In the phototherapy of inflammatory skin diseases, dermatologists also try to avoid the proinflammatory properties of UV radiation (e.g. the capability to induce sunburn) by choosing sub-erythemogenic doses. This clearly indicates that doses of UV light that do not induce sunburn still have profound effects on the skin. This applies not only to its short-term effects, but also to its long-term effects. A third and important aspect of photodermatology is the diagnosis and treatment of photosensitive or photo-aggravated skin disorders (see Ch. 86).

Spectrum of UV Light

The sun emits UV radiation as part of an electromagnetic spectrum (see Fig. 134.1). It is usually subdivided, rather arbitrarily, into UVA (400–315 nm), UVB (315–290 nm), and UVC (290–200 nm). UVA has been further subdivided into UVA1 (400–340 nm) and UVA2 (340–315 nm). More than 95% of the sun's UV radiation that reaches the earth's surface is UVA. Practically all of the UVC, and much of the UVB, are absorbed by the oxygen and ozone in the earth's atmosphere, so that UV radiation below 290 nm is virtually undetectable at ground level. Nevertheless, the remaining UV radiation can still be absorbed by biologic molecules (DNA, protein, lipids), and it can damage and kill unprotected cells.

To survive in our environment, all living organisms had to develop protective mechanisms in order to prevent UV-induced killing and to maintain the stability of their genome. Such defenses include the development of UV-absorbing surface layers, enzymatic and non-enzymatic antioxidative defenses, repair processes, and removal of damaged cells. Through evolution, humans have lost most of the UV-protective fur, which remains an effective UV-protector only on the scalp (of most individuals). Nevertheless, the human skin is quite effective in protecting the rest of the organism from the harmful effects of solar UV irradiation, since UV radiation does not penetrate any deeper than the skin. Within the skin, the depth of penetration of UV light is wavelength-dependent[1,2] – i.e. the longer the wavelength, the deeper the penetration (Fig. 85.1). While UVA readily reaches the dermis, including its deeper portions, most of the UVB is absorbed in the epidermis, and only a small proportion reaches the upper dermis. UVC, if it reached the earth's surface, would be absorbed or reflected predominantly in the stratum corneum and in upper layers of the epidermis.

Some of the UV light reaching the skin is absorbed by biomolecules, thus eliciting photochemical and photobiological responses. A light-absorbing molecule is called a chromophore. Upon absorption of the radiation's energy, this chromophore is elevated to an excited state. Ensuing photochemical reactions may either change the chromophore directly, or, through energy transfer in a so-called photosensitized reaction, indirectly change a molecule other than the chromophore[3]. Affected cells react, which in turn may lead to visible changes in exposed skin. When thinking about the biologic effects of different wavelengths in the different layers of the skin, it is necessary to consider that a particular wavelength can have a biologic effect even in a layer that it does not reach; for example, through secretion of a proinflammatory mediator in a higher layer.

Both short-term and long-term effects of exposure to UV light are wavelength-dependent[4]. However, when comparing the photobiologic

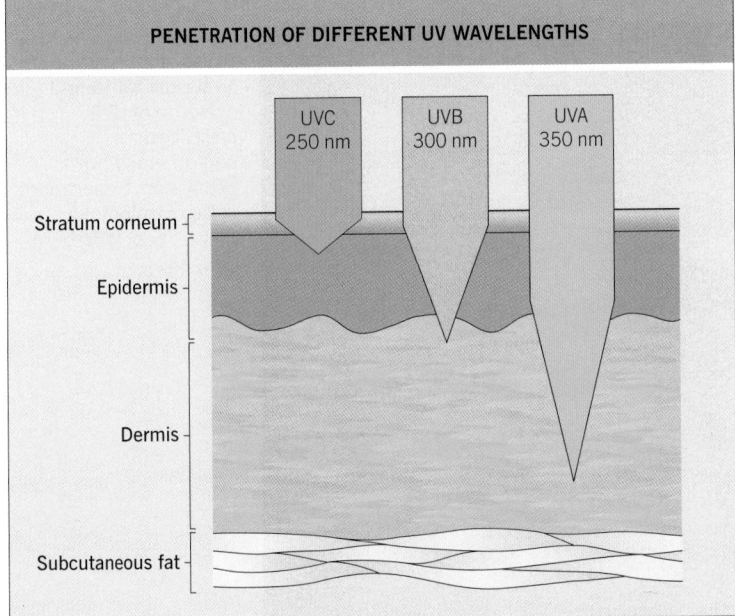

PENETRATION OF DIFFERENT UV WAVELENGTHS

UVC 250 nm · UVB 300 nm · UVA 350 nm

Stratum corneum · Epidermis · Dermis · Subcutaneous fat

Fig. 85.1 Depth of penetration of different wavelengths of UV light into human skin. Depth of penetration varies greatly with the thickness of the different skin layers and their composition (e.g. melanin content). The beginning of the wedge-shaped portion of the penetration symbol represents a decrease to approximately one-third of the incident energy density, and the tip of the symbol represents a decrease to approximately 1%. Figure not drawn to scale.

properties of UVB with those of UVA, it is important to remember that they are not two different entities, but rather a continuum of wavelengths, with gradually changing properties, and that the division between UVA and UVB is rather arbitrary.

Sunburn and Tanning

Visible, short-term effects of UV radiation on the skin include sunburn (solar erythema, possibly blister formation, desquamation) and tanning. Microscopic, short-term effects include inflammatory infiltrates, vasodilation, formation of sunburn cells, depletion of Langerhans cells, acanthosis and hyperkeratosis. On the cellular and molecular level, UV exposure induces a multitude of damage responses, including the induction of stress proteins, repair processes and cytokine production. In a dose-dependent manner, exposed cells can either undergo apoptosis (visible histologically as sunburn cells) or cease proliferating (cell cycle arrest) in order to undergo repair (see Ch. 107). Hyperproliferation may follow the initial growth arrest, visible histologically as epidermal thickening.

The ability to induce sunburn (Fig. 85.2) rapidly declines with increasing wavelength. For example, UV light with a wavelength of 360 nm is approximately 1000-fold less erythemogenic than light with a wavelength of 300 nm. A UVB-induced sunburn reaches its peak between 6 and 24 hours after exposure. An immediate erythema reaction is rarely observed. In contrast, after exposure to a high dose of UVA, an immediate erythema is regularly observed, followed by a distinct delayed erythema reaction after 6 to 24 hours. DNA is hypothesized to be the chromophore for the delayed erythema associated with UVB[5], whereas the responsible chromophore for UVA-induced erythema is not known.

The tanning response of human skin to sun exposure is biphasic and also wavelength-dependent. The immediate pigment darkening occurs during and immediately after exposure, and is due to alteration (e.g. oxidation) and redistribution of existing melanin. It is most prominent with UVA. Delayed tanning is usually the result of an exposure to UVB, and it peaks approximately 3 days after sun exposure. Fair skin (skin type II) usually tans only with UVB doses above the erythema threshold (only with prior sunburn). Darker skin (skin types III and higher) also has a significant tanning response to sub-erythemogenic doses (without prior sunburn). A UVB-induced tan is based on an increased number of melanocytes, increased melanin synthesis, increased arborization of

melanocytes, and increased transfer of melanosomes to keratinocytes (see Ch. 64). Here, it is necessary to emphasize that differences between UVA and UVB are gradual; for example, the shorter wavelengths of UVA (UVA2) exhibit tanning properties similar to those of UVB. However, a UVA-induced tan, such as from the use of a tanning bed (Fig. 85.3A), provides 5–10 times less protection against a sunburn from subsequent UV exposure than does a UVB-induced tan, probably due to the less pronounced epidermal thickening and hyperkeratosis that accompanies an UVA-induced tan.

An individual's tendency to develop sunburn and tanning after sun exposure has been used to categorize skin phototypes (see Table 134.3). These categories of an individual's susceptibility to short-term effects also correlate with the individual's susceptibility to long-term effects following sunlight exposure. In general, those individuals with a higher acute sun sensitivity are also more at risk for developing skin cancer after chronic UV exposure.

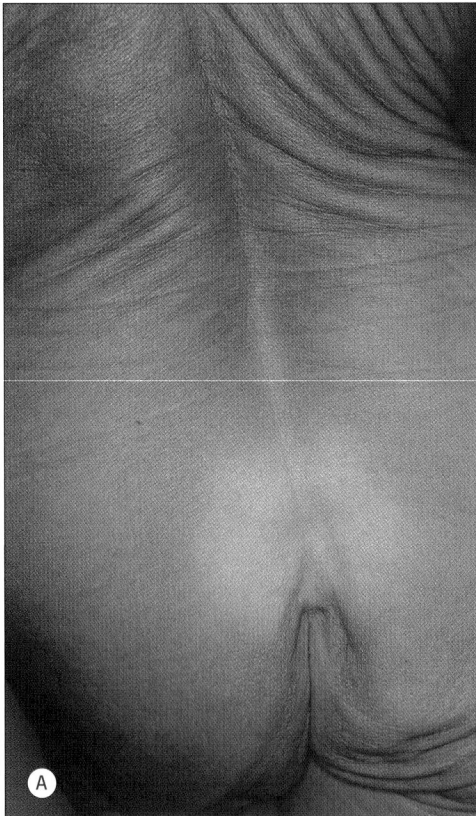

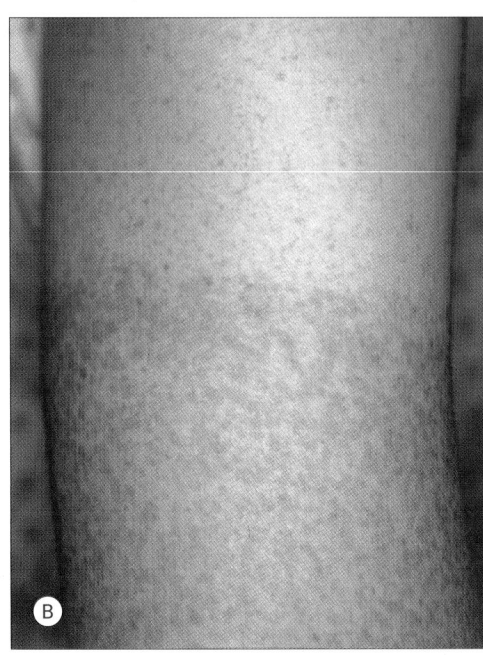

Fig. 85.3 Sequelae of exposure to UV light. A UVA-induced tan with reduced pigmentation within an area of relative ischemia; the patient was a habitual user of a UVA tanning bed. B Sharp demarcation of solar lentigines in a bicyclist who consistently over several years wore a tightly fitting spandex shirt. A, B, Courtesy of Jean L Bolognia MD.

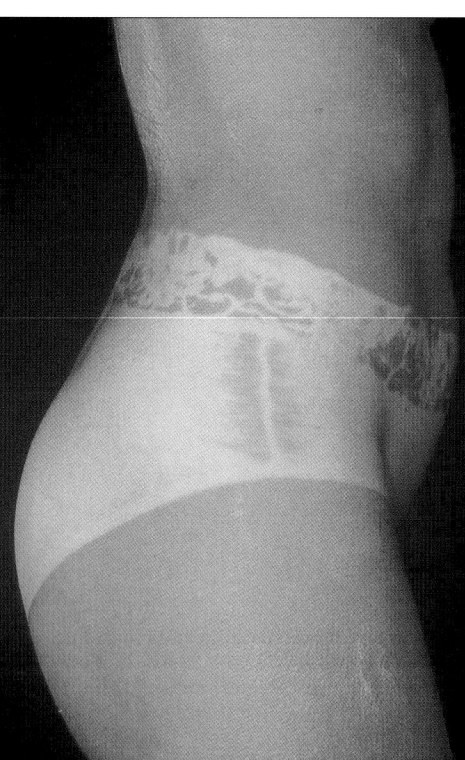

Fig. 85.2 Sunburn. Twenty-four hours after an accidental 10-fold overdose of UVB prescribed as phototherapy. With permission, Department of Dermatology, University of Würzburg, Germany.

Effects on the Cutaneous Immune System

A sunburn exemplifies the profound effect that UV light has on the skin's immune function, in this case a proinflammatory effect. Additional clinical examples of the proinflammatory properties of UV light include phototoxic and photoallergic reactions, other photodermatoses, and photoaggravation of inflammatory skin disorders (e.g. atopic dermatitis, psoriasis, pityriasis rubra pilaris). On the other hand, UV light also exerts immunosuppressive effects on the skin, exemplified by reactivation of herpes labialis after sun exposure, an increased risk of skin cancer in chronically immunosuppressed patients, and its therapeutic effect against inflammatory skin disorders. However, it is unlikely that there is a simple threshold between the UV doses that have proinflammatory and those that have anti-inflammatory effects. Proinflammatory, anti-inflammatory and immunomodulatory changes occur side-by-side within different arms of cellular and humoral immune reaction cascades, with varying dose–responses as well as modulation by wavelengths and many individual factors far beyond just the degree of skin pigmentation (skin types).

UV light-induced immunosuppression involves not only the areas of skin directly exposed to UV light, but also non-irradiated skin[6-8]. This systemic response includes development of tolerance to antigens applied to the skin after irradiation. The *local* effects are mediated by the ability of UV radiation to: (1) deplete the epidermis of Langerhans cells (or modulate their function); and (2) activate signaling cascades in keratinocytes and other skin cells, with release of a variety of cytokines (e.g. IL-10), neuropeptides and neuroendocrine hormones (e.g. α-MSH). *Systemic* immunosuppression and tolerance is mediated by regulatory T cells[8] and the release of immunosuppressive cytokines by UV-irradiated keratinocytes. Systemic immunosuppressive effects last for approximately 10 days.

Cellular photoreceptors that mediate the signaling that leads to UV-induced immune responses are: DNA (via formation of DNA damage [DNA photoproducts]); urocanic acid in the stratum corneum (via UV-induced isomerization from the trans- to the cis-isoform), and membrane lipids (via UV-induced alteration of the membrane redox potential). While the immunosuppressive effects of UVB are well established, the relative contribution of UVA to the immunomodulatory properties of solar UV radiation is still a matter of debate, but evidence is accumulating that UVA also has prominent effects.

Photoaging and Photocarcinogenesis

Long-term effects of chronic sun exposure include photoaging and photocarcinogenesis. In the case of photocarcinogenesis, UV exposure provides a one–two punch – not only does it generate DNA damage that leads to mutation formation and malignant transformation, but its immunosuppressive properties, including the induction of specific tolerance to UV-induced skin tumors, reduce the ability of the host immune-defense system to recognize and remove malignant cells[9]. UV irradiation also impairs immune surveillance against cells infected with oncogenic viruses (e.g. certain HPV types) and may thereby further promote skin cancer formation.

The advantage of reduced immune reactivity following exposure to UV light is the prevention of illicit (auto)-immune reactions to transiently UV-altered cells. Any shift in the balance between pro- and anti-inflammatory responses toward a more immunosuppressed state increases the risk of UV-induced tumor formation, as occurs in chronically immunosuppressed patients. However, tilting this balance toward proinflammatory responses increases the risk of developing photodermatoses or photoaggravated skin diseases such as lupus erythematosus. The critical nature of this balance is also exemplified by the observation that effective photoprotection commonly leads to spontaneous resolution of actinic keratoses, even though these precursor lesions have identifiable genetic changes that provide growth advantage over non-mutated cells (see Ch. 107). Lastly, the individual degree of UV-induced immune suppression correlates with an increased tumor risk.

In contrast to photocarcinogenesis, where the anti-inflammatory effects of UV light play a pivotal role, photoaging is characterized by a chronic inflammatory response to UV light. As photocarcinogenesis commonly occurs in photoaged skin, this further demonstrates the simultaneous occurrence of pro- and anti-inflammatory responses to

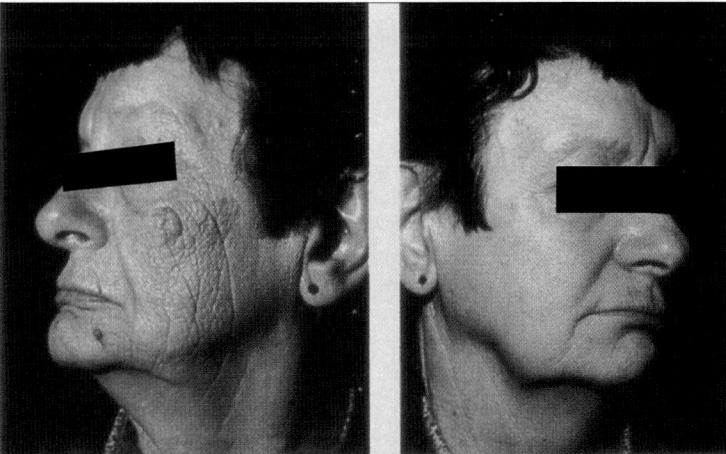

Fig. 85.4 Unilateral photoaging following 15 years of unilateral sun exposure through window glass. This individual had been working in the same office for 15 years, close to a window, with the left cheek always facing the window. Biopsy confirmed the diagnosis of nodular cutaneous elastosis with cysts and comedones (Favre–Racouchot disease). Since UVB does not penetrate window glass, this observation identifies UVA as an effective agent in photoaging. Reproduced with permission from Moulin G, Thomas L, Vigneau M, Fiere A. Un cas unilateral d'élastose avec kystes et comédons de Favre et Racouchot. Ann Dermatol Venereol. 1994;121:721–3.

UV light. Both processes, photoaging and photocarcinogenesis, usually require several years of sun exposure before clinical manifestations are apparent (Fig. 85.3B). However, initial pigmentary changes of photoaging can sometimes be seen just weeks or months after a sunburn (e.g. the large-sized lentigines of the upper back that follow a blistering sunburn).

Due to its ability to penetrate deeper into the dermis, UVA in particular is thought to play an important role in photoaging. Figure 85.4 depicts unilateral facial photoaging in an office worker whose face had been consistently side-on to the window during office hours for 15 years[10]. This case strikingly demonstrates the ability of UVA to induce photoaging, since only UVA, and not UVB, penetrates through window glass. The deeper penetration of UVA into the skin is significant for the process of photoaging, but it is not thought to be as important in photocarcinogenesis, since all UV-induced skin cancers (squamous cell carcinoma [SCC], basal cell carcinoma [BCC], and melanoma) arise from cells that reside within the epidermis, not from dermal cells. It is difficult to imagine that this difference (between epidermal and dermal cells) in their susceptibility to UV-induced carcinogenesis is due only to the more protected location of fibroblasts within the skin, given that fibroblasts are located just underneath the basal layer of epidermal cells. However, in mice, the predominant UV-induced skin cancers are fibrosarcomas. This suggests that the fibroblast is comparably susceptible to UV irradiation as the keratinocyte, and that it is mainly the thickness of the human epidermis that prevents the malignant transformation of the fibroblast.

PHOTOCARCINOGENESIS

UV-Induced Tumor Formation

It is well established that exposure of the skin to UV light is a major risk factor for the development of cutaneous melanoma and non-melanoma skin cancer[11]. It is a process that, like cancer in general, involves a stepwise accumulation of specific genetic changes in a single cell, with subsequent clonal expansion. Usually, it takes decades until a tumor arises. It is commonly accepted that UV-induced skin cancers (BCC, SCC and melanoma) develop along the photocarcinogenesis chain of events outlined in Figure 85.5. The three major steps are:
- DNA damage formation after UV exposure
- mutation formation following DNA damage formation
- malignant transformation following mutation formation (see below). There is limited information regarding which wavelengths of the UV spectrum are responsible for these effects. While the carcinogenic properties of short-wavelength UV light (UVC, UVB) have been well

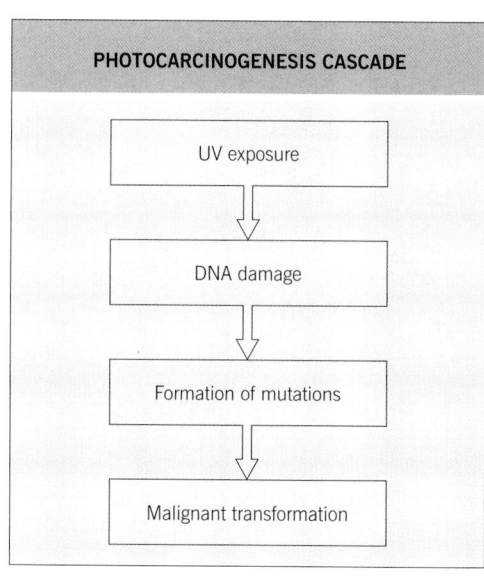

established for some time, UVA has long been thought to be harmless due to its relative inability to induce sunburn. In recent years, however, it has been shown that UVA is capable of inducing cutaneous SCC in mice. Subsequently, a photocarcinogenesis action spectrum for cutaneous SCC in mice was published, which demonstrated a steep decline in tumor rate with increasing wavelength[12]. This steep decline does not exclude a role for UVA in skin carcinogenesis, because natural sunlight contains much more UVA than UVB (depending on the time of day and weather: 20- to 100-fold more), which offsets at least some of the weaker effects of UVA. Additionally, UVA is less filtered by window glass or clothing, and it penetrates more effectively to the basal layer of the epidermis[2]; these two factors may serve to increase its relative contribution to the long-term effects of sunlight exposure.

Even less is known about the action spectrum for the induction of melanoma, the deadliest form of skin cancer. However, there are some indications that UVA may play a role[13]. These suggestions come from the following:

- Experiments in melanoma-susceptible fish, in which UVA was much more effective in inducing melanoma.
- Another animal model, the opossum *Monodelphis domestica*, in which not only UVB but also UVA induced melanoma precursor lesions.
- Meta-analyses of multiple retrospective studies and one large prospective study indicate that the use of tanning beds (which contain mostly high-dose UVA emitters) increases the risk for melanoma[14,14a].
- Reports that the use of sunscreens (which until recently contained no effective UVA filters) increased melanoma risk[15], possibly due to an increased exposure to unfiltered UVA.

However, more recently, a role for UVA in the pathogenesis of melanoma has been questioned, as only UVB, not UVA, induced melanoma in a transgenic mouse model[16].

Cutaneous SCC and lentigo maligna melanoma are associated with a high cumulative exposure to UV radiation, and they occur most commonly in chronically sun-exposed areas, such as the face, dorsal aspect of the hands, and extensor forearms. In contrast, the most common types of cutaneous melanoma (superficial spreading and nodular) usually arise in sites with intermittent sun exposure (e.g. the back in men and the lower legs in women), rather than in chronically sun-exposed areas, and they are associated with a history of sunburns. Several explanations for these phenomena have been proposed. One hypothesis suggests that melanocytes might be more prone to UV-induced mutagenesis following a single high dose of UV light, because of their relative inability to undergo apoptosis. Possibly due to high levels of antiapoptotic proteins such as Bcl-2, sunburn-induced apoptosis has not been described in melanocytes. Therefore, melanocytes with a high amount of DNA damage are more likely to survive than keratinocytes, which readily undergo apoptosis. Adaptive responses following repeated low-dose UV radiation, such as increased pigmentation or upregulation of DNA repair (see below for 'intrinsic protective mechanisms'), protect both melanocytes and keratinocytes against the

mutagenic assault from repeated low-dose UV exposures. However, in this situation, keratinocytes would be more prone to UV-induced mutagenesis, since they are proliferating more rapidly, especially after prior UV exposure, and they are, therefore, more likely to replicate damaged DNA. This could explain why keratinocytes are more vulnerable to the repeated low-dose UV irradiations of chronic sun exposure than are melanocytes[17], even though keratinocytes appear to have an increased ability to process UV-induced DNA damage (unpublished results, Rünger TM).

UV Induction of DNA Damage

Different wavelengths of UV light induce different types of DNA damage. UVC and UVB, but much less UVA, are capable of exciting the DNA molecule directly and subsequently generate DNA photoproducts[18]. Indeed, DNA is regarded as the chromophore for most of the biologic effects of UVB and UVC, including erythema, tanning, immuno-suppression, mutagenesis and carcinogenesis[5]. DNA photoproducts are dimers, formed by covalently binding two adjacent pyrimidines in the same polynucleotide chain. The two major types of pyrimidine dimers are cyclobutane dimers (Fig. 85.6) and 6,4-photoproducts (Fig. 85.7).

The focus in this chapter is on the long-term consequences of UV-induced DNA damage, mutagenesis and carcinogenesis. Following acute cellular injury, including DNA damage, cells initiate damage response pathways, which may result in cell cycle arrest, apoptosis, induction of DNA excision repair pathways, change in expression of cell surface proteins, secretion of cytokines, etc. This can explain how UV-induced DNA damage can result in acute effects, like erythema or immunosuppression. An upregulation of the transcription factor p53 plays a pivotal role in many of these cellular damage response pathways. However, the initial cellular sensor for the induction of damage response pathways is not clearly identified. For DNA damage, the unwinding and bending of the DNA double helix by, for example, DNA photoproducts is important for at least DNA damage recognition and initiation of DNA repair.

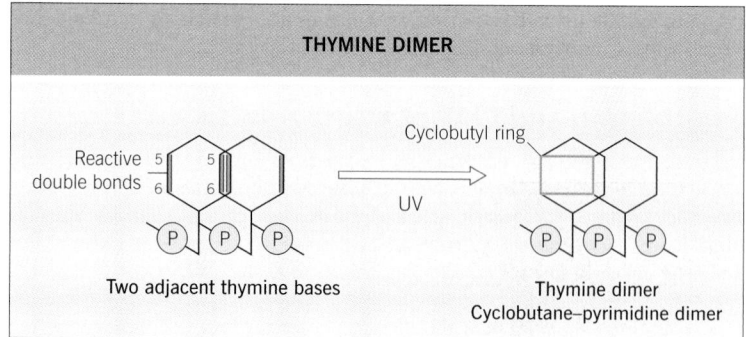

Fig. 85.6 Thymine dimer. Following excitation of the bases by UV light, a cyclobutane–pyrimidine dimer is formed by covalent linkage between two adjacent pyrimidines (here two thymine bases) and formation of a cyclobutyl ring.

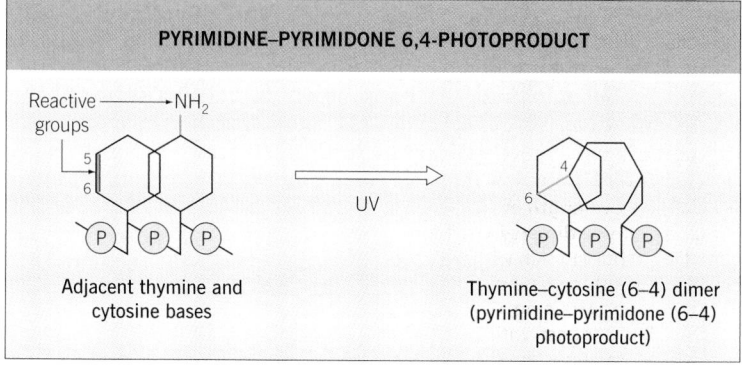

Fig. 85.7 Pyrimidine–pyrimidone 6,4-photoproduct. A pyrimidine–pyrimidone (6-4) photoproduct is formed by covalent linkage between C-6 and C-4 of two adjacent pyrimidines (here a thymine and a cytosine base), following excitation of the bases by UV light.

Cyclobutane–pyrimidine dimers (CPDs) are the most common DNA photoproduct formed by UV irradiation of the skin. They are generated upon saturation of the 5,6 double bonds and formation of a four-membered cyclobutyl ring (see Fig. 85.6). CPDs are observed at all possible dipyrimidine sites, with the thymine–thymine dimer (T-T) being the most common, followed by C-T and T-C dimers. C-C dimers are the least common. The formation of CPDs is not a random phenomenon: it is influenced by the sequence and conformational context of the affected DNA sequence.

The 6,4-photoproduct is a non-cyclobutane dipyrimidine photoproduct, which is formed upon covalent linkage between the C-6 position of one pyrimidine and the C-4 position of the 3′ adjacent pyrimidine (see Fig. 85.7). The T-C (6-4) dimer is the most common dimer of this type, but C-C and T-T dimers are also observed after UV irradiation. Upon further irradiation with UV wavelengths between 280 and 360 nm, the normal isomers of 6,4-photoproducts can be converted to their Dewar valence isomers, which are less mutagenic than the normal isomers but may still contribute to solar mutagenesis[19]. A few other rare DNA photoproducts have been described, such as complex purine lesions and pyrimidine hydrates, but their physiologic significance in the photobiology of human skin is unknown.

The absorption maximum of DNA is at 260 nm. This makes UVC the most effective wavelength for the induction of DNA photoproducts in naked DNA. However, in vivo, due to the absorption of shorter wavelengths in upper layers of the epidermis, 300 nm (UVB) is the most effective wavelength for inducing DNA photoproducts in the basal layer of the epidermis (which harbors the most relevant cells for skin carcinogenesis). Figure 85.8 demonstrates how 300 nm is much more effective than 290 nm in inducing cyclobutane T-T dimers in the basal layer of human epidermis[5]. While UVA can also generate a few pyrimidine dimers, its mutagenic properties have long been thought to be mediated via DNA lesions other than pyrimidine dimers. This is based on the observation that mutation frequencies per dimer increase with increasing wavelengths, in particular within the UVA range.

The UV-induced DNA damage discussed thus far results from the direct absorption of photons by bases of DNA. However, UV radiation can also damage DNA indirectly[3]. After absorption of photons by chromophores other than DNA, energy can be transferred either to DNA (type I photosensitized reaction) or to molecular oxygen, with reactive oxygen species in turn being able to damage DNA (type II photosensitized reaction). The indirect generation of oxidative DNA damage has been suggested to underlie UVA-induced mutagenesis and carcinogenesis, while the generation of a few pyrimidine dimers by UVA may involve a type I photosensitized reaction[20]. Of note, many of the biologic properties of UVA, including its toxicity to cells, are strictly dependent upon the presence of molecular oxygen[21], which points to a prominent role of reactive oxygen species. Although these reactive oxygen species are also formed by UVB, UVA has been shown to be responsible for almost all guanine oxidation products in DNA (see below) after exposure of cells to natural sunlight[22].

UV-induced reactive oxygen species include singlet oxygen and probably other non-radical and radical reactive oxygen species, such as hydrogen peroxide and the superoxide radical[23]. Even the highly reactive hydroxyl radical may be formed by a reaction of hydrogen peroxide with nuclear metals through a Fenton reaction. This oxidative stress affects not only DNA, but also membranes and proteins. The relative contribution of each (oxidative membrane damage, oxidative protein damage, oxidative DNA damage) to the different biologic effects of UV irradiation has not been well established. Singlet oxygen and the other reactive oxygen species react predominantly with guanine and generate several DNA changes, including the mutagenic and well-studied 7,8-dihydro-8-oxoguanosine (8-oxoG; Fig. 85.9).

Kielbassa et al.[24] published a UV action spectrum for the formation of dimers and oxidative guanine base modifications in mammalian cells (Fig. 85.10). Differences between the DNA-damaging properties of UVA, UVB and UVC are gradual, and only a few pyrimidine dimers are generated by the shorter wavelengths of UVA (UVA2: 315–340 nm). Young et al.[26] have shown that in vivo UVA (320 nm, 340 nm and 360 nm) can indeed induce pyrimidine dimers in human skin. This raises a question which remains a matter of debate[27] – are the mutagenic properties of UVA (in particular UVA1: 340–400 nm) really mediated by oxidative DNA damage or by the weak ability of UVA to form a few pyrimidine dimers (see Mutation Formation)?

Repair of UV-Induced DNA Damage

To counteract potentially mutagenic and cytotoxic effects, UV-induced DNA damage requires excision and replacement of damaged nucleotides by DNA repair pathways. No correction procedure is absolutely exact and error-free. If it were, UV-induced skin cancers would not occur in DNA repair-proficient individuals.

The bulky DNA photoproducts (pyrimidine dimers) are mutagenic, but they can be repaired by the nucleotide excision repair (NER) pathway. As exemplified by the hereditary disorder xeroderma pigmentosum (XP), a defect in this repair pathway increases UV sensitivity and UV mutagenesis in cells as well as non-melanoma and melanoma skin cancers in vivo[28,29] (Fig. 85.11). The NER pathway is now well understood, in part through the identification and characterization of the different XP genes. XP includes seven genetic complementation groups (XPA through XPG), which represent different proteins in the NER pathway (Table 85.1), in addition to a separate form, XP variant.

NER involves recognition of DNA damage, incision of the DNA strand containing a lesion, and DNA synthesis and ligation to replace

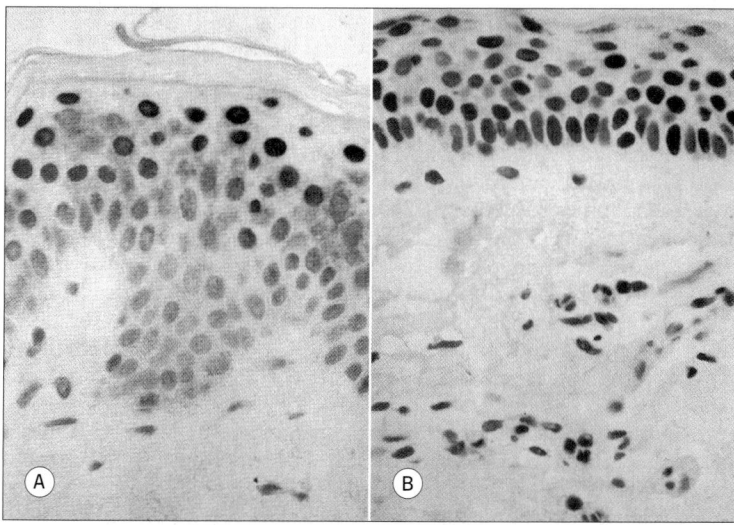

Fig. 85.8 A wavelength of 300 nm is more effective than one of 290 nm in inducing thymine dimers in the basal layer of the human epidermis. A After irradiation of human skin with monochromatic 290 nm UVB (2 MED) and staining with antithymine dimer antibodies, most cells in the basal layer show only blue counterstaining, while suprabasal layers demonstrate pronounced reactivity. B In contrast, with 2 MED of monochromatic 300 nm UVB, a pronounced immunostaining is also evident in the basal layer of the epidermis. Reproduced with permission from Young AR, Chadwick CA, Harrison GI, et al. The similarity of action spectra for thymine dimers in human epidermis and erythema suggests that DNA is the chromophore for erythema. J Invest Dermatol. 1998;111:982–8.

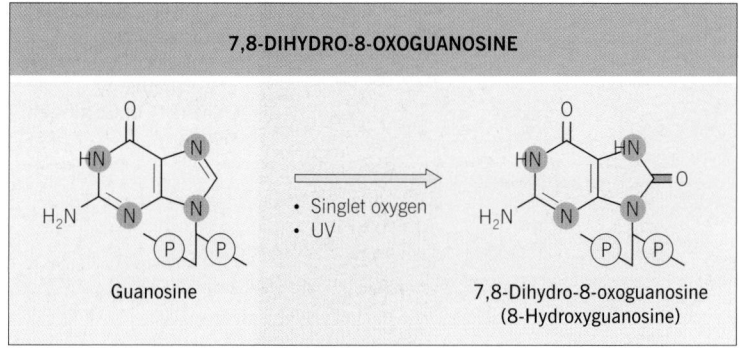

Fig. 85.9 7,8-Dihydro-8-oxoguanosine. 7,8-Dihydro-8-oxoguanosine (tautomer: 8-hydroxyguanosine) is an oxidation product of guanosine. It is formed by singlet oxygen, which is generated through a photosensitized reaction after excitation of a cellular chromophore by UV.

ACTION SPECTRUM FOR INDUCTION OF CYCLOBUTANE DIMERS AND OXIDATIVE GUANINE MODIFICATIONS

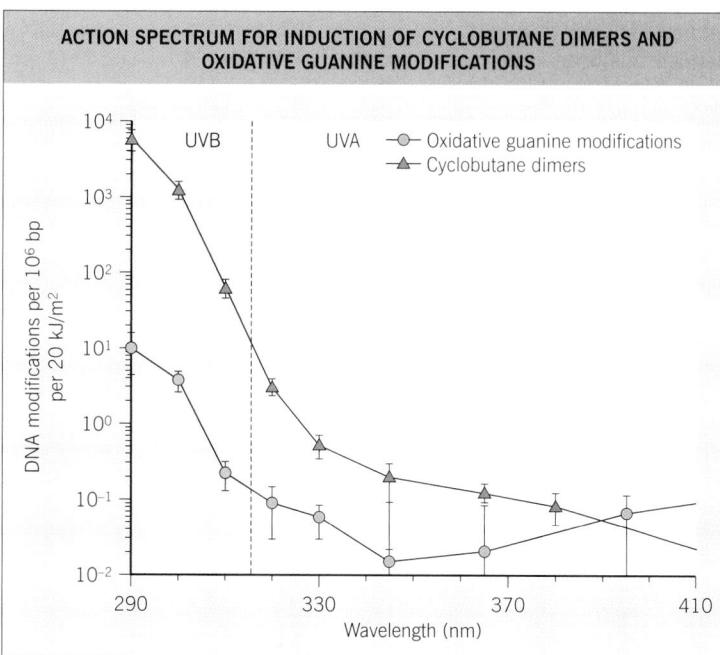

Fig. 85.10 Action spectrum for the induction of cyclobutane dimers and oxidative guanine modifications in Chinese hamster ovary cells. The number of DNA lesions was assessed by the ability of repair enzymes to incise DNA from cells irradiated with different wavelengths from a monochromator. The ability of UV light to induce cyclobutane dimers and oxidative DNA damage rapidly declines with increasing wavelengths, e.g., 320 nm UV light is approximately 1000-fold less capable of inducing cyclobutane dimers than is 290 nm UV light. This decline parallels well with the decline of skin cancer formation in mice from 300 to 340 nm (Utrecht–Philadelphia skin cancer action spectrum[9]). This decline does not mean that longer wavelengths do not contribute to photocarcinogenesis, because longer-wavelength UVA is much more abundant in natural sunlight than is UVB, which offsets at least some of the weaker effects of UVA. The second peak of oxidative base damage formation in the UVA range parallels with a second peak of skin cancer formation at 380 nm[9]. Since there is no second peak of cyclobutane dimer formation with UVA, this might indicate that oxidative base damage contributes more to skin cancer formation with UVA. More recent data[25,25a], however, indicates that it is not a different type of DNA damage (e.g. oxidative base damage) that explains this observation, but possibly a weaker cellular DNA damage response following UVA exposure.

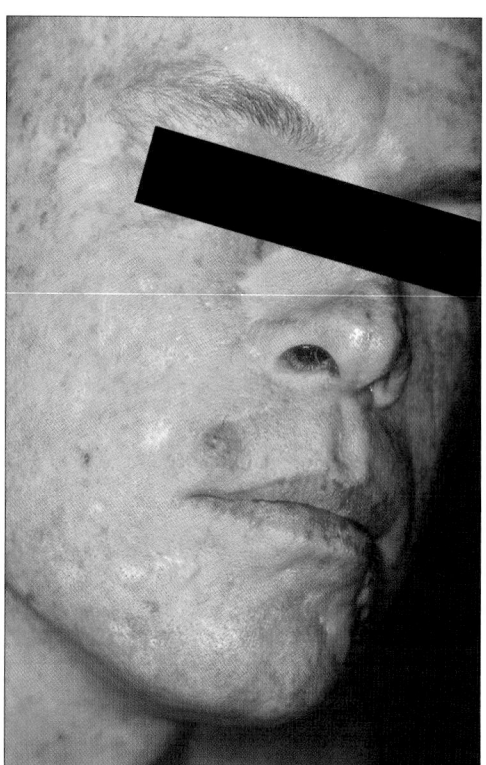

Fig. 85.11 Xeroderma pigmentosum. UV-exposed areas show the typical, irregular hypo- and hyperpigmented macules and surgical excision sites (more than 200 BCCs and SCCs had been removed). The nodule on the right cutaneous lip was diagnosed as an amelanotic melanoma metastasis. With permission, Department of Dermatology, University of Göttingen, Germany.

NUCLEOTIDE EXCISION REPAIR IN NON-TRANSCRIBED REGIONS

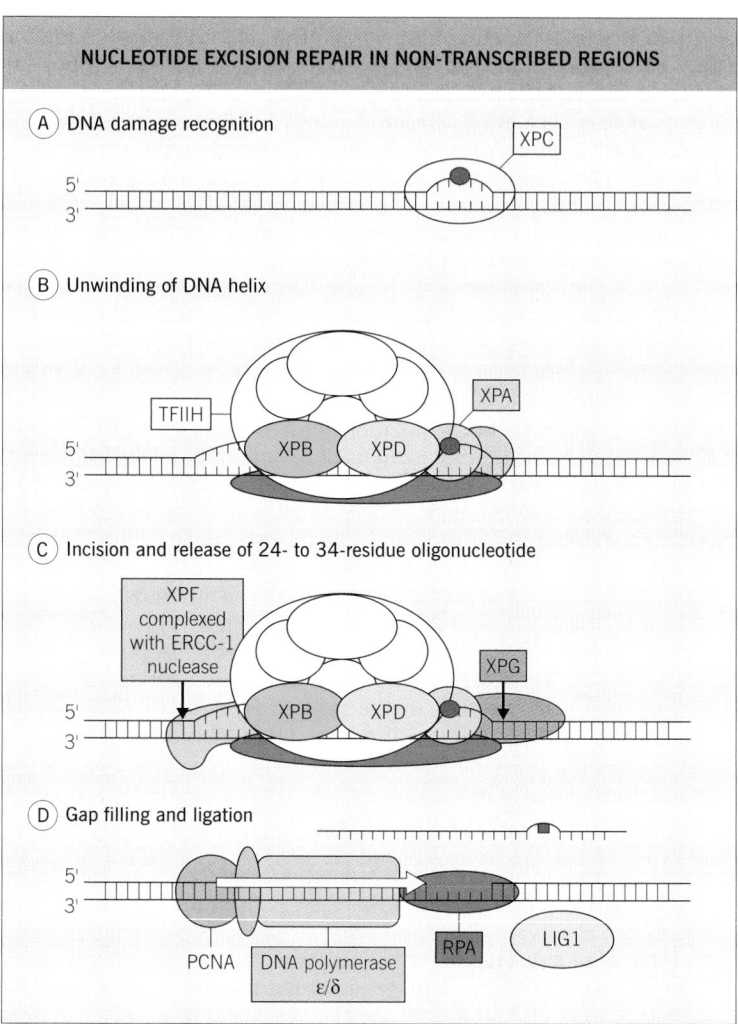

Fig. 85.12 Nucleotide excision repair in non-transcribed regions (global genome repair). This pathway repairs 'bulky' DNA lesions, such as pyrimidine dimers. **A** DNA damage recognition by XPC. **B** Formation of an open bubble around the lesion by the helicase activity of XPB and XPD. **C** Incision 5' and 3' of the lesion by the endonucleases XPF and XPG. **D** Repair synthesis and gap closing after release of a 24- to 34-residue oligonucleotide. LIG1, DNA ligase 1; PCNA, proliferating cell nuclear antigen; RPA, replication protein A; TFIIH, transcription factor IIH. Adapted with permission from Lindahl T, Wood RD. Quality control by DNA repair. Science. 1999;286:1897–905.

an excised oligonucleotide (24 to 32 residues). This is shown schematically in Figure 85.12. A key intermediate is an open, unwound structure formed around a DNA lesion in a reaction that uses the helicase activities of XPB and XPD. This creates sites for cutting by the endonucleases XPG on the 3' side of the lesion and the XPF–ERCC1 complex on the 5' side. A 24- to 32-residue oligonucleotide is released, and the gap is filled by DNA polymerase δ or ε and then sealed by DNA ligase 1. DNA damage recognition requires that the DNA photoproduct must distort (unwind and bend) the DNA helix. The different DNA photoproducts and their multiple different isoforms do that to varying degrees.

In active genes, the transcribed strand is corrected up to 5 to 10 times faster than the non-transcribed strand. For this transcription-coupled repair, all the same factors required for the repair of non-transcribed genes (global genome repair) are used, except for XPC. Unlike DNA replication and transcription, which take place in localized factories within cell nuclei, the multiple factors of NER diffuse freely, and they assemble only temporarily during repair. Although cells of some XP complementation groups usually exhibit a more impaired DNA repair than others (XPA, XPB, XPC and XPD), it is not possible to determine the affected DNA repair gene (XP complementation group) by the clinical phenotype alone. In addition, different mutations in the same gene can impair NER and/or the clinical phenotype to a varying degree.

Defects in NER are found not only in XP, but also in two other photosensitive disorders, Cockayne syndrome and the photosensitive

DEFICIENT DNA REPAIR GENES

Complementation group or inherited disorder	Function of affected gene product in DNA repair	Also associated with:
Nucleotide excision repair		
XPA	High affinity for injured DNA (single strands) Has many interactions with other NER proteins Might have a role in assembling the DNA repair machinery around the DNA lesion	–
XPB	Subunit of the transcription factor TFIIH Unwinds the DNA helix around the DNA lesion with its 3′→5′ helicase function	XP/CS*, TTD
XPC	DNA damage recognition Only required for global genome repair, not for transcription-coupled repair	–
XPD	Subunit of the transcription factor TFIIH like XPB Unwinds the DNA helix around the DNA lesion with its 5′→3′ helicase function	XP/CS*, TTD
XPE	Affinity for UV-damaged DNA Might have an auxiliary role in DNA damage recognition	–
XPF	5′-repair endonuclease The ERCC1/XPF complex cuts at the single-strand to double-strand transition 5′ of the DNA lesion	–
XPG	3′-repair endonuclease Cuts at the single-strand to double-strand transition 3′ of the DNA lesion Stablilizes TFIIH	XP/CS*
TTDA	Subunit of TFIIH (general transcription factor IIH, polypeptide 5) See XPB and XPD	
CSA	Only required for transcription-coupled repair Regulates recruitment of repair factors and chromatin remodelers upon stalling of RNA polymerase at the DNA lesion	–
CSB	Only required for transcription-coupled repair Regulates recruitment of repair factors and chromatin remodelers upon stalling of RNA polymerase at the DNA lesion	–
Translesional DNA synthesis		
XP variant	DNA polymerase-η Bypasses T–T dimers with correct insertion of two A residues	–

*Xeroderma pigmentosum/Cockayne syndrome overlap syndrome.

Table 85.1 Deficient DNA repair genes. Deficient DNA repair genes underlie xeroderma pigmentosum (XP) complementation groups XPA to XPG, trichothiodystrophy (TTD), Cockayne syndrome (CS), and XP variant. In addition, mutations in TTDN1, a protein that may have a role in maintaining cell cycle integrity, can lead to a nonphotosensitive form of TTD. ERCC1, excision repair cross complementing gene 1; NER, nucleotide excision repair; TFIIH, transcription

form of the brittle hair syndrome trichothiodystrophy[29]. These disorders are not cancer-prone, but sometimes have features that overlap with those of XP. It is remarkable how different mutations in the XPB, XPD and XPG genes are associated with specific clinical phenotypes, i.e. only XP or XP/Cockayne syndrome overlap or trichothiodystrophy (see Table 85.1). There is no clear correlation between disease phenotype and specific mutations or between the severity of the DNA repair defect and the clinical phenotype. The transcription/repair syndrome hypothesis has been put forward in an attempt to explain these various discrepancies. According to this hypothesis, mutations in XPD or XPB could affect the repair function of transcription factor IIH (TFIIH; see Fig. 85.12), resulting in photosensitivity and cancer development, and/or affect the transcription function of TFIIH, accounting for the typical phenotypes of trichothiodystrophy and Cockayne syndrome.

Individual cancer and skin cancer risks are determined not just by a pronounced NER deficiency, as in XP, but also by more subtle variations in DNA repair efficiency, e.g. as a consequence of polymorphisms in DNA repair genes[30,31]. Likewise, a decline in DNA repair efficiency with age has been linked to the increasing risk of skin cancer with advancing age[32].

Cells from patients with XP variant have an intact NER, yet a phenotype that is indistinguishable from the other XP complementation groups. Cells from these patients do not have a deficit in repairing DNA photoproducts, but a deficiency in what they do with unrepaired DNA photoproducts during replication (in the S phase of the cell cycle)[33]. Replicative DNA polymerases usually stall at unrepaired DNA lesions and detach from the DNA strand. For this situation, cells have a number of specialized DNA polymerases that are able to bypass different kinds of DNA damage and extend replication forks through damaged sites. Different polymerases perform this 'translesional DNA synthesis' with variable fidelity.

Due to a mutation in the pol-η gene, cells from patients with XP variant lack the particular ability of DNA polymerase-η to bypass T-T dimers with correct insertion of two A residues[34]. This indicates that NER does not always repair all DNA lesions and that the function of a high-fidelity translesional DNA polymerase is crucial for maintaining genomic stability (if cells enter S phase with unrepaired DNA damage). In cells from patients with XP variant, NER can remove most of the T-T dimers, but because polymerase-η is missing, any remaining dimers are more likely to be bypassed by polymerases that insert incorrect residues. This causes a UV-mutator phenotype. If DNA polymerase-η (or any other specialized translesional DNA polymerase) fails to bypass DNA damage during S phase, the cell is faced with a stalled replication fork. In these instances, DNA recombination repair, which utilizes strand invasion from the sister chromatid, can resolve the stalled replication fork. Recently, DNA recombination repair has been observed to also occur after exposure to UV irradiation[35].

In contrast to the bulky pyrimidine dimers, which can only be repaired by NER, the non-bulky oxidative DNA base modifications can be processed by base excision repair[28,36]. As the name implies, the initial step in base excision repair is the removal of a base rather than a nucleotide. This step is carried out by a DNA glycosylase, which removes the damaged DNA base by cleaving hydrolytically the base–deoxyribose glycosyl bond, leaving an apyrimidinic/apurinic (AP) site for further processing. This DNA glycosylase has substrate specificity for a particular kind of DNA base damage. The human DNA glycosylase 8-oxoG DNA glycosylase 1 has specificity for oxidized guanine bases, such as 8-oxoG (see above and Fig. 85.9), and it initiates processing of these lesions via base excision repair. Loss of this enzyme generates a cellular hypersensitivity to UVA, but does not increase UVA-associated mutation formation, further casting doubt regarding an important role for 8-oxoG in UVA mutagenesis[37].

Mutation Formation

Cancer development requires the accumulation of numerous genetic changes. UV induces mutations in several key genes involved in skin cancer development, e.g. *ras* oncogenes, *p53* and *PTCH* tumor suppressor genes. The *p53* tumor suppressor gene encodes a 53 kDa transcription factor that has a critical role in cell cycle regulation and induction of apoptosis after DNA damage[38]. Mutations in this gene can be found in most cutaneous SCCs and actinic keratoses (see Ch. 107). In addition, chronically sun-exposed skin harbors many keratinocyte clones with *p53* mutations, which are undetectable by light microscopy. This indicates that *p53* mutations are an early event in the pathogenesis of UV-induced cutaneous SCC. Most of these clones, and some of the actinic keratoses, regress after cessation of sun exposure. This indicates that loss of *p53* function through a *p53* mutation is not sufficient for malignant transformation, but that other mutations (probably many) need to accumulate in one cell, before this cell can undergo complete malignant transformation and develop into a tumor.

It is well established that different types of UV-induced damage can lead to the formation of a variety of different mutations, either during attempts by the cell to repair or to replicate these lesions. Most of the *p53* mutations in cutaneous SCCs and their precursors are C→T single base transition mutations at dipyrimidine sites[38]. Tandem CC→TT transition mutations are found in 10% of cutaneous SCCs. This spectrum of *p53* mutations is very different from *p53* mutations found in malignancies of internal organs; the latter do not have the preponderance of C→T mutations and have no CC→TT mutations. This, together with the fact that pyrimidine dimers most commonly cause C→T and some CC→TT mutations, provides convincing evidence for a crucial role of pyrimidine dimers in cutaneous photocarcinogenesis. Therefore, C→T, and especially CC→TT (Fig. 85.13), mutations have been termed 'signature mutations' for UV mutagenesis.

The mutagenic events that lead to the formation of melanoma are different, with *p53* mutations usually being an uncommon late event during tumor progression. With only a low frequency have C→T and CC→TT mutations been found in the melanoma suppressor gene *CDKN2A* (*INK4A*) of primary melanomas[39]. It remains unclear whether alterations in that gene represent early or late events in the pathogenesis of melanoma. If they were early events, only a small subset of melanomas could be regarded to be initiated by UV-induced pyrimidine dimers.

In melanomas and melanocytic nevi, a high frequency of T:A→A:T mutations at one particular site of *BRAF* has been described. Because these *BRAF* mutations have been found predominantly in melanomas from intermittently sun-exposed areas (and much less frequently in melanomas from unexposed areas or chronically UV-exposed areas), it has been suggested that this type of mutation is UV-induced[40]. However, such a mutation is not generated by any of the most common types of UV-induced DNA lesions. However, an unidentified, UV-induced thymine or adenine adduct might be responsible for these mutations.

Since many mutations are introduced during replication of damaged templates, and because pyrimidine dimers always form between adjacent pyrimidines, it is commonly thought that the transcribed strand is the site of the premutagenic DNA lesion. However, an example of ambiguity of strand assignment of the premutagenic lesion is the example of singlet oxygen-induced 8-oxoG, which can affect either the template (guanine in the DNA strand) or the substrate (guanine nucleotide)[41]. Extensive studies involving 8-oxoG have shown that it generates predominantly G→T transversions (by mispairing of the template 8-oxoG with adenine) or A→C transversions (by misincorporation of 8-oxoG as a substrate opposite adenine)[41].

As pointed out previously, UVB and UVA, the relevant wavelengths of UV light that reach the earth, produce a mixture of different types of DNA lesions, including the different DNA photoproducts and oxidative DNA damage. It is unclear to what degree these different forms of UV-induced DNA damage contribute to UV-induced mutations and

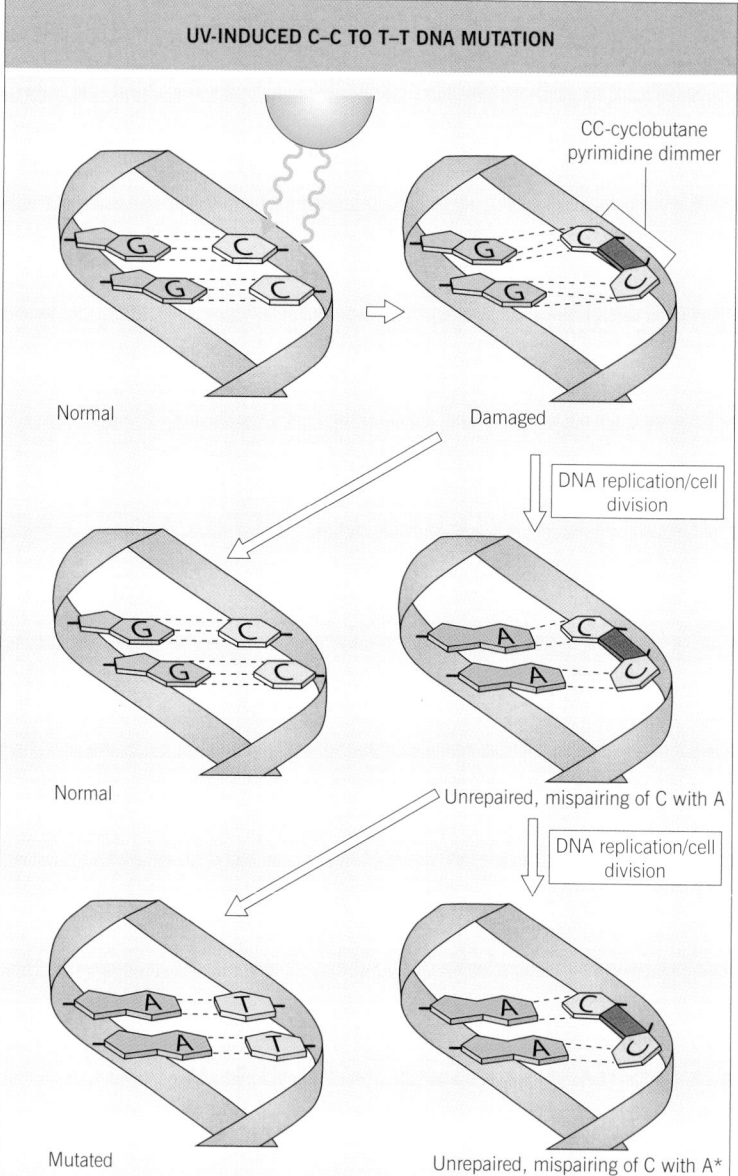

UV-INDUCED C–C TO T–T DNA MUTATION

Normal

Damaged — CC-cyclobutane pyrimidine dimmer

DNA replication/cell division

Normal

Unrepaired, mispairing of C with A

DNA replication/cell division

Mutated

Unrepaired, mispairing of C with A*

Fig. 85.13 UV-induced CC→TT DNA mutation. Following formation of a pyrimidine dimer between two adjacent cytosines and subsequent cell division, a CC→TT mutation results. This represents a UV signature mutation. *May give rise to more C→T mutations.

eventually to photocarcinogenesis. While there is little doubt that pyrimidine dimers cause many, and probably most, of the mutations induced by UVB, the contribution of oxidative DNA damage to mutation formation, especially that due to UVA, is still a matter of debate.

Several pieces of evidence, primarily from published mutation spectra in mammalian cells[42,43], suggest that the mechanisms of UVA-induced mutation formation are different from those of UVB-induced mutation formation. Until recently (see below), UVA-induced mutagenesis was most often attributed to a non-dimer type of DNA damage. Additional evidence for differences in UVA- and UVB-induced mutagenesis and carcinogenesis was provided by van Kranen et al.[44], who sequenced the *p53* gene of UVA-induced SCCs in mice. Less than 15% of these UVA-induced tumors carried *p53* mutations, very dissimilar to UVB-induced tumors, almost all of which carried *p53* mutations.

However, more recently, a comparison of UVB- and UVA-induced mutations in primary human skin cells revealed a striking similarity[25], raising the possibility of a very similar mechanism of mutation formation. In addition, several lines of evidence from observed mutation spectra point to pyrimidine dimers as the most important mutagenic DNA lesion, not just for UVB, but also for UVA. A less effective antimutagenic response, e.g. a less effective activation of p53 by UVA (as compared to UVB), might lead to a greater mutagenic potential for a UVA-induced pyrimidine dimer, as compared to a UVB-induced dimer[25a].

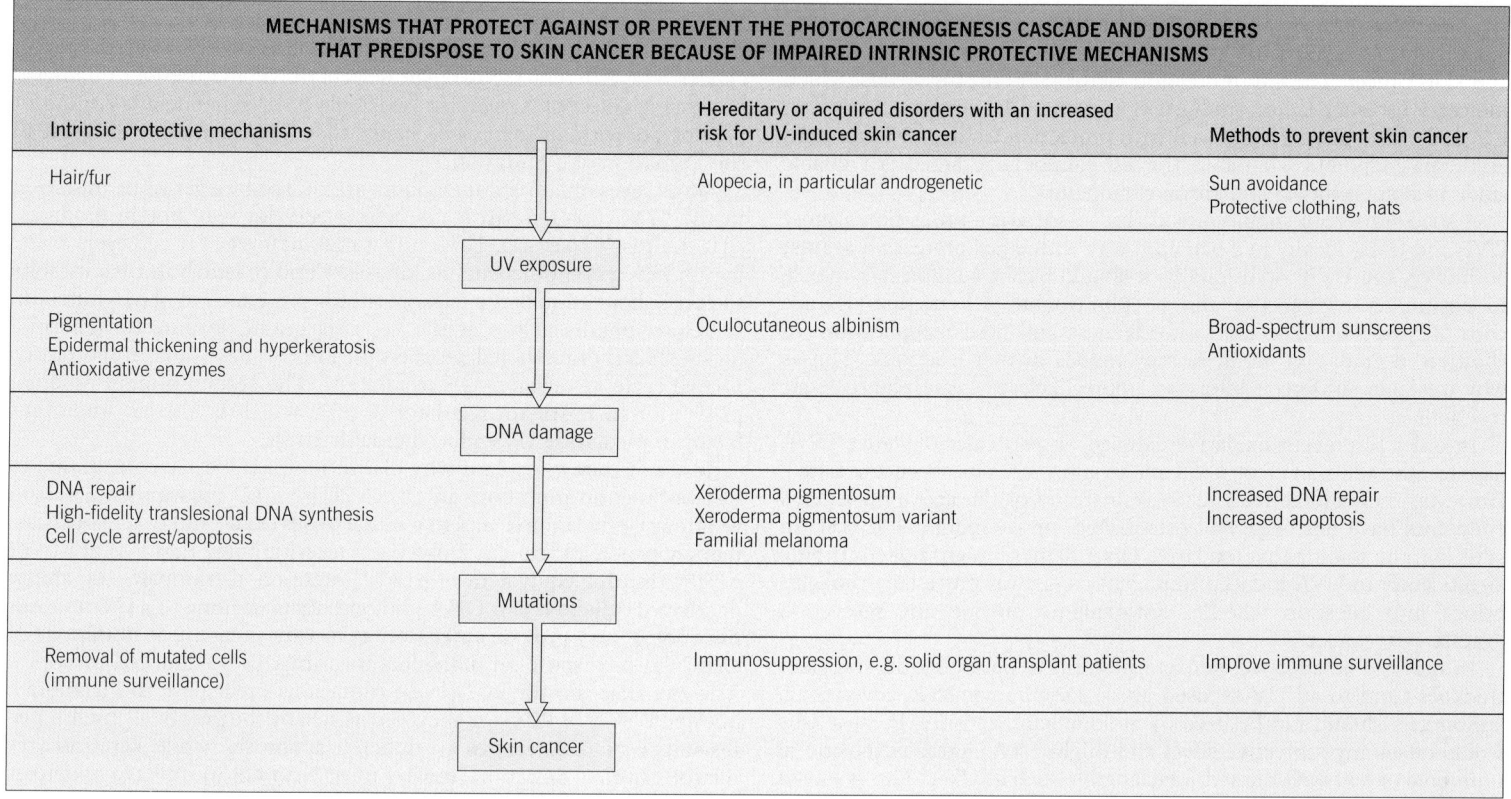

MECHANISMS THAT PROTECT AGAINST OR PREVENT THE PHOTOCARCINOGENESIS CASCADE AND DISORDERS THAT PREDISPOSE TO SKIN CANCER BECAUSE OF IMPAIRED INTRINSIC PROTECTIVE MECHANISMS

Intrinsic protective mechanisms	Hereditary or acquired disorders with an increased risk for UV-induced skin cancer	Methods to prevent skin cancer
Hair/fur	Alopecia, in particular androgenetic	Sun avoidance Protective clothing, hats
UV exposure		
Pigmentation Epidermal thickening and hyperkeratosis Antioxidative enzymes	Oculocutaneous albinism	Broad-spectrum sunscreens Antioxidants
DNA damage		
DNA repair High-fidelity translesional DNA synthesis Cell cycle arrest/apoptosis	Xeroderma pigmentosum Xeroderma pigmentosum variant Familial melanoma	Increased DNA repair Increased apoptosis
Mutations		
Removal of mutated cells (immune surveillance)	Immunosuppression, e.g. solid organ transplant patients	Improve immune surveillance
Skin cancer		

Fig. 85.14 Mechanisms that protect against or prevent the photocarcinogenesis cascade and disorders that predispose to skin cancer because of impaired intrinsic protective mechanisms. Several intrinsic mechanisms protect against the formation of skin cancer following UV exposure at different points of the photocarcinogenesis cascade of events. These mechanisms are impaired in disorders with increased risk for UV-induced skin cancer. Each step of the photocarcinogenesis cascade can be targeted for modification and reduction of skin cancer risk.

As a result, exposure to a pure UVA source, as in phototherapy (high-dose UVA1) or tanning parlors, might be more carcinogenic than exposure to a UVA source that also contains UVB, as the former will induce less of a protective damage response than will a mixed UVA/UVB irradiation.

Protection Against Photocarcinogenesis

To ensure that most of the damage inflicted by sun exposure will not lead to the formation of skin cancer, UV-exposed cells have several lines of defense against the photocarcinogenesis cascade (Fig. 85.14).

- In order to prevent DNA damage as a consequence of UV exposure, the epidermis has constitutive as well as inducible melanin. It can increase its thickness (which reduces UV exposure in the basal layer) and the epidermis contains antioxidative enzymes, which quench reactive oxygen species and reduce the formation of oxidative DNA damage[45]. Cellular melanin is a mixture of different polymerized pigments that absorb UV radiation (see Ch. 64). Illumination of the brown to black eumelanin generates the superoxide radical within the molecule, which is very rapidly scavenged. The red or yellow pheomelanin is a less effective radical scavenger; upon UV exposure, pheomelanin is degraded, with a net formation of superoxide. Therefore, pheomelanin is regarded as a photosensitizer, rather than a photoprotector like eumelanin.
- In order to prevent mutation formation after DNA damage has been introduced, cells have several different DNA repair systems (see above) as well as the ability to bypass DNA damage without inducing mutations. Cells also have the ability to halt proliferation (cell cycle arrest) in order to allow more time for repair, reducing the chance of replicating a damaged template, or they can die via apoptosis when they accrue overwhelming DNA damage.
- Even after mutations have fixed the inflicted damage for the lifetime of the affected cells, the organism still removes most of these cells, e.g. via immune surveillance.

Some of these protective mechanisms can be upregulated, facilitating an adaptive response to repeated UV 'attacks'. These include pigmentation, skin thickening, and antioxidant enzymes. DNA excision repair

can also be upregulated in a SOS-like response[46,47]. In contrast, immune surveillance is downregulated following UV exposures, likely contributing significantly to photocarcinogenesis (see above).

Exposure to UVA cannot be regarded as harmless, and dermatologists must warn not only against UVB but also UVA exposure. There are at least three areas where increased exposure to UVA might pose a public health risk.

- The use of high-dose UVA emitters for cosmetic purposes in tanning parlors is currently growing exponentially, and many researchers fear a second 'melanoma epidemic' for that reason. It is estimated that approximately 25 million Americans use tanning beds or sunlamps every year, especially teenagers and young adults.
- An increase in UVA exposure can also result from the use of sunscreens. According to Autier et al.[48], sunscreens are often used for their ability to prolong sun exposure. Since broad-spectrum sunscreens still do not filter UVA as efficiently as UVB, an increase in UVA exposure as a consequence of sunscreen use remains a problem.
- High-dose UVA1 phototherapy has been shown to be an effective treatment for atopic dermatitis, scleroderma, cutaneous T-cell lymphoma, and other dermatoses. However, the long-term risks of this treatment have not been established. Considering the possible role of UVA in the development of cutaneous melanoma, one must weigh the risks and benefits of the use of high-dose UVA1, especially in children.

In addition to the intrinsic protective mechanisms that counteract the chain of events leading to the formation of skin cancer, there are extrinsic protective agents and protective behaviors that can help individuals reduce their skin cancer risk (see Fig. 85.14).

In order to prevent or reduce UV irradiation of the skin, one can avoid the sun, especially around noontime, stay in the shade, wear protective clothing and/or wear sunscreens. Sunscreens are topical preparations that attenuate UV radiation before it enters the skin, by reflection, absorption or both (see Ch. 132). Reflectant products reflect UV from a film of inert metal particles, usually zinc oxide or titanium dioxide in a suitable vehicle. Absorbent sunscreens absorb UVB, UVA or both UVA and UVB into specific chemicals (UV filters) and re-emit the energy as insignificant quantities of heat.

Sunscreens protect not only against the acute skin injury of sunburn, but also against UV-induced immune suppression, photoaging and skin cancer. The sun protection factor (SPF) of sunscreens, which indicates by what factor sunburn is prevented by sunscreen use (see Ch. 132), does not correlate well with protection factors for other non-erythema endpoints. Therefore, the SPF cannot be regarded as a reliable guide to non-erythema and chronic endpoints[49].

A good sunscreen should provide broad-spectrum protection against UVB and UVA, ideally in a balanced way with equal protection against both UVA and UVB. Additionally, it should have a comfortable vehicle to ensure its regular use and be photostable. Filters that degrade with UV exposure lose their effectiveness and need reapplication. In addition, degradation products may induce further reactions. This is why unstable sunscreen filters are more likely to cause photoallergic reactions.

In order to prevent oxidative damage, in particular oxidative DNA damage, the addition of antioxidants to sunscreens has been advocated. However, their protective effects against any of the above-mentioned endpoints have not been well established, or are marginal at best. In addition, the finding that oxidative DNA damage might not contribute significantly to UVA-induced mutagenesis (as was previously thought) brings into question whether antioxidants provide any protection against skin cancer.

In order to be effective, sunscreens need to be applied in sufficient thickness and to all UV-exposed areas. Despite common advertising, sunscreens should not be used to prolong sun exposure, because this would offset any protective effect and might even increase exposure to unfiltered or less-well-filtered wavelengths, such as UVA. This is one of the explanations for the seemingly contradictory finding (in some studies) that the use of sunscreens might increase, rather than decrease, the incidence of skin cancer, especially melanoma[50].

Topical application of DNA repair enzymes has been shown to increase DNA repair in skin cells and to accelerate removal of DNA photoproducts. In patients with XP, such applications have been reported to reduce the occurrence of actinic keratoses[51]. This indicates that it may be possible to prevent the formation of mutations after the introduction of DNA photoproducts with the use of such 'enzymatic sunscreens'. Similarly, it may be possible in the future to accelerate or improve the removal of damaged or mutated cells (e.g. by increasing apoptosis of damaged cells) or to improve immune surveillance (e.g. by vaccination).

RELATED DISEASES

Many disorders with an increased risk of UV-induced skin cancer are characterized by a deficiency in the intrinsic protective mechanisms discussed above (see Fig. 85.14). For example, men with androgenetic alopecia have a much higher risk of developing skin cancers on the scalp than do men who have retained their UV-protective hair cover. Diminution or lack of protective melanin, as in oculocutaneous albinism, increases the amount of DNA damage in the basal layer of the epidermis after UV irradiation and, subsequently, the risk of skin cancer. The different DNA repair defects of XP and the DNA damage-processing defect of XP variant (see Table 85.1) generate a UV-mutator phenotype, with an increased chance that DNA damage will result in the formation of a mutation.

Some cases of familial melanoma are caused by a germline mutation in the CDKN2A (INK4A) locus, which encodes two protein products, p16 and p14ARF (see Ch. 107). Intact p16 induces a G1 cell cycle arrest by inhibiting cyclin-dependent kinases 4 and 6, which in turn inhibits the phosphorylation of the retinoblastoma protein. Loss of p16 function, therefore, entails a loss of the G1 checkpoint, leading to abnormal proliferation, unrestricted progression into S phase, and, importantly, no cell cycle arrest after UV irradiation. The second protein product, p14ARF, is an upstream regulator of p53, which is also an important factor in mediating UV-induced growth arrest.

It is not easy to explain why disruption of cell cycle control due to loss-of-function mutations in CDKN2A (INK4A) predisposes a person to primarily melanoma, and to a much lesser degree internal neoplasias, namely pancreatic cancer. However, a recent finding that loss of p16 or p19ARF (murine equivalent of p14ARF) function also impairs the ability of affected cells to repair DNA photoproducts (leading to a UV-mutator phenotype) may provide an answer as to why silencing or mutations of CDKN2A predispose an individual to primarily UV-induced tumors[52]. The fact that germline CDKN2A mutations predispose to melanoma, but not to SCC or BCC, might be explained by the previously mentioned resistance of melanocytes to undergo apoptosis, while keratinocytes require another mutation (mostly in p53) to fail to undergo apoptosis despite increased UV-induced DNA damage[53].

In addition to inducing apoptosis in cells with overwhelming UV-induced DNA damage, p53 protects against UV mutagenesis by inducing cell cycle arrest after UV-induced damage and by stimulating DNA repair by directly binding to DNA repair enzymes[54]. Consequently, loss of p53 function has been shown to result in a UV-mutator phenotype and reduced repair of UV-induced DNA damage. Li–Fraumeni syndrome is characterized by a germline mutation of the p53 gene, and predisposes to malignancies of various internal organs and possibly cutaneous melanoma[55].

Patients with the nevoid basal cell carcinoma syndrome, who develop multiple BCCs, especially in UV-exposed areas, harbor germline mutations in the PTCH gene. PTCH belongs to the Hedgehog signal transduction pathway that transmits extracellular growth and differentiation signals to the nucleus (see Ch. 107). While many of the PTCH mutations in sporadic BCCs are UV signature mutations (C→T and CC→TT), their frequency is lower than in p53, and it is unclear whether sporadic PTCH mutagenesis is purely UV-induced[56]. The latter speculation is supported by the clinical observation that a number of BCCs occur in relatively UV-protected sites, e.g. the inner canthus and the retro-auricular area.

REFERENCES

1. Anderson RR, Parrish JA. The optics of human skin. J Invest Dermatol. 1981;77:13–19.
2. Bruls WAG, Slaper H, van der Leun JC, Beurrens L. Transmission of human epidermis and stratum corneum as a function of thickness in the ultraviolet and visible wavelengths. Photochem Photobiol. 1984;40:485–95.
3. Piette J, Merville-Louis MP, Decuyper J. Damages induced in nucleic acids by photosensitization. Photochem Photobiol. 1986;44:793–802.
4. Soter NA. Acute effects of ultraviolet radiation on the skin. Semin Dermatol. 1990;9:11–15.
5. Young AR, Chadwick CA, Harrison GI, et al. The similarity of action spectra for thymine dimers in human epidermis and erythema suggests that DNA is the chromophore for erythema. J Invest Dermatol. 1998;111:982–8.
6. Ullrich SE. Mechanisms underlying UV-induced immune suppression. Mutat Res. 2005;571:185–205.
7. Schwarz T. Photoimmunosuppression. Photodermatol Photoimmunol Photomed. 2002;18:141–5.

8. Beissert S, Schwarz A, Schwarz T. Regulatory T cells. J Invest Dermatol. 2006;126:15–24.
9. de Gruijl FR. Ultraviolet radiation and tumor immunity. Methods. 2002;28:122–9.
10. Moulin G, Thomas L, Vigneau M, Fiere A. Un cas unilateral d'élastose avec kystes et comédons de Favre et Racouchot. Ann Dermatol Venereol. 1994;121:721–3.
11. International Agency for Research on Cancer. Solar and Ultraviolet Radiation. IARC Monographs on the Evaluation of Carcinogenic Risks to Humans, Vol. 55. Lyon: IARC, 1993.
12. de Gruijl FR, Sterenborg HJ, Forbes PD, et al. Wavelength dependence of skin cancer induction by ultraviolet irradiation of albino hairless mice. Cancer Res. 1993;53:53–60.
13. Rünger TM. Role of UVA in the pathogenesis of melanoma and non-melanoma skin cancer. Photodermatol Photoimmunol Photomed. 1999;15:212–16.
14. Gallagher RP, Spinelli JJ, Lee TK, et al. Tanning beds, sunlamps, and risk of cutaneous malignant melanoma.

Cancer Epidemiol Biomarkers Prevent. 2005; 14:562–6.
14b. Veierod MB, Weiderpass E, Thorn M, et al. A prospective study of pigmentation, sun exposure, and risk of cutaneous malignant melanoma in women. J Natl Cancer Inst. 2003;95:1530–8.
15. Autier P, Doré JF, Schifflers E, et al. Melanoma and use of sunscreens: an EORTC case-control study in Germany, Belgium, and France. The EORTC Melanoma Cooperative Group. Intl J Cancer. 1995;61:749–55.
16. De Fabo EC, Noonan FP, Fears T, Merlino G. Ultraviolet B but not ultraviolet A radiation initiates melanoma. Cancer Res. 2004;64:6372–6.
17. Gilchrest BA, Eller MS, Geller AC, Yaar M. The pathogenesis of melanoma induced by ultraviolet radiation. N Engl J Med. 1999;340:1341–8.
18. Friedberg EC, Walker GC, Siede W. DNA Repair and Mutagenesis. Washington: ASM Press, 1995.
19. Perdiz D, Grof P, Mezzina M, et al. Distribution and repair of bipyrimidine photoproducts in solar UV-irradiated mammalian cells. J Biol Chem. 2000;275:26732–42.

20. Douki T, Reynaud-Angelin A, Cadet J, Sage E. Bipyrimidine photoproducts rather than oxidative lesions are the main type of DNA damage involved in the genotoxic effect of solar UVA radiation. Biochemistry. 2003;42:9221–6.

21. Danpure HJ, Tyrrell RM. Oxygen-dependence of near UV (365 nm) lethality and the interaction of near UV and x-rays in two mammalian cell lines. Photochem Photobiol. 1976;23:171–7.

22. Kvam E, Tyrrell RM. Induction of oxidative DNA base damage in human skin cells by UV and near visible radiation. Carcinogenesis. 1997;18:2379–84.

23. Darr D, Fridovich I. Free radicals in cutaneous biology. J Invest Dermatol. 1994;102:671–5.

24. Kielbassa C, Roza L, Epe B. Wavelength dependence of oxidative DNA damage induced by UV and visible light. Carcinogenesis. 1997;18:811–16.

25. Kappes UP, Rünger TM. Short- and long-wave ultraviolet light (UVB and UVA) induce similar mutations in human skin cells. J Invest Dermatol. 2006;126:667–75.

25a. Rünger TM, Kappes UP. Mechanisms of mutation formation with long-wave ultraviolet light (UVA). Photodermatol, Photoimmunol, Photomed. 2007, in press.

26. Young AR, Potten CS, Nikaido O, et al. Human melanocytes and keratinocytes exposed to UVB or UVA in vivo show comparable levels of thymine dimers. J Invest Dermatol. 1998;111:936–40.

27. Douki T, Perdiz D, Grof P, et al. Oxidation of guanine in cellular DNA by solar UV radiation: biological role. Photochem Photobiol. 1999;70:184–90.

28. Lindahl T, Wood RD. Quality control by DNA repair. Science. 1999;286:1897–905.

29. de Boer J, Hoeijmakers JHJ. Nucleotide excision repair and human syndromes. Carcinogenesis. 2000;21:453–60.

30. Wei Q, Lee JE, Gershenwald JE, et al. Repair of UV light-induced DNA damage and risk of cutaneous malignant melanoma. J Natl Cancer Inst. 2003;95:308–15.

31. Blankenburg S, König IR, Moessner R, et al. Assessment of 3 xeroderma pigmentosum group C gene polymorphisms and risk of cutaneous melanoma: a case-control study. Carcinogenesis. 2005;26:1085–90.

32. Wei Q. Effect of aging on DNA repair and skin carcinogenesis: a minireview of population-based studies. J Investig Dermatol Symp Proc. 1998;3:19–22.

33. Woodgate R. A plethora of lesion-replicating DNA polymerases. Genes Dev. 1999;13:2191–5.

34. Johnson RE, Kondratick CM, Prakash S, Prakash L. hRAD30 mutations in the variant form of xeroderma pigmentosum. Science. 1999;285:263–5.

35. Dunn J, Potter M, Rees A, Rünger TM. Activation of the Fanconi anemia/BRCA pathway and recombination repair in the cellular response to solar ultraviolet light. Cancer Res. 2006;66:11140–7.

36. Demple B, Harrison L. Repair of oxidative damage to DNA: enzymology and biology. Ann Rev Biochem. 1994;63:915–48.

37. Kappes UP, Rünger TM. No major role for 7,8-dihydro-8-oxoguanine in ultraviolet light-induced mutagenesis. Radiat Res. 2005;164:440–5.

38. Wikonkal NM, Brash DE. Ultraviolet radiation induced signature mutations in photocarcinogenesis. J Investig Dermatol Symp Proc. 1999;4:6–10.

39. Peris K, Chimenti S, Fargnoli MC, et al. UV fingerprint CKDN2A but no p14ARF mutations in sporadic melanoma. J Invest Dermatol. 1999;112:825–6.

40. Maldonado JL, Fridlyand J, Patel H, et al. Determinants of BRAF mutations in primary melanomas. J Natl Cancer Inst. 2003;95:1878–90.

41. Cheng KC, Cahill DS, Kasai H, et al. 8-Hydroxyguanine, an abundant form of oxidative DNA damage, causes GT and AC substitutions. J Biol Chem. 1992;267:166–72.

42. Drobetsky EA, Turcotte J, Chateauneuf A. A role for ultraviolet A in solar mutagenesis. Proc Natl Acad Sci USA. 1995;92:2350–4.

43. Robert C, Muel B, Benoit A, et al. Cell survival and shuttle vector mutagenesis induced by ultraviolet A and ultraviolet B radiation in a human cell line. J Invest Dermatol. 1996;106:721–8.

44. van Kranen HJ, de Laat A, van de Ven J, et al. Low incidence of p53 mutations in UVA (365-nm)-induced skin tumors in hairless mice. Cancer Res. 1997;57:1238–40.

45. Halliwell B, Gutteridge JMC. Antioxidant defenses. In: Free Radicals in Biology and Medicine, 3rd edn. New York: Oxford University Press, 1999:105–245.

46. Francis MA, Rainbow AJ. UV-enhanced reactivation of a UV-damaged reporter gene suggests transcription-coupled repair is UV-inducible in human cells. Carcinogenesis. 1999;20:19–26.

47. Smith ML, Seo YR. P53 regulation of DNA excision repair pathways. Mutagenesis. 2002;17:149–56.

48. Autier P, Doré JF, Négrier S, et al. Sunscreen use and duration of sun exposure: a double-blind, randomized trial. J Natl Cancer Inst. 1999;91:1304–9.

49. Young AR, Walker SL. Sunscreens: photoprotection of non-erythema endpoints relevant to skin cancer. Photodermatol Photoimmunol Photomed. 1999;15:221–5.

50. Weinstock MA. Do sunscreens increase or decrease melanoma risk: an epidemiologic evaluation. J Investig Dermatol Symp Proc. 1999;4:97–100.

51. Yarosh D, Klein J, O'Conner A, et al. Effect of topically applied T4 endonuclease V in liposomes on skin cancer in xeroderma pigmentosum: a randomized study. Lancet. 2001;357:926–9.

52. Sarkar-Agrawal P, Vergilis I, Sharpless N, et al. Impaired processing of DNA photoproducts and ultraviolet hypermutability with loss of p16^{INK4a} or p19^{ARF}. J Natl Cancer Inst. 2004;96:1790–3.

53. Rünger TM, Vergilis I, Sarkar-Agrawal P, et al. How disruption of cell cycle regulating genes might predispose to sun-induced skin cancer. Cell Cycle. 2005;4:643–5.

54. Wang XW, Vermeulen W, Coursen JD, et al. The XPB and XPD DNA helicases are components of the p53-mediated apoptosis pathway. Genes Dev. 1996;10:1219–32.

55. Malkin D, Li FP, Strong LC, et al. Germ line p53 mutations in a familial syndrome of breast cancer, sarcomas, and other neoplasms. Science. 1990;250:1233–8.

56. Aszterbaum M, Beech J, Epstein E Jr. Ultraviolet radiation mutagenesis of hedgehog pathway genes in basal cell carcinoma. J Investig Dermatol Symp Proc. 1999;4:41–5.

Photodermatoses

Henry W Lim and John LM Hawk

86

All skin is photosensitive as a result of containing molecules of appropriate shape to absorb ultraviolet radiation (UVR) energy during exposure. The latter is then either re-emitted harmlessly as further radiation or diverted to power thermal chemical reactions which lead to molecular, cellular, tissue and clinical change, some repaired, some permanent. DNA is the most ubiquitous absorber, initiating UVR-induced changes including sunburning, tanning, hyperplasia, aging and carcinogenesis. On the other hand, only certain individuals develop abnormal reactions, otherwise known as the photodermatoses, as a result either of abnormal tissue responses following normal molecular absorption, or of normal responses following abnormal absorption (Table 86.1). An algorithmic guide to the diagnosis of cutaneous photosensitivity is provided in Figure 86.1.

ABNORMAL CUTANEOUS EFFECTS OF UVR EXPOSURE

Polymorphous light eruption is consistently the most common photodermatosis, based upon relative frequency analyses from photodermatology centers worldwide; it is followed (in decreasing order of frequency) by photoaggravated dermatoses, drug-induced photosensitivity, chronic actinic dermatitis and solar urticaria[1,2].

Of note, because of the relatively small number of patients afflicted with conditions discussed in this chapter, all treatment modalities mentioned are derived either from studies involving a series of patients or from anecdotal case reports.

Idiopathic, Probably Immunologically Based, Photodermatoses

This group of disorders is outlined in Table 86.2.

Polymorphous light eruption

Synonyms: ■ Polymorphic light eruption ■ Benign summer light eruption (one clinical form) ■ Juvenile spring eruption (one clinical form)

Key features

- The most common photodermatosis
- Presents with papules, vesicles or plaques within hours of sun exposure; lasts for a few days
- Most severe in the spring or early summer
- Action spectra: UVB, UVA and, rarely, visible light
- Management: photoprotection, narrowband (NB)-UVB, PUVA, antimalarials

Introduction

Polymorphous light eruption (PMLE) is a common, sunlight-induced eruption affecting individuals of all races[3]. Attacks are intermittent and follow minutes to hours (rarely days) of exposure of the skin to sunlight or artificial UVR. Non-scarring, pruritic, erythematous papules, papulovesicles, vesicles and/or plaques then develop minutes to hours later. The eruption is generally most severe in the spring or early summer, and it usually disappears completely during the winter.

CLASSIFICATION OF PHOTODERMATOSES
Abnormal tissue responses* following normal molecular absorption
• Idiopathic, probably immunologically based, disorders
• Defective DNA repair disorders
• Photoaggravated dermatoses
Normal tissue responses following abnormal molecular absorption
• Chemical- and drug-induced photosensitivity
– Exogenous
– Endogenous: cutaneous porphyrias, probably Smith–Lemli–Opitz syndrome
*Due to inherited or acquired defects.

Table 86.1 Classification of photodermatoses.

CLASSIFICATION OF IDIOPATHIC, PROBABLY IMMUNOLOGICALLY BASED, PHOTODERMATOSES
• Polymorphous light eruption
• Actinic prurigo
• Hydroa vacciniforme
• Chronic actinic dermatitis
• Solar urticaria

Table 86.2 Classification of idiopathic, probably immunologically based, photodermatoses.

History

PMLE was first described by Carl Rasch in 1900 and then mentioned again by Haxthausen in 1918.

Epidemiology

PMLE affects men and women of every race and all ages. The prevalence in the general population is inversely related to latitude, being highest in Scandinavia (22%), high in the UK and northern US (10–15%), and low in Australia (5%) and equatorial Singapore (around 1%)[3]. This may be due to the hardening phenomenon experienced by patients residing in sunny climates. Women are affected slightly more frequently than men, with the second and third decades being the most common times of onset.

Pathogenesis

Attacks of PMLE are produced by UVR (and perhaps, on occasion, by visible light) from sunlight or other sources such as tanning beds. Spring and summer sunlight in temperate regions is most efficient at inducing outbreaks, however, generally at lower than *minimal erythema* ('sunburning') *doses* (MEDs). Action spectra range from broadband UVB (BB-UVB) to UVA and rarely to visible irradiation. Photoprovocation studies have shown a positive response in 50% of patients to narrowband UVB (NB-UVB), 50% to BB-UVA, and 80% to both UVB and UVA[4].

PMLE appears to be a delayed-type hypersensitivity (DTH) response to undefined, endogenous, cutaneous photo-induced antigen(s)[3]. Timed biopsy specimens, following solar-simulated irradiation with doses that were approximately two-thirds of the MED, have shown perivascular infiltrates of primarily CD4+ T lymphocytes (within hours) and CD8+ cells (within days); an increased number of dermal and epidermal antigen-presenting cells has also been noted. Overall, this pattern is suggestive of a DTH response as is seen in allergic contact dermatitis

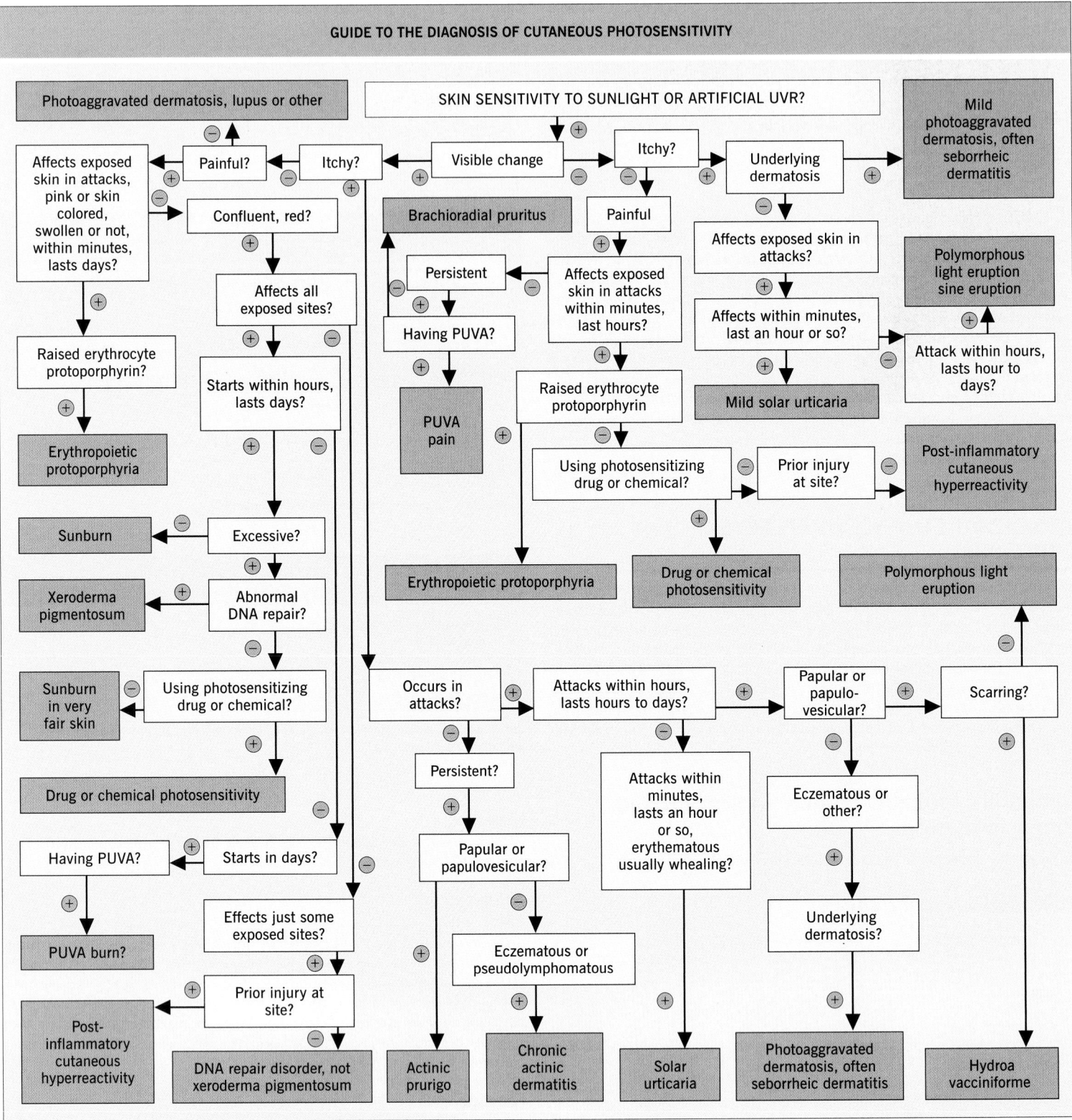

Fig. 86.1 Guide to the diagnosis of cutaneous photosensitivity. The diagnosis can generally be made from patient history and clinical findings, provided the titers of antinuclear antibodies and other LE-associated antibodies are normal.

and the tuberculin reaction. In addition, E-selectin, vascular cell adhesion molecule-1 (VCAM-1) and intercellular adhesion molecule-1 (ICAM-1) are expressed, as in other DTH responses. However, the UVR absorbers and antigens responsible for inducing PMLE have not been characterized.

Susceptibility to PMLE appears to be genetic, with perhaps 70% of the population having a 'tendency' for developing the condition but not all expressing it because of variations in penetrance[5]. In addition, the inherited abnormality appears to be a reduction in the normal UVR-induced suppression of the induction (but not the elicitation) of cutaneous DTH[6]. Specifically, in PMLE, there may be a lesser degree

of cutaneous immunosuppression following UV exposure (compared to healthy individuals), resulting in an enhanced response to putative photo-antigen(s) and the development of clinical lesions.

Clinical features

The appearance of PMLE is most common during the spring and early summer and follows minutes to hours (sometimes days, particularly on sunny vacations) of sun exposure. Outbreaks may also occur after exposure to snow-reflected sunlight during the winter or after the use of tanning beds. The eruption then develops minutes to hours later and lasts for one to several days or occasionally weeks, particularly with

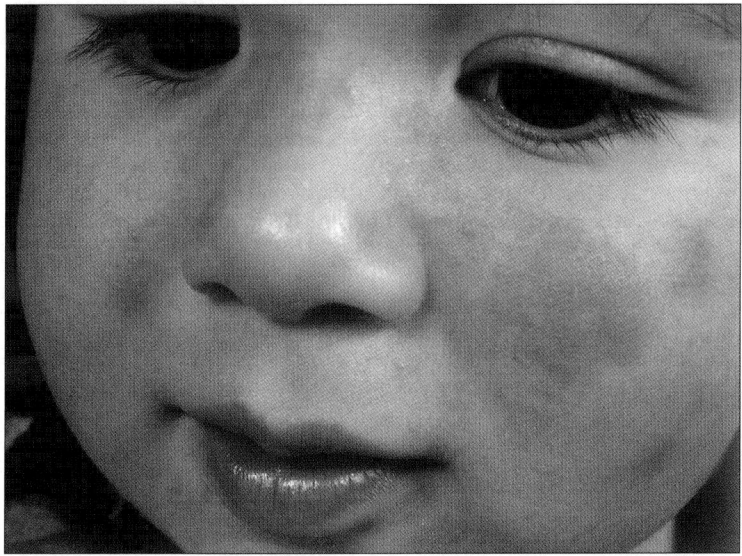

Fig. 86.2 **Polymorphous light eruption.** Edematous erythematous plaques on the cheeks in a young child.

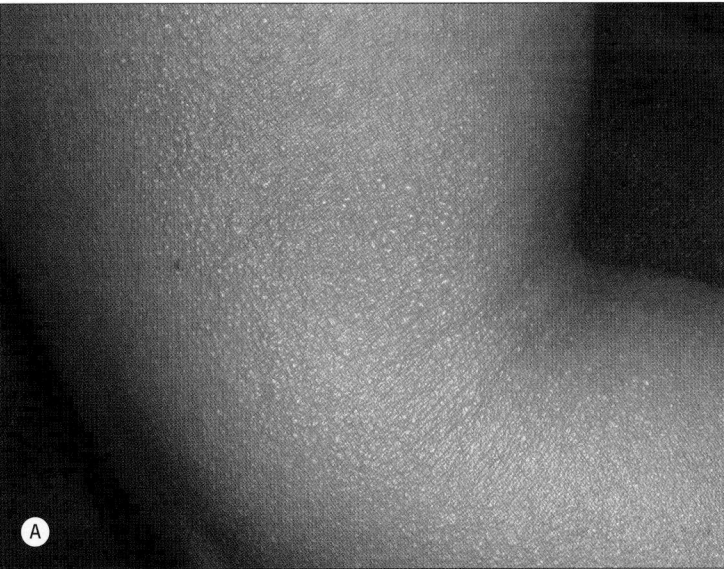

continuing exposure. However, the tendency for the eruption to occur often diminishes or ceases as the summer or a sunny vacation proceeds, a phenomenon described as 'hardening'.

In a symmetric and frequently patchy fashion, any, but usually not all, exposed skin is typically affected while other areas, especially those normally exposed to sunlight, are often spared. The distribution and nature of the eruption in a given patient are usually consistent. Areas commonly affected are the face, neck, outer aspect of the arms, and dorsal surface of the hands (Figs 86.2 & 86.3), but there may be more widespread involvement of sun-exposed sites (Fig. 86.4).

Lesions vary widely amongst patients, but are generally mildly pruritic, grouped, erythematous or skin-colored papules of varying sizes, not infrequently coalescing into large, smooth or unevenly surfaced plaques. In darkly pigmented individuals, the most common morphology is grouped, pinhead-sized papules in sun-exposed areas[7]. Vesicles, bullae, papulovesicles and confluent edematous swelling (particularly of the face) are also observed; uncommonly, erythema or only pruritus may occur. Occasionally, the helices of the ears, particularly in boys because their ears are relatively more exposed, may be principally affected, often with vesicles, in a form of PMLE sometimes referred to as 'juvenile spring eruption'. Rarely, covered sites may also be affected. General malaise, headache, fever, nausea and other symptoms rarely occur. PMLE may be lifelong; however, in a 32-year follow-up of 94 patients, the disease improved or resolved in 58% over a period of 16 years, and in 75% over a period of 32 years[8].

Pathology

There is variable epidermal spongiosis and a superficial and deep, perivascular and periappendageal, lymphohistiocytic dermal infiltrate (Fig. 86.5), often with scattered eosinophils and neutrophils. Significant papillary dermal edema occurs commonly[9]. Rarely, difficulty in distinction from cutaneous lupus may occur if interface changes are significant, or from lymphoma if the dermal inflammatory cell infiltrate is marked.

Differential diagnosis

The diagnosis of PMLE is suggested by its characteristic history, clinical findings, lack of circulating antinuclear and other lupus erythematosus (LE)-associated antibodies (e.g. anti-Ro; see Ch. 41), and normal porphyrin profile (see Ch. 49). Histologic findings are confirmatory and direct immunofluorescence is negative. Photoprovocative tests to induce lesions are helpful and may aid in patient management[4].

Up to 50% of predominantly photosensitive LE patients (including those with subacute cutaneous LE and LE tumidus) have symptoms consistent with PMLE. While the skin lesions in photosensitive LE are photoexacerbated, they can also occur without sun exposure and may be present in sun-protected areas. In contrast, lesions of PMLE are present almost exclusively in sun-exposed sites. Furthermore, lesions

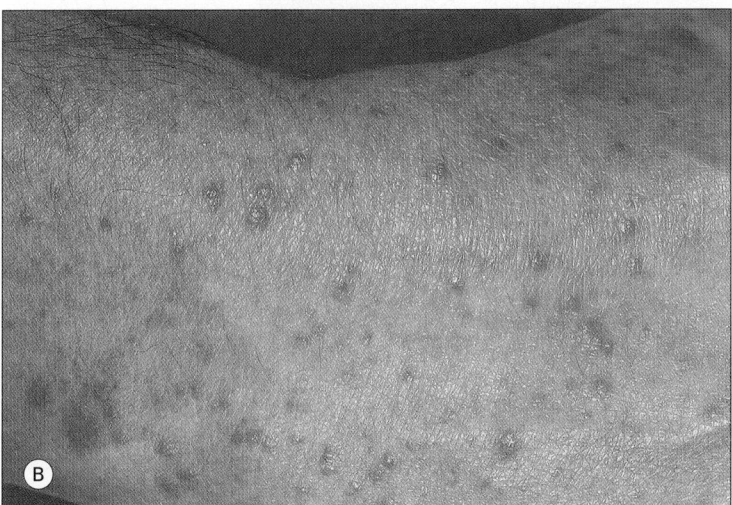

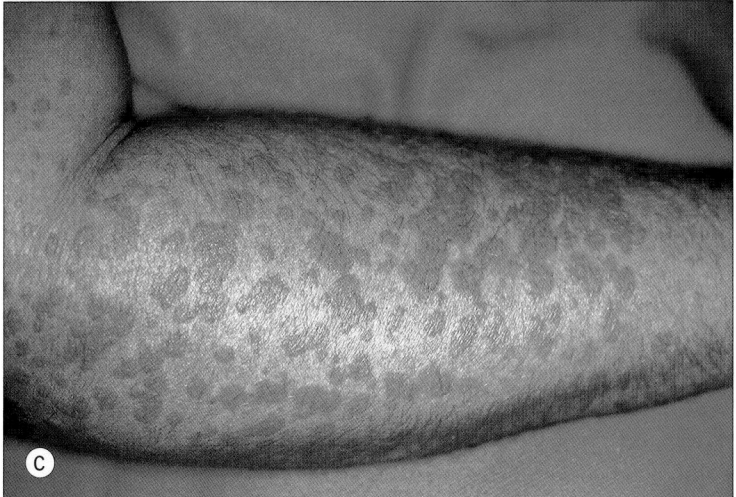

Fig. 86.3 **Polymorphous light eruption of the upper extremity.** Small papules (**A**), papulovesicles (**B**), and larger edematous papules and plaques (**C**).

of LE tend to last for weeks to months, whereas PMLE lesions, in the absence of further sun exposure, usually resolve within days.

Solar urticaria is distinguishable by its prompt onset, short 1- to 2-hour time course, and lesional morphology. Erythropoietic protoporphyria is typically markedly painful, there may be no inflammatory lesions, and an elevated red blood cell protoporphyrin concentration is detected. The light-exacerbated forms of atopic and seborrheic dermatitis are eczematous, while LE, which may rarely precede or coexist with

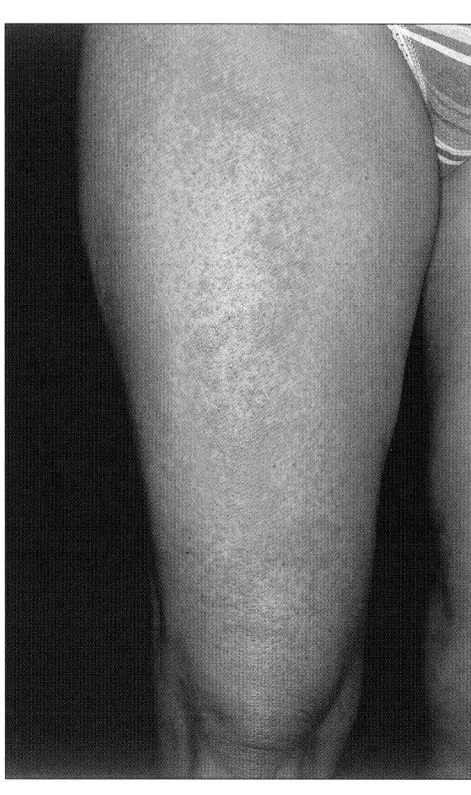

Fig. 86.4 Polymorphous light eruption of the thigh. Edematous papules becoming confluent into plaques. Courtesy of Jean L Bolognia MD.

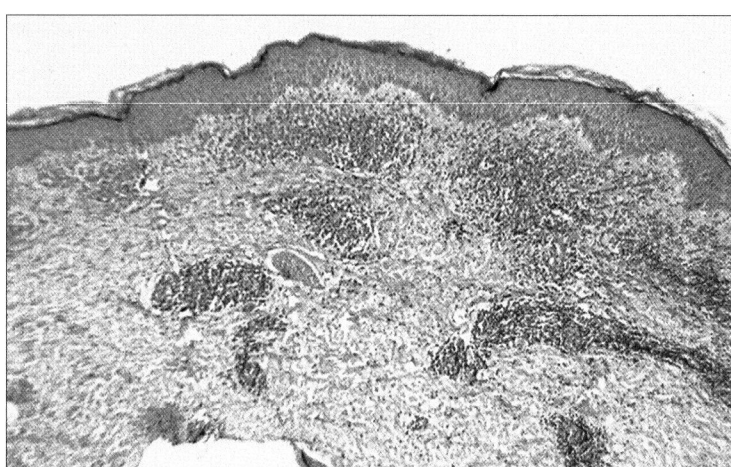

Fig. 86.5 Histology of polymorphous light eruption. The histology shows the characteristic perivascular mononuclear cell infiltration involving both the papillary and reticular dermis.

PMLE, is generally non-pruritic and demonstrates specific circulating and cutaneous immunologic abnormalities (see above). Finally, erythema multiforme, which may be photoaggravated, generally has different clinical and histologic features.

Treatment

PMLE in its milder forms may respond to photoprotection, consisting of sun avoidance, use of protective clothing, and regular application of high-SPF, broad-spectrum sunscreens (see Ch. 132). In patients with more severe disease, prophylactic, two to three times weekly sessions of NB-UVB phototherapy or psoralen photochemotherapy (PUVA) are usually effective[10]. For NB-UVB, an initial starting dose of 50–70% the MED for NB-UVB is recommended; the dose is then increased by 10–15% per treatment. For PUVA, 0.5–0.6 mg/kg of 8-methoxypsoralen is given 1 hour before UVA exposure; the starting UVA dose ranges from 0.5 to 3 J/cm², depending upon the skin phototype. The UVA dose is increased by 0.5 to 1.5 J/cm² per treatment. Oral prednisone (1 mg/kg) may be used during the initial 7–10 days of the treatment regimen, to minimize photoexacerbation. Treatment is usually initiated during the spring and an average of 15 treatments (about 5 weeks) is usually sufficient to induce hardening. Patients are then asked to

expose themselves to noonday sunlight for 15–20 minutes (without sunscreen) weekly for the remainder of the sunny season to maintain the hardened state.

Other treatment modalities which have been used with varying degrees of success include antimalarials (often only required from early spring to mid summer) and rarely, in severe cases, azathioprine or cyclosporine. High-potency topical corticosteroids and even brief courses of oral corticosteroids are also helpful in symptomatic patients.

Actinic prurigo

Synonyms: ■ Hutchinson's summer prurigo ■ Familial (or hereditary) polymorphous light eruption of American Indians ■ Hydroa aestivale

Key features

- Most commonly seen in Native Americans
- Childhood onset and may persist for years
- Papules and nodules with hemorrhagic crusts in sun-exposed sites
- Cheilitis and conjunctivitis are common in Native American patients
- Strong association with HLA-DR4, subtype DRB1*0407
- Management: photoprotection, NB-UVB, PUVA, thalidomide

Introduction

Actinic prurigo (AP) is a not uncommon sunlight-induced, pruritic, papular or nodular eruption. It involves uncovered and, to a lesser extent, covered skin, and lesions are often excoriated[3]. A similar condition, also known as hereditary or familial polymorphous light eruption, affects North, Central and South Americans of native or mixed race; the latter was first described in the 1960s and 1970s. AP may appear to be a persistent variant of the sometimes coexistent PMLE, but is clinically distinct.

History

AP was first described by Hutchinson in 1879, and then again by Haxthausen as a variant of PMLE in 1918.

Epidemiology

The disorder appears to occur in most parts of the world. It seems particularly common in Native Americans at all latitudes, especially among Mestizo (mixed American Indian and European) women. It is seen, but much less commonly, in the UK, continental Europe, Australia, Singapore and Japan.

In general, AP appears during childhood, more frequently in girls, and then often fades around adolescence; however, it may have an onset at, or persist to, any age[3,11]. Familial incidence is relatively common. In temperate climates, the eruption is usually the worst during the summer (rarely during the spring and fall or winter) and is often not clearly related to sun exposure. In patients living in Mexico and Central America, the eruption occurs year-round.

Pathogenesis

UVR exposure is the provocative factor in AP, in that the condition flares during the spring and summer and phototesting results are abnormal in approximately two-thirds of affected patients. About one-third react to UVB alone, one-third to both UVB and UVA, and a few to UVA alone, with the remainder having normal results[3,11].

The immunologic nature of this disease is supported by a study of Mestizo AP patients from Mexico, where the remarkable efficacy of thalidomide was associated with inhibition of TNF-α synthesis and modulation of interferon-γ-producing CD3⁺ cells[12]. The presence of a dense lymphocytic infiltrate and lymphoid follicles in lesional biopsy specimens from the lips plus an association with several HLA alleles provide further support for this concept[11].

AP may represent a persistent variant of PMLE, a contention supported by studies demonstrating that a higher-than-expected number of AP patients have first-degree relatives with PMLE[5]. A strong association with HLA-DR4, subtype DRB1*0407, has been observed in both patients from the UK[13] and Mestizo patients[11], and this could be the genetic factor that transforms PMLE into AP. Clinical conversion between AP and PMLE has been observed in the UK patients.

Clinical features

Erythematous papules or nodules, sometimes with hemorrhagic crusts, usually appear on all sun-exposed sites. Lesions sometimes have eczematous features or lichenification (due to associated pruritus); facial papules may heal with minute linear or pitted scars. The face (including the nose) and distal limbs are generally affected (Figs 86.6 & 86.7), but lesions can also develop in covered sites (Fig. 86.8). Cheilitis and conjunctivitis are common in Native Americans, and cheilitis may be the only clinical manifestation in up to 30% of Mestizo patients with AP[11].

Pathology

In early lesions, there is epidermal spongiosis, acanthosis and a dermal perivascular mononuclear cell infiltrate with occasional eosinophils, but, unlike in PMLE, papillary edema is usually absent[9,11]. Later, crusts, more pronounced acanthosis, variable lichenification, excoriations, focal dermal papillary fibrosis and a heavier mononuclear cell infiltrate can be seen (Fig. 86.9). These latter features resemble those of chronic dermatitis or prurigo nodularis. Dermal lymphoid follicles have been observed in biopsy specimens taken from the lips[11].

Differential diagnosis

The history and clinical features initially suggest the diagnosis, which is then supported by a lack of circulating antinuclear and other LE-associated antibodies (e.g. anti-Ro) as well as a normal porphyrin profile. Early lesional histology may occasionally help in narrowing the differential diagnosis, and direct immunofluorescence is negative. Photo-testing may confirm light sensitivity in up to two-thirds of patients, while solar-simulated or broad-spectrum exposure may on occasion induce a PMLE-like eruption. HLA typing is supportive of AP if DRB1*0401 (DR4) is demonstrated, and even more so if the DR4 subtype of DRB1*0407 is present.

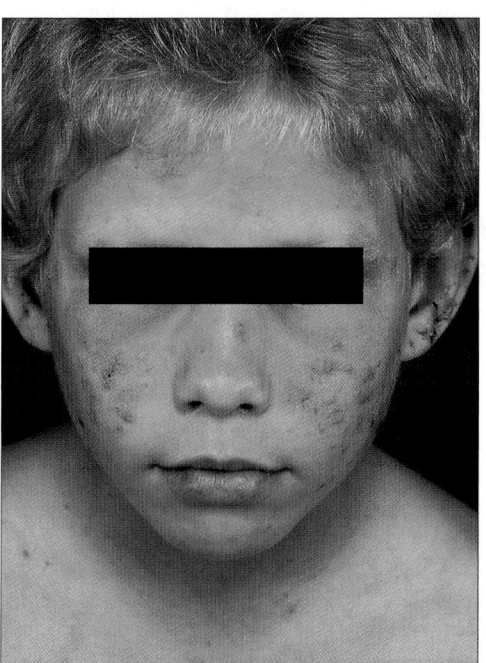

Fig. 86.6 Actinic prurigo. The clinical features are somewhat suggestive of polymorphous light eruption, but the lesions are persistent and the HLA type was that of actinic prurigo.

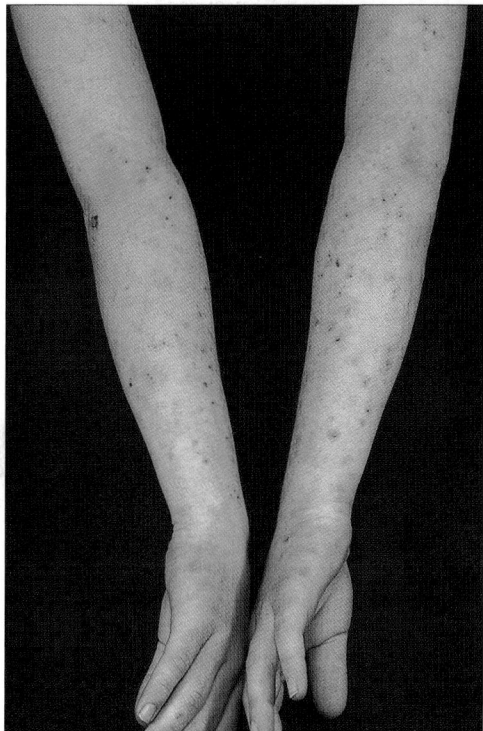

Fig. 86.7 Actinic prurigo. The arms show crusted papules that are denser distally; they are also worse in summer.

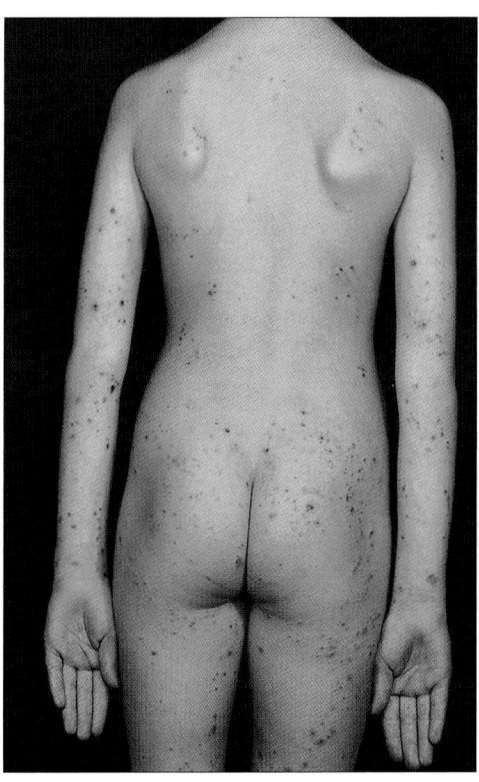

Fig. 86.8 Actinic prurigo. This patient with severe actinic prurigo has involvement of the buttocks.

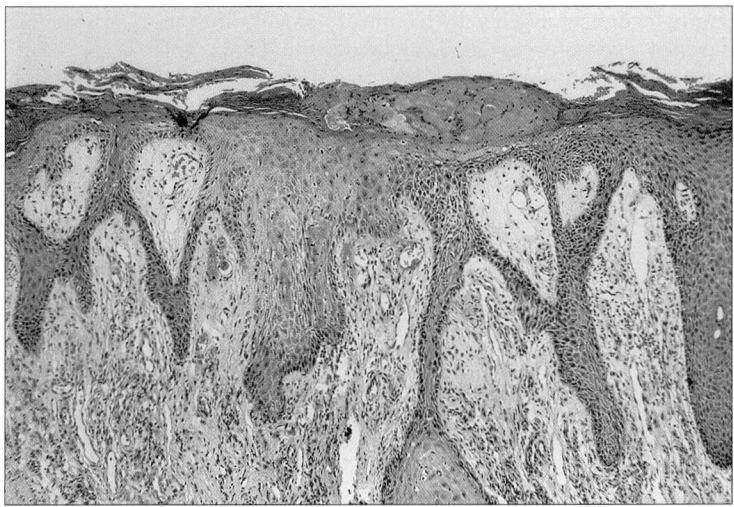

Fig. 86.9 Histology of an older lesion of actinic prurigo. Epidermal hyperplasia, scale-crust and a dermal mononuclear infiltrate are seen, but the overall picture is non-specific.

Insect bites are generally less persistent over time and scabies is diagnosed via skin scrapings. Prurigo nodularis lesions are not limited to sun-exposed skin and childhood porphyrias can be excluded by porphyrin assays.

Treatment

Photoprotection is always helpful. For milder disease, topical corticosteroids and topical tacrolimus may be used. NB-UVB or PUVA should be considered as the next step in the therapeutic ladder; the protocol is similar to that outlined for PMLE (see above). Resistant disease is best treated with oral thalidomide (50–100 mg nightly)[11,12], which is administered for several weeks until remission is achieved and then tapered to the lowest possible dose for maintenance. However, the risks of teratogenicity and peripheral neuropathy require very careful patient selection and supervision (see Ch. 130). Other medications that have been effective in smaller numbers of patients include pentoxifylline, antimalarials, oral corticosteroids, azathioprine and cyclosporine.

Hydroa vacciniforme

Synonym: ■ Bazin's hydroa vacciniforme

Key features

■ Rare, childhood-onset photodermatosis

■ Papules and vesicles, often with hemorrhagic crusts and associated with vacciniform scars

■ Epstein–Barr virus has been detected in some patients

■ Management: photoprotection, NB-UVB, PUVA

Introduction

Hydroa vacciniforme (HV) is a rare childhood-onset, sunlight-provoked disorder that is intermittent and leads to scarring.

History

The condition was first reported by Bazin in 1862.

Epidemiology

HV is well recognized in the US, UK, continental Europe and Japan, and very likely occurs elsewhere as well, apparently with a predilection for lightly pigmented individuals. Its rarity and lack of specific diagnostic tests (apart, perhaps, from its early histology) have made precise assessment of its distribution difficult. HV characteristically has its onset during childhood, affecting boys slightly more often than girls, and then it usually resolves during adolescence or early adulthood; a rare familial incidence has been noted[3,14].

Pathogenesis

Summer sunlight is generally required to provoke the eruption, although repeated exposures to artificial broadband UVA or UVB, or short-wavelength monochromatic UVA, may sometimes induce the eruption or an abnormal erythematous response[3,14]. Blood, urine and stool porphyrin concentrations, viral studies for herpes simplex or varicella-zoster, and antinuclear antibody titers are negative or normal. The exact nature of the reaction is unknown – perhaps it is a scarring variant of PMLE. The inducing molecular absorber also remains unknown.

There have been multiple reports from Asia, Mexico and Peru of the presence of Epstein-Barr virus (EBV) within cutaneous lesions of apparent HV, sometimes with disease progression to fatal EBV-associated natural killer (NK)/T-cell lymphoma or hemophagocytic syndrome[15,16]. In a recent Japanese series, T cells positive for EBV RNA were detected in lesional skin infiltrates from 94% of children with clinically typical HV (17/18; photoprovocation testing positive in 6, negative in 7 and not performed in 5) and 11/11 patients with severe HV-like eruptions associated with systemic symptoms, but 0/32 skin biopsy samples from patients with various other photodermatoses, inflammatory conditions and benign lymphoproliferative disorders[16a]. However, the relationship between EBV infection and true photosensitive

HV (as described herein) has yet to be established for other patient populations.

Clinical features

Symmetrical, clustered, pruritic or stinging erythematous macules appear within hours of summer sun exposure. They develop in some or all exposed sites, especially the face and dorsal aspect of the hands. These macules progress to tender papules and vesicles (Fig. 86.10) or bullae, which may be hemorrhagic. The latter umbilicate and often form hemorrhagic crusts over several days (Fig. 86.11). Weeks later, the crusts finally heal, leaving individual or confluent, sometimes telangiectatic, vacciniform scars (Fig. 86.12). Generalized malaise with fever or headache rarely accompanies the attacks.

Pathology

Progressive epidermal spongiosis precedes prominent reticular keratinocyte degeneration, intraepidermal vesiculation and confluent epidermal necrosis[9]; occasionally, there is focal upper dermal necrosis. Within the vesicles are fibrin and acute inflammatory cells. Early on, a perivascular lymphohistiocytic infiltrate is seen, followed by a

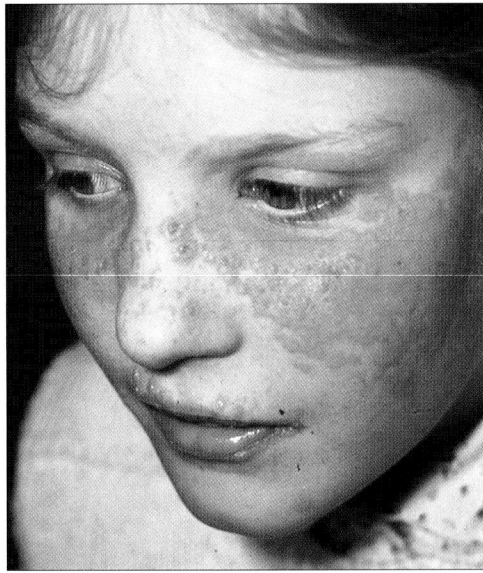

Fig. 86.10 Hydroa vacciniforme. There is an early, polymorphous light eruption-like appearance, but with vesicles around the mouth and umbilicated lesions on the nose.

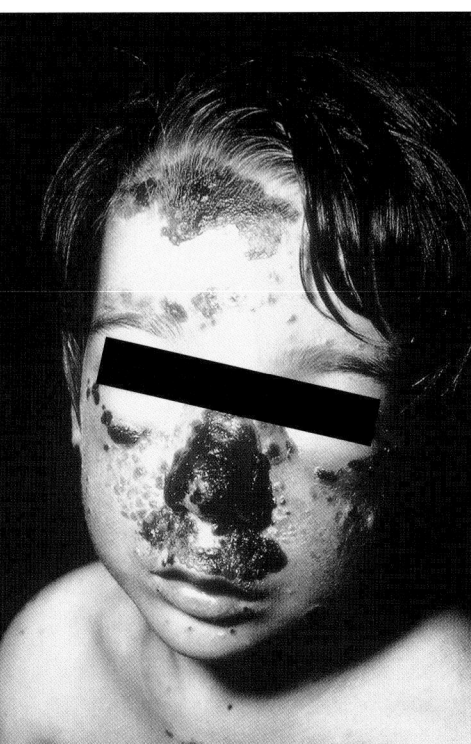

Fig. 86.11 Hydroa vacciniforme. A later, more severe example shows vesiculation with umbilication, but also marked hemorrhagic crusting.

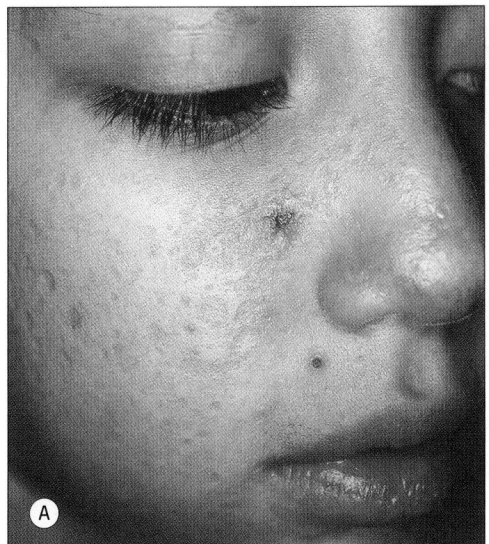

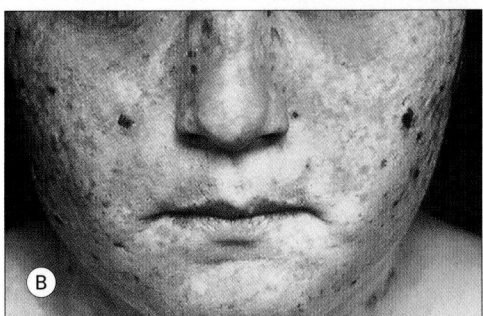

Fig. 86.12 Sequelae of hydroa vacciniforme. Repeated acute attacks can lead to scarring that is moderate (**A**) to severe (**B**). A, Courtesy of Jean L Bolognia MD.

neutrophilic invasion. Findings by direct immunofluorescence are non-specific.

Differential diagnosis

The diagnosis of HV is suggested by the typical history as well as the clinical and histologic findings. It is sometimes associated with abnormal erythematous or, rarely, vesicular phototest responses to monochromatic or broad-spectrum UVR exposure. Viral cultures, direct immunofluorescence findings, the porphyrin profile, urinary amino acid levels, and circulating antinuclear (and LE-related) antibody titers, complete blood count and hepatic profile are within normal limits or negative. In patients with HV-like eruptions associated with systemic EBV-related disease, the skin involvement typically becomes more severe with age and involves sun-protected as well as sun-exposed sites; additional features may include facial swelling, ulcerated nodular lesions, hypersensitivity to mosquito bites, high-grade fevers and hepatosplenomegaly. These individuals often have abnormal laboratory findings such as leukopenia, thrombocytopenia, elevated transaminases, increased NK lymphocytes and a high EBV DNA load (detected via polymerase chain reaction) in the peripheral blood, and a serologic pattern suggestive of chronic active EBV infection.

Treatment

HV is almost always refractory to treatment[3,14], but photoprotection is often useful in mild to moderate disease, until remission eventually develops. Anecdotally, and in small series, the following have been reported to be helpful: BB-UVB, NB-UVB, PUVA, β-carotene, antimalarials, azathioprine, thalidomide, cyclosporine, and dietary fish oil.

Chronic actinic dermatitis

Synonyms: ■ Photosensitivity dermatitis and actinic reticuloid (PD/AR) syndrome ■ Persistent light reaction ■ Actinic reticuloid (severe clinical variant) ■ Photosensitivity dermatitis (milder variant) ■ Photosensitive eczema (milder variant)

Key features

■ Persistent, chronic photodermatitis, usually in men >50 years of age

■ Eczematous papules and plaques with lichenification

■ Positive patch tests or photopatch tests a common finding

■ Probability of resolution: 10% in 5 years, 20% in 10 years

■ Management: photoprotection, low-dose PUVA, cyclosporine, azathioprine, mycophenolate mofetil, topical tacrolimus

Introduction

Chronic actinic dermatitis (CAD)[17,18] is a rare, persistent, often very distressing, dermatitis of uncovered and, to a lesser extent, covered skin. It is evoked by UVR and occasionally also visible light. CAD generally affects older men, more so during the summer. It likely represents a contact allergy-like DTH response against photo-induced endogenous allergen(s).

History

Reference to a condition suggestive of CAD was first made in 1933 by Haxthausen, and then in the 1960s by Wilkinson in the UK as well as Jillson & Baughman (who called it persistent light reaction) in the US. In 1969, Ive described its severe form, actinic reticuloid, followed soon thereafter by reports of two milder variants, photosensitive eczema and photosensitivity dermatitis. In 1979, the current global term, CAD, was introduced[17,19].

Epidemiology

CAD has been regularly observed in the UK, continental Europe, the US, Australia, Japan, Korea, India and the African continent.

Pathogenesis

CAD is eczematous, both clinically and histologically. It can be reproduced by exposure to UVB and/or UVA and/or visible light, often at doses below the MED. UVB represents the most common action spectrum[17,18]. The clinical and histologic appearance plus the dermal infiltrate of primarily CD8+ T lymphocytes and its pattern of adhesion molecule activation all resemble those of allergic contact dermatitis. This suggests that CAD is also a DTH response, perhaps against photo-induced cutaneous antigen(s) yet to be identified.

CAD most commonly affects older outdoor workers and enthusiasts, who commonly have a pre-existing allergic or photoallergic contact dermatitis to exogenous sensitizers, such as *Compositae* and sunscreens, respectively[17]. It therefore seems possible that chronic photodamage may ablate normal cutaneous immunosuppression in such individuals, while any contact dermatitis present may simultaneously further enhance cutaneous immune responsiveness against a weak endogenous antigen.

It should be noted that positive patch testing to *Compositae*, commonly observed in the UK patients, was not seen in patients evaluated in the US and Japan[20], perhaps reflecting a lack of exposure to this airborne allergen in patients from these regions.

Molecular absorbers and any inducing antigens have not been definitively determined, but DNA, RNA or associated molecules may be involved, in that the shape of the induction spectrum for the eczematous component of CAD almost always resembles that for sunburn inflammation, for which UVR absorption by DNA is responsible[17,21].

Clinical features

CAD occurs most often in temperate zones, affecting primarily older men of any race[17,18]; familial incidence has not been noted. The disorder may develop in previously normal skin, in patients with a prior history of dermatitis (in particular, photoallergic or allergic contact dermatitis), or perhaps rarely in the setting of oral drug photosensitivity or PMLE. Coexistent allergic contact sensitivity to ubiquitous, often airborne, chemicals such as plant antigens, fragrances or topical medications is also common. The photo-induced eruption is pruritic, patchy or confluent, and eczematous. Lichenification frequently occurs, while scattered or widespread, erythematous, shiny, infiltrated, pseudolymphomatous papules or plaques may develop in more severely affected individuals.

Lesions develop in sun-exposed sites (Figs 86.13–86.15). Frequently, the dermatitis has a sharp cut-off at the lines of clothing, often with sparing in the depths of skin furrows or of the upper eyelids, finger webs, or skin behind the ear lobes. Occasionally, eczematous changes of the palms and soles may also be present and eyebrow or scalp hairs may be stubbly or lost. Erythroderma can develop in severely affected patients. CAD generally persists for years, and it has been estimated that the probability of resolution is 10% over 5 years, 20% over 10 years, and 50% over 15 years[22].

Pathology

There is epidermal spongiosis and acanthosis, lymphocytic exocytosis, and a superficial and deep (often dense) perivascular lymphohistiocytic dermal cellular infiltrate[9]. The dermal infiltrate often contains eosinophils and plasma cells. In some biopsy specimens, erosions, focal epidermal necrosis, Pautrier microabscess-like epidermal cellular collections, dermal–epidermal junction fibrin deposition, dermal neutrophils and nuclear dust, vertically streaked papillary dermal collagen, and/or small, multinucleated dermal giant cells may be seen. In severe CAD, the dense infiltrate, epidermal lymphocyte exocytosis and frequent nuclear polymorphism may suggest the erroneous diagnosis of cutaneous T-cell lymphoma (CTCL).

Differential diagnosis

CAD is diagnosed on the basis of its clinical findings, histologic features, and abnormal erythematous or eczematous responses to photo-testing. The antinuclear (and LE-related) antibody titers and porphyrin profile are normal. Photoaggravated dermatoses are largely differentiated by their normal cutaneous irradiation responses and the characteristic clinical features of the primary disorder. In drug- and chemical-induced photosensitivity, evidence is usually present of exposure to an inducing substance (see below).

In rare instances, patients with CTCL (see Ch. 120) may demonstrate a CAD-like photosensitivity. However, phototesting abnormalities in CTCL patients are usually mild and are in the UVA range. In contrast to in CTCL, the infiltrates in CAD are predominantly CD8+ cells[17,18] and T-cell receptor gene rearrangement studies are negative. Erythrodermic CAD must be separated from other causes of erythroderma, if necessary by phototesting after the erythroderma has been controlled.

Treatment

Strict photoprotection and avoidance of relevant contact allergens are of primary importance. Of note, computer and television screens are safe. Museum film or other filters can be placed on home and car windows. Topical or intermittent oral corticosteroid therapy along with emollient use is generally needed. Therapy for refractory disease includes cyclosporine (3.5–5 mg/kg/day), azathioprine (1.0–2.5 mg/kg/day), mycophenolate mofetil (25–50 mg/kg/day), low-dose PUVA (with oral and topical corticosteroid cover for flares), and topical tacrolimus. These treatments are frequently used in combination[23].

Solar urticaria

Key features

- Urticaria following sun exposure, with lesions lasting <24 hours
- Female predominance and onset during the 4th and 5th decades of life
- Action spectrum: UVA, UVB, visible light, which may change over years
- May be associated with atopic dermatitis
- Estimated probability of resolution: 15% at 5 years, 25% at 10 years
- Management: photoprotection, antihistamines, low-dose UVA, PUVA

Introduction

Solar urticaria is a transient cutaneous eruption of wheals that appears almost immediately after exposure to UVR or visible radiation.

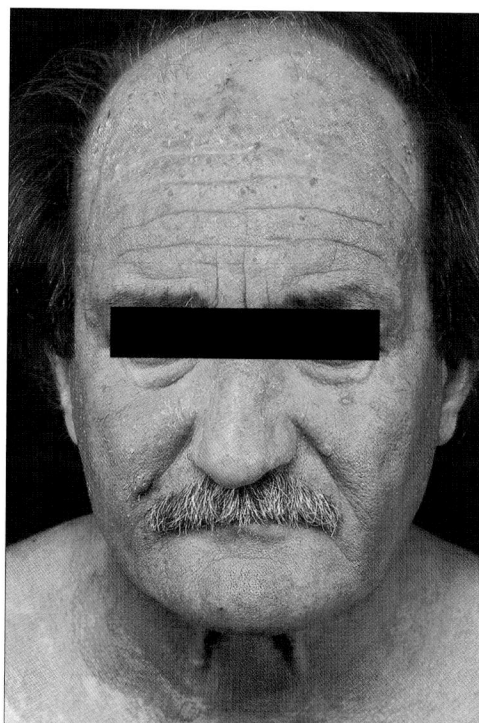

Fig. 86.13 Chronic actinic dermatitis. Somewhat infiltrated dermatitis of the face that is worse in the summer.

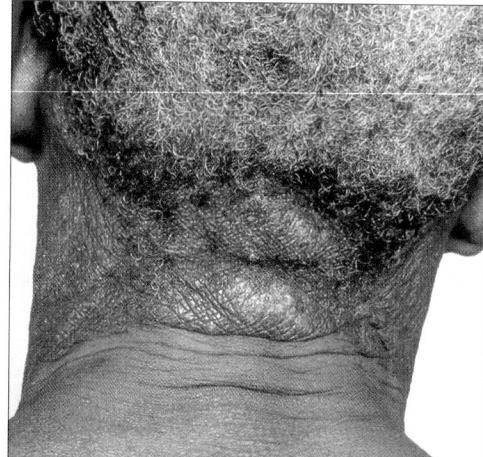

Fig. 86.14 Chronic actinic dermatitis. Lichenified eczematous changes of the posterior neck with a sharp cut-off at the collar in a patient with type V skin.

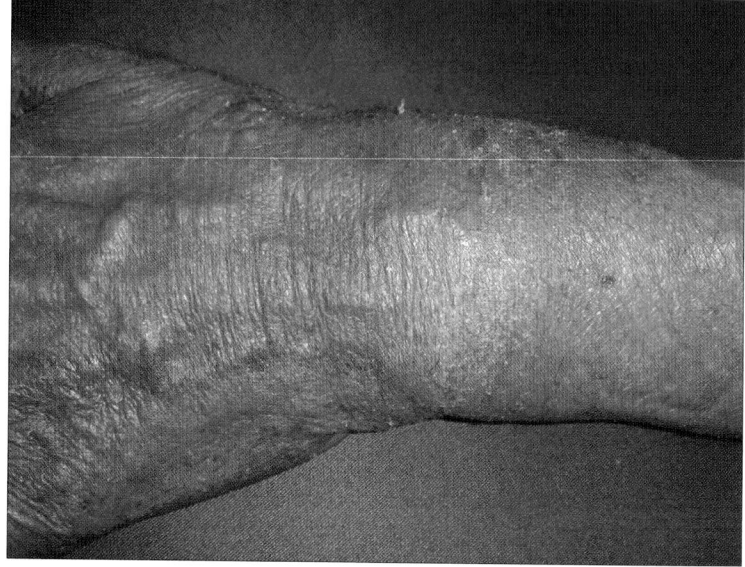

Fig. 86.15 Chronic actinic dermatitis. Lichenified eczematous changes of the dorsal aspects of the hand, with a sharp cut-off at the distal forearm.

History

One of the first reports of solar urticaria was in 1905 in a 47-year-old woman.

Epidemiology

Solar urticaria is a relatively uncommon disorder. In Tayside, Scotland, its prevalence has been estimated to be 3.1 per 100 000[24]. Both genders may be affected, but there is a female predominance. The peak age of onset is during the fourth or fifth decade of life. Solar urticaria is associated with atopic dermatitis in 20–50% of patients, and it may coexist with PMLE, CAD and other idiopathic dermatoses[24].

Pathogenesis

The pathogenesis is similar to that of other forms of urticaria (see Ch. 19), with mast cells playing a major role. However, the precise mechanism triggering their degranulation has not been fully elucidated. An IgE-mediated response to a photo-induced allergen is a possible mechanism, supported by observations that solar urticaria whealing can be induced by injections of autologous serum previously irradiated *in vitro* (and blocked by serum containing anti-IgE antibodies) as well as by the success of plasmapheresis in controlling the condition in some patients.

Clinical features

Patients generally present with whealing within minutes of sun exposure. Occasionally, erythema without urtication may occur (Fig. 86.16). As with other urticarias, lesions persist for less than 24 hours, but those of solar urticaria occur just on sun-exposed areas, especially the upper chest and outer aspects of the arms. Most patients note an accompanying pruritus, occasionally a burning sensation, and rarely pain, while severe attacks are occasionally associated with an anaphylactoid response that includes light-headedness, nausea, bronchospasm and syncope.

Solar urticaria is best classified based on its action spectrum, recognizing that the action spectrum may change over years[25]. The most common action spectrum is the visible light range, but the UVA and UVB regions or combinations thereof may also be responsible. Continued regular skin exposures to UVR sometimes decrease the likelihood of the development of urticaria in exposed sites, a phenomenon referred to as hardening. Solar urticaria inhibition spectra have also been detected in up to 70% of patients evaluated in Japan[26]. The probability of spontaneous resolution has been estimated to be 15% and 25% at 5 years and 10 years after onset, respectively[24].

There are several uncommon manifestations of this disorder. Patients with 'fixed solar urticaria' have disease limited to specific areas, presumably due to alterations to mast cells only at those sites[27]. Rarely,

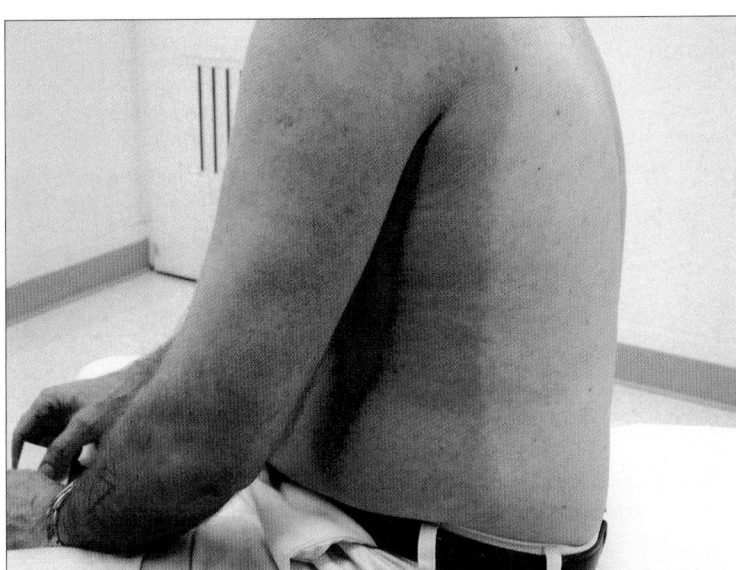

Fig. 86.16 Solar urticaria. Erythema and edema developed after driving for 1 hour. Notice sharp cut-off with no involvement of the non-sun-exposed portion of the back.

delayed solar urticaria has also been reported, in which lesions last longer than 24 hours; this disorder, by definition, should be considered to represent a form of PMLE. Drug-induced solar urticaria has been reported following patient exposure to chlorpromazine and tetracycline[26].

Pathology

The histologic findings of solar urticaria are similar to those of other urticarias – namely, mild dermal edema with a perivascular mixed neutrophilic and eosinophilic infiltrate; infiltration by mononuclear cells may also be seen. In addition, eosinophil major basic protein has been demonstrated in the dermis by immunofluorescence.

Differential diagnosis

The differential diagnosis includes other forms of urticaria (particularly heat urticaria), erythropoietic protoporphyria and PMLE. A clear history that the lesions of urticaria develop just following sunlight exposure should differentiate solar urticaria from idiopathic urticaria, while its separation from other physical urticarias may be accomplished by careful history taking and, if necessary, challenge with appropriate physical agents. Phototesting in affected patients generally results in whealing within minutes. The use of a water filter in front of any visible light source eliminates heat in order to exclude heat urticaria. Solar urticaria must also be differentiated from erythropoietic protoporphyria by determination of the porphyrin profile (see Ch. 49). Finally, PMLE can be distinguished by its frequent development within hours of sun exposure and its persistence for days, not hours. Exclusion of systemic LE using appropriate criteria is also warranted.

Treatment

Oral antihistamines are an integral component of the management of solar urticaria. Although patients with mild disease may occasionally respond to photoprotective measures, in many patients, this intervention is insufficient. A limiting factor for sunscreens is the observation that the action spectra in many patients are in the long UVA and visible light range, where, to date, there is no highly effective, commercially available sunscreen agent[28]. Graduated exposures to UVA or PUVA have been found to be helpful[29]. Antimalarials, cyclosporine, plasmapheresis, extracorporeal photopheresis, and IVIg have each been used with success in small numbers of resistant patients.

Inherited Disorders Characterized by Defective DNA Repair

The major disorders characterized by both defective DNA repair and photosensitivity are discussed below and outlined in Table 86.3. The underlying pathogenesis is reviewed in greater detail in Chapter 85. Four of the disorders are associated with defects in one of the nucleotide excision repair (NER) proteins: xeroderma pigmentosum, Cockayne syndrome, UV-sensitive syndrome, and the photosensitive form of trichothiodystrophy[30,31]. A fifth disorder with an NER defect, cerebro-oculo-facio-skeletal (COFS) syndrome has no associated photosensitivity, hence it will not be discussed.

Xeroderma pigmentosum
Introduction

Xeroderma pigmentosum (XP) is an autosomal recessive condition associated with a marked increase in the development of malignancies, especially cutaneous. Seven complementation groups and an XP variant have been delineated.

History

XP was first described by Hebra and Kaposi in 1874.

Epidemiology

XP has an estimated incidence of one per million in newborns in Western countries, and 1 per 40 000 to 100 000 newborns in Japan[32].

Pathogenesis

In XP, there are seven genetically different complementation groups (A to G), each associated with a different site of impairment in global genomic nucleotide excision repair (GG-NER), i.e. impairment in the

INHERITED PHOTOSENSITIVITY DISORDERS ASSOCIATED WITH DEFECTIVE DNA NUCLEOTIDE EXCISION REPAIR OR CHROMOSOME INSTABILITY					
Disorder	Clinical features	Inheritance	Photo-sensitivity	Action spectrum	Laboratory findings
Xeroderma pigmentosum (XP)	• 1 per million in Western countries; 1 per 40 000 to 100 000 newborns in Japan • Photosensitivity, early-onset lentigines (typically by 2 yrs of age) • Basal cell carcinomas, squamous cell carcinomas and melanomas in sun-exposed areas • Median age for development of first non-melanoma skin cancers: 8 yrs • Photophobia, keratitis, corneal opacification and vascularization • Neurologic abnormalities: hyporeflexia, deafness, seizures (most common in groups A and D; do not usually occur in XP variant) • XP variant patients usually have no neurologic problems • Support group: www.xps.org	AR	Yes	290–340 nm	• Complementation groups A to G: defective global genomic nucleotide excision repair (GG-NER) of UVR-induced DNA damage (e.g. pyrimidine dimers) from any part of the genome • XP variant: defective DNA polymerase-η, resulting in insertion of incorrect residue during replication of DNA with UVR-induced damage • Defective genes for all the XP groups have been identified • Cells are hypersensitive to killing by UVR
Cockayne syndrome (CS)	• Over 180 patients reported to date • Photosensitivity without pigmentary changes. Loss of adipose tissue, prominent ears, dental caries, thinning of skin and hair • Hypogonadism, stooped posture, joint contractures, short stature with extremely thin body habitus ('cachectic dwarfism'), microcephaly, mental retardation, deafness • Calcification of basal ganglia, demyelination, pigmentary retinal degeneration, osteoporosis • No increase in malignancies in 'pure' CS • CS type I: 80% of patients; onset at 2 years of age, progressive, mean age of death = 12.5 years due to respiratory problems • CS type II: symptoms at birth, life span = 6–7 years • CS type III: late onset, normal growth and development • Combined XP/CS: solar lentigines, skin cancers, pigmentary retinal degeneration, basal ganglion calcification • Support group: www.cockayne-syndrome.org	AR	Yes	Unclear	• Defective transcription-coupled nucleotide excision repair (TC-NER), which targets transcriptionally active regions of the genome • CS cells are defective in the repair of pyrimidine dimer photoproducts and oxidative DNA base modifications typically induced by UVB and UVA, respectively • Two complementation groups: CS-A (mutations in ERCC8) and CS-B (mutations in ERCC6); identical phenotypes • Mutations in XPB, XPD and XPG genes have been associated with combined XP/CS phenotypes
UV-sensitive syndrome (UVˢS)	• Fewer than 10 patients reported to date • Photosensitivity, solar lentigines; otherwise normal	AR	Yes	Unclear	• Similar to CS: defective TC-NER, normal GG-NER; however, unlike CS, patients with UVˢS only have defective in repair of UVB-induced photoproducts (not repair of oxidative damage) • Two complementation groups: mutations in ERCC6, and an undefined gene
Trichothiodystrophy (TTD)	• Over 100 patients reported to date • PIBI(D)S: photosensitivity, ichthyosis, brittle hair, intellectual impairment, decreased fertility, short stature • Other features: microcephaly, receding chin, protruding ears • No increase in malignancies	AR	Yes (in 50% of patients)	Unclear	• Hair shaft: alternating light and dark bands ('tiger tail banding'), trichoschisis, trichorrhexis nodosa-like changes, 'ribboning' • Reduction of cysteine-rich matrix proteins and low sulfur content in hair shafts • Mutations in XPD, XPB, general transcription factor IIH polypeptide 5 (GTF2H5 or TFB5), and C7orf11
Bloom syndrome	• Over 170 patients reported to date; most common among Ashkenazi Jews • Malar erythema and telangiectasias, café-au-lait macules and areas of hypopigmentation, elongated face with malar hypoplasia and prominent nose, short stature, diabetes mellitus, recurrent infections • Increased frequency of leukemia, lymphoma, GI adenocarcinoma • Normal intelligence • Men: sterile; women: reduced fertility • Patient registry: Bloom Syndrome Registry (see text)	AR	Yes	Unclear	• Decreased IgA, IgM, sometimes IgG • Mutations in BLM (RECQL3), resulting in chromosomal instability (increased sister chromatid exchanges, chromosomal breakage and rearrangement) • Quadriradial configurations in lymphocytes and fibroblasts are diagnostic

Table 86.3 **Inherited photosensitivity disorders associated with defective DNA nucleotide excision repair or chromosome instability.** AR, autosomal recessive.

Continued

INHERITED PHOTOSENSITIVITY DISORDERS ASSOCIATED WITH DEFECTIVE DNA NUCLEOTIDE EXCISION REPAIR OR CHROMOSOME INSTABILITY

Disorder	Clinical features	Inheritance	Photo-sensitivity	Action spectrum	Laboratory findings
Rothmund–Thomson syndrome	• Over 300 patients reported to date • Erythema, edema and vesicles on the cheeks and face during the first few months of life, followed by poikiloderma that also typically affects the dorsal aspect of the hands/forearms and the buttocks • Sparse hair (scalp, eyebrows, eyelashes), hypoplastic nails, acral keratoses (in adolescents and adults), short stature, skeletal (e.g. radial ray defects, osteoporosis) and dental abnormalities, juvenile cataracts, chronic diarrhea/vomiting during infancy, pituitary hypogonadism (may be associated with midface hypoplasia/'saddle nose') • Osteosarcoma (10–30%), squamous cell carcinoma (<5%; often acral) • Normal immune function, intelligence and lifespan (in the absence of malignancy)	AR	Transient (early childhood)	UVA	• Mutations in *RECQL4*; protein product is a DNA helicase • Genomic instability may account for propensity for malignancies

Table 86.3, cont'd Inherited photosensitivity disorders associated with defective DNA nucleotide excision repair or chromosome instability. AR, autosomal recessive.

removal of DNA damage from any place in the genome[30,32]. XP-A through -G represent different proteins in the NER pathway (see Fig. 85.12). It should be noted that different mutations in the *XPB*, *XPD* and *XPG* genes can be associated with different phenotypes – either XP or XP/Cockayne syndrome – and mutations in the *XPB* and *XPD* genes can also be associated with trichothiodystrophy (see below). XP variant, which has normal NER, is due to mutations in the gene that encodes DNA polymerase-η (also known as Pol η, Pol H or hRad30A). This enzyme is responsible for bypassing the unrepaired DNA photoproduct during DNA replication; mutations result in the insertion of erroneous residues during replication.

Phototesting in XP patients has shown the action spectrum for inflammatory erythema of the skin to be in the 290 to 340 nm range.

Clinical features
Patients usually have marked photosensitivity as well as the early onset of all major types of skin cancer (see Table 86.3). Starting from an early age, many patients also easily develop sunburns with erythema, edema and vesicles following minimal sun exposure. By the age of 2 years, practically all patients have developed solar lentigines. With continuing exposure, however, the skin gradually becomes xerotic, leading to the term 'xeroderma pigmentosum', or dry pigmented skin.

Actinic keratoses, basal cell carcinomas (BCCs), squamous cell carcinomas (SCCs) and, less frequently, melanomas then develop in sun-exposed sites, also prematurely (Fig. 86.17). The median age for initial non-melanoma skin cancer development in one study was 8 years of age[33]. SCC of the tip of the tongue has also been reported, presumably secondary to UVR exposure.

Ocular abnormalities are observed in ~40% of patients. Severe photophobia, keratitis, corneal opacification and vascularization are common ocular manifestations, while loss of eyelashes, ectropion, and SCC and melanoma of the UVR-exposed parts of the eyes are also frequently reported[33].

Approximately 20–30% of XP patients develop neurologic abnormalities, the most severe presentation being the DeSanctis–Cacchione syndrome, in which microcephaly, progressive mental retardation, retarded growth and sexual development, deafness, choreoathetosis, ataxia and quadriparesis may all occur. However, some XP patients develop a limited number of clinical manifestations, e.g. isolated hyporeflexia, progressive deafness. XP variant patients usually have no neurologic problems. Deep tendon reflex testing and routine audiometry are good screening tests for the presence of neurologic involvement. It has been postulated that these neurologic abnormalities are due to defective DNA repair in nerve cells, resulting in neuronal death. Patients with XP also have an approximately 10- to 20-fold increase in the incidence

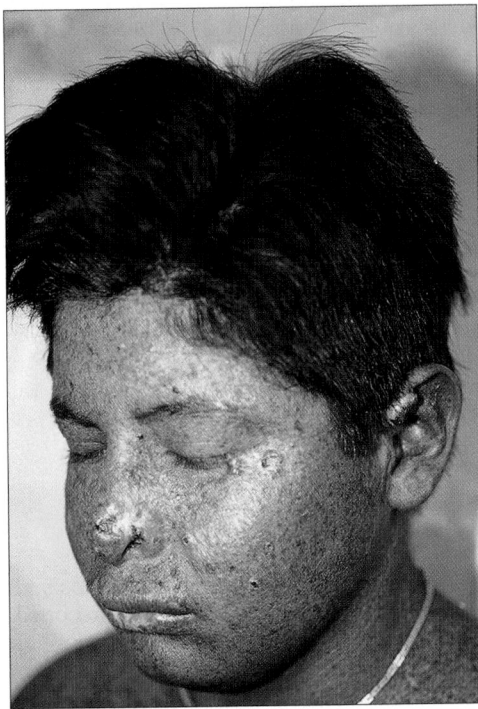

Fig. 86.17 Xeroderma pigmentosum. Multiple skin cancers and lentigines on the face of a 12-year-old Hispanic boy. Courtesy of Stanley Miller MD.

of internal malignancies, including tumors of the brain, lung, oral cavity, gastrointestinal tract, kidney and hematopoietic system.

Treatment
Management consists of extremely rigorous photoprotection. Oral calcium and vitamin D supplementation should be recommended for these patients[34]. Cryotherapy, electrodesiccation and curettage, and surgical excision are used to manage the pre-malignant and malignant skin tumors. Oral retinoids can be administered as chemopreventive agents, and, anecdotally, topical imiquimod has been reported to be useful. Topical application of bacterial DNA repair enzyme T4 endonuclease V (T4N5) formulated in a liposomal delivery vehicle has been successful in decreasing the development of actinic keratoses and BCCs[35].

Cockayne syndrome
Introduction
Cockayne syndrome is a rare photosensitivity disorder transmitted in an autosomal recessive fashion (see Table 86.3); to date, over 180 patients have been reported[36].

History
This entity was first described by Cockayne in 1936.

Epidemiology
Cockayne syndrome has been reported from the US, Europe and Japan.

Pathogenesis
Cells from affected patients are hypersensitive to killing by UVR[30]. However, the fundamental defect in NER in Cockayne syndrome is different from that of XP. In the former, there is defective transcription-coupled NER (TC-NER), which requires a subset of NER proteins plus additional factors and targets the transcriptionally active regions of the genome. The dysfunction results in the inability to recover RNA synthesis after exposure to UVR. In contrast, XP cells have defective global genomic NER (GG-NER; see above).

Cockayne syndrome cells have been shown to be defective in the repair of both cyclobutane pyrimidine dimer photoproducts and 8-oxoguanine (8-oxoG) photoproducts generated following UVB and UVA irradiation, respectively[36]. Repair of other oxidation-induced DNA lesions by TC-NER is also defective. In contrast to XP, there is no increase in cutaneous or internal malignancies in Cockayne syndrome. A possible explanation is that defective GG-NER, present in XP but not in Cockayne syndrome, is important in carcinogenesis.

There are two complementation groups with identical phenotypes: CS-A due to mutations in *ERCC8* (also known as *CSA*) and CS-B due to mutations in *ERCC6* (also known as *CSB*); CS-A is the more common group[36]. Several patients with an XP–Cockayne syndrome complex have also been reported (with mutations in *XPB*, *XPD* or *XPG*), typically demonstrating the solar lentigines and cutaneous neoplasms of XP, along with the pigmentary retinal degeneration and basal ganglia calcification of Cockayne syndrome[37].

Clinical features
Patients with Cockayne syndrome have been classified into three groups based upon severity of symptoms and age of onset (see Table 86.3)[36]. Unlike individuals with XP, these patients have photosensitivity without significant pigmentary changes, but the action spectrum of the photosensitivity has not been studied. Progressive signs of premature aging occur, as does growth failure affecting the weight more than the length (i.e. cachectic dwarfism).

Treatment
It consists of symptomatic treatment only.

UV-sensitive syndrome
UV-sensitive syndrome (UV^{s}S) is a rare, photosensitive, autosomal recessive disease; to date, fewer than 10 patients have been reported, mostly from Japan[38,39]. Clinically, patients present with lentigines, but no neurologic abnormalities, nor an increased frequency of skin or internal cancers. All patients have photosensitivity, although the action spectrum has not been studied. The molecular defects are summarized in Table 86.3.

Trichothiodystrophy
Introduction
Trichothiodystrophy (TTD) is an autosomal recessive disorder with over 100 patients reported to date (see Table 86.3)[40].

History
The term 'trichothiodystrophy' was coined by Price in the late 1970s.

Epidemiology
The disorder appears to occur worldwide and affects men and women.

Pathogenesis
TTD is associated with mutations in the genes encoding the XP-D and XP-B proteins of the NER pathway; recently, mutations in the gene that encodes TFB5, a newly discovered, tenth subunit of transcription factor II H (TFIIH), were identified in TTD[41]. In addition, mutations in chromosome 7 open reading frame 11 (*C7orf11*) were found to underlie a nonphotosensitive form of TTD.

Clinical features
TTD has heterogeneous clinical manifestations, and several previously described syndromes (e.g. Amish brittle hair, Marinesco–Sjögren, Sabinas, Pollitt, Tay and IBIDS) are probably part of its spectrum. Unlike XP, TTD is not associated with skin cancers, and pigmentary alterations are uncommon.

The clinical features of TTD are frequently described by the acronym PIBI(D)S[30]:

Photosensitivity: Photosensitivity has been reported in up to 50% of affected patients, but the action spectrum is not known. Most patients with photosensitivity can be assigned to the XP-D complementation group. It should be noted that *XPD* mutations associated with XP result in impaired NER function, while *XPD* mutations that underlie TTD lead to an *in vitro* basal transcription defect[42]; this may explain the lack of an association of skin cancer with TTD.

Ichthyosis: A non-bullous congenital ichthyosiform erythroderma phenotype is commonly observed during infancy, and patients occasionally present with a collodion membrane. The erythema tends to fade over time, eventuating in ichthyosis of variable severity (see Ch. 56).

Brittle hair: This is the hallmark of TTD and is present in most, but not all, patients[43]. By polarizing microscopy, hair shafts demonstrate alternating bright and dark bands ('tiger tail banding') (see Fig. 68.16). Light microscopic findings include an irregular contour, trichoschisis (transverse fractures through the shafts) and, sometimes, trichorrhexis nodosa-like features. Hair shafts are flattened and may fold like a ribbon ('ribboning'). There is a reduction in cysteine-rich matrix proteins, resulting in defective cross-linking of the intermediate keratin filaments and a low sulfur content within the hair shaft. This defect may also account for the brittle nails and the ichthyosis seen in TTD.

Intellectual impairment: Mental retardation, microcephaly and hypomyelination have all been associated with TTD.

Decreased fertility: This has been reported in patients of both sexes, but is not a prominent feature.

Short stature: Growth retardation is present to a varying degree.

Other manifestations include the characteristic facies (receding chin, protruding ears), sideroblastic anemia, eosinophilia, and liver angioendotheliomas.

Treatment
No specific treatment is available.

Inherited Disorders Characterized by Chromosomal Instability
Bloom syndrome

Synonym: ■ Congenital telangiectatic erythema

Introduction
Bloom syndrome is transmitted in an autosomal recessive fashion; to date, over 170 patients had been reported (see Table 86.3).

History
The condition was first reported by David Bloom, a New York City dermatologist, in 1954.

Epidemiology
Bloom syndrome is most frequently observed among Ashkenazi Jews, in whom a founder deletion/insertion mutation of the responsible gene (*BLM*) has been identified in about 1% of the population[44]. The disorder has also been observed in Japan[45].

Pathogenesis
The gene (*BLM*), on chromosome 15q26.1, is a member of the RECQ helicase family[44]. The functions of its protein product include unwinding DNA and maintaining genomic stability. Mutations in *BLM* result in an increased rate of spontaneous sister chromatid exchanges, chromosomal breakage and rearrangements. Quadriradial configurations of chromosomes in lymphocytes and fibroblasts are a diagnostic feature.

Clinical features

Beginning within the first few weeks of life, patients typically develop erythema and telangiectasias of the malar areas and occasionally the dorsal aspect of the hands and forearms. Café-au-lait macules with adjacent areas of hypopigmentation are common. While photoexacerbations have been reported, the action spectrum remains unclear. Growth delay and short stature are usually the most common reasons for parents to seek medical care. Other features include normal intelligence, diabetes mellitus, and immune deficiency resulting in chronic respiratory and gastrointestinal tract infections. Decreased circulating levels of IgA and IgM, sometimes with a concomitant decrease in IgG, are seen. Men are sterile due to defective sperm and women have reduced fertility[46].

Because of chromosomal instability, patients have a 150- to 300-fold increase in the frequency of malignancies, including leukemia, lymphoma and gastrointestinal adenocarcinoma[47]. The mean age for the development of leukemia is 22 years.

Treatment

Symptomatic management and photoprotection are the only treatment strategies. A patient registry is available (Bloom Syndrome Registry, Laboratory of Human Genetics, New York Blood Center, 310 East 67th St, New York, NY 10021, USA. Phone: 212-570-3075; Fax: 212-570-3195).

Rothmund–Thomson syndrome

Synonym: ■ Poikiloderma congenitale

Introduction

Rothmund–Thomson syndrome is a rare entity with autosomal recessive inheritance; to date, over 300 cases have been reported in the English literature[48] (see Table 86.3).

History

The disorder was first recognized by Auguste Rothmund, a German ophthalmologist, in 1868, before Sydney Thomson, a British dermatologist, described a similar entity in 1923. In 1957, William Taylor proposed the eponym 'Rothmund–Thomson syndrome'.

Epidemiology

Patients have been reported from the US, Canada, Central and South America, Europe, Australia, Japan and Israel.

Pathogenesis

The majority of patients with Rothmund–Thomson syndrome have mutations in the *RECQL4* gene[49]. The protein product is a DNA helicase, which unwinds DNA and stabilizes the genome. *RECQL4* is in the same gene family as *BLM* (Bloom syndrome). Mutations are thought to account for the increased susceptibility to cancers.

Clinical features

Patients typically present in the first few months of life with photo-distributed erythema, edema and vesicles on the cheeks and face, which may extend to involve the buttocks and extremities. Over months to years, poikiloderma develops. In one patient, the action spectrum of the photosensitivity was in the UVA range. Other features are summarized in Table 86.3.

Treatment

Treatment is symptomatic and preventative only.

Kindler Syndrome

Kindler syndrome is an autosomal recessive disorder with early-onset photosensitivity (average age = 2 years) that is due to loss-of-function mutations in *KIND1*[50-52]. This gene encodes a novel epidermal protein, kindlin-1, a membrane-associated structural/ signaling protein involved in linking the actin cytoskeleton to the extracellular matrix. The majority of patients have photosensitivity, with a decreased MED to UVB, and in some patients to UVA. Additional clinical findings are discussed in Chapter 62.

Photoaggravated Dermatoses

Key features

■ The underlying disease is exacerbated by exposure to sunlight

■ Phototesting is usually normal (with the exception of patients with LE)

■ Treatment focuses on the underlying disease; NB-UVB or PUVA, administered with caution, may be helpful in some patients

Introduction

A number of skin diseases that are not directly caused by UVR exposure may, in some patients, be worsened by it (Table 86.4). The reasons for such aggravation, however, have been poorly studied, with the exception of LE[53]. In patients with eczematous disorders, the presumed underlying pathogenic immunologic processes may be enhanced by UVR exposure, and perhaps disease- and UVR-induced inflammation may rarely summate directly to cause an exacerbation.

History

By the 1930s at the latest, the photoaggravation of dermatoses was formally recognized, especially in the case of psoriasis. The light exacerbation of viral exanthems was briefly evaluated in the 1950s and the action spectrum for lupus photosensitivity was studied extensively in the 1960s.

Epidemiology

This phenomenon appears to occur worldwide[2,54].

Clinical features

The basic dermatosis may be mildly or severely exacerbated by UVR exposure (Fig. 86.18), usually within minutes to hours. With sunlight avoidance, lesions gradually improve over a period of days to weeks. The UVR-exacerbated eruption may be limited to sites characteristic of the underlying condition, or, less commonly, involve all sun-exposed sites. Phototesting results are often normal, except in patients with LE. Occasionally, broad-spectrum irradiation may evoke the eruption.

Pathology

The histology is that of the underlying dermatosis.

Differential diagnosis

In general, photoaggravated dermatoses are recognized by the presence of the underlying skin disease (see Table 86.4). Differentiation from PMLE by history alone may be difficult. Clinically, the latter is typically

---

THE PHOTOAGGRAVATED DERMATOSES

- Acne vulgaris
- Atopic dermatitis
- Bullous pemphigoid
- Carcinoid syndrome
- Cutaneous T-cell lymphoma
- Dermatomyositis
- Disseminated superficial actinic porokeratosis
- Erythema multiforme
- Familial benign chronic pemphigus (Hailey–Hailey disease)
- Hartnup syndrome
- Keratosis follicularis (Darier disease)
- Lichen planus
- Lupus erythematosus
- Pellagra
- Pemphigus, including pemphigus foliaceus (erythematosus)
- Pityriasis rubra pilaris
- Psoriasis
- Reticular erythematous mucinosis (REM)
- Rosacea
- Seborrheic dermatitis
- Transient acantholytic dermatosis (Grover's disease)
- Viral infections, including herpes simplex, exanthems

Table 86.4 The photoaggravated dermatoses.

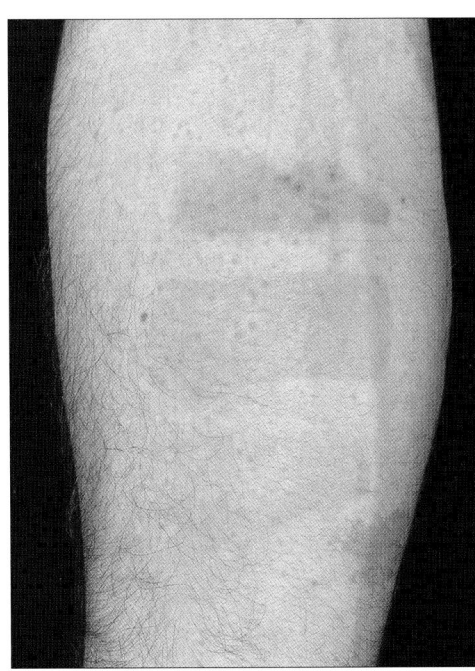

Fig. 86.18 Photoaggravated atopic dermatitis induced by the solar simulator. This was the appearance 24 hours after irradiation.

COMMON PHOTOTOXIC AND PHOTOALLERGIC AGENTS	
Common phototoxic agents	**Common photoallergic agents**

• Antiarrhythmics
  – Amiodarone
  – Quinidine
• Triazole antifungals
  – Voriconazole
• Diuretics
  – Furosemide
  – Thiazides
• Non-steroidal anti-inflammatory drugs
  – Nabumetone
  – Naproxen
  – Piroxicam
• Phenothiazines
  – Chlorpromazine
  – Prochlorperazine
• Psoralens
  – 5-Methoxypsoralen
  – 8-Methoxypsoralen
  – 4,5′,8-Trimethylpsoralen
• Quinolones
  – Ciprofloxacin
  – Lomefloxacin
  – Nalidixic acid
  – Sparfloxacin
• St. John's wort
  – Hypericin
• Tar (topical)
• Tetracyclines
  – Doxycycline
  – Demeclocycline
	Topical agents:
	• Sunscreens (e.g. oxybenzone, [benzophenone-3])
	• Fragrances
	  – 6-Methylcoumarin
	  – Musk ambrette
	  – Sandalwood oil
	• Antimicrobial agents
	  – Bithionol
	  – Chlorhexidine
	  – Fenticlor
	  – Hexachlorophene
	• Nonsteroidal anti-inflammatory drugs
	  – Diclofenac
	  – Ketoprofen
	• Phenothiazines
	  – Chlorpromazine
	  – Promethazine
	
	Systemic agents:
	• Antiarrhythmics
	  – Quinidine
	• Antifungal
	  – Griseofulvin
	• Antimalarial
	  – Quinine
	• Antimicrobials
	  – Quinolones (e.g. enoxacin, lomefloxacin)
	  – Sulfonamides
	• Non-steroidal anti-inflammatory drugs
	  – Ketoprofen
	  – Piroxicam

Table 86.5 Common phototoxic and photoallergic agents.

papular and pruritic, has negative lupus serology, and is often characterized by abnormal photoprovocation tests. It is important to note that PMLE may coexist with other dermatoses, in particular with photosensitive psoriasis. Photoaggravated atopic dermatitis, if widespread, may be confused with CAD; however, the latter patients have markedly positive phototest results. It is also important to distinguish UVR exacerbation of dermatoses from aggravation due to heat.

Treatment
Treatment consists primarily of topical or systemic therapy aimed at the underlying disorder. If significant photosensitivity persists, low-dose broad- or narrowband UVB or PUVA therapy (as for PMLE) may on occasion be effective. However, the latter is contraindicated in patients with LE or dermatomyositis, because systemic exacerbation may conceivably occur. Photoprotection is also important.

Chemical- and Drug-Induced Photosensitivity

Key features
- Phototoxicity is characterized by an exaggerated sunburn reaction and is usually caused by systemic agents
- Photoallergy presents with eczematous lesions and is most commonly associated with topical photoallergens
- The cutaneous porphyrias are an example of phototoxicity induced by endogenous agents
- Management consists of identification and avoidance of the offending agent

Exogenous
Introduction
Photosensitivity induced by exogenous agents can be divided into phototoxicity and photoallergy (Table 86.5). Phototoxicity is the result of direct tissue and cellular injury following UVR-induced activation of a phototoxic agent; theoretically, phototoxicity can be induced in every individual. In contrast, photoallergy is a delayed-type hypersensitivity response consisting of a sensitization phase, an incubation period of 7 to 10 days (following the first exposure), and a clinical reaction after any subsequent challenge; only previously sensitized individuals can develop a photoallergy.

History
Phototoxic agents have been used as medications from as early as 4000BC, with the inhabitants of Mesopotamia (and later the Indians and Egyptians) employing plant-derived psoralens for the treatment of leukoderma. In 1913, hematoporphyrin-induced phototoxicity was demonstrated by Meyer-Betz, while the current method of PUVA therapy was introduced in the 1970s. Photoallergy was first recognized in 1939 based on a classic study by Epstein on sulfanilamide.

Epidemiology
While the exact prevalence of phototoxicity and photoallergy in the general population is unknown, their frequency in photodermatology referral centers has ranged from 7% to 15% for phototoxicity and from 4% to 8% for photoallergy[1,2,54].

Pathogenesis
The pathogenesis of phototoxicity involves the generation of oxygen free radicals, superoxide anions, hydroxyl radicals and singlet oxygen, which leads to a host of cytotoxic effects. Other mechanisms of tissue damage include the generation of stable photoproducts (reported with chlorpromazine and tetracyclines), the formation of photoadducts (reported with psoralens), and the generation of inflammatory mediators (reported with porphyrins and demethylchlortetracycline)[55].

The pathogenesis of photoallergy is identical to that of allergic contact dermatitis, with the exception of the requirement for the presence of UVR to induce photoallergen formation.

Clinical features
Phototoxicity
Following cutaneous or systemic exposure to a phototoxic agent *and* appropriate UVR, phototoxicity develops within hours; for the vast majority of such agents, the action spectrum is in the UVA range. Erythema and edema as well as burning and stinging sensations characterize the initial presentation, with vesicles and bullae seen in severely affected patients. Phototoxic reactions due to oral medications resemble an exaggerated sunburn. These reactions resolve spontaneously with desquamation and hyperpigmentation.

Other less common manifestations of phototoxicity include pseudo-porphyria (frequently caused by non-steroidal anti-inflammatory drugs [NSAIDs], especially naproxen), photo-onycholysis (reported with tetracyclines and psoralens), slate-gray hyperpigmentation (reported with amiodarone, tricyclic antidepressants and diltiazem) (Fig. 86.19)[56], and lichenoid eruptions (seen with quinine and quinidine). Evolution of phototoxicity reactions into chronic actinic dermatitis (see above) has rarely been reported following exposure to thiazides, quinidine, quinine or simvastatin. The medications most commonly associated with phototoxicity are listed in Table 86.5.

5-Fluorouracil (5-FU), methotrexate and retinoids, three commonly used medications in dermatology, have been associated with 'photosensitivity'; however, none is associated with UVR-induced activation of the drug. UV-exacerbated erythema in patients receiving 5-FU usually occurs in sites with actinic keratoses. While no systematic phototesting study has been performed in patients taking 5-FU, this reaction most likely represents an exacerbation of 5-FU-induced cutaneous inflammation by UVR. Administration of methotrexate is known to occasionally cause a recurrence of UV-induced erythema. Phototesting in patients taking methotrexate has been normal[57], and the mechanism for the 'recall erythema' reaction remains unclear. Phototesting in patients taking isotretinoin or etretinate is also usually normal[58]. The propensity for these patients to develop UV-induced erythema is most likely due to retinoid-induced thinning of the stratum corneum.

Phytophotodermatitis is characterized by linear streaks of erythema that occur a day or so after contact with plants (frequently furocoumarin-containing) plus exposure to sunlight. Linear postinflammatory hyperpigmentation is a classic finding. Plants capable of inducing phyto-photodermatitis include yarrow, parsley, celery, parsnips, milfoil, lime, lemon and fig (see Ch. 18). Therefore, this condition most commonly occurs in individuals whose outdoor activities expose them to such plants (e.g. vegetable harvesters, bartenders).

Roofers and road workers may occasionally develop phototoxicity secondary to exposure to tar plus UVA from sunlight. St. John's wort (*Hypericum perforatum*), a product widely available in health food stores that is used to treat minor cuts, diarrhea, fever and depression, contains hypericin, a known phototoxic agent.

Photoallergy

In previously sensitized individuals, exposure to photoallergens plus sunlight results in the development of a pruritic eczematous eruption. In more severely affected patients, vesicles and bullae may develop (but less commonly than in phototoxic reaction). While there are clear differences between the clinical manifestations of phototoxicity versus photoallergy, such differences may not always be obvious, and careful history taking and examination are essential.

Currently, in the US, UK and France, sunscreen agents (especially benzophenone-3) are the most common cause of photoallergy, while NSAIDs are the leading photoallergen in the databank of the German, Austrian and Swiss Photopatch Test Group[59]. However, it should be noted that the actual prevalence of photoallergy amongst sunscreen users is very low. Other common photoallergens include fragrances and antibacterial products (Table 86.6; see Table 86.5).

Pathology

Phototoxicity is characterized by scattered necrotic keratinocytes ('sunburn' cells) and a dermal infiltrate composed primarily of lymphocytes and neutrophils. In contrast, photoallergy is characterized by a spongiotic dermatitis with a dermal lymphohistiocytic infiltrate, indistinguishable from other causes of spongiotic dermatitis.

Differential diagnosis

In order to arrive at a correct diagnosis of phototoxicity or photoallergy, careful history taking is essential. This should include a detailed history of any exposure to potential photosensitizers and determination of any seasonality to the eruption. Because glass thicker than $\frac{1}{4}$ inch (0.6 cm) filters UVB, an eruption following exposure to window glass-filtered light indicates that the action spectrum is in the UVA or visible light range. However, it should be noted that the newer glass used in commercial buildings and in the front and back wind-shield of cars has good protection against UVA (up to 380 nm) as well as UVB.

On physical examination, careful attention should be paid to the distribution of the lesions and whether there is sparing of photo-protected areas, e.g. postauricular and submental areas, skin beneath the lower lip and above the upper eyelid, nasolabial folds, and covered areas of the trunk and upper arms.

As noted previously, photoallergy is usually caused by topically applied agents, while phototoxicity is due to systemic compounds (see Table 86.5). While there are reports of systemic agents inducing photo-allergy, in general, this subject has not been well studied. For uncertain cases, both phototesting and photopatch testing should be performed. In patients with phototoxicity (who are still taking the responsible medication), phototesting frequently demonstrates a decreased MED to UVA, which is the absorption spectrum of the vast majority of photo-toxic agents. Phototesting in patients with photoallergy is usually normal.

Photoallergy can often be confirmed by photopatch testing, where duplicate sets of photoallergens are placed on the patient's back and one is irradiated with UVA, while the other is not. Interpretation of photopatch test results is shown in Figure 86.20.

An important entity in the differential diagnosis is airborne contact dermatitis. Potentially, all exposed sites can be involved, including the

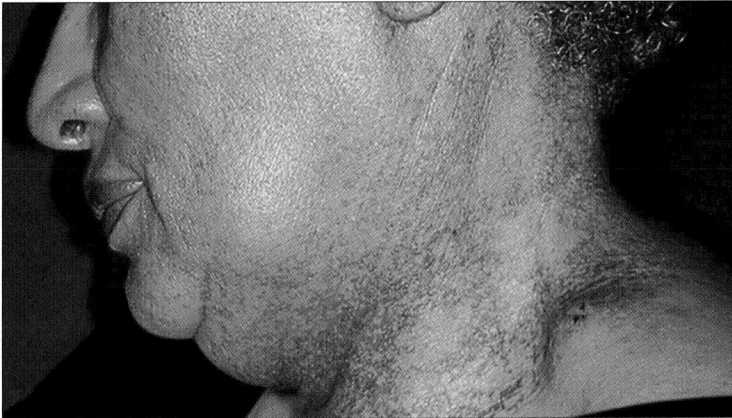

Fig. 86.19 Exogenous drug-induced photosensitivity and hyperpigmentation. Gray–brown reticulated patches involving the sun-exposed skin of a patient receiving diltiazem; note the sparing of the shoulder.

COMMONLY EMPLOYED PHOTOPATCH TEST AGENTS	
Substance	**Concentration (%)**
Sunscreen agents	
Octyl methoxycinnamate (octinoxate)	10
Benzophenone-3 (oxybenzone)	10
Octyl dimethyl PABA (padimate O)	10
Butyl methoxydibenzoylmethane (avobenzone)	10
4-Methylbenzylidene camphor (enzacamene)*	10
Benzophenone-4 (sulisobenzone)	10
Isoamyl methoxycinnamate*	10
Phenylbenzimidazole sulfonic acid (ensulizole)	10
Musk ambrette	1%
Tribromosalicylanilide	1
Sesquiterpene lactone mix	0.1%
Nonsteroidal anti-inflammatory agents**	
Naproxen	5
Ibuprofen	5
Diclofenac	1
Ketoprofen	2.5

*Not approved in the US.
**Observed as topical sensitizers primarily in Europe.

Table 86.6 Commonly employed photopatch test agents. Blue-shaded portions adapted from Bruynzeel DP, Ferguson J, Andersen K, et al. European Taskforce for Photopatch Testing. Photopatch testing: a consensus methodology for Europe. J Eur Acad Dermatol Venereol. 2004;18:679–82.

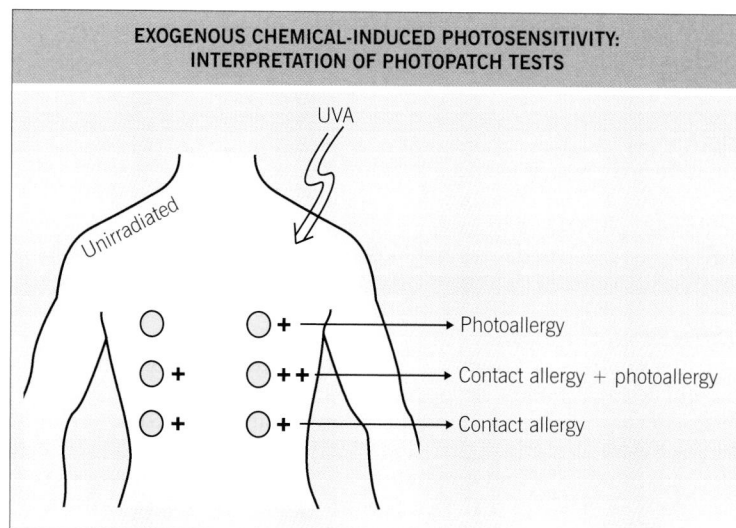

Fig. 86.20 **Exogenous chemical-induced photosensitivity.** This schematic demonstrates the interpretation of photopatch tests. The UVA dose is usually the lower of 5 J/cm², or 50% of the MED to UVA.

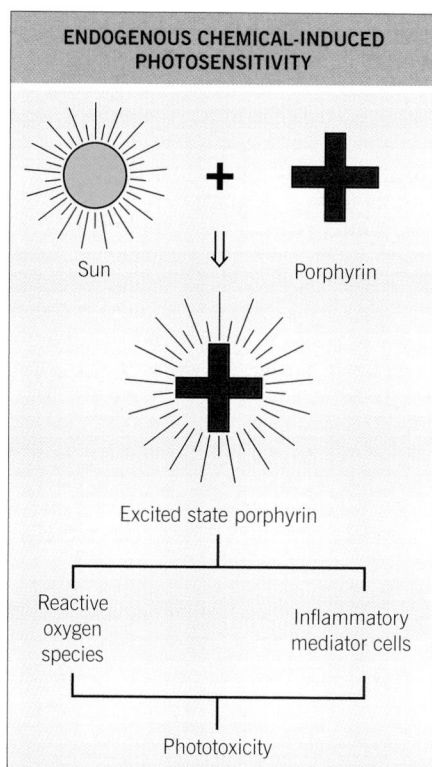

Fig. 86.21 **Endogenous chemical-induced photosensitivity.** The pathophysiology of phototoxicity as seen in the cutaneous porphyrias is shown.

upper eyelids, submental region and postauricular areas. Phototesting and photopatch testing are negative and history plus patch testing generally reveal the diagnosis.

Treatment
The identification and avoidance of any offending agent are essential. Other therapeutic measures include photoprotection from both UVB and UVA as well as the use of topical – and, in severe cases, systemic – corticosteroids for short durations. Compresses and systemic antihistamines may sometimes provide symptomatic relief.

Endogenous
The cutaneous porphyrias, discussed in Chapter 49, represent the most obvious examples of photosensitivity induced by endogenous agents. The mechanism of porphyrin-induced phototoxicity involves reactive oxygen species, the complement system, mast cells and neutrophils (Fig. 86.21).

Smith–Lemli–Opitz syndrome, a rare autosomal recessive disorder with early onset of photosensitivity to UVA, is probably another example[60]. Mutations in *DHCR7*, which encodes for 7-dehydrocholesterol reductase, result in an accumulation of 7-dehydrocholesterol. The mechanism of photosensitivity is unknown.

NORMAL CUTANEOUS EFFECTS OF UVR EXPOSURE

Key features

- Acute and subacute effects of UV exposure include erythema, pigment darkening, delayed tanning, epidermal hyperplasia, immunologic changes and vitamin D₃ synthesis
- Chronic effects include photoaging and photocarcinogenesis
- UVR has been implicated in the development of actinic keratoses, squamous cell carcinoma, basal cell carcinoma and melanoma
- UV effects are attenuated in individuals with more darkly pigmented skin

This discussion is limited to the clinical aspects of UVR, as the underlying mechanisms are reviewed in Chapter 85.

Acute and Subacute Effects
These effects are primarily a result of the absorption of UVR by DNA; the exception being vitamin D synthesis.

Inflammation/Erythema
Exposure to UVR leads to the acute inflammatory reaction of sunburn. Wavelengths around 300 nm are the most erythemogenic, with those between 260 and 280 nm a little less so. The lowest dose capable of inducing erythema, the so-called minimal erythema dose (MED), in individuals with Fitzpatrick skin type I is about 100 J/m² (10 mJ/cm²) for UVC (100–280 nm), 300 J/m² (30 mJ/cm²) for broadband UVB (280–315 nm), and 300 kJ/m² (30 J/cm²) for broadband UVA (315–400 nm).

In a few individuals, brief immediate erythema occurs within seconds of UVR exposure and lasts for minutes[61]. Otherwise, the typical delayed bright red appearance of sunburn develops confluently on all sufficiently exposed skin, beginning within 30 minutes to 8 hours, peaking at 12 to 24 hours and diminishing over hours to days in the case of UVB exposure. With UVC, the response is pinker in color and shorter in duration, starting within hours, peaking at 5 to 8 hours and fading over hours to a day or so; in the case of UVA, the reaction is deeper red in color, is usually more persistent, and often begins during irradiation before fading over hours to several days. After excessive exposure, edema and blistering may occur, which if widespread may lead to associated systemic symptoms such as chills and malaise. These reactions are generally followed by pruritus and desquamation for a period of days to 1 to 2 weeks.

Photoprotection is the best prevention[28]. However, once excessive UV exposure has occurred, treatment is symptomatic, requiring increased fluid intake and the use of soothing emollient creams or lotions as well as topical or oral non-steroidal or steroidal anti-inflammatory agents as soon as possible after irradiation. If the sunburn is severe or life-threatening, hospitalization and treatment as for thermal burns are necessary.

Pigment darkening and delayed tanning
Immediate, often grayish, tanning of irradiated skin that lasts for 10–20 minutes may occur within seconds of ~20–120 kJ/m² of UVA irradiation (and perhaps also short-wavelength visible light), particularly in more darkly pigmented individuals[61]. This phenomenon, known as *immediate pigment darkening*, results from photo-oxidative darkening and cellular redistribution of melanin within epidermal melanocytes. Pigmentation that persists for more than 2 hours after irradiation is referred to as *persistent pigment darkening*; it is brownish in color and lasts for up to 24 hours. Similar to immediate pigment darkening, persistent pigment darkening is due to oxidation of pre-existing melanin. Persistent pigment darkening then blends with *delayed*

tanning, which persists for weeks to months and develops in genetically competent individuals over hours to days following approximately: 400 J/m^2 of broadband UVB (a little higher than the MED, particularly in fair-skinned persons); 150–200 kJ/m^2 of broadband UVA (a little less than the MED); or 100 J/m^2 of UVC (about equal to the MED). As a result of delayed tanning, sunburning sensitivity is mildly decreased by a factor of two to four.

Epidermal hyperplasia

Hyperplasia lasting a month or so occurs over a period of hours to days following UVB or UVC (but generally not UVA) exposure. This is the result of a markedly increased cellular mitotic rate and DNA, RNA and protein synthesis, following several initial hours of inactivity[61]. Hyperplasia of the viable epidermis and thickening of the stratum corneum results in several-fold protection against later sunburning; this adds to, and may exceed, that simultaneously provided by delayed tanning, particularly in fair-skinned individuals.

Immunologic changes

Cutaneous UVB, UVC and, to some extent, UVA irradiation alters epidermal Langerhans cell function, generates suppressor T lymphocytes, and changes the cutaneous cytokine profile[62]. This topic is discussed in greater detail in Chapter 5.

Vitamin D$_3$ synthesis

UVB irradiation quickly converts epidermal 7-dehydrocholesterol into previtamin D$_3$ (see Ch. 51)[34]; the latter then isomerizes over days to vitamin D$_3$ (cholecalciferol). Vitamin D$_3$ is converted in the liver to 25-hydroxyvitamin D, and then in the kidneys to 1,25-dihydroxyvitamin D, its active form. UV-induced vitamin D$_3$ synthesis is maximal at suberythemogenic doses. Only low UVB doses over small amounts of skin on a regular basis are necessary to maintain sufficient circulating vitamin D concentrations; this amount of exposure is usually achievable through normal daily activities.

Other changes

On occasion, otherwise healthy subjects develop *photo-onycholysis* and increased skin fragility with blistering (*pseudoporphyria*) following intense exposure to sunlight or tanning beds. This may be due to photosensitization by normal levels of endogenous substances such as porphyrins. *Mid-dermal elastolysis* is characterized by patches of finely wrinkled skin and loss of elastic fibers in the mid-reticular dermis (see Ch. 49); its onset is frequently associated with intense UV exposure. *Brachioradial pruritus*, characterized by primary pruritus of the outer arm, is commonly associated with cervical radiculopathy; however, in many patients, UVR may act as a trigger of the symptoms (see Ch. 7).

Chronic Effects

Photoaging

Photoaging refers to cutaneous changes secondary to long-term exposure to sunlight. Characteristic clinical manifestations are outlined below.

Solar elastosis refers to thickening of the skin associated with a yellow discoloration and marked wrinkling in sun-exposed areas, most commonly on the face. Histologically, there is a marked increase in dermal elastosis. Similar changes occur on the posterior neck and are referred to as *cutis rhomboidalis nuchae* (Fig. 86.22A). This latter condition is characterized by deeper wrinkling and furrowing of the skin associated with a leathery texture.

A *solar lentigo* is a light brown to dark brown, even-colored or reticulated macule that occurs in sun-exposed areas. Although solar lentigines can be solitary, they are more often multiple. The dorsal aspects of the hands, extensor forearms, upper trunk and face are the most common sites for these lesions.

An *ephelide*, also known as a freckle, presents as a light brown to medium brown macule, usually less than 6 mm in diameter. They occur on exposed areas of the face, as well as the shoulders and the outer aspect of the arms. Numerous lesions are usually present.

Histologically, a solar lentigo is associated with elongation of the rete ridges and a mild increase in the number of melanocytes, while hyper-

pigmentation of the basal layer without elongation of the rete ridges is observed in an ephelide.

Poikiloderma of Civatte refers to reticulated red to red-brown patches with telangiectasias that spare perifollicular skin and occur most commonly on the lateral aspects of the neck of faired-skinned, frequently sun-exposed individuals (Fig. 86.22B). Characteristically, there is sparing of the central submental region. Mild atrophy and hyperpigmentation may also be present. Histologically, telangiectasias, dermal atrophy and irregular hyperpigmentation of the basal layer are observed.

In *Favre–Racouchot syndrome*, multiple large open comedones develop on the lateral and inferior aspects of the periorbital area (Fig. 86.22C). This is associated with marked solar elastosis of the surrounding skin. Histologically, there are dilated pilosebaceous openings and cyst-like spaces filled with horny material.

Colloid milium is characterized by translucent yellow papules that measure 1 to 3 mm in diameter. There are usually numerous, closely spaced lesions in chronically sun-exposed areas, especially the neck, face and dorsum of the hands. Histologically, homogeneous masses of colloid are present in the papillary dermis, which are PAS-positive and diastase-resistant.

Erosive pustular dermatosis of the scalp presents as sterile pustules, erosions and mild inflammation on a photodamaged bald scalp (Fig. 86.22D). It may be misdiagnosed as folliculitis or hypertrophic actinic keratoses, and the possibility of the Brunsting-Perry variant of cicatricial (mucous membrane) pemphigoid needs to be considered. Although response to treatment is variable, successful therapy with potent topical corticosteroids, topical tacrolimus, topical calcipotriol, oral isotretinoin, oral zinc sulfate and oral nimesulide (a NSAID that inhibits the respiratory burst of granulocytes) has been reported.

Photoaging in patients with skin of color

Photoaging is much less pronounced and has a delayed onset in individuals with more darkly pigmented skin[63]. Small seborrheic keratoses, melasma and mottled hyperpigmentation are common signs of photoaging in East Asians (Chinese, Japanese and Koreans); wrinkles are fine and do not appear before 50 years of age. South Asians (Indians, Pakistanis, Sri Lankans and Bangladeshis) often have darker skin; dyspigmentation and fine wrinkles are signs of photoaging. Lightly pigmented Latinos have changes similar to those seen in whites, while those with brown skin photoage in a manner similar to South Asians. Blacks, which include African-Americans, Afro-Caribbeans and individuals from Africa, have a wide range of Fitzpatrick skin types, from III to VI. Dyspigmentation is commonly seen and fine wrinkles appear late in life.

Photocarcinogenesis

Chronic sun exposure has been associated with the development of actinic keratoses, SCC, BCC and melanoma[64]. In the case of actinic keratoses, the use of sunscreens has been associated with a decrease in their development. SCCs tend to develop within sun-exposed areas in fair-skinned individuals, and people who migrated to Australia early in life have a higher risk of developing SCC than immigrants who arrived later in life, suggesting an important role for sun exposure. Several studies from Australia have also demonstrated an association between BCC and sun exposure. For example, the incidence of BCC was higher in native-born Australians than in immigrants, and a statistically significant association between *intermittent* sun exposure and the risk of BCC was reported.

Compared to BCC, the risk of developing SCC increases more steeply with age, suggesting that *continuous* exposure is more important in the formation of SCC. Consistent with these findings are the results of a 4.5-year study of 1621 subjects in Australia, which demonstrated that the regular use of sunscreens was associated a decreased number of new SCCs but not new BCCs[65].

There is also an association between chronic exposure to sunlight and cutaneous melanoma, especially lentigo maligna[64]. In two different mouse models, the action spectrum for the development of melanoma was found to be in the UVB range[66,67]. Nevus density, considered to be a surrogate for melanoma development, also correlates with degree of sun exposure[68,69], and in both men and women, lifetime UV exposure dose has been associated with increased risk for developing melanoma.

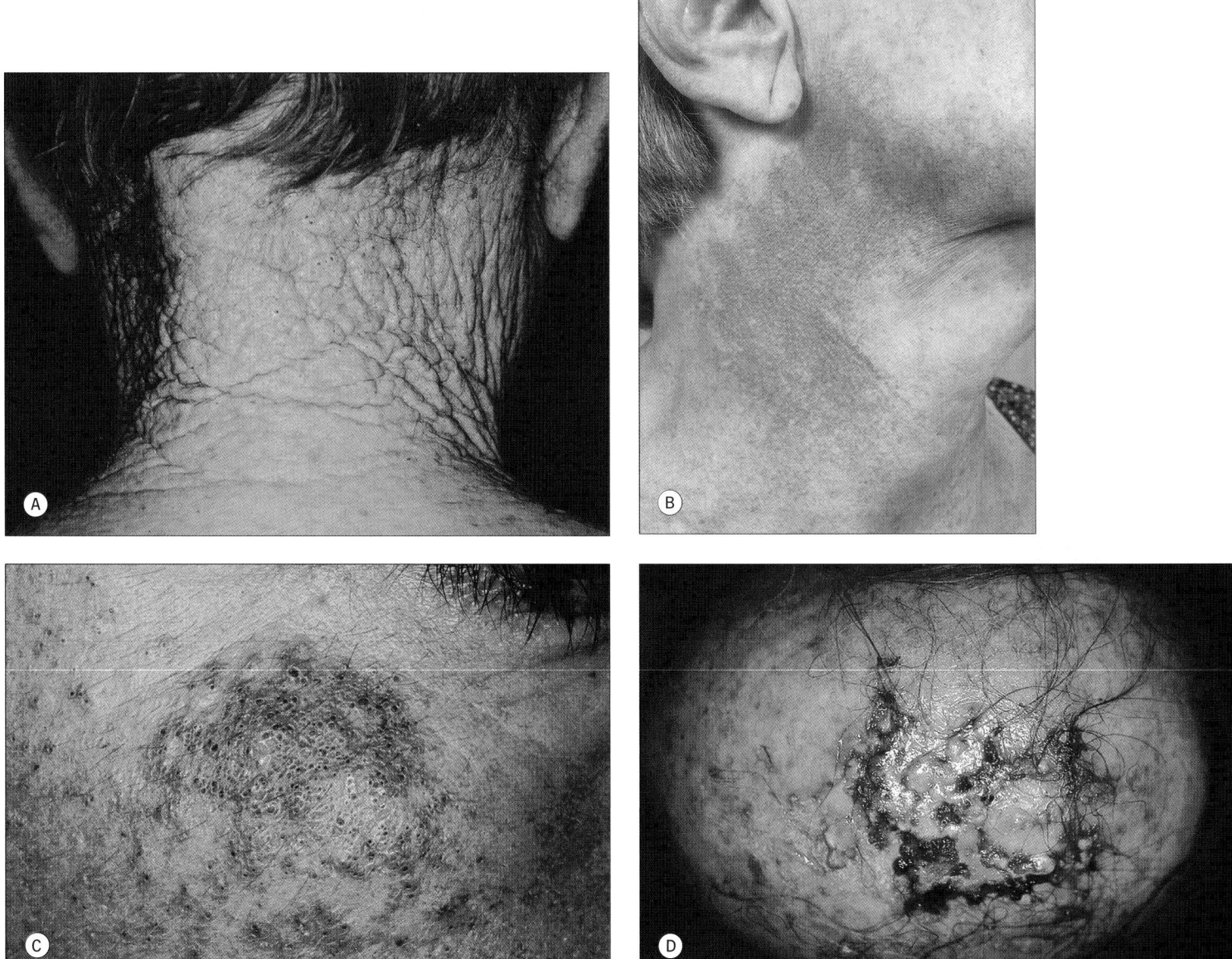

Fig. 86.22 Cutaneous signs of significant photoaging. A Cutis rhomboidalis nuchae with deep furrowing of the posterior neck. **B** Poikiloderma of Civatte with sparing of the anterior neck. **C** Multiple open comedones of the malar region in Favre–Racouchot syndrome. **D** Erosive pustular dermatosis of the bald scalp.

An analysis of data from the National Cancer Institute Surveillance, Epidemiology, and End Results (SEER) study concluded that fair-skinned individuals are at a higher risk for the development of melanoma. Additional analysis of cases of melanoma in the 2001 SEER database indicated that risk factors for pediatric melanoma included being white, being female, increasing age, and environmental UV radiation[70]. There are also multiple case-controlled studies demonstrating that blue eyes, blonde or red hair, and pale skin are risk factors for melanoma. Melanoma is also known to occur more commonly on the trunk in men and the lower extremities in women, sites of relative high sun exposure. In a study of cutaneous melanoma mortality, it was found that sun exposure, paradoxically, was associated with increased survival[71]; however, additional studies are needed to substantiate this finding.

Melanoma development in populations with more darkly pigmented skin has also been studied. An analysis of patients with cutaneous melanoma in the SEER database (1992–2001) concluded that a higher melanoma incidence was associated with an increased UV index and lower latitude only in non-Hispanic whites, not in black or Hispanic populations[72]. However, other studies in more darkly pigmented populations have shown that sun exposure indices were an important risk factor for melanoma development[73,74].

REFERENCES

1. Fotiades J, Soter NA, Lim HW. Results of evaluation of 203 patients for photosensitivity in a 7.3-year period. J Am Acad Dermatol. 1995;33:597–602.
2. Wong SN, Khoo LS. Analysis of photodermatoses seen in a predominantly Asian population at a photodermatology clinic in Singapore. Photodermatol Photoimmunol Photomed. 2005;21:40–4.
3. Norris PG, Hawk JLM. The idiopathic photodermatoses: polymorphic light eruption, actinic prurigo and hydroa vacciniforme. In: Hawk JLM (ed.). Photodermatology. London: Arnold, 1999:103–11.
4. Das S, Lloyd JJ, Walshaw D, Farr PM. Provocation testing in polymorphic light eruption using fluorescent ultraviolet (UV) A and UVB lamps. Br J Dermatol. 2004;151:1066–70.
5. McGregor JM, Grabczynska S, Vaughan RW, et al. Genetic modeling of abnormal photosensitivity in families with polymorphic light eruption and actinic prurigo. J Invest Dermatol. 2000;115:471–6.
6. Palmer RA, Hawk JLM, Young AR, Walker SL. The effect of solar-simulated radiation on the elicitation phase of contact hypersensitivity does not differ between controls and patients with polymorphic light eruption. J Invest Dermatol. 2005;124:1308–12.

7. Kontos A, Cusack C, Chaffins M, Lim HW. Polymorphous light eruption in African-Americans: pinpoint papular variant. Photodermatol Photoimmunol Photomed. 2002;18:303–6.

8. Hasan T, Ranki A, Jensen CT, Karvonen J. Disease associations in polymorphous light eruption. A long-term follow-up study of 94 patients. Arch Dermatol. 1998;134:1081–5.

9. Hawk JLM, Smith NP, Black MM. The photosensitivity disorders. In: Elder DE, Elenitsas R, Jaworsky C, Johnson B Jr (eds). Lever's Histopathology of the Skin. Philadelphia: Lippincott Williams & Wilkins, 2005:245–353.

10. Man I, Dawe RS, Ferguson J. Artificial hardening for polymorphic light eruption: practical points from ten years' experience. Photodermatol Photoimmunol Photomed. 1999;15:96–9.

11. Hojyo-Tomoka MT, Vega-Memije ME, Cortes-Franco R, Dominguez-Soto L. Diagnosis and treatment of actinic prurigo. Dermatol Ther. 2003;16:40–4.

12. Estrada-G I, Garibay-Escobar A, Nunez-Vazquez A, et al. Evidence that thalidomide modifies the immune response of patients suffering from actinic prurigo. Int J Dermatol. 2004;43:893–7.

13. Grabczynska SA, McGregor JM, Kondeatis E, et al. Actinic prurigo and polymorphic light eruption: common pathogenesis and the importance of HLA-DR4/DRB1*0407. Br J Dermatol. 1999;140:232–6.

14. Gupta G, Man I, Kemmett D. Hydroa vacciniforme: a clinical and follow-up study of 17 cases. J Am Acad Dermatol. 2000;42:208–13.

15. Ruiz-Maldonado R, Parrilla FM, Orozco-Covarrubias ML, et al. Edematous, scarring vasculitic panniculitis: a new multisystemic disease with malignant potential. J Am Acad Dermatol. 1995;32:37–44.

16. Cho KH, Lee SH, Kim CW, et al. Epstein-Barr virus-associated lymphoproliferative lesions presenting as a hydroa vacciniforme-like eruption: an analysis of six cases. Br J Dermatol. 2004;151:372–80.

16a. Iwatsuki K, Satoh M, Yamamoto T, et al. Pathogenic link between hydroa vacciniforme and Epstein-Barr virus-associated hematologic disorders. Arch Dermatol. 2006;142:587–95.

17. Menagé H du P, Hawk JLM. The idiopathic photodermatoses: chronic actinic dermatitis (photosensitivity dermatitis/ actinic reticuloid syndrome). In: Hawk JLM (ed.). Photodermatology. London: Arnold, 1999:127–42.

18. Lim HW, Morison W, Kamide R, et al. Chronic actinic dermatitis: an analysis of 51 patients evaluated in the United States and Japan. Arch Dermatol.1994;130:1284–9.

19. Hawk JLM, Magnus IA. Chronic actinic dermatitis – an idiopathic photosensitivity syndrome including actinic reticuloid and photosensitive eczema [proceedings]. Br J Dermatol. 1979;101(suppl. 17):24.

20. Lim HW, Cohen D, Soter NA. Chronic actinic dermatitis: results of patch and photopatch tests with Compositae, fragrances and pesticides. J Am Acad Dermatol. 1998;38:108–11.

21. Menagé H du P, Harrison GI, Potten CS, et al. The action spectrum for induction of chronic actinic dermatitis is similar to that for sunburn inflammation. Photochem Photobiol. 1995;62:976–9.

22. Dawe RS, Crombie IK, Ferguson J. The natural history of chronic actinic dermatitis. Arch Dermatol. 2000;136:1215–20.

23. Nousari HC, Anhalt GJ, Morison WL. Mycophenolate in psoralen-UV-A desensitization therapy for chronic actinic dermatitis. Arch Dermatol. 1999;135:1128–9.

24. Beattie PE, Dawe RS, Ibbotson SH, Ferguson J. Characteristics and prognosis of idiopathic solar urticaria: a cohort of 87 cases. Arch Dermatol. 2003;139:1149–54.

25. Ng JC, Foley PA, Crouch RB, Baker CS. Changes of photosensitivity and action spectrum with time in solar urticaria. Photodermatol Photoimmunol Photomed. 2002;18:191–5.

26. Uetsu N, Miyauchi-Hashimoto H, Okamoto H, Horio T. The clinical and photobiological characteristics of solar urticaria in 40 patients. Br J Dermatol. 2000;142:32–8.

27. Tuchinda C, Leenutaphong V, Sudtim S, Lim HW. Fixed solar urticaria induced by UVA and visible light: a report of a case. Photodermatol Photoimmunol Photomed. 2005;21:97–9.

28. Kullavanijaya P, Lim HW. Photoprotection. J Am Acad Dermatol. 2005;52:937–58.

29. Beissert S, Stander H, Schwarz T. UVA rush hardening for the treatment of solar urticaria. J Am Acad Dermatol. 2000;42:1030–2.

30. De Boer J, Joeijmakers JHJ. Nucleotide excision repair and human syndromes. Carcinogenesis. 2000;21:453–60.

31. Lehmann AR. DNA repair-deficient diseases, xeroderma pigmentosum, Cockayne syndrome and trichothiodystrophy. Biochimie. 2003;85:1101–11.

32. Moriwaki SI, Kraemer KH. Xeroderma pigmentosum – bridging a gap between clinic and laboratory. Photodermatol Photoimmunol Photomed. 2001;17:47–54.

33. Kraemer KH, Lee MM, Scotto J. Xeroderma pigmentosum: cutaneous, ocular, and neurologic abnormalities in 830 published cases. Arch Dermatol. 1987;123:241–50.

34. Lim HW, Gilchrest BA, Cooper KD, et al. Sunlight, tanning booths, and vitamin D. J Am Acad Dermatol. 2005;52:868–76.

35. Yarosh D, Klein J, O'Connor A, et al. Effects of topically applied T4 endonuclease V in liposomes on skin cancer in xeroderma pigmentosum: a randomized study. Xeroderma Pigmentosum Study Group. Lancet. 2001;357:926–9.

36. Spivak G. The many faces of Cockayne syndrome. Proc Natl Acad Sci USA. 2004;101:15273–4.

37. Nance MA, Berry SA. Cockayne syndrome: review of 140 cases. Am J Med Genet. 1992;42:68–84.

38. Horibata K, Iwamoto Y, Kuraoka I, et al. Complete absence of Cockayne syndrome group B gene product gives rise to UV-sensitive syndrome but not Cockayne syndrome. Proc Natl Acad Sci USA. 2004;101:15410–15.

39. Spivak G. UV-sensitive syndrome. Mutat Res. 2005;577:162–9.

40. Itin PH, Sarasin A, Pittelkow MR. Trichothiodystrophy: update on the sulfur-deficient brittle hair syndrome. J Am Acad Dermatol. 2001;44:891–920.

41. Giglia-Mari G, Coin F, Ranish JA, et al. A new, tenth subunit of TFIIH is responsible for the DNA repair syndrome trichothiodystrophy group A. Nat Genet. 2004;36:714–19.

42. Dubaele S, Proietti De Santis L, Bienstock RJ, et al. Basal transcription defect discriminates between xeroderma pigmentosum and trichothiodystrophy in XPD patients. Mol Cell. 2003;11:1635–46.

43. Liang C, Kraemer K, Morris A, et al. Characterization of tiger tail banding and hair shaft abnormalities in trichothiodystrophy. J Am Acad Dermatol. 2005;52:224–32.

44. Ellis NA, Groden J, Ye TZ, et al. The Bloom's syndrome gene product is homologous to RecQ helicases. Cell. 1995;83:655–66.

45. Kaneko H, Isogai K, Fukao T, et al. Relatively common mutations of the Bloom syndrome gene in the Japanese population. Int J Mol Med. 2004;14:439–42.

46. Bajoghli A. Bloom syndrome (congenital telangiectatic erythema). E-medicine. www.emedicine.com/derm/topic54.htm. (updated Feb 28, 2007)

47. German J. Bloom's syndrome. The first 100 cancers. Cancer Genet Cytogenet. 1997;93:100–6.

48. Wang LL, Levy LL, Lewis RA. Clinical manifestations in a cohort of 41 Rothmund-Thomson syndrome patients. Am J Med Genet. 2001;102:11–17.

49. Lindor NM, Furuichi Y, Kitao S, et al. Rothmund-Thomson syndrome due to RECQ4 helicase mutations: report and clinical and molecular comparisons with Bloom syndrome and Werner syndrome. Am J Med Genet. 2000;90:223–8.

50. Penagos H, Jaen M, Sancho MT, et al. Kindler syndrome in Native Americans from Panama: report of 26 cases. Arch Dermatol. 2004;140:939–44.

51. Siegel DH, Ashton GH, Penagos HG, et al. Loss of kindlin-1, a human homolog of the Caenorhabditis elegans actin-extracellular-matrix linker protein UNC-112, causes Kindler syndrome. Am J Hum Genet. 2003;73:174–87.

52. Jobard F, Bouadjar B, Caux F, et al. Identification of mutations in a new gene encoding a FERM family protein with a pleckstrin homology domain in Kindler syndrome. Hum Mol Genet. 2003;12:925–35.

53. Morison WL, Towne LE, Honig B. The photoaggravated dermatoses. In: Hawk JLM (ed.). Photodermatology. London: Arnold, 1999:199–212.

54. Crouch RB, Foley PA, Baker CS. Analysis of patients with suspected photosensitivity referred for investigation to an Australian photodermatology clinic. J Am Acad Dermatol. 2003;48:714–20.

55. Ferguson J. Photosensitivity due to drugs. Photodermatol Photoimmunol Photomed. 2002;18:262–9.

56. Scherschun L, Lee MW, Lim HW. Diltiazem-associated photodistributed hyperpigmentation. A review of 4 cases. Arch Dermatol. 2001;137:179–82.

57. Guzzo C, Kaidby K. Recurrent recall of sunburn by methotrexate. Photodermatol Photoimmunol Photomed. 1995;11:55–6.

58. Ferguson J, Johnson BE. Photosensitivity due to retinoids: Clinical and laboratory studies. Br J Dermatol. 1986;115:275–83.

59. Darvay A, White IR, Rycroft RJG, et al. Photoallergic contact dermatitis is uncommon. Br J Dermatol. 2001;145:597–601.

60. Anstey AV, Taylor CR. Photosensitivity in the Smith-Lemli-Opitz syndrome: the US experience of a new congenital photosensitivity syndrome. J Am Acad Dermatol. 1999;41:121–3.

61. Hönigsmann H. Erythema and pigmentation. Photodermatol Photoimmunol Photomed. 2002;18:75–81.

62. Kulms D, Schwarz T. 20 years after – milestones in molecular photobiology. J Invest Dermatol Symp Proc. 2002;7:46–50.

63. Halder RM, Richards GM. Photoaging in patients of skin of color. In: Rigel DS, Weiss RA, Lim HW, Dover JS (eds). Photoaging. New York: Marcel Dekker, 2004:55–63.

64. Lim HW, Robson KJ. Acute and chronic photodamage from solar radiation, phototherapy, and photochemotherapy. In: Krutmann J, Hönigsmann H, Elmets CA, Bergstresser PR (eds). Dermatological Phototherapy and Photodiagnostic Methods. Berlin: Springer-Verlag, 2001:279–302.

65. Green A, Williams G, Neale R, et al. Daily sunscreen application and betacarotene supplementation in prevention of basal-cell and squamous-cell carcinomas of the skin: a randomized controlled trial. Lancet. 1999;354:723–9.

66. DeFabo EC, Noonan FP, Fears T, Merlino G. Ultraviolet B but not ultraviolet A radiation initiates melanoma. Cancer Res. 2004;64:6372–6.

67. Yamazaki F, Okamoto H, Matsumura Y, et al. Development of a new mouse model (xeroderma pigmentosum a-deficient, stem cell factor-transgenic) of ultraviolet B-induced melanoma. J Invest Dermatol. 2005;125:521–5.

68. Wachsmuth RC, Turner F, Barrett JH, et al. The effect of sun exposure in determining nevus density in UK adolescent twins. J Invest Dermatol. 2005;124:56–62.

69. Bauer J, Buttner P, Wiecker TS, et al. Risk factors of incident melanocytic nevi: a longitudinal study in a cohort of 1232 young German children. Int J Cancer. 2005;115:121–6.

70. Strouse JJ, Fears TR, Tucker MA, Wayne AS. Pediatric melanoma: risk factor and survival analysis of the surveillance, epidemiology and end results database. J Clin Oncol. 2005;23:4735–41.

71. Berwick M, Armstrong BK, Ben-Porat L, et al. Sun exposure and mortality from melanoma. J Natl Cancer Inst. 2005;97:195–9.

72. Eide MJ, Weinstock MA. Association of UV index, latitude, and melanoma incidence in nonwhite populations – US Surveillance, Epidemiology, and End Results (SEER) program, 1992-2001. Arch Dermatol. 2005;141:447–81.

73. Lasithiotakis K, Kruger-Krasagakis S, Ioannidou D, et al. Epidemiological differences for cutanous melanoma in a relatively dark-skinned Caucasian population with chronic sun exposure. Eur J Cancer. 2004;40:2502–7.

74. Hu S, Ma F, Collado-Mesa F, Kirsner RS. UV radiation, latitude, and melanoma in US Hispanics and blacks. Arch Dermatol. 2004;140:819–24.

Environmental and Sports-related Skin Diseases

Michael L Smith

The skin is the primary interface with the environment. Humans are unique among the earth's creatures in their ability to manipulate the environment by manufacturing clothing, shelter, and heating and cooling devices to allow them to live in a variety of environmental extremes. Despite technologic advances that have allowed humans to live, work and play in most of the environments on the planet, deliberate or inadvertent exposure to those environments may subject individuals to injury. The following discussion will focus upon temperature-related skin diseases, water immersion injury, electrical burns, chemical injury, heavy metals in cutaneous disease, frictional and traumatic skin injury, sports-related dermatoses, and skin problems of instrumental musicians.

INJURY DUE TO HEAT EXPOSURE

Thermal Burns and Heat-Related Illnesses

Synonyms: ■ Thermal burns: burns ■ Heat-related illnesses: heat cramps, heat syncope, heat edema, heat exhaustion, heat stroke

Key features

- Assess depth of burn (i.e. first, second or third degree) and surface area involved
- Burn treatment includes prevention of infection, serial excisions and skin substitutes
- Heat-related illnesses occur when the body's thermoregulatory mechanisms fail; correction of fluid and electrolyte balance is critical in their management

Introduction

Humans, like all other mammals and all birds, are homeothermic organisms, maintaining their core body temperature within a narrow range by varying cutaneous and visceral blood flow. Normal core body temperatures vary between 36°C and 37.5°C (96.8°F and 99.5°F). At normal core temperature, cutaneous blood flow is about 4% of cardiac output or 250 ml/min. Alteration of the cutaneous blood flow is performed by the hypothalamus in a delicate balancing act between heat retention and loss. Cutaneous, muscle and spinal cord temperature sensors send signals to the preoptic area of the anterior hypothalamus. Communication with the posterior hypothalamus sets up thermoregulatory mechanisms of vasomotor control, sweating and shivering.

When prolonged exposure to a hot environment leads to an increase in core temperature, the subsequent decrease in sympathetic output results in peripheral vasodilation, allowing an increase in cutaneous blood flow of up to 6–8 l/min. Cholinergic output stimulates sweating. These changes allow radiant, conductive, convective and evaporative heat loss. In contrast, cold temperature exposure leads to increased sympathetic output with peripheral vasoconstriction. Countercurrent heat exchange between parallel arteries and veins further reduces heat loss to the skin, helping to conserve core heat. The behavioral response of shivering generates heat through muscular activity[1].

When the normal hypothalamic regulatory setpoint is overcome by extremes of temperature, pathologic conditions result (Table 87.1). The following discussion will explore heat-related illnesses and thermal burns. Heat-induced urticaria is covered in Chapter 19.

History

It is speculated that King Edward and his armored crusaders lost the final battle of the Holy Land because the Arab horsemen were adapted and dressed appropriately for the severe heat. Thermal burns, on the other hand, surely occurred with the prehistoric discovery of fire.

HEAT-RELATED ILLNESSES			
Condition	**Core temperature**	**Clinical features**	**Treatment**
Heat cramps	Normal	Painful spasm in large muscle groups, weakness, fatigue, N/V, **marked sweating**, tachycardia, ↑BP	Fluid and salt replacement
Heat syncope	Normal	Nausea, sighing, yawning, restlessness, fainting (brief)	Avoid standing still in heat, flex legs, lie down if prodrome, cool off, replace fluid
Heat edema	Normal	**Dependent edema** from vasodilatory pooling	None needed (self-limited)
Heat exhaustion	Normal to 39°C (102.2°F)	Weakness, dizziness, headache, N/V, irritability, dyspnea/hyperventilation, malaise, myalgias/muscle cramps, tachycardia, orthostatic hypotension, **profuse sweating, piloerection**, impaired judgment, syncope Hypernatremic form: thirst, rare cramps Hyponatremic form: fatigue, cramps, history of excessive free water intake, altered mental status	Intravenous fluids and electrolytes, sprinkle water and fan or use ice packs, rest, cool environment
Heat stroke	>40°C (104°F)	**Anhidrosis to profuse sweating**, ↓BP, N/V, diarrhea, altered mental status (profound), seizures, coma, cardiac arrhythmias, ↑ transaminases, rhabdomyolysis, acute renal failure, DIC, respiratory alkalosis Poor prognostic indicators: T >42.2°C (108°F); coma >2 h; AST >1000 (day 1)	Rapid lowering of core temperature to 38°C (100.4°F), intravenous hydration, intensive care unit

Table 87.1 **Heat-related illnesses**[1,2]. Cutaneous features are indicated in bold. AST, aspartate transaminase; BP, blood pressure; DIC, disseminated intravascular coagulation; N/V, nausea and vomiting; T, temperature.

Epidemiology

The frequency of heat-related illnesses is unknown, since milder forms resolve with simple measures. Heat-related illness accounted for more than 8000 deaths in the US between 1979 and 1999, and is responsible for 7% of wilderness deaths[1,2]. Risk factors are found in Table 87.2.

Burn injuries are far more common, occurring in 2 million people per year in the US alone, and resulting in 60 000 hospitalizations and 6000 deaths, half of which occur in children[3,4]. The male:female ratio is 2:1. The main sources of burns in children are scald, flame and electrical. Abuse or neglect may account for up to 20% of pediatric burns. Mortality rates have declined in recent years due to improved resuscitative and surgical management. In the 1940s, burns in children involving 50% body surface area (BSA) had a 50% mortality rate, whereas today, 50% of children with 90% BSA burns survive[3,4].

A unique form of burn injury is that due to fireworks, particularly sparklers[5]. In the US, fireworks account for over 12 000 emergency department visits annually. Blast injuries of the hand and eyes are seen in addition to burns.

Pathogenesis

Athletic activity can generate 800 to 1000 kcal/h of heat for prolonged periods. This results in a 1°C rise in core body temperature every 5 to 8 minutes. The normal thermoregulatory mechanisms dissipate this heat as it is generated. When the regulatory mechanisms fail, heat injury occurs. Heat illnesses are not defined by a specific temperature, but by the abnormal response to heat. *Heat cramps* are thought to be due to dilutional hyponatremia as free water, but not electrolytes, are replaced. *Heat syncope* is caused by decreased cerebral blood flow due to volume depletion, peripheral vasodilation and decreased vasomotor tone in poorly acclimatized or elderly individuals. *Heat exhaustion* is a result of volume and/or salt depletion. *Heat stroke* is the end result of thermoregulatory failure. Volume depletion leads to peripheral vasoconstriction, with reduced transfer of heat peripherally. This core heating leads to multiple organ failure[1].

Thermal burns occur when skin is exposed to infrared radiation (800 to 170 000 nm) from an external heat source with a temperature exceeding 44°C (111°F). Time and temperature curves have been developed to determine maximum thermal exposure times. Necrosis of the epidermis occurs in about 45 minutes at 47°C (117°F), but only 1 second at 70°C (158°F). Denaturation and coagulation of cellular proteins occur in thermal injury. Interstitial edema develops from altered osmotic pressure and capillary permeability. Several chemical mediators with vasoactive and tissue-destructive properties are released, including prostaglandins, bradykinin, serotonin, histamine, lipid peroxides and oxygen radicals[4].

Clinical features

Although heat-related illnesses are not primary skin diseases, they can present with cutaneous findings. Their clinical features are summarized in Table 87.1.

Thermal burns of the skin differ in their clinical presentation, depending upon the depth of injury (Table 87.3). Conventional nomenclature categorizes cutaneous burn wounds as *first degree* (superficial; limited to epidermis), *second degree* (partial thickness) and *third degree* (full thickness). Second-degree burns are further subdivided into superficial (Fig. 87.1) and deep variants. Burns involving deeper structures such as muscle are sometimes referred to as fourth-degree burns.

A definitive diagnosis of wound depth may not be possible for the first 24 to 72 hours because of vascular occlusive changes. Clinical and pathologic features of thermal burns are found in Table 87.3.

At sites where the dermis is thinner (ears, volar forearms, medial thighs, perineum), burns may be deeper than the initial presentation might suggest; this is also the case in the comparatively thinner skin of

RISK FACTORS FOR HEAT-RELATED ILLNESS
Occupational exposure
Age (elderly, young child)
Poverty
Insufficient acclimatization
Alcoholism
Mental illness
Medications (anticholinergics, phenothiazines, diuretics; see Table 40.9)
Medical conditions • Excessive fluid loss (fever, gastrointestinal fluid loss, diabetes insipidus, diabetes mellitus) • Suboptimal sweating (e.g. injuries/infarcts/tumors of the brain stem or spinal cord, ectodermal dysplasias; see Tables 40.8 and 40.10) • Excessive sweating (heart disease, chronic obstructive lung disease; see Tables 40.2 and 40.3) • Inadequate fluid intake (young child, mental retardation, elderly, dementia) • Decreased thirst (cystic fibrosis, other disorders with elevated sweat electrolytes; see Table 40.12) • Abnormal thermoregulation (prior heat illness, anorexia nervosa, malnutrition) • Obesity

Table 87.2 Risk factors for heat-related illness[1,2].

CLINICAL AND PATHOLOGIC FEATURES OF THERMAL BURNS			
Type	Depth	Clinical features	Pathology
First degree	Epidermis only	Pain, tenderness, erythema No blistering Heals without scar	Upper epidermal necrosis
Second degree – superficial	Epidermis and superficial dermis	Severe pain, tenderness, serous or hemorrhagic bullae, deep rubor, erosion and exudation Heals in 10–21 days with mild but variable scarring	More extensive epidermal necrosis with vertical elongation of keratinocytes Necrotic areas may have serous crust with neutrophils, fibrin and cellular debris Subepidermal bullae possible
Second degree – deep	Epidermis and most of dermis destroyed, including deep follicular structures	Intense pain but reduced sensation, deep red to pale and speckled in color Serosanguineous bullae and erosions May appear devitalized initially Prolonged healing time Hypertrophic scars and marked wound contracture	Destruction of entire epidermis, dermal collagen and most of adnexal structures Collagen bundles may be fused, with eosinophilic appearance Thrombosis of deep vessels common Granulation tissue present at junction of normal and injured tissue
Third degree	Full-thickness epidermal and dermal destruction	Dry, hard, charred, non-blanching, insensitive areas of coagulation necrosis Small lesions heal with significant scarring Most require surgical correction	Necrosis of entire epidermis and dermis, with extension into subcutis Inflammatory infiltrate at interface between burned and normal skin If scar forms, it exhibits hyalinized collagen, decreased elastic tissue, loss of arrector pili muscles

Table 87.3 Clinical and pathologic features of thermal burns[4,6,7].

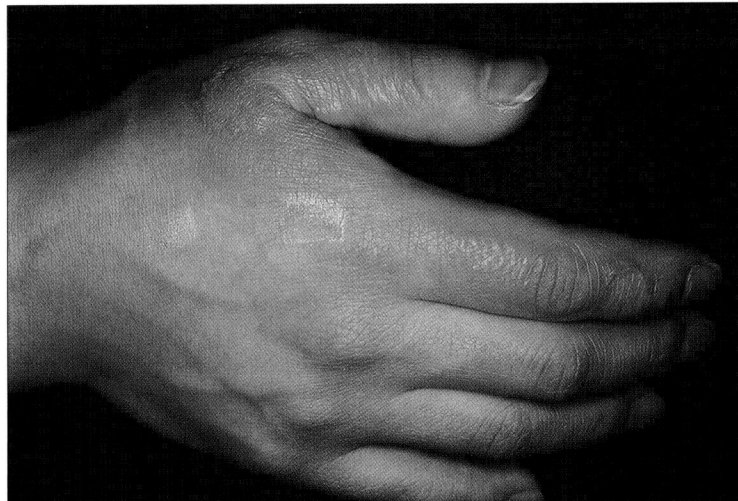

Fig. 87.1 Thermal burn. This superficial second-degree burn is characterized by bullae that contain serous fluid. Courtesy of Kalman Watsky MD.

children and the elderly. Wounds that appear dull red from entrapment of clot (denatured hemoglobin) imply full-thickness injury[8].

The severity of burn injuries is based upon depth and BSA involvement. BSA is estimated in adults by the 'rule of nines' (Fig. 87.2). This formula cannot be applied to children, since the head accounts for approximately 19% BSA in a 2-year-old, 15% in a 7-year-old, and 13% in a 12-year-old. Lund & Browder charts are useful for more accurate assessment of BSA involvement[4]. Initial evaluation should address airway and circulatory status; associated inhalation injury is seen in up to 25% of burn patients. Cardiovascular evaluation must address the issue of hypovolemic shock, regardless of burn severity. Urine output must be monitored because of the significant fluid loss and rhabdomyolysis that may compromise renal function[3,4].

Pathology

Pathologic features of thermal burns are summarized in Table 87.3.

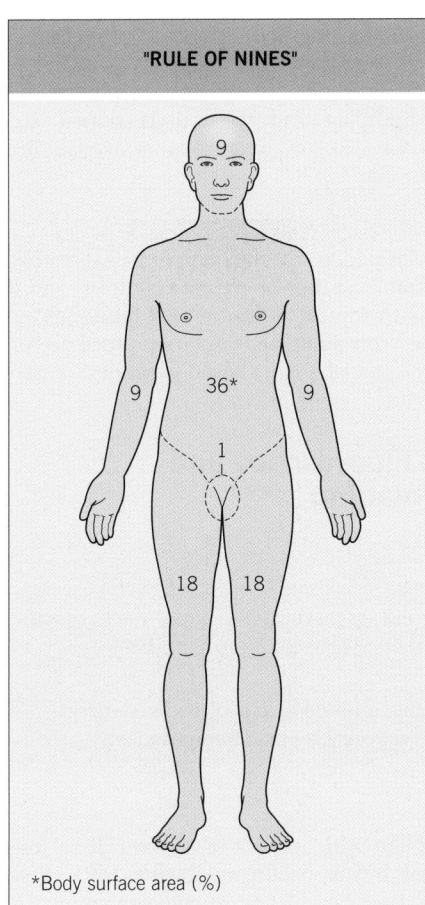

"RULE OF NINES"

9

9   36*   9

1

18   18

*Body surface area (%)

Fig. 87.2 Rule of nines. In adults, an estimate of burn extent is often based upon this surface area distribution chart. Infants and children have a relatively increased head:trunk surface area ratio.

Differential diagnosis

The differential diagnosis of heat injury is listed in Table 87.1. Although there is considerable overlap in clinical features, an important distinction is the degree of neurologic compromise. The most important diagnostic issue with thermal burns is the depth of the injury (see Table 87.3).

Treatment

Management of heat-related injuries involves removal from the hot environment, rest, rehydration, restoration of electrolyte balance, and evaluation of involved systems (Table. 87.1; see Lugo-Amador et al.[1] for more details).

Initial management of burn victims includes assessment of cardiopulmonary status as well as the extent and depth of the burn. Information regarding resuscitation of burn victims is beyond the scope of this text, but can be found in references 3, 4 and 7. Management of the burn wound should start with cool compresses to ease pain and reduce heat. Then, the wound should be cleaned gently to remove any foreign material. The next step is prevention of infection, followed by creation of a proper healing environment (see Ch. 141). Topical antimicrobial agents shown to be effective in burn wound care include silver sulfadiazine, mafenide acetate and silver nitrate. Silver sulfadiazine has gained wide acceptance for both pediatric and adult burn treatment. However, percutaneous absorption can lead to leukopenia. Also, silver sulfadiazine produces a pseudoeschar that may interfere with burn depth assessment. Superficial wounds may require little additional therapy[3,4,7].

Deeper burn wounds need more aggressive therapy, the most popular approach being serial excision. Third-degree burns are excised early, with indeterminate and deep second-degree wounds delayed until maximum depth and extent are known. Biologic dressings (e.g. pig skin, human allograft) were popular for several years, but have been largely displaced due to higher infection risk and poor healing. Newer skin substitutes such as acellular dermal matrix (AlloDerm®), bilaminar collagen-chondroitin sulfate and silicone (Integra®) and cultured epithelial autografts are gaining popularity[7,8] (see Ch. 145).

Erythema Ab Igne

Synonyms: ■ Toasted skin syndrome ■ Fire stains

Key features

- Localized areas of reticulated erythema and hyperpigmentation
- Chronic exposure to heat below the threshold for a thermal burn
- Commonly in lumbosacral region (heat applied to relieve pain) and shins (in regions without central heating in homes)
- Squamous atypia histologically
- Risk of cutaneous malignancy, particularly squamous cell carcinoma

Introduction

Chronic exposure to low levels of infrared heat can lead to the characteristic reticulated cutaneous pattern of erythema ab igne (EAI), with subsequent risk of malignant degeneration.

History

EAI, once a very common entity, was first described in the UK as a result of standing near stoves fired with peat. In the southern US, the custom of sitting around pot-bellied stoves to keep warm while socializing also led to its development. Although the advent of central heating in much of the industrialized world has led to a dramatic decline in incidence, creative cultural and therapeutic applications of various heating devices continue to induce EAI[9-11].

Epidemiology

In the past, EAI was seen up to ten times more frequently in women than in men. The vast majority of those affected were middle-aged or beyond. Risk factors include lack of central heating, occupations with close heat exposure, and medical conditions with symptoms relieved by heating or associated with decreased sensation.

Pathogenesis

Long-term exposure to heat below the threshold for thermal burn is the primary etiologic factor in EAI. The precise pathophysiology is unknown. Repeated exposure to heat below 45°C (113°F) produces reticulated erythema followed by hyperpigmentation in the same pattern[10]. Heat sources reported to cause EAI are found in Table 87.4.

Clinical features

The initial presentation is a transient macular erythema in a broad reticulated pattern that easily blanches. The entire size and shape often approximates that of the heat source. As the heat exposure continues over time, the erythema evolves into a dusky hyperpigmentation, with lesions fixed and no longer blanchable (Fig. 87.3). Epidermal atrophy may overlie the reticulated pigmentation. Later-stage lesions may become somewhat keratotic and bullae may appear. Lesions are

HEAT SOURCES REPORTED TO CAUSE ERYTHEMA AB IGNE	
• Heating pads	• Steam radiators
• Hot water bottles	• Car heaters
• Electric stove/heater	• Heated reclining chairs
• Open fires	• Heating blanket
• Coal stoves	• Hot bricks
• Peat fires	• Infrared lamps
• Wood stoves	• Microwave popcorn
	• Laptop computer

Table 87.4 Heat sources reported to cause erythema ab igne[9–11].

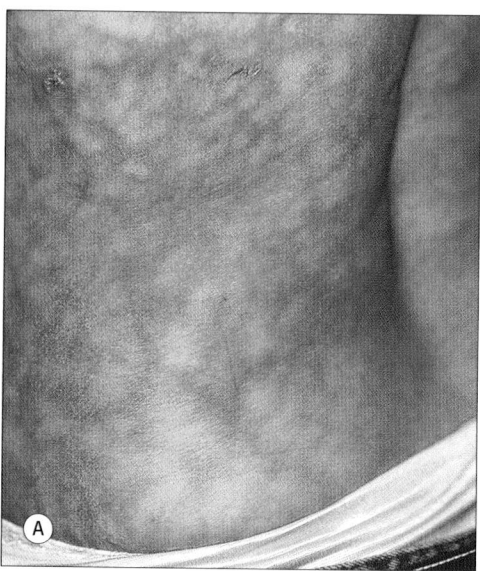

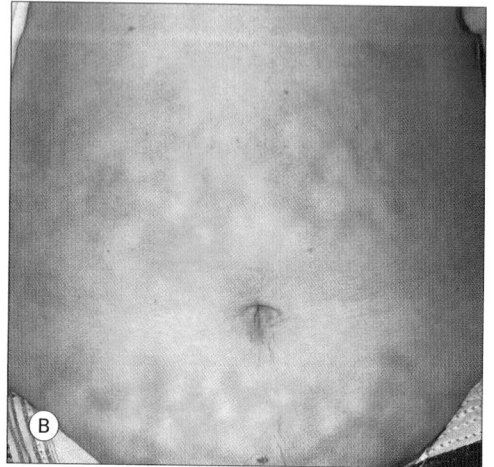

Fig. 87.3 Erythema ab igne. A Reticulated dusky hyperpigmentation due to chronic heat exposure. B Earlier phase with significant pink discoloration of the skin as well as hyperpigmentation. B, Courtesy of Jeffrey Callen MD.

characteristically asymptomatic, although a slight burning sensation is sometimes noted[9].

Once the heat source is identified, it is important to determine if it is being used to relieve pain and, if so, the cause of the pain. A lumbosacral location usually points to musculoskeletal disease or, less often, bony metastases. EAI of the abdomen, flank or mid-back may reflect an attempt to relieve pain from inflammation (e.g. pancreatitis, peptic ulcer disease) or malignancy (e.g. pancreatic, gastric). Symptoms of pain should prompt a thorough review of systems and consideration of a search for occult disease. An inquiry into occupation and hobbies is also important, as EAI can develop in exposed areas, e.g. the forearms of bakers, and the face or arms of glass blowers and foundry workers[9,10].

The possible development of cutaneous squamous cell carcinoma (SCC) or Merkel cell carcinoma represents the major long-term risk. The latent period may be 30 years or more. Apparently, the risk of developing SCC is highest with hydrocarbon-fueled heat exposures, e.g. 'peat fire cancers' on the shins of women, Japanese 'Kairo cancers' and Tibetan 'Kangri ulcers' due to coal-fired clothing warmers, and Chinese 'Kang cancers' from sleeping on coal-fire-heated bricks[9,10].

Pathology

The earliest histopathologic changes include epidermal atrophy, vasodilation and dermal pigmentation (both melanin and hemosiderin). As lesions progress, the epidermal atrophy becomes more pronounced, with flattening of the rete ridges. Focal hyperkeratosis and dyskeratosis are noted along with squamous atypia. Basal cell vacuolization has been reported and the dermal–epidermal junction may exhibit an interface dermatitis. The dermis appears thinned and sometimes edematous, with accumulation of abnormal elastic tissue and pigment as well as ectatic capillaries. Dermal capillaries may exhibit enlarged endothelial cells with hyperchromatic nuclei. Later lesions may also show basophilic degeneration of connective tissue. Hemosiderin deposition and prominent telangiectasias are seen most often in leg lesions. Ultrastructural evaluation also shows increased melanocyte dendritic processes, suggesting melanocyte activation[9,10,12].

Differential diagnosis

EAI needs to be distinguished from livedo reticularis, which is a temperature-sensitive vasculopathy (see Ch. 106) that favors the extremities but only occasionally develops associated hyperpigmentation. Cutis marmorata (see Ch. 106) and cutis marmorata telangiectatica congenita are less commonly considered in the differential diagnosis of EAI. The presence of telangiectasias along with atrophy and hyperpigmentation raises the possibility of poikiloderma and its various causes, e.g. cutaneous T-cell lymphoma (see Ch. 120), dermatomyositis (see Ch. 43) and several genodermatoses (see Ch. 62).

Treatment

Management consists primarily of removal of the offending heat source. The epidermal atypia is comparable to that of actinic keratoses, and it has been treated successfully with topical 5-fluorouracil (although no controlled trials of therapy have been published). As mentioned above, the use of heat to treat symptoms of pain should prompt a determination of the cause of this pain[9,10].

Burns Associated with Fluoroscopy and Magnetic Resonance Imaging

Key features

- MRI may produce first-, second- or third-degree burns due to metal or wire contact with skin, creating a closed-loop conduction system
- Fluoroscopy, particularly when repeatedly performed in patients with cardiovascular disease, may result in radiation-induced injury

Introduction

The radiologic literature is replete with reports of superficial to full-thickness thermal or electrical burns occurring during MRI. Risk factors for MRI burns are found in Table 87.5. In addition, there are

RISK FACTORS FOR BURNS DURING MAGNETIC RESONANCE IMAGING
ECG leads Monitoring cables Pulse oximeter Pins in halo fixation device Transdermal patches Metallic body piercing jewelry Tattoos Extremity skin-to-skin contact

Table 87.5 Risk factors for burns during magnetic resonance imaging[13-15].

reports in the radiologic and dermatologic literature of ulcerations on the back following repeated fluoroscopy[16-18].

Pathogenesis

Although the precise cause of MRI burns is unknown, the presence of both pulsed radiofrequency and pulsed magnetic gradient fields is thought to play a role. If an electrically conductive loop is formed between the patient and an electrode, patient and wiring, or even small areas of skin–skin contact, current can be produced by the changing magnetic flux, causing a thermal or electrical burn. Resistance at the skin surface may create a thermal injury, while contact with wiring in a capacitative coupling may create electrical injury. Alternatively, the burn may result from formation of a resonant conducting loop with an extended wire creating a resonant antenna, heating maximally at the antenna tip[13,19].

The mechanism behind fluoroscopy-induced radiodermatitis is related to the dose of radiation that is delivered. Repeated procedures are notorious for increasing the risk. Patients with diabetes mellitus, collagen vascular diseases or genetic defects involving repair of radiation-induced injury as well as individuals receiving chemotherapy appear to be more prone to developing this complication at lower doses of radiation.

Clinical features

Thermal burns appear soon after MRI, and may be partial to full thickness (see Table 87.3). The shape and size of the burns are determined by the conductor causing the injury (e.g. circular burns under ECG electrodes; figurate burns conforming to the shape of metallic wires or tattoo pigment deposition)[13,19].

Fluoroscopy-induced radiation dermatitis may be acute, but, as time passes and the acute injury resolves, the patient may continue to develop further changes, including epilation of hair, desquamation, permanent erythema and eventual ulceration (Fig. 87.4).

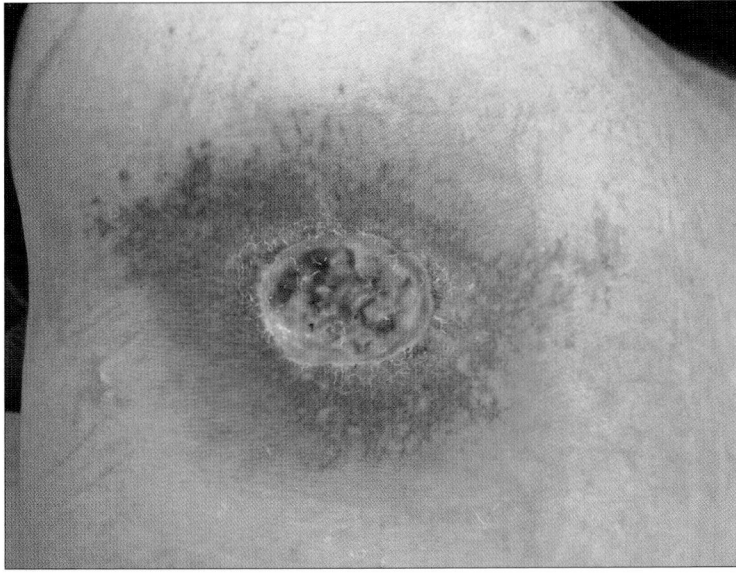

Fig. 87.4 Fluroscopy-induced radiation dermatitis. Courtesy of Jeffrey Callen MD.

Differential diagnosis

Because of the proximity of the MRI event to the detection of a burn injury, the diagnosis is generally straightforward. However, in the case of a tattoo burn, allergic contact dermatitis or foreign body granuloma formation within the tattoo may be considered. Timing of the event plus the sensation of a burn rather than pruritus should allow a distinction.

The differential diagnosis of fluoroscopy-induced disease includes fixed drug eruptions, morphea, contact dermatitis, herpes virus infection, impetigo and spider bites.

Treatment

Prevention of this injury by avoiding risk factors is ideal. However, when burns occur, they should be managed as any other thermal burn or, in the case of fluoroscopy-induced injury, by limiting the dose delivered.

Airbag Burns

Key features

- Deployment of airbags causes numerous cutaneous injuries, including frictional and blunt trauma, thermal burns and, possibly, chemical burns
- Friction due to contact with the bag, thermal burning from the bag and its released gases, and exposure to corrosive aerosol produce the injuries

Introduction

Automobile airbags provide additional crash protection, with a resulting reduction in driver and passenger fatalities by up to 31%. Although patented in 1953, US manufacturers only began installation of airbags in the mid-1970s. European airbag installation began in 1981. Since 1997, new cars in the US have been required to have airbags. By 1999, 45% of cars and 41% of trucks in the US were thought to be compliant. Despite the beneficial effect, numerous injuries have resulted from airbag deployment, including burns, abrasions and lacerations[20,21].

Pathogenesis

Airbag activation consists of detection, inflation and deflation phases. The sudden deceleration caused by impact triggers sensors in the front bumper to fire a sodium azide canister inside the nylon rubber bag. The sodium azide ignites with explosive release of hot nitrogen gas to inflate the bag in about 10 milliseconds at speeds exceeding 160 km/h. The hot nitrogen gas and other byproducts are then vented out the upper sides of the bag away from the occupant, thus deflating the bag. Vented aerosol contains nitrogen, carbon mono- and dioxides, sodium hydroxide, ammonia, nitric oxide, metallic oxides and other trace gases, creating a corrosive environment. Friction and pressure from the bag, heat from the bag and gases, and contact with the corrosive aerosol may produce injury[20-22].

Clinical features

The cutaneous injuries produced by airbag deployment are summarized in Table 87.6. Chemical burns occur rarely, but appear to be a result of skin exposure to small amounts of the corrosive alkaline aerosol. The aerosolized particles need to dissolve in a water layer such as tears or sweat before creating a corrosive injury. Of note, alkali burns of the skin may continue to deepen and extend over time, unless all the corrosive chemical is washed away[20-22].

Differential diagnosis

The pattern of injury and history of airbag deployment makes the diagnosis obvious. However, it is important to determine whether a burn injury is purely thermal or if it has a chemical component. Assessment of tissue pH and monitoring for continued extension of the burn help determine whether an alkali injury exists.

Treatment

Prevention is, of course, the most valuable therapy. Newer airbag design modifications include repositioning of the exhaust vents to direct the

AIRBAG INJURIES TO SKIN		
Type	**Frequency**	**Clinical features**
Abrasions/friction burns	64%	Patches of erythema or ecchymosis, typically with superficial erosion
Contusion	38%	Ecchymosis
Lacerations	18%	Variable severity
Thermal burns	8%	First and second degree most common (see Table 87.3) Localized full-thickness burn may result from metallic accessories or melted clothing Face and forearms, followed by hands, chest
Chemical burns	?	Painful superficial violaceous erythema and edema Partial to full thickness, often in splash pattern
Irritant dermatitis	?	Erythema and edema of upper chest, arms, face Burning or stinging sensation Desquamation and postinflammatory hyperpigmentation common

Table 87.6 Airbag injuries to skin[20–22].

escape of hot gases away from possible areas of skin contact. Seats should be positioned as far back from the airbag module as possible. Children too small to benefit from the adult three-point restraint should not be in the front passenger area. Children in any type of car seat or booster should never be put in the front seat. When a thermal or frictional injury occurs, local wound care and protection from secondary infection usually suffice.

Alkali burns require copious irrigation to dilute the corrosive substance. Acidic neutralization is contraindicated because of possible extension of injury by the resulting exothermic reaction. When the tissue pH is normal, local wound care is adequate.

INJURY DUE TO COLD EXPOSURE

Frostbite

Synonym: ■ Frost-nip

Key features

- Frostbite can occur when the skin temperature drops below about −2°C (28°F)
- Erythema, edema and numbness are replaced by marked hyperemia and pain
- Tissue freezing, vasoconstriction and inflammatory mediator release are central to the pathophysiology of frostbite
- Rapid rewarming in a warm water bath is the cornerstone of therapy

Introduction

Exposure to cold environments, whether during occupational or recreational activities, poses a risk of cold-related injury. Prolonged exposure may lead to hypothermia, frost-nip or frostbite. Hypothermia (i.e. a decline in core temperature below 35°C [95°F]) is a systemic process with minor cutaneous features and therefore will not be discussed in detail.

History

Cold injury predates recorded history – the quest for clothing, shelter and fire as protection from the elements must have preoccupied pre-

historic humans. Mass casualties from cold injury have been seen most often in military conflicts. For example, General George Washington lost as many men to the cold as to the British Army during the American Revolution. When Napoleon entered Eastern Europe his army had 385 000 soldiers, but only 3000 returned, in large part because he lost over 250 000 soldiers to cold-related death. During World War II, the German army on the Russian front experienced over 100 000 cold injuries, with some 15 000 requiring amputations[23,24].

Epidemiology

A 10-year retrospective assessment (1986 to 1995) of cold injury in members of the British Antarctic Survey found an incidence of 65.6 per 1000 per year seeking medical attention. Ninety-five percent had frostbite, 3% hypothermia and 2% cold water immersion foot. Superficial frostbite was the most common injury (74% of cases), and the face (nose and ears) was the most frequent site of involvement. Seventy-eight percent of the victims were injured during recreational activities. Although temperature and wind chill had no influence on severity of injury, the prevalence of cold injury increased with falling temperature, with a maximum prevalence at −25°C to −30°C (−13°F to −22°F). A major risk factor was prior cold injury[25].

Additional risk factors for frostbite are listed in Table 87.7.

Pathogenesis

The underlying pathophysiology of frostbite is a combination of freezing, vascular insufficiency (constriction and occlusion) and damage due to inflammatory mediators. As extremities cool, the 'hunting response of Lewis' (alternating vasoconstriction and vasodilation) occurs, ending with vasoconstriction. This tends to conserve the core temperature at the expense of the extremity, which tends toward ambient temperature. The head does not exhibit a vasoconstrictor response, except for the nose and ears. The trunk surface may cool a bit, but the core temperature is maintained. Frostbite is therefore unusual on the trunk or head (except the nose and ears), unless there is direct contact with ice or a refrigerant. The pathophysiologic stages of frostbite are summarized in Table 87.8, along with key clinical features[24,26].

Clinical features

Frostbite has been divided into four categories of severity, analogous to burn injuries. These are only recognizable upon rewarming. *Frost-nip* (first-degree frostbite) presents with erythema, edema, cutaneous anesthesia and transient pain (Fig. 87.5A). Full recovery is expected, with only mild desquamation. *Second-degree frostbite* is characterized by marked hyperemia, edema and blistering, with clear fluid in the bullae (Fig. 87.5B). Healing occurs, but many patients have long-term sensory neuropathy, often with significant cold sensitivity.

Third-degree frostbite consists of full-thickness dermal loss, with hemorrhagic bulla formation or development of waxy, dry, mummified skin. The latter features are poor prognostic indicators for tissue loss. *Fourth-degree frostbite* is a full-thickness loss of the entire part, with skin, muscle, tendon and bone damage. Injuries of this severity lead to amputation[24,26]. Some authors advocate simple designation as superficial or deep injury, with better prognostic accuracy.

RISK FACTORS FOR FROSTBITE
Alcohol consumption Psychiatric illness Drug abuse Vehicular trauma Vehicle mechanical failure Homelessness Fatigue Circulatory impairment Tobacco use Improper clothing High altitude

Table 87.7 Risk factors for frostbite[26].

	FOUR STAGES OF FROSTBITE	
Phase	Physiologic events	Clinical findings
I (cooling)	Cyclic vasoconstriction and vasodilation Extracellular ice formation (−2°C, 28°F) Intracellular ice crystal formation (if rapid freeze of >10°C or 18°F/min) Intravascular ice formation leads to erythrocyte sludging, vessel occlusion	Cool extremity Blanched appearance Numbness Hard, woody texture
II (thawing and rewarming)	Ice melts Dehydrated cells start to swell Loss of integrity of vessel walls, creating edema Vascular tone is compromised, leading to vasodilation Inflammatory mediator release leads to aggregation of platelets and leukocytes, causing thrombosis	Erythematous to violaceous color Intense pain Blisters form
III (extension of injury)	Thromboxane A2 levels increase Platelet and leukocyte aggregation extends into bordering tissue, creating vascular compromise	Blisters rupture
IV (resolution)	Tissue either re-epithelializes or desiccates and mummifies Vasomotor instability may persist indefinitely	Healing or amputation

Table 87.8 Four stages of frostbite[24].

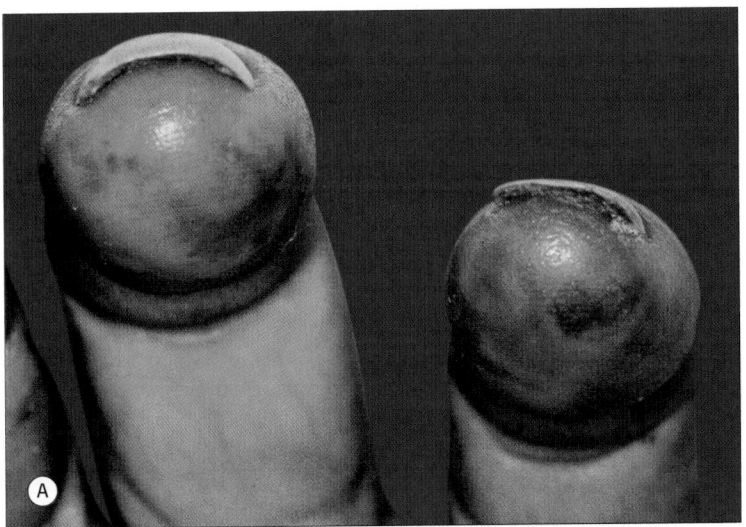

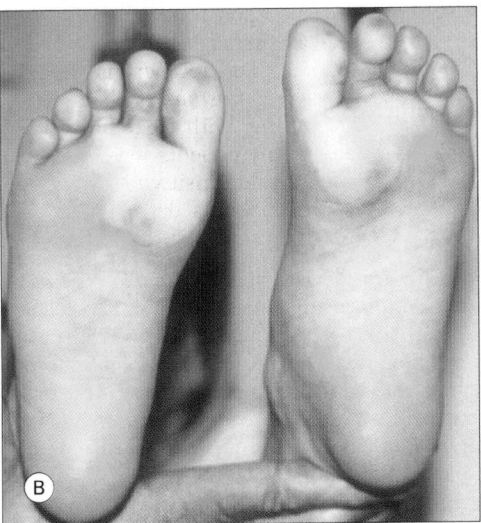

Fig. 87.5 Frostbite.
A Erythema, edema and hemorrhage are seen on the fingertips in a first-degree frostbite. **B** Bullae filled with clear fluid on the distal plantar surfaces in a second-degree frostbite.
B, Courtesy of Timothy Givens MD.

Pathology
Superficial dermal edema and subepidermal bulla formation are typical findings in frostbite. Vascular permeability leads to hemorrhage, most pronounced in deep injury. The epidermis and involved dermis become necrotic, with an inflammatory infiltrate and granulation tissue at the junction with normal tissue[6].

Differential diagnosis
Frostbite injuries should be readily recognizable, given exposure history and typical presentation. A greater diagnostic challenge is determination of the depth of the injury (see above). One possible diagnosis in the differential is cold water immersion foot (see Table 87.10).

Treatment
Fundamental therapeutic goals in frostbite are rapid rewarming, prevention of further cold exposure, and restoration of circulation. Once the patient is in a setting in which re-freezing cannot occur, rapid water bath rewarming is indicated. The water bath temperature should be about 40°C (104°F). Rubbing the frozen extremity with ice, using dry heat, and slow rewarming are all contraindicated. In the hypothermic patient with frostbite injury, it is important to complete fluid resuscitation and core rewarming before limb rewarming, to prevent sudden hypotension and shock. Routine wound care, protection of the frost-bitten part, and tetanus prophylaxis should then follow. Radiologic evaluation (MRI, bone scan, plain films) may help determine extent of injury and prognosis.

Additional therapeutic suggestions have been based on animal studies, case reports or small series. Because of increased blood viscosity and sludging, thrombolytic therapy (e.g. heparin, streptokinase, iloprost, limaprost) has been suggested. Superficial white (non-hemorrhagic) bullae may be debrided to avoid prolonged exposure to prostaglandins and thromboxanes in blister fluid. Aloe vera, a thromboxane inhibitor, has been shown to be useful as a topical agent in superficial frostbite. The problem of vasoconstriction has been addressed by sympathectomy, with the most impressive effect being prevention of re-injury with repeat exposure to cold conditions. Pentoxifylline has been found to be useful, as have anti-inflammatory agents such as methylprednisolone, methimazole and aspirin[24,26,27].

Pernio

Synonyms: ■ Chilblains ■ Perniosis ■ Kibes

Key features
- Cold-sensitive inflammatory disorder in which erythrocyanotic discoloration of acral skin is accompanied by a sensation of itching or burning
- Common trigger is exposure to cold, wet, non-freezing conditions
- Must be distinguished from chilblain lupus erythematosus and cold-sensitive blood dyscrasias
- Treat with nifedipine

Introduction
Pernio is an abnormal inflammatory response to cold, damp, non-freezing conditions[28]. It is most common in areas without central heating.

History

Over a hundred years ago, pernio/chilblains was apparently common enough in Europe and the UK that the condition was well recognized. In 1881, Piffard[29] described it quite well –

> This affection, so common in cold climates, affects, by preference, the face, hands, nose, and ears. It is characterized by redness, usually with a purplish tinge, together with more or less pain of a burning character giving little or no trouble during the summer, but causing inconvenience and suffering as cold weather sets in.

Epidemiology

Exposure to cold, wet conditions is the major risk factor for pernio. This condition is common in the UK and northwestern Europe, particularly in those whose homes lack central heating. Women, children and the elderly are most commonly affected. Elderly patients may have a prolonged course, while younger patients improve spontaneously[30–32].

Pathogenesis

The precise pathogenesis of pernio is unknown, but the condition is thought to have a vascular origin. In children, it may be associated with cryoglobulins or cold agglutinins[32].

Clinical features

Pernio presents with single or multiple erythematous to blue–violet macules, papules or nodules (Fig. 87.6). In severe cases, blistering and ulceration may be seen. Lesions are often symmetrically distributed on the distal toes and fingers, and less often on the heels, nose and ears. Deep pernio may be seen on the thighs, calves and buttocks as blue-erythrocyanotic plaques. Patients describe itching, burning or pain. Lesions often resolve in 1 to 3 weeks, except among elderly patients with venous insufficiency, in whom lesions can become chronic[31–34].

Pathology

Pernio has a non-specific histology consisting of dermal edema plus a superficial and deep lymphohistiocytic infiltrate with peri-eccrine accentuation. The infiltrate is composed predominantly of T lymphocytes. Necrotic keratinocytes and lymphocytic vasculitis have been noted[31].

Differential diagnosis

Idiopathic pernio needs to be distinguished from several other cold-induced syndromes (Table 87.9). The latter can be assessed by laboratory evaluation including: (1) complete blood count to exclude hemolytic anemia and myelomonocytic leukemia; (2) cryoglobulin, cold agglutinin and cryofibrinogen levels to eliminate cold-sensitive dysproteinemia; and (3) serum protein electrophoresis to exclude a monoclonal gammopathy. Chilblain lupus erythematosus (Hutchinson), whose clinical features are similar to pernio, typically exhibits histologic features compatible with discoid lesions of lupus erythematosus and occurs in a patient with serologic evidence of autoimmunity (e.g. positive antinuclear antibody screen). The diagnosis of lupus pernio (Besnier), which favors the nose, is confirmed by the presence of the histologic features of sarcoidosis[30,35].

Treatment

Adequate clothing and avoidance of cold, damp conditions are important preventive measures, as are keeping feet dry and avoidance of smoking. In a double-blind, placebo-controlled trial, nifedipine was found efficacious for the treatment of pernio. None of the nifedipine-treated patients relapsed, while all of the placebo-treated patients developed new lesions[36]. It is effective in about 70% of patients with pernio. Other anecdotal remedies include nicotinamide, phenoxybenzamine, sympathectomy and erythemogenic UVB phototherapy[30].

INJURY DUE TO WATER EXPOSURE

Immersion Foot

Synonyms: ■ Trench foot ■ Tropical jungle foot ■ Shelter foot ■ Paddy-field foot ■ Swamp foot ■ Jungle rot ■ Foxhole foot ■ Peripheral vasoneuropathy

Key features

- Injury occurs after continuous exposure of feet to moist, occluded conditions
- Cold water, warm water and tropical variants exist
- The underlying pathologic process is overhydration of the stratum corneum
- Neuropathy may persist indefinitely
- Feet exposed to immersion injury are more sensitive to re-injury

Introduction

Immersion injury occurs in either cold or warm environments when the feet are exposed to continuous moisture with no opportunity for intermittent drying. Severe injury may produce permanent peripheral neuropathy and long-term morbidity.

History

Soldiers on the Western Front in World War I spent extended periods of time in the cold, wet, muddy conditions of trench warfare. The Second World War produced another variant, with shipwrecked troops spending days in partially submerged lifeboats. The Korean conflict and the Vietnam War led to more variations and tremendous numbers of casualties. The most recent military experience with immersion foot occurred during the Falklands War. Civilian immersion foot also occurs singly or in small groups, particularly among the homeless[37–40].

Epidemiology

Susceptibility to immersion foot is widely variable. Use of sandals or open shoes, constant activity, thinner plantar stratum corneum, and intermittent air drying seem somewhat protective. Risk factors for immersion foot include: prolonged occupational or recreational exposure to wet conditions, immobility, constrictive clothing, dehydration, poor nutritional status, smoking, alcoholism, mental disturbances, drug abuse, peripheral vascular disease, uncontrolled diabetes, trauma, prolonged dependency of feet, and homelessness[37,39].

Pathogenesis

The underlying pathophysiology of all forms of immersion foot is overhydration of the stratum corneum. The permeability coefficient of

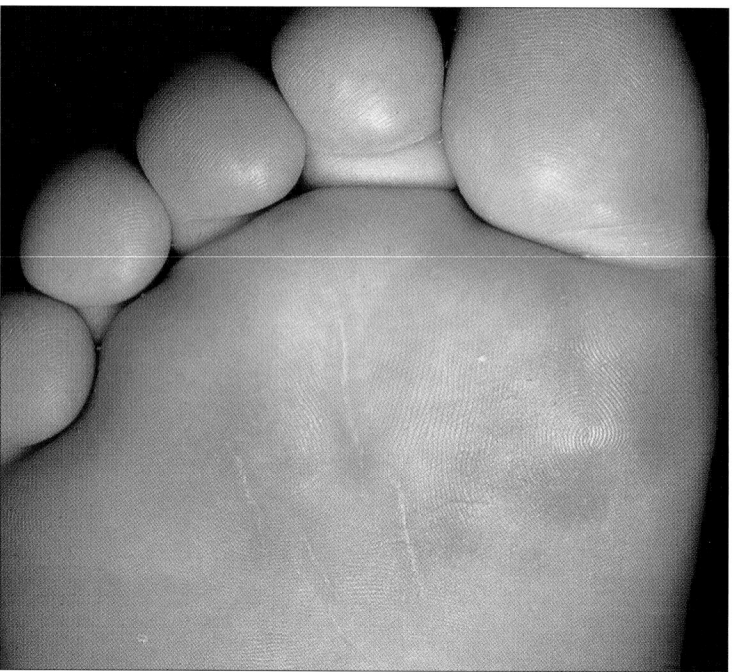

Fig. 87.6 Pernio. Areas of violaceous discoloration on the plantar surface of the foot and toes. Courtesy of Ronald P Rapini MD.

DIFFERENTIAL DIAGNOSIS OF SKIN LESIONS INDUCED BY NON-FREEZING COLD EXPOSURE

Disorder	Features	Possible associated conditions	Chapter reference
Acrocyanosis	Red to purple discoloration Hands and feet Painless	Erythromelalgia Cryoproteins Anorexia nervosa	106 24 51
Pernio	Erythrocyanotic Symmetric distribution Painful		87
Raynaud's phenomenon	Clearly demarcated pallor, followed by blue then red discoloration Idiopathic form usually does not ulcerate	AI-CTD Blood dyscrasias Drugs Trauma	44
Livedo reticularis	Bluish, broad reticulated patches May be idiopathic	AI-CTD Hematologic disorders Vascular occlusive diseases Infections Medications	106
Cold panniculitis	Erythematous indurated plaques, most often on cheeks Children Clears in 2 weeks		100
Cold urticaria	Cold-induced wheals May be idiopathic	Cryoproteins Infections Malignancies Familial cold autoinflammatory syndrome	19
Chilblain lupus	Cold-induced acral lesions Histologic features of lupus erythematosus Coexistent lupus erythematosus		42
'Pulling boat hands'	Rowing in cold, wet conditions Papules to vesicles Itching, burning, tenderness		
Retiform purpura due to cryoproteins*	Favors acral sites		24
Cryoglobulins	Cold serum protein precipitate	Plasma cell dyscrasias Lymphoproliferative disorders	
Cryofibrinogen**	Cold plasma protein precipitate	Infections Malignancies	
Cold agglutinins**	RBCs agglutinate in cold Occasional RBC lysis in cold	Infections (e.g. with *Mycoplasma*, EBV, CMV) Lymphoproliferative disorders	
Cold hemolysins**	RBC lysis in cold Paroxysmal hemoglobinuria	Infections (e.g. viral, syphilis)	

*Acrocyanosis, Raynaud's phenomenon, livedo reticularis and cold urticaria can also be observed in association with cryoproteins.
**Rarely cause cold-related occlusion syndromes.

Table 87.9 Differential diagnosis of skin lesions induced by non-freezing cold exposure[30–35]. AI-CTD, autoimmune connective tissue disease; CMV, cytomegalovirus; EBV, Epstein-Barr virus; RBC, red blood cell.

plantar skin is approximately ten times that of the dorsal foot skin, leading to increased water absorption. The plantar stratum corneum can absorb approximately 200% of its dry weight in water, with a proportionally higher absorption of fresh water than saline.

Cold water immersion foot (CWIF) is more severe due to the addition of cold-induced vasospasm. Because water conducts heat 23 times faster than air, the cold water immersion invokes 'thermo-protective' peripheral vasoconstriction. This creates hypoxic injury to nerves (initially large myelinated axons, but eventually all types) and muscle, with later injury to subcutaneous fat and blood vessels.

Warm water immersion foot (WWIF), on the other hand, results from severe hyperhydration of the stratum corneum, with subsequent maceration. Plantar skin temperature reaches body core temperature after about an hour in an impervious boot with 19°C (66°F) water. As the injury continues (tropical immersion foot, TIF), inflammatory changes develop and may progress to a lymphocytic vasculitis with vascular compromise and erythrocyte extravasation. Eventual involvement of the dorsal foot skin develops with striking inflammation. Secondary infection may develop in the compromised tissue after 3–4 days, further complicating management and worsening morbidity[24,37,38,41].

Clinical features

The clinical syndromes of immersion foot (Table 87.10) are divided into three variants: CWIF, WWIF, and TIF. Although the latter is sometimes viewed simply as a prolonged and more severe variant of WWIF, it will be discussed separately because prolonged warm water exposure does produce different clinical features.

Pathology

All forms of immersion foot demonstrate edema, thickening and fragmentation of the stratum corneum. Variable superficial dermal edema is noted. In more severe forms (CWIF, TIF), superficial dermal capillaries are narrowed due to edema or even frank lymphocytic vasculitis. CWIF produces much deeper damage in blood vessels (narrowing and fibrosis), muscle, nerves and bone.

Differential diagnosis

The differential diagnosis of immersion foot includes dermatophyte infection, cellulitis, pitted keratolysis, erythrasma, Gram-negative or complex toe web infections, and (occasionally in diabetics) candidiasis. The latter three conditions are usually confined to toe web spaces, and

		IMMERSION FOOT: COLD WATER, WARM WATER AND TROPICAL VARIANTS			
Variant	Exposure temperature	Exposure time	Clinical features	Complications	Duration
Cold water	15.5–21°C (60–70°F)	>7 days	Feet cold, heavy, stiff and numb May appear swollen Waxy white to mildly cyanotic Three phases after rewarming: 1. pre-hyperemic – feet cold, edematous and numb, with stocking anesthesia; purpura, blisters and necrosis possible; pulses not palpable 2. hyperemic – return of vascular and nerve function; tingling, pain and throbbing; increasing erythema and edema; skin anhidrotic, hot and painful to touch; ambulation difficult; vasomotor instability; dependent rubor, pallor upon elevation; bullae, intermittent cyanosis; infection risk high 3. post-hyperemic – cold sensitivity with digital blanching, intermittent edema, hyperhidrosis, persistent peripheral neuropathy	Infection Muscle atrophy Chronic venous stasis Joint contractures Trophic ulcers Myonecrosis Permanent axonal damage Bony changes such as hammer toe	Hours to days Up to 10 weeks Years
Warm water	15.5–32°C (60–90°F)	1–3 days	Thickening, softening and exaggerated wrinkling of soles (thicker soles worse) Ambulation painful ('walking on rope')		3 days
Tropical	21–32°C (70–90°F)	3–7 days	Prolonged warm water exposure In addition to plantar hyperhydration, dorsal foot becomes inflamed and edematous Pruritus, erythema and scattered vesicles Later purpura, brawny edema, maceration and scaling Fever, lymphadenopathy		>5 days

Table 87.10 Immersion foot: cold water, warm water and tropical variants[24,37,38].

dermatophytosis is usually more patchy, with fine scale and no significant maceration outside the web spaces. Pitted keratolysis can be distinguished by history and by the presence of punched-out tiny pits in the plantar surface of the forefoot and heel. Cellulitis is not limited at the immersion water mark, and can progress proximally.

Treatment

Prevention is the best treatment. Jungle boots have been shown to decrease the risk of WWIF when compared with thicker hiking boots. Once the condition develops, thorough and rapid drying is essential to restore function. CWIF patients must remain some distance from a heat source because the neuropathic insensitivity poses further risk of inadvertent thermal injury. WWIF can be prevented by frequent drying breaks and the use of silicone grease. The silicone is of no use in CWIF and has minimal value in TIF[38,40,41].

INJURY DUE TO ELECTRICITY

Electrical Burns

Key features

- The extent of an electrical burn injury may be much worse than the cutaneous contact burns suggest
- Contact point burns may be partial to full thickness
- Neurovascular, muscular and skeletal tissue may be damaged
- Lightning strikes can result in an erythematous, transient fern-like pattern on the skin

Introduction

Although electricity and lightning claim hundreds of lives each year, many more non-fatal injuries occur. The majority of electrical burns are work related, particularly among electricians, linesmen and construction workers. Children are also a major risk group, with low-voltage (<1000 V) injury more common under 6 years of age and high-voltage injury in older children and adolescents. A survey of 700 electrical injury admissions to Parkland Memorial Hospital over a 20-year period showed electric arc (flash burn, no current) injury to be the most

common (40%), followed by high voltage (38%), low voltage (20%), and lightning strikes (2%). Mortality was highest with lightning strikes[42].

Lightning injuries are most common in late spring through early fall. Most lightning strike victims are men (usually between 15 and 44 years of age) involved in outdoor activities. In the US, lightning-associated injuries occur most commonly in the south, Gulf Coast, Rocky Mountains, and Ohio, Mississippi and Hudson River Valleys[42,43].

Pathogenesis

The severity of an electrical injury depends upon the strength and frequency of the electrical field, the duration of exposure, path of current, and relative resistance of the tissue. Acute tissue damage by strong (high-voltage) low-frequency fields is due to holes punched in cell membranes (electroporation), Joule heating of the extracellular fluid, and cell membrane protein denaturation through electroconformational coupling. The thermal effects (i.e. Joule and dielectric) depend upon tissue resistance to the flow of current. For example, bone has the most resistance of any body tissue, therefore generating the most heat. Resistance then decreases through fat, tendon, skin, muscle, blood vessels, and, finally, nerves (least resistance). An additional indirect effect is a field-generated formation of free radicals with subsequent lipid peroxidation and membrane disruption[44,45].

Lightning injury follows similar electrothermal principles, but with three important differences: (1) current and voltage are massive, e.g. 30 000 to 50 000 A, and a difference between clouds and object of 2 million V/m; (2) the superheating of air through which the current passes to 30 000°K, creating a high-pressure thermoacoustic shock wave (thunder) that may generate 100 atm of air pressure locally; and (3) the creation of internal conduction loops as the large magnetic field passes through the body. Injury can occur from a radial spread of current after lightning strikes the ground, from a direct hit, from flashover (current around body), or from blast effect[43,46].

Clinical features

Electrical burns usually range from partial to full thickness, and high-tension burns often involve deep tissue, with the current damaging muscle, nerves and vessels. Erythema, edema and blisters (partial-thickness damage) may result from a current of 20 to 35 mA/mm² with an exposure time of 20 seconds (heats skin to 50°C) (Fig. 87.7). At a higher current of 75 mA/mm² with the same exposure time, the temperature could rise to 90°C, causing skin perforation and charring.

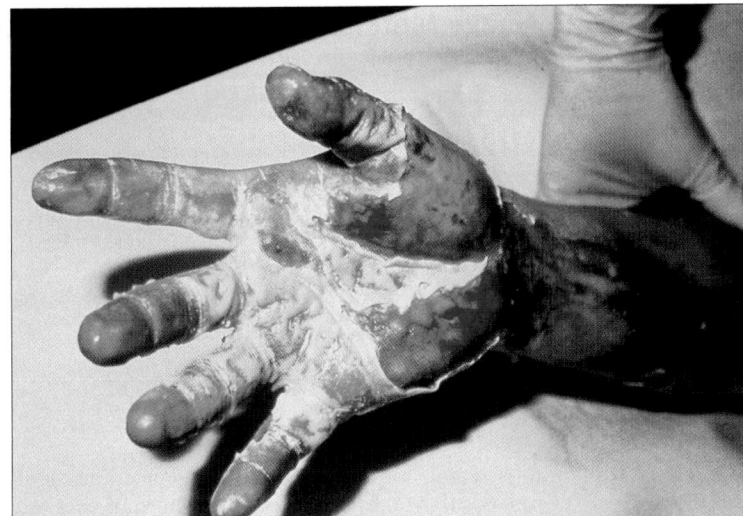

Fig. 87.7 Electrical burn. It is characterized by erythema, edema, bulla formation and sloughing of the necrotic epidermis. Courtesy of Timothy Givens MD.

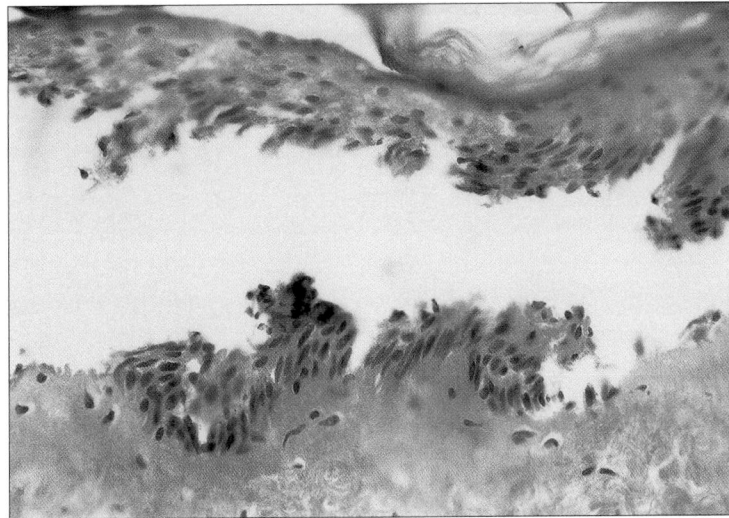

Fig. 87.8 Pathology of an electrical burn. Blistering seen in a biopsy from a patient who died of an electrical burn. Notice the elongated keratinocyte nuclei. Courtesy of Ronald P Rapini MD.

Identification of so-called 'entrance' and 'exit' wounds is of no value, since 60 Hz alternating current (AC) has current changing directions 120 times per second. More important is determination of the extent of skin and internal injury. In some cases, current may arc between body parts, creating 'kissing' wounds. High-voltage injuries may result in electroplating of skin with black metallic debris that leaves charred craters when removed. Additional thermal injury may occur when clothing or nearby items are ignited by an electrical arc[44,46].

Deep tissue injury can be considerably more severe than the cutaneous wounds might suggest. Muscle injury may be deceptively deep, since bone (with higher electrical resistance) retains heat more readily than other tissues. Edema in deep burns may result in compartment syndromes. High-tension AC and direct current (DC) can cause ventricular asystole, whereas low-tension AC, such as household current, is more likely to produce ventricular fibrillation, plus some patients develop chronic and recurrent arrhythmias. Considerable nerve, blood vessel and musculoskeletal injury may also be seen[44–46].

Lightning burns generally are more superficial due to the very brief contact. A unique pattern of skin lesions after a lightning strike is the 'lightning print', 'feathering' or Lichtenberg figures. These markings are erythematous, transient linear fern-like patterns that resolve in hours to days. While not a true burn, they are pathognomonic of lightning strike injury. Other cutaneous changes may include patchy mottling, erythema, blistering, full-thickness punctate skin loss, flash burns, thermal burns from ignited clothing, and contact burns from grounding. Although internal burn injuries are uncommon in lightning strikes because of the very brief duration, the internal electrical currents that are created are strong enough to cause cardiac arrest or seizures. Additional sequelae include profound neuromuscular shutdown (keraunoparalysis), confusion, temporary amnesia, deafness and blindness, and prolonged or permanent neurologic disturbances, e.g. peripheral sensory neuropathy[43,44].

Pathology

Electrical burns are characterized by epidermal necrosis, with cytoplasmic strands extending into the cavity between damaged and normal skin. Keratinocytes may be elongated vertically (Fig. 87.8), and collagen appears homogenized. Severe electrical burns destroy the entire skin, including the subcutis, often with accompanying necrosis of deeper blood vessel walls. The Lichtenberg figures after lightning injury display subcutaneous hemorrhage[6].

Treatment

Electrical injuries are very complex, often involving multiple organ systems, since any organ in the path of current can be damaged, and initial assessment may underestimate the extent of injury. Although full management of electrical burns should be carried out in level one trauma centers, initial management includes isolation of the patient from the power source, assessment of vital signs, cervical spine immobilization,

determination of contact points on the skin, and, if possible, venous access. For more details, see the section above on thermal burns.

One special circumstance should be noted. Toddlers who sustain oral commissure burns from biting into electrical cords are at risk for delayed bleeding. About 10–14 days after the burn, the eschar comes off, often exposing a damaged labial artery. Direct pressure will control the bleeding, pending definitive care[44–46].

Chemical Burns and Exposures

These entities are discussed in several chapters, including those on irritant contact dermatitis (Ch. 16), occupational dermatoses (Ch. 17), plant dermatoses (Ch. 18) and child abuse (Ch. 89).

INJURY DUE TO CHEMICAL EXPOSURE

Chemical Hair Discoloration

Synonyms: ■ Green hair ■ Chlorotrichosis

Key features

- Hair discoloration may be a voluntary cosmetic change or the result of a chemical or metal exposure
- Green hair may result from exposure to copper or selenium
- Most hair discoloration normalizes over time

Introduction

Decorative hair coloring has risen to new heights with the flamboyant artistry of the past two decades. Brilliant pink, green, purple, blue and orange, and myriad styles, from a buzz cut to dramatic multicolored spikes, adorn many of today's youths. Much of this is deliberate decoration, but hair discoloration at any age may be an inadvertent, and sometimes unwanted, occurrence as well.

History

Green hair among copper workers was noted as early as 1654. More recently, such discoloration has been attributed to swimming pools[47].

Epidemiology

Most patients with unwanted hair discoloration have blond or white hair, although black hair may become discolored as well. Risk factors include exposure to the substances in Table 87.11, in addition to frequent contact with chlorinated water (especially swimmers), use of

CAUSES OF UNINTENTIONAL HAIR DISCOLORATION		
Green	**Yellow to orange to golden**	**Purple**
• Copper • Selenium sulfide • Tar shampoo • Cobalt • Chromium • Nickel • Yellow mercuric oxide • Hypothyroidism* • Phenylketonuria*	• Tar shampoo • Anthralin • Minoxidil • Copper	• Alkalinized anthralin
*Speculative.		

Table 87.11 **Causes of unintentional hair discoloration**[47–50]. See Table 65.12 and Fig. 65.10 for causes of diffuse hypomelanosis of scalp hair.

an alkaline shampoo, dyeing, peroxide bleaching, and mechanical or sun-induced hair damage[47,48].

Pathogenesis

Green hair discoloration due to copper occurs when metallic copper is released from pipes under acidic conditions into domestic or swimming pool water, or when copper algicides or chlorination are used to sanitize swimming pools. Damage to the hair cuticle by permanent wave treatments, frequent water exposure and sunlight allow the copper to penetrate the hair more readily. The copper content of discolored green hair (or golden hair in Asian patients) is considerably higher than in non-discolored hair in the same individual. Increased systemic copper may lead to elevated levels in hair, but does not cause a greenish color change. The mechanism of selenium-induced green hair is unknown[47–49].

Yellowish hair discoloration appears to result from staining of lighter-colored hair, but the mechanisms are not known[50,51]. Nanko et al.[48] speculated that the golden color of Japanese swimmers' hair is due to water friction injury of the cuticle, allowing hypochlorous acid from the chlorination process to invade the cortex and degrade melanosomes. Copper seems to play a role as well, but the mechanism is uncertain.

Clinical features

The presenting concern is a progressive yellow to green discoloration of the hair. Scalp hair is the only hair involved, and the surface hair is more noticeably discolored than underlying hair.

Pathology

By electron microscopy, loss of the hair cuticle and wearing of the cortex layers were seen in discolored, golden hairs in Japanese swimmers[48]. In addition, there was a reduced number and density of melanosomes in the discolored hair relative to controls. X-ray spectrography demonstrated an increased chlorine content in both the discolored and normal hair of swimmers relative to controls, and a reduced sulfur content in only the discolored hairs.

Differential diagnosis

Hair discoloration is readily visible. The specific etiology and subsequent therapy needed may be determined by ascertaining the type of exposure (see Table 87.11) that led to the color change. For example, copper from cosmetic plant extracts and metallic eyeglass frames can produce green hair.

Treatment

Discontinuation of the offending exposure would seem the most prudent remedy. Numerous anecdotal remedies have been described, including hot oil, hydrogen peroxide, alkaline shampoos, penicillamine- or EDTA-based shampoos, commercial hair decolorizers, and hydroxyethyl diphosphonic acid[47].

Arsenical and Heavy Metal Dermatoses

Key features

- Chronic arsenic exposure may occur via drinking water contamination or occupational exposure
- Chronic arsenicism is characterized by mottled hyperpigmentation with areas of hypopigmentation, keratoses on the palms and soles (and other sites), and multiple non-melanoma skin cancers, particularly Bowen's disease
- Histologically, arsenical neoplasia is almost identical to actinic neoplasia

Introduction

Arsenic is a ubiquitous metal, ranking 20th in abundance among all the elements. Exposure occurs via drinking water, agricultural uses, ore mining, and medicinal applications. Chronic exposure poses significant health risks, including development of benign and malignant tumors (Table 87.12). The other toxic and heavy metals and their cutaneous impact are outlined in Table 87.13. Allergic contact dermatitis due to metals is covered in Chapter 15.

History

Medicinal effects of arsenic have been known since the days of Hippocrates and Galen. Early applications of arsenic included the treatment of psoriasis, eczema, pemphigus, urticaria, furuncles, warts, lupus, epitheliomas, syphilis, leprosy, molluscum contagiosum, and lichen rubor[29]. Even in the late 1800s, cutaneous side effects of arsenic exposure were noted, including pruritus, papulosquamous eruptions, and palmoplantar keratoses.

Chemical forms of therapeutic arsenic include Fowler's solution (liquor potassii arsenitis), arsenici bromidum, arsenici iodidum, Pearson's solution (liquor sodii arseniatis), arsenicum hydrogenisatum, Donovan's solution (liquor arseni et hydrargyri iodidi), and Asiatic pills (arsenic with opium or pepper)[29,62]. Apparently, Fowler's solution and Asiatic pills are the most widely used, with the latter still available in India and the Far East. Traditional Chinese medicine may continue to use inorganic arsenic. Most of the Western World has abandoned arsenicals, although treatment of asthma with Fowler's solution continued until the 1960s in parts of the US. Arsenic trioxide is now used therapeutically for acute promyelocytic leukemia[52,53].

Metallic arsenic has been consumed in large quantities by the arsenic eaters of the Swiss and Austrian Alps, believing that such consumption improved physical strength. Inorganic arsenic (the toxic form) is believed to have caused Napoleon's death during his second exile at St Helena[52].

Epidemiology

Accidental exposure to arsenic still occurs via contaminated drinking water in many areas of the world. Naturally contaminated drinking water is found in India, China, Taiwan, Chile, Argentina, Mexico, the Philippines, Bangladesh, Thailand and the US. Careless contamination of drinking water has resulted from mining of ores containing silver, gold, tin, copper, lead, tungsten, zinc and cobalt[52,53].

An estimated cumulative dose of arsenic capable of producing arsenical keratoses or skin cancer is about 0.5 to 1 g. Adverse effects have been noted when arsenic is in drinking water at a concentration of 0.4 to 0.6 mg/l. The current World Health Organization provisional guideline value and US Environmental Protection Agency limit is 0.01 mg/l. This was recently decreased from the previous limit of 0.05 mg/l, since cutaneous and internal cancers may develop with the latter level of exposure. However, no chronic skin changes have been noted with arsenic concentrations <0.017 mg/l in drinking water.

Chronic exposure to inorganic arsenic poses an increased risk for developing cancer (see Table 87.12). Trivalent inorganic arsenic is the most toxic form, with a latent period for chronic manifestations of 30 to 50 years[52,62]. Occupational exposure to arsenic may occur during the use of pesticides, herbicides or treated wood, and during electroplating, mining, smelting, wine making, carpentry, and manufacture of gallium arsenide computer microchips[52,62].

CLINICAL FEATURES OF ACUTE AND CHRONIC ARSENIC POISONING

ACUTE

Skin

- Flushing, erythema, facial edema, acrodynia, urticaria
- Loss of hair and nails
- Remaining nails show Mee's lines after 8 weeks

Gastrointestinal

- Nausea, vomiting, severe abdominal pain, profuse watery diarrhea, malabsorption

Neurologic

- Acute peripheral neuropathy
- May progress to Guillain–Barré-like ascending paralysis

Other

- Pancytopenia, metallic breath odor, cardiac arrhythmias, renal failure, respiratory failure

CHRONIC

Skin

- Hyperpigmentation of axillae, groin, nipples, palms, soles and pressure points, with superimposed guttate hypopigmentation ('raindrops on dusty road')
- Alopecia
- Arsenical keratoses – precancerous papules on palms and soles (Fig. 87.9)
  - Symmetric yellow punctuate corn-like papules measuring 2–10 mm
  - Favor thenar and hypothenar eminences, distal palms, lateral fingers, dorsal aspect of IP joints, weight-bearing plantar surfaces
  - Rarely on trunk, proximal extremities, eyelids, genitalia
  - May coalesce to plaques
- Blackfoot disease (vascular occlusive disease with blackening of skin)

Other

- Nasal septum perforation
- Peripheral neuropathy
- Bone marrow hypoplasia
- Gastrointestinal disturbance

Malignancies

- Bowen's disease
  - Any skin surface
  - If no HPV, occurrence on sun-protected skin might suggest arsenic exposure
  - Skin-colored to red papules that become keratotic
  - Scale-crust removal leaves red, moist, papillomatous base
  - Multiple lesions common
  - Invasive squamous cell carcinoma develops in 5–20%
- Squamous cell carcinoma
  - Arising in arsenical keratosis or Bowen's disease, has more aggressive behavior
  - Metastasis in one-third
- Basal cell carcinoma
  - Multiple, superficial, may resemble Bowen's disease
- Extracutaneous malignancies
  - Genitourinary, especially bladder
  - Lung
  - Liver

Table 87.12 Clinical features of acute and chronic arsenic poisoning[52–54]. HPV, human papillomavirus; IP, interphalangeal.

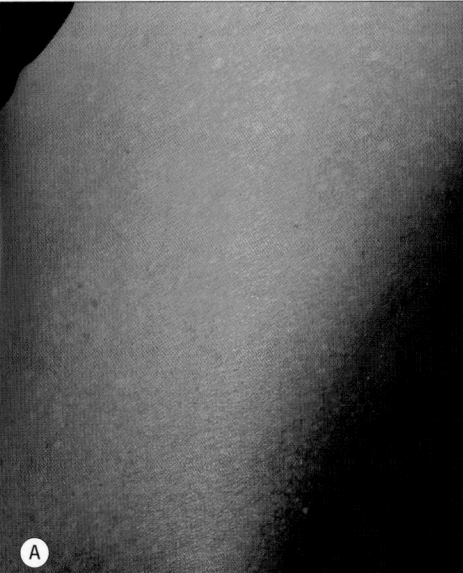
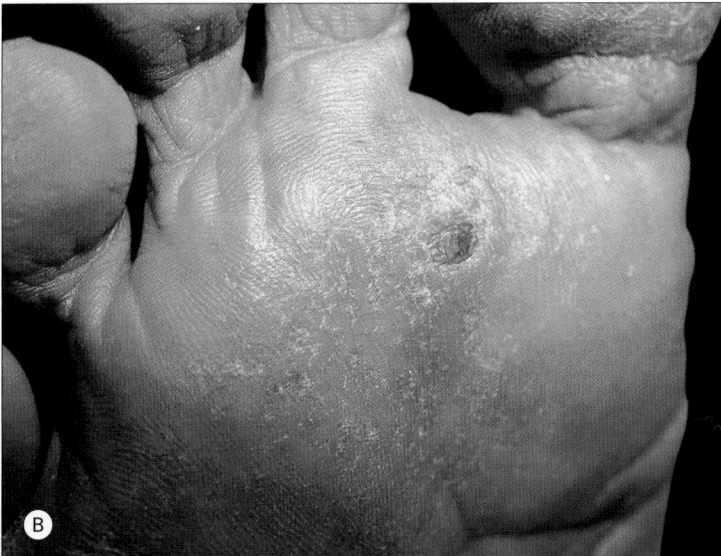
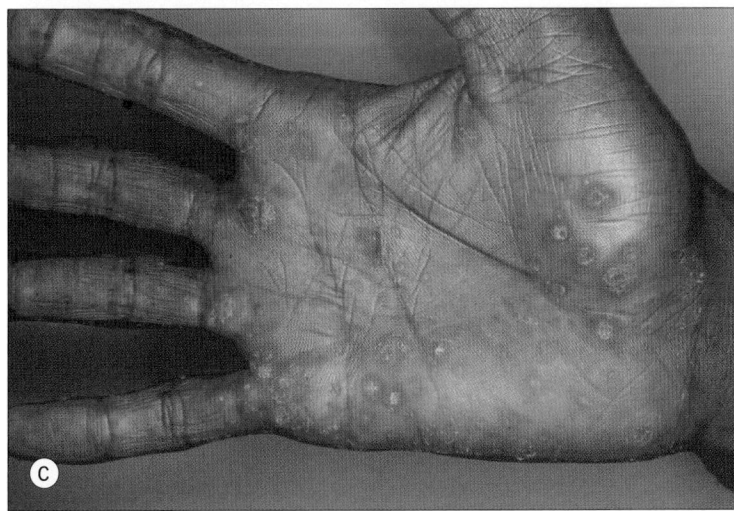

Fig. 87.9 Cutaneous manifestations of exposure to arsenic. A Guttate hypopigmentation superimposed on hyperpigmentation resembles 'raindrops on a dusty road'. B, C Arsenical keratoses on the plantar and palmar surface. A, Courtesy of John Steinbaugh MD. C, Courtesy of Jeffrey Callen MD.

Pathogenesis

Many of the toxic effects of arsenic are through interference with cellular respiration and uncoupling of oxidative phosphorylation. Arsenic can cause chromosomal alterations and gene amplification, induce sister chromatid exchanges, inhibit DNA repair, and transform mammalian cells *in vitro*. The precise mechanism of tumor promotion is unknown, but arsenic has been shown to modulate expression of several key transcription factors, including tumor suppressor p53, nuclear factor-κB, and activating protein-1[54].

Clinical features

Arsenic exposure can be divided into acute and chronic forms. Acute exposure (medicinal, homicidal, suicidal) produces myriad cutaneous and systemic features. Chronic arsenic exposure (drinking water, occupational) produces altered pigmentation, keratoses and substantial malignancy risk. See Table 87.12 for a summary of clinical features of acute and chronic arsenic poisoning.

Pathology

Arsenical keratoses exhibit marked hyperkeratosis with scattered parakeratosis and mild to moderate keratinocyte atypia. Vacuolation of keratinocytes may be noted and adnexal structures are spared. Basophilic

TOXIC AND HEAVY METALS AND THEIR CUTANEOUS IMPACT

Metal	Form	Cutaneous health hazards	Treatment and protection	IDLH*	Cancer risk
Aluminum	Alum, sulfates	Irritant contact dermatitis	Wash off	—	—
Antimony	Metal	Irritant contact dermatitis	Soap wash immediately	50 mg/m³	—
Arsenic	Inorganic	(see Table 87.12)	Avoidance, chelation	—	Lung, bladder and skin cancer
Barium	Chloride, nitrate	Irritant contact dermatitis, burns	Water flush immediately	50 mg/m³	—
Beryllium	Metal	Dermatitis, granulomas	—	—	Lung cancer
Bismuth	Telluride	Irritant contact dermatitis	Soap wash immediately	—	—
Boron	Borates, oxide	Erythema, irritant contact dermatitis	Soap wash, water flush	—	—
Cesium	Hydrate, hydroxide	Irritant contact dermatitis, burns	Water flush immediately	—	—
Chromium	Hexavalent	Allergic and irritant contact dermatitis, skin ulceration, burns; systemic absorption can lead to renal failure, hepatic failure, anemia, coagulopathy	Water flush promptly	—	Lung cancer
Cobalt	Metal dust	Dermatitis, diffuse nodular fibrosis	Soap wash	20 mg/m³	—
Copper	Metal dust	Dermatitis	Soap wash promptly	100 mg/m³	—
Gold	Elemental salts	Most common: lichen planus, lichenoid drug eruption, allergic contact dermatitis, eczematous dermatitis, PR-like eruption, pruritus, flushing, erosive stomatitis
Less common: chrysiasis, erythema nodosum, erythema multiforme, toxic epidermal necrolysis, exfoliative dermatitis	Avoid gold-laden liquor	—	—
Indium	Metal	Irritant contact dermatitis	Soap wash	—	—
Iron	Salts	Irritant contact dermatitis, mucosal irritation	Soap wash	—	—
Lead	Metal	Irritant contact dermatitis, gingival lead line	Soap wash promptly	100 mg/m³	—
Lithium	Hydride	Irritant contact dermatitis, burns	Brush off gently, DO NOT WASH	0.5 mg/m³	—
Magnesium	Carbonate	Irritant contact dermatitis	—	—	—
Manganese	Cyclopentadienyl tricarbonyl	Irritant contact dermatitis	Soap wash	—	—
Mercury	Elemental, inorganic, organic	Acrodynia, tattoo reaction (cinnabar), granuloma, exanthem, cutaneous hyperpigmentation, allergic and irritant contact dermatitis, baboon syndrome	Soap wash promptly	10 mg/m³ (elemental) 2 mg/m³ (organic)	—
Nickel	Elemental	Allergic contact dermatitis	Water wash immediately	10 mg/m³	Lung and nasal cancer
Osmium	Tetroxide	Irritant contact dermatitis	Soap wash immediately	1 mg/m³	—
Platinum	Metal	Irritant contact dermatitis	Soap wash	—	—
Selenium	Elemental, alloy	Irritant contact dermatitis, skin burns	Soap wash immediately	1 mg/m³	—
Silver	Metal	Argyria, irritant contact dermatitis, skin ulceration	Water flush	10 mg/m³	—
Tellurium		Dermatitis, garlic smell of sweat	Soap wash promptly	25 mg/m³	—
Thallium	Soluble	Alopecia, acneiform papules, hyperkeratotic plaques on hands and feet, Mee's lines	Water wash promptly	15 mg/m³	—
Tin	Metal, organic	Irritant contact dermatitis, skin burns, pruritus	Water flush immediately	100 mg/m³ (metal) 25 mg/m³ (organic)	—
Tungsten		Irritant contact dermatitis	Soap/water wash immediately	—	—
Uranium		Irritant contact dermatitis, skin burns	Soap/water wash immediately	10 mg/m³	Lung cancer
Vanadium	Dust, fume	Irritant contact dermatitis, green tongue	Soap wash promptly	—	—
Zinc	Chloride	Irritant contact dermatitis, skin burns (fixes tissue *in situ*), mucocutaneous hyperpigmentation	—	—	—

Concentration posing immediate danger to life and health (IDLH). Since 1979, the National Institute for Occupational Safety and Health (NIOSH) has not allowed detectable levels of known carcinogens. Therefore there are no values in the IDLH column for carcinogens.

Table 87.13 Toxic and heavy metals and their cutaneous impact[55–61]. PR, pityriasis rosea.

degeneration of dermal connective tissue is highly variable. There are no features that clearly distinguish arsenical keratoses from actinic keratoses.

Arsenical Bowen's disease exhibits the same epidermal histologic features as common Bowen's disease (see Ch. 108). Although the superficial type is most commonly observed, the basal cell carcinomas associated with arsenic can be any of the clinicopathologic subtypes (see Ch. 108)[52,62].

Differential diagnosis

Arsenical keratoses may resemble punctate palmoplantar keratoderma (including the porokeratotic variant) and verrucae vulgaris. Small pits are often noted when central keratotic plugs are removed from the papules in the inherited keratodermas, but not with arsenical keratoses. Family history and early onset are helpful in distinguishing palmoplantar keratodermas. In the nevoid basal cell carcinoma syndrome, there are persistent pits due to the localized absence of stratum corneum; additional clues are the characteristic facial features (see Section 18), odontogenic jaw cysts, and typical basaloid proliferative histology in the palmar pits.

Treatment

Chelation therapy is the mainstay of treatment for acute arsenicism. Dimercaprol (British anti-lewisite; BAL) is the most widely used agent. Other chelating agents reported efficacious include dimercaptosuccinic acid and dimercaptopanesulfonic acid. For chronic arsenicism, chelation has little value. Oral retinoids have been reported to reduce arsenical keratoses and decrease formation of arsenical basal cell carcinomas. Surgical extirpation, curettage, cryosurgery, topical chemotherapy and photodynamic therapy have been reported with some success. These treatments are all anecdotal or based upon small series[52,63].

FRICTIONAL AND TRAUMATIC INJURY TO THE SKIN

Corns and Calluses

> **Synonyms:** ■ Callosity ■ Tyloma ■ Clavus ■ Heloma ■ Heloma durum ■ Heloma molle ■ Intractable plantar keratosis

Key features

- Corns and calluses are keratotic lesions resulting from repeated trauma
- Ill-fitting footwear, bony protuberances and specific activities are contributing factors
- Hard corns are found on the dorsal aspects of the toes, while soft corns are in the interdigital web spaces
- Proper footwear and medical management usually suffice

Introduction

Repeated mechanical trauma to the feet, whether from poorly fitting footwear, anatomic differences, or work or leisure activities, produces hyperkeratosis. This otherwise natural protective response to injury may result in the formation of uncomfortable thickened areas of skin known as corns or calluses. Calluses are broad based, whereas corns are more narrowly based and sharply defined. Calluses also form on the hands from repeated trauma, but are usually asymptomatic[64].

Epidemiology

Risk factors for the development of corns and calluses on the feet include bony protuberances, abnormal biomechanical foot function, poorly fitted shoes, and repetitive trauma due to athletic activity[64].

Pathogenesis

Bony protuberances such as the condyles of metatarsal and phalangeal bones create outward pressure on the skin. Footwear and activities (walking, running) create counter pressure at these sites. The repeated

friction and pressure leads to hyperkeratosis. The latter further compromises the site by increasing pressure. The cycle of friction, pressure and thickening continues until a corn or callus develops[64].

Clinical features

Hard corns (heloma durum) are firm, small, dome-shaped papules with translucent central cores, found on the dorsolateral fifth toes and dorsal aspects of other toes. Soft corns (heloma molle) are painful keratoses in the interdigital web spaces. They often become macerated. Opposing toes may exhibit 'kissing lesions'. Broad keratotic plaques, often under the metatarsal heads, are calluses.

A unique callus is seen on the tip of the second (and sometimes third) toe, with associated transverse ridging, thickening and splinter hemorrhages in the nail. This is known as tennis toe (see Fig. 87.12) or center's callus. Also seen in gymnasts, soccer players, runners, football players and dancers, it results from sudden stops with repeated collision between toe tip and shoe. In many cases, the second toe is found to project further forward than the hallux[64,65].

Differential diagnosis

These common lesions rarely elude diagnosis, but must be distinguished from verruca vulgaris. Warts and corns interrupt dermatoglyphics, while calluses often demonstrate accentuated lines. Paring of a corn reveals a central translucent whitish yellow core, as opposed to the thrombosed capillaries and multiple bleeding points seen in a wart. Paring of a callus reveals layers of yellowish keratin, without the multiple punctate thrombosed capillaries of a mosaic plantar wart.

Treatment

Treatment should be directed toward both symptomatic relief and correction of the biomechanical conflict. Paring of the callosity, with removal of the corn's central core, provides prompt relief. Filing after warm water soaking can be performed periodically. Topical agents such as salicylic acid or urea help soften the callosity. Soft cushions (silicone sheet, sheepskin) reduce friction and improve comfort. Properly fitted footwear and the use of appropriate orthotics lead to long-term solutions. If all of these maneuvers fail, a plain film to look for exostoses and referral to orthopedic surgery may be indicated[64,65].

Black Heel and Palm

> **Synonyms:** ■ Talon noir ■ Tache noir ■ Calcaneal petechiae ■ Post-traumatic punctate intraepidermal hemorrhage

Key features

- Black macules on the palms or soles due to hemoglobin within the thickened stratum corneum
- Lesions are secondary to impact trauma and resolve with paring or time

Introduction

Black heel (or palm) is a post-traumatic intraepidermal hemorrhage seen most often in athletes. This harmless and self-healing process is a potential source of concern because of its dark black color.

History

Black heel was first described in 1961 by Crissey & Peachey[66] as calcaneal petechiae. A variety of subsequent reports under different monikers (see above) has led to confusion and debate over the proper nomenclature. The association with sports has been recognized since the beginning, with basketball the prototypical sport.

Epidemiology

Adolescents and young adults comprise the majority of patients with this entity. Sports participation is of paramount importance, particularly basketball, lacrosse, tennis, football, gymnastics and marching. Elderly patients with unusual palm and sole trauma may also be predisposed. Self-inflicted hammer injury can produce a similar clinical finding[67-69].

Pathogenesis

Black heel is a traumatic phenomenon thought to be due to shearing forces, often produced by sudden stopping or landing on the floor or ground. These shearing forces rupture papillary dermal blood vessels, with subsequent leakage of blood into the epidermis[69]. Hemoglobin resides in the stratum corneum for a longer transit time, and the position of the blood is out of reach of the phagocytic cells, maintaining the intact molecular structure of the hemoglobin[69,70].

Clinical features

The black or violet–black macules are asymptomatic and may be isolated or in clusters. They can form linear or horizontal arrays on the posterior or posterolateral aspect of the heel (Fig. 87.10A). Lesions are usually unilateral and favor the edge of the thick plantar keratin. Forefoot, toe and palmar (Fig. 87.10B) lesions have also been observed; in patients with thickened stratum corneum due to disorders of cornification, extrapalmoplantar lesions can be seen. Paring of the stratum corneum reveals red–brown to red–violet specks of dried blood.

Pathology

Hyperkeratosis with 'lakes of pigment'[69] within the stratum corneum form the characteristic histopathology. Iron stains may be negative (especially Prussian blue). Both the benzidine and Patent Blue V stains for hemoglobin are positive, perhaps because the intracorneal location has no phagocytic or proteolytic activity to allow formation of hemosiderin[69,70].

Differential diagnosis

The major entities in the differential diagnosis are cutaneous melanoma and verruca vulgaris. The ability to remove the lesion with gentle paring allows one to exclude a melanocytic lesion; positive staining for hemoglobin provides additional evidence. One author found the standard hemoccult test useful for confirming the presence of hemoglobin in parings[69].

Treatment

Once the diagnosis is ascertained, treatment is unnecessary.

Chondrodermatitis Nodularis Helicis

Synonyms: ■ Chondrodermatitis nodularis chronica helicis ■ Chondrodermatitis nodularis chronica helicis et antihelicis ■ Ear corn

Key features

- Exquisitely tender nodules appear on the pinnae
- Most patients have unilateral lesions and are over 50 years of age

Chondrodermatitis nodularis helicis (CNH) is a tender inflammatory process of the ear that was first described in 1915. Lesions are most common after age 40 years, with 94% of cases occurring in those between 50 and 80 years of age. Both men and women are affected, with men having more lesions on the helix, and women, the antihelix. Bilateral lesions are seen in 6–10% of patients. Several cases of childhood CNH have been reported[71,72].

Pathogenesis

The precise etiology of CNH is unknown. Predisposing factors include actinic damage, cold exposure, trauma, local ischemia, and, occasionally, radiotherapy. A suggested pathogenesis is that helical lesions begin with perichondritis or folliculitis, extending secondarily to the skin. On the contrary, antihelical lesions may begin with pressure-induced ischemia, involving the cartilage secondarily. These concepts remain speculative[72].

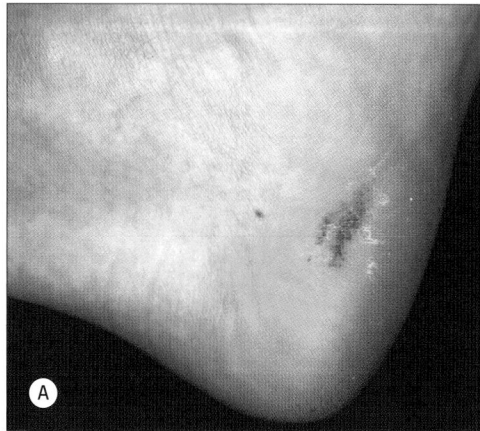

Fig. 87.10 Black heel and palm. A, B This black color is due to hemoglobin within the thickened stratum corneum. A, Courtesy of Jeffrey Callen MD. B, Courtesy of Jean L Bologna MD.

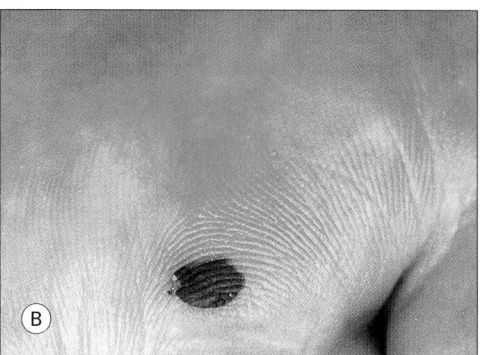

Clinical features

CNH presents as skin-colored to erythematous, dome-shaped nodules with central crusts or keratin-filled craters. Surrounding inflammation may be noted. The majority of lesions occur on the upper helical rim or the middle to lower antihelical rim; these sites often correspond to the outermost portions of the pinna. The lesions of CNH are often exquisitely tender to palpation (Fig. 87.11A), and sleeping on the side of the affected ear may be impossible[72,73].

Pathology

The epidermis exhibits a well-circumscribed area of acanthosis, parakeratosis and hypergranulosis. A central crater with epidermal disruption may be filled with a keratotic plug or dermal debris. The underlying dermis shows degenerative changes with acellular collagen, fibrosis (Fig. 87.11B) and variable lymphohistiocytic inflammation that is often granulomatous. Epithelioid cells may be present. The infiltrate extends into a thickened perichondrium[71-73].

Differential diagnosis

Lesions that are most commonly confused with CNH are squamous cell carcinomas, basal cell carcinomas, actinic keratoses, cutaneous horns and weathering nodules. Additional entities to consider include verrucae, keratoacanthomas, calcinosis cutis, gouty tophi, and reactive perforating collagenosis. Although the marked tenderness and characteristic locations point to the diagnosis of CNH, histologic evaluation may be necessary to confirm the diagnosis[72].

Treatment

A variety of treatment modalities have been suggested for CNH, although few controlled studies have been performed. Small series of patients treated with topical corticosteroids or topical antibiotics showed variable success. The use of specially designed pillows to relieve pressure is operator-dependent. Intralesional corticosteroid injections have been successful in some small series.

Numerous surgical approaches have been suggested, including cryosurgery, electrodesiccation and curettage, full-thickness excision, carbon dioxide laser ablation, and excision of skin with partial cartilage excision. Surgical excision seems to be the favored modality, although a paucity of data exists. A retrospective cohort study of 41 patients treated surgically and 15 patients treated conservatively (circular foam pad

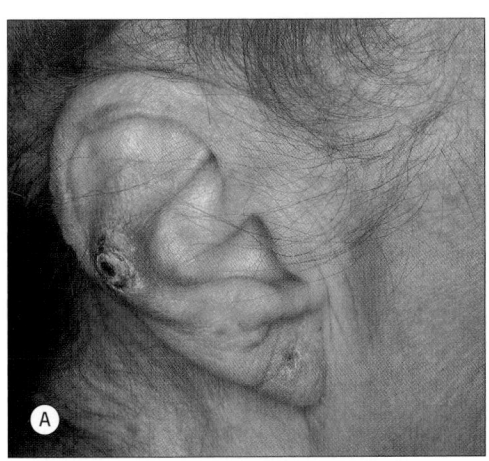

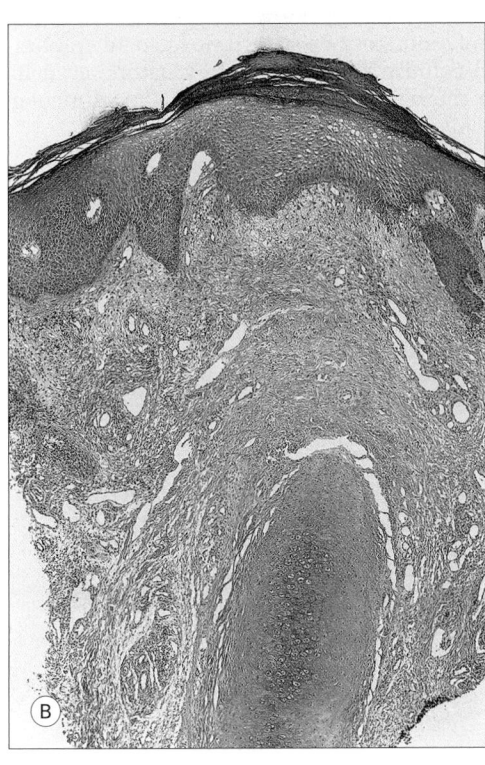

Fig. 87.11 Chondrodermatitis nodularis helicis. **A** Tender, erythematous papulonodule with central scale-crust on the mid antihelix of an older woman. This represented the site most susceptible to pressure-induced ischemia. **B** Central crust, epithelial hyperplasia, fibrosis, granulation tissue and degenerated cartilage are seen on histologic examination. A, Courtesy of Kalman Watsky MD. B, Courtesy of Ronald P Rapini MD.

Pathogenesis

Acanthoma fissuratum is thought to be due to pressure and friction created by eyeglass frames in the retroauricular sulcus or the upper lateral nose. Chronic irritation leads to collagen deposition. The collagen then appears to deteriorate, leading to local inflammation as a means of eliminating the abnormal collagen[77]. Additional factors that may contribute to the pathogenesis are composition and weight of the eyeglasses, roughness of the eyeglass frame, perspiration or local areas of dermatitis[76].

Clinical features

The classic lesion is a firm, skin-colored to erythematous nodule or plaque in the upper portion of the postauricular sulcus or upper lateral nose. The center of the lesion is characterized by the presence of a vertical groove or fissure. There may be occasional tenderness, serous discharge or slight hyperkeratosis. A surrounding inflammatory halo may be noted[75–77].

Pathology

The epidermis exhibits irregular acanthosis, most marked at the lesion's periphery. In some instances, the appearance may be that of pseudo-epitheliomatous hyperplasia. The central depression may show epidermal thinning or variable epidermal separation. Compact ortho-hyperkeratosis is noted over most of the lesion, with patchy areas of parakeratosis near the central groove. Dermal papillae exhibit dilated vessels and a moderately dense perivascular inflammatory infiltrate comprised of lymphocytes, histiocytes and plasma cells, with occasional neutrophils. Slight fibrosis may be noted in the superficial and mid dermis. Elastic tissue stains show no significant elastin within the nodule[75–77].

Differential diagnosis

These lesions are most commonly mistaken for basal cell or squamous cell carcinomas and, less often, keloids and CNH. Although histologic examination can readily exclude the cutaneous carcinomas, the presence of pseudoepitheliomatous hyperplasia may create some confusion. However, the cellular atypia of squamous cell carcinoma should be absent in acanthoma fissuratum.

Treatment

Lesions should clear within a few months of discontinuation, replacement or proper adjustment of the offending spectacles. Excision should be considered for persistent lesions. Anecdotal success of intralesional corticosteroids has been reported[75,76].

with headband) showed that 66% of the surgical and 87% of the non-surgical patients were healed at follow-up. Selection bias, small sample size and variable follow-up times were problematic. Additional controlled studies will be necessary before conclusions can be drawn regarding optimal therapy[72,73].

Acanthoma Fissuratum

Synonyms: ■ Granuloma fissuratum (of the ears) ■ Spectacle frame acanthoma ■ Eyeglass frame acanthoma

Key features

- Retroauricular nodules with a central vertical groove or fissure occur at the site of eyeglass frame contact
- Refitting of the spectacle frame leads to resolution

Ill-fitting eyeglass frames create a frictional injury in the postauricular sulcus or upper lateral nose leading to development of acanthoma fissuratum. The entity 'granuloma fissuratum' was first described by Epstein[74] in 1965 and the term was derived from an earlier report of a buccal mucosal lesion of that name. The term 'spectacle frame acanthoma' and the currently accepted designation 'acanthoma fissuratum' were added to the literature in the 1970s[75,76].

Weathering Nodules of the Ear

Key features

- Asymptomatic whitish papules (2 to 3 mm) along the helices of middle-aged or elderly Caucasian men
- Histologically, a fibrous tissue spur with cartilage metaplasia
- No treatment needed

Asymptomatic papules, known as weathering nodules, are seen on the helices of Caucasian men who have a history of significant cumulative sun exposure. The largest series published to date is that of Kavanagh et al.[78] All of their patients were Caucasian men who had significant outdoor sun exposure either at work or with hobbies. The median age was 79 years (range 44–91). A survey of 100 geriatric male inpatients in the same geographic area revealed that four had similar lesions.

Although the precise pathogenesis is unknown, the consistent history of sun exposure and the presence of actinic damage suggest a role for UV light.

Clinical features

Weathering nodules are white or skin-colored, and present along the free margin of the helix. They are bilateral and multiple in most patients. Multiple lesions create a scalloped appearance to the helical rim. Individual lesions are 2 to 3 mm in diameter and slightly elevated. Patients generally have significant actinic damage elsewhere[78].

Pathology

Epidermal atrophy, solar elastosis and telangiectasias occur over the nodule. The nodule itself is a fibrous tissue spur with cartilage metaplasia extending upward from disrupted perichondrium. The spur is connected to the underlying cartilage. No inflammation or epidermal disruption are noted[78].

Differential diagnosis

Alternative diagnostic considerations include CNH, elastotic nodules, granuloma annulare, rheumatoid nodules, amyloid, gouty tophi and calcinosis cutis. Chondrodermatitis occurs in a similar clinical setting, but can be distinguished by the presence of ulceration and tenderness clinically, and marked inflammatory changes histologically. Elastotic nodules of the ear occur more often on the anterior ear or antihelix. They are waxy, firm, mildly tender nodules. Microscopically, these lesions exhibit thick coalescing elastic fibers and amorphous basophilic masses. No cartilaginous changes are seen. Granuloma annulare and rheumatoid nodules consist of necrobiotic granulomas. The deposits of amyloid, uric acid and calcium have distinctive appearances and staining characteristics[78,79].

Treatment

Treatment is unnecessary, but Kavanagh et al.[78] note that two of their patients had received cryosurgery, with no local recurrence of the nodules.

Traumatic Auricular Hematoma

Synonyms: ■ Cauliflower ear ■ Wrestler's ear

Key features

- Trauma to the pinna avulses the anterior perichondrium from the underlying cartilage, then a subperichondrial hematoma can develop
- Drainage and replacement of the perichondrium can prevent development of fibroneocartilage

Introduction

Blunt trauma to the auricle can create a subperichondrial hematoma. If not corrected quickly, the hematoma will organize into a permanent disfiguring nodularity known as cauliflower ear. Therefore, early surgical correction is crucial.

History

Ancient Greek wrestlers were recognized by the stigma of a misshapen, thickened ear, the wrestler's 'ear-mark'. Similar ear injuries also are seen in boxers, rugby players, and piano movers. Early 20th century Hong Kong opium dens produced a similar finding as opium abusers slept for long periods on the wooden pillows. Although past generations of wrestlers lined up after competition to have their ears 'needled'[79], soft plastic protective headgear has been available for several decades[80].

Epidemiology

Traumatic auricular hematoma is seen almost exclusively in male athletes who participate in wrestling, boxing or rugby. Piano movers are at risk as well, due to pressure on the ear while lifting.

Pathogenesis

A glancing blow or twisting movement against the anterolateral pinna avulses the anterior perichondrium from the underlying cartilage. Adhesion between skin structures and perichondrium is apparently stronger than between perichondrium and cartilage. These shearing forces rupture vessels that then bleed into the subperichondrial or intracartilaginous space, creating the auricular hematoma[80]. Regardless of the location of the hematoma, there is agreement that, if left untreated, the hematoma will organize into a solid mass with subsequent production of fibroneocartilage. Fibroneocartilage formation begins 7–10 days after injury. Calcification may also ensue. Repeated injury produces the multinodular deformity known as cauliflower ear[81].

Clinical features

A painless to slightly tender swelling appears on the upper anterior aspect of the pinna in the scaphoid or triangular fossa after a glancing blow or twisting injury. If left untreated, the swelling persists and becomes firmer with time. The color varies from skin-colored to slightly bluish. No epidermal change is noted. Older lesions may feel soft and cystic or very firm[80,81].

Pathology

Histopathologic examination reveals a hematoma with fibrosis and foci of new cartilage formation. Older lesions may exhibit calcification and even ossification within the hematoma[80].

Differential diagnosis

The history of trauma and characteristic presentation readily help to establish a diagnosis. Other considerations include relapsing polychondritis, auricular pseudocyst and epidermoid cyst. Polychondritis should produce painful inflammatory episodes unrelated to trauma. Histologic features would confirm the inflammatory nature, even in the quiescent phase with thickening of the perichondrium. Auricular pseudocysts and epidermoid cysts are discussed in Chapter 110.

Treatment

Goals of treatment for auricular hematomas are evacuation of the hematoma, prevention of fluid reaccumulation, and maintenance of function and cosmesis. There is general consensus that treatment needs to proceed within 7 days (preferably the first 72 hours). Treatment modalities include aspiration, incision and drainage (with or without cartilage removal), and splinting to prevent recurrence[81]. Cochrane database investigators were unable to find controlled randomized or cohort studies to determine the best modality. Their conclusion was that there are no good data defining a best treatment, or even whether post-drainage treatment is needed[82].

SPORTS-RELATED DERMATOSES

Synonyms: ■ Tennis toe ■ Jogger's toe ■ Turf toe ■ Surfer's nodules ■ Surfer's knots ■ Jogger's nipple

Key features

- Cutaneous trauma produces abrasions, blistering, ecchymoses, callosities and unique sport-specific stigmata
- Allergic contact dermatitis in athletes is often due to rubber antioxidants and adhesives
- Cutaneous bacterial, viral and fungal infections occur more often in sports with close physical contact
- Existing dermatoses may be exacerbated by sports participation

Introduction

Participation in sports may be associated with many types of cutaneous injuries or infections. Most of these problems are minor inconveniences. The following discussion will be organized into: mechanical trauma (acute, chronic); exposure-related dermatoses; infections; and exacerbation of existing conditions.

History

Cutaneous injury has been an accepted consequence of athletic activity at least since ancient Greece. Stigmata such as the wrestler's 'ear-mark' have been viewed as marks of athletic prowess.

Epidemiology

Sports participation has shown a steady increase over the past 30 years. Along with the gain in popularity of athletic activity has come an increase in sports-related dermatoses and infections. For example, herpes simplex viral infections were seen in 2.6% of high school and 7.6%

Condition	Clinical features	Sports	Etiology/pathogenesis	Prevention/treatment
Friction blisters* (see Ch. 33)	Bullae and superficial erosions	Any	Friction or tangential impact to foot while in warm moist shoes	Frequent drying of feet, lubrication, proper shoe fit, drain blisters/leave roof
Contusion*	Ecchymosis	Any	Perpendicular mechanical trauma producing vascular damage	Padding
Subungual hematoma*		Running, tennis	Sudden impact of toe tip with end of shoe	Enlarged shoe toe box with proper arch and metatarsal support, drainage of hematoma may be needed
Black heel*	(See text)			
Turf toe*	Painful, erythematous, edematous hallux	Football, soccer	Acute dorsal and plantar tendonitis	Rest
Jogger's nipple*	Pain, erythema, fissuring, occasional bleeding	Running	Repeated friction of rough shirt fabric	Woman: jogging bra Man: taping, lubrication, semisynthetic or silk shirt
Callosities	(See text)	Many		
Tennis toe	Toe tip callus, nail thickening, subungual hyperkeratosis (Fig. 87.12)	Tennis, running	Repeated trauma of longest toe against inside of toe box	Proper shoe fit, enlarged toe box, improved arch support
Nail dystrophy	Onycholysis, hematoma, subungual hyperkeratosis, paronychia	Many	Repeated trauma to nails	Keeping nails trimmed
Fibrotic nodules (e.g. surfer's knots)	Thick fibrotic nodules on knees, knuckles, dorsal feet	Surfing, boxing, football, marbles	Chronic pressure over bony prominences	Padding, position change, prone rather than kneeling on surfboard
Piezogenic papules	Multiple asymptomatic to tender yellowish outpouchings on lateral aspect of heels when standing (Fig. 87.13)	Distance running, high-impact sports	Herniation of subcutaneous fat through small tears in lateral plantar fascia	None known
Runner's rump	Small ecchymoses in upper gluteal cleft	Running	Constant friction with each stride	Lubrication
Alopecia and hypertrichosis	Transient alopecia on forearms followed by hypertrichosis	Gymnastics	Frictional alopecia, compensatory regrowth	

*Acute injury.

Table 87.14 Frictional and mechanical dermatoses in athletes[86–89].

of collegiate wrestlers in the 1984 season, and 34% of wrestlers in a wrestling camp in 1989[83,84]. During the 1984–85 wrestling season, 60% of college and 52% of high school wrestlers had tinea corporis gladiatorum at some point[85].

Pathogenesis

The types of frictional and mechanical trauma that can lead to dermatoses in athletes are summarized in Table 87.14.

Acne mechanica is thought to occur when the local micro-environment of the skin is altered by a combination of pressure, heat, moisture (perspiration), friction and occlusion[86].

Exposure to heat and cold are discussed in other sections of this chapter. The pathogenetic mechanisms underlying pre-existing dermatoses that may be aggravated by athletic activity are discussed in the respective sections.

Clinical features

Acute or chronic mechanical trauma during sports activity creates unique cutaneous lesions summarized in Table 87.14.

In some patients, chronic friction on extensor extremities during the summer is thought to produce frictional lichenoid dermatitis (summertime pityriasis). This malady affects prepubertal children (mostly boys) and

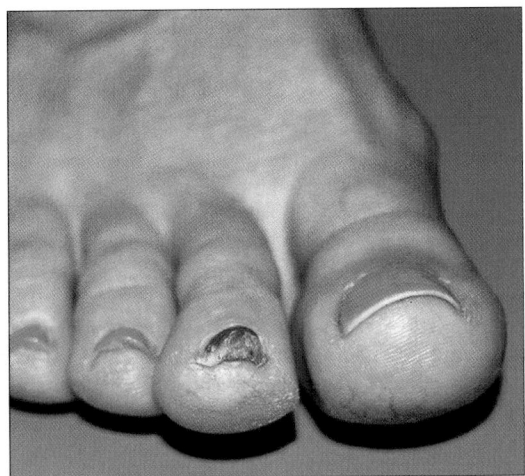

Fig. 87.12 Chronic 'tennis toe'. Chronic and repeated trauma of the longer second toe against the end of the tennis shoe toe box during sudden stops creates the distal callus formation and nail plate thickening known as tennis toe.

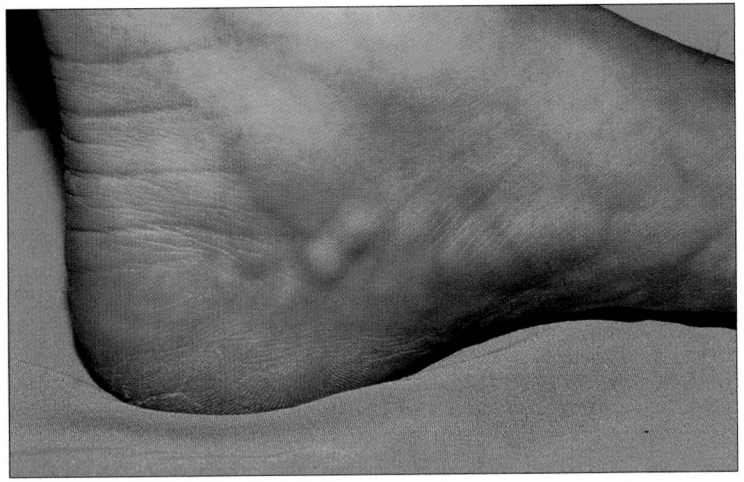

Fig. 87.13 Piezogenic papules. Yellowish outpouchings on the heel represent herniation of subcutaneous fat through the plantar fascia in this sometimes painful condition.

is characterized by irregular clusters of pale to skin-colored, flat-topped, lichenoid papules on the elbows, knees, dorsal metacarpophalangeal and interphalangeal joints, and extensor shins and forearms. Mild pruritus may develop, although most children are asymptomatic[88].

Another common finding in athletes is the presence of striae distensae, or stretch marks. These are most common in sports that emphasize strength training by weightlifting, such as body builders, football players, wrestlers and gymnasts. Striae are also seen in non-athletic settings such as Cushing's syndrome, obesity, pregnancy and overuse of corticosteroids. In addition, striae are thought to occur in 70% of adolescent girls and 40% of adolescent boys[86].

Environmental exposure creates additional challenges for the sports enthusiast, especially with activity during temperature extremes. Mountain climbers, skiers (downhill and Nordic), biathletes, winter hikers and others are at risk for cold injury (see above). Summer heat poses different risks such as heat exhaustion and heat stroke (see above). Water exposure in swimming, diving, snorkeling and scuba diving has intrinsic risks as well. Overhydration of the stratum corneum increases susceptibility to blisters, skin breakdown and cutaneous infection.

Allergic contact dermatitis is likely to be as common among athletes as the general population, but specific situations may arise from the use of specialized equipment. Erythema in the distribution of a swimmer's goggles or scuba mask ('mask burn') may be seen, and individuals with more severe reactions can also develop vesiculation, weeping, crusting, pruritus and pain. Rubber antioxidant allergy is known to occur in this setting, with mercaptobenzothiazole, tetramethylthiuram and para-phenylenediamine derivatives the major allergens. Rubber compounds in athletic shoes pose risks to individuals with contact sensitivity, particularly with thiourea, mercaptobenzothiazole and thiuram antioxidants. The resulting erythema, desquamation, vesiculation, fissuring, pain and pruritus of the feet can prove quite disabling for the athlete, particularly when alternative footwear without rubber (e.g. soccer cleats, baseball cleats) is not readily available. Adhesives in tape, benzoin, topical antiseptics and antibiotics, dyes and leather tanning agents also may be problematic in athletes[86,90].

Acne mechanica occurs commonly in athletes in whom occlusive uniforms or protective gear create the right microenvironment. Football players flare during the August pre-season practice with follicular papules, pustules and nodules on the forehead, preauricular areas, chin and shoulders, corresponding to forehead and ear pads of the helmet, chin strap and shoulder pads, respectively. Acne keloidalis of the lower occiput may be aggravated by the helmet as well. Other sports in which protective headgear may create acne mechanica include hockey, lacrosse and wrestling. Occlusive synthetic clothing of dancers and gymnasts, plastic benches of weight lifters, the golf bag shoulder strap, and the cradling of the shot against the neck in shot putters may also produce acne mechanica[86].

Heat, moisture, friction and contact with other athletes or various surfaces increase the risk of some infectious conditions (Table 87.15). Several common monikers attest to the frequent association, such as 'jock itch', 'herpes gladiatorum', 'athlete's foot' and 'swimmer's ear'. A recent report dealt with the risk of staphylococcal infections in football players within a professional team and noted that weight and turf injuries were risk factors and, therefore, linemen were more prone to developing this infection. However, epidemiologic study of the practices of the trainers and the use of whirlpool equipment demonstrated risks associated with poor hygienic practices[93,94].

The final issue of sports-related skin disease is aggravation of pre-existing conditions. Psoriasis, vitiligo and lichen planus may exhibit a Koebner phenomenon, flaring in areas of skin injury such as abrasions. Epidermolysis bullosa simplex of the Weber–Cockayne type is worsened by friction on the feet and hands, particularly in warm summer months (see Ch. 33). Photosensitive dermatoses may be exacerbated by outdoor sun exposure (see Ch. 86). Both cholinergic and exercise-induced urticaria may worsen with heavy physical exertion[87] (see Ch. 19). The American Academy of Pediatrics has created a useful guide on medical conditions affecting sports participation[95].

Pathology

Many of the friction-induced conditions discussed here have histologic features similar to callosities (see above). Surfer's nodules show hyper-keratosis and mild acanthosis of the epidermis with increased numbers of normal-appearing collagen bundles. The overall histologic appearance is similar to that of a collagenoma[96]. The infectious processes are covered in detail in their respective chapters, as are the existing dermatoses aggravated by sports participation.

Treatment

Therapy for the non-infectious conditions discussed in this section is based primarily upon anecdotal reports and small series, and is summarized in Table 87.14. Frictional lichenoid dermatitis responds to friction avoidance, the use of clothing to protect extensor surfaces, and moderate-potency topical corticosteroids[86–88]. Education and changes in practice behavior might aid in the prevention of infections in athletes.

MUSICAL INSTRUMENT-RELATED DERMATOSES

Synonyms: ■ Cellist's chest or knee ■ Clarinetist's cheilitis ■ Drummer's digit ■ Fiddler's neck ■ Flautist's chin ■ Garrod's pads ■ Guitar nipple ■ Harpist's fingers

Key features

- Cutaneous disorders in musicians include frictional injury, irritant and allergic contact dermatitis, hyperhidrosis, acne mechanica and vascular compromise
- Dermatoses tend to be recurrent unless the posture, use or contact can be avoided
- Identification of the mechanism of injury is critical for successful therapy

Introduction

Musicians have unique cutaneous reactions related to countless hours of practice and performance required to master their art. Skin and associated soft tissue and musculoskeletal changes are therefore not uncommon. The major categories of injury in musicians are contact dermatitis, repetitive motion injury and dysautonomia.

History

One of the first reports of an occupational dermatosis is reputed to be the recognition of fiddler's neck in 1713. About the same time, Italian physician Bernadino Ramazzini noted the peculiar distension and soft tissue laxity of the cheeks in horn players, and summarized the occupational problems of musicians[97].

Epidemiology

The injuries discussed below all require considerable devotion of time to practice and performance of the chosen instruments. Some of these conditions are considered marks of virtuosity, such as cellist's thumb. The impact of these conditions is greatest on professional musicians, although amateurs, and even beginners, may be afflicted[98].

Pathogenesis and clinical features

The clinical features and pathogenesis of dermatoses caused by musical instruments are summarized in Table 87.16.

Another common dermatosis that may occur in musicians is 'lip licker's' dermatitis, characterized by erythema, fissuring and scaling in wind instrument players. Intraoral hyperkeratosis of the lip or shallow erosions may develop in patients with dental irregularities or orthodontic appliances. Salivary abnormalities may interfere with performance with wind instruments. Xerostomia is devastating to the wind player (especially brass), while increased salivation is problematic for the recorder player. Sialolithiasis has been seen in association with fiddler's neck.

Sharing of mouthpieces may increase the risk of transmission of infections such as herpes simplex virus, Epstein-Barr virus, cytomegalovirus, and hepatitis A and B. Latent herpes simplex may be reactivated by the frictional trauma of wind instruments, with brass players

CUTANEOUS INFECTIONS IN ATHLETES

Condition	Common name	Clinical features	Organisms	Typical sport
Impetigo		Small vesicles to large bullae on glistening erythematous bases; honey-colored crusts	*Staphylococcus aureus*, β-hemolytic streptococci	Wrestling, European football (soccer), American football, swimming, gymnastics
Folliculitis		Erythematous follicular papules and pustules	*S. aureus*	Most sports
Hot tub folliculitis		Markedly erythematous, edematous follicular papulopustules, few in number, often involving axillae, breasts, pubic area and buttocks	*Pseudomonas aeruginosa*	Swimming; use of whirlpool, hot tub or Jacuzzi
Pseudomonas hot-foot syndrome		Tender nodules on soles	*P. aeruginosa*	Use of wading pool
Furuncles	Boils	Tender warm red nodules or abscesses on trunk or extremities	*S. aureus* (including MRSA)	Basketball, football, swimming
Erythrasma		Reddish-brown dry patches in axillae, groin or toe webs	*Corynebacterium minutissimum*	Most sports, especially with occlusive clothing
Pitted keratolysis	Toxic sock syndrome	Malodorous feet with plantar 1 to 3 mm punched-out erosions extending only through the stratum corneum of overhydrated skin	*Corynebacterium* spp., *Micrococcus (Kytococcus) sedentarius*	Running, tennis, basketball
Otitis externa	Swimmer's ear	Pruritus may be followed by pain, discharge, tenderness of the pinna, sensation of fullness and reduced hearing	*P. aeruginosa* most common; also streptococci, diphtheroids and staphylococci	Swimming, diving (atopics at risk)
Swimming pool granuloma		Firm acral red papules	*Mycobacterium marinum*	Swimming
Verruca vulgaris	Warts	Verrucous, keratotic papules and plaques	Human papillomavirus	Any that use locker-room showers or public pools
Herpes simplex viral infection	Herpes gladiatorum	Clustered vesicles on erythematous bases at point of skin-to-skin contact	Herpes simplex virus	Wrestling
Molluscum contagiosum		Shiny, umbilicated 2 to 3 mm papules at the skin contact site	Parapoxvirus	Wrestling, swimming
Tinea pedis	Athlete's foot	Maceration, scaling, pruritus in toe webs; or diffuse plantar erythema and scale	*Trichophyton rubrum*, *T. mentagrophytes*, *Epidermophyton floccosum*	Any sport
Tinea cruris	Jock itch	Annular to polycyclic erythema with scaly, active borders, perifollicular papules or pustules	Same as tinea pedis	Any sport
Tinea corporis	Tinea gladiatorum	Except for location, the same as tinea cruris	*Trichophyton* spp.	Wrestling
Seabather's eruption	Sea lice	Pruritic papules on areas covered by bathing suit	*Edwardsiella lineata*, *Linuche unguiculata*	Salt water swimming
Swimmer's itch	Cercarial dermatitis	Pruritic erythematous papules on exposed skin	Duck schistosome cercaria	Fresh water pond and lake swimming and wading

Table 87.15 Cutaneous infections in athletes[83,84,86,87,91,92].

DERMATOSES CAUSED BY MUSICAL INSTRUMENTS

Condition (synonym)	Clinical features	Pathogenesis	Associated instruments
Acne mechanica (fiddler's neck, clarinetist's cheilitis, flautist's chin)	Follicular papules and pustules, lichenification, hyperpigmentation	Repetitive friction and pressure, coupled with occlusion and moisture (sweat, saliva)	Violin, viola, clarinet, saxophone, flute
Cellist's chest	Sternal skin tenderness, erythema, edema, hyperpigmentation	Pressure and friction	Cello
Cellist's knee	Erythema, scale, callus and hyperpigmentation of left medial knee	Friction callus	Cello
Finger calluses	Hyperkeratotic callosities on fingertip pads	Repetitive friction	All strings
Drummer's digit	Vesicle or erosion on the radial aspect of the left ring finger distal and middle phalanx, followed by callus formation	Friction from holding left drumstick in classical position	Drums
Garrod's pads (violinist's pads)	Calluses on dorsal aspect of proximal interphalangeal joints of left index and middle fingers	Repeated extension and flexion of extensor tendon over tightly flexed joint	Violin, viola
Guitar nipple	Unilateral mastitis with erythema, edema, pain	Pressure and friction of guitar sound box pressed against chest	Guitar
Paronychia, onycholysis, subungual hemorrhage		Repeated trauma to nail apparatus	Piano, strings (especially playing pizzicato), harp, guitar

Table 87.16 Dermatoses caused by musical instruments[97,99,100].

tending to have upper lip lesions and woodwind players having lower lip lesions[101].

Hyperhidrosis of the palms may lead to corrosion of metal instruments or the inability to maintain proper contact with instrument keys or strings[99,102].

Allergic contact dermatitis associated with musical instruments is summarized in Table 87.17.

Pathology

Diagnosis of most of these conditions does not require histologic evaluation. However, fiddler's neck has been shown to exhibit epidermal hyperplasia with elongation of the rete ridges, follicular plugging, folliculitis and perifolliculitis, and epidermoid cyst formation[99].

Differential diagnosis

Fiddler's neck needs to be distinguished from localized cervical lymphadenitis, an inflamed epidermoid cyst, draining dental abscess, and acne mechanica from other causes (e.g. telephone, headset). Clinical history should suffice, along with the characteristic location and clinical features. For example, a dental abscess with fistula formation often leaves the area indented and bound to underlying structures.

Treatment

Discontinuation of the instrument is curative in almost all cases, but usually quite impractical. Professional musicians, in particular, need other options. Frictional injuries may be addressed with padding, or change in position of the instrument. Fiddler's neck, for example, seems less common if the dropping neck position is avoided. Anecdotal remedies for the treatment of fiddler's neck include astringents, benzoyl peroxide, keratolytics, tretinoin, topical erythromycin and application of French brandy.

ALLERGIC CONTACT DERMATITIS ASSOCIATED WITH MUSICAL INSTRUMENTS		
Sensitizer/contactant	**Skin distribution**	**Instrument**
Rosin/colophony (abietic acid)	Hands, face, neck	Violin, viola, cello, double bass
Rosewood	Lips, chin, cheek	Strings, reeds
Makassar ebony	Chin	Violin
Cocobolo wood	Lips	Recorder
African blackwood	Lips	Recorder, oboe
Nickel	Chin Fingers, hands Lips, chin	Violin Cello, sitar Flute, brass
Reed (perhaps only irritant)	Lips	Saxophone, clarinet
Propolis (bee glue)	Hands	Violin
Chromium	Hands	Harp, violin
Paraphenylenediamine	Chin	Violin, viola

Table 87.17 Allergic contact dermatitis associated with musical instruments[97,99,100,103].

Treatment of excess salivation with a transdermal scopolamine patch has been reported. Remedies for hyperhidrosis include topical aluminum-based drying agents, iontophoresis, β-adrenergic blocking agents (especially if the hyperhidrosis is due to 'stage fright'), calcium channel blockers and ganglionectomy (see Ch. 40). Anticholinergic therapy is not useful for many musicians because of the frequent side effects of dry mouth and blurred vision[97,99,100]. If allergic contact dermatitis is suspected, patch testing can be performed (see Ch. 15).

REFERENCES

1. Lugo-Amador NM, Rothenhaus T, Moyer P. Heat-related illness. Emerg Med Clin North Am. 2004;22:315–27.
2. AAP Committee on Sports and Fitness. Climatic heat stress and the exercising child and adolescent. Pediatrics. 2000;106:158–9.
3. Ramzy PI, Barret JP, Herndon DN. Thermal injury. Crit Care Clin. 1999;15:333–52.
4. Passaretti D, Billmire DA. Management of pediatric burns. J Craniofac Surg. 2003;14:713–18.
5. Fogarty BJ, Gordon DJ. Firework related injury and legislation: the epidemiology of firework injuries and the effect of legislation in Northern Ireland. Burns. 1999;25:53–6.
6. Weedon D. Skin Pathology. Edinburgh: Churchill Livingstone, 1997:504–6.
7. Bishop JF. Burn wound assessment and surgical management. Crit Care Nurs Clin North Am. 2004;16:145–77.
8. Baxter CR. Management of burn wounds. Dermatol Clin. 1993;11:709–14.
9. Tan S, Bertucci V. Erythema ab igne: an old condition new again. CMAJ. 2000;162:77–8.
10. Bilic M, Adams BB. Erythema ab igne induced by a laptop computer. J Am Acad Dermatol. 2004;50:973–4.
11. Donohue KG, Nahm WK, Badiavas E, Li L, Pedvis-Leftick A. Hot pop brown spot: erythema ab igne induced by heated popcorn. J Dermatol. 2002;29:172–3.
12. Cavallari V, Cicciarello R, Torre V, et al. Chronic heat-induced skin lesions (erythema ab igne): ultrastructural studies. Ultrastruct Pathol. 2001;25:93–7.
13. Karoo ROS, Whitaker IS, Garrido A, Sharpe DT. Full-thickness burns following magnetic resonance imaging: a discussion of the dangers and safety suggestions. Plast Reconstr Surg. 2004;114:1344–5.
14. Muensterer OJ. Temporary removal of navel piercing jewelry for surgery and imaging studies. Pediatrics. 2004;114:e384–6.
15. Karch AM. Don't get burnt by the MRI: transdermal patches can be a hazard to patients. Am J Nurs. 2004;104:31.

16. Koenig TR, Mettler FA, Wagner LK. Skin injuries from fluoroscopically guided procedures. II. Review of 73 cases and recommendations for minimizing dose delivered to the patient. AJR Am J Roentgenol. 2001;177:13–20.
17. Koenig TR, Wolff D, Mettler FA, Wagner LK. Skin injuries from fluoroscopically guided procedures. I. Characteristics of radiation injury. AJR Am J Roentgenol. 2001;177:3–11.
18. Miller DL, Balter S, Noonan PT, Georgia JD. Minimizing radiation-induced skin injury in interventional radiology procedures. Radiology. 2002;225:329–36.
19. Dempsey MF, Condon B. Thermal injuries associated with MRI. Clin Radiol. 2001;56:457–65.
20. Corazza M, Trincone S, Virgili A. Effects of airbag deployment: lesions, epidemiology and management. Am J Clin Dermatol. 2004;5:295–300.
21. Ulrich D, Noah E-M, Fuchs P, Pallua N. Burn injuries caused by air bag deployment. Burns. 2001;27:196–9.
22. Masaki F. A new category of contact burn resulting from air bag infusion. Burns. 2005;31:118–19.
23. Hamlet MP. An overview of medically related problems in the cold environment. Mil Med. 1987;152:393–6.
24. Meffert JJ. Environmental skin diseases and the impact of common dermatoses on medical readiness. Dermatol Clin. 1999;17:1–17.
25. Cattermole TJ. The epidemiology of cold injury in Antarctica. Aviat Space Environ Med. 1999;70:135–40.
26. Murphy JV, Banwell PE, Roberts AHN, McGrouther DA. Frostbite: pathogenesis and treatment. J Trauma. 2000;48:171–8.
27. Long WB, Edlich RF, Winters KL, Britt LD. Cold injuries. J Long Term Eff Med Implants. 2005;15:67–78.
28. Simon TD, Soep JB, Hollister JR. Pernio in pediatrics. Pediatrics. 2005;116:e472–5.
29. Piffard HG. A Treatise on the Materia Medica and Therapeutics of the Skin. New York: William Wood and Co., 1881:236.
30. Parlette EC, Parlette HL. Erythrocyanotic discoloration of the toes. Cutis. 2000;65:223–6.
31. Cribier B, Djeridi N, Peltre B, Grosshans E. A histologic and immunohistochemical study of chilblains. J Am Acad Dermatol. 2001;45:924–9.

32. Weston WL, Morelli JG. Childhood pernio and cryoproteins. Pediatr Dermatol. 2000;17:97–9.
33. Wanderer AA, Grandel KE, Wasserman SI, Farr RS. Clinical characteristics of cold-induced systemic reactions in acquired cold urticaria syndromes: recommendations for prevention of this complication and a proposal for a diagnostic classification of cold urticaria. J Allergy Clin Immunol. 1986;78:417–23.
34. Wigley FM, Flavahan NA. Raynaud's phenomenon. Rheum Dis Clin North Am. 1996;22:765–81.
35. Yazawa H, Saga K, Omori F, Jimbow K, Sasagawa Y. The chilblain-like eruption as a diagnostic clue to the blast crisis of chronic myelocytic leukemia. J Am Acad Dermatol. 2004;50(suppl. 1):42–4.
36. Rustin MH, Newton JA, Smith NP, Dowd PM. The treatment of chilblains with nifedipine: the results of a pilot study, a double-blind placebo-controlled randomized study and a long-term open trial. Br J Dermatol. 1989;120:267–75.
37. Wrenn K. Immersion foot. A problem of the homeless in the 1990s. Arch Intern Med. 1991; 151:785–8.
38. Zafren K. Clinical images: immersion injury. Wilderness Environ Med. 2000;11:269–71.
39. Oumeish OY, Parish LC. Marching in the army: common cutaneous disorders of the feet. Clin Dermatol. 2002;20:445–51.
40. Moore JK. Do jungle boots stop jungle rot? Wilderness Environ Med. 2004;15:230–3.
41. Humphrey W, Ellyson R. Warm water immersion foot: still a threat to the soldier. Mil Med. 1997;162:610–11.
42. Arnoldo BD, Purdue GF, Kowalske K, Helm PA, Burris A, Hunt JL. Electrical injuries: a 20-year review. J Burn Care Rehabil. 2004;25:479–84.
43. Edlich RF, Farinholt H-MA, Winters KL, Britt LD, Long WB. Modern concepts of treatment and prevention of lightning injuries. J Long Term Eff Med Implants. 2005;15:185–96.
44. Lee RC. Injury by electrical forces: pathophysiology, manifestations, and therapy. Curr Probl Surg. 1997;34:684–764.
45. Koumbourlis AC. Electrical injuries. Crit Care Med. 2002;30:S424–30.

46. Jain S, Bandi V. Electrical and lightning injuries. Crit Care Clin. 1999;15:319–31.

47. Sticherling M, Christophers E. Why hair turns green. Acta Derm Venereol (Stockh). 1993;73:321–2.

48. Nanko H, Mutoh Y, Atsumi R, et al. Hair-discoloration of Japanese elite swimmers. J Dermatol. 2000;27:625–34.

49. Fitzgerald EA, Purcell SM, Goldman HM. Green hair discoloration due to selenium sulfide. Int J Dermatol. 1997;36:238–9.

50. Rebora A, Guarrera M. Hair discoloration caused by minoxidil lotion. J Am Acad Dermatol. 1989;21:1314.

51. Rogers MJ, Whitefield M, Marks VJ. Yellow hair discoloration due to anthralin J Am Acad Dermatol. 1988;19:370–1.

52. Schwartz RA. Arsenic and the skin. Int J Dermatol. 1997;36:241–50.

53. Ratnaike RN. Acute and chronic arsenic toxicity. Postgrad Med J. 2003;79:391–6.

54. Tchounwou PB, Centeno JA, Patlolla AK. Arsenic toxicity, mutagenesis, and carcinogenesis – a health risk assessment and management approach. Mol Cell Biochem. 2004;255:47–55.

55. NIOSH Pocket Guide to Chemical Hazards. U.S. Department of Health and Human Services. Cincinnati: NIOSH Publications, 1997.

56. Russell MA, Langley M, Truett AP, et al. Lichenoid dermatitis after consumption of gold-containing liquor. J Am Acad Dermatol. 1997;36:841–4.

57. Boyd AS, Seger D, Vannucci S, et al. Mercury exposure and cutaneous disease. J Am Acad Dermatol. 2000;43:81–90.

58. Järup L. Hazards of heavy metal contamination. Br Med Bull. 2003;68:167–82.

59. Moreno-Ramirez D, Garcia-Bravo B, Pichardo AR, Rubio FP, Martinez FC. Baboon syndrome in childhood: easy to avoid, easy to diagnose, but the problem continues. Pediatr Dermatol. 2004;21:250–3.

60. Misra UK, Kalita J, Yadav RK, Ranjan P. Thallium poisoning: emphasis on early diagnosis and response to hemodialysis. Postgrad Med J. 2003;79:103–5.

61. Greenberg JE, Lynn M, Kirsner RS, Elgart GW, Hanly AJ. Mucocutaneous pigmented macule as a result of zinc deposition. J Cutan Pathol. 2002;29:613–15.

62. Schwartz, RA. Premalignant keratinocytic neoplasms. J Am Acad Dermatol. 1996;35:223–42.

63. Hall AH. Chronic arsenic poisoning. Toxicol Lett. 2002;128:69–72.

64. Freeman DB. Corns and calluses resulting from mechanical hyperkeratosis. Am Fam Physician. 2002;65:2277–80.

65. Adams B, Lucky A. A center's callosities. Cutis. 2001;67:141–2.

66. Crissey JT, Peachey JC. Calcaneal petechiae. Arch Dermatol. 1961;83:501.

67. Garcia-Doval I, de la Torre C, Losada A, Cruces MJ. Disseminated punctate intraepidermal haemorrhage: a widespread counterpart of black heel. Acta Derm Venereol. 1999;79:403.

68. Rashkovsky I, Safadi R, Zlotogorski A. Black palmar macules. Arch Dermatol. 1998;134:120–4.

69. Wilkinson DS. Black heel. A minor hazard of sport. Cutis. 1997;20:393–6.

70. Hafner J, Haenseler E, Ossent P, et al. Benzidine stain for the histochemical detection of hemoglobin in splinter hemorrhage (subungual hematoma) and black heel. Am J Dermatopathol. 1995;17:362–7.

71. Rogers NE, Farris PK, Wang AR. Juvenile chondrodermatitis nodularis helices: a case report and literature review. Pediatr Dermatol. 2003;20:488–90.

72. Oelzner S, Elsner P. Bilateral chondrodermatitis nodularis chronica helicis on the free border of the helix in a woman. J Am Acad Dermatol. 2003;49:720–2.

73. Moncrieff M, Sassoon EM. Effective treatment of chondrodermatitis nodularis chronica helicis using a conservative approach. Br J Dermatol. 2004;150:892–4.

74. Epstein E. Granuloma fissuratum of the ears. Arch Dermatol. 1965;91:621–2.

75. Benedetto AV, Bergfeld WF. Acanthoma fissuratum: histopathology and review of the literature. Cutis. 1979;24:225–9.

76. Cerroni L, Soyer HP, Chimenti S. Acanthoma fissuratum. J Dermatol Surg Oncol. 1988;14:1003–5.

77. Thomas MR, Sadiq HA, Raweily EAA. Acanthoma fissuratum. J Laryngol Otol. 1991;105:301–3.

78. Kavanagh GM, Bradfield JWB, Collins CMP, Kennedy CTC. Weathering nodules of the ear: a clinicopathological study. Br J Dermatol. 1996;135:550–4.

79. Requena L, Aguilar A, Sanchez Yus E. Elastic nodules of the ears. Cutis. 1989;44:452–4.

80. Giffin CS. Wrestler's ear: pathophysiology and treatment. Ann Plast Surg. 1992;28:131–9.

81. Henderson JM, Salama AR, Blanchaert RH. Management of auricular hematoma using a thermoplastic splint. Arch Otolaryngol Head Neck Surg. 2000;126:888–90.

82. Jones SE, Mahendran S. Interventions for acute auricular hematoma. Cochrane Database Syst Rev. 2004;(2):CD004166.

83. Becker TM. Herpes gladiatorum: a growing problem in sports medicine. Cutis. 1992;50:150–2.

84. Sevier TL. Infectious disease in athletes. Med Clin North Am. 1994;78:389–412.

85. Adams BB. Tinea corporis gladiatorum. J Am Acad Dermatol. 2002;47:286–90.

86. Metelitsa A, Barankin B, Lin AN. Diagnosis of sports-related dermatoses. Int J Dermatol. 2004;43:113–19.

87. Conklin RJ. Common cutaneous disorders in athletes. Sports Med. 1990;9:100–19.

88. Fisher AA. Sports-related cutaneous reactions: part I. Dermatoses due to physical agents. Cutis. 1999;63:134–6.

89. Biolcati G, Berlutti G, Bagarone A, Caselli G. Dermatological marks in athletes of artistic and rhythmic gymnastics.. Int J Sports Med. 2004; 25:638–40.

90. Fisher AA. Sports-related cutaneous reactions: part II. Allergic contact dermatitis to sports equipment. Cutis. 1999;63:202–4.

91. Nichols AW. Nonorthopaedic problems in the aquatic athlete. Clin Sport Med. 1999;18:395–411.

92. Nguyen DM, Mascola L, Bancroft E. Recurring methicillin-resistant staphylococcus aureus infections in a football team. Emerg Infect Dis. 2005;11:526–32.

93. Kazakova SV, Hageman JC, Matava M, et al. A clone of methicillin-resistant Staphylococcus aureus among professional football players. N Engl J Med. 2005;352:468–75.

94. Rihn JA, Posfay-Barbe K, Harner CD, et al. Community-acquired methicillin-resistant Staphylococcus aureus outbreak in a local high school football team unsuccessful interventions. Pediatr Infect Dis J. 2005;24:841–3.

95. American Academy of Pediatrics, Committee on Sports Medicine and Fitness. Medical conditions affecting sports participation. Pediatrics. 2001;107:1205–9.

96. Cohen PR, Eliezri YD, Silvers DN. Athlete's nodules: sports-related connective tissue nevi of the collagen type (collagenomas). Cutis. 1992;50:131–5.

97. Liu L, Hayden GF. Maladies in musicians. South Med J. 2002;95:727–34.

98. Fisher AA. Dermatitis in a musician. Part II: injuries to skin, soft tissue, and bone from musical instruments. Cutis. 1998;62:214–15.

99. Rimmer S, Spielvogel RL. Dermatologic problems of musicians. J Am Acad Dermatol. 1990;22:657–63.

100. Fisher AA. Dermatitis in a musician. Part I: allergic contact dermatitis. Cutis. 1998;62:167–8.

101. Fisher AA. Dermatitis in a musician. Part IV: physiologic, emotional, and infectious problems in musicians. Cutis. 1999;63:13–14.

102. Hoppman RA, Burke WA, Patrone NA. Hyperhidrosis in the performing artist. Med Probl Perform Art. 1988;3:60–2.

103. Lombardi C, Bottello M, Caruso A, Gargioni S, Passalacqua G. Allergy and skin diseases in musicians. Allerg Immunol (Paris). 2003;35:52–5.

Signs of Drug Abuse

Miguel Sanchez

88

INTRODUCTION

According to the Diagnostic and Statistical Manual of Mental Disorders, drug abuse is a non-conforming pattern of drug practice in a manner that deviates from medically recommended or socially accepted standards. Repeated drug abuse can progress to drug addiction, the result of drug-induced CNS changes that effect maladaptive alterations in spontaneous behavior and in the behavioral response to subsequent exposures to the drug. Drug addiction is associated with physical dependence, which denotes a syndrome with cognitive, behavioral and physiologic symptoms manifested by compulsive drug use, tolerance, and withdrawal symptoms upon discontinuation of a drug (Table 88.1).

A worldwide problem, drug abuse is directly responsible for minor to life-threatening and fatal illnesses and injuries, as well as adverse sociologic consequences (loss of occupational productivity and higher rates of poverty, crime, prison occupancy, domestic violence, child abuse or neglect) which increase the risk of infirmity and disability. According to the Office of National Drug Control Policy, the overall economic cost of drug abuse to American society during 2002 was estimated to be $180.8 billion, a 5.9% annual rate increase since 1992.

Illicit drug use may be suspected or diagnosed on the basis of cutaneous findings. In fact, the skin is the tissue most evidently affected by intravenous drug addiction[1]. The wide spectrum of complications result from local or systemic effects (including toxic or allergic) of the drug itself, adulterants or infectious agents. Polydrug use, especially involving the consumption of alcohol and drugs, is common among drug addicts[1].

Amphetamines

Amphetamines were initially sold as a non-prescription appetite suppressant and rapidly became a favorite street drug ('pep pills', 'Bennies'). Crystallized methamphetamine ('ice', 'crystal', 'glass', 'tina'), an addictive stimulant with a high potential for abuse and dependence, produces an even stronger 'rush' or 'flash' when injected intravenously or inhaled. Oral ingestion of tablets ('speed', 'meth', 'chalk') or snorting powder merely produces a profound sense of euphoria. Smoking the base form ('snot') extends the duration of the 'high' for up to 24 hours. Speed freaks (high-intensity abusers) progressively use the drug to remain euphoric and experience extreme weight loss, pale facial skin, sweating, body odor, discolored teeth, and scars or open sores on their bodies. 'Tweaking', continuous drug use without sleep for 3 to 15 days, is often associated with irritability, paranoia, violence, and frustration due to inability to recreate the euphoric high. Methylenedioxymethamphetamine (MDMA), also known as 'ecstasy', 'Adam', 'XTC', 'hug', 'beans', or 'love drug', is a synthetic stimulant and hallucinogen with a chemical structure similar to methamphetamine. It is a neurotoxin and even a few doses can cause permanent brain damage. High doses can cause malignant hyperthermia, leading to rhabdomyolysis, renal failure and cardiovascular collapse. A staple at raves and PNP ("party and play") parties where the emphasis is on sex and drugs, because they increase energy and reduce sexual inhibition, crystallized methamphetamine and MDMA have been associated with unprotected, promiscuous sexual activity and specially high risk of contracting sexually transmitted diseases.

Benzodiazepines

Benzodiazepines (including the long-acting diazepam) are among the most frequently prescribed medications in the US, as they are in the UK, where surveys indicate that approximately 10% of the population take benzodiazepine sedatives regularly. Although they are only mild euphoriants, benzodiazepines are commonly misused by polydrug addicts, alcoholics and recreational drug users. Benzodiazepines are ingested (often with alcohol), snorted or, occasionally, injected. Injectable temazepam is especially popular among opiate addicts as it enhances the euphoric effects of heroin. Although not approved in the US, flunitrazepam is very popular in many countries. In surveys, flunitrazepam is often preferred by opiate addicts over other benzodiazepines. Approximately ten times more potent than diazepam, the drug has been used to facilitate rape, as it produces social disinhibition, impaired motor skills, and blackout with memory loss, particularly when mixed with alcoholic beverages.

Cannabis

Cannabis ('marijuana', 'pot', 'herb', 'weed', 'ganja', 'Mary Jane') is the most frequently self-administered illicit drug. It is a mixture of dried shredded leaves and flowers of the *Cannabis sativa* plant, which contains the chemical delta-9-tetrahydrocannabinol (THC) and is usually smoked as a cigarette or through a pipe or bong. Marijuana cigarettes may be laced with other drugs, such as crack or heroin.

Cocaine

Cocaine ('coke', 'blow', 'toot', 'flake', 'snow') is an alkaloid stimulant and topical anesthetic which is extracted from the leaves of the *Erythroxylon coca* shrub. The $35 billion (per annum) cocaine industry has replaced coffee as Colombia's main export.

Crack ('base', 'rock', 'hubba', 'gravel'), a freebase form of cocaine, is more addictive than heroin. It is produced by dissolving cocaine in water and baking soda and then heating the mixture until it crystallizes. Cocaine is injected or snorted, while crack is smoked.

Gamma-hydroxybutyrate

Gamma-hydroxybutyrate (GHB), a 'party drug', is a rapid-acting CNS depressant popular among revelers for its relaxant, euphoric and purported aphrodisiac properties. GHB can mentally and physically paralyze a person as well as induce memory loss, and it is more often used than flunitrazepam as a 'rape drug'. Because it reportedly promotes muscle mass, it is commonly misused by bodybuilders.

Lysergic Acid Diethylamide

Lysergic acid diethylamide ('LSD', 'acid'), a popular hallucinogen, is manufactured from the lysergic acid found in ergot, a fungus that grows on rye and other grains. It is often sold in single-dose (20 to 80 μg) squares of blotter paper.

Opiates

Also known as diacetylmorphine, heroin ('junk', 'smack', 'horse', 'scag'), the fastest acting and strongest of all opiates, is three times

---

FEATURES OF DRUG DEPENDENCE

- Recurrent and excessive drug use which may result in tolerance and withdrawal
- Recurrent social, occupational, psychological or physical problems as a result of excessive drug use
- Failed attempts to control substance use

Table 88.1 **Features of drug dependence.**

more potent than morphine and still accounts for much of the illicit opiate abuse in the US. Because of its increased lipid solubility, it crosses the blood–brain barrier more rapidly, prompting a 'rush' within 7 to 8 seconds after intravenous injection or 10–15 minutes after being snorted or smoked. There has been a growing tendency to sniff, snort ('shabbang') or smoke ('chase the dragon') heroin rather than inject it intravenously ('shoot up') or subcutaneously ('skin pop'). Opiate addicts may alternate injections of heroin and cocaine (crisscrossing) or inject highly addictive 'speedballs' of the two drugs together. Methadone, an oral synthetic opioid with a half-life between 24 and 48 hours, is widely used as a substitute for heroin in narcotic treatment programs and for chronic pain. Opiates remain the leading cause of fatal overdoses, with methadone, which is increasingly being obtained through the Internet, becoming the single biggest killer. Fentanyl, a narcotic analgesic that is 50 to 100 times more potent than morphine, is particularly prone to overdosing. Buprenorphine, a more potent and longer-lasting analgesic than morphine, appears to act as a partial agonist of μ and κ opioid receptors, but tolerance with chronic use may not develop, presumably due to the lack of δ-agonist activity. Pentazocine is an orally administered benzomorphan opiate antagonist with a lower risk of drug dependence than opiates, but ingestion of pentazocine may precipitate withdrawal symptoms in persons physically dependent on opiates. However, when injected in combination with the antihistamine tripelennamine, the euphoric effects are similar to those produced by heroin.

Anabolic Steroids

Anabolic steroids promote the growth of skeletal muscle and the development of male sexual characteristics. They are ingested (oxandrolone, oxymetholone, stanozolol) or injected (nandrolone, testosterone, boldenone) intramuscularly by bodybuilders to increase muscle mass and by athletes to boost physical performance. Physical dependence can develop after habitual use. Higher risks for cardiovascular disease, hepatic disease, and infectious diseases (due to needle sharing) are among the long-term complications of anabolic steroid misuse.

PATHOPHYSIOLOGY OF ADDICTION

Administration of addictive drugs directly or indirectly produces high extracellular concentrations of dopamine in the nucleus accumbens and other regions of the mesolimbic system associated with modulating reward and pleasure responses. However, additional factors, such as dopamine-modulated changes in the frontal cortex and anterior cingulate areas, appear to be involved in incentive salience, craving, and compulsive use that determine the risk of becoming addicted to a drug. MRI studies have documented progressive losses of frontal lobe volume in cocaine-dependent as well as in heroin-dependent addicts. It is postulated that reductions in prefrontal processes promote unrestricted behaviors and stress-like reactions in which inhibitory performances are abated and stimulus-driven behaviors are intensified. Persons who are predisposed to compulsive behavior are at higher risk of chronic, repetitive and uncontrolled use of drugs.

Narcotics produce intense feelings of wellbeing and euphoria by stimulating μ and δ receptors. Amphetamines and cocaine bind to and block the transporters responsible for the reuptake of dopamine and noradrenaline into the presynaptic neurons, producing high levels of dopamine in the synapses. Amphetamines and cocaine suppress the prefrontal cortex inhibition of the amygdala, a structure that appears to potentiate the addictive responses to these drugs.

Eventually, chronic amphetamine abuse leads to dopamine depletion in the orbitofrontal cortex, the dorsolateral prefrontal cortex, and the amygdala. Barbiturates increase the resting potential of neurons and their propensity to fire by binding to a subset of GABA receptors that enhance the flow of chloride ions into postsynaptic neurons.

EPIDEMIOLOGY

Throughout the world, about 200 million people in 134 countries and territories (5% of the global population) use illicit drugs and approximately 13 million of them inject drugs[2]. As many as 78% of drug users live in developing nations. In 2004, the United Nations Office of Drugs

and Crime estimates that 29 million people misused amphetamines, 14 million cocaine and 13.5 million opiates[2]. Based on 2005 data from the US National Institute on Drug Abuse, the annual prevalence of illicit drug use has fallen by 10% among 12th-graders since the peak year in 1997, but the use of illicit drugs among young people in the US continues to be alarming (Table 88.2).

According to the US Drug Abuse Warning Network, of an estimated 106 million Emergency Department visits in 2004, about 941 000 were associated with use of illicit drugs (cocaine: 41%; marijuana: 23%; heroin: 17%; amphetamines: 11%). In 2000, approximately 10.6 million persons in the US used marijuana, 8.26 million using it as their only illicit drug. Estimates of numbers of individuals currently dependent on or abusing illicit drugs in the US are shown in Figure 88.1. The National Institute of Drug Abuse has estimated that at least 980 000 people in the US are currently addicted to opiates and that 5000–10 000 persons die as a result of intravenous drug overdose every year.

CLINICAL FEATURES

Scars

Intravenous drug users have a number of recognizable stigmata, which identify their habit to anyone with experience in illicit drug use[3]. The most prominent of these are 'skin tracks', which represent scarring and

SELF-REPORTED ALCOHOL AND ILLICIT DRUG USE AMONG HIGH SCHOOL SENIORS IN THE US	
Drug	Use within the past year (%)
Alcohol	66
Marijuana	32
Sedatives/tranquilizers	13
Stimulants	8
Opioids (other than heroin)	9
Hallucinogens	5
Cocaine	6
Inhalants	4
Anabolic steroids	2
Heroin	1

Table 88.2 Self-reported alcohol and illicit drug use among high school seniors in the US (2006). From the US Department of Justice, Bureau of Justice Statistics (www.ojp.usdoj.gov/bjs/dcf/du.htm).

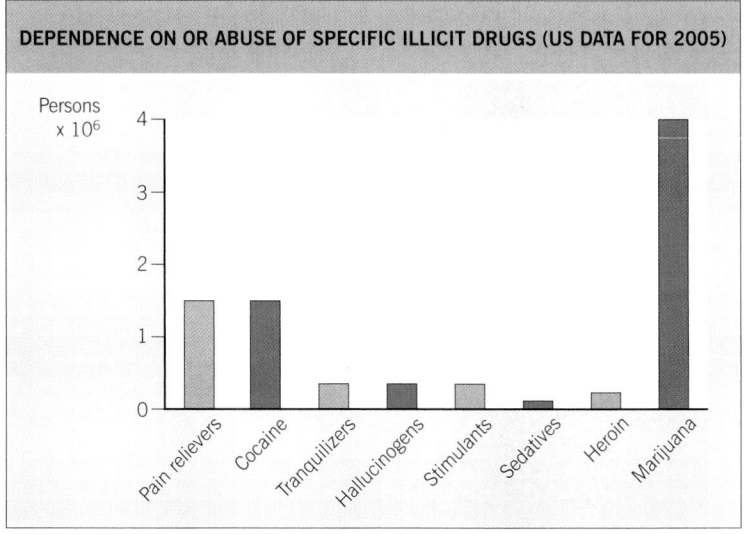

Fig. 88.1 Dependence on or abuse of specific illicit drugs during the past year (US data for 2005). Estimates in those 12 years of age or older. www.oas.samhsa.gov/NSDUH/2k5NSDUH/2k5results.htm

pigmentation of veins due to inflammation from repeated non-sterile injections and injections of irritating drugs and adulterants (Fig. 88.2). Early lesions in intravenous drug users consist of trails of punctures, crusted lesions and ecchymoses along the veins of an extremity[4]. Usually, the veins of the arms are initially used for injection and when these become scarred, drug is injected into the vessels of the hand, digits, wrist, lower extremities, neck, axillae and eventually into any visible vein or palpable artery[3]. Increasingly, parenteral drug users are injecting themselves in the legs, feet and groin in order to avoid the presence of scars on exposed parts of the body.

Tissue injury occurs from intradermal or subcutaneous injections and from accidental extravasation after intended injection into veins[4]. Drugs are injected subcutaneously and intradermally when patent vessels cannot be found. The resulting 'skin pop' scars are depressed, irregular, circular and often leukodermic (Fig. 88.3). In some users, indurated, hypertrophic, or keloidal scars form at these sites[3]. Drug users who cannot find intact veins may also rub powdered drugs into lacerations created with razor blades or knives.

Adulterants such as lactose, mannitol, dextrose, baking soda and flour are used to dilute heroin and other powder drugs[3]. Many adulterants, especially quinine and dextrose, are highly sclerosing and more damaging to tissue than pure heroin[1]. Quinine is a popular adulterant because it has a bitter taste similar to heroin and it accentuates the narcotic euphoria. It is destructive to lymphatics and repeated injections can lead to chronic, non-pitting hand edema.

Propoxyphene injections are so predisposing to thrombophlebitis and skin necrosis that even the most determined addict ceases use of the drug after only a few weeks (Table 88.3)[4]. Highly vasoconstrictive cocaine produces tissue ischemia, especially when extravasated. In fact, skin and muscle infarction have developed after inhalation of freebase cocaine[5]. Due to their alkalinity, barbiturates, when injected into the skin, cause tender, erythematous, indurated plaques, which break down into deep ulcers and frequently become infected. Injection of the antihistamine tripelennamine (pyribenzamine), usually injected in combination with pentazocine or another opioid, also induces tissue necrosis and ulceration. Pentazocine injection may cause brawny, sclerodermatous skin thickening and large, irregularly shaped, deeply penetrating ulcers that may extend to muscle (Fig. 88.4)[6]. Pentazocine-related cutaneous sclerosis develops more commonly in addicts with diabetes mellitus[6].

Fibrous myopathy, joint restriction, muscle contractures, brachial plexus neuropathy, inflexible ankylosis and suppurative tenosynovitis are musculoskeletal complications from intracutaneous and intravenous injections[1].

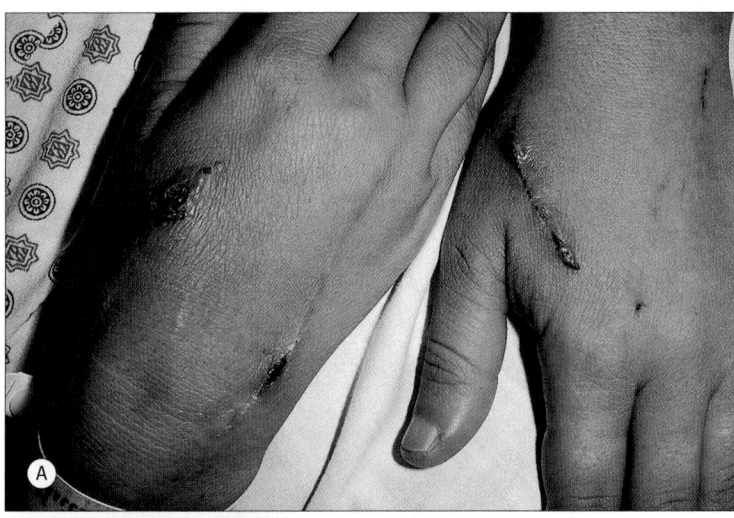
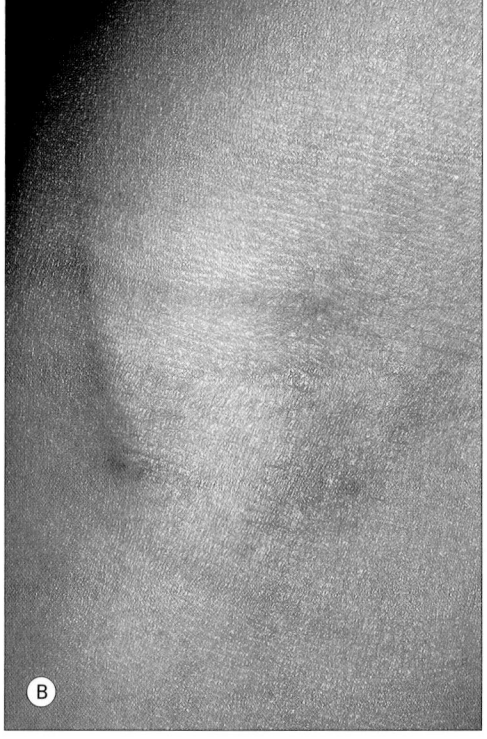

Fig. 88.2 Injection sites in an intravenous drug user. Linear hemorrhagic crusts are seen (A) as well as hyperpigmented skin tracts (B). Courtesy of Ronald P Rapini MD.

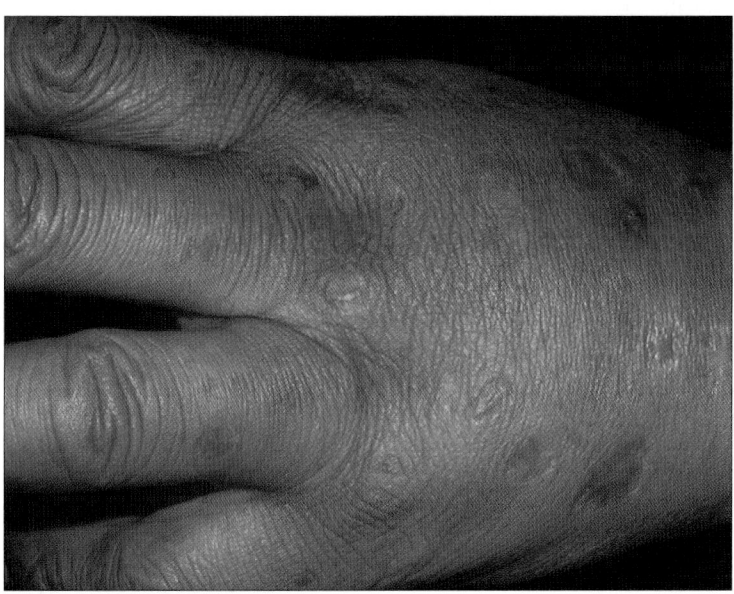

Fig. 88.3 Skin popping scars. Circular depressed 'skin pop' scars on the dorsal aspect of the fingers and hands.

Fig. 88.4 Atrophic depression and extensive calcification of the buttock from chronic abuse of pentazocine injections. Courtesy of Ronald P Rapini MD.

CUTANEOUS SIGNS OF DRUG ABUSE

Lesion type	Route(s)/associated drug(s)	Other associated signs
Skin tracks	iv	Lymphedema
Skin popping scars	sc or dermal	Lymphedema
Ulcerations	iv/propoxyphene iv/cocaine sc/barbiturates sc, im/pentazocine (± tripelennamine)	Circumferential pigmented bands
Sclerosis	sc, im/pentazocine sc/barbiturates sc/cocaine	
Palmar and digital hyperkeratosis	Smoking/crack cocaine	Madarosis Linear and circular black plaques on the fingers and palms Cuts and blisters on the lips
Nasal verrucae	Snorting/cocaine or heroin	Nasal irritation Septal perforation
Pseudoaneurysm	Arterial injection	Petechiae/purpura Reduced peripheral pulses
Cellulitis	iv, sc, intradermal	Osteomyelitis and pyogenic arthritis
Cutaneous *Pseudomonas* infection	iv, sc, intradermal/heroin sc/pentazocine ± tripelennamine	Folliculitis
Wound botulism (*Clostridium botulinum*, especially type A)	im, sc/black tar heroin or quinine-adulterated heroin	Lymphedema Skin popping scars
Excoriations & self-induced ulcers	Methamphetamine	Dry leathery skin Red dry nose Dental caries/loss of teeth Weight loss Paranoia
Formication or delusions of parasitosis	Cocaine Methamphetamine	
Pruritus	Heroin Cocaine (chronic) Methamphetamine	With heroin: Flushing Pseudoacanthosis nigricans
Papulopustular acneiform eruption	MDMA (ecstasy)	
Acne vulgaris	Anabolic steroids	Coarse skin Hirsutism Male and female pattern alopecia Increased hair growth in women Gynecomastia (in men) Testicular atrophy Clitoral enlargement
	Methamphetamine Marijuana	Excoriations
Perinasal and perioral irritant dermatitis	Sniffing of volatile solvents and inhalants	

Table 88.3 **Cutaneous signs of drug abuse.** im, intramuscular; iv, intravenous; MDMA, methylenedioxymethamphetamine; sc, subcutaneous.

Bacterial Infections

Unless they participate in needle exchange programs, hardcore parenteral drug users rarely use sterile techniques, which predisposes them to frequent infections (Table 88.4). Skin and soft tissue infections are the most common diseases for which drug addicts seek health care or are hospitalized[7-9]. Among 127 intravenous drug users, 40.9% developed cellulitis, 32.3% an abscess with cellulitis, 16.5% an abscess alone, 10.2% infected skin ulcers, 7.1% necrotizing fasciitis and 5.5%

INFECTIOUS COMPLICATIONS OF DRUG ABUSE

Type of infection	Organisms and/or associated features
Bacterial	
Abscesses and cellulitis	• *Staphylococcus aureus* > *Streptococcus* spp. > Gram-negative bacilli, anaerobes • Often polymicrobial • Lymphangitis is common • *Clostridium* infection (e.g. *C. botulinum* type A) with adulterated heroin (e.g. black tar skin popping) • *Pseudomonas aeruginosa* with pentazocine ± tripelennamine or heroin injections • *Eikenella corrodens* with methylphenidate injections (esp. into the femoral triangle)
Necrotizing fasciitis	• Polymicrobial in 60–85% of cases • Includes anaerobes in ~10%
Pyomyositis	
Septic thrombophlebitis	• Associated with endocarditis or pulmonary emboli
Septic arthritis	Increased likelihood of Gram-negative bacilli (esp. *Pseudomonas*)
Osteomyelitis	• In *Pott's puffy tumor*, frontal sinusitis leads to frontal bone osteomyelitis and a subgaleal abscess; may be complicated by an epidural abscess
Endocarditis	• *S. aureus* > *Streptococcus viridans* > Gram-negative (esp. *Pseudomonas*), polymicrobial • Often right-sided (e.g. tricuspid valve)
Fungal	
Candidiasis	• Disseminated candidiasis with pustular folliculitis; associated with injections of brown heroin • Septic arthritis, osteomyelitis, endocarditis (*C. parapsilosis*, *C. tropicalis*), septicemia ('fungemia syndrome')
Aspergillosis	• Pulmonary infections from contaminated marijuana • Dissemination and endocarditis may occur
Zygomycosis	• Cellulitic plaques or necrotic abscesses
Viral	
Hepatitis	• Hepatitis B viral infection may be associated with immune complex disease (e.g. arthritis, urticarial vasculitis) during the period of antigenemia • Syringe/needle sharing accounts for more than half of new cases of hepatitis C in the US
HIV	

Table 88.4 **Infectious complications of drug abuse.**

septic phlebitis with cellulitis[9]. The most common presentation of cellulitis is an erythematous, tender, warm, edematous, indurated plaque (see Ch. 74); however, only tenderness and edema may be apparent initially, and in more darkly pigmented skin, erythema may be difficult to appreciate.

Lymphangitis associated with skin infection is common. In addition, underlying osteomyelitis and pyogenic arthritis should be considered in cutaneous infections associated with injections. In some reports, up to one-third of hospitalized addicts with skin and soft tissue infections have an associated culture-proven bacteremia[3,9]. In a smaller subset, bacterial endocarditis develops, which is the most common systemic bacterial infection in intravenous drug users and accounts for 5% to 8% of hospitalizations[10] (see the discussion below).

The flora spectrum of street heroin does not correlate with the spectrum of bacteria causing infections in intravenous drug users[11]. Cellulitis is most frequently caused by *Staphylococcus aureus* and less often by streptococci[9,10]. However, bacterial cultures and sensitivity testing are indicated in order to identify those cutaneous infections due to Gram-negative bacteria, anaerobes or unusual organisms and to determine the most effective antibiotic regimen[11]. The combination of tripelennamine and pentazocine may promote the selective survival of *Pseudomonas aeruginosa*, and the use of quinine to adulterate heroin appears to predispose to *Clostridium* infection.

Wound botulism due to *Clostridium botulinum* type A occurs almost exclusively in drug addicts[12]. This particular infection is associated with parenteral injection, especially skin popping of black tar heroin, a form that derives its color from impurities during its manufacture and from adulterants. Black tar heroin is very hygroscopic and has a high water content, which supports the growth of organisms[13].

The spores of *C. botulinum* are not destroyed by heating the contaminated heroin and are inoculated into the subcutaneous tissue, where they germinate and produce toxin[13]. In the early stages, there is usually pain, tenderness and swelling, but a cellulitis or abscess may not be apparent. In cocaine snorters, the intranasal septum or paranasal sinuses may become infected. Botulism causes acute, usually descending and symmetric, flaccid paralysis with ophthalmoplegia, ptosis, or other cranial nerve dysfunction. The diagnosis is supported by conventional electromyography. Treatment consists of high-dose penicillin, antitoxin and respiratory support. *C. novyi* type A was responsible for an outbreak of severe infection with high mortality in drug users who injected heroin extravascularly.

Upper extremity infections require special attention. In a 5-year review of 103 patients with an upper extremity infection requiring admission, 92% had cellulitis, 80% edema and 33% ulceration at the site of injection. Seven percent presented with gangrene[11]. In addition, necrotizing cellulitis of the scrotum and penis has been reported in addicts who accidentally injected drugs into the femoral artery instead of the vein[14].

The popularity of skin popping has caused an increase in the incidence of abscesses among parenteral drug users. Abscesses from subcutaneous drug injection are often multilobulated, deep and have extensive necrosis, requiring exploration and debridement. Superficial abscesses often rupture spontaneously, leaving punched-out ulcers. A single pathogen is cultured in over 50% of cases, and more than one organism is present in 33% to 45%[9]. Fever and leukocytosis are not particularly reliable measures of severity, as they are absent in 50% and 57% of cases, respectively[9]. The injection of a cocaine and heroin mixture, or 'speedball', may predispose patients to develop abscesses by inducing soft tissue ischemia[15].

Any type of bacteria may be cultured from these abscesses, but the more common are *Staphylococcus aureus* (20–60%), *Streptococcus* species (25%) and Gram-negative bacilli (up to 25%). Anaerobic bacteria are common as well, especially in polymicrobial infections. In one study, anaerobic bacteria were recovered from two-thirds of abscesses, and in one-third of these, they were the only cultured organism[16]. *Eikenella corrodens*, an oral flora bacterium, has been cultured from some abscesses caused by injections of methylphenidate. Curiously, some abscesses develop months after a patient has ceased use of drugs. Abscesses may be contiguous with underlying bone in the setting of associated osteomyelitis. In intravenous drug users, acute or chronic osteomyelitis develops from contiguous infection in surrounding soft tissue, hematogenous seeding of bacteria or direct penetrating trauma from needles. The presence of osteomyelitis should be considered in anyone with continued pain after treatment of soft tissue infection or with soft tissue infections that recur or respond indolently to appropriate treatment with antibiotics. Cervical abscesses usually occur in the anterior cervical triangle, and may cause life-threatening complications such as mediastinitis, pneumomediastinum, airway obstruction, internal jugular vein thrombosis, and extension into the carotid sheath. Abscesses in the groin may present with only tenderness and edema. These abscesses can be deep and extensive, especially if they originate in the femoral triangle.

The degree of pain usually exceeds that anticipated from the clinical findings. Radiography may show soft tissue swelling or joint effusion. Sinography can delineate the extent of abscess cavity or fistula. MRI is superior to CT imaging in revealing the presence of fluid, as well as in the depiction of fluid and purulent collections in skin, joints or tendon sheaths, but both are valuable in confirming the presence of deep and groin abscesses[17]. It is crucial to be aware that necrotizing fasciitis with or without myositis can present as erythema (77%), fluctuance (20%), edema (20%) or induration (43%), clinically resembling a non-fluctuant abscess yet requiring extensive subfascial debridement[18]. Fever and leukocytosis are often present. In some cases, only swelling or inconspicuous cellulitis is apparent. However, severe pain, disproportionate to the physical findings, is present in 94% of cases[19]. If this complaint

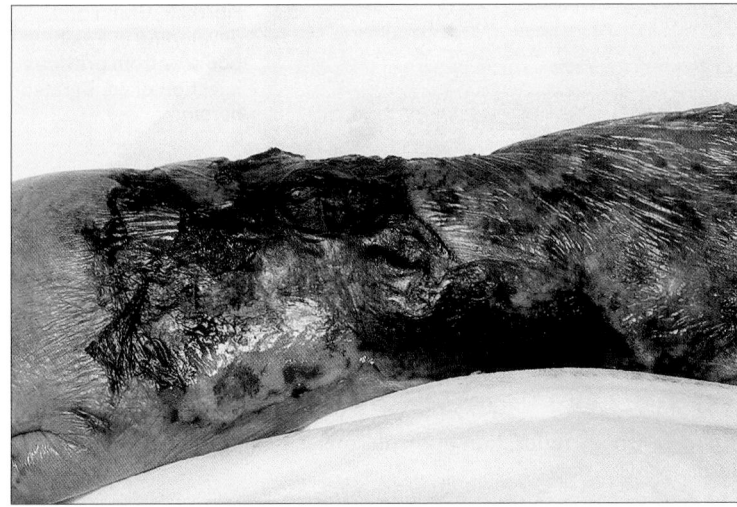

Fig. 88.5 Necrotizing fasciitis of the upper extremity with bulla formation and extensive tissue necrosis in an intravenous heroin user.

is disregarded or misinterpreted as a request for narcotics, the outcome can be devastating.

Notably, the classic cutaneous findings of necrotizing fasciitis, such as bullae (3%), tissue crepitance (3%) and skin necrosis (10%), are usually absent, and only present in a small minority of patients[18] (Fig. 88.5). For this reason, surgical exploration is mandatory in any parenteral drug user with cellulitis and unexplainable severe pain[20]. Any necrotic tissue should be debrided surgically, as the infection will progress in 75% of patients treated only with parenteral antibiotics[20]. Multiple organisms are cultured in 60% to 85% of cases, including anaerobes in 12% of patients. The presence of gas is not pathognomonic for *Clostridium* infection, as gas gangrene can also (but infrequently) be caused by other bacteria (e.g. usually mixed infections with *Enterococcus faecalis*, *Escherichia coli*, group G *Streptococcus*, *Klebsiella pneumoniae*, *Proteus vulgaris*, *Citrobacter diversus*, *Bacteroides bivius*, *Peptostreptococcus asaccharolyticus* or *Morganella morganii*).

Fungal Infections

Dermatophytosis is very common in addicts. Disseminated candidiasis associated with injections of brown heroin was reported in the 1980s and found to be caused by an overgrowth of yeast in the lemon juice used to dissolve heroin[21]. Initially, patients develop high fevers, rigors, headaches, myalgias and occasionally jaundice, but, at this stage, blood and urine cultures rarely demonstrate organisms. Usually after about a week, up to 90% of the patients developed pustular folliculitis and painful nodules in hair-bearing areas (scalp, moustache and beard)[21]. The lesions resemble bacterial folliculitis but potassium hydroxide examination and lesional biopsy specimens demonstrate the presence of yeast. Other complications included ocular disease (chorioretinitis, uveitis, endophthalmitis, episcleritis), monoarthritis, painful costal osteochondritis and pleuritis[21].

Unlike HIV infection, intravenous drug use is a predisposing factor for zygomycosis. The characteristic cutaneous lesion is a cellulitic plaque or abscess with extensive necrotic tissue.

Granulomas

Injection of hydrous magnesium silicate (talc) or starch can produce granulomatous responses (Fig. 88.6) in the walls of veins, deep dermis and subcutaneous tissue, resulting in the formation of firm, movable cutaneous nodules[22]. Talc is the main ingredient in some of the narcotic tablets that are crushed, diluted in liquid, and then injected. Talc granulomas may also develop in the lungs, liver, lymph nodes, spleen and bone marrow. Granulomas may not appear for 50 years after subcutaneous injection, because it is the conversion of silica to its colloidal form that stimulates the formation of granulomas[22]. Injection of sclerosing adulterants and drugs can produce tender and inflammatory nodules that ulcerate and heal with epidermal pigmentary

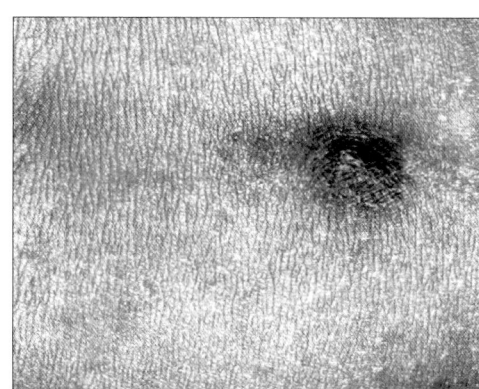

Fig. 88.6 Granuloma developing in a skin pop scar from previous injection of adulterated heroin.

changes, woody induration of the dermis and subcutaneous tissue, and retracted cicatrices.

Mucous Membrane Lesions

Snorting cocaine causes erythema of the nasal mucosa, nasal irritation, anosmia and rhinitis, and may lead to epistaxis, perforation of the nasal septum and osteolytic sinusitis. Nasal verrucae (snorters' warts) can also erupt in cocaine users. Less often, sniffing heroin causes these findings. A complex consisting of nasal collapse, septal perforation, palatal retraction, and pharyngeal wall ulceration has been described in cocaine snorters. Cuts and blisters on the lips from glass or metal smoking pipes have been noted in addicts who smoke crack cocaine, while ageusia, halitosis and repeated lip smacking are additional signs of cocaine abuse. There are reports of men applying cocaine powder on their glans penis to postpone ejaculation and of women rubbing cocaine on their genitals to enhance pleasure. These practices can lead to priapism, irritant dermatitis and even ulcerations.

Penile ulcers have developed after injections of heroin into the shaft veins. The labial mucosa may become dry in heroin or amphetamine users[3]. Amphetamine use may also cause dysgeusia and xerostomia.

Hardcore drug users frequently have marked dental and gingival disease due to poor hygiene (Fig. 88.7). Betel palm seeds (betel nuts) contain a narcotic stimulant and habitual chewing of these nuts, a practice in some areas of Southeast Asia, stains the teeth and is associated with the development of oral leukoplakia and submucous fibrosis. The addictive habit of chewing *Catha edulis* tree leaves, which contain the narcotic Qat, is popular in several African and Middle Eastern countries and produces oral keratotic white lesions in approximately 20% of users.

Red or 'bloodshot' eyes due to conjunctival vascular injection occurs with marijuana and sometimes with cocaine or phencyclidine (PCP) use. Repeated sniffing of volatile solvents and inhalants, such as butane gas, paint thinner, aerosol sprays, cleaning fluids and glues, can cause

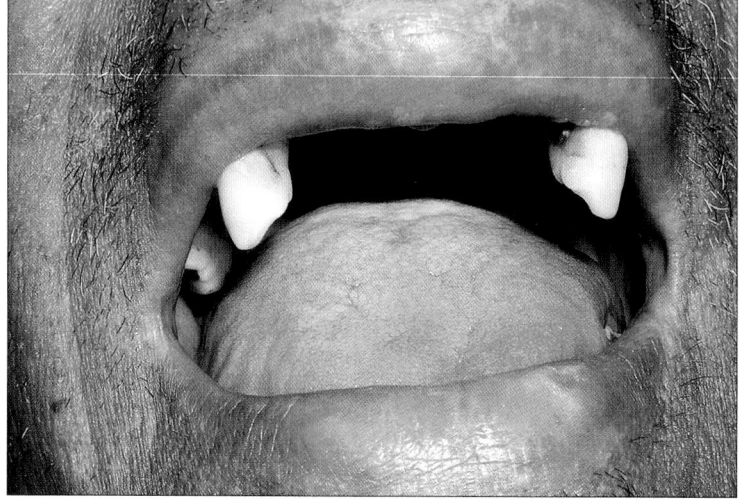

Fig. 88.7 Missing and carious teeth and inflamed gums are common physical findings in hardcore drug addicts.

nasal, labial, perioral and perinasal irritant dermatitis (sniffer's rash). The skin lesions may be discrete papules or erosions that are often confused with acne.

Burns

In addicts with an altered state of mind, burns are not uncommon, including those from lit matches, cigarettes, paraphernalia, and contact with fire during cooking. Cigarette burns, most commonly seen on the digits and sternum, occur from lit cigarettes, which the addict was holding or smoking before nodding off[3]. The necklace sign is produced by cigarette ashes, which fall on the neck when the smoking addict falls asleep. Singeing of the eyelashes and eyebrows, resulting in madarosis, may be caused by rising hot vapors during the smoking of crack cocaine. Crack addicts may also have linear and circular black plaques on the fingers and palms.

Ulcers

As has been previously described, ulcers can be caused by direct drug-related cutaneous, deep tissue or vascular injury, by accidental or incidental trauma, or by infection. When other venous accesses have been exhausted, drug users may attempt to inexorably maintain the granulation tissue with its rich vascular network of capillaries for injection of heroin or other drugs, resulting in chronic non-healing ulcers called 'shooter's patches'[23].

Formication

Prolonged use of cocaine may lead to the development of formication, tactile hallucinations during which the patient senses that insects are crawling on or under their skin ('coke bugs')[4]. Repetitive, stereotypical skin picking leading to excoriations and disfiguring skin ulcers on the face and extremities is a common finding in methamphetamine abusers. Not uncommonly, these individuals also feel that bugs are crawling under their skin, and cocaine or crystal methamphetamine use should be considered in anyone who presents with delusions of parasitosis as well as neurotic excoriations. Other signs of methamphetamine abuse are dry skin, itching with lichenification, unpleasant body odor, a red dry nose, sweating, weight loss, premature aging, rotting teeth, aggressive behavior and paranoia. Acne, especially the excoriée type, has been described.

Additional Cutaneous Findings

Circumferential, pigmented bands due to pressure from tourniquets are common in intravenous drug users with darkly pigmented skin. 'Soot tattoos' are produced by injections of residual carbon on the needle after flaming[4]. Self-induced tattoos have been considered a sign of drug abuse; however, the current popularity of tattoos and their pervasive presence in persons with present or past connections to street gangs have diminished the reliability of this sign[4]. Hyperkeratosis of the fingers and palms are common in heavy users of crack cocaine. Traumatic bullae at the site of injection are occasionally observed. Pressure erythema, bullae and ulcers (Fig. 88.8) develop in comatose patients after an overdose with barbiturates or other sedative drugs[5] (see Ch. 35).

The combination of chronic cocaine use coupled with marijuana inhalation often leads to very pruritic skin. The feeling of euphoria induced by heroin is frequently accompanied by skin flushing and itching, as well as a dry mouth, watery eyes and rhinorrhea. Generalized or focal, especially genital, itching during the euphoric stage following heroin administration has been named 'high pruritus'.

Hyperhidrosis is a common adverse effect of amphetamines or LSD. Within 30 to 90 minutes of LSD ingestion, the user feels a wide range of emotions, accompanied by sweating, increased body temperature, dry mouth, tremors and dilated pupils. Piloerection, paresthesias and flushing are manifestations of the somatic phase of LSD intoxication, while pseudohallucinations and synesthesias occur during the perceptual phase. Delusions and visual hallucinations occur at higher doses. Hypoesthesia is a common manifestation of low-dose exposure to PCP.

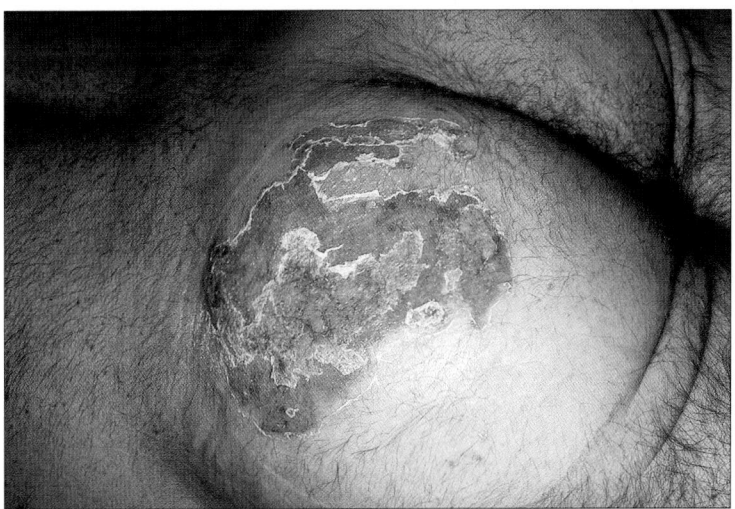

Fig. 88.8 Healing ulcer on the buttock due to prolonged coma from barbiturate overdose.

A small study comparing HIV-infected to non-HIV-infected drug addicts found that numerous HIV-associated skin diseases afflicted HIV-infected subjects (see Ch. 78), but only fungal infections were highly prevalent in the non-HIV-infected cohort[24]. However, a number of uncontrolled studies have described a higher prevalence of skin diseases among non-HIV-infected drug addicts. For example, seborrheic dermatitis may be more frequently diagnosed in chronic cocaine users, and eczemas, especially contact dermatitis, have been reported to occur more frequently in parenteral drug users[3]. Heroin addicts often have dry skin, which can become irritated and pruritic, and they may develop pseudoacanthosis nigricans.

In better-designed and controlled studies, there has been a correlation, with a relative risk factor as high as 8.1, between alcohol use and the development and exacerbation of large plaque psoriasis in men. However, there are no good studies evaluating psoriasis and drug abuse[25].

There have been scattered reports in habitual MDMA (ecstasy) users of a papulopustular, facial acneiform eruption, which may indicate a higher risk of severe adverse effects, such as hepatic damage. In some cases, the eruption responded to topical metronidazole[26]. Acne and other skin eruptions are anecdotally worsened by cannabis. Acne ranging from mild to cystic, especially on the trunk, is common among users of anabolic steroids. Other effects of anabolic steroid abuse include oily hair and skin, male and female pattern alopecia, increased hair growth in women, gynecomastia in men, coarse skin, testicular atrophy, clitoral enlargement, cardiovascular disease, peliosis hepatitis and liver cancer. Most are reversible if the abuser stops taking the drugs, but some are permanent.

Drug-Induced Reactions

As expected, hypersensitivity reactions to drugs, especially morbilliform eruptions, urticaria (opiates, barbiturates, amphetamines, marijuana), bullous eruptions, fixed drug reactions, leukocytoclastic vasculitis, Stevens-Johnson syndrome and toxic epidermal necrolysis occur more frequently in illicit drug users than in the general population (Table 88.5). In one study, dermatographism was found in 26% of patients comatose from a drug overdose. Angioedema due to barbiturates and heroin can cause eyelid as well as labial edema. Pigmented patches on the skin and mucous membranes may be extensive in addicts with fixed drug eruptions.

Vascular Lesions

The most common vascular lesions are ecchymoses and even hematomas over injected vessels. Petechiae may form distal to the placement of a tourniquet. Vascular compromise of the hands is common and is characterized by discoloration, edema and cold temperature. Severe arterial constriction or emboli can lead to gangrene and loss of digits or a limb. Intense burning pain is often experienced after self-administered intra-arterial injection of drugs. This is followed within hours by edema of the affected limb. Although the peripheral pulses usually remain strong, cyanosis and patches of livedo reticularis develop. The changes may progress to localized necrosis, and distal necrosis occurs in the most severe cases. Ischemia and ulceration can appear after injection of temazepam (as high as 100% when injected into the radial artery), barbiturates, cocaine, heroin, pentazocine, diazepam, amphetamine, sodium thiopental[11] and others. Other manifestations reported after accidental or intentional drug injections into the radial artery include purpuric and pustular nodules, presumably as a result of embolization, as well as palmar cyanosis and edema with or without ulceration.

Pseudoaneurysms result from infected injuries to arteries during intra-arterial injection of drugs ('hitting the pinkie') and are most common in the extremities and groin. The typical lesion is a tender, diffusely indurated, pulsatile mass with an associated bruit (50–60% of cases) and decreased peripheral pulses (25%). Local suppuration and petechiae and purpura are often present. Half will resolve with antibiotics alone, but expanding lesions require proximal ligation of the vessel, resection of the pseudoaneurysm, and appropriate drainage.

Mycotic aneurysms occur in 15% to 25% of patients with infective endocarditis, most frequently in the femoral artery. These aneurysms require immediate surgery.

In addition to arterial disease, cocaine can produce superficial or deep venous thromboses. Treatment consists of parenterally administered antibiotics, bed rest, elevation of the involved extremity, and anticoagulation, however, care must be taken to exclude a mycotic aneurysm, which can bleed[5], especially in the setting of anticoagulation. Distal thrombosis with extensive infarctive thigh lesions and associated hepatitis and glomerulonephritis has been reported following intravenous injection of cocaine into an arm vein.

Septic thrombophlebitis results in tender, swollen extremities with or without erythema. A tender cord may be present when the affected vein is superficial, but deep vein thrombophlebitis is easily misdiagnosed as cellulitis or an abscess, either of which may be an associated complication. Deep vein thromboses are diagnosed via Doppler ultrasonography.

DRUG-INDUCED CUTANEOUS REACTIONS					
	Opiates	Barbiturates	Amphetamines	Cocaine	Marijuana
Morbilliform eruption	✓	✓	✓		✓
Bullous eruption	✓	✓		✓	
Fixed drug eruption	✓	✓	✓		
Small vessel vasculitis	✓	✓	✓	✓	
Stevens–Johnson syndrome	✓	✓			
Toxic epidermal necrolysis	✓	✓			
Urticaria	✓	✓	✓	✓	✓

Table 88.5 Drug-induced cutaneous reactions.

Arteriovenous fistula-associated angiomatoid nodules (pseudo-Kaposi's sarcoma) in a patient with hepatitis B viral infection was reported as a possible complication of heroin use[27]. In addition, palpable purpura and tender nodules may appear as cutaneous manifestations of small and medium-sized vessel vasculitis due to hepatitis B or C viral infections or specific drugs (see Table 88.5). Repeated vascular injury and infection of the digits can cause irreversible contractures (camptodactyly) that resemble Dupuytren's disease.

Systemic Complications

Drug abuse may indirectly contribute to congenital cutaneous malformations and domestic violence (see Ch. 90). The estimated incidence of infective endocarditis, a major cause of mortality in this population, is 1.5 to 3.3 cases per 1000 injection-drug users per year[28]. Several cutaneous signs (arterial emboli, conjunctival hemorrhages, splinter hemorrhages, Janeway lesions and Osler nodes) may be present. The prevalence of HIV infection among intravenous drug users with infectious endocarditis is very high, ranging from 44% to 90%. The US Centers for Disease Control and Prevention estimates that 55–60% of AIDS cases among women and one-third of overall AIDS cases in the US are linked to injection-drug use or sex with partners who inject drugs.

Parenteral drug users are also at high risk for contracting other blood-borne viruses such as hepatitis B and C and human T-lymphotrophic virus types 1 and 2 (HTLV-1, HTLV-2). Approximately 60% of all new cases of hepatitis C infections in the US are attributed to syringe and needle sharing with an infected individual. In some user populations, transmission of hepatitis C occurs so rapidly that within 6 months of beginning drug use, one-third of users are infected, and within 2 years, up to 90% have contracted the infection[29].

Drug addicts have high prevalences of all sexually transmitted diseases, due to multiple partners, prostitution and failure to use condoms. However, narcotic abuse is a common cause of false-positive non-treponemal syphilis screening tests (e.g. VDRL, RPR). In these cases, treponemal tests (e.g. MHA-TP, FTA-ABS) will be non-reactive. In addicts who have had syphilis, both types of tests will be positive, but the titers of the non-treponemal test may not decrease rapidly after treatment.

Cocaine may initiate scleroderma in susceptible individuals or unmask it at an earlier age in those with subclinical disease. The localized cutaneous induration induced by cocaine injections is reversible. Cases of Henoch–Schönlein purpura, polyarteritis nodosa and necrotizing angiitis with renal and pulmonary disease have been associated with the use of heroin. Nephrotic syndrome from amyloidosis has been reported in heroin skin poppers and intravenous drug users with chronically draining skin lesions[30]. Some cases of toxic shock syndrome related to intravenous heroin abuse have been reported.

TREATMENT

A detailed discussion of the management of drug addiction is beyond the scope of this chapter. Approaches are summarized in Table 88.6 and discussed elsewhere in the literature[31]. Sensitivity and carefulness to avoid bias are essential when providing care for drug users. When providing care to persons suspected of drug addiction, it should be remembered that even admission of illicit drug use is difficult, as patients risk disapproval and overt or concealed rejection even from medical professionals.

The success of treatment efforts is variable, and, in general, successful recovery from drug addiction is a long-term process that often requires multiple attempts and many behavioral changes. The potential for relapse appears to persist indefinitely. Methamphetamine releases particularly high levels of dopamine in the brain. Because withdrawal symptoms are so intense, methamphetamine addicts are the

TREATMENT OF DRUG ADDICTION	
Drug	**Treatments**

Opiates	• Drug detoxification
	  – Office-based
	  – Inpatient
	  – Ultra-rapid under general anesthesia using naltrexone (plus clonidine, benzodiazepines and antiemetics)
	• Maintenance therapy
	  – Agonist (methadone, levomethadyl*)
	  – Partial agonist (long-acting buprenorphine)
	  – Antagonist (naltrexone)
	• Pharmacologic therapy for withdrawal (e.g. clonidine, lofexidine, guanfacine)
	• Additional measures (counseling, psychotherapy, acupuncture)

Cocaine	• Drug rehabilitation • Anticonvulsants (e.g. topiramate, tiagabine), dopamine agonists† (e.g. amantadine, bromocriptine, pergolide), antidepressants†, modafinil
Amphetamines	• Drug rehabilitation • Antidepressants (e.g. fluoxetine, imipramine, desipramine, mirtazapine), modafinil, antipsychotics (e.g. chlorpromazine, haloperidol, thioridazine)

*Withdrawn from the US market due to risk of cardiac arrhythmias.
†To date, no statistical evidence of benefit.

Table 88.6 Treatment of drug addiction.

hardest to treat. Continued or relapsing use of drugs can be monitored with drug screening.

The selection of antibiotics to treat skin infections should be guided by antibiotic sensitivities of the cultured organisms. With the emergence of community acquired methicillin-resistant *Staphylococcus aureus* (MRSA), appropriate cultures of lesions and wounds have become more imperative than ever. Broad-spectrum antibiotic regimens that cover *S. aureus* should be prescribed until antibiotic sensitivity results are available. Treatment of cellulitis consists of splinting, limb elevation and intravenous antibiotics. Inclusion of vancomycin or linezolid (for MRSA) and clindamycin (for anaerobes) in the antibiotic regimen has been recommended for hand infections and should also be considered in infections that may result in loss of limb or life[11]. Hand infections must be aggressively treated, in view of the 10% rate of amputation of digits or the hand in such cases[11].

Even with surgical plus aggressive medical treatment, the mortality rate of necrotizing fasciitis in drug addicts is approximately 20% and limb amputation is necessary in another 18%[18]. A decrease in mortality from 27% to 7% was reported with a protocol consisting of aggressive diagnosis, intense intravenous broad-spectrum antimicrobial therapy, supportive care, early subfascial debridement, and follow-up debridement of the wound in 8 to 12 hours until no further necrotic tissue had formed. Between two and four debridements were required[19].

Skin grafting of large ulcers may be necessary when healing does not occur with compression and appropriate dressings. Some substance abusers may deliberately sabotage the skin graft by injecting through it or into the vacuum (VAC) dressing tubing[32]. Recovered parenteral drug users often wear long sleeves and garments to hide the stigmata of their past addiction and may seek help in diminishing the appearance of these signs. Hypertrophic scars improve with intralesional injections of corticosteroids or interferon-α and pulsed dye laser treatments. Hyperpigmented scars require the use of pigment-specific lasers and bleaching agents, including hydroquinone. Tissue augmentation with hyaluronic acid, collagen or fat can improve the appearance of depressed scars. Such scars may also respond to low-fluency treatments with visible light lasers, which stimulate fibroblast proliferation.

REFERENCES

1. Del Giudice P. Cutaneous complications of intravenous drug abuse. Br J Dermatol. 2004;150:1–10.
2. World Drug Report. Volume 1. Analysis. New York: United Nations Office on Drugs and Crime, 2004.
3. Burnett JW. Drug abuse. Cutis. 1992;49:307–8.
4. Sim MG, Hulse G, Khong E. Injecting drug use and skin lesions. Aust Fam Phys. 2004;33:519–22.
5. Zamora-Quezada JC, Dinerman H, Stadecker MJ, Kelly JJ. Muscle and skin infarction after free-basing cocaine (crack). Ann Intern Med. 1988;108:564–6.
6. Furner BB. Parenteral pentazocine: cutaneous complications revisited. J Am Acad Dermatol. 1990;22:694–5.
7. Orangio GR, Pitlick SD, Della Latta P, et al. Soft tissue infections in parenteral drug abusers. Ann Surg. 1984;199:97–100.
8. White AG. Medical disorders in drug addicts: 200 consecutive admissions. J Am Med Assoc. 1973;223:1469–71.
9. Hasan SB, Albu E, Gerst PH. Infectious complications in IV drug abusers. Infect Surg. 1988;7:218–32.
10. Tuazon CU, Sheagren JN. Staphylococcal endocarditis in parenteral drug abusers: source of the organism. Ann Intern Med. 1975;82:788–90.
11. Smith DJ Jr, Busuito MJ, Velanovich V, et al. Drug injection injuries of the upper extremity. Ann Plast Surg. 1989;22:19–24.
12. MacDonald KL, Cohen ML, Blake PA. The changing epidemiology of adult botulism in the United States. Am J Epidemiol. 1986;124:794–9.
13. Centers for Disease Control and Prevention (CDC). Wound botulism – California, 1995. MMWR Morb Mortal Wkly Rep. 1995;44:889–92.
14. Alguire PC. Necrotizing cellulitis of the scrotum: a new complication of heroin addiction. Cutis. 1984;34:93–5.
15. Murphy EL, DeVita D, Liu H, et al. Risk factors for skin and soft-tissue abscesses among injection drug users: a case-control study. Clin Infect Dis. 2001;33:35–40.
16. Webb D, Thadepalli H. Skin and soft tissue polymicrobial infections from intravenous abuse of drugs. Western J Med. 1979;130:200–4.
17. Johnston C, Leogan MT. Imaging features of soft-tissue infections and other complications in drug users after direct subcutaneous infection ("skin popping"). Am J Roentgenol. 2005;182:1195–202.
18. Callahan TE, Schecter WP, Horn JK. Necrotizing soft tissue infection masquerading as cutaneous abscess following illicit drug injection. Arch Surg. 1998;133:812–18.
19. Sudarsky LA, Laschinger JC, Coppa GF, Spencer FC. Improved results from a standardized approach in treating patients with necrotizing fasciitis. Ann Surg. 1987;206:661–5.
20. Clark DD. Surgical management of infections and other complications resulting from drug abuse. Arch Surg. 1970;101:619–23.
21. Dupont B, Drouhet E. Cutaneous, ocular, and osteoarticular candidiasis in heroin addicts: new clinical and therapeutic aspects in 38 patients. J Infect Dis. 1985;152:577–91.
22. Posner DI, Guill MA III. Cutaneous foreign body granulomas associated with intravenous drug abuse. J Am Acad Dermatol. 1985;13:869–72.
23. Tice AD. An unusual, non-healing ulcer on the forearm. N Engl J Med 2002;347:1725–6.
24. Gaeta GB, Maisto C, Sichenze R, et al. Mucocutaneous diseases in drug addicts with or without HIV infection. A case-control study. Infection. 1994;22:77–80.
25. Del Giudice P, Vandenbos F, Boissy C, et al. Cutaneous complications of direct intraarterial injections in drug addicts. Acta Derm Venereol. 2005;85:451–2.
26. Wollina U, Kammler HJ, Hasselbarth N, et al. Ecstasy pimples – a new facial dermatosis. Dermatology. 1998;197:171–3.
27. Fimiani M, Miracco C, Bianciardi S, Andreassi L. Pseudo-Kaposi's sarcoma in a drug addict. Int J Dermatol. 1986;25:651–2.
28. Gordon RJ, Lowy FD. Bacterial infections in drug users. N Engl J Med. 2005;253:1945–54.
29. Garfein RS, Vlahov D, Galai N, et al. Viral infections in short-term injection drug users: the prevalence of the hepatitis C, hepatitis B, human immunodeficiency, and human T-lymphotropic viruses. Am J Public Health. 1996;86:655–61.
30. Neugarten J, Gallo GR, Buxbaum J, et al. Amyloidosis in subcutaneous heroin abusers ('skin poppers' amyloidosis'). Am J Med. 1986;81:635–40.
31. Principles of Drug Addiction Treatment: A Research Based Guide. National Institutes of Health, Publication no. 00-4180, July 2000.
32. Williams AM, Southern SJ. Conflicts in the treatment of chronic ulcers in drug addict – case series and discussion. Br J Plast Surg. 2005;58:997–9.

Signs of Drug Abuse

Skin Signs of Abuse

Sharon S Raimer and Ben G Raimer

89

Abuse among individuals, both physical and psychological, is a problem that may occur in any age group or culture. Although abuse is not limited to any particular group of individuals, this chapter will focus on abuse inflicted on those often least able to defend or provide for themselves or to correct or escape their situation without the recognition of the abuse by others: children and elders.

CHILD ABUSE

Synonym: ▪ Battered child syndrome

Key features

▪ Signs of physical abuse include: unexplained bruises; injuries of the thorax, abdomen, buttocks, genitals, chin, ears or neck; curvilinear marks; and cigarette burns or well-demarcated burns

▪ Signs of sexual abuse include attenuation, fresh tears or scars of the hymen and/or the anal margin extending out onto perianal skin

Introduction

Child abuse is a term used to encompass the broad spectrum of non-accidental maltreatment of children, including physical, emotional and sexual abuse, as well as neglect. Physical abuse is defined as a non-accidental injury of a child; the injury may be the result of a single abusive episode or may occur over a period of time. The abused child is often an infant. Younger children are at greater risk because they are demanding, non-verbal and defenseless. As many as 90% of abused children are younger than 10 years of age and more than 70% are 3 years of age or younger.

The parent may describe the child as a difficult child, which in fact may be true; however, the parents may attempt to intervene in a manner that is excessive and inappropriate. Premature infants, handicapped children, and children with behavioral problems appear to be at increased risk of abuse. Parents who abuse their children were often themselves abused as children. They are frequently immature and dependent individuals who are socially isolated. Often, they do not handle stress well, and a personal or family crisis may trigger an abusive episode. It is important that all physicians recognize signs of physical abuse in children, as abusive episodes tend to be repeated, and an intentionally injured child should be considered at high risk for the future occurrence of a severe physical injury.

Physical neglect is a failure to provide the necessities of life for a child, including nutrition, clothing, housing, medical care and safe supervision. Emotional abuse or neglect results when parents fail to provide a nurturing environment that permits the child to grow and reach his or her full potential.

Sexual abuse can be defined as the engaging of a child in a sexual activity that the child cannot comprehend, for which the child is developmentally unprepared and cannot give informed consent, and/or that violates the social and legal taboos of society[1]. The child's involvement is either coerced through physical threats or rewarded through bribes or misrepresentation of moral values. Sexual abuse may be assaultive or non-assaultive. Non-assaultive sexual abuse probably occurs frequently and most often goes unreported since there is usually little or no physical injury to the child. Assaultive sexual abuse, on the other hand, is characterized by physical injury and violence. Both types of sexual abuse may result in severe emotional trauma to the child.

History

Maltreatment of children has always existed, but Dr John Caffey, a pediatric radiologist, can probably be credited with initiating medical concern about child abuse with his description of six children who presented with skeletal fractures and associated subdural hematomas that were clearly related to trauma[2]. The immense importance of this problem was not generally recognized until 1962, when Kempe et al.[3] coined the term *battered child syndrome*, the findings of which include inadequately explained signs of trauma, multiple fractures at different stages of healing, and/or failure to thrive that responds to either nutritional therapy or placing the child in an emotionally supportive environment[3].

Epidemiology

Child abuse is a worldwide problem that occurs among all ethnic and racial groups and in families of all socioeconomic and educational levels, although, in the US, single-parent families with incomes below 200% of the poverty threshold have much higher probabilities of violence[4]. It does appear to occur more frequently when other problems such as unemployment, substance abuse, unplanned pregnancies or discord between parents increase the stress on individuals within the family. Boys are at greater risk for serious injury than are girls.

The perpetrator of sexual abuse is most often a person well known to the child, in most cases the natural father, followed in frequency by a stepfather or other close relative. Although girls are reported to be about three times more likely to be abused than are boys[5], a great deal of sexual abuse in boys may go undetected or unreported[6]. Epidemiologic studies have shown that the risk for sexual abuse rises during preadolescence[5]. Features related to family structure that have been associated with a small, but statistically significant, increase of sexual abuse are the presence of a stepfather in the household, children living without one or both of their natural parents, and children whose mothers are disabled, ill or extensively out of the home[5].

Clinical Features

Physical abuse

Physical abuse is frequently identified by *bruises* (Fig. 89.1) that may be located in areas not normally prone to accidental injury, most commonly the head and neck (particularly the face) followed by the buttocks, trunk and arms[7]. They often are large, multiple and occur in clusters. The shape of the bruises may help to identify the object with which the child was struck. Linear bruising is produced when an object such as a rod, stick or strap is used to strike a child. Hematomas and traumatic fractures of underlying bone may be present.

Loop marks are perhaps the single most characteristic finding in child abuse (Fig. 89.2). Such curvilinear marks are produced by small ropes, cords, electrical cords or belts and appear randomly over the body as a result of the striking of a struggling child[8].

Buckles from belts leave a characteristic imprint that can often be matched to the belt buckle used. Buckles inflict deep ecchymotic injury and can result in injury to underlying organs and bones.

Pinch marks, particularly on the ears or in the genital region of male children, should alert the examining physician to the possibility of abuse. Male toddlers rarely sustain bruises on the genitalia secondary to a fall.

Blunt trauma can be a very severe form of abuse that may or may not result in cutaneous lesions. Blunt trauma to the abdomen can

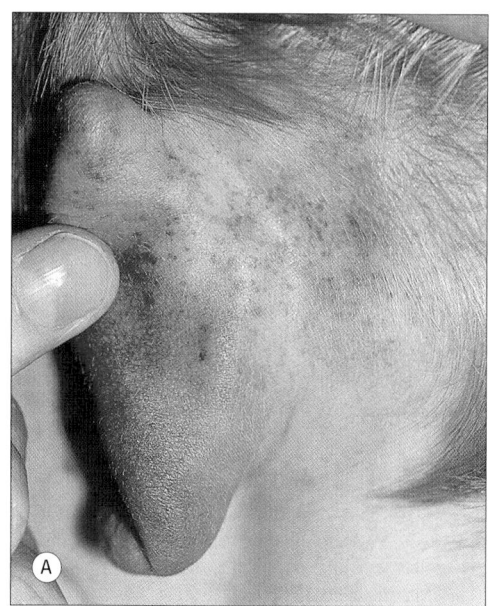

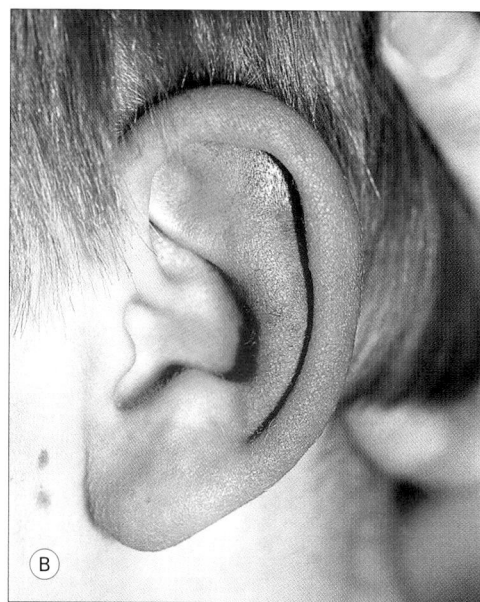

Fig. 89.1 Bruising and petechiae. A, B Bruising and petechiae of the pinna and post-auricular area in a 6-year-old boy consistent with a hand slap by an adult. C Complex bruising of the buttocks in a 3-week-old infant. From Hobbs CJ, Wynne JM. Physical Signs of Child Abuse. © 2001 WB Saunders.

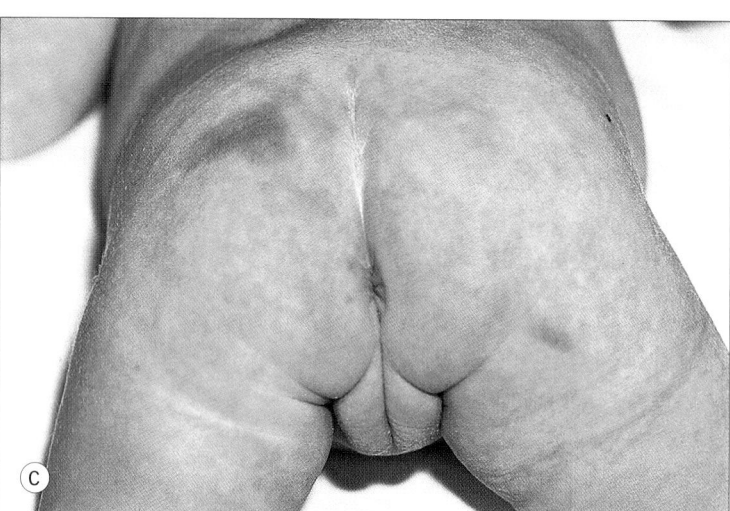

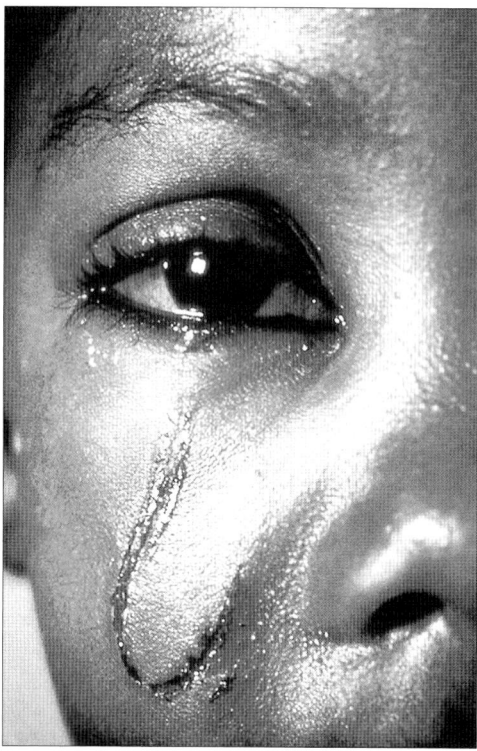

Fig. 89.2 Curvilinear mark on the cheek of a child from assault with an electric cord.

result in severe injury or even death of a child. Soft intra-abdominal organs are injured when they are slammed against the vertebral column by a kick or severe blow delivered to the abdomen. Blunt trauma in the form of slapping injury often leaves the imprint of the perpetrator's hand across the child's skin (Fig. 89.3). Capillaries break between the fingers, producing linear bruises outlining the blunt object (fingers).

Binding injuries are more likely to occur when the perpetrator is emotionally disturbed or psychotic. Acute binding injuries cause edema of the soft tissue around the wrists and ankles that may resemble rope burns with redness and warmth or abrasions (Fig. 89.4). Chronic binding injuries may result in bands of postinflammatory hyperpigmentation.

Traumatic alopecia results from the forceful pulling out of the scalp hair. The occipital region is the most common location. Acutely, when a large tuft of hair is pulled out, the underlying scalp may hemorrhage, with subsequent hematoma formation.

Human bite marks leave the indelible mark of the perpetrator and may serve to identify the abuser[9]. Adult human bite marks must be distinguished from those of a child since the healthy toddler may have numerous bite marks from his or her peers. Adult bites can be identified by the width of the dental arch (greater than 4 cm)[9]. Human bite marks differ from animal bites in that they produce a crushing type of injury, whereas typical animal bites result in puncture of the skin.

Thermal burns constitute an especially traumatic form of injury to the young child, and the abuser in such cases is likely to be suffering from a severe psychiatric disturbance. Cigarette burns represent a frequent form of thermal injury and tend to be randomly distributed

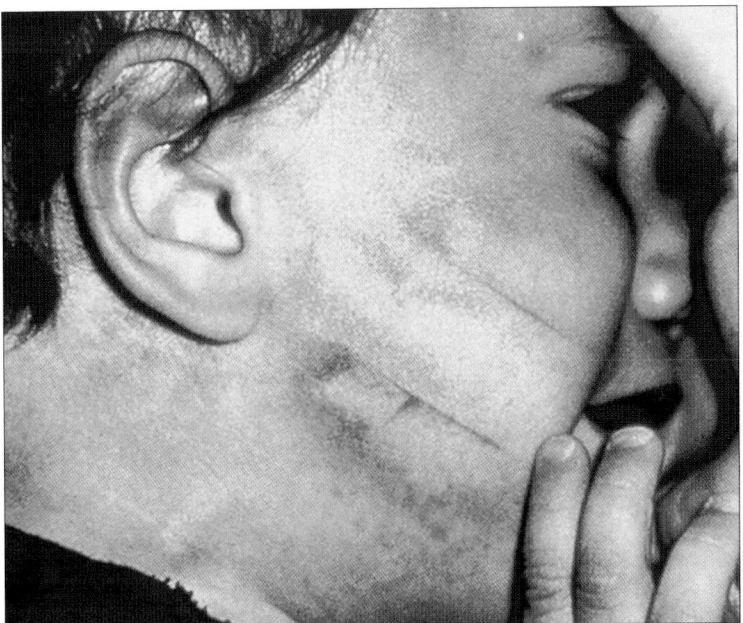

Fig. 89.3 Slap mark on the cheek. Ecchymoses that outline the fingers often can be matched to the perpetrator's hand.

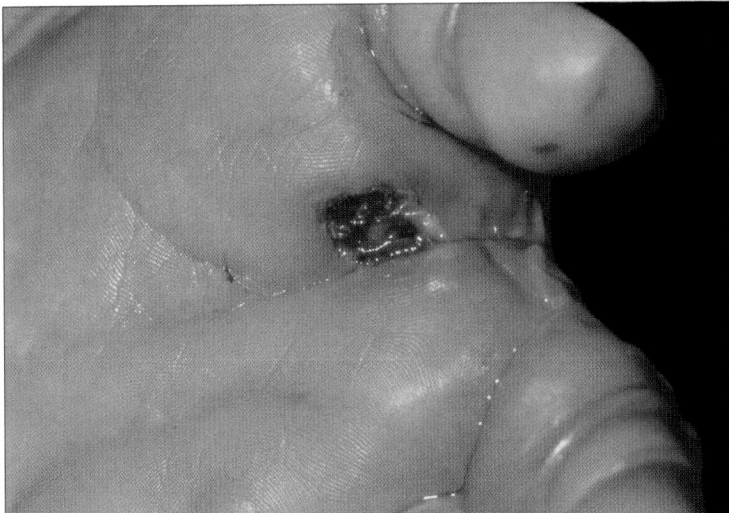

Fig. 89.5 Injury produced by a cigarette burn.

Fig. 89.6 Branding injury on the thigh from a fork.

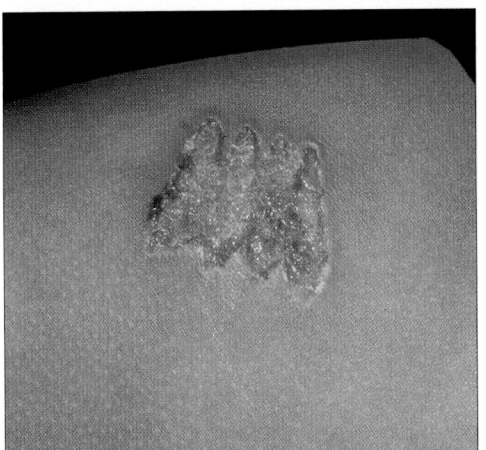

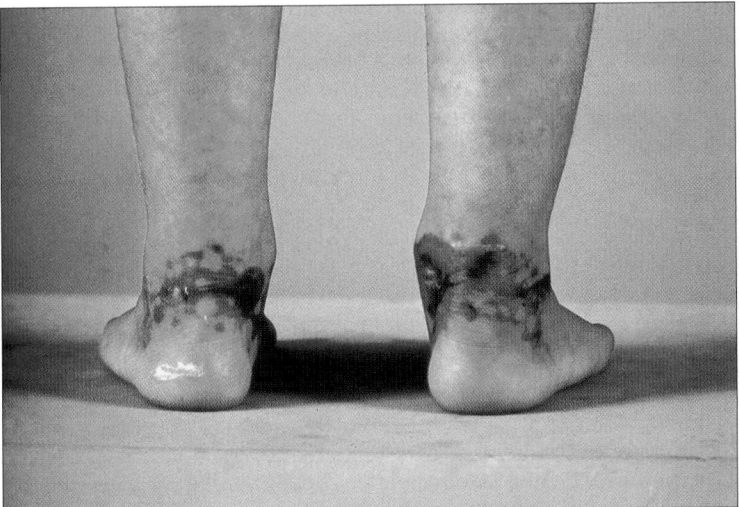

Fig. 89.4 Healing injury due to binding around the ankles.

Fig. 89.7 Burn injury from an iron.

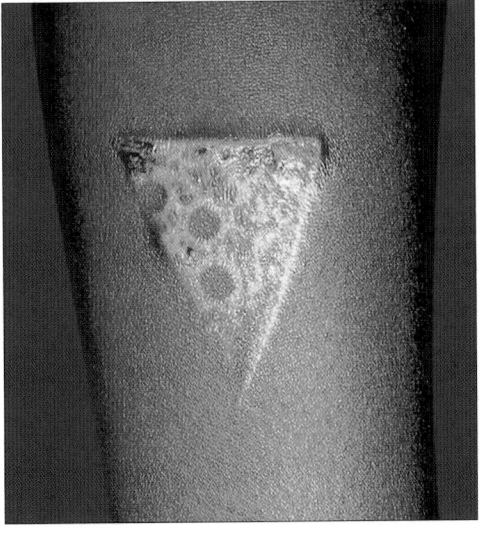

(Fig. 89.5). Branding injuries are also quite common, taking the shape of the heated object (Figs 89.6 & 89.7). Dunking scald injuries occur most often in infants and toddlers, and scalds on the buttocks may be associated with attempts to toilet train an infant. 'Donut-type sparing' may occur on the child's buttocks when the buttocks are held against a cooler tub or basin while the surrounding hot water scalds the remaining immersed skin. Dunking scalds of the extremities leave a characteristic 'stocking and glove' distribution with a very sharp demarcation of the burn (Fig. 89.8).

A child may present with skin signs of multiple types of physical abuse. Such a child may be severely injured at the time of presentation or, if not, should be considered at high risk for the future occurrence of a severe injury. Both acute and healing injuries are frequently present in chronically abused children.

Physical neglect

Physical neglect usually represents a constellation of findings obvious to most observers, including poor nutrition, hygiene and, at times, general health. The child may have old untreated injuries, dermatitis, and infestations of the skin and hair, and typically has not received required childhood immunizations.

Emotional deprivation

Emotional neglect or emotional deprivation accounts for at least one-half of the children placed under the pediatric diagnostic term *failure to*

thrive. These children fail to grow and develop in their home environment despite adequate caloric intake, while they thrive with food and stimulation in a hospital setting or foster home. There are no characteristic physical findings or diagnostic laboratory tests for these children. The diagnosis can be rendered only after other potential causes of failure to thrive have been excluded, and is usually confirmed when the child demonstrates 'catch-up' growth and development outside the disturbed home environment.

Sexual abuse

The diagnosis of child sexual abuse is based on the combined findings of the patient's history, physical examination and, when appropriate, laboratory tests. Children rarely fabricate reports of sexual abuse, and

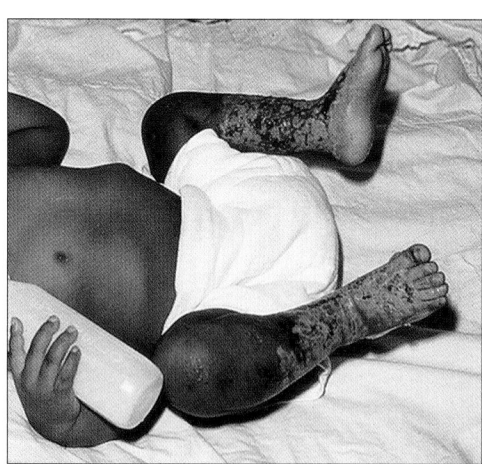

Fig. 89.8 Burn injury due to dunking in hot water by the father. Courtesy of Leo Litter MD.

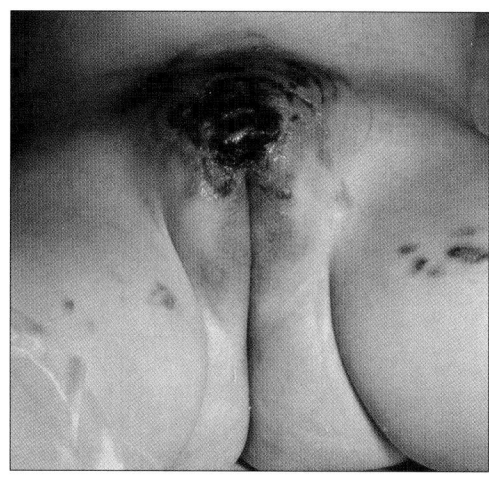

Fig. 89.9 Multiple erosions and ulcerations in child who was sexually abused. Courtesy of Ronald P Rapini MD.

PHYSICAL SIGNS OF CHILDHOOD SEXUAL ABUSE
Diagnostic
• Attenuation of the hymen with loss of tissue
• Fresh tears or scars of the hymen
• Anal margin extending out onto perianal skin
Suggestive
• Gaping hymenal opening
• Notch or concavity in posterior half of hymen
• Notch in anterior half of hymen (if asymmetric and associated with other abnormalities)
• Anal fissures
• Gaping of anal sphincter with mucosal prolapse
• Laxity of anal sphincter with edema ('tire sign')
• Dilated perianal veins
• Reflex anal dilatation

Table 89.1 Physical signs of childhood sexual abuse.

any such report by a child should be thoroughly investigated. Unfortunately, false accusations by parents involved in custody disputes have become increasingly common in recent years and are a burden to the medical and legal systems.

Physical signs that are diagnostic or suggestive of childhood sexual abuse are described in Table 89.1. However, physical findings may be absent following sexual abuse. Many types of sexual molestation such as fondling and oral sodomy may not leave physical findings. Even when injury occurs, healing in the anogenital area may be rapid and the result is very subtle or undetectable physical findings[10,11]. Acute findings that should alert the physician to the possibility of abuse include fresh genital (Fig. 89.9) or anal injuries without an adequate explanation to account for accidental trauma[12]. In the absence of a history of trauma or severe constipation, anal fissures or scarring may be suggestive of abuse. Pierce[13] reported that among 50 children with a strong history of anal abuse, 41 (82%) had anal fissures or scars. In contrast, only 2 of 81 children with no history of sexual abuse had fissures and none had scars.

The amount of data regarding normal physical findings in the genital area of female children is increasing rapidly. There is no documented case of an infant girl being born without a hymen[12]. Studies of newborns report that anterior hymenal clefts are common, but posterior clefts are not normally seen[12]. Anatomic features that are suggestive of penetration include narrowing of the posterior hymenal rim to less than 1 mm and complete hymenal clefts located between 5 and 7 o'clock[14]. Comparison of the transhymenal diameters in prepubertal girls with a history of penetration versus those without a history of sexual abuse showed that the first group had a significantly larger transverse opening when examined in the knee-chest position (5.6 vs. 4.6 mm), although there was extensive overlap between lthe two groups[15]. The presence of semen, sperm or acid phosphatase is indi-

cative of abuse, as is the presence of non-perinatally acquired syphilis, gonorrhea or HIV infection; other modes of acquiring HIV must also be excluded[12]. Perinatally acquired infections with *Chlamydia trachomatis* have been documented to persist as long as 28 months; therefore, infections with this organism in young children are not conclusive evidence of abuse.

Present evidence suggests that anogenital warts in children may be perinatally acquired, transmitted during the routine care of children, autoinoculated from other sites of infection, or acquired as a result of sexual abuse. Great variation exists in the incidence of documented or strongly suspected sexual abuse in recent studies of children with anogenital warts, ranging from a low of 6% of 31 children[16] to a high of 91% of 11 children[17]. In most studies, proven abuse is uncommon in children with anogenital warts who are younger than 3 years of age[18].

Differential Diagnosis

Although it may be difficult to differentiate abuse from accidental injury in a child, the distribution of injuries may be helpful. Children suspected of being abused have significantly more soft tissue injuries on the cheeks, trunk, genitalia and upper legs than accidentally injured children[7]. Labbe & Caouette[19] performed over 2000 skin examinations in 1467 normal children to determine the type and location of recent skin injuries. The majority of children over 9 months of age had at least one injury, usually a bruise, but 15 or more injuries was rare. The lower limbs were the most commonly involved sites. Less than 2% of the children had injuries to the thorax, abdomen, pelvis or buttocks, and less than 1% to the chin, ears or neck. Bruises were rare in infants who are not independently mobile. Therefore, injury in infants or in the locations mentioned above should arouse suspicion of the possibility of abuse.

In a retrospective study of medical records submitted to the National Pediatrics Trauma Registry in the US between 1988 and 1997, child abuse accounted for 10.6% of all blunt trauma in patients younger than 5 years of age[20]. Abused children were significantly younger and were more likely to have a pre-injury medical history and retinal hemorrhages than were children with accidental injuries. Abused children also were more likely to sustain intracranial, thoracic and abdominal injuries and to sustain very serious injuries. The child may present with skin signs of multiple types of physical abuse, and both acute and healing lesions may be present in chronically abused children.

In non-accidental burns, adults responsible for the child (and possibly the burn) frequently claim not to have witnessed the burning incident[21]. Relatives other than the adult responsible for the burn commonly bring the child to the hospital. A delay between injury and seeking medical care often occurs with inflicted burns.

There are several disorders – in particular, cutaneous disorders – that may be confused with child abuse (Table 89.2; Fig. 89.10). In addition, normal anatomy may be mistaken for childhood sexual abuse. Twenty-five percent of newborn girls have a white line or linea vestibularis in the posterior vestibule that could be confused with scar tissue produced by sexual abuse[22]. Other conditions that may be confused with sexual abuse are listed in Table 89.3.

CONDITIONS THAT CAN MIMIC CHILD ABUSE	
Condition	**Comments**
Bleeding into the skin (ecchymoses, purpura) • Multiple bruises due to platelet or clotting disorders • Ehlers–Danlos syndrome, especially the vascular type (type IV) • Bruising due to 'cupping' or cao gio (coin rubbing) • Vasculitis, particularly Henoch–Schönlein purpura and acute hemorrhagic edema of infancy	• Areas most commonly traumatized by children (e.g. shins, knees) • Common sites of trauma, especially shins • Primarily children from SE Asia (see Ch. 133) • Favors lower extremities and buttocks; associated edema and arthritis
Blue discoloration of skin mistaken as bruising • Dermal melanocytosis • Infantile hemangioma (deep) or vascular malformation	• Lack of progression of color to green or yellow; favors presacrum and back
Linear hyperpigmentation • Phytophotodermatitis	
Vesicles, bullae or erosions mistaken as non-accidental burns • Impetigo, ecthyma, blistering distal dactylitis • Erythema multiforme, fixed drug eruption • Bullous mastocytosis • Irritant contact dermatitis • Arthropod bite reaction • Moxibustion • Burn from a hot car seat or seat-belt buckle	 • e.g. laxative-induced irritant contact dermatitis mimicking an immersion burn • Primarily children from SE Asia (see Ch. 133)
Other • Osteogenesis imperfecta • Hair tourniquet	• Multiple fractures, blue sclerae

Table 89.2 Conditions that can mimic child abuse.

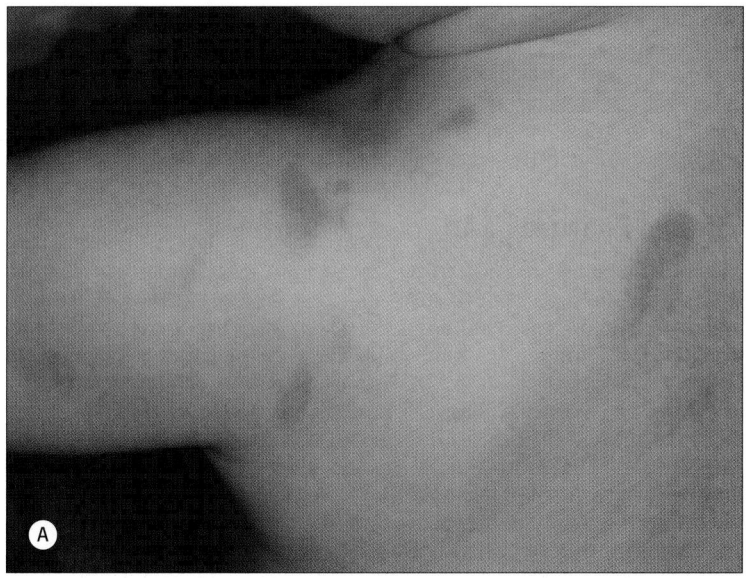

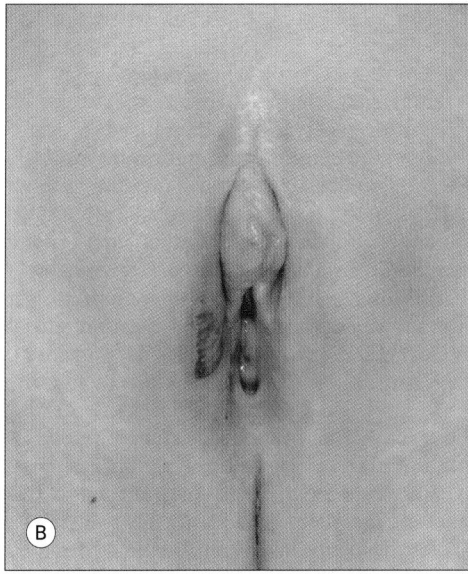

Fig. 89.10 Cutaneous disorders that may be misdiagnosed as physical or sexual abuse. A Linear hyperpigmented streaks on the back of a 2-year-old girl due to phytophotodermatitis; the parent had lime juice on her hand and touched the child. **B** Genital lichen sclerosus may have associated purpura or hemorrhagic bullae. Courtesy of Anthony J Mancini MD.

CONDITIONS OCCASIONALLY MISDIAGNOSED AS CHILDHOOD SEXUAL ABUSE

• Congenital anomalies
• Accidental injury
• Perianal streptococcal infection
• Lichen sclerosus (may be associated with purpura or hemorrhagic bullae)
• Genital vitiligo
• Localized vulvar bullous pemphigoid or other bullous diseases
• Crohn's disease
• Entities misdiagnosed as genital or perianal warts
  • Perianal pyramidal protrusion
  • Molluscum contagiosum
  • Pseudoverrucous papules and nodules due to encopresis or urinary incontinence
  • Perianal papillomatous lesions of Goltz syndrome

Table 89.3 Conditions occasionally misdiagnosed as childhood sexual abuse.

Evaluation and Management

When any lesion suspicious for abuse is present, the entire cutaneous surface of a child should be examined, as well as the oral, rectal and genital mucosae. If parents lack an explanation for a child's injuries, relate circumstances not compatible with the physical findings, describe activities of which a child is developmentally incapable, give differing stories or change their stories, child abuse should be suspected. Detailed records of any traumatic lesions should be made. If possible, photographs should be taken to characterize physical findings more precisely. During the examination, an attempt should be made to determine the age of individual lesions and to identify potentially associated injuries. A funduscopic examination to look for retinal hemorrhages, which can occur secondary to head trauma or after severe shaking of a child, should be done. In a child under 3 years of age, the presence of extensive, bilateral retinal hemorrhages raises a strong possibility of abuse[23]. An otoscopic examination of the ears to exclude hemotympanum should also be done. Skeletal surveys are usually recommended to evaluate for

EVALUATION AND MANAGEMENT OF SUSPECTED CHILD ABUSE
• Examine entire cutaneous surface as well as oral, rectal and genital mucosae • Detail any traumatic lesions in medical record • Photograph injuries whenever possible • Funduscopic examination for retinal hemorrhages • Otoscopic examination to exclude hemotympanum • Skeletal surveys in children under 6 years of age • Treatment of acute injury or infections • Report by telephone suspected abuse to local child protective services agency • Protection of the child from further injury while suspected abuse is being investigated • Long-term counseling for proven abuse

Table 89.4 Evaluation and management of suspected child abuse.

unsuspected fractures, especially in children under the age of 6 years. A summary of generally recommended steps in the evaluation and management of suspected abuse is provided in Table 89.4.

Acute injuries and infections should be treated and laboratory data obtained when appropriate. Most governments require physicians to report suspected physical abuse, neglect and sexual abuse of children. Healthcare providers reporting suspected abuse in good faith are usually provided with legal protection. Check with laws in your locale, and obtain legal advice if necessary. An initial report should be made by telephone, followed by a factual, non-accusatory written report to the local child protective services agency. The child should be protected from further injury while suspected abuse is being investigated. Abuse is often repeated if no intervention is made on behalf of the child. Therapy in the form of counseling should be obtained for abusive families.

When a child gives a history of sexual abuse or when specific physical findings for abuse are present, an immediate referral should be made to a child protective services agency. Whenever possible, the physical examination of a child suspected of being sexually abused should be done by a pediatrician or gynecologist experienced in evaluating children for possible abuse. Anogenital examination by multiple physicians should be avoided if possible, given the potential trauma this may impose on the child. When the history and/or physical findings suggest the possibility of oral, genital or rectal contact, appropriate cultures and serologic tests should be obtained. In the absence of a definitive history or physical findings, it seems most appropriate for experienced medical personnel to make the decision of whether sexual abuse is likely and referral to child protective services is warranted, since the potential negative impact of misdiagnosis on the family structure is substantial[24].

Victims of all types of abuse may suffer long-term psychologic consequences. Some children withdraw and develop feelings of worthlessness, helplessness, hopelessness and depression. Others exhibit aggressive and impulsive behavior and are at risk for delinquency, substance abuse, absenteeism from school or work, adolescent pregnancy, sexual promiscuity and prostitution. Abused children are more likely as adults to be abusive to their own children and spouses. Thus, long-term psychologic support for abused children is desirable.

In summary, the dermatologist may be the first physician to encounter the abused child, so it is important to be alert for possible abuse, perform the appropriate documentation and testing, and report it to the proper authorities. It is often necessary to enlist the help of a primary care physician or gynecologist experienced in the evaluation of abuse. A recent atlas by Hobbs & Wynne[25] provides additional information and many color illustrations.

ELDER ABUSE

Key features

■ Intentional actions that cause harm or create a serious risk of harm

■ Failure by a caretaker to satisfy the basic needs of an elder or to protect the elder from harm

TYPES OF ELDER ABUSE
Physical abuse Psychologic abuse Sexual assault Material exploitation Neglect

Table 89.5 Types of elder abuse.

Introduction

The establishment in 1997 of the International Network for the Prevention of Elder Abuse, with representatives from countries throughout the world, demonstrates that there is international concern about elder abuse[26]. Key features (listed above) of elder abuse have been defined by a panel convened by the US National Academy of Sciences[27]. Both clinical reports and most international legal statutes recognize the types of abuse listed in Table 89.5.

Risk Factors for Elder Abuse

Because of increased opportunities for contact and thus for conflict and tension, a shared living arrangement is a major risk factor for elder abuse[28,29]. People living alone are at lowest risk for abuse except for financial abuse, which is more likely to occur among elders who live alone[30]. Physical abuse is reported to occur more frequently in elders with dementia than in those without this disorder[31,32]. Social isolation has also been identified as a risk factor, with victims more likely to be isolated from friends and family (other than the person with whom they may be living) than are non-victims[26,33]. Pathologic characteristics of perpetrators of elder abuse include mental illness, particularly depression and alcohol abuse[34–36]. Additionally, people who abuse elders may be heavily dependent on the person they are abusing. In some cases, abuse stems from attempts by relatives (particularly adult offspring) to obtain the victim's resources[37].

Clinical Features and Assessment

Most of the physical indicators described in elder abuse are derived from anecdotal case reports and small case series. Lachs & Pillemer[26] have integrated these findings with their own experience and have developed a guideline for medical assessment of patients when elder abuse is suspected (Table 89.6). Special attention should be given to assessing the cognitive status of suspected abuse victims, as their ability to make decisions for themselves will affect possible subsequent interventions[26]. Unfortunately, abused elders may not always have findings clearly attributable to abuse. Conversely, older individuals may have findings that mimic abuse but which are actually a result of accidental injuries or chronic disease[26].

If elder abuse is suspected, a comprehensive assessment should be done by a provider with substantial clinical and psychosocial expertise. The patient should not be examined in the presence of the suspected abuser. The presence of other healthcare staff should be minimized, since many patients are ashamed to admit that they are victims of elder abuse[26]. Although direct questions about abuse are appropriate, the interviewer may prefer to begin with general questions about safety issues and the home environment. Attempts to elicit details about the nature, frequency and provoking factors of abuse are recommended[26].

The physician must use considerable caution in interacting with a suspected abuser. One of the risks of confronting an alleged abuser is that access to the elderly person may be lost. If the physician deems it necessary to interview a suspected abuser, an empathetic non-judgmental approach may be helpful[26].

Management

Because elder abuse is multifactorial, Lachs & Pillemer[26] have suggested potential interventions based on the context of abuse (Table 89.7). A multidisciplinary team involving physicians, nurses, social workers, elder care attorneys and, when appropriate, adult protection agencies

POTENTIAL FINDINGS IN ELDER ABUSE	
Behavior observations	• Withdrawal • Absence of eye contact with interviewer • Infantilizing of patient by caregiver • Functionally impaired patient who presents without designated caregiver
General appearance	• Hygiene, cleanliness and appropriateness of dress
Skin and mucous membranes	• Skin turgor, other signs of dehydration • Multiple abrasions in various stages of evolution • Wrist or ankle lesions suggestive of restraint use • Bruises (shape may suggest implement used) • Decubitus ulcers • Lack of care provided for established skin lesions • Infestations • Immersion burn (stocking/glove distribution)
Head and neck	• Traumatic alopecia (distinguishable from androgenetic alopecia on basis of distribution) • Scalp hematomas, lacerations, abrasions
Genitourinary	• Rectal or vaginal bleeding could indicate sexual abuse
Musculoskeletal	• Examination for occult fracture, pain • Observe gait • Fractures that are not explained by mechanisms of reported injury

Table 89.6 **Potential findings in elder abuse.** Adapted from Lachs MS, Pillemen K. Elder abuse. Lancet 2004;364:1263–72.

and law enforcement officials may be most effective in dealing with elder abuse. Specific interventions will depend on whether or not the abused person is willing to accept intervention. If the individual is willing to accept services, then education regarding elder abuse can be provided, a safety plan implemented (e.g. placement in a safe home), and the patient as well as family members referred to appropriate services. On the other hand, if intervention is refused, the physician must try to determine if the individual has the mental capacity to make that decision. When the patient lacks the mental capacity, conservatorship and an order of protection may be required, whereas if the patient has the ability to make decisions, then education, a potential safety plan, emergency phone numbers and a follow-up plan are provided.

In summary, dermatologists should remain vigilant in observing for physical signs of abuse in elderly patients, particularly in those

INTERVENTIONS FOR ELDER ABUSE	
Context of elder abuse	**Potential interventions**
Abuse potentially related to stress from caring for impaired family member	Respite services Adult daycare Caregiver education programs (e.g. on what constitutes abuse) Recruitment of other family, informal, or paid caregivers to share burden of care Psychotherapy for caregiver Treatment for depression Social integration of caregiver to reduce isolation
Violence related to substance or alcohol misuse	Referral to alcohol or drug misuse rehabilitation programs as appropriate
Violence related to behavioral problems associated with mental health	Treatment referral
Longstanding spousal violence	Marital counseling Support groups Shelter Orders of protection Victim advocacy
Abuse by aggressive dementia patient	Geriatric medical assessment of causes of underlying behavior
Financial exploitation by family members	Guardianship proceeding, power of attorney (transfer of legal authority) Protective services
Financial exploitation by paid caregiver	Referral to legal services Involvement of law enforcement Protective services

Table 89.7 **Interventions for elder abuse.** From Lachs MS, Pilleman K. Elder abuse. Lancet 2004;364:1263–72.

dependent on caregivers. Even though patients suspected of being abused should be evaluated, wherever possible, by individuals with expertise in elder abuse, the dermatologist may be the first healthcare provider to encounter or recognize the signs of abuse and therefore responsible for initiating the evaluation process for these fragile members of society.

REFERENCES

1. American Academy of Pediatrics Committee on Child Abuse and Neglect. Guidelines for the evaluation of sexual abuse of children. Pediatrics. 1991;87:254–60.
2. Caffey J. Multiple fractures in the long bones of infants suffering from chronic subdural hematoma. Am J Roentgenol Radium Ther. 1946;56:163–73.
3. Kempe CH, Silverman FN, Steele BF, Droegemueller W, Silver HK. The battered child syndrome. JAMA. 1962;181:17–24.
4. Berger LM. Income, family characteristics, and physical violence toward children. Child Abuse Negl. 2005;29:107–33.
5. Finkelhor D. Epidemiological factors in the clinical identification of child sexual abuse. Child Abuse Negl. 1993;17:67–70.
6. Holmes WC, Slap GB. Sexual abuse of boys. Definition, prevalence, correlates, sequelae and management. JAMA. 1998;280:1855–62.
7. Maguire S, Mann MK, Sibert J, Kemp A. Are there patterns of bruising in childhood which are diagnostic or suggestive of abuse? A systematic review. Arch Dis Child. 2005;90:182–6.
8. Raimer BG, Raimer SS, Hebeler JR. Cutaneous signs of child abuse. J Am Acad Dermatol. 1981;5:203–12.
9. Levine LJ. The solution of a battered-child homicide by dental evidence: report of a case. J Am Dent Assoc. 1973;87:1234–6.
10. McCann J, Voris J, Simon M. Genital injuries resulting from sexual abuse: a longitudinal study. Pediatrics. 1992;89:307–17.
11. Topley J, Thomas A, Hobbs C, Wynne J. Detection of child sexual abuse. Am J Obstet Gynecol. 2001;184:1043–5.
12. Bays J, Chadwick D. Medical diagnosis of the sexually abused child. Child Abuse Negl. 1993;17:91–110.
13. Pierce AM. Anal fissures and anal scars in anal abuse – are they significant? Pediatr Surg Int. 2004;20:334–8.
14. Johnson CF. Child sexual abuse. Lancet. 2004;364:462–70.
15. Berenson AB, Chacko MR, Wiemann CM, et al. Use of hymenal measurements in the diagnosis of previous penetration. Pediatrics. 2002;109:228–35.
16. Handley J, Hanks E, Armstrong K, et al. Common association of HPV 2 with anogenital warts in prepubertal children. Pediatr Dermatol. 1997;5:339–43.
17. Herman-Giddens ME, Gutman LT, Berson NL, and the Duke Child Protection Team. Association of coexisting vaginal infections and multiple abusers in female children with genital warts. Sex Transm Dis. 1988;15:63–7.
18. Cohen BA, Honig P, Androphy E. Anogenital warts in children. Clinical and virologic evaluation for sexual abuse. Arch Dermatol. 1990;126:1575–80.
19. Labbe J, Caouette G. Recent skin injuries in normal children. Pediatrics. 2001;108:271–6.
20. DiScala C, Sege R, Li G, Reece RM. Child abuse and unintentional injuries: a 10-year retrospective. Arch Pediatr Adolesc Med. 2000;154:16–22.
21. Greenbaum AR, Donne J, Wilson D, Dunn KW. Intentional burn injury: an evidence-based, clinical and forensic review. Burns. 2004;30:628–42.
22. Kellogg ND, Parra JM. Linea vestibularis: a previously undescribed normal genital structure in female neonates. Pediatrics. 1991;87:926–9.
23. Kivlin JD. Manifestations of the shaken baby syndrome. Curr Opin Ophthalmol. 2001;12:158–63.
24. Vorenberg E. Diagnosing child abuse. The cost of getting it wrong. Arch Dermatol. 1992;128:844–5.
25. Hobbs CJ, Wynne JM. Physical Signs of Child Abuse: A Colour Atlas, 2nd edn. London: WB Saunders, 2001.
26. Lachs MS, Pillemer K. Elder abuse. Lancet. 2004;364:1263–72.
27. Bonnie RJ, Wallace RB (eds). Elder Mistreatment: Abuse, Neglect, and Exploitation in an Aging America. Washington, DC: National Academies Press, 2002.
28. Pillemer K, Finkelhor D. The prevalence of elder abuse: a random sample survey. Gerontologist. 1988;28:51–7.
29. Lachs MS, Williams C, O'Brien S, Hurst L, Horwitz R. Risk factors for reported elder abuse and neglect: a nine-year observational cohort study. Gerontologist. 1997;37:469–74.
30. Choi NG, Kulick DB, Mayer J. Financial exploitation of elders: analysis of risk factors based on county adult protective services data. J Elder Abuse Negl. 1999;10:39–62.
31. Paveza GJ, Cohen D, Eisdorfer C, et al. Severe family violence and Alzheimer's disease: prevalence and risk factors. Gerontologist. 1992;32:493–7.
32. Pillemer K, Suitor JJ. Violence and violent feelings: what causes them among family caregivers? J Gerontol. 1992;47:S165–72.

33. Lachs MS, Berkman L, Fulmer T, Horwitz RI. A prospective community-based pilot study of risk factors for the investigation of elder mistreatment. J Am Geriatr Soc. 1994;42:169–73.

34. Homer AC, Gilleard C. Abuse of elderly people by their carers. BMJ. 1990;301:1359–62.

35. Reay AM, Browne KD. Risk factor characteristics in carers who physically abuse or neglect their elderly dependants. Aging Ment Health. 2001;5:56–62.

36. Anetzberger GJ, Korbin JE, Austin C. Alcoholism and elder abuse. J Interpers Viol. 1994;9:184–93.

37. Greenberg JR, McKibben M, Raymond JA. Dependent adult children and elder abuse. J Elder Abuse Negl. 1990;2:73–86.

Histiocytoses

Warren T Goodman and Terry L Barrett

OVERVIEW

The histiocytoses represent a group of proliferative disorders with a common progenitor cell in the bone marrow. Three 'histiocytes' of cutaneous importance are the Langerhans cell, which migrates to and from the epidermis and functions as a potent antigen-presenting cell (APC), the mononuclear cell/macrophage (sometimes called the 'true' histiocyte), which migrates to and from the dermis and has both phagocytic and APC properties, and the dermal dendrocyte, which may represent a reservoir of pluripotential mononuclear cells with both phagocytic and APC potential.

The dysfunction of these cells has led to a group of well-known but poorly understood disorders. For years, many of the histiocytoses were known by numerous names, reflecting the lack of understanding and agreement regarding their origin. Electron microscopy and the development of immunohistochemical stains have provided insight into these conditions. It is now clear that the histiocytoses are closely related entities, with Langerhans cell histiocytosis (LCH) representing one group of disorders and non-Langerhans cell histiocytosis (non-LCH) representing another.

Many believe that, within a given group, the various disorders simply represent different phases of disease along a spectrum. This is often supported by similar histologic and clinical findings amongst the disorders. In addition, differences in the immunophenotype of the non-LCH disorders are not clear. There appears to be significant staining variation between lesions of the same disorder, with immunophenotypic 'exceptions' very common. This chapter covers the most common and many of the rarer histiocytic disorders. The hemophagocytic syndromes are outlined in Table 90.1 and the malignant histiocytic disorders are beyond the scope of this chapter.

LANGERHANS CELL HISTIOCYTOSIS

Synonyms:
- Langerhans cell histiocytosis (LCH; class I histiocytosis, histiocytosis X), comprising:
    - Letterer–Siwe disease
    - Hand–Schüller–Christian disease
    - Eosinophilic granuloma
    - Congenital self-healing reticulohistiocytosis (Hashimoto–Pritzker disease)

Key features

- LCH is a clonal proliferative disorder
- LCH cells are S100- and CD1a-positive
- Ultrastructurally, intracytoplasmic Birbeck granules are seen
- Osteolytic bone lesions are common
- Diabetes insipidus is common

Introduction

Langerhans cell histiocytosis (LCH) is a clonal proliferative disease of Langerhans cells that express an immunophenotype positive for S100 and CD1a, and which contain cytoplasmic Birbeck granules. LCH represents a disease spectrum with four prominent but overlapping syndromes:
- Letterer–Siwe disease
- Hand–Schüller–Christian disease
- Eosinophilic granuloma
- Congenital self-healing reticulohistiocytosis (Hashimoto–Pritzker disease)

Disease expression ranges from mild, sometimes asymptomatic, single-organ involvement to severe, progressive multisystem disease

History

Letterer–Siwe disease, Hand–Schüller–Christian disease and eosinophilic granuloma were described in the early 20th century. In 1953, Lichtenstein[2] grouped the three disorders into a single entity which he called *histiocytosis X*. In 1978, Hashimoto & Pritzker[3] described the entity congenital self-healing reticulohistiocytosis. Immunologic and ultrastructural studies confirmed the relationship of the pathologic cells in histiocytosis X and congenital self-healing reticulohistiocytosis to Langerhans cells, providing a basis for the Writing Group of the Histiocyte Society[4], in 1987, to reclassify them as 'Langerhans cell histiocytoses'.

Epidemiology

LCH occurs worldwide and most commonly develops in children ages 1–3 years, though disease can develop at any age. The reported incidence of LCH varies widely. However, many authorities quote an annual incidence of at least 5 per million children, with the adult incidence suspected to be less than one-third that of children. LCH is more common in boys, with a male:female ratio of nearly 2:1. In adults, there may be a slight female predominance.

Some cases of LCH appear to be familial. A recent study demonstrated simultaneous development of LCH in four of five monozygotic twin pairs and in one of three dizygotic pairs[5]. Additionally, in two families with affected non-twin siblings, parental consanguinity was known in one and possible in the other.

Pathogenesis

The pathogenesis of LCH remains unknown. Viral and immunologic etiologies have long been considered, though no studies have thus far demonstrated a primary immune abnormality in patients with LCH, and there has been no consistent detection of viral genomes in LCH tissue. An extensive investigation utilizing PCR and *in situ* hybridization to identify nine possible viruses in LCH was performed by McClain et al[6]. In contrast to an earlier study, which detected human herpesvirus type 6 (HHV-6) genomes in LCH tissue, these investigators found no evidence linking the tested viruses to LCH.

Recent studies have demonstrated elevated levels of cytokines in lesions of patients with LCH. These have included TNF-α, interferon-γ, granulocyte–monocyte colony-stimulating factor (GM-CSF), interleukin (IL)-1, IL-2, IL-4 and IL-10, among others. While not known to be responsible for the development of disease, these cytokines and interleukins are thought to promote various disease-related symptoms and morbidity.

A genetic basis for LCH, either primary or secondary, now appears likely. As discussed previously, at least a small subset of LCH appears to be hereditary[5]. Secondly, several recent studies by different investigators demonstrated clonal CD1a+ histiocytes in all LCH tissue tested[7,8]. On the basis of these results, Willman et al.[7] proposed that LCH is likely a clonal neoplastic disorder with highly variable biologic behavior.

Clinical features

The four well-described variants of LCH have significant clinical overlap. However, many no longer attempt to differentiate between the

CLINICAL FEATURES OF THE HISTIOCYTOSES

Histiocytosis	Usual age	Most common mucocutaneous sites	Other findings
Langerhans cell histiocytoses			
Letterer–Siwe disease	0–2 years	Scalp, flexural areas, trunk	Visceral and bone lesions
Hand–Schüller–Christian disease	2–6 years	Scalp, flexural areas, trunk, gingiva	Diabetes insipidus, bone lesions, exophthalmos
Eosinophilic granuloma	7–12 years	Skin lesions rare	Bone lesions primarily
Congenital self-healing reticulohistiocytosis (Hashimoto–Pritzker disease)	Congenital	Widespread, localized, or single lesion	Spontaneous resolution
Non-Langerhans cell histiocytoses			
Primarily cutaneous, usually self-resolving			
Juvenile xanthogranuloma	0–2 years	Head and neck > upper trunk > extremities	Rare eye and visceral lesions
Benign cephalic histiocytosis	0–3 years	Face and neck > trunk and extremities	Usually none, spontaneous resolution
Giant cell reticulohistiocytoma	Adults	Head (solitary lesion)	None
Generalized eruptive histiocytoma	<4 and 20–50 years	Widespread (axial)	Spontaneous resolution
Indeterminate cell histiocytosis	Any	Widespread > face and neck	Uncommon visceral and bone lesions
Primarily cutaneous, often persistent/progressive			
*Papular xanthoma	Any	Generalized (discrete yellow papules and papulonodules with relative sparing of flexural sites)	None
*Progressive nodular histiocytoma	Any	Generalized (discrete yellow papules and nodules with prominent facial involvement)	May represent same entity as the progressive form of papular xanthoma[1]
Frequent systemic involvement			
Necrobiotic xanthogranuloma	17–60 years	Periorbital > other face, trunk, extremities	Paraproteinemia, hepatosplenomegaly, lymphoproliferative disease
Multicentric reticulohistiocytosis	30–50 years	Head; hands, elbows (over joints); mucosa (oral, nasopharyngeal)	Arthritis (often destructive), up to 30% with internal malignancy
Rosai–Dorfman disease	10–30 years	Eyelids and malar area	Massive lymphadenopathy in a subset of patients, fever, hypergammaglobulinemia; skin-limited form increasingly recognized
Xanthoma disseminatum	Any	Flexural areas to widespread > mucosa (oral, nasopharyngeal)	Diabetes insipidus
Systemic with rare skin involvement			
*Erdheim–Chester disease	Any	Periorbital area, scalp, trunk, extremities (yellow nodules and indurated plaques)	Bone lesions, exophthalmos, diabetes insipidus; involvement of the lungs, kidneys, adrenals, heart, CNS, retroperitoneum and testes

*Hemophagocytic lymphohistiocytosis (HLH; hemophagocytic syndrome)
• Primary (genetic; see Table 59.5)
  – Familial HLH‡, Chédiak–Higashi syndrome, Griscelli syndrome type 2, and X-linked lymphoproliferative syndrome
• Secondary (acquired)
  – Infection-associated (e.g. EBV, CMV)§
  – Malignancy-associated (e.g. T-cell lymphoma)
  – Macrophage activation syndrome associated with autoimmune connective tissue disease (e.g. Still's disease, systemic lupus erythematosus)
	Primary: 0–2 years
	Secondary: any
		Generalized (purpuric macules and papules, morbilliform eruptions, erythroderma, keratotic nodules) or acral (erythematous macules)†; malignancy-associated forms may present with lesions of cutaneous or subcutaneous T-cell lymphoma	Fever, hepatosplenomegaly, cytopenias, hypertriglyceridemia, hypofibrinogenemia, histologic evidence of hemophagocytosis (e.g. in the bone marrow, lymph nodes or spleen), low natural killer cell activity, hyperferritinemia, elevated soluble CD25 (plus evidence of infectious agent, malignancy or autoimmune connective tissue disease in secondary forms)

*Not covered in the body of the text.
†Skin biopsy specimens rarely demonstrate hemophagocytosis.
‡In the US, most commonly due to mutations in the gene that encodes perforin
§A list of infectious agents associated with HLH is available at www.cdc.gov/ncidod/eid/vol6no6/fisman_refs.htm.

Table 90.1 Clinical features of the histiocytoses. EBV, Epstein-Barr virus; CMV, cytomegalovirus.

various syndromes seen in LCH, recognizing that LCH is one disease with a wide clinical spectrum and a highly varied course. For historical context, the three classically described variants and the more recently recognized congenital self-healing reticulohistiocytosis are discussed here.

Letterer–Siwe disease is the acute diffuse form of LCH. It is a multisystem disease that nearly always develops prior to age 2 years, and commonly presents in children less than 1 year of age. Cutaneous involvement occurs in most patients as 1–2-mm pink to skin-colored papules, pustules and/or vesicles in the scalp, flexural areas of the neck, axilla and perineum, and on the trunk (Fig. 90.1). The lesions tend to coalesce and become tender. Scale and crust with secondary impetiginization, and the development of petechiae and purpura are common. Palmoplantar and nail involvement can occur. The eruption

is most often confused with seborrheic dermatitis, scabies, eczema, varicella and intertrigo.

During the course of the disease, many organs can become infiltrated by clonal LCH cells. However, only if the key functions of the organ are affected is such involvement of prognostic significance. Lung, liver, lymph node and bone involvement commonly occur at some point during the illness. Osteolytic bone lesions are painful, usually multiple, and most frequently affect the cranium. Occasionally, the hematopoietic system can be involved, with thrombocytopenia and anemia portending a poor prognosis.

Classically, Hand–Schüller–Christian disease represents the triad of diabetes insipidus, bone lesions and exophthalmos. These patients tend to have a chronic progressive course. For most, Hand–Schüller–Christian disease begins between the ages of 2 and 6 years. Patients

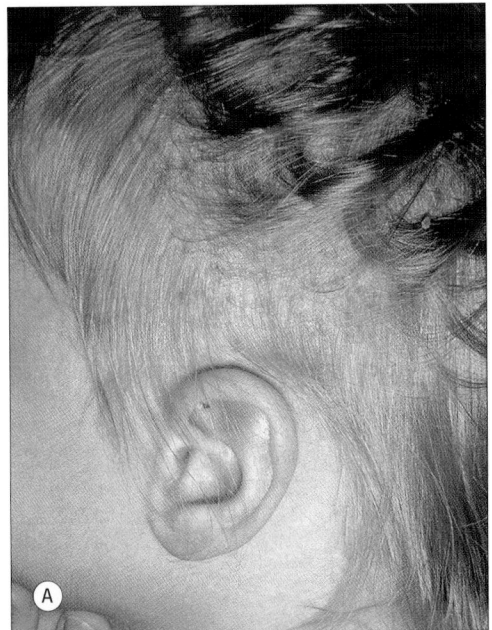

Fig. 90.1 Langerhans cell histiocytosis (Letterer–Siwe variant). A Scalp involvement may initially be diagnosed as seborrheic dermatitis; however, there are usually more discrete papules and crusting. **B** Erythematous, eroded plaques in the inguinal creases. **C** Advanced disease with widespread cutaneous involvement and prominent inguinal lymphadenopathy.

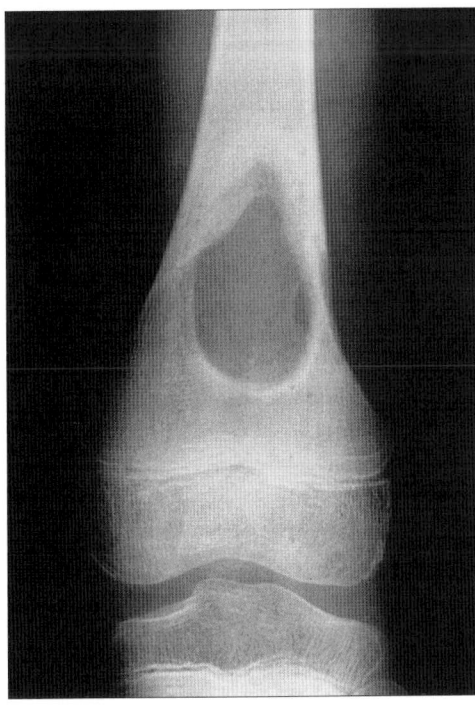

Fig. 90.2 Langerhans cell histiocytosis (eosinophilic granuloma of the bone). Radiography of the femur shows a large well-circumscribed osteolytic lesion. Courtesy of Edward McCarthy MD.

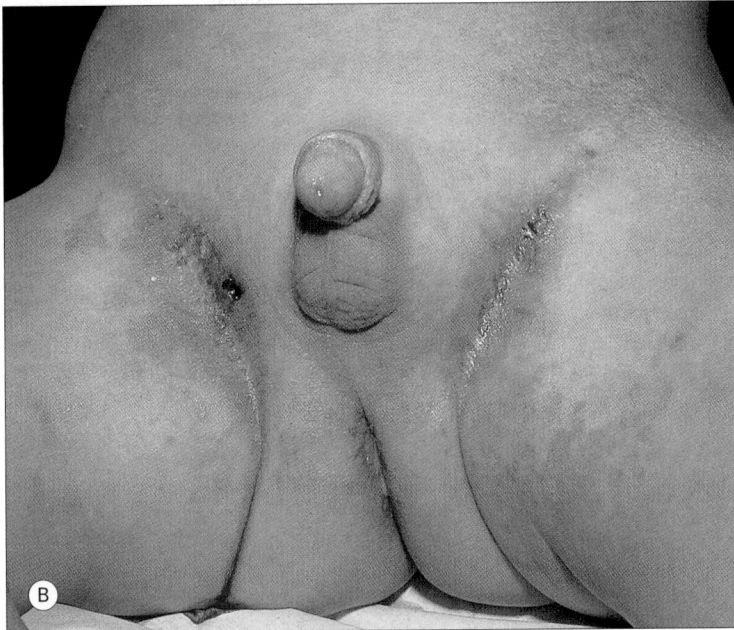

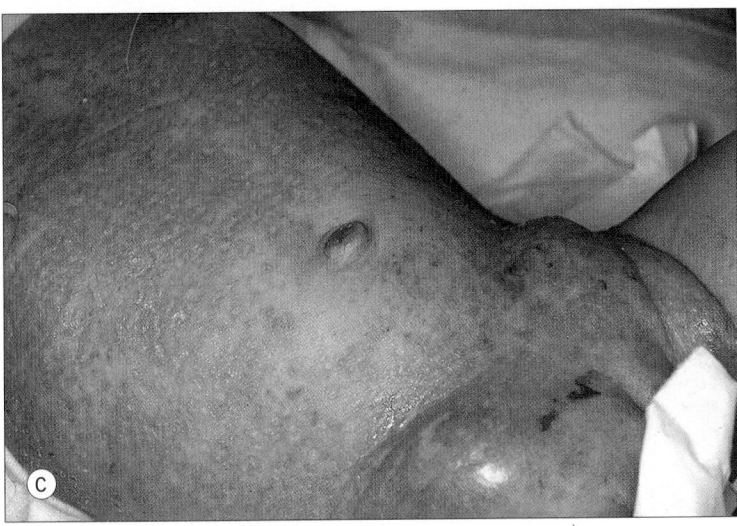

areas, with premature loss of teeth possible secondary to gingival lesions.

At least 80% of patients with Hand–Schüller–Christian disease develop bone lesions, the cranium being preferentially involved. Chronic otitis media occurs commonly in these patients and in patients with all forms of LCH. Diabetes insipidus, secondary to infiltration of the posterior pituitary by LCH cells, develops in approximately 30% of patients and is more common in those patients with cranial bone involvement. The chances of reversing the disease with radiation or chemotherapy are remote once symptoms develop. However, symptomatic treatment with vasopressin is effective.

Eosinophilic granuloma is a localized variant of LCH that generally affects older children, boys more than girls. Skin and mucous membrane lesions are rare, with a single asymptomatic granulomatous lesion of the bone the most common manifestation (Fig. 90.2). The cranium is most frequently affected, though lesions can also develop in the ribs, vertebrae, pelvis, scapulae and long bones. A spontaneous fracture or otitis media may be the first sign of disease.

Congenital self-healing reticulohistiocytosis (Hashimoto–Pritzker disease) is a variant of LCH which is generally limited to the skin and rapidly self-healing. It presents at birth or in the first few days of life with a characteristic eruption of widespread red to brown papulonodules. After several weeks, the lesions crust and involute. Solitary papules, nodules and vesicles have also been observed (Fig. 90.3). Mucous membrane lesions are rare, although systemic involvement has been reported. While congenital self-healing reticulohistiocytosis is considered a benign, self-resolving disorder, its relationship to other LCH variants suggests a cautious approach with respect to prognosis.

Adults rarely develop LCH but, when they do, the most commonly involved sites are the skin, lung and bone. Diabetes insipidus can also develop and, as in children, is more likely when bony involvement of the skull is present. Severe multisystem disease, classically referred to as Letterer–Siwe disease, is rare in adults. However, LCH can be a progressive disease in adults, especially when both bone and extraskeletal sites are involved.

Two patterns of associations between LCH and malignancy have been noted[9]. First, an increased incidence of solid tumors and leukemia has been noted in patients treated for their LCH. In 20 of 21 recently reported cases of acute lymphoblastic leukemia (ALL) or acute non-lymphoblastic leukemia (ANLL) occurring after treatment for LCH, treatment of the LCH had included chemotherapy, radiotherapy, or both. It was suspected that the increased incidence of leukemias in this group may have been secondary to the treatment for the LCH. In addition, multiple patients developed solid tumors in the fields of radiation therapy for their LCH.

with the complete triad are rare, as exophthalmos is uncommon and often a late finding. Approximately 30% of patients develop skin or mucous membrane lesions. While early cutaneous lesions are similar to those seen in Letterer–Siwe disease, older lesions may become xanthomatous. Ulcerative nodules may develop in the oral and genital

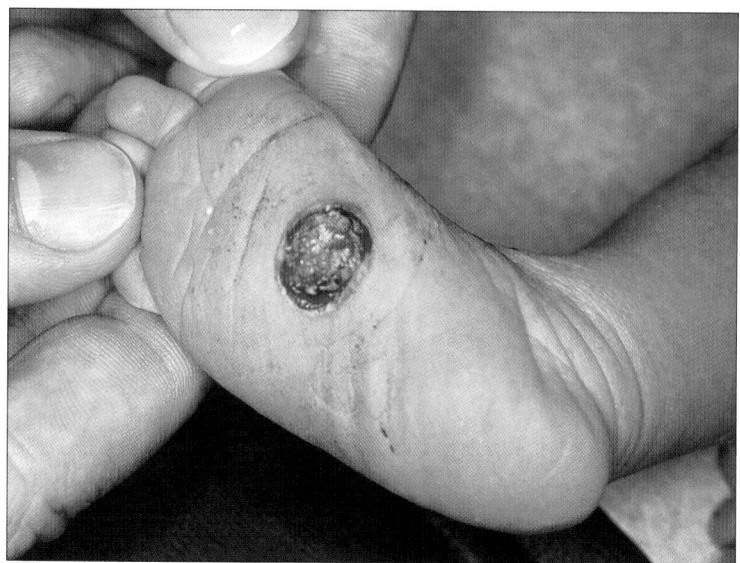

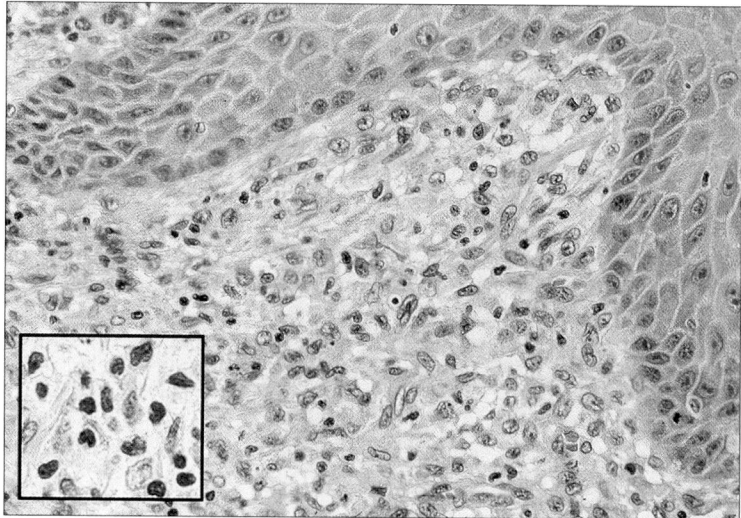

Fig. 90.4 Langerhans cell histiocytosis. Superficial dermal infiltrate of pleomorphic LCH cells. Many nuclei, as seen in the inset, show a classic reniform shape.

Fig. 90.3 Congenital self-healing reticulohistiocytosis (Hashimoto–Pritzker disease). Solitary eroded nodule on the plantar surface of a neonate. Courtesy of Richard Antaya MD.

Second, there may be an increased incidence of LCH developing in patients with ALL or solid tumors[9]. In 7 of 12 recently reported cases with both LCH and ALL, the leukemia preceded the LCH. There may also be an association between retinoblastoma and LCH. Of nine recently reported cases of solid tumors preceding LCH or developing concurrently with LCH, four were retinoblastomas[9].

The prognosis of patients with LCH varies dramatically. A high mortality rate is associated with multisystem disease, especially in children less than 2 years of age, and in any patient with multiorgan disease if the hematopoietic system, liver, lungs or spleen is involved. Even with aggressive treatment, mortality in this group of patients ranges from 38% to 54%[10]. Patients not falling into this category tend to do better. Nevertheless, progression or persistence of disease is common.

Pathology

Just as the clinical appearance of LCH is variable, so is the histologic appearance. In a typical papule, a proliferation of LCH cells is present in the papillary dermis (Fig. 90.4). These cells are large, 10–15 μm in diameter, with a reniform (kidney-shaped) nucleus. Usually, some epidermal infiltration by Langerhans cells is present, as well as interface changes. The dermal LCH cells are often admixed with eosinophils, neutrophils, lymphocytes and plasma cells. Mast cells may be present in large numbers. Secondary features such as crusting, pustule formation, hemorrhage or necrosis may obscure the characteristic LCH cell infiltrate. Older lesions that are no longer proliferative may appear granulomatous, xanthomatous or fibrous.

In nodular lesions of congenital self-healing reticulohistiocytosis, the histology may be identical to other variants of LCH. However, lesions with sheets of histiocytes with abundant eosinophilic cytoplasm,

Fig. 90.5 Immunohistochemistry of the histiocytoses.

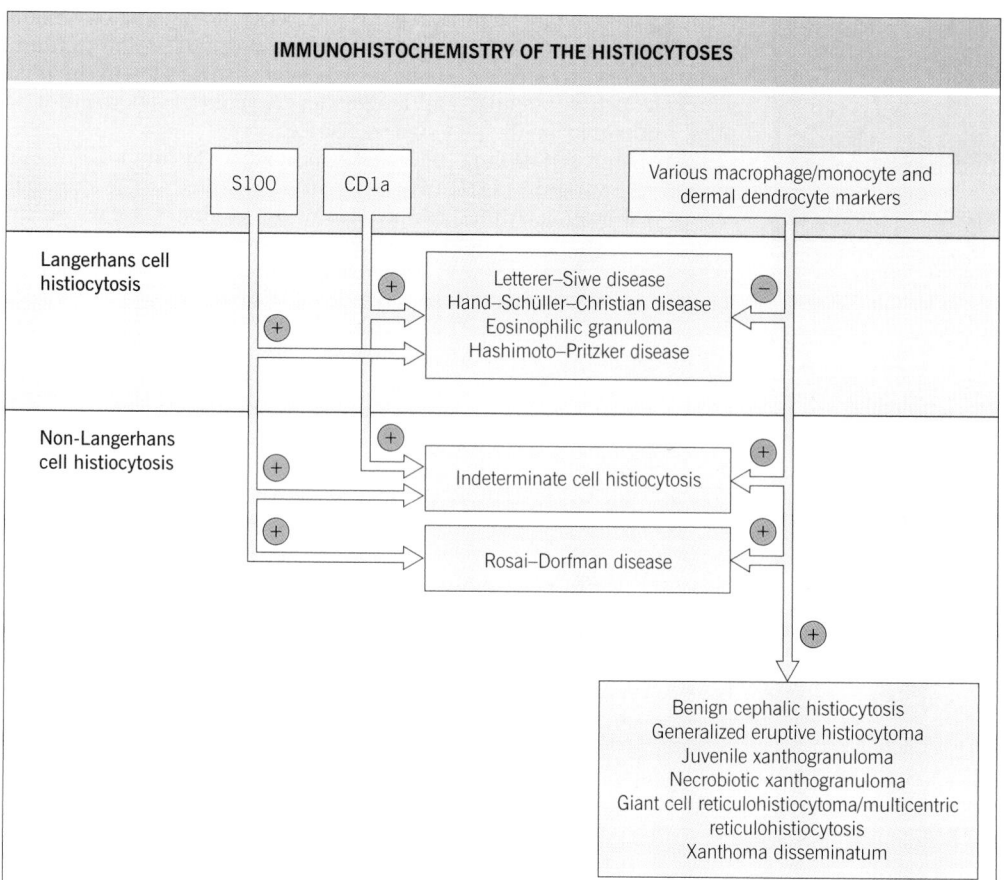

ANTIGENIC MARKERS OF THE HISTIOCYTOSES				
Histiocytic disorder	**S100**	**CD1a (OKT6)**	**CD68* (KP1/KiMP)**	**CD11b/CD11c/CD14/HAM56*/Mac387*/Factor XIIIa†**
Langerhans cell histiocytoses	+	+	–	
Juvenile xanthogranuloma			+	Variable
Benign cephalic histiocytosis			+	Variable
Giant cell reticulohistiocytoma			+	Variable
Generalized eruptive histiocytoma			+	Variable
Indeterminate cell histiocytosis	+	+	+	Variable
‡Papular xanthoma			+	Variable
‡Progressive nodular histiocytoma			+	Variable
Necrobiotic xanthogranuloma			+	Variable
Multicentric reticulohistiocytosis			+	Variable
Rosai–Dorfman disease	+	–	+	Variable
Xanthoma disseminatum			+	Variable

*Classic macrophage/monocyte markers.
†Classic dermal dendrocyte marker.
‡Not covered in the body of the text.

Table 90.2 Antigenic markers of the histiocytoses. Classical results are provided and results may vary in specific cases.

so-called 'reticulohistiocytes', intermixed with LCH cells and giant cells, have also been described. The cytoplasm of the reticulohistiocytes and the giant cells may have a 'ground glass' appearance, as in multicentric reticulohistiocytosis.

In soft tissue nodules or bone lesions, LCH cells are readily identifiable, especially during the proliferative phase of the process, as the aggregates tend to be larger. In these lesions, sheets of LCH cells may be found, and a few mitoses may be seen. Older bone lesions, on the other hand, may show only xanthomatous or fibrous changes. Early lesions should be biopsied when possible.

Langerhans cells are of bone marrow origin (see Ch. 5). Clonal LCH cells have a similar though not identical immunophenotype to Langerhans cells. Like Langerhans cells, LCH cells show positive immunostaining for CD1a and S100, and do not characteristically express factor XIIIa (a marker for dermal dendrocytes) or classic macrophage/monocyte markers such as CD68, Mac387 or HAM56 (Fig. 90.5; Table 90.2). ATPase, peanut lectin and α-D-mannosidase are positive in LCH cells, but staining for these is less often performed, as CD1a staining is more specific. Langerin (CD207), a transmembrane C-type lectin that serves as an endocytic receptor and induces Birbeck granule formation, is another highly specific Langerhans cell marker. Both Langerin and CD1a have important roles in the uptake, processing and presentation of non-peptide (e.g. lipid) antigens by Langerhans cells.

Electron microscopy demonstrates Birbeck granules, which are rod- or racquet-shaped cytoplasmic structures pathognomonic for Langerhans cells and LCH cells (Fig. 90.6). The percentage of cells with Birbeck granules in LCH lesions varies greatly and rarely they may not be detected. On average, approximately 50% of cells will demonstrate Birbeck granules. With the availability of CD1a and Langerin staining, electron microscopy is performed less frequently today than in the past.

Differential diagnosis

The clinical differential diagnosis is vast and includes seborrheic dermatitis, Darier disease, candidiasis, leukemia, lymphoma, multiple myeloma (bony lesions), urticaria pigmentosa, mycosis fungoides and the non-Langerhans cell histiocytoses (see Table 90.1). However, the characteristic histologic features of LCH will lead one to suspect the diagnosis, which is confirmed with the combination of positive immunostaining for CD1a, S100 and Langerin or demonstration of Birbeck granules on electron microscopy. The non-Langerhans cell histiocytoses do not contain Birbeck granules by electron microscopy, and, except for indeterminate cell histiocytosis and possibly Rosai–Dorfman disease, they do not characteristically express CD1a and S100. Additionally, the non-Langerhans cell histiocytoses demonstrate various macrophage markers (see Fig. 90.5, Table 90.2).

Older, less proliferative lesions, such as those often found in Hand–Schüller–Christian disease and eosinophilic granuloma, may appear

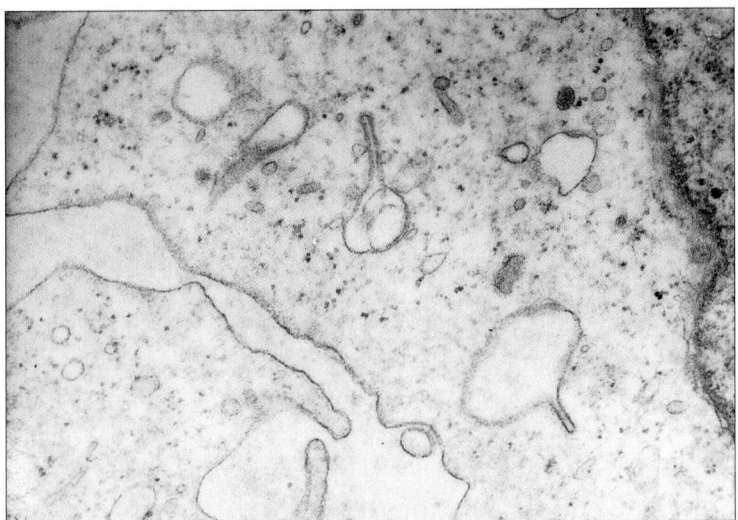

Fig. 90.6 Langerhans cell histiocytosis (Birbeck granules). Electron micrograph demonstrates classic racquet-shaped Birbeck granules in the cytoplasm of an LCH cell.

granulomatous, xanthomatous or fibrous. Here, a high index of suspicion based on the clinical findings and the radiologic appearance is required.

Treatment

All patients diagnosed with LCH should undergo evaluation of the hematologic, pulmonary, hepatic, renal and skeletal systems to determine the extent of disease. Further evaluation of the CNS and the bone marrow may be required. Treatment of LCH is dependent on the number of body systems involved and severity of involvement.

For mild single-system skin disease (if treatment is required), topical corticosteroids, topical antibacterial agents, PUVA, and topical nitrogen mustard (mechlorethamine) have been reported to be effective in case series, though each has well-known adverse effects that must be considered. For more extensive disease, thalidomide may be effective.

Localized bone lesions can be treated effectively with curettage. Symptomatic recurrent or new lesions, or those with a significant risk of fracture, cosmetic defect or functional abnormality, may require treatment with radiation. Treatment options for less problematic bone tumors include oral non-steroidal anti-inflammatory drugs (NSAIDs) and intralesional corticosteroid injections.

Multisystem disease has traditionally been treated with systemic therapy. To determine the most favorable treatment, the Histiocyte Society, in 1991, initiated the first international randomized prospective clinical trial: LCH-1[10]. This study compared the effectiveness of vinblastine to that of etoposide; each patient received a single dose of methylprednisolone at the onset of the trial. The vinblastine- and etoposide-based regimens were found to be equivalent with regard to disease response (58% vs. 65%, respectively), reactivation (61% vs. 55%), toxicity (47% vs. 58%) and survival (76% vs. 83%) as well as in prevention of disease-related permanent consequences such as diabetes insipidus, endocrinopathies (e.g. growth hormone deficiencies), orthopedic problems, hearing impairment, liver and lung failure, and CNS disease.

In addition, there were several important findings with regard to systemic disease. First, it was demonstrated that a failure to respond to treatment at 6 weeks was a predictor of poor outcome. Second, those patients with multisystem disease, but over 2 years of age at diagnosis *and* without involvement of the hematopoietic system, liver, lungs or spleen, had a 100% probability of survival. As a result, treatment regimens can be patient-specific. More aggressive therapy can be provided to those at high risk, whereas a more moderate, less hazardous protocol can be used for those patients at lower risk from their LCH. Information on additional trials for multisystem disease as well as for adults with single-system disease can be obtained at the website for the Histiocyte Society (www.histio.org/society/).

Perhaps the most significant shortcoming of treatment with either vinblastine or etoposide (plus an initial dose of methylprednisolone), as shown in LCH-1, was the high rate of reactivation of disease (58% ± 6%). For these patients, multidrug chemotherapy is an option. Additionally, small numbers of patients with reactivation of LCH have benefited from etanercept, cyclosporine or 2-chlorodeoxyadenosine. Imatinib mesylate was also reportedly beneficial in a case of multisystem LCH involving the brain which was unresponsive to radiation. For those with the most severe disease, bone marrow, hematopoietic stem cell, liver or lung transplantation may be required.

NON-LANGERHANS CELL HISTIOCYTOSES

Synonyms: ■ Class II histiocytosis ■ Non-X histiocytosis ■ Histiocytoses of mononuclear phagocytes other than Langerhans cells

Benign Cephalic Histiocytosis

Synonym: ■ Histiocytosis with intracytoplasmic worm-like bodies

Key features

- Infants <1 year of age most commonly affected
- Red to brown macules and papules of the face and neck
- Self-limiting disease, so no treatment required
- Ultrastructural finding: worm-like bodies

Introduction

Benign cephalic histiocytosis is a rare, self-limited histiocytic proliferative disorder of young children, primarily affecting the face.

History

Gianotti et al.[11], in 1971, described the condition as 'infantile histiocytosis with intracytoplasmic worm-like bodies', based upon findings of comma-shaped structures by ultrastructural studies. The disorder was renamed 'benign cephalic histiocytosis', based upon typical clinical findings, when it became clear that many histiocytic disorders had similar ultrastructural findings.

Epidemiology

Benign cephalic histiocytosis is rare, with approximately 40 cases having been described to date. The disorder typically begins by the age of 1 year and always within the first 3 years of life. There appears to

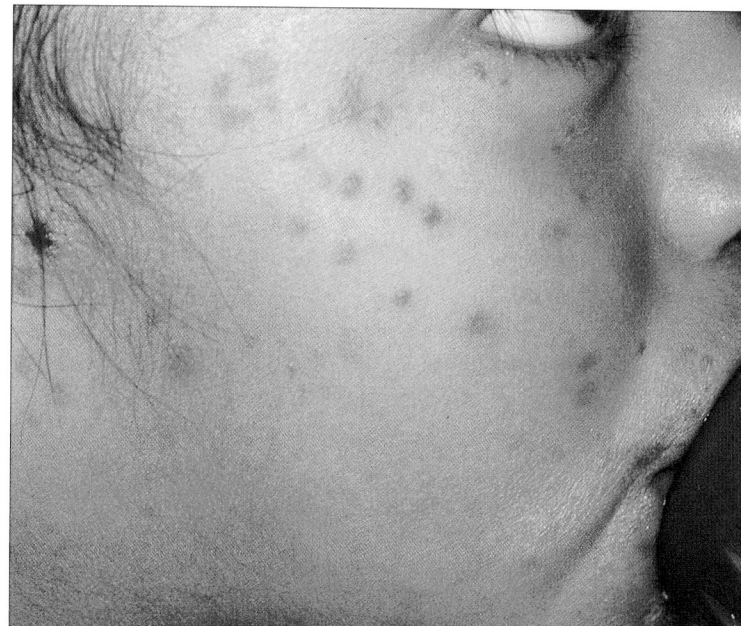

Fig. 90.7 Benign cephalic histiocytosis. Multiple brown papules on the face of a young child.

be no gender predilection[12]. One adult patient with T-cell lymphoma developed lesions similar to benign cephalic histiocytosis.

Pathogenesis

The pathogenesis of benign cephalic histiocytosis is not known. However, given a similar histopathology, ultrastructural appearance and immunohistochemical profile to juvenile xanthogranuloma and generalized eruptive histiocytoma, several investigators have suggested that benign cephalic histiocytosis may represent a variant of juvenile xanthogranuloma or generalized eruptive histiocytoma. Gianotti et al.[13], on the basis of a blinded histopathologic comparison that found great similarity between 14 benign cephalic histiocytosis, 25 juvenile xanthogranuloma, and 4 generalized eruptive histiocytoma specimens, believe that these three non-LCH self-healing histiocytoses should be viewed as a single disease with a spectrum of clinical features.

Clinical features

The eruption of benign cephalic histiocytosis is characterized by the evolution of 2–5-mm, red to red–brown macules and papules, first on the face (Fig. 90.7), with subsequent appearance on the ears and neck. Occasionally, lesions may develop on the trunk and arms, with infrequent involvement of the buttocks and thighs. The lesions spontaneously resolve after months or years. The papules flatten, become briefly hyperpigmented, and often disappear completely. Most children are otherwise healthy without involvement of the mucous membranes or internal organs. However, diabetes insipidus has recently been reported in a young girl with benign cephalic histiocytosis[14]. The course can be marked by exacerbations.

Pathology

Gianotti et al.[13] have described three histologic patterns in benign cephalic histiocytosis: a papillary dermal pattern, a diffuse pattern, and a lichenoid pattern. In the papillary dermal pattern, the most common form, the infiltrate is well defined and closely approaches the epidermis. The histiocytes are pleomorphic and have abundant eosinophilic cytoplasm, with hyperchromatic, sometimes indented nuclei and large nucleoli. There are scattered lymphocytes and a few eosinophils. In the diffuse pattern, pleomorphic histiocytes are rare, with most histiocytes being round and regular with minimal cytoplasm. The infiltrate is dispersed throughout the dermis. In the lichenoid pattern, small regular histiocytes and occasional lymphocytes are seen perivascularly and in the superficial dermis. In all forms, Touton cells are absent and foamy cells are rare or absent.

The histiocytes in benign cephalic histiocytosis express CD11b, CD14b, CD68, HAM56 and factor XIIIa (see Fig. 90.5, Table 90.2)[15,16].

Ultrastructural studies have demonstrated cytoplasmic comma-shaped bodies, worm-like particles, and desmosome-like junctions between histiocytes. The comma-shaped bodies and worm-like particles are also found in LCH, juvenile xanthogranuloma, generalized eruptive histiocytoma, and Rosai–Dorfman disease, so they are not as helpful diagnostically as originally thought.

Differential diagnosis

The differential diagnosis includes LCH and the non-LCH disorders, in particular juvenile xanthogranuloma. Like benign cephalic histiocytosis, juvenile xanthogranuloma most often occurs in children. However, dome-shaped nodules are more typical of juvenile xanthogranuloma, while macules and papules are more common in benign cephalic histiocytosis. Additionally, unlike benign cephalic histiocytosis, the lesions of juvenile xanthogranuloma are either widespread and numerous, or occur as one or several nodules. Juvenile xanthogranuloma is most often easily differentiated from benign cephalic histiocytosis by histopathology. Even in early juvenile xanthogranuloma or in the micronodular form of juvenile xanthogranuloma, where foamy cells are few to none, Touton cells can be found on step sections[13]. Touton cells are not seen in benign cephalic histiocytosis.

Generalized eruptive histiocytoma, though it has nearly identical histologic findings to benign cephalic histiocytosis, can be differentiated clinically. The former occurs most frequently in adults and lesions are widespread. LCH has a different immunohistochemical profile from benign cephalic histiocytosis, as well as Birbeck granules on electron microscopy.

Treatment

Benign cephalic histiocytosis is generally a self-limiting disorder and no treatment is needed. However, careful regular examinations of all patients with benign cephalic histiocytosis is recommended, as both exacerbations of the disease and diabetes insipidus can occur.

Generalized Eruptive Histiocytoma

Synonyms: ■ Eruptive histiocytoma ■ Generalized eruptive histiocytosis

Key features

- Adults affected more commonly than children
- Recurrent crops of numerous small red to brown papules
- Widespread axial distribution
- Self-limiting disease, so no treatment required

Introduction

Generalized eruptive histiocytosis is a very rare disorder, characterized by recurrent crops of small papules, axially distributed, which heal with hyperpigmented macules.

History

In the initial description of generalized eruptive histiocytoma in 1963, three adult patients were described by Winkelmann & Muller[17]. The disorder has also been described in children[18].

Epidemiology

Generalized eruptive histiocytoma is a very rare disease. Approximately 35 cases have been reported to date, with about one-third being children[18]. There may be a male predilection. Onset in adults is from the third to sixth decade. In children, onset is usually before age 4 years.

Pathogenesis

The cause of generalized eruptive histiocytoma is unknown. As discussed in the section on benign cephalic histiocytosis, several authors have suggested that generalized eruptive histiocytoma, benign cephalic histiocytosis, and juvenile xanthogranuloma may represent different expressions of the same disorder. Generalized eruptive histiocytoma-

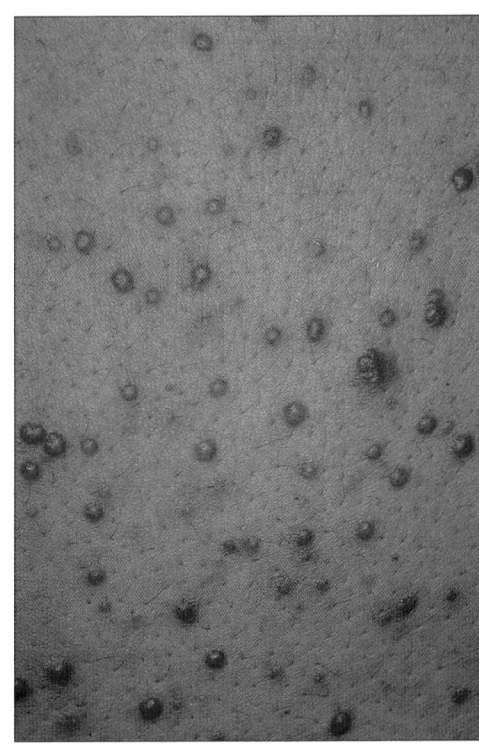

Fig. 90.8 Generalized eruptive histiocytoma. Multiple firm red papules on the trunk.

like presentations have been seen early in the course of other non-LCH disorders, leading some investigators to suggest that generalized eruptive histiocytoma may be an early, indeterminate stage of non-LCH[19].

Clinical features

The eruption is characterized by recurrent crops of red to brown papules. At each occurrence, hundreds of papules, less than 1 cm, are distributed on the face, trunk and proximal extremities (Fig. 90.8). In adults, there may be a symmetric arrangement of papules; mucosal surfaces are occasionally involved. Within several months, the lesions resolve completely or leave behind hyperpigmented macules or small scars. In the few reports involving children, papules are not arranged in a symmetric fashion, mucous membranes are not involved, and papules can become xanthomatous. Internal involvement has not been observed and the affected individuals are otherwise healthy.

Pathology

The superficial and mid dermis contain a nearly uniform infiltrate of histiocytes with a few lymphocytes. Rarely, a lichenoid pattern has been observed[13]. Xanthomatous cells are rare and giant cells have not been reported. The histiocytes stain for lysozyme, α_1-antitrypsin, CD11b, CD14b, Mac387, CD68 and factor XIIIa (see Fig. 90.5, Table 90.2)[20,21]. Ultrastructural studies demonstrate prominent cytoplasmic dense bodies, occasional worm-like bodies, and concentric laminated bodies.

Differential diagnosis

The differential diagnosis includes LCH, urticaria pigmentosa, and other non-LCH disorders. Of the latter, juvenile xanthogranuloma, xanthoma disseminatum, benign cephalic histiocytosis, and indeterminate cell histiocytosis may be particularly difficult to differentiate from generalized eruptive histiocytoma. While primary lesions of benign cephalic histiocytosis can appear clinically similar to generalized eruptive histiocytoma, and the histopathology seen in benign cephalic histiocytosis can be identical to that of generalized eruptive histiocytoma, benign cephalic histiocytosis occurs in children and is most often localized to the head and neck. Xanthoma disseminatum may initially resemble generalized eruptive histiocytoma, though the characteristic laryngeal, oral and eye lesions, the tendency for plaque formation, flexural distribution, and frequent diabetes insipidus are not found in generalized eruptive histiocytoma.

Juvenile xanthogranuloma is usually easily differentiated from generalized eruptive histiocytoma by histopathology. Even in early juvenile xanthogranuloma or the micronodular form of juvenile xanthogranuloma, where foamy cells are few to none, Touton cells can be found on step sections[13]. Touton cells are not seen in generalized eruptive histiocytoma. While indeterminate cell histiocytosis is clinically indistinguishable from generalized eruptive histiocytoma, the disorders show different histopathology, and lesional cells of indeterminate cell histiocytosis are S100- and CD1a-positive. LCH has a different immunohistochemical profile from generalized eruptive histiocytoma, as well as Birbeck granules by electron microscopy.

Treatment

No treatment is required as the disorder is self-limited and without systemic symptoms. However, careful follow-up of all patients with generalized eruptive histiocytoma is recommended as more serious forms of non-LCH, including xanthoma disseminatum, have been reported to develop in patients with generalized eruptive histiocytoma.

Indeterminate Cell Histiocytosis

Key features

■ Adults and children affected

■ Clinically indistinguishable from generalized eruptive histiocytoma

■ Immunophenotypic profile – antigenic markers of both LCH (S100⁺, CD1a⁺) and non-LCH (CD68⁺, etc.)

■ Usually self-limiting disease

Introduction

Indeterminate cell histiocytosis is a very rare proliferative disorder of histiocytes which displays both LCH and non-LCH immunophenotypic features. The majority of patients develop multiple lesions which are clinically indistinguishable from generalized eruptive histiocytosis.

History

Indeterminate cells were described in 1963, and a patient with features first recognized as indeterminate cell histiocytosis was reported by Wood et al.[22] in 1985. Approximately 20 cases have been reported to date in the literature. Indeterminate cells and indeterminate cell histiocytosis cells have a similar morphology to Langerhans cells and are further related as they express both S100 and CD1a antigens. However, they lack Birbeck granules ultrastructurally, and express several macrophage/monocyte markers.

Epidemiology

Indeterminate cell histiocytosis is extremely rare and has no apparent sexual predilection. The disorder occurs in adults, adolescents and infants, and a congenital form has also been reported.

Pathogenesis

The pathogenesis of indeterminate cell histiocytosis is unknown. However, it has most recently been speculated that indeterminate cells are dendritic cells en route from the skin to the regional lymph nodes. Therefore, indeterminate cell histiocytosis may represent a group of proliferating cells which have lost their capability to move as veiled cells from the skin through the lymphatics. The question has also been raised as to whether this disorder is actually a separate entity or represents various macrophage disorders identified at various time points in the inflammatory response[23].

Clinical features

While most cases of indeterminate cell histiocytosis have involved the trunk and extremities, isolated disease of the face and neck has been described. Both a generalized form and a solitary form have been documented. In the generalized form, cutaneous lesions usually begin as firm red to brown papules, each less than 1 cm. In the solitary form, there is a single soft erythematous lesion, approximately 1 cm in diameter. Ulceration can occur. As lesions age, they become brown to yellow. The course may wax and wane, though most patients experience a partial or complete regression of lesions.

Mucous membrane involvement has not been observed. However, ocular involvement has been described, and visceral involvement and

death have been reported in two instances. One infant developed an aggressive form of indeterminate cell histiocytosis with a fatal course. The disease initially presented in the bone and eventually spread to visceral organs and the skin[24]. To date, two cases have been associated with leukemia.

Pathology

Histology usually reveals a monomorphous infiltrate of vacuolated/xanthomatized mononuclear histiocytes throughout the entire dermis. Lymphocytes are either scattered throughout the infiltrate or clustered. Less common findings include epidermotropism, scattered reniform nuclei, multinucleated histiocytes, and spindle-shaped cells.

The immunophenotype of indeterminate cell histiocytosis demonstrates characteristics of *both* LCH and non-LCH. Lesional cells show expression of S100, CD1a, HAM56, CD68, Mac387, lysozyme, α_1-antitrypsin, HLA-DR, CD11c, CD14b and factor XIIIa (see Fig. 90.5, Table 90.2)[19,24,25]. The ultrastructural features of the histiocytes in indeterminate cell histiocytosis are similar to those seen in Langerhans cells except that no Birbeck granules are found.

Differential diagnosis

The clinical appearance of the cutaneous lesions of indeterminate cell histiocytosis is not unique. Similar-appearing papules in the same distribution can be found in generalized eruptive histiocytoma, juvenile xanthogranuloma (micronodular form), and congenital self-healing reticulohistiocytosis (see Table 90.1). When lesions of indeterminate cell histiocytosis are limited to the head and neck, benign cephalic histiocytosis also must be considered. The diagnosis of indeterminate cell histiocytosis can be suspected based upon histopathology. However, confirmation requires the histiocytic infiltrate to demonstrate immunophenotypic features of both LCH and non-LCH disorders, and to lack Birbeck granules ultrastructurally.

Treatment

Treatment of cutaneous lesions is not usually required as the condition is often self-limited and the lesions are asymptomatic. There are case reports of the beneficial effects of PUVA and 2-chlorodeoxyadenosine. Because visceral involvement and leukemia can occur, careful follow-up of all patients with indeterminate cell histiocytosis is recommended.

Juvenile Xanthogranuloma

Key features

■ Most common histiocytosis

■ Usually infants and young children with involvement of the head and neck region and upper body

■ Small and large nodular forms which acquire a yellow color as they mature

■ Ocular lesions can cause blindness

■ Rare association with both neurofibromatosis type 1 and juvenile myelomonocytic leukemia

■ Touton giant cell characteristic histologic finding

Introduction

Juvenile xanthogranuloma is a fairly common non-LCH, most often affecting infants and young children. Cutaneous lesions usually resolve and most patients have an otherwise unremarkable course. Ocular juvenile xanthogranuloma can lead to blindness and there is an association of juvenile xanthogranuloma with neurofibromatosis type 1 (NF1) and juvenile myelomonocytic leukemia.

History

The term 'juvenile xanthogranuloma' was suggested by Helwig & Hackney[26] in 1954 based upon histologic findings of xanthomatous histiocytes and giant cells. However, multiple cases of juvenile xanthogranuloma, under different names, had been reported during the first half of the 20th century. The first case of juvenile xanthogranuloma was reported in 1905 by Adamson[27], who named the disorder 'congenital xanthoma multiplex'.

Epidemiology

Juvenile xanthogranuloma is a fairly common disorder and the most common histiocytic disease of childhood[28]. However, the true incidence may be underestimated, as many lesions, especially those which are solitary and small, may be unrecognized. In childhood there is a male predominance of approximately 1.5:1; no sex predilection is noted in adults. A significant majority of reported patients are Caucasian. Almost 75% of cases appear during the first year of life, with over 15% being noted at birth. Juvenile xanthogranuloma is rare in adults, in whom its peak incidence is in the late twenties to early thirties, though lesions have been reported in the elderly. Most adult patients have solitary lesions.

Pathogenesis

The cause of juvenile xanthogranuloma is not known; however, it is often suggested that the condition is reactive with histiocytes possibly responding to a traumatic or infectious stimulus. The reason for the progressive lipidation of histiocytes in the absence of hyperlipidemia is not clear. However, it has been shown that the uptake of low-density lipoprotein and the synthesis of cholesterol within macrophages in adult patients with xanthogranuloma is increased[29]. As discussed in the section on benign cephalic histiocytosis, several authors have suggested that generalized eruptive histiocytoma, benign cephalic histiocytosis, and juvenile xanthogranuloma may represent different expressions of the same disorder.

Clinical features

Gianotti & Caputo[30] described two common clinical variants of juvenile xanthogranuloma: a small nodular form and large nodular form. Patients with the small nodular form, also known as the micro-nodular form, can present with many pink to red–brown, dome-shaped papules, 2–5 mm in diameter. The lesions are widely scattered on the upper part of the body and rapidly become yellow. In contrast, the more common large nodular form is characterized by one or a few nodules 1–2 cm in diameter. Both forms frequently coexist.

The most common location for juvenile xanthogranuloma is the head and neck (Fig. 90.9), followed by the upper torso, the upper extremities and the lower extremities. Oral juvenile xanthogranuloma is rare and usually presents as a solitary yellow nodule on the lateral aspect of the tongue or the midline of the hard palate. Unusual morphologic presentations include keratotic, pedunculated, subcutaneous, clustered, plaque-like and giant lesions.

Extracutaneous lesions have been reported in many organs, the eye being most commonly affected. Visceral, bone and CNS involvement is rare, although to date two deaths have been attributed to the disease.[31] The lung is the second most frequent extracutaneous site of disease. Ocular juvenile xanthogranuloma is almost always unilateral and develops in less than 0.5% of patients with cutaneous lesions. However,

approximately 40% of patients with ocular juvenile xanthogranuloma have cutaneous lesions, always multiple, at the time of diagnosis[32]. Ocular involvement usually occurs before 2 years of age and often affects the iris. Hyphema (hemorrhage into the anterior chamber) and glaucoma are serious complications which can result in blindness. Early referral to an ophthalmologist for evaluation and possible treatment is important.

A well-recognized association exists between juvenile xanthogranuloma and café-au-lait macules. Some of these patients have a family history of NF1, while others fulfill the clinical criteria for NF1. Another well-known association is that of juvenile xanthogranuloma and juvenile myelomonocytic leukemia. Patients with NF1 also have an increased risk of developing juvenile myelomonocytic leukemia. A so-called 'triple association' consisting of juvenile xanthogranuloma, NF1 and juvenile myelomonocytic leukemia has been observed in several patients, and patients with juvenile xanthogranuloma and NF1 have at least a 20-times increased risk of developing juvenile myelomonocytic leukemia[33]. Other forms of leukemia have also been reported in association with juvenile xanthogranuloma.

In the majority of patients with disease limited to the skin, the course is self-limited and benign. These patients are otherwise in good health and lesions usually regress within 3–6 years. Hyperpigmentation, mild atrophy, or anetoderma may remain.

Pathology

Typically, nodules demonstrate a well-demarcated dense infiltrate of histiocytes in the superficial dermis in small lesions, extending into the subcutis in larger lesions. There is often loss of the rete ridges, and ulceration occurs in some cases. Early lesions usually demonstrate monomorphous histiocytes with abundant eosinophilic cytoplasm. In mature lesions, the histiocytes develop lipid in their cytoplasm, creating a foamy 'xanthomatous' appearance. Touton giant cells are a characteristic finding (Fig. 90.10). Lymphocytes, eosinophils and plasma cells are also scattered throughout the infiltrate. Variants without Touton giant cells or with many spindle cells have been reported, but serial sections may reveal rare giant cells[13]. A rare lichenoid pattern has also been reported[13].

Juvenile xanthogranuloma histiocytes stain positively for HAM56, CD68 and factor XIIIa (see Fig. 90.5, Table 90.2)[34]. Some cases have shown expression of S100; CD1a is usually negative. By electron microscopy, comma-shaped bodies, lipid vacuoles, cholesterol clefts, and myeloid bodies have been observed in the histiocytes.

Differential diagnosis

The major diagnostic dilemmas occur with the other non-LCH disorders and LCH. Some examples of adult xanthogranuloma have been reported to have a similar clinical presentation, histology and immunophenotype to giant cell reticulohistiocytoma[35]. Clinical distinctions

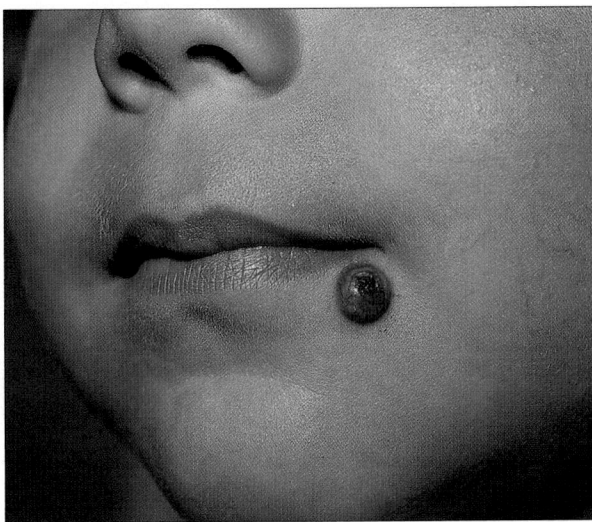

Fig. 90.9 Juvenile xanthogranuloma. Red–brown nodule with central yellow color that had been present for 5 months. Courtesy of Anthony J Mancini MD.

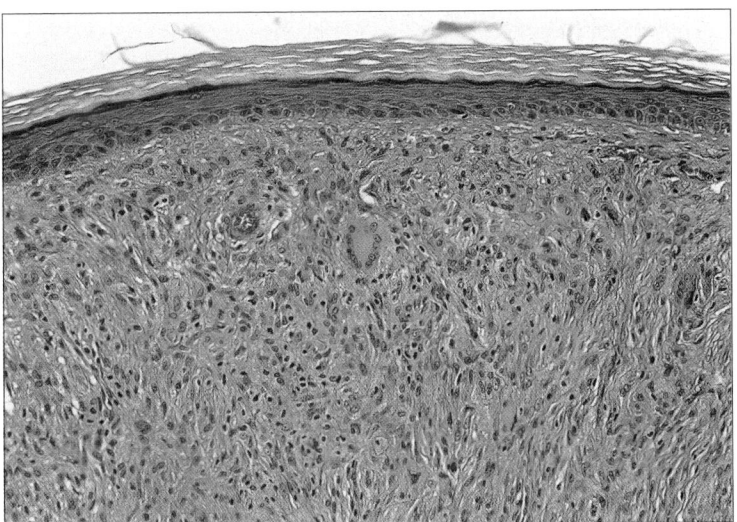

Fig. 90.10 Juvenile xanthogranuloma. Dermal histiocytic infiltrate mixed with lymphocytes and scattered Touton giant cells. Touton giant cells have a 'wreath-like' arrangement of nuclei within the cell. Identical histologic findings are seen in xanthoma disseminatum.

between juvenile xanthogranuloma and either benign cephalic histiocytosis or generalized eruptive histiocytoma are discussed in their respective sections (see above). Juvenile xanthogranuloma is usually easily differentiated from both benign cephalic histiocytosis and generalized eruptive histiocytoma by histopathology, since only juvenile xanthogranuloma has Touton giant cells.

The lesions of indeterminate cell histiocytosis are not yellowish and are S100- and CD1a-positive. While xanthoma disseminatum and juvenile xanthogranuloma cannot be differentiated by histopathology, mucous membrane lesions are uncommon in juvenile xanthogranuloma. Additionally, diabetes insipidus is common in xanthoma disseminatum and to date has been reported but once in juvenile xanthogranuloma. Finally, xanthoma disseminatum tends to develop later in life than juvenile xanthogranuloma, the lesions tend to be widespread and confluent, and the condition is often persistent or progressive.

LCH can always be differentiated from juvenile xanthogranuloma by the use of immunostains, and Birbeck granules are not found in juvenile xanthogranuloma. In the case of a single (or few) immature lesions, molluscum contagiosum can usually be excluded by its clinical appearance or examination of expressed contents. Differentiation from a Spitz nevus, fibrous histiocytoma, keloid or pyogenic granuloma may require histopathologic examination.

Treatment

Due to the self-limiting nature of the eruption, no treatment is required. Occasionally, lesions are removed for cosmetic concerns, despite the anticipated spontaneous resolution. While ocular lesions often require intervention (e.g. topical corticosteroids for iris lesions, excision for limbal lesions), sites of systemic involvement can be followed without treatment unless their location interferes with normal function. For patients in the latter group, various chemotherapeutic regimens, radiotherapy, high-dose corticosteroids, and cyclosporine have been tried in isolated case reports[36]. Given the possibility of spontaneous involution, however, it is difficult to gauge response to treatment.

Necrobiotic Xanthogranuloma

Synonym: ■ Necrobiotic xanthogranuloma with paraproteinemia

- ■ Average age of onset is the sixth decade
- ■ Firm nodules and plaques with a yellow hue; may develop ulcerations
- ■ Most common site of involvement is the periorbital region
- ■ Multisystem disease includes hepatosplenomegaly and ocular involvement
- ■ An IgG monoclonal gammopathy is seen in at least 80% of patients
- ■ Increased risk of plasma cell dyscrasias and lymphoproliferative disorders

---

Introduction

Necrobiotic xanthogranuloma is a rare, progressive multisystem histiocytic disease characterized by destructive cutaneous and subcutaneous lesions, an increased risk of plasma cell dyscrasias and lymphoproliferative disorders, and a strong association with paraproteinemia.

History

Necrobiotic xanthogranuloma was characterized in 1980 by Kossard & Winkelmann[37]. Their original eight patients demonstrated yellowish plaques, subcutaneous nodules, and an associated dysproteinemia. These authors also noted several reports published prior to 1980 representing unrecognized cases of necrobiotic xanthogranuloma.

Epidemiology

Necrobiotic xanthogranuloma is a rare disorder. In 1992, Mehregan & Winkelmann[38] reported their 32 patients with necrobiotic xanthogranuloma and reviewed the 16 reported cases from the world literature. Men and women are affected approximately equally. The average age

of onset is the sixth decade; the youngest patient to date to develop necrobiotic xanthogranuloma was 17 years of age.

Pathogenesis

The strong association of necrobiotic xanthogranuloma with paraproteinemia has led to several hypotheses regarding the pathogenesis of necrobiotic xanthogranuloma. The paraprotein has been suspected either to be the primary inciting agent or to act as a cofactor in eliciting a giant cell granulomatous reaction. Nevertheless, the pathogenesis of necrobiotic xanthogranuloma is as yet unknown.

Clinical features

Cutaneous lesions, typically multiple, have appeared in all cases (Fig. 90.11). The classic skin lesion is an asymptomatic indurated papule, nodule or plaque with a yellow 'xanthomatous' hue. Other features can include telangiectasias, atrophy, ulceration of lesions and scarring, with scars being common sites for development of new lesions.

The periorbital region is the most common site of involvement. The trunk, remainder of the face, and proximal extremities are also frequently involved. Approximately 50% of patients have ophthalmic manifestations, which include orbital masses, ectropion, ptosis, conjunctival lesions, keratitis and scleritis, episcleritis, anterior uveitis, and proptosis[39].

A hallmark feature of necrobiotic xanthogranuloma is the associated paraproteinemia, an IgG monoclonal gammopathy, which is found in at least 80% of cases. Other common findings include hepatomegaly, splenomegaly, an increased ESR, leukopenia, hypocomplementemia, and underlying myeloma or plasma cell dyscrasia. Less commonly, cryoglobulinemia and/or an underlying lymphoproliferative disorder are observed. Of the 48 patients described by Mehregan & Winkelmann[38], multiple myeloma was found in eight, lymphoproliferative disorders in two, and a plasma cell proliferative disorder in nine. Postmortem examination has demonstrated involvement of multiple organ systems, with endocardial necrobiotic xanthogranuloma found in most cases.

Ugurlu et al.[40] examined the outcomes of 26 patients with ocular and systemic manifestations of necrobiotic xanthogranuloma. Ten of their patients developed multiple myeloma, a plasma cell dyscrasia

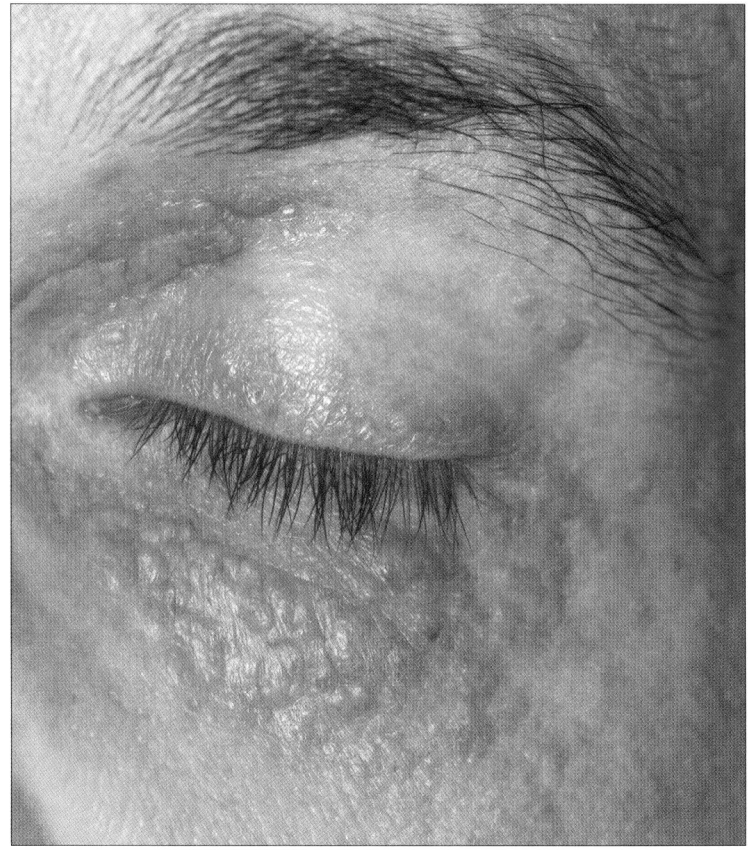

Fig. 90.11 Necrobiotic xanthogranuloma. Yellow–brown papules and plaques in a periorbital distribution in a patient with chronic lymphocytic leukemia. Such lesions may initially be mistaken for xanthelasma. Courtesy of Kalman Watsky MD.

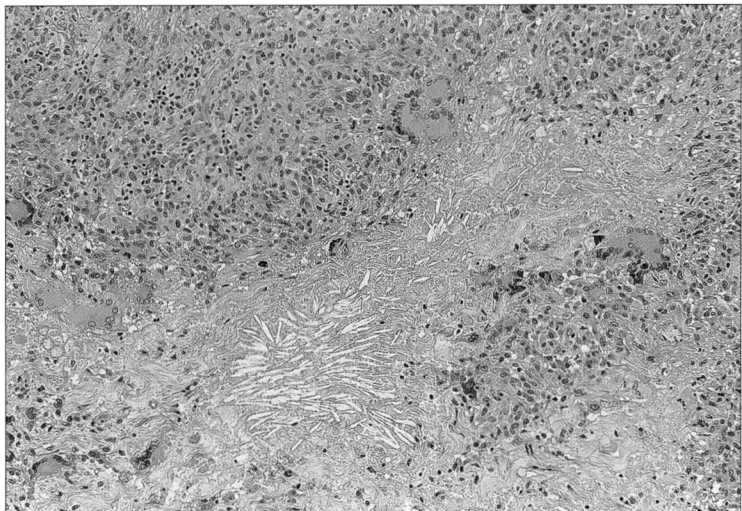

Fig. 90.12 Necrobiotic xanthogranuloma. A necrobiotic area contains cholesterol clefts. Surrounding this area are many bizarre multinucleated giant cells.

or a lymphoproliferative disorder. The associated malignancy often developed after the onset of cutaneous manifestations and did not tend to be aggressive. Overall survival was 100% at 10 years and 90% at 15 years. A poorer survival rate was noted in a study of 22 patients by Finan & Winkelmann[41]. Two patients died of multiple myeloma within 10 years, and three others died of various solid tumor malignancies.

Pathology

Classic, non-ulcerated lesions have a normal epidermis and superficial dermis. A palisading xanthogranuloma is found in the middle dermis extending through the panniculus (Fig. 90.12). The granulomas consist of histiocytes, foam cells, lymphoid follicles, plasma cells and giant cells with zones of necrobiosis. Cholesterol clefts are found in areas of 'necrobiosis' (altered collagen, in which there appears to be necrosis, loss of collagen bundle integrity, and nuclear debris). A prominent feature is the presence of both Touton giant cells and large, bizarre foreign body giant cells. These cells are found scattered within the granuloma and often at the margins of areas of necrobiosis. Histiocytic cells stain positively for lysozyme, CD68, Mac387 and CD11b (see Fig. 90.5, Table 90.2)[38,40,42].

Differential diagnosis

The clinical differential diagnosis includes necrobiosis lipoidica, granuloma annulare and xanthelasma, non-LCH disorders (xanthoma disseminatum, multicentric reticulohistiocytosis, juvenile xanthogranuloma), and sarcoidosis. However, most of these disorders can be excluded on the basis of morphology, distribution pattern, histologic features and associated systemic manifestations (if any). Overall, normolipemic plane xanthoma (see Ch. 91) is most closely related to necrobiotic xanthogranuloma. Both have a yellow hue, are associated with a paraproteinemia, usually have normal serum lipids, and demonstrate an upper body distribution pattern. However, normolipemic plane xanthoma has a much stronger association with multiple myeloma, and the plaques lack induration and rarely ulcerate[43]. Uncommonly, necrobiosis, cholesterol clefts and Touton giant cells can be seen in normolipemic plane xanthoma, making histologic differentiation from necrobiotic xanthogranuloma difficult.

Treatment

No controlled clinical studies are available regarding the treatment of necrobiotic xanthogranuloma. Resolution or improvement of skin lesions has been seen in some patients treated with low-dose chlorambucil, melphalan or cyclophosphomide (± systemic corticosteroids), radiation therapy, CO_2 laser, and plasmapheresis. With rare exceptions, topical and locally injected corticosteroids have been tried with minimal or no benefit; in case series, systemic corticosteroids (including pulsed high-dose dexamethasone) have resulted in improvement in some patients. Ugurlu et al.[40] noted a 42% rate of recurrence for excised lesions, and recommended avoidance of surgical removal if possible.

Reticulohistiocytosis

Synonyms for giant cell reticulohistiocytoma: ■ Solitary reticulohistiocytosis ■ Solitary reticulohistiocytoma

Key features

- Clinical spectrum ranges from a single lesion to multicentric reticulohistiocytosis with systemic involvement
- All forms are seen primarily in adults
- Papules and nodules favor the head, hands and elbows; periungual papules have been likened to 'coral beads'
- 50% of patients develop mucous membrane lesions (oral and nasopharyngeal)
- Multicentric reticulohistiocytosis is associated with a destructive arthritis and, in some patients, solid-organ malignancies
- Histiocytes have a characteristic 'ground glass' appearance

Introduction

The reticulohistiocytoses are a rare group of closely related non-Langerhans cell histiocytoses which most commonly affect adults. The spectrum of disease ranges from a solitary cutaneous form to multicentric reticulohistiocytosis, a disease with both cutaneous and systemic features. Well-developed lesions demonstrate a classic histopathology consisting of mononucleated and multinucleated giant cells with a 'ground glass' appearance.

History

Giant cell reticulohistiocytoma, an isolated cutaneous tumor sometimes referred to as solitary reticulohistiocytoma, was first reported in 1950 by Zac[44]. The term multicentric reticulohistiocytosis was introduced by Goltz & Laymon[45] in 1954 to define those cases with both cutaneous and systemic manifestations. Familial histiocytic dermatoarthritis, described in 1973, is a very rare variant of multicentric reticulohistiocytosis, characterized by a familial occurrence and associated glaucoma, uveitis and cataracts[46].

Epidemiology

All forms of reticulohistiocytoses occur predominantly in Caucasian adults, pediatric cases being exceptionally rare. Multicentric reticulohistiocytosis is uncommon, occurring most frequently in women during the fourth decade. Giant cell reticulohistiocytoma occurs in young adults and has no sexual predilection.

Pathogenesis

The pathogenesis of the reticulohistiocytoses is unknown. However, it has been speculated that it represents an abnormal histiocytic response to various stimuli. Mycobacteria have been suggested as a possible trigger for multicentric reticulohistiocytosis. In one old study, 56% of multicentric reticulohistiocytosis patients had a positive tuberculin skin test[47]. Multicentric reticulohistiocytosis has also been reported to respond to antituberculosis treatment. However, confirmation of mycobacteria in skin nodules is lacking. Others have suggested that the histiocytic response in multicentric reticulohistiocytosis is an immunologic process related to an underlying autoimmune or neoplastic disorder.

The cause of giant cell reticulohistiocytoma is even less clear. Some lesions are believed to occur after trauma. Cerio et al.[35] referred to giant cell reticulohistiocytoma synonymously with the solitary or eruptive adult form of xanthogranuloma.

Clinical features

Giant cell reticulohistiocytoma presents as a single, asymptomatic, yellow to red nodule. It can develop at any cutaneous site but is thought to favor the head. The patients are otherwise healthy and lesions tend to spontaneously resolve. Rarely, multiple cutaneous lesions develop without any evidence of systemic disease. Nodules are generally less than 1 cm.

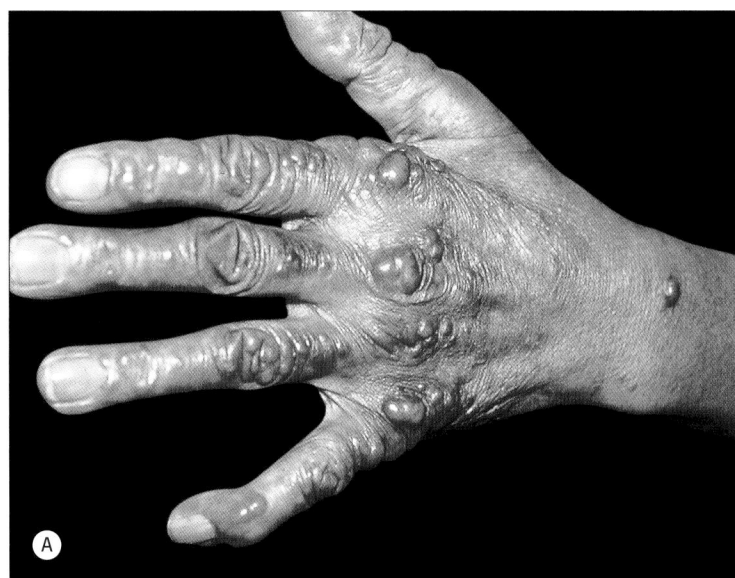

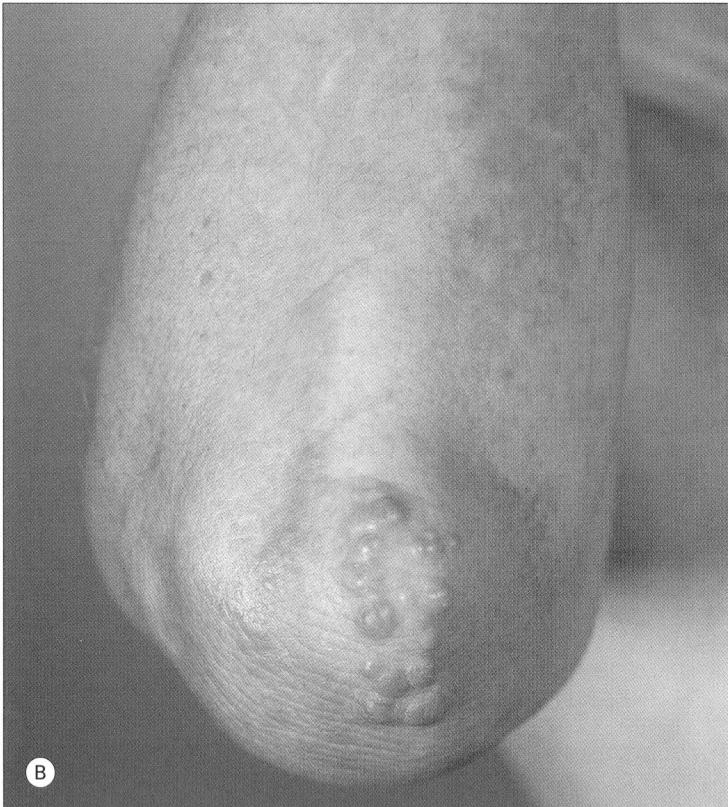

Fig. 90.13 Multicentric reticulohistiocytosis. A Grouped firm red–brown papules on the dorsal surface of the fingers, hand and wrist in this 73-year-old African-American woman. Courtesy of Susan D Laman MD. **B** Grouped pink papulonodules on the elbow in a second patient. Courtesy of Jean L Bolognia MD.

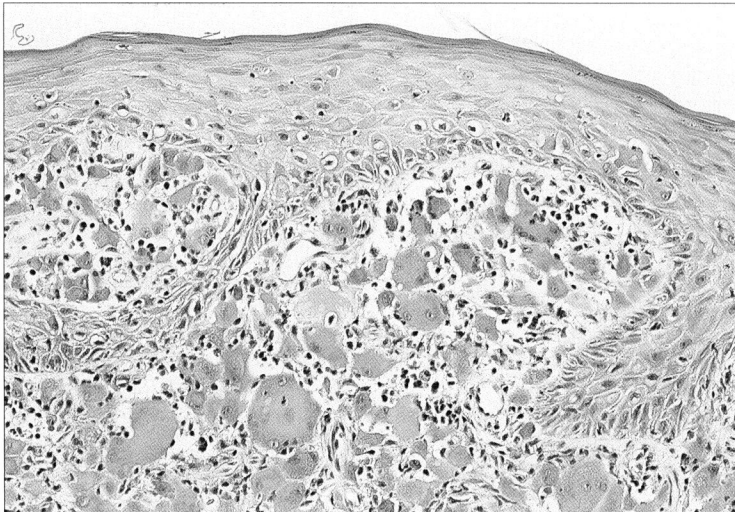

Fig. 90.14 Reticulohistiocytosis. Light microscopy: numerous mononucleated and multinucleated histiocytes extending from the papillary tips into the deep dermis. These histiocytes have abundant eosinophilic, finely granular cytoplasm, creating a 'ground glass' appearance.

Multicentric reticulohistiocytosis is a disease characterized by cutaneous and mucous membrane reticulohistiocytomas and severe arthropathy. There is an association with hyperlipidemia, positive tuberculin skin test, systemic vasculitis, and autoimmune disease. Up to 28% of multicentric reticulohistiocytosis patients have reportedly had an associated malignancy, with bronchial, breast, stomach and cervical carcinomas being most common. An elevated ESR and anemia have been noted in approximately half of patients, and one-third demonstrate hypercholesterolemia. Occasionally, IgG hypergammaglobulinemia and cryoglobulinemia have been observed. Fever and weight loss can occur.

Cutaneous lesions range from a few millimeters to 2 cm and are skin-colored to red, brown or yellow. Lesions tend to be acrally distributed. Favored sites include the head, hands, fingers, ears, and articular regions of the limbs (Fig. 90.13). Small papules aligned along the periungual regions result in a characteristic 'coral bead' appearance. Approximately one-half of patients develop papules and nodules of the oral, pharyngeal and nasal mucosa. Less common findings include a 'leonine facies' secondary to severe facial involvement, periarticular rheumatoid-like nodules, an initial photodistribution, and secondary nail changes.

A 6–8-year course of symmetric, erosive arthritis of multiple joints is common and there is progression to arthritis mutilans in 45% of cases. The joints of the fingers and hands, as well as the knees and wrists, are most commonly involved, though any joint may be affected. Cartilaginous destruction of the nose and ears can lead to facial disfigurement. Rarely, there is histiocytic involvement of the heart, eye, lungs, thyroid, liver, kidney, muscle, salivary gland and/or bone marrow. The disease spontaneously remits in 5–10 years, though patients are often left with significant disability.

Pathology

Many believe that the histopathology of giant cell reticulohistiocytoma and multicentric reticulohistiocytosis is identical. Well-developed lesions demonstrate a dermal infiltrate of lymphocytes and histiocytes, with occasional plasma cells and eosinophils. The histiocytes have a characteristic appearance. They are both mononuclear and multi-nuclear, with abundant eosinophilic, homogenous, and finely granular cytoplasm, creating a 'ground glass' effect (Fig. 90.14). Multinucleated cells demonstrate nuclei arranged haphazardly, aligned at the periphery, or clustered in the center.

Giant cell reticulohistiocytoma and multicentric reticulohistiocytosis histiocytes stain positively for lysozyme and α_1-antitrypsin and also express CD68, CD11b, CD14 and HAM56 (see Fig. 90.5, Table 90.2)[35,48]. S100 is most often negative. Several case reports have shown positive staining for factor XIIIa, though Zelger et al.[49] found that factor XIIIa was positive in cases of giant cell reticulohistiocytoma and negative in multicentric reticulohistiocytosis lesions.

Differential diagnosis

The nodule of giant cell reticulohistiocytoma is not clinically distinctive. Other conditions presenting with a single nodule must be considered, such as solitary adult xanthogranuloma, Spitz nevus, adnexal tumor, dermatofibroma and atypical fibroxanthoma. Histo-pathology is required for diagnosis. Some examples of adult xanthogranuloma have been reported to have a similar clinical presentation, histology and immunophenotype to giant cell reticulohistiocytoma[35].

Multicentric reticulohistiocytosis must be differentiated from the other histiocytoses, with juvenile xanthogranulomas, generalized eruptive histiocytosis, and cutaneous Rosai–Dorfman disease presenting the greatest challenge. In addition to different distribution patterns and histopathology, the early age of onset of juvenile xanthogranuloma and the recurrent crops of papules of generalized eruptive histiocytosis aid in distinguishing these entities. When present, the erosive arthritis points to the diagnosis of multicentric reticulohistiocytosis. Occasionally, the combination of arthritis plus nodules overlying joints leads to the misdiagnosis of rheumatoid arthritis. The clinical differential diagnosis also includes papular mucinosis and, when there is an initial photo-distribution, dermatomyositis.

Treatment

Surgical excision of giant cell reticulohistiocytoma is curative. Most systemic therapy for multicentric reticulohistiocytosis has not been effective. Although not in controlled clinical trials, NSAIDs, oral corticosteroids, azathioprine, cyclophosphamide and chlorambucil have been tried, but with limited or no benefit. However, there are multiple case reports of substantial benefit with methotrexate, either alone or in combination with cyclophosphamide and corticosteroids[50]. Alendronate and inhibitors of TNF-α have recently been shown to be of value in isolated cases.

Rosai–Dorfman Disease

Synonym: ■ Sinus histiocytosis with massive lymphadenopathy

Key features

- Children and young adults are most commonly affected
- Although massive, painless bilateral cervical lymphadenopathy is characteristic, extranodal sites can be the sole manifestation
- Cutaneous lesions occur in a minority of cases (10%), are usually multiple, and are clinically non-specific
- Fever and IgG polyclonal hypergammaglobulinemia are often seen
- In the lymph nodes and the skin, emperipolesis is a common histologic feature

Introduction

Rosai–Dorfman disease is an uncommon, often protracted, histiocytic proliferative disorder. It is characterized by massive but painless bilateral cervical lymphadenopathy, fever, anemia, elevated ESR, neutrophilia and a polyclonal hypergammaglobulinemia. Cutaneous lesions occur in a minority of cases, are usually multiple, and are clinically non-specific.

History

Sinus histiocytosis with massive lymphadenopathy was described as a distinct entity by Rosai & Dorfman[51] in 1969. However, the eponymous designation 'Rosai–Dorfman disease' is more appropriate as some cases have demonstrated extranodal lesions as the sole manifestation of the condition[52].

Epidemiology

For a time, there was a repository for cases of Rosai–Dorfman disease, rather than a registry in the true sense. In 1990, the repository contained 423 patients; almost 600 cases had been reported by 1995[53,54]. Rosai–Dorfman disease has a widespread geographic distribution. It occurs most commonly in children and young adults and is more frequently seen in male patients. In 1990, an equal percentage of white and black patients, 44% of each, were in the registry[53]. Although Rosai–Dorfman disease has been documented in many areas of the world, a higher incidence has been noted in the West Indies. Congenital disease, onset in the elderly, and disease in siblings and identical twins have been reported.

Pathogenesis

The etiology of Rosai–Dorfman disease has not been identified, though a viral pathogenesis has been postulated. *In situ* hybridization for EBV has failed to demonstrate evidence for active or latent EBV infection. In a similar study of lymph node specimens utilizing *in situ* hybridization for HHV-6 sequences, seven of nine cases demonstrated positive results for the HHV-6 genome[55]. However, HHV-6 has been frequently found in many reactive and infectious disorders of lymphoid tissue. Its finding in lymphoid tissue of Rosai–Dorfman disease, therefore, is non-specific[56]. More recently, it has been suggested that Rosai–Dorfman disease may be closely related to autoimmune lymphoproliferative syndrome, an inherited disorder associated with defects in Fas-mediated apoptosis (see Table 59.5)[57].

Clinical features

While Rosai–Dorfman disease is often an indolent, self-limited disease, a protracted course marked by remissions and exacerbations occurs in many patients. The characteristic clinical feature is massive, painless, bilateral cervical lymphadenopathy. However, any nodal site may be involved, unilateral involvement may occur, and an absence of lymph node involvement has been reported in multiple patients. Fever is a frequent occurrence and most cases demonstrate an elevated ESR and an IgG polyclonal hypergammaglobulinemia. A common finding is mild anemia, though severe anemia has occurred. Neutrophilia is occasionally seen. There are multiple reports of non-Hodgkin lymphoma occurring in association with Rosai–Dorfman disease.

Immune disorders occur in approximately 15% of patients with Rosai–Dorfman disease. Anti-red blood cell autoantibodies and joint disease are the most common findings. Patients with immunologic abnormalities have an unfavorable prognosis. Ten of 14 fatal cases were noted to have some form of immune dysfunction[58]. Other unfavorable prognostic signs include disseminated nodal disease or involvement of the liver, kidney or lower respiratory tract.

Over 40% of patients with Rosai–Dorfman disease have at least one extranodal site of involvement. The most common extranodal sites are the skin and soft tissue, the eyelid and orbit, the upper respiratory tract, major salivary glands, CNS and bone. However, virtually any organ can be involved.

Cutaneous involvement occurs in approximately 10% of cases, and the skin may be the only organ involved. Cutaneous lesions are often multiple and appear as non-specific red to red–brown or xanthomatous macules, papules, nodules or plaques (Fig. 90.15). Panniculitis has also been reported. The eyelids and malar regions are frequent sites of involvement.

Pathology

Rosai–Dorfman disease, or sinus histiocytosis with massive lymphadenopathy, is a disease which had been characterized by specific findings in the affected lymph nodes. However, consistent and unique histologic and immunohistochemical findings in the skin make diagnosis possible even in cases without lymph node involvement.

Affected lymph nodes demonstrate dilated sinuses containing neutrophils, lymphocytes, plasma cells, and histiocytes with large vesicular nuclei and abundant cytoplasm. A characteristic though not unique feature is emperipolesis, or the taking up of intact lymphocytes and plasma cells by the histiocytes. Neutrophils and red cells can also be internalized in a similar fashion.

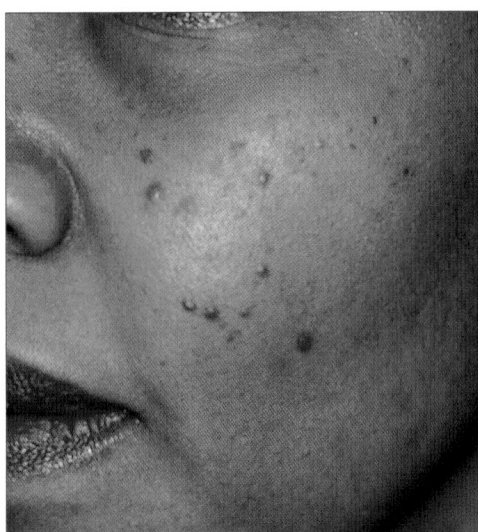

Fig. 90.15 Cutaneous Rosai–Dorfman disease. Discrete, dome-shaped papules.

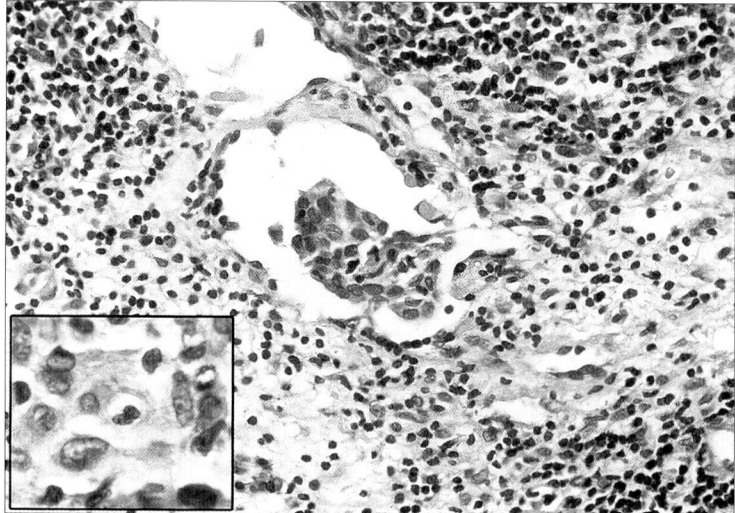

Fig. 90.16 Rosai–Dorfman disease. Large histiocytes are located inside a dermal lymphatic. Surrounding the lymphatic are numerous histiocytes and groups of lymphocytes. The inset shows a histiocyte which has engulfed several lymphocytes (emperipolesis).

Cutaneous lesions demonstrate a dense dermal infiltrate of histiocytes with scattered lymphocytes, plasma cells and neutrophils (Fig. 90.16). The histiocytes have large vesicular nuclei, small nucleoli, and abundant foamy, eosinophilic cytoplasm with feathery borders. Emperipolesis is a constant finding. Occasional findings include foamy histiocytes within dilated lymphatics, thick-walled venules with surrounding plasma cells, lymphoid aggregates, fibrosis and multinucleate histiocytes.

Rosai–Dorfman disease histiocytes stain positively for S100, CD11c, CD14, CD68, laminin 5 and lysozyme (see Fig. 90.5, Table 90.2)[59]. Mac387 is occasionally expressed and examples positive for factor XIIIa have been reported. With the exception of one study from 1994[60], CD1a expression in Rosai-Dorfman disease has been shown to be negative.

Differential diagnosis

Given the clinically non-specific cutaneous lesions found in Rosai–Dorfman disease, the differential diagnosis includes the other histiocytoses, sarcoidosis, infectious processes, and other infiltrative disorders. The diagnosis of cutaneous Rosai–Dorfman disease is based upon the combination of characteristic histologic and immunohistochemical findings. The differential diagnosis of massive lymphadenopathy includes Hodgkin lymphoma, non-Hodgkin lymphoma, chronic lymphocytic leukemia, metastases, infectious lymphadenopathies, and Kikuchi's disease. Rosai–Dorfman disease is differentiated by a typical combination of clinical and laboratory findings plus confirmatory histology and immunohistochemistry.

Kikuchi's disease, or histiocytic necrotizing lymphadenitis, is a self-limited condition of unknown etiology characterized by fever and tender, usually cervical, lymphadenopathy. It is more common in Asia and generally affects young women. Oral prednisone has been an effective treatment[61]. While the lymph node swelling and fever seen in Kikuchi's disease may mimic that seen in Rosai–Dorfman disease, patients with Kikuchi's disease have a normal white blood cell count, ESR and hematocrit. Histology of affected lymph nodes in Kikuchi's disease is markedly different from that seen in Rosai–Dorfman disease. The former is characterized by necrotic foci and a cellular population of large blastic lymphocytes and histiocytes. Engulfing of apoptotic bodies by the histiocytes is a prominent feature.

Treatment

Many lesions are asymptomatic and heal spontaneously, thus not requiring treatment. When treatment is indicated due to destructive lesions, disseminated disease or lesions causing physical compromise, radiotherapy, surgical excision, systemic corticosteroids, and alkylating agents have been used with some success[62]. There are also a few isolated reports of improvement with thalidomide. However, due to the rarity of the disorder, there have been no controlled trials.

Xanthoma Disseminatum

Synonym: ■ Disseminated xanthosiderohistiocytosis

Key features

- Classic triad of cutaneous xanthomas, mucous membrane xanthomas and diabetes insipidus
- Symmetric distribution
- Flexural and intertriginous involvement
- Upper airway lesions

Introduction

Xanthoma disseminatum is a rare, normolipemic, histiocytic proliferative disorder affecting the skin, mucous membranes and, frequently, the hypothalamus and pituitary, leading to transient diabetes insipidus.

History

Four cases of 'xanthomatosis disseminata' were described by Montgomery & Osterberg[63] in 1938. A review and characterization of the disorder was provided by Altman & Winkelmann[64] in 1962.

Epidemiology

Xanthoma disseminatum is a rare condition, with approximately 100 cases reported cases by 1995[65]. Men are more commonly affected than women. Age of onset ranges from 8 months to 85 years, though more than 60% of patients develop the disease before age 25 years.

Pathogenesis

The etiology of xanthoma disseminatum is unknown. As most patients have normal lipid levels, it has been suggested that xanthoma disseminatum represents a reactive proliferative disorder of histiocytes with secondary accumulation of lipid.

Clinical features

Patients with xanthoma disseminatum may demonstrate the triad of cutaneous xanthomas, xanthomas of mucous membranes, and diabetes insipidus. The primary xanthomatous lesion is a yellow, red or brown papule. The onset of disease is marked by the eruption of hundreds of papules, symmetrically arranged, on the face and in the flexural and intertriginous areas of the trunk and proximal extremities (Fig. 90.17). The lesions tend to cluster into well-formed, potentially disfiguring plaques (Fig. 90.18). Older lesions may become atrophic.

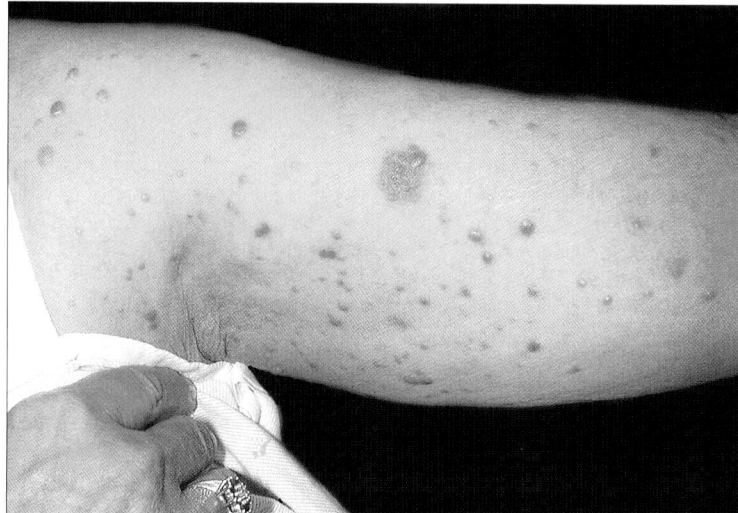

Fig. 90.17 Xanthoma disseminatum. Flexural involvement is common. In this patient, multiple red–yellow papules are seen in the axilla, as well as on the shoulder and proximal arm. Courtesy of Grant J Anhalt MD.

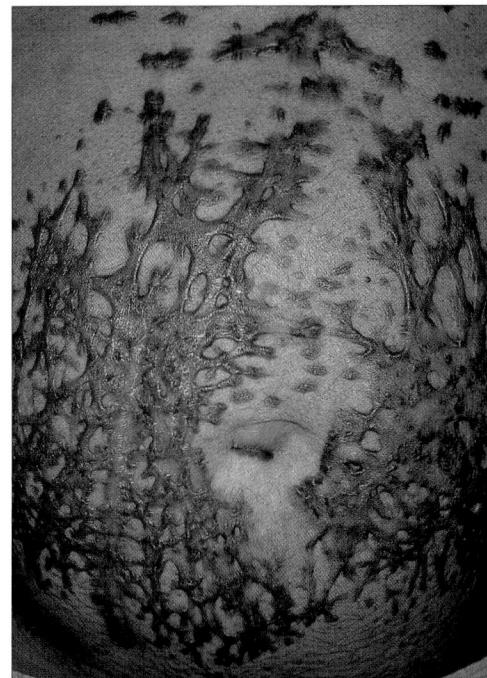

Fig. 90.18 Xanthoma disseminatum. Sclerotic form of xanthoma disseminatum in a patient who developed multiple myeloma.

Mucous membrane lesions are found in 40–60% of patients with xanthoma disseminatum, the upper airway and oral mucosa being commonly involved. Corneal and conjunctival lesions can threaten vision. CNS involvement of the hypothalamus and pituitary stalk results in diabetes insipidus in 40% of patients. This is usually mild, transient, and sensitive to vasopressin. Rare associations with xanthoma disseminatum have included plasma cell dyscrasia, monoclonal gammopathy and thyroid disorders.

Caputo et al.[65] have suggested that patients follow one of three clinical courses: (1) a rare self-healing form with spontaneous resolution of lesions; (2) the common persistent form in which lesions may never resolve; and (3) the very rare progressive form with organ dysfunction and CNS involvement. Mortality has been associated with CNS involvement outside the pituitary and hypothalamus[66].

Pathology

In the early stages, there is a dense dermal infiltrate of histiocytes with few foamy cells or other inflammatory cells. Fully developed lesions, however, demonstrate many foam cells and scattered histiocytes, lymphocytes, plasma cells, Touton cells and neutrophils. When intercellular accumulation of iron, or siderosis, is a prominent feature, the disorder has been called 'disseminated xanthosiderohistiocytosis'. However, like the other histologic features of xanthoma disseminatum, siderosis is also found in juvenile xanthogranuloma and cannot be used to distinguish between the two entities. Xanthoma disseminatum histiocytes stain for lysozyme and α_1-antitrypsin and also express CD68, CD11b, CD14, CD11c and factor XIIIa (see Fig. 90.5, Table 90.2)[65,67].

Differential diagnosis

The disorder most closely related to xanthoma disseminatum is juvenile xanthogranuloma. Mucous membrane lesions and diabetes insipidus are important diagnostic features of xanthoma disseminatum. While xanthoma disseminatum and juvenile xanthogranuloma cannot be differentiated by histopathology, mucous membrane lesions are rare in juvenile xanthogranuloma, and, to date, diabetes insipidus has been reported but once in juvenile xanthogranuloma. In contrast to xanthoma disseminatum, juvenile xanthogranuloma tends to develop in children less than 2 years of age, the lesions tend to be few in number, and the disorder tends to resolve completely over 3–6 years.

Diabetes insipidus is common in LCH, though the clinical lesions, histology, immunophenotype and ultrastructural findings of LCH are completely different from those of xanthoma disseminatum. Bone lesions, very common in LCH, are rare in xanthoma disseminatum. Other conditions easily differentiated on clinical and/or histopathologic bases from xanthoma disseminatum include eruptive xanthoma (see Ch. 91), generalized eruptive histiocytoma, papular xanthoma, and multicentric reticulohistiocytosis.

Treatment

As xanthoma disseminatum is a rare disease, there are no controlled trials for systemic therapy. Radiotherapy has been used to control airway obstructive disease. For cutaneous and mucosal lesions, oral corticosteroids have not been of value, while the effectiveness of clofibrate has been mixed. Cyclophosphamide has been effective in the control of mucosal lesions[65]. Cutaneous lesions have been treated by CO_2 laser, dermabrasion, radiotherapy, electrocoagulation, intralesional corticosteroids, cryotherapy and surgical excision.

REFERENCES

1. Caputo R, Passoni E, Cavicchini S. Papular xanthoma associated with angiokeratoma of Fordyce: considerations on the nosography of this rare non-Langerhans cell histiocytoxanthomatosis. Dermatology 2003;206:165–8.
2. Lichtenstein L. Histiocytosis X: integration of eosinophilic granuloma of bone, "Letterer-Siwe disease" and "Hand-Schüller-Christian" disease as related manifestations of a single nosologic entity. Arch Pathol. 1953;56:84–102.
3. Hashimoto K, Pritzker MS. Electron microscopic study of reticulohistiocytoma. An unusual case of congenital self-healing reticulohistiocytosis. Arch Dermatol. 1973;107:263–70.
4. Chu A, D'Angio GJ, Favara BE, et al. Histiocytosis syndromes in children. Lancet. 1987;2:41–2.
5. Arico M, Nichols K, Whitlock JA, et al. Familial clustering of Langerhans cell histiocytosis. Br J Haematol. 1999;107:883–8.
6. McClain K, Jin H, Gresik V, et al. Langerhans cell histiocytosis: lack of a viral etiology. Am J Hematol. 1994;47:16–20.
7. Willman CL, Busque L, Griffith BB, et al. Langerhans'-cell histiocytosis (histiocytosis X) – a clonal proliferative disease. N Engl J Med. 1994;331:154–60.
8. Yu RC, Chu C, Buluwela L, et al. Clonal proliferation of Langerhans cells in Langerhans cell histiocytosis. Lancet. 1994;343:767–8.
9. Egeler RM, Neglia JP, Arico M, et al. The relation of Langerhans cell histiocytosis to acute leukemia, lymphomas, and other solid tumors. Hematol Oncol Clin North Am. 1998;12:369–78.

10. Gadner G, Grois N, Arico M, et al. A randomized trial of treatment for multisystem Langerhans' cell histiocytosis. J Pediatr. 2001;138:728–34.
11. Gianotti F, Caputo R, Ermacora E. Singulière histiocytose infantile à cellules avec particules vermiformes intracytoplasmiques. Bull Soc Fr Dermatol Syphiliogr. 1971;78:232–3.
12. Jih DM, Salcedo SL, Jaworsky C. Benign cephalic histiocytosis: a case report and review. J Am Acad Dermatol. 2002;47:908–13.
13. Gianotti R, Alessi E, Caputo R. Benign cephalic histiocytosis: a distinct entity or a part of a wide spectrum of histiocytic proliferative disorders of children? Am J Dermatopathol. 1993;15:315–19.
14. Weston WL, Travers SH, Mierau GW, et al. Benign cephalic histiocytosis with diabetes insipidus. Pediatr Dermatol. 2000;17:296–8.
15. Gianotti F, Caputo R, Ermacora E, et al. Benign cephalic histiocytosis. Arch Dermatol. 1986;122:1038–43.
16. Zelger BG, Zelger B, Steiner H, et al. Solitary giant xanthogranuloma and benign cephalic histiocytosis – variants of juvenile xanthogranuloma. Br J Dermatol. 1995;133:598–604.
17. Winkelmann RK, Muller SA. Generalized eruptive histiocytoma: a benign papular histiocytic reticulosis. Arch Dermatol. 1963;88:586–96.
18. Wee SH, Kim HS, Chang SN, et al. Generalized eruptive histiocytoma: a pediatric case. Pediatr Dermatol. 2000;17:453–5.
19. Sidoroff A, Zelger B, Steiner H, et al. Indeterminate cell histiocytosis – a clinicopathological entity with features

of both X- and non-X histiocytosis. Br J Dermatol. 1996;134:525–32.
20. Caputo R, Ermacora E, Gelmetti C, et al. Generalized eruptive histiocytoma in children. J Am Acad Dermatol. 1987;17:449–54.
21. Repiso T, Roca-Miralles M, Kanitakis J, et al. Generalized eruptive histiocytoma evolving into xanthoma disseminatum in a 4-year-old boy. Br J Dermatol. 1995;132:978–82.
22. Wood GS, Hu CH, Beckstead JH, et al. The indeterminate cell proliferative disorder: report of a case manifesting as an unusual cutaneous histiocytosis. Dermatol Surg Oncol. 1985;11:1111–19.
23. Ratzinger G, Burgdorf WH, Metze D, et al. Indeterminate cell histiocytosis: fact or fiction? J Cutan Pathol. 2005;32:552–60.
24. Flores-Stadler EM, Gonzalez-Crussi F, Greene M, et al. Indeterminate-cell histiocytosis: immunophenotypic and cytogenetic findings in an infant. Med Pediatr Oncol. 1999;32:250–4.
25. Manente L, Cotellessa C, Schmitt I, et al. Indeterminate cell histiocytosis: a rare histiocytic disorder. Am J Dermatopathol. 1997;19:276–83.
26. Helwig EB, Hackney VC. Juvenile xanthogranuloma (nevoxantho-endothelioma). Am J Pathol. 1954;30:625–6.
27. Adamson NF. Congenital xanthoma multiplex in a child. Br J Dermatol. 1905;17:222.
28. Caputo R. Juvenile xanthogranuloma. In: Text Atlas of Histicytic Syndromes: A Dermatological Perspective. London: Martin Dunitz, 1998:39–58.

29. Bergman R, Aviram M, Shemer A, et al. Enhanced low-density lipoprotein degradation and cholesterol synthesis in monocyte-derived macrophages of patients with adult xanthogranulomatosis. J Invest Dermatol. 1993;101:880–2.

30. Gianotti F, Caputo R. Histiocytic syndromes: a review. J Am Acad Dermatol. 1985;13:383–404.

31. Freyer DR, Kennedy R, Bostrom BC, et al. Juvenile xanthogranuloma: forms of systemic disease and their clinical implications. J Pediatr. 1996;129:227–37.

32. Chang MW, Frieden IJ, Good W. The risk of intraocular juvenile xanthogranuloma: survey of current practices and assessment of risk. J Am Acad Dermatol. 1996;34:445–9.

33. Zvulunov A, Barak Y, Metzker A. Juvenile xanthogranuloma, neurofibromatosis, and juvenile chronic myelogenous leukemia. World statistical analysis. Arch Dermatol. 1995;131:904–8.

34. Marrogi AJ, Dehner LP, Coffin CM, et al. Benign cutaneous histiocytic tumors in childhood and adolescence, excluding Langerhans' cells proliferations. A clinicopathologic and immunohistochemical analysis. Am J Dermatopathol. 1992;14:8–18.

35. Cerio R, Spaull J, Oliver GF, et al. A study of factor XIIIa and Mac 387 immunolabeling in normal and pathological skin. Am J Dermatopathol. 1990;12:221–33.

36. Hernandez-Martin A, Baselga E, Drolet BA, et al. Juvenile xanthogranuloma. J Am Acad Dermatol. 1997;36:355–67.

37. Kossard S, Winkelmann RK. Necrobiotic xanthogranuloma. Australas J Dermatol. 1980;21:85–8.

38. Mehregan DA, Winkelmann RK. Necrobiotic xanthogranuloma. Arch Dermatol. 1992;128:94–100.

39. Robertson DM, Winkelmann RK. Ophthalmic features of necrobiotic xanthogranuloma with paraproteinemia. Am J Ophthalmol. 1984;97:173–83.

40. Ugurlu S, Bartley GB, Gibson LE. Necrobiotic xanthogranuloma: long-term outcome of ocular and systemic involvement. Am J Ophthalmol. 2000;129:651–7.

41. Finan MC, Winkelmann RK. Necrobiotic xanthogranuloma with paraproteinemia. A review of 22 cases. Medicine. 1986;65:376–88.

42. Stork J, Kodetova D, Vosmik F, et al. Necrobiotic xanthogranuloma presenting as a solitary tumor. Am J Dermatopathol. 2000;22:453–6.

43. Williford PM, White WL, Jorizzo JL, et al. The spectrum of normolipemic plane xanthoma. Am J Dermatopathol. 1993;15:572–5.

44. Zac FG. Reticulohistiocytoma ("ganglioneuroma") of the skin. Br J Dermatol Syphilol. 1950;62:351–5.

45. Goltz RW, Laymon CW. Multicentric reticulohistiocytosis of the skin and synovia. Arch Dermatol Syphilol. 1954;69:717–30.

46. Zayid I, Farraj S. Familial histiocytic dermatoarthritis: a new syndrome. Am J Med. 1973;54:793–800.

47. Barrow MV, Holubar K. Multicentric reticulohistiocytosis. A review of 33 patients. Medicine. 1969;48:287–305.

48. Gorman JD, Danning C, Schumacher HR, et al. Multicentric reticulohistiocytosis: case report with immunohistochemical analysis and literature review. Arthritis Rheum. 2000;43:930–8.

49. Zelger B, Cerio R, Soyer HP, et al. Reticulohistiocytoma and multicentric reticulohistiocytosis. Histopathologic and immunophenotypic distinct entities. Am J Dermatopathol. 1994;16:577–84.

50. Rentsch JL, Martin EM, Harrison LC, et al. Prolonged response of multicentric reticulohistiocytosis to low dose methotrexate. J Rheumatol. 1998;25:1012–15.

51. Rosai J, Dorfman RF. Sinus histiocytosis with massive lymphadenopathy. A newly recognized benign clinicopathological entity. Arch Pathol. 1969;87:63–70.

52. Weedon D. Rosai-Dorfman disease. In: Skin Pathology. New York: Churchill Livingstone, 1997:865–96.

53. Foucar E, Rosai J, Dorfman R. Sinus histiocytosis with massive lymphadenopathy (Rosai-Dorfman disease): review of the entity. Semin Diagn Pathol. 1990; 7:19–73.

54. Rosai J. Lymph nodes. In: Ackerman's Surgical Pathology, 8th edn. St. Louis: Mosby, 1996:1694–5.

55. Levine PH, Jahan N, Murari P, et al. Detection of human herpesvirus 6 in tissues involved by sinus histiocytosis with massive lymphadenopathy (Rosai-Dorfman disease). J Infect Dis. 1992;166:291–5.

56. Sumiyoshi Y, Kikuchi M, Ohshima K, et al. Human herpesvirus-6 genomes in histiocytic necrotizing lymphadenitis (Kikuchi's disease) and other forms of lymphadenitis. Am J Clin Pathol. 1993;99:609–14.

57. Maric I, Pittaluga S, Dale JK, et al. Histologic features of sinus histiocytosis with massive lymphadenopathy in patients with autoimmune lymphoproliferative syndrome. Am J Surg Pathol. 2005;29:903–11.

58. Foucar E, Rosai J, Dorfman RF. Sinus histiocytosis with massive lymphadenopathy. An analysis of 14 deaths occurring in a patient registry. Cancer. 1984;54:1834–40.

59. Paulli M, Rosso R, Kindl S, et al. Immunophenotypic characterization of the cell infiltrate in five cases of sinus histiocytosis with massive lymphadenopathy (Rosai-Dorfman disease). Hum Pathol. 1992;23:647–54.

60. Paulli M, Feller AC, Boveri E, et al. Cathepsin D and E co-expression in sinus histiocytosis with massive lymphadenopathy (Rosai-Dorfman disease) and Langerhans' cell histiocytosis: further evidences of a phenotypic overlap between these histiocytic disorders. Virchows Arch. 1994;424:601–6.

61. Jang YJ, Park KH, Seok HJ. Management of Kikuchi's disease using glucocorticoid. J Laryngol Otol. 2000;114:709–11.

62. Olsen EA, Crawford JR, Vollmer RT. Sinus histiocytosis with massive lymphadenopathy. Case report and review of a multisystemic disease with cutaneous infiltrates. J Am Acad Dermatol. 1988;18:1322–32.

63. Montgomery H, Osterberg AE. Xanthomatosis. Correlation of clinical, histopathologic and chemical studies of cutaneous xanthoma. Arch Derm Syphilol. 1938;37:373–402.

64. Altman J, Winkelmann RK. Xanthoma disseminatum. Arch Dermatol. 1962;86:582–96.

65. Caputo R, Veraldi S, Grimalt R, et al. The various clinical patterns of xanthoma disseminatum. Considerations on seven cases and review of the literature. Dermatology. 1995;190:19–24.

66. Hammond RR, Mackenzie IRA. Xanthoma disseminatum with massive intracranial involvement. Clin Neuropathol. 1995;14:314–21.

67. Zelger B, Cerio R, Orchard G, et al. Histologic and immunohistochemical study comparing xanthoma disseminatum and histiocytosis X. Arch Dermatol. 1992;128:1207–12.

Xanthomas

W Trent Massengale and Lee T Nesbitt Jr

91

Key features

- Cutaneous xanthomas can signal the presence of an underlying hyperlipidemia or monoclonal gammopathy
- An understanding of basic lipid metabolism provides insight into the underlying hyperlipoproteinemias as well as the formation of xanthomas
- The major forms of xanthomas associated with hyperlipidemia are: eruptive, tuberous, tendinous and plane (including xanthelasma)
- Normolipemic plane xanthomas occur in association with monoclonal gammopathies
- Histologically, lipid-laden macrophages (foam cells) are seen in the dermis
- Prompt recognition and proper treatment can lead to xanthoma resolution as well as prevention of potentially life-threatening complications

Introduction

Cutaneous xanthomas develop as a result of intracellular and dermal deposition of lipid. One of the major distinguishing clinical features of xanthomatous tissue is a characteristic yellow to orange hue. Lesions may present with a variety of morphologies, from macules and papules to plaques and nodules. As discussed below, the morphology and anatomic location of the lesions can suggest the type of underlying lipid disorder or presence of a paraproteinemia.

Xanthomas can exist in the setting of primary or secondary disorders of lipid metabolism. Early recognition of these lesions can make a significant impact on the diagnosis, management and prognosis of patients who suffer from an underlying disease. It is therefore important for dermatologists to become familiar with the basic concepts of lipid metabolism and the associated disease states, as well as be able to recognize the often pathognomonic lesions that can point to a specific underlying disease state.

Epidemiology

Hyperlipidemia is quite common in the general population. In North America alone, it is estimated that over 100 million people currently have an elevated serum cholesterol level >200 mg/dl. Despite the large number of people who suffer from hyperlipidemia, only a minority will develop cutaneous xanthomas. It is not always possible to predict who will develop xanthomas, because the exact mechanism by which they form is not yet fully understood. It is believed they result from the permeation of circulating plasma lipoproteins through dermal capillary blood vessels followed by phagocytosis of the lipoproteins by macrophages, forming lipid-laden cells known as foam cells[1]. However, the precise steps and their regulation are still an area of investigation.

Pathogenesis

There is strong evidence to support the theory that the lipids found in the various xanthomas are the same as those in the circulation[2]. The majority of plasma lipids are transported in complex structures known as lipoproteins. The basic structure of the lipoprotein allows the delivery of triglycerides and cholesterol to peripheral cells for their metabolic needs. This structure consists of a hydrophilic outer shell and a hydrophobic core. The outer shell consists of phospholipids, free cholesterol,

and non-covalently linked specialized proteins known as apolipoproteins or apoproteins (apo). The inner core contains triglycerides and cholesterol esters.

Lipoproteins differ in their core lipid content. Triglycerides are the major core lipids in chylomicrons and very-low-density lipoproteins (VLDLs), while cholesterol esters dominate the core of low-density lipoproteins (LDLs), high-density lipoproteins (HDLs), and remnants of chylomicrons and VLDLs. The apoproteins found in the outer shell can also differ amongst the various lipoproteins (Table 91.1). These proteins serve several important functions, such as mediating the binding of lipoproteins to their respective receptors in target organs and activating enzymes involved in their metabolism.

There are two major pathways of lipoprotein synthesis (Fig. 91.1A). The exogenous pathway begins with dietary fat intake. Through the action of pancreatic lipase and bile acids, dietary triglycerides are degraded to fatty acids and monoglycerides. After absorption by the intestinal epithelium, the triglycerides are reformed and packaged with a small amount of cholesterol esters into the central core of a chylomicron. The outer shell of the chylomicron consists of phospholipids, free cholesterol, and several apoproteins, including B-48, E, A-I, A-II and C-II.

Chylomicrons then enter the lymphatics and eventually the systemic circulation via the thoracic duct. Once in the circulation, hydrolysis of the core triglycerides occurs, releasing free fatty acids to the peripheral tissues. This is mediated through the action of the enzyme lipoprotein lipase that is bound to capillary endothelium. The activation of the lipoprotein lipase system is complex and involves not only hormones such as insulin, but also apoproteins such as C-II, located on the lipoprotein outer surface.

After hydrolysis of approximately 70% of the original triglyceride content, a chylomicron 'remnant' exists. The central core now contains predominantly cholesterol ester that has been acquired from circulating HDL molecules. The chylomicron remnant is taken up in the liver by specialized high-affinity apo B-100/E receptors that recognize the apoproteins E_3 or E_4 on its outer shell. Once in the liver, the remaining lipids enter hepatic storage and apoproteins such as B-48 are degraded.

The endogenous pathway begins with the hepatic formation of VLDL particles. The central core of the VLDL consists primarily of triglycerides. The triglycerides are derived from circulating free fatty

IMPORTANT APOPROTEINS		
Apoprotein	**Lipoprotein association**	**Function and comments**
A-I	Chylomicrons, HDLs	Major protein of HDL; activates *lecithin:cholesterol acyltransferase* (LCAT)
B-48	Chylomicrons, chylomicron remnants	Unique marker for chylomicrons
B-100	VLDLs, IDLs and LDLs	Major protein of LDL; binds to LDL receptor
C-II	Chylomicrons, VLDLs, IDLs and HDLs	Activates lipoprotein lipase
E (at least 3 alleles [E2, E3, E4])	Chylomicrons, chylomicron remnants, VLDLs, IDLs and HDLs	Binds to LDL receptor

Table 91.1 Important apoproteins. HDL, high-density lipoprotein; IDL, intermediate-density lipoprotein; LDL, low-density lipoprotein; VLDL, very-low-density lipoprotein.

1411

EXOGENOUS AND ENDOGENOUS PATHWAYS OF LIPOPROTEIN SYNTHESIS AND SITES OF DYSFUNCTION THAT LEAD TO THE MAJOR FORMS OF HYPERLIPIDEMIA

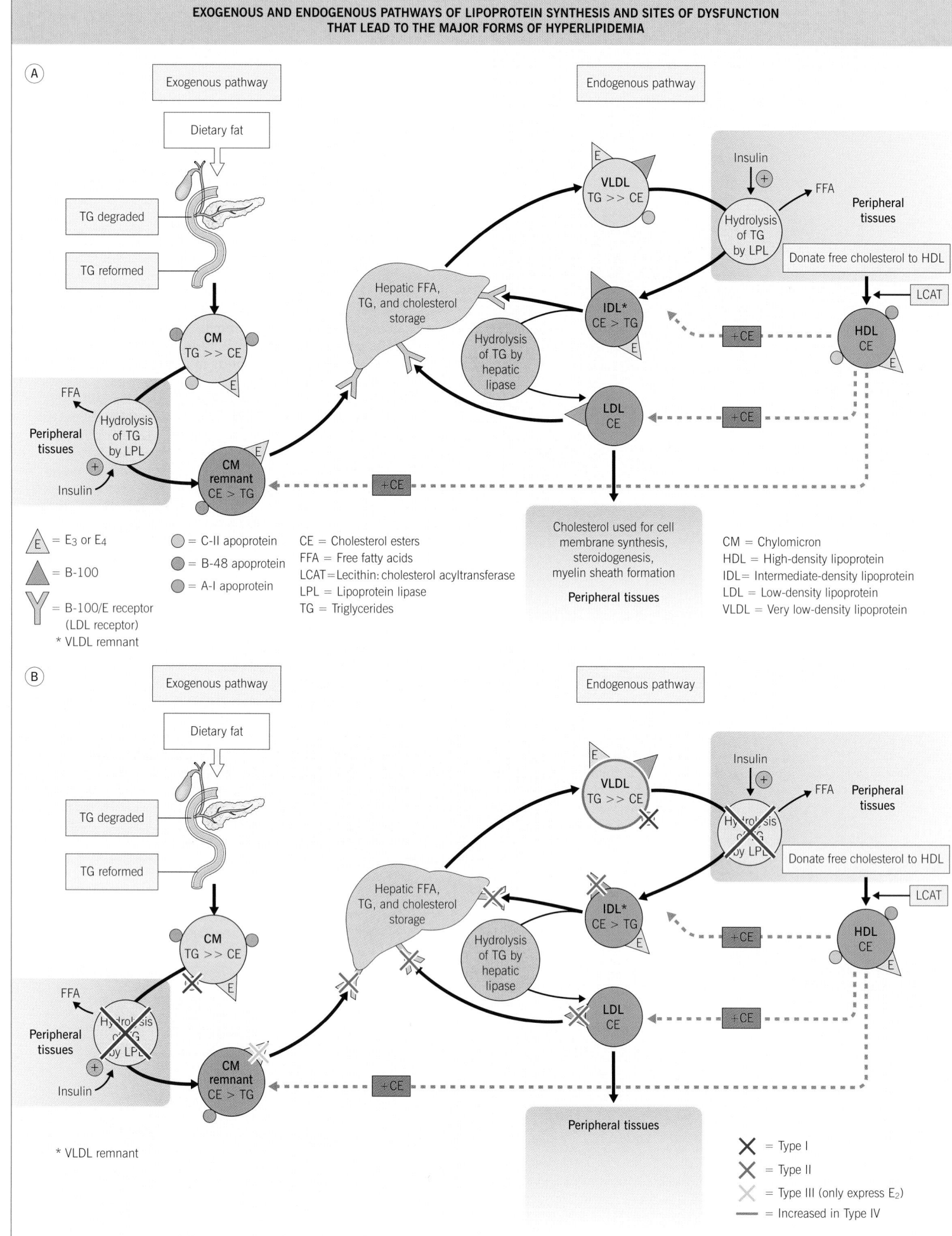

Fig. 91.1 Exogenous and endogenous pathways of lipoprotein synthesis (A) and sites of dysfunction that lead to the major forms of hyperlipidemia (B). Lipoprotein lipase (LPL) is activated by the C-II apoprotein.

acids and hepatic triglyceride stores. Important apoproteins found on the outer shell include B-100, E, and C-II. In a fashion similar to the chylomicron, lipoprotein lipase mediates hydrolysis of the VLDL molecule, removing the majority of its triglyceride content, and cholesterol esters are acquired from HDL molecules. Lipoprotein lipase activation requires the presence of apo C-II on the VLDL outer shell. After removal of the majority of the triglyceride content, the VLDL 'remnant', also known as an intermediate-density lipoprotein (IDL), can then be taken up in the liver by apo B-100/E receptors and degraded. IDLs that escape uptake by the hepatocyte are stripped of their remaining core triglycerides by extracellular hepatic lipases and enter the circulation as LDLs.

The LDL contains predominantly cholesterol ester in its central core and expresses B-100 on its surface. LDL delivers the cholesterol ester to peripheral tissues, where it can be converted to free cholesterol. Cholesterol has several important functions in the body, such as being an essential component of cell membrane bilayers. It is also important in the production of the myelin sheath of nerves, adrenal and gonadal steroidogenesis, and the production of bile acids. Hepatocytes play the major role in the catabolism of LDLs. Their uptake is mediated through the high-affinity apo B-100/E receptor found on the cell surface of the hepatocytes. Free cholesterol in excess of metabolic needs is re-esterified for storage.

HDLs serve several important functions in cholesterol metabolism. One of the primary functions of HDLs is the removal of cholesterol from the peripheral tissues. During this process, free cholesterol and phospholipids are transferred from the cell membranes of peripheral cells to the HDL molecules. The free cholesterol is then esterified by the enzyme lecithin:cholesterol acyltransferase, or LCAT. This enzyme requires the presence of the HDL apoprotein A-I. HDL molecules then transfer the cholesterol esters to other lipoproteins such as LDLs or remnants of chylomicrons and VLDLs for transportation back to the liver.

The liver plays the central role in the overall cholesterol economy. Hepatic intracellular cholesterol levels have a direct impact on the activity of HMG-CoA reductase, the rate-limiting enzyme of cholesterol synthesis, and on the expression of the high-affinity apo B-100/E receptor. When intracellular cholesterol levels are low, HMG-CoA reductase becomes activated and high-affinity apo B-100/E receptor expression increases. The increase in high-affinity receptors leads to increased uptake of cholesterol-containing lipoproteins such as chylomicron remnants, IDLs and LDLs. This is followed by the lowering of plasma cholesterol levels. As discussed later, this mechanism will be the basis for many of the pharmacologic interventions aimed at lowering cholesterol agents.

Clinical Features

Due to the complexity of cholesterol homeostasis, there are several possible ways in which hyperlipidemia may occur. Genetic mutations can affect important enzymes, receptors or receptor ligands, with such defects leading to the overproduction of lipoproteins or the inhibition of their clearance (Fig 91.1B). Each possible defect would lead to a different abnormal lipid profile.

In 1965, Lees & Frederickson[3] published a system for classifying various disorders of lipid metabolism based upon the electrophoretic migration of the serum lipoproteins present. This system for phenotyping hyperlipoproteinemias is used today in a modified form (Table 91.2). There have also been advances with regard to the underlying pathogenesis of several of the hyperlipidemic syndromes. In the sections that follow, the clinical features of the different types of xanthomas will be discussed, as well as the disorders in which they are found. Descriptions of the lipid disorders will reference not only the Frederickson classification system but also the specific molecular defects when possible.

Eruptive xanthomas

Eruptive xanthomas appear as erythematous to yellow papules, approximately 1 to 4 mm in diameter. They are usually distributed on the extensor surfaces of the extremities, buttocks and hands (Figs 91.2 & 91.3). Early in their development, lesions may have an inflammatory halo (likely due to their triglyceride component), which may be accompanied by tenderness and pruritus. The Koebner phenomenon has been reported to occur with eruptive xanthomas[6].

Eruptive xanthomas can be seen in the setting of primary or secondary hypertriglyceridemia. Triglyceride levels in patients with eruptive xanthomas often exceed 3000 to 4000 mg/dl. In the Frederickson classification of hyperlipidemias, hypertriglyceridemia can be seen in type I (elevated chylomicrons), type IV (elevated VLDLs) and type V (elevated chylomicrons and VLDLs).

IMPORTANT HYPERLIPOPROTEINEMIAS				
Type	Pathogenesis	Laboratory findings	Clinical findings	
			Skin (types of xanthoma)	Systemic
Type I (familial LPL deficiency, familial hyperchylomicronemia)	(a) Deficiency of LPL (b) Production of abnormal LPL (c) Apo C-II deficiency	Slow chylomicron clearance Reduced LDL and HDL levels Hypertriglyceridemia	Eruptive	No increased risk of coronary artery disease
Type II (familial hypercholesterolemia or familial defective apo B-100)	(a) LDL receptor defect (b) Reduced affinity of LDL for LDL receptor (c) Accelerated degradation of LDL receptor due to missense PCSK9 mutations*	Reduced LDL clearance Hypercholesterolemia	Tendinous, tuberoeruptive, tuberous, plane (xanthelasma, intertriginous areas, interdigital web spaces†)	Atherosclerosis of peripheral and coronary arteries
Type III (familial dysbetalipoproteinemia, remnant removal disease, broad beta disease, apo E deficiency)	Hepatic remnant clearance impaired due to apo E abnormality; patients only express the apo E2 isoform that interacts poorly with the apo E receptor	Elevated levels of chylomicron remnants and IDLs Hypercholesterolemia Hypertriglyceridemia	Tuberoeruptive, tuberous, plane (palmar creases) Tendinous	Atherosclerosis of peripheral and coronary arteries
Type IV (endogenous familial hypertriglyceridemia)	Elevated production of VLDL associated with glucose intolerance and hyperinsulinemia	Increased VLDLs Hypertriglyceridemia	Eruptive	Frequently associated with type 2 non-insulin-dependent diabetes mellitus, obesity, alcoholism (see Fig. 91.4)
Type V	Elevated chylomicrons and VLDLs due to unknown cause	Decreased LDLs and HDLs Hypertriglyceridemia	Eruptive	Diabetes mellitus

*Almost exclusively in African-Americans[4,5].
†Said to be pathognomonic for homozygous state.

Table 91.2 Important hyperlipoproteinemias. Apo, apolipoprotein; HDL, high-density lipoprotein; IDL, intermediate-density lipoprotein; LDL, low-density lipoprotein; LPL, lipoprotein lipase; PCSK9, proprotein convertase subtilisin kexin 9; VLDL, very-low-density lipoprotein.

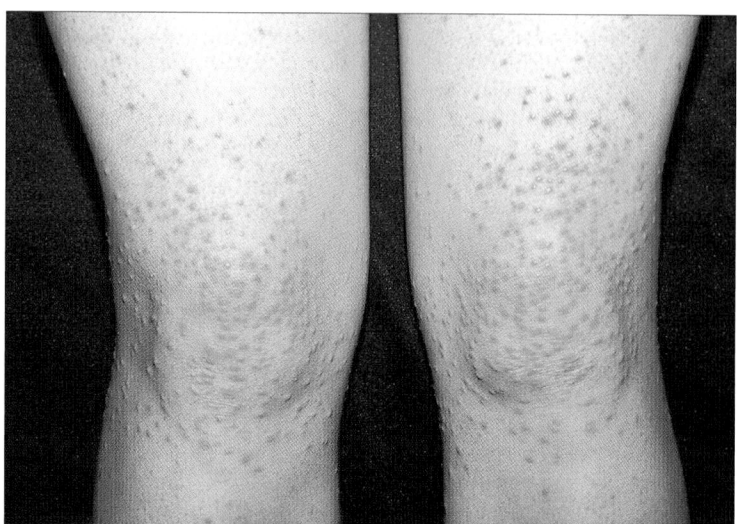

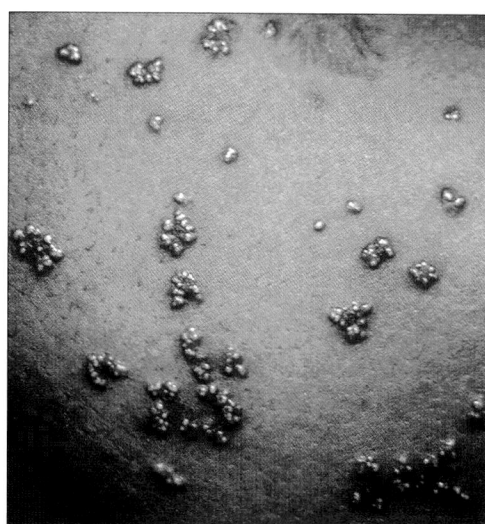

Fig. 91.3 **Eruptive xanthomas.** Note the yellowish hue and 'mulberry' pattern in a patient with Frederickson type IV disease.

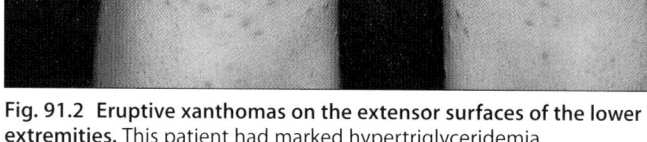

Fig. 91.2 **Eruptive xanthomas on the extensor surfaces of the lower extremities.** This patient had marked hypertriglyceridemia.

One reason for elevated triglyceride levels is failure to remove such lipids from the circulation. Deficient activity of lipoprotein lipase will lead to accumulation of triglyceride-rich chylomicrons and VLDLs. This can be related to abnormalities in the enzyme itself, as in *lipoprotein lipase deficiency (chylomicronemia syndrome)*, or in other controlling factors such as *dysfunctional apoprotein C-II* or impaired insulin activity (Fig. 91.4)[7,8].

Another reason for increased triglyceride levels is hepatic overproduction of triglyceride-rich lipoproteins via the endogenous pathway. In *endogenous familial hypertriglyceridemia*, a genetic defect exists that causes the liver to respond abnormally to dietary carbohydrates and insulin, with overproduction of hepatic VLDLs. The result is a Frederickson type IV pattern of hypertriglyceridemia. Secondary acquired defects in lipoprotein lipase activity, such as those due to diabetes mellitus, are not uncommon in these patients. With this second insult, the lipoprotein lipase system can become saturated and, as a result, no longer handles dietary lipids, leading to chylomicron elevations as well. This pattern is classified as a Frederickson type V phenotype.

Environmental factors and underlying diseases commonly exacerbate genetic defects of triglyceride metabolism, leading to worsening of the hypertriglyceridemia with eruptive xanthoma formation. Such factors include obesity, high caloric intake, diabetes mellitus, alcohol abuse, oral estrogen replacement and retinoid therapy. The resultant pattern usually leads to a Frederickson type IV phenotype. Oral retinoid therapy with acitretin, isotretinoin and especially bexarotene can elevate triglyceride levels through the elevation of hepatic VLDL secretion. With isotretinoin, this finding seems to be more prevalent in genetically predisposed individuals and may signal an increased risk for future hypertriglyceridemia and metabolic syndrome.

The treatment of eruptive xanthomas involves the identification and treatment of the underlying causes of the hypertriglyceridemia (see Fig. 91.4). Failure to recognize and treat the patient with hypertriglyceridemia could lead to complications of acute pancreatitis or atherosclerosis. Dietary and pharmacologic lowering of the circulating triglycerides to reasonable levels will result in the prompt resolution of the eruptive lesions.

Tuberous/tuberoeruptive xanthomas

Tuberoeruptive and tuberous xanthomas are clinically and pathologically related and often described as being on a continuum. Tuberoeruptive xanthomas present as pink–yellow papules or nodules on extensor

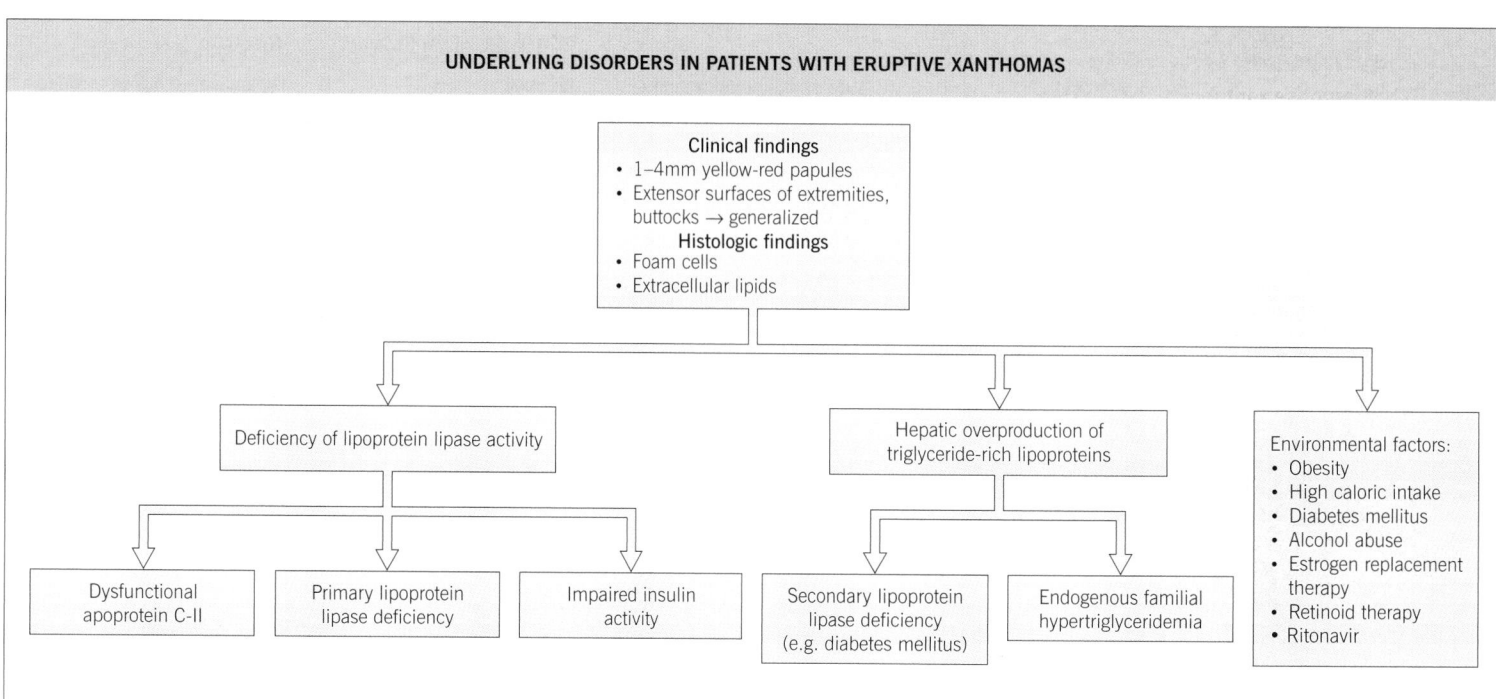

Fig. 91.4 **Underlying disorders in patients with eruptive xanthomas.**

surfaces, especially the elbows and knees (Fig. 91.5). Tuberous lesions are noted to be larger than tuberoeruptive lesions and may exceed 3 cm in diameter (Fig. 91.6). Together, these lesions can be seen in hypercholesterolemic states such as *dysbetalipoproteinemia* (Frederickson type III) and *familial hypercholesterolemia* (Frederickson type II; see below). In contrast to eruptive xanthomas, tuberous xanthomas are usually slow to regress following institution of appropriate therapy.

Dysbetalipoproteinemia, or broad beta disease, is a genetic disorder of lipid metabolism that is inherited in an autosomal dominant fashion. It is caused by the presence of an isoform of apo E, mainly apo E_2, that is a poor ligand for the high-affinity apo B-100/E receptor. This results in the poor hepatic uptake of chylomicron and VLDL remnants. As a result, both the serum levels of cholesterol and triglycerides are elevated. The cutaneous lesions that are most characteristic of this disease are tuberous or tuberoeruptive xanthomas (present in 80% of patients) and plane xanthomas of the palmar creases (*xanthoma striatum palmare*), which are present in two-thirds of the patients[10].

Tendinous xanthomas

Tendinous xanthomas are firm, smooth, nodular lipid deposits that can affect the Achilles tendons (Fig. 91.7) or the extensor tendons of the hands (Fig. 91.8), knees or elbows. The overlying skin is normal in appearance. Ultrasound can help in the diagnosis of subtle lesions of the Achilles tendon by demonstrating hypoechoic nodules or an increase in the anteroposterior diameter of the tendon[11]. The presence of tendinous xanthomas is almost always a clue to an underlying disorder

of lipid metabolism. Lipid disorders that have been associated with this type of xanthoma include familial hypercholesterolemia, dysbetalipoproteinemia, and hepatic cholestasis (Table 91.3).

Tendinous xanthomas are most frequently seen in the setting of *familial hypercholesterolemia*. This disorder results from a deficiency of normal LDL receptors on cell membranes, which leads to the poor hepatic clearance of circulating LDLs and, therefore, elevated LDL cholesterol levels (Frederickson type II). This condition is inherited in an autosomal dominant fashion with a high degree of penetrance. Homozygotes can have LDL cholesterol levels of 800 to 1000 mg/dl with widespread atherosclerosis and the appearance of xanthomas during

SECONDARY HYPERLIPIDEMIA – UNDERLYING DISORDERS
• Diabetes mellitus
• Cholestasis
– Primary biliary cirrhosis (often plane xanthomas, including palmar)
– Biliary atresia
• Hypothyroidism
• Nephrotic syndrome

Table 91.3 Secondary hyperlipidemia – underlying disorders.

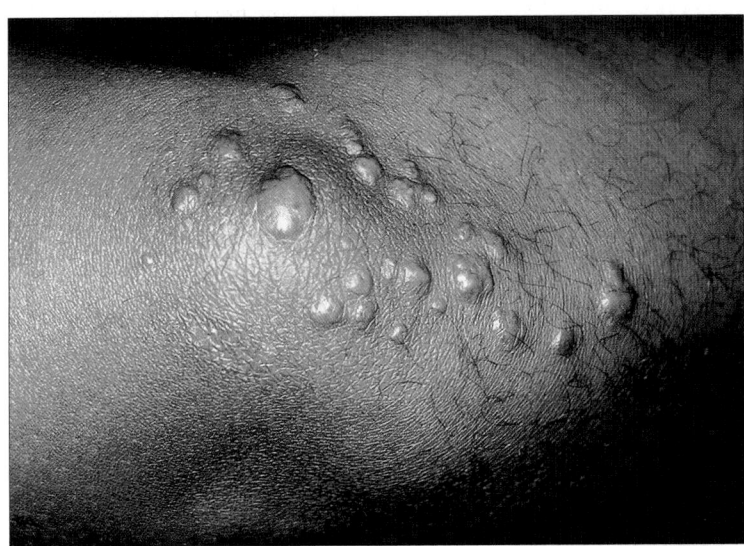

Fig. 91.5 **Tuberoeruptive xanthomas of the elbow.** Note the yellowish hue.

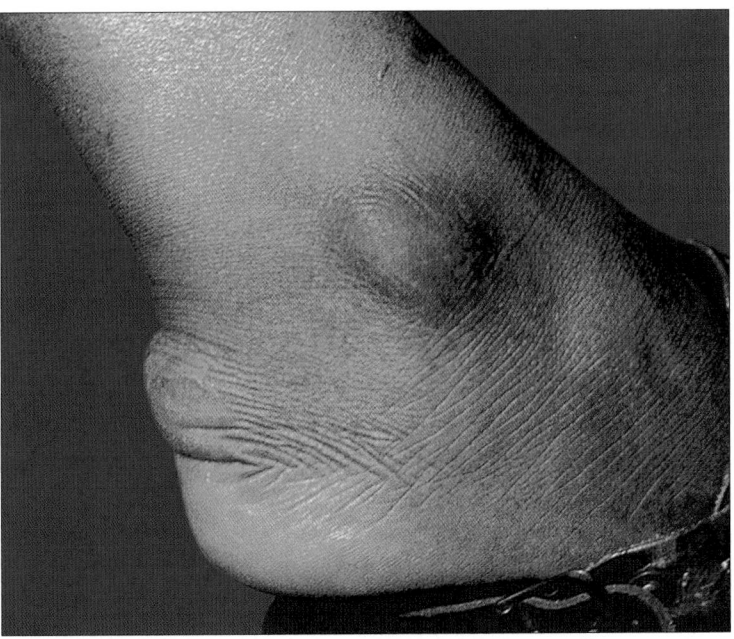

Fig. 91.7 **Tendinous xanthoma.** Linear swelling of the Achilles area, representing a tendinous xanthoma in a patient with dysbetalipoproteinemia.

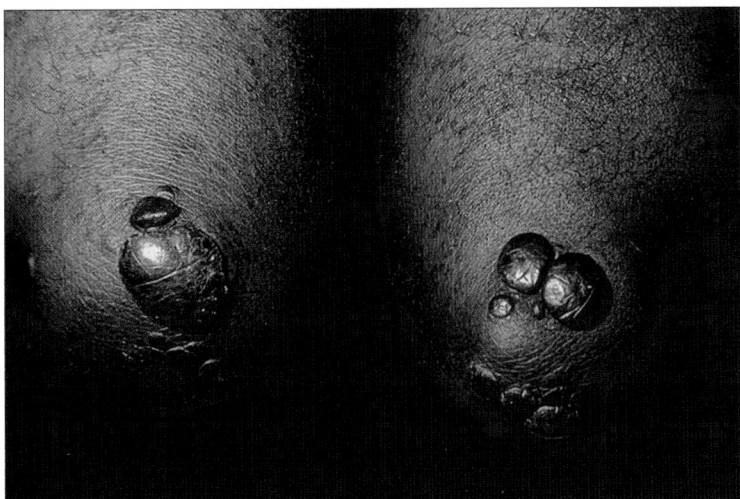

Fig. 91.6 **Nodular tuberous xanthomas of the elbows.** This form occurred in a young patient with familial hypercholesterolemia.

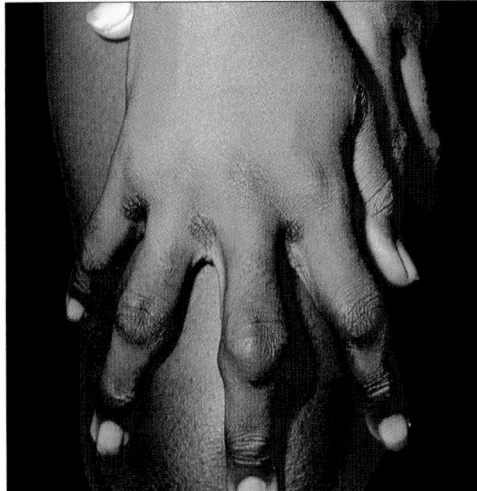

Fig. 91.8 **Tendinous xanthomas of the fingers in a patient with homozygous familial hypercholesterolemia.** Note intertriginous plane xanthomas of the web spaces.

the first decade of life. Heterozygosity for the disorder is more common and is estimated to occur in 1 in 500 individuals in the US. The types of xanthomas seen in this disorder include tendinous, tuberous, tubero-eruptive, and plane (including xanthelasma). Because of its relatively common occurrence, patients with tendinous xanthomas are more likely to have the heterozygous form of the disease than the rare homozygous state. Plane xanthomas of the intertriginous web spaces of the fingers are thought to be pathognomonic for the homozygous condition (see Fig. 91.8)[12].

A closely related disorder, known as *familial defective apolipoprotein B-100*, has been described. In this dominantly inherited genetic disorder, the LDL receptor is normal. However, there is decreased affinity of LDL for the LDL receptor because the mutation affects its apo B-100 ligand. Patients may present with identical clinical findings as in familial hypercholesterolemia, although usually not as severe. The value of distinguishing this disorder from familial hypercholesterolemia may become important from a therapeutic standpoint, especially when future treatments become directed more toward correcting LDL receptor function[13].

Rarely, tendinous xanthomas can develop in the absence of a lipoprotein disorder. Two examples are *cerebrotendinous xanthomatosis* and *β-sitosterolemia*. In cerebrotendinous xanthomatosis, an enzymatic defect exists in the bile acid synthetic pathway, leading to the abnormal accumulation of an intermediate known as cholestanol. This intermediate is deposited in most tissues, including the brain, and can also form tendinous xanthomas[14]. In β-sitosterolemia, an abnormal accumulation of plant sterols occurs, leading to tendinous xanthoma formation.

Plane xanthomas and xanthelasma

Plane xanthomas are seen as yellow to orange, non-inflammatory macules, papules, patches and plaques. They can be circumscribed or diffuse. Their location can vary and the site often serves as a clue to the particular underlying disease state. For example, intertriginous plane xanthomas may occur in the antecubital fossae (Fig. 91.9) or the web spaces of the fingers (see Fig. 91.8), where they are almost pathognomonic for homozygous familial hypercholesterolemia[12]. Plane xanthomas of the palmar creases, or *xanthoma striatum palmare* (Fig. 91.10), are almost diagnostic for dysbetalipoproteinemia, especially when accompanied by tuberous xanthomas[15].

Xanthelasma, or *xanthelasma palpebrarum*, are commonly observed plane xanthomas of the eyelids (Fig. 91.11). Although the presence of xanthelasma warrants investigation for hyperlipidemia, the latter is present in only about one-half of the patients with these lesions. Younger patients with xanthelasma, or those with a strong family history of hyperlipidemia and xanthelasma, are more likely to have an underlying lipid disorder and should be appropriately screened.

Plane xanthomas of cholestasis may occur as a complication of diseases such as biliary atresia or primary biliary cirrhosis. In these conditions, unesterified cholesterol begins to accumulate in the blood, leading to plane xanthoma formation. The lesions often begin as localized plaques of the hands and feet, but can become generalized.

Plane xanthomas can also occur in a normolipemic patient, where they may signal the presence of an underlying monoclonal gammopathy (Fig. 91.12), including that due to multiple myeloma or a lymphoproliferative disorder such as B-cell lymphoma or Castleman's disease (see Ch. 119). This type of xanthoma can also be seen in patients with chronic myelomonocytic leukemia. In gammopathy-associated plane xanthomas, monoclonal IgG is thought to bind to circulating LDL, rendering the antibody–LDL complex more susceptible to phagocytosis by macrophages[16]. Favored locations include the neck, upper trunk, flexural folds and periorbital region.

Verruciform xanthomas

Verruciform xanthomas are asymptomatic, planar or verrucous solitary plaques averaging 1 to 2 cm in diameter. They occur primarily in the mouth (Fig. 91.13), but sometimes in anogenital (including the scrotum) or periorificial sites. There is usually no associated hyperlipidemia and the lesions persist for years. Histologically, there is usually hyperkeratosis, acanthosis, papillomatosis and foamy macrophages limited to the submucosa or dermal papillae.

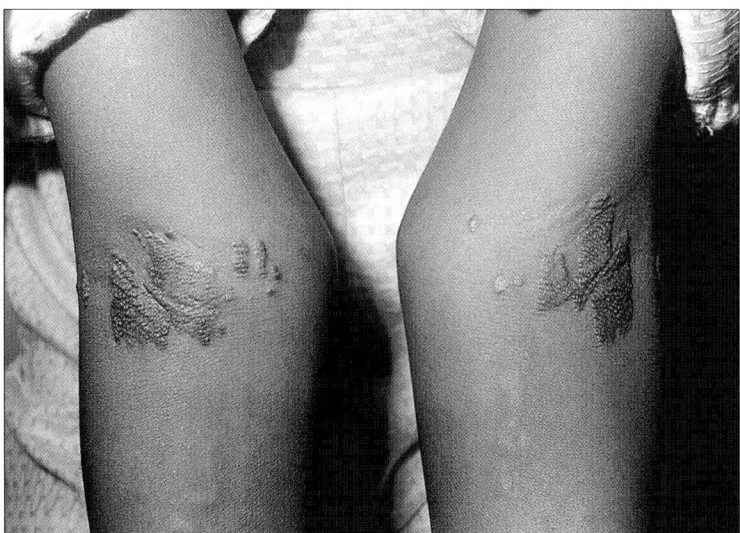

Fig. 91.9 Plane xanthomas of the antecubital fossae in a young patient with homozygous familial hypercholesterolemia.

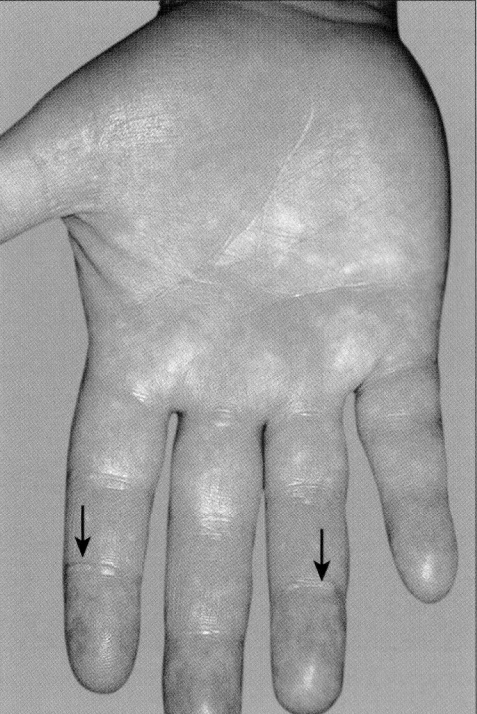

Fig. 91.10 Plane xanthomas of the palmar creases (arrows) in a patient with dysbetalipoproteinemia. They are seen in approximately two-thirds of patients with this disorder.

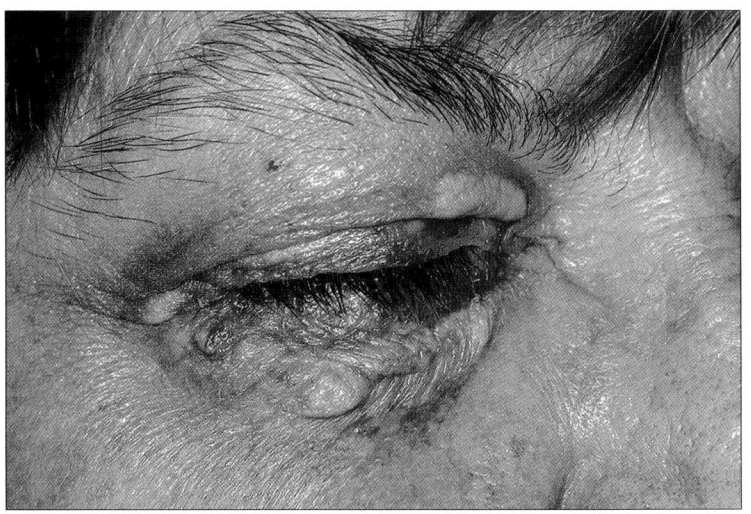

Fig. 91.11 Xanthelasma palpebrarum with typical yellowish hue.

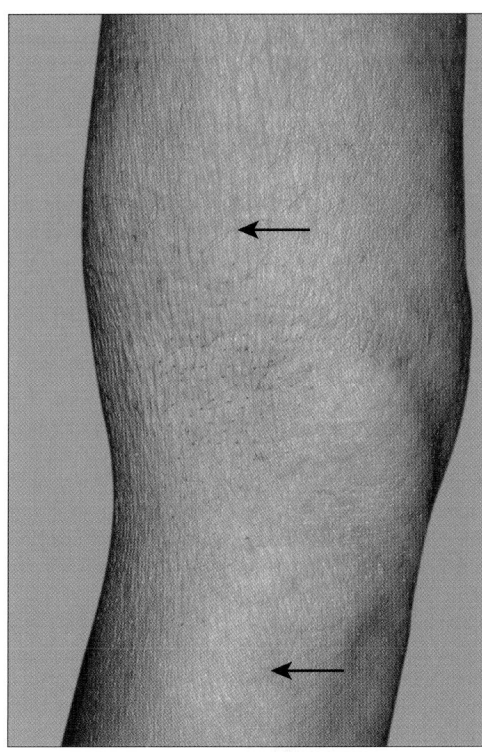

Fig. 91.12 Plane xanthoma in a patient with a monoclonal IgG gammopathy. These lesions can be subtle clinically; arrows point to the edge of the xanthoma.

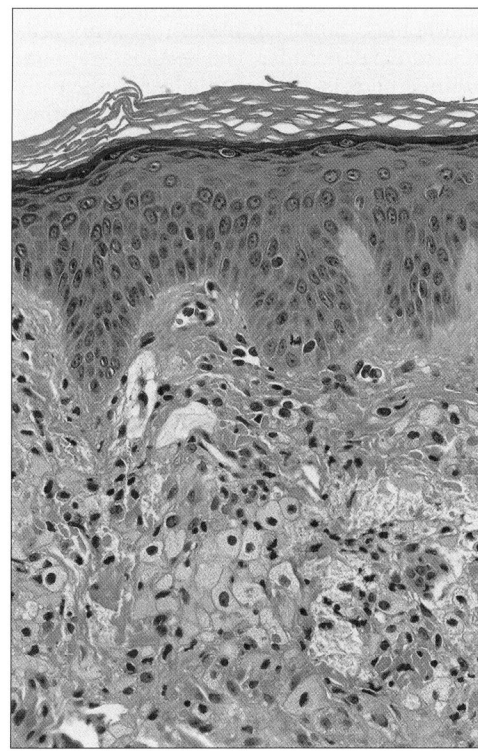

Fig. 91.14 Histology of a xanthoma. Foamy macrophages are seen in the dermis. Courtesy of Ronald P Rapini MD.

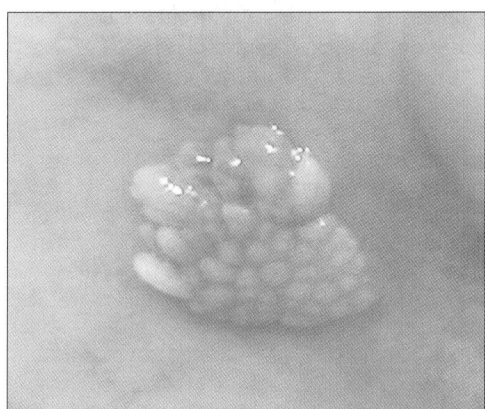

Fig. 91.13 Verruciform xanthoma of the oral mucosa. Courtesy of Kishore Shetty DDS.

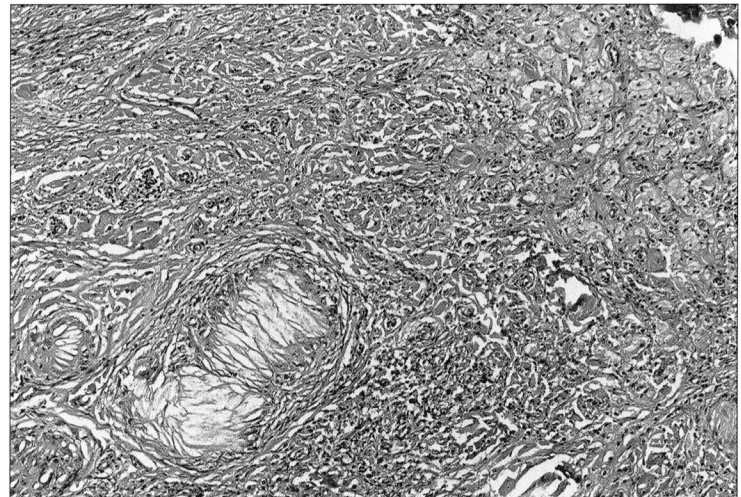

Fig. 91.15 Histology of a tuberous xanthoma. Fibrosis as well as foamy macrophages and cholesterol clefts are present. Courtesy of Ronald P Rapini MD.

These lesions are also seen in the setting of lymphedema, epidermolysis bullosa and GVHD, as well as within cutaneous lesions of the X-linked dominant disorder *c*ongenital *h*emidysplasia with *i*chthyosiform erythroderma and *l*imb *d*efects (CHILD) syndrome. The latter is due to mutations in the *NSDHL* gene, which encodes 3β-hydroxysteroid dehydrogenase, an enzyme involved in cholesterol biosynthesis (see Ch. 56). In a recent molecular study of sporadic verrucous xanthomas, two of nine lesions were found to have a missense somatic mutation in exon 6 of the *NSDHL* gene (only exons 4 and 6 were examined) which differed from the mutations seen in CHILD syndrome[17]. The possibility was raised that enzymatic dysfunction leads to an excess formation and accumulation of lipid storage droplets, followed by formation of lipid-laden dermal macrophages.

Another hypothesis suggests that the foam cells could be due to damage to the epithelium much in the same way as the amyloid deposits within the dermal papillae in lichen amyloidosis. The few foam cells beneath the epithelium may be subtle and easy to miss, in which case they may be confused histologically with warts and other papillomatous conditions. Surgery is generally curative.

Pathology

The characteristic histologic finding in xanthomas is the foam cell. Foam cells consist of macrophages that contain imbibed lipid within their cytoplasm (Fig. 91.14). All xanthomas contain dermal infiltrates of lipid, but they may vary in the degree of lipid content, the inflammatory infiltrate, the amount and location of the infiltrate, and the presence of extracellular lipid. The histologic appearance of xanthomas is somewhat altered by routine processing, as formalin fixation can remove deposits of lipid and leave artifactual clefting. Polarized microscopy can be used to detect lipid material in the dermal infiltrates, as cholesterol esters are doubly refractile.

Eruptive xanthomas contain lipid deposits in the reticular dermis. Of note, early in lesion development, foam cells are relatively small in number and size. The initial inflammatory infiltrate is mixed, containing both neutrophils and lymphocytes. As increased lipidization occurs, the appearance of the lesion becomes more typical of a xanthoma, but foam cells remain fewer in number compared with other types of xanthomas. Extracellular lipids are present in the dermis, which are seen as artifactual clefts filled with a wispy faint blue–gray material.

Tuberous xanthomas demonstrate large aggregates of foam cells in the dermis, often accompanied by fibrosis but without a large number of inflammatory cells (Fig. 91.15). Tendinous xanthomas have a similar histology but the foam cells are even larger in size. Cholesterol esters are present in these lesions and can be seen with polarized microscopy.

Plane xanthomas such as xanthelasma can have a unique histologic appearance. The foam cells in this type of xanthoma are more superficial than in other types of xanthomas. Small aggregates of foam cells are often present in the superficial dermis. The lesions are non-inflammatory and have minimal fibrosis. With xanthelasma, there are often clues as to the location of the lesion, such as a thin epidermis, fine vellus hair follicles, and striated muscle fibers that are characteristic of the eyelid.

Differential Diagnosis

A selection of the diseases included in the differential diagnosis of xanthomas is listed in Table 91.4.

Treatment

The treatment of xanthomas associated with hyperlipidemia requires the identification of the underlying lipoprotein disorder and other possible exacerbating factors. A multidisciplinary approach is often required to manage these complex patients. In addition to dietary measures, there are several lipid-lowering pharmacologic agents available to help lower lipid levels in patients with primary and secondary hyperlipidemia. The main classes of lipid-lowering agents include HMG-CoA reductase inhibitors, bile acid-binding resins, nicotinic acid, probucol, and fibric acid derivatives. Correction of the underlying lipid disorder leads to the eventual resolution of the xanthomas in many patients. Xanthomas that have grown slowly over years, such as tendinous and tuberous xanthomas, are often slow to regress, whereas eruptive xanthomas may disappear within weeks of aggressive therapy.

Dietary measures are important components of successful lipid-lowering therapy. Decreasing total caloric intake and the achievement of ideal body weight alone can make a significant impact on lipid levels in some patients. Dietary fat restriction to less than 30% of total caloric intake should be attempted. Monounsaturated fats such as olive oil should comprise the majority of the fat intake. Alcohol avoidance is essential, especially in patients with hypertriglyceridemia.

The HMG-CoA reductase inhibitors (often referred to as 'statins') represent a major class of drugs used to treat hypercholesterolemia. They work via competitive inhibition of the rate-limiting enzyme of hepatic cholesterol synthesis, HMG-CoA reductase. This inhibition leads to the depletion of hepatocellular stores of cholesterol. Hepatic LDL receptors that bind apo B-100/E are then upregulated, directly lowering circulating LDL levels. VLDL remnants, which are LDL precursors, are also removed by the increase in B-100/E-binding receptors, leading to further decreases in LDL levels. VLDL synthesis by the endogenous lipid pathway is also reduced. The end result is a 25–45% decrease in LDL levels and a 25% decrease in VLDL levels. HDL levels

are affected positively, with a 10% increase. These agents are useful in many lipid disorders such as heterozygous familial hypercholesterolemia, as well as in diabetes mellitus, nephrotic syndrome and other diseases associated with hypercholesterolemia. Importantly, LDL levels are not significantly affected in patients with homozygous familial hypercholesterolemia, since LDL receptor function is totally lacking.

Although the use of HMG-CoA reductase inhibitors is considered safe, there are several important adverse affects. These include elevations in hepatic transaminases and myopathy. The risk for myopathy may be increased by the simultaneous administration of other medications such as cyclosporine, erythromycin, nicotinic acid and fibrates. Warfarin levels may also be increased with concurrent administration. Drug-induced dermatomyositis has been reported in patients on HMG-CoA reductase inhibitors[18].

Inhibitors of cholesteryl ester transfer protein (CETP) represent another, newer class of lipid-lowering drugs. An example would be torcetrapib. These inhibitors increase circulating levels of HDLs and it was hoped that they could be combined with an HMG-CoA reductase inhibitor. However, a 60% increase in deaths, in particular cardiovascular, in patients on combination therapy (as compared to a statin alone) led to termination of clinical trials.

Bile acid-binding resins are useful agents for the lowering of LDL cholesterol. They act by binding to bile acids in the small intestine, preventing their reabsorption in the terminal ileum. With the enhancement of bile acid secretion, the liver must increase its synthesis of bile acids from cholesterol. The subsequent decrease in hepatic cholesterol stores leads to increased numbers of high-affinity LDL receptors on the hepatocyte surface as well as increased HMG-CoA reductase activity. Although an increase in cholesterol synthesis partially negates the overall lowering of cholesterol, the ultimate result is a 10–35% decrease in total LDL levels. This lowering can be further enhanced by the addition of an HMG-CoA reductase inhibitor or nicotinic acid.

The bile acid-binding resins are the safest systemic agents available for hypercholesterolemia. They are used effectively in the treatment of heterozygous familial hypercholesterolemia, but, like the HMG-CoA reductase inhibitors, they are ineffective in the homozygous condition. Resins can elevate triglyceride levels, especially in patients with dysbetalipoproteinemia and pre-existing hypertriglyceridemia. The most notable side effects are patient intolerance to the gritty texture of the powder and gastrointestinal upset. Importantly, the resins can affect the absorption of other medications such as digitalis, thyroxine and warfarin.

Nicotinic acid or niacin is a water-soluble B-complex vitamin with lipid-lowering properties. Its primary effect is to lower VLDL synthesis and therefore LDL levels. Lipoprotein lipase activity is also enhanced, which facilitates lowering of plasma triglyceride levels. Nicotinic acid raises HDL levels by unknown mechanisms. The overall effect of niacin therapy is a rapid decrease in triglyceride levels of 20–80%, a slower decrease in LDL levels of 10–15%, and a 20–30 mg/dl increase in HDL.

Niacin may be used alone or in combination with the HMG-CoA reductase inhibitors or bile acid-binding resins. Complicating its administration is a poor side-effect profile. Intense flushing and pruritus are commonly experienced. Hepatic dysfunction and the ability to worsen glucose intolerance are also potential adverse effects. As mentioned above, when used in combination with the HMG-CoA reductase inhibitors, the potential for myopathy and rhabdomyolysis is increased. Cutaneous side effects include acanthosis nigricans, hyperpigmentation and xerosis[19]. Niacin is most commonly used either as part of combination therapy for familial hypercholesterolemia or to treat severe hypertriglyceridemia refractory to fibric acid derivatives in order to prevent pancreatitis.

Probucol is a drug that has both lipid-lowering and antioxidant effects. Although it lowers plasma LDL levels, it has no effect on plasma triglyceride levels and can lower HDL levels significantly, which limits its therapeutic usefulness. However, it is the only agent that can lower cholesterol levels in patients with homozygous familial hypercholesterolemia, presumably through mechanisms independent of LDL receptors[20]. It also can have a dramatic effect on the resolution of tendon and plane xanthomas[21,22]. This effect on xanthomas is thought to be due (at least in part) to the antioxidant properties of probucol. It is generally considered safe and well tolerated, with few drug interactions.

DIFFERENTIAL DIAGNOSIS OF XANTHOMAS
• Eruptive xanthomas
– Non-Langerhans cell histiocytoses
Xanthoma disseminatum
Papular xanthoma
Generalized eruptive histiocytomas
Indeterminate cell histiocytosis
Rosai–Dorfman disease
Juvenile xanthogranuloma (micronodular form)
– Xanthomatous lesions of Langerhans cell histiocytosis
– Disseminated granuloma annulare
• Tuberous xanthomas
– Erythema elevatum diutinum
– Multicentric reticulohistiocytosis
• Tendinous xanthomas
– Giant cell tumor of the tendon sheath
– Rheumatoid nodule
– Subcutaneous granuloma annulare
• Xanthelasma
– Syringomas
– Necrobiotic xanthogranuloma
– Adult-onset asthma and periocular xanthogranuloma (AAPOX)
– Sebaceous hyperplasia

Table 91.4 Differential diagnosis of xanthomas.

Fibric acid derivatives such as gemfibrozil, fenofibrate and clofibrate are most useful for the treatment of hypertriglyceridemia. Although not completely clear, their primary mechanism of action seems to involve the activation of lipoprotein lipase in peripheral tissues such as muscle. They also decrease VLDL synthesis by suppression of the endogenous lipid pathway. Patients affected by dysbetalipoproteinemia often show dramatic improvement in lipid levels, with resolution of their tuberous and palmar xanthomas, after beginning treatment with fibric acid derivatives[23]. In patients with severe hypertriglyceridemia and chylomicronemia syndrome, this class of drugs helps to lower triglyceride levels and prevent pancreatitis, as well as eruptive xanthoma formation. Fibric acid derivatives inhibit the cytochrome P-450 3A4 system. Because of this inhibition, important dermatologic drug interactions could occur, such as increased plasma bexarotene or cyclosporine levels.

Xanthomas, particularly xanthelasma, can be treated surgically by excision or destructive methods. When xanthelasma excision is performed, it may be followed by suture or second intention healing[24]. Reported destructive methods for xanthelasma include laser surgery (CO_2, pulsed-dye or erbium:YAG lasers), chemical agents such as trichloroacetic acid, and cryosurgery[25–28]. Despite the initial success of the chosen method, the lesions often recur. Surgical excision has also been employed in the management of tendinous xanthomas. This can be technically difficult, however, as the lipid deposits may be intertwined with the involved tendon[29].

REFERENCES

1. Parker F. Normocholesterolemic xanthomatosis. Arch Dermatol. 1986;122:1253–7.
2. Cruz PD Jr, East C, Bergstresser PR. Dermal, subcutaneous, and tendon xanthomas: diagnostic markers for specific lipoprotein disorders. J Am Acad Dermatol. 1988;19:95–111.
3. Lees RS, Frederickson DS. The differentiation of exogenous and endogenous hyperlipemia by paper electrophoresis. J Clin Invest. 1965;44:1968–77.
4. Abifadel M, Varret M, Rabès J-P, et al. Mutations in PCSK9 cause autosomal dominant hypercholesterolemia. Nat Genet. 2003;34:154–6.
5. Cohen J, Pertsemlidis A, Kotowski IK, et al. Low LDL cholesterol in individuals of African descent resulting from frequent nonsense mutations in PCSK9. Nat Genet. 2005;37:161–5.
6. Goldstein GD. The Koebner response with eruptive xanthomas. J Am Acad Dermatol. 1984;10:1064–5.
7. Santamarina-Fojo S. The familial chylomicronemia syndrome. Endocrinol Metab Clin North Am. 1998;27:551–67.
8. Breckenridge WC, Alaupovic P, Cox DW, Little JA. Apolipoprotein and lipoprotein concentrations in familial apolipoprotein C-II deficiency. Atherosclerosis. 1982;44:223–35.
9. Rodondi N, Darioli R, Ramelet AA, et al. High risk for hyperlipidemia and the metabolic syndrome after an episode of hypertriglyceridemia during 13-cis retinoic acid therapy for acne: a pharmacogenetic study. Ann Intern Med. 2002;136:582–9.
10. Parker F. Xanthomas and hyperlipidemias. J Am Acad Dermatol. 1985;13:1–30.

11. Bude RO, Adler RS, Bassett DR. Diagnosis of Achilles tendon xanthoma in patients with heterozygous familial hypercholesterolemia: MR vs sonography. AJR Am J Roentgenol. 1994;162:913–17.
12. Sethuraman G, Thappa DM, Karthikeyan K. Intertriginous xanthomas – a marker of homozygous familial hypercholesterolemia. Indian Pediatr. 2000;37:338.
13. Rauh G, Keller C, Kormann B, et al. Familial defective apolipoprotein B100: clinical characteristics of 54 cases. Atherosclerosis. 1992;92:233–41.
14. Bel S, Garcia-Patos V, Rodriguez L, et al. Cerebrotendinous xanthomatosis. J Am Acad Dermatol. 2001;45:292–5.
15. Alam M, Garzon MC, Salen G, Starc TJ. Tuberous xanthomas in sitosterolemia. Pediatr Dermatol. 2000;17:447–9.
16. Daoud MS, Lust JA, Kyle RA, Pittelkow MR. Monoclonal gammopathies and associated skin disorders. J Am Acad Dermatol. 1999;40:507–35.
17. Mehra S, Li L, Fan CY, et al. A novel somatic mutation of the 3β-hydroxysteroid dehydrogenase gene in sporadic cutaneous verruciform xanthoma. Arch Dermatol. 2005;141:1263–7.
18. Dourmishev AL, Dourmishev LA. Dermatomyositis and drugs. Adv Exp Med Biol. 1999;455:187–91.
19. Stals H, Vercammen C, Peeters C, Morren MA. Acanthosis nigricans caused by nicotinic acid: case report and review of the literature. Dermatology. 1994;189:203–6.
20. Yamamoto A, Matsuzawa Y, Yokoyama S, et al. Effects of probucol on xanthomata regression in familial hypercholesterolemia. Am J Cardiol. 1986;57:29H–35H.

21. Fujita M, Shirai K. A comparative study of the therapeutic effect of probucol and pravastatin on xanthelasma. J Dermatol. 1996;23:598–602.
22. Kajinami K, Nishitsuji M, Takeda Y, et al. Long-term probucol treatment results in regression of xanthomas, but in progression of coronary atherosclerosis in a heterozygous patient with familial hypercholesterolemia. Atherosclerosis. 1996; 120:181–7.
23. Kuo PT, Wilson AC, Kostis JB, et al. Treatment of type III hyperlipoproteinemia with gemfibrozil to retard progression of coronary artery disease. Am Heart J. 1988;116:85–90.
24. Eedy DJ. Treatment of xanthelasma by excision with secondary intention healing. Clin Exp Dermatol. 1996;21:273–5.
25. Ullmann Y, Har-Shai Y, Peled IJ. The use of CO_2 laser for the treatment of xanthelasma palpebrarum. Ann Plast Surg. 1993;31:504–7.
26. Schonermark MP, Raulin C. Treatment of xanthelasma palpebrarum with the pulsed dye laser. Lasers Surg Med. 1996;19:336–9.
27. Mannino G, Papale A, De Bella F, et al. Use of Erbium:YAG laser in the treatment of palpebral xanthelasmas. Ophthalmic Surg Lasers. 2001; 32:129–33.
28. Hawk JL. Cryotherapy may be effective for eyelid xanthelasma. Clin Exp Dermatol. 2000;25:351.
29. Bozentka DJ, Katzman BM. Two cases of surgically treated hand tendon xanthomas. Am J Orthop. 2001;30:337–9.

Non-infectious Granulomas

92

Amy Howard and Clifton R White Jr

INTRODUCTION

The diseases considered in this chapter are unified by similar histologic findings despite having disparate, often unknown, causes. Granulomatous dermatitis may be defined as having an inflammatory cutaneous infiltrate in which histiocytes are the preponderant inflammatory cells. While numerous non-infectious cutaneous eruptions fall within this broad definition, cutaneous sarcoidosis is the prototype of granulomatous dermatitis. Many conditions mimic the appearance of sarcoidosis, including cutaneous Crohn's disease as well as certain foreign body reactions. Granuloma annulare, the closely related annular elastolytic giant cell granuloma (actinic granuloma), and necrobiosis lipoidica are the best-known examples of palisaded granulomatous dermatitis. Each will be discussed in this chapter (Fig. 92.1 & Table 92.1).

SARCOIDOSIS

Synonyms/subsets: ■ Löfgren's syndrome – erythema nodosum, hilar adenopathy, fever, arthritis ■ Heerfordt's syndrome – parotid gland enlargement, uveitis, fever, cranial nerve palsy ■ Darier–Roussy disease – subcutaneous sarcoidosis

Key features

- A systemic granulomatous disorder of unknown origin that most commonly involves the lungs
- Cutaneous manifestations of sarcoidosis are seen in up to one-third of patients, and they may be the first clinical sign of the disease
- Red–brown to violaceous papules and plaques appear most often on the face, lips, neck, upper back and extremities
- Variants of sarcoidosis include subcutaneous, lupus pernio and ulcerative
- Erythema nodosum is a non-specific inflammatory skin finding associated with acute, transient sarcoidosis
- Histologically, sarcoidosis is characterized by non-caseating epithelioid granulomas, usually without surrounding lymphocytic inflammation (i.e. 'naked' granulomas)

History

Sarcoidosis was described initially by Sir Jonathan Hutchinson in 1875 and cutaneous sarcoidosis (lupus pernio) by Besnier in 1889. Caesar Boeck first coined the term 'multiple benign sarkoid' in 1899.

CLINICAL FEATURES OF THE MAJOR GRANULOMATOUS DERMATITIDES						
	Sarcoidosis*	**Classic granuloma annulare****	**Necrobiosis lipoidica**	**AEGCG**	**Cutaneous Crohn's disease**	**Rheumatoid nodule**
Average age (years)	25–35, 45–65	<30	30	50–70	35	40–50
Sex predilection	Female	Female	Female	None	Female	Male[†]
Racial/ethnic predilection in US	African–American	None	None	Caucasian	Ashkenazi Jews	None
Sites	Symmetric on face, neck, upper trunk, extremities	Hands, feet, extensor aspects of extremities	Anterior and lateral aspects of distal lower extremities	Face, neck, forearms (sites of chronic sun exposure)	Genital areas, lower > upper extremities	Juxta-articular areas, especially elbows, hands, ankles, feet
Appearance	Red to red–brown papules and plaques; occasionally annular	Papules coalescing into annular plaques	Plaques with elevated borders, telangiectasias centrally	Annular plaques	Dusky erythema and swelling, ulceration	Skin-colored, firm, mobile subcutaneous nodules
Size of lesions	0.2 to >5 cm	1–2 mm papules, <5 cm annular plaques	3 to >10 cm	1–6 cm	Variable	1–3 cm
No. of lesions	Variable	1–10	1–10	1–10	1–5	1–10
Associations	Systemic manifestations of sarcoidosis; interferon-α therapy for hepatitis C viral infection	Rare diabetes mellitus, HIV infection, malignancy	Diabetes mellitus	Actinic damage	Intestinal Crohn's disease	Rheumatoid arthritis
Special clinical characteristics	Occasional central atrophy and hypopigmentation; development within scars	Central hyperpigmentation	Yellow-brown atrophic centers, ulceration	Central atrophy and hypopigmentation	Draining sinuses and fistulae	Occasional ulceration, especially at sites of trauma

*Clinical variants include lupus pernio and subcutaneous (Darier-Roussy), psoriasiform, ichthyosiform, angiolupoid and ulcerative sarcoidosis.
**Clinical variants include generalized, micropapular, nodular, perforating, subcutaneous and patch GA.
[†]Although rheumatoid arthritis has a female:male ratio of 2–3:1.

Table 92.1 Clinical features of the major granulomatous dermatitides. AEGCG, annular elastolytic giant cell granuloma; HIV, human immunodeficiency virus.

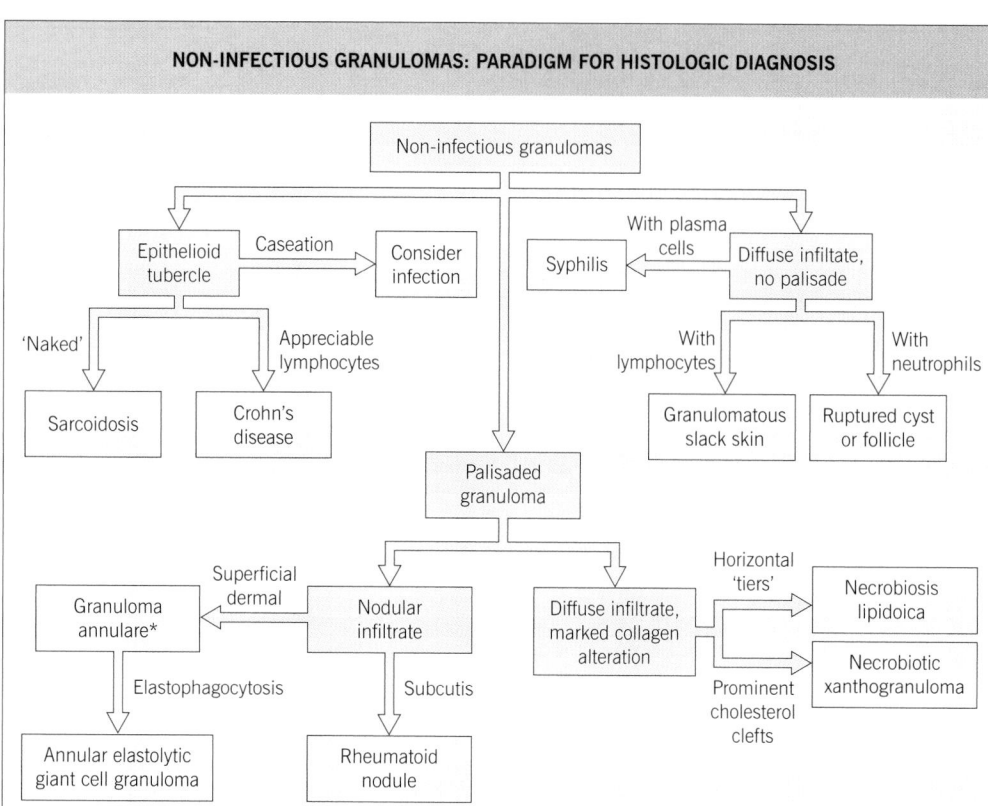

Fig. 92.1 Non-infectious granulomas: paradigm for histologic diagnosis. Interstitial granulomatous dermatitis and palisaded neutrophilic and granulomatous dermatitis may represent an additional diagnostic consideration (see Table 92.2). *May also have a patchy dermal interstitial pattern without palisades, or subcutaneous palisades with more mucin than rheumatoid nodules.

Epidemiology

Sarcoidosis, which occurs in patients of all races, all ages, and both sexes, is characterized by a bimodal age distribution, with peaks between 25 and 35 years and then again between 45 and 65 years in women. In the US, there is an increased incidence of sarcoidosis in African-Americans, ranging from 35.5 to 64 per 100 000. Sarcoidosis in African-Americans tends to be more acute and severe than in other races. African-American women in the fourth decade of life have the highest incidence, occurring with a rate of 107 per 100 000. The incidence in Caucasians in the US ranges between 10 and 14 per 100 000. Worldwide, the incidence of sarcoidosis is highest in Sweden (64 per 100 000) and the UK (20 per 100 000) and lowest in Spain and Japan (both 1.4 per 100 000). A greater number of patients with new-onset sarcoidosis are reported in the winter and spring[1].

Pathogenesis

Sarcoidosis is a multisystem granulomatous disease characterized by hyperactivity of the cell-mediated immune system. Specifically, upregulation of CD4+ T-helper cells of the Th1 subtype occurs following antigen presentation by monocytes bearing MHC class II molecules, which initiates formation of epithelioid granulomas in a variety of tissue types[2]. Increased production of Th1 cytokines, including interleukin 2 (IL-2) and interferon-γ (IFN-γ), leads to B-cell stimulation and hypergammaglobulinemia. Monocyte chemotactic factor (MCF), produced by activated T-helper cells, attracts monocytes from the circulation into peripheral tissues. Compartmentalization of granuloma-forming T lymphocytes and monocytes in peripheral tissues leads to lymphopenia and decreased delayed-type hypersensitivity to common antigens (anergy), most pronounced during the initial stages of sarcoidosis.

The identity of the antigen responsible for the cascade of events leading to granuloma formation in patients with sarcoidoses remains uncertain. Some investigators propose an autoimmune etiology, while others have searched for an infectious cause. The latter is suggested by the observation that sarcoidal granulomas have developed in patients receiving organ transplants from donors with sarcoidosis. Mycobacterial DNA sequences have been identified in lung tissue, peripheral blood, skin, and cerebrospinal fluid in some studies of patients with sarcoidosis but not in others[3]. Sarcoidosis patients do not develop fulminant infectious symptoms when placed on immunosuppressive agents, which argues against a purely infectious etiology. In addition, mycobacteria have not been cultured from sarcoidal tissues. Possible viral causes of sarcoidosis, including human herpesvirus-8, have been postulated but not proven[4]. Sarcoidal lesions have been reported in HIV-infected patients upon immune restoration when given highly active antiretroviral therapy. However, no evidence of infection with *Mycobacterium tuberculosis* could be identified in these sarcoidosis-like lesions[5].

Genetic susceptibility to sarcoidosis has been associated with HLA-1, HLA-B8 and HLA-DR3 alleles[6]. Polymorphisms in the gene encoding angiotensin-converting enzyme (ACE) have also been identified in patients with sarcoidosis. An environmental trigger for the disease is suggested by seasonal clustering of sarcoidosis with erythema nodosum in the spring. Occupational associations have been recorded in health-care workers, firemen, and navy personnel on aircraft carriers[3].

While the etiologic agent has remained elusive, the immuno-pathogenesis of the disease has been elucidated by studying the cutaneous reaction produced by injection of a tissue suspension prepared from sarcoidal spleen. The suspension (Kveim–Siltzbach antigen) causes characteristic non-caseating granuloma formation in the skin of patients with sarcoidosis, and although this skin test is rarely performed in the US, it can help confirm the diagnosis. Immunohistochemical studies have demonstrated a predominance of CD4+ helper T cells and a paucity of CD8+ suppressor T cells, B cells, and immunoglobulin deposition in the cutaneous granulomas. Peripheral blood monocytes are present in tissue for the first several days, but then transform into epithelioid histiocytes and multinucleated giant cells[2].

Clinical Features

Up to a third of patients with systemic sarcoidosis develop skin lesions, which may be the first or only clinical manifestation of the disease. Cutaneous sarcoidosis most commonly manifests as papules and plaques, often red–brown in color (Fig. 92.2A). Papules may be flat-topped in appearance. Sarcoidal lesions favor the face, lips, neck, upper trunk and extremities (Figs 92.2B and 92.2C), and are fairly symmetric in distribution. Lesions classically are dermal without scale, although epidermal change occasionally gives a psoriasiform appearance to lesions. Less common presentations include hypopigmentation, sub-cutaneous nodules, ichthyosis (Fig. 92.2D), alopecia and ulcerations; erythroderma and erythema multiforme are rare manifestations. A

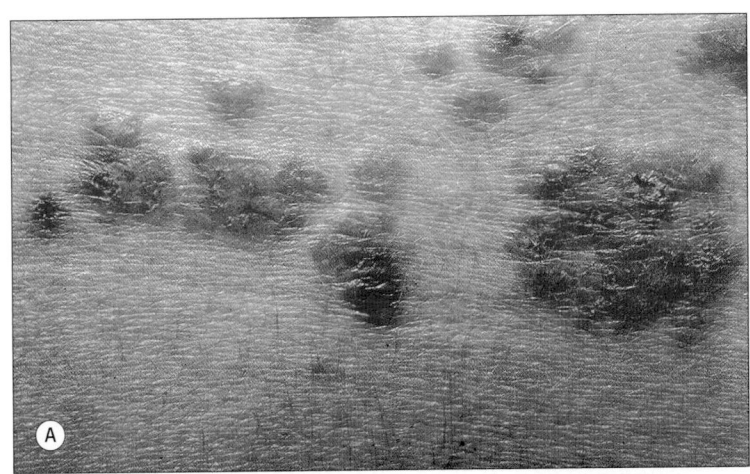

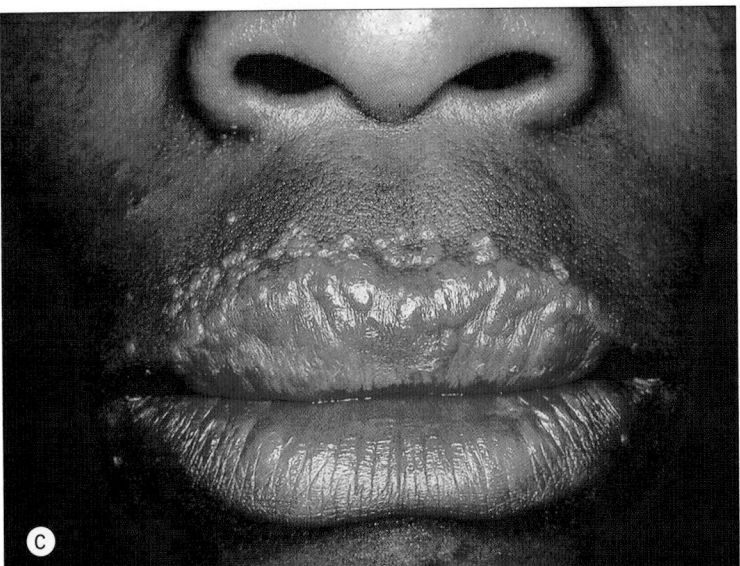

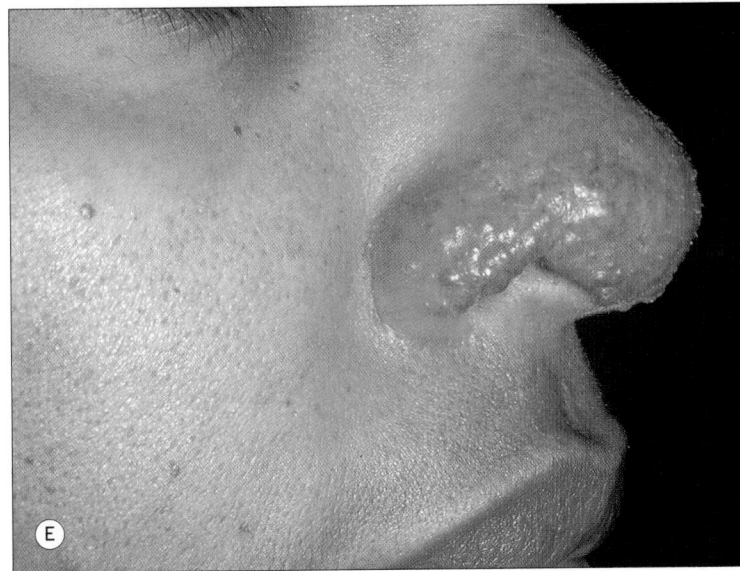

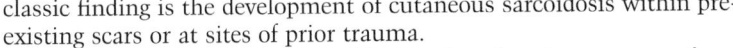

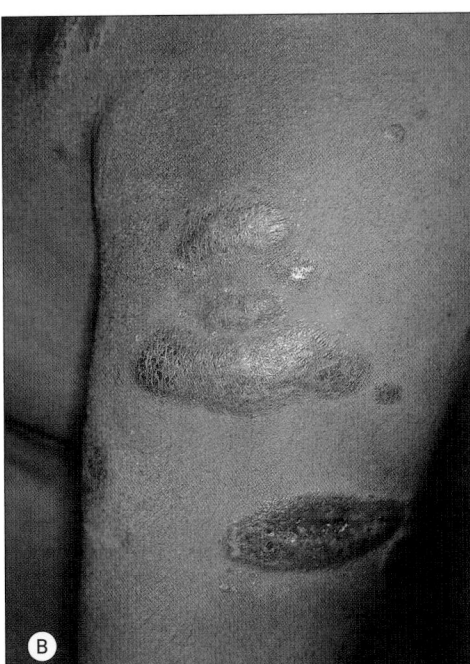

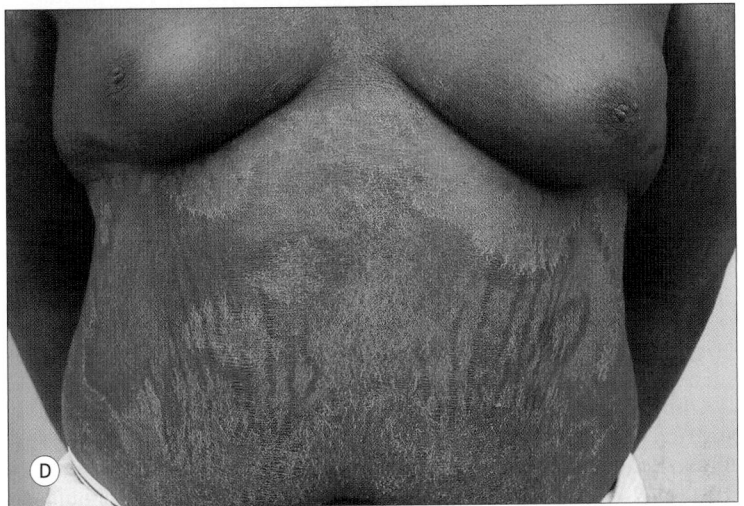

Fig. 92.2 Sarcoidosis.
A Cutaneous sarcoidosis usually consists of papules and plaques with a typical reddish-brown color.
B Hyperpigmented plaques, some of which have scale. **C** Lesions often favor the lips and perioral region. **D** An ichthyosiform presentation is less common. **E** Coalescing violaceous papules on the nose in lupus pernio; note the notching of the nasal rim. D, Courtesy of Jean L Bolognia MD.

classic finding is the development of cutaneous sarcoidosis within pre-existing scars or at sites of prior trauma.

Although many lesions are red–brown in color, they can vary from yellow–brown to erythematous (especially in lightly pigmented skin) to violaceous; the latter color is often associated with lupus pernio. Upon diascopy, in which pressure induces blanching, the lesions are said to have the color of 'apple jelly' (Fig. 92.3); this finding is usually easier to appreciate in lightly pigmented skin. Individual plaques can develop central clearing leading to an annular configuration or they can contain prominent telangiectasias (angiolupoid sarcoidosis).

Variants of sarcoidosis include Darier–Roussy disease and lupus pernio. Patients with Darier–Roussy sarcoidosis present with painless, firm, mobile nodules without epidermal involvement. This variant represents sarcoidosis limited to the subcutaneous tissue. Lupus pernio is characterized by papulonodules and plaques, primarily affecting areas most affected by cold (i.e. pernio), including the nose, ears and cheeks; there is often a beaded appearance along the nasal rim (Fig. 92.2E). Recognition of lupus pernio is important because of its association with chronic sarcoidosis of the lungs (approximately 75% of patients) and of the upper respiratory tract (approximately 50% of patients). In addition, cystic lesions in bone of the distal phalanges are seen more frequently. Although most skin lesions of sarcoidosis are asymptomatic and, with treatment, resolve without scarring, lupus pernio is often the exception[7].

The most important non-specific cutaneous manifestation of sarcoidosis is erythema nodosum. Erythema nodosum is associated with subacute, transient sarcoidosis that usually resolves spontaneously and generally does not require systemic corticosteroid therapy. In general, there are no additional cutaneous manifestations. Biopsy specimens from erythema nodosum lesions show a granulomatous septal panniculitis (see Ch. 100). Sarcoidosis manifesting as erythema nodosum with hilar adenopathy, fever, migrating polyarthritis, and acute iritis is termed Löfgren's syndrome.

Nail changes can be seen in sarcoidosis, including clubbing, subungual hyperkeratosis, and onycholysis. Oral sarcoidosis may affect the mucosa, gingival tissue, tongue, hard palate, and major salivary glands. Heerfordt's syndrome (i.e. uveoparotid fever) includes parotid

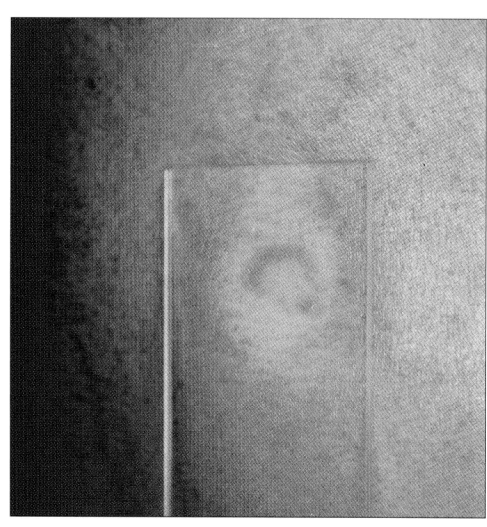

Fig. 92.3 Sarcoidosis. With diascopy, a yellow-brown, 'apple jelly' color is seen.

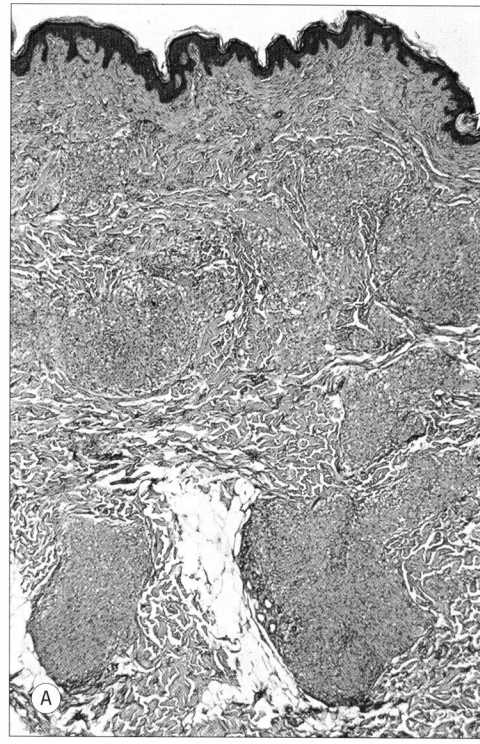

Fig. 92.4 Sarcoidosis. A Scanning power of cutaneous sarcoidosis demonstrating nodular aggregates of epithelioid histiocytes forming tubercles filling the dermis and extending into the subcutaneous tissue. **B** Higher power of a sarcoidal tubercle with a sparse admixture of lymphocytes ('naked tubercle').

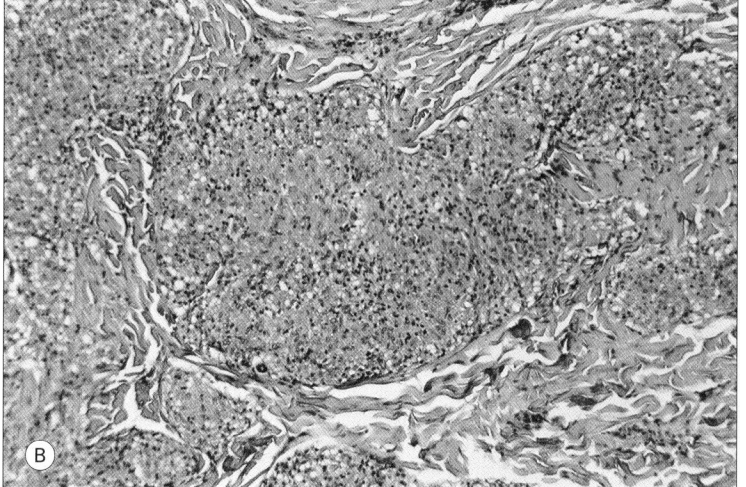

gland enlargement, uveitis, fever, and cranial nerve palsies, usually of the facial nerve.

Systemic manifestations of sarcoidosis are protean. Lung disease occurs in approximately 90% of patients, ranging from alveolitis to granulomatous infiltration of the alveoli, blood vessels, bronchioles, pleura and fibrous septa[8]. The end stage of pulmonary sarcoidosis is fibrosis with bronchiolectasis and 'honeycombing' of the lung parenchyma. Hilar and/or paratracheal lymphadenopathy, which is usually asymptomatic unless associated with parenchymal lung disease, occurs in 90% of patients.

Granulomatous inflammation also occurs in the liver, spleen and bone, as well as the kidney, gastrointestinal tract (upper and lower) and peripheral lymph nodes. Additional sites include the central and peripheral nervous systems, muscle, heart, endocrine glands (e.g., pituitary, thyroid) and bone marrow. Occasionally, there is involvement of the ear, breast, and male and female reproductive systems. Ocular sarcoidosis may present with granulomatous inflammation of the iris, ciliary body, choroid, retina, optic nerve, conjunctiva or lacrimal glands.

Childhood sarcoidosis is rare, and usually presents with a triad of arthritis, uveitis and cutaneous lesions along with constitutional symptoms. Peripheral adenopathy is also often present, but pulmonary involvement is less common than in adults. Sarcoidosis should be considered in the differential diagnosis of any childhood illness with arthritis, especially if ocular symptoms are present.

Hypercalcemia is present in up to 10% of patients, and it is believed to be due to increased calcitriol synthesis by sarcoidal histiocytes. Subsequent hypercalciuria and nephrocalcinosis may lead to renal failure. Lymphopenia, leukopenia and an elevated ESR can be seen in up to 40% of patients.

Pathology

The histopathologic hallmark of sarcoidosis is the presence of superficial and deep dermal epithelioid cell granulomas (Fig. 92.4) with minimal or absent associated lymphocytes or plasma cells ('naked tubercles'). Central caseation is usually absent, although fibrinoid deposition may be observed in up to 10% of cases. Multinucleated histiocytes ('giant cells') are usually of the Langhans type, with nuclei arranged in a peripheral arc or circular fashion. The giant cells may contain eosinophilic stellate inclusions known as asteroid bodies or rounded laminated basophilic inclusions known as Schaumann bodies. Asteroid bodies (Fig. 92.5) represent engulfed collagen, whereas Schaumann bodies likely represent degenerating lysosomes. Neither finding is specific for sarcoidosis.

A range exists within the histologic spectrum of sarcoidosis, from the characteristic tubercles with little surrounding lymphocytic inflammation to unusual cases with dense lymphocytic and plasmocytic infiltrates around and within the nodular histiocytic aggregates. Occasionally, these aggregates may extend into the subcutaneous fat, producing the clinical features of Darier–Roussy sarcoidosis and fibrosing panniculitis[9].

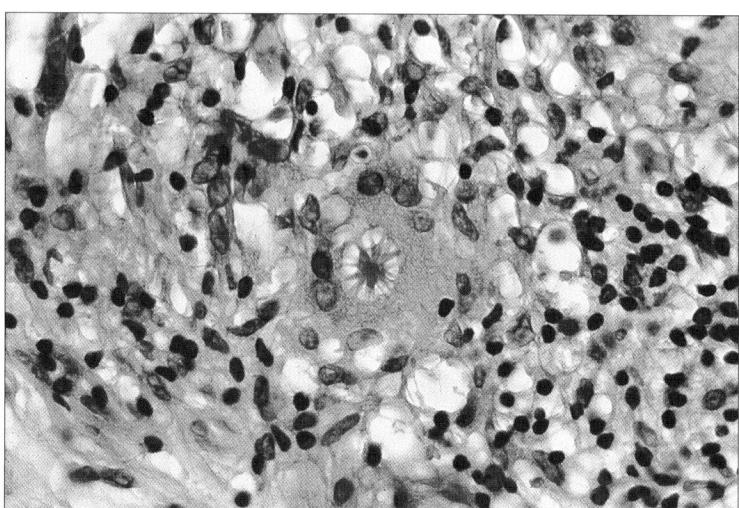

Fig. 92.5 Sarcoidosis. High magnification demonstrating an asteroid body within the cytoplasm of a multinucleated epithelioid histiocyte in cutaneous sarcoidosis.

Diagnosis

Sarcoidosis is a diagnosis of exclusion, both clinically and histologically. In order to establish the diagnosis, a supportive clinical history must be accompanied by the histologic presence of non-caseating granulomas in at least one organ system. Radiologic findings include hilar and/or paratracheal lymph node enlargement with or without pulmonary infiltrates on chest radiography. High resolution CT scans of the chest are more sensitive than radiographs in detecting parenchymal and nodal disease and may be used to delineate active inflammation from fibrosis. Pulmonary function tests reveal restrictive lung disease, with decreased vital capacity, residual volume, total lung capacity, and diffusing capacity. Musculoskeletal radiographs may show joint effusions and cystic lesions in the small bones of the hands and feet. The granulomatous lesions of the gastrointestinal tract can be indistinguishable from Crohn's disease or Whipple's disease on biopsy.

Serologically, elevated antinuclear antibody titers occur in approximately 30% of patients. The serum angiotensin-converting enzyme (ACE) level is elevated in about 60% of patients; it has a false-positive incidence of 10%, making it a more useful test for monitoring disease progression than for establishing the diagnosis. Most patients exhibit lymphopenia, with a decreased CD4+:CD8+ ratio of circulating lymphocytes. Five percent of patients have non-hemolytic anemia, and one-quarter have eosinophilia. The ESR is elevated in two-thirds of patients and hypercalcemia may be present (see above).

Like syphilis, sarcoidosis is a great mimic and the clinical and differential diagnosis depends upon the type of presenting clinical lesions. For example, a list of other disorders apart from sarcoidosis that present with annular lesions is given in Table 20.1. Papules, nodules and plaques may be non-specific in clinical appearance, dictating biopsy, and then the differential diagnosis rests upon the histopathologic findings.

The histologic differential diagnosis is broad, and includes multiple infections that lead to granulomatous inflammation. Special stains for acid-fast and fungal organisms should be obtained. When clinically appropriate, tissue culture should be performed. In tuberculoid leprosy, clues to the diagnosis include inflammation within and around peripheral nerves (where acid-fast *Mycobacterium leprae* occasionally may be demonstrated with a Fite stain), elongated tubercles (reflecting nerve involvement), and denser collections of lymphocytes and plasma cells around the tubercles. Lupus vulgaris is the form of cutaneous tuberculosis most difficult to distinguish from sarcoidosis histologically, due to the difficulty demonstrating organisms in this variant. Histologic features of lupus vulgaris include caseation necrosis within the central portion of tubercles, denser collections of peripheral lymphocytes, and epidermal changes, such as ulceration or pseudoepitheliomatous hyperplasia, and usually allow its distinction from sarcoidosis.

Other histologic mimics include foreign body reactions to zirconium, beryllium, silica, and tattoo ink. Special laboratory techniques, including histochemical, microincineration or spectrophotometric examinations, may be required to identify the causative agents in zirconium and beryllium granulomas (see Ch. 93). Specimens should be polarized to exclude birefringent foreign material as a causative agent, although up to 20% of known sarcoidal granulomas will have foreign material present within them. This observation is particularly common in lesions from the elbows and knees. Therefore, the dermatologic diagnoses of foreign body granuloma and sarcoidosis are not mutually exclusive[10].

In addition, granulomatous mycosis fungoides, Hodgkin disease, granulomatous rosacea, cutaneous Crohn's disease, Blau syndrome, cheilitis granulomatosa (see Ch. 70) and the sarcoidal reaction to an underlying lymphoma can have histologic appearances similar to sarcoidosis. The histologic differences between sarcoidosis, granuloma annulare, necrobiosis lipoidica, annular elastolytic giant cell granuloma, rheumatoid nodule and interstitial granulomatous dermatitis are outlined in Table 92.2.

Treatment

Corticosteroids, either in topical, intralesional or systemic form, are the mainstay of therapy for systemic sarcoidosis (Table 92.3). Therapy is guided by disease severity and progression. The typical oral prednisone dose for systemic disease is 1 mg/kg/day for 4–6 weeks, followed by a slow taper over months to years as dictated by the pulmonary disease, sarcoidosis of the upper respiratory tract, ocular disease or other internal manifestations. Cutaneous sarcoidosis that is major in terms of disfigurement may respond to lower doses of prednisone, including every-other-day regimens[11]. Hydroxychloroquine (200–400 mg/day) and chloroquine (250–500 mg/day) can be effective in controlling skin manifestations of sarcoidosis, particularly chronic disease. Other reported therapeutic agents for cutaneous disease include methotrexate

	Sarcoidosis	Granuloma annulare	Necrobiosis lipoidica	AEGCG	Cutaneous Crohn's disease	Rheumatoid nodule[†]	Interstitial granulomatous dermatitis[†]	Palisading neutrophilic and granulomatous dermatitis[†]
HISTOLOGIC FEATURES OF THE MAJOR GRANULOMATOUS DERMATITIDES								
Typical location	Superficial and deep dermis*	Superficial and mid dermis*	Entire dermis, subcutis	Superficial and mid dermis	Superficial and deep dermis	Deep dermis, subcutis	Mid and deep dermis	Entire dermis
Granuloma pattern	Tubercle with few peripheral lymphocytes ('naked')	Palisading or interstitial	Diffuse palisading and interstitial; horizontal 'tiers'	Palisading, irregular	Tubercle with surrounding lymphocytes	Palisading	Palisading in small 'rosettes'	Palisading; prominent neutrophils and leukocytoclasia
Necrobiosis (altered collagen)	No	Yes ('blue')	Yes ('red')	No	No	Yes ('red')	Yes ('blue')	Yes ('blue')
Giant cells	Yes	Variable	Yes	Yes	Yes	Yes	Variable	Variable
Elastolysis	No	Variable	Variable	Yes	No	No	Variable	Variable
Elastophagocytosis	No	No	No	Yes	No	No	No	No
Asteroid bodies	Yes	Variable	Variable	Yes	No	No	Variable	Variable
Mucin	No	Yes	Minimal	No	No	Variable	Minimal	Variable
Extracellular lipid	No	Variable	Yes	No	No	Variable	No	No
Vascular changes	No	Variable	Yes	No	No	Yes	No	Yes

*Subcutaneous variant can also occur.
[†]See Chapter 45.

Table 92.2 Histologic features of the major granulomatous dermatitides. AEGCG, annular elastolytic giant cell granuloma.

TREATMENT OF CUTANEOUS SARCOIDOSIS

Topical, intralesional or systemic corticosteroids (2)
Topical calcineurin inhibitors (3)
Minocycline (2)
Systemic hydroxychloroquine or chloroquine (2)
Intralesional chloroquine (3)
Allopurinol (3)
Isotretinoin (3)
Methotrexate (2)
PUVA (3)
Thalidomide (2)
TNF-α inhibitors (infliximab, adalimumab) (3)
Mycophenolate mofetil (3)
Surgical excision (3)
Pulsed dye or CO₂ laser (3)
Systemic tacrolimus or cyclosporine* (3)

Table 92.3 Treatment of cutaneous sarcoidosis. Key to evidence-based support: (1) prospective controlled trial; (2) retrospective study or large case series; (3) small case series or individual case reports. TNF, tumor necrosis factor. *May worsen cutaneous disease.

(10–25 mg weekly), thalidomide (50–300 mg/day), isotretinoin (1 mg/kg/day for 3–8 months), minocycline (200 mg/day) and allopurinol (100–300 mg/day)[11–16]. Infliximab and adalimumab have been reported to improve systemic and cutaneous sarcoidosis as has etanercept; however, a phase II trial of the latter was terminated early due to adverse events (e.g. lymphoproliferative disorders). Benefit from leflunomide has also been reported[17].

Other treatments for cutaneous disease include superpotent topical corticosteroids with or without occlusion, intralesional triamcinolone (3–10 mg/ml every month), and PUVA[18,19]. Pulsed-dye and CO₂ laser treatments may be effective for lupus pernio, but there is also a report of laser therapy worsening a patient's disease[20,21]. Surgical excisions with grafting have been performed for ulcerative sarcoidosis[22].

GRANULOMA ANNULARE

Synonym: ▪ Pseudorheumatoid nodule (subcutaneous granuloma annulare variant)

Key features

▪ Small grouped papules assuming an annular configuration often in a symmetrical and acral distribution

▪ Seen primarily in children and young adults

▪ Clinical variants include localized, generalized, micropapular, nodular, perforating, patch and subcutaneous forms

▪ Reports of an association with diabetes mellitus are controversial

▪ Histopathologic specimens show infiltrative or palisading granulomatous dermatitis with focal degeneration of collagen and elastin and deposition of mucin

History

Calcott Fox first described 'ringed eruption of the fingers' in 1895. Radcliffe-Crocker called this entity granuloma annulare in 1902.

Epidemiology

Two-thirds of patients with granuloma annulare (GA) are less than 30 years of age. The female-to-male ratio is approximately 2:1 in this common disease.

Pathogenesis

The etiology of GA is unknown. Trauma, insect bite reactions, tuberculin skin testing, sun exposure, PUVA therapy, and viral infections have all been proposed as inciting factors[23,24]. Based on the T-cell subpopulations identified in GA lesions, a delayed-type hypersensitivity reaction to an unknown antigen has been postulated as the precipitating event[25]. Morphologic similarities to tuberculosis suggest that GA is caused by a Th1 inflammatory reaction, with IFN-γ-producing lymphocytes eliciting matrix degradation[26]. These lymphocytes release cytokines, including macrophage inhibitor factor, that cause monocytes to accumulate in the dermis and release lysosomal enzymes that can degrade connective tissue[27]. One ultrastructural study found that the main alteration in GA is elastic fiber degeneration and suggested that this disease is primarily a disorder of elastic tissue injury[28]. Familial cases of GA have been reported, including cases in identical twins, and an association may exist between generalized GA and HLA-Bw35[29]. Vessel-based mixed inflammatory cell infiltrates with endothelial swelling are sometimes detected in routine histopathologic specimens, and immunofluorescence studies of GA may show vessel-based deposits of immunoreactions, but a role for these findings in the pathogenesis of this disease has not been established.

Clinical Features

GA is a benign, usually self-limited cutaneous disease that classically presents as arciform to annular plaques located on the extremities of young people (Fig. 92.6A)[24]. The approximate distribution of GA lesions is 60% isolated to the hands and arms, 20% on the legs and feet, 7% on both upper and lower extremities, 5% on the trunk, and 5% on the trunk plus other areas[30]. Facial lesions are rare. The plaques may be skin-colored, pink or violaceous in color, and, upon close inspection, are found to be composed of individual small papules measuring a few millimeters in diameter (Fig. 92.6B). These lesions are usually asymptomatic. Solitary umbilicated papules or nodules may also occur, especially on the fingers.

Generalized GA, which occurs in up to 15% of patients, is characterized by myriad small skin-colored to pink-violet papules in a symmetric distribution on the trunk and extremities. Some of these papules may coalesce to form small annular plaques (Fig. 92.7). Generalized GA has a later age of onset, poorer response to therapy, and an increased prevalence of the HLA-Bw35 allele. In one study of 100 patients with generalized GA, 45% had lipid abnormalities, including hypercholesterolemia, hypertriglyceridemia, or both[31].

Perforating GA presents clinically as small papules with central umbilications, crusts or focal ulcerations on the dorsal hands and fingers (Fig. 92.8). This variant represents up to 5% of GA cases, and exhibits transepidermal elimination of degenerating collagen histologically[32].

Deep dermal or *subcutaneous* GA manifests as large, painless, skin-colored nodules which may be mistaken for rheumatoid nodules, leading to the term pseudorheumatoid nodule. It has a predilection for children in the first 5 to 6 years of life. Typical locations include the palms, hands, anterior tibial surfaces and feet, as well as the buttocks, scalp and, rarely, the eyelids[24]. As many as 50% of patients with deep GA lesions also have associated classic lesions.

Patch GA is a distinct variant that is characterized by patches of erythema on the extremities and trunk. Symmetrical lesions on the dorsum of the feet usually present as macular (i.e. 'patch') disease. It may lack an annular configuration, but it displays the classic histopathologic findings of interstitial GA described below, allowing for the diagnosis to be made microscopically.

GA has been described as a paraneoplastic granulomatous reaction to solid organ tumors, Hodgkin disease, non-Hodgkin lymphoma and granulomatous mycosis fungoides[33–36]. In these patients, the clinical pattern is frequently atypical, with painful lesions in unusual locations, including the palms and soles.

Many reports supporting or refuting the association of GA with diabetes mellitus have been published. In a retrospective study of 84 patients, 12% were found to have diabetes mellitus, and these patients were more likely to suffer from chronic relapsing GA than were non-diabetic patients[37]. In a larger retrospective study of 1383 patients, diabetes mellitus was diagnosed in 21% of patients with generalized GA, compared with 9.7% of patients with localized GA[31].

Classic GA and perforating GA may occur in herpes zoster scars[38]. Atypical variants of GA have been associated with HIV infection[39].

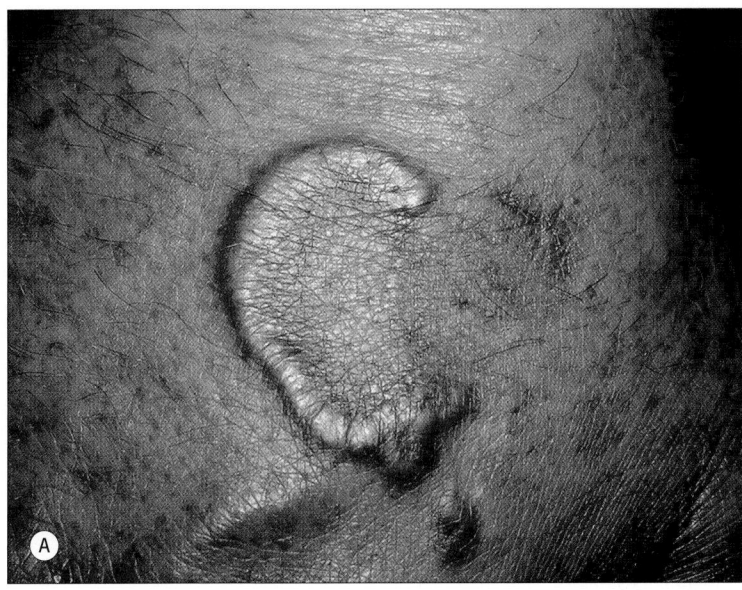

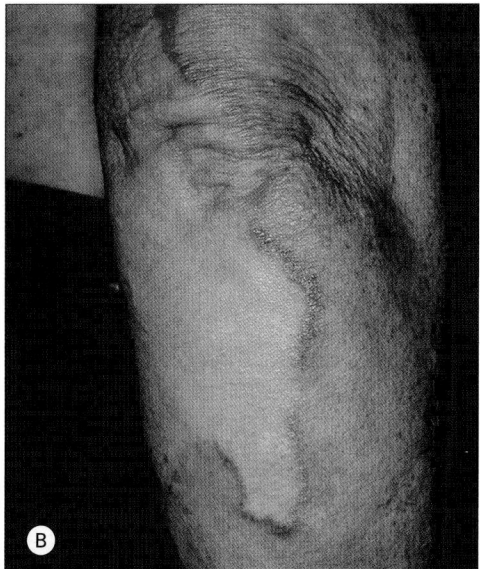

Fig. 92.6 **Granuloma annulare.** Clinical appearance of granuloma annulare consisting of papules coalescing into an arciform plaque on the dorsum of the hand (**A**) and the extensor arm (**B**). Note the red–brown color of previously involved skin.

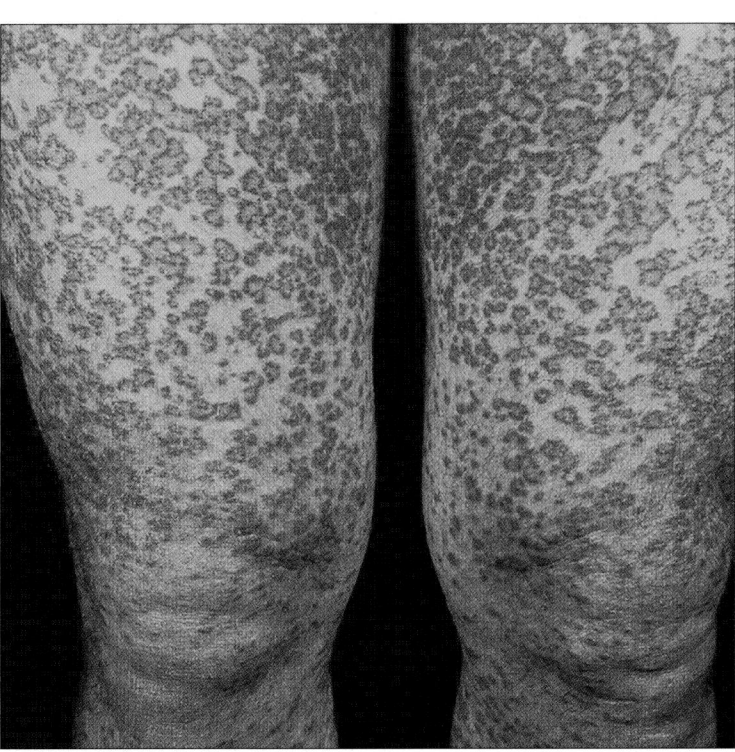

Fig. 92.7 **Disseminated granuloma annulare.** Numerous papules and small annular plaques.

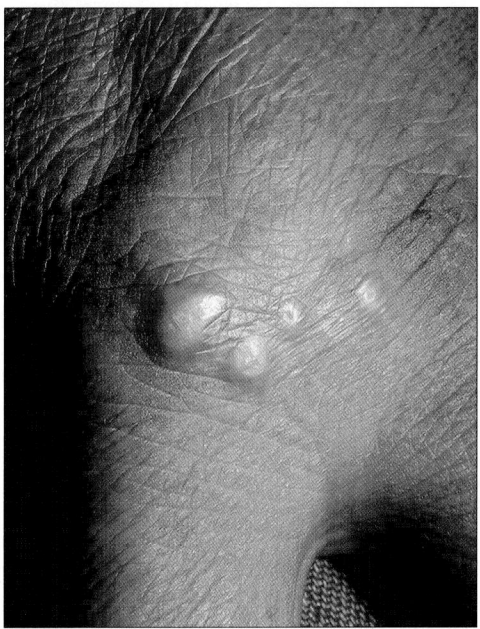

Fig. 92.8 **Perforating granuloma annulare.** Papules can have a central keratotic plug or umbilication. Courtesy of Ronald P Rapini MD.

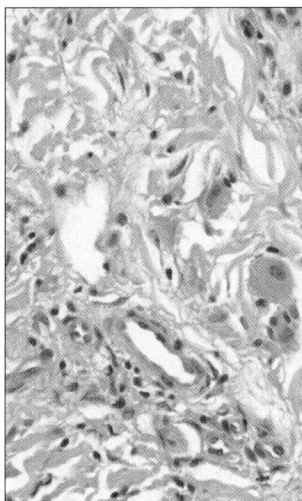

Fig. 92.9 **Granuloma annulare, interstitial pattern.** Note the interstitial macrophages and perivascular lymphocytes. Courtesy of Ronald P Rapini MD.

Pathology

GA is a granulomatous dermatitis characterized by focal degeneration of collagen and elastic fibers, mucin deposition, and a perivascular and interstitial lymphohistiocytic infiltrate in the upper and mid dermis. The key to the histopathologic diagnosis of GA is the identification of histiocytes in one of three patterns. The most common (accounting for approximately 70% of cases) is the infiltrative or interstitial pattern (Fig. 92.9), in which scattered histiocytes are distributed between collagen fibers. Degeneration of collagen fibers is minimal, but granular, basophilic mucin deposition between collagen bundles can be highlighted with Alcian blue and colloidal iron stains[27]. The second pattern (25% of cases) is more obvious and is easier to diagnose. It consists of one to several palisading granulomas with central connective tissue degeneration surrounded by histiocytes and lymphocytes (Fig. 92.10). Mucin is abundant in the center of the palisaded granuloma, and fibrin, neutrophils and nuclear dust may also be present. The final pattern is

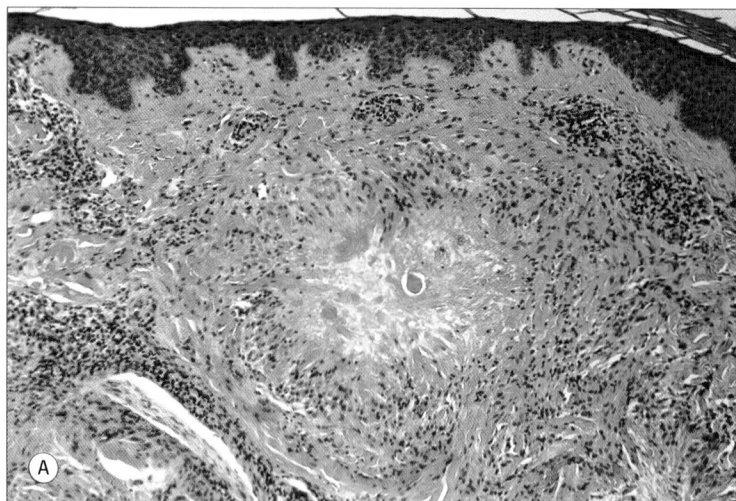

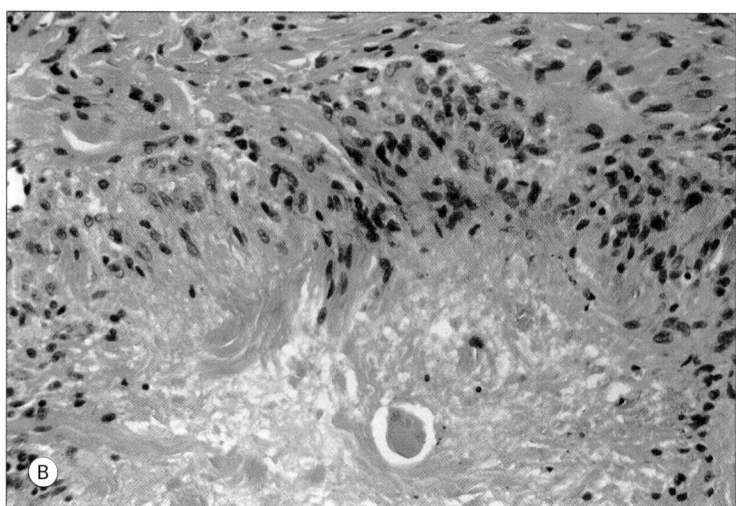

Fig. 92.10 Granuloma annulare (GA), palisaded pattern. A GA at scanning magnification demonstrating epithelioid histiocytes forming a nodule in the upper dermis. The histiocytes are arranged in palisaded fashion with adjacent more darkly staining perivascular lymphocytes. **B** Higher power reveals epithelioid histiocytes palisaded around anuclear dermis characterized by altered collagen and pallor due to deposition of acid mucopolysaccharide (mucin).

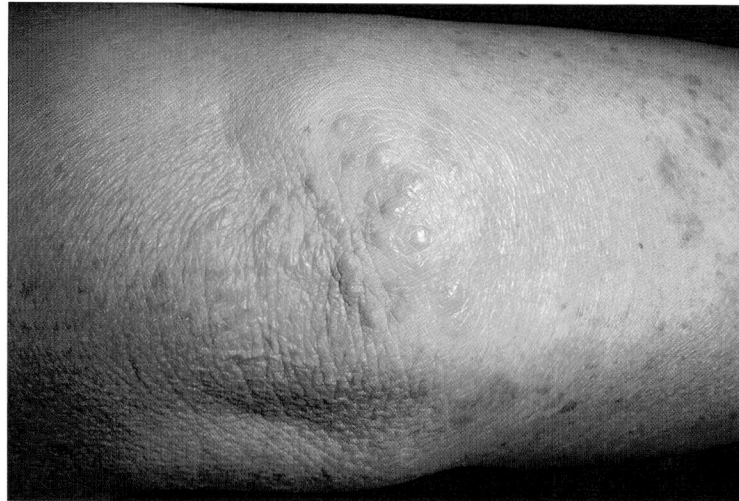

Fig. 92.11 Papular granuloma annulare of the elbow. The clinical diagnosis can be more difficult when annular plaques are not present. Courtesy of Ronald P Rapini MD.

rare, and it consists of epithelioid histiocytic nodules that can resemble cutaneous sarcoidosis.

Increased mucin can be detected in approximately 70% of biopsy specimens from GA lesions. The sensitivity of detection is increased by using at least two different mucin stains, such as colloidal iron or Alcian blue. Elastic tissue is reduced or absent in the histiocytic aggregates in approximately 20% of generalized GA and 35% of localized GA cases[40]. Collagen degeneration is more common in localized GA than in generalized GA[40]. Elastophagocytosis is occasionally noted, but is not a prominent histopathologic feature in GA.

On ultrastructural study, the collagen fiber degeneration in GA consists of collagen fiber swelling, loss of periodic banding, fragmentation, and dissolution of fiber structure with replacement by a granular and finely fibrillar material. Collagen degeneration is more common in localized GA than in generalized GA[40]. Elastophagocytosis is occasionally noted, but is not a prominent histopathologic feature in GA.

Vascular changes in GA are variable, but include fibrin, C3 and IgM deposition in vessel walls (detected by direct immunofluorescence) and occlusion of vascular lumina[41]. One study found that vasculitic disease of leukocytoclastic, granulomatous or thrombogenic types within lesions of GA was predictive of associated systemic disease[42] and the possibility of palisading neutrophilic and granulomatous dermatitis (as a reflection of disorders such as rheumatoid arthritis or Wegener's granulomatosis) needs to be considered.

In deep GA, the histologic changes are usually of the palisaded granulomatous type and extend into the deep dermis or subcutaneous fat. In perforating GA, there is a superficial histiocytic infiltrate with transfollicular and/or transepidermal elimination of granulomatous inflammation.

Diagnosis

GA is diagnosed based on its clinical and histopathologic features – there are no laboratory tests which aid in confirming the diagnosis. When the diagnosis of deep GA versus rheumatoid nodule is in question, a rheumatoid factor level identifies patients at risk for the latter. Rheumatoid nodules also demonstrate fibrin rather than mucin histologically.

The differential diagnosis for conventional GA includes the annular entities listed in Table 20.1. While lesions of GA seldom show epidermal changes such as scale, annular lichen planus and tinea might still be considered. Annular lichen planus is characterized by flat-topped, violaceous plaques with overlying Wickham's striae, while tinea can be excluded by KOH examination of associated scale. Arcuate and annular plaques of mycosis fungoides, sarcoidosis or borderline leprosy may also simulate GA, requiring biopsy for definitive diagnosis.

Papular GA (Fig. 92.11) can simulate arthropod bites, secondary syphilis, xanthomas, and non-X-histiocytoses such as eruptive histiocytomas (see Ch. 90). Subcutaneous GA can be clinically similar to rheumatoid nodules, the nodules of rheumatic fever, epithelioid sarcoma, subcutaneous sarcoidosis, and deep granulomatous infections. Rheumatoid nodules usually occur in the setting of arthritis and high-titer rheumatoid factor. Rheumatic fever nodules occur in the context of a febrile illness, arthritis and a new heart murmur. Perforating GA must be differentiated from perforating collagenosis, perforating folliculitis, Kyrle's disease, elastosis perforans serpiginosa, keratoacanthoma and pityriasis lichenoides et varioliformis acuta, based on histopathologic findings[24]. Importantly, none of these conditions favor the digits.

The clinical and histologic differences between GA, sarcoidosis, necrobiosis lipoidica, annular elastolytic giant cell granuloma, rheumatoid nodule and interstitial granulomatous dermatitis are outlined in Tables 92.1 & 92.2. The histopathologic differential diagnosis of GA also includes morphea, cutaneous T-cell lymphoma, xanthomas and epithelioid sarcoma.

Treatment

Given the self-limited and benign nature of GA, reassurance and clinical observation may be the treatment of choice for localized, asymptomatic disease. High-potency topical corticosteroids with or without occlusion and intralesional corticosteroid injections are the usual first-line local therapies. Other cutaneous treatment modalities include cryosurgery, PUVA or UVA1 therapy, and CO_2 laser treatment (Table 92.4)[43–46]. Intralesional recombinant human IFN-γ was used successfully in three patients at a dose of 2.5×10^5 IU/lesion on seven consecutive days and then three times per week for 2 weeks; however, side effects and cost may be difficult to justify[47].

TREATMENT OF GRANULOMA ANNULARE

Topical corticosteroids (3)
Intralesional corticosteroids (2)
Topical calcineurin inhibitors (3)
Topical imiquimod (3)
Cryosurgery (2)
Hydroxychloroquine or chloroquine (2)
Pentoxifylline (3)
Niacinamide (nicotinamide) (3)
Intralesional interferon (2)
5-lipoxygenase inhibitor (zileuton) plus vitamin E* (3)
Dapsone (3)
Isotretinoin (3)
PUVA or UVA-1 (2)
Cyclosporine (3)
TNF-α inhibitors (3)
Efalizumab (anti-CD11a) (3)
Fumaric acid esters (3)
Chlorambucil (3)
Photodynamic therapy with topical 5-aminolevulinic acid (3)
CO_2 laser (3)
Scarification or surgery (3)

Doses of 2400 mg po qd (zileuton) and 400 IU po qd (vitamin E).

Table 92.4 Treatment of granuloma annulare. Key to evidence-based support: (1) prospective controlled trial; (2) retrospective study or large case series; (3) small case series or individual case reports.

Systemic agents are reserved for severe cases, and include niacinamide (nicotinamide; 500 mg three times daily)[48], isotretinoin (0.5–0.75 mg/kg/day)[49], antimalarials (chloroquine 3 mg/kg/day or hydroxychloroquine 6 mg/kg/day)[31,50], dapsone (100 mg/day)[51] and pentoxifylline[52]. Use of more toxic and/or expensive therapies are controversial, but reports exist for cyclosporine (3–4 mg/kg/day for 3 months)[53,54], chlorambucil[55], etretinate[56] and topical 5-aminolevulinic acid photodynamic therapy[57] being beneficial in individual or small groups of patients. Use of etanercept is reported to be variably successful[58]. However, no large, randomized, double-blind, placebo-controlled studies have been performed to support the use of these systemic medications.

Spontaneous resolution of GA occurs within 2 years in 50% of cases, but there is a 40% recurrence rate. The recurrent lesions tend to occur at the original sites, but clear more rapidly (80% within 2 years). The duration of untreated lesions has been reported to range from a few weeks to several decades[59].

NECROBIOSIS LIPOIDICA

Synonym: ■ Necrobiosis lipoidica diabeticorum

Key features

■ Plaques with violaceous to red–brown, palpable peripheral rims and yellow–brown atrophic centers with telangiectasias

■ The most common site is the shins

■ Ulceration can occur following trauma

■ The proportion of patients with diabetes mellitus varies from 14% to 65%

■ Pathogenesis is unknown

■ Pathology shows palisading granulomatous dermatitis with a 'layered' appearance, often with perivascular plasma cells

History

First called 'dermatitis atrophicans diabetica' by Oppenheim in 1929, the condition was renamed necrobiosis lipoidica diabeticorum (NLD)

by Urbach in 1932. The first non-diabetic patient with NLD was described in 1935 by Goldsmith, generating the more general term necrobiosis lipoidica, which is currently preferred. Nonetheless, the abbreviation NLD is ingrained in the lexicon.

Epidemiology

In a study of 171 patients, Muller & Winkelmann found that diabetes mellitus, usually type 1, was found in approximately 65% of patients with NLD[60]. An additional 12–15% of patients with NLD demonstrated abnormal glucose tolerance tests. In addition, over half of the patients with no evidence of diabetes and a normal glucose tolerance test reported a positive family history of glucose intolerance[60,61]. A more recent retrospective study of 65 patients with NLD seen in a dermatology outpatient clinic found that only 11% had diabetes mellitus at the time of presentation. An additional 11% were later diagnosed with impaired glucose tolerance or diabetes[62].

There is no proven connection between a patient's level of glycemic control and the likelihood of developing NLD lesions, but diabetic patients with NLD do appear to have a higher rate of diabetes-related complications such as peripheral neuropathy, retinopathy and limited joint mobility[63]. Only 0.03% of patients with diabetes have NLD. The female-to-male ratio is approximately 3:1.

Pathogenesis

The cause of NLD remains unknown. There is no HLA linkage. Immunologically mediated vascular disease has been suggested as the primary cause of the altered collagen seen in NLD, and this hypothesis is supported by the presence of immunoreactants deposited in vessel walls of lesional as well as uninvolved skin in patients with NLD[64]. Ullman & Dahl[65] also found evidence for immune complex vasculitis in NLD. It is also postulated that the microangiopathic vessel changes seen in diabetic patients could contribute to the development of collagen degeneration and subsequent dermal inflammation. Elevated plasma fibronectin, factor VIII-related antigen, and α_2-macroglobulin levels have been detected in patients with NLD, but the significance of these findings has not been determined[66]. Theories regarding abnormally elevated platelet adhesion, increased thromboxane A_2 production, and increased blood viscosity within NLD lesions remain speculative.

Some investigators consider NLD to be primarily a disease of collagen, with inflammation occurring as a secondary event. Anticollagen antibodies have been detected in patients with both NLD and GA, but no significant increase in antibody levels as compared with control patients has been demonstrated[67]. The concentration of collagen is decreased in NLD lesions, and electron microscopy reveals a loss of the cross-striations of collagen fibrils and significant variation in the diameter of individual fibrils. Fibroblasts cultured from NLD lesions synthesize less collagen than their counterparts from unaffected skin[68]. Overhydration of collagen due to hyperglycemia can lead to increased collagen cross-linking and stiffness, but it is unclear if this phenomenon occurs in NLD.

Clinical Features

NLD presents clinically with yellow–brown, atrophic, telangiectatic plaques surrounded by raised, violaceous rims, typically in the pretibial region (Fig. 92.12). The lesions start as small, firm, red–brown papules that gradually enlarge and then develop central epidermal atrophy. Lesions are often multiple and occur with bilateral symmetry. Ulceration occurs in 35% of lesions (see Fig. 52.16), usually following minor trauma. Less typical anatomic locations for NLD include the upper extremities, face and scalp, where the lesions may be more annular or serpiginous in configuration and are less atrophic.

Decreased sensation to pinprick and fine touch, hypohidrosis and partial alopecia can be found within NLD plaques. Boulton et al[63] found decreased S100 staining within cutaneous nerves in the inflammatory plaques and postulated that degenerative changes in these nerves could account for the loss of sensation. In contrast, the cutaneous nerves in GA demonstrate normal S100 staining patterns. Although the lesions of NLD are typically asymptomatic, some patients report

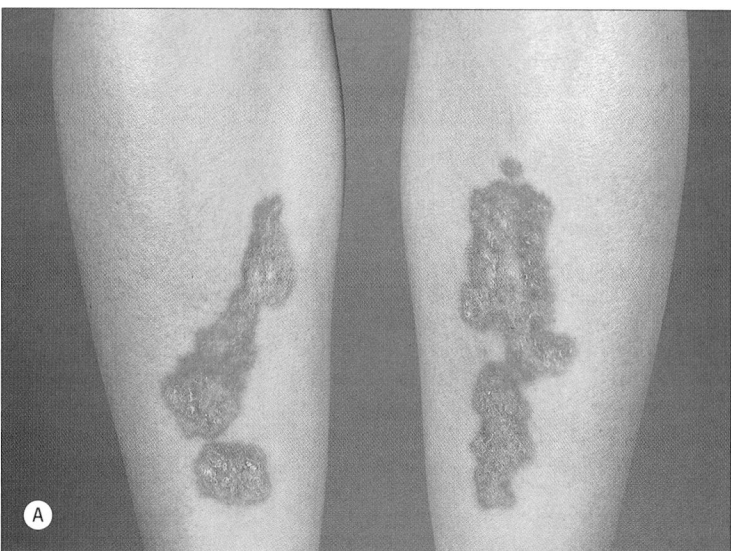

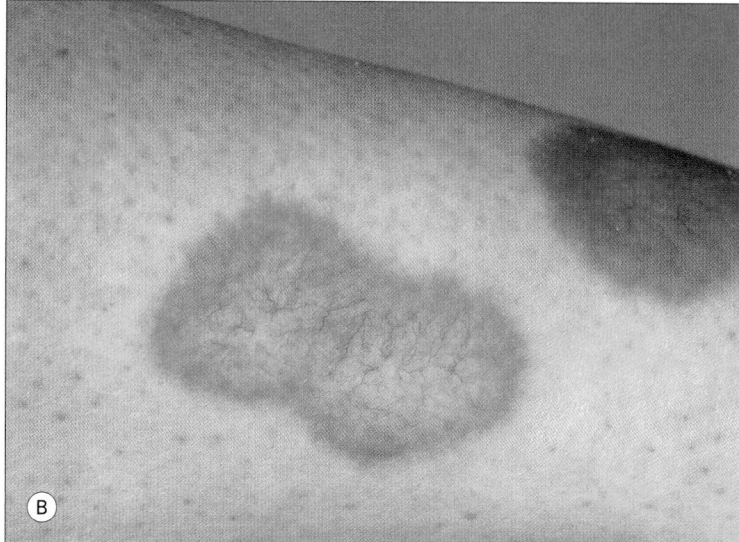

Fig. 92.12 **Necrobiosis lipoidica. A** Pink–brown atrophic plaques on the shins. **B** Annular plaques with central telangiectasias.

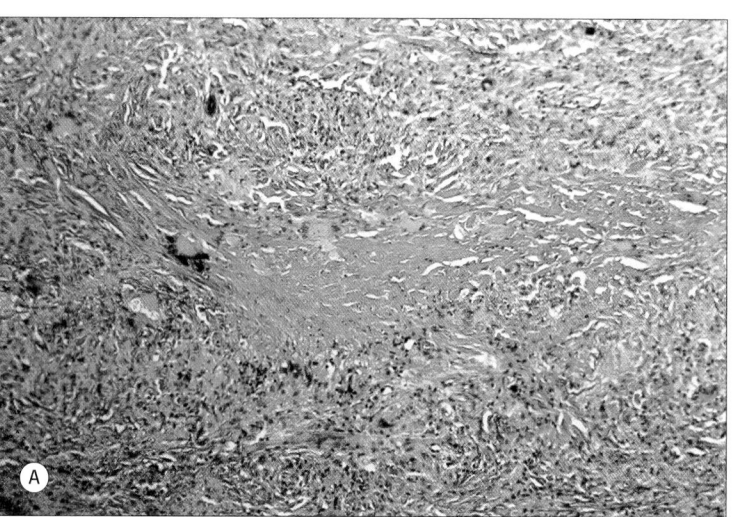

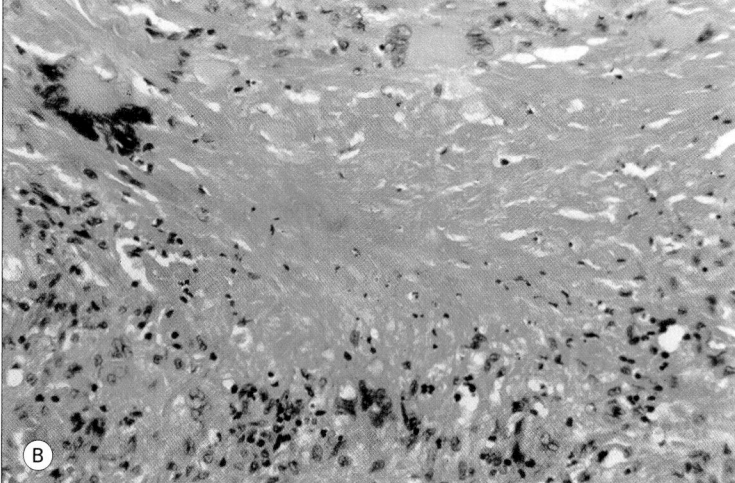

Fig. 92.13 **Necrobiosis lipoidica. A** Biopsy of necrobiosis lipoidica reveals epithelioid histiocytes, some of them multinucleated, arranged in palisaded fashion throughout the dermis and extending into subcutaneous fat septae. **B** Higher power of necrobiosis lipoidica reveals altered collagen surrounded by palisaded histiocytes.

pruritus, dysesthesia or pain. Lesions that ulcerate after trauma or from transepidermal elimination of altered collagen and elastic fibers can be very painful. Rarely, squamous cell carcinoma has been reported to develop within lesions of NLD[69].

Pathology

Biopsy specimens, particularly from the palpable inflammatory borders, reveal a diffuse palisaded and interstitial granulomatous dermatitis (Fig. 92.13), with 'layered' tiers of granulomatous inflammation aligned parallel to the skin surface involving the entire dermis and extending into the subcutaneous fat septae. The epidermis is normal or atrophic. There is a superficial and deep perivascular infiltrate that is predominantly lymphocytic but also contains plasma cells and occasionally eosinophils. The granulomatous inflammation includes multinucleated histiocytes but no asteroid bodies.

Focal loss of elastic tissue can be demonstrated in areas of connective tissue sclerosis. Between the layers of inflammatory cells, there are horizontal tiers of degenerated collagen, exhibiting fibers of irregular size and shape. Extracellular lipid deposition in these foci can be identified only by histopathologic examination of frozen sections with an oil red O stain. This is seldom done from a practical standpoint. In contrast to GA, there is no significant mucin deposition in the center of the palisading granulomas.

Both NLD and GA may have foci of leukocytoclasia in early lesions, but NLD shows more prominent endothelial cell swelling, fibrosis and

hyalinization, which can lead to blood vessel wall thickening or even endarteritis obliterans. The vessel walls often contain a PAS-positive, diastase-resistant material suggesting neutral glycosaminoglycans[66].

NLD occasionally presents with less sclerotic collagen and more typical epithelioid cell granulomas rather than the horizontally tiered pattern of altered collagen and palisaded granulomatous inflammation described above. Vascular changes are rare, and this form of NLD is felt to have a weaker association with diabetes mellitus than the classic lesions[66].

Immunofluorescent studies of NLD lesions have yielded conflicting results, and are not performed routinely. Ullman & Dahl[65] found C3, fibrinogen, IgM and IgA deposited around dermal blood vessels, and Quimby et al.[64] reported vascular deposition of C3, fibrin and IgM in both lesional and non-lesional skin. However, Laukkanen et al.[70] found positive immunofluorescence in only four out of 14 lesional skin biopsies. Fibrin is consistently found deposited in areas of altered collagen[71].

Diagnosis

Clinically, the differential diagnosis of NLD includes primarily GA, necrobiotic xanthogranuloma, sarcoidosis, diabetic dermopathy and stasis dermatitis. Additional entities in the differential diagnosis include various forms of panniculitis (erythema nodosum and several variants of panniculitis which histologically show lobular panniculitis), granulomatous infections (e.g. leprosy, tertiary syphilis, dimorphic fungal infections), morphea, lichen sclerosus and sclerosing lipogranuloma.

Lesions of GA and sarcoidosis generally do not exhibit the same degree of atrophy, telangiectasias or yellow–brown color as NLD lesions, although prominent telangiectasias can be present in angiolupoid sarcoidosis and can occur following injections of triamcinolone. If sarcoidosis is suspected, a chest radiograph to search for bilateral hilar adenopathy may be helpful. Of note, NLD and sarcoidosis may coexist in the same patient[72]. The typical location of GA on the distal extremities, including the hands and feet, may be helpful in distinguishing it from NLD. Necrobiotic xanthogranuloma is characterized by yellow, indurated, often periorbital (among other sites) plaques, and it is associated with a paraproteinemia. The lesions of diabetic dermopathy and stasis dermatitis are both located on the shins, but the former are macular and hyperpigmented rather than yellow. The latter usually has an eczematous presentation with associated varicose veins, edema, hyperpigmentation, lipodermatosclerosis and sometimes ulcers.

Erythema nodosum occurs on the lower extremities (often of young women) as slightly elevated dusky erythematous nodules. It is distinguishable from NLD by the painful quality of the nodules, the subcutaneous location of lesions, and a lack of epidermal atrophy or ulceration. One or more red nodules that may ulcerate and scar characterize nodular vasculitis, but these nodules are typically located on the posterior legs of women rather than on the shin (see Ch. 100).

The injection of substances such as paraffin, cottonseed oil, sesame oil or beeswax may cause plaque-like indurations with ulcerations mimicking NLD, but the ensuing lesions of sclerosing lipogranuloma are rarely located on the legs. Leprosy has many clinical manifestations, including a few anesthetic hypopigmented plaques with elevated borders (tuberculoid leprosy), but it can be distinguished based on clinical and histologic findings.

The major entity in the histopathologic differential diagnosis for NLD is GA. Whereas the inflammation in NLD is diffuse and involves the entire dermis extending into subcutaneous fat septae, GA is patchy with discrete foci of granulomatous inflammation amid areas of uninvolved dermis. There is usually deposition of mucin within areas of granulomatous inflammation in GA but not in NLD. In general, NLD has more giant cells, plasma cells, vascular changes, collagen degeneration, and extracellular lipid deposition than GA.

Necrobiotic xanthogranuloma can be differentiated from NLD histologically by the presence of abundant cholesterol clefts in necrobiotic xanthogranuloma. One case report described NLD with prominent cholesterol clefts and transepithelial elimination of cholesterol crystals through hair follicles[73]. Transepidermal elimination of elastic fibers has also been reported and should not be misconstrued with entities such as elastosis perforans serpiginosa[74].

Treatment

No treatment for NLD has proven to be effective in large, double-blind, placebo-controlled studies. In patients with diabetes mellitus, control of blood glucose levels usually does not have a significant effect on the course of NLD. Spontaneous remission after an average of 8 to 12 years was observed in only 17% of 171 patients with NLD in one study[60].

First-line therapy includes potent topical corticosteroids for early lesions and intralesional corticosteroids injected into the active borders of established lesions. Boulton et al.[63] found that in clinically active NLD lesions, the histologic changes can extend well into normal-appearing skin. Based on this finding, they advocated the injection of intradermal corticosteroids into a rim of clinically normal skin around expanding plaques in an effort to halt disease progression. In addition, 5-week courses of systemic corticosteroids were found to be effective in a series of six patients with an average follow-up period of 7 months, but this will elevate serum glucose[75].

Other therapies are directed at increasing fibrinolysis or decreasing platelet aggregation and thromboxane A_2 synthesis in order to decrease microangiopathy and vascular thrombosis seen in lesions of NLD. Stanozolol, inositol niacinate (inositol nicotinate), nicofuranose, ticlopidine hydrochloride and pentoxifylline are all agents that have been used towards this end in anecdotal reports or uncontrolled case series. The use of stanozolol is limited by its potential hepatotoxicity, and ticlopidine can cause agranulocytosis. A 16-patient controlled trial of aspirin (40 mg/day) versus placebo showed no significant difference

between the groups[76]. A 12-patient controlled trial of aspirin (300 mg three times daily) plus dipyridamole (75 mg three times daily) versus placebo also showed no significant effects of treatment[77]. Perilesional heparin injection has been reported in the Russian literature[78].

Niacinamide (500 mg three times daily) has been used with some success in both NLD and GA, and it is postulated to inhibit the release of lymphokines and decrease macrophage migration[66]. Topical tretinoin (0.025% gel twice daily) decreased lesional atrophy in one case[79]. Systemic cyclosporine was successfully used to treat a total of four patients with severe, ulcerating NLD on the lower legs[80,81]. Other reported therapies include topically applied granulocyte–macrophage colony-stimulating factor (GM-CSF), bovine collagen[82], topical PUVA[83,84], UVA1 phototherapy[85], mycophenolate mofetil (500 mg twice daily)[86], thalidomide[87] and etanercept[88].

If surgical therapy becomes necessary for severe ulcerations that are refractory to medical treatment, excision to deep fascia or periosteum must be performed to minimize the chance of recurrence. Split-thickness skin grafting is performed following excision.

ANNULAR ELASTOLYTIC GIANT CELL GRANULOMA

Synonyms: ■ Actinic granuloma ■ Giant cell elastophagocytosis ■ Miescher's granuloma of the face ■ Atypical (annular) necrobiosis lipoidica of the face and scalp

Key features

- Asymptomatic annular plaques, predominantly on the head and neck and other sun-exposed areas
- Borders of plaques are elevated and erythematous, while the central areas are slightly atrophic and hypopigmented
- Histopathology is characterized by non-palisading granulomas with foreign body type multinucleated giant cells, histiocytes and lymphocytes
- Elastic fibers are absent in the central portion of lesions, and some elastic fibers are found within giant cells
- No collagen alteration, mucin or lipid deposition, or vascular changes are seen histopathologically

History

O'Brien[89] described the entity known as actinic granuloma in 1975 but attributed the first description of this disease to Georgouras in 1964. O'Brien used 'actinic' in the name of this disorder because he believed that its etiology was linked to ultraviolet and infrared radiation. This nosologic theory was rejected by Hanke et al.[90] whose patients did not all demonstrate significant solar elastosis histologically but otherwise fit O'Brien's clinical and histopathologic descriptions. These authors coined the descriptive term annular elastolytic giant cell granuloma in 1979. Upon review of the literature, both O'Brien and Hanke realized that the diseases they were describing had previously been reported under other names, including atypical necrobiosis lipoidica of the face and scalp[91], Miescher's granuloma of the face[92], and possibly granuloma multiforme[93].

Epidemiology

Annular elastolytic giant cell granuloma is an uncommon disease that occurs predominantly in middle-aged women, at least 30 years of age but usually over 40. Patients have been reported from several areas of the world, including Australia, the UK, the US, the Caribbean, and Africa.

Pathogenesis

Debate exists as to whether annular elastolytic giant cell granuloma is a distinct clinical entity or a variant of GA[94,95]. Its pathogenesis is not understood, but it may be related to inflammation precipitated by actinic damage. Specifically, O'Brien postulated that 'a state of auto-aggression develops in relation to the damaged [elastic] fibers', in an attempt to repair or remodel damaged skin[89]. T lymphocytes involved in annular elastolytic giant cell granuloma are predominantly of the helper-inducer subset, suggesting that the pathogenesis may involve a cell-mediated immunologic response to a weakly antigenic determinant on altered elastotic fibers[95]. However, Hanke et al.[90] noted that elastic tissue was also destroyed in classic GA and NLD, and that this may be a secondary event caused by the granulomatous inflammation rather than a precipitating one. A few patients with annular elastolytic giant cell granuloma as well as diabetes mellitus, NLD and/or sarcoidosis have been reported.

Clinical Features

Annular elastolytic giant cell granuloma presents with large annular plaques with raised erythematous borders (3–5 mm) and slightly atrophic, hypopigmented central regions that are distributed mainly in sun-exposed areas (Fig. 92.14). The sites of predilection include the neck, face, chest and arms. Early on, skin-colored or pink papules may be identified singly or in small groups before they coalesce into annular plaques. Scale is rarely observed. There is no yellow color, telangiectasias or alopecia in the lesions as there is in NLD. Individual lesions measure 1–10 cm in diameter, and the total number of lesions is generally less than ten. Patients are usually asymptomatic, although pruritus has been reported. A single plaque lasts for months to years, after which spontaneous remission may occur, leaving mottled dyspigmentation or normal-appearing skin[89].

Pathology

Sections through the raised border of an annular elastolytic giant cell granuloma lesion show a non-palisading granulomatous infiltrate of histiocytes, foreign body type multinucleated giant cells with haphazardly arranged nuclei, and lymphocytes in the mid to upper dermis, with an absence of altered collagen, mucin or lipid deposition[96]. Elastic fibers are identified adjacent to and within the giant cells, giving rise to the term elastophagocytosis. Asteroid bodies that stain like elastic fibers with acid orcein are observed within the multinucleated giant cells. These findings are not specific for annular elastolytic giant cell granuloma, but they are seen less frequently in other granulomatous conditions such as GA and NLD. Elastin tissue stains, such as the Verhoeff-van Gieson stain, show a characteristic complete absence of elastic fibers in the areas affected by granulomatous inflammation (Fig. 92.15). Normal quantities of elastin are seen in the deeper dermis. Sections from previously involved skin show normal elastic and elastotic fibers around a well-demarcated zone of dermis that remains free of elastic tissue staining.

There are no vascular changes other than a sparse perivascular lymphocytic infiltrate. Basophilic solar elastosis may be present, and was observed in all of O'Brien's patients with actinic granuloma. The epidermis may be normal or slightly thinned. Direct immunofluorescence studies for fibrin, C3, IgG, IgM and IgA are negative.

Occasionally, histiocytes and epithelioid cells form tubercles that are indistinguishable from sarcoid nodules.

Diagnosis

The diagnosis of annular elastolytic giant cell granuloma is based on the characteristic clinical appearance and histopathologic findings outlined above. There are no helpful laboratory tests. The clinical differential diagnosis includes the annular variants of the diseases outlined in Table 92.1, as well as erythema annulare centrifugum (different distribution), annular lichen planus and secondary syphilis (central hyperpigmentation), tinea corporis and granulomatous infections. Granuloma multiforme (Mkar disease) clinically resembles annular elastolytic giant cell granuloma, but it occurs in Africa and has prominent collagen alteration surrounded by palisading granulomas on biopsy. Therefore, it may be a variant of GA rather than annular elastolytic giant cell granuloma.

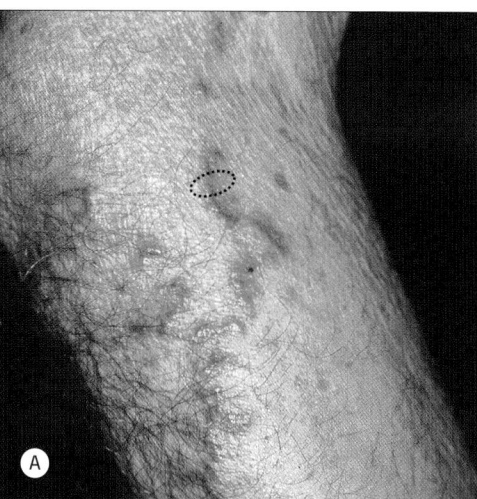

Fig. 92.14 **Annular elastolytic giant cell granuloma (actinic granuloma).** The border resembles granuloma annulare but the central portion is hypopigmented and/or atrophic (**A, B**). A biopsy specimen that includes the area outlined in A would contain the three characteristic histologic zones: absence of elastic fibers, granulomatous inflammation, and normal skin. B, Courtesy of Kalman Watsky MD.

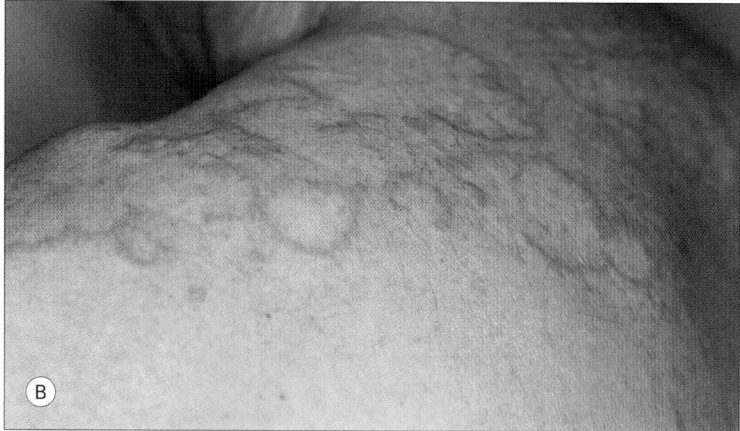

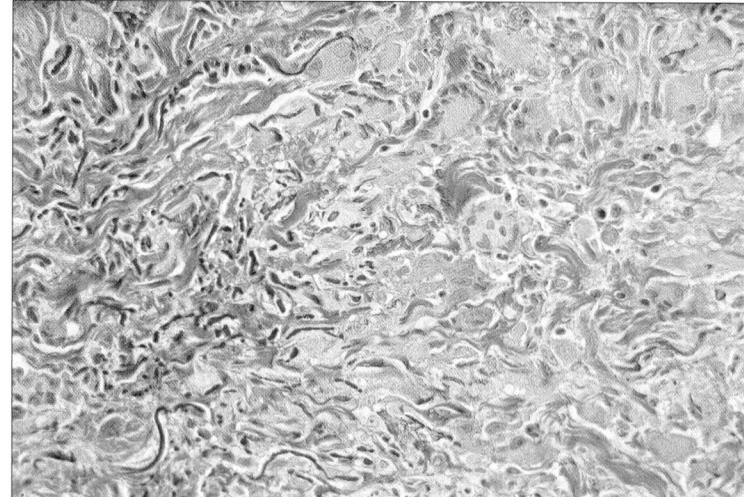

Fig. 92.15 **Annular elastolytic giant cell granuloma (actinic granuloma).** Loss of elastic fibers (black) is seen amid the granulomatous infiltrate (yellow). The remaining collagen is stained red (Verhoeff-van Gieson stain). Courtesy of Ronald P Rapini MD.

Other entities in the histologic differential diagnosis include granulomatous slack skin, mid-dermal elastolysis, anetoderma and cutis laxa. Special stains for acid-fast bacilli and fungal organisms should be performed to exclude an infectious granulomatous process such as tuberculosis, leprosy or deep fungal infections.

Treatment

Annular elastolytic giant cell granuloma is a persistent condition that responds poorly or inconsistently to topical or intralesional corticosteroids, PUVA therapy and antimalarial drugs[97]. Case reports of one patient who responded well to 8 weeks of cyclosporine (5 mg/kg/day) and one patient who responded to 16 weeks of chloroquine therapy (200–400 mg/day) exist in the literature[98,99]. Excision of lesions followed by partial-thickness skin grafting has been performed with no recurrence at 15 months of follow-up[100], but this would rarely be required. Cryotherapy, cauterization and methotrexate were reported to be ineffective in reports of single cases.

CUTANEOUS CROHN'S DISEASE

Synonym: ■ Metastatic Crohn's disease

Key features

- Erythematous plaques, often on the buttock and genital skin
- Cutaneous non-caseating granulomatous lesions that are not contiguous with intestinal Crohn's disease have been referred to as 'metastatic'
- Approximately 20% of patients have cutaneous lesions without preceding diagnosis of gastrointestinal Crohn's disease

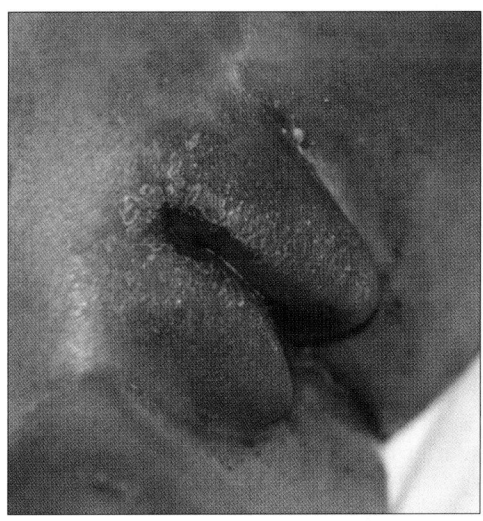

Fig. 92.16 **Cutaneous Crohn's disease.** Note the swelling and violaceous discoloration of the labia majora in this prepubescent girl. Courtesy of Joseph L Jorizzo MD.

History

Crohn's disease, first described in 1932, is characterized by segmental granulomatous inflammation of the intestinal tract and frequently involves cutaneous tissues as well.

Epidemiology

Crohn's disease usually begins between the second and fourth decades of life. Mucosal and skin findings occur in 20–45% of patients[101], and include distant cutaneous (metastatic) Crohn's disease, contiguous perianal Crohn's disease, oral Crohn's disease, reactive dermatologic diseases (including erythema nodosum and pyoderma gangrenosum) and nutritional skin changes[102]. Cutaneous Crohn's disease has been reported in children[103].

Cutaneous Crohn's disease is relatively rare, with fewer than 100 cases reported in the literature. Two-thirds of the patients are women, and the mean age of onset is 34.5 years. Fewer than 20 cases have been reported in children. Approximately 20% of the reported cases had skin disease that preceded the diagnosis of intestinal Crohn's disease by 3 months to 8 years.

Pathogenesis

Cutaneous Crohn's disease is seen in association with or preceding intestinal Crohn's disease. A number of genetic abnormalities which can lead to an exaggerated T-cell response to certain commensal enteric bacteria and defective microbial clearance, including after breaks in the mucosal barrier or an alteration in the balance in gut flora (dysbiosis), have been linked to Crohn's disease. The protein products of these genes have several functions including regulation of NFκB function (e.g. *CARD15*, *PPARG*) and structural integrity of epithelial cells (e.g. *DLG5*). Like psoriasis, Crohn's disease is a predominantly TH1- and TH17-mediated disease, and elevated levels of IL-23 and IL-17 are present within involved tissues[103a].

Clinical Features

Cutaneous Crohn's disease may be either genital or extra-genital, with genital involvement found in approximately two-thirds of children and one-half of adults. Labial or scrotal erythema and swelling are the usual presenting signs[104] (Fig. 92.16). Non-genital disease presents with dusky erythematous plaques, often followed by ulceration with undermined edges, draining sinuses and fistulae, and scarring. These lesions have been observed on the lower extremities and soles (38%), abdomen and trunk (24%), upper extremities and palms (15%), face and lips (11%), flexural areas (8%), and in a generalized distribution (4%)[102,105].

Perianal lesions, which may extend to the adjacent perineum, buttocks or abdomen, consist of ulcers, fissures, sinus tracts or vegetating plaques[106]. These are seen in approximately one-third of patients with intestinal Crohn's disease. Abdominal surgical sites, such as laparotomy scars, colostomies and ileostomies, may also be sites of Crohn's inflammation. For semantic purposes, these lesions are considered to be 'contiguous' Crohn's disease rather than 'metastatic' Crohn's disease, but show the same non-caseating granulomatous infiltrates on histopathologic examination.

Oral lesions occur in 5–20% of patients with Crohn's disease, and these may consist of cobblestoning of the buccal mucosa, tiny gingival nodules, small aphthae-like ulcers, linear ulcerations, angular cheilitis and ulceration, pyostomatitis vegetans, gingival hyperplasia, cheilitis granulomatosa, diffuse oral swelling, or indurated fissuring of the lower lip. Histologically, 90% of oral lesions associated with Crohn's disease contain granulomas[106]. Other reactive cutaneous manifestations of Crohn's disease include cutaneous polyarteritis nodosa, erythema nodosum, erythema multiforme, finger clubbing, leukocytoclastic vasculitis, epidermolysis bullosa acquisita, palmar erythema, a pustular response to trauma (pathergy), and pyoderma gangrenosum. Zinc deficiency may cause an acrodermatitis enteropathica-like syndrome in patients with severe Crohn's disease[102].

There is no consistent correlation between the appearance of skin lesions and intestinal Crohn's disease activity. Cutaneous Crohn's disease is more commonly associated with colorectal rather than small intestinal disease.

Pathology

The cutaneous and oral lesions of Crohn's disease consist of nodular, non-caseating epithelioid tubercles with surrounding lymphocytes in the superficial and deep dermis, sometimes extending into the subcutaneous fat. There are a few scattered multinucleated Langhans-type giant cells and a sparse perivascular lymphohistiocytic infiltrate. The histopathologic changes are the same as those seen in intestinal lesions.

Diagnosis

Clinically, the differential diagnosis of cutaneous Crohn's disease includes other granulomatous disorders such as cutaneous sarcoidosis, mycobacterial infections, deep fungal infections and foreign body reactions. Other infections, such as actinomycosis or cellulitis, may mimic cutaneous Crohn's disease. Ulcerated lesions may be misdiagnosed as pyoderma gangrenosum. In the case of genital swelling and ulcerations, one must consider granuloma inguinale, schistosomiasis, hidradenitis suppurativa, and chronic lymphedema due to obstruction[105]. Tissue cultures, chest radiographs, tuberculin skin tests and endoscopic findings may add helpful information and allow the diagnosis to be made with increased certainty. The presence of lymphadenopathy, splenomegaly, and pulmonary or ocular symptoms would favor a diagnosis of sarcoidosis.

The histologic picture of cutaneous Crohn's disease is, at times, indistinguishable from other granulomatous diseases with tuberculoid features, including the lupus vulgaris lesion from *M. tuberculosis*. In the latter, central necrosis within tubercles is a helpful distinguishing clue. Differentiating cutaneous Crohn's disease from sarcoidosis can also be challenging, although Crohn's disease usually has denser lymphocytic collections. Zirconium and beryllium granulomas, other foreign body granulomas, and infectious granulomas must all be considered in the histologic differential diagnosis. Special stains for acid-fast bacilli and fungal organisms should be obtained, and all skin biopsies should be polarized to look for foreign bodies.

Treatment

Cutaneous Crohn's disease tends to be chronic, and its severity is not related to the condition of the patient's intestinal disease. Oral metronidazole is an effective treatment (250 mg three times daily), and is frequently paired with topical or intralesional corticosteroids. Systemic agents reported for the treatment of cutaneous Crohn's disease include oral corticosteroids, sulfasalazine, azathioprine, 6-mercaptopurine, and the TNF-α inhibitors infliximab and now adalimumab[107]. Surgical excision of lesions is often complicated by wound dehiscence and disease recurrence.

FOREIGN BODY GRANULOMAS (see also Ch. 93)

Key features

- The most common cause of a foreign body granuloma is rupture of a follicle or cyst
- Inflammation may be either a suppurative and diffuse granulomatous dermatitis or a nodular mononuclear granulomatous dermatitis
- Clues to the inciting foreign body should be sought by polarizing the specimen and searching for cornified cells, tattoo pigment, suture remnants, splinter material, etc.

REFERENCES

1. Demirkok SS, Basaranoglu M, Akbilgic O Seasonal variation of the onset of presentations in stage 1 sarcoidosis. Int J Clin Pract. 2006;60:1443–50.
2. Kataria YP, Holter JF. Immunology of sarcoidosis. Clin Chest Med. 1997;18:719–39.
3. English JC, Patel PJ, Greer KE. Sarcoidosis. J Am Acad Dermatol. 2001;44:725–43.
4. DiAlberti L, Piattelli A, Artese L, et al. Human herpesvirus 8 in sarcoid tissues. Lancet. 1997;350:1655–61.
5. Lassalle S, Selva E, Hofman V, et al. Sarcoid-like lesions associated with the immune restoration inflammatory syndrome in AIDS: absence of polymerase chain reaction detection of Mycobacterium tuberculosis in granulomas isolated by laser capture microdissection. Virchows Arch 2006;449:689–96.
6. Martinetti M, Tinelli C, Kolek V, et al. The sarcoidosis map: a joint survey of clinical and immunogenetic findings in two European countries. Am J Respir Crit Care Med. 1995;152:557–64.
7. Yanardag H, Pamuk ON, Pamuk GE. Lupus pernio in sarcoidosis: clinical features and treatment outcomes of 14 patients. J Clin Rhematol. 2003;9:72–6.
8. Sheffield EA. Pathology of sarcoidosis. Clin Chest Med. 1997;18:741–54.
9. Resnik KS. Subcutaneous sarcoidosis histopathologically manifested as fibrosing granulomatous panniculitis. J Am Acad Dermatol. 2006;55:918–19.
10. Marcoval J, Mana J, Moreno A, et al. Foreign bodies in granulomatous cutaneous lesions of patients with systemic sarcoidosis. Arch Dermatol. 2001;137:427–30.
11. Russo G, Millikan LE. Cutaneous sarcoidosis: diagnosis and treatment. Compr Ther. 1994;20:418–22.
12. Baughman RP, Lower EE. Steroid-sparing alternative treatments for sarcoidosis. Clin Chest Med. 1997;18:853–64.
13. Voelter-Mahlknecht S, Benex A, Metzger S, Fierlbeck G. Treatment of subcutaneous sarcoidosis with allopurinol. Arch Dermatol. 1999;135:1560–1.
14. Lee JB, Koblenzer PS. Disfiguring cutaneous manifestation of sarcoidosis treated with thalidomide: a case report. J Am Acad Dermatol. 1998;39:835–8.
15. Georgiou S, Monastirli A, Pasmatzi E, Tsambaos D. Cutaneous sarcoidosis: complete remission after oral isotretinoin therapy. Acta Derm Venereol. 1998;78:457–9.
16. Bachelez H, Senet P, Cadranel J, et al. The use of tetracyclines for the treatment of sarcoidosis. Arch Dermatol. 2001;137:69–73.
17. Pinto P, Dougados M. Leflunomide in clinical practice. Acta Reumatol Port. 2006;31:215–24.
18. Liedtka JE. Intralesional chloroquine for the treatment of cutaneous sarcoidosis. Int J Dermatol. 1996;35:682–3.
19. Patterson JW, Fitzwater JE. Treatment of hypopigmented sarcoidosis with 8-methoxypsoralen and long wave ultraviolet light. Int J Dermatol. 1982;21:476–80.

20. Goodman MM, Alpern K. Treatment of lupus pernio with the flashlamp pulsed dye laser. Lasers Surg Med. 1992;12:549–51.
21. Green JJ, Lawrence N, Heymann WR. Generalized ulcerative sarcoidosis induced by therapy with the flashlamp-pumped pulsed dye laser. Arch Dermatol. 2001;137:507–8.
22. Collison DW, Novice F, Banse L, et al. Split-thickness skin grafting in extensive ulcerative sarcoidosis. J Dermatol Surg Oncol. 1989;15:679–83.
23. Mills A, Chetty R. Auricular granuloma annulare. A consequence of trauma? Am J Dermatopathol. 1992;14:431–3.
24. Muhlbauer JE. Granuloma annulare. J Am Acad Dermatol. 1980;3:217–30.
25. Buechner SA, Winkelmann RK, Banks PM. Identification of T-cell subpopulations in granuloma annulare. Arch Dermatol. 1983;119:125–8.
26. Fayyazi A, Schweyer S, Eichmeyer B, et al. Expression of IFN-gamma, coexpression of TNF-alpha and matrix metalloproteinases and apoptosis of T lymphocytes and macrophages in granuloma annulare. Arch Dermatol Res. 2000;292:384–90.
27. Umbert P, Winkelmann RK. Histologic, ultrastructural, and histochemical studies of granuloma annulare. Arch Dermatol. 1977;113:1681–6.
28. Hanna WM, Moreno-Merlo F, Andrighetti L. Granuloma annulare: an elastic tissue disease? Case report and literature review. Ultrastruct Pathol. 1999;23:33–8.
29. Friedman-Birnbaum R, Haim S, Gideone O, Barzilai A. Histocompatibility antigens in granuloma annulare. Br J Dermatol. 1978;98:425–8.
30. Cronquist SD, Stashower ME, Benson PM. Deep dermal granuloma annulare presenting as an eyelid tumor in a child, with review of pediatric eyelid lesions. Pediatr Dermatol. 1999;16:377–80.
31. Dabski K, Winkelmann RK. Generalized granuloma annulare: clinical and laboratory findings in 100 patients. J Am Acad Dermatol. 1989;20:39–47.
32. Penas PF, Jones-Caballero M, Fraga J, Sanchez-Perez J, Garcia-Diez A. Perforating granuloma annulare. Int J Dermatol. 1997;36:340–8.
33. Barksdale SK, Perniciaro C, Halling KC, Strickler JG. Granuloma annulare in patients with malignant lymphoma: clinicopathologic study of thirteen new cases. J Am Acad Dermatol. 1994;31:42–8.
34. Ono H, Yokozeki H, Katayama I, Nishioka K. Granuloma annulare in a patient with malignant lymphoma. Dermatology. 1997;195:46–7.
35. Cohen PR. Granuloma annulare associated with malignancy. Southern Med J. 1997;90:1056–9.
36. Wong WR, Yang LJ, Kuo TT, Chan HL. Generalized granuloma annulare associated with granulomatous mycosis fungoides. Dermatology. 2000;200:54–6.
37. Studer EM, Calza AM, Saurat JH. Precipitating factors and associated diseases in 84 patients with granuloma annulare: a retrospective study. Dermatology. 1996;193:364–8.

38. Ohata C, Shirabe H, Takagi K, Kawatsu T. Granuloma annulare in herpes zoster scars. J Dermatol. 2000;27:166–9.
39. O'Moore EJ, Nandawni R, Uthayakumar S, et al. HIV-associated granuloma annulare (HAGA): a report of six cases. Br J Dermatol. 2000;142:1054–6.
40. Dabski K, Winkelmann RK. Generalized granuloma annulare: histopathology and immunopathology. J Am Acad Dermatol. 1989;20:28–39.
41. Dahl MV, Ullman S, Goltz RW. Vasculitis in granuloma annulare: histopathology and direct immunofluorescence. Arch Dermatol. 1977;133:463–7.
42. Magro CM, Crowson AN, Regauer S. Granuloma annulare and necrobiosis lipoidica tissue reactions as a manifestation of systemic disease. Hum Pathol. 1996;27:50–6.
43. Blume-Peytavi U, Zouboulis CC, Jacobi H, et al. Successful outcome of cryosurgery in patients with granuloma annulare. Br J Dermatol. 1994;130:494–7.
44. Muchenberger S, Schopf E, Simon JC. Phototherapy with UV-A-1 for generalized granuloma annulare [letter]. Arch Dermatol. 1997;133:1605.
45. Setterfield J, Huilgol SC, Black MM. Generalised granuloma annulare successfully treated with PUVA. Clin Exp Dermatol. 1999;24:458–60.
46. Rouilleault P. CO2 laser and granuloma annulare [letter]. J Dermatol Surg Oncol. 1988;14:120.
47. Weiss JM, Muchenberger S, Schopf E, Simon JC. Treatment of granuloma annulare by local injections with low-dose recombinant human interferon gamma. J Am Acad Dermatol. 1998;39:117–19.
48. Ma A, Medenica M. Response of generalized granuloma annulare to high-dose niacinamide. Arch Dermatol. 1983;119:836–9.
49. Ratnavel RC, Norris PG. Perforating granuloma annulare: response to treatment with isotretinoin. J Am Acad Dermatol. 1995;32:126–7.
50. Simon M Jr, von den Driesch P. Antimalarials for control of disseminated granuloma annulare in children. J Am Acad Dermatol. 1994;31:1064–5.
51. Steiner A, Pehamberger H, Wolff K. Sulfone treatment of granuloma annulare. J Am Acad Dermatol. 1985;13:1004–8.
52. Rubel DM, Wood G, Rosen R, Jopp-McKay A. Generalised granuloma annulare successfully treated with pentoxifylline. Australas J Dermatol. 1993;34:103–8.
53. Fiallo P. Cyclosporin for the treatment of granuloma annulare [letter]. Br J Dermatol. 1998;138:369–70.
54. Filotico R, Vena GA, Coviello C, Angelini G. Cyclosporin in the treatment of generalized granuloma annulare. J Am Acad Dermatol. 1994;30:487–8.
55. Kossard S, Winkelmann RK. Low-dose chlorambucil in the treatment of generalized granuloma annulare. Dermatologica. 1979;158:443–50.
56. Asano Y, Saito A, Idezuki T, Igarashi A. Generalized granuloma annulare treated with short-term

administration of etretinate. J Am Acad Dermatol. 2006;54:s245–7.

57. Kim YJ, Kang HY, Lee ES, Kim YC. Successful treatment of granuloma annulare with topical 5-aminolaevulinic acid photodynamic therapy. J Dermatol. 2006;33:642–3.

58. Kreuter A, Altmeyer P, Gambichler T. Failure of etanercept therapy in disseminated granuloma annulare. Arch Dermatol. 2006;142:1236–7.

59. Wells RS, Smith MA. The natural history of granuloma annulare. Br J Dermatol. 1963;75:199–205.

60. Muller SA, Winkelmann RK. Necrobiosis lipoidica diabeticorum. A clinical and pathological investigation of 171 cases. Arch Dermatol. 1966; 93:272–81.

61. Muller SA, Winkelmann RK. Necrobiosis lipoidica diabeticorum. Results of glucose-tolerance tests in nondiabetic patients. J Am Med Assoc. 1966; 195:433–6.

62. O'Toole EA, Kennedy U, Nolan JJ, et al. Necrobiosis lipoidica: only a minority of patients have diabetes mellitus. Br J Dermatol. 1999;140:283–6.

63. Boulton AJM, Cutfield RG, Abouganem D, et al. Necrobiosis lipoidica diabeticorum: a clinicopathologic study. J Am Acad Dermatol. 1988;18:530–7.

64. Quimby SR, Muller SA, Schroeter AL. The cutaneous immunopathology of necrobiosis lipoidica diabeticorum. Arch Dermatol. 1988;124:1364–71.

65. Ullman S, Dahl MV. Necrobiosis lipoidica. An immunofluorescence study. Arch Dermatol. 1977;113:1671–3.

66. Lowitt MH, Dover JS. Necrobiosis lipoidica. J Am Acad Dermatol. 1991;25:735–48.

67. Evans CD, Pereira RS, Yuen CT, Holden CA. Anti-collagen antibodies in granuloma annulare and necrobiosis lipoidica. Clin Exp Dermatol. 1988;13:252–4.

68. Oikarinen A, Mortenhumer M, Kallioinen M, Savolainen ER. Necrobiosis lipoidica: ultrastructural and biochemical demonstration of a collagen defect. J Invest Dermatol. 1987;88:227–32.

69. Lim C, Tschuchnigg M, Lim J. Squamous cell carcinoma arising in an area of long-standing necrobiosis lipoidica. J Cutan Pathol. 2006;33:581–3.

70. Laukkanen A, Fraki JE, Vaatainen N, et al. Necrobiosis lipoidica: clinical and immunofluorescent study. Dermatologica. 1986;172:89–92.

71. Nieboer C, Kalsbeek GL. Direct immunofluorescence studies in granuloma annulare, necrobiosis lipoidica and granulomatosis disciformis Miescher. Dermatologica. 1979;158:427–32.

72. Graham-Brown RA, Shuttleworth D, Sarkany I. Coexistence of sarcoidosis and necrobiosis lipoidica of the legs – a report of two cases. Clin Exp Dermatol. 1985;10:274–8.

73. De la Torre C, Losada A, Cruces MJ. Necrobiosis lipoidica: a case with prominent cholesterol clefting and transepithelial elimination. Am J Dermatopathol. 1999;21:575–7.

74. McDonald L, Zanolli MD, Boyd AS. Perforating elastosis in necrobiosis lipoidica diabeticorum. Cutis. 1996;57:336–8.

75. Tappeiner G. Necrobiosis lipoidica: treatment with systemic corticosteroids. Br J Dermatol. 1992;126:542–5.

76. Beck H, Bjerring P, Rasmussen I, et al. Treatment of necrobiosis lipoidica with low-dose acetylsalicylic acid. Acta Derm Venereol. 1985;65:230–4.

77. Statham B, Finlay AY, Marks R. A randomized double blind comparison of an aspirin dipyridamole combination versus a placebo in the treatment of necrobiosis lipoidica. Acta Derm Venereol. 1981;61:270–1.

78. Wilkin JK. Perilesional heparin injections for necrobiosis lipoidica. J Am Acad Dermatol. 1983; 8:904.

79. Heymann WR. Necrobiosis lipoidica treated with topical tretinoin. Cutis. 1996;58:53–4.

80. Smith K. Ulcerating necrobiosis lipoidica resolving in response to cyclosporine-A. Dermatol Online J. 1997;3:2.

81. Darvay A, Acland KM, Russell-Jones R. Persistent ulcerated necrobiosis lipoidica responding to treatment with cyclosporin. Br J Dermatol. 1999; 141:725–7.

82. Spencer EA, Nahass GT. Topically applied bovine collagen in the treatment of ulcerative necrobiosis lipoidica diabeticorum. Arch Dermatol. 1997;133:817–18.

83. Patel GK, Harding KG, Mills CM. Severe disabling Koebnerizing ulcerated necrobiosis lipoidica successfully managed with topical PUVA. Br J Dermatol. 2000;143:668–9.

84. McKenna DB, Cooper EJ, Tidman MJ. Topical psoralen plus ultraviolet A treatment for necrobiosis lipoidica. Br J Dermatol. 2000;143:1333–5.

85. Beattie PE, Dawe RS, Ibbotson SH, Ferguson J. UVA1 phototherapy for treatment of necrobiosis lipoidica. Clin Exp Dermatol. 2006;31:235–8.

86. Reinhard G, Lohmann F, Uerlich M, et al. Successful treatment of ulcerated necrobiosis lipoidica with mycophenolate mofetil. Acta Derm Venereol. 2000;80:312–13.

87. Kukreia T, Petersen J. Thalidomide for the treatment of refractory necrobiosis lipoidica. Arch Dermatol. 2006;142:20–2.

88. Zeichner JA, Stern DW, Lebwohl M. Treatment of necrobiosis lipoidica with the tumor necrosis factor antagonist etanercept. J Am Acad Dermatol. 2006;54:s120–1.

89. O'Brien JP. Actinic granuloma: an annular connective tissue disorder affecting sun- and heat-damaged (elastotic) skin. Arch Dermatol. 1975;111:460–6.

90. Hanke CW, Bailin PL, Roenigk HM. Annular elastolytic giant cell granuloma. J Am Acad Dermatol. 1979;1:413–21.

91. Dowling GB, Wilson-Jones E. Atypical (annular) necrobiosis lipoidica of the face and scalp. Dermatologica. 1967;135:11–26.

92. Mehregan AH, Altman J. Miescher's granuloma of the face. Arch Dermatol. 1973;107:62–4.

93. Leiker DL, Kok SH, Spaas JAJ. Granuloma multiforme. Int J Lepr. 1964;32:368–76.

94. MacGrae JD. Actinic granuloma. A clinical, histopathological and immunocytochemical study. Arch Dermatol. 1986;122:43–7.

95. Regaz A, Ackerman AB. Is actinic granuloma a specific condition? Am J Dermatopathol. 1979;1:43–53.

96. Tock CL, Cohen PR. Annular elastolytic giant cell granuloma. Cutis. 1998;62:181–7.

97. Lim KB, Phay KL. Annular elastolytic giant-cell granuloma. Int J Dermatol. 1987;26:463–4.

98. Tsutsui K, Hirone T, Kubo K, Matsui Y. Annular elastolytic giant cell granuloma: response to cyclosporin A. J Dermatol. 1994;21:426–9.

99. Ozkaya-Bayazit E, Buyukbabani N, Baykal C, et al. Annular elastolytic giant cell granuloma: sparing of a burn scar and successful treatment with chloroquine. Br J Dermatol. 1999;140:525–30.

100. Schwarz T, Lindlbauer R, Gschnait F. Annular elastolytic giant cell granuloma. J Cutan Pathol. 1983;10:321–6.

101. Repiso A, Alcantara M, Munoz-Rosas C, et al. Extraintestinal manifestations of Crohn's disease: prevalence and related factors. Rev Esp Enferm Dig. 2006;98:510–17.

102. Burgdorf W. Cutaneous manifestations of Crohn's disease. J Am Acad Dermatol. 1981;5:689–95.

103. Pinna AL, Atzori L, Ferreli C, Aste N. Cutaneous Crohn disease in a child. Pediatr Dermatol. 2006;23:49–52.

103a. Balfour Sartor R. Mechanisms of disease: pathogenesis of Crohn's disease and ulcerative colitis. Nat Clin Pract Gastroenterol Hepatol. 2006;3:390–407.

104. Gonzalez-Guerra E, Angulo J, Vargas-Machuca I, Farina C, Martin L, Requena L. Cutaneous Crohn's disease causing deformity of the penis and scrotum. Acta Derm Venereol. 2006;86:179–80.

105. Ploysangam T, Heubi JE, Eisen D, et al. Cutaneous Crohn's disease in children. J Am Acad Dermatol. 1997;36:697–704.

106. McCallum DI, Kinmont PDC. Dermatologic manifestations of Crohn's disease. Br J Dermatol. 1968;80:1–8.

107. Rispo A, Scarpa R, DiGirolamo E, et al. Infliximab in the treatment of extra-intestinal manifestations of Crohn's disease. Scand J Rheumatol. 2005;34:387–91.

Foreign Body Reactions

MA Abdallah

Key features

- Foreign body reactions represent inflammatory responses to inorganic and high-molecular-weight organic materials that have been introduced into the skin and are variably resistant to degradation
- Routes of introduction can vary from accidental or self-inflicted to surgical procedures and topical application of medications
- The most common clinical presentation is red to red–brown papules, nodules or plaques (with or without ulceration) that are due to granulomatous inflammation
- Less common presentations of foreign body reactions include lichenoid or pseudolymphomatous, and a fistula or draining wound

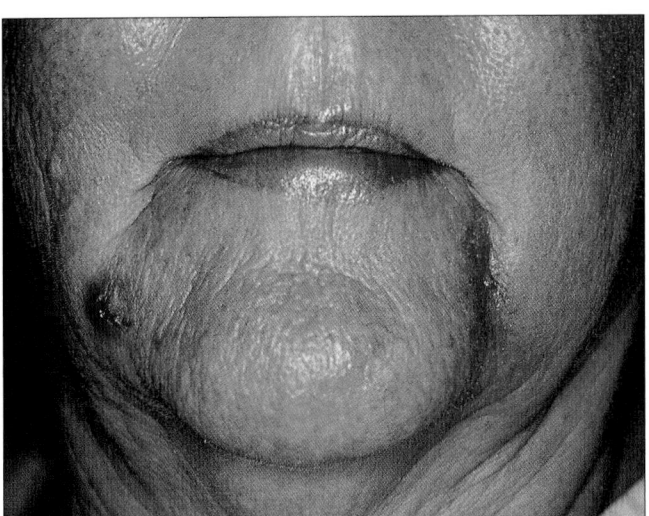

Fig. 93.1 Granulomatous reaction to collagen injection.

GENERAL CONSIDERATIONS

Definition

Literally, any material – living or non-living – introduced into the body is a 'foreign body' and is treated by our defense mechanisms as 'non-self' in order to elicit the appropriate response. Such a broad definition also includes infective agents, but they are covered elsewhere (see Chs 73–84). This chapter will focus on non-living materials that have been introduced into the dermis or subcutis[1-3]. They represent inorganic compounds or organic material of high molecular weight that resist degradation by the body's inflammatory cells or their products. Foreign bodies reported to elicit skin reactions are listed in Table 93.1.

Routes of Entry

Accidental

Accidental inoculation with foreign bodies may occur during various activities such as gardening (wood splinters, cactus spines) or swimming and diving (coelenterate envenomation, sea urchin spines), or it may result accidentally, such as in blast injury (silica particles) or motor vehicle accidents.

Surgical procedures

Contamination of wounds by talc or starch powders used for lubrication of surgical gloves may incite a foreign body reaction. Surgical sutures can also cause a foreign body response. Histologically, suture granulomas are commonly seen in excisional specimens of previously sampled cutaneous tumors.

Iatrogenic

Foreign material implanted into the skin for the purpose of tissue augmentation (fillers), such as silicone, bovine collagen (Fig. 93.1) or hyaluronic acid, can induce reactions in some individuals (see Ch. 158). Paraffin is still being used illegally for tissue augmentation, and cases of paraffin reactions can also occur after the application of paraffin-containing materials such as nasal packs[4].

Tattooing

Tattooing is the introduction of an exogenous pigment into the dermis, either deliberately or accidentally, resulting in permanent discoloration of the skin.

Topical application

Deodorants and anti-pruritus preparations containing zirconium oxide applied to the skin surface may cause foreign body reactions. Of note, zirconium lactate was generally banned in 1978.

Self-inflicted

Self-administered intravenous injections, a common practice among drug addicts, may lead to the introduction of foreign material into the skin.

Pathogenesis

The initial tissue response to most foreign substances involves an accumulation of neutrophils which usually fail to deal properly with the foreign body. Its persistence attracts monocytes and local tissue macrophages that engulf the foreign material and become activated. Engulfed material may resist degradation and remain sequestered within the macrophages. Activated macrophages secrete a variety of specific biologically active substances, e.g. cytokines, that attract additional macrophages and blood monocytes. The formation of a chronic granuloma represents an attempt by the body to sequester a persistent indigestible material. Individual macrophages may become larger (epithelioid histiocytes) or fuse to form multinucleated foreign body giant cells. The infiltrate also contains T lymphocytes and fibroblasts. The pathogenesis of other patterns of reactions, e.g. lichenoid, pyogenic granuloma-like, pseudolymphomatous, remains speculative.

Clinical Features

The host response and, consequently, the clinical presentations of foreign body implantation are variable (Tables 93.2 and 93.3). An acute inflammatory response occurs shortly after the entry of the foreign material. This may resolve, to be followed weeks, months or even years later by a chronic inflammatory response. Although the latter may have a variety of clinical presentations, red to red–brown papules, nodules and plaques (with or without ulceration) are the most common. Over time, the lesions may become firmer due to fibrosis. The pattern and arrangement of the cutaneous lesions will correspond to the route of inoculation, and observation of this patterning, in association with relevant patient history, is crucial.

CLASSIFICATION OF FOREIGN BODIES ACCORDING TO THEIR ORIGINS AND ROUTES OF ENTRY		
Origin		**Route of entry**
Non-biologic (inorganic/metallic compounds)		
	Tattoo inks	Decoration Cosmetic Accidental Iatrogenic
	Paraffin	Tissue augmentation Topical paraffin-containing preparations
	Silicone (polydimethyl siloxane) liquid or gel	Tissue augmentation
	Silica	Wound contamination Blast injuries
	Talc	Surgical procedures Wound contamination Umbilical stump contamination Intravenous injection of self-prepared drugs
	Zirconium	Topical application: deodorants, antipruritus medications
	Beryllium	Laceration by broken fluorescent lamps (historical) Inhalation
	Aluminum	Subcutaneous injection of aluminum-containing vaccines
	Zinc	Subcutaneous injection of insulin–zinc preparations
	Other synthetic fillers, e.g. poly-L-lactic acid, polymethylmethacrylate	Tissue augmentation
Biologic		
Produced in the skin but normally isolated from body's defense mechanisms	Hair keratin (see Ch. 39)	Ruptured follicle or cyst* Ingrown hair Barber's sinus
	Nail keratin	Ingrown nail Accidental
Produced by other living organisms	Bovine collagen	Tissue augmentation
	Hyaluronic acid	Tissue augmentation
	Starch	Surgical procedures
	Cactus spines	Accidental Occupational
	Jellyfish and corals	Accidental Swimming or diving
	Sea urchin spines (see Ch. 84)	Accidental Swimming or diving
	Silk sutures	Surgical procedures
Miscellaneous	Corticosteroids	Intralesional injection
	Sutures (less frequently nylon or polypropylene)	Surgical procedures

Most common cause of a foreign body reaction in the skin.

Table 93.1 Classification of foreign bodies according to their origins and routes of entry.

CLINICAL PRESENTATIONS OF FOREIGN BODY REACTIONS	
Clinical presentation	**Foreign substance**
Erythema, induration, papules, nodules (with or without ulceration)	Tattoo inks, paraffin, silicone, silica, beryllium (local), starch, fillers (e.g. bovine collagen)
Sarcoidosis-like granulomatous papules	Tattoo inks, talc, zirconium, beryllium (systemic), fillers (e.g. bovine collagen, hyaluronic acid)
Pyogenic granuloma-like lesions	Talc, keratin (ingrown nail)
Pseudofolliculitis barbae, acne keloidalis nuchae	Keratin
Pruritic lichenoid papules and plaques (often in an irregular linear pattern)	Tattoo inks, jellyfish and coral stings
Abscess	Bovine collagen, zinc, paraffin, keratin (pilonidal disease)
Sinus tract/fistula	Suture, keratin (pilonidal disease, barber's sinus)
Persistent subcutaneous nodules at injection site	Aluminum, fillers containing synthetic particles (see Table 93.3)
Photoallergic eczematous reaction	Tattoo ink containing cadmium sulfide (yellow), cadmium selenide (red) or azo dyes (yellow, red)

Table 93.2 Clinical presentations of foreign body reactions.

In addition to nodules and plaques, other forms of foreign body reaction include pyogenic granuloma-like lesions[5], lichenoid lesions[6,7], and a chronic draining fistula or wound[8].

Pathology

Apart from the acute reaction to the trauma that accompanies the introduction of the foreign body, a chronic reaction is the usual response (see Table 93.3). Although different patterns of chronic local tissue reactions have been described, including lichenoid[6], chronic inflammatory and pseudolymphomatous[9], the most common is the granulomatous type of reaction[10,11] (Table 93.4). Granulomas that develop as a reaction to foreign bodies are of two major types:

- allergic (immunologic)
- non-allergic ('foreign body').

The allergic type is characterized by the presence of groups of individual epithelioid histiocytes associated with variable numbers of lymphocytes and fewer multinucleated Langhans-type giant cells[11]. In the non-immunologic type, the foreign body giant cell (Fig. 93.2) is the most conspicuous component of the infiltrate, which also contains histiocytes, lymphocytes and other inflammatory cells.

A histologic decision as to whether a granuloma is of the foreign body type or of the allergic type is not always possible and different patterns may be seen in the same section. It is of note that foreign body reactions in patients infected with HIV are different, with abundant individual macrophages, but no giant cells, suggesting an immunologic dysfunction[12]. The foreign material inciting a reaction may be detected in conventional H&E sections or may require special procedures for its identification (see Table 93.3).

Diagnosis

Foreign body reactions should be considered in the differential diagnosis of localized inflammatory nodules and plaques, especially when there is a persistent draining wound or sinus. Occasionally, they appear as pyogenic granulomas or localized lichenoid papules. Clinical morphology

CLINICAL AND HISTOPATHOLOGIC FEATURES OF FOREIGN BODY REACTIONS					
Foreign body	Clinical presentations	Histologic reaction patterns	Other distinctive features	Birefringent	Other detection methods
Tattoo inks	Erythema, induration, papules, nodules Lichenoid papules and plaques Eczematous dermatitis (including photoallergic reactions)	Foreign body or (with certain dyes) sarcoidal granulomas Lichenoid dermatitis Spongiotic dermatitis Pseudolymphoma Pseudoepitheliomatous hyperplasia Non-specific chronic inflammation	Pigment granules scattered throughout the infiltrate, extra- and intracellular (macrophages)		EDXA
Paraffin	Firm nodules, indurated plaques Ulceration or abscess formation	Foreign body granulomas between cavities	'Swiss cheese' appearance Positive fat stains (e.g. oil red O)		IRS (non-processed tissue)
Silicone	Erythema, induration Nodules, ulcers Often appears after years	Foreign body granulomas between cavities	'Swiss-cheese' appearance* Histiocytes may be foamy Negative fat stains		EDXA Radio-opaque on X-ray
Silica	Nodules, indurated plaques within scar Disseminated papules (blast injuries) Prolonged incubation period	Granulomas (sarcoidal > foreign body)	Colorless crystals, extra- and intracellular	✓	IRS or EDXA
Talc	Sarcoid-like papules Thickening and erythema of an old scar Involvement of intertriginous zones, iv injection sites Umbilical stumps Pyogenic granuloma-like	Sarcoidal or foreign body granulomas Pyogenic granuloma-like	Needle-shaped or round talc crystals: clear, blue–green or yellow–brown	✓	EDXA
Zirconium	Persistent, soft, brownish papules Involvement of axillary skin	Sarcoidal granulomas			EDXA
Beryllium, local skin reaction	Nodule, ulcer	Caseating granulomas			EELS
Beryllium, systemic	Widely scattered papules (<1% of cases)	Sarcoidal granulomas			Bronchoalveolar lavage
Aluminum	Persistent subcutaneous nodules at injection site	Granulomas with peripheral lymphocytes and eosinophils Pseudolymphoma			EDXA
Zinc	Furuncles at injection sites	Early: dense neutrophilic infiltrate Late: granulomas and fibrosis	Rhomboidal crystals	✓	EDXA
Bovine collagen	Induration and erythema Papules and nodules Abscesses Localized tissue necrosis (early; due to vascular disruption)	Palisaded granulomas containing many foreign body giant cells Diffuse granulomatous pattern Associated lymphocytes, eosinophils, plasma cells and neutrophils	Pale-staining aggregates of implanted collagen		Immunoperoxidase staining with anti-bovine collagen type I antibodies
Hyaluronic acid	Induration and erythema Papules and nodules Abscesses	Foreign body granulomas Associated eosinophils and neutrophils	Amorphous basophilic material Stains with Alcian blue		

*With injection of particulate silicone (e.g. Bioplastique®), cystic spaces contain jagged, translucent, non-birefringent particles.

Table 93.3 Clinical and histopathologic features of foreign body reactions. The order of the entities in this table corresponds to that in the text. EDXA, energy dispersive X-ray analysis; EELS, electron energy loss spectroscopy; IRS, infrared spectrophotometry; iv, intravenous. *Continued*

CLINICAL AND HISTOPATHOLOGIC FEATURES OF FOREIGN BODY REACTIONS

Foreign body	Clinical presentations	Histologic reaction patterns	Other distinctive features	Birefringent	Other detection methods
Fillers containing synthetic particles (see Table 158.6)	Induration and erythema Papules and nodules Abscesses	Foreign body granulomas with cystic spaces	Various types of particles within cystic spaces*,†: • Round (polymethylmethacrylate; [Artefill®]) • Irregular polygonal (poly[hydroxyl] ethylmethacrylate [DermaLive®]) • Irregular 'spiky' (poly-L-lactic acid [Sculptra®/ New-Fill®])	✓ (Sculptra®)	
Starch	Papules, nodules	Foreign body granulomas	Ovoid basophilic starch granules PAS-positive	✓	
Cactus	Dome-shaped, skin-colored papules with a central black dot	Early: neutrophils Late: sarcoidal or foreign body granulomas	Spines, extra- and intracellular (giant cells) PAS-positive	✓	
Jellyfish, corals, sea urchin spines	Pruritic lichenoid papules and plaques (onset 2–3 weeks after exposure) Linear, zig-zag and whip-like (flagellate) patterns of erythema/edema (early), hyperpigmentation or lichenoid papules (late)	Lichenoid dermatitis	Calcite crystals (sea urchin spines)	✓ (sea urchin spines)	
Keratin	Pseudofolliculitis/acne keloidalis nuchae Pyogenic granuloma-like lesions, ingrown nails Pilonidal disease	Foreign body granulomas	Other inflammatory cells	✓	
Intralesional corticosteroids	Skin-colored to yellow–white papules or nodules develop at the site of a previous intralesional injection of corticosteroid The incubation period varies between weeks to months	Foreign body granulomas	Pale bluish material on H&E		
Suture	Wound appears inflamed, red, edematous (or develops papules or nodules) and opens to form a fistula	Foreign body granulomas		✓	

*With injection of particulate silicone (e.g. Bioplastique®), cystic spaces contain jagged, translucent, non-birefringent particles.
†Irregularly shaped particles are more likely to incite a granulomatous response than smooth-surfaced particles; DermaLive® is not available in the US.

Table 93.3, cont'd Clinical and histopathologic features of foreign body reactions. The order of the entities in this table corresponds to that in the text. EDXA, energy dispersive X-ray analysis; EELS, electron energy loss spectroscopy; IRS, infrared spectrophotometry; iv, intravenous.

HISTOPATHOLOGIC REACTIONS TO FOREIGN BODIES

Histopathologic reaction	Foreign substance
Foreign body granuloma (non-allergic)	Tattoo ink, paraffin, silicone, silica, talc, starch, cactus, keratin, intralesional corticosteroids, sutures
Sarcoidal granuloma (allergic)	Tattoo ink, silica, talc, zirconium, cactus
Tuberculoid granuloma with caseation	Beryllium (local reaction)
Palisaded granulomas containing many foreign body giant cells	Bovine collagen
Cavities surrounded by granulomatous reaction ('Swiss cheese' appearance)	Paraffin, silicone
Lichenoid dermatitis	Tattoo ink, jellyfish and corals
Pyogenic granuloma-like	Talc, keratin
Pseudolymphomatous	Tattoo ink, aluminum
Chronic non-specific inflammation	Tattoo ink
Neutrophilic infiltrate	Early reaction to cactus and zinc

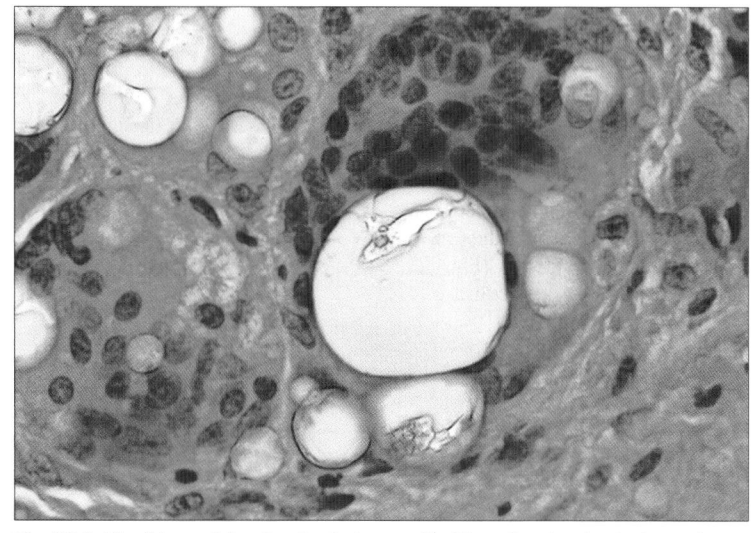

Fig. 93.2 Birefringent foreign body is engulfed by a foreign body type giant cell with the typical haphazard array of nuclei. Courtesy of Thomas D Horn MD.

Table 93.4 Histopathologic reactions to foreign bodies.

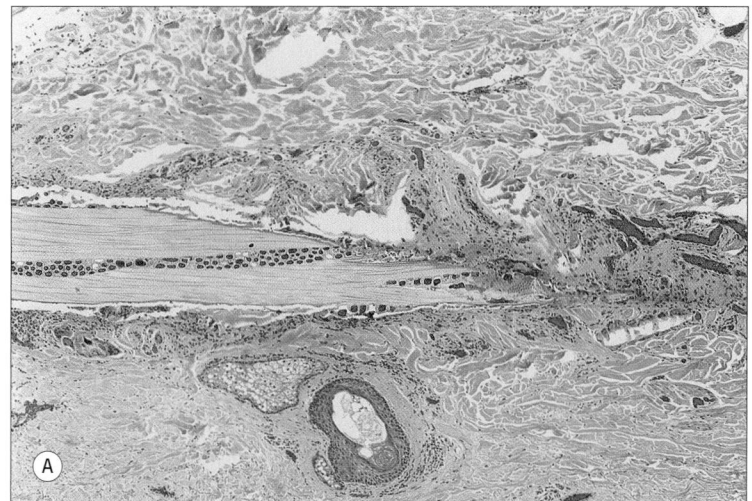

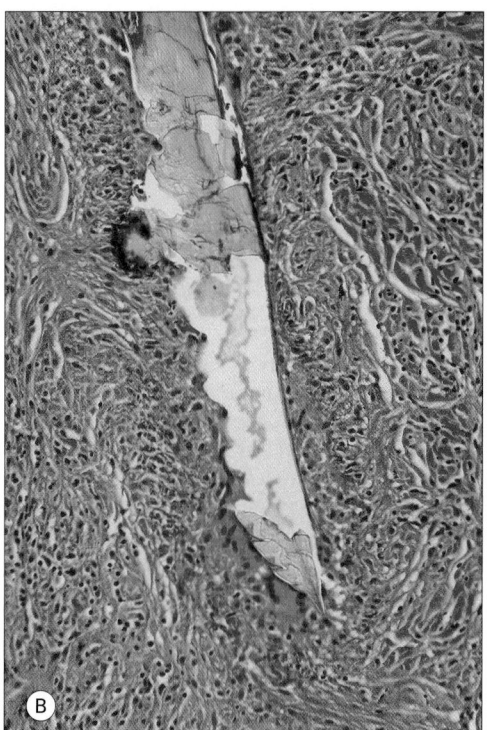

Fig. 93.3 Granulomatous foreign body reactions. Wood splinter (**A**) versus bee stinger (**B**). A, Courtesy of Ronald P Rapini MD.

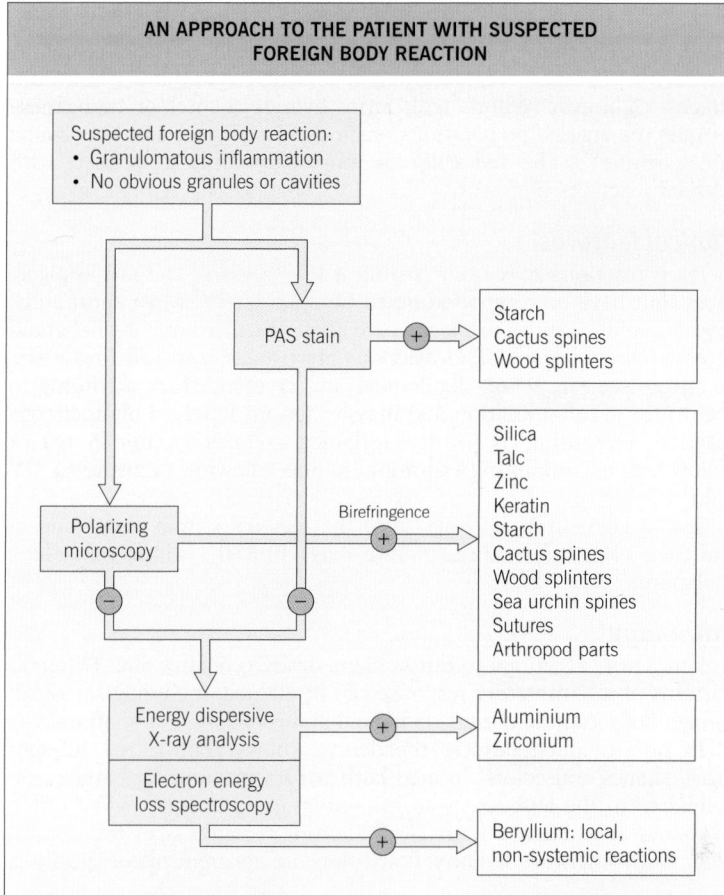

AN APPROACH TO THE PATIENT WITH SUSPECTED FOREIGN BODY REACTION

Fig. 93.4 An approach to the patient with suspected foreign body reaction.

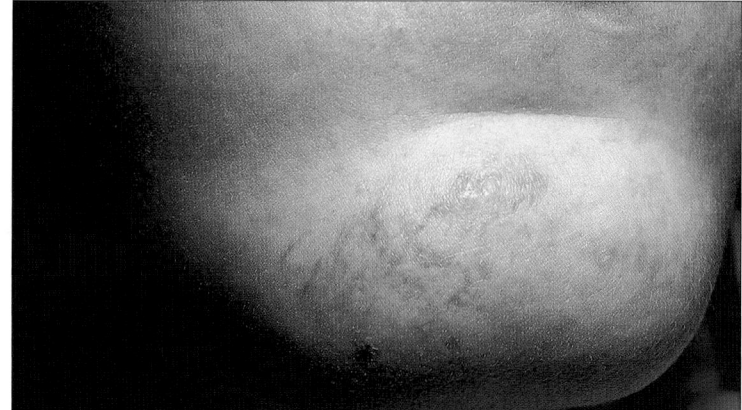

Fig. 93.5 Traumatic tattoo of the chin. Bluish discoloration and slight erythema, predominantly due to silica. Courtesy of Ronald P Rapini MD.

is usually not distinctive, and a thorough history is indispensable for arriving at the correct diagnosis.

Imaging techniques such as plain radiography, ultrasonography, CT scanning and MRI are of little practical value in visualizing small cutaneous foreign bodies, even if the foreign body is radio-opaque.

Histologic examination confirms the granulomatous nature of the lesion and rare foreign bodies may show distinctive microscopic features in H&E-stained sections (Fig. 93.3). However, special procedures are usually required for an accurate diagnosis, e.g. PAS staining and microscopic examination with polarized light (Fig. 93.4). Wood splinters, fungi and starch stain with PAS, while nylon suture material, wood, talc and starch powder are doubly refractile with polarized light.

Identification of the chemical nature of the foreign body requires sophisticated physicochemical procedures that necessitate special processing of the tissue sample and are available in only a few research centers. Energy dispersive X-ray analysis (EDXA), electron energy loss spectroscopy (EELS), laser microprobe mass analysis, and infrared spectrophotometry are examples (see Table 93.3).

To summarize, accurate identification of a foreign body reaction depends on a high index of suspicion, thorough history taking, and histologic examination using routine staining, PAS staining and polarized microscopy.

FOREIGN BODY REACTIONS TO INORGANIC AND METALLIC COMPOUNDS

Tattoo

A tattoo may occur accidentally or deliberately for cosmetic and decorative purposes. Accidental tattooing results from unintentional deposition of exogenous pigmented substances such as asphalt, graphite or carbon within injured skin (Fig. 93.5). Automobile, bicycle and skating accidents as well as puncture wounds are the most common causes of traumatic tattoos. In decorative tattooing, the pigment is introduced into the dermis with needles or a tattoo gun to create various pictures, group-identity symbols, or writings. The motif differs according to the culture of the society and the purpose for which it is created. Cosmetic tattoos are also done to define lip contours, replace eyeliner, or hide an abnormality in skin color. Iatrogenic tattoo may remain after the use of ferrous subsulfate (Monsel's solution) for hemostasis.

Tattoos often contain a number of pigments that are combined to create different hues. These may be inorganic salts of metals, such as mercury in cinnabar (red, becoming historical), cobalt (blue), chromium (green), cadmium (yellow, red), ferric hydrate (ochre) or manganese (purple), or organic preparations, such as sandalwood and brazilwood and carmine[10]. The red color is most commonly associated with nodular reactions (Fig. 93.6).

Clinical features

Delayed reactions may occur within a few weeks of the tattoo placement, but have been reported up to 17 years later[13]. Most commonly, erythematous nodules or plaques are seen, but there may be lichenoid or eczematous lesions. The reactions are usually confined to the site of tattoo (see Fig. 93.6). Tenderness and erythema vary according to the degree of inflammation and may be absent. Rarely, a photoallergic reaction, presenting as pruritic inflamed nodules, occurs in red or yellow tattoos containing cadmium sulfide following exposure to UV light[13].

Tattoo pigments may migrate to the regional lymph nodes and at the time of lymph node sampling may clinically mimic metastatic melanoma.

Pathology

Inflammatory reactions to tattoo pigment are generally rare. Different patterns of inflammatory response can be elicited, including sarcoidal, foreign body granulomatous, lichenoid and pseudolymphomatous[9].

In non-inflamed tattoos, the dermis shows granules of different sizes, shapes and colors, located both within macrophages and extracellularly, in the absence of an inflammatory infiltrate[14]. Most tattoo pigments appear black with H&E staining, regardless of the clinical color, but sometimes red or yellow colors are apparent histologically.

Diagnosis and differential diagnosis

The presence of inflammatory lesions confined to the site of a tattoo suggests the diagnosis. The differential diagnosis includes other inflammatory disorders that may arise in tattoos, e.g. sarcoidosis. Inoculation of certain infectious agents may mimic pigment-induced inflammation within a tattoo. Identification of the causative pigment is generally unnecessary unless further tattooing is anticipated. Other causes of dermal pigmentation include melanin, hemosiderin, lipofuscin, silver, gold, minocycline, amiodarone and chlorpromazine. Special stains to identify melanin and iron (hemosiderin) may be useful, along with electron microscopy.

Treatment

Although many therapeutic modalities for tattoo removal have been used, some of them resulted in significant scarring. Nowadays, lasers

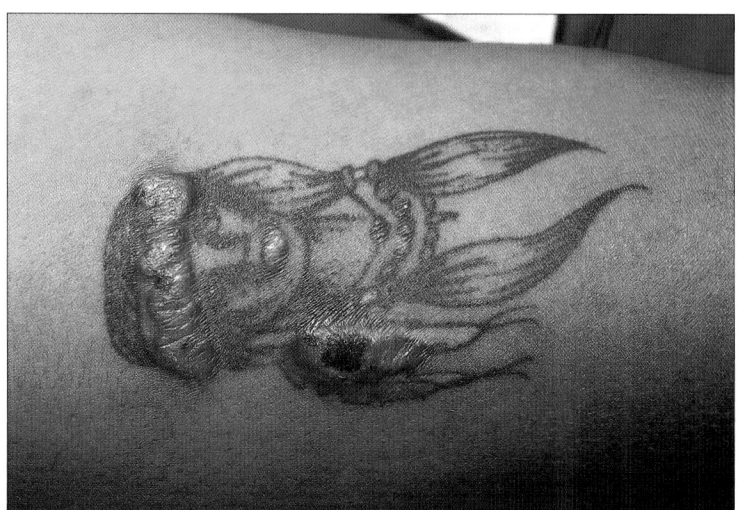

Fig. 93.6 Granulomas due to allergic reaction to the red (cinnabar) portions of a tattoo. Over the past several years, cinnabar (mercuric sulfide) has been gradually replaced by cadmium selenide (cadmium red), ferric hydrate (sienna or red ochre) and organic compounds. Courtesy of Ronald P Rapini MD.

(e.g. Q-switched ruby, alexandrite and Nd:YAG, see Table 137.2) represent the primary treatments, allowing selective destruction of chromophores while leaving adjacent collagen intact. The specific type of laser chosen depends on the tattoo ink colors and the wavelengths to which they best respond[15] (see Ch. 137). Several wavelengths are necessary to treat multicolored tattoos optimally.

Surgical excision is the main alternative in treatment of inflamed tattoos. Topical corticosteroids are often ineffective, but intralesional corticosteroids can be tried; laser therapy is ill advised because of the risk of inducing a systemic reaction, following release of pigment from macrophages, in the already sensitized patient[15].

Paraffin (Sclerosing Lipogranuloma)

Paraffin, being a mineral oil, is not hydrolyzed by tissue lipases and is treated by the body as a foreign substance. Augmentation of body contour by local injection of paraffin, though banned in most countries, is still performed in some areas of the world and is mostly done by non-medical personnel. Accidental paraffinoma of the orbit and palpebrum has been reported following intraoperative placement of paraffin-impregnated gauze packs within the nasal cavity.

Clinical features

In those cases due to injected paraffin, the genitalia and breast are the most common sites of involvement. Clinically, non-tender firm nodules and indurated plaques are seen, sometimes with ulceration or abscess formation and involvement of subcutaneous tissue (see Ch. 100). The interval between the time of injection and the development of lesions may span many years.

Pathology

The dermis shows a characteristic 'Swiss cheese' appearance due to the presence of numerous ovoid or round cavities where the paraffin resided prior to processing. The tissue between the cavities shows fibrotic connective tissue and a cellular infiltrate composed of macrophages, variable numbers of multinucleated foreign body giant cells, and lymphocytes. Some of the macrophages have foamy cytoplasm. In specially processed tissue, the foreign material stains with fat stains[16], though less intensely than neutral fats, helping to differentiate paraffinoma from reactions to silicone, which also have numerous cavities but will not stain.

Treatment

Excision with appropriate tissue reconstruction is the only means of therapy.

Silicone

Silicone (polydimethyl siloxane), either in its liquid form or as silicone gel-filled implants, is used for tissue augmentation, and, in some patients, its use has been followed by foreign body reactions.

Clinical features

Silicone gel-filled implants are widely used for breast augmentation and reconstruction after mastectomy and may be followed, usually after months or years, by the formation of cutaneous nodules and plaques at the site. Silicone is also employed to correct HIV-related lipoatrophy. Silicone reaches the dermis if the capsule ruptures as a result of trauma or there is leakage from the capsule[17]. Nodular foreign body granulomatous reactions evolve some years after rupture or leakage[17], and can slowly progress, resulting in sclerosis and ulceration of involved skin. Spread of the leaked gel from the implant down into the arm or abdominal wall has been reported and leads to the development of nodules distant from the site of the implant.

Similar nodules and indurated plaques, sometimes with ulceration, have been seen following injections of liquid silicone into the subcutaneous tissue[18].

In the literature, there are anecdotal reports of patients in whom autoimmune connective tissue diseases such as scleroderma and systemic lupus erythematosus developed after breast augmentation with silicone-filled prostheses. However, carefully controlled epidemiologic studies have not supported a causal link.

Pathology

A biopsy specimen is critical to establishing the diagnosis. Histologic sections have a 'Swiss cheese' appearance due to the presence of silicone-filled cavities surrounded by histiocytes, lymphocytes and eosinophils. The histiocytes may be foamy or multinucleated. Fibrous tissue within the areas separating the cavities is also seen. In contrast to paraffinomas, the cavity contents do not stain with lipid stains.

Treatment

Excision of persistent symptomatic lesions is recommended.

Silica

Wounds or penetrating injuries accidentally contaminated with silica (silicon dioxide) contained in sand, soil, rocks and glass may be followed some years later by the formation of a foreign body reaction. The period between inoculation and development of a reaction may be as long as 25 years. This extended 'incubation' period is due to the very slow release of colloidal silica (the only form capable of inciting a reaction) from the large particles of silica introduced into the body[19]. Reactions to silica are thought to be due to a delayed-type hypersensitivity response.

Clinical features

At first, the wound heals, but then papules, nodules or indurated plaques develop within the scar years later (Fig. 93.7). Multiple disseminated lesions may follow trauma produced by explosion of land mines and bombs[19]. Macrocheilitis was described following a road accident occurring 25 years prior to the development of the foreign body reaction[20].

Pathology

The dermis contains multiple nodular aggregates of granulomas, usually sarcoidal and less often foreign body, separated by strands of connective tissue. Langhans and foreign body type giant cells are usually numerous in both types of nodule. Colorless crystals may be observed within the cytoplasm of the giant cells or lying free in the interstitium. These bodies are birefringent when examined with polarized microscopy.

Differential diagnosis

Granulomatous lesions occurring at the site of an old scar may mimic systemic sarcoidosis clinically and histologically[21]. The presence of foreign material within a sarcoidal granuloma does not exclude sarcoidosis, since some granulomas of sarcoidosis appear to be attracted to old scars. Examination under polarized light will identify silica crystals, but byproducts of histiocyte metabolism are known to crystallize rarely.

Treatment

Excision of persistent symptomatic lesions is recommended. Spontaneous resolution of silica granuloma, though reported, is exceptional.

Talc

Talc (hydrous magnesium silicate) that contaminates wounds, erosions, umbilical stumps or intravenous puncture sites is another important cause of foreign body reactions. Because of its widespread use, it is a common cause of foreign body granulomas. Talc is a component of many dusting powders and antibiotic powders and is still preferred by some surgeons as a lubricant for surgical gloves. The use of talc powder following bathing, and for babies and for drying intertriginous areas, is a firmly rooted ritual in traditional body care in many parts of the world.

Despite repeated warnings in the medical literature, dusting raw umbilical stumps with antibiotic powders containing talc was reported to be the most frequent cause of umbilical granulomas[5]. Talc may also enter the skin through abrasions and fissures, particularly in intertriginous areas in obese persons who apply talc powder liberally[22]. Tablet forms of medications contain, in addition to the pharmacologically active material, talc as a filler to hold the tablet together. Tablets are frequently crushed and suspended in solutions by drug addicts to be used for intravenous injections[23], and foreign body reactions may

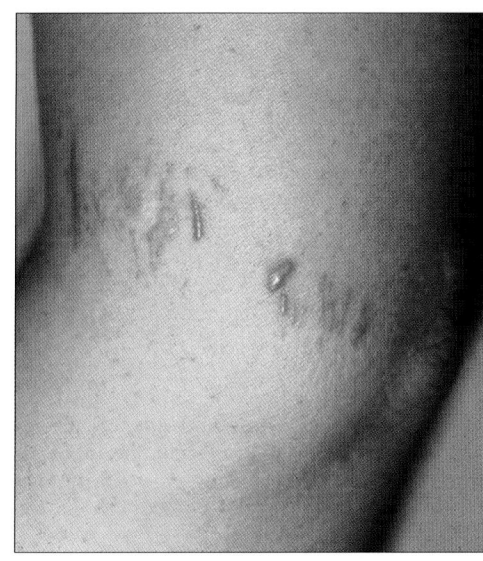

Fig. 93.7 Silica granulomas. Courtesy of Kenneth Greer MD.

develop at intravenous injection sites. Talc may also reach the lungs by inhalation (usually occupational) or through injections of self-prepared drugs.

Clinical features

As with reactions to other forms of silica, the lesions usually take a long time to appear. The clinical appearance is varied: it may take the form of erythematous papules or nodules suggestive of sarcoidosis, or appear as thickening and erythema of an old scar. Despite the long latency period, the diagnosis should be considered, especially when lesions appear in certain sites, e.g. umbilicus in infants, inguinal area in patients with a history of intertrigo, injection sites in intravenous drug addicts.

Pathology

The histologic features may be similar to those of sarcoidosis or non-caseating tuberculosis. Alternatively, there may be granulomatous inflammation consisting of histiocytes and foreign body giant cells. A few of these cells may contain clear, blue–green or yellow–brown needle-shaped or round crystals. Under polarized light, talc crystals appear as white birefringent particles[5]. A picture simulating a pyogenic granuloma plus giant cells has also been described[5].

Treatment

Excision of persistent symptomatic lesions is recommended.

Zirconium

Some zirconium salts are components of antiperspirant preparations as well as over-the-counter preparations used in the treatment of allergic contact dermatitis. Sodium zirconium lactate was the first salt incriminated as a cause of foreign body reaction and was banned in the late 1970s. Subsequently, zirconium oxide and aluminum–zirconium complex have also been shown to be capable of producing the same reaction. Development of the granulomas represents a delayed-type hypersensitivity reaction to zirconium[24].

In sensitized individuals, persistent soft red–brown papules appear in areas to which zirconium-containing preparations were applied. The axillary skin is the most frequently affected site.

Histologically, non-caseating granulomas resembling a sarcoidal reaction are seen[24]. The small size of the zirconium particles does not allow their detection with polarized light microscopy; however, energy dispersive X-ray analysis can prove their presence (see Table 93.3).

Beryllium

In the past, beryllium-containing compounds were widely used in the manufacture of fluorescent light tubes, and industrial exposure resulted in serious systemic and local complications. As a result, their use was discontinued.

Occupational inhalation of beryllium particles results in systemic berylliosis, in which the primary pathology is in the lung and skin involvement is rare (<1%). The cutaneous granulomas of systemic berylliosis consist of widely scattered papules with no secondary changes. Laceration or puncture of the skin by broken fluorescent tubes used to result in local cutaneous berylliosis. Wounds heal slowly and are followed by persistent erythema, swelling, induration and possible ulceration.

Histologically, cutaneous lesions of systemic berylliosis are indistinguishable from sarcoidosis. Local berylliosis, on the other hand, has a caseating tuberculoid pattern[11]. In systemic berylliosis, bronchio-alveolar lavage is recommended for diagnosis.

Aluminum

Rare hypersensitivity reactions to the aluminum adjuvant in vaccines and hyposensitization immunotherapy do occur. Persistent subcutaneous granulomatous nodules appear at the site of injection several months after vaccination[25]. Histologically, granuloma formation with central granular debris surrounded by a histiocytic mantle is seen. A dense lymphoid infiltrate with eosinophils is present at the periphery[25]. Topical application of aluminum chloride for hemostasis produces a stippled appearance within macrophages in the healing wound.

Zinc

A zinc-induced granuloma at the site of an injection is a rare complication of zinc-containing insulin[26]. Sterile furuncles develop at the injection sites and eventually heal with atrophic scars. Histologically, an initial stage characterized by a dense neutrophilic infiltrate is followed by granuloma formation that ends in fibrosis. By polarizing microscopy, birefringent rhomboid crystals are seen. Zirconium, beryllium, aluminum and zinc granulomas may be surgically excised if they are symptomatic.

REACTIONS TO ORGANIC AND BIOLOGIC PRODUCTS

Injectable Bovine Collagen

Bovine collagen implants have been widely used for the correction of facial rhytides, dermal contour deformities and soft tissue defects (see Ch. 158). There are two preparations: Zyderm® (a purified, pepsin-digested suspension of bovine dermal collagen) and Zyplast® (a more durable and less antigenic form cross-linked with glutaraldehyde). Due to the animal origin of the product, skin testing is required before treatment, and a positive test is an absolute contraindication to further use. Despite negative testing, a small proportion of treated patients still develop a local reaction after injection. Two types of reaction have been reported: non-immunogenic and immunogenic.

Clinical features

Non-immunogenic reactions cause localized tissue necrosis, which occurs shortly after implantation; such reactions are probably the result of local vascular interruption. Two-thirds of local necrotic events have occurred in the glabellar area[27].

The most common hypersensitivity reaction is the development of induration and erythema at the treatment site. It usually resolves spontaneously in less than a year. Rarely, abscesses ensue as a manifestation of hypersensitivity to bovine collagen (4 in 10 000 cases) and they may persist for several weeks. Periods of remission and exacerbation may occur, ranging from 1 to more than 24 months[27].

Questions have been raised regarding a possible relationship between injectable collagen and the development of polymyositis and dermatomyositis. Carefully controlled studies have found no supporting evidence.

Pathology

Compared with normal collagen, the implanted bovine collagen is paler staining and less fibrillar. It lacks birefringence on polarized microscopy. The inflammatory reaction may assume a palisaded pattern with many foreign body giant cells, or it may be a more diffuse granulomatous reaction with an admixture of other inflammatory cells (see Table 93.3).

Treatment

Intralesional corticosteroids are recommended for inflammatory reactions. Abscesses may be drained prior to injection.

Hyaluronic Acid and Other Soft Tissue Augmentation Materials

The incidence of foreign body reactions from hyaluronic acid used for tissue augmentation is much lower (0.42%) than that reported for bovine collagen (3–4%)[28]. The injected sites are firm, tender, edematous and erythematous, and evolve into abscess formation. This reaction begins approximately 6 to 8 weeks after hyaluronic acid injection. Spontaneous resolution occurs in 6 to 24 weeks. The reaction responds to intralesional injections of corticosteroid or hyaluronidase[29]. Reactions to multiple other soft tissue augmentation materials are discussed in Chapter 158 and Table 93.3.

Starch

Granulomas may result from the contamination of wounds with starch used as a lubricant for surgical gloves.

Pathology

Foreign body granulomas with multinucleated giant cells are seen. Starch granules appear as ovoid basophilic structures. They react with PAS and are birefringent in polarized light[30].

Cactus

Accidental implantation of cactus spines into the skin results from contact with cacti in gardens and fields. Occupational exposure occurs in persons peeling and selling prickly pear fruit, especially in the Middle East and Latin America. Most of the reported cases are due to contact with the genus *Opuntia*[31].

At the time of injury, acute inflammation occurs and eventually evolves into a typical foreign body reaction. The lesions occur primarily on the hands and fingers as clusters of dome-shaped, skin-colored papules with a central black dot, sometimes called sabra dermatitis. This often resembles scabies or fiberglass dermatitis.

Pathology

Two types of granulomatous reaction have been described: an allergic reaction consisting of epithelioid cells and Langhans type and foreign body type giant cells[31], as well as foreign body type granulomas[11]. The granulomas occupy the entire dermis, surrounding spine fragments which stain intensely red with PAS. Wood splinters and thorns of other plant origin have a similar suppurative or granulomatous reaction. Most splinters appear brown with a rectangular pattern of cell walls (see Fig. 93.4A). Fungal hyphae may be present within the plant material, but they seldom invade the surrounding dermis in the healthy host.

Reactions to Cnidaria (Coelenterata)

Members of the phylum Cnidaria (Coelenterata) include jellyfish, corals and sea anemones (see Ch. 84). Almost all cnidarians possess nematocysts, or stinging capsules. Each nematocyst contains toxins and a coiled thread-like apparatus with a barbed end that functions as a flexible syringe. When the nematocyst comes in contact with the victim, the barbed end of the thread-like organ is discharged and the toxin is injected into the skin.

Clinical features

Jellyfish and coral stings elicit similar cutaneous reactions: an early primary irritant toxic reaction in all exposed persons, and a delayed-type hypersensitivity reaction in a small percentage. A sharp burning pain is felt and, within minutes, the affected area becomes erythematous and edematous and may form blisters. The acute response may be accompanied by an immediate-type hypersensitivity reaction including urticaria, angioedema and even anaphylaxis. The lesions resolve, leaving postinflammatory hyperpigmentation in a streaky flagellate fashion corresponding to where the coral or jellyfish brushed the skin. In some

Pseudofolliculitis barbae and acne keloidalis nuchae

Pseudofolliculitis barbae (see Ch. 39) is a foreign body inflammatory reaction surrounding a hair following shaving or plucking. The condition affects mainly those with curly hair, with an incidence of more than 50% among blacks. Certain inherent properties of the hairs in affected individuals, namely curled flattened elliptical forms, play an important pathogenetic role. Because the shaft is curved, it grows back toward the skin surface. The flattened elliptical hair shaft when shaved develops a pointed tip, which facilitates re-entry of the hair into the skin. A foreign body reaction to keratin results in the development of inflammatory papules and pustules that result in hyperpigmentation or small keloidal scars[8].

Pseudofolliculitis also affects women who regularly remove hair from the pubic, axillary and leg regions by plucking or shaving. This is a common practice in many countries throughout the world. Papules containing embedded hairs, pustules and cysts develop in affected areas, often resolving with significant postinflammatory hyperpigmentation (see Ch. 39).

Treatment

Apart from cessation of shaving or laser epilation of the affected areas, all therapeutic modalities are unrewarding. For further details, see Chapters 39 and 137.

Pilonidal sinus

Most cases of pilonidal sinus (see Ch. 39) occur in the sacrococcygeal region. Much less often it is seen in the umbilical region[8] and, rarely, interdigitally in barbers[32].

Sacrococcygeal pilonidal sinuses may be asymptomatic (debris-filled pit) or present as a draining sinus or an acute abscess. The condition is more common in young men. There is often an underlying cyst with associated granulation tissue, fibrosis and frequently tufts of hairs. Excisional specimens reveal a sinus tract extending into the subcutaneous tissue and dermis, surrounded by chronic inflammation. Hairs are found in the sinuses in three-quarters of the cases[33].

Small, asymptomatic, or slightly tender openings in the interdigital web spaces of the hands have been observed in barbers. The lesions are caused by the penetration of short hairs into the interdigital spaces, inciting an inflammatory foreign body granuloma. The clinical course is usually self-limited but can be complicated by repeated infections, which may require surgical excision of the involved area[32]. Histologically, a sinus tract lined by epidermis and containing one or several hairs is seen. Hairs extending deeper than the sinus tract incite a foreign body reaction.

Intralesional Corticosteroids

Foreign body reactions to intralesional corticosteroids are quite rare despite the widespread use of this treatment modality. Reactions result from failure of the injected material to disperse in the usual manner or from incomplete absorption, leaving a small residuum that evokes a foreign body reaction[34].

Histologically, pools of granular, lightly stained material surrounded by a histiocytic and foreign body granulomatous infiltrate are seen in the dermis. Cellular reactions are absent around sites of recent injections[34].

Suture Granuloma

Nylon and polypropylene sutures used in contemporary surgery are relatively inert (see Ch. 144), but most other materials regularly produce chronic inflammation and granuloma formation. The incubation period varies from weeks[35] to years[36].

The incision site may appear inflamed, red and edematous. A fistula may develop, through which the suture material is extruded. Inflammation persists until the suture material is totally removed.

Histologically, granulomatous inflammation of various types is seen surrounding suture material: foreign body, histiocytic, palisading, or a combination thereof[35,36]. Transepidermal elimination of the suture material occurs[35].

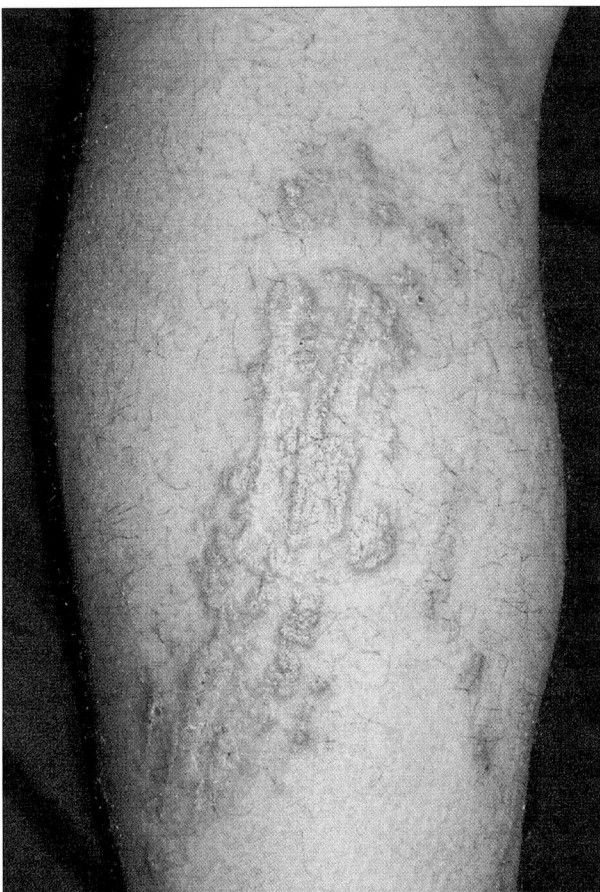

Fig. 93.8 Coral envenomation. Delayed lichenoid reaction on the calf. The patient accidentally contacted a coral reef and developed acute dermatitis that resolved, to be followed 3 weeks later by this severely itchy eruption that responded favorably to intralesional triamcinolone injection.

individuals, new lesions appear a few weeks later at previously involved sites (average 3 weeks)[7]. The latter are severely pruritic shiny lichenoid papules and plaques and are arranged in a number of patterns, including linear, zig-zag and whip-like (Fig. 93.8).

Pathology

The lesions that comprise the delayed response have a lichenoid tissue reaction.

Treatment

First aid includes soaking the site in hot, but not scalding, water (denatures proteins). Subsequent use of topical potent corticosteroids, antihistamines and systemic corticosteroids is controversial. Treatment of acute reactions is reviewed in Chapter 84. Intralesional corticosteroids are the most effective therapy for delayed-type hypersensitivity reactions.

Keratin

In addition to ruptured epidermoid cysts, dermatologic foreign body reactions to keratin are involved in three common, distressing conditions that occur in otherwise healthy young persons: pseudofolliculitis, ingrown nails and sacrococcygeal pilonidal sinus disease.

Keratin, normally sequestered from the body's immune mechanisms by the surrounding epithelium, is treated as foreign if it directly contacts the dermis. This may happen as a result of ruptured hair follicles, epidermoid cysts or acne lesions, or because of external keratin sources, e.g. ingrown hairs or nails, or through accidental entry of hairs into the interdigital skin especially of barbers and dog groomers.

REFERENCES

1. Del Rosario RN, Barr RJ, Graham BS, Kaneshiro S. Exogenous and endogenous cutaneous anomalies and curiosities. Am J Dermatopathol. 2005;27:259–67.
2. Jaworsky C. Analysis of cutaneous foreign bodies. Clin Dermatol. 1991;9:157–78.
3. Lammers RL, Magill T. Detection and management of foreign bodies in soft tissue. Emerg Med Clin North Am. 1992;10:767–81.
4. Feldmann R, Harms M, Chavaz P, et al. Orbital and palpebral paraffinoma. J Am Acad Dermatol. 1992;26:833–5.
5. McCallum DI, Hall GF. Umbilical granulomata – with particular reference to talc granuloma. Br J Dermatol. 1970;83:151–6.
6. Hindson C, Foulds I, Cotterill J. Laser therapy of lichenoid red tattoo reaction. Br J Dermatol. 1995;133:665–6.
7. Addy JH. Red sea coral contact dermatitis. Int J Dermatol. 1991;30:271–3.
8. Halder RM. Pseudofolliculitis barbae and related disorders. Dermatol Clin. 1988;6:407–12.
9. Ploysangam T, Breneman DL, Mutasim DF. Cutaneous pseudolymphomas. J Am Acad Dermatol. 1998;38:877–95.
10. Sowden JM, Byrne JP, Smith AG, et al. Red tattoo reactions: X-ray microanalysis and patch-test studies. Br J Dermatol. 1991;124:576–80.
11. Hirsh BC, Johnson WC. Pathology of granulomatous diseases. Foreign body granulomas. Int J Dermatol. 1984;23:531–8.
12. Smith KJ, Skelton HG III, Yeager J, et al. Histologic features of foreign body reactions in patients infected with human immunodeficiency virus type 1. The Military Medical Consortium for Applied Retroviral Research. J Am Acad Dermatol. 1993;28:470–6.

13. Goldstein M. Mercury-cadmium sensitivity in tattoos. A photoallergic reaction in red pigment. Ann Intern Med. 1967;67:984–9.
14. Abel EA, Silberberg I, Queen D. Studies of chronic inflammation in a red tattoo by electron microscopy and histochemistry. Acta Derm Venereol. 1972;52:453–61.
15. Kilmer SL. Laser treatment of tattoos. Dermatol Clin. 1997;15:409–17.
16. Urbach F, Wine SS, Johnson WC, et al. Generalized paraffinoma (sclerosing lipogranuloma). Arch Dermatol. 1971;103:277–85.
17. Raso DS, Greene WB, Harley RA, Maize JC. Silicone deposition in reconstruction scars of women with silicone breast implants. J Am Acad Dermatol. 1996;35:32–6.
18. Mastruserio DN, Pesqueira MJ, Cobb MW. Severe granulomatous reaction and facial ulceration occurring after subcutaneous silicone injection. J Am Acad Dermatol. 1996;34:849–52.
19. Mesquita-Guimaraes J, Azevedo F, Aguiar S. Silica granulomas secondary to the explosion of a land mine. Cutis. 1987;40:41–3.
20. Harms M, Masouye I, Saurat JH. Silica granuloma mimicking granulomatous cheilitis. Dermatologica. 1990;181:246–7.
21. Marcoval J, Moreno A, Mana J. Foreign bodies in cutaneous sarcoidosis. J Cutan Pathol. 2004;31:516.
22. Pucevich MV, Rosenberg EW, Bale GF, et al. Widespread foreign-body granulomas and elevated serum angiotensin-converting enzyme. Arch Dermatol. 1983;119:229–34.
23. Posner DI, Guill MA III. Cutaneous foreign body granulomas associated with intravenous drug abuse. J Am Acad Dermatol. 1985;13:869–72.

24. Skelton HG III, Smith KJ, Johnson FB, et al. Zirconium granuloma resulting from an aluminum zirconium complex: a previously unrecognized agent in the development of hypersensitivity granulomas. J Am Acad Dermatol. 1993;28:874–6.
25. Cominos D, Strutton G, Busmanis I. Granulomas associated with tetanus toxoid immunization. Am J Dermatopathol. 1993;15:114–17.
26. Jordaan HF, Sandler M. Zinc-induced granuloma – a unique complication of insulin therapy. Clin Exp Dermatol. 1989;14:227–9.
27. Hanke CW, Higley HR, Jolivette DM, et al. Abscess formation and local necrosis after treatment with Zyderm or Zyplast collagen implant. J Am Acad Dermatol. 1991;25:319–26.
28. Lowe NJ, Maxwell CA. Hyaluronic acid skin fillers: adverse reactions and skin testing. J Am Acad Dermatol. 2001;45:930–3.
29. Born T. Hyaluronic acids. Clin Plast Surg. 2006;33:525–38.
30. Leonard DD. Starch granulomas. Arch Dermatol. 1973;107:101–3.
31. Suzuki H, Baba S. Cactus granuloma of the skin. J Dermatol. 1993;20:424–7.
32. Zerboni R, Moroni P, Cannavo SP, et al. Interdigital pilonidal sinus in barbers. Med Lav. 1990;81:138-41.
33. Sondenaa K, Pollard ML. Histology of chronic pilonidal sinus. APMIS. 1995;103:267–72.
34. Bhawan J. Steroid-induced 'granulomas' in hypertrophic scar. Acta Derm Venereol. 1983;63:560–3.
35. Goette DK. Transepithelial elimination of suture material. Arch Dermatol. 1984;120:1137–8.
36. Marcus VA, Roy I, Sullivan JD, et al. Necrobiotic palisading suture granulomas involving bone and joint: report of two cases. Am J Surg Pathol. 1997;21:563–5.

Biology of the Extracellular Matrix

Leena Bruckner-Tuderman

94

Key features

- Extracellular matrices (ECMs) represent specifically organized structural networks of collagens, elastin, glycoproteins and proteoglycans that have distinct structural roles and specific functional properties in all tissues

- They are biologically active, interact with cells, and regulate their functions during development, regeneration and normal tissue turnover

- Mutations in ECM genes cause a broad spectrum of human diseases, from Ehlers–Danlos syndrome to epidermolysis bullosa, and components of the ECM are targeted in autoimmune diseases, e.g. bullous pemphigoid, bullous systemic lupus erythematosus, lichen sclerosus

- The collagen family contains 28 different subtypes. All collagens consist of three polypeptide chains, α-chains, which are folded into a triple helix. In each chain, every third amino acid is glycine (Gly), and thus a sequence of an α-chain can be expressed as $(Gly-X-Y)_n$. A hallmark of collagens is the presence of hydroxyproline (Hyp) in the Y position of this repeat sequence. Collagens are expressed in all tissues of the human body, and distinct sets of collagens co-polymerize into highly organized suprastructures, e.g. fibrils and filaments, in a tissue-specific manner

- Elastin provides tissues with their elasticity. Elastin monomers contain repetitive hydrophobic sequences and are highly cross-linked. The cross-links between several individual molecules provide for both elasticity and insolubility of the elastic fibers, which can be stretched by 100% or more and still return to their original form. In addition to elastin, the elastic fibers in the dermis also contain a microfibrillar component which attaches the fibers to the surrounding structures.

INTRODUCTION

The different types of extracellular matrix (ECM) represent specifically organized assemblies of matrix macromolecules including collagens, elastin, glycoproteins and proteoglycans (Table 94.1). Characteristically, the macromolecules aggregate into insoluble suprastructures with a high degree of order at successive hierarchic levels[1,2]. Each of these structures is tissue-specific and adapted to the particular needs of a given tissue. At first glance, the major constituents are often similar in functionally diverse ECM. However, different types of quantitatively minor molecular components associate with major elements into tissue-specific suprastructural arrays determined by their relative compositions. The matrix suprastructures may be likened to alloys, each having metallurgic properties that differ from each other and those of the pure metals (Fig. 94.1).

Individual matrix macromolecules are usually large oligomers composed of one or several polypeptides. Intimate contacts between the subunits are formed by coiled-coil structures, such as the collagen triple helix or supercoiled α-helices comprised of three or more polypeptides. In addition, large matrix macromolecules can be regarded as linear sequences of structural modules that are similar in a large variety of proteins[3,4]. The modules can be recognized by several cellular receptors, but receptor clustering will be determined in a tissue-specific manner and the response may be different in different tissues.

Our knowledge of the matrix macromolecules has expanded drastically in recent years due to the great power of both molecular genetics and proteomics. A multitude of molecules have been characterized at both protein and gene levels, and their expression, regulation, tissue specificity and functions have been discerned[1-4]. The genes encoding ECM molecules are obvious candidate genes for heritable matrix disorders affecting many tissues, including the skin. To date, mutations in over 40 different genes have been identified that underlie heritable ECM disorders in humans and mice.

The assembled ECM structures are generally adhesive; and tissue-specific cells, leukocytes, tumor cells, and even microorganisms can adhere to the ECM. Through integrin-mediated interactions with the cells, matrix molecules control cell proliferation, differentiation and

COMPONENTS OF THE EXTRACELLULAR MATRIX	
Collagens (28 types)	Laminins (15 types)
Elastin	Proteoglycans (Table 94.3)
Fibrillins (2 types)	Glycoproteins (Table 94.4)
LTBPs (4 types)	Integrins
Fibulins* (5 types)	Modifying enzymes

Fibulins are believed to function as intra-molecular bridges that stabilize ECM structural networks (e.g. elastic fibers, microfibrils or basement membrane structures).

Table 94.1 Components of the extracellular matrix (ECM). The dermal ECM components belong to several protein superfamilies. The molecules assemble into mixed fibrils and networks in a tissue-specific manner. Several enzymes are involved in the biosynthesis and modification of ECM assemblies. Integrins are the main cellular receptors for the ECM. LTBP, latent TGF-β binding protein.

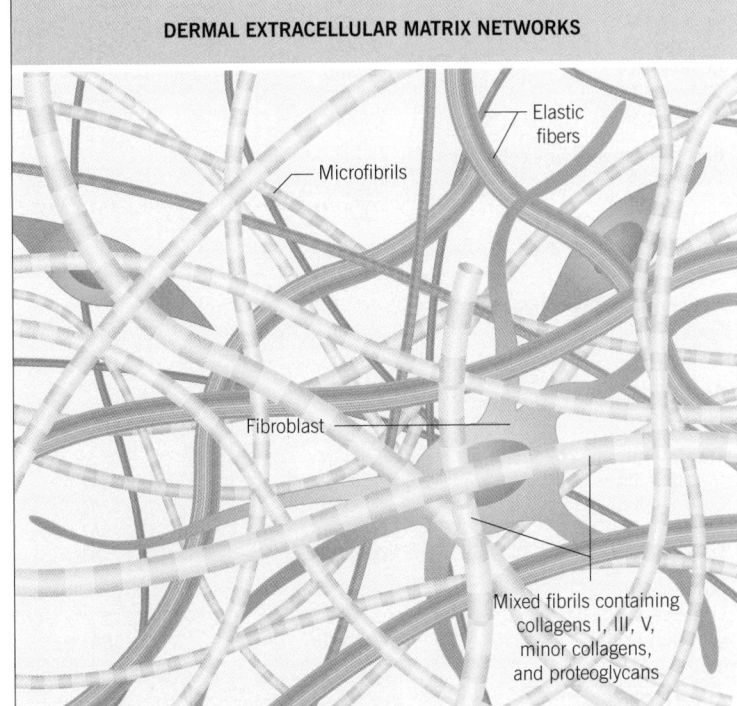

DERMAL EXTRACELLULAR MATRIX NETWORKS

Elastic fibers
Microfibrils
Fibroblast
Mixed fibrils containing collagens I, III, V, minor collagens, and proteoglycans

Fig. 94.1 Dermal extracellular matrix networks. Different molecules polymerize into distinct fibril networks and, within the mesh of the networks, cells are embedded in the amorphous extrafibrillar matrix. The fibril networks interact with each other, with the extrafibrillar matrix and with the cells. The former have a dual function, i.e. support of the tissue and regulation of cellular functions.

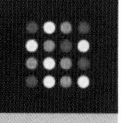

migration, especially during development and regenerative processes. Without contact with the ECM, many cells undergo apoptosis. Furthermore, the ECM can function as a reservoir for information; certain ECM proteoglycans and proteins bind growth factors (e.g. TGF-β) and release and activate them as needed to control cellular functions.

STRUCTURE AND FUNCTION OF THE EXTRACELLULAR MATRIX

Collagens

The collagen family of proteins plays an important role in maintaining the integrity of most tissues. The family currently includes 28 proteins formally defined as collagens (Table 94.2). They contain at least 43 distinct polypeptide chains, each encoded by a different gene, and more than 15 other proteins have a collagen-like domain (e.g. macrophage scavenger receptor 1 and 2, ectodysplasin, pulmonary surfactant proteins)[5].

Collagen triple helix

All collagen molecules consist of three polypeptide chains, known as α-chains, which are folded into a collagen triple helix. In some collagens,

the α-chains are identical (homotrimers), while others contain two or three different α-chains (heterotrimers). In each polypeptide chain, every third amino acid is glycine (Gly), and so the sequence of an α-chain can be expressed as $(Gly-X-Y)_n$, where X and Y represent other amino acids and n varies according to the length of the α-chain. A high number of proline (Pro) and hydroxyproline (Hyp) residues are in the X and Y positions, respectively, and hydrogen bonds between the hydroxyl groups of Hyp contribute to the stability of the helix. The prototype collagen (type I) has an uninterrupted Gly-X-Y repeat sequence that is almost 1000 amino acid residues in length, and this forms a rigid, rod-like structure with a diameter of 1.5 nm and length of 300 nm. In some collagens, the $(Gly-X-Y)_n$ repeats are interrupted by one or more amino acids. The interruptions may be numerous and longer than the $(Gly-X-Y)_n$ repeats, and they provide the molecule with flexibility, which is important for the specific functions of a given collagen type (see below).

Biosynthesis of collagens

Collagen biosynthesis involves a number of post-translational modifications (Fig. 94.2). Some collagens are first synthesized as procollagen molecules that have propeptide extensions at either their N- or their C-terminus, or at both ends. The main intracellular steps in collagen biosynthesis include the following:

	THE COLLAGEN FAMILY OF PROTEINS		
Type	Chains	Gene	Tissue distribution
Fibril-forming collagens			
Collagen I	$α_1(I), α_2(I)$	COL1A1, COL1A2	Skin, most ECM
Collagen II	$α_1(II)$	COL2A1	Cartilage, vitreous humor
Collagen III	$α_1(III)$	COL3A1	Skin (including fetal skin), lung, vasculature
Collagen V	$α_1(V), α_2(V), α_3(V)$	COL5A1, COL5A2, COL5A3	Skin, with collagen I heterotypic fibrils
Collagen XI	$α_1(XI), α_2(XI), α_3(XI)$	COL11A1, COL11A2, COL11A3	With collagen II heterotypic fibrils
Collagen XXIV*	$α_1(XXIV)$	COL24A1	Developing bone and cornea
Collagen XXVII*	$α_1(XXVII)$	COL27A1	Cartilage, eye, ear, lung
FACITs			
Collagen IX	$α_1(IX), α_2(IX), α_3(IX)$	COL9A1, COL9A2, COL9A3	With collagen II heterotypic fibrils
Collagen XII	$α_1(XII)$	COL12A1	Skin, tissues containing collagen I
Collagen XIV	$α_1(XIV)$	COL14A1	Skin, tissues containing collagen I
Collagen XVI	$α_1(XVI)$	COL16A1	Skin, many tissues
Collagen XIX	$α_1(XIX)$	COL19A1	Basement membranes, fetal muscle
Collagen XX	$α_1(XX)$	COL20A1	Skin, cornea, cartilage, tendon
Collagen XXI	$α_1(XXI)$	COL21A1	Many tissues, including skin
Collagen XXII*	$α_1(XXII)$	COL22A1	Tissue junctions
Collagen XXVI*	$α_1(XXVI)$	COL26A1	Testis, ovary
Basement membrane collagen			
Collagen IV	$α_1(IV), α_2(IV), α_3(IV),$ $α_4(IV), α_5(IV), α_6(IV)$	COL4A1, COL4A2, COL4A3, COL4A4, COL4A5, COL4A6	All basement membranes, isoforms vary Skin: $α_1(IV), α_2(IV), α_5(IV),$ and $α_6(IV)$
Microfibrillar collagens			
Collagen VI	$α_1(VI), α_2(VI), α_3(VI)$	COL6A1, COL6A2, COL6A3	Skin, other microfibril-containing tissues
Network-forming collagens			
Collagen VIII	$α_1(VIII), α_2(VIII)$	COL8A1, COL8A2	Skin, subendothelial matrices
Collagen X	$α_1(X)$	COL10A1	Hypertrophic cartilage
Anchoring fibril collagen			
Collagen VII	$α_1(VII)$	COL7A1	Skin, mucous membranes, cornea
Transmembrane collagens			
Collagen XIII	$α_1(XIII)$	COL13A1	Skin, many tissues
Collagen XVII	$α_1(XVII)$	COL17A1	Skin, mucous membranes, cornea
Collagen XXIII*	$α_1(XXIII)$	COL23A1	Lung, cornea, brain, skin, tendon, kidney
Collagen XXV*	$α_1(XXV)$	COL25A1	Brain, neurons
Multiplexins			
Collagen XV	$α_1(XV)$	COL15A1	Many tissues; parent molecule of restin[†]
Collagen XVIII	$α_1(XVIII)$	COL18A1	Many tissues, including skin, subendothelial matrices; parent molecule of endostatin[†]
Novel collagens			
Collagen XXVIII	$α_1(XXVIII)$	COL28A1	Schwann cells; fetal skin and calvaria

*Classification based upon cDNA sequence.
[†]Inhibitors of angiogenesis.

Table 94.2 The collagen family of proteins. Although the structures of collagens types XXII–XXVIII have been predicted from their cDNA sequences, their protein structures have not yet been characterized in detail. ECM, extracellular matrix; FACITs, fibril-associated collagens with interrupted triple helices.

- cleavage of signal peptides
- hydroxylation of certain Pro and lysine (Lys) residues to 4-Hyp, 3-Hyp, and hydroxylysine (Hyl)
- glycosylation of some of the Hyl residues to galactosyl-Hyl and glucosylgalactosyl-Hyl
- glycosylation of certain asparagine residues
- association of the α-chains in a specific manner
- formation of intra- and interchain disulfide bonds
- folding of the triple helix.

After the chains have become associated, and after approximately 100 Hyp residues have been formed in each chain, a nucleus of the triple helix forms (usually in the C-terminal region) and the triple helix propagates towards the other end of the molecule in a zipper-like fashion[5]. The procollagen molecules are then transported from the endoplasmic reticulum across the Golgi apparatus without leaving the lumen of the Golgi cisternae. During this transport, the molecules begin to aggregate laterally, and form early fibrils ready for secretion[6]. The extracellular steps in the biosynthesis include cleavage of the N- and/or C-terminal propeptides, assembly into suprastructures with other collagens and non-collagenous components, and formation of covalent cross-links.

The specific enzymes involved in the biosynthesis of collagens include prolyl-4-hydroxylase and prolyl-3-hydroxylase, which hydroxylate Pro residues to Hyp, and lysyl hydroxylase, which hydroxylates Lys residues to Hyl. These enzymes require O_2, Fe^{2+}, α-ketoglutarate and ascorbate as cofactors for the reactions. In the rough endoplasmic reticulum, glycosyltransferases add up to 10 glucosylgalactosyl disaccharides onto the α-chains, depending on the collagen type. The intracellular enzymes modify all collagen chains[5]. The extracellular processing enzymes have a higher substrate specificity. Procollagen N-proteinase cleaves the N-propeptide of procollagens I and II. This enzyme is a member of the disintegrin and metalloproteinase (ADAM) proteinase family, and was designated as ADAMTS-2[7]. Procollagen C-proteinase cleaves the C-propeptide of collagens I, II, III, V and VII. It is a member of the tolloid proteinase family and is called bone morphogenetic protein-1 (BMP-1), since it was initially co-purified with other BMPs from bone extracts[8]. Cross-linking between collagen molecules involves the ε-amino groups of Lys and Hyl and is catalyzed by lysyl oxidase, a copper-requiring enzyme[5]. Another enzyme that catalyzes cross-linking of at least some collagens is tissue transglutaminase. Collagen VII-containing anchoring fibrils in the skin appear to be transaminated, and collagen VII serves as a substrate for tissue transglutaminase-2 *in vitro*[9].

The collagen family of proteins

The length and continuity of the triple helical domains vary amongst the collagen types. For practical purposes, the collagens have been divided into groups according to their ability to form supramolecular aggregates (Fig. 94.3). These are:

- fibril-forming collagens: types I, II, III, V, XI, and, based on gene structure, XXIV and XXVII
- fibril-associated collagens with interrupted triple helices (FACITs): types IX, XII, XIV, XVI, XIX, XX, XXI, XXII and XXVI
- basement membrane collagens: different isoforms of type IV
- microfibrillar collagens: type VI
- network-forming collagens: types VIII and X
- anchoring fibril collagen: type VII
- collagens with transmembrane domains: types XIII, XVII, XXIII and XXV
- collagens with multiple triple helix domains and interruptions, i.e. multiplexins: types XV and XVIII
- novel collagens that have not yet been characterized in detail: type XXVIII.

More information on the collagens in each group is found in Table 94.2 and in Refs 10–13. Full discussion of the structure and functions of all collagen types is beyond the scope of this chapter, and the reader is referred to recent reviews on the subject[1–5,14,15].

Collagens of the skin

Collagens represent 75% of the dry weight and 20–30% of the volume of the dermis. At least 12 different collagens in the skin polymerize into distinct suprastructures and have specific functions in the dermis as well as in the epidermal and vascular basement membranes. 'Pure'

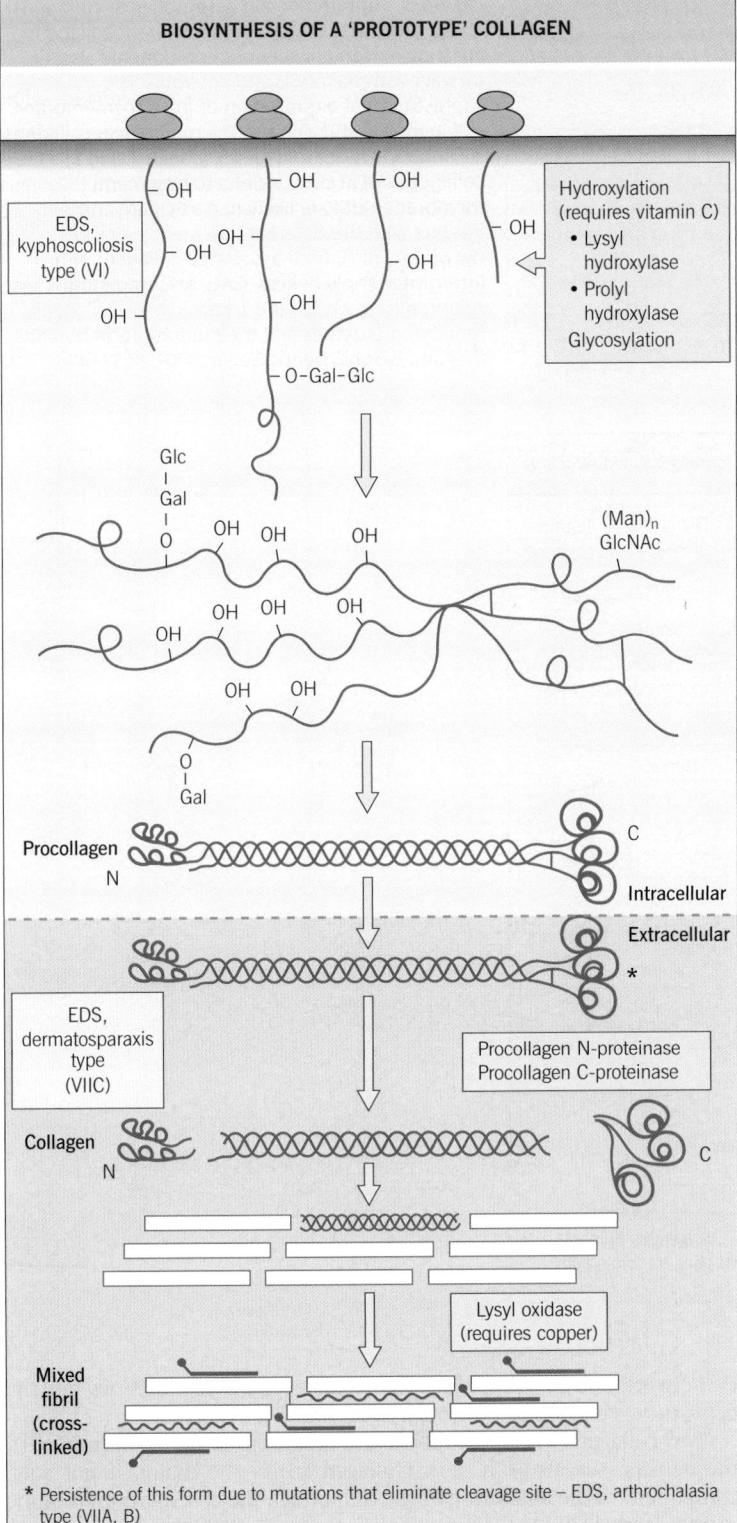

Fig. 94.2 Biosynthesis of a 'prototype' collagen. The procollagen α-chains are synthesized in the rough endoplasmic reticulum. Already during the synthesis of the nascent polypeptide, certain prolyl and lysyl residues are hydroxylated and modified by glycosylation. Three α-chains associate to form a trimer and fold into a triple helix. The newly formed triple helical procollagen is secreted into the extracellular space, where the N- and C-terminal propeptides are cleaved by specific proteases. The mature collagen molecules assemble to form mixed fibrils with other collagens and non-collagenous molecules. The suprastructures are stabilized by covalent cross-links. EDS, Ehlers–Danlos syndrome. Adapted from Myllyharju J, Kivirikko KI. Collagens, modifying enzymes and their mutations in humans, flies and worms. Trends Genet. 2004;20:33–43.

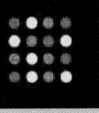

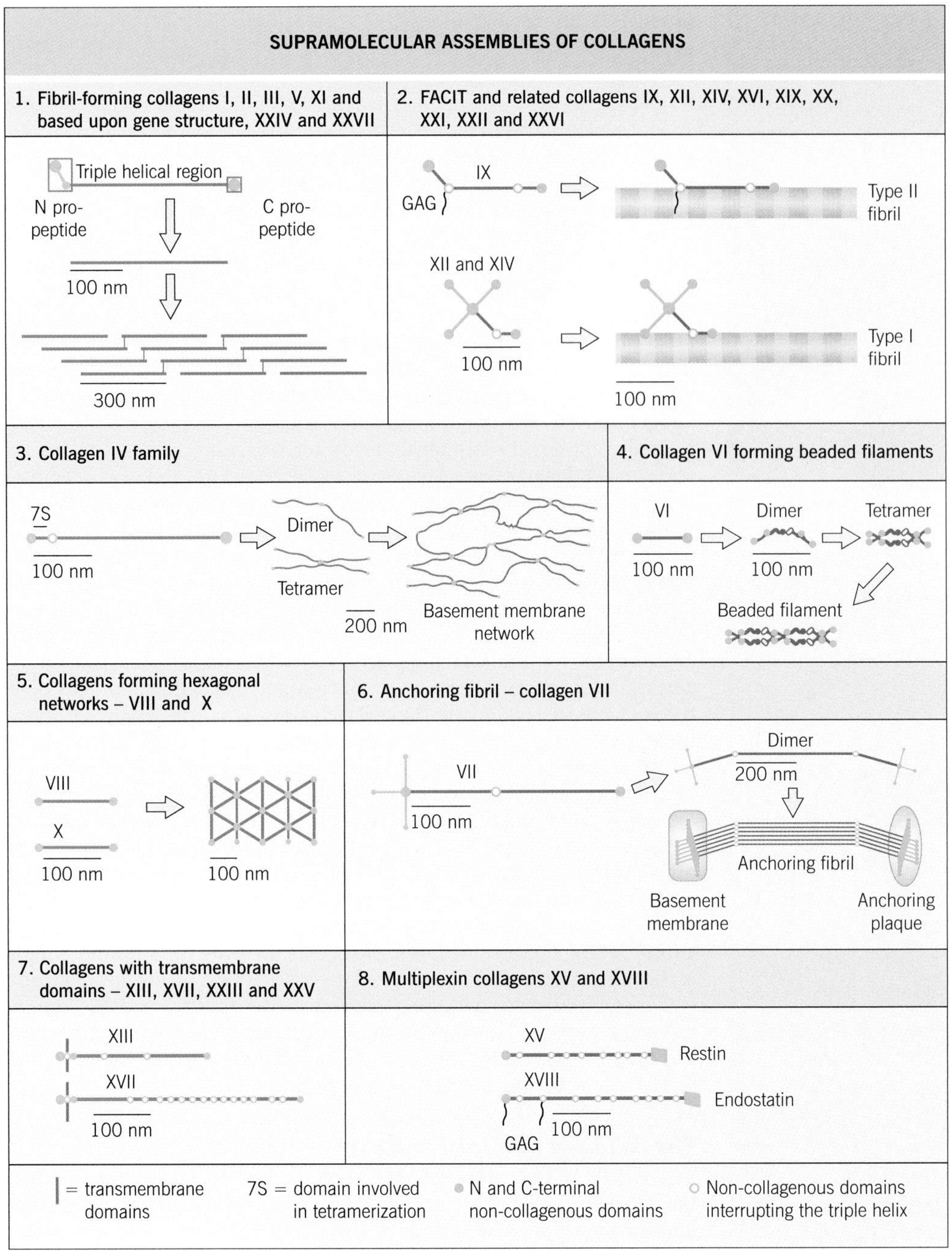

SUPRAMOLECULAR ASSEMBLIES OF COLLAGENS

1. Fibril-forming collagens I, II, III, V, XI and based upon gene structure, XXIV and XXVII

Triple helical region

N pro-peptide   C pro-peptide

100 nm

300 nm

2. FACIT and related collagens IX, XII, XIV, XVI, XIX, XX, XXI, XXII and XXVI

IX

GAG

Type II fibril

XII and XIV

100 nm

Type I fibril

100 nm

3. Collagen IV family

7S

100 nm

Dimer

Tetramer

Basement membrane network

200 nm

4. Collagen VI forming beaded filaments

VI   Dimer   Tetramer

100 nm   100 nm

Beaded filament

5. Collagens forming hexagonal networks – VIII and X

VIII

100 nm

X

100 nm

100 nm

6. Anchoring fibril – collagen VII

VII

100 nm

Dimer

200 nm

Anchoring fibril

Basement membrane   Anchoring plaque

7. Collagens with transmembrane domains – XIII, XVII, XXIII and XXV

XIII

XVII

100 nm

8. Multiplexin collagens XV and XVIII

XV   Restin

XVIII   Endostatin

GAG   100 nm

| = transmembrane domains

7S = domain involved in tetramerization

● N and C-terminal non-collagenous domains

○ Non-collagenous domains interrupting the triple helix

Fig. 94.3 Supramolecular assemblies of collagens. The suprastructures formed by different collagens are shown. Non-collagenous components also interact with the fibrils and networks. The suprastructural organization of the transmembrane collagens XIII and XVII and the multiplexin collagens XV and XVIII is not known yet (panels 7 and 8). These collagens are in close vicinity to basement membranes and are likely to participate and/or interact with the different basement membrane networks. FACIT, fibril-associated collagens with interrupted triple helices; GAG, glycosaminoglycans. Adapted from Myllyharju J, Kivirikko KI. Collagens, modifying enzymes and their mutations in humans, flies and worms. Trends Genet. 2004;20:33–43.

collagen fibrils do not exist; these fibrils are always mixtures of several collagens and other molecules, e.g. proteoglycans. Classic, ultrastructurally recognizable, cross-banded fibrils in the dermis contain collagens I, III, V, XII and XIV. The characteristic cross-banding (Fig. 94.4) with periodicity of 64 nm results from precise lateral packing of the different collagens within the fibrils (see Fig. 94.3). Collagen I is the major component of the fibrils, and the amount of other collagens varies. For example, during embryonic development and wound repair, the content of collagen III is higher than in the steady-state situation. Collagen VI, a highly glycosylated and disulfide-bonded collagen, is a component of almost all tissues, including the skin. *In vitro*, it polymerizes to form beaded filaments (see Fig. 94.3), but *in vivo* in the dermis, the ultrastructure of the collagen VI fibrils is reminiscent of microfibrils. Expression studies have shown that collagens XX–XXII are also expressed in the skin[5,10].

The collagen IV molecules in different basement membranes contain genetically distinct but structurally homologous α-chains. Six different α-chains have been identified so far. The existence of three major networks – namely, α_1/α_2-containing, $\alpha_3/\alpha_4/\alpha_5$-containing, and $\alpha_1/\alpha_2/\alpha_5/\alpha_6$-containing networks – has been established[5]. The chain composition is determined by the non-collagenous NC1 domains, and the α-chains are linked to each other by covalent interactions through these domains (see Fig. 94.3). In the skin, the α_1/α_2-containing collagen

IV network dominates within the dermal–epidermal junction, but the $\alpha_1/\alpha_2/\alpha_5/\alpha_6$-containing network is also likely to be present[5].

Two collagens are essential for the cohesion of the epidermis with the dermis (see also Ch. 33). Collagen VII is the major, if not sole, component of the anchoring fibrils that attach the basement membrane to the dermal ECM. Collagen XVII is a component of the anchoring filaments that bind the basal keratinocytes to the basement membrane. It is a transmembrane collagen in type II orientation with a long extracellular domain containing a multiply-interrupted triple helix. The ectodomain can be shed from the cell surface by transmembrane proteases[15], a process important for regulation of cell adhesion and migration. The basal epidermal keratinocytes also express a second transmembrane collagen, type XIII, which is a component of focal contacts.

The vascular basement membranes in the skin contain yet other collagens – namely, collagens VIII and XVIII. Collagen VIII builds hexagonal networks below the endothelial basement membranes (see Fig. 94.3) and, thus, structurally strengthens the vascular wall. Collagen XVIII is localized at the dermal side of basement membranes. It has been the focus of much attention, since its C-terminal fragment, endostatin (see Fig. 94.3), which is proteolytically released from the collagen molecule, inhibits angiogenesis and tumor growth in experimental models[16].

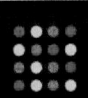

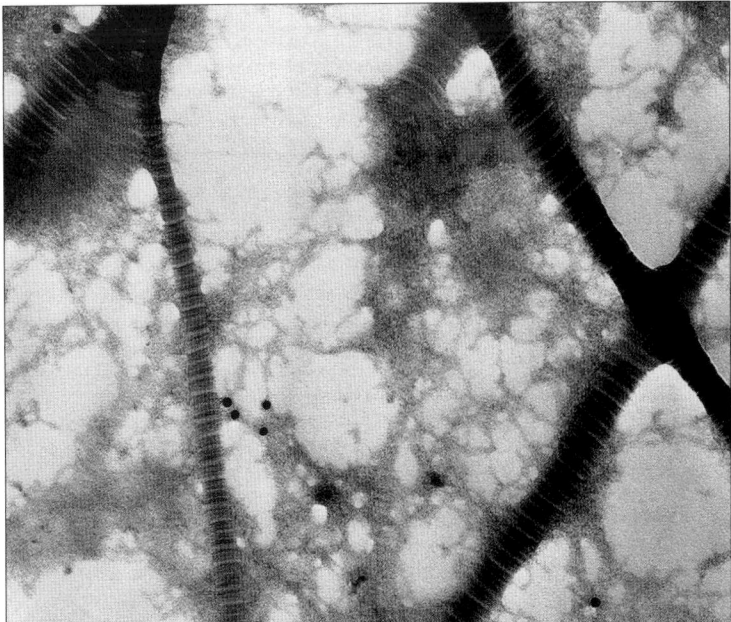

Fig. 94.4 Fibrillar and filamentous networks extracted from human skin. The large cross-banded fibrils represent dermal mixed fibrils containing collagens I, III, V, other minor collagens, and decorin (a proteoglycan). The cross-banding has a characteristic periodicity of 64 nm. The filamentous network in the background contains microfibrillar and basement membrane components. In this immunoelectron photomicrograph, the black dots are colloidal gold particles coupled to anti-collagen IV antibodies, indicating that basement membrane networks are strongly associated with the dermal fibrillar networks. Courtesy of Dr Uwe Hansen.

Most collagens in the skin are products of dermal fibroblasts. Exceptions include the epithelial collagens VII and XVII synthesized by epidermal keratinocytes, and collagens VIII and XVIII, which are produced by endothelial cells. Several genetic and acquired diseases are associated with abnormalities of skin collagens or the enzymes processing them (see Tables 94.5 & 94.6, and discussion below).

Elastin and Elastic Fibers

The elasticity of many tissues, including the skin, is based on the structure of elastic fibers, which come in different compositions. A characteristic property of elastic fibers is that they can be stretched by 100% or more and still return to their original form. The elastic fibers in the dermis are composed of microfibrillar (see below) and amorphous components. Biochemical analyses have clarified the molecular constitution of the 'oxytalan fibers' and 'elaunin fibers', which were previously defined on the basis of histologic staining properties. The 'oxytalan fibers' contain the microfibrillar component in the absence of the amorphous component; the 'elaunin fibers' represent the microfibrillar component in the presence of small amounts of the amorphous component; and the microfibrillar component in the presence of abundant amorphous component represents the elastic fibers of the dermis. In the papillary dermis, the microfibrils insert into the basement membrane in a perpendicular orientation and extend into the dermis, where they gradually merge with the elastic fibers that form a plexus parallel to the dermal–epidermal junction. These fibers appear to be continuous with the elastic fibers deep within the reticular dermis. The gradient of an increasing amorphous component from the basal lamina into the reticular dermis may represent a system of increasingly mature elastic fibers.

The stretchable amorphous component consists of elastin, a highly cross-linked protein[17]. The elastin monomer tropoelastin contains repetitive modules of the hydrophobic amino acid residues (Val-Gly-Val-Pro-Gly)$_n$. It exists in several different splice variants, depending on the tissue. Ala- and Lys-rich repeats form critical cross-linking domains and may interrupt the basic repetitive structure. Lysyl oxidase, the same copper-dependent enzyme that catalyzes collagen cross-linking, catalyzes oxidative deamination of Lys to form allysine, an aldehyde that reacts with other allysine residues and/or unmodified Lys residues

to form desmosine cross-links. The cross-links between several individual elastin molecules account for both the elasticity and insolubility of the elastic fibers.

Microfibrils

In the uppermost dermis, the microfibrils (10 to 12 nm in diameter) emerge from the basement membrane zone, traverse the papillary dermis perpendicularly, and merge with a horizontal elastic fiber system in the reticular dermis. Their main component is fibrillin 1, a large protein that polymerizes to form beaded microfilaments *in vitro*[18] and interacts with perlecan in the epidermal basement membrane to attach the microfibrils to the dermal–epidermal junction zone[19]. Fibrillins are glycoproteins, more than 2800 amino acid residues in length, and they contain both epidermal growth factor (EGF) and cysteine (Cys) repeats. The EGF repeats bind calcium, which is required for stabilization of the protein. Other microfibrillar or microfibril-associated components, depending on the tissue, include fibrillin 2, microfibril-associated glycoproteins (MAGPs), latent TGF-β binding proteins (LTBPs), fibulins[20] and collagen XVI[21]. It is hypothesized that fibrillin 2 guides elastogenesis, whereas fibrillin 1 provides force-bearing structural support[17,18].

Latent TGF-β binding proteins, members of the fibrillin/LTBP superfamily, are high-molecular-weight glycoproteins characterized by EGF-like repeats and 8-Cys repeats. Four different LTBPs have been identified, and they all associate with the small latent complex of TGF-β (Fig. 94.5). Confocal laser scanning microscopy of the *in situ* distribution of LTBP-1 and latent TGF-β$_1$ in normal human skin and skin regenerating from cultured keratinocyte autografts localized the LTBP-1/latent TGF-β$_1$ complex to fibrillin-containing microfibrils (Fig. 94.6). Both LTBP-1 and latent TGF-β$_1$ were already present during the earliest stages of the *de novo* formation of the microfibrillar apparatus in the papillary dermis[22]. LTBPs contain multiple proteinase-sensitive sites, providing the means to solubilize the large latent complex from ECM structures, and both soluble and ECM-associated forms are known to exist. An important consequence of this is LTBP-mediated deposition and targeting of latent, activatable TGF-β into different ECMs. Thus, the fibrillin-containing microfibrils in the dermis serve not only as a force-bearing element and scaffolding for elastin deposition in the dermis, but also as an important repository for latent TGF-β in the skin (see below for discussion of TGF-β function)[22].

Confocal laser scanning microscopy of normal skin has also disclosed collagen XVI to be associated with microfibrils. The collagen co-localizes with fibrillin 1 below the basement membrane zone and in the papillary dermis, but not in deeper layers of the dermis[21], indicating that it contributes to the structural integrity of the dermal–epidermal junction by interacting with the microfibrillar apparatus. *In vitro*, keratinocytes and fibroblasts produce collagen XVI; therefore, both cells are also likely sources of this protein *in vivo*.

The Extrafibrillar Matrix

The dermal fibril networks and cells are embedded in an amorphous extrafibrillar material that binds water and provides the hydrated consistency of the skin. Previously, this amorphous material was presumed to be biologically unstructured and inert and was called the 'ground substance'. This prediction turned out to be incorrect: the extrafibrillar matrix is molecularly and structurally diverse, highly organized, and biologically active. It contains a number of proteoglycans and glycoproteins, hyaluronic acid, and water. Its functions are variable and adapted to the biologic needs of each tissue. For example, during embryonic development, water-binding proteoglycans and glycosaminoglycans form a hydrated milieu for cell migration and proliferation. During development and tissue remodeling, glycoproteins of the extrafibrillar matrix are essential for formation of the correct tissue architecture.

Glycosaminoglycans (GAGs) are polysaccharides of sulfated and acetylated sugars with negative charges that can bind large amounts of ions and water. Usually, GAGs are bound to proteins with a serine hydroxyl group and form a proteoglycan (Fig. 94.7)[23]. However, the most prominent and ubiquitous *protein-free* GAG is hyaluronic acid, a giant polysaccharide composed of thousands of N-acetylglucosamine/glucuronic acid disaccharides. Proteoglycans differ remarkably in their

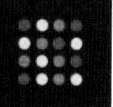
REGULATION OF TRANSFORMING GROWTH FACTOR-β (TGF-β) ACTIVITY

Pro-TGF-β

Cleavage*

Large latent complex
Small latent complex
TGF-β latency associated peptide
TGF-β
Latent TGF-β binding protein

N   C

Secretion**

Intracellular

Extracellular

Protease

Fibrillin 1-containing microfibrils

ECM proteins

N   C   N   C

Release of soluble large latent complex

Active TGF-β

Thrombospondin 1
Fibrillin 1 fragment

Fibrosis

Fig. 94.5 Regulation of transforming growth factor-β (TGF-β) activity. TGF-β is synthesized as an inactive homodimeric propeptide, pro-TGF-β. After cleavage, mature TGF-β is sequestered in an inactive form via its continued association (now noncovalent) with the latency-associated peptide (LAP; forming the small latent complex) and covalent linkage of the LAP to the latent TGF-β binding protein (LTBP; forming the large latent complex). In addition, the large latent complex becomes attached to the extracellular matrix (ECM) via covalent linkage of the LTBP N-terminus with ECM proteins and noncovalent association of the LTBP C-terminus with fibrillin 1 (a member of the LTBP/fibrillin superfamily). Solubilization of the large latent complex from the ECM can occur via proteolytic cleavage of susceptible hinge regions within the LTBP and disruption of the fibrillin 1-LTBP interaction by fibrillin 1 fragments. Binding of ECM glycoproteins such as thrombospondin 1 to the LAP results in the release of active TGF-β that can bind to its receptors and promote fibrosis. *Both intracellular and (more recently) extracellular cleavage has been reported; cleavage can occur before or after association with LTBP. **Small latent complexes and pro-TGF-β may also be secreted. Adapted from August P, Suthanthiran M. Transforming growth factor beta signaling, vascular remodeling, and hypertension. N Engl J Med. 2006;354:2721–3.

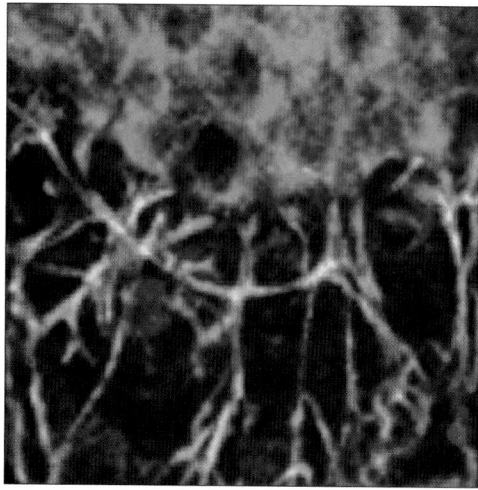

Fig. 94.6 Microfibrils in the papillary dermis. Confocal scanning microscopy of microfibrils which emerge from the epidermis and traverse the papillary dermis perpendicularly. The immunostaining is with antibodies to fibrillin 1 (red) and latent TGF-β complex (green). The orange–yellow color demonstrates co-localization of both proteins on the microfibrils. Note that the epidermal keratinocytes contain latent TGF-β. Courtesy of Dr Michael Raghunath. See also Raghunath et al. 1998[22].

protein content and the number, type and length of their GAG side chains (Table 94.3). Four different proteoglycan-bound GAGs are known: chondroitin sulfate, dermatan sulfate, keratan sulfate and heparan sulfate. Versican is the most important proteoglycan in the dermis (see Fig. 94.7). It is associated with the elastic fiber system and forms huge complexes with hyaluronic acid, which provide the skin with its tautness[23]. Versican can be synthesized by fibroblasts, smooth muscle cells, and epithelial cells.

Perlecan is a major heparan sulfate proteoglycan found in all basement membranes, including the epidermal basement membrane[24]. Small leucine-rich proteoglycans typically contain a protein core of Leu-rich repeats and Cys-bonded loops, with only one or two GAG chains[23]. Decorin has multiple functions; for example, it binds to collagen fibrils and TGF-β. Biglycan is a cell surface proteoglycan that also binds TGF-β. Fibromodulin regulates formation of collagen-containing fibrils. Other small leucine-rich proteoglycans, such as lumican and keratocan, are also found in the skin[23]. Syndecans are transmembrane heparan sulfate proteoglycans that are present on most cell types[25]. They regulate a variety of biologic processes, ranging from coagulation cascades, lipase binding and activity, and cell adhesion to the ECM and subsequent cytoskeletal organization, to infection of cells with microorganisms[25]. Particularly interesting are indications that syndecans and other ECM molecules are active in outside-in cell signaling[26]. Syndecans 1, 2 and 4 are expressed in the skin and can be found in keratinocytes, dendritic cells and fibroblasts.

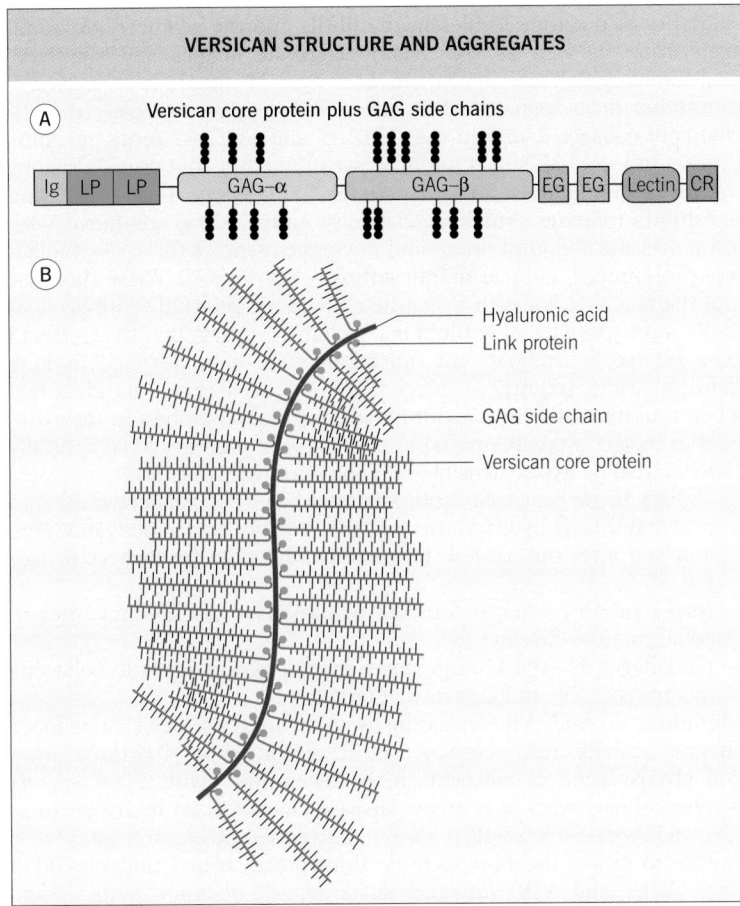

VERSICAN STRUCTURE AND AGGREGATES

A Versican core protein plus GAG side chains

| Ig | LP | LP | GAG-α | GAG-β | EG | EG | Lectin | CR |

B

Hyaluronic acid
Link protein
GAG side chain
Versican core protein

Fig. 94.7 Versican structure and aggregates. A The core protein contains several structural motifs important for glycosaminoglycan (GAG) and ligand binding. The N-terminal immunoglobulin-type repeat (Ig) is followed by two consecutive link-protein type modules (LP), which are involved in mediating the binding of the core protein to hyaluronic acid. The GAG binding domain, which comes in tissue-specific alternative splice variants, GAG-α and/or GAG-β, carries the GAG side chains. It is followed by structural motifs, including two EGF-like repeats (EG), a C-type lectin domain (Lectin), and a complement regulatory protein-like module (CR). **B** In the dermis, versican can form huge aggregates with hyaluronic acid (red). The core protein (blue), which carries a number of GAG side chains (black), is bound to hyaluronic acid via its link-protein domain (green; LP module in the scheme in panel A). The aggregates can bind large amounts of water, and thus provide for the tautness of the skin. Adapted from Iozzo RV. Matrix proteoglycans: from molecular design to cellular function. Ann Rev Biochem. 1998;67:609–52.

Laminins and Other Glycoproteins

Laminins, a family of basement membrane molecules with 15 distinct members, are expressed in all tissues except bone and cartilage. Each laminin molecule is a trimer consisting of an α-, a β- and a γ-chain; the composition and combinations of the three chains vary depending on the particular type[27]. In the skin, the epithelial basement membrane contains laminins 5, 6 and 10, and the vascular basement membrane contains laminins 8 and 10. The structure, biologic functions and genetic defects of the laminins of the skin are discussed in more detail in Chapters 29 and 33. Very recently, a new nomenclature based on the chain composition was proposed for the laminins[28], e.g. laminin 5 which is composed of α_3, β_3, and γ_2 chains is referred to as laminin 332.

The ECMs also contain a number of other glycoproteins, such as fibronectin, vitronectin, thrombospondins, matrilins and tenascins, which exert important functions in many tissues (Table 94.4). A detailed discussion of all of these is outside the scope of this chapter and, therefore, the reader is referred to recent reviews on these ECM components[29–31].

Functions of the Extracellular Matrix

Structural role of the extracellular matrix

In the past, the ECM was regarded as a gross structural scaffold that gave organs their shape and consistency. Recent investigations have

---

PROTEOGLYCANS OF THE SKIN

Proteoglycan	Gene/location	Size of the core protein (kDa)	GAG side chains (number)
Versican	CSPG2/5q13.2	265–370, splice variants	Chondroitin/dermatan sulfate (10–30)
Perlecan	HSPG2/1p36	400–467	Heparan/chondroitin sulfate (3)
Decorin*	DCN/12q23	40	Chondroitin/dermatan sulfate (1)
Fibromodulin*	FMOD/1q32	42	Keratan sulfate (2–3)
Lumican*	LUM/12q21.3–22	38	Keratan sulfate (3–4)
Keratocan*	KERA/12q22	38	Keratan sulfate (3–5)
Biglycan*	BGN/Xq28	40	Chondroitin/dermatan sulfate (2)
Syndecans 1, 2, 4	SDC1/2p24.1 SDC2/8q22–24 SDC4/20q12–13	35–120	Heparan/chondroitin sulfate (3–5)

*Small leucine-rich proteoglycan.

Table 94.3 Proteoglycans of the skin.

GLYCOPROTEINS OF THE SKIN

Glycoproteins	Key functions
Fibronectin	Cell adhesion and migration
Vitronectin	Cell adhesion and migration
Thrombospondins (4 types)	Cell-to-cell and cell-to-matrix communication
Matrilins (4 types)	Matrix assembly, cell adhesion
Tenascins (3 types)	Regulation of cellular function

Table 94.4 Glycoproteins of the skin.

---

extended and refined our knowledge on the structural aspects and have demonstrated that a broad spectrum of ECM suprastructures is used for distinct structural roles and specific functional properties[1–5]. For example, corneal stroma contains stacked sheets of parallel fibrils with a uniform and small diameter. In each consecutive layer, the fibrils are oriented almost perpendicularly to the adjacent layers, rendering the tissue resistant to high tensile forces in two dimensions and, at the same time, allowing undisturbed penetration of visible light. Tendons contain rope-like bundles of parallel, thick fibrils to facilitate transmission of muscular forces to skeletal elements. Basement membranes are sheets with limited tensile strength but homogeneous and tissue-specific surface properties that allow for particular cell attachments and, thereby, determine metabolism and barrier functions within the skin[24,27]. In the dermis, ECM networks (consisting of collagens, elastin, fibrillins, fibulins and proteoglycans) are embedded in the water-binding extrafibrillar matrix, securing the elasticity, resilience and tautness of the skin[5,17–20,29–31]. At the dermal–epidermal junction, specific basement membrane-associated aggregates, the anchoring complexes, ensure strong adhesion of the epidermis and the dermis and, as a result, they provide resistance against external shearing forces[32].

Regulation of cellular functions

In addition to their structural roles, the ECMs are biologically active. *In vitro* studies and transgenic and knockout mouse models (see Ch. 4) have demonstrated the importance of the ECMs as potent regulators of cellular functions during development, regeneration, wound healing, inflammation and tumorigenesis. ECM macromolecules can influence a multitude of events, such as cell adhesion and migration, organization of the cytoskeleton and cell shape, cell division, differentiation and polarization, and apoptosis.

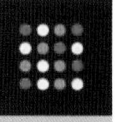
Cells use different receptors to recognize signals from the ECM, such as integrins or cell surface proteoglycans[26,33]. The family of β_1 integrins represents the most common class of matrix receptors. The α-subunit of the integrin determines the ligand specificity for the individual matrix proteins, but the affinity and the specificity seem to vary. Some integrins recognize only one ligand, while others can bind to several matrix proteins.

The ECM signals from outside can have different effects on the cell. For example, they can induce clustering of integrins on the cell surface and lead to formation of protein complexes between the cytoplasmic domains of the integrins and the cytoskeleton, thus influencing cell shape. Alternatively, the activation of integrins by ECM signals induces signal transduction pathways including focal adhesion kinase (pp^{125}FAK), paxillin and tensin, or microtubule-associated protein (MAP) kinase-mediated regulation of transcription, cell proliferation or differentiation. A further level of regulation of integrin-mediated ECM signaling results from the regulation of integrin activation through divalent cations, phospholipids or other agents[26,33].

Growth factors of the TGF-β family are potent regulators of ECM formation, in addition to their immunomodulatory and regulatory roles in cell growth. They are secreted from cells as latent complexes containing TGF-β and its propeptide latency-associated peptide (LAP). In most cells, LAP is covalently linked to LTBP, forming the large latent complex (see Fig. 94.5). The secreted large latent complexes associate covalently with the ECM proteins via the N-termini of the LTBPs. TGF-β can be released from the complexes by various matrix-degrading proteinases released from fibroblasts or inflammatory cells. In addition to the LTBPs, several other ECM molecules can bind to TGF-β and modulate its activity, such as thrombospondin or the core proteins of the proteoglycans decorin, biglycan and fibromodulin[23,25,27,29].

RELATED DISEASES

Molecular studies of ECM diseases, and the genes and proteins involved, have produced a wealth of information regarding the normal biology of the ECM[5,32]. Putative functions for many matrix macromolecules were found for the first time, or confirmed, when mutations in their genes were defined in diseases. For example, functions of the minor fibrillar collagens V, IX and XI in controlling the collagen fibril diameter have been ultimately proven via studies of animal or human genetic disorders. The fundamental roles of collagen VII and collagen XVII in dermal–epidermal adhesion became clear when absence of these proteins was observed in patients with hereditary epidermolysis bullosa (EB), and mutations in the corresponding genes were defined[32]. Genetic ECM diseases with skin manifestations are listed in Table 94.5, and their molecular mechanisms and pathophysiology are delineated below. The clinical features of the different subtypes of Ehlers–Danlos syndrome (EDS), cutis laxa and pseudoxanthoma elasticum are discussed in Chapter 97, and the hallmarks of the different EB subtypes in Chapter 33.

Ehlers–Danlos syndromes

The quantitatively major components within the collagen fibrils found in the ECM of many tissues, such as skin, tendon, bone or cartilage, are collagens I, II and III[5]. These proteins, together with minor collagens, types V, IX, XI, XII and XIV, are expressed in a tissue-specific manner[1,3,5], and mutations in the corresponding genes have been shown to result in distinct abnormalities in different organs[5]. Mutations and haploinsufficiency of the COL3A1 gene encoding collagen III are causative for EDS type IV (vascular type), the most severe form of EDS[34], with symptoms of thin translucent skin, arterial fragility, bruising, and delayed wound healing. The disease can lead to sudden death from rupture of large arteries. A large number of mutations, including amino acid substitutions, deletions, RNA-splicing defects and null alleles, have been described. Mutations in the COL3A1 gene have also been found in a subset of patients with arterial aneurysms, but very few other tissue manifestations[5].

Alterations in several genes encoding minor fibrillar collagens have been discerned as causative in severe connective tissue diseases, suggesting pivotal functions for these quantitatively minor components. The α_1- and the α_2-chains of collagen V co-polymerize with collagens I and III and have a role in the control of fibrillogenesis. They limit the

solubility of macromolecules in the fibrils and the geometry of lateral aggregation as well as the overall aggregate shapes and sizes[1,5,14]. Consistent with this concept, in EDS types I and II (classic types), mutations have been found in the COL1A1 gene encoding the α_1-chains of collagen I, and in the COL5A1 and COL5A2 genes encoding the α_1- and α_2-chains of collagen V, with the latter mutations accounting for approximately 50% of patients[34]. EDS type I is severe, and it exhibits extreme skin hyperelasticity and fragility, combined with atrophic scars and joint laxity, and EDS type II shows the same, though less pronounced, clinical manifestations (Fig. 94.8A). These findings, and the fact that collagen V is a heterotrimeric molecule consisting of α_1(V) and α_2(V) with or without α_3(V) chains, suggest that the COL5A3 gene is also a candidate for mutations still to be detected in EDS families. More recently, a novel EDS-associated gene was identified when mutations in the gene for tenascin-X, a glycoprotein in the extrafibrillar matrix, were discovered in families with recessive EDS, clinically characterized by hyperextensible skin and joint hypermobility[35].

Collagens are post-translationally modified by several enzymes:
- prolyl and lysyl hydroxylases convert Pro and Lys residues into Hyp and Hyl after the nascent polypeptides have been synthesized (see Fig. 94.2)
- lysyl oxidase participates in the oxidation of Lys residues prior to collagen cross-linking
- procollagen N- and C-proteinases process procollagens to collagens by removing N- and C-terminal propeptides.

Mutations in the gene encoding lysyl hydroxylase lead to reduced enzyme activity and, subsequently, to abnormal lysyl hydroxylation and glycosylation of collagens in many families with EDS type VI (kyphoscoliosis type), a recessive disease characterized by hyperextensible and fragile skin as well as lax joints, scoliosis and ocular fragility[5,14,34]. Failure to cleave the N-propeptide from procollagen I underlies EDS types VIIA and VIIB (arthrochalasia types), disorders with severe joint hypermobility, including dislocations. The persistence of the propeptide on the collagen molecules drastically alters fibrillogenesis, and the fibrils become thin and highly irregular in diameter[5,34]. The mutations in the COL1A1 and COL1A2 genes, causing EDS types VIIA and VIIB, are often splice-site mutations that cause exon skipping and elimination of the cleavage site for ADAMTS-2 in the proα_1(I) or proα_2(I) chain[5,14]. Mutations in the gene for ADAMTS-2 are the underlying cause of EDS type VIIC (dermatosparaxis type; Fig. 94.8B), in which, similarly to EDS VIIA and VIIB, procollagen N-propeptides persist and sterically disturb polymerization of the collagen fibrils in the skin and other tissues. A clearly reduced procollagen proteinase activity has been found to result from different mutations[14].

Cutis laxa

Cutis laxa is a relatively rare ECM disease characterized by genetic heterogeneity and clinical variability[14]. In all cases, the primary diagnostic feature is loose, hyperextensible skin with decreased resilience and elasticity, leading to an appearance of 'too large skin' and of premature aging (Fig. 94.8C). The skin changes are often accompanied by extracutaneous manifestations, including pulmonary emphysema, bladder diverticula and pulmonary artery stenosis. Histologically, there is marked fragmentation or diminution of elastic fibers.

In a few families with autosomal dominant cutis laxa, elastin mutations have been identified[36]. For example, a frameshift mutation in the ELN gene was predicted to replace the C-terminus of elastin by a nonsense sequence; mRNA and immunoprecipitation studies demonstrated that the mutant allele was expressed. By electron microscopy, abnormal branching and fragmentation in the amorphous elastin component was observed, and immunocytochemistry showed reduced elastin deposition in the elastic fibers and fewer microfibrils in the dermis. These observations suggest that the mutant protein was synthesized, secreted, and incorporated into the elastic matrix, where it altered the architecture of the elastic fibrils[36]. More recent investigations have identified mutations in the gene that encodes fibulin-5 in patients with autosomal recessive and autosomal dominant forms of cutis laxa as well as mutations in the gene that encodes fibulin-4 in those with autosomal recessive cutis laxa, indicating genetic heterogeneity[37].

Some other inherited disorders are characterized by secondary effects on elastin deposition or degradation[14,18,38]. For example, elastic fibers are prematurely degraded due to unregulated elastase activity in

GENETIC EXTRACELLULAR MATRIX DISEASES OF THE SKIN

Protein	Gene	OMIM	Disease	Phenotypic features in the skin* and other organs
Collagen I (α_1- & α_2-chains)	COL1A1	#130060	EDS, arthrochalasia (type VIIA)	Skin hyperextensibility and fragility, joint hypermobility, congenital hip dislocation[†]
		#130000	EDS, classic (type I)	See below
	COL1A2	#130060	EDS, arthrochalasia (type VIIB)	Skin hyperextensibility and fragility, joint hypermobility, congenital hip dislocation[†]
		#225320	EDS, cardiac valvular	Cardiac valve defects, otherwise similar to classic EDS (see below)
Collagen III	COL3A1	#130050	EDS, vascular (type IV)	Thin, fragile skin with extensive bruising, arterial fragility[‡]
Collagen V (α_1- & α_2-chains)	COL5A1 COL5A2	#130000, 130010	EDS, classic (type I – severe; type II – milder)	Skin hyperextensibility and fragility, joint hypermobility
Collagen VI	COL6A1, COL6A2	#254090	Ullrich disease	Puffy skin, distal joint hypermobility, muscular dystrophy
Collagen VII	COL7A1	#131750, 226600	Dystrophic epidermolysis bullosa	Skin blistering
Collagen XVII	COL17A1	#226650	Junctional epidermolysis bullosa	Skin blistering
Fibrillin 1	FBN1	#154700	Marfan syndrome	Striae atrophicae, characteristic body habitus, aortic dilation/dissection[‡]
Elastin	ELN	#123700	Cutis laxa, AD	Lax, redundant skin
Fibulin-4	FBLN4	#219100	Cutis laxa, AR	Lax, redundant skin; emphysema and arterial anomalies
Fibulin-5	FBLN5	#123700, 219100	Cutis laxa, AD and AR	Lax, redundant skin; emphysema and arterial anomalies (AR form)
Laminin β1	LAMB1	#150240	Cutis laxa, neonatal marfanoid	Lax, redundant skin; arachnodactyly, joint contractures, emphysema
Tenascin-X	TNXB	#606408 #130020	EDS, AR due to tenascin-X deficiency EDS, hypermobility (type III)	Skin hyperextensibility, joint hypermobility Variable skin hyperextensibility, joint hypermobility with recurrent dislocations
Extracellular matrix protein-1	ECM1	#247100	Lipoid proteinosis	Hyalin deposition in the dermis and submucosal tissues, hoarse voice, intracranial calcifications
TGF-β receptors 1 & 2	TGFRB1, TGFRB2	#609192	Loeys–Dietz syndrome (type I)	Translucent skin, aortic aneurysms, arterial tortuosity, craniofacial and skeletal anomalies, joint hypermobility[‡]
ABCC6 transporter	ABCC6	#177850, 264800	Pseudoxanthoma elasticum	Yellowish papules, lax skin, retinal angioid streaks, cardiovascular disease
ATPase, Cu^{2+}-transporting, α-polypeptide	ATP7A	#304150	Occipital horn syndrome	Lax skin, tortuous arteries, joint hypermobility, occipital exostoses
Glucose transporter 10	GLUT10	#208050	Arterial tortuosity syndrome	Hyperextensible or lax skin, telangiectasias on the cheeks, tortuous arteries, joint hypermobility
Lysyl hydroxylase	PLOD1	#225400	EDS, kyphoscoliosis (type VI)	Skin hyperextensibility and fragility, ocular fragility, joint hypermobility, scoliosis
ADAMTS-2 (procollagen N-proteinase)	ADAMTS2	#225410	EDS, dermatosparaxis (type VIIC)	Sagging, doughy, fragile skin; characteristic facies
Galactosyl transferase-I	B4GALT7	#130070	EDS, progeroid	Skin hyperextensibility, joint hypermobility, progeroid facies, osteopenia, mental and growth retardation
Filamin A (actin-binding protein 280)	FLNA	#300537	EDS, periventricular nodular heterotopia variant	Variable skin hyperextensibility, aortic dilation, periventricular nodular heterotopia, joint hypermobility

*Also elastosis perforans serpiginosa in EDS and pseudoxanthoma elasticum.
[†]A phenotype with features of both EDS and osteogenesis imperfecta has also been reported.
[‡]TGF-β receptor mutations can lead to phenotypes that mimic Marfan syndrome (TGFBR2) or vascular EDS (type II Loeys–Dietz syndrome; TGFBR1 or TGFBR2).

Table 94.5 Genetic extracellular matrix diseases of the skin. Lax, redundant skin can also be observed in Costello syndrome (due to *HRAS* gene mutations; also features deep palmoplantar creases, periorificial papillomas, acanthosis nigricans, mental and growth retardation, and increased risk of malignancies such as rhabdomyosarcoma) and hereditary gelsolin amyloidosis (due to mutations in the gene encoding gelsolin; also features corneal dystrophy and polyneuropathy). AD, autosomal dominant; ADAM, a disintegrin and metalloproteinase; AR, autosomal recessive; EDS, Ehlers–Danlos syndrome; TGF, transforming growth factor.

patients with α_1-antitrypsin deficiency and some forms of acquired atrophoderma. Decreased or aberrant deposition of elastic fibers in certain tissues is characteristic of Marfan syndrome (see below).

Marfan syndrome

The other structural component of elastic fibers is fibrillin. Fibrillin 1 is the major component of 10–12 nm microfibrils in the skin. The highly homologous fibrillin 2 exhibits different spatial and temporal expression during development, and the functional relationship between the two molecules is not fully understood. Fibrillin 1 mutations are causative in Marfan syndrome, an autosomal dominant disorder with variable connective tissue weakness of the skin as well as skeletal, ocular and cardiovascular systems[18,38]. The cutaneous manifestations include thin and slightly hyperextensible skin, elastosis perforans serpiginosa, and striae atrophicae. It is likely that in Marfan syndrome, dominant-negative effects cause remarkable structural and functional disturbances of elastic fibers and microfibrils, explaining the reduced fibrillin staining observed in *in vitro* immunofluorescence studies. Fibrillin binds calcium, and mutations at the calcium-binding sites may affect the conformation of individual molecules and perturb their ability to

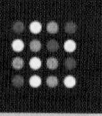

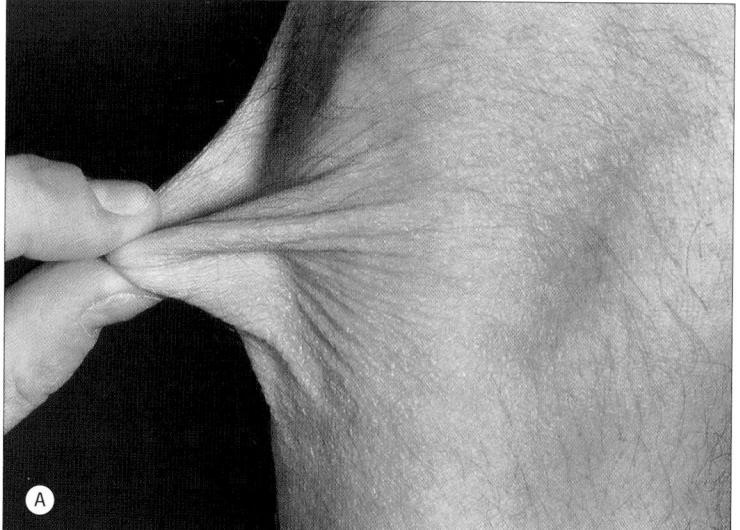

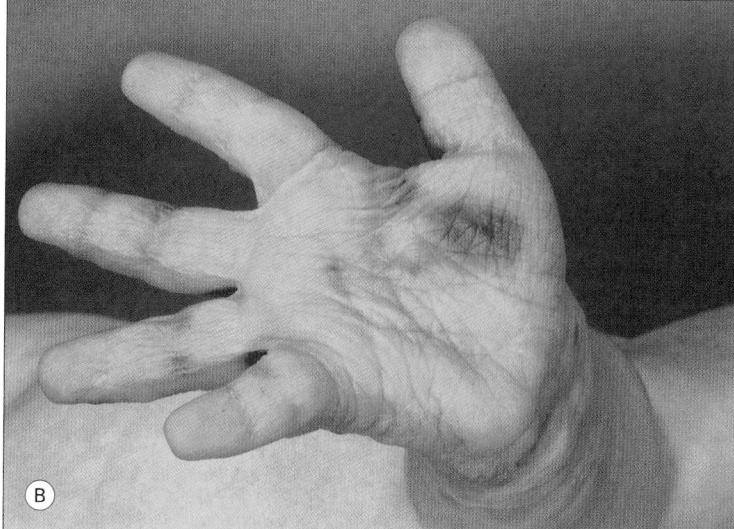

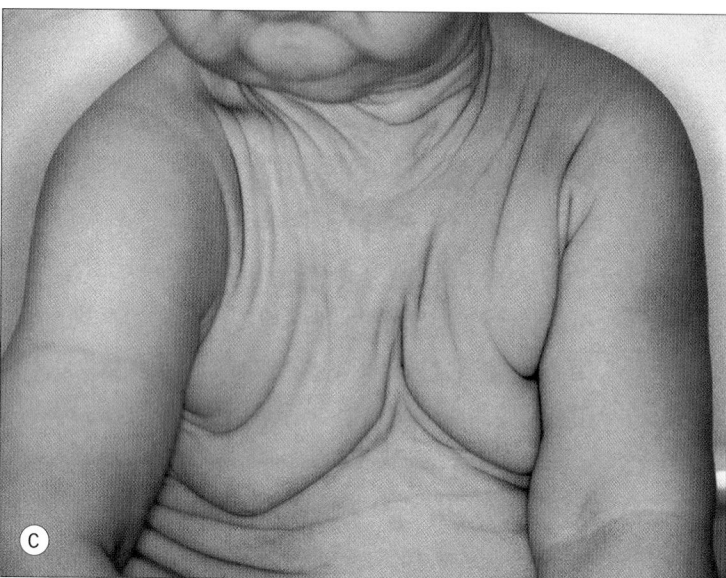

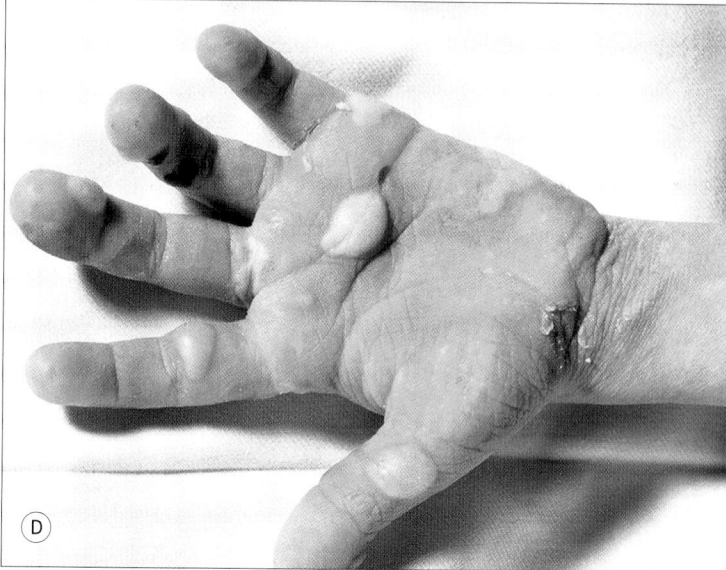

Fig. 94.8 Phenotypic manifestations of genetic extracellular matrix defects. A Ehlers–Danlos syndrome type II with slightly overstretchable skin results from mutations in the collagen V genes. **B** Dermatosparaxis showing fragile skin with purpura and a 'doughy' texture due to mutations in the gene for ADAMTS-2. **C** Autosomal dominant cutis laxa is associated with mutations in the elastin gene. **D** Junctional epidermolysis bullosa with skin blisters after minimal friction can be caused by mutations in the collagen XVII gene. B, Courtesy of Julie V Schaffer MD.

bind this cation[18,38]. Mutations in the gene encoding fibrillin 2 lead to a Marfan syndrome-like disease called congenital contractural arachnodactyly (skeletal abnormalities in the absence of ocular and cardiovascular features)[38]. In addition to fibrillins, defects in the genes encoding other microfibrillar proteins are likely to be found in ECM disorders.

Heterozygous mutations in the gene encoding the TGF-β receptor 2 have been identified in patients with a Marfan syndrome-like phenotype[39]. The newly recognized Loeys–Dietz syndrome is also caused by heterozygous mutations in the genes encoding TGF-β receptors 1 and 2. Type I Loeys–Dietz syndrome is characterized by aortic aneurysms, generalized arterial tortuosity, craniofacial and skeletal anomalies, joint laxity and translucent skin, whereas type II Loeys–Dietz syndrome presents with a phenotype similar to that of EDS type IV (vascular type; including easy bruising and atrophic scarring)[40]. This phenotypic overlap is not surprising considering the association between fibrillin-containing microfibrils and latent TGF-β (see above) and the role of TGF-β in regulating collagen expression.

Pseudoxanthoma elasticum

Pseudoxanthoma elasticum (PXE) is a heritable disorder characterized by dermal, vascular and ocular lesions that result from the accumulation of morphologically abnormal and mineralized elastic fibers in these tissues. The skin manifestations – yellowish papules and plaques, and laxity of the skin – are the most prevalent symptom of PXE and often

the first sign of the disorder. The accumulation of abnormal calcified elastic fibers in the mid dermis underlies the visible changes. Vascular calcification and retinal angioid streaks, the other hallmarks of PXE, result from fragmentation and calcification of the elastic components of either the media and intima or Bruch's membrane, respectively.

PXE has been considered a prototypic heritable ECM disorder affecting the elastic fiber system, and, therefore, mutations were sought in the genes for structural ECM proteins. Unexpectedly, mutations responsible for PXE were found in a gene that encodes the ATP-binding cassette (ABC) subfamily C member 6 (ABCC6) transporter, also known as 'multidrug resistance-associated protein 6' (MRP6)[41]. *ABCC6* encodes a 165 kDa transmembrane protein that is predominantly expressed in the liver and the kidney. It is not known which molecule(s) the transmembrane protein transports. Similarly, the relationship between aberrant ABCC6 activity and extracellular changes in PXE tissues remains to be elucidated. This information, together with clinical observations suggesting environmental, hormonal and/or dietary modulation of the disease, raises the intriguing possibility that PXE is primarily a metabolic disorder with secondary changes of the ECM suprastructures in particular tissues.

Epidermolysis bullosa

Epidermolysis bullosa (EB) is a name coined for a diverse group of hereditary blistering skin diseases characterized by dermal–epidermal separation and cutaneous blister formation after minimal trauma.

Mutations in the collagen VII gene, *COL7A1*, are the underlying cause of dystrophic EB. Collagen VII is a component of the anchoring fibrils that are abnormal in this EB subtype. The tissue separation occurs at the level of the anchoring fibrils, and it leads to scarring as a consequence of blister formation. Patients with very severe forms of recessive dystrophic EB are nullizygotes harboring mutations that lead to premature termination codons[32]. As a consequence, anchoring fibrils and collagen VII are absent from the skin. Localized, milder forms of dystrophic EB are associated with missense mutations in the *COL7A1* gene. Such mutations often exert dominant-negative effects, since structurally aberrant collagen VII molecules are assembled and incorporated into the anchoring fibrils, rendering them functionally inadequate[32].

Collagen XVII, a homotrimeric transmembrane collagen localized to the hemidesmosomes of the basal keratinocytes, is a component of the epidermal anchoring complex. Mutations in the *COL17A1* gene encoding the α_1(XVII) chains have been identified in patients with junctional EB, an EB subtype characterized by dermal–epidermal separation within the basement membrane. Many patients are compound heterozygotes or homozygotes carrying null alleles of *COL17A1*, and they exhibit a characteristic phenotype with generalized cutaneous blistering, nail dystrophy, dental anomalies, and gradual early loss of scalp hair (Fig. 94.8D). In analogy to collagen VII diseases, patients with missense mutations exhibit milder clinical phenotypes[42].

Laminin 5, a heterotrimeric molecule consisting of an α-, a β- and a γ-chain, is the major structural component of the anchoring filaments that attach the hemidesmosomes into the epidermal basement membrane. The filaments secure epidermal adhesion by binding on one side to $\alpha_6\beta_4$ integrin on the cell surface and on the other side to collagen VII of the anchoring fibrils. Like defects of collagen XVII, mutations in the genes encoding the three polypeptide chains of laminin 5 cause junctional EB. The most severe form, Herlitz junctional EB, results from null mutations and complete lack of laminin 5 in the skin. Missense mutations are associated with milder forms of the disease[14,42].

Other hereditary matrix diseases with skin symptoms

Scleroatonic muscular dystrophy (Ullrich disease) is caused by mutations in the *COL6A1* and *COL6A2* genes encoding the α_1(VI) and α_2(VI) chains of collagen VI[14]. This collagen forms beaded filaments/microfibrils in several tissues, including muscle and skin. Not much is known about the molecular mechanisms of this disease, but the extramuscular symptoms – an abnormal puffy consistency of the skin and joint hyperlaxity – likely reflect abnormalities of the microfibrillar networks in the dermis and synovia.

Recent studies have identified mutations in the gene for the extracellular matrix protein-1 (ECM-1) as the cause of lipoid proteinosis, an inherited multiorgan disease with profound disorder of the ECM and accumulation of 'hyalinized material' in many tissues, including the dermis[41]. Practically nothing is known about the functions of ECM-1, a 85 kD glycoprotein, except that it binds fibulin[43].

Extracellular matrix components as autoantigens

Acquired autoimmune diseases are associated with immunologic abnormalities and the formation of autoantibodies to nuclear components or structural proteins in certain tissues. Several ECM components are targeted in autoimmune diseases affecting the kidney, cartilage or skin (Table 94.6). Classic autoantigens are the α_3-chain of collagen IV in Goodpasture syndrome[44], collagen II in relapsing polychondritis, and collagens VII and XVII in the autoimmune blistering skin diseases EB acquisita[32] and bullous pemphigoid[15], respectively.

Antibodies to fibrillin 1 have been described in a significant percentage of Choctaw Native American and Japanese scleroderma patients, but not as often in other populations[45]. A recent study showed that when native, correctly folded fibrillin 1 was the antigen utilized in the assays, no antibody reactivity was demonstrable in the serum of Caucasian scleroderma patients[46]. The target protein in lipoid proteinosis, ECM-1, is the autoantigen in lichen sclerosus, an inflammatory skin disease with atrophy and hyalinization of the dermis[47].

The immunodominant epitopes within the above molecules are often localized to one or several distinct structural domains and, therefore, recombinant domains can be employed for precise diagnostic testing. The role of the autoantibodies in the etiopathology of the dis-

EXTRACELLULAR MATRIX COMPONENTS AS TARGETS IN AUTOIMMUNE DISEASES		
Disease	**Autoantigen**	**Biologic and clinical features**
Goodpasture syndrome	Collagen IV, α_3 chain	Glomerulonephritis, pneumonitis with hemoptysis
Relapsing polychondritis, arthritis	Collagen II; IX	Chondritis of ear, larynx and trachea; arthritis
Pemphigoid, bullous and cicatricial	Collagen XVII; laminin 5	Skin blistering
Epidermolysis bullosa acquisita	Collagen VII	Skin blistering, fragility
Bullous systemic lupus erythematosus (LE)	Collagen VII	Skin blistering with underlying systemic LE
Scleroderma*	Fibrillin 1; PDGF receptor	Skin fibrosis
Lichen sclerosus*	Extracellular matrix (ECM) protein-1	Inflammation, epidermal atrophy, hyalinization of the dermis

*Not confirmed in large patient cohorts.

Table 94.6 Extracellular matrix components as targets in autoimmune diseases. PDGF, platelet-derived growth factor.

orders is not fully understood, but it is feasible that binding of the antibodies to the ECM components disturbs their supramolecular aggregation or ligand binding, which in turn leads to functional deficiency and to corresponding clinical symptoms.

Other acquired matrix abnormalities

A number of changes in the dermal ECM occur during aging and in acquired disorders such as scleroderma, scurvy or keloids. Biologic hallmarks of skin aging include reduction in the content of hyaluronic acid in the dermis, clumping of elastic fibers, and reduction and weakening of different collagen fibril networks, leading to lax and wrinkled skin. These processes are enhanced by UV irradiation, which generates oxygen radicals and induces inflammation and subsequent degradation of the ECM. Weakened ECM, disturbed wound healing, and a bruising tendency are characteristics of scurvy, a disease resulting from an insufficient supply of ascorbic acid (vitamin C). This vitamin is an essential cofactor for two enzymes, prolyl and lysyl hydroxylase, which modify collagens during their biosynthesis and are required for cross-linking[5]. Fibrotic, thickened skin in scleroderma reflects excessive ECM in the dermis. The reasons for the accumulation remain elusive; inflammation-mediated upregulation of ECM synthesis (via TGF-β) and downregulation of matrix metalloproteinases (see Ch. 141) have been postulated as causative mechanisms in scleroderma (see Ch. 44).

A keloid is an overgrowth of dense fibrous tissue that develops in the skin as a result of trauma. The cellularity of keloids is increased, and the ECM shows abnormal thin fibrils that are haphazardly organized in dense nodules. Various abnormalities of collagen biosynthesis have been measured in keloid fibroblasts *in vitro*, but the molecular mechanisms leading to excessive ECM accumulation still remain unclear. A genetic predisposition for keloid formation seems to exist. Among Caucasians, 5–10% of individuals with keloids have a positive family history; among Africans, the prevalence is much higher.

Animal Models

A number of connective tissue disease models have been produced in mice via targeted mutations. In many cases, the mouse models have produced new insights into pathomechanisms and allowed assessment of abnormalities in the various stages of development of human ECM diseases. In the future, they may become valuable in testing gene therapy approaches for these diseases. Mice with a targeted mutation in one collagen V gene had thin and fragile skin, and, by electron microscopy, disorganized and less tightly packed fibrils were seen in the skin, reminiscent of human EDS[34]. This animal model established the collagen V genes as candidate genes for EDS and preceded the detection of human mutations. A tenascin-X-deficient mouse reproduced the symptoms of human recessive EDS, i.e. greatly disturbed biomechanical properties of the skin, but no or milder joint abnormalities[48].

For fibrillin 1, transgenic mouse models[49] have been used to discern genotype–phenotype correlations. They revealed that the phenotype is determined by the degree of the functional impairment. Haploinsufficiency, or expression of small amounts of a product with dominant-negative potential, is associated with mild Marfan syndrome-like phenotypes, whereas high levels of expression of a dominant-negative-acting protein lead to severe phenotypes[49].

Targeted ablation of the elastin gene in mice resulted in significant vascular changes reminiscent of human supravalvular aortic stenosis. The mice died of an obstructive arterial disease, which resulted from subendothelial cell proliferation and reorganization of smooth muscle, suggesting that elastin has a role in regulating cellular proliferation. The phenotype of heterozygous mice also suggested that human supravalvular aortic stenosis is caused by functional hemizygosity of the elastin gene, a fact that was confirmed by mutational analysis in humans[49]. Unfortunately, no information on the skin phenotype in these mice was reported.

Collagen VII-deficient mice have recapitulated the clinical, genetic, immunohistochemical and ultrastructural characteristics of recessive dystrophic EB in humans and in inbred sheep[32]. The mice exhibited extensive cutaneous blistering and died during the first 2 weeks of life, probably due to complications arising from the blistering[50]. These animals did not provide significant information regarding recessive dystrophic EB pathogenesis, but they may become useful for testing cutaneous gene therapy approaches in the future.

Mice harboring a targeted disruption of the decorin gene had fragile skin with markedly reduced tensile strength. Ultrastructural analysis revealed abnormal fibril morphology in the skin and tendons, with coarser fibers and irregular fiber outlines. These findings pointed to a fundamental role for decorin in regulating collagen fibril formation *in vivo*[51]. Mice with a disrupted syndecan 4 gene are viable, fertile and macroscopically indistinguishable from wild-type littermates. However, they have a significant wound-healing defect and exhibit impaired angiogenesis within wound granulation tissue, suggesting that syndecan 4 is an important cell surface receptor in wound healing and angiogenesis[52].

Abnormalities in collagen-processing enzymes also occur spontaneously in animals. Like human EDS type VIIC, bovine dermatosparaxis is a recessively inherited connective tissue disorder, characterized by extreme fragility and droopiness of the skin as well as joint laxity. Both the human and the bovine disease result from an absence of ADAMTS-2 activity; the latter is the enzyme that excises the N-propeptide of procollagens I and II. In one strain of dermatosparactic calves, the *ADAMTS2* gene mutation was a 17 base-pair deletion, which changed the reading frame and led to a premature termination codon[5,34].

Potential for Biologically Valid Molecular Therapies

Clarification of molecular mechanisms underlying ECM disorders forms a basis for novel therapeutic approaches. Diseases well suited for such therapies include several forms of EB, in particular those with a lack of collagen VII, collagen XVII or laminin 5. Based on our present knowledge of the relevant molecular and biologic aspects, protein-, cell- and gene-based therapies seem possible. Attempts to treat dystrophic EB with collagen VII and junctional EB with laminin 5 have been reported[53–55]. For example, because of its simplicity, direct intradermal injection of recombinant human collagen VII seems an attractive approach to treat dystrophic EB, and, indeed, one group reported successful correction of the dystrophic EB phenotype in mice by this method[56]. However, it remains unclear as to which molecular form and conformation collagen VII can be injected, how the collagen homes to the dermal–epidermal junction, and how long it or its specific aggregates (the anchoring fibrils) will remain stable and functional in the skin. Delivering gene-corrected cells or vectors expressing the missing protein will have the advantage of continuous production of collagen VII in the skin[57].

An advantage of ex-vivo keratinocyte gene therapy is the fact that although potential systemic side effects cannot be anticipated, in case of unexpected negative effects, the transplant and the genetically manipulated cells are easy to remove. Gene transfer into human keratinocytes *in vitro* has been successfully performed in many laboratories; however, stable transfection and expression of correctly folded proteins still prove challenging[53,54]. Nonetheless, a great breakthrough was recently achieved in the treatment of one individual with junctional EB via transplantation of genetically modified epidermal stem cells transfected with the cDNA for laminin 5[54a]. For the treatment of dominant disorders, other strategies must be employed for silencing the expression of the mutated alleles; for example, antisense oligonucleotides or ribozymes (see Ch. 4).

Better understanding of molecular and cellular disease mechanisms has recently disclosed an unexpected pharmacologic approach to the treatment of Marfan syndrome[58]. Excessive TGF-β signaling was found to contribute to certain disease manifestations, such as aortic aneurysms and impaired alveolar septation, and the use of TGF-β antagonists in a mouse model of Marfan syndrome prevented or partially reversed these symptoms. Particularly interesting in this context is the drug losartan, an angiotensin II type 1 receptor antagonist, which also demonstrated the above effects. Losartan is already commercially available as a medication for hypertension and it may show promise in the prevention of severe complications of Marfan syndrome[58].

Future development of successful therapies will also depend on the progress in our understanding of 'alloy' formation by matrix macromolecules. This involves not only the mechanisms of aggregate formation but also the structural characteristics unique for each alloy. Furthermore, functional redundancies of molecular components within the aggregates will have to be defined in greater detail than at present. This endeavor will be facilitated not only by the analysis of aggregate formation by matrix macromolecules or their mixtures *in vitro*, but also by the elucidation of further genetic defects and their consequences in animal or human diseases, as well as the generation of transgenic animals as models for human disorders. This combined information will help us to understand and treat not only inherited ECM diseases but also many common disorders currently considered as acquired.

REFERENCES

1. Birk DE, Bruckner P. Collagen suprastructures. Top Curr Chem. 2005;247:185–205.
2. Ezura Y, Chakravarti S, Oldberg A, et al. Differential expression of lumican and fibromodulin regulate collagen fibrillogenesis in developing mouse tendons. J Cell Biol. 2000;151:779–88.
3. Fitzgerald J, Bateman JF. Is there an evolutionary relationship between WARP (von Willebrand factor A-domain-related protein) and the FACIT and FACIT-like collagens? FEBS Lett. 2003;552:91–4.
4. Ricard-Blum S, Ruggiero F. The collagen superfamily: from the extracellular matrix to the cell membrane. Pathol Biol (Paris). 2005;53:430–2.
5. Myllyharju J, Kivirikko KI. Collagens, modifying enzymes and their mutations in humans, flies and worms. Trends Genet. 2004;20:33–43.

6. Canty EG, Kadler KE. Procollagen trafficking, processing and fibrillogenesis. J Cell Sci. 2005;118:1341–53.
7. Colige A, Ruggiero F, Vandenberghe I, et al. Domains and maturation processes that regulate the activity of ADAMTS-2, a metalloproteinase cleaving the aminopropeptide of fibrillar procollagens type I-III and V. J Biol Chem. 2005;280:34397–408.
8. Steiglitz BM, Kreider JM, Frankenburg EP, et al. Procollagen C proteinase enhancer 1 genes are important determinants of the mechanical properties and geometry of bone and the ultrastructure of connective tissues. Mol Cell Biol. 2006;26:238–49.
9. Raghunath M, Hopfner B, Aeschlimann D, et al. Cross-linking of the dermo-epidermal junction of skin regenerating from keratinocyte autografts. Anchoring

fibrils are a target for tissue transglutaminase. J Clin Invest. 1996;98:1174–84.
10. Koch M, Schulze J, Hansen U, et al. A novel marker of tissue junctions: collagen XXII. J Biol Chem. 2004;279:22514–21.
11. Banyard J, Bao L, Zetter BR. Type XXIII collagen, a new transmembrane collagen identified in metastatic tumor cells. J Biol Chem. 2003;278:20989–94.
12. Boot-Handford RP, Tuckwell DS, Plumb DA, et al. A novel and highly conserved collagen (pro(alpha)1(XXVII)) with a unique expression pattern and unusual molecular characteristics establishes a new clade within the vertebrate fibrillar collagen family. J Biol Chem. 2003;278:31067–77.
13. Veit G, Kobbe B, Keene DR, et al. Collagen XXVIII, a novel von Willebrand factor A domain-containing protein with

many imperfections in the collagenous domain. J Biol Chem. 2006;281:3494–504.

14. Royce P, Steinmann B (eds). Connective Tissue and its Heritable Disorders. Molecular, Genetic and Medical Aspects, 2nd edn. New York: Wiley-Liss Inc, 2002.

15. Franzke C-W, Bruckner P, Bruckner-Tuderman L. Collagenous transmembrane proteins: recent insights into biology and pathology. J Biol Chem. 2005;280:4005–8.

16. Marneros AG, Olsen BR. Physiological role of collagen XVIII and endostatin. FASEB J. 2005;19:716–28.

17. Kozel BA, Rongish BJ, Czirok A, et al. Elastic fiber formation: a dynamic view of extracellular matrix assembly using timer reporters. J Cell Physiol. 2006;207:87–96.

18. Ramirez F, Sakai LY, Dietz HC, et al. Fibrillin microfibrils: multipurpose extracellular networks in organismal physiology. Physiol Genomics. 2004;19:151–4.

19. Tiedemann K, Sasaki T, Gustafsson E, et al. Microfibrils at basement membrane zones interact with perlecan via fibrillin-1. J Biol Chem. 2005;280:11404–12.

20. Timpl R, Sasaki T, Kostka G, et al. Fibulins: a versatile family of extracellular matrix proteins. Nat Rev Mol Cell Biol. 2003;4:479–89.

21. Grässel S, Unsöld C, Schäcke H, et al. Collagen XVI is expressed by human dermal fibroblasts and keratinocytes and is associated with the microfibrillar apparatus in the upper papillary dermis. Matrix Biol. 1999;18:309–17.

22. Ramirez F, Sakai LY, Rifkin DB, et al. Extracellular microfibrils in development and disease. Cell Mol Life Sci. E-publication prior to print, DOI 10.1007/s00018-007-7166-z.

23. Iozzo RV. Matrix proteoglycans: from molecular design to cellular function. Annu Rev Biochem. 1998;67:609–52.

24. Iozzo RV. Basement membrane proteoglycans: from cellar to ceiling. Nat Rev Mol Cell Biol. 2005;6:646–56.

25. Woods A. Syndecans: transmembrane modulators of adhesion and matrix assembly. J Clin Invest. 2001;107:935–41.

26. Tkachenko E, Rhodes JM, Simons M. Syndecans: new kids on the signalling block. Circ Res. 2005;96:488–500.

27. Miner JH, Yurchenco PD. Laminin functions in tissue morphogenesis. Annu Rev Cell Dev Biol. 2004;20:255–84.

28. Aumailley M, Bruckner-Tuderman L, Carter WG, et al. A simplified laminin nomenclature. Matrix Biol. 2005;24:326–32.

29. Adams JC, Lawler J. The thrombospondins. Int J Biochem Cell Biol. 2004;36:961–8.

30. Hsia HC, Schwarzbauer JE. Meet the tenascins: multifunctional and mysterious. J Biol Chem. 2005;280:26641–4.

31. Wagener R, Ehlen HW, Ko YP, et al. The matrilins – adaptor proteins in the extracellular matrix. FEBS Lett. 2005;579:3323–9.

32. Bruckner-Tuderman L, Höpfner B, Hammami-Hauasli N. Biology of anchoring fibrils: lessons from dystrophic epidermolysis bullosa. Matrix Biol. 1999;18:43–54.

33. Pannu J, Trojanowska M. Recent advances in fibroblast signaling and biology in scleroderma. Curr Opin Rheumatol. 2004;16:739–45.

34. Malfait F, de Paepe A. Molecular genetics in classic Ehlers-Danlos syndrome. Am J Med Genet C Semin Med Genet. 2005;139:17–23.

35. Schalkwijk J, Zweers MC, Steijlen PM, et al. A recessive form of the Ehlers-Danlos syndrome caused by tenascin-X deficiency. N Engl J Med. 2001;345:1167–75.

36. Milewicz DM, Urban Z, Boyd C. Genetic disorders of the elastic fiber system. Matrix Biol. 2000;19:471–80.

37. Markova D, Zhou Y, Ringpfeil F, et al. Genetic heterogeneity of cutis laxa: a heterozygous tandem duplication within the fibulin-5 (FBLN5) gene. Am J Hum Genet. 2003;72:998–1004.

38. Kielty CM, Sherratt MJ, Marson A, et al. Fibrillin microfibrils. Adv Protein Chem. 2005;70:405–36.

39. Mizuguchi T, Collod-Beroud G, Akiyama T, et al. Heterozygous *TGFBR2* mutations in Marfan syndrome. Nat Genet. 2004;36:855–60.

40. Loeys BL, Schwarze U, Holm T, et al. Aneurysm syndromes caused by mutations in the TGF-β receptor. N Engl J Med. 2006;355:788–98.

41. Ringpfeil F. Selected disorders of connective tissue: pseudoxanthoma elasticum, cutis laxa, and lipoid proteinosis. Clin Dermatol. 2005;23:41–6.

42. Uitto J, Richards G. Progress in epidermolysis bullosa: genetic classification and clinical implications. Am J Med Genet C Semin Med Genet. 2004;131C:61–74.

43. Fijimoto N, Terlizzi J, Brittingham R, et al. Extracellular matrix protein 1 interacts with the domain III of fibulin-1C and 1D variants though its central tandem repeat 2. Biochem Biophys Res Commun. 2005;333:1327–33.

44. Wang XP, Fogo AB, Colon S, et al. Distinct epitopes for anti-glomerular basement membrane Alport alloantibodies and Goodpasture autoantibodies within the noncollagenous domain of alpha3(IV) collagen: a Janus-faced antigen. J Am Soc Nephrol. 2005;16:3563–71.

45. Tan FK, Wang N, Kuwana M et al. Association of fibrillin 1 single-nucleotide polymorphism haplotypes with systemic sclerosis in Choctaw and Japanese populations. Arthritis Rheum. 2001;44:893–901.

46. Brinckmann J, Hunzelmann N, El-Hallous E, et al. Absence of autoantibodies against correctly folded recombinant fibrillin-1 protein in systemic sclerosis patients. Arthritis Res Ther. 2005;7:R1221–6.

47. Oyama N, Chan I, Neill SM, et al. Autoantibodies to extracellular matrix protein 1 in lichen sclerosus. Lancet. 2003;362:118–23.

48. Egging DF, van Vlijmen I, Starcher B, et al. Dermal connective tissue development in mice: an essential role for tenascin-X. Cell Tissue Res. 2006;323:465–74.

49. Dietz HC, Mecham RP. Mouse models of genetic diseases resulting from mutations in elastic fiber proteins. Matrix Biol. 2000;19:481–8.

50. Heinonen S, Männikkö M, Klement JF, et al. Targeted inactivation of the type VII collagen gene (Col7a1) in mice results in severe blistering phenotype: a model for recessive dystrophic epidermolysis bullosa. J Cell Sci. 1999;112:3641–8.

51. Danielson KG, Baribault H, Holmes DF, et al. Targeted disruption of decorin leads to abnormal collagen fibril morphology and skin fragility. J Cell Biol. 1997;136:729–43.

52. Echtermeyer F, Streit M, Wilcox-Adelman S, et al. Delayed wound repair and impaired angiogenesis in mice lacking syndecan-4. J Clin Invest. 2001;107:R9–14.

53. Ortiz-Urda S, Lin Q, Yant SR, et al. Sustainable correction of junctional epidermolysis bullosa via transposon-mediated nonviral gene transfer. Gene Ther. 2003;10:1099–104.

54. Baldeschi C, Gache Y, Rattenholl A, et al. Genetic correction of canine dystrophic epidermolysis bullosa mediated by retroviral vectors. Hum Mol Genet. 2003;12:1897–905.

54a. Mavilio F, Pellegrini G, Ferrari S, et al. Correction of junctional epidermolysis bullosa by transplantation of genetically modified epidermal stem cells. Nature Med. 2006;12:1397–1402.

55. Woodley DT, Krueger GG, Jorgensen CM, et al. Normal and gene-corrected dystrophic epidermolysis bullosa fibroblasts alone can produce type VII collagen at the basement membrane zone. J Invest Dermatol. 2003;121:1021–8.

56. Woodley DT, Keene DR, Atha T, et al. Injection of recombinant human type VII collagen restores collagen function in dystrophic epidermolysis bullosa. Nat Med. 2004;10:693–5.

57. Ferrari S, Pellegrini G, Matsui T, et al. Gene therapy in combination with tissue engineering to treat epidermolysis bullosa. Expert Opin Biol Ther. 2006;6:367–78.

58. Habashi JP, Judge DP, Holm TM, et al. Losartan, an AT1 antagonist, prevents aortic aneurysm in a mouse model of Marfan syndrome. Science. 2006;312:117–21.

Perforating Diseases

Ronald P Rapini

95

Synonyms: ■ Hyperkeratosis follicularis et parafollicularis in cutem penetrans: Kyrle's disease ■ Acquired perforating dermatosis: acquired reactive perforating collagenosis, acquired reactive perforating dermatosis, perforating disorder of uremia

Key features

- Group of disorders with transepidermal elimination of collagen, elastic tissue or necrotic connective tissue
- Papules or nodules with keratotic plugs
- Elastosis perforans serpiginosa is associated with genetic diseases or penicillamine administration and involves elastic tissue; lesions are typically annular and most commonly occur on the neck
- Reactive perforating collagenosis occurs after minor trauma, involves collagen, and often involves the upper extremities
- Acquired perforating dermatosis is almost always associated with diabetes mellitus or the pruritus of renal failure; it favors the lower extremities of adults
- UV light therapy is the most effective treatment for acquired perforating dermatosis

INTRODUCTION

The perforating diseases (Table 95.1) are a group of papulonodular skin disorders characterized by keratotic plugs or crusts in which dermal connective tissue 'perforates' or is eliminated through the epidermis. There are two prototypic perforating diseases, both of which can be inherited. They are reactive perforating collagenosis (RPC), in which primarily collagen fibers perforate the epidermis[1], and elastosis perforans serpiginosa (EPS), in which primarily elastic fibers perforate. The third major perforating disease is acquired perforating dermatosis, which

usually develops during adulthood in association with diabetes mellitus and/or the pruritus of renal failure[2]. Many textbooks traditionally list 'perforating folliculitis' as the fourth perforating disease[3], but, in the opinion of the author, this seems unjustified. It does not appear to be a specific entity, since perforation or rupture of follicles occurs in a wide variety of diseases classified as folliculitis, regardless of whether the pathogenesis involves bacteria, fungi, *Demodex* mites, physical trauma or other mechanisms.

Some authorities have expanded the concept of the preceding so-called 'primary' perforating diseases to include a variety of unrelated 'secondary' perforating disorders in which transepidermal elimination of a substance occurs as a secondary component of a primary dermatosis (Table 95.2). As in most of the preceding perforating disorders, the epidermis often becomes hyperplastic, eventually surrounds the material to be extruded, and subsequently causes the material's elimination via normal keratinocyte maturation. Some of these disorders are discussed elsewhere in this text and involve perforation of endogenous substances[4,5], exogenous foreign material, infectious organisms, granulomas, and even neoplastic cells.

HISTORY

In 1916, Kyrle reported a diabetic woman with generalized hyperkeratotic nodules, which he called hyperkeratosis follicularis et parafollicularis in cutem penetrans. Lutz first described EPS as keratosis follicularis serpiginosa in 1953, and, in 1955, Miescher described the histologic findings, naming it elastoma intrapapillare perforans verruciforme. Mehregan, Schwartz & Livingood reported the first child with RPC in 1967. Mehregan & Coskey expanded the concept of perforating disease to include perforating folliculitis in their article in 1968.

EPIDEMIOLOGY

The perforating diseases are found worldwide, without any clear racial predilection. The very rare childhood form of RPC is commonly familial, and childhood EPS is occasionally familial. Although the exact

MAJOR PERFORATING DISEASES					
Disease	Incidence	Time of onset	Location	Perforating substance	Associations
Reactive perforating collagenosis (RPC), inherited	Very rare	Childhood	Arms, hands, sites of trauma	Collagen	None
Elastosis perforans serpiginosa (EPS)	Rare, M>F	Childhood, young adulthood; variable with penicillamine-induced	Neck, face, arms, other flexural areas	Elastic tissue	Genetic diseases (see Fig. 95.13), penicillamine
Perforating folliculitis	Common	Young adulthood	Trunk, extremities	Necrotic material	May simply be ordinary folliculitis with follicular rupture, i.e. not a specific entity
Acquired perforating dermatosis, includes acquired RPC, Kyrle's disease* and, occasionally, acquired EPS	Common (10% of dialysis patients)	Adulthood	Legs or generalized	Necrotic material, collagen or, uncommonly, elastic tissue	Diabetes, renal disease, pruritus, rarely liver disease; may be end stage of perforating folliculitis
Perforating periumbilical calcific elastosis	Very rare, more common in black women	Adulthood	Abdomen, periumbilical	Calcified elastic tissue	Multiparity

*In the opinion of some authors.

Table 95.1 Major perforating diseases.

SECONDARY PERFORATING DISEASES
Endogenous substances
Chondrodermatitis nodularis helicis
Hematomas
Perforating pseudoxanthoma elasticum[4]
Perforating calcinosis[5]
Gout
Exogenous foreign material
Silica
Wood splinters
Infectious diseases/organisms
Chromoblastomycosis
Botryomycosis
Spirochetes
Granulomas
Perforating granuloma annulare (Fig. 92.8)
Necrobiosis lipoidica
Sarcoidosis
Neoplastic cells
Melanoma
Paget's disease
Mycosis fungoides

Table 95.2 Secondary perforating diseases.

inheritance pattern for both is still uncertain, isolated inherited EPS may have an autosomal dominant pattern. EPS affects nearly four times more men than women, but the sex distribution is about equal in RPC and acquired perforating dermatosis. Perforating folliculitis is said to be more common in women. In patients receiving dialysis, acquired perforating dermatosis is rather common, with a prevalence rate of about 10%[6].

PATHOGENESIS

The precise pathogenesis for the perforating disorders is unknown. It is unlikely that dermal connective tissue or hair shafts actively perforate into the epithelium, so some have argued that 'transepidermal elimination' is a more accurate term. The term 'perforating' is embedded in the dermatologic lexicon, however, and is easier to say. Epithelium becomes hyperplastic and eventually surrounds the abnormal connective tissue, just as it appears to do with wood splinters or other foreign bodies. In acquired perforating dermatosis, pruritus probably leads to chronic scratching, which results in epithelial hyperplasia, as in prurigo nodularis. Indeed, many of the patients have common prurigo nodules in addition to classic perforating lesions.

Primary perforating diseases may be due to either genetic or acquired abnormalities of collagen or elastic fibers. However, attempts to identify specific abnormalities, e.g. non-enzymatic glyco-oxidation of collagen, have to date been inconclusive. In EPS as well as some cases of acquired perforating dermatosis (in which elastic fibers were perforating), interactions between elastin and elastin receptors on keratinocytes have been observed[7].

Fibronectin levels have been shown to be increased in the serum of patients with diabetes mellitus and uremia, and it has also been found to be increased in the skin at sites of perforating lesions[8]. This may be significant, since fibronectin plays a role in epithelial cell signaling, locomotion and differentiation. It binds to type IV collagen (the type found in basement membranes) and to keratinocytes, and may incite epithelial proliferation and perforation. In one study of RPC, the investigators demonstrated that it was type IV collagen that was being transepidermally eliminated[9]. Increased expression of TGF-β_3 has also been observed in the epidermis and dermis near the sites of perforation in RPC, but this enhanced expression occurs in general wound healing reactions as well[10].

Other proposed pathomechanisms include abnormal vitamin A or D metabolism, enzyme release from neutrophils[11], microangiopathy

related to diabetes, and an imbalance in the expression of metalloproteinases and their tissue inhibitors. Deposition of substances such as uric acid, hydroxyapatite, silicon[12] or other materials[13] has also been implicated in the pathogenesis of perforating disorders.

CLINICAL FEATURES

Reactive Perforating Collagenosis

RPC is a rare familial disorder that begins during childhood. After superficial trauma, patients develop keratotic papules that reach a size of 5–8 mm over the following 3–4 weeks (Fig. 95.1). The Koebner phenomenon may occur, in which injury to the skin results in the formation of new lesions, often in a linear distribution. Koebnerization is more commonly observed with RPC than with the other perforating disorders, but it has been reported with all of them. Arms and hands are the most common sites of involvement in RPC. The papules tend to spontaneously resolve over 6–8 weeks. Verrucous perforating collagenoma (*collagenome perforant verruciformé*) is a very rare non-familial variant of RPC in which severe trauma to the skin results in verrucous papules with transepidermal elimination of collagen[14]. Acquired RPC that begins during adulthood has also been described, especially in association with diabetes mellitus or renal insufficiency, but these cases are best classified as acquired perforating dermatosis, even though the histopathology can be identical to the inherited form of RPC.

Elastosis Perforans Serpiginosa

EPS is a rare disorder beginning during childhood or early adulthood. About 40% of cases occur in association with other genetic disorders, including Down syndrome, Ehlers–Danlos syndrome, osteogenesis imperfecta, Marfan syndrome (Fig. 95.2), pseudoxanthoma elasticum, Rothmund–Thomson syndrome, and acrogeria[15]. Very rare cases of EPS associated with renal failure (clearly more rarely encountered than the acquired form of RPC) are best classified as acquired perforating dermatosis. EPS has also been reported to be induced by the drug penicillamine, which disrupts desmosine cross-links within elastin (see Ch. 97)[16]. Lesions of EPS are keratotic 2–5 mm papules that tend to be arranged in a serpiginous or annular pattern, most commonly on the lateral neck (Fig. 95.3), but also on the face, arms (Fig. 95.4) or other flexural areas. The rings of papules may reach several centimeters in diameter. Most patients experience no symptoms or only mild pruritus. Like RPC, the lesions may spontaneously resolve, but they tend to persist longer, often for several years.

Acquired Perforating Dermatosis and Kyrle's Disease

Acquired perforating dermatosis has been used as a catch-all term for those examples of perforating disease arising in adults, usually in

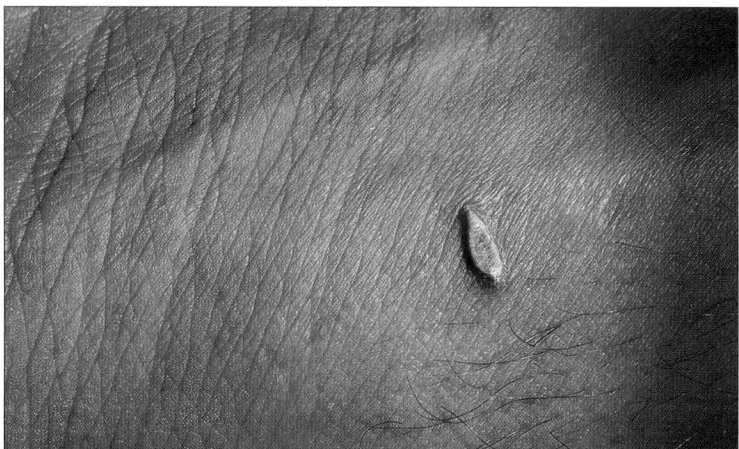

Fig. 95.1 **Reactive proliferating collagenosis.** This keratotic papule on the upper extremity followed minor trauma in a healthy man who had developed similar papules since childhood.

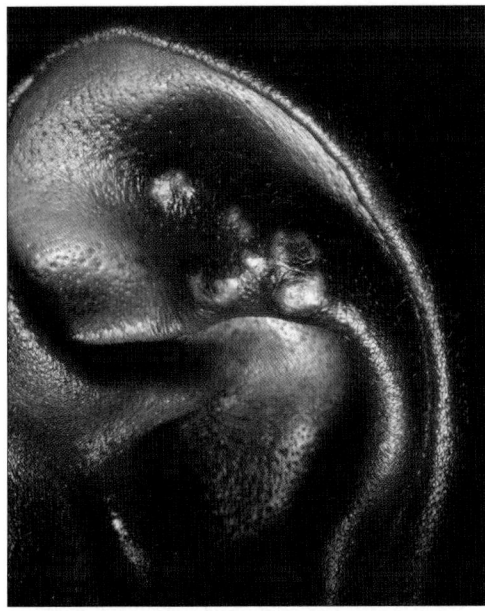

Fig. 95.2 **Elastosis perforans serpiginosa in the setting of Marfan syndrome.** Annular papules and plaques developed on the ear.

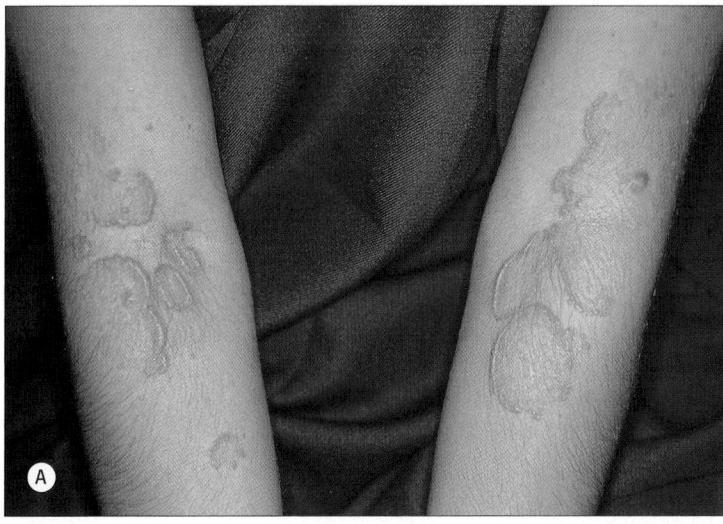

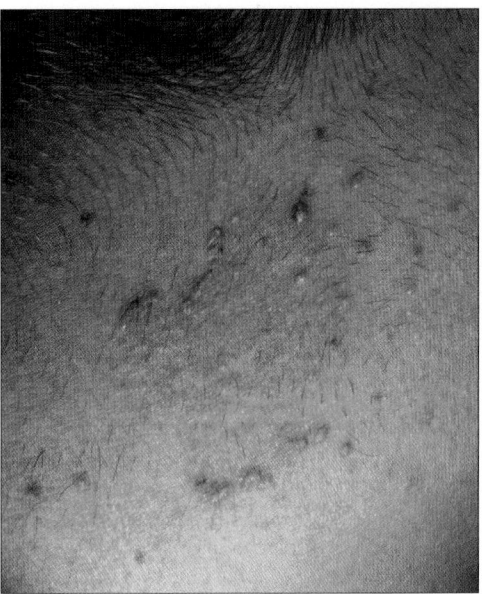

Fig. 95.3 **Elastosis perforans serpiginosa.** Papules arranged in an annular configuration on the neck.

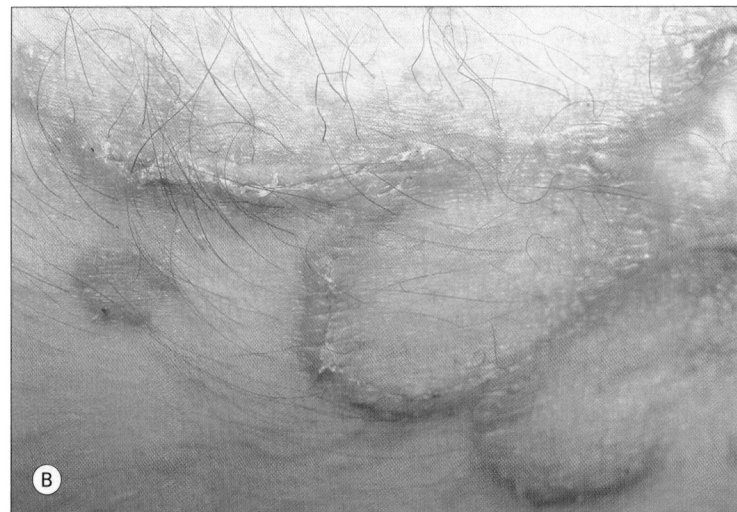

Fig. 95.4 **Penicillamine-induced elastosis perforans serpiginosa. A** Multiple annular plaques favoring the antecubital fossae. **B** Closer view with foci of hyperkeratosis at sites of transepidermal elimination.

association with diabetes mellitus and/or the pruritus of renal failure[2]. It has rarely been reported to occur with the pruritus of liver disease or internal malignancy. Acquired perforating dermatosis occurs most commonly on the legs (Fig. 95.5), but generalized or widely scattered papules or nodules can be seen (Figs 95.6 & 95.7). Largely on the basis of their histologic findings, patients with acquired perforating dermatosis have been variably designated in the literature as having RPC[17], EPS[2], perforating folliculitis[13] or perforating pseudoxanthoma elasticum[18]. Since the pathologic findings vary from lesion to lesion in the same patient, it seems unwise to subclassify patients in this way. Since some, but not necessarily all, of these lesions appear to be follicular, and since manipulation of the lesions by patients frequently alters the histologic changes, the term 'acquired perforating dermatosis' was proposed to encompass all of these cases. Furthermore, since Kyrle had used the phrase 'follicularis et parafollicularis' to emphasize that not all lesions were proved to be centered on follicles, the eponym Kyrle's disease has been used synonymously with acquired perforating dermatosis by some authorities[2]. However, others do not consider Kyrle's disease to be an entity, or prefer to define it as merely representing the presence of end-stage excoriated hyperplastic nodules of folliculitis[2].

Perforating Periumbilical Calcific Elastosis

This disorder is characterized by keratotic papules on the abdomen, especially the periumbilical area of multiparous black women (Fig. 95.8)[19].

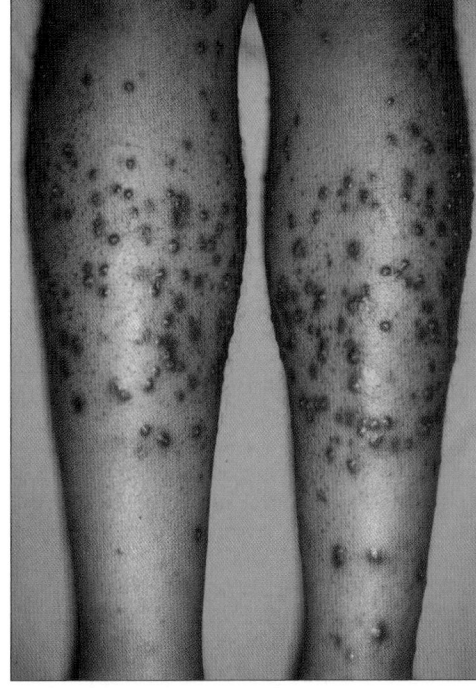

Fig. 95.5 **Acquired perforating dermatosis.** Numerous papules and nodules on the legs in a patient with both renal failure and diabetes mellitus.

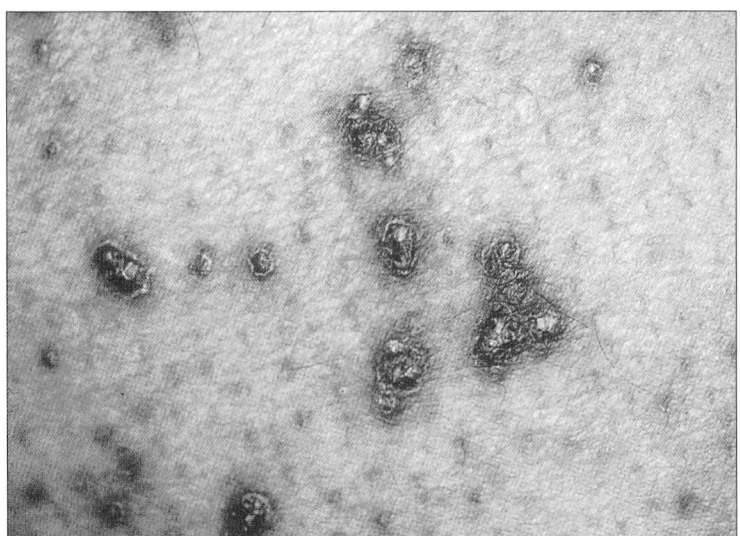

Fig 95.6 **Acquired perforating dermatosis.** Keratotic papules on the arm of a diabetic woman on hemodialysis. Note the central keratotic core which is sometimes dislodged by the patient.

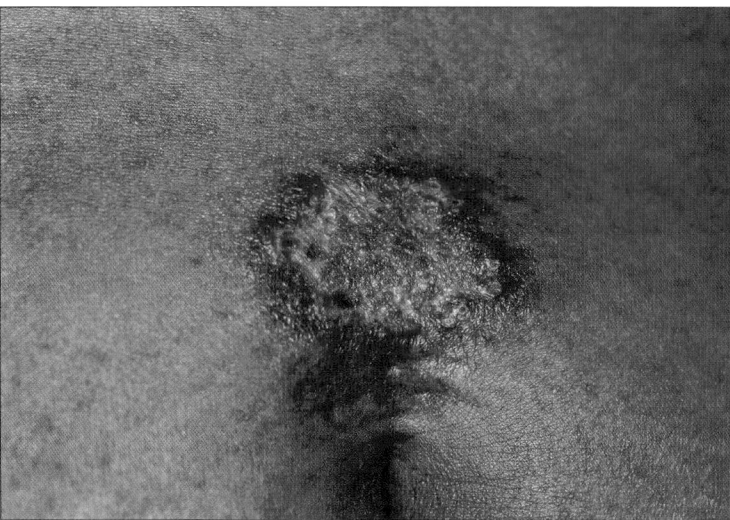

Fig. 95.8 **Perforating periumbilical calcific elastosis.** When a biopsy was performed from the elevated edge of this supraumbilical plaque in a multiparous African-American woman, resistance was felt, as well as a grinding sound.

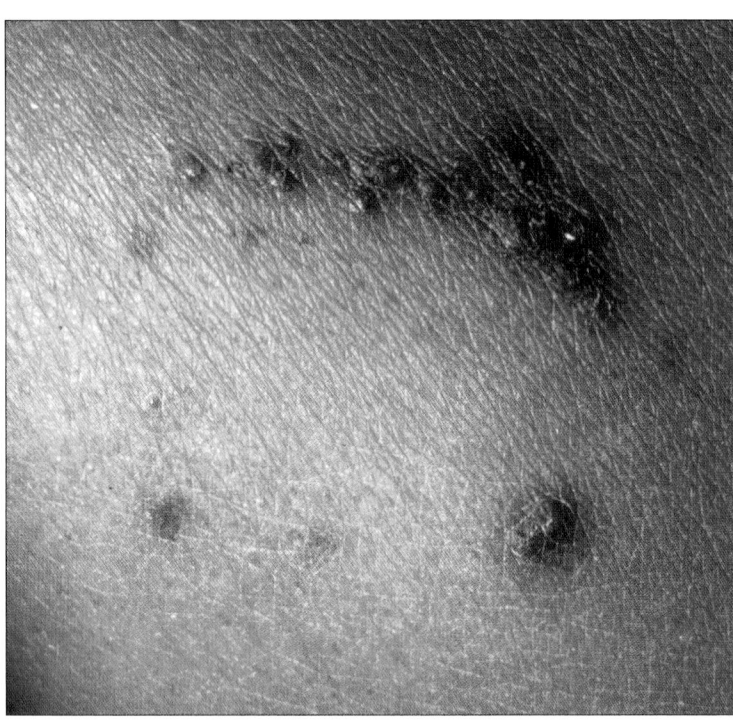

Fig. 95.7 **Acquired perforating dermatosis.** Note the linear arrangement of the keratotic papules (Koebner phenomenon).

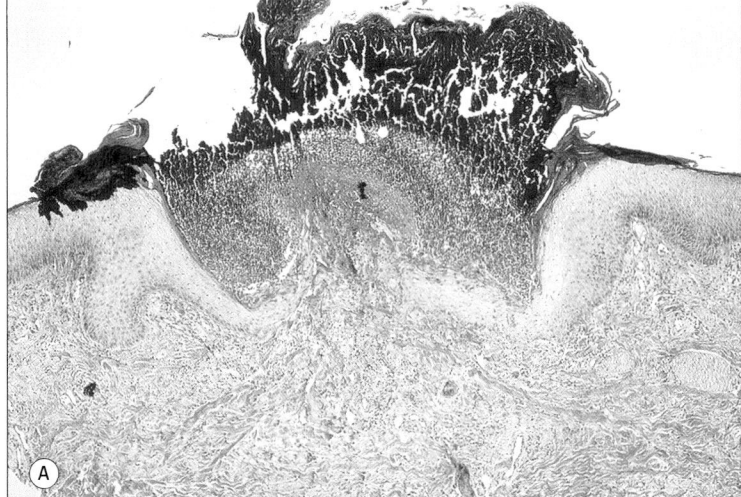

Fig 95.9 **Acquired reactive perforating collagenosis. A** Scanning view of a crusted keratotic plug in a patient whose biopsy showed perforating collagen fibers. **B** Higher magnification demonstrating collagen fibers extending through the epidermis (arrows) into the crusted plug.

Transepidermal elimination of calcified elastic fibers is observed, but there is no clinical evidence of the disorder pseudoxanthoma elasticum. Similar transepidermal elimination has been observed in patients who treated their dermatitis with a commercially available calcium salt water normally used for making bean curd[20].

PATHOLOGY

In all the perforating diseases, there is a plug of crusting or hyperkeratosis, with variable parakeratosis, depending upon the stage of the lesion (Fig. 95.9A). Sections from multiple levels through the tissue may need to be examined to find the site of perforation. Some lesions may have aggregates of neutrophils in the dermis, while older lesions, particularly those of EPS, tend to have lymphocytes, macrophages or multinucleated giant cells in the dermis at the site of perforation. In RPC, collagen fibers are seen within the plug or within the epidermis

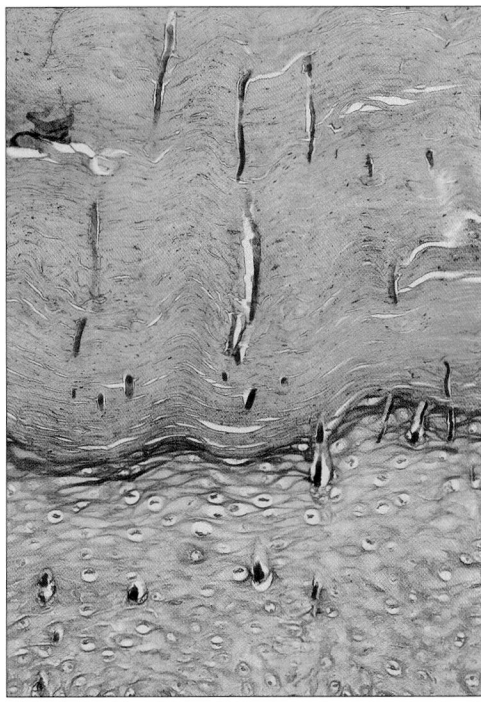

Fig. 95.10 Reactive perforating collagenosis. Transepidermal elimination of red collagen fibers through the spinous layer and into the stratum corneum (Verhoeff–van Gieson stain).

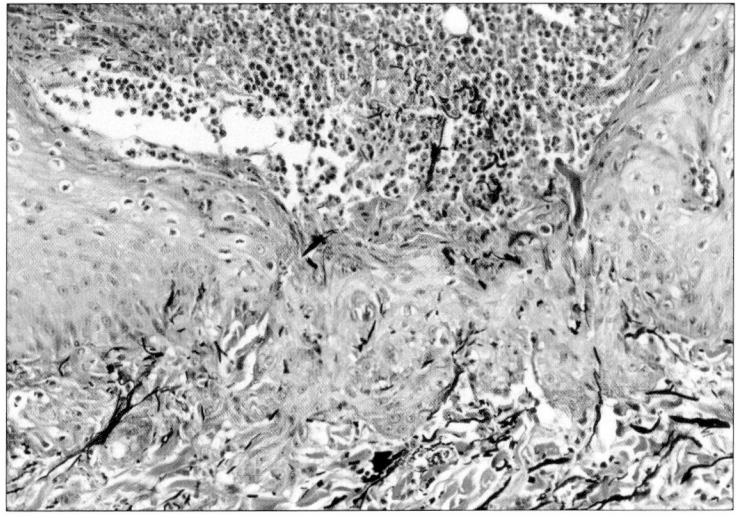

Fig 95.12 Acquired perforating dermatosis. Transepidermal elimination of both collagen (red) and elastic fibers (black) into a crust with many neutrophils is seen (Verhoeff–van Gieson stain).

(Figs 95.9B & 95.10). In EPS, elastic fibers are seen instead, in the same location (Fig. 95.11). In RPC, the dermal connective tissue adjacent to the plug appears unremarkable, while, in EPS, an increased amount of brightly eosinophilic elastic tissue is often present in the superficial dermis. The Verhoeff–van Gieson stain is most helpful, because collagen fibers appear red and elastic fibers appear black (Fig. 95.12). However, in EPS, the elastic fibers higher up in the epidermis may lose their ability to stain black. In penicillamine-induced EPS, characteristic 'lumpy-bumpy' elastic fibers with lateral buds resembling a 'bramble bush' are seen in both lesional and non-lesional skin.

Biopsy findings in acquired perforating dermatosis vary according to the stage of evolution of the lesion. The histology may be identical to childhood RPC or EPS, or perforating folliculitis. In other cases, it may be less specific, with amorphous degenerated material within the perforations. This material often cannot be clearly identified as collagen or elastic fibers, but sometimes both are present (see Fig. 95.12)[2].

DIFFERENTIAL DIAGNOSIS

The differential diagnosis includes other disorders characterized by papules or nodules with central keratotic plugs or crusts (Table 95.3).

DIFFERENTIAL DIAGNOSIS OF PERFORATING DISEASES

Reactive perforating collagenosis and acquired perforating dermatosis

Excoriations from a variety of causes (prurigo simplex)
Prurigo nodularis
Folliculitis
Arthropod bites
Perforating of exogenous foreign material
Perforating of endogenous substances
Multiple keratoacanthomas
Dermatofibromas
If Koebner phenomenon, psoriasis, lichen planus, verrucae

Elastosis perforans serpiginosa (resembles other annular diseases; see Ch. 20)

Granuloma annulare ⎤
Tinea   ⎦ Common annular diseases
Sarcoidosis
Actinic granuloma (annular elastolytic giant cell granuloma)
Perforating pseudoxanthoma elasticum
Porokeratosis
Discoid lupus erythematosus

Table 95.3 Differential diagnosis of perforating diseases.

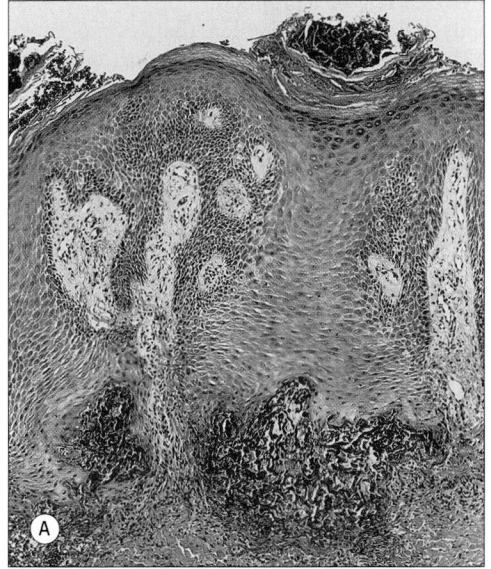

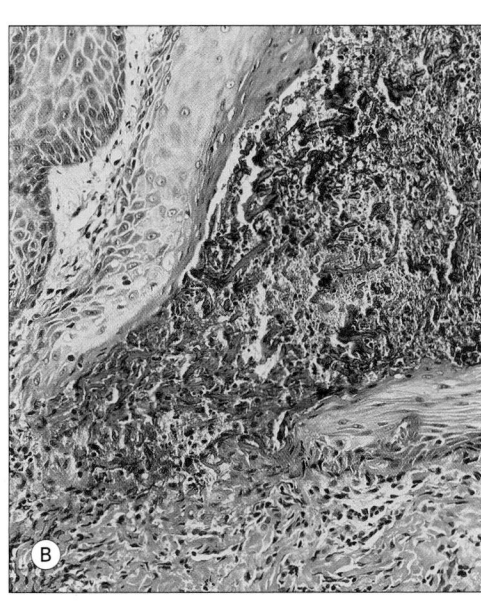

Fig. 95.11 Elastosis perforans serpiginosa.
A Hyperplastic epidermis clutches the increased dermal elastic fibers like a claw. **B** Transepidermal elimination of neutrophils and elastic fibers from the dermis through a channel in the epidermis.

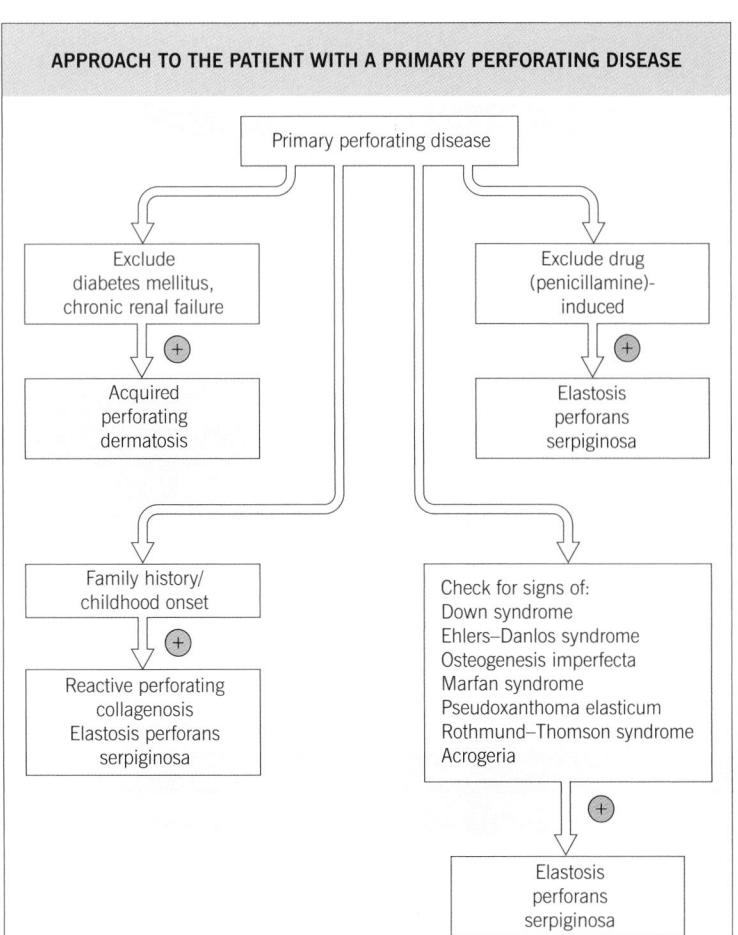

APPROACH TO THE PATIENT WITH A PRIMARY PERFORATING DISEASE

Fig. 95.13 Approach to the patient with a primary perforating disease.

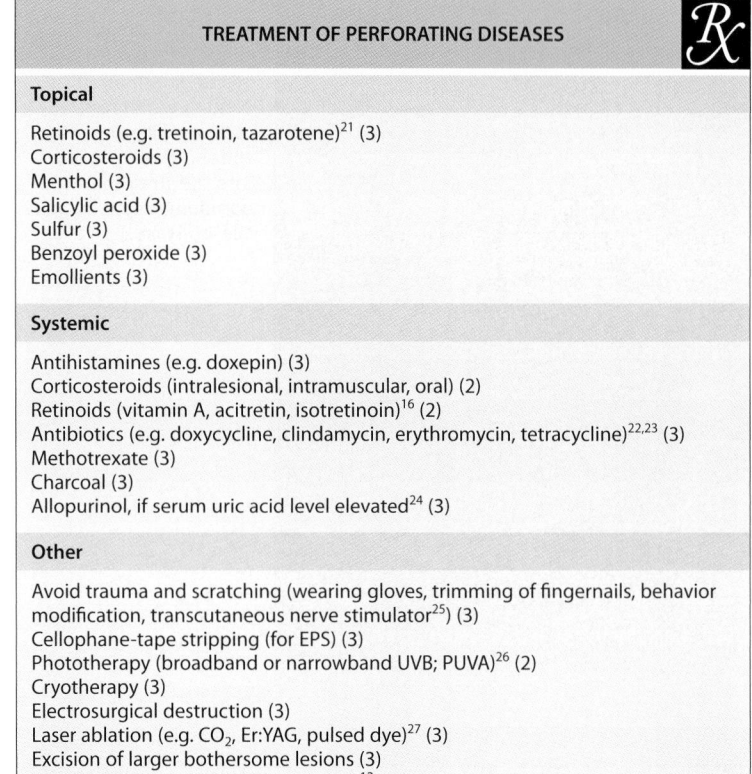

TREATMENT OF PERFORATING DISEASES

Table 95.4 Treatment of perforating diseases. Key to evidence-based support: (1) prospective controlled trial; (2) retrospective study or large case series; (3) small case series or individual case reports.

When the Koebner phenomenon occurs, other disorders that can also arise in a linear pattern should be considered, e.g. psoriasis, lichen planus and verrucae. EPS may be confused with other disorders that are annular or serpiginous (see Ch. 20), but usually the individual keratotic plugs within the ring make it distinctive. Since many patients with acquired perforating dermatosis have coexisting folliculitis and prurigo nodularis, it is important to realize that these patients may have multiple different types of lesions at different stages of development and that a biopsy of just one lesion may not be representative of the entire process. Figure 95.13 provides an algorithm for the approach to the patient with a primary perforating disorder.

TREATMENT

Table 95.4 summarizes the various treatments that have been reported, most of which are anecdotal. There have been no well-designed studies of therapeutic interventions. The inherited forms of RPC and EPS generally remain mild and localized and are therefore not so problem-atic. Local measures may be successful, but some authors have declared treatment to be largely ineffective. The patient with mild RPC may be satisfied to simply avoid trauma and wait for lesions to resolve spontaneously.

EPS may be treated with local cryotherapy, tangential excision, electro-surgical destruction, or cellophane tape stripping. Aggressive treatment is more likely to result in scarring. As with RPC, spontaneous resolution of lesions makes it difficult to evaluate therapies.

Treatment of generalized acquired perforating dermatosis or extensive perforating folliculitis is often difficult. Antihistamines are marginally helpful, as are most other typical 'pruritus treatments' (see Ch. 7). Phototherapy (broadband or narrowband UVB or PUVA) is a particu-larly good choice for patients with renal disease, since it often relieves their coexisting pruritus. Other therapies that are sometimes helpful include intralesional corticosteroids[6] and oral[14] or topical[6] retinoids. Anecdotally, some patients have attributed rapid improvement to a change in the type of dialysis tubing or equipment employed, or even an alteration in the methods used during the actual dialysis procedure (personal observation). Occasional dialysis patients with acquired perforating dermatosis have been cured after renal transplantation[12].

REFERENCES

1. Flannigan SA, Tucker SB, Rapini RP. Recurrent hyperkeratotic papules from superficial trauma: reactive perforating collagenosis (RPC). Arch Dermatol. 1985;121:1554–5, 1557–8.
2. Rapini RP, Herbert AA, Drucker CR, et al. Acquired perforating dermatosis. Evidence of combined transepidermal elimination of both collagen and elastic fibers. Arch Dermatol. 1989;125:1074–8.
3. Rubio FA, Herranz P, Robayna G, et al. Perforating folliculitis: report of a case in an HIV-infected man. J Am Acad Dermatol. 1999;40:300–2.
4. Kazakis AM, Parish WR. Periumbilical perforating pseudoxanthoma elasticum. J Am Acad Dermatol. 1988;19:384–8.
5. Enelow TJ, Huang W, Williams CM. Perforating papules in chronic renal failure. Metastatic calcinosis cutis with transepidermal elimination. Arch Dermatol. 1998;134:98–9, 101–2.
6. Morton CA, Henderson IS, Jones MC, et al. Acquired perforating dermatosis in a British dialysis population. Br J Dermatol. 1996;135:671–7.
7. Fujimoto N, Tajima S, Ishibashi A. Elastin peptides induce migration and terminal differentiation of cultured keratinocytes via 67kDa elastin receptor in vitro. J Invest Dermatol. 2000;115:633–9.
8. Bilezikci B, Seckin D, Demirhan B. Acquired perforating dermatosis in patients with chronic renal failure: a possible role for fibronectin. J Eur Acad Dermatol Venereol. 2003;17:230–2.
9. Herzinger T, Schirren CG, Sander CA, et al. Reactive perforating collagenosis – transepidermal elimination of type IV collagen. Clin Exp Dermatol. 1996;21:279–82.
10. Kawakami T, Soma Y, Mizoguchi M, Saito R. Immunohistochemical analysis of transforming growth factor-[beta]3 expression in acquired reactive perforating collagenosis. Br J Dermatol. 2001; 144:197–8.
11. Zelger B, Hintner H, Aubock J, et al. Acquired perforating dermatosis. Transepidermal elimination of DNA material and possible role of leukocytes in pathogenesis. Arch Dermatol. 1991;127:695–700.
12. Saldanha LF, Gonick HC, Rodriguez HJ, et al. Silicon-related syndrome in dialysis patients. Nephron. 1997;77:48–56.
13. Haftek M, Euvrard S, Kanitakis J, et al. Acquired perforating dermatosis of diabetes mellitus and renal failure: further ultrastructural clues to its pathogenesis. J Cutan Pathol. 1993;20:350–5.

14. Delacretaz J, Gattlen JM. Transepidermal elimination of traumatically altered collagen. Report of three cases and consideration on the relationship between 'collagenome perforant verruciformé' and reactive perforating collagenosis. Dermatologica. 1976;152:65–6.

15. Mehta RK, Burrows NP, Payne CM, et al. Elastosis perforans serpiginosa and associated disorders. Clin Exp Dermatol. 2001;26:521–4.

16. Ratnavel RC, Norris PG. Penicillamine-induced elastosis perforans serpiginosa treated successfully with isotretinoin. Dermatology. 1994;189:81–3.

17. Faver IR, Daoud MS, Su WP. Acquired reactive perforating collagenosis. Report of six cases and review of the literature. J Am Acad Dermatol. 1994;30:575–80.

18. Nickoloff BJ, Noodleman R, Abel EA. Perforating pseudoxanthoma elasticum associated with chronic renal failure and hemodialysis. Arch Dermatol. 1985;121:1321–2.

19. Lopes LC, Lobo L, Bajanca R. Perforating calcific elastosis. J Eur Acad Dermatol Venereol. 2003;17:206–7.

20. Lee SJ, Jang JW, Lee WC, et al. Perforating disorder caused by salt-water application and its experimental induction. Int J Dermatol. 2005;44:210–14.

21. Outland JD, Brown TS, Callen JP. Tazarotene is an effective therapy for elastosis perforans serpiginosa. Arch Dermatol. 2002;138:169–71.

22. Brinkmeier T, Schaller J, Herbst RA, Frosch PJ. Successful treatment of acquired reactive perforating collagenosis with doxycycline. Acta Derm Venereol. 2002;82:393–5.

23. Kasiakou SK, Peppas G, Kapaskelis AM, Falagas ME. Regression of skin lesions of Kyrle's disease with clindamycin: implications for an infectious component in the etiology of the disease. J Infect. 2005;50:412–16.

24. Iyoda M, Hayashi F, Kuroki A, et al. Acquired reactive perforating collagenosis in a nondiabetic hemodialysis patient: successful treatment with allopurinol. Am J Kidney Dis. 2003;42:E11–13.

25. Chan LY, Tang WY, Lo KK. Treatment of pruritus of reactive perforating collagenosis using transcutaneous electrical nerve stimulation. Eur J Dermatol. 2000;10:59–61.

26. Ohe S, Danno K, Sasaki H, et al. Treatment of acquired perforating dermatosis with narrowband ultraviolet B. J Am Acad Dermatol. 2004;50:892–4.

27. Saxena M, Tope WD. Response of elastosis perforans serpiginosa to pulsed CO_2, Er:YAG, and dye lasers. Dermatol Surg. 2003;29:677–8.

Morphea and Lichen Sclerosus

Martin Röcken and Kamran Ghoreschi

Morphea and lichen sclerosus are inflammatory skin diseases that ultimately evolve into two distinct modes of scar formation. Morphea affects primarily the dermis and may extend to subcutaneous structures. Lichen sclerosus is most often a disease of the genital mucosa and affects the epidermis and superficial dermis. Neither one leads to significant involvement of internal organs and both may be manifestations of chronic GVHD. Because of the multiple dissimilarities, morphea and lichen sclerosus will be addressed separately. The therapy of both diseases will be discussed together.

MORPHEA

Synonyms: ▪ Localized scleroderma ▪ Circumscribed scleroderma ▪ Linear scleroderma ▪ Scleroderma en coup de sabre

Key features

- Asymmetric sclerotic plaques, usually 2–15 cm in diameter
- Active lesions can have a lilac border, while inactive lesions often become hyperpigmented
- The sclerosus may extend deeply into the fat or underlying structures, causing disability
- There is no associated systemic disease
- Often progresses for several years, then regresses

INTRODUCTION

Morphea is a clinically distinct inflammatory disease, primarily of the dermis and subcutaneous fat, which ultimately leads to a scar-like sclerosis. Because the small vessel changes, the inflammatory infiltrate and the ultimate structural modifications are identical in morphea and systemic sclerosis, the local cascade of inflammatory events is probably similar. The two diseases are distinct entities that can easily be distinguished based on clinical features. Raynaud's phenomenon is regularly present in systemic sclerosis and not associated with morphea. Morphea has an asymmetric patchy or linear distribution. It never starts as symmetric sclerosis of the hands and fingers that extends progressively toward the proximal upper extremity, and it does not involve the internal organs. Although generalized morphea may resemble early diffuse scleroderma, the presence in the latter condition of Raynaud's phenomenon, digital sclerosis, and involvement of the gastrointestinal tract and the lung generally allows separation of systemic sclerosis from morphea.

Morphea is usually a relatively harmless disease. However, in about 10% of the patients, scar formation may lead not only to the usual disfigurement but also to significant contractures or growth retardation and handicaps the affected individuals for their entire life[1]. Thus, prompt treatment is indicated in most patients in whom morphea affects more than the superficial dermis. Either bath PUVA or UVA1 therapy (30–60 J/cm^2) is currently the most promising approach in the authors' opinion and can improve morphea in about 60% of patients. For rapidly progressive disabling disease, weekly methotrexate combined with pulsed, high-dose corticosteroids has recently been advocated by other clinical investigators.

HISTORY

A condition of thickened skin was first mentioned by Hippocrates, the famous physician living on the Greek island of Kos, around 400 BC. The term scleroderma is derived from the Greek words *skleros* (hard or indurated) and *derma* (skin). The first description of a generalized 'hardness' of the skin in a young woman, retrospectively assumed to represent diffuse scleroderma, was by an Italian physician, Carlo Curzio, in 1753. Almost one century passed before new scleroderma-like diseases, some with involvement of internal organs, were reported; in 1847, the French physician Gintrac coined the term 'sclérodermie'[2]. Thomas Addison has been credited with the first detailed report on morphea, which he called Alibert's keloid syndrome, in 1854[3]. In 1924, Matsui[4] described the typical histopathologic changes of scleroderma, including the increase in collagen and thickening of vessel walls in involved skin. O'Leary & Nomland[5] elaborated the distinctive features of systemic sclerosis versus morphea in an extensive clinical study in 1930.

EPIDEMIOLOGY

Even though morphea has been long recognized as a well-defined entity, few population-based studies have been published. One of the best analyses is a survey from Olmsted County, Minnesota, that attempted to register all patients with the disorder from 1960 to 1993[6]. During this period, the incidence, i.e. the number of newly diagnosed patients, was 27 per million inhabitants. The incidence appears to be increasing slightly[1]. According to the Olmsted County study, 56% of patients had plaque-type morphea, 20% linear, 13% generalized and 11% deep morphea.

The prevalence (total number of affected patients per million) increases with age. It is approximately 500 per million at age 18 and 2200 at age 80 years[1]. The disease is more prevalent in women than in men (2.6 to 1), with the exception of linear morphea, which has no gender preference. In the Olmsted County study, morphea was diagnosed in 82 patients, and in 28, the disease started before age 18 years[6]. Data published on the incidence and prevalence of morphea seem to reflect an underestimation, as they critically depend on clinician assessment and include a referral bias. For example, a British pediatric rheumatology unit described a total of 58 children, 16 with linear morphea, 31 with other forms of morphea and 11 with generalized scleroderma[7]. In contrast, a pediatric dermatology center in Warsaw evaluated 301 children with linear morphea and 118 with other types of morphea, but only seven with systemic sclerosis[8].

Morphea is very rarely life-threatening, and in the Olmsted County study, the survival rate of patients with morphea was not significantly different from that of the general population. In 11% of the patients, substantial disability occurred. This is of particular concern since disability occurs primarily with linear morphea, the entity that starts before age 18 in two-thirds of the affected individuals[6].

PATHOGENESIS

Autoantibodies are usually as prevalent in morphea as in the general population, except for the following: (1) an increased prevalence of anti-single strand (ss)DNA, -topoisomerase IIα, -phospholipid, -fibrillin 1 and -histone antibodies in patients with morphea, especially anti-ssDNA antibodies in the linear form and the remainder in generalized (more so than linear) morphea (see Ch. 41); and (2) high titers of antinuclear antibodies (ANA) in juvenile patients with linear morphea

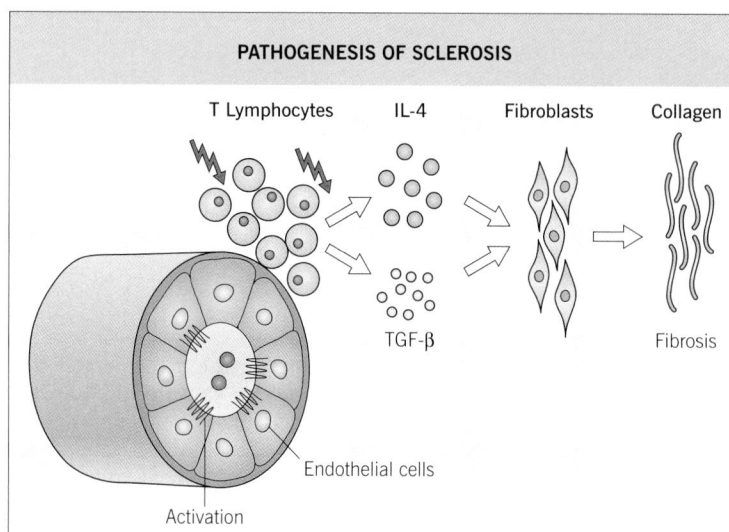

Fig. 96.1 Pathogenesis of sclerosis. Three components are involved during the formation of sclerosis: vascular damage, lymphocyte activation and altered connective tissue production. IL, interleukin; TGF, transforming growth factor.

and individuals with generalized morphea[9]. Neither histology nor immunohistology of a single lesion will distinguish between morphea and systemic sclerosis. In most clinicopathologic reviews, it is assumed that the two diseases are triggered by distinct events. However, the development of sclerosis following the initiating event seems to follow a common pathway. It is therefore assumed here that the pathogenic steps leading to systemic sclerosis also contribute to the development of morphea, so they will be included in this discussion.

Currently, sclerosis of the skin is thought to involve three major, closely connected components: vascular damage, activated T cells and altered connective tissue production by fibroblasts (Fig. 96.1)[10].

Vascular Changes

A prominent feature of advanced sclerosis is a reduction in the number of capillaries. Studies performed in systemic sclerosis suggest that microvascular injury is a very early – and perhaps even the primary – event. Endothelial cell markers such as endothelin-1, soluble vascular cell adhesion molecule-1 (sVCAM-1), soluble E-selectin (sE-selectin), and vascular endothelial growth factor (VEGF) are elevated in the sera of patients with systemic sclerosis[11]. Serum levels of sVCAM-1 and sE-selectin are also higher in localized scleroderma, all these findings indicating endothelial activation[12]. The morphologic changes principally affect capillaries and small arterioles 50–500 μm in diameter. The initial changes include expression of adhesion molecules and endothelial swelling, followed by thickening of the basement membrane and intimal hyperplasia.

Control of Fibroblast Function by T-Cell-Derived Cytokines

Pioneering work by Leroy[13,14] showed that fibroblasts isolated from sclerotic tissue produce increased amounts of collagen (types I, II and III) as well as other extracellular matrix proteins when they are cultured *in vitro*. Importantly, fibroblasts maintain this phenotype for weeks over several passages. This raised the question as to whether scleroderma results from an inborn or an acquired error in collagen metabolism within fibroblasts[15]. Today, most data favor the concept that abnormal collagen production is due to instructions from surrounding cells. T lymphocytes are one group of cells that have at least the capacity to modify collagen synthesis by fibroblasts via the cytokines they secrete. This may be relevant, as T lymphocytes are regularly present, at least in a perivascular location and especially at the leading edge of developing sclerosis (see Fig. 96.1).

Pathologically enhanced production of collagen (types I, II, III) as well as other extracellular matrix proteins is induced by two T-cell-derived cytokines, interleukin-4 (IL-4) and transforming growth factor β (TGF-β). IL-4 is produced by CD4⁺ T lymphocytes (T helper cells)

following differentiation toward a Th2 phenotype (see Ch. 5) and can directly enhance TGF-β production by T cells and other cells[16]. On the other hand, pathologic production of collagen (types I, II, III) and other extracellular matrix proteins can be significantly suppressed by interferon-α (IFN-α) or IFN-γ[17]. IFN-γ is also produced by CD4⁺ T lymphocytes, but only after differentiation toward a Th1 phenotype. CD4⁺ T cells are not a source of IFN-α, but IFN-α is one of the major mediators capable of directing T-cell differentiation toward a Th1 phenotype[16].

CD4⁺ T cells tend to differentiate toward a Th2 phenotype when continuously stimulated through the T-cell receptor (TCR). In T cells stimulated through the TCR, IL-4 itself is the most potent force in driving T-cell differentiation toward a Th2 phenotype. As the Th2 cytokine IL-4 enhances pathologic collagen production by fibroblasts and induces recruitment of eosinophils (which are regularly found in the early inflammatory phase of morphea and systemic sclerosis), it is believed that immune responses dominated by IL-4- and TGF-β-producing cells are critically involved in the development of skin sclerosis. This concept is supported by clinical and experimental data:

1 *In situ* analysis of progressing inflammatory margins of skin sclerosis has revealed predominantly IL-4 expression[18].
2 Early treatment of scleroderma-developing mice with anti-IL-4 antibodies prevented scleroderma[19].
3 Acitretin or isotretinoin can inhibit TGF-β production and consequently reduce pathologic collagen synthesis by fibroblasts. Importantly, preliminary data suggest that both retinoids can improve sclerosis in patients with sclerodermoid GVHD or systemic sclerosis.

Another therapeutic approach to morphea would be to shift from IL-4-dominated Th2 responses to IL-4-deficient, IFN-γ-dominated Th1 responses. A series of placebo-controlled clinical trials that tested the efficacy of IFN-γ or IFN-α in morphea had negative results[20]. As increasing evidence suggests a critical role for these cytokines in the development of sclerosis, it remains unclear whether the type I and II interferons tested were really ineffective. Perhaps establishment of more effective cytokine-based therapies for morphea and possibly systemic sclerosis requires a more detailed understanding of cytokine actions *in vivo*.

Lastly, when scleroderma fibroblasts are compared to control fibroblasts, there are differences in intracellular signaling proteins. Examples include constitutive phosphorylation and activation of p38 mitogen-activated protein kinase (MAPK) in scleroderma fibroblasts as well as higher levels of Ha-Ras protein in association with an elevated production of reactive oxygen species (ROS)[21,22]. The intracellular level and/or activity of these proteins in scleroderma fibroblasts may contribute to collagen production and development of fibrosis. Interestingly, in one study, antibodies to Cu/Zn superoxide dismutase (SOD) were observed in the sera of 89% of patients with localized scleroderma and almost 100% of those with generalized morphea[23]. These autoantibodies may impair SOD activity, resulting in enhanced ROS production, again pointing to the involvement of oxidative stress in the pathogenesis of scleroderma.

Animal Model and Genetics

An animal model used to study pathogenic events in scleroderma is the tight skin (TSK) mouse (Fig. 96.2). It is currently considered to be the best animal model for scleroderma. A partial duplication of the fibrillin 1 gene may be responsible for the increased synthesis and accumulation of collagen in the skin and internal organs of TSK mice. TSK mice not only have increased collagen deposits, but the collagen fibers are reduced in length and amounts of hydroxyproline are increased in the dermis, as is the case in morphea and systemic sclerosis. Moreover, the mice have high antibody titers against topoisomerase I or fibrillin 1, similar to patients with systemic sclerosis or morphea, respectively. One major difference is that vessels remain uninvolved in TSK mice. This does not exclude the possibility that small vessel disease may initiate or contribute to scleroderma in humans, it simply demonstrates that sclerosis of the skin can develop in the presence of apparently normal vessels[24]. The phenotype can be transferred from diseased animals to healthy syngeneic mice via bone marrow cells (see Fig. 96.2).

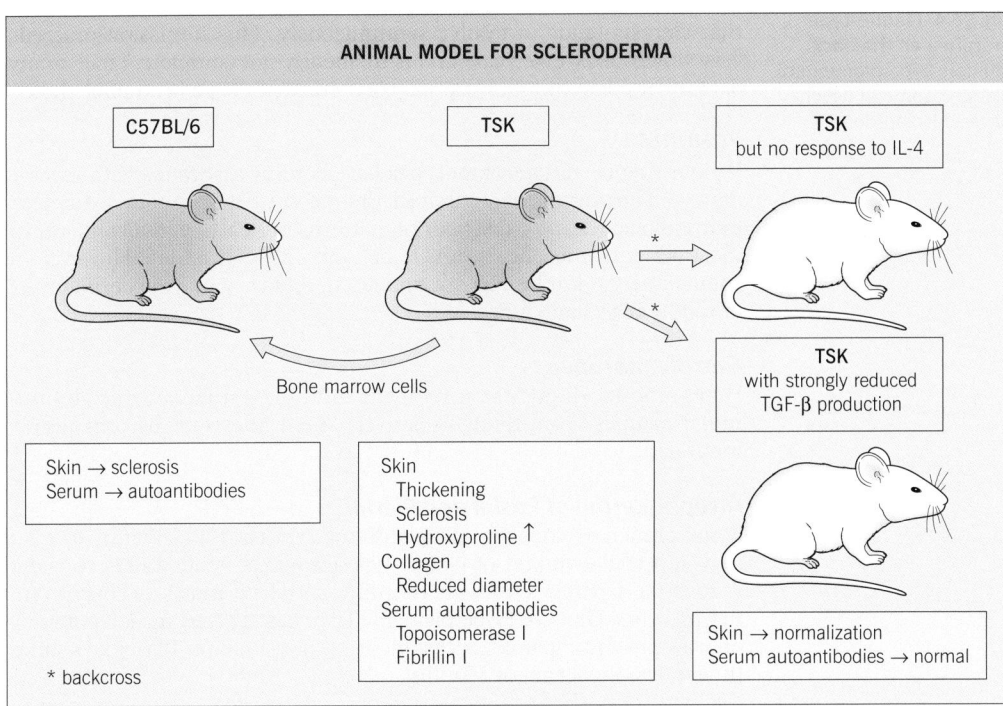

Fig. 96.2 Animal model for scleroderma. Transfer of scleroderma phenotype from diseased animals (TSK mice) to healthy syngeneic mice (C57BL/6) by bone marrow cells. Lack of tight skin and autoantibody production by back-crossing TSK mice with mice that cannot respond to IL-4 or mice that produce minimal amounts of TGF-β. TSK, tight skin strain of mice. IL, interleukin; TGF, transforming growth factor.

Fibroblasts from TSK mice have elevated IL-4 receptor α expression and it has been suggested that IL-4 plays a role in their increased expression of type I collagen[25]. Back-crossing the TSK mice onto a genetic background that either can not respond to IL-4 or is deficient in producing TGF-β prevents skin sclerosis in TSK mice. Moreover, this back-cross normalizes collagen length, skin thickness and hydroxyproline content and prevents antibody formation to topoisomerase I (see Fig. 96.2)[24]. In addition, a promising new therapeutic intervention based upon CpG motifs containing oligodeoxynucleotides (ODN) has been reported. Intramuscular injections of CpG ODN which promoted IL-12 production and Th1 responses while simultaneously suppressing IL-4 production prevented skin fibrosis in TSK mice when administered at a young age[26].

Besides the phenotypic similarities, more recent data have suggested that the genetic locus associated with the TSK phenotype is also associated with the risk of developing scleroderma, at least in Choctaw-Americans and Japanese. Microsatellite markers have shown that the susceptibility locus is on chromosome 15q in a region of 2-cM that contains the fibrillin 1 gene.

Triggering Events

Most immunologic (cytokine regulation) and metabolic (altered collagen synthesis) studies were designed to understand systemic sclerosis, and the question remains as to whether they can also explain focal, asymmetric inflammation and sclerosis of the skin. The major discriminating factor between morphea and systemic sclerosis might be the triggering event, with morphea caused by a local trigger within the skin, and systemic sclerosis initiated by some general trauma, such as physical stress to the blood vessels during rapid temperature changes.

These questions initiated the search for potential triggers and studies of diseases that share clinical features with morphea and scleroderma. One intensively investigated area was the potential role of infection with *Borrelia burgdorferi* or related pathogenic species. Arguments in favor of an association were that morphea progresses with an erythematous ring similar to erythema migrans following *B. burgdorferi* infection, and that morphea may improve with penicillin therapy. The isolation of *B. burgdorferi* from the urine or the skin of some selected patients with morphea originally supported this speculation[27,28]. Moreover, some groups identified mRNA specific for *Borrelia* species in morphea. However, larger studies by several groups from different countries found that morphea lesions normally do not contain mRNA for *B. burgdorferi* or related strains and the prevalence of antibodies against *B. burgdorferi* is similar in patients with and without morphea[29,30].

CLINICAL FEATURES

Morphea can be subdivided into four major entities: plaque morphea, linear morphea, generalized (disabling) morphea, and inflammatory syndromes leading to superficial or deep sclerosis of the skin that resembles morphea (i.e. morpheaform). Importantly, patients do not have Raynaud's phenomenon or involvement of internal organs, except underlying muscle, fascia and bone involvement in linear morphea. In rare patients, clinically insignificant fibrosis of the lung or slightly reduced esophageal motility is detectable radiographically or by scintigraphy. Clinically relevant involvement of internal organs is only observed in certain types of pseudoscleroderma (see Ch. 44).

Clinical Manifestations

Plaque-type morphea is the most frequent variant. The classical lesion starts insidiously as a slightly elevated erythematous or violaceous, somewhat edematous plaque that undergoes centrifugal expansion (Fig. 96.3). It is generally asymptomatic and therefore frequently goes unnoticed by the patient. The central part of the progressing lesion starts to transform into sclerotic, scar-like tissue. Depending on the depth of the sclerosis, the skin becomes progressively indurated. Centrally, it can acquire a shiny white color, and peripherally, a violaceous or

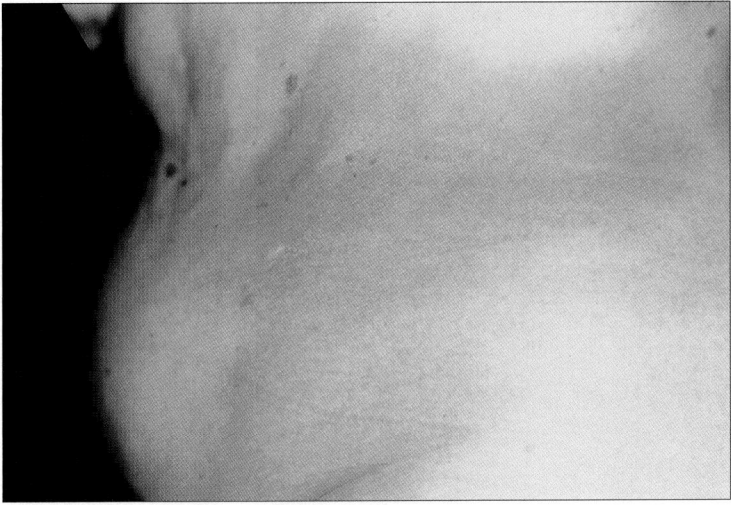

Fig. 96.3 Early inflammatory plaque-type morphea of the trunk. Early stage lesion presenting as an erythematous edematous plaque.

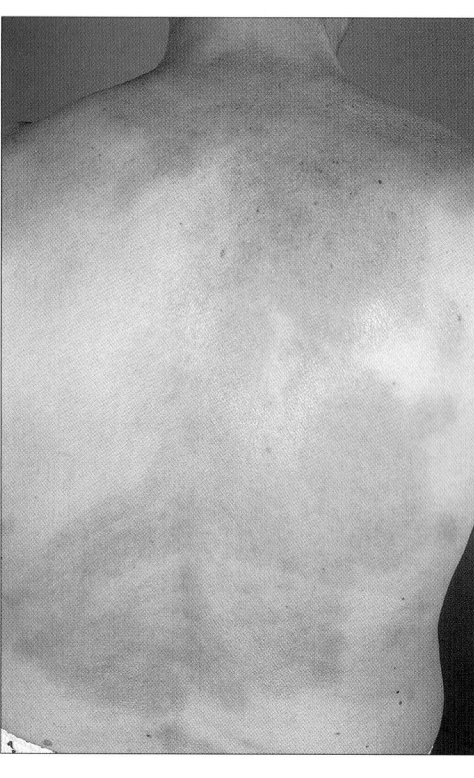

Fig. 96.4 Plaque-type morphea on the back. Multiple hyperpigmented plaques, some of which have a lilac border.

the sclerosis tends to resolve spontaneously. This remission proceeds very slowly, may take years and is frequently not complete. Since many patients are lost to follow-up, no clear statistics have been published.

Variants

Various manifestations of morphea have become associated with specific names. They do not really reflect unique entities, but rather different morphologic features, distribution patterns or depth of involvement. In most patients, morphea seems to be randomly distributed. However, in some patients, the lesions are unilateral, and they may be dermatomal or follow Blaschko's lines.

Guttate morphea

Here, morphea presents primarily as multiple, rather superficial nummular plaques. Even though relatively small, they may become deeply indurated.

Atrophoderma of Pasini and Pierini

Some clinicians consider atrophoderma of Pasini and Pierini to be a very superficial variant of plaque-type morphea, while others consider it to be a separate entity in the differential diagnosis of 'burnt-out' morphea (see Ch. 99). Hyperpigmented patches are seen most commonly on the posterior trunk; occasionally, lesions follow Blaschko's lines (linear atrophoderma of Moulin).

Deep morphea

This variant, also known as 'solitary morphea profunda', reflects a sclerosing inflammation that affects mainly the deep dermis and subcutaneous fat and may even involve underlying structures (e.g. the fascia) (Fig. 96.5). Patients normally develop a single or few hard plaques of the deep tissue that may impair the motility of the skin; ultimately, lesions may calcify leading to deep osteoma cutis[31]. Because of the location of the sclerosis, individual lesions can share some clinical features with eosinophilic fasciitis.

Nodular or keloid morphea

Here, the inflammation of the dermis leads to thick, keloid-like nodules (Fig. 96.6) or streaks, clinically indistinguishable from indurated keloids.

Bullous morphea

In some patients, especially those where sclerosis of the skin is associated with diffuse, rapidly progressive edema, lymphoceles may result

'lilac' ring. Postinflammatory hyperpigmentation often dominates over the white sclerosis (Fig. 96.4).

Skin structures such as hairs and sweat glands are frequently lost. Some patients complain of itch, but it is often a consequence of the associated 'xeroderma' rather than a genuine manifestation of morphea. Once the 'lilac' ring vanishes, the lesion's progression also halts; the progressing margin may be difficult to appreciate, especially in linear sclerosis.

The plaques of morphea are usually between 2 and 15 cm in diameter, multiple and asymmetric, but there is marked variation. Lesions may enlarge significantly or remain stable in size (see Figs 96.3 & 96.4). The trunk is a common location for this variant.

The course of morphea is variable. In most patients, morphea progresses over 3–5 years and then arrests. Rarely, patients have relapsing disease for more than 5 years. At the end of the progression,

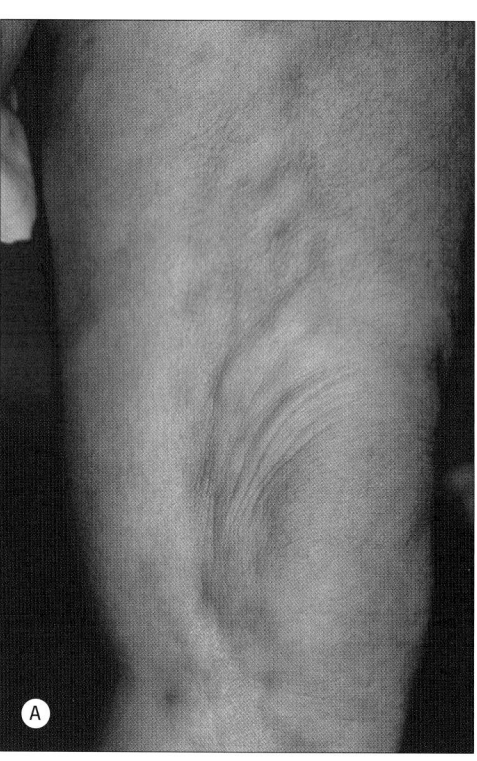

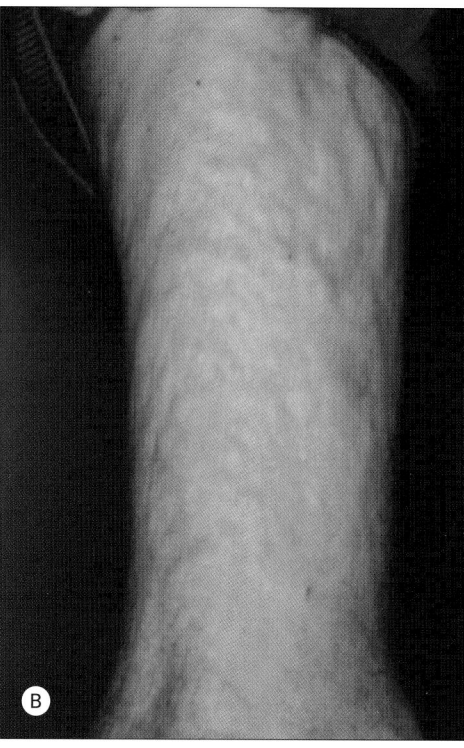

Fig. 96.5 Comparison of deep morphea and eosinophilic fasciitis. A Note the 'pseudo-cellulite' appearance of the involved skin of the thigh in deep morphea. **B** In eosinophilic fasciitis, the level of fibrosis is also deep, resulting in a similar clinical appearance.

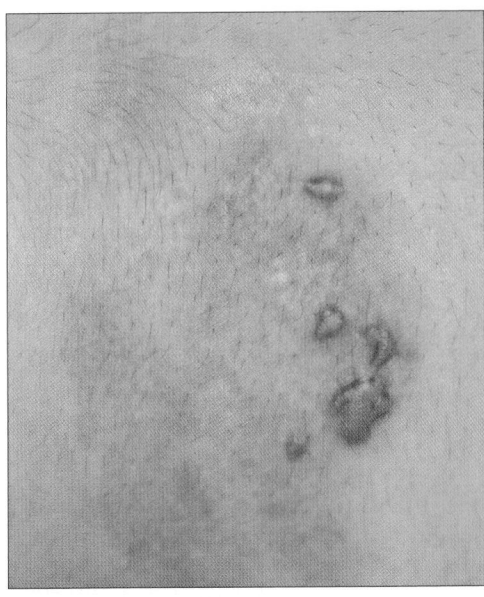

Fig. 96.6 Keloid morphea. Elevated, firm pink papulonodules arising within an area of hyperpigmented induration. Courtesy of Jean L Bolognia MD.

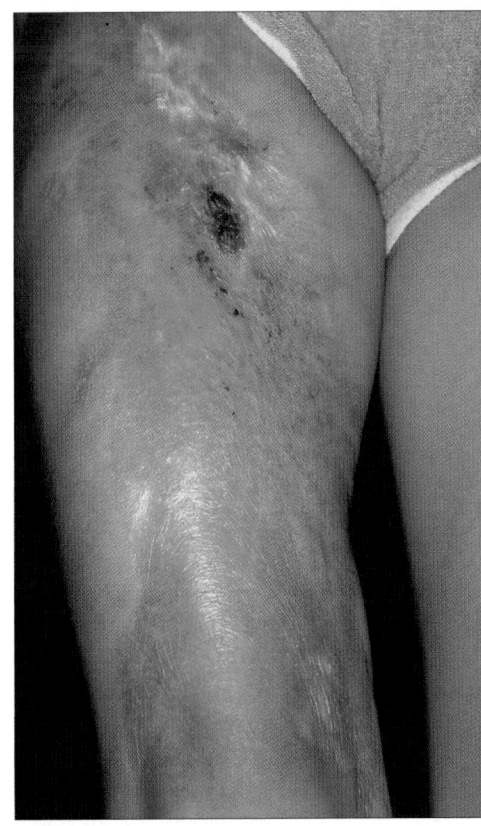

Fig. 96.8 Linear morphea of the leg. The differential diagnosis includes linear melorheostosis which is associated with underlying candlewax-like linear hyperostosis.

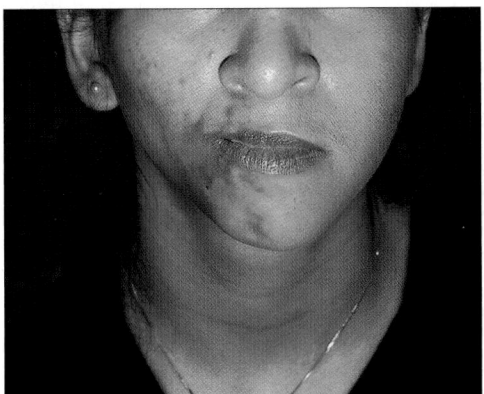

Fig. 96.7 Parry–Romberg syndrome. Hyperpigmentation and loss of subcutaneous tissue is seen, leading to facial asymmetry. Courtesy of Ronald P Rapini MD.

from stasis of lymphatic fluid and may appear as bullae. This is rarely a feature of plaque-type morphea. It seems to be more frequent in generalized, disabling morphea or sclerodermoid GVHD. Bullous morphea has to be separated from mechanical blisters that may occur in the central scar and are secondary to impaired mechanical stability of the dermal–epidermal junction.

Linear Morphea and Parry–Romberg Syndrome

Linear morphea is different from plaque morphea, with respect to age of onset, distribution, clinical outcome and serologies. Morphea *en coup de sabre* (sabre hit) is linear morphea of the forehead. Hemifacial atrophy, or Parry–Romberg syndrome, is probably a very severe variant of linear morphea, but it may be a separate entity (Fig. 96.7). It shows little or no sclerosis and may affect the entire distribution of the trigeminal nerve, including the eye and the tongue. One distinct aspect of linear morphea is the frequent association with high titers of ANA, including in children (see above). The reason remains enigmatic, as the histology or biochemical analysis of an individual lesion is indistinguishable from that of classical plaque morphea.

Linear morphea may present initially as a linear erythematous, inflammatory streak, but more frequently it begins as a harmless-appearing lesion of plaque-type morphea that extends longitudinally as a series of plaques that join to form a scar-like band that may severely impair the mobility of the affected limb (Fig. 96.8). Linear morphea tends to involve the underlying fascia, muscle and tendons. This leads not only to muscle weakness but also to a shortening of the muscles and fascia that impairs joint motility. Linear morphea is especially dangerous when extending over joints, as this almost invariably results in disabling joint immobilization. In some patients, involvement is somewhat circular rather than linear and results in progressive atrophy of the limb similar to the Parry–Romberg variant of facial morphea.

The *en coup de sabre* type of morphea represents linear morphea of the head. It is normally unilateral and extends from the forehead into the frontal scalp. It may start either as a linear streak or as a row of small plaques that coalesce. A paramedian location is more common than a median location. Like plaque morphea, it may initially be surrounded by a discrete lilac ring that extends longitudinally and may reach the eyebrows, nose and even the cheeks. The waning inflammation leaves a linear, hairless crevice that in some patients is more sclerotic, while in others is more atrophic (Fig. 96.9).

En coup de sabre morphea can also involve the underlying muscles and osseous structures. Rarely, the inflammation and sclerosis progress to involve the meninges and even the brain, creating a potential focus for seizures. Alternatively, very slowly progressing inflammation, indistinguishable from the inflammatory process of linear morphea, leads to gradual involution of the skin, fatty tissues and underlying bones.

Generalized or Disabling Morphea

Rarely, plaque morphea is rapidly progressive, where multiple enlarging plaques appear simultaneously and coalesce until they involve nearly the entire integument. Rather, this variant normally begins insidiously on the trunk as plaque morphea. A single lesion is indistinguishable from classical plaque morphea, except it does not stop expanding. Just as in the central form of systemic sclerosis, the plaques rapidly coalesce and affect the entire trunk, often only sparing the nipples. The sclerosis may involve the extremities down to the hands (presenting initially as puffy edema). Progressive sclerosis of the skin may result in disabling constrictions that even cause difficulty in breathing due to impaired thorax mobility and inflammation of the intercostal muscles. Although an aggressive therapeutic approach is recommended, the disease is usually persistent given its often limited response.

Morphea in Childhood

About 20% of those with morphea are children and teenagers[32]. The female to male ratio in juvenile localized scleroderma is about 2:1, with a mean age of disease onset of 7 years[33]. Linear morphea is more of a problem, as two-thirds of the patients with this variant are younger than 18 years when it develops. Also, in young children and adolescents, linear morphea often leads to growth retardation in the affected limb. Thus, if left untreated, linear morphea may result not only in stiff joints but also in permanent limb asymmetry from unilateral hypoplasia (Fig. 96.10). Linear morphea that is indistinguishable from the

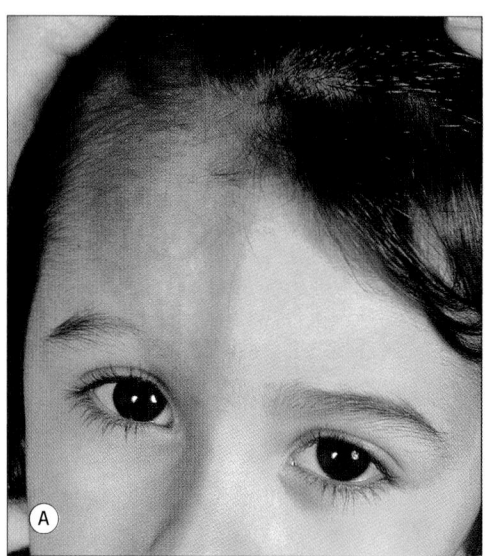

Fig. 96.9 Morphea en coup de sabre. Paramedian depressions (**A**) are more common than midline involvement (**B**).

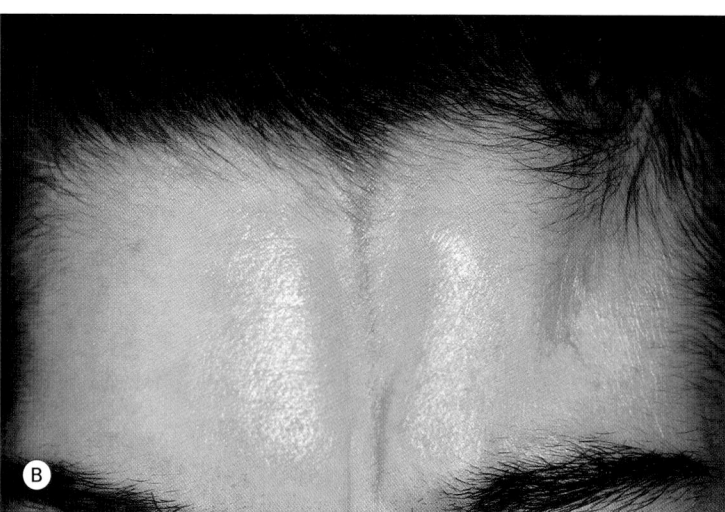

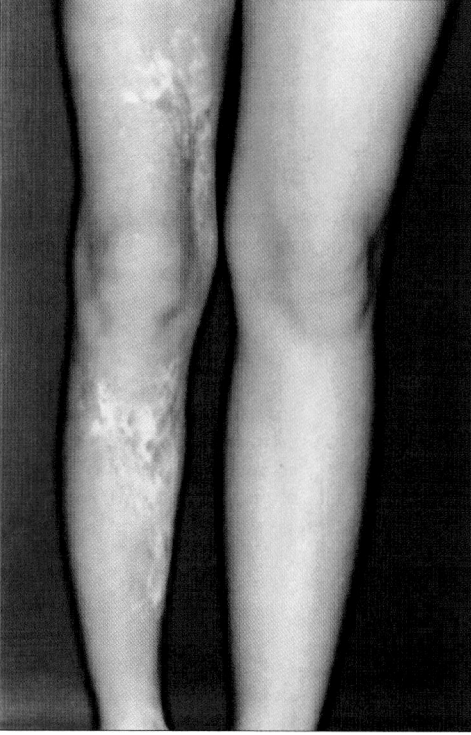

Fig. 96.10 Linear morphea of the leg in a child. Unilateral hypoplasia as a result of untreated linear morphea.

lying muscles and contractures of the involved joints. The disease tends to extend from the trunk to the hands and feet. Periodontal atrophy may occur, but there is only slight involvement of the esophagus and lung.

Importantly, in a large multicenter study of children with morphea (n=750, 85% of whom had linear morphea or Parry–Romberg syndrome), 22% had extracutaneous findings that were primarily articular (11%), neurologic (4%) and ocular (2%)[33]. Neurologic and ocular involvement were observed primarily in those with linear scleroderma of the scalp and face or Parry–Romberg syndrome.

LABORATORY FINDINGS

Laboratory abnormalities are not a prominent feature of morphea, except for generalized and linear morphea. The ESR and serum protein levels are usually normal, but eosinophilia may occur, especially during early active phases of the disease. The presence of ANA or antibodies to ssDNA and histones are unusual in patients with plaque-type morphea. They are more frequent in linear and generalized morphea, where ANA can be found in high titers in 40–80% of patients[34,35]. About 40% of children and adolescents with localized scleroderma (linear and deep forms more so than plaque or generalized types) have elevated ANA titers[33,36]. In addition to the markers of inflammation, procollagen type 1 carboxy-terminal propeptide is elevated in about 30% of patients; the serum levels have correlated with the extent of the skin involvement[37].

PATHOLOGY

The histology of scleroderma depends on two factors: the stage of the disease (early inflammatory margin or central sclerosis) and the depth to which the disease extends. In most situations, morphologic changes are best seen at the border between the dermis and subcutaneous fat. Specimens for histology must include subcutaneous fat and it is important to note whether the biopsy is taken from the inflammatory border or from the fibrotic center (Fig. 96.11).

At the inflammatory border, vascular changes are relatively discrete by light microscopy. Vessel walls show endothelial swelling and edema. Capillaries and small arterioles are surrounded by an infiltrate that contains primarily CD4+ T cells and sometimes eosinophils, plasma cells and mast cells (see Fig. 96.11).

In later stages, the inflammatory infiltrate wanes and ultimately disappears completely, except in some areas of the subcutaneous fat. The epidermis is basically normal in appearance, but the rete ridges may be diminished, leaving a flattened dermal–epidermal junction. Edema is no longer visible in the dermis and upper subcutis. Capillaries and small vessels are significantly reduced in number, and homogeneous collagen bundles with decreased space between the bundles replace most structures. At this stage, collagen bundles in the reticular dermis appear densely packed, as evidenced by a more intense eosinophilic staining, and are aligned parallel to the dermal–epidermal junction. Eccrine glands appear atrophic, and lonely sweat ducts transverse the thickened dermis. The underlying subcutis is homogenized and hyalinized.

Morphea profunda affects primarily the deep subcutaneous tissue. Following the inflammatory phase, extensive sclerosis and hyalinization extend into the underlying fascia. Involvement of the underlying fascia is obligatory in deep morphea and is also frequently observed in linear and generalized types of morphea. In these patients, the fascia and even the underlying muscles (frequently vacuolated) are involved in the process of progressive sclerosis, characterized by replacement of the differentiated tissue by collagen bundles.

MORPHEAFORM (AND SCLERODERMOID) INFLAMMATORY SYNDROMES

Some entities (e.g. sclerosis secondary to exposure to bleomycin, vinyl chloride or epoxy resin) that are characterized by acrosclerosis and Raynaud's phenomenon have a clinical presentation similar to scleroderma (i.e. sclerodermoid or pseudoscleroderma), while others present with circumscribed plaques similar to morphea (i.e. morpheaform). The former are discussed in Chapter 44 and the latter are discussed

idiopathic variant can also follow allogeneic hematopoietic stem cell transplantation.

Disabling pansclerotic morphea of children is similar to generalized morphea of the adult. It usually starts before age 14 years and tends to cause lifelong severe disability due to persistent atrophy of the under-

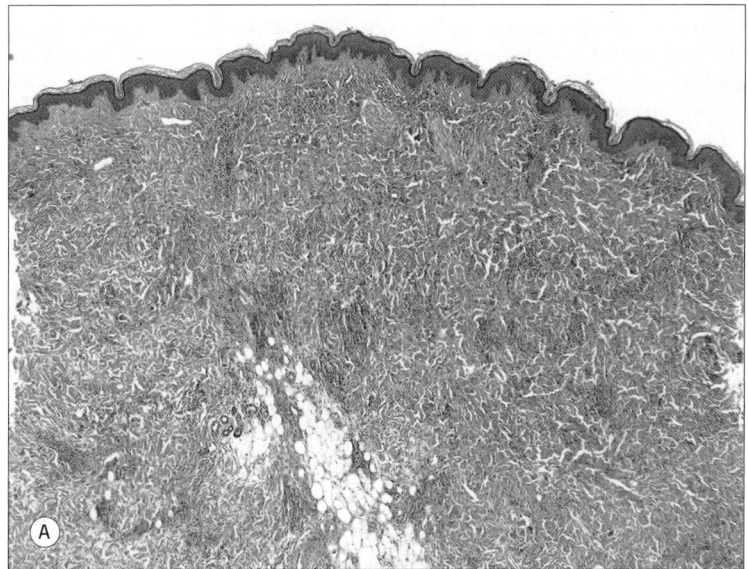

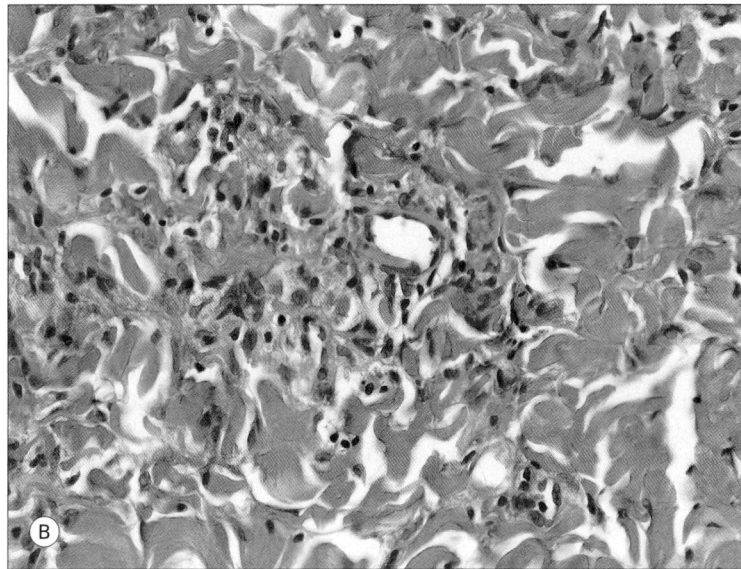

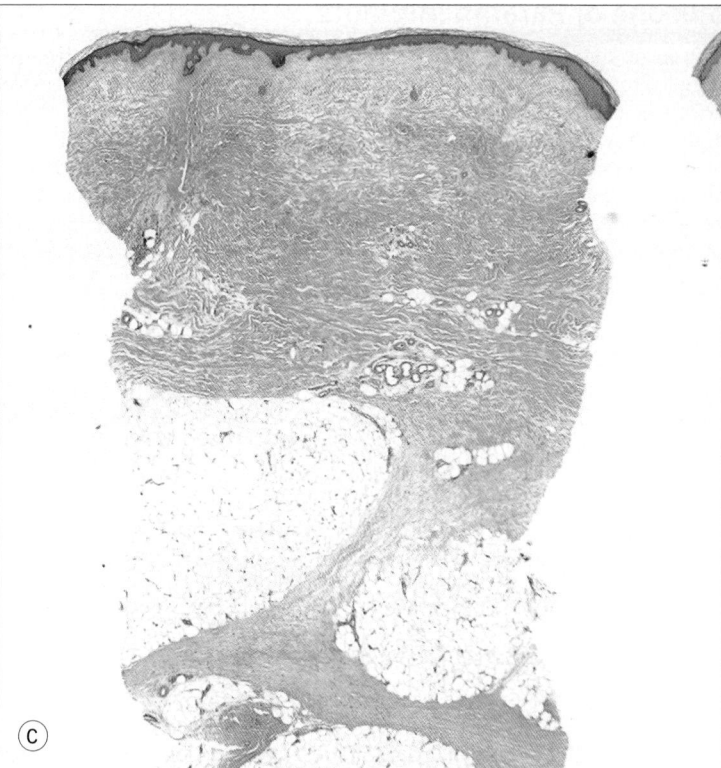

Fig. 96.11 Histology of morphea. Overview (**A**) with thickening of the dermis and perivascular infiltrates of lymphocytes and plasma cells (**B**). **C** Advanced sclerosis of the entire dermis extending into the fat with thickened collagen bundles and 'trapped' eccrine glands.

DIFFERENTIAL DIAGNOSIS OF MORPHEAFORM SKIN LESIONS
Morphea (plaque-type, linear, generalized* or deep*)
Chronic graft-versus-host disease*
Lichen sclerosus (may coexist with morphea)
Lipodermatosclerosis*
Sclerosis at injection sites[†]
• Vitamin K₁ (Texier's disease) or vitamin B₁₂
• Silicone or paraffin implants
• Interferon-β
• Glatiramer
• Enfuvirtide
• Bleomycin (intralesional therapy)
• Opioids (e.g. pentazocine, ketobemidone, methadone)
Chemical/toxin exposures
• Aromatic/chlorinated hydrocarbons (e.g. benzene or toluene at sites of contact with skin)*
• Nephrogenic systemic fibrosis (possibly induced by gadolinium)*
• Toxic oil syndrome (historical)*
Radiation-induced morphea
Porphyria (porphyria cutanea tarda, hepatoerythropoietic porphyria, congenital erythropoietic porphyria)
Muckle–Wells syndrome
Winchester syndrome*
Asymmetric childhood scleredema/stiff skin syndrome*
Linear melorheostosis
Reflex sympathetic dystrophy*
Morpheaform sarcoidosis
Cutaneous metastases (e.g. carcinoma *en cuirasse*)

*Can overlap with sclerodermoid disorders, which are outlined in Table 44.6; in particular, deep morphea and eosinophilic fasciitis may have a similar appearance.
[†] Systemic medications for which there have been reports of an association with morpheaform lesions include bleomycin, bromocriptine, ethosuximide, valproic acid, appetite suppressants and penicillamine.

Table 96.1 Differential diagnosis of morpheaform skin lesions.

below and presented in Table 96.1. There are also clinical disorders that may have either type of clinical presentation, such as toxic oil syndrome. Confusion arises when the term sclerodermoid is used to describe circumscribed plaques, as is often done in GVHD.

While a variety of inflammatory diseases ultimately lead to superficial or deep sclerosis of the skin, their exact relationship to morphea is enigmatic. Some of these diseases are preceded by or associated with eosinophilia in blood or tissue. Infiltration by eosinophils may be of unknown etiology, as in eosinophilic fasciitis, or it may reflect an immune reaction to a defined toxic insult or antigenic stimulus, as in the L-tryptophan syndrome (eosinophilia myalgia syndrome), toxic oil syndrome, or GVHD following hematopoietic stem cell transplantation. Lastly, since certain exogenous drugs or chemicals, endogenous metabolites or X-ray irradiation induce sclerosis at the site of tissue injury in only a subset of individuals, this suggests that unique metabolic events and innate or adaptive immune responses to these compounds determine the individual's susceptibility to develop sclerosis.

Chronic Venous Insufficiency

Chronic venous insufficiency that persists for many years leads to sclerosis in association with chronic hypoxia. Lipodermatosclerosis (hypodermitis sclerodermiformis) is discussed in Chapter 100. Induration often begins above the medial malleolus and, over time, may extend both proximally and circumferentially, eventually leading to an 'inverted wine bottle' configuration. Lipodermatosclerosis may also involve the pannus.

Vitamin K₁ Injections (Texier's Disease)

Injection of oil-soluble vitamin K₁ rarely causes a strictly localized, deep eosinophilic fasciitis that is indistinguishable from morphea profunda[38]. It may ultimately resolve with atrophy of the dermis and/or subcutis.

Silicone or Paraffin Implants

It is suspected that injection of silicone or liquid paraffin in reconstructive surgery may cause chronic inflammation that results in morphea-like sclerosis at the site of injection[39]. The belief that these substances can cause more generalized inflammation and trigger systemic diseases such as systemic sclerosis, eosinophilic fasciitis or mixed connective tissue disease was not substantiated when meta-analyses were performed[40]. Despite this, the debate continues as to whether or not systemic disease occurring after silicone injections or leaky silicone implants simply reflects coincidence[41].

Porphyrias

Porphyria cutanea tarda can lead to morphea-like sclerosis in UV-exposed sites, such as the face, hairless scalp, dorsal aspects of the hands, and the upper chest (see Ch. 49). Histology and electron microscopy findings may resemble morphea except for the presence of PAS-positive deposits around dermal blood vessels. It remains unanswered as to whether the sclerosis is the consequence of chronic UV-induced damage or whether increased levels of uroporphyrins or mast cell-derived products stimulate exaggerated collagen synthesis[42].

Radiation-Induced Morphea

Radiation-induced morphea is characterized by marked sclerosis, erythema and pigmentary changes occurring within the radiation field or even beyond it. The incidence of radiation-induced morphea is about 1 in 500 patients and it is seen primarily in patients treated for breast carcinoma. Predictive risk factors for the development of radiation-induced morphea are unknown and disease onset can occur even several years after radiation therapy. In addition to the changes of radiation dermatitis, histopathology demonstrates perivascular and subcutaneous inflammation together with dermal fibrosis and collagen deposition.

Graft-versus-Host Disease

The incidence of chronic GVHD, a major long-term side effect of allogeneic hematopoietic stem cell transplantation, is still high and occurs in at least half of transplanted patients. The skin is frequently involved in both acute and chronic GVHD, and the clinical spectrum of GVHD is reviewed in Chapter 12. Chronic cutaneous GVHD may resemble lichen planus, morphea, eosinophilic fasciitis or lichen sclerosus[43], but not systemic sclerosis. However, the latter three presentations have been grouped under the heading 'sclerodermoid'. In the past, sclerodermoid GVHD was usually preceded by lichenoid GVHD, but nowadays, because of rapid reductions in immunosuppression and the use of donor lymphocyte infusions (to induce graft-versus-tumor effects in patients with recurrent disease), sclerodermoid GVHD may appear *de novo*.

All variants of morphea can develop: plaque-type, linear or generalized that nearly encases the entire patient. As in idiopathic morphea, the nipples are normally spared. Progressive disease can lead to lymphedema that may even cause bullae which give rise to poorly healing ulcers. If left untreated, isolated plaques can increase in number and become confluent, and patients may become severely handicapped due to almost complete immobilization[44]. Chronic GVHD can also present with a clinical picture nearly identical to eosinophilic fasciitis[45], and the diagnosis can be established by MRI without a need to perform a fascial biopsy.

DIFFERENTIAL DIAGNOSIS

In addition to the other morpheaform and sclerodermoid conditions discussed above, the most important entity in the differential diagnosis is systemic sclerosis (see Ch. 44). Absence of Raynaud's phenomenon and lung or esophageal involvement is characteristic of morphea. The other common considerations are lichen sclerosus and keloids; however, the former can coexist with morphea. Dupuytren's contracture and camptodactyly, a benign ulnar deviation of the fourth and fifth finger, can be clinically distinguished from linear morphea[46].

Scleredema leads to diffuse woody induration of the upper back and neck. Symmetric tightness and induration of acral sites can be seen in insulin-dependent diabetes with cheiroarthropathy, also referred to as waxy skin and stiff joints[47]. In children, progeria and premature aging syndromes need to be distinguished from Parry–Romberg syndrome, but the latter is unilateral. Additional entities in the sclerodermoid differential diagnosis (e.g. scleromyxedema and nephrogenic systemic fibrosis) are listed in Table 44.6.

LICHEN SCLEROSUS

Synonyms: ■ Lichen sclerosus et atrophicus ■ Kraurosis vulvae ■ Balanitis xerotica obliterans (lichen sclerosus of the penis)

Key features

- Sclerotic white plaques with epidermal atrophy and, in extramucosal sites, follicular plugging
- Most commonly affects female or male genitalia, less often non-genital skin
- May cause scarring of the vaginal introitus or phimosis
- Severe pruritus may occur
- No systemic manifestations

INTRODUCTION

Lichen sclerosus is a clinically distinct inflammatory disease primarily of the superficial dermis that leads to white scar-like atrophy. In non-genital skin, lichen sclerosus may itch and be cosmetically disturbing. Genital lichen sclerosus causes both dryness and severe, persistent pruritus, and it often leads to progressive atrophy and functional impairment. Phimosis and scarring of the vaginal introitus are the most frequent complications.

HISTORY

Francois Henri Hallopeau's report on a 'lichen plan atrophique' in 1887 is considered to be the first description of lichen sclerosus. The typical histopathologic changes of lichen sclerosus et atrophicus were published by Ferdinand Jean Darier in 1892[48]. Unna, Westberg, von Zumbusch and others elucidated the clinical features of lichen sclerosus in various case reports[49–51]. This contributed to the panoply of terms, such as white spot disease or lichen albus, an aspect that complicates any literature survey. Lichen sclerosus in the genital area was first described in women by Breisky as kraurosis vulvae[52]. Forty years later, lichen sclerosus of the glans penis was described by Stühmer as balanitis xerotica obliterans[53]. Today, lichen sclerosus, the term proposed by the International Society for the Study of Vulvar Disease, is most frequently used[54,55].

EPIDEMIOLOGY

Lichen sclerosus is relatively uncommon, even though the exact prevalence is unknown. It occurs at all ages, seems to be similar in all races, and is said to be more common in women than in men, but the reported female to male ratio varies widely among the different studies (from 10:1 to 1:1)[54,55].

In both sexes, the anogenital area is affected in at least 85% of the patients. However, the best epidemiologic studies concentrate on vulvar disease, and the extragenital manifestations of the disease have not always been evaluated. Since lichen sclerosus of non-genital skin frequently causes no symptoms, it is likely that the prevalence of extragenital lichen sclerosus is underestimated.

Prospective and retrospective studies in adult patients suggest that lichen sclerosus is one of the most common causes of symptomatic vulvar disease. Lichen sclerosus was the second most common diagnosis in an Australian study (13% of 141 consecutive patients)[56] and lichen sclerosus was diagnosed in 19.2% of 500 patients during a 5-year period in a New York vulvar clinic[57]. In women, the peak incidence is during the fifth and sixth decades. The second peak in female patients occurs in girls between 8 and 13 years of age. Among prepubertal girls with vulvar disease, the relative frequency of lichen sclerosus is similar to that in adults (18% of 130 prepubertal girls)[58]. Extragenital lichen sclerosus is rare in children. In boys and men, lichen sclerosus frequently leads to phimosis and was diagnosed in 14 of 100 prepubertal boys undergoing circumcision for phimosis[59]. Similar data were reported from a London dermatology department, where 52 of 357 male patients with genital skin disease had lichen sclerosus[60].

PATHOGENESIS

As in most inflammatory diseases, genetic predisposition contributes to the development of lichen sclerosus, as it may be found in monozygotic or non-identical twins. In addition, association with the MHC class II antigen HLA-DQ7 was observed in a relatively large study[61]. The existence of a susceptibility gene for sclerosis in this region of the MHC is underlined by the finding that the same region is associated with an increased risk of autoimmune diseases[62]. Even though inflammation seems essential for initiation and progression of lichen sclerosus, the mechanisms leading to subsequent sclerosis remain speculative.

Perhaps with the exception of autoantibodies against extracellular matrix protein 1 (ECM-1), no specific immunologic parameters have been identified in patients' sera that clearly correlate with either risk of disease or disease activity. IgG autoantibodies against ECM-1 are found in 80% of patients with lichen sclerosus and the latter may act as autoantigen[63]. Even though there is no correlation with extent of disease, detection of such antibodies may be helpful for diagnosis. Oxidative stress may play a role in the pathogenesis of lichen sclerosus, based upon analysis of lesional skin that showed lipid peroxidation of epidermal basal cell layers, oxidative DNA damage and oxidative protein damage[64].

CLINICAL FEATURES

Lichen sclerosus is a disease that can affect both the extragenital skin and the anogenital region. Lichen sclerosus of the oral cavity, the palms or soles is rare. In the oral mucosa, bluish white papules up to 5 mm in diameter may occur on the buccal mucosa or under the tongue. They can lead to superficial scar-like atrophy or erosions.

Extragenital lichen sclerosus normally does not cause symptoms except for dryness and associated pruritus. The lesions occur primarily on the trunk and the proximal extremities. Predilection sites include the neck (Fig. 96.12), shoulders, flexor surfaces of the wrists, and sites of physical trauma or continuous pressure (e.g. the shoulder or hip). The periorbital area and scalp are rarely affected.

It is unusual to see extragenital disease during its early phases when single lesions begin as polygonal, bluish white, shiny, slightly elevated, interfollicular papules. Papules may coalesce into patches or large plaques. Within weeks, they develop the scar-like atrophy.

Most patients present with slightly sclerotic, white scar-like lesions that are guttate, aggregated or coalescent into a shiny, livid to ivory, relatively soft scar with a wrinkled surface. At sites of continuous pressure, a very superficial parchment-like sclerotic scar and skin atrophy may develop.

In more advanced stages, telangiectasias or follicular plugging can be seen (Fig. 96.13A). The flattened interface of the epidermis and dermis results in fragility of the dermal–epidermal junction; therefore, lichen sclerosus is occasionally complicated by the occurrence of bullae that tend to become hemorrhagic (Fig. 96.13B).

In women, the vulva and the perianal region are commonly involved. Although the disease may be symptom-free, it frequently causes severe pruritus and soreness. These symptoms may be considerable and lead to dysuria, dyspareunia, or pain upon defecation (often manifesting as constipation in children). Lichen sclerosus begins as a slightly elevated, sharply demarcated area of erythema, which can be slightly eroded

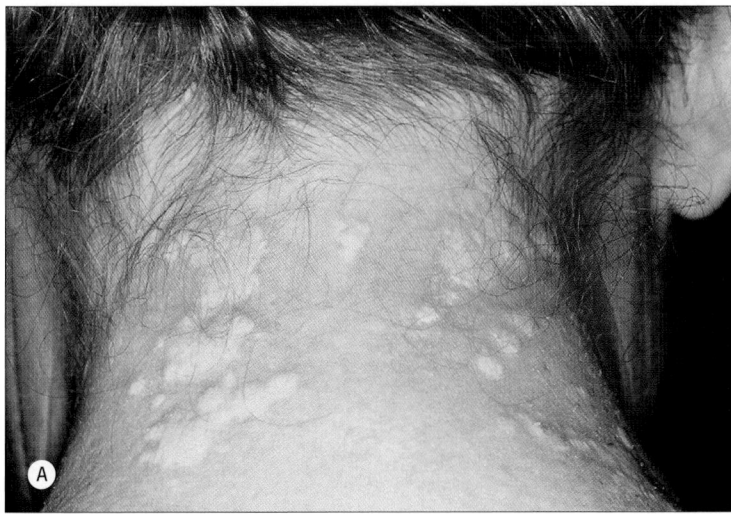
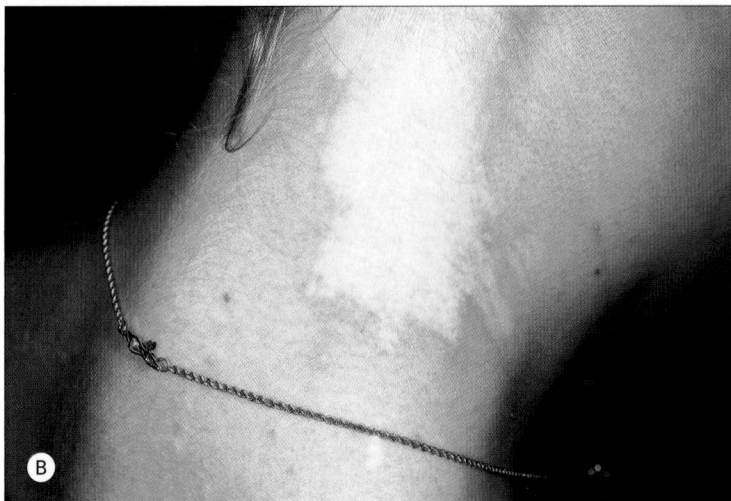

Fig. 96.12 **Lichen sclerosus of the neck.** Papules and small plaques (**A**) versus a large coalescent plaque (**B**).

(Fig. 96.14). The area evolves into a dry, hypopigmented sclerotic lesion. Atrophy may not only affect the epidermis, but can lead to severe shrinkage of the labia majora and especially labia minora and clitoris. In extreme cases, obliteration of the vulva occurs. Sexual intercourse can become impossible. In women, genital lichen sclerosus frequently presents as a lesion that encircles both the perianal region and the genitalia (figure-of-eight configuration).

In the beginning, genital lichen sclerosus may present with a bruised, bluish color resembling post-traumatic hemorrhage. In girls, the bruised appearance and erosions of lichen sclerosus may be misdiagnosed as sexual abuse. Careful examination, perhaps with confirmation of the diagnosis by histology, is mandatory. They can coexist and sexual abuse may (although rarely) trigger the onset of lichen sclerosus as a Koebner phenomenon. False accusations can be as problematic or traumatic to the child and family as overlooking child abuse.

In boys and men, acquired phimosis or recurrent balanitis are the presenting features, and perianal involvement is very rare. Itching and soreness are common. On the glans and the inner aspect of the foreskin, lichen sclerosus starts as sharply demarcated, sometimes slightly bluish erythematous lesions, occasionally with erosions. This inflammation tends to evolve into an atrophic white sclerotic scar (Fig. 96.15). The constriction may cause pain on erection and, at advanced stages, dysuria and urinary obstruction. If the foreskin is affected, lichen sclerosus invariably leads to phimosis with the risk of paraphimosis, which may lead to almost complete occlusion of the glans. Many boys and men first present when the phimosis impairs repositioning of the foreskin; in these situations, diagnosis depends on histology. Progressive disease can be associated with poorly healing ulcers of the glans. Recurrence of lichen sclerosus commonly occurs at the site of a circumcision.

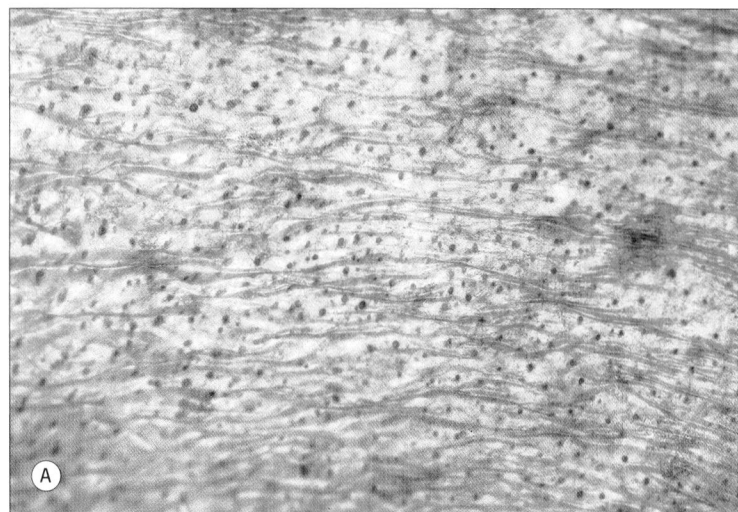

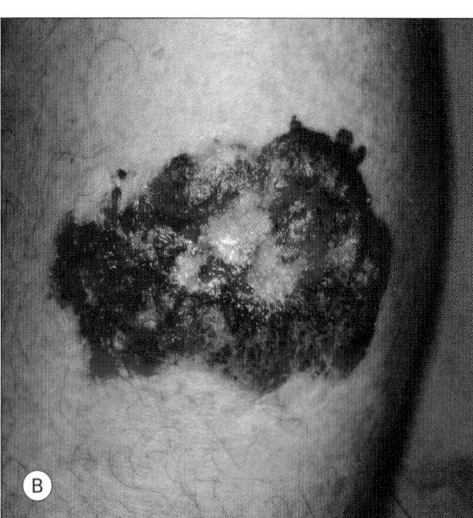

Fig. 96.13 Lichen sclerosus. Follicular plugging in a plaque of lichen sclerosus on the back of a patient with chronic GVHD (**A**). Hemorrhagic bullae on the leg (**B**). **A** Courtesy of Jean L Bolognia M.D.

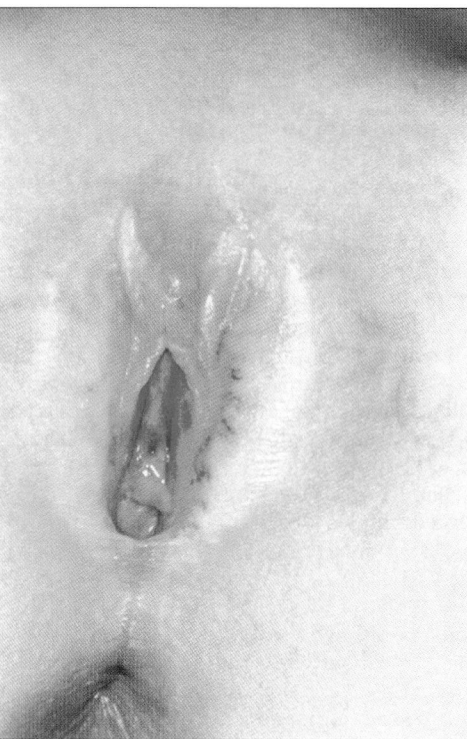

Fig. 96.14 Vulvar lichen sclerosus. Centrally, there is erythema with superficial erosion and purpura. More peripherally, white plaques with a wrinkled surface are seen. Note fissuring of the perineum.

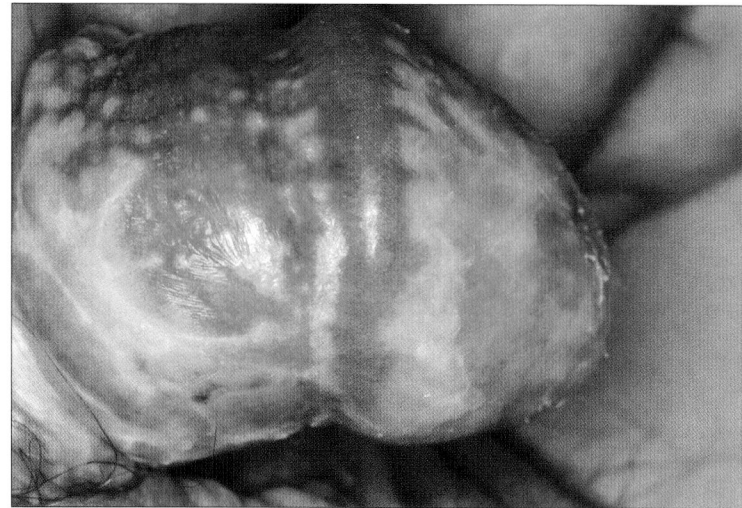

Fig. 96.15 Lichen sclerosus of the penis (balanitis xerotica obliterans). Note the areas of hypopigmentation, erosion and scarring.

very difficult to establish a useful meta-analysis. Most data suggest that lichen sclerosus is not intrinsically precancerous, but that it has to be considered as chronic scar continuously exposed to a humid milieu, where carcinogenesis may be promoted[54,55].

PATHOLOGY

Lichen sclerosus has a specific histologic pattern. In the beginning, superficial dermal edema dominates, associated with a band-like lymphocytic infiltrate beneath that zone. The epidermis is thinned, with orthohyperkeratosis and vacuolar degeneration of the basal layer. Hyperkeratosis is especially pronounced at follicular openings and may lead to plugging. The vacuolar degeneration at the dermal–epidermal interface and the flattening of the rete ridges predisposes to the development of blisters, which may become hemorrhagic. The most important changes are found in the superficial dermis, where the pale staining reflects homogenized dermal collagen (Fig. 96.16) and extreme edema in early stages. Loss of elastic fibers is typical for lichen sclerosus and is not found in morphea. Clefting and hemorrhage within homogenized papillary dermis is often seen.

The inflammatory infiltrate is especially pronounced during early phases along the zone of hyalinization and consists of lymphocytes (CD3+, CD4+, CD8+), macrophages and mast cells. In older lesions, the mononuclear infiltrate is reduced and sparse, and patchy islands of mononuclear cells are dispersed within the hyalinized dermis. Ultrastructural studies reveal shortened collagen fibers.

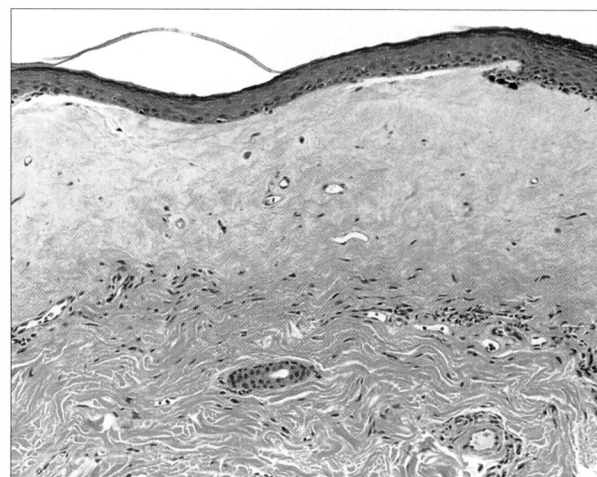

Fig. 96.16 Histology of lichen sclerosus. Homogenized papillary dermis with lymphocytic infiltrate beneath that zone is classic. A flattened dermal–epidermal junction is also seen.

An open question is whether genital lichen sclerosus is a precancerous condition. Interpretation and comparison of the data are complicated by two factors: some of the patients reported as developing cancer had previously received X-ray therapy for the disease or had previous dysplasia due to human papillomavirus (HPV) infection. It is therefore

DIFFERENTIAL DIAGNOSIS

The most important entity in the differential diagnosis for extragenital lichen sclerosus is morphea, and for genital lichen sclerosus in girls and boys, is sexual abuse[65]. In adults, genital lichen sclerosus may mimic erythroplasia of Queyrat or erosive lichen planus (see Ch. 72). They have to be excluded either clinically or histologically. Biopsies may also be required to exclude malignant transformation, especially when lichen sclerosus is superinfected by potentially carcinogenic HPV-16 or HPV-18. A past history of allogeneic hematopoietic stem cell transplant points to chronic GVHD.

TREATMENT OF MORPHEA AND LICHEN SCLEROSUS

Various therapeutic modalities have been reported for lichen sclerosus and morphea (Table 96.2). Most reports are based on single or limited observations or, occasionally, larger numbers of patients but without controls. Well-designed, randomized controlled trials are rare. Meta-analysis of the literature suggests that some treatments are well established and effective in a majority of patients while others seem to be effective in only a small number of patients. These approaches should be considered separately from suggestions that rely on a single observation and others that require more substantial investigation.

Phototherapies

Phototherapy for morphea was first described in 1994[66], and, since then, the efficacy has been confirmed by more than 25 publications[67,68]. Due to the nature of phototherapy, placebo-controlled studies can not be performed. Nonetheless, little doubt exists as to the efficacy of this therapy, as untreated morphea normally progresses over 3–5 years and then regresses very slowly over years. More rapid spontaneous improvement occurs in a small minority of patients[6]. The clinical course is definitely different in patients receiving either bath PUVA therapy or UVA1. If 36 treatments of bath PUVA therapy at slightly suberythematous doses or 36 treatments of UVA1 with 20–60 J/cm^2 are given, morphea either completely resolves or markedly improves in at least 60% of the patients[69] (Fig. 96.17). Even low-dose UVA photo-therapy (i.e. 5 or 10 J/cm^2) may improve morphea[70]. One trial reported improvement of cutaneous sclerosis in all those patients who received 20 treatments with medium-dose UVA1 (48 J/cm^2)[71].

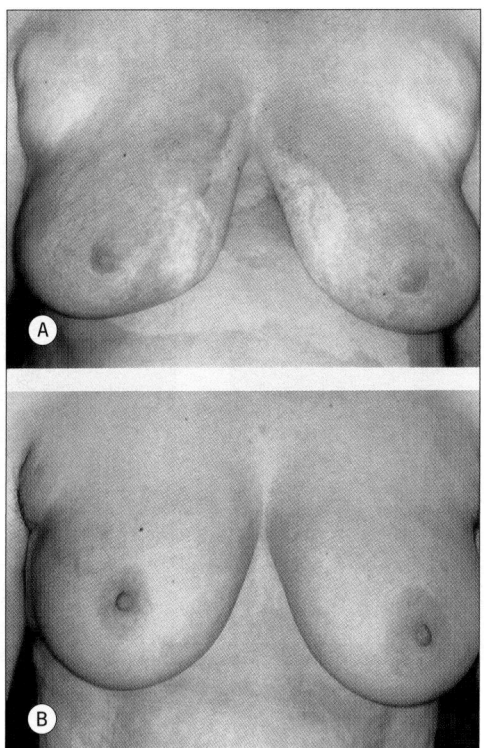

Fig. 96.17 Phototherapy of morphea. Disseminated morphea on the trunk before (**A**) and after PUVA bath photochemotherapy (**B**).

		Morphea		Lichen sclerosus	
	Treatment modalities	**Efficacy**	**Level of evidence**	**Efficacy**	**Level of evidence**
Local	Topical corticosteroids	+	3	+++ (ultrapotent)	1
	Intralesional corticosteroids	+	3	++	2
	Topical calcineurin inhibitors	+ (under occlusion)	3	+	2
	Vitamin A analogues	+	3	+	2
	Vitamin D analogues	+	3	+	3
	Testosterone	No experience		0	1
	Progesterone	No experience		0	1
	Intralesional interferon-γ	0	1	No experience	
Systemic	Penicillin	++ (approx. 5% of patients)	3	No experience	
	Hydroxy-/chloroquine	No experience		+	3
	Corticosteroids	+	3	+	3
	Vitamin A analogues	+	3	++	1
	Vitamin D analogues	0	1	+	3
	Cyclosporine	0	3	No experience	
	Penicillamine	++	3	No experience	
	Methotrexate	++	2	No experience	
Phototherapy	Oral photochemotherapy	++	3	+	3
	Bath photochemotherapy	+++	2	++	3
	Cream photochemotherapy	++	3	+	3
	UVA1	+++	2	++	2
	Photodynamic therapy	+	3	++	3
	Extracorporeal photopheresis	+	3	No experience	
Others	CO$_2$ laser	No experience		++	3
	Surgery	Selected patients		Selected patients	
	Physical therapy	Important		–	–

Table 96.2 Treatment of morphea and lichen sclerosus. +++, Highly effective; ++, effective; +, moderately effective; 0, low efficacy or ineffective. 1, prospective controlled trial; 2, retrospective study or large case series; 3, small case series or individual case reports.

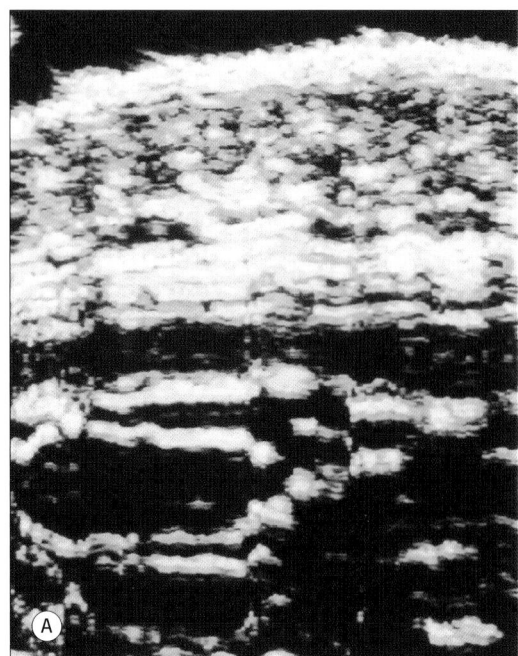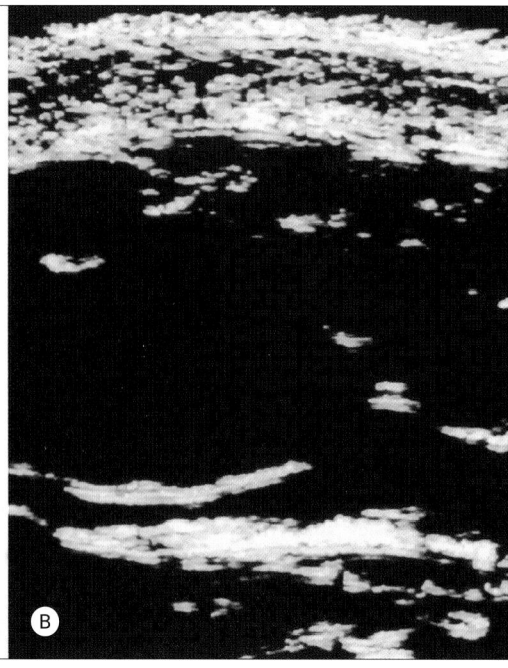

Fig. 96.18 High-frequency ultrasound (20 MHz) of a morphea plaque. Before (**A**) and after PUVA bath photochemotherapy (**B**), showing reduction of corium thickness and hyperechoic bands of connective tissue.

Both photochemotherapy and UVA1 induce expression of matrix metalloproteinase 1, a collagenase that reduces procollagen and collagen within the skin. The regression of morphea can be objectively documented by measuring skin thickness and skin density by 20 MHz ultrasound (Fig. 96.18) or by histology[68,72,73]. Both phototherapies seem to be effective in all types of morphea except for morphea profunda. Less experience exists with extensive linear or pansclerotic morphea, but these types may also improve with either mode of phototherapy[74]. Our impression is that UVA1 more efficiently silences the erythematous phase and progression of morphea, while both treatments are similarly effective in resolving the scar-like sclerosis of more advanced disease.

Photochemotherapy has been most frequently performed as bath PUVA therapy[75]. Few reports exist on treatment of single patients with either cream PUVA or systemic PUVA[74]; these treatments have not been compared with the other two modes of phototherapy (i.e. bath PUVA, UVA1). In particular, the relative efficacy of oral PUVA should be further studied.

Another open question is the ideal dose for UVA1 therapy; one group suggested that single treatment doses of 130 J/cm^2 of UVA1 were superior to lower doses[72]. However, all other studies were performed with either low (20 J/cm^2) or medium doses (30–60 J/cm^2) of UVA1 and reported similar efficacy. In agreement with these reports, we have observed that 36 treatments with 30 J/cm^2 of UVA1 markedly improve morphea in the majority of patients. Importantly, in responding patients, the morphea continues to improve beyond the end of the therapy. Thus, therapy can be terminated after 36 treatments, even if the sclerosis has not yet completely resolved. The only exception seems to be linear scleroderma, which may require significantly more treatments. In our experience, selected patients who fail to respond to one mode of phototherapy may benefit from a switch to another therapy. Thus, if a patient does not improve within 4 months with one type of phototherapy (e.g. bath PUVA), a new therapy cycle should be initiated utilizing another mode of phototherapy (e.g. UVA1).

Much less experience exists with regard to phototherapy for lichen sclerosus. Based upon observations in a small number of patients with extragenital lichen sclerosus, bath or cream PUVA therapy or UVA1 therapy may induce clearance in some selected patients; similar results have been reported for genital lichen sclerosus. For example, a preliminary study reported clinical improvement in ten patients with extragenital lichen sclerosus following 40 treatments with low-dose UVA1 (20 J/cm^2)[76]. Based upon our experience with extragenital lichen sclerosus, phototherapy seems less effective than in morphea. More detailed studies are required and phototherapy may be an alternative in selected patients who respond poorly to topical corticosteroids and/or calcineurin inhibitors.

In morphea, extracorporeal photopheresis has brought contradictory results. The associated costs and the invasiveness are very high. The efficacy of UVA1 or photochemotherapy clearly seems to be superior.

New trials are investigating the role of photodynamic therapy for localized scleroderma and lichen sclerosus. Preliminary data from a prospective study showed that photodynamic therapy, using 5-aminolevulinic acid before irradiation, can significantly relieve the symp-toms of vulvar lichen sclerosus[77]. While photodynamic therapy may also lead to improvement in morphea, this therapy needs further investigation.

Topical Therapies
Corticosteroids
Retrospective and prospective studies have clearly documented that ultrapotent topical corticosteroids are highly effective in the treatment of genital lichen sclerosus. In the majority of these studies, clobetasol propionate 0.05% cream was applied for 12–24 weeks[78]. Clinical improvement was confirmed by histopathology. Safety and efficiency of clobetasol in the treatment of genital lichen sclerosus were documented for all age groups and in both sexes[79,80]. Nearly all the patients with vulvar lichen sclerosus responded to ultrapotent topical corticosteroids, and amongst those who improved, about 20% experienced complete clearance[81]. However, topical glucocorticoids do not cure the disease and relapses may occur.

Major side effects were not found, even with long-term and maintenance use of clobetasol. Therefore, potent topical corticosteroids represent first-line therapy for genital lichen sclerosus, including in children (Fig. 96.19). Alternatively, corticosteroids such as triamcinolone can be injected intralesionally[82]. Of note, vulvar squamous cell carcinoma appeared to develop primarily in untreated or irregularly treated vulvar lichen sclerosus lesions[83].

The benefit of topical corticosteroids in the treatment of morphea is questionable. Ultrapotent topical corticosteroids may be useful for reducing inflammation in superficial active lesions. Similarly, intralesional injection of triamcinolone into the margins may reduce or prevent progression. Topical corticosteroids are ineffective in resolving sclerosis.

Calcineurin inhibitors
The macrolide immunosuppressants pimecrolimus (1% cream) and tacrolimus (0.1% ointment) have been used as topical treatments for vulvar lichen sclerosus. Even though the total number of published case reports is limited, these therapies seem to be effective. However, long-term safety and efficacy studies as well as randomized trials comparing these agents with clobetasol propionate have yet to be done[84].

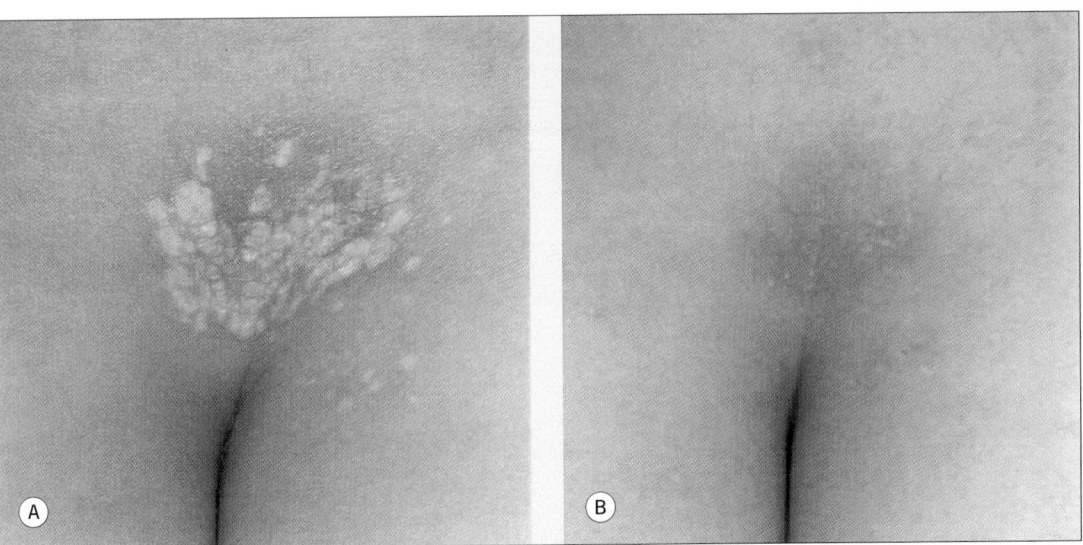

Fig. 96.19 Ultrapotent topical corticosteroids in the treatment of lichen sclerosus in a 12-year-old girl. Before (**A**) and after topical application of clobetasol propionate 0.05% cream for 5 months (**B**).

Vitamin derivatives

Derivatives of vitamin D and vitamin A are still under study in morphea. *In vitro*, calcipotriol inhibits the proliferation of cultured fibroblasts and topical calcipotriene 0.005% ointment has been used for the treatment of morphea[85]. Single reports have described improvement of both vulvar lichen sclerosus and morphea when treated with topical vitamin A derivatives. All of these observations require confirmation by controlled studies.

Hormones

For years, topical testosterone or progesterone preparations were frequently used in the treatment of genital lichen sclerosus. In sharp contrast to ultrapotent topical corticosteroids, no evidence has been found for the efficacy of these agents. Controlled clinical studies have clearly shown that none of these hormone preparations has clinical benefit in lichen sclerosus[86]. In one study, 2% testosterone propionate was even less effective than petrolatum ointment[87].

Systemic Treatments

Immunosuppression

Oral corticosteroids (methylprednisolone 1–2 mg/kg/day) may be helpful in the inflammatory stages of morphea, especially in some patients with either rapidly progressive linear or disabling morphea, but corticosteroids do not improve established sclerosis. Alternatively, 15–20 mg/week of methotrexate seems to be helpful in the acute phase of morphea[88]. Based on experience with other autoimmune diseases, some authors favor the combination of methotrexate and glucocorticoids, especially in rapidly progressive disabling types of morphea[89]. Clinical data from a recent prospective pilot study confirmed the therapeutic effectiveness of methotrexate (15 mg/week) combined with pulsed high-dose intravenous methylprednisolone (1 g 3 days per month)[90]. Placebo-controlled studies are still lacking, but the potential benefit documented in systemic sclerosis suggests that immunosuppression for several months, perhaps up to 1 year, may be indicated.

In contrast, cyclosporine has not been shown to be effective. Furthermore, cyclosporine should not be combined with any form of phototherapy. As the latter are currently the most effective therapies for morphea, this drug should be avoided.

Systemic immunosuppression is normally not indicated for lichen sclerosus.

Penicillin and its derivatives

Regression of morphea or systemic sclerosis during prolonged treatment with penicillin or penicillamine has been observed in adults and in children[91]. Penicillin in the range of 30×10^6 IU/day for 3–4 weeks is helpful in a few patients (about 5%); these occasionally responsive patients have been documented by several authors. In addition, the response is reproducible in previously responsive individuals who relapse. Penicillamine seems to be similarly effective but is used less often because of its potential side effects.

In lichen sclerosus, neither penicillin nor other antibiotics nor penicillamine are helpful.

Vitamin derivatives

Treatment with the vitamin A derivatives etretinate or acitretin at doses of 10–50 mg/day is effective in localized scleroderma or lichen sclerosus[92,93]. Importantly, the response can only be assessed after several months of therapy. Retinoids can inhibit TGF-β, one of the key cytokines that promote collagen synthesis by fibroblasts (see Fig. 96.1). Retinoids are also effective in certain pseudoscleroderma disorders such as 'sclerodermoid' GVHD.

The other vitamin derivative investigated for the treatment of morphea is calcitriol. 1,25-dihydroxyvitamin D_3 has pronounced anti-inflammatory effects, and it modulates fibroblast growth as well as TGF-β[94]. Despite promising case reports, a double-blind, placebo-controlled study did not confirm the clinical efficacy of oral calcitriol in morphea[95].

Cytokines

As IFN-γ and IFN-α normalize pathogenic collagen production by fibroblasts *in vitro*, both cytokines have been tested for the treatment of morphea. Controlled studies did not demonstrate efficacy for either of these cytokines in the reversal of sclerosis[20].

Physical Therapies

Expert and long-standing physiotherapy is obligatory for patients in whom morphea threatens to impair mobility. In the case of persistent contractures, reconstructive surgery may be needed. Similarly, surgical revision may be needed in linear or *en coup de sabre* morphea. Circumcision is the treatment of choice for genital lichen sclerosus leading to phimosis, and reconstructive surgery is mandatory.

REFERENCES

1. Mayes MD. Classification and epidemiology of scleroderma. Semin Cutan Med Surg. 1998;17:22–6.
2. Gintrac E. Note sur la sclérodermie. Rev Med Chir. 1847;2:263.
3. Addison T. On the keloid of Alibert, and on true keloid. Med Chirurg Trans. 1854;37:27.
4. Matsui S. Über die Pathologie und Pathogenese von Sclerodermia universalis. Mitt Med Fakult Univ Tokyo. 1924;31:55.
5. O'Leary PA, Nomland R. A clinical study of one hundred and three cases of scleroderma. Am J Med Sci. 1930;180:95.
6. Peterson LS, Nelson AM, Su WP, et al. The epidemiology of morphea (localized scleroderma) in Olmsted County 1960–1993. J Rheumatol. 1997;24:73–80.
7. Vancheeswaran R, Black CM, David J, et al. Childhood-onset scleroderma: is it different from adult-onset disease. Arthritis Rheum. 1996;39:1041–9.

8. Blaszczyk M, Janniger CK, Jablonska S. Childhood scleroderma and its peculiarities. Cutis. 1996; 58:141–4,148–52.

9. Takehara K, Sato S. Localized scleroderma is an autoimmune disorder. Rheumatology. 2005;44:274–9.

10. Abraham DJ, Varga J. Scleroderma: from cell and molecular mechanisms to disease models. Trends Immunol. 2005;26:587–95.

11. Kuryliszyn-Moskal A, Klimiuk PA, Sierakowski S. Soluble adhesion molecules (sVCAM-1, sE-selectin), vascular endothelial growth factor (VEGF) and endothelin-1 in patients with systemic sclerosis: relationship to organ systemic involvement. Clin Rheumatol. 2005; 24:111–16.

12. Yamane K, Ihn H, Kubo M, Yazawa N, et al. Increased serum levels of soluble vascular cell adhesion molecule 1 and E-selectin in patients with localized scleroderma. J Am Acad Dermatol. 2000;42:64–9.

13. Leroy EC. Connective tissue synthesis by scleroderma skin fibroblasts in cell culture. J Exp Med. 1972;135:1351–62.

14. Leroy EC. Increased collagen synthesis by scleroderma skin fibroblasts in vitro: a possible defect in the regulation or activation of the scleroderma fibroblast. J Clin Invest. 1974;54:880–9.

15. Jimenez SA, Hitraya E, Varga J. Pathogenesis of scleroderma. Collagen. Rheum Dis Clin North Am. 1996;22:647–74.

16. Röcken M, Racke M, Shevach EM. IL-4-induced immune deviation as antigen-specific therapy for inflammatory autoimmune disease. Immunol Today. 1996;17:225–31.

17. Serpier H, Gillery P, Salmon-Ehr V, et al. Antagonistic effects of interferon-gamma and interleukin-4 on fibroblast cultures. J Invest Dermatol. 1997;109:158–62.

18. Salmon-Ehr V, Serpier H, Nawrocki B, et al. Expression of interleukin-4 in scleroderma skin specimens and scleroderma fibroblast cultures. Potential role in fibrosis. Arch Dermatol. 1996;132:802–6.

19. Ong C, Wong C, Roberts CR, et al. Anti-IL-4 treatment prevents dermal collagen deposition in the tight-skin mouse model of scleroderma. Eur J Immunol. 1998;28:2619–29.

20. Hunzelmann N, Anders S, Fierlbeck G, et al. Double-blind, placebo-controlled study of intralesional interferon gamma for the treatment of localized scleroderma. J Am Acad Dermatol. 1997;36:433–5.

21. Ihn H, Yamane K, Tamaki K. Increased phosphorylation and activation of mitogen-activated protein kinase p38 in scleroderma fibroblasts. J Invest Dermatol. 2005;125:247–55.

22. Svegliati S, Cancello R, Sambo P, et al. Platelet-derived growth factor and reactive oxygen species (ROS) regulate Ras protein levels in primary human fibroblasts via ERK1/2: amplification of ROS and Ras in systemic sclerosis fibroblasts. J Biol Chem. 2005;280:36474–82.

23. Nagai M, Hasegawa M, Takehara K, Sato S. Novel autoantibody to Cu/Zn superoxide dismutase in patients with localized scleroderma. J Invest Dermatol. 2004;122:594–601.

24. McGaha T, Saito S, Phelps RG, et al. Lack of skin fibrosis in tight skin (TSK) mice with targeted mutation in the interleukin-4R alpha and transforming growth factor-beta genes. J Invest Dermatol. 2001;116:136–43.

25. McGaha TL, Le M, Kodera T, et al. Molecular mechanisms of interleukin-4-induced up-regulation of type I collagen gene expression in murine fibroblasts. Arthritis Rheum. 2003;48:2275–84.

26. Shen Y, Ichino M, Nakazawa M, et al. CpG oligodeoxynucleotides prevent the development of scleroderma-like syndrome in tight-skin mice by stimulating a Th1 immune response. J Invest Dermatol. 2005;124:1141–8.

27. Aberer E, Neumann R, Lubec G. Acrodermatitis chronica atrophicans in association with lichen sclerosus et atrophicans: tubulo-interstitial nephritis and urinary excretion of spirochete-like organisms. Acta Derm Venereol. 1987;67:62–5.

28. Aberer E, Klade H, Stanek G, Gebhart W. Borrelia burgdorferi and different types of morphea. Dermatologica. 1991;182:145–54.

29. Wienecke R, Schlupen EM, Zochling N, Neubert U, Meurer M, Volkenandt M. No evidence for Borrelia burgdorferi-specific DNA in lesions of localized scleroderma. J Invest Dermatol. 1995;104:23–6.

30. Weide B, Schittek B, Klyscz T, et al. Morphoea is neither associated with features of Borrelia burgdorferi infection, nor is this agent detectable in lesional skin by polymerase chain reaction. Br J Dermatol. 2000;143:780–5.

31. Whittaker SJ, Smith NP, Jones RR. Solitary morphoea profunda. Br J Dermatol. 1989;120:431–40.

32. Vierra E, Cunningham BB. Morphea and localized scleroderma in children. Semin Cutan Med Surg. 1999;18:210–25.

33. Zulian F, Vallongo C, Woo P, et al. Localized scleroderma in childhood is not just a skin disease. Arthritis Rheum. 2005;52:2873–81.

34. Falanga V, Medsger TA Jr, Reichlin M, Rodnan GP. Linear scleroderma. Clinical spectrum, prognosis, and laboratory abnormalities. Ann Intern Med. 1986;104:849–57.

35. Ruffatti A, Peserico A, Rondinone R, et al. Prevalence and characteristics of anti-single-stranded DNA antibodies in localized scleroderma. Comparison with systemic lupus erythematosus. Arch Dermatol. 1991;127:1180–3.

36. Zulian F, Athreya BH, Laxer R, et al. Juvenile localized scleroderma: clinical and epidemiological features in 750 children. An international study. Rheumatology (Oxford). 2006;45:614–20.

37. Kikuchi K, Sato S, Kadono T, et al. Serum concentration of procollagen type I carboxyterminal propeptide in localized scleroderma. Arch Dermatol. 1994;130:1269–72.

38. Texier L, Gendre P, Gauthier O, et al. Scleroderma-like hypodermitis of the buttock due to intramuscular injection of drugs combined with vitamin K 1. Ann Dermatol Syphiligr. 1972;99:363–71.

39. Kumagai Y, Shiokawa Y, Medsger TA Jr, Rodnan GP. Clinical spectrum of connective tissue disease after cosmetic surgery. Observations on eighteen patients and a review of the Japanese literature. Arthritis Rheum. 1984;27:1–12.

40. Janowsky EC, Kupper LL, Hulka BS. Meta-analyses of the relation between silicone breast implants and the risk of connective-tissue diseases. N Engl J Med. 2000;342:781–90.

41. Cooper C, Dennison E. Do silicone breast implants cause connective tissue disease? BMJ. 1998;316:403–4.

42. Doyle JA, Friedman SJ. Porphyria and scleroderma: a clinical and laboratory review of 12 patients. Australas J Dermatol. 1983;24:109–14.

43. Schaffer JV, McNiff JM, Seropian S, et al. Lichen sclerosus and eosinophilic fasciitis as manifestations of chronic graft-versus-host disease: expanding the sclerodermoid spectrum. J Am Acad Dermatol. 2005;53:591–601.

44. Aractingi S, Chosidow O. Cutaneous graft-versus-host disease. Arch Dermatol. 1998;134:602–12.

45. Janin A, Socie G, Devergie A, et al. Fasciitis in chronic graft-versus-host disease. A clinicopathologic study of 14 cases. Ann Intern Med. 1994;120:993–8.

46. McFarlane RM, Classen DA, Porte AM, Botz JS. The anatomy and treatment of camptodactyly of the small finger. J Hand Surg. 1992;17:35–44.

47. Rosenbloom AL, Silverstein JH. Connective tissue and joint disease in diabetes mellitus. Endocrinol Metab Clin North Am. 1996;25:473–83.

48. Darier J. Lichen plan scléreux. Ann Derm Syph. 1892;23:833.

49. Unna PG. Karenblattförmige Sklerodermie. Lehrbuch der speziellen path Anatomie. Berlin: A Hirschwald, 1894:112.

50. Westberg F. Ein Fall mit weissen Flecken einhergehender, bisher nicht bekannter Dermatose. Monatschr Prakt Dermatol. 1901;33:355.

51. von Zumbusch LR. Über lichen albus, eine bisher unbeschriebene Erkrankung. Arch Dermatol Syph. 1906;82:339.

52. Breisky A. Über kraurosis vulvae. Z. Heilkd. 1885;6:69–80.

53. Stühmer A. Balanitis xerotica obliterans (post operationem) und ihre Beziehungen zur Kraurosis glandis et praeputii penis. Arch Derm Syph. 1928;156:613.

54. Meffert JJ, Davis BM, Grimwood RE. Lichen sclerosus. J Am Acad Dermatol. 1995;32:393–416.

55. Powell JJ, Wojnarowska F. Lichen sclerosus. Lancet. 1999;353:1777–83.

56. Fischer GO. The commonest causes of symptomatic vulvar disease: a dermatologist's perspective. Australas J Dermatol. 1996;37:12–18.

57. Heller DS, Randolph P, Young A, et al. The cutaneous-vulvar clinic revisited: a 5-year experience of the Columbia Presbyterian Medical Center Cutaneous-Vulvar Service. Dermatology. 1997;195:26–9.

58. Fischer G, Rogers M. Vulvar disease in children: a clinical audit of 130 cases. Pediatr Dermatol. 2000;17:1–6.

59. Chalmers RJ, Burton PA, Bennett RF, et al. Lichen sclerosus et atrophicus. A common and distinctive cause of phimosis in boys. Arch Dermatol. 1984;120:1025–7.

60. Mallon E, Hawkins D, Dinneen M, et al. Circumcision and genital dermatoses. Arch Dermatol. 2000;136:350–4.

61. Marren P, Yell J, Charnock FM, et al. The association between lichen sclerosus and antigens of the HLA system. Br J Dermatol. 1995;132:197–203.

62. Powell J, Wojnarowska F, Winsey S, et al. Lichen sclerosus premenarche: autoimmunity and immunogenetics. Br J Dermatol. 2000;142:481–4.

63. Oyama N, Chan I, Neill SM, et al. Autoantibodies to extracellular matrix protein 1 in lichen sclerosus. Lancet. 2003;362:118–23.

64. Sander CS, Ali I, Dean D, et al. Oxidative stress is implicated in the pathogenesis of lichen sclerosus. Br J Dermatol. 2004;151:627–35.

65. Powell J, Wojnarowska F. Childhood vulval lichen sclerosus and sexual abuse are not mutually exclusive diagnoses. BMJ. 2000;320:311.

66. Kerscher M, Volkenandt M, Meurer M, et al. Treatment of localised scleroderma with PUVA bath photochemotherapy. Lancet. 1994;343:1233.

67. Kerscher M, Dirschka T, Volkenandt M. Treatment of localised scleroderma by UVA1 phototherapy. Lancet. 1995;346:1166.

68. Kerscher M, Meurer M, Sander C, et al. PUVA bath photochemotherapy for localized scleroderma. Evaluation of 17 consecutive patients. Arch Dermatol. 1996;132:1280–2.

69. Ghoreschi K, Rocken M. Phototherapy of sclerosing skin diseases. Dermatology. 2002;205:219–20.

70. El-Mofty M, Mostafa W, El-Darouty M, et al. Different low doses of broad-band UVA in the treatment of morphea and systemic sclerosis. Photodermatol Photoimmunol Photomed. 2004;20:148–56.

71. de Rie MA, Enomoto DN, de Vries HJ, et al. Evaluation of medium-dose UVA1 phototherapy in localized scleroderma with the cutometer and fast Fourier transform method. Dermatology. 2003;207:298–301.

72. Stege H, Berneburg M, Humke S, et al. High-dose UVA1 radiation therapy for localized scleroderma. J Am Acad Dermatol. 1997;36:938–44.

73. Gruss C, Reed JA, Altmeyer P, et al. Induction of interstitial collagenase (MMP-1) by UVA-1 phototherapy in morphea fibroblasts. Lancet. 1997;350:1295–6.

74. Scharffetter-Kochanek K, Goldermann R, Lehmann P, Holzle E, Goerz G. PUVA therapy in disabling pansclerotic morphoea of children. Br J Dermatol. 1995;132:830–1.

75. Lüftl M, Degitz K, Plewig G, Röcken M. Psoralen bath plus UV-A therapy. Possibilities and limitations. Arch Dermatol. 1997;133:1597–603.

76. Kreuter A, Gambichler T, Avermaete A, et al. Low-dose ultraviolet A1 phototherapy for extragenital lichen sclerosus: results of a preliminary study. J Am Acad Dermatol. 2002;46:251–5.

77. Hillemanns P, Untch M, Prove F, et al. Photodynamic therapy of vulvar lichen sclerosus with 5-aminolevulinic acid. Obstet Gynecol. 1999;93:71–4.

78. Lorenz B, Kaufman RH, Kutzner SK. Lichen sclerosus. Therapy with clobetasol propionate. J Reprod Med. 1998;43:790–4.

79. Lindhagen T. Topical clobetasol propionate compared with placebo in the treatment of unretractable foreskin. Eur J Surg. 1996;162:969–72.

80. Dahlman-Ghozlan K, Hedblad MA, von Krogh G. Penile lichen sclerosus et atrophicus treated with clobetasol dipropionate 0.05% cream: a retrospective clinical and histopathological study. J Am Acad Dermatol. 1999;40:451–7.

81. Cooper SM, Gao XH, Powell JJ, Wojnarowska F. Does treatment of vulvar lichen sclerosus influence its prognosis? Arch Dermatol. 2004;140:702–6.

82. Mazdisnian F, Degregorio F, Palmieri A. Intralesional injection of triamcinolone in the treatment of lichen sclerosus. J Reprod Med. 1999;44:332–4.

83. Renaud-Vilmer C, Cavelier-Balloy B, Porcher R, et al. Vulvar lichen sclerosus: effect of long-term topical application of a potent steroid on the course of the disease. Arch Dermatol. 2004;140:709–12.

84. Goldstein AT, Marinoff SC, Christopher K. Pimecrolimus for the treatment of vulvar lichen sclerosus: a report of 4 cases. J Reprod Med. 2004;49:778–80.

85. Cunningham BB, Landells ID, Langman C, et al. Topical calcipotriene for morphea/linear scleroderma. J Am Acad Dermatol. 1998;39:211–15.

86. Cattaneo A, De Marco A, Sonni L, et al. Clobetasol vs. testosterone in the treatment of lichen sclerosus of the vulvar region. Minerva Ginecol. 1992;44:567–71.

87. Sideri M, Origoni M, Spinaci L, Ferrari A. Topical testosterone in the treatment of vulvar lichen sclerosus. Int J Gynaecol Obstet. 1994;46:53–6.

88. Seyger MM, van den Hoogen FH, van Vlijmen-Willems IM, et al. Localized and systemic scleroderma show different histological responses to methotrexate therapy. J Pathol. 2001;193:511–16.

96

Morphea and Lichen Sclerosus

89. Uziel Y, Feldman BM, Krafchik BR, et al. Methotrexate and corticosteroid therapy for pediatric localized scleroderma. J Pediatr. 2000;136:91–5.

90. Kreuter A, Gambichler T, Breuckmann F, et al. Pulsed high-dose corticosteroids combined with low-dose methotrexate in severe localized scleroderma. Arch Dermatol. 2005;141:847–52.

91. Falanga V, Medsger TA Jr. D-penicillamine in the treatment of localized scleroderma. Arch Dermatol. 1990;126:609–12.

92. Samsonov VA, Gareginian SA. Tigazon in the therapy of patients with circumscribed scleroderma. Vestn Dermatol Venerol. 1990;(11):17–20.

93. Bousema MT, Romppanen U, Geiger JM, et al. Acitretin in the treatment of severe lichen sclerosus et atrophicus of the vulva: a double-blind, placebo-controlled study. J Am Acad Dermatol. 1994;30:225–31.

94. Oyama N, Iwatsuki K, Satoh M, Akiba H, Kaneko F. Dermal fibroblasts are one of the therapeutic targets for topical application of 1 alpha,25-dihydroxyvitamin D3: the possible involvement of transforming growth factor-beta induction. Br J Dermatol. 2000;143:1140–8.

95. Hulshof MM, Bouwes Bavinck JN, Bergman W, et al. Double-blind, placebo-controlled study of oral calcitriol for the treatment of localized and systemic scleroderma. J Am Acad Dermatol. 2000;43:1017–23.

Heritable Disorders of Connective Tissue

Franziska Ringpfeil and Jouni Uitto

97

Key features

- Heritable connective tissue disorders with skin involvement comprise a phenotypically diverse group of conditions
- Skin involvement may signify the presence of underlying internal involvement, as exemplified by cardiovascular and ocular manifestations in pseudoxanthoma elasticum or pulmonary emphysema in patients with cutis laxa
- The molecular bases of many of the heritable connective tissue disorders have recently become known and include specific mutations in genes encoding structural connective tissue proteins, such as various collagens and components of elastic fibers, as well as an ABC-cassette membrane transporter
- Identification of specific mutations allows for improved classification and prognostication, more accurate genetic counseling, presymptomatic and prenatal testing, and carrier detection in families at risk for recurrence

Introduction

Heritable skin diseases can manifest as a spectrum of abnormalities with a variable degree of cutaneous involvement. At one end of the spectrum, the clinical findings may be minimal and limited to the skin, while at the other end of the spectrum, the cutaneous manifestations may be part of a multiorgan pathology causing considerable morbidity and even mortality[1,2]. Many of the genetic skin diseases have continued to pose a clinical challenge to the practicing dermatologist, in part due to their rarity and in part because of the complexity and variability of the phenotypic manifestations. This diagnostic dilemma has been compounded by the complexity of the traditional classifications, often riddled with eponyms. Furthermore, many of these conditions have not been well defined at the clinical, histopathologic and/or ultrastructural level, and the understanding of their molecular bases has been incomplete.

With the advent of molecular biology in general, and with the advances made by the human genome project, tremendous progress has been made towards understanding the molecular bases of genodermatoses. In fact, there are currently over 200 distinct genes that harbor mutations which underlie the phenotypic manifestations characteristic of heritable skin diseases[2]. An example of a group of disorders in which significant progress in molecular understanding has recently been made is the heritable disorders affecting the extracellular matrix of connective tissue.

The connective tissue meshwork is critical for developmental organogenesis and homeostatic maintenance of tissues, with complex protein assembly and cell–matrix interactions. In the connective tissue of the skin, the principal fibrillar components of the extracellular matrix are the fiber networks consisting of collagen and elastic fibers (see Ch. 94). The genetic heterogeneity of collagen, a family of closely related structural proteins, and the complexity of elastic fibers, which consist of elastin and a number of associated microfibrillar proteins, have been recently recognized. Such knowledge has allowed the identification of critical metabolic and structural features that are a prerequisite for normal physiologic functions of these proteins.

Consequently, primary genetic defects that impact on collagen and elastic fibers can result in abnormalities that manifest clinically as a heritable disorder of connective tissue. Examples of such primary inherited conditions affecting collagen and elastic fibers are Ehlers–Danlos syndrome (EDS) and cutis laxa (CL), respectively. In addition to primary genetic defects in the genes encoding the structural components of collagen and elastin, or enzymes modifying these proteins, the fiber structures can be perturbed by genetically unrelated pathologic processes. An example of the latter, which can be considered a secondary connective tissue disorder, is pseudoxanthoma elasticum (PXE).

This chapter will highlight the progress made in heritable disorders of connective tissue by detailed discussions of EDS, PXE and CL. Marfan syndrome, homocystinuria, osteogenesis imperfecta, and Buschke–Ollendorff syndrome are briefly described in Table 97.1. For other heritable disorders of connective tissue, see Pulkkinen et al.[2] and Steinmann & Royce[3] as well as Table 94.5.

EHLERS–DANLOS SYNDROME

Synonym: ■ Cutis hyperelastica

Key features

- Defects in various collagens (e.g. types I, III, V) and tenascin-X, as well as enzymes involved in post-translational modification of collagen
- Both autosomal dominant and autosomal recessive inheritance patterns
- Cutaneous features include hyperextensible and fragile skin, poor wound healing, molluscoid pseudotumors, and bruising
- Systemic features include joint hypermobility, scoliosis and, in the 'vascular' subtype, a significant risk of spontaneous arterial, intestinal or uterine rupture

History

A survey of the literature reveals descriptions of patients with features of Ehlers–Danlos syndrome (EDS) as early as the mid 1600s, while the first comprehensive description of the systemic nature of this condition was published in 1892 by Tschernogobow[4]. Drs Ehlers and Danlos, Danish and French dermatologists, respectively, contributed to the clinical description in the early 1900s, and this clinical constellation became known as the Ehlers–Danlos syndrome in 1936. The genetic nature of EDS was noted in 1949, and soon thereafter it was suggested that the phenotype resulted from defects in the collagen meshwork. The genetic heterogeneity of EDS became evident in the 1960s, and the first molecular defects in collagen synthesis were described in 1972.

Until recently, EDS was divided into as many as 11 distinct subtypes (types I–XI) based upon clinical and molecular features. In 1997, a consensus conference was held and a revised nosology was proposed[5] (Table 97.2). Currently, the molecular basis of most major forms of EDS is known[6,7].

Epidemiology

A relatively large number of individuals in the general population may have features suggestive of EDS, such as loose-jointedness, and they are

ADDITIONAL HERITABLE DISORDERS OF CONNECTIVE TISSUE

Disease	Cutaneous findings	Extracutaneous manifestations	Inheritance	Associated gene/protein product
Marfan syndrome	Striae distensae, elastosis perforans serpiginosa, decreased subcutaneous fat on extremities	Skeletal abnormalities (e.g. disproportionately long limbs, arachnodactyly), lens subluxations (upward), cardiovascular abnormalities (e.g. dilation/dissection of ascending aorta)	AD	*FBN1*/fibulin-1 (a microfibrillar protein)*
Homocystinuria	Malar flush, livedo reticularis, diffuse pigmentary dilution	Marfanoid habitus, lens subluxations (downward), venous and arterial thrombosis, mental retardation	AR	*CBS*/cystathionine synthase enzyme deficiency (resulting in increased plasma homocysteine†); rarely, methylenetetrahydrofolate reductase, 5-methyltetrahydrofolate-homocysteine methyltransferase, or 5-methyltetrahydrofolate-homocysteine methyltransferase reductase deficiency (enzymes that convert homocysteine back to methionine)
Osteogenesis imperfecta	Thin skin	Bone fragility, blue sclerae, dentinogenesis imperfecta (in a subset of patients)	AD	*COL1A1, COL1A2*/type I collagen defects
Buschke–Ollendorff syndrome	Connective tissue nevi	Osteopoikilosis	AD	*LEMD3*/LEM domain-containing 3, an antagonist of bone morphogenic protein (BMP) and TGF-β signaling

*TGF-β receptor (TGFBR2) mutations can lead to a phenotype that mimics Marfan syndrome.
†Elevated plasma homocystine and homocysteine can be detected in patients with homocystinuria (but only homocysteine in hyperhomocysteinemia).

Table 97.1 Additional heritable disorders of connective tissue. AD, autosomal dominant; AR, autosomal recessive.

CLASSIFICATION OF EHLERS–DANLOS SYNDROME

EDS type*	Traditional classification†	Clinical features	Inheritance	Mutated gene/protein
Classic	I, II	Hyperextensible skin, joint hypermobility, atrophic scars, easy bruising, absence of the inferior labial and lingual frenula	AD‡, AR‡	*COL5A1, COL5A2*/α₁- and α₂-chains of type V collagen; *TNXB*/tenascin-X Rarely, *COL1A1*/α₁-chain of type I collagen
Hypermobility	III	Joint hypermobility, pain, dislocations, absence of inferior labial and lingual frenula	AD	*TNXB*/tenascin-X (~10% of affected individuals, predominantly female)
Vascular	IV	Thin skin, arterial, gastrointestinal or uterine rupture, marked bruising, small joint hypermobility, characteristic facies	AD	*COL3A1*/α₁-chain of type III collagen
Kyphoscoliosis	VI	Hypotonia, joint laxity, congenital scoliosis, ocular fragility	AR	*PLOD1*/lysyl hydroxylase§
Arthrochalasia	VIIA, VIIB	Severe joint hypermobility with congenital bilateral hip dislocation, scoliosis, easy bruising	AD	*COL1A1, COL1A2*/α₁- and α₂-chains of type I collagen
Dermatosparaxis	VIIC	Severe skin fragility, sagging and redundant skin that is soft and doughy, easy bruising	AR	*ADAMTS2*/procollagen N-peptidase
Other¶	V, VIII, X			
	EDS, cardiac valvular	Cardiac valve defects, otherwise similar to classic EDS (see above)	AR	α₂-chain of type I collagen
	EDS, progeroid	Skin hyperextensibility, joint hypermobility, progeroid facies, osteopenia, mental and growth retardation	AR	*B4GALT7*/galactosyl transferase-1
	EDS, periventricular nodular heterotopia variant	Variable skin hyperextensibility, aortic dilation, periventricular nodular heterotopia, joint hypermobility	XD	*FLNA*/filamin A (actin-binding protein 280)

*According to the 1997 Villefranche Consensus Meeting[5].
†Replaced by the Consensus classification[5].
‡The classic forms due to type V collagen mutations are inherited in an autosomal dominant (AD) fashion, while those caused by tenascin-X deficiency are autosomal recessive (AR).
§Analysis of the urine for an increased deoxypyridinoline:pyridinoline ratio can be used as a screening test for kyphoscoliosis-type EDS.
¶The previous EDS types IX and XI have been reclassified as occipital horn syndrome, a disorder allelic with Menkes disease (see Ch. 62), and familial joint hypermobility syndrome, respectively.

Table 97.2 Classification of Ehlers–Danlos syndrome (EDS). AD, autosomal dominant; ADAMTS2, a disintegrin-like and metalloprotease domain with thrombospondin type 1 motifs 2; AR, autosomal recessive; COL, collagen; PLOD1, procollagen-lysine 1, 2-oxoglutarate 5-dioxygenase 1; XD, X-linked dominant.

often encountered in certain ethnic groups (e.g. in several African populations). However, more stringent diagnostic criteria that include findings in the skin and joints at a minimum, limit the incidence of EDS to approximately 1 in 5000. Although all forms of EDS cause considerable morbidity, only one subtype, the vascular type (previously type IV EDS), causes premature demise of affected individuals[8].

Pathogenesis

EDS is a clinically and genetically heterogeneous group of connective tissue disorders caused by defects in the collagen meshwork. Progress in the basic understanding of the biosynthetic pathways of collagen fibril formation has been fundamental in elucidating the pathogenetic mechanisms of different EDS variants (Fig. 97.1). The collagen family is now known to consist of as many as 28 distinct proteins with differential tissue distributions[9] (see Ch. 94). Each collagen member consists of three polypeptides, the so-called α-chains, which are synthesized as precursor molecules, pro-α-chains; each trimeric collagen molecule may be either a homotrimer or heterotrimer (i.e. consisting of the same versus two or three different kinds of polypeptides, respectively). As a result, there are well over 40 genetically different pro-α-chains, each being a distinct gene product[9].

The pathogenesis of EDS involves at least three mechanisms affecting different stages of collagen biosynthesis; these include: (1) deficiency of collagen processing enzymes; (2) dominant-negative effects of mutant collagen α-chains; and (3) haploinsufficiency. These general mechanisms are applicable to different subtypes of EDS, and the precise phenotype is dependent upon the nature of the mutations and the type of collagen being affected.

Lysyl hydroxylase deficiency, caused by mutations in the corresponding gene, PLOD, results in reduced hydroxylysine content of collagen polypeptides and an altered cross-linking profile of collagen fibrils. This leads to the recessively inherited kyphoscoliosis type of EDS (previously known as type VI). Mutations affecting another collagen processing enzyme, procollagen N-peptidase (encoded by the ADAMTS2 gene) that is responsible for the cleavage of amino-terminal propeptides from triple-helical type I procollagen, result in the formation of irregular and thin collagen fibrils with reduced mechanical properties. The collagen fibrils appear 'hieroglyphic' in cross-section and contain type I collagen with an intact N-propeptide, termed pN-collagen. Procollagen N-peptidase deficiency leads to the recessively inherited dermatosparaxis type of EDS (previously known as type VIIC).

Dominant-negative effects leading to EDS are caused by mutations in different collagen genes, including those encoding α-chains of type I (COL1A1, COL1A2), type III (COL3A1) and type V (COL5A1, COL5A2) collagens. Characteristically, these types of genetic lesions are splicing mutations resulting in an in-frame deletion of a single exon, or missense mutations resulting in a glycine substitution in the collagenous domain. Since the expression levels of these 'mutated' polypeptides is the same as for the normal chains and they are incorporated into the polymeric collagen molecules, they affect the triple helix formation and/or thermal stability of the collagen triple helices by a dominant-negative mechanism. The presence of these abnormal chains results in defective secretion of collagen molecules, and, as a consequence, the collagen fibrils are structurally abnormal and reduced in amounts.

Haploinsufficiency is caused by loss-of-function mutations, frequently premature termination codon mutations. These types of mutations often result in unstable mRNA due to accelerated mRNA decay, and this leads to an absence of the corresponding polypeptide. Haploinsufficiency can also be caused by missense mutations, which lead to the synthesis of polypeptides that are unable to incorporate into collagen triple helices. Haploinsufficiency results in the synthesis of only 50% of the normal amount of collagen molecules, and this is not enough to form fully functional collagen fibrils.

COLLAGEN BIOSYNTHESIS, SECRETION AND FIBRIL ASSEMBLY – RELATIONSHIP OF PATHOLOGY TO THE MAJOR SUBTYPE OF EHLERS-DANLOS SYNDROME

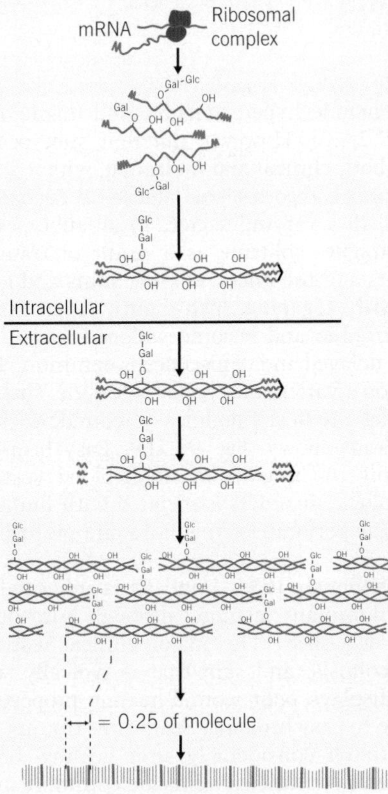

Physiology		Pathology	EDS subtype (mode of inheritance)
	Synthesis, hydroxylation and glycosylation of pro-α polypeptides of type I, III and V collagens	Lysyl hydroxylase deficiency results in reduced hydroxylysine content and altered cross-linking profile	Kyphoscoliosis (AR)
	Formation of interchain S-S bonds at the carboxyl ends followed by triple helix formation	Dominant-negative mutations or haploinsufficiency in COL3A1 affect triple helix formation, thermal stability, and secretion of type III collagen molecules	Vascular type (AD)
	Secretion of procollagen	Dominant-negative mutations in the recognition sites for procollagen N-peptidase in COL1A1 and COL1A2 prevent cleavage of amino-terminal propeptides	Arthrochalasia (AD)
	Removal of propeptides by specific proteases	Loss-of-function mutations in procollagen-N-peptidase result in the formation of only thin collagen fibrils	Dermatosparaxis (AR)
	Fibril assembly	Dominant-negative mutations in COL5A1 and COL5A2 or haploinsufficiency in COL5A1 result in abnormal or reduced amount of collagen fibrils	Classical type (AD)
		Absence of tenascin-X leads to reduced collagen fibril density	Classical type (AR)
	Stabilization of fibrils by intermolecular cross-linking		

Fig. 97.1 **Collagen biosynthesis, secretion and fibril assembly – relationship of pathology to the major subtype of Ehlers–Danlos syndrome.** AD, autosomal dominant; AR, autosomal recessive; Glc-Gal, glucosyl-galactosyl residue attached to the hydroxyl group (OH) of lysine residues; S-S bonds, disulfide bonds.

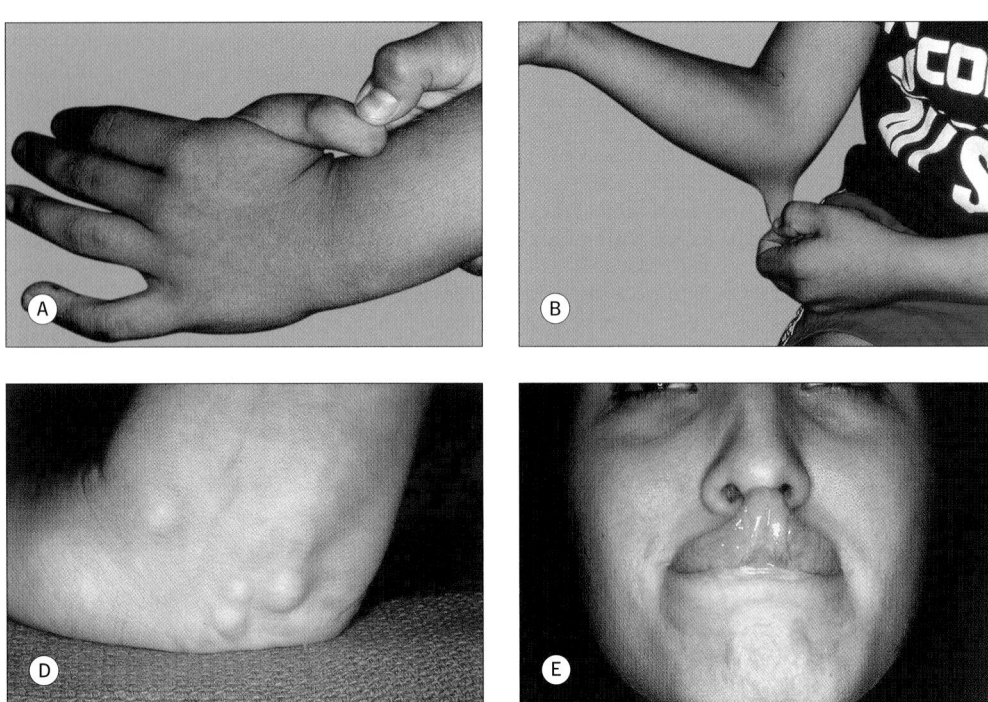

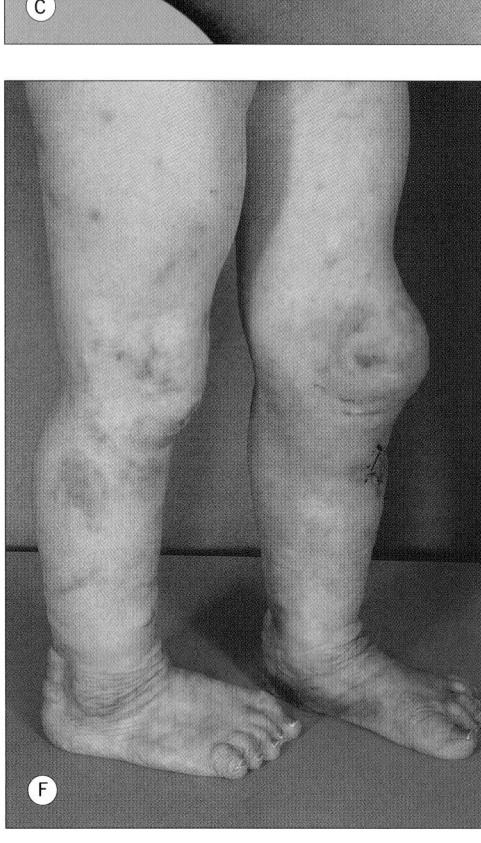

Fig. 97.2 Clinical features of Ehlers–Danlos syndrome (EDS). Patients with classic EDS demonstrating joint hypermobility (**A**), hyperextensible skin (**B**), a widened atrophic scar (**C**), molluscoid pseudotumors (**D**) and Gorlin's sign (**E**). Extensive bruising on the shins in a patient with dermatosparaxis (**F**); similar changes can be seen in vascular EDS. F, Courtesy of Julie V Schaffer MD.

The vascular type of EDS (previously known as type IV) can be caused by both dominant-negative mutations in *COL3A1* and haplo-insufficiency of type III collagen, an important component of arterial and intestinal walls, and less abundant component in dermal connective tissue. Yet, the reduced amount of type III collagen leads to small and variably sized dermal collagen fibrils and thinning of the dermis, emphasizing the pivotal role of type III collagen in fibrillogenesis.

The classic type of EDS (previously known as types I and II) can be caused by both dominant-negative mutations in *COL5A1* and *COL5A2* as well as haploinsufficiency of type V collagen (*COL5A1*). It has been estimated that 30–50% of all classic EDS cases are caused by a haploinsufficiency of type V collagen. The role of type V collagen in collagen fibrillogenesis is to limit fibril diameter, and consequently, reduced amounts of type V collagen could explain the approximately 25% increase in fibril diameter as observed by electron microscopy. Mutations in the genes encoding the pro-α-chains of type I collagen (*COL1A1*, *COL1A2*) that correspond to the cleavage site of procollagen N-peptidase result in the dominantly inherited arthrochalasia type of EDS (previously known as types VIIA and VIIB), while procollagen N-peptidase deficiency leads to dermatosparaxis (previously known as type VIIC), a recessively inherited condition.

The role of tenascin-X in the pathogenesis of EDS became evident when a patient with adrenal hyperplasia and classic EDS was found to harbor a contiguous gene deletion encompassing the *CYP21* gene that encodes steroid 21-hydroxylase and the tenascin-X gene (*TNX*)[7]. Since tenascin-X is expressed in the tissues affected in EDS, i.e. skin, tendons, muscle and blood vessels, and since tenascin-X is developmentally associated with collagen fibrils[10], it was reasonable to propose that this protein is somehow involved in the pathogenesis of EDS in such patients. Subsequently, it was found that tenascin-X was absent in the fibroblast culture medium and serum of a number of EDS patients due to null mutations in both alleles of the *TNX* gene, thus verifying that tenascin-X deficiency is an autosomal recessive disorder leading to EDS with features similar to those of the classic type of EDS[11]. The pathoetiologic role of tenascin-X has also been confirmed by the development of *TNX* null mice ('knockout mice'; see Ch. 4), which exhibit progressive hyperextensibility and reduced tensile strength of their skin[12].

Clinical Features

The general features of EDS include hyperextensible and fragile skin and loose-jointedness (Fig. 97.2A,B). However, different subtypes of EDS have additional features, both clinical and molecular, which allow their classification into six distinct categories (see Table 97.2; Fig. 97.3). The skin findings are present, to a varying degree, in all subtypes of EDS[3]. Typically, the skin is fragile, splitting as a result of trauma, particularly over pressure points and the knees, elbows, shins and forehead. The wounds present with a gaping, 'fish-mouth' appearance, and the resulting scars are atrophic and become widened with time (Fig. 97.2C). Wound healing is delayed and dehiscence is common. The areas of repeated trauma develop a variety of secondary lesions, such as molluscoid pseudotumors, which are fleshy nodules of redundant skin, usually found on the knees and elbows (Fig. 97.2D). Easy bruising is a common finding, reflecting the fragility of small blood vessels. A number of unusual dermatologic disorders associated with (but not specific to) EDS include elastosis perforans serpiginosa and piezogenic papules.

The *classic type of EDS* (previously types I and II) is inherited in most cases in an autosomal dominant fashion, although autosomal recessive families have been described. The major clinical features include hypermobile joints, scoliosis, and skin that is typically soft, velvety, hyperextensible and displays poor wound-healing properties. The dermis is fragile and prone to easy bruising. Scars after trauma are thin and atrophic and can stretch considerably after healing, often having a 'cigarette paper' appearance. Varicose veins are common, as is Gorlin's sign (Fig. 97.2E). A significant number of classic EDS patients have cardiac defects, including mitral valve prolapse; pes planus in which the entire sole touches the ground is also quite common.

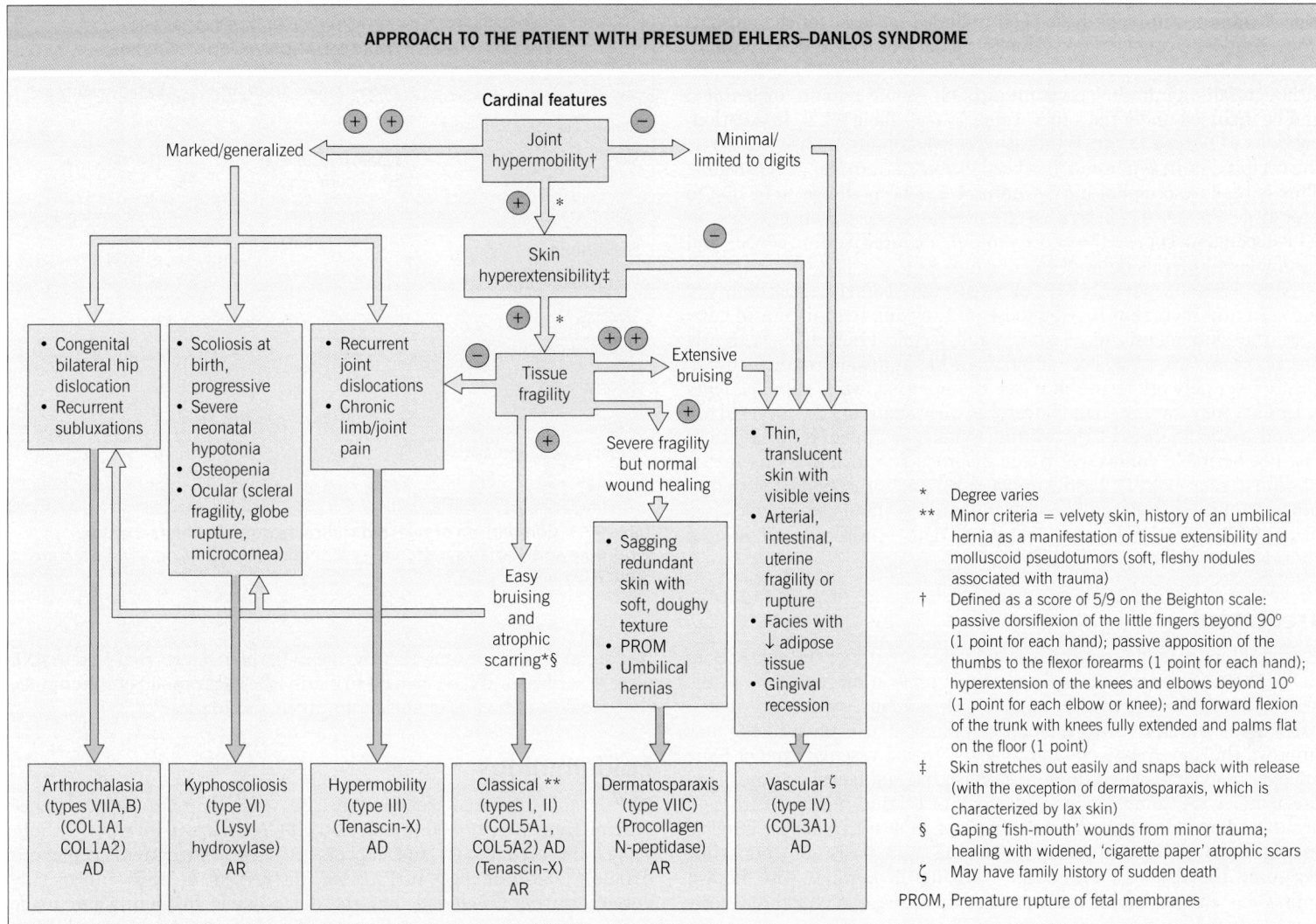

Fig. 97.3 Approach to the patient with presumed Ehlers–Danlos syndrome. AD, autosomal dominant; AR, autosomal recessive.

The *hypermobility type of EDS* (previously type III) has an autosomal dominant inheritance pattern. The prominent clinical features are generalized joint hypermobility and hyperextensible, smooth and velvety skin. Other features include recurrent joint dislocations which can cause chronic joint and limb pain as well as eventually osteoarthritic changes.

The *vascular type of EDS* (previously type IV) is inherited in an autosomal dominant fashion. These patients have thin, translucent skin, and they have a high risk for arterial, intestinal and uterine ruptures[13]. Spontaneous arterial rupture has the highest incidence in the third or fourth decade of life, but may occur much earlier. Extensive bruising is a common feature. These patients often have a characteristic facial appearance, with a thin, pinched nose, thin lips, hollow cheeks, and prominent 'staring' eyes due to decreased periorbital adipose tissue.

The *kyphoscoliosis type of EDS* (previously type VI) is inherited in an autosomal recessive fashion. Major diagnostic features are generalized joint laxity, severe muscular hypotonia at birth (leading to delayed gross motor development), progressive kyphoscoliosis which is apparent at birth, and scleral fragility which can lead to rupture of the ocular globe. Less frequent clinical features are tissue fragility, atrophic scars, easy bruising, a marfanoid habitus, microcornea and osteopenia.

The *arthrochalasia type of EDS* (previously types VIIA and VIIB) is inherited in an autosomal dominant fashion. The major clinical features include severe generalized joint hypermobility with recurrent subluxations and congenital bilateral hip dislocation. In addition, patients may also present with hyperextensible skin, tissue fragility, atrophic scars, easy bruising, muscle hypotonia, kyphoscoliosis and mild osteopenia.

The *dermatosparaxis type of EDS* (previously type VIIC) is an autosomal recessive disorder with the major clinical features being severe skin fragility and sagging, redundant skin. These features are associated with soft and doughy skin, easy bruising (Fig. 97.2F), premature rupture of fetal membranes and, occasionally, large umbilical or inguinal hernias. Additional findings include delayed closure of fontanels, distinctive facies with puffy eyelids and micrognathia, blue sclerae, gingival hyperplasia, abnormal dentition and short limbs.

Pathology

Histopathologic examination of the skin may provide clues to a connective tissue disorder when a thinned reticular dermis and reduced and disorganized collagen fibrils are seen, but, in general, the histopathology is not diagnostic. Non-specific increases in elastic fibers have been reported, particularly in areas of trauma, which form molluscoid pseudotumors. Electron microscopy often shows the presence of collagen fibrils with variable diameters and occasional large fibrils with an irregular contour. Characteristic hieroglyphic fibrils can be encountered in the dermatosparaxis type of EDS. With immunohistochemistry, demonstration of an accumulation of type III collagen intracellularly may be helpful in pointing to the vascular type of EDS. In general, the diagnosis of EDS is clinical, and a subtype can be confirmed by the demonstration of specific collagen defects (see Fig. 97.1), particularly in the case of the vascular type of EDS[13]. Tenascin-X deficiency can be demonstrated by an ELISA of a serum sample[11].

Differential Diagnosis

The revised classification scheme identifies six distinct categories of EDS, based on pathognomonic descriptions and molecular diagnostics[5]. Several previously described but exceedingly rare subtypes of EDS, including type V (X-linked variant), type VIII (periodontitis type) and type X (fibronectin type), have been excluded (at least for the present) from diagnostic considerations due to the lack of a clear description of the clinical features and the precise molecular basis. These patients, although falling into the spectrum of EDS, should remain unclassified and be included under the 'other' category (see Table 97.2). In addition, previous EDS type IX, an X-linked recessive condition, also known as the occipital horn syndrome, has been excluded from the EDS category. This is because occipital horn syndrome has been shown to be due to mutations in the same gene as Menkes disease, which encodes an ATP-dependent copper transport protein. Reduced serum copper and ceruloplasmin levels point to the diagnosis.

Although some patients with EDS have marked hyperextensibility of the skin and their skin may be loose and sagging reminiscent of cutis laxa, the skin retains its elasticity and recoil. Thus, EDS is clearly distinct from cutis laxa, a condition resulting from abnormalities in the elastic fiber network in the skin (see below). Also, while some patients with EDS may have marfanoid features, these patients do not regularly exhibit other findings of the Marfan syndrome (Table 97.3), a clearly distinct heritable connective tissue disorder due to mutations in the fibrillin-1 gene (FBN1). Lastly, unusual variants of EDS related to dysfunction of galactosyl transferase-1 or filamin A should be excluded (see Table 97.2), as should type II Loeys–Dietz syndrome and arterial tortuosity syndrome (see Table 94.5).

Treatment

Currently, no specific treatment is available for any of the subtypes of EDS. The most important intervention is prevention of trauma to the skin, such as the use of shin guards and avoidance of contact sports. Meticulous surgical care, including prolonged use of sutures, may improve the appearance of surgical scars. In the vascular type of EDS, affected individuals are at high risk of arterial and bowel ruptures, and pregnancies are complicated by the risk of uterine rupture. Early and accurate diagnosis of the vascular type of EDS is critical for surgical management of catastrophic events, and is a basis for counseling regarding the risk of pregnancies[13]. Finally, in families with known mutations and at risk for recurrence of the disease, prenatal diagnosis can be offered.

PSEUDOXANTHOMA ELASTICUM

Synonym: ■ Grönblad–Strandberg syndrome

Key features

■ An autosomal recessive disorder characterized by clumped and distorted elastic fibers with deposits of calcium

■ Mutations in the *ABCC6* gene disrupt the function of the ABC-cassette transporter MRP6

■ Cutaneous features include yellowish skin papules, 'cobblestoning' and redundant folds in flexural sites

■ Angioid streaks due to breaks in the calcified elastic lamina of Bruch's membrane can result in loss of visual acuity

■ Calcification of elastic fibers in medium-sized arteries leads to claudication, hypertension, angina and myocardial infarctions

History

The French dermatologist Balzer first described the skin manifestations of pseudoxanthoma elasticum (PXE) in association with elastic degeneration of the skin and heart in 1884[14], followed by a similar case report by Chauffard 5 years later[15]. After extensive examination of these two cases, Darier coined the name 'pseudo-xanthome élastique' in 1896 to differentiate this condition from xanthomas (hence pseudo-xanthoma)[16]. In the late 1920s, Grönblad[17] and Strandberg[18] recognized the association of the characteristic skin manifestations with angioid streaks, while the cardiovascular manifestations were fully appreciated

COMPARISON OF SELECTED CLINICAL FEATURES IN EHLERS–DANLOS SYNDROME AND MARFAN SYNDROME

	Ehlers–Danlos syndrome	Marfan syndrome
Molluscoid pseudotumors	++	–
Skin	Hyperextensibility, 'fish-mouth' scars	Striae distensae
Joint hypermobility	++ (often severe)	+ (mild–moderate)
Easy bruising	++	–
Pectus excavatum	–	++
Scoliosis	+	++
High-arched palate	–	++
Ectopia lentis	+	++
Myopia	+	++
Mitral valve abnormalities	+	++
Stature	Short, normal or tall	Tall

Table 97.3 **Comparison of selected clinical features in Ehlers–Danlos syndrome and Marfan syndrome.** ++, common feature; +, occasional feature; –, not a feature.

two decades later[19]. More recently, the molecular defects that lead to PXE were described and have helped to clarify the exact mode of inheritance that previously had been subject to much speculation[20,20a].

Epidemiology

PXE is an autosomal recessive disease with estimates of prevalence ranging from 1 in 25 000 to 1 in 100 000. It occurs in all races without geographic predilection and appears to have a slight female preponderance[21]. Skin changes of PXE are not present at birth and usually develop during childhood, but the diagnosis is frequently not made until serious systemic or ocular complications develop in the third or fourth decade of life.

Pathogenesis

Inactivating mutations in the *ABCC6* gene on the short arm of chromosome 16 can be identified in the majority of patients with PXE. *ABCC6* encodes MRP6, an ABC-cassette transporter with a high degree of sequence homology to the multidrug resistance-associated proteins. MRP6 is expressed in the membrane of hepatocytes and renal cells and probably serves as an efflux pump. Unlike other members of this protein family, MRP6 does not seem to confer any significant chemotherapy resistance; however, there may be some functional overlap in that MRP6 is believed to play a role in cellular detoxification.

Although the physiologic or pathologic substrates of this ATP-dependent transporter are still unknown and, thus far, no abnormality in the plasma or serum has been identified, faulty or aberrant expression of MRP6 in PXE is hypothesized to result in an accumulation of substances with an affinity for elastic fibers[22]. Subsequent clumping and distortion of these elastic fibers in target organs then leads to deposition of calcium and other minerals. These secondary changes impair the proper function of elastin and elastic fibers in the mid and deep dermis, the media and intima of mid-sized arteries, and Bruch's membrane in the eye, where characteristic clinical and histopathologic changes occur.

Clinical Features

PXE typically affects the elastic fiber network of three organ systems – the skin, eyes and cardiovascular system. There is tremendous variability in severity even among siblings, and occasionally, only one or two of these organ systems show signs of the disease.

PXE owes its name to the characteristic cutaneous findings, which bear some resemblance to xanthomas and represent the most uniform feature amongst all affected individuals. Discrete, flat, yellowish papules

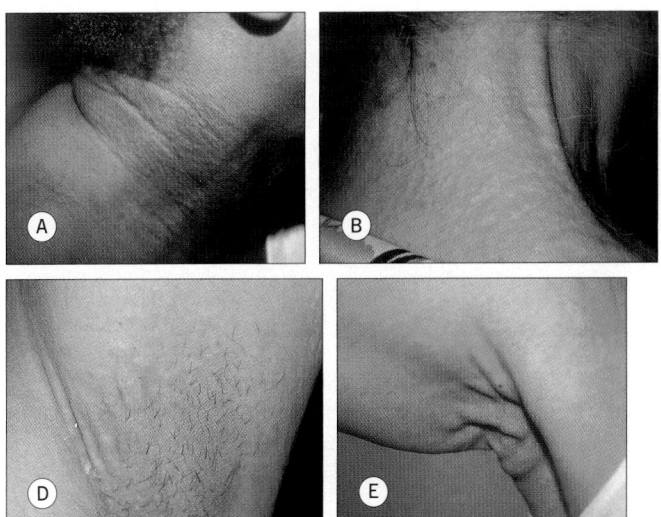

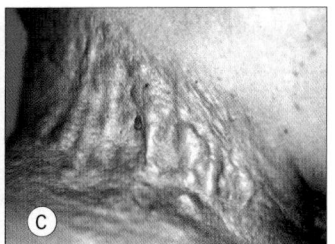

Fig. 97.4 Clinical features of pseudoxanthoma elasticum. Yellowish papules and plaques on the neck (**A, B**). Firm, calcified plaques within longstanding skin lesions (**C**). Skin-colored papules and mild redundancy in the axilla (**D**). Sagging skin in the axilla (**E**).

appear in flexural areas, most commonly during the first or second decade of life. The lateral neck is usually affected first (Fig. 97.4A,B). Over time, these papules progress and coalesce to form cobblestone-like plaques, giving rise to a 'plucked chicken skin' appearance. Depending on the extent of the disease, other flexural sites such as the antecubital and popliteal fossae, the wrists, axillae and groin become affected, and involvement of non-flexural sites may be observed in extensive cases. Increased physical stress on the elastic fiber network, as is common for the neck and skin folds, may perhaps permit injury mediated by MRP6 dysfunction. This theory is supported by the fact that skin involvement may be seen after excessive weight gain in non-predilection sites such as around the umbilicus in multiparous women (not to be confused with perforating periumbilical calcific elastosis, a localized, acquired, purely cutaneous PXE-like condition [see Ch. 95 and Table 97.4]). In some patients without typical skin manifestations but with other findings suggestive of PXE, such as angioid streaks, a diagnosis may be confirmed by a biopsy of a pre-existing scar[23].

With advanced disease, significant calcium deposits may present as firm papules or plaques (Fig. 97.4C), and may occasionally extrude from the skin in 'perforating PXE'. Loss of recoil due to impaired function of the elastic fiber network often leads to sagging of the skin, which is most notable in the axillae (Fig. 97.4D,E) and groin. Mucosal involvement is most prominent on the inner aspect of the lower lip (Fig. 97.5), and presents in a similar fashion to the skin lesions with yellow papules. Prominent mental (chin) creases represent an additional cutaneous sign of PXE, occurring in two-thirds of affected individuals less than 30 years of age and the vast majority of older patients.

While the cutaneous findings present primarily a cosmetic problem and do not interfere with normal activities, ophthalmologic complications are often quite debilitating. The majority of patients with PXE have angioid streaks (Fig. 97.6), and after the age of 30, their prevalence approaches 100%[21]. While angioid streaks may be detected as early as in the first decade of life, they usually become symptomatic only after trauma to the eye. Angioid streaks result from breaks in the calcified elastic lamina of Bruch's membrane, which is derived from the retina and the choroid plexus. These fractures can lead to neovascularization from choriocapillaries, and subsequent leakage of newly formed vessels may lead to hemorrhage and scarring. Ultimately, these pathologic changes cause progressive loss of visual acuity and, rarely, legal blindness.

DIFFERENTIAL DIAGNOSIS OF PSEUDOXANTHOMA ELASTICUM			
Disorder	**Patient characteristics**	**Clinical features**	**Histologic features**
Actinic elastosis	History of chronic sun exposure; lightly pigmented skin; middle-aged and older adults	Yellow to gray, thickened, lax, finely to coarsely wrinkled skin; photodistribution on the lateral forehead, neck, dorsal aspect of the forearms	Masses of basophilic, amorphous, degenerated elastic fibers in the papillary and upper reticular dermis
Late-onset focal dermal elastosis	7th–9th decades	Multiple 1–3 mm yellow papules; may coalesce; neck, axillae, groin, antecubital and popliteal fossae	Increased normal-appearing elastic fibers in the mid and deep reticular dermis
Elastoderma	3rd–4th decades	Localized areas of lax, pendulous skin; neck, trunk, arm	Increased normal- and abnormal-appearing elastic fibers throughout the dermis, extending into the subcutis
Perforating periumbilical calcific elastosis*	Multiparous black women; 5th–8th decades†	Plaque composed of coalescing keratotic papules (most apparent at the periphery); periumbilical area‡	Transepidermal elimination of calcified, distorted elastic fibers
PXE-like papillary dermal elastolysis§	6th–9th decades; primarily women	Multiple 2–3 mm yellow or skin-colored papules coalescing to form plaques with a cobblestone appearance; neck, flexor forearms, axillae, lower abdomen, inframammary folds	Decreased elastic tissue in a band-like distribution in the papillary dermis, with fragmentation and clumping of elastic fibers
White fibrous papulosis of the neck§	5th–9th decades; Japanese men, Caucasian women	Multiple 2–3 mm whitish papules; neck > upper trunk	Thickened collagen bundles and decreased elastic fibers in the papillary and mid reticular dermis

*Also referred to as periumbilical perforating PXE.
†Occasionally associated with an increased calcium-phosphate product in the setting of chronic renal failure.
‡Similar lesions have been reported on the breasts.
§Within the spectrum of fibroelastolytic diseases of the skin.

Table 97.4 Differential diagnosis of pseudoxanthoma elasticum (PXE). The differential diagnosis also includes PXE-like skin lesions in patients receiving D-penicillamine, after local exposure to saltpeter, and in longstanding end-stage renal disease. In addition, the possibility of underlying β-thalassemia and sickle cell anemia needs to be considered.

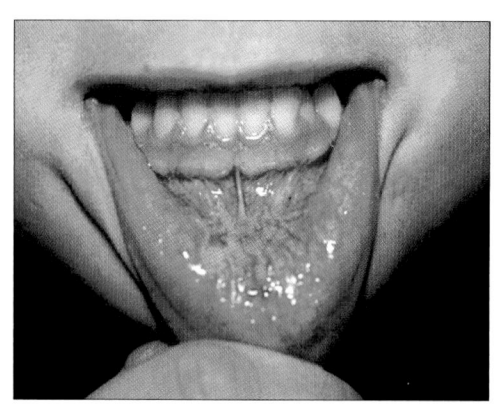

Fig. 97.5 Mucosal lesions in pseudoxanthoma elasticum. Yellow papules on the inner aspect of the lower lip.

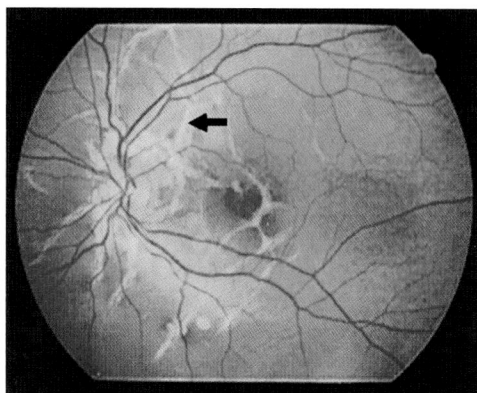

Fig. 97.6 Funduscopic appearance of angioid streaks in pseudoxanthoma elasticum. Broad, lightly colored streaks (arrow) represent the angioid streaks.

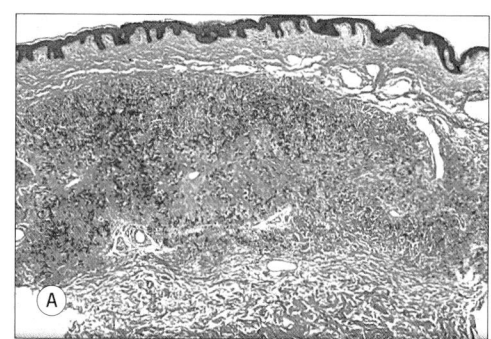

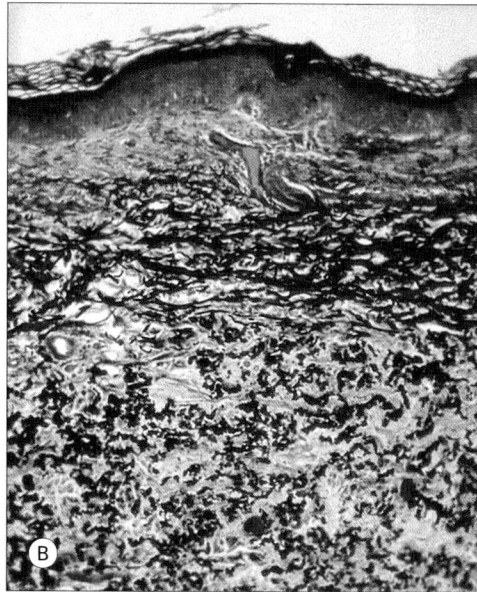

Fig. 97.7 Histopathology of pseudoxanthoma elasticum (PXE). **A** Purple clumps in the mid and deep reticular dermis in H&E-stained sections represent calcium deposits on elastic fibers in advanced PXE. **B** Verhoeff–van Gieson elastic stain can reveal black-staining, irregularly clumped elastic fibers in earlier disease.

It should be noted that angioid streaks, although characteristic for PXE, are not pathognomonic. They can be encountered in a variety of metabolic and heritable disorders, including Paget's disease of the bone, sickle cell anemia, thalassemia, EDS, and lead poisoning, as well as in the setting of age-related degeneration of Bruch's membrane. Mottling of the retinal pigment epithelium (*peau d'orange*) is the most prevalent ophthalmologic finding in PXE, and, less commonly, macular degeneration, optic drusen and 'owl's eyes' (paired hyperpigmented spots) may be detected.

PXE affects primarily mid-sized arteries, predominantly of the extremities, where progressive calcification of the elastic media and intima leads to the formation of atheromatous plaques[24]. As a result, intermittent claudication, loss of peripheral pulses, renovascular hypertension, angina pectoris and myocardial infarction are frequent sequelae that occur at a much younger age than in the unaffected population. There is an increased incidence of cerebral ischemic attacks but not of aneurysms[25]. Mitral valve prolapse is also a common finding[26], easily diagnosed by echocardiography. Calcified blood vessels of the gastric and intestinal mucosa may have an increased propensity for rupture and hemorrhage leading to gastrointestinal bleeding, particularly from the stomach[21]. The aforementioned vascular symptoms often cause significant morbidity and may even result in early death. PXE does not affect the lung, liver or kidneys.

Pathology

While there is no epidermal alteration or cellular infiltrate, characteristic light microscopic changes of the skin consist of distorted, fragmented elastic fibers in the mid and deep reticular dermis. In advanced cases, calcium deposits on these altered elastic fibers are visible in H&E-stained sections as purple clumps (Fig. 97.7A). Similar changes are observed in the media of mid-sized arteries. In early disease, stains for elastin (Verhoeff–van Gieson; Fig. 97.7B) and calcium (von Kossa) are sometimes necessary to visualize the characteristic alterations in the elastic fibers. An increased deposition of matrix proteins with a high degree of affinity for calcium is observed on an ultrastructural level; these proteins include osteonectin, fibronectin and vitronectin, as well as alkaline phosphatase and bone sialoprotein[27]. Serum levels of calcium and phosphate are normal[21].

Differential Diagnosis

Although typical skin lesions of PXE are quite characteristic and easily diagnosed in young patients, actinic damage within chronically sun-exposed sites in older individuals may clinically mimic the yellowish, lax plaques. However, the latter involves the neck, but not the axillae or groin. The differential diagnosis also includes late-onset focal dermal elastosis, elastoderma, perforating periumbilical calcific elastosis, and fibroelastolytic diseases of the skin (PXE-like papillary dermal elastolysis and white fibrous papulosis of the neck) (see Table 97.4)[28,29].

PXE-like skin lesions in predilection sites and with similar histologic features have been observed in patients receiving D-penicillamine[30], after local exposure to saltpeter[31,32], in longstanding end-stage renal disease[33] and in L-tryptophan-induced eosinophilia myalgia syndrome[34]. In patients with penicillamine-induced PXE-like skin changes, the von Kossa stain is negative, indicating no calcification of the abnormal fibers, whereas in saltpeter exposure and end-stage renal disease, it is positive. Ophthalmologic and cardiovascular findings are absent and the skin lesions may resolve after correction of the underlying disorder. Penicillamine interferes with desmosine cross-links between elastin molecules (see below).

A PXE-like phenotype is present in up to 20% of the patients with β-thalassemia (Greek population) or sickle cell anemia[35]. They may have characteristic cutaneous involvement as well as angioid streaks and vascular stigmata, but none of their unaffected siblings have signs of PXE and mutations in *ABCC6* have not been detected. The etiology remains unclear because there is no obvious genetic link between these disorders. In addition, PXE-like skin lesions have been encountered in amyloid elastosis, but histopathology reveals deposition of amyloid and no evidence of elastic fiber abnormality[36]. Recently, PXE-like clinical and histopathologic findings have been encountered in CL patients in association with multiple coagulation factor deficiency (see below).

Treatment

Appropriate management of PXE requires a multispecialty approach. After confirmation of the diagnosis by skin biopsy from an affected area or a predilection site, patients should undergo baseline ophthalmologic and cardiovascular examinations. Cutaneous manifestations of PXE present a considerable aesthetic problem, but no specific therapy is currently available. If sagging of the skin is prominent, reconstructive surgery may provide temporary relief[37].

Ophthalmologic care includes biannual or annual funduscopy, regular use of an Amsler grid, and prevention of retinal hemorrhage through avoidance of head trauma, heavy straining and smoking. A diet rich in antioxidants and the use of sunglasses are recommended. Laser photocoagulation is the only treatment proven effective for choroidal neovascularization, but this modality is hampered by a high recurrence rate (65%)[38]. Macular translocation, an experimental approach, may be considered if bleeding has occurred as a result of extensive neovascularization[39].

Emphasis should be placed on preventative medicine and a healthy lifestyle with respect to the cardiovascular complications resulting from calcification of blood vessels. Regular exercise, weight control, avoidance of smoking and excessive alcohol consumption, and treatment of hypercholesterolemia and hypertension are essential. Although it has been suggested that increased serum calcium exacerbates calcium deposition in patients with PXE[40], dietary restriction of calcium is not recommended until further studies become available. Calcium intake should be moderate but adequate for age. The role of EDTA chelation therapy, which aims at binding calcium and other minerals, is controversial because of serious side effects in addition to its unproven clinical efficacy[41]. Although platelet inhibitors may increase the severity of gastrointestinal bleeds, low-dose therapy with acetylsalicylic acid may occasionally be indicated to prevent the risk of myocardial infarction and to treat intermittent claudication. Pentoxifylline, cilostazol and clopidogrel are also helpful in some patients with intermittent claudication.

In families with known mutations, genetic analysis is available for presymptomatic testing, carrier detection and prenatal diagnosis.

CUTIS LAXA

Synonyms: ■ Dermatochalasia ■ Dermatomegaly ■ Generalized elastolysis ■ Generalized elastorrhexis

Key features

- Loss and fragmentation of elastic fibers in the skin and, in some patients, in other tissues such as the lung and gastrointestinal tract
- Both heritable (autosomal dominant or recessive) and acquired forms
- Loose, sagging skin with reduced elasticity and resilience
- Extracutaneous manifestations include pulmonary emphysema, hernias and diverticuli

History

Historically, cutis laxa (CL) was often confused with EDS, until 1923, when F Parkes Weber noted the clinical differences between these two conditions[4]. The internal involvement and the systemic nature of CL were elucidated by Goltz and co-workers[42], who emphasized the phenomenon of generalized elastolysis in some patients.

Epidemiology

The heritable forms of CL are relatively rare and no precise estimate of their prevalence or incidence is available. There appears to be no racial or ethnic predilection, and the inheritance can be autosomal dominant or autosomal recessive. A number of cases of CL are acquired and have a late onset.

Pathogenesis

CL is a primary disorder of the elastic fiber network and can involve multiple tissues, including the skin. With regard to the heritable forms

of CL, recent discoveries have begun to provide insight into the underlying pathogenesis. Initially, fibulin-5 'knockout' mice (see Ch. 4) were noted to develop a phenotype remarkably similar to human CL[43,44]. Specifically, the mice developed disorganized elastic fibers, with resulting loose skin, vascular abnormalities and emphysematous lungs. Fibulin-5 is a calcium-dependent, elastin-binding protein that localizes to the surface of elastic fibers in vivo. Subsequently, fibulin-5 mutations were described in families with an autosomal recessive form of CL, as well as in a sporadic case with evidence of an autosomal dominant form of CL[45,46].

In addition, specific mutations in the elastin gene (*ELN*) have been observed in several families with an autosomal dominant form of CL[47–49]. These mutations were interpreted to be 'dominant-acting' and responsible for qualitative and quantitative defects in elastin, resulting in the CL phenotype. Lastly, a recessively inherited mutation in the fibulin-4 gene was described in a patient with a CL syndrome, suggesting that fibulin-4 is also necessary for elastic fiber formation[50].

Consistent with the notion that mutations in the elastin gene can be found in some cases of CL, it has been demonstrated that elastin mRNA steady-state levels are reduced in fibroblasts from patients with severe congenital forms of the disease[51]. In some cases, elastin expression is essentially undetectable or clearly less than 10% of the level noted in healthy unrelated controls. Although the reason for reduced steady-state levels of elastin mRNA could be multiple (e.g. reduced rate of transcription or decreased stability of the transcript), the end result would be the same, i.e. less elastin protein being synthesized in the skin and other tissues affected in these patients.

An alternate mechanism for the development of CL is enhanced degradation of the elastic fibers[52]. Proteolytic mechanisms are presumably also involved in some of the patients with acquired, late-onset forms of CL. In this latter group, extensive sagging of the skin develops, with little or no evidence of internal organ involvement, and the patients frequently have experienced an allergic reaction, e.g. a drug reaction, which within the ensuing weeks or months can result in a prematurely aged appearance and sagging of the skin. In cases of inflammatory cutaneous reactions, a possible explanation for the development of CL is that inflammatory cells, such as polymorphonuclear leukocytes and monocyte-macrophages, contain powerful elastases which become activated and are released from these cells into the extracellular milieu, resulting in proteolytic degradation of the elastic fibers[53]. Furthermore, immunopathogenetic mechanisms may play a role in a small subset of patients, as evidenced by IgG and IgA deposits in lesional skin or paraproteinemia[54]. In addition, there may be an underlying genetic susceptibility for the development of acquired CL, e.g. missense alleles in the elastin and fibulin-5 genes[55].

Finally, CL-like cutaneous changes as well as elastosis perforans serpiginosa and PXE-like changes have been observed in patients treated for a prolonged period with high-dose D-penicillamine for conditions such as Wilson's disease or cystinuria. D-Penicillamine can interfere with elastin cross-linking by two mechanisms. Firstly, D-penicillamine is a copper chelator and can result in low serum copper levels, which in turn reduce the activity of lysyl oxidase, the enzyme required for the oxidative deamination of lysine to allysine, a necessary step for elastin cross-linking[56]. Secondly, D-penicillamine can chemically block the allysine and lysine residues that come together to form desmosine cross-links. As a result of these actions, the newly synthesized elastin molecules do not become stably cross-linked. Instead, they are subject to rapid proteolysis, thus precluding the synthesis of functional elastic fibers.

Clinical Features

Clinically, CL is characterized by loose and sagging skin with reduced elasticity and resilience that often gives the affected patient an appearance of premature aging (Figs 97.8 & 97.9A). These cutaneous findings can be present at birth and progress steadily throughout life. In some patients, the clinical findings are limited to the skin, and the phenotype can be primarily of cosmetic concern. In other patients, however, the cutaneous findings are associated with a number of xtracutaneous manifestations, including pulmonary emphysema, umbilical and inguinal hernias, and gastrointestinal and vesico-urinary tract diverticuli. The extracutaneous manifestations, particularly the

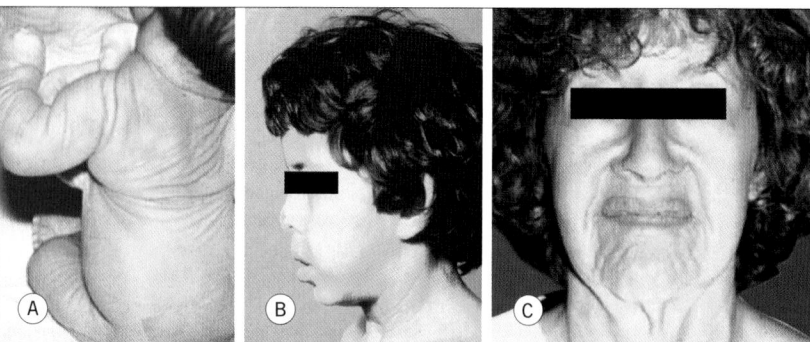

Fig. 97.8 Clinical features in cutis laxa. Loose and sagging skin in a newborn (**A**), a sagging jowl in a 4-year-old boy (**B**), and prematurely aged appearance of a 30-year-old woman (**C**). Adapted with permission from Uitto J, Pulkkinen L. Heritable disorders affecting the elastic tissues: cutis laxa, pseudoxanthoma elasticum and related disorders. In: Rimoin DL, Connor JM, Pyeritz RE (eds). Emery and Rimoin's Principles and Practice of Medical Genetics, 3rd edn. London: Churchill Livingstone, 2002.

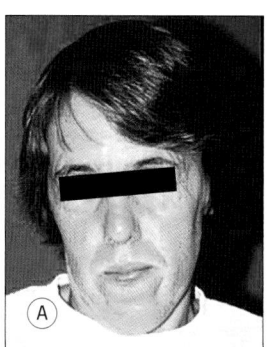
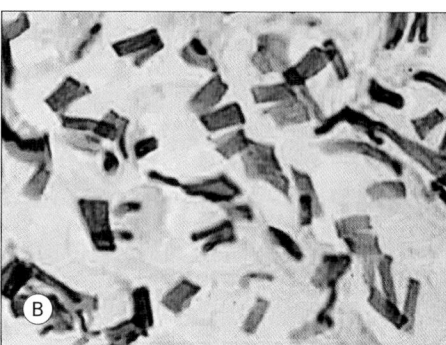

Fig. 97.9 Clinical and histologic features in cutis laxa. A Premature aging appearance of a 15-year-old patient. **B** Histopathology of the skin depicts fragmentation of dermal elastic fibers (orcein stain). Adapted with permission from Uitto J, Pulkkinen L. Heritable disorders affecting the elastic tissues: cutis laxa, pseudoxanthoma elasticum and related disorders. In: Rimoin DL, Connor JM, Pyeritz RE (eds). Emery and Rimoin's Principles and Practice of Medical Genetics, 3rd edn. London: Churchill Livingstone, 2002.

ACQUIRED CUTIS LAXA: CLINICAL PRESENTATIONS AND ASSOCIATED CONDITIONS	
Presentations	**Associations**
Generalized • Postinflammatory • Paraneoplastic • α_1-antitrypsin deficiency • Drug-induced • Idiopathic Localized • Postinflammatory • Paraneoplastic • α_1-antitrypsin deficiency • Drug-induced	Inflammatory conditions • Urticaria • Angioedema • Rheumatoid arthritis • Systemic lupus erythematosus • Erythema multiforme • Sweet's syndrome (Marshall's syndrome) • Nephrotic syndrome • Celiac disease • Dermatitis herpetiformis Infectious diseases • *Borrelia burgdorferi* Hematologic disorders • Plasma cell dyscrasias, including multiple myeloma (especially acral) • Congenital hemolytic anemia Drugs • Penicillin (hypersensitivity) • Penicillamine

Table 97.5 Acquired cutis laxa: clinical presentations and associated conditions.

pulmonary complications, can cause considerable morbidity and mortality[42]. In rare cases, CL is associated with congenital hemolytic anemia of unknown origin[57].

CL-like skin can also be observed in individual cases when there is no family history of the disorder and the disease has a late onset. These acquired late-onset forms of CL are phenotypically very similar, if not indistinguishable, from milder, heritable forms of CL. Acquired CL may occur without an identifiable cause, present as a paraneoplastic phenomenon, or follow prior inflammation of the skin (Table 97.5). In the latter situation, the inflammatory reaction is followed by progressive sagging of the skin, which can be extensive and lead to a prematurely aged appearance. Generalized skin involvement is most commonly observed in acquired CL. Rarely, localized CL develops predominantly around the eyes (blepharochalasis) or on the distal extremities, particularly the palms and soles. In a sense, anetoderma may be considered a variant of localized CL.

Pathology

In the skin of patients with CL, the characteristic histologic feature is a loss or fragmentation of elastic fibers (Fig. 97.9B). In the newborn with severe congenital CL, the elastic fibers can essentially be absent. In several cases of late-onset CL, the elastic fibers were present but fragmented and physiologically non-functional. Electron microscopy confirms an irregular fragmentation of the fiber structure. In some patients, elastic fiber abnormalities have been shown to be accompanied by alterations in collagen fibers. The changes in collagen, however, are likely a reflection of an overall perturbation in the extracellular matrix of the connective tissue due to altered mechanical properties of the skin, with the primary defect clearly residing in the elastic fibers.

Differential Diagnosis

Clinical findings consistent with CL can be part of the normal aging process of the skin or they can be seen in association with other heritable connective tissue disorders, particularly certain variants of EDS. In the latter patients, the primary pathology resides in the collagen meshwork, and these individuals should not be diagnosed as having CL. The diagnosis of CL should be reserved specifically for those conditions in which abnormalities in the structure or quantity of elastic fibers can be demonstrated by routine histopathology or electron microscopy. Furthermore, in EDS, the skin is hyperextensible but still elastic and displays normal recoil. In PXE, the skin can also be loose and sagging without recoil; however, the primary papular lesions at the predilection sites clearly distinguish this disorder from CL.

Mid-dermal elastolysis (see Ch. 99) is a condition initially reported as an acquired, non-inflammatory disease in young adults with a pathognomonic histopathologic finding of a band-like loss of elastic fibers in the mid dermis. Clinically, these patients present with fine wrinkling of the skin, usually apparent within large areas on the upper arms and upper back[58]. As a rule, there is no family history and the clinical findings are often accentuated in sun-exposed areas. These individuals do not have internal organ involvement. A proposal has been made to divide mid-dermal elastolysis into inflammatory and non-inflammatory variants[59]. However, since preceding inflammation may have already subsided in some cases, and only the sequelae of the inflammatory reaction are evident at later stages, this distinction may not have any etiologic or pathomechanistic significance. Anetoderma, or localized sagging of the skin, may be the end stage of an antecedent inflammatory process of the skin, and it is histologically and ultrastructurally identical to CL. It may be regarded as a variant of acquired localized CL. Finally, loose and sagging skin with CL and PXE-like changes has been encountered in patients with vitamin K-dependent coagulation factor deficiency and mutations in the *GGCX* gene[60].

A number of rare conditions with elastin abnormalities and some features reminiscent of CL are included in the differential diagnosis[56]. These include de Barsy syndrome, Michelin tire baby syndrome, hereditary gelsolin amyloidosis, and Costello syndrome. However, the clinical features and associated findings clearly distinguish these from CL[56]. Lastly, a neonatal marfanoid form of CL can present with lax skin as well as emphysema and arachnodactyly.

Treatment

The redundant and sagging skin may be of major cosmetic concern to patients with CL, and reconstructive surgery can provide a dramatic improvement with significant psychosocial benefit. Tissue fragility is not a major problem, as in EDS, and the scars heal normally with normal tensile strength. However, sagging may reoccur, necessitating additional surgical procedures. The associated internal organ involvement requires appropriate care through a multidisciplinary approach.

REFERENCES

1. Sybert VP. Genetic Skin Disorders. Oxford Monographs on Medical Genetics, No. 33. Oxford: Oxford University Press, 1997.
2. Pulkkinen L, Ringpfeil F, Uitto J. Progress in heritable skin diseases: molecular bases and clinical implications. J Am Acad Dermatol. 2002;47:91–104.
3. Steinmann B, Royce PM. Connective Tissue and Its Heritable Disorders. Molecular Genetic, and Medical Aspects. New York: Wiley-Liss, 1993.
4. McKusick VA. Heritable Disorders of Connective Tissue, 4th edn. St Louis: Mosby, 1972.
5. Beighton P, De Paepe A, Steinmann B, et al. Ehlers-Danlos syndromes: revised nosology, Villefranche, 1997. Ehlers-Danlos National Foundation (USA) and Ehlers-Danlos Support Group (UK). Am J Med Genet. 1998;77:31–7.
6. Burrows NP. The molecular genetics of the Ehlers-Danlos syndrome. Clin Exp Dermatol. 1999;24:99–106.
7. Mao JR, Bristow J. The Ehlers-Danlos syndrome: on beyond collagens. J Clin Invest. 2001;107:1063–9.
8. Pyeritz RE. Ehlers-Danlos syndrome. N Engl J Med. 2000;342:730–2.
9. Myllyharju J, Kivirikko KI. Collagens and collagen-related diseases. Ann Med. 2001;33:7–21.
10. Burch GH, Bedolli MA, McDonough S, et al. Embryonic expression of tenascin-X suggests a role in limb, muscle, and heart development. Dev Dyn. 1995; 203:491–504.
11. Schalkwijk J, Zweers MC, Steijlen PM, et al. A recessive form of the Ehlers-Danlos syndrome caused by tenascin-X deficiency. N Engl J Med. 2001;345:1167–75.
12. Mao JR, Taylor G, Dean WB, et al. Tenascin-X deficiency mimics Ehlers-Danlos syndrome in mice through alteration of collagen deposition. Nat Genet. 2002;30:421–5.
13. Pepin M, Schwarze U, Superti-Furga A, Byers PH. Clinical and genetic features of Ehlers-Danlos syndrome type IV, the vascular type. N Engl J Med. 2000;342:673–80.
14. Balzer F. Recherches sur les charactères anatomiques du xanthelasma. Arch Physiol. 1884;4:65–80.
15. Chauffard MA. Xanthelasma disséminé et symmétrique sans insuffiçiance hépatique. Bull Soc Med Hop Paris. 1889;6:412–19.
16. Darier J. Pseudo-xanthome élastique. IIIe Congrès Intern de Dermat de Londres. 1896;5:289–95.
17. Grönblad E. Angioid streaks – pseudoxanthoma elasticum. Acta Ophthalmol. 1929;7:329.
18. Strandberg J. Pseudoxanthoma elasticum. Z Haut Geschlechtskr. 1929;31:689–94.
19. Carlborg U. Study of circulatory disturbances, pulse wave velocity and pressure pulses in large arteries in cases of pseudoxanthoma elasticum and angioid streaks: a contribution to the knowledge of function of the elastic tissue and the smooth muscles in larger arteries. Acta Med Scand. 1944;151:1–209.
20. Ringpfeil F, Lebwohl MG, Christiano AM, Uitto J. Pseudoxanthoma elasticum: mutations in the MRP6 gene encoding a transmembrane ATP-binding cassette (ABC) transporter. Proc Natl Acad Sci USA. 2000;97:6001–6.
20a. Ringpfeil F, McGuigan K, Fuchsel L, et al. Pseudoxanthoma elasticum is a recessive disease characterized by compound heterozygosity. J Invest Derm. 2006;126:782–6.
21. Neldner KH. Pseudoxanthoma elasticum. Clin Dermatol. 1988;6:1–159.
22. Uitto J, Pulkkinen L, Ringpfeil F. Molecular genetics of pseudoxanthoma elasticum: a metabolic disorder at the environment-genome interface? Trends Mol Med. 2001;7:13–17.
23. Lebwohl M, Phelps RG, Yannuzzi L, et al. Diagnosis of pseudoxanthoma elasticum by scar biopsy in patients without characteristic skin lesions. N Engl J Med. 1987;317:347–50.
24. Goodman RM, Smith EW, Paton D, et al. Pseudoxanthoma elasticum: a clinical and histopathological study. Medicine (Baltimore). 1963;42:297–334.
25. van den Berg JS, Hennekam RC, Cruysberg JR, et al. Prevalence of symptomatic intracranial aneurysm and ischaemic stroke in pseudoxanthoma elasticum. Cerebrovasc Dis. 2000;10:315–19.
26. Lebwohl MG, Distefano D, Prioleau PG, et al. Pseudoxanthoma elasticum and mitral-valve prolapse. N Engl J Med. 1982;307:228–31.
27. Contri MB, Boraldi F, Taparelli F, et al. Matrix proteins with high affinity for calcium ions are associated with mineralization within the elastic fibers of pseudoxanthoma elasticum dermis. Am J Pathol. 1996;148:569–77.
28. Lewis KG, Bercovitch L, Dill SW, Robinson-Bostom L. Acquired disorders of elastic tissue: Part I. Increased elastic tissue and solar elastosis syndromes. J Am Acad Dermatol. 2004;51:1–21.
29. Lewis KG, Bercovitch L, Dill SW, Robinson-Bostom L. Acquired disorders of elastic tissue: Part II. Decreased elastic tissue. J Am Acad Dermatol. 2004;51:165–85.
30. Bolognia JL, Braverman I. Pseudoxanthoma-elasticum-like skin changes induced by penicillamine. Dermatology. 1992;184:12–18.
31. Nielsen AO, Christensen OB, Hentzer B, et al. Salpeter-induced dermal changes electron-microscopically indistinguishable from pseudoxanthoma elasticum. Acta Derm Venereol. 1978;58:323–7.
32. Christensen OB. An exogenous variety of pseudoxanthoma elasticum in old farmers. Acta Derm Venereol. 1978;58:319–21.
33. Nickoloff BJ, Noodleman FR, Abel EA. Perforating pseudoxanthoma elasticum associated with chronic renal failure and hemodialysis. Arch Dermatol. 1985;121:1321–2.
34. Mainetti C, Masouye I, Saurat JH. Pseudoxanthoma elasticum-like lesions in the L-tryptophan-induced eosinophilia-myalgia syndrome. J Am Acad Dermatol. 1991;24:657–8.
35. Aessopos A, Farmakis D, Loukopoulos D. Elastic tissue abnormalities resembling pseudoxanthoma elasticum in beta thalassemia and the sickling syndromes. Blood. 2002;99:30–5.
36. Sepp N, Pichler E, Breathnach SM, et al. Amyloid elastosis: analysis of the role of amyloid P component. J Am Acad Dermatol. 1990;22:27–34.
37. Viljoen DL, Bloch C, Beighton P. Plastic surgery in pseudoxanthoma elasticum: experience in nine patients. Plast Reconstr Surg. 1990;85:233–8.
38. Lim JI, Bressler NM, Marsh MJ, Bressler SB. Laser treatment of choroidal neovascularization in patients with angioid streaks. Am J Ophthalmol. 1993;116:414–23.
39. Roth DB, Estafanous M, Lewis H. Macular translocation for subfoveal choroidal neovascularization in angioid streaks. Am J Ophthalmol. 2001;131:390–2.
40. Hamamoto Y, Nagai K, Yasui H, Muto M. Hyperreactivity of pseudoxanthoma elasticum-affected dermis to vitamin D3. J Am Acad Dermatol. 2000;42:685–7.
41. Frishman WH. Chelation therapy for coronary artery disease: panacea or quackery? Am J Med. 2001;111:729–30.
42. Goltz RW, Hult AM, Goldfarb M, Gorlin RJ. Cutis laxa. A manifestation of generalized elastolysis. Arch Dermatol. 1965;92:373–87.
43. Nakamura T, Lozano PR, Ikeda Y. Fibulin-5/DANCE is essential for elastogenesis in vivo. Nature. 2002;415:171–5.
44. Yanagisawa H, Davis EC, Starcher BC, et al. Fibulin-5 is an elastin-binding protein essential for elastic fibre development in vivo. Nature. 2002;415:168–71.
45. Loeys B, Van Maldergem L, Mortier G, et al. Homozygosity for a missense mutation in fibulin-5 (FBLN5) results in a severe form of cutis laxa. Hum Mol Genet. 2002;11:2113–18.
46. Elahi E, Kalhor R, Banihosseini SS, et al. Homozygous missense mutation in fibulin-5 in an Iranian autosomal recessive cutis laxa pedigree and associated haplotype. J Invest Dermatol. 2006;126:1506–9.
47. Tassabehji M, Metcalfe K, Hurst J, et al. An elastin gene mutation producing abnormal tropoelastin and abnormal elastic fibers in a patient with autosomal dominant cutis laxa. Hum Mol Genet. 1998;7:1021–8.
48. Zhang MC, He L, Giro M, et al. Cutis laxa arising from frameshift mutations in exon 30 of the elastin gene (ELN). J Biol Chem. 1999;274:981–6.
49. Rodriguez-Revenga L, Iranzo P, Badenas C, et al. A novel elastin gene mutation resulting in an autosomal dominant form of cutis laxa. Arch Dermatol. 2004;140:1135–9.
50. Hucthagowder V, Sausgruber N, Kim KH, et al. Fibulin-4: a novel gene for an autosomal recessive cutis laxa syndrome. Am J Hum Genet. 2006;78:1075–80.
51. Olsen DR, Fazio MJ, Shamban AT, et al. Cutis laxa: reduced elastin gene expression in skin fibroblast cultures as determined by hybridizations with a homologous cDNA and an exon 1-specific oligonucleotide. J Biol Chem. 1988;263:6465–7.
52. Anderson LL, Oikarinen AI, Ryhänen L, et al. Characterization and partial purification of a neutral protease from the serum of a patient with autosomal recessive pulmonary emphysema and cutis laxa. J Lab Clin Med. 1985;105:537–46.
53. Shapiro SD. Matrix metalloproteinase degradation of extracellular matrix: biological consequences. Curr Opin Cell Biol. 1998;10:602–8.
54. Krajnc I, Rems D, Vizjak A, Hodl S. Acquired generalized cutis laxa with paraproteinemia (IgG lambda). Immunofluorescence study, clinical and histologic findings with review of the literature. Hautarzt. 1996;47:545–9.
55. Hu Q, Reymond J-L, Pinel N, et al. Inflammatory destruction of elastic fibers in acquired cutis laxa is associated with missense alleles in the elastin and fibulin-5 genes. J Invest Dermatol 2006;126:283–90.
56. Uitto J, Pulkkinen L. Heritable disorders affecting the elastic tissues: cutis laxa, pseudoxanthoma elasticum and related disorders. In: Rimoin DL, Connor JM, Pyeritz RE (eds). Emery and Rimoin's Principles and Practice of Medical Genetics, 3rd edn. London: Churchill Livingstone, 2002.
57. Anderson CE, Finklestein JZ, Nussbaum E, et al. Association of hemolytic anemia and early-onset pulmonary emphysema in three siblings. J Pediatr. 1984;105:247–51.
58. Rao BK, Endzweig CH, Kagen MH, et al. Wrinkling due to mid-dermal elastolysis: two cases and literature review. J Cutan Med Surg. 2000;4:40–4.
59. Grossin M, Maghraoui S, Crickx B, Belaich S. The spectrum of dermal elastolysis. J Am Acad Dermatol. 1993;29:506–7.
60. Vanakker OM, Martin L, Gheduzzi D, et al. Pseudoxanthoma elasticum-like phenotype with cutis laxa and multiple coagulation factor deficiency represents a separate genetic entity. J Invest Dermatol. 2007;127:584–7.

Dermal Hypertrophies

98

Claude S Burton and Vaishali Escaravage

HYPERTROPHIC SCARS AND KELOIDS

Synonym: ■ Keloidal scar

Key features

- Normal scars are preceded by injury, immediate in onset, flat and asymptomatic
- Hypertrophic scars are raised and confined to the wound margin. They have a good response to treatment
- Keloids extend beyond the wound margin and are delayed in onset. They seldom resolve spontaneously, and their response to treatment is often poor

Introduction

Animals have evolved a way of healing injured tissue that works remarkably well in most instances. While some species possess the ability to regenerate injured or missing tissue, this is seldom the case in humans. For cutaneous wounds beyond the second trimester of fetal development, only the epidermis is truly regenerative. Any injury that extends into the dermis will always heal with a scar. In humans, as well as several other species, cutaneous wounds on occasion heal with exuberant scarring, far in excess of what we consider to be a 'normal' scar, resulting in a process known as hypertrophic scarring. For an unfortunate few, the scar will extend far beyond the original injury, resulting in a lesion commonly referred to as a keloid, from the Greek word *chele*, or crab claw. Both hypertrophic scarring and keloids can produce significant discomfort and disfigurement. An understanding of their similarities and differences, and a comparison with the normal healing process, has provided several options for the management of patients with either of these conditions.

History

Presumably, aberrant wound healing that produces hypertrophic scarring and keloid formation has evolved with our species. Descriptions of hypertrophic scars and keloids were found among the hieroglyphics of ancient Egyptians, though we first credit the use of the word keloid to Alibert, who described the claw-like extensions of spontaneous keloids in the early 19th century.

Epidemiology

Keloids and hypertrophic scars occur worldwide in all skin types. The more darkly pigmented the skin, the higher the risk is for keloid formation. Incidence rates for keloids as high as 16% have been reported in a predominantly black population[1,1a]. Women and men are equally likely to develop keloids, though women have historically outnumbered men in series that included earlobe piercing-induced keloids[2]. While keloids have been reported in people of all ages, they are uncommon among small children and the elderly. There is often a familial tendency for developing hypertrophic scars and keloids. A recent review of 14 pedigrees suggested an autosomal dominant mode of inheritance with incomplete clinical penetrance and variable expression[3], although earlier reviews implied the inheritance pattern was autosomal recessive. Two very rare syndromes that include the spontaneous development of keloids are the Rubinstein–Taybi and Goeminne syndromes.

Pathogenesis

The pathogenesis of hypertrophic scarring and keloid formation is unknown. Vigorous study of cutaneous wound healing reveals an extraordinarily complex hierarchy of events (see Ch. 141), representing a plethora of opportunities for wound healing misadventure. The key stages in the wound healing process and potential pathways to the development of keloids and hypertrophic scars are illustrated in Figure 98.1.

Upon injury, hemostasis is the skin's first teleologic order of business, as platelets quickly react to plug bleeding vessels, and fibrin polymerizes throughout the region of injury. An inflammatory phase, characterized by the migration of neutrophils, macrophages and lymphocytes, follows shortly thereafter. Numerous cytokines, released by injured and disturbed tissues, platelets and cellular migrants, initiate a host of synthetic events in which angiogenesis and fibrogenesis occur. The defect is rapidly closed by tissue proliferation, followed by re-epithelialization. In acute surgical wounds without tension, healing proceeds quickly enough to allow suture removal within a week in most cases, though the breaking strength of the wound at this point is only 5–10% of the skin's original strength. Over the next 6–12 months, the wound undergoes significant remodeling. This period is characterized by matrix deposition and collagen synthesis and cross-linking, resulting in the establishment of a mature scar approximating 80% of the original tissue strength[4].

The hypertrophic scar and keloid, in contrast, depart early from this orderly sequence and rarely involute spontaneously. The reasons for this are not known but events known to trigger inflammation –

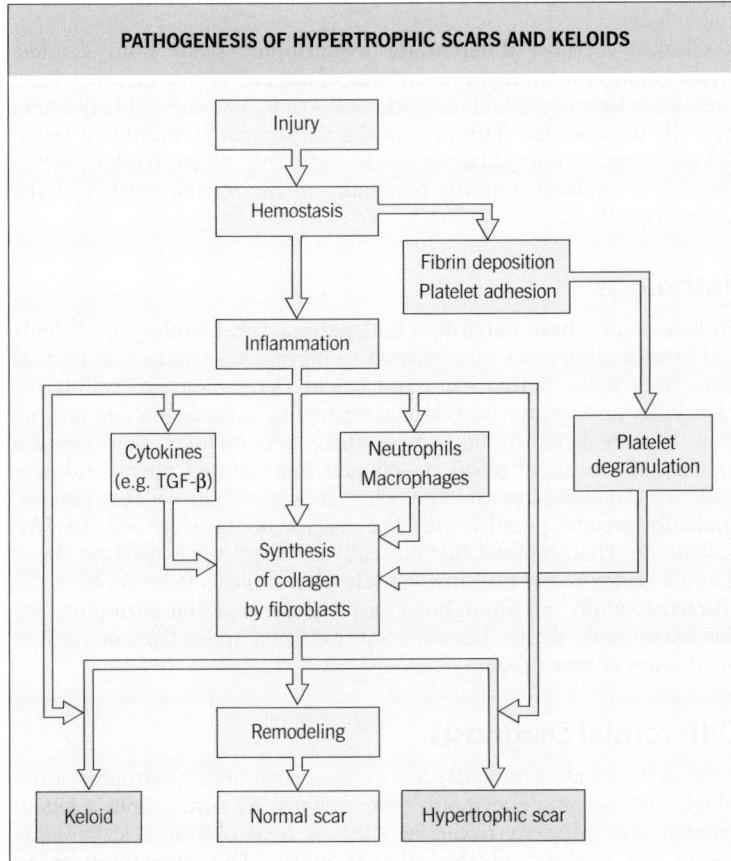

Fig. 98.1 **Pathogenesis of hypertrophic scars and keloids.**

including infection, excessive wound tension, and foreign material – are implicated in the keloidal response. Melanin-producing melanocytes may play a role, since, to date, keloids have not been reported in patients with oculocutaneous albinism, and keloids occur with increasing frequency in individuals with more darkly pigmented skin. Mast cells are numerous in both hypertrophic scars and keloids, and mast cell mediators are known to upregulate collagen synthesis and likely contribute to excessive deposition.

Transforming growth factor-β (TGF-β) has emerged as a likely candidate molecule for inducing scar and keloid formation. Both TGF-β_1 and TGF-β_2 are highly expressed in keloid-derived fibroblasts compared with normal control fibroblasts. The synthesis of a number of extracellular matrix components is stimulated by TGF-β_1, and keloid fibroblasts are particularly sensitive to exposure to TGF-β_2[5]. In addition, injection of genetically modified human fibroblasts that overexpress TGF-β_1 into athymic mice leads to the formation of keloid-like nodules[6].

Especially exciting is the observation that fetal wounds (prior to the third trimester) heal *without* scarring[7]. Scrutiny of the differences between adult and fetal wound healing suggests that both inflammation and cytokines unique to adult wound healing are likely to play a prominent role in the development of hypertrophic scars and keloids (Table 98.1).

Clinical Features

Hypertrophic scars and keloids have many features in common (Table 98.2). Both are raised, initially pink-to-purple lesions that are often painful, pruritic, or both (Fig. 98.2). The overlying epidermis is typically smooth, and the dermal portion of the lesion is firm to palpation. Both types of lesions are disfiguring (Fig. 98.3) and may inhibit normal motion of adjacent tissues. Hypertrophic scars and keloids may appear anywhere on the body, but they are especially frequent on the earlobes, upper trunk, and the deltoid region. Wounds in areas of tension are especially prone to keloid formation, and it is reported that keloids transplanted to areas of low tension subsequently resolve[8]. Keloids are very unusual on the central face, eyelids and genitalia.

Both types of lesions are precipitated by trauma, although keloids have the unique ability to develop without apparent injury. A variety of cutaneous insults, including acne (Fig. 98.4), infections (Fig. 98.5), burns and piercings, may precede the onset of both hypertrophic scars and keloids.

Clinical features differentiate hypertrophic scars from keloids. Hypertrophic scars remain in the area of original injury, and they have a tendency toward gradual resolution over time. Resolution of erythema typically precedes the flattening of the scar by many months or years. Keloids migrate into adjacent tissue with very active borders, while showing a tendency towards regression in the central portion of the lesion (Fig. 98.6).

Pathology

Ehrlich et al.[9] have carefully characterized the histology of keloids and hypertrophic scars as compared to normal scar tissue and normal skin. Both hypertrophic scars and keloids have increased cellularity, vascularity and connective tissue compared to normal skin and normal scar. Within hypertrophic scars, there are nodules that contain myofibroblasts, small blood vessels and fine collagen fibers, and over time, these nodules become somewhat thinner and the collagen bundles gradually become parallel with the surface of the skin (Fig. 98.7A). Keloids are characterized histologically by large, thick collagen fibers that are composed of multiple, closely packed fibrils (Figs 98.7B & C). Ultrastructurally, an amorphous extracellular material surrounds the fibroblastic cells within keloids[9]. Subepidermal appendages are absent in all types of scar tissue.

Differential Diagnosis

Perhaps the greatest difficulty lies in distinguishing hypertrophic scars, which may become enormous, from keloids. By convention, a keloid extends into adjacent tissue, whereas a hypertrophic scar remains within the confines of the original injury. The sclerotic form of xanthoma disseminatum may be confused with keloids clinically but

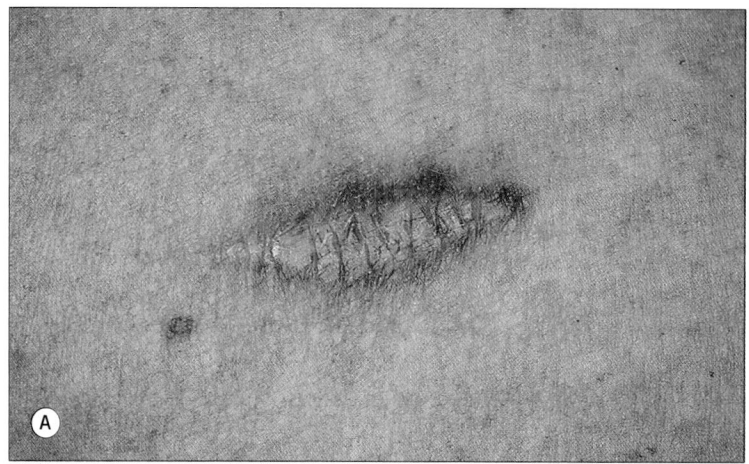

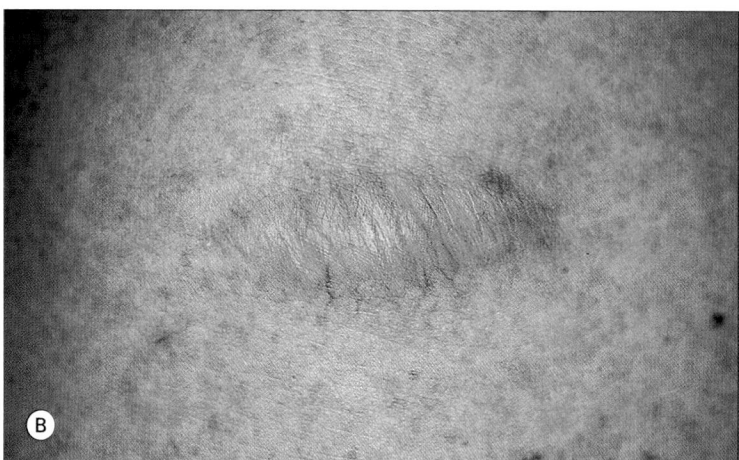

Fig. 98.2 Hypertrophic scars. A A 5-month-old scar that is still pink. **B** A 1-year-old scar that is hypopigmented. Courtesy of Jean L Bolognia MD.

DIFFERENCES IN ADULT VERSUS FETAL WOUND HEALING		
	Adult	**Fetal**
Fluid environment	No	Yes
Sterile environment	No	Yes
Inflammation	Yes	No
Scar formation	Yes	No
PO$_2$ (mmHg)	>60	20

Table 98.1 Differences in adult versus fetal wound healing.

KEY FEATURES OF NORMAL, HYPERTROPHIC AND KELOID SCARS			
	Normal scar	**Hypertrophic scar**	**Keloid**
Preceded by injury	Yes	Yes	Not always
Onset	Immediate	Immediate	Delayed
Erythema	Temporary	Prominent	Varies
Profile	Flat	Raised	Raised
Symptomatic	No	Yes	Yes
Confined to wound margin	Yes	Yes	No
Increased mast cells	No	Yes	Yes
Contains myofibroblasts	N/A	Yes	No
Spontaneous resolution	N/A	Sometimes, gradual	Rare
Treatment response	N/A	Good	Poor

Table 98.2 Key features of normal, hypertrophic and keloid scars.

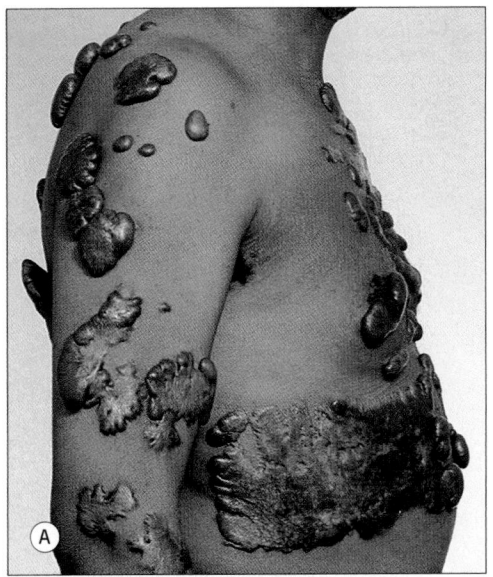
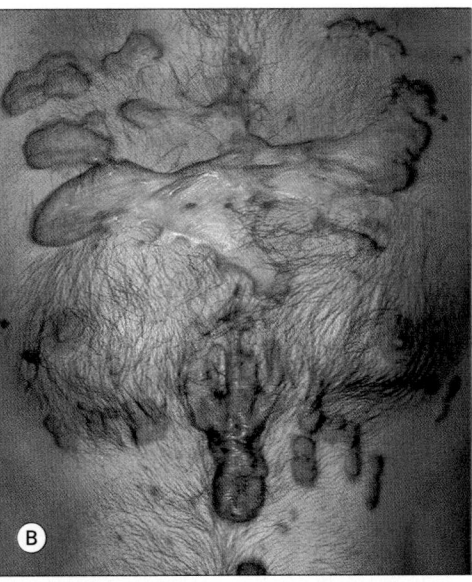

Fig. 98.3 Spontaneous generalized keloids. Extensive spontaneous keloids in a patient with darkly pigmented skin (**A**) and a patient with lightly pigmented skin (**B**).

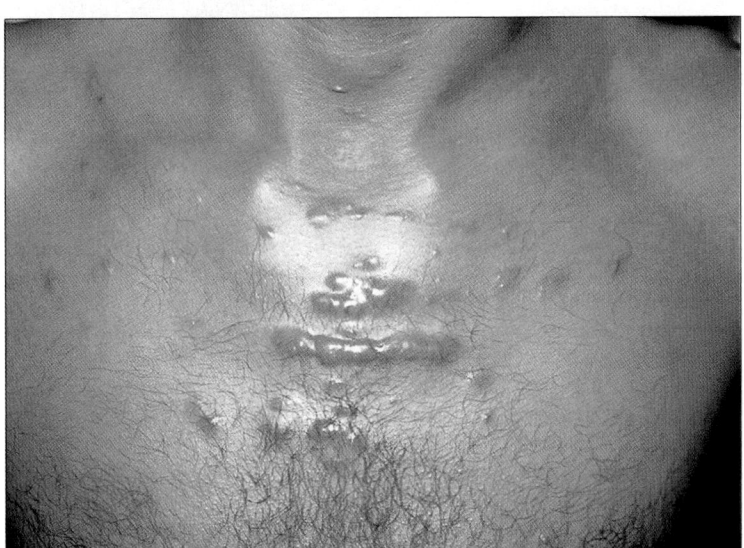

Fig. 98.4 Acne-induced keloids.

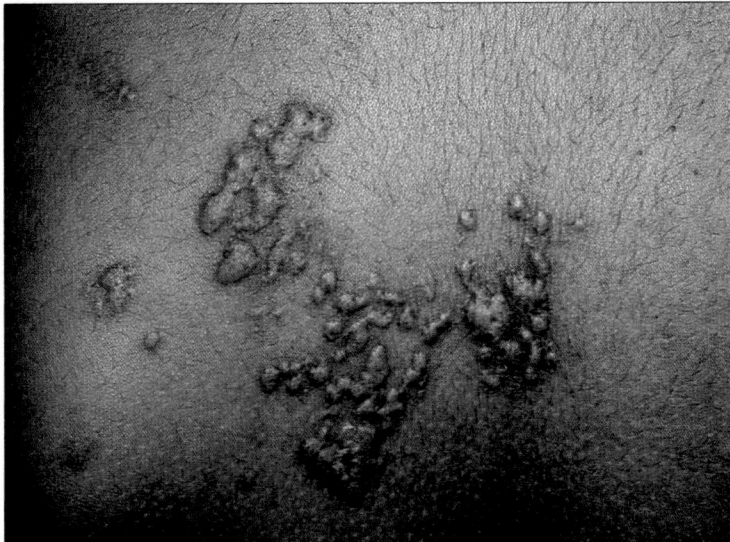

Fig. 98.5 Hypertrophic scarring following an episode of herpes zoster. Elevated scars are limited to the area of infection.

not histologically (see Ch. 90) – as may lobomycosis (keloidal blastomycosis; lacaziosis), which is due to infection with *Lacazia loboi*. There are also keloidal forms of scleroderma and morphea, in addition to the rare presentation of carcinoma en cuirasse as keloidal nodules and keloidal plaques on the lower extremities of patients with type IV Ehlers-Danlos syndrome.

Treatment

Treatment of hypertrophic scars and keloids is often challenging. Because keloids can prove especially recalcitrant, new therapies are constantly emerging. The treatment strategies for hypertrophic scars and keloids do overlap (Table 98.3), and they will be discussed together. Oftentimes, several strategies are combined.

Intralesional corticosteroids are the most commonly used therapy for hypertrophic scars and keloids. In an uncontrolled study of triamcinolone acetonide monotherapy in 17 keloidal scars, Darzi and colleagues[10] reported 71% of treated keloids were fully flattened at 10 years and the remaining 29% experienced partial flattening. The dose injected varied depending upon the size of the keloid (1–12 cm² in this series), with a range of 20–120 mg triamcinolone acetonide injected over four sessions.

Surgery is a useful approach for hypertrophic scars, which may not recur, but it is inadvisable for most keloids, where the eventual recurrence rate is reported to be in excess of 80%. The abysmal response to surgery as monotherapy for keloids has led to the combination

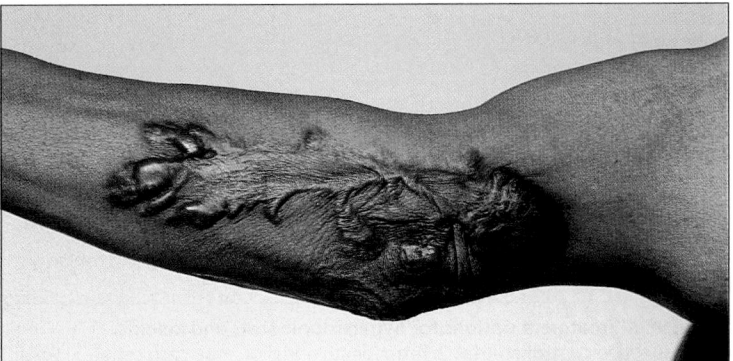

Fig. 98.6 Keloid scarring. Note the extension of the keloid scar into the normal tissue and the central involution.

of surgical procedures to debulk the lesion with other modalities to prevent recurrence. Berman & Flores[11] reviewed their surgical experience in the removal of 124 keloids from 74 patients followed for an average of 7 months. Of note, 83% of the lesions had been previously treated. Postoperatively, patients received triamcinolone acetonide injections (10–40 mg/ml for a mean of 1.4 treatments), no injections, or interferon-α-2b injections (1 × 10⁶ U in 0.1 ml/linear cm per treatment) on the day of surgery and, in some cases, again 1 week later with five million units. Recurrence rates were similar in the triamcinolone

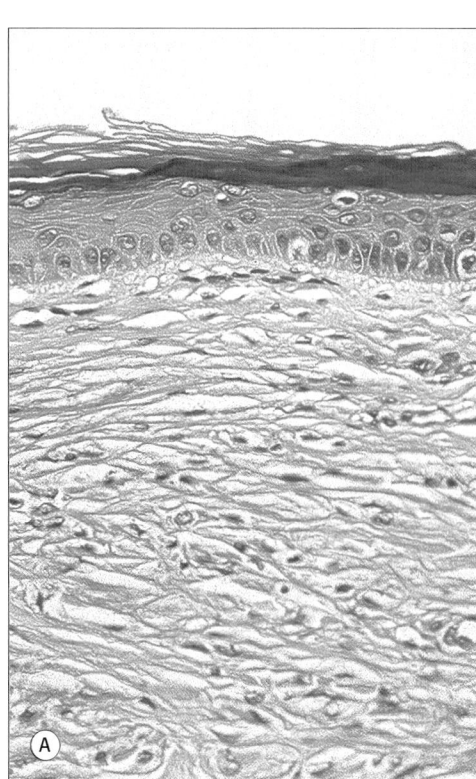
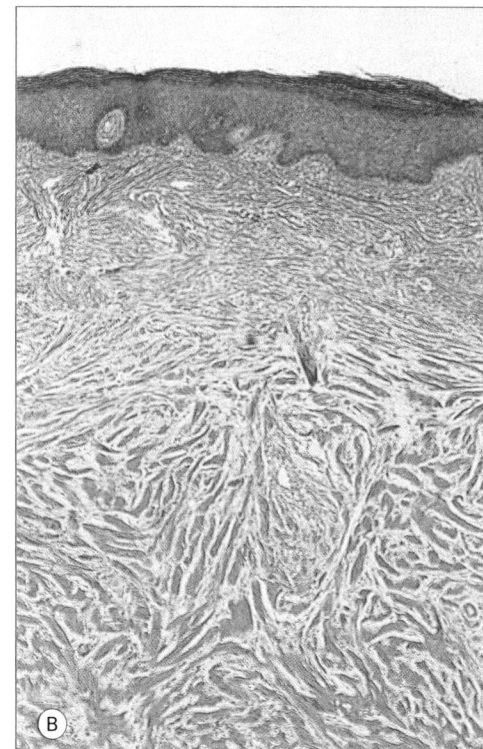
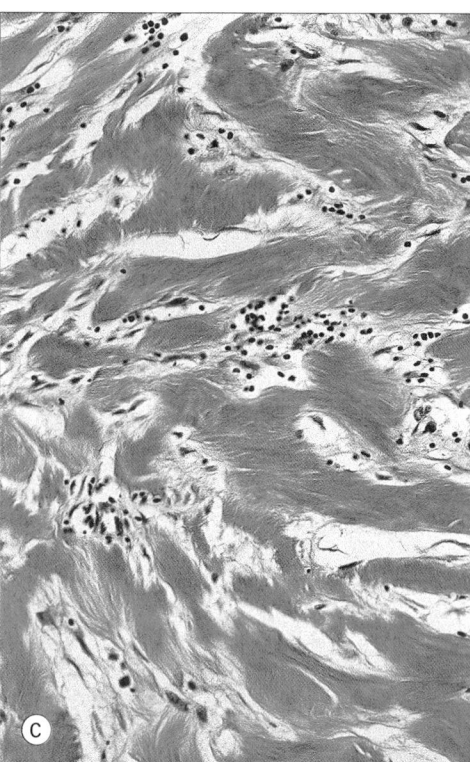

Fig. 98.7 Histopathology of a hypertrophic scar and a keloid. A Hypertrophic scar. **B** Keloid. **C** Keloid close-up. Courtesy of Thomas Cummings MD.

TREATMENT OPTIONS FOR HYPERTROPHIC SCARS AND KELOIDS ℞			
Treatment	Study	HS	K
Excision	2	√	√*
Triamcinolone acetonide (intralesional injection)	1	√	√†
Interferon-α-2b (intralesional injection)	1		√†,‡
Silicone gel sheets	2	√	√
Laser (flashlamp-pumped pulsed dye)	1	√	√
Radiation	2		√*
Topical imiquimod	2		√*
5-Fluorouracil (intralesional injection)	2	√†	√†
Cryotherapy	2	√†	√†,§
Pressure	2	√	√†
Topical tacrolimus	3		√
Topical retinoids	3	√	√
Intralesional verapamil	2		√*

*As a component of combined therapy.
†Alone or as a component of combined therapy.
‡Several controlled studies have shown no benefit.
§One small, unblinded, controlled study showed a significant benefit of combination cryotherapy and intralesional triamcinolone over either alone.

Table 98.3 Treatment options for hypertrophic scars and keloids. 1, prospective controlled trial; 2, retrospective trial or large case series; 3, small series or individual case reports. Radiofrequency treatment was found to have no effect (3). HS, hypertrophic scars; K, keloids.

group and the group that received no injections, at 58% and 51.2%, respectively. The interferon group fared much better, with a recurrence rate of only 18.7%.

However, results from several controlled studies as well as smaller series using interferon-α-2b alone or following excision have not been as promising (including inferior results compared to intralesional corticosteroids), even though keloid-derived fibroblasts have been shown to dramatically decrease their collagen production, decrease glycosaminoglycan (GAG) synthesis, and increase collagenase activity after exposure

to interferon-α-2b[12]. In a controlled clinical trial where patients served as their own controls, keloids injected with interferon-α-2b three times per week decreased in volume by 30.4% at 22 days[13]. While such short-term improvement is encouraging, long-term results would be more significant, given the high relapse rate for keloids.

Radiation has also been combined with surgery to prevent recurrence of keloids following excision. In a retrospective series that reviewed the outcome of 126 keloids in 83 patients who had received postoperative radiation, Klumpar et al.[14] reported an overall improvement rate of 83%. Complete flattening was noted in 68% and flattening to less than 2 mm in height in an additional 11%. The majority of patients received a median cumulative dose of 28 Gy (range, 4–40 Gy) over a period of days (most often 2 or 3 consecutive days) immediately following excision. Radiation for keloids has a remarkable safety record; however, two instances of breast cancer have been reported in women receiving radiation for keloids[15].

5-Fluorouracil (5-FU), a pyrimidine analogue with antimetabolite activity, has also been used with some success in both hypertrophic scars and keloids. Fitzpatrick[16] described his experience injecting 5-FU into inflamed hypertrophic scars and keloids in 'over 1000' individuals during a 9-year period. Patients received injections one to three times per week initially and less often as they cleared, often in combination with triamcinolone acetonide injections and/or flashlamp-pumped pulsed dye laser therapy. Favorable responses were noted in 'most' patients, with no significant side effects. However, in general, the results with keloids are less impressive. For example, in an open-label study of 20 patients with keloids who received once-weekly intralesional 5-FU (50 mg/ml; 0.2 to 0.4 ml/cm^2) for an average of seven treatments, 17 (85%) experienced ≥50% improvement. Unfortunately, recurrence was noted in 47% (9 of 19) of those who had responded within 1 year[17]. Pain (20 of 20), hyperpigmentation (20 of 20) and tissue sloughing (6 of 20) were the major side effects.

Based upon the findings of increased expression of the *gli-1* oncogene in keloids (but not in normal scar tissue) and inhibition of its expression *in vitro* by rapamycin, the possibility was raised that rapamycin or related analogues (e.g. tacrolimus) might lead to improvement of keloids[18]. However, to date, no controlled trials have been published demonstrating a significant beneficial effect.

The epidermis overlying keloids has been shown to produce increased amounts of vascular endothelial growth factor (VEGF)[19]. This may provide an explanation for the beneficial effects of interferon (given its antiangiogenic properties) or drugs such as imiquimod that can induce interferon production. This would be in addition to interferon's effect on collagen and GAG synthesis (see above). In a small, non-randomized trial involving 10 patients who had undergone surgical excision of their keloids, 5% imiquimod cream was applied nightly for 8 weeks; at the 24-week follow-up examination, no regrowth of any keloids was noted[20]. Lastly, the possibility exists that imiquimod upregulates genes associated with apoptosis and this plays a role in keloid regression[21].

Several controlled clinical trials have established the usefulness of flashlamp-pumped pulsed dye laser (PDL) therapy for hypertrophic scars (Fig. 98.8). Utilizing one-half of the patient's median sternotomy scar as a control, 16 individuals were treated on two occasions (6–8 weeks apart), at 585 nm for 450 µs with a spot size of 5 mm and a fluence per pulse of 6.5–7.25 J/cm². Using blinded evaluators plus measurements of scar size and color, all treated scars improved after 6 months of follow-up, compared with untreated control sites[22]. In prospective studies of ten patients with keloids (in which they served as their own controls), immunohistochemical analyses of biopsy specimens prior to and 1 week after PDL therapy (wavelength 585 nm, pulse duration 450 µs, spot size 5 mm, mean fluence 14 J/cm²) demonstrated: (1) a threefold increase in ERK (extracellular signal related kinase) expression; (2) a twofold increase in p38 kinase expression; (3) a downregulation of TGF-β_1 expression (see Pathogenesis); and (4) an upregulation of matrix metalloproteinase-13 activity (which increases the degradation of connective tissue)[23,24]. Of note, both ERK and p38 are subgroups of mitogen-activated protein kinases which regulate apoptosis, cell growth and differentiation.

Topical silicone gel sheeting is another approach to hypertrophic scars and keloids. The proposed mechanism of action is reduced water vapor loss, which decreases capillary activity, leading to reduced collagen deposition. This therapy is relatively easy to use, safe, and reasonably well tolerated. In a meta-analysis of 13 controlled trials (n = 559), silicon gel sheeting reduced the incidence of hypertrophic scarring in people prone to scarring (RR 0.46, 95% CI 0.21 to 0.98) and improved scar elasticity (RR 8.60, 95% CI 2.55 to 29.02), but the studies were felt to be highly susceptible to bias[25].

Based upon *in vitro* studies utilizing keloid-derived fibroblasts, future therapies may involve increasing the production of prostaglandin E2 (an antifibrogenic molecule) locally[26]; inhibiting the TGF-β/Smad-signaling pathway (important in epithelial–mesenchyme interactions in keloids) via the flavonoid quercetin; using a transcriptional factor decoy against AP-1 to suppress TGF-β_1-induced type I collagen gene expression; inhibiting activin-A (a member of the TGF-β family) via follistatin[26a]; and inhibiting the major mechanical signal transduction pathway with the ERK inhibitor U0126[27].

RELATED CONDITIONS

Introduction

In addition to hypertrophic scars and keloids, an excess of collagen deposition is also seen in the group of diseases known as the fibromatoses (see Ch. 116). In this section, the most common fibromatosis, Dupuytren's contracture, will be discussed as well as cutis verticis gyrata, juvenile hyaline fibromatosis, and infantile systemic hyalinosis.

Dupuytren's Contracture

Synonyms: ■ Palmar fibromatosis ■ Dupuytren's disease/diathesis

Key features

- Thickening of the palmar and digital fascia
- Flexion contracture of affected digits
- Myofibroblast proliferation followed by excess collagen synthesis
- Surgical approaches correct deformity and restore function

History

In 1777, Henry Cline discovered that thickening of the palmar fascia produced this characteristic contracture and, 2 years later, proposed palmar fasciotomy as a cure.

Epidemiology

Dupuytren's contracture is common in Caucasians of northern European ancestry, and it is rare in darkly pigmented populations. The prevalence approaches 30% in individuals over 60 years of age in Norway. The condition affects middle-aged to older people of both sexes, although men are affected about a decade earlier than women. Familial associations suggest an autosomal dominant inheritance, but sporadic cases are common. The lesion is associated with other fibromatoses, including Peyronie's disease, plantar fibromatosis (Ledderhose's disease), and knuckle pads (see Ch. 116). The condition has also been associated with alcoholism and diabetes.

Pathogenesis

Fibrogenic cytokines (e.g. TGF-β_1 and TGF-β_2) are thought to be involved in the genesis of Dupuytren's contractures. They are able to induce the growth of fibroblasts and their differentiation into myofibroblasts, in addition to stimulating the production of extracellular matrix.

Clinical features

Patients often present late in the course of their disease with flexion contractures of the affected digits. Most often, lesions develop in an ulnar distribution, and the ring finger is most commonly affected. The disorder begins with a nodule in the fascia of the palm, which grows at varying rates to produce a cord, and then it contracts, producing a flexion contracture (Fig. 98.9).

Pathology

Biopsy of the nodular lesion reveals a proliferation of myofibroblasts, which subsequently align along lines of tension. As the cord develops, there is collagen thickening and myofibroblasts disappear.

Differential diagnosis

Although usually a straightforward diagnosis, one must consider ganglion cysts, giant cell tumors of the tendon sheath, soft-tissue sarcomas, calluses and tenosynovitis.

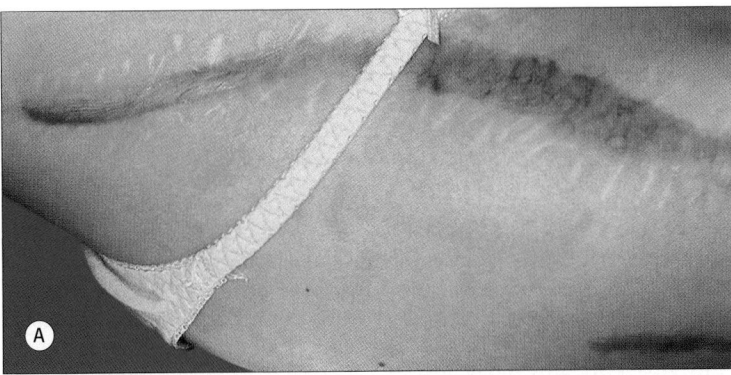
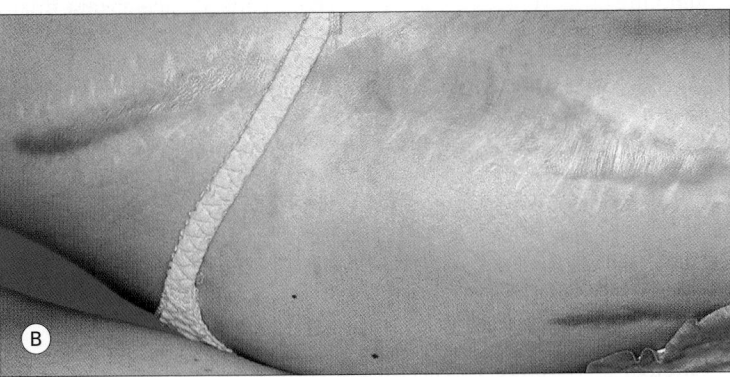

Fig. 98.8 Flashlamp-pumped pulsed dye laser treatment. Hypertrophic scar before (**A**) and after (**B**) treatment with a flashlamp-pumped pulsed dye laser.

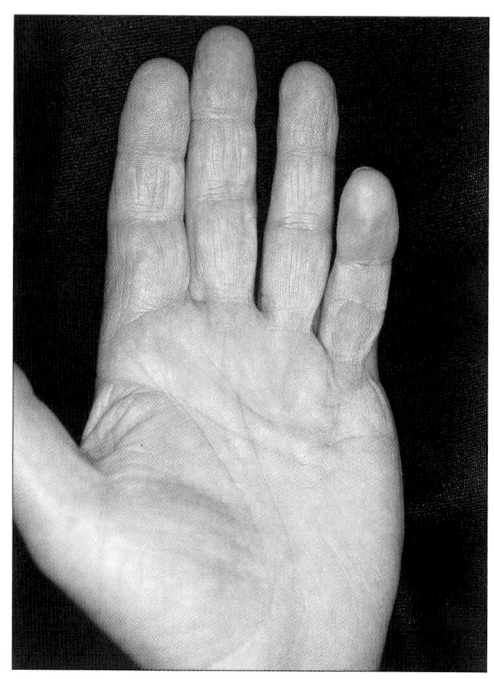

Fig. 98.9 Dupuytren's contracture. There is greater involvement of the 5th finger than the 4th finger. Fibrotic cords can be felt and are accentuated by extension of the digits. Eventually, flexion contractures develop. Courtesy of Jean L Bolognia MD.

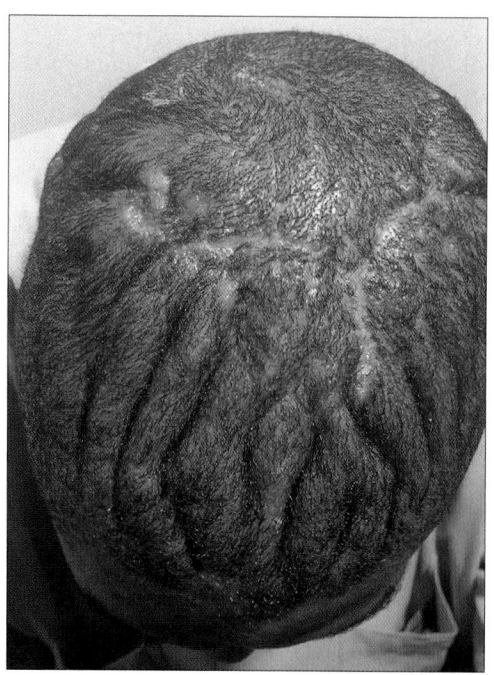

Fig. 98.10 Cutis verticis gyrata. Cerebriform folding of the skin of the scalp. Erythema in the posterior grooves is related to a previous superinfection.

Treatment

Surgical approaches are the mainstay of therapy. Fasciectomy releases the joint contracture in most cases. Postoperative splinting and range-of-motion exercises are important for a good outcome, and recurrences are common. Complications of Dupuytren's contracture include nerve injury, loss of joint mobility, and the development of reflex sympathetic dystrophy[28].

Cutis Verticis Gyrata

Key features

- Hypertrophy and folding of the scalp
- Primary (idiopathic) form seen almost exclusively in males, with an onset at puberty
- Face not affected as in pachydermoperiostosis
- Underlying disorders in the secondary form include acromegaly, Turner syndrome and myxedema

Clinical features

In primary cutis verticis gyrata, overgrowth of the scalp develops at puberty and progresses to produce symmetric gyrate or cerebriform folding of the skin (Fig. 98.10). The folds are usually aligned in an anterior–posterior direction on the crown and vertex and are soft to spongy on palpation. Terminal hair density may be reduced on the folds, but not in the furrows. Primary cutis verticis gyrata can be subdivided into essential (isolated) and non-essential (associated with neurologic and/or ophthalmologic abnormalities) forms, both of which have a male predominance. Secondary cutis verticis gyrata is less common and has a more equal sex distribution. Onset of the latter varies from birth to adulthood and secondary forms may be asymmetric, depending on the underlying etiology (Table 98.4).

Pathology

Biopsy specimens from cutis verticis gyrata typically show increased dermal collagen in otherwise normal-appearing skin.

Differential diagnosis

An extensive congenital cerebriform melanocytic nevus of the scalp can have the appearance of cutis verticis gyrata. One must differentiate the latter from pachydermoperiostosis, which is associated with facial involvement and thickening of the skin on the hands and feet as well as clubbing of the digits[29]. Furrowed skin on the scalp, forehead, preauricular areas, neck, trunk, palms and soles in association with

CUTIS VERTICIS GYRATA – DISEASE ASSOCIATIONS
Primary essential
• None
Primary non-essential
• Neurologic abnormalities (e.g. mental retardation, seizures)
• Ophthalmologic abnormalities (e.g. cataracts, optic atrophy)
Secondary
• Acromegaly
• Myxedema (including cretinism)*
• Insulin resistance
• Turner and Noonan syndromes (following resolution of intrauterine lymphedema)*
• Fragile X syndrome
• Klinefelter syndrome
• Hereditary neuralgic amyotrophy
• Tuberous sclerosis
• Paraneoplastic due to metastatic carcinoma
Increased dermal mucin may also be observed.

Table 98.4 Cutis verticis gyrata – disease associations.

acanthosis nigricans, craniosynostosis and a prominent umbilical stump characterizes Beare–Stevenson cutis gyrata syndrome, an autosomal dominant condition caused by mutations in the fibroblast growth factor receptor 2 (*FGFR2*) gene. Dissecting cellulitis of the scalp, Darier disease or extensive AL amyloid deposition can lead to cerebriform folds of skin resembling cutis verticis gyrata. Less often, cutis verticis gyrata might be confused with a plexiform neurofibroma, nevus lipomatosus, connective tissue nevus, aggregated cylindromas, acanthosis nigricans or cutaneous leukemic infiltrates.

Treatment

This unusual morphologic syndrome is generally asymptomatic, and it requires no treatment.

Juvenile Hyaline Fibromatosis and Infantile Systemic Hyalinosis

Synonyms: ■ Murray–Puretic–Drescher syndrome ■ Fibromatosis hyalinica multiplex juvenilis ■ (Juvenile) systemic hyalinosis

Key features

- Rare, allelic autosomal recessive disorders
- Usually present during infancy or early childhood
- Clinical features include papulonodular lesions (favoring the ears, scalp, neck, hands and periorificial areas), gingival hypertrophy and flexion contractures of large joints; infantile systemic hyalinosis represents a more severe variant with internal organ involvement
- Mutations in the gene that encodes capillary morphogenesis protein-2 (CMG2) are responsible for both disorders
- Treatment consists of excision of nodules and gingivae as needed, but lesions often recur

Introduction

Both juvenile hyaline fibromatosis (JHF) and infantile systemic hyalinosis (ISH) are rare autosomal recessive genodermatoses characterized by hyaline accumulation in the dermis. They are allelic disorders, i.e. due to mutations in the same gene, but differ with regard to severity and involvement of internal organs (Table 98.5). It has been proposed that JHF and ISH exist within a continuum of disease with varying phenotypic expression[30].

History

As early as 1873, Murray had described a condition which he termed 'molluscum fibrosum'. In 1972, Kitano et al.[31] renamed the disorder 'juvenile hyaline fibromatosis'.

Epidemiology

Both JHF and ISH are rare disorders that present during infancy or early childhood. As expected given the autosomal recessive inheritance pattern, both sexes are equally affected.

Pathogenesis

The gene that encodes capillary morphogenesis protein 2 (CMG2) resides on chromosome 4q21. CMG2 is an integrin-like cell surface receptor that binds laminins and type IV collagen, and it is thought to play a role in cell–matrix and cell–cell interactions. Mutations in this gene can lead to both JHF and ISH. Missense and other in-frame mutations that affect the cytoplasmic domain cause JHF, whereas truncating mutations and missense mutations that affect the extracellular protein-binding domain cause ISH[32]. However, the exact pathophysiology is still unclear.

Clinical features

Initially, firm papules and nodules develop on the scalp, ears (Fig. 98.11), neck and face (particularly perinasal and perioral regions) as well as the perianal area; papulonodules also favor the hands. Affected children are of normal intelligence, but often suffer severe physical handicap from joint contractures and tumors. Gingival hyperplasia and osteolytic bone lesions may also occur. Infantile systemic hyalinosis is a more severe variant that is characterized by hyaline deposits in multiple internal organs, recurrent infections and, in most cases, death during early childhood.

Pathology

An increased number of fibroblasts are embedded in a hyalinized connective tissue stroma that is homogeneous, amorphous and acidophilic (stains positively with PAS)[31]. Mononuclear cells and CD68+, osteoclast-like, giant cells are also present in a perivascular location. Additional findings include intracytoplasmic and extracellular eosinophilic globules; over time, the lesions tend to become more paucicellular[33].

Differential diagnosis

Winchester syndrome and nodulosis–arthropathy–osteolysis (NAO) syndrome share clinical features with JHF and ISH (e.g. nodules, joint contractures, osteopenia)[33]. The former are allelic autosomal recessive disorders due to mutations in the gene that encodes matrix metallo-proteinase-2 (MMP2). Additional findings include coarse facies and hypertrichosis. Painful nodules on the palms and soles are observed

	Juvenile hyaline fibromatosis	Infantile systemic hyalinosis
Age of onset	Childhood (<5 years old)	Infancy
Cutaneous findings:		
• Firm, pearly papules (favoring the perinasal area and ears)	+	+
• Verrucous perianal nodules	+	+
• Firm nodules/tumors (favoring the scalp, neck, hands and trunk)	+	–
• Reddish-blue to brown plaques overlying extensor surfaces of joints	–	+
• Diffusely thickened skin	–	+
Gingival hypertrophy	+	+
Joint contractures	+	+
Osteopenia	+	+
Persistent diarrhea	–	+
Recurrent infections	–	+
Visceral involvement	–	+
Normal mental development	+	+
Survival into adulthood	+	–

CLINICAL FEATURES OF JUVENILE HYALINE FIBROMATOSIS VERSUS INFANTILE SYSTEMIC HYALINOSIS

Table 98.5 Clinical features of juvenile hyaline fibromatosis versus infantile systemic hyalinosis.

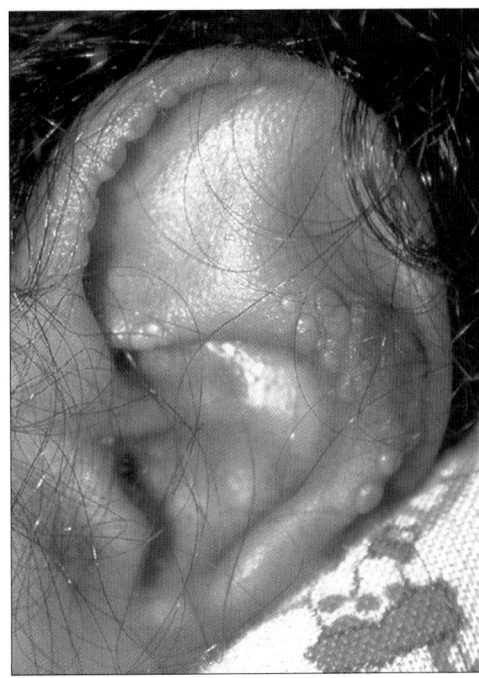

Fig. 98.11 Juvenile hyaline fibromatosis.

in NAO syndrome, whereas thickened, hyperpigmented skin and gingival hypertrophy characterize Winchester syndrome. Histologically, both conditions feature a proliferation of fibroblasts and thickened collagen bundles extending from the deep reticular dermis to the subcutaneous fat.

Treatment

Unfortunately, treatment options for JHF and ISH are limited. Surgical excision of nodules and gingival hypertrophy, as well as release of contractures can be performed, but lesions often recur. Physiotherapy may slow the progression of joint contractures[33]. Injections of corticosteroids into fibromas have met with limited success. Systemic interferon-α-2b therapy was reported to improve the skin lesions, gingival hypertrophy and joint contractures in one patient.

REFERENCES

1. Kim WJH, Levinson H, Gittes GK, Longaker MT. Molecular mechanisms in keloid biology. In: Garg HG, Longaker MT (eds). Scarless Wound Healing. New York: Marcel Dekker, 2000:161–71.

1a. Alhady SM, Sivanantharajah K. Keloids in various races. A review of 175 cases. Plast Reconstr Surg. 1969; 44:564–6.

2. Niessen FB, Spauwen PH, Schalkwijk J, Kon M. On the nature of hypertrophic scars and keloidal scars: a review. Plast Reconstr Surg. 1999;104:1435–58.

3. Marneros AG, Norris JEC, Olsen BR, Reichenberger E. Clinical genetics of familial keloids. Arch Dermatol. 2001;137:1429–34.

4. Ehrlich HP. Collagen considerations in scarring and regenerative repair. In: Garg HG, Longaker MT (eds). Scarless Wound Healing. New York: Marcel Dekker, 2000:99–113.

5. Smith P, Mosiello G, Deluca L, et al. TGF-beta2 activates proliferative scar fibroblasts. J Surg Res. 1999; 82:319–23.

6. Campaner AB, Ferreira LM, Gragnani A, et al. Upregulation of TGF-beta1 expression may be necessary but is not sufficient for excessive scarring. J Invest Dermatol. 2006;126:1168–76.

7. Shaw AM. Recent advances in embryonic wound healing. In: Garg HG, Longaker MT (eds). Scarless Wound Healing. New York: Marcel Dekker, 2000:227–37.

8. Calnan JS, Copenhagen HJ. Autotransplantation of keloid in man. Br J Surg. 1967;54:330–5.

9. Ehrlich HP, Desmouliere A, Diegelmann RF, et al. Morphological and immunochemical differences between keloid and hypertrophic scar. Am J Pathol. 1994;145:105–13.

10. Darzi MA, Chowdri NA, Kaul SK, Khan M. Evaluation of various methods of treating keloids and hypertrophic scars: a 10-year follow-up study. Br J Plast Surg. 1992;45:374–9.

11. Berman B, Flores F. Recurrence rates of excised keloids treated with postoperative triamcinolone acetonide injections or interferon alfa-2b injections. J Am Acad Dermatol. 1997;37:755–7.

12. Berman B, Duncan MR. Short-term keloid treatment *in vivo* with human interferon alfa-2b results in a selective and persistent normalization of keloidal fibroblast collagen, glycosaminoglycan, and collagenase production *in vitro*. J Am Acad Dermatol. 1989;21:694–702.

13. Granstein RD, Rook A, Flotte TJ, et al. A controlled trial of intralesional recombinant interferon-gamma in the treatment of keloidal scarring. Clinical and histologic findings. Arch Dermatol. 1990;126:1295–302.

14. Klumpar DI, Murray JC, Anscher M. Keloids treated with excision followed by radiation therapy. J Am Acad Dermatol. 1994;31:225–31.

15. Botwood N, Lewanski C, Lowdell C. The risks of treating keloids with radiotherapy. Br J Radiol. 1999; 72:1222–4.

16. Fitzpatrick RE. Treatment of inflamed hypertrophic scars using intralesional 5-FU. Dermatol Surg. 1999;25:224–32.

17. Kontochristopoulos G, Stefanaki C, Panagiotopoulos A, et al. Intralesional 5-fluorouracil in the treatment of keloids: an open clinical and histopathologic study. J Am Acad Dermatol. 2005;52:474–9.

18. Kim A, DiCarlo J, Cohen C, et al. Are keloids really 'gli-loids'? High-level expression of *gli-1* oncogene in keloids. J Am Acad Dermatol. 2001;45:707–11.

19. Gira AK, Brown LF, Washington CV, et al. Keloids demonstrate high-level epidermal expression of vascular endothelial growth factor. J Am Acad Dermatol. 2004;50:850–3.

20. Berman B, Villa A. Imiquimod 5% cream for keloid management. Dermatol Surg. 2003;29:1050–1.

21. Jacob SE, Berman B, Nassiri M, Vinvek V. Topical application of imiquimod 5% cream to keloids alters expression genes associated with apoptosis. Br J Dermatol. 2003;149(suppl. 66):62–5.

22. Alster TS, Williams CM. Treatment of keloid sternotomy scars with 585 nm flashlamp-pumped pulsed dye-laser. Lancet. 1995;345:1198–2000.

23. Kuo YR, Wu WS, Jeng SF, et al. Activation of ERK and p38 kinase mediated keloid fibroblast apoptosis after flashlamp pulsed-dye lased treatment. Lasers Surg Med. 2005;36:31–7.

24. Kuo YR, Wu WS, Jeng SF, et al. Suppressed TGF-beta1 expression is correlated with up-regulation of matrix metalloproteinase-13 in keloid regression after flashlamp pulsed-dye laser treatment. Lasers Surg Med. 2005;36:38–42.

25. O'Brien L, Pandit A. Silicon gel sheeting for preventing and treating hypertrophic and keloid scars. Cochrane Database Systemic Rev 2006;(1):CD003826.

26. Hayashi T, Nishihira J, Koyama Y, et al. Decreased prostaglandin E2 production by inflammatory cytokine and lower expression of EP2 receptor result in increased collagen synthesis in keloid fibroblasts. J Invest Dermatol. 2006;126:990–7.

26a. Mukhopadhyay A, Chan SY, Lim IJ, et al. The role of the activin system in keloid pathogenesis. Am J Physiol – Cell Physiol. 2007;292:C1331–8.

27. Wang Z, Fong KD, Phan TT, et al. Increased transcriptional response to mechanical strain in keloid fibroblasts due to increased focal adhesion complex formation. J Cell Physiol. 2006;206:510–17.

28. Weinzweig N, Culver JE, Fleegler EJ. Severe contractures of the proximal interphalangeal joint in Dupuytren's disease: combined fasciectomy with capsuloligamentous release versus fasciectomy alone. Plast Reconstr Surg. 1996;97:560–6.

29. Oikarinen A, Palatsi R, Kylmaniemi M, et al. Pachydermoperiostosis: analysis of the connective tissue abnormality in one family. J Am Acad Dermatol. 1994;31:947–53.

30. Shehab ZP, Raafat F, Proops DW. Juvenile hyaline fibromatosis. Int J Pediatr Otorhinolaryngol. 1995;33:179–86.

31. Kitano Y, Horiki M, Aoki T, et al. Two cases of juvenile hyaline fibromatosis: some histological, electron microscopic and tissue culture observations. Arch Dermatol.1972;106:877–83.

32. Hanks S, Adams S, Douglas J, et al. Mutations in the gene encoding capillary morphogenesis protein 2 cause juvenile hyaline fibromatosis and infantile systemic hyalinosis. Am J Hum Genet. 2003;73:791–800.

33. Thomas JE, Moossavi M, Mehregan DR, et al. Juvenile hyaline fibromatosis: a case report and review of the literature. Int J Dermatol. 2004;43:785–9.

Atrophies of Connective Tissue

Catherine Maari and Julie Powell

99

Atrophies of the skin that are due to a diminution or loss of collagen and/or elastic fibers are discussed in this chapter. The areas of involvement can be quite large, as in mid-dermal elastolysis, or punctate, as in follicular atrophoderma. In most disorders, the underlying pathogenesis remains to be discovered.

MID-DERMAL ELASTOLYSIS

Key features

- Uncommon disorder with areas of fine wrinkling
- Usually affects Caucasian middle-aged women
- Selective loss of elastic tissue in the mid dermis

Introduction

Mid-dermal elastolysis is a rare acquired disorder of elastic tissue. It is characterized clinically by diffuse fine wrinkling, most often located on the trunk, neck and arms. Histologically, a clear band of elastolysis is present in the mid dermis.

History

In 1977, Shelley & Wood reported the first case of 'wrinkles due to idiopathic loss of mid-dermal elastic tissue'. Their patient, a 42-year-old woman, had circumscribed areas of fine wrinkles that gave her an inappropriately aged appearance[1].

Epidemiology

To date, approximately 60 cases have been reported in the literature. The vast majority of patients are Caucasian women between the ages of 30 and 50 years[2].

Pathogenesis

The cause of the acquired elastic tissue degeneration in mid-dermal elastolysis is still unclear. Exposure to UV light is thought to be a major contributing factor in the degeneration of elastic fibers[3] (as in annular elastolytic giant cell granuloma). Other possible mechanisms include defects in the synthesis of elastic fibers, autoimmunity against elastic fibers, and damage to elastic fibers via the release of elastase by inflammatory cells or fibroblasts. More recent studies have suggested that an altered balance between matrix metalloproteinases (MMPs) and tissue inhibitors of metalloproteinases (TIMPs) may be playing a role, in addition to CD34+ dendritic fibroblasts[4].

Clinical features

Mid-dermal elastolysis is characterized by well-circumscribed or larger diffuse areas of fine wrinkling (Fig. 99.1). The wrinkles themselves usually follow cleavage lines. Discrete perifollicular papules can be seen in some patients, with the site of the central hair follicle being indented. Inconstant features include erythematous patches and telangiectasias. Although in the majority of cases there is no history of a prior inflammatory dermatosis, some patients do report previous mild to moderate erythema and, rarely, the elastolysis is preceded by episodes of urticaria or granuloma annulare.

The sites of predilection are the trunk, lateral neck and upper extremities. Once the patches of wrinkling have appeared, they usually remain stationary. They are asymptomatic and give the skin a prematurely aged appearance. The affected areas usually have normal pigmentation and no associated scaling, induration or herniation. There is neither associated systemic involvement nor a family history of similar lesions.

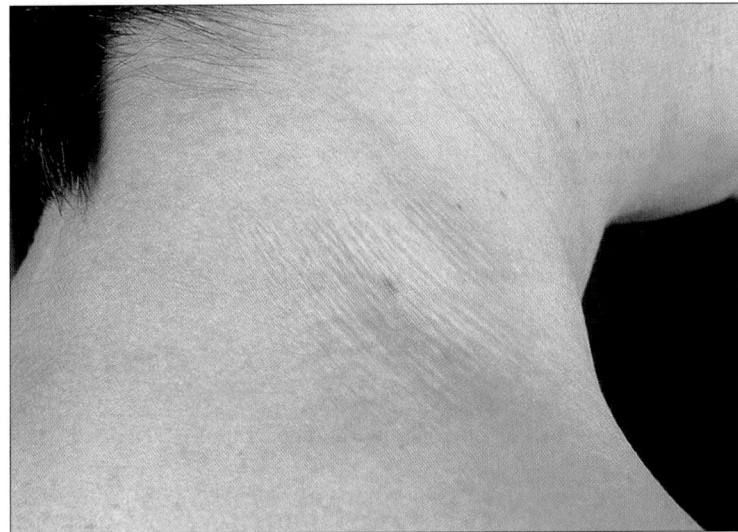

Fig. 99.1 Mid-dermal elastolysis. Well-circumscribed area of fine wrinkling on the neck of a middle-aged woman. Courtesy of Richard Dubuc MD.

Pathology

The epidermis is normal in appearance and, occasionally, a mild perivascular infiltrate is noted in the dermis. Elastic tissue stains, such as Verhoeff–van Gieson or Weigert's stain, reveal a selective loss of elastic fibers in the mid dermis (Fig. 99.2). There is preservation of normal elastic tissue in the superficial papillary dermis above, in the reticular dermis below, and along adjacent hair follicles. The preservation of elastic tissue around the hair follicles explains the perifollicular papules that can be seen in some cases.

By electron microscopy, phagocytosis of normal as well as degenerated elastic fiber tissue by macrophages has been observed[5].

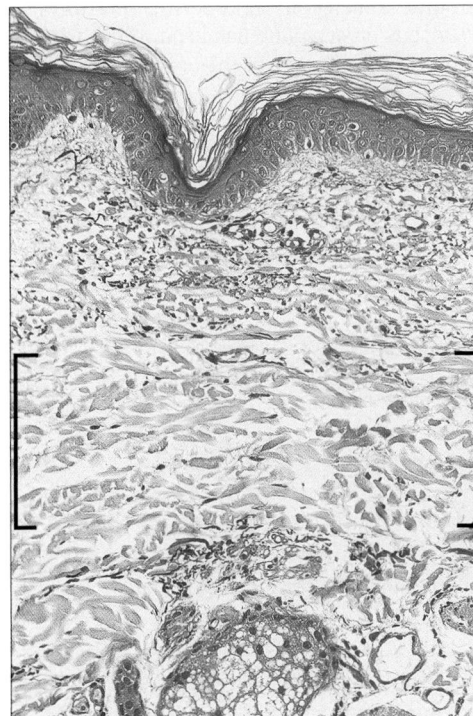

Fig. 99.2 Histology of mid-dermal elastolysis. Note selective loss of elastic fibers in the mid dermis (brackets). Normal elastic tissue is preserved in the superficial papillary dermis and in the reticular dermis (Weigert's stain). Courtesy of Danielle Bouffard MD.

DISORDERS OF ELASTIC TISSUE			
Condition	Clinical findings	Site of predilection	Pathology
Anetoderma	Multiple circumscribed areas of flaccid skin; lesions are often elevated (protruding), but can be macular or depressed	Usually on trunk	Focal or complete loss of elastic tissue in the papillary and/or mid-reticular dermis
Mid-dermal elastolysis	Diffuse areas of fine wrinkling and occasional perifollicular papules in middle-aged women	Trunk, arms and lateral neck	Selective loss of elastic fibers within the mid dermis in a band-like pattern
Pseudoxanthoma elasticum (see Ch. 97)	Yellowish coalescing skin papules, 'cobblestoning', and redundant folds in flexural sites; associated ocular and cardiovascular involvement	Lateral neck, axillae, and groin; scars	Calcified and clumped elastic fibers in the mid dermis
Cutis laxa (see Ch. 97)	Loose, sagging skin folds resulting in prematurely aged appearance. Hereditary or acquired. Internal organ involvement, e.g. pulmonary, in hereditary form	Eyelids, cheeks, neck, shoulder girdle and abdomen	Diminished and fragmented elastic fibers throughout the dermis
Elastosis perforans serpiginosa (see Ch. 95)	Small keratotic papules arranged in arcuate or serpiginous patterns. Association with various syndromes (Down syndrome being the most frequent) and with penicillamine treatment	Lateral neck and antecubital fossae	Thickened elastic fibers are extruded from the dermis through a transepidermal channel

Table 99.1 Disorders of elastic tissue. For additional entities, see Tables 94.5, 97.4 and 97.5.

Differential diagnosis

Mid-dermal elastolysis must be differentiated from the other disorders of elastic tissue such as anetoderma, pseudoxanthoma elasticum (see Ch. 97) and cutis laxa (Table 99.1).

Clinically, anetoderma is characterized by smaller soft macules and papules that herniate upon palpation, as opposed to diffuse wrinkling; histologically, elastolysis can occur in the papillary and/or mid reticular dermis in anetoderma (see below). Patients with cutis laxa have loose, redundant skin, hanging in folds, and histologic examination shows elastolysis that frequently involves the entire dermis. There is also a form of postinflammatory elastolysis and cutis laxa that was originally described in young girls of African descent. An inflammatory phase consisting of indurated plaques or urticaria, malaise and fever preceded the diffuse wrinkling, atrophy and severe disfigurement. Insect bites may be the trigger for the initial inflammatory lesions[6].

Less often, mid-dermal elastolysis is confused with solar elastosis or perifollicular elastolysis. Solar elastosis differs by its onset in an older age group, restriction to only sun-exposed areas, yellowish color and coarser wrinkling, as well as by hyperplasia of abnormal elastic fibers and basophilic degeneration of the collagen in the papillary dermis. Perifollicular elastolysis leads to a selective and almost complete loss of the elastic fibers that surround hair follicles, compared with preservation of elastic fibers around follicles in mid-dermal elastolysis. Elastase-producing *Staphylococcus epidermidis* has been found within the hair follicles and is the presumed etiology of this condition[7].

Treatment

Currently, there is no effective treatment for mid-dermal elastolysis. Sunscreens, colchicine, retinoic acid and vitamin E have been tried without success[2].

ANETODERMA

Synonym: ■ Macular atrophy; anetoderma maculosa; anetoderma maculosa cutis; atrophia maculosa cutis

Key features

- Circumscribed 1–2 cm areas of flaccid skin, which may be elevated, macular or depressed
- Both inflammatory and non-inflammatory forms of primary anetoderma occur
- Secondary anetoderma is associated with infectious and inflammatory cutaneous disorders as well as tumors
- Focal dermal defect of elastic tissue

Introduction

The term 'anetoderma' is derived from *anetos*, the Greek word for slack, and *derma* for skin. Anetoderma is an elastolytic disorder characterized by localized areas of flaccid skin, which may be depressed, macular or papular; the latter can reflect herniation of the subcutaneous tissue. Anetoderma may be idiopathic or associated with an inflammatory disorder of the skin.

History

The first case of primary inflammatory anetoderma was reported by Jadassohn in 1892, and it occurred in a 23-year-old woman who had depressed pink-to-red lesions on her elbows that were noted to have an atrophic, wrinkled appearance[8]. A year previously, Schweninger & Buzzi described a 29-year-old woman with multiple, sac-like tumors that demonstrated herniation upon palpation; the lesions were located on the trunk and upper extremities but lacked inflammation[9].

Epidemiology

Several hundred cases of anetoderma have been reported in the world literature since the original report. The lesions usually occur in young adults between 15 and 25 years of age and more frequently in women than men.

Pathogenesis

The pathogenesis of anetoderma is not known. These lesions could be considered unusual scars, since scars also have decreased elastic tissue. The loss of dermal elastin may reflect an impaired turnover of elastin, caused by either increased destruction or decreased synthesis of elastic fibers. There are a number of proposed explanations for the focal elastin destruction, e.g. the release of elastase from inflammatory cells, the release of cytokines such as interleukin-6, an increased production of progelatinases A and B[10], and the phagocytosis of elastic fibers by macrophages. In addition, immunologic mechanisms may play a role in anetoderma and may explain the associated findings of antiphospholipid antibodies, antinuclear antibodies, false-positive serologic testing for syphilis or *Borrelia*, and positive direct immunofluorescence (see below).

Primary anetoderma occurs when there is no underlying associated disorder, and it arises within clinically normal skin. It can be classified into two major forms: those with preceding inflammatory lesions (the Jadassohn–Pellizzari type) and those without preceding inflammatory lesions (the Schweninger–Buzzi type) (Table 99.2). This clinical classification is primarily of historical interest, since the two types of lesions can coexist in the same patient and their histopathology is often the same (i.e. inflammation has been observed in both types of lesions); the presence or absence of clinical inflammation at the onset of the disease is not related to prognosis[11]. Although the vast majority of cases are sporadic, familial anetoderma has been described and is usually not associated with pre-existing lesions[12].

CLASSIFICATION OF ANETODERMA	
Primary anetoderma	• Jadassohn–Pellizzari type: preceding inflammatory lesions • Schweninger–Buzzi type: no preceding inflammatory lesions
Secondary anetoderma	• To a primary dermatosis • To a systemic disease
Familial anetoderma	

Table 99.2 Classification of anetoderma.

Clinical features

The characteristic lesions are flaccid circumscribed areas of slack skin that are a reflection of a marked reduction or absence of dermal elastic fibers; they can appear as depressions, wrinkling or sac-like protrusions (Fig. 99.3). These atrophic lesions can vary in number from a few to hundreds, and they measure 1–2 cm in diameter and are skin-colored to blue–white in color. The skin surface can be normal in appearance or wrinkled, and a central depression may be seen. Coalescence of smaller lesions can give rise to larger herniations.

The examining finger sinks into a distinct pit with sharp borders as if into a hernia ring. The bulge reappears when the pressure from the finger is released. This 'buttonhole' sign is identical to the one seen in neurofibromas.

Predilection sites for these asymptomatic lesions are the chest, back, neck and upper extremities. They usually develop in young adults, and new lesions often continue to form for many years as the older lesions fail to resolve.

True secondary anetoderma implies that the characteristic atrophic lesion has appeared in the same site as a previous specific skin lesion (see Fig. 99.3B). Some authors also consider lesions associated with an underlying disease (e.g. HIV infection, antiphospholipid antibody syndrome) as secondary anetoderma; however, in this instance, the atrophic areas do not necessarily develop within areas of known inflammation. The numerous and heterogeneous dermatoses associated with secondary anetoderma as an endpoint are listed in Table 99.3. The clinical features are the same as those of primary anetoderma.

SECONDARY ANETODERMA – ASSOCIATED CONDITIONS	
Infectious	• Varicella • Folliculitis • Syphilis • Molluscum contagiosum • Tuberculosis • Lepromatous leprosy • HIV infection • Acrodermatitis chronica atrophicans • Post-hepatitis B immunization
Drugs	• Penicillamine
Inflammatory	• Acne vulgaris • Mastocytosis • Lichen planus • Granuloma annulare • Juvenile xanthogranuloma • Sarcoidosis • Cutaneous lymphoid hyperplasia (lymphocytoma cutis) • Prurigo nodularis
Autoimmune	• Discoid and systemic lupus erythematosus • Antiphospholipid syndrome
Tumors and depositions	• Pilomatricoma • Melanocytic nevi • Dermatofibroma • Involuted infantile hemangioma • Nodular amyloidosis • Plasmacytoma* • Immunocytoma* • Xanthomas

Table 99.3 Secondary anetoderma – associated conditions. *Under current WHO-EORTC classification, considered forms of marginal zone B-cell lymphoma.

Anetoderma has also been described in premature infants and, in some cases, it may have been related to the use of cutaneous monitoring leads or adhesives[13].

In patients with anetoderma, a variety of systemic abnormalities have been reported, including ocular, endocrinologic, bony, cardiac, pulmonary and gastrointestinal. Because there has been no consistency

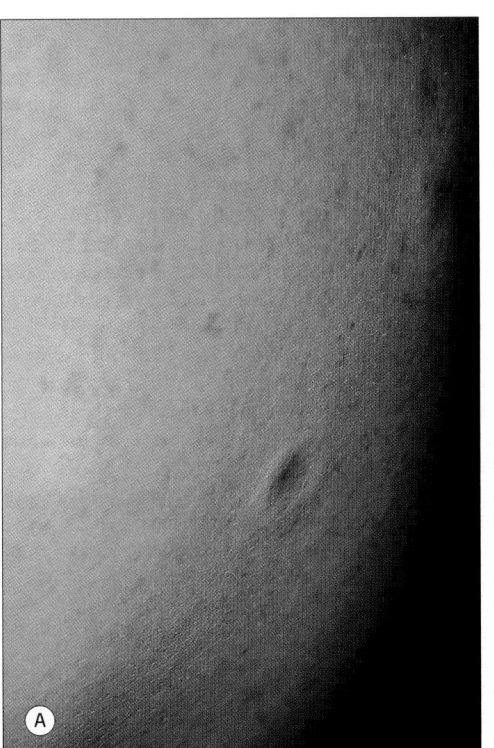
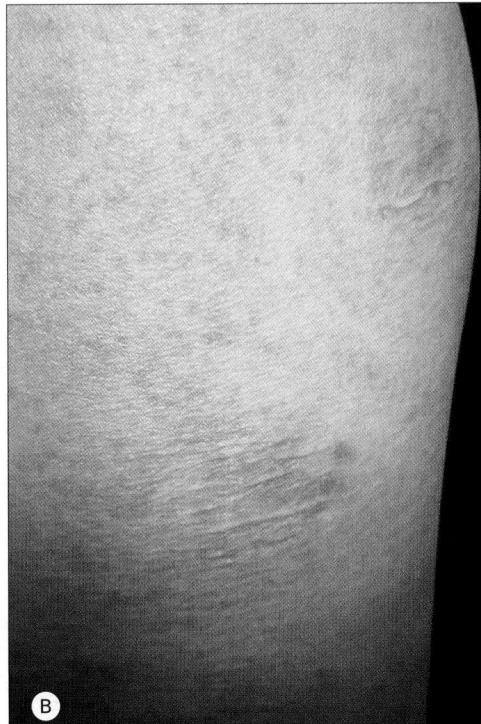
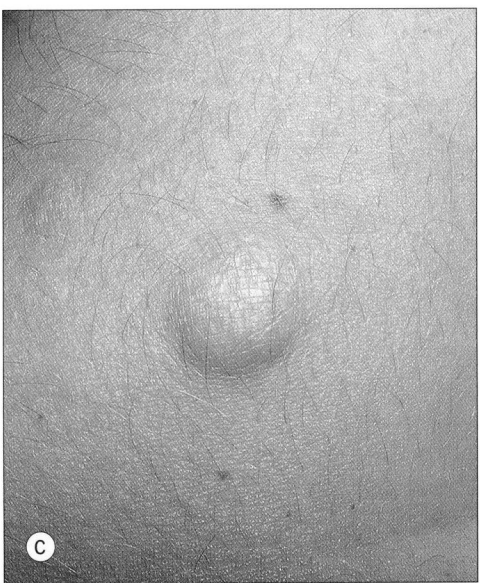

Fig. 99.3 Anetoderma – primary and secondary. A Small, flaccid, sac-like protrusion on the back; note the central depression. **B** Circumscribed patches of anetoderma at sites of previous cutaneous sarcoidosis; note the wrinkling. **C** Soft, skin-colored papule that herniates upon palpation. C, Courtesy of Ronald P Rapini MD.

with regard to these associated abnormalities, they are probably coincidental, although the possibility exists that they may reflect a more generalized elastolytic disorder that has yet to be defined.

Pathology

In routinely stained sections, the collagen within the dermis of affected skin appears normal. Perivascular lymphocytes are often present but do not correlate with clinical findings of inflammation. Monoclonal antibody studies have shown that the majority of lymphocytes in these infiltrates are helper T cells.

The predominant abnormality (as revealed by elastic tissue stains) is a focal, more or less complete loss of elastic tissue in the papillary and/or mid-reticular dermis. There are usually some residual abnormal, irregular and fragmented elastic fibers (Fig. 99.4)[14]. Plasma cells and histiocytes with occasional granuloma formation can be seen.

Direct immunofluorescence sometimes shows linear or granular deposits of immunoglobulins and complement along the dermal–epidermal junction or around the dermal blood vessels in affected skin[15]. However, this finding is not used diagnostically.

Electron microscopy demonstrates that the elastic fibers are fragmented and irregular in shape and occasionally they are engulfed by macrophages.

Differential diagnosis

Anetoderma must be differentiated from other disorders of elastic tissue such as mid-dermal elastolysis (see Table 99.1) as well as atrophodermas (see below). However, the major differential diagnosis consists of post-traumatic scars and papular elastorrhexis. The latter is an acquired disorder characterized by firm, white, non-follicular papules that measure 1–4 mm in diameter and are evenly scattered on the trunk. The lesions usually appear during adolescence or early adulthood. Histology demonstrates focal degeneration of elastic fibers and normal collagen. There are no associated extracutaneous abnormalities. This disorder is believed by some authors to be a variant of connective tissue nevi[16] or an abortive form of the Buschke–Ollendorff syndrome[17], while others think that these lesions represent papular acne scars[18]. They are differentiated from anetoderma by being firm and non-compressible.

Less often, anetoderma is confused with nevus lipomatosus or focal dermal hypoplasia (Goltz syndrome). Nevus lipomatosus superficialis of Hoffman and Zurhelle presents as a clustered group of soft, skin-colored to yellow nodules, usually located on the lower trunk and present since birth (see Ch. 117). Histology shows ectopic mature lipocytes located within the dermis. The lesions (be it telangiectasia, vermiculate dermal atrophy, hypopigmentation, hyperpigmentation, or fatty herniation/hamartoma) of Goltz syndrome are in a linear array along the lines of Blaschko (see Ch. 61). Histologically, a decrease in dermal content is seen as well as extension or deposition of subcutaneous fat into the dermis.

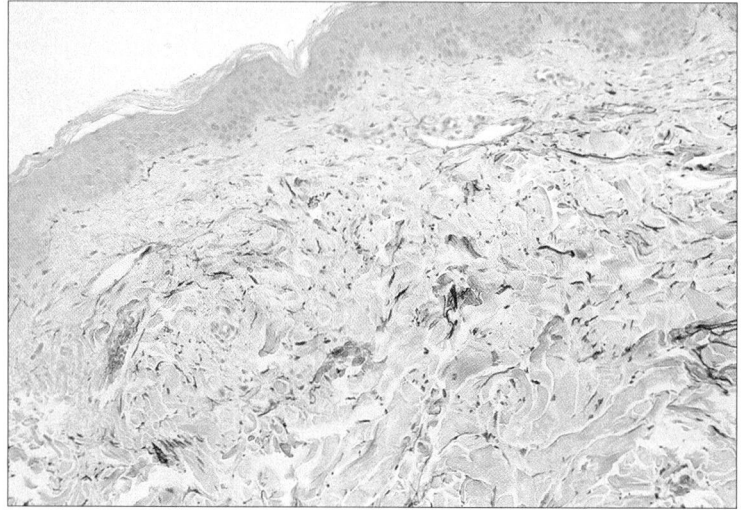

Fig. 99.4 Histology of anetoderma. A decrease of elastic fibers in both the papillary and reticular dermis (Weigert's stain).

Treatment

Various therapeutic modalities have been tried, but have not resulted in improvement of existing atrophic lesions; these include intralesional injections of triamcinolone and systemic administration of aspirin, dapsone, phenytoin, penicillin G, vitamin E and inositol niacinate. Some authors have reported improvement with hydroxychloroquine. Surgical excision in patients with limited lesions may be helpful.

STRIAE

Synonym: ■ Striae distensae; striae atrophicans; 'stretch marks'; linear atrophy

Introduction

Striae are a very common condition in all age groups. They are linear atrophic depressions of the skin that form in areas of dermal damage produced by stretching of the skin. They are associated with various physiologic states, including puberty, pregnancy, growth spurts, rapid weight gain or loss, obesity[19], and disorders that lead to hypercortisolism.

History

Striae were first described by Roederer in 1773, and the first histologic descriptions were made by Troisier & Menetrier in 1889.

Epidemiology

Striae are very common and usually develop between the ages of 5 and 50 years. They are seen more commonly in Caucasians, and striae occur about twice as frequently in women as in men. They commonly develop during puberty, with an overall incidence of 25–35%[20], or during pregnancy, with an incidence of approximately 75%[21].

Pathogenesis

Factors leading to the development of striae have not been fully elucidated. Striae distensae are a reflection of 'breaks' in the connective tissue that lead to dermal atrophy. A number of factors, including hormones (particularly corticosteroids), mechanical stress and genetic predisposition, appear to play a role.

Clinical features

Striae are usually multiple, symmetric, well-defined linear atrophic lesions that often follow the lines of cleavage. They are usually more of a cosmetic concern, but rarely they can ulcerate. Initially, striae appear as red-to-violaceous elevated lines that can be mildly pruritic and are called striae rubra (Fig. 99.5). Over time, the color gradually fades, and the lesions become atrophic, with the skin surface exhibiting a fine wrinkled appearance. These striae alba are usually permanent, but they may fade somewhat over time[20]. The striae can measure several centimeters in length and a few millimeters to a few centimeters in width.

During puberty, striae appear in areas where there is a rapid increase in size. In girls, the most common sites are the thighs, hips, buttocks and breasts, whereas in boys, they are seen on the shoulders, thighs and lumbosacral region (Fig. 99.6). Other less common sites include the abdomen, upper arms, neck and axillae.

Striae distensae are a common finding on the abdomen, and less so on the breasts and thighs, of pregnant women, especially during the last trimester. They are more common in younger primigravidas than in older pregnant women. One study showed that striae gravidarum are statistically significant predictors of lacerations during vaginal delivery[22]. More recently, the presence of striae was found to be a risk factor for the development of pelvic relaxation and clinical prolapse[23].

The striae associated with systemic corticosteroid therapy and Cushing's syndrome can be larger and more widely distributed (see Ch. 52). Flexural and intertriginous areas are particularly at risk for developing striae from the use of topical corticosteroids.

Atrophic striae may become elevated and even 'worm-like' in the setting of severe edema, including lymphedema. In addition, there are

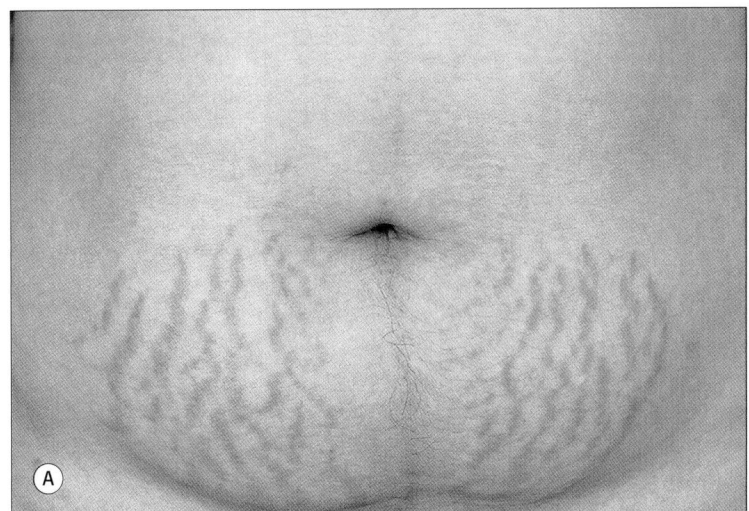

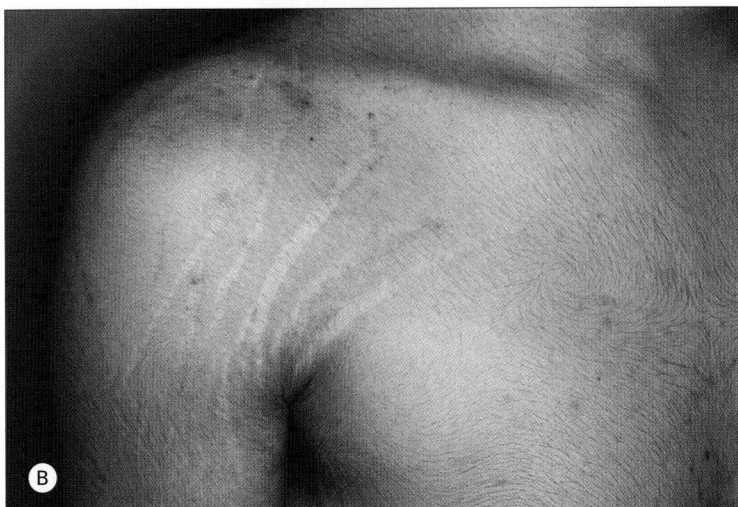

Fig. 99.5 Striae. A Linear erythematous lesions on the abdomen (striae rubra). **B** Atrophic linear lesions of striae alba in a teenager. B, Courtesy of Kalman Watsky MD.

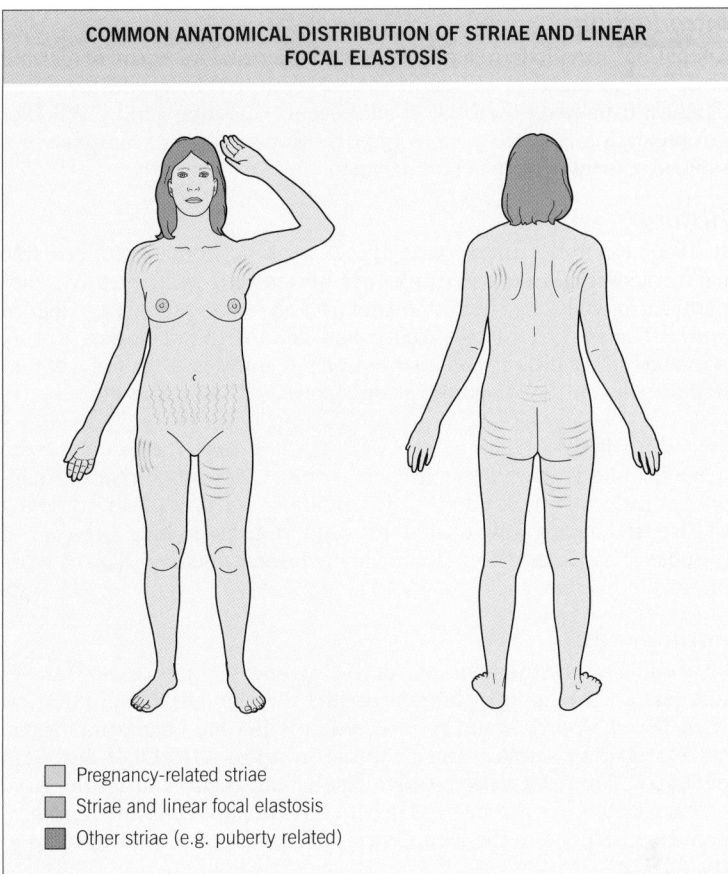

COMMON ANATOMICAL DISTRIBUTION OF STRIAE AND LINEAR FOCAL ELASTOSIS

☐ Pregnancy-related striae
☐ Striae and linear focal elastosis
☐ Other striae (e.g. puberty related)

Fig. 99.6 Common anatomic distribution of striae and linear focal elastosis. Striae associated with pregnancy are in green and linear focal elastosis is in blue.

diseases such as pruritic urticarial papules and plaques of pregnancy that begin within striae.

Pathology

Histologic findings depend upon the stage of evolution of the striae at the time the biopsy is performed. The epidermis can be normal during the early stages, but eventually it becomes flattened and atrophic with blunted rete ridges. The dermal thickness is decreased, as is the collagen in the upper dermis. The collagen bundles are thinned and lie parallel to the epidermis, but they are also arranged transversely to the direction of the striae. Alterations in elastic fibers are variable, but dermal elastin can be fragmented, and specific elastin staining can demonstrate a marked reduction in visible elastin content compared with adjacent normal dermis[24]. There is an absence of both hair follicles and other appendages.

Differential diagnosis

The diagnosis of striae distensae is usually straightforward, but the differential diagnosis does include linear focal elastosis (elastotic striae), an entity first described by Burket et al. in 1989[25]. Linear focal elastosis is characterized by rows of yellow, palpable, striae-like bands on the lower back. Unlike striae, the lesions are raised and yellow rather than depressed and white. Elderly men are most commonly affected, although such lesions have been described in teenagers. Linear focal elastosis is probably not an uncommon condition. Histologically, there is a focal increase in the number of elongated or fragmented elastic fibers as well as a thickened dermis. It is postulated that linear focal elastosis may represent an excessive regenerative process of elastic fibers and could be viewed as a keloidal repair of striae distensae[26].

Treatment

Striae distensae have no medical consequences, but they are frequently distressing to those afflicted. As stretch marks tend to improve spontaneously over time, the usefulness of treatments that have been tested without case controls is difficult to assess. Treatment of early-stage striae with tretinoin 0.1% cream can improve their appearance, and its application has been shown to decrease the length and width of striae[27]. Other topical treatments, including 0.05% tretinoin/20% glycolic acid and 10% L-ascorbic acid/20% glycolic acid, may also improve the appearance of stretch marks[28]. Several lasers have been used to treat striae: the 585 nm pulsed dye laser has been shown to result in some improvement in the appearance of striae rubra, but it has no effect on striae alba; secondary pigmentary alterations in darker skin are a concern[29]. Improvement in the leukoderma of striae alba was noted with the 308 nm excimer laser, but maintenance treatment was required to sustain the cosmetic benefit[30].

IDIOPATHIC ATROPHODERMA OF PASINI AND PIERINI

Synonym: ▪ Sclérodermie atrophique d'emblée; morphea plana atrophica; dyschromic and atrophic variation of scleroderma

Key features

▪ Brown-to-blue depressed patches, usually on the posterior trunk
▪ 'Cliff-drop' or abrupt transition from normal to diseased skin
▪ Lesions are asymptomatic and lack induration
▪ Disorder lasts for many years but has a benign course

Introduction

Idiopathic atrophoderma of Pasini and Pierini is a form of dermal atrophy that presents as one or several sharply demarcated depressed patches, usually on the back of adolescents or young adults. Whether atrophoderma is an atypical, primarily atrophic form of morphea or a separate distinct entity is still debated.

History

In 1923, Pasini described a case of a 21-year-old woman with atrophic cutaneous lesions on the trunk that he reported as progressive idiopathic atrophoderma[31]. In 1936, and over the subsequent years, Pierini and associates extensively studied and defined the condition and its possible link to morphea. This prompted Canizares et al.[32] in 1958 to rename this entity 'idiopathic atrophoderma of Pasini and Pierini'.

Epidemiology

This disorder is more frequently encountered in women than in men, with a ratio of 6:1 in adults[33]. It usually starts insidiously in young individuals during the second or third decade of life. However, a number of cases have been described in children younger than 13 years of age.

Pathogenesis

The etiology of atrophoderma of Pasini and Pierini remains as yet unknown. Some authors have suggested the possible role of infection with *Borrelia burgdorferi*, as in acrodermatitis chronica atrophicans, since a positive serology can be found in up to 40–50% of European patients[34]. However, false-positive results can occur, and results have varied widely. Given some overlap between atrophoderma and morphea, perhaps insights into the pathogenesis of the latter will provide clues to the former.

Clinical features

Lesions usually appear on the trunk, especially on the back and lumbosacral region, followed in frequency by the chest, arms and abdomen[34]. The face, hands and feet are usually spared. The distribution is often symmetric and bilateral, but a linear pattern along Blaschko's lines has been described (atrophoderma of Moulin; see Ch. 66).

The lesions are single or multiple and usually round or ovoid, ranging in size from a few centimeters to patches covering large areas of the trunk. They are usually asymptomatic and lack inflammation. When lesions coalesce, they can form large irregular patches. The patches usually have a brown color (Fig. 99.7), but some are more blue to violet in color. The surface of the skin is normal in appearance, as is the consistency upon palpation. There is a lack of cutaneous induration or sclerosis.

The borders or edges of these lesions are sharply defined, and they are usually described as abrupt 'cliff-drop' borders ranging from 1 to 8 mm in depth, although they can have a gradual slant[32]. These depressed patches have a characteristic appearance and give the impression of inverted plateaus, or, if multiple lesions are present, they can have the appearance of Swiss cheese. The lesions are even more apparent when present on the back, because the dermis is thicker in this area. Occasionally, deep blood vessels may be seen running through the depressed patches.

The skin surrounding the patches is normal in appearance, and there is no erythema or lilac ring as in morphea. However, typical lesions of morphea, lichen sclerosus and atrophoderma have been observed to occur simultaneously in the same patient (but in different areas), supporting the view that these conditions are related[35]. In addition, sclerodermatous changes can occasionally appear years later in the center of the depressed lesions, leading to a white, shiny induration[32]. In a series of 139 patients, 17% had a white induration in the central portions of their atrophic lesions, and, in 22%, superficial plaques of morphea coexisted in sites separate from the atrophic foci[33].

The course of this benign disease is progressive, and lesions can continue to appear for decades before reaching a standstill. Transformation to generalized morphea has not been observed.

Pathology

In general, the histologic picture is generally not diagnostic, so the diagnosis is primarily a clinical one. The epidermis is usually normal

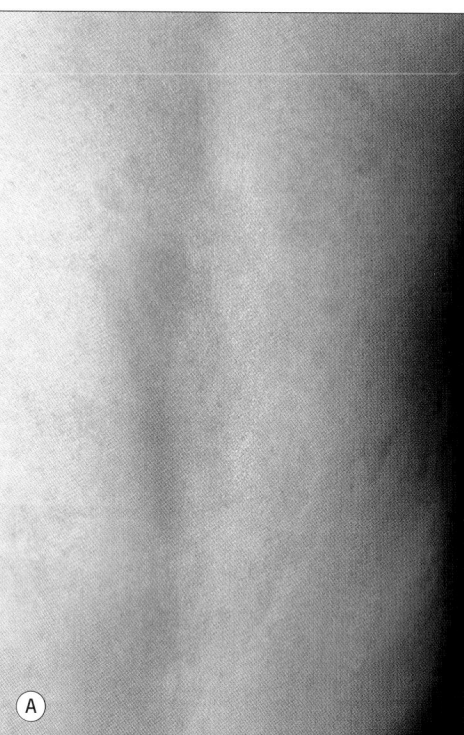

Fig. 99.7 Atrophoderma of Pasini and Pierini. A Multiple depressed, slightly hyperpigmented patches on the back. **B** Coalescent hyperpigmented patches on the abdomen. **A** Courtesy of Catherine C McCuaig MD.

or slightly atrophic. Pigmentation of the basal layer may be increased. A perivascular infiltrate consisting of T cells and histiocytes may be seen. Collagen bundles in the mid and reticular dermis show varying degrees of homogenization and clumping. Dermal thickness is eventually reduced when compared with adjacent normal skin[36]. Dermal atrophy is difficult to evaluate on a punch biopsy, but it can be more easily demonstrated if an elliptical biopsy is taken in an area that includes the cliff-drop border and is then sectioned longitudinally to show the transition between normal and lesional skin. MRI performed in one patient with atrophoderma of Pierini and Pasini showed that the clinical depression was not secondary to subcutaneous atrophy[37]. Some irregular clumping and loss of elastic fibers were described in earlier case reports[32] but, in most series, no abnormality has been observed with elastic tissue stains[33,34]; therefore, this is not of diagnostic value. The appendages are usually preserved.

If sclerodermatous changes appear in pre-existing patches, the histology reveals varying degrees of collagen sclerosis resembling morphea. Direct immunofluorescence may show non-specific IgM and C3 staining in the dermal papillary blood vessels in early lesions or at the dermal–epidermal junction[38].

Differential diagnosis

Since the original description, there has been much debate over whether idiopathic atrophoderma of Pasini and Pierini is a distinct entity or an atrophic, non-indurated, perhaps 'burnt-out' variant of morphea (see

Ch. 96). Active lesions of morphea present as indurated, often hyperpigmented plaques with a characteristic peripheral lilac rim.

Although atrophoderma of Pasini and Pierini lacks sclerosis[33–35,38], its relationship to morphea is favored by its striking clinical and histologic similarities to the atrophy seen at sites of regressing plaques of morphea. To some, the different course and outcome of atrophoderma of Pierini and Pasini as compared with morphea justifies preservation of a distinct name.

Anetoderma, also an atrophic dermal process, is easily differentiated by palpation and histology, which shows a loss of elastic fibers in the dermis (as opposed to a loss of collagen).

Treatment

The natural course of the disease is often protracted (10–20 years) but self-healing, making the evaluation of therapy difficult. No treatment has been proven effective. In view of the possibility of an underlying *Borrelia* infection, penicillin has been used to treat atrophoderma of Pasini and Pierini, but the results have been inconclusive. A retrospective evaluation of 25 patients treated with oral penicillin (2 million IU/day) or oral tetracycline (500 mg three times daily) for 2–3 weeks in one study showed clinical improvement and no evidence of new active lesions in 20 of the 25 patients. In the same study, four of six patients who did not receive treatment also had no evidence of progressive disease[34].

In one case, the Q-switched alexandrite laser was effective in diminishing the hyperpigmentation by 50% after three treatment sessions[39].

FOLLICULAR ATROPHODERMA

Follicular atrophoderma refers to dimple-like depressions at the follicular orifices. It can occur as an isolated defect of limited extent, in association with a variety of disorders in which hair follicles are plugged with keratin, or with rare genodermatoses.

In 1944, Miescher described follicular atrophoderma in an 8-year-old girl with atypical chondrodystrophy[40]. Six years later, Curth also used the term follicular atrophoderma (although there was no evidence of follicular atrophy but rather follicular agenesis) and further reported in 1978 on the genetics of follicular atrophoderma[41].

Clinical features

Distinctive ice-pick depressions around hair follicles can be seen most commonly on the back of the hands and feet or on the cheeks. These pitted scars are often present at birth or during childhood. A family history may be present. Follicular atrophoderma can be associated with Bazex syndrome or with Conradi–Hünermann–Happle syndrome. When the lesions are found exclusively on the cheeks, the term 'atrophoderma vermiculatum' applies. Atrophoderma vermiculatum can in turn be associated with the various disorders discussed in the next section.

Atrophoderma Vermiculatum

Atrophoderma vermiculatum, a disorder limited to the face, has been described under a variety of names, including ulerythema acneforme, acne vermoulante, atrophoderma reticulata symmetrica faciei, folliculitis ulerythema reticulata, folliculitis ulerythemosa, and honeycomb atrophy ('ulerythema' means scar plus redness and 'vermiculatum' means worm-eaten).

Atrophoderma vermiculatum is a condition that can: (1) occur sporadically; (2) be inherited as an autosomal dominant disorder; (3) be part of a group of related diseases that are referred to as 'keratosis pilaris atrophicans' (see Table 39.2); or (4) be associated with various syndromes.

Multiple symmetric inflammatory papules on the cheeks, presumably centered around hair follicles, may precede the atrophic lesions. These papules then go on to become pitted, atrophic and depressed scars in a reticulated or honeycomb pattern (Fig. 99.8). The severity of erythema varies, as does the presence of milia and horny follicular plugs. These lesions can extend to the forehead and preauricular regions. This condition usually has its onset during childhood or, less often, around puberty. Both sexes appear to be equally affected[42]. It usually has a slow progressive course.

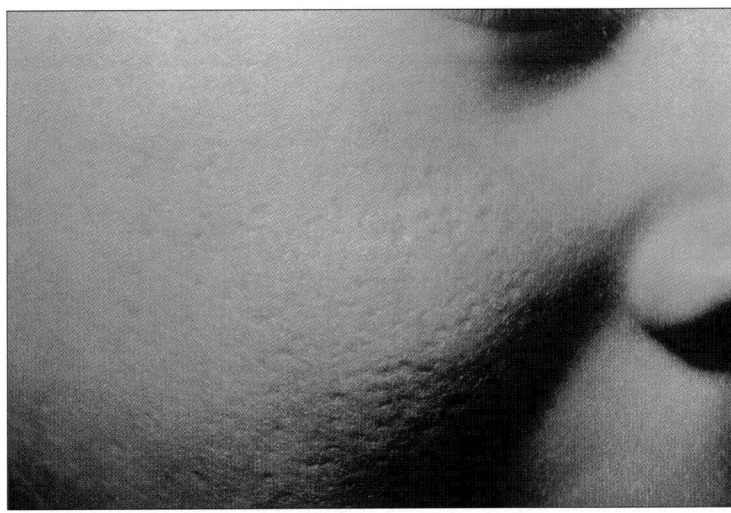

Fig. 99.8 Atrophoderma vermiculatum. Multiple small pitted scars on the cheek of a young girl. Note the honeycomb pattern on the lower inner cheek; the skin is said to appear 'worm-eaten'. Courtesy of Robert Hartman MD.

Atrophoderma vermiculatum can be associated with a group of closely related disorders referred to as keratosis pilaris atrophicans (see Table 39.2)[43]. This group also includes keratosis follicularis spinulosa decalvans and ulerythema ophryogenes. These conditions are characterized by keratotic follicular papules, variable degrees of inflammation, and secondary atrophic scarring. Ulerythema ophryogenes (or keratosis pilaris atrophicans faciei) differs from atrophoderma vermiculatum by affecting primarily the lateral portion of the eyebrows (ophryogenes) in the form of erythema, follicular papules and alopecia. The inheritance pattern is autosomal dominant with incomplete penetrance, and progression usually ceases after puberty. Keratosis follicularis spinulosa decalvans begins during childhood as keratotic follicular papules on the malar area and progresses to involve the eyebrows, scalp and extremities, with associated scarring alopecia. In most patients, this disorder is inherited in an X-linked recessive fashion.

The underlying pathogenesis in atrophoderma vermiculatum as well as the other disorders in the keratosis pilaris atrophicans group appears to be abnormal follicular hyperkeratinization. The latter occurs in the upper third of the hair follicle, leading to obstruction of the growing hair shaft and production of chronic inflammation. The end result is scarring below the level of obstruction.

Histopathology is usually not very helpful and shows dilated follicles, sometimes associated with plugging, inflammation and sclerosis of dermal collagen.

The various syndromes that include atrophoderma vermiculatum are the Rombo syndrome (milia, telangiectasias, basal cell carcinomas [BCCs], hypotrichosis, acral cyanosis and, rarely, trichoepitheliomas), Nicolau–Balus syndrome (syringomas and milia), Tuzun syndrome (scrotal tongue) and, finally, the Braun–Falco–Marghescu syndrome (palmoplantar hyperkeratosis and keratosis pilaris).

The differential diagnosis of atrophoderma vermiculatum includes atrophia maculosa varioliformis cutis, keratosis pilaris rubra of the cheeks and, in older adults, erythromelanosis faciei.

This disorder is primarily a cosmetic problem. Various topical treatments, including emollients, corticosteroids, tretinoin and keratolytics, have shown no consistent benefit. In some instances, systemic isotretinoin has been shown to stop progression and to induce remission[43]. Dermabrasion, laser therapy (e.g. CO_2 and 585 nm pulsed dye) and fillers (e.g. collagen, hyaluronic acid, autologous fat) are other options for improving the appearance of the atrophic scars[44].

Bazex Syndrome

Bazex, Dupré and Christol first described this genodermatosis in 1964, not to be confused with the other disease called Bazex syndrome (acrokeratosis paraneoplastica) in which hyperkeratotic plaques of the ears, nose, cheeks, hands, feet and knees are associated with carcinomas of the upper aerodigestive tract (see Ch. 52).

The Bazex syndrome discussed in this section is characterized by follicular atrophoderma, multiple BCCs, hypotrichosis, and localized hypohidrosis (above the neck). It is inherited in an X-linked dominant fashion, and the gene has been linked to Xq24–q27[45]. Additional reported findings include facial hyperpigmentation, milia, hair shaft dystrophy and multiple genital trichoepitheliomas. Systemic manifestations are absent.

The follicular atrophoderma, described as multiple ice-pick marks or patulous follicles, is found most commonly on the dorsal aspect of the hands, but can also be seen on the feet, lower back, elbows and, rarely, the face; it is usually present at birth or appears during childhood. No abnormalities of the elastic fibers have been found (nor any evidence of atrophy of the epidermis, hair or dermis), making the term 'follicular atrophoderma' a misnomer. The histopathology usually shows hair follicles that are abnormally wide, plugged and surrounded by an inflammatory cell infiltrate. Sweat glands can be absent.

The BCCs occur primarily on the face and they can resemble melanocytic nevi; the age of onset varies from 9 to 50 years of age. To date, less than 20 families with this form of Bazex syndrome have been described.

The differential diagnosis includes other genodermatoses with multiple BCCs: nevoid basal cell carcinoma syndrome (Gorlin syndrome), an autosomal dominant disorder due to mutations in the *PTCH* gene, and Rombo syndrome, an autosomal dominant disorder characterized by BCCs, atrophoderma vermiculatum, milia, hypotrichosis, acrocyanosis and, occasionally, trichoepitheliomas.

X-Linked Dominant Chondrodysplasia Punctata

This disorder is also known as Conradi–Hünermann–Happle syndrome or chondrodysplasia calcificans congenita. It is an X-linked dominant disorder that occurs almost exclusively in girls, since it is usually lethal in hemizygous males. This form of chondrodysplasia punctata results from mosaicism for mutations in the gene on the X chromosome that encodes the emopamil binding protein[46]. The clinical manifestations include an ichthyosiform scaling erythroderma patterned along the lines of Blaschko that usually resolves during the first year of life and is replaced by bands of follicular atrophoderma[47]. Hyperpigmentation, cataracts, scarring alopecia, saddle-nose deformity, asymmetric limb reduction defects, and stippled calcifications of the epiphyses can be seen (see Ch. 56). Within ichthyosiform areas in newborns, keratotic follicular plugs containing dystrophic calcification is a distinctive histopathologic feature[46].

ATROPHIA MACULOSA VARIOLIFORMIS CUTIS

Atrophia maculosa varioliformis cutis was first described by Heidingsfeld in 1918[48] and is not as rare as the number of published cases would suggest. It consists of small round 'varioliform' and linear facial depressions that are asymptomatic (Fig. 99.9)[49]. It occurs spontaneously on the cheeks and occasionally involves the forehead or chin. There is a gradual increase in the number of lesions, but in the absence of preceding trauma, acne or inflammatory lesions. A familial variant has been described. Pachydermodactyly and extrahepatic biliary atresia have been associated findings, but this association is probably fortuitous. The pathogenesis is unknown.

The histologic changes include a depression of the epidermis and normal collagen fibers, but a slightly decreased number of elastic fibers. There is usually little or no inflammation. The differential diagnosis includes simple scars, which can be differentiated by history and the presence histologically of dermal fibrosis, and atrophoderma vermiculatum, which is harder to differentiate but can present with inflammatory papules that are followed by pitted scars, usually has a honeycombed (rather than sharply linear) pattern, and is usually centered on hair follicles. There is no known treatment to prevent the occurrence of these lesions.

PIEZOGENIC PEDAL PAPULES

Piezogenic pedal papules were first described by Shelley & Rawnsley in 1968[50]. This term is somewhat of a misnomer as piezogenic means 'producing pressure', when in fact these lesions are produced by

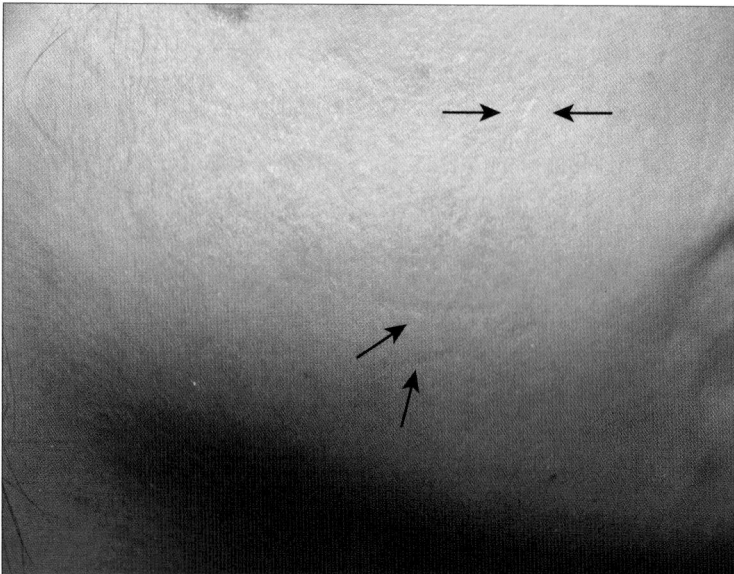

Fig. 99.9 Atrophia maculosa varioliformis cutis. Multiple linear scar-like depressions (between and above arrows) with no history of trauma. Courtesy of Jean L Bolognia MD.

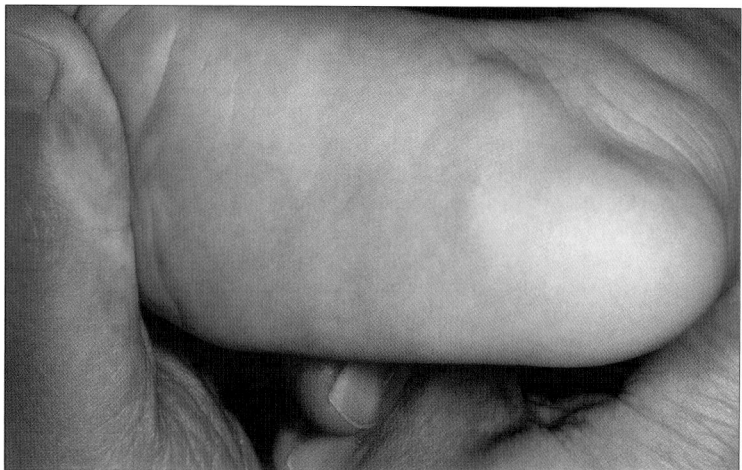

Fig. 99.10 Pedal papules of infancy. Soft nodules on the medial and plantar surfaces of the foot. Courtesy of Julie V Schaffer MD.

pressure. It is postulated that pressure induces herniation of fat through connective tissue in the dermis of the heels.

These papules are common enough in the general population to be considered normal and have also been described in association with Ehlers–Danlos syndrome and Prader–Willi syndrome. An infantile variant characterized by larger nodules on the medial aspect of the heel (present without weight-bearing) has recently been reported (Fig. 99.10)[51].

Skin-colored papules and nodules are seen on the sides of the heels (see Ch. 87); they are induced by weight-bearing and disappear when the leg is raised. The lesions are usually asymptomatic, but pain has been described during weight-bearing, and, in these cases, an orthopedic shoe or surgical excision may help.

OTHER ATROPHIES OF THE CONNECTIVE TISSUE

Many systemic conditions (scleroderma, lupus erythematosus, dermatomyositis) and genodermatoses (poikiloderma congenitale, dyskeratosis congenita, Cockayne syndrome, Hallermann–Streiff syndrome) have skin atrophy as an associated finding. Lichen sclerosus is discussed in Chapter 96, progeria in Chapter 62, Ehlers–Danlos syndrome and cutis laxa in Chapter 97, and acrodermatosis chronica atrophicans in Chapter 73. Cutaneous atrophy is also a well-known complication of prolonged use of either systemic or topical corticosteroids (see Ch. 125).

Atrophies of Connective Tissue

1. Shelley WB, Wood MG. Wrinkles due to idiopathic loss of mid-dermal elastic tissue. Br J Dermatol. 1977;97:441–5.
2. Patroi I, Annessi G, Girolomoni G. Mid-dermal elastolysis: a clinical, histologic, and immunohistochemical study of 11 patients. J Am Acad Dermatol. 2003;48:846–51.
3. Snider RL, Lang PG, Maize JC. The clinical spectrum of mid-dermal elastolysis and the role of UV light in its pathogenesis. J Am Acad Dermatol. 1993;28:938–42.
4. Gambichler T, Breuckmann F, Kreuter A, et al. Immunohistochemical investigation of mid-dermal elastolysis. Clin Exp Dermatol. 2004;29;192–5.
5. Harmon CB, Su WPD, Gagne EJ, et al. Ultrastructural evaluation of mid-dermal elastolysis. J Cutan Pathol. 1994;21:233–8.
6. Verhagen AR, Woederman MJ. Post-inflammatory elastolysis and cutis laxa. Br J Dermatol. 1975;92:183–90.
7. Varadi DP, Saqueton AC. Perifollicular elastolysis. Br J Dermatol. 1970;83:143–50.
8. Jadassohn J. Uber eine eigenartige form von 'atrophica maculosa cutis'. Arch Dermatol Syphilol. 1892;24:342–58.
9. Schweninger E, Buzzi F. Multiple benign tumor-like new growths of the skin. In: Internationaler Atlas Selltener Hautkrankheiten, plate 15. Leipzig: L Voss, 1891.
10. Venencie PY, Bonnefoy A, Gogly B, et al. Increased expression of gelatinases A and B by skin explants from patients with anetoderma. Br J Dermatol. 1997;137:517–25.
11. Venencie PY, Winkelmann RK, Moore BA. Anetoderma: clinical findings, associations, and long-term follow-up evaluations. Arch Dermatol. 1984;120:1032–9.
12. Thomas JE, Mehregan DR, Holland J, et al. Familial anetoderma. Int J Dermatol. 2003;42:75–7.
13. Prizant TL, Lucky AW, Frieden IJ, et al. Spontaneous atrophic patches in extremely premature infants. Anetoderma of prematurity. Arch Dermatol. 1996;132:671–4.
14. Venecie PY, Wilkelmann RK. Histopathologic findings in anetoderma. Arch Dermatol. 1984;120:1040–4.
15. Bergman R, Friedman-Birnbaum R, Hazaz B, et al. An immunofluorescence study of primary anetoderma. Clin Exp Dermatol. 1990;15:124–30.
16. Sears J, Stone M, Argenyi Z. Papular elastorrhexis: a variant of connective tissue nevus: case reports and review of the literature. J Am Acad Dermatol. 1988;19:409–4.
17. Schirren H, Schirren C, Stolz W, et al. Papular elastorrhexis: a variant of dermatofibrosis lenticularis disseminata (Buschke-Ollendorff syndrome). Dermatology. 1994;189:368–72.

18. Wilson B, Dent C, Cooper P. Papular acne scars: a common cutaneous finding. Arch Dermatol. 1990;126:797–800.
19. Garcia-Hidalgo L, Orozco-Topete R, Gonzalez-Barranco J, et al. Dermatoses in 156 obese adults. Obes Res. 1999;7:299–302.
20. Ammar NM, Rao B, Schwartz RA, et al. Adolescent striae. Cutis. 2000;65:69–70.
21. Muzaffar F, Hussain I, Haroon TS. Physiologic skin changes during pregnancy: a study of 140 cases. Int J Dermatol. 1998;37:429–31.
22. Wahman AJ, Finan MA, Emerson SC. Striae gravidarum as a predictor of vaginal lacerations at delivery. South Med J. 2000;93:873–6.
23. Salter SA, Batra RS, Rohrer TE, et al. Striae and pelvic relaxation: two disorders of connective tissue with a strong association. J Invest Dermatol. 2006;126:1745–8.
24. Arem A, Ward Kisher C. Analysis of striae. Plast Reconst Surg. 1980;65:22–9.
25. Burket JM, Zelickson AS, Padilla RS. Linear focal elastosis (elastotic striae). J Am Acad Dermatol. 1989;20;633–6.
26. Hashimoto K. Linear focal elastosis: keloidal repair of striae distensae. J Am Acad Dermatol. 1998;39:309–13.
27. Kang S. Topical tretinoin therapy for management of early striae. J Am Acad Dermatol. 1998;39:S90–2.
28. Ash K, Lord J, Zukowski M, McDaniel D. Comparison of topical therapy for striae alba (20% glycolic acid/0.05% tretinoin versus 20% glycolic acid/10% L-ascorbic acid). Dermatol Surg. 1998;24:849–56.
29. Jimenez GP, Flores F, Berman B, Gunja-Smith Z. Treatment of striae rubra and striae alba with the 585-nm pulsed-dye laser. Dermatol Surg. 2003;29:362–5.
30. Alexiades-Amenakas MR, Bernstein LJ, Friedman PM, Geronemus RG. The safety and efficacy of the 308-nm excimer laser for pigment correction of hypopigmented scars and striae alba. Arch Dermatol 2004;140:955–60.
31. Pasini A. Atrophoderma idiopathica progressiva. Gior Ital Derm Sif. 1923;58:785.
32. Canizares O, Sachs PM, Jaimovich L, Torres VM. Idiopathic atrophoderma of Pasini and Pierini. Arch Dermatol. 1958;77:42–60.
33. Kencka D, Blaszczyk M, Jablonska S. Atrophoderma Pasini-Pierini is a primary atrophic abortive morphea. Dermatology. 1995;190:203–6.
34. Buechner SA, Rufli T. Atrophoderma of Pasini and Pierini: clinical and histopathologic findings and antibodies to Borrelia burgdorferi in thirty-four patients. J Am Acad Dermatol. 1994;30:441–6.
35. Wakelin SH, James MP. Zosteriform atrophoderma of Pasini and Pierini. Clin Exp Dermatol. 1995;20:244–6.

36. Yokoyama Y, Akimoto S, Ishikawa O. Disaccharide analysis of skin glycosaminoglycans in atrophoderma of Pasini and Pierini. Clin Exp Dermatol. 2000;25:436–40.
37. Franck JM, Macfarlan D, Silvers ON, Katz BE, Newhouse J. Atrophoderma of Pasini and Pierini: atrophy of dermis or subcutis? J Am Acad Dermatol. 1995;32:122–3.
38. Berman A, Berman GD, Kinnkelmann RK. Atrophoderma (Pasini-Pierini): findings on direct immunofluorescent, monoclonal antibody, and ultrastructural studies. Int J Dermatol. 1988;27:487–90.
39. Arpey CJ, Patel DS, Stone MS, et al. Treatment of atrophoderma of Pasi and Pierini-associated hyperpigmentation with Q-switched alexandrite laser: a clinical, histologic, and ultrastructural appraisal. Lasers Surg. 2000;27:206–12.
40. Miescher G. Atypische Chondrodystrophie, Typus morquino kombiniert mit follikularer atrophodermie. Dermatologica. 1944;89:38–51.
41. Curth HO. The genetics of follicular atrophoderma. Arch Dermatol. 1978;114:1479–83.
42. Frosch P, Brumage M, Schuster-Pavlovic C, Bersch A. Atrophoderma vermiculatum: case reports and review. J Am Acad Dermatol. 1988;18:538–42.
43. Callaway SR, Lesher JL. Keratosis pilaris atrophicans: case series and review. Pediatr Dermatol. 2004;21:14–17.
44. Handrick C, Alster T. Laser treatment of atrophoderma vermiculata. J Am Acad Dermatol. 2001;44:693–5.
45. Vabres P, Lacombe D, Rabinowitz LG, et al. The gene for Bazex-Dupré-Christol syndrome maps to chromosome Xq. J Invest Dermatol. 1995;105:87–91.
46. Hoang MP, Carder KR, Pandya AG, Bennettt MJ. Ichthyosis and keratotic follicular plugs containing dystrophic calcification in newborns: distinctive histopathologic features of X-linked dominant chondrodysplasia punctata (Conradi-Hünermann-Happle syndrome). Am J Dermatopathol. 2004;26:53–8.
47. Jacyk WK. What syndrome is this? X-linked dominant chondroplasia punctata (Happle syndrome). Pediatr Dermatol. 2001;18:442–4.
48. Heidingsfeld ML. Atrophia maculosa varioliformis cutis. J Cutan Dis. 1918;36:285–8.
49. Kuflik JH, Schwartz RA, Becker KA, Lambert WC. Atrophia maculosa varioliformis cutis. Int J Dermatol. 2005;44:864–6.
50. Shelley WB, Rawnsley JM. Painful feet due to herniation of fat. JAMA. 1968;205:308–9.
51. Greenberg S, Krafchik BR. Infantile pedal papules. J Am Acad Dermatol. 2005;53:333–4.

Panniculitis

James W Patterson

100

INTRODUCTION

Panniculitis is diagnostically challenging for dermatologists and pathologists. Terminology is difficult, partly because various names have been applied to the same disorder (e.g. nodular vasculitis and erythema induratum), and partly because new discoveries have resulted in the introduction of new terms and the abandonment of others. For example, cases that might have previously been classified as Weber–Christian disease may now be categorized as α_1-antitrypsin deficiency panniculitis, lupus panniculitis or pancreatic panniculitis. From a clinical standpoint, many forms of panniculitis of diverse etiologies closely resemble one another, presenting as tender erythematous subcutaneous nodules. Some panniculitides can be a manifestation of different disease processes (erythema nodosum is the classic example), and, even if the type of panniculitis is correctly identified, this is only the first step in a series of clinical and laboratory investigations required to determine the underlying cause. From a pathologic standpoint, the subcutaneous fat responds to a variety of different insults in a limited number of ways, and, therefore, histopathologic differences among the various forms of panniculitis may be subtle. Management can also be difficult, since there are often at least two therapeutic desiderata:

- specific treatment of the panniculitis
- treatment of the underlying illness.

In this chapter, these issues will be addressed by introducing a schema for the classification of these disorders, recommending an approach to the histopathologic diagnosis, and providing information about the specific forms of panniculitis and their management.

Table 100.1 provides a working classification of the forms of panniculitis. The categories are determined partly by clinical characteristics such as location (Fig. 100.1), partly by histopathology, and partly by etiology. A word should be said about *septal* versus *lobular* panniculitis. These are largely artificial constructs, since there is no purely septal or purely lobular panniculitis. Certain forms of panniculitis can be characterized as having predominantly septal involvement, and this finding can provide a useful clue to diagnosis when combined with other clinical and histopathologic features.

Table 100.2 provides an approach to the histopathologic diagnosis of an unknown case of panniculitis. When performing a biopsy in a patient with panniculitis, it is absolutely critical that the specimen include a generous portion of subcutaneous fat. Excisional biopsies carried through the subcutis or narrow incisional biopsies that incorporate a broad expanse of subcutaneous fat are preferable to punch biopsies.

CLASSIFICATION OF THE PANNICULITIDES
Predominantly septal panniculitis
• Erythema nodosum   Erythema nodosum migrans (subacute nodular migratory panniculitis)
• Panniculitis of morphea/scleroderma
• Alpha₁-antitrypsin deficiency panniculitis*
Lobular and mixed septal–lobular panniculitis
• With vasculitis involving larger subcutaneous vessels   Erythema induratum (nodular vasculitis)
• With necrosis as an early finding   Pancreatic panniculitis

• With needle-shaped clefts within lipocytes
  Sclerema neonatorum
  Subcutaneous fat necrosis of the newborn
  Poststeroid panniculitis

• Associated with connective tissue disease
  Lupus erythematosus panniculitis (lupus profundus)
  Panniculitis of dermatomyositis

• Lipodystrophic panniculitis (see Ch. 101)
  Lipoatrophy
  Lipohypertrophy

• Traumatic panniculitis
  Cold panniculitis (popsicle panniculitis, Haxthausen's disease)
  Sclerosing lipogranuloma (including grease gun granuloma)
  Panniculitis due to other injectable substances
  Panniculitis due to blunt trauma

• Lipodermatosclerosis
• Infection-induced panniculitis

• Malignancy-related panniculitis
  Cytophagic histiocytic panniculitis/subcutaneous panniculitis-like T-cell lymphoma spectrum
  Malignant subcutaneous infiltrates

Descriptions vary; some authors regard this as a lobular or mixed septal–lobular panniculitis.

Table 100.1 Classification of the panniculitides. The categories for classification of panniculitis are determined partly by clinical characteristics such as location and associated diseases and partly by histopathology.

ERYTHEMA NODOSUM

Synonyms: ▪ Erythema contusiformis ▪ Erythema nodosum migrans (variant form, see below)

Key features

- Painful, erythematous subcutaneous nodules
- Usually distributed symmetrically over pretibial areas; occasionally elsewhere
- In later stages, lesions acquire a bruise-like appearance
- May be accompanied by fever, arthralgias and malaise
- Associated with a wide variety of systemic disorders

Introduction

Erythema nodosum is probably the best-known form of panniculitis, as well as the most common. It typically presents as an acute eruption of erythematous, tender subcutaneous nodules over the pretibial areas bilaterally. It is widely regarded as a delayed hypersensitivity response to a variety of antigenic challenges[1], although the mechanisms of its development are more complex than this statement would indicate. Histopathologically, it is the prototype of a 'septal' panniculitis. Identification and treatment of the underlying disorder, if found, is of primary importance, but therapy directed toward the lesions themselves is also an option.

History

At the beginning of the 18th century, Robert Willan gave the first clear description of erythema nodosum and provided its name in his famous work, *On Cutaneous Disease*[2,3].

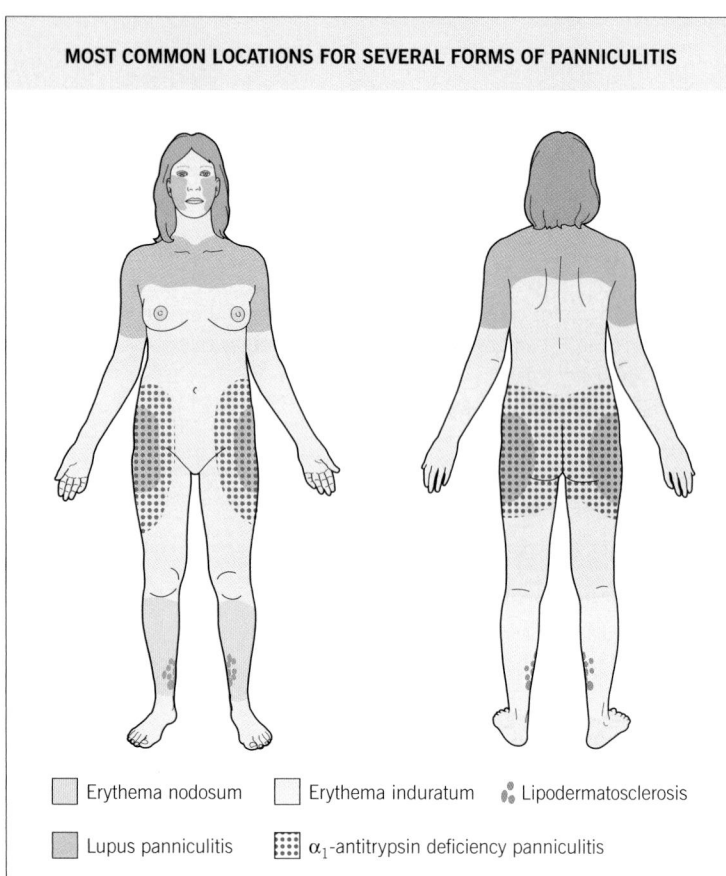

MOST COMMON LOCATIONS FOR SEVERAL FORMS OF PANNICULITIS

| | Erythema nodosum | | Erythema induratum | | Lipodermatosclerosis |
| | Lupus panniculitis | | α_1-antitrypsin deficiency panniculitis | | |

Fig. 100.1 Most common locations for several forms of panniculitis.

AN APPROACH TO THE HISTOPATHOLOGIC DIAGNOSIS OF PANNICULITIS

Histopathologic aspects to consider	Conclusions
Look for the 'center of gravity' of the infiltrate	Recommended originally by Pinkus, the purpose is to determine whether or not the inflammatory process is centered in the subcutis (favoring a primary panniculitis), in the dermis, or in the fascia (in which case the panniculitis may be a secondary manifestation of a deeper inflammatory process)
Determine if the panniculitis is predominantly septal, predominantly lobular, or mixed	Generally, a predominantly septal panniculitis narrows the diagnostic considerations (see Table 100.1). If the panniculitis is lobular or mixed, look for other distinguishing features
Determine if there is vasculitis involving a medium-sized vessel, in the face of a lobular or mixed panniculitis	This is characteristic of **erythema induratum (nodular vasculitis)**
Look for fat necrosis with saponification and 'calcium soap' formation	This is a feature of **pancreatic panniculitis**
Look for needle-shaped clefts within lipocytes	Their presence favors a diagnosis of **sclerema neonatorum, subcutaneous fat necrosis of the newborn,** or **poststeroid panniculitis**
Determine if the panniculitis has a lymphoplasmacytic predominance	This tends to be a feature of **panniculitis due to connective tissue disease,** including lupus erythematosus
Check for a 'central nidus' of inflammation or evidence of a needlestick injury Look for vacuolated spaces or foreign material	These are clues to **traumatic panniculitis**. Polarization microscopy can be helpful
Look for membranocystic changes in the subcutis	This change is characteristic of (though not pathognomonic for) **lipodermatosclerosis**
Determine if the panniculitis is associated with substantial cellular necrosis, vascular proliferation, hemorrhage, sweat gland necrosis, or neutrophilic aggregates	These changes are often encountered in **infection-induced panniculitis**. Tissue cultures and special stains for organisms may be indicated
Determine if the infiltrating cells are particularly monotonous or atypical in appearance, or if there are large cells with cytophagic activity	Consideration should be given to **malignant infiltration** or **cytophagic histiocytic panniculitis.** Immunohistochemical staining may be indicated

Table 100.2 An approach to the histopathologic diagnosis of panniculitis.

Epidemiology

Erythema nodosum can occur at any age, in both sexes, and in all racial groups. It is more common among women and is more frequently observed during the second through fourth decades of life[4,5]. The relative ranking of underlying causes may vary according to geographic location, for example, areas where *Coccidioides immitis* is endemic and regions where Behçet's disease is more prevalent.

Pathogenesis

Erythema nodosum has been considered a delayed hypersensitivity response to a variety of antigenic stimuli, including bacteria, viruses and chemical agents[1,6]. Llorente et al.[7] observed expression of mRNA for Th1 cytokines (interferon-γ, interleukin-2) in the skin lesions and peripheral blood of patients with erythema nodosum; a Th1 pattern of cytokine synthesis is associated with delayed hypersensitivity-type reactions. However, a complex series of intermediate steps is involved in the development of these lesions. A variety of adhesion molecules and inflammatory mediators appear to be associated with the disease. For example, vascular cell adhesion molecule-1 (VCAM-1), platelet endothelial cell adhesion molecule-1 (PECAM-1), HLA-DR and E-selectin are expressed on endothelial cells, while intercellular adhesion molecule-1 (ICAM-1), very late antigen-4 (VLA-4), L-selectin and HLA-DR are expressed by inflammatory cells in erythema nodosum lesions[8].

Neutrophils are frequently numerous in early lesions, and it has been shown that a higher percentage of circulating neutrophils in patients with erythema nodosum leads to the production of reactive oxygen intermediates; these intermediates in turn may provoke inflammation and tissue damage[9]. Support for a pathogenic role for these cells and molecules is provided by studies of the effects of colchicine. This inhibitor of neutrophil chemotaxis is useful in treating inflammatory lesions of Behçet's disease and non-Behçet's-related erythema nodosum[10]. Among other effects, colchicine has been shown to diminish L-selectin expression on the neutrophil surface, inhibit E-selectin-mediated endothelial adhesiveness for neutrophils, and diminish stimulated expression of ICAM-1 on endothelium (see Ch. 102)[8]. Other indirect evidence for the role of inflammatory cells and mediators includes a report of erythema nodosum following treatment with granulocyte colony-stimulating factor[11] and the response of erythema nodosum lesions to treatment with anti-TNF agents[12].

A wide variety of precipitating factors has been linked with erythema nodosum. Infectious causes are common, particularly upper respiratory infections (both streptococcal and non-streptococcal). Other commonly reported causes include sarcoidosis, inflammatory bowel disease and certain medications. Table 100.3 lists the most well-known causes or associations as reported in several clinical series[4,5,13].

Clinical features

Erythema nodosum presents with bilateral, tender, erythematous nodules. These arise in crops and the most common site is the shins (Fig. 100.2). Other locations are occasionally involved, particularly the thighs and forearms[4]. Nodules may also appear on the trunk, neck and face[3], but this is sufficiently rare that development of lesions in these locations should prompt consideration of other diagnoses. Unlike other forms of panniculitis, ulceration is not a feature of erythema nodosum. Systemic symptoms may occur that are not necessarily related to a specific coexisting systemic disorder; these include arthritis, arthralgia, fever and malaise[3].

CAUSES OF ERYTHEMA NODOSUM

Incidence	Cause	Comments
Most common	Idiopathic	Still the largest single category, accounting for a third to a half of cases
	Streptococcal infections, especially of the upper respiratory tract	The largest single infectious cause
	Other infectious associations: Bacterial gastroenteritis – *Yersinia* > *Salmonella*, *Campylobacter* Viral upper respiratory tract infections Coccidioidomycosis	Overall, infection may account for a third or more of cases Erythema nodosum is associated with a lower incidence of disseminated disease
	Drugs	Especially estrogens and oral contraceptive pills; also sulfonamides, penicillin, bromides, iodides
	Sarcoidosis*	10–20% of cases in some series
	Inflammatory bowel disease	Crohn's disease has a stronger association with erythema nodosum than does ulcerative colitis
Uncommon	Less common infectious associations: Brucellosis *Chlamydia pneumoniae* or *trachomatis* *Mycoplasma pneumoniae* Tuberculosis Hepatitis B[†] Histoplasmosis	
	Neutrophilic dermatoses: Behçet's disease Sweet's syndrome	'Erythema nodosum' in Behçet's disease more closely resembles erythema induratum (nodular vasculitis)
	Pregnancy	
Rare	Rare infectious associations: Gonorrhea Meningococcemia *Escherichia coli* Pertussis Syphilis Cat-scratch disease HIV infection Blastomycosis Giardiasis	*Erythema nodosum leprosum* is a different disease that is characterized by a cutaneous small vessel vasculitis
	Malignancy, most often acute myelogenous leukemia, Hodgkin disease	May overlap with Sweet's syndrome

*Löfgren's syndrome is an acute, spontaneously resolving form of sarcoidosis characterized by erythema nodosum, hilar lymphadenopathy, fever, polyarthritis and uveitis.
[†] Erythema nodosum secondary to the hepatitis B vaccine has also been reported.

Table 100.3 Causes of erythema nodosum.

Because of its close association with a variety of disorders, erythema nodosum is an important skin sign of systemic disease. For example, its development may precede or accompany a flare of inflammatory bowel disease[14]. It may also have some value as a prognostic indicator in certain conditions. For example, erythema nodosum is associated with a protective effect against disseminated disease in patients with coccidioidomycosis, and it is closely associated with more benign and self-limited forms of sarcoidosis[1,15]. Nevertheless, a significant percentage of cases – more than one-third – have no known disease association, even when followed for a year or more[5]. Clinical or laboratory

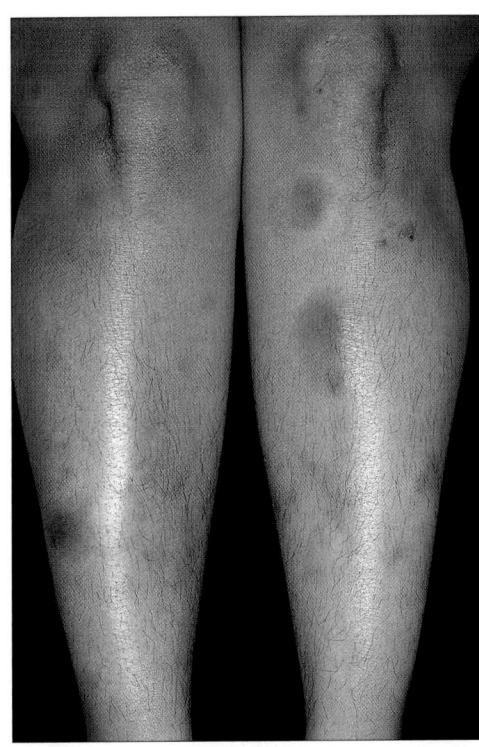

Fig. 100.2 Erythema nodosum. Erythematous nodules located bilaterally on the shins. Courtesy of Kenneth E Greer MD.

FINDINGS SUGGESTIVE OF A SYSTEMIC CAUSE FOR ERYTHEMA NODOSUM

- Synovitis
- Diarrhea
- Abnormal chest X-ray
- Preceding upper respiratory tract infection
- Elevated antistreptolysin O and/or anti-DNase B titers
- Positive tuberculin skin test

Table 100.4 Findings suggestive of a systemic cause for erythema nodosum.

data that tend to predict that a case of erythema nodosum may be secondary to a systemic disease are listed in Table 100.4.

Erythema nodosum lesions usually last a few days or weeks and then slowly involute, without scar formation. Discoloration suggestive of a bruise may be seen as erythema subsides. More chronic forms do occur, some of which show a tendency toward migration or centrifugal spread; the latter have been termed subacute nodular migratory panniculitis or erythema nodosum migrans (see below). Up to one-third of cases of erythema nodosum recur. Annual recurrences are particularly common among idiopathic cases[13].

Pathology

Erythema nodosum is the prototypic septal panniculitis, but this should not be taken to imply that histopathologic changes are entirely confined to subcutaneous septa[15a]. Biopsy specimens of early lesions tend to show edematous septa and mild lymphocytic infiltrates (Fig. 100.3). Neutrophils may predominate in early lesions[8], and a variant with a predominance of eosinophils has been reported[16]. True vasculitis of the type seen in leukocytoclastic vasculitis is not demonstrable, and erythema nodosum is not generally regarded as a vasculitic process. However, 'secondary' vasculitis may be observed in lesions containing relatively heavy mixed or neutrophil-rich inflammatory infiltrates. Thrombophlebitis has been reported, and this change is apparently more frequent in erythema nodosum lesions associated with Behçet's disease[6,8].

In early lesions, one may also find Miescher's microgranulomas, a characteristic if not pathognomonic feature of erythema nodosum. These are small collections of histiocytes, found within septa or at a septal–lobular interface, that tend to surround neutrophils or small cleft-like spaces[3]. Reported variations in the frequency of these granulomas in erythema nodosum[3,17] may result in part from differences in definition, in the acceptance of subtle changes, and in the rigor of the search. Miescher's microgranulomas can also be observed in older

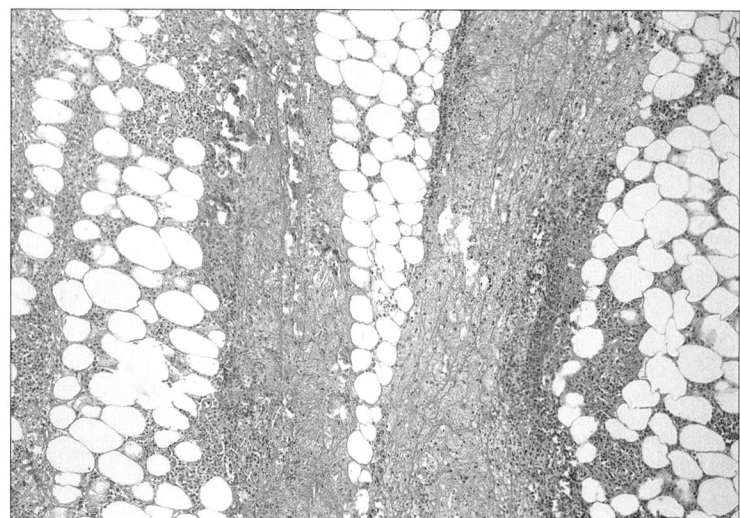

Fig. 100.3 Erythema nodosum. Septa are widened and edematous, and infiltrated by lymphocytes and neutrophils.

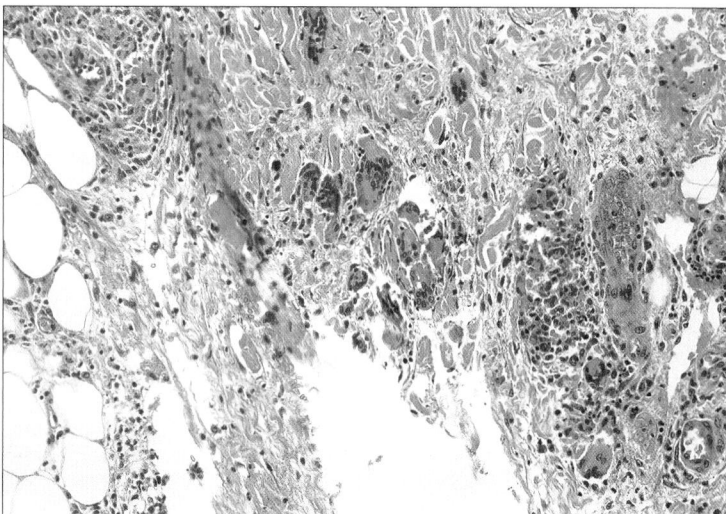

Fig. 100.4 Erythema nodosum. Miescher's microgranulomas within septa. Multinucleated giant cells surround cleft-like spaces.

THERAPEUTIC LADDER FOR ERYTHEMA NODOSUM
Discontinue possible causative medications
Treatment of underlying infectious diseases
Bed rest and leg elevation
Non-steroidal anti-inflammatory drugs (NSAIDs) (3)
Potassium iodide (2)
Colchicine (3) (esp. in the setting of Behçet's disease)
Prednisone (3)
Dapsone (3)
Hydroxychloroquine (3)
Mycophenolate mofetil (3)
Infliximab (3) (esp. in the setting of inflammatory bowel disease)
Thalidomide (3) (esp. in the setting of inflammatory bowel disease)*
Cyclosporine (3) (esp. in the setting of Behçet's disease)

May transiently exacerbate erythema nodosum associated with Behçet's disease.

Table 100.5 Therapeutic ladder for erythema nodosum. Key to evidence-based support: (1) prospective controlled trial; (2) retrospective trial or large case series; (3) small series or individual case reports.

USE OF POTASSIUM IODIDE (KI)
Saturated solution of potassium iodide (SSKI)
• 1000 mg/ml

• Droppers are supplied with calibrations for:
  0.3 ml (300 mg)*
  0.6 ml (600 mg)

• In adults and older children, common dose = 300 mg tid po with starting dose = 150–300 mg tid
• In infants and young children, common dose = 150 mg tid
• SSKI should be diluted in water or juice to try to minimize the bitter aftertaste
• Crystallization may occur with cold temperatures, but rewarming and shaking dissolves the crystals; discard if solution turns yellow–brown
Side effects of SSKI
• Acute – nausea, bitter eructation, excessive salivation, urticaria, angioedema, cutaneous small vessel vasculitis
• Chronic – enlargement of salivary and lacrimal glands, acneiform eruption, iododerma, hypothyroidism, hyperkalemia, occasionally hyperthyroidism

0.3 ml = 10 drops from the calibrated dropper supplied with SSKI.

Table 100.6 Use of potassium iodide (KI).

lesions, at which point the constituent cells have evolved into the appearance of epithelioid and multinucleated giant cells (Fig. 100.4).

As lesions progress, the septa become widened and contain a mixed, partly granulomatous infiltrate. These cells infiltrate the periphery of fat lobules in a lace-like configuration. The extent of lobular involvement varies, and in some cases can be prominent[8]. Nevertheless, in the case of a lobular panniculitis without the characteristic septal changes, a diagnosis of erythema nodosum should be made with caution. There is also frequently a mild to moderate perivascular lymphocytic infiltrate in the overlying dermis. In later stages, the septa become fibrotic, partly replacing the fat lobules. Residual granulomas and lipophages can be observed, and vascular proliferation may be present[3]. Over the long term, a remodeling process takes place that usually results in minimal residual scarring[3].

Differential diagnosis

The clinical picture of an acute eruption of tender subcutaneous nodules over both shins in a young person is highly characteristic of erythema nodosum. However, when lesions are few in number, located in sites other than the lower legs, or of longer duration (>6 weeks), erythema nodosum can be difficult to distinguish from other forms of panniculitis. Lesions of erythema induratum (nodular vasculitis) can resemble those of erythema nodosum, but they tend to occur on the posterior aspect of the lower legs and may ulcerate. Ulceration is also a feature of pancreatic panniculitis, which occurs more frequently in other locations (although still favoring the lower legs), is more likely to be accompanied by arthritis and serositis, and is associated with elevated serum amylase and lipase levels.

Histopathologically, the picture of a predominantly septal panniculitis usually limits the differential diagnosis and tends to exclude those conditions that are chiefly lobular or mixed. Pancreatic panniculitis may show predominantly septal changes in its earliest stages[18], but, eventually, these lesions exhibit the characteristic fat necrosis, with saponification and 'ghost cell' formation. Infection-induced panniculitis can sometimes mimic erythema nodosum, but there are often more extensive neutrophilic infiltrates, cellular necrosis (including sweat gland necrosis), vascular proliferation, and hemorrhage[19]. Special staining for organisms and microbiologic studies may be helpful if infection is a serious consideration.

Treatment

Treatments most often recommended for uncomplicated erythema nodosum include bed rest, salicylates, and non-steroidal anti-inflammatory drugs (NSAIDs; Table 100.5)[2,14]. Potassium iodide has been used with success, with adult dosages ranging from 300 to 1500 mg/day (Table 100.6)[2,20]. Improvement may be seen within 2 weeks. Potassium iodide may work through inhibition of cell-mediated immunity, as well as through inhibition of neutrophil chemotaxis and suppression of neutrophil-generated oxygen intermediates[2]. In light of this treatment response, reports of erythema nodosum *triggered* by potassium iodide seem contradictory.

Treatment of erythema nodosum is influenced by underlying conditions. Thus, colchicine is useful in management of erythema nodosum that accompanies Behçet's disease[8]. Various treatments for inflammatory bowel disease are also effective in managing coexistent erythema nodosum[12]. Agents that have been employed in these circumstances include systemic corticosteroids, hydroxychloroquine, cyclosporine, thalidomide and infliximab[21]. NSAIDs are to be avoided in treating the erythema nodosum of inflammatory bowel disease, since these may trigger a flare of the bowel disease or compromise maintenance therapy[14].

Subacute Nodular Migratory Panniculitis

Synonyms: ▪ Erythema nodosum migrans ▪ Chronic erythema nodosum

Key features

▪ Nodules on the lower extremities that migrate or undergo centrifugal spread, with central clearing

▪ Often unilateral

▪ Most cases are idiopathic; occasionally associated with streptococcal infection or thyroid disease

▪ More chronic course than typical erythema nodosum

Clinical features

This condition was first described by Bafverstedt in 1954[22] and was named subacute nodular migratory panniculitis by Vilanova & Piñol Aguade in 1956[23]. Some of its clinical and microscopic characteristics are similar to chronic erythema nodosum, and it is believed by many to represent a variant of the latter[3,22]; however, others consider it to be a separate disorder[24]. Subacute nodular migratory panniculitis is seen predominantly in women, is often unilateral, and is characterized by nodules that migrate or expand in a centrifugal manner (with central clearing)[3] and may assume a yellowish or morpheaform appearance[25]. Lesions tend to be less tender than those of classic erythema nodosum. There are few, if any, associated systemic symptoms[22], though arthralgias have been reported and the erythrocyte sedimentation rate may be elevated[23]. Most cases are idiopathic, but some are associated with streptococcal infection (as evidenced by elevated antistreptolysin O and anti-DNase B titers) or thyroid disease[24].

Pathology

Microscopically, the changes are those of a chronic septal panniculitis[25]. However, in contrast to more classic forms of chronic erythema nodosum, subacute nodular migratory panniculitis shows greater septal thickening, more prominent granulomatous inflammation along the borders of widened subcutaneous septa, absence of phlebitis, and rare hemorrhage[24].

Treatment

Untreated, subacute nodular migratory panniculitis can last for months or years. However, treatment with potassium iodide is usually effective, resulting in clearing of lesions within several weeks[25].

MORPHEA/SCLERODERMA PANNICULITIS

(See also Chs 44 & 96.)

Clinical features

Both morphea and scleroderma (systemic sclerosis) can affect the subcutaneous fat (Table 100.7), which is the primary site of involvement in deep morphea (morphea profunda)[26]. Subcutaneous extension also occurs in variants such as disabling pansclerotic morphea of childhood, generalized morphea, and linear morphea. In addition, eosinophilic fasciitis can involve the subcutaneous fat as well as the fascia[27]. These syndromes may be associated with peripheral eosinophilia, polyclonal gammopathy, and serologic abnormalities[27,28]. Fleischmajer et al.[29] proposed that the sclerosing process in scleroderma is initiated by the changes that take place in the subcutis.

Pathology

Table 100.7 outlines the microscopic changes in morphea and scleroderma. These conditions are associated with septal panniculitis (Fig. 100.5). Lymphocytes and plasma cells predominate[27,30-32], although macrophages and eosinophils may be present. In some cases, the number of plasma cells is striking[30]. Inflammatory changes are generally less prominent in scleroderma, in which lymphoid follicles typically do not occur[31]. In late stages of morphea, the subcutis is largely replaced by hyalinized connective tissue, often accompanied by changes of lipoatrophy[32].

CLINICAL AND MICROSCOPIC FEATURES OF CONNECTIVE TISSUE PANNICULITIS				
Disorder	**Clinical presentation**	**Lesion distribution**	**Relation to systemic disease**	**Histopathology of panniculitis**
Morphea and scleroderma	Indurated plaques	Extremities, trunk	Occurs in scleroderma, but usually more pronounced in morphea	Septal, with thickening and mucin deposition; inflammation especially at dermal–subcutaneous interface; lymphocytes and plasma cells; lymphoid follicles in morphea*
Lupus panniculitis	Tender, subcutaneous nodules and plaques; may have overlying discoid lupus lesions	Face (especially cheeks), upper arms, shoulders, hips, trunk	Only minority of cases associated with systemic lupus erythematosus	Lobular or mixed lobular/septal; mucin deposition; hyaline necrosis of lobules; lymphocytes and plasma cells; nodular lymphocytic aggregates or lymphoid follicles
Dermatomyositis	Indurated, painful plaques and nodules; may ulcerate	Buttocks, abdomen, thighs, arms	Can arise in patients with established dermatomyositis or precede other disease manifestations	Lobular or mixed lobular/septal; fat necrosis; lipomembranous changes; sometimes calcification; lymphocytes and plasma cells; sometimes nodular lymphocytic aggregates
Annular atrophic connective tissue panniculitis of the ankles	Subcutaneous atrophy, which may be preceded by induration and tenderness	Circumferential bands around the ankles	Patients often have antinuclear antibodies and/or autoimmune conditions such as thyroiditis or rheumatoid arthritis	Lobular or mixed lobular/septal lymphohistiocytic panniculitis with areas of fat necrosis
Atrophic connective tissue panniculitis	Erythematous, indurated plaques that resolve with subcutaneous atrophy	Favors extremities; may be widespread	As above	As above

*Less often than in lupus panniculitis.

Table 100.7 Clinical and microscopic features of connective tissue panniculitis. Based on references 27 & 30–32. Forms of connective tissue panniculitis with overlapping features have also been described, such as sclerodermic linear lupus panniculitis.

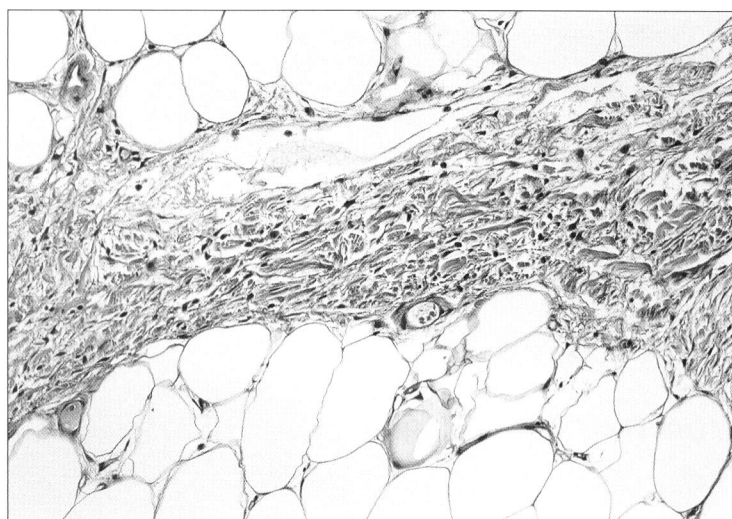

Fig. 100.5 Morphea panniculitis. Septal thickening, mucin deposition, and mild lymphocytic infiltration.

Differential diagnosis

The combination of septal panniculitis with lymphoplasmacytic predominance and dermal and subcutaneous sclerosis is unique, and this helps to separate morphea/scleroderma panniculitis from other septal forms of panniculitis. Differentiation among the several variants outlined above is more difficult, requiring clinical data for accurate classification. Sclerosis with lesser degrees of subcutaneous inflammation characterizes scleroderma, while a predominance of fascial involvement with extension into the subcutis is more typical of eosinophilic fasciitis.

ALPHA₁-ANTITRYPSIN DEFICIENCY PANNICULITIS

Synonym: ■ Alpha₁-protease (proteinase) deficiency panniculitis

Key features

■ Erythematous, painful subcutaneous nodules or plaques that often ulcerate and drain

■ Associated with α_1-antitrypsin deficiency; patients with the most severe disease are homozygotes for the Z allele of the *SERPINA1* gene (PiZZ)

■ A characteristic histologic finding is liquefactive necrosis of dermis and subcutaneous septa, but lobular or mixed septal–lobular changes with neutrophils may occur

Introduction

Alpha₁-antitrypsin deficiency is a well-established but uncommon cause of panniculitis. The most severely affected individuals, with markedly decreased levels of the protease inhibitor, are most prone to the development of ulcerating neutrophilic panniculitis. Recognition of the disorder is important not only in the selection of appropriate therapy, but also in addressing other manifestations of the disease and dealing with its genetic aspects.

History

Alpha₁-antitrypsin deficiency is an inborn error of metabolism that was first delineated by Eriksson and others in the early 1960s[33]. In 1972, Warter and colleagues identified members of a family with α_1-antitrypsin deficiency and 'Weber–Christian syndrome'. Subsequent investigations have linked the associated clinical and microscopic findings to known effects of protease inhibitor deficiency.

Epidemiology

No apparent racial or geographic prevalence has been noted for α_1-antitrypsin deficiency panniculitis. The incidence of the disease is approximately equal in men and women[34,35]. Age of onset ranges from infancy to the eighth decade of life[35].

Pathogenesis

Alpha₁-antitrypsin, a glycoprotein produced in the liver, is the most abundant circulating *ser*ine *p*rotease *in*hibitor (serpin). The more than 120 different alleles of the gene that encodes this protein (*SERPINA1*; formerly known as *PI*) are divided into categories based upon the electrophoretic mobility of their protein products (M=medium, S=slow, Z=very slow). The most common protease inhibitor (Pi) phenotype is MM (homozygous for M alleles), which is associated with normal serum levels of α_1-antitrypsin (120–200 mg/dl)[36]. Heterozygotes with one copy of the S or Z allele have mild to moderate deficiencies of the inhibitor (PiMS and PiMZ; prevalences of 1–3% in Caucasian populations). Patients who are homozygous for the Z allele (PiZZ; prevalence of 1:1500–1:5000 in Caucasian populations) have severe α_1-antitrypsin deficiency, with serum levels in the range of 20–45 mg/dl. In these individuals, most of the aberrant α_1-antitrypsin protein accumulates in the endoplasmic reticulum of hepatocytes, and the small amounts that enter the circulation have decreased function and a tendency to form inactive polymers that may stimulate neutrophil chemotaxis[37].

Alpha₁-antitrypsin acts upon a wide range of proteolytic enzymes that play a direct role in degradation of tissues, including trypsin, collagenase and elastase[38]. It also has important effects on immune function, e.g. inhibition of membrane-bound serine proteases involved in the activation of lymphocytes and macrophages[39]. It may also inhibit complement activation, both through a direct effect on complement-related proteases[40] and by inhibiting the neutrophil proteases that activate enzymes of the complement system[41].

In addition to panniculitis, the consequences of α_1-antitrypsin deficiency include chronic liver disease with cirrhosis (resulting from retention of the molecule in the liver), emphysema, pancreatitis, membranoproliferative glomerulonephritis, rheumatoid arthritis, C-ANCA (cytoplasmic antineutrophil cytoplasmic antibody)-positive vasculitis, other cutaneous vasculitides, and angioedema (resulting from deficiency of the protease inhibitor)[34,41]. The initiating event in individuals who develop panniculitis is not always clear; trauma appears to play a role in some cases. A postpartum flare of disease has been reported in genetically susceptible individuals. This is attributed to the estrogen-promoted increase in protease inhibitor levels during pregnancy, followed by a precipitous decline to subnormal levels postpartum[42]. Absence of the α_1-antitrypsin protease inhibitor results in activation of lymphocytes and macrophages, lack of restraint upon the complement cascade, release of chemotactic factors, accumulation of neutrophils with release of their proteolytic enzymes, and consequent attack upon fat and nearby connective tissues[37,38]. The subcutis may be particularly vulnerable to this process, since the abundant fatty acids make nearby elastin more susceptible to proteolytic degradation[41].

Clinical features

Large, erythematous to purpuric, tender nodules or plaques appear in a variety of sites (Fig. 100.6), especially the lower trunk and proximal extremities (flanks, buttocks and thighs)[34,37,38]. Ulcers develop that may be deep and necrotic, accompanied by an oily discharge[35,37,38]. Migration of lesions has been reported[34]. A history of antecedent trauma can be elicited in approximately one-third of cases[35]. Some patients with panniculitis also have fever, pleural effusions and pulmonary emboli[35]. The clinical course of the panniculitis is often prolonged, and lesions are resistant to therapy. Healing is accompanied by scarring and subcutaneous atrophy[35]. The most severe manifestations arise in those with profound protease inhibitor deficiency (PiZZ), although the panniculitis can also occur in heterozygotes[34].

Pathology

Descriptions of the pathology of α_1-antitrypsin deficiency panniculitis have varied. Early, there is a neutrophilic panniculitis, followed rapidly by necrosis and destruction of fat lobules[38]. Splaying of neutrophils between collagen bundles in the reticular dermis has been described as an early clue to the diagnosis[43]. Dissolution of dermal collagen, with resultant liquefactive necrosis and separation of fat lobules from adjacent septa, is a principal change in most cases[44]. Another characteristic feature is the presence of 'skip areas' of normal fat adjacent to foci of

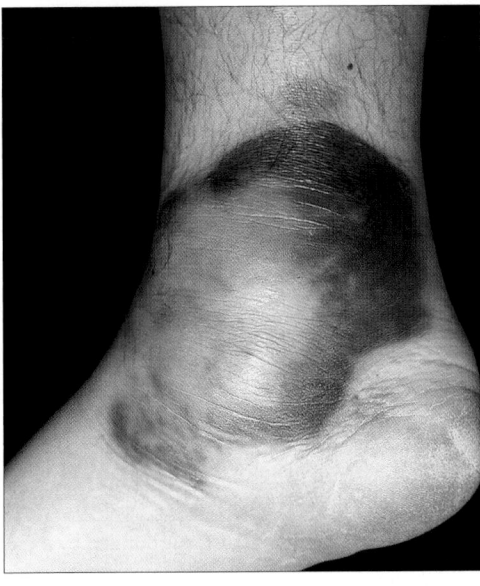

Fig. 100.6 Alpha$_1$-antitrypsin deficiency panniculitis. Purpuric nodules on the ankle. Courtesy of Kenneth E Greer MD.

severe necrotizing panniculitis[38]. Chronic inflammation and hemorrhage may be present at the periphery of areas of involvement[38]. Although small vessel vasculitis has been described[45], most authors have not found evidence for *primary* leukocytoclastic vasculitis, although there may be evidence for lymphocytic vasculitis, *secondary* vasculitis in areas of heavy neutrophilic infiltration, or thrombosis[38]. In individuals with intermediate levels of protease inhibitor deficiency, lipophage and giant cell accumulation may be prominent[38]. Lesions heal with scarring and obliteration of fat lobules.

Views differ on whether α_1-antitrypsin deficiency panniculitis should be regarded as a primarily septal or lobular panniculitis. Clearly, involvement of fat lobules can be significant, and as a result some authors have labeled the process a lobular panniculitis. On the other hand, some descriptions have emphasized early inflammation of septal vessels[45], collagenolysis of the fibrous septa[44], and prominent septal fibrosis in late-stage lesions[43,45].

Differential diagnosis

Clinically, the degrees of inflammation, ulceration and drainage associated with α_1-antitrypsin deficiency panniculitis may actually raise a differential diagnosis more focused upon ulcerative skin disorders. The presence of ulcers with geometric patterns supports a diagnosis of factitial panniculitis. The ulcers associated with α_1-antitrypsin deficiency generally lack the necrotic, 'undermined' borders associated with pyoderma gangrenosum[38].

Su et al.[38] have extensively reviewed the microscopic differential diagnosis for this disorder. Entities that are of particular importance for consideration include traumatic (factitial) panniculitis, infection-induced panniculitis, pancreatic panniculitis and erythema induratum (nodular vasculitis). Each of these can be associated with infiltrates that include neutrophils and varying degrees of necrosis, yet each has other distinct findings (see below). In the appropriate clinical settings, subcutaneous Sweet's syndrome and rheumatoid arthritis-associated neutrophilic lobular panniculitis may represent additional diagnostic considerations.

Treatment

Treatments that are usually ineffective include corticosteroids, immunosuppressants, cytotoxic agents, colchicine, danazol and hydroxychloroquine[34,38]. Doxycycline is sometimes effective, particularly in mild cases; one suggested dosage schedule is 200 mg twice daily for 3 months[40,46]. Dapsone may also be beneficial in mild cases, by suppressing neutrophil migration and inhibiting oxidation reactions induced by myeloperoxidase[34]. Reduction of alcohol intake has been recommended, since ethanol (as a hepatotoxin) may precipitate α_1-antitrypsin-associated hepatitis[41].

The most effective therapeutic measure is replacement of α_1-antitrypsin via intravenous infusions. Dosages are generally 60 mg/kg per week, administered over a period of 3 to 7 weeks[34,35,47]. Improvement is relatively rapid, and clearing of the panniculitis can occur after three weekly doses[34,47]. Recurrences are possible when α_1-antitrypsin levels fall below 50 mg/dl[34] but these typically respond to further replacement therapy. Other successful treatments have included plasma exchange[45] and liver transplantation[34].

ERYTHEMA INDURATUM

Synonyms: ■ Nodular vasculitis ■ Erythema induratum of Bazin or Bazin's disease (tuberculous etiology) ■ Erythema induratum of Whitfield (non-tuberculous etiology)

Key features

- Erythematous nodules or plaques, usually on posterior lower legs of young to middle-aged women
- Ulceration and drainage may occur
- Microscopic features of lobular or mixed panniculitis with evidence for vasculitis involving arteries or veins
- Well-established association with tuberculosis, but similar lesions can be idiopathic or induced by other infectious agents or drugs

Introduction

Erythema induratum is a condition characterized by nodules on the lower extremities, which may ulcerate and drain. Originally classified as a tuberculid, its relationship to tuberculosis in a subset of patients has been solidified by several more recent studies detecting mycobacterial DNA in cutaneous lesions.

History

Erythema induratum was first described by Ernest Bazin in 1861. It was generally regarded as a tuberculid because of a strong association with tuberculosis, though Koch's postulates could not be fulfilled. In 1945, Montgomery and colleagues proposed the term *nodular vasculitis* for cases with similar clinical and pathologic features that were not of tuberculous origin. Since the early 1970s, erythema induratum and nodular vasculitis have generally been considered as synonyms referring to a clinicopathologic entity with several possible causes, one of which is tuberculosis. The detection of mycobacterial DNA in cutaneous lesions has confirmed a tuberculous origin in some patients[48]. There are some clinicians, however, who prefer to use the term nodular vasculitis when referring to individuals with a non-tuberculous etiology.

Epidemiology

In erythema induratum, an overwhelming female predominance is observed, but men can also develop the disease[49]. There is no apparent racial predilection, and although there is a wide age range among affected patients, the mean is between 30 and 40 years[49]. Erythema induratum of tuberculous etiology occurs more frequently in populations with a high prevalence of tuberculosis.

Pathogenesis

As mentioned, there has been a strong association of some cases with tuberculosis. This has now been substantiated by the detection of mycobacterial DNA in skin lesions by PCR[48,50-53]. Specific primers can be used to distinguish *M. tuberculosis* complex DNA from that of other mycobacterial pathogens[53]. Non-tuberculous cases have been related to other infectious agents (e.g. *Nocardia*[19]) or to drugs (e.g. propylthiouracil[54]). An example of erythema induratum in association with 'red fingers' syndrome was described in a patient with chronic hepatitis C infection[55].

Although it has been suggested that erythema induratum results from an immune complex-mediated vasculitis[49], most investigators believe that the process represents a type IV, cell-mediated response to an antigenic stimulus[56]. Biopsy specimens show a predominance of T lymphocytes, macrophages and dendritic cells, including Langerhans cells[49,57,58]. One study of peripheral blood mononuclear cells from a

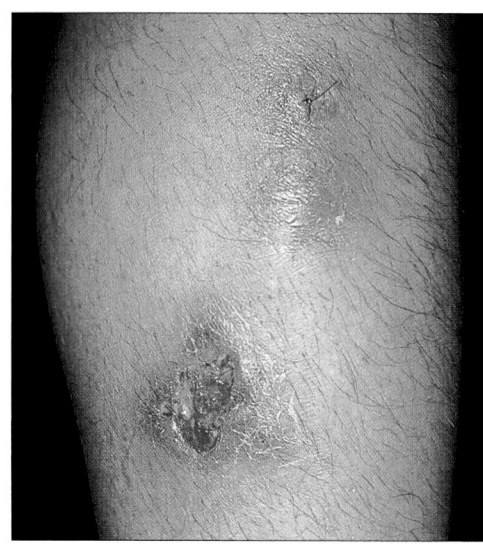

Fig. 100.7 Erythema induratum. Nodular lesions on the lower leg, with evidence of ulceration. Courtesy of Kenneth E Greer MD.

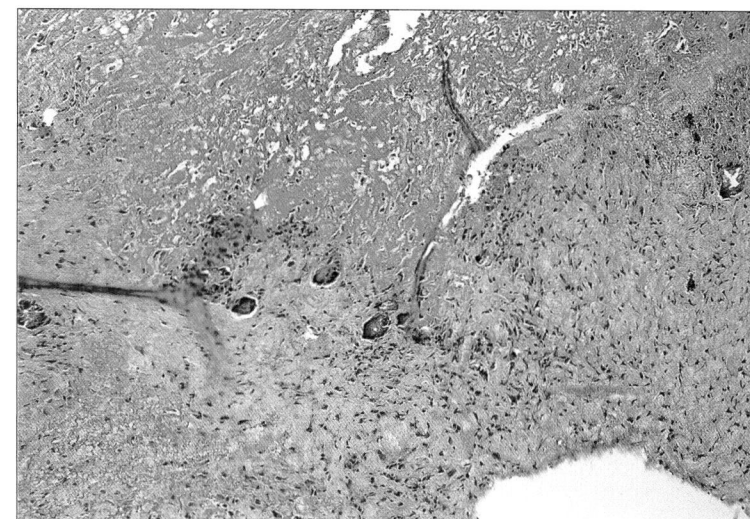

Fig. 100.9 Erythema induratum. Zone of caseous necrosis surrounded by a palisade of macrophages and multinucleated giant cells.

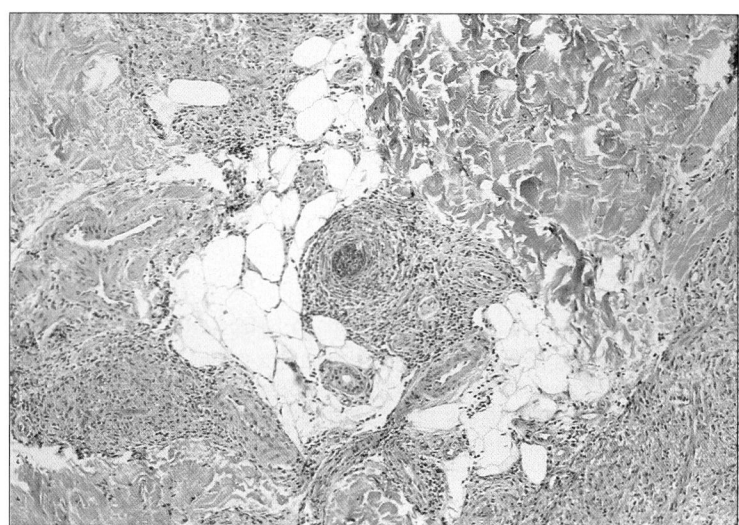

Fig. 100.8 Erythema induratum. Vasculitis involving a medium-sized vessel in the subcutis.

patient with erythema induratum and active tuberculosis showed a high proliferative response to purified protein derivative (PPD) and marked production of interferon-γ, suggesting a pathogenic role for these PPD-specific T cells in a delayed hypersensitivity response to mycobacterial antigens[59].

Clinical features

Erythema induratum is characterized by tender, erythematous to violaceous nodules and plaques that most often develop on the lower legs, especially the calves[57,58]. Lesions have also been observed on the feet, thighs, buttocks and arms[49,51]. Annular arrangements of nodules have been described in *M. tuberculosis*-related cases[60]. Ulceration can occur (Fig. 100.7). Lesions are persistent, tend to heal with scarring, and are prone to recurrence[49,57,61]. In erythema induratum associated with *M. tuberculosis*, there may be clinical and radiographic evidence for active tuberculosis and positive skin tests to PPD. Clinical differences between tuberculous and non-tuberculous cases are minor.

Pathology

Erythema induratum is a lobular or mixed septal/lobular panniculitis. Inflammation is mixed, including neutrophils, lymphocytes, histiocytes and multinucleated giant cells. Vasculitis is frequently present and can involve small- or medium-sized vessels (Fig. 100.8). It may be predominantly neutrophilic[57], lymphocytic[61], or granulomatous. Necrosis with a coagulative or caseous appearance may be present, sometimes with palisading granulomas[57] (Fig. 100.9). Necrosis has been described in both tuberculous and non-tuberculous cases, and the incidence

and degree of necrosis are greater in those cases that are positive for *M. tuberculosis* DNA by PCR methods[50]. However, this finding is absent in over half of cases.

Differential diagnosis

Infection-induced panniculitis tends to show a more prominent neutrophilic component, granular basophilic necrosis, sweat gland necrosis and proliferation of small vessels, and organisms may be identified on special staining. Lupus panniculitis tends to be less granulomatous, has a prominent lympho-plasmacellular infiltrate, may show mucin deposits, and sometimes has overlying epidermal and dermal changes typical for lupus erythematosus. Both polyarteritis nodosa and thrombophlebitis tend to show inflammation limited to the immediate perivascular zone, in contrast to the extensive lobular panniculitis often encountered in erythema induratum. Histologically, perniosis can be difficult to distinguish from erythema induratum, but there is typically a history of cold exposure[57], and on microscopic examination the vessels often show 'fluffy edema' of their walls.

Treatment

Treatment should be directed at the underlying cause, if found. This includes multi-drug antituberculous therapy for those cases associated with *M. tuberculosis* (see Ch. 74)[60]. Appropriate antimicrobial therapy is indicated for other infection-related cases, and possible inciting medications should be discontinued. Other helpful therapies have included corticosteroids, NSAIDs, potassium iodide, tetracycline, gold[61] and mycophenolate mofetil[61a]. Supportive care includes bed rest, bandages, gradient support hose, and avoidance of aggravating factors such as smoking.

PANCREATIC PANNICULITIS

Synonyms: ▪ Pancreatic fat necrosis ▪ Enzymatic panniculitis

Key features

- ▪ Subcutaneous nodules, sometimes accompanied by fever, arthritis or abdominal pain
- ▪ Associated with pancreatic disorders, including acute and chronic pancreatitis and pancreatic carcinoma
- ▪ Mixed septal/lobular panniculitis featuring 'ghost cell' formation and the deposition of basophilic material due to saponification of fat by calcium salts
- ▪ Treatment primarily directed towards the underlying pancreatic disorder

Introduction

Pancreatic panniculitis is an uncommonly reported complication of pancreatic disease. In addition to the symptoms associated with fat necrosis, its chief importance is as a sign of a significant systemic disorder, particularly because the panniculitis may be recognized prior to detection of the underlying pancreatic disease.

History

Chiari first described pancreatic panniculitis in 1883. By 1999, fewer than 100 cases had been reported[62,63].

Epidemiology

Panniculitis develops in up to 2% of patients with pancreatic disorders[64]. No geographic, racial or sex predilections have been reported.

Pathogenesis

There is considerable evidence that the enzymes lipase, amylase and trypsin are involved in producing the lesions of pancreatic panniculitis[62,65]. Elevated enzyme levels have been detected in blood[63,64], urine[62], and skin lesions, even in the absence of detectable pancreatic disease. Lipase has the clearest relationship with the panniculitis, with a number of cases showing elevated serum lipase levels but normal amylase levels[63]. Amylase levels tend to peak 2–3 days after eruption of the skin lesions and return to normal 2–3 days after regression of the lesions. Trypsin and perhaps amylase may act by promoting increased permeability of vessel walls, thereby permitting lipase to hydrolyze neutral fat to form glycerol and free fatty acids, with resulting fat necrosis and inflammation[63,64]. Venous stasis may promote this process, possibly explaining the predilection for the lower extremities. Enzyme levels may not completely explain the changes of pancreatic panniculitis[66]; immunologic factors probably also play a role.

Clinical features

Subcutaneous nodules develop in association with acute or chronic pancreatitis, pancreatic carcinoma (acinar cell > other types [e.g. neuroendocrine carcinomas]), pancreatic pseudocysts, pancreas divisum, or traumatic pancreatitis[63,65,67]. Panniculitis developing in individuals with chronic pancreatitis is often associated with a pancreaticoportal fistula, and, in some of these patients, an acinar cell carcinoma can be found. Panniculitis may precede detection of pancreatic disease by 1–7 months[64,64], and, in the case of pancreatic carcinoma, its onset may signal the presence of metastatic disease[63,64].

In pancreatic panniculitis, subcutaneous nodules develop, most often on the legs (Fig. 100.10) but also on the abdomen, chest, arms and scalp[63,64]. Erythematous, edematous, sometimes painful lesions arise singly or in crops and may migrate. They can become fluctuant and

ulcerate, discharging an oily material[63]. Panniculitis may also involve visceral fat, including the omentum and peritoneum[63]. Associated findings include fever, abdominal pain, inflammatory polyarthritis, ascites and pleural effusions[63]. The association of subcutaneous nodules, polyarthritis and eosinophilia is known as Schmid's triad, and it is associated with a poor prognosis. Some patients have radiographic evidence of multiple lytic areas involving cortical bone near large joints. Cutaneous lesions may involute within a period of weeks, leaving hyperpigmented scars. In acute pancreatitis, the panniculitis resolves as the acute inflammatory phase passes[63]. However, lesions may also persist and expand until the underlying pancreatic abnormality has been treated.

Pathology

Pancreatic panniculitis may begin as a septal panniculitis[18], but, with progression, the lesion takes on the appearance of a lobular or mixed septal/lobular process. Even in early stages, fat necrosis with liquefaction and microcyst formation is observed[62,65,66]. Lipocytes lose their nuclei and develop thick, shadowy walls, forming the characteristic 'ghost cells'. Saponification of fat by calcium salts results in deposition of granular or homogeneous basophilic material (Fig. 100.11). Neutrophils, occasional eosinophils, macrophages and multinucleated giant cells are sometimes present and may encroach upon the septa. Fibrosis and lipoatrophy are seen in late stages as the process resolves.

Differential diagnosis

Clinically, the nodules of pancreatic panniculitis can resemble those of a number of other forms of panniculitis. Ulceration and discharge would argue against erythema nodosum, and an association with fever, polyarthritis and abdominal pain should raise suspicion of associated pancreatic disease. Serum amylase and lipase levels, if elevated, may also be helpful. Histologic evidence of 'ghost cell' formation and saponification of fat distinguishes pancreatic panniculitis from other panniculitides. Eosinophilic 'hyaline necrosis' is seen in lupus panniculitis, rather than granular or homogeneous basophilic necrosis typical of pancreatic panniculitis.

Treatment

Although supportive measures such as compression and elevation can be helpful, effective management of pancreatic panniculitis is dependent upon treatment of underlying pancreatic disease. In chronic pancreatitis, a pancreatic duct stent can be used to relieve obstruction, or, if a fistula or cyst is involved, biliary bypass surgery can be undertaken if simple drainage measures are unsuccessful. Octreotide, a synthetic somatostatin-like polypeptide, can be used to inhibit pancreatic enzyme production[63]. Resection of pancreatic cancer may be followed by regression of the panniculitis.

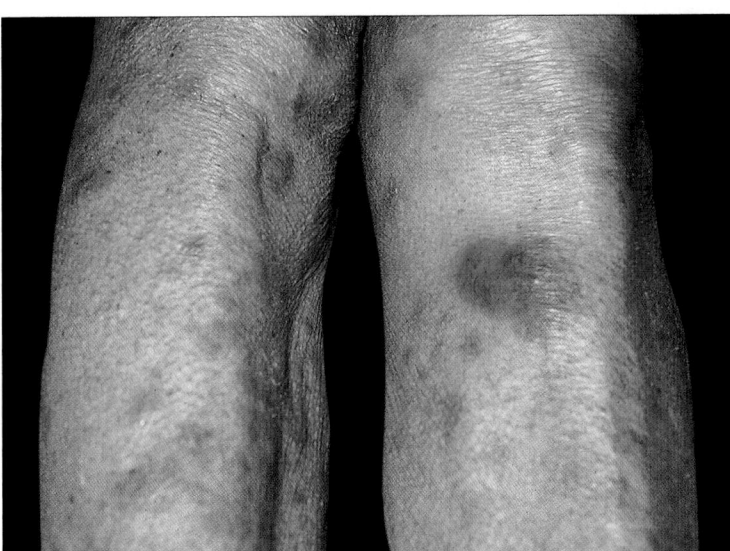

Fig. 100.10 Pancreatic panniculitis. Nodules on the legs. Courtesy of Kenneth E Greer MD.

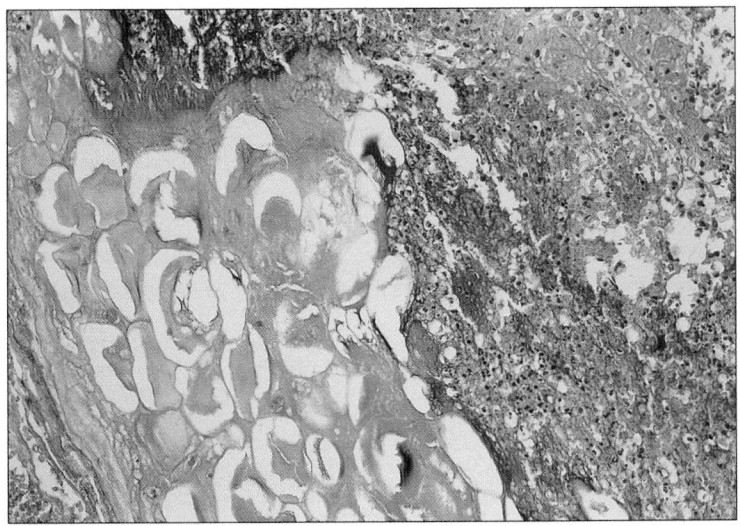

Fig. 100.11 Pancreatic panniculitis Neutrophilic inflammation, cellular necrosis, and deposition of homogeneous basophilic material due to saponification of fat by calcium salts.

SCLEREMA NEONATORUM, SUBCUTANEOUS FAT NECROSIS OF THE NEWBORN, AND POSTSTEROID PANNICULITIS

There are three entities – sclerema neonatorum, subcutaneous fat necrosis of the newborn, and poststeroid panniculitis – that are characterized histologically by formation of needle-shaped clefts within lipocytes. In contrast to adult fat, the subcutaneous fat of infants is thought to be prone to crystal formation because of a higher content of saturated fatty acids, including palmitic and stearic acids, and a relatively lower content of unsaturated fatty acids, such as oleic acid[68]. This increased saturated to unsaturated fatty acid ratio results in a higher melting point for stored fat and promotes crystallization under certain conditions. Microsized crystals (type A) apparently do not produce an inflammatory response; they are actually common (in a widely dispersed form) in healthy infants 6 months of age or less, but are more numerous in sclerema neonatorum. Larger, type B crystals that tend to be arranged in rosettes are capable of eliciting a granulomatous response; these crystal types are most often seen in subcutaneous fat necrosis of the newborn and poststeroid panniculitis[68,69]. Crystallization and defects in fat mobilization account for the clinical findings in these disorders.

Sclerema Neonatorum

Key features

- Arises in premature infants
- Skin is diffusely cold, rigid, and board-like
- Microscopically, needle-shaped clefts are present within lipocytes with minimal inflammation
- Affected infants are often hypothermic and may have a variety of other medical problems; early death is common

History

Sclerema neonatorum was first recognized in 1722 by Uzembenzius, although the classic description is usually attributed to Underwood (1784). Ballantyne provided an early description of the histopathologic changes, and Knopfelmacher noted the presence of needle-shaped crystals in subcutaneous tissue in 1897.

Epidemiology

Sclerema neonatorum presents most often in premature, debilitated infants, usually during the first week of life. There is a slight male predominance, with no substantial difference in death rates between the sexes[70].

Pathogenesis

In infants who develop sclerema, crystallization and hardening of fat occur in the setting of an increased saturated:unsaturated fatty acid ratio and a defective ability to mobilize fatty acids. Precipitating factors, which may include subcutaneous ischemia due to perinatal asphyxia as well as hypothermia, are listed in Table 100.8[68,71].

Clinical features

The clinical features are outlined in Table 100.8[68,70,72]. Rapid hardening of the subcutaneous tissues leads to firm, rigid skin over most of the body. Low admission weight and temperature as well as hemorrhagic phenomena portend a particularly poor prognosis[70].

Pathology

Table 100.8 outlines the microscopic features. Inflammation is usually sparse, and most of the needle-shaped clefts are found within lipocytes rather than within giant cells (Fig. 110.12)[68,72]. At a later stage, thickened connective tissue bands may be the only histologic finding[72].

Differential diagnosis

In contrast to sclerema neonatorum, subcutaneous fat necrosis of the newborn is a localized process with a favorable prognosis; histologically, the latter is distinguished by more prominent inflammation

PANNICULITIDES WITH NEEDLE-SHAPED CLEFTS IN THE SUBCUTIS						
Condition	Patient characteristics	Onset	Cutaneous findings	Associated systemic findings	Histopathology	Possible precipitating factors
Sclerema neonatorum	Severely ill premature neonates	First week of life	Widespread, diffuse hardening, sparing only the genitalia, palms and soles; cool, waxy, rigid and board-like skin with livid, mottled discoloration	Respiratory difficulties, congestive heart failure, intestinal obstruction, diarrhea; death, usually from septicemia, in three-fourths of cases	Needle-shaped clefts in lipocytes; septal thickening; inflammation sparse to absent (few neutrophils, eosinophils, macrophages or multinucleated giant cells may be seen)	Hypothermia, perinatal asphyxia, defective complement activity, dehydration
Subcutaneous fat necrosis of the newborn	Full-term neonates	First 2–3 weeks of life	Circumscribed, erythematous, indurated subcutaneous nodules favoring the cheeks, shoulders, back, buttocks, thighs; may become fluctuant	Hypercalcemia (onset may be delayed for several months), thrombocytopenia, hypertriglyceridemia	Lobular panniculitis with neutrophils, lymphocytes, macrophages; needle-shaped clefts in a radial array within lipocytes and giant cells; sometimes foci of calcification, hemorrhage	Hypothermia, hypoglycemia (e.g. due to gestational diabetes), perinatal hypoxemia (e.g. due to meconium aspiration, placenta previa, umbilical cord prolapse, pre-eclampsia), birth trauma
Poststeroid panniculitis	Children (ages 1–14 years)	1–40 days* after cessation of high-dose systemic corticosteroid therapy	Firm red plaques on cheeks, arms, trunk; small and discrete or large and confluent lesions; pruritic, tender or asymptomatic	Underlying conditions treated with systemic corticosteroids have included leukemia, cerebral edema, nephrotic syndrome, secretory diarrhea, acute rheumatic fever	Lobular panniculitis with lymphocytes, macrophages, multinucleated giant cells; needle-shaped clefts in lipocytes and giant cells	Follows rapid corticosteroid withdrawal

Usually within 10 days.

Table 100.8 **Panniculitides with needle-shaped clefts in the subcutis.**

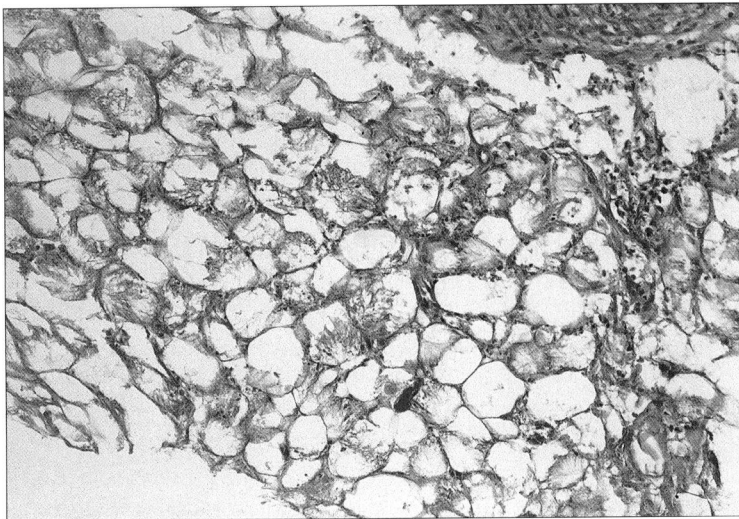

Fig. 100.12 Sclerema neonatorum. Needle-shaped clefts within lipocytes, in the absence of inflammation.

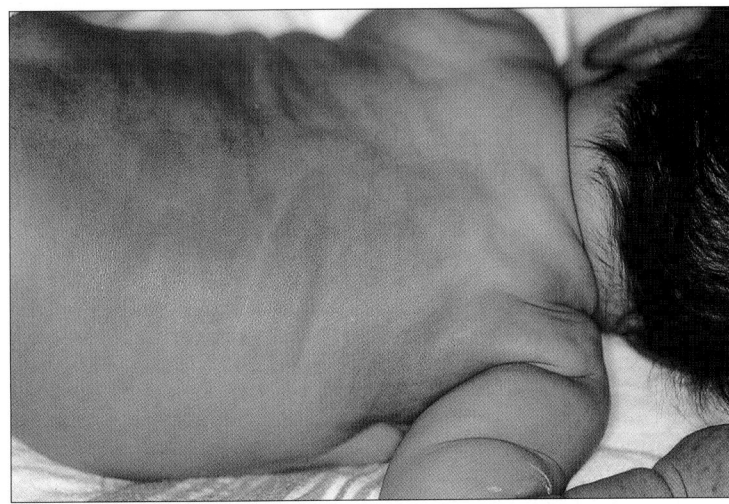

Fig. 100.13 Subcutaneous fat necrosis of the newborn. Indurated plaques on the trunk.

and localization of needle-shaped clefts within giant cells. Scleredema neonatorum is a condition seen in premature infants with congenital heart disease. In this disorder, the skin is distended and wax-like, and on biopsy the dermis appears edematous, with increased amounts of mucin[68]. Other conditions that can present with diffusely indurated skin in the neonatal period include stiff skin syndrome (usually favoring the trunk, buttocks and thighs), restrictive dermopathy and Hutchinson–Gilford progeria.

Treatment

Attempts to treat this disorder are disappointing[70]. Management includes treatment of sepsis, ventilatory support, correction of fluid and electrolyte imbalances, and maintenance of body temperature[68,73]. Exchange transfusions may be of value in selected instances[68,73]. Systemic corticosteroids are of questionable value[68,70].

Subcutaneous Fat Necrosis of the Newborn

Key features

- Development of one or more mobile, firm, subcutaneous nodules or plaques during the newborn period
- Sometimes associated with hypercalcemia or thrombocytopenia
- Granulomatous, lobular panniculitis with needle-shaped clefts in lipocytes and giant cells
- Prognosis is usually favorable; spontaneous resolution is common

Introduction

In contrast to sclerema neonatorum, subcutaneous fat necrosis is a localized process. Although complications can arise, particularly in relation to hypercalcemia, most cases resolve spontaneously.

History

At the beginning of the 20th century, Fabyan described 'abscesses' that spontaneously resorbed, and provided the first microscopic description of subcutaneous fat necrosis.

Epidemiology

Subcutaneous fat necrosis of the newborn typically occurs in full-term neonates during the first 2 to 3 weeks of life[74].

Pathogenesis

It is believed that a variety of stresses imposed upon fetal fat, with its high ratio of saturated to unsaturated fatty acids, results in crystallization, adipocyte injury, and granulomatous inflammation. Hypothermia is one potential eliciting factor, as illustrated by a case of subcutaneous fat necrosis that developed as a complication of hypothermic cardiac

surgery[75]. Other proposed causes are listed in Table 100.8[68,74,76]. The role of birth trauma has been questioned, since many cases have occurred in infants delivered by cesarian section[74].

Clinical features

The clinical features are outlined in Table 100.8[68,74]. Smooth, circumscribed, mobile, red to violaceous, subcutaneous nodules or plaques develop, sometimes in a symmetrical fashion[68,74] (Fig. 100.13). The areas of fat necrosis have been detected by CT[77] or MRI[78].

Some cases are associated with hypercalcemia or thrombocytopenia, and the former may develop 1–4 months after the onset of the skin lesions[76]. It is believed that the hypercalcemia results from extrarenal production of 1,25-dihydroxyvitamin D_3 (calcitriol) by activated macrophages (expressing 1-α hydroxylase) within areas of granulomatous panniculitis, which stimulates calcium absorption from the gut and mobilization from the bones[74,79]. The mechanism for thrombocytopenia may be local sequestration in the subcutis, as studies have shown normal bone marrow findings and resolution of the platelet abnormality as the inflammatory process resolves[80]. Spontaneous resolution of lesions is the rule, sometimes in association with lipoatrophy. Deaths have been reported in patients with associated hypercalcemia[80].

Pathology

The microscopic changes are outlined in Table 100.8. Needle-shaped clefts are observed within lipocytes and giant cells (Fig. 100.14). The crystals are doubly refractile and stain with oil red O[68]. Occasionally, needle-shaped clefts are not evident in otherwise typical cases.

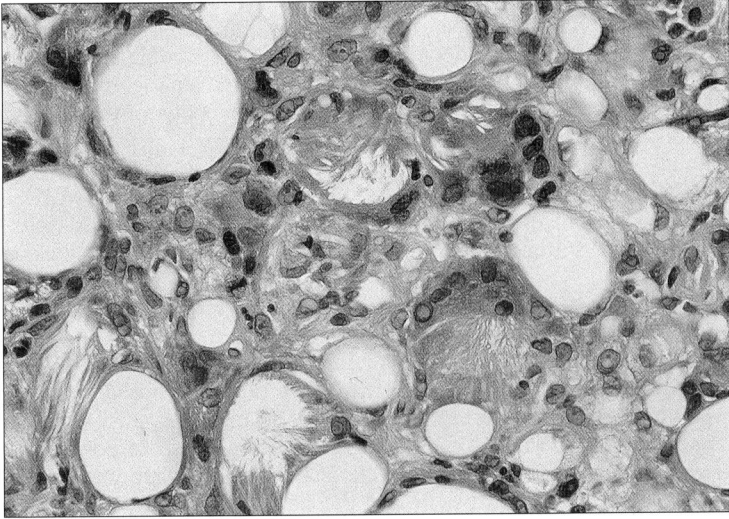

Fig. 100.14 Subcutaneous fat necrosis of the newborn. Needle-shaped clefts in a radial configuration are present within giant cells.

Differential diagnosis

The extensive cutaneous involvement in sclerema neonatorum is usually clinically distinguishable from the localized, self-limited process of subcutaneous fat necrosis; histologically, inflammation in sclerema is minimal. Poststeroid panniculitis is microscopically indistinguishable from subcutaneous fat necrosis, but arises in a different clinical setting (see below).

Treatment

Since many lesions resolve spontaneously, the emphasis is on supportive care. Systemic corticosteroids may be indicated to control the inflammation in severe cases[68]. Serial monitoring of calcium levels (for at least 4 months) is important. Hypercalcemia is managed by hydration, dietary restriction of both calcium and vitamin D, calcium-wasting diuretics (e.g. furosemide), calcitonin and bisphosphonates (e.g. etidronate, pamidronate)[74,76,81]. Corticosteroids may be helpful in managing hypercalcemia, by interfering with the metabolism of vitamin D to calcitriol, and by inhibiting calcitriol production by macrophages[76].

Poststeroid Panniculitis

Key features

- A rare complication of rapid systemic corticosteroid withdrawal
- Subcutaneous nodules develop on the cheeks, arms and trunk
- Lesions resolve spontaneously or when corticosteroids are readministered
- Pathology consists of granulomatous lobular panniculitis with needle-shaped clefts in lipocytes and giant cells

History

In 1956, Smith & Good[82] reported 11 children with acute rheumatic fever who were treated with large doses of corticosteroids with rapid taper. Five children developed pruritic, erythema nodosum-like lesions.

Epidemiology

Poststeroid panniculitis is a disorder of children. It occurs in an older age group than either sclerema neonatorum or subcutaneous fat necrosis of the newborn, with reported ages ranging from 20 months to 14 years[83].

Pathogenesis

Poststeroid panniculitis occurs after rapid withdrawal of systemic corticosteroids, including oral prednisone, dexamethasone, and intravenous methylprednisolone. Cumulative dosages for those patients receiving prednisone have ranged from 2000 to 6000 mg[83]. The precise mechanism by which the panniculitis arises is not known.

Clinical features

Patients who have developed this form of panniculitis received corticosteroid therapy for a variety of conditions[82–85], including those listed in Table 100.8. Lesions appear 1 to 40 days after rapid corticosteroid withdrawal (see Table 100.8) and disappear spontaneously over a period of months to a year[84].

Pathology

Microscopic changes are outlined in Table 100.8[84]. Needle-shaped clefts, some with a 'starburst' pattern, can be identified within lipocytes or giant cells.

Differential diagnosis

A less nodular presentation involving the cheeks can mimic non-panniculitic disorders such as erythema infectiosum, atopic dermatitis, lupus erythematosus or facial cellulitis. The microscopic changes in these conditions would be quite different from those of poststeroid panniculitis. Cold panniculitis has clinical and microscopic similarities, but the history of cold exposure and the lack of needle-shaped clefts on biopsy permits distinction. The microscopic changes of poststeroid panniculitis are virtually identical to those of subcutaneous fat necrosis

of the newborn, although calcification and hemorrhage are more commonly observed in the latter condition. Clinical history is decisive.

Treatment

Since spontaneous resolution is the rule, treatment is usually unnecessary. Readministration of corticosteroids followed by a more gradual taper may be helpful[84].

LUPUS ERYTHEMATOSUS PANNICULITIS (LUPUS PANNICULITIS)

Synonyms: ■ Lupus profundus ■ Subcutaneous lupus erythematosus

Key features

- Tender subcutaneous nodules and plaques arising on the face, proximal extremities, and trunk
- Associated with chronic cutaneous (discoid) lupus erythematosus in at least one-third of patients; less often associated with systemic lupus erythematosus (10–15% of patients)
- Often precedes onset of other manifestations of lupus erythematosus
- Characteristic microscopic changes include lobular panniculitis with hyaline necrosis and a predominantly lymphoplasmacytic infiltrate; nodular aggregates of lymphocytes are common
- Overlying epidermal or dermal changes of lupus erythematosus are frequently present

History

Kaposi first described the clinical characteristics of lupus panniculitis in 1869. In 1940, it was recognized as a manifestation of lupus erythematosus (LE) by Irgang. Lupus panniculitis was firmly established as a specific subtype of LE in a 1956 paper by Arnold[86].

Epidemiology

Lupus panniculitis constitutes a small subset of all cases of LE, representing 2–3% of this group[87]. It usually occurs in adults, with a median age of onset of 30–40 years[88]. Children can also develop lupus panniculitis, and an association with neonatal lupus has been described[86]. There is a predominance among women, with a female:male ratio ranging from 2:1 to 4:1[28,88]. Sometimes there is a family history of either LE or another autoimmune connective tissue disease[87].

Pathogenesis

The autoimmune basis of lupus panniculitis is thought to be similar to that of other types of LE (see Ch. 42). The cells comprising the infiltrates of lupus panniculitis are T lymphocytes and macrophages[89]. Lupus panniculitis (often with a childhood onset and widespread distribution) has been described in patients with partial C4 deficiency[90]. This complement deficiency causes defective opsonization of immune complexes, which may play a role in the pathogenesis of the disease[90].

Clinical features

Lupus panniculitis presents with tender subcutaneous nodules and plaques that may arise in crops (see Table 100.7). A history of trauma can sometimes be elicited. Lesions tend to develop on the face, upper arms, hips and trunk (Fig. 100.15). The lack of involvement of the distal extremities is noteworthy[88]. Changes in the overlying skin range from a light pink color to those of chronic cutaneous (discoid) LE (e.g. scaling, follicular plugging, dyspigmentation, telangiectasias, atrophy and scarring). At times, findings of discoid LE are too subtle to be recognized clinically but can be seen on microscopic examination of biopsy specimens. The overlying skin may also be 'tethered' to the subcutaneous nodule or plaque, creating a surface depression, and ulceration occasionally occurs. Lupus panniculitis has a chronic, relapsing clinical course[91]. It usually eventuates in subcutaneous atrophy, which can be disfiguring (see Ch. 42).

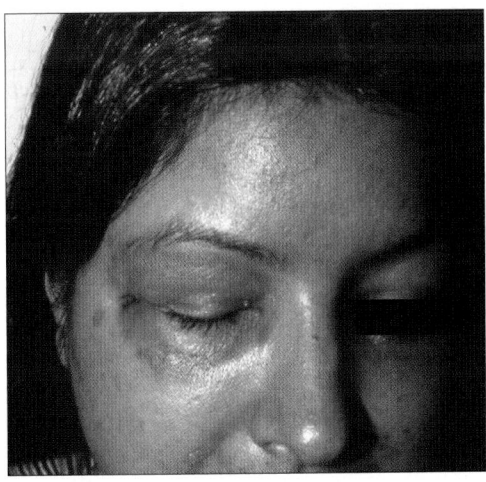

Fig. 100.15 Lupus panniculitis. Erythematous plaque involving the orbital area.

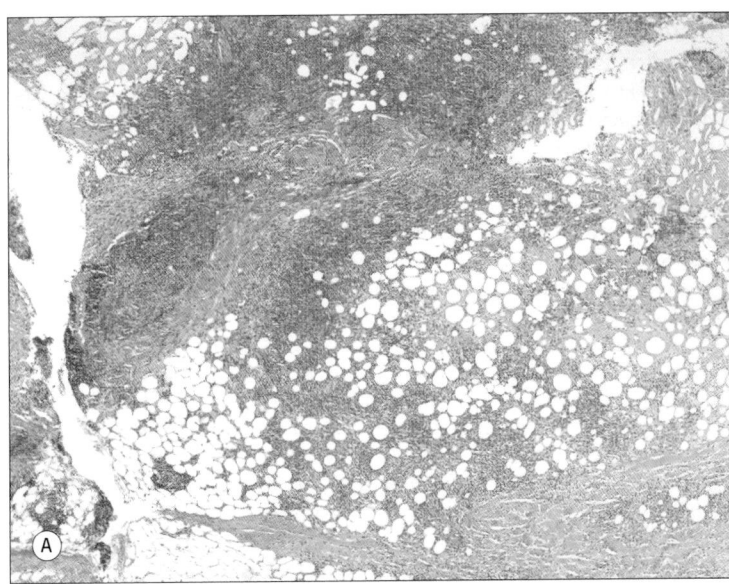

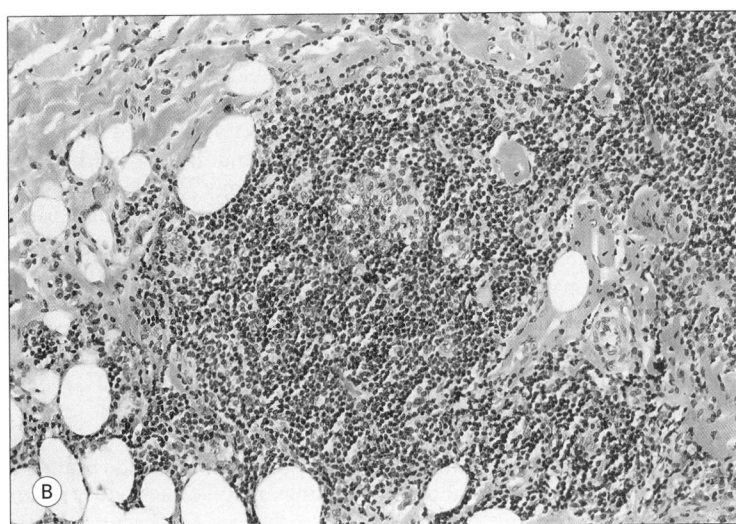

Fig. 100.16 Lupus panniculitis. A Low-power view showing a septal and lobular panniculitis with hyaline necrosis of fat lobules. **B** High-power view of a nodular aggregate of lymphocytes in the subcutis with lymphoid follicle configuration.

Lupus panniculitis often occurs prior to other manifestations of LE and in the absence of other autoimmune connective tissue diseases[88]. For example, lesions of discoid LE have developed up to 10 years after the appearance of the panniculitis. However, manifestations of systemic LE or discoid LE can also occur long before (or at the same time as) the panniculitis[28]. There is a closer relationship of lupus panniculitis to chronic cutaneous LE than to systemic LE. Coexistent discoid lesions are observed in at least one-third of patients, whereas only 10–15% meet the diagnostic criteria for systemic LE[88,92]. Most individuals in the latter group have relatively mild systemic manifestations, usually arthralgias or Raynaud's phenomenon[87]. It is common for patients to have low-titer antinuclear antibodies; they can also have other circulating autoantibodies (including those targeting double-stranded DNA or extractable nuclear antigens), leukopenia, hypocomplementemia, and elevated erythrocyte sedimentation rates[32,87].

Pathology
Lupus panniculitis is a predominantly lobular process with a variable degree of inflammation (Fig. 100.16). The characteristic microscopic changes (e.g. hyaline necrosis of the fat lobules) are outlined in Table 100.7. Granulomas can occur and tend to encroach upon the septa, but they are usually not prominent. Other features include lymphocytic vasculitis and mucin or calcium deposition[32].

The subcutaneous findings alone are considered sufficiently characteristic to permit a diagnosis of lupus panniculitis. However, overlying epidermal or dermal changes of chronic cutaneous LE occur in a half to two-thirds of cases and are also helpful diagnostically[89,92,93]. With direct immunofluorescence, a positive lupus band can be identified in the overlying skin in a high percentage of cases, even in those where the histopathologic changes are non-specific[93].

Differential diagnosis
Clinically, lesions of lupus panniculitis can resemble other forms of panniculitis. The rarity of involvement of the distal extremities helps to distinguish it from conditions such as erythema nodosum and erythema induratum. It should also be remembered that other forms of subcutaneous inflammation may occur in patients with LE, including erythema nodosum, thrombophlebitis, pancreatic panniculitis, and juxta-articular, rheumatoid nodule-like lesions.

Microscopically, lupus panniculitis can resemble the panniculitis associated with morphea and dermatomyositis (see Table 100.7), traumatic panniculitis (which often has evidence of foreign material) and, in its later stages, localized lipoatrophy due to other etiologies[87,91]. Overlying epidermal or dermal changes of LE, when present, can be of help in excluding other forms of panniculitis. However, a vacuolar interface dermatitis and abundant dermal mucin together with a lobular lymphocytic infiltrate have been described in cases of subcutaneous panniculitis-like T-cell lymphoma (see below). A lack of prominent CD8[+] T cells or cytophagia as well as the presence of lymphoid follicles with reactive germinal centers, a mixed infiltrate with conspicuous plasma cells, and a polyclonal T-cell receptor gene rearrangement can help to establish a diagnosis of lupus panniculitis in patients lacking additional cutaneous or systemic manifestations of LE[94].

Treatment
Antimalarials are frequently used to treat lupus panniculitis, and they produce improvement in most patients[88]. Addition of a second antimalarial may prove useful in patients who do not respond to a single agent[91]. In view of the chronic, relapsing nature of the disease, treatment may be required for several years[87].

Systemic corticosteroids, when used, are often restricted to initial phases of the disease[87]. Other systemic therapies include dapsone, cyclophosphamide and thalidomide[88,90]. Overlying discoid lesions, if present, can be treated with potent topical or intralesional corticosteroids.

PANNICULITIS OF DERMATOMYOSITIS

Key features
- An uncommon manifestation of dermatomyositis
- Incidental microscopic changes of panniculitis (in the absence of clinical lesions) are seen more often
- Can precede or follow other manifestations of dermatomyositis
- Microscopically, it is a lobular or mixed panniculitis with lymphoplasmacytic predominance
- Usually responds well to therapy

Introduction

Panniculitis is a rare but established clinical manifestation of dermatomyositis. However, there is some evidence that microscopic involvement of subcutaneous fat without overt clinical features of panniculitis is more common.

Clinical features

The characteristic lesions are persistent, indurated, painful plaques and nodules that may ulcerate and lead to lipoatrophy (see Table 100.7)[95]. They can arise in the setting of established dermatomyositis[95] or represent the first manifestation of the disease[96]. The other clinical and laboratory features and the incidence of malignancy in affected individuals appear to be similar to those of dermatomyositis patients without panniculitis[95]. It has been suggested that panniculitis is a favorable prognostic sign, as good responses to therapy have generally been reported[97]. However, partial or generalized lipoatrophy without preceding clinical lesions of panniculitis (occasionally accompanied by increased abdominal fat) occurs in up to one-quarter of patients with juvenile dermatomyositis, and it is often associated with metabolic abnormalities such as hypertriglyceridemia and insulin resistance (see Ch.101).

Pathology

The microscopic features are outlined in Table 100.7. Lymphocytic vasculitis has been described, and fat necrosis has been noted in several reports[95,98]. Lipomembranous changes have been observed in some cases (see section on lipodermatosclerosis), and lesions with lipomembranous changes may be resistant to therapy[95]. Calcification is variable and is an expected finding in cases of dermatomyositis associated with calcinosis of deep soft tissues and skeletal muscle[27]. Vacuolar alteration of the basal layer of the overlying epidermis has been reported[95,99], and the dermis may be edematous or mucinous with perivascular lymphocytic inflammation[97]. Direct immunofluorescence is negative for deposits along the dermal–epidermal junction[95], although immunoreactants have been detected in vessel walls[97].

Differential diagnosis

Lupus panniculitis is more likely to show hyaline necrosis and lymphoid nodules, but clinical and laboratory findings may be needed to make a distinction. Overlying poikilodermatous changes can occur in both diseases, but lupus is more likely to show appendageal involvement and is associated with positive basement membrane zone fluorescence.

Treatment

Treatments include prednisone, methotrexate, azathioprine, cyclosporine and intravenous immunoglobulin[95–97]. Panniculitis lesions have shown variable responses to hydroxychloroquine[99].

TRAUMATIC PANNICULITIS

Key features

- Inflammation in the subcutis resulting from external injury
- The injurious event may be accidental, purposeful or iatrogenic, and it may be a manifestation of an underlying psychiatric disturbance
- A variety of histopathologic changes are observed, depending upon the inciting agent
- Identification of foreign material is of greatest help in diagnosis

Introduction

Extrinsic injury of varying types can produce panniculitis. There are four broad categories: cold panniculitis (Haxthausen's disease), sclerosing lipogranuloma, panniculitis due to other injectable substances or therapies, and panniculitis due to blunt trauma.

History

Cold panniculitis was reported by Lemez in 1928, when he noted that newborns and infants up to 6 months of age were particularly susceptible to cold injury, as demonstrated by the production of a subcutaneous nodule following application of an ice cube[100]. In 1941, Haxthausen described a condition occurring in small children a few days after exposure to cold, consisting of firm infiltrated nodules of the cheeks and chin. A similar type of cold injury due to popsicles was reported by Epstein & Oren in 1970[101].

Injection of foreign lipid material into the skin for cosmetic or other purposes has been performed for centuries[102]. In 1950, Smetana & Bernhard reported 14 cases of what they termed *sclerosing lipogranuloma* of the male genitalia. They believed it was an endogenous process, but subsequent studies demonstrated the presence of mineral oil in similar cases[102].

Epidemiology

Infants and small children are most at risk for cold panniculitis. A form of the disease also occurs on the thighs of young women who are equestrians[103]. Sclerosing lipogranuloma of the male genitalia is seen mostly in young adults[104]. A sclerosing, pseudosclerodermatous panniculitis has been reported following megavoltage radiation for metastatic carcinoma[105] and as a radiation recall reaction after cyclophosphamide therapy[106].

Pathogenesis

Cold injury to fat favors small children, due in part to a higher ratio of saturated to unsaturated fatty acids that results in a higher solidification point for infantile fat[107]. Cold injury is also related to fluctuations in blood flow that occur with declining temperatures (the 'hunting phenomenon'), ice crystal formation, and the changes that occur with thawing[107]. Injections of oils (and associated impurities) are known for producing subcutaneous inflammation. Substances include mineral oil (paraffin) as well as camphor, cottonseed and sesame oils. Even medical-grade silicone may contain impurities, and, since encapsulation of this material is desirable when used for cosmetic purposes, fibrosis-inducing substances such as olive oil or castor oil are often added[102]. Injected substances responsible for factitial panniculitis have included milk and feces.

Panniculitis has been produced by numerous therapeutic agents, such as meperidine, morphine, tetanus antitoxoid, pentazocine, phytonadione (vitamin K)[108], povidone[109], aurothioglucose[110], interleukin-2 (IL-2)[111] and bovine collagen[112]. In addition to the foreign body response elicited by many of these agents, other immune mechanisms may also be involved. With blunt trauma, granulomas contain material that may be derived from breakdown of erythrocyte membranes[113].

Clinical features

In cold panniculitis (including popsicle panniculitis), erythematous, firm nodules develop, particularly on the cheeks and chin[107,114]. In equestrian cold panniculitis, erythematous to violaceous, tender plaques appear on the thighs following exposure to cold while wearing tight-fitting clothing[103] (Fig. 100.17).

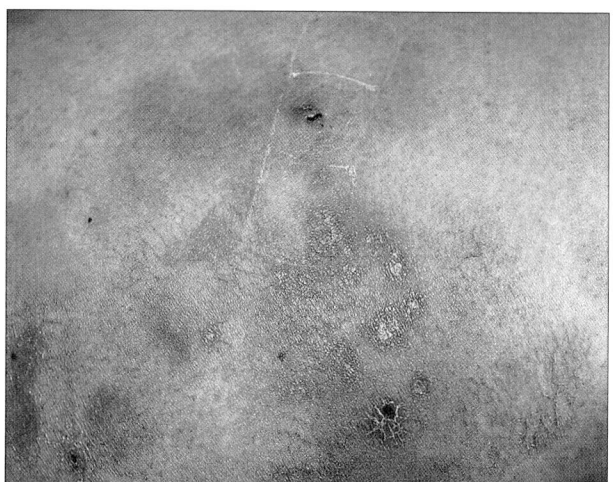

Fig. 100.17 Cold panniculitis. Erythematous, violaceous plaques on the thighs of a young woman with equestrian cold panniculitis. Courtesy of Kenneth E Greer MD.

In lipogranuloma, nodules are sometimes migratory and can be accompanied by varying degrees of swelling, erythema, abscess formation, lymphangitis and fibrosis[102]. The term *sclerosing lipogranuloma* often refers to lesions arising on the male genitalia due to self-injection of oily materials (see Ch. 93). There has also been a report of a sclerosing lipogranuloma that apparently resulted from topical application of a vitamin E cream[115]. In several Japanese patients, Y-shaped induration of the scrotum (in which exogenous lipids could not be detected) was described as eosinophilic sclerosing lipogranuloma[116]. Patients with sclerosing lipogranuloma frequently deny self-injection, making diagnosis difficult. Another variant of lipogranuloma is the *grease gun granuloma*, which results from accidental firing of the grease gun used by mechanics. This results in formation of a verrucous nodule, often on the dorsum of the hand[117].

Inflamed nodules with varying degrees of pain and fibrosis have been observed in other forms of panniculitis due to injection, with the distribution of lesions sometimes providing a clue to their cause. A dramatic example of this is *Texier's disease*, a panniculitis due to phytonadione (vitamin K) injections. In this disorder, sclerotic lesions with lilac-colored borders form on the buttocks and thighs in a configuration resembling a 'cowboy gunbelt and holster'[108]. Lesions due to blunt trauma often have an ecchymotic character and involve locations such as the arm or hand[113].

Pathology

Table 100.9 outlines the microscopic changes in various forms of traumatic panniculitis[104–106,117]. In addition, sclerosing lipogranuloma is discussed in Chapter 93.

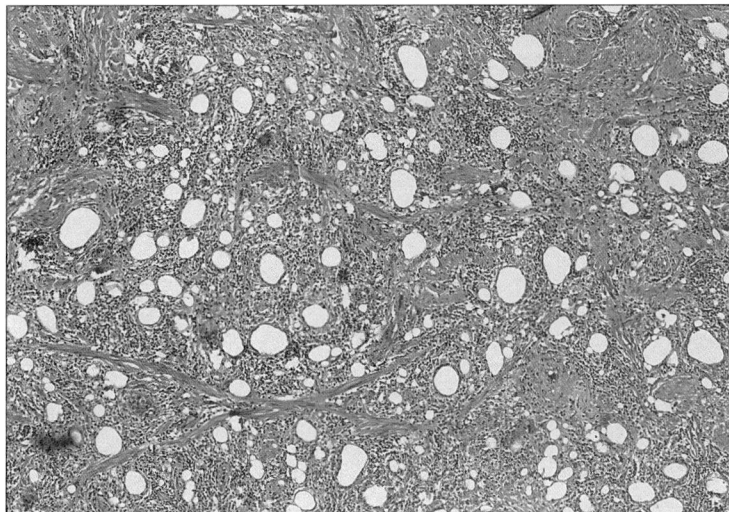

Fig. 100.18 Oil granuloma. Numerous vacuolated spaces, in this case due to grease gun injury.

Differential diagnosis

In cold panniculitis, the absence of needle-shaped clefts in lipocytes and location of the most intense inflammation near the dermal–subcutaneous interface help to distinguish this condition from subcutaneous fat necrosis of the newborn. In sclerosing lipogranuloma and related lipogranulomas, the large vacuoles found in the dermis and subcutis are distinctive. Radiographs are sometimes useful in differentiating lipogranulomas from silicone granulomas, since only the latter are radio-opaque[118]. Mineral oil in non-processed tissue can be identified by infrared spectrophotometry[117].

Panniculitis due to injectable substances can be diagnosed when foreign material (often identified by polarization microscopy) is present. Cases with acute inflammation and necrosis may resemble infection-induced panniculitis, and, in fact, infection may accompany injection panniculitis[119]; special stains and cultures for organisms (including atypical mycobacteria) are useful in this regard. Sclerosing traumatic panniculitis (e.g. that due to phytonadione or pentazocine injections) may resemble morphea clinically, but would not present as a septal panniculitis histologically.

Treatment

Treatment of these disorders mainly involves removal of the inciting stimulus and eradication of any associated infection. Intralesional or systemic corticosteroids can be helpful in controlling the inflammation and they have been used in the management of sclerosing lipogranuloma[102,120] and granulomatous panniculitis due to bovine collagen injections[112]. Surgical excision may also be an option for sclerosing lipogranuloma[102].

LIPODERMATOSCLEROSIS

Synonyms: ▪ Hypodermitis sclerodermiformis ▪ Sclerosing panniculitis ▪ Chronic panniculitis with lipomembranous changes

Key features

▪ Erythema, induration and hyperpigmentation involving one or both lower legs, usually in a setting of chronic venous insufficiency

▪ Both septal and lobular panniculitis; lipomembranous changes are common, particularly in chronic lesions

Introduction

Erythema, induration and pigmentary changes have been known for many years to be associated with venous insufficiency. Because of the variety of clinical appearances and histopathologic findings that can occur at different stages of the disease, a number of diagnostic terms

---

MICROSCOPIC FEATURES OF TRAUMATIC PANNICULITIS		
Condition	**Microscopic features**	**Special considerations**
Cold panniculitis	Septal/lobular inflammation, especially at the dermal–subcutaneous border and periadnexally; lymphocytes, neutrophils, foamy macrophages, poorly developed granulomas; mucin, adipocyte necrosis, microcysts	Needle-shaped clefts are not observed
Lipogranuloma	*Sclerosing lipogranuloma* – granulomatous lobular panniculitis with marked fibrosis and numerous round or oval vacuoles of various sizes in the dermis and subcutis, producing a 'Swiss cheese' appearance (Fig. 100.18); nodular aggregates of lymphocytes, plasma cells, eosinophils, macrophages or giant cells often present *Grease gun granuloma* – also pseudoepitheliomatous hyperplasia	Exogenous oils within the vacuoles can be identified in frozen sections stained with oil red O, silver bromide and osmium tetroxide
Injection-induced panniculitis	Central nidus of subcutaneous inflammation; sometimes fibrosis* or polarizing foreign material	Povidone panniculitis shows gray–blue material within macrophages on routine staining that also stains with Congo red and chlorazol-fast pink
Blunt trauma	Organizing hematoma, focal granuloma	Deposits of mucopolysaccharides and iron can be seen
Postirradiation or radiation recall panniculitis	Deep fibrosis, mixed inflammation	Inflammation includes lymphocytes, plasma cells, histiocytes, eosinophils

*Especially with phytonadione (vitamin K) and pentazocine injections; lipid-containing vacuoles, fat necrosis, foam cells, thrombosis and endarteritis are also observed in the latter.

Table 100.9 Microscopic features of traumatic panniculitis.

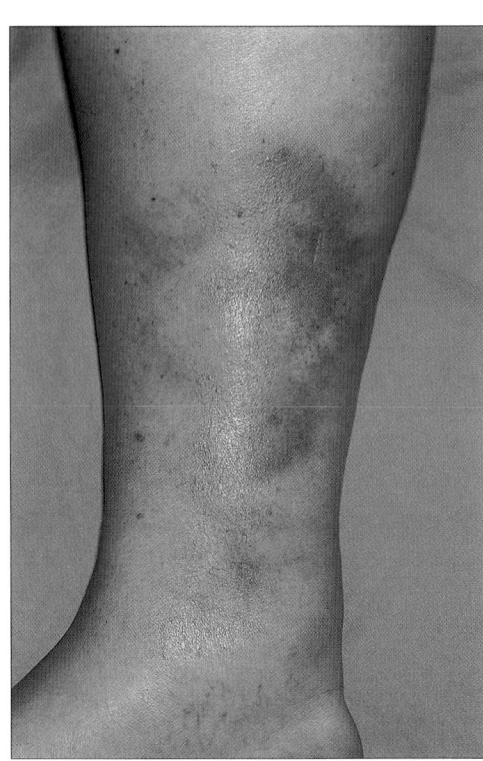

Fig. 100.19 Lipodermatosclerosis. Sclerotic plaque on the lower leg. Courtesy of Kenneth E Greer MD.

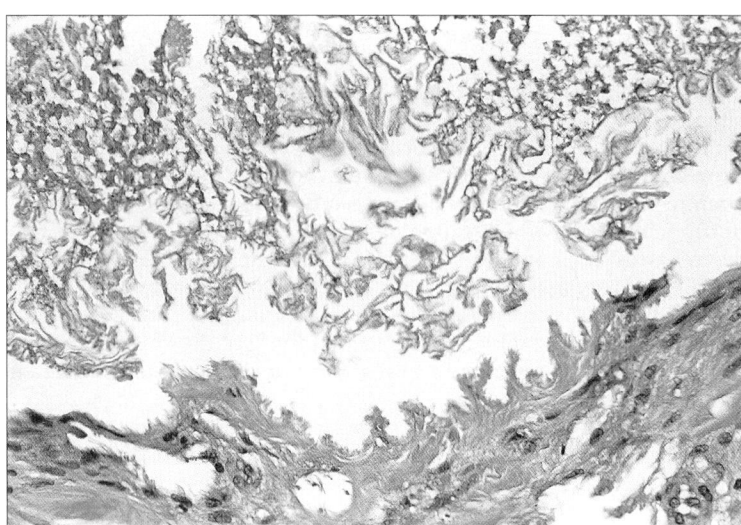

Fig. 100.20 Lipodermatosclerosis. Lipomembranous change, consisting of cystic formation with elaborate papillary configurations.

have been employed to explain the changes. Recently, the various manifestations of this panniculitis have been consolidated under the heading of *lipodermatosclerosis* or *sclerosing panniculitis*.

History

The cutaneous sequelae of venous insufficiency have long been recognized. In 1955, Huriez drew attention to a related indurated lesion, which he termed *hypodermitis sclerodermiformis*[121].

Epidemiology

Most patients are women over the age of 40 years, but cases appearing after the age of 75 years have also been reported[122,123].

Pathogenesis

There is considerable evidence for venous insufficiency in patients with lipodermatosclerosis[124], and fibrinolytic abnormalities are also present in these individuals. Venous hypertension leads to a compromised ability to reduce foot vein pressure during exercise. This results in increased capillary permeability, which causes leakage of fibrinogen, its polymerization to form fibrin cuffs around vessels, impedance of oxygen exchange, and tissue anoxia (see Ch. 105)[123]. Pericapillary fibrin deposits can be seen in uninvolved, clinically normal extremities of patients with healed venous ulcers of the opposite extremity, suggesting that this abnormality precedes the clinical changes of lipodermatosclerosis[125]. Additional factors contributing to the pathogenesis may include protein C and S deficiencies[126], local stimulation of collagen synthesis[123], and obesity.

Clinical features

The acute phase of lipodermatosclerosis presents with pain, warmth, erythema, and some induration, most often located on the medial lower leg above the malleolus. Other dependent sites such as the lower aspect of the abdominal pannus can also develop lipodermatosclerosis. At this point, the changes are relatively diffuse[123]. In the chronic phase, there is marked sclerosis of the dermis and subcutis, resulting in induration that is sharply demarcated from the adjacent normal skin (Fig. 100.19). Hyperpigmentation due to hemosiderin deposition may also be present[122]. These features give the affected leg the appearance of an inverted wine bottle[127].

Pathology

Early lesions show mid-lobular ischemic necrosis, a lymphocytic infiltrate in the septa that rims the fat lobules, variable degrees of capil-

lary congestion and thrombosis, and hemorrhage with hemosiderin deposition. With progression, there is septal thickening, hyaline sclerosis involving lipocytes, lipophage formation, and mixed inflammatory cell infiltrates[122]. Advanced lesions show marked septal sclerosis and lipomembranous change in the face of markedly reduced inflammation.

Lipomembranous change has been emphasized as a key feature in lipodermatosclerosis[128,129]. This consists of thickened, undulating membranes that form cysts and papillary configurations (Fig. 100.20). The membranes are believed to result from degenerated cell membranes of lipocytes and/or macrophages. The material comprising the membranes is ceroid, an oxidation product of unsaturated fatty acids[130].

Pericapillary fibrin can be demonstrated in lesions of lipodermatosclerosis with phosphotungstic acid–hematoxylin stain or by immunofluorescent methods[128]. Dermal changes include fibrosis, tortuous thick-walled veins, and superficial and deep perivascular inflammation[122]. Biopsy should be avoided if the diagnosis is obvious, since poor wound healing and ulceration frequently result. When necessary, a thin elliptical excision should be obtained from the margin of a lesion.

Differential diagnosis

Difficulties in clinical diagnosis arise most often in early lesions, when the process is more diffuse and erythematous. At this stage, consideration is often given to cellulitis, erythema nodosum, or erythema induratum[122,123,127]. Persistence of a lesion, association with stasis changes, and lack of response to antimicrobials suggest the correct diagnosis, perhaps aided by studies of venous function[124].

As induration develops and progresses, differentiation from morphea and scleromyxedema may be necessary. In morphea, subcutaneous involvement is predominantly septal, and lipophagic and lipodystrophic changes are not as prominent as they are in lipodermatosclerosis[122]. Lipomembranous changes, when present, can be of great diagnostic help; however, these findings can occur in a variety of other conditions, including lupus and dermatomyositis panniculitis, liposarcoma, erythema nodosum, and diabetic dermopathy[130].

Treatment

Leg elevation and consistent compression therapy are the mainstays of treatment for lipodermatosclerosis[123]. Traditional anti-inflammatory therapies are usually ineffective in this condition[122], although intralesional corticosteroids may be of benefit when used in conjunction with compression therapy. Good results have been reported in early disease with the anabolic steroid stanozolol (2–5 mg twice daily)[123]. This agent enhances fibrinolysis, and it has been shown to reduce pain, extent of involvement, and induration of the skin. However, side effects of sodium retention, lipid profile abnormalities, hepatotoxicity and virilization in women limit its use. Oxandrolone, an anabolic steroid with less hepatotoxicity and fewer androgenic effects, represents another therapeutic option[127]. Other reported treatments include ultrasound, pentoxifylline, fasciotomy and phlebectomy[123,129,131].

INFECTION-INDUCED PANNICULITIS

Synonym: Infective panniculitis

Key features

- A wide variety of infectious agents has been reported to produce panniculitis
- Some degree of immunosuppression is common, but not invariable
- Histopathologic findings vary, but often include mixed septal/lobular panniculitis, neutrophilic infiltration, hemorrhage and necrosis
- Special staining and culture studies can provide definitive diagnosis

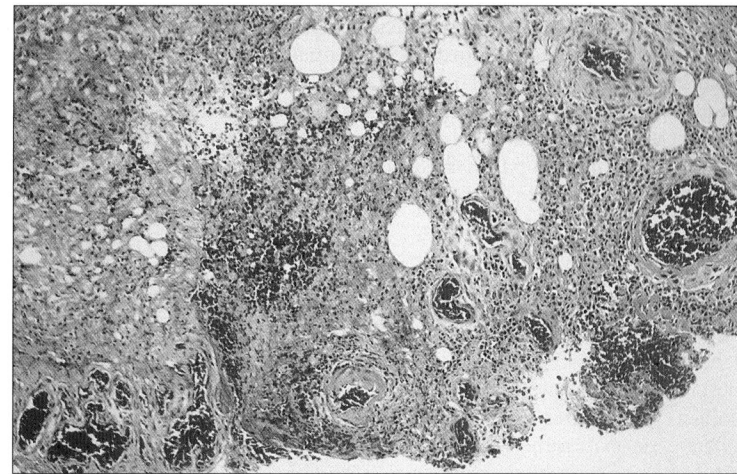

Fig. 100.21 Infection-induced panniculitis. Bacterial panniculitis, showing heavy neutrophilic inflammation, basophilic necrosis, vascular proliferation, and hemorrhage.

Introduction

Panniculitis can result from a distant focus of infection (a classic example being erythema nodosum) or panniculitis can be *directly* induced by an infectious agent. The latter can produce a variety of clinical and microscopic appearances, although there are some features that infection-induced lesions have in common, regardless of the etiologic agent.

History

Multiple case reports of panniculitis directly caused by infectious agents have been published[132,133], but most early studies of deep skin infections did not focus upon the changes in the subcutaneous fat. In 1989, Patterson et al.[19] studied 15 patients with infection-induced panniculitis, with an emphasis on the histopathologic features in the subcutis. Since that time, additional reports of panniculitis due to infection have appeared.

Epidemiology

There appears to be no age, sex or racial predilection among cases of infection-induced panniculitis. Many of these patients are immunosuppressed[19,134] or have predisposing medical conditions such as diabetes mellitus[132].

Pathogenesis

In this group of disorders, infectious agents are considered to be directly responsible for the panniculitis. Some of the reported microorganisms include Gram-positive and Gram-negative bacteria[135–137], mycobacteria[19,133], and fungi including dermatophytes[138], dimorphic fungi[132], opportunistic fungi[134,139] and *Candida* species[19,140].

Involvement of the subcutis can result from direct inoculation or septicemia. Other potential modes of spread include transfascial from an enteric source, in the case of abdominal panniculitis[135], or via 'persorption', a proposed mechanism by which *Candida* migrates across intact endothelium from the gut to a subcutaneous site[140]. Immunosuppression is common, but not invariable, among individuals with infection-induced panniculitis.

Clinical features

Patients develop local swelling and erythema. There may be one or more fluctuant nodules that ulcerate and drain. Lesions on the legs and feet are common, but sites of involvement may also include the gluteal region, abdomen, axillary area, arm or hand. Underlying conditions include diabetes mellitus, leukemias or solid tumors, autoimmune connective tissue disease, AIDS and organ transplantation.

Pathology

Individual cases can mimic other primary forms of panniculitis. Common changes (regardless of the infectious agent) include a mixed septal/lobular panniculitis, neutrophilic infiltration, vascular proliferation, hemorrhage, and necrosis that involves lipocytes, inflammatory cells and eccrine sweat coils[19] (Fig. 100.21). In the rickettsial disease Q fever, there may be a 'doughnut-like' granulomatous lobular panniculitis, in which fibrin and inflammatory cells form a ring around a central clear space; similar changes have been found in the liver and bone marrow of patients with Q fever[141].

Differential diagnosis

Fluctuant, ulcerating nodules also occur in pancreatic panniculitis, traumatic panniculitis and α_1-antitrypsin deficiency panniculitis. Clinical and laboratory data can usually permit distinction. Of note, traumatic panniculitis may be accompanied by infection. Examples of infection-induced panniculitis with predominantly septal involvement or with large vessel vasculitis could be confused with acute erythema nodosum or erythema induratum, respectively. Special stains for organisms and cultures are keys to the diagnosis. In one study, special stains were positive for organisms in 14 of 15 cases[19].

Treatment

Treatment consists of appropriate antimicrobial therapy. Surgery may be indicated for isolated lesions caused by grain-forming fungi or bacteria, such as mycetoma or botryomycosis[138]. A more radical surgical approach has been used successfully in treating abdominal panniculitis due to enteric bacteria[135].

CYTOPHAGIC HISTIOCYTIC PANNICULITIS

Synonym: Subcutaneous panniculitis-like T-cell lymphoma with cytophagocytosis (may exist on the same disease spectrum)

Key features

- Subcutaneous nodules, which may be accompanied by fever, hepatosplenomegaly, pancytopenia, liver failure, intravascular coagulation and a hemorrhagic diathesis
- Many cases are associated with lymphoma, particularly subcutaneous panniculitis-like T-cell lymphoma
- Non-fatal cases exist, in which systemic signs and symptoms are lacking
- Microscopic features of lobular panniculitis with cytophagocytosis by benign-appearing 'histiocytes' (macrophages)

Introduction

Initial reports of cytophagic histiocytic panniculitis focused on the cytophagic activity demonstrated by 'histiocytes' (more accurately termed macrophages) and upon a possible relationship to forms of 'malignant histiocytosis'. With the evolution of immunophenotyping and genetic techniques, it has become apparent that many cases are associated with lymphoma, particularly T-cell lymphoma. In fact, cytophagic histiocytic panniculitis may be part of a spectrum of disease that includes subcutaneous panniculitis-like T-cell lymphoma[142,143]. At the same time, 'benign' forms of cytophagic histiocytic panniculitis, fatal cases in which a diagnosis of lymphoma cannot be proven, and examples associated with lupus erythematosus suggest that under certain circumstances other factors may be capable of producing the lesions of cytophagic panniculitis. The concept of cytophagic histiocytic panniculitis is currently in evolution.

History

In 1980, Winkelmann & Bowie[144] reported five patients with cytophagic panniculitis and a fulminant clinical course. Previously, there had been individual reports of clinically similar cases that had been labeled 'Weber–Christian disease'. Gonzales and colleagues[145] first described T-cell lymphoma involving subcutaneous tissue as a distinct subset of peripheral T-cell lymphoma, associated with a hemophagocytic syndrome. However, several authors have described non-fatal cases of cytophagic histiocytic panniculitis that lacked evidence for an associated lymphoma[146,147].

Epidemiology

The disorder tends to affect young to middle-aged adults[142,144], although children and teenagers with this disease have also been reported[142,148]. Cytophagic histiocytic panniculitis occurs in both men and women, and cases have been reported from Asia and Europe as well as the US.

Pathogenesis

Accumulating evidence indicates that many patients with cytophagic histiocytic panniculitis have a T-cell lymphoma (see Ch. 120). The relationship is particularly close with subcutaneous panniculitis-like T-cell lymphomas, which can have either an α/β or γ/δ phenotype[142,145]. In the 2005 WHO/EORTC classification of cutaneous lymphomas[149], tumors expressing an α/β phenotype are referred to as subcutaneous panniculitis-like T-cell lymphomas *sui generis*, whereas cases with a γ/δ phenotype are included in the group of peripheral T-cell lymphomas, not otherwise specified (NOS). Morphologically similar tumors have expressed natural killer cell (CD56) phenotypes or have proved to be B-cell lymphomas[143]. However, other examples of cytophagic histiocytic panniculitis, both fatal and non-fatal, have not been shown to be lymphomas[147]. Latent EBV infection has been detected in subcutaneous panniculitis-like T-cell lymphoma with hemophagocytosis, but not in fatal or non-fatal cases of cytophagic histiocytic panniculitis without lymphoma[147,150].

Examples of cytophagic histiocytic panniculitis have been reported in association with lupus erythematosus[151,152], and a hemophagocytic syndrome has long been associated with a number of infectious agents (see Ch. 90)[143]. Therefore, while it is possible that some 'non-lymphoma' cases of cytophagic histiocytic panniculitis may escape our current methods of detection and over time prove to be lymphoma[153], it is also possible that some cases may be of non-neoplastic origin. Whatever the origin in a particular case, the cytophagic activity probably results from generation of cytokines such as interferon-γ, tumor necrosis factor-α and interleukin-1β. Monocytes and endothelial cells activated by these cytokines are also capable of generating procoagulant molecules that contribute to the hypercoagulable state and organ failure associated with this form of panniculitis[143,154].

Clinical features

Patients develop skin-colored to erythematous, sometimes painful subcutaneous nodules or diffuse ill-defined hemorrhagic plaques on the extremities and trunk (Fig. 100.22). Ulceration or persistent drainage following biopsy can occur[144,147,155]. There may be few associated symptoms in those with benign forms of the disease (other than swelling and transient fever), and these cases tend to follow a chronic course[147]. More fulminant forms of the disease are associated with persistent fever, hepatosplenomegaly, mucosal ulcers, serosal effusions, pancytopenia, intravascular coagulation and liver failure. A hemorrhagic diathesis and death may ensue[156].

Pathology

There is a mixed septal/lobular panniculitis, sometimes with foci of fat necrosis. Lymphocytes tend to predominate, but there are also

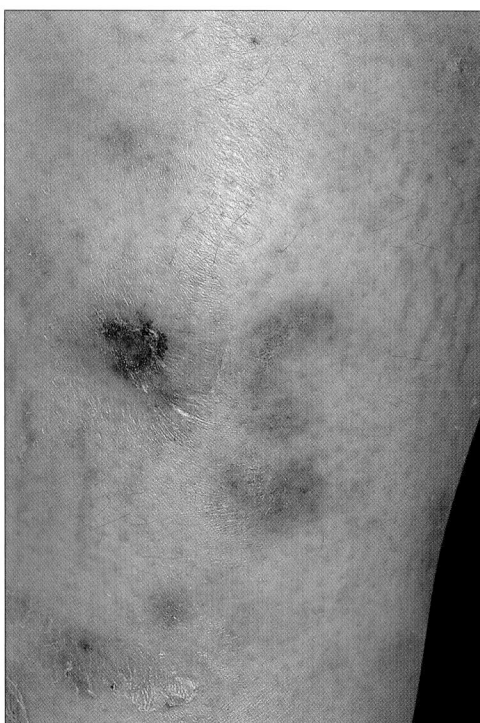

Fig. 100.22 Cytophagic histiocytic panniculitis. Subcutaneous nodules with purpura. Courtesy of Kenneth E Greer MD.

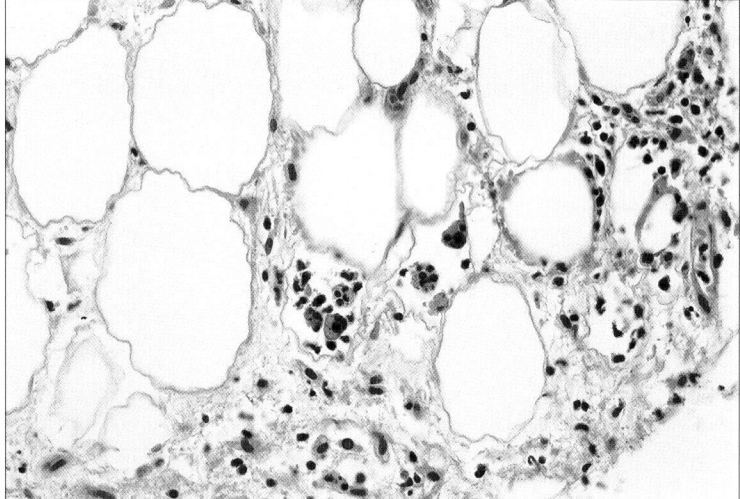

Fig. 100.23 Cytophagic histiocytic panniculitis. Macrophages engaged in cytophagic activity. Some of them have the appearance of 'bean bag cells'.

macrophages, neutrophils and plasma cells[157,158]. Macrophages, some of them enlarged but not otherwise atypical, contain erythrocytes, lymphocytes or karyorrhectic debris. These are often described as 'bean bag cells'[157,158] (Fig. 100.23). Atypical lymphoid cells can usually be identified in those cases associated with subcutaneous panniculitis-like T-cell lymphoma, and a diagnosis of lymphoma can be supported by immunophenotyping or gene rearrangement studies. In rapidly progressive or fatal cases, cytophagic changes can be seen in other organs, including lymph nodes, spleen, liver and bone marrow (leading to pancytopenia)[142].

Differential diagnosis

The clinical features of the more florid cases are diagnostic, while the subcutaneous nodules occurring in 'benign' forms of the disease can be confused with other forms of panniculitis. Biopsy is usually definitive, because of the characteristic feature of cytophagocytosis. More problematic is the question of whether a given patient with cytophagic histiocytic panniculitis has a lymphoma or a non-neoplastic disorder. Immunophenotyping and genotypic studies are helpful in this regard, but, even in the face of negative results, an evolving lymphoma is still possible[143,153].

Treatment

Treatments for cytophagic histiocytic panniculitis have included prednisone, cyclosporine and dapsone[142]. Cytotoxic chemotherapy with hematopoietic cell rescue has been recommended for aggressive disease[159]. Patients with subcutaneous panniculitis-like T-cell lymphoma have been managed with a variety of forms of combination chemotherapy, particularly the CHOP regimen (cyclophosphamide, doxorubicin, vincristine, prednisone)[142], but prolonged remissions are uncommon.

MALIGNANT SUBCUTANEOUS INFILTRATES

Malignant infiltrates may involve the subcutis, mimicking the clinical and microscopic appearance of panniculitis. The best known of these is subcutaneous panniculitis-like T-cell lymphoma, in which cytophagia is usually prominent[159a]. As mentioned above, examples of subcutaneous B-cell lymphoma[160] and lymphoma with a natural killer cell phenotype[161,162] have also been reported. Other lymphomas, leukemias and metastatic solid tumors may infiltrate the subcutis. For example, a case of melanophagic panniculitis that obscured foci of metastatic melanoma has been reported[163]. Clinical information is crucial in such cases. Histopathologic clues include the recognition of significant pleomorphism or monotony among infiltrating cells in the subcutis, infiltration between collagen bundles of the dermis or around adnexal structures, and supporting immunohistochemical studies. The diagnosis of subcutaneous panniculitis-like T-cell lymphoma can be elusive. Individuals who initially presented as non-specific panniculitis with lipomembranous changes[164] or with interface dermatitis and other features suggesting lupus panniculitis have been described[165].

OTHER CONSIDERATIONS IN THE DIAGNOSIS OF PANNICULITIS

Weber–Christian Disease

This condition, also known as 'relapsing febrile non-suppurative panniculitis', was described by Weber, Christian, and others in the 1920s. It has been said to consist of recurrent subcutaneous nodules that heal with depression of the overlying skin. Involvement of peri-visceral fat, systemic symptoms, and sometimes a fatal outcome have been reported. Microscopically, there are three phases, consisting of an acute neutrophilic lobular panniculitis, subacute adipocyte necrosis and foam cell formation, and chronic fibrosis. Unfortunately, these changes are recapitulated in a wide variety of panniculitides and, therefore, must be considered non-specific. Doubts about the existence of Weber–Christian disease as a specific nosologic entity were raised at least as early as the 1960s. This view has been supported by subsequent studies in which cases initially bearing this designation have been reclassified as erythema nodosum, lipodermatosclerosis, traumatic panniculitis, cytophagic histiocytic panniculitis, α_1-antitrypsin deficiency panniculitis, or lupus panniculitis[62,166]. While definitely of historic interest, most authorities recommend that the term 'Weber–Christian disease' be abandoned in favor of more specific diagnostic entities.

Painful Plantar Erythema (Idiopathic Palmoplantar Hidradenitis; Plantar Panniculitis)

The sudden onset of painful erythematous nodules on the soles and, less frequently, the palms in otherwise healthy children characterizes *idiopathic palmoplantar hidradenitis*, a self-limited form of neutrophilic eccrine hidradenitis that may be precipitated by mechanical and thermal trauma (see Ch. 40)[167,168]. Painful plantar erythema can also be a manifestation of several forms of panniculitis (e.g. erythema nodosum, cold panniculitis) as well as traumatic plantar urticaria, vasculitis and the 'pseudomonas hot-foot syndrome'.

Crystal Deposition Diseases Associated With Panniculitis

There are several disorders characterized by crystal deposition that can present as panniculitis. In *calciphylaxis*, calcium is deposited in small vessels of the subcutis (of arteriolar or lesser size), in association with fat necrosis and varying degrees of inflammation (see Ch. 50). A similar necrotizing panniculitis can occur due to vascular deposits of calcium oxalate in patients with *hyperoxaluria* (see Ch. 24)[169]. In *hyperuricemia* (gout), sodium urate crystals can be deposited in the subcutis (see Ch. 48).

REFERENCES

1. Braverman IM. Protective effects of erythema nodosum in coccidioidomycosis. Lancet. 1999;353:168.
2. Cohen PR, Holder WR, Rapini RP. Concurrent Sweet's syndrome and erythema nodosum: a report, world literature review and mechanism of pathogenesis. J Rheumatol. 1992;19:814–20.
3. White WL, Hitchcock MG. Diagnosis: erythema nodosum or not? Semin Cutan Med Surg. 1999;18:47–55.
4. Cribier B, Caille A, Heid E, et al. Erythema nodosum and associated diseases. A study of 129 cases. Int J Dermatol. 1998;37:667–72.
5. Garcia-Porrua C, Gonzalez-Gay MA, Vazquez-Caruncho M, et al. Erythema nodosum: etiologic and predictive factors in a defined population. Arthritis Rheum. 2000;43:584–92.
6. Honma T, Bang D, Lee S, et al. Ultrastructure of endothelial cell necrosis in classical erythema nodosum. Hum Pathol. 1993;24:384–90.
7. Llorente L, Richaud-Patin Y, Alvarado C, et al. Elevated Th1 cytokine mRNA in skin biopsies and peripheral circulation in patients with erythema nodosum. Eur Cytokine Netw. 1997;8:67–71.
8. Senturk T, Aydintug O, Kuzu I, A et al. Adhesion molecule expression in erythema nodosum-like lesions in Behçet's disease. A histopathological and immunohistochemical study. Rheumatol Inl. 1998;18:51–7.
9. Kunz M, Beutel S, Brocker E. Leucocyte activation in erythema nodosum. Clin Exp Dermatol. 1999;24:396–401.
10. Wallace SL. Erythema nodosum treatment with colchicine. JAMA. 1967;202:1056.
11. Nomiyama J, Shinohara K, Inoue H. Erythema nodosum caused by the administration of granulocyte colony-stimulating factor in a patient with refractory anemia. Am J Hematol. 1994;47:333.
12. Winter HS. Treatment of pyoderma gangrenosum, erythema nodosum, and aphthous ulcerations. Inflamm Bowel Dis. 1998;4:71.
13. Mert A, Ozaras R, Tabak F, Pekmezci S, Demirkesen C, Ozturk R. Erythema nodosum: an experience of 10 years. Scand J Infect Dis. 2004;36:424–7.
14. Hanauer SB. How do I treat erythema nodosum, aphthous ulcerations, and pyoderma gangrenosum? Inflamm Bowel Dis. 1998;4:70; discussion 78.
15. Arsura EL, Kilgore WB, Ratnayake SN. Erythema nodosum in pregnant patients with coccidioidomycosis. Clin Infect Dis. 1998;27:1201–3.
15a. Thurber S, Kohler S. Histopathologic spectrum of erythema nodosum. J Cutan Pathol. 2006;33:18–26.
16. Winkelmann RK, Frigas E. Eosinophilic panniculitis: a clinicopathologic study. J Cutan Pathol. 1986;13:1–12.
17. Sanchez Yus E, Sanz Vico MD, de Diego V. Miescher's radial granuloma. A characteristic marker of erythema nodosum. Am J Dermatopathol. 1989;11:434–42.
18. Ball NJ, Adams SP, Marx LH, et al. Possible origin of pancreatic fat necrosis as a septal panniculitis. J Am Acad Dermatol. 1996;34:362–4.
19. Patterson JW, Brown PC, Broecker AH. Infection-induced panniculitis. J Cutan Pathol. 1989;16:183–93.
20. Horio T, Imamura S, Danno K, et al. Potassium iodide in the treatment of erythema nodosum and nodular vasculitis. Arch Dermatol. 1981;117:29–31.
21. Banks PA, Present DH. Treatment of erythema nodosum, aphthous stomatitis, and pyoderma gangrenosum in patients with IBD. Inflamm Bowel Dis. 1998;4:73.
22. Bafverstedt B. Erythema nodosum migrans. Acta Derm Venereol. 1954;34:181–93.
23. Vilanova X, Piñol Aguade J. Subacute nodular migratory panniculitis. Br J Dermatol. 1959;71:45–50.
24. de Almeida Prestes C, Winkelmann RK, Su WP. Septal granulomatous panniculitis: comparison of the pathology of erythema nodosum migrans (migratory panniculitis) and chronic erythema nodosum. J Am Acad Dermatol. 1990;22:477–83.
25. Ross M, White GM, Barr RJ. Erythematous plaque on the leg. Vilanova's disease (subacute nodular migratory panniculitis). Arch Dermatol. 1992;128:1644–5, 1647.
26. Su WP, Person JR. Morphea profunda. A new concept and a histopathologic study of 23 cases. Am J Dermatopathol. 1981;3:251–60.
27. Winkelmann RK. Panniculitis in connective tissue disease. Arch Dermatol. 1983;119:336–44.
28. Peters MS, Su WP. Eosinophils in lupus panniculitis and morphea profunda. J Cutan Pathol. 1991;18:189–92.
29. Fleischmajer R, Damiano V, Nedwich A. Alteration of subcutaneous tissue in systemic scleroderma. Arch Dermatol. 1972;105:59–66.
30. Vincent F, Prokopetz R, Miller RA. Plasma cell panniculitis: a unique clinical and pathologic presentation of linear scleroderma. J Am Acad Dermatol. 1989;21:357–60.
31. Fleischmajer R, Nedwich A. Generalized morphea. I. Histology of the dermis and subcutaneous tissue. Arch Dermatol. 1972;106:509–14.
32. Patterson JW. Differential diagnosis of panniculitis. Adv Dermatol. 1991;6:309–29.
33. Eriksson S. Alpha 1-antitrypsin deficiency: lessons learned from the bedside to the gene and back again. Historic perspectives. Chest. 1989;95:181–9.
34. O'Riordan K, Blei A, Rao MS, et al. Alpha 1-antitrypsin deficiency-associated panniculitis: resolution with intravenous alpha 1-antitrypsin administration and liver transplantation. Transplantation. 1997;63:480–2.
35. Pittelkow MR, Smith KC, Su WP. Alpha-1-antitrypsin deficiency and panniculitis. Perspectives on disease relationship and replacement therapy. Am J Med. 1988;84:80–6.
36. American Thoracic Society/European Respiratory Society statement: standards for the diagnosis and

management of individuals with alpha-1 antitrypsin deficiency. Am J Respir Crit Care Med. 2003;168:818–900.

37. Irvine C, Neild V, Stephens C, et al. Alpha-1-antitrypsin deficiency panniculitis. J R Soc Med. 1990;83:743–4.

38. Su WP, Smith KC, Pittelkow MR, et al. Alpha 1-antitrypsin deficiency panniculitis: a histopathologic and immunopathologic study of four cases. Am J Dermatopathol. 1987;9:483–90.

39. Arora PK, Miller HC, Aronson LD. Alpha 1-antitrypsin is an effector of immunological stasis. Nature. 1978;274:589–90.

40. Breit SN, Penny R. The role of alpha 1 protease inhibitor (alpha 1 antitrypsin) in the regulation of immunologic and inflammatory reactions. Aust NZ J Med. 1980;10:449–53.

41. Smith KC, Pittelkow MR, Su WP. Panniculitis associated with severe alpha 1-antitrypsin deficiency. Treatment and review of the literature. Arch Dermatol. 1987;123:1655–61.

42. Yesudian PD, Dobson CM, Wilson NJ. α1-Antitrypsin deficiency panniculitis (phenotype PiZZ) precipitated postpartum and successfully treated with dapsone. Br J Dermatol. 2004;150:1222–3.

43. Geller JD, Su WP. A subtle clue to the histopathologic diagnosis of early alpha 1-antitrypsin deficiency panniculitis. J Am Acad Dermatol. 1994;31:241–5.

44. Hendrick SJ, Silverman AK, Solomon AR, et al. Alpha 1-antitrypsin deficiency associated with panniculitis. J Am Acad Dermatol. 1988;18:684–92.

45. Viraben R, Massip P, Dicostanzo B, et al. Necrotic panniculitis with alpha-1 antitrypsin deficiency. J Am Acad Dermatol. 1986;14:684–7.

46. Humbert P, Faivre B, Gibey R, et al. Use of anti-collagenase properties of doxycycline in treatment of alpha 1-antitrypsin deficiency panniculitis. Acta Derm Venereol. 1991;71:189–94.

47. Furey NL, Golden RS, Potts SR. Treatment of alpha-1-antitrypsin deficiency, massive edema, and panniculitis with alpha-1 protease inhibitor. Ann Intern Med. 1996;125:699.

48. Degitz K, Messer G, Schirren H, et al. Successful treatment of erythema induratum of bazin following rapid detection of mycobacterial DNA by polymerase chain reaction [letter]. Arch Dermatol. 1993;129:1619–20.

49. Cho KH, Lee DY, Kim CW. Erythema induratum of Bazin. Int J Dermatol. 1996;35:802–8.

50. Baselga E, Margall N, Barnadas MA, et al. Detection of Mycobacterium tuberculosis DNA in lobular granulomatous panniculitis (erythema induratum-nodular vasculitis). Arch Dermatol. 1997;133:457–62.

51. Chuang YH, Kuo TT, Wang CM, et al. Simultaneous occurrence of papulonecrotic tuberculide and erythema induratum and the identification of Mycobacterium tuberculosis DNA by polymerase chain reaction. Br J Dermatol. 1997;137:276–81.

52. Schneider JW, Jordaan HF, Geiger DH, et al. Erythema induratum of Bazin. A clinicopathological study of 20 cases and detection of Mycobacterium tuberculosis DNA in skin lesions by polymerase chain reaction. Am J Dermatopathol. 1995;17:350–6.

53. Tan SH, Tan BH, Goh CL, et al. Detection of Mycobacterium tuberculosis DNA using polymerase chain reaction in cutaneous tuberculosis and tuberculids. Int J Dermatol. 1999;38:122–7.

54. Wolf D, Ben-Yehuda A, Okon E, et al. Nodular vasculitis associated with propylthiouracil therapy. Cutis. 1992;49:253–5.

55. Gimenez-Garcia R, Sanchez-Ramon S, Sanchez-Antolin G, Velasco Fernandez C. Red fingers syndrome and recurrent panniculitis in a patient with chronic hepatitis C. J Eur Acad Dermatol Venereol. 2003;17:692–4.

56. Ollert MW, Thomas P, Korting HC, et al. Erythema induratum of Bazin. Evidence of T-lymphocyte hyperresponsiveness to purified protein derivative of tuberculin: report of two cases and treatment. Arch Dermatol. 1993;129:469–73.

57. Schneider JW, Jordaan HF. The histopathologic spectrum of erythema induratum of Bazin [see comments]. Am J Dermatopathol. 1997;19:323–33.

58. Smolle J, Kneifel H. S-100-protein-positive dendritic cells in nodular vasculitis. Dermatologica. 1986;172:139–43.

59. Koga T, Kubota Y, Kiryu H, et al. Erythema induratum in a patient with active tuberculosis of the axillary lymph node: IFN-gamma release of specific T cells. Eur J Dermatol. 2001;11:48–9.

60. Jacinto SS, Nograles KB. Erythema induratum of bazin: role of polymerase chain reaction in diagnosis. Int J Dermatol. 2003;42:380–1.

61. Shaffer N, Kerdel FA. Nodular vasculitis (erythema induratum): treatment with auranofin. J Am Acad Dermatol. 1991;25:426–9.

61a. Taverna JA, Radfar A, Pentland A, et al. Case reports: nodular vasculitis responsive to mycophenolate mofetil. J Drugs Dermatol. 2006;5:992–3.

62. Forstrom T, Winkelmann RK. Acute, generalized panniculitis with amylase and lipase in skin. Arch Dermatol. 1975;111:497–502.

63. Heykarts B, Anseeuw M, Degreef H. Panniculitis caused by acinous pancreatic carcinoma. Dermatology. 1999;198:182–3.

64. Francombe J, Kingsnorth AN, Tunn E. Panniculitis, arthritis and pancreatitis. Br J Rheumatol. 1995;34:680–3.

65. Bennett RG, Petrozzi JW. Nodular subcutaneous fat necrosis. A manifestation of silent pancreatitis. Arch Dermatol. 1975;111:896–8.

66. Berman B, Conteas C, Smith B, et al. Fatal pancreatitis presenting with subcutaneous fat necrosis. Evidence that lipase and amylase alone do not induce lipocyte necrosis. J Am Acad Dermatol. 1987;17:359–64.

67. Preiss JC, Faiss S, Loddenkemper C, Zeitz M, Duchmann R. Pancreatic panniculitis in an 88-year-old man with neuroendocrine carcinoma. Digestion. 2002;66:193–6.

68. Fretzin DF, Arias AM. Sclerema neonatorum and subcutaneous fat necrosis of the newborn. Pediatr Dermatol. 1987;4:112–22.

69. Proks C, Valvoda V. Fatty crystals in sclerema neonatorum. J Clin Pathol. 1966;19:193–5.

70. Milunsky A, Levin SE. Sclerema neonatorum: a clinical study of 79 cases. S Afr Med J. 1966;40:638–41.

71. Mogilner BM, Alkalay A, Nissim F, et al. Subcutaneous fat necrosis of the newborn. Clin Pediatr (Phila). 1981;20:748–50.

72. Pasyk K. Sclerema neonatorum. Light and electron microscopic studies. Virchows Arch A Pathol Anat Histol. 1980;388:87–103.

73. Ferguson CK. Care of the infant with sclerema neonatorum. JOGN Nurs. 1983;12:391–4.

74. Burden AD, Krafchik BR. Subcutaneous fat necrosis of the newborn: a review of 11 cases. Pediatr Dermatol. 1999;16:384–7.

75. Chuang SD, Chiu HC, Chang CC. Subcutaneous fat necrosis of the newborn complicating hypothermic cardiac surgery. Br J Dermatol. 1995;132:805–10.

76. Hicks MJ, Levy ML, Alexander J, et al. Subcutaneous fat necrosis of the newborn and hypercalcemia: case report and review of the literature. Pediatr Dermatol. 1993;10:271–6.

77. Norton KI, Som PM, Shugar JM, et al. Subcutaneous fat necrosis of the newborn: CT findings of head and neck involvement. AJNR Am J Neuroradiol. 1997;18:547–50.

78. Anderson DR, Narla LD, Dunn NL. Subcutaneous fat necrosis of the newborn. Pediatr Radiol. 1999;29:794–6.

79. Bachrach LK, Lum CK. Etidronate in subcutaneous fat necrosis of the newborn. J Pediatr. 1999;135:530–1.

80. Wolach B, Raas-Rothschild A, Vogel R, et al. Subcutaneous fat necrosis with thrombocytopenia in a newborn infant. Dermatologica. 1990;181:54–5.

81. Khan N, Licata A, Rogers D. Intravenous bisphosphonates for hypercalcemia accompanying subcutaneous fat necrosis: a novel treatment approach. Clin Pediatr. 2001;40:217–19.

82. Smith RT, Good RA. Sequelae of prednisone treatment of acute rheumatic fever. Clin Res Proc. 1956;4:156–7.

83. Roenigk HH Jr, Haserick JR, Arundell FD. Poststeroid panniculitis. Arch Dermatol. 1964;90:387–91.

84. Silverman RA, Newman AJ, LeVine MJ, et al. Poststeroid panniculitis: a case report. Pediatr Dermatol. 1988;5:92–3.

85. Reichel M, Diaz Cascajo C. Bilateral jawline nodules in a child with a brain-stem glioma. Poststeroid panniculitis. Arch Dermatol. 1995;131:1448–9, 1451–2.

86. Nitta Y. Lupus erythematosus profundus associated with neonatal lupus erythematosus [see comments]. Br J Dermatol. 1997;136:112–14.

87. Peters MS, Su WP. Lupus erythematosus panniculitis. Med Clin North Am. 1989;73:1113–26.

88. Martens PB, Moder KG, Ahmed I. Lupus panniculitis: clinical perspectives from a case series. J Rheumatol. 1999;26:68–72.

89. Riccieri V, Sili Scavalli A, Spadaro A, et al. Lupus erythematosus panniculitis: an immunohistochemical study. Clin Rheumatol. 1994;13:641–4.

90. Burrows NP, Walport MJ, Hammond AH, et al. Lupus erythematosus profundus with partial C4 deficiency responding to thalidomide. Br J Dermatol. 1991;125:62–7.

91. Chung HS, Hann SK. Lupus panniculitis treated by a combination therapy of hydroxychloroquine and quinacrine. J Dermatol. 1997;24:569–72.

92. Ng PP, Tan SH, Tan T. Lupus erythematosus panniculitis: a clinicopathologic study. Int J Dermatol. 2002;41:488–90.

93. Sanchez NP, Peters MS, Winkelmann RK. The histopathology of lupus erythematosus panniculitis. J Am Acad Dermatol. 1981;5:673–80.

94. Massone C, Kodama K, Salmhofer W, et al. Lupus erythematosus panniculitis (lupus profundus): clinical, histopathological, and molecular analysis of nine cases. J Cutan Pathol. 2005;32:396–404.

95. Lee MW, Lim YS, Choi JH, et al. Panniculitis showing membranocystic changes in the dermatomyositis. J Dermatol. 1999;26:608–10.

96. Solans R, Cortes J, Selva A, et al. Panniculitis: a cutaneous manifestation of dermatomyositis. J Am Acad Dermatol. 2002;46(5 suppl.):S148–50.

97. Molnar K, Kemeny L, Korom I, et al. Panniculitis in dermatomyositis: report of two cases. Br J Dermatol. 1998;139:161–3.

98. Neidenbach PJ, Sahn EE, Helton J. Panniculitis in juvenile dermatomyositis. J Am Acad Dermatol. 1995;33:305–7.

99. Ghali FE, Reed AM, Groben PA, et al. Panniculitis in juvenile dermatomyositis. Pediatr Dermatol. 1999;16:270–2.

100. Lemez L. Beitrag zur Pathogenese der subcutanen Fettgewebsnekrose Neugeborener (Sog. Sclerodermia neonatorum) an der Hand. Einer Kalterreaktion des subcutanen Fettgewebes bei Neugeborenen und jungen Sauglingen. Zeitung der Kinderheilkunden. 1928;46.

101. Epstein EH Jr, Oren ME. Popsicle panniculitis. N Engl J Med. 1970;282:966–7.

102. Behar TA, Anderson EE, Barwick WJ, et al. Sclerosing lipogranulomatosis: a case report of scrotal injection of automobile transmission fluid and literature review of subcutaneous injection of oils. Plast Reconstr Surg. 1993;91:352–61.

103. Beacham BE, Cooper PH, Buchanan CS, et al. Equestrian cold panniculitis in women. Arch Dermatol. 1980;116:1025–7.

104. Oertel YC, Johnson FB. Sclerosing lipogranuloma of male genitalia. Review of 23 cases. Arch Pathol Lab Med. 1977;101:321–6.

105. Carrasco L, Moreno C, Pastor MA, et al. Postirradiation pseudosclerodermatous panniculitis. Am J Dermatopathol. 2001;23:283–7.

106. Borroni G, Vassallo C, Brazzelli V, et al. Radiation recall dermatitis, panniculitis, and myositis following cyclophosphamide therapy: histopathologic findings of a patient affected by multiple myeloma. Am J Dermatopathol. 2004;26:213–16.

107. Rajkumar SV, Laude TA, Russo RM, et al. Popsicle panniculitis of the cheeks. A diagnostic entity caused by sucking on cold objects. Clin Pediatr (Phila). 1976;15:619–21.

108. Pang BK, Munro V, Kossard S. Pseudoscleroderma secondary to phytomenadione (vitamin K1) injections: Texier's disease. Australas J Dermatol. 1996;37:44–7.

109. Kossard S, Ecker RI, Dicken CH. Povidone panniculitis. Polyvinylpyrrolidone panniculitis. Arch Dermatol. 1980;116:704–6.

110. McCain J, West TW, Vasey FB, et al. Intramuscular aurothioglucose (Solganal) leading to panniculitis. J Rheumatol. 1993;20:1632–3.

111. Baars JW, Coenen JL, Wagstaff J, et al. Lobular panniculitis after subcutaneous administration of interleukin-2 (IL-2), and its exacerbation during intravenous therapy with IL-2. Br J Cancer. 1992;66:698–9.

112. Garcia-Domingo MI, Alijotas-Reig J, Cistero-Bahima A, et al. Disseminated and recurrent sarcoid-like granulomatous panniculitis due to bovine collagen injection. J Investig Allergol Clin Immunol. 2000;10:107–9.

113. Winkelmann RK, Barker SM. Factitial traumatic panniculitis. J Am Acad Dermatol. 1985;13:988–94.

114. Hultcrantz E. Haxthausen's disease. Cold panniculitis in children. J Laryngol Otol. 1986;100:1329–32.

115. Foucar E, Downing DT, Gerber WL. Sclerosing lipogranuloma of the male genitalia containing vitamin E: a comparison with classical 'paraffinoma'. J Am Acad Dermatol. 1983;9:103–10.

116. Takihara H, Takahashi M, Ueno T, et al. Sclerosing lipogranuloma of the male genitalia: analysis of the lipid constituents and histological study. Br J Urol. 1993;71:58–62.

117. Henrichs WD, Helwig EB. Grease gun granulomas. Mil Med. 1986;151:78–82.

118. Claudy A, Garcier F, Schmitt D. Sclerosing lipogranuloma of the male genitalia: ultrastructural study. Br J Dermatol. 1981;105:451–6.

119. Oh C, Ginsberg-Fellner F, Dolger H. Factitial panniculitis and necrotizing fasciitis in juvenile diabetes. Diabetes. 1975;24:856–8.

120. Robenzadeh A, Don PC, Davis I, et al. Sclerosing lipogranuloma secondary to supposed vitamin E injection for facial rejuvenation: successful treatment with intralesional steroids. Dermatol Surg. 1998;24:1036–7.

121. Huriez C. Ulceres de jambes et troubles trophiques d'origine veineuse (donnes tirees de l'etude d'un millier d'ulcereux hospitalises). Rev Pract. 1955;5:2703–21.

122. Jorizzo JL, White WL, Zanolli MD, et al. Sclerosing panniculitis. A clinicopathologic assessment. Arch Dermatol. 1991;127:554–8.

123. Kirsner RS, Pardes JB, Eaglstein WH, et al. The clinical spectrum of lipodermatosclerosis. J Am Acad Dermatol. 1993;28:623–7.

124. Greenberg AS, Hasan A, Montalvo BM, et al. Acute lipodermatosclerosis is associated with venous insufficiency. J Am Acad Dermatol. 1996;35:566–8.

125. Stacey MC, Burnand KG, Bhogal BS, et al. Pericapillary fibrin deposits and skin hypoxia precede the changes of lipodermatosclerosis in limbs at increased risk of developing a venous ulcer. Cardiovasc Surg. 2000;8:372–80.

126. Falanga V, Bontempo FA, Eaglstein WH. Protein C and protein S plasma levels in patients with lipodermatosclerosis and venous ulceration. Arch Dermatol. 1990;126:1195–7.

127. Segal S, Cooper J, Bolognia J. Treatment of lipodermatosclerosis with oxandrolone in a patient with stanozolol-induced hepatotoxicity. J Am Acad Dermatol. 2000;43:558–9.

128. Alegre VA, Winkelmann RK, Aliaga A. Lipomembranous changes in chronic panniculitis. J Am Acad Dermatol. 1988;19:39–46.

129. Demitsu T, Okada O, Yoneda K, et al. Lipodermatosclerosis – report of three cases and review of the literature. Dermatology. 1999;199:271–3.

130. Ishikawa O, Tamura A, Ryuzaki K, et al. Membranocystic changes in the panniculitis of dermatomyositis. Br J Dermatol. 1996;134:773–6.

131. Goldman MP. The use of pentoxifylline in the treatment of systemic sclerosis and lipodermatosclerosis: a unifying hypothesis? J Am Acad Dermatol. 1994;31:135–6.

132. Maioriello RP, Merwin CF. North American blastomycosis presenting as an acute panniculitis and arthritis. Arch Dermatol. 1970;102:92–6.

133. Sanderson TL, Moskowitz L, Hensley GT, et al. Disseminated Mycobacterium avium-intracellulare infection appearing as a panniculitis. Arch Pathol Lab Med. 1982;106:112–14.

134. Guynes RD, Huey RL, McMullan MR, et al. Case records of the Department of Medicine University of Mississippi Medical Center. Acute panniculitis secondary to fungal infection, most likely Aspergillus species. J Miss State Med Assoc. 1996;37:610–15.

135. Nauta RJ. A radical approach to bacterial panniculitis of the abdominal wall in the morbidly obese. Surgery. 1990;107:134–9.

136. Palmeiro Fernandez G, Sanchez Burson J, Martinez Gomez W, Atanes Sandoval A. [Xanthomonas maltophilia in a case of mixed infectious panniculitis]. Med Clin (Barc). 1992;98:516.

137. Pao W, Duncan KO, Bolognia JL, et al. Numerous eruptive lesions of panniculitis associated with group A streptococcus bacteremia in an immunocompetent child. Clin Infect Dis. 1998;27:430–3.

138. Farnsworth GA. Case for diagnosis. Panniculitis, pyogranulomatous, diffuse, severe, with numerous fungal aggregates; etiology consistent with deep dermatophytosis. Mil Med. 1990;155:618, 622.

139. Skaria AM, Chavaz P, Hauser C. [Metastatic aspergillus panniculitis in blast transformation of a myelodysplastic syndrome and agranulocytosis]. Hautarzt. 1995;46:579–81.

140. Ginter G, Rieger E, Soyer HP, et al. Granulomatous panniculitis caused by Candida albicans: a case presenting with multiple leg ulcers. J Am Acad Dermatol. 1993;28:315–17.

141. Galache C, Santos-Juanes J, Blanco S, Rodriguez E, Martinez A, Soto J. Q fever: a new cause of 'doughnut' granulomatous lobular panniculitis. Br J Dermatol. 2004;151:685–7.

142. Marzano AV, Berti E, Paulli M, Caputo R. Cytophagic histiocytic panniculitis and subcutaneous panniculitis-like T-cell lymphoma: report of 7 cases. Arch Dermatol. 2000;136:889–96.

143. Wick MR, Patterson JW. Cytophagic histiocytic panniculitis – a critical reappraisal. Arch Dermatol. 2000;136:9224.

144. Winkelmann RK, Bowie EJ. Hemorrhagic diathesis associated with benign histiocytic, cytophagic panniculitis and systemic histiocytosis. Arch Intern Med. 1980;140:1460–3.

145. Gonzalez CL, Medeiros LJ, Braziel RM, et al. T-cell lymphoma involving subcutaneous tissue. A clinicopathologic entity commonly associated with hemophagocytic syndrome. Am J Surg Pathol. 1991;15:17–27.

146. Barron DR, Davis BR, Pomeranz JR, et al. Cytophagic histiocytic panniculitis. A variant of malignant histiocytosis. Cancer. 1985;55:2538–42.

147. Craig AJ, Cualing H, Thomas G, et al. Cytophagic histiocytic panniculitis – a syndrome associated with benign and malignant panniculitis: case comparison and review of the literature. J Am Acad Dermatol. 1998;39:721–36.

148. Yanagawa T, Yokoyama A, Noya K, et al. Cytophagic histiocytic panniculitis evolving into total lipodystrophy. South Med J. 1990;83:1323–6.

149. Willemze R, Jaffe ES, Burg G , et al. WHO-EORTC classification for cutaneous lymphomas. Blood. 2005;105:3768–85.

150. Iwatsuki K, Harada H, Ohtsuka M, Han G, Kaneko F. Latent Epstein-Barr virus infection is frequently detected in subcutaneous lymphoma associated with hemophagocytosis but not in nonfatal cytophagic histiocytic panniculitis [letter; comment]. Arch Dermatol. 1997;133:787–8.

151. Tsukahara T, Fujioka A, Horiuchi Y, et al. A case of cytophagic histiocytic panniculitis with sicca symptoms and lupus nephritis. J Dermatol. 1992;19:563–9.

152. Tsukahara T, Horiuchi Y, Iidaka K. Cytophagic histiocytic panniculitis in systemic lupus erythematosus. Hiroshima J Med Sci. 1995;44:13–16.

153. Sajben FP, Schmidt C. Subcutaneous T-cell lymphoma: a case report and additional observations. Cutis. 1996;58:297–302.

154. Okamura T, Niho Y. Cytophagic histiocytic panniculitis – what is the best therapy? Intern Med. 1999;38:224–5.

155. Willis SM, Opal SM, Fitzpatrick JE. Cytophagic histiocytic panniculitis. Systemic histiocytosis presenting as chronic, nonhealing, ulcerative skin lesions. Arch Dermatol. 1985;121:910–13.

156. Crotty CP, Winkelmann RK. Cytophagic histiocytic panniculitis with fever, cytopenia, liver failure, and terminal hemorrhagic diathesis. J Am Acad Dermatol. 1981;4:181–94.

157. White JW Jr, Winkelmann RK. Cytophagic histiocytic panniculitis is not always fatal. J Cutan Pathol. 1989;16:137–44.

158. Hytiroglou P, Phelps RG, Wattenberg DJ, Strauchen JA. Histiocytic cytophagic panniculitis: molecular evidence for a clonal T-cell disorder. J Am Acad Dermatol. 1992;27:333–6. Erratum in: J Am Acad Dermatol 1992;27:900.

159. Koizumi K, Sawada K, Nishio M, et al. Effective high-dose chemotherapy followed by autologous peripheral blood stem cell transplantation in a patient with the aggressive form of cytophagic histiocytic panniculitis. Bone Marrow Transplant. 1997;20:171–3.

159a. Aguilera P, Mascaro JM Jr, Martinez A, et al. Cutaneous gamma/delta T-cell lymphoma: a histopathologic mimicker of lupus erythematosus profundus (lupus panniculitis). J Am Acad Dermatol. 2007;56:643–7.

160. Matsuoka LY. Neoplastic erythema nodosum. J Am Acad Dermatol. 1995;32:361–3.

161. Yamashita Y, Tsuzuki T, Nakayama A, et al. A case of natural killer/T cell lymphoma of the subcutis resembling subcutaneous panniculitis-like T cell lymphoma. Pathol Int. 1999;49:241–6.

162. Dargent JL, Roufosse C, Delville JP, et al. Subcutaneous panniculitis-like T-cell lymphoma: further evidence for a distinct neoplasm originating from large granular lymphocytes of T/NK phenotype. J Cutan Pathol. 1998;25:394–400.

163. Pierard GE. Melanophagic dermatitis and panniculitis. A condition revealing an occult metastatic malignant melanoma. Am J Dermatopathol. 1988;10:133–6.

164. Weenig RH, Ng CS, Perniciaro C. Subcutaneous panniculitis-like T-cell lymphoma: an elusive case presenting as lipomembranous panniculitis and a review of 72 cases in the literature. Am J Dermatopathol. 2001;23:206–15.

165. Cassis TB, Fearneyhough PK, Callen JP. Subcutaneous panniculitis-like T-cell lymphoma with vacuolar interface dermatitis resembling lupus erythematosus panniculitis. J Am Acad Dermatol. 2004;50:465–9

166. White JW Jr, Winkelmann RK. Weber-Christian panniculitis: a review of 30 cases with this diagnosis. J Am Acad Dermatol. 1998;39:56–62.

167. Buezo GF, Requena L, Fraga Fernandez J, et al. Idiopathic palmoplantar hidradenitis. Am J Dermatopathol. 1996;18:413–16.

168. Rabinowitz LG, Cintra ML, Hood AF, Esterly NB. Recurrent palmoplantar hidradenitis in children. Arch Dermatol. 1995;131:817–20.

169. Somach SC, Davis BR, Paras FA, et al. Fatal cutaneous necrosis mimicking calciphylaxis in a patient with type 1 primary hyperoxaluria. Arch Dermatol. 1995;131:821–3.

Lipodystrophies

101

Jacqueline M Junkins-Hopkins, Alison Sharpe Avram and Mathew Avram

Synonyms: Lipodystrophy: lipoatrophy, lipohypertrophy

Key features

- Lipoatrophy is characterized by a paucity or complete absence of fat that may be generalized, partial or localized, and may be familial or acquired
- Lipodystrophy and lipoatrophy often coexist, and the terms are often used interchangeably, with lipodystrophy implying a redistribution of fat, in part due to a hypertrophic compensation of the non-atrophic fat
- Lipodystrophy syndromes are a heterogeneous group of disorders that are characterized by lipoatrophy and fat accumulation in characteristic body distribution patterns
- Fat is a metabolically active organ, thus fat loss is associated with metabolic derangements, which parallel the extent and duration of lipoatrophy.
- Patients with lipodystrophy typically develop the metabolic syndrome, which includes insulin resistance, diabetes mellitus, hyperinsulinemia, hypertriglyceridemia, cardiovascular disease and fatty liver. This association has provided insights into the pathogenesis of coronary artery disease and diabetes mellitus
- Generalized and partial lipodystrophy syndromes present in conjunction with systemic associations, including medical complications of the metabolic syndrome, hormonal abnormalities, organ dysfunction, anabolic syndrome, glomerulonephritis and autoimmune disorders
- A distinct syndrome of peripheral lipoatrophy, central and visceral obesity, breast hypertrophy, dorsocervical pad enlargement, hyperlipidemia and insulin resistance occurs in patients with HIV infection undergoing treatment with highly active antiretroviral therapy (HAART)
- Isolated or localized lipoatrophy can occur at the site of medication injection, trauma or pressure, in association with autoimmune connective tissue disease, following certain pannicultic inflammatory or neoplastic processes, or due to idiopathic causes
- Microscopically, there may be a complete absence of subcutaneous fat or a decrease in adipocyte size and number. An inflammatory panniculitis may be seen in early disease

Introduction

Lipodystrophy is the term that describes a heterogeneous group of diseases characterized by fat loss and fat accumulation within a given body distribution pattern. Adipose tissue has crucial metabolic and endocrine functions, in addition to having a role in mechanical protection. The loss of peripheral subcutaneous fat and a compensatory accumulation of visceral fat is closely associated with insulin resistance, diabetes mellitus, hyperlipidemia (including hypertriglyceridemia), hypertension and coronary artery disease. These metabolic abnormalities and their sequelae are now referred to as the metabolic syndrome[1] and they underscore the important metabolic and endocrine functions of fat, in its role as a diverse and crucial body organ.

Lipodystrophy is subtyped based upon its distribution, in conjunction with inheritance patterns and genetic mutations, age of onset and systemic manifestations (Fig. 101.1 & Table 101.1). Based upon distribution pattern, lipodystrophy may be subdivided into three major groups: (1) generalized; (2) partial (extensive, but not generalized); and (3) localized (limited to an isolated area).

Localized lipodystrophy is a commonly encountered form of lipoatrophy, which may be due to medication injection, previous surgery, trauma or panniculitis (see Ch. 100). Nowadays, lipodystrophy due to highly active antiretroviral therapy (HAART) is the most common non-localized subtype. It is important for dermatologists to recognize this drug effect and associated metabolic syndrome, as there are profound social, psychological and medical implications. The dermatologist is also likely to occasionally encounter partial lipodystrophy that may be associated with glomerulonephritis or with autoimmune diseases such as dermatomyositis or lupus erythematosus. Finally, there are several rare genetic syndromes that will be discussed (see Table 101.1).

History

Mitchell, in 1885, reported the first case of lipoatrophy in a patient with partial lipodystrophy of the upper body[2]. Acquired generalized lipodystrophy was first reported by Ziegler in 1928[3], and the metabolic disturbances associated with this condition were further detailed by Lawrence in 1946[4]. Berardinelli first described congenital generalized lipodystrophy in 1954[5], and Seip further delineated the manifestations of both the congenital[6] and acquired forms[7]. In the early 1900s, Barraquer[8] and Simons[9] separately described a syndrome of progressive lipodystrophy that bears their name. Gellis et al.[10] (1958) first described the association of partial lipodystrophy with renal disease and Ozer et al.[11] (1973) reported the first case of familial partial lipodystrophy. In the 1970's, unique variants of localized lipodystrophy were described[12–14], while HAART-related lipodystrophies were first reported in 1998[15,16]. Winkelmann and colleagues contributed greatly to our understanding of the histology of localized lipoatrophy[17]. Currently, investigators are focusing on the molecular and genetic basis of adipocyte function and dysfunction, as it relates to lipodystrophy.

Pathogenesis

The adipocyte functions as an endocrine organ via its secretion of hormones and adipocytokines, such as leptin[18], TNF-α, interleukin (IL)-6 and adiponectin. Altered expression and activity of these factors play a role in insulin homeostasis and other metabolic changes seen in lipodystrophic syndromes[19,20].

Adiponectin, a product of the *apM1* gene[21,22], is expressed in and secreted exclusively by differentiated adipocytes. It plays a positive role in regulating insulin sensitivity and glucose and lipid homeostasis. Plasma adiponectin levels are inversely correlated with fasting insulin levels and insulin resistance[23]. Serum adiponectin and leptin levels are reduced in murine models of lipoatrophy with insulin resistance[24], as well as in humans with congenital and acquired lipodystrophies, or HIV/HAART-related lipodystrophy[25–28]. Of note, infusion of leptin reverses insulin resistance in mouse models with deficient messenger RNAs encoding leptin[29].

Destruction or inadequate differentiation of adipocytes may result in a cascade of hormonal and metabolic consequences. For instance, hyperphagia, reduced leptin levels, and deficiency in leptin signaling associated with generalized lipodystrophy results in an increased carbohydrate load, triglyceride accumulation in the muscle and liver, and, ultimately, insulin resistance, diabetes and hepatic steatosis[30].

Lastly, a transgenic mouse model expressing a truncated version of nuclear sterol regulatory element-binding protein-1c (SREBP-1c) in adipose tissue exhibits features of generalized lipodystrophy tissue (see below)[31]. The exact mechanisms of adipocyte deficiency or destruction have

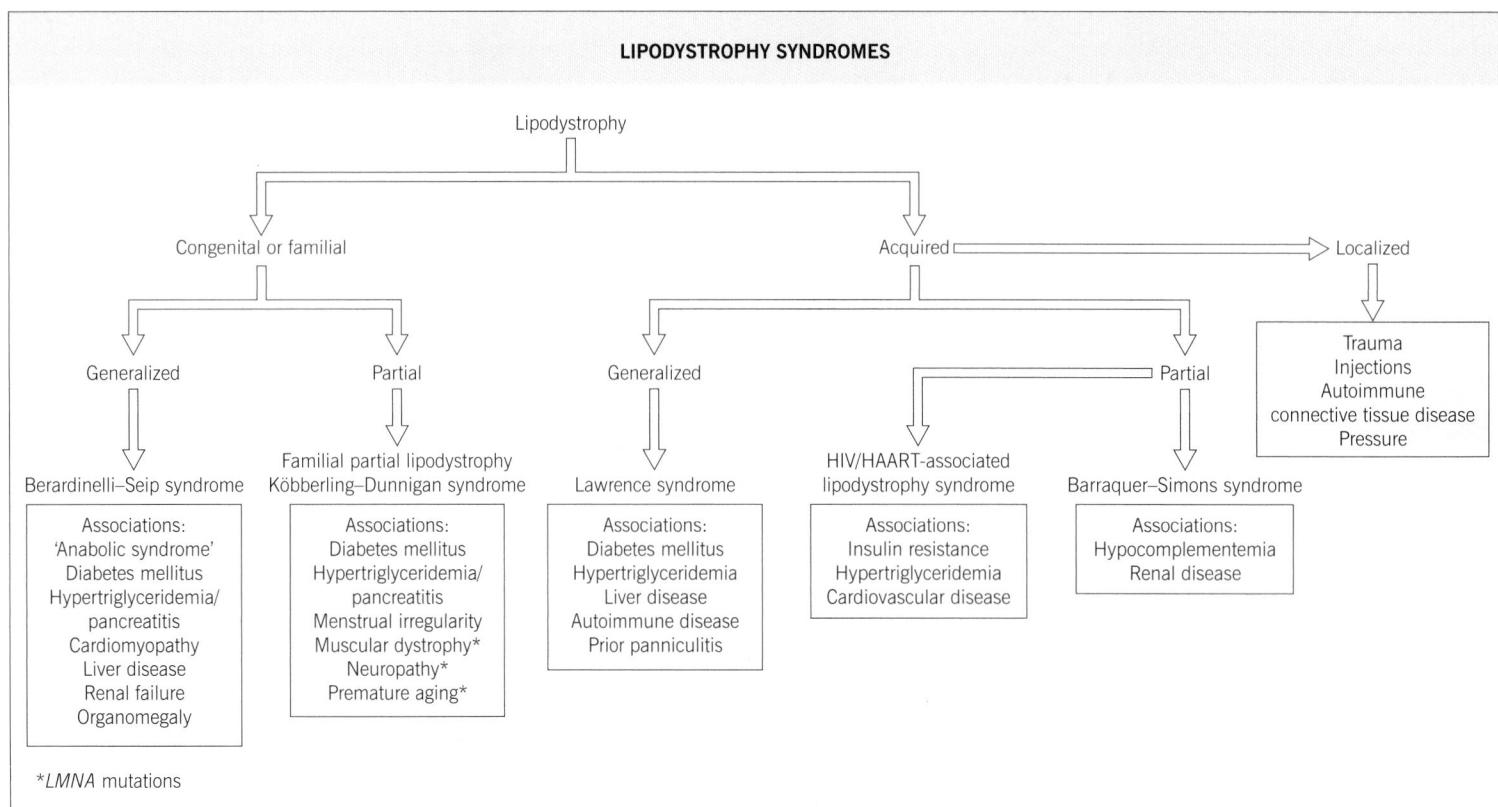

Fig. 101.1 Lipodystrophy syndromes.

not completely been established. The pathogenesis is heterogeneous, reflecting the different subtypes of disease, and includes genetic and immunologic factors, as outlined below.

Congenital generalized lipodystrophy (Berardinelli–Seip syndrome)

Congenital generalized lipodystrophy (CGL) is an autosomal recessive disorder, and to date two molecular genetic subtypes have been described, Berardinelli-Siep congenital lipodystrophy type 1 (BSCL1; mutations in AGPAT2) and type 2 (BSCL2; mutations in BSCL2) (see Table 101.1). As some patients do not have mutations in either gene, presumably additional pathogenetic mechanisms are involved. In type 1, mutations in the gene encoding 1-acylglycerol-3-phosphate O-acyltransferase 2 (AGPAT2) on chromosome 9q34 have been found in patients from several pedigrees with CGL[32]. AGPAT2, which is prominent in omental adipose tissue, is an enzyme involved in the synthesis of triglycerides and phospholipids; thus, aberrant AGPAT2 enzyme activity may cause lipodystrophy by reducing the synthesis of triglycerides in adipose tissue[32].

In type 2 CGL, several large pedigrees have mutations in the BSCL2 gene on chromosome 11q13. The function of the protein product of this gene is unknown[32].

The metabolic and clinical features of BSCL1 and BSCL2 demonstrate phenotypic heterogeneity[33]. There is also allelic heterogeneity at the BSCL2 locus, as mutations in this gene have been identified in families with Silver syndrome and distal hereditary motor neuropathy type II or V[34].

Acquired generalized lipodystrophy (Lawrence syndrome)

There is no known genetic defect. A third of patients have an antecedent autoimmune disease or viral or bacterial infection, but a causal relationship with the latter has not been established. Twenty-five percent of cases of acquired generalized lipodystrophy are heralded by panniculitis (see Table 101.1)[35,36].

The preceding panniculitis and the frequent association of autoimmune disease imply immunologically mediated fat cell lysis. As with the other forms of lipodystrophy, most patients have low serum levels of leptin and adiponectin[28].

Familial partial lipodystrophy (including Dunnigan variety, Köbberling variety)

Familial partial lipodystrophy (FPLD) is a heterogeneous group of autosomal dominantly inherited disorders, and three major groups have been described. The most prevalent subtype is the Dunnigan variety, or FPLD2, which has been linked to LMNA on chromosome 1q21–22[37]. LMNA encodes lamins A and C, and missense mutations in LMNA occur in patients with partial lipodystrophy[38]. Mutations in LMNA alter plasma leptin concentration, and heterozygotes with a LMNA mutation have decreased plasma leptin and increased fasting plasma insulin and C-peptide levels[39]. Lamins belong to the intermediate filament family of proteins that compose the nuclear lamina. Thus, adipocyte loss associated with LMNA mutations is felt to possibly be due to disruption of nuclear function resulting in cell death or to a disruption of the interaction between lamins and transcription factors such as SREBP-1c[40].

Overexpression of lamin A inhibits lipid accumulation, triglyceride synthesis and expression of adipogenic markers. The former has also been associated with inhibition of expression of peroxisome proliferator-activated receptor-γ2 (PPARγ2) and GLUT4[41].

FPLD2 belongs to a group of laminopathies that include muscular dystrophy, cardiomyopathy, neuropathies, and syndromes of premature aging (see Table 62.8). The clinical phenotype/syndrome is determined by the site and type of LMNA mutations[42,43].

FPLD subtype 3 (FPLD3) results from heterozygous missense mutations in PPARG which encodes PPARγ[44]. The PPAR protein plays an essential role in adipogenesis, but the complete pathogenesis remains unclear[36]. Fat redistribution is more extreme in FPLD2 compared to FPLD3, although clinical features and metabolic disturbances are greater in FPLD3, suggesting that PPARG mutations may have additional direct effects[45].

Partial lipodystrophy may also be seen in association with mandibuloacral dysplasia, an autosomal recessive syndrome, associated with a mutation in the LMNA gene (type A)[46,47], or with mutations in the gene (ZMPSTE24) which encodes a zinc metalloproteinase involved in post-translational proteolytic processing of prelamin A (type B). The latter has been associated with severe mandibuloacral dysplasia, premature aging and generalized lipodystrophy[48].

Syndrome	Age of onset	Sex	Genetics	Distribution of fat changes	Metabolic derangements	Systemic associations	Systemic complications
Congenital generalized lipodystrophy (Berardinelli–Seip syndrome)	Birth	F=M	AR **Type 1:** *AGPAT2* (9q34) **Type 2:** *BSCL2* (11q13)	↓ Fat: face, trunk, extremities, visceral	+++: IR, DM, ↑TG; anabolic syndrome; ↑ metabolic rate	None preceding	Hypertrophic cardiomyopathy, liver failure/ cirrhosis, organomegaly, acute pancreatitis, proteinuric nephropathy (see Table 101.4)
Acquired generalized lipodystrophy (Lawrence syndrome)	Childhood to puberty	F>M 3:1	None known	↓ Fat: face, trunk, extremities	++: IR, DM, ↑TG (correlates with the degree of lipodystrophy)	1/3 have a preceding autoimmune disease (e.g. juvenile dermatomyositis, Sjögren's syndrome) or infection; 25% have a preceding panniculitis	Liver failure/ cirrhosis, proteinuric nephropathy
Familial partial lipodystrophy (Köbberling–Dunnigan syndrome)	Puberty	F>M	AD **Type 2:** *LMNA* (lamin A/C; 1q21.2) **Type 3:** *PPARG* (3p25)	**Type 1 (Köbberling):** ↓ fat on extremities ± trunk, face spared **Type 2 (Dunnigan):** ↓ fat on extremities ± trunk, ↑ fat on face/neck (double chin), muscular hypertrophy **Type 3:** ↓ fat on extremities/buttocks (less severe than type 2); trunk/viscera spared	IR, DM, ↑TG, ↓HDL (more severe in type 3 than type 2)	None preceding	Acute pancreatitis, hepatic steatosis/cirrhosis, menstrual abnormalities
Acquired partial lipodystrophy (Barraquer–Simons syndrome)	Childhood or puberty (median 8–10 y) Rarely adults	F>M 3:1	Sporadic or AD *LMNB2* (Lamin B2; 19p13.3)	↓ Fat: face → cephalothoracic spread to medial thighs, buttocks ↑ Fat: hips and legs Hemilipodystrophic variants	Rare IR, DM, ↑TG	Often preceded by a febrile illness >1/3 have mesangiocapillary glomerulonephritis, C3 nephritic factor and hypocomplementemia Autoimmune disease	Sequelae of renal abnormalities
HIV/HAART-associated lipodystrophy syndrome	2 months–2 y after initiation of combination antiretroviral therapy Adults>children	M=F overall, F>M central adiposity	None known	↓ Fat: face, extremities ↑ Fat: central (trunk/ viscera), dorso-cervical ('buffalo hump'), breasts Lipomas (e.g. pubic)	++: IR, ↑TG, ↑LDL, ↓HDL; ± DM	HIV infection	Cardiovascular disease

Table 101.1 Lipodystrophy syndromes. *AGPAT2*, 1-acylglycerol-3-phosphate O-acyltransferase-2; AR, autosomal recessive; AD, autosomal dominant; *BSCL2*, Bernardinelli-Seip congenital lipodystrophy 2 (Seipin); chol, cholesterol; DM, diabetes mellitus; HAART, highly active antiretroviral therapy; HDL, high-density lipoproteins; HIV, human immunodeficiency virus; LDL, low-density lipoproteins; IR, insulin resistance; PI, protease inhibitor; *PPARG*, peroxisome proliferator-activated receptor-γ; TG, triglycerides.

Mesangiocapillary glomerulonephritis type 2 (MCGN II) has been reported in a case of partial lipodystrophy caused by a mutation in the *LMNA* gene, suggesting that partial lipodystrophy of both the sporadic and familial subtypes may predispose to this condition and that the observed renal and complement abnormalities may be secondary to other factors associated with lipodystrophy[49].

Acquired partial lipodystrophy syndrome (Barraquer–Simons syndrome)

This occurs sporadically or may be autosomal dominant. Subcutaneous fat is often lost acutely after a viral illness. The exact pathogenesis is not known, but may be related to adipsin, a protein produced by adipocytes which is identical to factor D (a component of the alternative complement pathway), and C3 nephritic factor (C3NeF), an IgG autoantibody against an alternative pathway enzyme. There is dysregulated activation of the alternative pathway, associated with C3NeF binding to the rate-limiting C3 convertase enzyme (C3bBb). This results in unopposed activation of the alternative complement pathway and excessive consumption of C3, and complement-dependent lysis of adipocytes. Regional differences in factor D expression parallel the regional distribution of adipocyte loss in partial lipodystrophy, which

may explain the cephalocaudal distribution of fat. Renal cells also express complement components, and a similar mechanism of complement-mediated injury may be responsible for the MCGN II seen in these patients[50,51].

Recently, mutations in *LMNB2* have been described in four patients with acquired partial lipodystrophy[52].

Localized lipoatrophy

The pathogenesis of localized lipoatrophy is heterogeneous. Lipoatrophic plaques may be the result of direct sequelae of pyogenic abscesses, various lobular panniculitides, localized connective tissue diseases such as lupus profundus and morphea, or panniculitic lymphoma. Atrophic connective tissue disease panniculitis is associated with systemic evidence of various autoimmune disorders such as systemic lupus erythematosus or dermatomyositis, implying an immunologic mechanism. Iatrogenic causes include complications of injected medications, including insulin (especially the non-human form), corticosteroids, antibiotics (especially penicillin G), iron, heparin, vaccines (including the diphtheria–pertussis–tetanus vaccine), and growth hormone[53]. Growth hormone may produce a direct lipolytic effect. The causes may be multifactorial, such as inflammatory responses to the

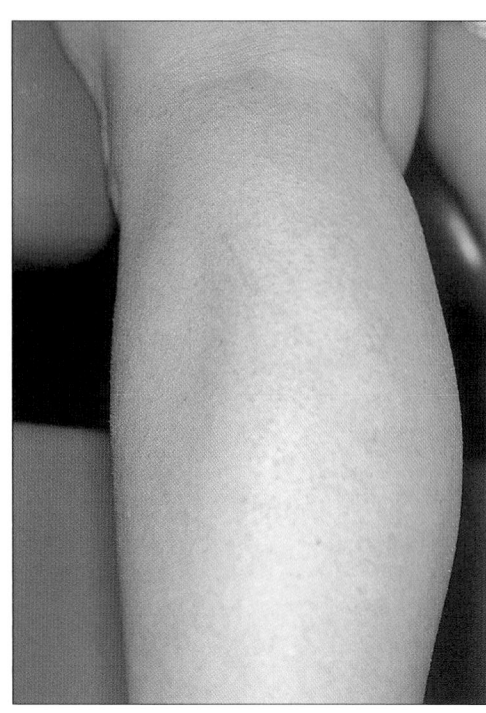

Fig. 101.2 Localized lipoatrophy of the upper lateral calf. A common finding in women due to crossing the legs while seated. Courtesy of Jean L Bolognia MD.

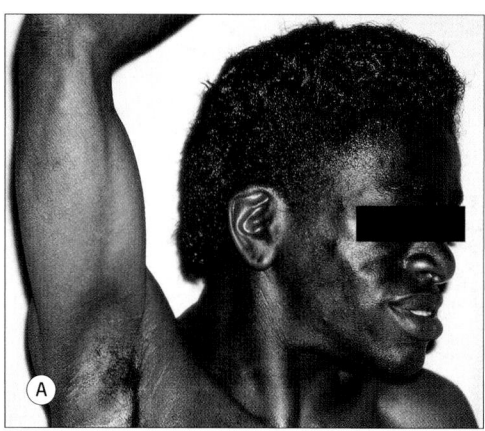

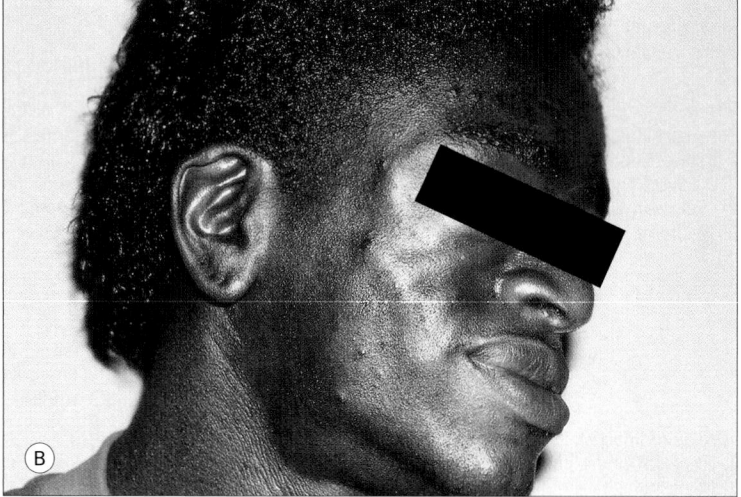

Fig. 101.3 Congenital generalized lipodystrophy syndrome in a patient with a strong family history. A Extensive acanthosis nigricans, facial and extremity lipodystrophy, and muscular habitus. **B** Close-up view demonstrating loss of Bichat's fat pad and buccal fat. Courtesy of Kenneth E Greer MD, University of Virginia.

injected medicines and/or trauma. Panniculitis at the injection site may precede localized lipoatrophy due to glatiramer[54]. Subcutaneous injections of methotrexate may cause semicircular lipoatrophy[55].

Lipoatrophia semicircularis may represent repetitive trauma or pressure-induced changes, due to constant or intermittent pressure such as leaning against a desk or chair edge[56], basin, bathtub or counter, or from tight-fitting jeans or girdles. Support for microtrauma is demonstrated by resolution of the lesions when trauma is avoided, and the occurrence of similar lesions in multiple employees in the same workplace[57]. Others have implicated local hyperproduction of TNF-α by macrophages[58]. Localized lipoatrophy of the upper and lateral calf is commonly observed in women who cross their legs when seated (Fig. 101.2).

Up to 60% of involutional lipoatrophy (see below) may be associated with prior local injections, suggesting a trauma-related phenomenon[59,60]. Lipophagocytizing macrophages seen on electron microscopy suggest an initial stimulation by injectable material[59,61]; typically, an active foreign body reaction is absent. Perivascular mononuclear infiltrates and vascular immunoreactants near insulin injections suggest a localized immune response[59,61,62].

Lipodystrophia centrifugalis abdominalis infantalis is usually idiopathic, but has been reported to be associated with mechanical trauma or focal infection.

Foreign body inflammatory reactions due to material injected for cosmetic purposes may result in lipoatrophy[63].

Clinical Features

Congenital generalized lipodystrophy

CGL (Berardinelli–Seip syndrome) is quite rare, with an estimated prevalence of less than 1 case in 10 million. As an autosomal recessive disorder, there is often consanguity. Both subtypes are characterized by generalized loss or absence of metabolically active subcutaneous fat from birth, resulting in a cadaveric facies and distinctive muscular-appearing body habitus (Fig. 101.3). Features of anabolic syndrome are evident in early childhood (Table 101.2). There is also a deficiency of bone marrow and visceral fat. Type 2 also lacks mechanical fat, in addition to metabolically active fat. The inability to store sufficient fat in the adipocytes results in the metabolic syndrome (see Ch. 52), which becomes more profound in puberty[7,64]. Hepatosplenomegaly is typical, and may be associated with umbilical herniation. Ketone-resistant diabetes is evident by adolescence, but the hyperinsulinemia can be detected as early as infancy. Enlarged genitalia are especially seen in women, and may be associated with polycystic ovarian syndrome and infertility. Dermatologic sequelae (see Table 101.2) include acanthosis nigricans, which is noted by adolescence and may be extensive. Mild

mental retardation and hypertrophic cardiomyopathy may be present, particularly with type 2. Serious medical complications and metabolic derangements include cirrhosis from fatty liver, premature atherosclerosis, sequelae of diabetes, pancreatitis from hypertriglyceridemia, and a high mortality rate from hypertrophic cardiomyopathy. The mean age of death is 32 years.

Acquired generalized lipodystrophy

To date, approximately 80 cases of acquired generalized lipodystrophy (AGL; Lawrence–Seip or Lawrence syndrome) have been reported in the English literature. New diagnostic criteria for AGL have been proposed, as well as a subclassification into three subtypes (Table 101.3).

Lipoatrophy develops insidiously and typically does not become apparent until childhood (usually before 15 years of age), but rarely presents after age 30 years. It occurs approximately three times more often in women. About one-third to one-half of cases are preceded by a systemic illness, such as viral or bacterial infection, autoimmune disease (e.g. thyroiditis) or connective tissue disease[64]. Features of AGL are similar to those of the congenital variant, but are of later onset and milder (Figs 101.4 & 101.5). Marrow fat is preserved and the latter feature may be helpful in differentiating these two subtypes. The distribution and severity of fat loss is heterogeneous, and may be localized to the face and extremities. The palms and/or soles are involved in 30–50% of patients, and approximately half may have painful callosities. Loss of peripheral fat as well as perinephric and intra-abdominal fat can be documented by MRI scans. The values of total body fat usually range from 0.3% to 15%.

Panniculitis may precede the lipoatrophy in the type 1 variant and there may be an overlap in the panniculitic and autoimmune varieties. Progression may occur rapidly or over an extended period. When the lipodystrophy becomes generalized, the systemic abnormalities become manifest. Occasionally, lipoatrophy may not be clinically recognized until after the glucose or insulin abnormalities manifest.

The metabolic syndrome is similar to that with CGL (but less severe), in contrast to the liver sequelae, which are often lethal. The latency before the development of frank diabetes (typically non-ketotic)

FEATURES OF CONGENITAL GENERALIZED LIPODYSTROPHY

Lipodystrophic features

- Lack of Bichat's fat pad in the preauricular region, resulting in a cadaveric facies
- MRI studies show near total absence of subcutaneous fat and other metabolically active adipose tissues
- Preservation of fat deposits in 'mechanical' sites (Type I): orbit, palms, soles, tongue, breasts, vulva and in periarticular and epidural regions
- Muscular body habitus due to the extreme paucity of subcutaneous fat

Anabolic syndrome

- Muscular hypertrophy with prominent superficial veins
- Acromegalic facial and acral features
- Voracious appetite
- Increased basal metabolic rate
- Heat intolerance
- Accelerated growth with a normal to slightly increased adult height
- Advanced bone and dental age
- Osteosclerotic and lytic skeletal changes
- Masculine features in females (clitoromegaly rare)
- Enlarged genitalia (usually limited to infancy and childhood)

Metabolic disturbances

- Insulin resistance and severe fasting or postprandial hyperinsulinemia from early infancy
- Insulin levels may decrease after several years, due to exhaustion of pancreatic β cells
- Very insulin-resistant diabetes mellitus: noted at puberty with growth cessation
- Impaired glucose tolerance is noted around age 8–10
- Hypertriglyceridemia and sequelae (chylomicronemia, pancreatitis)
- Hyperlipidemia accelerates at puberty (with growth cessation)
- Low HDL cholesterol levels (accurate assessment may be hindered by the increased TGs)
- Low plasma leptin levels, corresponding to decreased body fat

Dermatologic manifestations

- Acanthosis nigricans (AN), often early onset and widespread
- Hypertrichosis, including increased (often curly) scalp hair at birth
- Hyperhidrosis
- Coarse skin on the upper body
- Hyperkeratotic epidermal papillomatosis (may represent an exaggerated form of AN)
- Xanthomas

Gynecologic disturbances

- Oligomenorrhea
- Polycystic ovaries
- Infertility (females)

Organomegaly and organ dysfunction

- Hypertrophic cardiomyopathy (often fatal)
- Fatty liver, hepatomegaly, cirrhosis, liver failure
- Organomegaly: tonsils and adenoids, lymph nodes, spleen, kidneys, adrenals, pancreas, ovaries
- Central nervous system abnormalities: hypothalamic–pituitary dysfunction, ventricular dilation, below average intelligence, +/– mild mental retardation
- Proteinuric nephropathy

Table 101.2 Features of congenital generalized lipodystrophy[7,64]. TG, triglyceride; HDL, high-density lipoprotein.

ACQUIRED GENERALIZED LIPODYSTROPHY: PROPOSED DIAGNOSTIC CRITERIA AND SUBTYPES

Essential criterion

Selective loss of fat involving large regions of the body beginning after birth (usually by adolescence)

Supportive criteria

Clinical

- Loss of subcutaneous fat from the palms and soles
- Acanthosis nigricans
- Hepatosplenomegaly
- Panniculitis prior to onset (by clinical history or histologic confirmation; see below)
- Associated autoimmune diseases (see below)

Laboratory

- Diabetes mellitus or impaired glucose tolerance
- Severe hyperinsulinemia (fasting and/or postprandial)
- Increased serum triglyceride and/or decreased HDL cholesterol levels
- Reduced serum leptin and/or adiponectin levels
- Anthropomorphic or MRI evidence of large regions of fat loss
- MRI evidence of preserved bone marrow fat

Subtypes

Panniculitic variant (type 1)

- Preceding panniculitis; lipoatrophy may be noted upon its resolution, in the center of expanding annular lesions or at distant sites
- Mean age of onset is 7 years; slight female predominance (~1.5-fold)
- Associated symptoms include low-grade fever, malaise, arthralgias and abdominal pain
- May be associated with autoimmune diseases (see below)
- Relatively mild metabolic derangements and leptin abnormalities
- Histopathologic evaluation reveals a lymphohistiocytic subcutaneous infiltrate ± granulomatous foci

Autoimmune variant (type 2)

- Concurrent or prior autoimmune disease without preceding panniculitis; associated with juvenile dermatomyositis, Sjögren's syndrome > juvenile idiopathic arthritis, vitiligo, chronic urticaria/angioedema and autoimmune thyroiditis, hepatitis or hemolytic anemia
- Mean age of onset is 15 years; female predominance (~3-fold)
- Hepatomegaly is invariably present; hypertriglyceridemia and diabetes mellitus occur in most patients
- Laboratory abnormalities may be observed without clinical evidence of autoimmune disease, including antinuclear, anti-smooth muscle, anti-glomerular basement membrane, anti-salivary duct, antimitochondrial and anti-adrenal/ovary/placenta/testis antibodies

Idiopathic (type 3)

- No evidence of panniculitis or autoimmune disease
- Mean age of onset is 20 years (range, <2–60 years); female predominance (~3-fold)

Table 101.3 Acquired generalized lipodystrophy: proposed diagnostic criteria and subtypes. Adapted from reference 35.

is shorter than with the congenital variant, approximately 4 years after the loss of fat. If preceded by panniculitis, there may be less severe fat loss and a lower prevalence of diabetes and hypertriglyceridemia than with other two varieties (see Table 101.3)[35]. The anabolic syndrome is variable and less prominent; its severity is less striking when the condition starts in later childhood or adulthood. Hepatic steatosis often begins in childhood, and results in a higher incidence rate of hepatomegaly, cirrhosis and liver-related mortality, especially due to variceal bleeds, in AGL than in CGL. Gynecologic abnormalities include true or pseudo-clitoromegaly (due to fat loss), polycystic ovarian syndrome, and menstrual irregularities. Premature coronary artery disease and carotid or peripheral vascular disease may occasionally be seen. Renal and CNS abnormalities are usually absent. Dermatologic features, in addition to panniculitis and lipoatrophic areas, include acanthosis nigricans, localized or generalized hyperpigmentation, eruptive xanthomas, telangiectases, mild palmar/plantar keratoderma, and hair abnormalities, including mild hirsutism, curly hair and occasional alopecia. The acanthosis nigricans begins in childhood and involves the neck, axillae, groin, umbilicus and nipples. Associated autoimmune diseases include juvenile dermatomyositis, Sjögren's syndrome, vitiligo, chronic urticaria and angioedema.

Familial partial lipodystrophy

Familial partial lipodystrophy (FPLD) was initially referred to as Köbberling–Dunnigan syndrome[65], named after Dunnigan and Köbberling, who outlined the clinical characteristics of large Scottish[66] and German[67] pedigrees with familial syndromes of partial lipodystrophy, respectively. FPLD is now defined by genetic mutations and clinical phenotype (see Table 101.1), and designated as FPLD1 (previously Köbberling type), FPLD2 (previously Dunnigan type[65,68]), and FPLD3 (previously Dunnigan type, with *PPARG* mutations). These differ from the other forms of inherited lipodystrophy in that the onset is in puberty and the face is spared of lipoatrophy[64].

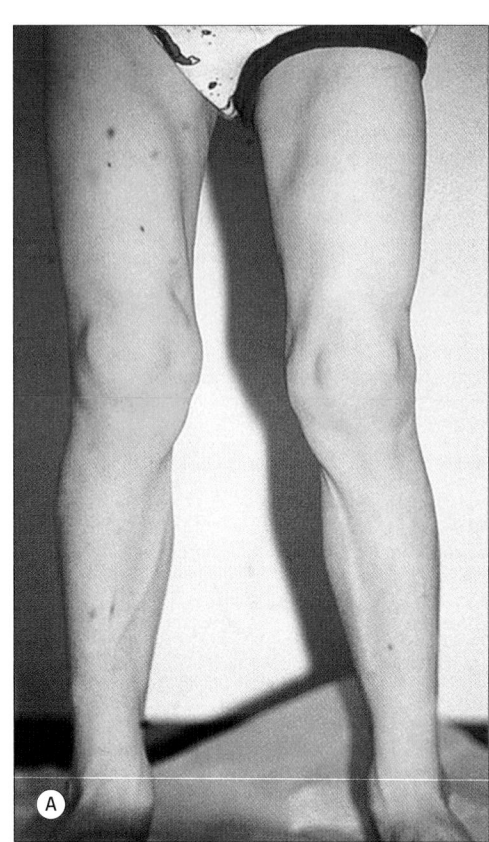

Fig. 101.4 A child with acquired generalized lipodystrophy and thyroiditis. A There is prominent lower extremity lipodystrophy, with muscular features and prominent veins. B The buttock is also involved. Courtesy of Julie Allee MD.

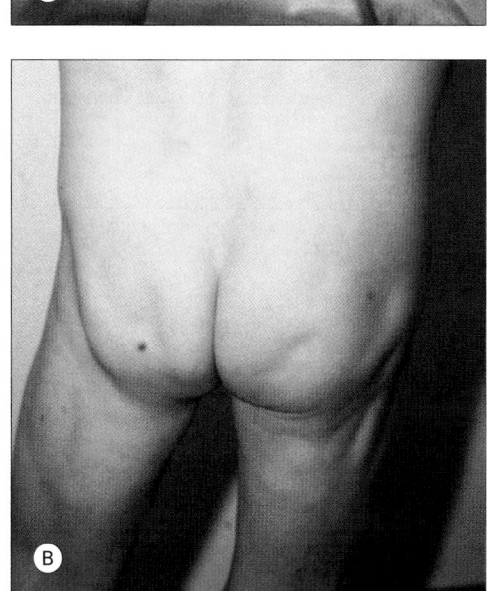

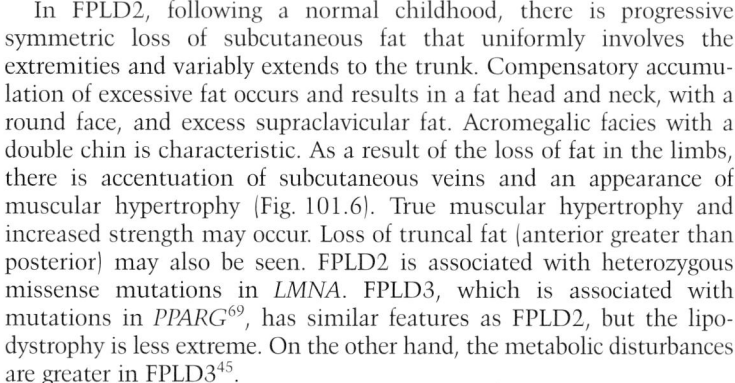

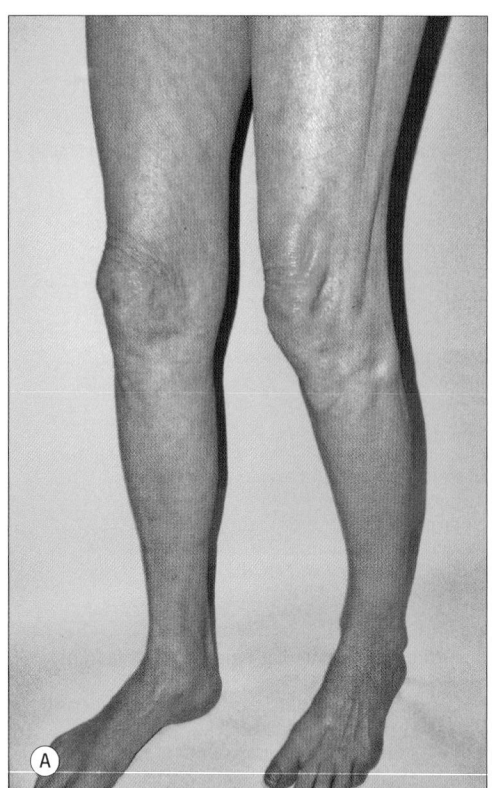

Fig. 101.5 Acquired generalized lipodystrophy. A There is loss of subcutaneous fat, resulting in a muscular appearance of the legs and accentuation of the veins and tendons. B There is obvious accentuation of the tendons in areas of fat loss.

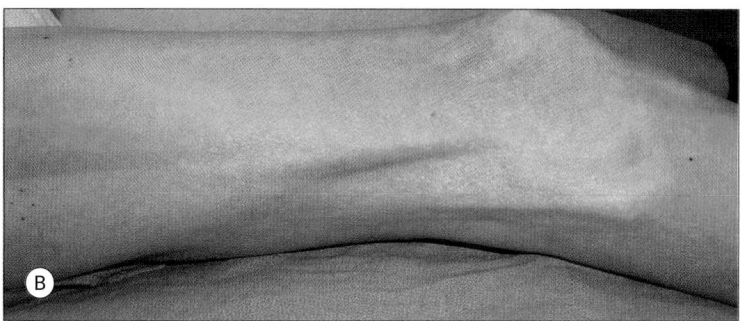

In FPLD2, following a normal childhood, there is progressive symmetric loss of subcutaneous fat that uniformly involves the extremities and variably extends to the trunk. Compensatory accumulation of excessive fat occurs and results in a fat head and neck, with a round face, and excess supraclavicular fat. Acromegalic facies with a double chin is characteristic. As a result of the loss of fat in the limbs, there is accentuation of subcutaneous veins and an appearance of muscular hypertrophy (Fig. 101.6). True muscular hypertrophy and increased strength may occur. Loss of truncal fat (anterior greater than posterior) may also be seen. FPLD2 is associated with heterozygous missense mutations in *LMNA*. FPLD3, which is associated with mutations in *PPARG*[69], has similar features as FPLD2, but the lipodystrophy is less extreme. On the other hand, the metabolic disturbances are greater in FPLD3[45].

FPLD1 is less well characterized, but differs from FPLD2 and FPLD3 by the absence of fat accumulation in the face and neck. The loss of fat is restricted to the lower extremities, and patients may have excessive truncal fat.

Metabolic disturbances in familial partial lipodystrophy are similar to those in the generalized lipodystrophy syndromes. The glucose

intolerance occurs in young adulthood. The severity ranges from mild to severe. Acute pancreatitis, steatosis and cirrhosis may occur, and death may result from complications of diabetes mellitus, premature cardiovascular disease or hypertrophic cardiomyopathy. Dermatologic manifestations include tuberous xanthomas, acanthosis nigricans and hirsutism. Gynecologic abnormalities include menstrual abnormalities, polycystic ovaries, and fat hypertrophy of the labia majora.

The prevalence of FPLD is less than 1 in 15 million[64]. At least 15 families with the Dunnigan variety of this syndrome are known. Nearly all of the patients have light complexions. Only a few pedigrees with the Köbberling variety have been reported.

Familial partial lipodystrophy with mandibuloacral dysplasia[64] is a rare variant of partial lipodystrophy characterized by mandibular and clavicular hypoplasia, short stature, high-pitched voice, and ectodermal abnormalities of the skin, teeth, nails and hair. There are multiple craniofacial defects, including dental overcrowding and bird-like facies with prominent eyes and a beaked nose. Skeletal abnormalities include osteolysis of clavicles, acro-osteolysis, delayed closure of cranial sutures and joint contractures. Cutaneous abnormalities include mottled hyperpigmentation, alopecia, atrophy of extremity skin and nail dysplasia. Less common findings include sensorineural hearing loss, delayed puberty, high-arched palate and cutaneous calcinosis. Features of the metabolic syndrome are also seen in these patients. The disorder is usually associated with mutations in *LMNA* or *ZMPSTE24* (see Pathogenesis), although some patients have not had mutations detected[69].

Acquired partial lipodystrophy

Acquired partial lipodystrophy (Barraquer–Simons syndrome, progressive lipodystrophy, cephalothoracic lipodystrophy) is the most common type

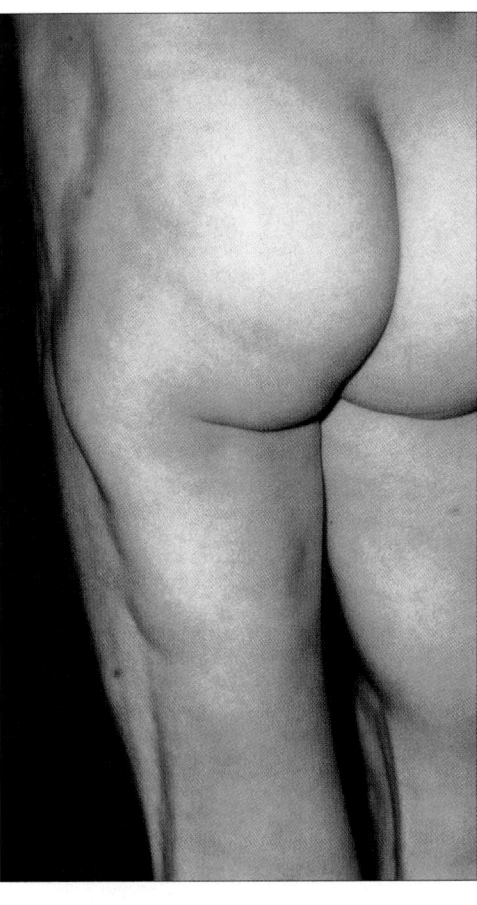

Fig. 101.6 Lipoatrophy, demonstrating involvement of the limbs with muscular features. Courtesy of William D James MD.

years. Physical findings may be apparent by the teen years, although the onset may be delayed until 40 years of age. Women are affected three times more often than men.

The face is usually first affected, with sunken eyes due to loss of retro-orbital and periorbital tissue, and loss of Bichat's fat pad, resulting in a progeria-like or cadaveric appearance. The hips and legs tend to be spared, and often demonstrate fat hypertrophy, especially in women. Growth delay or stunted growth is not characteristic.

MCGN II with nephritic syndrome, seen in one-fifth to one-third of patients, may occur many years, usually about eight, after the onset of lipodystrophy. C3 nephritic factor (C3NeF), low levels of C3, and complement dysfunction are seen in nearly all of the patients. As the low C3 level predisposes these patients to recurrent *Neisseria meningitidis* infections, prophylactic antibiotics may be required.

Metabolic syndrome is less common than in other lipodystrophies, but acanthosis nigricans, menstrual abnormalities, hirsutism, insulin resistance, type 2 diabetes mellitus, and hyperlipidemia may be seen. Other associations include autoimmune disease such as juvenile dermatomyositis[70], scleroderma, systemic lupus erythematosus, pernicious anemia, hypothyroidism, celiac disease, dermatitis herpetiformis, temporal arteritis and small vessel vasculitis. An association of acquired partial lipodystrophy with chronic sclerodermatous GVHD[71], POEMS syndrome[72] and extrinsic allergic alveolitis[73] have recently been reported. CNS abnormalities such as mental retardation, epilepsy, and sensorineural deafness have been observed[74].

Rare cases of acquired partial lipodystrophy may occur that do not fit well into the Barraquer–Simons clinical phenotype. These patients should be monitored for the features of metabolic syndrome and evaluated for the associated autoimmune diseases.

Localized lipoatrophy

Localized lipoatrophy presents as one or multiple depressed areas (i.e. indentations), usually on the proximal extremities, ranging from under a few centimeters to greater than 20 cm in diameter.

Drug-induced lipodystrophy may be accompanied by local lipohypertrophy. Multifocal lipoatrophy due to intravenous corticosteroid use has been described. The drugs that most commonly lead to lipodystrophy are discussed in the Pathogenesis section.

Involutional lipoatrophy is an idiopathic lipoatrophy characterized clinically by non-inflammatory focal loss of fat. There is a strong predominance of women reported in the literature[60]. Focal oval areas of lipoatrophy, 2 to 8 cm in diameter, occur predominantly on the buttocks and proximal extremities, especially the upper arm, corresponding to locations frequently used as injection sites. Scalp lesions may occur at sites of treated alopecia areata. However, lipoatrophy may occur without prior injection.

of non-localized lipodystrophy other than HAART-related lipodystrophy. It has been reported worldwide, with approximately 250 patients described in the literature[64].

Three phenotypic subtypes have been noted: (1) fat loss in the upper half of the body; (2) fat loss in the upper half of the body, with hypertrophy of adipose tissue in the lower half; and (3) hemilipodystrophy, where one half of the face or body is affected.

Lipodystrophy begins in childhood or pre-puberty (median age of diagnosis, 8–10 years), at times after a viral illness; it is characterized by a symmetric and insidious but progressive loss of subcutaneous fat in a cephalocaudal fashion starting on the face (Fig. 101.7) and scalp, and extending down to the pelvic girdle and mid thighs. Progression usually occurs within a 1–2-year period, but may occur over many

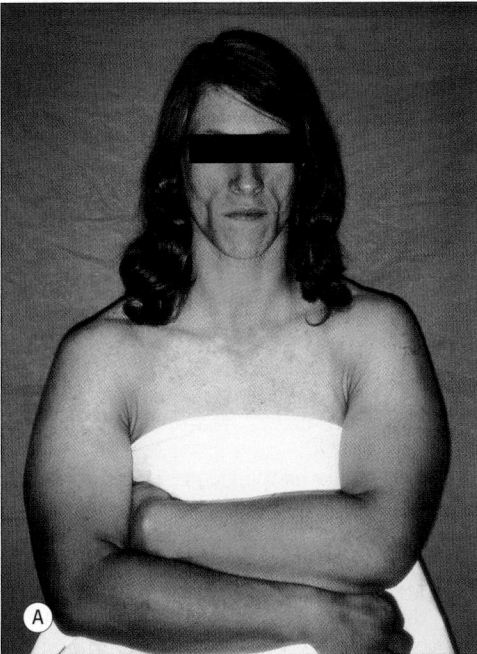
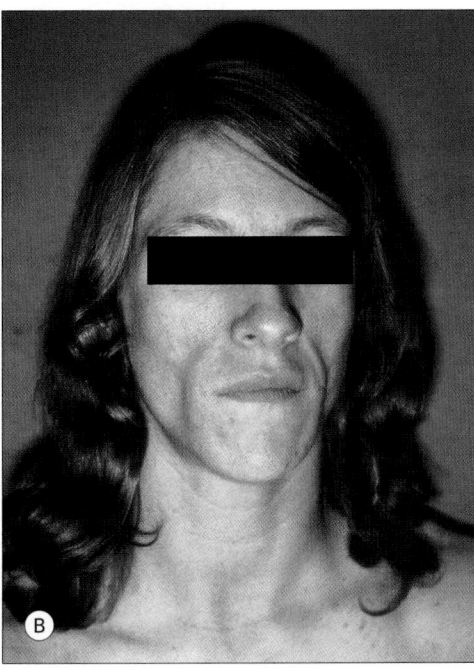

Fig. 101.7 Acquired partial lipodystrophy syndrome in a patient with nephritic factor and renal disease. A Lipoatrophic features are most prominent on the face. **B** Closer view, demonstrating marked loss of buccal fat. Axillary acanthosis nigricans is present. Courtesy of Kenneth E Greer MD.

Atrophic connective tissue panniculitis[75] is rare, and often occurs on the upper or lower extremities. In 'pure' cases of this condition, there is no prior clinical inflammation although there is lymphocytic panniculitis on biopsy. In other patients, the lipoatrophy may be the direct result of clinical panniculitis[76]. This is common on the head and neck or proximal extremities if associated with lupus profundus (Fig. 101.8). Other associated autoimmune diseases include thyroiditis, juvenile idiopathic arthritis, vitiligo, and insulin-dependent diabetes mellitus.

Lipoatrophia semicircularis (semicircular lipoatrophy) has been reported in around 100 patients[57], most of whom have been women in their 20s to 30s[56]. Rarely, it has been reported in children[77]. The prevalence in males (and in general) may be underestimated, since the condition may go unnoticed. It presents as symmetric, asymptomatic 2–4 cm linear horizontal depressions on the anterolateral thighs. Infrequent presentations include two or three parallel depressions, a unilateral distribution, or symptoms of cramps, pain after sports, heavy legs, or a burning sensation. The lesions usually appear over a few weeks and spontaneously resolve between 9 months to 4 years. The lipoatrophy may recur. MRI can assist in differentiating this from an inflammatory panniculitis[78].

Annular lipoatrophy[79] presents with a deep, persistent, pseudo-sclerotic band approximately 9–11 cm in length that encircles the arm or ankle. More extensive lesions have recently been reported that were 14–16 cm in length[80]. It may be preceded by tenderness and swelling of the limb, or associated with discomfort and arthritis. This entity may represent a variant or end-stage presentation of atrophic connective tissue disease panniculitis. Thus, there may be patients with associated autoimmune diatheses[80].

More than 100 cases of *lipodystrophia centrifugalis abdominalis infantalis* (centrifugal lipodystrophy) have been reported from Japan and Southeast Asia, as well as Europe[81]. Age of onset is usually before 3 years, with more than 90% of patients presenting by age 5 years. Although lipodystrophia centrifugalis abdominalis infantalis affects mainly Asian children, it may occasionally occur in Caucasians[82] and in adults[83]. There is a well-demarcated area of lipoatrophy with a periphery of erythema and scale on the trunk or abdomen, associated with regional lymphadenopathy. Ulceration may occur in the depressed area. The lipoatrophy begins in the groin region (and may include the genitalia) in about 80% of patients, and in the axillary region in about 20% of patients; it spreads onto the abdomen or chest, respectively, in a centrifugal fashion. Less common locations include the face, sacrolumbar region and neck, mimicking progressive lipodystrophy[84]. The lesions progress slowly over several years, then improve or resolve spontaneously by age 13 years[81]. Rarely, the disorder may persist into adulthood.

Progressive hemifacial atrophy (Parry–Romberg syndrome)[85] may be considered a form of severe morphea (see Ch. 96), and may be accompanied by atrophy of the underlying cartilage and bone, with potential ophthalmologic and dental consequences.

Non-progressive late-onset linear hemifacial lipoatrophy occurs on the malar cheek, mostly in the elderly population[86].

Becker's nevus-associated localized lipoatrophy has been reported in at least two patients[87].

Inflammatory reactions due to material injected for cosmetic purposes or due to self-inflicted injections of foreign material can lead to lipoatrophy which may be associated with scarring and dyschromia[63].

Pathology

Generalized lipodystrophy and some forms of *partial lipodystrophy* have a near or complete absence of subcutaneous fat, with the dermis and fascia in direct opposition[88]. When present, the adipocytes are markedly reduced in number and size, and are arranged in small groups surrounded by abundant connective tissue. In some cases, biopsies will appear to show no overt abnormality, except an increased amount of collagen, which has replaced the subcutaneous fat; the adipose tissue may appear normal in early disease.

Some biopsies show lobular panniculitis (Fig. 101.9), especially in cases of *acquired generalized lipoatrophy*. Localized lipodystrophy may be inflammatory or non-inflammatory, and even in cases without panniculitis, biopsies of early lesions may show inflammation.

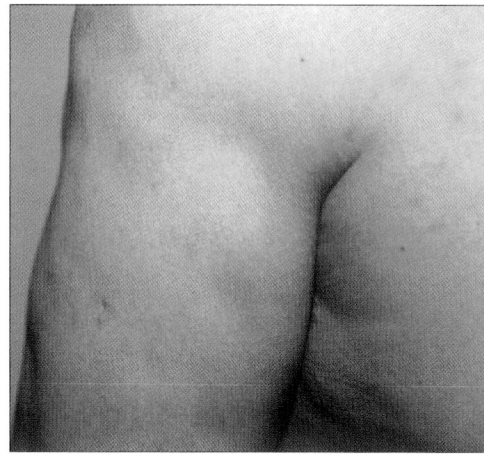

Fig. 101.8 Lipoatrophy secondary to lupus panniculitis. Circular depressions on the upper arm.

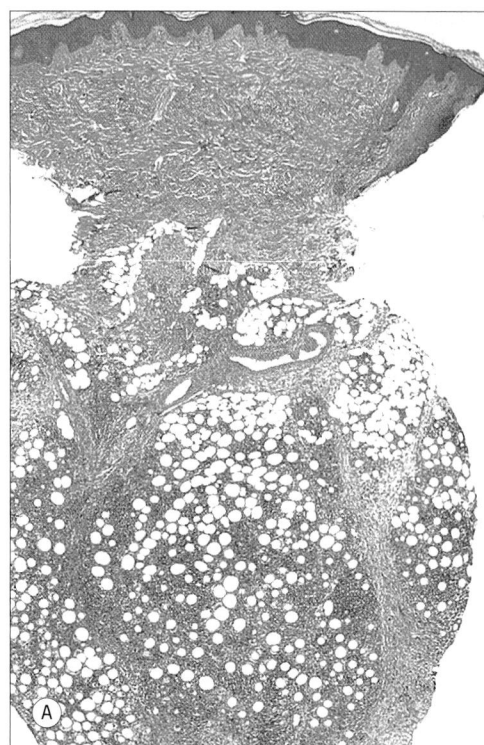

Fig. 101.9 Skin biopsy from a child with acquired generalized lipodystrophy demonstrating pre-atrophic inflammatory changes. A Scanning power demonstrates a lobular panniculitis. **B** High power reveals the panniculitis to be composed of lymphocytes, histiocytes, multinucleated giant cells, lipophages and phagocytized mucopolysaccharide. There is microcystic alteration of fat cells.

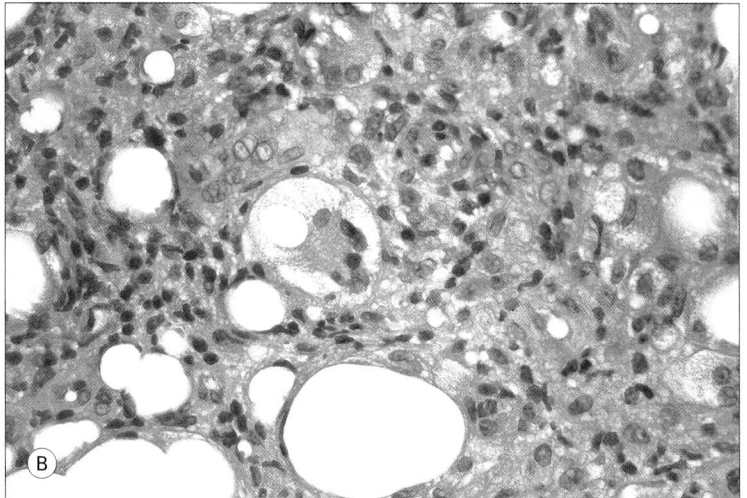

Involutional lipoatrophy can have two histologic presentations, both of which are characterized by small lobules with a reduction in size and number of fat cells[59]. The lobules may be composed of faintly acidophilic small fat cells that retract from the surrounding connective tissue, they often have an eosinophilic appearance (Fig. 101.10). This change is more prominent at the periphery of the depression, with the depressed area showing tiny acidophilic fat cells with distinct margins,

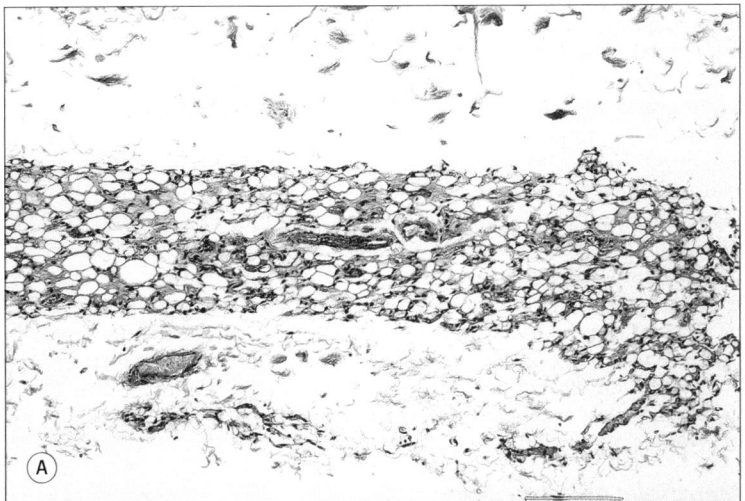

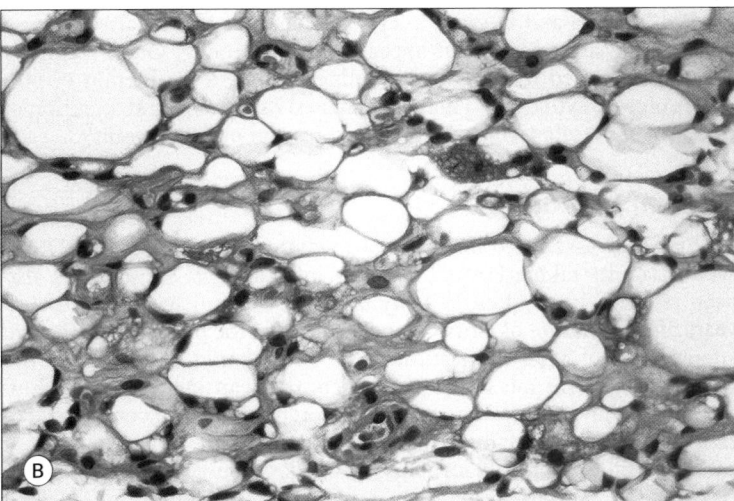

Fig. 101.10 Skin biopsy of involutional lipoatrophy secondary to injected corticosteroid. A There is marked diminution and collapse of the fat lobule, without inflammation. **B** Higher power demonstrates decreased size of fat cells with eosinophilic thickened cell walls with a hyalinized and mucinous stroma.

similar to embryonic fat. Inflammation is absent to sparsely mononuclear. A second type, with indistinguishable clinical features, shows small atrophic adipocytes with a normal fat cell membrane surrounded by prominent vasculature. At scanning magnification, the lobules are collapsed, oriented parallel with the skin surface, and are surrounded by a prominent capillary network. Acid mucopolysaccharide deposition within the fat lobules and fibrosis of the septae may be seen.

Birefringent non-crystalline foreign material may be demonstrated; however, foreign body giant cells and lipophages are typically absent in both types (by light microscopy of routinely stained sections). CD68+ macrophages can be demonstrated with immunohistochemical staining[60]. They appear as histiocytes with yellow–gray material, which is positive for acid mucopolysaccharide. Ultrastructural studies have also shown lysosomally active macrophages within the connective tissue and adjacent to lipocytes and they may contain degenerated lipid[59]. At the edge of insulin-injection-associated lipoatrophy[59], perivascular mononuclear cells in the upper dermis have been reported, along with vascular deposition of IgM, C3 and/or fibrin, but a frank inflammatory response to injectable material is not seen.

Semicircular lipoatrophy is rarely biopsied, and when examined, there have not been consistent abnormalities described. Biopsies have shown partial loss of fatty tissue, which has been replaced by collagen, or hemorrhage without significant fat inflammation, suggesting trauma[89].

Annular lipoatrophy of the ankles shows changes of a mixed lobular panniculitis with fat necrosis and a dense inflammatory cell infiltrate, composed of lymphocytes, histiocytes, plasma cells and lipidized foreign body giant cells.

Biopsies of the well-developed areas of *lipodystrophia centrifugalis abdominalis infantilis* show a diminution of subcutaneous fat with scant or absent inflammation. The surrounding areas of erythema have a moderate or marked lymphohistiocytic infiltrate in the subcutaneous fat. There may be increased dermal collagen within the subcutis. The few adipocytes that are seen may show myxoid changes[84].

Differential Diagnosis

There are a variety of other complex syndromes that present with lipoatrophy along with many other physical and systemic features. A detailed discussion of these syndromes is beyond the scope of this chapter.

The excessive fat accumulation seen in patients with familial partial lipodystrophy (Dunnigan variety) and protease inhibitor-induced lipodystrophy could be confused with Cushing's syndrome. Acromegaly can have overlapping features with generalized lipodystrophy.

In an infant with generalized lipodystrophy, the following conditions should also be considered:

- *Leprechaunism* (Donohue syndrome) is included in some lipodystrophy classifications, as the patients present with generalized lipodystrophy, severe insulin resistance, acanthosis nigricans and hirsutism. In contrast to CGL, these patients have a distinct elfin facies, severe intrauterine growth retardation, prominent nipples, loose skin, a mutation in the insulin receptor gene, and death in infancy[90].
- *SHORT syndrome* (short stature, *h*yperextensible joints, *o*cular depression, *R*ieger anomaly [iridocorneal mesodermal dysgenesis], and *t*eething delay) is also included in some lipodystrophy classifications, as there is congenital lipoatrophy of the face and upper body. This is distinguished by the above-outlined associated abnormalities, intrauterine growth retardation, delayed bone age, and a dysmorphic facies which includes a triangular shape, micrognathia, deep set eyes (not sunken) and anteverted ears. Carbohydrate metabolic abnormalities are rare to absent[91].
- *Progeria-type syndromes* are characterized by limb lipoatrophy, cardiovascular disease and diabetes, but they are accompanied by muscle wasting, sclerodermatous changes, cataracts and other signs of premature aging. Some of the progeric syndromes have *LMNA* mutations similar to those associated with FPLD, and may be considered as part of a broader group of disorders, termed laminectomies (see Table 62.8).
- In *Cockayne syndrome*, lipoatrophic changes are accompanied by growth delay, retinal abnormalities, photosensitivity and defects in DNA repair (see Ch. 86).
- *AREDYLD syndrome*: congenital generalized lipoatrophic diabetes is associated with an acrorenal field defect and ectodermal dysplasia[92].

Localized lipodystrophies should be differentiated from initial phases of progressive lipodystrophy, morphea, and atrophoderma of Pasini and Pierini. Although there is overlap amongst the various types of localized lipodystrophy, the distribution and morphology combined with a history of injections, the presence clinically or histologically of panniculitis, and associated autoimmune disorders may aid in the diagnosis.

Poland's syndrome is a rare congenital disorder consisting of unilateral partial or total absence of a breast and/or pectoralis major muscle, and ipsilateral symbrachydactyly, which may simulate lipoatrophy[93]. Lastly, MRI can help to differentiate loss of fat from other causes of localized depressions of the skin.

Treatment

Management issues for lipodystrophy syndromes are threefold: (1) cosmetic concerns; (2) metabolic derangements; and (3) systemic associations. The approach to therapy may differ, depending on the cause of the lipodystrophy.

Treatment options for the physical aspects of lipodystrophy are limited (see below). Localized lipodystrophy may resolve spontaneously, depending on the etiology and/or subtype. In trauma-induced cases, in particular lipoatrophia semicircularis, the depressions may normalize over a period of weeks[56]. Switching to purified human insulin may improve insulin lipoatrophy, but it may take 1–3 years[94].

Surgical treatment has had variable and limited success. Persistent facial lipoatrophy may be amenable to flaps[95,96]. Soft tissue augmentation using a variety of permanent and non-permanent fillers may be helpful (see Ch. 158). Solid synthetic volumetric midfacial implants, made using computer-aided design and manufacturing technology[97], may offer a more durable correction of the defects. A thoughtful assessment of possible long-term complications of permanent fillers is always mandatory prior to treatment. Fat transplantation via lipoinjection may help facial defects[98].

Medical therapy therapy is directed predominantly at the metabolic derangements, but may offer some benefit for the lipodystrophic features. Treatment with the thiazolidinedione troglitazone, a ligand for PPAR-γ[99], or rosiglitazone, another PPAR-γ agonist[100], may provide some benefit in limited patients, but the mild benefits may not outweigh the side effects.

Therapy has also been targeted at the adipokine abnormalities, such as leptin deficiency. Treatment with recombinant methionyl human leptin (r-metHuLeptin) for generalized lipodystrophy has resulted in an improvement of glycemic control, hyperlipidemia and hepatomegaly. Adverse effects include treatment-limiting proteinuria and nephropathy[30]. Improvement has been documented after only 4 months of therapy[101]. In addition to correcting the metabolic derangements, leptin replacement may assist in appetite regulation.

Nutritional alteration, exercise, and pharmacologic intervention can alter the degree of hyperlipidemia and hyperglycemia, and should be employed to avoid the associated morbidity and mortality. Endocrinologic consultation is beneficial.

Acquired partial lipodystrophy

Management of patients with acquired partial lipodystrophy should include initial evaluation and continued monitoring for autoimmune disease (such as lupus and dermatomyositis), thyroid disease and renal disease. The latter should include evaluation for proteinuria, low C3, and C3 nephritic factor (C3NeF), and, if necessary, renal biopsy to exclude MCGN.

The presence of neutralizing antibodies against C3NeF in IVIg has led to treatment of a patient with MCGN II and C3NeF with IVIg, with encouraging results[102].

Genetic counseling should be considered for the familial variants.

HIV/HAART-RELATED LIPODYSTROPHY

Pathogenesis

HIV treatment with HAART, specifically protease inhibitors (PI) plus reverse transcriptase inhibitors, which may be either nucleoside analogues (NRTI) or non-nucleoside analogues (NNRTI), may induce peripheral lipoatrophy and/or central lipohypertrophy[103–105]. Fat loss and fat accumulation may occur together as overlapping syndromes or

independently, and likely have distinct pathogenic pathways, reflecting a complex combination of drug-induced phenomena, viral-related effects, and host-specific features[106].

Proposed mechanisms for HAART-induced subcutaneous fat loss include: (1) impaired pre-adipocyte differentiation and increased adipocyte apoptosis[107–110]; (2) impaired insulin-stimulated lipogenesis and increased lipolysis[110–112], leading to decreased adipocyte size; and (3) mitochondrial toxicity[113,114] (Table 101.4 & Fig. 101.11). NRTI-induced alterations in mitochondrial biogenesis may contribute to increased lipolysis, increased TNF-α, reduced secretion of adiponectin, reduced adipocyte differentiation, and increased apoptosis[113]. The pathogenesis is similar to that of multiple symmetrical lipomatosis type I, which may also be mediated by mitochondrial dysfunction[114].

It is not clear whether central lipohypertrophy is a direct drug effect or a secondary response to subcutaneous lipoatrophy, serving as an alternative site for fat storage[113].

Metabolic abnormalities

PI-induced insulin resistance is reproducible in experimental models *in vitro*, *ex vivo* and *in vivo*[111]. The mechanisms for impaired glucose homeostasis are unclear, but appear multifactorial[111]. One hypothesis suggests impaired insulin signaling due to altered production of pro-inflammatory cytokines. There is increased expression and secretion of IL-6 and TNF-α, as well as reduced expression of adiponectin[110].

Clinical Features

HIV/HAART-associated lipodystrophy syndrome (HIV/HAART LDS) is seen in adults taking HAART for HIV infection[106,115,116], but has also been reported in children[117]. Body fat changes are detected months to years after initiation of HAART, and are seen in the presence of effective suppression of viral replication[116,118]. One should be aware of the associated adverse metabolic parameters that can increase the risk of cardiovascular disease[119] as well as the potential for poor compliance to HAART due to the stigmatizing cosmetic aspect[120].

Universally accepted data about its incidence, prevalence, associated risk factors, pathogenesis and response to treatment are lacking because a single case definition for the 'syndrome' has not yet been established[106,115]. Thus, the prevalence of lipodystrophy in the literature has varied widely, from 2% to 84%[115]. Problems in characterizing body fat changes have also made it difficult to understand the role of antiretroviral drugs.

Definitions of HIV/HAART LDS have been proposed by two multicenter studies[103,121]. A definition for body composition changes introduced by the HIV Lipodystrophy Case Definition Study[103] (Table 101.5) is 80% sensitive and specific but is too cumbersome for use in clinical practice. Patient self-report in concert with physician examination still remains the earliest and best indicator of body shape change. The Fat Redistribution and Metabolic Changes in HIV

MECHANISMS OF HIGHLY ACTIVE ANTIRETROVIRAL THERAPY (HAART)-ASSOCIATED LIPOATROPHY			
	HIV drugs implicated	**Drug-induced effect**	**Cellular response**
↓ Adipocyte differentiation*	PIs, NRTIs	Defect in lamin A/C processing and/or RXR-PPAR-γ heterodimer activation decreases function of SREBP-1c & other downstream transcription factors	↓ Production of new mature fat cells → ↓ fat cell number
↑ Adipocyte apoptosis*	PIs, NRTIs	↑ TNF-α signaling (as well as mechanism described above for ↓ differentiation)	↑ Fat cell death → ↓ fat cell number
↑ Lipolysis*	PIs, NRTIs	↓ Expression of perilipin	↑ Release of stored TGs as FFAs and glycerol into circulation → ↓ fat cell size
↓ Lipogenesis	PIs, NRTIs	↓ Expression and function of lipogenic SREBP-1c	↓ FFA uptake by adipocytes → ↓ fat cell size
Mitochondrial toxicity	NRTIs	Inhibition of mitochondrial DNA polymerase-γ	↑ Catabolic pathways (lipolysis), altered production of hormones and cytokines (↓ adiponectin, ↑ TNF-α), ↓ adipocyte differentiation, ↑ adipocyte apoptosis

Table 101.4 Mechanisms of highly active antiretroviral therapy (HAART)-associated lipoatrophy. From references 107, 108, 110–114. *Also represent sequelae of mitochondrial toxicity. FFA, free fatty acids; HIV, human immunodeficiency virus; LRP, low-density lipoprotein receptor-related protein; NRTI, nucleoside reverse transcriptase inhibitor; PI, protease inhibitor; PPAR-γ, peroxisome proliferator-activated receptor-γ; RXR, retinoid X receptor; SREBP-1c, sterol regulatory element binding protein-1c; TG, triglycerides; TNF-α, tumor necrosis factor-α.

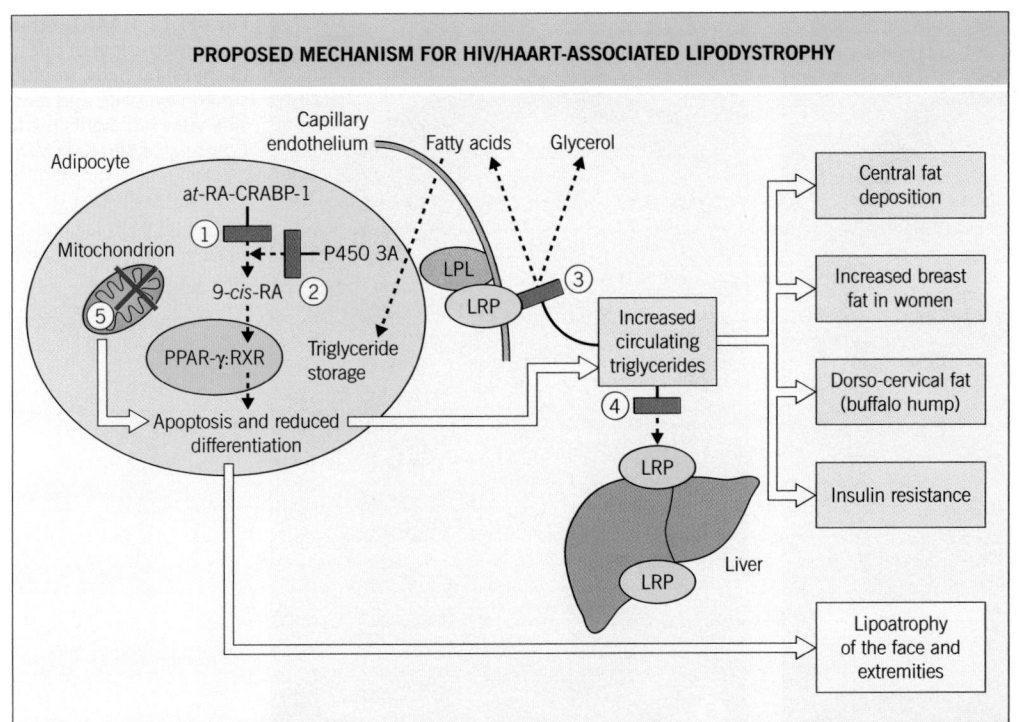

PROPOSED MECHANISM FOR HIV/HAART-ASSOCIATED LIPODYSTROPHY

Fig. 101.11 Proposed mechanism of HIV/HAART-associated lipodystrophy syndrome. Decreased activation of the retinoid X receptor (RXR)-peroxisome proliferator-activated receptor (PPAR)-γ heterodimer may occur via: (1) direct binding of protease inhibitors (PIs) to cytoplasmic retinoic acid binding protein type 1 (CRABP-1), preventing conversion of all-*trans*-retinoic acid (at-RA) to 9-*cis*-RA that can bind the RXR; or (2) PI inhibition of P450 isoforms needed to metabolize at-RA to 9-*cis*-RA. This can lead to apoptosis and reduced differentiation of peripheral adipocytes, producing lipoatrophy of the face and extremities. Lipids, now unable to be stored in these adipocytes, are released. Low-density lipoprotein receptor-related protein (LRP) present on capillary endothelium (in a complex with lipoprotein lipase) and in the liver may also be inhibited by PIs, resulting in: (3) reduced cleavage of fatty acids from circulating triglycerides; and (4) decreased hepatic uptake of chylomicrons. Of note, CRABP-1 and LRP have partial homology to the catalytic site of the HIV-1 protease that is targeted by PIs. The cascade of metabolic events from increased circulating triglycerides includes fat redistribution (with increased storage in the abdomen, breast and dorsocervical region) and insulin resistance. Lastly, nucleoside reverse transcriptase inhibitor-induced mitochondrial toxicity (5) may contribute to apoptosis and abnormal differentiation of adipocytes. HAART, highly active antiretroviral therapy. Adapted from Carr A. HIV protease inhibitor-related lipodystrophy syndrome. Clin Infect Dis. 2000;30:S135–42.

Infection (FRAM) study is a cross-sectional study that is assessing body fat changes[121].

HIV/HAART has been described as a syndrome of combined peripheral fat loss with simultaneous central fat accumulation with associated metabolic disturbances[118]. *Peripheral lipoatrophy* refers to: (1) loss of subcutaneous facial fat – in particular, loss of buccal, parotid, and preauricular (Bichat) fat pads – resulting in prominent zygomata, sunken eyes, deepened and redundant melolabial folds and a cachectic facies (Fig. 101.12); and/or (2) diffuse lipoatrophy of the upper and lower extremities (resulting in a muscular appearance; Fig. 101.13) as well as the buttocks[118]. *Central lipohypertrophy* refers to: (1) accumulation of visceral abdominal fat (omental, mesenteric, retroperitoneal), resulting in abdominal protrusion ('protease paunch' or 'Crix belly', in reference to Crixivan®) and abdominal fullness or discomfort; and/or (2) increased fat deposition in the dorsocervical fat pad ('buffalo hump'),

breasts (resulting in gynecomastia in men, larger breasts in women), anterior neck and/or lateral mandibular region, in lipomata, and within the muscle and liver[104,118,119].

The concept of one redistribution syndrome of lipoatrophy with reciprocal lipohypertrophy has recently been challenged[104,105,121–123]. Results from the FRAM study demonstrate that subcutaneous lipoatrophy, but not lipohypertrophy, is the dominant morphologic pattern[104,105,122,124]. In comparison to HIV patients without clinical fat loss, HIV-infected patients with lipoatrophy were found to have less fat in both peripheral and visceral compartments[104,105,123]. In response to these observations, current studies are reporting the prevalence and incidence of peripheral lipoatrophy and central lipohypertrophy separately[115].

HIV/HAART was initially considered a PI-mediated disease, but the use of NRTIs has been identified as an independent and significant risk factor for the development of lipodystrophy, the duration of their use being predictive of the severity of the peripheral lipoatrophy. Different drugs likely produce distinct clinical syndromes of fat redistribution[106]. For example, PIs are more likely associated with central fat hypertrophy as well as the metabolic derangements reported with the syndrome, whereas treatment with NRTIs (stavudine in particular) is a stronger independent risk factor for the development of peripheral fat wasting and lipoatrophy. Multiple NRTI-induced complications related to mitochondrial toxicity, including myopathy, polyneuropathy, liver steatosis, pancreatitis, hyperlactatemia, bone marrow toxicity and a Fanconi-like syndrome, may occur simultaneously[114].

The most common significant risk factors for the development of either lipoatrophy or lipohypertrophy are age (>40 years), disease severity at the onset of therapy (CD4 count <200/μl; higher nadir viral load), and longer duration of therapy with either PIs and/or NRTIs[106,116]. White race is a predictor for lipoatrophy, but not lipohypertrophy[106]. The risk of developing lipoatrophy is higher in individuals with less subcutaneous fat pre-HAART, whereas fat accumulation is more likely in those with more fat at baseline[125]. Combination therapy using two NRTIs and a PI has a strong association with severe lipoatrophy[119].

VARIABLES INCLUDED IN CASE DEFINITION OF HIV LIPODYSTROPHY	
Demographic	• Sex • Age • Duration of HIV infection • HIV clinical stage
Clinical	• Waist/hip circumference ratio
Metabolic	• Anion gap • HDL cholesterol
Body composition	• Leg fat • Trunk/limb fat ratio • Intra-abdominal/subcutaneous abdominal fat ratio

Table 101.5 Variables included in case definition of HIV lipodystrophy. Adapted from Carr A, et al. and the HIV Lipodystrophy Case Definition Study Group. An objective case definition of lipodystrophy in HIV-infected adults: a case-control study. Lancet 2003;361:726–35.

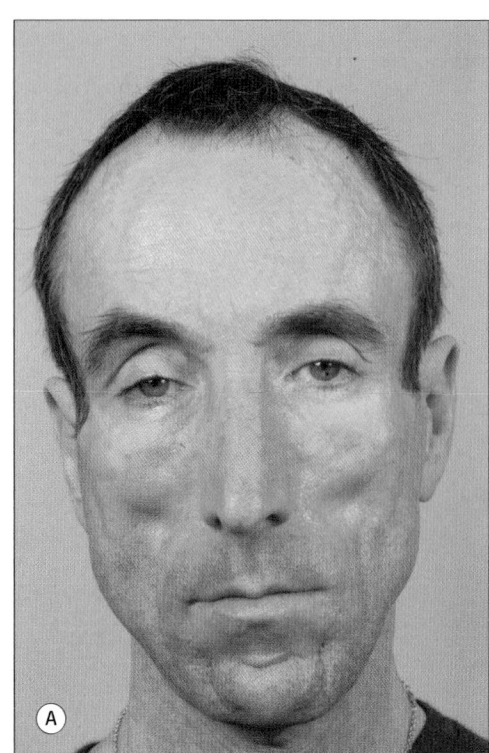 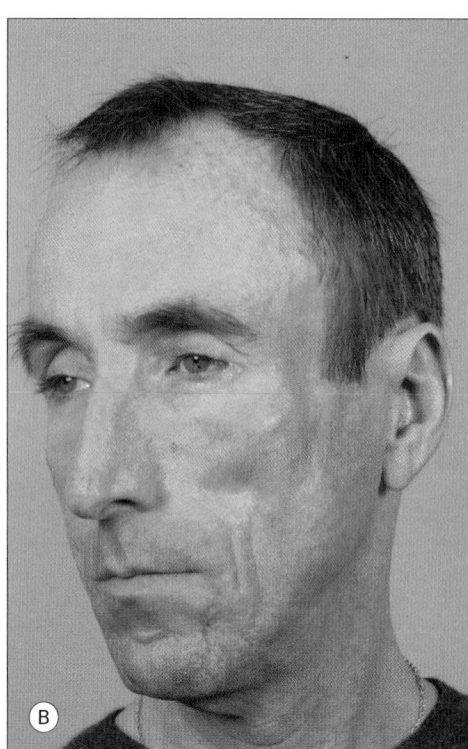

Fig 101.12 HAART-induced lipodystrophy. A There is symmetric loss of buccal, parotid, and preauricular (Bichat's) fat pads, resulting in prominent zygomata, sunken eyeballs, and a cachectic appearance. **B** The side view highlights the loss of temporal fat. Courtesy of Ken Katz MD, FDA.

When the clinical fat loss syndrome is present, women and men have less fat in both peripheral and central sites (see above). Men with HIV have a lower risk of presenting with lipohypertrophy than do women[104–106,126]. HIV-infected women tend to have more fat in central sites (both subcutaneous and visceral) compared to uninfected controls even when the lipoatrophy syndrome is not present[105]. Of note, HIV-infection alone may be associated with diminished subcutaneous adipose[104,105] and lipodystrophy has also been described in treatment-naive patients[116]. The body fat changes in HIV disease, therefore, reflect multiple etiologies: drug-related phenomena, including type of anti-retroviral therapy used, viral-induced effects, and other host factors.

Metabolic complications associated with long-term use of HAART have been well described[119]. The most commonly reported abnormalities include dyslipidemia, insulin resistance, type 2 diabetes mellitus, hyperlactinemia, and bone disorders, such as osteopenia, osteoporosis and avascular necrosis. Recent evidence suggests that an imbalance between trunk and limb fat, rather than absolute measures of fat loss and gain, correlate best with the development of adverse metabolic parameters[124].

Up to 60% of HAART users with lipodystrophy developed hyper-triglyceridemia (>200 mg/dl) with prolonged use of antiretroviral therapy[127]. With the initiation of HAART, low-density lipoprotein levels may stabilize or normalize, but high-density lipoprotein levels decline with prolonged duration of therapy.

Hyperinsulinemia is commonly seen[119] and impaired glucose tolerance has been reported in more than 35% of HIV-infected individuals. Diabetes mellitus is approximately three times more likely to develop in HIV-infected men receiving combination HAART[128].

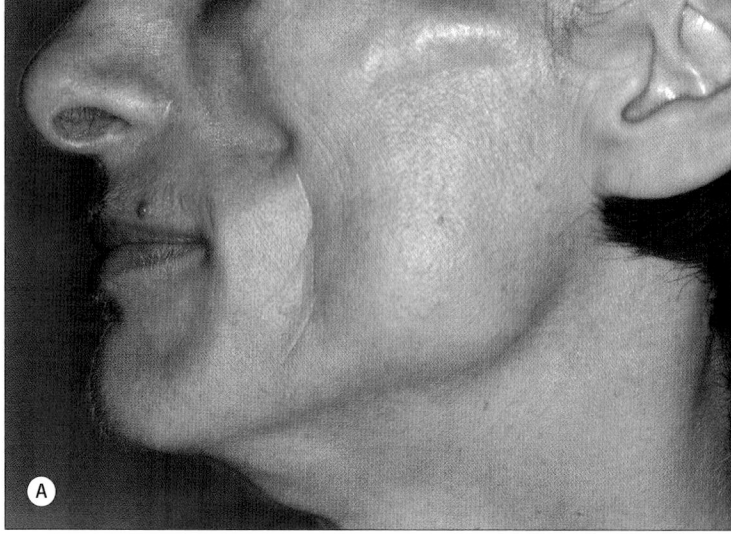 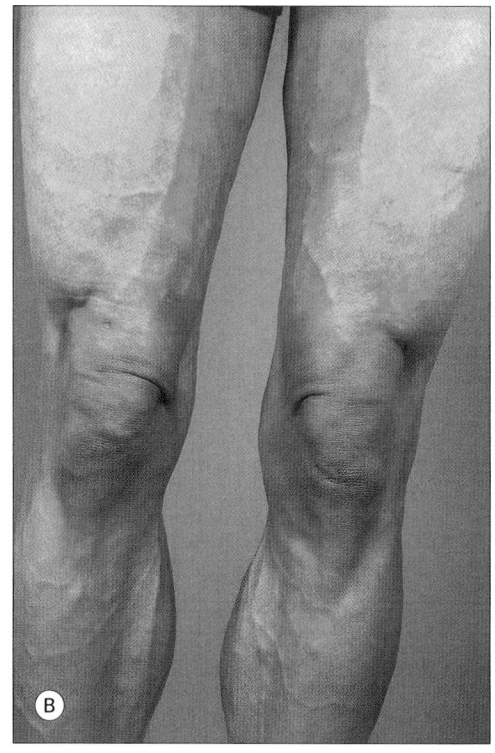

Fig. 101.13 HIV-associated lipodystrophy. A Marked indentation of the medial cheek. **B** Lower extremities with prominent veins and defined musculature. A, Courtesy of Kalman Watsky MD.

The Data Collection on Adverse Events of Anti-HIV Drugs (DAD) study found an increase in the relative risk of cardiovascular disease with increased duration of HAART[129]. There was a 26% increase in the rate of myocardial infarction per year of exposure to combination antiretroviral therapy during the first 4–6 years of use.

Treatment

When treating HIV/HAART LDS, consideration should be given to potential drug interactions, the side-effect profile of medical therapies, and consequences of manipulating the antiviral medications[119,130,131]. None of the medical therapies have shown consistent efficacy in reversing lipodystrophy, and often have limiting side effects. These treatments include insulin-sensitizing agents, hormonal therapies (growth hormone, growth hormone-releasing hormone and testosterone), statins, and the dietary supplement uridine. A multidisciplinary approach, utilizing medical and surgical interventions, is most beneficial[132].

HIV-associated lipoatrophy

Switching to a less toxic antiviral agent is recommended. Replacing PIs with NRTIs is not effective, and may actually worsen peripheral fat loss in some patients[133,134]. Newly designed PIs, such as atazanavir, an azapeptide PI, did not appear to induce HAART LDS when given in combination with NRTIs during a 48-week trial[135]. Cessation of NRTIs will improve limb fat mass, but results in virologic failure, unless substituted[119]. For example, switching from the NRTI stavudine to either abacavir or tenofovir reverses fat loss and improves metabolic parameters without compromising viral control[136].

Results of studies evaluating the efficacy of thiazolidinediones (TZDs) in correcting lipoatrophy in HIV/HAART LDS are inconclusive[119,130,131]. Although TZDs are associated with improved insulin resistance, rosiglitazone, in particular, causes unfavorable increases in serum cholesterol and triglycerides[119,137].

Surgical and injectable treatment options can be helpful, but are expensive and require multiple visits to obtain and maintain the desired cosmetic effect[138,139]. Autologous fat transplantation, although effective, requires overcorrection to compensate for loss of injected volume[139,140]. Limitations include insufficient donor fat for large defects and high rates of reabsorption within the first month[140].

Poly-L-lactic acid, a synthetic biodegradable polymer, is approved by the Food and Drug Administration (FDA) as an injectable intradermal implant to correct HAART-associated facial lipoatrophy[139,141]. Intradermal injections every 2 weeks for three sessions can significantly increase dermal thickness at 24 weeks, without serious adverse events. Duration of the correction is approximately 2 years[141]. Side effects include temporary edema, nodules, hematoma and rare cases of anaphylaxis.

HIV-associated fat accumulation

Switching from a PI to an alternative antiretroviral agent does not reverse visceral fat accumulation[131]. Exercise may reduce overall fat and truncal fat in HIV-infected individuals with central fat accumulation[142]. Metformin decreases visceral fat and improves insulin sensitivity in HIV patients with truncal obesity and hyperinsulinemia[119,131], but subcutaneous fat is also reduced, so it should be avoided in those with clinical lipoatrophy[119]. Although metformin has limited benefit on fat changes and metabolic parameters in HIV patients with normal glucose tolerance, it enhances the benefit of exercise in HIV-infected individuals with insulin resistance and body fat changes[143]. Recombinant human growth hormone (hGH), 4–6 mg/day subcutaneously for 12 to 16 weeks, may be of benefit for those with increased visceral fat and/or a buffalo hump, but is not recommended for patients with lipoatrophy because it can lead to decreased peripheral fat[119,131]. Other potential side effects include joint pain, fluid retention and glucose intolerance. Growth hormone-releasing factor may offer similar improvements of lipohypertrophy, without the adverse side effects[144].

Liposuction or surgical excision of the buffalo hump and other localized areas of subcutaneous fat accumulation produce good short-term results[119,131]. Although fat tissue may reaccumulate within a few months[145], favorable long-term effects have been reported[146].

Metabolic derangements

The metabolic derangements in HIV/HAART may be severe and unresponsive to intervention. Routine assessment of fasting lipids in patients on long-term PI therapy is recommended. Statins, commonly used for hyperlipidemia, are metabolized by the cytochrome P450 (CYP) 3A4 isoenzyme, which is inhibited by PIs. Although pravastatin or rosuvastatin is the preferred treatment, atorvastatin, which has a lower affinity for CYP3A4, is another option. Fibric acid derivatives, such as gemfibrozil or fenofibrate, are recommended for hypertriglyceridemia. Patients should be closely monitored for liver and muscle toxicity when on antilipemic agents. Diet and exercise may improve metabolic parameters and improve cardiovascular risk[119,131].

REFERENCES

1. Hegele RA. Phenomics, lipodystrophy, and the metabolic syndrome. Trends Cardiovasc Med. 2004;14:133–7.
2. Mitchell SW. Singular case of absence of adipose matter in the upper half of the body. Am J Med Sci. 1885;90:105–6.
3. Zeigler LH. Lipodystrophies: report of seven cases. Brain. 1928;51:147–61.
4. Lawrence RD. Lipodystrophy and hepatomegaly with diabetes, lipaemia and other metabolic disturbances. Lancet. 1946;1724–31.
5. Berardinelli W. An undiagnosed endocrinometabolic syndrome: report of 2 cases. J Clin Endocrinol Metab. 1954;14:193–204.
6. Seip M. Lipodystrophy and gigantism with associated endocrine manifestations: a new diencephalic syndrome? Acta Paediatr Scand. 1959;48:555–74.
7. Seip M, Trygstad O. Generalized lipodystrophy, congenital and acquired (lipoatrophy). Acta Paediatr Suppl. 1996;413:2–28.
8. Barraquer L. Histore clinique d'un cas d'atrophie du tissu celluloadipeux. Neurolog Zentralblatt. 1907;26:1072.
9. Simons A. Eine seltnen trophoneurose: 'lipodystrophia progressiva'. Z Ges Neurol Psychiat. 1911;5:29–38.
10. Gellis SS, Green S, Walker D. Chronic renal disease in children. Am J Dis Child. 1958;96:605–11.
11. Ozer FL, Lichtenstein JR, Kwiterovich PO, McKusick VA. A new genetic variety of lipodystrophy. Clin Res. 1973;21:533.
12. Imamura S, Yamada M, Ikeda T. Lipodystrophia centrifugalis infantalis. Arch Dermatol. 1971;104:291–8.

13. Imamura A, Yamada M, Yamamoto K. Lipodystrophia centrifugalis infantalis. J Am Acad Dermatol.1984;11:203–9.
14. Gschwandtner WR, Münzberger H. Lipoatrophia semicircularis: ein beitrag zu bandförmig-circulören atrophien des subcutanen fettgewebes im extremitötenbereich. Hautarzt. 1974;25:222–7.
15. Carr A, Samaras K, Burton S, et al. A syndrome of peripheral lipodystrophy, hyperlipidemia and insulin resistance in patients receiving HIV protease inhibitors. AIDS. 1998;12:F51–8.
16. Viraben R, Aquilina C. Indinavir-associated lipodystrophy. AIDS. 1998;12:F37–9.
17. Peters MS, Winkelmann RK. The histopathology of localized lipoatrophy. Br J Dermatol. 1986; 114:27–36.
18. Wauters M, Considine RB, van Gaal LF. Human leptin: from an adipocyte hormone to an endocrine mediator. Eur J Endocrinol. 2000;143:293–311.
19. Vigouroux C, Maachi M, Nguyen TH, et al. Serum adipocytokines are related to lipodystrophy and metabolic disorders in HIV-infected men under antiretroviral therapy. AIDS. 2003;17:1503–11.
20. Lagathu C, Kim M, Maachi M, et al. HIV antiretroviral treatment alters adipokine expression and insulin sensitivity of adipose tissue in vitro and in vivo. Biochimie. 2005;87:65–71.
21. Kissebah AH, Sonnenberg GE, Myklebust J, et al. Quantitative trait loci on chromosomes 3 and 17 influence phenotypes of the metabolic syndrome. Proc Natl Acad Sci USA. 2000;97:14478–83.
22. Vionnet N, Hani El-H, Dupont S, et al. Genomewide search for type 2 diabetes-susceptibility genes in

French whites: evidence for a novel susceptibility locus for early-onset diabetes in chromosome 3q27-qter and independent replication of a type 2-diabetes locus on chromosome 1q21-q24. Am J Hum Genet. 2000;67:1470–80.
23. Weyer C, Funahashi T, Tanaka S, et al. Hypoadiponectinemia in obesity and type 2 diabetes: close association with insulin resistance and hyperinsulinemia. J Clin Endocrinol Metab. 2001;86:1930–5.
24. Yamauchi T, Kamon J, Waki H, et al. The fat-derived hormone adiponectin reverses insulin resistance associated with both lipoatrophy and obesity. Nat Med. 2001;7:941–6.
25. Pardini VC, Victoria IM, Rocha SM, et al. Leptin levels, β-cell function, and insulin sensitivity in families with congenital and acquired generalized lipoatrophic diabetes. J Clin Endcrinol Metab. 1998;83:503–8.
26. Addy CL, Gavrila A, Tsiodras S, Brodovicz K, Karchmer AW, Mantzoros CS. Hypoadiponectinemia is associated with insulin resistance, hypertriglyceridemia, and fat redistribution in human immunodeficiency virus-infected patients treated with highly active actiretroviral therapy. J Clin Endocrinol Metab. 2003;88:627–36.
27. Nagy S, Tsiodras S, Martin L, et al. Leptin is independently associated with lipodystrophy in HIV-1 infected patients treated with HAART. Clin Infect Dis. 2003;36:795–802.
28. Haque WA, Shimomura I, Matsuzawa Y, Garg A. Serum adiponectin and leptin levels in patients with lipodystrophies. J Clin Endcrinol Metab. 2002;87:2395–8.

29. Shimomura I, Hammer RE, Ikemoto S, et al. Leptin reverses insulin resistance and diabetes mellitus in mice with congenital lipodystrophy. Nature. 1999;401:73–6.

30. Javor ED, Cochran EK, Musso C, Young JR, Depaoli AM, Gorden P. Long-term efficacy of leptin replacement in patients with generalized lipodystrophy. Diabetes. 2005;54:1994–2002.

31. Shimomura I, Hammer RE, Richardson RE, et al. Insulin resistance and diabetes mellitus in transgenic mice expressing nuclear SREBP-1c in adipose tissue: model for congenital generalized lipodystrophy. Genes Dev. 1998;12:3182–94.

32. Agarwal AK, Garg A. Genetic basis of lipodystrophies and management of metabolic complications. Annu Rev Med. 2006;57:297–311.

33. Gomes KB, Pardini VC, Ferreira AC, Fernandes AP. Phenotypic heterogeneity in biochemical parameters correlates with mutations J Inherit Metab Dis. 2005;28:1123–31.

34. van de Warrenburg BP, Scheffer H, van Eijk JJ, et al. BSCL2 mutations in two Dutch families with overlapping Silver syndrome-distal hereditary motor neuropathy Neuromuscul Disord. 2006; 16:122–5.

35. Misra A, Garg A. Clinical features and metabolic derangements in acquired generalized lipodystrophy: case reports and review of the literature. Medicine (Baltimore). 2003;82:129–46.

36. Billings JK, Milgraum SS, Gupta AK, Headington JT, Rasmussen JE. Lipoatrophic panniculitis: a possible autoimmune inflammatory disease of fat: report of three cases. Arch Dermatol. 1987;123:1662–6.

37. Peters JM, Barnes R, Bennett L, et al. Localization of the gene for familial partial lipodystrophy (Dunnigan variety) to chromosome 1q21-22. Nat Genet. 1998;18:292–5.

38. Shackleton S, Lloyd DJ, Jackson SNJ, et al. LMNA, encoding lamin A/C, is mutated in partial lipodystrophy. Nat Genet. 2000;24:153–6.

39. Hegele RA, Cao H, Huff MW, Anderson CM. LMNA R482Q mutation in partial lipodystrophy associated with reduced plasma leptin concentration. J Clin Endocrinol Metab. 2000;855:3089–93.

40. Lloyd DJ, Trembath RC, Shackleton S. A novel interaction between lamin A and SREBP1: implications for partial lipodystrophy and other laminopathies. Hum Mol Genet. 2002;11:769–77.

41. Boguslavsky RL, Stewart CL, Worman HJ. Nuclear lamin A inhibits adipocyte differentiation: implications for Dunnigan-type familial partial lipodystrophy. Hum Mol Genet. 2006;15:653–63.

42. Garg A, Vinaitheerthan M, Weatherall PT, Bowcock AM. Phenotypic heterogeneity in patients with familial partial lipodystrophy (Dunnigan variety) related to the site of missense mutations in lamin A/C gene. J Clin Endocrinol Metab. 2001;86:59–65.

43. Garg A, Speckman RA, Bowcock AM. Multisystem dystrophy syndrome due to novel missense mutations in the amino-terminal head and alpha-helical rod domain of the lamin A/C gene. Am J Med. 2002;112:549–55.

44. Agarwal AK, Garg A. A novel heterozygous mutation in peroxisome proliferator-activated receptor-gamma gene in a patient with familial partial lipodystrophy. J Clin Endocrinol Metab. 2002;87:408–11.

45. Francis GA, Li G, Casey R, et al. Peroxisomal proliferator activated receptor-gamma deficiency in a Canadian kindred with familial partial lipodystrophy type 3 (FPLD3).BMC Med Genet. 2006;7:3.

46. Novelli G, Muchir A, Sangiuolo F, et al. Mandibuloacral dysplasia is caused by a mutation in LMNA-encoding lamin A/C. Am J Hum Genet 2002;71:426–31.

47. Simha V, Agarwal AK, Oral EA, Fryns JP, Garg A. Genetic and phenotypic heterogeneity in patients with mandibuloacral dysplasia-associated lipodystrophy. J Clin Endocrinol Metab. 2003; 88:2821–4.

48. Agarwal AK, Fryns JP, Auchus RJ, Garg A. Zinc metalloproteinase, ZMPSTE24, is mutated in mandibuloacral dysplasia. Hum Mol Genet. 2003;12:1995–2001.

49. Owen KR, Donohoe M, Ellard S, et al. Mesangiocapillary glomerulonephritis type 2 associated with familial partial lipodystrophy (Dunnigan-Kobberling syndrome). Nephron Clin Pract. 2004;96:c35–8.

50. Mathieson PW, Peters DK. Lipodystrophy in MCGN type II: the clue to links between the adipocyte and the complement system. Nephrol Dial Transplant. 1997;12:1804–6.

51. Williams DG. C3 nephritic factor and mesangiocapillary glomerulonephritis. Pediatr Nephrol. 1997;11:96–8.

52. Hegele RA, Cao H, Liu DM, et al. Sequencing of the reannotated LMNB2 gene reveals novel mutations in patients with acquired partial lipodystrophy Am J Hum Genet. 2006;79:383–9.

53. Buyukgebiz A, Aydin A, Dundar B. Localized lipoatrophy due to recombinant growth hormone therapy in a child with 6.7 kilobase gene deletion isolated growth hormone deficiency. J Pediatr Endocrinol Metab. 1999;12:85–7.

54. Soos N, Shakery K, Mrowietz U. Localized panniculitis and subsequent lipoatrophy with subcutaneous glatiramer acetate (Copaxone) injection for the treatment of multiple sclerosis. Am J Clin Dermatol. 2004;5:357–9.

55. Haas N, Henz BM, Bunikowski R, Keitzer R.. Semicircular lipoatrophy in a child with systemic lupus erythematosus after subcutaneous injections with methotrexate. Pediatr Dermatol. 2002;19:432–5.

56. DeGroot AC. Is lipoatrophia semicircularis induced by pressure? Br J Dermatol. 1994;131:887–90.

57. Gómez-Espejo C, Pérez-Bernal A, Camacho-Martínez F. A new case of semicircular lipoatrophy associated with repeated external microtraumas and review of the literature. J Eur Acad Dermatol Venereol. 2005;19:459–61.

58. Becker C, Barbulescu K, Hildner K, Meyer zum Buschenfelde KH, Neurath MF. Activation and methotrexate-mediated suppression of the TNF alpha promoter in T cells and macrophages. Ann N Y Acad Sci. 1998;859:311–14.

59. Dahl PR, Zalla MJ, Winkelmann RK. Localized involutional lipoatrophy: a clinicopathologic study of 16 patients. J Am Acad Dermatol. 1996;35:523–8.

60. Yamamoto T, Yokozeki H, Nishioka K. Localized involutional lipoatrophy: report of six cases. J Dermatol. 2002;29:638–43.

61. Zalla MJ, Winkelmann RK, Gluck OS. Involutional lipoatrophy: macrophage-related involution of fat lobules. Dermatology. 1995;191:149–53.

62. Sasaki T, Kanbara T, Inayama Y. Do mucin-phagocytosing histiocytes in localized lipoatrophy have any primary pathogenetic importance? Br J Dermatol. 1999;140:976–8.

63. Bechara FG, Rotterdam S, Stücker M, et al. A case of localized bilateral lipodystrophy associated with self-injection of xenogenous material. J Dermatol. 2003;30:924–6.

64. Garg A. Lipodystrophies. Am J Med. 2000;108:143–52.

65. Köbberling J, Dunnigan MG. Familial partial lipodystrophy: two types of an X linked dominant syndrome, lethal in the hemizygous state. J Med Genet. 1986;23:120–7.

66. Dunnigan MG, Cochrane MA, Kelly A, Scott JW. Familial lipoatrophic diabetes with dominant transmission: a new syndrome. Q J Med. 1974;49:33–48.

67. Köbberling J, Willms B, Kettermann R, Creutzfeldt W. Lipodystrophy of the extremities: a dominantly inherited syndrome associated with lipoatrophic diabetes. Humangenetik. 1975;29:111–20.

68. Garg A, Peshock RM, Fleckenstein JL. Adipose tissue distribution pattern in patients with familial partial lipodystrophy (Dunnigan variety). J Clin Endocrinol Metab. 1999;84:170–4.

69. Garg A. Acquired and inherited lipodystrophies. N Engl J Med. 2004;350:1220–34.

70. Kavanaugh G, Colaco B, Kennedy CT. Juvenile dermatomyositis associated with partial lipoatrophy. J Am Acad Dermatol. 1993;28:348–51.

71. Rooney DP, Ryan MF. Diabetes with partial lipodystrophy following sclerodermatous chronic graft vs .host disease. Diabet Med. 2006;23:436–40.

72. Caramaschi P, Biasi D, Lestani M, Chilosi M. A case of acquired partial lipodystrophy associated with POEMS syndrome. Rheumatology. 2003;42:488–90.

73. Winhoven SM, Hafejee A, Coulson IH. An unusual case of an acquired acral partial lipodystrophy (Barraquer-Simons syndrome) in a patient with extrinsic allergic alveolitis. Clin Exp Dermatol. 2006;31:594–6.

74. Spranger S, Spranger M, Tasman AJ, et al. Barraquer-Simons syndrome (with sensorineural deafness): a contribution to the differential diagnosis of lipodystrophy syndromes. Am J Med Genet. 1997;71:397–400.

75. Peters MS, Winkelmann RK. Localized lipodystrophy (atrophic connective tissue disease panniculitis). Arch Dermatol. 1980;116:1363–8.

76. Mirza B, Muir J, Peake J, Whitehead K. Connective tissue panniculitis in a child with vitiligo and Hashimoto's thyroiditis. Australas J Dermatol. 2006;47:49–52.

77. Haas N, Henz BM, Bunikowski R, KeitzerR. Semicircular lipoatrophy in a child with systemic lupus erythematosus after subcutaneous injections with methotrexate. Pediatr Dermatol. 2002;19:432–5.

78. Ogino J, Saga K, Tamagawa M, Akutsu Y. Magnetic resonance imaging of semicircular lipoatrophy. Dermatology. 2004;209:340–1.

79. Rongioletti F, Rebora A. Annular and semicircular lipoatrophies: report of three cases and review of the literature. J Am Acad Dematol. 1989;20:433–6.

80. Dimson OG, Esterly NB. Annular lipoatrophy of the ankles. J Am Acad Dermatol. 2006;54:S40–2.

81. Imamura S. Skin diseases first described in Japan. Clin Dermatol. 1999;17:117–26.

82. Caputo R. Lipodystrophia centrifugalis sacralis infantilis. A 15-year-follow-up observation. Acta Derm Venereol. 1989;69:442–3.

83. Payne CMER, Harper JI, Farthing CE, Branfort AC, Staughton RE. Lipodystrophia centrifugalis. Br J Dermatol. 1985;113(suppl.):100–1.

84. Tay YK, Ong BH. Localized lipodystrophy in a child. Pediatr Dermatol. 2002;19:365–7.

85. Tollefson MM, Witman PM. En coup de sabre morphea and Parry-Romberg syndrome: a retrospective review of 54 patients. J Am Acad Dermatol. 2007;56:257–63.

86. Sonnino M, Ribuffo D, Piovano L, Cigna E, Scuderi N. Nonprogressive, late onset atrophy of the cheek [Italian]. Minerva Chir. 2000;55;881–5.

87. Cox NH. Becker's naevus of the thigh with lipoatrophy: report of two cases. Clin Exp Dermatol. 2002;27:27–8.

88. Taylor WB, Honeycutt WM. Progressive lipodystrophy and lipoatrophic diabetes. Arch Dermatol. 1961;84:31–6.

89. Nagore E, Sánchez-Motilla JM, Rodriguez-Serna M, Vilata JJ, Aliaga A, Lipoatrophia semicircularis – a traumatic panniculitis: report of seven cases and review of the literature. J Am Acad Dermatol. 1998;39:879–81.

90. Kosztolányi G. Leprechaunism/Donohue syndrome/insulin receptor gene mutations: a syndrome delineation story from clinicopathological description to molecular understanding. Eur J Pediatr. 1997;156:253–5.

91. Sorge G, Ruggieri M, Polizzi A, Scuderi A, Di Pietro M. SHORT syndrome: a new case with probable autosomal dominant inheritance. Am J Med Genet.1996;61:178–81.

92. Breslau-Siderius EJ, Toonstra J, Baart JA, et al. Ectodermal dysplasia, lipoatrophy, diabetes mellitus, and amastia: a second case of the AREDYLD syndrome. Am J Med Genet. 1992;14:374–7.

93. Inaloz HS, Gursoy S, Madenci E, Kirtak N. Minor Poland's syndrome mimicking localized lipoatrophy. J Dermatol. 2002;29:815–17.

94. Herold DA, Albrecht G. Local lipohypertrophy in insulin treatment. Hautarzt. 1993;44:40–2.

95. Goossens S, Coessens B. Facial contour restoration in Barraquer-Simons syndrome using two free TRAM flaps: presentation of two case reports and long-term follow-up. Microsurgery. 2002;22:211–18.

96. Guelinckx PJ, Sinsel NK. Facial contour restoration in Barraquer-Simons syndrome using two free anterolateral thigh flaps. Plast Reconstr Surg. 2000;105:1730–6.

97. Binder WJ, Bloom DC. The use of custom-designed midfacial and submalar implants in the treatment of facial wasting syndrome. Arch Facial Plast Surg. 2004;6:394–7.

98. Wolfort FG, Centrulo CL, Nevarre DR. Suction-assisted lipectomy for lipodystrophy syndromes attributed to HIV-protease inhibitor use. Plast Reconstr Surg. 1999;104:1820–1.

99. Arioglu E, Duncan-Morin J, Sebring N, et al. Efficacy and safety of troglitazone in the treatment of lipodystrophy syndromes. Ann Intern Med. 2000;133:263–74.

100. Ludtke A, Heck K, Genschel J, et al. Long-term treatment experience in a subject with Dunnigan-type familial partial lipodystrophy: efficacy of rosiglitazone. Diabet Med. 2005;22:1611–13.

101. Oral EA, Simha V, Ruiz E, et al. Leptin-replacement therapy for lipodystrophy. N Engl J Med. 2002;346:570–8.

102. Levy Y, George J, Yona E, Shoenfeld Y. Partial lipodystrophy, mesangiocapillary glomerulonephritis, and complement dysregulation. An autoimmune phenomenon. Immunol Res. 1998;18:55–60.

103. Carr A, Emery S, Law M, Puls R, Lundgren JD, Powderly WG: HIV Lipodystrophy Case Definition Study Group. An objective case definition of lipodystrophy in HIV-infected adults: a case-control study. Lancet 2003;361:726–35.

104. Study of Fat Redistribution and Metabolic Change in HIV Infection (FRAM). Fat distribution in men with HIV infection. J Acquir Immune Defic Syndr. 2005;40:121–31.

105. Study of Fat Redistribution and Metabolic Change in HIV Infection (FRAM). Fat distribution in women with HIV infection. J Acquir Immune Defic Syndr. 2006;42:562–71.

106. Lichtenstein KA. Redefining lipodystrophy syndrome. J Acquir Immune Defic Syndr. 2005;39:395–400.

107. Domingo P, Vidal F, Domingo JC, et al. Tumor necrosis factor alpha in fat redistribution syndromes associated with combination antiretroviral therapy in HIV-1-infected patients: potential role in subcutaneous adipocyte apoptosis. Eur J Clin Invest. 2005;35:771–80.

108. Caron M, Auclair M, Sterlingot H, Kornprobst M, Capeau J. Some HIV protease inhibitors alter lamin A/C maturation and stability, SREBP-1 nuclear localization and adipocyte differentiation. AIDS. 2003;17:2437–44.

109. Capanni C, Mattioli E, Columbaro M, et al. Altered pre-lamin A processing is a common mechanism leading to lipodystrophy. Hum Mol Genet. 2005;14:1489–502.

110. Grigem S, Fischer-Posovszky P, Debatin KM, Loizon E, Vidal H, Wabitsch M. The effect of the HIV protease inhibitor ritonavir on proliferation, differentiation, lipogenesis, gene expression and apoptosis of human preadipocytes and adipocytes. Horm Metab Res. 2005;37:602–9.

111. Rudich A, Ben-Romano R, Etzion S, Bashan N. Cellular mechanisms of insulin resistance, lipodystrophy and atherosclerosis induced by HIV protease inhibitors. Acta Physiol Scand. 2005;183:75–88.

112. El Hadri K, Glorian M, Monsempes C, et al. In vitro suppression of the lipogenic pathway by the nonnucleoside reverse transcriptase inhibitor efavirenz in 3T3 and human preadipocytes or adipocytes. J Biol Chem. 2004;279:15130–41.

113. Villarroya F, Domingo P, Giralt M. Lipodystrophy associated with highly active anti-retroviral therapy for HIV infection: the adipocyte as a target of anti-retroviral-induced mitochondrial toxicity. Trend Pharmacol Sci. 2005;26:88–93.

114. Pinti M, Salomoni P, Cossarizza A. Anti-HIV drugs and the mitochondria. Biochim Biophys Acta. 2006;1757:700–7.

115. Tien P, Grunfeld C. What is HIV-associated lipodystrophy? Defining fat distribution changes in HIV infection. Curr Opin Infect Dis. 2004;17:27–32.

116. Miller J, Carr A, Emery S, et al. HIV lipodystrophy: prevalence, severity and correlates of risk in Australia. HIV Med. 2003;4:293–301.

117. European Paediatric Lipodystrophy Group. Antiretroviral therapy, fat redistribution and hyperlipidaemia in HIV-infected children in Europe. AIDS. 2004;18:1443–51.

118. Carr A, Samaras K, Thorisdottir A, Kaufmann GR, Chisholm DJ, Cooper DA. Diagnosis, prediction, and natural course of HIV-1 protease-inhibitor-associated lipodystrophy, hyperlipidaemia, and diabetes mellitus: a cohort study. Lancet. 1999;353:2093–9.

119. Grinspoon S, Carr A. Cardiovascular risk and body-fat abnormalities in HIV-infected adults. N Engl J Med. 2005;352:48–62.

120. Duran S, Saves M, Spire B, et al. Failure to maintain long-term adherence to highly active antiretroviral therapy: the role of lipodystrophy. AIDS. 2001;15:2441–4.

121. Tien PC, Benson C, Zolopa AR, Sidney S, Osmond D, Grunfeld C. The Study of Fat Redistribution and Metabolic Change in HIV Infection (FRAM): methods, design, and sample characteristics. Am J Epidemiol. 2006;163:860–9.

122. Tien P, Cole S, Williams C, et al. Incidence of lipoatrophy and lipohypertrophy in the Women's Interagency HIV Study. J Acquir Immune Defic Syndr. 2003;34:461–6.

123. Mallon P, Miller J, Cooper D, Carr A. Prospective evaluation of the effects of antiretroviral therapy on body composition in HIV-1 infected men starting therapy. AIDS. 2003;17:971–9.

124. Hansen AB, Lindegaard B, Obel N, et al. Pronounced lipoatrophy in HIV-infected men receiving HAART for more than 6 years compared with the background population. HIV Med. 2006;7:38–45.

125. Jacobson DL, Knox T, Spiegelman D, Skinner S, Gorbach S, Wanke C. Prevalence of, evolution of, and risk factors for fat atrophy and fat deposition in a cohort of HIV-infected men and women. Clin Infect Dis. 2005;40:1837–45.

126. Galli M, Veglia F, Angarano G, et al. Gender differences in antiretroviral drug-related adipose tissue alterations: women are at higher risk than men and develop particular lipodystrophy patterns. J Acquir Immune Defic Syndr. 2003;34:58–61.

127. Friis-Møller N, Weber R, Reiss P, et al. Cardiovascular disease risk factors in HIV patients – association with antiretroviral therapy: results from the DAD study. AIDS. 2003;17:1179–93.

128. Brown TT, Cole SR, Li X, et al. Prevalence and incidence of pre-diabetes and diabetes in the Multicenter AIDS Cohort Study. In: Proceedings of the 11th Conference on Retroviruses and Opportunistic Infections, San Francisco, February 8-11, 2004:73 (abstract).

129. The Data Collection on Adverse Events of Anti-HIV Drugs (DAD) Study Group. Combination antiretroviral therapy and the risk of myocardial infarction. N Engl J Med. 2003;349:1993–2003.

130. Morse CG, Kovacs JA. Metabolic and skeletal complications of HIV infection: the price of success. JAMA. 2006;296:844–54.

131. Wohl DA, McComsey G, Tebas P, et al. Current concepts in the diagnosis and management of metabolic complications of HIV infection and its therapy. HIV/AIDS. 2006;43:645–53.

132. Guaraldi G, Orlando G, Squillace N, et al. Multidisciplinary approach to the treatment of metabolic and morphologic alterations of HIV-related lipodystrophy. HIV Clin Trials. 2006;7:97–106.

133. Carr A, Hudson J, Chuah J, et al. HIV protease inhibitor substitution in patients with lipodystrophy: a randomized, controlled, open-label, multicentre study. AIDS. 2001;15:1811–22.

134. van der Valk M, Allick G, Weverling GJ, et al. Markedly diminished lipolysis and partial restoration of glucose metabolism, without changes in fat distribution after extended discontinuation of protease inhibitors in severe lipodystrophic human immunodeficient virus-1-infected patients. J Clin Endocrinol Metab. 2004;89:3554–60.

135. Jemsek JG, Arathoon E, Arlotti M, et al. Body fat and other metabolic effects of atazanavir and efavirenz, each administered in combination with zidovudine plus lamivudine, in antiretroviral-naive HIV-infected patients. Clin Infect Dis. 2006;42:273–80.

136. Moyle GJ, Sabin CA, Cartledge J, et al. A randomized comparative trial of tenofovir DF or abacavir as replacement for a thymidine analogue in persons with lipoatrophy. AIDS. 2006;20:2043–50.

137. Feldt T, Oette M, Kroidl A, et al. Evaluation of safety and efficacy of rosiglitazone in the treatment of HIV-associated lipodystrophy syndrome. Infection. 2006;34:55–61.

138. Guaraldi G, Orlando G, de Fazio D, et al. Comparison of three different interventions for the correction of HIV-associated facial lipoatrophy: a prospective study. Antivir Ther 2005;10:753–9.

139. Mest DR, Humble G. Human immunodeficiency virus-associated facial lipoatrophy: a review. Cosmet Dermatol. 2006;19:62–6.

140. Serra-Renom JM, Fontdevila J. Treatment of facial fat atrophy related to treatment with protease inhibitors by autologous fat injection in patients with human immunodeficiency virus infection. J Plast Reconstr Surg. 2004;114:551–5.

141. Moyle GJ, Brown S, Lysakova L, Barton SE. Long-term safety and efficacy of poly-L-lactic acid in the treatment of HIV-related facial lipoatrophy. HIV Med. 2006;7:181–5.

142. Roubenoff R, Schmitz H, Bairos L, et al. Reduction of abdominal obesity in lipodystrophy associated with human immunodeficiency virus infection by means of diet and exercise: case report and proof of principle. Clin Infect Dis. 2002;34:390–3.

143. Driscoll SD, Meininger GE, Ljungquist K, et al. Differential effects of metformin and exercise on muscle adiposity and metabolic indices in human immunodeficiency virus-infected patients. J Clin Endocrinol Metab. 2004;89:2171–8.

144. Falutz J, Allas S, Kotler D, et al. A placebo-controlled, dose-ranging study of a growth hormone releasing factor in HIV-infected patients with abdominal fat accumulation. AIDS. 2005;19:1279–87.

145. Piliero PJ, Hubbard M, King J, Faragon JJ. Use of ultrasonography-assisted liposuction for the treatment of human immunodeficiency virus-associated enlargement of the dorsocervical fat pad. HIV/AIDS. 2003;37:1374–7.

146. Gervasoni C, Ridolfo AL, Vaccarezza M, et al. Long-term efficacy of the surgical treatment of buffalo hump in patients continuing antiretroviral therapy. AIDS. 2004;18:574–6.

Vascular Biology

102

Michael Detmar and Satoshi Hirakawa

Key features

- Cutaneous blood vessels and lymphatic vessels play important roles in skin inflammation and tumor progression
- Vascular endothelial growth factor (VEGF) and placental growth factor (PlGF) are major skin angiogenesis factors
- Expression of VEGF and PlGF by keratinocytes is upregulated in psoriasis, healing wounds and cutaneous squamous cell carcinomas
- VEGF-C and VEGF-D induce skin lymphangiogenesis via interaction with VEGF receptor-3 on lymphatic endothelium. Inactivating VEGF receptor-3 mutations have been found in congenital lymphedema
- Cutaneous lymphatic vessels can be specifically visualized in skin sections due to their selective expression of the transcription factor Prox1 and of the hyaluronan receptor LYVE-1

INTRODUCTION

The blood vessels of the skin are involved in the control of body temperature and provide a conduit for the supply of nutrients and oxygen to the skin and for the rapid disposal of metabolic waste products. Recent scientific progress in the field of vascular biology has provided ample evidence that both blood vessels and lymphatic vessels also play essential roles in the development and progression of skin tumors, in the mediation and perpetuation of cutaneous inflammation, as well as in physiologic processes such as tissue repair and hair follicle growth. An increased knowledge about markers for specific types of vessels, together with the identification of key molecules that control vascular growth and function, has led to an in-depth understanding of the mechanisms that control the function of the cutaneous vascular system in health and disease, with important implications for the development of novel therapeutic strategies for the treatment of skin diseases.

STRUCTURE AND FUNCTION OF CUTANEOUS BLOOD VESSELS

Blood vessels are essential in order to: supply sufficient oxygen and nutrients to the skin, maintain normal tissue homeostasis and function, and meet the increased nutritional needs of the skin in various pathologic conditions. Blood flows from arteries and arterioles through capillary loops to postcapillary venules and veins. For practical and didactic purposes, the vascular system of the skin has been divided into a superficial and a deep vascular plexus (Fig. 102.1), with additional vascular networks surrounding sweat glands and hair follicles. The architecture of the cutaneous vascular system varies in different areas of the body. In the presence of pronounced epidermal rete ridges, such as in the skin overlying the extensor aspects of the joints or on the palms and soles, straight capillary loops extend into the elongated dermal papillae. In contrast, rete ridge formation and papillary loop formation are less pronounced in the abdominal skin. In fact, it appears that the shape of the papillary microvessels exactly reflects the three-dimensional architecture of the epidermal rete ridges, with only one loop within each papilla[1]. The inner diameter of papillary blood vessels averages between 5 and 10 μm. In contrast to the idealized architectural model of the cutaneous vascular system, vascular perfusion studies (Fig. 102.2) and immunofluorescent studies (Fig. 102.3) reveal a rather continuous, sometimes irregular meshwork of interconnecting

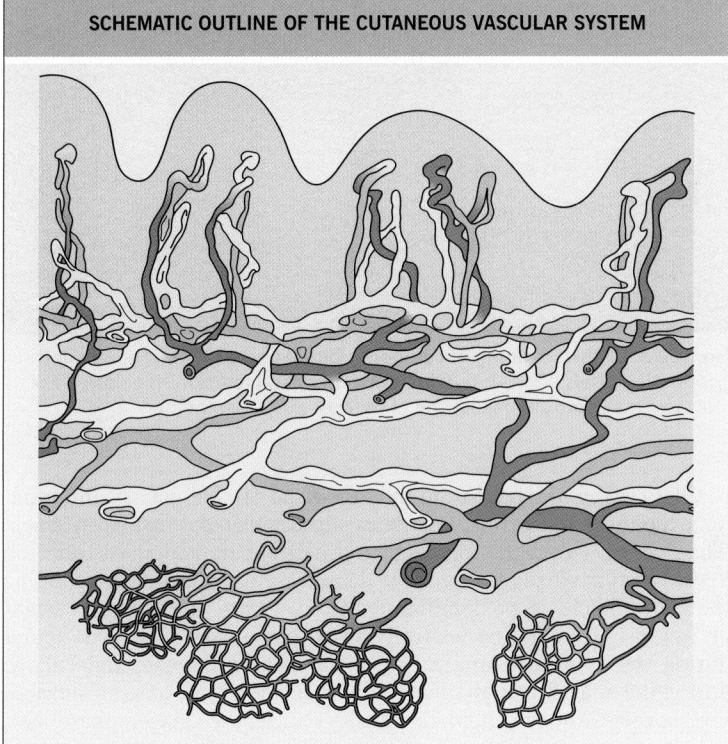

SCHEMATIC OUTLINE OF THE CUTANEOUS VASCULAR SYSTEM

Fig. 102.1 Schematic outline of the cutaneous vascular system. The superficial vascular plexus feeds vessels in the dermal papillae; arteries (red) and veins (blue) are closely associated with lymphatic vessels (yellow).

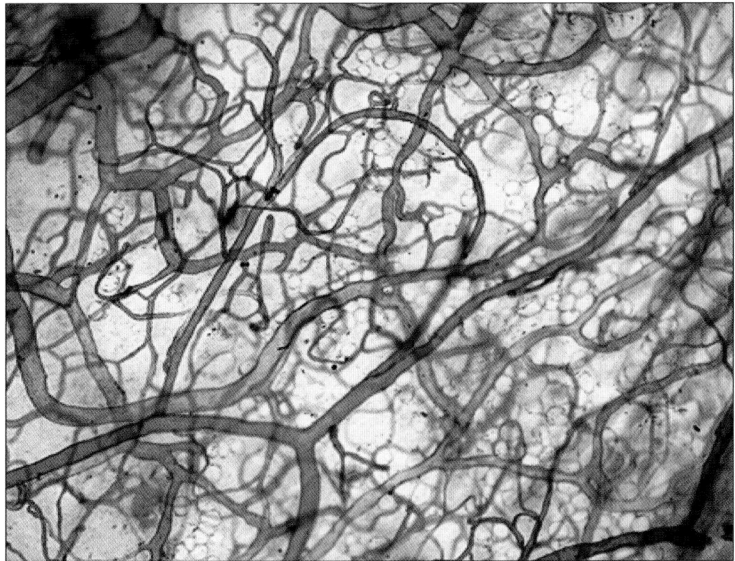

Fig. 102.2 Intravascular perfusion of murine skin with the lectin *Leucopersicon esculentum.* The perfusion highlights dense irregular vascular networks.

cutaneous blood vessels. Consistently, blood vessels are found immediately below the non-vascularized epidermis and surrounding anagen hair follicles.

It has been thought that hair follicles and other skin appendages are predominantly supplied from the lower vascular plexus, whereas the

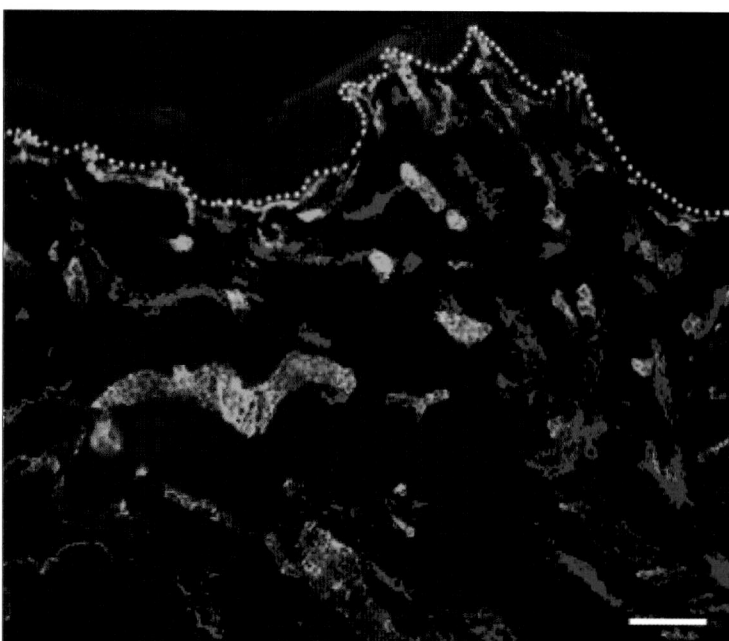

Fig. 102.3 Distinct staining of cutaneous blood vessels (PAL-E; green) and lymphatic vessels (LYVE-1; red) in human neonatal foreskin. The dotted line indicates the approximate location of the basement membrane.

papillary vessels originate from the superficial vascular plexus. Immuno-histochemical and perfusion studies suggest that the frequently single blood vessel within the mesenchymal hair papilla is derived from the lower vascular plexus, whereas the dense vascular network surrounding the hair follicle is predominantly derived from the upper vascular plexus (Fig. 102.4). The relatively small blood vessels that are found during the telogen resting phase of the follicle elongate and enlarge during the anagen growth phase, and then extend towards the subcutis together with the growing hair follicle. During the catagen phase, hair follicle involution is associated with regression of perifollicular blood vessels and with increased rates of endothelial cell apoptosis[2]. Whereas the richness of the follicular blood supply depends on the size of the hair follicles, recent studies suggest that, conversely, the extent of perifollicular vascularization may directly influence the size of the hair follicles[2].

In addition to its importance for the nutritional support of the skin, the cutaneous vasculature also plays a systemic role in regulating body temperature and blood pressure. Arterioles possess precapillary muscular sphincters that, upon contraction, can shunt the blood via arteriovenous anastomoses directly to venules, thereby bypassing the

capillary networks. Arteriovenous anastomoses are frequently found in the fingertips, where they form the glomi or glomus bodies[1]. Glomi show autonomous innervation and are able, via modulation of their muscular contraction levels, to control peripheral blood flow. The density and importance of arteriovenous anastomoses in other body areas remains unclear.

All blood vessels contain a continuous inner monolayer of flat endothelial cells that are surrounded, on the external side, by a continuous basement membrane. Smaller vessels contain a second, sometimes discontinuous layer of perivascular cells, called pericytes, which are also surrounded by a basement membrane. Pericytes play an important role in the maintenance of mature blood vessels, and detachment of pericytes from endothelial cells is an early event during sprouting angiogenesis (outgrowth of new capillaries from pre-existing blood vessels). Arterioles and venules are also surrounded by pericytes, which can be visualized by staining for α-smooth muscle actin and desmin. The walls of most arterioles and larger venules and veins contain contractile smooth muscle cells that are surrounded by a basement membrane. Vascular basement membranes contain collagen types IV, XV and XVIII, laminin, fibronectin, and other extracellular matrix proteins. Electron microscopy studies have shown that the basement membrane of endothelial cells in the arterial side of the cutaneous vasculature is rather homogeneous, whereas multilayered basement membranes have been described surrounding venous capillaries[3].

At the ultrastructural level, vascular endothelial cells are characterized by tight junctions between neighboring cells and by a specialized organelle, the rod-shaped Weibel–Palade body (Fig. 102.5), which serves as a storage organelle for the coagulation factor von Willebrand factor, also known as factor VIII-related antigen. Weibel–Palade bodies also contain P-selectin, tissue plasminogen activator, angiopoietin-2 and endothelin-1. Activation of endothelial cells by proinflammatory cytokines or pro-angiogenic factors readily leads to translocation of these storage organelles to the cell membrane, with consecutive enhanced membrane expression of P-selectin and release of von Willebrand factor. Other characteristic ultrastructural features include caveolae (minute invaginations) of the membrane surface, pinocytotic vesicles, and the formation of vesiculo-vacuolar organelles (VVOs)[4]. Circulating macro-molecules cross the endothelium through interendothelial cell gaps and transendothelial cell pores, some of which arise from VVOs. Endothelial cell fenestrations, areas with direct apposition of the endothelial cell membranes without intervening cytoplasm, are rarely seen in normal skin except in angiogenic perifollicular blood vessels during the growth phase of the hair follicle. However, fenestrated endothelial cells are frequently seen in skin diseases with pronounced angiogenesis and vascular hyperpermeability, including psoriasis[5].

Several markers for blood vascular endothelial cells have been identified (see Table 102.3). However, some of these markers (e.g. CD31, CD34) can also be detected on other dermal cells such as lymphatic

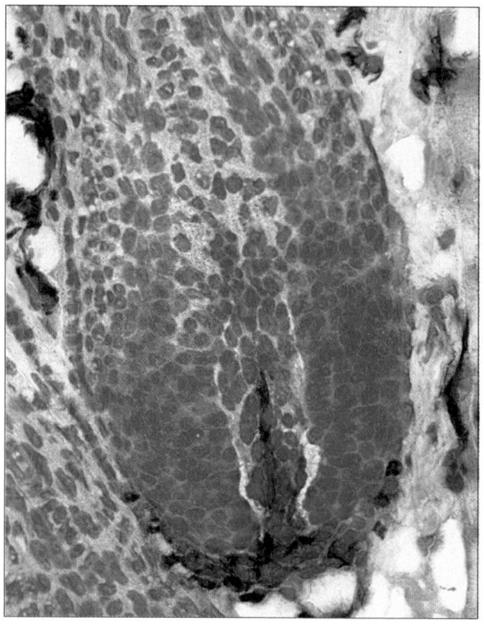

Fig. 102.4 Blood supply of the hair follicle. A single vascular loop extends into the dermal papilla of the hair follicle, while a mesh of blood vessels surrounds the anagen hair follicle (CD31 stain).

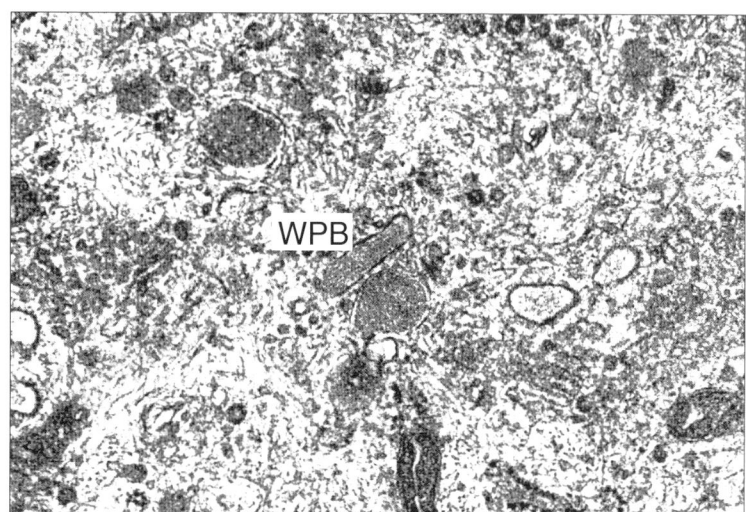

Fig. 102.5 Ultrastructural visualization of a rod-shaped Weibel–Palade body (WPB) within the cytoplasm of a human endothelial cell.

endothelial cells (CD31) or fibrocytes (CD34). In normal skin, the most specific markers for cutaneous blood vessels appear to be CD34 and PAL-E (see Fig. 102.3). Double immunofluorescence stains for the pan-endothelial cell marker CD31 (PECAM-1) and for the lymphatic vascular endothelium-specific hyaluronan receptor LYVE-1 also allow for the selective visualization of LYVE-1-negative blood vessels in the skin (see Fig. 102.16). In addition, differential immunostains for CD31 and vascular basement membrane markers such as laminin (see Fig. 102.14), collagen IV and collagen XVIII can also be used to visualize cutaneous blood vessels[6].

VASCULAR DEVELOPMENT

During embryogenesis, the first blood vessels are formed through vasculogenesis, the differentiation of undifferentiated angioblasts into endothelial cells that form a primitive vascular network. Angioblasts originate from blood islands in the extraembryonic mesoderm of the yolk sac. Blood islands are clusters of epithelioid cells; the outer cells differentiate into angioblasts, whereas the inner cells differentiate into primitive hematopoietic cells, suggesting that both cell types originate from a common embryonic precursor cell, the hemangioblast[7], which is formed from earlier precursor cells under the influence of fibroblast growth factors (Fig. 102.6). Hemangioblasts already express the high-affinity receptor for vascular endothelial growth factor (VEGF), vascular endothelial growth factor receptor-2 (VEGFR-2; KDR [human]; Flk-1 [murine]; see Fig. 102.8); under experimental conditions, early VEGFR-2-positive cells can give rise to both endothelial cells and blood cells[8].

Angioblasts develop under the influence of stimulation by VEGF and express several vascular endothelial cell markers, including the Tie-1 and Tie-2 receptors, vascular endothelial (VE)-cadherin, and the high-affinity VEGF receptors 1 (Flt-1), 2 (KDR) and 3 (Flt-4). Angioblasts within the embryo appear along the anterior intestinal portal and along the lateral edges of the somites, later coalescing to form the dorsal aorta and the large vessel primordia of the body. Angioblasts are highly migratory 'prevascular' endothelial cells and are found throughout the embryo with the exception of tissues such as cartilage and epithelia[7].

When angioblasts form a lumen, they become endothelial cells with a polarized phenotype and production of a basal lamina. Interactions of integrin receptors on the endothelial surface with the basement membrane are of paramount importance for the formation of the primordial vascular plexus, and establishment of interendothelial adherence junctions requires the vascular endothelial cadherin VE-cadherin. The early vascular system consists of sinusoidal capillaries that are arranged in a polygonal honeycomb pattern (see Fig. 102.6). The primordial vascular plexus then becomes surrounded by mesenchymal cells that give rise to pericytes and vascular smooth muscle cells. In a next step, under the influence of VEGF, angiopoietins (see Fig. 102.7) and ephrins, profound remodeling of the primordial vascular plexus takes place. Remodeling involves both the formation and the regression of blood vessels and apoptosis of vascular endothelial cells.

Angiogenesis, the sprouting of new blood vessels from existing primordial vessels, represents the major mechanism for new blood vessel formation. In addition, intussusception, the non-sprouting generation of new blood vessels, involves the formation of intravascular endothelial pillars, leading to the division of the vascular lumen and to the formation of a new vascular space. The Tie-2 receptor tyrosine kinase, expressed on vascular endothelial cells, plays a crucial role in vascular sprouting and remodeling during early embryonic angiogenesis. Angiopoietin-1 (Ang-1) activates the Tie-2 receptor, whereas Ang-2 can act as an inhibitor of Ang-1[9]. Studies in genetic mouse models suggest that Ang-1 is involved in vessel maturation, whereas Ang-2 may either promote angiogenesis, in the presence of VEGF, or lead to vessel regression, in the absence of VEGF (Fig. 102.7).

Ephrin–Eph receptor interactions, via bidirectional signaling, also play an important role in vascular remodeling and in the determination of vascular identity. Ephrin B2 is specifically expressed by arterial endothelium, whereas its receptor, Eph-B4, is expressed by venous endothelium. Both molecules are involved in the definition of boundaries between arterial and venous endothelial cells. Additional molecules are involved in the control of embryonic angiogenesis and vascular remodeling, including transforming growth factor-β (TGF-β), its low-affinity receptor endoglin, and activin receptor-like kinase-1. Platelet-derived

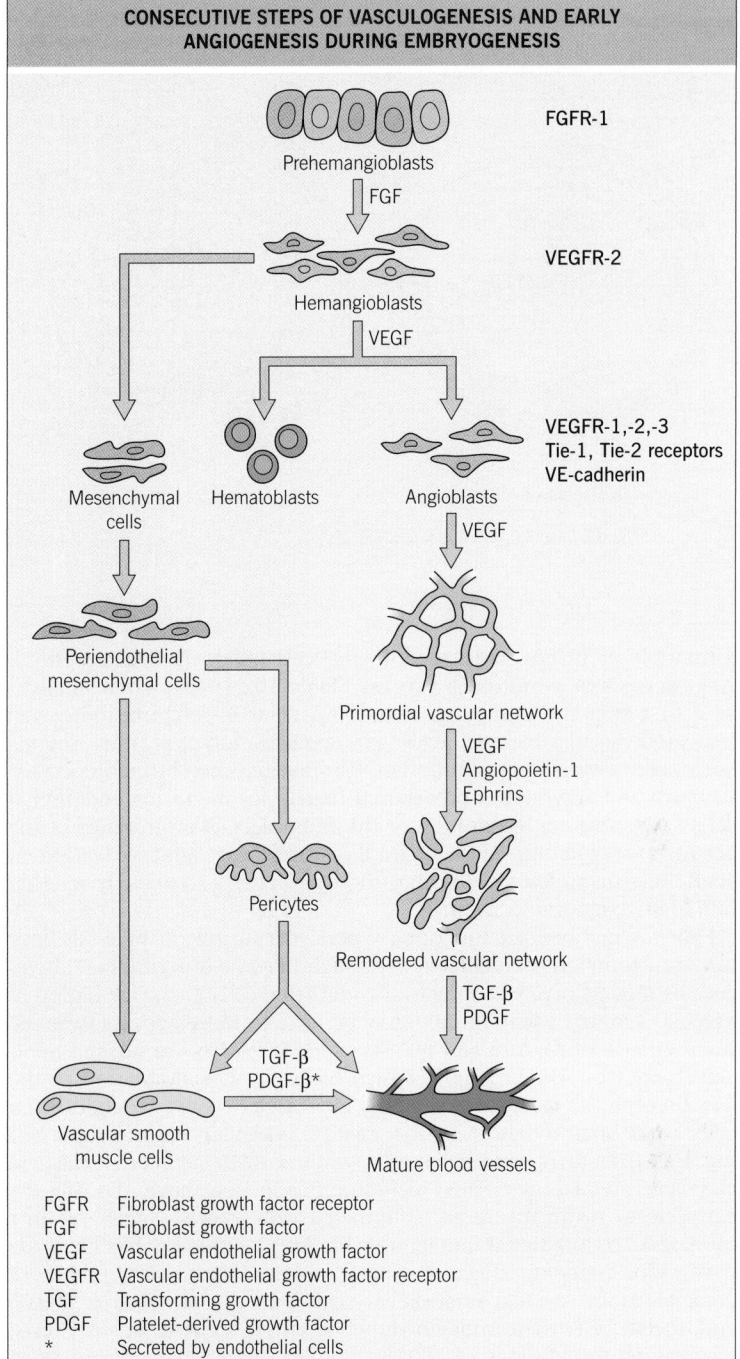

CONSECUTIVE STEPS OF VASCULOGENESIS AND EARLY ANGIOGENESIS DURING EMBRYOGENESIS

FGFR	Fibroblast growth factor receptor
FGF	Fibroblast growth factor
VEGF	Vascular endothelial growth factor
VEGFR	Vascular endothelial growth factor receptor
TGF	Transforming growth factor
PDGF	Platelet-derived growth factor
*	Secreted by endothelial cells

Fig. 102.6 **Consecutive steps of vasculogenesis and early angiogenesis during embryogenesis: formation and remodeling of primordial vascular networks.**

growth factor-β (PDGF-β), secreted by endothelial cells, plays a critical role in the recruitment and differentiation of pericytes and periendothelial smooth muscle cells that contribute to the stability of mature blood vessels[10].

Regulation of Skin Angiogenesis

Angiogenesis is a common feature of developing skin during embryogenesis. In contrast, the blood vessels in healthy adult skin are predominantly quiescent, with the exception of the cyclic expansion and involution of perifollicular blood vessels during the hair cycle[2]. However, adult skin retains the capacity for brisk initiation of angiogenesis during wound healing, in the setting of inflammation, and during neoplastic growth. Angiogenesis occurs as: (1) the sprouting outgrowth of new capillaries from pre-existing postcapillary venules; or (2) non-sprouting remodeling of pre-existing blood vessels either through circumferential growth/vascular enlargement or through the

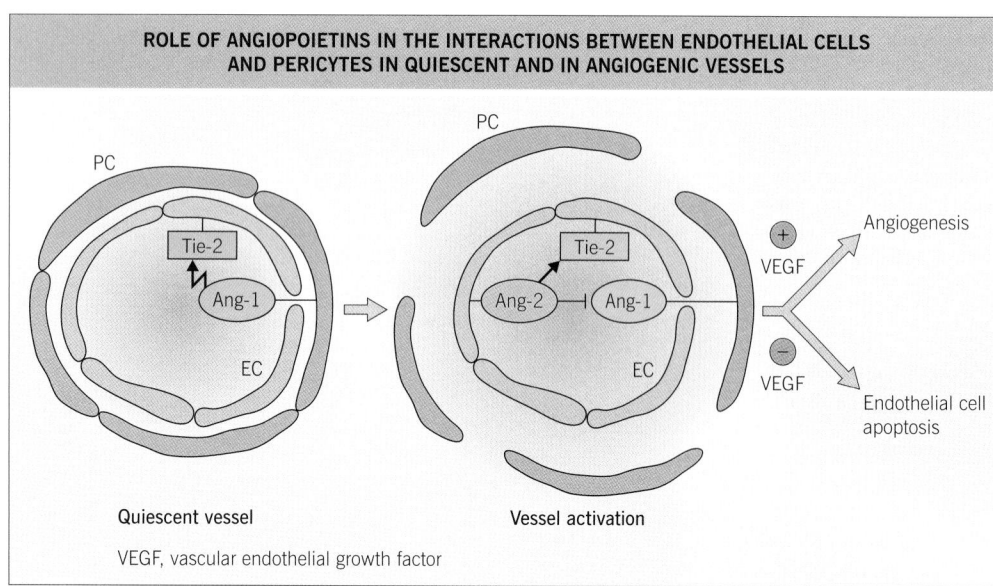

ROLE OF ANGIOPOIETINS IN THE INTERACTIONS BETWEEN ENDOTHELIAL CELLS AND PERICYTES IN QUIESCENT AND IN ANGIOGENIC VESSELS

PC

Tie-2

Ang-1

EC

Quiescent vessel

PC

Tie-2

Ang-2 ⊣ Ang-1

EC

Vessel activation

+ VEGF → Angiogenesis

− VEGF → Endothelial cell apoptosis

VEGF, vascular endothelial growth factor

Fig. 102.7 Role of angiopoietins in the interactions between endothelial cells and pericytes in quiescent and in angiogenic vessels. Activation of the endothelial Tie-2 receptor by pericyte (PC)-derived angiopoietin-1 (Ang-1) is thought to result in vessel maturation. Upregulation of angiopoietin-2 (Ang-2) in angiogenic endothelial cells (EC) blocks the vessel-stabilizing effect of pericyte-derived Ang-1 via the endothelial Tie-2 receptor.

formation of intravascular endothelial cell pillars (intussusception). Angiogenesis is a multistep process (Table 102.1) that often involves as a first step the induction of microvascular hyperpermeability, i.e. increased vascular leakage, leading to extravasation of plasma proteins such as fibrinogen and prothrombin. Fibrinogen is then further processed to fibrin and serves as a provisional matrix for migrating endothelial cells[11], whereas the generation of thrombin acts as an initiator of the extrinsic coagulation cascade, leading to cleavage and activation of several matrix proteins[12]. Together, these processes lead to the generation of a highly angiogenic stroma.

The distinct biologic functions of pericytes during angiogenesis have not been completely elucidated. Although in some experimental angiogenesis models pericytes may lead endothelial cells in the formation of vascular sprouts, a major function of pericyte coverage appears to be the maintenance of mature and quiescent blood vessels. In normal adult skin, pericytes secrete Ang-1, which leads to phosphorylation of the Tie-2 receptor (a receptor exclusively expressed on vascular endothelial cells) and maintenance of the mature vascular architecture (see Fig. 102.7). In turn, endothelial cells secrete growth factors that mediate the recruitment of pericytes, including PDGF (see above). During the early stages of angiogenesis, endothelial cells express high amounts of Ang-2, a functional antagonist of Ang-1, thereby blocking the maturation-inducing effect of Ang-1 and leading to detachment of pericytes from vascular endothelial cells[13]. In the presence of VEGF, endothelial cells then undergo the consecutive steps of angiogenesis, whereas in the absence of VEGF, vascular endothelial cells undergo apoptosis (see Fig. 102.7). Both VEGF and Ang-2 expression are upregulated in angiogenic skin diseases, including psoriasis, and keratinocyte-derived VEGF and placental growth factor (PlGF; see below) both potently induce the expression of Ang-2 in dermal microvascular endothelial cells.

The vascular basement membrane serves as a natural barrier that prevents sprouting of endothelial cells from quiescent, non-angiogenic vessels. An early step in the angiogenic response involves the degradation of vascular basement membrane components such as collagen type IV through the concerted action of activated proteases, including matrix metalloproteinase (MMP)-2 and MMP-9. Integrin receptors on the surface of endothelial cells, in particular the $\alpha_1\beta_1$, $\alpha_2\beta_1$ and $\alpha_v\beta_3$

integrins, then interact with either native or degraded matrix molecules (e.g. collagen type I, fibronectin) in order to facilitate endothelial cell migration[14–16]. The migration of endothelial cells in the skin is directed towards a gradient of angiogenesis factors that are most commonly produced by the epidermis, but that can also be secreted by macrophages. Endothelial cells then undergo a series of cell divisions, promoted by potent angiogenesis factors such as VEGF and basic fibroblast growth factor. Finally, endothelial cells form vascular lumina and mature new blood vessels with basement membrane and pericyte coverage.

In normal skin, vascular quiescence is maintained by the dominant influence of potent endogenous angiogenesis inhibitors over angiogenic stimuli, whereas angiogenesis is induced by increased secretion of angiogenic factors and/or by downregulation of angiogenesis inhibitors. Several factors that control angiogenesis in the skin have been recently identified. The major skin angiogenesis factor, vascular endothelial growth factor (VEGF), was originally discovered as vascular permeability factor (VPF), due to the activity of tumor cell-conditioned media to induce accumulation of ascites fluid[17]. VEGF is a homodimeric, heparin-binding glycoprotein occurring in at least four isoforms of 121, 165, 189 and 201 amino acids, due to alternative splicing. VEGF binds to two type III tyrosine kinase receptors that are expressed predominantly on vascular endothelial cells, Flt-1/VEGF receptor-1 (VEGFR-1) and KDR/Flk-1/VEGFR-2 (Fig. 102.8). In addition, VEGF165 also binds to the neuropilin receptor on endothelial and other cells.

In vitro, VEGF acts as a specific mitogen for human dermal microvascular endothelial cells and also induces endothelial cell migration towards several extracellular matrices, partly through upregulation of the collagen receptors $\alpha_1\beta_1$ and $\alpha_2\beta_1$ on endothelial cells[16]. *In vivo*, VEGF enhances microvascular permeability and angiogenesis. VEGF is expressed at low levels in normal epidermis, whereas healing wounds and skin diseases associated with angiogenesis and vascular hyperpermeability, particularly psoriasis, show prominent upregulation of VEGF expression by epidermal keratinocytes[18]. The expression and biologic activity of VEGF are controlled by several distinct molecular mechanisms. Hypoxia and low intracellular glucose concentrations result in transcriptional activation (via hypoxia-inducible factors) and stabilization of VEGF mRNA. Skin hypoxia directly leads to upregulation of VEGF expression by epidermal keratinocytes, dermal fibroblasts and dermal endothelial cells. Hypoxia also induces upregulation of the VEGF receptor Flt-1/VEGFR-1 on microvessels, suggesting the existence of an autocrine pro-angiogenic loop. This mechanism likely is important in the induction of epidermal VEGF expression during wound healing and in areas of skin cancers adjacent to tumor necrosis[19].

Keratinocyte VEGF expression is also induced by several growth factors that mediate epidermal hyperplasia. In psoriasis, healing wounds and squamous cell carcinomas, TGF-α and other ligands of the epidermal growth factor receptor are released by suprabasal keratinocytes. In an autocrine loop, these growth factors induce hyperplasia of the epidermis. Simultaneously, they induce VEGF gene expression and

THE STEPWISE INDUCTION OF ANGIOGENESIS

1. Induction of microvascular hyperpermeability
2. Enzymatic degradation of vascular basement membrane and interstitial matrix
3. Endothelial cell migration
4. Endothelial cell proliferation
5. Formation of mature blood vessels

Table 102.1 The stepwise induction of angiogenesis.

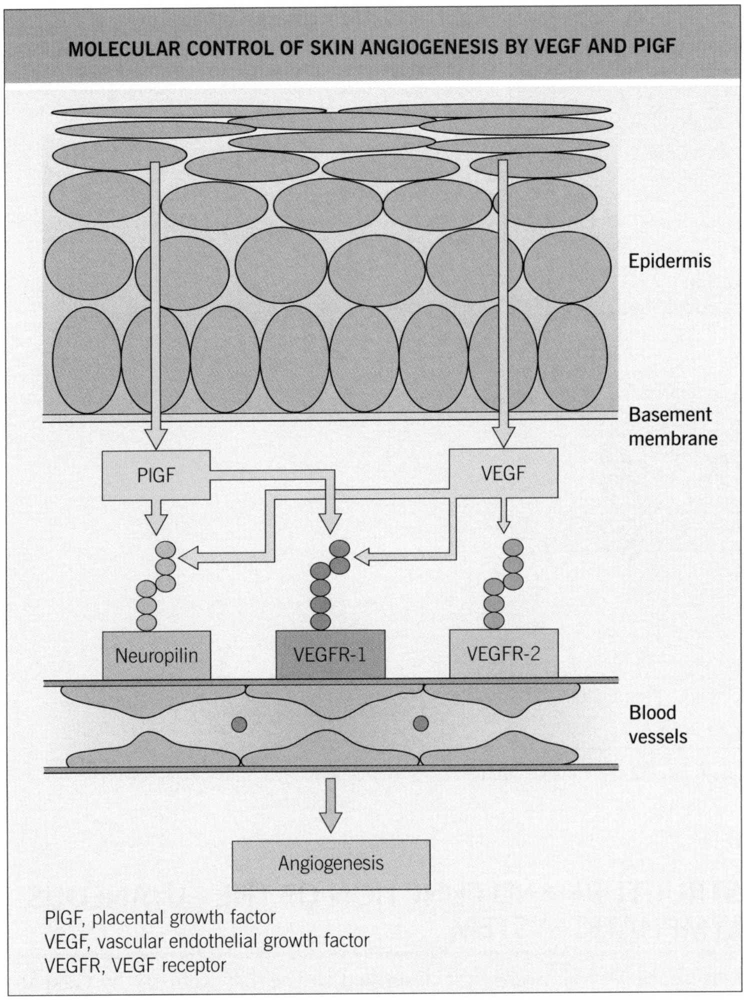

MOLECULAR CONTROL OF SKIN ANGIOGENESIS BY VEGF AND PIGF

PIGF, placental growth factor
VEGF, vascular endothelial growth factor
VEGFR, VEGF receptor

Fig. 102.8 Molecular control of skin angiogenesis by vascular endothelial growth factor (VEGF) and placental growth factor (PIGF).

protein secretion by epidermal keratinocytes, which lead to paracrine induction of angiogenesis through interaction with VEGF receptors on cutaneous microvessels (see Fig. 102.8). This mechanism links epidermal hyperplasia with increased vascularization, thereby providing enhanced vascular support to meet the enhanced nutritional needs of proliferating keratinocytes. It also provides a molecular explanation for the previously reported association of thickened acanthotic epidermis with elongated capillary vessels[1]. Several other growth factors that stimulate keratinocyte proliferation, including keratinocyte growth factor and hepatocyte growth factor, have recently joined the group of VEGF-inducing molecules.

The biologic importance of epidermis-derived VEGF for cutaneous angiogenesis *in vivo* has been confirmed in transgenic mouse models, using the keratin 14 promoter to selectively target expression of murine VEGF164 to basal epidermal keratinocytes and to keratinocytes of the outer root sheath of the hair follicle[20]. VEGF transgenic mice are characterized by elongated and tortuous dermal blood vessels that are hyperpermeable to circulating plasma proteins. VEGF-overexpressing mice are unable to downregulate experimentally induced cutaneous inflammation and develop chronic inflammatory skin lesions that closely resemble those of human psoriasis[21].

The majority of human cancers studied thus far are characterized by overexpression of VEGF by tumor cells and by overexpression of VEGF receptors on tumor-associated blood vessels; blocking of VEGF function inhibits angiogenesis and suppresses tumor growth *in vivo*. VEGF also promotes skin carcinogenesis, since antibody inhibition of the VEGF receptor Flk-1/VEGFR-2 prevented squamous cell carcinoma invasion[22], and selective overexpression of VEGF in epidermal keratinocytes resulted in enhanced tumor development and metastasis[23].

Placental growth factor (PlGF) is a recently identified new member of the VEGF family of angiogenesis factors, with considerable sequence homology with VEGF. PlGF occurs in at least three different isoforms

of 149 (PlGF-1), 170 (PlGF-2) and 221 (PlGF-3) amino acids. Both PlGF-1 and PlGF-2 are expressed in human skin. Similar to VEGF, the expression of PlGF is upregulated in cutaneous squamous cell carcinomas, in epidermal keratinocytes at the advancing wound edge, and in the hyperplastic psoriatic epidermis. In contrast to VEGF, PlGF does not activate VEGFR-2 (KDR), but selectively binds to VEGFR-1 (see Fig. 102.8). In addition, the heparin-binding isoform PlGF-2, but not PlGF-1, binds to the neuropilin receptor. Recent evidence from genetic mouse models indicates that: (1) PlGF and VEGF act in synergy to induce angiogenesis and vascular leakage; (2) PlGF exerts proinflammatory effects; and (3) the presence of PlGF is essential for distinct VEGF effects to occur[24,25]. A number of additional pro-angiogenic molecules are upregulated in angiogenic skin conditions, including interleukin-8, platelet-derived growth factors, fibroblast growth factors and angiogenic chemokines. However, the distinct contributions of each of these factors to the cutaneous vascular response remain to be characterized in more detail.

Thrombospondin (TSP)-1 and TSP-2 are major endogenous inhibitors of skin angiogenesis and are expressed in normal human skin. Thrombospondins are matricellular proteins that mediate interactions between extracellular matrix molecules and cellular integrin receptors (Fig. 102.9). TSP-1, a 450 kD modular, homotrimeric glycoprotein, contains a procollagen homology region, three properdin-like type I repeats, three epidermal growth factor-like repeats, and seven Ca^{2+}-binding repeats. TSP-1 is involved in a large number of biologic processes, including proliferation, migration and differentiation of various cell types; moreover, TSP-1 inhibits endothelial cell proliferation *in vitro* and angiogenesis *in vivo*. In normal human skin, TSP-1 is expressed by dermal cells and by epidermal keratinocytes, and it is deposited in the dermo-epidermal basement membrane zone, contributing to the barrier that prevents ingrowth of blood vessels into the epidermis. In contrast, TSP-1 expression is downregulated in squamous cell carcinomas of the skin. Reintroduction of the *TSP-1* gene into squamous cell carcinomas inhibits tumor growth in mice, associated with inhibition of tumor angiogenesis and enhanced tumor cell necrosis[26]. The potential mechanisms by which TSP-1 inhibits skin angiogenesis include the induction of endothelial cell apoptosis through specific interactions with the endothelial CD36 receptor, the activation of latent TGF-β, and the inhibition of matrix metalloproteinase activity. Overexpression of TSP-1 in the skin of transgenic mice results in impaired granulation tissue formation and wound vascularization, delayed and reduced skin carcinogenesis, and diminished photodamage induced by chronic UVB irradiation of the skin[27].

A second member of the thrombospondin gene family, TSP-2, is also expressed in normal human skin and acts as an endogenous inhibitor of angiogenesis. The expression of TSP-2 is downregulated in epithelial squamous cell carcinoma cells, whereas a strong upregulation of TSP-2

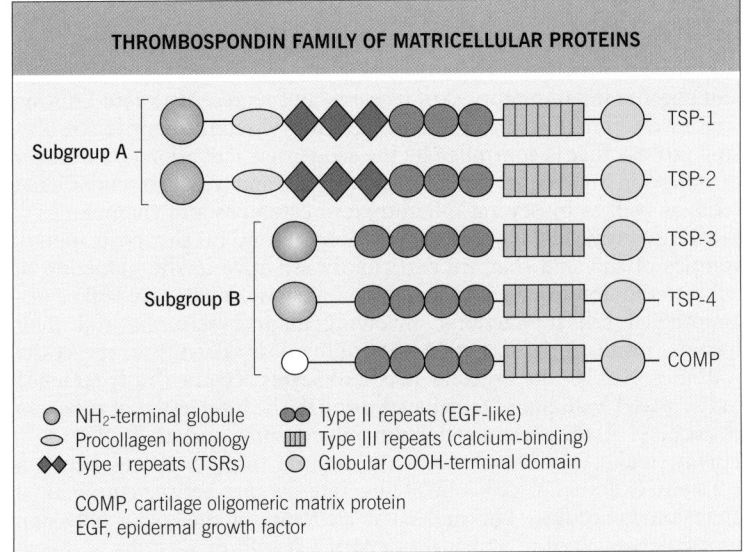

THROMBOSPONDIN FAMILY OF MATRICELLULAR PROTEINS

Subgroup A: TSP-1, TSP-2
Subgroup B: TSP-3, TSP-4, COMP

- NH₂-terminal globule
- Procollagen homology
- Type I repeats (TSRs)
- Type II repeats (EGF-like)
- Type III repeats (calcium-binding)
- Globular COOH-terminal domain

COMP, cartilage oligomeric matrix protein
EGF, epidermal growth factor

Fig. 102.9 The thrombospondin (TSP) family of matricellular proteins. TSP-1 and TSP-2 are potent endogenous inhibitors of skin angiogenesis.

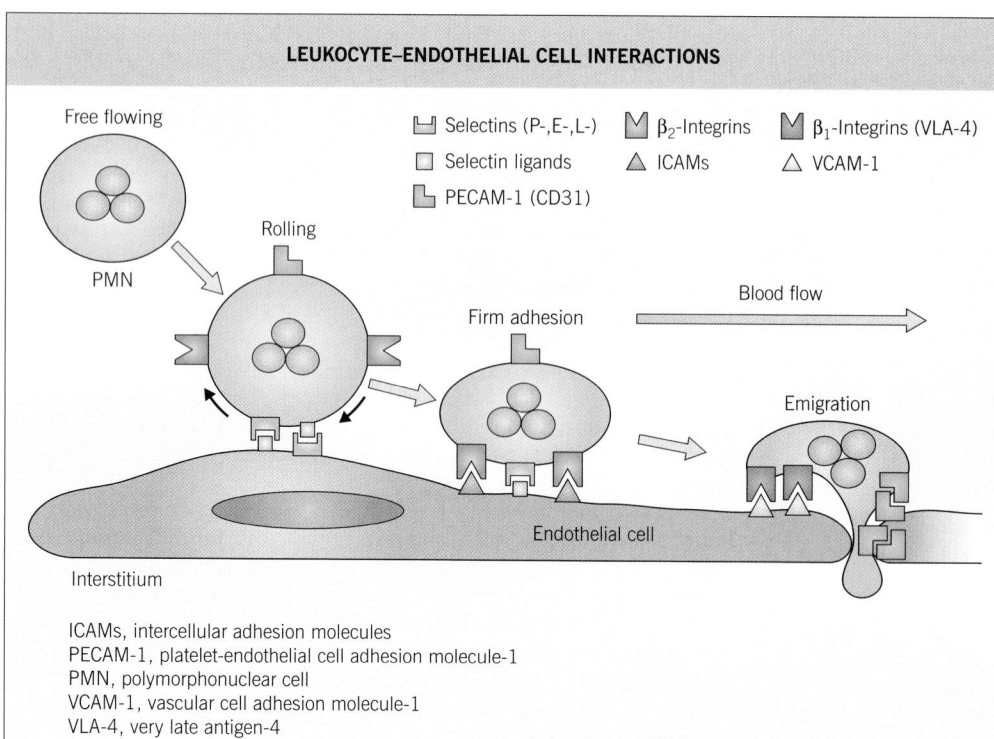

LEUKOCYTE–ENDOTHELIAL CELL INTERACTIONS

ICAMs, intercellular adhesion molecules
PECAM-1, platelet-endothelial cell adhesion molecule-1
PMN, polymorphonuclear cell
VCAM-1, vascular cell adhesion molecule-1
VLA-4, very late antigen-4

Fig. 102.10 The multistep process of leukocyte–endothelial cell interactions that leads to leukocyte recruitment into inflamed skin.

is found in the mesenchymal stroma during skin carcinogenesis, representing a natural tumor defense mechanism[28]. Mice that are deficient in TSP-2 show increased skin vascularization, enhanced and prolonged inflammatory reactions, and enhanced skin carcinogenesis, confirming the important role of endogenous TSP-2 in the control of skin angiogenesis. Accordingly, genetic overexpression of TSP-2 protects from skin cancer development and inhibits the growth of established skin cancers.

A number of additional endogenous inhibitors of angiogenesis are likely involved in the maintenance of normal vascular quiescence in the skin, most prominently interferons. Moreover, antiangiogenic activity has been reported for several cleavage products of molecules that are expressed in the vascular basement membrane, including fragments of collagens type IV (tumstatin), XV, and XVIII (endostatin). The potential contribution of these molecules to the antiangiogenic environment in normal skin remains to be established.

Regulation of Leukocyte–Endothelial Cell Interactions

Accumulation of leukocytes in the skin is a prominent feature of acute and chronic inflammatory skin diseases and represents a rate-limiting step in the inflammatory response. Leukocyte recruitment is a multi-step process that is controlled by the sequential activation of a number of adhesion molecules on both leukocytes and vascular endothelial cells, as well as by several inflammatory cytokines and chemokines[29]. Predominantly, leukocyte extravasation occurs in the postcapillary venules of the skin that are particularly sensitive to the induction of adhesion molecules. As a first step, relatively weak adhesive leukocyte–endothelial cell interactions, involving distinct selectins and their ligands, result in the tethering and rolling of leukocytes on the vessel wall (Fig. 102.10). In a second step, leukocytes become firmly attached to the vessel wall, mainly mediated through the interaction of adhesion molecules of the immunoglobulin superfamily and their ligands[30]. Finally, leukocytes migrate into the dermis through spaces between adjacent endothelial cells, involving interactions between junctional adhesion molecules. The molecular structure of the major adhesion molecules involved in leukocyte–endothelial cell interactions is shown in Figure 102.11, and the localization, ligand binding specificity, and function of each adhesion molecule are summarized in Table 102.2.

STRUCTURE AND FUNCTION OF THE CUTANEOUS LYMPHATIC SYSTEM

Lymphatic vessels were first described in the 17th century by Gasparo Aselli as 'lacteae venae' (milky veins). The cutaneous lymphatic system develops in parallel with the blood vascular system through a process termed lymphangiogenesis, and lymphatic vessels are not present in avascular structures such as epidermis, hair and nails[31]. The lymphatic system is composed of a vascular network of thin-walled capillaries that drain protein-rich lymph from the extracellular space and play an important role in the maintenance of normal tissue pressure[32]. Lymphatic vessels also play an important role in mediating the trafficking of immune cells from the skin to the regional lymph nodes, and in the metastatic spread of cutaneous malignancies[32a].

Lymphatic capillaries are lined by a continuous single-cell layer of overlapping endothelial cells and lack a continuous basement membrane. Lymph returns to the venous circulation via the larger lymphatic collecting vessels, which contain a muscular and adventitial layer as well as numerous valves, and the thoracic duct. The lymphatic vessels of the skin form two horizontal plexuses. The superficial plexus collects lymph from lymphatic capillaries that can extend into the dermal papillae and is located in close vicinity to the superficial cutaneous arterial plexus. Vertical lymphatic vessels connect the superficial plexus with the larger collecting vessels in the lower dermis and upper subcutis, whereas few lymphatics are found within the subcutis (see Fig. 102.1). The deep lymphatic vessels are located below the deep arterial system and contain valves to ensure unidirectional fluid transport.

In normal human skin and during tissue repair, lymphatic vessels connect with other lymphatic vessels, but not with blood vessels, and lymphatic endothelial cells remain separated from blood vascular endothelial cells during tube formation of co-cultured cells *in vitro*[33]. Whereas specific ephrins and their Eph receptors have been detected on arteries and veins, the molecular mechanisms that mediate lymphatic identity and homeotypic interactions remain to be identified. The structure of the cutaneous lymphatics is dependent on the structure of the skin at a particular site and can vary significantly. Lymphatic vessels have a regular, uniform shape where the skin is firm and thick, whereas the shapes are more variable in regions where the skin is thin and loose. Certain areas, such as the fingers, the palms and soles, the scrotum and the foreskin appear to have a more abundant lymphatic network.

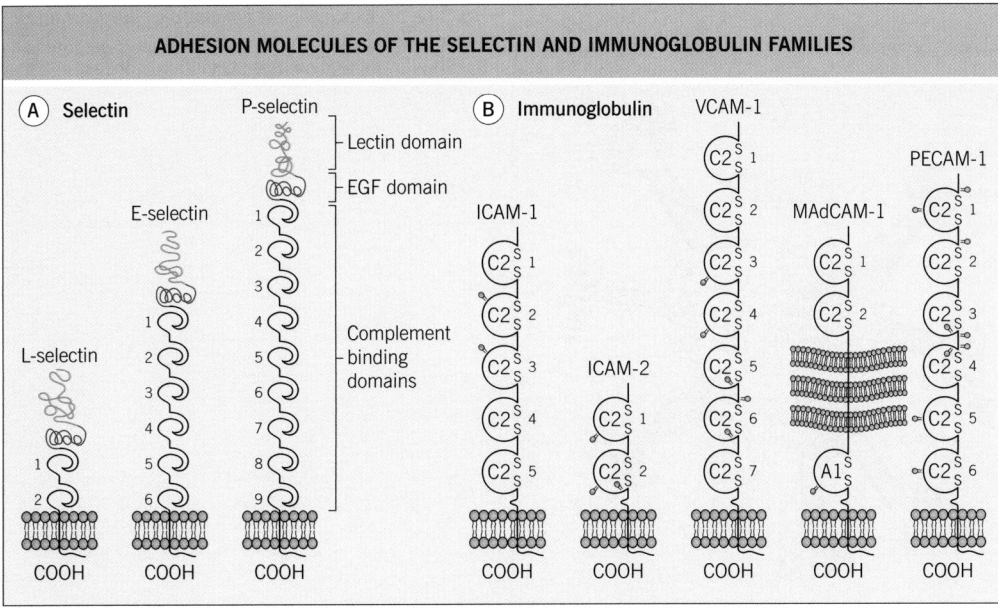

Fig. 102.11 Adhesion molecules of the selectin (A) and immunoglobulin (B) families. EGF, epidermal growth factor; MAdCAM, mucosal addressin cell adhesion molecule; ICAM, intercellular adhesion molecule; PECAM, platelet-endothelial cell adhesion molecule; VCAM, vascular cell adhesion molecule.

MAJOR ADHESION MOLECULES INVOLVED IN LEUKOCYTE–ENDOTHELIAL CELL INTERACTIONS: CELL-TYPE SPECIFIC EXPRESSION, LIGANDS AND FUNCTION

Adhesion molecule	Cell type	Ligands	Function
Integrin family			
LFA-1 (CD11a/CD18)	Leukocytes	ICAM-1, ICAM-2	Adhesion, emigration
Mac-1 (CD11b/CD18)	Granulocytes, monocytes	ICAM-1, iC3b	Adhesion, emigration
VLA-4 (CD49d/CD29)	Lymphocytes, monocytes, eosinophils, basophils	VCAM-1	Adhesion
Selectin family			
E-selectin (CD62E)	Endothelial cells	L-selectin, CLA, SSEA-1	Rolling
P-selectin (CD62P)	Endothelial cells	L-selectin, PSGL-1	Rolling
L-selectin (CD62L)	Leukocytes	E-selectin, CD14, P-selectin, GlyCAM, MAdCAM	Rolling
Ig supergene family			
ICAM-1 (CD54a)	Endothelial cells, monocytes	LFA-1, Mac-1, CD43	Adhesion, emigration
ICAM-2 (CD102)	Endothelial cells	LFA-1	Adhesion, emigration
VCAM-1 (CD106)	Endothelial cells	VLA-4	Adhesion
PECAM-1 (CD31)	Endothelial cells	PECAM-1	Adhesion, emigration

Table 102.2 Major adhesion molecules involved in leukocyte–endothelial cell interactions: cell-type specific expression, ligands and function. CLA, cutaneous lymphocyte-associated antigen; ICAM, intercellular adhesion molecule; LFA, lymphocyte function-associated antigen; MAdCAM, mucosal addressin cell adhesion molecule; PECAM, platelet-endothelial cell adhesion molecule; PSGL, P-selectin glycoprotein ligand; SSEA, stage-specific embryonic antigen; VCAM, vascular cell adhesion molecule; VLA, very late activation antigen.

Lymphatic capillaries respond to increased tissue fluid content by widening their lumina (Fig. 102.12), an action mediated by anchoring filaments that connect the lymphatic endothelial cells with the surrounding interstitium. In normal skin, the majority of lymphatic vessels are collapsed. Whereas elevation of the interstitial pressure up to +2 mmHg results in distention of lymphatic vessels and in increased lymph flow, higher interstitial fluid pressure results in edema formation. The detection of enlarged lymphatics in the skin, however, does not allow predictions about their function, because overextended lymphatics can be dysfunctional, as in some types of lymphedema.

The first concept of lymphatic development was hypothesized by Sabin, who proposed, based upon ink injection experiments, that isolated primitive lymph sacs originate from endothelial cells that bud from the veins during early development[34]. The peripheral lymphatic system originates from the primary lymph sacs and spreads by endothelial sprouting into the surrounding tissues and organs, where local capillaries are formed. As an alternative, it has been proposed that the primary lymph sacs arise in the mesenchyme, independent of the veins, and secondarily establish venous connections. Recent experimental evidence has supported the venous origin of the lymphatic system in mammals[31]. The homeobox gene *Prox1* is a specific marker for lymphatic endothelial cells and is first expressed, during embryonic development, in a polarized manner by a subset of venous endothelial cells that consequently bud off from the cardinal veins, migrate through the tissues, and finally form lymphatic vessels (Fig. 102.13). Accordingly, Prox1 deficiency results in complete absence of a lymphatic system in mice, among other defects[35].

Until very recently, studies of the lymphatic system have been hampered by the lack of specific markers that reliably distinguish lymphatic from blood vascular endothelial cells. The endothelial marker PECAM-1 (platelet-endothelial cell adhesion molecule-1, CD31) is expressed by both blood vessel and lymphatic endothelial cells, although the expression levels are lower in lymphatics. Because of the absence or only rudimentary formation of a basement membrane, lymphatic vessels can be visualized by differential immunostaining for both CD31 and basement membrane components, such as collagen types IV and XVIII or laminin (Fig. 102.14). Similarly, double stains for both CD31 and the specific blood vascular marker PAL-E (only

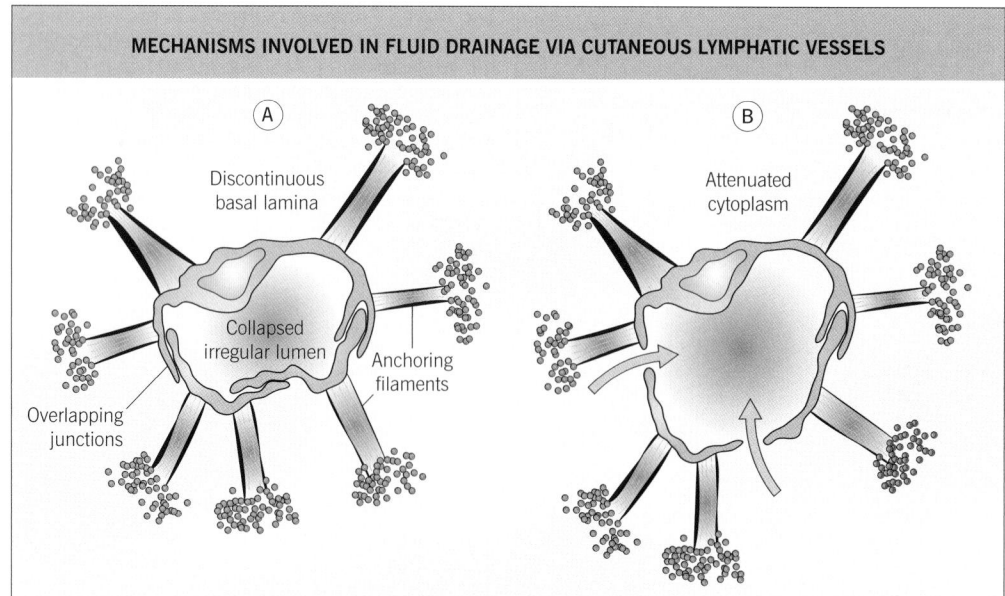

MECHANISMS INVOLVED IN FLUID DRAINAGE VIA CUTANEOUS LYMPHATIC VESSELS

Ⓐ

Discontinuous basal lamina

Collapsed irregular lumen

Anchoring filaments

Overlapping junctions

Ⓑ

Attenuated cytoplasm

Fig. 102.12 Mechanisms involved in fluid drainage via cutaneous lymphatic vessels. A Normal skin. **B** Skin with increased interstitial fluid content.

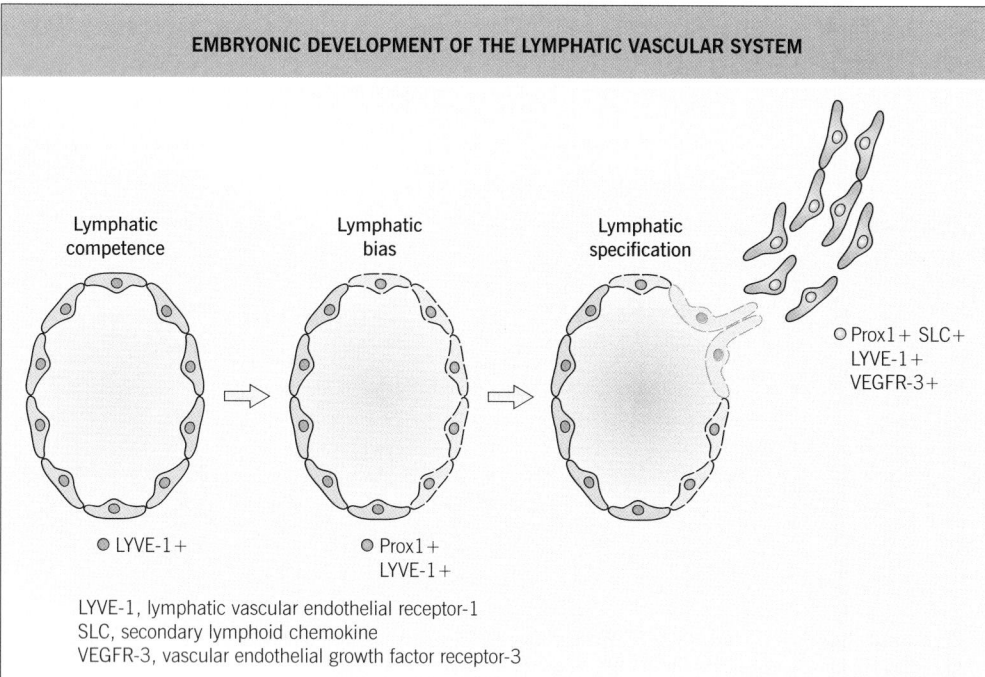

EMBRYONIC DEVELOPMENT OF THE LYMPHATIC VASCULAR SYSTEM

Lymphatic competence

Lymphatic bias

Lymphatic specification

◯ Prox1+ SLC+
LYVE-1+
VEGFR-3+

◯ LYVE-1+

◯ Prox1+
LYVE-1+

LYVE-1, lymphatic vascular endothelial receptor-1
SLC, secondary lymphoid chemokine
VEGFR-3, vascular endothelial growth factor receptor-3

Fig. 102.13 Embryonic development of the lymphatic vascular system.

detectable on frozen sections; see Fig. 102.3) or the blood vascular marker CD34 can be used to specifically detect lymphatic vessels in the skin.

Recently, several new markers have been identified that are predominantly expressed by lymphatic endothelial cells in the skin (Table 102.3)[31]. VEGFR-3 (vascular endothelial growth factor receptor-3, Flt-4) is expressed on lymphatic vessels in normal skin and serves as a receptor for the lymphangiogenesis factors VEGF-C and VEGF-D (Fig. 102.15). Podoplanin, a surface glycoprotein, has been recently described as a novel marker for the lymphatic vasculature in normal skin, and podoplanin deficiency results in congenital lymphedema formation in mice. Desmoplakin, a cytoplasmic protein that attaches intermediate filaments to the plasma membrane in epithelial cells, has also been reported to be a marker of the lymphatic endothelium[36].

The lymphatic vascular endothelial hyaluronan receptor (LYVE-1), a CD44 homologue, was recently identified as a specific cell-surface protein of lymphatic endothelial cells and macrophages[37]. Whereas some specialized blood vascular endothelial cells that are involved in hyaluronic acid metabolism, including sinusoidal endothelial cells

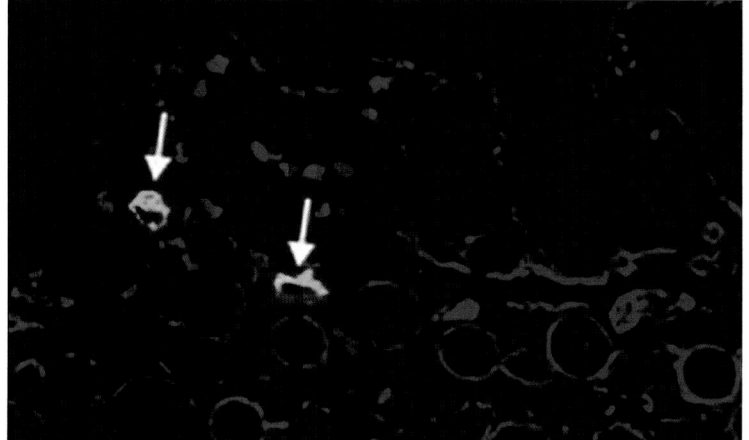

Fig. 102.14 Double-immunofluorescence stain for the lymphatic marker LYVE-1 (green) and the basement membrane component laminin (red) reveals basement membranes (red) and lymphatic vessels (green; arrows).

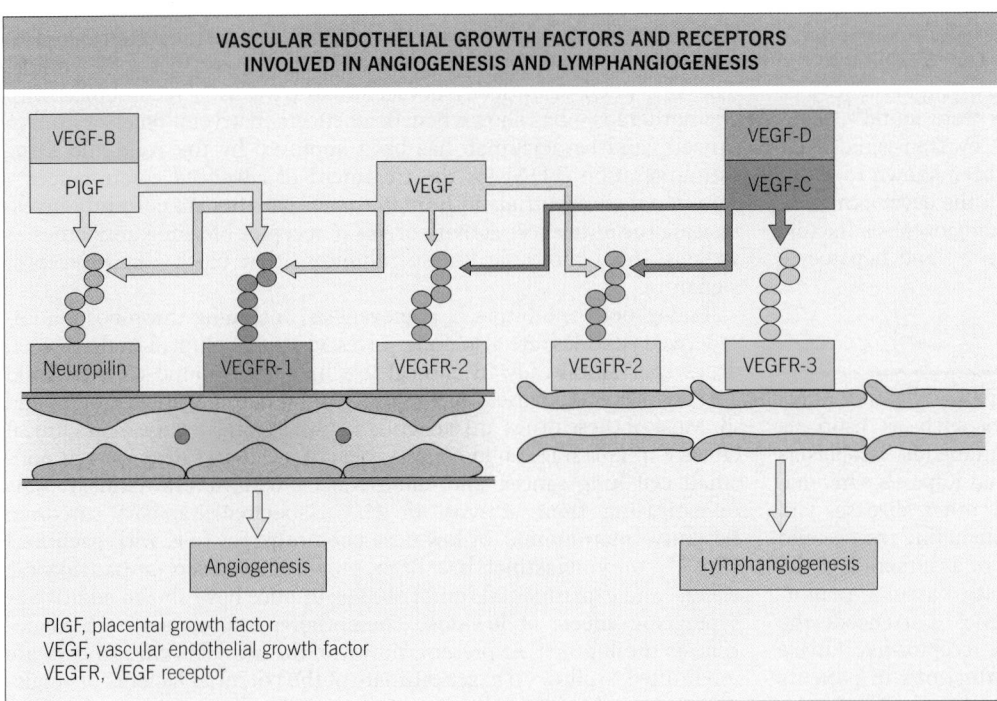

VASCULAR ENDOTHELIAL GROWTH FACTORS AND RECEPTORS INVOLVED IN ANGIOGENESIS AND LYMPHANGIOGENESIS

PIGF, placental growth factor
VEGF, vascular endothelial growth factor
VEGFR, VEGF receptor

Fig. 102.15 Vascular endothelial growth factors and their receptors involved in angiogenesis and lymphangiogenesis. VEGF is also known as VEGF-A.

MARKERS FOR LYMPHATICS AND FOR BLOOD VESSELS		
Marker	**Lymphatics**	**Blood vessels**
CD31 (PECAM-1)	+	++
CD34	–	+
PAL-E	–	+
Collagen type IV	–	+
Collagen type XVIII	–	+
Laminin	(+)	++
VEGFR-1	–	+
VEGFR-2	+	+
VEGFR-3	+	–
Podoplanin	++	–
SLC/CCL21	+	–
LYVE-1	++	–
Prox1	+	–
M2A oncofetal antigen*	+	–

*Detected by the D2-40 monoclonal antibody.

Table 102.3 Markers for lymphatics and for blood vessels. LYVE-1, lymphatic vascular endothelial receptor-1; PAL-E, pathologische anatomie Leiden-endothelium; PECAM-1, platelet-endothelial cell adhesion molecule-1; Prox1, prospero-related homeobox 1; SLC, secondary lymphoid chemokine; VEGFR, vascular endothelial growth factor receptor.

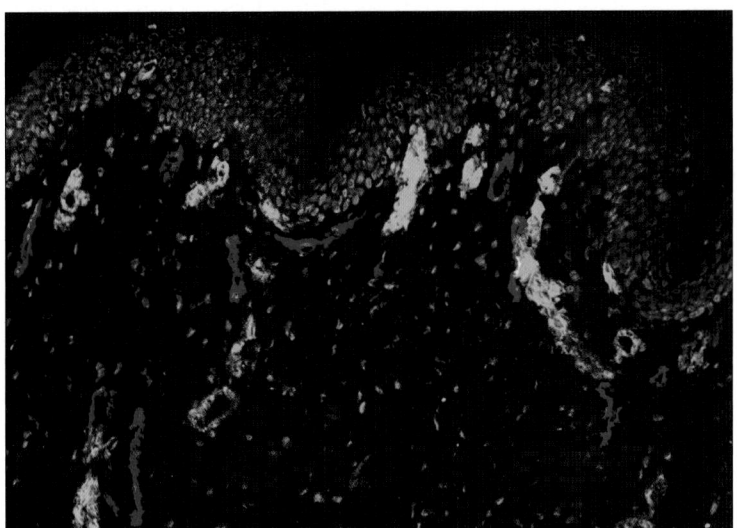

Fig. 102.16 Specific immunofluorescence staining of CD31-positive blood vessels (green) that are LYVE-1-negative and of CD31-positive/LYVE-1-positive lymphatic vessels (red) in human foreskin. Nuclei are stained blue.

in the liver, also express LYVE-1, its expression is highly specific for lymphatics in most organs, including the skin (Fig. 102.16). One has to keep in mind, however, that most of the markers discussed here, including VEGFR-3 and LYVE-1, are also expressed by distinct subsets of leukocytes such as dermal dendritic cells and/or macrophages.

Secondary lymphoid chemokine (SLC; also termed CCL21) is specifically produced by lymphatic endothelial cells in the skin and binds to the CC chemokine receptor-7 (CCR-7) on dendritic cells and lymphocytes. It serves an important role as a guidance molecule for the migration of dendritic and other cells via the lymphatics to the lymph nodes. Expression of CCR-7 in human melanoma cells resulted in increased lymph node metastasis of experimental melanomas in mice, suggesting that tumor cells may be able to take advantage of natural immune response mechanisms to further their metastatic spread[38]. Conversely, the chemokine receptor D6 – a receptor for several pro-inflammatory chemokines, including RANTES, monocyte chemotactic protein (MCP)-1 and MCP-3 – has been detected on lymphatic vessels, but not on blood vessels[39]. The homeobox gene *Prox1* is the earliest marker for lymphatic endothelial cells during embryonic development and its specific expression is maintained by cutaneous lymphatic endothelial cells in the adult. Functional inactivation of Prox1 in mice leads to complete absence of a lymphatic system, and Prox1 appears to be the most specific marker for lymphatic vascular differentiation in the skin[31].

Until recently, the molecules regulating growth and function of lymphatic vessels have remained unknown. Within the past several years, two new members of the VEGF family of angiogenesis factors have been identified that are distinguished by their capacity to stimulate lymphangiogenesis. Both VEGF-C and VEGF-D activate the receptor tyrosine kinase VEGFR-3 (Flt-4) on lymphatic endothelial cells and, after cleavage, the receptor tyrosine kinase VEGFR-2 (KDR) that is expressed on blood vessels and lymphatic endothelium. Transgenic mice with targeted overexpression of either VEGF-C or VEGF-D in the skin were characterized by hyperplastic cutaneous lymphatic vessels, whereas no major abnormalities of blood vessels were found[40]. Conversely, blockade of both VEGF-C and VEGF-D by transgenic over-expression of a soluble VEGFR-3 in the skin has been shown to result in absence of a cutaneous lymphatic system and in the development of lymphedema[41]. Very recently, additional lymphangiogenesis factors have been identified, including VEGF-A[23], Ang-1[42,43] and hepatocyte growth factor[44].

RELATED DISEASES

Angiogenesis is a characteristic feature of tissue repair and of numerous diseases, including inflammatory skin disorders such as psoriasis and contact dermatitis, blistering diseases, cutaneous neoplasias including squamous cell carcinoma, melanoma and Kaposi's sarcoma, and infantile hemangiomas. Moreover, several other diseases are characterized by prominent visible blood vessels, including rosacea and basal cell carcinoma. Genetic mutations that lead to dysfunction of the vascular Tie-2 receptor have been associated with vascular malformations (see Ch. 104), and mutations in the genes that encode the low-affinity TGF-β receptor endoglin and activin receptor-like kinase (ALK)-1 lead to the formation of vascular malformations in patients with hereditary hemorrhagic telangiectasia types I and II[45]. Recent studies indicate that there might be an angiogenetic disposition, and specific single-nucleotide polymorphisms of the *VEGF-A* gene have been associated with more severe psoriasis[46]. Lastly, VEGF-C has been identified as a growth factor for HIV-associated Kaposi's sarcomas that strongly express Flt-4/VEGFR-3, and infection of blood vascular endothelial cells with the Kaposi sarcoma-associated herpes virus leads to their genetic reprogramming and to the adoption of a lymphatic endothelial cell phenotype[47].

Impairment of lymphatic function leads to the development of a number of diseases, most prominently to lymphedema of the skin, with associated impaired immune function and fibrotic changes[32,48]. Heterozygous inactivating missense mutations of the gene encoding VEGFR-3, the receptor for the lymphangiogenesis factors VEGF-C and VEGF-D, have been found in families affected by primary lymphedema (Milroy disease), which is characterized by chronic swelling of the extremities[49]. *VEGFR-3* mutations were also found in *Chy* mutant mice, the murine equivalent of Milroy disease, and both virus-mediated VEGF-C gene therapy[50] and delivery of VEGF-C protein have been shown to induce generation of functional lymphatic vessels in injured skin, indicating possible novel therapeutic strategies for congenital or acquired lymphedemas.

In lymphedema–distichiasis, lymphatic vessel function fails because of mutations affecting the function of the forkhead transcription factor FOXC2[51], and mutations in the transcription factor gene *SOX18* underlie recessive and dominant forms of hypotrichosis–lymphedema–telangiectasia[52]. Finally, tumor-associated lymphangiogenesis has been found to increase the risk of sentinel lymph node metastasis and to reduce overall survival in human melanomas[53,54]. In summary, the recent progress in our understanding of the molecular mechanisms that control blood vascular and lymphatic development and function have led to novel insights into the pathogenesis of a number of skin diseases with vascular involvement, as well as to the development of novel therapeutic approaches to treat these diseases.

CURRENT TRENDS IN ANTIANGIOGENESIS

A large number of experimental studies have shown that the induction of angiogenesis is essential for tumor progression and that inhibition of blood vessel growth inhibits malignant tumor growth and metastasis in mice. Based upon these findings, inhibition of tumor angiogenesis has become a main target of anticancer strategies. Despite the identification of several distinct tumor angiogenesis factors, including interleukin-8 and basic fibroblast growth factor, the majority of current antitumor angiogenesis therapies are aimed at inhibiting the bioavail-

ability or the receptor signaling of VEGF-A, generally considered to represent the major angiogenic factor in the majority of solid tumors. The anti-VEGF-A antibody bevacizumab (Avastin®) – combined with chemotherapy – has shown beneficial effects in several types of human cancers, and bevacizumab has been approved by the Food and Drug Administration (FDA) for the treatment of advanced colon cancer[55]. Additional clinical trials in human cancer patients are currently investigating the anticancer activity of VEGF receptor-blocking antibodies as well as small molecule kinase inhibitors that block VEGF receptor signaling.

Endogenous inhibitors of angiogenesis, including thrombospondin-1-derived peptides, are also under investigation in clinical trials. Several drugs that are already in clinical use have been found to exert mild antiangiogenic activities, including thalidomide and interferon-α and -β. Most of these drugs are currently being investigated for their clinical efficacy in late-stage solid cancers such as head and neck cancer, non-small cell lung cancer, and colon cancer, with several clinical trials investigating their activity in HIV-associated Kaposi's sarcoma. Recently, 'metronomic' or low-dose chemotherapy (e.g. with paclitaxel [Taxol®] or vinblastine) has been proposed to exert antiangiogenic effects, and experimental tumor studies in mice have shown additive or synergistic effects of low-dose chemotherapy combined with angiogenesis inhibitors[56]. At present, however, the available clinical data are too limited to allow an exact estimate of the potential benefits of single-agent or combined antiangiogenic therapy for distinct types of cancer. The recent discovery of active tumor lymphangiogenesis and its correlation with cancer metastasis[56a] suggests that, at least in some types of cancer, antilymphangiogenic therapy might provide a novel strategy[6].

Although the efficacy of antiangiogenic therapy in the treatment of advanced melanoma or cutaneous squamous cell carcinoma still remains unclear, an increasing number of non-malignant skin diseases have emerged as potential targets for treatments aimed at vascular endothelium. Infantile hemangiomas represent benign vascular hyper-proliferations and have been found to respond, at least in part, to treatment with interferon-α; additional vascular lesions that might respond to antiangiogenic treatment include angiokeratomas and kaposiform hemangioendotheliomas. Psoriasis is characterized by vascular enlargement and activation, and recent experimental data suggest that blockade of epidermal-derived VEGF might represent a novel therapeutic strategy. In fact, pulsed dye laser therapy has been used to effectively treat psoriatic skin lesions, predominantly by targeting cutaneous blood vessels. Similarly, telangiectasias, in particular in rosacea, would appear to represent prime targets for antiangiogenic therapy. Recent reports suggest that blockade of angiogenesis and vascular activation might also represent a novel approach for preventing UVB-induced skin damage[57] as well as multistep skin carcinogenesis, indicating the potential use of angiogenesis inhibitors for chemoprevention. Because systemic inhibition of angiogenesis might cause considerable side effects, including hypertension, proteinuria and interference with reproductive functions, the challenge and opportunity for dermatology will be to develop topical angiogenesis inhibitors that will be able to penetrate the skin but not reach potentially toxic systemic levels.

In addition to these potential dermatologic applications, antiangiogenesis has become a promising new therapeutic approach in ophthalmology. Diabetes mellitus is frequently associated with intraocular neovascularization, and new blood vessel growth is the principal cause of visual loss in the wet form of age-related macular degeneration, the most common cause of blindness in Western countries. Intravitreal injection of VEGF inhibitors has been successfully used to prevent progression of this disease and has been approved for clinical use by the FDA. Other potential applications of antiangiogenesis include diseases of the female reproductive tract such as polycystic ovary syndrome, endometriosis and ovarian hyperstimulation syndrome. The potential side effects of chronic, systemic angiogenesis inhibition are at present not well characterized and, therefore, it is difficult to predict whether systemic antiangiogenic therapies will be used for non-malignant conditions in the future. However, increasing evidence suggests that tissue repair, including cutaneous wound healing, is not critically dependent on unimpaired angiogenesis.

REFERENCES

1. Ryan TJ. Cutaneous circulation. In: Goldsmith LA (ed.). Biochemistry and Physiology of the Skin. New York: Oxford University Press, 1983:817–77.
2. Yano K, Brown LF, Detmar M. Control of hair growth and follicle size by VEGF-mediated angiogenesis. J Clin Invest. 2001;107:409–17.
3. Braverman IM, Yen A. Ultrastructure of the human dermal microcirculation. II. The capillary loops of the dermal papillae. J Invest Dermatol. 1977;68:44–52.
4. Dvorak HF, Brown LF, Detmar M, Dvorak AM. Vascular permeability factor/vascular endothelial growth factor, microvascular hyperpermeability, and angiogenesis. Am J Pathol. 1995;146:1029–39.
5. Braverman IM, Sibley J. Role of the microcirculation in the treatment and pathogenesis of psoriasis. J Invest Dermatol. 1982;78:12–17.
6. Skobe M, Hawighorst T, Jackson DG, et al. Induction of tumor lymphangiogenesis by VEGF-C promotes breast cancer metastasis. Nat Med. 2001;7:192–8.
7. Flamme I. Molecular biology of vasculogenesis and early angiogenesis. In: Rubanyi GM (ed.).Angiogenesis in Health and Disease: Basic Mechanisms and Clinical Applications. New York: Marcel Dekker, 2000:1–30.
8. Nishikawa SI, Nishikawa S, Hirashima M, et al. Progressive lineage analysis by cell sorting and culture identifies FLK1+VE-cadherin+ cells at a diverging point of endothelial and hemopoietic lineages. Development. 1998;125:1747–57.
9. Davis S, Yancopoulos GD. The angiopoietins: Yin and Yang in angiogenesis. Curr Top Microbiol Immunol. 1999;237:173–85.
10. Armulik A, Abramsson A, Betsholtz C. Endothelial/pericyte interactions. Circ Res. 2005;97:512–23.
11. Dvorak HF. Tumors: wounds that do not heal. Similarities between tumor stroma generation and wound healing. N Engl J Med. 1986;315:1650–9.
12. Senger DR. Molecular framework for angiogenesis: a complex web of interactions between extravasated plasma proteins and endothelial cell proteins induced by angiogenic cytokines. Am J Pathol. 1996;149:1–7.
13. Holash J, Maisonpierre PC, Compton D, et al. Vessel cooption, regression, and growth in tumors mediated by angiopoietins and VEGF. Science. 1999;284:1994–8.
14. Brooks PC, Clark RA, Cheresh DA. Requirement of vascular integrin alpha v beta 3 for angiogenesis. Science. 1994;264:569–71.
15. Senger DR, Ledbetter SR, Claffey KP, et al. Stimulation of endothelial cell migration by vascular permeability factor/vascular endothelial growth factor through cooperative mechanisms involving the alphavbeta3 integrin, osteopontin, and thrombin. Am J Pathol. 1996;149:293–305.
16. Senger DR, Claffey KP, Benes JE, et al. Angiogenesis promoted by vascular endothelial growth factor: regulation through alpha1beta1 and alpha2beta1 integrins. Proc Natl Acad Sci USA. 1997;94:13612–17.
17. Senger DR, Galli SJ, Dvorak AM, et al. Tumor cells secrete a vascular permeability factor that promotes accumulation of ascites fluid. Science. 1983;219:983–5.
18. Detmar M, Brown LF, Claffey KP, et al. Overexpression of vascular permeability factor/vascular endothelial growth factor and its receptors in psoriasis. J Exp Med. 1994;180:1141–6.
19. Detmar M. Molecular regulation of angiogenesis in the skin. J Invest Dermatol. 1996;106:207–8.
20. Detmar M, Brown LF, Schon MP, et al. Increased microvascular density and enhanced leukocyte rolling and adhesion in the skin of VEGF transgenic mice. J Invest Dermatol. 1998;111:1–6.
21. Kunstfeld R, Hirakawa S, Hong YK, et al. Induction of cutaneous delayed-type hypersensitivity reactions in VEGF-A transgenic mice results in chronic skin inflammation associated with persistent lymphatic hyperplasia. Blood. 2004;104:1048–57.
22. Skobe M, Rockwell P, Goldstein N, et al. Halting angiogenesis suppresses carcinoma cell invasion. Nat Med. 1997;3:1222–7.
23. Hirakawa S, Kodama S, Kunstfeld R, et al. VEGF-A induces tumor and sentinel lymph node lymphangiogenesis and promotes lymphatic metastasis. J Exp Med. 2005;201:1089–99.
24. Carmeliet P, Moons L, Luttun A, et al. Synergism between vascular endothelial growth factor and placental growth factor contributes to angiogenesis and plasma extravasation in pathological conditions. Nat Med. 2001;7:575–83.
25. Oura H, Bertoncini J, Velasco P, et al. A critical role of placental growth factor in the induction of inflammation and edema formation. Blood. 2003;101:560–7.
26. Streit M, Velasco P, Brown LF, et al. Overexpression of thrombospondin-1 decreases angiogenesis and inhibits the growth of human cutaneous squamous cell carcinomas. Am J Pathol. 1999;155:441–52.
27. Yano K, Oura H, Detmar M. Targeted overexpression of the angiogenesis inhibitor thrombospondin-1 in the epidermis of transgenic mice prevents ultraviolet-B-induced angiogenesis and cutaneous photo-damage. J Invest Dermatol. 2002;118:800–5.
28. Hawighorst T, Velasco P, Streit M, et al. Thrombospondin-2 plays a protective role in multistep carcinogenesis: a novel host anti-tumor defense mechanism. EMBO J. 2001;20:2631–40.
29. Robert C, Kupper TS. Inflammatory skin diseases, T cells, and immune surveillance. N Engl J Med. 1999;341:1817–28.
30. Panes J, Granger DN. Leukocyte-endothelial cell interactions: molecular mechanisms and implications in gastrointestinal disease. Gastroenterology. 1998;114:1066–90.
31. Oliver G, Detmar M. The rediscovery of the lymphatic system: old and new insights into the development and biological function of the lymphatic vasculature. Genes Dev. 2002;16:773–83.
32. Witte MH, Bernas MJ, Martin CP, Witte CL. Lymphangiogenesis and lymphangiodysplasia: from molecular to clinical lymphology. Microsc Res Tech. 2001;55:122–45.
32a. Cueni L, Detmar M. New insights into the molecular control of the lymphatic vascular system and its role in disease. J Invest Dermatol. 2006;126:2167–77.
33. Kriehuber E, Breiteneder-Geleff S, Groeger M, et al. Isolation and characterization of dermal lymphatic and blood endothelial cells reveal stable and functionally specialized cell lineages. J Exp Med. 2001;194:797–808.
34. Sabin FR. On the origin of the lymphatic system from the veins and the development of the lymph hearts and thoracic duct in the pig. Am J Anat. 1902;1:367–91.
35. Wigle JT, Harvey N, Detmar M, et al. An essential role for Prox1 in the induction of the lymphatic endothelial cell phenotype. EMBO J. 2002;21:1505–13.
36. Ebata N, Nodasaka Y, Sawa Y, et al. Desmoplakin as a specific marker of lymphatic vessels. Microvasc Res. 2001;61:40–8.
37. Jackson DG, Prevo R, Clasper S, Banerji S. LYVE-1, the lymphatic system and tumor lymphangiogenesis. Trends Immunol. 2001;22:317–21.
38. Wiley HE, Gonzalez EB, Maki W, et al. Expression of CC chemokine `7 and regional lymph node metastasis of B16 murine melanoma. J Natl Cancer Inst. 2001;93:1638–43.
39. Nibbs RJ, Kriehuber E, Ponath PD, et al. The beta-chemokine receptor D6 is expressed by lymphatic endothelium and a subset of vascular tumors. Am J Pathol. 2001;158:867–77.
40. Veikkola T, Jussila L, Makinen T, et al. Signalling via vascular endothelial growth factor receptor-3 is sufficient for lymphangiogenesis in transgenic mice. EMBO J. 2001;20:1223–31.
41. Makinen T, Jussila L, Veikkola T, et al. Inhibition of lymphangiogenesis with resulting lymphedema in transgenic mice expressing soluble VEGF receptor-3. Nat Med. 2001;7:199–205.
42. Tammela T, Saaristo A, Lohela M, et al. Angiopoietin-1 promotes lymphatic sprouting and hyperplasia. Blood. 2005;105:4642–9.
43. Morisada T, Oike Y, Yamada Y, et al. Angiopoietin-1 promotes LYVE-1-positive lymphatic vessel formation. Blood. 2005;105:4649–56.
44. Kajiya K, Hirakawa S, Ma B, et al. Hepatocyte growth factor promotes lymphatic vessel formation and function. EMBO J. 2005;24:2885–95.
45. Marchuk DA. Genetic abnormalities in hereditary hemorrhagic telangiectasia. Curr Opin Hematol. 1998;5:332–8.
46. Young HS, Summers AM, Bhushan M, et al. Single-nucleotide polymorphisms of vascular endothelial growth factor in psoriasis of early onset. J Invest Dermatol. 2004;122:209–15.
47. Hong YK, Foreman K, Shin JW, et al. Lymphatic reprogramming of blood vascular endothelium by Kaposi sarcoma-associated herpesvirus. Nat Genet. 2004;36:683–5.
48. Ryan TJ. The lymphatics of the skin. In: Jarrett A (ed.). Physiology and Pathophysiology of the Skin. New York: Academic Press, 1978:1755–811.
49. Karkkainen MJ, Ferrell RE, Lawrence EC, et al. Missense mutations interfere with VEGFR-3 signalling in primary lymphoedema. Nat Genet. 2000;25:153–9.
50. Saaristo A, Tammela T, Timonen J, et al. Vascular endothelial growth factor-C gene therapy restores lymphatic flow across incision wounds. FASEB J. 2004;18:1707–9.
51. Petrova TV, Karpanen T, Norrmen C, et al. Defective valves and abnormal mural cell recruitment underlie lymphatic vascular failure in lymphedema distichiasis. Nat Med. 2004;10:974–81.
52. Irrthum A, Devriendt K, Chitayat D, et al. Mutations in the transcription factor gene SOX18 underlie recessive and dominant forms of hypotrichosis-lymphedema-telangiectasia. Am J Hum Genet. 2003;72:1470–8.
53. Dadras SS, Paul T, Bertoncini J, et al. Tumor lymphangiogenesis: a novel prognostic indicator for cutaneous melanoma metastasis and survival. Am J Pathol. 2003;162:1951–60.
54. Dadras SS, Lange-Asschenfeldt B, Velasco P, et al. Tumor lymphangiogenesis predicts melanoma metastasis to sentinel lymph nodes. Mod Pathol. 2005; 18:1232–42.
55. Ferrara N, Hillan KJ, Novotny W. Bevacizumab (Avastin), a humanized anti-VEGF monoclonal antibody for cancer therapy. Biochem Biophys Res Commun. 2005;333:328–35.
56. Kerbel RS, Kamen BA. The anti-angiogenic basis of metronomic chemotherapy. Nat Rev Cancer. 2004;4:423–36.
56a. Hirakawa S, Brown LF, Kodama S, et al. VEGF-C-induced lymphangiogenesis in sentinel lymph nodes promotes tumor metastasis to distant sites. Blood. 2007;109: 1010–7.
57. Hirakawa S, Fujii S, Kajiya K, et al. Vascular endothelial growth factor promotes sensitivity to ultraviolet B-induced cutaneous photodamage. Blood. 2005;105:2392–9.

Infantile Hemangiomas

Maria C Garzon

103

Synonyms: ■ Hemangioma of infancy ■ Hemangioma ■ Vascular tumor

Key features

- The most common soft tissue tumor of infancy
- Benign endothelial cell neoplasms
- Demonstrate a typical growth pattern characterized by early proliferation followed by gradual, spontaneous involution
- Distinct histopathologic and immunohistochemical features that differentiate them from other vascular anomalies in children
- May be associated with systemic malformations when occurring at certain anatomic sites, e.g. face, neck and lumbosacral area
- Treatment choice, if any, depends on multiple factors and must be tailored to each individual patient

INTRODUCTION

Infantile hemangiomas are benign proliferations of endothelial tissue, and are the most common tumors arising in the neonatal period. They are characterized by significant postnatal growth during the first several months of life, followed by slow spontaneous involution over the ensuing years. This natural history differentiates them from vascular malformations (see Ch. 104 & Fig. 104.1). During the past decade, as mechanisms governing growth and regulatory pathways of normal vascular development have been elucidated, new insights into the pathophysiology of common infantile hemangiomas have been described.

HISTORY

The terms 'infantile hemangioma' and 'hemangioma of infancy' are now used to describe a specific group of vascular tumors that arise during infancy and demonstrate characteristic clinical and histologic features. Infantile hemangiomas have been recognized in the medical literature for centuries, and they have been given various names such as *nevus maternus, angioma simplex, angioma cavernosum, angiodysplasia, strawberry nevus* and *capillary hemangioma*[1]. Despite early attempts to make distinctions between different types of vascular birthmarks, the term hemangioma was frequently applied to a wide variety of vascular anomalies including vascular malformations. 'Hemangioma' thus became a generic term used to describe both congenital and acquired vascular lesions, without consideration of differences in their biologic behavior.

One of the most important developments in the study of vascular birthmarks was the suggestion and acceptance of a biologic classification scheme. In 1982, Mulliken & Glowacki[2] first proposed that vascular birthmarks should be classified according to their biologic and clinical behavior. The International Society for the Study of Vascular Anomalies modified the classification slightly in 1996 (Table 103.1)[3].

Under this classification scheme, vascular birthmarks are divided into two broad categories: *vascular tumors* and *vascular malformations*. Vascular tumors are characterized by cellular proliferation and include infantile hemangiomas, the later-onset pyogenic granuloma, and other rare vascular tumors that may arise during infancy or early childhood, including tufted angioma and kaposiform hemangioendothelioma (Table 103.2; see Ch. 114). Vascular malformations, on the other hand, are believed to represent errors in vascular morphogenesis. They are

VASCULAR BIRTHMARKS IN CHILDREN		
	Infantile hemangioma	**Vascular malformation**
Clinical	• Usually absent at birth (often precursor lesion present, occasionally fully formed) • Rapid proliferation • Spontaneous involution over years	• Usually evident at birth • Slow expansion, proportionate with growth • Persists into adulthood
Epidemiology	More common in: • Girls (3–5:1) • Premature infants • Infants of mothers post chorionic villus sampling	No gender or gestation predilection
Pathology	**Proliferating:** endothelial cell hyperplasia, lobule formation, mast cells, prominent basement membrane **Involuting:** fibrofatty tissue replacement, decreased mast cells	Dependent upon type, often irregular vascular channels
Immunohistochemistry	GLUT1-, Lewis Y antigen-, merosin-, FcγRII-positive	GLUT1-, Lewis Y antigen-, merosin-, FcγRII-negative

Table 103.1 Vascular birthmarks in children.

frequently noted during the neonatal period, but, unlike infantile hemangiomas, they do not rapidly proliferate in the first year of life nor do they resolve spontaneously (see Table 103.1). Vascular malformations are characterized by the type of dysplastic vessels they contain and their flow properties (see Ch. 104).

Adopting specific terminology has allowed investigators to better categorize vascular birthmarks and predict their clinical behavior and prognosis. The biologic classification was expanded to include unique histopathologic and immunohistochemical features that aid in distinguishing infantile hemangiomas from other vascular tumors (see Table 103.1). Unfortunately, despite the wide acceptance of the biologic classification scheme, nosologic confusion still persists in the medical community as well as in the literature. A review of genetic reference texts found the term hemangioma to be used imprecisely with great frequency[4].

EPIDEMIOLOGY

Infantile hemangioma is the most common tumor in infancy. The majority of lesions are noted within the first several weeks of life and occur overall in 10–12% of infants by the first year of life. Early investigators noted an incidence of 1–2.5% in the immediate newborn period. Infantile hemangiomas may occur more commonly in Caucasian infants than in other racial groups, but this predilection has been variably reported[5]. They are clearly more common in girls than in boys, with a reported female:male ratio of 2–5:1[6–8]. Moreover, severe complicated hemangiomas have been observed more frequently in girls, with a 7:1 ratio[9]. Hemangiomas also appear more often in premature infants, occurring in 23–30% of infants with birth weights less than 1000 g and 15% of infants with birth weights between 1000 and 1500 g[5,10]. There is a threefold increased incidence in infants born following chorionic villus sampling compared to those born following amniocentesis or

BIOLOGIC CLASSIFICATION OF VASCULAR BIRTHMARKS

Vascular tumors

- Infantile hemangioma
- Congenital hemangioma
- Kaposiform hemangioendothelioma
- Tufted angioma
- Pyogenic granuloma
- Congenital hemangiopericytoma
- Spindle cell hemangioma

Vascular malformations

- Capillary malformations (slow flow)
- Venous malformations (slow flow)
  - Typical
  - With glomus cells
- Lymphatic malformations (slow flow)
  - Macrocystic
  - Microcystic
- Arteriovenous malformations (fast flow)
- Combined malformations (slow or fast flow)

Table 103.2 Biologic classification of vascular birthmarks.

without a history of instrumentation[11]. A recent multicenter, prospective cohort study of over 1000 infants from the US with infantile hemangiomas examined demographic and epidemiologic factors. When the data were compared to National Vital Statistics data for children born in the US in 2002, several important differences were noted. Infants in the study population were more likely to be female, Caucasian race, low birth weight, premature and of multiple gestation. Mothers of infants with hemangiomas were more likely to be of advanced maternal age[12].

Infantile hemangiomas typically arise sporadically, although Margileth & Museles[13] reported a 10% incidence of familial cases in their 1965 series. The frequency with which hemangiomas occur in the general population makes it difficult to assess the true familial incidence. Rare familial occurrence of infantile hemangiomas has been reported in six kindreds demonstrating autosomal dominant segregation. Some of these families included members who also had vascular malformations. Genetic mapping was performed on these kindreds in the hope of elucidating a candidate gene that could be involved in the pathogenesis of infantile hemangioma (see below)[14,15].

PATHOGENESIS

The pathogenesis of infantile hemangiomas is not clearly defined, although recent advances in the understanding of normal vascular development have provided some clues (see Ch. 102). The latter consists of a series of complex processes that leads to new vessel formation and remodeling. Angiogenesis refers to the process by which new vessels form. Hemangiomas are believed to represent localized areas of abnormal angiogenesis. Several hypotheses have been proposed to explain their pathogenesis, but no single hypothesis accounts for all aspects of their development.

The origin of hemangioma endothelial cells is unknown, but several hypotheses exist. Hemangioma endothelial cells may represent human microvascular endothelial cells in which a somatic mutation has occurred, leading to the differences in behavior that characterize hemangioma endothelial cells as compared to normal microvasculature. Another hypothesis is that extrinsic factors such as abnormalities in other cell types in the hemangioma's environment, for instance, monocytes, fibroblasts, mesenchymal cells, adipocytes and mast cells, cause normal microvasculature endothelial cells to undergo aberrant proliferation, leading to hemangioma formation. It has also been suggested that hemangioma cells could be of placental origin, owing to their shared immunohistochemical phenotype with placental endothelium. Another theory is that hemangiomas may arise from immature endothelial progenitor cells[16,17]. Several of these hypotheses are discussed in greater detail below.

Recent data suggest that hemangioma endothelial cells represent a clonal expansion of cells in which a somatic mutation in a gene or genes

that play a significant role in vascular growth or regulatory pathways has occurred[18]. In hemangiomas, mutations in several genes involved in the vascular endothelial growth factor (VEGF) signaling pathway (e.g. VEGF receptors) as well as the gene that encodes Tie-2 have been noted. However it remains to be determined whether these mutations are the direct cause of the hemangioma phenotype[17,19,20]. Initial analysis of several pedigrees of familial hemangiomas revealed linkage to chromosome 5q[14]. Subsequent analysis of sporadic hemangiomas then demonstrated loss of heterozygosity of 5q (see Ch. 53), further supporting the possibility that somatic mutations play a role in hemangioma formation[21]. It has also been speculated that mutational events lead to altered expression of genes that affect angiogenesis as well as genes that appear to have no obvious effect on blood vessel development but may interfere with other normal physiologic functions such as thyroid hormone levels[22].

Immunohistochemical analysis of hemangioma tissue has demonstrated that infantile hemangiomas express markers that are shared by human placenta. North and co-workers[23] reported that glucose transporter protein-1 (GLUT1) is expressed by infantile hemangiomas during all phases of their development (proliferating, involuting, involuted) and is not expressed by vascular malformations and other vascular tumors. Moreover, other placenta-associated vascular antigens, including merosin, FcγRII and Lewis Y antigen, are present in hemangioma specimens and placental chorionic villi and absent in microvessels of normal skin and subcutis[24]. It has been speculated that hemangiomas may originate from invading angioblasts that aberrantly differentiate toward a placental phenotype in the skin or subcutaneous tissue. Local factors and loss of mechanisms controlling intrauterine angiogenesis might also contribute to hemangioma development. An alternative explanation offered by these investigators is that hemangiomas arise from embolized placental cells[24]. These hypotheses, however, have been challenged by other data, specifically a finding in which immunohistochemical analysis of hemangiomas for placental trophoblastic markers was negative[25].

Hemangiomas have been studied during different phases of their growth cycle in an attempt to gain an insight into the mechanisms that govern growth and involution. Researchers noted that in the proliferative phase, hemangiomas elaborate markers of proliferation, such as proliferating cell nuclear antigen (PCNA) and increased levels of the growth factors VEGF and basic fibroblast growth factor (bFGF)[26–28]. Angiogenesis mediators, including monocyte chemoattractant protein-1 and the adhesion molecules E-selectin and ICAM-3, are also expressed at high levels in hemangiomas[29–32]. In addition, proteins involved in extracellular matrix remodeling, including the enzymes urokinase and type IV collagenase, type VI collagen, fibronectin, vitronectin and laminin, are expressed during the proliferating phase[22,26,33,34]. Increased levels of urinary matrix metalloproteinases, proteins that play an important role in extracellular matrix remodeling, are noted in patients with active (proliferating) and extensive infantile hemangiomas[35]. Immunophenotyping of endothelial cells from proliferating hemangioma tissue for vascular lineage-specific markers demonstrated expression of lymphatic endothelial hyaluronan receptor-1 (LYVE-1). This marker is then lost or significantly reduced during the involuting phase. These findings suggest that proliferating hemangiomas may be arrested in an early developmental stage of vascular differentiation. Such a phenotype may contribute to the rapid growth pattern seen in the proliferating phase[36].

The molecular characteristics of proliferating hemangiomas were investigated by analyzing mRNA expression patterns for a variety of genes whose products are important for angiogenesis, including the angiopoietin/Tie receptor signaling pathway[20] (see Ch. 102). This signaling pathway plays an important role in normal blood vessel development and maintenance, and activation of the pathway can lead to abnormal angiogenesis[37]. Specifically, activating mutations in the gene for Tie-2 are found in a subset of families with inherited venous malformations[38]. Tie-2 expression is increased and there is an enhanced response to angiopoietin-1 and dysregulated expression of angiopoietin-2 in hemangioma endothelial cells[39]. This suggests that alterations in this pathway may be involved in the pathogenesis of infantile hemangiomas. Local factors are also believed to play a significant role in hemangioma proliferation. Investigators have noted that hemangioma growth correlates with hyperplasia of the adjacent epidermis, with the epidermis elaborating angiogenic factors (e.g. VEGF, bFGF). Moreover, the epidermis overlying the hemangiomas lacks expression of the angiogenesis inhibitor interferon-β[39].

Recent data have provided some interesting clues regarding factors governing the transition from proliferation to involution. Indoleamine 2,3-dioxygenase (IDO) enzyme activity (which degrades tryptophan and is important in maintaining T-cell function) was noted during the proliferating phase of hemangiomas. IDO activity is also present in the placenta, where it is believed to protect the fetus from rejection. IDO mRNA is upregulated during the proliferating phase of hemangiomas and downregulated during involution. It is expressed by macrophages and dendritic cells but not in normal endothelial cells. One hypothesis is that increased IDO activity protects the hemangioma from rejection during its proliferating phase and that IDO activity decreases as involution occurs[17,40].

Additional factors governing the involution of hemangiomas are poorly understood. Involuting hemangiomas do not express the increased levels of angiogenic factors that are found in proliferating lesions[26,31,32]. Levels of tissue inhibitor of metalloproteinase-1, an angiogenesis inhibitor, are increased during involution[26]. Interferon-regulated genes are upregulated in involuting hemangiomas, providing evidence that these genes play a role in the regression of infantile hemangiomas[41]. Studies have also demonstrated that apoptosis is increased during involution of a hemangioma and this correlates with clinical regression of the tumor[42,43]. Inhibitors of apoptosis are upregulated during proliferation and factors believed to promote apoptosis are elevated in involuting hemangiomas[42,44].

Despite the frequency of infantile hemangiomas, their pathogenesis remains incompletely understood. It appears likely that several mechanisms under the control of multiple genes, in addition to local effects, play a role in their development, growth and involution.

CLINICAL FEATURES

Presentation

The majority of infantile hemangiomas have a typical presentation and growth pattern. Most lesions do not become apparent until the first few weeks of life, although the incidence of congenital hemangiomas reported in the literature varies, ranging from 15% to 60%[8,45]. Within the group of hemangiomas noted in the immediate newborn period, there are several distinct subgroups: (1) hemangioma precursor lesions; (2) typical hemangiomas that are fully formed in the neonate and demonstrate the same natural history as those that arise later; and (3) a rare subset of congenital hemangiomas that demonstrate intrauterine proliferation, little if any postnatal growth, and then either early rapid involution in postnatal life or incomplete or absent involution. This third group of lesions has been termed rapidly involuting congenital hemangioma (RICH), non-involuting congenital hemangioma (NICH) and non-progressive hemangioma. These lesions are discussed later in this chapter.

The higher reported incidences of hemangiomas noted at birth probably represent the inclusion of precursor lesions that may be noted by an experienced examining physician. Telangiectasias surrounded by a border of pallor, pink macules, and blue bruise-like patches are the most common precursor lesions (Fig. 103.1). Pink patches and macules may mimic a capillary malformation, and repeat examination is essential to confirm the diagnosis (Fig. 103.2). Rarely, an area of ulceration on the lip or perineum may herald the onset of an infantile hemangioma, and in a newborn infant these lesions may be confused with bacterial or viral infections. Biopsy of the ulcerated lesion may not be clearly diagnostic of an infantile hemangioma, but continued observation of the site as the infant matures usually clarifies the diagnosis[46].

Hemangiomas may occur anywhere on the skin and mucosal surfaces[12]. The clinical appearance of a hemangioma is determined by its location within the skin and subcutaneous tissues. Superficial hemangiomas are located in the superficial dermis and are bright red in color during their proliferating phase. The surface is finely lobulated 'like that of unpolished shagreen leather' and the term 'strawberry' hemangioma has been used to describe them. The majority of superficial hemangiomas are small focal lesions (Fig. 103.3). Less common and perhaps more worrisome is the larger, diffuse, plaque-type or segmental pattern of superficial hemangioma. These lesions may begin as erythematous

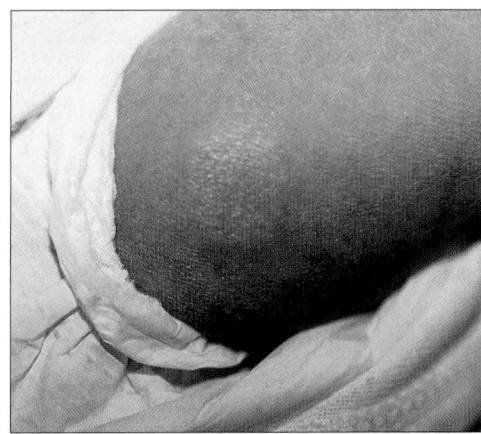

Fig. 103.1 Hemangioma precursor. The lesion has a 'bruised' appearance.

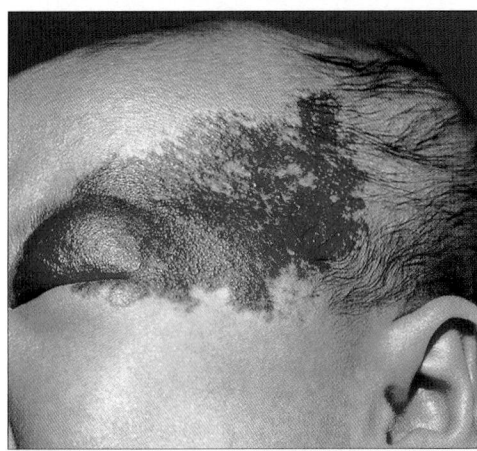

Fig. 103.2 Superficial hemangioma mimicking a capillary malformation.

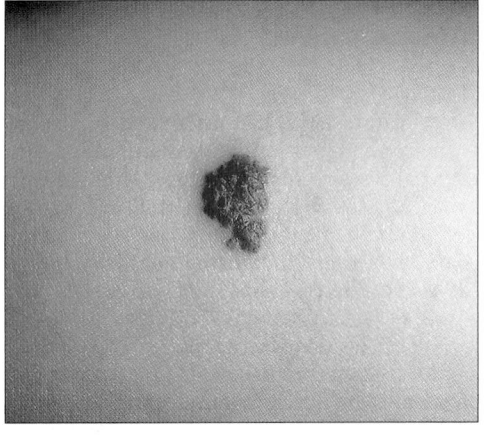

Fig. 103.3 Superficial hemangioma. Note the bright red color and finely lobulated surface. Courtesy of Ronald P Rapini MD.

patches that are either confluent or reticulated. Within a few weeks, erythematous papules and plaques arise on the surface.

Deep hemangiomas are located in the deep dermis and/or subcutis. They usually are not apparent in the immediate newborn period but are recognized at several weeks of age. They present as warm blue–purple masses with minimal or no overlying skin changes (Fig. 103.4), making them more difficult to diagnose than superficial or mixed hemangiomas[47]. The presence of dilated veins or telangiectasias overlying a deep hemangioma provides a clue that the lesion is of vascular origin. Larger deep hemangiomas often have significant arterial blood supply during their peak growth phase. A bruit may be felt on physical examination, and high flow on Doppler ultrasonography can raise the possibility of an arteriovenous malformation. Detailed imaging studies will help to clarify the diagnosis. A number of hemangiomas will show features of both superficial and deep components. During the proliferating phase, a well-delineated superficial vascular plaque overlying a less well-defined deeper component often characterizes mixed hemangiomas.

Superficial hemangiomas are the most common type of hemangioma, representing approximately 50–60% of cases. Mixed or combined superficial and deep hemangiomas are observed in 25–35% of cases and deep

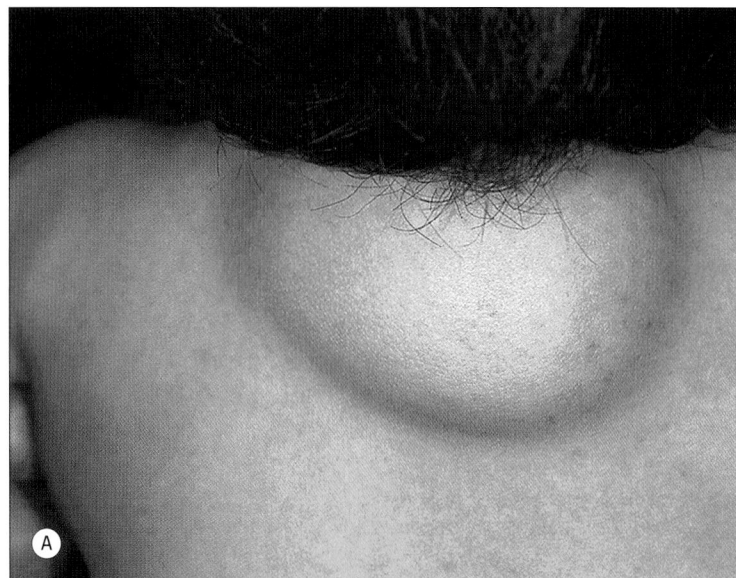

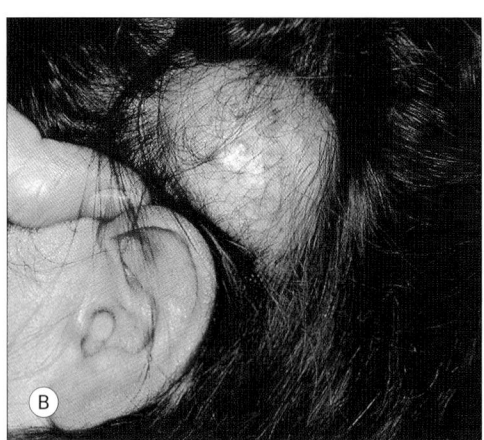

Fig. 103.4 Deep hemangiomas. Note the skin-colored to bluish hue with scattered telangiectasias. A, Courtesy of Anthony J Mancini MD.

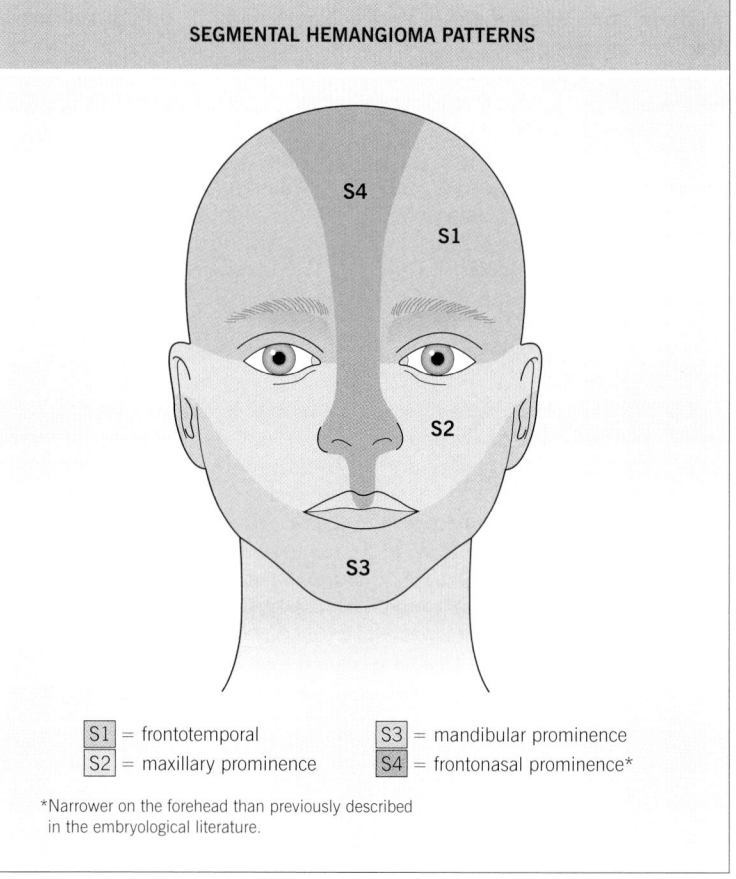

SEGMENTAL HEMANGIOMA PATTERNS

S1 = frontotemporal	S3 = mandibular prominence
S2 = maxillary prominence	S4 = frontonasal prominence*

*Narrower on the forehead than previously described in the embryological literature.

Fig. 103.5 Segmental hemangioma patterns. Based upon a prospective study (n = 165) of image analyses of hemangiomas[50]. Adapted with permission from Haggstrom AN, Lammer EJ, Schneider RA, et al. Patterns of infantile hemangiomas: new clues to hemangioma pathogenesis and embryonic facial development. Pediatrics. 2006;117:698–703.

hemangiomas in 15%[6]. Investigators have also attempted to classify hemangiomas based on their configuration and distribution (see below). Well-circumscribed focal lesions are most commonly seen. In addition, most hemangiomas are solitary, although multiple lesions may occur and can herald systemic hemangiomatosis.

Several recent studies have characterized hemangiomas based upon the pattern of involvement in the skin and subcutaneous tissues, and found that these features may be useful for predicting prognosis[48,49]. Pattern subtypes include: (1) *focal* lesions that appear to arise from a single focus; and (2) *segmental* lesions that have a diffuse pattern and appear to arise from a broad area or developmental unit (the terms 'plaque-like' or 'diffuse' are also used to describe this latter group). In some cases it is difficult to classify lesions and they are designated as *indeterminate*. It is thought that segmental lesions correlate with a higher incidence of associated systemic anomalies, including PHACES syndrome, spinal dysraphism, and gastrointestinal and genitourinary anomalies[49]. A recent study attempted to define segmental hemangiomas based upon clinically observed patterns and to relate the observed patterns to previously described developmental patterns. Investigators identified four primary segments, which they called S1 to S4 (Fig. 103.5). Large segmental hemangiomas involving the periorbital area did not consistently follow the described patterns. Incomplete involvement of segments was also noted. The authors hypothesized that the patterns provide useful clues to the pathogenesis of facial hemangiomas and facial development[50].

Natural History

Natural history studies have documented the typical growth pattern of infantile hemangiomas. Three phases are observed: proliferation, involution and involuted. Proliferation and involution coexist in the first months of life, with proliferation predominating. Infantile hemangiomas classically proliferate for a period of several months and

deep lesions may proliferate for up to 1 year. During the proliferating phase, the hemangioma may become warmer and firmer in texture, and the surface of superficial hemangiomas may appear tense. During the proliferative phase, mixed and deep hemangiomas often feel firmer with crying or activity. Involution may begin as early as the first year of life and continues for several years. A color change from a deep red to gray–purple (Fig. 103.6) and a flattening of the surface are often the earliest signs of involution in a superficial hemangioma. Parents often notice that the superficial plaque breaks apart into smaller islands before clearing. As the tumor involutes, the mass becomes less firm and assumes a fatty consistency. During involution, larger lesions demonstrate less fluctuation in consistency and size with crying and activity[5,51].

Natural history studies of untreated hemangiomas demonstrate that 30% of lesions involute by 3 years of age, 50% by 5 years, 70% by 7 years, and over 90% by 9 years[5,8,51]. Residual lesions following involution are of varying cosmetic significance. Some hemangiomas involute completely, while others may leave atrophic, fibrofatty or telangiectatic residua (Fig. 103.7). Predicting whether the residual lesion will be of cosmetic significance is one of the most challenging aspects of hemangioma management.

Complications

The majority of hemangiomas are small lesions that require little or no intervention. However, certain hemangiomas may be problematic owing to their size, location or association with other anomalies. The age of the patient and the growth pattern of the hemangioma are crucial factors in predicting complications.

Ulceration

Significant bleeding is a rare complication of proliferating hemangiomas; however, ulceration is the most common complication, occurring in up to 10% of all infantile hemangiomas[51a]. Most bleeding episodes are

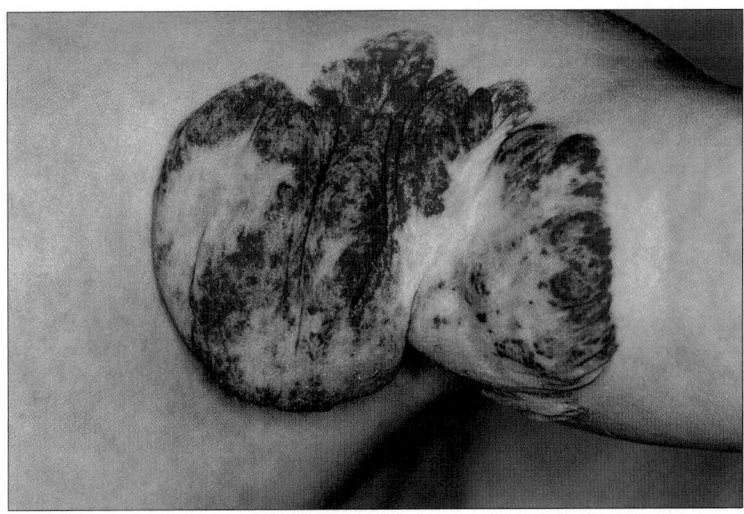

Fig. 103.6 Hemangioma during involution. Note the lightening (gray color) and softening of the hemangioma during involution.

minor and can be controlled with firm pressure. Ulceration is more common on the lip and neck or in the anogenital region, but may occur at any location (Fig. 103.8). Ulceration appears to occur more commonly within large, mixed (superficial and deep) and segmental hemangiomas[51a]. In addition to causing pain, ulcers increase the risk of infection and result in scarring with textural change of the affected area. The management of ulcerated hemangiomas may be challenging and will be addressed separately in this chapter[52].

Size
Large hemangiomas may distort normal tissues, interfere with normal function, and lead to significant long-term complications because of residual masses. In addition, high-output congestive heart failure may complicate the course of large hemangiomas. There is a greater risk of this latter life-threatening complication in visceral hemangiomas, especially those located in the liver.

Regionally-significant hemangiomas
Even small lesions may cause short- or long-term complications if they arise in vulnerable locations[53]. Periocular hemangiomas are often associated with ophthalmologic complications (Fig. 103.9). They may cause visual abnormalities by obstructing the visual axis as they proliferate or by invading the orbital musculature, which can lead to light-deprivation amblyopia and strabismus. Most commonly, periocular hemangiomas cause astigmatism by compressing the globe and deforming the cornea, which results in asymmetric refractive errors. Lesions located on the upper lid are most problematic, but visual obstruction can complicate lesions on the lower lid as well. Proptosis is a rare presentation of an orbital hemangioma and may develop gradually or quite suddenly. In these cases, the diagnosis of hemangioma may be difficult to establish clinically when a cutaneous lesion is not present. Infantile hemangiomas associated with proptosis may cause corneal exposure after the mass has involuted. All infants with periocular hemangiomas should be evaluated by an ophthalmologist at baseline and closely thereafter during the proliferative stage[54–56].

Hemangiomas located on the nasal tip are particularly challenging. Deep and mixed hemangiomas can distort the underlying cartilage and leave significant fibrofatty residua. The resultant 'Cyrano-nose' deformity may require reconstructive surgery. In rare cases, superficial hemangiomas

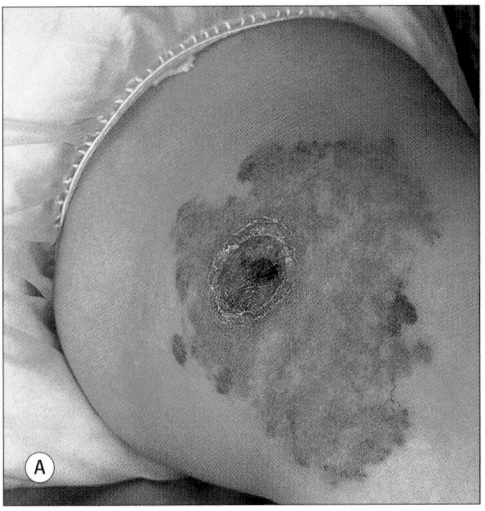
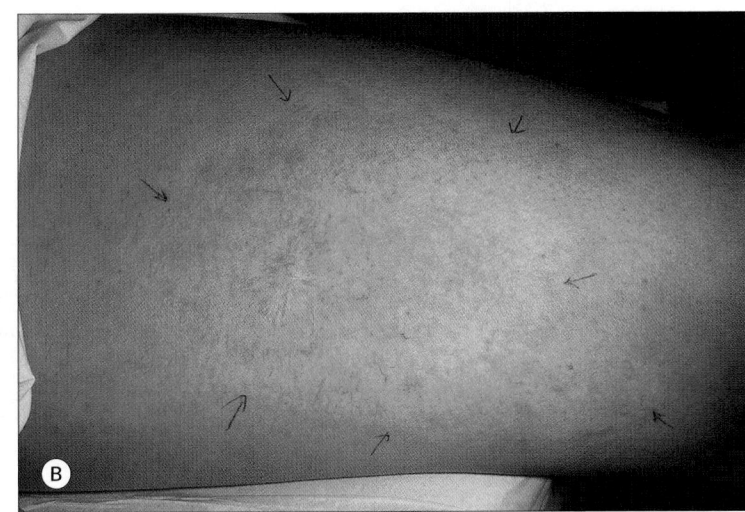
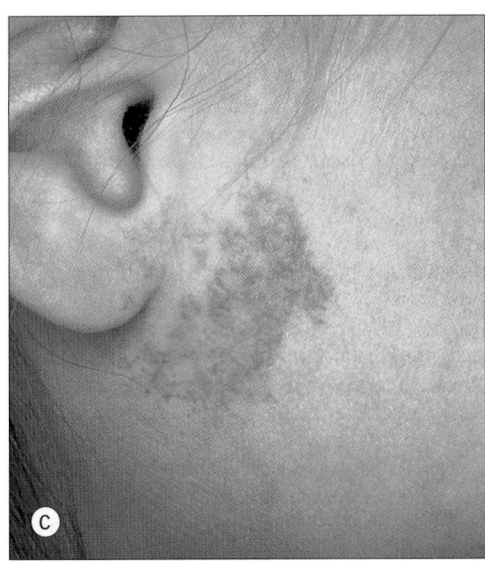
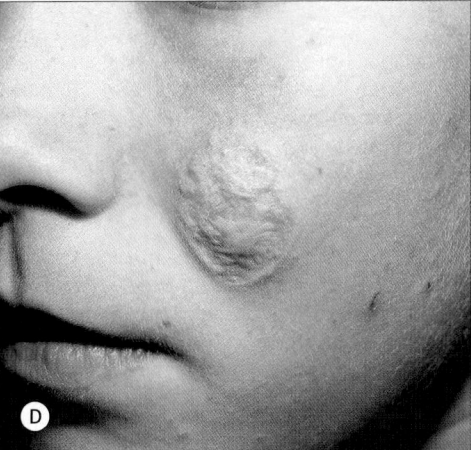

Fig. 103.7 Residua of hemangiomas.
A, B Minimal hypopigmentation (arrows) and a circular scar at site of ulceration in the same patient 20 years later; **C** telangiectasias; and **D** atrophy and fibrofatty changes. A, B, D, Courtesy of Ronald P Rapini MD.

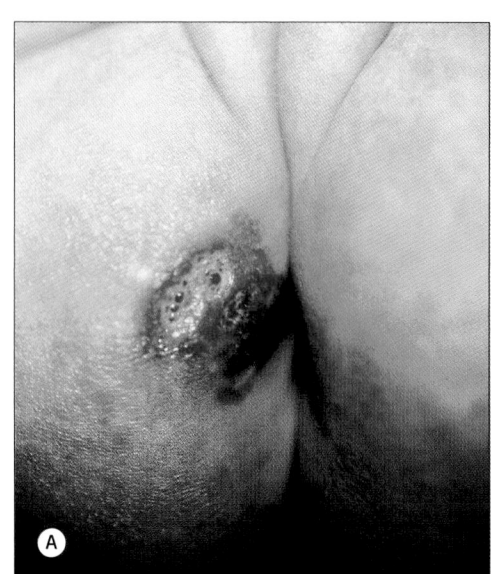

Fig. 103.8 Ulcerated hemangiomas.
A Ulcerated hemangioma in the perineum. **B** Ulcerated mixed hemangioma on the upper back.

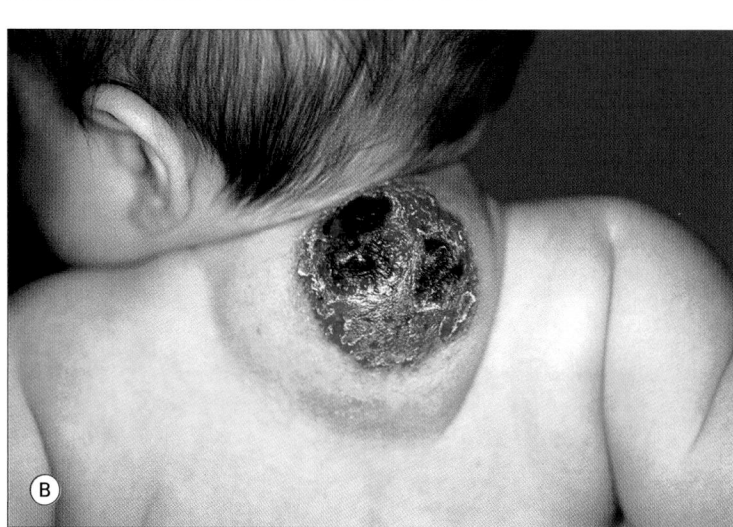

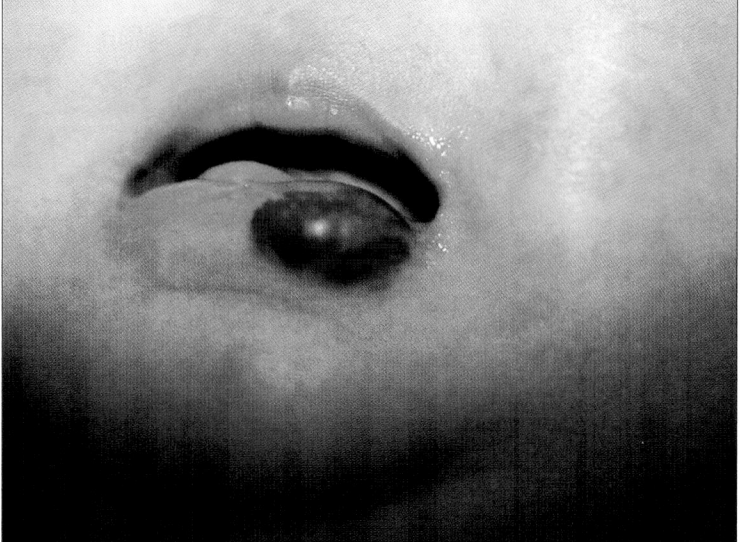

Fig. 103.9 Hemangioma obstructing the visual axis. This patient also had associated laryngeal involvement requiring a tracheostomy. Courtesy of Ronald P Rapini MD.

Fig. 103.10 Lip hemangioma crossing the vermilion border.

located along the columella may ulcerate and lead to textural changes and scarring.

Lip hemangiomas are often superficial or mixed lesions; painful ulceration is common as they proliferate, which leads to feeding difficulties. Local factors, including recurrent trauma and the commensal bacterial flora, may lead to an increased incidence of this complication. Even small hemangiomas crossing the vermilion border (Fig. 103.10) may leave significant cosmetic residua.

Hemangiomas located on the pinna may ulcerate and become infected, increasing the risk of scarring and distortion of normal structures. Conductive hearing loss can result from obstruction of the external auditory canal by a hemangioma[5].

Hemangiomas located on the breast pose a particular challenge to the clinician. There is little information in the literature regarding their course and management, and therefore it is often difficult to predict the ultimate outcome. Proliferation of a hemangioma may affect the underlying breast bud and residual masses may lead to the appearance of breast asymmetry. Moreover, lesions complicated by ulceration may result in permanent scarring. Early surgical intervention is ill advised as it may ultimately affect normal breast development.

Anogenital hemangiomas are often complicated by ulceration and infection, and local management may be difficult in this location. Affected infants often experience painful urination and defecation. Large plaque and mixed hemangiomas of the limbs may be complicated by ulceration, and when they resolve, residual masses that cause size discrepancy can remain.

Hemangiomas and extracutaneous involvement

Large cervicofacial hemangiomas, specifically segmental lesions, pose a particular challenge. They occur more frequently in female children (7:1) and are often associated with other congenital anomalies[9]. They may present as segmental plaque-type lesions or deep masses. The association between hemangiomas and structural and vascular CNS anomalies was recognized over 20 years ago[57]. Since then, other characteristic congenital anomalies have been identified. The acronym PHACES syndrome was recently coined to describe these anomalies *(P, posterior fossa and other brain malformations; H, hemangioma; A, arterial anomalies typically of the aortic branches [aortic branch vessels]; C, cardiac defects and coarctation of the aorta; E, eye anomalies; S, sternal defects and supraumbilical raphe)* (Fig. 103.11). However, the syndrome often presents incompletely[58–60]. Infants with large facial hemangiomas and intracranial vascular anomalies may also be at increased risk for developing progressive cerebrovascular disease and should have periodic neurologic assessments[60].

Lower facial or 'beard' hemangiomas are markers of laryngeal hemangiomatosis and the risk can be estimated by the extent of cutaneous involvement (Fig. 103.12)[61]. Symptoms caused by airway obstruction can appear at several weeks or months of life, well after the cutaneous hemangioma has become apparent[61]. Therefore, infants with lower facial hemangiomas of concern should be referred promptly for otolaryngologic evaluation. Hemangiomas located in the lumbosacral

PHACES SYNDROME

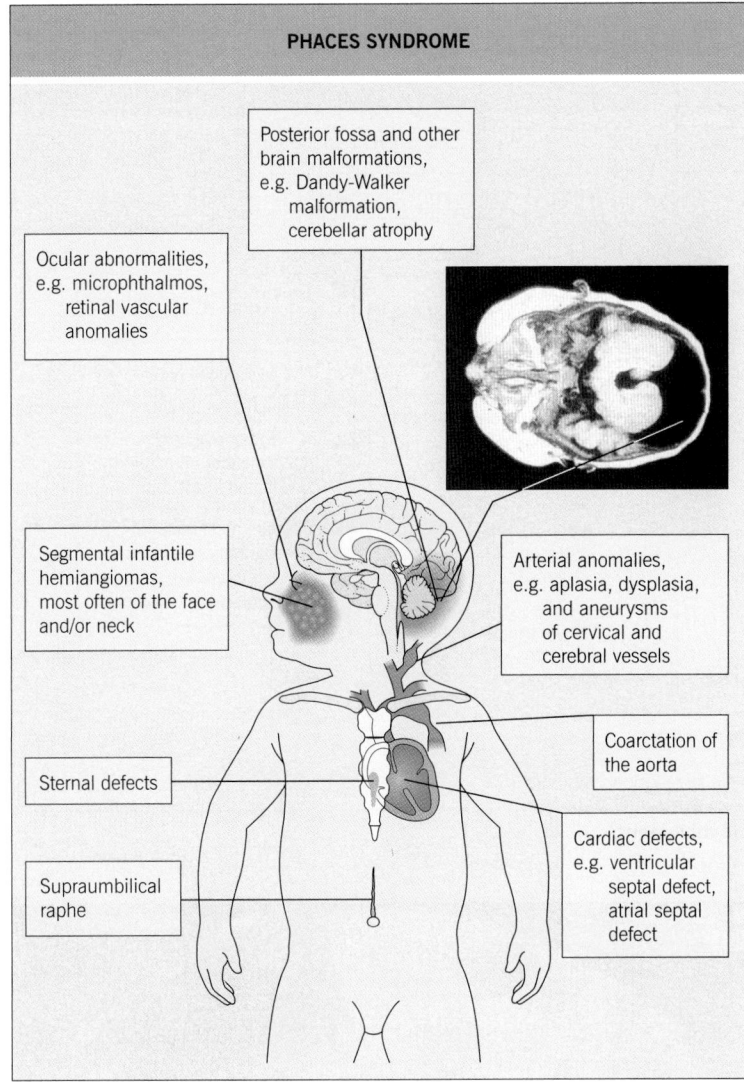

Posterior fossa and other brain malformations, e.g. Dandy-Walker malformation, cerebellar atrophy

Ocular abnormalities, e.g. microphthalmos, retinal vascular anomalies

Segmental infantile hemangiomas, most often of the face and/or neck

Arterial anomalies, e.g. aplasia, dysplasia, and aneurysms of cervical and cerebral vessels

Sternal defects

Coarctation of the aorta

Cardiac defects, e.g. ventricular septal defect, atrial septal defect

Supraumbilical raphe

Fig. 103.11 PHACES syndrome. Major clinical features are illustrated.

HEMANGIOMAS IN A 'BEARD'

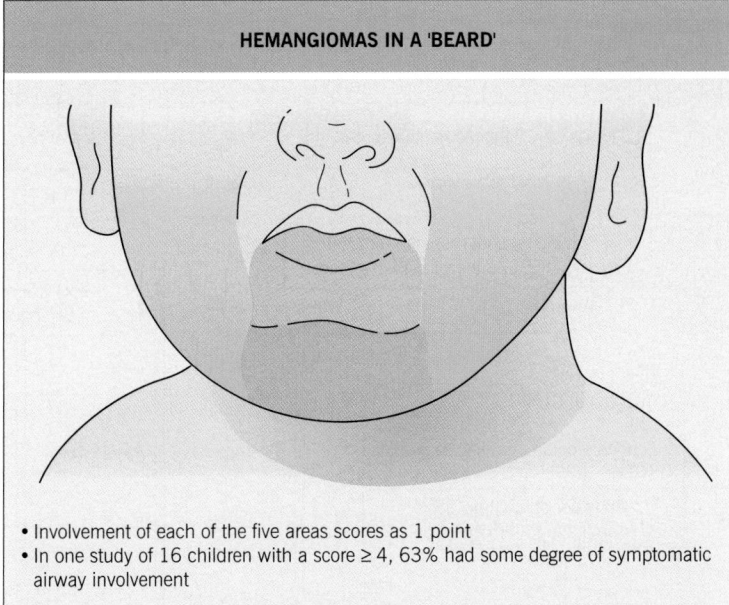

- Involvement of each of the five areas scores as 1 point
- In one study of 16 children with a score ≥ 4, 63% had some degree of symptomatic airway involvement

Fig. 103.12 Anatomic sites of hemangiomas that are in a 'beard' distribution. Adapted, with permission, from Orlow SJ, Isakoff MS, Blei F. Increased risk of symptomatic hemangiomas of the airway in association with cutaneous hemangiomas in a "beard" distribution. J Pediatr. 1997;131:643–6.

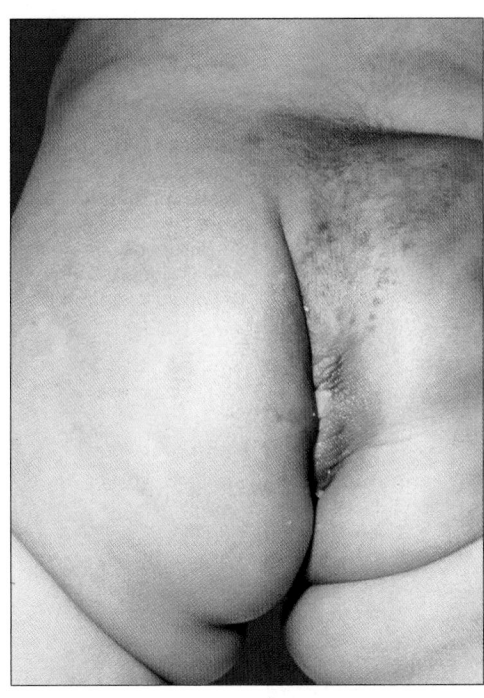

Fig. 103.13 Lumbosacral hemangioma associated with tethered cord. Photograph courtesy of Ilona Frieden MD.

area may be a marker for underlying occult spinal dysraphism (Fig. 103.13). In addition, other malformations, including imperforate anus, rectovesical/rectovaginal/rectoscrotal fistulae, skeletal anomalies and renal anomalies, may occur in association with lumbosacral hemangiomas. MRI is a reliable method of screening for such abnormalities[62,63] (Fig. 103.14).

Multiple lesions occur in 10–25% of infants with hemangiomas and may indicate visceral hemangiomatosis[64]. *Diffuse neonatal hemangiomatosis* is a term used to describe infants with multiple cutaneous and systemic hemangiomas[65]. *Benign neonatal hemangiomatosis* is the term reserved for infants with multiple cutaneous lesions without evident visceral hemangiomas[66]. Most infants with multiple lesions will present with small superficial hemangiomas (Fig. 103.15), ranging from a few millimeters to a few centimeters in diameter. There is no consensus regarding the number of cutaneous hemangiomas that need to be present to suspect visceral involvement, and several to over 100 lesions may be seen. Evaluation for visceral involvement is often recommended in infants with five or more lesions. It should be noted that visceral hemangiomatosis may occur without cutaneous lesions.

The liver, gastrointestinal tract, lungs and CNS are the most common sites of internal involvement in diffuse neonatal hemangiomatosis[65–67] (Fig. 103.16). Hemangiomas may also develop within mucosal surfaces and the eyes. Cutaneous and hepatic hemangiomas can be diagnosed by prenatal ultrasonography as early as 32 weeks' gestation[68]. Infants with diffuse neonatal hemangiomatosis and hepatic hemangiomatosis have a high incidence of cardiac failure[69]. Among infants with hepatic hemangiomatosis, the presence of arteriovenous or arterioportal shunts or portovenous fistulae is associated with greater morbidity[70]. Other complications include gastrointestinal bleeding, hydrocephalus,

visceral hemorrhage and ocular abnormalities[71]. Congenital anomalies similar to those described in patients with large facial hemangiomas and PHACES syndrome (see above) have rarely been reported in infants with multiple hemangiomas, including absent corpus callosum, sternal agenesis, median abdominal raphe, tricuspid atresia and coarctation of the aorta[72,73].

It is well recognized that visceral hemangiomas can occur in infants with multiple small cutaneous lesions; however, they may also occur in infants with solitary, large hemangiomas. In addition to laryngeal hemangiomatosis, hepatic, gastrointestinal and CNS hemangiomatosis may arise in infants with hemifacial and neck hemangiomas[9]. Extracutaneous hemangiomatosis has been observed in infants with segmental hemangiomas associated with PHACES syndrome as well as large cutaneous hemangiomas in non-facial sites[74,75].

Recently, investigators noted increased levels of iodothyronine deiodinase, an enzyme that deactivates thyroid hormone, in proliferating hemangiomas. This may lead to hypothyroidism in infants with large proliferative-phase lesions[76]. Moreover, the hemangiomas causing the

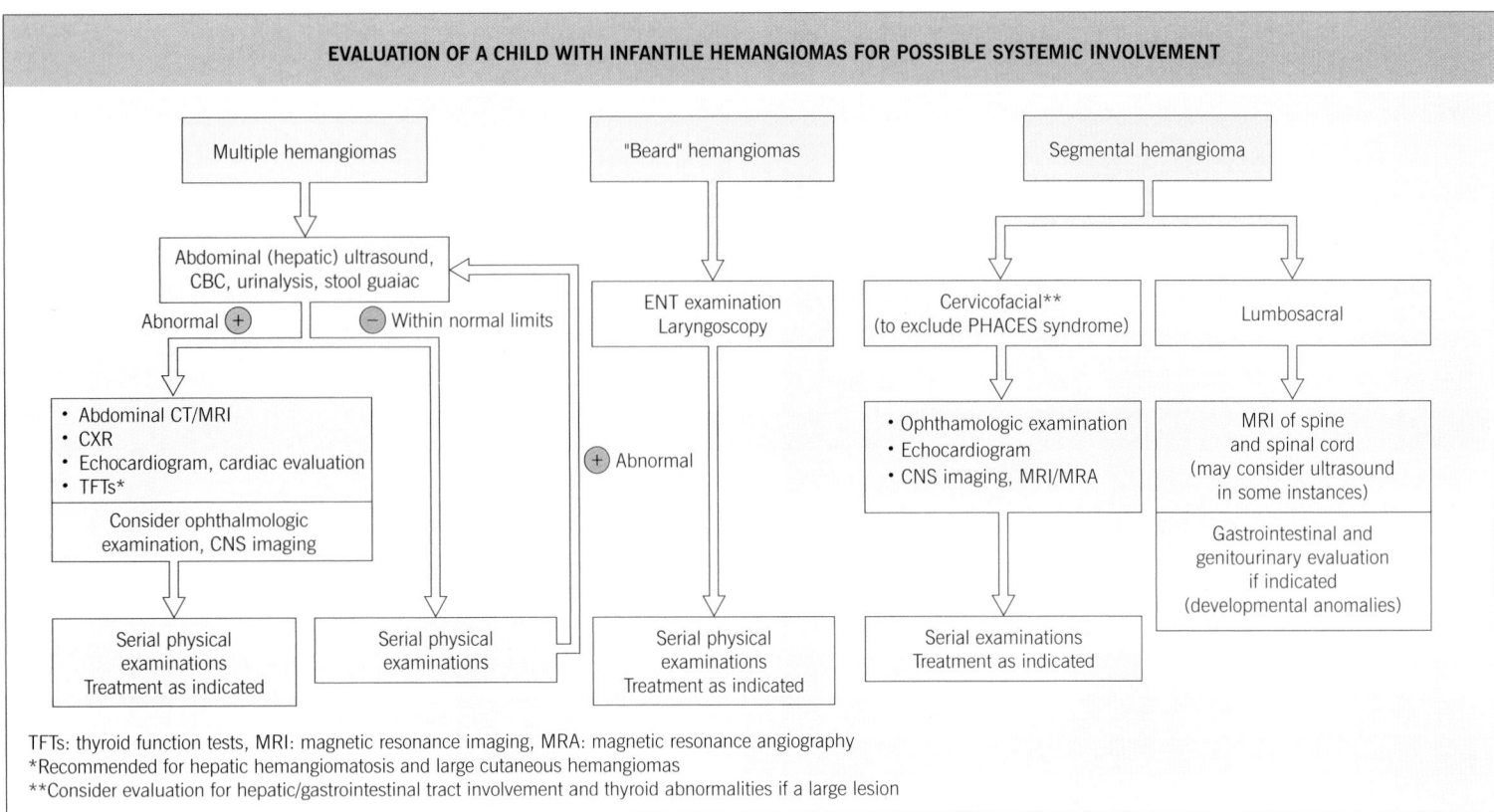

TFTs: thyroid function tests, MRI: magnetic resonance imaging, MRA: magnetic resonance angiography
*Recommended for hepatic hemangiomatosis and large cutaneous hemangiomas
**Consider evaluation for hepatic/gastrointestinal tract involvement and thyroid abnormalities if a large lesion

Fig. 103.14 Evaluation of a child with infantile hemangioma for possible systemic involvement.

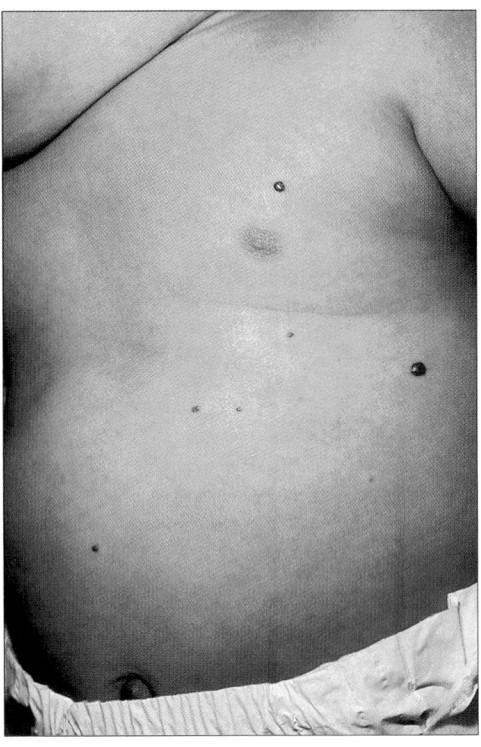

Fig. 103.15 Diffuse neonatal hemangiomatosis. Note the multiple small superficial hemangiomas. Courtesy of Ronald P Rapini MD.

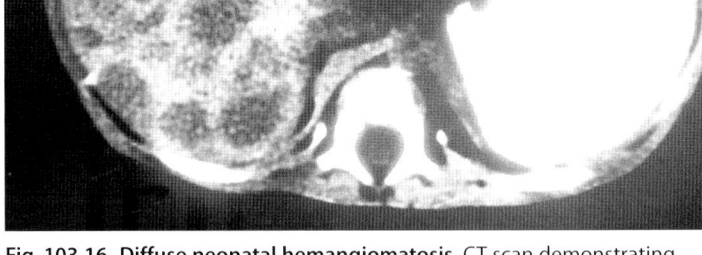

Fig. 103.16 Diffuse neonatal hemangiomatosis. CT scan demonstrating multiple hepatic hemangiomas. Courtesy of Amy Paller MD.

hypothyroidism may not be causing any other complications. The hypothyroidism may be difficult to correct, but, as the tumor regresses, it resolves. Screening for hypothyroidism in the immediate neonatal period is inadequate, as hemangiomas are often not present or in their peak proliferative phase at that time. The majority of reported cases have been associated with hepatic hemangiomatosis; however, type 3 iodothyronine deiodinase activity has been noted in cutaneous hemangiomas. Consequently, it has been recommended that children with large cutaneous hemangiomas or hepatic hemangiomatosis undergo evaluation of thyroid function[76,77].

Diffuse neonatal hemangiomatosis is a life-threatening disorder with reported mortality rates of 30–80% with various treatment regimens[67,69]. Infants with multiple cutaneous hemangiomas need to be monitored closely with careful periodic physical examinations for signs or symptoms of visceral involvement. Radiologic evaluation including ultrasonography, CT and/or MRI may be indicated to assess for systemic involvement (see Fig. 103.14). Periodic re-evaluation with these modalities is often employed to monitor progression and response to treatment. Not all infants with hepatic hemangiomatosis require treatment, but it is often difficult to determine those who will at initial presentation. Typically, infantile hemangiomas located within the viscera follow the same course of proliferation and involution as cutaneous lesions. Close monitoring for complications is essential.

Congenital Hemangioma

Infrequently, infants will present with a fully developed hemangioma in the immediate newborn period. This rare tumor undergoes significant intrauterine growth, little if any postnatal growth, and rapid involution within the first year of life. This subset of hemangiomas has been called *rapidly involuting congenital hemangioma (RICH)* or *congenital non-progressive hemangioma*. Recent evidence suggests that these tumors demonstrate some features that are clinically, histologically and immunohistochemically distinct from infantile hemangiomas[45,78,79]. RICHs are equally common in boys and girls. Intrauterine growth may be noted by prenatal ultrasonography as early as 12 weeks' gestation and prenatal Doppler ultrasonography may reveal high vascularity and fast flow[78,79]. At birth, the tumor can present as a raised violaceous tumor with prominent radiating veins, a hemispheric tumor surrounded by a pale rim with surface telangiectasias, or a firm, pink to violaceous tumor that is often located on the lower extremity. Superimposed milia and hypertrichosis are occasionally noted. Ulceration, hemorrhage and necrosis can occur within the tumor and rapid regression is evident within the first year of life[3,78] (Fig. 103.17). North and co-workers[45] used the term 'congenital non-progressive hemangioma' to describe these lesions because early excision of their specimens did not permit them to observe whether rapid involution occurred.

Another very rare type of congenital hemangioma has been described as the *non-involuting congenital hemangioma (NICH)*. These lesions occur slightly more often in male infants and are well developed at birth. They typically present as well-circumscribed, erythematous to blue–violet masses or plaques surrounded by a pale or bluish rim with overlying telangiectasia. They are warm to palpation and grow proportionately with the child, unlike infantile hemangiomas. The lesions may worsen somewhat with maturity and do not involute spontaneously. The diagnosis is often established retrospectively after the lesion is excised when involution fails to occur. The histologic and immunohistochemical features of congenital hemangiomas differ from

those of typical infantile hemangiomas (Table 103.3), but some overlap does exist (see below)[45,79]. It remains unclear whether NICH represents a distinct histopathologic entity or whether it is a variant of RICH[80]. In addition, it has been suggested that these rare congenital hemangiomas and common infantile hemangiomas may be variations of a single entity[79,81].

Kasabach–Merritt Syndrome

Kasabach–Merritt syndrome (KMS) is the association of a vascular tumor with a thrombocytopenic coagulopathy. Kasabach and Merritt reported the first case in 1940 and classified the tumor as a 'capillary hemangioma'. For decades thereafter it was assumed that thrombocytopenic coagulopathy was a rare complication occurring in typical hemangiomas[82]. However, data have shown that the tumors associated with this life-threatening complication are not typical infantile hemangiomas. Rather, the histopathologic features of the tumors most commonly associated with KMS are those of kaposiform hemangioendothelioma and tufted angioma[83,84].

Infants with KMS present in the first several months of life with a rapidly enlarging mass associated with thrombocytopenia and coagulopathy. This syndrome is equally common in boys and girls. The mass is often a superficial plaque or mass (Fig. 103.18), but deep lesions within the mediastinum, neck or retroperitoneum may occur. The clinical appearance of the tumor prior to the development of KMS is quite variable. Some patients will have plaques that are skin-colored, red or violaceous, while others have masses that resemble lymphatic malformations. Many of these tumors are noted at birth. The

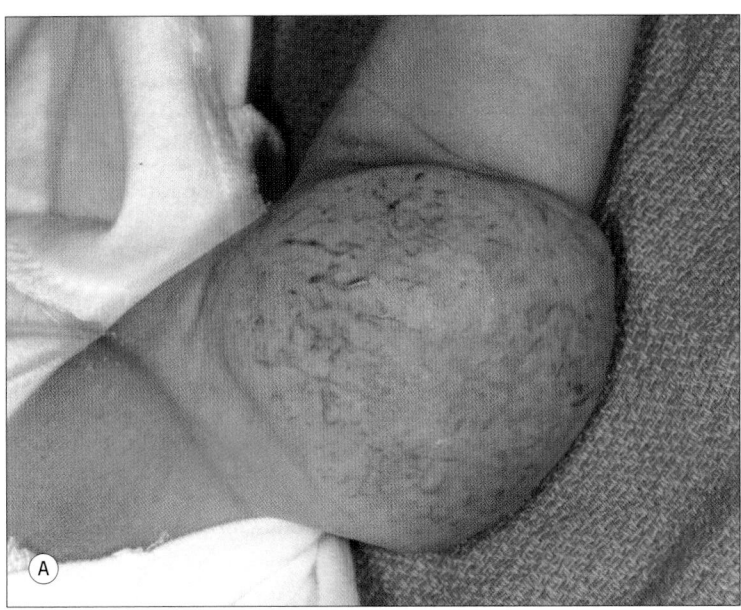
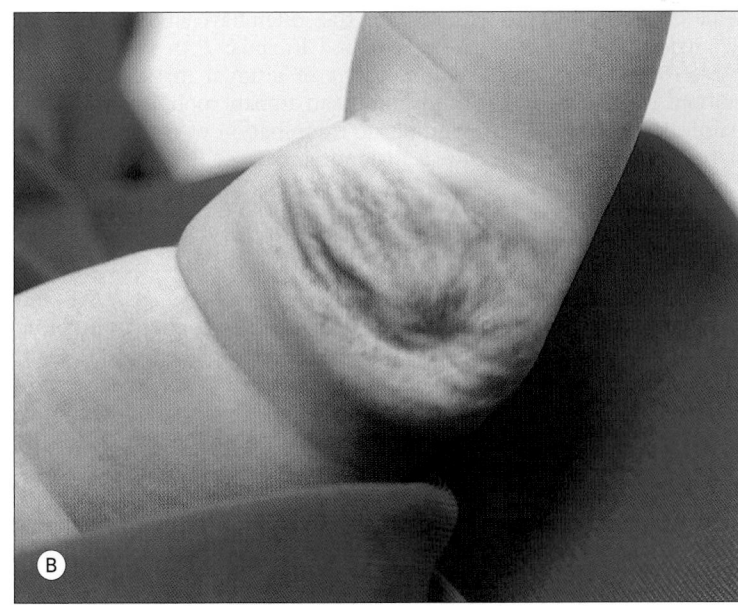

Fig. 103.17 Rapidly involuting congenital hemangioma (RICH) in a neonate. A Violaceous tumor on the upper extremity with surface telangiectasias. **B** Spontaneous involution at 5 months of age, with fibrofatty residua. Courtesy of Annette Wagner MD.

KEY FEATURES OF INFANTILE AND CONGENITAL HEMANGIOMAS		
Infantile hemangioma	**Rapidly involuting congenital hemangioma (RICH)/ congenital non-progressive hemangioma**	**Non-involuting congenital hemangioma (NICH)**
Absent, precursor or present at birth	Fully developed at birth	Fully developed at birth
Rapid postnatal proliferation	Intrauterine proliferation	Proportionate growth
Slow spontaneous involution	Rapid involution after the first year	Do not involute spontaneously
More common in girls	Equal prevalence or slightly more common in girls	Slightly more common in boys
Lobular endothelial proliferation during proliferative phase; fibrofatty tissue during involution	Capillary lobules within fibrotic stroma containing thin-walled vessels, hemosiderin	Lobules of small, thin-walled vessels with large central vessel; dilated, dysplastic veins between lobules; 'hobnailed' endothelial cells lining intralobular vessels
GLUT1-, Lewis Y antigen-positive	GLUT1-, Lewis Y antigen-negative	GLUT1-negative

Table 103.3 **Key features of infantile and congenital hemangiomas.**

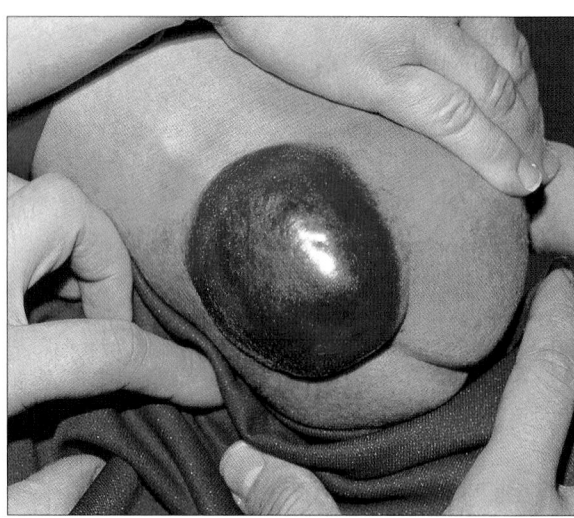

Fig. 103.18 Kasabach–Merritt syndrome in a 1-week-old boy. He had a kaposiform hemangioendothelioma. Courtesy of Anthony J Mancini MD.

counterparts. The findings from MRI, Doppler sonography and CT of the various phases of hemangiomas as well as in KMS are listed in Table 103.4.

MRI is the most useful imaging study for helping to define the extent and tissue characteristics of vascular tumors, and the use of contrast can help to differentiate an infantile hemangioma from other tumors. If MRI does not confirm the diagnosis of infantile hemangioma or there are concerns regarding a possible malignancy, histologic examination of the tumor is recommended. MRI can also be used to determine the presence of hemangiomas within internal organs and other structural anomalies, including CNS malformations and arterial anomalies[86].

Rapidly involuting congenital hemangiomas (RICH) may demonstrate distinct radiographic features. Although they can be diagnosed by prenatal ultrasonography during the second and third trimester, misdiagnosis in the prenatal period is common. The differential diagnosis for these lesions includes other vascular anomalies such as lymphatic malformations and arteriovenous malformations[87]. Postnatal ultrasonographic evaluation of RICH reveals uniformly hypoechoic lesions mostly confined to the subcutaneous fat. Diffuse vascularity is typical, with vessels showing venous flow or low resistance arterial flow signals[88].

Doppler evaluation of a non-involuting congenital hemangioma (NICH) routinely demonstrates fast-flow vessels. MRI reveals features similar to infantile hemangioma[80]. MRI of vascular tumors associated with KMS show diffuse soft tissue masses that enhance after contrast administration (see Table 103.4). Some authors feel that the MRI findings in kaposiform hemangioendothelioma are distinct. Ill-defined margins, involvement of multiple tissue planes, overlying cutaneous thickening, edema, subcutaneous stranding and signal voids caused by hemosiderin deposits may help to differentiate them from infantile hemangioma[84].

coagulopathy may develop early or late during the first year of life. When the coagulopathy develops, the tumor enlarges and becomes indurated, and petechiae and purpura are noted.

Tumors associated with KMS do not respond as well to treatment as do typical infantile hemangiomas. The coagulopathy may persist for months to years, and once the initial episode resolves, residual masses are common. Worsening of the residual mass occurs with maturity in some patients. Residual masses following KMS may look like a port-wine stain with papules within it and they often have a fibrotic texture. Telangiectatic streaks with swelling and irregular firm subcutaneous masses are other clinical presentations of residual masses. Residual tumors involving muscles and joints can impair mobility and cause painful contractures. Histopathologic examination of residual masses has revealed features of tufted angioma and/or KHE with prominent fibrosis[85].

Radiologic Features

Diagnostic radiologic techniques including ultrasonography, CT and MRI play an important role in the diagnosis and evaluation of infantile hemangiomas. Most superficial and mixed infantile hemangiomas can be diagnosed based upon their clinical features. However, imaging may be useful for defining the extent and depth of the deep component of mixed lesions. Radiologic evaluation is particularly helpful for confirming the diagnosis of deep infantile hemangiomas that lack superficial changes. It is important to consider the phase of growth when assessing hemangiomas radiographically, because proliferating hemangiomas demonstrate different characteristics than their involuting and involuted

PATHOLOGY

Infantile Hemangioma

The histopathologic features of infantile hemangioma correlate with the stage of hemangioma development (see Tables 103.1 & 103.3). Infantile hemangiomas may extend from the superficial dermis to the deep subcutaneous tissue, and in some locations there may be involvement of surrounding tissues such as salivary glands and muscle. Biopsy specimens obtained from superficial and deep lesions show the same features. Well-defined non-encapsulated masses composed of proliferating plump endothelial cells and pericytes characterize proliferating hemangiomas (Fig. 103.19). Small vascular lumens may be noted focally throughout the tumor mass, but lumen formation may be more difficult to appreciate in early proliferating lesions. Reticulin staining demonstrates the reticulin fibers surrounding the endothelial cells and PAS staining highlights the basement membrane beneath the endothelial channels.

IMAGING FINDINGS IN SELECTED PEDIATRIC VASCULAR TUMORS						
Lesion	**MRI**				**Doppler sonography**	**CT**
	T1 weighted	Contrast enhancement	T2 weighted	Gradient		
Infantile hemangioma Proliferating	STM, iso- or hypointense to muscle Flow voids	Uniform intense enhancement	Lobulated STM Increased signal Flow voids	HFV within and around STM	Discrete STM containing HFV Decreased arterial resistance	Uniformly enhancing STM Dilated feeding and draining vessels
Involuting	Variable fat content	As above	Variable fat content	As above	As above	Variable fat content
Involuted	High signal (fat)	No enhancement	Decreased signal (fat)	No HFV	Echogenic avascular STM	Fat density No enhancement
Kasabach–Merritt syndrome	Diffuse STM STT and skin thickening	Diffuse enhancement	Diffuse increased signal SQ stranding	Mildly dilated in/around STM	Diffuse infiltrating STM with HFV	Diffuse enhancing STM SQ stranding

Table 103.4 Imaging findings in selected pediatric vascular tumors. HFV, high-flow vessels; SQ, subcutaneous; STM, soft tissue mass; STT, soft tissue thickening. Adapted with permission from Burrows et al. Diagnostic imaging in the evaluation of vascular birthmarks. Dermatol Clin. 1998;16:455–88[86].

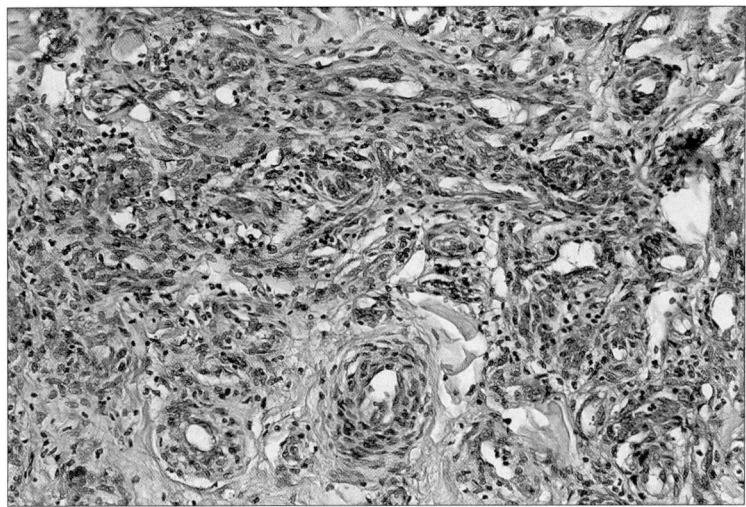

Fig. 103.19 Histologic features of a proliferating hemangioma. Collections of endothelial cells and pericytes are seen, as well as the formation of vascular lumens. Courtesy of Ronald P Rapini MD.

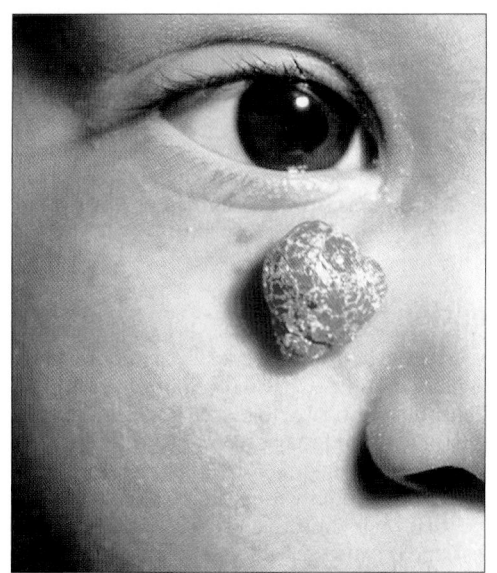

Fig. 103.20 Pyogenic granuloma mimicking an infantile hemangioma. Courtesy of Vincent P Beltrani MD.

Later in the proliferating stage, lobules of endothelial masses separated by fibrous septae become more prominent. Larger feeding and draining vessels are noted within the septae, and mitotic figures and apoptotic bodies may be noted within the tumor mass. Although abnormal mitotic figures are not typical of proliferating hemangiomas, some authors have noted that mitotic activity and mild nuclear pleomorphism may be present in infantile hemangiomas and should not be a cause for concern if other typical histopathologic features are also present. An increased number of mast cells may be present within a proliferating hemangioma.

As the lesion matures, proliferation ceases and involution progresses, and, in some lesions, histologic features of both growth phases may be evident. The involuting phase is marked by flattening of the endothelium and reduced numbers of mitotic figures. Eventually, the vessels decrease in number and lose their tightly packed appearance, and fibrofatty tissue separates the vessels within and between lobules. The feeding and draining vessels within the septae may persist, but mast cells decrease in number. Involuted lesions reveal fibrofatty tissue and a few persistent vessels at sites where tumor lobules and septae previously existed.

Immunohistochemical analysis is useful for confirming the diagnosis of infantile hemangioma. Erythrocyte-type glucose transporter protein-1 (GLUT1) is a protein that is normally restricted to vessels with blood–tissue barrier functions, such as the brain and placenta. A high level of GLUT1 immunoreactivity is present in the endothelia within infantile hemangiomas at all phases of development. GLUT1 staining is absent in other types of vascular tumors and vascular malformations. In addition, other placenta-associated vascular proteins, including FcγRII, merosin and Lewis Y antigen, are present in infantile hemangiomas and are absent in vascular malformations and pyogenic granulomas. Moreover, these placental markers are absent in normal vessels of the skin and subcutis[23,34].

Histologically and immunophenotypically, congenital hemangiomas have several features that are distinct from infantile hemangiomas (see Table 103.3). These include striking lobularity with densely fibrotic stroma, stromal hemosiderin deposits, focal thrombosis and sclerosis of capillary lobules, lack of infiltration of surrounding tissues, fewer mast cells, and the coexistence of proliferating vasculature with multiple thin-walled vessels. Moreover, congenital hemangiomas lack immunoreactivity to GLUT1 and Lewis Y antigen[45,79]. Some tumors do, however, demonstrate zones of involution[79].

DIFFERENTIAL DIAGNOSIS

Superficial and mixed hemangiomas are usually diagnosed based upon their characteristic clinical features. Hemangioma precursors and early proliferating lesions may sometimes be misdiagnosed as capillary malformations or telangiectasias. Deep lesions provide a greater challenge and radiographic evaluation may be helpful in clarifying the diagnosis.

A number of other entities may masquerade as deep hemangiomas in infants, including vascular malformations (particularly venous, lymphatic or combined venous–lymphatic malformations; see Ch. 104), kaposiform hemangioendothelioma and tufted angioma. Other rare vascular tumors seen in young children include infantile hemangiopericytoma, spindle cell hemangioma and congenital eccrine angiomatous hamartoma. Pyogenic granulomas occur quite commonly in children and may mimic a hemangioma. They typically arise after the first few months of life and are pedunculated lesions (Fig. 103.20).

A congenital fibrosarcoma may mimic a hemangioma because the former are often firm and blue–purple in color and may have ectatic superficial veins. In addition, some patients with this malignancy present with disseminated intravascular coagulation, which further confuses the clinical picture. Rhabdomyosarcoma, neuroblastoma, primitive neuroectodermal tumor and dermatofibrosarcoma protuberans are other examples of neoplasms that may present as deep soft tissue masses. Additional entities that may be mistaken for a hemangioma include: infantile myofibromatosis, which can present as a solitary red to pink plaque or mass; lipoblastoma, a rare benign tumor of immature fat cells that presents as an enlarging mass; and nasal glioma, often presenting as a congenital blue mass on the bridge of the nose. Radiographic studies, especially MRI, may be useful in differentiating these tumors from a hemangioma. However, if the diagnosis is not clarified by clinical and radiographic examinations, or if the lesions are atypical, then histologic examination is indicated.

TREATMENT

Infantile hemangiomas manifest with a spectrum of clinical severity. The best approach to their management remains controversial and needs to be individualized. There is no universal approach to management, and most therapeutic recommendations are based on anecdotal experience. In the last few decades there has been an attempt to identify subgroups of infantile hemangiomas that carry a greater risk of developing complications, and indications for active intervention have been summarized[89]. By recognizing that not all hemangiomas are the same, physicians and parents can make educated choices regarding the possible interventions. The major goals of management include: (1) preventing or reversing life- or function-threatening complications; (2) treating ulcerations; (3) preventing permanent disfigurement; (4) minimizing psychosocial distress to the patients and their families; and (5) avoiding overly aggressive, potentially scarring procedures for lesions that have a strong probability of involuting without significant residua[90].

Aggressive interventions such as early surgery, extensive cryosurgery and radiotherapy were employed during the first half of the 20th century to manage these lesions. Outcomes were often poor, with a significant potential for adverse effects[91]. The pendulum swung in the latter half of the 20th century to a policy that has been called 'benign neglect' when it was recognized that spontaneous involution offered a better outcome in many cases when compared to aggressive therapy. It has been recognized, however, that benign neglect is inadequate even in cases that do not require active intervention. A slightly different approach, which has been termed 'active non-intervention', is more appropriate[92]. In addition, increased experience with modalities such as systemic corticosteroids and lasers has provided clinicians with more therapeutic options.

Active Non-intervention

Small hemangiomas that carry an excellent prognosis for spontaneous resolution with good cosmetic outcome are usually managed without active intervention. Physicians must recognize that even small, seemingly trivial lesions are troubling to parents and may cause significant distress. Parents of children with facial hemangiomas demonstrate reactions similar to those seen in parents of children with permanent deformities. Moreover, many parents feel that their concerns have been inadequately addressed, and, when questioned, expressed dissatisfaction with their medical care[92]. Use of the internet has increased parental access to information about hemangiomas and their treatment, and although this source provides information of variable scientific quality, it has become a source from which many parents receive what they perceive to be correct information.

'Active non-intervention' encompasses a strategy of actively discussing information that parents have learned about hemangiomas and their treatment. Indications for treatment, types of therapy and why they are or are not indicated for their child must be reviewed. Close observation with periodic photography to monitor the hemangioma is essential. Reviewing photographic examples of the evolution of hemangiomas is helpful for families. Many parents are fearful of bleeding and ulceration; therefore, reviewing the care for superficial bleeding or ulceration up front, in anticipation of these potential complications, is worthwhile.

Management of Ulceration

Ulceration is the most frequent complication of infantile hemangiomas. Management should be directed at healing the ulceration, preventing infection and reducing pain. A recent review of 60 infants with ulcerations found that multiple modalities were often used concurrently, and that no single therapy proved most effective[52]. The authors advocated an approach that focused on four major areas: local wound care, treatment of infection, specific therapies (e.g. pulsed dye laser, corticosteroids) and pain management. Superficial ulcerations can frequently be managed with local wound care. Saline or Burow's solution compresses may be used to gently debride thick crusts, and topical antibiotics such as mupirocin and bacitracin ointments are applied, followed by application of occlusive dressings.

In open trials, some investigators have found metronidazole gel to be useful for ulcers in intertriginous and moist areas such as the perineum. Although the safety of metronidazole gel has not been established in young children, systemic metronidazole has been used safely to treat parasitic infections in this age group. Kim et al.[52] calculated that it would require relatively large amounts of topical gel to reach systemic levels of the drug or toxicity from its propylene glycol vehicle; nonetheless, they recommended limited application of small amounts of metronidazole gel when it is used in this setting. Oral antibiotics are often prescribed to treat ulcerated hemangiomas for presumed infection. Antibiotics that cover staphylococci and streptococci, such as first-generation cephalosporins, are commonly employed (see Ch. 127). A bacterial culture should be obtained from the wound. Occlusive dressings such as Duoderm®, Duoderm Extra Thin®, Vigilon® or Omniderm® can be applied after application of the topical antibiotic at sites that are amenable (see Ch. 145). Thin hydrocolloid dressings are often favored because of the ease of application and the ability to leave them in place for a few days. Petrolatum-impregnated gauze may also be used for perineal ulcers but needs to be changed frequently. Compression dressings such as Coban® elastic bandage are useful for extremity hemangiomas, but parents should be instructed in the proper application of these dressings.

A variety of modalities that are used to treat hemangiomas for other indications may be useful for treating ulcerations. These include systemic or intralesional corticosteroids and interferon (discussed below). Laser therapy may also be useful for ulcerated hemangiomas. Argon and Nd:YAG lasers were used in earlier series, but more recently the flashlamp-pumped pulsed-dye laser has been the one most widely used for the treatment of ulcerated and non-ulcerated hemangiomas. Some uncontrolled studies demonstrated healing of ulcerations and resolution of pain after two to three treatments with the pulsed-dye laser performed at 2-week intervals[93-96]. However, others observed mixed results, with 50% showing improvement and 5% experiencing worsening of the ulceration[52]. Excisional surgery may be considered as a means to manage small or pedunculated ulcerated lesions.

Improvement of chronically ulcerated, treatment-resistant facial and genital hemangiomas was observed after application of 0.01% becaplermin (recombinant platelet-derived growth factor) gel[97,98]. This preparation is approved for the treatment of diabetic ulcers in adults and is not approved for use in children. Its mechanism of action includes promotion of angiogenesis, which raises questions regarding the potential for stimulation of growth and worsening of hemangiomas. Further studies are indicated to determine the effectiveness and safety of this modality.

An important consideration in the treatment of the child with an ulcerated hemangioma is pain, which is a commonly associated symptom. Local wound care, and especially occlusive dressings, can provide some pain relief. Oral acetaminophen and topical lidocaine ointment may also help to alleviate the discomfort, although the latter must be used sparingly to prevent systemic lidocaine toxicity. In some patients, narcotic analgesics (e.g. acetaminophen with codeine) may be necessary for short periods of time. Eutectic mixture of local anesthetics is not recommended for the treatment of ulcerated hemangiomas because it should not be applied to eroded or ulcerated skin[52].

Corticosteroid Therapy

Systemic corticosteroids, usually prednisolone or prednisone, are the mainstay of treatment for life- or function-threatening hemangiomas. They are also used to treat hemangiomas that are highly likely to cause disfigurement and for those that are persistently ulcerated. The mechanism of action of corticosteroids is this setting is not entirely clear, although they are believed to alter cellular function by regulating cytokine expression[99]. A recent review of the literature found systemic corticosteroids to be effective in 84% of patients with infantile hemangiomas[100].

Dosage recommendations, duration of therapy, tapering schedules and monitoring guidelines vary widely and no single standard exists. Initial dosages of prednisone (or its equivalent) of 2–3 mg/kg/day are most commonly used[53]. However, some authors have advocated higher dose regimens of 3–5 mg/kg/day[101] because it is speculated that larger doses result in higher response rates. Treatment is usually maintained at these doses until cessation of growth or shrinkage occurs, and is followed by a gradual taper. The taper schedule is determined by a variety of factors, including the age of the patient, hemangioma growth rate, reason for treatment, presence of adverse effects and rebound growth. The latter may occur if steroids are discontinued while the hemangioma is still in its proliferating phase, and should not be interpreted as a treatment failure but, rather, underscores the importance of recognizing the growth pattern of the hemangioma when making therapeutic decisions.

A recent literature review used strict inclusion and exclusion criteria to assess the effectiveness of systemic corticosteroids in lesions that were felt to be true proliferating infantile hemangiomas[100]. A mean dose of 2.9 mg/kg/day was used over a mean period of 1.8 months before tapering, with a response rate of 84%. Doses exceeding 3 mg/kg/day resulted in a response rate of 94% but with a greater incidence of adverse effects. Overall, few major adverse effects were reported in the clinical series included in this review. An earlier review of 62 children who received prednisone or prednisolone at an initial dosage of 2–3 mg/kg/day tapered over a mean period of 7.9 months demonstrated a low incidence of serious side effects[102]. Several adverse reactions can occur in children receiving corticosteroids, including cushingoid facies, personality changes (irritability and disruption of sleep patterns), gastrointestinal symptoms, and decreased growth rate (height and weight); however, the majority of children experience catch-up growth after cessation of therapy. In a series of 22 children with hemangiomas who were treated with systemic corticosteroids, hypertension and hypothalamic–pituitary–adrenal (HPA) axis suppression were frequently observed[103]. Immunosuppression and serious life-threatening infections are other potential side effects, but they are rarely reported. Recently, *Pneumocystis jiroveci* (*carinii*) pneumonia was reported in a 3-month-old child receiving systemic corticosteroids for an airway hemangioma[104].

Another concern in children treated with systemic corticosteroids is the administration of live-virus vaccines. A dose of ≥2 mg/kg/day of prednisone or ≥20 mg/day in children weighing more than 10 kg, particularly if given for more than 2 weeks, is considered by many to be sufficient to raise safety concerns about such vaccine administration. The American Academy of Pediatrics' Committee on Infectious Disease has published specific guidelines regarding their administration, and recommends that the administration of live-virus vaccines be avoided while an infant is receiving corticosteroids at these doses and until they have been discontinued for at least 1 month[105].

Recently, concerns have been raised about neurotoxicity in very premature infants treated with corticosteroids for other indications[106]. There is currently no evidence of similar effects in term infants, but this finding raises questions about long-term side effects. Randomized controlled studies are needed to determine the optimal dosage regimen of corticosteroids needed to achieve response with the lowest incidence of adverse effects.

Intralesional corticosteroids

Intralesional corticosteroids are usually used to treat well-localized lesions, such as small lip hemangiomas. Systemic absorption likely occurs, but is believed to be less than with oral corticosteroids when small lesions are treated. As with oral corticosteroids, there is no well-established dosage regimen. Concentrations of triamcinolone acetonide between 5 and 40 mg/ml have been reported in the literature[52,107,108]. Shorter-acting corticosteroid preparations, such as dexamethasone or betamethasone acetate, are sometimes administered in combination with triamcinolone. It is recommended that the total maximum dose of triamcinolone not exceed 3–5 mg/kg per treatment session[53]. The interval between treatment sessions is also not well established. Some patients require repeat treatments at approximately monthly intervals, while others respond after a single treatment. The need for repeat therapy will depend upon the stage of proliferation of the hemangioma.

The use of intralesional corticosteroids to treat periorbital hemangiomas is controversial[109]. Reports of serious complications, including retinal and ophthalmic artery occlusion leading to permanent vision loss, as well as local atrophy and necrosis, have limited the use of this modality at this anatomic site[108,110,111]. A recent study found that injection pressures during administration of corticosteroids into periorbital hemangiomas routinely exceeded systemic arterial pressures, and this could lead to embolization of corticosteroid particles into the ocular circulation from retrograde arterial flow. The authors recommended limiting the volume of corticosteroid administered and performing indirect ophthalmoscopy on all patients receiving injections of corticosteroids in the orbital or periorbital area[112]. Intralesional corticosteroid injections into hemangiomas may also result in HPA axis suppression, although the overall incidence is unknown. Since this complication is probably related to the dosage (and concentration) of corticosteroid administered, it is of particular concern in those children receiving higher doses[113]. Concerns have also been raised regarding the potential for neurotoxicity in neonates who experience excessive exposure to benzyl alcohol, the preservative commonly found in corticosteroid preparations used for injection.

Topical corticosteroids

A few case reports and one larger case series of 34 patients utilized an ultrapotent class I topical corticosteroid to treat periocular hemangiomas. A decrease in the size of the hemangioma was observed, and there was an absence of significant side effects. The efficacy of topical corticosteroids in reducing refractive error is unclear. Further studies are needed to assess the effectiveness of this modality and to identify the subset of hemangiomas that would be most amenable to such treatment[114–117].

Other Topical Therapies

There are a few reports in which 5% imiquimod cream was used to treat proliferating hemangiomas. This compound, used primarily for the treatment of genital warts and cutaneous neoplasia, has immune-modifying and antiangiogenic activity[118,119]. Erosion of the hemangioma surface may be a complication of this particular therapy[17]. Further studies are needed to assess the effectiveness of this modality and to identify the subset of hemangiomas that would be most amenable to such treatment.

Other Systemic Medications

Recombinant interferon-α (2a and 2b) has been used to treat infantile hemangiomas (Fig. 103.21). It appears to inhibit angiogenesis and has been reported to successfully treat life- and function-threatening

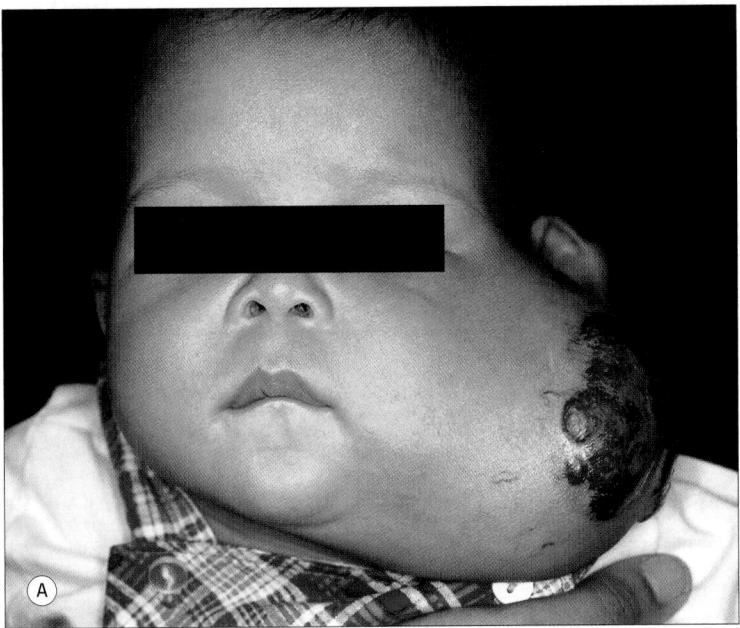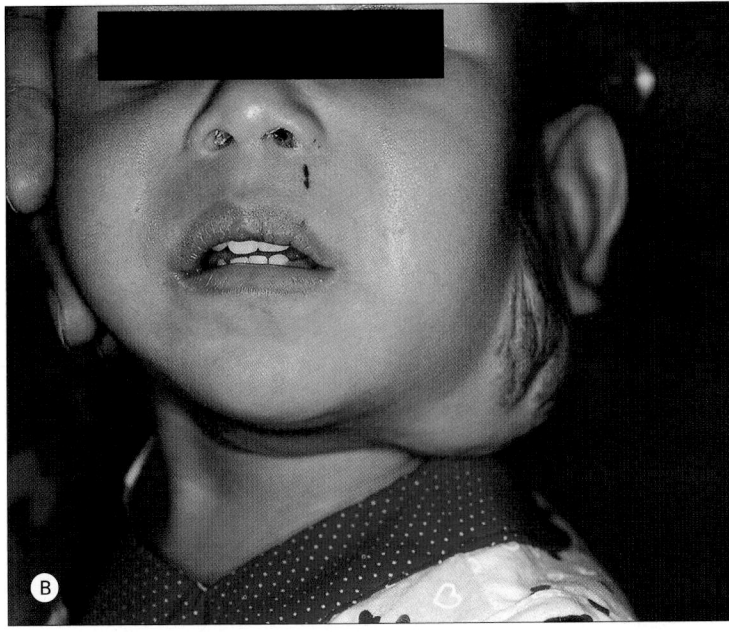

Fig. 103.21 Infantile hemangioma. A An enormous infantile hemangioma of the left cheek, ear and neck despite systemic corticosteroids (2.5 mg/kg/day for 2–3 months) and complicated by high-output congestive heart failure. **B** Eleven months after institution of interferon-α (3 million U/m²/day SC) for 8 months. Courtesy of Richard Antaya MD.

hemangiomas that have been resistant to corticosteroid therapy[120–122]. Interferon-α is typically administered as a daily subcutaneous injection, and dosages between 1 million and 3 million U/m²/day are most commonly employed. Unlike corticosteroids, where a response to treatment may be evident within several days of beginning therapy, it may take weeks to appreciate an improvement with interferon. Adverse effects include fever, irritability, diarrhea, neutropenia, elevated transaminases and skin necrosis[121–123].

The most worrisome side effect of interferon-α in infants is spastic diplegia, which was reported in 5 of 26 patients treated with interferon-α-2a in one series[124]. Three patients in this series had persistent neurologic impairment following discontinuation of therapy and two improved; neurotoxicity did not appear to be dose-related. In another series of infants treated with interferon-α-2b, 10 of 43 patients had abnormal neurologic examinations, one of whom had spastic diplegia[123]. Owing to this worrisome adverse effect, interferon should be reserved for life-threatening infantile hemangiomas that have been resistant to corticosteroids, and baseline neurologic assessment and serial examinations are essential.

Vincristine is a chemotherapeutic agent that has been used widely for the treatment of childhood neoplasms. It is a vinca alkaloid that interferes with microtubule formation during mitosis by inhibiting tubulin. *In vitro*, it induces apoptosis of tumor and endothelial cells[125]. There are reports in the literature of its use to treat hemangiomas and vascular tumors that are unresponsive to corticosteroids, as well as the Kasabach–Merritt syndrome. Toxicities include peripheral neuropathy, constipation, jaw pain, and, rarely, anemia and leukopenia. Placement of a central venous catheter is favored to administer the medication, and participation of a pediatric oncologist/hematologist is advisable. Further studies are needed to determine its effectiveness, incidence of adverse reactions, and optimal dosage regimens for the treatment of infantile hemangiomas[125–129].

Surgery

Flashlamp-pumped pulsed-dye laser (PDL) is effective for the treatment of capillary malformations. PDL with wavelengths of 585 and 595 nm and pulse durations of 450 microseconds or 1.5 milliseconds are the systems most commonly used for this treatment. In the case of hemangiomas, laser therapy appears to be most effective for superficial lesions[130–132]. Hemangiomas with deep dermal or subcutaneous involvement may show lightening of the superficial portion, but treatment does not appear to alter the growth pattern of the deeper component[133]. Multiple treatment sessions, usually every few weeks, are required during the proliferating phase to improve the lesion and prevent rebound growth. Treatments are generally well tolerated and adverse reactions are usually minor, including pigmentary alteration, atrophic scarring and ulceration.

However, a randomized controlled study of early PDL treatment of uncomplicated infantile hemangiomas found no significant difference in the number of children with complete clearance of their hemangiomas at 1 year of age compared to the untreated control group. In the PDL-treated infants, redness was improved, but they were more likely to develop cutaneous atrophy and hypopigmentation than were the untreated cohort[134]. In addition, severe ulceration and scarring have been reported in young infants with large superficial hemangiomas following early laser treatment[135].

The PDL is effective for the treatment of telangiectasias that may be present on the surface of involuting and involuted hemangiomas. Other laser sources that have been used to treat infantile hemangiomas include the argon and Nd:YAG lasers. These lasers appear to carry a higher risk of scarring but may be more effective for deeper lesions. Percutaneous treatment utilizing bare fiber Nd:YAG has been reported for deep hemangiomas.

Surgical excision is usually employed to treat involuted or partially involuted lesions in order to remove fibrofatty tissue and redundant skin. The optimal timing for surgery is controversial and dependent upon many factors, including the location and size of the lesion. Surgical excision during the active proliferating phase is controversial and reserved for specific situations, such as a function-threatening periorbital hemangioma that has failed to respond to pharmacologic therapy or in which pharmacologic therapy is believed to pose a greater risk to the patient than surgical excision. Other situations where surgery may be appropriately considered include pedunculated lesions for which resection will be inevitable and small, persistently ulcerated lesions that have failed more conservative therapy. Excision is considered in preschool children for involuting lesions when they are located in a cosmetically sensitive area (e.g. nasal tip, lip). The ultimate management goal is to achieve as normal an appearance as possible without significant scarring. Therefore, just as with other treatment modalities, the surgical management of infantile hemangiomas needs to be individualized.

Arterial embolization has been used to treat life-threatening hemangiomas that are causing high-output congestive heart failure. It may be used concurrently with other modalities and prior to surgical resection in some cases[136].

Cryosurgery has also been used to treat infantile hemangiomas[137–138]. Contact cryosurgery is the method most commonly employed, and it is used mostly in Europe and Latin America. The majority of case reports demonstrate complete or partial regression of the superficial component of the hemangioma. Adverse effects include scar formation, pigment alteration and infection.

Management of Kasabach–Merritt Syndrome

Kasabach–Merritt syndrome (KMS) is a life-threatening disorder and a medical emergency. The associated vascular tumors respond less consistently to treatment than do infantile hemangiomas. Systemic corticosteroids, interferon-α, chemotherapeutic agents including vincristine and cyclophosphamide, ticlopidine and aspirin have been used alone and in combination with a variable response rate[85]. A recent retrospective case series suggested that some patients may be successfully managed with vincristine[139]. Surgical excision, embolization and radiation have also been used to treat some patients[125,140], and supportive care is mandatory. Platelet transfusions may lead to enlargement of the tumor and worsening of the coagulopathy, owing possibly to angiogenic growth factors present in these blood products[141].

REFERENCES

1. Mulliken, JB. Classification of vascular birthmarks. In: Mulliken JB, Young AE (eds). Vascular Birthmarks: Hemangiomas and Malformations. Philadelphia: WB Saunders, 1988:24–37.
2. Mulliken JB, Glowacki J. Hemangiomas and vascular malformations in infants and children: a classification based on endothelial characteristics. Plast Reconstr Surg. 1982;69:412–20.
3. Enjolras O, Mulliken J. Vascular tumors and vascular malformations, new issues. Adv Dermatol. 1998;13:375–423.
4. Hand JL, Frieden IJ. Vascular birthmarks of infancy; resolving nosologic confusion. Am J Med Genet. 2002;108:257–64.
5. Mulliken JB. Diagnosis and natural history of hemangiomas. In: Mulliken JB, Young AE (eds). Vascular

Birthmarks: Hemangiomas and Malformations. Philadelphia: WB Saunders, 1988:41–62.
6. Esterly NB. Cutaneous hemangiomas, vascular stains and malformations, and associated syndromes. Curr Probl Dermatol. 1995;7:69–107.
7. Finn MC, Glowacki J, Mulliken JB. Congenital vascular lesions: clinical application of a new classification. J Pediatr Surg. 1983;18:894–900.
8. Moroz B. Long-term follow-up of hemangiomas in children. In: Williams HB (ed.). Symposium on Vascular Malformations and Melanotic Lesions. St. Louis: CV Mosby, 1983:162–71.
9. Enjolras O, Gelbert F. Superficial hemangiomas: associations and management. Pediatr Dermatol. 1997;14:173–9.
10. Amir J, Metzker A, Krikler R, Reisner SH. Strawberry

hemangioma in preterm infants. Pediatr Dermatol. 1986;3:331–2.
11. Burton BK, Schulz CJ, Angle B, Burd LI. An increased incidence of hemangiomas in infants born following chronic villus sampling (CVS). Prenat Diagn. 1995;15:209–14.
12. Hemangioma Investigator Group: Haggstrom AN, Drolet BA, Baselga E, et al. Prospective study of infantile hemangiomas: Demographic, prenatal and perinatal characteristics. J Pediatr. 2007; 150:291–4.
13. Margileth AM, Museles M. Cutaneous hemangiomas in children: diagnosis and conservative management. J Am Med Assoc. 1965;194:523–6.
14. Blei F, Walter J, Orlow SJ, Marchuk DA. Familial segregation of hemangiomas and vascular

malformations as an autosomal dominant trait. Arch Dermatol. 1998;134:718–22.
15. Walter, JW, Blei F, Anderson JL, et al. Genetic mapping of a novel familial form of infantile hemangioma. Am J Med Genet. 1999;82:77–83.
16. Yu Y, Flint AF, Mulliken JB, Wu JK, Bischoff J. Endothelial progenitor cells in infantile hemangioma. Blood. 2004;103:1373–5.
17. Frieden IJ, Haggstrom AN, Drolet BA, et al. Infantile hemangiomas: current knowledge, future directions. Proceedings of a research workshop on infantile hemangiomas, April 7-9, 2005, Bethesda, Maryland, USA. Pediatr Dermatol. 2005;22:383–406.
18. Boye E, Ying Y, Paranya G, et al. Clonality and altered behavior of endothelial cells from hemangioams. J Clin Invest. 2001;107:745–52.
19. Walter JW, North PE, Waner M, et al. Somatic mutation of vascular endothelial growth factor receptors in juvenile hemangioma. Genes Chromosomes Cancer. 2002:33:295–303.
20. Yu Y, Brown LF, Mulliken JB, Bischoff J. Increased Tie2 expression, enhanced response to angiopoietin-1, and dysregulated angiopoietin-2 expression in hemangioma-derived endothelial cells. Am J Pathol. 2001;159:2271–80.
21. Berg JN, Walter JW, Thisanagayam U, et al. Evidence for loss of heterozygosity of 5q in sporadic hemangiomas: are somatic mutations involved in hemangioma formation? J Clin Pathol. 2001;54:249–52.
22. Bischoff J, Mulliken JB. Discussion of Hasan Q, Tan ST. Altered mitochondrial cytochrome *b* gene expression during the regression of hemangioma. Plast Recontr Surg. 2001;108:1477–8.
23. North PE, Waner M, Mizeracki A, Mihm MC. GLUT1: a newly discovered immunohistochemical marker for juvenile hemangiomas. Hum Pathol. 2000;31:11–22.
24. North PE, Waner M, Mizeracki A, et al. A unique microvascular phenotype shared by juvenile hemangiomas and human placenta. Arch Dermatol. 2001;137:559–70.
25. Bree AF, Siegfried E, Sotelo-Avila C, Nahass G. Infantile hemangiomas: speculation on placental trophoblastic origin. Arch Dermatol. 2001;137:573–7.
26. Takahashi K, Mulliken JB, Kozakewich HPW, et al. Cellular markers that distinguish the phases of hemangiomas during infancy and childhood. J Clin Invest. 1994;93:2357–64.
27. Chang J, Most D, Bresnick S, et al. Proliferative hemangiomas: analysis of cytokine gene expression and angiogenesis. Plast Reconstr Surg. 1999;103:1–9.
28. Zhang L, Lin X, Wang W, et al. Circulating level of vascular endothelial growth factor in differentiating hemangioma from vascular malformation patients. Plast Reconstr Surg. 2005;116:200–4.
29. Isik FF, Rand RP, Gruss JS, et al. Monocyte chemoattractant protein-1 mRNA expression in hemangiomas and vascular malformations. J Surg Res. 1996;61:71–6.
30. Salcedo R, Ponce ML, Young HA, et al. Human endothelial cells express CCR2 and respond to MCP-1: direct role of MCP-1 in angiogenesis and tumor progression. Blood. 2000;96:34–40.
31. Kraling BM, Razon MJ, Boon LM, et al. E-selectin is present in proliferating endothelial cells in human hemangiomas. Am J Pathol. 1996;148:1181–91.
32. Verkarre V, Patey-Mariaud de Serre N, Vazeux R, et al. ICAM-3 and E-selectin endothelial cell expression differentiate two phases of angiogenesis in infantile hemangiomas. J Cutan Pathol. 1999;26:17–24.
33. Jang YC, Arumugam S, Ferguson M, et al. Changes in matrix composition during the growth and regression of human hemangiomas. J Surg Res. 1998;80:9–15.
34. Tan ST, Velickovic M, Ruger BM, Davis BF. Cellular and extracellular markers of hemangioma. Plast Reconstr Surg. 2000;106:529–38.
35. Marler JJ, Fishman SJ, Kilroy SM, et al. Increased levels of urinary matrix metalloproteinases parallels the extent and activity of vascular anomalies. Pediatrics. 2005;116:38–45.
36. Dadras SS, North PE, Bertoncini J, et al. Infantile hemangiomas are arrested in an early developmental vascular differentiation state. Mod Pathol. 2004;17:1068–79.
37. Sato TN, Tozawa Y, Deutsch U, et al. Distinct roles of the receptor tyrosine kinases Tie-1 and Tie-2 in blood vessel formation. Nature. 1995;376:70–4.
38. Vikkula M, Boon LM, Carraway KL, et al. Vascular dysmorphogenesis caused by an activating mutation in the receptor tyrosine kinase TIE2. Cell. 1996;87:1181–90.
39. Bielenberg DR, Bucana CD, Sanchez R, et al. Progressive growth of infantile cutaneous hemangiomas is directly correlated with hyperplasia and angiogenesis of adjacent epidermis and inversely correlated with expression of the endogenous angiogenesis inhibitor, IFN-beta. Int J Oncol. 1999;14:401–8.
40. Ritter MR, Moreno SK, Dorrell MI, et al. Identifying potential regulators of infantile hemangioma progression through large-scale expression analysis: a possible role of the immune system and indoleamine 2,3 dioxygenase (IDO) during involution. Lymphat Res Biol. 2003:1:291–9.
41. Ritter MR, Dorrell MI, Edmonds J, et al. Insulin-like growth factor 2 and potential regulators of hemangioma growth and involution identified by large-scale expression analysis. Proc Natl Acad Sci USA. 2002;99:7455–60.
42. Mancini AJ, Smoller BR. Proliferation and apoptosis within juvenile capillary hemangiomas. Am J Dermatopathol. 1996;18:505–14.
43. Razon MJ, Kraling BM, Mulliken JB, Bischoff J. Increased apoptosis coincides with onset of involution in infantile hemangiomas. Microcirculation. 1998;5:189–95.
44. Hasan Q, Ruger BM, Tan ST, et al. Clusterin/apoJ expression during the development of hemangiomas. Hum Pathol. 2000;31:691–7.
45. North PE, Waner M, James CA, et al. Congenital nonprogressive hemangiomas: a distinct clinicopathologic entity unlike infantile hemangioma. Arch Dermatol. 2002;137:1607–20.
46. Liang MG, Frieden IJ. Perineal and lip ulcerations as the presenting manifestation of hemangioma of infancy. Pediatrics. 1997;99:256–9.
47. Martinez-Perez D, Fein, N, Boon L, Mulliken JB. Not all hemangiomas look like strawberries: uncommon presentations of the most common tumor of infancy. Pediatr Dermatol. 1995;12:1–6.
48. Waner M, North PE, Scherer KA, et al. The nonrandom distribution of facial hemangiomas. Arch Dermatol. 2003;139:869–75.
49. Chiller KG, Passaro D, Frieden IJ. Hemangiomas of infancy: clinical characteristics, morphologic subtypes and their relationship to race, ethnicity and sex. Arch Dermatol. 2002;138:1567–76.
50. Haggstrom AN, Lammer EJ, Schneider RA, et al. Patterns of infantile hemangiomas: new clues to hemangioma pathogenesis and embryonic facial development. Pediatrics. 2006;117:698–703.
51. Bowers RE, Graham EA, Tomlinson KM. The natural history of the strawberry nevus. Arch Dermatol. 1960;82:667–80.
51a. Hemangioma Investigator Group: Chamlin SL, Haggstrom AN, Drolet BA, et al. Multicenter prospective study of ulcerated hemangiomas. J Pediatr. 2007; in press. 2007.
52. Kim HJ, Colombo M, Frieden IJ. Ulcerated hemangiomas: clinical characteristics and response to therapy. J Am Acad Dermatol. 2001;44:962–72.
53. Drolet BA, Esterly NB, Frieden IJ. Hemangiomas in children. N Engl J Med. 1999;341:173–81.
54. Haik BG, Jakobiec F, Ellsworth RM, et al. Capillary hemangiomas of the lid and orbit: an analysis of the clinical features and therapeutic results in 101 cases. Ophthamology. 1979;86:760–89.
55. Robb R. Refractive errors associated with hemangiomas of the eyelids and orbit in infancy. Am J Ophthamol. 1977;83:52–8.
56. Ceisler EJ, Santos L, Blei F. Periocular hemangiomas: what every physician should know. Pediatr Dermatol. 2004;21:1–9.
57. Pascual-Castroviejo I. Vascular and nonvascular intracranial malformations associated with external capillary hemangiomas. Neuroradiology. 1978;16:82–4.
58. Frieden IJ, Reese V, Cohen D. PHACE syndrome: the association of posterior fossa brain malformations, hemangiomas, arterial anomalies, coarctation of the aorta and cardiac defects, and eye abnormalities. Arch Dermatol. 1996;132:307–11.
59. Metry DW, Dowd CF, Barkovich AJ, Frieden IJ. The many faces of PHACE syndrome. J Pediatr. 2001; 139:470.
60. Burrows PE, Robertson RL, Mulliken JB, et al. Cerebral vasculopathy and neurologic sequelae in infants with cervicofacial hemangioma: report of eight patients. Radiology. 1998;207:601–7.
61. Orlow SJ, Isakoff MS, Blei F. Increased risk of symptomatic hemangiomas of the airway in association with cutaneous hemangiomas in a 'beard' distribution. J Pediatr. 1997;131:643–6.
62. Albright AL, Gartner C, Wiener ES. Lumbar cutaneous hemangiomas as indicators of tethered spinal cords. Pediatrics. 1989;83:977–80.
63. Goldberg NS, Herbert AA, Esterly NB. Sacral hemangiomas and multiple congenital abnormalities. Arch Dermatol. 1986;122:684–7.
64. Achauer BM, Chang C, Vander Kam VM. Management of hemangiomas of infancy: review of 245 patients. Plast Reconstr Surg. 1997;99:1301–8.
65. Holden KR, Alexander F. Diffuse neonatal hemangiomatosis. Pediatrics. 1970;46:411–21.
66. Stern JK, Wolf JE, Jarratt M. Benign neonatal hemangiomatosis. J Am Acad Dermatol. 1981;4:442–5.
67. Golitz LE, Rudikoff J, O'Meara OP. Diffuse neonatal hemangiomatosis. Pediatr Dermatol. 1986;3:145–52.
68. Sheu B, Shyu M, Ling Y, et al. Prenatal diagnosis and corticosteroid treatment of diffuse neonatal hemangiomatosis. J Ultrasound Med. 1994;13:495–9.
69. Boon LM, Burrows PE, Paltiel HJ, et al. Hepatic vascular anomalies in infancy: a twenty-seven year experience. J Pediatr. 1996;129:346–54.
70. Kassarjian A, Zurakowski D, Dubois J, et al. Infantile hepatic hemangiomas: clinical and imaging findings and their correlation with therapy. AJR Am J Roentgenol. 2004;182:785–95.
71. Fishman SJ, Burrows PE, Mulliken JB. Gastrointestinal manifestations of vascular anomalies in childhood: varied etiologies require multiple therapeutic modalities. J Pediatr Surg. 1998;33:1163–7.
72. Geller JD, Topper SF, Hashimoto K. Diffuse neonatal hemangiomatosis: a new constellation of findings. J Am Acad Dermatol. 1991;24:816–18.
73. Wong CH, Wright JG, Silove ED, et al. A new syndrome of multiple hemangiomas, right dominant double aortic arch, and coarctation. J Thorac Cardiovasc Surg. 2001;121:1207–9.
74. Hughes JA, Hill V, Patel K, et al. Cutaneous hemangioma: prevalence and sonographic characteristics of associated hepatic hemangioma. Clin Radiol. 2004;59:273–80.
75. Metry DW, Hawrot A, Altman C, et al. Association of solitary, segmental hemangiomas of the skin with visceral hemangiomatosis. Arch Dermatol. 2004;140:591–6.
76. Huang SA, Tu HM, Harney JW, et al. Severe hypothyroidism caused by type 3 iodothyronine deiodinase in infantile hemangiomas. N Engl J Med. 2000;343:185–9.
77. Konrad D, Ellis G, Perlman K. Spontaneous regression of severe acquired hypothyroidism associated with multiple liver hemangiomas. Pediatrics. 2003;112:1424–6.
78. Boon, LM, Enjolras O, Mulliken JB. Congenital hemangioma: evidence of accelerated involution. J Pediatr. 1996;128:329–35.
79. Berenguer B, Mulliken JB, Enjolras O, et al. Rapidly involuting congenital hemangioma: clinical and histopathologic features. Pediatr Dev Pathol. 2003;6:495–510.
80. Enjolras O, Mulliken JB, Boon LM, et al. Noninvoluting congenital hemangioma: a rare cutaneous vascular anomaly. Plast Reconstr Surg. 2001;107:1647–54.
81. Mulliken JB, Enjolras O. Congenital hemangiomas and infantile hemangioma: missing links. J Am Acad Dermatol. 2004;50:875–82.
82. Kasabach HH, Merritt KK. Capillary hemangioma with extensive purpura, report of a case. Am J Dis Child. 1940;59:1063–70.
83. Enjolras O, Wassef M, Mazoyer E, et al. Infants with Kasabach-Merritt syndrome do not have 'true' hemangiomas. J Pediatr. 1997;130:631–40.
84. Sarkar M, Mulliken JB, Kozakewich HPW, et al. Thrombocytopenic coagulopathy (Kasabach-Merritt phenomenon) is associated with kaposiform hemangioendothelioma and not with common infantile hemangioma. Plast Reconstr Surg. 1997;100:1377–86.
85. Enjolras O, Mulliken JB, Wassef M, et al. Residual lesions after Kasabach-Merritt phenomenon in 41 patients. J Am Acad Dermatol. 2000;42:225–35.
86. Burrows PE, Laor T, Paltiel H, et al. Diagnostic imaging in the evaluation of vascular birthmarks. Dermatol Clin. 1998;16:455–88.
87. Marler JJ, Fishman SJ, Upton J, et al. Prenatal diagnosis of vascular anomalies. J Pediatr Surg. 2002;37:318–26.
88. Rogers M, Lam A, Fischer G. Sonographic findings in a series of rapidly involuting congenital hemangiomas (RICH). Pediatr Dermatol. 2002;19:5–11.
89. Frieden IJ, Eichenfield LF, Esterly NB, Geronemus R, Mallory SB. Guidelines of care for hemangiomas of infancy. J Am Acad Dermatol. 1997;37:631–7.

90. Frieden IJ. Which hemangiomas to treat and how? Arch Dermatol. 1997;133:1593–5.

91. Mulliken JB. Treatment of hemangiomas. In Mulliken JB, Young AE (eds). Vascular Birthmarks: Hemangiomas and Malformations. Philadelphia: WB Saunders, 1988:77–103.

92. Tanner JL, Dechert MP, Freiden IJ. Growing up with a facial hemangioma: parent and child coping and adaptation. Pediatrics. 1998;101:446–51.

93. Achauer BM, Vander Kam VM. Ulcerated anogenital hemangioma of infancy. Plast Reconstr Surg. 1991;87:861–6.

94. Morelli JG, Tan OT, Weston WL. Treatment of ulcerated hemangiomas with the pulsed tunable dye laser. Am J Dis Child. 1991;145:1062–4.

95. Scheepers JH, Quaba AA. Does the pulsed tunable dye laser have a role in the management of infantile hemangiomas? Observations based on 3 years' experience. Plast Reconstr Surg. 1995;95:305–12.

96. David LR, Malek MM, Argenta LC. Efficacy of pulse dye laser therapy for the treatment of ulcerated hemangiomas: a review of 78 patients. Br J Plast Surg. 2003;56:317–27.

97. Sugarman JL, Mauro TM, Frieden IJ. Treatment of an ulcerated hemangioma with recombinant platelet-derived growth factor. Arch Dermatol. 2002; 138:314–16.

98. Metz BJ, Rubenstein MC, Levy ML, et al. Response of ulcerated perineal hemangiomas of infancy to becaplermin gel, a recombinant human platelet-derived growth factor. Arch Dermatol. 2004; 140:867–70.

99. Hasan Q, Tan ST, Gush J, et al. Steroid therapy of a proliferating hemangioma: histochemical and molecular changes. Pediatrics. 2000;105:117–20.

100. Bennett ML, Fleischer AB Jr, Chamlin SL, Frieden IJ. Oral corticosteroid use is effective for cutaneous hemangiomas: an evidence-based evaluation. Arch Dermatol. 2001;137:1208–13.

101. Sadan N, Wolach B. Treatment of hemangiomas of infants with high doses of prednisone. J Pediatr. 1996;128:141–6.

102. Boon LM, MacDonald DM, Mulliken JB. Complications of systemic corticosteroid therapy for problematic hemangioma. Plast Reconstr Surg. 1999;104:1616–23.

103. George ME, Sharma V, Jacobson J, et al. Adverse effects of systemic glucocorticosteroid therapy in infants with hemangiomas. Arch Dermatol. 2004;140:963–9.

104. Aviles R, Boyce TG, Thompson DM. Pneumocystis carinii pneumonia in a 3-month-old infant receiving high-dose corticosteroid therapy for airway hemangiomas. Mayo Clin Proc. 2004;79:243–5.

105. Pickering LK (ed). Red Book: Report of the Committee on Infectious Diseases, 26th edn. Elk Grove Village, IL: American Academy of Pediatrics, 2003:75.

106. Halliday HL. The effect of postnatal steroids on growth and development. J Perinat Med. 2001;29:281–5.

107. Chen MT, Yeong EK, Horng SY. Intralesional corticosteroid therapy in proliferating head and neck hemangiomas: a review of 155 cases. J Pediatr Surg. 2000;35:420–3.

108. Egbert JE, Schwartz GS, Walsh AW. Diagnosis and treatment of ophthalmic artery occlusion during an intralesional injection of corticosteroid into an eyelid capillary hemangioma. Am J Ophthamol. 1996;121:638–42.

109. Kushner BJ. Hemangiomas. Arch Ophthamol. 2000;118:835–6.

110. Schorr N, Seiff SR. Central retinal artery occlusion associated with periocular corticosteroid injection for juvenile hemangioma. Ophthamol Surg. 1986;17:229–31.

111. Sutula FC, Glover AT. Eyelid necrosis following intralesional corticosteroid injection for capillary hemangioma. Ophthamol Surg. 1987;18:103–5.

112. Egbert JE, Paul S, Engel WK, Summers CG. High injection pressure during intralesional injection of corticosteroids into capillary hemangiomas. Arch Ophthamol. 2001;119:677–83.

113. Goyal R, Watts P, Lane CM, et al. Adrenal suppression and failure to thrive after steroid injections for periocular hemangioma. Ophthalmology. 2004;111:389–95.

114. Elsas FJ, Lewis AR. Topical treatment of periocular capillary hemangioma. J Pediatr Opthalmol Strabismus. 1994;31:153–6.

115. Cruz OA, Zarnegar SR, Myers SE. Treatment of periocular capillary hemangioma with topical clobetasol propionate. Ophthalmology. 1995;102:2012–15.

116. Garzon MC, Lucky AW, Hawrot A, et al. Ultrapotent topical corticosteroid treatment of hemangiomas of infancy. J Am Acad Dermatol. 2005;52:281–6.

117. Ranchod TM, Frieden IJ, Fredrick DR. Corticosteroid treatment of periorbital haemangioma of infancy: a review of the evidence. Br J Ophthalmol. 2005; 89:1134–8.

118. Sidbury R, Neuschler N, Neuschler E, et al. Topically applied imiquimod inhibits vascular tumor growth in vivo. J Invest Dermatol. 2003;121:1205–9.

119. Hazen PG, Carney JF, Engstrom CW, et al. Proliferating hemangioma of infancy: successful treatment with topical 5% imiquimod cream. Pediatr Dermatol. 2005;22:254–6.

120. Ezekowitz R, Mulliken JB, Folkman J. Interferon alfa-2a treatment for life threatening hemangiomas of infancy. N Engl J Med. 1992;326:1456–63.

121. Chang E, Boyd A, Nelson CC, et al. Successful treatment of infantile hemangiomas with interferon - alfa-2b. J Pediatr Hematol Oncol. 1997;19:237–44.

122. Tamayo L, Ortiz D, Orozco-Covarrubias L, et al. Therapeutic efficacy of interferon alfa-2b in infants with life-threatening giant hemangiomas. Arch Dermatol. 1997;133:1567–71.

123. Hershon DJ, Carman L, Belanger S, et al. Toxicity profile of interferon alfa-2b in children: a prospective evaluation. J Pediatr. 1999;135:782–5.

124. Barlow C, Priebe C, Mulliken JB, et al. Spastic diplegia as a complication of interferon alfa-2a treatment of hemangiomas of infancy. J Pediatr. 1998;132:527–30.

125. Adams DM. The nonsurgical management of vascular lesions. Facial Plast Clin North Am. 2001;9:601–8.

126. Payarols P, Masferrer P, Bellvert G. Treatment of life-threatening hemangiomas with vincristine. N Engl J Med. 1995;333:69.

127. Hu B, Lachman R, Phillips J, et al. Kasabach-Merritt syndrome-associated kaposiform hemangioendothelioma successfully treated with cyclophosphamide, vincristine, and actinomycin D. J Pediatr Hematol Oncol. 1998;20:567–9.

128. Moore J, Lee M, Garzon M, et al. Effective therapy of a vascular tumor of infancy with vincristine. J Pediatr Surg. 2001;36:1273–6.

129. Fawcett SL, Grant I, Hall PN, et al. Vincristine as a treatment for a large haemangioma threatening vital functions. Br J Plast Surg. 2004;57:168–71

130. Ashinoff R, Geronemus RG. Capillary hemangiomas and treatment with flash lamp-pumped pulsed dye laser. Arch Dermatol. 1991;127:202–5.

131. Garden JM, Bakus AD, Paller AS. Treatment of cutaneous hemangiomas by the flashlamp-pumped pulsed dye laser: prospective analysis. J Pediatr. 1992;120:555–60.

132. Hohenleutner S, Badur-Ganter E, Landthaler M, Hohenleutner U. Long-term results in the treatment of childhood hemangioma with the flashlamp-pumped pulsed dye laser: an evaluation of 617 cases. Lasers Surg Med. 2001;28:273–7.

133. Ashinoff R, Geronemus RG. Failure of the flashlamp-pumped pulsed dye laser to prevent progression to deep hemangioma. Pediatr Dermatol. 1993;10:77–80.

134. Batta K, Goodyear HM, Moss C, Williams HC, Hiller L, Waters R. Randomised controlled study of early pulsed dye laser treatment of uncomplicated childhood haemangiomas: results of a 1-year analysis. Lancet. 2002;360:521–7.

135. Witman PM, Wagner AM, Scherer K, Waner M, Frieden IJ. Complications following pulsed dye laser treatment of superficial hemangiomas. Lasers Surg Med. 2006;38:116–23.

136. Burrows PE, Lasjaunias PL, Ter Brugge KG, Flodmark O. Urgent and emergent embolization of lesions of the head and neck in children: indications and results. Pediatrics. 1987;80;386–94.

137. Cremer H. Cryosurgery for hemangiomas. Pediatr Dermatol. 1998;15:173–9.

138. Reischle S, Schuller-Petrovic S. Treatment of capillary hemangiomas of early childhood with a method of cryosurgery. J Am Acad Dermatol. 2000;42:809–13.

139. Haisley-Royster C, Enjolras O, Frieden IJ, et al. Kasabach-Merritt phenomenon: a retrospective study of treatment with vincristine. J Pediatr Hematol Oncol. 2002;24:459–62. Erratum in: J Pediatr Hematol Oncol. 2002;24:794.

140. Drolet BA, Scott LA, Esterly NB, Gosain AK. Early surgical intervention in a patient with Kasabach-Merritt phenomenon. J Pediatr. 2001;138:756–8.

141. Phillips WG, Marsden JR. Kasabach-Merritt syndrome exacerbated by platelet transfusion. J R Soc Med. 1993;86:231–2.

Vascular Malformations

104

Odile Enjolras

Synonyms: ■ Mature angiomas; angiodysplasias; vascular birthmarks ■ Capillary malformation (CM): port-wine stain, nevus flammeus, telangiectasia ■ Venous malformation (VM): cavernous angioma, cavernous hemangioma, phlebectasia ■ Lymphatic malformation (LM): lymphangioma, lymphangioma circumscriptum, lymphangioma simplex, cystic hygroma, cavernous lymphangioma ■ Arteriovenous malformation (AVM): cirsoid aneurysm, cirsoid hemangioma

Key features

- Although both types were once called 'angiomas', vascular malformations clearly differ from vascular tumors seen in infants and children
- In slow-flow malformations, capillaries, veins or lymphatic channels are anomalous and malformed; the majority are either present at birth or become evident within a few months or years
- In fast-flow malformations, there is arteriovenous shunting; they tend to become evident later in life, sometimes in adulthood
- All vascular malformations are lifelong and may worsen, creating cosmetic consequences and functional impairment
- The most endangering group is arteriovenous malformations

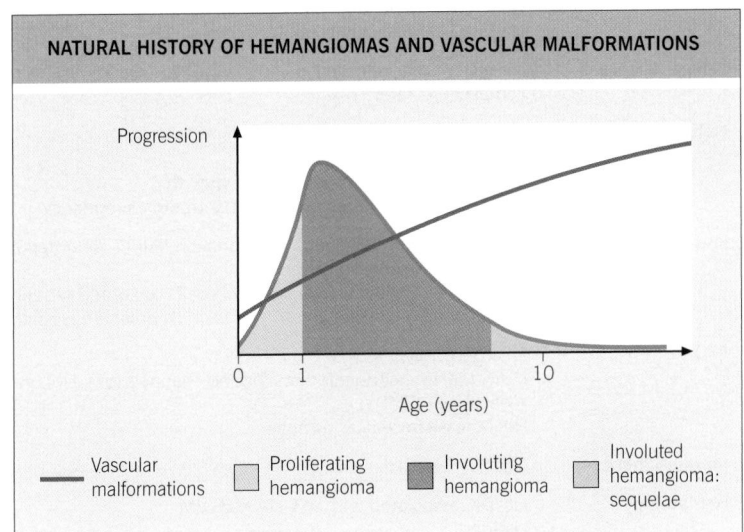

NATURAL HISTORY OF HEMANGIOMAS AND VASCULAR MALFORMATIONS

Fig. 104.1 Natural history of hemangiomas and vascular malformations.

INTRODUCTION

According to the classification system adopted by the International Society for the Study of Vascular Anomalies (ISSVA), there are two types of vascular anomalies: vascular tumors (the most common one is the infantile hemangioma) and vascular malformations[1,2] (Table 104.1). Vascular malformations are localized defects of vascular morphogenesis, likely caused by dysfunction in pathways regulating embryogenesis and vasculogenesis. It is not clear whether true angiogenesis occurs in some of these lesions, explaining their propensity to worsen, thicken, and even expand. Vascular malformations have a quiescent endothelium, and they do not exhibit the markers of proliferation seen in hemangiomas of infancy during their proliferating phase[3,4] (Fig. 104.1). Therefore, because vascular malformations are not truly proliferating lesions, with cellular hyperplasia, the suffix 'oma' (meaning 'tumor') has been deemed inaccurate[3,4] (thus, the terms 'angioma', 'lymphangioma' and 'hemangioma' are no longer used to describe vascular malformations).

Vascular malformations are subcategorized depending on the predominant anomalous channels and flow characteristics: slow-flow or fast-flow. A slow-flow vascular malformation may be:

- capillary (CM), i.e. port-wine stain
- venous (VM): a misnomer for this entity is 'cavernous hemangioma', a term also used to describe deep infantile hemangiomas
- lymphatic (LM): this category includes microcystic lesions (lymphangioma circumscriptum), or those with macrocystic channels (cystic hygroma).

A fast-flow vascular malformation combines arterial anomalies and arteriovenous shunting creating the nidus of an arteriovenous malformation (AVM).

Some patients have complex-combined vascular malformations, anatomically delineated as capillary-venous malformation (CVM), capillary-lymphatic malformation (CLM), capillary-lymphatic-venous malformation (CLVM), lymphatic-venous malformation (LVM), capillary-arteriovenous malformation (C-AVM) and lymphatic-arteriovenous malformation (L-AVM), depending on the association. A few lesions provide evidence for overlap (e.g. both spindle cell hemangio-mas and VM in patients with Maffucci syndrome, pyogenic granulomas superimposed on CM or AVM) or coexistence of vascular tumors and vascular malformations (e.g. association of hemangiomas and VM, LM, or CM).

Vascular malformations occur in any body part and any organ system. They are easily identified in skin and mucous membranes. Some are deeply invasive down to muscles, bones or joints. A number of them are within visceral locations. They may appear as localized, purely vascular anomalies of varying size or occur within a segmental distribution or as disseminated multifocal lesions. Vascular malformations may also be part of a complex syndrome in combination with other defects, e.g. Klippel–Trenaunay syndrome.

Vascular malformations never regress. They persist and worsen over time if not treated. Subcategorization into CM, LM, VM and AVM is very important for management, since diagnostic interventions as well as treatment will differ depending on the specific type. In the majority of patients, a multidisciplinary team is required to provide the best chance of improvement. Cure is rarely achievable. A realistic aim is improvement, that is, to minimize the consequences of cosmetic, and often disabling function-threatening, lesions. Many of these patients, particularly those with VM and AVM, will require long-term management and follow-up, from childhood well into adulthood.

HISTORY

Medical literature addressing vascular malformations begins in the early 19th century. Originally, lesions and syndromes were described based on clinical features. Many authors played a major role in their description, including Virchow, Trélat, Monod, Klippel, Trenaunay, Weber, Sturge, Bockenheimer, Maffucci and Bell. In the mid-20th century, Malan first tried to classify these anomalies. Unfortunately, pathologists and physicians involved in clinical medicine or surgery did not work together; consequently, the multiple nomenclatures have become an important obstacle to communication amongst those involved in treating these patients. In 1976, John B Mulliken (a plastic surgeon in the US), Anthony E Young (a vascular surgeon in the UK) and Jean-Jaques Merland (a neuro-interventional radiologist in France) joined forces to convene the Workshop on Vascular Anomalies. The ISSVA, created in 1992 after 16 years of these Workshops, is dedicated to analyzing the clinical, radiologic, biologic[3,4] and pathologic[5]

DIFFERENCES BETWEEN VASCULAR MALFORMATIONS AND INFANTILE HEMANGIOMAS		
Characteristics	**Vascular malformations**	**Infantile hemangiomas**
Clinical data	CM: red, macular during infancy VM: blue, compressible, fills with dependency LM: vesicles or large cysts AVM: four stages, from dormant (stage 1) to more serious ones: stage 1 – dormant: red, warm, often macular stage 2 – expansion; warm mass with thrill stage 3 – destruction stage 4 – cardiac failure	Premonitory markers at birth in 50% of cases: red telangiectatic or white 'anemic' macules Superficial hemangioma: bright red 'strawberry' mark (during the proliferative phase) Deep hemangioma: rubbery mass under normal or bluish skin
Sex prevalence	No gender preponderance Female:male ratio 1:1	Female preponderance Female:male ratio 3:1 to 6:1
Natural history	Persistent, lifelong Present at birth in a majority Slow worsening or commensurate growth AVMs experience flares with puberty, trauma, pregnancy	Postnatal proliferation over months Slow involution over years Stable involuted stage
Radiology	Slow-flow VM or LM gives hypersignal on MRI T2-weighted images Slow-flow VM: phleboliths Fast-flow AVM: flow voids on MRI T1- or T2-weighted sequences Fast-flow AVM: arteriovenous shunts on Doppler ultrasound	Well-defined mass Some flow voids on MRI T1-weighted sequences (high-flow vessels)
Pathology	Enlarged vessels (CM) *or* Distorted, interconnected malformed channels (VM, LM) *or* AV fistulae (AVM) No increase in cellular turnover	Lobular dense proliferation of endothelial cells forming capillaries with tiny lumens Increase in cellular turnover can be demonstrated by using markers of proliferation (PCNA, collagenase, urokinase, UEA, bFGF, VEGF)
Immunophenotype	GLUT-1-negative	GLUT-1-positive
Hematology	LIC/DIC associated with VM, LM and LVM Lifelong Treatment of flares is low-molecular-weight heparin	(Kasabach–Merritt syndrome is not linked to hemangiomas, but to different types of vascular tumors: kaposiform hemangioendothelioma [KHE] or tufted angioma [TA], both of which are Glut-1-negative; see Ch. 114)
Molecular biology	A few known mutated genes mapped and identified in familial vascular malformations (see Table 104.2)	Rare families with autosomal dominant inheritance and loss of heterozygosity of 5q Clonality in some hemangiomas Mutation (somatic) of *VEGFR-3* and *VEGFR-2* in some hemangiomas

Table 104.1 Differences between vascular malformations and infantile hemangiomas. AVM, arteriovenous malformation; bFGF, basic fibroblast growth factor; CM, capillary malformation; DIC, disseminated intravascular coagulation; LIC, localized intravascular coagulation; LM, lymphatic malformation; PCNA, proliferating cell nuclear antigen; UEA, *Ulex europaeus* agglutinin; VEGF, vascular endothelial growth factor; VM, venous malformation.

characteristics of vascular lesions and improving diagnosis and treatment via multidisciplinary and international collaboration.

EPIDEMIOLOGY

Little is known regarding the exact prevalence of vascular malformations in the general population. The most common types are CM, then VM, and the least common are AVM. Vascular malformations have no gender prevalence. They appear to be less frequent in African, African-American and Asian patients.

PATHOGENESIS

Vasculogenesis is the initial embryologic process that creates the primitive vascular plexus. Then angiogenesis, the secondary sprouting of mesoderm-derived endothelial cells, forming new vessels from existing ones, generates most blood and lymphatic vessels. Endothelial differentiation, recruitment of smooth muscle cell precursors to ensheathe endothelial cells and build vessel walls, and, finally, changes in channel size, morphology and rheology create capillaries, veins and arteries. Vascular malformations are likely caused by changes in the expression and function of proteins involved in the cascade of events implicated in the development of vascular channels.

This heterogeneous group of disorders represents alterations in formation and growth of blood or lymphatic vessels. Dysfunction in signaling processes that regulate migration, differentiation, maturation, adhesion and survival of the cells of vascular walls must occur. Of note, markers of cellular proliferation are not elevated in vascular malformations[4]. In the cephalic region of the embryo, mural cells associated with endothelial cells come from the neural crest; therefore, vascular malformations such as Sturge–Weber syndrome or Bonnet–Dechaume–Blanc syndrome (Wyburn–Mason syndrome) are likely caused by a somatic mutation in the embryo's anterior neural crest or adjacent cephalic mesoderm. Rare familial cases of vascular malformations allow mapping of these inherited lesions to precise chromosomal locations, identification of the disease-causing mutations in the associated gene(s), discovery of the function of the encoded proteins, and clarification of the role the dysfunction plays in complex regulatory pathways (Table 104.2). It remains to be seen if sporadic vascular malformations, which are far more frequent than familial ones, are caused by the same gene mutations. Such research brings hope of replacement gene therapy or of currently unimaginable novel ways of therapy[6–9].

CLINICAL FEATURES

Distinctive clinical features characterize each type of vascular malformation. With the expertise of multidisciplinary vascular clinics, more than 90% of vascular malformations can be correctly categorized on the basis of clinical features. This helps in the selection of the best investigational tools, avoiding redundant assessments with often unnecessary diagnostic imaging techniques. Non-invasive studies such as ultrasonography and Doppler ultrasonography, and MRI, as well as series of magnetic resonance arteriography and magnetic resonance venography, sufficiently analyze the vast majority of CM, VM or LM. AVM is the only group of vascular malformations requiring a more invasive evaluation including arteriography (Table 104.3).

Capillary Malformation

Two types of CM exist: port-wine stains and telangiectasia. They may be the most obvious cutaneous or mucocutaneous sign of a complex syndrome, such as Sturge–Weber syndrome. An approach to the evaluation of a patient with a presumed CM of the head and neck region is shown in Figure 104.2.

CURRENT STATUS OF MOLECULAR GENETICS OF VASCULAR ANOMALIES

Vascular malformation	Mode of inheritance	Mutated gene(s)	Type of mutation	Protein and function
Familial CMVM, multiple cutaneous and mucosal venous malformations	AD	*TEK* (9p21)	Gain-of-function	TIE-2/TEK – an endothelial cell-specific tyrosine kinase receptor
Osler–Weber–Rendu; hereditary hemorrhagic telangiectasia (HHT)	AD	HHT1: *ENG* (9q3) HHT2: *ACVRL1* (12q13)	Loss-of-function	Endoglin and activin receptor-like kinase 1 (ALK1) – two TGF-β receptors with roles in vessel wall integrity
Juvenile polyposis with HHT	AD	*SMAD4* (18q21.1)	Loss-of-function	SMAD4 tumor suppressor protein – role in TGF-β signaling
Hereditary lymphedema type I (familial congenital; Milroy disease)	AD	*FLT4* (5q34)	Loss-of-function	VEGFR-3 – a tyrosine kinase receptor in lymphatic vessels
Hereditary lymphedema type II (late-onset; Meige lymphedema) and lymphedema–distichiasis syndrome	AD	*FOXC2* (16q22–24)	Loss-of-function	Forkhead family transcription factor C2
Hypotrichosis–lymphedema–telangiectasia	AR, AD	*SOX18* (20q13.33)	Loss-of-function	SRY–box 18 transcription factor
Cerebral capillary malformations (familial cerebral cavernomas)	AD	CCM1: *KRIT1* (7q21–22)* CCM2: *CCM2* (7p13) CCM3: *PDCD10* (3q26.1)	Loss-of-function	KRIT-1 interacts with KREV-1, RAP-1A and malcavernin (the *CCM2* gene product) – roles in MAPK and integrin signaling
CADASIL	AD	*NOTCH3* (19q12)	Loss-of-function in a subset of cases	Accumulation of NOTCH-3 protein in vascular smooth muscle cells
Familial glomangiomatosis (glomuvenous malformations)	AD	*GLMN* (1p21–22)	Loss-of-function (germline plus second hit within lesions)	Glomulin protein is a component of a multiprotein complex – role in vascular morphogenesis
Ataxia–telangiectasia	AR	*ATM* (11q22–23)	Loss-of-function	ATM protein is similar to phosphoinositol-3 kinase – regulates cell cycle, DNA repair, p53
Capillary malformation-arteriovenous malformation	AD	*RASA1*	Loss-of-function	p120-Ras-GAP protein – involved in signaling by growth factor receptors

*Including patients with hyperkeratotic cutaneous capillary-venous malformation.

Table 104.2 Current status of molecular genetics of vascular anomalies. AD, autosomal dominant; AR, autosomal recessive; CADASIL, cerebral autosomal dominant arteriopathy with subcortical infarcts and leukoencephalopathy; MAPK, mitogen-activated protein kinase; TGF-β, transforming growth factor-β; VEGFR-3, vascular endothelial growth factor receptor-3; VM, venous malformation.

INVESTIGATIVE TOOLS AND WHEN TO USE THEM

Tool	Vascular lesion			
	Capillary malformation	*Lymphatic malformation*	*Venous malformation*	*Arteriovenous malformation*
Ultrasonography	+/–	++++	+++	++++
Computed tomography	–	++	++	++
MRI, MRA, MRV	–	+++	+++++	+++
Arteriography	–	–	–	++++
Phlebography	–	–	+/–	–
Lymphography	–	+/–	–	–
Biopsy	+/–	+/–	–	–

Table 104.3 Investigative tools and when to use them. MRA, magnetic resonance arteriography; MRI, magnetic resonance imaging; MRV, magnetic resonance venography.

Port-wine stain

Port-wine stains (PWSs) are easily recognized on physical examination. They create well-demarcated red macular stains. Port-wine stain is not the correct term for the frequent mid-face (forehead, glabella, tip of the nose and philtrum; Fig. 104.3A), eyelid, and nape or occiput capillary stains, which may disappear spontaneously between 1 and 3 years of age. The facial capillary stains more commonly fade than do those in the nape area. They are referred to as nevus simplex, or salmon patch, evanescent macule, angel kiss or 'aigrette' on the forehead and stork bite on the nape.

PWSs often create rather large red patches, and their growth is commensurate with the child's growth. They can be localized or follow a segmental distribution. Some are extremely diffuse and multifocal. They never follow the lines of Blaschko. Facial PWSs are often distributed according to what has classically been considered the sensory trigeminal nerve distribution, with three areas recognized: V1 (ophthalmic: forehead and upper eyelid), V2 (maxillary region; Fig.104.3B) and V3 (mandibular region). Over time, those affecting the V2 and V3 areas will often develop a more pronounced red hue, changing from pink (at birth) to deep purple (in adulthood). Affected skin commonly thickens and develops nodularity and pyogenic granulomas (Fig. 104.4). Histologically, dilated capillaries and ectasias increase in number, occupying a deeper portion of the reticular dermis. In a group of 173 patients with PWSs[10], thickening was observed in 11% (median age 32 years), while nodularity was present in 24% (median age 44 years) and both hyperplastic skin changes occurred in 6% (median age 45 years). In parallel, the upper jaw may enlarge in all three planes (Fig. 104.5). This asymmetric overgrowth of the maxilla creates an open-bite deformity in

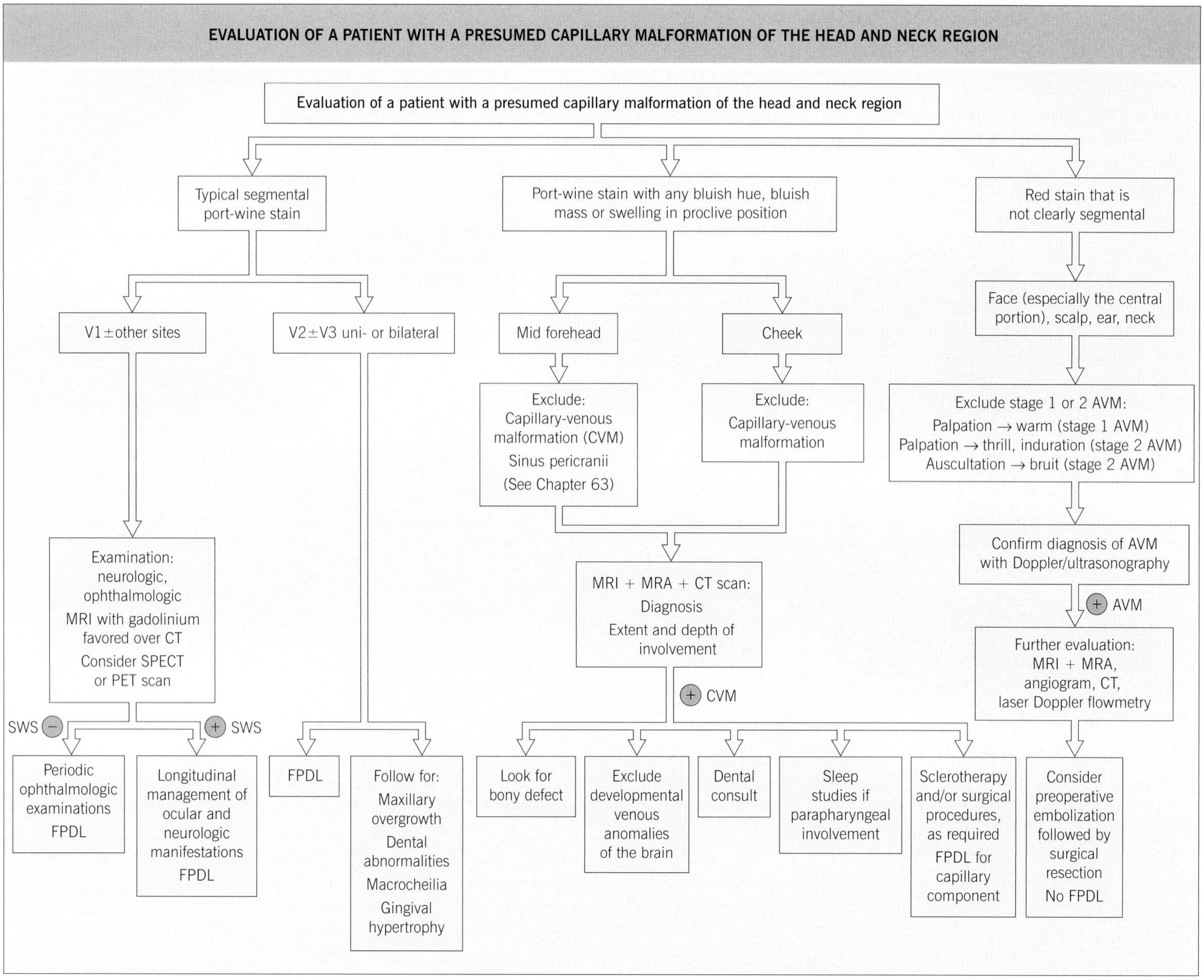

EVALUATION OF A PATIENT WITH A PRESUMED CAPILLARY MALFORMATION OF THE HEAD AND NECK REGION

Evaluation of a patient with a presumed capillary malformation of the head and neck region

Typical segmental port-wine stain

Port-wine stain with any bluish hue, bluish mass or swelling in proclive position

Red stain that is not clearly segmental

V1 ± other sites

V2 ± V3 uni- or bilateral

Mid forehead

Cheek

Face (especially the central portion), scalp, ear, neck

Exclude:
Capillary-venous malformation (CVM)
Sinus pericranii
(See Chapter 63)

Exclude:
Capillary-venous malformation

Exclude stage 1 or 2 AVM:
Palpation → warm (stage 1 AVM)
Palpation → thrill, induration (stage 2 AVM)
Auscultation → bruit (stage 2 AVM)

Examination:
neurologic, ophthalmologic
MRI with gadolinium favored over CT
Consider SPECT or PET scan

MRI + MRA + CT scan:
Diagnosis
Extent and depth of involvement

Confirm diagnosis of AVM with Doppler/ultrasonography

(+) AVM

Further evaluation:
MRI + MRA, angiogram, CT, laser Doppler flowmetry

(+) CVM

SWS (−)   (+) SWS

Periodic ophthalmologic examinations
FPDL

Longitudinal management of ocular and neurologic manifestations
FPDL

FPDL

Follow for:
Maxillary overgrowth
Dental abnormalities
Macrocheilia
Gingival hypertrophy

Look for bony defect

Exclude developmental venous anomalies of the brain

Dental consult

Sleep studies if parapharyngeal involvement

Sclerotherapy and/or surgical procedures, as required
FPDL for capillary component

Consider preoperative embolization followed by surgical resection
No FPDL

Fig. 104.2 Evaluation of a patient with a presumed capillary malformation of the head and neck region. AVM, arteriovenous malformation; CT, computed tomography; FPDL, flashlamp-pumped pulsed dye laser; MRA, magnetic resonance arteriography; MRI, magnetic resonance imaging; PET, positron emission tomography; SPECT, single photon emission computed tomography; SWS, Sturge–Weber syndrome.

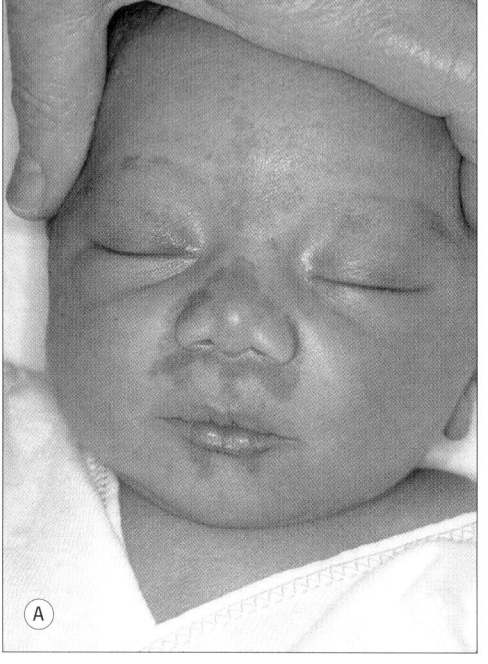

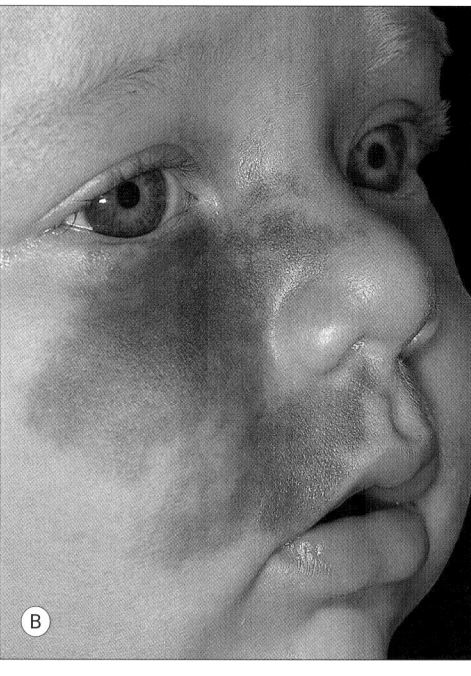

Fig. 104.3 Salmon patch versus port-wine stain (PWS) in a V2 distribution. A Involvement of the central face in a symmetric pattern is common with a salmon patch; such lesions fade over the first few years of life but are sometimes misdiagnosed as a capillary malformation (PWS). **B** In this young infant with a PWS, the skin is smooth. This lesion will be persistent.

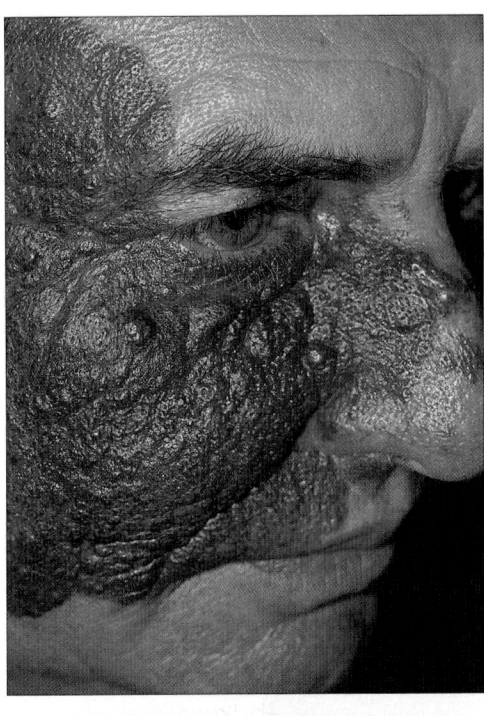

Fig. 104.4 Port-wine stain in a V2 distribution in an adult. Hyperplasia and nodularity are prominent.

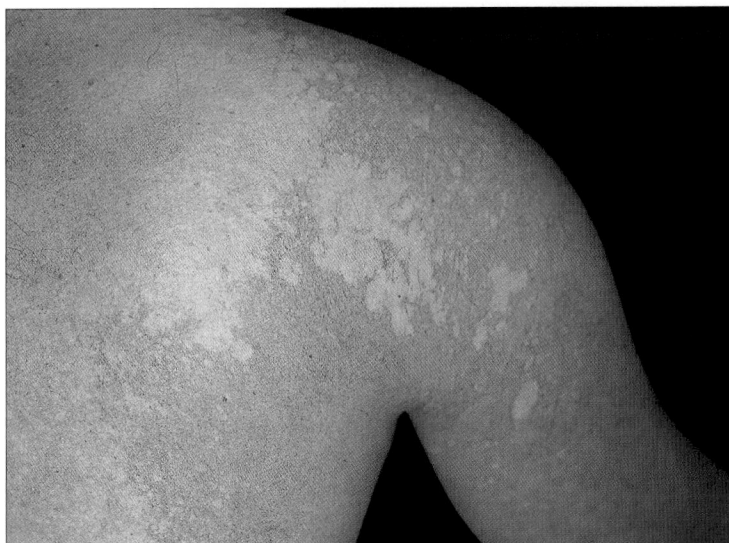

Fig. 104.6 Phakomatosis pigmentovascularis type 2b (with Sturge–Weber syndrome). A capillary malformation and nevus anemicus are intermingled on the shoulder of this man.

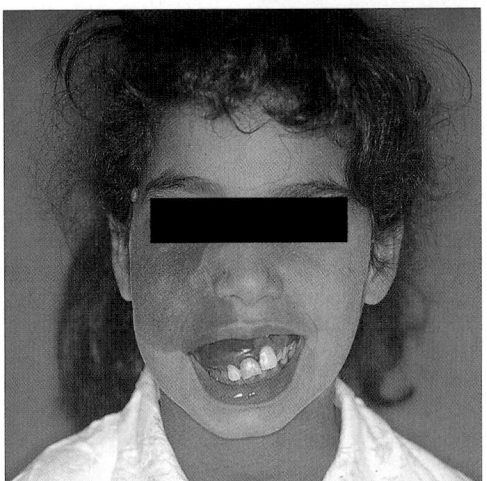

Fig. 104.5 Port-wine stain in a V2 distribution. Note the enlarged gingiva on the right and overgrowth of the right maxilla.

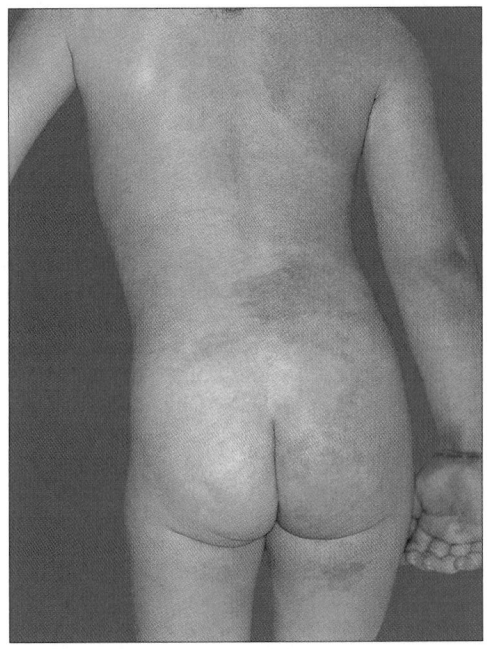

Fig. 104.7 Phakomatosis pigmentovascularis type 2a. Extensive capillary malformation and dermal melanocytosis are seen.

the adolescent. Gums and lips, when involved, may also enlarge, resulting in macrocheilia with lip incompetence or an epulis with bleeding of gingiva. Hypertrophic skin changes are very rare in PWSs of the trunk and limbs.

PWSs are congenital in the vast majority of patients. However, acquired PWSs developing primarily in adolescents or adults have been reported, and, in some patients, trauma may have played a role[11].

A CM can be admixed with a network of white round macules of nevus anemicus (Fig. 104.6), a phenomenon referred to as vascular twin spotting. A CM associated with a nevus anemicus and extensive aberrant Mongolian spots (dermal melanocytosis; Fig. 104.7) represents the most common of the types of *phakomatosis pigmentovascularis (PPV)*:

- Type 1: CM + epidermal nevus
- Type 2: CM + dermal melanocytosis ± nevus anemicus
- Type 3: CM + nevus spilus ± nevus anemicus
- Type 4: CM + dermal melanocytosis + nevus spilus ± nevus anemicus.

These types are further subdivided into those with only skin anomalies (subtype a) and those with skin plus systemic abnormalities (subtype b), for example, ocular nevus of Ota, Sturge–Weber syndrome, Klippel–Trenaunay syndrome. A fifth type of PPV has been proposed that combines cutis marmorata telangiectatica congenita with dermal melanocytosis, and the existence of type 1 PPV has been questioned.

A midline PWS of the lumbosacral, dorsal or nape areas may be a hallmark for *occult spinal dysraphism*, especially if it is associated with other markers of dysraphism, such as a pit, dimple, sinus, tail-like fibroma, hypertrichosis, lipoma, deviation of the gluteal cleft, congenital scar or melanocytic nevus[12,13]. In patients with clinically suspected dysraphism, ultrasound is a useful technique in infants less than 3–5 months of age, but MRI is the most sensitive study; myelography is no longer necessary.

When a child has a PWS and develops atopic dermatitis, more conspicuous lesions of eczema develop in areas of skin affected by the CM.

Syndromic capillary malformations
Sturge–Weber syndrome

Sturge–Weber syndrome (SWS) is a sporadic neurologic disorder in which a facial CM is associated with ipsilateral ocular and leptomeningeal anomalies. The facial PWS typically involves the area known as V1 trigeminal (skin of the forehead and upper eyelid)[14]. It may be more extensive, extending unilaterally or bilaterally over the face (Fig. 104.8). Some patients also have large PWSs of the extremities and trunk, and a small number have associated Klippel–Trenaunay syndrome (a slow-flow CLVM with overgrowth of the affected limb). Sturge–Weber syndrome may also occur in the setting of phakomatosis pigmentovascularis. Ocular involvement may be detected at birth because of buphthalmos (congenital glaucoma). Acute glaucoma with a cloudy cornea can be an infantile emergency. Usually, however, increased eye

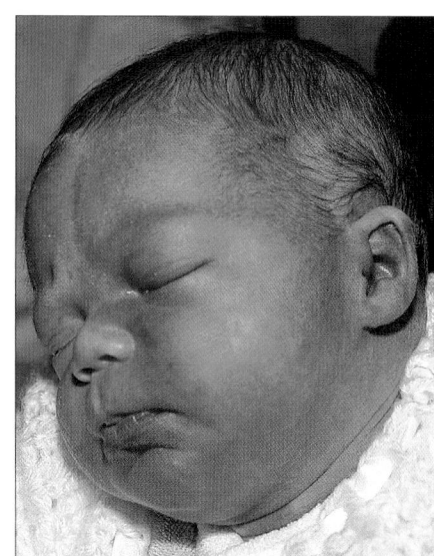

Fig. 104.8 Infant at risk for Sturge–Weber syndrome. Port-wine stain with involvement of V1 as well as V2 and V3.

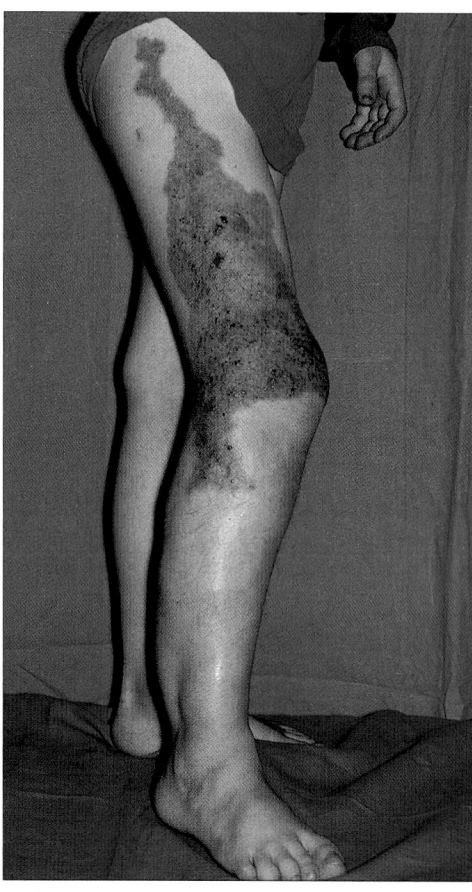

Fig. 104.9 Klippel–Trenaunay syndrome. Geographic capillary stain of the thigh with lymphatic vesicles, dilated incompetent veins, and enlarged lower limb.

pressure develops slowly. Glaucoma may become obvious only in late childhood; thus, periodic lifelong assessment of visual function and eye pressure is mandatory. A diffuse choroidal vascular malformation may also be present in the affected eye. If not treated and controlled, glaucoma results in visual field defects and visual loss.

Neurologic symptoms are due to the presence of a CVM within the pia mater, ipsilaterally to the V1 PWS. The occipital region is the most common location, but the leptomeningeal vascular lesion may be more extensive. Neurologic consequences include seizures, either affecting the side of the body opposite the brain vascular anomaly or generalized. Focal partial sensory or motor seizures, temporal lobe seizures and absence seizures may occur. Epilepsy typically develops in the first year of life[15] and sometimes the seizures are very difficult to control with anticonvulsants, especially early on. Additional findings include contra-lateral hemiparesis or hemiplegia, developmental delays in motor and cognitive skills, emotional and behavioral problems, attention deficits and migraine headaches. In association with the leptomeningeal slow-flow vascular malformation, cerebral atrophy and convoluted calcifi-cations develop.

Between 10% and 15% of infants with V1 PWS have the ocular and neurologic abnormalities of SWS. The risk of SWS is higher with a bilateral PWS[14a]. The cause of the disorder is unknown; all three tissues involved in SWS – namely, all the cellular components of the V1 facial skin (except for the endothelial cells), the ocular choroid, and the pia mater – are cephalic neural crest derivatives, originating from a common precursor in the anterior neural primordium. A somatic mutation has been hypothesized, occurring in an early precursor cell, prior to migration of embryonic neural crest derivatives. Regionalization of the cephalic neural crest cells to specific areas of the face is not very strict, explaining some fluidity in the final phenotypic expression of the facial vascular lesions. This is obvious when considering the varying limits between the so-called V1 and V2 PWS at the internal and external eyelid canthus (V1–V2 watershed).

Ocular and neurologic evaluation is mandatory in at-risk infants with a V1 PWS. CT with iodinated contrast and MRI with gadolinium enhancement can detect the pial and brain lesions, as well as the frequently enlarged ipsilateral choroid plexus. Gyriform calcifications develop in childhood and are clearly visible by plain radiography and CT. Before 6 months of age, MRI may demonstrate an advanced myelination in the involved hemisphere. Functional cerebral imaging[1], such as SPECT (single photon emission computed tomography, which evaluates the regional cerebral blood flow) or PET (positron emission tomography, which images the metabolism of glucose), permits a more precise evaluation of the location of brain lesions and their consequences.

Klippel–Trenaunay syndrome

Klippel–Trenaunay syndrome (KTS) is a limb CVM or CLVM with progressive overgrowth of the affected extremity. In some patients, there are additional findings, including lipomatosis, lymphedema, and intestinal or urinary vascular lesions. By colonoscopy or capsule video-endoscopy, extensive dilated venous channels and capillary patches (as well as lymphatic microcystic lesions) can be seen in the gastrointes-tinal tract; occasionally there is associated bleeding. The cutaneous stain (a CM) presents either as the very common blotchy capillary stain that is pink to purple in color and in an apparently haphazard distri-bution over the affected extremity, or it presents at birth as a geographic stain on the lateral aspect of the thigh, knee and leg. Superimposed on the geographic CM (Fig. 104.9), purple or clear vesicles (representing angiokeratomas or associated lymphatic anomalies) appear[16]. KTS with a geographic stain has a worse prognosis with respect to limb over-growth and complications, e.g. thromboses. Ultrasonography and color Doppler ultrasonography document vascular anomalies well. MRI can delineate the extent of tissue involvement. Lymphoscintigraphy may be indicated.

Proteus syndrome

Proteus syndrome is characterized by a progressive course and a mosaic distribution of the associated anomalies (see Ch. 61)[17]. The latter include asymmetric disproportionate overgrowth with orthopedic con-sequences (partial gigantism, hyperostoses of the skull, megaspondylo-dysplasia with scoliosis, facial or cranial hemihypertrophy), cerebriform connective tissue nevus of the soles and palms, benign hamartomatous lesions in a haphazard distribution (lipomas, epidermal nevi, hyper-pigmented macules, patchy dermal hypoplasia and regional absence of fat), a distinctive facial phenotype and slow-flow vascular anomalies (CM, varicose veins and macrocystic LM).

Telangiectasia

Telangiectasias (see Ch. 106) are capillary-type dilated blood vessels that appear as small, punctate, stellar, or linear red lesions. They may be widespread, unilateral, and linear, and in certain inherited disorders they favor particular anatomic sites (see below). In *angioma serpiginosum* (Hutchinson type), there are clusters of tiny telangiec-tasias, often in an annular or serpiginous pattern. The lesions tend to favor an extremity. There is both a congenital and an acquired form of *unilateral nevoid telangiectasia*. This disorder is seen primarily in women and the telangiectasias are usually on the face, neck, chest and arms. The smallest telangiectasias often have a prominent halo of vasoconstriction. The lesions of *hereditary benign telangiectasia* mimic those of hereditary hemorrhagic telangiectasia (HHT), but in the absence of epistaxis or any type of visceral hemorrhage; the disorder is slowly progressive, beginning early in life.

Cutis marmorata telangiectatica congenita

Cutis marmorata telangiectatica congenita (CMTC) is a distinctive cutaneous vascular syndrome with an obvious reticulated pattern to the vascular anomalies. They more commonly affect one or several limbs and the corresponding quadrant of the trunk. The reticulated pattern is persistent (unlike cutis marmorata) (Fig.104.10), dark purple, and intermingled with telangiectasias and, occasionally, atrophic depressions in the same net-like pattern. The latter are prominent over the joints and they may ulcerate, resulting in scarring. Phlebectasia (linear blue venous dilations) may also be seen. The most dramatic changes occur in the first year and lesions taper thereafter. However, persistence of some violaceous reticulated capillary network is a common finding[18]. Up to 50% of patients have been reported to have associated abnormalities, particularly orthopedic, ocular, neurologic and other vascular abnormalities; they occur primarily in diffuse CMTC, whereas localized mono- or dimelic CMTC have either no associated anomalies or only hypotrophy of the affected limb[19,20]. Hypoplasia in girth, usually not in length, can be obvious in infants with a single extremity affected (see Fig. 104.10). In Adams–Oliver syndrome, characterized by distal transverse limb defects as well as scalp skin and skull defects (aplasia cutis congenita), CMTC or a reticulate CM may be seen. Macrocephaly–CMTC syndrome often manifests with a reticulate PWS rather than true CMTC; additional features include a vascular stain of the philtrum, hemihypertrophy and syndactyly (especially of the second and third toes)[21]. Lastly, CMTC has been described in infants with neonatal lupus erythematosus.

Hereditary hemorrhagic telangiectasia

Hereditary hemorrhagic telangiectasia (HHT; Osler–Weber–Rendu disease) is a dominantly inherited autosomal disorder with late-onset penetrance characterized by skin, mucous membrane and visceral telangiectasias, recurrent epistaxis, and visceral hemorrhages (especially gastrointestinal). The telangiectasias actually represent AVMs, explaining their propensity to bleed. Phenotypes vary (even between affected members of a given family) with regard to age of onset and clinical symptoms[22–25]. The first manifestation of HHT is epistaxis, and it occurs in children, usually by puberty; hemorrhages of the gastrointestinal and genitourinary tracts occur later in life and often present as iron deficiency anemia[25]. Telangiectases appear most commonly on the face, lips, tongue, palms and fingers (including periungual). The dark red telangiectases are either round and slightly elevated, or they have an ill-defined border and stellate appearance.

Arteriovenous fistulas and malformations are not rare, as demonstrated by screening evaluations of asymptomatic patients with HHT: an estimated 30% have hepatic AVMs, 30% pulmonary AVMs, and 10–20% cerebral AVMs[25]. Pulmonary AVMs result in hypoxemia, hemorrhages, and an absence of capillary bed filtering with a risk of cerebral events (e.g. cerebral abscesses or stroke due to paradoxical emboli). Embolization of pulmonary AVMs is recommended[25]. In addition to hepatic AVMs, patients may have hepatic fibrosis and atypical cirrhosis; accompanying coagulation abnormalities increase the risk of hemorrhage.

It is not clear whether phenotype–genotype correlations can be established in HHT, but there may be a higher prevalence of pulmonary AVMs in HHT1[23]. To date, mutations in two genes have been identified – mutations in *ENG* (endoglin gene) lead to HHT1 and mutations in *ACVRL1* (*ALK1*) cause HHT2 (see Table 104.2). There are reports, however, of families with HHT not linked to the two known genes[24].

Ataxia–telangiectasia

Ataxia–telangiectasia is an autosomal recessive disorder that occurs in 1 in 40 000 births and is due to mutations in both copies of the *ATM* gene (see Ch. 59). Ataxia is the initial symptom, which usually presents during early childhood (after 15 months of age) and is eventually present in 98% of patients. Telangiectases appear after 4–6 years of age, primarily on the conjunctivae, face and ears, in up to 96% of patients[25]. A deficiency of IgA and IgG explains the frequent sinus and bronchial infections. These patients are at high risk for the development of lymphomas, leukemia and breast cancer. High levels of circulating α-fetoprotein are found in affected children. Heterozygote carriers of one copy of a mutated *ATM* gene also have an increased risk of developing cancers, including breast cancer.

Angiokeratomas

Angiokeratomas (see Ch. 106) consist of ectasias of dermal capillaries with an acanthotic and hyperkeratotic overlying epidermis. These dark red to purple papular vascular anomalies can present as a wide range of lesions varying in size, depth and location. The two most common types are solitary papular angiokeratoma and angiokeratoma of the scrotum and vulva. The former is often found on the lower extremity, and it may be mistaken for cutaneous melanoma. In *angiokeratoma circumscriptum*, clusters of ectasias form a plaque or linear lesion, usually on an extremity, and present at birth. Congenital hyperkeratotic vascular anomalies resembling angiokeratoma circumscriptum but with a deeper dermal component consisting of small, thick-walled blood vessels (larger than normal capillaries) have been referred to as 'verrucous hemangiomas'; such lesions behave clinically as vascular malformations, although low-level expression of proliferative markers and GLUT-1 was described in a recent series[25a]. Grouped tiny lesions are also seen in *angiokeratoma of Mibelli*, which favors the toes, fingers, knees and elbows.

As the name implies, *angiokeratoma corporis diffusum* is characterized by more widespread lesions, and it may be associated with hereditary lysosomal storage disorders such as *Fabry disease*[26] (X-linked recessive; deficiency of α-galactosidase A, accumulation of globotriaosylceramide) and α-1 fucosidase deficiency (see Table 62.5)[27]. In addition, angiokeratomas (and microcystic lymphatic lesions) may develop on the surface of the geographic CM frequently located on the lateral aspect of the thigh in Klippel–Trenaunay syndrome. A distinctive *hyperkeratotic cutaneous capillary-venous malformation* (HCCVM) occurs in a small subgroup of patients with inherited cerebral capillary malformations (CCMs), also referred to as *familial cerebral cavernomas*; these patients have a high risk of cerebral hemorrhage. In some families, the cutaneous lesion has represented a sign of brain involvement, as CCMs co-segregated with HCCVMs[28]. In one such family, a mutation in *CCM1*, which is located on 7q21–22 and encodes the protein KRIT-1, was observed (see Table 104.2).

Sinusoidal hemangioma

Sinusoidal 'hemangioma' is a misnomer for a lesion that is in fact a vascular malformation with various clinical presentations. It may

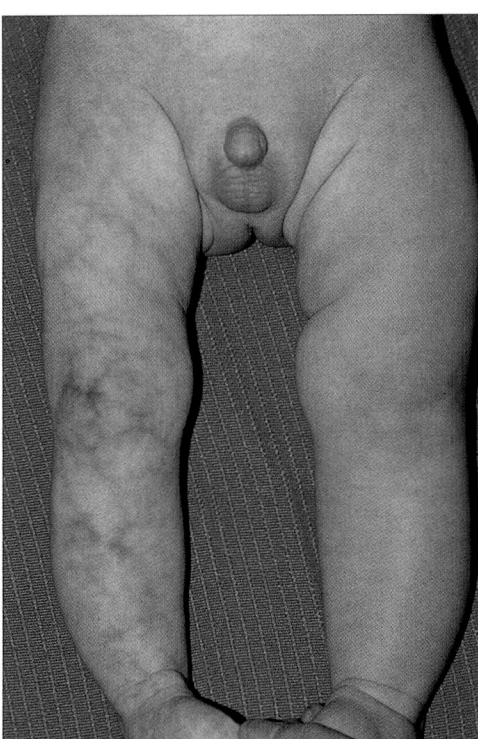

Fig. 104.10 Cutis marmorata telangiectatica congenita with hypoplasia of affected limb.

present as nodules, often in the breast area or extremities, or as large firm bulging facial masses beneath normal-appearing skin; the latter have an aggressive and invasive course[29]. Diagnosis is based on distinctive pathologic features: well-circumscribed nodules with a lobular architecture composed of very large, thin-walled, blood-filled, densely packed channels with scanty fibrous stroma between them.

Venous Malformation

VM consists of an often poorly recognized, puzzling group of vascular malformations commonly confused with deep growing hemangiomas in children, or with Klippel–Trenaunay syndrome when they involve a full extremity[1]. VMs are easily recognized clinically thanks to their blue or blue–purple hue; lesions are soft and compressible. They usually occur in a segmental distribution, although some patients develop multiple VMs scattered on the skin and mucous membranes, a finding more common in familial forms with autosomal dominant inheritance. Sporadic cases are more common than inherited forms. VMs are best evaluated using T2-weighted MRI[30] (Fig. 104.11 & Tables 104.1 and 104.3).

Cephalic venous malformation

These relatively common lesions lead to cosmetic and functional problems that increase from birth to adulthood. They develop in facial and neck skin, lips, and oral mucous membranes (cheeks, tongue, and floor of the mouth). VMs permeate deeper structures, such as muscles, infratemporal fossa, buccal fat pad in the cheek, and orbit. In all of these locations, VMs swell and enlarge when the head is in a proclive or declive position. Swelling is tender, and, with time, distortion of facial features becomes conspicuous. A lip VM rapidly enlarges the normal size of the lip; labial incompetence occurs if the whole lip is involved, or commissural displacement develops if the lesion affects half of the labial vermilion border. Due to a mass effect, VMs in the cheek and mouth interfere with the growth of the jaws, creating a shift of the dental midline and progressive, usually lateral, open-bite deformity. This cosmetic and functional problem (Fig. 104.12) requires specific management of the dental malalignment after the child has secondary teeth or during adulthood. Orbital VMs may communicate with cheek VMs through the sphenomaxillary fissure. An orbital VM swells and shrinks depending on the position of the head; this changing volume, getting bigger and smaller many times a day, over the years, will progressively broaden the orbital bones and eventually the patient gets an enophthalmic appearance when standing. However, there is no visual dysfunction.

Patients with parapharyngeal and laryngeal VMs should be monitored with overnight sleep studies if they are known to snore and to feel tired in the morning. These patients are often found to have a severe sleep apnea syndrome. This puts them at high risk of sudden death during sleep. In these patients, multiple procedures of direct puncture of the lesions and sclerotherapy with Ethibloc® or pure

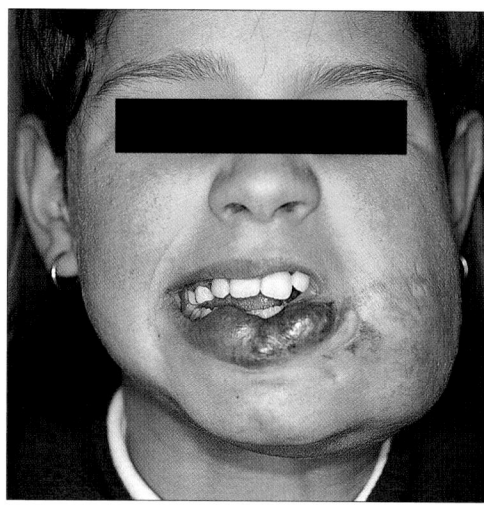

Fig. 104.12 **Venous malformation of cheek and lip.** The typical blue color and distortion of facial features with an open bite are seen.

ethanol is required. A tracheotomy is often needed temporarily, because of the secondary inflammatory reaction.

Patients with extensive cephalic VMs can have associated brain vascular anomalies. In my experience, 25% of these patients have developmental venous anomalies (DVAs). These anomalies are present in less than 1% of the general population, and they are easily detected by CT or MRI. They were once called 'venous angiomas', a misnomer as they are not true vascular malformations; DVAs are uncommon trajectories of the brain venous drainage system, usually with enlarged deep venous channels. They do not entail risk of cerebral hemorrhage, but they may cause headaches; DVAs do not need treatment, as they represent well-functioning venous drainage. They just require detection to avoid misdiagnosis. Of note, patients with cephalic VMs are not at increased risk of having cerebral vascular malformations of the so-called cavernoma type.

Patients with extensive cephalic VMs may also have bony defects underlying vascular anomalies of the scalp, frontal and orbital regions. In my experience, these bony defects occur in more than 20% of cases. They may be small or large, and they need to be detected before any decision is made regarding sclerotherapy of an overlying VM, to avoid dangerous embolic migration through the pathologic bone.

Trunk and limb venous malformation

VMs of the trunk and limbs have cosmetic consequences: the blue color of the skin (Fig. 104.13) and swelling of soft tissues. They also have functional consequences, as they are often deeply invasive, spreading through muscles and penetrating joints[31]. VMs create spongy masses due to ectatic saggy venous channels, and these are easily emptied by elevating and massaging the affected region. Bright white hypersignals are seen in MRI T2-weighted images, clearly delineating the VMs from host tissues. Limb VMs may progressively alter underlying bones; osteoporosis, diaphyseal thinning, lytic lesions and bony distortion have all been described. Pathologic fractures may occur with minimal trauma.

Muscle involvement creates episodes of pain after motion and in the morning, with the pain linked to thromboses inside the slow-flow channels. These thromboses lead to phlebolith formation (round calcifications detected on plain radiographs). A chronic localized intravascular coagulopathy (low serum fibrinogen, elevated D-dimers, moderately low platelet count)[31] is common, and it explains thromboses and pain. Joint involvement is associated with pain and sudden tense swelling due to effusions, hemarthrosis, and intermittent and recurrent joint block. In the most extensive intrasynovial VMs of the knee or elbow, recurrent hemarthrosis results in cartilage alteration and permanent flexion contracture of the joint. Symptoms usually begin before 10 years of age. A common error is to misdiagnose extensive limb VMs as Klippel–Trenaunay syndrome. The latter does not have muscle and joint involvement. On the other hand, overgrowth is rare with limb VMs (undergrowth of the extremity is more common). VMs in the lower extremity may also affect the genitalia, in both girls and boys. Trunk VMs commonly penetrate the parietal muscles, and they may reach the pleura by infiltrating intercostal spaces. Paraspinal muscular VMs are often discovered because of pain.

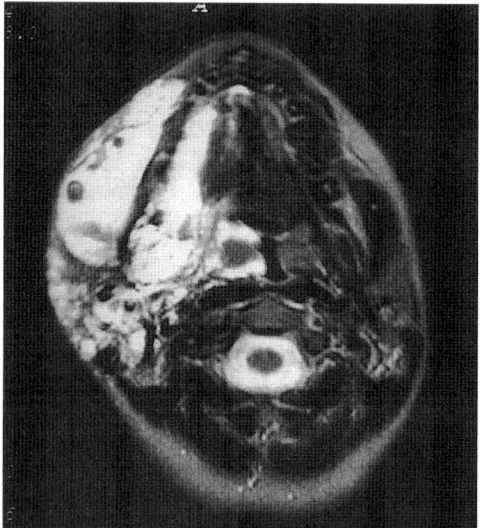

Fig. 104.11 **T2-weighted sequence of MRI clearly shows venous malformation (VM) in the neck (white hypersignals).** The black dots in the white areas of VMs are phleboliths.

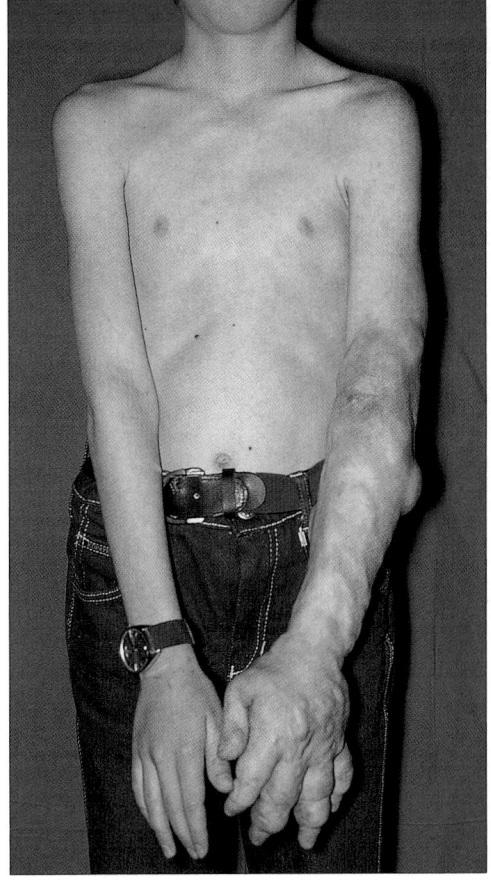

Fig. 104.13 Venous malformation involving the skin and muscles of an entire arm. Excess slack, blue skin is prominent in involved fingers, and swelling is obvious in the dependent position.

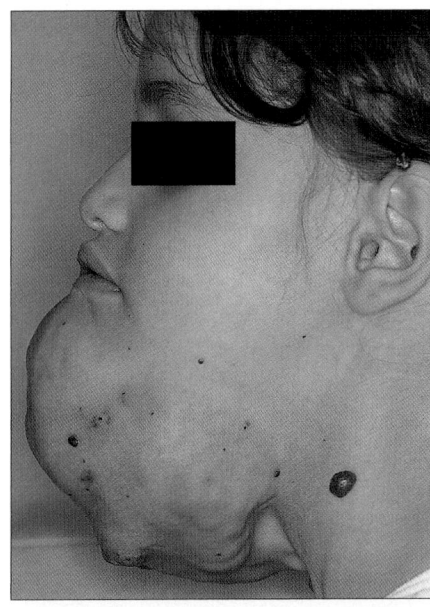

Fig. 104.14 Bean syndrome. Small blue venous nodules are superimposed on a large subcutaneous venous malformation in this girl.

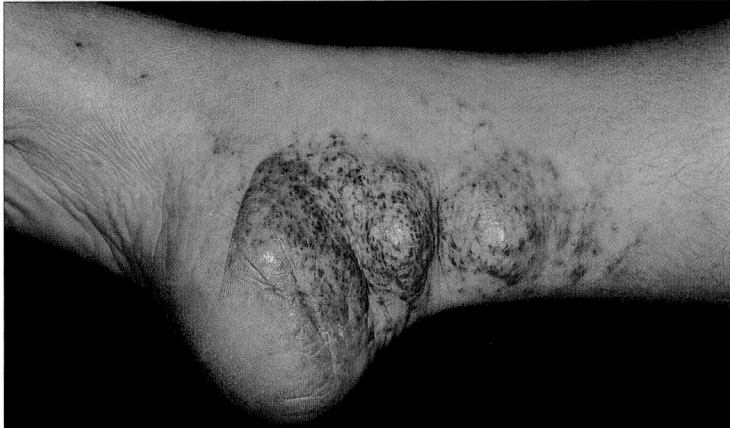

Fig. 104.15 Plaque-type segmental extremity glomangiomas (glomuvenous malformations).

Syndromes associated with venous malformations

Familial cutaneous and mucosal venous malformation (CMVM, OMIM 600195) is an autosomal dominantly inherited type of VM, with multiple lesions affecting the skin, oral mucosa, and muscles. The mutated gene, *TEK*, has been cloned and the locus mapped to 9p21[6,7] (see Table 104.2). Of note, patients have 'gain-of-function' mutations that result in activation of a tyrosine kinase receptor (TIE-2/ TEK). Unlike individuals with Bean syndrome, these patients do not develop visceral lesions; specifically, they do not develop intestinal VMs. In the past, there was some confusion between the two syndromes, but patients with Bean syndrome do not have *TEK* mutations.

Blue rubber bleb nevus syndrome (Bean syndrome) is a sporadic disease with widely distributed dark blue papules and nodules and soft skin-colored compressible protuberances ('rubber blebs') as well as large VM (Fig. 104.14) or LVM. Gastrointestinal lesions are documented by upper endoscopy and colonoscopy; hemorrhages from these lesions create iron-deficiency anemia. Other sites of visceral involvement (CNS, lungs, heart) are less common. Bean syndrome should not be confused with CMVM.

Glomangiomas and familial glomangiomatosis, now known as *glomuvenous malformations*, represent the association of VM with rows of glomus cells around the distorted venous channels (see Ch. 114). They occur as small solitary lesions (the nail bed is a common location; usually sporadic), widely scattered blue–purple round nodules, or, less commonly, in a segmental distribution (Fig. 104.15)[31a]. In contrast to classic VM, glomuvenous malformations tend to be hyperkeratotic and painful when palpated, are only partially compressible, and typically do not involve viscera or affect joints. Infrequently there is mucosal involvement (e.g. deep intraoral lesions) or superficial invasion of muscles. Multiple lesions are usually familial (OMIM 138000). In our experience, approximately two-thirds of patients with glomuvenous malformations but only 1% of those with other VMs have a family history of similar lesions[32]. The mutated gene in glomuvenous malformations, *GLMN*, resides on 1p21 (see Table 104.2)[8,32,32a].

Maffucci syndrome combines blue or skin-colored nodules (VMs) and enchondromas. These multiple enchondromas are similar to those of Ollier disease, and they have orthopedic and cosmetic consequences. They appear more commonly in the extremities; however, cephalic

lesions may occur with severe neuro-ophthalmologic outcomes. Histologically, the skin lesions demonstrate features of both a VM and a vascular tumor, the spindle cell hemangioma (Fig. 104.16) (see Ch. 114). The syndrome is rare and sporadic.

Lymphatic Malformation

Lymphatic anomalies such as lymphedema and lymphatic malformations (LMs) correspond to opposite aspects of an anomalous lymphatic network. Lymphedema results from hypoplasia or aplasia of lymphatic channels and nodes, whereas LMs are due to hyperplasia of the lymphatic network. Lymphatic anomalies may be microcystic, macrocystic or combined. They are superficial (skin and mucous membranes) or deep and visceral (less than 10% of cases).

Lymphedema

Patients with lymphedema accumulate lymph fluid in their affected extremities, and rare cases also have cephalic involvement. These patients are at risk for bacterial infections and septicemia. Diffuse lymphedema is often associated with intestinal lymphangiectasias and exudative enteropathy or pleural effusions.

Lymphedema is congenital or acquired (see Ch. 105). It may occur in the setting of either *Turner syndrome* or *Noonan syndrome*. Congenital forms may manifest later in life, from childhood to adulthood. A number of congenital forms (one-third) have a family history with an autosomal dominant inheritance pattern. Hereditary lymphedema – i.e. *Milroy disease* (congenital; type I; MIM153100) and *Meige lymphedema* (late-onset; type II; MIM153200) – have been associated with mutations in the genes that encode vascular endothelial growth factor receptor 3 and forkhead family transcription factor C2, respectively

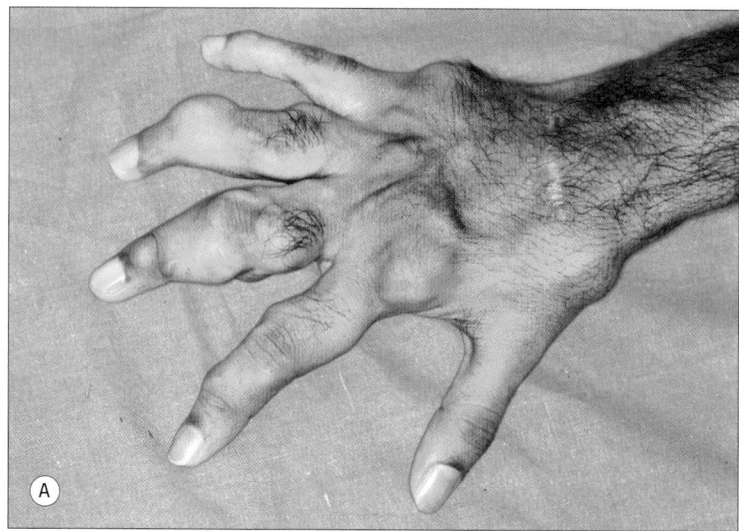

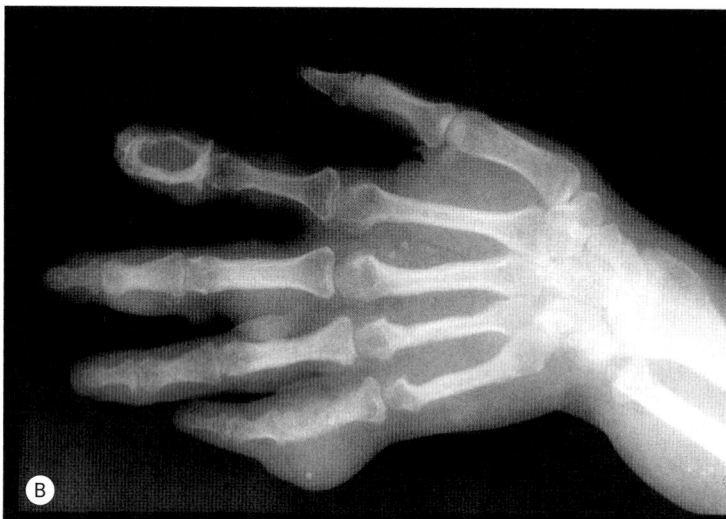

Fig. 104.16 Maffucci syndrome. A Both nodular venous malformations and enchondromas distort the hand. **B** A radiograph demonstrates an enchondroma and multiple phleboliths.

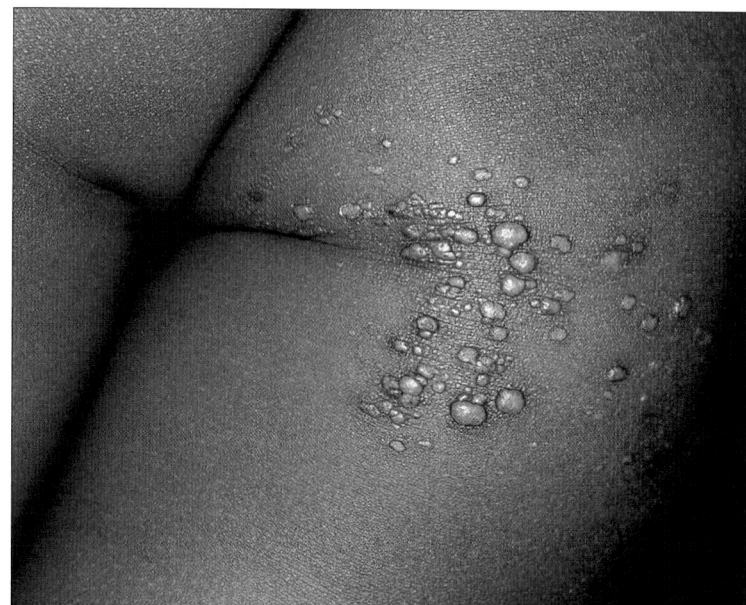

Fig. 104.17 Microcystic lymphatic malformation showing a cluster of papulovesicles.

(see Table 104.2 and Ch. 102). More complex familial syndromes with lymphedema have also been described. *Hennekam syndrome,* an autosomal recessive disorder, is characterized by lymphedema of the lower extremities, intestinal lymphangiectasias and facial anomalies. *Njolstad syndrome* combines lymphedema of the limbs and face with congenital pulmonary lymphangiectasias, with hydrops fetalis in some cases. *Aagenaes syndrome* combines lymphedema and infantile cholestasis.

Macrocystic lymphatic malformation

Macrocystic LMs represent collections of interconnected, large lymphatic cysts lined by a thin endothelium, commonly called cystic hygromas in the literature. The most common locations are the neck, axilla and lateral chest wall. Prenatal detection by ultrasound is possible as early as the 4th month of pregnancy. Some of the cases diagnosed prenatally are associated with karyotype abnormalities or malformation syndromes (Down syndrome, Turner syndrome, Noonan syndrome) and possibly with teratogenic agents. There are no gender differences.

Diagnosis of a macrocystic LM is usually easily made clinically, as it appears as a large translucent soft mass under normal skin. It is confirmed by ultrasound, CT or MRI, as well as by direct puncture and cytologic analysis of the fluid. Multiple cysts may exist. Hemorrhage inside a cyst creates sudden swelling, and the mass becomes tense, firm, purple or yellowish, and tender.

Microcystic lymphatic malformation

Dermatologists and ENT surgeons commonly see microcystic LMs. They represent aggregations of ill-defined, abnormal, microscopic lym-

phatic channels. The most common presentation, occurring anywhere on the skin, is a plaque with crops of clear or hemorrhagic vesicles scattered on its surface (Fig. 104.17), varying in size and number over time. The lesions may be misdiagnosed as molluscum contagiosum or warts. Additional clinical findings are swelling and intermittent bruising. Lesions are often much more extensive than clinically expected from the number of vesicles visible. Intermittent lymph leakage from the superficial vesicles can be troublesome, as can inflammatory flares, infections, and erysipelatous reactions after small wounds in the affected region. In the mouth (a common location), multiple vesicles with fragile roofs are filled with clear or milky fluid or blood. They may involve large areas of the mucosal surfaces of the cheek, tongue, and floor of the mouth. By MRI, lesions of microcystic LM are characterized by hypersignals in T2-weighted sequences.

Combined microcystic and macrocystic lymphatic malformation

In some diffuse cervicofacial LMs, bony involvement is common, as evidenced on pathologic specimens[33]. Bilateral LMs create mandibular overgrowth and prognathism in most patients, with anterior open-bite deformities and class III abnormal occlusal planes. When only one side of the face is affected, maxillary and mandibular deformities induce cross bite and displacement of the midline. In the case of intraoral LM, inflammatory flares or spontaneous bleeding occur during common ENT infections. This can result in sudden expansion of lesions, particularly those in the tongue.

In some patients with massive micro- and macrocystic LMs in the mouth plus parapharyngeal, tongue base, and laryngeal extensions, flares create airway compromise requiring tracheotomy. The majority of children with bulky LM in the mouth experience a number of local infections, sometimes with subsequent cellulitis or even severe septicemia. Dental caries are common, with loss of teeth. Speech impairment is frequent, particularly during flares of macroglossia. Mastication and swallowing may also be affected. Massive cervicofacial LMs have a poor lifetime prognosis, being both function-threatening and life-threatening[34].

In the orbital region, combined micro- and macrocystic LMs are intraconal or extraconal or both. They can lead to swelling, pain, infections, chemosis, strabismus and amblyopia. During flares or bleeding, they may cause proptosis in addition to a risk of visual loss.

On the trunk and limbs, rare combined micro- and macrocystic LMs severely worsen as the child grows; on serial MRI, there is an obvious 'opening' of new large cysts over a several-year period. Small wounds of the feet are easily infected, resulting in worsening of the lesions due to inflammatory reactions (just as in patients with limb lymphedema). Careful hygiene of the limbs is mandatory. In these patients, a chronic localized intravascular coagulopathy (low serum fibrinogen, elevated D-dimers, moderately low platelet count) is common, and this is responsible for painful hemorrhagic episodes within the lesions, requiring low-molecular-weight heparin therapy.

Arteriovenous Malformation

AVMs are vascular malformations with direct communications (AV shunting) between arteries and veins creating a nidus (AV nidus). They are rare, with no gender preference, and they constitute the most endangering group of vascular anomalies. Schobinger's staging was adopted by the ISSVA in order to classify AVMs according to their clinical severity[2,35].

- Stage 1 (quiescent, dormant stage): the lesion is macular or slightly infiltrated, red, and warm, mimicking a PWS (Fig. 104.18) or involuting/involuted hemangioma.
- Stage 2 (expansion): lesions are warm masses with throbbing and thrills over dilated draining veins; ultrasound easily confirms the presence of AV fistulae (Fig. 104.19).
- Stage 3 (destruction): in addition to signs and symptoms of stage 2, this stage is characterized by necrosis, ulcers, hemorrhages, and, occasionally, lytic bone lesions (Fig. 104.20).
- Stage 4 combines cardiac decompensation with stage 2 or 3 clinical symptoms.

In 40% of patients, AVMs are congenital and visible at birth; however, they may appear later in life, seemingly acquired. The most common location is cephalic (70% of cases in my experience; Fig. 104.21). Flares are common, in girls as well as in boys, during puberty (75% of

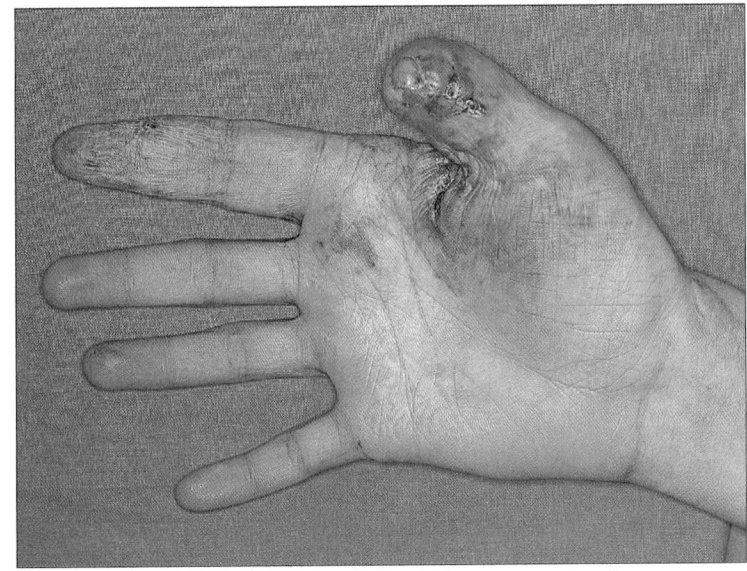

Fig. 104.20 Arteriovenous malformation in necrotic stage 3. Shortening of the phalanx and miniaturization of the nail announce the unavoidable amputation of the finger.

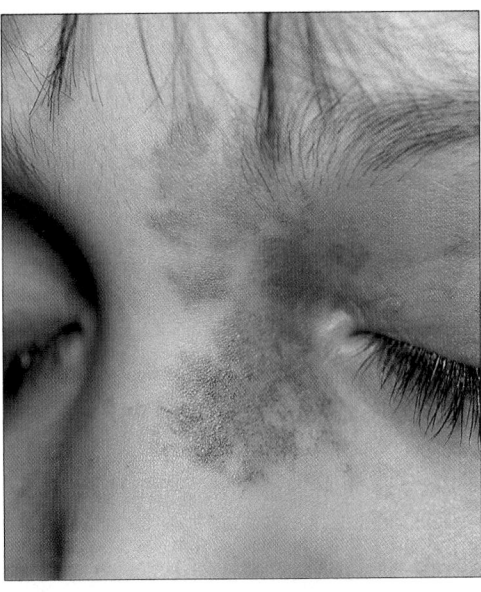

Fig. 104.18 Arteriovenous malformation in dormant stage 1, mimicking a port-wine stain. Doppler ultrasound confirmed the existing shunt.

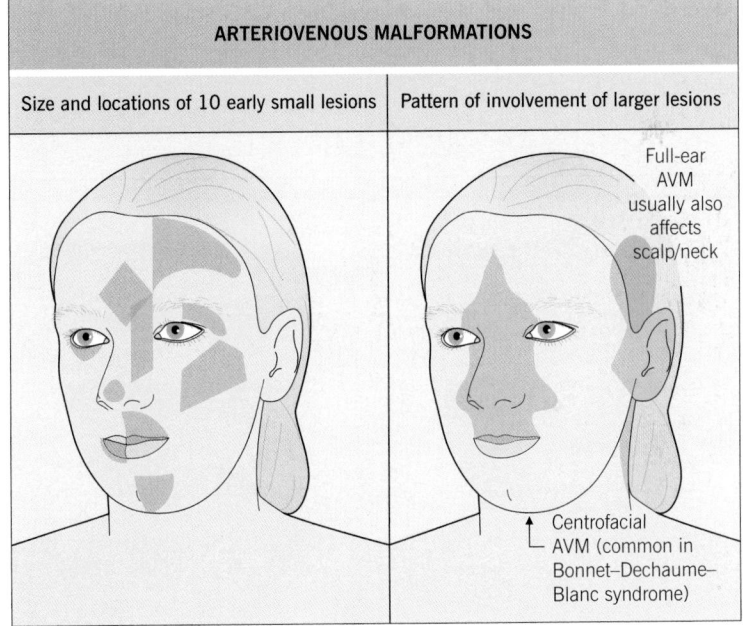

ARTERIOVENOUS MALFORMATIONS

Size and locations of 10 early small lesions	Pattern of involvement of larger lesions

Full-ear AVM usually also affects scalp/neck

Centrofacial AVM (common in Bonnet–Dechaume–Blanc syndrome)

Fig. 104.21 Arteriovenous malformations – sizes, locations and patterns.

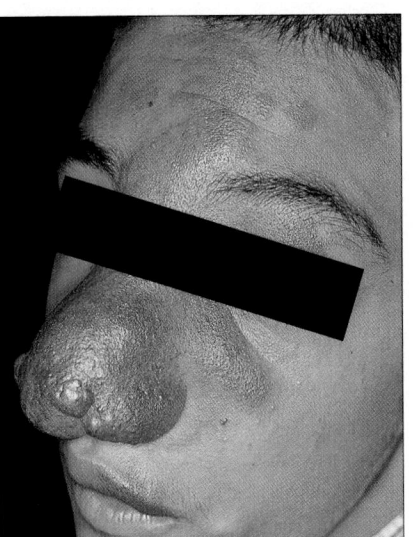

Fig. 104.19 Arteriovenous malformation in expansion stage 2. This boy has metameric Bonnet–Dechaume–Blanc syndrome (Wyburn–Mason syndrome) involving the centrofacial skin, the retina and brain.

patients); pregnancy may induce worsening of AVMs (25% of women), as can trauma[35]. In an analysis of 65 patients with cephalic AVMs (unpublished personal data): 39 were centrofacial; seven were hemifacial; four affected the scalp, ten the forehead, and ten the ear. Stage 3 cephalic AVMs are disfiguring and function- or even life-threatening lesions. Stage 3 AVMs of the extremities or of the ear[36] may lead to amputation. These situations are too often precipitated by ill-adapted treatments, for example, arterial or venous ligatures, partial excision, and proximal (not selective and distal) embolization.

The diagnosis of clinically suspected AVM is confirmed by ultrasound[37]. For a full evaluation of these lesions, MRI, CT (for possible bony lesions) and arteriography are required before assessing prognosis and therapeutic management.

Syndromes associated with arteriovenous malformations
Cobb syndrome

This is a very rare metameric skin, spinal, and vertebral AVM. The spinal AVM results in neurologic deficits, primarily paraparesis and paraplegia during young adulthood, due to a mass effect of the expanding AVM on the spinal cord and subarachnoid hemorrhage. The spinal AVM is intramedullary or extends to the meninges. It may involve the vertebral body and the soft tissues of the same metamere(s). Skin lesions, from red or red–brown cutaneous stains mimicking a PWS (in fact a stage 1 AVM) to throbbing masses with dilated veins and thrills, are present in only 20% of patients with spinal AVMs. The cutaneous AVM may be congenital or develop later in life after the onset of neurologic signs. Angiograms and MRI[38] establish the presence of the spinal AVM. Endovascular embolization of the spinal AVM can dramatically improve the prognosis.

Parkes Weber syndrome

This rare association of overgrowth of the affected limb in length and girth, often with multiple arteriovenous fistulae, must be differentiated from Klippel–Trenaunay syndrome. There is often, in association, excess fat, a capillary stain, and lymphatic anomalies. Bone lytic lesions and cardiac failure can occur. The prognosis is poor after puberty.

Bonnet–Dechaume–Blanc syndrome (or Wyburn–Mason syndrome)

This is a rare metameric AVM extending from the craniofacial to the orbital regions and brain. Some patients express the full spectrum of the malformation, while others have incomplete forms of the disease[39]. The brain AVM may remain asymptomatic or manifest itself as seizures or hemiparesis/hemiplegia. In my experience (in a study conducted at Lariboisière Hospital, Paris, with Monique Boukobza MD) with 12 such patients between 5 and 51 years of age, the disabling facial AVM was either a thick warm red stain mimicking a CM (stage 1 AVM), or a typical stage 2 or stage 3 AVM with a vascular mass, throbbing and a thrill. The locations were: facial midline in three (see Fig. 104.19); hemifacial in three; and both hemifacial and midfacial in six. Four of our 12 patients had orbital AVMs (therefore, an inconstant finding) and the brain lesions (present in all 12) were located in the chiasm in eight, choroid plexus in four, and thalamus in four; a dural AVM was present in two; four of the 12 patients had had a cerebral hemorrhage. In the series from Bhattacharya et al.[39] of 15 patients with this syndrome, orbital involvement was present in all but one, and it consisted of an AVM of the optic nerve (13/15), retina (11/15), thalamus (9/15) and chiasm-hypothalamus (9/15). Patients had various symptoms, from reduced visual acuity or fields to blindness. Other craniofacial complications are recurrent epistaxis, nasal obstruction and gingival hemorrhages.

Capillary malformation-arteriovenous malformation

In this newly recognized syndrome (see Table 104.2), a single AVM or Parkes Weber syndrome is associated with multiple small, round or oval CMs with an ill-defined pale border in a haphazard distribution, most often on the extremities[9]. Some affected individuals present with multiple CMs but no obvious high-flow lesion[39a].

PATHOLOGY

The histologic characteristics of the four major types of vascular malformations[5,40] are illustrated in Figure 104.22.

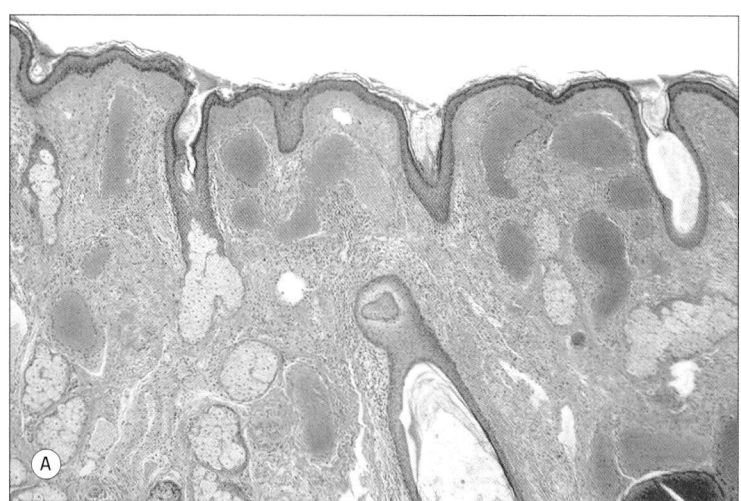
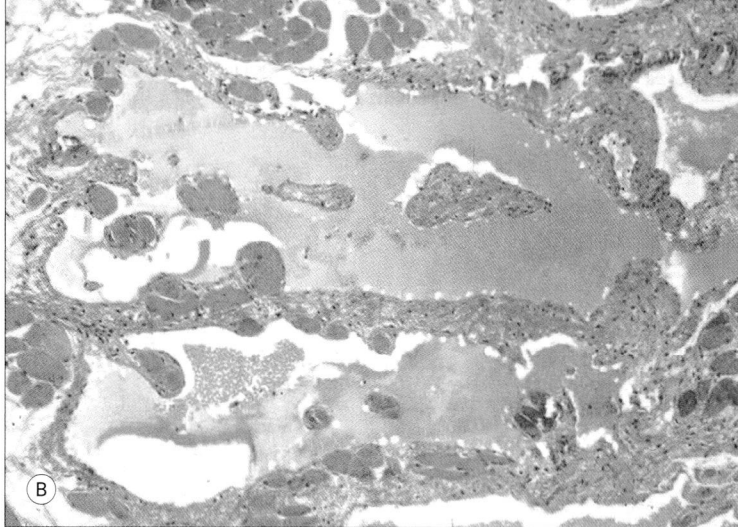
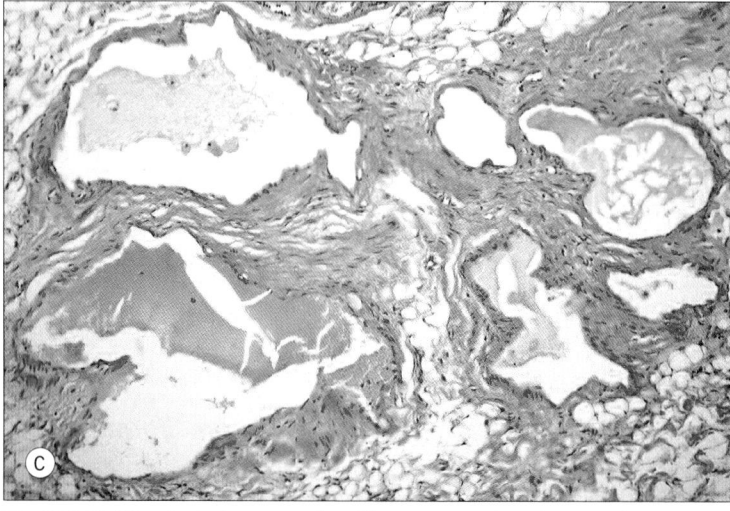
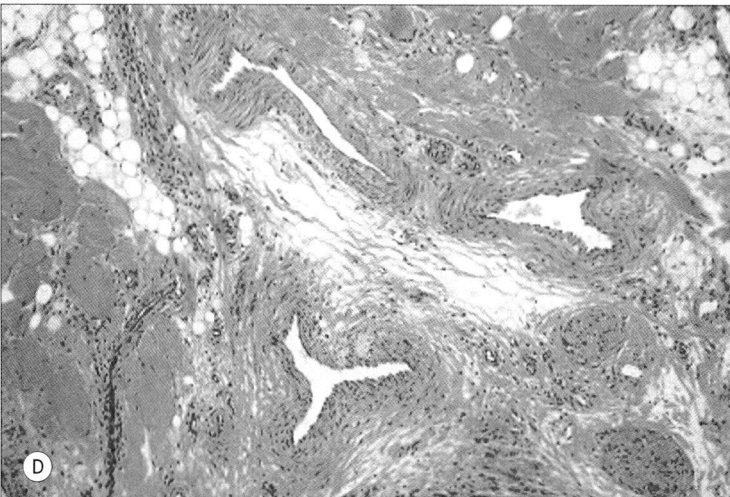

Fig. 104.22 Histologic features of capillary, venous, lymphatic and arteriovenous malformations. A Capillary malformation in an adult that was thickened and nodular. An increased number of dilated capillaries are present throughout the dermis. **B** Venous malformation. Note the large, thin-walled, irregularly anastomosing channels dissecting the normal connective tissue. **C** Lymphatic malformation. The large lymphatic channels are located here in the subcutaneous fat. **D** Arteriovenous malformation. The irregularly shaped, thick-walled vessels are randomly distributed within the dermis. Courtesy of Dr M Wassef.

Capillary Malformation

A CM is composed of ectatic capillaries within the papillary and reticular dermis, lined by a flat continuous endothelium. In some patients, there is a clear increase in the number of malformed capillaries. The thickening of affected facial skin is due to a progressive increase in the diameter of the capillaries, involvement of the dermis and subcutis, fibrosis of the dermis, and, in some patients, venous channels in the subcutis.

Venous Malformation

A VM has large convoluted and interconnected anomalous venous channels dissecting the normal connective tissues, surrounding normal vessels and nerves, and threading their way through normal host structures (e.g. muscles, sweat glands). Organized thrombi, phleboliths (round calcifications) and Masson's papillary endothelial hyperplasia are frequently observed. Anomalous vessels of a VM have a continuous flat endothelium and a thin basement membrane. Their walls have discontinuous media due to foci with a relative lack or absence of smooth muscle cells.

Lymphatic Malformation

LMs of the microcystic type ('lymphangioma') exhibit enlarged distorted irregular lymphatic channels with varying numbers of smooth muscle cells in their walls and a very thin endothelium, sometimes barely visible. Some larger polyhedral lymphatic vessels may exhibit valves, and they are usually separated by fibrous septa. The lymphatic clefts dissect the host connective tissues. Hyperkeratotic epidermis may overly some clusters of dermal lymphatic vesicles. LMs of the macrocystic type ('hygroma') are composed of large lymphatic cisterns, often interconnected with thinner channels. Vesicles and large cysts in LMs usually contain watery, yellowish or pink fluid, lymphocytes, and macrophages; however, hemorrhage can be seen.

Arteriovenous Malformation

AVMs have blood vessels with irregularly thickened walls, usually randomly distributed in the dermis and other involved tissues. Direct communications between vessels with different elastic components, probably arteries and veins, may be seen, and they represent the AV shunting. A capillary component is obvious histologically, and it may have a lobular architecture or dissect the surrounding muscles. In the papillary dermis overlying an AVM nidus, numerous branching capillaries are commonly observed.

DIFFERENTIAL DIAGNOSIS

Occasionally, inflammatory disorders and neoplasms are misdiagnosed as vascular anomalies. Errors in diagnosis amongst the vascular anomalies are usually made when signs, for example, morphology, color, distribution, palpation characteristics (softness vs firmness, increased warmth, thrill) or auscultation results (presence or absence of bruit) are not synthesized with the symptoms and natural history of the lesion. The color (red or blue) of a lesion and the location of a mass underneath normal skin can represent potentially misleading clinical signs.

Some patients with the clinical diagnosis of PWS actually have erythematous lesions of lupus erythematosus or plaque-type angiofibroma. Because of their deep blue color, cases of nevus of Ota and Ito and extensive Mongolian spots (either isolated or as part of phakomatosis pigmentovascularis) have been misdiagnosed as VMs. Masses beneath normal skin erroneously diagnosed as macrocystic LM include:

- in infants or children: lipoblastoma, teratoma, bronchogenic cyst, branchial cyst, thyroglossal duct cyst, infantile myofibromatosis of intramuscular location, and infantile hemangiopericytoma with a central cyst
- in adults: cases of B-cell lymphoma in the parotid area.

An infantile hemangiopericytoma rapidly growing in the cheek may be misdiagnosed as an AVM because of fast-flow characteristics on ultrasound, Doppler ultrasound, and arteriography; however, MRI will indicate a tumor with high-flow vessels, and a biopsy establishes the diagnosis.

In adults with Crohn's disease, lymphangiectasias may develop in the anogenital region (particularly in women); they are indistinguishable from microcystic tissue-infiltrating LMs.

Telangiectasia macularis eruptiva perstans, a type of mastocytosis seen mainly in adults, may mimic a CM. Profuse telangiectasias of the face and neck were reported in aluminum workers; they may look like CM, but they are acquired. Profuse linear telangiectases of the thorax have been reported in HIV-positive homosexual young men[41].

TREATMENT

Obviously, vascular malformations are a heterogeneous group of lesions and no single treatment exists.

Capillary Malformation

Both PWSs and telangiectasias are currently best treated with flashlamp-pumped pulsed dye lasers[42] (FPDL; see Ch. 137). This treatment of PWSs has been reported as very effective, with few adverse reactions, and this was confirmed by many authors in the 1990s; however, not all lesions respond well[43,44]. Areas with a poor response (despite numerous treatment sessions) have been identified, including the malar areas of the face and the distal limbs. The treatment is safe, with a low risk of atrophic or hypertrophic scars, hypopigmentation, or postinflammatory hyperpigmentation; when the latter occurs, it usually resolves over a 6- to 12-month period[43]. Patients less than 1 year old tend to respond better, particularly if their PWS is small (less than 20 cm²)[44]. It seems that early intervention in infants less than 1 year of age using a modified FPDL with a longer wavelength, broader pulse width, higher energy fluence (11–12 J/cm²) and dynamic cooling spray can result in better lightening or clearing of PWSs, with minimal risk of adverse effects[45]. The cryogen spray delivered prior to each pulse of FPDL also has some anesthetic effect, and this, combined with the use of EMLA® cream (lidocaine 2.5%, prilocaine 2.5%) under occlusion for 2 hours before the laser treatment procedure, limits the use of general anesthesia in children.

Patients with a PWS and pigmented skin (skin phototype V) may have side effects such as hypo- or hyperpigmentation and scarring more frequently than do patients with lighter skin types; however, they should not be excluded from FPDL treatment, as some of them may achieve a good response[46]. Recurrences and re-darkening of the stain after cessation of treatment has been reported[46a]. However, when recurrent and non-recurrent lesions were compared, no differences with regard to the size of the lesions or energy densities used for therapy were observed. Relapses are less common in the younger age group, suggesting that the age at the beginning of the therapy may influence the outcome[47]. Psychological distress of parents of children with facial PWS seems to be alleviated when laser treatments begin early in life, before school age. This gives their children a better chance for a healthy psychological development.

Facial and gingival PWSs with hyperplastic changes need specific management. The cobblestone appearance of the V2 skin or nose may require excision or dermabrasion before the FPDL treatment. Orthodontic management and orthognathic surgery may be indicated when there is gaping between teeth and open-bite deformities. Correction of macrocheilia during adolescence or adulthood will restore fully competent lips.

Treatment of a patient with Sturge–Weber syndrome is multidisciplinary; anticonvulsants are the mainstay of the neurologic treatment regimen. Phenobarbital may interfere with the development of cognitive functions in infants, so the recommended drugs are carbamazepine, benzodiazepines or, in countries where it is licensed, vigabatrin (not available in the US). In selected patients with uncontrolled severe seizures, surgery (including focal resection, callosotomy or hemispherectomy) is considered. Glaucoma responds to medications or surgical treatment[16]. PWS treatment with the PDL can begin in infancy. Psychological support for the patient and family is important because of the psychosocial impact and emotional distress linked to the presence of the facial PWS, poor control of seizures, and the variety of problems encountered by and with a mentally impaired child or adolescent[17]. In the US, since 1987, the Sturge–Weber Foundation

(SWF) has actively supported parents, affected children and adults, and also professionals through grants for medical research.

Venous Malformation

From a cosmetic and functional point of view, satisfactory treatment of a cephalic VM requires multiple procedures, over several years, by adolescence and young adulthood. Percutaneous sclerotherapy[48] with pure ethanol or Ethibloc® (a mixture of zein, sodium amidotrizoate, oleum papaveris, propylene glycol and ethanol) (for deeper lesions), or sclerosants commonly used for varicose veins (for superficial blue lesions), is combined with surgical excisions. Most commonly, surgical procedures address the oral region, including lip harmonization, naso-labial cutaneous and muscular surgery, commissuroplasty, and orthognathic surgery after orthodontic treatment to correct gaping between the teeth. The aim is to maintain facial symmetry, to save facial muscular functions, and to restore the dynamics of the smile. Limb VMs may benefit from sclerotherapy and resection, however, many of them are too extensive and invasive, and elastic stockings to prevent swelling and pain may be the only advisable treatment. Control of the chronic coagulopathy requires low-molecular-weight heparin therapy[31].

Lymphatic Malformations

Microcystic LMs are excised with direct linear closure, if they are not too extensive; larger lesions require either split-thickness grafts or inflation of skin expanders before resection, to allow an adequate covering of the surgical wound. A macrocystic LM is best treated initially with percutaneous sclerotherapy. A number of sclerosing agents have been used, including killed bacteria (picibani®; OK-432®), Ethibloc®, pure ethanol and doxycycline, each of them creating an inflammatory reaction with subsequent fibrosis and shrinking of the treated cysts. Procedures can be repeated as long as necessary. A surgical approach is a second-line therapy, if sclerotherapy fails or gives incomplete results. Severe, extensive, combined LMs may be unmanageable[48a].

Arteriovenous Malformations

Head and neck stage 2 and 3 AVMs are widely excised after careful preoperative embolization (using either the arterial route alone or both arterial and direct puncture approaches) to prevent excessive intra-operative bleeding. In many of these patients, direct linear closure is impossible and reconstruction will require skin grafts or free tissue transfer[2]. Free vascularized flaps, and notably a large latissimus dorsalis micro-anastomosed free flap, may be used to cover the surgical defect. This technique gives good functional results, but cosmetic sequelae are also important. Subtotal excision frequently results in rapid progression of the AVM, with recruitment of adjacent vessels and apparently true angiogenesis. Conservative management is usually recommended for stage 1 and early stage 2 lesions, if postsurgical cosmetic results might be worse than the lesion itself. However, resection of these early stages has been recommended in order to prevent further progression.

Embolization alone usually cannot cure a superficial AVM. The best embolic agent is pure ethanol, but it poses substantial risks during and after anesthesia, depending on the injected dose[49]. Embolization is indispensable when a complication, usually hemorrhage, occurs, and it may be a life-saving treatment. Distal upper or lower extremity AVMs are rarely controlled long term by embolotherapy, alone or in association with nidus resection; complicated lesions with extreme pain, necrosis, ulcerations and bleeding may require amputation.

A *complex-combined* vascular malformation of the limbs requires a specially tailored management plan, depending on the location and associated symptoms. Long-term orthopedic evaluation and follow-up is a major component of the supportive care plan for lower extremity lesions during the growth period. Vascular treatments – for example, laser, sclerotherapy of varicose veins or varicose vein surgery in Klippel–Trenaunay syndrome, and arterial embolization and resection of the AV nidus in Parkes Weber syndrome – rarely give satisfactory results. Elastic stockings and a compensatory shoe-lift are indispensable. Epiphysiodesis is considered, before the end of the growth period, to allow correction of leg-length discrepancy in Klippel–Trenaunay syndrome, but it can worsen the vascular disease in Parkes Weber syndrome[50].

REFERENCES

1. Enjolras O, Mulliken JB. Vascular tumors and vascular malformations (new issues). Adv Dermatol. 1997;13:375–423.
2. Kohout MP, Hansen M, Pribaz JJ, et al. Arteriovenous malformations of the head and neck: natural history and management. Plast Reconstr Surg. 1998;102:643–5.
3. Mulliken JB, Glowacki J. Hemangiomas and vascular malformations in infants and children: a classification based on endothelial characteristics. Plast Reconstr Surg. 1982;69:412–22.
4. Takahashi K, Mulliken JB, Kozakewich HP, et al. Cellular markers that distinguish the phases of hemangioma during infancy and childhood. J Clin Invest. 1994;93:2357–64.
5. Wassef M, Enjolras O. Les malformations vasculaires superficielles: classification et histopathologie. Ann Pathol. 1999;19:253–64.
6. Vikkula M, Boon LM, Mulliken JB. Molecular basis of vascular anomalies. Trends Cardiovasc Med. 1998;8:281–92.
7. Vikkula M, Boon LM, Carraway KL III, et al. Vascular dysmorphogenesis caused by an activating mutation in the receptor tyrosine kinase TIE2. Cell. 1996; 87:1181–90.
8. Irrthum A, Brouillard P, Enjolras O, et al. Linkage disequilibrium narrows locus for venous malformation with glomus cells (VMGLOM) to a single 1.48 Mbp YAC. Eur J Hum Genet. 2001;9:34–8.
9. Eerola L, Boon LM, Mulliken JB, et al. Capillary malformation-arteriovenous malformation: a new clinical and genetic disorder caused by *RASA1* mutations. Am J Hum Genet. 2003;73:1240–9.
10. Klapman MH, Yao JF. Thickening and nodules in port-wine stains. J Am Acad Dermatol. 2001;44:300–2.
11. Adams BB, Lucky AW. Acquired port-wine stains and antecedent trauma: case report and review of the literature. Arch Dermatol. 2000;136:897–9.
12. Tavafoghi V, Ghandchi A, Hambrick GW Jr, et al. Cutaneous signs of spinal dysraphism. Report of a patient with a tail-like lipoma and review of 200 cases in the literature. Arch Dermatol. 1978;114:573–7.
13. Guggisberg D, Hadj-Rabia S, Viney C, et al. Skin markers of occult spinal dysraphism in children. A review of 54 cases. Arch Dermatol. 2004;140:1109–15.
14. Enjolras O, Riché MC, Merland JJ. Facial port-wine stains and Sturge-Weber syndrome. Pediatrics. 1985;76:48–51.
14a. Mazereeuw-Hautier J, Syed S, Harper J. Bilateral facial capillary malformation associated with eye and brain abnormalities. Arch Dermatol 2006;142:994–8.
15. Kramer U, Kahana E, Shorer Z, et al. Outcome of infants with Sturge-Weber syndrome and early onset seizures. Dev Med Child Neurol. 2000;42:756–9.
16. Maari C, Frieden IJ. Klippel-Trenaunay syndrome: the importance of "geographic stains" in identifying lymphatic disease and risk of complications. J Am Acad Dermatol. 2004;51:391–8.
17. Turner JT, Cohen MM, Biesecker LG. Reassessment of the Proteus syndrome literature: application of diagnostic criteria to published cases. Am J Med Genet. 2004;130A:111–22.
18. Enjolras O. Cutis marmorata telangiectatica congenita. Ann Dermatol Venereol. 2001;128:161–6.
19. Devillers ACA, de Waard-van der Spek FB, Oranje AP. Cutis marmorata telangiectatica congenita: clinical features in 35 cases. Arch Dermatol. 1999;135:34–8.
20. Ben Amitai D, Fichman S, Merlob P, et al. Cutis marmorata telangiectatica congenita: clinical findings in 85 patients. Pediatr Dermatol. 2000;17:100–4.
21. Gerritsen MJP, Steijlen PM, Brunner HG, Rieu P. Cutis marmorata telangiectatica congenita: report of 18 cases. Br J Dermatol. 2000;142:366–9.
22. McDonald JE, Miller FJ, Hallam SE, et al. Clinical manifestations in a large hereditary hemorrhagic telangiectasia (HHT) type 2 kindred. Am J Med Genet. 2000;14:320–7.
23. Cymerman U, Vera S, Pece BN, et al. Identification of hereditary hemorrhagic telangiectasia type 1 in newborns by protein expression and mutation analysis of endoglin. Pediatr Res. 2000;47:24–35.
24. Wallace GM, Shovlin CL. A hereditary haemorrhagic telangiectasia family with pulmonary involvement is unlinked to the known HHT genes, endoglin and ALK-1. Thorax. 2000;55:685–90.
25. Begbie ME, Wallace GMF, Shovlin CL. Hereditary haemorrhagic telangiectasia (Osler-Weber-Rendu syndrome). A view from the 21st century. Postgrad Med J. 2003;79:18–24.
25a. Tennant LB, Mulliken JB, Perez-Atayde AR, Kozakewich HP. Verrucous hemangioma revisited. Pediatr Dermatol. 2006;23:208–15.
26. Brady RO, Schiffmann R. Clinical features of and recent advances in therapy for Fabry disease. JAMA. 2000;284:2771–5.
27. Fleming C, Rennie A, Fallowfield M, McHenry PM. Cutaneous manifestations of fucosidosis. Br J Dermatol. 1997;136:594–7.
28. Labauge P, Enjolras O, Bonerandi JJ, et al. An association between autosomal dominant cerebral cavernomas and a distinctive hyperkeratotic capillaro-venous cutaneous vascular malformation in 4 families. Ann Neurol. 1999;45:250–4.
29. Enjolras O, Wassef M, Brocheriou-Spelle I, et al. L'hémangiome sinusoidal, un diagnostic histologique. Ann Dermatol Venereol. 1998;125:575–80.
30. Trop I, Dubois J, Guibaud L, et al. Soft-tissue venous malformations in pediatric and young adult patients: diagnosis with Doppler US. Radiology. 1999;212:841–5.
31. Mazoyer E, Enjolras O, Laurian C, et al. Coagulation abnormalities associated with extensive venous malformations of the limbs. Clin Haematol Oncol 2002;24:243–51.
31a. Mallory SB, Enjolras O, Boon LM, et al. Congenital plaque-type glomuvenous malformations presenting in childhood. Arch Dermatol. 2006;142:892–6.
32. Boon LM, Mulliken JB, Enjolras O, et al. Glomuvenous malformation (glomangioma) and venous

malformation: distinct clinicopathologic and genetic entities. Arch Dermatol. 2004;140:971–6.

32a. Brouillard P, Ghassibe M, Penington A, et al. Four common glomulin mutations cause two thirds of glomuvenous malformations ('familial glomangiomas'): evidence for a founder effect. Online Report. J Med Genet. 2005;42:e13.

33. Padwa BL, Hayward PG, Ferraro NF, Mulliken JB. Cervicofacial lymphatic malformation: clinical course, surgical intervention, and pathogenesis of skeletal hypertrophy. Plast Reconstr Surg. 1995;95:951–60.

34. Hartl DM, Roger G, Denoyelle F, et al. Extensive lymphangioma presenting with upper airway obstruction. Arch Otolaryngol Head Neck Surg. 2000;126:1378–82.

35. Enjolras O, Logeart I, Gelbert F, et al. Malformations artérioveineuses: étude de 200 cas. Ann Dermatol Venereol. 2000;127:17–22.

36. Wu JK, Bisdorff A, Gelbert F, et al. Auricular arteriovenous malformation: evaluation, management, and outcome. Plast Reconstr Surg. 2005;115:985–95.

37. Paltiel HJ, Burrows PE, Kozakewich HPW, et al. Soft-tissue vascular anomalies: utility of US for diagnosis. Radiology. 2000;214:747–54.

38. Binkert CA, Kollas SS, Valavanis A. Spinal cord vascular disease: characterization with fast three-dimensional contrast-enhanced MR angiography. Am J Neuroradiol. 1999;20:1785–93.

39. Bhattacharya JJ, Luo CB, Suh DC, et al. Wyburn-Mason or Bonnet-Dechaume-Blanc as cerebrofacial arteriovenous metameric syndromes (CAMS). Intervent Neuroradiol. 2001;7:5–17.

39a. Boon LM, Mulliken JB, Vikkula M. RASA1: variable phenotype with capillary and arteriovenous malformations. Curr Opin Genet Dev. 2005;15:265–9.

40. Requena L, Sangueza OP. Cutaneous vascular anomalies. Part I. Hamartomas, malformations, and dilatation of preexisting vessels. J Am Acad Dermatol. 1997;37:523–49.

41. MacFarlane DF, Gregory N. Telangiectases in human immunodeficiency virus-positive patients. Cutis. 1994;53:79–80.

42. Tan OT, Sherwood K, Gilchrest BA. Treatment of children with port-wine stains using the flashlamp-pulsed tunable dye laser. N Engl J Med. 1989;320:416–21.

43. Seukeran DC, Collins P, Sheehan-Dare RA. Adverse reactions following pulsed tunable dye laser treatment of port wine stains in 701 patients. Br J Dermatol. 1997;136:725–9.

44. Nguyen CM, Yohn JJ, Huff C, et al. Facial port wine stains in childhood: prediction of the rate of improvement as a function of the age of the patient, size and location of the port wine stain and the number of treatments with the pulsed dye (585nm) laser. Br J Dermatol. 1998;138:821–5.

45. Geronemus RG, Quintana AT, Lou WW, et al. High-fluence modified pulsed dye laser photocoagulation with dynamic cooling of port-wine stains in infancy. Arch Dermatol. 2000;136:942–3.

46. Sommer S, Sheehan-Dare RA. Pulsed dye laser treatment of port-wine stains in pigmented skin. J Am Acad Dermatol. 2000;42:667–71.

46a. Huikeshoven M, Koster PHL, de Borgie CAJM, et al. Redarkening of portwine stains 10 years after pulsed dye laser treatment. N Eng J Med. 2007;356:1235–40.

47. Michel S, Landthaler M, Hohenleutner U. Recurrence of port-wine stains after treatment with the flashlamp-pumped pulsed dye laser. Br J Dermatol. 2000;143:1230–4.

48. Berenguer B, Burrows PE, Zurakowski D, et al. Sclerotherapy of craniofacial venous malformations: complications and results. Plast Reconstr Surg. 1999;104:1–15.

48a. Okazaki T, Iwatani S, Yanai T, et al. Treatment of lymphangioma in children: our experience of 128 cases. J Pediatr Surg. 2007;42:386–9.

49. Mason KP, Michna E, Zurakowski D, et al. Serum ethanol levels in children and adults after ethanol embolization or sclerotherapy for vascular anomalies. Radiology. 2000;217:127–32.

50. Enjolras O, Chapot R, Merland JJ. Vascular anomalies and the growth of limbs: a review. J Pediatr Orthop B. 2004;13:349–57.

Ulcers

Tania Phillips

Key features

- The history should include onset, course, symptoms, exacerbating and alleviating factors, past medical history, family history, social history, travel and medications
- Important aspects of the physical examination include location, size and shape of the ulcer, characteristics of the ulcer edge and base, and associated physical findings
- Helpful laboratory tests include vascular studies, blood tests, cultures and biopsy
- A biopsy of non-healing chronic ulcers is indicated to exclude carcinoma or other underlying diseases
- In addition to local care, therapy of ulcers should aim to correct or treat the underlying cause:
  - Venous insufficiency: compression
  - Arterial insufficiency: surgery
  - Neuropathic or pressure ulcer: relief of pressure
  - Infection: antibiotics
  - Neoplasm: surgery, chemotherapy, radiotherapy
  - Vasculopathy: treat the underlying cause of the occlusive disorder
  - Vasculitis or other inflammatory process (e.g. pyoderma gangrenosum): corticosteroids, immunosuppressive agents
- A key factor in therapy is the promotion of wound healing:
  - Debridement: mechanical, enzymatic, autolytic
  - Dressings: maintain a moist wound environment
  - Infection control: antibiotics
  - Skin grafting or skin substitutes
  - Growth factors

INTRODUCTION

Leg and pressure ulcers represent a significant portion of the burden of skin disease, and they affect the healthcare system in terms of skilled medical intervention, cost of supplies, and patient suffering. Identifying patients at risk and initiating appropriate measures are important preventive steps. This chapter addresses current concepts regarding definitions, epidemiology, pathogenesis, clinical features, differential diagnosis, and management of the most common types of leg ulcers and pressure ulcers.

A wound is any break in skin integrity causing loss of anatomic structure and function, and it may be the result of internal and/or external pathologic processes. An ulcer is a wound with loss of epidermal and dermal layers, in contrast to an erosion, which is a loss of the epidermal layer only. Wounds may be classified as acute or chronic[1]. Acute wounds are usually repaired in an orderly and timely manner (see Ch. 141), and anatomic and functional integrity are maintained once the wound is healed. Chronic wounds remain in a persistent inflammatory and/or proliferative state and accumulate components, e.g. metalloproteinases, collagenase and elastase, which prematurely degrade collagen and growth factors. This chronic inflammatory state impairs wound healing[2,2a]. The most common chronic cutaneous wounds

include venous, arterial and neuropathic leg ulcers, which are reviewed in the first part of this chapter. Another common type of chronic wound is the pressure ulcer, which is discussed in the second part of this chapter.

HISTORY

Therapies for open wounds can be traced back to over 3500 years ago, and they have evolved into the myriad of wound dressings commercially available today. The Edwin Smith papyrus (1615 BC) described the application of a fresh piece of meat to a wound, followed by an ointment composed of honey and grease. Hippocrates (460–375 BC) cleansed wounds with seawater or wine and then allowed them to 'breathe' without any bandages or topical agents. Celsus (30 BC–50 AD) also did not endorse any special dressings for wounds, although for patients insistent on applying something, he recommended 'barabarum', composed of alum, verdigris, litharge, dried pitch, dried pine resin, oil and vinegar, covered with a linen bandage. Guy de Chauliac (1300–1367) suggested applying egg whites and wine to wounds, and Ambroise Pare (1510–1590) used egg yolks, rose oil and turpentine. Cesare Magati in 1616, and later Vincenz von Kern (1760–1829), recommended bandages moistened with plain water as wound dressings[3].

Lord Joseph Lister (1827–1912) introduced antimicrobial therapy and inhibited microbial growth with bandages soaked in crude carbolic acid. William Stewart Halsted (1852–1912) originated the silver foil dressing in 1896. In 1948, Oscar Gilje applied adhesive tape to wounds and discovered improved healing, which he attributed to bacteriostatic and occlusive effects. By 1958, Odland discovered that an unbroken blister healed more rapidly than a broken one, and in 1962 Winter demonstrated that wounds in domestic pigs re-epithelialized faster under occlusion with polyethylene film, thus marking the origin of occlusive dressings. Similar beneficial effects of occlusion in human wounds were demonstrated in 1963 by Hinman and colleagues[3].

LEG ULCERS

Chronic leg ulcers are open wounds, often below the knee, which fail to heal within a period of 6 weeks[4]. Although they can have numerous causes, most leg ulcers are secondary to venous insufficiency, arterial disease, neuropathy or a combination of these factors (Table 105.1). Other conditions that can cause leg ulcers are listed in Figure 105.1[5,5a].

EPIDEMIOLOGY

In the US, approximately 2.5 million people suffer from leg ulcers and an estimated 2 million workdays per year are lost because of leg ulcers[6]. The incidence and prevalence of these problems increase as the population ages[7]. The current annual direct cost of skin ulcers and wound healing in the US is estimated at $8–10 billion. Approximately 1.5 million skin grafts or amputations are required per year for ulcerations of the lower extremities[5]. Venous disease is responsible for approximately 72% of leg ulcers, whereas 22% have a mixed venous and arterial etiology[8]. Only about 6% are due to pure arterial disease.

Venous Ulcers

The exact prevalence of venous leg ulcers is unknown, but European studies have reported prevalence rates ranging from 0.18% to 1%[4,9–13]. In the US, it is estimated that between 600 000 and 2.5 million individuals are affected[7]. Prevalence increases with age, as demonstrated by

COMPARISON OF CLINICAL FINDINGS IN THE THREE MAJOR TYPES OF LEG ULCERS

	Venous	Arterial	Neuropathic/mal perforans*
Location	Medial malleolar region	Pressure sites Distal points (toes)	Pressure sites
Morphology	Irregular borders	Dry, necrotic base 'Punched out'	'Punched out'
Surrounding skin	Pigmentation secondary to hemosiderin Lipodermatosclerosis	Shiny atrophic skin with hair loss	Thick callus
Other physical examination findings	Varicosities Leg/ankle edema ± Stasis dermatitis ± Lymphedema	Weak/absent peripheral pulses Prolonged capillary refill time (>3–4 s) Pallor on leg elevation (45° for 1 min) Dependent rubor	Peripheral neuropathy with decreased sensation ± Foot deformities

*Most commonly due to diabetes mellitus.

Table 105.1 Comparison of clinical findings in the three major types of leg ulcers. Adapted with permission from Phillips TJ, Dover JS. Leg ulcers. J Am Acad Dermatol. 1991;25:965–87.

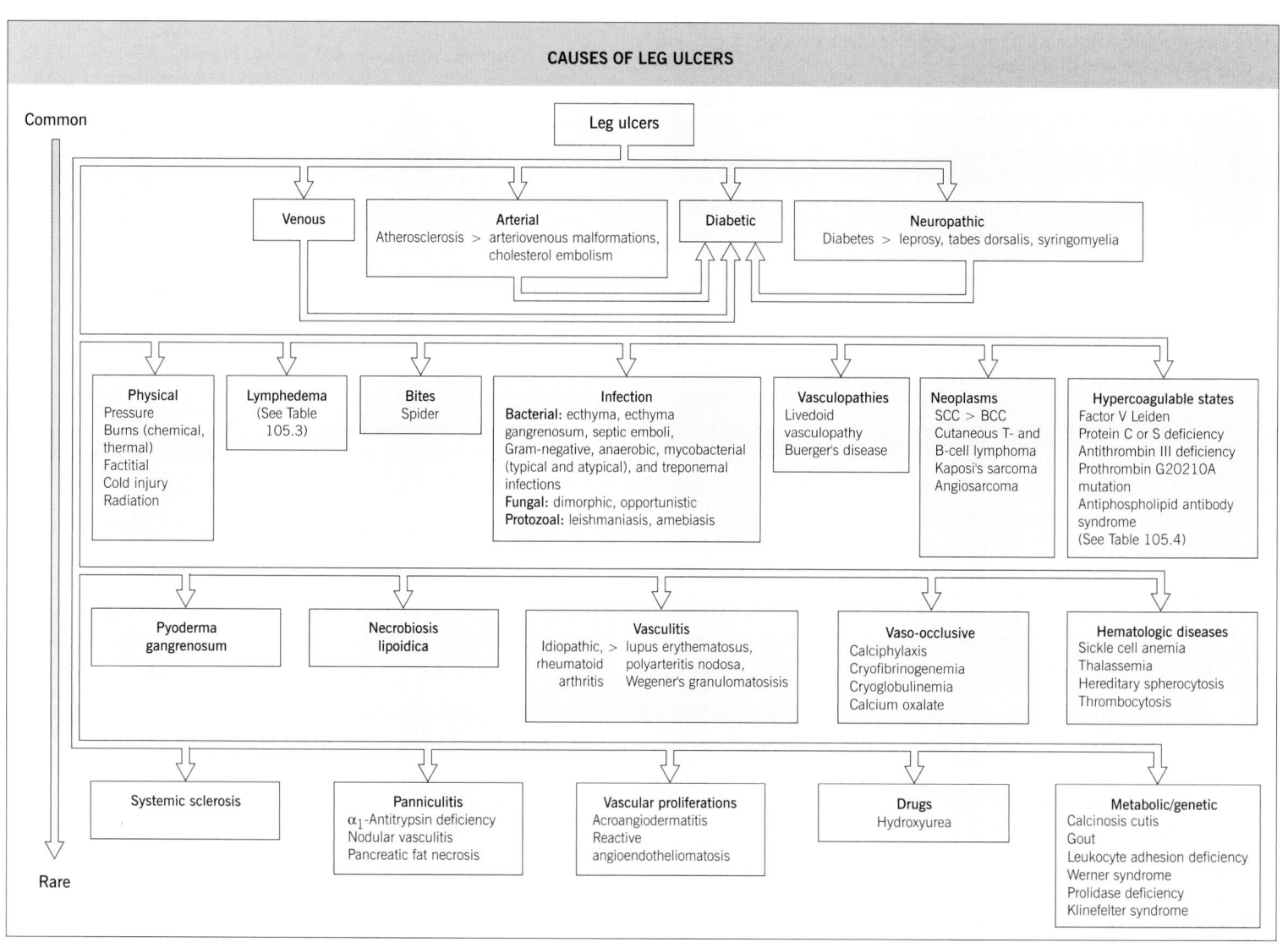

Fig. 105.1 Causes of leg ulcers.

one study which found that >85% of those affected were over 64 years of age[4]. Risk factors for the development of leg ulcers include obesity and a history of significant leg injury, deep venous thrombosis and/or phlebitis[5,14,15]. In addition, the factor V Leiden mutation is more prevalent in patients with venous ulcers than in the general population. The incidence of venous ulcers is equal in men and women[16].

The recurrence rate can be over 70%, especially in ulcers of more than 1 year's duration. Other factors associated with poor prognosis include a large wound area, the presence of fibrin on more than 50% of

the wound surface, an ankle–brachial pressure index (ABI) of less than 0.8, and a history of venous ligation or venous stripping[17].

Arterial Ulcers

The prevalence of peripheral arterial disease is approximately 10% in the general population over the age of 45 years. Major risk factors are age >40 years, cigarette smoking and diabetes mellitus. Hyperlipidemia, hypertension, hyperhomocysteinemia, male gender, and sedentary lifestyle are also important risk factors. Peripheral arterial disease increases the risk of death from cardiovascular causes even in the absence of a history of a myocardial infarction or ischemic stroke[18].

Neuropathic and Diabetic Ulcers

The most common cause of neuropathic foot ulcers in the US is diabetes mellitus. Approximately 20% of the 16 million people in the US known to have diabetes will develop an ulcerated foot at some time during their lifetime[19]. Of these, 15–25% will require an amputation[20]. The major cause of non-traumatic lower-extremity amputations in the US is in fact non-healing diabetic foot ulcers, which are responsible for 85% of all amputations[21]. Risk factors include male gender, diabetes for >10 years, poor glucose control, and associated cardiovascular, retinal or renal complications[21]. Other causes of peripheral neuropathy that are associated with neuropathic ulcers include spinal cord lesions, spina bifida, alcohol abuse, medications and leprosy.

PATHOGENESIS

Venous Ulcers

Venous ulcers are often secondary to venous reflux and/or calf muscle pump dysfunction[5,22]. Normally, the calf muscle pumps venous blood towards the heart, distally to proximally against gravity, and from the superficial to deep venous systems (Fig. 105.2)[5]. Competent one-way valves are essential for blood to flow to the heart without reflux. As calf muscles contract, the deep venous system empties and a decrease in the deep venous pressure occurs (see Fig. 155.4). As calf muscles relax, blood flows from the superficial veins through the perforating veins into the deep veins. In calf muscle pump dysfunction, the expected decrease in the venous pressure during exercise does not occur and 'venous hypertension' results. Another term for this situation is 'venous insufficiency'. It may occur with neuromuscular dysfunction, after deep venous thrombosis and/or thrombophlebitis, or with combinations of these factors[5].

The mechanism by which venous insufficiency results in ulceration is still not entirely clear, although there are a number of theories. Burnand et al.[23] postulated that distension of the capillary bed caused by venous insufficiency leads to a leakage of fibrinogen from the distended dermal capillaries. This fibrinogen then polymerizes to form fibrin cuffs, which accumulate around capillaries and deprive the surrounding tissue of oxygen and other nutrients (Fig. 105.3). This process ultimately leads to the formation of an ulcer[24]. Pericapillary fibrin cuffs have been demonstrated in patients with venous ulcers; however, it has been shown that venous ulcers will heal in spite of these cuffs[25]. Falanga & Eaglstein[26] postulated that growth factors are trapped by fibrinogen and other leaked macromolecules, such as albumin and α_2-macroglobulin. In the trapped state, these factors are unavailable for tissue repair. A third hypothesis is the theory of white cell trapping, which suggests that leukocytes adhere to the vascular endothelium, causing tissue ischemia and vascular damage by releasing mediators such as collagenase, free radicals and tumor necrosis factor (TNF), thereby resulting in increased vascular permeability and the release of fibrinogen into the pericapillary tissue[27,28].

A more recent theory states that fibroblasts present in chronic wounds such as venous ulcers become senescent and may be unable to participate in an appropriate wound healing response[29]. Harmful effects of wound fluid and its components on cellular function are also being investigated[2].

Arterial Ulcers

In arterial disease, progressive narrowing of the arterial lumen occurs as a result of accumulated cholesterol plaques, cells, matrix fibers and tissue debris. As the arterial lumen becomes progressively narrowed, blood flow gradually becomes obstructed and collateral vessels form. Insufficient arterial blood supply and/or thrombosis leads to tissue ischemia, necrosis and, ultimately, ulceration. Other causes of arterial leg ulcers include cholesterol emboli (Fig.105.4), vasospastic disease (e.g. Raynaud's), and trauma or hypothermia (e.g. frostbite)[5].

Neuropathic and Diabetic Ulcers

Neuropathy and peripheral vascular disease are probably the most important etiologic factors in the development of diabetic foot ulcers[30]. Distal symmetric neuropathy is present in over 80% of diabetic patients with foot lesions[31]. The actual mechanism by which diabetes mellitus damages blood vessels and nerves is not well understood; however, progression of neuropathy and nephropathy is known to be associated

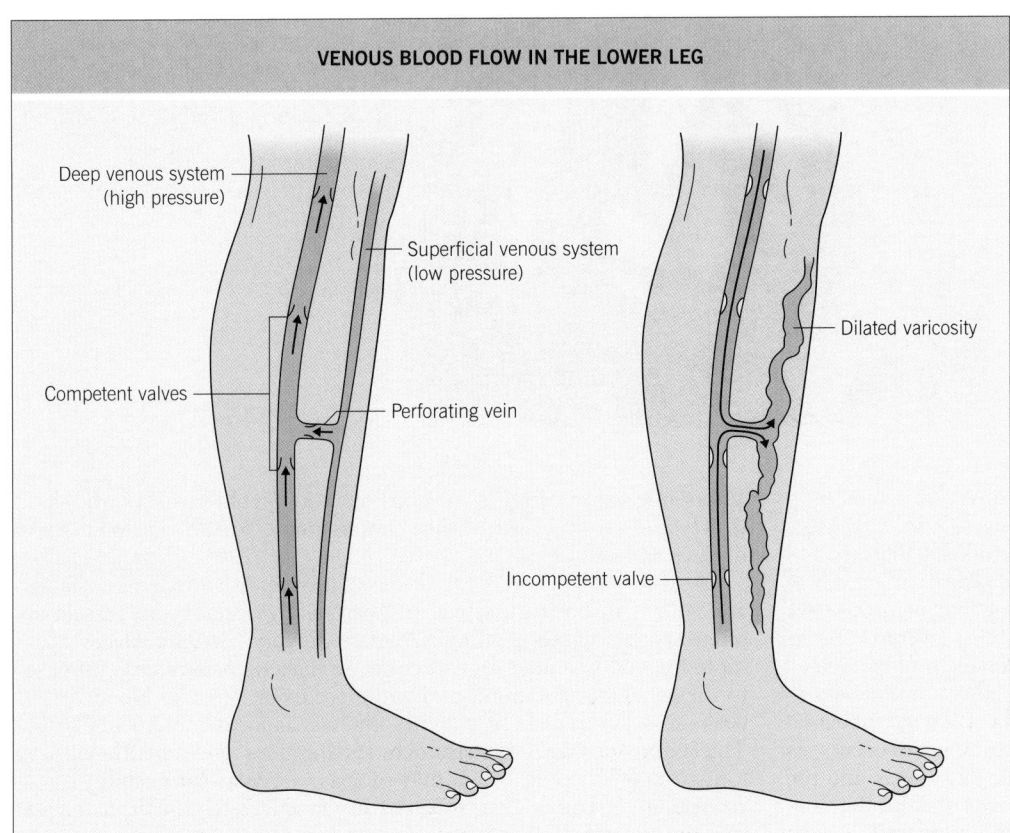

VENOUS BLOOD FLOW IN THE LOWER LEG

Deep venous system (high pressure)

Superficial venous system (low pressure)

Competent valves

Perforating vein

Dilated varicosity

Incompetent valve

Fig. 105.2 Venous blood flow in the lower leg. Normally, the calf muscle pumps venous blood towards the heart distally to proximally against gravity, and from the superficial to deep venous systems. Venous ulcers are often secondary to venous reflux and/or calf muscle pump dysfunction. In calf muscle pump dysfunction, the expected decrease in the venous pressure during exercise does not occur and 'venous hypertension' occurs.

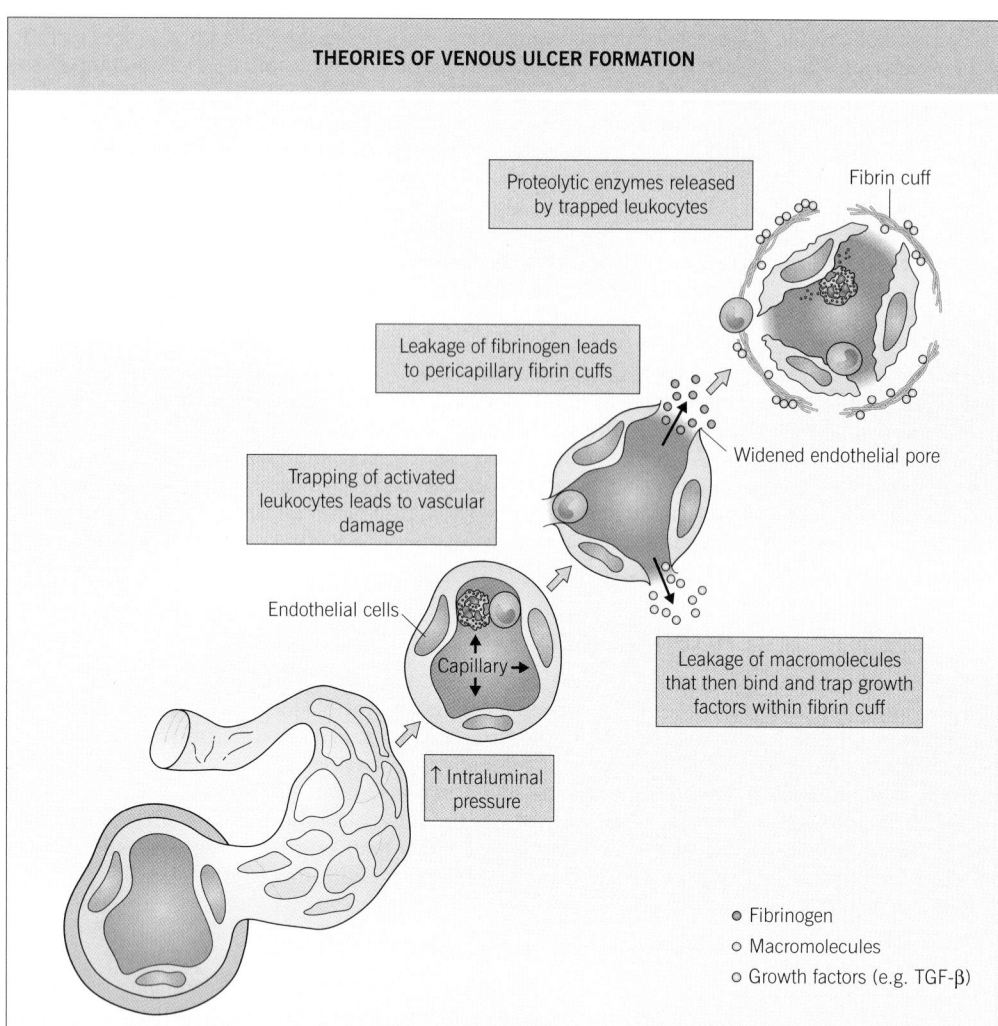

THEORIES OF VENOUS ULCER FORMATION

Proteolytic enzymes released by trapped leukocytes

Fibrin cuff

Leakage of fibrinogen leads to pericapillary fibrin cuffs

Trapping of activated leukocytes leads to vascular damage

Widened endothelial pore

Endothelial cells

Capillary →

Leakage of macromolecules that then bind and trap growth factors within fibrin cuff

↑ Intraluminal pressure

● Fibrinogen
○ Macromolecules
○ Growth factors (e.g. TGF-β)

Fig. 105.3 Theories of venous ulcer formation. The theories include the presence of pericapillary cuffs due to leakage of fibrinogen, binding of growth factors by leaked molecules, and the trapping of leukocytes with subsequent vascular damage.

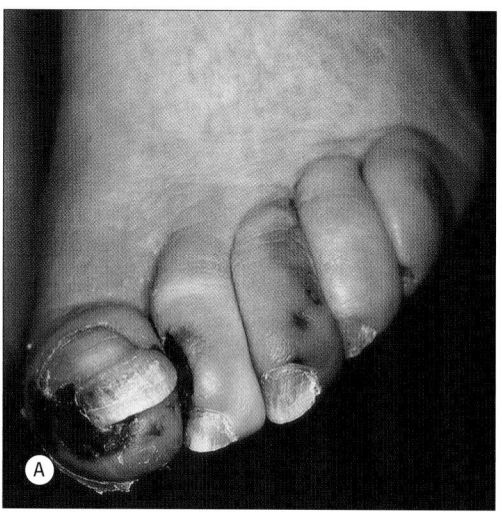

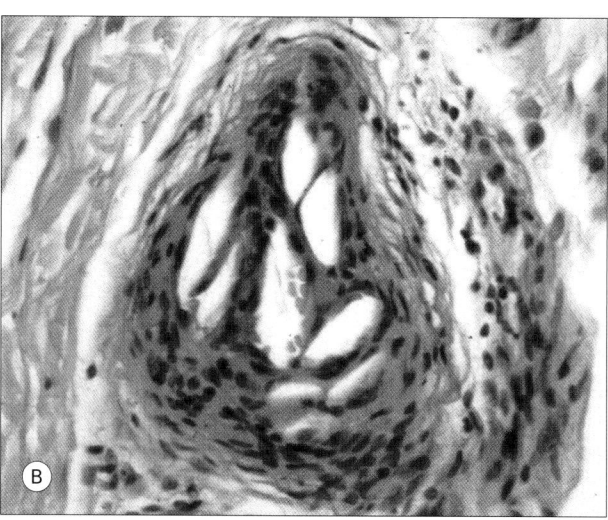

Fig. 105.4 Cholesterol emboli. A Ischemia of the toes and necrosis with early ulcer formation. **B** Histologically, intravascular clefts are observed within the vessel lumen due to dissolution of cholesterol crystals during fixation. B, Courtesy of Norbert Sepp MD.

with hemoglobin A1C (HbA1C) levels over 9%. HbA1C is a good indicator of glycemic control during the previous 90 days. A level of 3–6% is considered normal, and 7–8% reflects well-controlled diabetes[21].

Neuropathy can cause a loss of protective pain sensation as well as motor dysfunction leading to the development of foot deformities[30]. Foot deformities develop when extrinsic muscles overpower the atrophied intrinsic muscles of the foot (that are preferentially affected by motor neuropathy), causing the skin overlying bony prominences to be more prone to ulceration. Repetitive trauma, namely increased pressure, shearing and frictional forces, to bony prominences occurs, as there is loss of protective sensation. Although the toes, heels and the plantar surfaces overlying the metatarsal heads are at risk for developing ulcerations, it is the latter that most commonly ulcerate[20]. Lastly,

autonomic neuropathy is responsible for hypohidrosis of the foot, which leads to dry, brittle skin that is prone to the development of fissures and calluses[30].

Large vessels are affected in diabetics as well. Atherosclerotic changes are evident in both the tibial and peroneal vessels. Pedal vessels are often spared, which facilitates bypass surgery. Arterial ulcers occur more frequently and at an earlier age in diabetic patients as compared to the general population[5], and while occlusion of small blood vessels does not occur in diabetic patients, there is abnormal microcirculation. Thickening of capillary basement membranes and endothelial gap formation both occur, which may increase vascular permeability[5].

Wound healing is also impaired in diabetics, as growth factor and cytokine activity as well as collagen synthesis are abnormal[30]. In addition, HbA1C levels over 12% alter leukocytic functions such as chemotaxis, adherence, phagocytosis, and intracellular bactericidal activity, thereby predisposing the patient to infections[21,32].

CLINICAL FEATURES

A thorough history and physical examination are essential in elucidating the cause of an ulcer and should be performed prior to embarking upon therapy[33] (Tables 105.1 & 105.2). Figure 105.1 gives an overview of the causes of leg ulcers[33].

Venous Ulcers

Patients with venous ulcers often complain of limb heaviness, aching and/or swelling which are associated with standing and are worse at the end of the day. Shoes may become more tightly fitting in the evening. These symptoms of edema are often relieved by elevation of the limb[5]. Varicose veins of varying severity may be present. Yellow to red–brown discoloration and petechiae, secondary to hemosiderin within macrophages and extravasated red blood cells, respectively, are commonly observed in the surrounding skin. Melanin deposition sometimes also occurs. Eczematous changes (venous or stasis dermatitis) with scaling, redness, pruritus, and occasionally crusting, are almost invariably present (Fig.105.5). Chronic venous ulcer patients often suffer from allergic contact dermatitis to a variety of topical medications[22].

Lipodermatosclerosis is a common finding and represents fibrosed subcutaneous tissues (Fig. 105.6; see Ch. 100). The affected skin feels firm, indurated and 'woody', and severe lipodermatosclerosis has been associated with poor wound healing. Early or 'acute' lipodermatosclerosis presents with diffuse indurated erythema that is warm and extremely tender and may be misdiagnosed as cellulitis or erythema nodosum. An 'inverted champagne bottle' leg, in which the proximal leg swells as a result of chronic venous obstruction and the lower leg constricts because of fibrosis and loss of subcutaneous fat, represents advanced disease[25]. Lipodermatosclerosis can also develop in the dependent portions of the pannus along with chronic ulcers and lymphedema (Fig. 105.7).

Atrophie blanche (livedoid vasculopathy; livedoid vasculitis) appears as smooth, ivory white atrophic plaques of sclerosis with multiple telangiectasias (primarily at the periphery of the plaques) and surrounding brown discoloration; these changes are present in up to 40% of patients with chronic venous insufficiency. In addition, there can be painful ulcerations of varying sizes with smaller lesions often having overlying hemorrhagic crusts (Fig. 105.8). Nearly all patients with atrophie blanche show signs of venous hypertension, although the condition has been associated with several causes of hypercoagulability, e.g. antiphospholipid syndrome (see Ch. 24)[34].

Venous ulcers may be single or multiple. They are typically larger than non-venous ulcers (see Fig. 105.5) and can involve the entire circumference of the leg[22]. These ulcers are most often located along the course of the long saphenous vein where it is most superficial, i.e. in the gaiter area of the leg, extending from the lower medial calf to just below the medial malleolus (see Fig. 105.6)[22]. Venous ulcers are generally irregularly shaped and shallow in depth (relative to surface area), and have edges that are usually flat or sloping. The wound bed is most often covered with a yellow fibrinous exudate which, when removed, reveals a healthy red granulation tissue base[5].

Lymphedema

Venous hypertension may occur simultaneously with lymphedema, and sometimes the two may be clinically indistinguishable. In a normal leg, the lymphatic channels run parallel to the venous blood vessels and may become incompetent and dilated with repeated tissue injury due

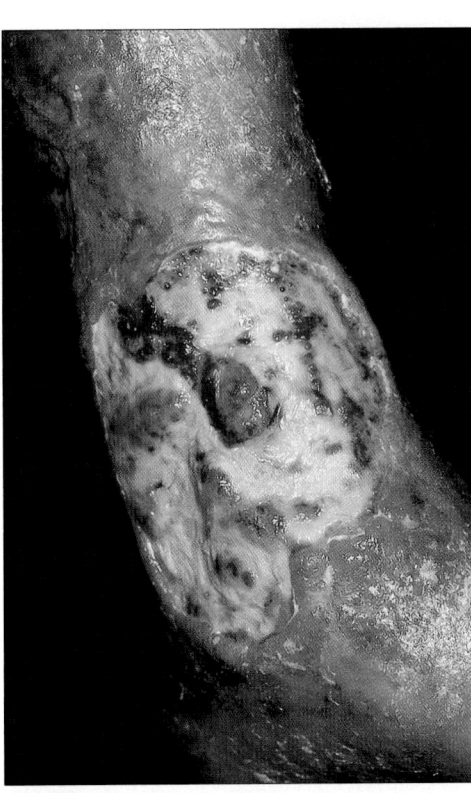

Fig. 105.5 Venous ulcer and stasis dermatitis. Note the erythema, crusting and scaling of the skin surrounding the ulcer of the medial malleolus. Granulation tissue is seen in approximately 15% of the ulcer bed.

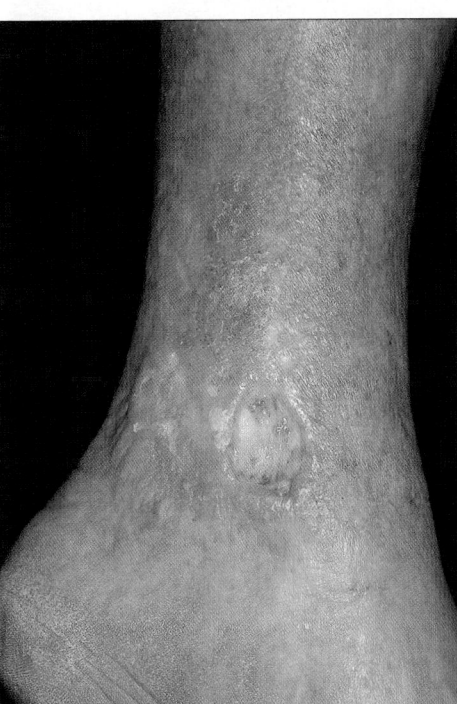

Fig. 105.6 Venous ulcer of the medial malleolus. This is a common site for this type of ulcer. Induration due to lipodermatosclerosis, hemosiderin deposition, and atrophie blanche scars were present in the surrounding skin. Courtesy of Jean L Bolognia MD.

POINTS TO INCLUDE IN THE HISTORY AND PHYSICAL EXAMINATION OF PATIENTS WITH A LEG ULCER	
History	**Physical examination**

• Onset and clinical course of ulcer
• Symptoms, including those of vascular disease or neuropathy
• Alleviating factors
• Exacerbating factors
• Past medical history, e.g. diabetes mellitus, ASCVD, autoimmune CTD
• Family history
• Medications, topical and systemic
• Personal habits (e.g. smoking, alcohol intake)
	General, emphasizing the following:
	• Ulcer characteristics
	  – Location and size
	  – Morphology, including depth, shape, border and base
	  – Surrounding skin, e.g. edema, dermatitis, fibrosis, cellulitis, necrosis
	• Peripheral pulses
	• Capillary refill time
	• Evidence of peripheral neuropathy
	• Deep tendon reflexes

Table 105.2 Points to include in the history and physical examination of patients with a leg ulcer. ASCVD, atherosclerotic cardiovascular disease; CTD, connective tissue disease. Adapted with permission from Kanj LF, Phillips TJ. Management of leg ulcers. Fitpatrick's J Clin Dermatol. 1994;Sept/Oct:52–60.

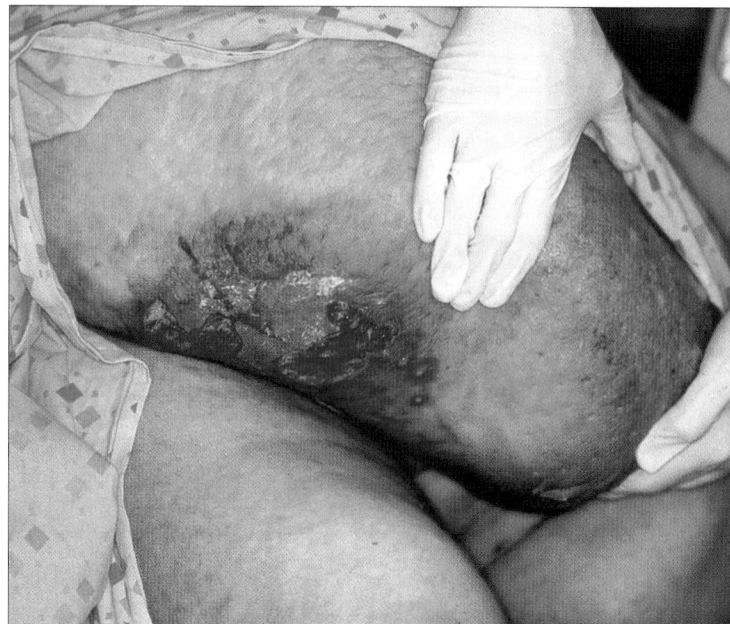

Fig. 105.7 Lipodermatosclerosis, chronic ulceration and lymphedema of the dependent portion of the pannus. The changes are similar to those seen on the distal lower extremities.

to infections (e.g. cellulitis) or venous ulcers. The term 'lymphedema' refers to the accumulation of lymph fluid within extravascular tissues, and it is classified into primary and secondary forms (Table 105.3).

Primary lymphedema is further classified according to the age at which the disorder presents. Congenital lymphedema is either present at birth or appears within the first 2 years of life (Fig. 105.9). Lymphedema praecox typically manifests at the time of puberty, whereas lymphedema tarda usually presents after the age of 35 years[35]. The protein constituents of static lymph fluid can cause inflammation and subsequent tissue fibrosis. In patients with lymphedema, the overlying skin may develop cobblestoning as well as a verrucous or mossy appearance. The differential diagnosis of lymphedema includes lipedema, in which there is bilateral swelling of the lower extremities but sparing of the feet.

Elephantiasis nostras is a complication of chronic lymphedema and is characterized by hyperkeratosis, verrucous changes and fibrosis (Fig. 105.10), as well as massive enlargement of the affected body part, usually the lower legs or scrotum. Other sites that may be affected are amputation stumps and the abdominal pannus, and rarely the periorbital area or the oral mucosa. Synonyms for elephantiasis nostras include mossy leg, lymphangitis recurrens elephantogenica, and elephantiasis nostras verrucosa. 'Nostras' means 'of our region', and the term is often used to designate the non-filiarial form of elephantiasis.

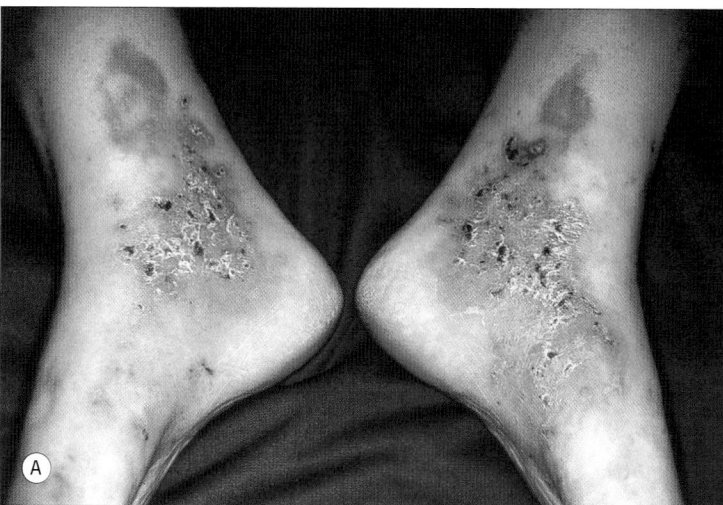

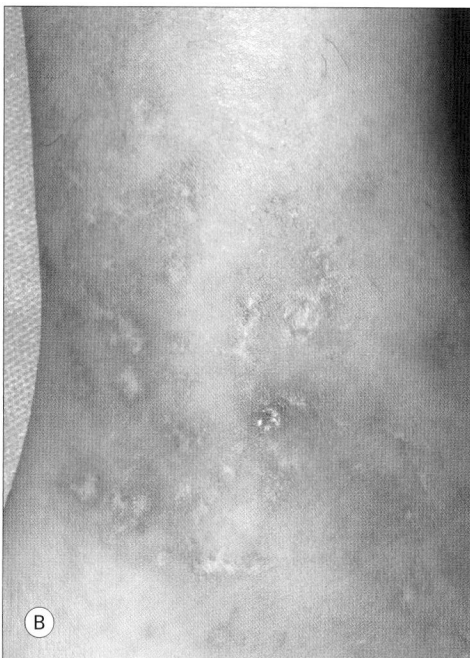

Fig. 105.8 Livedoid vasculopathy. A Multiple hemorrhagic crusts and small painful ulcers associated with brown discoloration due to hemosiderin. **B** Stellate, porcelain-white atrophic scars with peripheral telangiectatic papules, referred to as atrophie blanche. B, Courtesy of Julie V Schaffer MD.

CAUSES OF LYMPHEDEMA	
Primary lymphedema	**Secondary lymphedema**
Congenital lymphedema (presents at birth or within first 2 years of life) • Congenital aplasia of the thoracic duct • Hypoplasia of peripheral lymphatics • Congenital abnormalities of the abdominal or thoracic lymphatics • Hereditary (Nonne-Milroy) – AD; caused by *VEGFR3 (FLT4)* mutations in some families • Turner syndrome • Noonan syndrome	• Recurrent lymphangitis and cellulitis • Parasitic infections, e.g. filariasis • Lymph node dissection, e.g. for melanoma or breast cancer • Malignant obstruction, e.g. lymphoma, Kaposi's sarcoma, retroperitoneal sarcoma • Radiation injury • Obesity • Surgical excisions, e.g. mastectomy, prostatectomy • Acne vulgaris and acne rosacea (midface) • Granulomatous disease
Lymphedema praecox (presents around puberty) • Hereditary (Meige; lymphedema-distichiasis syndrome; yellow nail syndrome) – AD; caused by *FOXC2* mutations in some families • Hypotrichosis-lymphedema-telangiectasia syndrome – AD or AR; caused by *SOX18* mutations	
Lymphedema tarda (presents after age 35 years)	

Table 105.3 Causes of lymphedema. AD, autosomal dominant.

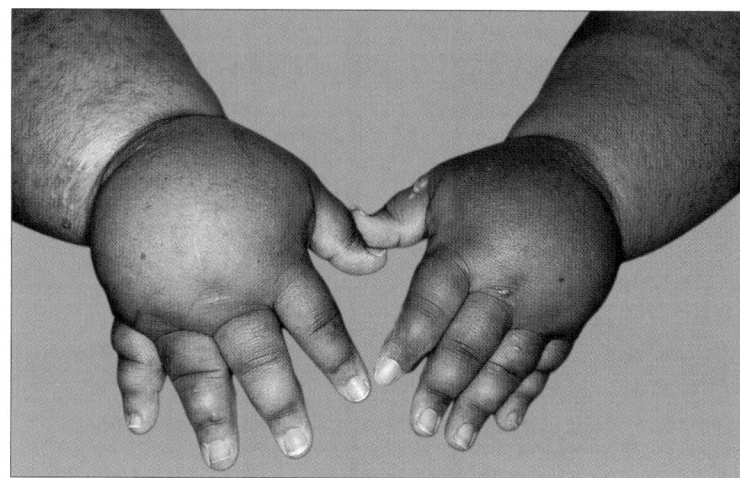

Fig. 105.9 Bilateral primary lymphedema due to Milroy disease.

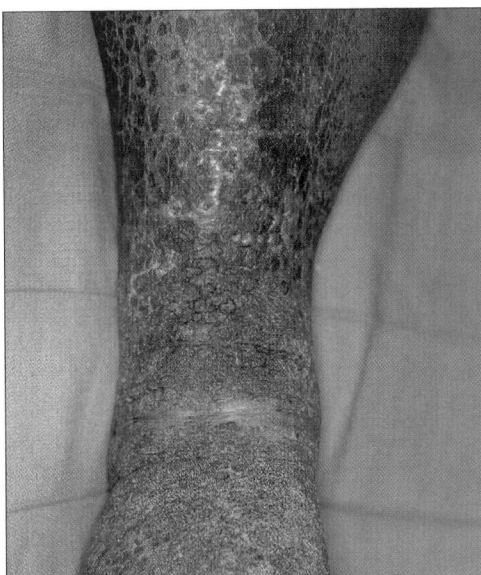

Fig. 105.10 Elephantiasis nostras due to combined lymphedema and venous insufficiency.

Improvement of the associated cutaneous changes was observed in three obese patients following the administration of an oral retinoid[36].

Arterial Ulcers

Approximately one-third of patients with peripheral arterial disease experience claudication, defined as pain in one or both legs upon walking, primarily affecting the calves. The pain is relieved by rest. Claudication is characteristic of arterial insufficiency, and, in more advanced disease, patients may suffer from rest pain and tend to keep the limb in a dependent position[18]. Peripheral pulses are poor. Capillary refill time, obtained by compressing the tip of the great toe until it blanches and then releasing the pressure, is sluggish (>3–4 seconds)[5]. Color change in the limbs with alteration in position indicates ischemia. For example, an ischemic leg becomes pale after being elevated at 45° for 1 minute. Rubor then appears after a delay of more than the normal 10–15 seconds once the leg is placed in a dependent position. It begins in the feet and spreads proximally. The leg becomes bright pink or red in color. It is believed that the greater the arterial insufficiency, the greater the intensity and extent of the rubor and also the longer the venous filling time[5]. In some patients, ulcers due to arterial insufficiency will show diffuse dermal angiomatosis histologically.

Arterial ulcer pain is often severe and difficult to relieve. Ulcers usually occur over a bony prominence, such as the toes or ankle, and often develop after minor trauma. The shape varies, but may follow the outline of traumatic pressure. Arterial ulcers are typically round, with sharply demarcated borders (Fig. 105.11). There is little or no granulation tissue and the base of the wound bed may be dry and covered with necrotic debris. Exposure of tendons or deep tissues also suggests an arterial etiology. The surrounding skin may appear normal, or it can be dry, cold, shiny and hairless. There may be a loss of subcutaneous tissue, muscle wasting and atrophic skin of the lower calf and foot. Toenails may be thickened. Audible bruits may be present over the femoral artery and the distal vessels, and peripheral pulses may be diminished or absent[5].

The ankle–brachial pressure index (ABI) is calculated by dividing the ankle systolic pressure by the higher of the two systolic pressures obtained from the brachial arteries in both arms. In the absence of arterial occlusive disease, the ankle pressure should be equal to the arm pressure. An ABI slightly greater than or equal to 1 is usually normal. An ABI of 0.5 to 0.8 usually indicates occlusive arterial disease. These patients often complain of claudication with exercise. If the ABI is <0.5, there is severe obstructive occlusive disease, and these patients often have pain at rest. The ABI in diabetic patients or in those with calcified vessels can be misleadingly high. When necessary, Doppler segmental pressures can be used to identify the presence, location and severity of arterial occlusive disease. Those with evidence of inadequate arterial blood flow should be referred to a vascular surgeon[37].

Neuropathic and Diabetic Ulcers

Neuropathic ulcers

Patients with neuropathic ulcers may complain of burning, numbness, itching, needle-like pain and/or paresthesias of the distal extremities, but the ulcer is typically asymptomatic[5]. The Semmes–Weinstein monofilament is utilized to test cutaneous perception, as sensory neuropathy is common in diabetics. A 4.17 monofilament is normally felt in a person with intact sensation. It is equivalent to 1 g of linear pressure. If a 5.07 monofilament (equivalent to 10 g of linear pressure) cannot be detected, the patient is considered to have lost protective sensation[31,34]. The sites that are tested are shown in Figure 105.12.

Classic locations for neuropathic ulcers are pressure sites, e.g. the plantar surface overlying the first and fifth metatarsal heads, the plantar surface of the great toe (Fig. 105.13), and the heel. Neuropathic ulcers often appear 'punched out', with a thick rim of callus surrounding the ulcer[5]. There may be dryness and fissuring of the surrounding skin secondary to hypo- or anhidrosis from autonomic impairment.

Because motor neuropathy affects the small intrinsic muscles of the foot, the predominance of the extrinsic muscles then leads to cocked-up toes and prominent metatarsal heads. Distortion of the protective fat pads of the foot, which normally distribute pressure evenly over the surface of the foot, leads to increased pressure on the plantar surface, and hence increased susceptibility to ulceration[21].

Diabetic ulcers

As stated previously, neuropathy and peripheral vascular disease are probably the most important etiologic factors in the development of diabetic foot ulcers[30]. However, pulse examination in diabetic patients

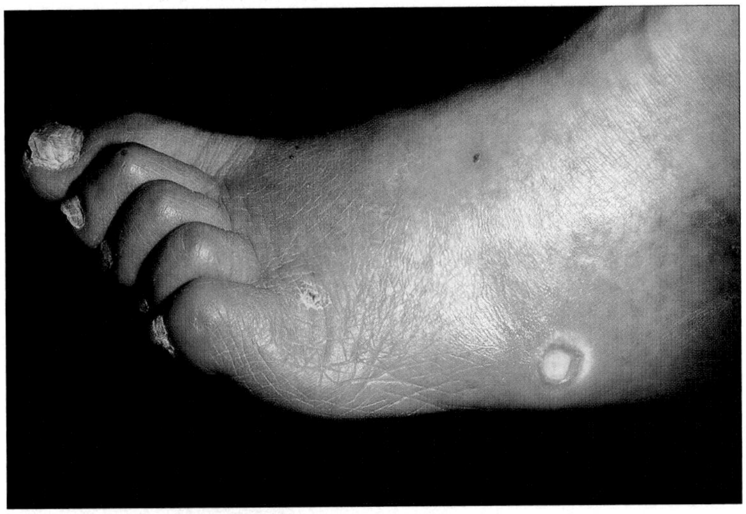

Fig. 105.11 Arterial ulcer. The punched-out appearance and surrounding smooth shiny skin are common features. Courtesy of Ronald P Rapini MD.

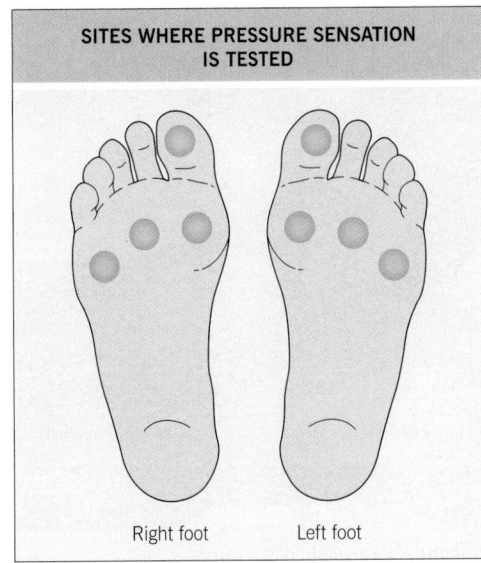

SITES WHERE PRESSURE SENSATION IS TESTED

Right foot   Left foot

Fig. 105.12 Sites where pressure sensation is tested. These sites are the same as those at risk for the development of neuropathic ulcers.

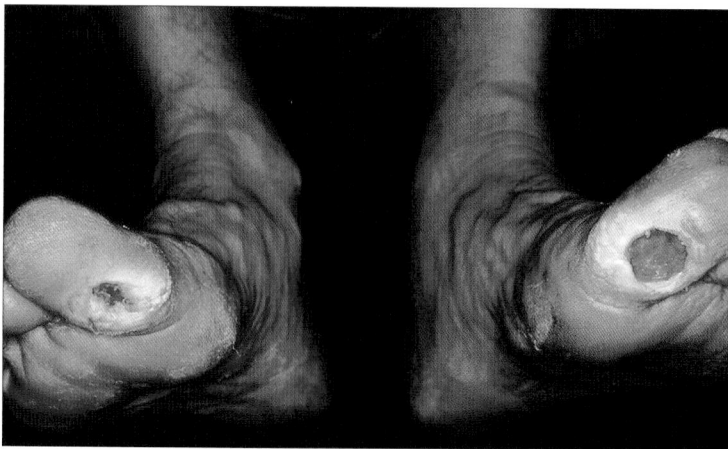

Fig. 105.13 Mal perforans. Neuropathic ulcerations at pressure points on the plantar surface of the great toes in a patient with diabetic neuropathy. Note the thick rim of callus.

is less reliable because of the calcification of arteries[31]. Atherosclerosis is suggested if there is pallor on limb elevation, rubor with dependency, delayed toe capillary refill, shiny atrophic skin, thickened toenails or absence of toe hair (see above). All of these changes are caused by poor perfusion to the feet[5,34]. A history of claudication may be elicited[21]. In diabetics, occlusion of the tibial and peroneal arteries is common, resulting in an ischemic foot but a strong popliteal pulse[5]. Non-invasive vascular studies frequently underestimate the severity of arterial disease in the diabetic patient because of medial calcification of the arteries (see above). While conventional contrast arteriography was routinely performed if ischemic disease were suspected[34], nowadays magnetic resonance angiography and contrast tomographic angiography represent alternative non-invasive techniques.

DIFFERENTIAL DIAGNOSIS

Although the three major types of leg ulcers are venous, arterial and neuropathic (see Table 105.1), there are additional more unusual causes of lower-extremity ulcers (see Fig. 105.1; Fig. 105.14). Atypical features or lack of response to appropriate therapy should lead to re-evaluation and widening of the differential diagnosis.

Acroangiodermatitis (of Mali)

Acroangiodermatitis, also known as pseudo-Kaposi's sarcoma, is characterized by violaceous patches and plaques that usually appear on the extensor surfaces of the distal lower extremities (Fig. 105.15) as well as the dorsal aspects of the feet. Rarely, there is plantar involvement. This condition is most commonly seen in association with chronic

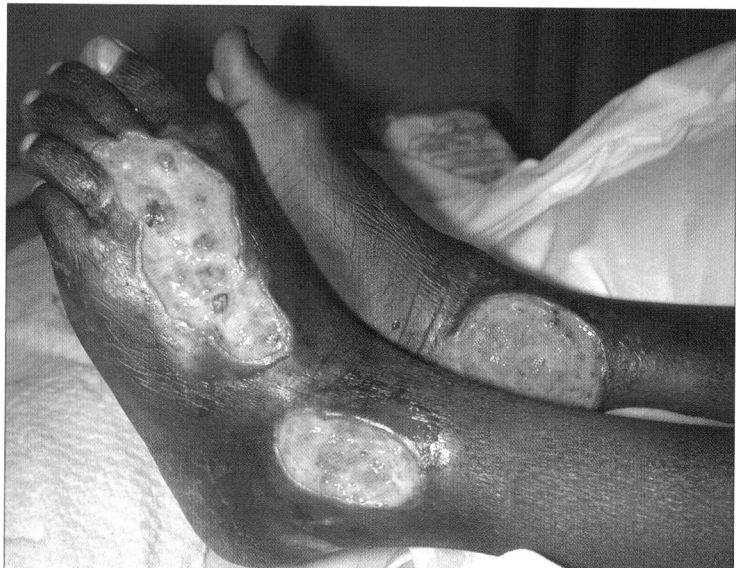

Fig. 105.14 Multiple ulcers secondary to sickle cell anemia.

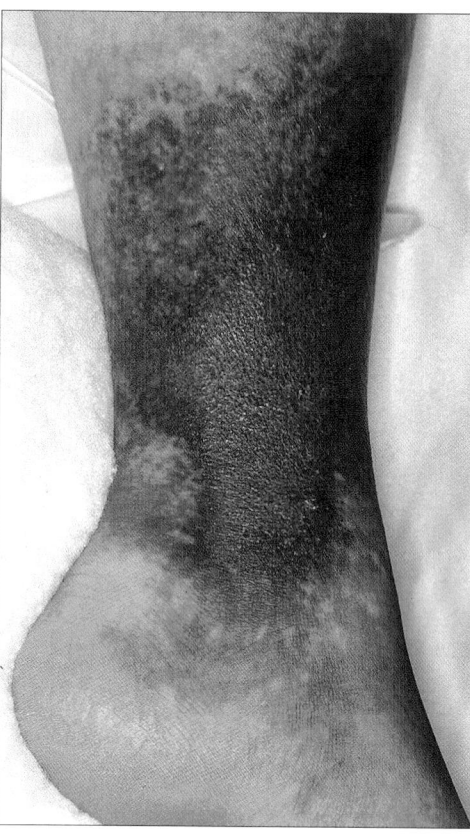

Fig. 105.15 Acroangiodermatitis (pseudo-Kaposi's sarcoma). Violaceous plaque in a patient with venous hypertension. Histologically, these lesions can resemble Kaposi's sarcoma.

venous hypertension and less often with an arteriovenous malformation or fistula[38,39]. As a result, the surrounding skin frequently exhibits changes associated with the former, e.g. hemosiderin deposition. Lesions may progress in size or become painful, and they can even ulcerate.

Although the precise etiology is unknown, it is postulated that chronic tissue hypoxia from chronic edema induces neovascularization and fibroblast proliferation. The histologic features overlap with those of Kaposi's sarcoma, e.g. proliferation of capillaries and fibroblasts, extravasated erythrocytes and dermal siderophages. However, vascular slits, spindle cells and nuclear atypia are not present. Clinicopathologic correlation is often necessary to establish the diagnosis of acroangiodermatitis.

Cryofibrinogenemia

In cryofibrinogenemia, there is a circulating protein that precipitates when the plasma is cooled. The cryoprecipitate is composed of fibrin, fibrinogen, fibronectin (cold-insoluble protein), albumin, immuno-globulins and other plasma proteins[40]. It may be idiopathic (primary/essential) or secondary to a malignancy (e.g. lymphoma), autoimmune connective tissue disease or infection[41]. However, the actual mechanism of formation of cryofibrinogen is not known. Cryofibrinogenemia usually presents with purpura, livedo reticularis, ecchymoses or leg ulcers that are refractory to standard therapy.

For the diagnosis of cryofibrinogenemia, blood must be collected in an anticoagulated tube (preferably with sodium citrate) which is kept and then centrifuged at 37°C. This prevents both the clot from consuming the fibrinogen as well as the cryofibrinogen from precipitating, either of which could lead to a falsely low or falsely negative result. In biopsy specimens, there are precipitation complexes of fibrin, fibrinogen and fibronectin which occlude small vessels[42]. The precipitate is seen as dense eosinophilic intravascular deposits with variable surrounding inflammation. Stanozolol has been shown to produce significant improvement in patients with cryofibrinogenemia, but relapses may occur[42]. If stanozolol is unavailable, other anabolic steroids with fibrinolytic effects (e.g. oxandrolone) may be beneficial.

Buerger's disease

Buerger's disease (thromboangiitis obliterans) is an inflammatory and occlusive condition that affects small to medium-sized arteries and veins. The etiology of this condition is not known, but it has been hypothesized that it might represent an autoimmune process triggered

EVALUATION FOR HYPERCOAGULABILITY

Disorder	%*	Screening tests	Potential confounding conditions
Inherited			
Factor V Leiden	5	Activated protein C (APC) resistance**	(Warfarin, heparin, OCP, pregnancy, ↑ factor VIII level, lupus anticoagulant)**
	5	Factor V Leiden mutation (AD)	–
Prothrombin G20210A	2	Prothrombin G20210A mutation (AD)	–
Hyperhomocysteinemia	>5	↑ Homocysteine level (may have homozygous *MTHFR* C677T mutation > heterozygous *CBS* mutation)	Deficient folate, B_{12} or B_6; older age, smoking
Protein C deficiency	0.3	↓ Protein C activity (AD)	Warfarin, OCP, pregnancy, liver disease, ↑ factor VIII level, lupus anticoagulant
Protein S deficiency	0.05	↓ Free protein S antigen level and/or activity (AD)	Warfarin, OCP, pregnancy, liver disease, ↑ factor VIII level, lupus anticoagulant, acute thrombosis
Antithrombin III deficiency	0.1	↓ Antithrombin III activity (AD)	Heparin, liver disease, acute thrombosis
Excess factor VIII	10	↑ Factor VIII level	Acute phase response, OCP, pregnancy, old age
Excess fibrinogen	ND	↑ Fibrinogen level	Acute phase response, pregnancy, smoking, older age
Dysfibrinogenemia	ND	↓ Functional fibrinogen; ↑ thrombin time	Recent birth, liver disease
Excess factor IX or XI	ND	↑ Factor IX or XI level	Warfarin (factor IX)
Plasminogen deficiency	ND	↓ Plasminogen	–
Excess plasminogen activator inhibitor-1 (PAI-1)	ND	↑ PAI-1	Wide range of normal values
	10	*PAI* 4G/4G polymorphism	–
Excess lipoprotein (a)	10	↑ Lipoprotein (a) level	–
Tissue factor pathway inhibitor (TFPI)	10	↓ TFPI	–
Thrombin-activatable fibrinolysis inhibitor	ND	↑ Thrombin-activatable fibrinolysis inhibitor	–
Thrombomodulin deficiency	ND	↓ Thrombomodulin	–
Acquired			
Lupus anticoagulant†	ND	↑ RVVT (dilute), sensitive PTT, or kaolin clotting time‡	Warfarin, heparin
Anticardiolipin antibodies†	ND	IgG or IgM anticardiolipin antibodies at moderate-high levels, on ≥2 occasions ≥6 weeks apart	Various infectious diseases
Cryoglobulinemia, type I	ND	Type I cryoglobulins present	–
Anti-β₂-glycoprotein I antibodies†	ND	Anti-β₂-glycoprotein I antibodies present	–
Cryofibrinogenemia	ND	Cryofibrinogens present	Acute phase response

*Approximate percentage of general population with the defect.
**Factor V Leiden accounts for ~95% of patients with APC resistance when the latter is assessed by 'second generation' assays, which are not limited by most potential confounding conditions.
†Antiphospholipid antibodies.
‡Confirmed by: (1) failure to correct the prolonged coagulation time in mixing studies; and (2) correction with the addition of excess phospholipids.

Table 105.4 Evaluation for hypercoagulability. Shaded areas represent first-tier screening tests. The initial laboratory evaluation should also include a complete blood count with differential and platelet count, examination of a peripheral blood smear, erythrocyte sedimentation rate, activated partial thromboplastin time (PTT), and hepatic and renal function panels. Testing for antineutrophil cytoplasmic antibodies (ANCA) can be considered for patients with retiform purpura, as ANCA-positive vasculitides occasionally present with minimally inflammatory lesions. Additional inherited causes of hypercoagulability include polymorphisms in the genes encoding the endothelial protein C receptor, the protein Z-dependent protease inhibitor, and E-selectin. AD, autosomal dominant; CBS, cystathionine, β-synthase; MTHFR, methylenetetrahydrofolate reductase; ND, not determined; OCP, oral contraceptive pills; RVVT, Russell viper-venom time.

by tobacco. Clinical findings include asymmetric coldness of the extremities and impaired or absent peripheral arterial pulses; the characteristic arteriographic findings are an abrupt occlusion or tapering of vessels and a corkscrew appearance of collaterals. Criteria that point to the diagnosis of Buerger's disease include a history of smoking, an age <50 years, an absence of atherosclerotic risk factors other than smoking, infrapopliteal occlusions, upper limb involvement and migratory thrombophlebitis[43–45].

Laboratory Investigations

A routine complete blood count may help in diagnosing infection, anemia or polycythemia. Glucose levels should be checked to exclude diabetes mellitus. Measurements of serum albumin, transferrin, ferritin, vitamin A, vitamin C, and trace elements such as zinc can uncover nutritional deficiencies that affect wound healing[5,46]. Additional laboratory tests that may be helpful include an erythrocyte sedimentation rate; measurements of protein C, protein S and antithrombin III; and screening for lupus anticoagulant, antinuclear, anticardiolipin and anti-β₂-glycoprotein antibodies, resistance to activated protein C/factor V Leiden mutation, cryoglobulins, cryofibrinogen, rheumatoid factor, and hepatitis B or C viral infections[47,48]. This latter set is most useful when biopsy specimens demonstrate vasculitis or bland thrombi (see Chs 24 & 25). Table 105.4 outlines an approach to the evaluation of hypercoagulability.

Bacterial culture and sensitivities provide a guideline for antibiotic therapy in patients with cellulitis or sepsis. Biopsy or curettage of the ulcer should be performed to obtain tissue samples for culture, helping to differentiate between colonization versus infection ($>10^5$ organisms per gram of tissue)[25,48]. Tissue for mycobacterial and fungal cultures should also be obtained if the ulcer has not begun to heal after 3 months of treatment. Histologic evaluation can help to exclude malignancy, vasculitis or panniculitis. Deep wedge biopsies that include the ulcer margin and bed are preferred. However, if this is not possible, biopsy specimens should be obtained from several areas in order to avoid sampling error[25].

Patients with chronic leg ulcers commonly have superimposed allergic contact dermatitis, and, if this is suspected, they should undergo patch testing. Common offending allergens include topical antibacterial agents such as neomycin and bacitracin, lanolin, and preservatives such as parabens[25].

Non-invasive vascular studies, such as color duplex scanning, provide information about superficial, communicating and deep venous systems (see Ch. 155, Table 155.2), as well as information regarding arterial systems. Photoplethysmography (PPG) and air plethysmography (APG) are other non-invasive tests that are used less often. These tests measure the degree of venous reflux and the efficiency of the calf muscle pump. Invasive phlebographic studies such as venography are only rarely recommended as an investigation prior to vascular surgery[5a,22,48].

A plain radiograph may be considered if osteomyelitis is suspected. However, it is insensitive, especially in early osteomyelitis. Additional studies include a three-phase bone scan, MRI (as sensitive as bone scan for acute disease, with better anatomic detail and specificity), and CT scan (for chronic disease). If blood cultures are negative, needle aspiration of pus or a bone biopsy is performed for microbiologic studies before initiation of antibiotics.

TREATMENT

Venous Ulcers

The primary role of treatment is to reverse the effects of venous hypertension. The simplest method is leg elevation above the level of the heart. However, leg elevation must often be combined with compression therapy (Fig. 105.16). Compression devices include stockings (Table 105.5), bandages (Unna boot and multilayer), orthotics, and pneumatic compression (Table 105.6).

It is important to measure the ABI to exclude arterial occlusive disease. An ABI of less than 0.8 indicates the presence of arterial disease, and caution should be exercised when applying compression. In patients with an ABI of less than 0.5, compression is contraindicated. Patients

CLASSES OF COMPRESSION STOCKINGS		
Class	Pressure at the ankle	Indication
I	20–30 mmHg	Simple varicose veins Mild edema Leg fatigue
II	30–40 mmHg	Moderate edema Severe varicosities Moderate venous insufficiency
III	40–50 mmHg	Severe edema Severe venous insufficiency Post-thrombotic lymphedema
IV	50–60 mmHg	Elephantiasis

Table 105.5 Classes of compression stockings. Adapted with permission from Phillips TJ. Current approaches to venous ulcers and compression. Dermatol Surg. 2001;27:611–21.

with a reduced ABI should be evaluated by a vascular surgeon. It is also important to document if the patient is diabetic, as the ABI can be inaccurate in these patients (see above).

Graduated sustained compression reduces pressure in the superficial venous system and increases venous return to the heart. The pressure difference between the capillaries and the tissue is decreased, thereby improving edema[22]. The optimal pressure necessary to overcome venous hypertension is not well defined, but it is generally agreed to be 35–40 mmHg at the ankle.

Either non-elastic or elastic compression systems may be utilized (see Ch. 145). Non-elastic bandages mostly act as a support system. They provide high pressure with muscle contraction (i.e. walking) and minimal pressure at rest. Because they require muscle activity in order to be effective, they are not recommended for non-ambulatory patients. The Unna boot is a moist, zinc-impregnated paste bandage. It is the prototype of the non-elastic bandage. An adherent elastic wrap (e.g. Coban™) can be applied as a second layer over the Unna boot. Care should be taken to apply the Unna boot correctly; if it is applied improperly, it can exert abnormal pressure and impair circulation, leading to skin necrosis, new ulcerations, and even gangrene[25].

Multilayer elastic compression bandages are an alternative to the Unna boot (see Ch. 145). They provide sustained pressure and conform to the leg better than the Unna boot. There are three classes of elastic bandages, depending on the amount of pressure they exert (Table 105.7). A legging orthotic with multiple adjustable Velcro® straps (from the instep to the knee) is useful in patients who cannot apply compression stockings. Intermittent pneumatic compression pumps are useful in patients in whom edema does not respond to conventional compression bandages or stockings[8].

Patients should be encouraged to wear graduated compression stockings for the rest of their lives to prevent ulcer recurrence. Compression should be applied immediately upon arising from bed and removed at bedtime. There are four classes of graduated compression stockings, which are based on the amount of ankle compression (see Table 105.5)[8]. The elasticity of stockings decreases with washing and wearing, so they should be replaced at least every 6 months[22].

Several groups have reported that by the third or fourth week of compression therapy, it can be predicted whether or not an ulcer will heal[49–51]. After 4 weeks of treatment, the log healing rate, the log wound area ratio, and the percent change in wound area represent valid surrogate markers for anticipated wound healing following 12 and 24 weeks of care. In general, wounds that heal by 40–50% by 4 weeks of therapy will go on to heal completely. Patients who are compliant with compression therapy have significantly improved ulcer healing rates, with decreased rates of recurrence.

Topical treatment
Dressing selection, maintaining a moist wound, and autolytic debridement
A moist wound environment accelerates healing compared to air exposure[52,53]. Wound dressings that sustain a moist environment are usually composed of synthetic polymers that are fashioned into fibers,

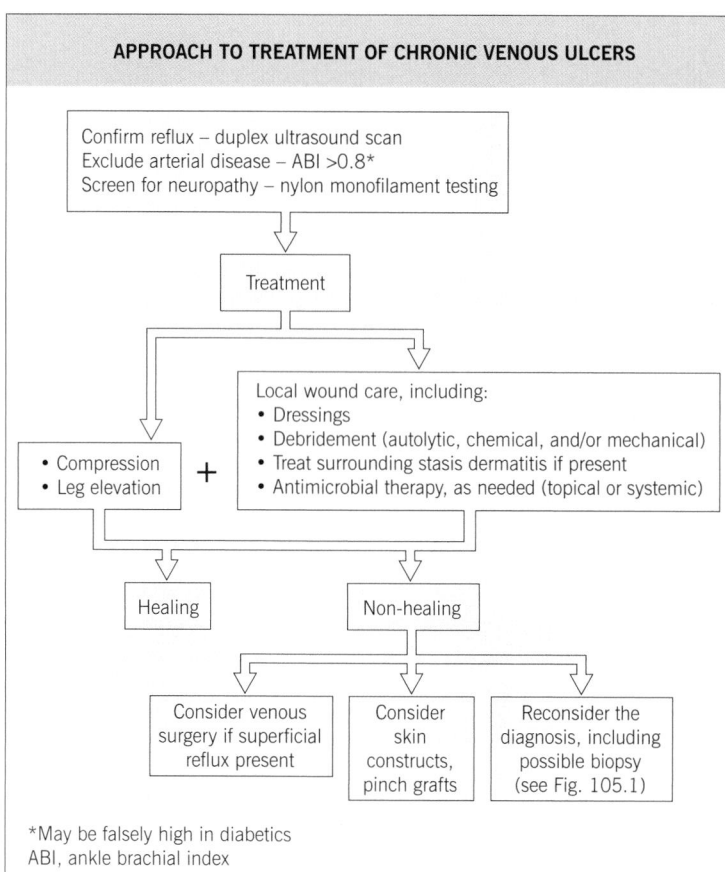

Fig. 105.16 Approach to the treatment of chronic venous ulcers.

TYPES OF COMPRESSION THERAPY

Bandage	Advantages	Disadvantages
Elastic wraps	Inexpensive Can be reused	Often applied incorrectly by the patient Tend to unravel Do not maintain sustained compression Lose elasticity after washing
Self-adherent wraps	Self-adherent Maintain compression	Expensive Cannot be reused
Unna boot	Comfortable Protects against trauma Full maintenance of ambulatory outpatient status Minimal interference with regular activities Substitutes for a failing pump	Pressure changes over time Needs to be applied by well-trained physicians and nurses Does not accommodate highly exudative wounds
Four-layer bandage	Comfortable Can be left in place for 7 days Protects against trauma Maintains a constant pressure for 7 days because of the overlap and elasticity of the bandages Useful for highly exudative wounds	Need to be applied by well-trained physicians and nurses Expensive
Graduated compression stockings	Reduce the ambulatory venous pressure Increase venous refilling time Improve calf pump function Different types of stockings accommodate different types of legs Dressings underneath can be changed frequently	Often cannot monitor patient compliance Difficult to put on
Orthotic device	Adjustable compression Sustained pressure Easily put on and removed Comfortable	Expensive Bulky appearance
Compression pump	Augments venous return Improves hemodynamics and microvascular functions Enhances fibrinolytic activity Prevents postoperative thromboembolic complications in high-risk patients	Expensive Requires immobility for a few hours per day

Table 105.6 Types of compression therapy. Adapted with permission from Choucair M, Phillips TJ. Compression therapy. Dermatol Surg. 1998;24:141–8.

CLASSES OF COMPRESSION BANDAGES

Class	Properties
Class I	Light-weight and conforming Stretch and simple dressing retention properties
Class II	Also known as short stretch bandages Act like rigid, non-elastic bandages Used for light support
Class III • Class IIIA • Class IIIB • Class IIIC	Light compression bandages Moderate compression bandages Extra-high performance Achieve 40 mmHg at the ankle Useful for: • Severe varicosities • Severe edema • Postphlebitic syndrome

Table 105.7 Classes of compression bandages.

RECOMMENDED DRESSINGS ACCORDING TO CHRONIC ULCER TYPE

Type of ulcer	Dressing recommended
Venous Heavy exudate	Foam Alginate Hydrofiber*
Moderate exudate	Hydrocolloid Foam
Mild exudate	Hydrogel Hydrocolloid
Malodorous	Foam Alginate Hydrocolloid Charcoal
Recalcitrant	Tissue-engineered skin equivalents
Arterial	Hydrogel
Neuropathic Moist granulating	Hydrogel Alginate Hydrofiber*
Dry necrotic	Hydrogel Hydrocolloid
Pressure Stage I	Film (to reduce friction) Thin hydrocolloid
Stages II and III	Hydrocolloid Foam Hydrogel Debriding agent
Stage IV (undermined borders, cavities or sinuses)	Alginate Hydrofiber* Debriding agent

*A highly absorbent dressing composed of carboxymethylcellulose fibers.

Table 105.8 Recommended dressings according to chronic ulcer type. Adapted with permission from Bello YM, Phillips TJ. Therapeutic dressings. Adv Dermatol. 2000;16;253–70.

mats, wafers or membranes that are semipermeable to gases (oxygen, carbon dioxide) and moisture, but are impermeable to liquids. This characteristic defines them as semi-occlusive. The term 'semi-occlusive' is often used interchangeably with the term 'occlusive', although the latter implies a total lack of permeability. These dressings create and/or maintain a moist local environment by capturing transpired moisture vapor or liquid drainage from the wound and holding it at the surface. Five basic types of occlusive dressings are available, each with its own advantages and disadvantages. These include hydrogels, alginates, hydrocolloids, foams and films (see Ch. 145, Table 145.2)[53]. Based on the characteristics of the different types of ulcers, specific dressings are recommended (Table 105.8)[3].

Chemical and mechanical debridement

Standard venous ulcer care incorporates debridement of necrotic and fibrinous debris to allow for the formation of good granulation tissue and adequate re-epithelialization. Enzymatic debriding agents include collagenase (Santyl®) and papain (e.g. Panafil®, Accuzyme®). Mechanical debridement is most commonly accomplished via the use of either surgical instruments or wet-to-moist saline dressings. The major concern regarding mechanical debridement is the non-discriminatory removal of viable tissue along with necrotic material. Topical lidocaine gel or cream or lidocaine/prilocaine cream under occlusion often provides helpful anesthesia before performance of surgical debridement. In a controlled prospective trial, sharp debridement was shown to

Table 105.9 Treatment of venous leg ulcers – summary of clinical trials.

accelerate venous ulcer healing[54] (Table 105.9). Debridement should be performed cautiously (if at all) in arterial occlusive disease, because it may cause further tissue ischemia[25,58].

Antiseptics and antibiotics

Antiseptics such as chlorhexidine, povidone-iodine, acetic acid and sodium hypochlorite are not recommended for open wounds as they are cytotoxic and likely to impair epithelialization and delay healing. Although 0.25% acetic acid is often used in wounds that are heavily infected with *Pseudomonas*, its ability to significantly reduce bacterial counts has not been proven[25]. Some topical antibiotics, such as neomycin, polymyxin B and bacitracin (all three contained in Neosporin®) as well as gentamicin, may cause contact dermatitis, and rarely anaphylaxis[59,60]. If severe contact dermatitis develops, a short course of systemic corticosteroids may be indicated. Mupirocin and topical erythromycin rarely lead to sensitization, but to date their effects on wound healing have not been documented. Benzoyl peroxide has antimicrobial properties and the 20% lotion was found to enhance wound healing when applied to chronic wounds under occlusion; however, wound contraction is inhibited by 20% benzoyl peroxide lotion[25]. Metronidazole gel may be used to control odor in wounds and retapamulin can also be used as a topical antibiotic.

A cadexomer-iodine polymer is also available that absorbs wound exudate and slowly releases bacteriocidal iodine from dextran beads (see Ch. 145)[61]. In addition, controlled-release silver dressings provide an antimicrobial barrier effective against methicillin-resistant *Staphylococcus aureus* (MRSA), *Candida albicans* and *Pseudomonas aeruginosa*. These dressings, composed of nanocrystalline silver layered into a polyurethane material, are non-cytotoxic to the wound[61].

Growth factors

Growth factors are important regulatory peptides that promote cell growth and synthetic activity and also modify cell migration and differentiation. A topical recombinant human platelet-derived growth factor (becaplermin) is approved by the Food and Drug Administration (FDA) as an adjunctive treatment for diabetic neuropathic ulcers[62]. Of the family of keratinocyte growth factors, only palifermin is currently approved and it is indicated for reduction of mucositis due to chemotherapy or radiation.

Bone marrow cells

In a case series of three patients with chronic non-healing wounds, application of cultured bone marrow cells to the wound bed facilitated healing[63].

Topical corticosteroids

Venous (stasis) dermatitis often improves with compression, moisturizers and the short-term use of mid-potency topical corticosteroid ointments. This can be followed by maintenance therapy with hydrocortisone 2.5% ointment several times per week. If acute dermatitis is present with weeping and oozing, open wet dressings may be helpful.

Systemic treatment
Antibiotics

The majority of chronic leg ulcers are colonized or contaminated by a variety of microorganisms. The most common isolates are *S. aureus*, *P. aeruginosa* and enterobacteria. Uncomplicated venous ulcers without

evidence of cellulitis or systemic infection will not benefit from antibiotic therapy. However, the presence of more than 10^5 bacteria per gram of tissue may impede wound healing, and systemic antibiotics should be considered. Cellulitis presents with erythema, swelling, warmth, tenderness and/or fever and requires appropriate systemic antibiotic therapy[22].

Pentoxifylline

Pentoxifylline is a substituted xanthine derivative with fibrinolytic and antithrombotic activities. Although the actual mechanism of action is uncertain, it is also thought to reduce leukocyte adhesion to the vascular endothelium and decrease production of TNF-α by lymphocytes. Pentoxifylline as an adjunct to compression therapy for venous ulcers has been the subject of several trials that have reported conflicting results[64,65]. In one trial, 800 mg three times daily accelerated the healing rate of venous ulcers and was more effective than the standard dose of 400 mg three times daily. Side effects include gastrointestinal upset and dizziness[66].

Stanozolol or other anabolic steroids

Anabolic steroids with fibrinolytic properties may be beneficial in the treatment of acute and chronic lipodermatosclerosis as well as leg ulcers caused by cryofibrinogenemia[22]. However, no effect on the rate of venous ulcer healing has been documented. Side effects include sodium retention, edema, hypertension, hirsutism, acne, hepatic dysfunction, lipid abnormalities and dysmenorrhea.

Physical modalities

With regard to enhancing wound healing, the therapeutic efficacies of hyperbaric oxygen, infrared light, UV light, ultrasound and laser have not been sufficiently established. Therefore, they can not be recommended as routine adjuvant therapy. However, electrical stimulation was recommended by the Agency for Healthcare Research and Quality for stages II, III and IV pressure ulcers which have been recalcitrant to standard therapy (see next section). Hydrotherapy may help to clean wounds, but it does not replace aggressive debridement. Additional treatments, such as constant tension approximation or vacuum-assisted and warming therapies, have not been adequately evaluated in controlled clinical trials.

Surgery
Pinch grafts

This technique is suitable only for small ulcers, as it is time consuming. Thin, superficial pinch grafts are harvested from the anterior thigh using a 3–4-mm trephine and then placed dermis-side down on the ulcer bed, spaced several millimeters apart from one another. This procedure can be performed on an outpatient basis[25].

Split-thickness skin grafts (STSGs)

STSGs have been successfully used for the treatment of chronic leg ulcers and can be performed under local, spinal or general anesthesia. A dermatome set at a predetermined depth is used at the donor site (see Ch. 148). Meshed grafts are useful for large, highly exudative ulcers because they allow fluid to escape through the graft interstices[22,25].

Engineered skin constructs
Epidermal or dermal grafts

Epidermal grafts can be derived from the patient's own skin (autografts) or from allogeneic donors (allografts), but only the former are currently commercially available (see Ch. 145). Cultured allogeneic keratinocytes derived from neonatal foreskins presumably stimulate re-epithelialization and the formation of granulation tissue by releasing growth factors and by acting as a moist wound dressing. However, evidence of their therapeutic effectiveness for chronic ulcers that have failed to respond to conservative treatment is anecdotal, as large randomized controlled studies have yet to be performed[67,68]. Dermal grafts can be xenogenic (e.g. porcine or bovine collagen) or allogeneic (e.g. cultured neonatal foreskin fibroblasts within a mesh) (see Ch. 145).

Composite grafts

Commercially available bilayered skin constructs, or cultured human skin equivalents (HSEs), are composed of an epidermal layer of keratinocytes derived from human neonatal foreskin and a dermal layer containing bovine type 1 collagen seeded with cultured human fibroblasts. Melanocytes, mast cells, cells involved in the immune response (e.g. Langerhans cells, lymphocytes, macrophages and endothelial cells) as well as various skin structures (e.g. blood vessels, lymphatics, nerves and adnexal structures) are absent.

In a multicenter, randomized, prospective study of 275 patients with venous leg ulcers, 63% of the patients in the group treated with an HSE plus compression had complete healing within 6 months, compared to 49% in the group using compression alone (p = 0.02). The median time to complete healing was 61 days for the HSE group and 181 days for the control group (p = 0.003). No significant differences in rates of ulcer recurrence were observed over a 12-month follow-up period. In another randomized, prospective study involving ulcers of greater than 1 year's duration, complete healing occurred within 6 months in 34 patients (47%) treated with an HSE and in nine patients (19%) treated with active control (compression alone). Apligraf® is FDA-approved for the treatment of venous and diabetic foot ulcers that fail to heal despite adequate clinical evaluation and treatment[57,68], while OrCel® is approved for STSG donor sites (see Ch. 145).

Saphenous vein surgery
There is evidence from European studies that in patients with pure superficial venous insufficiency (15–40% of venous ulcer patients), surgical intervention reduced venous ulcer recurrence rates. Superficial vein surgery (ligation or sclerosis of the long and short saphenous systems, with or without communicating vein ligation or sclerosis) was shown to decrease the rate of recurrence only if the deep veins were competent[22]. In one randomized controlled study, 500 venous ulcer patients received compression, either alone or in combination with superficial vein surgery. Overall healing rates at 24 weeks were similar in the two groups (65%), but 12-month ulcer recurrence rates were significantly reduced in the compression plus surgery group versus compression alone (12% and 28%, respectively)[56].

Radical excision of the ulcer bed, the fibrotic suprafascial tissues and the diseased superficial and perforating veins, as well as coverage of the large tissue defect with a free flap, has been successfully performed in a few cases. However, the magnitude of the surgical procedure limits its widespread application[69].

Arterial Ulcers

The main goal of therapy is the re-establishment of an adequate arterial supply[54]. Patients should be referred to a vascular surgeon for assessment and revascularization by angioplasty or bypass surgery. The patient is encouraged to eat a low-cholesterol diet, reduce or discontinue smoking, lose weight, and maintain control of contributory factors such as hypertension, diabetes mellitus and hyperlipidemia. In addition to lipid-lowering drugs (e.g. HMG-CoA reductase inhibitors ['statins'])[18], antiplatelet drugs may be prescribed. Exercise encourages the development of collateral circulation, and elevation of the head of the bed by 4–6 inches improves arterial flow[54].

Although the data are not conclusive, aspirin is recommended as a primary antiplatelet drug for preventing ischemic events in patients with peripheral arterial disease. Clopidogrel (Plavix®), an inhibitor of ADP-induced platelet aggregation, has FDA approval for this purpose and may be more effective than aspirin. Cilostazol (Pletal®), an inhibitor of phosphodiesterase III, has been found to improve both pain-free and maximal treadmill walking distances. In addition, several propionyl L-carnitines are currently being explored for the treatment of claudication and arterial leg ischemia[18]. To date, there is no evidence that PGE$_1$ or pentoxifylline improve arterial ulcer healing, and, in the future, gene therapy with growth factors, such as VEGF, may prove useful.

Additional interventions include providing adequate pain control, keeping the limbs warm, and good local wound management. Hyperbaric oxygen therapy can be used to improve tissue perfusion in patients who are slow to heal despite revascularization or who are not candidates for this procedure.

Neuropathic and Diabetic Ulcers

Management of neuropathic ulcers includes aggressive debridement, treatment of associated arterial disease, offloading of pressure, resto-

ration of circulation to the lower extremity when necessary, and assessment and treatment of infection[30]. Figure 105.17 provides an algorithm for the overall management and prevention of neuropathic foot ulcers in patients with diabetes mellitus. The risk of ulceration and amputation may be reduced by two-thirds by education and preventative measures (Table 105.10)[5].

The cause of most diabetic foot ulcers is repetitive trauma[19]. For these patients, orthotic devices are utilized which permit ambulation while decreasing pressure at the site of the wound. Small and shallow ulcers may be managed successfully with felted foam inserts. Total contact casting is frequently used for neuropathic ulcers in ambulatory patients. Diabetic patients with foot deformities need therapeutic footwear that accommodates all of their foot deformities and provides cushioning[30].

Calluses can increase local pressure by up to 30%. Ulcer management therefore includes aggressive debridement of devitalized tissue and surrounding callus as well as sterile dressings and frequent inspection. The wound needs to be free of all infected and necrotic tissue. Surgical debridement should be performed until good granulation tissue is apparent[30].

The standard of care recommended by the American Diabetes Association is saline-moistened gauze, which should be changed two to three times daily. Hydrogen peroxide, chlorhexidine and astringents should be avoided, as they interfere with wound healing. For dry necrotic ulcers, hydrocolloid dressings and hydrogels can maintain a moist wound environment while providing some autolytic debridement (see Table 105.8). Enzymatic debridement agents and mechanical debridement (Fig. 105.18) are utilized to remove necrotic tissues. For moist granulating ulcers, the alginates and absorptive dressings absorb drainage well while maintaining a moist wound environment.

Becaplermin gel – topically applied recombinant platelet-derived growth factor – is FDA-approved as an adjunctive treatment for patients with diabetic neuropathic foot ulcers[30]. The composite graft Apligraf® (see above) is also FDA-approved as an adjunct for the treatment of diabetic foot ulcers. Data from a prospective, randomized, controlled multicenter clinical trial (n = 208) revealed that 56% of ulcers treated with the HSE healed within 12 weeks, compared to 38% with standard treatment alone; complete healing was achieved after an average of 65 days and 90 days, respectively[30]. Thirdly, both porcine collagen (Oasis®) and a human fibroblast-derived dermal substitute (Dermagraft™) have been approved by the FDA for the treatment of diabetic foot ulcers. In a randomized controlled trial, 314 patients were randomized to conventional therapy versus the latter dermal substitute. By week 12, 30% of the dermal substitute-treated patients had healed versus 18% of control patients treated with standard care[70].

Arterial insufficiency is a pathogenic factor in up to 60% of diabetic patients with non-healing ulcers and in 45% of those undergoing major amputations[30]. Atherosclerotic occlusion in diabetic patients characteristically involves the distal tibial and peroneal arteries. Typically, foot vessels are spared, especially the dorsalis pedis artery[5].

INSTRUCTIONS FOR THE PATIENT WITH A DIABETIC OR NEUROPATHIC ULCER

1. Stop smoking, control blood sugar levels, and lose weight if overweight.
2. Inspect feet daily for blisters, scratches, and red areas. If your vision is impaired, get someone to do this for you.
3. Wash your feet daily in warm water. Dry carefully between the toes.
4. Apply petroleum jelly to dry areas of skin but not between the toes.
5. Always test water temperature before bathing.
6. Inspect the insides of your shoes before putting them on.
7. Do not remove corns or apply strong chemicals to your feet.
8. Cut nails straight across.
9. See your podiatrist regularly.
10. Wear properly fitting shoes. New shoes should be worn for 1–2 hours daily only. Check your feet for red spots afterwards.
11. Avoid open-toed sandals and pointed shoes.
12. Never walk barefoot.
13. If you develop any breaks in the skin or blisters, inform your doctor.
14. See your doctor regularly.

Table 105.10 Instructions for the patient with a diabetic or neuropathic ulcer. Adapted with permission from Levin M, O'Neal ME. The Diabetic Foot. St Louis: Mosby, 1988.

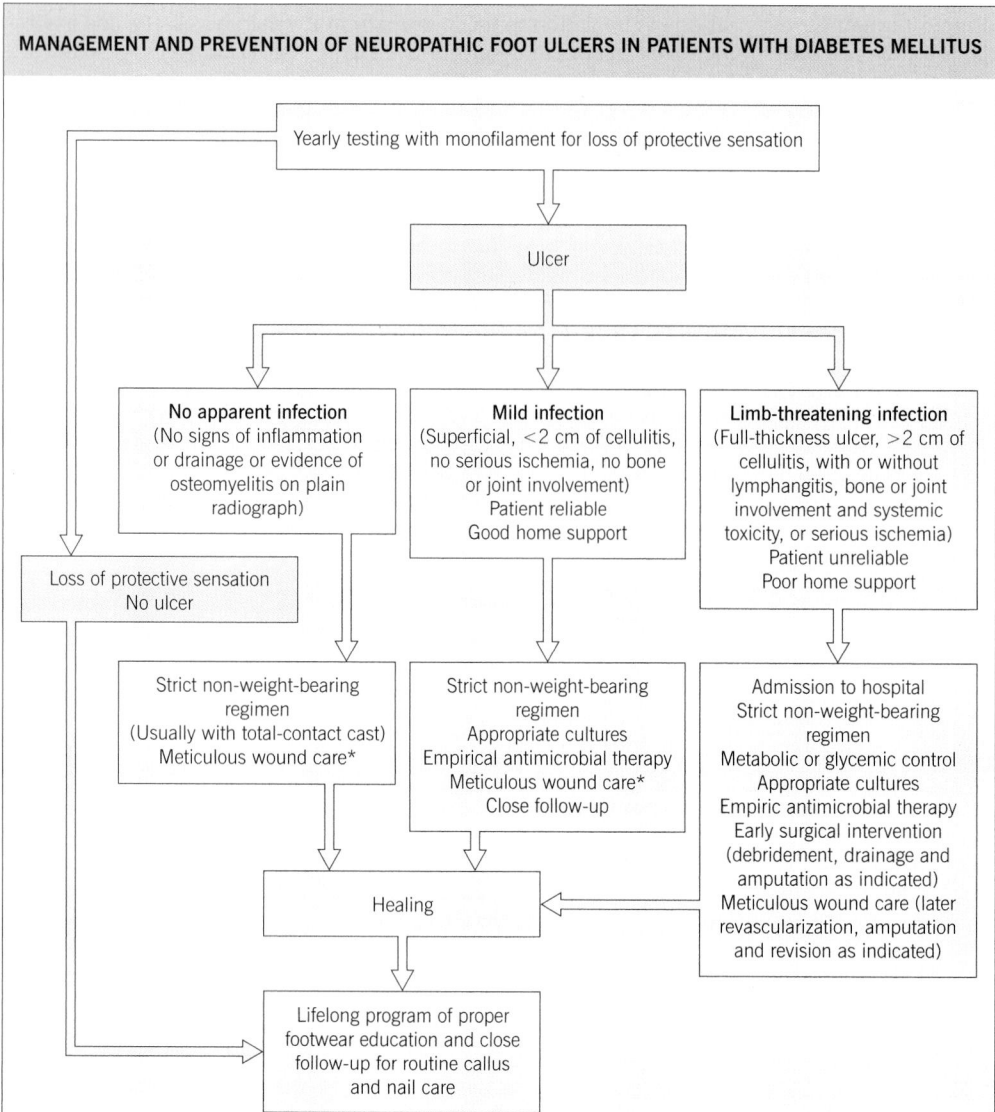

MANAGEMENT AND PREVENTION OF NEUROPATHIC FOOT ULCERS IN PATIENTS WITH DIABETES MELLITUS

Yearly testing with monofilament for loss of protective sensation

Ulcer

No apparent infection
(No signs of inflammation or drainage or evidence of osteomyelitis on plain radiograph)

Mild infection
(Superficial, <2 cm of cellulitis, no serious ischemia, no bone or joint involvement)
Patient reliable
Good home support

Limb-threatening infection
(Full-thickness ulcer, >2 cm of cellulitis, with or without lymphangitis, bone or joint involvement and systemic toxicity, or serious ischemia)
Patient unreliable
Poor home support

Loss of protective sensation
No ulcer

Strict non-weight-bearing regimen
(Usually with total-contact cast)
Meticulous wound care*

Strict non-weight-bearing regimen
Appropriate cultures
Empirical antimicrobial therapy
Meticulous wound care*
Close follow-up

Admission to hospital
Strict non-weight-bearing regimen
Metabolic or glycemic control
Appropriate cultures
Empiric antimicrobial therapy
Early surgical intervention (debridement, drainage and amputation as indicated)
Meticulous wound care (later revascularization, amputation and revision as indicated)

Healing

Lifelong program of proper footwear education and close follow-up for routine callus and nail care

Fig. 105.17 Management and prevention of neuropathic foot ulcer in patients with diabetes mellitus. *Including debridement of the keratotic rim of the ulcer. Reproduced with permission from Caputo et al. Current concepts: assessment and management of foot disease in patients with diabetes. N Engl J Med. 1994;331:845–60.

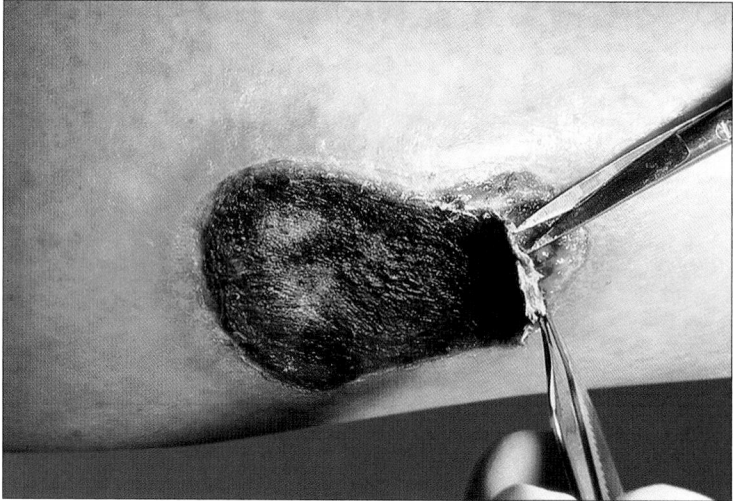

Fig. 105.18 Debridement of black eschar from a diabetic ulcer. Courtesy of Ronald P Rapini MD.

Non-invasive vascular laboratory tests frequently underestimate the extent and severity of arterial insufficiency in diabetic patients (see above). If serious ischemia is suspected, arteriography or magnetic resonance angiography of the lower extremity, including the foot vessels, should be performed. The decision to perform vascular surgery depends upon the severity of the vascular impairment. Other considerations include the risks associated with surgery and the potential for rehabilitation. Revascularization can be as safe as a major amputation and less costly[30].

Wound infections may be superficial or deep and are most often caused by *S. aureus* or streptococci. Limb-threatening infections are usually polymicrobial, involving aerobic Gram-positive cocci, Gram-negative bacilli (e.g. *Escherichia coli*, *Klebsiella* species and *Proteus* species), and anaerobes (e.g. *Bacteroides* species and peptostreptococci). All crusted areas of an ulcer should be unroofed and the wound explored with a metal probe to determine the depth and extent of tissue destruction. If the wound can be probed to bone, osteomyelitis is very likely and should be assessed as outlined in Laboratory Investigations. If bone cannot be reached by probing and the plain radiograph does not suggest osteomyelitis, further evaluation depends upon the degree of clinical suspicion for osteomyelitis Radiography can be repeated in 2 weeks and further imaging studies (e.g. bone scan, MRI) performed[30].

PRESSURE ULCERS

INTRODUCTION

Pressure ulcers are areas of tissue necrosis caused by unrelieved pressure to soft tissues compressed between a bony prominence and an external surface for a prolonged period of time. Synonyms for 'pressure' ulcers exist, such as bed sores, pressure sores, decubitus ulcers and ischemic ulcers (with the latter term also used to refer to arterial ulcers). The term 'decubitus' is derived from the Latin word meaning 'to lie down', as it was previously thought that these ulcers resulted only from prolonged recumbency. However, because the prolonged application of

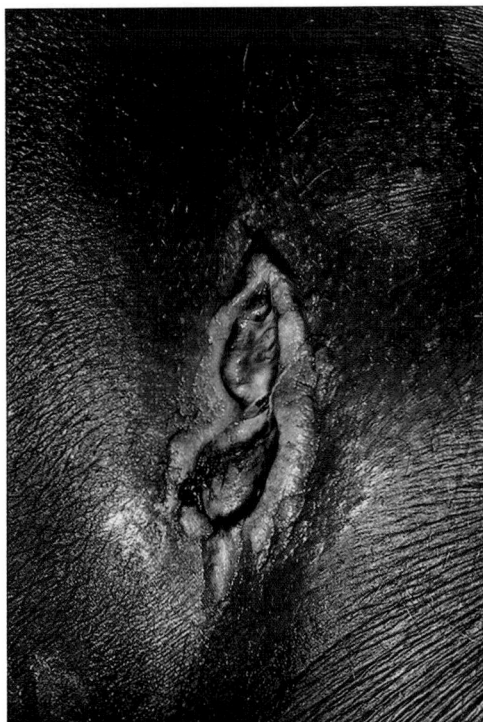

Fig. 105.19 Sacral decubitus ulcer. Courtesy of Ronald P Rapini MD.

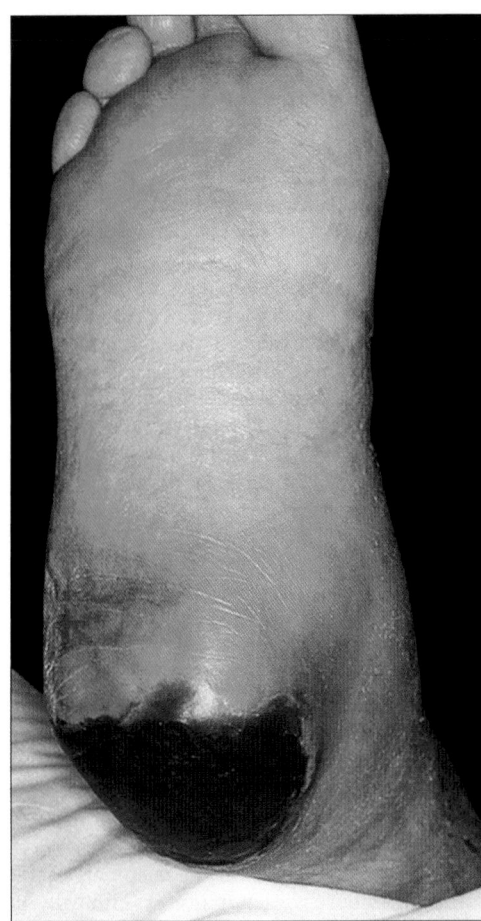

Fig. 105.20 Black eschar of the heel at site of pressure necrosis.

pressure in any position can result in ulceration, 'pressure ulcer' is the most appropriate term to use. The most common bony prominences involved are the sacrum (Fig. 105.19), ischial tuberosities, greater trochanters, heels (Fig. 105.20), and lateral malleoli[71] (Fig. 105.21).

EPIDEMIOLOGY

Approximately 1.5–3 million people in the US are afflicted with pressure ulcers. The annual cost is estimated to be $5 billion[71]. The US Department of Health and Human Services reports that approximately 10% of all hospitalized patients and 25% of nursing home patients have pressure ulcers, most of which develop during the first few weeks of hospitalization. Although the majority of pressure ulcers develop in a hospital setting, approximately 20% develop at home. An estimated 70% occur in patients over 70 years of age. Ninety-five percent of all pressure ulcers are located on the lower portion of the body: 65% in the pelvic area and 30% on the lower limbs. Risk factors

that predispose to the development of pressure ulcers include prolonged immobility, sensory deficit, circulatory disturbance, and poor nutrition[71].

PATHOGENESIS

Subcutaneous tissues are at greater risk for pressure injury. The four major etiologic factors involved in the development of pressure ulcers are pressure, shearing forces, friction and moisture. Each of these factors is significant in its own right. However, when all four are combined, their effect on the skin is even more damaging and ulceration becomes almost inevitable[71].

Fig. 105.21 Most common sites for pressure ulcers.

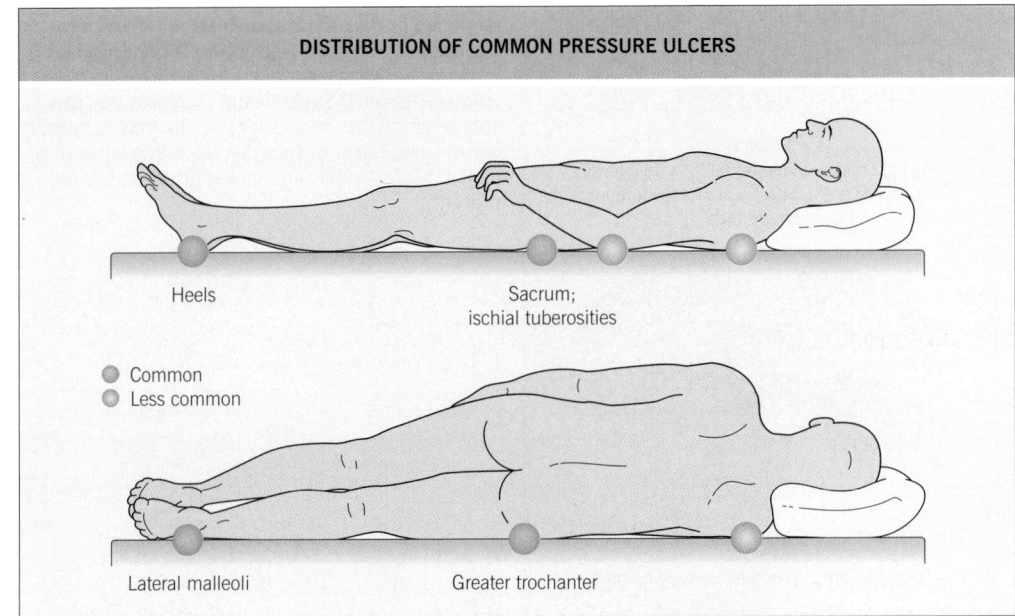

DISTRIBUTION OF COMMON PRESSURE ULCERS

Heels

Sacrum; ischial tuberosities

● Common
● Less common

Lateral malleoli

Greater trochanter

Pressure

Pressure, or force per area, has been considered the single most important etiologic factor in this type of ulcer formation. External pressure is generally concentrated over bony prominences. Normal capillary pressure usually ranges between 12 and 32 mmHg. Pressures over 32 mmHg raise interstitial pressure, compromising oxygenation and microcirculation. There is an inverse time–pressure curve, with slow ulcer formation at low pressures and rapid ulcer formation at high pressures of 70 mmHg or more. When a patient lies on a hospital mattress, pressures of 150 mmHg can be generated. Several studies have shown that the duration as well as the degree of pressure is an important parameter in determining the extent of tissue damage. For example, a constant pressure of 70 mmHg for 2 hours leads to tissue death. If, however, pressure is intermittently relieved, minimal changes occur. Highest interstitial pressures occur at the bone–muscle interface, with less damage at the dermal–epidermal level. Thus, deep tissue trauma can occur with relatively little superficial damage to alert caregivers to the extent of tissue injury[71].

Shearing Forces

Shearing forces result from the sliding and relative displacement of two apposing surfaces. Although externally applied pressure is more effective than shear alone in reducing skin arteriolar blood flow, these two factors can combine to enhance vascular occlusion. The size and grade of a pressure ulcer are also influenced by shearing forces. When the head of a supine patient is raised more than 30°, shearing forces occur in the sacral and coccygeal areas. Sliding of the torso transmits pressure to the sacrum and deep fascia, although the outer sacral skin is fixed because of friction with the bed. Vessels in the deep part of the superficial fascia angulate and thrombose, which manifests clinically as undermining of the ulcer. Shearing forces are accentuated by the lack of tensile strength in the subcutaneous tissue, which renders it more vulnerable to mechanical forces[71].

Friction and Moisture

Friction is the force that resists relative motion between two surfaces in contact. It is produced when a bedridden patient is dragged across the bed sheets. Damage to the protective stratum corneum enhances skin ulceration by compromising the skin barrier. Moist environments are created from perspiration and fecal and/or urinary incontinence, and, if long-term, can increase the risk of pressure ulcer formation fivefold[71].

CLINICAL FEATURES

Many classification systems exist to categorize pressure ulcers, but in this chapter we discuss the one that the National Pressure Ulcer Advisory Panel (NPUAP) (1989) employs. The ulcers do not necessarily progress sequentially from stage I to stage IV, nor do they necessarily heal from stage IV to stage I (Fig. 105.22)[72].

- *Stage I*: non-blanchable erythema of intact skin. This finding is the heralding sign of impending skin ulceration. For darker-skinned individuals, other signs may be indicators, including warmth, edema, discoloration of the skin, and induration[71,72].
- *Stage II*: partial-thickness skin loss involving the epidermis, dermis, or both. This superficial lesion presents as an erosion, blister or shallow ulcer[71,72].
- *Stage III*: full-thickness skin loss in which the subcutaneous tissue is damaged or necrotic; it may extend down to, but does not include, the underlying fascia. This deep lesion presents as a crater-like ulcer and sometimes involves adjacent tissue[71,72].
- *Stage IV*: full-thickness skin loss and extensive tissue necrosis; destruction extending to muscle, bone or supporting structures such as tendons or joint capsules. Undermining or sinus tracts can be present[71,72].

Limitations are evident in classifying pressure ulcers with this system. Stage I ulcers may be superficial or they may signal deeper tissue damage, and they are not always reliably assessed, especially in darkly

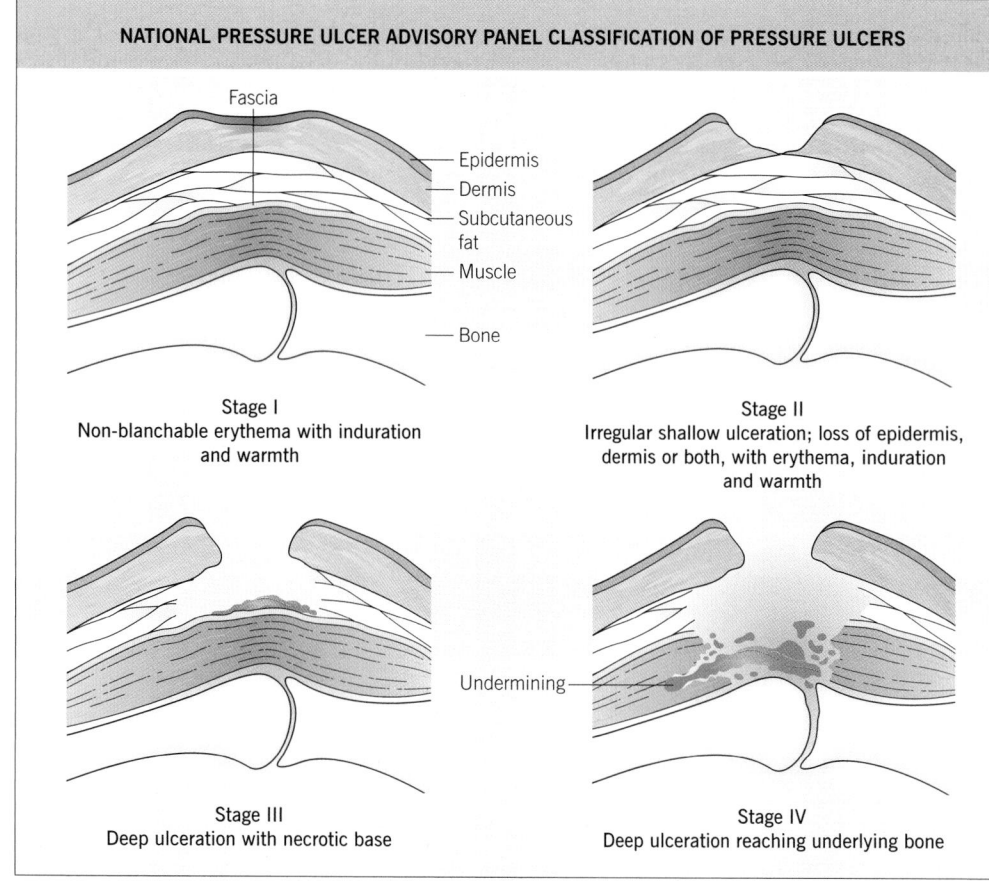

Fig. 105.22 **National Pressure Ulcer Advisory Panel classification of pressure ulcers. A** Stage I: non-blanchable erythema of intact skin. This lesion is the heralding sign of impending skin ulceration. For darker-skinned individuals, other signs may be indicators and include warmth, edema, discoloration of the skin, and induration. **B** Stage II: partial-thickness skin loss involving the epidermis, dermis or both. This superficial lesion presents as an abrasion, blister or shallow crater. **C** Stage III: full-thickness skin loss, in which subcutaneous tissue is damaged or necrotic and may extend down into, but not including, the underlying fascia. This deep lesion presents as a crater and sometimes involves adjacent tissue. **D** Stage IV: full-thickness skin loss and extensive tissue necrosis, destruction to muscle, bone, or supporting structures such as a tendon or joint capsule. Undermining or sinus tracts can be present.

NATIONAL PRESSURE ULCER ADVISORY PANEL CLASSIFICATION OF PRESSURE ULCERS

Fascia

Epidermis
Dermis
Subcutaneous fat
Muscle

Bone

Stage I
Non-blanchable erythema with induration and warmth

Stage II
Irregular shallow ulceration; loss of epidermis, dermis or both, with erythema, induration and warmth

Undermining

Stage III
Deep ulceration with necrotic base

Stage IV
Deep ulceration reaching underlying bone

pigmented skin. Adequate evaluation may also be hampered by the presence of an eschar, which should be debrided for full assessment[71].

Most pressure ulcers, regardless of the setting, are partial thickness (stages I–II) and are located on the sacrum or coccyx. The second most common site is the heels.

PATHOLOGY

In the earliest clinically recognizable stage of *blanchable* erythema, the superficial dermal capillaries and venules dilate. Mild to moderate edema appears in the papillary dermis in association with a mild perivascular lymphocytic infiltrate. The epidermis, pilosebaceous structures and reticular dermis remain normal. This scenario is in contrast to *non-blanchable* erythema, where there is red blood cell engorgement of capillaries and venules, platelet thrombi, and hemorrhage into the papillary dermis. Although the epidermis still appears normal, sweat gland and subcutaneous fat degeneration is often present[71].

Early lesions have crusting or erosion of the epidermis. Subepidermal separation can occur with formation of a subepidermal bulla. The epidermis, sweat glands and hair follicles may be normal or necrotic. In early ulceration, the epidermis is lost and the dermal papillae are often identifiable. Acute inflammation of the papillary and reticular dermis is seen. Chronic ulcers show a diffusely fibrotic dermis with loss of appendages. On their surface, they can have a hemorrhagic crust containing acute inflammatory cells or a thin zone of coagulation necrosis. In the black eschar stage, full-thickness destruction of the skin occurs. General dermal architecture is preserved, but there is obliteration of cellular detail. Histopathologic studies demonstrate that early pressure damage first involves deeper structures, and thus what is initially seen as localized surface erythema may actually be the 'tip of the iceberg'[71].

TREATMENT

Pressure on the ulcer should be relieved. This can be accomplished by frequent position changes. In addition, a variety of support surfaces, such as air- or liquid-filled flotation devices and foam products, as well as positioning devices such as pillows and foam wedges, are used to relieve pressure. Ulcer care is critical, and the general principles discussed in other sections of this chapter may be applied to pressure ulcer management. Briefly, debridement may be via mechanical, enzymatic and/or autolytic means. Wounds should be cleansed as nontraumatically as possible, and normal saline is preferred to cytotoxic agents such as hydrogen peroxide or povidone-iodine. As always, bacterial colonization and infection must be monitored. Dressings should provide a moist, but not macerated, environment and occlusive dressings are often utilized.

In addition to local wound care, management of pressure ulcers should address the general condition of the patient, including ensuring adequate nutrition, education, pain management, and the provision of psychosocial support. Causes of immobility and systemic conditions that interfere with wound healing or decrease tissue perfusion must be considered, including congestive heart failure, diabetes and/or spastic paresis. In general, stage I, II, and III pressure ulcers are more likely to heal with local therapy, whereas stage IV ulcers, particularly over the ischial tuberosities, often require surgical intervention. Adjuvant therapies such as laser, ultrasound, hyperbaric oxygen, and UV irradiation are being investigated and are not yet standard recommendations. The application of growth factors, cultured keratinocyte grafts and skin substitutes is promising, but these are also still in the investigational stage.

REFERENCES

1. Lazarus GS, Cooper DM, Knighton DR, et al. Definitions and guidelines for assessment of wounds and evaluation of healing. Arch Dermatol. 1994;130:489–93.
2. Phillips TJ, Al-Amoudi HO, Leverkus M, Park HY. Effect of chronic wound fluid on fibroblasts. J Wound Care. 1998;7:527–32.
2a. Chen WYJ, Rogers AA. Recent insights into the causes of chronic leg ulceration in venous disease and implications on other types of chronic wounds. Wound Rep Reg. 2007;15:434–49.
3. Bello YM, Phillips TJ. Therapeutic dressings. Adv Dermatol. 2000;16:253–71.
4. Nelzen O, Bergquist D, Lindhagen A, Hallbook T. Chronic leg ulcers: an underestimated problem in primary health care among elderly patients. J Epidemiol Commun Health. 1991;45:184–7.
5. Phillips TJ, Dover JS. Leg ulcers. J Am Acad Dermatol. 1991;25:965–87.
5a. Bergan JJ, Schmid-Schonbein GW, Coleridge Smith PD, Nicolaides AN, et al. Chronic venous disease. NEJM;2006;335:488–98.
6. Phillips T, Stanton B, Provan A, Lew R. A study of the impact of leg ulcers on quality of life: financial, social, and psychological implications. J Am Acad Dermatol. 1994;31:49–53.
7. Phillips TJ. Chronic cutaneous ulcers: etiology and epidemiology. J Invest Dermatol. 1994;102:38S–41S.
8. Phillips TJ. Current approaches to venous ulcers and compression. Dermatol Surg. 2001;27:611–21.
9. Hansson C, Andersson E, Swanbeck G. Leg ulcer epidemiology in Gothenburg. Acta Chir Scand. 1988;544(suppl.):12–16.
10. Cornwall JV, Dore CJ, Lewis JD. Leg ulcers: epidemiology and aetiology. Br J Surg. 1986;73:693–6.
11. Baker SR, Stacey MC, Jopp-McKay AG, et al. Epidemiology of chronic venous ulcers. Br J Surg. 1991;78:864–7.
12. Hallbook T. Leg ulcer epidemiology. Acta Chir Scand. 1988;544(suppl.):17–20.
13. Callam MF, Ruckley CV, Harper DR, Dale JJ. Chronic ulceration of the leg: extent of the problem and provision of care. Br Med J (Clin Res Ed). 1985;290:1855–6.
14. McGuckin M, Stineman MG, Goin JE (eds). Venous Leg Ulcer Guideline. Philadelphia: University of Pennsylvania, 1997.

15. Scott TE, LaMorte WW, Gorin DR, Menzoian JO. Risk factors for chronic venous insufficiency: a dual case-control study. J Vasc Surg. 1995;22:622–8.
16. Baker SR, Jopp-McKay AG, Hoskin SE, Thompson PJ. Epidemiology of chronic venous ulcers. Br J Surg. 1991;78:864–7.
17. Margolis DM, Berlin JA, Strom BL. Risk factors associated with the failure of a venous ulcer to heal. Arch Dermatol. 1999;135:920–6.
18. Hiatt WR. Medical treatment of peripheral arterial disease and claudication. N Engl J Med. 2001;344:1608–21.
19. Pham HT, Rich J, Veves A. Wound healing in diabetic foot ulceration: a review and commentary. Wounds. 2000;12:79–81.
20. American Diabetes Association. Consensus Development Conference on Diabetic Foot Wound Care, Boston, MA, 7-8 April 1999.
21. Browne AC, Sibbald RG. The diabetic neuropathic ulcer: an overview. Ostomy Wound Manage. 1999; 45(1A suppl.):6S–20S.
22. Valencia IC, Falabella A, Kirsner RS, Eaglstein WH. Chronic venous insufficiency and venous leg ulceration. J Am Acad Dermatol. 2001;44:401–21.
23. Burnand KG, Whimster I, Naidoo A, Browse NL. Pericapillary fibrin in the ulcer-bearing skin of the leg: the cause of lipodermatosclerosis and venous ulceration. Br Med J (Clin Res Ed). 1982;285:1071–2.
24. Falanga V, Kirsner R, Katz MH, et al. Pericapillary fibrin cuffs in venous ulceration. Persistence with treatment and during ulcer healing. J Dermatol Surg Oncol. 1992;18:409–14.
25. Ouahes N, Phillips TJ. Leg ulcers. Curr Probl Dermatol. 1995;7:109–42.
26. Falanga V, Eaglstein WH. The trap hypothesis of venous ulceration. Lancet. 1993;341:1006–8.
27. Coleridge-Smith PD, Thomas P, Scurr JH, Dormandy JA. Causes of venous ulceration: a new hypothesis. Br Med J (Clin Res Ed). 1988;296:1726–7.
28. Gourdin FW, Smith JG Jr. Etiology of venous ulceration. South Med J. 1993;86:1142–6.
29. Mendez MV, Raffetto JD, Phillips TJ, Menzoian JO, Park HY. The proliferative capacity of neonatal skin fibroblasts is reduced after exposure to venous ulcer wound fluid: a potential mechanism for senescence in venous ulcers. J Vasc Surg. 1999;30:734–43.

30. Caputo GM, Cavanagh PR, Ulbrecht JS, et al. Assessment and management of foot disease in patients with diabetes. N Engl J Med. 1994;331:854–60.
31. Kumar S, Fernando DJ, Veves A, Knowles EA, Young MJ, Boulton AJ. Semmes-Weinsten monofilaments: a simple, effective and inexpensive screening device for identifying diabetic patients at risk of foot ulceration. Diabetes Res Clin Pract. 1991;13:63–7.
32. Naghibi M, Smith RP, Baltch AL, et al. The effect of diabetes mellitus on chemotactic and bactericidal activity of human polymorphonuclear leukocytes. Diabetes Res Clin Pract.1987;4:27–35.
33. Kanj LF, Phillips TJ. Management of leg ulcers. Fitzpatrick's J Clin Dermatol. 1994;Sept/Oct:52–60.
34. Sumpio BE. Foot ulcers. N Engl J Med. 2000;343:787–93.
35. Rockson SG. Lymphedema. Am J Med. 2001;110:288–95.
36. Zouboulis CC, Biczo S, Gollnick H, et al. Elephantiasis nostras verrucosa: beneficial effect of oral etretinate therapy. Br J Dermatol. 1992;127:411–16.
37. Vowden K, Vowden P. Doppler and the ABPI; how good is our understanding? J Wound Care. 2001;10:197–202.
38. De Villez RL, Roberts LC. Acroangiodermatitis of Mali. South Med J. 1984;77:255–8.
39. Lyle WG, Given KS. Acroangiodermatitis (pseudo-Kaposi's sarcoma) associated with Klippel-Trenauney syndrome. Ann Plast Surg. 1996;37:654–6.
40. Beightler E, Diven DG, Sanchez RL, Solomon AR. Thrombotic vasculopathy associated with cryofibrinogenemia. J Am Acad Dermatol. 1991;24:342–5.
41. Bello YM, Khachmoune A, Stefanato CM, Phillips TJ. Diagnostic dilemmas – cryofibrinogenemia. Wounds. 2000;12:76–8.
42. Kirsner RS, Eaglstein WH, Katz MH, Kerdel FA, Falanga V. Stanazol causes rapid pain relief and healing of cutaneous ulcers caused by cryofibrinogenemia. J Am Acad Dermatol. 1993;28:71–4.
43. Mishima Y. Thromboangiitis obliterans (Buerger's disease). Int J Cardiol. 1996;54(suppl.):185–7.
44. Shionoya S. Diagnostic criteria of Buerger's disease. Int J Cardiol. 1998;66(suppl.):243–5.
45. Olin JW. Thromboangiitis obliterans (Buerger's disease). N Engl J Med. 2000;343:864–9.
46. Levenson SM, Seifter E. Dysnutrition, wound healing, and resistance to infection. Clin Plast Surg. 1977;4:375–88.

47. Bello YM, Phillips TJ. Management of venous ulcers. J Cutan Med Surg. 1998;3(suppl. 1): S1-6–12.

48. Ongenae KC, Phillips TJ. Leg ulcer management. Emerg Med. 1993;25:45–53.

49. Kantor J, Margolis DJ. A multicentre study of percentage change in venous leg ulcer area as a prognostic index of healing at 24 weeks. Br J Dermatol. 2000;142:960–4.

50. Phillips TJ, Machado F, Trout R, et al. Prognostic indicators in venous ulcers. J Am Acad Dermatol. 2000;43:627–30.

51. Goslen JB. Wound healing for the dermatologic surgeon. J Dermatol Surg Oncol. 1988;14:959–72.

52. Dyson M, Young SR, Hart J, et al. Comparison of the effects of moist and dry conditions on the process of angiogenesis during dermal repair. J Invest Dermatol. 1992;99:729–33.

53. Ovington LG. Wound care products: how to choose. Adv Skin Wound Care. 2001;14:259–64.

54. Williams D, Enoch S, Miller D, et al. Effect of debridement using curette on recalcitrant nonhealing venous leg ulcers. A concurrently controlled, prospective cohort study. Wound Repair Regen. 2005,13;131–7.

55. Cullum N, Nelson EA, Fletcher AW, Sheldon TA. Compression for venous leg ulcers (Cochrane Review). In: The Cochrane Library, Issue 2, 2004. Oxford: Update Software.

56. Barwell JR, Davies CE, Deacon J, et al. Comparison of surgery and compression with compression alone in chronic venous ulceration (ESCHAR study): randomized controlled trial. Lancet. 2004;363;1854–9.

57. Falanga V, Margolis D, Alvares O, et al. Rapid healing of venous ulcers and lack of clinical rejection with an allogeneic cultured human skin equivalent. Arch Dermatol. 1998;134:293–300.

58. Phillips TJ. Successful methods of treating leg ulcers. Postgrad Med.1999;105:159–74.

59. Phillips TJ, Rogers GS, Kanj LF. Case report: bacitracin anaphylaxis. J Geriatr Dermatol. 1995;3:83–5.

60. Katz BE, Fisher N. Bacitracin: a unique topical antibiotic sensitizer. J Am Acad Dermatol. 1987;17:1016–24.

61. Bello YM, Falabella AF, Carbalho HD, Nayyar G, Kirsner RS. Infection and wound healing. Wounds. 2001;13:127–31.

62. Choucair MM, Phillips TJ. What is new in clinical research in wound healing? Dermatol Clin. 1997;15:45–58.

63. Badievas EV, Falanga V. Treatment of chronic wounds with bone marrow-derived cells. Arch Dermatol. 2003;139:510–16.

64. Colgan MP, Dormandy JA, Jones PN, et al. Oxpentifylline treatment of venous ulcers of the leg. BMJ. 1990;300:972–5.

65. Dale JJ, Ruckley CV, Harper DR, et al. Randomized, double blind placebo controlled trial of pentoxyfylline in the treatment of venous leg ulcers. BMJ. 1999;319:875–8.

66. Falanga V, Fujitana RM, Diaz C, et al. Systemic treatment of venous leg ulcers with high doses of pentoxifylline: efficacy in a randomized, placebo-controlled trial. Wound Repair Regen. 1999;7:208–13.

67. Phillips TJ. New skin for old: developments in biological skin substitutes. Arch Dermatol. 1998;134:344–9.

68. Phillips TJ. Biologic skin substitutes. J Dermatol Surg Oncol. 1993;19:794–800.

69. Falanga V. Care of venous leg ulcers. Ostomy Wound Manage. 1999;45(suppl.):33S–43S.

70. Marston W, Hanft J, Norwood P, Pollak R. The safety and efficacy of Dermagraft in improving the healing of chronic diabetic foot ulcers: results of a prospective randomized trial. Diabetes Care. 2003;261:1701–5.

71. Kanj LF, Wilking SVB, Phillips TJ. Pressure ulcers. J Am Acad Dermatol. 1998;38:517–36.

72. Bergstrom, N, Allman, RM, Alvarez OM, et al. Treatment of pressures ulcers. Clinical Practice Guideline, No 15. Publication No. 95-0652, Dec 1994. Rockville: US Department of Health and Human Services.

Other Vascular Disorders

106

Christopher Baker and Robert Kelly

Chapter Contents

INTRODUCTION

This chapter will cover several disorders of the skin vasculature, including livedo reticularis, flushing and erythromelalgia, as well as vascular ectasias such as telangiectasias and angiokeratomas. Some of the diseases described here are important skin signs of systemic disease, while others are incidental findings. Additional disorders of blood vessels are covered elsewhere, e.g. infantile hemangiomas (Ch. 103), vascular malformations (Ch. 104), and vascular neoplasms and proliferations (Ch. 114).

LIVEDO RETICULARIS

Key features

- A common physiologic finding consisting of a mottled reticulated vascular pattern
- May occur secondarily due to an underlying disease, e.g. autoimmune connective tissue disease
- The pattern varies depending on the underlying cause
- Appropriate investigations depend on the clinical context and associated findings

Introduction

Livedo reticularis (LR) is an extremely common finding and usually results from a physiologic vasospastic response to cold exposure. Among normal healthy individuals, the predisposition to LR will vary. It can also be a reflection of a number of underlying systemic diseases. LR resulting from any cause can vary to some degree with changes in external temperature. Physiologic LR will usually disappear with warming and reappear with cooling. Other variants may persist to varying degrees with warming.

History

The term 'livedo reticularis' was first used by Hebra over a century ago to describe a violaceous skin discoloration caused by an abnormality of the cutaneous circulation. Renault (1883) and later Unna (1896) and Spalteholz (1927) suggested that a cone arrangement of the cutaneous microvasculature served as an explanation for the occurrence and pattern of LR[1].

Pathogenesis

LR results from alterations in blood flow through the cutaneous microvasculature system (Fig. 106.1). The latter consists of arterioles that are

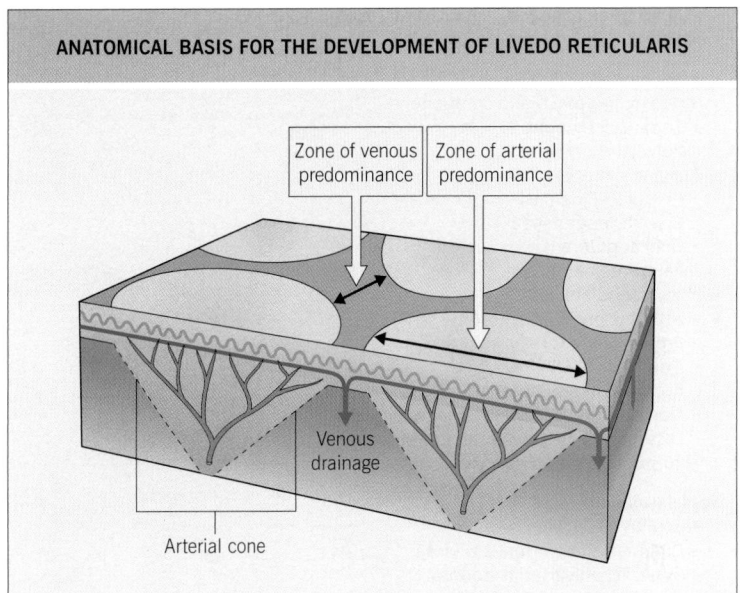

ANATOMICAL BASIS FOR THE DEVELOPMENT OF LIVEDO RETICULARIS

Fig. 106.1 Anatomical basis for the development of livedo reticularis.

oriented perpendicularly to the skin surface. The vessels then divide into capillary beds that in turn drain into a subpapillary plexus. It has been proposed that this arrangement of vessels gives rise to a series of 1 to 3 cm cones with the ascending arteriole at the apex of each cone. At the edge of the cone, the venous plexus is more prominent and the arterial bed is diminished. Any process that either reduces blood flow to and through the skin or reduces drainage of blood out of the skin will result in the accumulation of deoxygenated blood in the venous plexus, leading to the clinical appearance of LR[1-3].

There are a number of causes of LR (Table 106.1) and the clinical pattern of LR can vary with the nature of the underlying cause. A complete fine network is indicative of alterations in blood flow caused by vasospasm or by factors within the blood that alter the viscosity and the flow through the vessels. Vessel wall pathology and intraluminal obstruction are more likely to result in a patchy distribution of LR, depending on the distribution of the underlying pathology.

Livedo racemosa (Fig. 106.2) refers to a distinct pattern of LR consisting of a large branching pattern that is usually situated on the trunk and proximal limbs. It is generally indicative of Sneddon's syndrome, which is associated with multiple strokes that lead to progressive neurologic impairment[4]. Similar findings may also be seen in the antiphospholipid antibody syndrome (APS)[5].

Clinical Features

Congenital livedo reticularis

Cutis marmorata telangiectatica congenita

Cutis marmorata telangiectatica congenita (CMTC) is characterized by a persistent reticulated vascular pattern that is often limited to one extremity (see. Ch. 104) but can be more widespread. Lesions are usually noted at birth, and, when the trunk is involved, there may be a sharp cut off at the midline. Associated anomalies include other vascular birthmarks, limb asymmetry and, occasionally, neurologic or ocular abnormalities[6,7]. Cutaneous vascular changes can improve during the first few years of life, with 20% of patients showing complete resolution.

CAUSES OF LIVEDO RETICULARIS
Congenital livedo reticularis
• Cutis marmorata telangiectatica congenita
Acquired livedo reticularis
Vasospasm
• Cutis marmorata/physiologic livedo reticularis
• Primary (idiopathic) livedo reticularis
• Autoimmune connective tissue diseases (e.g. SLE)
• Raynaud's phenomenon/disease
Intravascular/reduced flow
• Increased normal blood components
– Thrombocythemia
– Polycythemia vera
• Abnormal proteins
– Cryoglobulinemia
– Cryofibrinogenemia
– Cold agglutinins
– Paraproteinemia
• Hypercoagulability
– Antiphospholipid syndrome
– Protein S and C deficiencies
– Antithrombin III deficiency
– Factor V Leiden mutation
– Homocystinuria, hyperhomocysteinemia
– Disseminated intravascular coagulation
• Thrombotic thrombocytopenic purpura
Vessel wall pathology
• Vasculitis
– Cutaneous polyarteritis nodosa
– Systemic polyarteritis nodosa
– Cryoglobulinemic vasculitis
– Autoimmune connective tissue disease-associated vasculitis (e.g. rheumatoid arthritis, SLE, Sjögren's syndrome)
• Calciphylaxis
• Sneddon's syndrome
• Livedoid vasculopathy (also intraluminal obstruction)
Vessel obstruction
• Embolic
– Cholesterol emboli
– Septic emboli
– Atrial myxoma
– Nitrogen (decompression sickness)
– Carbon dioxide arteriography
• Thrombosis (see above)
• Hyperoxaluria
Other
• Medications (e.g. amantadine, norepinephrine, interferon)
• Infections (e.g. hepatitis C [vasculitis], *Mycoplasma* [cold agglutinins], syphilis)
• Neoplasms (e.g. pheochromocytoma)
• Neurologic disorders (e.g. reflex sympathetic dystrophy, paralysis)
• Moyamoya disease

Table 106.1 **Causes of livedo reticularis.** SLE, systemic lupus erythematosus.

PATTERN OF LIVEDO RETICULARIS VERSUS LIVEDO RACEMOSA

(A) Livedo reticularis   (B) Livedo racemosa

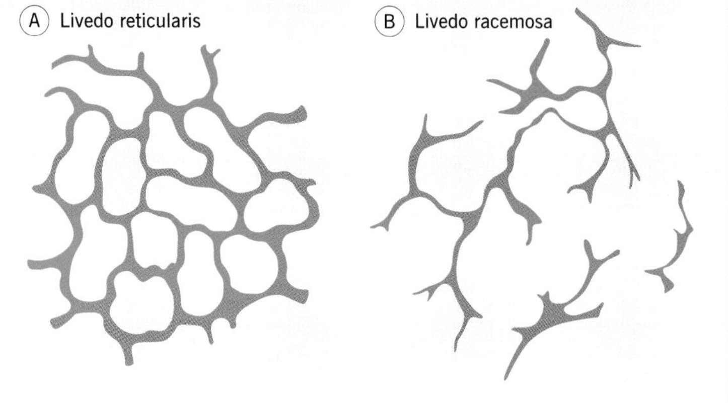

Fig. 106.2 **Pattern of livedo reticularis (A) versus livedo racemosa (B).**

Acquired livedo reticularis
Livedo reticularis without systemic associations
Physiologic livedo reticularis/cutis marmorata
These terms are synonymous and refer to a normal pattern of LR that occurs in response to cold (Fig. 106.3A). It is often more marked in neonates, infants and young children[2,3]. In adults, it may be associated with a tendency towards acrocyanosis and chilblains.

Primary/idiopathic livedo reticularis
This refers to a persistent fine network of LR that is often widespread, particularly on the lower extremities. While there is some fluctuation with temperature, the LR will usually persist with warming (Fig. 106.3B). It is due to persistent vasospasm of arterioles and is not secondary to any underlying cause. However, primary LR is a diagnosis of exclusion and it is important to consider secondary causes (see Table 106.1). This is especially true when the LR is extensive[2,3].

Livedo reticularis secondary to systemic disease
Livedo reticularis due to vasospasm
Vasospasm is the most common cause of LR, including that seen in association with autoimmune connective tissue diseases (CTD; Fig. 106.3C). Reflecting a vasospastic tendency, it occurs more commonly in patients with Raynaud's phenomenon.

Livedo reticularis due to intraluminal pathology
Blood viscosity can be increased either by the presence of abnormal proteins (e.g. cryoglobulins[8], cryofibrinogens, cold agglutinins, paraproteins) or by an increase in quantities of normal blood components (e.g. polycythemia vera[9] or thrombocytosis). A fine, evenly distributed pattern of LR is usually seen. Hypercoagulable states can also be associated with LR, including the APS[10] and protein C[11], protein S or antithrombin III deficiencies[12]. LR of the lower extremities is often seen in patients with neurologic conditions that lead to immobility of the lower limbs and stasis.

Livedo reticularis due to vessel wall pathology
Vasculitis is the most common cause of vessel wall pathology associated with LR. In general, LR will only occur if medium-sized arterioles at the dermal–subcutaneous border or in the deep dermis are affected. Cutaneous polyarteritis nodosa (PAN) always involves these vessels and is therefore invariably associated with LR[13]. Systemic PAN, cryoglobulinemic vasculitis and autoimmune CTD-related vasculitis may also affect these arterioles. The pattern of LR seen is usually a larger network that may be continuous or patchy depending on the distribution of vessel involvement.

Calciphylaxis consists of calcium deposition in the walls of blood vessels (see Ch. 50). It is most commonly seen in the setting of chronic renal failure complicated by hyperparathyroidism. It may initially commence with LR that becomes purpuric and subsequently necrotic (Fig. 106.4).

Sneddon's syndrome is a rare syndrome consisting of widespread livedo racemosa (Fig. 106.5A) in conjunction with multiple cerebral ischemic episodes leading to progressive neurologic impairment[4,5]. It remains uncertain as to whether the vascular pattern results from vasculopathy, vasculitis or coagulopathy, but characteristic changes are seen within affected vessels (Fig. 106.5B; see below).

Livedo reticularis due to intraluminal obstruction
This can result from either emboli (e.g. cholesterol emboli derived from atheromata[14]) or thromboses within vessels (e.g. APS, heparin or warfarin necrosis). Intracellular crystal deposition is seen in hyperoxaluria and this also gives rise to luminal obstruction and LR[15]. A patchy, discontinuous-pattern LR is seen with intraluminal obstruction and it may subsequently become purpuric with areas of infarction and necrosis.

A combination of intraluminal obstruction and vessel wall pathology is seen in livedoid vasculopathy. This is an uncommon condition that is sometimes associated with LR. It consists of multiple recurrent painful ulcers on the lower extremities that heal slowly with residual atrophie blanche. Histologically, vessel lumina are filled with hyaline thrombi, and fibrinoid material is also present in the walls of these vessels and in the perivascular stroma[16].

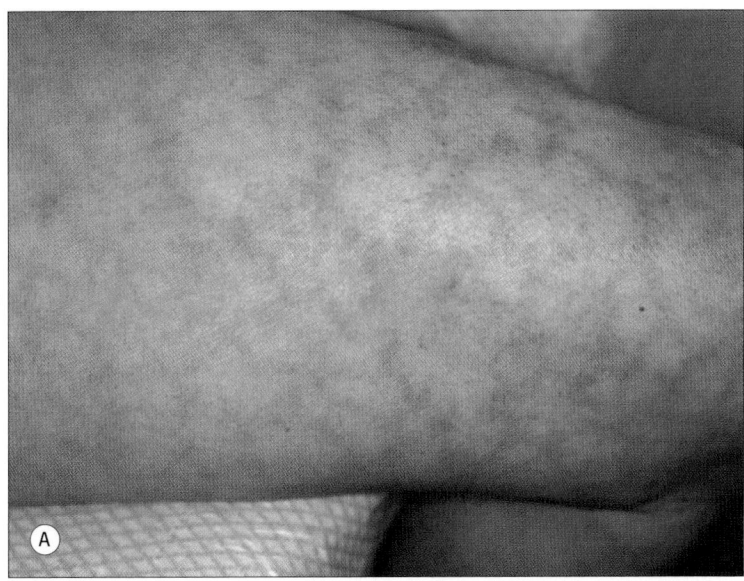

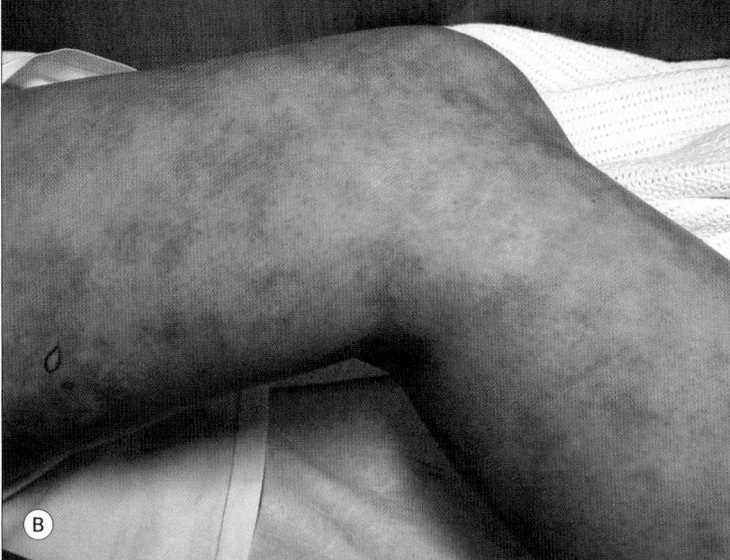

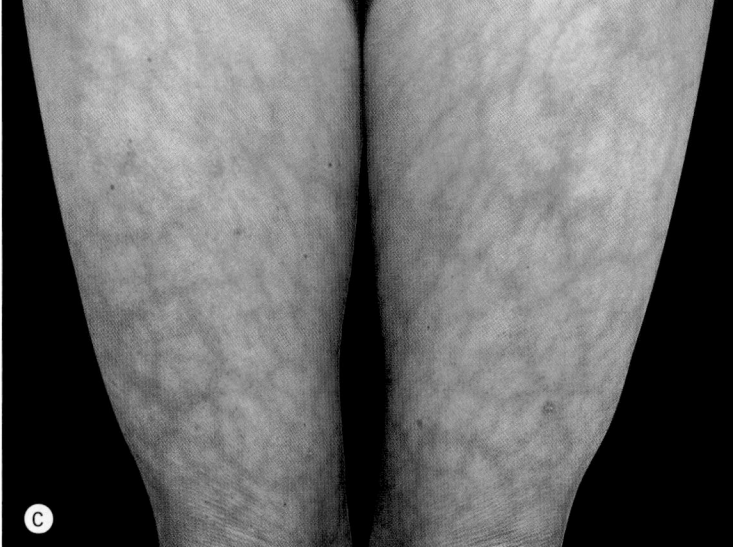

Fig. 106.3 Livedo reticularis. A An even net-like pattern is seen on the thigh in physiologic livedo reticularis. **B** In primary (idiopathic) livedo reticularis, the pattern persists with warming. **C** Livedo reticularis in a patient with lupus erythematosus. C, Courtesy of Jeff Callen MD.

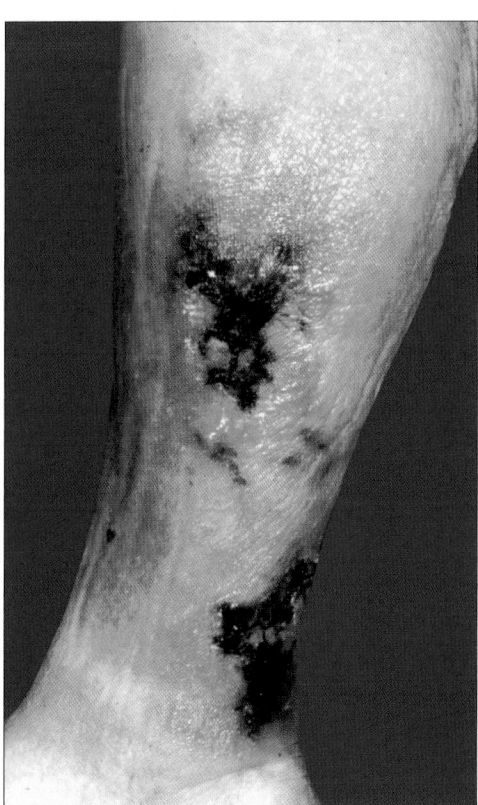

Fig. 106.4 Reticulate purpura and cutaneous necrosis due to calciphylaxis. These patients also often have areas of livedo reticularis. Courtesy of Norbert Sepp MD.

Other causes of livedo reticularis

There are numerous causes of LR cited in the literature, and, in most, one of the above mechanisms can generally be implicated. The other causes include drugs such as amantadine[17] and norepinephrine, as well as infections. The latter can lead to: the production of cryoglobulins, cold agglutinins or antiphospholipid antibodies; the induction of immune vasculitis; or septic vasculitis or septic emboli. Neoplasms may also be associated with LR via hypercoagulability or paraproteinemia as well as vasospasm (e.g. pheochromocytoma). LR may also be seen in several neurologic conditions (e.g. reflex sympathetic dystrophy) as a result of vasospasm or vasodilation (this is in addition to stasis arising from immobility).

Differential Diagnosis

Erythema ab igne is a heat-induced skin disease that begins as a reversible LR, then, with continued heat exposure, evolves into a fixed reticulated hyperpigmentation in the same pattern. Various cutaneous eruptions may have a reticulated pattern and might be confused with LR, including reticulated erythematous mucinosis (favors mid central trunk) and some viral exanthems (e.g. erythema infectiosum). Poikilodermatous conditions may also have a reticulate pattern (e.g. mycosis fungoides, dermatomyositis or GVHD); however, the presence of epidermal changes and telangiectasias will help distinguish these conditions from LR.

Pathology

The histology of LR varies depending on the underlying cause. In idiopathic or physiologic forms resulting from vasospasm, no abnormality will be evident. With secondary causes of LR, a number of abnormalities may be seen, including vasculitis, calcium deposition within vessel walls (calciphylaxis), intravascular eosinophilic plugging (monoclonal cryoglobulinemia), intraluminal thromboses (hypercoagulable states), cholesterol clefting (cholesterol emboli) and crystal deposition (oxalosis). In Sneddon's syndrome, vessel walls demonstrate endothelial inflammation and subendothelial myointimal hyperplasia with partial or complete occlusion of affected arterioles (see Fig. 106.5B). In order to locate the histopathologic changes, it is necessary to sample the affected arterioles. A moderately large elliptical biopsy from the non-discolored skin in the center of the net pattern is necessary and serial sectioning may be required.

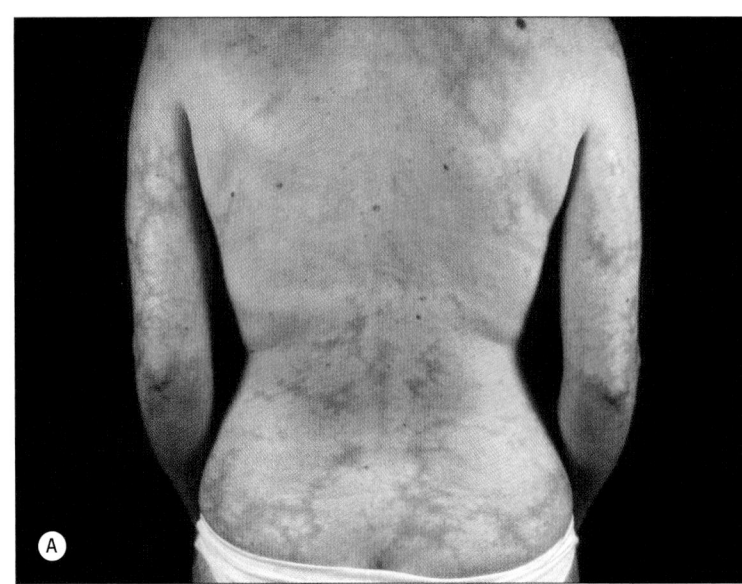

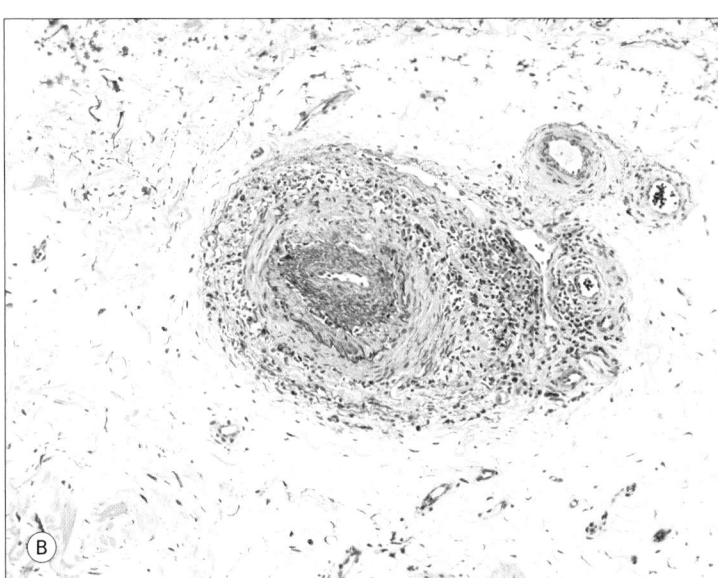

Fig. 106.5 Sneddon's syndrome. A The characteristic irregular, broken, branching pattern as seen on the back and arms. **B** Connective tissue stain showing a subcutaneous artery with subendothelial proliferation of smooth muscle leading to almost complete luminal occlusion.

CAUSES OF FLUSHING
• Physiologic
• Exogenous agents (see Table 106.3)
• Menopause
• Neurologic disorders
• Anxiety
• Autonomic dysfunction
• Tumors (e.g. hypogonadal pituitary tumors)
• Migraine
• Frey's syndrome (auriculotemporal syndrome)
• Systemic diseases
• Carcinoid syndrome
• Mastocytosis
• Pheochromocytoma
• Medullary carcinoma of the thyroid
• Thyrotoxicosis
• POEMS syndrome
• Pancreatic tumors (e.g. VIPomas)
• Prostaglandin-secreting renal cell carcinoma

Table 106.2 Causes of flushing.

EXOGENOUS AGENTS THAT CAN CAUSE FLUSHING
• Alcohol
• Drugs
• Angiotensin-converting enzyme (ACE) inhibitors
• Calcium channel blockers
• Calcitonin
• Chlorpropamide*
• Cholinergic agonists (e.g. pilocarpine)
• Cyclosporine
• Disulfiram*
• Fumaric acid esters
• Gold ('nitritoid reactions')
• Hydralazine
• Nicotinic acid
• Nitrates (e.g. glyceryl trinitrate)
• Opiates
• Prostaglandins
• Sildenafil, tadalafil, vardenafil
• Tamoxifen
• Foods
• Spoiled scombroid fish
• Foods additives
• Monosodium glutamate (MSG), sodium nitrite, sulfites
*With alcohol intake.

Table 106.3 Exogenous agents that can cause flushing.

Treatment

LR is a clinical sign and does not require treatment per se. It is unresponsive to treatments such as vascular laser therapy or vasodilatory medications. Underlying causes require identification and appropriate treatment.

FLUSHING

Key features

■ Flushing is a physiologic response, but in an exaggerated form causes clinical symptoms

■ Common triggers (e.g. heat, emotion, exercise and some foods) will exacerbate flushing of any cause

■ Causes of excessive flushing include exogenous medications, menopause, neurologic disorders and systemic diseases

Introduction

Flushing is the term used to describe transient and episodic reddening of the skin, most commonly of the face, and less often the neck, ears and upper chest. It is the visible sign of a generalized increase in cutaneous blood flow. The greater visibility and capacitance of the superficial cutaneous vasculature of the face and adjacent areas accounts for the limited distribution[18]. In the evaluation of an affected patient, there are a number of causes to consider, including underlying systemic disorders (Table 106.2).

Pathogenesis

An increase in cutaneous blood flow occurs with relaxation of vascular smooth muscle. This may occur via the autonomic nervous system[19] (usually leading to active vasodilation), endogenous vasoactive agents (such as histamine and serotonin) or exogenous agents (Table 106.3). Alcohol-induced flushing may result from both the direct effect of alcohol and cutaneous vasodilation from elevated blood levels of acetaldehyde; the latter occurs in those with alcohol dehydrogenase deficiency (prevalent in Asians) and in the 'disulfiram reaction' induced by some medications. Flushing from fermented alcoholic drinks may be caused by vasoactive substances such as tyramine[20]. Vasodilation mediated by the autonomic nervous system is often accompanied by eccrine sweating due to a direct effect on both sweat glands and blood vessels (wet flush)[21]. Direct vasodilation by vasoactive agents is usually not associated with increased sweating (dry flush).

Clinical Features

Blushing is a common emotionally triggered form of flushing associated with embarrassment and anxiety and is considered an exaggerated physiologic response. *Physiologic flushing* also occurs as part of normal thermoregulation in response to heat or exercise. *'Hot flashes'* refer to flushing associated with menopause, which lasts for a few minutes and is usually associated with sweating[22]. Flushing of any cause may be exacerbated or triggered by a number of common factors such as heat, hot drinks, exercise, anxiety, food additives and alcohol. Affected patients often report a feeling of heat and burning of the skin during episodes and find the color change a social hinderance. Some patients become anxious that they will flush at inopportune times and this further exacerbates the problem. Repeated flushing may lead to fixed erythema, telangiectasias and rosacea.

Those carcinoid tumors that secrete vasoactive agents (e.g. serotonin) are associated with the carcinoid syndrome (Table 106.4). Flushing, often severe, is present in the majority of cases of carcinoid syndrome[23] and may be precipitated by the common triggers of flushing. The classic 'carcinoid flush' seen with approximately 10% of midgut tumors (small intestine, appendix, proximal colon), lasts minutes and consists of erythema and pallor as well as a cyanotic hue. Of note, liver metastases are required. Type III gastric carcinoid tumors are associated with a pruritic patchy bright red flush admixed with white patches, which is probably mediated by histamine. Bronchial tumors are associated with a prolonged (hours to days) intensely red to purple flush. Hindgut tumors (distal colon, rectum) are rarely, if ever, associated with the carcinoid syndrome and flushing, even with liver metastases.

An approach to the clinical assessment of flushing and relevant investigations are listed in Table 106.5.

Differential Diagnosis

Fixed erythema, and sometimes telangiectasia, of the face and neck are seen in fair-skinned individuals with photodamage as well as patients with seborrheic dermatitis, photosensitivity disorders or autoimmune CTD. Affected individuals may complain of the persistent redness and burning of the skin rather than actual flushing. Rosacea may be associated with pronounced flushing, but, usually, fixed erythema, papulopustules, edema and/or telangiectasia are present to some degree.

Treatment

The clinician should consider and eliminate any suspected exogenous cause (see Table 106.3). Underlying systemic causes, although rare, should be considered (see Table 106.2). Triggers of flushing are likely to be clinically relevant in most cases and should be avoided where possible. Non-selective β-blockers (e.g. nadolol, propranolol) or clonidine may be effective in idiopathic flushing. Anxiolytics may be helpful, particularly if emotional symptoms or anxiety are evident. Menopausal flushing may respond to hormone replacement therapy, clonidine or selective serotonin reuptake inhibitors (SSRIs). In troublesome cases unresponsive to these measures, transthoracic endoscopic sympathectomy may be considered.

ERYTHROMELALGIA

Synonyms: ▪ Erythermalgia ▪ Erythralgia

Key features

- Characterized by painful burning and erythema of the distal extremities (lower > upper)
- Precipitated by heat and relieved by cooling
- May be idiopathic, familial or arise secondarily due to an underlying condition. Thrombocythemia is the most well recognized associated disorder

SIGNS AND SYMPTOMS OF THE CARCINOID SYNDROME

- Cutaneous
  - Flushing
  - Vascular rosacea-like changes
  - Pellagra
  - Edema and induration of the face > extremities
- Bronchospasm
- Diarrhea
- Cardiac dysfunction (right-sided)
- Hypotension
- Peptic ulcers

Table 106.4 **Signs and symptoms of the carcinoid syndrome.**

CLINICAL APPROACH TO THE EVALUATION OF FLUSHING

1. Identify provocative factors
   - Direct questioning
   - Patient diary (food, medications, activities)

2. Check for associated symptoms
   - Sweating
   - Urticaria
   - Diarrhea
   - Bronchospasm

3. Investigation
   Not required in all cases
   Indicated if flushing
   - Of sudden or recent onset
   - Severe
   - Associated with systemic symptoms

   Investigations to consider
   - Complete blood count with differential and platelets
   - Thyroid function tests
   - Serum tryptase, histamine and/or chromogranin A levels; plasma free metanephrines
   - 24-hour urine collection for
     - Serotonin metabolites such as 5-hydroxyindole acetic acid (5-HIAA)
     - Fractionated metanephrines
     - Histamine metabolites such as methylimidazole acetic acid (MIAA)
   - CT/MRI scans; somatostatin receptor scintigraphy (using radiolabeled analogue of somatostatin)

4. Elimination
   - Exclude suspected drugs and food additives

Table 106.5 **Clinical approach to the evaluation of flushing.**

Introduction

Erythromelalgia (EM) is an episodic condition characterized by a burning sensation, erythema and increased skin temperature. It affects acral sites, particularly the lower extremities. There are three major forms, including:

- Type 1 associated with thrombocythemia
- Type 2 primary or idiopathic form
- Type 3 associated with underlying causes other than thrombocythemia.

History

The term 'erythromelalgia' was first coined by Mitchell in 1878. It was used to describe redness (erythos), involvement of extremities (melos), and pain (algos). The diagnostic criteria were established by Thompson[24] in 1979: (1) burning pain in the extremities; (2) pain aggravated by warming; (3) pain relieved by cooling; (4) erythema of affected skin; and (5) increased temperature of affected skin.

Epidemiology

In Norway, the estimated incidence of EM is 0.25/100 000 with a prevalence of 2/100 000[25]. While types 1 and 3 usually appear during adulthood, type 2 may appear in childhood and may be familial. The female:male incidence varies from 2:1 to almost 3:1. In one study, the mean age of onset was 56 years (range, 5–91years) with 4% having their symptoms begin in childhood.

Pathogenesis

The pathogenesis of EM is not completely understood and may vary depending on the underlying cause and between different patient subgroups. In patients with thrombocythemia, it is likely to be related to both increased numbers of platelets as well as abnormalities in platelet function. Of note, an explanation for why type 1 EM does not respond to heparin or warfarin is that the microthrombi that form do not require thrombin activation[26]. In other types of EM, changes in vascular dynamics may be a factor. It has been proposed that hyperemia results from increased blood flow through arteriovenous shunts with a resultant reduction in blood flow within nutritional vessels, thus leading to cutaneous hypoxia[25,27]. Another proposed mechanism is vasoconstriction as occurs in Raynaud's phenomenon, but in EM it is followed by a prolonged phase of hyperemia[28]. Some investigators have suggested that temperature-triggered release of vasoactive substances and chemical pain mediators may play a role.

Recently, mutations in the *SCN9A* gene, which encodes the voltage-gated sodium channel alpha subunit Na(v)1.7, have been detected in patients with primary familial EM[29]. Na(v)1.7 produces threshold currents and is expressed within sensory neurons including nociceptors. Mutations lead to lowered thresholds and 'over-excitability' of pain-signaling sensory neurons[29a] while at the same time producing 'under-excitability' of sympathetic neurons. However, there exist additional families that are not linked to chromosome 2q31–32 (site of the *SCN9A* gene), suggesting genetic heterogeneity[30].

Associations in secondary EM include myelodysplastic syndromes, diabetes mellitus, peripheral vascular disease, vasculitis, systemic lupus erythematosus and other autoimmune CTDs.

Clinical Features

EM is characterized by burning, erythema and warmth of acral sites (Fig. 106.6). Attacks most commonly occur late in the day, last through the night, and frequently impair sleep. The symptoms are usually episodic, though occasionally may be continuous. The feet are involved in 90% of patients, whereas the hands are affected in 25%. Less commonly, there is also involvement of the head and neck. Type 1 EM may be unilateral and is more frequently associated with progression to ischemic necrosis. In contrast, the idiopathic type is more likely to be

bilateral. The pain is precipitated by minor elevations in temperature between 32°C and 36°C. Other exacerbating factors include exercise, standing, walking, fever, and limb dependency. Cooling and limb elevation generally reduce the symptoms.

The affected areas will often appear red and swollen. Other findings include acrocyanosis, livedo reticularis, facial flushing, cutaneous necrosis, and ulceration. In up to 40% of patients, the limb may appear normal between attacks. Prolonged immersion in water may lead to extensive maceration and contribute to ulcer formation.

Prognosis is variable. In one long-term study, approximately 30% of patients fell into each of three categories: worsening, no change, and improvement. A further 10% had complete resolution of their symptoms[31].

Pathology

In type 1 EM, vessels may show intimal proliferation and occlusive thrombosis. In general, however, biopsies are not required and histology is non-specific.

Differential Diagnosis

Chronic regional pain syndrome (CRPS; reflex sympathetic dystrophy) may sometimes have features similar to EM. Abnormal warmth, erythema and burning pain may be seen in both, but CRPS does not have the characteristic close relationship to temperature and tends to be constant rather than episodic. Peripheral neuropathy may also cause tingling and burning and may require differentiation by nerve conduction studies. Calcium channel blockers and mushroom poisoning as well as occlusive vascular diseases such as thromboangiitis obliterans may be associated with EM-like symptoms. It is important to consider underlying causes of EM, in particular chronic myeloproliferative disorders, as EM may be the first sign of the latter.

Treatment

Although numerous treatments have been reported as possible therapies for EM, no single therapy is consistently effective and many cases can prove difficult to control. The assistance of a specialist pain clinic can be valuable. Various methods of cooling the limbs during attacks, such as fans, wet dressings, and ice packs wrapped in towels, should be explored and have often already been tried by the time of presentation. Frequent periods of leg elevation can be helpful in both reducing discomfort and reducing leg edema, whereas prolonged periods of leg dependency should be avoided. Simple oral analgesia is also important.

Aspirin can be effective for type 1 EM and treatment for the thrombocythemia with medications such as hydroxyurea should also be considered. Topical therapies include 10% capsaicin and lidocaine patches, while possible oral medications include SSRIs (e.g. venflaxine), tricyclic antidepressants (e.g. amitriptyline), anticonvulsants (e.g. gabapentin), calcium channel blockers (e.g. diltiazem), sodium channel blocking agents (e.g. flecainide) and the prostaglandin analogue misoprostol. Several intravenous therapies have been used for more severe cases, including nitroprusside, prostaglandin E1, and lidocaine (combined with oral mexiletine). More invasive approaches include epidural infusions of bupivacaine and opiates, lumbar sympathetic blocks and bilateral lumbar sympathectomies[32]. Oral medications should be tried initially, but more invasive procedures may be necessary for more severe cases.

TELANGIECTASIAS

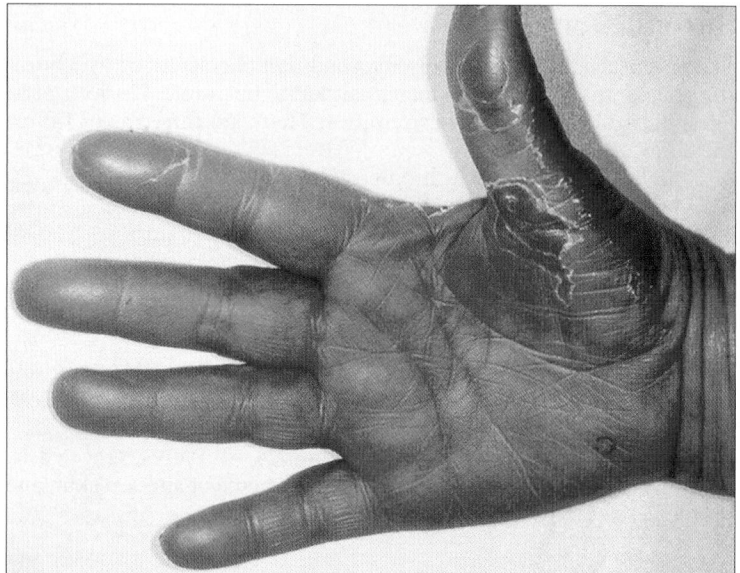

Fig. 106.6 Erythromelalgia. A red, hot and painful hand. In addition, there is a superficial erosion on the hypothenar eminence. Courtesy of Agustin Alomar MD.

Key features

- Telangiectasia is due to persistently dilated dermal vessels and not angiogenesis

- Can occur as a primary process, a result of cutaneous damage, or secondary to systemic disease

Introduction

Telangiectasia refers to abnormal, small, persistently dilated blood vessels visible in the skin (Fig. 106.7). Individual vessels can be discerned and range in color from light red to deep purple and will usually empty with pressure. They occur as a result of vascular dilation rather than new vessel growth and are thought to arise from capillaries, venules or small arteriovenous malformations. Telangiectasias are seen in a range of clinical settings (Table 106.6).

Treatment is often not required; however, options include cosmetic camouflage, light or fine wire diathermy, injection sclerotherapy, and laser or intense pulse light therapies.

Spider Telangiectasia

| Synonyms: ■ Nevus araneus ■ Spider nevus ■ Spider angioma |

This localized lesion has a slightly raised central red papule (which often becomes more prominent with time) and multiple small, radiating, dilated vessels[33] (Fig. 106.8). The lesion can vary from several millimeters to more than a centimeter in diameter. They are commonly located on the face, neck, upper trunk and hands.

Spider telangiectasias represent a form of telangiectasia with a central feeding arterial vessel. They are usually seen in otherwise healthy individuals, especially women and children. Lesions, often multiple, commonly occur with pregnancy, liver disease and oral contraceptive pills (OCPs). Spontaneous resolution may occur, especially after pregnancy. Treatment options include electrosurgery or vascular lasers.

Generalized Essential Telangiectasia

This widespread and progressive telangiectasia is a primary disorder that typically affects adult women but may commence in childhood. The limbs are affected, especially the legs, with sheets of telangiectasias[34,35]. The trunk may be involved at a later stage.

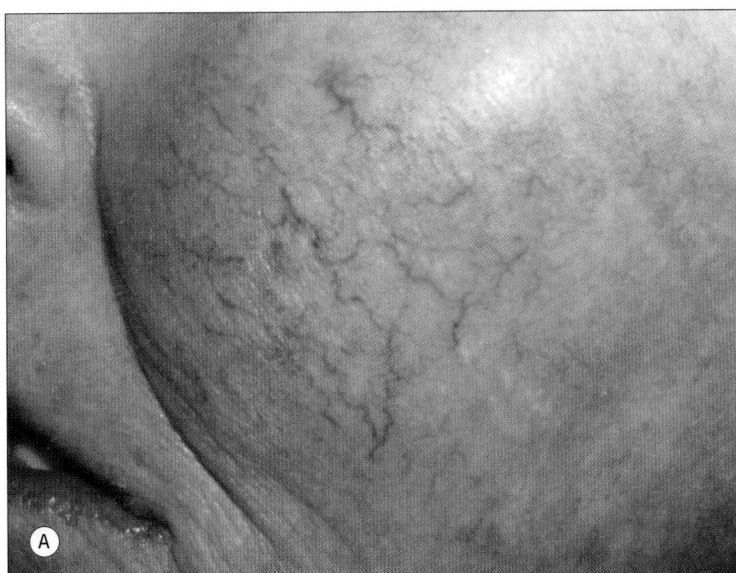

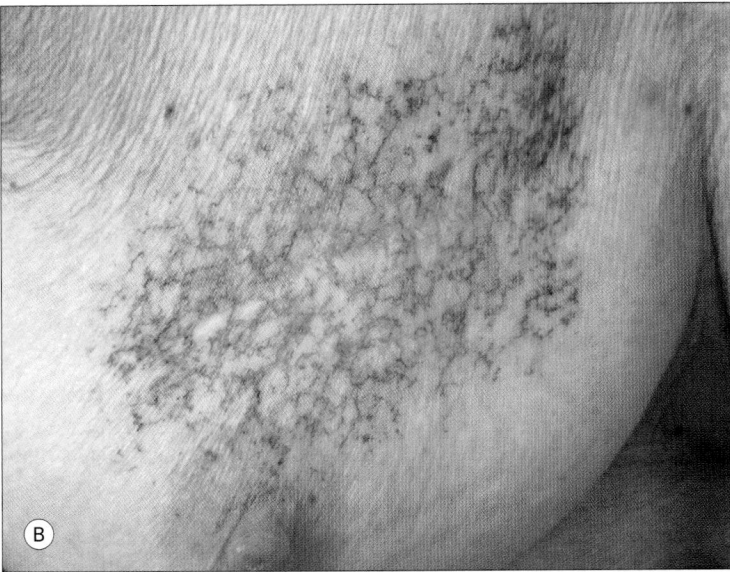

Fig. 106.7 Telangiectasias. A Sun-induced telangiectasias on the cheek. **B** Prominent telangiectasias on the breast following radiation therapy.

CAUSES OF TELANGIECTASIAS

Primary

- Generalized essential telangiectasia
- Unilateral nevoid telangiectasia
- Angioma serpiginosum
- Spider telangiectasias (also associated with estrogen excess)
- Hereditary benign telangiectasia*
- Costal fringe

Secondary to physical changes or damage

- Photodamage
- Post radiation therapy
- Traumatic
- Venous hypertension

Skin disease

- Telangiectatic rosacea
- Incipient or involuted infantile hemangiomas
- Poikiloderma vasculare atrophicans

Hormonal/Metabolic

- Estrogen-related
  - Liver disease
  - Pregnancy
  - Exogenous estrogens
- Corticosteroids

Systemic conditions

- Carcinoid syndrome
- Mastocytosis (telangiectasia macularis eruptiva perstans)
- Autoimmune connective tissue diseases
  - Lupus erythematosus
  - Dermatomyositis
  - CREST syndrome/systemic sclerosis
- Mycosis fungoides
- B-cell lymphomas
- Angiolupoid sarcoidosis
- Graft-versus-host disease (in the context of poikiloderma)
- HIV infection

Congenital malformations and genodermatoses

- Cutis marmorata telangiectatica congenita
- Klippel–Trenaunay syndrome
- Hereditary hemorrhagic telangiectasia
- Ataxia–telangiectasia
- Hypotrichosis–lymphedema–telangiectasia syndrome
- Rombo syndrome
- Bloom syndrome
- Rothmund–Thomson syndrome
- Poikiloderma with neutropenia
- Dyskeratosis congenita
- Xeroderma pigmentosum
- Goltz syndrome (in Blaschko's lines)
- GM1-gangliosidosis (also associated with angiokeratoma corporis diffusum)
- Prolidase deficiency

Childhood onset of multiple punctate, linear or arborizing telangiectasias favoring sun-exposed areas of the face and upper extremities; the vermilion lips and palate are occasionally affected, but there is no visceral involvement.

Table 106.6 Causes of telangiectasias.

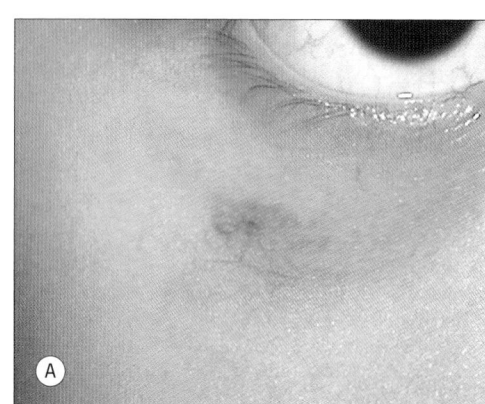

Fig. 106.8 Spider angiomas. A Central arteriole with radiating telangiectatic 'legs' on the cheek of a young child. **B** Multiple lesions in a jaundiced patient with liver disease. A, Courtesy of Phillip Bekhor MD. B, Courtesy of Ronald P Rapini MD.

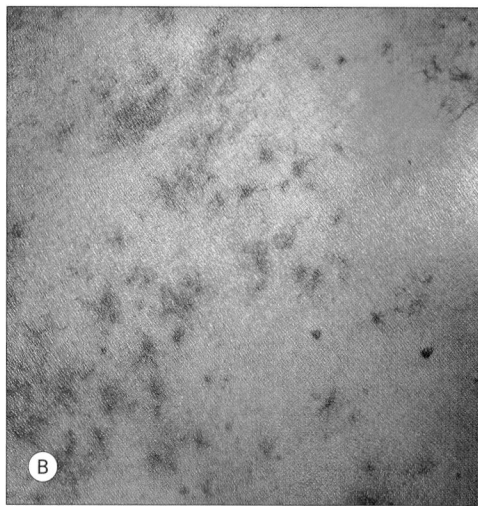

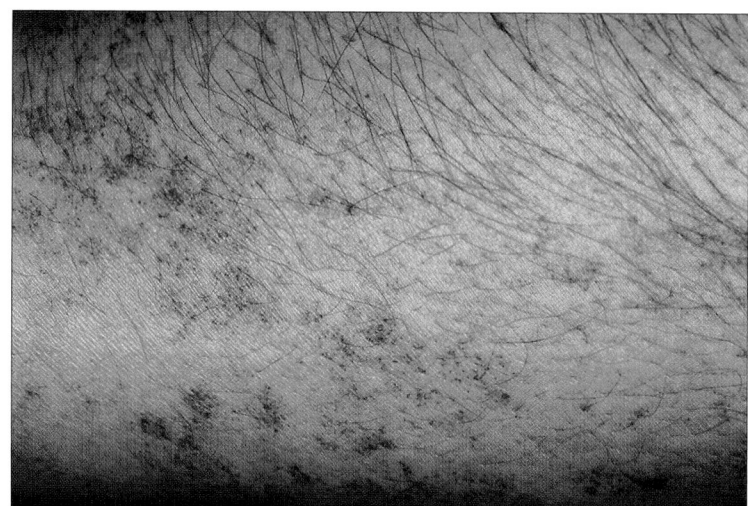

Fig. 106.10 Angioma serpiginosum. Grouped dark red puncta on the arm in a serpiginous pattern.

Unilateral Nevoid Telangiectasia

Telangiectasias in this condition are usually confined to the trigeminal or upper cervical dermatomes (Fig. 106.9) and may follow Blaschko's lines[36,37]. Congenital and acquired forms are recognized. It has been proposed that an increase in estrogen receptors on blood vessels in affected areas and/or an increase in estrogen levels is causative. Situations of relative estrogen excess such as pregnancy, puberty and liver disease are associated with the acquired form.

Angioma Serpiginosum

Angioma serpiginosum is a rare vascular disorder with a characteristic appearance[38,39]. It is usually sporadic, but familial cases have been

reported. Typically, the condition affects females and commences during the first two decades of life. Lesions consist of multiple small, asymptomatic, non-palpable, deep-red to purple puncta occurring in small clusters and sheets (Fig. 106.10). The arrangement and extension of the lesions may produce a serpiginous pattern. The extremities are most commonly affected, initially with a unilateral distribution; over months to years, the involvement may become more widespread. The palms, soles and mucous membranes are not involved.

The puncta represent dilated non-inflamed capillaries in the dermal papillae. These can be seen with dermoscopy. Incomplete blanching occurs with pressure, but lesions are not purpuric. The differential diagnosis includes pigmented purpuric eruptions, particularly Majocchi's variant (purpura annularis telangiectoides), which is more likely to be bilateral and on biopsy has lymphocytes and extravasated erythrocytes. Treatment is not necessary, but lesions can be improved with the pulsed dye laser.

Hereditary Hemorrhagic Telangiectasia

Synonym: ■ Osler–Weber–Rendu disease

Hereditary hemorrhagic telangiectasia (HHT) is an autosomal dominant condition in which there are multiple mucocutaneous and gastrointestinal telangiectasias (which are actually arteriovenous malformations) as well as variable visceral involvement (lung, liver and CNS). The diagnosis may first be suspected in children who have repeated episodes of epistaxis; however, the initial presentation may be during the second or third decades of life. The characteristic mat-like and papular telangiectasias on the mucous membranes are first seen during adolescence[40]. Cutaneous lesions usually appear after puberty or even later in life.

Lesions, which increase in size and number as the patient ages, are most commonly seen on the face, tongue, lips, nasal mucosa, hands and fingertips. They frequently occur throughout the gastrointestinal tract and may result in obvious hemorrhage or iron deficiency. Hemorrhage from vascular lesions in the lung, liver, CNS, spleen and urinary tract may occur, as well as paradoxical emboli due to pulmonary arteriovenous malformations.

HHT can result from mutations in at least two different genes (to date, *HHT1* and *HHT2*), which encode endoglin and ALK-1, respectively. Both of these glycoproteins are TGF-β receptors expressed by vascular endothelium, and they are thought to play a role in angiogenesis and vessel wall integrity.

Treatment of the vascular lesions may not be required. Destructive treatments such as diathermy, cautery or laser may be used to treat individual lesions. Surgical management or embolization may be required for uncontrolled hemorrhage from mucosal lesions or complications arising from visceral lesions.

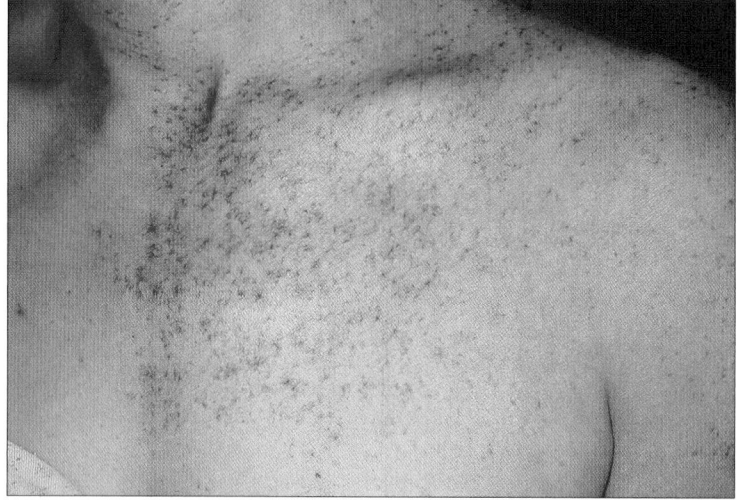

Fig. 106.9 Unilateral nevoid telangiectasia. Note the segmental, unilateral distribution pattern of the telangiectasias. Courtesy of Robert Hartman MD.

Ataxia–Telangiectasia

Synonym: ■ Louis-Bar syndrome

Ataxia–telangiectasia was first described by Louis-Bar in 1941. It is an autosomal recessive disorder characterized by cerebellar ataxia, chromosomal instability (frequent translocations between chromosomes 7 and 14), growth retardation, oculocutaneous telangiectasias, pulmonary infections (including bronchiectasis), immunodeficiency and the development of lymphomas[41].

It is covered in more detail in Chapter 59. Linear telangiectasias first appear in the bulbar conjunctivae between 3 and 6 years of age. Cutaneous telangiectasias favor the head and neck region, and they are most common on the malar prominences, ears and eyelids in addition to the popliteal and antecubital fossae. Patients may have poikiloderma (hypopigmentation, hyperpigmentation, atrophy, telangiectasia), premature hair graying, and decreased subcutaneous fat.

ANGIOKERATOMAS

Key features

■ Small, dark, vascular and variably hyperkeratotic lesions that result from dilation of superficial vessels

■ Angiokeratoma circumscriptum is a capillary–lymphatic malformation

■ Angiokeratoma corporis diffusum results from several lysosomal storage disorders and is associated with systemic manifestations

Introduction

Angiokeratomas are well-circumscribed vascular lesions consisting of superficial vascular ectasia and hyperkeratosis[42]. Five variants have been recognized. With the exception of angiokeratoma circumscriptum (which represents a capillary–lymphatic malformation), angiokeratomas result from ectatic dilation of pre-existing vessels in the papillary dermis.

Clinical Features

Solitary or multiple angiokeratomas

These occur most commonly as a small, warty, black papule on the lower extremities, but may occur anywhere on the body (Fig. 106.11). The lesions are thought to result from injury/trauma to or chronic irritation of the wall of a venule in the papillary dermis. Solitary lesions may be confused with melanoma due to their dark color. Dermoscopy will readily distinguish between these two entities.

Angiokeratomas of the scrotum and vulva

Synonym: ■ Angiokeratoma of Fordyce

These angiokeratomas may arise in the second or third decade but are most commonly seen in older age groups. The lesions are red to black in color, may be single or multiple, and arise along superficial vessels (Fig. 106.12). In some patients, they may be associated with thrombophlebitis, varicoceles and inguinal hernias. Vulvar lesions may be associated with vulvar varicosities, hemorrhoids, OCPs, or increased venous pressure during pregnancy.

Angiokeratoma corporis diffusum

This disorder is characterized by the development of multiple, often clustered angiokeratomas, usually in a bathing trunk distribution. Lesions vary in number (from only a few to many) and usually begin to appear during late childhood or adolescence. X-linked recessive Fabry disease is the best known entity with this clinical presentation and results from a deficiency of the lysosomal enzyme α-galactosidase A (see Ch. 62). This leads to the accumulation of the neutral glycolipid

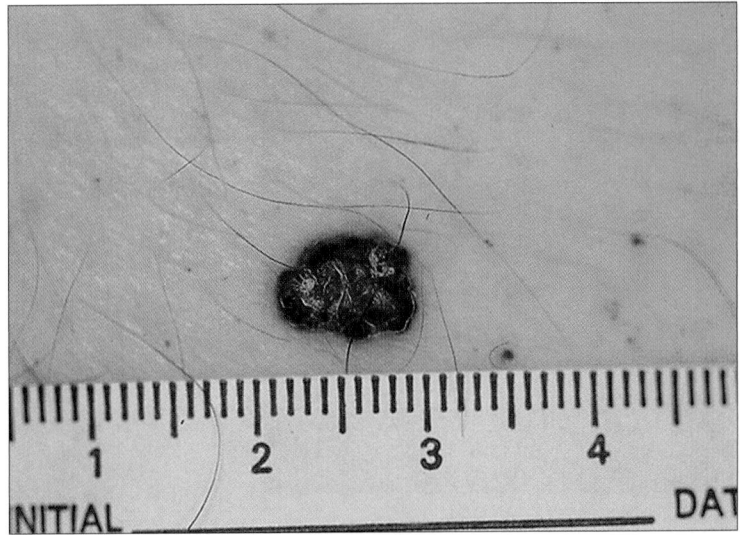

Fig. 106.11 Solitary angiokeratoma. Because of their dark color, these lesions may resemble cutaneous melanoma. Dermoscopy will readily distinguish between these two entities. Courtesy of Jean L Bolognia MD.

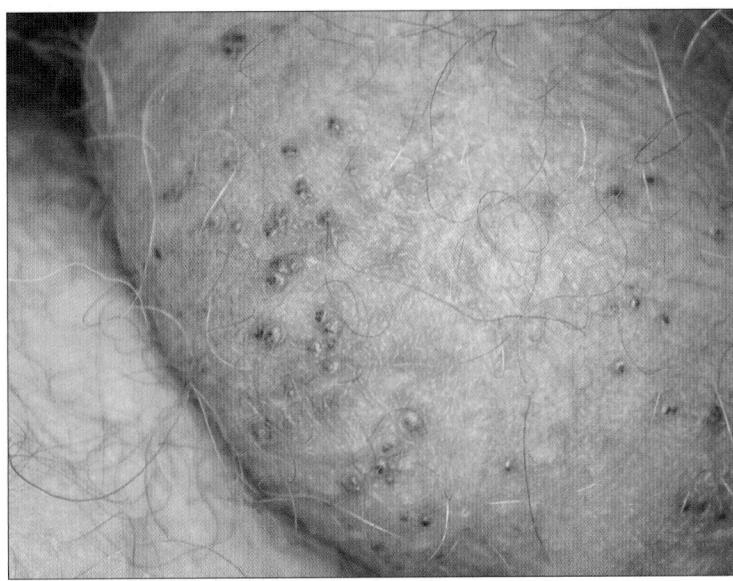

Fig. 106.12 Scrotal angiokeratomas. These lesions typically arise along superficial vessels.

ceramide trihexidose within lysosomes of multiple cell types. Other enzyme deficiencies associated with angiokeratoma corporis diffusum are outlined in Table 62.5.

Angiokeratoma of Mibelli

Lesions usually develop between the ages of 10 and 15 years and are most commonly situated on the dorsal and lateral aspects of the fingers and toes. They may also occur on the dorsa of the hands and feet and rarely on the elbows and knees. They may be associated with chilblains and acrocyanosis. In rare instances, ulceration of the fingertips may occur. There is a familial predisposition and the disorder may be transmitted in an autosomal dominant fashion with variable penetrance.

Angiokeratoma circumscriptum

This entity usually develops during infancy or childhood as either a plaque of multiple discrete papules (Fig. 106.13) or hyperkeratotic papules and nodules that often become confluent. They occur on the trunk, arms or legs and are unilateral in most patients. There is a female predominance.

Pathology

Marked dilatation of the papillary dermal vessels is seen in association with an acanthotic, variably hyperkeratotic epidermis. Elongated rete

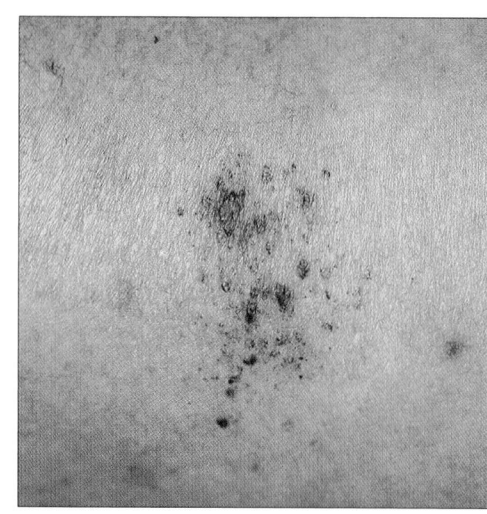

Fig. 106.13 **Angiokeratoma circumscriptum.** These grouped red–violet papules had been present since childhood. Courtesy of Jean L Bolognia MD.

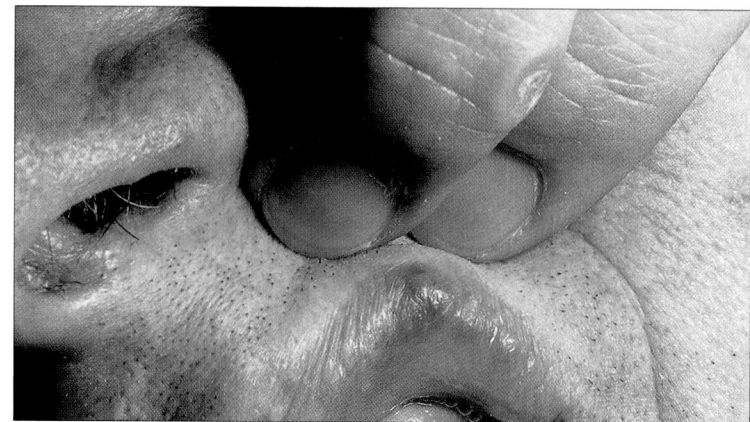

Fig. 106.14 **Venous lake on the lip.** The lesion is soft and, with compression, can be emptied of most of its blood content. Courtesy of Ronald P Rapini MD.

ridges may partially or completely enclose vascular channels, and a collarette may be present at the margin of the lesions. In Fabry disease, vacuoles can be detected in endothelial cells and pericytes. The amount of glycolipid is small and may be difficult to detect in routinely prepared sections. However, the deposits are PAS-positive and Sudan black-positive and these stains can therefore assist in diagnosis. They can also be demonstrated by electron microscopy.

Differential Diagnosis

Angiokeratomas should be distinguished from other vascular lesions. In particular, darkly colored or thrombosed angiokeratomas may resemble cutaneous melanoma.

Treatment

Patients may request removal for cosmetics reasons. This may be achieved by shave excision, diathermy or laser therapy, the choice of which would largely depend on the size of the lesion.

VENOUS LAKES

Venous lakes are small, dark blue, slightly elevated, soft lesions that are predominantly localized on the lips (Fig. 106.14), ears or face of elderly persons. They can usually be emptied of most of their blood content by persistent pressure[43,44]. Pathologically, venous lakes represent telangiectasias in the dermis. Either a great, dilated venule or several communicating dilated spaces that contain erythrocytes are seen. Thrombosis is sometimes present. Optional treatment with electrosurgery or a hemoglobin-targeting laser is usually effective.

NEVUS ANEMICUS

Nevus anemicus is a congenital pale area of skin, most commonly found on the upper trunk. These patches have an irregular border and an average diameter of 5–10 cm. Within the body of the lesion, local blood vessels are very sensitive to endogenous catecholamines and are permanently vasoconstricted[45]. The border and extent of the lesion become imperceptible with pressure (or diascopy) sufficient to cause blanching of surrounding skin. Conversely, application of heat or an ice cube will often accentuate the lesion; the border becomes hyperemic during warming, while the lesion stays pale (Fig. 106.15). The pale appearance of the lesion rather than an absence of pigmentation and the results of the above clinical maneuvers allow nevus anemicus to be differentiated from vitiligo and nevus depigmentosus, respectively.

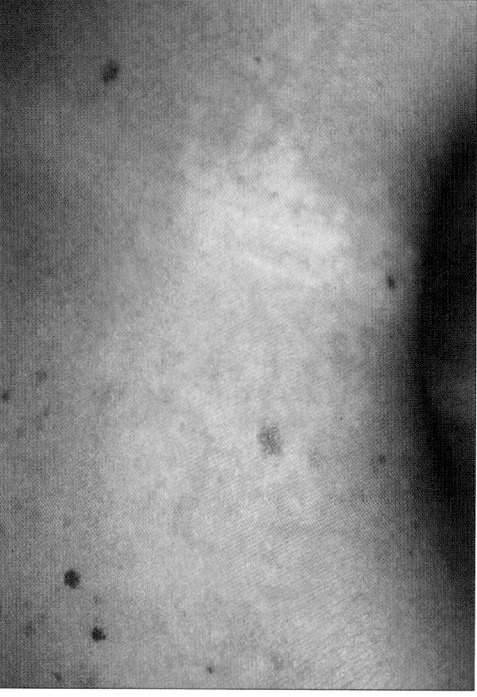

Fig. 106.15 **Nevus anemicus.** Area of vasoconstriction with irregular borders. Courtesy of Jean L Bolognia MD.

Interestingly, islands of sparing may be present within the lesion, and skin transplanted within the nevus anemicus retains the characteristics of the donor site (donor dominance). No histologic abnormalities have been reported. No treatment is required or effective.

BIER SPOTS (ANGIOSPASTIC MACULES)

These were first described by Bier in 1898 and represent a pattern of vascular mottling consisting of white macular areas surrounded by a red to occasionally blue cyanotic background. Bier spots most commonly occur on the arms and legs of young adults but may also occur on the trunk. They may be induced by venous congestion and can be elicited by placing a limb in a dependant position or by placing a tourniquet around a limb. The spots disappear with limb elevation or release of the tourniquet. As with nevus anemicus, the border of the lesions becomes imperceptible with pressure (diascopy). The vascular pattern is thought to result from a benign physiological response consisting of vasoconstriction. Bier spots have also been associated with pregnancy and cryoglobulinemia.

1. Fleischer AB Jr, Resnick SD. Livedo reticularis. Dermatol Clin. 1990;8:347–54.

2. Gibbs MB, English JC, Zirwas MJ. Livedo reticularis: an update. J Am Acad Dermatol. 2005;52:1009–19.

3. Dowd PM. Reactions to cold. In: Burns T, Breathnach S, Cox N, Griffiths C (eds). Textbook of Dermatology, 7th edn. Blackwell Science, 2004:23.7–23.12.

4. Francés C, Piette JC. The mystery of Sneddon syndrome: relationship with antiphospholipid syndrome and systemic lupus erythematosus. J Autoimmun. 2000;15:139–43.

5. Francés C, Papo T, Wechsler B, et al. Sneddon syndrome with or without antiphospholipid antibodies: a comparative study in 46 patients. Medicine (Baltimore). 1999;78:209–19.

6. Devillers AC, de Waard-van der Spek FB, Oranje AP. Cutis marmorata telangiectatica congenita: clinical features in 35 cases. Arch Dermatol. 1999;135:34–8.

7. Gerritsen MJP, Steijlen PM, Brunner HG, Rieu P. Cutis marmorata telangiectatica congenita: report of 18 cases. Br J Dermatol. 2000;142:366–9.

8. Speight EL, Lawrence CM. Reticulate purpura, cryoglobulinaemia and livedo reticularis. Br J Dermatol. 1993;129:319–23.

9. Filo V, Brezová D, Hlavčák P, Filová A. Livedo reticularis as a presenting symptom of polycythemia vera. Clin Exp Dermatol. 1999;24:428.

10. Gibson GE, Su WPD, Pittelkow MR. Antiphospholipid syndrome and the skin. J Am Acad Dermatol. 1997;36:970–82.

11. Weir NU, Snowden JA, Greaves M, Davies-Jones GAB. Livedo reticularis associated with hereditary protein C deficiency and recurrent thromboembolism. Br J Dermatol. 1995;132:283–5.

12. Donnet A, Khalil R, Terrier G, et al. Cerebral infarction, livedo reticularis, and familial deficiency in antithrombin-III. Stroke. 1992;23:611–12.

13. Bauzá A, España A, Idoate M. Cutaneous polyarteritis nodosa. Br J Dermatol. 2002;146:694–9.

14. Rosman HS, Davis TP, Reddy D, Goldstein S. Cholesterol embolization: clinical findings and implications. J Am Coll Cardiol. 1990;15:1296–9.

15. Spiers EM, Sanders DY, Omura EF. Clinical and histologic features of primary oxalosis. J Am Acad Dermatol. 1990;22:952–6.

16. Yamamoto M, Danno K, Shio H, Imamura S. Antithrombotic treatment in livedo vasculitis. J Am Acad Dermatol. 1988;18:57–62.

17. Sladden MJ, Nicolaou N, Johnston GA, Hutchinson PE. Livedo reticularis induced by amantadine. Br J Dermatol. 2003;149:655–80.

18. Wilkin JK. Why is flushing limited to a mostly facial cutaneous distribution? J Am Acad Dermatol. 1988;19:309–13.

19. Freeman R, Waldorf HA, Dover JS. Autonomic neurodermatology (Part II): Disorders of sweating and flushing. Semin Neurol. 1992;12:394–407.

20. Mooney E. The flushing patient. Int J Dermatol. 1985;24:549–54.

21. Wilkin JK. The red face: flushing disorders. Clin Dermatol. 1993;11:211–23.

22. Wilkin JK. Flushing reactions. Recent Adv Dermatol. 1983;6:157–87.

23. Hurst E, Heffernan M. Cutaneous changes in the flushing disorders and the carcinoid syndrome. In: Freedberg I, Eisen A, Wolff K, et al. (eds). Dermatology in General Medicine, 6th edn. New York, NY: McGraw-Hill 2003:1673–5.

24. Thompson GH, Hahn G, Rang M. Erythromelalgia. Clin Orthop Rel Res. 1979:144:249–54.

25. Kvernebo K. Erythromelalgia: a condition caused by microvascular arteriovenous shunting. Vasa. 1998;Suppl. 51:1–40.

26. van Genderen PJ, Lucas IS, van Strik R, et al. Erythromelalgia in essential thrombocythemia is characterized by platelet activation and endothelial cell damage but not by thrombin generation. Thromb Haemost. 1996;76:333–8.

27. Mork C, Asker CL, Salerud EG, Kvernebo K. Microvascular arteriovenous shunting is a probable pathogenetic mechanism in erythromelalgia. J Invest Dermatol. 2000;114:643–6.

28. Berlin AL, Pehr K. Coexistence of erythromelalgia and Raynaud's phenomenon. J Am Acad Dermatol. 2004;50:456–60.

29. Yang Y, Wang Y, Li S, et al. Mutations in SCN9A, encoding a sodium channel alpha subunit, in patients with primary erythermalgia. J Med Genet. 2004; 41:171–4.

29a. Choi JS, Dib-Hajj SD, Waxman SG. Inherited erythermalgia: limb pain from an S4 charge-neutral Na channelopathy. Neurology. 2006;67:1563–7.

30. Burns TM, Te Morsche RH, Jansen JB, Drenth JP. Genetic heterogeneity and exclusion of a modifying locus at 2q in a family with autosomal dominant primary erythermalgia. Br J Dermatol. 2005;153:174–7.

31. Davis MDP, O'Fallon WM, Rogers RS III, Rooke TW. Natural history of erythromelalgia. Arch Dermatol. 2000;136:330–6.

32. Cohen JS. Erythromelalgia: new theories and new therapies. J Am Acad Dermatol. 2000;43:841–7.

33. Bean WB. Vascular Spiders and Related Lesions of the Skin. Oxford: Blackwell Scientific, 1958.

34. Rothe MJ, Grant-Kels JM. Nomenclature of the primary telangiectasias. Int J Dermatol. 1992;31:320.

35. McGrae JD Jr, Winkelmann RK. Generalized essential telangiectasia: report of a clinical and histochemical study of 13 patients with acquired cutaneous lesions. J Am Med Assoc. 1963;185:909–13.

36. Wilken JK. Unilateral dermatomal superficial telangiectasia. Arch Dermatol. 1984;120:579–80.

37. Uhlin SR, McCarty KS Jr. Unilateral nevoid telangiectatic syndrome: the role of estrogen and progesterone receptors. Arch Dermatol. 1983;119:226–8.

38. Hunt SJ, Santa Cruz DJ. Acquired benign and 'borderline' vascular lesions. Dermatol Clin. 1992;10:97–115.

39. Marriott PJ, Munro DD, Ryan T. Angioma serpiginosum: familial incidence. Br J Dermatol. 1975;93:701–6.

40. Abrahamian LM, Rothe MJ, Grant-Kels JM. Primary telangiectasia of childhood. Int J Dermatol. 1992;31:307–13.

41. Smith LL, Conerly SL. Ataxia-telangiectasia or Louis-Bar syndrome. J Am Acad Dermatol. 1985;12:681–96.

42. Requena L, Sangueza OP. Cutaneous vascular anomalies. Part I. Hamartomas, malformations, and dilatation of preexisting vessels. J Am Acad Dermatol.1997;37:523–49.

43. Bean WB, Walsh JR. Venous lakes. Arch Dermatol. 1956;74:459–63.

44. Alcalay J, Sandbank M. The ultrastructure of cutaneous venous lakes. Int J Dermatol. 1987;26:645–6.

45. Mountcastle EA, Diestelmeier MR, Lupton GP. Nevus anemicus. J Am Acad Dermatol. 1986;14:628–32.

Principles of Tumor Biology and Pathogenesis of BCCs and SCCs

107

Fredrik Pontén, Joakim Lundeberg and Anna Asplund

Key features

- Oncogenes act in a dominant fashion and gain-of-function results in increased proliferation
- Tumor suppressor genes act in a recessive fashion and loss of normal function results in uncontrolled growth
- The *p53* gene, the most frequently mutated gene in human cancer, controls signaling pathways involved in cell division and apoptosis
- The p53 protein is a general sensor of cytotoxic stress, and normal function counteracts acquisition of genetic alterations
- The *PTCH* gene controls proliferation and differentiation, and disruption of normal function is required for the development of basal cell carcinoma (BCC)
- BCCs, the most frequent cancer in humans, grow in skin that contains hair follicles, arise without precursors, and show no sign of progression
- BCCs are stroma-dependent and are locally invasive without producing metastasis (with rare exceptions)
- Squamous cell carcinomas (SCCs) arise in chronically sun-exposed skin and originate from epidermal keratinocytes
- SCC develops through a series of progressive stages including actinic keratosis, invasive cancer and eventual metastasis

INTRODUCTION

No definition of cancer is entirely satisfactory from a cell biology point of view, despite the fact that cancer is essentially a cellular disease, characterized by a transformed cell population with net cell growth and antisocial behavior. Microscopic evaluation of a tissue section taken from an excised skin tumor remains the gold standard for determining the diagnosis of skin cancer. Analysis of genomic DNA, transcribed genes and expressed proteins adds important information to the histologic features detected by light microscopy. In the future, diagnosis and prognostic information and choice of treatment will most likely be based upon a synoptic evaluation of morphology in conjunction with an analysis of nucleic acids and proteins. Even today, evolving knowledge based on the human genome sequence and biochemical pathways, including signaling within and between cells, enables us to dissect some of the mechanisms that underlie different stages in tumor formation as well as the variation of phenotypes which define the different types of cancer.

Carcinogenesis

Malignant transformation represents the transition to a malignant phenotype and is based on irreversible genetic alterations. Although not formally proven, malignant transformation takes place in one cell from which a subsequently developed tumor originates (the clonality of cancer dogma). Carcinogenesis is the process by which cancer is generated and is generally accepted to include multiple events which ultimately lead to growth of a malignant tumor[1]. This multistep process includes several rate-limiting steps, representing the addition of mutations and possibly also epigenetic events, which eventually lead to the formation of cancer (after various stages of precancerous proliferation).

The most common forms of cancer arise in somatic cells and are predominantly of epithelial origin (skin, prostate, breast, colon and lung), followed by cancers originating from hematopoietic lineage (leukemia and lymphoma) and mesenchymal cells (sarcomas). The stepwise changes involve an accumulation of errors (mutations) in vital regulatory pathways that control cell division, social behavior and cell death. Each of these changes provides a selective Darwinian growth advantage compared to surrounding cells, resulting in a net growth of the tumor cell population. A certain degree of genomic instability is probably required to attain a sufficient number of mutations. The spontaneous mutation rate is not high enough to explain the speed with which a cancer develops and thus tumor cells display a 'mutator phenotype' with a higher mutation rate compared to neighboring normal cells. Decreased efficiency in DNA repair systems is one important mechanism leading to a 'mutator phenotype'[2].

Knowledge of the events involved in carcinogenesis has been obtained from experimental cell culture and animal studies, as well as from clinicopathologic studies in humans. Information regarding cellular, molecular and genetic changes that represent tumor initiation and progression can be linked to histopathologic correlations. Primary genetic alterations leading to initiation of cancer can be identified and validated in experimental systems, but in clinical investigations, this is not feasible. Progression is ascribed to the events that occur after malignant transformation and can in part be defined by histology. This multistep model includes defined stages of tumor development accompanied by features that include multiple genetic and epigenetic events involving different signal pathways. Specific changes in DNA, signifying different steps in cancer development, were first described for colorectal cancer[2a]. This model illustrates distinct genetic hits acquired during the passage from normal epithelium to metastatic cancer and provides support for the multi-hit carcinogenesis hypothesis.

The hallmarks of cancer have also been described from a functional perspective and consist of a number of molecular, biochemical and cellular traits that are shared by most human cancers. Six traits have been proposed and include self-sufficiency with regard to growth signals, insensitivity to antigrowth signals, evasion of apoptosis, limitless replicative potential, sustained angiogenesis, and tissue invasion/ metastasis[3]. Self-sufficiency with regard to growth signals can be achieved by activation of oncogenes. Loss of function of tumor suppressor genes results in uncontrolled proliferation due to insensitivity to antigrowth signals. Evasion of apoptosis can be accomplished via inactivation of the *p53* tumor suppressor gene and production of survival factors. Constitutively active telomerase can render limitless replicative potential. The production of vascular endothelial growth factors results in sustained angiogenesis, and inactivation of cellular adhesion molecules, e.g. E-cadherin, facilitates the cell migration necessary for tissue invasion and metastasis. The order in which these capabilities are acquired is not static and varies between different forms of cancer.

Several traits can be achieved through a single genetic change, whereas a certain trait may require several genetic alterations. For example, inactivation of the *p53* tumor suppressor gene can result in insensitivity to antigrowth signals, resistance to apoptosis and increased angiogenesis. In addition, impairment of cell cycle control and apoptotic pathways contributes to the 'mutator phenotype'. In individuals predisposed to cancer at an early age, certain traits result from alterations in the germline and are thus carried in every cell. Xeroderma pigmentosum ('mutator phenotype'; mutations in nuclear excision repair genes; Ch. 85), familial melanoma (defect in cell cycle control; *CDKN2A [INK4A]* mutations), Li–Fraumeni syndrome (defect in cell

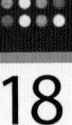

cycle control/apoptosis; *p53* mutations) and Gorlin syndrome (defect in control of proliferation/differentiation; *PTCH* gene mutations) are examples of how mutations within single genes in the germline result in this phenomenon.

The Cell Cycle

Normal cell growth and cell mass are influenced by several internal factors, including signals which regulate proliferation, differentiation and cell death. These factors are in part triggered by blood supply and the external environment, including soluble molecules as well as matrix–cell and cell–cell contacts. Proliferation involves DNA replication and mitosis in a series of events termed the cell cycle (Fig. 107.1). In normally dividing cells, the first gap (G_1 phase, 8–30 h) prepares the cell for DNA synthesis (S phase, 8 h). The G_1 gap includes a connection to a resting state (G_0 phase) representing quiescent cells capable of entering into G_1 after appropriate stimuli. Certain cells that exit the cell cycle and enter G_0 phase are destined for terminal differentiation or senescence, irreversibly locked out of the cell cycle. After S phase, reorganization of the chromatin occurs in a second gap (G_2 phase, 3 h) prior to mitosis (M, 1 h). Differentiation, which has a reciprocal correlation to proliferation, takes place in G_0 after exit from G_1.

Three primary checkpoints (G_1, G_2 and M), which act to ensure successful cell division, have been identified in the cell cycle (see Fig. 107.1)[4]. Regulation of these G_1, G_2 and M transitions involves three major protein families: cyclins, cyclin-dependent kinases (CDKs) and cyclin-dependent kinase inhibitors (CKIs). CDKs regulate the phosphorylation of key proteins involved in cell cycle progression, e.g. the retinoblastoma (Rb) protein. The concentration and balance of cyclins versus CKIs in turn regulate CDK activity. CDKs are activated by mitogenic growth factors and are removed by ubiquitin-mediated proteolysis in a cyclic manner correlating to the different phases of the cell cycle.

The G_1 transition is a critical one and is regulated by a complex interplay of macromolecules influenced by growth factors, hormones and cell contacts. The key factor is the degree of phosphorylation of Rb. If, at the G_1 checkpoint, Rb is underphosphorylated, then cell proliferation is blocked and the cell is arrested in G_1. The repression can be reversed by CDK-mediated phosphorylation. This phosphorylation/dephosphorylation cycle can thus reversibly regulate cell cycle progression and rate of proliferation.

There are two major families of CKIs, and both are involved in the G_1 checkpoint. The family of inhibitors of CDK4, also referred to as INK4, consists of p15, p16, p18 and p19; these inhibitors specifically bind to CDK4 and CDK6. The other family of CKIs is less specific with respect to the type of CDK they bind and includes the general CDK-cyclin complex inhibitors p21, p27 and p57. Expression of these CKIs is in part tissue-specific.

The *CDKN2A* (*INK4A*) gene locus, which is involved in familial melanoma (see Ch. 113), has an extraordinary feature; it encodes two different mRNAs by shifting the reading frame (hence the term ARF or alternative reading frame) and these two mRNAs are independently regulated. As a result, the two protein products (p16 and p14^ARF) have different amino acid sequences and different functions. p16 is a CKI that blocks Rb phosphorylation, whereas p14^ARF binds MDM2, resulting in an increase in p53 through interference with the p53–MDM2 feedback loop. Thus, both p16 activation and p14^ARF activation lead to cell cycle arrest through different pathways and their dysfunction can lead to cell proliferation. In carcinomas, cyclin and CKI alterations are common, whereas activating mutations in CDKs are rare, e.g. only a few families with familial melanoma have been described with mutations in *CDK4*. p53 and Rb alterations are also common events in human cancer.

Oncogenes

Qualitative or quantitative changes in regulatory proteins that participate in normal signaling pathways have been implicated in carcinogenesis, and the genes that encode them are frequently denoted as 'cancer genes'. Increase of gene function (oncogenes) as well as loss of gene function (tumor suppressor genes) will affect cell proliferation and can lead to uncontrolled growth. These two categories of genes, and their encoded proteins, represent the functional features that drive carcinogenesis at a molecular level. Oncogenes, described by a three-letter code (*ras*, *myc*, *src*, *fos*) are genes that gain oncogenic or transforming potential as a result of genetic changes[5].

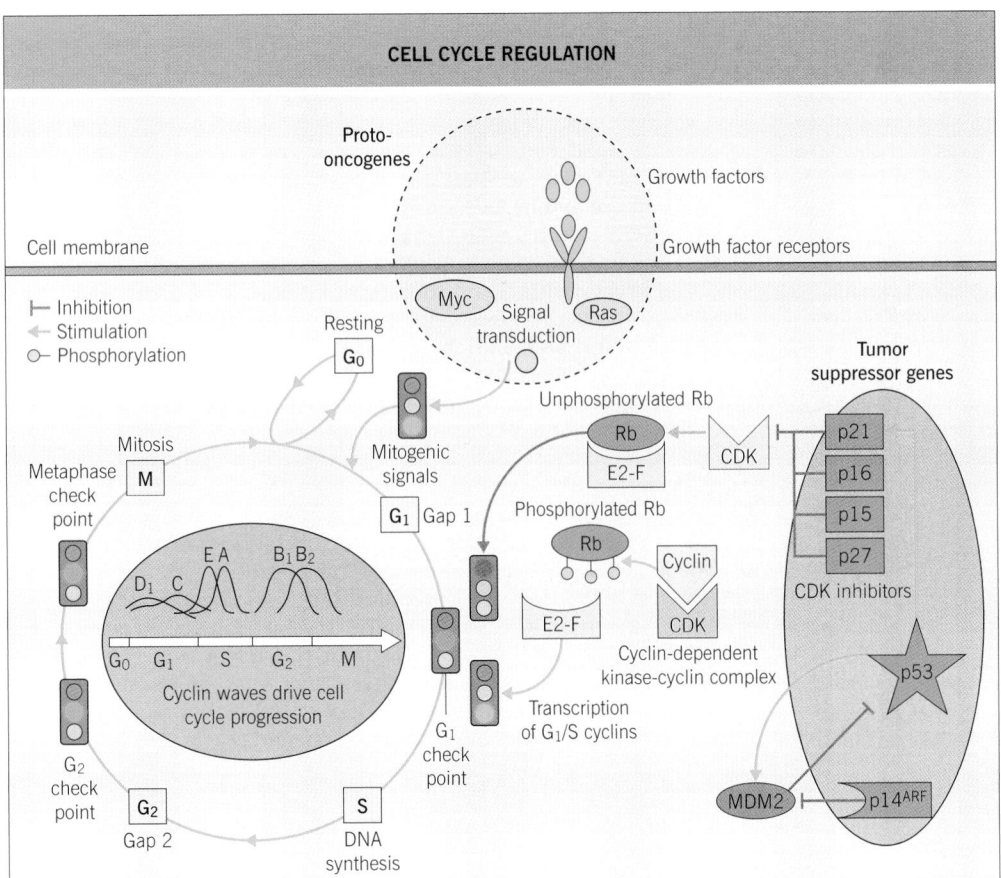

Fig. 107.1 Cell cycle regulation. Cyclin waves, an underlying mechanism for cell cycle progression, are illustrated inside the cell cycle. Proto-oncogenes acting as driving forces on the cell cycle (green traffic lights), are depicted in green. Tumor suppressor genes, regulating the G_1 checkpoint (red traffic light) of the cell cycle, are depicted in red. Yellow traffic light symbols represent checkpoints in the cell cycle.

A non-mutated oncogene is often referred to as a 'proto-oncogene' and it encodes a protein that is part of the necessary network for regulating cell division. Proto-oncogenes convert to oncogenes by mutations in their coding region (altered gene product) or regulatory sequences (increased product) or by gene rearrangement, i.e. gene amplification or translocation (increased and/or altered product) (Fig. 107.2). Point mutations in coding sequences can occur early in tumor development and drive proliferation. Gene amplification is common in advanced cancer, but is infrequent in the early stages of carcinogenesis. More than 100 oncogenes have been identified that participate in diverse regulatory pathways that control cell fate (Table 107.1).

Extracellular signals determine if cells move from a quiescent state into a proliferative state. These signals are transmitted into the cell through transmembrane structures that have distinct features (e.g. receptors) and the signals are then propagated into the nucleus by a multitude of interacting pathways (i.e. signal transduction). The signal molecules can be diffusable growth factors, extracellular matrix components or cell–cell adhesion/interaction molecules with either stimulatory or inhibitory effects. Autocrine (within a cell), paracrine (between neighboring cells) and endocrine (between distant cells) signals can all contribute to the regulation of growth stimulation. Increased production of growth factors and growth factor receptors is frequently observed in cancer cells and this results in an autocrine loop leading to enhanced cell division[6]. Upon ligand binding, growth receptors mediate signals via tyrosine kinases or serine/threonine kinases on the cytosolic

EXAMPLES OF ONCOGENES AND TUMOR SUPPRESSOR GENES IMPLICATED IN CARCINOGENESIS

Gene			Protein product	
Name	Function	Chromosome	Location	Function
sis	Oncogene	22	Extracellular	Platelet-derived growth factor (PDGF)
ras	Oncogene	11	Membrane	GTPase
src	Oncogene	20	Cytoplasm/membrane	Tyrosine kinase
raf	Oncogene	3	Cytoplasm/membrane	Serine/threonine kinase
myc	Oncogene	8	Nucleus	Transcription factor
fos	Oncogene	14	Nucleus	Transcription factor
Rb	Suppressor gene	13	Nucleus	Cell cycle regulator
p53	Suppressor gene	17	Nucleus	DNA repair, apoptosis
bcl-2	Suppressor gene	18	Mitochondria	Apoptosis

Table 107.1 **Examples of oncogenes and tumor suppressor genes implicated in carcinogenesis.**

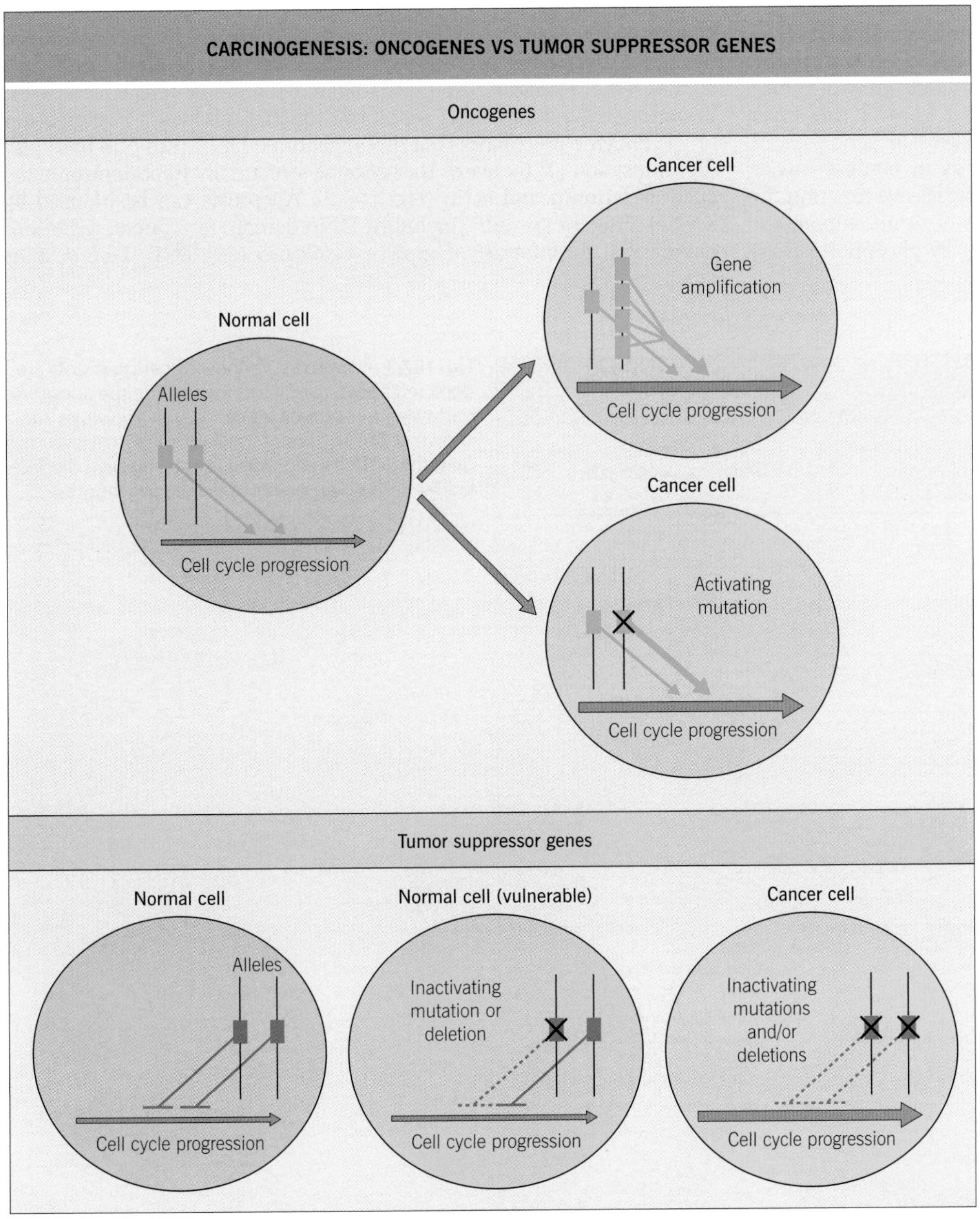

Fig. 107.2 **Carcinogenesis: oncogenes vs tumor suppressor genes.** An oncogene acts as an accelerator on the cell cycle to increase cell proliferation. Oncogenes are proto-oncogenes that have acquired activating mutations or gene amplifications. Oncogenes function in a dominant fashion, meaning that activating alterations in only one allele are sufficient for the gene to gain oncogenic potential. A tumor suppressor gene acts as a brake on the cell cycle to decrease cell proliferation. Tumor suppressor genes are inactivated by mutations in both alleles. Tumor suppressor genes function in a recessive manner, meaning that a mutation in only one allele is not sufficient for loss of gene function.

side of the membrane. Cancer cells can also alter receptor activity via 'activating' mutations in the genes that encode the receptors, thus generating constitutively active, ligand-independent receptor molecules (e.g. KIT in mastocytosis).

The *ras* proto-oncogene, which is mutated in approximately 40% of human cancers, plays a key role in signal transduction pathways between the cell membrane and the nucleus, communicating signals to a number of effector pathways. The *ras* family members are *H-ras*, *K-ras* and *N-ras*, and the 21 kDa Ras protein is a GTP-binding protein with latent GTPase activity, active when bound to GTP and inactive when GTP is hydrolyzed to GDP. The *ras* oncogene acts as a multifunctional modulator capable of redirecting input signals from growth receptors to alternative pathways. The end result of the signal cascade following *ras* activation is increased transcription due to an alteration in the quantity or function of nuclear transcription factors.

Tumor Suppressor Genes

For oncogenes, a change in one of the two inherited alleles leads to a gain-of-function that is dominant (over that of the unaffected allele). In contrast, tumor suppressor genes act in a recessive manner, i.e. a mutation in one allele has no effect (see Fig. 107.2). The biologic consequence of a recessive mutation becomes apparent when the second, normal (wild-type) allele is lost. Loss of this allele is termed loss of heterozygosity (LOH) and represents alteration from a heterozygous to a homozygous state for a gene. Several tumor suppressor genes have been identified through analysis of LOH in different chromosomal regions.

The tumor suppressor genes are limited in number and have proved to be of critical importance in human carcinogenesis. In contrast to the diverse interactions of oncogenes converging to stimulate growth, tumor suppressor genes act by inhibiting proteins that control cell cycle progression. Inactivation of both alleles of a suppressor gene (one of which may be inherited in an inactivated state as in familial cancer syndromes) is required to inactivate the normal repressive function. In normal cells, inactivation of the protein products of tumor suppressor genes is achieved via binding to other proteins or by phosphorylation.

In tumor cells, inactivation is often due to mutations, insertions and/or deletions (allelic loss).

The Rb protein serves as a classic example for examining the functions of tumor suppressor genes. Underphosphorylated Rb protein blocks proliferation in normal cells by binding to, and thereby inactivating, a transcription factor (E2F) necessary for propagation of the cell cycle (see Fig. 107.1). Serine/threonine phosphorylation of the Rb protein disrupts this binding, releasing E2F and enabling cell cycle progression. Genes that control the levels of Rb phosphorylation (e.g. *CDKN2A*) act as tumor suppressor genes and are often affected in cancer[7].

Lastly, the *p53* gene is frequently inactivated by a point mutation, and as opposed to classic tumor suppressor genes (that act in a recessive manner), *p53* mutations can act in a dominant-negative manner (see Ch. 53). This is because the p53 protein is a tetramer protein and oligomerization of a mutant allele product and a normal allele product results in an inactive protein.

Apoptosis

An equilibrium between proliferation and cell death is essential for normal homeostasis, and an imbalance can lead to abnormal growth. Cell death is important for tissue remodeling during embryogenesis and for maintaining homeostasis in normal adult tissues. Cell death is equally crucial for the removal of damaged cells, and this can occur via two different mechanisms – necrosis or apoptosis. Necrosis involves poor nutrient supply leading to membrane disruption and cell lysis without *de novo* protein synthesis.

In contrast, apoptosis is regulated and requires mRNA and protein synthesis. Microscopically, apoptosis is characterized by the appearance of apoptotic bodies composed of cell membrane remnants and condensed chromatin[8]. Apoptosis-related proteases, termed caspases, become activated and affect signal transduction pathways by activation of: (1) enzyme precursors that digest genomic DNA into 200 base pair (bp) units; and (2) proteases that degrade structurally important proteins such as laminin and actin (Fig. 107.3). Apoptosis can be induced by several different stimuli[9], including DNA damage (e.g. due to radiation, chemicals), withdrawal of growth cytokines (e.g. EGF, TGF-α, IGF,

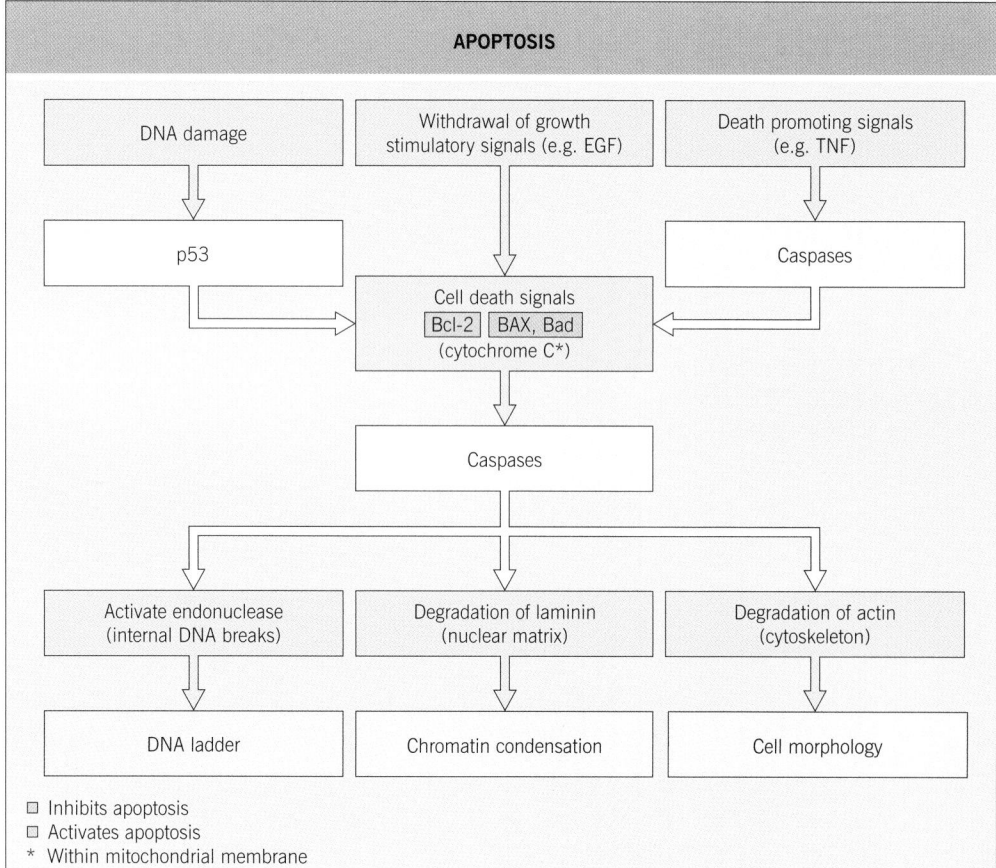

Fig. 107.3 **Apoptosis.** Various triggering events are depicted above the factors involved in the apoptotic pathways. Consequences of induced apoptosis are shown at the bottom of the figure. Fragmentation of genomic DNA by endonucleases results in a discrete ladder of DNA fragments of decreasing lengths.

PDGF) and death-promoting agents (e.g. TNF) (see Fig. 107.3). Conflicts between different signaling pathways can also provoke apoptosis.

Independent of triggering apoptotic stimuli, apoptosis converges into a common series of molecular events that lead to irreversible morphologic changes and ultimately cell death. The regulation of apoptosis is under the strict control of proteins, including Bcl-2, BAX and Bad families that are capable of regulatory cross-talk by heterodimerization of protein subunits. The mitochondrial membranes contain proteins that either activate apoptosis (BAX, Bad) or inhibit apoptosis (Bcl-2). Overexpression of the survival factor Bcl-2 blocks apoptosis and thus protects the cells against radiation and chemotherapeutic agents, consequently complicating treatment of cancer cells overexpressing Bcl-2 (e.g. follicular lymphoma). The p53 protein activates transcription of *BAX* and inhibits transcription of *bcl-2*, the net result favoring apoptosis. Thus, the p53 protein is a key factor for integrating pathways regulating DNA synthesis, DNA repair and apoptosis.

Limitless Replicative Potential

The number of mutations in a cell increases with time and partially explains the increasing risk for acquiring cancer as we age. The increased number of mutations is evident in normal cultured cells, which undergo approximately 60–70 doublings before reaching senescence and then death as a consequence of accumulating mutations and telomere shortening. Senescent cells are viable, but they are incapable of proliferation. During senescence, abnormal chromosomes accumulate and the telomere sequences diminish, eventually resulting in a crisis that leads to apoptosis.

The progressive erosion of telomere sequences (50–100 bp per mitosis) through successive cycles of replication eventually precludes protection of the ends of the chromosomes (see Ch. 66). This facilitates end-to-end chromosomal fusions, resulting in karyotypic disarray and then apoptosis. Carcinogenesis involves disruption of these normal apoptotic events, yielding limitless replicative potential for the tumor cells. For example, tumor cells frequently exhibit increased levels of telomerase, the enzyme required for maintenance of telomere sequences in normal cells[10]; this leads to retention of telomeres irrespective of the number of cell divisions. Between 85% and 90% of all cancers show increased levels of telomerase.

Angiogenesis

Formation of new blood vessels (angiogenesis) is essential for tumor mass expansion, in order to provide adequate levels of oxygen and nutrients[11]. Endothelial cells are normally quiescent, with low proliferation rates and mitoses rarely being observed (aside from the setting of wound healing). Angiogenesis (see Ch. 102) is initiated by growth factors, e.g. fibroblast growth factor (FGF) and vascular endothelial growth factor (VEGF), acting in a paracrine fashion and stimulating local endothelial proliferation. Sprouts from surrounding vasculature migrate toward the tumor via protease-mediated remodeling of extracellular matrix (e.g. serine proteases and metalloproteinases) and thereby establish new matrix–cell contacts. Of note, cancer cells express increased levels of VEGF and FGF. Inhibitors of angiogenesis, e.g. angiostatin, endostatin and thrombospondin, have been identified in plasma and extracellular matrix. Because thrombospondin is activated by p53, inactivation of p53 facilitates angiogenesis.

Invasion/Metastasis

Cell–cell interactions and extracellular glycoprotein matrix recognition are achieved by four classes of membrane-bound receptors, consisting of integrins, cadherins, selectins and members of the immunoglobulin family. All of these cellular adhesion molecules have an extracellular domain that binds ligands, leading to a conformational change in the cytoplasmic tail of the receptor. Upon ligand binding, internal regions of the receptors bind to specific cytoplasmic proteins influencing various pathways involved in proliferation, cell migration, differentiation and apoptosis. The extracellular ligands for integrins are matrix components composed of collagen, fibronectin or laminin (see Table 55.4). Cadherins bind to cadherins present on adjacent cells and selectins bind to carbohydrate chains. The extracellular ligands for the immuno-

globulin family include integrins and immunoglobulins expressed on adjacent cells.

Disruption of tissue organization is a hallmark of cancer and is the result of alterations in cellular adhesion receptors resulting in selective growth advantage. In cell cultures, dysregulation of cell adhesion pathways underlies anchorage-independent growth. Metastases from epithelial cancers often lose E-cadherin expression, facilitating the escape of cells from the primary site to other locations. E-cadherin expression can be inactivated by hypermethylation of regulatory regions as well as mutations in the coding sequence. Alternatively, inactivation occurs through proteolysis of the extracellular domain of E-cadherin or mutations in the gene encoding E-cadherin's intracellular ligand, β-catenin.

Signaling from normal neighboring cells, e.g. fibroblasts and endothelial cells, appears to be equally important for the growth of a tumor and is often induced by signals from the tumor cells. Reciprocal release of abundant growth-stimulating signals creates amplifying loops enabling growth of both the tumor and its cognate stroma. Inflammatory cells have also been shown to be involved in a similar cross-talk between normal and malignantly transformed cells.

In humans, the most common cancers are basal cell carcinoma (BCC) and squamous cell carcinoma (SCC), often termed 'non-melanoma skin cancer'. Although BCCs and SCCs possess many similar features, there are fundamental biologic differences, justifying a distinction between the two and rendering 'non-melanoma skin cancer' a poor conceptual term. In the remainder of this chapter, BCC and SCC will be described with an emphasis on the similarities and the differences between their tumor biology. Disruption of the Hedgehog–Patched signaling pathway is closely linked to development of BCC and the *p53* gene is often mutated in both BCC and SCC. The *Patched* (*PTCH*) and *p53* genes will serve as a model to illustrate some of the basic features of epithelial skin carcinogenesis.

STRUCTURE AND FUNCTION OF *p53*

Background

The *p53* tumor suppressor gene was first described in 1979 and was initially erroneously classified as an oncogene due to its ability to transform cells. The wild-type p53 protein is involved in a multitude of cellular events and illustrates the complex molecular machinery within a cell[12]. The p53 protein is regarded as the 'guardian of the genome'[13] as it protects DNA integrity in response to cytotoxic stress, including radiation. Protection is achieved by management of signaling pathways that regulate cell cycle progression, DNA repair and apoptotic cell death. The ability of p53 to induce apoptosis by transactivation of target genes is critical for its function as a tumor suppressor gene (see Fig. 107.3).

Inactivation of the p53 protein destabilizes the genome in general and enables mutations to become manifest due to the diminution of the protein's normal functions. Aside from genomic alterations, p53 protein can also be inactivated by binding to other proteins, such as the viral proteins adenovirus E1B, human papillomavirus E6 and the SV40 T-antigen.

The *p53* Gene, Protein and Regulation

The *p53* gene is located on the long arm of chromosome 17 and contains 11 exons spanning some 20 000 bp of genomic sequence. The gene encodes a 53 kDa nuclear phosphoprotein of 393 amino acid residues. Four functional domains involved in the regulation of transcription, DNA binding, oligomerization and auto-inhibition can be recognized (Fig. 107.4). Transcription is indirectly regulated within the transactivation domain (42 amino acid residues) either by binding to other proteins or by phosphorylation. For example, the nuclear protein MDM2 is capable of inactivating wild-type p53 protein by binding to the transactivation domain. Subsequent to binding to MDM2, p53 is degraded via the ubiquitin-mediated proteolysis pathway. In normal cells containing latent p53 protein bound to MDM2, the half-life of p53 is approximately 2 minutes.

Interaction between MDM2 and the p53 protein is dependent upon phosphorylation of the p53 transactivation domain as well as

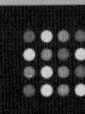

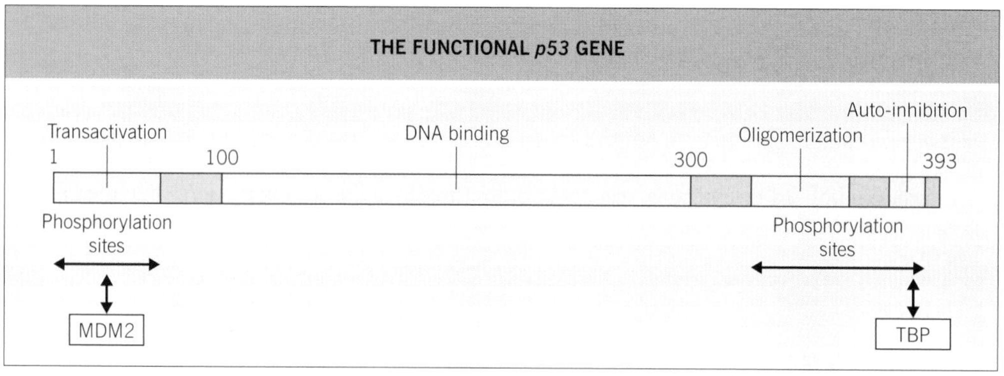

Fig. 107.4 The functional *p53* gene. There are four functional domains and they are involved in transactivation, sequence-specific DNA binding, oligomerization and auto-inhibition. Binding sites for MDM2 and TBP proteins are noted. TBP, TATA box-binding protein.

interactions with other proteins. Upon DNA damage, serine protein kinases are activated that readily phosphorylate p53 and release it from MDM2 binding. Up to a 100-fold increased cellular content of functional p53 is thus obtained without a requirement for protein synthesis. p53 protein is a transcription factor for MDM2, thus creating a feedback loop between p53 and MDM2. MDM2 protein levels are further regulated by binding to the $p14^{ARF}$ protein (see Fig. 107.1), which translocates MDM2 to the nucleolus and thus prevents MDM2–p53 interaction.

The structure of the DNA-binding domain has been shown to consist of a scaffold with three loops (Fig. 107.5). The first loop binds to the major groove of the target DNA sequence. The second loop has contact with the minor groove, and the third loop stabilizes the second loop via a zinc atom. The majority (80–90%) of detected *p53* mutations involve the sequence-specific DNA-binding domain. The distribution of reported mutations is shown in Figure 107.6 and depicts a number of hot spots within this region.

The p53 protein requires a tetramer configuration for DNA binding. The oligomerization domain is responsible for assembly of the protein. Because both normal and mutant allele products can be assembled together, this leads to the dominant-negative phenotype (see Ch. 53) that is characteristic of the mutant p53 protein. The auto-inhibitory domain of 30 basic amino acid residues is thought to block the DNA-binding domain and can be removed by phosphorylation or binding to other proteins such as TATA box-binding proteins (TBP).

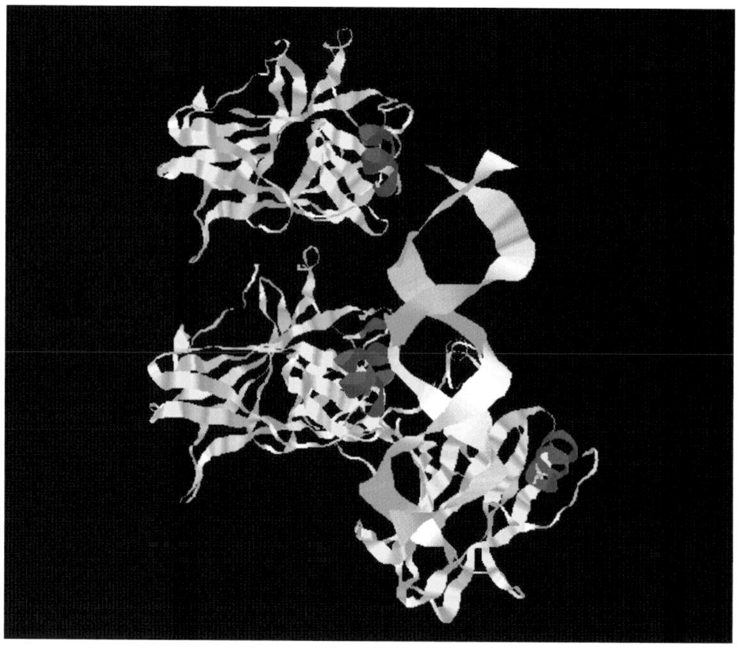

Fig. 107.5 Three-dimensional view of the p53 protein. Three units of the normally tetramerized active p53 are shown surrounding the DNA double helix. The β-sheets are shown in yellow and α-helices are depicted in red. From Sayle RA, Milner-White EJ. RASMOL: biomolecular graphics for all. Trends Biochem Sci. 1995;20:374; Cho Y, et al. Crystal structure of a p53 tumor suppressor-DNA complex: understanding tumorigenic mutations. Science. 1994;265:346–55.

The p53 protein exerts its effects predominantly (but not exclusively) at the level of transcription. Genes that increase their transcription due to interaction with p53 contain a promotor (response) element for binding to the p53 tetramer (Table 107.2). The transactivation domain of p53 can also recruit additional transcription factors required for transcription. In addition, the p53 protein can inhibit the transcription of genes lacking a p53 response element. This inhibition is executed in an indirect manner in which p53 binds to transcription factors required for these genes. The latter is achieved by binding between the C-terminal auto-inhibitory domain of p53 and TATA box-binding transcription factors.

The Cellular Response to DNA Damage

p53 is a general sensor of cytotoxic stress and can be activated by several types of DNA insults that create single- and double-strand breaks as well as cyclobutane pyrimidine dimers and 6-4 photoproducts, e.g. chemicals or gamma and UV radiation[14] (see Ch. 85). In response to DNA damage, the level of p53 protein increases rapidly within the cell and exerts multiple, complex functions, including protection of DNA integrity and cellular proofreading[15]. The former involves cell cycle arrest at G_1 in order to facilitate the repair of damaged DNA prior to cell division. The pathway downstream of p53 involves upregulation of p21, which, in turn, inhibits cyclin-dependent kinases and subsequent phosphorylation of Rb protein (see Fig. 107.1). Underphosphorylated Rb protein binds the transcription factor E2F and prevents the cell from entering into the S phase. Cellular proofreading involves apoptosis as a response to irreversible damage of genomic DNA and prevents survival of cells with severe genetic alterations. Sunburn cells in the epidermis represent apoptotic keratinocytes and can frequently be observed in normal skin subjected to sunburn.

Mutated *p53*

The *p53* gene is the most frequently altered gene in human cancer. A majority of *p53* mutations are missense mutations leading to an altered amino acid sequence. Missense mutations are primarily found in the

EXAMPLES OF GENES WHERE TRANSCRIPTION IS INFLUENCED BY THE P53 TETRAMER		
Gene (protein)	**Regulation**	**Function**
p21 (p21)	Activation	Proliferation
GADD45 (GADD45)	Activation	Proliferation
bax (BAX)	Activation	Apoptosis
thrombospondin (Thrombospondin)	Activation	Angiogenesis
mdm2 (MDM2)	Inhibition	Regulatory
bcl-2 (Bcl-2)	Inhibition	Apoptosis
fos (Fos)	Inhibition	Proliferation
jun (Jun)	Inhibition	Proliferation

Table 107.2 Examples of genes where transcription is influenced by the p53 tetramer.

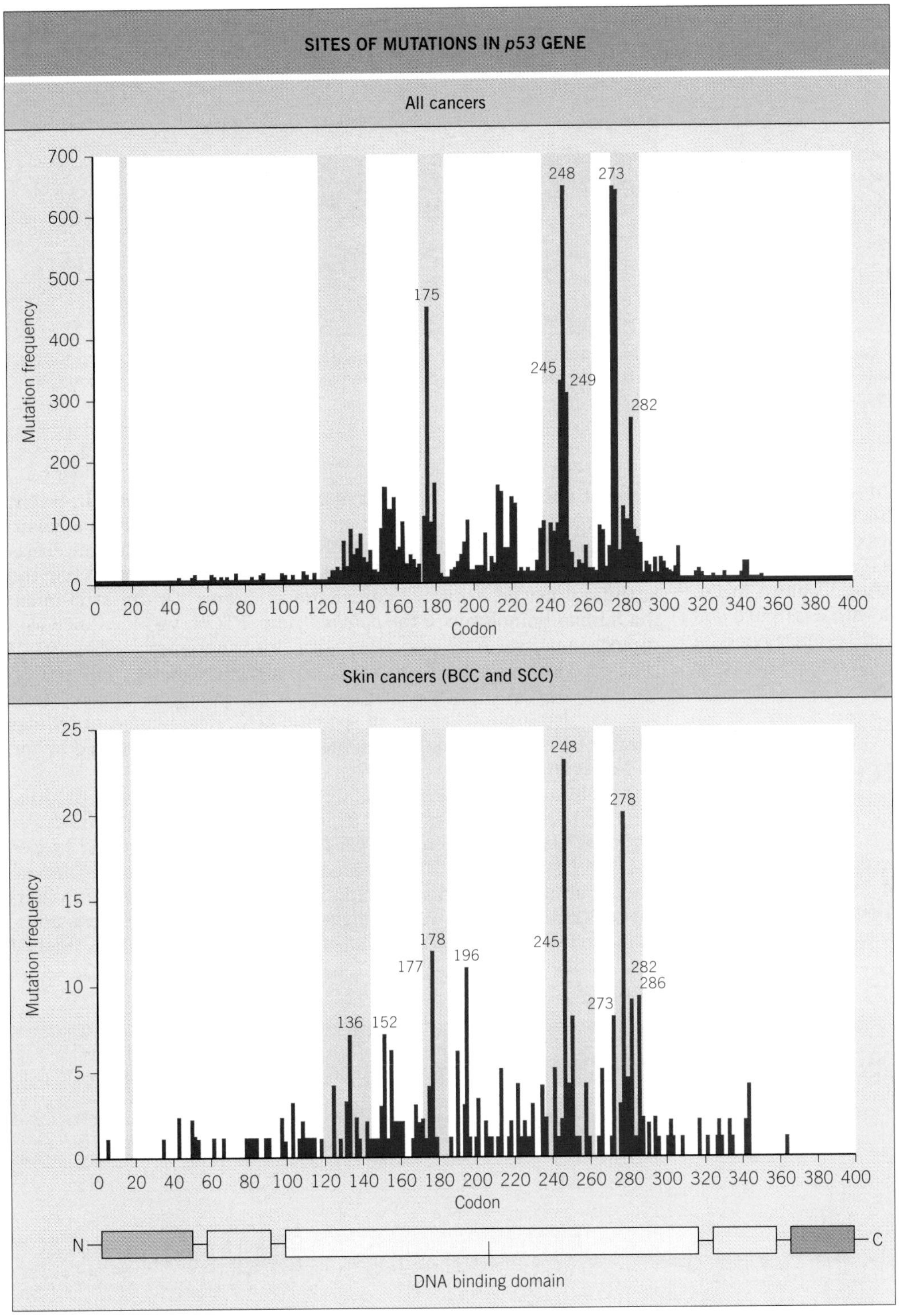

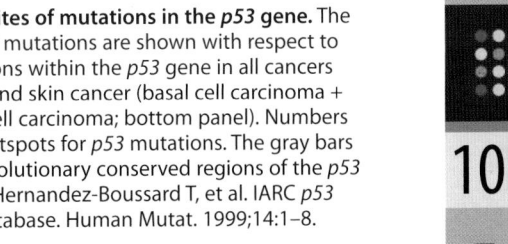

SITES OF MUTATIONS IN *p53* GENE

All cancers

[Graph: x-axis "Codon" from 0 to 400; y-axis "Mutation frequency" from 0 to 700. Labeled hotspot peaks at codons 175, 245, 248, 249, 273, 282.]

Skin cancers (BCC and SCC)

[Graph: x-axis "Codon" from 0 to 400; y-axis "Mutation frequency" from 0 to 25. Labeled hotspot peaks at codons 136, 152, 177, 178, 196, 245, 248, 273, 278, 282, 286.]

DNA binding domain

Fig. 107.6 Sites of mutations in the *p53* gene. The frequency of mutations are shown with respect to specific codons within the *p53* gene in all cancers (top panel) and skin cancer (basal cell carcinoma + squamous cell carcinoma; bottom panel). Numbers represent hotspots for *p53* mutations. The gray bars represent evolutionary conserved regions of the *p53* gene. From Hernandez-Boussard T, et al. IARC *p53* mutation database. Human Mutat. 1999;14:1–8.

DNA-binding domain between codons 112 and 286 (see Fig. 107.6). The sequence-specific DNA-binding capacity is diminished by exchange of amino acid residues in direct contact with DNA or indirectly by destabilization of the protein scaffold and loops necessary for appropriate DNA binding. The mutation spectra vary depending on the type of cancer; however, certain hot spots have been identified at codons 175, 245, 248, 249, 273 and 282, with a slight variation in skin cancer (see Fig. 107.6). Mutations in the DNA-binding domain do not affect oligomerization; thus, mutant p53 can still form tetramers with normal p53 protein derived from the intact *p53* allele. The formed heterodimers are, however, incapable of binding to promotor sequences.

The addition of small peptides (corresponding to the C-terminal domain) has the potential to disrupt the auto-inhibitory binding of the C-terminal region to the DNA-binding domain of the mutant heterodimers and thereby reactivate the function of mutated p53. This observation may be exploited in future therapeutic strategies. Mutant

p53 protein also has an extended half-life as compared with wild-type protein, since the MDM2/ubiquitin degradation pathway is less efficient, a property that is used as a semiquantitative surrogate marker for altered p53 in immunohistologic examination of tumors.

Clandestine proliferations of keratinocytes overexpressing p53 protein are evident in normal, chronically sun-exposed skin of Caucasians[16,17]. The pattern and degree of overexpression are distinctly different from the dispersed pattern of p53-immunoreactive keratinocytes following a single exposure of UV irradiation (Fig. 107.7). These epidermal p53 clones, which consist of histologically normal keratinocytes, have been shown to harbor a missense *p53* mutation in at least 70% of analyzed cases. The number and size of epidermal p53 clones increase with age and are abundant in facial skin. These clones appear in clinically normal skin and are also frequently detected adjacent to actinic keratoses, SCCs and BCCs[18]. Epidermal p53 clones can also be experimentally induced in mice by chronic exposure to UVB.

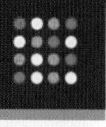

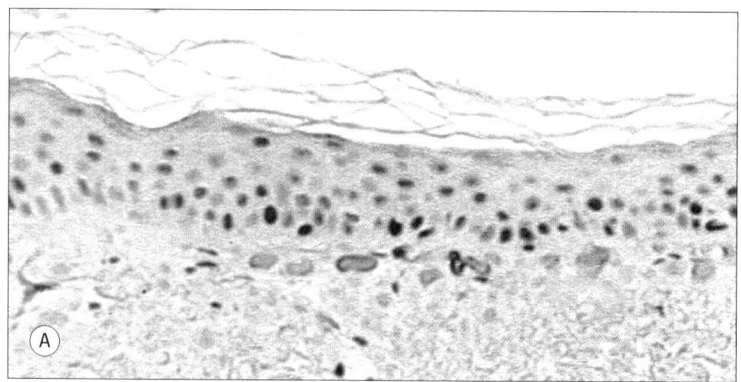
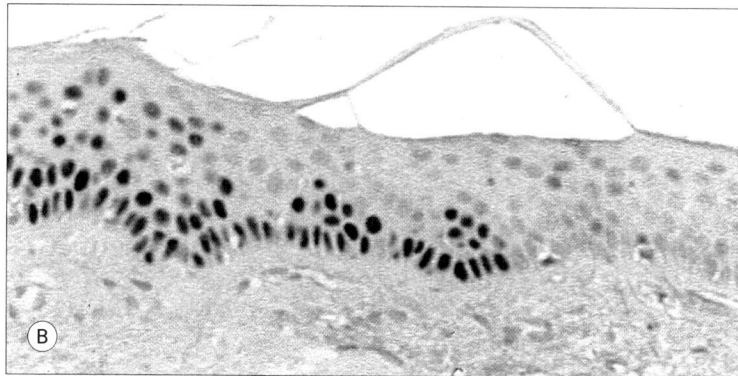

Fig. 107.7 p53 immunoreactivity. Photomicrographs of two different patterns of p53 immunoreactivity found in normal skin. **A** Dispersed pattern of p53 positivity representing a normal reactive response to DNA damage (e.g. single exposure to UVB). **B** Epidermal p53 clone representing a clonal expansion of morphologically normal keratinocytes with a *p53* mutation. The latter is seen in chronically sun-exposed skin.

The risk of an epidermal clone progressing into a carcinoma is small, and this risk has been estimated to be 1:8300 to 1:40 000 per individual[19]. The mechanism by which these clones enlarge and prevail is their relative resistance to UV-induced apoptosis, i.e. normal adjacent keratinocytes retain a higher probability of undergoing apoptosis due to repetitive sun exposure compared to keratinocytes with a mutated *p53* gene[20]. These epidermal p53 clones may very well be forerunners of skin cancer, although a clear relationship to skin cancer has yet to be proven.

STRUCTURE AND FUNCTION OF PATCHED

Background

The Hedgehog signaling pathway plays a key role during normal development, regulating both proliferation and cell fate. Initially, *patched* and *hedgehog* genes were identified in *Drosophila melanogaster*, where members of this complex signaling pathway were found to act as segment polarity genes involved in embryonic development. In recent years, it has become evident that an impairment of genes and pathways controlling development is also deeply involved in driving tumorigenesis and cancer development[21]. When screening candidate genes for the hereditary nevoid basal cell carcinoma syndrome (Gorlin syndrome), the human homologue of the *patched* gene, *PTCH*, was identified as a tumor suppressor gene associated with this syndrome[22,23]. The *PTCH* gene encodes a receptor that mediates Hedgehog signaling (Fig. 107.8). Later studies have shown that inactivating mutations in the *PTCH* gene are also common events in sporadic BCC. The significant cellular effects of Hedgehog signaling are mediated by proteins encoded by the *GLI* gene family.

The human Hedgehog signaling pathway is complex, with three identified *hedgehog* genes (*sonic hedgehog*, *indian hedgehog* and *desert hedgehog*), two *PTCH* genes (*PTCH1* and *PTCH2*) and three *GLI* genes (*GLI1*, *GLI2* and *GLI3*). The encoded proteins within these families are similar, although they display variations in expression levels in different cells and tissues as well as slightly different modes of interactions. In the following section, a simplified scheme using Hedgehog, Patched

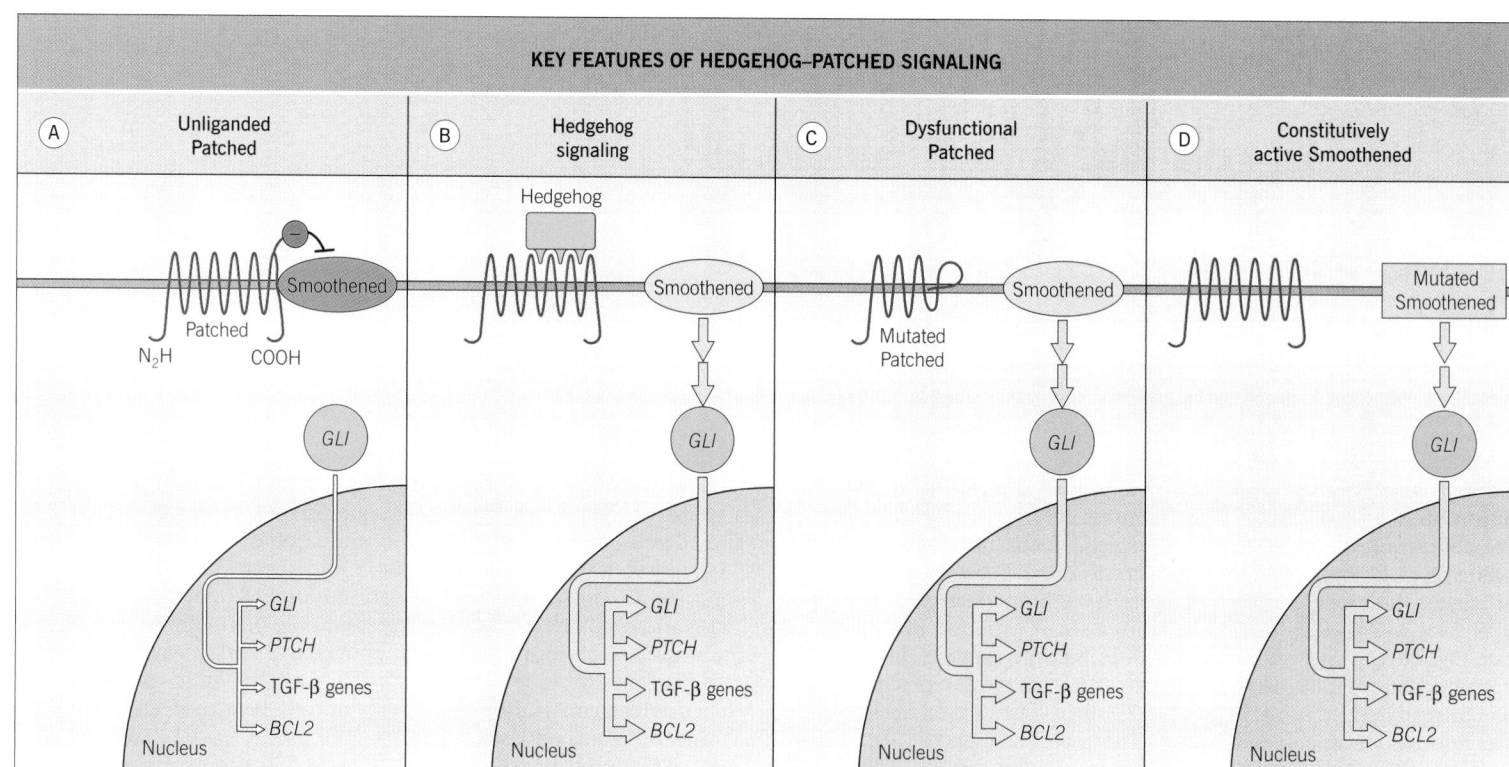

Fig. 107.8 Key features of Hedgehog–Patched signaling. A Unbound Patched silences Smoothened (SMO) signaling. **B** As Hedgehog binds to its receptor (Patched), the repression of SMO is removed and signals are transduced via Gli to the nucleus. **C** Inactivating mutations in *PTCH* simulate Hedgehog binding and result in constitutive activation of Gli and downstream target genes. **D** An activating mutation in *SMO* results in constitutive signaling to Gli and downstream target genes.

and Gli as common denominators will be used to illustrate interactions and effects in this important pathway.

PTCH Gene

The human *PTCH* gene was cloned and identified in 1996. Positional cloning was used to search the region within 9q22.3 in order to identify the gene responsible for Gorlin syndrome. The gene is 35 kb in length and consists of 23 exons; *PTCH* cDNA has an open reading frame of 4242 nucleotides, and Northern blot analyses have shown that different transcripts exist with alternative 5′ ends. The different transcripts have been identified in human epidermis.

PTCH Protein Product (Patched)

The protein product of the human *PTCH* gene is the sonic hedgehog (SHH) receptor, which is an integral membrane protein with 12 predicted transmembrane regions and two large extracellular loops as well as a putative sterol-sensing domain. The protein is a putative glycoprotein consisting of 1236 amino acid residues and both the amino- and carboxy-terminal portions have an intracellular location containing numerous potential phosphorylation sites. Patched protein normally binds a seven transmembrane G-protein receptor named Smoothened (SMO). SMO has been shown to be constitutively active when not bound to Patched (see Fig. 107.8).

Normal Function of Patched

By controlling proliferation, differentiation and cell fate, the SHH–Patched signaling pathway is deeply involved in normal embryonic development. Preserved normal signaling is crucial for morphogenesis, and disruption of the pathway is lethal in mice. The balance of gene expression in different cell populations is critical for normal development in general and of particular importance for normal development of the CNS. The induced downstream genes play key roles in epithelial–mesenchymal interactions.

Patched function is mediated via release of suppression on SMO. SMO signaling is then transduced and executed through the transcription factor Gli (see Fig. 107.8). Active Gli serves as a transcription factor for *GLI* itself as well as inducing transcription of *PTCH*, thus creating a negative feedback loop. Other genes induced through the SHH–Patched signaling pathway include members of the *TGF-β* gene family and *bcl-2*.

TGF-β inhibits growth of epithelial cells and promotes cell differentiation, whereas its effect on mesenchymal cells is growth stimulation. Bone morphogenic proteins (TGF-β family proteins) play a key role in the development of cartilage and bone as well as the induction of hair follicles during embryogenesis. Of note, skeletal malformations are a common feature in Gorlin syndrome. In adult tissues, TGF-β proteins are dynamically expressed in hair follicles (including the surrounding mesenchyme) and have been implicated in the cyclic growth of hair, including remodeling of the extracellular matrix surrounding hair follicles. Bcl-2 protein is a well-known suppressor of apoptosis (see above) and is commonly expressed in BCC.

Regulation of Patched

Knowledge about genes and molecules involved in SHH–Patched signaling has been obtained mainly by genetic analyses in *Drosophila*. The signaling pathway is well conserved, although with increasing complexity, from insects to vertebrates, including humans. The SHH–Patched signaling pathway induces transcription of *PTCH* itself, creating a negative feedback loop for *PTCH*. Unliganded Patched interacts with and suppresses signaling by the co-receptor SMO. SHH signaling accordingly induces transcription of target genes by opposing the repressive activity of Patched. In other words, when SHH binds to the receptor Patched, repression of SMO is relieved and downstream target genes are induced. In a simplified scheme (see Fig. 107.8B), secreted SHH proteins bind to the receptor protein Patched and upon binding to the ligand, Patched dissociates from its co-receptor Smoothened.

Inactivating mutations of *PTCH* simulate SHH signaling due to the failure of mutated Patched protein to suppress SMO (see Fig. 107.8C).

The loss of negative autoregulation leads to increased transcription of non-functional *PTCH* mRNA. In carcinogenesis, several lines of evidence (including experiments using transgenic mice) suggest that the critical cellular effect is stimulation of proliferation as opposed to differentiation, and that this effect is mediated by upregulation of Gli.

PTCH Mutations

An early onset of multiple BCCs is a hallmark of Gorlin syndrome. The *PTCH* gene is mutated in patients with Gorlin syndrome and thus strongly linked to the development of BCCs. Additional features that constitute Gorlin syndrome include skeletal abnormalities, jaw cysts, macrocephaly and palmoplantar pits. A majority of the germline mutations in *PTCH* are truncating, suggesting that haploinsufficiency underlies the developmental abnormalities. Both alleles of *PTCH* are often inactivated in both familial and sporadic cases of BCC, as would be expected for a classic tumor suppressor gene. Most tumors where *PTCH* is inactivated display a truncating mutation in one allele and deletion of the other allele, i.e. loss of heterozygosity (LOH). Alternatively, point mutations in both alleles can occur in tumors without a LOH in the *PTCH* locus.

Constitutive activation of SHH signaling by inactivating mutations in *PTCH* or activating mutations in *SMO* appear to be required, and possibly also sufficient, for development of BCC. Disruption of the SHH–Patched pathway has also been found in other tumors such as medulloblastoma, as well as ovarian and cardiac fibromas, which are common in patients with Gorlin syndrome. In addition, *PTCH* mutations have been found in sporadic trichoepitheliomas, bladder carcinoma and SCC of the esophagus. Mutational analysis has shown that two-thirds of reported mutations were truncating or affected splicing. Mutations, including missense mutations, are spread over the entire gene, without any particular hotspot region.

STRUCTURE AND FUNCTION OF BCC

Sun exposure and anatomic site appear to be of etiologic importance in the development of BCC. Intermittent, recreational sun exposure more so than cumulative UV radiation is a significant risk factor[24]. The development of BCCs is restricted to skin containing pilosebaceous units. The fact that BCCs commonly develop on the face, and in particular on the nose, suggests that anatomic site, i.e. specific areas of skin that contain a higher number of target progenitor cells, plays an important role. Analogous to other malignancies, BCC appears to have a capacity for infinite growth and spontaneous regression is not a feature. Sophisticated studies of tumor biology have been sparse due to difficulties in establishing good experimental models, and *in vitro* culture of BCC cells from explanted tumors has in general been unsuccessful. Transplantation of BCC into athymic mice has been more successful, although extensive studies of long-term effects have been sparse. The recent development of strategies using transgenic mice as a model to study BCC has been rewarding, especially with regard to elucidating the role of different components in the SHH–Patched signaling pathway[25,25a].

Precursors

Perhaps the most striking feature of BCCs is that tumors virtually never develop metastases. BCCs appear resistant to tumor progression and there are no known precursors (with the possible exception of p53 clones)[26]. Although tumors can grow for many years in the setting of sustained exposure to mutagenic UV radiation, the tumors remain indolent. Non-aggressive forms of BCC, such as superficial and nodular BCC, appear to develop *de novo* and continue to grow without progressing to more aggressive forms of BCC. Aggressive forms of BCC, e.g. morpheaform or sclerosing BCC, also show an unusual genomic stability, with a persistent pattern of locally invasive growth and tissue destruction, but without progression to metastatic disease. This also holds true for BCCs that develop in xeroderma pigmentosum patients where there is a high number of unrepaired mutations. It is unclear why BCC cells are resistant to acquiring additional genetic hits leading to more autonomous growth.

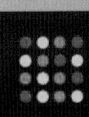

Cancer

BCC is a tumor with unique growth characteristics. It is dependent on a specific loose connective tissue stroma for its continued growth, and one hypothesis for the inability of a BCC to transform into a metastasizing tumor is an unconditional dependence on a stroma produced by dermal fibroblasts. In an experiment where autotransplantation of BCC with and without its cognate stroma was performed, it became evident that BCC devoid of its stroma failed to proliferate and instead differentiated into keratin-filled cysts[27].

The loose connective tissue stroma that characteristically surrounds nests of BCC cells consists of dermal fibroblasts and thin collagen fibers. The cross-talk between tumor cells and mesenchymal cells of the cognate stroma simulates the epithelial–stromal interactions found in normal developing and adult cycling hair follicles. One example of this involves the PDGF system, where the growth factor receptors for PDGF are upregulated in BCC stroma whereas the ligand PDGF is mainly expressed in tumor cells.

The invasive nature of BCCs can be explained in part by proteolytic activity of the tumor. Increased expression of enzymes such as metalloproteinases and collagenases, which degrade pre-existing dermal tissue and facilitate spread of tumor cells, can be found in both BCC cells and stromal cells.

Microscopically, BCCs often appear as multicentric tumors. In superficial BCCs, nests of tumor cells connected to the basal cell layer of the overlying epidermis appear as discontinuous buds of tumor cells. Recent studies based on microdissection, gene amplification and gene sequencing have shown that BCCs develop as a monoclonal proliferation consistent with a unicellular origin. Interestingly, BCCs often consist of subclones (Fig. 107.9). Using p53 mutations as a marker for clonality, it was shown that different parts of a tumor share a common mutation but differ with respect to second, third or even fourth mutations within the two alleles of the p53 gene[28]. The precise background required for a selection of additional p53 mutations is not known. It is possible that a first mutation in the p53 gene allows for a slight growth advantage and that additional mutations generate tumor cells with an even higher level of selective growth advantage due to the different and complex roles that p53 plays in cell cycle control, apoptosis and DNA repair.

Although BCC appears as a tumor with extraordinary genomic stability, a large number of tumors are aneuploid. Analyses of LOH have shown allelic loss of chromosome 9q, while LOH involving other chromosomes was observed infrequently[29]. Of note, the gene most often altered in BCCs is the *PTCH* gene, which is located on chromosome 9q. Two out of three BCCs show LOH and/or truncating mutations in the *PTCH* gene. In tumors where the *PTCH* gene is intact, other mutations such as activating mutations in *SMO* (20%) have been detected. Accumulating data suggest that a sufficiently elevated expression level of Gli, by homozygous inactivation of *PTCH* or by activating mutations of *SMO*, in a responding cell is necessary and perhaps also sufficient to drive the formation of BCC. Constitutive SHH signaling has also been demonstrated to be required for growth of *established* BCCs (see Fig. 107.8)[30].

The second most common genetic alteration found in BCCs is point mutations in the *p53* gene. *p53* mutations appear early during carcinogenesis and at least 50% of BCCs have a mutated *p53* gene. The vast majority of *p53* mutations are missense mutations that carry a UV signature (see Ch. 85)[31]. In many BCCs, both *p53* alleles are affected by point mutations, unlike the more common combination of a point mutation and a deletion (LOH) observed in most other solid tumors. The role of *p53* mutations in the carcinogenesis of BCCs could be based on the expansion of the number of target cells, i.e. epidermal p53 clones, susceptible to transformation.

Mutations in the *CDKN2A* (*INK4A*) locus, which encodes both p16 and p14[ARF] (see above), have also been detected in a smaller number of sporadic BCCs. In contrast to tumor suppressor genes (e.g. *PTCH*, *p53*), oncogenes appear to play a lesser role in the development of BCC. *ras* genes are the most studied oncogenes and the frequency of *ras* mutations in BCC has varied between 0 and 30%, depending on the study. Alterations in other oncogenes and tumor suppressor genes have only sporadically been recorded.

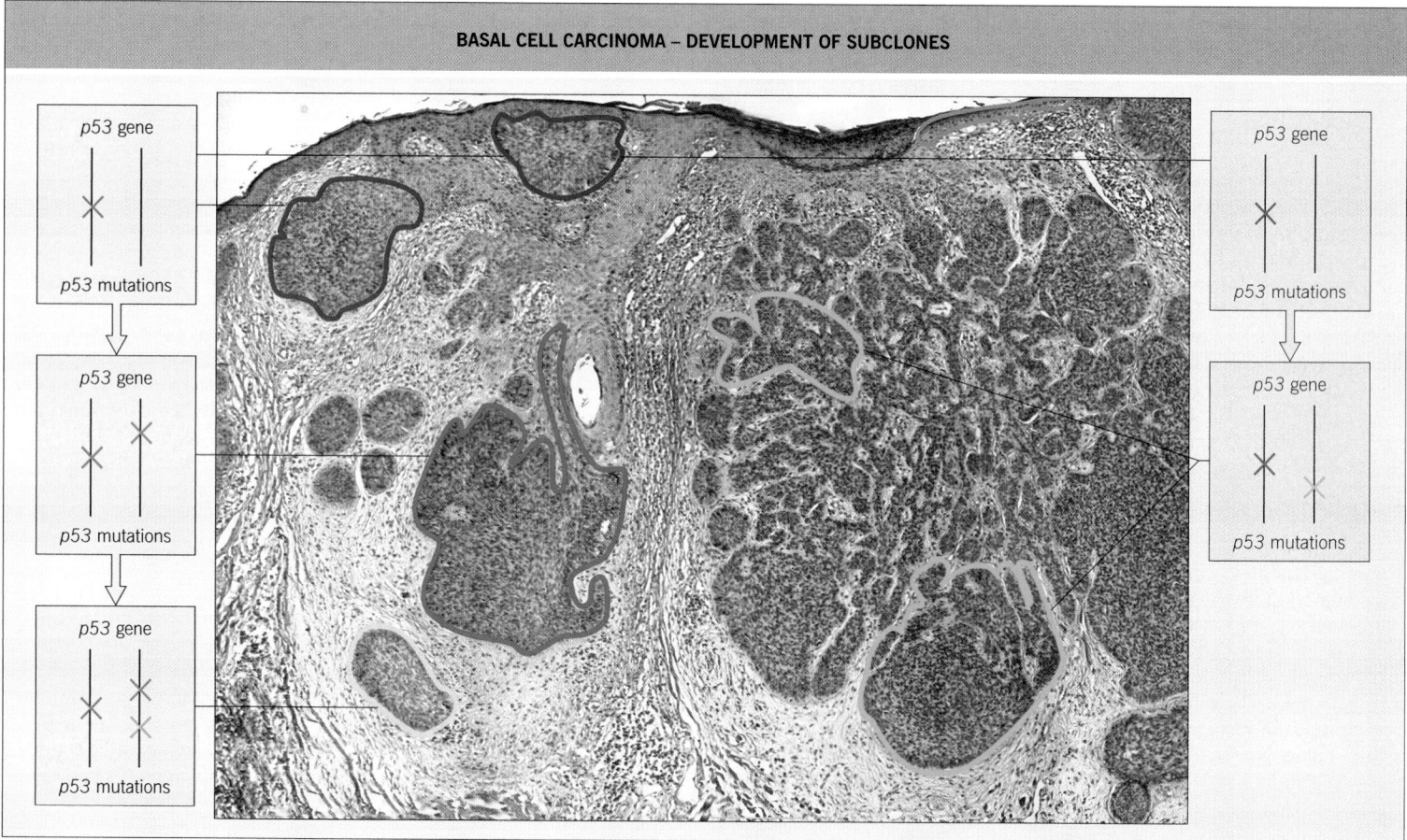

BASAL CELL CARCINOMA – DEVELOPMENT OF SUBCLONES

Fig. 107.9 Basal cell carcinoma (BCC) – development of subclones. A common *p53* mutation (red cross) is found in different parts of the tumor. Despite indistinguishable morphology, different parts of individual BCCs have acquired additional mutations in the *p53* gene (blue, orange and green crosses). Boxes illustrate the two *p53* alleles. Note normal *p53* status (outlined in orange) in overlying epidermal keratinocytes.

Limitless replicative potential is essential for the malignant phenotype, and telomere maintenance is also evident in BCCs, due to high telomerase activity. Interestingly, BCCs express equal or higher levels of telomerase when compared to high-grade malignancies. The presence of intact DNA repair genes is also of critical importance. The detrimental effect of insufficient repair of UV-induced DNA damage is well illustrated in patients with xeroderma pigmentosum, who develop numerous BCCs at an early age.

Metastasis

Although BCCs virtually never metastasize, there have been a few reports in the literature of BCCs that developed metastases, and the incidence has been estimated to be 1:1000 to 1:35 000. It appears as if these rare cases represent aggressive tumors with perineural spread of tumor cells. Lymph node metastasis followed by lung and bone metastasis is the most common progression. The diagnosis has been based on morphology, and the possibility that some of these cases represent poorly differentiated variants of SCCs cannot be excluded.

In summary, BCC is a common, locally invasive tumor of the skin, for which UV radiation and alterations in the *PTCH* gene are important etiologic factors. BCC is stroma-dependent for its growth, arises without precursors, and shows continuous growth without progression to metastatic disease.

STRUCTURE AND FUNCTION OF SCC

UV solar radiation is also a major etiologic factor in the development of cutaneous SCC. The cumulative dose of UV radiation received over time is a significant risk factor, in contrast to the more complex relationship between BCC and sun exposure early in life or cutaneous melanoma and sunburns[24]. SCC of the skin is a 'classic cancer', as it has precursor lesions, tumor progression and the potential to develop metastatic disease[32]. SCC can develop in different regions of the skin as well as other sites lined by squamous epithelia, e.g. mouth, esophagus, vagina. The biology of cutaneous SCC differs in part from that of SCCs that arise in other tissues. In particular, SCC in areas of chronically sun-exposed skin exhibits a relatively indolent behavior and the development of metastases is infrequent (less than 5%). The nature of SCCs arising at mucocutaneous interfaces, e.g. lips, genitalia and perianal area, appears to be more aggressive, with a higher risk of metastases. SCC also arises in tissues where squamous cell metaplasia occurs, e.g. the lung, cervix, salivary glands.

Precursors

The current opinion regarding cutaneous SCC is that the cancer is derived from a single transformed cell of keratinocytic lineage[26]. The precise genetic events and number of mutations required for malignant transformation are unknown. However, cutaneous SCC develops through the addition of genetic alterations leading to a selective growth advantage. In this scheme of events, several stages can be defined. An attractive model (supported by studies in hairless mice) includes epidermal p53 clones as forerunners to squamous cell dysplasia (Fig. 107.10)[33]. According to the dogma, slight dysplasia precedes moderate and severe dysplasia (which is seen in SCC *in situ*) and invasive SCC then develops from carcinoma *in situ*. Further genetic alterations and selection leads to the final stage, where a locally invasive SCC gives rise to metastases in regional lymph nodes and distant organs.

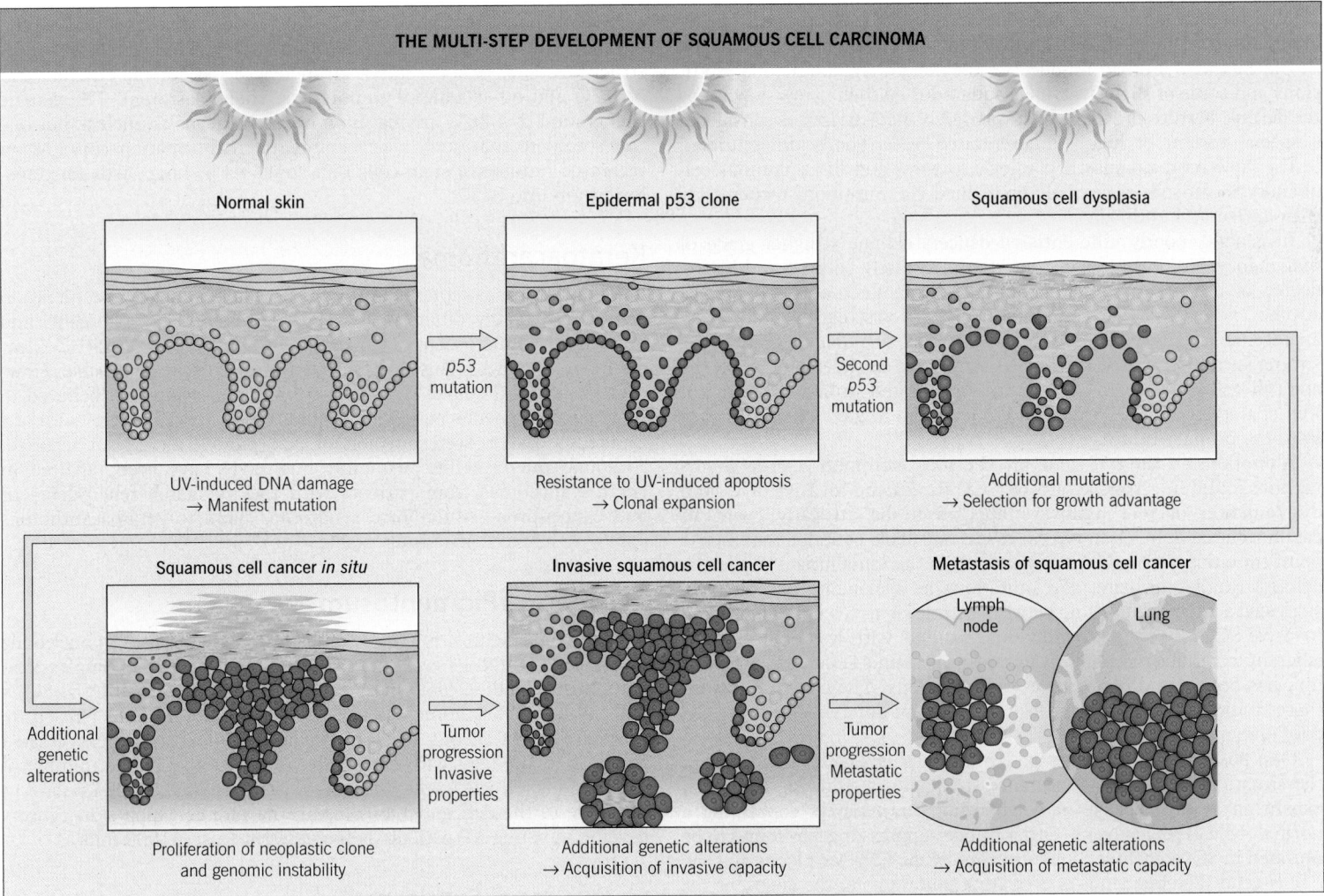

Fig. 107.10 The multistep development of squamous cell carcinoma. UV irradiation of normal skin induces mutations in keratinocytes and facilitates clonal expansion of keratinocytes with a mutated *p53* gene. Additional mutations (including a second *p53* mutation) that affect genes controlling proliferation, cell migration and cell death provide for selective growth advantage and cause genomic instability. The final result is metastatic tumor cells, capable of growing in regional lymph nodes and internal organs.

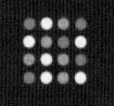

Clinical precursor lesions associated with cutaneous SCC include actinic keratoses and Bowen's disease. Microscopically, actinic keratoses display signs of chronic sun damage, i.e. solar elastosis and a slight to severe grade of squamous cell dysplasia within the epidermis, especially in its lowermost portions. Bowen's disease also displays squamous cell dysplasia, which is full-thickness and often high-grade. Actinic keratoses are exceedingly common in chronically sun-exposed skin of older Caucasians. Lesions occur primarily on the face, hairless scalp, dorsal aspects of the hands, and helices of the ears (primarily in men). The risk for an individual actinic keratosis to progress into an invasive cancer is low, probably less than 1 in 1000 per year[26]. The risk of SCC *in situ* progressing to invasive cancer is considered to be higher.

Cancer

UV solar radiation is accepted as a major risk factor for SCC. Numerous experiments using chemical multistage carcinogenesis models have been performed in mice, yielding SCC-like tumors. A typical protocol consists of a single application of an initiating compound, e.g. 7,12-dimethylbenz[a]anthracene (DMBA), which leads to irreversible activating mutations in *ras* genes within basal cells of the epidermis. In a second step, repetitive doses of a tumor-promoting agent, e.g. 12-O-tetradecanoylphorbol 13-acetate (TPA), induces a hyperproliferative response. Through partly epigenetic mechanisms, this leads to the development of squamous cell papillomas. Conversion of benign papillomas into malignant SCCs then involves a number of chromosome and gene alterations required for the acquisition of the malignant phenotype. UV radiation can act as both an initiating factor and a tumor-promoting factor in such models. Agents associated with human SCC include chemical agents, e.g. petroleum oils, coal tar, soot and arsenic, and physical agents, e.g. UV and ionizing irradiation, or the combination of both.

Invasive SCCs can have different degrees of differentiation. Highly differentiated tumors show features of keratinization and often invade the dermis with a broad rounded tumor margin. Papillomatous extensions and cords of slightly atypical squamous epithelia grow down into the dermis. Verrucous SCC, which very rarely metastasizes, is considered a special variant of highly differentiated SCC. Poorly differentiated SCCs show more anaplastic cytologic features and the squamous cell phenotype can sometimes only be verified via immunohistochemistry with antikeratin antibodies.

In general, poorly differentiated cancers exhibit a higher grade of malignancy. However, biologic behavior can rarely be predicted by the degree of differentiation alone. SCC is dependent on a supportive stroma, as are all other solid tumors, and a vasculature induced by angiogenic signals is needed for the tumor to enlarge. Unlike the stroma surrounding a BCC, the SCC stroma is considered non-specific and cell–cell interactions between tumor cells and stromal cells are not well characterized. SCC thus has the potential to grow at sites distant from the primary tumor.

Alterations in the *p53* gene are the most common genetic abnormalities found in actinic keratoses, SCC *in situ* and invasive SCC, and dysregulation of p53 pathways appears to be an early event in carcinogenesis of SCC. In typical cases, one allele contains a missense point mutation with a UV signature, while the remaining *p53* allele is deleted. Studies utilizing *p53* mutations as a clonality marker have suggested a direct relationship between actinic keratoses, SCC *in situ* and invasive SCC. By studying individual patients with lesions (e.g. SCC) adjacent to various morphologic entities (e.g. actinic keratoses), a genetic link has been found between coexisting lesions. The conclusion from these studies is that coexisting lesions represent different stages in SCC development.

One possible role for early *p53* mutations in SCCs (analogous to the situation in BCCs) is resistance to apoptosis, allowing for clonal expansion at the expense of neighboring keratinocytes containing a normal (wild-type) *p53* gene. Other tumor suppressor genes found to be mutated in SCCs include different exons of the *CDKN2A* locus and the *PTCH* gene. The frequency of activating mutations in the oncogene *ras* ranges from 10% to 50%.

Loss of heterozygosity has been studied in different chromosomes, and unlike the case in BCC, where LOH is mainly restricted to chromosome 9q, actinic keratoses and SCCs demonstrate a more widespread LOH

pattern with deletions in several chromosomes, e.g. 3p, 9p, 9q, 13q, 17p and 17q[34]. SCCs appear to have a higher degree of genomic instability compared with BCCs, and 25–80% of SCCs are aneuploid. Precancerous lesions such as actinic keratoses and Bowen's disease appear to have an even higher degree of genomic instability, since aneuploid cell populations are frequently found in such lesions.

Metastasis

SCC has the potential for developing metastatic disease, although this appears to occur rather infrequently. The proportion of SCCs in chronically sun-exposed skin that give rise to metastases is in the order of 1 in 20 or less. SCCs at mucocutaneous borders, including the lip (which by definition is a sun-exposed site), have a higher rate of progression to metastatic disease, with an up to 30% risk of developing metastasis. Most metastases are found in regional lymph nodes, but distant hematogenous spread can also be observed.

In summary, SCC arising in chronically sun-exposed skin is a common tumor for which cumulative sun exposure is an important etiologic factor. SCC arises through a series of stages involving precursor lesions, such as actinic keratoses, and can with time develop metastatic disease.

RELATED DISEASES

Adnexal Tumors

Tumors that mimic cutaneous appendageal differentiation display a multitude of different phenotypes (see Ch. 111). A majority of these tumors are benign, although malignant counterparts do exist. The degree of differentiation allows these tumors to be distinguished from BCC and SCC. In one sense, BCCs can be thought of as undifferentiated adnexal tumors. An organoid nevus, e.g. nevus sebaceus of Jadassohn, represents a cutaneous malformation that includes pilosebaceous structures. Such lesions harbor an increased risk for the development of BCC and other adnexal tumors (e.g. trichoblastoma). The genetic background of a BCC arising in an organoid nevus is unclear, but one can speculate that such a developmental malformation contains an increased number of stem cells that could act as target cells for transformation into BCC.

Keratoacanthoma

Keratoacanthomas represent tumors characterized by the proliferation of atypical, highly differentiated squamous epithelia. Clinically, and even more so microscopically, keratoacanthomas resemble SCC. Clear distinction from a highly differentiated SCC is often impossible. However, the clinical course is usually benign and lesions are believed to undergo spontaneous regression if not excised. Sporadic cases with *p53* mutations and/or overexpression of p53 protein have been reported. Although microsatellite instability and LOH have been reported in keratoacanthomas from patients with the mismatch repair-deficient and cancer-prone Muir–Torre syndrome, sporadic keratoacanthomas appear to be more genetically stable.

Xeroderma Pigmentosum

Xeroderma pigmentosum (XP) is caused by inherited defects in nucleotide excision repair (NER) genes (see Ch. 85), resulting in a complex skin pathology including lentigines, epidermal hyperplasias, BCCs, SCCs and cutaneous melanomas triggered by exposure to the sun. This entire spectrum of cutaneous disease can be described as an exaggerated response to UV light with early onset of a vastly increased number of skin lesions, which would otherwise occur in small numbers late in life. Due to the deficient DNA repair, the rate at which skin cancers develop in young XP patients is increased at least a 1000-fold.

Li–Fraumeni Syndrome

The Li–Fraumeni syndrome is a rare familial cancer syndrome where germline mutations of the *p53* gene play an important role. The syndrome is characterized by an autosomal dominant inheritance

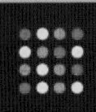

pattern and affected individuals display an early onset of various tumors, including breast cancer, brain tumors, osteosarcoma and leukemia. However, skin cancer is not a typical feature of Li–Fraumeni syndrome, despite the fact that *p53* mutations are frequently observed in BCCs and SCCs.

Gorlin Syndrome

The most common inherited disorder associated with BCCs is the Gorlin syndrome (see above); it is transmitted in an autosomal dominant fashion. Affected individuals have a wide range of developmental anomalies, including skeletal abnormalities, craniofacial dysmorphism and macrocephaly. Multiple BCCs with an early onset are a hallmark of the syndrome that also includes features such as odontogenic

keratocysts, palmoplantar pits and calcification of the falx cerebri. In addition to BCCs, patients have an increased incidence of medulloblastomas, meningiomas, ovarian fibromas and ovarian cancer, as well as cardiac fibromas. Germline mutations in the *PTCH* gene are found in a vast majority of patients with this syndrome.

Bazex Syndrome

Bazex syndrome is a rare genodermatosis characterized by follicular atrophoderma and the early onset of multiple BCCs. The responsible gene has been linked to Xq24–q27 and there is no male-to-male transmission. It should not be confused with acrokeratosis paraneoplastica, also known as Bazex syndrome, which occurs most commonly in the setting of carcinomas of the upper aerodigestive tract (see Ch. 52).

REFERENCES

1. Kinzler KW, Vogelstein B. Life (and death) in a malignant tumour [news; comment]. Nature. 1996;379:19–20.
2. Loeb LA. Mutator phenotype may be required for multistage carcinogenesis. Cancer Res. 1991;51:3075–9.
2a. Vogelstein B, Fearon ER, Hamilton SR, et al. Genetic alterations during colorectal-tumor development. N Engl J Med. 1988;319:525–32.
3. Hanahan D, Weinberg RA. The hallmarks of cancer. Cell. 2000;100:57–70.
4. Kastan MB. Checkpoint Controls and Cancer, Vol. 29. New York: Cold Spring Harbor Laboratory Press, 1997.
5. Land H, Parada LF, Weinberg R. Cellular oncogenes and multistep carcinogenesis. Science. 1983;222:771–8.
6. Heldin CH, Westermark B. Growth factors: mechanism of action and relation to oncogenes. Cell. 1984;37:9–20.
7. Cordon-Cardo C. Mutation of cell cycle regulators. Biological and clinical implications for human neoplasia. Am J Pathol. 1995;147:545–60.
8. Kerr JF, Wyllie AH, Currie AR. Apoptosis: a basic biological phenomenon with wide-ranging implications in tissue kinetics. Br J Cancer. 1972;26:239–57.
9. Evan G, Littlewood T. A matter of life and cell death. Science. 1998;281:1317–22.
10. Harley CB, Futcher AB, Greider CW. Telomeres shorten during ageing of human fibroblasts. Nature. 1990;345:458–60.
11. Hanahan D, Folkman J. Patterns and emerging mechanisms of the angiogenic switch during tumorigenesis. Cell. 1996;86:353–64.
12. Levine AJ. p53, the cellular gatekeeper for growth and division. Cell. 1997;88:323–31.
13. Lane DP. p53, guardian of the genome. Nature. 1992;358:15–16.
14. Harris C. Structure and function of the p53 tumor suppressor gene: clues for rational cancer therapeutic strategies. J Natl Cancer Inst. 1996;16:1442–55.
15. Brash DE. Cellular proofreading. Nat Med. 1996; 2:525–6.

16. Jonason AS, Restifo RJ, Spinelli HM, et al. Frequent clones of p53-mutated keratinocytes in normal human skin. Proc Natl Acad Sci USA. 1996;93:14025–9.
17. Pontén F, Berne B, Ren Z, et al. Ultraviolet light induces expression of p53 and p21 in human skin; effect of sunscreen and constitutive p21 expression in skin appendages. J Invest Dermatol. 1995;105:402–6.
18. Backvall H, Asplund A, Gustafsson A, et al. Genetic tumor archeology: microdissection and genetic heterogeneity in squamous and basal cell carcinoma. Mutat Res. 2005;571:65–79.
19. Rebel H, Kram N, Westerman A, et al. Relationship between UV-induced mutant p53 patches and skin tumours, analysed by mutation spectra and by induction kinetics in various DNA-repair-deficient mice. Carcinogenesis. 2005;26:2123–30.
20. Zhang W, Remenyik E, Zelterman D, et al. Escaping the stem cell compartment: sustained UVB exposure allows p53-mutant keratinocytes to colonize adjacent epidermal proliferating units without incurring additional mutations. Proc Natl Acad Sci USA. 2001;98:13948–53.
21. Toftgard R. Hedgehog signalling in cancer. Cell Mol Life Sci. 2000;57:1720–31.
22. Hahn H, Wiking C, Zaphiropoulos PG, et al. Mutations of the human homolog of Drosophila patched in the nevoid basal cell carcinoma syndrome. Cell. 1996;85:841–51.
23. Johnson RL, Rothman AL, Xie J, et al. Human homolog of patched, a candidate gene for the basal cell nevus syndrome. Science. 1996;272:1668–71.
24. Armstrong BK, Kricker A. The epidemiology of UV induced skin cancer. J Photochem Photobiol B. 2001;63:8–18.
25. Hahn H, Wojnowski L, Miller G, et al. The patched signaling pathway in tumorigenesis and development: lessons from animal models. J Mol Med. 1999;77:459–68.

25a. Mao J, Ligon KL, Rakhlin EY, et al. A novel somatic mouse model to survey tumorigenic potential applied to the hedgehog pathway. Cancer Res. 2006;66:10171–8.
26. Pontén J. Precancer: Biology, Importance and Possible Prevention, Vol. 32. New York: Cold Spring Harbor Laboratory Press, 1998.
27. van Scott EJV, Reinertson RP. The modulating influence of stromal environment on epithelial cells studied in human autotransplants. J Invest Dermatol. 1961;36:109–17.
28. Pontén F, Berg C, Ahmadian A, et al. Molecular pathology in basal cell cancer with p53 as a genetic marker. Oncogene. 1997;15:1059–67.
29. Teh MT, Blaydon D, Chaplin T, et al. Genomewide single nucleotide polymorphism microarray mapping in basal cell carcinomas unveils uniparental disomy as a key somatic event. Cancer Res. 2005;65:8597–603.
30. Hutchin ME, Kariapper MS, Grachtchouk M, et al. Sustained Hedgehog signaling is required for basal cell carcinoma proliferation and survival: conditional skin tumorigenesis recapitulates the hair growth cycle. Genes Dev. 2005;19:214–23.
31. Brash DE, Rudolph JA, Simon JA, et al. A role for sunlight in skin cancer: UV-induced p53 mutations in squamous cell carcinoma. Proc Natl Acad Sci USA. 1991;88:10124–8.
32. de Gruijl FR, van Kranen HJ, Mullenders LH. UV-induced DNA damage, repair, mutations and oncogenic pathways in skin cancer. J Photochem Photobiol B. 2001;63:19–27.
33. Kramata P, Lu YP, Lou YR, et al. Patches of mutant p53-immunoreactive epidermal cells induced by chronic UVB irradiation harbor the same p53 mutations as squamous cell carcinomas in the skin of hairless SKH-1 mice. Cancer Res. 2005;65:3577–85.
34. Quinn AG, Healy E, Rehman I, et al. Microsatellite instability in human non-melanoma and melanoma skin cancer. J Invest Dermatol. 1995;104:309–12.

Actinic Keratosis, Basal Cell Carcinoma and Squamous Cell Carcinoma

108

Darrell S Rigel, Clay J Cockerell, John Carucci and James Wharton

Synonyms: ■ Solar keratosis and senile keratosis are non-preferred synonyms for actinic keratosis (solar keratosis is abbreviated to SK, causing confusion with seborrheic keratosis) ■ Bowen's disease – squamous cell carcinoma *in situ* ■ Basal cell epithelioma and rodent ulcer are antiquated synonyms for basal cell carcinoma ■ Basal cell nevus syndrome is a non-preferred synonym for nevoid basal cell carcinoma syndrome (Gorlin syndrome)

Key features

- Non-melanoma skin cancer (NMSC) is the most common malignancy in humans
- Although most NMSCs are related to UV light exposure, other factors include exposure to ionizing radiation, arsenic or organic chemicals, human papillomavirus infection, immunosuppression, and genetic predisposition
- Prevention efforts are aimed at lowering incidence and mortality
- NMSC, if neglected or inappropriately managed, can cause significant morbidity and even death
- Surgery is the mainstay of treatment, but promising new modalities include immunomodulators, photodynamic therapy, and drugs that address genetic defects

INTRODUCTION

Non-melanoma skin cancer (NMSC) is the most common cancer in humans. Approximately 75–80% of NMSCs are basal cell carcinomas (BCCs) and up to 25% are squamous cell carcinomas (SCCs). Although BCC rarely metastasizes and thus rarely causes death, it can result in significant morbidity if not correctly diagnosed and managed. SCC of the skin, if not diagnosed and treated early, can lead to significant morbidity and mortality. Actinic keratosis (AK), the most commonly treated neoplasm in humans, is a potential precursor to SCC. Because the incidence of NMSC continues to rise, these neoplasms represent a significant health problem from the standpoint of patients' wellbeing and from the perspective of healthcare expenditures.

HISTORY

In 1775, Sir Percivall Pott noted an etiologic relationship between SCC and chimney soot exposure in his short treatise *Chirurgical Observations Relative to the Cancer of the Scrotum*. During the industrial revolution, links to arsenic, coal tar, shale oil and creosote were also identified. In the late 1800s, Paul Unna noted a connection to UV light, when he described skin cancer development in chronically sun-exposed sites in sailors.

Evidence of the nevoid basal cell carcinoma syndrome, consisting of jaw cysts, syndactyly and bifid ribs, has been identified in Egyptian mummies almost 4000 years old. In the 1850s H Lebert first used the term 'rodent ulcer' to describe untreated BCCs of long duration. Several years later, Sir Jonathan Hutchinson published a review of 42 cases of BCCs, identifying the tumor as a single entity with many different clinical and histologic forms. Krompecher first suggested BCC arose from the cells of the basal layer of the epidermis. Other theories were proposed regarding the site of origin of this tumor, including the hair follicle and other appendageal structures. Some authors hypothesized that a BCC was not a carcinoma but rather a nevoid tumor or hamartoma or that a BCC was derived from immature pluripotential cells which formed continuously during one's lifetime.

EPIDEMIOLOGY

NMSC occurs worldwide in all races. It is estimated that 2 million cases of NMSC were diagnosed in the US in 2004[1]. There are more skin cancers in the US population than there are all other cancers combined and it is estimated that one in five Americans will develop skin cancer during their lifetime[2] (over 95% will be NMSC). The most important factor related to development of these neoplasms appears to be skin phenotype (Table 108.1), but other factors also play a significant role. For example, the incidence of NMSC is about ten times higher in white versus Hispanic men and five times higher in white versus Hispanic women[12].

The exact incidence of NMSC may be difficult to determine due to issues such as diagnostic accuracy and diagnostic criteria (e.g. differentiation between AKs and SCC *in situ*). In addition, deriving precise data on NMSC is hampered by the fact that these neoplasms are not routinely included in state cancer registries (which often rely upon hospital data). Even if NMSCs were included, they would still be significantly underreported, given the number treated in private offices.

The amount of average annual UV radiation correlates with the incidence of skin cancer (Fig. 108.1). There is also a direct relationship between the incidence of NMSC and latitude (Table 108.2) in that the closer individuals are to the equator, the greater their exposure to UV

INFLUENCE OF SKIN COLOR ON EPIDEMIOLOGY OF NMSC		
Characteristic	**Lightly pigmented individuals**	**Darkly pigmented individuals**
NMSC incidence	230 per 100 000	3.4 per 100 000
BCC:SCC ratio	4:1	1:1.1
BCC male:female ratio	1.5:1	1.3:1
SCC male:female ratio	2:1–5:1	1.3:1
% of BCCs developing in the head and neck region	60–80	90
% of SCCs developing in the head and neck region	65	35
% of SCCs developing in scars and chronic non-healing ulcers	<2	30–40
NMSC incidence rates	Increasing	?
NMSC mortality rates	Decreasing	Decreasing
% of skin cancer deaths due to NMSC in persons <50 years of age	10	70
% of skin cancer deaths due to NMSC in persons >85 years of age	55	60

Table 108.1 Influence of skin color on epidemiology of non-melanoma skin cancer (NMSC). BCC, basal cell carcinoma; SCC; squamous cell carcinoma. From refs 3–11.

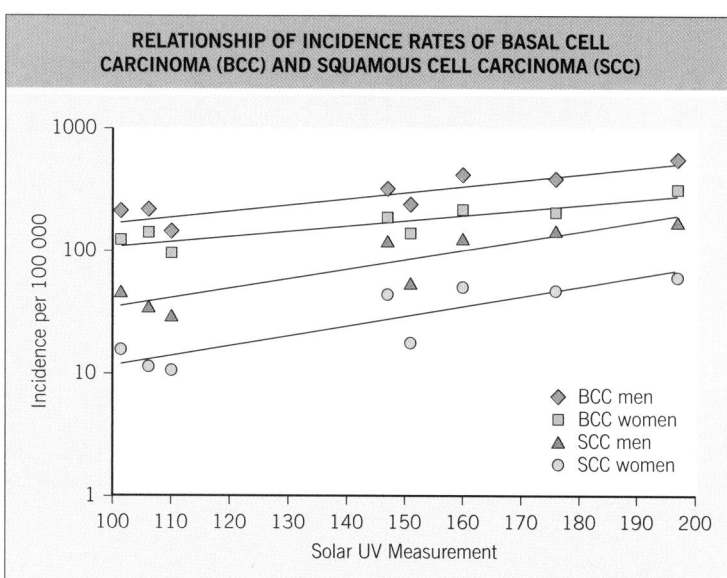

Fig. 108.1 Relationship of incidence rates of basal cell carcinoma (BCC) and squamous cell carcinoma (SCC) to estimated ambient erythemal UV radiation as measured in ten cities in the US. From Armstrong BK, Kricker A. J Photochem Photobiol B. 2001;63:8–18.

INCIDENCE RATES PER YEAR (PER 100 000) OF BASAL CELL CARCINOMA AND SQUAMOUS CELL CARCINOMA BY GEOGRAPHIC LOCATION		
Geographic location	**Basal cell carcinoma (men/women)**	**Squamous cell carcinoma (men/women)**
Finland	49/45	9/5
Switzerland	52/38	16/8
The Netherlands	53/38	…
United Kingdom	112/54	32/6
United States (overall)	247/150	65/24
New Hampshire	159/87	32/8
Rochester, Minnesota	175/124	63/23
Hawaii	576/298	153/92
Southern Arizona	935/497	270/112
Nambour, Australia	2074/1579	1035/472

Table 108.2 Incidence rates per year (per 100 000) of basal cell carcinoma and squamous cell carcinoma by geographic location. Data are from refs 5 & 12; refers to Caucasian populations.

radiation. In Australia, the cumulative risk by age 70 years of having at least one NMSC is 70% for men and 58% for women. Incidence of NMSC increases with age (Fig. 108.2). In those under 40 years of age, a majority of NMSC is found in women, but, by age 80, the incidence in men exceeds women by a 2–3:1 ratio[12].

AKs are most often found in fair-skinned individuals, but can be seen in all races. AKs are so common that they accounted for 3 million annual visits to dermatologists in the US during the early 1990s. In the UK, incidence rates for AKs are approximately 15 times those for BCC and SCC. Over 80% of AKs occur on the head, neck and upper extremities (dorsal hands and forearms). AKs develop much more often in individuals with a prior history of AKs, with increasing age, and in men. AKs are also markers for an increased risk for developing invasive NMSC[13].

The demographics of SCC are similar to those of AKs, with the majority of SCC occurring on the head, neck and upper extremities[14]. In lighter-skinned populations, the degree of UV exposure is related to SCC development. On the other hand, in darker-skinned populations, the pathogenesis of SCC may be unrelated to sun exposure, but rather may relate to chronic irritation or injury. SCC is found more frequently in men (3:1 male:female) and the incidence increases dramatically with age[12] (see Fig. 108.2).

The incidence of SCC has been rising worldwide in all age groups over the last several decades at an estimated 3–10% per year, with over

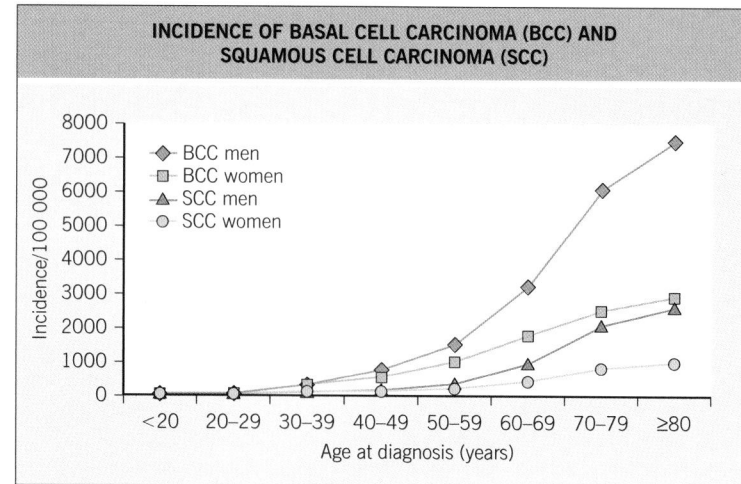

Fig. 108.2 Incidence of basal cell carcinoma (BCC) and squamous cell carcinoma (SCC) by age and gender.

250 000 cases of invasive SCC diagnosed annually in the US. Similar incidence trends have been noted worldwide.

Weinstock[15] reported an age-adjusted mortality rate for confirmed cases of SCC in Rhode Island of 0.26/100 000. SCC-associated mortality is higher in whites and older persons. Men have a 3:1 greater SCC mortality rate compared to women[15]. SCCs located on the ear, lip and genitalia appear to have a higher risk of death. While melanoma among whites is responsible for 90% of skin cancer deaths before 50 years of age, in adults over 85 years of age, the majority of skin cancer deaths are attributable to SCC[4].

BCC is the most common skin cancer in humans. Men generally have higher rates of BCC than do women (1.5–2:1)[16]. BCC occurs most frequently on the head and neck in both genders[12]. Women have a greater frequency of BCC on the lower extremities while men have more ear lesions. These trends may relate to fashion differences, including clothing and hairstyle. BCC is becoming increasingly more common on the trunk and limbs.

The incidence of BCC is increasing. Over the last 30 years, incidence rates are estimated to have risen between 20% and 80%. In the US, a disproportionate increase in young women has been observed. Similar increases in incidence rates have been noted worldwide, with the incidence doubling in Finland and Switzerland and increasing in Wales by 50% over the past two decades.

Incidence rates for BCC also increase with age and the median age at diagnosis is 68 years. In Queensland, Australia, age-adjusted incidence rates for BCC are 2074 and 1579 per 100 000 per year for men and women, respectively – the highest rates for any specific cancer ever reported. In this geographic location, SCC occurred at half the rate of BCC among men and at about one-third the rate among women.

Mortality from BCC is quite rare and can occur in immunocompromised patients. Cases of metastatic BCC are more likely from tumors with aggressive histologic patterns (morpheaform, infiltrating, metatypical, basosquamous). Perineural space invasion may be an indicator of aggressive disease. Metastases often involve regional lymph nodes, lungs, bone and skin[17]. The mean age at the time of death is higher than with SCC and the age-adjusted mortality rate for BCC has been estimated at 0.12 per 100 000. Mortality risk is related to increasing age, Caucasian race and male gender (>2× compared to women).

PATHOGENESIS

See Chapter 107.

RISK FACTORS (Table 108.3)

Exposure to Carcinogenic Agents

UV radiation

The vast majority of NMSCs are related to UV light exposure. For SCCs, the major pattern is chronic long-term exposure; however, for

BCCs, the pattern appears to be slightly different, with intermittent intense episodes of burning being more important. Sun exposure early in life appears to have a greater influence on subsequent skin cancer risk than at a later age. As is the case with melanoma, persons born in UV-intense environments such as Australia have an increased risk of developing skin cancer compared to those born in Northern Europe who then emigrated to such locales at age 10 years or older (Fig. 108.3).

Tanning lamp usage

Several studies have demonstrated an increased risk for the development of NMSC in those who are exposed to artificial sources of UV radiation. Intentional tanning has been shown to increase the risk of SCC development[18] and Karagas et al.[19] demonstrated that any use of tanning devices was associated with an odds ratios of 2.5 for SCC and 1.5 for BCC, even after adjustment for history of sunburns, sunbathing and sun exposure. In one study, women with BCCs had on average twice as many visits to tanning beds than did matched controls[20].

Therapeutic UV exposure

Persons with psoriasis have been shown to be at increased risk for the development of NMSC. While long-term follow-up of psoriasis patients who underwent UV and tar (Goekerman) therapy found no increase in NMSC risk, long-term PUVA therapy was associated with a significant, dose-related risk of SCC development (adjusted relative risk = 8.6 for an accumulated exposure of between 100 and 337 treatments)[21]. With prolonged therapy, a slightly increased risk for BCC development was noted as well. PUVA-induced immunosuppression may play a role.

Ionization radiation

Exposure to ionizing radiation leads to a threefold increased risk of NMSC[22]. The risk is in proportion to the radiation dose. Larger fractionated doses (>12–15 Gy) are thought to be necessary to induce tumor formation, so the risk with a given total dose may be less if a larger number of smaller fractionated doses are given. Most SCCs and BCCs that occur after exposure to ionizing radiation have a long latency period of up to several decades, with most cases occurring ~20 years after the initial exposure.

Treatment of tinea capitis with radiation (prior to the discovery of effective systemic anti-fungal medications) has been linked to the development of multiple BCCs. In a study of 2224 children given X-ray therapy for tinea capitis (compared to a control group of 1380 tinea capitis patients given only topical medications), the relative risk for developing BCC of the head and neck among irradiated Caucasians was 3.6[23]. BCCs have been observed in radiation fields following treatment of port-wine stains and Hodgkin disease as well as after accidental exposure[24].

Chemical exposures

Multiple organic chemicals have been associated with an increased risk for the development of NMSC (Table 108.4). Occupational chemical exposures which can lead to skin cancer most commonly involve pesticides, asphalt, tar and polycyclic aromatic hydrocarbons, and

RISK FACTORS FOR THE DEVELOPMENT OF BASAL CELL CARCINOMAS AND SQUAMOUS CELL CARCINOMAS		
	SCC	BCC
Environmental exposures		
Cumulative/occupational sun exposure	+	
Intermittent/recreational sun exposure		+
Other exposures to UV light (PUVA, tanning beds)	+	+
Ionizing radiation	+	+
Chemicals (arsenic)	+	(+)
Human papillomavirus	+	
Cigarette smoking	+	
Pigmentary phenotype		
Fair skin	+	+
Always burns, never tans	+	+
Freckling	+	+
Red hair	+	+
Genetic syndromes		
Xeroderma pigmentosum	+	+
Oculocutaneous albinism	+	(+)
Epidermodysplasia verruciformis	+	
Dystrophic epidermolysis bullosa (primarily recessive)	+	
Ferguson–Smith syndrome	+	
Muir–Torre syndrome	+*	(+)*
Nevoid basal cell carcinoma syndrome		+
Bazex and Rombo syndromes		+
Predisposing clinical settings		
Chronic non-healing wounds	+	
Longstanding discoid lupus erythematosus, lichen planus (erosive) or lichen sclerosus	+	
Porokeratosis (especially linear)	+	
Nevus sebaceus		+†
Immunosuppression		
Organ transplantation	+	(+)
Other (e.g. chronic lymphocytic leukemia treated with fludarabine, AIDS patients with HPV infection)	+	

*Both SCCs (keratoacanthoma type) and BCCs typically have sebaceous differentiation.
†More often trichoblastomas.

Table 108.3 Risk factors for the development of basal cell carcinomas (BCCs) and squamous cell carcinomas (SCCs). HPV, human papillomavirus.

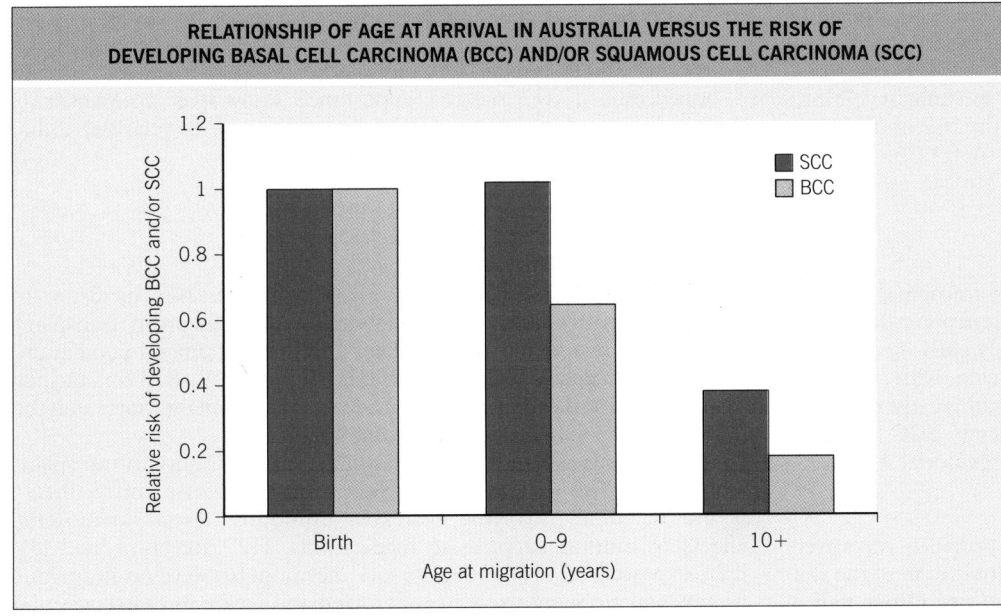

RELATIONSHIP OF AGE AT ARRIVAL IN AUSTRALIA VERSUS THE RISK OF DEVELOPING BASAL CELL CARCINOMA (BCC) AND/OR SQUAMOUS CELL CARCINOMA (SCC)

Fig. 108.3 Relationship of age at arrival in Australia versus the risk of developing basal cell carcinoma (BCC) and/or squamous cell carcinoma (SCC).

CHEMICALS ASSOCIATED WITH THE DEVELOPMENT OF NON-MELANOMA SKIN CANCER
Agent
Mineral oil
Coal tar
Soot
Polychlorinated biphenyls
Arsenic
4,4' bipyridyl
Psoralen (plus UVA)
Nitrogen mustard

Table 108.4 Chemicals associated with the development of non-melanoma skin cancer. Based on ref. 25.

typically result in SCC. NMSCs induced by chemical exposures are usually localized, most often on the arms, and usually multiple[26].

Arsenic is a well-defined cause of SCC (see Ch. 87). A clue to arsenic exposure is the presence of palmoplantar arsenical keratoses. The SCCs that arsenic induces are often multiple[27]. Increasing evidence indicates that arsenic acts as a tumor promoter by modulating the signaling pathways responsible for cell growth[28]. BCC has been reported with extensive arsenic exposure. The typical latency period from exposure to clinical appearance of NMSC is 20–40 years[29].

Occupational risk factors

Persons with outdoor occupations have a higher risk for developing NMSC. Airline pilots, who are exposed to ionizing radiation at flight attitudes, have been shown to have an elevated risk for both BCC and SCC[30]. Other occupations associated with an increased risk for NMSC include textile workers, sailors, locomotive engineers and agricultural workers.

Human papillomavirus infection

Human papillomavirus infection (HPV)(see Ch. 78), especially with oncogenic strains such as 16 or 18, is associated with SCC development. This is especially true in the anogenital and periungual regions, in the setting of HIV infection, and in the case of the verrucous carcinoma subtype of SCC. HPV also plays a role in SCC development in organ transplant recipients.

Other risk factors

Other possible risk factors include residence at high altitudes, dietary fat intake, tobacco abuse[31], thermal burns and chronic ulcers.

Genetic Syndromes Associated with Increased NMSC Risk

Xeroderma pigmentosum

Xeroderma pigmentosum (XP) consists of a group of autosomal recessive disorders characterized by defects in unscheduled DNA repair (see Ch. 85). NMSC and melanoma occur with a markedly increased frequency in these individuals if they are exposed to sunlight. NMSCs appear at an early age (median age, 8 years) and the risk of NMSC in affected individuals who are <20 years of age is 4800 times that of the general population. Strict UV avoidance for life can significantly decrease NMSC formation.

Oculocutaneous albinism

Oculocutaneous albinism is comprised of a group of autosomal recessive disorders in which there is a variable degree of pigmentary dilution of the skin, eyes and hair (see Ch. 65). At a relatively early age, NMSC, especially SCC, and cutaneous melanoma develop with increased frequency. As in XP, strict sun avoidance for life can greatly minimize tumor development. However, metastatic cutaneous SCC is still a significant problem in areas of the world such as equatorial Africa.

Epidermodysplasia verruciformis

Epidermodysplasia verruciformis (EDV) is a rare, primarily recessively inherited disorder in which there is widespread colonization of the skin by HPVs of multiple subtypes (see Ch. 78). One-third to one-half of

patients will develop SCCs as adults, usually in sun-exposed regions, and several decades earlier than is typical of SCC development in the general population. Aggressive biologic behavior, including perineural spread, metastases and death, have been reported. HPV subtypes most frequently identified in the SCCs that arise in EDV patients are 5, 8 and 47.

Dystrophic epidermolysis bullosa

Dystrophic epidermolysis bullosa associated with significant scarring can result from both dominant and recessive mutations in the type VII collagen gene. SCCs more commonly appear in the recessive forms, where it is the most common cause of death. Tumors usually develop during the third to fifth decades of life, are frequently multiple, and show aggressive behavior in terms of recurrences and metastases. Whether this aggressive biologic behavior is due to tumor development within scars and chronic non-healing wounds, to specific mutations in the type VII collagen gene, or to elevated levels of basic fibroblast growth factor is uncertain.

Nevoid basal cell carcinoma syndrome

Nevoid basal cell carcinoma syndrome is a rare, autosomal dominant disorder, in which the underlying genetic defect is a mutation in the human *PTCH* gene[32]. Major manifestations (occurring in more than half of all patients) include multiple BCCs, palmar and plantar pits, odontogenic keratocysts of the jaws, skeletal abnormalities, and calcification of the falx cerebri (see Table 71.1). BCCs can number from a few to thousands, making treatment decisions difficult. Tumor development appears to be related to sun exposure, as BCCs develop most frequently in sun-exposed sites and are rare in darkly pigmented individuals. The clinical course of the lesions (which often have the appearance of melanocytic nevi or acrochordons) is usually indolent prior to puberty. Thereafter, individual lesions enlarge and ulcerate, like typical BCCs in the general population. Individuals with nevoid basal cell carcinoma syndrome are exquisitely sensitive to ionizing radiation. Hundreds of tumors have developed in children within radiation ports following treatment for medulloblastoma. Tumor development begins several years after the radiation therapy, and the BCCs that develop can grow aggressively, even in the prepubertal period.

Bazex syndrome and Rombo syndrome

Bazex syndrome is a rare condition, consisting of follicular atrophoderma (usually occurring as circumscribed areas on the dorsal aspect of the hands and feet), hypotrichosis, localized hypohidrosis, milia, epidermoid cysts, and multiple, primarily facial, BCCs. Genetic transmission in most families appears to occur in an X-linked dominant fashion. Sometimes leading to confusion, there is a completely different Bazex syndrome (acrokeratosis paraneoplastica), in which psoriasiform plaques of the fingers, toes, ears and nose are often associated with SCC of the upper aerodigestive tract. In the follicular atrophoderma form of Bazex syndrome, BCCs develop in the second decade of life and frequently have a trichoepithelioma-like histologic appearance.

The so-called Rombo syndrome has many of the features of Bazex syndrome. Keratosis pilaris-like lesions of the cheeks can give rise to a honeycombed, worm-eaten appearance known as atrophoderma vermiculatum. Patients often have hypotrichosis, blepharitis, milia, peripheral vasodilation with cyanosis, and BCCs.

Immunosuppression
Organ transplantation

Organ transplant recipients have a markedly increased incidence of NMSC, primarily SCC. The incidence of BCC in organ transplant recipients is five to ten times greater than in the general population, while the incidence of SCC is 40–250 times greater. Risk factors include skin type, cumulative sun exposure, age at transplantation, and the degree and the length of immunosuppression.

SCC is a significant cause of morbidity and mortality in transplant recipients[33]. The pathogenesis of skin cancer in transplant recipients is multifactorial, involving decreased immunity, direct carcinogenic effects of immunosuppressive medications, HPV infection, and UV light exposure. Transplant recipients are prone to develop numerous lesions and are more likely to suffer local and regional recurrences and

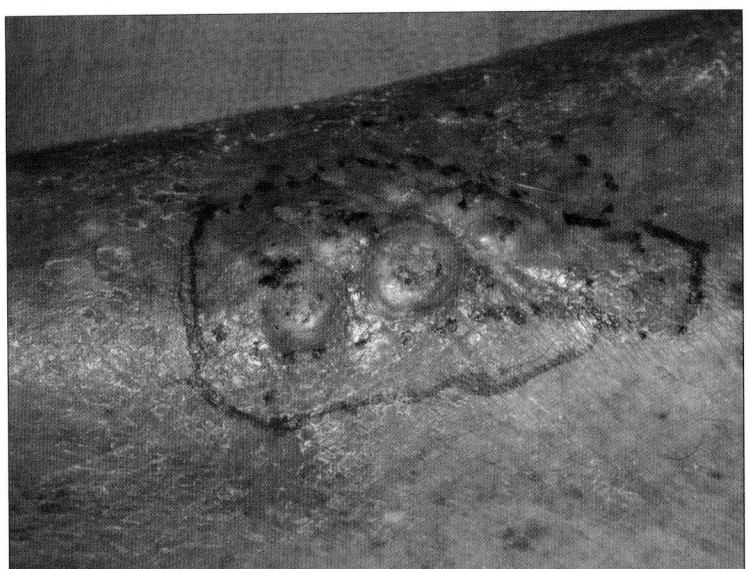

Fig. 108.4 Recurrent squamous cell carcinoma in a patient who had received a solid-organ transplant.

metastases[33] (Fig.108.4). AKs and SCCs begin to appear with increasing frequency several years after transplantation. Lesions are often multiple, and usually develop in sun-exposed areas. HPV DNA is found in approximately 70–90% of transplant-associated SCCs. Tumors from transplant recipients contain HPV strains that occur in common benign cutaneous warts (HPV types 1 and 2), epidermodysplasia verruciformis (HPV 5 and others), high-risk oncogenic warts (HPV types 16 and 18) and low-risk oncogenic genital warts (HPV types 6 and 11). Sometimes, several HPV types are detected within a single tumor.

In one series of renal transplant patients from the US, 5% of the patients died of skin cancer. In another series of heart transplant patients from Australia, 27% died of skin cancer. Two-thirds of these deaths are due to SCC. Patients who receive hematopoietic transplants do not experience this marked increase in skin cancer incidence, presumably because of a shorter duration of immunosuppression.

HIV infection

Patients with HIV infection are at increased risk for the development of several cancers, including cutaneous SCC[34]. The incidence of HPV-related SCC of the anus is significantly increased in this population. Serial examinations and anal cytologies are recommended for surveillance. The biologic behavior of these SCCs can be aggressive.

Immunosuppressive drugs

Use of immunosuppressive drugs, other than for organ transplantation as discussed previously, also increases the risk for the development of NMSC (particularly SCC). Risk of SCC development is directly related to length of immunosuppressive drug usage. In one study, the risk of SCC was significantly increased among recipients of oral glucocorticoids (odds ratio = 2.31) and the risk of BCC was also elevated (odds ratio = 1.49)[35].

Risk of additional cancers

Persons with an initial BCC and SCC are at increased risk for the development of additional BCCs and SCCs, compared to the general population. NMSC patients are also at increased risk for developing melanoma[36]. In addition, persons with a history of NMSC are at increased risk for developing and dying from other (non-skin) cancers[37].

ACTINIC KERATOSIS AND SQUAMOUS CELL CARCINOMA

Clinical Features

Actinic keratosis

AKs were initially described as solar keratoses (due to their suspected cause) and senile keratoses (due to the age of onset). The term 'actinic keratosis' is relatively recent. The term actinic keratosis is preferred over solar keratosis, partly because the abbreviation SK also stands for seborrheic keratosis.

AKs have historically been characterized as being 'precancerous' or 'premalignant' because the atypical keratinocytes within these lesions are confined to the epidermis. There is no risk of metastasis until these lesions evolve into invasive carcinoma. An alternative minority view is that it is not accurate to deem them 'premalignant' because they are malignant in the same sense as Bowen's disease (SCC *in situ*) or intra-epithelial melanoma (melanoma *in situ*). The likelihood of an invasive SCC evolving from a given AK has been estimated to occur at a rate of 0.075–0.096% per lesion per year. Thus, for a person with 7.7 AKs, the average number present on the skin of an affected individual, SCC would develop at a rate of 10.2% over 10 years. Other estimates are even higher, with rates of 13–20% over a 10-year period (if the lesions were left untreated). These rates are similar to those that have been determined for intraepithelial neoplasia of other sites. In the uterine cervix, approximately 15% of all untreated low and moderate grade cervical intraepithelial neoplasia lesions (CIN I and II) will progress to carcinoma *in situ* (CIN III) and to more advanced carcinoma involving deeper tissues if left untreated. This process generally occurs over 10 to 20 years, although in some patients this interval may be as short as 6 months. Because of this continuum of progression of AKs in the skin, the analogous term keratinocytic intraepithelial neoplasia (KIN I, II and III) has been proposed, but has not gained widespread use.

AKs are some of the most frequently encountered lesions in clinical practice. They present on sun-damaged skin of the head, neck, upper trunk and extremities (Fig. 108.5). Individuals most at risk include the elderly, those with lighter skin types and those with a history of chronic sun exposure. The primary lesion is a rough erythematous papule with white to yellow scale. Patients may report tenderness. AKs may range in size from a few millimeters to large confluent patches several centimeters in diameter, especially in heavily sun-exposed individuals. One of the earliest signs is slight erythema with almost imperceptible scale, although some lesions are devoid of visible erythema and present only as slight scale with indistinct borders. A clue to their presence is background solar damage, i.e. dyspigmentation, telangiectasia and wrinkling. Advanced lesions are typically thicker and well defined with more visible hyperkeratosis and erythema. Lesions typically are clustered in areas of highest sun exposure, such as the tops of the ears, upper forehead, nasal bridge, malar eminences, dorsal hands, extensor forearms, and scalp in bald individuals.

Any region of the body can be affected if enough actinic damage has occurred. Visual inspection is best performed with simultaneous palpation to detect lesions that may not be readily apparent. This is especially true in individuals with heavy background erythema from chronic sun exposure or rosacea. Tenderness on palpation should alert the clinician to the possibility that the lesion has evolved into carcinoma. Clinical subtypes of AKs include the classic variant already described, hyperplastic (or hyperkeratotic), pigmented, lichenoid, atrophic, bowenoid, 'cutaneous horn' and actinic cheilitis.

Hyperkeratotic AKs are easily identified on visual inspection as papules and plaques with scale or scale-crust and an erythematous base (Fig. 108.5D). The erythematous base often extends beyond the overlying hyperkeratosis. The hyperkeratotic scale can become white or yellow–brown over time. Patients often find these lesions annoying due to their thickness. Sometimes, distinction from SCC can be difficult and biopsy is warranted. Occasionally, hyperkeratotic AKs may develop cutaneous horns which manifest as columns of thick cornified material that protrude above the skin. These should be biopsied to exclude the possibility of underlying malignancy, as approximately 15% of cutaneous horns have invasive SCC at their bases[38].

Pigmented AKs, sometimes called superficial pigmented AKs (SPAK), is a subtype that often lacks associated erythema and has a hyper-pigmented or reticulated appearance. These lesions can at times be difficult to distinguish from reticulated seborrheic keratoses, lentigines, or even the lentigo maligna subtype of melanoma. Dermoscopy may be a useful adjunct in these situations. Clinical clues are the location on sun-exposed skin, background solar changes, and hyperkeratosis that is sometimes appreciable by palpation. In cases in which the diagnosis is questionable, a biopsy is required to exclude the possibility of melanoma.

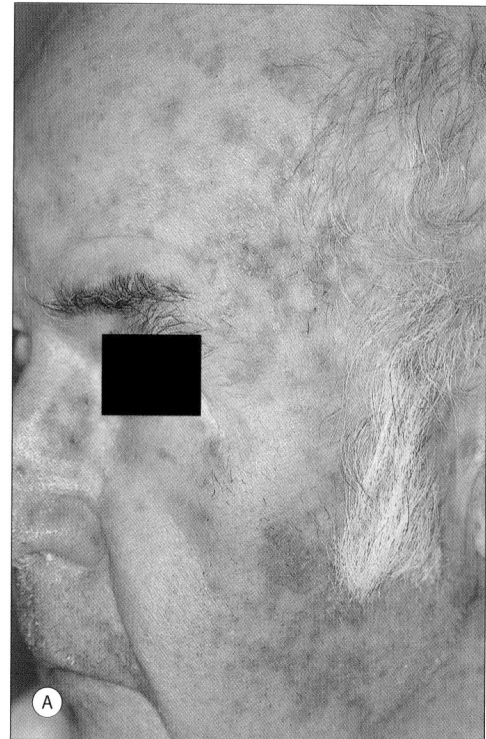
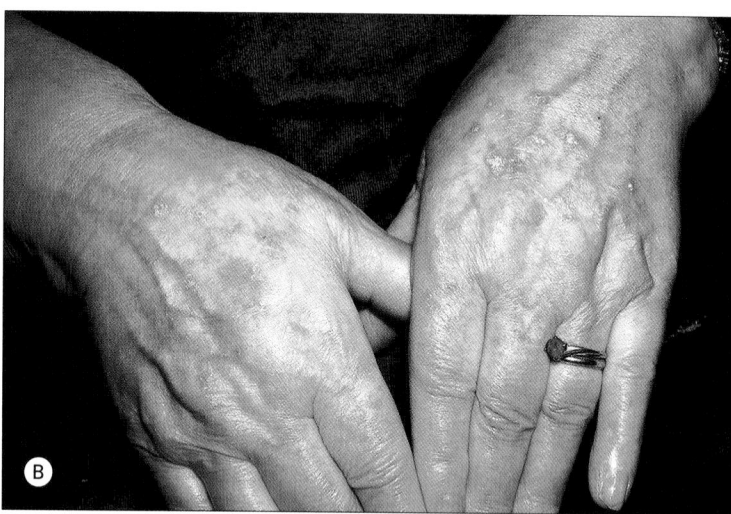
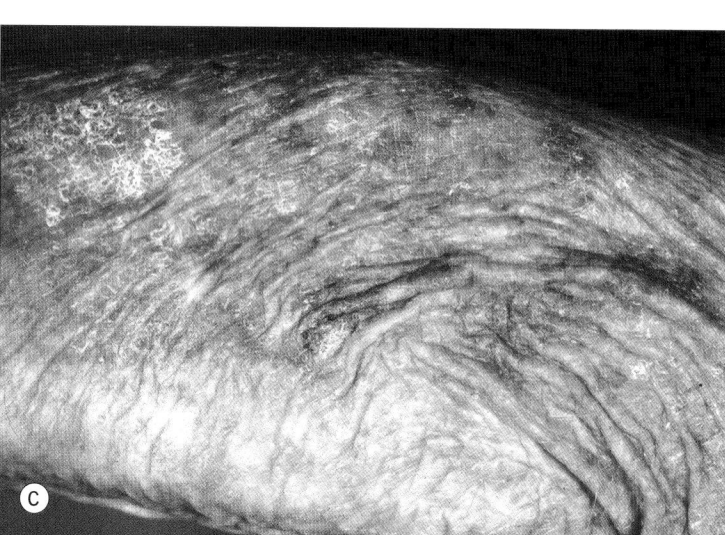
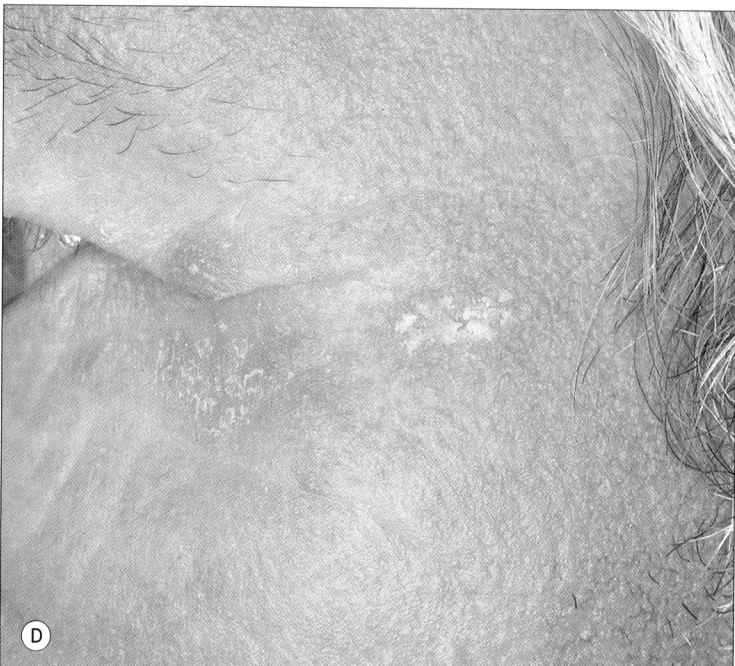

Fig. 108.5 Actinic keratoses. A Multiple actinic keratoses (AKs) on the face, varying in size from a few millimeters to over a centimeter, which have become inflamed following application of 5-fluorouracil. **B** AKs on the dorsal hands. **C** AKs on the forearm; note the severe background photodamage. **D** Two facial AKs, one of which is hypertrophic with thick scale overlying an erythematous base. Bowen's disease was excluded in the larger lesion via histologic examination. A, Courtesy of Kalman Watsky MD. B, Courtesy of Stanely Miller MD.

Lichenoid AK is characterized histologically by the presence of a dense band-like inflammatory infiltrate. Clinically, this lesion is similar to the classic form of AK but has more erythema surrounding the base of the lesion. Patients may relate pruritus or tenderness that coincides with the onset of the lichenoid infiltrate in a pre-existing AK.

Atrophic AKs usually have minimal surface change but are appreciated as erythematous, slightly scaling patches that are found on histologic examination to have an atrophic epidermis.

Actinic cheilitis is the term used to describe the characteristic changes that occur on the lower lip of heavily sun-exposed individuals. Actinic cheilitis may resemble the classic form of AK, with well-demarcated erythematous scaling papules and patches, or have a more diffuse erythema and scale that encompasses the entire lower lip. These lesions may present as leukoplakia and should be biopsied to exclude the possibility of SCC when clinical distinction is not possible.

Squamous cell carcinoma *in situ*

SCC *in situ* is commonly called Bowen's disease. The most common presentation of SCC *in situ* is an erythematous scaling patch or slightly elevated plaque (Fig. 108.6B, Fig. 108.7) that arises on sun-exposed skin of an elderly individual (Fig 108.6A). Lesions may be crusted. Bowen's

disease may arise *de novo* or from a pre-existing AK. The head and neck, followed by the extremities and trunk, are the most common sites.

Clinical distinction of SCC *in situ* from AK, superficial BCC, psoriasis and nummular eczema may at times be difficult. Generally, AKs are smaller lesions. Superficial BCCs often have a more translucent quality and slight elevation to the leading edge. Patients with psoriasis and diffuse actinic damage can pose a real diagnostic dilemma, as concomitant psoriatic papules and plaques may clinically resemble AKs and Bowen's disease.

Arsenic-induced SCC *in situ* resembles the classic variety clinically but has a marked tendency to be multifocal and arise on non-sun-exposed areas of the trunk. Associated findings include palmoplantar keratoses and guttate hypopigmentation superimposed on hyperpigmentation (see Ch. 87).

Bowenoid papulosis is a term used when histologic changes of SCC *in situ* are found within genital warts, usually due to infection with an oncogenic strain such as HPV-16 or -18. Dermatologists often prefer to use this term when multiple papules are present, as opposed to calling all of them SCC *in situ*, because the lesions behave like typical condyloma acuminata, rarely becoming invasive. Clinically, they appear similar to venereal warts, but are more likely to be pigmented. The

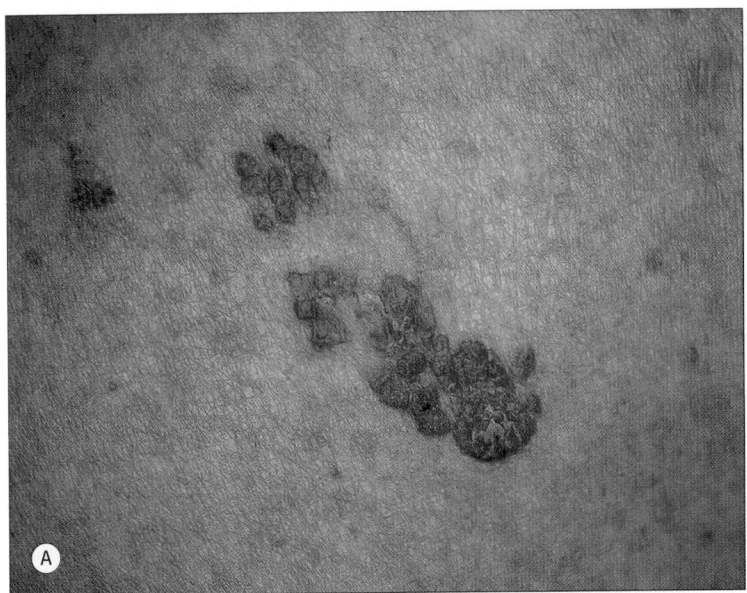

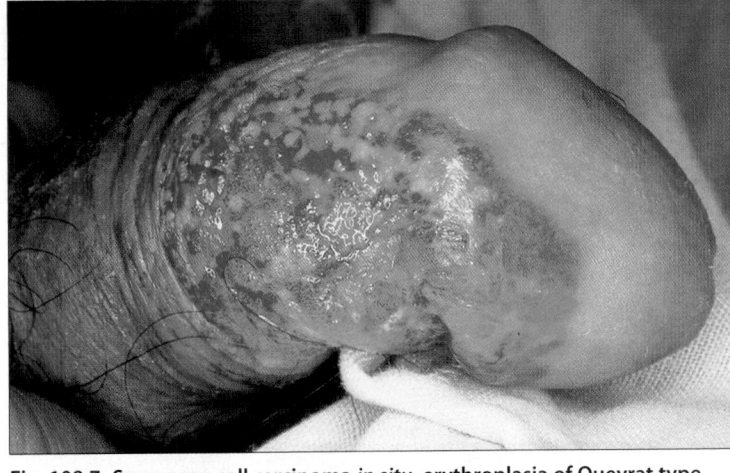

Fig. 108.7 Squamous cell carcinoma *in situ*, erythroplasia of Queyrat type. Large, eroded erythematous plaque with well-demarcated borders. The lesion began on the shaft of the penis.

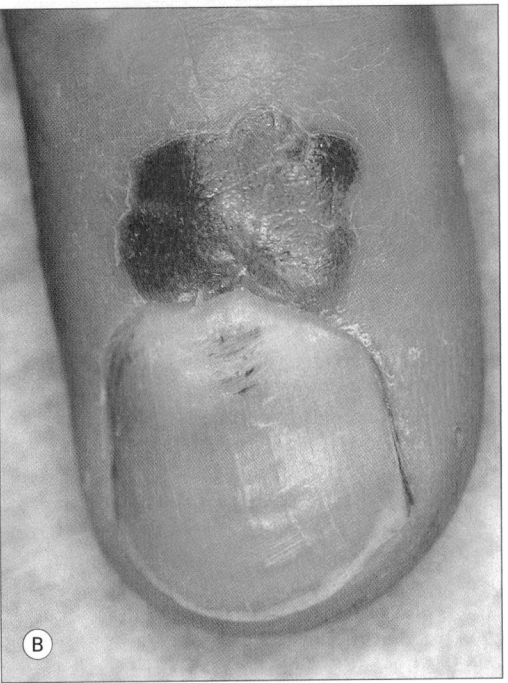

Fig. 108.6 Squamous cell carcinoma *in situ*, Bowen's type. A Scaly red plaque on the chest with skip areas. **B** Bright-red, well-demarcated plaque on the proximal nail fold with associated nail dystrophy. The latter may be associated with oncogenic strains of HPV.

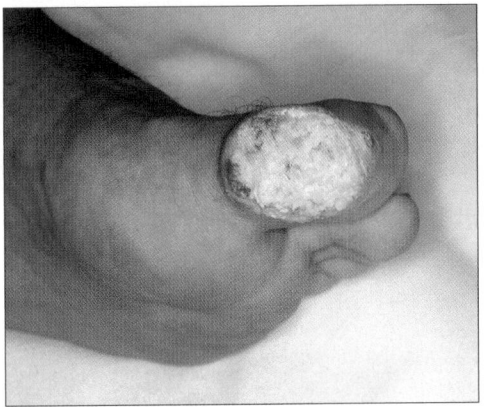

Fig. 108.8 Verrucous carcinoma. Large keratotic and ulcerated plaque on the great toe. The lesion was originally diagnosed as a plantar wart.

Lesions arising in scars and sites of inflammation are perhaps the most prone to metastasize[39].

SCC may resemble BCC, atypical fibroxanthoma, neuroendocrine carcinoma, amelanotic melanoma, adnexal tumors, prurigo nodularis, verruca and irritated seborrheic keratosis.

Keratoacanthoma

Keratoacanthomas (KAs) are usually considered to be a variant of SCC, but sometimes are considered to be benign, especially when lesions spontaneously regress or occur as multiple lesions in one of the syndromes cited below (Fig. 108.11)[40]. Typically, a rapidly enlarging papule evolves into a sharply circumscribed crateriform nodule with a keratotic core over a period of a few weeks and then may resolve slowly over months to leave an atrophic scar[40]. Most lesions occur on the head or sun-exposed areas of the extremities, with or without symptoms of pain or tenderness.

There are several distinct clinical presentations of KA, including solitary, multiple, grouped, giant, subungual, intraoral, multiple spontaneously regressing (Ferguson–Smith), multiple non-regressing, generalized eruptive (Grzybowski), keratoacanthoma centrifugum marginatum, KAs associated with Muir–Torre syndrome (sebaceous neoplasms and gastrointestinal carcinoma), and KAs associated with chemical exposure, immunosuppression[29] and HPV infection[41]. KAs have been noted in increased number in individuals exposed to tar-containing products.

By far the most common presentation is the solitary KA. While most of these tumors are small (5 to 15 mm), some KAs (e.g. keratoacanthoma centrifugum marginatum; see Fig. 108.11D) may reach several centimeters in diameter, persist for months before resolution, and heal with prominent scarring. Grouped KAs may show a greater tendency for slow resolution, while subungual KAs have been associated with underlying bony destruction.

The Ferguson–Smith syndrome is an autosomal dominant condition. Multiple KAs develop in sun-exposed regions, usually beginning in the

term is not favored by some other specialists, such as gynecologists. Whether this entity represents true SCC *in situ*, or is a histologic stimulant, is a matter of debate.

Other variants of SCC *in situ* include a pigmented variant often found on individuals with darker skin types and a verrucous form. Pigmented SCC *in situ* may be mistaken for a melanocytic lesion and verrucous SCC *in situ* may simulate a verruca clinically.

Invasive squamous cell carcinoma

The common clinical presentation of invasive SCC is an erythematous keratotic papule or nodule that arises within a background of sun-damaged skin. There is often a history of tenderness as the lesion slowly or rapidly enlarges to become more nodular. The degree of hyperkeratosis is variable, but, in general, is more pronounced than that seen in AK or in SCC *in situ*. Some lesions become so hyperkeratotic that clinical distinction from hypertrophic AK or verruca is impossible (Fig. 108.8). Lesions may ulcerate. Tumors may have an exophytic and an endophytic (invasive) component (Fig. 108.9).

Sites of chronic trauma, scars (Marjolin's ulcer), inflammation, radiation or chemical exposure have also been known to develop SCC. The metastatic potential of individual SCCs tends to be relatively low, especially in the solar-induced forms, although high-risk sites for metastasis include the lip and ear (Fig. 108.10). The incidence of metastasis also increases with size and with immunosuppression.

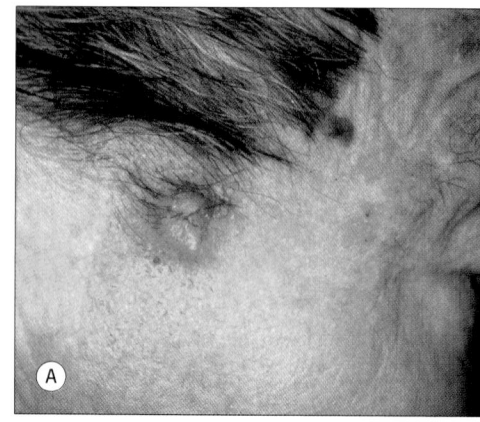
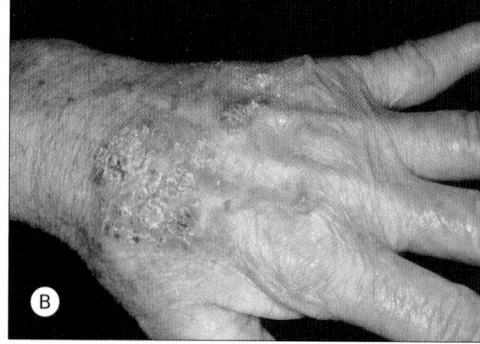
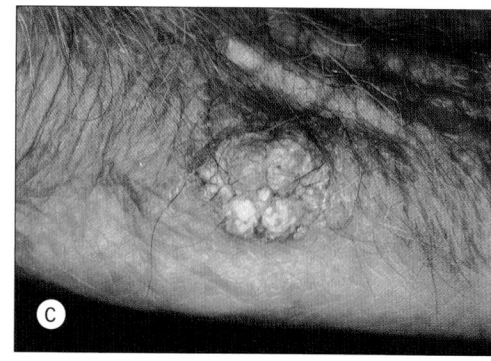
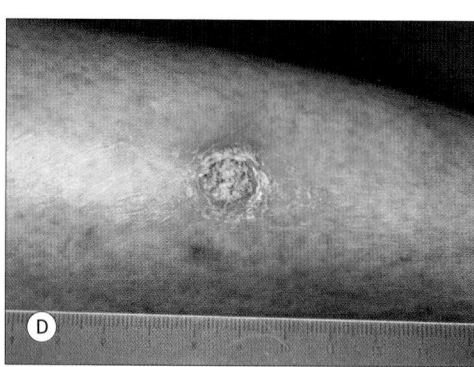
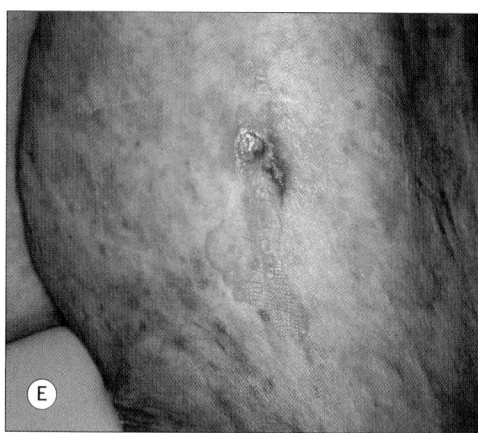

Fig. 108.9 Squamous cell carcinomas (SCCs).
A Smooth-surfaced erythematous nodule in the preauricular area. **B** Large scaly plaque developing in a background of photodamage and actinic keratoses on the dorsal hand. **C** Hyperkeratotic nodule on the dorsolateral hand. **D** Eroded and keratotic nodule that developed rapidly at a site of trauma on the leg. **E** Pink verrucous plaque arising within a burn scar. D, Courtesy of Jean L Bolognia MD.

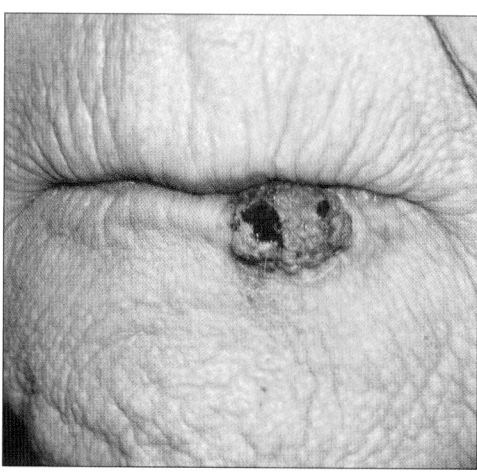

Fig. 108.10 Squamous cell carcinoma (SCC) of the lower lip. The patient subsequently died from metastatic SCC. Note the severe solar elastosis.

third decade of life. Lesions typically regress over weeks to months, but rare examples of metastases have been reported.

Multiple KAs of the Grzybowski type present as thousands of papules resembling milia which develop rapidly and may slowly resolve over a period of months[40]. Patients often have scarring, ectropion and a mask-like facies.

Pathology

Actinic keratosis

Several histologic variants have been described, including pigmented, acantholytic, atrophic, bowenoid, lichenoid, hypertrophic and actinic cheilitis types. All are characterized by atypical keratinocytic proliferation confined to the epidermis (Fig. 108.12).

Microscopic changes consist of partial-thickness atypical keratinocytes displaying nuclear pleomorphism, and disordered maturation from a small basal keratinocyte to progressively flattening squame at upper epidermal levels. The lesion may be acanthotic, often with increased numbers of buds protruding into the papillary dermis, or atrophic with loss of rete ridges. The basal layer often appears more basophilic than normal, a consequence of crowding of atypical keratinocytes. Hyperkeratosis and parakeratosis are seen. Acrosyringia and acrotrichia are often uninvolved with atypical keratinocytes, resulting in orthokeratosis at the ostia of these structures. This produces a characteristic pattern of alternating ortho- and parakeratosis, often referred to as the 'flag' sign, since the stratum corneum can also alternate between a more eosinophilic and basophilic hue. AKs are almost always associated with solar elastosis in the dermis. Merkel cell hyperplasia may accompany these changes.

The keratinocytic atypia of an AK is confined to a partial-thickness of the epidermis, as opposed to full-thickness atypia in SCC *in situ*. Diagnostic difficulty arises when the presence of small foci of full-thickness atypia occur in a lesion with otherwise characteristic features of AK. Some pathologists may use the term 'bowenoid AK' in this setting. In a follicular AK (proliferative AK), the atypical keratinocytes can extend down an adnexal structure, but this is more commonly seen in SCC *in situ*. In hyperkeratotic AKs, marked hyperkeratosis with associated parakeratosis is evident. If pronounced, this can lead to cutaneous horn formation. Pigmented AKs additionally show basilar pigmentation in a pattern similar to a solar lentigo. Lichenoid lesions demonstrate a marked band of lymphocytes in the papillary dermis at the dermal–epidermal junction. Actinic cheilitis is present on paramucosal skin, usually the lower lip, and may or may not show accompanying inflammation.

Squamous cell carcinoma in situ

SCC *in situ* (Bowen's disease), by definition, demonstrates full-thickness atypia of epidermal keratinocytes over a broad zone (Fig. 108.13). Nuclear pleomorphism and apoptosis are often more florid than in AK and mitoses are frequent. The epidermis may become atrophic or hyperplastic, and a horn may develop. The neoplasm more commonly extends down the adnexa than in AK. Diffuse confluent parakeratosis is more often observed than the focal parakeratosis more commonly seen in AK.

A number of different histologic variants have been described. The 'pagetoid' variant demonstrates large keratinocytes with abundant pale-staining cytoplasm scattered throughout the epidermis, simulating melanoma *in situ* or Paget's disease (see Fig. 72.16). Immunohistochemistry may be necessary to make a distinction, although the location of the lesion on sun-damaged skin (as opposed to Paget's disease), the presence of desmosomal spines, and the presence of many apoptotic cells can be helpful. Another subtype is the pigmented variant, in which there is abundant melanin in the epidermis.

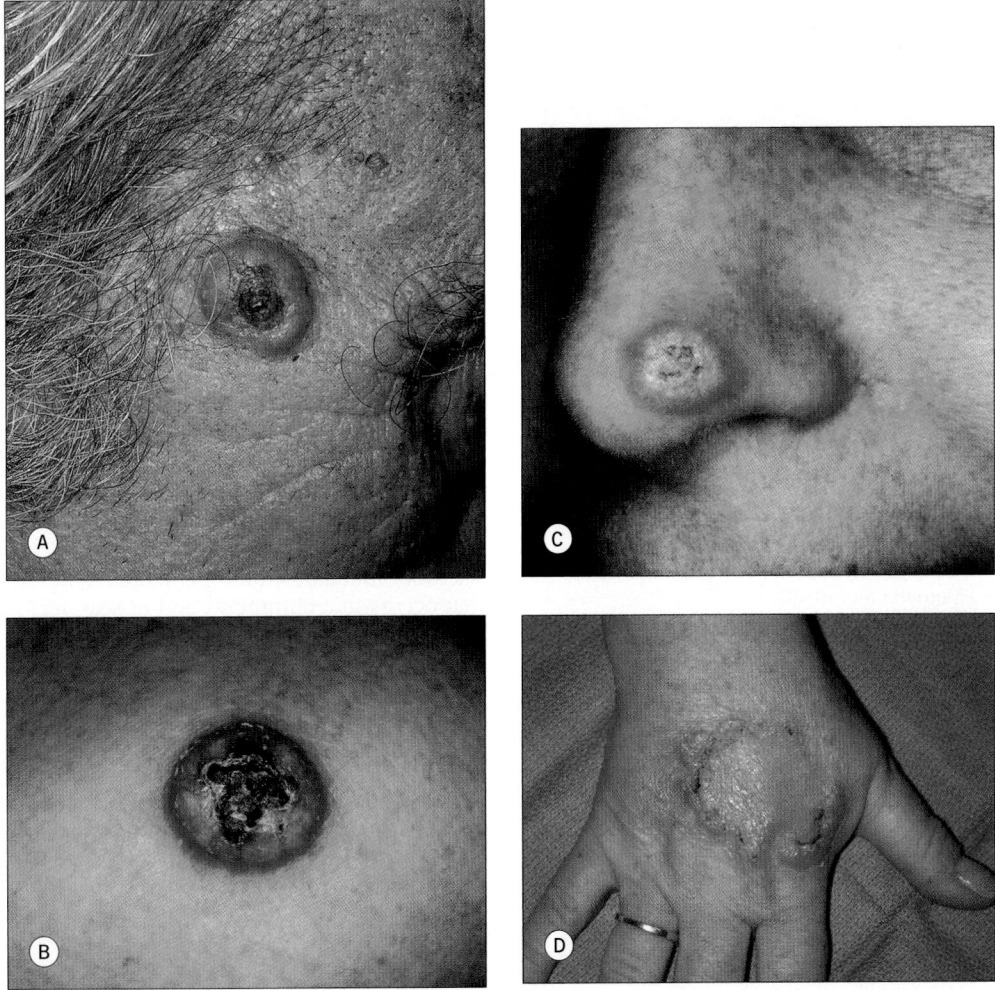

Fig. 108.11 Keratocanthomas. A, B Erythematous crateriform nodules with a rolled border and central keratotic core. The lesions arise rapidly and may be tender. Note the yellow color representing neutrophils in B. **C** A well-developed keratotic core may not be present in longer-standing lesions. **D** Progressive peripheral expansion and central involution leaving atrophy characterize keratoacanthoma centrifugum marginatum.

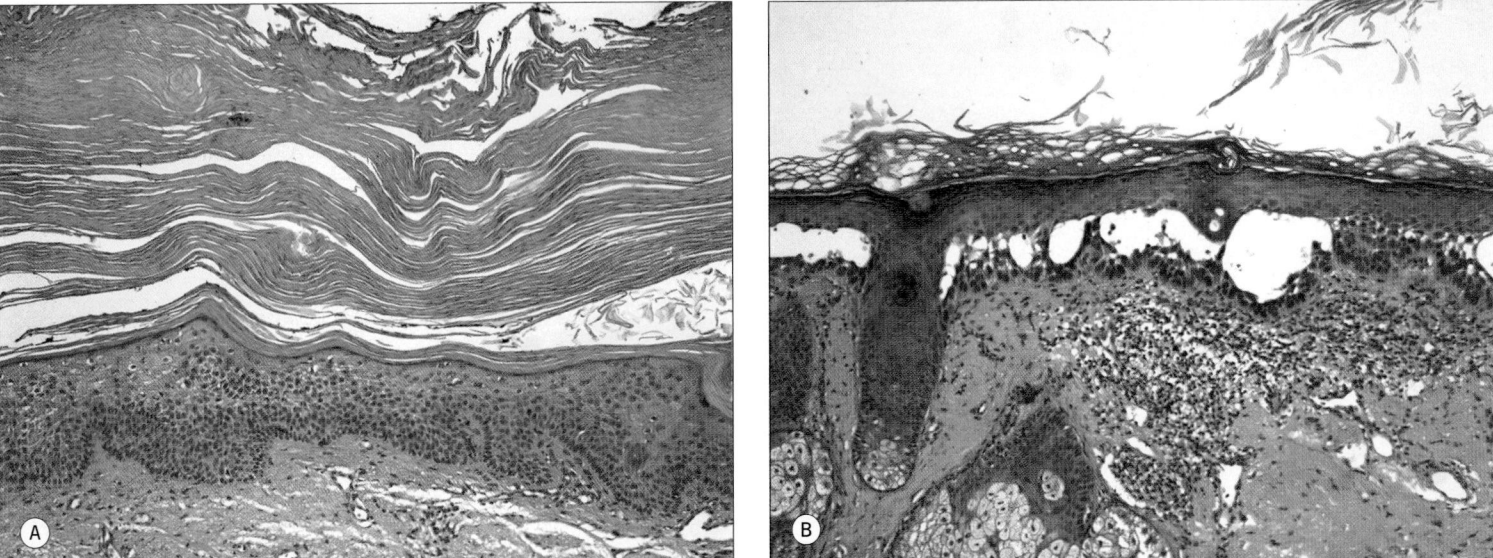

Fig. 108.12 Actinic keratoses. A hypertrophic variant with marked hyperkeratosis (**A**) and an acantholytic variant (**B**). Note the solar elastosis in the dermis. Courtesy of Thomas D Horn MD.

Invasive squamous cell carcinoma

Well-differentiated SCC generally arises in the setting of epidermal changes consistent with AK. There is a downward proliferation of lobules and detached islands of glassy, brightly eosinophilic keratinocytes containing nuclei with some degree of pleomorphism and mitosis (Fig. 108.14A). Nucleoli may be prominent. Intercellular bridges (desmosomes) are often apparent, along with keratin pearls and apoptotic cells. The degrees of nuclear atypia and cellular differentiation vary within and among tumors (Fig. 108.14B). The pink quality of the cytoplasm arises from abundant high-molecular-weight keratin.

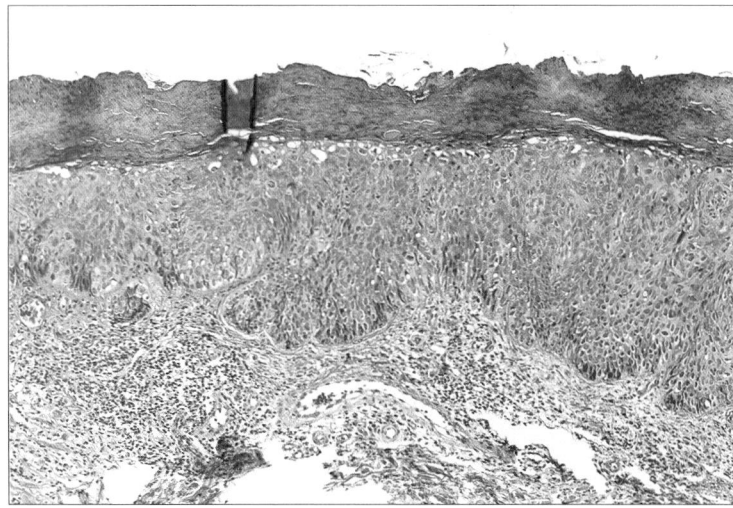

Fig. 108.13 Histology of Bowen's disease (squamous cell carcinoma *in situ*). Keratinocytic atypia of the entire epidermal thickness is seen with significant pleomorphism and crowding of cells, as well as scattered mitotic figures at suprabasal levels. Courtesy of J Margaret Moresi MD.

Invasion is seen as detached tumor islands lying free within the dermis at varying levels. A polymorphous inflammatory infiltrate may be present.

Less commonly, invasive SCC arises from SCC *in situ*. In this instance, detached islands of tumor in the dermis have a strikingly similar appearance to the cells comprising the full-thickness epidermal atypia.

Poorly differentiated SCCs display progressive and overlapping features ending in highly infiltrative spindle cell tumors lacking overt keratinization (Fig. 108.14C). Perineural infiltration and sclerotic stromal change become more common in these forms. Poorly differentiated tumors (cytokeratin-positive) generally require immunohistochemistry to distinguish them from spindled melanoma (generally S100-positive), atypical fibroxanthoma (CD68-positive) and leiomyosarcoma (smooth muscle actin-positive).

There are several variants of SCC. The acantholytic SCC (Fig. 108.14D) possibly has a worse prognosis. A similar variant is the adenoid (pseudoglandular) SCC, in which pseudoglandular spaces are sometimes related to acantholysis as opposed to true duct formation. Other variants include bowenoid, SCC with overlying cutaneous horn, sclerotic, mucinous, and pigmented SCC. Marjolin's ulcer is an SCC that occurs in a chronic wound or scar, including from a burn. Neurotropic SCCs behave in a more aggressive manner, with local recurrence rates approaching 50%[39].

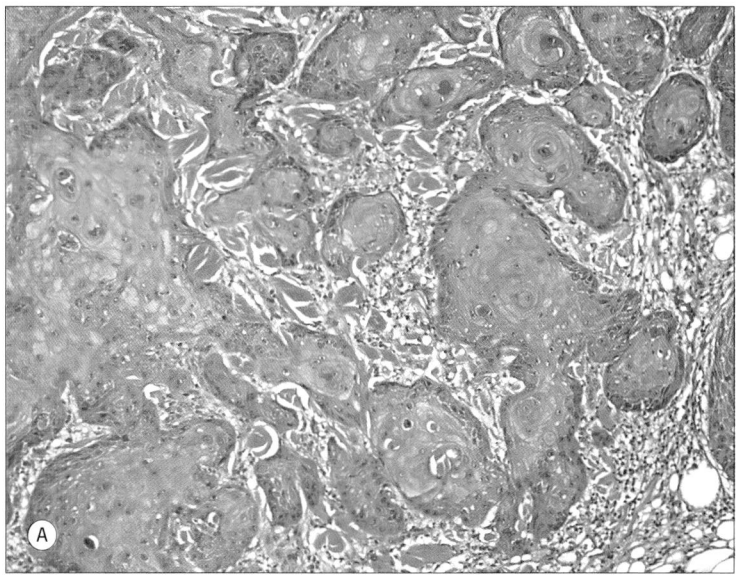

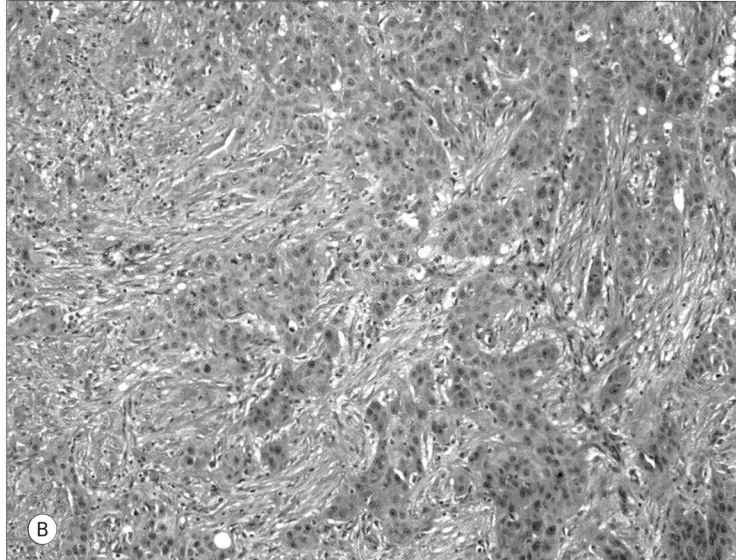

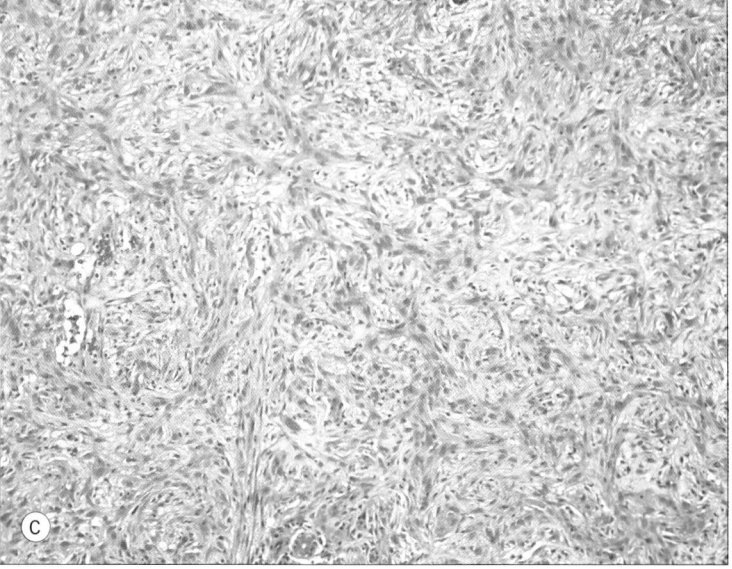

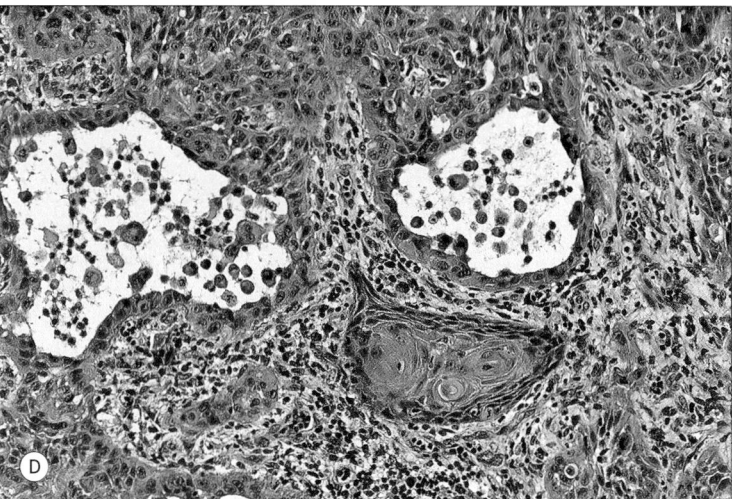

Fig. 108.14 Squamous cell carcinoma: range of histologic findings. Well-differentiated with abundant eosinophilic keratinization (**A**); moderately differentiated with more nuclear atypia and less eosinophilic keratinization (**B**); poorly differentiated with prominent nuclear atypia and the least keratinization (**C**); and acantholytic with acantholysis within invasive islands (**D**). A–C, Courtesy of Tom Horn MD; D, Courtesy of Ronald P Rapini MD.

Verrucous carcinoma

Verrucous carcinoma is defined as a massive well-differentiated variant of carcinoma in which the proliferating tumor is large, pale, glassy and well differentiated. However, this term is not correctly used for any SCC that has a warty appearance. Cytologic atypia is minimal, and the tumors have a pushing border as opposed to an infiltrating invasive edge. They can be associated with HPV infection, and a distinction between a verrucous carcinoma and a large wart can be difficult. The difference mainly depends upon the massiveness and depth of the lesion. Verrucous carcinoma is usually locally destructive but typically does not metastasize. Three subtypes have been described. Epithelioma cuniculatum appears on the soles, arising from a plantar wart (see Fig. 108.8). Cuniculatum refers to a rabbit burrow appearance, since crevices appear in these lesions. Giant condyloma of the genitals is known as a Buschke–Lowenstein tumor. Oral florid papillomatosis is the form of verrucous carcinoma found in the mouth. Some authorities consider subungual keratoacanthoma to be a fourth type of verrucous carcinoma (other KAs share the tendency to have pale glassy epithelial proliferation, but typically have a cornified plug in the center).

Keratoacanthoma

A KA typically has a volcano architecture. The tumor is comprised of well-differentiated keratinocytes with a brightly eosinophilic glassy cytoplasm surrounding a core filled with cornified material (Fig. 108.15). An inflammatory infiltrate of lymphocytes, and often eosinophils, is usually present. Small intratumoral abscesses of neutrophils are common. Elastic fibers are often seen within the epithelium at the base of the lesion. As the lesion regresses, the dome-shaped architecture flattens and fibrosis develops at the base of the lesion. Cytologic atypia is minimal in a KA. If hyperchromatic nuclei or abnormal mitoses are prominent, then the diagnosis of an ordinary invasive SCC is made instead.

Histologic simulators of SCC

There are a number of histologic simulators of SCC, including irritated seborrheic keratosis, verruca vulgaris, warty dyskeratoma, inverted follicular keratosis, prurigo nodularis, hypertrophic lichen planus, hypertrophic lupus erythematosus, atypical mycobacterial or 'deep' fungal infections, granular cell tumor, and pseudocarcinomatous hyperplasia of a healing wound. Architectural pattern and recognition of cellular and nuclear features of malignancy are critical in establishing a diagnosis. In some cases, only clinical correlation allows a distinction between SCC and some of these conditions.

BASAL CELL CARCINOMA

Clinical Features

No universally accepted classification exists for BCC and at least 26 different subtypes have been described[42]. Attempts have been made to classify lesions based on growth pattern or along lines of differentiation, but this has not gained universal acceptance. Variants of BCC include nodular, superficial, morpheaform, cystic, basosquamous, micronodular, and fibroepithelioma of Pinkus.

Nodular basal cell carcinoma

This is the most common variant of BCC, accounting for approximately 60% of all primary BCCs. Nodular BCC presents as a raised, translucent papule or nodule with telangiectasias, and has a propensity for the face (Fig. 108.16). As the lesion enlarges, ulceration may occur. Pigmented BCC is a variant of nodular BCC, usually with a few flecks of brown pigment (Fig. 108.17A). However, the tumor may be completely black or blue–black and may be difficult to differentiate from nodular melanoma (Fig. 108.17B). Nodular BCCs may reach a large size and extend deeply, destroying an eyelid, nose or ear. In large lesions, tissue destruction and ulceration may dominate the picture, so that the inexperienced clinician may not recognize the true nature of the ulcer.

Superficial basal cell carcinoma

Superficial BCC commonly presents as an erythematous macule or thin plaque, and it may be difficult to differentiate clinically from AK, SCC in situ, or a benign inflammatory lesion (Fig. 108.18). Although this common variant of BCC is more often found on the trunk and extremities, the head and neck also may be affected. The mean age at diagnosis of 57 years is younger than in other BCCs[43]. Areas of

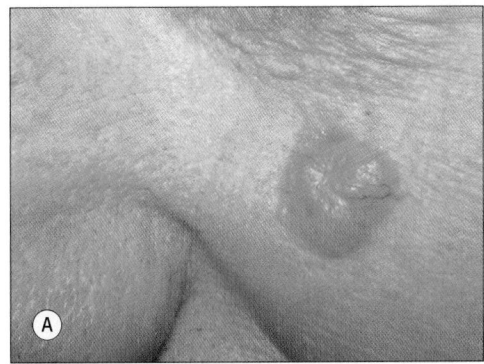
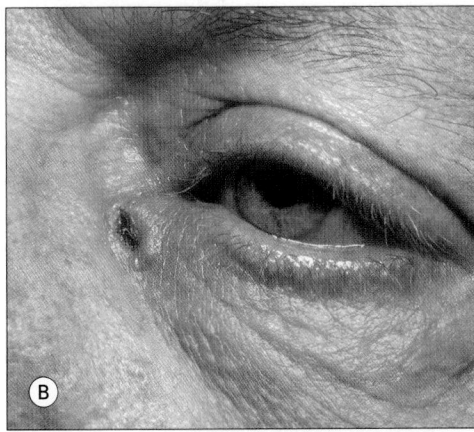
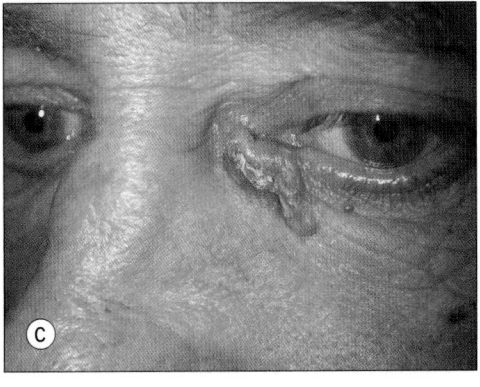

Fig. 108.16 Nodular basal cell carcinoma. A Translucent papulonodule with prominent telangiectasias on the infraorbital cheek. **B** Classic presentation with rolled border and central hemorrhagic crust of the medial canthus. **C** More advanced lesion. A, Courtesy of Stanley J Miller MD.

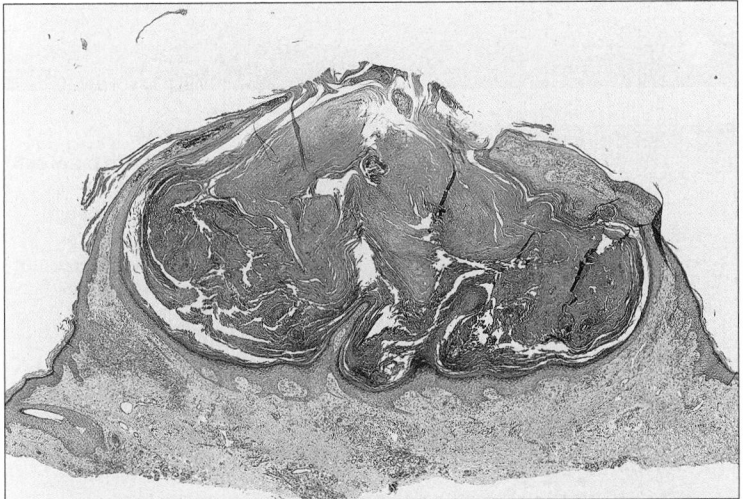

Fig. 108.15 Histology of keratoacanthoma. Note the keratin-filled crater. Courtesy of Ronald P Rapini MD.

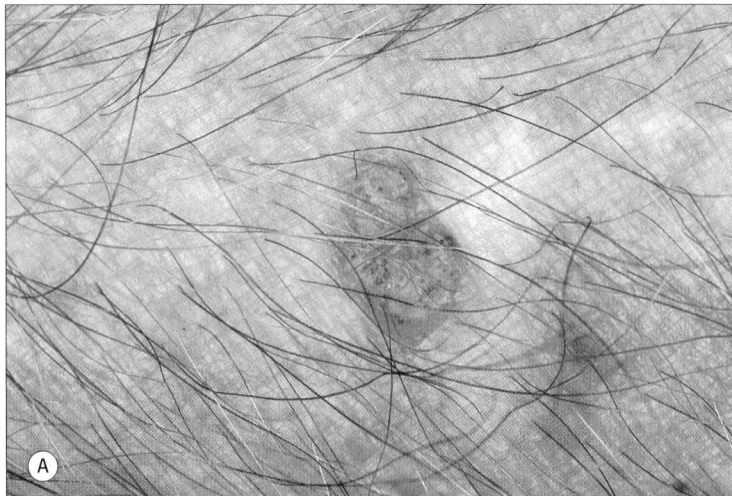

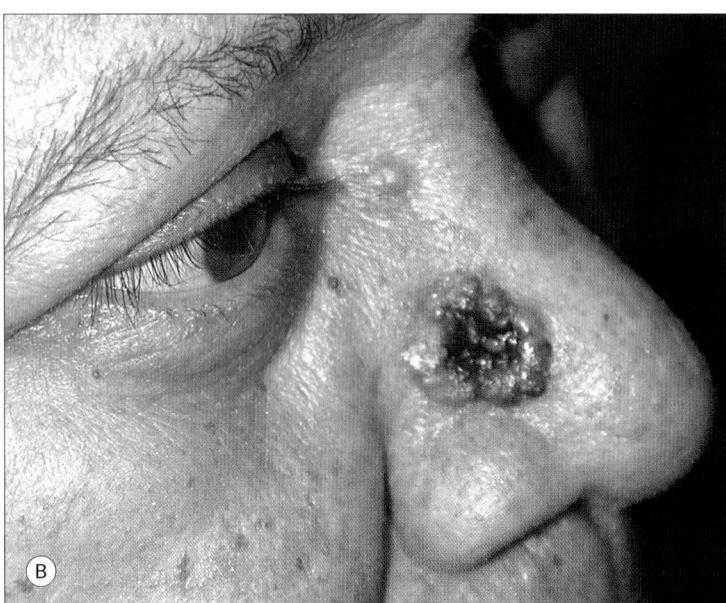

Fig. 108.17 Pigmented basal cell carcinoma. A Randomly distributed foci of pigment are often observed. **B** Occasionally, the pigmentation is more diffuse. Such lesions may have a clinical appearance similar to that of a melanoma.

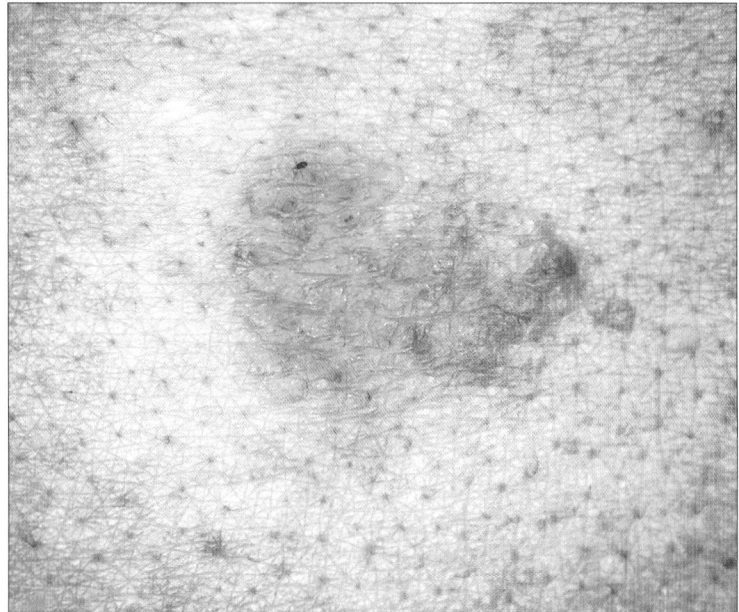

Fig. 108.18 Superficial basal cell carcinoma. An erythematous plaque that may resemble dermatitis. The trunk is a common location for this type of basal cell carcinoma. Courtesy of Rhonda Pomerantz MD.

spontaneous regression characterized by atrophy and hypopigmentation may be present. The diameter of the lesion varies from a few millimeters to several centimeters. Multiple lesions may be present. Variable amounts of pigment can be present, which may lead to confusion with a melanocytic lesion. The growth pattern is primarily horizontal, but these tumors can become deeply invasive, with induration, ulceration, and nodule formation. Extensive subclinical lateral spread accounts for the significant recurrence rate of these tumors after routine surgical treatment.

Morpheaform basal cell carcinoma

Morpheaform BCC derives its name from an appearance similar to a plaque of morphea. Sometimes, sclerosing or infiltrating BCC is used as a synonym, but these terms are viewed differently by different authors. This tumor presents as a flat, slightly atrophic lesion, or as a plaque without well-demarcated borders. It is often difficult to differentiate from a scar (Fig. 108.19A). Typically, the lesion is indurated and red or whitish in color (Fig 108.19B), and there may be overlying telangiectasia. The actual size of the cancer is often much greater than the clinical extent of the tumor. Occasionally, metastatic carcinoma, particularly breast cancer, may be misdiagnosed clinically and histologically as a morpheaform BCC.

Cystic basal cell carcinoma

Cystic BCCs have a clear or blue–gray appearance and exude a clear fluid if punctured or cut. If the lesion is in the periorbital area, it may be confused with a hidrocystoma. Cystic degeneration in a BCC often is not clinically obvious and thus the lesion may sometimes appear to be a typical nodular BCC.

Basosquamous carcinoma

Basosquamous carcinoma (metatypical BCC) is a tumor that has basaloid histologic features as well as eosinophilic squamoid features of SCC. Basosquamous carcinoma may behave biologically more like SCC than BCC and is more aggressive and destructive in its behavior, more likely to metastasize, and it is more likely to recur after treatment[44].

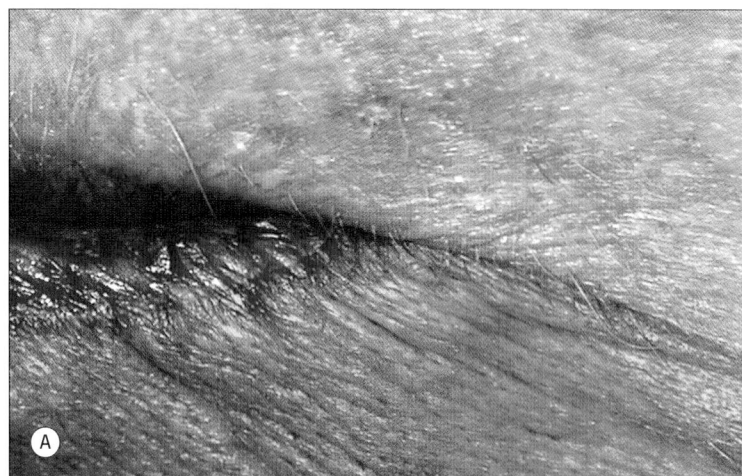

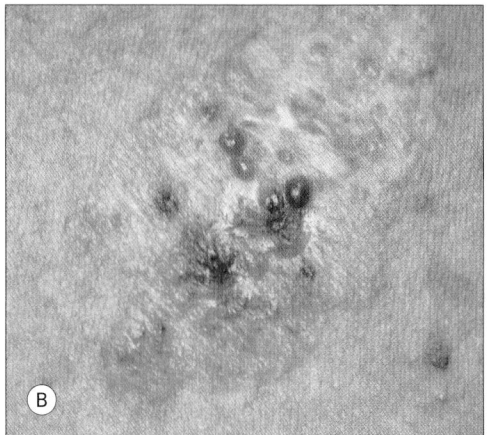

Fig. 108.19 Morpheaform basal cell carcinoma. A The lip lesion was indurated and had a scar-like appearance. **B** Recurrent tumor 2 years post-microscopically controlled surgery. Note the scar-like appearance and overlying erythematous and pigmented papulonodules.

It has been estimated that this variant constitutes 1% of all NMSC. When metastases occur, they may have the same microscopic appearance as the original tumor or may resemble a poorly differentiated SCC. The incidence of metastases with this variant of BCC has been estimated to be 9–10%.

Micronodular basal cell carcinoma

This is a histologic term used when BCCs have smaller tumor aggregates infiltrating the dermis. The designation should be used sparingly and only for more aggressive tumors. Micronodular BCCs are notorious for their destructive behavior, subclinical spread, and high recurrence rate. Clinically, they may present as macules, papules, or slightly elevated plaques and may be difficult to differentiate from nodular BCC.

Fibroepithelioma of Pinkus

This is a rare variant of BCC which usually presents as a pink plaque on the lower back. It may be difficult to distinguish clinically from amelanotic melanoma, but has unique histologic features. The typical lesion is a smooth, slightly pink nodule or plaque that may be pedunculated (Fig. 108.20).

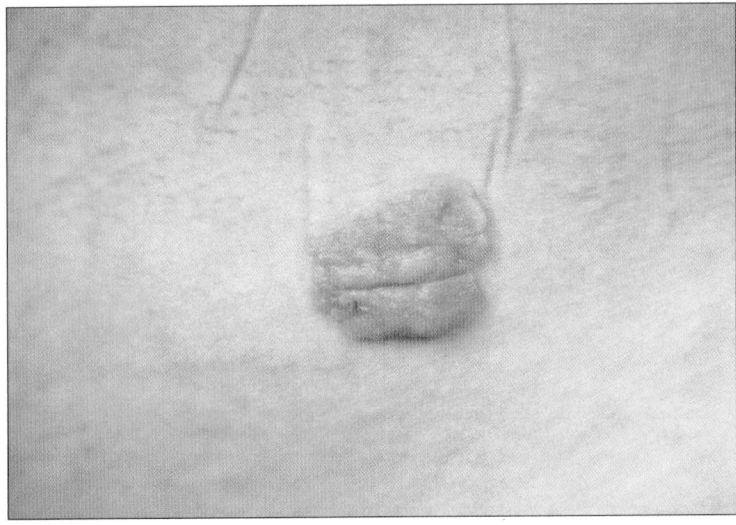

Fig. 108.20 Fibroepithelioma of Pinkus. Soft, skin-colored, sessile plaque on the lower back.

Pathology

BCCs have in common proliferations of basaloid keratinocytes in various configurations with a variable fibromyxoid stroma. Epidermal origin is usually evident and an inflammatory infiltrate is variably present. The cells are characterized by large, relatively uniform nuclei and scant cytoplasm. Cellular borders are indistinct and desmosomes are inapparent. Apoptotic cells are common. The fibromyxoid stroma is intimately associated with the tumor islands, often showing increased cellularity. A characteristic feature of BCC is retraction of the stroma around the tumor islands, creating microscopically visible clefts (Fig. 108.21). Although this feature may not be seen in all instances, it is useful when present and aids in differentiating histologic simulators.

In nodular BCC (see Fig. 108.21C,D), large, round or oval islands of basaloid keratinocytes extend from the epidermis into the dermis. Usually, an epidermal origin is apparent. Overlying ulceration with an associated inflammatory response may be present. Peripheral palisading is usually prominent and peritumoral clefts are often conspicuous in nodular BCC. Centrally, the nuclei lack organization and are more randomly distributed. In larger tumor islands, central areas of necrosis may develop, leading to the formation of cystic spaces. True cystic or nodulocystic BCCs form on the basis of mucin pools within the tumors (see Fig. 108.21E). Micronodular BCCs are composed of tumor islands much smaller than those of nodular BCC. The cellular features are similar (see Fig. 108.21F,G).

Superficial BCCs (see Fig. 108.21A,B) are characterized by small, superficially located buds of basaloid cells extending no more deeply than the papillary dermis, with or without clefting. In a given two-dimensional plane of section, there are skip areas along the epidermis, hence the synonym superficial multifocal BCC. There is evidence that many of these multifocal buds connect in a net-like pattern, so most are not truly multifocal.

Keratotic BCCs or BCCs with follicular differentiation contain small keratinized cysts that lack a granular layer within the aggregates of neoplastic cells. These lesions display differentiation towards hair follicle structures. They can be difficult to differentiate from trichepithelioma or other follicular adnexal neoplasms. Prominent clefting between the palisaded tumor islands and stroma, and a myxoid rather than fibrocellular stroma characterize the BCC. Infundibulocystic BCC may appear similar but usually has a more anastomosing pattern of tumor nests.

Pigmented BCCs (see Fig. 108.21D) usually have the overall architecture of a nodular BCC but may have other patterns as well. They contain aggregates of melanin, often irregularly dispersed, and melanocytes. Melanophages are frequently dispersed within the dermis.

Morpheaform, sclerosing and infiltrative BCCs share histologic features (see Fig. 108.21H). A common finding is a pattern of strands of basaloid keratinocytes extending between collagen bundles. These tumor islands may be composed of very few cells and may surround nerves. A peripheral palisaded pattern of tumor cells is absent and stromal retraction is also frequently not evident.

Fibroepithelioma of Pinkus (Fig. 108.22) is a variant characterized by thin anastomosing strands and cords of tumor cells projecting downward from the epidermis and embedded in a fibrous stroma. Peripheral palisading is less prominent, as is peritumoral retraction. In the differential diagnosis are eccrine syringofibroadenoma and reticulated seborrheic keratosis.

The diagnosis of basosquamous carcinoma has been variably defined and applied. To some, an admixture of typical BCC with zones of keratinization (with higher-molecular-weight keratin) is meant, while to others, basosquamous carcinoma consists of the admixture of features typical for BCC and SCC. To some extent, use of the term may reflect diagnostic uncertainty between BCC and SCC. The diagnosis should be made sparingly, and not for any BCC that has some increased keratinization. In particular, BCCs that are prone to keratinize more in the bed of an ulcer should not be designated as basosquamous if other portions of the lesion away from the ulcer are clearly basaloid.

Other basaloid tumors may simulate BCC (Table 108.5). Basaloid tumors are those with small darkly staining nuclei and scant cytoplasm, resembling basal cells of the epidermis. Adnexal neoplasms in particular (see Ch. 111) cause the most difficulty. Basaloid induction within dermatofibromas and nevus sebaceus also simulate BCC histologically.

TREATMENT

The National Comprehensive Cancer Network (NCCN) has established guidelines of care for NMSCs. Their guidelines are not strictly evidence-based, but developed through consensus by a working group of clinician experts who review, interpret and synthesize the existing literature. The current version of these guidelines can be found at *http://www.nccn.org/professionals/physician_gls/PDF/nmsc.pdf*. Recommendations are depicted in Figures 108.23 & 108.24.

Evaluation and risk assessment

Evaluation of a suspected NMSC requires a history, physical examination and biopsy of the suspicious lesion. The history should assess duration, rate of growth, and any prior therapy, as well as any personal or family history of prior skin cancers. Localized neurologic symptoms, although rare, may suggest the possibility of perineural involvement. Any history of prior radiation therapy to the area should be elicited. Current medical problems, medications and allergies should be reviewed. Evidence of immunosuppression (i.e. organ transplantation, underlying hematologic malignancy, immunosuppressive medications or HIV infection) should be determined, and any of the risk factors listed in Table 108.6 identified.

Physical examination should include observation and palpation of a tumor to determine exact location and size, and whether it appears to have any connection to underlying structures such as muscle, cartilage or bone. How well or poorly defined the tumor borders are, whether there is physical evidence of prior surgery or other treatment modality

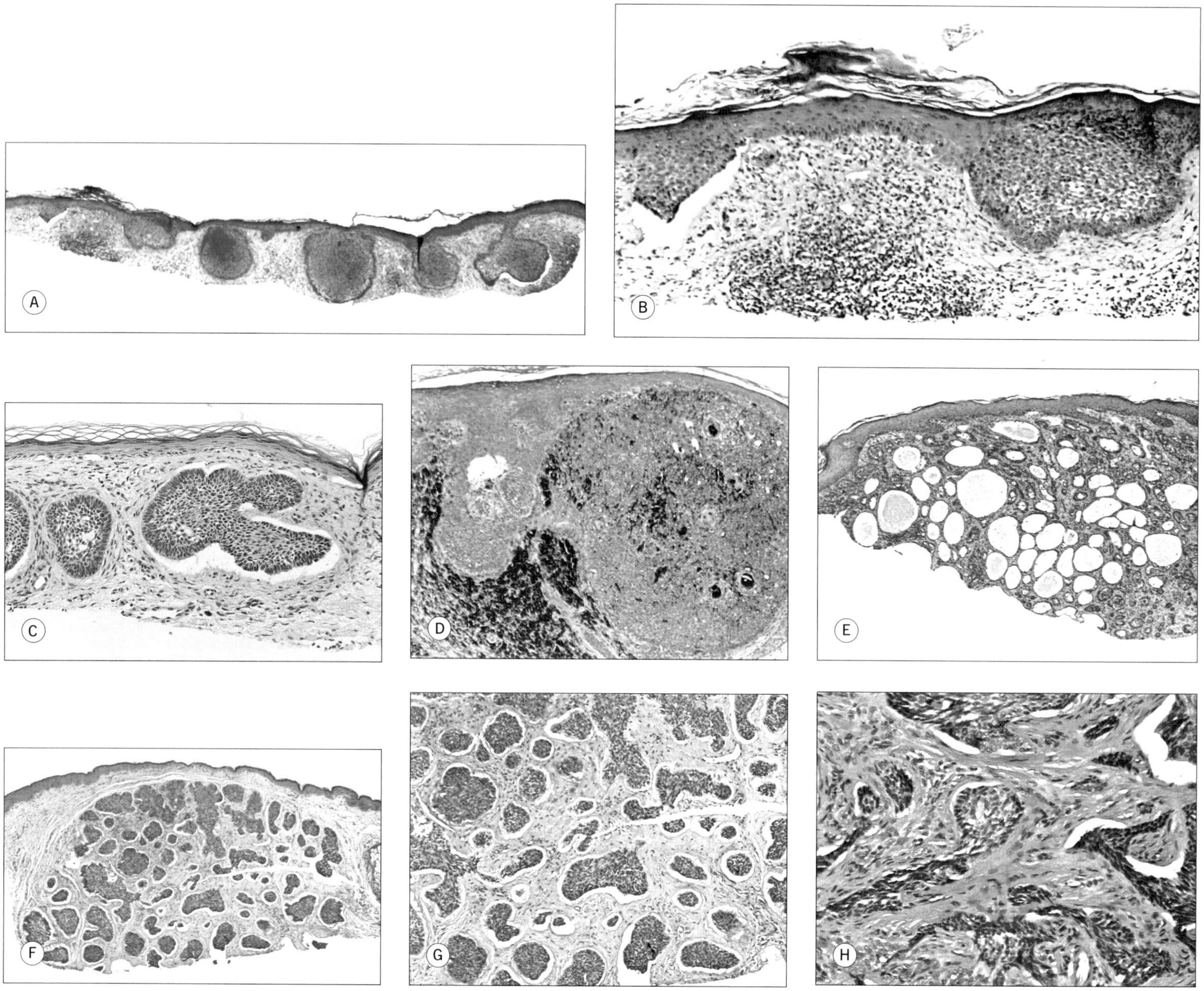

Fig. 108.21 Histology of various types of basal cell carcinoma. A, B Superficial type with multiple basaloid buds, nuclear palisading, and stromal retraction. **C** Nodular type with peripheral palisading and stromal retraction. **D** Pigmented nodular type with brown melanin pigmentation within the tumor and the stroma. **E** Nodulocystic type. **F, G** Micronodular type. **H** Morpheaform type. C, Courtesy of Ronald P Rapini MD.

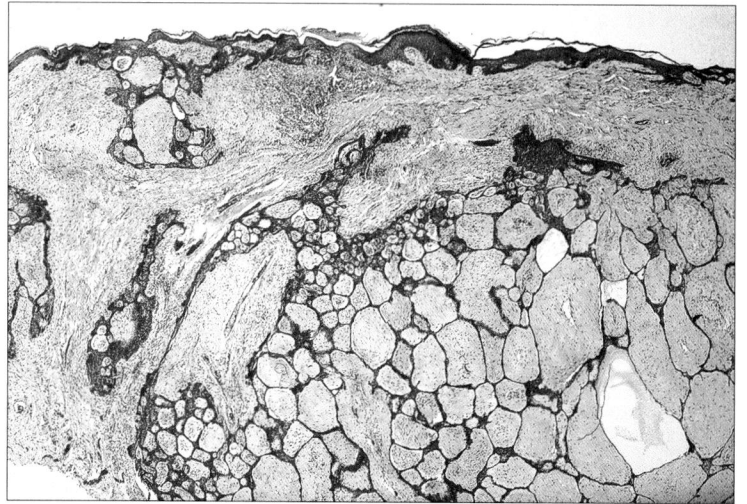

Fig. 108.22 Fibroepithelioma of Pinkus. This variant of basal cell carcinoma has delicate reticulated basaloid strands in a pale stroma. Courtesy of Ronald P Rapini MD.

(indicating the possibility of recurrence), and development within a site of chronic inflammation or scar should all be assessed. Careful inspection of the surrounding skin to exclude the presence of satellite lesions is necessary, as is examination of the draining lymph nodes, especially for high-risk tumors, since in transit[46] and distant metastases[47] are more common in these patients. In all patients, a full skin examination is required, to exclude other cutaneous malignancies.

Skin cancers are often identifiable visually by an experienced clinician. Nevertheless, a properly performed biopsy is essential to the diagnosis and management of the skin cancer. Numerous biopsy techniques, including excisional, incisional, shave, saucerization and punch, may be employed (see Ch. 146). When there is doubt about the diagnosis, a biopsy should be done prior to definitive treatment. For obvious skin cancers, sometimes a tissue specimen can be sent at the same time as definitive therapy. If a superficial process (such as superficial BCC or SCC *in situ*) is suspected, or if shallow therapy (such as curettage and electrodesiccation) is being contemplated, a shave biopsy is usually adequate to establish a diagnosis. AKs are often treated without prior biopsy unless invasive NMSC is suspected. In most other instances, a punch biopsy that extends to subcutaneous fat is preferred. The biopsy report should include an assessment of histologic subtype in both BCC and SCC, and degree of differentiation in SCC. Perineural

HISTOLOGIC SIMULANTS OF BASAL CELL CARCINOMA

	Major distinguishing features
Adenoid cystic carcinoma	Cribriform pattern, EMA-positive
Basaloid follicular hamartoma	Multiple small papules, positive family history
Cloacogenic carcinoma	Anal location
Desmoplastic trichoepithelioma	Keratin cysts, no stromal retraction around basaloid strands
Eccrine carcinoma	Small sweat ducts
Folliculocentric basaloid proliferation	Focal follicular budding
Merkel cell carcinoma	Punctate keratin (CK20-positive) in cytoplasm plus EMA expression
Metastatic breast carcinoma	History, single filing, EMA expression
Microcystic adnexal carcinoma	Keratin cysts, absent stromal retraction, ductal differentiation
Mucinous carcinoma	Pools of mucin with floating basaloid islands
Ameloblastoma	Location in mouth
Sebaceous carcinoma	Oil red O-positive sebocytes on histochemical staining
Trichoepithelioma	Horn cysts, absent stromal retraction, papillary mesenchymal bodies, peritumoral CD34 positivity; positive family history when multiple

Table 108.5 **Histologic simulants of basal cell carcinoma.** EMA, epithelial membrane antigen.

RISK FACTORS FOR RECURRENCE OF NMSC

	Low risk	High risk
Clinical risk factors		
Location/size	Area L <20 mm Area M <10 mm Area H <6 mm	Area L ≥20 mm Area M ≥10 mm Area H ≥6 mm
Borders	Well defined	Poorly defined
Primary vs recurrent	Primary	Recurrent
Immunosuppression	Negative	Positive
Tumor at site of prior radiation therapy	Negative	Positive
Tumor at site of chronic inflammatory process (SCC only)	Negative	Positive
Rapidly growing tumor (SCC only)	Negative	Positive
Neurologic symptoms: pain, paresthesia, paralysis (SCC only)	Negative	Positive
Pathologic risk factors		
Perineural involvement	Negative	Positive
Subtype (BCC only)	Nodular, superficial	Micronodular, infiltrating, sclerosing
Degree of differentiation (SCC only)	Well differentiated	Moderately or poorly differentiated
Adenoid, adenosquamous or desmoplastic (SCC only)	Negative	Positive
Depth: Clark level or thickness (SCC only)	I, II, III or <4 mm	IV, V or ≥4 mm

Area L: low risk for recurrence: trunk, extremities.
Area M: middle risk for recurrence: cheeks, forehead, neck, scalp.
Area H: high risk for recurrence: 'mask areas' of face (central face, eyelids, eyebrows, periorbital, nose, lips, chin, mandible, preauricular and postauricular skin/sulci, ear, temple), genitalia, hands and feet.

Table 108.6 **Risk factors for recurrence of non-melanoma skin cancer.** BCC, basal cell carcinoma; SCC, squamous cell carcinoma. Adapted from Miller SJ. The National Comprehensive Cancer Network guidelines of care for nonmelanoma skin cancers. Dermatol Surg. 2000;26:289–92.

or vascular involvement should be indicated. In SCC, histologic assessment of tumor depth, as either an anatomic estimate of depth or an actual measurement of tumor thickness in millimeters, appears to be prognostically useful. This is often not included in the standard biopsy report and requires sampling past the base of the tumor.

Using these results, stratification of a specific tumor into a low- or high-risk category may be made (see Table 108.6). High-risk tumors, particularly SCCs, need to be treated aggressively[48]. For larger and deeper tumors, the possible need for multispecialty collaboration or preoperative imaging studies should be considered. On the basis of this assessment, a rational therapeutic plan is designed. As always, the particular factors of the individual case and the patient's and physician's preferences help to guide this decision-making process. Because of the risk of post-therapeutic tumor recurrence and the elevated risk for subsequent NMSC and melanoma, patients with NMSC are typically followed regularly for life.

Standard excision

Standard surgical excision is effective for most primary BCCs; however, cure rates are inferior to those achieved with Mohs surgery in the case of recurrent BCC, infiltrative BCC, and BCC from high-risk anatomic sites (see Table 108.6). It has been demonstrated that 4 mm margins are adequate for removal of BCC in 98% of cases of non-morpheaform BCC <2 cm in diameter. For facial lesions, simple excision with narrow margins is often not adequate for effective removal[49]. High-risk SCC requires 6 mm margins, with size >2 cm, poor differentiation, invasion to fat, and location in high-risk areas associated with a greater risk of subclinical tumor extension.

Curettage with electrodesiccation

Curettage with electrodesiccation is frequently used by dermatologists to treat BCCs. Cure rates as high as 97–98% have been reported[50], but careful selection of appropriate smaller lesions that are not deep is necessary. Curettage and electrodesiccation can be used for small SCCs *in situ* and well-differentiated primary SCCs <1 cm in diameter. Honeycutt & Jansen reported a 99% cure rate for 281 SCCs after a 4-year follow-up[51]. In this study, two recurrences were noted in lesions >2 cm in diameter.

Curettage alone

The use of electrodesiccation (often dogmatically done sequentially three times after curettage three times) in the treatment of BCC may lead to hypertrophic scarring and poor cosmetic result. Barlow et al.[52] reported that 302 biopsy-proven BCCs treated by a single investigator with curettage alone had a 5-year cure rate of 96%, with minimal complications (hypopigmentation, scarring). Tumors involving more than 50% of the deep edge of the shave biopsy specimen had an increased risk of recurrence.

Mohs micrographic surgery

Mohs surgery (see Ch. 150) results in superior histologic verification of complete removal, can allow maximum conservation of tissue, and remains cost-effective when compared to some excisions (such as in a surgicenter or hospital operating room) or radiation therapy for NMSC. Rowe and colleagues reported a recurrence rate for BCC treated with Mohs surgery of only 1% over 5 years. This was superior to all other modalities, including excision (10%), curettage and dessication (7.7%), radiation therapy (8.7%), and cryotherapy (7.5%). Of course, these percentages vary by the study, the physician involved, and the types of lesions selected for inclusion. Comparisons between different studies are difficult, but Mohs surgery clearly has the highest cure rate when all tumor types are included. In a similar study of treatment of *recurrent* BCC, Mohs surgery showed a long-term recurrence rate of 5.6%. Once again, this was superior to all other modalities, including excision (17.4%), radiation therapy (9.8%), and curettage with electrodesiccation (40%). Mohs surgery is the preferred treatment for morpheaform,

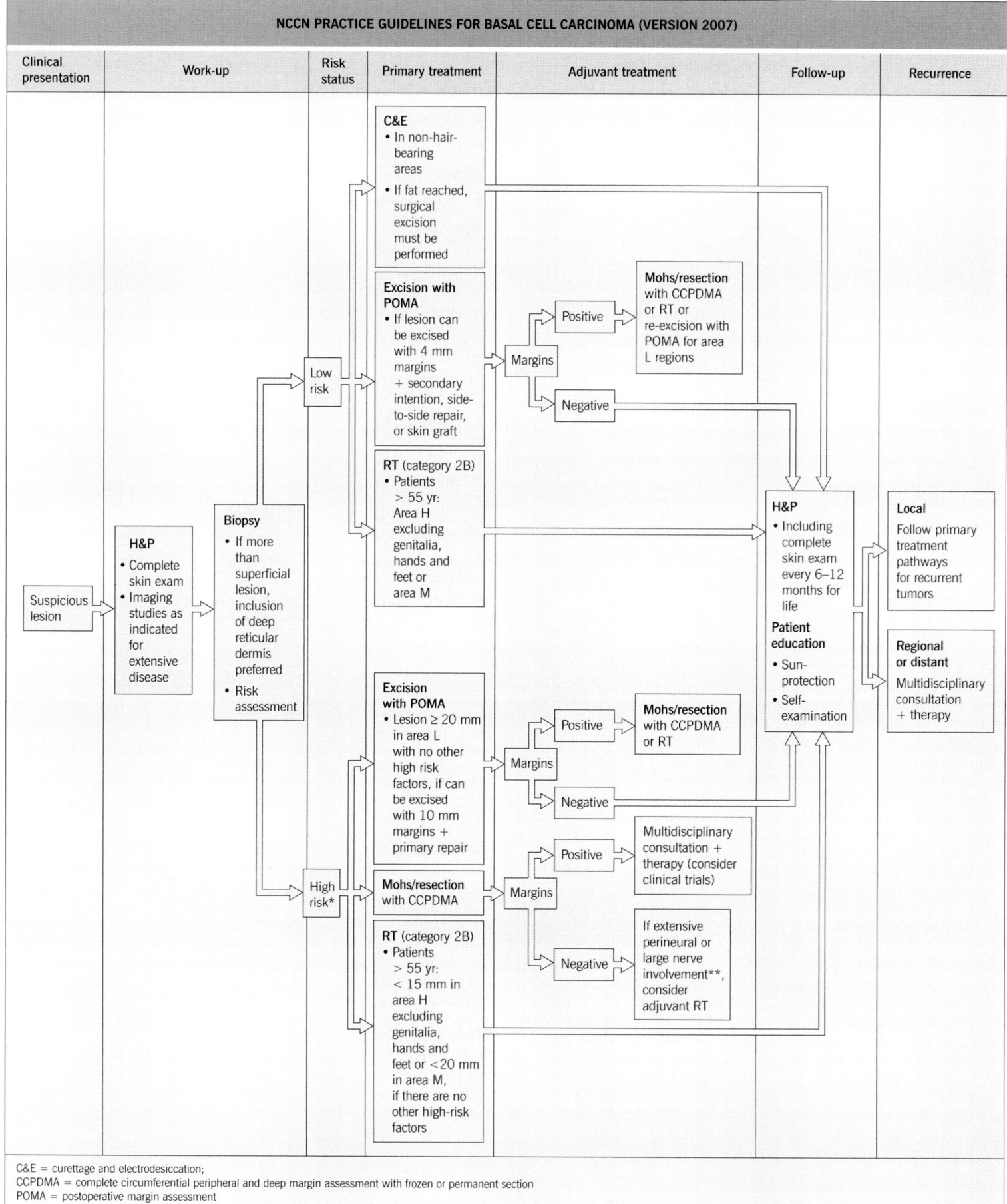

NCCN PRACTICE GUIDELINES FOR BASAL CELL CARCINOMA (VERSION 2007)

Clinical presentation	Work-up	Risk status	Primary treatment	Adjuvant treatment	Follow-up	Recurrence

Suspicious lesion

H&P
• Complete skin exam
• Imaging studies as indicated for extensive disease

Biopsy
• If more than superficial lesion, inclusion of deep reticular dermis preferred
• Risk assessment

Low risk

C&E
• In non-hair-bearing areas
• If fat reached, surgical excision must be performed

Excision with POMA
• If lesion can be excised with 4 mm margins + secondary intention, side-to-side repair, or skin graft

RT (category 2B)
• Patients > 55 yr: Area H excluding genitalia, hands and feet or area M

Margins → Positive → **Mohs/resection** with CCPDMA or RT or re-excision with POMA for area L regions

Margins → Negative

High risk*

Excision with POMA
• Lesion ≥ 20 mm in area L with no other high risk factors, if can be excised with 10 mm margins + primary repair

Margins → Positive → **Mohs/resection** with CCPDMA or RT

Margins → Negative

Mohs/resection with CCPDMA

Margins → Positive → Multidisciplinary consultation + therapy (consider clinical trials)

Margins → Negative

RT (category 2B)
• Patients > 55 yr: < 15 mm in area H excluding genitalia, hands and feet or <20 mm in area M, if there are no other high-risk factors

If extensive perineural or large nerve involvement**, consider adjuvant RT

H&P
• Including complete skin exam every 6–12 months for life

Patient education
• Sun-protection
• Self-examination

Local
Follow primary treatment pathways for recurrent tumors

Regional or distant
Multidisciplinary consultation + therapy

C&E = curettage and electrodesiccation;
CCPDMA = complete circumferential peripheral and deep margin assessment with frozen or permanent section
POMA = postoperative margin assessment

Fig. 108.23 National Comprehensive Cancer Network (NCCN) practice guidelines, version 2007, for basal cell carcinoma. *Any high-risk factor places the patient in a high-risk category. **If large nerve involvement, consider MRI to evaluate and rule out skull involvement. Area L, low risk for recurrence: trunk, extremities; Area M, middle risk for recurrence: cheeks, forehead, neck, scalp; Area H, high risk for recurrence: 'mask areas' of face (central face, eyelids, eyebrows, periorbital, nose, lips, chin, mandible, preauricular and postauricular skin/sulci, ear, temple), genitalia, hands and feet; RT, radiation therapy.

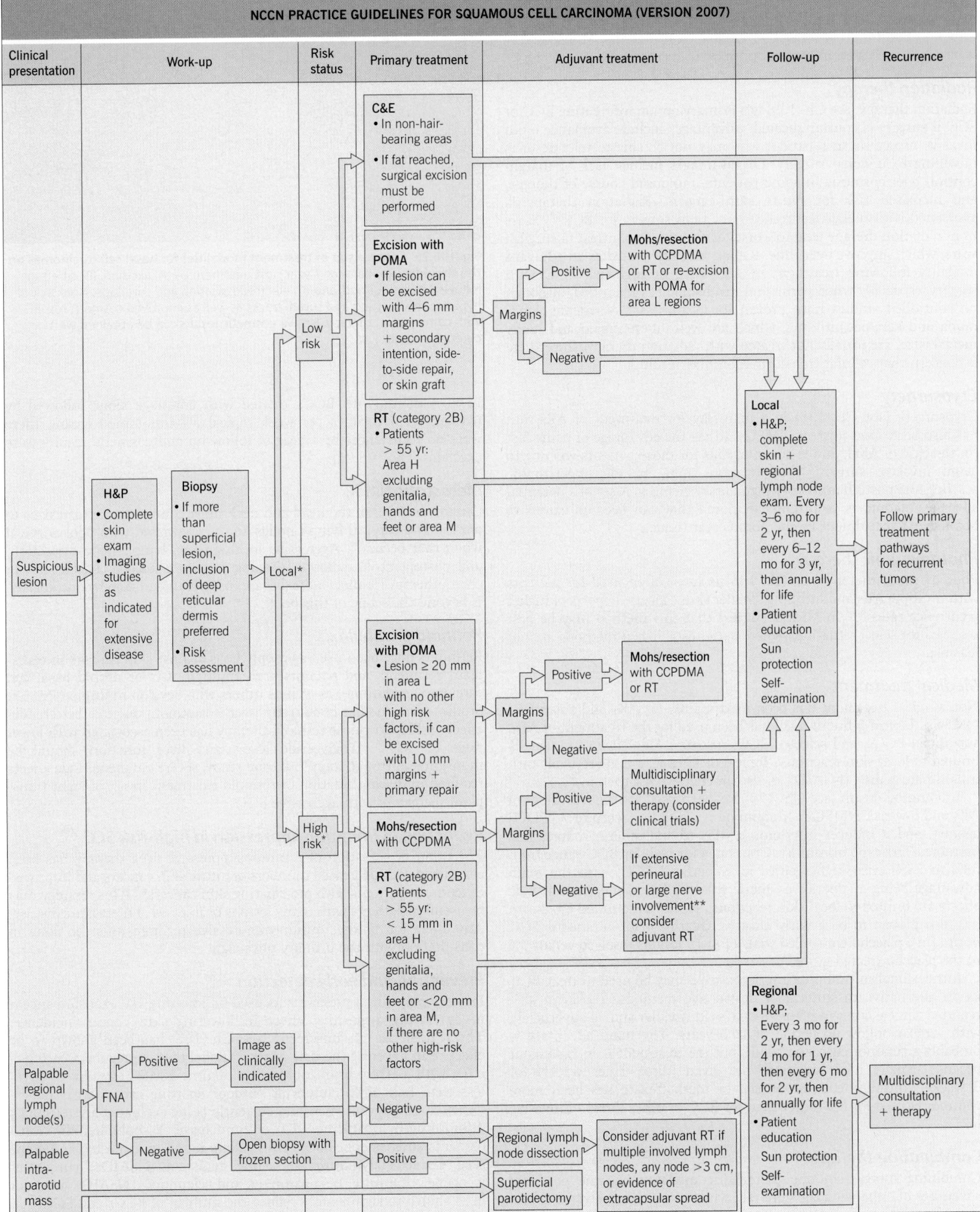

Fig. 108.24 National Comprehensive Cancer Network (NCCN) practice guidelines, version 2007, for squamous cell carcinoma. *Any high-risk factor places the patient in a high-risk category. **If large nerve involvement, consider MRI to evaluate and rule out skull involvement. Area L, low risk for recurrence: trunk, extremities; Area M, middle risk for recurrence: cheeks, forehead, neck, scalp; Area H, high risk for recurrence: 'mask areas' of face (central face, eyelids, eyebrows, periorbital, nose, lips, chin, mandible, preauricular and postauricular skin/sulci, ear, temple), genitalia, hands and feet; C&E, curettage and electrodessication; CCPDMA, complete circumferential peripheral and deep margin assessment with frozen or permanent section; POMA, postoperative margin assessment; RT, radiation therapy.

Actinic Keratosis, Basal Cell Carcinoma and Squamous Cell Carcinoma

recurrent, poorly delineated, high-risk (defined earlier), or incompletely removed BCC, and for those sites in which tissue conservation is imperative and there is a need for reliable clear margins. Mohs surgery is similarly indicated in cases of primary or recurrent SCC.

Radiation therapy

Radiation therapy (see Ch. 139) is a primary option for treating BCC or SCC if surgery is contraindicated. Advantages include avoidance of an invasive procedure in a patient who may not be able to tolerate or is unwilling to undergo surgery. Disadvantages include lack of margin control, poor cosmesis in some patients, prolonged course of therapy, and increased risk for future skin cancers. Radiation therapy is associated with higher recurrence rates than surgery for BCC[53]. Scars from radiation therapy tend to worsen with time, in contrast to surgical scars, which improve over time. Radiation is often used as an adjuvant modality following treatment of aggressive or high-risk SCC with surgery, especially when perineural involvement is identified, although no controlled studies have proven its usefulness[54]. Verrucous carcinoma and keratoacanthoma, which are well differentiated and rarely metastasize, are usually not treated with radiation therapy, since there is concern that cellular transformation may result.

Cryosurgery

Cryosurgery (see Ch. 138) is a mainstay for treatment of AKs, but has also been used to treat NMSCs. It has the advantage of being fast (in the case of AKs), and is advantageous for those patients wishing to avoid invasive surgery. Complications may include hypertrophic scarring and postinflammatory pigmentary changes. A serious potential adverse outcome is recurrent carcinoma that can become extensive because of concealment by the fibrous scar tissue.

Photodynamic therapy

Photodynamic therapy (see Ch. 135) is most often used for patients with multiple AKs and multiple smaller skin cancers. Reports of higher recurrence rates[55,56] in NMSC suggest that this method may be best reserved for select situations where better-established methods are not feasible.

Medical treatment

Non-surgical treatment has been used mainly for AKs and superficial NMSCs. Topical 5-fluorouracil has been used for the treatment of AKs, superficial BCCs, and selected SCCs *in situ*[57]. Side effects are usually limited to local skin reactions. Topical diclofenac, a non-steroidal anti-inflammatory drug (NSAID), is also an effective AK therapy[58].

Imiquimod cream (see Ch. 129) has been used for the treatment of AKs and low-risk NMSC[59]. Imiquimod is a Toll-like receptor 7 (TLR7) agonist, and it induces interferon-α (IFN-α) and other cytokines and promotes Th1-type immunity. Cure rates for nodular BCC range from 53% to 75%, with higher cures for superficial BCC, with the main advantage being a superior cosmetic result[60]. In general, adverse side effects are limited to local skin reactions. Topical imiquimod 5% cream has also proven to be a fairly effective treatment for cutaneous SCC *in situ*; in a placebo-controlled trial, 11 of 15 lesions resolved versus 0% in the placebo-treated group[61].

Intralesional injection of interferon-α-2b may be used to treat BCC as an alternative to surgical or destructive methods. Tucker et al.[62] reported clinical cures in 95 of 98 BCCs (51 nodular and 44 superficial), with a mean follow-up period of 10.5 years. The main advantage is probably a superior cosmetic result, but the treatment is inconvenient because usually nine injections are given (three times weekly for 3 weeks). Intralesional fluorouracil or methotrexate has been more commonly used for KA rather than for BCC or other forms of invasive SCC.

Combination therapy

Combining more than one therapeutic modality has the potential advantage of enhancing the cure rate while minimizing adverse effects and maximizing cosmetic results. Topical 5-fluorouracil cream or 5% imiquimod cream has been used to pretreat BCC sites prior to Mohs surgery, leading to a decrease in the eventual wound size[63]. Imiquimod cream has also been used in conjunction with topical fluorouracil cream for the treatment of SCC *in situ* in transplant recipients.

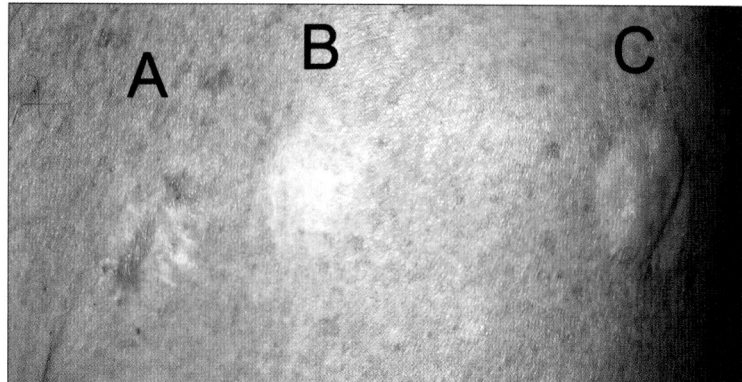

Fig. 108.25 Comparison of treatment modalities for basal cell carcinomas on the shoulder. Appearance 1 year post treatment by (A) excision, (B) curettage followed by imiquimod, and (C) electrodessication and curettage. Note lack of hypertrophic scarring and suture tracks as well as improved cosmetic result with combination therapy. Similar cosmetic results can be obtained with curettage alone.

In 20 patients with BCCs treated with curettage alone followed by 6 weeks of five times per week topical 5% imiquimod cream, there were no recurrences at 1 year of follow-up and cosmetic results were excellent (Fig. 108.25).

Metastatic NMSC

Cutaneous SCC of the head and neck most commonly metastasizes to parotid and cervical lymph nodes and is associated with poor survival when that occurs[64]. Aggressive local surgery, lymph node dissection, and postoperative radiation therapy are often needed. Discussion of chemotherapy for metastatic disease, usually undertaken by oncologists, is beyond the scope of this book.

Retinoid prophylaxis

Retinoids have been used as prophylaxis against skin cancers in transplant recipients and patients with multiple KAs or nevoid basal cell carcinoma syndrome, as well as others who develop multiple NMSCs. Studies favor the use of acitretin over isotretinoin due to a better side-effect profile. Low-dose retinoid therapy has been associated with lower rates of SCC[65]. Triglyceride levels and liver function should be monitored during therapy[66]. In one study, severe cutaneous side effects resulted in discontinuation of retinoid treatment in six of eight transplant recipients with aggressive SCC.

Reduction of immunosuppression in high-risk SCC

Reduction or cessation of immunosuppressive drug therapy has been associated with decreased numbers of future skin cancers and improved outcome in patients with pre-existing skin cancers[67]. This strategy may be useful in patients with many lesions or in cases of metastatic disease. Any alteration of the immunosuppressive regimen must be done in consultation with the primary physician.

Prevention and early detection

Primary prevention programs focused on lowering UV exposure appear to be having a positive effect in lowering skin cancer incidence. The regular use of sunscreens (see Ch. 132) has been shown to be effective in lowering the risk. Marks[68] noted that the regular wearing of a hat with a 10 cm brim could lower lifetime NMSC rates by 40%, yet less than half of spectators at outdoor sporting events wear hats[69]. Other chemopreventive agents currently being evaluated are retinoids, difluoromethylornithine, T4 endonuclease V, polyphenolic antioxidants such as epigallocatechin gallate found in green tea and grape seed extract, silymarin, isoflavone genistein, NSAIDs, curcumin, lycopene, vitamin E, beta-carotene, and selenium[70]. NSAIDs have not been shown to significantly reduce the number of BCCs and SCCs[71].

Since less than 20% of medical students receive training in skin cancer examination[72], programs need to be developed to educate medical professionals in order to increase NMSC diagnostic skills. New noninvasive diagnostic techniques such as reflectance confocal microscopy may lead to enhanced diagnostic accuracy in the future[73].

108

REFERENCES

1. Madan V, Hoban P, Strange RC, Fryer AA, Lear JT. Genetics and risk factors for basal cell carcinoma. Br J Dermatol. 2006;154(suppl. 1):5–7.
2. Rigel DS, Friedman RJ, Kopf AW. Lifetime risk for development of skin cancer in the U.S. population: current estimate is now 1 in 5. J Am Acad Dermatol. 1996;35:1012–13.
3. Hannuksela-Svahn A, Pukkala E, Karvonen J. Basal cell skin carcinoma and other nonmelanoma skin cancers in Finland from 1956 through 1995. Arch Dermatol. 1999;135:781–6.
4. Weinstock MA. Death from skin cancer among the elderly: epidemiologic patterns. Arch Dermatol. 1997;133:1207–9.
5. Stern RS. The mysteries of geographic variability in nonmelanoma skin cancer incidence [editorial]. Arch Dermatol. 1999;135:843–4.
6. Halder RM, Bridgeman-Shah S. Skin cancer in African Americans. Cancer. 1995;75:667–73.
7. Alam M, Ratner D. Cutaneous squamous cell carcinoma. N Engl J Med. 2001;344:975–83.
8. Halder RM, Bang KM. Skin cancer in blacks in the United States. Dermatol Clin. 1988;6:397–405.
9. Bang KM, Halder RM, White JE, Sampson CC, Wilson J. Skin cancer in black Americans: a review of 126 cases. J Natl Med Assoc. 1987;79:51–8.
10. Kwa RE, Campana K, Moy RL. Biology of cutaneous squamous cell carcinoma. J Am Acad Dermatol. 1992;42:S8–S10.
11. Fewkes J. Do dark-skinned people get skin cancer? Skin Cancer Found J. 1999;11:33–4.
12. Harris RB, Griffith K, Moon TE. Trends in the incidence of nonmelanoma skin cancers in southeastern Arizona, 1985–1996. J Am Acad Dermatol. 2001;45:528–36.
13. Chen GJ, Feldman SR, Williford PM, et al. Clinical diagnosis of actinic keratosis identifies an elderly population at high risk of developing skin cancer. Dermatol Surg. 2005;31:43–7.
14. Lebwohl M. Actinic keratosis: epidemiology and progression to squamous cell carcinoma. Br J Dermatol. 2003;149(suppl. 66):31–3.
15. Weinstock MA. Controversies in the public health approach to keratinocyte carcinomas. Br J Dermatol. 2006;154(suppl. 1):3–4.
16. Scrivener Y, Grosshans E, Cribier B. Variations of basal cell carcinomas according to gender, age, location and histopathological subtype. Br J Dermatol. 2002;147:41–7.
17. Ting PT, Kasper R, Arlette JP. Metastatic basal cell carcinoma: report of two cases and literature review. J Cutan Med Surg. 2005;9:10–15.
18. Hemminki K, Zhang H, Czene K. Time trends and familial risks in squamous cell carcinoma of the skin. Arch Dermatol. 2003;139:885–9.
19. Karagas MR, Stannard VA, Mott LA, Slattery MJ, Spencer SK, Weinstock MA. Use of tanning devices and risk of basal cell and squamous cell skin cancers. J Natl Cancer Inst. 2002;94:224–6.
20. Boyd AS, Shyr Y, King LE Jr. Basal cell carcinoma in young women: an evaluation of the association of tanning bed use and smoking. J Am Acad Dermatol. 2002;46:706–9.
21. Stern RS, Liebman EJ, Vakeva L. Oral psoralen and ultraviolet-A light (PUVA) treatment of psoriasis and persistent risk of nonmelanoma skin cancer. PUVA Follow-up Study. J Natl Cancer Inst. 1998;90:1278–84.
22. Lichter MD, Karagas MR, Mott LA, Spencer SK, Stukel TA, Greenberg ER. Therapeutic ionizing radiation and the incidence of basal cell carcinoma and squamous cell carcinoma. The New Hampshire Skin Cancer Study Group. Arch Dermatol. 2000;136:1007–11.
23. Shore RE, Moseson M, Xue X, Tse Y, Harley N, Pasternack BS. Skin cancer after X-ray treatment for scalp ringworm. Radiat Res. 2002;157:410–18.
24. Stante M, Salvini C, De Giorgi V, Carli P. Multiple synchronous pigmented basal cell carcinomas following radiotherapy for Hodgkin's disease. Int J Dermatol. 2002;41:208–11.
25. Yuspa SH. Cutaneous chemical carcinogenesis. J Am Acad Dermatol. 1986;15:1031–44.
26. Lei U, Masmas TN, Frentz G. Occupational non-melanoma skin cancer. Acta Derm Venereol. 2001;81:415–17.

27. Dorfner B, Baum C, Voigtlander V. Multiple superficial basal cell carcinomas following chronic ingestion of sodium hydrogen carbonate containing arsenic. Hautarzt. 2002;53:542–5.
28. Simeonova PP, Luster MI. Mechanisms of arsenic carcinogenicity: genetic or epigenetic mechanisms? J Environ Pathol Toxicol Oncol. 2000;19:281–6.
29. Wong SS, Tan KC, Goh CL. Cutaneous manifestations of chronic arsenicism: review of seventeen cases. J Am Acad Dermatol. 1998;38:179–85.
30. Ott C, Huber S. The clinical significance of cosmic radiation in aviation. Schweiz Rundsch Med Prax. 2006;95:99–106.
31. Freiman A, Bird G, Metelitsa AI, Barankin B, Lauzon GJ. Cutaneous effects of smoking. J Cutan Med Surg. 2004;8:415–23.
32. Kimonis VE, Goldstein AM, Pastakia B, et al. Clinical manifestations in 105 persons with nevoid basal cell carcinoma syndrome. Am J Med Genet. 1997;69:299–308.
33. Berg, D, Otley CC. Skin cancer in organ transplant recipients: epidemiology, pathogenesis, and management. J Am Acad Dermatol. 2002;47:1–17; quiz 18–20.
34. Clifford GM, Polesel J, Rickenbach M, et al. Cancer risk in the Swiss HIV Cohort Study: associations with immunodeficiency, smoking, and highly active antiretroviral therapy. J Natl Cancer Inst. 2005;97:425–32.
35. Karagas MR, Cushing GL Jr, Greenberg ER, Mott LA, Spencer SK, Nierenberg DW. Non-melanoma skin cancers and glucocorticoid therapy. Br J Cancer. 2001;85:683–6.
36. Marghoob AA, Slade J, Salopek TG, et al. Basal cell and squamous cell carcinomas are important risk factors for cutaneous malignant melanoma. Screening implications. Cancer. 1995;75(suppl.):707–14.
37. Nugent Z, Demers AA, Wiseman MC, et al. Risk of second primary cancer and death following a diagnosis of nonmelanoma skin cancer. Cancer Epidemiol Biomarkers Prev. 2005;14:2584–90.
38. Yu RH, Pryce DW, MacFarlane AQ, Stewart TW. A histopathological study of 643 cutaneous horns. Br J Dermatol.1991;24:449–52.
39. Rowe DE, Carroll RJ, Day CL. Prognostic factors for local recurrence, metastasis, and survival rates in squamous cell carcinoma of the skin, ear, and lip. J Am Acad Dermatol. 1992;26:976–90.
40. Schwartz RA. Keratoacanthoma. J Am Acad Dermatol. 1994;30:1–19.
41. Norgauer J, Rohwedder A. Human papillomavirus and Grzybowski's generalized eruptive keratoacanthomas. J Am Acad Dermatol. 2003;49:771–2.
42. Wade TR, Ackerman AB. The many faces of basal-cell carcinoma. J Dermatol Surg Oncol. 1978;4:23–8.
43. McCormack CJ, Kelly JW, Dorevitch AP. Differences in age and body site distribution of the histological subtypes of basal cell carcinoma. A possible indicator of differing causes. Arch Dermatol. 1997;133:593–6.
44. Costantino D, Lowe L, Brown DL .Basosquamous carcinoma – an under-recognized, high-risk cutaneous neoplasm: case study and review of the literature. Br J Plast Surg. 2006;59:424–8.
45. Miller SJ. The National Comprehensive Cancer Network guidelines of care for nonmelanoma skin cancers. Dermatol Surg. 2000;26:289–92.
46. Carucci JA, Martinez JC, Zeitouni NC, et al. In-transit metastasis from primary cutaneous squamous cell carcinoma in organ transplant recipients and nonimmunosuppressed patients: clinical characteristics, management, and outcome in a series of 21 patients. Dermatol Surg. 2004;30:651–5.
47. Martinez JC, Otley CC, Stasko T, et al. Defining the clinical course of metastatic skin cancer in organ transplant recipients: a multicenter collaborative study. Arch Dermatol. 2003;139:301–6.
48. Stasko T, Brown MD, Carucci JA, et al. Guidelines for the management of squamous cell carcinoma in organ transplant recipients. Dermatol Surg. 2004;30:642–50.
49. Kimyai-Asadi A, Alam M, Goldberg LH, et al. Efficacy of narrow-margin excision of well-demarcated primary facial basal cell carcinomas. J Am Acad Dermatol. 2005;53:464–8.

50. Spiller WF, Spiller RF. Treatment of basal cell epithelioma by curettage and electrodesiccation. J Am Acad Dermatol. 1984;11:808–14.
51. Honeycutt WM, Jansen GT. Treatment of squamous cell carcinoma of the skin. Arch Dermatol. 1973;108:670–2.
52. Barlow JO, Zalla M, Kyle A, et al. Treatment of basal cell carcinoma with curettage alone. J Am Acad Dermatol. 2006;54:1039–45.
53. Bath FJ, Bong J, Perkins W, Williams HC. Interventions for basal cell carcinoma of the skin. Cochrane Database Syst Rev. 2003;(2):CD003412.
54. Barrett TL, Greenway HT Jr, Massullo V, Carlson, C. Treatment of basal cell carcinoma and squamous cell carcinoma with perineural invasion. Adv Dermatol. 1993;8:277–304; discussion 305.
55. Marmur, ES, Schmults, CD, Goldberg, DJ. A review of laser and photodynamic therapy for the treatment of nonmelanoma skin cancer. Dermatol Surg. 2004;30:264–71.
56. Rhodes LE, de Rie M, Enstrom Y, et al. Photodynamic therapy using topical methyl aminolevulinate vs surgery for nodular basal cell carcinoma: results of a multicenter randomized prospective trial. Arch Dermatol. 2004;140:17–23.
57. Jorizzo JL, Carney PS, Ko WT, et al. Fluorouracil 5% and 0.5% creams for the treatment of actinic keratosis: equivalent efficacy with a lower concentration and more convenient dosing schedule. Cutis. 2004;74:18–23.
58. Nelson C, Rigel D, Smith S, et al. Phase IV, open-label assessment of the treatment of actinic keratosis with 3.0% diclofenac sodium topical gel (Solaraze). J Drugs Dermatol. 2004;3:401–7.
59. Saldanha G, Fletcher A, Slater, DN. Basal cell carcinoma: a dermatopathological and molecular biological update. Br J Dermatol. 2003;148:195–202.
60. Peris K, Campione E, Micantonio T, et al. Imiquimod treatment of superficial and nodular basal cell carcinoma: 12-week open-label trial. Dermatol Surg. 2005;31:318–23.
61. Patel G, Goodwin R, Chawla BA, et al. Imiquimod 5% cream monotherapy for cutaneous squamous cell carcinoma in situ (Bowen's disease): a randomized, double-blind, placebo-controlled trial. J Am Acad Dermatol. 2006;54:1025–32.
62. Tucker S, Polasek JW, Perri AJ, Goldsmith EA. Long-term follow-up of basal cell carcinomas treated with perilesional interferon alfa 2b as monotherapy. J Am Acad Dermatol. 2006;54:1033–8.
63. Ceilley RI, Del Rosso JQ. Current modalities and new advances in the treatment of basal cell carcinoma. Int J Dermatol. 2006;45:489–98.
64. Moore BA, Weber RS, Prieto V, et al. Lymph node metastases from cutaneous squamous cell carcinoma of the head and neck. Laryngoscope. 2005;11:1561–7.
65. Harwood CA, Leedham-Green M, Leigh IM, Proby CM. Low-dose retinoids in the prevention of cutaneous squamous cell carcinomas in organ transplant recipients: a 16-year retrospective study. Arch Dermatol. 2005;141:456–64.
66. Neuhaus IM, Tope WD. Practical retinoid chemoprophylaxis in solid organ transplant recipients. Dermatol Ther. 2005;18:28–33.
67. Otley CC, Maragh SL. Reduction of immunosuppression for transplant-associated skin cancer: rationale and evidence of efficacy. Dermatol Surg. 2005;31:163–8.
68. Marks R. Photoprotection and prevention of melanoma. Eur J Dermatol. 1999;9:406–12.
69. Rigel AS, Lebwohl MG. Hat-wearing patterns in persons attending baseball games. J Am Acad Dermatol. 2006;54:918–19.
70. Wright TI, Spencer JM, Flowers FP. Chemoprevention of nonmelanoma skin cancer. J Am Acad Dermatol. 2006;54:933–46.
71. Grau MV, Baron JA, Langholz B, et al Effect of NSAIDs on the recurrence of nonmelanoma skin cancer. Int J Cancer. 2006;119:682–6.
72. Moore MM, Geller AC, Zhang Z, et al. Skin cancer examination teaching in US medical education. Arch Dermatol. 2006;142:439–44.
73. Agero AL, Busam KJ, Benvenuto-Andrade C, et al. Reflectance confocal microscopy of pigmented basal cell carcinoma. J Am Acad Dermatol. 2006;54:638–43.

Benign Epidermal Tumors and Proliferations

109

Clay J Cockerell and Fiona Larsen

Chapters Contents

SEBORRHEIC KERATOSIS

Key features

- Common benign lesions, typically begin to appear during the fourth decade of life
- Solitary or multiple, tan to black, macular, papular or verrucous lesions
- Often have a waxy, velvety or verrucous, 'stuck-on' appearance
- May occur anywhere except mucous membranes, palms and soles
- Large variation in clinical appearance and may simulate melanocytic neoplasms
- In the very rare sign of Leser–Trélat, an abrupt increase in size or number of seborrheic keratoses is associated with an internal malignancy

Introduction

Seborrheic keratoses (SKs) are common benign skin lesions that are almost ubiquitous among older individuals. They only occur on hair-bearing skin, invariably sparing the mucosal surfaces and the palms and the soles. SKs appear on the face, neck and trunk (especially the upper back), as well as the extremities.

Many clinical and histologic variants of SK have been described and although they are usually easily recognized clinically, some lesions may prove difficult to diagnose by inspection alone so that biopsy for histopathologic examination may be required. This is especially true when there is a history of recent change or if there is inflammation.

Larger dark lesions are sometimes biopsied when there is concern about the possibility of melanoma.

History

The date of the initial description of SKs is uncertain. In 1927, Frudenthal delineated their clinical and histologic features.

Epidemiology

An apparent familial predisposition with a postulated autosomal dominant inheritance with incomplete penetrance has been described for the development of SKs. Despite their frequent occurrence, there are few statistics on prevalence, gender or racial predilection, or geographic distribution. Almost all epidemiologic studies have noted SKs as coincidental findings. They have been reported to be more common in Caucasian populations and to affect men and women with equal incidence[1]. Their appearance prior to the fourth decade is uncommon. Usually, additional lesions develop throughout the course of the life of the individual.

Pathogenesis

Although SKs are common in areas covered by clothing, sun exposure has been implicated in their development. Supporting evidence comes from the more frequent occurrence and earlier age of onset of SKs in individuals residing in tropical climates. An Australian study found a higher prevalence of SKs within sun-exposed areas such as the head and neck in contrast to non-sun-exposed areas in the same subjects. The authors also reported a more frequent occurrence and an earlier age of onset in their Australian study group population compared to a UK study group[2].

Based upon analysis of androgen receptor polymorphism, a recent study demonstrated a clonal origin in over half of lesions evaluated, suggesting a neoplastic as opposed to hyperplastic origin[3]. An alteration in the distribution of epidermal growth factor receptors has also been proposed as a cause. In irritated SKs, apoptosis within areas of squamous differentiation has been implicated as a cause of the irritation[4]. Recently, somatic activating mutations in the gene that encodes fibroblast growth factor receptor 3 have been demonstrated within SKs[4a].

Although SKs are often clinically verrucous, human papillomavirus (HPV) has been detected infrequently, except in lesions in the genital region. It is likely that these latter lesions actually represent condyloma acuminatum, as the two entities may appear similar both clinically and histologically[5].

Clinical Features

Occasionally solitary, SKs more commonly present as multiple, pigmented, sharply marginated lesions. They may be macules, papules or even plaques, depending on their stage of development (Fig. 109.1). Even within the same lesion there may be a great variation in color. They are usually light brown but may appear waxy yellow to brown–black in color. SKs typically evolve from a macule and may progress to become papular or verrucous. Keratotic plugging with follicular prominence, a velvety surface, a 'stuck-on' appearance and/or hyperkeratotic scale are helpful features in distinguishing SKs from other pigmented lesions. Individual lesions may be of any size but usually

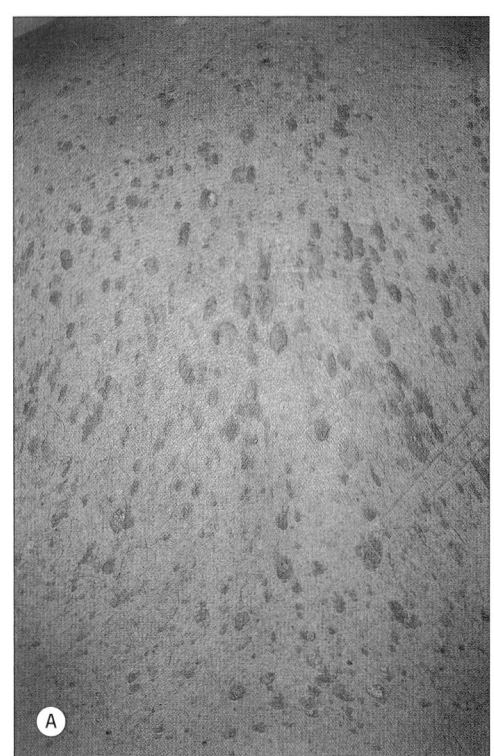

Fig. 109.1 Seborrheic keratoses. A Multiple seborrheic keratoses on the back in a pattern that has been likened to raindrops. **B** Sharply demarcated, pigmented papule and plaques with a papillomatous surface and horn pseudocysts. Note the 'stuck-on' appearance. A, Courtesy of Jean L Bologna MD.

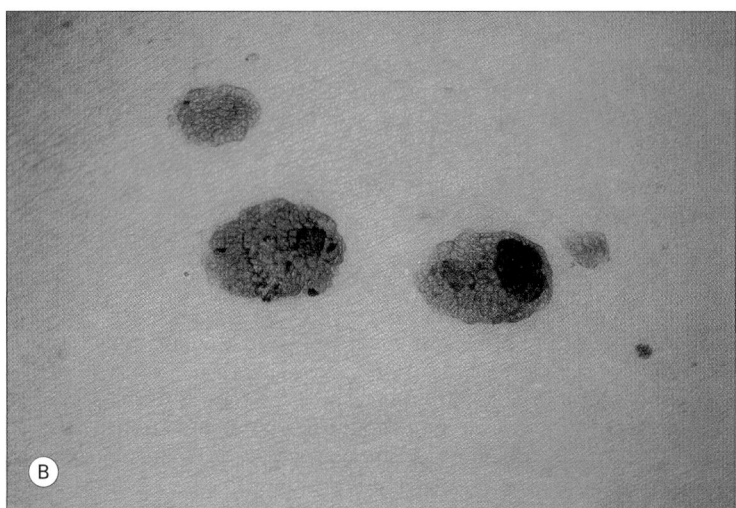

study identified only SCC *in situ* when 4310 cases accessioned as SK clinically were evaluated histologically. SCC *in situ* was seen histologically in 60 of these specimens (1.4%)[10]. In another investigation, 4.6% of SCCs were clinically diagnosed as SKs, and in some of these, features of SK were seen in association with the SCC. The 'collision' theory, when two distinct neoplasms develop separately at the same site, was entertained as a possible cause for this occurrence, especially given the prevalence of both of these lesions in the population at large[8]. Others believe that BCCs and SKs are both derived from the infundibular portion of the hair follicle, cells of which could evolve into either neoplasm, and in some cases, both concurrently.

The sign of Leser–Trélat is a rare cutaneous marker of internal malignancy (in particular gastric or colonic adenocarcinoma, breast carcinoma, and lymphoma). It is considered to be a paraneoplastic cutaneous syndrome characterized by an abrupt and striking increase in the number and/or size of SKs occurring before, during or after an internal malignancy has been detected[11–13]. Associated pruritus has been documented in over 40% of cases and the majority of the lesions are located on the back, followed by the extremities, face and abdomen[14,15]. Malignant acanthosis nigricans, another paraneoplastic syndrome, may appear at the same time or shortly after the sign of Leser–Trélat in approximately 20% of patients[14]. Rarely, in other conditions such as inflammatory dermatoses (see Ch. 11) and pregnancy[16,17], an abrupt appearance or increase in the number and size of SK lesions has also been reported.

The sign of Leser–Trélat was first described in 1900. Its validity as a reliable marker of internal malignancy has been challenged, given the frequency of both neoplasia and SKs in the elderly population, in whom the condition is usually observed[15]. Its description is also loosely defined, which is problematic as there are no standards that quantify the number of lesions required for the diagnosis. The few studies investigating SKs and their link with internal malignancy have largely been inconclusive. One retrospective review examined 1752 consecutive patients with the diagnosis of SK, and of these, 62 individuals were diagnosed with an internal malignancy within 1 year before or after the diagnosis of SK. Of those 62 patients, six patients presented with findings consistent with the sign of Leser–Trélat. However, an age- and sex-matched control group demonstrated similar findings[18].

The pathogenesis of the sign of Leser–Trélat is uncertain, but it is thought to be related to secretion of a growth factor by the neoplasm which leads to epithelial hyperplasia[14]. To qualify as a paraneoplastic process, the cutaneous findings need to coincide with the presence of the malignancy, resolving when the primary tumor is excised or successfully treated and reappearing with its recurrence or metastasis.

Pathology

There are at least six histologic types of SK: acanthotic, hyperkeratotic, reticulated, irritated, clonal, and melanoacanthoma. Different histologic features are often present in the same lesion, resulting in diverse appearances. There are varying degrees of hyperkeratosis, acanthosis and papillomatosis. Horn pseudocysts, the product of cross-sectioned epidermal invaginations, are highly characteristic, though not invariably present. Generally, the base of an SK lies on a flat horizontal plane flanked by normal epidermis. The characteristic acanthosis is the result of an accumulation of benign squamous and basaloid keratinocytes, typically projecting outward and upward in an irregular fashion. The sharp demarcation at the base of most lesions has been called the 'string' sign. The marked papillomatosis and hyperkeratosis are often likened to 'church spires' with shadows of retained cornified material at their peaks.

The squamous cells of many SKs are representative of those found in the normal-appearing epidermis, but some SKs may contain basaloid cells that have a smaller size, uniform appearance and large oval-shaped nuclei. When slight intercellular edema is present, intercellular bridges are easily visualized. Cytologic atypia is usually not a feature of most SKs. Mild keratinocyte atypia and mitotic figures, when present, are usually associated with irritation and inflammation. The papillary dermis in most instances is unremarkable.

The *acanthotic* SK is the most common histologic type. It usually presents as a smooth-surfaced, dome-shaped papule. Slight hyperkeratosis and papillomatosis are often present, while the greatly

measure about 1 cm in diameter. They may become quite large, i.e. greater than 5 cm in diameter. Lesions may become inflamed due to rupture of the small pseudocysts they contain, or from trauma or rarely from infection with microorganisms such as *Staphylococcus aureus*. Although usually asymptomatic, traumatized or inflamed lesions may become tender, pruritic, erythematous, crusted and, rarely, pustular.

'Spontaneous regression', although observed, is not a common feature of SKs, even following inflammation. Conditions associated with an abrupt 'flare' of lesions followed by regression include pregnancy, coexisting inflammatory dermatoses (in particular erythroderma) and malignancy[6].

Seborrheic Keratosis and Malignancy

Instances of malignant neoplasms arising within and adjacent to SKs were reported as early as 1932[7]. Invasive squamous cell carcinoma (SCC), cutaneous melanoma, basal cell carcinoma (BCC), keratoacanthoma, and SCC *in situ* have all been observed in association with SKs. This likely represents a coincidental neoplasm developing in adjacent skin, although it is possible that the various cell types present in an SK could develop into their respective neoplasms. In theory, the basaloid cells could give rise to BCC, the spinous cells to SCC, and melanocytes to melanoma[7]. BCC is thought to be the most frequent neoplasm seen in association with SKs[7–9], although one prospective

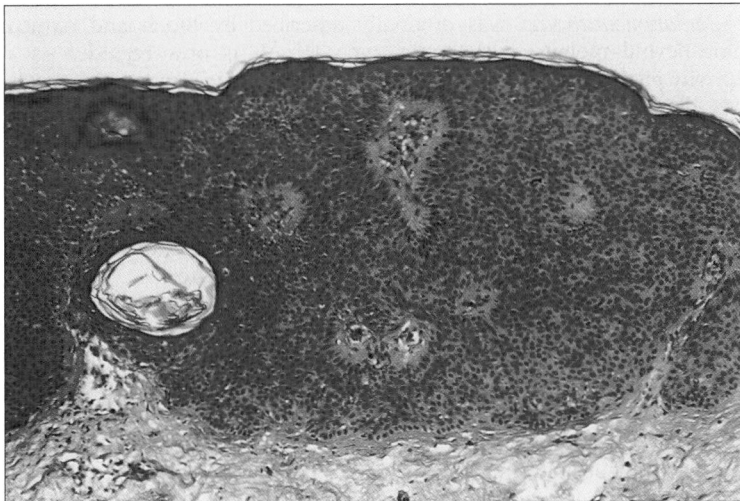

Fig. 109.2 Seborrheic keratosis, acanthotic type. The thickened epidermis consists of basaloid cells. A horn pseudocyst is present.

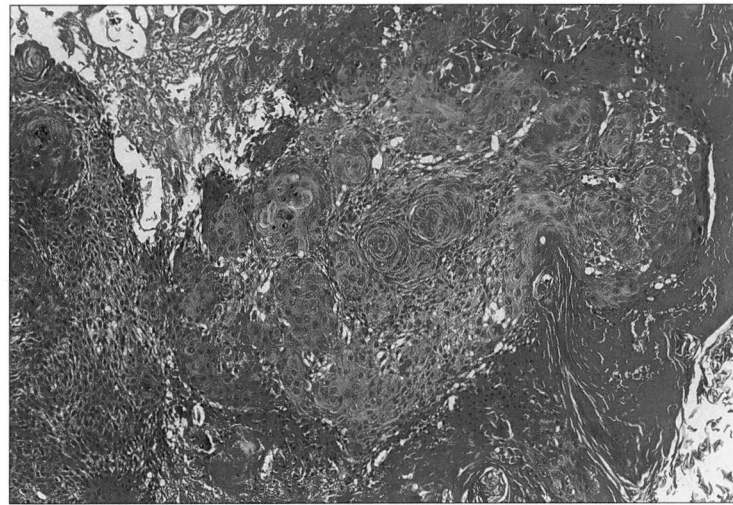

Fig. 109.4 Seborrheic keratosis, irritated type. The cells are less basaloid than in other types of seborrheic keratosis, and there are prominent squamous eddies.

thickened epidermis typically contains a preponderance of basaloid cells (Fig. 109.2). Papillae may be narrow in some lesions, while others may be composed of interwoven aggregates of epithelial cells surrounding islands of connective tissue in a retiform pattern. Invaginated horn pseudocysts are most prevalent in this variant. Melanin is often increased in the acanthotic type of SK; it is primarily concentrated in keratinocytes and is transferred from neighboring melanocytes. Deeply pigmented lesions contain abundant melanin in basaloid cells.

The *hyperkeratotic* type of SK, also known as a digitated, serrated or papillomatous type, is almost the morphologic reverse of the acanthotic type. There is acanthosis but there is more prominent hyperkeratosis and papillomatosis. A preponderance of squamous cells relative to basaloid cells is seen. Abundant pigmentation is unusual, and keratinizing pseudocysts are observed less frequently than in acanthotic SKs. The hyperkeratotic type is the variant often described as having epidermal projections resembling 'church spires', a finding also seen in acrokeratosis verruciformis.

The *reticulated* or *adenoid* type of SK is characterized histologically by delicate strands of epithelium that extend from the epidermis in an interlacing pattern (Fig. 109.3). They are composed of a double row or more of basaloid cells that may be hyperpigmented. Horn pseudocysts, although less common than in the acanthotic variant, may be observed.

A lymphoid infiltrate is often present in the dermis of *inflamed* or *irritated* SKs. It may be perivascular, diffuse or lichenoid. Spongiosis is often present and there may be necrosis of keratinocytes. Squamous eddies are common findings as well (Fig. 109.4). These consist of

whorls of eosinophilic keratinocytes. Irritated SKs often lack the sharply demarcated horizontal base seen with most SKs.

Differential Diagnosis

Most SKs are easily identified clinically, although there are entities that may have a similar appearance (Fig. 109.5). Conditions thought to be variants of SKs include dermatosis papulosa nigra, stucco keratoses and inverted follicular keratoses. They are discussed in this chapter under their respective headings. The clinical differential diagnosis includes acrochordon, verruca vulgaris, condyloma acuminatum, acrokeratosis verruciformis, tumor of the follicular infundibulum, eccrine poroma, Bowen's disease, SCC, solar lentigo, melanocytic nevus and melanoma.

Clinical differentiation between macular SKs, solar lentigines, and melanocytic neoplasms such as melanoma may at times be impossible. Solar lentigines are neither hyperkeratotic nor elevated and some are considered to represent an incipient reticulated type of SK. Over time, these lesions can develop into SKs as the buds of pigmented basaloid cells become thicker and there is greater acanthosis. Dermoscopy may be useful in distinguishing these entities.

A recent review of 20 cases of verrucous melanoma demonstrated how difficult it may be to distinguish between benign and malignant tumors. Of interest, 50% of these verrucous melanomas were thought to represent SKs clinically and a histopathologic diagnosis of a benign nevus was assigned to 10%. A broad spectrum of histopathologic findings, including hyperkeratosis, pseudoepitheliomatous hyperplasia, asymmetry and exophytic papillomatous growth pattern, were present in these cases[19].

Acanthotic and irritated types of SK should be delineated from eccrine poroma. On occasion, SKs may demonstrate 'poroid' differentiation. Clinically, poromas are skin-colored, brown, pink or sometimes red papules or nodules that may be pedunculated and multilobular. Histologically, poromas are comprised of homogeneous, small basophilic cells with a delicate fibrovascular stroma and narrow ductal lumina with eosinophilic, PAS-positive, diastase-resistant cuticles (see Ch. 111).

Differentiation between an irritated SK, an SCC *in situ* (Bowen's disease) and SCC may require histopathologic examination. An irritated SK may be misdiagnosed as a carcinoma if atypia is present. Although squamous eddies may be abundant in both tumors, there should be no evidence of involvement of the dermis in irritated SKs. Bowen's disease demonstrates a preponderance of atypical keratinocytes with vacuolated cytoplasm, close crowding of nuclei, abundant mitoses and parakeratosis. The adnexal epithelium is also involved.

Clonal SKs are considered by some to represent a variant of irritated SK. The clonal, or nested, type of SK is characterized by having well-defined nests of loosely packed cells in the epithelium. This Borst–Jadassohn pattern is also seen in some examples of Bowen's disease. The nests are composed predominantly of variably sized keratinocytes that are often paler than adjacent cells and have a uniform appearance. They may also contain melanocytes.

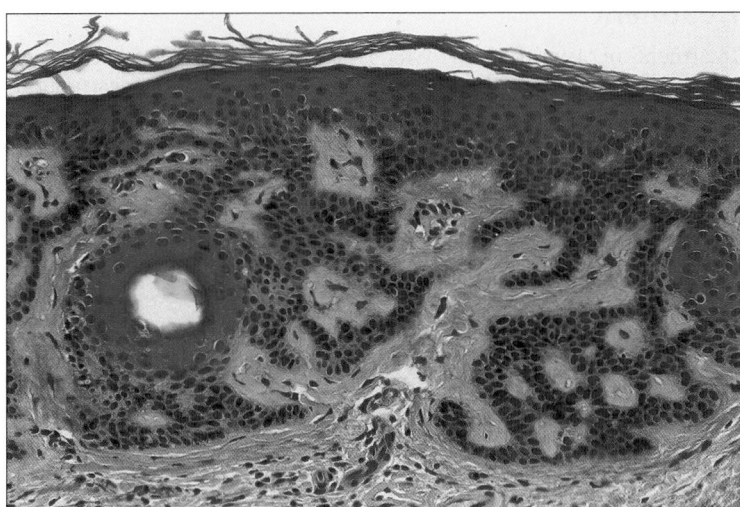

Fig. 109.3 Seborrheic keratosis, reticulated type. The basaloid cells are organized in a reticulated architecture.

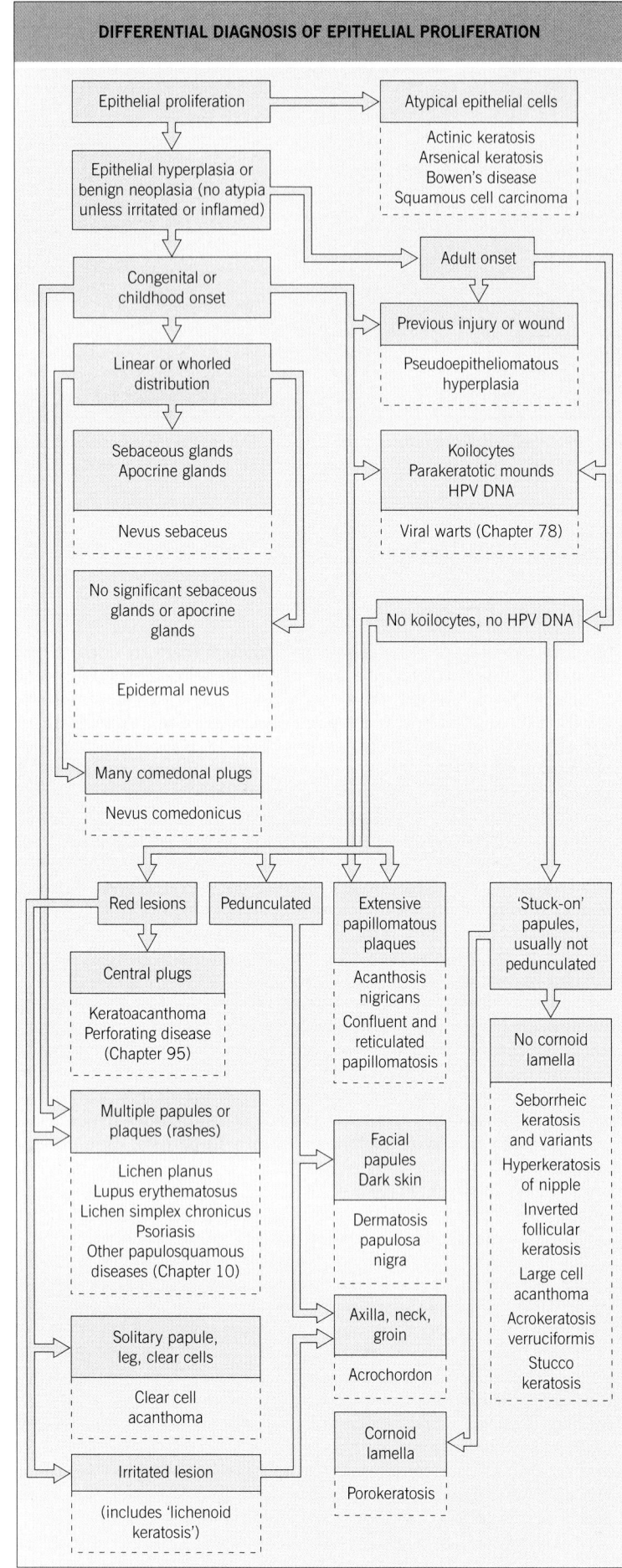

DIFFERENTIAL DIAGNOSIS OF EPITHELIAL PROLIFERATION

Fig. 109.5 Differential diagnosis of epithelial proliferation.

Melanoacanthoma was originally described by Bloch and named 'non-nevoid melano-epithelioma, type 1'[20]. It is now regarded as a heavily pigmented SK by most authorities. In this variant, melanocytes are distributed throughout the lesion. Although the keratinocytes contain melanin, the bulk of the pigment is present within melanocytes, many of which also have long dendrites[21]. Although the melanocytes are prominent, there is no significant increase in their number. The heavy pigmentation of melanoacanthoma has been explained by the blockage of transfer of melanin to keratinocytes perhaps leading to an increase in the amount of melanin within melanocytes.

Intraoral melanoacanthoma or melanoacanthosis was first described in 1979. These lesions bear a striking clinical resemblance to the melanoacanthoma type of SK. Histologically, they are distinct from the cutaneous variant by having only minimal epithelial hyperplasia. Their histologic features are most like those of a heavily pigmented lentigo simplex, with a proliferation of dendritic melanocytes within the basal layer of the epithelium[22].

Verruca and condyloma acuminatum are hyperplasias caused by HPV. Both can clinically mimic SKs but differ in that they most frequently occur in younger individuals. Verrucae often present as rough papules with red or black dots that represent dilated or thrombosed capillary loops at the tips of the underlying dermal papillae. Verrucae favor acral locations, while condylomata acuminata occur in the genital region and rarely on the buccal mucosa. HPV has been reported in anogenital lesions with histologic features of SK[23] (see above). Koilocytic changes of perinuclear vacuolization with nuclear pyknosis in the superficial epidermis may not be present in some verrucae, but are helpful if present. An SK generally tends to be oriented in a more horizontal than vertical fashion, often has horn pseudocysts, and lacks koilocytes.

Tumor of the follicular infundibulum is distinguished from an SK by a superficial distinct plate-like epithelial proliferation. The latter consists of multiple slender epidermal connections composed of basaloid or pale cells, without as much hyperkeratosis as an SK. The reticulated type of SK has a similar pattern but lacks the distinct plate-like growth. Lightly pigmented SKs can easily be mistaken for an acrochordon, which has a pedunculated shape and is usually smoother and smaller in size.

Other conditions with papillated epidermal hyperplasia histologically are readily distinguished on a clinical basis. Some of these include acanthosis nigricans, epidermal nevus, and confluent and reticulated papillomatosis. Epidermal nevi tend to follow Blaschko's lines, appearing in a linear arrangement on the extremities and a whorled pattern on the trunk. Although histologic sections of epidermal nevi typically exhibit acanthosis and hyperkeratosis, they usually lack the pseudocysts seen in many SKs. Epidermal nevi are also usually apparent at birth or shortly thereafter, unlike SKs, which are seen in adults.

Acrokeratosis verruciformis of Hopf has a 'church spire' configuration similar to that described for hyperkeratotic SK[24], but it is an autosomal dominant disorder (see Ch. 58) and lesions are usually limited to the distal extremities.

Treatment

Treatment of asymptomatic SKs is largely performed for cosmetic reasons. Symptomatic lesions are usually removed by destruction, curettage or shave excision. The most common method of destruction is cryotherapy. Other methods include laser vaporization (pulsed CO_2, erbium:YAG) or electrodesiccation.

DERMATOSIS PAPULOSA NIGRA

Key features

- Most common in individuals of African descent with darkly pigmented skin
- Multiple hyperpigmented papules of the face
- Considered to be a variant of SK
- Cryotherapy can result in hypopigmentation; best treatment is scissor snip, curettage or electrodesiccation, when desired

Introduction

Dermatosis papulosa nigra (DPN) is characterized by the presence of multiple, hyperpigmented, sessile to filiform, smooth-surfaced papules measuring from 1 to 5 mm, typically occurring on the face of darkly pigmented individuals (Fig. 109.6).

History

DPN was first described by Castellani in 1925 based on his observations during visits to Central America and Jamaica.

Epidemiology

DPN has a strong familial predisposition and has been reported to have an incidence in selected study populations ranging from 10% to 77%. This variability in incidence may be a reflection of sampling, as lighter-skinned blacks are affected less commonly[25]. In addition to those with African heritage, the condition has also been reported in Filipinos, Vietnamese, Europeans and Mexicans[25]. Rarely, it may be seen in children. Women are twice as likely to be affected as men. DPN is not related to any systemic disease or syndrome.

Pathogenesis

The cause of DPN is unknown. It tends to have an earlier age of onset than that of SKs, but otherwise is similar and probably is a variant of SK. Others view it as a variant of multiple fibroepithelial papillomata (acrochordons). There are ongoing molecular studies evaluating the potential role of circulating growth factors and receptor interactions in the development of DPN.

Clinical Features

Pigmented papules are distributed symmetrically across the malar eminences and forehead. Less often, lesions are on the neck, chest and back. The papules usually appear during adolescence, gradually increasing in size and number over time, and peaking in the sixth decade.

Pathology

DPN is characterized by acanthosis, papillomatosis and hyperkeratosis in a pattern quite similar to the acanthotic type of SK. Horn pseudocysts, however, are not a common feature.

Differential Diagnosis

The differential diagnosis of DPN includes primarily multiple SKs and acrochordons. Occasionally, melanocytic nevi, lentigines, verrucae, trichoepitheliomas, trichilemmomas, follicular hamartomas, syringomas and angiofibromas might be considered clinically.

Treatment

Treatment of DPN is generally performed only for cosmetic purposes, although individual lesions may be troublesome. Care should be exercised to avoid treatments that may result in dyspigmentation, so it may be best at first to only treat a small number of lesions. Snip excision with scissors, curettage and light electrodesiccation are the most common treatment modalities. Hypopigmentation after cryotherapy can be particularly problematic, since melanocytes are more sensitive to freeze damage than are keratinocytes.

STUCCO KERATOSIS

Synonym: ■ Keratosis alba

Key features

- Gray–white papules or small plaques
- Typically on the lower extremities of older adults, especially the ankles
- Lesions are 'stuck on' and, when scraped off, there is minimal bleeding
- Probably is a white variant of SK

Introduction

Stucco keratoses are discrete gray–white papules and small plaques that are hard and opaque, the latter reflecting focal accumulations of cornified material. They are usually distributed symmetrically below the knee, especially on the dorsal and lateral aspects of the foot and ankle (Fig. 109.7). Occasionally, they may also be noted on the thighs and the forearms.

History

Koscard was the first to characterize stucco keratoses in 1958 based on his observations in 24 affected men in an Australian study group of 240 geriatric participants. The term stucco keratosis was coined by Koscard

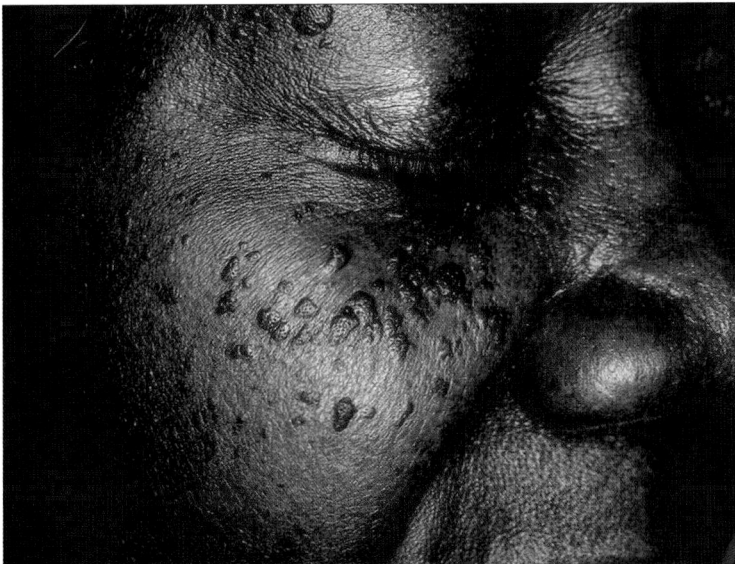

Fig. 109.6 Dermatosis papulosis nigra. Multiple hyperpigmented papules with typical location on the cheeks.

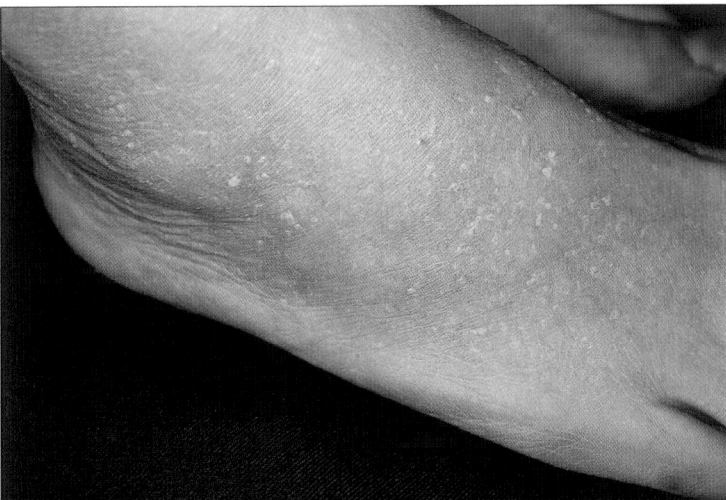

Fig. 109.7 Stucco keratoses. Multiple gray–white keratotic papules on the ankle and dorsal foot. Courtesy of Jean L Bolognia MD.

in 1966, alluding to its 'stuck-on' appearance. Although early accounts of stucco keratoses described elastotic changes in the upper dermis, this has been shown to represent solar elastosis.

Epidemiology

There is no familial predilection for stucco keratoses. They are noted more frequently during cold winter months, which is probably a manifestation of their being more overt with lower humidity and dry skin. They are seen most commonly in middle-aged to elderly individuals and are usually first observed after the age of 40. Men are four times more likely to be affected than women. Most patients are Caucasian, although information regarding racial or ethnic background is minimal. There are no known associated diseases or syndromes.

Pathogenesis

The cause of stucco keratosis remains unknown. Histochemical studies suggest an acquired focal abnormality of keratinization. Ultrastructural examination has revealed no viral particles[26]. However, one immunocompetent patient with extensive stucco keratoses was shown to have multiple HPV types within various lesions using PCR technology[27]. The significance of this finding is not known, as HPV is purported to occur in about 20% of normal skin specimens[28].

Sun exposure has been proposed to be a factor in the formation of stucco keratosis, as most affected individuals present with manifestations of solar damage. However, this may be a reflection of the age and phototype of the patients. Heat and petroleum products such as tar have also been implicated.

Clinical Features

Gray–white papules or small plaques are typically present on the lower extremities of older adults. Lesions on the upper extremity are less common and the palms and soles are not involved. The papules may number in the hundreds. They are usually small, measuring from 1 to 4 mm, but individual plaques may be as large as a few centimeters. Occasionally, brown, pink and deep yellow shades have been described. The lesions may be scraped or flicked off the skin surface with a fingernail and there is usually minimal, if any, bleeding. A collarette of dry scale may remain.

Pathology

Stucco keratoses display prominent orthokeratotic hyperkeratosis and papillomatosis, often imparting a peaked 'church spire' pattern. Acanthosis is usually present, but to a lesser degree than in some SKs. The granular layer may be thickened. Horn cysts are usually absent and cytologic atypia is not a feature.

Differential Diagnosis

Stucco keratoses may resemble SKs, acrokeratosis verruciformis of Hopf, epidermodysplasia verruciformis, or verrucae plana. SKs tend to be larger and pigmented with a surface that appears 'greasy', in contrast to stucco keratoses, which are smaller and have a dry, rough surface. Histologically, stucco keratoses resemble hyperkeratotic SKs and acrokeratosis verruciformis. All three may demonstrate papillomatosis and digitation, giving an appearance similar to 'church spires' under the microscope. Acrokeratosis verruciformis differs from stucco keratoses in that it is an autosomal dominant disorder and involves the dorsal aspects of the hands.

Treatment

As with SKs, treatment is generally for cosmetic reasons, although symptomatic lesions may require removal. Curettage, or local destruction with cryosurgery or electrodesiccation, are the usual forms of treatment. Some lesions soften with application of urea, lactic or α-hydroxy acids, or retinoid preparations, although these agents do not usually lead to their removal.

INVERTED FOLLICULAR KERATOSIS

Key features

- Asymptomatic, firm, white–tan to pink papule
- Typically solitary; most commonly on the face and neck of middle-aged and older adults
- Benign endophytic variant of irritated SK
- Histologically, squamous eddies and inflammation are common

History

Helwig was the first to delineate the features of inverted follicular keratosis (IFK) in 1955.

Epidemiology

IFK is seen most commonly in middle-aged to older Caucasian individuals. Men are affected twice as frequently as women.

Pathogenesis

In 1963, Duperrat & Mascaro proposed that the tumor was derived from the infundibulum of the hair follicle, although the cause is unclear.

Clinical Features

IFK is typically an asymptomatic, firm, white–tan to pink papule. It is found on the face in approximately 85% of cases, in particular on the cheek and upper lip. Other sites within the head and neck region are also affected. IFKs are usually less than 1 cm in diameter, but rarely they may reach up to 8 cm. They are typically stable and persistent lesions, but may regress.

Pathology

IFK exhibits an endophytic, somewhat bulbous proliferation of eosinophilic keratinocytes with basaloid or squamous differentiation (Fig. 109.8). The keratinocyte proliferation seems to surround one or several follicular canals that open to the surface. There may be inflammation. Squamous eddies are commonly seen.

Differential Diagnosis

The clinical differential diagnosis of IFK includes verruca, SK, trichilemmoma and other follicular adnexal tumors, BCC and SCC. Trichilemmoma has a predominance of clear cells, often with a palisade of basal cells and a thickened basement membrane. Rare mitotic figures may be appreciated in IFK, but overt cellular atypia as in SCC is absent.

ACROKERATOSIS VERRUCIFORMIS

Key features

- Multiple skin-colored, small, warty papules on the dorsal aspect of the hands and feet
- Rare autosomal dominant disorder of keratinization, often associated with Darier disease
- 'Church spire' hyperkeratosis, papillomatosis and acanthosis

Clinical Features

Acrokeratosis verruciformis of Hopf is a rare autosomal dominant disorder, and it is often recognized during early childhood. Multiple skin-colored, small, warty papules appear on the dorsal aspect of the

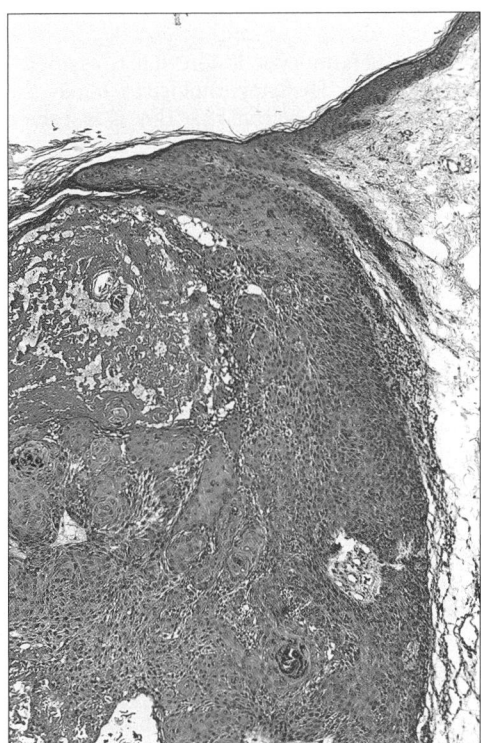

Fig. 109.8 Inverted follicular keratosis. An endophytic proliferation of keratinocytes with prominent squamous eddies is seen.

Introduction

First described by Degos in 1962, clear cell acanthoma is an uncommon red papule or plaque of the leg that may be suspected by astute clinicians, but usually a biopsy is required to establish the diagnosis.

Epidemiology

Clear cell acanthoma shows no sexual predilection and generally develops during middle-age, peaking in incidence by 50 to 60 years of age. It has not been described in children and neither an ethnic nor racial preference has been identified. Familial predisposition is rare, although there is one report of a French kinship with multiple affected family members having disseminated lesions[29].

Pathogenesis

The etiology of clear cell acanthoma is unknown. It was once thought to be induced by crude coal tar and UV light, although research has failed to demonstrate any link with environmental trauma, drugs, toxic substances or viruses. Given its abundant clear cytoplasm, it was originally thought to exhibit eccrine differentiation, although immuno-histochemical and ultrastructural findings are more consistent with trichilemmal differentiation or features of the interfollicular epidermis[30,31]. It may be regarded as a variant of SK in which there are abundant glycogen-containing keratinocytes[32].

Others have proposed that clear cell acanthoma may actually be a localized, non-specific, reactive inflammatory dermatosis. Several benign hyperproliferative dermatoses, including psoriasis, share a cytokeratin staining pattern similar to that seen in clear cell acanthoma. Furthermore, similarities in the histopathologic features between psoriasis and clear cell acanthoma suggest a common abnormality in the maturation of keratinocytes[33]. However, clear cell acanthomas do not develop following trauma and do not exhibit koebnerization, suggesting they are not simply a variant of localized psoriasis.

Clinical Features

Clear cell acanthoma presents as an erythematous, rounded papule or plaque that appears 'stuck on' similar to an SK (Fig 109.9A)[34]. A 'wafer-like' scale is often appreciated, especially at the periphery[35]. The majority of clear cell acanthomas are solitary papules on the legs, but they may be found on the face, forearm, trunk and inguinal region. Lesions are almost always asymptomatic. Occasionally they are slightly eroded and a serous exudate may be present on the surface. There is often prominent vascularity that occasionally simulates a pyogenic granuloma, although the erythema can be blanched with application of pressure.

Clear cell acanthomas usually develop slowly, most commonly over a period of 2–10 years. They range in size from 0.3 to 2 cm in diameter, although rarely larger lesions have been reported, one of which had a diameter of 6 cm. Multiple lesions are rare, with only about 25 cases reported in the English literature, and these may either be few in number or numerous and widespread[36]. Disseminated forms have been categorized as either discrete (<12 lesions) or eruptive (>30 lesions)[37]. One patient had approximately 400 lesions[36]. Multiple lesions show a predilection for the lower extremities and may occur in conjunction with SKs, some forms of ichthyosis, and varicose veins[36]. Clear cell acanthomas with cystic, pigmented and polypoid features have been described, but these are uncommon. They have also been noted to develop in areas of pre-existing dermatoses, epidermal nevi, after trauma and following insect bites[38]. SCC *in situ* has also been rarely documented in association with clear cell acanthoma.

hands and feet and less commonly the extensor surfaces of the fore-arms and legs. It is often seen in patients with Darier disease (see Ch. 58), and patients with acrokeratosis verruciformis can have small, keratin-filled depressions on the palms and soles, as well as nail involvement. These observations are not surprising given that both Darier disease and acrokeratosis verruciformis can be due to mutations in the gene *ATP2A2* (see Fig. 58.1).

Pathology

There is hyperkeratosis, papillomatosis and acanthosis, often with hyperpigmentation. The hyperkeratosis may be quite prominent, and this lesion is often described as having a 'church spire' configuration similar to that described for hyperkeratotic SK and stucco keratosis.

Differential Diagnosis

Histologic features similar to SK include hyperkeratosis, papillomatosis and acanthosis as well as some degree of hyperpigmentation. Clinicopathologic correlation is necessary to distinguish between these disorders. The name acrokeratosis verruciformis should not be confused with the unrelated epidermodysplasia verruciformis, a form of HPV infection (see Ch. 78) which usually has koilocytosis and cytologic atypia.

Treatment

Treatment is similar to that described for SKs and stucco keratoses.

CLEAR CELL ACANTHOMA

Synonym: ■ Degos' acanthoma

Key features

- Uncommon, usually solitary, papule or plaque on the leg
- Lesions are blanchable, erythematous and discrete; they may have attached 'wafer-like' scale at their periphery
- Psoriasiform histology with well-demarcated zone containing clear to pale keratinocytes that stain positively with PAS

Pathology

Clear cell acanthoma displays a zone of sharply demarcated thickened epidermis with regular psoriasiform hyperplasia composed of enlarged pale keratinocytes (Fig. 109.9B). The epidermis is eroded and neutrophils extend from the papillary dermis into the stratum spinosum, aggregating

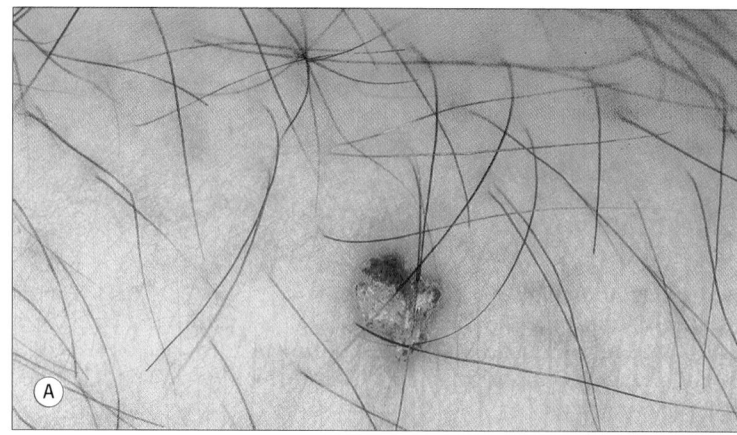

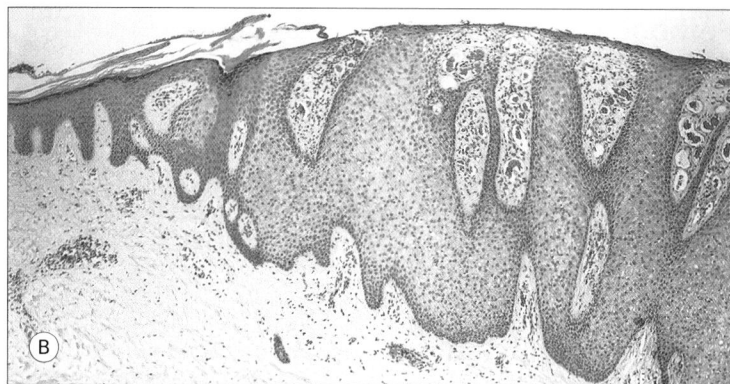

Fig. 109.9 **Clear cell acanthoma. A** An erythematous papule on the distal lower extremity; note the peripheral scale and erosion in the superior position. **B** A psoriasiform epidermis contains large pale keratinocytes. A, Courtesy of Jean L Bolognia MD. B, Courtesy of Ronald P Rapini MD.

in the overlying thin crust. The granular layer is diminished. PAS stains the pale cytoplasm of the keratinocytes red. The material that stains with PAS is diastase-sensitive, confirming it is glycogen. Electron microscopy also demonstrates abundant glycogen within the cytoplasm. Epidermal rete ridges are elongated. The dermis contains dilated blood vessels and sparse perivascular lymphocytes.

Differential Diagnosis

Clear cell acanthoma may be clinically confused with a pyogenic granuloma, traumatized hemangioma, dermatofibroma, verruca, BCC, SCC, amelanotic melanoma, inflamed SK, or psoriasis. Other clear cell neoplasms may occasionally cause confusion histologically, although the overall psoriasiform pattern of a clear cell acanthoma usually allows for distinction. Trichilemmomas usually appear on the face and consist of an inwardly growing lobule of pale keratinocytes lacking other features of psoriasis. The sebocytes of sebaceous neoplasms have a multiloculated cytoplasm containing lipid instead of glycogen, and are positive with oil red O or epithelial membrane antigen.

Treatment

Simple destruction or excision is adequate for removal. Shave excision or curettage combined with electrofulguration is a common form of treatment. Most lesions do not recur.

LARGE CELL ACANTHOMA

Key features

- Small, skin-colored, hyper- or hypopigmented papule or plaque
- Located on sun-exposed skin of older individuals
- Likely a variant of solar lentigo or SK

Introduction

Large cell acanthoma is a benign keratinocytic lesion that is asymptomatic and often ignored[39,40]. Some dermatopathologists make the diagnosis frequently, while others do not believe that this is a specific entity.

History

Pinkus first described the lesion in 1967 during a lecture on benign epidermal neoplasms where he coined the term. He published his observations in 1970, noting its resemblance to solar keratosis[41].

Epidemiology

Large cell acanthoma is seen most commonly on sun-damaged skin of middle-aged to elderly individuals, with ages at diagnosis ranging from 28 to 89 years, and a mean age in the mid-60s. Women have a slightly higher incidence and most affected patients are Caucasian[41].

Pathogenesis

The pathogenesis of large cell acanthoma is unknown. Genetic studies have demonstrated low-grade aneuploidy, a finding typically associated with malignancy. Nevertheless, large cell acanthoma has generally been considered to be clinically benign. Some investigators have proposed that it is a variant of Bowen's disease[42]. Still others classify it as a variant of solar lentigo in a stage evolving into a reticulated SK or lichen planus-like keratosis[43].

Clinical Features

Large cell acanthoma characteristically presents as an asymptomatic, sharply demarcated, solitary, skin-colored, hyper- or hypopigmented papule or plaque on the face or neck, including the eyelid[44]. It also may be found on the upper or lower extremities and the trunk[42]. Rarely, multiple lesions scattered on the extremities are observed.

As it is asymptomatic and often ignored, the time to diagnosis is quite variable, ranging from 3 months to 15 years[39,40].

Pathology

Histologically, large cell acanthomas are well demarcated, with uniform large keratinocytes with abundant cytoplasm and enlarged nuclei. Mild cytologic atypia may be appreciated. There is variable hyperkeratosis, epidermal rete ridge elongation, papillomatosis, or basal layer hyperpigmentation. Some lesions have minimal hyperkeratosis with flattened rete ridges and only small dermal papillae[42].

Differential Diagnosis

The differential diagnosis includes solar lentigo, solar keratosis, SK, Bowen's disease and melanoma.

Treatment

Shave or simple excision as well as destruction are options.

POROKERATOSIS

Key features

- At least five clinical variants of porokeratosis are recognized
- The prototype, porokeratosis of Mibelli, is a plaque that appears during infancy or childhood
- Disseminated superficial actinic porokeratosis (DSAP) is the most common type, with multiple thin papules appearing most commonly on the legs of adult women
- Linear porokeratosis develops during infancy or childhood and follows the lines of Blaschko

- Punctate porokeratosis appears during or after adolescence as 1–2 mm papules of the palms and soles
- Porokeratosis palmaris et plantaris disseminata (PPPD) is a variation of punctuate porokeratosis, with lesions also present on other areas of the body
- Some forms are inherited in autosomal dominant fashion, but many patients have no family history
- A thread-like raised hyperkeratotic border is characteristic
- Histologically, a thin column of parakeratosis, the cornoid lamella, is seen in all variants and corresponds to the raised hyperkeratotic border seen clinically
- Development of SCC is possible but rare

Introduction

Porokeratosis presents as a hyperkeratotic papule or plaque, with an annular appearance due to its thread-like elevated border that expands centrifugally. The disorder was erroneously named porokeratosis because the column of parakeratosis known as the cornoid lamella was initially described as being present over a sweat pore, which of course is a fixed structure that cannot expand peripherally. At least five types of porokeratosis have been recognized. The different varieties of porokeratosis are likely related, as evidenced by reports of more than one type of porokeratosis developing in the same patient[45] and in multiple members of an affected family[46].

History

In 1893, Mibelli first described what is now considered classic porokeratosis: one to several discrete plaques that may occur anywhere on the skin or mucous membranes, usually appearing during infancy or childhood. That same year, Respighi reported a superficial and disseminated form of the disease. Descriptions of linear porokeratosis first appeared in 1918. Disseminated superficial actinic porokeratosis (DSAP) was detailed by Chernosky in 1966. Guss, in 1971, was the first to report porokeratosis palmaris et plantaris disseminata (PPPD). In 1977, Rahbari proposed that punctate porokeratosis be added to the group of diseases already classified as variations of porokeratosis.

Epidemiology

Porokeratosis is sometimes inherited as an autosomal dominant disorder, but most cases appear to be sporadic. Porokeratosis of Mibelli affects boys more than girls, but DSAP is more common in women. PPPD is inherited in an autosomal dominant manner yet is twice as common in males than in females, perhaps reflecting an environmental factor. DSAP is more common in Caucasians and is rare in blacks. Linear porokeratosis has been reported in monozygotic twins[47], and it has been seen in families with other types of porokeratosis (see below)[48], but a specific heritable pattern has thus far not been identified.

Pathogenesis

Although porokeratosis is thought to be a disorder of keratinization, the definitive pathogenesis remains unclear. An old hypothesis set forth by Reed proposes that lesions of porokeratosis represent an expanding mutant clone of keratinocytes. In Reed's view, the characteristic cornoid lamella, seen histologically, represents the border between normal epidermis and the mutant clone of cells. A dermal lymphocytic infiltrate beneath the cornoid lamella or in the central zone of the lesion is considered to be an immunologic response. Supporting this theory is the finding of abnormal DNA ploidy in keratinocytes of porokeratosis[49]. Triggering factors such as UV exposure[50] or immunosuppression due to AIDS[51] or organ transplantation[52] may induce porokeratosis in individuals who are genetically predisposed to developing abnormal clones of keratinocytes. A second, less accepted, theory suggests that the dermal lymphocytic infiltrate may be directed against an unidentified epidermal antigen and that this population of inflammatory cells releases mediators that provide a mitotic stimulus for epidermal cells[53]. A relationship between porokeratosis and HPV has not been established.

Clinical Features

Classic porokeratosis of Mibelli is a rare condition, beginning during infancy or childhood as an asymptomatic, small, brown to skin-colored keratotic papule that gradually enlarges over a period of years to form a plaque that may measure several centimeters in diameter. There is a raised, sharply demarcated, keratotic, thready border with a longitudinal furrow (Fig. 109.10A). The center of the lesion may be hyperpigmented, hypopigmented, atrophic and/or anhidrotic. Lesions may occur anywhere on the body, including mucous membranes, but the extremities are most frequently involved. Multiple lesions may appear, but they are almost always regionally localized and unilateral. It can be inherited in an autosomal dominant fashion.

Disseminated superficial porokeratosis and disseminated superficial actinic porokeratosis (DSAP) are actually more common than the Mibelli type. Small asymptomatic or mildly pruritic keratotic papules, usually ranging from 2 to 7 mm in diameter, appear during the third to fourth decades of life. They are often skin-colored to pink or red in color. As the lesions progress, they expand radially, and the older, central area becomes atrophic while the well-demarcated border develops a thin, elevated, furrowed keratotic rim (Fig. 109.10B,C). Lesions occur in a more widespread pattern than other types of porokeratosis. Disseminated superficial porokeratosis usually involves the extremities bilaterally and symmetrically, sparing the palms, soles and mucous membranes, while the actinic form (DSAP) occurs exclusively in sunexposed areas, most commonly the legs below the knees.

A majority of patients with DSAP report that the lesions become more prominent and erythematous during the summer[54]. Chernosky coined the term DSAP to distinguish this variant from the non-actinic disseminated superficial porokeratosis. He was able to induce lesions by exposing patients to UV light. Other investigators have not been able to reproduce these results and have questioned whether these lesions are really actinically induced. While many patients with DSAP have involvement of the shins and extensor forearms without involvement on other areas of sun damage (analogous to idiopathic guttate hypomelanosis), there are individuals with widespread involvement who clearly have sparing of non-sun-exposed sites. In addition, there are case reports of patients with psoriasis receiving UVB or PUVA treatments developing DSAP. DSAP may resemble and coexist with actinic keratoses, but, unlike actinic keratoses, DSAP almost always involves the legs and rarely the face whereas patients with actinic keratoses on the legs almost always have them on the face as well[55].

Linear porokeratosis arises in infancy or childhood, and it consists of one or more plaques that are similar in appearance to classic porokeratosis; however, the plaques follow the lines of Blaschko, most commonly on the extremities (Fig. 109.10D). Some patients have both DSAP and linear porokeratosis and the latter may represent loss-of-heterozygosity (i.e. type 2 mosaicism; see Table 61.5).

PPPD is uncommon and individual lesions resemble those of porokeratosis of Mibelli except they are smaller and have a less pronounced keratotic border. They may be asymptomatic or pruritic, and generally arise during childhood or adolescence. As the name suggests, the palms and soles are initially affected, but any surface, including mucous membranes, may be involved.

Punctate porokeratosis is the most difficult type to recognize clinically because of the small size of the lesions. It appears during adolescence or adulthood as small 'seed-like' keratotic papules with a peripheral raised rim on the palms and/or soles[56] (Fig. 109.10E). It may clinically resemble punctate keratoderma, Darier disease, Cowden disease and arsenical keratoses, but a biopsy will usually confirm the diagnosis of punctate porokeratosis with its characteristic cornoid lamella. However, parakeratotic columns can be seen in spiny keratoderma in which the lesions resemble the spines of an old-fashioned music box.

Development of SCC in lesions of porokeratosis has been reported in all variants except the punctate form. Lesions in older patients, those of longstanding duration, and linear variants all have higher rates of malignant degeneration. DSAP has the lowest risk of malignant change[57]. SCC generally appears as a papule or plaque arising in contiguity with the individual lesion of porokeratosis, leading to asymmetry.

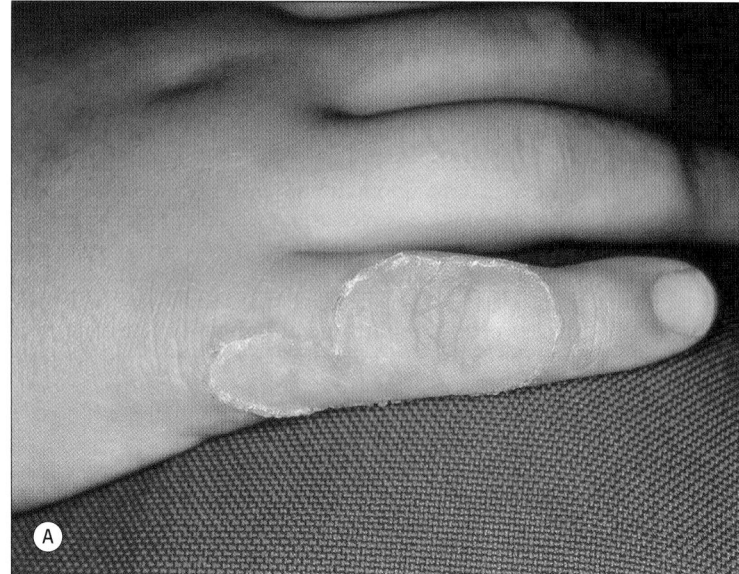
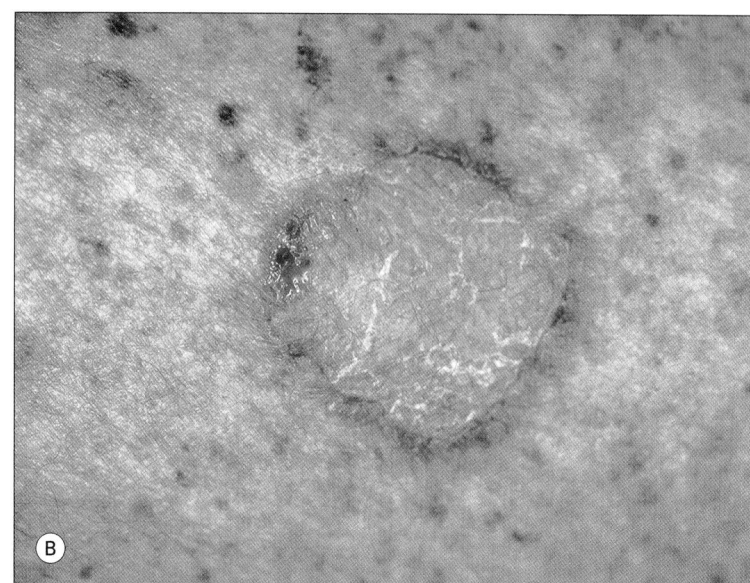
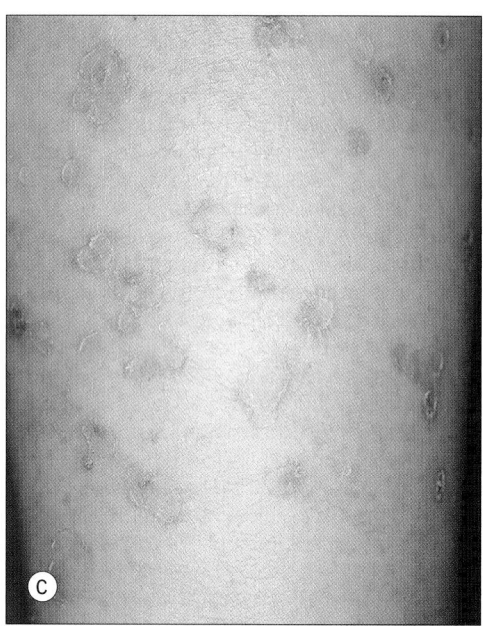
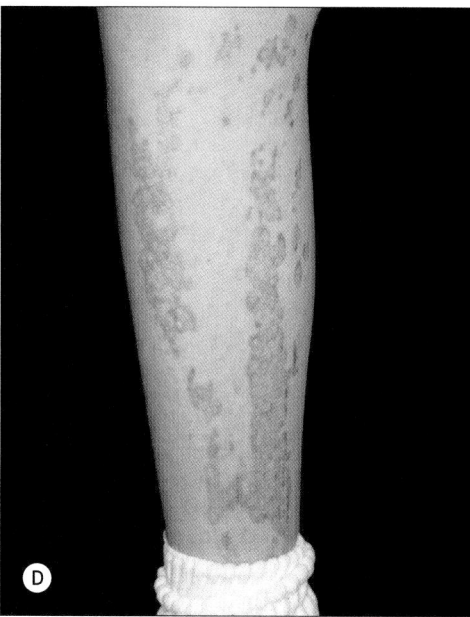
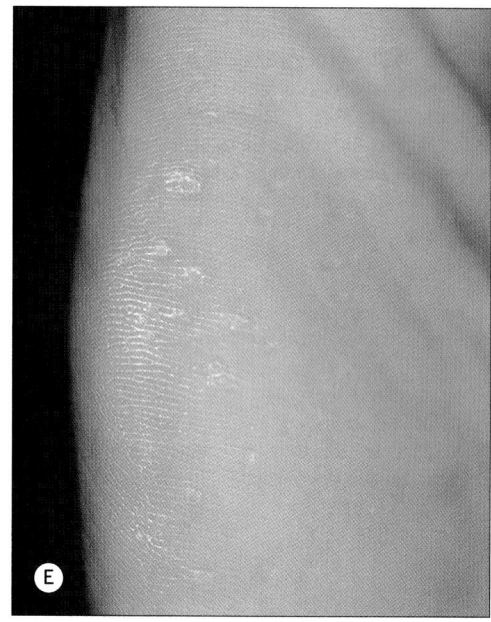

Fig. 109.10 Porokeratoses. A Porokeratosis of Mibelli on the hand of a child. **B** Actinic porokeratosis in a renal transplant patient with significant solar damage. Note the narrow, elevated rim. **C** Multiple lesions of disseminated superficial actinic porokeratosis (DSAP) with obvious peripheral keratotic rims. **D** Several streaks of linear porokeratosis on the lower extremity. **E** Multiple lesions of punctate porokeratosis on the palm. B, C Courtesy of Jean L Bolognia MD.

Pathology

Identification of the cornoid lamella is the *sine qua non* for the histologic diagnosis of porokeratosis, although it may be seen in other conditions such as verruca vulgaris and actinic keratosis. It is characterized by a thin column of tightly packed parakeratotic cells extending from an invagination of the epidermis through the adjacent stratum corneum, often protruding above the surface of the adjacent skin (Fig. 109.11). Under the cornoid lamella, the granular layer is either absent or markedly attenuated, but it is of normal thickness in other areas of the lesion. Dyskeratosis and pyknotic keratinocytes with perinuclear edema are present in the spinous layer beneath the cornoid lamella. The superficial portion of the cornoid lamella trails toward the center of the lesion in a pattern that has been likened to smoke coming out of a moving train as the 'clone' of epidermal cells advances centrifugally. The cornoid lamella corresponds to the clinically observed raised hyperkeratotic border. The clinician should include this portion of the lesion in the biopsy to establish the diagnosis. Sometimes, cornoid lamellae are found in multiple locations throughout the lesion in addition to the periphery. The invagination from which the cornoid lamella extends is less pronounced in varieties other than classic porokeratosis of Mibelli. Corresponding with the less prominent border

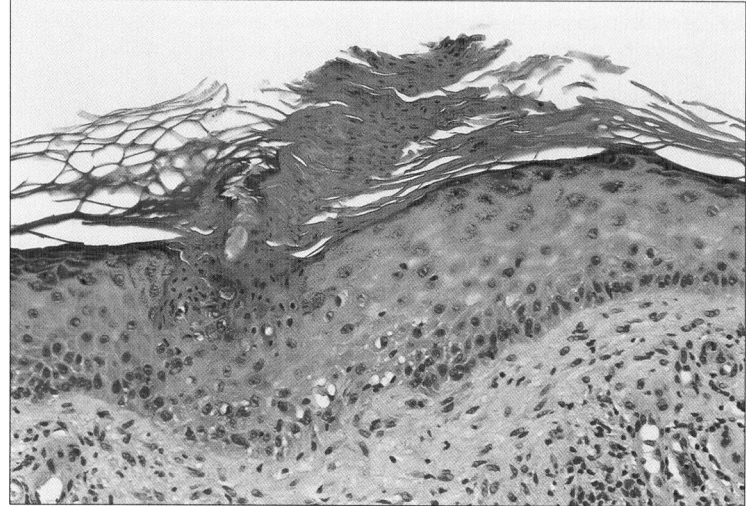

Fig. 109.11 Porokeratosis. The cornoid lamella, a narrow column of parakeratotic cells, is the typical histologic feature of porokeratosis. Note the absence of the granular layer beneath the cornoid lamella.

seen in DSAP, the cornoid lamella in DSAP often does not protrude above the surface of the adjacent stratum corneum. The epidermis in the central portion of the porokeratotic lesion may be normal, hyperplastic or atrophic, with effacement of rete ridges. The dermis contains lymphocytes that may be perivascular, localized beneath the cornoid lamella, or lichenoid in the central portion of the lesion.

Differential Diagnosis

Porokeratosis can resemble other annular lesions (see Table 20.1) as well as actinic keratoses. Linear porokeratosis may be confused with other linear lesions (see Ch. 61) such as inflammatory linear epidermal nevus, incontinentia pigmenti (stage II) and linear lichen planus, none of which have a cornoid lamella. Cornoid lamellae can be found in actinic keratoses, but, in the latter, partial epidermal cytologic atypia is invariably present. Verruca vulgaris often has mounds of parakeratosis that are sometimes identical to cornoid lamellae, but koilocytosis is usually present along with other histologic features of warts. Porokeratotic eccrine ostial and dermal duct nevus is a separate entity (see Ch. 111).

Treatment

Cryotherapy[54], topical 5-fluorouracil (5-FU)[55], topical retinoids in combination with 5-FU, topical imiquimod, CO_2 and other lasers, shave excision, curettage, linear excision[58], and dermabrasion[59] have all been used with variable degrees of success in treating porokeratosis. The abnormal clone of keratinocytes must be destroyed lest lesions recur. Porokeratosis is more difficult to eradicate than both actinic keratoses and SKs. In widespread or refractory lesions, administration of oral acitretin may be beneficial, although the disease will recur following its discontinuation[60].

EPIDERMAL NEVUS

Synonym: ■ Nevus verrucosus

Key features

- Onset usually within the first year of life with 'nervus' referring to a hamartoma of the epidermis and papillary dermis
- Most commonly, hyperpigmented papillomatous papules and plaques appear in a linear array along Blaschko's lines
- In nevus unius lateris (unilateral) and ichthyosis hystrix (bilateral), there are multiple lesions in streaks and whorls
- Patients with epidermal nevus syndrome have associated abnormalities, especially of the musculoskeletal and neurologic systems

Introduction

The word nevus (plural, nevi) is derived from Latin and, as currently used, has three definitions: (1) a congenital lesion (birthmark) or lesion arising early in life; (2) a benign tumor of melanocytes; or (3) a hamartoma. The latter is a benign malformation with an excess or deficiency of structural elements normally found in the affected area (e.g. epidermis, connective tissue, adnexa). In most hamartomas, one element is predominant.

Epidemiology

The incidence of epidermal nevus is estimated to be 1 in 1000 infants. The majority of epidermal nevi develop sporadically, although familial cases have been reported[61,62]. Males and females are equally affected.

Pathogenesis

Epidermal nevi are thought to originate from pluripotent cells in the basal layer of the embryonic epidermis. While mosaicism is thought to be responsible for most epidermal nevi (see Ch. 61), until recently only those nevi associated histologically with epidermolytic hyperkeratosis or acantholytic dyskeratosis had been shown to be due to genetic mosaicism (i.e. mutations in KRT1 and KRT10 versus ATP2A2 that are limited to involved epidermis). In 2006, mosaicism for activating mutations in the gene that encodes fibroblast growth factor receptor 3 (FGFR3) were demonstrated in 'common' epidermal nevi (i.e. those with acanthosis, papillomatosis and hyperkeratosis; see Table 61.7)[63]. Of note, similar germline mutations in FGFR3 lead to skeletal dysplasia syndromes associated with acanthosis nigricans. The possibility exists that additional genetic mutations in keratinocytes or fibroblasts within epidermal nevi may be detected in the future, including those that encode proteins involved in differentiation or growth factor receptors.

While these lesions are classically referred to as 'epidermal' nevi, the hamartomatous process also involves at least some portion of the dermis, especially the papillary dermis. This is evident when treatment directed purely at destruction of the epidermis fails to eradicate the lesion, which invariably recurs unless there is ablation or destruction of the upper dermis.

Clinical Features

In a review of 131 patients with epidermal nevi, the age of onset ranged from birth to 14 years, with 80% occurring within the first year of life[64]. They may occasionally appear during adulthood[65]. Epidermal nevi most commonly present as a single linear lesion, but sometimes multiple unilateral or bilateral linear plaques are seen. Most lesions consist of well-circumscribed, hyperpigmented, papillomatous papules or plaques that are usually asymptomatic. The earliest lesions may be macular and confused with linear and whorled nevoid hypermelanosis. Rarely, epidermal nevi are hypopigmented. Once developed, the nevi may thicken and become more verrucous, especially over joints and in flexural areas such as the neck. Lesions occur most commonly on the trunk, extremities or neck[64] and their size and distribution are highly variable. Epidermal nevi follow Blaschko's lines (see Ch. 61) and may have an abrupt midline demarcation.

Nevus verrucosus is a term used for localized lesions that have a warty appearance. Nevus unius lateris, first named in 1863 by von Baerensprung, is a variant in which there are extensive unilateral plaques, often involving the trunk. Ichthyosis hystrix (systematized epidermal nevus) is a variant with extensive bilateral involvement, also usually on the trunk[66].

Epidermal nevus syndrome, a concept proposed by Solomon and Esterly in 1968, is diagnosed when epidermal nevi occur in combination with other developmental anomalies (see Ch. 61). These abnormalities most commonly involve the neurologic or musculoskeletal systems. Excluding cutaneous manifestations, a study of 119 patients with epidermal nevi found that 33% had abnormalities in one organ system, 6% in two, 5% in three, and 5% in five or more.

Pathology

At least ten histologic patterns have been observed in epidermal nevi, and more than one may be present in the same lesion[67,68]. Virtually all are characterized by epidermal hyperplasia, hyperkeratosis, acanthosis, papillomatosis, and variable parakeratosis. Other findings, such as epidermolytic hyperkeratosis and focal acantholytic dyskeratosis, may be prominent features. Inflammatory linear verrucous epidermal nevus (ILVEN) may have clinical and histologic features very similar to psoriasis (see the following section).

Neoplasms such as BCC, SCC and keratoacanthoma may rarely develop in association with epidermal nevi. This malignant change occurs less commonly in epidermal nevus than in the closely related nevus sebaceus. Malignancy in epidermal nevus, when it does occur, typically develops after puberty[69]. Examples of BCC arising in epidermal and sebaceous nevus may actually be trichoblastomas, representing a manifestation of the hamartomatous nature of the neoplasm[70-72].

Differential Diagnosis

Nevus sebaceus (see Ch. 111), usually found on the head instead of the trunk or extremities, can be considered a subtype of epidermal nevus with additional hamartomatous components of sebaceous and apocrine glands accompanying the papillomatous epidermis. Organoid nevi combine features of both epidermal nevus and nevus sebaceus, with variation often depending upon anatomic site (e.g. head and neck versus trunk). Lichen striatus is an acquired lesion, has less papillomatosis and acanthosis as well as more dyskeratosis and spongiosis, and does not persist indefinitely. There are other nevoid conditions that are distributed along Blaschko's lines and therefore may simulate epidermal nevi, depending on the type and degree of epidermal proliferation. Examples include porokeratotic eccrine ostial and dermal duct nevus, linear lichen planus and X-linked dominant chondrodysplasia punctata. Small lesions must be distinguished from SKs, verrucae vulgares and psoriasis, especially if there is Koebner phenomena.

Treatment

Infants and children with epidermal nevi, particularly multiple or extensive lesions, require a thorough evaluation for systemic abnormalities in conjunction with a pediatrician (see Ch. 61). Full-thickness surgical excision is curative, but recurrence is common when only the epidermis is removed (e.g. by shave excision or curettage). Surgical excision of larger lesions can be complicated by hypertrophic scars or keloid formation[73]. Topical therapy such as corticosteroids, retinoic acid, tars, anthralin, 5-fluorouracil and podophyllin have all been used, but they are of limited benefit. Chronic therapy with oral retinoids has been reported to be effective at decreasing the thickness of systematized epidermal nevi, although it does not result in resolution. Laser ablation may also be undertaken, but, to be effective, it must induce scar and fibrosis of at least the papillary dermis. Therefore, this treatment is often not cosmetically acceptable to patients and test sites are recommended.

INFLAMMATORY LINEAR VERRUCOUS EPIDERMAL NEVUS

Synonym: ■ Dermatitic epidermal nevus

Key features

- Linear, psoriasiform papules or plaques, usually on one extremity
- 75% of nevi appear before the age of 5 years
- Four times more common in girls
- Usually persists for years despite attempts at treatment
- Histologically, psoriasiform hyperplasia with alternating parakeratosis and orthokeratosis

Introduction

Inflammatory linear verrucous epidermal nevus (ILVEN) is a relatively rare, linear, psoriasiform plaque that usually presents during childhood.

History

Altman & Mehregan are credited with the first description of ILVEN in 1971[74].

Pathogenesis

The definitive cause is unknown. As it bears some resemblance to psoriasis histologically, some believe that the two conditions share a common pathogenesis[75]. Involucrin, a structural component of mature squamous epithelium, is expressed in ILVEN in increased amounts within the orthokeratotic epithelium, but is minimally expressed within keratinocytes underlying areas of parakeratosis. However, in psoriasis, involucrin is expressed in all layers of the epidermis except the basal layer[76]. While there are similarities to psoriasis, others propose that ILVEN represents a clonal dysregulation of keratinocyte growth[75].

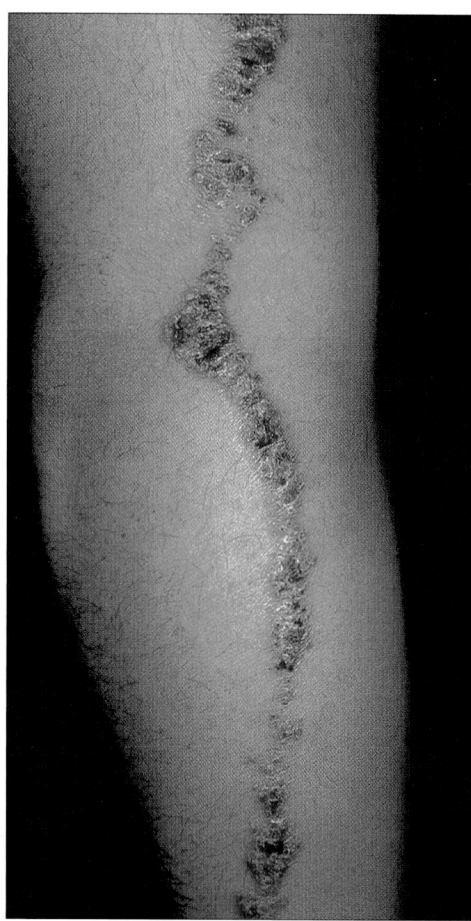

Fig. 109.12 Inflammatory linear verrucous epidermal nevus (ILVEN). Linear erythematous scaly plaque with a psoriasiform appearance on the leg.

Clinical Features

ILVEN has a psoriasiform appearance and may be associated with significant pruritus. Scaly, erythematous papules coalesce to form a linear plaque, usually on a limb (Fig. 109.12), although occasionally the trunk may be involved. Lesions are almost always unilateral. The left leg is reportedly more frequently affected than the right[74]. In 75% of patients, the age of onset is before the age of 5 years. Isolated instances of adult onset have been reported[77] and, rarely, there may be a familial predisposition. ILVEN has a 4:1 female-to-male predilection. Most lesions spontaneously resolve by adulthood[78]. A possible association of ILVEN with arthritis has been described[79].

Pathology

The psoriasiform histology of ILVEN correlates with its psoriasiform clinical appearance. Epidermal rete ridges are elongated, and broad zones of parakeratosis without an underlying granular layer alternate abruptly with depressed regions of orthokeratosis and hypergranulosis (Fig. 109.13). There is often exocytosis of lymphocytes and neutrophils into the spongiotic papillomatous epidermis and occasionally Munro's microabscesses may be seen.

Differential Diagnosis

At least three other variants of epidermal nevi with inflammation have been described, including lichenoid epidermal nevus, psoriasis superimposed on an epidermal nevus, and epidermal nevi in congenital hemidysplasia with ichthyosiform nevus and limb defects (CHILD) syndrome (see Ch. 56). Lichenoid epidermal nevus is typically a verrucous plaque with a lichenoid lymphocytic dermal infiltrate. It is debatable whether lichenoid epidermal nevus truly represents linear lichen planus. The age of onset, distribution, lack of development of additional lesions of psoriasis over time, resistance to therapy, and lack of family history are all features of ILVEN. Patients with linear (nevoid) psoriasis can have or develop classic plaques of psoriasis elsewhere.

It has been suggested that ILVEN may be a form fruste of CHILD syndrome because rarely ipsilateral skeletal anomalies are seen in

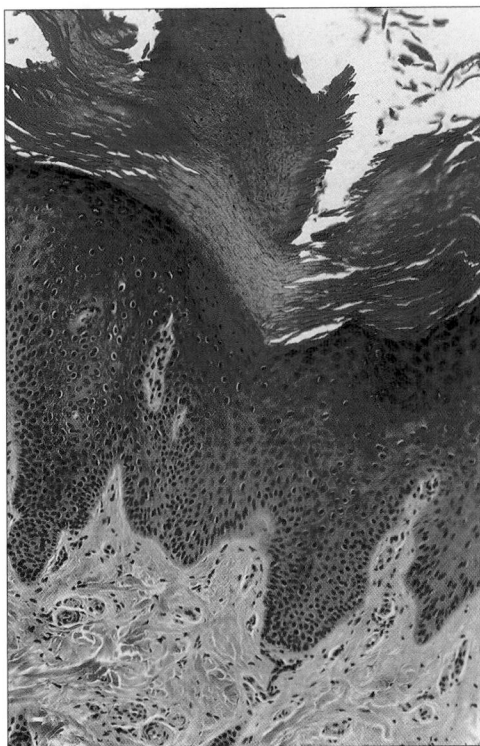

Fig. 109.13 Inflammatory linear verrucous epidermal nevus (ILVEN). The epidermis is acanthotic, and zones of parakeratosis devoid of a granular layer alternate with zones of orthohyperkeratosis.

Introduction

Nevus comedonicus is a rare hamartoma of the pilosebaceous unit resulting in numerous dilated, keratin-filled comedones.

History

Kofmann, in 1895, was the first to delineate the features of nevus comedonicus. In 1914, White attempted to change the name to 'nevus follicularis keratosis' as he considered the comedo-like lesions not to represent true comedones, as sebaceous glands were either rudimentary or absent in most cases.

Epidemiology

Approximately half of the cases of nevus comedonicus are evident at birth, with others appearing during childhood, usually before the age of 10 years. Onset in adulthood, albeit rare, is often associated with irritation or trauma. There is no racial or sexual predilection. Although most cases arise sporadically, familial clustering has been reported[85].

Pathogenesis

Nevus comedonicus is thought to represent growth dysregulation affecting the mesodermal portion of the pilosebaceous unit. The epithelial-lined invaginations, incapable of forming mature terminal hairs and sebaceous glands, accumulate a soft cornified ostial product resulting in a comedo-like plug. In 1998, *FGFR2* mutations were detected in a nevus comedonicus and not in the adjacent normal skin, providing evidence for genetic mosaicism (see Table 61.7)[86].

Clinical Features

There is usually a single circumscribed area or linear streak composed of clusters of dilated follicular ostia that contain firm, darkly pigmented, cornified material. Occasionally, multiple linear plaques may be seen with midline demarcation. Their size is variable and they can range from a few centimeters in diameter to extensive lesions affecting half of the body. The site most commonly affected is the face, followed by the trunk, neck and upper extremity. These nevi may also arise in areas that are devoid of hair follicles such as the palms, soles and glans penis. When present on the elbows and knees, lesions can be verrucous in appearance. Inflammatory papules and cysts can be admixed with the comedones. Hormonal influences of puberty often worsen the condition.

Pathology

Nevus comedonicus consists of grouped undeveloped hair follicles, presenting as dilated invaginations filled with cornified debris devoid of hair shafts. Epidermolytic hyperkeratosis may sometimes be present in the follicular epithelium.

Differential Diagnosis

Many skin conditions present with comedones, and these must be differentiated from nevus comedonicus. Infantile acne typically presents on the face between the ages of 3 and 24 months. The comedones, pustules and papules in this disorder are not linear, and they are self-limited. Chloracne is associated with exposure to toxins that lead to the formation of comedones, generally located on both sides of the face and commonly behind the ears.

Familial dyskeratotic comedones is a rare autosomal dominant disorder in which comedones arise during childhood or adolescence and are widely scattered on the trunk and extremities without a linear configuration. Histologically, acantholytic dyskeratosis in the comedo wall is seen.

The dilated pore nevus resembles nevus comedonicus clinically but differs histologically by containing dilated follicular cysts. Porokeratotic eccrine ostial duct nevi also may be confused with nevus comedonicus, especially when the latter involves the palms or soles. These lesions are comprised of dilated eccrine ducts containing parakeratotic debris. The

patients with ILVEN. Also, although large areas of ichthyosiform erythema characteristically involve one-half of the body with an affinity for skin folds (ptychotropism), patients with CHILD syndrome can have linear keratotic plaques along Blaschko's lines that have an appearance similar to ILVEN. CHILD syndrome differs histologically from ILVEN in that it has features of verruciform xanthoma with elongated dermal papillae and cells with foamy cytoplasm in the upper papillary dermis[80] as well as ultrastructurally, vacuoles within the cells of the lower stratum corneum.

Treatment

As with other epidermal nevi, ILVEN is difficult to treat. Treatments that are successful in psoriasis are only partially effective for ILVEN[79]. Surgical excision is effective but results in scarring. The pulsed dye laser (see Ch. 136) has been used successfully in some cases. Its mechanism of action is thought to involve destruction of small blood vessels in the papillary dermis that supply the overlying epidermis[81]. Combination therapy with topical tretinoin and 5-fluorouracil creams has also been employed with beneficial results, but long-term success can only be achieved with maintenance therapy[82]. Topical synthetic derivatives of vitamin D_3, such as calcipotriol, may also be partially effective[83,84]. There are anecdotal reports of improvement with etanercept.

Arthritis in association with ILVEN, although rare, can lead to significant morbidity. Early recognition is critical. Treatment is the same as for psoriatic arthritis[79].

NEVUS COMEDONICUS

Synonym: ■ Comedo nevus

Key features

- Benign hamartoma, usually arising before the age of 10 years
- Multiple grouped comedones in a linear array, most commonly on the face, trunk or neck
- Histologically, underdeveloped hair shafts and epidermal invaginations containing a keratin plug

keratinocyte cytoplasm is typically vacuolated and the granular layer is absent.

Treatment

As with other epidermal nevi, treatment of nevus comedonicus is problematic. Localized lesions can be surgically excised, although it is often difficult to excise larger lesions. Manual comedo extraction, dermabrasion, and the use of keratolytic agents (e.g. salicylic acid, tretinoin and ammonium lactate[87]) may be helpful, but they are not curative. Isotretinoin is not usually recommended owing to the long-term treatment required, but it may be beneficial in preventing cyst formation. Antibiotics may be necessary to treat secondary infections.

EPIDERMOLYTIC ACANTHOMA

Key features

- Discrete keratotic papules in adults, with epidermolytic hyperkeratosis seen histologically
- Two varieties: an isolated form and a disseminated form

Epidemiology

Epidermolytic acanthomas may appear any time during adulthood. No particular race or gender is favored. There are no reports of familial epidermolytic acanthoma.

Pathogenesis

Because its clinical and histologic features may resemble those of verrucae, a viral origin was originally suspected, but HPV DNA has not been detected in skin lesions[88]. Gene mutations and exogenous factors such as UV light, other viruses[89], and trauma[89a] have all been suggested as causes of acquired epidermolytic hyperkeratosis. Other theories include increased keratinocyte metabolic activity or aberrant keratin gene expression[90].

Clinical Features

Isolated epidermolytic acanthoma was initially described in 1970, while the disseminated form was described in 1973. Both the solitary and disseminated forms present as pigmented keratotic papules that may resemble verrucae or SKs. Individual lesions are generally 1 cm or less in diameter. Isolated epidermolytic acanthoma may appear on any body site. Lesions are discrete but they may occur in clusters and still be considered to represent the isolated variant. The disseminated form has a predilection for the trunk, especially the back[91]; it has also been reported in the genital region. Lesions are usually asymptomatic, but they may be pruritic.

Pathology

The histologic pattern of epidermolytic hyperkeratosis (Fig. 109.14) consists of four components:
- clear spaces of varying size surrounding nuclei in the stratum spinosum and stratum granulosum
- indistinct cellular boundaries consisting of reticulated, lightly staining material
- a markedly thickened granular zone containing an increased number of small and large, irregularly shaped, basophilic keratohyaline-like bodies
- compact hyperkeratosis.

The basal layer is normal. Epidermolytic acanthoma generally demonstrates more papillomatosis than is typically seen in other conditions with the histologic pattern of epidermolytic hyperkeratosis. There is often a slight superficial perivascular lymphocytic infiltrate in the dermis.

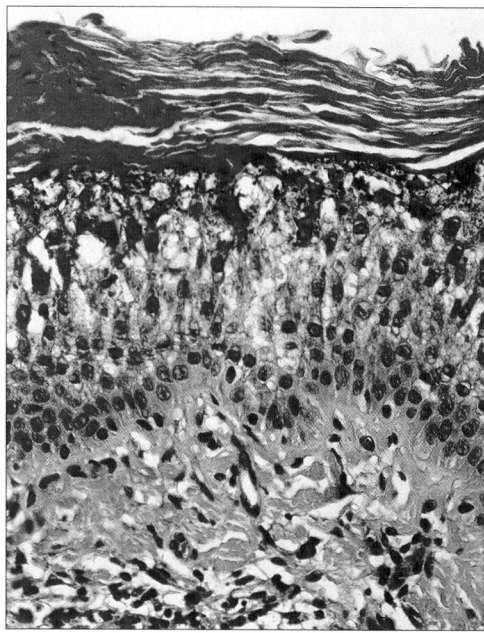

Fig. 109.14
Epidermolytic hyperkeratosis. There is clearing of the cytoplasm of keratinocytes, coarsening of keratohyaline granules, and overlying hyperkeratosis.

Differential Diagnosis

Conditions resembling epidermolytic acanthoma clinically include verrucae and SKs. Because the former does not have a characteristic clinical appearance, the diagnosis is not usually made until after a biopsy is performed. Epidermolytic hyperkeratosis is a histologic finding common to several conditions, including bullous congenital ichthyosiform erythroderma, some epidermal nevi, and Vörner's palmoplantar keratoderma, and it is seen incidentally in normal skin and in lesions such as follicular cysts, SKs, atypical nevi, actinic keratoses and cutaneous horns[91].

Treatment

Treatment is not required as the lesions are benign. Destruction, shave excision or linear excision is successful, although recurrence may follow superficial removal.

FLEGEL'S DISEASE

Synonym: ■ Hyperkeratosis lenticularis perstans

Key features

- Very rare disorder, possibly autosomal dominant inheritance
- Multiple keratotic papules with a disc-like appearance in a symmetric distribution
- Predilection for the dorsal aspect of the feet and the distal extremities of adults

Introduction

In 1958, Flegel described this rare disorder in which asymptomatic, disc-shaped keratotic papules appear most commonly on the distal extremities of adults. The name hyperkeratosis lenticularis perstans refers to the disc or lens shape (lenticularis) of the papules and their persistent nature (perstans).

Epidemiology

Flegel's disease is possibly inherited in an autosomal dominant pattern, although it also presents sporadically. Lesions are usually not evident until mid-to-late adulthood, but they have been described in individuals as young as 13 years of age[92,93]. No racial predilection has been reported.

Pathogenesis

Lamellar granules (Odland bodies) have been shown to be either absent or altered on electron microscopic examination[94]. The lipid byproducts within lamellar granules influence stratum corneum desquamation, and, if they are absent or abnormal, hyperkeratosis may develop.

Clinical Features

Flegel's disease is characterized by numerous symmetric keratotic papules (Fig. 109.15A). Lesions are most commonly observed on the dorsal aspect of the feet and the distal arms and legs, including the palms and soles. Lesions of the pinna and oral mucosa have also been documented. Individual papules are small, typically measuring from 1 to 5 mm in size. There is attached scale which may be more prominent at the peripheral margin. Removal of this scale can result in bleeding. Although most lesions are asymptomatic, patients occasionally complain of pruritus. While most lesions are small papules, those on the palms or soles often appear as fine pits. Flegel's disease has been

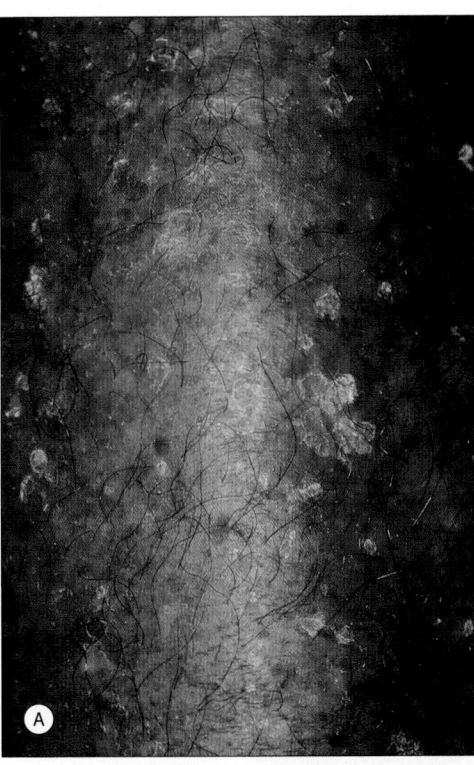

Fig. 109.15 Flegel's disease (hyperkeratosis lenticularis perstans). A Multiple symmetric keratotic papules are seen on the shins. **B** The spinous layer is markedly thinned, and there is a lichenoid infiltrate and obvious hyperkeratosis.

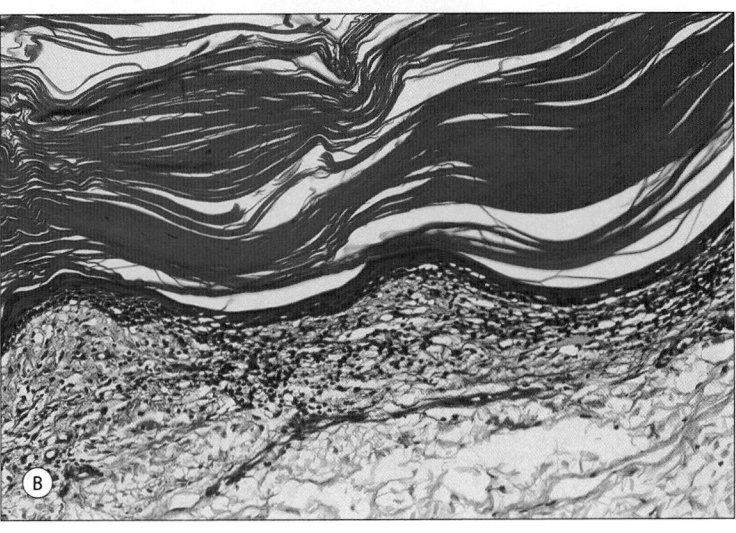

reportedly associated with endocrine disorders such as diabetes mellitus and hyperthyroidism[95].

Pathology

The papules consist of a discrete zone of orthohyperkeratosis, contrasting with the normal basket-weave cornified layer of the surrounding normal epidermis in most locations. There is often focal parakeratosis and hypogranulosis. The thin atrophic stratum spinosum is often sharply indented or depressed at its lateral margin (Fig. 109.15B). A lichenoid infiltrate of lymphocytes is often present in the papillary dermis, along with dilated blood vessels[95a].

Differential Diagnosis

Stucco keratoses present as whitish-gray papules on the legs, but they typically do not bleed easily when scraped off and histologically there is papillomatosis not atrophy of the epidermis. There is no inflammation unless lesions have become irritated. Perforating disorders (see Ch. 95) such as Kyrle's disease have more prominent central keratotic plugs instead of disc-shaped hyperkeratosis, and there is a transepidermal elimination of connective tissue. With the exception of perforating granuloma annulare, perforating diseases rarely, if ever, occur on the palms or soles. Disseminated superficial actinic porokeratosis usually occurs on the legs, and a cornoid lamella is present. Other lichenoid diseases (see Ch. 12) can resemble the dermal changes in Flegel's disease, but the clinical presentation allows differentiation.

Treatment

Treatment of Flegel's disease is problematic as lesions tend to resist all but destructive therapy. Application of topical 5-fluorouracil cream is moderately effective, although it may not be well tolerated because of irritation. Other options include PUVA in combination with calcipotriol. Oral administration of retinoids has been attempted with inconsistent results.

CUTANEOUS HORN

Key features

- Clinical term for a firm, white to yellow, conical, markedly hyperkeratotic papule, plaque or nodule
- Most common in sun-exposed areas and arising from a hyperkeratotic actinic keratosis
- SCC is present at the base of the lesion in up to 20% of patients
- Other common causes include verruca and SK

Clinical Features

Cutaneous horn (cornu cutaneum) is a clinical term for a firm, white to yellow, conical, keratotic papule or plaque ranging from a few millimeters to several centimeters in size (Fig. 109.16). These lesions result from abnormal accumulation of keratin in an elongated, vertically oriented column overlying an abnormality of the underlying spinous layer. Cutaneous horns may arise anywhere on the body, but sun-exposed areas are the most common locations. Men are affected more frequently than women. Individuals with a fair complexion and the elderly are particularly predisposed[96].

Pathology

A cutaneous horn consists of hyperkeratosis and parakeratosis associated with variable acanthosis, usually in association with the atypical keratinocytes of an actinic keratosis. Up to 20% of cutaneous horns arise over *in situ* or invasive SCCs[96]. Other lesions that may give rise to cutaneous horns include verruca and SK. Less common are other epithelial neoplasms, including tumors derived from follicular epithelium,

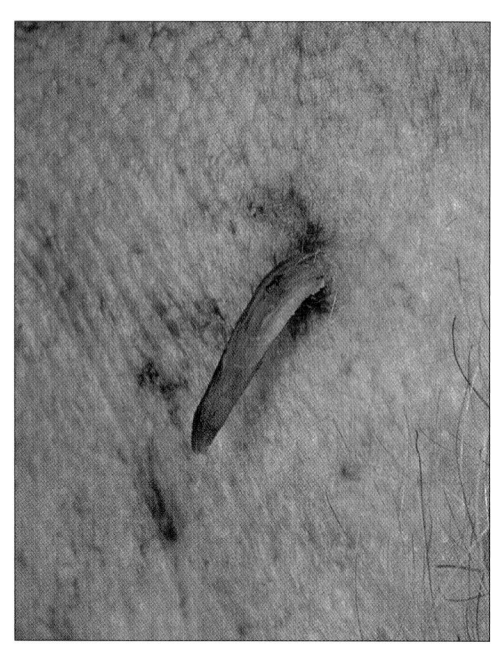

Fig. 109.16 Cutaneous horn. This cutaneous horn arose from an actinic keratosis.

especially trichilemmoma. A keratoacanthoma may produce a horn, but usually there is more of an endophytic keratinous plug.

Treatment

Shave excision with local destruction is the most common treatment. This must be done deeply enough to allow the pathologist to see the dermis beneath the horn in order to evaluate the possibility of dermal involvement by invasive carcinoma. Excision to adipose is best when invasion is suspected. In that case, induration of the dermis is detected, as opposed to the thickness related only to the horn. Treatment of malignant lesions otherwise is as described in Chapter 108. Cryotherapy alone may fail because the base may not be adequately treated unless the horn is pared first.

LICHENOID KERATOSIS

Synonyms: ▪ Lichen planus-like keratoses (LPLK) ▪ Solitary lichen planus ▪ Solitary lichenoid keratosis (SLK) ▪ Benign lichenoid keratosis (BLK)

Key features

- A solitary, pink to red–brown, scaly papule, most common on the upper chest or forearms
- Histologically, it appears almost identical to lichen planus but is distinguished by clinical correlation
- Represents an inflammatory stage of a solar lentigo, actinic keratosis, or SK

History

In 1966, two independent groups reported lesions with the histologic features of lichen planus but, unlike lichen planus, they occurred as solitary asymptomatic lesions. These two groups referred to these lesions as solitary lichen planus and solitary lichen planus-like keratosis.

Epidemiology

Eighty-five percent of lichenoid keratoses (LKs) develop between the ages of 35 and 65 years[97]. Women are diagnosed with the condition twice as frequently as men, and the vast majority of lesions are seen in Caucasians.

Pathogenesis

LKs have been thought to represent inflammation of a benign lentigo, actinic keratosis, or SK. Because at least half of the lesions are related to 'precancerous' actinic keratoses, the term lichenoid keratosis is preferred over the term benign lichenoid keratosis. Lesions are best referred to as lichenoid actinic keratosis when there is significant keratinocyte cytologic atypia or other classic features of an actinic keratosis, and as irritated SK when a lichenoid infiltrate is associated with other features of an SK. The authors prefer to use the term BLK only when the lesion is associated with a lentigo, with no evidence of actinic keratosis or SK.

Increased numbers of Langerhans cells have been observed in the epidermis of LKs. This has led to the suggestion that the lichenoid infiltrate of lymphocytes is secondary to a stimulus from Langerhans cells after their processing of an unidentified epidermal antigen. This mechanism is similar to that proposed for lichen planus.

Clinical Features

LKs occur almost exclusively as solitary pink to red–brown, often scaly, papules ranging from 0.3 to 1.5 cm in diameter (Fig. 109.17A). An astute clinician can oftentimes suspect the diagnosis before the biopsy is performed. LK most closely resembles a BCC, and for this reason, these lesions are frequently biopsied. They are usually asymptomatic, although occasionally patients complain of slight pruritus or stinging[98]. The most common sites are the forearm and upper chest, with less frequent occurrence on the shins (in women) and other chronically sun-exposed sites.

Pathology

LK has a lichenoid infiltrate composed mainly of lymphocytes with scattered histiocytes (Fig. 109.17B). Eosinophils and plasma cells are

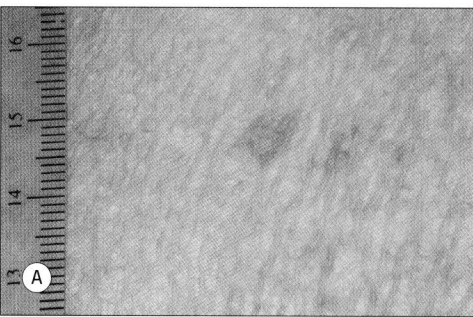

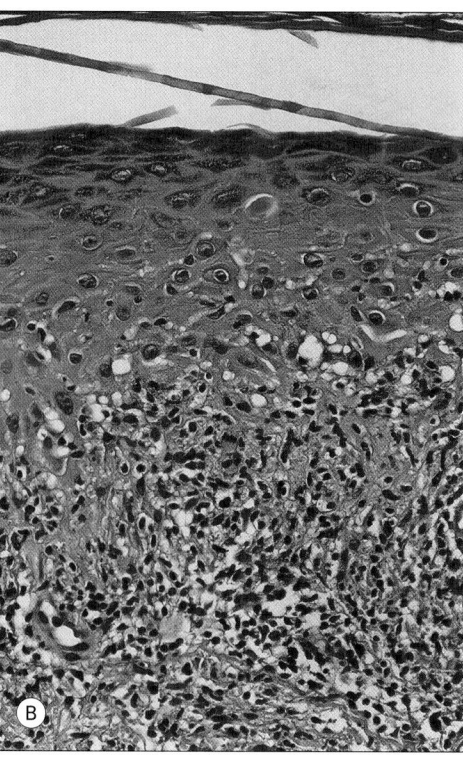

Fig. 109.17 Solitary lichenoid keratosis. A A flat-topped, thin, pink papule that arises in photodamaged skin. **B** A lichenoid infiltrate obscures the dermal–epidermal junction. The keratinocytes at the junction show vacuolar alteration. A necrotic keratinocyte (Civatte body) is seen in the upper epidermis. A, Courtesy of Jean L Bolognia MD.

sometimes present. All other elements of an interface dermatitis are observed, including basal vacuolar alteration, melanin incontinence, and colloid bodies. When melanin incontinence is prominent, and the lesion is clinically pigmented, sometimes the term pigmented lichenoid keratosis is used. Parakeratosis may be seen, unlike typical lichen planus. Sometimes there is frank separation of the epidermis from the infiltrate in the dermis, giving rise to a subepidermal blister or cleft. Basal cell proliferation is absent, and keratinocyte atypia is either mild or absent. Changes of a solar lentigo are often present at the periphery of the specimen. In some cases, a macular SK is observed.

LKs may undergo regression, and histologically, the appearance of a regressed keratosis may be confused with other regressing tumors, especially melanoma. The regressed LK usually displays a loosely fibrotic papillary dermis with scattered lymphocytes and melanophages. Regressed melanoma typically has a dense band of melanophages with lymphocytes and dilated blood vessels. There is also usually a thin epidermis overlying effaced rete ridges. In states of partial regression, remaining histologic clues to the proper diagnosis remain. The end stages of both tumors may not be distinguishable. Careful search for elements of superficial BCC is also advisable.

Differential Diagnosis

Frequently cited clinical impressions include BCC, Bowen's disease, actinic keratosis, irritated SK, melanoma (including amelanotic), and nevus. A recent change in pigmentation of a lesion often leads the clinician to suspect an atypical melanocytic nevus or melanoma[97]. There is frequently melanin incontinence in the dermis associated with the vacuolar alteration of the basal cell layer and damage to melanocytes. The pathologist must take care to ensure that the lichenoid infiltrate is not obscuring melanoma *in situ* or even melanoma involving the superficial dermis, as these tumors may become heavily inflamed.

LK resembles other conditions with a band-like inflammatory (lichenoid) reaction pattern, including lichen planus, 'lichenoid' lupus erythematosus, and lichenoid fixed drug reactions. Clinical correlation is very useful in excluding these conditions. Although lichen planus may be virtually identical to LK histologically, there is usually more wedge-shaped hypergranulosis and less parakeratosis in lichen planus. Clinically, in contrast to lichen planus, LK occurs as a single lesion in an overwhelming majority of patients.

Differential Diagnosis

Once the diagnosis of LK is made, no further therapy is necessary. Any remaining lesion may be destroyed by any method.

ACANTHOSIS NIGRICANS

Acanthosis nigricans is discussed in detail in Chapter 52. The clinical presentation is that of hyperpigmented velvety plaques on the neck and in the axillae, as well as sometimes in other areas. It arises in association with obesity, diabetes mellitus, other endocrinopathies, as a side effect of certain drugs, or as a manifestation of an underlying visceral malignancy. Acanthosis nigricans is not a true epidermal neoplasm. Histologically, it may be misinterpreted as SK, acrochordon, epidermal nevus, or other papillomatous epithelial proliferation, unless appropriate clinical correlation is provided. Acanthosis nigricans has overlapping clinical features with confluent and reticulated papillomatosis. The sign of Leser–Trélat (see above) may also appear with acanthosis nigricans, especially when it is a harbinger of an internal malignancy.

CONFLUENT AND RETICULATED PAPILLOMATOSIS

Synonym: ■ Confluent and reticulated papillomatosis of Gougerot and Carteaud

Key features

- Onset typically during puberty
- Multiple brown verrucous papules or patches in a confluent and/or reticulated pattern, most commonly on the central chest and upper abdomen
- Oral minocycline is effective in approximately 50% of patients

History

Confluent and reticulated papillomatosis of Gougerot and Carteaud (CARP) was first described in 1927.

Epidemiology

The typical onset of CARP is during puberty. Young women are affected 2.5 times more frequently than young men, and blacks are twice as likely to have CARP as whites. Occurrence of CARP is mostly sporadic, although familial cases have been reported[99].

Pathogenesis

Some think CARP may be caused by an endocrine imbalance, especially insulin resistance, because of its association with conditions such as obesity, menstrual irregularities and diabetes mellitus as well as pituitary and thyroid disorders. In addition, there is a clinical resemblance to acanthosis nigricans. However, most patients are otherwise healthy. Another hypothesis is that CARP is a disorder of keratinization. This theory arose because a number of patients have been successfully treated with topical and systemic retinoids[100]. An abnormal host response to *Malassezia furfur* has also been suggested, because this organism is sometimes prevalent within areas of involvement in its yeast (and, less often, hyphal) forms and because treatment with topical selenium sulfide has sometimes been successful[101]. The majority of cases, however, demonstrate no evidence of *M. furfur* proliferation.

Clinical Features

The initial lesions of CARP are 1–2 mm papules, first appearing in the intermammary area or less frequently the interscapular or epigastric regions. Lesions rapidly enlarge to 4–5 mm and become brown, hyperkeratotic, verrucous papules or patches. The papules coalesce and become confluent centrally and reticulated peripherally (Fig. 109.18). Involvement of the neck, shoulders, and back can develop. Oral lesions have not been reported. The eruption is asymptomatic or rarely mildly pruritic.

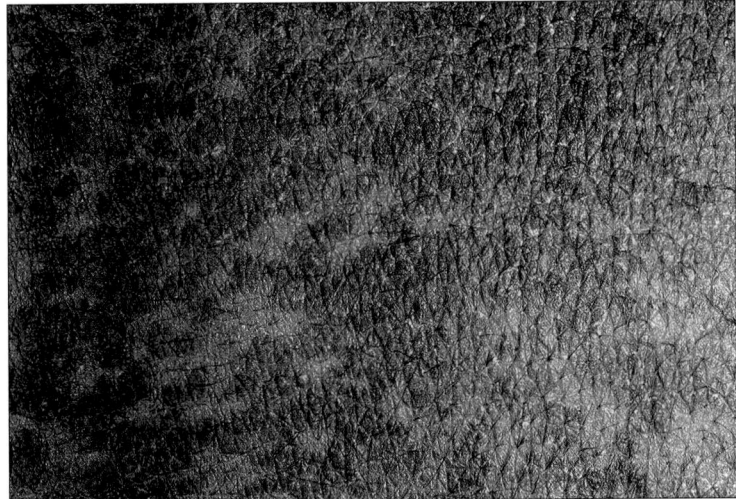

Fig. 109.18 Confluent and reticulated papillomatosis. Multiple hyperpigmented verrucous papules form a reticulated pattern at the periphery (right) and are largely confluent at the center of the affected area (left).

Pathology

There is hyperkeratosis, acanthosis and papillomatosis. Sparse superficial perivascular lymphocytes are also seen. A characteristic feature is the club-shaped, bulbous epidermal rete ridges that protrude slightly into the papillary dermis with pigment at their bases ('dirty feet').

Differential Diagnosis

CARP can clinically resemble acanthosis nigricans, pseudoacanthosis nigricans, Darier disease and tinea versicolor. Acanthosis nigricans has thicker, more velvety plaques involving intertriginous areas; it also lacks the reticulated pattern of CARP. Although pseudoacanthosis nigricans, like CARP, has a predilection for darkly pigmented individuals, it is characteristically associated with weight gain and disappears with weight loss. Tinea versicolor may be related to CARP because of its brownish scale and association with *M. furfur*, but it is neither reticulated nor papillomatous.

Histologically, CARP may be misinterpreted as an SK, acrochordon, epidermal nevus, acanthosis nigricans, or other papillomatous epithelial proliferation, unless appropriate clinical information is provided.

Treatment

Treatment of CARP is often frustrating because it may not respond to therapeutic interventions or recurs after cessation of therapy. No single agent has been uniformly successful at providing long-term resolution. Temporary improvement has been reported with the use of various antibiotics, isotretinoin[102], etretinate[100] and acitretin as well as topical salicylic acid, hydroquinone, antifungals[101], and 5-fluorouracil[101]. Oral minocycline has been reported to be effective in about 50% of patients. Many reported no recurrences, while others experienced disease-free intervals for up to 18 months[103]. Oral retinoids are no more successful than oral antibiotics at maintaining a disease-free state, and, given their potential for causing hypertriglyceridemia and teratogenicity, they are generally considered to be second- or third-line agents.

WARTY DYSKERATOMA

Key features

- Uncommon, usually solitary papule or nodule with a central keratotic plug
- Usually located on the head or neck
- Acantholytic dyskeratosis seen at the base and sides of a cup-like epidermal invagination

Introduction

Warty dyskeratoma is an uncommon solitary papule or nodule usually found on the head or neck with a comedo-like plug and acantholysis with dyskeratosis histologically.

History

Helwig coined the term 'isolated Darier's disease' in 1954. Three years later, the lesion was given the name warty dyskeratoma to indicate its solitary verrucous nature.

Epidemiology

Warty dyskeratoma is uncommon and demonstrates no genetic predisposition. It is more prevalent in men, usually appearing between the fifth and seventh decades of life. It is seen more commonly in Caucasians[104].

Pathogenesis

The pathogenesis of the acantholytic dyskeratosis in warty dyskeratomas has not been elucidated, although abnormal adhesion of keratinocytes

has been demonstrated. Now that the gene responsible for Darier disease has been cloned, abnormalities in the function of its protein product could potentially be investigated in related entities like warty dyskeratoma.

Clinical Features

Warty dyskeratoma presents as a solitary, rarely multiple, verrucous, often crusted, skin-colored to red–brown papule or nodule with a central pore and a keratotic plug. Lesions grow slowly, and they are located most commonly on the scalp, cheek, temple, forehead, post-auricular area and nose. Lesions have been found beneath the nail plate and in the mouth, especially on the hard palate and alveolar ridge. Warty dyskeratomas typically range in size from several millimeters to 2 cm in diameter.

Most warty dyskeratomas are asymptomatic, but patients may rarely complain of pruritus or burning. Bleeding and discharge of foul-smelling cornified material may occur. Warty dyskeratoma has been reported to coexist with other skin lesions, including verruciform xanthoma, actinic keratosis, SCC, BCC and adnexal carcinomas. Malignant degeneration in warty dyskeratoma has not been reported[104].

Pathology

Warty dyskeratoma is well circumscribed, and usually involves at least one dilated pilosebaceous unit (Fig. 109.19). There is a central cup-like invagination lined with epithelium displaying acantholysis and individual cell necrosis, corps ronds and grains, most closely resembling Darier disease. The central crater is filled with cornified debris. Villous-like papillae, sometimes composed of only a single layer of basal cells, often project upward from the invaginated hyperplastic base.

Differential Diagnosis

Warty dyskeratoma may resemble other epithelial neoplasms and proliferations such as verruca, epidermal inclusion cyst, SK, hypertrophic actinic keratosis and SCC. Histologically, other conditions with suprabasilar acantholytic dyskeratosis must be excluded, such as Darier disease, Grover's disease, Hailey–Hailey disease, solitary acantholytic keratosis, acantholytic actinic keratosis, and acantholytic SCC (Fig. 109.20). Most of these are quite different clinically.

Treatment

Warty dyskeratoma is benign, so treatment depends upon the clinical situation. Most lesions are biopsied to exclude the possibility of a malignancy. Excision is curative.

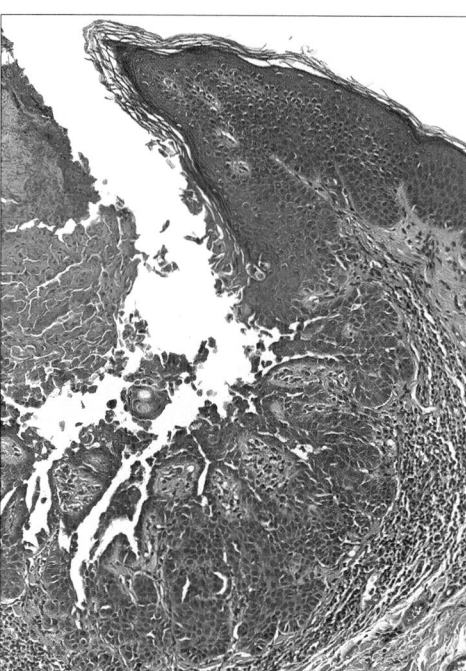

Fig. 109.19 Warty dyskeratoma. A portion of a cup-shaped lesion is shown. The central keratotic plug is seen on the left. The lower portion of the cup is occupied by numerous villi with acantholytic epithelium.

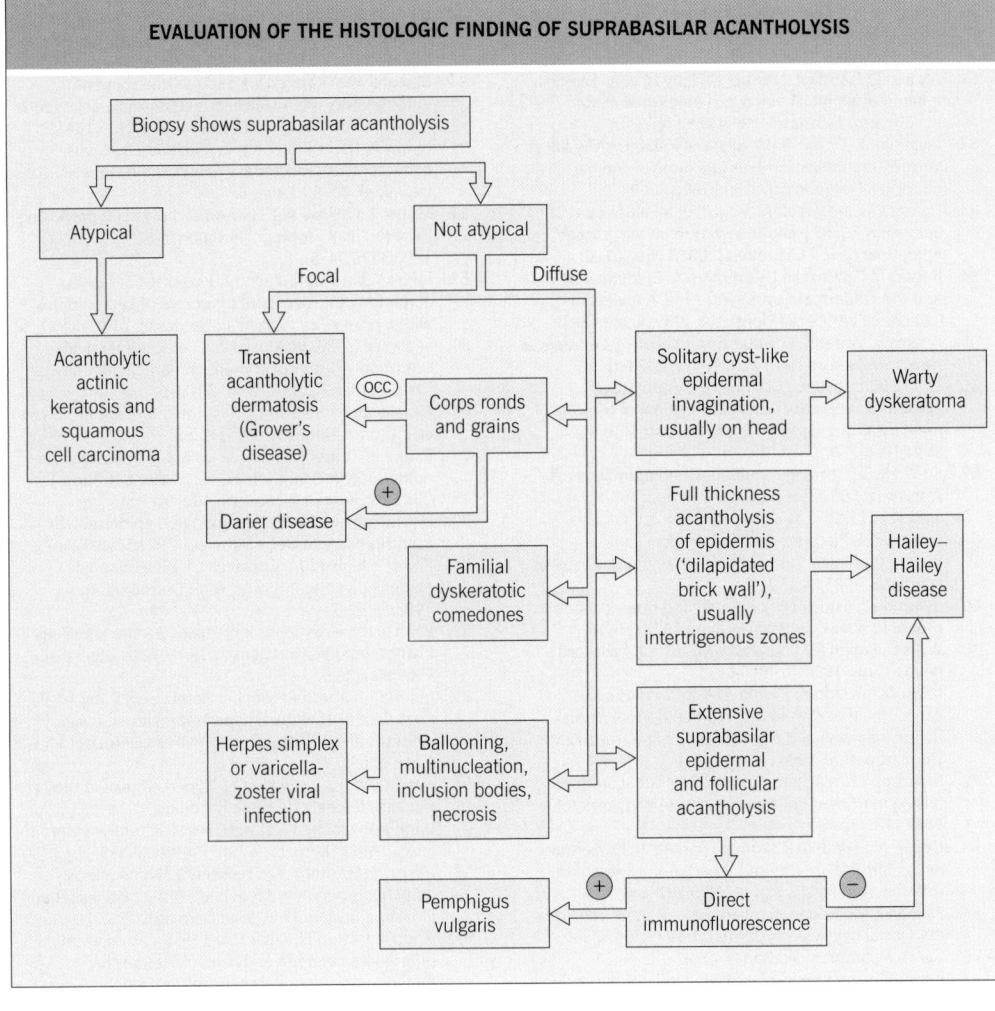

EVALUATION OF THE HISTOLOGIC FINDING OF SUPRABASILAR ACANTHOLYSIS

Fig. 109.20 Evaluation of the histologic finding of suprabasilar acantholysis. occ, occasional.

REFERENCES

1. Verhagen ARHB, Koten JW, Chaddah VK, Patel RI. Skin diseases in Kenya: a clinical and histopathological study of 3,168 patients. Arch Dermatol. 1968;98:577–86.
2. Yeatman J, Kilkenny M, Marks R. The prevalence of seborrhoeic keratoses in an Australian population: does exposure to sunlight play a part in their frequency? Br J Dermatol. 1997;137:411–14.
3. Nakamura H, Hirota S, Adachi S, et al. Clonal nature of seborrheic keratosis demonstrated by using the polymorphism of the human androgen receptor locus as a marker. J Invest Dermatol. 2001;116:506–10.
4. Pesce C, Scalora S. Apoptosis in the areas of squamous differentiation of irritated seborrheic keratosis. J Cutan Pathol. 2000;27:121–3.
4a. Hafner C, Hartmann A, van Oers JMM, et al. FGFR3 mutations in seborrheic keratoses are already present in flat lesions and associated with age and localization. Mod Pathol. 2007;20:895–903.
5. Leonardi C, Zhu W, Kinsey W, Penneys N. Seborrheic keratoses from the genital region may contain human papillomavirus DNA. Arch Dermatol. 1991; 127:1203–6.
6. Winkelmann R. Superficial spreading (and disappearing) seborrheic keratosis. Cutis. 1999;63:235–7.
7. Cascajo C, Reichel M, Sanchez J. Malignant neoplasms associated with seborrheic keratoses. An analysis of 54 cases. Am J Dermatopathol. 1996;18:278–82.
8. Rao B, Freeman R, Poulos E, et al. The relationship between basal cell epithelioma and seborrheic keratosis. A study of 60 cases. J Dermatol Surg Oncol. 1994;20:761–4.
9. Zabel R, Vinson R, McCollough M. Malignant melanoma arising in a seborrheic keratosis. J Am Acad Dermatol. 2000;42:831–3.
10. Sloan J, Jaworsky C. Clinical misdiagnosis of squamous cell carcinoma in situ as seborrheic keratosis. A prospective study. J Dermatol Surg Oncol. 1993;19:413–16.
11. Vielhauer V, Herzinger T, Korting HC. The sign of Leser-Trélat: a paraneoplastic cutaneous syndrome that facilitates early diagnosis of occult cancer. Eur J Med Res. 2000;5:512–16.
12. Heaphy MR Jr, Millns JL, Schroeter AL. The sign of Leser-Trélat in a case of adenocarcinoma of the lung. J Am Acad Dermatol. 2000;43:386–90.
13. Grob JJ, Rava MC, Gouvernet J, et al. The relation between seborrheic keratoses and malignant solid tumours. A case-control study. Acta Derm Venereol. 1991;71:166–9.
14. Yeh J, Munn S, Plunkett T, et al. Coexistence of acanthosis nigricans and the sign of Leser-Trélat in a patient with gastric adenocarcinoma: a case report and literature review. J Am Acad Dermatol. 2000;42:357–62.
15. Schwartz R. Sign of Leser-Trélat. J Am Acad Dermatol. 1996;35:88–95.
16. Schwengle L, Rampen F. Eruptive seborrheic keratoses associated with erythrodermic pityriasis rubra pilaris: possible role of retinoid therapy. Acta Derm Venereol. 1988;68:443–5.
17. Garcia R, Bishop M. The rapid onset of seborrheic keratosis of the breast during pregnancy. J Assoc Mil Dermatol. 1977;3:13–14.
18. Lindelof B, Sigurgeirsson B, Melander S. Seborrheic keratoses and cancer. J Am Acad Dermatol. 1992;26:947–50.
19. Blessing K, Evans AT, al-Nafussi A. Verrucous naevoid and keratotic malignant melanoma: a clinico-pathological study of 20 cases. Histopathology. 1993;23:453–8.
20. Mishima Y, Pinkus H. Benign mixed tumor of melanocytes and malpighian cells. Arch Dermatol. 1960;81:539–50.
21. Simón P, Requena L, Sánchez E. How rare is melanoacanthoma? Arch Dermatol. 1991;127:583–4.
22. Tomich C, Zunt S. Melanoacanthosis (melanoacanthoma) of the oral mucosa. J Dermatol Surg Oncol. 1990;16:231–6.
23. Li J, Ackerman A. 'Seborrheic keratoses' that contain human papillomavirus are condylomata acuminata. Am J Dermatopathol. 1994;16:398–405.
24. Schueller W. Acrokeratosis verruciformis of Hopf. Arch Dermatol. 1972;106:81–3.
25. Grimes P, Arora S, Minus H, Kenney J. Dermatosis papulosa nigra. Cutis. 1983;32:385–6, 392.
26. Shall L, Marks R. Stucco keratoses. A clinico-pathological study. Acta Derm Venereol. 1991;71:258–61.
27. Stockfleth E, Rowert J, Arndt R, et al. Detection of human papillomavirus and response to topical 5% imiquimod in a case of stucco keratosis. Br J Dermatol. 2000;143:846–50.
28. Astori G, Lavergne D, Benton C, et al. Human papillomaviruses are commonly found in normal skin of immunocompetent hosts. J Invest Dermatol. 1998;110:752–5.
29. Balus L, Cainelli T, Cristiani R, et al. Multiple familial clear cell acanthoma. Ann Dermatol Venereol. 1984;111:665–6.
30. Hashimoto T, Inamoto N, Nakamura K, et al. Involucrin expression in skin appendage tumours. Br J Dermatol. 1987;117:325–32.
31. Akiyama M, Hayakawa K, Watanabe Y, et al. Lectin-binding sites in clear cell acanthoma. J Cutan Pathol. 1990;17:197–201.
32. Kwittken J. Clear cell acanthoma: a metabolic variant of seborrheic keratosis. Mt Sinai J Med. 1980;47:49–51.
33. Finch TM, Tan CY. Clear cell acanthoma developing on a psoriatic plaque: further evidence of an inflammatory aetiology? Br J Dermatol. 2000;142:842–4.
34. Degos R, Civatte J. Clear-cell acanthoma. Experience of 8 years. Br J Dermatol. 1970;83:248–54.
35. Fine R, Chernosky M. Clinical recognition of clear-cell acanthoma (Degos'). Arch Dermatol. 1969; 100:559–63.
36. Innocenzi D, Barduagni F, Cerio R, et al. Disseminated eruptive clear cell acanthoma – a case report with

review of the literature. Clin Exp Dermatol. 1994;19:249–53.

37. Naeyaert J, de Bersaques J, Geerts M, et al. Multiple clear cell acanthomas. A clinical, histological, and ultrastructural report. Arch Dermatol. 1987;123:1670–3.

38. Yamasaki K, Hatamochi A, Shinkai H, et al. Clear cell acanthoma developing in epidermal nevus. J Dermatol. 1997;24:601–5.

39. Sanchez Yus E, de Diego V, Urrutia S. Large cell acanthoma. A cytologic variant of Bowen's disease? Am J Dermatopathol. 1988;10:197–208.

40. Rabinowitz A, Inghirami G. Large-cell acanthoma. A distinctive keratosis. Am J Dermatopathol. 1992;14:136–8.

41. Pinkus H. Epidermal mosaic in benign and precancerous neoplasia (with special reference to large-cell acanthoma). Acta Dermatol (Kyoto). 1970;65:75–81.

42. Sanchez Yus E, del Rio E, Requena L. Large-cell acanthoma is a distinctive condition. Am J Dermatopathol. 1992;14:140–8.

43. Roewert H, Ackerman A. Large-cell acanthoma is a solar lentigo. Am J Dermatopathol. 1992;14:122–32.

44. Chevez P, Patrinely J, Font R. Large-cell acanthoma of the eyelid. Report of two cases. Arch Ophthalmol. 1991;109:1433–4.

45. Dover JS, Phillips TJ, Burns DA. Disseminated superficial actinic porokeratosis: coexistence with other porokeratotic variants. Arch Dermatol. 1986;122:887–9.

46. Lucker GP, Steiflen PM. The coexistence of linear and giant porokeratosis associated with Bowen's disease. Dermatology. 1994;189:78–80.

47. Guillot P. Porokeratose de Mibelli lineaire chez des jumelles monozygotes. Ann Dermatol Venereol. 1991;118:519–24.

48. Commens CA, Shumack SP. Linear porokeratosis in two families with disseminated superficial actinic porokeratosis. Pediatr Dermatol. 1987;4:209–14.

49. Otsuka F, Chi HI, Shima A. Cytological demonstration of abnormal DNA ploidy in the epidermis of porokeratosis. Arch Dermatol Res. 1988;230:61–3.

50. Cockerell CJ. Induction of disseminated superficial actinic porokeratosis by phototherapy for psoriasis. J Am Acad Dermatol. 1991;24:301–2.

51. Kanitakis J. Disseminated superficial porokeratosis in a patient with AIDS. Br J Dermatol. 1994;131:284–9.

52. Fields LL. Rapid development of disseminated superficial porokeratosis after transplant induction therapy. Bone Marrow Transplant. 1995;15:993–5.

53. Raychaudhuri SP, Smoller BR. Porokeratosis in immunosuppressed and nonimmunosuppressed patients. Int J Dermatol. 1992;31:781–2.

54. Shumack SP, Commens CA. Disseminated superficial actinic porokeratosis: a clinical study. J Am Acad Dermatol. 1989;20:1015–22.

55. McDonald SG, Peterka ES. Porokeratosis (Mibelli): treatment with topical 5-fluorouracil. J Am Acad Dermatol. 1983;8:107–10.

56. Rahbari H, Cordero A, Mehregan A. Punctate porokeratosis. A clinical variant of porokeratosis of Mibelli. J Cutan Pathol. 1977;4:338–41.

57. Sasson M, Krain A. Porokeratosis and cutaneous malignancy: a review. Dermatol Surg. 1996; 22:339–42.

58. Rabbin PE, Baldwin HE. Treatment of porokeratosis of Mibelli with CO$_2$ laser vaporization versus surgical excision with split-thickness skin graft: a comparison. J Dermatol Surg Oncol. 1993;19:199–202.

59. Spencer JM, Katz BE. Successful treatment of porokeratosis of Mibelli with diamond fraise abrasion. Arch Dermatol. 1992;128:1187–8.

60. Goldman GD, Milstone LM. Generalized linear porokeratosis treated with etretinate. Arch Dermatol. 1995;131:496–7.

61. Alsaleh Q, Nanda A, Hassab-el-Naby H, et al. Familial inflammatory linear verrucous epidermal nevus (ILVEN). Int J Dermatol. 1994;33:52–4.

62. Goldman K, Don P. Adult onset of inflammatory linear verrucous epidermal nevus in a mother and her daughter. Dermatology. 1994;189:170–2.

63. Hafner C, van Oers JMM, Vogt T, et al. Mosaicism of activating FGFR3 mutations in human skin causes epidermal nevi. J Clin Invest. 2006;116:2201–6.

64. Rogers M, McCrossin I, Commens C. Epidermal nevi and the epidermal nevus syndrome. A review of 131 cases. J Am Acad Dermatol. 1989;20:476–88.

65. Adams B, Mutasim D. Adult onset verrucous epidermal nevus. J Am Acad Dermatol. 1999;41:824–6.

66. Loff H, Bardenstein D, Levine M. Systematized epidermal nevi: case report and review of clinical manifestations. Ophthal Plast Reconstr Surg. 1994;10:262–6.

67. Su W. Histopathologic varieties of epidermal nevus. A study of 160 cases. Am J Dermatopathol. 1982;4:161–70.

68. Submoke S, Piamphongsant T. Clinico-histopathological study of epidermal naevi. Australas J Dermatol. 1983;24:130–6.

69. Solomon L, Esterly N. Epidermal and other congenital organoid nevi. Curr Probl Pediatr. 1975;6:1–56.

70. Willis D, Rapini RP, Chernosky ME. Linear basal cell nevus. Cutis. 1990;46:493–4.

71. Levin A, Amazon K, Rywlin A. A squamous cell carcinoma that developed in an epidermal nevus. Report of a case and a review of the literature. Am J Dermatopathol. 1984;6:51–5.

72. Braunstein B, Mackel S, Cooper P. Keratoacanthoma arising in a linear epidermal nevus. Arch Dermatol. 1982;118:362–3.

73. Dellon AL, Luethke R, Wong L, Barnett N. Epidermal nevus: surgical treatment by partial-thickness skin excision. Ann Plast Surg. 1992;28:292–6.

74. Altman J, Mehregan A. Inflammatory linear verrucose epidermal nevus. Arch Dermatol. 1971;104:385–9.

75. Welch M, Smith K, Skelton H, et al. Immunohistochemical features in inflammatory linear verrucous epidermal nevi suggest a distinctive pattern of clonal dysregulation of growth. Military Medical Consortium for the Advancement of Retroviral Research. J Am Acad Dermatol. 1993;29:242–8.

76. Ito M, Shimizu N, Fujiwara H, et al. Histopathogenesis of inflammatory linear verrucose epidermal naevus: histochemistry, immunohistochemistry and ultrastructure. Arch Dermatol Res. 1991;283:491–9.

77. Kawaguchi H, Takeuchi M, Ono H, et al. Adult onset of inflammatory linear verrucous epidermal nevus. J Dermatol. 1999;26:599–602.

78. Morag C, Metzker A. Inflammatory linear verrucous epidermal nevus: report of seven new cases and review of the literature. Pediatr Dermatol. 1985;3:15–18.

79. Al-Enezi S, Huber A, Krafchik B, et al. Inflammatory linear verrucous epidermal nevus and arthritis: a new association. J Pediatr. 2001;138:602–4.

80. Happle R. How many epidermal nevus syndromes exist? A clinicogenetic classification. J Am Acad Dermatol. 1991;25:550–6.

81. Altster T. Inflammatory linear verrucous epidermal nevus: successful treatment with the 585 nm flashlamp-pumped pulsed dye laser. J Am Acad Dermatol. 1994;31:513–14.

82. Kim J, Chang M, Shwayder T. Topical tretinoin and 5-fluorouracil in the treatment of linear verrucous epidermal nevus. J Am Acad Dermatol. 2000;43:129–32.

83. Gatti S, Carrozzo AM, Orlandi A, et al. Treatment of inflammatory linear verrucous epidermal naevus with calcipotriol. Br J Dermatol. 1995;132:837–9.

84. Mitsuhashi Y, Katagiri Y, Kondo S. Treatment of inflammatory linear verrucous epidermal naevus with topical vitamin D3. Br J Dermatol. 1997;136:134–5.

85. Patrizi A, Neri I, Fiorentini C, Marzaduri S. Nevus comedonicus syndrome: a new pediatric case. Pediatr Dermatol. 1998;15:304–6.

86. Munro CS, Wilkie AO. Epidermal mosaicism producing localised acne: somatic mutation in FGFR2. Lancet. 1998;352:704–5.

87. Inoue Y, Miyamoto Y, Ono T. Two cases of nevus comedonicus: successful treatment of keratin plugs with a pore strip. J Am Acad Dermatol. 2000;43:927–9.

88. Leonardi C, Zhu W, Kinsey W, et al. Epidermolytic acanthoma does not contain human papillomavirus DNA. J Cutan Pathol. 1991;18:103–5.

89. Metzler G, Sonnichsen K. Disseminated epidermolytic acanthoma. Hautarzt. 1997;48:740–2.

89a. Banky JP, Turner RJ, Hollowood K. Multiple scrotal epidermolytic acanthomas; secondary to trauma? Clin Exp Dermatol. 2004; 29: 489–91.

90. Hirone T, Fukushiro R. Disseminated epidermolytic acanthoma. Acta Derm Venereol. 1973;53:393–402.

91. Knipper JE, Hud JA, Cockerell CJ. Disseminated epidermolytic acanthoma. Am J Dermatopathol. 1993;15:70–2.

92. Bean S. Hyperkeratosis lenticularis perstans: a clinical, histopathologic, and genetic study. Arch Dermatol. 1969;99:705–9.

93. Miranda-Romero A, Sanchez Sambucety P, Bajo del Pozo C, et al. Unilateral hyperkeratosis lenticularis perstans (Flegel's disease). J Am Acad Dermatol. 1998;39:655–7.

94. Jang K, Choi J, Sung K, et al. Hyperkeratosis lenticularis perstans (Flegel's disease): histologic, immunohistochemical, and ultrastructural features in a case. Am J Dermatopathol. 1999;21:395–8.

95. Pearson LH, Smith JG, Chalker DK. Hyperkeratosis lenticularis perstans (Flegel's disease): case report and literature review. J Am Acad Dermatol. 1987;16:190–5.

95a. Ando K, Hattori H, Yamauchi Y. Histopathological differences between early and old lesions of hyperkeratosis lenticularis perstans (Flegel's disease). Am J Dermatopathol. 2006;28:122–6.

96. Korkut T, Tan NB, Oztan Y. Giant cutaneous horn: a patient report. Ann Plast Surg. 1997;39:654–5.

97. Berger TG, Graham JH, Goette DK. Lichenoid benign keratosis. J Am Acad Dermatol. 1984;11:635–8.

98. Prieto VG, Casal M, McNutt NS. Lichen planus-like keratosis: a clinical and histologic reexamination. Am J Surg Pathol. 1993;259–63.

99. Henning JP, de Wit RFE. Familial occurrence of confluent and reticulated papillomatosis. Arch Dermatol. 1981;117:809–10.

100. Buynzeel-Koomen CAFM, de Wit RFE. Confluent and reticulated papillomatosis successfully treated with aromatic etretinate. Arch Dermatol. 1984;120:1236–7.

101. Nordby AC, Mitchell AJ. Confluent and reticulated papillomatosis responsive to selenium sulfide. Int J Dermatol. 1986;25:194–9.

102. Lee MP, Stiller MJ, McClain SA, et al. Confluent and reticulated papillomatosis: response to high-dose oral isotretinoin therapy and reassessment of epidemiologic data. J Am Acad Dermatol. 1994;31:327–31.

103. Chang SN, Kim SC, Lee SH, Lee WS. Minocycline treatment for confluent and reticulated papillomatosis. Cutis. 1996;57:454–7.

104. Tanay A, Mehregan A. Warty dyskeratoma. Dermatologica. 1969;138:155–64.

Cysts

Mary Seabury Stone

110

Key features

- Many different types of cutaneous cysts have been described
- Cutaneous cysts present as circumscribed dermal or subcutaneous papules or nodules
- Histologic features of the cyst lining and the anatomic location determine the type of cyst
- Cysts may be lined by stratified squamous epithelium, non-stratified squamous epithelium, or no epithelium at all
- Treatment of cysts, when indicated, is primarily surgical

INTRODUCTION

Cysts are common cutaneous lesions. Patients with cysts may present to clinicians because of medical or cosmetic concerns, or due to discomfort from mechanical irritation or inflammation of the cyst. The definitive diagnosis of a cyst requires histologic examination, as many other dermal and subcutaneous tumors can form cyst-like nodules. Cysts can be classified by anatomic location (as they may occur in virtually any organ of the body), by embryologic derivation, or by histologic features. As the histologic features determine the definitive diagnosis, that scheme will be used in this chapter, which is limited to cutaneous cysts.

True cysts have an epithelial lining that may be composed of stratified squamous epithelium or other forms of epithelia. Some 'cysts' have no epithelial lining at all. Cutaneous cysts can be divided into three main categories based on the presence or absence and composition of the cyst wall (Table 110.1; Fig. 110.1). Many non-dermatologists refer to epidermoid and pilar cysts as 'sebaceous cysts', believing erroneously that the hydrated white keratinized contents of many epithelial-lined cysts is of sebaceous origin. The only true sebaceous cyst is the steatocystoma. Because of the confusion, the term 'sebaceous cyst' is best avoided.

CYSTS WITH A LINING OF STRATIFIED SQUAMOUS EPITHELIUM

Epidermoid Cyst

Synonyms: ■ Infundibular cyst ■ Epidermal cyst ■ Epidermal inclusion cyst

Epidermoid cysts are the most common cutaneous cysts. They can occur anywhere on the skin, but they are most common on the face and upper trunk. These lesions are well-demarcated dermal nodules, and may have a clinically visible central punctum representing the follicle from which the cyst is derived (Fig. 110.2). They range from a few millimeters to several centimeters in diameter. Tiny superficial epidermoid cysts are known as milia (see below). Epidermoid cysts derive from the follicular infundibulum (hence the synonym infundibular cysts; Fig. 110.3). They may be primary, or they may arise from disrupted follicular structures or traumatically implanted epithelium (hence the synonym epidermal 'inclusion' cyst). As follicular disruption is important in the pathogenesis of many epidermoid cysts, multiple epidermoid cysts may occur in individuals with a history of significant acne vulgaris. Multiple cysts may also occur in the setting of Gardner syndrome (familial adenomatous polyposis) and in nevoid basal cell carcinoma

Category	Type	Most common location
Stratified squamous epithelium	Epidermoid cyst	Face; upper trunk
	Milium	Face (women, infants)
	Trichilemmal cyst	Scalp
	Proliferating trichilemmal cyst	Scalp (older women)
	Proliferating epidermoid cyst	Pelvic (anogenital)
	Vellus hair cyst	Trunk (chest)
	Steatocystoma	Trunk; axillae; groin
	Cutaneous keratocyst	No characteristic location
	Pigmented follicular cyst	Face (men)
	Dermoid cyst	Face along embryonic fusion planes, e.g. lateral eyebrow (infants)
	Ear pit cyst	Preauricular
	Pilonidal cyst	Upper gluteal cleft; sacrococcygeal area
Non-stratified squamous epithelium	Hidrocystoma	
	• Eccrine	Face
	• Apocrine	Face (eyelid margin)
	Bronchogenic cyst	Suprasternal notch (infants)
	Thyroglossal duct cyst	Midline anterior neck
	Branchial cleft cyst	Lateral neck; preauricular; mandibular (teenagers, young adults)
	Cutaneous ciliated cyst	Lower extremities (young women)
	Ciliated cyst of the vulva	Labia majora
	Median raphe cyst	Ventral glans of penis
	Omphalomesenteric duct cyst	Umbilical; periumbilical
Absence of epithelium	Mucocele	Oral mucosa (lower labial)
	Digital mucous cyst	Dorsal aspect of distal phalanx of finger
	Ganglion	Wrist
	Pseudocyst of the auricle	Scaphoid fossa of the ear (adult men)
	Cutaneous metaplastic synovial cyst	Sites of surgical trauma

Table 110.1 **The three main categories of cutaneous cyst.**

syndrome[1,2]. Multiple scrotal cysts may lead to scrotal calcinosis via dystrophic calcification[4]. Non-inflamed epidermoid cysts are usually asymptomatic, but, with pressure, cysts contents may be expressed that may have an objectionable odor. Rupture of the cyst wall can result in an intensely painful inflammatory reaction, and this is a common reason for presentation to a physician's office (Fig. 110.4). Development of a basal cell carcinoma or squamous cell carcinoma within an epidermoid cyst is a very rare event[5].

Pathology

Histologic examination shows a cystic cavity filled with laminated keratin lined by a stratified squamous epithelium including a granular layer (Fig. 110.5). A surrounding inflammatory response with both acute and chronic granulomatous inflammation may be seen as evidence of prior rupture. In individuals with Gardner syndrome, some cysts show, as a characteristic feature, columns of pilomatricoma-like shadow cells projecting into the cyst cavity[1].

Treatment

If treatment is desired, excision is curative. Removal may be accomplished by simple excision, or incision and expression of the cyst contents and wall through the surgical defect. If the entire cyst wall is

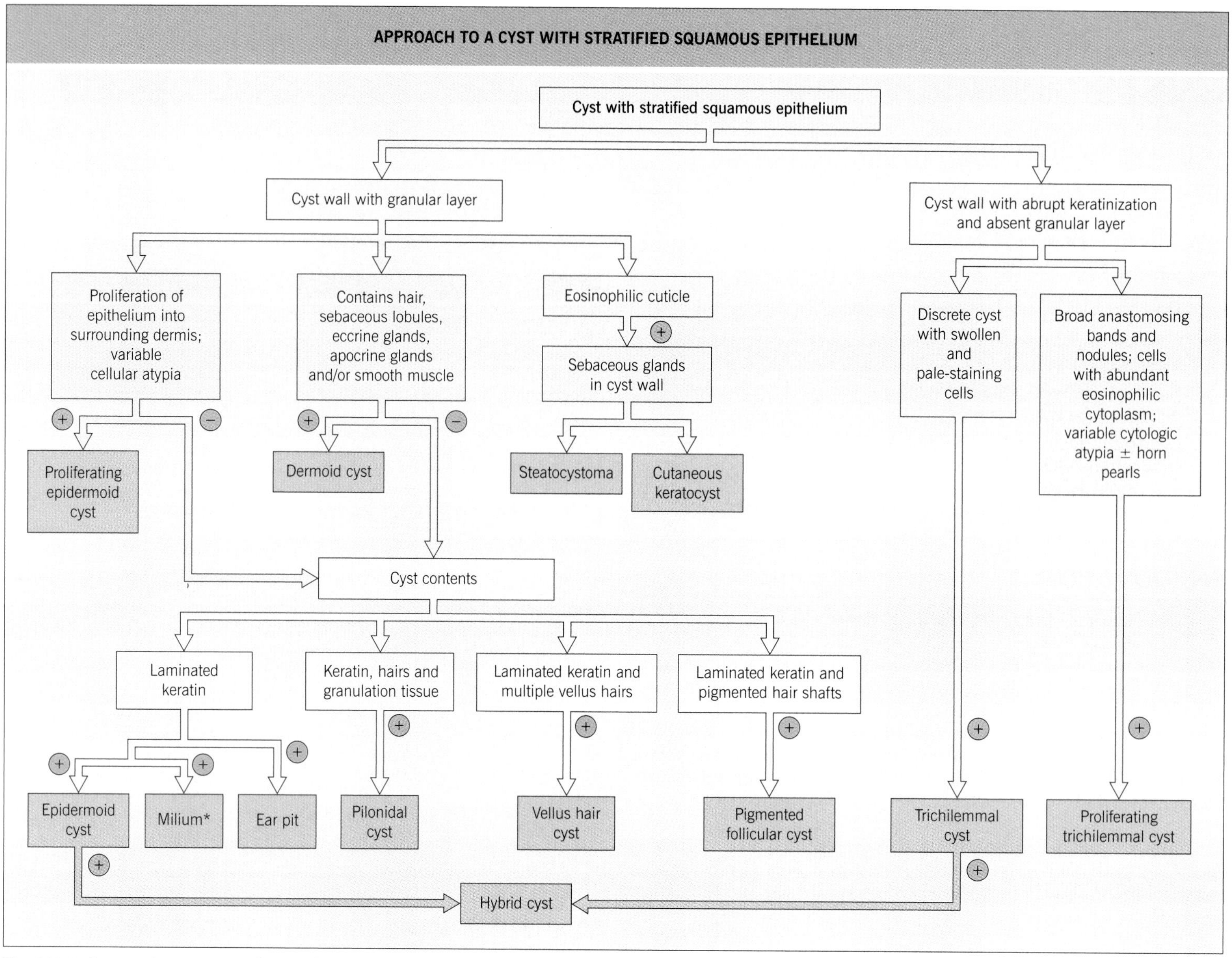

APPROACH TO A CYST WITH STRATIFIED SQUAMOUS EPITHELIUM

Cyst with stratified squamous epithelium

Cyst wall with granular layer

Cyst wall with abrupt keratinization and absent granular layer

Proliferation of epithelium into surrounding dermis; variable cellular atypia

Contains hair, sebaceous lobules, eccrine glands, apocrine glands and/or smooth muscle

Eosinophilic cuticle

Discrete cyst with swollen and pale-staining cells

Broad anastomosing bands and nodules; cells with abundant eosinophilic cytoplasm; variable cytologic atypia ± horn pearls

Sebaceous glands in cyst wall

Proliferating epidermoid cyst

Dermoid cyst

Steatocystoma

Cutaneous keratocyst

Cyst contents

Laminated keratin

Keratin, hairs and granulation tissue

Laminated keratin and multiple vellus hairs

Laminated keratin and pigmented hair shafts

Epidermoid cyst

Milium*

Ear pit

Pilonidal cyst

Vellus hair cyst

Pigmented follicular cyst

Trichilemmal cyst

Proliferating trichilemmal cyst

Hybrid cyst

Fig. 110.1 Approach to a cyst with stratified squamous epithelium. *Diameter 1–2 mm.

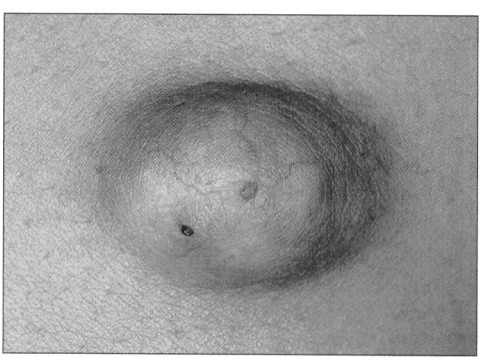

Fig. 110.2 Epidermoid cyst. Typical clinical appearance of an epidermoid cyst. Pores are present in this example.

not removed, the cyst may recur. Inflamed epidermoid cysts may require incision and drainage, and, occasionally, antibiotic therapy. Intralesional triamcinolone may be helpful in speeding the resolution of the inflammation.

Milium

Milia are small epidermoid cysts and are quite common, occurring at all ages of life. Milia present as 1–2 mm white to yellow subepidermal papules. Between 40% and 50% of infants will have milia, most commonly on the face. Most milia in newborns will resolve spontaneously in the first 4 weeks of life. Milia in newborns may also occur on the hard palate (Bohn's nodules) or on the gum margins (Epstein's pearls). These also resolve spontaneously. Milia may occur as a primary phenomenon, especially on the face, or as secondary phenomena following blistering processes or superficial ulceration from trauma or cosmetic procedures. Milia may also occur in areas of topical corticosteroid-induced atrophy[6].

Milia en plaque is characterized by multiple milia within an erythematous edematous plaque. Milia en plaque most often occurs in the postauricular area, but may also occur on or anterior to the ear[7]. Persistent widespread milia in infancy may be seen as part of hereditary trichodysplasia (Marie–Unna hypotrichosis) or oral-facial-digital syndrome type 1, an X-linked disorder that is lethal in males, in which milia are associated with facial and skull malformations, cleft lip and palate, a lobulated tongue, mental retardation, and polycystic kidneys; areas of alopecia follow the lines of Blaschko on the scalp. Milia are also seen in the setting of a number of other syndromes, including the basal cell carcinoma-associated syndromes, Rombo syndrome and Bazex syndrome.

Pathology

Histologic features are those of a small epidermoid cyst with a stratified squamous epithelial lining including a granular layer and laminated keratin cyst contents.

Treatment

Milia may be removed by incising the epidermis over the milium with a needle, scalpel or lancet and expressing the milium. The latter can be

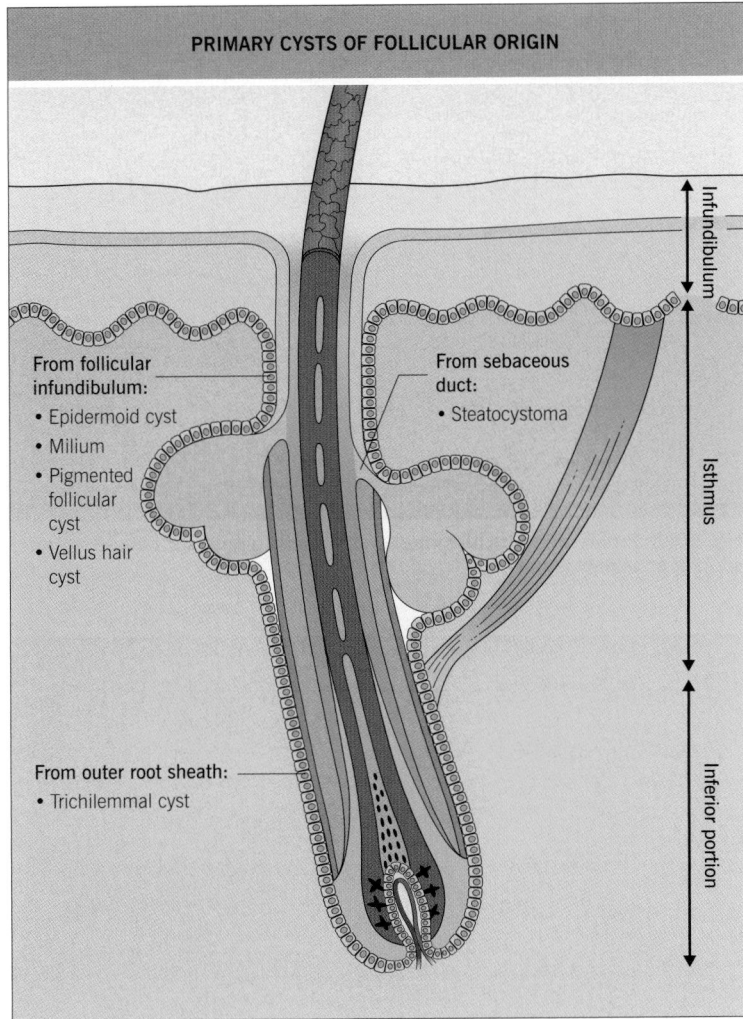

PRIMARY CYSTS OF FOLLICULAR ORIGIN

Infundibulum

Isthmus

Inferior portion

From follicular
infundibulum:
• Epidermoid cyst
• Milium
• Pigmented
  follicular
  cyst
• Vellus hair
  cyst

From sebaceous
duct:
• Steatocystoma

From outer root sheath:
• Trichilemmal cyst

Fig. 110.3 Primary cysts of follicular origin. Anatomic origin of cysts derived from the pilosebaceous unit. Adapted from Requena L, Sanchez Yus E. Follicular hybrid cysts. An expanded spectrum. Am J Dermatopathol. 1991;13:228–33.

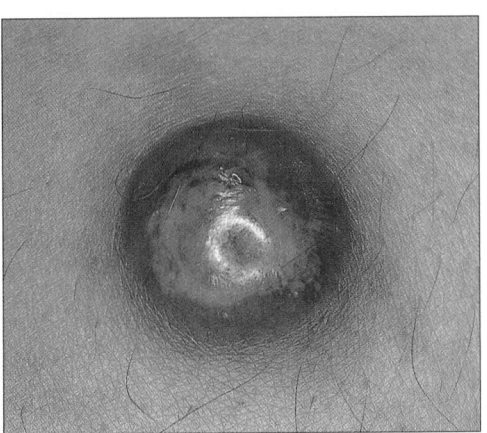

Fig. 110.4 Inflamed epidermoid cyst. Such painful inflammatory reactions to cyst rupture are a frequent cause for presentation to a physician.

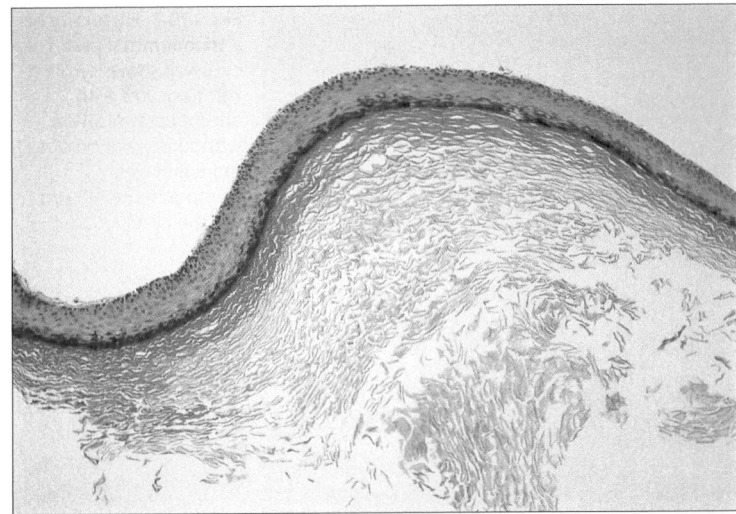

Fig. 110.5 Histology of an epidermoid cyst. The cyst wall shows epidermal keratinization including a granular layer. Laminated keratin cyst contents are seen.

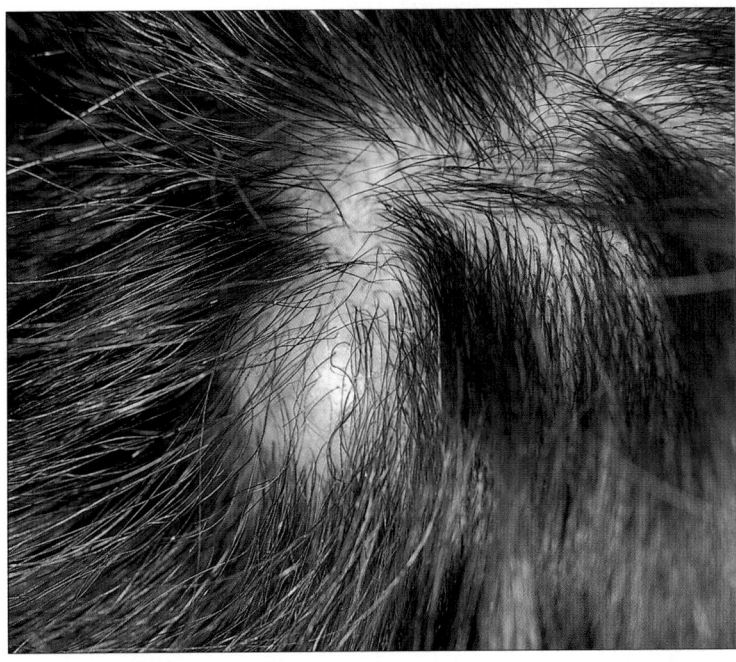

Fig. 110.6 Trichilemmal cyst. Trichilemmal cysts are most commonly seen on the scalp.

aided by the use of a comedo extractor. Laser ablation and electro-desiccation are also reported options. For multiple facial milia, topical retinoid therapy may be helpful in reducing the number of milia and aiding in the ease of removal. Milia en plaque may respond to oral minocycline[7].

Trichilemmal Cyst

Synonyms: ■ Pilar cyst ■ Wen ■ Isthmus–catagen cyst

Trichilemmal cysts are clinically indistinguishable from epidermoid cysts, but they are fourfold to fivefold less common. Ninety percent of trichilemmal cysts are located on the scalp (Fig. 110.6). They may

be solitary, but frequently they are multiple. Trichilemmal cysts may be inherited as an autosomal dominant trait. Trichilemmal cyst walls show keratinization analogous to that of the outer root sheath of the hair follicle at the isthmus and the sac surrounding catagen and telogen hairs (hence the synonym isthmus–catagen cyst).

Pathology

Histologically, trichilemmal cysts are lined by stratified squamous epithelial cells without visible intracellular bridges that become swollen and pale close to the cystic cavity and show abrupt keratinization without an intervening granular layer (Fig. 110.7). The cyst contents consist of homogeneous eosinophilic material that frequently shows foci of calcification. A foreign body giant cell response may surround the cyst if prior wall rupture has occurred.

Treatment

Treatment is by excision. Trichilemmal cysts typically 'deliver' themselves through an incision without rupture more easily than do epidermoid cysts, and, therefore, the distinction between a trichilemmal cyst and an epidermoid cyst can often be correctly made at the time of excision.

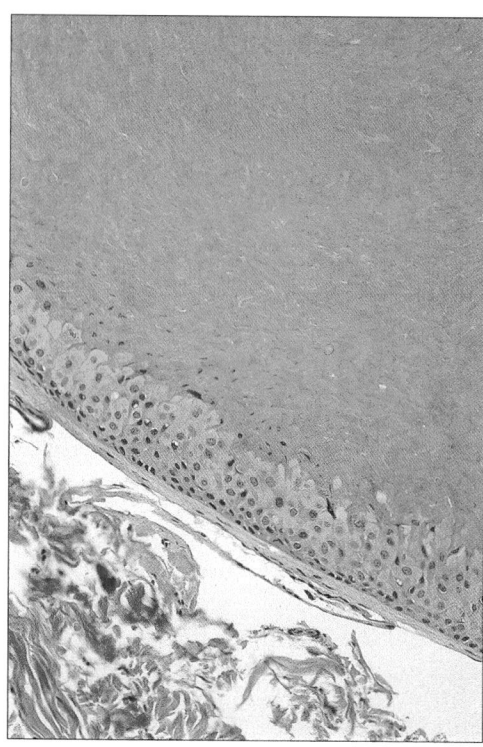

Fig. 110.7 Histology of a trichilemmal cyst. The cyst wall shows swollen keratinocytes with abrupt keratinization without formation of a granular layer. Homogeneous keratin fills the cyst.

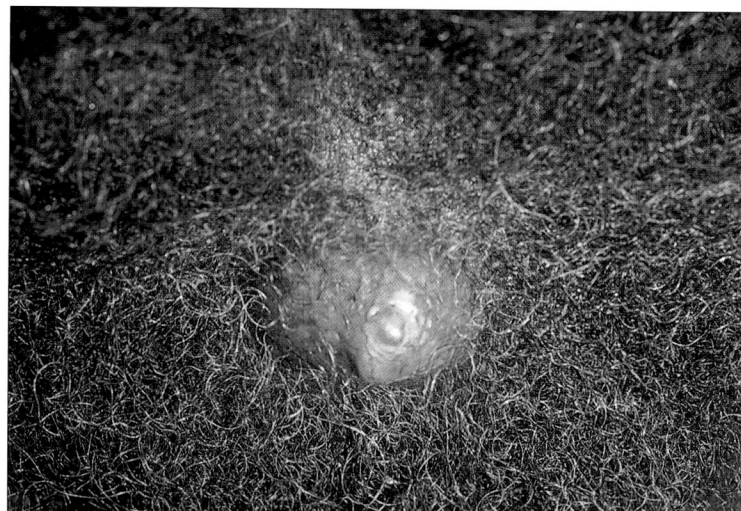

Fig. 110.8 Proliferating trichilemmal cyst. An enlarging cystic nodule on the scalp of an elderly female.

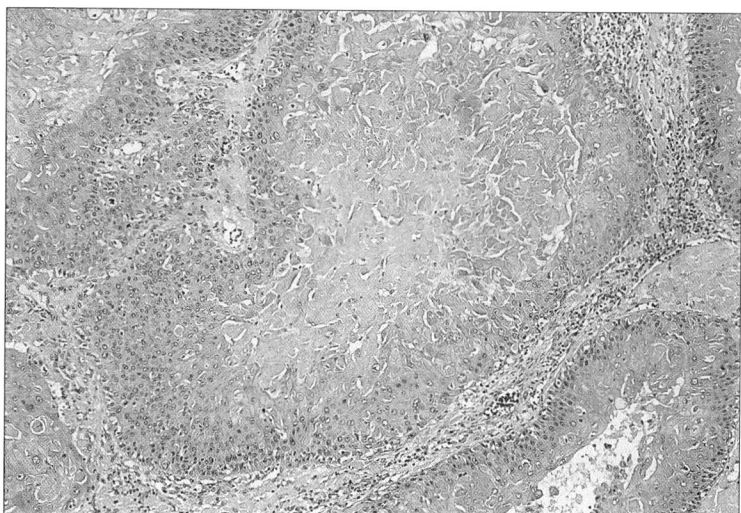

Fig. 110.9 Histology of a proliferating trichilemmal cyst. Irregular bands and nodules of squamous epithelium show central areas of abrupt keratinization.

Proliferating Trichilemmal Cyst

Synonyms: ■ Proliferating trichilemmal tumor ■ Pilar tumor
■ Proliferating follicular cystic neoplasm

A proliferating trichilemmal cyst classically occurs as a slow-growing nodule on the scalp of an elderly woman (Fig. 110.8). In fact, 90% occur on the scalp, and 84% occur in women with a median age of 63 years[8]. Proliferating trichilemmal cysts vary in size from a few millimeters to up to 25 cm in diameter. These tumors generally behave in a benign fashion, although, on occasion, aggressive local growth with recurrences and metastases has been observed[8]. Extremely rarely, spindle cell carcinomas may develop within a proliferating trichilemmal cyst[9,10]. Distant metastases are rare in proliferating trichilemmal cysts, but over 30 such cases have been reported[11]. Whether a proliferating trichilemmal cyst is a benign pseudomalignancy in which a squamous cell carcinoma may develop or a variant of squamous cell carcinoma is an area of controversy[12].

Pathology

The histologic features of proliferating trichilemmal cyst consist of broad anastomosing bands and nodules of squamous epithelium. The epithelium shows a proliferation of cells with abundant eosinophilic cytoplasm showing abrupt keratinization forming dense homogeneous keratin that fills cystic spaces. There may be areas of epidermoid keratinization with formation of horn pearls (Fig. 110.9) as well as areas of foreign body giant cell reaction. One-quarter of cases show an epidermal connection[8]. Cytologic atypia may vary markedly. Most tumors show well-circumscribed, pushing borders surrounded by compressed collagen. The lack of infiltrative growth into the surrounding stroma and abrupt trichilemmal keratinization helps in differentiation from squamous cell carcinoma. Areas of marked atypia and infiltrative borders are features of a potential for aggressive behavior[13].

Treatment

Treatment is by complete surgical excision.

Proliferating Epidermoid Cysts

Synonym: ■ Proliferating epithelial cyst

Proliferating epidermoid cysts were first described in detail in 1995[8]. Unlike proliferating trichilemmal cysts, proliferating epidermoid cysts are reported more commonly in men and only 20% occur on the scalp. They range in size from 0.4 to 15 cm. In the 30 patients reported by Sau et al.[8] for whom follow-up was available, 20% of the cysts recurred, some multiple times, and one patient died of intractable local disease. None of the patients developed metastatic disease.

Pathology

Histologically, almost half of cases show an epidermal connection, usually with a narrow opening or connection to a dilated follicle. Most tumors show areas of typical epidermoid cyst wall. In addition, areas of squamous proliferation with squamous eddy formation are seen, with formation of a granular layer and production of loose laminated keratin. The epithelium tends to proliferate peripherally into the surrounding dermis, rather than centrally as seen in proliferating trichilemmal cysts. Degrees of cellularity and atypia are variable, and frank carcinomatous change with an infiltrative growth pattern may be seen.

Treatment

Treatment is by complete surgical excision.

Vellus Hair Cysts

Vellus hair cysts, described by Esterly, Fretzin & Pinkus in 1977[14], most commonly present as numerous tiny dome-shaped papules, ranging

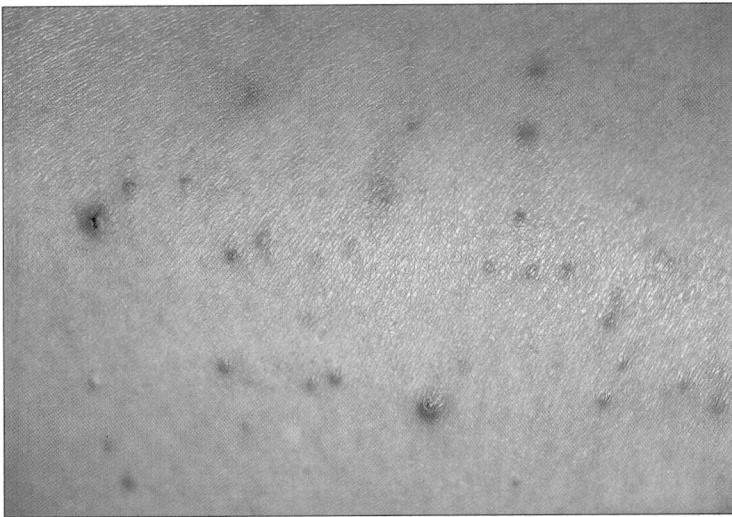

Fig. 110.10 Eruptive vellus hair cysts. Pigmented small papules seen on the thigh of a young woman.

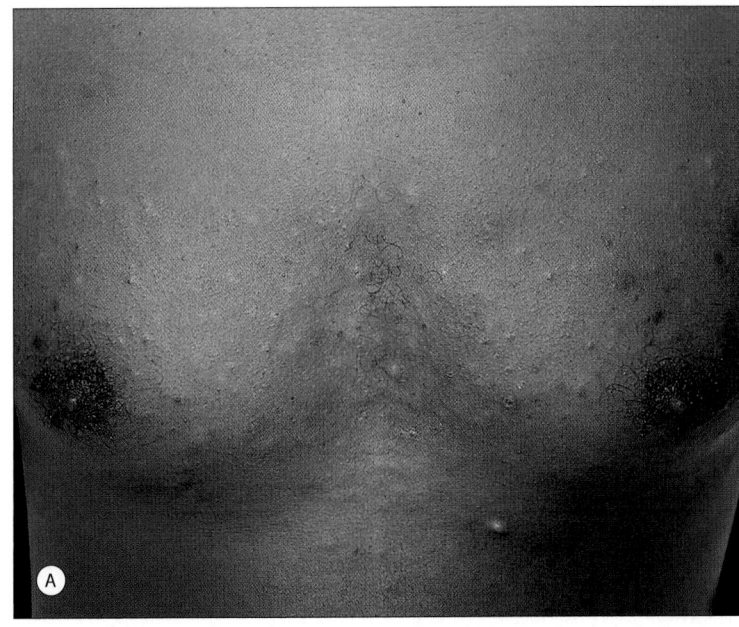

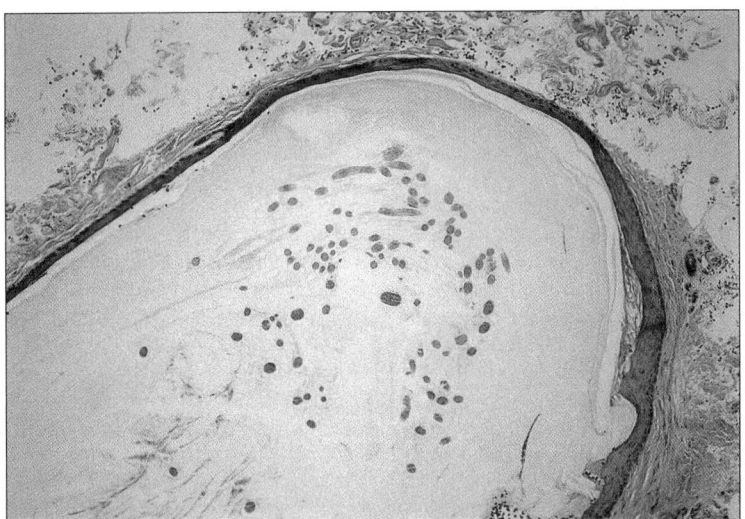

Fig. 110.11 Histology of a vellus hair cyst. A small cyst shows epidermoid keratinization of the cyst wall and numerous vellus hairs in the lumen.

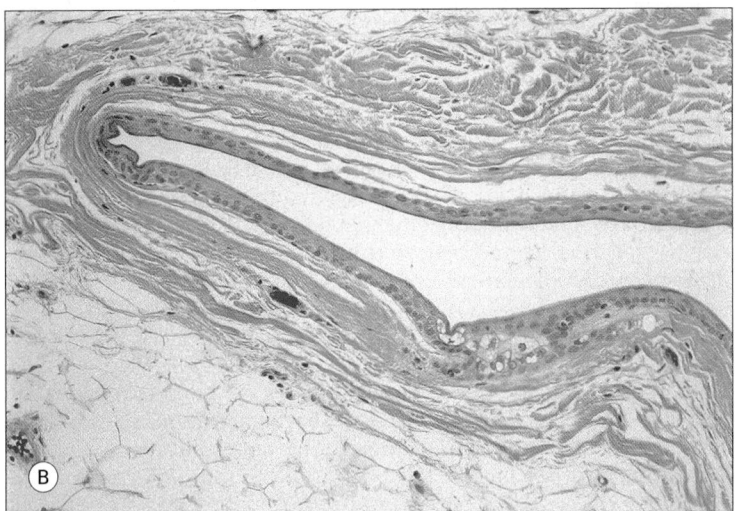

Fig. 110.12 Steatocystoma multiplex. A Numerous cystic nodules are seen on the trunk. **B** Histology of steatocystoma. A flattened sebaceous lobule is seen in the cyst wall, which is lined by a thin eosinophilic cuticle. The clinical differential diagnosis includes an umbilical (pyogenic) granuloma and urachal cyst/remnant.

from skin-colored to darkly pigmented (Fig. 110.10). They are most commonly located on the trunk, and they may be inherited in an autosomal dominant pattern. Multiple lesions are known as 'eruptive' vellus hair cysts; occasionally, solitary cysts are seen. Although some lesions may resolve via transepidermal elimination of cyst products, most lesions persist indefinitely[15]. Vellus hair cysts may become inflamed but, in general, they are asymptomatic except for cosmetic concerns.

Eruptive vellus hair cysts may be seen in conjunction with steatocystoma multiplex, and both types of cysts have been reported in the setting of pachyonychia congenita (type 2). Each of these entities has been associated with mutations in the gene that encodes keratin 17[16]. The latter is expressed in the nail bed, hair follicles and sebaceous glands, but not in stratified squamous epithelium[17].

Pathology

Histologically, one sees a small cystic structure lined by stratified squamous epithelium with epidermoid keratinization. The cysts contain loose laminated keratin and numerous vellus hairs (Fig. 110.11). A follicle may be found entering the lower portion of the cyst.

Treatment

Vellus hair cysts may be treated by a number of modalities, including incision and drainage, needle evacuation, topical retinoic or lactic acid, and laser ablation.

Steatocystoma

Steatocystomas occur as single (steatocystoma simplex) or multiple (steatocystoma multiplex) lesions. They tend to be a few millimeters to a centimeter in diameter and appear as cysts in the dermis that drain oily fluid if punctured. Steatocystomas are most numerous on the chest (Fig. 110.12A) and in the axillae and groin. There are unusual facial and acral variants as well as a rare congenital linear form. Steatocystomas persist indefinitely, and they are usually asymptomatic except for cosmetic concerns.

Steatocystoma multiplex is inherited as an autosomal dominant condition, and is due to mutations in the keratin 17 gene. It may occur in association with eruptive vellus hair cysts and pachyonychia congenita type 2, also caused by keratin 17 (as well as K6b) defects[17].

Pathology

Biopsy specimens show a dermal cyst lined by a thin stratified squamous epithelium, with a granular layer surmounted by a thin, irregular, corrugated eosinophilic cuticle. Small sebaceous lobules are found in or immediately adjacent to the cyst wall (Fig. 110.12B).

Treatment

Lesions can be excised or incised with removal of the cyst wall.

Cutaneous Keratocyst

Cutaneous keratocysts have been reported primarily in patients with the nevoid basal cell carcinoma syndrome. Their clinical appearance is similar to epidermoid cysts and there is no characteristic clinical location.

Pathology

These cysts have a stratified squamous epithelial wall with a granular layer and an eosinophilic cuticle, like a steatocystoma. However, no associated sebaceous lobules are seen[18].

Follicular Hybrid Cyst

Synonym: ▪ Hybrid cyst

Follicular hybrid cysts are not distinctive clinically, but rather represent a histologic variant of cysts with a stratified squamous lining in which there is transition in the cell wall between epidermoid keratinization and trichilemmal or pilomatrical keratinization[3,19]. They were originally described by Brownstein[19].

Pigmented Follicular Cyst

Pigmented follicular cysts, described by Mehregan & Medenica[20], are solitary and occur primarily on the face of men. They are often deeply pigmented, and may be confused clinically with a nevus.

Histologically, these cysts have a pore-like connection to the epidermis, are lined by stratified squamous epithelium including a granular layer, and contain pigmented hair shafts. The clinical presentation, epidermal connection, and pigmented hair shafts distinguish the pigmented follicular cyst from vellus hair cysts.

Dermoid Cyst

Cutaneous dermoid cysts typically present in an infant along an embryonic fusion plane as a discrete, subcutaneous nodule. Dermoid cysts are usually 1–4 cm in diameter. The most common location is around the eyes (see Fig. 63.2).

Pathology

Histologically, dermoid cysts are lined by stratified squamous epithelium including a granular layer. They contain other normal cutaneous structures such as hair, sebaceous lobules, eccrine glands, apocrine glands, or smooth muscle.

Treatment

Treatment is by excision. However, as the differential diagnosis includes neural heterotopias, imaging studies may be appropriate prior to excision to exclude a connection to the CNS (see Ch. 63).

Ear Pit

Synonyms: ▪ Preauricular cyst ▪ Congenital auricular fistula
▪ Preauricular fistula

Ear pits are congenital defects, and they may present as a true cystic nodule or an invagination in the preauricular area (Fig. 110.13). During development, the ear is formed by the fusion of six tubercles: three each from the first two branchial arches. Preauricular cysts reflect defective embryologic fusion with epithelial entrapment. These defects are relatively common, occurring in approximately 0.5–1% of the normal population, and they may be transmitted in an autosomal dominant fashion[21]. Ear pits are usually unilateral and right-sided. Infection with tenderness and purulent drainage may prompt presentation to a physician.

Although ear pits are usually not associated with other significant abnormalities, the former are seen in conjunction with deafness or

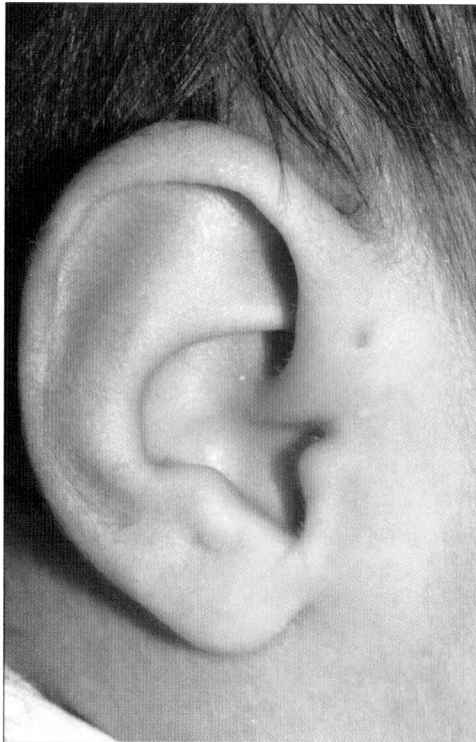

Fig. 110.13 Ear pit. Courtesy of Julie V Schaffer MD.

deafness plus renal anomalies in the branchio-otic syndrome and branchio-oto-renal dysplasia, respectively. Ear pits are also seen in a number of other congenital syndromes associated with additional major morphologic anomalies, including Treacher Collins–Franceschetti syndrome, Goldenhar syndrome, Lowry–MacLean syndrome and cat-eye syndrome[22].

Pathology

Histologically, preauricular pits or cysts are lined by stratified squamous epithelium with a granular layer.

Treatment

If removal is desired, simple excision is curative. Although most ear pits are incidental findings, in a newborn, a physical examination to exclude one of the associated syndromes and an evaluation for hearing loss is indicated. Infected lesions may require antibiotic therapy.

Pilonidal Cyst

Synonyms: ▪ Pilonidal sinus ▪ Pilonidal disease ▪ Barber's interdigital pilonidal sinus (when located in the interdigital spaces)

Pilonidal cysts typically present as an inflamed, painful cystic swelling in the upper gluteal cleft or sacrococcygeal area, but they have been described in many other locations. They are most common in men (at a ratio of 3–4:1) and in Caucasians. Pilonidal cysts are uncommon in individuals with darkly pigmented skin and practically non-existent in Asians. They occur most commonly in hirsute individuals[23]. Pilonidal cysts typically present near the end of the first decade of life and were a significant source of morbidity and hospitalization during World War II[23].

The etiology of pilonidal cysts and sinuses has been a controversial issue. Some authors have argued that they are congenital, essentially representing a dermoid cyst, whereas most authors now believe that the vast majority of lesions are acquired, representing a foreign body response to entrapped hair. A pilonidal cyst can be seen as part of the 'follicular inclusion tetrad' which consists of acne conglobata, hidradenitis suppurativa, perifolliculitis capitis abscedens et suffodiens, and pilonidal cyst (see Ch. 39). Persistent exogenous hairs in the interdigital space of barbers or dog groomers may incite an encompassing epidermal proliferation, giving rise to a pilonidal cyst.

Pathology

Histologic features are those of an epidermal lined cyst or sinus tract. Cyst cavities are lined with granulation tissue and mixed inflammation, with hair and keratin debris.

Treatment

Treatment is surgical and may include excision, marsupialization, or incision and curettage.

CYSTS LINED WITH NON-STRATIFIED SQUAMOUS EPITHELIUM

Hidrocystoma

> **Synonyms:** ■ Cystadenoma ■ Sudoriferous cyst ■ Moll's gland cyst

Hidrocystomas typically present as translucent, skin-colored to bluish cysts on the face, although they may occur in other sites. Hidrocystomas are traditionally divided into apocrine and eccrine hidrocystomas by histologic features, and as solitary (Smith type) or multiple (Robinson type). The traditional division of hidrocystomas into eccrine and apocrine types is somewhat controversial since immunohistochemical studies have shown that this distinction is not always reliably made by light microscopy, as some 'eccrine' hidrocystomas in fact express apocrine antigens[24].

Apocrine hidrocystomas are usually solitary, whereas eccrine hidrocystomas may be solitary or multiple and are occasionally quite numerous (Figs 110.14 & 110.15). Eccrine hidrocystomas can enlarge with heat exposure or during the summer and regress with cooler temperatures. In general, eccrine hidrocystomas are thought to develop from cystic dilation of eccrine ducts due to retention of eccrine secretions, while apocrine hidrocystomas are thought to represent adenomas of apocrine sweat gland coils[24]. Apocrine hidrocystomas are sometimes referred to as cystadenomas, although some authors reserve this term for lesions with prominent papillomatous hyperplasia histologically[25]. Lesions along the lower eyelid margin are also known as Moll's gland cysts.

Pathology

Histologically, apocrine hidrocystomas are unilocular to multilocular dermal cysts lined by one to several layers of epithelial cells that show bulbous protrusions ('snooting') and luminal decapitation secretion (Fig. 110.16). Similarly lined papillary projections may extend into the cyst lumen. Histologic features of eccrine hidrocystomas are those of a uniloculate cyst containing clear fluid, lined by two layers of cuboidal to flattened epithelium (Fig. 110.17). Apocrine hidrocystomas express human milk-fat globulin antigen, while 'true' eccrine hidrocystomas do not. Hidrocystomas that appear by light microscopy to be eccrine include a subset of lesions that mark immunohistochemically as apocrine hidrocystomas, despite a flattened wall[24].

Treatment

Hidrocystomas may be removed by simple excision, electrodesiccation or CO_2 laser. Multiple eccrine hidrocystomas may also be treated with daily application of topical 1% atropine in aqueous solution, although lesions reappear within days of discontinuing therapy[26]. Hidrocystomas may be associated with certain syndromes of ectodermal dysplasia, including Schöpf–Schulz–Passarge syndrome.

Bronchogenic Cyst

Cutaneous bronchogenic cysts are most commonly found in the suprasternal notch and, rarely, on the anterior neck or chin (see Fig. 63.2). A fistulous tract may connect to the epidermis. Rarely, they present as

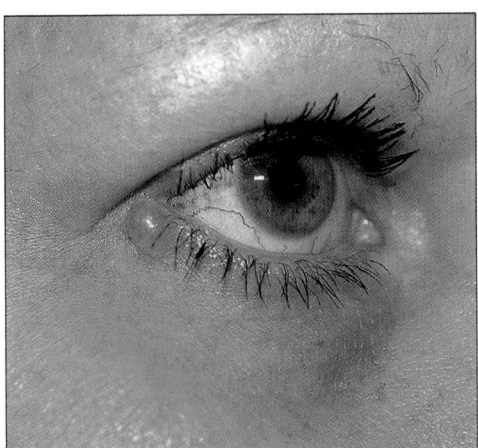

Fig. 110.14 Apocrine hidrocystoma. A single bluish translucent papule is seen on the lower lid.

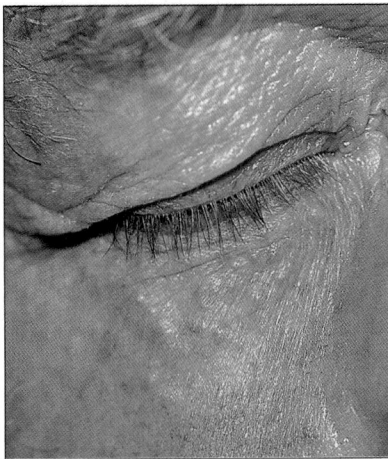

Fig. 110.15 Eccrine hidrocystoma. Numerous translucent papules are seen on the lower lid and upper cheek.

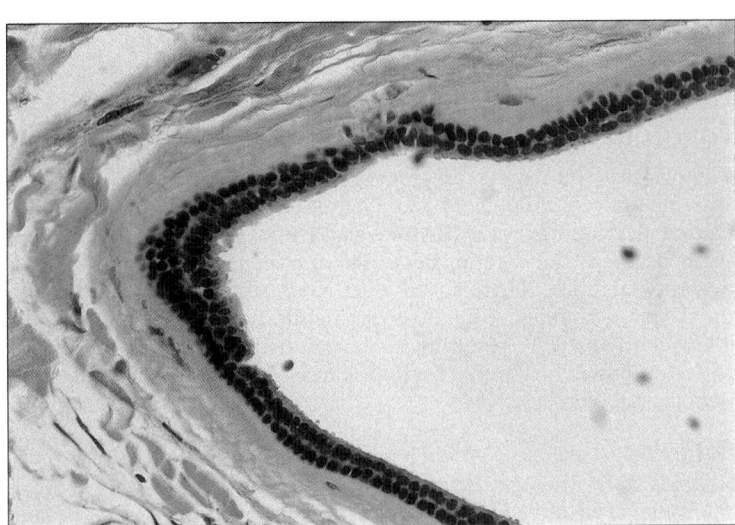

Fig. 110.16 Histology of apocrine hidrocystoma. The cyst wall shows typical apocrine decapitation secretion.

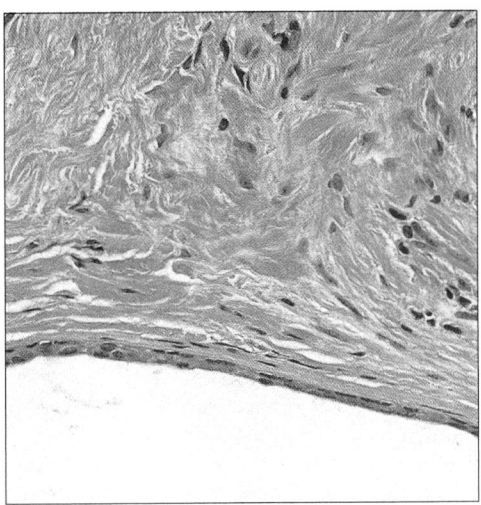

Fig. 110.17 Histology of eccrine hidrocystoma. Two layers of flattened epithelium form the cell wall.

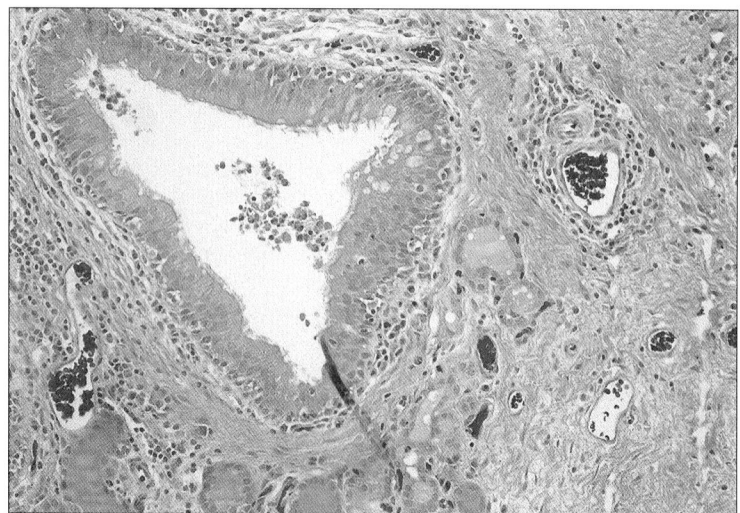

Fig. 110.18 Histology of thyroglossal duct cyst. Thyroid follicles are seen adjacent to a cyst lined by ciliated epithelium.

a pedunculated growth[27]. Bronchogenic cysts are solitary, and they are typically found at birth. Malignant transformation is very rare. They represent respiratory epithelium sequestered during embryologic development of the tracheobronchial tree.

Pathology

Bronchogenic cysts are lined by pseudostratified ciliated columnar epithelium with interspersed goblet cells. The cyst wall often contains smooth muscle and mucous glands, and, rarely, cartilage.

Treatment

Treatment is by excision.

Thyroglossal Duct Cyst

Thyroglossal duct cysts present as midline cystic nodules on the anterior neck in children or young adults (see Ch. 63 and Fig. 63.2). During development, the thyroid gland descends from the floor of the pharynx to the anterior neck. The tract it forms is known as the thyroglossal duct. Thyroglossal duct cysts arise from remnants of the thyroglossal duct. A tract connecting these cysts to the hyoid bone is frequently present, resulting in characteristic movement of the cyst with swallowing. Rarely, thyroid carcinoma may originate in a thyroglossal duct cyst[28].

Pathology

Histologically, thyroglossal duct cysts may be lined with cuboidal, columnar or stratified squamous epithelium and may contain some ciliated columnar cells. The characteristic histologic feature is the presence of thyroid follicles, characterized by low cuboidal cells surrounding homogeneous pink material, in the cyst wall (Fig. 110.18).

Treatment

Treatment is surgical, with excision of the cyst and any residual tract.

Branchial Cleft Cyst

> **Synonyms:** ■ Lymphoepithelial cyst ■ Lateral cervical cyst

Branchial cleft cysts occur in the preauricular area, mandibular region, or along the anterior border of the sternocleidomastoid muscle (see Ch. 63 and Fig. 63.2). The origin of these cysts is controversial. There are two major theories regarding their origin:
- they arise from branchial cleft remnants
- they represent cystic alteration of embryologic epithelium or tonsillar epithelium within cervical lymph nodes[29].

Branchial cleft cysts most commonly present in the second or third decade. Infection of these cysts is a frequent cause of presentation to a physician.

Pathology

Histologically, these cysts are lined by stratified squamous epithelium or by pseudostratified ciliated columnar epithelium, and they are surrounded by lymphoid tissue.

Treatment

Treatment is by excision of the cyst and its associated tract after delineation of the extent of the lesion by CT or MRI[30].

Cutaneous Ciliated Cyst

> **Synonyms:** ■ Cutaneous müllerian cyst ■ Cutaneous ciliated cystadenoma

Cutaneous ciliated cysts are uncommon cysts that typically occur on the lower extremities of young women, although a few cases have been reported in men. They are usually a few centimeters in diameter and, on rupture, drain clear to amber fluid. The histogenesis of these cysts is controversial. Most authors have suggested a müllerian duct origin. However, the few cases in men have led to the alternative hypothesis of ciliated metaplasia of eccrine glands (in at least some cases)[31].

Pathology

Histologically, cutaneous ciliated cysts may be unilocular or multiloculated. The cyst wall is composed of simple cuboidal to columnar ciliated epithelium that frequently shows papillary projections into the cyst lumen. The lining resembles that seen in the fallopian tube.

Treatment

Excision is curative.

Ciliated Cyst of the Vulva

> **Synonyms:** ■ Paramesonephric mucinous cyst of the vulva ■ Cutaneous müllerian cyst

Ciliated cysts of the vulva represent müllerian heterotopias, and they are located, as their name implies, on the vulva, most commonly on the labia majora. They usually measure between 1 and 3 cm in diameter.

Pathology

Histologically, these cysts are lined by simple columnar ciliated cells with basally located nuclei and abundant mucin within the cytoplasm. Small papillary infoldings of the wall may be seen. The cyst wall markedly resembles uterine endocervix[32]. It has been suggested that both this cyst and the cutaneous ciliated cyst should be called cutaneous müllerian cysts, as their presumed origin is the same[32].

Treatment

Treatment is by excision.

Median Raphe Cyst

> **Synonym:** ■ Apocrine cystadenoma of the penis

Median raphe cysts are solitary and usually only a few millimeters in diameter, although they may extend over several centimeters linearly. They occur in young men on the ventral aspect of the penis, most commonly on or near the glans. These cysts are thought to develop from aberrant urethral epithelium, but do not connect to the urethra[33].

Pathology

Histologically, median raphe cysts are lined by stratified columnar epithelium (one to four cell layers thick) without a connection to the overlying epithelium. Occasional mucin-containing cells are seen in the lining. Very rarely, a ciliated lining has been observed[34].

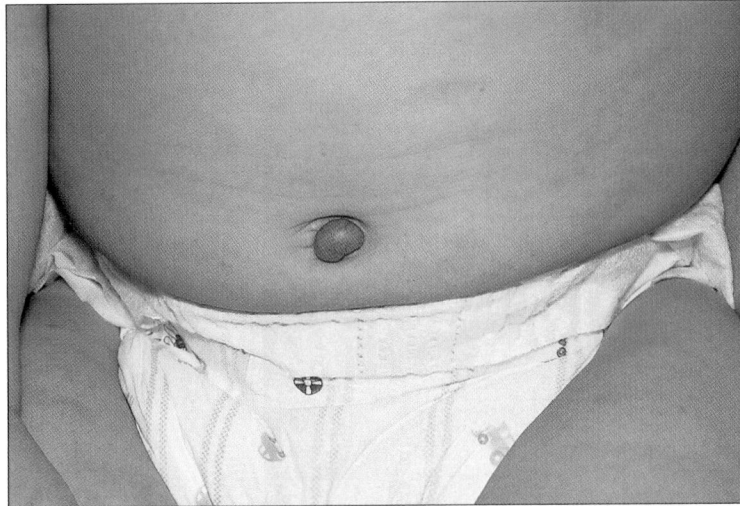

Fig. 110.19 Omphalomesenteric duct cyst. This pink papule in the umbilicus of this infant showed gastrointestinal epithelium histologically. The clinical differential diagnosis includes an umbilical (pyogenic) granuloma and urachal cyst/remnant.

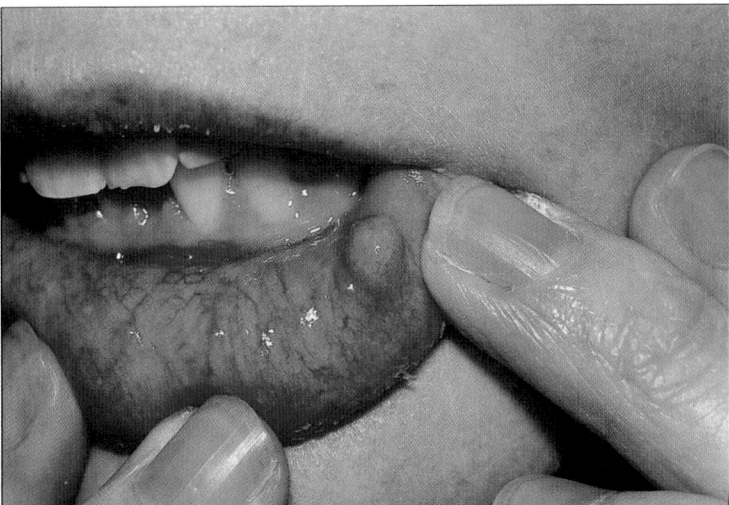

Fig. 110.20 Mucocele. A bluish translucent papule on the lower mucosal lip.

Treatment

Excision is curative.

Omphalomesenteric Duct Cyst

> Synonyms: ■ Vitelline cyst ■ Omphalomesenteric duct remnant

Omphalomesenteric duct cysts represent a developmental defect in the closure of the omphalomesenteric duct. The omphalomesenteric duct is the fetal connection between the midgut and the yolk sac. It is usually obliterated and loses its intestinal attachment by 6 weeks of gestation[35]. Remnants of this duct may occur anywhere along its course between the intestines and the umbilicus. The spectrum of defects resulting from this faulty closure includes Meckel's diverticulum, umbilical-enteric fistulae, umbilical sinuses and omphalomesenteric duct cysts (internal or external); the latter can present as an umbilical polyp (Fig. 110.19).

Pathology

These lesions are characterized histologically by ectopic gastrointestinal mucosa and must be distinguished from umbilical metastases of gastrointestinal adenocarcinomas.

Treatment

Management of omphalomesenteric duct cysts includes appropriate radiologic studies to exclude communication to the gastrointestinal tract prior to surgical excision.

CYSTS WITHOUT AN EPITHELIAL LINING

Mucocele

> Synonyms: ■ Mucous cyst of oral mucosa ■ Ranula (when located on the floor of the mouth)

Mucoceles occur most frequently on the lower labial mucosa, but they also occur on the floor of the mouth, buccal mucosa, and tongue. They appear as dome-shaped, bluish, translucent papules or nodules of a few millimeters to over a centimeter in diameter (Fig. 110.20). They arise as a result of disruption of minor salivary ducts. This disruption leads to an accumulation of mucinous material, a reactive inflammatory response, and the development of surrounding granulation tissue.

A variant of mucocele, superficial mucocele, presents as a clear tense vesicle that is a few millimeters in diameter. Superficial mucoceles are most commonly found on the retromolar pad, posterior buccal mucosa, and soft palate. These lesions are short-lived, asymptomatic and recurrent. They may be confused clinically with an immunobullous or viral process[36].

Pathology

Biopsy specimens of mucoceles show one or several spaces in the connective tissue filled with mucinous material without an epithelial lining, but surrounded by chronic inflammation, mucin-containing macrophages, and granulation tissue. A salivary duct may be seen at the periphery of these findings. Adjacent minor salivary glands may show chronic inflammation and fibrosis. The mucinous material is sialomucin, and the latter contains both neutral and acid mucopolysaccharides, which stain with PAS (diastase-resistant) and with Alcian blue or colloidal iron, respectively.

Histologically, the variant superficial mucocele shows a subepithelial vesicle filled with mucin and a surrounding sparse to moderate mixed inflammatory infiltrate. Salivary gland ducts are seen opening into the vesicle or immediately adjacent to the vesicle.

Treatment

Mucoceles may resolve spontaneously. If they do not, treatment options include excision, marsupialization, electrodesiccation, intralesional corticosteroid injection, cryosurgery, and CO_2 laser therapy.

Digital Mucous Cyst

> Synonym: ■ Cutaneous myxoid cyst

Digital mucous cysts most commonly occur on the dorsal surface of the distal phalanx of the finger. Toe lesions are less commonly observed. A characteristic depressed nail deformity may be seen distal to the cyst (Fig. 110.21). These cysts appear bluish in color and drain clear gelatinous material when punctured. The etiology of digital mucous cysts is controversial, with some authors stating that they are degenerative in origin while others believe they extend from the distal interphalangeal joint space. A pedicle connecting the cyst to the adjacent joint space can usually be demonstrated[37].

Pathology

Histologically, clefts are seen in the dermis without an epithelial lining. The clefts and the surrounding loose connective tissue contain abundant acid mucopolysaccharides, which can be highlighted by Alcian blue or colloidal iron stains.

Treatment

Resolution may be seen after intralesional injection of corticosteroids. Repeated puncture and drainage of a digital mucous cyst leads to resolution in up to 72% of patients[38]. Surgical excision may give even

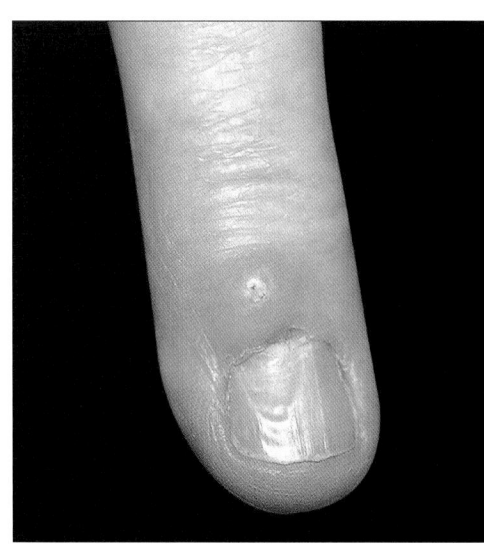

Fig. 110.21 Digital mucous cyst. A translucent papule on the dorsal distal phalanx of the finger causing a depression in the nail plate.

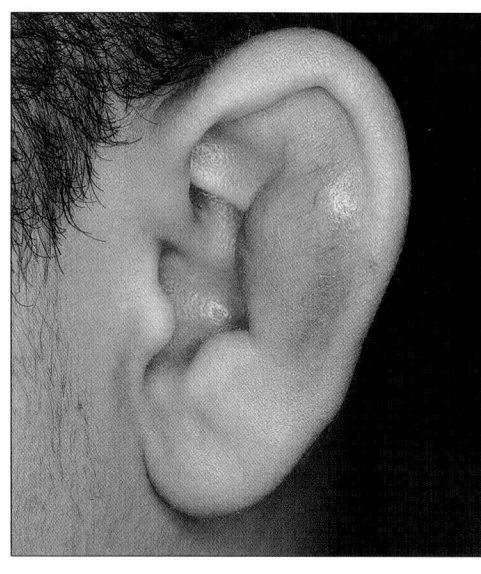

Fig. 110.22 Pseudocyst of the auricle. Erythematous firm nodule on the ear.

higher success rates. De Berker & Lawrence[37] reported a technique for identification and ligature of the connection to the joint capsule. This technique was curative in 94% of finger lesions and 57% of those on the toes.

Ganglion

> **Synonyms:** ▪ Ganglion cyst ▪ Synovial cyst

Ganglia are soft cystic masses up to 4 cm in diameter that most commonly occur on the dorsal aspect of the wrist; they may also be found on the volar wrist or fingers, the dorsal aspect of the feet, or the knees. Ganglia rarely develop on the lateral elbow or anterior shoulder. They occur more commonly in women and may cause discomfort with activity, impairment of mobility, or cosmetic concerns. Ganglia are frequently attached to a tendon sheath or the joint capsule, but usually do not communicate with the joint space[39]. The mucin present within a ganglion is thought to be produced by local fibroblasts.

Pathology

Myxoid change is seen in the connective tissue that ultimately forms cystic spaces. These spaces coalesce into a dominant cystic space lined by fibrous tissue, sometimes with a synovial lining.

Treatment

Early lesions may respond to several weeks of compression therapy, such as that achieved with a padded coin secured by an elastic bandage[39]. Other options include aspiration plus intralesional corticosteroid injection or excision. Recurrences are common, even with excisional therapy.

Pseudocyst of the Auricle

> **Synonyms:** ▪ Endochondral pseudocyst ▪ Cystic chondromalacia
> ▪ Intracartilaginous cyst

Pseudocyst of the auricle usually arises in the scaphoid fossa of the ear of a middle-aged man. Lesions are usually unilateral. They present as a painless swelling (Fig. 110.22), and they tend to arise over the course of a few weeks. The etiology of pseudocyst of the auricle is unknown, but the presence of a potential space during embryogenesis and chronic trauma have been suggested.

Pathology

Biopsy specimens show a cavity within the auricular cartilage (without an epithelial lining) that contains clear fluid. Fibrous tissue and granulation tissue may be found in the cavity as well. The cartilage lining the cavity may show degenerative changes. No inflammation is seen within the cartilage, a distinguishing feature from relapsing polychondritis, which is frequently in the clinical differential diagnosis.

Treatment

Treatment options include aspiration, with or without intralesional injection of corticosteroids, as well as incision and drainage with destruction of the cavity. Each of these modalities should be followed by pressure dressings[40,41].

Cutaneous Metaplastic Synovial Cyst

Cutaneous metaplastic synovial cysts typically present as a solitary tender subcutaneous nodule, although multiple lesions have been reported[42]. They occur primarily in areas of prior trauma, particularly prior surgical trauma. Frequently, the preoperative diagnosis is that of a suture granuloma.

Pathology

A cystic cavity is seen in the dermis that is not lined by epithelium. The cavity may communicate to the overlying epidermis via fistulae. Variably cellular villous structures mimicking hyperplastic synovium protrude into the cavity. These villi are covered with a fibrinous exudate. The base of the villi tends to merge with surrounding scar tissue.

Treatment

Excision is curative.

REFERENCES

1. Cooper PH, Fechner RE. Pilomatricoma-like changes in the epidermal cysts of Gardner's syndrome. J Am Acad Dermatol. 1983;8:639–44.
2. Gorlin RJ. Nevoid basal cell carcinoma syndrome. Dermatol Clin. 1995;13:113–25.
3. Requena L, Sanchez Yus E. Follicular hybrid cysts. An expanded spectrum. Am J Dermatopathol. 1991;13:228–33.
4. Sha V, Shet, T. Scrotal calcinosis results from calcification of cysts derived from hair follicles: A series

of 20 cases evaluating the spectrum of changes resulting in scrotal calcinosis. Am J Dermatopathol. 2007;29:172–175.
5. Lopez-Rios F, Rodriguez-Peralto JL, Castano E, Benito A. Squamous cell carcinoma arising in a cutaneous epidermal cyst: case report and literature review. Am J Dermatopathol. 1999;21:174–7.
6. Langley RG, Walsh NM, Ross JB. Multiple eruptive milia: report of a case, review of the literature, and a classification. J Am Acad Dermatol. 1997;37:353–6.

7. Keohane SG, Beveridge GW, Benton EC, et al. Milia en plaque – a new site and novel treatment. Clin Exp Dermatol. 1996;21:58–60.
8. Sau P, Graham JH, Helwig EB. Proliferating epithelial cysts. Clinicopathological analysis of 96 cases. J Cutan Pathol. 1995;22:394–406.
9. Alvarez-Quinones M, Garijo MF, Fernandez F, et al. Malignant aneuploid spindle-cell transformation in a proliferating trichilemmal tumour. Acta Derm Venereol. 1993;73:444–6.

10. Mori O, Hachisuka H, Sasai Y. Proliferating trichilemmal cyst with spindle cell carcinoma. Am J Dermatopathol. 1990;12:479–84.

11. Lopez-Rios F, Rodriguez-Peralto JL, Aguilar A, et al. Proliferating trichilemmal cyst with focal invasion: report of a case and a review of the literature. Am J Dermatopathol. 2000;22:183–7.

12. Mones JM, Ackerman AB. Proliferating trichilemmal cyst is squamous cell carcinoma. Dermatopathology: Practical & Conceptual. 1998;4:295–310.

13. Ye J, Nappi O, Swanson PE, et al. Proliferating pilar tumors: a clinicopathologic study of 76 cases with a proposal for definition of benign and malignant variants. Am J Clin Pathol. 2004;122:566–74.

14. Esterly NB, Fretzin DF, Pinkus H. Eruptive vellus hair cysts. Arch Dermatol. 1977;113:500–3.

15. Bovenmyer DA. Eruptive vellus hair cysts. Arch Dermatol. 1979;115:338–9.

16. Tomkova H, Fujimoto W, Arata J. Expression of keratins (K10 and K17) in steatocystoma multiplex, eruptive vellus hair cysts, and epidermoid and trichilemmal cysts. Am J Dermatopathol. 1997;19:250–3.

17. McLean WH, Rugg EL, Lunny DP, et al. Keratin 16 and keratin 17 mutations cause pachyonychia congenita. Nat Genet. 1995;9:273–8.

18. Cassarino DS, Linden KG, Barr RJ. Cutaneous keratocyst arising independently of the nevoid basal cell carcinoma syndrome. Am J Dermatopathol. 2005;27:177–8.

19. Brownstein MH. Hybrid cyst: a combined epidermoid and trichilemmal cyst. J Am Acad Dermatol. 1983;9:872–5.

20. Mehregan AH, Medenica M. Pigmented follicular cysts. J Cutan Pathol. 1982;9:423–7.

21. Scheinfeld NS, Silverberg NB, Weinberg JM, Nozad V. The preauricular sinus: a review of its clinical presentation, treatment, and associations. Pediatr Dermatol. 2004;21:191–6.

22. McKusick VA (ed). OMIM™ Online Mendelian Inheritance in Man. National Center for Biotechnology Information. www.ncbi.nlm.nih.gov/Omim/

23. da Silva JH. Pilonidal cyst: cause and treatment. Dis Colon Rectum. 2000;43:1146–56.

24. de Viragh PA, Szeimies RM, Eckert F. Apocrine cystadenoma, apocrine hidrocystoma, and eccrine hidrocystoma: three distinct tumors defined by expression of keratins and human milk fat globulin 1. J Cutan Pathol. 1997;24:249–55.

25. Glusac EJ, Hendrickson MS, Smoller BR. Apocrine cystadenoma of the vulva. J Am Acad Dermatol. 1994;31:498–9.

26. Sanz-Sanchez T, Dauden E, Perez-Casas A, et al. Efficacy and safety of topical atropine in treatment of multiple eccrine hidrocystomas. Arch Dermatol. 2001;137:670–1.

27. Miller OF III, Tyler W. Cutaneous bronchogenic cyst with papilloma and sinus presentation. J Am Acad Dermatol. 1984;11:367–71.

28. Dedivitis RA, Guimaraes AV. Papillary thyroid carcinoma in thyroglossal duct cyst. Int Surg. 2000;85:198–201.

29. Golledge J, Ellis H. The aetiology of lateral cervical (branchial) cysts: past and present theories. J Laryngol Otol. 1994;108:653–9.

30. Thaller SR, Bauer BS. Cysts and cyst-like lesions of the skin and subcutaneous tissue. Clin Plast Surg. 1987;14:327–40.

31. Fontaine DG, Lau H, Murray SK, et al. Cutaneous ciliated cyst of the abdominal wall: a case report with a review of the literature and discussion of pathogenesis. Am J Dermatopathol. 2002;24:63–6.

32. Kurban RS, Bhawan J. Cutaneous cysts lined by nonsquamous epithelium. Am J Dermatopathol. 1991;13:509–17.

33. Asarch RG, Golitz E, Sausker WF, Kreye GM. Median raphe cysts of the penis. Arch Dermatol. 1979;115:1084–6.

34. Fernandez Acenera MF, Garcia-Gonzales J. Median raphe cyst with ciliated cells: report of a case. Am J Dermatopathol. 2003;251:175–6.

35. Larralde de Luna M, Cicioni V, Herrera A, et al. Umbilical polyps. Pediatr Dermatol. 1987;4:341–3.

36. Jensen JL. Superficial mucoceles of the oral mucosa. Am J Dermatopathol. 1990;12:88–92.

37. de Berker D, Lawrence C. Ganglion of the distal interphalangeal joint (myxoid cyst): therapy by identification and repair of the leak of joint fluid. Arch Dermatol. 2001;137:607–10.

38. Epstein E. A simple technique for managing digital mucous cysts. Arch Dermatol. 1979;115:1315–16.

39. Soren A. Clinical and pathologic characteristics and treatment of ganglia. Contemp Orthop. 1995;31:34–8.

40. Schulte KW, Neumann NJ, Ruzicka T. Surgical pearl: the close-fitting ear cover cast – a noninvasive treatment for pseudocyst of the ear. J Am Acad Dermatol. 2001;44:285–6.

41. Secor CP, Farrell HA, Haydon RC III. Auricular endochondral pseudocysts: diagnosis and management. Plast Reconstr Surg. 1999;103:1451–7.

42. Singh SR, Ma AS, Dixon A. Multiple cutaneous metaplastic synovial cysts. J Am Acad Dermatol. 1999;41:330–2.

Adnexal Neoplasms

Timothy H McCalmont

111

Chapter Contents

Key features

- Terminology and classification of adnexal tumors has varied considerably according to different authorities
- Various combinations of follicular, sebaceous, apocrine and eccrine differentiation occur commonly
- Many tumors traditionally classified as eccrine are more commonly apocrine

The nosology of adnexal neoplasms has been confused for decades, and much of the mystification stems from a lack of logical classification. Classification schemes and inferences regarding lineage have often been contradictory, which stems from the fact that broad conclusions regarding lineage and classification have been based on morphologic and enzyme histochemical attributes of uncertain specificity[1].

The crucial embryologic principle to keep in mind when considering adnexal neoplasms is that the development of the eccrine apparatus is distinct from the folliculosebaceous-apocrine unit. Eccrine glands develop directly from the embryonic epidermis in the early months of fetal development[2]. Hair follicles arise directly from the epidermis at much the same time, but the development of follicles differs from the development of eccrine glands in that mesenchymal cells, precursors of the follicular papilla, descend jointly into the dermis with the developing epithelial elements. Subsequently, sebaceous and apocrine glands and their ducts begin to develop as secondary structures, elaborating from bulges on the side of the developing follicle.

These ontogenetic relationships reflect relationships that can be observed repetitively in clinical disease[1]. As one would expect from ontogeny, follicular, sebaceous and apocrine differentiation commonly occur conjointly, and combinations of eccrine and folliculosebaceous differentiation probably do not exist.

The topographic distribution of adnexal structures also offers insight into logical classification. There is striking variation in anatomic distribution among adnexal neoplasms, and some of these differences hold implications with respect to a logical assignment of lineage. Consider poroma, designated for decades as an eccrine neoplasm. Poroma develops commonly on the palms and soles, sites rife with eccrine structures[3,4]. The fact that poroma also occurs on glabrous skin supports tabulation of poroma as an eccrine neoplasm.

Microscopy and other morphologic tools also play a role in the assessment of lineage. For some lines of differentiation, the meanings attributed to specific microscopic findings are indisputable. The presence of cells with coarsely vacuolated cytoplasm and scalloped nuclei is a generally accepted correlate of sebaceous differentiation. There is consensus that follicular differentiation is established if a proliferation contains basaloid cells resembling the follicular bulb and adjacent mesenchymal cells resembling the papilla. Other unequivocal marks of follicular differentiation include 'shadow' cells and a palisade of pallid cells with an adjacent thickened basement membrane, an attribute of the trichilemma (follicular outer sheath). There are no attributes that clearly permit recognition of eccrine or apocrine differentiation.

NEOPLASMS AND PROLIFERATIONS OF FOLLICULAR LINEAGE

Follicular and Folliculosebaceous-apocrine Hamartomas

Hamartomas are benign proliferations composed of cellular elements, normal to a given site, in aberrant proportion. A congenital hamartoma, such as nevus sebaceus, is properly referred to as a *nevus*. Hamartomas can also be acquired, in the event of which they present clinically as a tumor, although such lesions do not represent authentic neoplasms.

Proliferations of the folliculosebaceous-apocrine unit are commonly 'hamartomatous' and sometimes represent authentic hamartomas, rather than true neoplasms. As the folliculosebaceous-apocrine unit is in a sense hamartomatous, incorporating multiple cellular components such as follicular epithelial, follicular mesenchymal, sebaceous and apocrine cells, the fact that it yields proliferations of microscopically diverse composition is not surprising. Indeed, many follicular neoplasms that we consider neoplasms, such as trichoblastoma, have integral stroma, and thus the distinction between hamartoma and neoplasm is sometimes blurred.

Hair follicle nevus
Introduction
Hair follicle nevi are authentic hamartomas, usually congenital, in which hairs and the follicles that ensheathe them have abnormal morphology or size or are present in increased numbers.

Clinical features
Hair follicle nevus, also known as *vellus hamartoma*, presents as a small papule from which fine hairs protrude evenly from the surface, often located on the face and commonly in the vicinity of the ear[5]. The pattern of an *accessory tragus* overlaps with that of hair follicle nevus, and some clinicians have suggested the two entities are the same[6,7]. *Nevus pilosus* designates hamartomas characterized by closely set, thick, scalp-like hairs.

Pathology
Microscopically, hair follicle nevi display a domed surface from which closely set but normally formed vellus follicles protrude. Depending upon the type of biopsy obtained, the microscopic pattern may closely resemble normal skin. Accessory tragi exhibit an identical pattern superficially, but are uniquely identifiable if a segment of underlying hyaline cartilage can be found deep within the specimen, usually at the level of the subcutis. Nevus pilosus is characterized by closely set terminal follicles.

Treatment
No therapy is required; conservative complete excision can be considered for cosmesis. In the evaluation of a hair follicle nevus or accessory tragus in a small child, it is important to counsel the parents of the infant that the relative size of the lesion will diminish with time. Thus, the child will grow much faster than the lesion, and by late childhood, the nevus may be inconspicuous.

Trichofolliculoma
Introduction
Often regarded as a hair follicle 'tumor', trichofolliculoma does not represent an authentic neoplasm. Rather, the term designates a group of follicular hamartomas in which fully formed follicular structures emanate from a central space, which is sometimes cystically dilated.

Clinical features
Trichofolliculoma presents as a papule or nodule, commonly involving the face, scalp, or sometimes the upper trunk (Fig. 111.1). Most examples are not clinically distinctive and receive the clinical diagnosis of basal cell carcinoma (BCC) or nevus. Sometimes, a central follicular ostium or punctum may be identifiable, and a small tuft of hairs may protrude from the surface. Rarely, the clinical presentation will be as a large nodule or as a cyst.

Pathology
The prototypical microscopic pattern of a trichofolliculoma consists of a central cystic space with infundibular (epidermoid) cornification, containing laminated orthokeratotic material. Sometimes, a few cross-

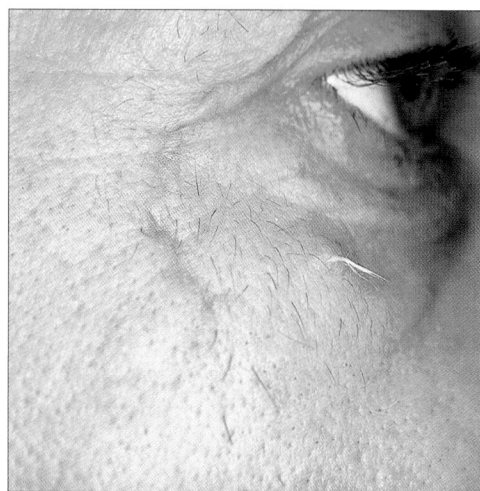

Fig. 111.1 Trichofolliculoma. Wispy vellus hairs emerge from a skin-colored papule with a dilated central pore.

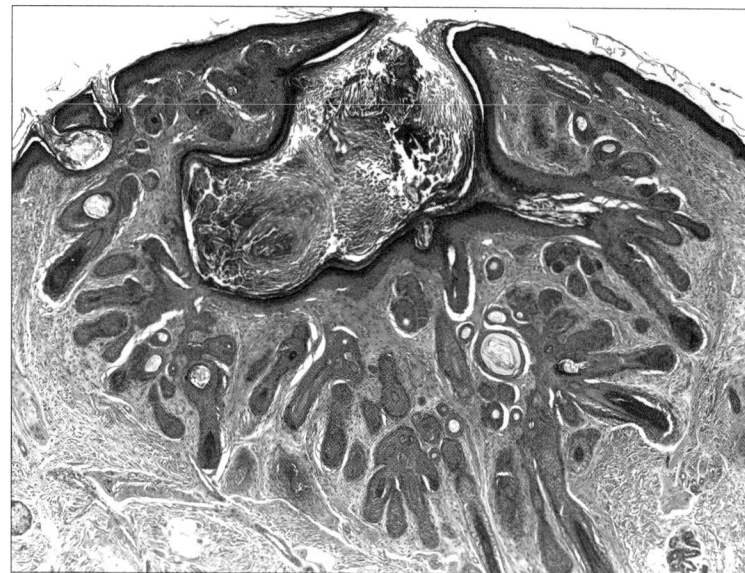

Fig. 111.2 Trichofolliculoma, viewed at scanning magnification. There is a central patulous follicular infundibulum, from which fully formed or nearly fully formed follicles radiate.

sections of hair shafts are also identifiable within the cyst lumen. Relatively well-developed and nearly normally formed vellus follicles protrude in radial fashion from the central cyst (Fig. 111.2). The follicles usually display a bulb and papilla peripherally, with inner and outer sheath and isthmic differentiation evident centrally, and often the germinative component of the follicle is increased in prominence or 'abortive' (basaloid) follicles may be seen. The entire structure, including the central cystic space and the radiating follicles, is enveloped by a highly vascularized, fibrocytic (angiofibroma-like) stroma.

The radiating follicles are frequently cut on tangent, which contributes to the great variation in microscopic patterns, and sometimes additional sections through the paraffin block are required to demonstrate fully diagnostic findings. If fully differentiated and well formed, the radiating follicles may be accompanied by sebaceous lobules[8]. When sebaceous lobules are conspicuous, the hamartoma can be referred to as a *sebaceous trichofolliculoma*. This diagnostic embellishment is not of any known additional clinical significance.

The term *folliculosebaceous cystic hamartoma* has been applied to a group of large nodular and cystic lesions described independently from trichofolliculoma[9–11]. These lesions are characterized by a central cyst with infundibular keratinization from which follicular and sebaceous structures emanate, and the investing stroma may be fibrocytic or myxoid and often contains adipocytes. Rather than a unique clinico-pathologic entity, is seems likely that folliculosebaceous cystic hamartoma represents a large cystic sebaceous trichofolliculoma[9].

Treatment
Trichofolliculoma is a benign lesion, and no treatment is required. If a trichofolliculoma is discovered by biopsy, there is no need for further re-excision of the site.

Fibrofolliculoma, perifollicular fibroma and trichodiscoma
Introduction
Much like trichofolliculoma, fibrofolliculoma does not represent an authentic neoplasm. Rather, the term designates a type of follicular hamartoma in which thin strands of follicular cells emanate from a central structure, and the complex epithelial structure is encompassed by highly vascularized, fibrocytic stroma. Perifollicular fibroma and trichodiscoma were described independently (as distinct entities) but are probably best thought of as purely stromal proliferations on the same spectrum as fibrofolliculoma.

Clinical features
Fibrofolliculomas (Fig. 111.3), perifollicular fibromas and trichodiscomas are not clinically distinctive. All present as small, skin-colored papules, commonly involving the face, scalp, or sometimes the upper trunk. The papules commonly present in multiplicity. When multiple lesions

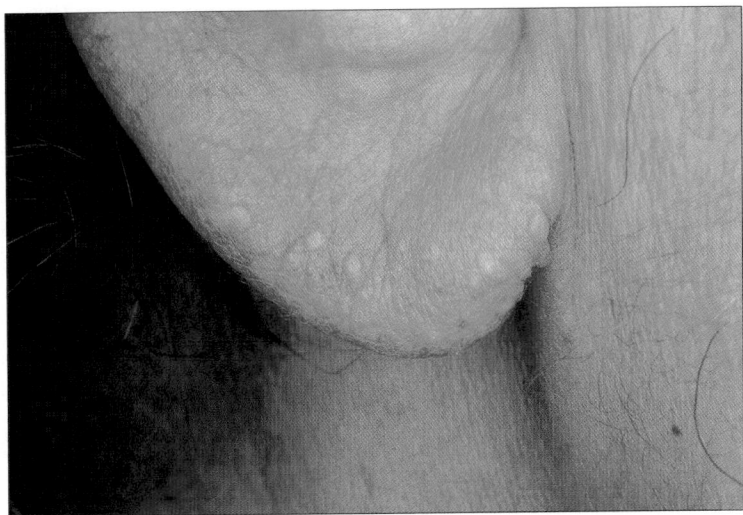

Fig. 111.3 Fibrofolliculoma. Several skin-colored papules are present on the ear.

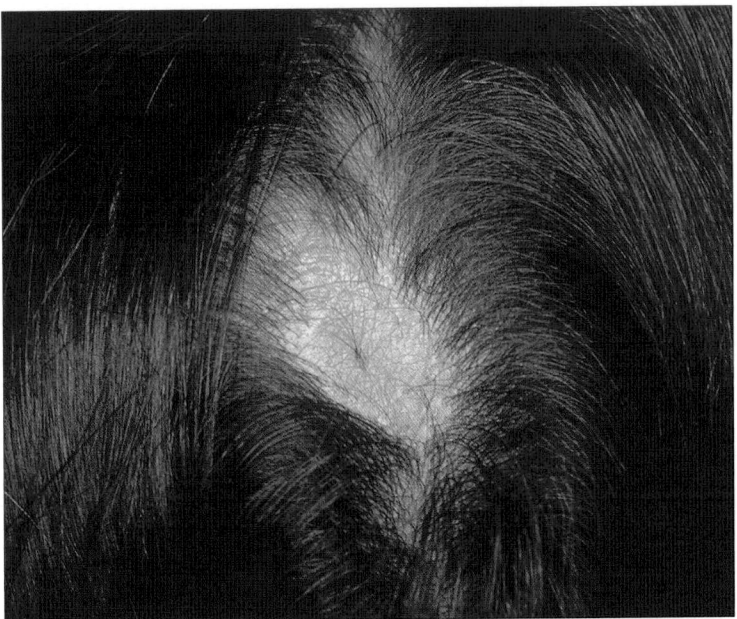

Fig. 111.4 Nevus sebaceus. Yellow–pink verrucous plaque on the scalp. Note the alopecia.

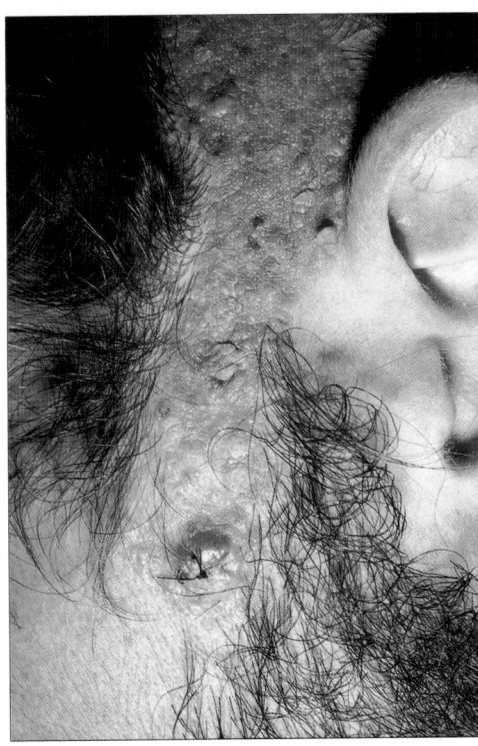

Fig. 111.5 Nevus sebaceus. Yellow–brown verrucous plaque in which a bluish 'basal cell carcinoma' developed. Courtesy of Ronald P Rapini MD.

are present, strong considerations should be given to the possibility of the Birt–Hogg–Dube syndrome (see Ch. 62). This is an autosomal dominant condition in which fibrofolliculomas, trichodiscomas and acrochordons appear on the face, neck and chest. There is an association with renal cell carcinoma and other renal tumors, colonic adenomas, pulmonary cysts, medullary carcinoma of the thyroid, and connective tissue nevi.

Pathology

At low magnification, fibrofolliculoma displays slender strands of follicular epithelial cells that emanate from a central follicular structure, typically at the level of the follicular isthmus. Usually, the strands are composed of cells with a slightly basaloid appearance, and sometimes small clusters of sebocytes are identifiable. The entire structure is enveloped by a highly vascularized, fibrocytic (angioma-like) stroma.

Perifollicular fibroma represents a proliferation that consists almost exclusively of stroma (identical with the stromal component of fibro-folliculoma and angiofibroma), with spindled and stellate cells arrayed amongst thickened collagen bundles with a proportionate number of intervening delicate, thin-walled vascular channels. Sometimes, a concurrent component of follicular epithelial hyperplasia is identifiable, although the epithelial component is never as striking as that observed in fibrofolliculoma. Trichodiscoma was thought by Pinkus to represent a unique proliferation with differentiation toward the 'haarscheibe' or 'hair disk', which is probably a mythical structure. More recently, trichodiscomas have been interpreted as fibrofolliculomas or peri-follicular fibromas in which the proliferation of spindled cells is accompanied by loose, myxoid stroma.

Treatment

Fibrofolliculomas, perifollicular fibromas and trichodiscomas are all benign and require no surgical treatment. Superficial electrodesiccation, carbon dioxide laser ablation or dermabrasion can be attempted to eradicate multiple lesions.

Nevus sebaceus
Introduction

Described by Jadassohn and also known as *organoid nevus*, nevus sebaceus is commonly thought of as a sebaceous malformation and is typically the first entity discussed in chapters describing sebaceous neoplasms. In truth, nevus sebaceus is not a sebaceous proliferation but a hamartoma that exhibits follicular, sebaceous and apocrine malformation to varying degrees[12].

Clinical features

Nevus sebaceus is a classical *nevus* or congenital malformation. The lesion is usually only slightly raised and subtly discernible at birth (Fig. 111.4). Nevus sebaceus involves the scalp or face commonly, sometimes involves the neck, and only rarely involves the trunk. The lesions are distributed along the lines of Blaschko and are arrayed in a linear configuration, although this may be difficult to appreciate if small. If on

the scalp, the nevus will remain hairless or mostly so as the infant's hair grows around it. During childhood, the lesion typically remains stable or thickens slightly and assumes a slightly yellow or orange hue. Upon reaching adolescence, progressive thickening occurs and the surface becomes pebbly, and in some individuals, the lesion may develop a verrucous surface.

It is well established that nevus sebaceus is a fertile field for the development of secondary adnexal neoplasms, most commonly benign but sometimes malignant[13–16]. A generation of dermatologists and dermatologic surgeons have been taught that secondary BCC develops in 10% or more of these lesions over time, although this figure is poorly substantiated and the vast majority of these 'carcinomas' represent follicular germinative (trichoblastic) proliferations with no malignant potential (Fig. 111.5); the actual occurrence of BCC in nevus sebaceus is less than 1% of cases[14]. Historically, the most common benign neoplasm to develop secondarily in nevus sebaceus was thought to be syringocystadenoma papilliferum (papillary syringadenoma), but more recent analysis indicates that trichoblastoma holds this role[13,14]. Other relatively common secondary neoplasms include trichilemmoma (including the desmoplastic variant), sebaceous adenoma, apocrine adenoma and poroma. Only rarely does secondary sebaceous carcinoma or apocrine carcinoma arise in a nevus sebaceus. This consequence probably only occurs in longstanding or neglected lesions, but can be a source of mortality.

Pathology

Nevus sebaceus is a malformation, and the principal malformation is of individual folliculosebaceous units. The microscopic pattern in an infantile nevus sebaceus can be quite subtle, particularly if the biopsy specimen includes only lesional skin, as the malformed follicular units are small and differ only subtly from normal. During childhood, the diagnosis remains a relatively subtle one. In an excisional specimen from the scalp during childhood, the tiny misshapen lesional follicles provide a stark contrast to the normal terminal follicles at the periphery of the biopsy. Small apocrine glands may be identifiable in the superficial subcutis in a specimen of sufficient depth. The surface epidermis also gradually thickens throughout early childhood and becomes progressively more papillated, assuming a pattern identical to that of an epidermal nevus by early adolescence.

At adolescence, nevus sebaceus displays a pattern identical to that of an epidermal nevus, with papillated epidermal hyperplasia, interanastomosis of rete, and a coarsely fibrotic papillary dermis. There may be enlarged sebaceous lobules that appear to emanate from the dermal–epidermal junction and buds of follicular germinative cells may jut from the junctional zone as well (Fig. 111.6). The underlying follicular units remain smallish and appear distorted, but their sebaceous lobules increase in prominence. Dilated glandular structures with inspissated secretion are commonly identifiable in the reticular dermis.

In adulthood, the microscopic pattern remains relatively stable. Some patients develop exaggerated verrucous epidermal hyperplasia with a microscopic pattern identical to verruca vulgaris. This alteration is probably not induced by papillomavirus, although this has not been comprehensively studied. As noted previously, secondary neoplasms are common, and trichoblastoma, trichilemmoma and syringocystadenoma are frequently observed in this context[13,14]. Indeed, the association between syringocystadenoma and nevus sebaceus is so strong that when the diagnosis of syringocystadenoma is offered microscopically, careful scrutiny is warranted to ascertain whether the diagnosis of nevus sebaceus can be derived from the same specimen.

Treatment

As noted previously, BCC (and occasionally other types of carcinoma) was alleged to develop in nevus sebaceus in 10% or more of cases, and this risk of 'malignant transformation' was used as justification for complete excision. In truth, the risk of development of carcinoma appears to be closer to 1%[16]. However, the risk for the development of a secondary neoplasm (such as syringocystadenoma or trichoblastoma) in the milieu of nevus sebaceus is relatively high, although virtually all such neoplasms are benign. In addition, it is clear that nevus sebaceus becomes increasingly verrucous and unsightly over time. Most patients will not tolerate such unattractive lesions, given their predilection for occurrence on the head or neck.

In light of this, conservative complete excision of nevus sebaceus to adipose or galea is warranted in many cases. Lesions within the scalp may be difficult to follow clinically and extirpation will prevent the development of occult secondary changes. For facial lesions, consideration should be given to excision during childhood, before the development of secondary verrucous changes and at a time when the risk of scarring is minimal. The excisional margins can probably be minimal. Removal by shave or laser ablation is usually not successful.

Mixed tumor (chondroid syringoma)
Introduction

Cutaneous mixed tumor, also known as *chondroid syringoma*, represents an acquired hamartoma with folliculosebaceous-apocrine differentiation that has been generally interpreted as a form of adnexal adenoma (neoplasm) since the time of its original description. Despite this legacy, mixed tumor is clearly best classified as a hamartoma. The stroma of mixed tumor is always abundant and generally comprises over half of the surface area of a given lesion in conventional microscopic sections, and the epithelial component is often heterogeneous[17]. An analogy has been made between cutaneous mixed tumor and mixed tumor (pleomorphic adenoma) of the salivary gland. While the comparison has some validity, it is important to note that pleomorphic adenoma of the salivary gland often functions as a neoplasm in a biologic sense, with a tendency for local recurrence if incompletely extirpated and the potential for evolution to malignancy. In contrast, cutaneous mixed tumor is an indolent process virtually devoid of proliferative capacity and rarely recurs after enucleation.

Clinical features

The clinical presentation of mixed tumor is not distinctive (Fig. 111.7). The lesions present as cutaneous nodules, most commonly on the head and neck and occasionally involving the upper trunk, axillary or inguinal areas, or genital skin.

Pathology

At low magnification, mixed tumor is a well-circumscribed nodule that resides partially within the deep reticular dermis and the subcutis. A 'biphasic' pattern is clearly apparent, with epithelial structures enveloped by abundant stroma that often comprises more than half of the area of a given microscopic section. The enveloping stroma varies considerably in composition within a given lesion and among different lesions[17]. There is always a prominent collagenous component to the stroma.

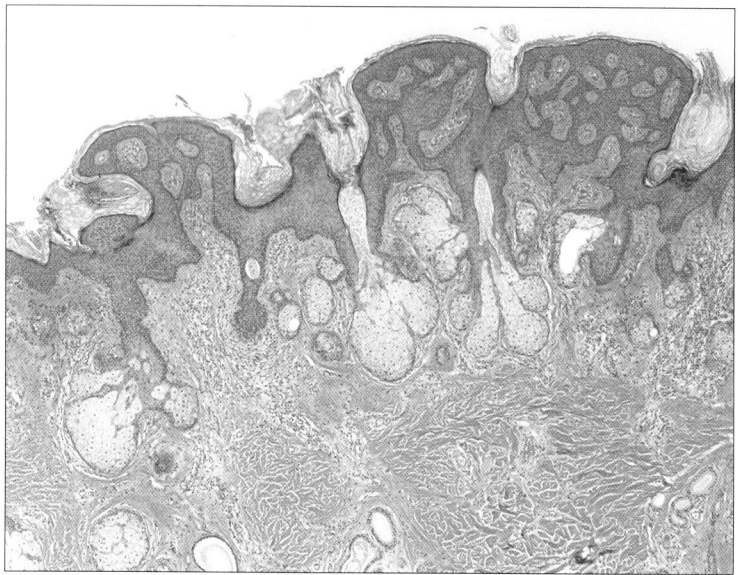

Fig. 111.6 Nevus sebaceus. Medium magnification reveals expansion of the epidermis in a papillated fashion, much like the pattern of an epidermal nevus, jointly with adnexal malformation, with enlarged sebaceous lobules and clusters of follicular germinative cells positioned along the dermal–epidermal junction.

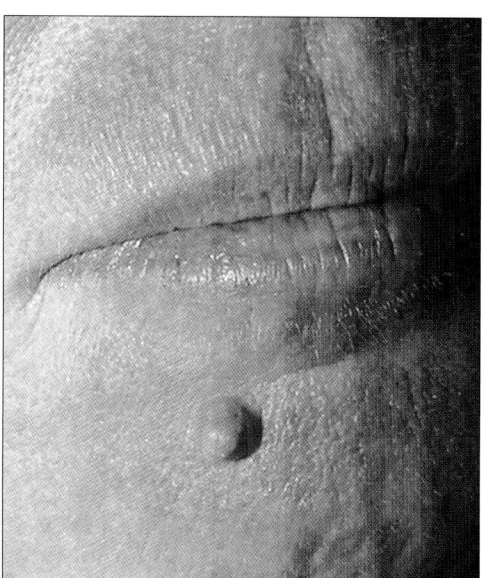

Fig. 111.7 Chondroid syringoma. Nodule of chin. Courtesy of Ronald P Rapini MD.

Myxoid areas are common, as are clusters of adipocytes. Despite the implications of the name, mature hyaline cartilage is present in the stroma in less than half of patients.

The epithelial component of mixed tumor displays two primary patterns. Most mixed tumors demonstrate a pattern with large branching tubules arrayed in an interanastomosing fashion, and these tubules are usually lined by columnar apocrine cells with an obvious 'decapitation' pattern at the luminal border; this pattern has been commonly referred to as 'apocrine' mixed tumor[18] (Fig. 111.8). Much less commonly, mixed tumors demonstrate a pattern with small tubules or ducts, some of which may have a central cuticle (Fig. 111.9). Such lesions are sometimes termed 'eccrine' mixed tumor. However, it seems most likely that all mixed tumors are hamartomas of folliculosebaceous-apocrine lineage, and that the epithelial component can be arrayed either as large branching tubules or as small ducts or as a mixture of the two.

In addition to ducts and tubules, the epithelial component of mixed tumor commonly includes follicular and sebaceous attributes[17,19]. Follicular differentiation can consist of small clusters of follicular germinative cells, lobules of outer sheath cells, cystic foci with isthmic or infundibular keratinization and clusters of 'shadow' cells, reflecting matrical differentiation. Small clusters of sebocytes can also be found within mixed tumors, usually in lesions that also display follicular differentiation.

Treatment

Mixed tumor is a benign process with little proliferative capacity. Most lesions are treated by simple enucleation, and the risk for persistence/recurrence is minimal. In contrast to mixed tumors of salivary origin, there is no need for excision with generous margins.

Neoplasms and Proliferations with Follicular Germinative Differentiation

Trichoepithelioma/trichoblastoma
Introduction

Trichoepithelioma and trichoblastoma are terms that refer to benign neoplasms with mostly follicular germinative differentiation[20].

In historical perspective, the term 'trichoepithelioma' is older, and represents the name ascribed to a solitary lesion of the familial multiple form of trichoepithelioma (epithelioma adenoides cysticum). The designation 'trichoblastoma' was coined more recently, and was originally applied to neoplasms that showed follicular bulbar differentiation almost exclusively; lesions of this type have also been referred to as 'immature trichoepitheliomas'[21]. Although the term 'trichoepithelioma' is still used, the designation 'trichoblastoma' has evolved to be an overarching label for benign proliferations with follicular germinative differentiation[20]. Thus, in the current dermatologic and dermatopathologic lexicon, trichoepithelioma could be considered to be a variant of trichoblastoma.

Many authors have described subtle variations within the spectrum of follicular germinative neoplasms, utilizing terms such as trichogerminoma, trichoblastic fibroma, and lymphadenoma (adamantinoid trichoblastoma)[20]. For the purposes of this discussion, these variations will be considered as microscopic variations within the spectrum of trichoblastoma and not as unique clinicopathologic entities.

Clinical features

Classical trichoepithelioma usually presents as a skin-colored papule or small nodule on the face or upper trunk, and lesions have a special predilection for the nose (Fig. 111.10). When in multiplicity (epithelioma adenoides cysticum or Brooke's disease), the density of lesions is always greatest in the central face. The gene for Brooke's disease has been mapped to 9p21; the disease can be cosmetically troublesome, but there are no other associated anomalies[22]. Lesions described historically as 'trichoblastoma' were commonly larger, deeper and more nodular than classical trichoepithelioma.

Pathology

All trichoepitheliomas and trichoblastomas share in common the architectural attributes of a benign neoplasm – namely, relative symmetry, sharp circumscription and a lack of substantial cytologic atypicality.

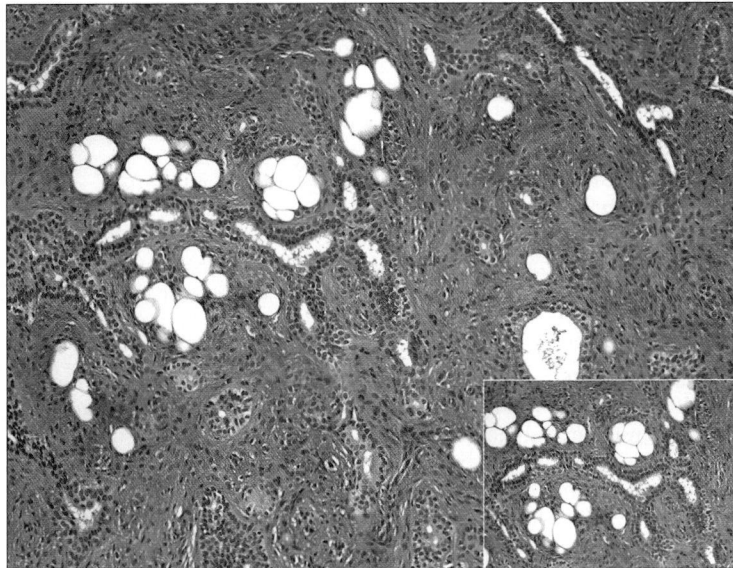

Fig. 111.8 Mixed tumor (chondroid syringoma) with overt apocrine differentiation. At medium magnification, there is a hamartomatous pattern, with large branching tubules arrayed within a mucinous stroma that contains lipocytes. Conspicuous apocrine differentiation with a 'decapitation' pattern is evident in the inset.

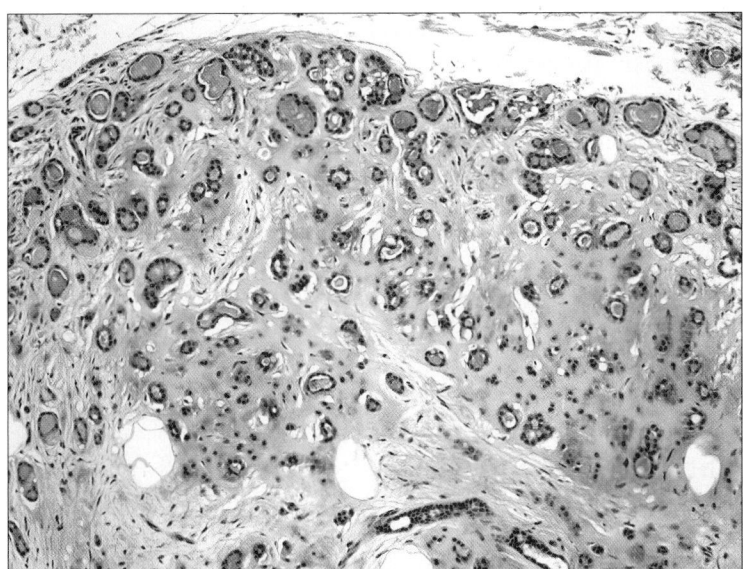

Fig. 111.9 Mixed tumor (chondroid syringoma) with ductal differentiation. This pattern, commonly referred to as the 'eccrine' type of mixed tumor, shows small syringoma-like ducts positioned in ample stroma reminiscent of hyaline cartilage.

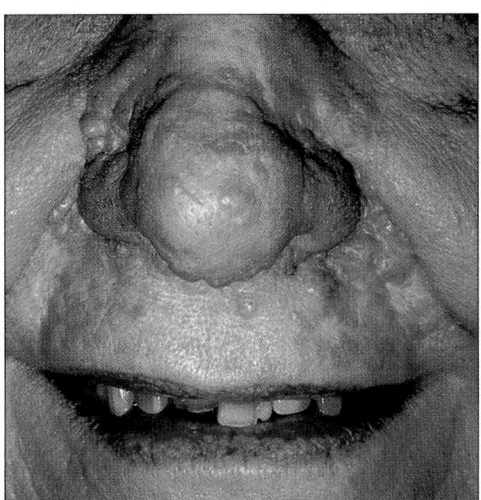

Fig. 111.10 Trichoepithelioma. Numerous skin-colored papules on the mid-face.

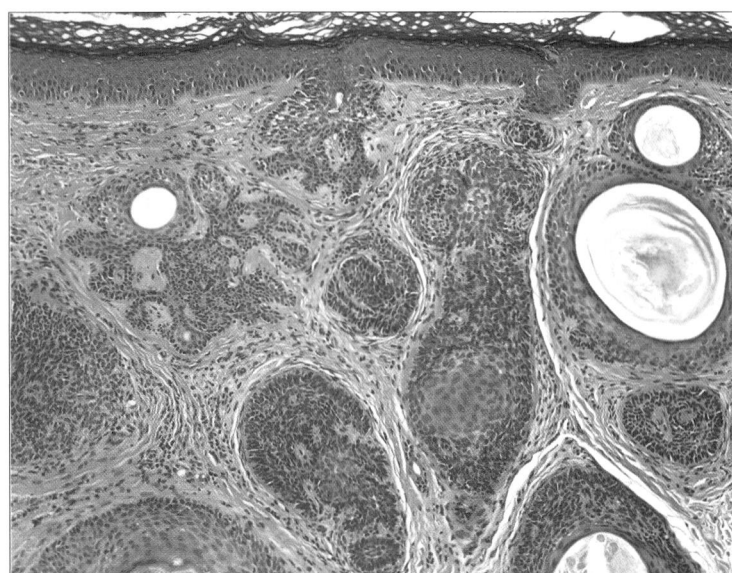

Fig. 111.11 Trichoepithelioma (trichoblastoma). This 'classical' trichoepithelioma is composed mostly of clusters of follicular germinative cells but also shows superficial follicular differentiation, with small keratinizing cystic spaces. Note that clefts within the proliferation are between stromal elements, in contrast to the clefts between tumor and stroma that are characteristic of basal cell carcinoma.

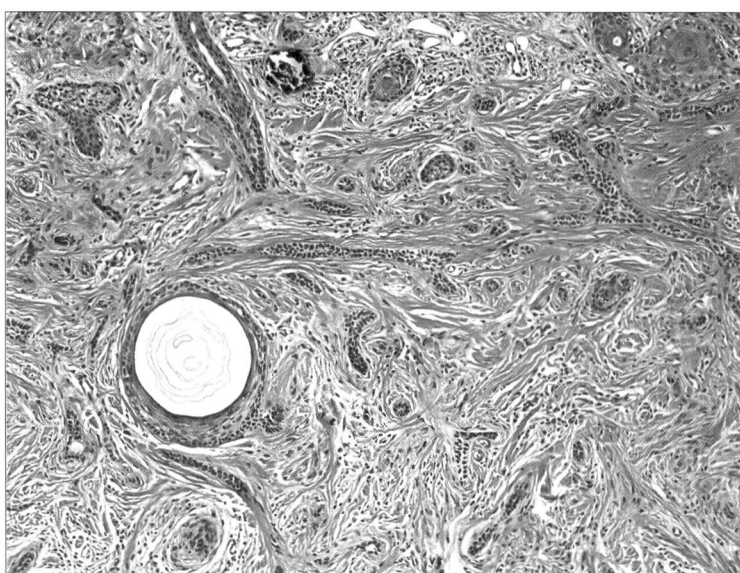

Fig. 111.12 Desmoplastic trichoepithelioma. It is composed of thin strands of basaloid (follicular germinative) cells, arrayed in sclerotic stroma. Much like conventional trichoepithelioma, there are foci of superficial follicular keratinization.

In addition, all trichoblastomas and trichoepitheliomas are linked by a predominance of follicular germinative (basaloid) cells with enveloping fibrocytic stroma that varies in degree[20,23]. In classical trichoepithelioma, the fibrocytic stroma is conspicuous and constitutes as much as half of the cellularity of the lesion in a given cross-section. In contrast, in a trichoblastoma, there may be a vast predominance of follicular germinative cells, arrayed as either small or large nodules, with only scant intervening sclerotic stroma. The fibrocytic stroma typically maintains tightly adherent contact to the neoplastic follicular germinative cells[23]. This is in distinct contrast to the pattern of BCC, in which clefts between basaloid cells and stromal elements serve as a clue to the diagnosis.

In classical trichoepithelioma, the follicular germinative cells are arrayed as small clusters or as reticulate and cribriform cords of basaloid cells (Fig. 111.11). There are usually foci of pronounced bulbar differentiation, emulating the follicular bulb and papilla; these structures have been referred to as 'papillary mesenchymal bodies'[23,24]. Classical trichoepithelioma does not usually show solely follicular germinative differentiation, but also exhibits superficial follicular differentiation to varying degrees, as seen by small cornifying cystic spaces with surrounding pinkish keratinocytes, reflecting infundibular or isthmic differentiation.

In small or large nodular patterns of trichoblastoma, papillary mesenchymal bodies may be inconspicuous and superficial follicular differentiation is usually absent. A nodular trichoblastoma is usually composed mostly of follicular germinative cells with little stroma, and the microscopic pattern from low magnification consists of a well-circumscribed array of closely packed cells with a distinctly basaloid appearance. *Trichoblastic fibroma* is a designation used to characterize small nodular trichoblastomas with conspicuous fibrocytic stroma, sometimes constituting over 50% of the lesion[25–27]. Papillary mesenchymal bodies may be conspicuous in trichoblastic fibroma. In either classical trichoepithelioma or trichoblastoma, other patterns of differentiation can occasionally be found with close scrutiny. There may be small clusters of sebocytes, reflecting a component of sebaceous differentiation, and ductal differentiation (presumably apocrine) may also be noted.

Treatment
Trichoblastoma is a benign adnexal neoplasm, and, as such, there is no imperative for surgical treatment. However, multiple facial trichoblastomas can be cosmetically disabling and many affected patients desire some type of intervention. Because of the number of lesions, conventional excision is not usually indicated. Other ablative approaches, including laser or electrosurgical destruction, have been employed with some success[28,29].

Desmoplastic trichoblastoma (desmoplastic trichoepithelioma)
Introduction
Originally described as 'sclerosing epithelial hamartoma', desmoplastic trichoepithelioma represents a variant of trichoblastoma with extensive stromal sclerosis (desmoplasia)[30]. It can be misinterpreted as sclerosing BCC.

Clinical features
The stereotypical presentation of desmoplastic trichoepithelioma is as a firm skin-colored to erythematous annular plaque with a central dell or depression, usually on the upper cheek of a woman[30]. Most examples do not exceed 1 cm in diameter. Nearly all desmoplastic trichoepitheliomas are solitary. Multiple lesions are quite rare.

Pathology
Desmoplastic trichoepitheliomas are composed of cords of basaloid cells, often two cells wide, arrayed interstitially amongst strikingly thickened collagen bundles[20,30] (Fig. 111.12). The lesions are relatively circumscribed and are usually confined to the upper two-thirds of the reticular dermis, although this is difficult to appreciate in biopsies *en parte*. Small cystic foci of isthmic or infundibular keratinization may be present in the upper dermis, and if these cystic spaces constitute the predominant pattern of the lesion, the pattern can be interpreted as *trichoadenoma*. The cornifying cysts can rupture and elicit a granulomatous reaction, and small interstitial foci of calcification may also be identified[20,30].

Treatment
Desmoplastic trichoepithelioma is a benign lesion that holds no risk for the development of carcinoma, if the diagnosis is definitive. Small incomplete biopsies may cause uncertainty about excluding sclerosing BCC or microcystic adnexal carcinoma, and re-excision or resampling may be necessary for a definitive diagnosis or complete eradication in uncertain cases.

Neoplasms and Proliferations with Matrical Differentiation
Pilomatricoma
Introduction
Pilomatricoma (pilomatrixoma, trichomatrioma, calcifying epithelioma of Malherbe) is a benign neoplasm or cyst typified by follicular matrical cornification. It has now been demonstrated that mutations in *CTNNB1*, the gene that encodes for β-catenin, are present in matrical neoplasms generally, including pilomatricomas[31]. Beta-catenin is a

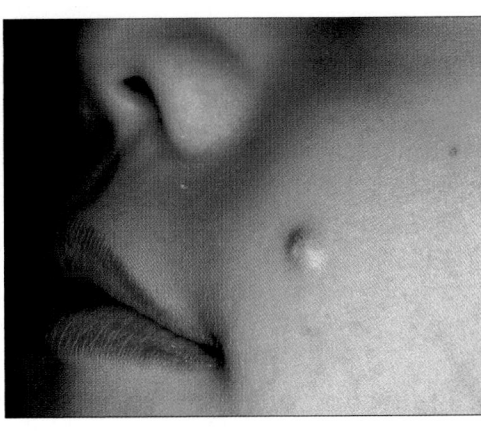

Fig. 111.13
Pilomatricoma. A nodule on the cheek of a child.

signaling pathway effector that influences cell differentiation and proliferation, and mutations in β-catenin are thought to be present in pilomatricomas generally.

Clinical features

Pilomatricoma usually presents as a solitary skin-colored to faint-blue nodule or cyst; rarely, multiple lesions are evident[32]. The nodules are typically firm, a reflection of the calcification that commonly accompanies these lesions and the fibrosis and inflammation they elicit (Fig. 111.13). Pilomatricomas may develop on any non-glabrous surface, but most occur on the head or upper trunk[33]. Most common in childhood and adolescence, pilomatricomas may occur at any age and can simulate BCC clinically and microscopically when occurrence is in later adulthood. Occasionally, the dermis overlying a pilomatricoma will develop anetoderma[34]. The nodules may become inflamed and erythematous.

Pathology

The microscopic pattern of an early evolving pilomatricoma is frequently that of a cyst with matrical cornification. The wall of the cyst is composed of basaloid matrical cells, with an abrupt transition to central eosinophilic cornified matrical cells in which barely discernible nuclear outlines ('ghosts') remain. Sometimes, pink trichohyalin granules, implying matrical cornification, are identifiable at the transition point. The central anucleate cornified cells are commonly referred to as 'ghost' cells or 'shadow' cells.

In fully developed pilomatricomas, a cystic configuration is commonly lost, and solid collections of basaloid matrical cells and 'shadow' cells are present in varying degrees (Fig. 111.14). The cornified matrical cells elicit considerable fibrosis and granulomatous inflammation, which can become the predominant microscopic pattern, especially in longstanding lesions. Matrical cells have a proliferative capacity as high as any human

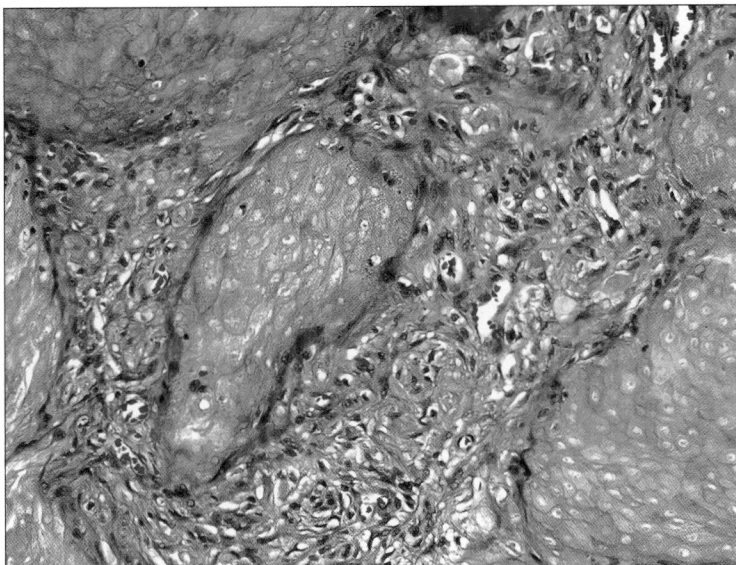

Fig. 111.14 Pilomatricoma. At high magnification, this longstanding example is notable for anucleate keratinized matrical cells ('shadow' cells) and a surrounding granulomatous reaction.

tissue and can display a considerable number of mitotic figures, and pilomatricomas with a predominance of basaloid cells can be misinterpreted as carcinoma, especially if the basaloid cells are arrayed irregularly in a background of fibrosis, creating a pattern that simulates invasion. In late lesions, basaloid matrical cells may be entirely absent, and only small clusters of shadow cells, buried in a background of fibrosis and granulomatous inflammation, may remain as evidence of the preceding pilomatricoma. Calcification and ossification also ensue in late lesions.

Treatment

Pilomatricoma is a benign lesion that is usually treated by simple enucleation. A pilomatricoma may recur after limited excision. If multiple recurrences are observed, complete excision (with negative margins) should be performed to exclude the possibility of pilomatrical carcinoma.

Pilomatrical carcinoma
Introduction

Pilomatrical (matrical) carcinoma is an uncommon form of carcinoma that exhibits matrical cornification, similar to pilomatricoma[35]. Much like its benign counterpart, mutations in the *CTNNB1* gene (coding for β-catenin) are common in matrical carcinoma[31]. This suggests a common initial pathogenesis for pilomatricoma and matrical carcinoma, and also suggests that there is some risk for matrical carcinoma developing from a conventional pilomatricoma.

Clinical features

Matrical carcinoma is typically a disease of adulthood, and lesions typically develop on the head and neck (often in the retroauricular area). Although a pathogenic link with UV light has not been established, most matrical carcinomas develop on severely sun-damaged skin. If a diagnosis of matrical carcinoma is offered in a child or young adult at an age when the diagnosis is unlikely, the case should be re-evaluated with the possibility of pilomatricoma reconsidered.

Pathology

Much like pilomatricoma, matrical carcinomas include both basaloid matrical cells and cornified cells. In contrast to pilomatricoma, the basaloid matrical cells usually have considerable nuclear pleomorphism and an infiltrative pattern is usually apparent, especially in excisional biopsies. There may be considerable squamous cornification as well, and parts of a given lesion may resemble conventional squamous cell carcinoma (SCC), with basaloid matrical cells only focally apparent.

Matrical carcinoma should be distinguished microscopically from BCC with matrical differentiation[36,37]. The latter entity represents a carcinoma in which typical BCC comprises the bulk of the lesion, but small foci of matrical cornification (with shadow cells) are identifiable. The clinical behavior of this variant is thought to be identical to conventional BCC.

Treatment

Matrical carcinoma is a low-grade form of adnexal carcinoma that poses some risk for metastasis, although this risk is believed to be low[35]. Complete extirpation with negative margins is the standard of care.

Neoplasms and Proliferations with Follicular Sheath (Trichilemmal) Differentiation

Trichilemmoma
Introduction

Trichilemmoma (tricholemmoma) constitutes a form of benign adnexal neoplasm with differentiation mostly toward the follicular outer sheath[38]. Some have averred that trichilemmoma is merely a pattern of viral wart based upon findings in conventional microscopic sections[20]. However, molecular analysis has generally not revealed papillomavirus DNA sequences in these lesions, and thus a viral causation seems unlikely[39].

Clinical features

Trichilemmomas may arise as simple or as multiple[38,40] papules or small nodules that usually hold similar coloration to surrounding normal skin and only rarely are pigmented. Individual lesions may display hyperkeratosis or a verrucous surface. Most are distributed on the central face, especially the nose or upper lip, but the papules can occur at any non-glabrous site. Trichilemmomas can also present on genital skin and simulate the clinical pattern of a condyloma, especially if multiple. Trichilemmoma may occur as a secondary neoplasm within the milieu of *nevus sebaceus*; the variant form known as 'desmoplastic' trichilemmoma is especially common in this context[41].

Multiple trichilemmomas typically present on facial or genital skin. Multiple trichilemmomas are a common manifestation of Cowden syndrome (see Ch. 62)[38,42]. In addition to trichilemmomas, characteristic cutaneous manifestations of Cowden disease include sclerotic ('hypocellular') fibromas and acrokeratosis verruciformis[43]. Systemic consequences of Cowden disease include adenocarcinoma, most commonly of the breast, thyroid gland or gastrointestinal tract.

Pathology

Microscopically, trichilemmomas are typically small circumscribed and lobular or multilobular proliferations composed mostly of pallid, glycogen-containing outer sheath cells, often with a broad connection to the surface epidermis[38,40,42]. A papillated surface is common, and there may be marked verrucous hyperplasia with hypergranulosis, simulating the pattern of a verruca in a superficial biopsy. Squamous eddies are also common. There is a palisade of small, compact basal keratinocytes at the periphery of a lobule, usually with an adjacent thickened basement membrane that is PAS-D (periodic acid–Schiff with diastase)-positive (Fig. 111.15).

In desmoplastic trichilemmoma, small angular clusters of tumor cells are arrayed in an infiltrative pattern with enveloping sclerotic stroma, creating a microscopic pattern that resembles invasive carcinoma[41,44,45]. Most commonly, a desmoplastic focus is accompanied or surrounded by areas of conventional trichilemmoma that serve as the basis for accurate pathologic diagnosis, but the pattern can be quite deceptive in partial or superficial biopsies.

Treatment

Trichilemmoma is a benign adnexal neoplasm with limited proliferative capacity. After recognition by biopsy, no further treatment is needed, unless desired by the patient or there is uncertainty of the diagnosis. Since superficial biopsies of solitary lesions can resemble actinic keratosis or superficial SCC, complete removal may be indicated. Cryotherapy, electrosurgical destruction, shave, curettage or excision may be used.

Trichilemmal carcinoma

This malignant counterpart to trichilemmoma is characterized as invasive lesions composed in part of glycogen-containing clear cells,

similar to cells of the follicular outer sheath. If a thickened, PAS-positive prominent basement membrane can be identified peripheral to areas of clear cell change, it is probably of considerable diagnostic significance. Many of these carcinomas show considerable accompanying keratinization and thus there is considerable overlap with lesions that have been pigeonholed as clear cell SCC.

Treatment

Trichilemmal carcinoma is a low-grade carcinoma with low metastatic potential. These lesions are probably best considered equivalent to SCC and treated as such.

Neoplasms and Proliferations with Superficial Follicular (Infundibular and Isthmic) Differentiation

Tumor of follicular infundibulum (isthmicoma)

Introduction

This benign lesion is best known as *tumor of follicular infundibulum (TFI)* or *infundibuloma*, but the designation *isthmicoma* is more apt, as the proliferation shows mostly follicular isthmic differentiation.

Clinical features

TFI prototypically presents clinically as subtle macules, or thin papules or plaques[14,46]. They are skin-colored or sometimes slightly hypopigmented and may appear slightly atrophic[14,46]. Many examples are diagnosed incidentally within skin cancer excision specimens and no known clinical lesion was even identifiable. TFI may occur in multiplicity, and patients with this presentation may defy diagnosis for a time because of the subtlety of both the clinical and the microscopic findings[46–49]. Patients with multiple atrophic-appearing TFI may display a clinical pattern reminiscent of disseminated superficial porokeratosis. TFI is occasionally present in Cowden disease[14].

Pathology

TFI consists of a plate-like proliferation of eosinophilic isthmic keratinocytes arrayed in reticulate fashion in the superficial dermis, in broad but intermittent continuity with both the surface epidermis and existent follicular structures[14,46]. Most of the constituent keratinocytes have cytoplasm similar to keratinocytes of the follicular isthmus, follicles in catagen phase, or the cells of an isthmic (pilar) cyst (Fig. 111.16). The keratinocytes are paler than those of the surface epidermis, and sometimes a few scattered apoptotic or dyskeratotic keratinocytes are present. Some lesions will display trichilemmal foci in which pallid keratinocytes or a thickened basement membrane can be found, and

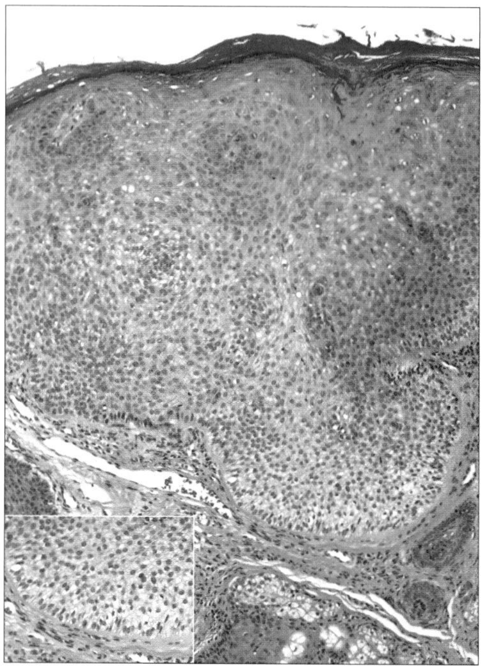

Fig. 111.15 Trichilemmoma. This benign neoplasm with follicular differentiation shows a verrucous surface with hypergranulosis. This pattern, which is commonly present, has suggested to some that these lesions may be induced by papillomavirus. The inset shows follicular outer sheath differentiation, with pale keratinocytes surrounded by a palisade of small basal cells, adjacent to which is a densely eosinophilic thickened basement membrane.

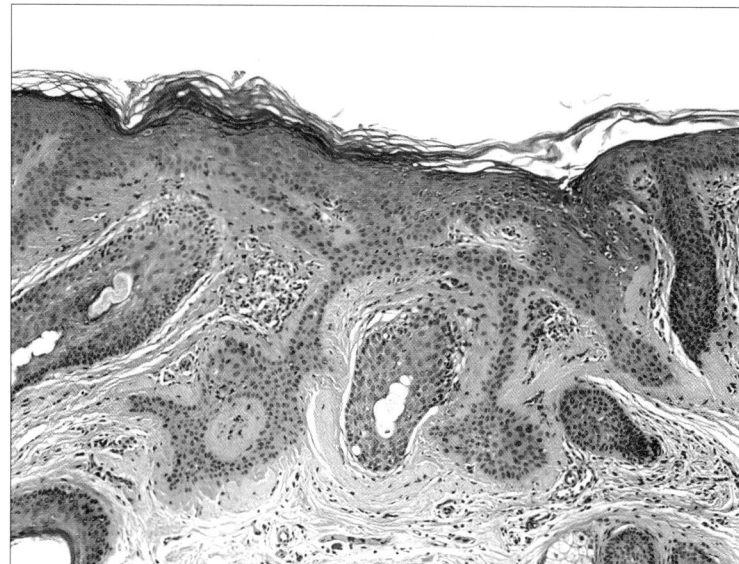

Fig. 111.16 Tumor of follicular infundibulum (TFI). The microscopic pattern of TFI is subtle, resembling reticulated seborrheic keratosis. Strands of pale eosinophilic keratinocytes display multifocal attachment to the epidermal surface and also commonly interconnect with existent follicular structures.

occasionally a 'hybrid' lesion with mixed features of TFI and trichilemmoma may be encountered. Sometimes, small buds of follicular germinative cells may jut from the undersurface of TFI.

Rarely, small clusters of sebocytes may be found within TFI[50]. Sebaceous or apocrine ducts have also been documented[49].

Treatment

TFI is a benign adnexal proliferation with negligible proliferative capacity. If desired, they may be removed by cryotherapy, shave, or electrosurgical destruction. For multiple lesions, superficial laser ablation can be considered[46].

Trichoadenoma (trichoadenoma of Nikolowski)
Introduction

The term *trichoadenoma* is a misnomer, as there are no adenomas of strictly follicular lineage; the hair follicle is not a structure that exhibits glandular differentiation. Trichoadenoma is a benign follicular neoplasm that consists mostly of small cystic spaces that exhibit infundibular and isthmic differentiation, enveloped by sclerotic stroma[51].

Clinical features

The clinical presentation of trichoadenoma is not distinctive. The neoplasm presents as a skin-colored papule or small plaque.

Pathology

At low magnification, the neoplasm is usually positioned in the superficial dermis. Cornifying cysts with infundibular or isthmic keratinization comprise the bulk of the proliferation[51]. The sclerotic stroma is often accompanied by thin strands of basaloid cells, similar to the cords of basaloid cells observed in desmoplastic trichoepithelioma (Fig. 111.17). The degree of microscopic overlap between trichoadenoma and desmoplastic trichoepithelioma can be striking. Indeed, these names may describe the same tumor.

Treatment

Trichoadenoma is a benign adnexal neoplasm with negligible proliferative capacity. No further treatment is necessary if the histologic diagnosis is certain, unless the patient desires removal.

Proliferating pilar tumor (proliferating follicular-cystic neoplasm)
Introduction

Known for decades as *proliferating pilar tumor (PPT)* or *proliferating pilar cyst*, the designation *proliferating follicular-cystic neoplasm (PFCN)* was proposed by Ackerman as a more apt designation[20]. This term describes a group of nodular and, occasionally, cystic neoplasms characterized microscopically by abrupt keratinization, similar to the pattern observed at the follicular isthmus, in an isthmic (pilar) cyst, or in a follicle in catagen phase[52]. In the past, it was known that PPT could simulate SCC microscopically, but the entity was generally regarded as a benign process, although it was recognized that, occasionally, locally destructive behavior could occur[52].

Recently, this concept has been called into question, and a proposal has been issued that PFCN represents a mix of benign and malignant neoplasms grouped together under one rubric[20]. The proposal further iterates that a 'benign' PFCN should be designated as a *proliferating follicular-cystic acanthoma*, while a 'malignant' PFCN should be designated as *proliferating follicular-cystic squamous cell carcinoma*. As some examples of PFCN share features in common with carcinoma, including clinical characteristics such as locally destructive behavior, microscopic characteristics such as nuclear atypicality, and molecular characteristics such as aberrations in ploidy, it is clear that this proposal holds some merit[53–55]. However, as most PFCNs are circumscribed microscopically and the patients who harbor them follow a benign clinical course, it seems premature at this time to reclassify the entire entity as a variant of SCC.

Clinical features

PPT presents as a nodule, usually no more than a few centimeters in size, although there have been reports of lesions exceeding 20 cm in diameter. The lesions can develop in men or in women, with a female predominance. Roughly 90% of cases arise in the scalp, probably as a reflection of the density of follicles at that locale. The prototypical presentation is as a nodule on the scalp of an elderly woman. The lesions are usually well circumscribed but may be multinodular. Their circumscription is reflected in smooth borders and the fact that lesions generally 'shell out' from adjacent tissues during surgical excision.

Pathology

PPT consists of a large, sharply circumscribed nodule that resides in the deep reticular dermis and subcutis or in the subcutaneous compartment exclusively[52]. Because of their large size, the laboratory commonly receives fragmented specimens. Both solid and cystic patterns are usually evident at low magnification, with cystic areas exhibiting the pattern of an isthmic (pilar) cyst. The constituent keratinocytes are mostly isthmic keratinocytes with dense eosinophilic cytoplasm, and the centers of both solid and cystic areas display an abrupt transition to compact keratin, usually with little intervening granular layer (Fig. 111.18). Rarely, shadow cells, implying matrical keratinization, can be found.

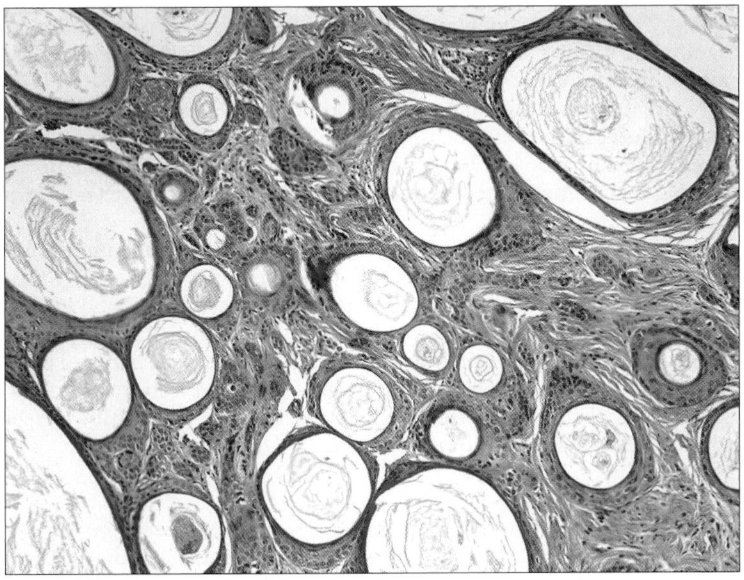

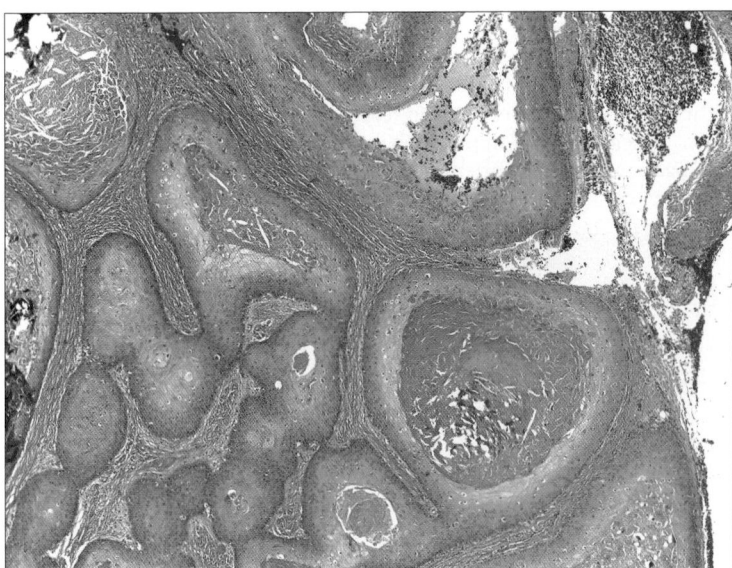

Fig. 111.17 Trichoadenoma. This lesion consists almost exclusively of small keratinizing cystic spaces. There are also a few strands of basaloid cells and sclerotic stroma, similar to the pattern observed in desmoplastic trichoepithelioma.

Fig. 111.18 Proliferating follicular-cystic neoplasm. This complex multicystic neoplasm shows abrupt keratinization, similar to the pattern exhibited at the follicular isthmus. Although it can be difficult to determine whether these lesions are benign or malignant, this example was well circumscribed and was eradicated by simple enucleation.

Keratinized areas may exhibit secondary calcification. There may be focal necrosis.

The degree of cytologic atypicality varies among lesions and amongst different areas of a given lesion. Commonly, the neoplastic cells contain enlarged vesicular nuclei with prominent nucleoli and some degree of nuclear hyperchromasia, and mitotic figures are usually identified, but overtly anaplastic nuclear features are usually not present. Since some examples of PPT represent low-grade forms of carcinoma, tumors with marked cytologic atypicality, extensive necrosis, a lack of circumscription, or extraordinary numbers of mitotic figures should be interpreted cautiously[53,55].

Treatment

As noted, some examples of PPT may represent carcinoma. If a lesion has been enucleated in its entirety or near entirety, is circumscribed, and lacks substantial cytologic atypism, then additional surgical therapy is probably not necessary and close clinical follow-up should suffice. If a given lesion lacks circumscription, shows substantial cytologic atypism or necrosis, or has been sampled *en parte*, then complete excision is warranted, as carcinoma remains a concern.

NEOPLASMS AND PROLIFERATIONS WITH SEBACEOUS DIFFERENTIATION

Sebaceous hyperplasia

Introduction
Sebaceous hyperplasia does not represent a true neoplasm. It represents benign enlargement of the sebaceous lobule around a follicular infundibulum.

Clinical features
Sebaceous hyperplasia is relatively common and presents with one or multiple yellowish, occasionally telangiectatic papules, usually on the central or upper face (Fig. 111.19) and sometimes on the upper trunk. Commonly, the clinical lesions display a central dell that corresponds to a central follicular infundibular ostium. 'Beaded lines' represent a unique expression of sebaceous hyperplasia in which a linear array of hyperplastic sebaceous lobules is present, usually in the vicinity of the clavicle or on the neck[56]. Biopsy is occasionally indicated to exclude BCC.

Pathology
The sebaceous gland in sebaceous hyperplasia shows normal morphology, with a thin rim of seboblastic cells surrounding the remainder of the gland, composed of mature sebocytes. The enlarged sebaceous lobules usually circumferentially surround a central infundibulum.

Treatment
If treatment is desired, lesions can be removed or diminished by shave, light electrosurgical destruction, cryotherapy, or laser ablation[57]. Long-term topical retinoid application may be beneficial. Oral isotretinoin has been utilized for patients with extensive disfiguring lesions.

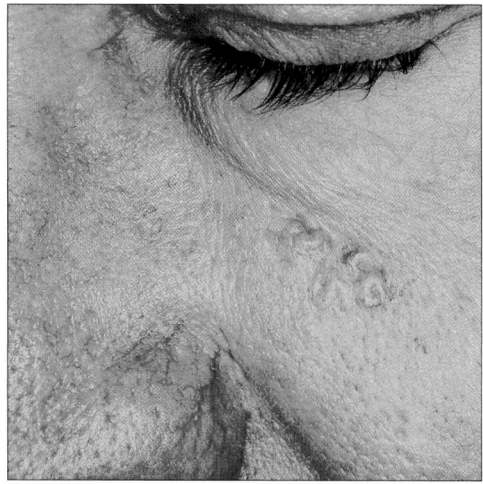

Fig. 111.19 Sebaceous hyperplasia. Skin-colored to yellowish papules with a central dell.

Sebaceous adenoma, sebaceous epithelioma and sebaceoma
Introduction
The term 'adenoma' designates a benign neoplasm with glandular differentiation, and any benign proliferation with predominance of sebaceous differentiation can be grouped under this rubric. Commonly, the term sebaceous adenoma has been applied to superficial benign sebaceous neoplasms with a predominance of mature 'sebocytic' differentiation, while sebaceous epithelioma and sebaceoma have been applied to sebaceous neoplasms with a predominance of 'seboblastic' cells.

Practically speaking, the term sebaceous epithelioma is inherently confusing, as the diagnosis has been utilized in different ways by different authorities. To some, a sebaceous epithelioma represents a low-grade form of sebaceous carcinoma or BCC with focal sebaceous differentiation. Others have utilized the term to describe benign sebaceous lesions (or sebaceous proliferations of uncertain potential) in which a preponderance of 'seboblastic' differentiation occurs. We believe that the term sebaceous epithelioma should be abandoned.

Troy & Ackerman[58] coined *sebaceoma* as an alternative to describe a group of benign sebaceous proliferations that were generally more deeply situated than superficial sebaceous adenomas and in which a vertically oriented microscopic pattern was identifiable. In this chapter, the term *sebaceous adenoma* is used in broad fashion to encompass both superficial proliferations with mostly sebocytic differentiation (superficial sebaceous adenoma) and larger nodular proliferations with mostly seboblastic differentiation (sebaceoma).

Clinical features
Sebaceous adenomas present clinically as papules or nodules, usually less than a centimeter in diameter, distributed on the head or neck and sometimes on the upper trunk. The lesions are not clinically distinctive except when there is a yellowish color, which is often not apparent. Superficial sebaceous adenomas are usually relatively small and papular, while 'sebaceomas' may present as a deep nodule or 'cyst'[58,59]. Multiple sebaceous neoplasms, especially cystic ones, may serve as a presenting sign of the Muir–Torre syndrome, characterized also by multiple keratoacanthomas and visceral carcinomas, especially colonic adenocarcinoma[60,61].

Pathology
Superficial sebaceous adenoma is usually captured in continuity with the surface epidermis and is relatively small and circumscribed. The relative proportions of basaloid seboblastic cells and mature sebocytic cells varies, but mature sebocytes usually predominate. Seboblasts comprise a multilayer of cells at the periphery of each lobule of adenoma, with sebocytes positioned centrally. Mitotic figures can be found in seboblastic cells but are usually not conspicuous. Necrosis is not usually evident in an adenoma unless the lesion has been traumatized. Significant degrees of necrosis, whether of single cells or *en masse*, raises concern for the possibility of carcinoma.

Nodular sebaceous adenoma (sebaceoma) is usually more deeply situated, often involving the deep reticular dermis and sometimes the superficial subcutis[58]. The lesions are sharply circumscribed in an excisional specimen, but this may be difficult to fully appreciate in a biopsy *en parte*.

Seboblasts usually predominate in nodular sebaceous adenoma, and, sometimes, sebocytic differentiation may be only focal, yielding a microscopic pattern not unlike large nodular trichoblastoma (Fig. 111.20). If sebaceous differentiation is only focal, then epithelial membrane antigen (EMA) immunoperoxidase staining can be considered as a diagnostic supplement. EMA specifically labels mature sebocytes in the normal sebaceous gland and can also be utilized to identify foci of sebaceous differentiation in neoplasms.

Treatment
Once a definite microscopic diagnosis has been achieved, no further treatment is obligatory. It is often difficult to establish the circumscription of lesions captured in superficial or partial biopsies. Complete excision of such lesions is appropriate to exclude the possibility of BCC with sebaceous differentiation or sebaceous carcinoma. Deeply situated lesions of Muir–Torre syndrome are particularly prone to rapid growth and may behave like carcinomas. Evaluation of patients with just

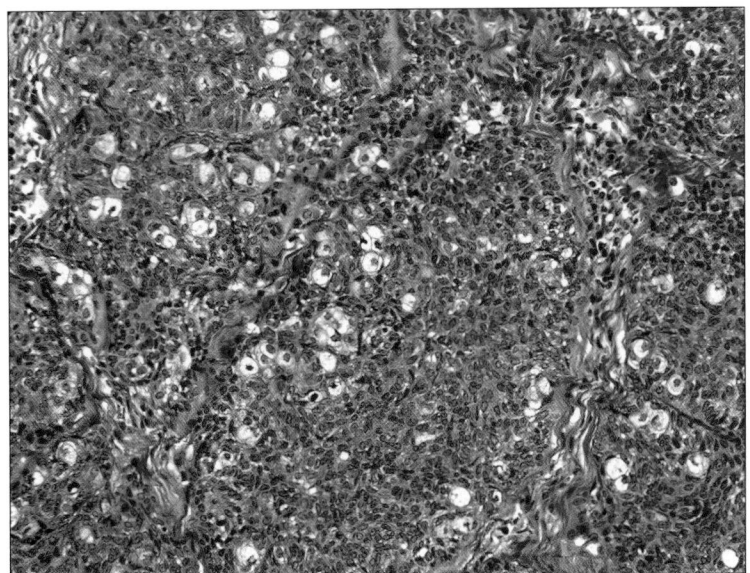

Fig. 111.20 Sebaceous adenoma (sebaceoma). This high-magnification view shows a background of basaloid seboblastic cells punctuated by scattered mature sebocytes with coarsely vacuolated cytoplasm. The neoplasm was large but sharply circumscribed at low magnification.

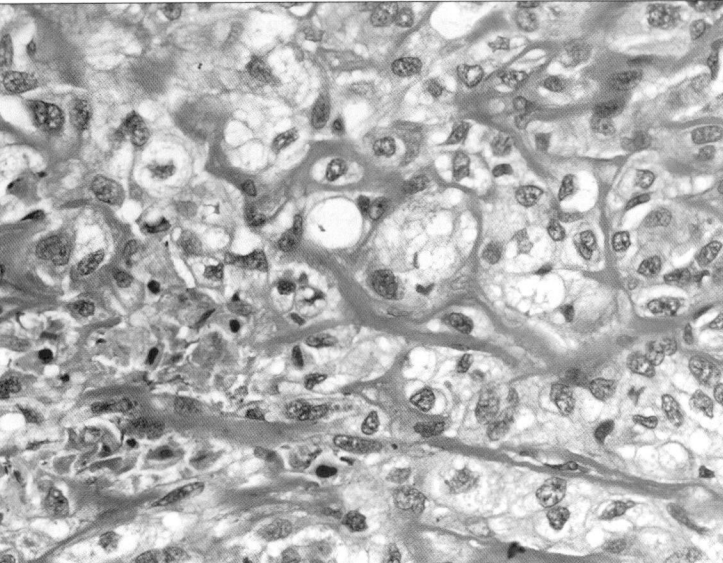

Fig. 111.21 Sebaceous carcinoma. At high magnification, there are cells with atypical nuclei and ample coarsely vacuolated cytoplasm. There are also many necrotic cells with pyknotic nuclei.

one sebaceous adenoma of any type for colonic adenocarcinoma is recommended.

Sebaceous carcinoma

Introduction
The term sebaceous carcinoma designates an adenocarcinoma with sebaceous differentiation. By historical convention, these carcinomas have been separated into ocular and extraocular types. Extraocular sebaceous carcinoma is thought to hold a graver prognosis, although the data behind this belief are old and have been questioned[62].

Clinical features
The clinical presentation of sebaceous carcinoma is not distinctive. Typical clinical lesions include erythematous nodules or plaques that may be ulcerated or crusted and only occasionally display yellowish coloration. More commonly, the lesions display an erythematous or pearly morphology that is indistinguishable from common forms of non-melanoma skin cancer. Ocular lesions are very commonly misdiagnosed as blepharitis or ocular rosacea.

Sebaceous carcinomas commonly develop in the periorbital area, but also develop elsewhere on the head and neck and less commonly on the trunk. Carcinomas from the trunk commonly display a nodular pattern, and superficial biopsies from such lesions may be deceptive and can be misinterpreted as sebaceous adenoma[62]. Sebaceous carcinoma can occur in patients with Muir–Torre syndrome, but the identification of a sebaceous carcinoma alone is not sufficient to diagnose the syndrome[60]. However, any unusual sebaceous neoplasm other than sebaceous hyperplasia, whether carcinomatous or not, is probably sufficient provocation for consideration of the disease.

Pathology
Sebaceous carcinoma exhibits asymmetry, a lack of circumscription, and areas with an infiltrative pattern. In nodular sebaceous carcinoma, cells are arrayed as large nests and lobules. In infiltrative sebaceous carcinomas, jagged nests and thin strands are found. Sebaceous carcinoma can involve the surface epidermis or conjunctiva, in a pagetoid pattern, especially in ocular lesions[63,64]. This can be confused with Bowen's disease or melanoma.

The degree of sebaceous differentiation in sebaceous carcinoma varies greatly, as does the degree of nuclear atypicality (Fig. 111.21). Some carcinomas display obvious sebaceous differentiation, while other examples may be composed mostly of neoplastic cells with a squamous or basaloid appearance, with sebaceous differentiation only focally apparent.

Stains for lipid, such as oil red O or Sudan black, have been utilized in the past as a tool to confirm sebaceous differentiation through labeling of cytoplasmic fat. However, such stains have little routine practical applicability, as they require the use of frozen sections, as lipid is extracted from tissue during the preparation of conventional formalin-fixed, paraffin-embedded sections. EMA immunoperoxidase staining remains the best supplemental test for confirmation of sebaceous differentiation. When authentic sebaceous differentiation is present, a positive reaction consists of EMA labeling of cytoplasm in a coarsely vacuolated pattern.

Crateriform or cystic sebaceous neoplasms that display a clinical and microscopic pattern reminiscent of keratoacanthoma are uncommon lesions that probably represent low-grade carcinomas[60]. Sebaceous neoplasms with a keratoacanthoma-like pattern probably only occur in the context of Muir–Torre syndrome.

Treatment
Sebaceous carcinoma is an adnexal carcinoma with significant metastatic potential. The primary treatment remains surgical extirpation. Although the risk of metastatic disease was formerly believed to be high, particularly for ocular carcinomas, the data contained within many older reports may be skewed by inclusion of carcinomas diagnosed late in their evolution. Extensive disease of the eye has been treated with ocular enucleation, especially when ocular conjunctival involvement was present. The metastatic potential of both superficial sebaceous carcinoma and sebaceous carcinoma with an infiltrative pattern may be limited, although additional study will be necessary to fully establish this.

NEOPLASMS AND PROLIFERATIONS WITH APOCRINE DIFFERENTIATION

In most textbooks, adnexal neoplasms with glandular and ductular differentiation have been rigorously separated into eccrine and apocrine neoplasms. Commonly, the distinction was based upon enzyme histochemical data, an imprecisely applied technique that is no longer readily available. Discrimination has also been based upon conventional microscopic assessment, a useful but imprecise tool, at least for the distinction of eccrine and apocrine attributes.

A few authorities have responded to this difficulty by grouping apocrine and eccrine neoplasms together, in recognition of the fact that it is impossible to determine whether a given lesion, such as a given syringoma, is of apocrine or eccrine lineage. In the sections that follow, the traditional categorization as 'apocrine' or 'eccrine' will be maintained, but areas of overlap will be expressly noted. For entities such as syringoma, poroma and hidradenoma, which can be of either apocrine or eccrine lineage, the presentation will be included in the discussion of apocrine lesions.

Benign Neoplasms and Proliferations with Apocrine Ductular and Tubular Differentiation

Syringoma

Introduction

The designation 'syringoma' refers to a group of benign adnexal neoplasms with mostly ductal ('syringeal') differentiation. Historically, syringomas have been interpreted as neoplasms of eccrine lineage[65,66]. The term syringoma can be used to describe neoplasms of either apocrine or eccrine lineage, and it is currently impossible to judge the lineage of any given neoplasm, other than by its context.

Clinical features

A syringoma is manifest clinically as a 2- to 4-mm, firm, skin-colored papule (Fig. 111.22). Syringomas commonly present in multiplicity and may be eruptive[67,68]. The lesions are removed from women more commonly than men, although it is not entirely clear that this represents gender predilection rather than biopsy selection bias due to cosmetic or social factors.

Syringomas may occur at any site on the body, but are prone to occur in the periorbital area, especially the eyelids. Sometimes, lesions involve the upper trunk or genital skin[67–69]. Eruptive syringomas most commonly involve the trunk, but may involve the extremities, including the palms and soles. Acral syringomas are those that are most clearly of eccrine lineage, as the acini of glabrous skin are exclusively eccrine[70].

Pathology

From scanning magnification, a syringoma is small, symmetric and well circumscribed, and is usually confined to the superficial dermis. The surrounding stroma is sclerotic. The epithelial component of the

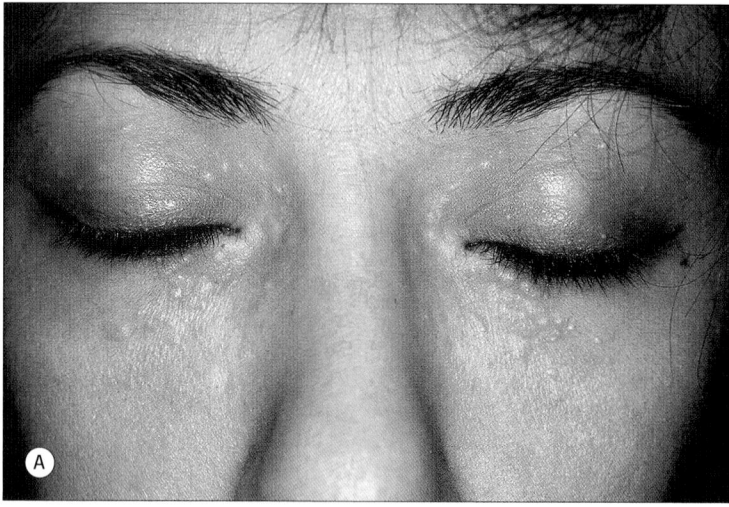

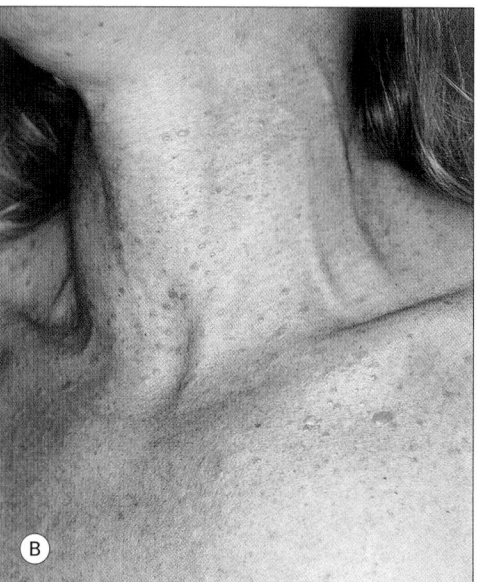

Fig. 111.22 **Syringomas.** **A** Aggregated skin-colored papules on the eyelids. **B** Multiple skin-colored to pink, smooth papules on the neck and upper chest. The lesions favor the ventral surface of the trunk, a distribution pattern referred to as 'en demicuirasse'. B, Courtesy of Jean L Bolognia MD.

proliferation is composed of cells with pale or pinkish cytoplasm, arrayed as nests and tubules of relatively uniform size. Depending upon the exact plane of section, the nests of a syringoma vary in shape, and some nests may assume a morphology that resembles a comma or a tadpole (Fig. 111.23). Tubular areas exhibit ductular differentiation, with central lumina lined by a compact eosinophilic cuticle. Typically, half or more of the nests in a given plane of section with show central ductal differentiation.

Usually, a syringoma lacks keratinization, although, at times, superficial cornification can be seen in a lesion that abuts the dermal–epidermal junctional zone or in a lesion that has been traumatized. Syringomas also typically lack evidence of follicular differentiation. If either follicular differentiation or keratinization is identified, other differential diagnostic possibilities should be strongly considered. The combination of superficial cornification, poor circumscription, and extension into the deep reticular dermis (or subcutis) favors microcystic adnexal carcinoma over syringoma. A lesion with strands of basaloid cells, focal superficial cornification, and focal calcification probably represents desmoplastic trichoepithelioma rather than syringoma. If there are only cornifying cysts present, with a lack of authentic ductal differentiation, then the most likely diagnosis is trichoadenoma.

Treatment

Syringoma is a benign adnexal neoplasm with negligible proliferative capacity. After definitive diagnosis, no further surgical intervention is needed, unless sclerosing BCC or microcystic adnexal carcinoma is a clinicopathologic consideration. Syringomas may be treated with careful application of trichloroacetic acid, cryotherapy, punch excision, or electrosurgical destruction, with variable results. This can be difficult in the most common situation, when multiple lesions are present on eyelids. Disseminated lesions can be cosmetically disabling and therapeutically challenging, and laser ablation might be the best choice[71].

Poroma

Introduction

The term 'poroma' refers to a group of benign adnexal neoplasms with 'poroid' or terminal ductal differentiation. Like syringomas, poromas have been interpreted historically as neoplasms of eccrine lineage, mostly because of enzyme histochemical findings of dubious specificity[65,66]. The words 'eccrine' and 'poroma' have become seemingly inextricably linked in the dermatologic lexicon, and thus poromas are often referred to as 'eccrine' in reflexive fashion. Poroma can be a proliferation of either apocrine or eccrine lineage[72–75]. Eccrine poromas and apocrine poromas probably occur in nearly equal numbers.

The term *acrospiroma* is used by some authorities as a synonym for poroma, and is used by other authorities as a broad designation that encompasses both poroma and hidradenoma.

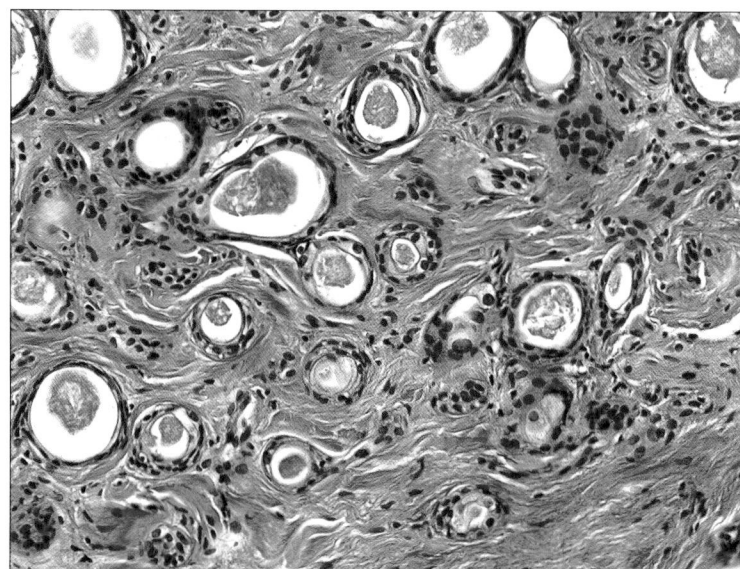

Fig. 111.23 **Syringoma.** This superficial adnexal neoplasm consists of nests of cells with pale cytoplasm positioned within sclerotic stroma. Many nests show central ductal differentiation with a compact eosinophilic cuticle.

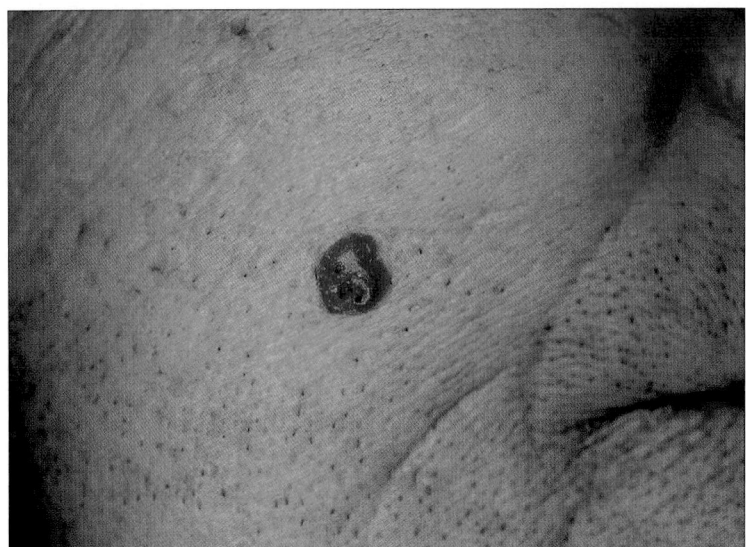

Fig. 111.24 Poroma. A biopsy specimen is necessary to establish a definitive diagnosis.

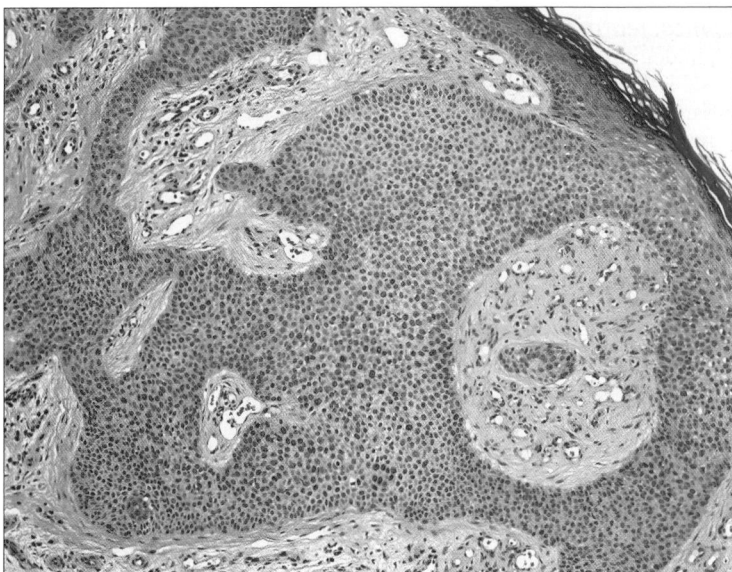

Fig. 111.25 Poroma, juxta-epidermal pattern. This poroma displays a pattern common to both eccrine and apocrine poroma. There are interanastomosing cords composed of small compact 'poroid' cells, and the intervening stroma is highly vascularized and resembles granulation tissue.

Clinical features

Poromas usually present as solitary papules, plaques or nodules (Fig. 111.24)[3]. When sessile vascular plaques surrounded by indented moats appear on the palms and soles, an astute dermatologist can strongly suspect the diagnosis. They can appear on any cutaneous surface, where they are less readily identified as poromas clinically. The scalp is another common site, with or without an associated nevus sebaceus[13]. Presumably, poromas arising secondarily within nevus sebaceus represent apocrine poromas. Occasionally, a poroma will be pigmented. Poromas commonly display highly vascularized stroma, and a clinical pattern suggestive of pyogenic granuloma is common, especially in poromas that involve acral skin. Rarely, multiple poromas will develop, either in an acral or in a widespread distribution, a clinical pattern referred to as poromatosis.

Pathology

The principal finding in all forms of poroma consists of a circumscribed proliferation of compact cuboidal keratinocytes with small monomorphous nuclei and scant eosinophilic cytoplasm. Poromas can be confined to the epidermis (intraepidermal poroma), a pattern known historically as hidroacanthoma simplex; can occur in broad continuity with the epidermis, with extension into the papillary dermis (juxta-epidermal poroma; Fig. 111.25); or can develop wholly (or nearly so) within the dermis (intradermal poroma; Fig. 111.26), a pattern known historically as dermal duct tumor[3]. Only the juxta-epidermal and intradermal types of poroma are notable for granulation tissue-like stroma.

The degree of ductal differentiation varies greatly in individual neoplasms. Some poromas display innumerable foci in which poroid cells form small ductal spaces lined by a compact eosinophilic cuticle. In other lesions, ducts may be difficult to identify, and those can resemble seborrheic keratoses. The latter does not occur on the palms and soles, however. Carcinoembryonic antigen (CEA) immunostaining, which labels the luminal surface of both apocrine and eccrine ducts, can be employed as a tool to confirm the presence of ductal differentiation. Poromas may occasionally display tubular (rather than ductular) foci in which a central cuticle is lacking. If such tubular foci are lined by columnar cells with a 'decapitation' pattern at their luminal border, a presumptive diagnosis of apocrine poroma can be offered.

At times, a poroma may display striking clear cell change. The constituent nuclei in such lesions are small but are surrounded by ample pale cytoplasm. Poromas are an exception to the rule that necrosis *en masse* is a clue to a malignancy. For reasons that are not entirely clear, poromas commonly display small collections of cells in coagulation necrosis. In malignant tumors, necrosis is usually a consequence of rapid growth (growth beyond the capacity of perfusion), but this is an unlikely explanation for necrosis in poroma, in which cellular proliferation is low. Poromas may occasionally display foci of sebaceous

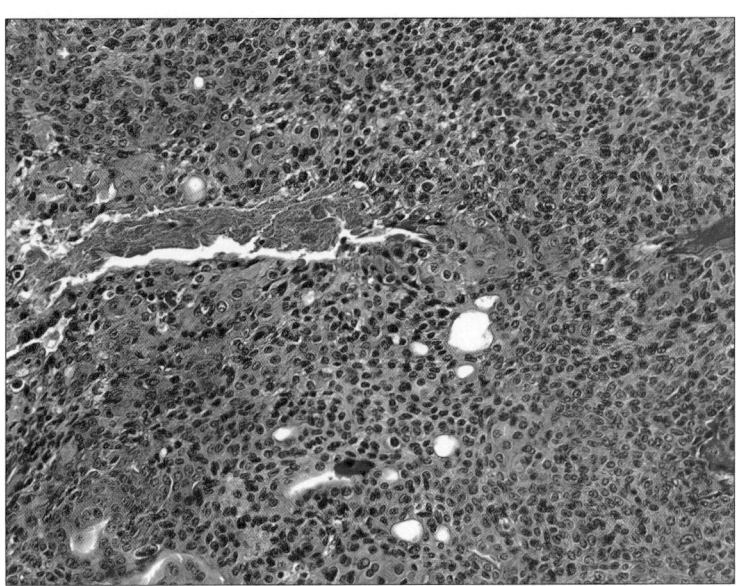

Fig. 111.26 Poroma, intradermal pattern. At low magnification, this lesion was a well-circumscribed dermal nodule. This high magnification shows conspicuous foci of ductal differentiation and also a focus of necrosis en masse, a finding common to poroma that is uncommon in other benign neoplasms.

differentiation, usually consisting of clusters of mature sebocytes near the lesion base[72,76,77].

Treatment

Poroma is a benign adnexal neoplasm, so treatment is optional. Superficial lesions may be treated by shave or electrosurgical destruction. Superficial or deeper lesions may also be treated with excision to adipose.

Hidradenoma
Introduction

Hidradenoma is a form of benign adnexal neoplasm that is a close relative of poroma, but is usually characterized by cells with ample cytoplasm, is never intraepidermal, and does not have a broad-base connection to the epidermis. Some authorities use the broad designation *acrospiroma* to refer to both hidradenoma and poroma jointly. Although commonly classified as an eccrine neoplasm, hidradenomas are currently thought to be of either apocrine or eccrine lineage[65,66]. Hidradenoma is probably of apocrine lineage most of the time[78].

Clinical features

Hidradenoma lacks any distinctive clinical attributes and is only diagnosable by biopsy. The lesion presents as a solitary dermal or subcutaneous nodule; sometimes, a cystic quality or a small amount of serous drainage can be detected.

Pathology

Hidradenomas are mostly dermal neoplasms with a nodular, sharply circumscribed pattern when viewed at low magnification. Some hidradenomas may display a juxta-epidermal pattern superficially with multifocal attachment to the epidermis, much like poroma. Although the stroma of hidradenoma is commonly sclerotic and may contain ectatic vessels, usually the granulation tissue-like quality that typifies the stroma of a poroma is not present. The cells of hidradenoma are large with ample cytoplasm but uniform nuclei, which are generally somewhat larger than the nuclei of poroma. Overt clear cell change ('clear cell' hidradenoma) is common, as is cystic degeneration ('solid-cystic' hidradenoma)[79,80] (Fig. 111.27). Ductal differentiation can be found with scrutiny, although the degree of ductal differentiation may be minimal. Some lesions contain tubules lined by columnar cells with a decapitation pattern along their luminal border; such lesions can be designated as apocrine hidradenoma without question. Not surprisingly, hybrid lesions with features of both hidradenoma and poroma can be encountered, and thus a judgment regarding the 'closest fit' must sometimes be made; the hybrid term *poroid hidradenoma* has also been applied to such lesions[81].

Treatment

Hidradenoma is a benign adnexal neoplasm. Complete conservative excision is curative.

Apocrine adenoma
Introduction

Any benign neoplasm with apocrine differentiation, including poroma and hidradenoma, could be grouped under the broad roof of this rubric. On a practical basis, only adenomas with conspicuous glandular differentiation are included in this category. Usually, these neoplasms exhibit abundant apocrine epithelium and a conspicuous decapitation pattern, where part of the cytoplasm pinches off into a lumen. Apocrine adenomas may present with a tubular or papillary microscopic pattern or a combination of the two. Entities within this conglomeration include *tubular adenoma, papillary adenoma, syringocystadenoma papilliferum* and *hidradenoma papilliferum*. The latter entity, also known as *papillary hidradenoma*, is a source of potential semantic confusion with conventional hidradenoma. Papillary hidradenoma (hidradenoma papilliferum) is an apocrine adenoma that usually exhibits a pronounced papillary pattern with apocrine epithelium lining the constituent papillae. In contrast, conventional hidradenoma (acrospiroma) exhibits a mostly solid pattern with focal ductal and tubular differentiation, with apocrine epithelium in tubular areas, sometimes.

Tubular, papillary or tubulopapillary adenomas with conspicuous apocrine differentiation may develop within the parenchyma or secretory apparatus of the breast. Apocrine adenomas in continuity with the nipple commonly exhibit a tubulopapillary pattern and have been referred to as *erosive adenomatosis*[82–84]. In addition to a tubulopapillary pattern, apocrine adenomas of the nipple may display small foci with solid and cribriform patterns, but usually necrosis is not identifiable. As such lesions are usually solitary, as erosive changes are commonly not present, and as the designation erosive adenomatosis is somewhat provocative, it is probably best to employ the simple term 'nipple adenoma' in this context. The distinction between nipple adenoma and ductal adenocarcinoma can sometimes be challenging, and consultation with an experienced breast pathologist should be sought in difficult cases.

Clinical features

The presentation of tubular or papillary adenoma is not distinctive. These tumors present as smooth papules or nodules, and biopsy is required for diagnosis.

Syringocystadenoma papilliferum presents as a papule or plaque, almost exclusively on the head or neck (Fig. 111.28). Syringocystadenomas

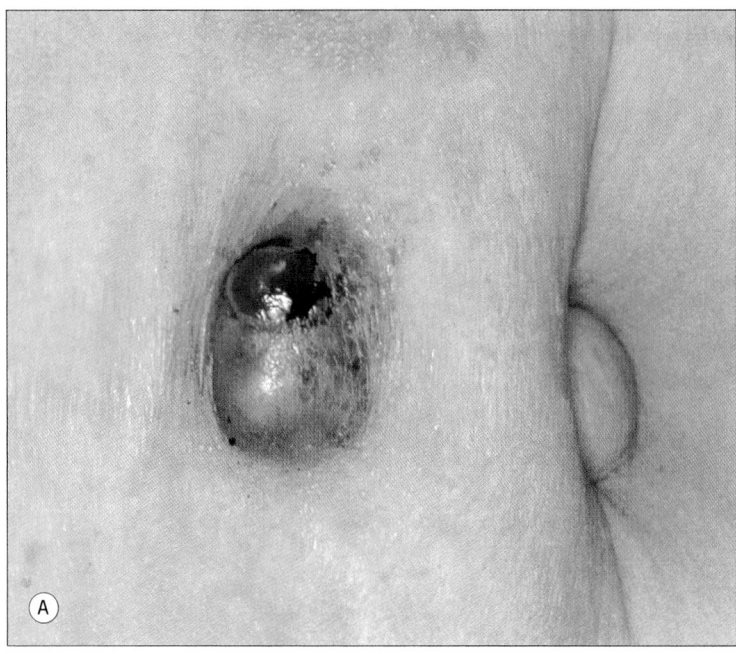

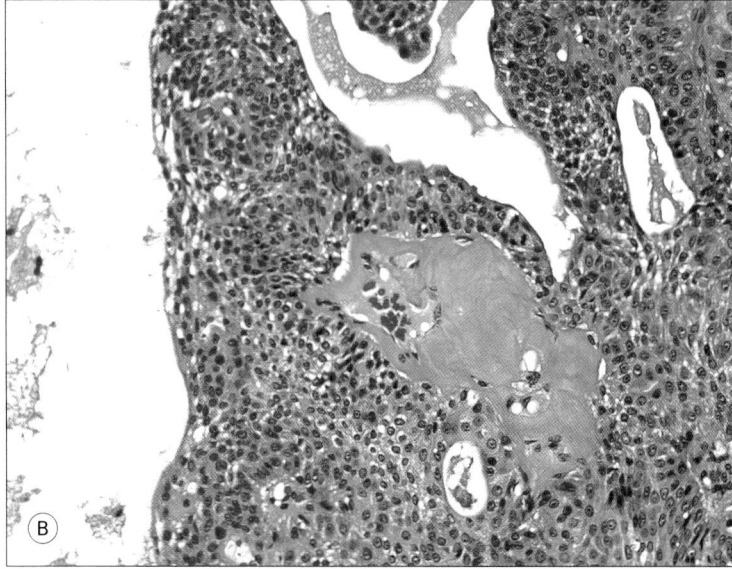

Fig. 111.27 Hidradenoma. A Solitary violaceous nodule on the abdomen with serous drainage. **B** This well-circumscribed nodule is composed of cells with small uniform nuclei and ample cytoplasm that often is pale or shows overt clear cell change. A cystic focus is present; lesions that display prominent cystic change have been referred to as 'solid-cystic' hidradenoma.

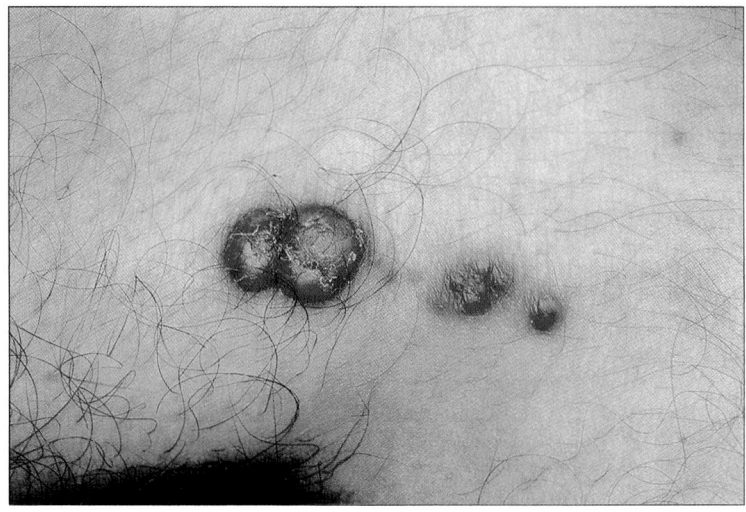

Fig. 111.28 Syringocystadenoma papilliferum. Grouped keratotic papules and nodules.

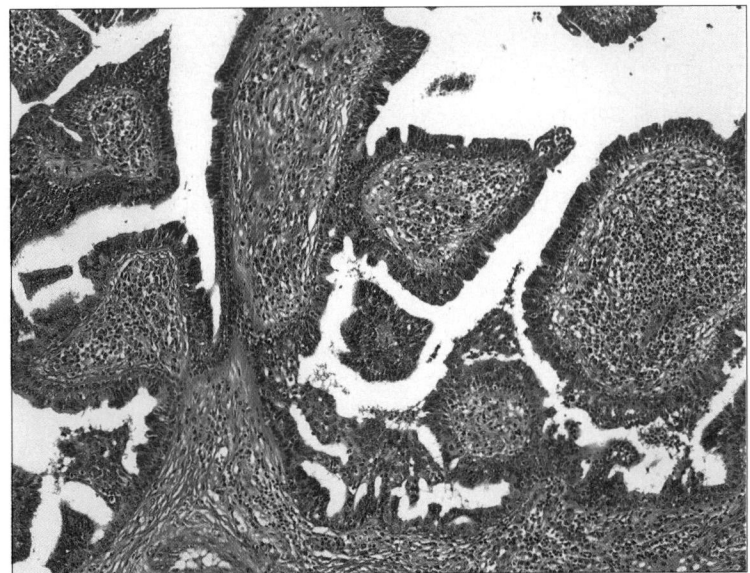

Fig. 111.29 Syringocystadenoma papilliferum. This neoplasm consists of papillary foci lined by columnar cells that usually display overt apocrine differentiation. The dermal cores of papillae are usually stuffed with lymphocytes and many plasma cells.

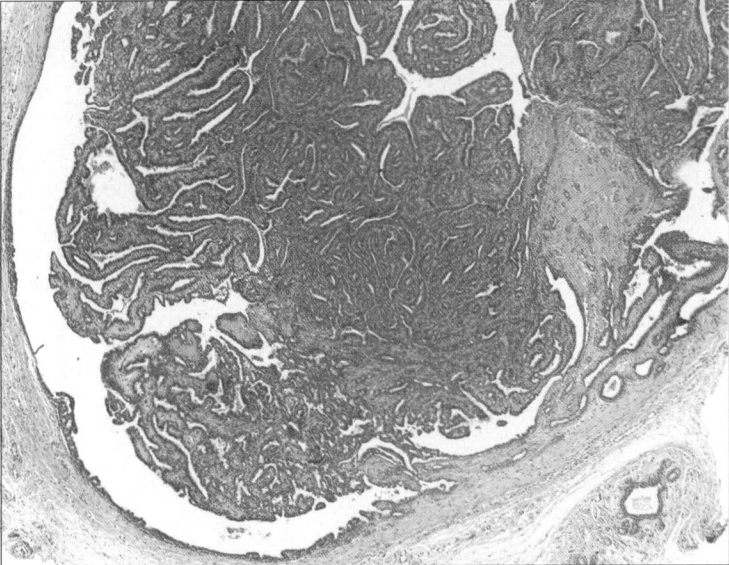

Fig. 111.30 Hidradenoma papilliferum. This well-circumscribed dermal nodule is composed of fronds and papillae with a connective tissue core lined by a bilayer of cells, with columnar apocrine cells positioned above a cuboidal monolayer of myoepithelial cells.

usually exhibit a crusted surface that may ooze serosanguinous fluid; this is a reflection of the fact that the papillae of a syringocystadenoma are in continuity with the epidermal surface, permitting extrusion of secretory products. Most papillary syringoadenomas present on the scalp in association with nevus sebaceus[13,85].

Hidradenoma papilliferum usually presents as a smooth dermal or subcutaneous nodule, usually no more than a centimeter in diameter. Most papillary hidradenomas arise on the vulva, but development within skin of the breast, axilla and inguinal or perianal areas has also been documented[86].

Pathology
At low magnification, tubular and papillary adenomas are usually well-circumscribed neoplasms positioned within the dermis, the superficial subcutis, or a combination of the two. Adenomas with a tubular pattern are composed mostly of rounded glandular spaces that vary in size and are lined by one or several layers of cuboidal cells with pale cytoplasm and small nuclei. Most spaces have small lumina and some display columnar apocrine cells apically. Papillary adenomas contain conspicuous tufts, with luminal cells that display an apocrine pattern. A combination of tubular and papillary patterns is not uncommon.

Papillary syringocystadenoma (syringocystadenoma papilliferum) is distinctive for its wide papillary fronds that are in continuity with the surface squamous epithelium. Syringocystadenomas are only rarely cystic. The fronds are lined by a bilayer, with basal cuboidal cells and apical columnar apocrine cells, and the cores of fronds virtually always contain a dense infiltrate of lymphocytes and plasma cells (Fig. 111.29). A plasmacytic infiltrate commonly accompanies neoplasms of apocrine lineage, and thus the mere presence of plasma cells in a given lesion is not sufficient to confirm a diagnosis of syringocystadenoma, although a plasmacytic infiltrate can be used as a clue to the identification of foci of apocrine differentiation.

At low magnification, papillary hidradenoma (hidradenoma papilliferum) consists of a well-circumscribed nodule within the dermis, usually without the connection to the surface and the prominent plasma cells seen in syringocystadenoma papilliferum. Both tubules and papillary fronds are usually present, and broad elongated fronds with delicate fibrous cores are usually identifiable. Both tubules and fronds are usually lined by a bilayer, with basal cuboidal 'myoepithelial' cells and apical apocrine cells, and the apical cells usually display a conspicuous 'decapitation' pattern (Fig. 111.30). At least some of the basal layer cells represent authentic myoepithelial cells with contractile function, and labeling of the myoepithelial layer through immunoperoxidase staining for actin filaments can sometimes be of diagnostic value in the distinction from adenocarcinoma, as adenocarcinomatous tubules typically lack a myoepithelial layer.

Treatment
Apocrine adenomas are completely benign lesions. Complete conservative excision is curative.

Undifferentiated Neoplasms of Apocrine Lineage
Most adnexal neoplasms contain foci of differentiation that may be rudimentary, but is nonetheless interpretable as representing normal structures. Thus, while trichoblastoma is in general 'undifferentiated', it contains foci such as papillary mesenchymal bodies that render the lesion recognizable as a proliferation of follicular germinative lineage. This principle holds true for most other forms of adnexal neoplasms. However, two entities, spiradenoma and cylindroma, display either a lack of differentiation or differentiation not readily identifiable as indicative of a normal structure. Both spiradenoma and cylindroma occasionally display tubular foci with a decapitation luminal pattern, suggesting apocrine lineage, but mostly these neoplasms display uninterpretable differentiation and thus are included in this section as 'undifferentiated' neoplasms.

Spiradenoma
Definition
The term *spiradenoma* connotes a form of undifferentiated or poorly differentiated but benign adnexal neoplasm that has been historically designated as a tumor of eccrine lineage, although reassessment indicates an apocrine process[65,66]. Both spiradenoma and cylindroma occasionally display tubular differentiation with a 'decapitation' pattern, as would be expected in an apocrine neoplasm. Spiradenoma not uncommonly occurs jointly with cylindroma and both occur jointly with trichoepithelioma/trichoblastoma; the most parsimonious explanation for this complex juxtaposition is that both spiradenoma and cylindroma are of folliculosebaceous-apocrine lineage[87,88]. Both spiradenoma and cylindroma occur jointly with trichoblastoma in the Brooke–Spiegler syndrome, again implying kinship rather than disparate lineage. Spiradenoma has never been observed on glabrous skin; if spiradenoma were truly 'eccrine', occurrence on the palm or sole would be the rule and not the exception.

Clinical features
Spiradenoma typically presents as a dermal or subcutaneous papule or nodule on nearly any location; extraordinary lesions may achieve a diameter of several centimeters. Sometimes, spiradenomas are painful (see differential diagnosis for painful dermal nodules in the first introductory chapter of this text). The clinical lesions are not distinctive and biopsy is required for diagnosis, although an astute dermatologist

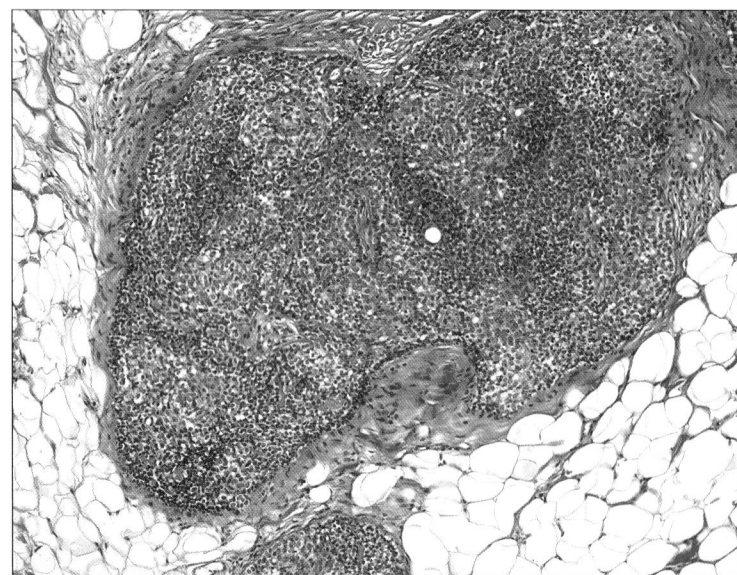

Fig. 111.31 Spiradenoma. This subcutaneous nodule shows multinodular basaloid aggregates with the typical trabecular pattern. Darkly staining cells line trabeculae and pale cells with pink cytoplasm are present in their centers, superimposed with lymphocytes.

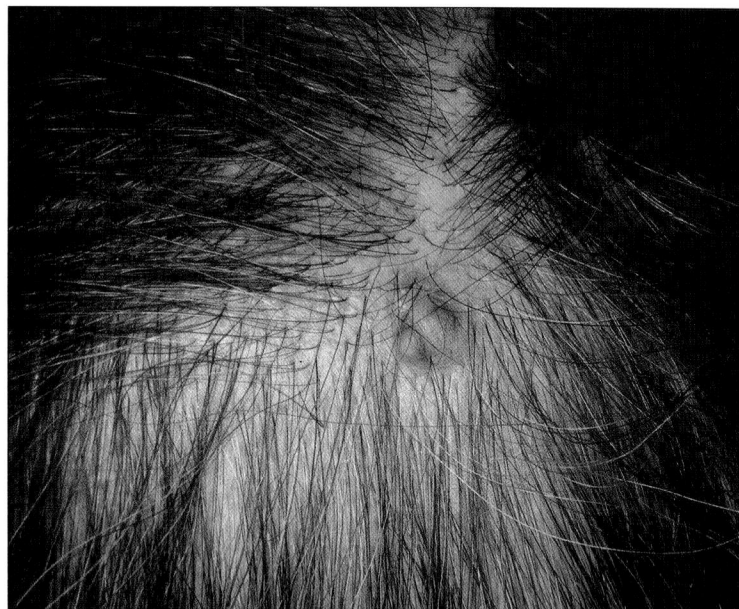

Fig. 111.32 Cylindroma. While numerous tumors aggregated on the scalp are called turban tumors, solitary lesions usually present as smooth erythematous nodules.

can suspect the diagnosis in the setting of a painful nodule with a slightly bluish hue. Spiradenomas may occur in multiplicity and in concert with cylindroma and trichoblastoma, and multiple lesions should prompt consideration of a diagnosis of Brooke–Spiegler syndrome.

Pathology
At low magnification, spiradenoma assumes a multinodular pattern, with relatively large nodules positioned within the dermis and subcutis. Although the nodules may be asymmetrically distributed, each is sharply circumscribed. The nodules are composed of basaloid cells without obvious differentiation, although tubular apocrine foci can be observed on occasion. With closer scrutiny, individual nodules exhibit a trabecular internal morphology, with compact basophilic cells lining the borders of trabeculae and larger cells with paler cytoplasm within their centers. Usually, small lymphocytes are scattered throughout trabecular areas (Fig. 111.31). Some 'giant' spiradenomas develop cystic areas of degeneration or striking vascular ectasia as secondary events. Compact eosinophilic basement membrane material, arrayed either as PAS-positive small 'droplets' or as circumferential bands, can occasionally be found within spiradenoma, although these deposits are more commonplace in cylindroma. Spiradenoma can occur jointly with cylindroma, at least some of the time[87,88].

Treatment
Spiradenoma is a benign adnexal neoplasm. Despite its 'basaloid' microscopic appearance, spiradenoma holds negligible proliferative capacity and recurrence is uncommon after simple enucleation or conservative excision.

Cylindroma
Introduction
The term *cylindroma* describes a form of undifferentiated or poorly differentiated adnexal neoplasm that has sometimes been interpreted as an 'eccrine' process but has mostly been interpreted as a neoplasm of apocrine lineage.

Clinical features
Cylindromas can present singly or in multiplicity and are not clinically distinctive; a biopsy specimen is required for diagnosis (Fig. 111.32). Solitary lesions commonly involve the head and neck area, especially the scalp, and can also develop on skin of the trunk or genitalia. Multiple cylindromas may coalesce and form giant mosaic plaques on the scalp, referred to as 'turban' tumor[89–91]. The recognition of multiple cylindromas should prompt consideration of the Brooke–Spiegler syn-

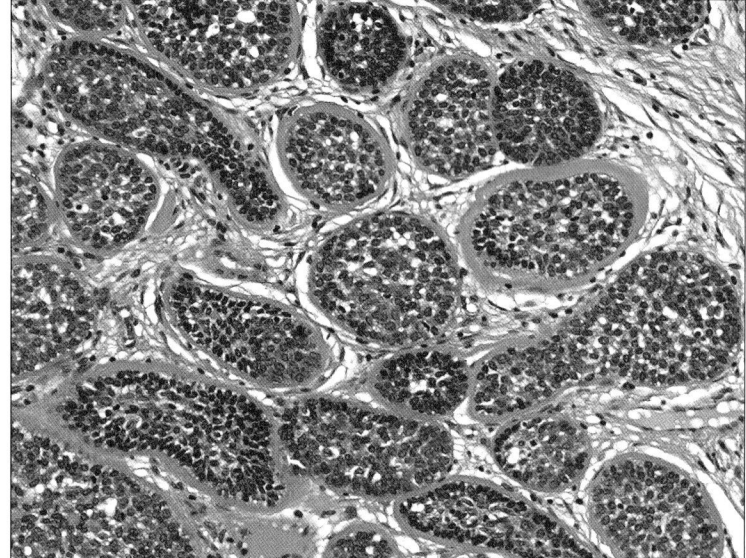

Fig. 111.33 Cylindroma. Nests of basaloid cells in a jigsaw puzzle-like pattern. Many nests are circumferentially enveloped by a dense eosinophilic cylinder of basement membrane material.

drome, an autosomal dominant condition, some examples of which are associated with the *CYLD* gene on chromosome 16q.

Pathology
At low magnification, cylindroma consists of sharply circumscribed nodules arrayed within the dermis, with extension into the underlying subcutis commonly. The nodules are composed of nests of basaloid cells in close apposition, arrayed in a complex pattern that has been likened to a jigsaw puzzle. A rim of densely eosinophilic, PAS-positive basement membrane material commonly envelops the individual nests, and 'droplets' of similar composition are often scattered in the centers of the small nests (Fig. 111.33). Foci of ductular and apocrine tubular differentiation can sometimes be found, but are not conspicuous.

Treatment
Cylindroma is a benign adnexal proliferation. Despite its 'basaloid' microscopic appearance, cylindroma holds negligible proliferative capacity and recurrence is uncommon after complete excision.

Carcinomas of apocrine lineage
Introduction

Adnexal carcinomas with tubular and ductular differentiation (adnexal adenocarcinomas) are relatively uncommon, and their rarity has contributed to confusion with respect to diagnosis, classification and therapy. Adnexal carcinomas can develop *de novo* or they can arise in association with other benign adnexal neoplasms. The semantics of carcinomas that arise in association with benign neoplasms has been problematic, as there has been a historical tendency to create a nomenclature by referring to a form of carcinoma by the name of its benign analogue with the addition of the adjective 'malignant'. This author prefers porocarcinoma and spiradenocarcinoma over the terms malignant poroma and malignant spiradenoma.

For some types of adnexal carcinoma, such as spiradenocarcinoma or cylindrocarcinoma, the adenocarcinomas that develop from the benign neoplasm typically lack a decisive pattern of differentiation and are only specifically diagnosable through recognition of the residual benign lesion. A spiradenocarcinoma in the absence of spiradenoma will likely only be recognizable as poorly differentiated adenocarcinoma. Some forms of adnexal adenocarcinoma, such as porocarcinoma, display distinctive differentiation that is recognizable in a de-novo lesion or in a carcinoma that developed within an existent tumor.

Clinical features

In general, the presentation of adnexal adenocarcinomas is not distinctive. Patients who develop adnexal carcinoma within an existent benign neoplasm often relate a history of recent rapid (sometimes explosive) enlargement of a previously stable, longstanding plaque or nodule (Fig. 111.34). Ulceration and bleeding are common associated findings. De-novo adnexal adenocarcinoma presents as a plaque or nodule, and biopsy and microscopy are required for diagnosis.

Perhaps the most is known about the presentation of *microcystic adnexal carcinoma* (MAC), a low-grade form of adnexal carcinoma (also known as *sclerosing sweat duct carcinoma*) that has been carefully evaluated in several large series[92]. MAC typically presents in young or middle-aged adults, most commonly in women, and lesions slowly enlarge over years and are often misdiagnosed prior to the time of definitive recognition (Fig. 111.35)[92]. The most common location is the lip. Curiously, a left-sided predominance was noted in the largest series from the US, suggesting that UV light exposure (from driving) might be contributory to carcinogenesis, much like common forms of non-melanoma skin cancer.

Pathology

All forms of adnexal adenocarcinoma share architectural attributes of malignancy, such as asymmetry, lack of circumscription, and an infiltrative pattern. There is considerable variability in the degree of cytologic atypicality, and no standard exists for the grading of these neoplasms. Some forms of adnexal carcinoma may display overtly anaplastic cytomorphology, while other carcinomas, such as MAC or syringomatous carcinoma, display very subtle nuclear atypism.

Syringomatous carcinoma refers to a rare form of carcinoma with distal ductular differentiation[93,94]. Syringomatous carcinoma may be of either apocrine or eccrine lineage. Syringomatous carcinoma is characterized by poor circumscription and an infiltrative pattern at low magnification, and is composed of small nests and tubules of pale cells with central cuticulated ducts. The degree of nuclear atypicality is usually modest, and thus a superficial biopsy, which hides the lack of circumscription, can lead to misinterpretation as syringoma. Syringomatous carcinoma has only been observed as a de-novo malignancy.

MAC is a close relative of syringomatous carcinoma that is distinctive for biphasic or multiphasic differentiation. MAC displays a ductal component identical to that of syringomatous carcinoma, coupled with follicular and (sometimes) sebaceous differentiation[92,95] (Fig. 111.36). The follicular component of MAC consists most notably of small cystic ('microcystic') foci with follicular infundibular and isthmic keratinization, similar to the superficial follicular keratinization observed in desmoplastic trichoepithelioma or trichoadenoma. Areas resembling the follicular outer sheath may also be present. Extensive infiltration of the reticular dermis and perineural extension of tumor cells are common findings. Although desmoplastic trichoepithelioma

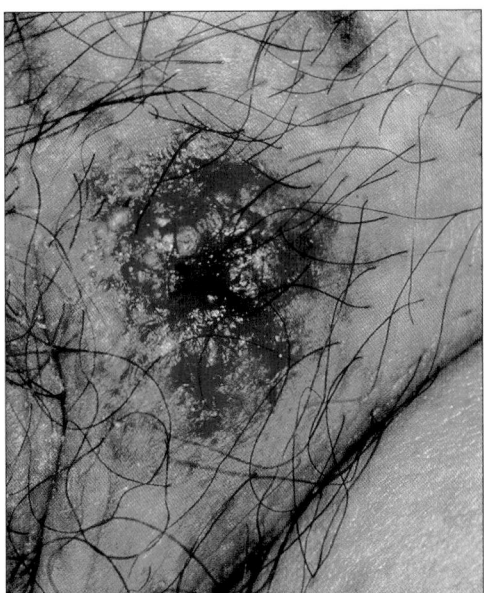

Fig. 111.34 Porocarcinoma. Rapid growth and erosion or ulceration accompany this malignant adnexal tumor.

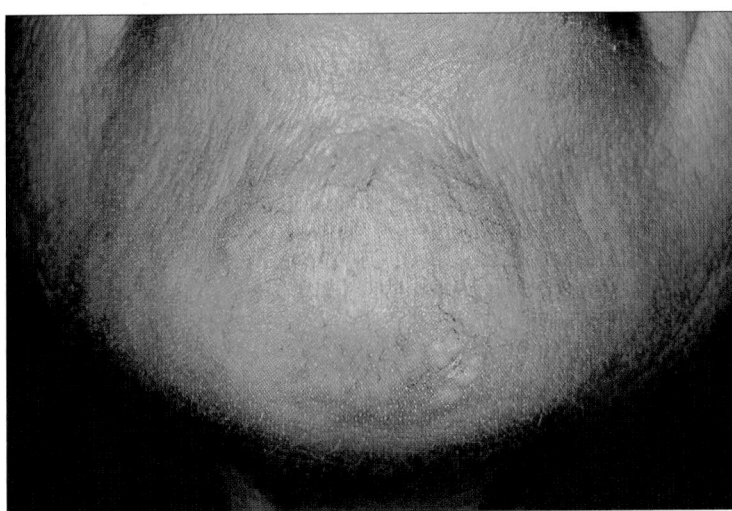

Fig. 111.35 Microcystic adnexal carcinoma. This tumor presents as a slowly expanding, firm plaque.

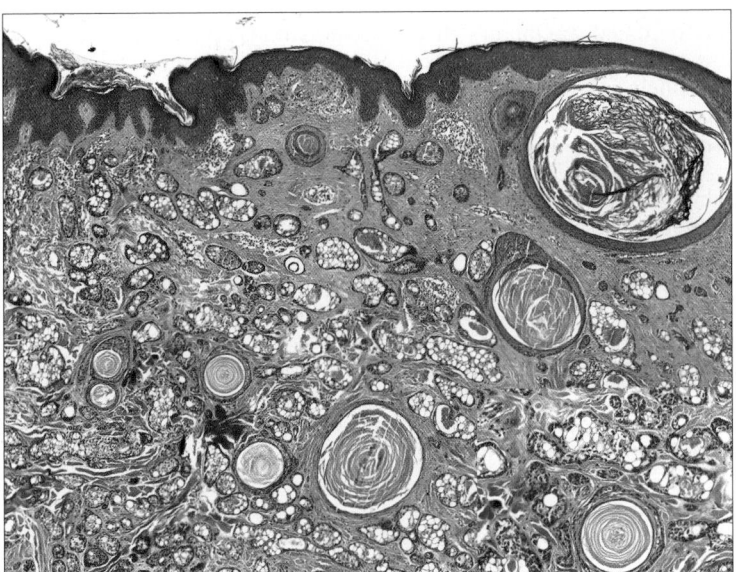

Fig. 111.36 Microcystic adnexal carcinoma. This deeply infiltrative carcinoma shows a biphasic microscopic pattern, with both ductular differentiation and superficial follicular keratinization. The high-magnification inset shows conspicuous ductal differentiation without cytologic atypism, which sometimes leads to misdiagnosis as a benign lesion.

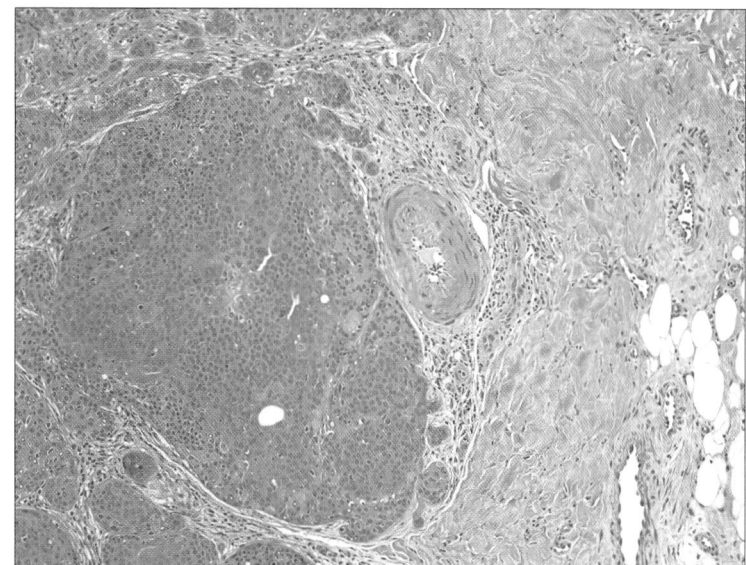

Fig. 111.37 Porocarcinoma. There are irregularly shaped nests of neoplastic cells that infiltrate deeply, with this image obtained at the level of the superficial subcutis. The largest nest shows central foci of ductular differentiation.

and MAC exhibit overlapping features and both are characterized by foci of superficial follicular keratinization, follicular germinative (basaloid) cells are a hallmark of trichoepithelioma but are essentially never present in MAC.

Porocarcinoma may develop *de novo* or in association with an existent poroma[96]. Like poroma, porocarcinoma may be of apocrine or eccrine lineage, and it is generally impossible to determine the exact lineage of any given tumor. Some examples of porocarcinoma display little cytologic atypism and thus close attention must be paid to other attributes of malignancy, and small or partial biopsies may defy exact diagnosis. However, the degree of cytologic atypism is variable[94,97]. The neoplasm is composed of nests of eosinophilic or pallid cuboidal cells that infiltrate the dermis, and ductal differentiation is usually conspicuous (Fig. 111.37). Porocarcinoma may display intraepidermal growth, with a 'pagetoid' pattern within the epidermis in some cases[94,97].

Hidradenocarcinoma may develop *de novo* or in association with an existent hidradenoma. Hidradenocarcinoma may be of apocrine or eccrine lineage. Cases reported in the older literature were notable for the presence of marked clear cell change, much like clear cell hidradenoma.

Spiradenocarcinoma and *cylindrocarcinoma* are usually poorly differentiated carcinomas that develop *de novo* or more commonly in association with an existent spiradenoma or cylindroma[98–100]. Both are extremely rare and may come to medical attention late in their course, as their evolution within longstanding stable lesions may contribute to a delay in pursuit of care by the patient.

Adenoid cystic carcinoma is a type of relatively undifferentiated adnexal carcinoma that resembles micronodular BCC but is generally distinctive for the presence of cribriform (net-like) glandular differentiation and a paucity of accompanying myxoid stroma. Primary cutaneous adenoid cystic carcinomas have been misinterpreted as metastatic lesions. Although initially postulated to represent a type of eccrine carcinoma, most authorities believe the entity represents a neoplasm of apocrine lineage. Adenoid cystic carcinoma tends to display considerable local invasiveness and most examples remain confined to the skin over years or even decades, but metastasis to lymph nodes and parenchymal organs can also rarely occur[101].

Treatment

As a rule, adnexal adenocarcinomas are low-grade forms of carcinoma that are locally invasive but pose a low risk for metastasis. Metastasis has been documented, but such reports are uncommon. Many adnexal carcinomas that yield metastatic spread are large lesions, or lesions that were diagnosed late in their evolution. Surgical extirpation, including Mohs micrographic surgery, remains the primary therapeutic modality. Careful microscopic classification is crucial to developing experience

with larger groups of histopathologically homogeneous lesions to enable careful assessment of natural history as well as proper medical and surgical care.

NEOPLASMS AND PROLIFERATIONS WITH ECCRINE DIFFERENTIATION

Eccrine nevus (hamartoma)

Nevi or malformations with an eccrine glandular component are extremely uncommon. The clinical morphology is not distinctive. Some lesions are alleged to maintain function of the eccrine apparatus, which can manifest clinically as mucinous discharge or localized hyperhidrosis.

Microscopically, the judgment as to whether eccrine glands are normal in number or increased can be difficult, especially in a partial biopsy. The absolute number of eccrine units is increased and the constituent units are of increased size in eccrine nevi. The surrounding stroma may be exclusively fibrotic or may include adipocytes. When the stroma also harbors an increase in small vascular channels, the designation eccrine angiomatous hamartoma can also be applied.

So-called porokeratotic eccrine ostial and dermal duct nevi are probably not eccrine nevi at all. These lesions are typically congenital and present as papules or plaques on the hands or feet, with punctate hyperkeratosis. The focal hyperkeratosis corresponds to cornoid lamellae that are often situated within acanthotic acrosyringia (Fig. 111.38). Eccrine acini are qualitatively and quantitatively normal in porokeratotic nevi, suggesting that these lesions should not be classified as a form of adnexal nevus. From the standpoint of nosology, these lesions probably fit best on the spectrum of epidermal nevi.

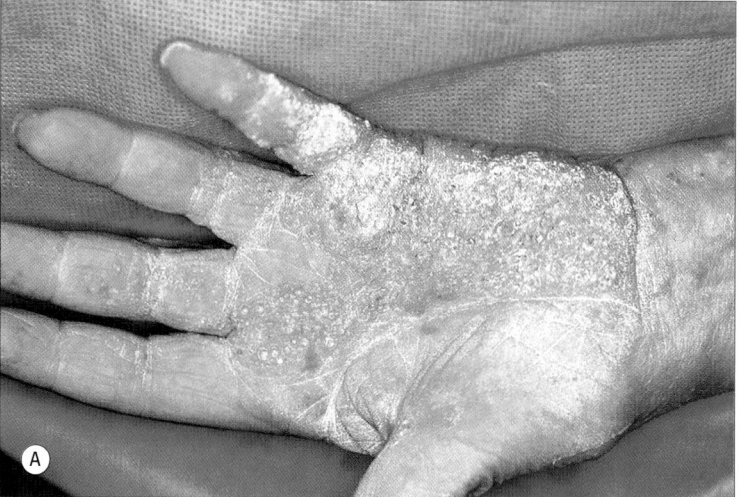

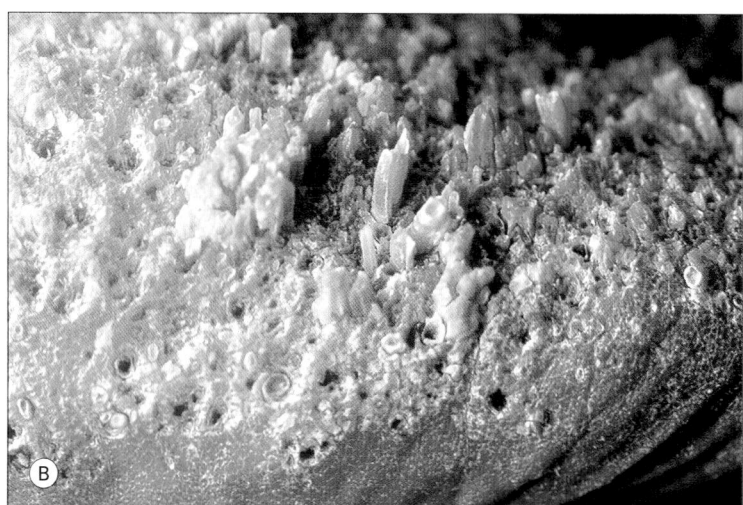

Fig. 111.38 Porokeratotic eccrine ostial and dermal duct nevus. Markedly hyperkeratotic spines arise from dilated eccrine ostia, corresponding to the histologic findings of coronoid lamellae.

Treatment

Eccrine nevi are benign and require no treatment, but excision can be performed if desired.

Papillary adenoma and adenocarcinoma
Introduction

The concept of *papillary adenoma* was put forth under the designation *aggressive digital papillary adenoma* in a report from the Armed Forces Institute of Pathology[102–104]. These neoplasms are uncommon and occur on acral skin of the fingers, toes, palms and soles, a topographic restriction suggestive of eccrine lineage. Papillary adenoma was deemed 'aggressive' because the neoplasms were prone to local recurrence if not completely excised, and some lesions were found to erode bone or infiltrate adjacent soft tissue[103]. Some lesions classified as aggressive papillary adenoma have metastasized[104], so that now it is unclear whether there is a spectrum that includes both adenomas and adeno-carcinomas, or whether all acral papillary lesions represent carcinomas.

Clinical features

Papillary adenoma/adenocarcinoma presents as a solitary nodular lesion in an adult of any age. Some lesions are large, up to several centimeters in diameter. There is a male predilection. The lesions may be deeply situated and can impinge upon or erode underlying bone. The metastatic route appears to be hematogenous, and metastases involving the lung are common.

Pathology

The neoplasms are extraordinarily cellular and display a combination of solid and papillary areas and are occasionally cystic[103]. A cribriform pattern can occasionally be found. Some lesions within this spectrum present with a largely cribriform or tubular configuration; the designation 'tubulopapillary' carcinoma can be employed in this context. Irrespective of the architecture of the lesion, its constituent cells have hyperchromatic nuclei and relatively little cytoplasm, and mitotic

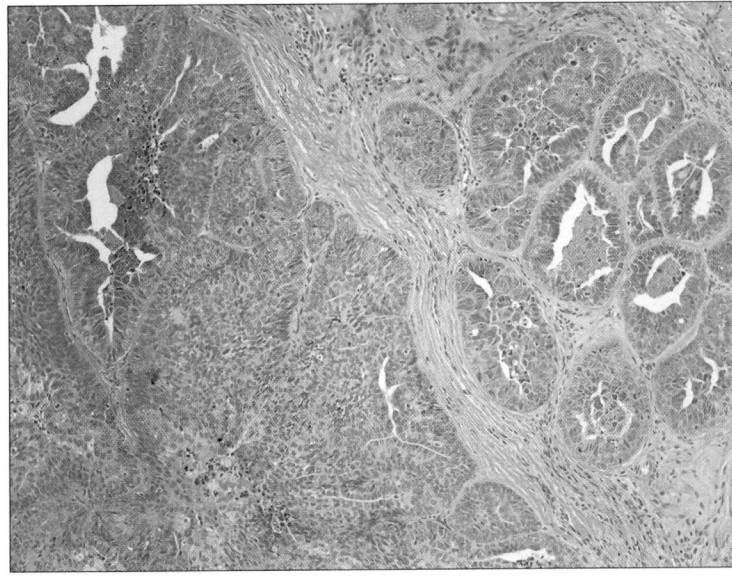

Fig. 111.39 Papillary adenocarcinoma of the digit. Solid, tubular and papillary foci, with small foci of necrosis. Mitotic figures are easily identified.

figures are usually readily identifiable (Fig. 111.39). There may be necrosis, both of individual cells or *en masse*. The enveloping stroma is commonly sclerotic. In overtly malignant lesions, vascular invasion or infiltration of bone may be observed.

Treatment

It is difficult to predict the clinical course based upon the microscopic pattern. Complete surgical extirpation of papillary 'adenoma' or adeno-carcinoma with negative margins remains the standard of care.

REFERENCES

1. McCalmont TH. A call for logic in the classification of adnexal neoplasms. Am J Dermatopathol. 1996;18:103–9.
2. Montagna W. Embryology and anatomy of the cutaneous adnexa. J Cutan Pathol. 1984;11:350–1.
3. Hyman AB, Brownstein MH. Eccrine poroma. An analysis of forty-five new cases. Dermatologica. 1969;138:29–38.
4. Brownstein MH, Shapiro L. The sweat gland adenomas. Int J Dermatol. 1975;14:397–411.
5. Labandeira J, Peteiro C, Toribio J. Hair follicle nevus: case report and review. Am J Dermatopathol. 1996;18:90–3.
6. Ban M, Kamiya H, Yamada T, Kitajima Y. Hair follicle nevi and accessory tragi: variable quantity of adipose tissue in connective tissue framework. Pediatr Dermatol. 1997;14:433–6.
7. Brownstein MH, Wanger N, Helwig EB. Accessory tragi. Arch Dermatol. 1971;104:625–31.
8. Plewig G. Sebaceous trichofolliculoma. J Cutan Pathol. 1980;7:394–403.
9. Schulz T, Hartschuh W. Folliculo-sebaceous cystic hamartoma is a trichofolliculoma at its very late stage. J Cutan Pathol. 1998;25:354–64.
10. Kimura T, Miyazawa H, Aoyagi T, Ackerman AB. Folliculosebaceous cystic hamartoma. A distinctive malformation of the skin. Am J Dermatopathol. 1991;13:213–20.
11. Bolognia JL, Longley BJ. Genital variant of folliculosebaceous cystic hamartoma. Dermatology. 1998;197:258–60.
12. Prioleau PG, Santa Cruz DJ. Sebaceous gland neoplasia. J Cutan Pathol. 1984;11:396–414.
13. Jaqueti G, Requena L, Sanchez Yus E. Trichoblastoma is the most common neoplasm developed in nevus sebaceus of Jadassohn: a clinicopathologic study of a series of 155 cases. Am J Dermatopathol. 2000;22:108–18.
14. Cribier B, Grosshans E. Tumor of the follicular infundibulum: a clinicopathologic study. J Am Acad Dermatol. 1995;33:979–84.
15. Alessi E, Wong SN, Advani HH, Ackerman AB. Nevus sebaceus is associated with unusual neoplasms. An atlas. Am J Dermatopathol. 1988;10:116–27.

16. Cribier B, Scrivener Y, Grosshans E. Tumors arising in nevus sebaceus: a study of 596 cases. J Am Acad Dermatol. 2000;42:263–8.
17. Akasaka T, Onodera H, Matsuta M. Cutaneous mixed tumor containing ossification, hair matrix, and sebaceous ductal differentiation. J Dermatol. 1997;24:125–31.
18. Hassab-el-Naby HM, Tam S, White WL, Ackerman AB. Mixed tumors of the skin. A histological and immunohistochemical study. Am J Dermatopathol. 1989;11:413–28.
19. Gianotti R, Coggi A, Alessi E. Cutaneous apocrine mixed tumor: derived from the apocrine duct of the folliculo-sebaceous-apocrine unit? Am J Dermatopathol. 1998;20:53–5.
20. Ackerman AB, Reddy VB, Soyer HP. Neoplasms with Follicular Differentiation, 2nd edn. New York: Ardor Scribendi, 2001:1109.
21. Zaim MT. 'Immature' trichoepithelioma. J Cutan Pathol. 1989;16:287–9.
22. Harada H, Hashimoto K, Ko MS. The gene for multiple familial trichoepithelioma maps to chromosome 9p21. J Invest Dermatol. 1996;107:41–3.
23. Bettencourt MS, Prieto VG, Shea CR. Trichoepithelioma: a 19-year clinicopathologic re-evaluation. J Cutan Pathol. 1999;26:398–404.
24. Brooke JD, Fitzpatrick JE, Golitz LE. Papillary mesenchymal bodies: a histologic finding useful in differentiating trichoepitheliomas from basal cell carcinomas. J Am Acad Dermatol. 1989;21:523–8.
25. Escalonilla P, Requena L. Plaque variant of trichoblastic fibroma. Arch Dermatol. 1996;132:1388–90.
26. Altman DA, Mikhail GR, Johnson TM, Lowe L. Trichoblastic fibroma. A series of 10 cases with report of a new plaque variant. Arch Dermatol. 1995;131:198–201.
27. Requena L, Renedo G, Sarasa J, et al. Trichoblastic fibroma. J Cutan Pathol. 1990;17:381–4.
28. Sajben FP, Ross EV. The use of the 1.0 mm handpiece in high energy, pulsed CO$_2$ laser destruction of facial adnexal tumors. Dermatol Surg. 1999;25:41–4.
29. Shaffelburg M, Miller R. Treatment of multiple

trichoepithelioma with electrosurgery. Dermatol Surg. 1998;24:1154–6.
30. Brownstein MH, Shapiro L. Desmoplastic trichoepithelioma. Cancer. 1977;40:2979–86.
31. Lazar AJ, Calonje E, Grayson W, et al. Pilomatrix carcinomas contain mutations in CTNNB1, the gene encoding beta-catenin. J Cutan Pathol. 2005;32:148–57.
32. Demircan M, Balik E. Pilomatricoma in children: a prospective study. Pediatr Dermatol. 1997;14:430–2.
33. Danielson-Cohen A, Lin SJ, Hughes CA, et al. Head and neck pilomatrixoma in children. Arch Otolaryngol Head Neck Surg. 2001;127:1481–3.
34. Shames BS, Nassif A, Bailey CS, et al. Secondary anetoderma involving a pilomatricoma. Am J Dermatopathol. 1994;16:55–60.
35. Hardisson D, Linaves MD, Cuevas-Santos, J, Contreas F. Pilomatrix carcinoma: a clinicopathologic study of six cases and review of the literature. Am J Dermatopathol. 2001;23:394–401.
36. Ambrojo P, Aguilar A, Simon P, et al. Basal cell carcinoma with matrical differentiation. Am J Dermatopathol. 1992;14:293–7.
37. Aloi FG, Molinero A, Pippione M. Basal cell carcinoma with matrical differentiation. Matrical carcinoma. Am J Dermatopathol. 1988;10:509–13.
38. Brownstein MH. Trichilemmoma. Benign follicular tumor or viral wart? Am J Dermatopathol. 1980;2:229–31.
39. Leonardi CL, Zhu WY, Kinsey WH, Penneys NS. Trichilemmomas are not associated with human papillomavirus DNA. J Cutan Pathol. 1991;18:193–7.
40. Brownstein MH, Shapiro L. Trichilemmoma. Analysis of 40 new cases. Arch Dermatol. 1973;107:866–9.
41. Roson E, Gomez Centeno P, Sanchez-Aguiler D, et al. Desmoplastic trichilemmoma arising within a nevus sebaceus. Am J Dermatopathol. 1998;20:495–7.
42. Brownstein MH, Mehregan AH, Bikowski JB, et al. The dermatopathology of Cowden's syndrome. Br J Dermatol. 1979;100:667–73.
43. Requena L, Gutierrez J, Sanchez Yus E. Multiple sclerotic fibromas of the skin. A cutaneous marker of Cowden's disease. J Cutan Pathol. 1992;19:346–51.

44. Hunt SJ, Kilzer B, Santa Cruz DJ. Desmoplastic trichilemmoma: histologic variant resembling invasive carcinoma. J Cutan Pathol. 1990;17:45–52.

45. Tellechea O, Reis JP, Baptista AP. Desmoplastic trichilemmoma. Am J Dermatopathol. 1992;14:107–4.

46. Vin-Christian K, Grekin R, McCalmont T. Hypopigmented papules of the cheeks, neck, and shoulders. Arch Dermatol. 1999;135:463–4, 466–7.

47. Kolenik SA 3rd, Bolognia JL, Castiglione FM Jr, Longley BJ. Multiple tumors of the follicular infundibulum. Int J Dermatol. 1996;35:282–4.

48. Kossard S, Finley AG, Poyzer K, Kocsard E. Eruptive infundibulomas. A distinctive presentation of the tumor of follicular infundibulum. J Am Acad Dermatol. 1989;21:361–6.

49. Horn TD, Vennos EM, Bernstein BD, Cooper PH. Multiple tumors of follicular infundibulum with sweat duct differentiation. J Cutan Pathol. 1995;22:281–7.

50. Mahalingam M, Bhawan J, Finn R, Stefanato CM. Tumor of the follicular infundibulum with sebaceous differentiation. J Cutan Pathol. 2001;28:314–17.

51. Rahbari H, Mehregan A, Pinkus A. Trichoadenoma of Nikolowski. J Cutan Pathol. 1977;4:90–8.

52. Brownstein MH, Arluk DJ. Proliferating trichilemmal cyst: a simulant of squamous cell carcinoma. Cancer. 1981;48:1207–14.

53. Sethi S, Singh UR. Proliferating trichilemmal cyst: report of two cases, one benign and the other malignant. J Dermatol. 2002;29:214–20.

54. Sleater J, Beers B, Stefan M, et al. Proliferating trichilemmal cyst. Report of four cases, two with nondiploid DNA content and increased proliferation index. Am J Dermatopathol. 1993;15:423–8.

55. Lopez-Rios F, Rodriguez-Peralto JR, Aguilar A, et al. Proliferating trichilemmal cyst with focal invasion: report of a case and a review of the literature. Am J Dermatopathol. 2000;22:183–7.

56. Finan MC, Apgar JT. Juxta-clavicular beaded lines: a subepidermal proliferation of sebaceous gland elements. J Cutan Pathol. 1991;18:464–8.

57. Bader RS, Scarborough DA. Surgical pearl: intralesional electrodesiccation of sebaceous hyperplasia. J Am Acad Dermatol. 2000;42:127–8.

58. Troy JL, Ackerman AB. Sebaceoma. A distinctive benign neoplasm of adnexal epithelium differentiating toward sebaceous cells. Am J Dermatopathol. 1984;6:7–13.

59. Misago N, Narisawa Y. Rippled-pattern sebaceoma. Am J Dermatopathol. 2001;23:437–43.

60. Rutten A, Burgdorf W, Hugel H, et al. Cystic sebaceous tumors as marker lesions for the Muir-Torre syndrome: a histopathologic and molecular genetic study. Am J Dermatopathol. 1999;21:405–13.

61. Misago N, Narisawa Y. Sebaceous neoplasms in Muir-Torre syndrome. Am J Dermatopathol. 2000;22:155–61.

62. Wick MR, Goellner JR, Wolfe JT 3rd, Su WP. Adnexal carcinomas of the skin. II. Extraocular sebaceous carcinomas. Cancer. 1985;56:1163–72.

63. Kohler S, Rouse RV, Smoller BR. The differential diagnosis of pagetoid cells in the epidermis. Mod Pathol. 1998;11:79–92.

64. Nguyen GK, Mielke BW. Extraocular sebaceous carcinoma with intraepidermal (pagetoid) spread. Am J Dermatopathol. 1987;9:364–5.

65. Hashimoto K, Lever WF. Histogenesis of skin appendage tumors. Arch Dermatol. 1969;100:356–69.

66. Hashimoto K, Lever WF. Skin appendage tumors. Arch Dermatol. 1970;101:252–3.

67. Patrizi A, Neri I, Marzaduri S, et al. Syringoma: a review of twenty-nine cases. Acta Derm Venereol. 1998;78:460–2.

68. Soler-Carrillo J, Estrach T, Mascaro JM. Eruptive syringoma: 27 new cases and review of the literature. J Eur Acad Dermatol Venereol. 2001;15:242–6.

69. Di Lernia V, Bisighini G. Localized vulvar syringomas. Pediatr Dermatol. 1996;13:80–1.

70. Garcia C, Krunic AL, Grichnik J, et al. Multiple acral syringomata with uniform involvement of the hands and feet. Cutis. 1997;59:213–14, 216.

71. Goyal S, Martins CR. Multiple syringomas on the abdomen, thighs, and groin. Cutis. 2000;66:259–62.

72. Harvell JD, Kerschmann RL, LeBoit PE. Eccrine or apocrine poroma? Six poromas with divergent adnexal differentiation. Am J Dermatopathol. 1996;18:1–9.

73. Azma M, Tawfik O, Casparian JM. Apocrine poroma of the breast. Breast J. 2001;7:195–8.

74. Groben PA, Hitchcock MG, Leshin B, et al. Apocrine poroma: a distinctive case in a patient with nevoid basal cell carcinoma syndrome. Am J Dermatopathol. 1999;21:31–3.

75. Kamiya H, Oyama Z, Kitajima Y. 'Apocrine' poroma: review of the literature and case report. J Cutan Pathol. 2001;28:101–4.

76. Lee NH, Lee SH, Ahn SK. Apocrine poroma with sebaceous differentiation. Am J Dermatopathol. 2000;22:261–3.

77. Mahalingam M, Byers HR. Intra-epidermal and intra-dermal sebocrine adenoma with cystic degeneration and hemorrhage. J Cutan Pathol. 2000;27:472–5.

78. Gianotti R, Alessi E. Clear cell hidradenoma associated with the folliculo-sebaceous-apocrine unit. Histologic study of five cases. Am J Dermatopathol. 1997;19:351–7.

79. Wolff K, Winkelmann RK, Decker RH. Solid-cystic hidradenoma: an enzyme histochemical, biochemical, and electron microscopic study. Acta Dermatol Kyoto Engl Ed. 1968;63:309–22.

80. Ohnishi T, Watanabe S. Histogenesis of clear cell hidradenoma: immunohistochemical study of keratin expression. J Cutan Pathol. 1997;24:30–6.

81. Requena L, Sanchez M. Poroid hidradenoma: a light microscopic and immunohistochemical study. Cutis. 1992;50:43–6.

82. Brownstein MH, Phelps RG, Magnin PH. Papillary adenoma of the nipple: analysis of fifteen new cases. J Am Acad Dermatol. 1985;12:707–15.

83. Diaz NM, Palmer JO, Wick MR. Erosive adenomatosis of the nipple: histology, immunohistology, and differential diagnosis. Mod Pathol. 1992;5:179–84.

84. Miller L, Tyler W, Maroon M, et al. Erosive adenomatosis of the nipple: a benign imitator of malignant breast disease. Cutis. 1997;59:91–2.

85. Koga T, Kubota Y, Nakayama J. Syringocystadenoma papilliferum without an antecedent naevus sebaceous. Acta Derm Venereol. 1999;79:237.

86. Vang R, Cohen PR. Ectopic hidradenoma papilliferum: a case report and review of the literature. J Am Acad Dermatol. 1999;41:115–18.

87. Goette DK, McConnell MA, Fowler VR. Cylindroma and eccrine spiradenoma coexistent in the same lesion. Arch Dermatol. 1982;118:274–4.

88. Michal M, Lamovec J, Mukensnabl P, Pizinger K. Spiradenocylindromas of the skin: tumors with morphological features of spiradenoma and cylindroma in the same lesion: report of 12 cases. Pathol Int. 1999;49:419–25.

89. Nerad JA, Folberg R. Multiple cylindromas. The 'turban tumor'. Arch Ophthalmol. 1987;105:1137.

90. Freedman AM, Woods JE. Total scalp excision and auricular resurfacing for dermal cylindroma (turban tumor). Ann Plast Surg. 1989;22:50–7.

91. Reingold IM, Keasbey LE, Graham JH. Multicentric dermal-type cylindromas of the parotid glands in a patient with florid turban tumor. Cancer. 1977;40:1702–10.

92. Chiller K, Passaro D, Scheuller M, et al. Microcystic adnexal carcinoma: forty-eight cases, their treatment, and their outcome. Arch Dermatol. 2000;136:1355–9.

93. Hoppenreijs VP, Reuser TT, Mooy CM, et al. Syringomatous carcinoma of the eyelid and orbit: a clinical and histopathological challenge. Br J Ophthalmol. 1997;81:668–72.

94. Urso C, Bondi R, Paglierani M, et al. Carcinomas of sweat glands: report of 60 cases. Arch Pathol Lab Med. 2001;125:498–505.

95. Nickoloff BJ, Fleischmann HE, Carmel J, et al. Microcystic adnexal carcinoma. Immunohistologic observations suggesting dual (pilar and eccrine) differentiation. Arch Dermatol. 1986;122:290–4.

96. Spencer DM, Bigler LR, Hearne DW, et al. Pedal papule. Eccrine porocarcinoma (EPC) in association with poroma. Arch Dermatol. 1995;131:211, 214.

97. Robson A, Greene J, Ansari N, et al. Eccrine porocarcinoma (malignant eccrine poroma): a clinicopathologic study of 69 cases. Am J Surg Pathol. 2001;25:710–20.

98. Granter SR, Seeger K, Calonje E, et al. Malignant eccrine spiradenoma (spiradenocarcinoma): a clinicopathologic study of 12 cases. Am J Dermatopathol. 2000;22:97–103.

99. Biernat W, Wozniak L. Spiradenocarcinoma: a clinicopathologic and immunohistochemical study of three cases. Am J Dermatopathol. 1994;16:377–82.

100. Durani BK, Kurzen H, Jaeckel A, et al. Malignant transformation of multiple dermal cylindromas. Br J Dermatol. 2001;145:653–6.

101. Kato N, Yasukawa K, Onozuka T. Primary cutaneous adenoid cystic carcinoma with lymph node metastasis. Am J Dermatopathol. 1998;20:571–7.

102. Smith KJ, Skelton HG, Holland TT. Recent advances and controversies concerning adnexal neoplasms. Dermatol Clin. 1992;10:117–60.

103. Kao GF, Helwig EB, Graham JH. Aggressive digital papillary adenoma and adenocarcinoma. A clinicopathological study of 57 patients, with histochemical, immunopathological, and ultrastructural observations. J Cutan Pathol. 1987;14:129–46.

104. Duke WH, Sherrod TT, Lupton GP. Aggressive digital papillary adenocarcinoma (aggressive digital papillary adenoma and adenocarcinoma revisited). Am J Surg Pathol. 2000;24:775–84.

Benign Melanocytic Neoplasms

Raymond L Barnhill and Harold Rabinovitz

112

Chapter Contents

EPHELIDES

Synonym: ■ Freckles

Key feature

- Small, well-circumscribed, pigmented macules found only on sun-exposed skin of individuals with fair skin

Epidemiology

Ephelides are common in individuals with blond or red hair[1–6]. They are not present at birth, but usually appear in the first 3 years of life. Since freckling can be seen in some families over generations, autosomal dominant inheritance is likely[1–3].

Pathogenesis

Hyperpigmentation in ephelides is the result of increased sun-induced melanogenesis and transport of an increased number of fully melanized melanosomes from melanocytes to keratinocytes.

Clinical Features

Ephelides occur only on sun-exposed areas of the body, mainly on the face, the dorsal aspects of the arms, and the upper part of the chest and the back. They are not found on mucous membranes. Ephelides are well demarcated and round, oval or irregular in shape. They are usually 1 to 3 mm in diameter, but some may be larger. Depending on the intensity of sun exposure, ephelides vary in color from light to dark brown, but almost never become as dark as lentigines or junctional nevi. They may increase in number and distribution and show a tendency to confluence, but they decrease later in life. Ephelides are benign and show no propensity for malignant transformation[4]. While they are not a direct precursor of melanoma, ephelides are a marker of UV-induced damage and, hence, a marker for increased risk of UV-induced neoplasia[5]. In a study of 195 patients diagnosed with melanoma in England, the density of freckles on the face and arms was found to be more strongly associated with melanoma than the number of nevi. When adjusted for other factors (nevi, sunburns, skin type), those with a high freckle density had an odds ratio of 6.0 for developing melanoma compared with those without freckles. Some ephelides may represent a subtype of solar lentigo[5].

Pathology

The epidermis exhibits a normal configuration. The keratinocytes show an increase in melanin content, predominantly in the basal cell layer[6]. Occasionally, melanophages are seen in the papillary dermis. The number of melanocytes in ephelides does not differ significantly from normal. The melanocytes in ephelides are larger and have more branching of dendrites and a higher dopa positivity than those in the adjacent normal epidermis, apparently indicating greater functional activity.

Differential Diagnosis

Ephelides must be distinguished from simple lentigines, solar lentigines, café-au-lait macules and junctional nevi. In general, ephelides are lighter in color than simple lentigines, are located on sun-exposed skin, and are responsive to solar exposure. In contrast, simple lentigines may occur on any site and are persistent. Table 112.1 compares ephelides and solar lentigines. Café-au-lait macules are usually solitary and larger than ephelides.

Treatment

Since darkening of ephelides depends on UV radiation, sun exposure should be minimized and sunscreens should be used. The bleaching action of hydroquinone and topical retinoids may be beneficial; however, it is difficult to achieve an even clinical effect. Cryotherapy can lighten ephelides. Superficial pigmented lesions such as ephelides can be effectively treated with any of the pigment-specific, pulsed lasers. Note that with the destructive therapies, any resulting dyspigmentation can be more disturbing to the patient than the original lesion.

CAFÉ-AU-LAIT MACULES

Key features

- Well-circumscribed, uniformly light to dark brown macules or patches averaging 2–5 cm in adults
- Usually noted during infancy or early childhood
- Associated with several syndromes, but found in 10–20% of the normal population

Epidemiology

Café-au-lait macules (CALM) can occur as an isolated lesion or as multiple lesions. Multiple lesions are sometimes a marker for multi-

COMPARATIVE CLINICAL FEATURES OF EPHELIDES AND SOLAR LENTIGINES		
	Ephelides (freckles)	**Solar lentigines**
Epidemiology		
Age of appearance	Early childhood	By 20–30 years (I, II)
Skin color	Light pigmentation	Light to dark pigmentation
Hair color	Often red or blond hair	Any type
Skin phototype	More common in I, II	More common in I and II, but also in III and IV
History		
Precipitating factors	Bursts of high-intensity sun exposure convert latent predetermined melanocytes to permanent freckles	Repeated sun exposure over time changes a cluster of melanocytes
Duration of lesions	Fade without sun exposure	Persist for life
Relation to season	Much darker in summer, fade in winter and over time with aging	May darken in summer but do not fade in winter
Heredity	Probably autosomal dominant	No data
Physical examination		
Type of lesion	Macule	Macule
Size	1–5 mm	5–15 mm or larger
Color	Light or medium brown	Medium or dark brown
Shape	Round to oval	Oval to stellate
Border	Smooth to jagged	Smooth to jagged
Distribution	Favor the face, forearms and back; rare on the dorsal aspect of the hands	Sites of chronic sun exposure, especially the face, arms (including dorsal aspect of the hands) and upper trunk
Electron microscopy		
	Melanocytes between freckle macules contain pheomelanosomes	Large melanosome complexes within keratinocytes

Table 112.1 Comparative clinical features of ephelides and solar lentigines. I, II, III, IV = skin phototypes (see Ch. 134).

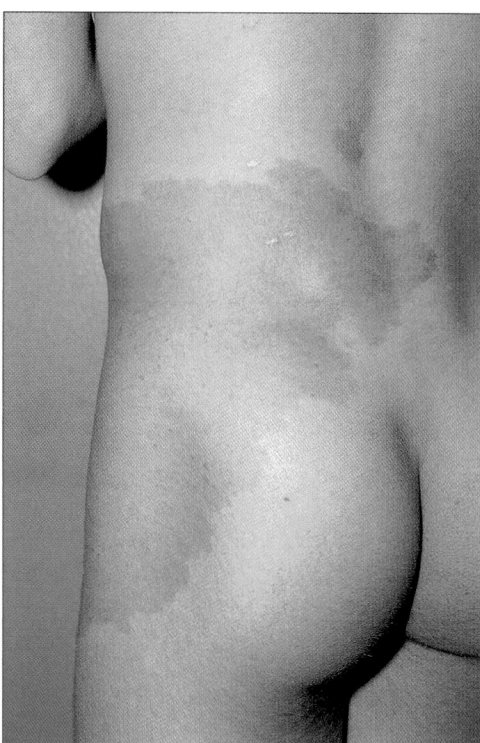

Fig. 112.1 Café-au-lait macule. Large tan patch in a geographic pattern on the lateral trunk. The patient did not have McCune–Albright syndrome.

located anywhere on the body, except the mucous membranes. CALM are usually 2.0 to 5.0 cm in diameter in adults, but may vary from freckle-like lesions <2 mm to patches >20 cm in size. CALM grow proportionately to body growth and remain stable in size after body growth has ceased. They demonstrate no tendency toward malignancy. Isolated CALM are very common within the general population and are rarely associated with an underlying systemic disorder. Multiple CALM are relatively rare (0.25–0.5%) in the general population and should alert the physician to the possibility of an associated disease (see Fig. 60.11).

Compared with neurofibromatosis, the CALM of McCune–Albright syndrome are typically fewer in number, larger, darker and may follow Blaschko's lines, with a linear or segmental configuration[11]. They favor the forehead, nuchal area, sacrum and buttocks. They also tend to be unilateral, often involving the same side as the bone lesions and situated in proximity. They can, however, be indistinguishable both clinically and histologically from CALM in neurofibromatosis. Axillary freckling does not occur in McCune-Albright syndrome.

Pathology

Light microscopy shows a normally configured epidermis with a slightly increased melanin content in the basilar keratinocytes. The adnexal epithelium is spared of hyperpigmentation, and melanophages are rarely found in the dermis. In dopa-stained epidermis from most patients with neurofibromatosis, the density of melanocytes is higher in both CALM and normal adjacent skin, in comparison with healthy individuals. The melanocytic density in isolated CALM of otherwise normal persons, however, is usually less than in surrounding skin. Melanin macroglobules (large pigment particles) may be found in CALM and are not specific for neurofibromatosis, since they are occasionally found in isolated CALM without underlying disease and occur in several other conditions such as simple lentigines, Becker's nevus, congenital nevi, dysplastic nevi, and sometimes even normal skin. By electron microscopy, the melanosomes are usually dispersed singly in melanocytes and are usually homogeneous, electron dense, and ellipsoidal when fully melanized[8,12,13].

Differential Diagnosis

Hyperpigmented macules or patches that might be confused with CALM include linear nevoid hyperpigmentation (pigmentary mosaicism), early nevus spilus (before the nevi have appeared), Becker's melanosis

system disease in various syndromes[7,8] (see Table 60.4). Single CALM are found in 10% to 20% of the normal population, and up to 1% of healthy young adults have up to three CALM. They may be present at birth, but usually become clinically obvious during early childhood and increase proportionately in size with age. Their prevalence increases through infancy and childhood and decreases in adults. African-Americans show an increased prevalence compared with Caucasians.

Pathogenesis

The hyperpigmentation observed in CALM is due to increased melanogenesis and an increased melanin content in keratinocytes. However, the basic defect leading to this localized pigmentary disturbance has not yet been elucidated. In patients with McCune-Albright syndrome, mosaicism for activating mutations in the gene that encodes $G_s\alpha$ has been suggested (see Ch. 64).

Clinical Features

The term café-au-lait refers to the lesion's characteristic homogeneous color of coffee with milk, which can be light to dark brown. CALM are completely macular, often have an overall oval morphology, and the margins are well defined and usually regular (Fig. 112.1)[9,10]. They may be (without obvious hypertrichosis), mastocytomas, postinflammatory hyperpigmentation and phytophotodermatitis. Smaller lesions may resemble lentigines or acquired melanocytic nevi while larger lesions may be confused with relatively flat congenital melanocytic nevi.

Treatment

CALM have never been reported to undergo malignant change. Hydroquinone bleaching products and sun protection will have no effect of CALM. A variety of lasers have been used to treat CALM with variable success[14,15]. The risks of laser surgery include transient hyperpigmentation or hypopigmentation, slight scarring, permanent hyperpigmentation, incomplete clearance, and especially recurrence. Typically, between 1 and 14 treatments are required, and responses are difficult to predict. For instance, of 12 CALM treated with a Q-switched ruby laser in one study, 50% developed repigmentation by 6 months follow-up. Responses to frequency-doubled Nd:YAG are also quite variable. In contrast, complete clearance of 34 CALM using a pulsed dye laser for 4–14 treatments, with no recurrences at 12 months follow-up, was noted in another study.

BECKER'S MELANOSIS

Synonyms: ■ Becker's nevus ■ Becker's pigmentary hamartoma ■ Nevoid melanosis ■ Pigmented hairy epidermal nevus

Key features

- Unilateral, hyperpigmented and often hypertrichotic patch or slightly elevated plaque
- Usually on the shoulder of male patients
- Onset during adolescence

Epidemiology

Becker's melanosis has been described in all races[16]. Although it is usually acquired, some cases are congenital. The lesions most often appear in the second and third decades of life and are six times more common in males than in females. Familial occurrence has been reported. In one study, the prevalence among 19 302 army recruits ages 17 to 26 years was 0.52%.

Pathogenesis

The pathogenesis of Becker's melanosis remains unclear. It is believed to be an organoid hamartoma of ectodermally and mesodermally derived tissues. An increase in androgen receptors and probable heightened sensitivity to androgens have been postulated. The latter characteristics would explain its onset during or after puberty, as well as its clinical and histologic manifestations, which include hypertrichosis, dermal thickening, acne and hypertrophic sebaceous glands. Androgen stimulation could also explain the accentuated smooth muscle elements often found in the dermis of Becker's melanosis[17].

Clinical Features

The onset of Becker's melanosis is usually noted in the second or third decade of life, sometimes following intense sunbathing. The lesions commonly have a unilateral distribution and involve an upper quadrant of the anterior or posterior chest plus the shoulder, but they also have been described on the forehead, face, neck, lower trunk, extremities (Fig. 112.2) and buttocks[16]. Normally, Becker's melanosis appears as single lesion, but multiple lesions have occasionally been reported. Becker's melanosis ranges from a few to >15 centimeters in diameter and the most common configuration is block-like, although linear patterns have been described.

The hyperpigmentation varies from uniformly tan to dark brown and the lesions are well demarcated, but the margins are usually

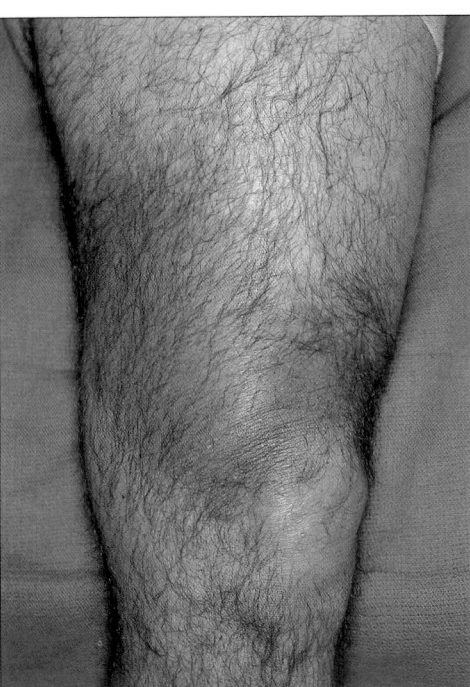

Fig. 112.2 Becker's melanosis (nevus). Large patch of hyperpigmentation on the leg which is medium brown in color. These lesions may be misdiagnosed as café-au-lait macules or congenital melanocytic nevi, especially when they do not occur on the upper trunk. Courtesy of Jean L Bolognia MD.

irregular. The center of the lesion may show slight thickening and corrugation of the skin. Hypertrichosis usually develops after the hyperpigmentation, and the hairs become coarser and darker with time. Sometimes, the hypertrichosis is subtle and can only be appreciated by comparison with the contralateral side. The hypertrichosis and pigmentation may not overlap completely.

Firmness to palpation may point to an associated smooth muscle hamartoma. In some patients, perifollicular papules may be a sign of coexistent proliferation of the muscular arrectores pilorum. Acneiform lesions strictly limited to the area of hyperpigmentation have been reported. Normally, Becker's melanosis is asymptomatic, but some patients report pruritus. After development, the lesion may enlarge slowly for a year or two but then remains stable in size. The color can fade with time, but hypertrichosis usually persists.

Becker's melanosis is a benign lesion, and malignant transformation has not been reported. In contrast to the hyperplasia of the ectodermal and mesodermal tissues in Becker's melanosis, occasional developmental abnormalities have been associated with Becker's melanosis and are generally hypoplastic in nature. These abnormalities include hypoplasia of the ipsilateral breast, areola, nipple and arm, ipsilateral arm shortening, lumbar spina bifida, thoracic scoliosis and pectus carinatum, as well as enlargement of the ipsilateral foot. Accessory scrotum and supernumerary nipples have also been reported. In cases of Becker's melanosis with associated abnormalities, the male:female ratio is reversed to 2:5 in comparison with patients with Becker's melanosis without abnormalities[18].

Pathology

There is variable papillomatosis, acanthosis and hyperkeratosis[16]. Regular elongation of the rete ridges and hyperplasia of the pilosebaceous unit may be observed. The melanin content of the keratinocytes is increased, whereas the number of melanocytes is normal or only slightly increased, without nesting. Melanophages may be found in the papillary dermis. A concomitant smooth muscle hamartoma is often, but not invariably, present in the dermis.

Differential Diagnosis

The differential diagnosis primarily includes CALM, congenital melanocytic nevus, plexiform neurofibroma and congenital smooth muscle hamartoma. The latter tends to be smaller in size but some authors consider Becker's melanosis and congenital smooth muscle hamartoma to be two ends of a clinical spectrum. A congenital melanocytic nevus, plexiform neurofibroma and congenital smooth muscle hamartoma can all have cutaneous hyperpigmentation and hypertrichosis. The presence of multiple CALM and axillary freckling can be helpful in establishing the diagnosis of neurofibromatosis, and unlike Becker's melanosis, CALM do not have corrugation on side-lighting. In an occasional patient, histologic evaluation is required, especially if the lesion is in an unusual location and there is an associated smooth muscle hamartoma.

Treatment

Patients with Becker's melanosis should be examined for soft tissue and bony abnormalities. Electrolysis, waxing, camouflage makeup, and laser treatments may be recommended. The hyperpigmented component has been successfully treated with Q-switched ruby and frequency-doubled Nd:YAG[19], but recurrence rates are high. The hypertrichosis can be addressed with one of several lasers designed for this purpose (see Ch. 137).

SOLAR LENTIGINES

Synonyms: ■ Lentigo senilis ■ Liver spot ■ Old age spot ■ Senile freckle

Key feature

■ Tan to dark brown or black macules due to exposure to ultraviolet (UV) irradiation

Epidemiology

Solar lentigines are found in 90% of the Caucasian population older than 60 years, and their incidence increases with advancing age[20,21]. They can also be found in younger individuals after acute or chronic sun exposure. Lentigines are more common in Caucasians, but also occur in Asians. Inherited patterned lentiginosis favors more lightly pigmented African-Americans.

Pathogenesis

Solar lentigines result from epidermal hyperplasia with variable proliferation of melanocytes and accumulation of melanin in keratinocytes in response to chronic UV radiation exposure. Associated mutations have not been elucidated.

Clinical Features

Solar lentigines are well-circumscribed, round, oval or irregularly shaped macules that vary in color from tan to dark brown or black. More lightly pigmented lesions are usually homogeneous (Fig. 112.3), whereas darker ones tend to have a mottled appearance. Solar lentigines almost always appear as multiple lesions. They usually vary from about 3 mm to 2 cm in diameter and demonstrate a tendency towards confluence. Solar lentigines occur on sun-exposed areas, predominantly the dorsal aspects of hands and forearms, the face, the upper chest and back.

Solar lentigines have an irregular border and a reticulated pigment pattern when examined by tangential lighting and hand lens magnification. They may also be visible under Wood's lamp illumination when not apparent in normal light. The dermoscopic features of a solar lentigo may include the following: a diffuse light brown structureless area, sharply demarcated and/or moth-eaten borders, fingerprinting, and a reticular pattern with thin lines that are occasionally short and interrupted[22] (Fig. P1; Appendix). A particular variant that may be termed sunburn, hypermelanotic, or 'ink spot' solar lentigo is characterized by a striking jet-black color and a stellate outline.

Solar lentigines may develop at almost any age and may fade slightly with age or after the cessation of UV exposure. Most, however, persist indefinitely. The development of melanocyte cytologic atypia in solar lentigines on occasion suggests a relationship of solar lentigines to lentigo maligna, but clear progression to lentigo maligna has not been established. Solar lentigines have been shown to be an independent risk

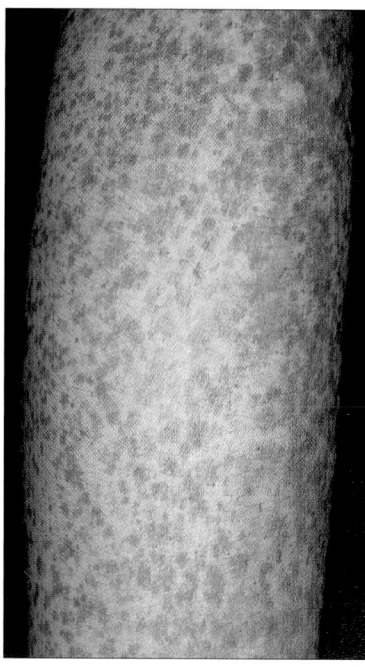

Fig. 112.3 Solar lentigines. Numerous light brown macules, some of which have an irregular border, on chronically sun-exposed skin. Courtesy of Jean L Bolognia MD.

factor for the development of melanoma. Histologic overlap suggests that solitary lichen planus-like keratosis and reticulated seborrheic keratosis can evolve from solar lentigines.

Associated diseases and special forms

PUVA (psoralen + ultraviolet A) lentigo is a well-defined hyperpigmented macule that commonly develops in individuals undergoing long-term PUVA chemotherapy (see Ch. 134). About 50% of PUVA-treated patients develop PUVA lentigines after an average of 5 to 7 years of photochemotherapy. The frequency and severity of the lesions are positively correlated with greater numbers of treatments, age of starting therapy, and male sex. There is a negative association with skin phototypes V and VI. In contrast to typical solar lentigines, PUVA lentigines also occur in sun-protected skin subjected to PUVA treatment. These lesions usually exhibit darker pigmentation and more of a stellate appearance in contrast to solar lentigines. PUVA lentigines often persist years beyond the discontinuation of PUVA therapy. Histologically, the PUVA-induced lesions display lentiginous hyperplasia of large melanocytes that often exhibit mild cytologic atypia. On ultrastructural examination, the melanosomes in PUVA lentigines are usually larger in comparison with the melanosomes in solar lentigines[20]. Patients treated with PUVA should be monitored for the development of melanoma. Solar lentigines are also found in patients with *xeroderma pigmentosum* (see Ch. 62), a rare genetic disease in which clinical and cellular hypersensitivity to UV radiation and defective DNA repair are associated with skin malignancies.

Pathology

The rete ridges often have club-shaped or bud-like extensions and branching or fusing of rete ridges, forming a reticulated pattern (Fig. 112.4). The epidermis between the rete ridges may appear thinned. There is increased basal layer pigmentation, especially in the basaloid cells of the rete ridges. In some (but not all) cases, the melanocytes are increased in number. Melanocytes in dopa-stained sections of solar lentigines exhibit increased melanogenesis, and these cells have more numerous as well as longer and thicker dendritic processes than the melanocytes of normal skin. The superficial dermis often contains melanophages and occasionally a mild perivascular infiltrate of lymphocytes. Electron microscopic studies reveal abundant melanosome complexes in keratinocytes which appear to be larger than in normal surrounding skin[21].

Differential Diagnosis

The differential diagnosis of solar lentigines includes ephelides, macular seborrheic keratoses, simple lentigines, pigmented actinic keratoses,

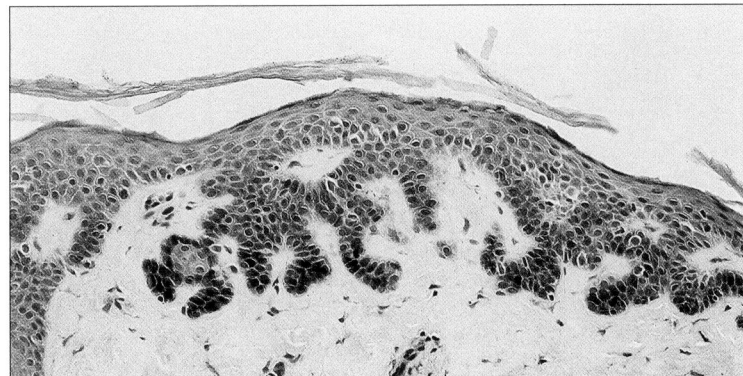

Fig. 112.4 Histology of a solar lentigo. Hyperpigmented elongated rete ridges with a diffuse increase in non-nested melanocytes, in addition to solar elastosis. Courtesy of Ronald P Rapini MD.

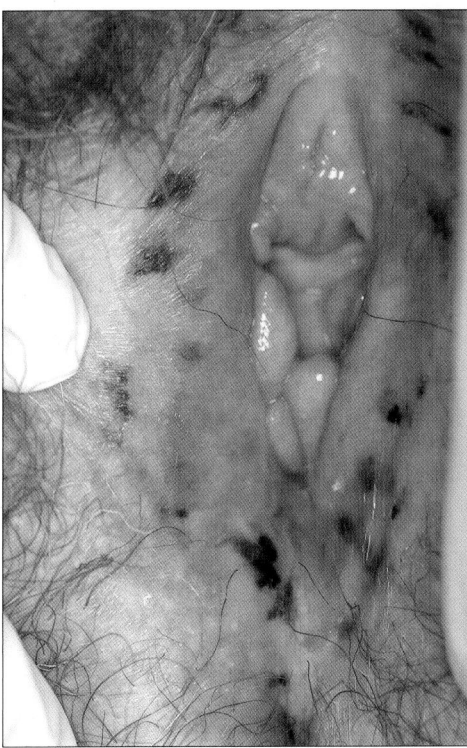

Fig. 112.5 Anogenital lentiginosis. Biopsy of the darkest lesion (at 7 o'clock) showed no cellular atypia. Over a period of ten years, several of the macules faded. Courtesy of Jean L Bolognia MD.

lentigo maligna, junctional melanocytic nevi and large cell acanthomas. Table 112.1 outlines the similarities and differences between solar lentigines and ephelides. There is essentially a continuum extending from solar lentigo to macular varieties of seborrheic keratosis. Demonstration of a keratotic surface with horn cysts is consistent with seborrheic keratosis. Pigmented actinic keratosis is more likely to have a scaly, rough surface. Lentigo maligna often exhibits greater variation in pigmentation and irregularity of borders compared with solar lentigo. Simple lentigines are often smaller and more heavily pigmented than solar lentigines, and arise in childhood with less relationship to UV exposure.

Treatment

Patients with PUVA lentigines should be monitored for the development of melanoma. Although a solar lentigo is a benign lesion of cosmetic concern only, it is an indication of chronic UV exposure which dictates monitoring of the patient for non-melanoma skin cancer and melanoma. Bleaching agents (e.g. hydroquinone) are not effective. Cryotherapy and laser surgery have been shown to be equally effective, but caution must be used to prevent post-treatment dyspigmentation. Preventive measures include sunscreens, physical barriers and limitation of sun exposure[21].

LENTIGO SIMPLEX AND MUCOSAL MELANOTIC LESIONS

Synonyms: ■ Simple lentigo ■ Lentiginosis ■ Genital lentiginosis ■ Melanosis ■ Mucosal melanotic macule

Key feature

■ A lentigo simplex is a brown macule with an early age of onset (as compared with a solar lentigo) and little or no relationship to sun exposure

Epidemiology

The frequency of lentigo simplex in children and adults is unknown. Lentigines are found in all races and seem to occur equally in both sexes. Isolated lesions may be present at birth, more commonly in darkly pigmented than lightly pigmented newborns. In darkly pigmented races, lentigo simplex is the most common histologic pattern for pigmented lesions in acral cutaneous sites. Lentigines simplex may increase in number during childhood or puberty and sometimes occur in an eruptive form called lentiginosis with or without obvious precipitating factors. After melanocyte activation, lentigo simplex is the most common histology in matrix biopsies of longitudinal melanonychia (see Ch. 70).

Oral melanotic macules are found primarily in adults over 40 years of age. Some authors report a slight female predilection, whereas others describe both sexes being affected equally. The most common sites are the vermilion border, followed by the gingiva, the buccal mucosa and the palate. Up to 30% of melanomas in the oral cavity of Caucasians are preceded by melanosis for several months or years. Sixty-six percent of infiltrative oral melanomas in Japanese individuals arise in association with oral melanosis. The labial (lip) melanotic macule usually appears between the second and fourth decades of life and has a strong predilection for white women.

The incidence of lentiginosis or melanosis of the female genital area is probably higher than reported. For example, 15% of 106 females between the ages of 16 and 42 years had genital 'nevi', and in a study of 100 random autopsies, three cases showed melanosis of the genitalia, and all three were elderly women. Most lesions are found on the labia minora (Fig. 112.5), but they can occur as well on the labia majora, the vaginal introitus, the cervix, the periurethral area and the perineum. In general, lentiginosis and melanosis of the female genitalia are benign conditions; atypia is uncommon, and progression to melanoma has not been reported.

In a study of 10 000 men between 17 and 25 years of age, 14.2% were noted to have 'pigmented nevi' of the genitalia[23]. It is uncertain what proportion represented penile lentiginosis or melanosis since no clinical descriptions or histologic studies were reported. In the literature, the ages of patients with penile lentiginosis or melanosis range from 15 to 72 years. The lesions occurred on the glans penis and penile shaft.

The incidence of conjunctival melanosis is unknown, but it can be assumed that primary acquired melanosis is a precursor lesion of melanoma in this area, since a significant number of conjunctival melanomas are associated with it. Lentigo simplex occasionally develops in scars following excision of cutaneous melanoma.

Pathogenesis

An increased number of melanocytes in the basal layer of the epidermis leads to an increased production of melanin, resulting in hyperpigmented macules. The cause of lentigo simplex is unknown, but the appearance of similar macules in disorders affecting other tissues of neuroectodermal origin, such as Carney complex, may indicate a genetic alteration in neural crest-derived cells. Some penile lesions have been reported to follow injury, irritation or PUVA therapy. In women, hormonal factors are thought to play a role. Acral lentigines may be influenced by genetic factors, since they are frequently found in darkly pigmented individuals.

Clinical Features

Lentigines simplex are light brown to black, homogeneous pigmented macules occurring anywhere on the body, including mucous membranes and palmoplantar skin, without any predilection for sun-exposed areas. They are well circumscribed, round or oval, have regular borders, and are usually less than 5 mm (often <3 mm) in diameter. Lesions on the mucous membranes frequently have irregular, ill-defined borders and mottled non-homogeneous pigmentation with areas devoid of pigment (see Fig. 112.5). The latter may be several centimeters in diameter and may resemble early melanoma. Lentigines simplex occur as solitary or multiple lesions. Generalized lentigines may be an isolated phenomenon without an underlying disease, either present at birth or appearing during childhood or adulthood, or it may be a sign of a genetic disorder (Table 112.2).

In contrast to lentigo simplex occurring on the skin, lesions on mucous membranes can slowly increase in size over months to years, with or without changes in the degree of pigmentation. The relationship between acral or anogenital lentigines and acrolentiginous melanoma requires more investigation.

Special forms and associated syndromes

Multiple lentigines may or may not be associated with other systemic manifestations. Synonyms for the *LEOPARD syndrome* include multiple lentiginosis syndrome, progressive cardiomyopathic lentiginosis and cardiocutaneous syndrome, as well as generalized lentigo and generalized lentiginosis. The acronym LEOPARD refers to: *l*entigines, *e*lectrocardiographic conduction defects, *o*cular hypertelorism, *p*ulmonary stenosis, *a*bnormalities of genitalia, *r*etardation of growth and *d*eafness. The latter syndrome is an autosomal dominant disorder with high penetrance and variable expressivity. Multiple lentigines are present at birth or appear during early infancy and may increase in number during childhood. The lesions occur on both sun-exposed and sun-protected sites, including genitalia, palms and soles. Variants of this syndrome with incomplete expression have been described as well as a syndrome of 'arterial dissection' with lentiginosis (see Table 112.2).

The *Carney complex* is an autosomal dominant syndrome characterized by multiple lentigines and multiple neoplasias, including: myxomas of the skin, heart (atrial) and breast; psammomatous melanotic schwannoma; epithelioid blue nevi of skin and mucosae; growth hormone-producing pituitary adenomas; and testicular Sertoli cell tumors. Components of the Carney complex have been described previously as the *NAME* (*n*evi, *a*trial myxoma, *m*yxoid neurofibroma, *e*phelides) and *LAMB* (*l*entigines, *a*trial myxoma, *m*ucocutaneous myxoma, *b*lue nevi) syndromes.

The *Peutz–Jeghers syndrome* is an autosomal dominant disorder characterized by mucocutaneous lentigines which are present at birth or appear during childhood in combination with intestinal polyposis. The skin lesions are predominantly perioral and periorbital, as well as involving the ventral aspects of the hands and feet. Mucosal lesions may affect the palate, tongue, buccal mucosa, and conjunctivae. The majority entity in the differential diagnosis is Laugier-Hunziker syndrome (Fig. 112.6).

Pathology

Lentigo simplex exhibits increased numbers of melanocytes in the basal layer of elongated epidermal rete ridges. Increased melanin in the basal layer and sometimes even in the upper layers of the epidermis and stratum corneum is commonly observed. Melanophages and a mild inflammatory infiltrate are often present in the superficial dermis.

Lesions on mucous membranes, including the lips, show acanthosis with or without elongation of the rete ridges (Fig. 112.7). Slight melanocytic hyperplasia is usually observed, but may be absent. Hyperkeratosis, telangiectasia, activated fibroblasts, and large dendritic melanocytes are described in labial melanotic macules. Some acral and mucosal lesions have been reported to exhibit cytologic atypia of the melanocytes. Melanin macroglobules have been described in lentigo simplex on ultrastructural examination. They are found within melanocytes, but

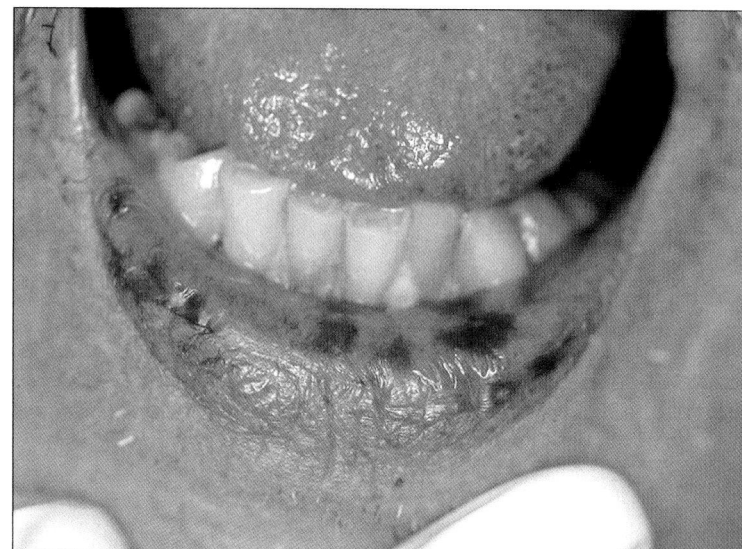

Fig. 112.6 Labial lentigines. Multiple hyperpigmented macules on the lower lip in a patient with Laugier–Hunziker syndrome. Additional lesions are present on the tongue. Peutz–Jeghers syndrome can have a similar clinical appearance.

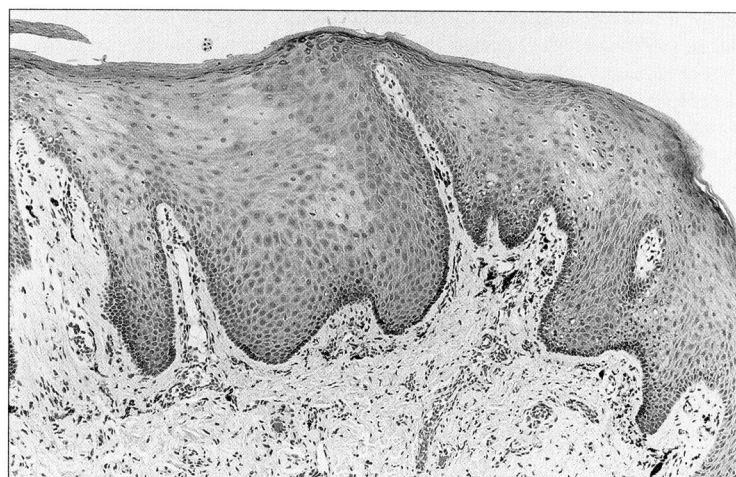

Fig. 112.7 Histology of a labial lentigo (melanotic macule). Hyperpigmented rete ridges are broader than in the average lentigo.

also in keratinocytes and melanophages. These are not specific for lentigo simplex, since they have been described in other pigmented lesions (see above).

Differential Diagnosis

The differential diagnosis of the solitary lentigo simplex involves primarily the junctional and relatively flat forms of compound melanocytic nevus, solar lentigo and ephelis. In some instances, cutaneous melanoma, pigmented spindle cell nevus, hemangioma and cutaneous hemorrhage might enter into the differential diagnosis.

Although there is a continuum from simple lentigo to junctional melanocytic nevus, the simple lentigo is distinguished from melanocytic nevi by the absence of distorted skin markings when viewed with side-lighting. Lentigo simplex is often smaller than a melanocytic nevus, but histopathologic examination may be required for discrimination. Lentigo simplex is usually distinguished from a solar lentigo by its smaller size, symmetry, uniform pigmentation, and lack of relationship to sun-exposed sites. However, this clinical distinction may not be possible in some instances.

Treatment

In general, there is no need to treat benign-appearing lentigo simplex. Lesions on acral or mucous membranes should be evaluated carefully and, if clinically atypical, should be considered for biopsy to assess melanocytic atypia. Patients with both generalized and localized

Disorder	Comments	Disorder	Comments
Generalized		**Localized**	
LEOPARD syndrome	• Autosomal dominant inheritance; mutations in *PTPN11* gene • Lentigines present in infancy/early childhood • Café-noir macules • EKG changes (conduction defects, hypertrophic cardiomyopathy), ocular hypertelorism, pulmonary stenosis, abnormal genitalia, growth retardation and deafness	*Head and neck (including oral mucosa) ± acral*	
		Peutz–Jeghers syndrome	• Autosomal dominant inheritance; mutations in *STK11* gene • Lentigines favor perioral region#, oral mucosa+ and hands; longitudinal melanonychia • Multiple hamartomatous GI polyps • Pancreatic carcinoma; ovarian (adenoma malignum)/testicular tumors
Generalized lentigines	• Autosomal dominant inheritance; mapped to 4q21.1-q22.3 • Café-au-lait macules		
Deafness plus lentiginosis*	• ? Forme fruste of LEOPARD syndrome	Bandler syndrome*	• Autosomal dominant inheritance • Distribution of lentigines similar to Peutz–Jeghers • GI bleeding with small intestine hemangiomas rather than polyps
Carney complex (NAME/LAMB syndrome)	• Autosomal dominant inheritance; mutations in *PRKAR1A* gene • Major findings in the Table legend • Pigmented nodular adrenocortical disease; myxoid mammary fibroadenomas; testicular (calcifying Sertoli cell), thyroid, and pituitary tumors; psammomatous melanotic schwannomas		
		Laugier–Hunziker syndrome	• Similar distribution of lentigines as in Peutz–Jeghers, including lips, oral mucosa and digits • Longitudinal melanonychia and genital melanosis
Arterial dissection plus lentiginosis	• ? Inheritance pattern • Cutaneous lentigines with onset in childhood • Dissection of aortic, internal carotid and vertebral arteries	Cantú (hyperkeratosis-hyperpigmentation) syndrome	• Autosomal dominant inheritance • Punctate palmoplantar keratoderma • Multiple small (1 mm) macules on the face, forearms, hands/feet
Gastrocutaneous syndrome*	• Autosomal dominant inheritance; see Table 60.4 for details	Cowden disease	• Autosomal dominant inheritance; mutations in *PTEN* gene • Periorificial and acral pigmented macules (see Table 62.3)
Tay syndrome*	• ? Autosomal recessive inheritance • Growth retardation, mental retardation; triangular face; cirrhosis; trident hands • Café-au-lait macules; premature canities; vitiligo	Centrofacial lentiginosis	• Autosomal dominant inheritance • Lentigines in a butterfly distribution on the nose, cheeks > forehead, eyelids, upper lip • Onset in infancy; increase in number in childhood • Possibly associated with neuropsychiatric illness and osseous anomalies
Pipkin syndrome*	• Autosomal dominant inheritance • Nystagmus; strabismus		
		Inherited patterned lentiginosis	• Autosomal dominant inheritance • African-Americans with light brown skin • Pigmented macules appear in early childhood • Present on central face and lips > buttocks, elbows, hands/feet • Occasional oral mucosal involvement
		Cronkhite-Canada syndrome	• Typically affects older men • Lentigines of buccal mucosa, face, hands/feet • Alopecia (diffuse, non-scarring), nail dystrophy, intestinal polyposis
		Genital	
		Bannayan-Riley-Ruvalcaba syndrome	• Autosomal dominant inheritance; mutations in *PTEN* gene • Penile > vulvar pigmented macules (see Table 62.3)
		Lentiginosis perigenito-axillaris	• Genital and acral pigmented macules
		'Photodistribution'	
		Xeroderma pigmentosum	• Autosomal recessive inheritance; mutations in genes encoding proteins that repair UV-induced DNA damage • Lentigines favor, but are not limited to, chronically sun-exposed sites • Multiple skin cancers
		Segmental	
		Partial unilateral lentiginosis	• Multiple lentigines in a segmental distribution • Café-au-lait macules in same distribution

*To date, observed in a single family
#may fade
+persists

Table 112.2 Disorders associated with multiple lentigines. EKG, electrocardiogram; GI, gastrointestinal; LEOPARD, *l*entigines/*E*CG abnormalities/ocular hypertelorism/pulmonary stenosis/abnormalities of genitalia/retardation of growth/deafness syndrome; NAME, *n*evi/*a*trial myxoma/*m*yxoid neurofibroma/*e*phelides syndrome; LAMB, *l*entigines/*a*trial myxoma/*m*ucocutaneous myxoma/*b*lue nevi syndrome. Adapted from Bolognia JL. Disorders of hypopigmentation and hyperpigmentation. In: Harper J, Oranje A, Prose N (eds). Textbook of Pediatric Dermatology. Oxford: Blackwell Science. 2nd edn. 2006;997–1040.

lentiginosis should undergo investigation to exclude systemic disease (see Table 112.2).

DERMAL MELANOCYTOSIS

Synonyms: ■ Congenital dermal melanocytosis ■ Mongolian spot

Key features

- Lumbosacral blue to blue-gray patch present at birth
- More common in Asians
- Usually resolves during childhood
- Sparse dendritic melanocytes in the deeper dermis

Epidemiology

Dermal melanocytosis is usually present at birth or appears within the first weeks of life; rarely lesions appear after early childhood[24–26]. Both sexes seem to be affected equally. Dermal melanocytosis usually regresses in early childhood, but can persist and was seen in 4.1% of 9996 Japanese males between 18 and 22 years of age. It occurs in all races, with a frequency in one study of 100% in Malaysians, 90–100% in Mongolians, Japanese, Chinese and Koreans, 87% in Bolivian Indians, 65% of blacks in Brazil, 17% of whites in Bolivia, but only 1.5% of whites in Brazil. The racial differences in the frequency of this abnormality suggest that genetic factors influence survival of dermal melanocytes (see Ch. 64). Microscopically, histologic findings consistent with dermal melanocytosis can be found in 100% of newborns, irrespective of race[24,25].

Pathogenesis

The blue color in dermal melanocytosis is secondary to melanocytes in the middle to lower dermis. Melanocytes appear in the dermis in the 10th week of gestation, and then either migrate into the epidermis or undergo cell death, except for melanocytes in the dermis of the scalp, extensor aspects of the distal extremities, and the sacral area. The latter is the most common site for dermal melanocytosis. The bluish coloration of dermal melanocytosis results from the Tyndall phenomenon: dermal pigmentation appears blue because of decreased reflectance in the longer-wavelength region compared with the surrounding skin. Longer wavelengths, such as red, orange and yellow, are not reflected, compared with the shorter-wavelengths of blue and violet, which are reflected[26].

Clinical Features

The classic location is the sacrococcygeal and lumbar areas and the buttocks, followed by the back (Fig. 112.8). Dermal melanocytosis may consist of a single or multiple patches and usually involves <5% of the body surface area. The lesions are macular and have a round, oval or angulated shape. The size varies from a few to more than 20 cm. The color varies from light blue to dark blue to blue gray. Extrasacral (aberrant) variants tend to be more persistent and there is overlap amongst persistent and adult-onset dermal melanocytosis, nevus of Ito and patch blue nevus. Extensive dermal melanocytosis should raise the possibility of phakomatosis pigmentovascularis types II and IV (see Ch. 104). When CALM and satellite melanocytic nevi reside within areas of dermal melanocytosis, there may be a rim that lacks dermal melanocytes around each lesion (see Fig 112.8).

Pathology

Bipolar dendritic melanocytes are dispersed singly in the lower half or two-thirds of the dermis. These melanocytes are dopa-positive and lie parallel to the epidermis between the collagen bundles without disturbing the normal architecture of the skin. Occasionally, persistent dermal melanocytosis has the histology of a blue nevus with involve-

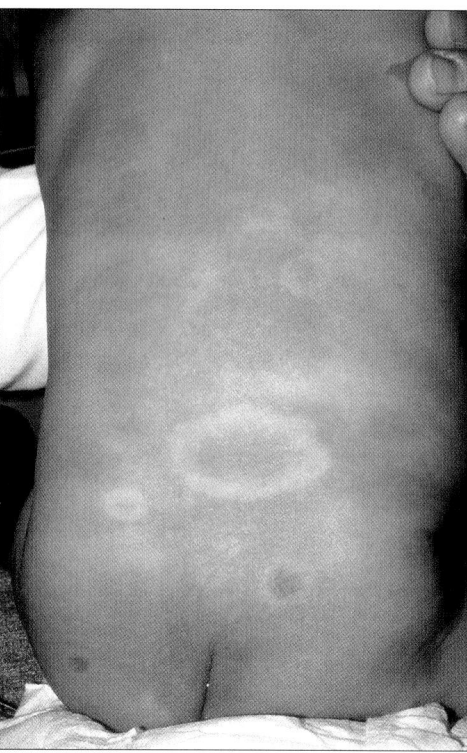

Fig. 112.8 Dermal melanocytosis (Mongolian spots) in a child with neurofibromatosis 1. Surrounding each café-au-lait macule there is an absence of the characteristic blue discoloration.

ment of the subcutis, muscle and fascia by melanocytes. On electron microscopy, dermal melanocytosis shows fully developed melanocytes with exclusively mature, electron-dense melanosomes and very few premelanosomes.

Differential Diagnosis

The differential diagnosis of congenital dermal melanocytosis includes primarily nevus of Ota, nevus of Ito, and patch blue nevus. The latter has many names in the literature including dermal melanocyte hamartoma, acquired dermal melanocytosis and acquired linear dermal melanocytosis. The differential also includes vascular malformation or hemangioma and a contusion. The distinctive clinical presentation of dermal melanocytosis generally allows easy distinction from all the entities listed above. Nonetheless, occurrence of dermal melanocytosis in other anatomic locations may suggest other processes. Some cases of so-called persistent dermal melanocytosis may in fact represent variants of nevus of Ito or related conditions.

Treatment

Persistent lesions may be treated with cover-up cosmetics or lasers (see Nevus of Ota).

NEVUS OF OTA AND RELATED CONDITIONS

Synonyms: ■ Nevus fuscoceruleus ophthalmomaxillaris ■ Oculodermal melanocytosis ■ Congenital melanosis bulbi ■ Melanosis bulborum and aberrant dermal melanocytosis ■ Progressive melanosis oculi, persistent aberrant dermal melanocytosis ■ Oculomucodermal melanocytosis

Key features

- Blue–brown unilateral or occasionally bilateral facial patch
- More common in Asians and blacks
- More dermal dendritic melanocytes than in congenital dermal melanocytosis, but less than in blue nevus

Epidemiology

Nevus of Ota occurs predominantly in more darkly pigmented individuals, especially in Asians and blacks, but has been described in whites as well. About 80% of all reported cases have been in women; however, this figure may be somewhat skewed as a result of a greater cosmetic concern in women. Nevus of Ota is seen in about 0.4% to 0.8% of all Japanese dermatologic patients. No epidemiologic studies on the frequency in whites are available at this time. The lesion has two peaks of onset: the first (about 50% to 60% of all cases) in infancy before the age of 1 year, with the majority present at birth, and the second (40% to 50%) around puberty. Onset between the ages of 1 and 11 years and after 20 years is unusual. Although rare familial forms of nevus of Ota have been reported, the condition is generally not considered hereditary.

Pathogenesis

The blue to blue-gray color in nevus of Ota is due to melanin-producing melanocytes in the dermis. The larger concentration of melanocytes in nevus of Ota in comparison with congenital dermal melanocytosis is thought to indicate a hamartoma. The possibility of a hormonal influence in women has been raised.

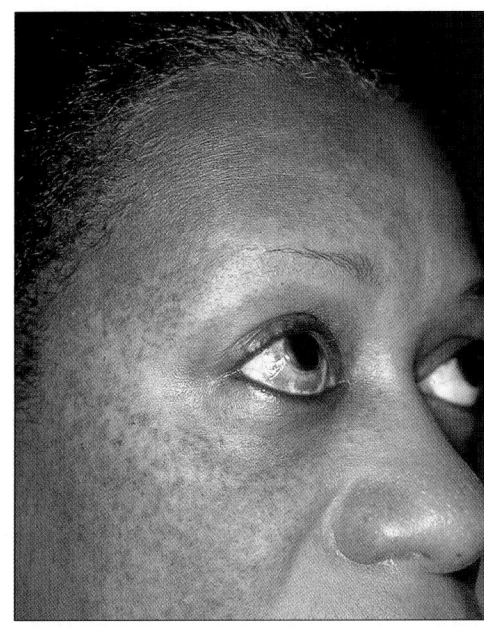

Fig. 112.9 Nevus of Ota (oculodermal melanocytosis). Unilateral blue–gray discoloration of the face, which is either mottled or confluent. There is also involvement of the sclera.

Clinical Features

Nevus of Ota is usually characterized by a confluence of individual macules varying from pinhead-sized to several millimeters in diameter. The shape of the individual macules may be round, oval or serrated, whereas the overall appearance is that of an irregularly demarcated and often mottled patch. The overall size varies from a few centimeters to extensive unilateral and occasionally bilateral involvement (Fig. 112.9). The color varies from shades of tan and brown to gray, blue, black and purple.

Nevus of Ota is usually unilateral and favors the distribution of the first two branches of the trigeminal nerve. The periorbital area, temple, forehead, malar area, earlobe, pre- and retroauricular regions, nose and conjunctivae are the most common sites of involvement. A characteristic feature, which is seen in about two-thirds of patients, is the involvement of the ipsilateral sclera; rarely, nevus of Ota affects the cornea, iris, fundus oculi, retrobulbar fat, periosteum, retina and optic nerve. Iris mammillations and glaucoma have been reported, but vision is usually not impaired. Other frequent sites of involvement are the tympanum (55%), nasal mucosa (30%), pharynx (25%) and palate (20%). Occasionally, the external auditory canal, mandibular area, lips, neck and thorax are involved. In 5% to 15% of patients, the lesion is bilateral.

Nevus of Ota may extend over time and it persists lifelong. Fluctuations in the intensity of the color have been described, especially in association with periods of hormonal flux such as menstruation, puberty or menopause.

Malignancies arising in nevi of Ota are rare. As of 1998, ten cases of cutaneous melanoma arising within a nevus of Ota had been reported in the literature. These typically presented in Caucasian patients as new subcutaneous nodules and did not adhere to the ABCD rules of melanoma[27]. Other tumors such as atypical and borderline cellular blue nevi also have been described[28]. Multiple examples of primary melanoma of the choroid, orbit, iris, chiasma and meninges have been observed in association with nevus of Ota that exhibited eye involvement. It is one of the entities that can have associated neuromelanosis. Glaucoma may affect 10% of patients with nevus of Ota[29].

Related conditions

Nevus of Ito (synonym: *N. fuscoceruleus acromiodeltoideus*) differs from nevus of Ota mainly in its area of involvement; the former corresponds to the distribution of the posterior supraclavicular and cutaneous brachii lateralis nerves (which encompasses the supraclavicular, scapular or deltoid regions). The clinical and histologic picture is the same as in nevus of Ota. There is a mottled appearance with bluish and brownish macules. Nevus of Ito may occur as an isolated lesion or in association with an ipsilateral or bilateral nevus of Ota. *Acquired nevus of Ota-like macules* (Hori's nevus) are characterized by bilateral blue-gray to gray-brown macules of the zygomatic area (less often the

forehead, upper outer eyelids and nose). Mainly Chinese or Japanese women ranging in age from 20 to 70 years have been reported with this condition. The eye and oral mucosa are not involved. It may also be misdiagnosed as melasma. A *patch blue nevus* (synonym: dermal melanocyte hamartoma, acquired dermal melanocytosis) presents as a diffusely gray-blue area that may have superimposed darker macules. The age of onset and sites of involvement vary, with some lesions having a linear distribution.

Pathology

The non-infiltrated areas in nevus of Ota show pigmented, elongated, dendritic melanocytes scattered among the collagen bundles. In comparison with dermal melanocytosis, the cells are more numerous and are located in the upper third of the reticular dermis. Occasionally, cells are found in the papillary dermis or even deep in the subcutaneous fat.

Hypermelanosis of the lower epidermis and an increase in basilar melanocytes may occur. The dopa reactivity of the melanocytes in nevus of Ota varies: slightly pigmented cells are often strongly reactive, whereas heavily pigmented melanocytes often are not reactive. The negative reaction in heavily pigmented melanocytes indicates that all melanogenic enzymes have been consumed. Melanocytes can be found clustering around blood vessels and sweat and sebaceous glands; occasionally, they are seen in vessel walls or in sweat ducts. Raised or infiltrated areas show a larger number of dendritic melanocytes forming cellular aggregates or clumps resembling blue nevi histologically.

Differential Diagnosis

The differential diagnosis of nevus of Ota and related conditions includes congenital dermal melanocytosis (Mongolian spot), blue nevus (patch or plaque), melasma, partial unilateral lentiginosis (when it involves the face), a nevus spilus that develops blue nevi, vascular malformations and ecchymosis. Congenital dermal melanocytosis differs from nevus of Ota and other dermal melanocytoses primarily because of anatomic location in the lumbosacral region and spontaneous regression during childhood.

Common blue nevus is distinguished from other dermal melanocytoses because it is a well-circumscribed, slightly elevated or papular lesion measuring less than 1 cm in greatest diameter[30]. Melasma of the face may exhibit a brown-gray color but is distinguished from nevus of Ota by sparing of sun-protected sites and absence of mucous membrane involvement.

Treatment

Nevus of Ota and nevus of Ota-like macules have been treated successfully by Q-switched ruby, alexandrite and Nd:YAG lasers[31]. Although malignant changes are rare in patients with nevus of Ota, patients with eye involvement should be followed more carefully, since the majority of associated melanomas are ocular in origin. Suspicious lesions, especially a new subcutaneous nodule, should be biopsied. An ophthalmologist should be consulted to screen for glaucoma and ocular melanomas. Any complaint of neurologic symptoms requires further investigation.

BLUE NEVUS AND ITS VARIANTS

Synonyms: ■ Blue nevus of Jadassohn–Tièche ■ Nevus bleu ■ Blue neuronevus ■ Dermal melanocytoma

Key features

- Blue to blue–black firm papule or nodule often with onset in childhood or adolescence
- Aggregates of dermal, dendritic, heavily pigmented melanocytes

Epidemiology

Blue nevi are usually acquired and have their onset most commonly in childhood and adolescence, although up to a quarter arise in middle-aged adults. A congenital common blue nevus is unusual but approximately 25% of cellular blue nevi are congenital.

Pathogenesis

Blue nevi consist of benign tumors of dermal melanocytes[32–37]. In general, melanocytes disappear from the dermis during the second half of gestation, but some residual melanin-producing cells remain in the scalp, sacral region, and dorsal aspect of the distal extremities. These are the sites where blue nevi most commonly occur (see above). The blue coloration of these nevi is the result of the Tyndall phenomenon.

Clinical Features

Common blue nevi

Common blue nevi are well-circumscribed, dome-shaped papules, blue, blue–gray or blue–black in color (Fig. 112.10). They are usually 0.5 to 1.0 cm in diameter, rarely larger. The lesions may occur anywhere, but about 50% are found on the dorsal aspect of the hands and feet, with the face and scalp being other common sites. Usually, the nevi are solitary, but they may be multiple or agminated or may arise with a nevus spilus or plaque blue nevus. Concentric, target-like lesions (target blue nevus) have been described as well. Dermoscopically, a blue nevus is characterized by homogeneous blue–gray to blue–black pigmentation (Fig. P2).

Cellular blue nevi

Cellular blue nevi are blue to blue–gray or black nodules or plaques, generally 1 to 3 cm in diameter but sometimes larger (Fig. 112.11). Their surface is smooth but sometimes irregular. The most common sites are the buttocks, sacrococcygeal area and scalp, followed by the face and feet. Congenital cellular blue nevi, some with satellite lesions, have been reported, as have benign or malignant cellular blue nevi arising in congenital melanocytic nevi. The ratio of common blue nevus to cellular nevus is at least 5:1.

Malignant blue nevi (cutaneous melanoma arising in or having features of blue nevus)

Malignant blue nevi are rare forms of cutaneous melanoma most commonly arising in cellular blue nevi. They tend to show progressive enlargement, often measuring several centimeters in diameter, and have a multinodular or plaque-like appearance. The scalp is the most common site of occurrence and lymph nodes are the most common sites of metastasis. Malignant blue nevi can arise in a previously benign cellular blue nevus, in a nevus of Ota or Ito, or *de novo*.

Blue nevi have been described in the vagina, the cervix, the prostate, the spermatic cord and the lymph nodes. Over time, hypopigmentation can appear centrally with common blue nevi. Cellular blue nevi and atypical variants, especially on the scalp, may undergo malignant change, but the incidence is unknown. Epithelioid blue nevi are sometimes a feature of Carney complex; the latter may be indistinguishable histologically from pigmented epithelioid melanocytoma.

Pathology

The *common* or *ordinary blue nevus* is composed of elongated and often slightly wavy melanocytes with long, branching dendrites (see Fig. 112.10). The melanocytes, with their long axes parallel to the epidermis, lie grouped or in bundles in the upper and mid dermis. Occasionally, they extend into the subcutaneous tissue or approach the epidermis, but do not alter it. Most of the melanocytes are filled with numerous fine melanin granules, often completely obscuring their nuclei and often extending into their dendrites. Variable numbers of melanin-laden

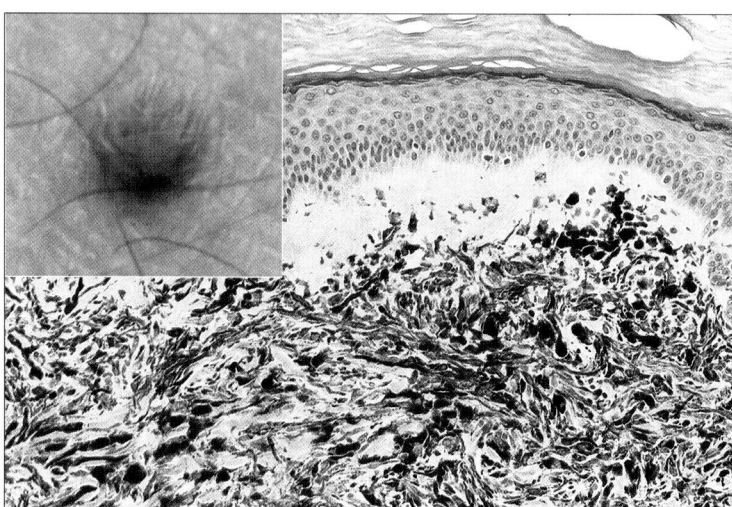

Fig. 112.10 Common blue nevus. Histologically, there are heavily pigmented dermal spindled melanocytes and melanophages; they are denser than in dermal melanocytosis or nevus of Ota. Clinically, a well-circumscribed, small, blue, dome-shaped papule is usually seen (inset).

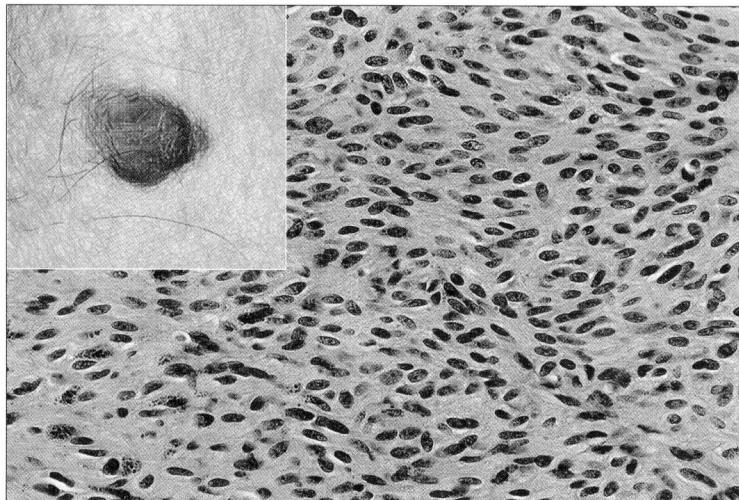

Fig. 112.11 Cellular blue nevus. Histologically, there are plump spindled melanocytes devoid of melanin pigment and arranged in bundles. Clinically, a thick blue plaque is often seen (inset). Inset, Courtesy of Jean L Bolognia MD.

macrophages are also present. The amount of collagen is usually increased, giving the lesion a fibrotic appearance.

In the *cellular blue nevus*, one often observes deeply pigmented dendritic melanocytes as in a common blue nevus associated with nests and fascicles of spindle-shaped cells with abundant pale cytoplasm containing little or no melanin (see Fig. 112.11). The aggregates of spindle cells may be arranged in intersecting bundles extending in various directions, a disposition resembling the storiform pattern of neurofibroma. Penetration of rounded, well-defined cellular islands into subcutaneous tissue is frequently noted. Some of the cells may appear atypical, with nuclear pleomorphism accompanied by multinucleated giant cells, rare mitoses and inflammatory infiltrates.

Occasionally, lymph nodes draining the anatomic site of a cellular blue nevus contain atypical cells. The foci found either in the marginal sinuses or in the capsule are usually small, discrete and peripherally located. They may result from passive transport or represent arrested migration from the neural crest. These 'benign metastases' are found in 5% of the reported cases of cellular blue nevi. Electron microscopy reveals that the spindle-shaped cells in cellular blue nevi contain melanosomes with little or no melanization. Melanin production in these cells and transition to bipolar dendritic nevus cells have been documented.

Atypical cellular blue nevi demonstrate one or more of the following features compared to conventional cellular blue nevi: larger size (e.g. >1 or 2 cm), asymmetry, ulceration, infiltrating features, cytological atypia, mitoses and necrosis[38]. Such lesions have been associated with lymph node metastases and evolution to frank melanoma. These lesions require further study since their biologic potential is difficult to predict.

Combined blue nevi (melanocytic nevi with phenotypic heterogeneity) have the pathology of common or cellular blue nevi in combination with a junctional, compound, dermal, or (rarely) spindle and epithelioid nevus/tumor. This is found in about 1% of all excised melanocytic nevi. They are most common on the face and usually resemble other blue nevi, but sometimes there is a blue–black focus within an otherwise typical nevus.

Deep penetrating nevus is probably a variant of cellular blue nevus and is closely related to plexiform pigmented spindle cell nevus. Pleomorphic spindle cells and variably present epithelioid cells push vertically into the deep dermis or fat.

Differential Diagnosis

The differential diagnosis of a common blue nevus includes traumatic tattoo, combined nevus, vascular lesions including venous lake and angiokeratoma, sclerosing hemangioma, primary and metastatic melanoma, atypical nevus, pigmented spindle cell nevus, dermatofibroma, papular pigmented basal cell carcinoma, glomus tumor and apocrine hidrocystoma. For cellular blue nevus, especially with satellitosis, malignant blue nevus needs to be considered and when the lesion is on the face, nevus of Ota. Blue nevi also need to be distinguished from a cutaneous neurocristic hamartoma, a complex proliferation of nevus cells, schwann cells and pigmented dendritic and spindled cells.

Treatment

Blue nevi that are <1 cm in diameter, are clinically stable, without atypical features and are located in a typical anatomic site do not require removal. On the other hand, histologic evaluation should be strongly considered for lesions appearing *de novo*, multinodular or plaque-like lesions, or changing lesions. Cellular blue nevi probably should be resected completely in order to prevent recurrence and misdiagnosis as malignant blue nevus and also because of their risk for malignant transformation (albeit rare).

COMMON ACQUIRED MELANOCYTIC NEVI

Synonyms: ■ Nevocellular nevus ■ 'Mole'

Key features

■ Junctional nevus is a brown to black macule with melanocytic nests at the junction of the epidermis and dermis

■ Intradermal nevus is a skin-colored or light brown papule with nests of melanocytes in the dermis

■ Compound nevus is a brown papule with combined histologic features of junctional and intradermal nevi

Epidemiology

The natural history of acquired melanocytic nevi is not well documented[39,40]. The prevalence of nevi is related to age, race, and perhaps genetic and environmental factors. A few nevi are present in early childhood, but they increase in number, reaching a peak in the third decade of life; they tend thereafter to disappear with increasing age. There is a period of particularly rapid development of nevi at puberty. In general, the greatest numbers of nevi are observed among individuals ages 20 to 29 years. A study in Scotland noted that in the first decade of life females had an average of three nevi and males two nevi. For the age interval 20 to 29 years, women and men had mean nevus counts of 33 and 22, respectively. There was a progressive decline thereafter, with women having a mean of six nevi and men four nevi in the seventh decade of life. No substantial differences between men and women have been noted for the prevalence of nevi. Caucasians in general have greater numbers of nevi than do darker-skinned groups, i.e. African-Americans and Asians. Furthermore, a greater prevalence of nevi is associated with lighter skin color in whites. The frequency of melanocytic nevi on the palms and soles, nail beds and conjunctivae is also related to race; nevi on these surfaces are more prevalent in blacks and Asians than in whites. Mean acral nevus counts for Africans in Uganda were 11, versus 2 to 8 for African-Americans.

Genetic factors may be operative in the prevalence of nevi: increased numbers of nevi have been shown to cluster in families, especially in those with familial melanoma. Although an autosomal dominant mode of inheritance has been postulated for clinically atypical nevi in hereditayr melanoma families, the pattern of inheritance may be more complex. Environmental factors such as sun exposure influence the development of melanocytic nevi. There is some evidence that individuals residing in sunny climates have a greater prevalence of melanocytic nevi compared with persons living in more temperate zones, but more objective evidence is needed to establish this relationship.

Pathogenesis

Melanocytic nevi are thought to originate from cells, termed melanoblasts, that migrate from the neural crest to the epidermis. Nevi are hypothesized to result from the proliferation of slightly altered melanocytes or 'nevus cells' within the epidermis, producing junctional nevi. It is believed that such nevus cells subsequently migrate into the dermis, giving rise to compound nevi and ultimately dermal nevi when there are no longer residual nevus cells within the epidermis. Nevi are thought to be either developmental malformations (hamartomas) or benign proliferations with some growth advantage over surrounding basilar melanocytes. Factors leading to the onset of melanocytic nevi are poorly understood but could include the genetic influences alluded to earlier and environmental agents, principally UV exposure (Table 112.3).

Clinical Features

Melanocytic nevi are well-circumscribed, round or ovoid lesions, generally measuring from 2 to 6 mm in diameter. They appear orderly and symmetric overall. Although many nevi display slight asymmetry, the borders are usually regular and well defined. The junctional nevus is a macular lesion with slight accentuation of skin markings visible with side-lighting. Junctional nevi are also characterized by a uniform, medium to dark brown color (Fig. 112.12A). The dermoscopic features of a junctional nevus include a uniform pigment network thinning out towards the periphery (Fig. P3). Compound nevi show variable degrees of elevation and in general somewhat lighter shades of brown than do

TRIGGERS FOR THE DEVELOPMENT AND/OR GROWTH OF MELANOCYTIC NEVI
Light exposure
• Sun exposure leading to multiple or severe sunburns*
• Intermittent intense sun exposure (e.g. on sunny holidays)
• Chronic moderate sun exposure (e.g. residence at lower latitudes)
• Neonatal phototherapy
Cutaneous injury
Blistering processes (other than severe sunburns)
• Toxic epidermal necrolysis/Stevens-Johnson syndrome*
• Epidermolysis bullosa – junctional (particularly generalized atrophic benign)>recessive dystrophic>recessive simplex*
• Bullae secondary to sulfur mustard gas exposure*
• Severe sunburn*
Scarring processes
• Lichen sclerosus[†]
Systemic immunosuppression
• Chemotherapy, particularly for childhood hematologic malignancies*,[†,‡]
• Allogeneic bone marrow transplantation[‡]
• Solid organ transplantation, particularly renal*,[‡]
• Human immunodeficiency viral infection/acquired immunodeficiency syndrome*
• Chronic myelogenous leukemia*
• Anti-tumor necrosis factor therapy*,[‡]
Increased hormone levels
• Pregnancy*,[§]
• Growth hormone (increased size, not number, of nevi)
• Addison disease*
• Thyroid hormone*
Other
• Atopic dermatitis in children (conflicting results in different studies)
• Postoperative fever*
• Seizures or electroencephalographic abnormalities*

*Eruptive nevi have been reported.
[†]An increased number of atypical nevi may also be seen.
[‡]Nevi have a predilection for the palms and soles.
[§]Relative immunosuppression may also play a role; an increase in the size or number of nevi has not been clearly demonstrated for pregnant women in general.

Table 112.3 Triggers for the development and/or growth of melanocytic nevi. Adapted from Schaffer JV, Bolognia JL. The biology of melanocytic nevi. In: Nordlund JJ, Boissy RE, Hearing VJ, et al. (eds). The Pigmentary System: Physiology and Pathophysiology. 2nd edn. Oxford: Blackwell Publishing. 2006;1092–125.

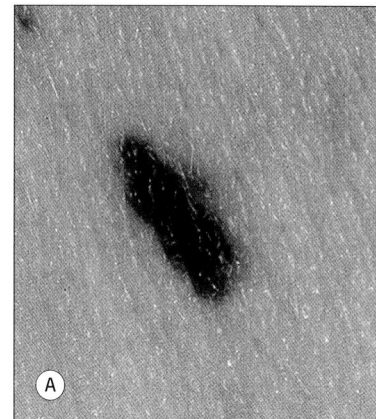
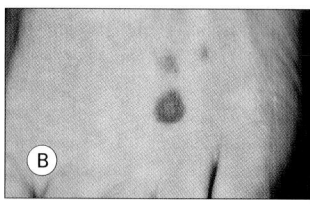
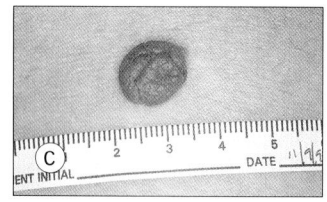

Fig. 112.12 Acquired melanocytic nevi. A Junctional nevus – dark brown macule. **B** Compound nevus – symmetric light to medium brown papule. **C** Intradermal nevus – soft tan papule. B, C, Courtesy of Jean L Bolognia MD.

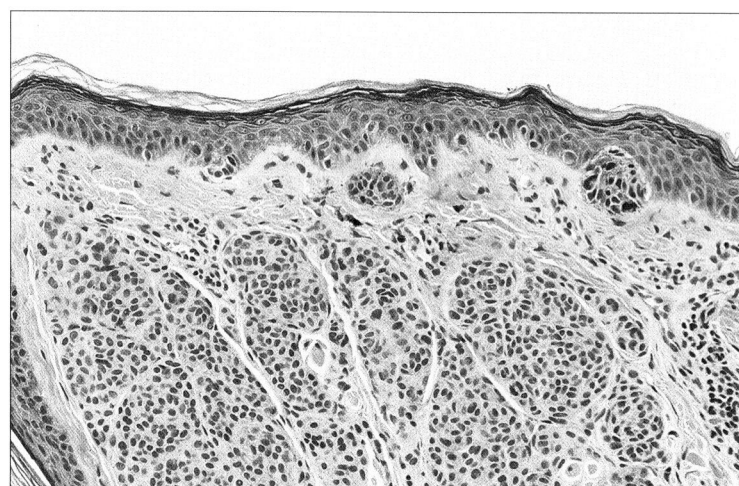

Fig. 112.13 Histology of a compound nevus. Nests of melanocytes in the dermis and at the dermal–epidermal junction. Courtesy of Ronald P Rapini MD.

junctional nevi (Fig. 112.12B). Dermoscopically, they are characterized by a globular architecture with multiple round ovoid globules sometimes forming a cobblestone pattern. Dermal nevi (Fig. 112.12C) are usually more elevated and show lighter shades of brown or even skin-colored tones compared with compound nevi. The dermoscopic features of an intradermal nevus predominantly consist of focal globules or globular-like structures. In addition, there may be pale to whitish structureless areas and fine linear or comma vessels (Fig. P4).

However, it should be emphasized that there is clinical and dermoscopic overlap among all three types of nevi. Dermal nevi and, to a lesser degree, compound nevi may be dome-shaped or papillomatous. Nevi may have a verrucous surface simulating that of a seborrheic keratosis. Many nevi contain hairs that are coarse and dark compared with those in surrounding skin. Nevi of the palms and soles are often macular or only slightly raised, have regular and well-defined borders, and show uniform or linear brown coloration (see below). Melanocytic nevi of the nail bed usually present as uniformly pigmented brown to dark brown longitudinal bands (melanonychia striata) with regular and distinct margins.

An important aspect of melanocytic nevi is their relationship to melanoma. A significant proportion of melanoma patients report the prior presence of a longstanding melanocytic nevus at the site of melanoma development. Histologic studies also have documented that approximately one-third of melanomas are associated with nevus

remnants. An increased number of melanocytic nevi marks increased melanoma risk.

Pathology

Melanocytic nevi contain intraepidermal or dermal collections of nevus cells or both (Fig. 112.13). The cells within the junctional nests have round, ovoid or fusiform shapes and are arranged in cohesive nests. In the superficial dermis, the cells in general have epithelioid cell characteristics and contain amphophilic cytoplasm and, frequently, granular melanin. The nuclei have uniform chromatin with a slightly clumped texture. Deeper in the dermis, there is a diminished content of cytoplasm, such that the cells resemble lymphocytes; they are frequently arranged in linear cords. There may be a further transition to cells separated by fine connective tissue and assuming a spindled configuration, similar to fibroblasts or Schwann cells.

Differential Diagnosis

The differential diagnosis of melanocytic nevi includes the entire gamut of pigmented and skin-colored lesions (see the Introduction chapter). Raised nevi, potentially confused with seborrheic keratoses, generally do not exhibit the rough, verrucoid surface and pseudo-horn cysts of a seborrheic keratosis. Dermatofibromas are usually differentiated from nevi by their very firm consistency, 'dimpling', and preference for the lower extremities. Both neurofibromas and fibroepithelial polyps may be indistinguishable from skin-colored or slightly pigmented, pedunculated dermal nevi. In general, typical melanocytic nevi are distinguishable from atypical nevi and melanoma by smaller size, overall symmetry and orderly appearance, homogeneous coloration and regular, well-defined borders. Furthermore, red, blue, gray and black colors are not usually seen in common acquired nevi and should alert one to a potentially atypical lesion.

Treatment

The indications for removing melanocytic nevi are as follows: (1) a changing lesion; (2) atypical clinical appearance suspicious for melanoma; (3) cosmetic reasons; and (4) repeated irritation. Beyond these indications, there is no reason to remove nevi on a routine basis.

HALO NEVUS

Synonyms: ■ Leukoderma acquisitum centrifugum ■ Sutton's nevus ■ Perinevoid vitiligo

Key features

■ White halo around a nevus

■ Most common on the upper back in teenagers with an increased number of nevi

■ Lymphocytes infiltrate the nevus

Epidemiology

Halo nevi generally affect individuals under the age of 20 years, with a mean age of approximately 15 years. In one series, the ages ranged from 3 to 42 years. The overall incidence of halo nevi in individuals under age 20 is probably less than 1%. There is no difference in incidence between males and females. In general, those patients with halo nevi have an overall increased number of melanocytic nevi. Approximately 20% of individuals with halo nevi have vitiligo; they are less often associated with melanoma and atypical (dysplastic) nevi. The natural history of halo nevi has not been well documented. However, in general, the onset of a ring of depigmentation is thought to occur over a period of weeks to months. The central nevus occasionally persists or, more likely, undergoes involution over a matter of months to years.

Pathogenesis

The basis for the development of a halo of depigmentation is thought to be either: (1) an immune response against antigenically altered nevus cells associated with tumor progression (dysplasia); or (2) a cell-mediated and/or humoral (antibody-mediated) reaction against non-specifically altered nevomelanocytes and possible cross-reactivity with nevo-melanocytes at a distant site or sites. The first hypothesis holds that all halo nevi are atypical, and thus the immunologic response is one associated with tumorigenesis. The second notion holds that halo nevi are the result of a host response directed against non-specifically altered nevomelanocytes in response to a physical, chemical or other insult or perhaps result from an autoimmune pathogenesis, as in vitiligo. The second is favored nowadays.

The basis for nevus cell destruction in halo nevi is poorly understood. Both humoral and cellular immunologic factors have been implicated. Copeman and colleagues were the first to show that individuals with regressing halo nevi have antibodies directed against melanoma cells. These antibodies also have been noted in patients with primary melanoma who have not developed metastases, but not in individuals with other types of conventional nevi. It also has been found that lymphocytes isolated from patients with halo nevi and from melanoma patients are cytotoxic to melanoma cells in culture. It is not known whether the preceding observations are important in the pathogenesis of halo nevi or are merely epiphenomena. As discussed below, the central nevus component of active halo nevi is usually associated with a dense mononuclear cell infiltrate, while the peripheral white halo has little or no such infiltrate. The mechanisms responsible for the white halo are even less well understood than other aspects of the pathogenesis of halo nevi. Presumably, the destruction of melanocytes in this zone is secondary to the diffusion of a cytotoxic factor.

Clinical Features

Halo nevi are characterized by a central melanocytic nevus component that may be relatively flat or raised and dark brown to pink in color. The nevus may exhibit surface scale or crusting. The central nevus is surrounded by a well-circumscribed annulus of hypo- or depigmented skin (Fig. 112.14A). Erythema occasionally precedes the development of the depigmented halo. In typical halo nevi, the central nevus commonly measures 3 to 6 mm in longest diameter, has regular and well-defined borders and has homogeneous coloration. The white halo is usually symmetric with a uniform width that may vary from a few millimeters up to several centimeters (uncommon). A Wood's lamp

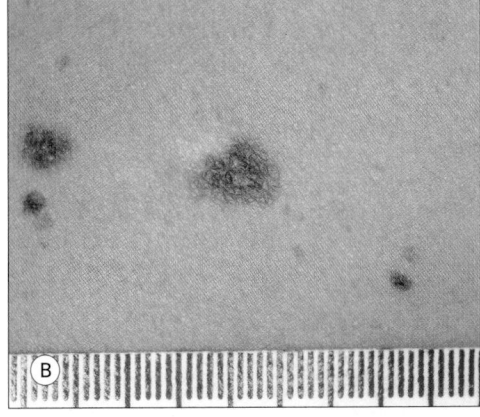

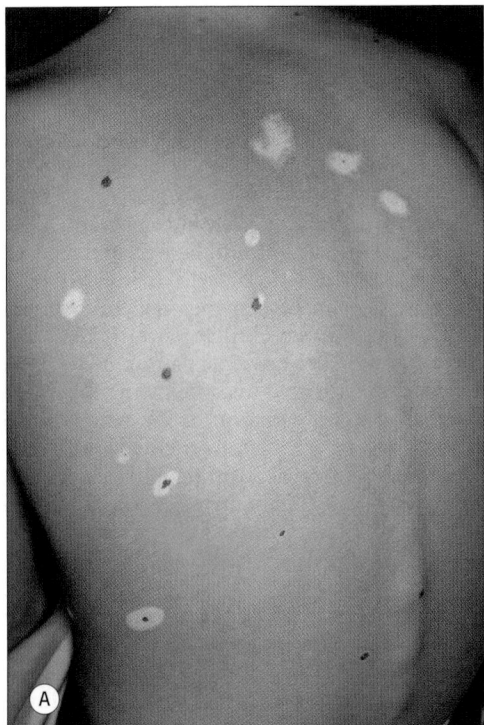

Fig. 112.14 Halo melanocytic nevi. A Stage I (central brown nevus), II (central pink nevus), III (depigmented macule), and early IV (partially repigmented) halo nevi are present. Multiple halo nevi are seen most commonly in children and young adults with numerous nevi. **B** A benign compound nevus with an asymmetric halo. B, Courtesy of Jean L Bolognia MD.

may enhance or discern the halo. Dermoscopically, it is characterized by a symmetric white structureless area surrounding the remaining structures of the nevus (Fig. P5).

Halo nevi are most typically located on the upper back, but may be found in any location. Approximately 25% to 50% of affected individuals have two or more halo nevi. Rarely, large numbers of halo nevi occur, sometimes with rapid onset. After the development of a halo nevus, its subsequent course is variable. The central nevus may persist indefinitely (and the halo repigment), but usually it regresses leaving a white macule. The central nevus may first become irregular or pink in color. Complete repigmentation of the skin is seen in the vast majority of patients, but the process may take years.

A relationship to vitiligo, melanoma and atypical nevi has been well documented. Multiple halo nevi may be a sign of an ocular or cutaneous melanoma elsewhere, especially in older adults.

Pathology

The halo nevus may be junctional, compound or dermal. In the fully evolved stages, the central nevus is associated with a well-circumscribed, dense, almost band-like infiltrate of mononuclear cells, almost exclusively lymphocytes and histiocytes, which occupies the papillary dermis and penetrates nests of nevus cells. The latter change is so prominent that nevus cells are difficult to distinguish from surrounding lymphoid cells. Degenerating nevus cells can sometimes be identified in this zone.

Differential Diagnosis

Common acquired melanocytic nevi with the halo phenomenon must be distinguished from: (1) other melanocytic proliferations with halos, such as congenital nevi, atypical melanocytic nevi, blue nevi, Spitz nevi and primary melanoma or melanoma metastases; and (2) non-melanocytic lesions with halos, such as dermatofibromas, seborrheic keratoses, flat warts, molluscum contagiosum, basal cell carcinoma, lichen planus, psoriasis and sarcoidosis. An asymmetric, irregular halo may be seen with melanoma, as compared with the symmetry usually found in a halo nevus, but asymmetry does not equate with malignancy (see Fig. 112.14B). Other attributes such as size usually >1 cm, irregular or notched borders, and striking irregularity of color typify melanoma. However, halo nevi are exceedingly more common than halo primary melanomas, especially in adolescents.

Treatment

The treatment of patients with halo nevi is individualized and depends on the clinical setting. All persons with halo nevi should be questioned for a personal or family history of cutaneous melanoma, atypical nevi and vitiligo. The individual halo nevus or nevi should be inspected carefully for any asymmetry or features suspicious for atypical melanocytic nevus or melanoma. The patient also should undergo a comprehensive skin examination for evidence of other halo nevi, atypical nevi, melanoma or vitiligo. If no clinical atypicality is observed, the patient should be followed with periodic skin examinations. In general, clinically atypical halo nevi should be examined histologically. Halo nevi with a benign, orderly clinical appearance need not be removed. Individuals beyond age 40 years with halo nevi should be examined carefully for melanoma (ocular and cutaneous).

MELANOCYTIC NEVI OF GENITAL AND FLEXURAL SKIN

Key feature

- These nevi sometimes have atypical histologic changes, making a distinction from melanoma difficult

Clinical Features

Melanocytic nevi occurring on genital sites, especially the vulva, are thought to have rather distinctive histopathologic features compared to most nevi from non-genital sites[41–43]. However, similar nevi may occur in other locations such as the scrotum, perineum, umbilicus or axilla[43]. In general, premenopausal women (ages 14 to 40 years) present with this type of vulvar lesion[41]. These nevi appear to be uncommon, perhaps accounting for less than 10% of nevi removed, but these data could be biased by selectional factors. A recent series of 36 cases suggests that these nevi may be elevated, but more than half were clinically flat. Such nevi are often larger in size (mean 5.9 mm with a range of about 2 to 24 mm) than non-genital ordinary nevi, usually have fairly regular borders, and often have a complex mahogany color, i.e. an admixture of tan, brown and red[42].

Pathology

In general, these nevi are characterized by an overall symmetry, frequent absence of lateral extension of intraepidermal melanocytic components beyond the dermal nevus elements (if present), and are well circumscribed[41–43]. Many have mushroom-like polypoidal morphology with the rather distinctive junctional elements overlying a prominent dermal nevus component. The most notable features include architectural and cytologic features similar to the atypical melanocytic nevus (see below).

Differential Diagnosis

The differential diagnosis of vulvar and related nevi is primarily that of melanoma and Spitz nevus. Vulvar melanoma tends to occur in older women (average age approximately 65 years) compared to genital nevi. Patients with lichen sclerosus may have histologically benign but clinically atypical nevi of the vulva.

MELANOCYTIC NEVUS OF ACRAL SKIN

Synonyms: ■ Melanocytic nevus with intraepidermal ascent of cells (MANIACS) ■ Acral nevus

Key feature

- About one-third of these nevi have intraepidermal upward migration of melanocytes and other architectural changes that can resemble melanoma

Clinical Features

Acral nevi are usually macular or only slightly elevated. They may display uniform brown or dark brown color, but often have linear striations (Fig. P6). The characteristic dermoscopic features of benign melanocytic nevi of the palms and soles are due to the unique anatomy of acral skin. The palms and soles consist of parallel ridges (mountains) and furrows (valleys). The intraepidermal eccrine ducts pass through the ridges (Fig. 112.15). In benign melanocytic nevi, the nests of nevus cells are situated around the furrows. The three major dermoscopic patterns seen in benign melanocytic nevi are the parallel furrow, the lattice-like, and the fibrillar pattern. The parallel furrow pattern is the most common dermoscopic pattern in acral melanocytic nevi. It consists of parallel pigmented lines following the furrows or valleys. The lattice-like pattern is a variation of the parallel furrow pattern (see Fig. P6). It consists of parallel pigmented lines following the furrows and crossing the furrows, forming a lattice. The fibrillar pattern consists of numerous finely pigmented filaments perpendicular to the furrows[44].

Pathology

Many of the same features as described for common acquired nevi of other sites are also applicable for acral nevi. They are usually relatively small (<5–6 mm), well-circumscribed and symmetric compound nevi. On occasion, the junctional nests of acral nevi are somewhat enlarged, but they usually have a fairly uniform round or oval shape and are

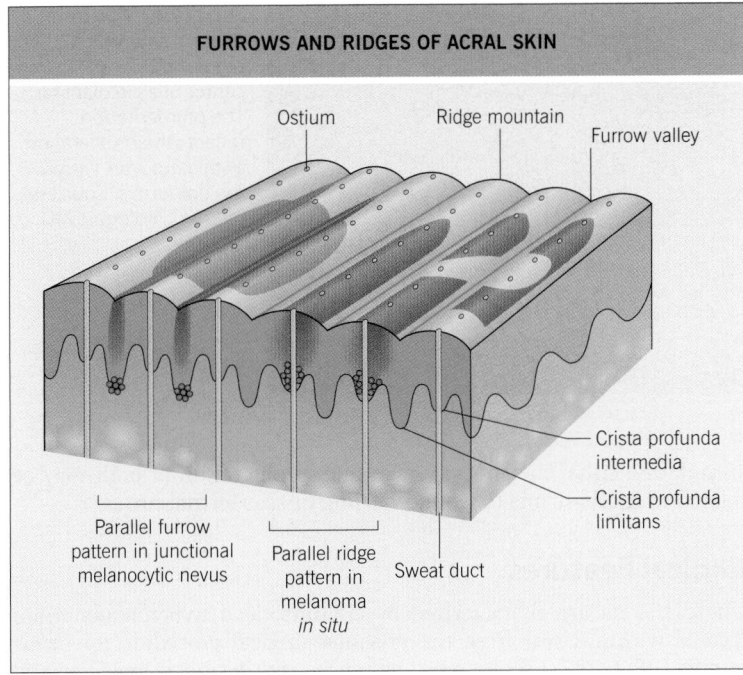

FURROWS AND RIDGES OF ACRAL SKIN

Fig. 112.15 Furrows and ridges of acral skin.

similar in size and spacing. Lentiginous melanocytic proliferation and some degree of upward migration of melanocytes are features commonly observed in acral nevi[45]. One should be cautious in over-interpreting the latter changes unless prominent architectural disorder and cytologic atypia are also present. The dermal component of acral nevi is often characterized by round nests of type A cells.

NEVUS SPILUS

Synonyms: ■ Speckled lentiginous nevus ■ Zosteriform lentiginous nevus

Key features

- Tan patch with superimposed 'speckles' that develop over time
- The darker macules and papules vary from junctional and compound nevi to Spitz and blue nevi
- Lighter brown background has the histology of lentigo simplex

Epidemiology

There is some controversy as to whether nevus spilus is congenital or acquired and this is explained in part by the initial appearance of a nevus spilus – a uniformly tan-colored, CALM-like patch. There is evidence to suggest that nevus spilus is a type of congenital melanocytic nevus. A nevus spilus was noted in approximately 2% of white adults in one

series. Males and females are equally affected. Familial cases have not been reported[46].

Pathogenesis

The nevus spilus may have a segmental or zosteriform distribution (designated *speckled zosteriform lentiginous nevus* by some), suggesting a localized 'field defect'. Although there are several case reports of twins who both displayed a nevus spilus, it is unclear how nevus spilus might differ in pathogenesis from other melanocytic nevi[47]. A nevus spilus has been likened to a garden of melanocytes in which any type of nevus can develop, simultaneously or sequentially.

Clinical Features

These lesions most commonly affect the trunk and extremities. The tan macular area commonly ranges from 1 to 4 cm in diameter (Fig. 112.16). The darker speckles are approximately 1 to 6 mm in greatest diameter and may be macular or papular. Larger varieties of nevus spilus may be unilateral, segmental or follow Blaschko's lines and can involve a substantial portion of skin, e.g. an entire extremity or half the trunk[47–49]. A nevus spilus persists indefinitely and increased degrees of speckling over time have been documented by serial photography. There are reports of cutaneous melanoma arising within a nevus spilus and on occasion melanocytic dysplasia has been noted in the nevus spilus adjacent to the site of melanoma development[50,51].

Pathology

The tan macule or patch of nevus spilus is characterized by lentiginous melanocytic hyperplasia associated with elongated epidermal rete ridges. The hyperpigmented macular foci are also characterized by lentiginous melanocytic hyperplasia, whereas the papular foci represent junctional, compound, blue, Spitz, and/or atypical nevi. Histologic features associated with congenital melanocytic nevi can also be seen.

Differential Diagnosis

Agminated nevi (junctional, compound > Spitz, blue) represent the major entity in the differential diagnosis. However, agminated nevi are not superimposed on a tan patch. Sometimes Wood's lamp examination is required to make the distinction.

Treatment

Because of reports of cutaneous melanoma developing in nevus spilus, it seems advisable that individuals be followed on a periodic basis (photography may be helpful). Areas of change or atypicality in a nevus spilus should be evaluated by biopsy or excision, as is appropriate for other atypical melanocytic lesions.

PARTIAL UNILATERAL LENTIGINOSIS

Synonym: ■ Segmental lentiginosis

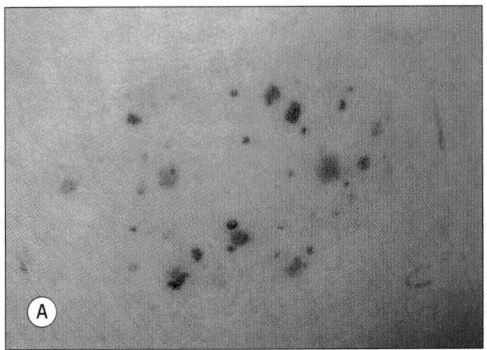
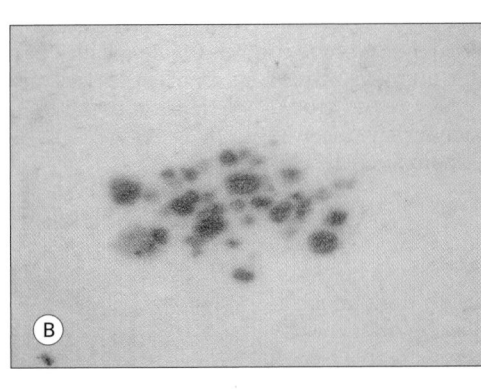

Fig. 112.16 Nevus spilus (speckled lentiginous nevus) versus agminated nevi. A Multiple brown macules and papules superimposed upon a tan patch. **B** Grouped brown macules and papules in the absence of background hyperpigmentation. A, B, Courtesy of Jean L Bolognia MD.

Key feature

- Segmental clustering of lentigines

Epidemiology

The prevalence of partial unilateral lentiginosis in the general population is not established, but it is probably rare. There is no known predilection for sex or race.

Pathogenesis

As with nevus spilus, the segmental distribution of this lesion suggests a developmental abnormality of melanocytes.

Clinical Features

The onset of this lesion may be during infancy or in childhood. The individual macules are well circumscribed and vary from about 2 to 10 mm in greatest diameter. The distribution is segmental and unilateral and facial lesions may have ocular involvement. In contrast to nevus spilus, there is no background hyperpigmentation and the lesion may expand in a wavefront-like manner. Also, CALM may be present. Progression to cutaneous melanoma has not been reported.

Pathology

The individual macules demonstrate lentiginous melanocytic hyperplasia in association with elongated epidermal rete ridges, as in lentigo simplex. Nests of nevus cells are not present.

Differential Diagnosis

Segmental lentiginosis is distinguished from nevus spilus by the absence of a tan macular background and nevus elements. Segmental lentiginosis differs from agminated nevi by the lack of nevus-cell nesting in the epidermis, dermis or both.

Treatment

Laser therapy may be tried, but recurrence is an issue.

RECURRENT MELANOCYTIC NEVUS

Synonym: ■ Pseudomelanoma

Key features

- Recurrent melanocytic nevi are fairly common following shave excision
- Heavily pigmented melanocytes proliferate in the epidermis, often with upward migration, and may resemble melanoma histologically

Epidemiology

According to Park et al.[52], recurrent nevi are noted most often in relatively young women (85% of cases, since greater numbers of nevi are removed from women). They are usually noted on the trunk, followed by the head and neck area. Most of the recurrences have followed a shave excision, at an estimated rate of 10–30%; approximately 50% of cases were noted to recur within 6 months[52].

Pathogenesis

The recurrence of melanocytic nevi is thought to result from an intra-epidermal proliferation of residual melanocytes, possibly from nearby sweat ducts, hair follicles or intraepidermal melanocytes. Trophic factors

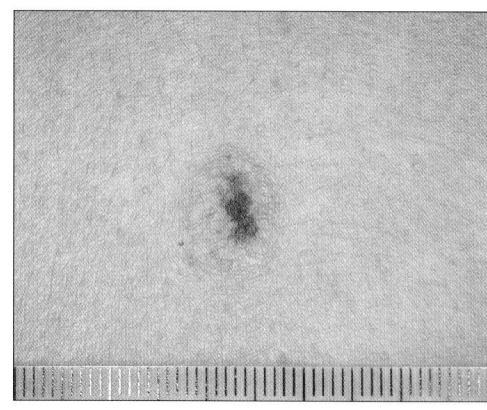

Fig. 112.17 Recurrent nevus. Dark brown pigmentation within the center of a circular scar. The pigmentation reflects the proliferation of melanocytes within the epidermis. Courtesy of Jean L Bolognia MD.

stimulating either melanocyte migration, proliferation or both may be related to mechanisms of wound healing or scar formation.

Clinical Features

These lesions are characterized by circumscribed hyperpigmentation located within a scar from the previous surgical procedure for nevus removal (Fig. 112.17). In most instances, the lesion is macular and exhibits variable irregularity of borders and pigment pattern. Stippling, mottling and a perifollicular distribution may be observed. Most recurrent nevi measure 2 to 5 mm in diameter. The dermoscopic features of persistent nevi are sometimes difficult to distinguish from melanoma. As a general rule, in recurrent nevi, the pigment will not extend beyond the white scarred area (Fig. P7). Most recurrent nevi are stable for years after development and then may fade. No increased melanoma risk has been associated with recurrent nevi.

Pathology

Corresponding to the clinical features, one frequently observes intra-epidermal melanocytic proliferation confined to the area above a dermal scar. The epidermis usually exhibits effacement of the rete pattern and variable lentiginous or nested proliferation of melanocytes. Often, the cells contain abundant melanin and relatively uniform nuclei. However, occasionally, low-grade cytologic atypia is noted. Upward migration of epidermal melanocytes may occur. Frequently, there are residual dermal nevus cells beneath the superficial dermal scar.

Differential Diagnosis

The differential diagnosis of recurrent nevus includes recurrent atypical melanocytic nevi, lentiginous melanocytic proliferations developing in melanoma scars, and recurrent melanoma. In general, recurrent melanocytic nevus is confined to the area of the surgical scar, appears within 6 months of surgery, and exhibits a banal histologic picture. Recurrent atypical nevi may have greater cytologic atypia than conventional recurrent nevi. Clinical features suggesting melanoma include irregular pigmentation, recurrence beyond the confines of the surgical scar, and a longer interval until recurrence (>6 months).

Treatment

Establishing that a previous surgical procedure has occurred is integral to the diagnosis. Review of the previous biopsy specimen is mandatory if any atypicality is noted histologically. Excision of a recurrent nevus is not necessary unless abnormal clinical features are present, e.g. extension of the lesion beyond the surgical scar.

SPITZ (SPINDLE AND EPITHELIOID CELL) NEVUS/TUMOR

Synonyms: ■ Spitz's juvenile melanoma ■ Benign juvenile melanoma

Key features

- Red or pigmented papule or nodule, usually in children or young adults
- Prominent epithelioid and/or spindled melanocytes
- Mimic of melanoma histologically

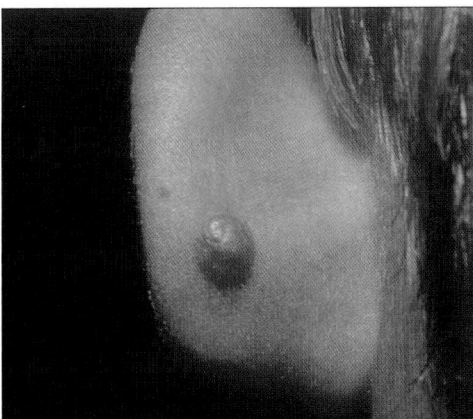

Fig. 112.18 Spitz nevus. Red dome-shaped papule on the ear of a child. Courtesy of Ronald P Rapini MD.

Epidemiology

The prevalence of Spitz nevus in the general population has not been documented accurately. However, among melanocytic lesions that have been surgically excised, approximately 1% exhibit the histologic characteristics of Spitz nevus. In data from Australia, it has been estimated that Spitz nevus accounts for 1.4 cases per 100 000 population, as compared with an annual incidence of 25.4 melanomas per 100 000 population. Spitz nevi are most commonly acquired, but as many as 7% may be congenital. Spitz nevi occur in all age groups but are uncommon beyond the ages of 40 to 50 years. In the series of Weedon & Little, 33% of affected individuals were between the ages of 10 and 20 years, and 31% were older than 20 years of age. Men and women are equally affected.

Pathogenesis

No particular etiologic factors that might account for the characteristic histologic changes found in these nevi have been identified. Widespread eruptive Spitz nevi have been associated with HIV infection, Addison's disease, chemotherapy, pregnancy, puberty and trauma. The eruption of Spitz nevi with pregnancy and puberty suggests that dormant nevi may become hormonally activated. Many Spitz nevi, however, have no identified precipitating cause. To date, no mutations in *BRAF* have been detected in Spitz nevi, in contrast to common melanocytic nevi (e.g. dermal).

Clinical Features

Spitz nevi vary in size from 2 mm to 2 cm or more, with an average diameter of approximately 8 mm[53–62]. Most commonly, they are well-circumscribed, dome-shaped papules or nodules varying in color from pink to tan to dark brown (Fig. 112.18). Generally, the color is homogeneous and the margins are well defined. The surface topography may be smooth or, in some instances, verrucous. Relatively flat, polypoid and pedunculated morphologies have also been described. Occasional lesions may have erosions and scale-crust. Telangiectasia is also a frequent finding.

Although Spitz nevi may involve any part of the body, the head and neck area is probably the most common site, accounting for 42% of lesions in one series. There is a rather even distribution of lesions over the upper extremities, lower extremities and trunk. In most instances, there is a history of recent onset, but a small percentage of nevi have been present for many years. Multiple Spitz nevi may occur in an agminated (grouped) or disseminated pattern. Disseminated Spitz nevi may number in the hundreds, erupt suddenly, and involve the entire integument except for the palms, soles and mucous membranes. The papules tend to be polymorphous, affect adults, and spontaneously regress over several years. To date, no cases of malignant degeneration of grouped or disseminated Spitz nevi have been reported. Disseminated Spitz nevi have been associated with seizures and electroencephalographic abnormalities.

Agminated (grouped) Spitz nevi are characterized by varying numbers of individual, raised nevi occurring in a localized or segmental distribution, and arising in otherwise clinically normal skin. There has been some confusion in the literature where lesions arising with a CALM-like tan background have been referred to as agminated Spitz nevi; however, these lesions would be better termed Spitz nevi within a nevus spilus (speckled lentiginous nevus). Solitary or multiple spindle and epithelioid cell proliferations developing within a large congenital nevi exhibit the features of typical Spitz nevi.

Pigmented spindle cell nevus (see below) is classified by some authors as a subtype of Spitz nevus.

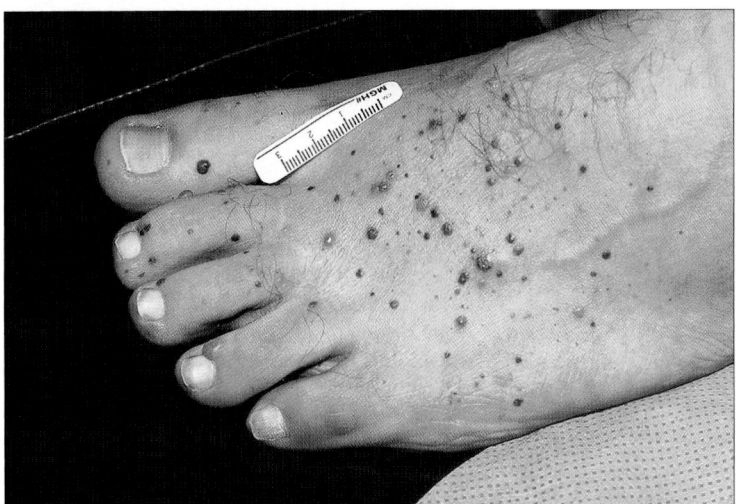

Fig. 112.19 Agminated Spitz nevi. The grouped papules have arisen on normally pigmented skin.

Atypical Spitz nevi refer to lesions demonstrating one or more (usually a constellation of) features that deviate from conventional Spitz nevi. The features may include large size (e.g. >1 cm in diameter), asymmetry, deep involvement of the dermis or subcutis, ulceration, easily found dermal mitoses (>2–3 mitoses/mm²), especially deep, significant pagetoid spread, prominent confluence and high cellular density of melanocytes in the dermis, and lack of maturation. A grading protocol for atypical Spitz nevi in childhood and adolescence has been formulated (Table 112.4). Recent work using comparative genomic hybridization and fluorescence *in situ* hybridization techniques have identified copy number increases of chromosome 11p and *HRAS* mutations in subgroups of atypical Spitz nevi. However, more studies are needed before the identification of such mutations can be used to predict the biologic behavior of Spitz nevi.

Malignant or metastasizing Spitz nevi are exceedingly rare lesions with features of atypical Spitz nevi that have been reported to result in a single regional lymph node metastasis, but no subsequent disease progression. Since such lesions are only rarely encountered, they have not been sufficiently studied to know their biologic nature and how (and if) they differ from conventional melanomas.

Pathology

Typically, these lesions display striking nests of large epithelioid cells, spindle cells or both (Fig. 112.20A), usually extending from the epidermis into the reticular dermis in an inverted-wedge configuration. The closely apposed nests of cells within a uniformly hyperplastic epidermis often contribute to a so-called 'raining-down' appearance (Fig. 112.20B). Both mononuclear and multinucleate giant epithelioid cells are frequently observed. These cells extend into the subjacent dermis as both single cells and as nests or fascicles. In general, there is orderly infiltration of the dermal collagen by these nests or cells with so-called maturation, i.e. gradual diminution of nuclear and cellular

ASSESSMENT OF ATYPICAL SPITZ NEVUS (TUMOR) IN CHILDREN AND ADOLESCENTS FOR RISK FOR METASTASIS	
Parameter	Score
Age (years)	
0–10	0
11–17	1
Diameter (mm)	
0–10	0
>10	1
Involvement of subcutaneous fat	
Absent	0
Present	2
Ulceration	
Absent	0
Present	2
Mitotic activity (mm²)	
0–5	0
6–8	2
≥9	5

Table 112.4 **Assessment of atypical Spitz nevus (tumor) in children and adolescents for risk for metastasis.** Total score and risk for metastasis: 0–2, low risk; 3–4, intermediate risk; 5–11, high risk.

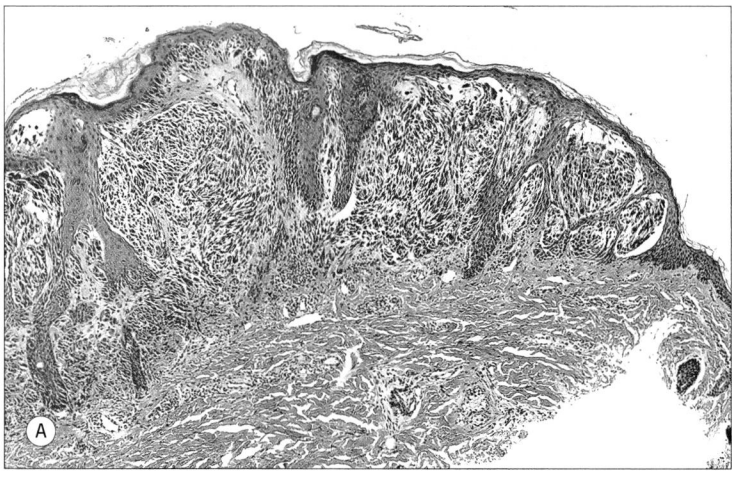

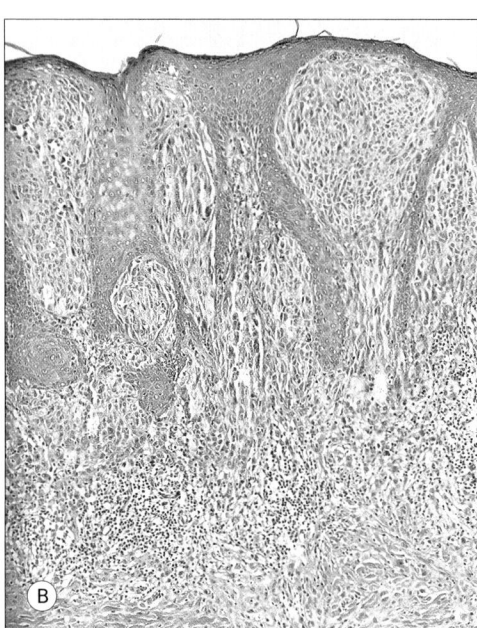

Fig. 112.20 **Histology of Spitz nevus. A** Sharply demarcated proliferation of spindled and epithelioid melanocytes, with clefts around nests and epithelial hyperplasia. **B** 'Raining-down' effect of melanocytes from a hyperplastic epidermis. A, B, Courtesy of Ronald P Rapini MD.

sizes. The individual cells usually have abundant cytoplasm that stains slightly bluish or pink and nuclei with open chromatin patterns. Rather uniform nucleoli are usually also noted. Occasional bizarre cytologic features, necrotic cells and mitotic figures are found within even the most banal lesions.

Differential Diagnosis

The clinical differential diagnosis of Spitz nevi is wide and includes other melanocytic nevi, particularly dermal nevi, hemangiomas, pyogenic granuloma, verrucae, molluscum contagiosum, juvenile and adult xanthogranulomas, dermatofibroma, mastocytoma and adnexal tumors. The fundamental diagnostic problem is the histologic differentiation of Spitz nevus from cutaneous melanoma. The latter distinction is one of the most difficult problems in all of pathology and at present is subjective, based on the experience of the pathologist, and the careful weighing of a number of clinical and histopathologic parameters summarized in Table 112.5.

Treatment

Because of the frequent diagnostic difficulty in classifying these lesions, histologic evaluation of the entire lesion is mandatory. Furthermore, recurrence rates as high as 7% to 16% have resulted from incompletely excised lesions. In the authors' opinion, complete excision with margins free of tumor is recommended for all Spitz nevi. However, there are clinicians who reserve this recommendation for lesions with any atypical features (clinically or histologically) or Spitz nevi in adults. Margins of approximately 1 cm are advised for markedly atypical variants. It is also advisable that patients with atypical lesions have periodic evaluation every 6 to 12 months. Although controversial, sentinel lymph biopsy may be considered for markedly atypical lesions with Breslow thicknesses of 1 mm or greater.

PIGMENTED SPINDLE CELL NEVUS

Synonyms: ■ Pigmented spindle cell tumor of Reed ■ Pigmented variant of Spitz nevus

Key features

■ Dark brown to black macule or papule, usually less than 6 mm

■ Found in children or young adults

■ They are a spindle cell variant of Spitz nevus

Epidemiology

Pigmented spindle cell nevi occur less frequently than other forms of spindle and epithelioid cell nevi[63,64]. A few have been noted at birth; however, the mean age at diagnosis is 25 years (the age range in one series was 3 to 66 years). Women are affected more often than men. Pigmented spindle cell nevi are most commonly located on the extremities (70% of cases in one study), with the thigh being the most frequent site. About 20% of pigmented spindle cell nevi are found on the trunk, and 9% occur in the head and neck area.

Pathogenesis

As with other melanocytic nevi, the pigmented spindle cell nevi are thought to be derived from cells migrating from the neural crest. The reasons for the prominent spindle cell features are not understood.

Clinical Features

The pigmented spindle cell nevus is usually a relatively flat or slightly raised, well-circumscribed lesion averaging about 3 mm in diameter (range 1.5 to 10 mm). The color is usually dark brown or black and is homogeneous (Fig. P8). The most common dermoscopic patterns include

Parameter	Spitz nevus	Melanoma
Age	Young age, especially <10 years, favors a benign process	Exceedingly rare under age 10 years (pre-pubertal); outnumber Spitz nevi in patients of ages >30 to 40 years
Anatomic site	Head and neck > extremities (especially thighs) are preferential sites, but may occur anywhere	Most often on the trunk (back) in men and distal lower extremities in women; favor intermittently sun-exposed skin, but may occur anywhere
Size	Often <5–6 mm, usually <10 mm	Often >6 mm, but early lesions may be smaller; large size favors melanoma
Symmetry	Usually symmetric	Increasing asymmetry favors melanoma
Architecture	Dome-shaped, plaque-like, wedge-shaped in dermis, plexiform	Heterogeneous and complex (with exceptions)
Circumscription	Usually well demarcated with peripheral junctional nests	Often poorly demarcated ending in single-cell patterns
Maturation	Overall reduction in cellular density with depth; orderly dispersion and regular spacing of nests and cells among collagen bundles with depth; nests become progressively smaller and finally resulting in single melanocytes at the base of lesion; cells and nuclei also diminish in size with depth	Little or no maturation; confluence of melanocytes is not lost with depth; irregular spacing and disorderly arrangements of cells
Pagetoid spread	Less frequent than in melanoma; orderly; often confined to the epidermis over the central part of the lesion; nested patterns may be more frequent than single cells	Common; disorderly; the melanoma cells often reach the granular layer; higher cellular density
Zonation	Uniformity of cytologic features across horizontal strata of lesion	Heterogeneity of features
Mitotic figures in dermal component	Limited in number, superficial, usually not atypical	Greater in number, deeply located, atypical
Cytologic features	Abundant ground-glass or opaque cytoplasm; polyangular, rhomboidal; occasional dendrites	Variable amount of cytoplasm; often granular or 'dusty' and abundant in epithelioid cells, scant cytoplasm in spindled cells
Nuclear features	Enlarged nuclei; uniform dispersed chromatin pattern; nucleoli may be prominent but usually uniform; reniform, multilobulated, multinucleate and giant bizarre forms occur	Pleomorphism; often high nuclear to cytoplasmic ratios; hyperchromatism; prominent variable nucleoli commonly multiple; thickened nuclear membranes

Table 112.5 Comparison of Spitz nevus and melanoma.

the following: a dark structureless area almost to the periphery of the lesion, a central dark structureless area with symmetric pseudopods or radial streaming (starburst pattern), and/or a peripheral globular pattern (see Fig. P8). Irregularity of pigmentation is not common but may be found in atypical variants of pigmented spindle cell nevi. There is often a history of recent development or alteration. In one study, lesions had been present, on average, for about 6 months, although some were of longstanding duration. There is usually no family history of melanoma or atypical nevi.

The natural history is largely unknown. As has been mentioned, the vast majority of pigmented spindle cell nevi have been present for only a short time, usually less than a year. Congenital forms of pigmented spindle cell nevi, although uncommon, have been recognized. The occurrence of atypical varieties of pigmented spindle cell nevi and the presence of remnants of pigmented spindle cell nevi in association with cutaneous melanoma are circumstantial evidence that pigmented spindle cell nevi can undergo rare transformation to cutaneous melanoma. In long-term (mean 8.8 years) follow-up of 15 patients with excised pigmented spindle cell nevi, there was no evidence of recurrence. In our experience, these lesions have almost never recurred. Thus, unless a lesion has been incompletely excised, recurrence strongly suggests an atypical process, possibly cutaneous melanoma.

Pathology

The pigmented spindle cell nevus displays a well-circumscribed and orderly appearance. The lesions are usually only slightly raised and are confined to the epidermis, but may involve the papillary dermis. The lesion is typified by fascicles of uniform, slender spindle cells that are closely aggregated (Fig. 112.21). The cells usually contain fine, granular melanin. The nuclei contain delicate chromatin and small inconspicuous nucleoli and have an overall monotonous appearance. There may be clefting about the intraepidermal fascicles. Numerous melanophages are usually present in the papillary dermis. Upward migration of nevus cells throughout the epidermis is sometimes noted, but these are usually confined to the lower half of the epidermis. Atypical variants

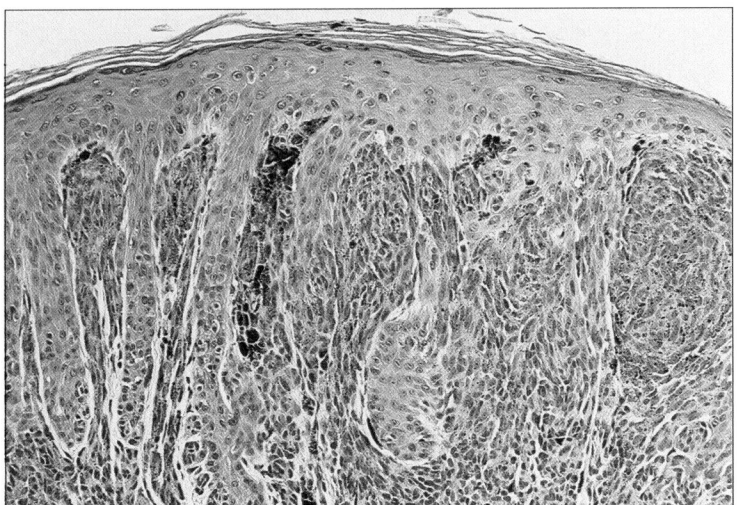

Fig. 112.21 Histology of a pigmented spindle cell nevus. Closely aggregated, uniform, slender spindle cells. Courtesy of Ronald P Rapini MD.

exhibit prominent single-cell hyperplasia extending peripherally along the basal layer of the epidermis and in a pagetoid pattern throughout the epidermis. Cytologic atypia also may be present in a varying degree in these atypical variants.

Differential Diagnosis

The differential diagnosis of pigmented spindle cell nevi includes early melanoma, atypical nevus, blue nevus, angiokeratoma and pigmented basal cell carcinoma. In general, the borders of pigmented spindle cell nevi are regular and well defined. The color is also homogeneous in most instances. However, atypical forms of pigmented spindle cell nevi may exhibit irregularity of borders and color. Histopathologic examination is essential for diagnosis. It must be stressed, however, that the clinicopathologic presentation of typical pigmented spindle cell nevi is distinctive. Its history is that of a recently developed or changing, small, well-circumscribed, black lesion on the thigh of a young woman (usually in her twenties). These lesions are usually conspicuous for the absence of any other pigmented lesions on the body.

Treatment

The proper treatment of pigmented spindle cell nevi is complete excision with clear margins. The reason for this recommendation is to prevent recurrence, since the pathology of recurring lesions may be alarming and difficult to distinguish from melanoma. For pigmented spindle cell nevi with atypical features, wider surgical margins are advised. For example, we advocate resection margins of 5 to 10 mm for markedly atypical forms of pigmented spindle cell nevus. Periodic follow-up, i.e. every 6 to 12 months, is also strongly advised for patients with atypical variants of pigmented spindle cell nevus.

ATYPICAL (DYSPLASTIC) MELANOCYTIC NEVUS

Synonyms: ■ B-K mole ■ Atypical nevus ■ Atypical mole ■ Clark's nevus ■ The mole of FAMM (familial atypical mole and melanoma syndrome) ■ 'Dysplastic' melanocytic nevus ■ Nevus with architectural disorder

The US National Institutes of Health Consensus Conference held in January 1992 has recommended that the histologic term 'nevus with architectural disorder' replace dysplastic melanocytic nevus

Key features

- A controversial clinical designation for various nevi that have morphologic changes such as asymmetry, irregular borders and color variation

- Also a controversial pathologic term used for nevi with certain architectural changes and/or cytologic atypia

- The relationship to melanoma is complex

History

Since the description of atypical or 'dysplastic' melanocytic nevi in the setting of melanoma-prone families over 20 years ago and subsequently in individuals outside such kindreds, these lesions have remained highly controversial. This has largely resulted from the failure to reach consensus about the nature of these lesions, an inability to formulate precise criteria for recognition, and finally a lack of understanding about their biologic significance. Specifically, this relates to criteria for individual

lesions and for the so-called 'dysplastic nevus syndrome', i.e. how many clinically atypical melanocytic nevi are needed and what are the minimal essential gross morphologic criteria needed for diagnosis of an individual lesion. One particular problem dating back to the original studies on atypical melanocytic nevi ('dysplastic nevi') in hereditary kindreds has been the tendency to consider that the histopathologic diagnosis of atypical melanocytic nevi ('dysplastic nevus') is the gold standard; whereas it has been shown that the histopathologic features ascribed to atypical melanocytic nevi ('dysplastic nevi') lack specificity (see below).

Many studies have established that irrespective of histology, melanoma risk is directly related to numbers of ordinary nevi (>50 or 100 on the total skin surface) as well as the presence and number of atypical nevi, as defined by size (e.g. >5, 6 or 8 mm), irregular or ill-defined borders, variation in color, macular component, etc. (Tables 112.6 & 112.7)[64a–64e]. Despite the seemingly logical conclusion that histopathologically atypical nevi should be associated with increased melanoma risk, only limited data thus far have shown such a relationship. Furthermore, studies examining the relationship between clinically atypical melanocytic nevi and histopathologic atypical melanocytic nevi have showed a poor correlation. Therefore the 'dysplastic' nevus cannot be considered a distinct clinicopathologic entity. At present, melanoma risk assessment of patients is based almost solely on gross morphologic parameters of nevi, i.e. total numbers of nevi on the skin surface and the presence and number of clinically atypical melanocytic nevi, along with other factors such as personal or family history of melanoma.

Therefore, at present, atypical melanocytic nevi undoubtedly encompass a large and heterogeneous group of nevi:

- nevi with atypical clinical features, which have been termed simply 'atypical nevi'; in general, these atypical nevi can simulate melanoma; this group of nevi should include not only 'atypical' or 'dysplastic' nevi, but also some congenital and combined melanocytic, as well as Spitz/pigmented spindle cell nevi;
- nevi with abnormal histopathologic features;
- nevi with *both* abnormal clinical and histopathologic features;
- nevi with histopathologic features that are equivocal or of unknown significance.

MELANOCYTIC NEVUS PHENOTYPES		
	Common pattern	**Atypical pattern**
Number	None to few (<25) nevi	Many (>50) nevi
Size	<5 mm	Variable: small to large, often several >5 mm
Color	Uniform, homogeneous color	Some to many nevi with irregular or haphazard color, erythema
Borders	Well circumscribed	Irregular or ill-defined borders

Table 112.6 Melanocytic nevus phenotypes.

MELANOMA RISK ASSOCIATED WITH CLINICALLY ATYPICAL MELANOCYTIC NEVI: COMPARISON OF OCCURRENCE IN MELANOMA PATIENTS VERSUS CONTROLS					
Study	**Country**	**Definition**	**Melanoma patients (%)**	**Controls (%)**	**Relative risk**
Roush et al. and Nordlund et al.	Australia	>5 mm, irregular border, and haphazard pigmentation	34	7	7.7
MacKie et al.	Scotland	>5 mm and either irregular pigmentation or inflammation	38	20	2.1–4.5*
Holly et al.	US	At least 3 of 6 criteria: ill-defined border, irregular border, irregular pigmentation, >5 mm, erythema, accentuated skin margins	55	17	3.8–6.3†
Halpern et al.	US	>4 mm, macular component, variegation of color, and irregular or indistinct border	39	7	8.8
Garbe et al.	Germany	At least 3 of 5 criteria: >5 mm, irregular margins, ill-defined border, color variation, macular and papular components	45	5	7

*Relative risk for one or two atypical nevi, 2.1; for three or more atypical nevi, 4.5.
†Relative risk for one to five atypical nevi, 3.8; for six or more atypical nevi, 6.3.

Table 112.7 Melanoma risk associated with clinically atypical melanocytic nevi: comparison of occurrence in melanoma patients versus controls[64a–64e].

The latter group of nevi may demonstrate findings that may be reactive or proliferative in nature rather than neoplastic[65–105].

Epidemiology

Estimates of the incidence of atypical melanocytic nevi cover a wide range, as would be expected since they are related to a lack of consensus about definitions. Most estimates are in the 5% range, but estimates as high as 53% have been reported for the US population.

The atypical melanocytic nevi may be single or multiple. In the general population, atypical melanocytic nevi may arise in a 'sporadic' fashion, i.e. without a history of familial melanoma, versus in the setting of a family history of atypical moles and/or melanoma. In the context of a family history of melanoma, there is agreement that they indicate some increase in melanoma risk, while there is controversy about the risk in the absence of family history.

Sporadic atypical melanocytic nevi may occur at any time, while persons with a family history of atypical melanocytic nevi and/or melanoma usually manifest their atypical lesions by the end of the second decade. In contrast to common acquired moles that tend to appear in clusters around puberty, atypical melanocytic nevi may appear, even in an eruptive fashion, as late as the sixth decade.

Correlation of atypical melanocytic nevi, family history, and melanoma has been documented in a study of 14 melanoma kindreds. This study followed 401 individuals for an average of 4 years each; 40 new melanomas were noted in family members who had atypical melanocytic nevi. Histologic contiguity of the atypical melanocytic nevi to the melanomas was reported frequently by the authors, but, nonetheless, must be considered a controversial finding. In another study of 234 melanomas (familial and sporadic), histologic contiguity of atypical melanocytic nevi and cutaneous melanoma was again observed frequently. These descriptions also tend to corroborate clinical observations of atypical-appearing nevi juxtaposed with melanoma. Continuing investigations of the much more common sporadic atypical melanocytic nevi and their relation to melanoma are needed. The development of melanoma in association with an individual atypical melanocytic nevus in the sporadic setting seems to be an uncommon event and difficult to clearly document.

Clinical Features

Nevi as described below can occur anywhere on the cutaneous or mucosal surfaces of Caucasians as well as on the acral and mucosal surfaces of other races. Of note, other authors believe that distinct atypical melanocytic proliferations apart from atypical melanocytic nevi occur on acral and mucosal sites. As outlined in Table 112.8, atypical melanocytic nevi occupy an intermediate position on the continuum of common nevi on the one hand and cutaneous melanoma on the other hand. At one end of the spectrum, atypical melanocytic nevi overlap with common nevi, and at the other end, with melanoma. No single feature is diagnostic of atypical melanocytic nevi; rather, a constellation of clinical findings is required for their recognition (Figs P9–P11). However, the greater the number of clinical abnormalities present, the greater is the likelihood that the lesion will prove to be histologically atypical, but there are many exceptions. As indicated in Table 112.8, the following gross morphologic features are commonly observed in atypical melanocytic nevi:

- *Asymmetry*: atypical melanocytic nevi often lack mirror-image symmetry. Greater asymmetry suggests greater likelihood of atypicality.
- *Size*: atypical melanocytic nevi may be of any size but generally range from 3 to 15 mm in greatest diameter. There is generally a positive correlation between increasing size and likelihood of atypia.
- *Borders*: atypical melanocytic nevi often exhibit irregular and ill-defined borders, but not typically the notched or scalloped borders of melanoma.
- *Coloration*: atypical melanocytic nevi often have many colors. They commonly exhibit irregularity of pigmentation with two or three shades of brown, e.g. tan, brown and dark brown. They may also have areas that are skin-colored, pink, gray or brown-black. Some atypical melanocytic nevi present with fairly uniform coloration and an erythematous appearance (Fig. 112.22).

Atypical melanocytic nevi most frequently involve the trunk and also show a striking (though less common) predilection for the scalp and for doubly covered areas of the body (breasts in women and bathing-trunk area in men). Their numbers may range from one or two to hundreds. When multiple large lesions are present, their prominence and variation are noteworthy. When multiple, lesions tend to be randomly and widely dispersed over the body surface, sometimes locally forming patterns such as linear tracts, clusters or figurate arrays (Fig. 112.23).

The overwhelming majority of atypical melanocytic nevi are clinically stable. However, there is definite evidence that some lesions eventuate in cutaneous melanoma. There are a number of studies documenting alterations in DNA content, cytogenetic alterations, and reactivity of atypical melanocytic nevi with monoclonal antibodies directed against various melanocyte-associated antigens. The progressive abnormalities in DNA content, cytogenetic alterations and the increased reactivity with melanocyte-associated antigens have been correlated with progressive degrees of histologic atypia. These latter findings suggest a progression of atypical melanocytic nevi toward melanoma, but atypical melanocytic nevi are not inevitable precursors to melanoma.

Pathology

Prototypic atypical melanocytic nevi are described as having several noteworthy architectural features (Fig. 112.24). Such nevi are often larger (commonly >5 to 6 mm in diameter), are more poorly circumscribed, are slightly more asymmetric, are relatively flat, particularly

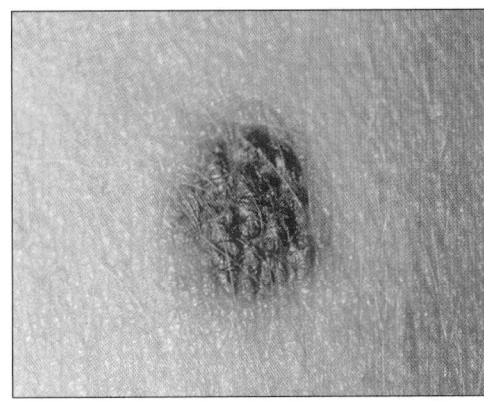

Fig. 112.22
Erythematous variant of atypical melanocytic nevus.

CLINICAL CHARACTERISTICS OF COMMON ACQUIRED NEVI, ATYPICAL MELANOCYTIC NEVI AND CUTANEOUS MELANOMA			
Characteristic	Common acquired nevi	Atypical nevi	Cutaneous melanoma
Size	<5–6 mm	3–15 mm	Any size, but tend to be greater than 5 mm
Border	Regular, well defined	Irregular, ill defined (continuum)	More irregular, very ill defined (continuum)
Symmetry	Symmetric	Some asymmetry (continuum)	Greater asymmetry (continuum)
Coloration	Homogeneous, regular	Somewhat haphazard (continuum)	Haphazard (more complexity) (continuum)
Colors	Tan to dark brown, skin-colored	Tan to dark brown, black, pink; occasionally gray, blue, white	Tan to dark brown, black, pink, red, gray, blue, white

Table 112.8 Clinical characteristics of common acquired nevi, atypical melanocytic nevi and cutaneous melanoma.

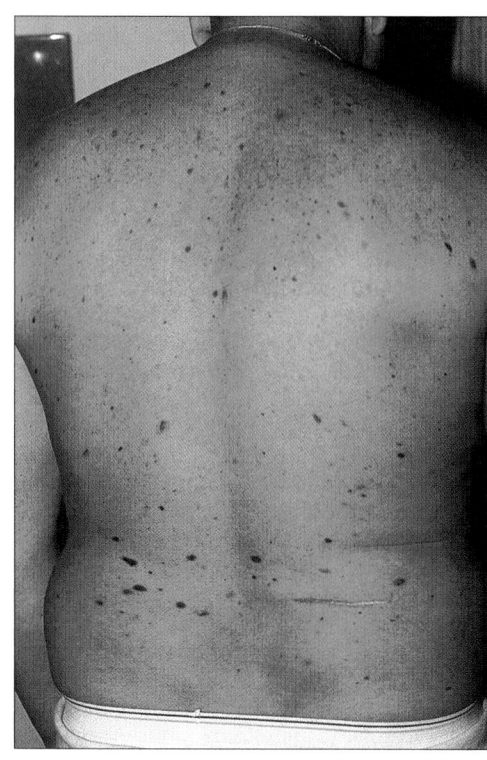

Fig. 112.23 Atypical melanocytic nevi. Multiple pigmented macules and papules of varying sizes on the back.

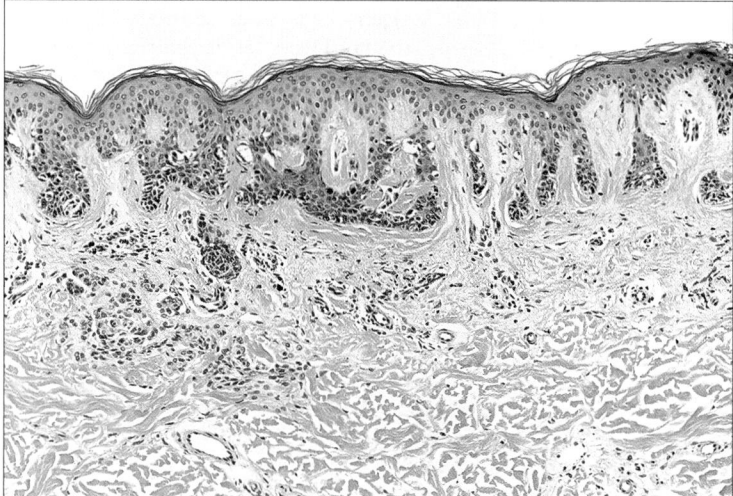

Fig. 112.24 Histology of an atypical melanocytic nevus. Elongated rete ridges, bridging between rete ridges, fibroplasia, and sparse lymphocytes are features. Cytologic atypia is usually mild. Courtesy of Ronald P Rapini MD.

at the peripheries of the lesion, and often show heterogeneity as compared to ordinary nevi. In atypical melanocytic nevi, the junctional nests frequently extend beyond the dermal component (the 'shoulder' phenomenon).

Of particular importance are abnormalities of the intraepidermal component. This architectural or organizational disorder occurs in two patterns that are often present simultaneously to a varying extent. The first is lentiginous melanocytic proliferation that is almost always associated with elongate epidermal rete ridges. In general, the basilar melanocytes are concentrated in the lowermost portions of the rete ridges, and the frequency of basilar melanocytes varies greatly, e.g. from one melanocyte per one to two keratinocytes to the melanocytes replacing the basilar keratinocytes and resulting in a confluent, clustered, or multilayered cellular appearance.

The second pattern includes nests of melanocytes irregularly disposed along and between the rete ridges in a more haphazard fashion as compared to ordinary nevi. These nests vary in size and shape, are frequently elongate, commonly have their long axes oriented along the dermal–epidermal junction, and contain variable numbers of cells. Colliding nests of melanocytes frequently fuse or 'bridge'. Dyscohesion

of cells within these nests is also common; this feature contrasts with the cohesive appearance of junctional nests of melanocytes in ordinary nevi. Often, atypical melanocytic nevi have a higher density or concentration of melanocytes in the intraepidermal component than do banal nevi, and this may be a helpful feature in their recognition.

Atypical melanocytic nevi with the latter two patterns usually exhibit cytologic atypia of their melanocytes. Such change is variable and discontinuous; it encompasses a wide spectrum of lesions, from those in which only a small percentage of cells demonstrate nuclear atypia to those in which most cells are atypical, and it often shows a general correlation with the degree of architectural abnormality present in the particular lesion. Pleomorphism of the nuclei (i.e. variation in size, shape and staining properties) is perhaps the most characteristic attribute of the nuclear changes in atypical melanocytic nevi. However, nuclear enlargement and hyperchromatism also occur. The cells are also frequently typified by a perinuclear clear space resulting from cytoplasmic shrinkage, an artifact of tissue processing. Criteria for grading the degree of cytologic atypia and even architectural abnormality have been proposed, but there is currently no consensus about grading.

Atypical melanocytic nevi may also contain a proliferation of atypical epithelioid melanocytes that resembles the epithelioid melanocytes in some forms of melanoma. It is characterized by prominent junctional nests of cells that are predominantly epithelioid in appearance, with round nuclei and finely granular melanin in their cytoplasm. The cells may also be disposed singly along the dermal–epidermal junction, with occasional pagetoid spread. Epithelioid cell proliferation may occur in a normal epidermis or in a hyperplastic epidermis. The normal epidermal rete ridge pattern is retained.

Cytologically, the melanocytes are enlarged and have variable degrees of nuclear enlargement, pleomorphism, hyperchromatism and, occasionally, prominent nucleoli. When these cells are in nests, they show some dyscohesion, but on the whole fill the nests completely. Mixtures of these intraepidermal patterns are common.

The dermal component of atypical melanocytic nevi may be composed of typical nevus cells, such as those in any acquired nevus, or of cells that may exhibit atypia. In addition to the abnormal proliferative patterns described above, other frequent alterations, particularly changes related to host response, characterize intermediate nevi. Two forms of collagenous change occur in the papillary dermis. Most common is a condensation of dense, acellular collagen around the elongate epidermal rete; this is known as concentric eosinophilic fibrosis. A less common pattern consists of delicately layered, or laminated, collagen subjacent to the rete tips with fibroblasts disposed along the laminated collagen fibers in a linear array. This pattern is referred to as lamellar fibroplasia. A mixture of the two collagen patterns is not uncommon.

Lymphocytic infiltrates, which usually are distributed in a perivascular fashion and less commonly in a band-like pattern, are also frequent in atypical melanocytic nevi. Finally, atypical melanocytic nevi usually have prominent vascularity throughout the papillary dermis, which is secondary to dilation and hypertrophy of existing vascular channels, rather than significant angiogenesis. The histopathologic criteria for atypical melanocytic nevi are still evolving, and, as already mentioned, many questions relating to the histopathology of these lesions are still unanswered.

Differential Diagnosis

The differential diagnosis of pigmented lesions approximately 4 to 15 mm in size includes both melanocytic and keratinocytic lesions. Among melanocytic proliferations, the principal diagnostic considerations lie among common acquired nevi, small congenital nevi, and cutaneous melanoma. The atypical melanocytic nevus can be identified successfully because of its haphazard, irregular coloration, including hues of pink, tan, brown and even black, and its irregularity in shape. The other nevic lesions either show symmetry and/or uniformity of coloration or, when irregularly colored, show orderly gradations or patterns of pigmentation.

Dermoscopy may also play an important role in evaluating atypical melanocytic nevi. Although atypical melanocytic nevi may clinically resemble melanoma, many of these lesions fall into one of the benign dermoscopic melanocytic patterns (see Fig. P9). The features employed to evaluate a melanocytic nevus include colors, symmetry and organization. Benign melanocytic lesions tend to have few colors and are symmetric with regard to the distribution of colors and structures. Organization refers to the distribution of structures in a lesion. When these structures are symmetrically distributed and there are less than three colors (light brown, dark brown, and black) noted, they create a pattern seen in many benign lesions. The most common benign patterns are reticular, globular and homogeneous. In addition, there are the subset patterns of reticular–homogeneous, reticular–globular and globular–homogeneous (see Fig. P9)[106].

Of particular note, a subset of atypical melanocytic nevi may demonstrate a 'malignant' melanocytic dermoscopic pattern (see Fig. P10). These lesions often have many colors and are asymmetric and disorganized with respect to a non-uniform distribution of colors and structures. It is recommended that these lesions be biopsied.

Finally, another subset of atypical melanocytic nevi is characterized by uncertain melanocytic dermoscopic patterns. Just as the clinical and histologic features of atypical melanocytic nevi are a continuum, so too are the features with dermoscopy (see Fig. P11). These lesions should either be serially monitored or undergo biopsy.

Pigmented seborrheic keratoses, solar lentigines, lichen planus-like keratoses, pigmented actinic keratoses, pigmented Bowen's disease and basal cell carcinoma may exhibit pink, tan, brown or dark brown coloration.

Treatment

As within any area of medicine, the physician is first obliged to do no harm. Such an approach is particularly germane to patients with atypical melanocytic nevi, in order to avoid overly aggressive procedures, surgery and follow-up. Common sense should prevail at all times and consideration given as to whether the intervention will have any impact on potentially reducing mortality from melanoma. Treatment depends, first, on whether the patient presents with one or a few nevi or with numerous nevi and whether there is a personal history of melanoma, and then on whether there exists a familial setting of atypical melanocytic nevi and/or melanoma. A gradient of melanoma risk has been clearly established for these various subsets of patients. Melanoma risk is probably continuous and increases with progressive increases in numbers of nevi, clinical atypia of nevi, and personal and familial occurrence of atypical nevi and melanoma.

Regardless of the risk group, any pigmented lesion suspicious for melanoma and any persistently and significantly changing lesion should in the authors' opinion be excised completely with approximately 2 mm margins for histopathologic examination. Some authors have advocated

'deep' shave excision (saucerization) for superficial lesions, as long as the base of the lesion is removed. As opposed to partial punch biopsy, the latter allows for assessment of the overall architecture of the lesion and leads to less sampling error. A helpful rule of thumb in following patients with many atypical melanocytic nevi is to search for lesions that clearly stand out as different from the patient's other (baseline) nevi; such lesions should be examined carefully. It should be kept in mind that new nevi continue to develop and nevi may enlarge and change with time in young individuals. One must use common sense in assessing such normal evolution of nevi and not be overly aggressive in removing such nevi. It is not mandatory to remove clinically atypical nevi simply to confirm or exclude atypical melanocytic nevi histologically. An acceptable practice is to follow such patients on a regular schedule with a total body skin examination plus dermoscopy, baseline photography, and digital dermoscopy as preferred by the clinician. The frequency of follow-up examinations is individualized and is based on the previously mentioned risk factors, i.e. numbers and clinical atypia of nevi, lesion stability, and personal and family history of melanoma (Fig. 112.25).

For patients having clinically suspicious lesions removed, narrow surgical margins are advised. If 'severe' cytologic atypia is present in the lesion, re-excision is recommended because of frequent overlap with melanoma *in situ*. For atypical melanocytic nevi with lesser degrees of melanocytic atypia, the question of re-excision for a nevus not completely removed is controversial. One reason for the latter statement is that there is currently no consensus about the grading of atypia in nevi or sufficient data about the significance of melanocytic atypia in nevi. However, as with any melanocytic lesion, it is important to know if the lesion has been adequately sampled and also if the lesion was considered to be clinically atypical. If lesions are 'slightly' atypical, no re-excision is recommended, as long as no residuum of the nevus is clinically apparent. If lesions are 'moderately' atypical and present in the margins, even when no residual lesion is clinically obvious, a re-excision with clear margins might be considered.

In general, follow-up of patients with multiple atypical nevi, especially in the context of a personal or family history of melanoma, should be every 3 to 12 months, depending on the clinical situation. One should consider documentation of nevi by body charts and clinical photography, as judged appropriate, with periodic updating. The authors have found that individual photographs of the most atypical or difficult-to-follow nevi are particularly helpful. Additional tools such as dermoscopy and/or digital imaging devices may be useful diagnostic aids.

Finally, individuals presenting with atypical melanocytic nevi should have a family history taken for the presence of atypical melanocytic nevi and/or melanoma. First-degree blood relatives should be examined both for documentation and to assess and potentially diminish their own risks of developing melanoma.

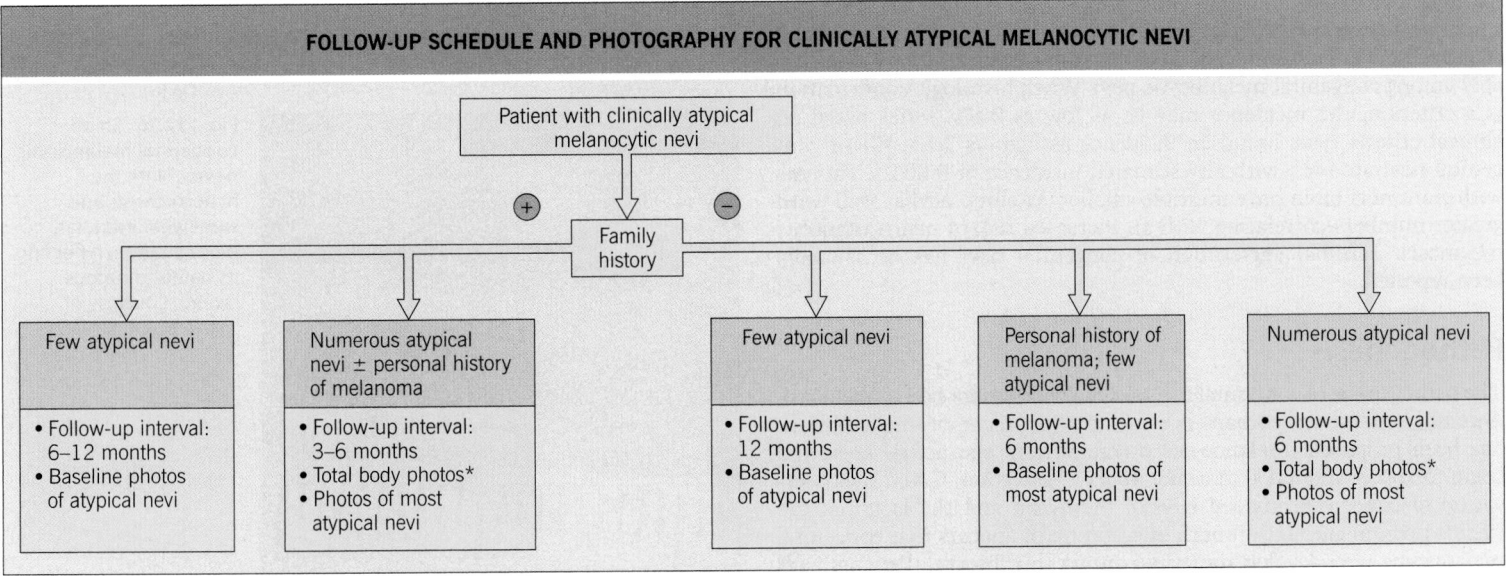

Fig. 112.25 Follow-up schedule and photography for clinically atypical melanocytic nevi. *Advocated by some authors, but not standard of care.

CONGENITAL MELANOCYTIC NEVUS

Key features

- Small congenital nevi are less than 1.5 cm in diameter
- Medium congenital nevi are between 1.5 and 19.9 cm in diameter
- Only the large (or giant) congenital nevi 20 cm or more in diameter (in adults) have a significantly higher risk for developing melanoma than do ordinary nevi

Introduction

Congenital melanocytic nevi are melanocytic nevi present at birth. They consist of proliferations of benign melanocytes that may be intra-epidermal, dermal or both. Rarely, lesions appear after birth or within 2 years that are not otherwise remarkably different from congenital nevi and are therefore referred to as *congenital nevus tardive*. Some congenital melanocytic nevi may be just a few millimeters in size and appear clinically indistinguishable from common acquired nevi. In general, congenital melanocytic nevi are classified as small, intermediate- or medium-sized, and large or giant. For practical purposes, small congenital nevi are <1.5 cm in greatest diameter. Intermediate- or medium-sized congenital nevi are from 1.5 to 19.9 cm in greatest diameter. Large (or giant) congenital nevi are 20 cm or more (in adults; 9 cm on the scalp and 6 cm on the trunk in newborns) and often cover large areas of the body such as the arm, scalp, or even the entire dorsal surface from the scalp to the feet. Some authors base the distinction between small, intermediate and large congenital nevi on their ease of removal. In this scheme, small congenital nevi generally may be removed by simple excision, intermediate congenital melanocytic nevi often require staged excisions for closure, and giant nevi often cannot be removed or require multiple staged excisions.

Neurocutaneous melanosis is a rare congenital syndrome charac-terized by: (1) the presence of either a large (>20 cm) congenital melano-cytic nevi, or multiple (>3) usually smaller congenital melanocytic nevi (or both), in association with meningeal melanosis or melanoma; (2) an absence of cutaneous melanoma except in patients with histologically benign meningeal lesions; and (3) an absence of meningeal melanoma except in patients with histologically benign cutaneous lesions[107–126].

Epidemiology

Estimates of the incidence of congenital nevi are imprecise since dis-tinctions between relatively 'small' congenital melanocytic nevi and acquired nevi are not well defined and histologic patterns vary consider-ably among congenital melanocytic nevi. When histologic confirmation is a criterion, the incidence may be as low as 0.6%; series based on clinical criteria have found an incidence as high as 2.5%. Giant con-genital nevi are rare, with an estimated incidence of 0.005%. Patients with giant nevi often have multiple smaller (satellite) nevi as well, with greater numbers correlating with an increased risk of neurocutaneous melanosis. Familial aggregation of congenital nevi has occasionally been reported.

Pathogenesis

The pathogenesis of congenital melanocytic nevi has not been established. A *de novo* mutation, perhaps in a melanocyte precursor (melanoblast), has been proposed. Melanocytes originate from the neural crest and begin to appear in fetal skin before 40 days' gestation. Given the obser-vation of congenital divided nevi of the eyelid and the fact that the eyelids open in the sixth month of gestation, it appears that congenital melanocytic nevi develop sometime during this interval. Patients with either a large congenital nevus or multiple satellite-like lesions should

be thought of as having a systemic disease as nevus cells can be found in sites beyond the skin and central nervous system such as the retroperitoneum.

Clinical Features

Congenital melanocytic nevi of the small and intermediate types are usually round or oval and fairly symmetric (Fig. P12). These lesions are usually slightly raised at birth and may be tan in color. They may or may not have associated hypertrichosis, and perifollicular hypo- or hyperpigmentation may be seen. Some congenital melanocytic nevi have rugose or pebbly surfaces. Lesions that begin as slightly raised tend with age to become more elevated; color darkening and the assumption of a verrucous appearance are also common. After an initial darkening during the first year or so of life, some congenital melanocytic nevi may become lighter in color with aging. In addition, congenital nevi can develop the halo phenomenon (see above) and occasionally, congenital nevi completely regress, even without forming a halo. As hamartomas, congenital nevi can exhibit asymmetry and variation in color (Fig. 112.26), develop papules and nodules (e.g. proliferative nodules), and undergo change over time; however, histologic examination of any concerning areas is recommended.

The dermoscopic structures seen in congenital nevi may include the following: globules, diffuse background pigmentation (structureless), milia-like cysts, hypertrichosis, hyphae-like structures and perifollicular pigment changes. Congenital nevi have repeatable dermoscopic patterns. The most common patterns are the reticular, globular, reticular–globular (see Fig. P12), diffuse brown pigmentation, and multicomponent. The multicomponent pattern is often difficult to distinguish from melanoma and requires either monitoring or biopsy.

Varying numbers of so-called satellite congenital melanocytic nevi often accompany giant congenital melanocytic nevi (Fig. 112.27). In one study, at least 80% of patients with large congenital melanocytic nevi had satellite congenital melanocytic nevi. Such lesions typically resemble small or medium-sized congenital melanocytic nevi. Of note, some patients present with multiple satellite-like lesions in the absence of a large congenital nevus (see Fig. 112.27A), and these individuals are also at risk for neurocutaneous melanosis.

Neurocutaneous melanosis

In one series of 33 patients with neurocutaneous melanosis associated with large congenital melanocytic nevi (>20 cm), all nevi had a posterior axial location (involving the head, neck, back and/or buttocks); 31 of 33 patients had satellite nevi. In another study, 80% had posterior axis involvement and 55% had more than 20 satellite nevi. Neurocutaneous melanosis is divided into symptomatic and asymptomatic (noted on screening MRI). Symptomatic neurocutaneous melanosis presents with signs and symptoms of increased intracranial pressure, often due to hydrocephalus or mass effect, and it is associated with a poor prognosis. By MRI, there are several presentations of neurocutaneous melanosis including: (1) multiple obvious postgadolinium-enhancing masses; (2) diffusely thickened leptomeninges noted by gadolinium enhancement;

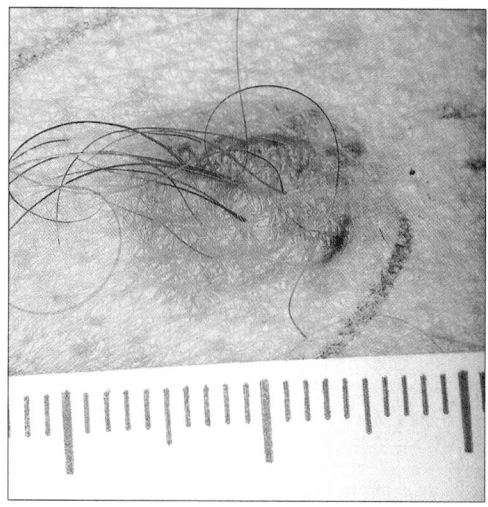

Fig. 112.26 Small congenital melanocytic nevus. Note the hypertrichosis and somewhat irregular pigmentation, reflecting its hamartomatous nature. Courtesy of Jean L Bolognia MD.

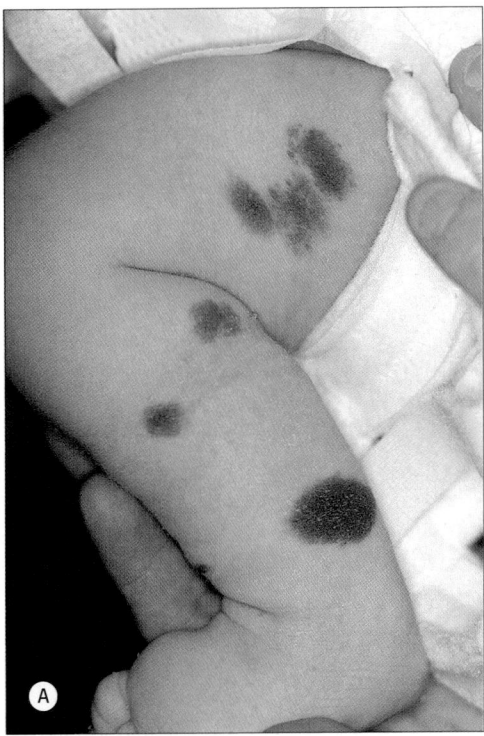

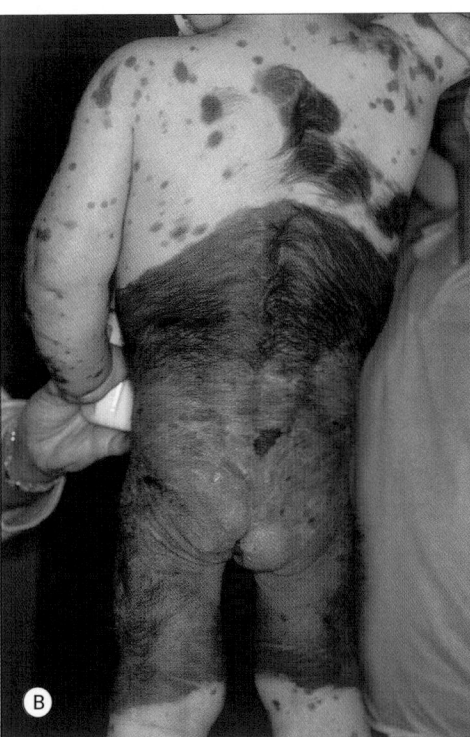

Fig. 112.27 Congenital melanocytic nevi. **A** Multiple medium-sized nevi. The patient had 25–30 such lesions. This presentation can be associated with neurocutaneous melanosis. **B** Large congenital nevus in an axial location with numerous satellite nevi, some of which have hypertrichosis. This patient died of intractable ascites due to the migration of benign melanocytes from the brain to the peritoneal cavity via his VP shunt. A, Courtesy of Jean L Bolognia MD.

and (3) focal areas of increased signal on T1-weighted images. The first two forms are associated with a poor prognosis.

Melanoma

Although all sizes of congenital melanocytic nevi may be associated with melanoma, historical estimates of melanoma risk have been exaggerated because of referral bias and misdiagnosis of atypical melanocytic proliferations that develop in congenital melanocytic nevi as melanoma. The potential risk is probably related to size of the congenital melanocytic nevi, i.e. the larger the nevus, the greater the risk. At present it is thought that the melanoma risk associated with small congenital melanocytic nevi is low and probably not much more than that associated with acquired nevi. A prospective study of 230 medium-sized congenital melanocytic nevi in 227 patients, followed on average for 6.7 years, failed to document the development of a single case of melanoma. Similarly, in a longitudinal cohort study of 265 patients with medium-sized congenital melanocytic nevi, none developed melanoma. Thus, in general, the latter studies suggest that medium- (and small-) sized congenital melanocytic nevi are not associated with significantly increased risk for melanoma.

On the other hand, recent studies have confirmed substantial melanoma risk linked to large or giant (>20 cm) congenital melanocytic nevi. In the same cohort study referred to above, Swerdlow, English & Qiao[114] estimated that patients with congenital melanocytic nevi >20 cm had a standardized morbidity ratio of 1224 for the development of melanoma. In a prospective study of 92 patients with large/giant congenital melanocytic nevi[120], three patients developed melanoma in extracutaneous sites (brain, CNS, retroperitoneum) during follow-up averaging 5.4 years. The latter authors calculated the cumulative 5-year life-table risk for melanoma to be 4.5%. The standardized morbidity ratio, which was calculated to be 239, was highly significant.

In a study of 289 patients with large congenital melanocytic nevi culled from the world literature[121], 34 patients (12%) developed primary cutaneous melanoma within their nevi. All of the patients developing these melanomas had congenital melanocytic nevi in an axial location, i.e. the head and neck and/or trunk. No melanomas were associated with an extremity or satellite congenital melanocytic nevus. The median age at diagnosis of melanoma was 4.6 years (range: birth to 52 years; average age: 13.2 years). Twenty-one patients developed primary melanomas in the CNS; all of the latter patients had neurocutaneous melanosis and large congenital melanocytic nevi in a posterior axial location. The median age at diagnosis was 3 years (range: 1 month to 50 years; average age: 11.6 years) for the latter group. An additional 10 patients presented with metastatic melanoma with unknown primary. All of the latter patients had axial congenital melanocytic nevi. A more recent study, based on a database of 1008 patients with large congenital melanocytic nevi or multiple medium-sized congenital melanocytic nevi, found a significantly lower risk than in previous publications: 2.9% developed cutaneous melanoma associated with 0.8% deaths.

When a cutaneous melanoma develops in a relatively small congenital melanocytic nevus, it appears most commonly at the dermal–epidermal junction in a fashion similar to that of other conventional melanomas. However, up to two-thirds of cutaneous melanomas arising in larger congenital melanocytic nevi develop in the dermis, subcutaneous fat, or deeper as a distinct nodule. Rarely, other malignant tumors may arise in these lesions, including neurogenic sarcomas, fibrosarcomas, leiomyosarcomas, rhabdomyosarcomas, osteogenic sarcomas and liposarcomas.

Leptomeningeal melanomas can arise in patients with neurocutaneous melanosis and most commonly involve the frontal and temporal lobes. As expected, these melanomas have a very poor prognosis.

Pathology

In contrast to common acquired nevi, which are confined to the papillary and upper reticular dermis, congenital nevi may exhibit infiltration of the lower reticular dermis, subcutaneous fat, fascia, and even deeper (Fig. 112.28). It is characteristic to observe nevus cells in a single-cell array throughout the middle or lower reticular dermis and even extending into the septa of the subcutis. Especially helpful is the presence of nevus cells surrounding (cuffing) and within the walls of blood vessels, within appendages such as hair follicles and sweat glands, and within cutaneous nerves, particularly when observed in the lower half of the reticular dermis. Nevus cells may be found in the papillae and epithelium of hair follicles, in the sebaceous glands, in arrector pili muscles, and in the eccrine ducts of the lower dermis. There is often diminished cellularity (or maturation) with depth in the dermis. Uncommonly, congenital melanocytic nevi may show striking neural differentiation suggesting a peripheral nerve sheath tumor such as a neurofibroma. Structures resembling Meissner's corpuscles, Verocay bodies, or neuroid tubules may be observed. Neurocutaneous melanosis is defined by the proliferation of benign 'melanotic cells' (a term used to avoid a more precise designation such as melanocyte or melanoblast) in the meninges. This melanosis may involve the convexities and base of the brain, the ventral surfaces of the pons, medulla, and upper cervical and lumbosacral spinal cord.

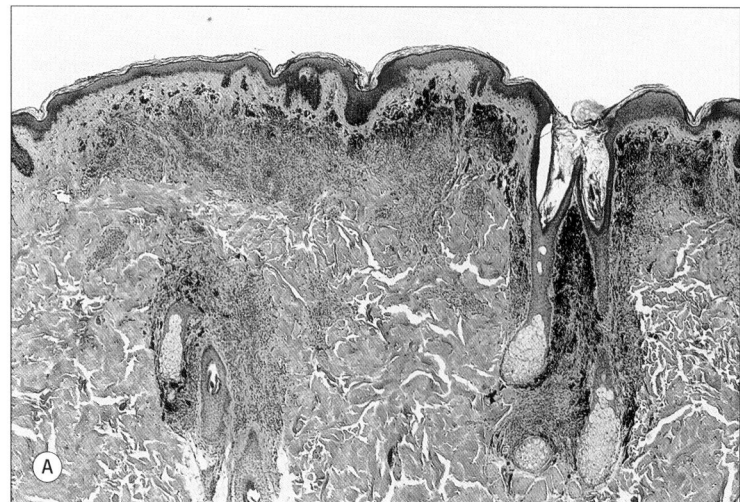

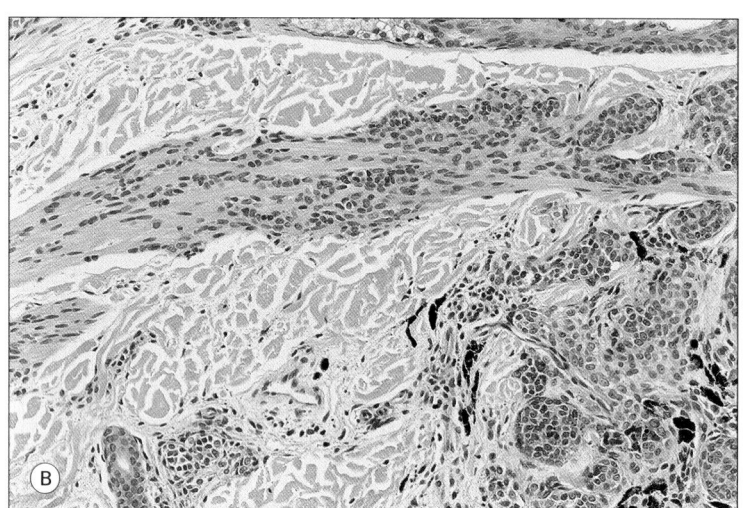

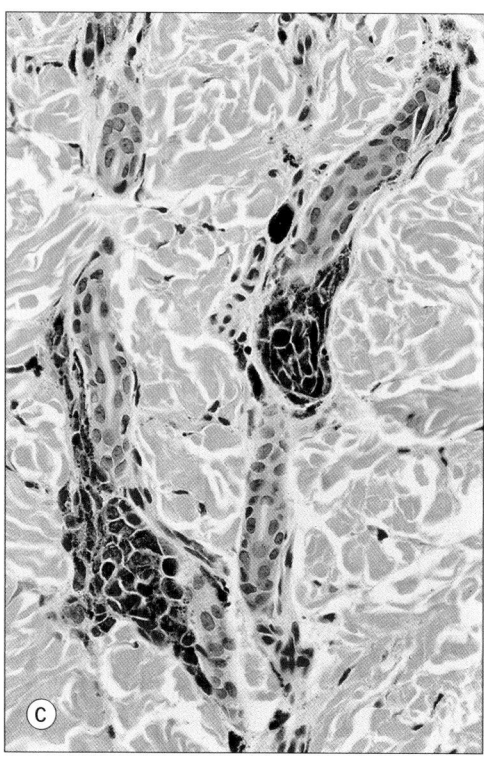

Fig. 112.28 Histology of a congenital melanocytic nevus. A Scanning view with nests extending down adnexal structures. **B** Melanocytes often extend in a single-file pattern and invade an arrector pili muscle here. **C** Melanocytes extending along sweat ducts. A–C, Courtesy of Ronald P Rapini MD.

Differential Diagnosis

Although giant congenital melanocytic nevi are quite distinctive, occasionally they are confused with plexiform neurofibromas as the latter can have both hyperpigmentation and hypertrichosis. The differential diagnosis of small congenital nevi includes congenital smooth muscle hamartoma, atypical nevus, and melanoma. For medium-sized congenital nevi, an additional entity to consider is Becker's melanosis. Of course, the possibility of melanoma exists for any clinically atypical area (e.g. darkening, nodularity) within a congenital nevus.

Treatment

The treatment of congenital melanocytic nevi is primarily related to two factors: their increased risk for progression to melanoma and their cosmetically disfiguring appearance. The decision to remove a congenital nevus is individualized and based on melanoma risk, age of the individual, anatomic location (proximity to vital structures), presence or absence of neurocutaneous melanosis, cosmetic outcome, and complexity of removal. The routine excision of uniform-appearing small- and medium-sized congenital nevi no longer seems justified, because of low melanoma risk. An acceptable alternative to surgical excision is baseline photography and yearly follow-up.

The treatment of giant congenital nevi is more problematic, since melanoma risk is present from birth. If such giant nevi are to be excised, most authorities recommend delaying the procedure for at least six months so as to decrease the risk from general anesthesia. Since the prognosis of patients with symptomatic neurocutaneous melanosis is so poor, surgical removal of large congenital melanocytic nevi should be delayed in such individuals. MRI of the CNS should be considered for neonatal patients with large posterior axial congenital melanocytic nevi and with multiple satellite nevi, in order to screen for neurocutaneous melanosis. For patients with asymptomatic neurocutaneous melanosis, repeat scans and individualized care is indicated.

In the past, dermabrasion was sometimes performed resulting in a more lightly pigmented and less elevated congenital nevus. More recently, especially in Europe, repeat curettage performed during the first few weeks of life (when there is a cleavage plane in the upper dermis) has led to similar results. Scarring and prolonged healing in the case of large lesions are the drawbacks.

As mentioned above, when melanoma supervenes in a large congenital nevus, it may involve the dermal or subcutaneous component and be difficult to detect early. Cutaneous melanoma arising in the smaller types of congenital melanocytic nevi usually begins in the epidermis and can be detected more readily.

REFERENCES

1. Bataille V, Snieder H, MacGregor AJ, Spector T. Genetics of risk factors for melanoma: an adult twin study of nevi and freckles. J Natl Cancer Inst. 2000;92:457–63.
2. McLean DI, Gallagher RP. 'Sunburn' freckles, café-au-lait macules, and other pigmented lesions of schoolchildren: the Vancouver Mole Study. J Am Acad Dermatol. 1995; 32:565–70.
3. Brues AM. Linkage of body build with sex, eye color and freckling. Am J Hum Genet. 1950;2:215–39.
4. Bliss JM, Ford D, Swerdlow AJ, et al. Risk of cutaneous melanoma associated with pigmentation characteristics and freckling: systematic overview of 10 case-control studies. Int J Cancer. 1995;62:367–76.
5. Rhodes AR, Albert LS, Barnhill RL, Weinstock MA. Sun-induced freckles in children and young adults: a correlation of clinical and histopathologic features. Cancer. 1991;67:1990–2001.

6. Breathnach AS. Melanocyte distribution in forearm epidermis of freckled human subjects. J Invest Dermatol. 1957;29:253–61.
7. Landau M, Krafchik BR. The diagnostic value of café-au-lait macules. J Am Acad Dermatol. 1999;40:877–90.
8. Nakagawa H, Hori Y, Sato S, Fitzpatrick TB, Martuza RL. The nature and origin of the melanin macroglobule. J Invest Dermatol. 1983;83:134–9.
9. Korf BR. Diagnostic outcome in children with multiple café au lait spots. Pediatrics. 1992;90:924–7.
10. Sigg C, Pelloni F, Schnyder UW. Frequency of congenital nevi, nevi spili and café-au-lait spots and their relation to nevus count and skin complexion in 939 children. Dermatologica. 1990;180:18–23.
11. Rieger E, Kofler R, Borkenstein M, et al. Melanotic macules following Blaschko's lines in McCune-Albright syndrome. Br J Dermatol. 1994;130:215–20.
12. Jimbow K, Szabo G, Fitzpatrick TB. Ultrastructure of giant pigment granules (macromelanosomes) in the cutaneous pigmented macules of neurofibromatosis. J Invest Dermatol. 1973;61:300–9.
13. Silvers DN, Greenwood RS, Helwig EB. Café-au-lait spots without giant pigment granules: occurrence in suspected neurofibromatosis. Arch Dermatol. 1974;110:87–8.
14. Carpo GB, Grevelink JM, Grevelink SV. Laser treatment of pigmented lesions in children. Semin Cutan Med Surg. 1999;18:233–43.
15. Goldberg DJ. Laser treatment of pigmented lesions. Dermatol Clin. 1997;15:397–407.
16. Cohen PR. Becker's nevus. Am Fam Physician. 1988;37:221–6.
17. Danari R, Konig A, Salhi A, Bittar M, Happle R Becker's nevus syndrome revisited. J Am Acad Dermatol. 2004:51:965–9.
18. Glinick SE, Alper JC, Bogaars H, Brown JA. Becker's melanosis: associated abnormalities. J Am Acad Dermatol. 1983;9:509–14.
19. Tse Y, Levine VJ, McClain SA, Ashinoff R. The removal of cutaneous pigmented lesions with the Q-switched ruby laser and the Q-switched Nd:YAG laser: a comparative study. J Dermatol Surg Oncol. 1994;20:795–800.
20. Rhodes AR, Harrist TJ, Momtaz TK. The PUVA-induced pigmented macule: a lentiginous proliferation of large, sometimes cytologically atypical, melanocytes. J Am Acad Dermatol. 1983;9:47–58.
21. Todd MM, Rallis TM, Gerwels JW, Itata TR. A comparison of three lasers and liquid nitrogen in the treatment of solar lentigines. Arch Dermatol. 2000;136:841–6.
22. Wang SQ, Rabinovitz H, Oliviero MC. Dermoscopic patterns of solar lentigines and seborrheic keratosis. In: Marghoob AA, Braun B, Kopf AW (eds). Atlas of Dermoscopy. London: Taylor & Francis, 2005:60–71.
23. Barnhill RL, Albert LS, Shama SK, et al. Genital lentiginosis: a clinical and histopathologic study. J Am Acad Dermatol. 1990;22:453–6.
24. Cordova A. The Mongolian spot. Clin Pediatr. 1981;20:714–19.
25. Kikuchi I. The biological significance of the Mongolian spot. Int J Dermatol. 1989;28:513–14.
26. Gilchrest BA, Fitzpatrick TB, Anderson RR, Parrish JA. Localization of melanin pigmentation in the skin with Wood's lamp. Br J Dermatol. 1977;96:245–8.
27. Patel BC, Egan CA, Lucius RW, et al. Cutaneous malignant melanoma and oculodermal melanocytosis (nevus of Ota): report of a case and review of the literature. J Am Acad Dermatol. 1998;38:862–5.
28. Balmaceda CM, Fetell RM, O'Brien JL, Housepian EH. Nevus of Ota and leptomeningeal melanocytic lesions. Neurology. 1993;43:381–6.
29. Teekhasaenee C, Ritch R, Rutnin U, Leelawongs N. Ocular findings in oculodermal melanocytosis. Arch Ophthalmol. 1990;108:1114–20.
30. Chan HH, Leung RS, Ying SY, et al. A retrospective analysis of complications in the treatment of nevus of Ota with the Q-switched alexandrite and Q-switched Nd:YAG lasers. Dermatol Surg. 2000;26:1000–6.
31. Chan HH, Ying SY, Ho WS, et al. An in vivo trial comparing the clinical efficacy and complications of Q-switched 755 nm alexandrite and Q-switched 1064 nm Nd:YAG lasers in the treatment of nevus of Ota. Dermatol Surg. 2000;26:919–22.
32. Goldenhersh MA, Savin RC, Barnhill RL, Stenn KS. Malignant blue nevus. J Am Acad Dermatol. 1988;19:712–22.
33. Gonzalez-Campora R, Galera-Davidson H, Vazquez-Ramirez FJ, Diaz-Cano S. Blue nevus: classical types and related entities. A differential diagnostic review. Pathol Res Pract. 1994;190:627–35.
34. Hendricks WM. Eruptive blue nevi. J Am Acad Dermatol. 1981;4:50–3.
35. Hendrickson MR, Ross JC. Neoplasms arising in congenital giant nevi. Am J Surg Pathol. 1981;5:109–35.
36. Lambert WC, Brodkin RH. Nodal and subcutaneous cellular blue nevi: a pseudometastasizing pseudomelanoma. Arch Dermatol. 1984;120:367–70.
37. Temple-Camp CR, Saxe N, King H. Benign and malignant cellular blue nevus: a clinicopathological study of 30 cases. Am J Dermatopathol. 1988;10:289–96.
38. Tran TA, Carlson JA, Barsaca PC, Mihm MC. Cellular blue nevus with atypia (atypical cellular blue nevus): a clinicopathologic study of nine cases. J Cutan Pathol. 1998;25:252–8.
39. Maize JC, Foster G. Age-related changes in melanocytic naevi. Clin Exp Dermatol. 1979;4:49–58.
40. Armstrong BK, English DR. The epidemiology of acquired melanocytic naevi and their relationship to malignant melanoma. In: Elwood JM (ed.). Melanoma and Naevi. Basel: Karger, 1988:27–47.
41. Clark WH Jr, Hood AF, Tucker MA, Jampel RM. Atypical melanocytic nevi of the genital type with a discussion of reciprocal parenchymal-stromal interactions in the biology of neoplasia. Hum Pathol. 1998;29:S1–S24.
42. Rongioletti F, Ball RA, Marcus R, Barnhill RL. Histopathological features of flexural melanocytic nevi: a study of 40 cases. J Cutan Pathol. 2000;27:215–17.
43. McCalmont TH, Brinsko R, LeBoit PE. Melanocytic acral nevi with intraepidermal ascent of cells (MANIACs): a reappraisal of melanocytic lesions from acral sites. J Cutan Pathol. 1991;18:378.
44. Grin, CM, Saida, T. Pigmented nevi of the palms and soles. In: Marghoob AA, Braun B, Kopf AW (eds). Atlas of Dermoscopy. London: Taylor & Francis, 2005:271–9.
45. Boyd AS, Rapini RP. Acral melanocytic neoplasms: a histologic analysis of 158 lesions. J Am Acad Dermatol. 1994;31:740–5.
46. Nguyen KQ, Pierson DL, Rodman OG. Mosaic speckled lentiginous nevi. Cutis. 1982;30:65–8.
47. Rhodes AR. Neoplasms: benign neoplasias, hyperplasias, and dysplasias of melanocytes. In: Fitzpatrick TB, Eisen AZ, Wolff K, Freedburg IM, Austen KF (eds). Dermatology in General Medicine, 4th edn. New York: McGraw-Hill, 1993:996–1077.
48. Cohen HJ, Minkin W, Frank SB. Nevus spilus. Arch Dematol. 1970;102:433–7.
49. Falo LD, Sober AJ, Barnhill RL. Evolution of nevus spilus. Dermatology. 1994;189:382–3.
50. Rhodes AR, Mihm MC Jr. Origin of cutaneous melanoma in a congenital dysplastic nevus spilus. Arch Dermatol. 1990;29:500–5.
51. Weinberg JM, Schutzer PJ, Harris RM, et al. Melanoma arising in nevus spilus. Cutis. 1998;61:287–9.
52. Park HK, Leonard DD, Arrington JH 3rd, Lund HZ. Recurrent melanocytic nevi: clinical and histologic review of 175 cases. J Am Acad Dermatol. 1987;17:285–92.
53. Bastian BC, Wesselmann U, Pinkel D, Leboit PE. Molecular cytogenetic analysis of Spitz tumors shows clear differences to melanoma. J Invest Dermatol. 1999;113:1065–9.
54. Dawe RS, Wainwright NJ, Evans AT, Lowe JG. Multiple widespread eruptive Spitz naevi. Br J Dermatol. 1998;138:872–4.
55. Duvic M, Lowe L, Rapini RP, et al. Eruptive dysplastic nevi associated with human immunodeficiency virus infection. Arch Dermatol. 1989;125:397–401.
56. Lancer H, Muhlbauer JE, Sober AJ. Multiple agminated spindle cell nevi: unique clinical presentation and review. J Am Acad Dermatol. 1983;8:707–11.
57. Schaffer JV, Bolognia JL. The clinical spectrum of pigmented lesions. Clin Plast Surg. 2000;27:391–408, viii.
58. Spatz A, Calonje E, Handfield-Jones S, Barnhill RL. Spitz tumors in children: a grading system for risk stratification. Arch Dermatol. 1999;135:282–9.
59. Spatz A, Peterse S, Fletcher CDM, Barnhill RL. Plexiform Spitz nevus/tumor: an intradermal Spitz nevus/tumor with plexiform growth pattern. Am J Dermatopathol. 1999;21:542–6.
60. Spitz S. Melanomas of childhood. Am J Pathol. 1948;24:591–609.
61. Barnhill RL, Mihm MC Jr. The pigmented spindle cell naevus and its variants: distinction from melanoma. Br J Dermatol. 1989;121:717–25.
62. Barnhill RL, Barnhill MA, Berwick M, Mihm MC Jr. The histologic spectrum of pigmented spindle cell nevus: a review of 120 cases with emphasis on atypical variants. Hum Pathol. 1991;22:52–8.
63. Ackerman AB, Mihara L. Dysplasia, dysplastic melanocytes, dysplastic nevi, the dysplastic nevus syndrome, and the relation between dysplastic nevi and malignant melanomas. Hum Pathol. 1985;16:87–91.
64. Bale SJ, Dracopoli NC, Tucker MA, et al. Mapping the gene for hereditary cutaneous malignant melanoma-dysplastic nevus to chromosome 1p. N Engl J Med. 1989;320:1367–72.
64a. Roush GC, Nordlund JJ, Forget B, et al. Independence of dysplastic nevi from total nevi in determining risk for nonfamilial melanoma. Prev Med. 1988;17:273–9.
64b. Nordlund JJ, Kirkwood J, Forget BM, et al. Demographic study of clinically atypical (dysplastic) nevi in patients with melanoma and comparison subjects. Cancer Res. 1985;45:1855–61.
64c. MacKie RM, Freudenberger T, Aitchison TC. Personal risk-factor chart for cutaneous melanoma. Lancet. 1989;2:487–90.
64d. Holly EA, Kelly JW, Shpall SN, Chiu SH. Number of melanocytic nevi as a major risk factor for malignant melanoma. J Am Acad Dermatol. 1987;17:459–68.
64e. Halpern AC, Guerry D 4th, Elder DE, et al. Dysplastic nevi as risk markers of sporadic (nonfamilial) melanoma. A case-control study. Arch Dermatol. 1991;127:995–9.
65. Bale SJ, Chakravarti A, Greene MH. Cutaneous malignant melanoma and familial dysplastic nevi: evidence for autosomal domination and pleiotropy. Am J Hum Genet. 1986;38:188–96.
66. Barnhill RL. Current status of the dysplastic melanocytic nevus. J Cutan Pathol. 1991;18:147–59.
67. Barnhill RL, Roush GC. Correlation of clinical and histopathologic features in clinically atypical melanocytic nevi. Cancer. 1991;67:3157–64.
68. Clark WH Jr, Elder DE, Guerry D 4th, et al. A study of tumor progression: the precursor lesions of superficial spreading and nodular melanoma. Hum Pathol. 1984;15:1147–65.
69. Clark WH Jr, Reimer RR, Greene M, et al. Origin of familial malignant melanomas from heritable melanocytic lesions. 'The B-K mole syndrome.' Arch Dermatol. 1978;114:732–8.
70. Clemente C, Cochran AJ, Elder DE, et al. Histopathologic diagnosis of dysplastic nevi: concordance among pathologists convened by the World Health Organization Melanoma Programme. Hum Pathol. 1991;22:313–19.
71. Elder DE, Goldman LI, Goldman SC, et al. Dysplastic nevus syndrome: a phenotypic association of sporadic cutaneous melanoma. Cancer. 1980; 46:1787–94.
72. Friedman RJ, Heilman ER, Rigel DS, Kopf AW. The dysplastic nevus: clinical and pathologic features. Dermatol Clin. 1985;3:239–49.
73. Greene MH, Clark WH Jr, Tucker MA, et al. High risk of malignant melanoma in melanoma-prone families with dysplastic nevi. Ann Intern Med. 1985;102:458–65.
74. Crutcher WA, Sagebiel RW. Clinical diagnosis of dysplastic melanocytic nevi. J Am Acad Dermatol. 1986;14:1044–52.
75. Kraemer KH, Greene MH, Tarone R, et al. Dysplastic nevi and cutaneous melanoma risk. Lancet. 1983;2:1076–7.
76. Piepkorn M, Meyer LJ, Goldgar D, et al. The dysplastic melanocytic nevus: a prevalent lesion that correlates poorly with clinical phenotype. J Am Acad Dermatol. 1989;20:407–15.
77. Rhodes AR, Harrist TJ, Day CL, et al. Dysplastic melanocytic nevi in histologic association with 234 primary cutaneous melanomas. J Am Acad Dermatol. 1983;9:563–74.
78. van Haeringen A, Bergman W, Nelan MR, et al. Exclusion of the dysplastic nevus syndrome (DNS) locus from the short arm of chromosome 1 by linkage studies in Dutch families. Genomics. 1989;5:61–4.
79. Weinstock MA, Barnhill RL, Rhodes AR, et al. Reliability of the histopathologic diagnosis of melanocytic dysplasia. Arch Dermatol. 1997;133:953–8.
80. Roush GC, Barnhill RL, Duray PH, et al. Diagnosis of the dysplastic nevus in different populations. J Am Acad Dermatol. 1986;14:419–25.
81. Barnhill RL, Roush GC, Titus-Ernstoff L, et al. Comparison of nonfamilial and familial melanoma. Dermatology. 1992;184:2–7.
82. Duray PH, DerSimonian R, Barnhill RL, et al. An analysis of interobserver recognition of the histopathologic features of dysplastic nevi from a mixed group of nevomelanocytic lesions. J Am Acad Dermatol. 1992; 27:741–9.

83. Mihm MC Jr, Barnhill RL, Sober AJ, Hernandez MH. Precursor lesions of melanoma: do they exist? Semin Surg Oncol. 1992;8:358–65.

84. Sober AJ, Kang S, Barnhill RL. Discerning individuals at elevated risk for cutaneous melanoma. Clin Dermatol. 1992;10:15–20.

85. Barnhill RL. Melanocytic nevi and tumor progression: perspectives concerning histomorphology, melanoma risk, and molecular genetics. Dermatology. 1993;187:86–90.

86. Duncan LM, Berwick MA, Bruijn JA, et al. Histopathologic recognition and grading of dysplastic melanocytic nevi: an inter-observer agreement study. J Invest Dermatol. 1993;100(suppl.);318S–21S.

87. Kenet RO, Kang S, Kenet BJ, et al. Clinical diagnosis of pigmented lesions using digital epiluminescence microscopy: grading protocol and atlas. Arch Dermatol 1993;129:157–74.

88. Roush GC, Dubin N, Barnhill RL. Prediction of histologic melanocytic dysplasia from clinical observation. J Am Acad Dermatol. 1993;29:555–62.

89. Titus-Ernstoff L, Barnhill RL, Duray PH, et al. Dysplastic nevi in relation to superficial spreading melanoma. Cancer Epidemiol Biomarkers Prev. 1993;2:99–101.

90. Kang S, Barnhill RL, Mihm MC Jr, et al. Melanoma risk in individuals with clinically atypical nevi. Arch Dermatol. 1994;130:999–1001.

91. Piepkorn MW, Barnhill RL, Cannon-Albright LA, et al. A multiobserver, population-based analysis of histologic dysplasia in melanocytic nevi. J Am Acad Dermatol. 1994;30:707–14.

92. Schmidt B, Hollister K, Weinberg D, Barnhill RL. Analysis of melanocytic lesions by DNA image cytometry. Cancer. 1994;73:2971–7.

93. Titus-Ernstoff L, Duray PH, Ernstoff MS, et al. Dysplastic nevi in association with multiple primary melanoma. Cancer Res. 1988;48:1016–18.

94. Gruber SB, Barnhill RL, Stenn KS, Roush GC. Nevomelanocytic proliferations in association with cutaneous malignant melanoma: a multivariate analysis. J Am Acad Dermatol. 1989;21:773–80.

95. Barnhill RL, Roush GC. Histopathologic spectrum of clinically atypical melanocytic nevi: studies of nonfamilial melanoma, II. Arch Dermatol. 1990;126:1315–18.

96. Barnhill RL, Roush GC, Duray PH. Correlation of histologic architectural and cytoplastic features with nuclear atypia in atypical (dysplastic) nevomelanocytic nevi. Hum Pathol. 1990;21:51–8.

97. Barnhill RL, Kiryu H, Sober AJ, Mihm MC Jr. Frequency of dysplastic nevi among nevomelanocytic lesions submitted for histopathologic examination: time trends over a 37-year period. Arch Dermatol. 1990;126:463–5.

98. Annesi G, Cattaruzza MS, Abeni D. Correlation between clinical atypia and histologic dysplasia in acquired melanocytic nevi. J Am Acad Dermatol. 2001;45:77–85.

99. Blessing K. Benign atypical naevi: diagnostic difficulties and continued controversy. Histopathology. 1999;34:189–98.

100. Shea CR, Vollmer RT, Prieto VG. Correlating architectural disorder and cytological atypia in Clark (dysplastic) melanocytic nevi. Hum Pathol. 1999;30:500–5.

101. Pozo L, Naase M, Cerio R, et al. Critical analysis of histologic criteria for grading atypical (dysplastic) melanocytic nevi. Am J Clin Pathol. 2001;115:194–204.

102. Slade J, Marghoob AA, Salopek TG, et al. Atypical mole syndrome: risk factor for cutaneous malignant melanoma and implications for treatment. J Am Acad Dermatol. 1995;32:479–94.

103. Garbe C, Buttner P, Weiss J, et al. Risk factors for developing cutaneous melanoma and criteria for identifying persons at risk: multicenter case-control study of the central malignant melanoma registry of the German Dermatological Society. J Invest Dermatol. 1994;102:695–9.

104. Garbe C, Buttner P, Weiss J, et al. Associated factors in the prevalence of more than 50 common melanocytic nevi, atypical melanocytic nevi, and actinic lentigines: multicenter case-control study of the central malignant melanoma registry of the German Dermatological Society. J Invest Dermatol. 1994;102:700–5.

105. Marghoob AA, Kopf AW, Rigel DS, et al. Risk of cutaneous malignant melanoma in patients with 'classic' atypical-mole syndrome: a case-control study. Arch Dermatol. 1994;130:993–8.

106. Hoffman-Wellenhof R, Blum A, Wolf IH, et al. Dermoscopic classification of atypical melanocytic nevi. Arch Dermatol. 1992;137:1575–80.

107. Castilla EE, da Graca Dutra M, Orioli-Parreiras IM. Epidemiology of congenital pigmented naevi: incidence rates and relative frequencies. Br J Dermatol. 1981;104:307–15.

108. Everett MA. Histopathology of congenital pigmented nevi. Am J Dermatopathol. 1989;1:11–12.

109. Illig L, Weidner F, Hundeiker M, et al. Congenital nevi less than or equal to 10 cm as precursors to melanoma. Arch Dermatol. 1985;121:1274–81.

110. Lanier VC, Pickrell KL, Georgiade NG. Congenital giant nevi: clinical and pathological considerations. Plast Reconstr Surg. 1976;58:48–54.

111. Lorentzen M, Pers M, Bretteville-Jensen G. The incidence of malignant transformation in giant pigmented nevi. Scand J Plast Reconstr Surg. 1977;71:163–7.

112. Rhodes AR. Congenital nevomelanocytic nevi: histologic patterns in the first year of life and evolution during childhood. Arch Dermatol. 1986; 122:1257–62.

113. Rhodes AR, Sober AJ, Day CL, et al. The malignant potential of small congenital nevocellular nevi: an estimate of association based on a histologic study of 234 primary cutaneous melanomas. J Am Acad Dermatol. 1982;6:230–41.

114. Swerdlow AJ, English JSC, Qiao Z. The risk of melanoma in patients with congenital nevi: a cohort study. J Am Acad Dermatol. 1995;32:595–9.

115. Shpall S, Frieden I, Chesney M, Newman T. Risk of malignant transformation of congenital melanocytic nevi in blacks. Pediatr Dermatol. 1994;11:204–8.

116. Barnhill RL, Aguiar M, Cohen C, et al. Congenital melanocytic nevi and DNA content: an analysis by flow and image cytometry. Cancer. 1994;74:2935–43.

117. Bouffard D, Barnhill RL, Mihm MC Jr, Sober AJ. Very late metastasis (27 years) of cutaneous malignant melanoma arising in a halo giant congenital nevus. Dermatology. 1994;189:162–6.

118. Barnhill RL, Fleischli M. Pathology of congenital melanocytic nevi in infants less than a year of age. J Am Acad Dermatol. 1995;33:780–5.

119. Sahin S, Levin L, Kopf AW, et al. Risk of melanoma in medium-sized congenital melanocytic nevi: a follow-up study. J Am Acad Dermatol. 1998;39:428–33.

120. Marghoob AA, Schoenbach SP, Kopf AW, et al. Large congenital melanocytic nevi and the risk for the development of malignant melanoma. A prospective study. Arch Dermatol. 1996;132:170–5.

121. DeDavid M, Orlow SJ, Provost N, et al. A study of large congenital melanocytic nevi and associated malignant melanomas: review of cases in the New York University Registry and the world literature. J Am Acad Dermatol. 1997;36:409–15.

122. Dawson HA, Atherton DJ, Mayou B. A prospective study of congenital melanocytic naevi: progress report and evaluation after 6 years. Br J Dermatol. 1996;134:617–23.

123. DeDavid M, Seth JO, Provost N, et al. Neurocutaneous melanosis: clinical features of large congenital melanocytic nevi in patients with manifest central nervous system melanosis. J Am Acad Dermatol. 1996;35:529–38.

124. Kadonaga JN, Frieden IJ. Neurocutaneous melanosis: definition and review of the literature. J Am Acad Dermatol. 1991;24:747–55.

125. Agero ALC, Benvenuto-Andrade C, Dusza SW, et al. Asymptomatic neurocutaneous melanocytosis in patients with large congenital melanocytic nevi: a study of cases from an Internet-based registry. J Am Acad Dermatol. 2005;53:959–65.

126. Bett BJ. Large or multiple congenital melanocytic nevi: occurrence of cutaneous melanoma in 1008 persons. J Am Acad Dermatol. 2005;52:793–7.

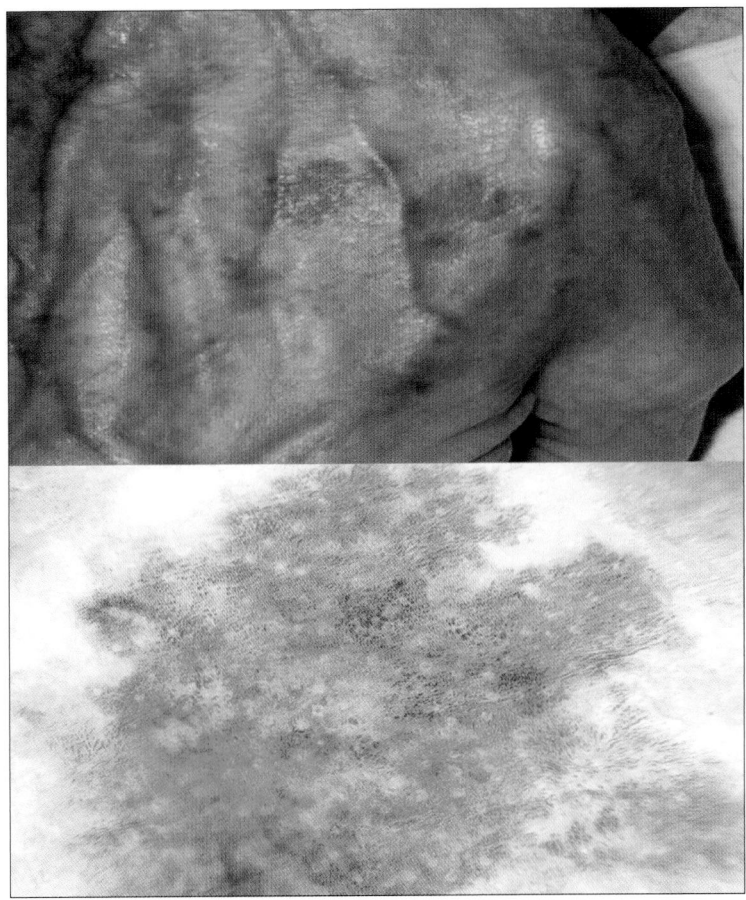

Fig. P1 Solar lentigines. Sharply demarcated, uniform, tan macules on sun-exposed skin. Dermoscopically, moth-eaten borders, fingerprinting, and a reticular pattern with thin lines, short and interrupted

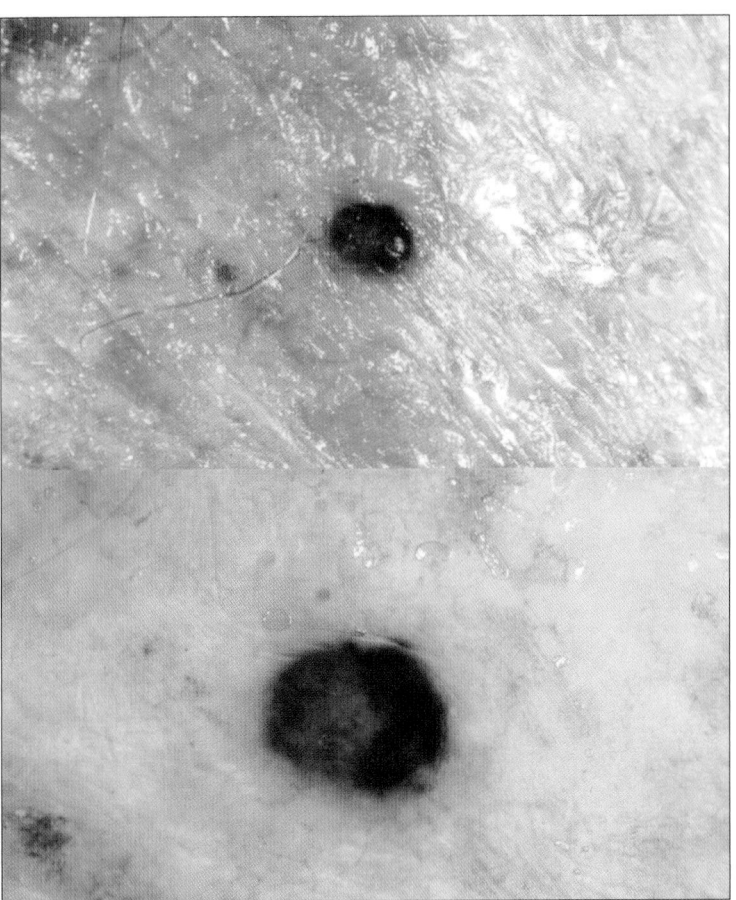

Fig. P2 Common blue nevus. A well-circumscribed, small, blue, dome-shaped papule on the dorsum of the hand. Dermoscopically, a homogeneous blue–gray to blue–black pigmentation.

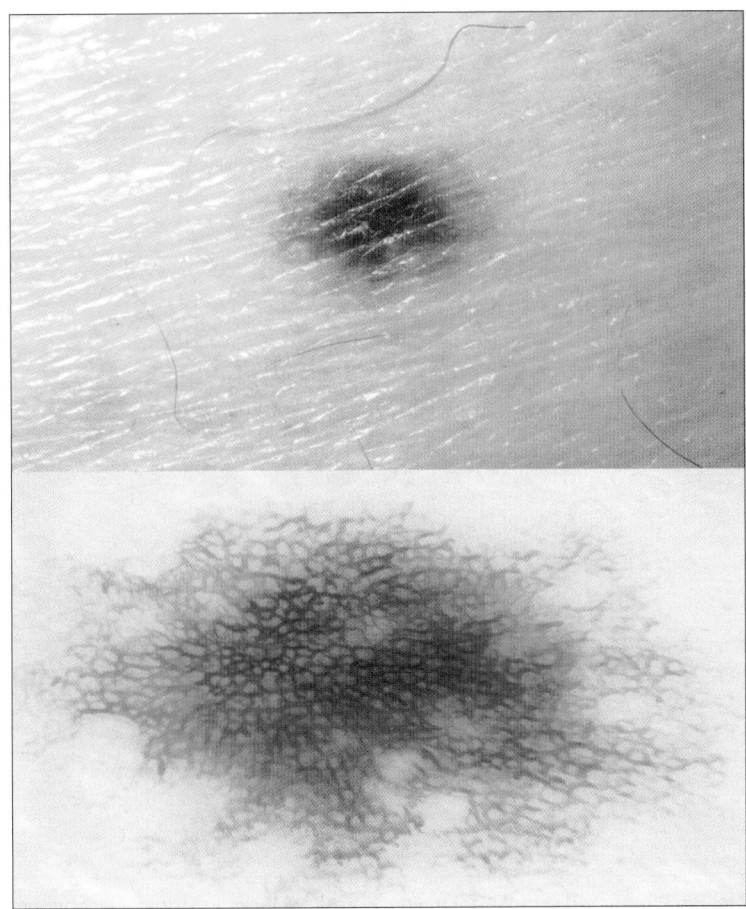

Fig. P3 Junctional nevus. Clinically, a brown macule with central hyperpigmentation. Dermoscopically, a uniform pigment network.

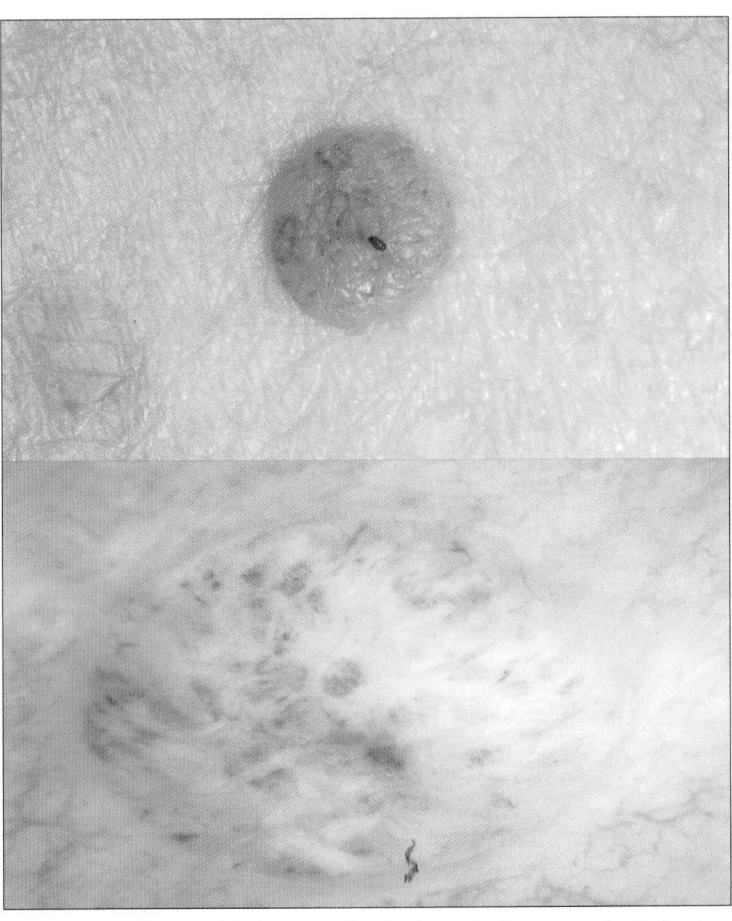

Fig. P4 Dermal nevus. A light tan, soft, raised papule. Dermoscopically, focal globular-like structures, whitish structureless areas, and fine comma vessels.

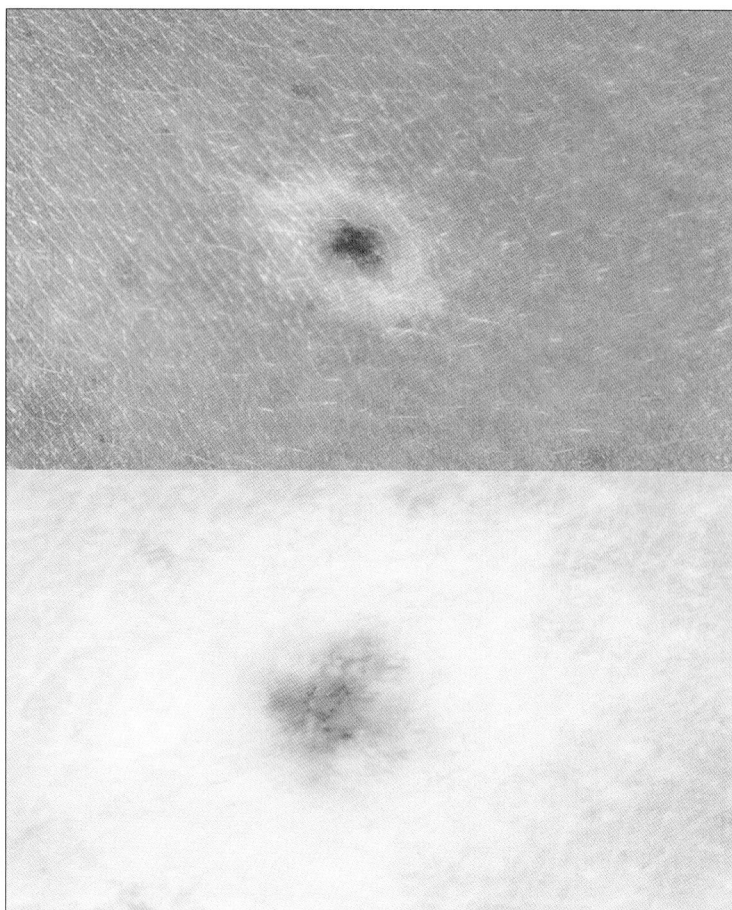

Fig. P5 Halo nevus. A depigmented macular halo surrounding a central dark brown papule. Dermoscopically, a symmetric white structureless area surrounding the remaining network of the nevus.

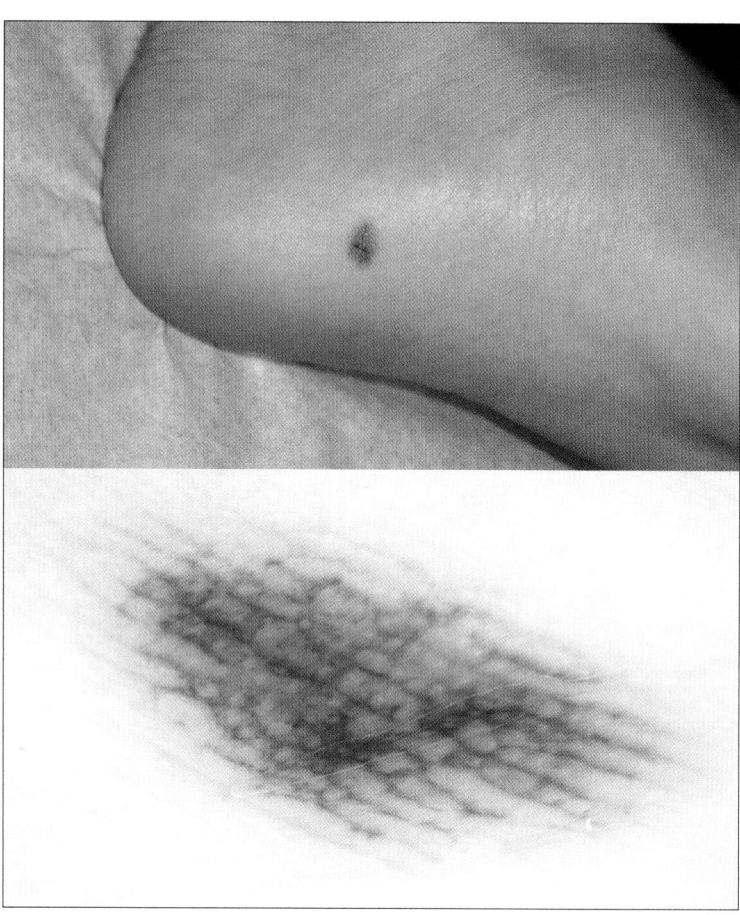

Fig. P6 Melanocytic nevus of acral skin. A brown macule on the sole of the foot. Dermoscopically, a lattice-like pattern.

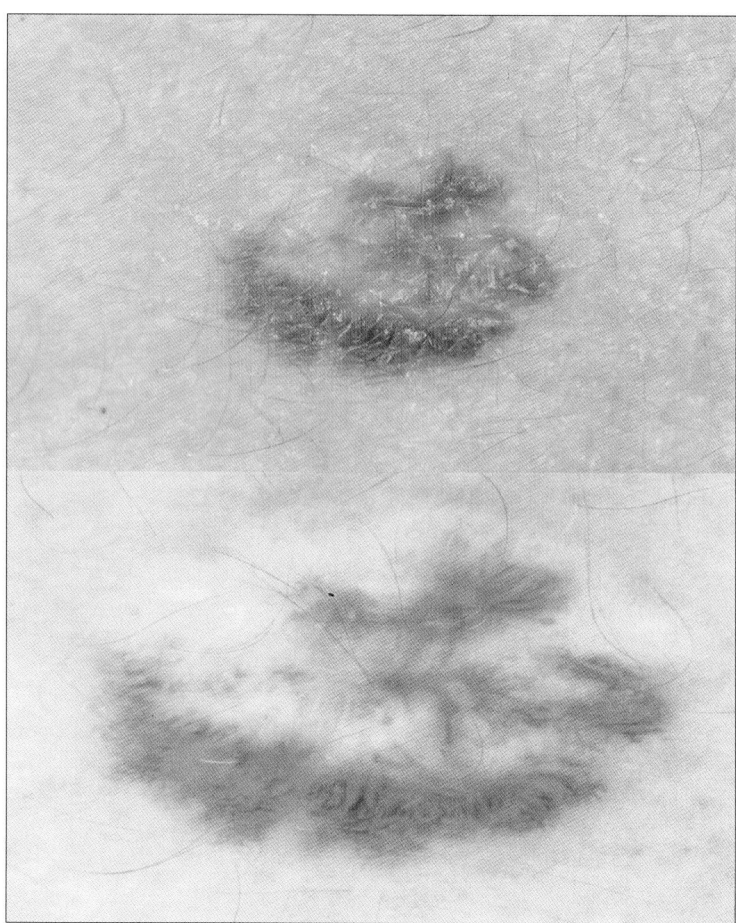

Fig. P7 Recurrent melanocytic nevus. A brown papule with areas of scarring. Dermoscopically, asymmetric pigmentation within the confines of the scar.

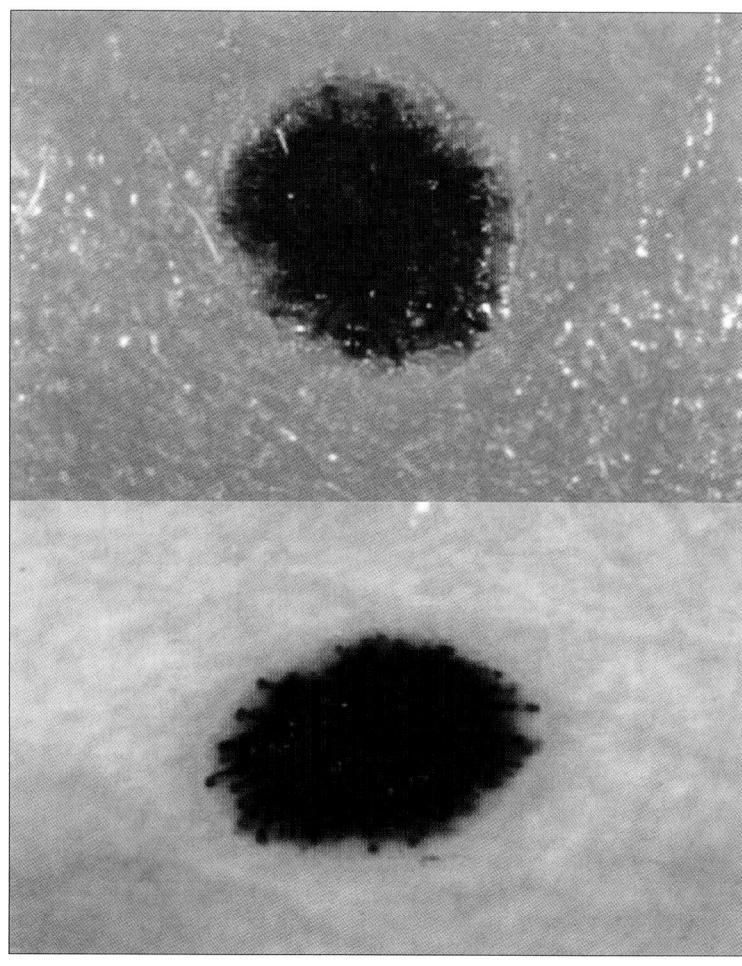

Fig. P8 Pigmented spindle cell nevus. A small, well-circumscribed, dark brown to black papule. Dermoscopically, a central dark structureless area with symmetric pseudopods.

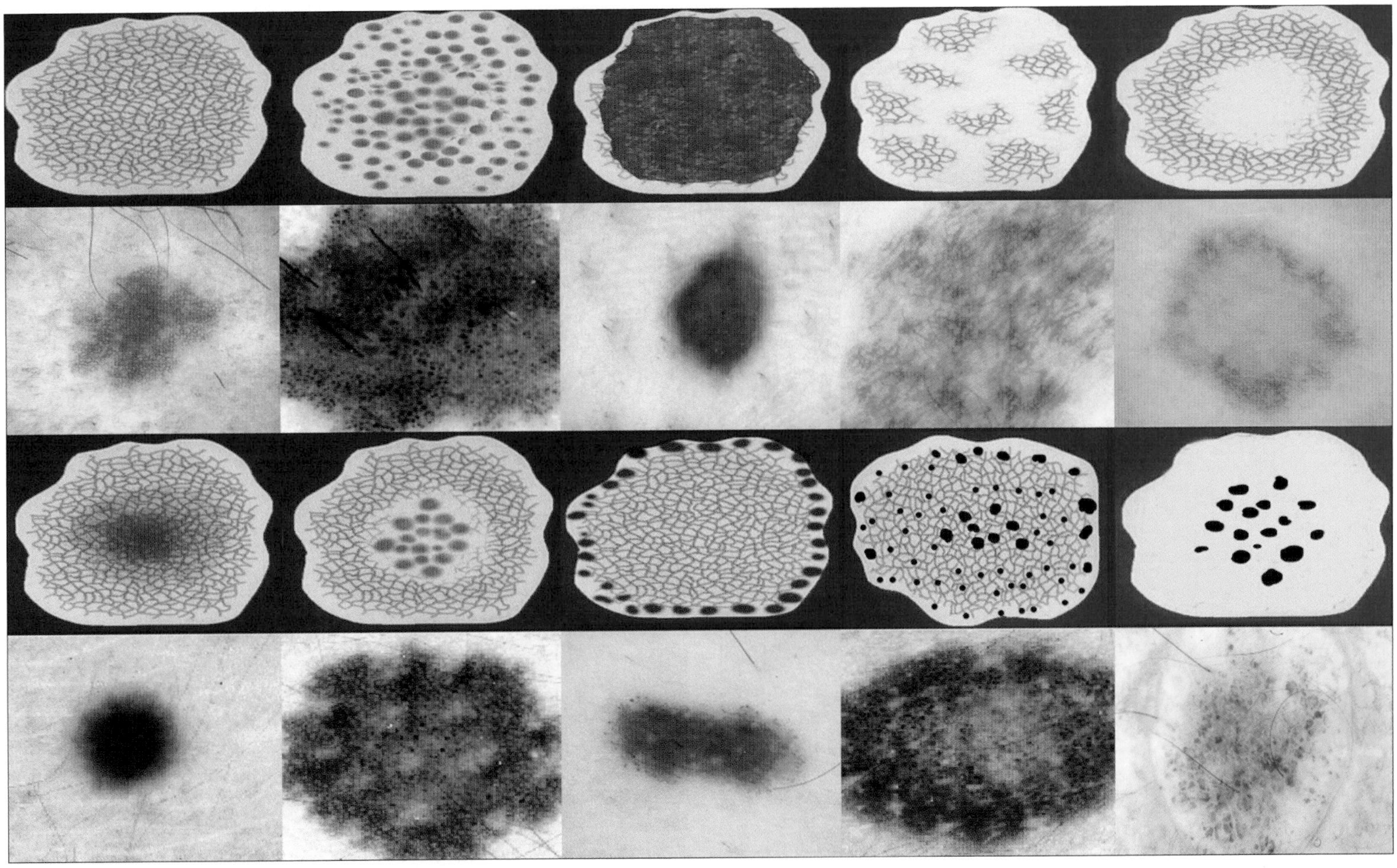

Fig. P9 Atypical melanocytic nevi with dermoscopic patterns commonly seen in benign melanocyic nevi. Courtesy of the AAD dermoscopy group.

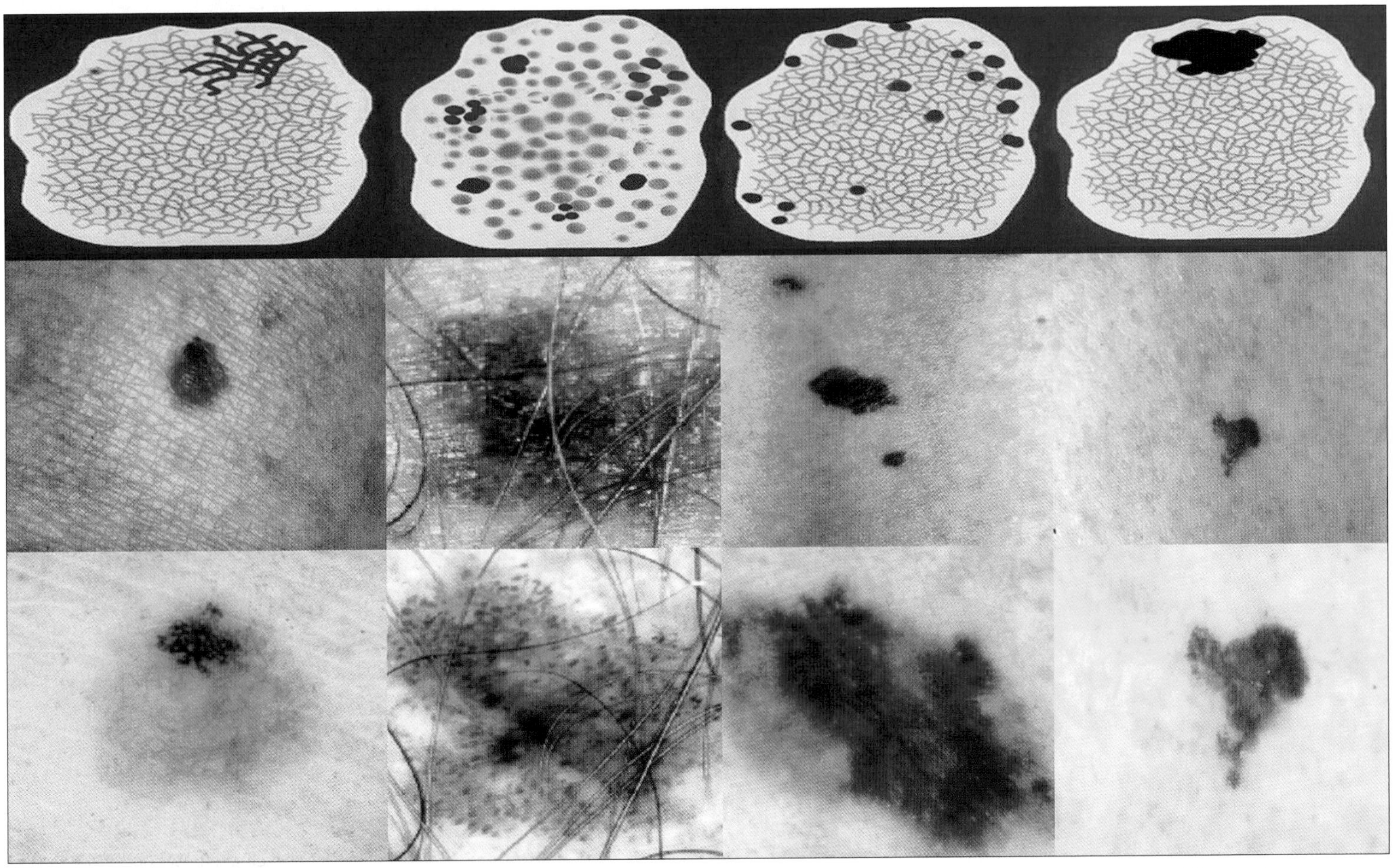

Fig. P10 Atypical melanocytic nevi with dermoscopic patterns often associated with melanoma. From top to bottom, schematic, normal illumination, and dermoscopy. Courtesy of the AAD dermoscopy group.

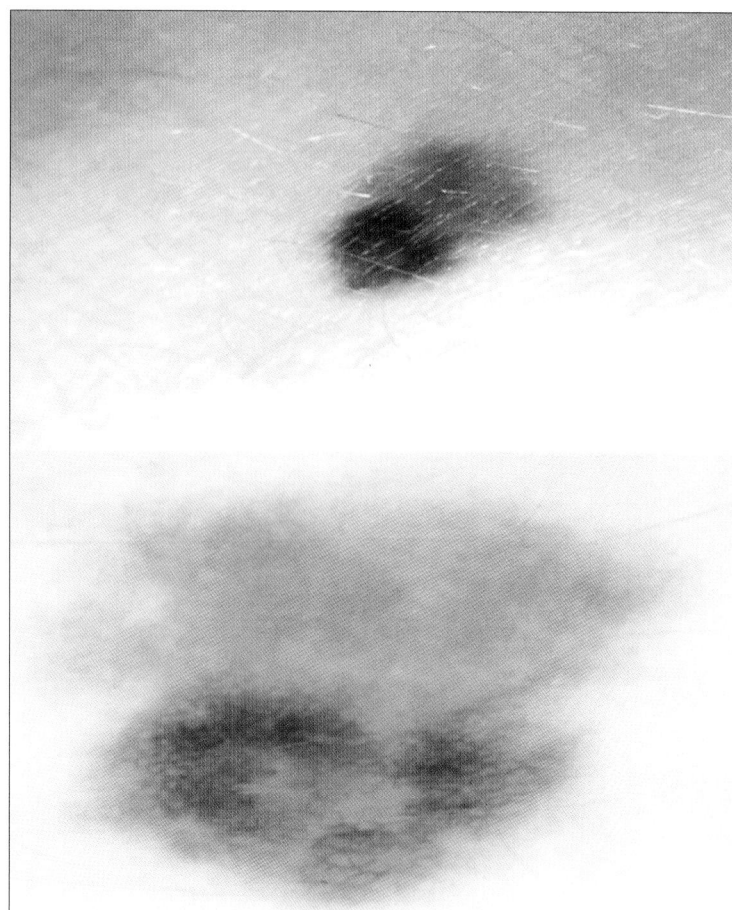

Fig. P11 Clinically atypical melanocytic nevus. The two-component dermoscopy pattern is seen with uncertain lesions.

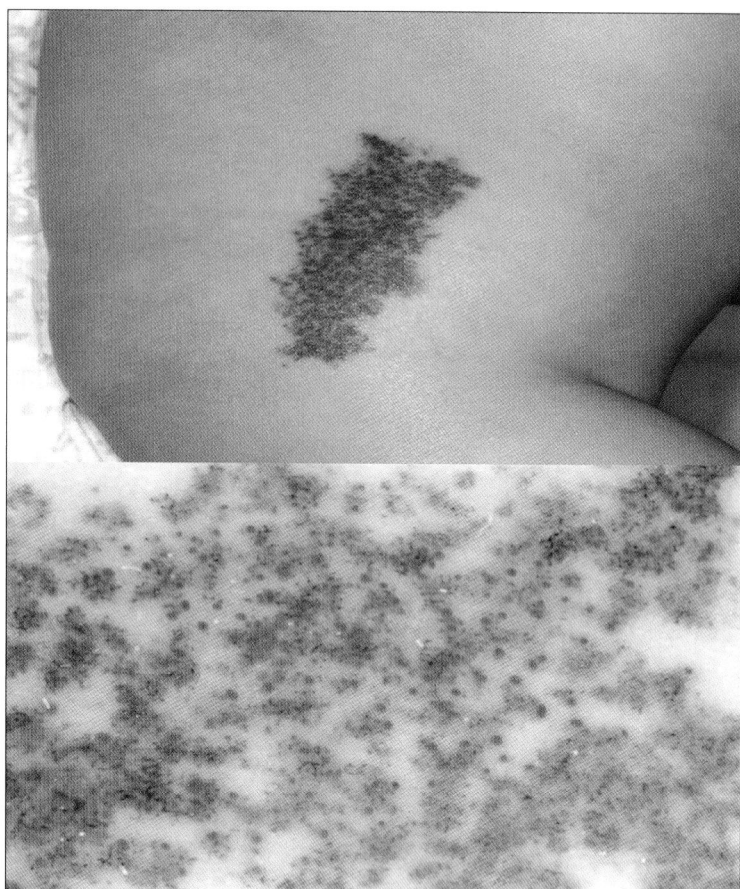

Fig. P12 Medium-sized congenital nevus. Dermoscopically, a globular pattern with hyphae-like structures.

Melanoma

Frank O Nestle and Allan C Halpern

113

Key features

- Melanoma is a malignant tumor arising from melanocytes
- The incidence and mortality rates of melanoma have been increasing in recent decades
- Death from melanoma occurs at a younger age than for other solid tumors
- Early detection is an important goal in melanoma management
- Appropriate surgical treatment of low-risk melanoma (<1 mm Breslow depth) with 1 cm margins will cure patients in at least 90% of cases

INTRODUCTION

Melanoma is a malignancy arising from melanocytes. Its incidence and overall mortality rates have been rising in recent decades[1]. Melanoma is among the most common forms of cancer in young adults[2]. It therefore represents a substantial public health problem. Up to one-fifth of patients develop metastatic disease, which usually is associated with death. However, early detection and appropriate excision leads to a cure rate of over 90% in low-risk (<1 mm Breslow depth) melanoma patients. Innovative early detection programs, in combination with improved diagnostic tools and new immunologic and molecularly targeted treatments for advanced stages of the disease, may influence the outcome of the disease in the future.

MOLECULAR PATHOGENESIS

Techniques in molecular epidemiology and genetics are advancing our understanding of melanoma pathogenesis. Ongoing research is continuing to elucidate the interplay between genetic predisposition and sun exposure in the development of melanoma, which often develops through a stepwise pathway of tumor progression[3]. These studies support the notion that there are biologic subsets of melanoma that vary in their pathogenesis, genetic profile, and etiologic relationship to sun exposure[4,5]. Such studies hold significant promise for improvements in melanoma risk assessment, prevention, and targeted therapy.

Genetic Predisposition to Melanoma

Germline genetic mutations and polymorphisms can predispose individuals to melanoma. The genes involved range from the rare high-penetrance genes responsible for some familial clustering of melanoma to the very common pigmentation genes responsible for the relative propensity to melanoma among fair-skinned individuals[6]. The major high-penetrance melanoma susceptibility gene locus associated with familial melanoma is *CDKN2A*. The locus encodes two distinct protein products, p16 and p14^{ARF} (the latter through an *alternative reading frame*), that exert regulatory effects on cell cycle progression through the retinoblastoma protein (Rb) and p53 pathways, respectively (Fig. 113.1A)[7,8]. Germline *CDKN2A* mutations are observed in about 25% of familial melanoma kindreds[9]. While tests for these *CDKN2A* mutations have been commercialized and have been advocated by some in the field, it is the recommendation of the International Melanoma Genetics Consortium that at present genetic testing for *CDKN2A* mutations should be done only as part of research protocols[10,11].

The major phenotypic factors associated with melanoma risk are melanocytic nevi, skin color, and skin type. Large numbers of common nevi and the presence of atypical nevi are strong risk factors for melanoma. While a 'nevus phenotype' appears to be largely genetically determined with a modulating effect of sun exposure, no specific nevus susceptibility genes have been identified[12]. Among pigmentation genes, the melanocortin-1 receptor (MC1-R; Fig. 113.1B) gene has been found to correlate with melanoma risk above and beyond clinically apparent skin phenotype[13].

Melanocytic Tumor Progression

As noted below, melanoma is commonly divided into major subsets that have varied clinical and histologic appearance and differing epidemiologic associations with skin color, sun exposure and anatomic site. Molecular studies (e.g. comparative genomic hybridization [CGH] analysis, mutational analysis of *p53* and *BRAF*) support the notion of biologically distinct – as yet, poorly defined – subsets of the disease that vary in their relationship to anatomic site, sun exposure and nevus phenotype[5,14].

A number of melanomas arise in clinically and histologically recognizable precursor lesions. For example, superficial spreading melanomas can arise within melanocytic nevi, whereas acral and mucosal melanomas may arise in precursor lentiginous melanocytic hyperplasias. The development of cellular atypia and pleomorphism within such lesions may represent intermediate steps of melanocytic tumor progression[3]. This paradigm of stepwise tumor progression has prompted studies of the genetic pathways and biologic mechanisms involved in melanoma pathogenesis. Recent advances have focused on the roles of stem cells, cell cycle control, senescence and apoptosis in the development of melanoma. Studies of hair graying have helped to elucidate the roles of the melanocyte master transcriptional regulator MITF in melanocyte stem cell maintenance and differentiation[15,16] while studies of somatic genetic mutations in melanomas and nevi have identified several cellular pathways critical for nevogenesis and malignant transformation. Major pathways that have been implicated include the Rb pathway (e.g. CKDN2A, CDK4), the p53 pathway (e.g. p53, p14^{ARF}), the PI3K/AKT pathway and, most importantly, the RAS/MAPK pathway (e.g. 20–30% of melanomas have activating *NRAS* mutations and 55–60% have *BRAF* mutations; see Fig. 113.1B). Studies indicate significant genetic heterogeneity among melanomas; for example, in one study, cutaneous melanomas arising in sites that were intermittently exposed to the sun had mutations in *BRAF* (59%) much more frequently than did other types of melanomas (e.g. mucosal [11%] or acral [23%]). There is also evidence that genes with relevance to developmental pathways for melanocytes are playing an important role in melanoma metastasis[17]. The impact of these genetic alterations is being further studied using *in vivo* mouse models that permit manipulation of the expression of multiple melanoma-associated genes in the presence or absence of UV exposure[18–20]. Improvements in our understanding of the molecular mechanisms of melanoma development derived from these studies are beginning to shape strategies for melanoma risk assessment, prevention, diagnosis, and molecularly targeted therapies.

HOST IMMUNE RESPONSE TO MELANOMA

Clinical observations such as incomplete or complete regression of melanoma (Fig. 113.2), occurrence of vitiligo-like depigmentation and halo nevi, as well as a higher rate of melanoma in immunosuppressed patients point to the fact that melanoma is an immunogenic tumor[21]. Studies of melanoma have played a central role in understanding recognition and rejection of tumors by the host immune system. The

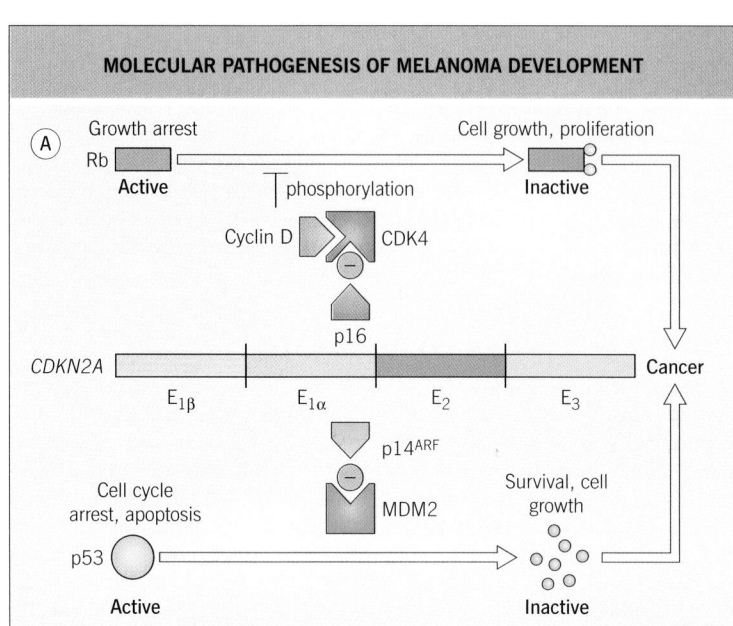

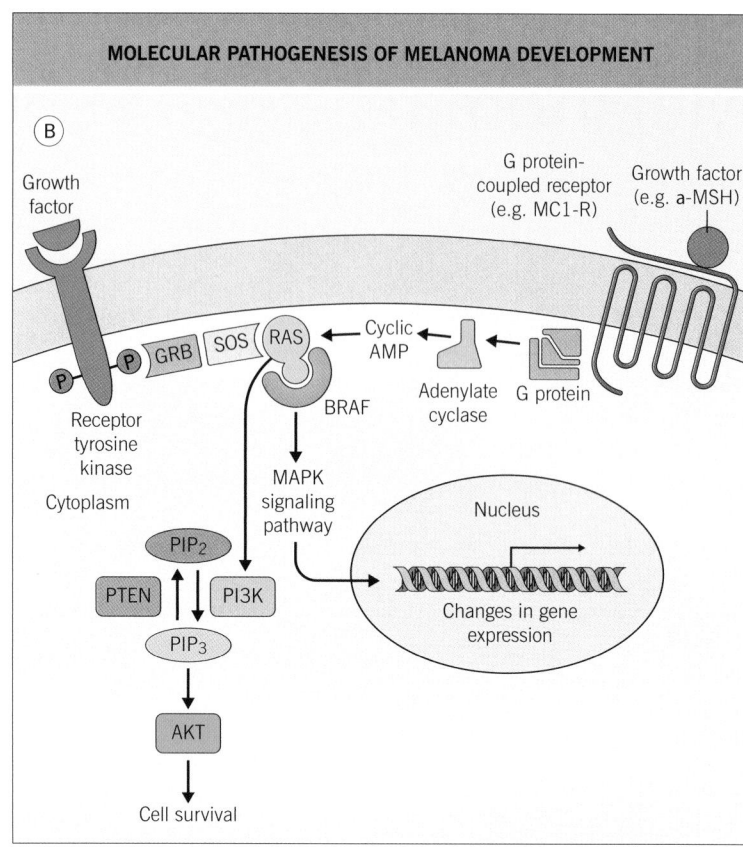

MOLECULAR PATHOGENESIS OF MELANOMA DEVELOPMENT

Fig. 113.1 Molecular pathogenesis of melanoma development. A *CDKN2A* (*INK4a*) encodes two separate protein products, p16 and p14^ARF, which are both negative regulators of cell cycle progression. The p16 protein executes its effects by competitive inhibition of cyclin-dependent kinase 4 (CDK4). CDK4 interacts with cyclin D and phosphorylates the 'master gatekeeper' retinoblastoma protein (Rb). Phosphorylation of Rb will lead to S-phase progression and, ultimately, cellular division and proliferation. An intact p16 protein is essential for cell cycle arrest. The net effect of a *CDKN2A* mutation with loss of p16 function is an increase in the likelihood that mutagenic DNA escapes repair before cell division. The second gene product, p14^ARF, binds to MDM2 and regulates melanocyte growth through effects on the p53 ('guardian of the genome') pathway. MDM2 accelerates the destruction of p53. The net effect of a *CDKN2A* mutation with loss of p14^ARF function is decreased p53 function with enhanced growth/survival of altered cells. **B** The mitogen-activated protein kinase (MAPK) signaling pathway is classically activated by ligand binding to receptor tyrosine kinases, but it can also be stimulated by increased intracellular cAMP resulting from ligand binding to G protein-coupled receptors such as the melanocortin-1 receptor (MC1-R). RAS initiates the MAPK cascade by phosphorylating BRAF. The majority of melanocytic nevi and melanomas have somatic activating *BRAF* or *NRAS* mutations. The phosphatidylinositol 3-kinase (PI3K)/AKT cascade, which promotes cell survival, is negatively regulated by the PTEN tumor suppressor protein and can be stimulated by RAS (via cross-talk with the MAPK pathway). PIP2, phosphatidylinositol diphosphate; PIP3, phosphatidylinositol triphosphate; PTEN, phosphatase and tensin homologue deleted on chromosome 10.

molecular characterization of melanoma antigens recognized by autologous T cells or antibodies was clearly a scientific breakthrough[22,23].

Major melanoma antigens recognized include: (1) mutated tumor antigens (e.g. mutated p16 [CDKN2A]); (2) shared tumor-specific antigens of the cancer/testis family (e.g. MAGE-1, -3, NY-ESO-1); and

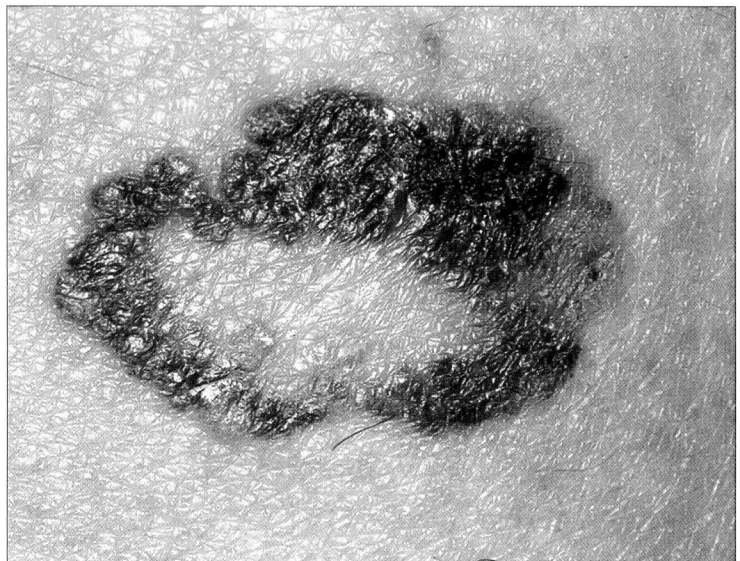

Fig. 113.2 Melanoma with regression. Note asymmetry, variegation in color, and uneven surface. The lighter zone is a reflection of regression.

(3) cell type-specific differentiation antigens (e.g. tyrosinase, gp100, Melan-A/MART-1). The expression pattern of the majority of these antigens may be followed *in situ* at the protein level using monoclonal antibodies. In an extensive immunohistochemical study, 44% of primary melanomas expressed MAGE-3, while 88% and 94% expressed Melan-A/MART-1 and tyrosinase, respectively[24]. These proteins are processed inside the cell and presented on the melanoma cell surface as MHC/peptide complexes (see Ch. 5). CD8+ cytotoxic T cells recognize these antigens and, if appropriately activated, are able to kill such tumor cells in an MHC-dependent manner through release of cytotoxic granules (e.g. perforin and granzyme B) or activation of Fas/tumor necrosis factor (TNF) pathways. CD8+ T cells are believed to be the major effector cells in an anti-melanoma-specific immune response, but CD4+ helper T cells as well as antibodies also play a critical role. Activation of melanoma-specific CD8+ T cells is dependent on the migration of tumor antigen-loaded professional antigen-presenting cells (dendritic cells) from the tumor site to a draining lymph node (Fig. 113.3). Here, melanoma antigens are presented to CD8+ T cells in the presence of costimulatory molecules, which is the decisive step in CD8+ T cell activation. This immunosurveillance system often fails in melanoma patients, but may be activated or replaced by specific immunotherapies (see section Immunotherapy).

Since melanoma is an immunogenic tumor, a variety of immune escape mechanisms may be found in advanced tumors. These include loss of tumor-specific antigens, loss of MHC class I molecules, as well as secretion of immuno-inhibitory cytokines such as interleukin (IL)-10 and TGF-β[25]. Downregulation of the melanoma-specific immune response might also involve naturally occurring CD4+CD25+ regulatory T cells, inducible IL-10-producing regulatory T cells, or negative

ANTIMELANOMA IMMUNE RESPONSE

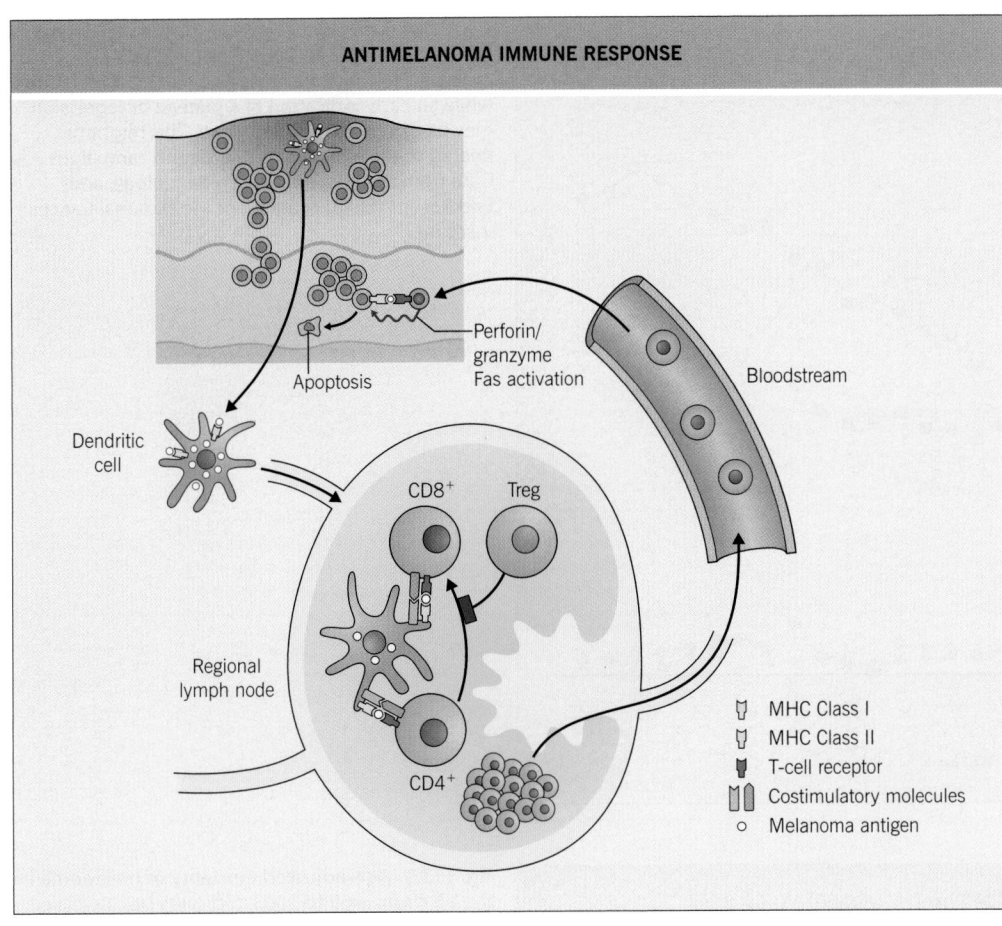

Dendritic cell

Apoptosis

Perforin/ granzyme Fas activation

Bloodstream

Regional lymph node

CD8⁺   Treg

CD4⁺

MHC Class I
MHC Class II
T-cell receptor
Costimulatory molecules
o Melanoma antigen

Fig. 113.3 Antimelanoma immune response involves migration of dendritic cells into secondary lymphoid organs. Activation of melanoma-specific CD8⁺ T cells is dependent on the migration of tumor antigen-loaded professional antigen-presenting cells (dendritic cells) from the tumor site to a draining lymph node. Here, melanoma antigens are presented to CD8⁺ T cells in the presence of costimulatory molecules (as well as to CD4⁺ helper T cells), which serves as the decisive step of CD8⁺ T-cell activation. Activated T cells upregulate chemokine receptors and adhesion molecules, which enables them to enter tissue sites where metastases are located. Downregulatory signals are delivered to the immune system through naturally occurring or inducible regulatory T cells as well as via the cell surface receptor CTLA-4. Whereas melanoma immunotherapy has focused on enhancing activation of cytotoxic T cells, in the future inhibition of immunosuppression, e.g. by T regulatory cells, may become a therapeutic strategy.

signals delivered via cell surface CTLA-4 (see Fig. 113.3)[26]. New insights into mechanisms of melanoma-specific host immune response and immune escape have set the stage for innovative approaches to melanoma immunotherapy (see section Immunotherapy).

EPIDEMIOLOGY

The incidence and mortality rates of melanoma have been increasing in recent decades in all parts of the world from which reliable cancer registration data can be obtained, and this represents a substantial public health problem[1]. The annual incidence rates have been increasing in the order of 3–7% in fair-skinned populations, but mortality rates have increased at a significantly lower rate. This has been attributed to improved early detection as evidenced by the diagnosis of thinner lesions over this time period[27]. While the increase in melanoma mortality, albeit small, belies a true increase in biologically aggressive disease, detection pressure may be contributing indolent disease to the pool of incident cases[28].

The melanoma incidence rate in Australia is the highest worldwide, exceeding 50 per 100 000 individuals in Queensland in 2002 (http://www.health.qld.gov.au). Yet, cohort analysis of both the incidence and mortality rates for melanoma in Australia revealed that the overall rise was not observed in all age groups. In the younger cohorts, who might have been influenced by public health campaigns over the previous 20 years, both incidence and mortality were falling[29]. In Europe, the rate of increase began in the 1950s in the more affluent European countries and has been in part attributed to greater opportunity for travel to southern European countries for sunbathing. Hope for an end to the melanoma epidemic has been seen in the UK, where melanoma mortality fell in young women in spite of a general increase in mortality[30]. Similar trends of falling melanoma incidence in young US women have been questioned as a possible artifact attributable to delays in reporting[31].

In the US, it is estimated that in the year 2005, 59 000 Americans were diagnosed with melanoma and 7700 died of the disease, indicating that nearly every hour an American dies from melanoma[2]. US melanoma incidence has increased from 1 per 100 000 to 15 per 100 000 over the last 40 years (Fig. 113.4). This 15-fold increase is more rapid than for

any other malignancy. Similarly, in the UK in 2001, the melanoma incidence rate (number of new cases per 100 000 population) was 12.4 (7321 persons), with a mortality rate (number of deaths per 100 000 population) of 3 (1766 persons) (http://www.cancerresearchuk.org/).

In contrast to women, mortality rates are still increasing in men (Fig. 113.5). Importantly, deaths from melanoma occur at a younger age than for most other cancers, and melanoma is among the most common types of cancer in young adults[32].

In conclusion, melanoma is a significant public health problem. Public health campaigns of the past 25 years have increased awareness of melanoma and the risks of sun exposure. This change in awareness has been paralleled by a rapidly growing incidence of thin melanomas in most age cohorts and a small rise in overall melanoma mortality. Continued efforts in primary prevention (i.e. sun protection) and secondary prevention (i.e. early detection) are warranted. Further scientific advances in our ability to distinguish between biologically aggressive and indolent melanomas are required to direct our strategies for melanoma prevention and assess the impact of our efforts.

RISK FACTORS

Recognition of risk factors for the development of melanoma is important for public health and clinical care. Identification of high-risk cohorts improves the efficiency and efficacy of public health efforts. Individual risk assessment influences clinical decision making regarding the threshold for biopsy, prevention counseling, and surveillance. Risk factors may be divided into three categories: genetic factors, environmental factors, and phenotypic manifestations of gene/environment interactions (Table 113.1).

Genetic Factors

As noted above, genetic susceptibility to melanoma relates to the inheritance of a sun-sensitive genotype or specific melanoma susceptibility genes. The former can be ascertained by assessment of skin color and skin type (i.e. ability to tan and susceptibility to sunburn). The latter tends to be reflected in a family history of melanoma. For epidemiologic studies, 'familial melanoma' has been variably defined. Some authors

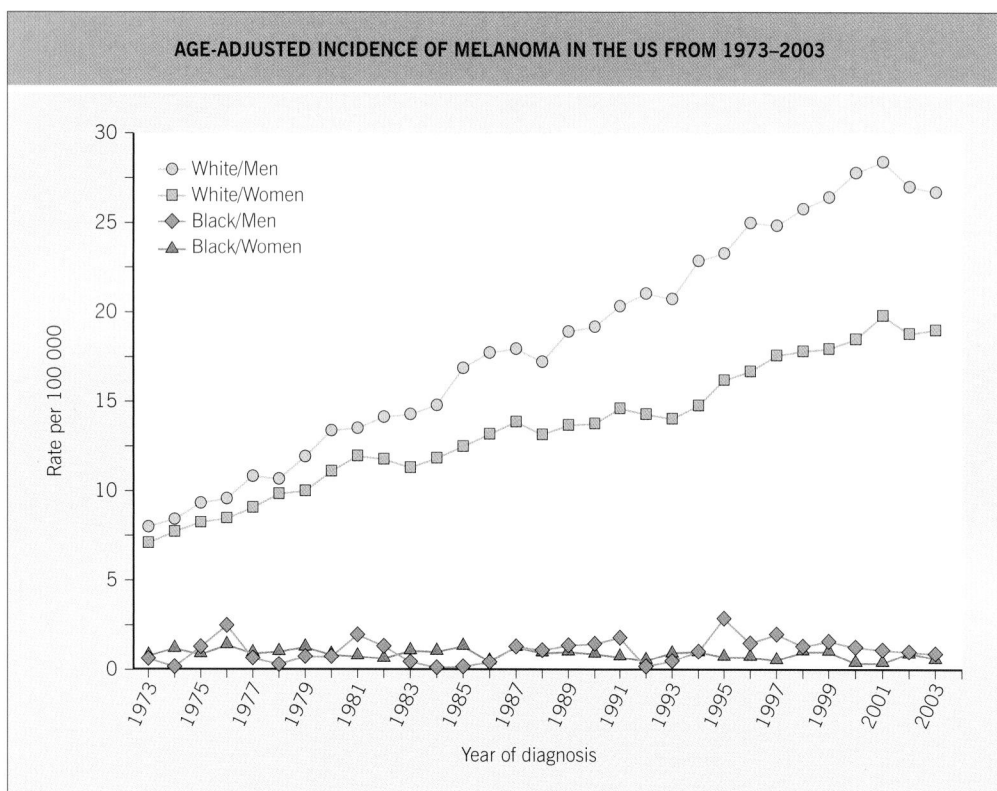

Fig. 113.4 Age-adjusted incidence of melanoma in the US from 1973 to 2003. The incidence has increased for both the male and female population, while an early indication of a plateau or regression may be observed in recent years. This might be related to the effects of public health campaigns. Data from the Surveillance, Epidemiology, and End Results (SEER) program of the National Cancer Institute.

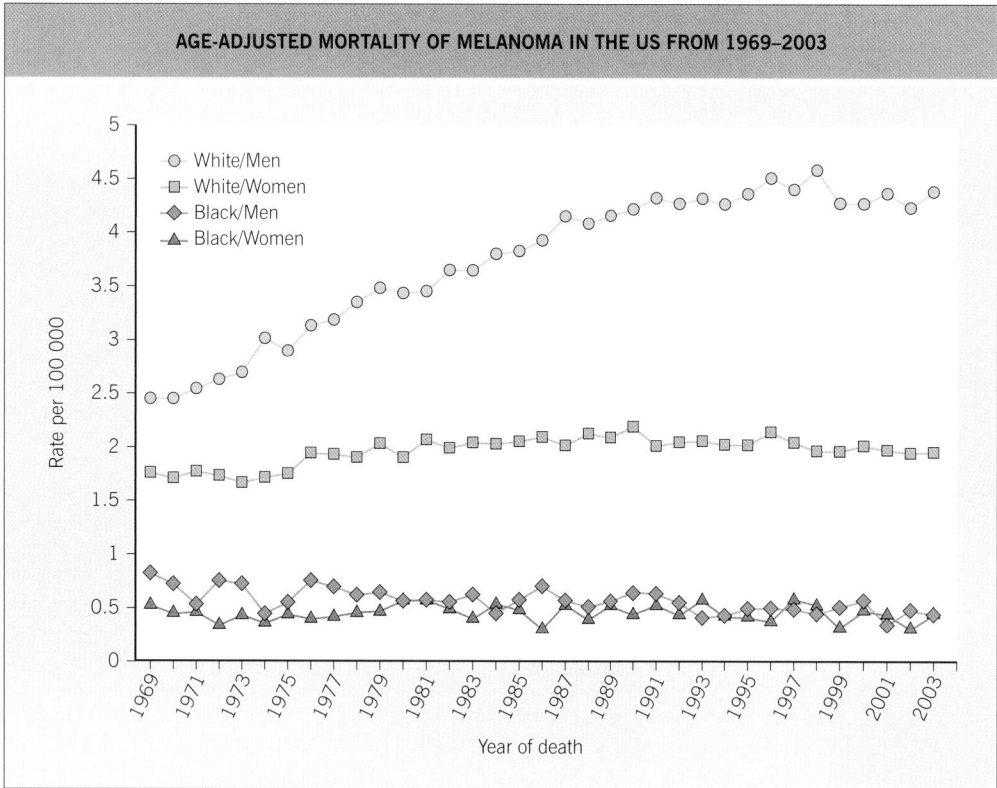

Fig. 113.5 Age-adjusted mortality of melanoma in the US from 1969 to 2003. Mortality has increased, especially for the male population in contrast to the female population. Data from the Surveillance, Epidemiology, and End Results (SEER) program of the National Cancer Institute.

apply the term to kindreds with two or more affected blood relatives, regardless of degree of relatedness. Others require two affected first-degree relatives. In clinical practice, a family history of melanoma in a single first-degree relative or in multiple more distant relatives should be considered an indication of possible high-risk genetic susceptibility. As noted above, genetic testing for melanoma susceptibility is not currently warranted outside of research protocols.

Environmental Factors

The main environmental risk factor for melanoma is excessive exposure of fair-skinned individuals to UV irradiation, primarily in the form of natural sunlight. Accordingly, latitude is a risk factor for melanoma, with proximity to the equator conferring increased risk. However, the exact wavelengths and pattern of exposure that cause melanoma are not yet well established. Intermittent high-intensity exposure of unacclimatized fair skin is a greater risk factor for melanoma than is cumulative chronic sun exposure[33]. This concept stems in part from the counterintuitive observation that outdoor workers experience lower melanoma rates than do indoor workers at a similar latitude. Intense intermittent sun exposure is most closely associated with melanomas of the trunk and legs that manifest with a superficial spreading histology and tend to occur in patients with atypical and/or an increased number of nevi. The less common lentigo maligna of chronically sun-exposed

RISK FACTORS FOR THE DEVELOPMENT OF MELANOMA

Genetic factors

- Family history of atypical (dysplastic) nevi or melanoma
- Lightly pigmented skin
- Tendency to burn, inability to tan
- Red hair color
- DNA repair defects (e.g. xeroderma pigmentosum)

Environmental factors

- Intense intermittent sun exposure
- Sunburn
- Residence in equatorial latitudes

Phenotypic expressions of gene/environment interactions

- Melanocytic nevi:
  – Increased total number
  – Multiple atypical (dysplastic)
  – Congenital (particularly large axial lesions with multiple satellites)
- Ephelides
- Personal history of melanoma

Table 113.1 Risk factors for the development of melanoma.

skin tends to occur in older individuals and is associated with the presence of actinic keratoses and solar lentigines[34]. The use of tanning beds is also thought to contribute to melanoma risk[35]. Studies of the contribution of tanning beds to melanoma risk are complicated by the varied light sources, recall bias, and the strong association between tanning bed use and outdoor tanning behaviors.

Phenotypic Factors Reflecting Gene/Environment Interactions

The strongest phenotypic risk factors for melanoma are those that reflect both genetic susceptibility and environmental exposure: melanocytic nevi and ephelides (freckles). Compelling evidence indicates that patients with increased numbers of benign melanocytic nevi have an increased risk for the development of melanoma. *Atypical (dysplastic) nevi* that are larger than 5 mm in diameter and darkly and/or irregularly pigmented with ill-defined borders are stronger risk factors for melanoma than are common nevi (see Ch. 112)[36]. Several lines of evidence indicate that nevi are largely genetically determined, with sun exposure playing a significant modifying role in nevus development[12]. In the population at large, atypical nevi are markers of moderately increased melanoma risk. In the less common setting of familial melanoma/dysplastic nevus syndrome (also known as the familial atypical mole and melanoma syndrome), defined as families with dysplastic nevi and two or more blood relatives with melanoma, the estimated penetrance of melanoma in affected family members approaches 85% by age 48 years[37]. Patients with a history of previous melanoma in the absence of atypical nevi are at a 3–5% risk of developing a second primary melanoma.

Ephelides (freckles) are another phenotypic manifestation of sun exposure in genetically susceptible individuals. In the population at large, they are associated with a two- to threefold relative risk for melanoma[38]. In the rare genetic syndrome of xeroderma pigmentosum, defective DNA repair of UV-induced mutations is associated with numerous solar lentigines and a very high risk of melanoma.

ULTRAVIOLET RADIATION AND PHOTOPROTECTION

Epidemiologic studies implicate intense intermittent exposure of unacclimatized skin to sunlight as a major factor in the induction of cutaneous melanoma[33] (see above). Epidemiologic studies linking sunburn(s) in childhood to melanoma development are consistent with experiments with genetically engineered mice, in which a single dose of sunburn-inducing UV radiation administered to neonates, but not adults, is sufficient to induce tumors that are reminiscent of human melanoma[39].

Transgenic mouse models as well as models utilizing human skin transplanted to mice imply a pivotal role for UVB radiation in melanoma genesis[20,40]. However, in contrast to non-melanoma skin cancers, in which there are often distinctive UVB-induced mutations in the *p53* gene, melanomas do not demonstrate signature UVB mutations. This has led to the supposition that UVA may play an important role in melanoma. Experiments involving the *Xiphophorus* fish and South American opossum models indicate that UVA may play a role in melanoma formation[41,42]. The fact that, in Norway, a higher melanoma to non-melanoma skin cancer ratio parallels a higher UVA to UVB ratio, also implicates UVA radiation in the etiopathogenesis of melanoma. The hypothesis that UVA contributes to the etiology of melanoma has significant implications for public health recommendations regarding the use of UVA-emitting tanning beds and the relative importance of UVA protection in the design and selection of sunscreens[41].

Sun Protection

Given the strength of the data linking sun exposure to melanoma and the lack of other identified causative agents, primary prevention of melanoma is appropriately focused on sun protection. It is generally accepted that intentional sun seeking and tanning behaviors should be avoided. The best strategies for minimizing incidental occupational and recreational sun exposure have been hotly debated. While commonly recommended, avoidance of outdoor midday activities is, for the most part, impractical, and public acceptance of sun-protective wide-brimmed hats and long-sleeved clothing has been very limited. As a result, sunscreens have gained popularity as a form of sun protection. Several retrospective epidemiologic studies have raised concerns about the utility of sunscreens for melanoma prevention, with some suggesting that sunscreens might even contribute to melanoma risk[43]. However, a quantitative review of epidemiologic studies of sunscreens and melanoma concluded that earlier studies suggesting a possible increased melanoma risk associated with sunscreen use suffered from failure to correct for confounding factors[44]. The review also noted that while a few studies suggested a protective effect of sunscreen use against melanoma, the majority did not. The failure of these retrospective studies to demonstrate a protective effect of sunscreens has been attributed to confounding factors, the limited efficacy of earlier-generation sunscreens at blocking UVA, and the incorrect use of sunscreens. It has indeed been demonstrated that sunscreens are seldom applied as directed and that sunscreens are often used as an aid to tanning[45]. Modern high-SPF, broad-spectrum sunscreens are very effective at blocking both UVA and UVB and have been shown to influence the development of nevi in children, suggesting that they should play a role in preventing melanoma if used correctly and consistently[46].

TYPES OF PRIMARY MELANOMAS

Four major subtypes (growth patterns) of primary cutaneous melanoma have been historically differentiated. These include: (1) superficial spreading melanoma; (2) nodular melanoma; (3) lentigo maligna melanoma; and (4) acral lentiginous melanoma (Table 113.2)[47]. It should be noted that these clinical subtypes do not predict prognosis independently of other factors such as the measured depth of invasion (Breslow depth) or ulceration. This histologic classification may be supplanted by the recognition of molecularly distinct subsets of melanoma in the future.

Superficial Spreading Melanoma

Superficial spreading melanoma (SSM) is the most common type of cutaneous melanoma in fair-skinned individuals (Fig. 113.6) and is diagnosed most frequently between the ages of 30 and 50 years. It accounts for approximately 70% of all melanomas and occurs at any site, but is most frequently seen on the trunk of men and the legs of women. It begins as an asymptomatic brown to black macule with color variations and irregular, notched borders. SSM can arise *de novo* or in a pre-existing nevus (Fig. 113.7). When *in situ* the melanoma is usually macular with an irregular outline and variable pigmentation

DIFFERENT TYPES OF PRIMARY CUTANEOUS MELANOMA

Type of melanoma	Frequency (%)	Site	Radial growth	Special features
Superficial spreading melanoma	60–70	Any site, preference for lower extremities (women), trunk (men and women)	Yes	More pagetoid spread, less solar elastosis
Nodular melanoma	15–30	Any site, preference for trunk, head, neck	No	Nodule with more rapid vertical growth
Lentigo maligna melanoma	5–15	Face, especially nose and cheeks	Yes	Slower growth over years within sun-damaged skin
Acral lentiginous melanoma	5–10	Palms, soles, nail unit	Yes	Most common melanoma type in patients with darker skin types

Table 113.2 Different types of primary cutaneous melanoma.

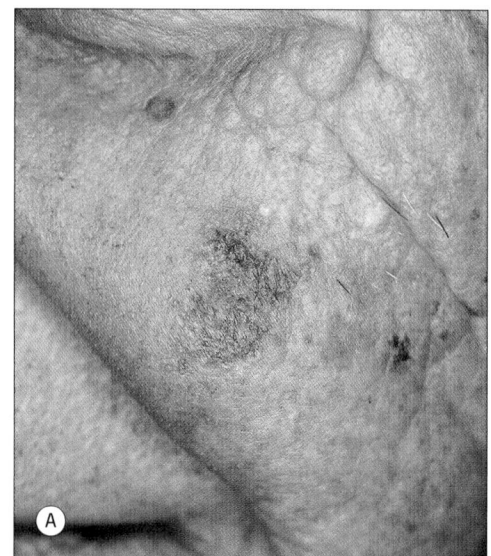

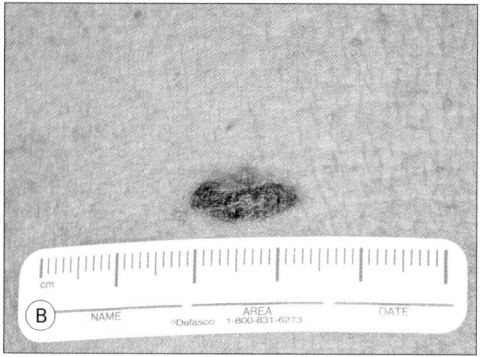

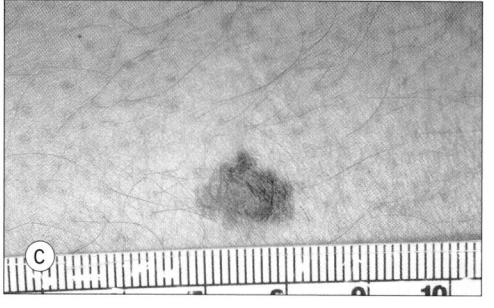

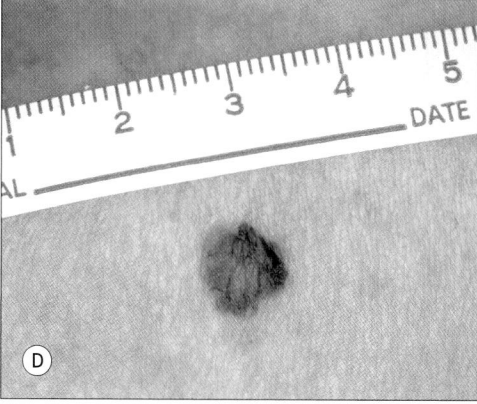

Fig. 113.6 **Early superficial spreading melanomas.**
A–D All of these lesions demonstrate asymmetry due to variation in color and irregularity in outline. In addition, there is pink discoloration in **D**. A–C were less than 0.5 mm in thickness and **D** was 0.8 mm. B, Courtesy of Kalman Watsky MD. C & D, Courtesy of Jean L Bolognia MD.

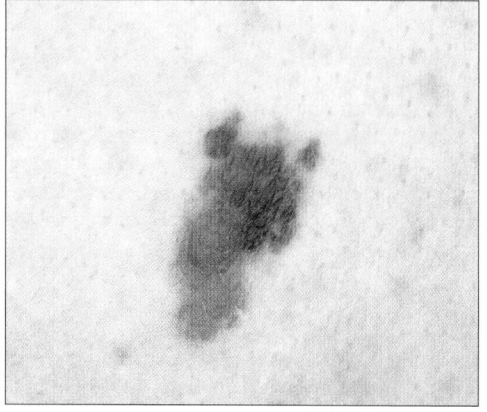

Fig. 113.7 **Superficial spreading melanoma arising within a compound melanocytic nevus.** Note the irregular outline and variable pigmentation.

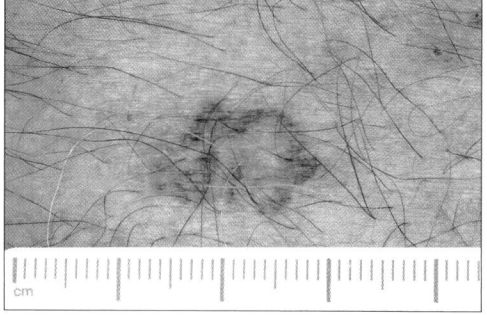

Fig. 113.8 **Melanoma *in situ*.** Asymmetry due to variation in color and irregularity in outline. There is evidence of hypopigmentation due to regression centrally. Courtesy of Kalman Watsky MD.

(Fig. 113.8). SSMs may have a diameter ≤5 mm (Fig. 113.9). After a typically slow horizontal (radial) growth phase limited to the epidermis or focally in the papillary dermis, a rapid vertically oriented growth phase, which presents clinically with the development of a papule or nodule, can then occur. In up to two-thirds of tumors, regression (visible as gray, hypo- or depigmentation) of part of the lesion is observed (see Fig. 113.2), reflecting the interaction of the host immune system with the progressing tumor. About half of these melanomas arise in a pre-existing nevus[48]. The likelihood of an individual nevus progressing to melanoma is exceedingly low.

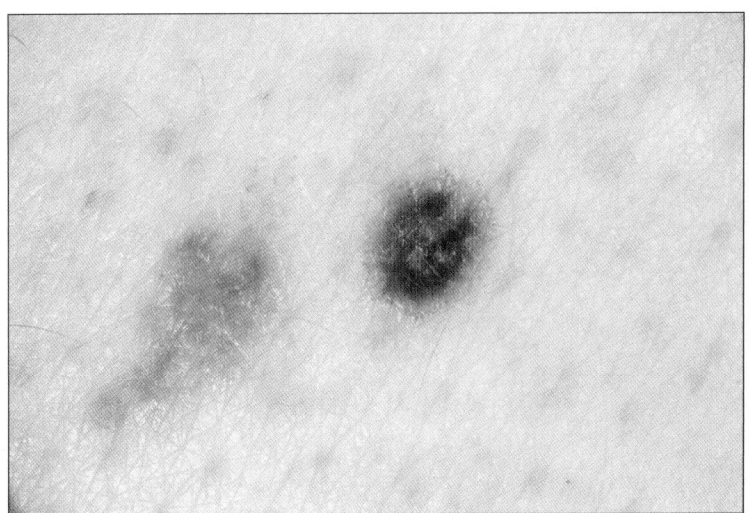

Fig. 113.9 Minimally invasive melanoma (Breslow depth 0.3 mm) with a diameter less than 5 mm.

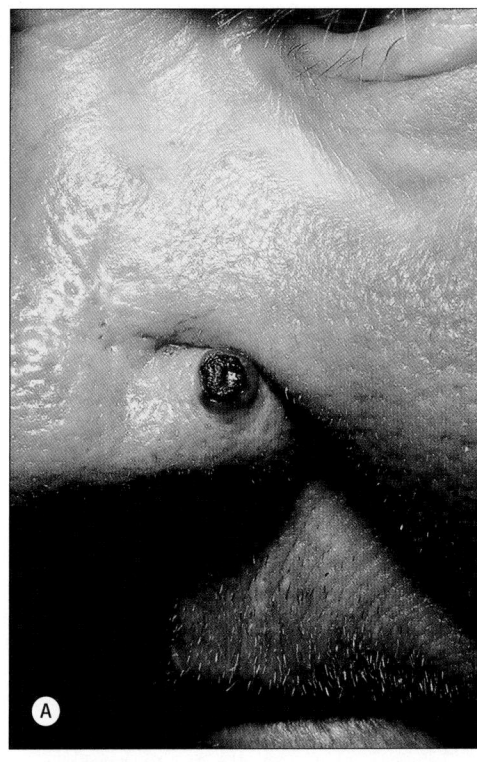

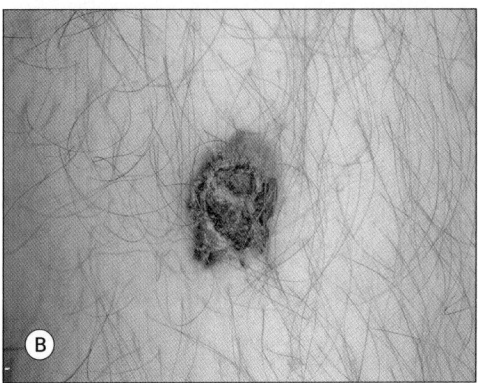

Fig. 113.10 Nodular melanomas. A Ulcerated black nodule on the nose. B Blue–black nodule with hemorrhagic crust. A, Courtesy of Ronald P Rapini MD.

Nodular Melanoma

Nodular melanoma is the second most common type of cutaneous melanoma in fair-skinned individuals and is diagnosed most frequently in patients in their sixth decade of life. It accounts for approximately 15% to 30% of all melanomas and occurs at any body site, but is most frequently seen on the trunk, head and neck. NMs are observed more frequently in men than in women. They usually present as a blue to black, but sometimes pink to red-colored, nodule which may be ulcerated or bleeding and has developed rapidly over months (Fig. 113.10). Nodular melanoma is believed to arise as a *de novo* vertical growth phase tumor without the pre-existing horizontal growth phase that characterizes the other histologic types. They tend to be diagnosed at a thicker, more advanced stage, with an associated poorer prognosis. The incidence of nodular melanoma has remained fairly stable in recent decades[49].

Lentigo Maligna Melanoma

Lentigo maligna melanoma represents a minority of cutaneous melanomas (up to 15%) and is diagnosed most frequently in the seventh decade of life. It occurs on chronically sun-damaged skin, most commonly on the face, with a preference for the nose and cheek. It usually develops as a slowly growing, asymmetric, brown to black macule with color variation and an irregular, indented border (Fig. 113.11). Invasive lentigo maligna melanoma arises in a precursor lesion termed lentigo maligna (*in situ* melanoma in sun-damaged skin). It has been estimated that 5% of lentigo malignas progress to invasive melanoma[50]. Because these lesions typically arise within a background of severely sun-damaged skin, it can be difficult to distinguish lentigo maligna from the atypical melanocytic hyperplasia seen in severely sun-damaged skin[51].

Acral Lentiginous Melanoma

Acral lentiginous melanoma (ALM) is a relatively uncommon type of cutaneous melanoma and is diagnosed most frequently in the seventh decade of life. It typically occurs on the palms and soles or in and around the nail apparatus. ALM accounts for approximately 5% to 10% of all melanomas and the incidence of ALM is similar across racial/ethnic groups. It represents a disproportionate percentage of melanomas diagnosed in blacks (up to 70%) and Asians (up to 45%) as a result of the relative paucity of sun-related melanomas in these groups[52].

ALM typically presents as an asymmetric, brown to black macule with color variation and irregular borders (Fig. 113.12). A disproportionate percentage of ALMs are diagnosed at an advanced stage. This is likely the result of the difficulty of clinically distinguishing many ALMs from benign lesions and traumatic skin changes, as well as an elevated threshold for biopsy due to the morbidity associated with surgery at acral sites. Melanoma of the nail matrix can present as longitudinal melanonychia (Fig. 113.13) or as hyperpigmentation

extending onto the hyponychium or beyond the lateral or proximal nail fold (see Ch. 70). The possibility of melanoma should be considered for all pigmented nail bands in fair-skinned individuals, especially if they are darkly pigmented and/or have a width ≥3mm (see Table 70.8). In blacks, the prevalence of pigmented nail bands increases with age, exceeding 75% by age 30 years[53]. Even so, a widening, irregularly pigmented, or irregularly shaped nail band requires biopsy of the nail matrix (see Ch. 149).

OTHER MELANOMA VARIANTS

There are melanomas that may present with unusual manifestations. Some of these are defined by clinical features, others by histologic findings.

Amelanotic Melanomas

Fortunately, the overwhelming majority of melanomas are pigmented, aiding in visual diagnosis. Melanomas lacking clinically evident pigment are termed 'amelanotic' (Fig. 113.14). All four histologic subtypes of melanoma discussed above can occur as amelanotic variants that largely defy clinical diagnosis. Amelanotic SSMs, nodular melanomas and lentigo maligna melanomas are often biopsied due to clinical suspicion of basal cell carcinoma. Amelanotic ALMs are especially challenging and may be mistaken for warts or squamous cell carcinoma. Amelanotic melanomas do not differ from pigmented melanomas in terms of prognosis or therapy.

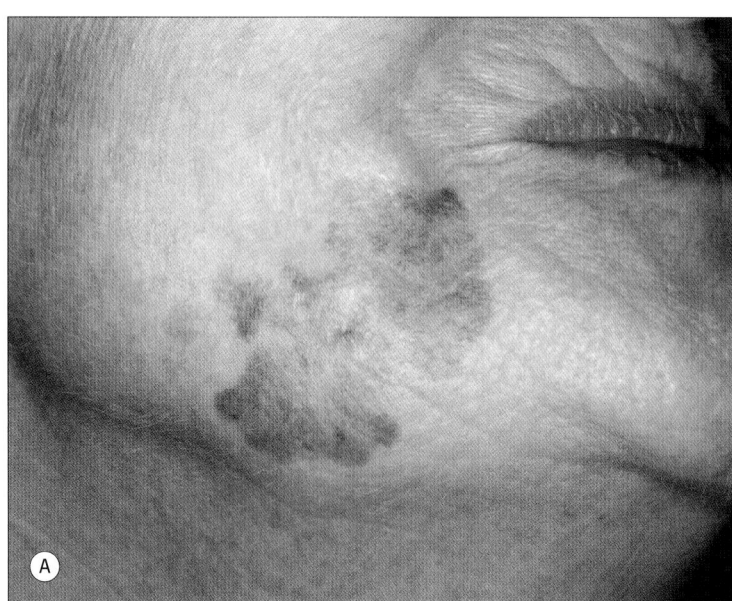

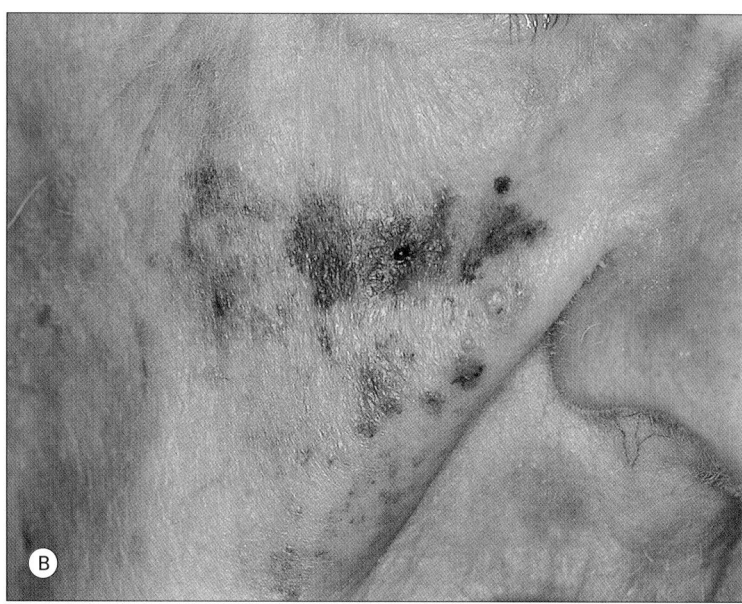

Fig. 113.11 Lentigo maligna versus lentigo maligna melanoma. A Large-sized brown patch with mild variation in color representing lentigo maligna. **B** Similarly sized lesion, but with marked variation in color and topography. There was invasion to a depth of 1.1 mm within the blue–gray papules. B, Courtesy of Kalman Watsky MD.

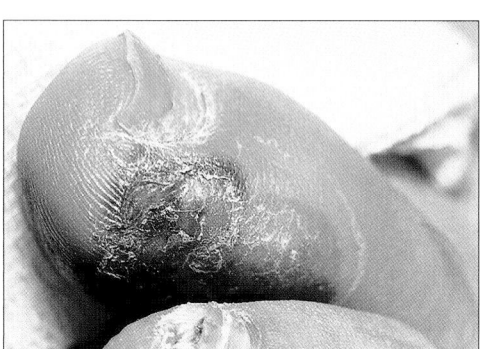

Fig. 113.12 Acral lentiginous melanoma. This lesion on the great toe could be mistaken for a traumatically induced injury. Courtesy of Ronald P Rapini MD.

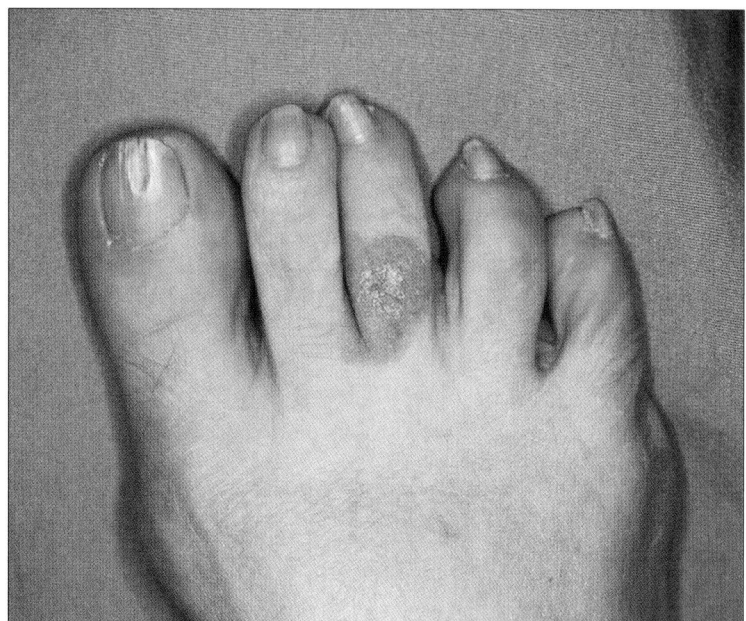

Fig. 113.14 Amelanotic nodular melanoma. Pink, slightly scaly, thick plaque on the dorsal aspect on the third toe. Melanoma may not be the initial clinical diagnosis for such lesions.

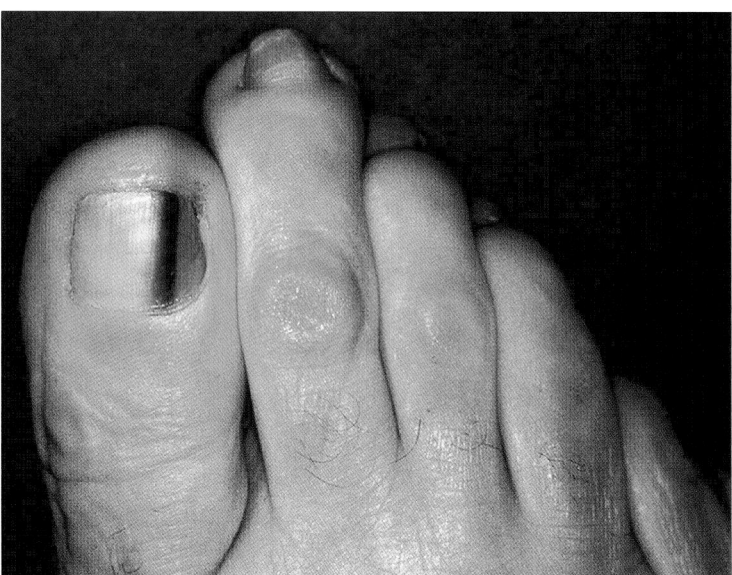

Fig. 113.13 Melanoma *in situ* of the nail. Darkly pigmented band in the nail bed and matrix.

Melanoma with features of a Spitz nevus ('spitzoid' melanoma)

This variant shows histologic features suggestive of Spitz nevus (Fig. 113.16) with overall symmetry and a dermal nodule of epithelioid melanocytes that do not mature with progressively deeper dermal extension. Other important histologic clues that point to the diagnosis of melanoma are sheets of atypical melanocytes in the dermis and mitotic figures at the base of the lesion (see Ch. 112). While several approaches have been taken to distinguish spitzoid melanomas from benign Spitz nevi (e.g. immunohistochemistry, CGH analysis), some of these lesions continue to defy definitive histologic diagnosis[55].

Nevoid Melanomas

These melanomas do not display clinically distinct features, creating diagnostic difficulty because they may resemble a Spitz nevus or an acquired or congenital melanocytic nevus (Fig. 113.15)[54]. Two histologic types of nevoid melanoma are recognized and are described below.

Melanoma with small nevus-like cells (small cell melanoma)

This tumor contains variably-sized, large nests of small melanocytes with hyperchromatic nuclei and prominent nucleoli. Mitoses are generally found throughout the dermal tumor.

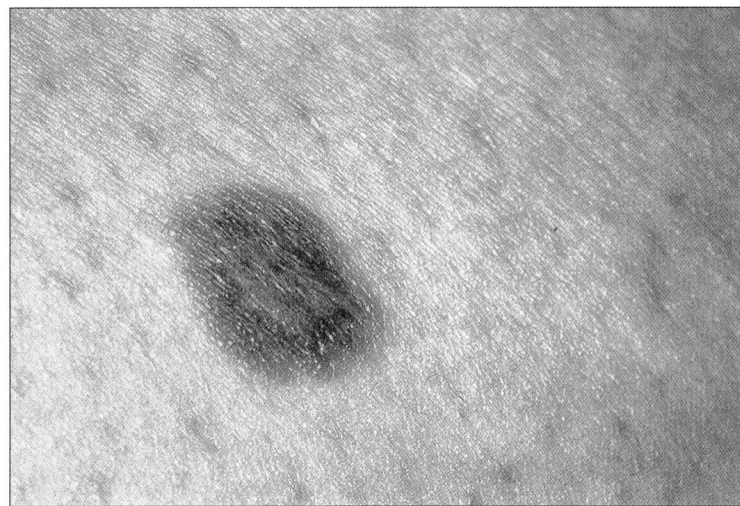

Fig. 113.15 **Nevoid melanoma.** The patient developed metastases from this red–brown plaque.

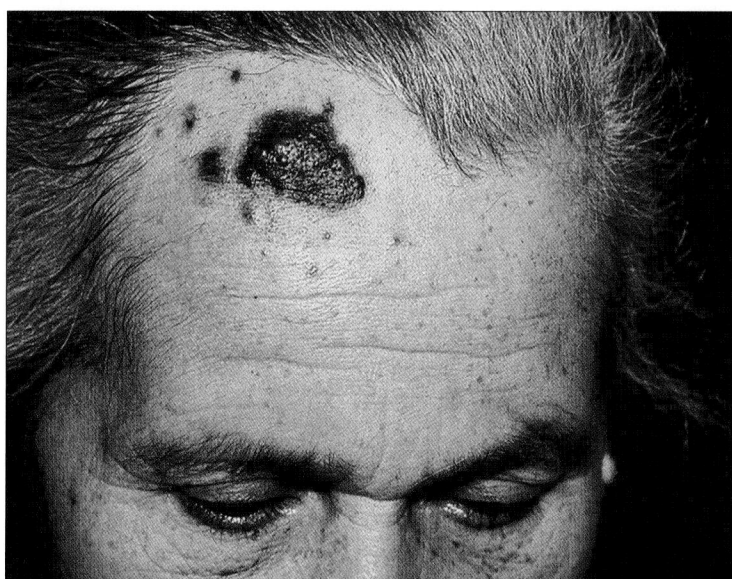

Fig. 113.17 **Melanoma in association with a cellular blue nevus (malignant blue nevus).** Satellite metastases are also present.

Malignant Blue Nevus

Malignant blue nevus is a rare dermal tumor of melanocytes, most commonly located on the head and particularly the scalp (Fig. 113.17). It appears as a blue–black, deeply situated nodule, generally >1 cm in diameter. Histologically, elements of a benign cellular blue nevus are associated with nodular areas of atypical spindle-shaped and bipolar dendritic melanocytes, mitotic figures, necrosis, and melanophages[56]. The clinical course is characterized by a high rate of recurrence and metastasis.

Desmoplastic/Spindled/Neurotropic Melanoma

While this type of melanoma is histologically defined, the typical clinical lesion consists of a skin-colored, red or brown-black nodule or plaque, usually in sun-exposed sites. It may arise *de novo*, but more commonly arises in conjunction with a lentigo maligna, ALM or mucosal radial growth phase melanoma. Deep tissue samples are necessary to establish the diagnosis (Fig. 113.18), as superficial portions of the tumor show subtle or non-diagnostic findings which may be mistaken for the fibrosis of a scar or other spindle cell neoplasms. Metastasis to lymph nodes is uncommon, but the tumor is highly infiltrative and, thus, locally aggressive, with recurrence being common after incomplete excision. While these tumors do have significant potential for distant metastasis, conventional T staging tends to overestimate the likelihood for metastasis of these tumors, which are typically quite deep at the time of diagnosis[57].

Clear Cell Sarcoma: Melanoma of Soft Parts

Clear cell sarcoma most often presents on the distal extremities of adolescents and young adults. The tumors usually arise in association with tendons and aponeuroses, and they are composed of nests and fascicles of oval to spindled cells with vesicular nuclei, basophilic nucleoli, and eosinophilic to clear cytoplasm. Multinucleated giant cells and melanin can frequently be seen. Despite its unique clinical and histologic presentation, several lines of evidence, including immuno-histochemical studies, presence of melanosomes on electron microscopy and gene profiling, support the classification of clear cell sarcoma as a subset of melanoma[58]. The clinical course of these lesions resembles that of other soft tissue sarcomas, with a high likelihood of regional and distant metastasis.

Animal-Type Melanoma

Animal-type melanoma is characterized by nodules and fascicles of epithelioid melanocytes with pleomorphic nuclei and striking hyperpigmentation, dendritic cells, numerous melanophages and, sometimes, an inflammatory infiltrate of lymphocytes[59]. Clinically, blue to jet-black plaques or nodules have been described. The prognostic features are not well known. Metastases have been observed in several patients. It is so named because histopathologically it resembles melanocytic neoplasms seen in white or gray horses.

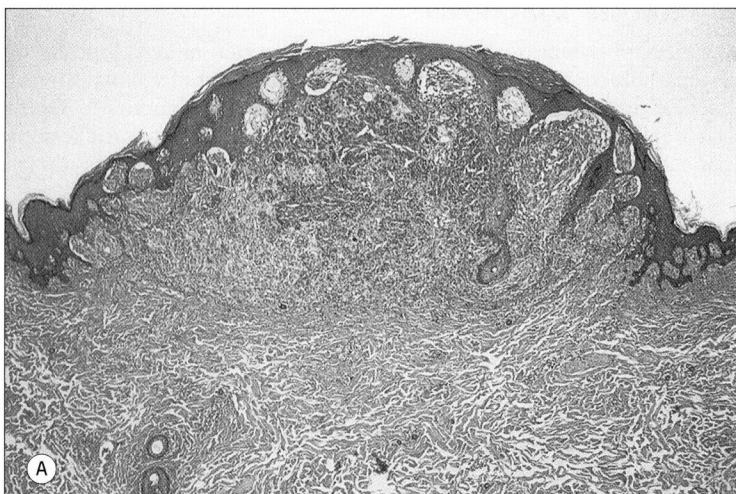

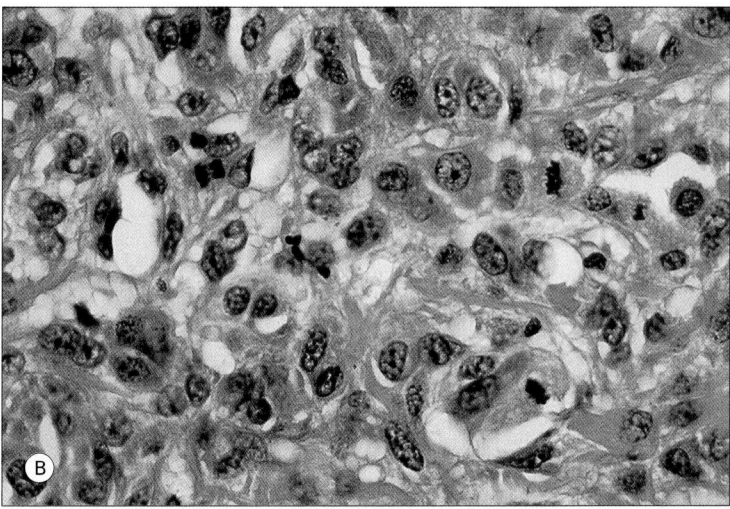

Fig. 113.16 **Histopathology of a melanoma mimicking a Spitz nevus.** This neoplasm could be misdiagnosed as a Spitz nevus because the lesion is symmetrical and well circumscribed. This is a melanoma because: nests of melanocytes have become confluent with formation of sheets; there is no distinct maturation of melanocytes; nuclei of melanocytes are atypical; and melanocytes are in mitosis at the base of the neoplasm.

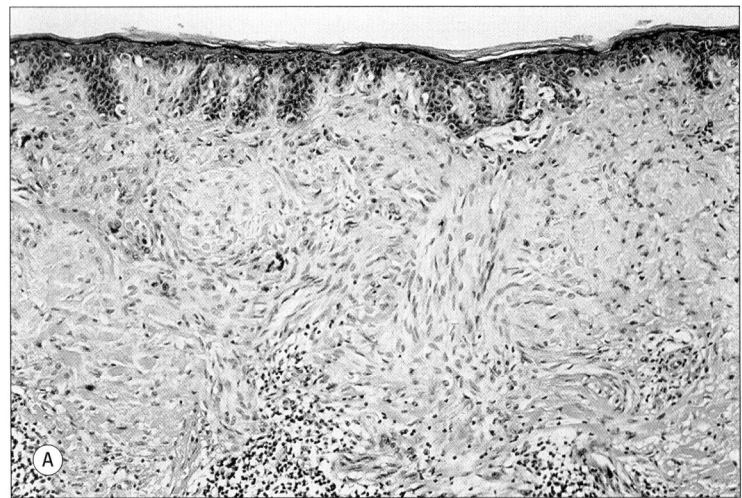

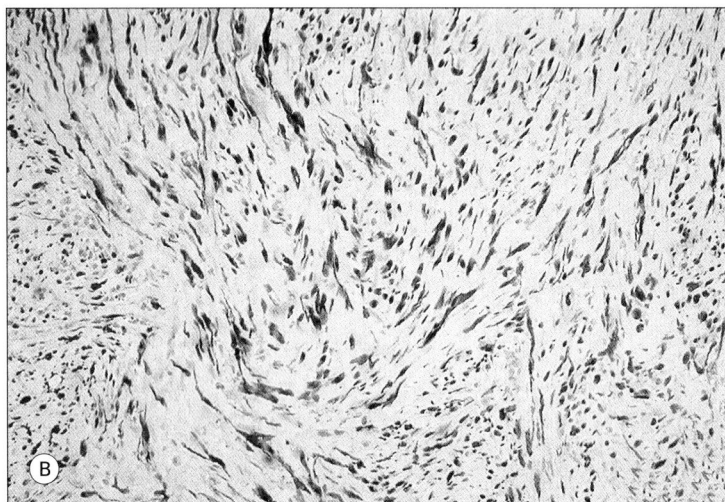

Fig. 113.18 Histopathology of desmoplastic melanoma. A Loosely textured spindle cells in focally fibroblastic stroma. In the epidermis there are changes of melanoma *in situ* with proliferation of atypical melanocytes. Note the lymphoid infiltrates. **B** S100-positive spindle cells within the dermis.

Ocular Melanoma

Primary ocular melanomas, which are relatively rare (5% of all melanomas), can be divided into conjunctival melanomas and uveal melanomas (iris, choroidal and ciliary body melanomas). Less is known about the pathogenesis of these tumors. Patients with dysplastic nevus syndrome have an increased number of conjunctival and uveal nevi. Although a true association between dysplastic nevus syndrome and ocular melanoma is controversial, it has been suggested that patients with ocular melanoma have an increased risk of developing cutaneous melanoma[60]. Patients, especially Caucasians, with melanosis oculi (nevus of Ota) may be at higher risk for uveal melanoma. The prognostic features and the treatment of ocular melanoma differ from those of cutaneous tumors[61].

Mucosal Melanoma

Mucosal melanomas are rare lesions that may occur in the mouth, nasopharynx, larynx, vagina and anus. They tend to occur near the mucocutaneous junctions of squamous and columnar epithelia and account for less than 4% of melanomas. As many as 35% of mucosal melanomas are reportedly amelanotic, further complicating an innately difficult clinical diagnosis[62]. Not surprisingly, these tumors tend to be diagnosed at a locally advanced stage with associated poor prognosis.

MELANOMA AND PREGNANCY

During pregnancy, levels of hormones and growth factors that stimulate melanocytes are elevated and increased pigmentation occurs in some patients. More than 10% of women experience darkening of melanocytic nevi during the first 3 months of pregnancy[63]. However, an association between hormonal changes during pregnancy and development of melanoma or worsening of the prognosis of an existing melanoma has not been demonstrated[64,65]. Transplacental metastases may arise in pregnant women with melanoma. Surgery with local anesthesia is the treatment of choice in pregnant patients with stage I or II melanoma (see Table 113.8). In more advanced stages, discussions with the patient of the advantages and disadvantages of immunotherapy and chemotherapy are advised. There have been no studies demonstrating an adverse effect of hormonal contraception on melanoma development[66]. In women with a history of high-risk melanoma, it may be reasonable to wait 2 years after diagnosis before becoming pregnant, because two-thirds of recurrences occur within this time period.

CHILDHOOD MELANOMA

Childhood melanoma is very rare. Approximately 2% of melanomas occur in patients younger than 20 years of age, and 0.3% in those younger than 14 years[67]. The risk factors for melanoma in children parallel those in adults. The exceedingly rare conditions of xeroderma pigmentosum and giant congenital nevi contribute minimally to the prepubertal incidence of melanoma. Histologically, childhood melanomas may resemble those of adults, but small cell melanomas and melanomas with features of Spitz nevus are reported to be more common in this age group[68]. As noted above, the differentiation of melanoma from Spitz nevi with atypical features remains a major challenge. Overall survival and prognosis seems to be stage-dependent and similar to that in adults[69]. Treatment follows the same rationale as in adults, with the aim of early detection and appropriate resection of the primary melanoma.

DIAGNOSIS

Early detection is a key factor in improving survival from melanoma. The clinical diagnosis of cutaneous melanoma continues to be based on simple visual inspection. A history of change in the color, shape or size of a pigmented skin lesion over the course of months is the most sensitive clinical sign for melanoma. Public awareness campaigns have highlighted the ABCD's of melanoma: **A**symmetry, **B**order irregularity, **C**olor variegation, and **D**iameter greater than 5 mm. These have recently been joined by '**E**' for 'evolving' to connote the importance of change as mentioned above[70]. In the clinical setting, it is essential to elicit a history of changing lesions and to do a complete skin examination, as melanoma can arise on any cutaneous surface. High-risk individuals with a personal or family history of melanoma, many nevi, and/or dysplastic nevi should undergo longitudinal dermatologic evaluation.

Differential Diagnosis

A variety of conditions may simulate melanoma, either clinically or histopathologically, or both. Awareness of these simulators is of great practical importance to avoid over-diagnosis of melanoma[71]. Tables 113.3 and 113.4 list several melanocytic and non-melanocytic lesions that can mimic melanomas.

Dermoscopy

Most melanocytic lesions of the skin can be correctly diagnosed based on unaided clinical observation. That said, certain melanocytic and non-melanocytic tumors may prove to be diagnostically challenging. Dermoscopy, also known as skin surface microscopy or epiluminescence microscopy (ELM), is a helpful non-invasive tool in this setting (Fig. 113.20)[72].

Classic dermoscopic examination is performed with a fluid interface (mineral oil, alcohol or water) and a hand-held lens, stereomicroscope, camera or digital imaging system that makes direct contact with the skin. The process eliminates surface reflection and renders the cornified layer translucent, so that morphologic structures within the epidermis, the dermal–epidermal junction, and the superficial dermis can be better

MELANOCYTIC LESIONS THAT SIMULATE MELANOMAS CLINICALLY AND/OR HISTOPATHOLOGICALLY
• Acral nevi
• Ancient nevi
• Black (hypermelanotic) nevi
• Blue nevi and variants
• Clonal nevi
• Combined nevi
• Congenital nevi biopsied shortly after birth
• Deep penetrating nevi
• Atypical (dysplastic, Clark's) nevi
• Halo nevi
• Hyperplasia of melanocytes in sun-damaged skin
• Melanocytic proliferation overlying a benign neoplasm*
• Longitudinal melanonychia
• Melanosis of mucosal regions
• Nevi arising within areas of lichen sclerosus
• Nevi exposed to UV radiation
• Nevi in genital regions (including milk-line nevi and flexural nevi)
• Nevi in patients with epidermolysis bullosa
• Nevi on or around the ear
• Pigmented streaks in melanoma scars*
• Proliferating nodules in giant congenital nevi in neonates
• Recurrent (persistent) nevi
• Reticulated (ink-spot) lentigo*
• Spitz nevi and variants
*These are not melanocytic diseases strictu sensu.

Table 113.3 Melanocytic lesions that simulate melanomas clinically and/or histopathologically[71].

NON-MELANOCYTIC SIMULATORS OF MELANOMA
• Paget's disease
• Extramammary Paget's disease
• Pigmented epidermotropic metastasis of breast carcinoma
• Epidermotropic neuroendocrine carcinoma
• Bowen's disease (pagetoid or pigmented)
• Pagetoid reticulosis
• 'Clear-cell' artefacts around keratinocytes
• Complete regression of skin tumors other than malignant melanoma (e.g. lichen planus-like keratosis, halo nevi)
• Pigmented basal cell carcinoma
• Pigmented actinic keratosis
• Dermatofibroma
• Seborrheic keratosis
• Pigmented poroma and pigmented porocarcinoma
• Pigmented pilomatricoma
• Subungual hematoma
• Black heel (hemorrhage in stratum corneum caused by trauma) (Fig. 113.19)
• Pyogenic granuloma
• Tinea nigra
• Thrombosed hemangioma, angiokeratoma

Table 113.4 Non-melanocytic simulators of melanoma[71].

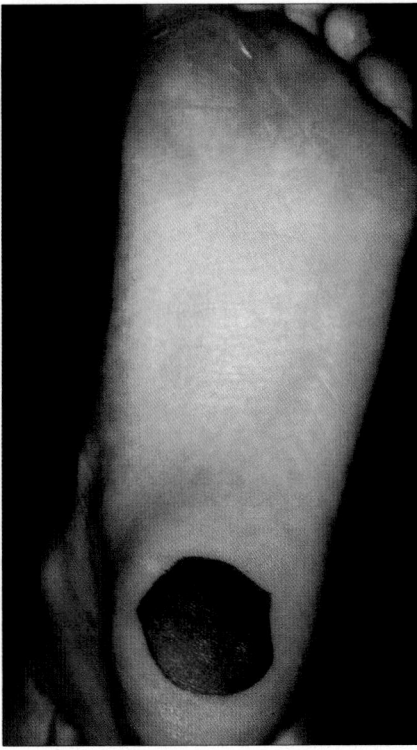

Fig. 113.19 Black heel. Traumatically induced hemorrhage within the stratum corneum simulating acral melanoma.

visualized. An alternative form of dermoscopy utilizes polarized light to eliminate the surface reflection without use of a liquid interface or direct skin contact. The magnifications of these instruments range from sixfold to 100-fold. The most widely used dermoscope provides a tenfold magnification and is sufficient for routine assessment of pigmented skin lesions. The most important practical application for dermoscopy is differentiation of the early stages of melanoma from benign lesions. Differentiation of melanocytic tumors in general from non-melanocytic pigmented skin lesions such as seborrheic keratosis, pigmented basal cell carcinoma and vascular proliferations is usually quite easy[72].

The dermoscopic evaluation of pigmented lesions of the skin relies on a crucial step known as the two-step dermoscopy algorithm. First, the observer needs to determine whether the lesion under investigation is of melanocytic origin or not. For a lesion to be considered melanocytic, it needs to have at least one of the following dermoscopic structures/features: network, streaks, aggregated globules, homogeneous blue pigment, or parallel pattern (acral lesions). If the lesion does not possess one of the aforementioned melanocytic features, then it needs to be evaluated further to determine if it has any dermoscopic characteristics consistent with other entities. However, if the lesion does not have any features of a melanocytic lesion *and* it does not have any features of one of the aforementioned non-melanocytic tumors, then, by default, the lesion is considered of melanocytic origin. Once a lesion is deemed to be of melanocytic origin, the second step of the two-step dermoscopy algorithm is executed. The second step helps to differentiate between benign nevi and melanoma. To this end, multiple algorithms have been created, including pattern analysis, the ABCD rule, Menzies method, and the 7-point check-list, among others, which assist the clinician in deciding which lesions require a biopsy[73].

The main dermoscopic criteria for melanoma can be broken down into global features, patterns and local features (Table 113.5). Global features of melanoma include dermoscopic asymmetry and the presence of multiple colors. Patterns seen under dermoscopy include reticular, globular, reticular–globular, homogeneous, reticular–homogeneous, and starburst. In melanoma, the most common patterns are the multi-component pattern (three or more dermoscopic structures distributed asymmetrically), asymmetric starburst pattern, and non-specific pattern (does not fit one of the known benign patterns). Lastly, the presence of any of the following local features should raise concern of melanoma: atypical network, streaks, atypical dots or globules, irregular blood vessels, regression structures and blue–white veil.

Photographically Assisted Evaluation

In high-risk patients, especially those with complex mole patterns, baseline photographs can be a helpful adjunct in the identification of new and changing lesions[74]. The advent of digital photography and computerized image archives have improved the practicality of this approach. The availability of baseline images for comparison permits the detection of melanomas that are growing or changing without manifesting obvious melanoma characteristics, while simultaneously avoiding the excision of stable, albeit clinically concerning, atypical nevi[75]. Videodermoscopy permits the serial evaluation of individual pigmented lesions for change.

PATHOLOGY

Pathology remains the gold standard for melanoma diagnosis. While most melanomas are readily distinguished from melanocytic nevi based on the criteria enumerated in Table 113.6, many melanocytic lesions remain diagnostically challenging despite the advent of immunohisto-chemical and molecular techniques. There is significant variability in

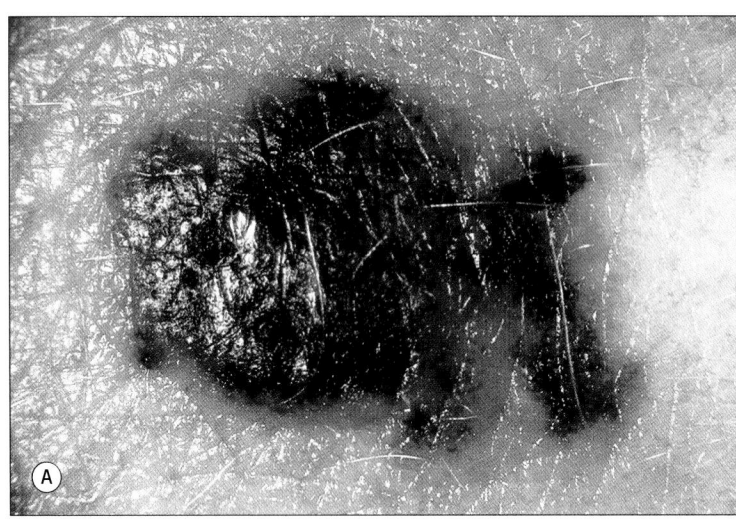
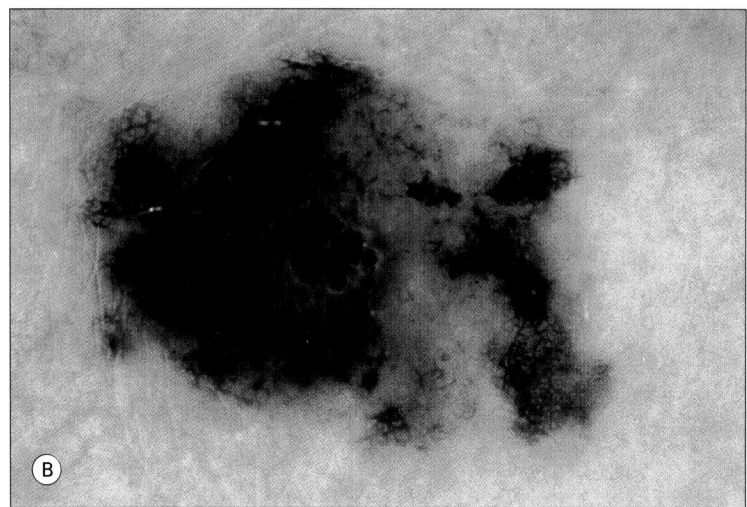

Fig. 113.20 Dermoscopy. This pair of images from an invasive melanoma illustrates the clinical appearance (**A**) and the same lesion viewed with dermoscopy (**B**). Note the multicomponent pattern with an atypical pigment network, black dots, irregular streaks, focally a blue-whitish veil and a white regression zone with hairpin vessels. All these dermoscopic criteria are suggestive of a melanoma.

DERMOSCOPIC CRITERIA AND THEIR CORRESPONDING HISTOPATHOLOGIC FEATURES			
Criterion	**Morphological definition**	**Associated histopathologic changes**	**Diagnosis**
Pigment network	Network of brownish lines over a diffuse tan background	Pigmented rete ridges	Melanocytic lesion
Typical network	Brown-colored, regularly meshed and narrowly spaced network	Regular and elongated rete ridges	Benign melanocytic lesion
Atypical network	Black, brown or gray network with irregular meshes and thick lines	Irregular and broadened rete ridges	Melanoma
Dots/globules	Black, brown and/or gray, round to oval, variably sized structures regularly or irregularly distributed within the lesion	Pigment aggregates within the stratum corneum, epidermis, dermo-epidermal junction or papillary dermis	If regular: benign melanocytic lesion; if irregular: melanoma
Streaks	Irregular, linear structures not clearly combined with pigment network lines at the margins	Confluent junctional nests of melanocytes	Melanoma
Blue-whitish veil	Irregular, confluent, gray-blue to whitish-blue diffuse pigmentation	Acanthotic epidermis with focal hypergranulosis above sheets of heavily pigmented melanocytes in the dermis	Melanoma
Blotches	Black-, brown- and/or gray-colored areas with regular or irregular shape/distribution	Hyperpigmentation throughout the epidermis and/or upper dermis	If regular: benign melanocytic lesion; if irregular: melanoma
Regression structures	White (scar-like) areas, blue (pepper-like) areas or combinations of both	Thickened papillary dermis with fibrosis and/or variable amounts of melanophages	Melanoma
Milia-like cysts	White-yellowish, roundish dots	Intraepidermal horn globules, also called horn pseudocysts	Seborrheic keratosis (occasionally observed in papillomatous melanocytic nevi)
Comedo-like openings	Brown-yellowish, round to oval or even irregularly shaped, sharply circumscribed structures	Keratin plugs situated within dilated follicular openings	Seborrheic keratosis
Leaf-like areas	Brown-gray to gray-black patches revealing a leaf-like configuration	Pigmented, solid aggregations of basaloid cells in the papillary dermis	Basal cell carcinoma
Red-blue lacunas	Sharply demarcated, roundish to oval areas with a reddish, red-bluish, or red-black color	Dilated vascular spaces situated in the upper dermis	Vascular lesion
Vascular structures	Comma-like vessels Arborizing vessels Hairpin vessels Dotted or irregular vessels		Benign melanocytic lesion Basal cell carcinoma Seborrheic keratosis Melanoma

Table 113.5 Dermoscopic criteria and their corresponding histopathologic features. With permission from Argenziano & Soyer, Lancet Oncol. 2001;2:443–9. © 2001 Elsevier.

the application of diagnostic criteria for thin and *in situ* melanomas among pathologists[77].

It has been proposed that melanomas progress through two phases[78]. The first is the *radial (horizontal) growth phase* (RGP), characterized by centrifugal spread of neoplastic melanocytes within the epidermis and infiltration of the papillary dermis by single cells or small nests. The second, *vertical growth phase* (VGP), is characterized by the presence of dermal nests/nodules of atypical melanocytes that are larger than and/or cytologically distinct from their intraepidermal counterparts. It has been further postulated that the RGP lacks metastatic potential even in the presence of dermal invasion, whereas the VGP correlates with the capacity for metastasis. The major histologic types of melanoma described above differ regarding the presence and appearance of the RGP.

CRITERIA FOR HISTOPATHOLOGIC DIAGNOSIS OF MELANOMA

Architectural pattern

- Asymmetry
- Poor circumscription of intraepidermal melanocytic component
- Silhouette of tumor base is uneven (except in nevoid melanoma)
- No maturation of melanocytes with progressive descent into the dermis
- Nests of melanocytes within the epidermis are not equidistant from one another
- Nests of melanocytes vary in size and shape
- Some nests of melanocytes become confluent
- Scatter of melanocytes above the dermal–epidermal junction
- Melanocytes arranged as solitary units predominate over nests within the epidermis
- Melanocytes in some nests are not cohesive
- Melanocytes extend down adnexal epithelium
- Sheets of melanocytes within the dermis
- Nests at base of lesions are occasionally large

Cytomorphology

- Atypical melanocytes (with pleomorphic nuclei)
- Mitotic figures
- Necrotic melanocytes

Other features

- Signs of regression
- Actinic elastosis
- 'Dusty' melanin within tumor cells
- Melanin is not distributed in a uniform fashion
- Plasma cells at the base of the lesion

Table 113.6 Criteria for histopathologic diagnosis of melanoma. Adapted from Ackerman A, Cerroni L, Kerl H. Pitfalls in Histopathologic Diagnosis of Malignant Melanoma. Philadelphia: Lea & Febiger, 1994.

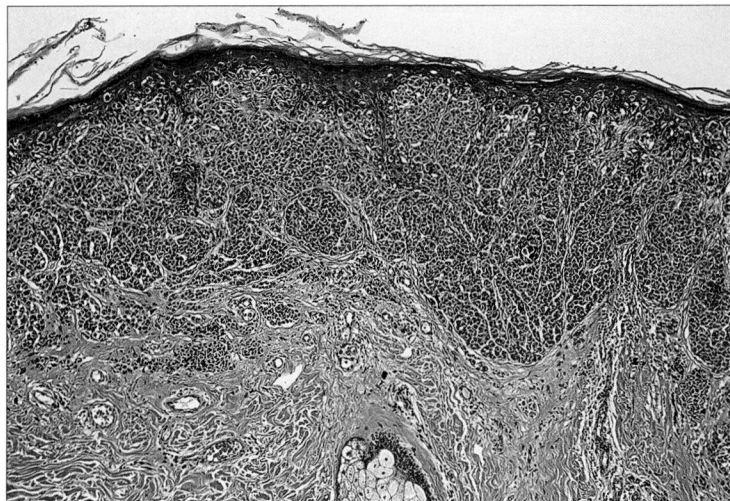

Fig. 113.21 Pathology of melanoma. Pagetoid melanocytes organized as solitary units and nests varying in size and shape are present throughout the entire epidermis. Neoplastic melanocytes extend into the dermis. There is absence of maturation at deeper levels of the dermis.

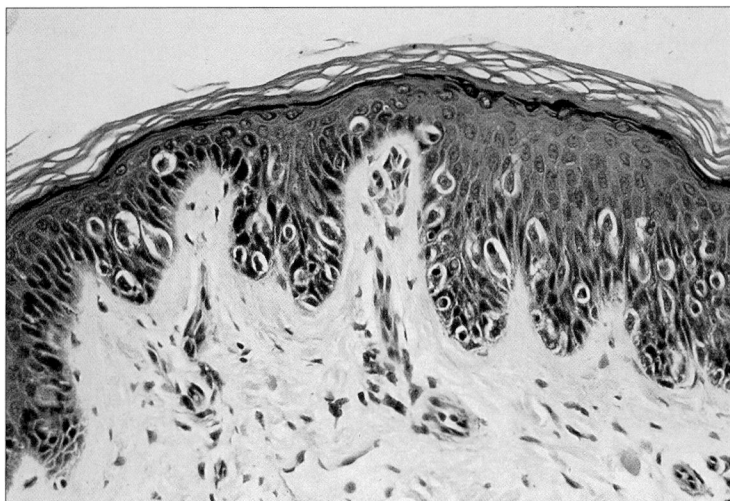

Fig. 113.22 Pathology of melanoma *in situ*. Increased number of melanocytes with atypical nuclei not only in the basal zone, but also at the upper levels of the epidermis.

A typical melanoma (Fig. 113.21)[47,76] is asymmetrical, poorly circumscribed and characterized by nests of melanocytes within the epidermis that are not equidistant from one another, vary in size and shape, and have become confluent in foci. Melanocytes present as solitary units within the epidermis predominate over nests. Some solitary melanocytes and nests of melanocytes are found well above the dermal–epidermal junction, at times extending into the upper epidermis, even the cornified layer. These findings define melanoma *in situ* (Fig. 113.22). One element of this histologic asymmetry is the observation of these intraepidermal changes away from the invasive intradermal component. Similar findings are present in the adnexal epithelium of pilosebaceous units and eccrine ducts. Within the dermis, nests of melanocytes do not become smaller with progressive descent (absence of maturation). In parallel, nuclei of melanocytes do not become smaller.

Nests of melanocytes within the dermis also vary in size and shape and become confluent, sometimes forming sheets of cells. The base of the neoplasm is uneven. Melanin is sometimes more plentiful at the base than at the surface of the neoplasm. Frequently, an infiltrate of lymphocytes can be observed. The neoplastic melanocytes show a wide spectrum of cytomorphologic features, including spindled, pagetoid, small and large round-shaped, polygonal, multinucleate and dendritic characteristics. Certain cytologic features of the melanocytes are more common in particular anatomic sites than in others. For example, the finding of increased numbers of intraepidermal atypical melanocytes with elongated branching dendritic processes is a very helpful diagnostic sign of early melanomas of the palms and soles.

Melanocytic atypia is defined by nuclear features including nuclear enlargement, variability in nuclear size, irregularity of nuclear shape, basophilia/hyperchromatism, and the presence of prominent nucleoli. Even in highly anaplastic tumors, the intranuclear pseudoinclusions typical of benign melanocytic tumors may be identified. Mitotic figures in the dermal component of benign melanocytic tumors are distinctly uncommon. In melanoma, atypical mitotic forms with tripolar and other bizarre configurations may be observed in addition to more typical ones. The absence of mitotic figures in the dermal component of a melanocytic tumor does not exclude the diagnosis of melanoma.

Lentigo maligna melanoma differs from the stereotypical melanoma by its presence on sun-damaged skin of older patients, and the tendency to have little pagetoid spread within the epidermis. The atypical melanocytes are commonly present within the epithelium of adnexal structures, especially along the outer root sheath of hair follicles (Fig. 113.23). The invasive component is more often composed of spindle cells. Desmoplastic stromal change and neurotropism of tumor cells are additional findings. Epidermal atrophy and signs of solar elastosis are often observed in the upper dermis.

ALM often has a proliferation of atypical melanocytes within the basal layer of a hyperplastic epidermis. Atypical melanocytes are also arranged singly and in irregularly shaped nests, at all levels of the epidermis ('pagetoid scatter'), with predominance of single cells. In the cornified layer, numerous melanocytes and melanin granules are usually found in a diffusely scattered distribution (Fig. 113.24). Notably, melanomas in volar and subungual sites display strikingly dendritic melanocytes.

Microstaging

Of the histologic features of a primary melanoma, the Breslow tumor thickness (depth of invasion) is the strongest predictor of survival. Melanoma thickness is measured in millimeters from the top of the granular cell layer of the epidermis (or base of an ulcer) to the deepest point of tumor penetration, using an ocular micrometer (Fig. 113.25).

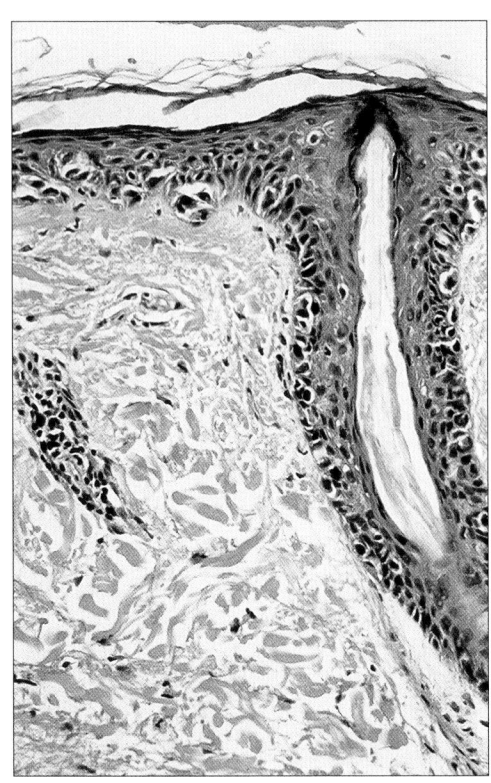

Fig. 113.23 Pathology of melanoma *in situ* on sun-exposed surfaces. Atypical melanocytes both singly and in small nests within the epidermis and the follicular epithelium.

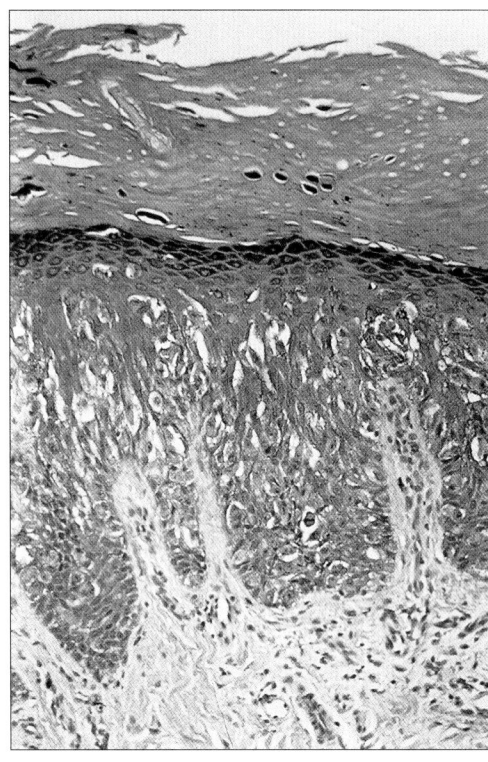

Fig. 113.24 Melanoma *in situ* on the plantar surface of a foot. Atypical melanocytes are scattered throughout the hyperplastic epidermis including the horny layer. Note the presence of dendritic melanocytes.

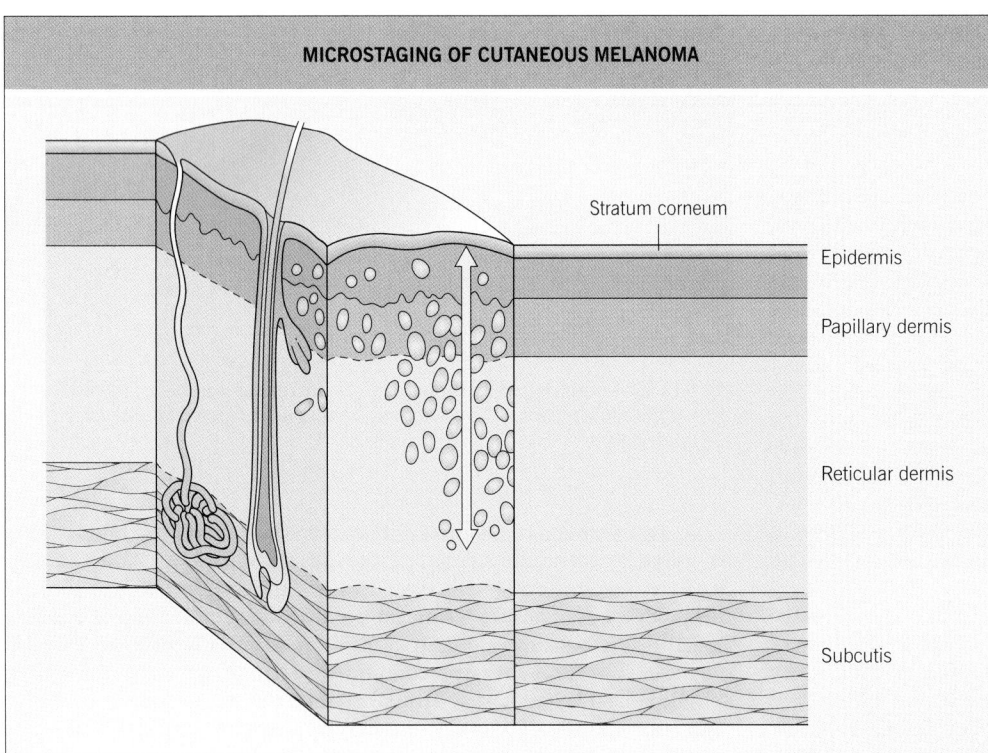

MICROSTAGING OF CUTANEOUS MELANOMA

Stratum corneum

Epidermis

Papillary dermis

Reticular dermis

Subcutis

Fig. 113.25 Microstaging of cutaneous melanoma. Breslow's method: measure from the granular layer of the epidermis to the deepest part of the tumor.

In addition to tumor thickness, a number of other histologic features, including ulceration, Clark level of invasion[47], presence of tumor-infiltrating lymphocytes, mitoses/mm^2, regression, vascular invasion and microscopic satellites, should be noted. Tumor thickness and ulceration are major determinants of T stage in the current staging system. Ulceration is defined as the absence of an intact epidermis overlying a major portion of the primary tumor, based on microscopic examination. Clark levels relate the depth of invasion of melanoma cells to the different anatomic layers of the skin: level I is confined to the epidermis (*in situ*); level II invades the papillary dermis; level III fills the papillary dermis to the junction with the superficial reticular dermis; level IV invades the reticular dermis; and level V invades the fat. In the current staging system, the Clark level is used to distinguish between stage Ia and Ib lesions. Tumor regression, which can occur in up to 40% of thin melanomas, has been proposed by some researchers to be of prognostic significance, but this has not been confirmed by others[79]. Table 113.7 outlines the currently recommended features that should be included in the histopathologic report of a cutaneous melanoma[80].

Immunohistology

While the majority of melanomas are diagnosed on routine histology, immunohistochemical studies can be helpful in the assessment of diagnostically difficult cases of primary melanoma as well as the assessment of metastatic tumors of unknown origin. A wide range of

HISTOPATHOLOGIC REPORTING OF CUTANEOUS MELANOMA

Diagnosis
Thickness (Breslow depth)
Mitoses/mm^2
Level of invasion (Clark)
Regression, tumor-infiltrating lymphocytes, presence of plasma cells
Ulceration
Vascular invasion
Microscopic satellites
Associated nevus
Margins

Table 113.7 Histopathologic reporting of cutaneous melanoma. The World Health Organization has also recommended notation of radial or vertical growth phase.

melanoma-associated antigens have been identified for which immuno-histochemical reagents have been developed. Melanocyte differentiation antigens gp100/HMB45, tyrosinase and Melan-A/MART-1 are useful for distinguishing cells of melanocytic lineage from other tumor types, for visualizing the full extent of lesional cells of a primary melanoma, and for identification of minute foci of melanoma in sentinel lymph node biopsies. Staining for S100, a calcium-binding protein, has high sensitivity for melanocytes and melanoma, but this protein is also expressed in Langerhans cells, eccrine glands, Schwann cells, chondrocytes and adipose tissue. S100 is the most reliable marker for identifying the spindled component of a melanoma. HMB45, which recognizes the melanosome-specific glycoprotein gp100 has high specificity for melanocytes and nevus cells, but its utility is limited by its heterogeneous staining pattern and limited sensitivity, with false-negative rates of up to 35%. Similarly, the more specific differentiation antigens tyrosinase, Melan-A/MART-1, etc. have limited sensitivity. The use of panels of these antibodies improves sensitivity and specificity, but remains diagnostically imperfect, even when used in combination with a host of melanoma progression markers[81].

STAGING

Prior staging systems have categorized melanoma into local, regional or distant disease, which strongly correlates with survival (Fig. 113.26). Greater use of the sentinel lymph node biopsy (SLNB; see section on

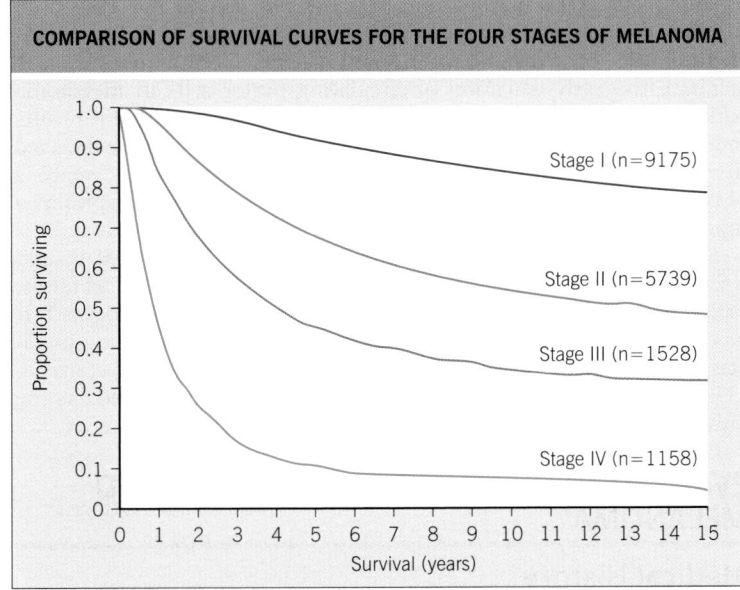

Fig. 113.26 Fifteen-year survival curves for the four stages of melanoma. Survival of localized melanoma (stage I and II), regional metastases (stage III) and distant metastases (stage IV) are compared. The numbers in parentheses are patients from the AJCC melanoma staging database used to calculate the survival rates. The differences between the curves are significant ($p < 0.05$). Reproduced from Balch et al. Journal of Clinical Oncology 2001;19:3635–3648. Reprinted with permisson from the Americam Society of Clinical Oncology.

MELANOMA TNM CLASSIFICATION

T classification	Thickness	Ulceration status
T1	≤1.0 mm	a: Without ulceration and level II/III b: With ulceration or level IV/V
T2	1.01–2.0 mm	a: Without ulceration b: With ulceration
T3	2.01–4.0 mm	a: Without ulceration b: With ulceration
T4	>4.0 mm	a: Without ulceration b: With ulceration
N classification	**Number of metastatic nodes**	**Nodal metastatic mass**
N1	1 node	a: Micrometastasis* b: Macrometastasis†
N2	2–3 nodes	a: Micrometastasis* b: Macrometastasis† c: In-transit met(s)/satellite(s)§ without metastatic node(s)
N3	4 or more metastatic nodes, matted nodes, or in-transit met(s)/satellite(s)§ with metastatic node(s)	
M classification	**Site**	**Serum lactate dehydrogenase**
M1a	Distant skin, subcutaneous or nodal metastases	Normal
M1b	Lung metastases	Normal
M1c	All other visceral metastases Any distant metastasis	Normal Elevated

*Micrometastases are diagnosed after sentinel or elective lymphadenectomy.
†Macrometastases are defined as clinically detectable nodal metastases confirmed by therapeutic lymphadenectomy or when nodal metastasis exhibits gross extracapsular extension.
§In-transit metastases are >2 cm from the primary tumor but not beyond the regional lymph nodes, while satellite lesions are within 2 cm of the primary.

Table 113.8 Melanoma TNM classification. Adapted from Balch CM, Buzaid AC, Soong SJ, et al. Final version of the American Joint Committee on Cancer staging system for cutaneous melanoma. J Clin Oncol. 2001;19:3635–48. Reprinted with permission from the American Society of Clinical Oncology.

Sentinel lymph node biopsy) has increased the sensitivity of detecting micrometastatic lymph node disease, necessitating a revision of older staging classifications. A new tumor-node-metastases (TNM) staging system was introduced by the American Joint Committee on Cancer (AJCC) in 2000, critically evaluated by the European Organization for Research and Treatment of Cancer (EORTC) Melanoma Group[84], and revised in 2001 based on a 17 600-melanoma-patient database derived from 13 cancer centers and melanoma cooperative groups (Table 113.8)[83]. With the publication of the sixth edition of the AJCC Cancer Staging Manual in 2002, this classification is now in use.

The most important modifications are: (1) the noted gradations for tumor thickness are ≤1 mm, 1 to 2 mm, 2 to 4 mm, and >4 mm; (2) Clark level of invasion is used only for further defining T1 melanomas; (3) microscopic ulceration has been added as a major prognostic factor of the primary tumor; (4) local recurrence, satellite disease, and in-transit metastases are now all classified together as regional stage III disease because of similar prognosis; (5) size of the involved lymph node as a prognostic factor has been eliminated and replaced with the number of positive nodes; (6) the presence of an elevated serum lactate dehydrogenase (LDH) level is used in the metastasis (M) category; and (7) the site of distant metastases is of importance for prognosis.

The revised AJCC staging system is outlined in Table 113.9 along with predicted survival by stage. A distinction between low-risk stage I

STAGE GROUPINGS FOR CUTANEOUS MELANOMA							
	Survival (%)*	Clinical staging[†]			Pathologic staging[‡]		
		T	N	M	T	N	M
0		Tis	N0	M0	Tis	N0	M0
IA	95	T1a	N0	M0	T1a	N0	M0
IB	90	T1b T2a	N0	M0	T1b T2a		
IIA	78	T2b T3a	N0	M0	T2b T3a	N0	M0
IIB	65	T3b T4a	N0	M0	T3b T4a	N0	M0
IIC	45	T4b	N0	M0	T4b	N0	M0
III[§]		Any T	N1 N2 N3	M0			
IIIA	66				T1-4a T1-4a	N1a N2a	M0
IIIB	52				T1-4b T1-4b T1-4a T1-4a T1-4a/b	N1a N2a N1b N2b N2c	M0
IIIC	26				T1-4b T1-4b Any T	N1b N2b N3	M0
IV	7.5–11	Any T	Any N	Any M1	Any T	Any N	Any M1

*Approximate 5-year survival (%), modified from Balch et al.[83]
[†]Clinical staging includes microstaging of the primary melanoma and clinical/radiologic evaluation for metastases. By convention, it should be used after complete excision of the primary melanoma with clinical assessment for regional and distant metastases.
[‡]Pathologic staging includes microstaging of the primary melanoma and pathologic information about the regional lymph nodes after partial or complete lymphadenectomy. Pathologic stage 0 or stage IA patients are the exception.
[§]There are no stage III subgroups for clinical staging.

Table 113.9 Stage groupings for cutaneous melanoma. Adapted from Balch CM, Soong SJ, Gershenwald JE, et al. Prognostic factors analysis of 17 600 melanoma patients: validation of the American Joint Committee on Cancer melanoma staging system. 2001;19:3622–34 and adapted from Balch CM, Buzaid AC, Soong SJ, et al. Final version of the American Joint Committee on Cancer staging system for cutaneous melanoma. J Clin Oncol. 2001;19:3635–48. Reprinted with permission from the American Society of Clinical Oncology.

MAJOR INDEPENDENT PROGNOSTIC FACTORS FOR SURVIVAL IN MULTIVARIATE ANALYSES	
Prognostic factor	Commentary
Tumor thickness	≤1 mm low risk, >1 mm higher risk melanoma
Ulceration	Worse prognosis with ulceration
Age	Higher age with worse prognosis
Sex	Only for localized disease, males with poorer prognosis
Anatomic site	Trunk, head and neck with poorer prognosis than extremities
Number of involved lymph nodes	Cut-off points: 1, 2–3, 4 or more lymph nodes
Regional lymph node tumor burden	Macroscopic (palpable) nodal metastases with poorer prognosis than microscopic (non-palpable) nodal metastases
Site of distant metastases	Visceral metastases with poorer prognosis than non-visceral (skin, subcutaneous, distant lymph nodes)

Table 113.10 Major independent prognostic factors for survival in multivariate analyses[82].

or more lymph nodes with clinically apparent metastases[82]. Major prognostic factors in this group are the number of metastatic lymph nodes and the tumor burden. Tumor burden is reflected by whether the nodal metastases are clinically occult (as detected by sentinel or elective lymph node dissection) or clinically palpable.

In stage IV patients, the major prognostic factor is the site of distant metastases, with a poorer prognosis for visceral than non-visceral (e.g. skin, subcutaneous, and distant lymph node) metastases. The median survival time for stage IV patients in a recent study was 7.5 months; the estimated 5-year survival rate was 6%[88]. The main variables that predicted survival were initial site of metastases, disease-free interval before distant metastases, and stage of disease preceding distant metastases. Patients with cutaneous, nodal or gastrointestinal metastases had a median survival of 12.5 months (estimated 5-year survival rate, 14%); with pulmonary metastases, the median survival was 8.3 months (estimated 5-year survival rate, 4%); and patients with metastases to the liver, brain or bone had a median survival of 4.4 months (estimated 5-year survival rate, 3%). Up to 9% of metastatic melanoma patients present with an unidentified primary tumor. This finding is not in itself a negative prognostic indicator.

There has been a longstanding search for melanoma-specific tumor markers (biomarkers) that would determine prognosis. Reverse transcription (RT) of tyrosinase mRNA and specific cDNA amplification to facilitate the early detection of circulating tumor cells in melanoma patients has been reported as a promising tool. However, recent results indicate that a low amount of tyrosinase-specific transcripts is detected in only a small subset of stage IV patients, suggesting that the analysis of tyrosinase mRNA in peripheral blood samples was not helpful as a prognostic marker or monitoring tool in these melanoma patients[89].

Serum levels of S100-β, melanoma-inhibiting activity (MIA), and 5-S-cysteinyldopa, as well as conventional variables such as LDH levels, have been analyzed for monitoring of advanced melanoma patients[90]. It has been reported that the highest sensitivities for determining metastasis were found with S100-β and MIA (91% and 88%, respectively). LDH had the highest specificity (92%) and LDH was identified as the only statistically significant marker for progressive disease[91].

EVALUATION OF A PATIENT WITH SUSPECTED MELANOMA

Medical History

A thorough medical history should be taken, focusing especially on risk factors for the development of melanoma (see above), such as a personal or family history of melanoma, skin type I/II (see Ch. 134), extensive tanning bed use, childhood history of sunburns, large number of melanocytic nevi, presence of atypical melanocytic nevi, presence of large congenital melanocytic nevi, genetic syndromes with skin cancer

PROGNOSIS

The prognosis of a patient with melanoma is dependent on stage at diagnosis. Prognosis for patients with localized melanoma and no nodal or distant metastases is generally good. In addition to the microstaging variables discussed above, clinical variables with prognostic significance in stage I/II disease include sex, age and anatomic site[82,85,86] (Table 113.10). For example, women with stage I/II disease tend to have a better survival rate than men. Location of the primary melanoma on the trunk, head or neck portends a poorer prognosis than a location on the extremities. Advancing age is inversely related to survival from melanoma. Multivariate models for survival from stage I/II melanoma have been developed that take these clinical features into consideration[87].

Stage III melanoma patients are a heterogeneous group with respect to their risk for distant metastases and melanoma-specific mortality. The 5-year survival rates range from 69% for patients with non-ulcerated melanomas who had a single clinically occult nodal metastasis to a low of 13% for patients with ulcerated primary melanomas and four

patients with a Breslow depth of ≤1 mm and higher-risk stage II patients with a Breslow depth of >2 mm is made. Involvement of regional lymph nodes (stage III) or distant metastases (stage IV) is associated with increasingly worse prognosis. This staging system may not accurately reflect variants of melanoma such as desmoplastic, mucosal or ocular melanoma.

predisposition (e.g. xeroderma pigmentosum), and iatrogenic (immuno-suppressive drugs used in transplant medicine or extended PUVA therapy) or acquired (e.g. HIV) immunosuppression. A detailed history of the specific lesion in question should be obtained. Was the lesion present at birth? Did the lesion develop in a pre-existing mole? Did it change in size or shape? Did it change in color or ulcerate? Was there itching or bleeding? What is the time course of change? Are there systemic symptoms such as weight loss, fatigue, headache or cough?[92] Other family members should be screened if either melanoma or atypical melanocytic nevi are present. All at-risk individuals should be educated about the clinical features of melanoma and about sun protection measures (see Ch. 132). Suggested follow-up intervals for high-risk individuals are considered in Chapter 112.

Skin Investigation and Clinical Diagnosis

The American Cancer Society uses the ABCD mnemonic (see above). A specificity of 0.88 and sensitivity of 0.73 has been reported if two out of three of the following characteristics are noted: irregular outline, diameter greater than 6 mm, and color variegation[93]. A pigmented lesion that stands out as atypical within the context of surrounding nevi should arouse suspicion of melanoma regardless of specific findings. This has been called the 'ugly duckling' sign[94]. Even expert clinicians misdiagnose melanoma in up to one-third of cases and only histologic examination can provide definitive diagnosis[95]. Dermoscopy increases diagnostic sensitivity when used by dermatologists formally trained in the use of this technique, but may decrease diagnostic accuracy in dermatologists not formally trained in its application[96] (see above). Any lesion suspicious of being melanoma should undergo biopsy. Excisional biopsy is the preferred method of biopsy, as it prevents sampling error (e.g. missing a focus of melanoma arising in a precursor benign lesion) and enables the pathologist to assess the overall architecture of the lesion and accurately microstage the tumor. There are, however, instances when a partial or shave biopsy may be appropriate, as in large lesions occurring in surgically sensitive areas or lesions for which the index of suspicion is low. Examination of lymph node basins and palpation of the abdomen for hepatosplenomegaly should be routinely performed.

Laboratory Investigations and Imaging

Evidence is accumulating that routine imaging studies including chest radiography and blood work have limited, if any, value in the initial evaluation of asymptomatic patients with primary cutaneous melanoma 4 mm or less in thickness[97]. An American Academy of Dermatology task force recommended that these initial imaging studies and blood work should be optional and most appropriately directed based on findings of a thorough medical history and physical examination[98]. In a study involving more than 200 asymptomatic patients with localized melanomas initially examined with chest radiography, the true-positive radiograph rate for lung metastases was 0% with a false-positive rate of 7%[97]. Unnecessary investigations are costly, may lead to patient anxiety, and are unlikely to influence outcome. Exceptions to obtaining imaging and blood chemistry studies on asymptomatic patients with primary melanoma include thickness >4 mm and in the setting of multidisciplinary referral centers conducting prospective studies.

Investigation of stage III/IV melanoma patients includes radiologic investigations such as MRI of the brain and CT of the chest, abdomen and pelvis. The most significant advance in imaging technology for early detection of metastases is whole body positron emission tomography (PET) using 18F-fluorodeoxyglucose (FDG)[99]. It is based on the assumption that melanoma metastases have a higher metabolic rate than normal tissue and utilize more glucose. The accuracy of nodal staging can be significantly improved by adding PET to the pre-therapeutic diagnostic procedures[100]. A meta-analysis of the existing literature regarding PET determined an overall sensitivity of 92% and an overall specificity of 90%[101]. However, in a selected patient population, FDG-PET was found to be inferior to CT for diagnosing lung and liver metastases[102], especially for lung nodules <1 cm in diameter.

The combination of FDG-PET with CT- or ultrasound-guided fine-needle aspiration (FNA) can increase the sensitivity of both methods[103]. FNA is used in the cytologic diagnosis of melanoma metastases, often in combination with immunohistochemistry with melanoma-specific antibodies, but should not be used for the diagnosis of primary melanoma. In a study in 330 melanoma patients with metastasis, 739 FNAs were performed with a sensitivity of 97.9% and a specificity of 100%[104]. FNA is especially useful in combination with ultrasound or CT for lymph node, lung and liver metastases.

MANAGEMENT

Management of the Primary Melanoma (Stage I and II)

Biopsy techniques: As noted above, a lesion that is clinically suspicious for melanoma should ideally undergo an excisional biopsy with narrow margins (such as 2 mm). Although there is evidence that an incisional biopsy does not adversely affect survival[105], this approach should be an exception and reserved for cases in which the tumor is too large to be excised, or when it is impractical to perform an excision (e.g. of the nail unit). The biopsy should be interpreted by a physician experienced in the microscopic diagnosis of melanocytic lesions. FNA cytology should not be used to assess the primary tumor[98].

Wide local excision of the primary site: Following histologic diagnosis, the primary melanoma site should be re-excised with an appropriate margin determined by the Breslow depth (Table 113.11). The rationale of an excisional margin is based on the capacity of melanoma cells to migrate away from the tumor origin. Melanoma may extend wider or deeper than is visibly apparent. The major goal is to prevent local recurrence or persistent disease. A World Health Organization (WHO) randomized trial indicated that 1 cm excisional margins are safe and effective for melanoma with a Breslow depth <1 mm[106]. A controversy persists about the effectiveness of 1 cm excisional margins for melanomas 1 to 2 mm deep, since there was a trend to local recurrence in this group in the WHO trial[107]. Several reports, including the American Academy of Dermatology Guidelines of Care for Primary Melanoma, have recommended 1 cm margins for melanoma <2 mm in depth[98,108,109]. A randomized trial for intermediate-thickness melanoma (1 to 4 mm deep) demonstrated that 2 cm margins were as effective as 4 cm margins in preventing local recurrences[110]. For this group of melanoma patients, local recurrence was associated with a high mortality rate. Ulceration of the primary melanoma is the most significant prognostic factor heralding an increased risk for local recurrence. To date, there are no informative randomized trials that determine the optimal margins of excision for melanoma >4 mm in thickness or *in situ* melanoma. Current recommendation are excision margins of 0.5 cm for *in situ* melanoma and 2 to 3 cm for melanoma >4 mm in depth[98,111].

Further investigative efforts will likely alter the standards of care over time. Margins of excision are also dictated by surgically difficult anatomic sites such as the distal extremities, the mucous membranes or the face, and, in many instances, an individualized surgical approach must be undertaken[112]. Some recommendations, such as excision to the underlying fascia, are based on questionable anatomic concepts[113]. No randomized trials have compared this approach to excision to the deep subcutaneous fat[113].

SURGICAL TREATMENT OF PRIMARY MELANOMA		
Thickness	Excision margins (cm)	Comments
In situ	0.5	No randomized studies; lentigo maligna of the face might be treated with radiotherapy in specialized centers
<1 mm	1.0	AAD task force suggests a 1 cm margin for melanomas <2 mm[98]
1–4 mm	2.0	AAD task force suggests a 2 cm margin for melanomas ≥2 mm[98]
>4 mm	2.0–3.0	No randomized studies

Table 113.11 **Surgical treatment of primary melanoma.** In the case of lentigo maligna, Wood's lamp examination can aid in defining the lesion and some authors suggest 1 cm margins for this variant of melanoma when it is >1 cm in diameter. AAD, American Academy of Dermatology.

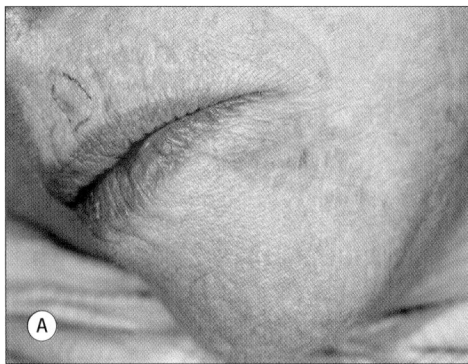

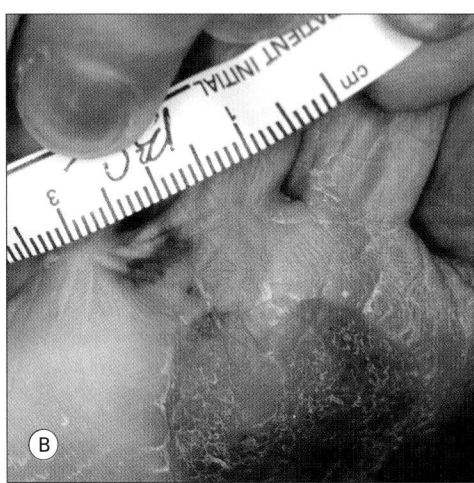

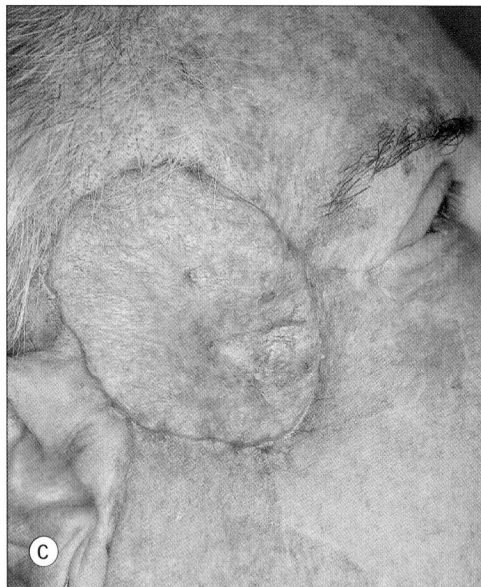

Fig. 113.27 Local recurrences of cutaneous melanoma. A Recurrent lentigo maligna along upper lateral margin of the excision on the chin; inked lesion on central upper lip is actinic keratosis. **B** Recurrent *in situ* acral lentiginous melanoma at the 10 o'clock position on the split-thickness skin graft. **C** Amelanotic nodular recurrence of a desmoplastic melanoma within the skin graft. A–C, Courtesy of Jean L Bolognia MD.

Data exist to indicate that definitive surgical treatment may be safely delayed for 3 weeks after an excisional biopsy without adversely influencing the 5-year survival rate[114]. Longer time periods may still be permissible, although the upper limit is unknown.

Follow-up is indicated because of the risk of developing a second primary melanoma (estimated at 3.5–4.5%)[115–117] as well as local relapse and/or metastasis from the original tumor[90]. There is little evidence to support specific follow-up intervals, but the American Academy of Dermatology task force recommends follow-up one to four times per year for 2 years after diagnosis, depending on the thickness of the lesion and other risk factors such as a melanoma family history, and then one to two times per year thereafter[98]. Follow-up interventions usually include medical history, clinical examination, and laboratory/radiologic tests as indicated by signs and symptoms. Patients should be educated in sun protection and the performance of routine skin self-examination.

Local Recurrences

Local recurrence is defined as any recurrence within 2 cm of the excisional surgical scar of a primary melanoma[83]. Recurrence results from extension of the primary tumor or intralymphatic spread. The overall risk of recurrence is approximately 4%, and is increased in thicker or ulcerated tumors as well as in head and neck and distal leg locations (Fig 113.27)[118]. Ultra-late recurrence (>15 years) may occur in melanoma, although without identifiable risk factors[119]. Local recurrence is strongly associated with the development of in-transit, regional and distant metastases but is not an independent prognostic indicator of survival in multivariate analysis[118]. There is evidence that patients with local recurrence, satellites and in-transit metastases all have a similar outcome[120]. There is no evidence that patient survival is adversely affected if local recurrence results from inadequate excision of the primary melanoma (i.e. persistent disease) provided that the residual *in situ* or radial growth-based tumor is promptly re-excised and provided there is no distant disease at the time[113]. Development of local recurrence in melanomas <4 mm thick is often due to inadequate surgical treatment[121].

In a population-based study, local recurrence had no major detrimental effect on survival[122]. However in a recent contradictory study, local recurrence was associated with a high mortality rate[110]. Patterns of treatment failure after local recurrence suggest that patients may benefit from aggressive loco-regional therapy[123]. Surgical resection with a wide margin (up to 3 cm depending on the anatomic site) is the most common and effective therapy. In selected patients, isolated limb perfusion which has high regional response rates for the treatment of in-transit metastases (Fig. 113.28) may be considered[124].

Management of Regional Metastatic Melanoma (Stage III)

Metastatic spread of melanoma is often regional and confined to the site of the primary melanoma and its draining lymph nodes. Metastasis may manifest as a clinically occult lymph node micrometastasis, as a rapidly growing clinically evident macrometastasis, or as in-transit metastasis.

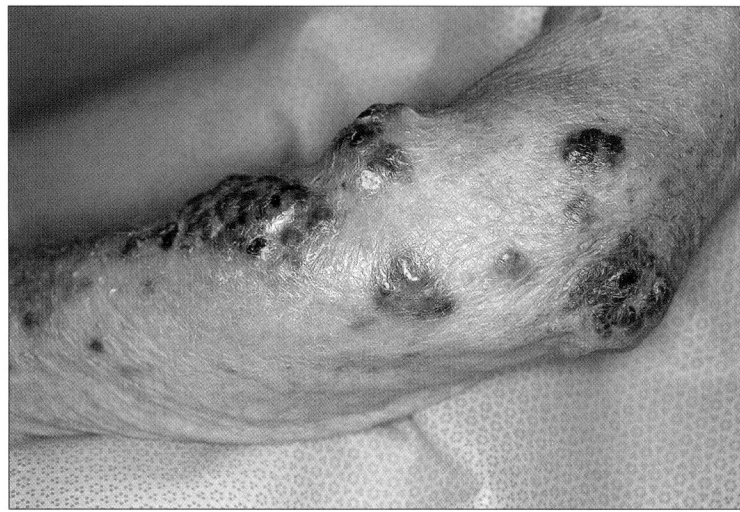

Fig 113.28 In-transit metastases of melanoma. Multiple large blue–black nodules along the lymphatics. Courtesy of Jean L Bolognia MD.

Elective lymph node dissection

Approximately 20% of patients with a cutaneous melanoma that is >1 mm in depth plus no evidence (clinically or radiologically) of detectable nodal disease at presentation show microscopic involvement[125]. On the basis of a presumed migration of melanoma cells in an orderly fashion towards the draining lymph node, surgical resection of regional lymph nodes in all patients with intermediate- and high-risk tumors was once recommended and was referred to as 'elective lymph node dissection (ELND)'. ELND was postulated to be especially beneficial for patients with microscopic disease of the lymph nodes by preventing spread of tumor cells to internal organs. An opposing view was that excision of lymph node metastases might impair the body's immune response to melanoma[126]. There is significant morbidity associated with ELND, such as postoperative lymphedema, wound infection, hematomas and seromas. While one retrospective trial suggested a benefit from ELND in intermediate-risk melanoma patients[127], four other multi-center randomized prospective trials in patients with primary melanoma did not show a survival benefit for patients treated with ELND plus wide re-excision as compared to wide re-excision alone[128–131]. A further randomized trial did not show any benefit of immediate dissection of regional nodes in patients with a melanoma >1.5 mm in depth[132]. Hence, the weight of the evidence indicates that ELND should not be performed in patients with primary melanoma.

Sentinel lymph node biopsy

As noted above, only a minority (~20%) of patients who underwent ELND in the past had micrometastatic disease in the lymph nodes. A less traumatic procedure to identify regional metastatic disease was devised based on similar concepts – namely, progression of metastatic disease through the lymphatic system before widespread dissemination[133]. The so-called sentinel lymph node biopsy (SLNB) is based on the finding that the cutaneous site of the melanoma drains to one or more lymph node basins and particularly to one (or two but rarely more) lymph node, the sentinel node, which is the first site of deposition of metastatic cells. The concept and its utility are also based on the ability to accurately identify this node. The draining lymph node basins for a given melanoma site and the approximate location of the sentinel node within that basin are identified and marked on the overlying skin preoperatively during lymphoscintigraphy performed in the nuclear medicine suite. Intraoperatively, typically in conjunction with the wide local excision, ^{99m}technetium sulfur colloid and blue dye are injected into the skin surrounding the melanoma biopsy site. A small incision is made at the previously marked site overlying the sentinel node and a hand-held gamma counter and visual inspection are used to identify the 'hot, blue' sentinel node(s) which is selectively biopsied and examined by serial sectioning using H&E stains combined with immunohistochemistry (S100, HMB45). If metastatic melanoma is identified, then a complete regional lymph node dissection is undertaken.

Training and experience are important in SLNB. SLNB performed with blue dye plus a radiocolloid is more accurate (99.1%) than SLNB performed with blue dye alone (95.2%). Evidence exists that at least 30 SLNBs are required to gain the appropriate skill level[134]. Numerous studies have documented the accuracy of this procedure for identifying nodal metastases. A randomized trial provided further evidence that lymphatic mapping and SLNB accurately reflect the status of the regional nodal basin[135]. This study also reported a low rate of tumor recurrence (11%) in sentinel node-negative patients. In 80% of these cases, occult micrometastases were later identified by serial sectioning and appropriate immunohistochemistry using S100 and HMB45 monoclonal antibodies. The use of RT-PCR to examine sentinel nodes for mRNA of melanoma-associated proteins such as tyrosinase or Melan-A/MART-1 might increase sensitivity of detection. In one study, tyrosinase transcripts were detected in 36–52% of stage I and II melanoma patients with negative sentinel nodes by histopathology alone. Importantly, the recurrence rate was significantly higher in patients with histologically negative sentinel nodes who were found to be positive by RT-PCR than in patients with negative results by both techniques[136]. Unanswered questions such as the clinical importance of RT-PCR-positive sentinel nodes as well as the effect of adjuvant therapy in patients with negative sentinel nodes will hopefully be answered by ongoing prospective trials[137].

Based on current data, there are four potential reasons to perform SLNB. First, SLNB is a staging tool that provides valuable prognostic information for patients and physicians to guide subsequent treatment decisions. Second, SLNB identifies patients with metastatic lymph nodes for early therapeutic lymph node dissection (see below). Third, SLNB identifies patients who might be candidates for adjuvant therapy with interferon-α (IFN-α). Fourth, results of SLNB can serve as a stratification criterion to enter more homogeneous patients into adjuvant clinical trials[138]. Indeed, the AJCC recommends that all patients with a primary melanoma >1.0 mm in tumor thickness have nodal staging with sentinel lymphadenectomy before entry into melanoma clinical trials[82].

From the perspective of staging, the widespread use of SLNB is causing a stage migration resulting in a growing number of stage III melanoma patients with diverse outcomes. The 5-year survival rates for stage III melanoma patients range from 69% for patients with non-ulcerated melanomas who had a single clinically occult nodal metastasis to 13% for patients with an ulcerated melanoma and four or more clinically apparent nodal metastases as detected by therapeutic lymphadenectomy[82].

From a therapeutic perspective, there is little evidence that early dissection in sentinel node-positive patients affords improved survival compared to dissection performed when clinically detectable nodes develop. One study suggested that further node dissection in patients with positive lymph nodes might be beneficial[132]. However, a randomized trial in patients with newly diagnosed melanoma that examined the contribution of SLNB to clinical outcome did not show an impact on overall survival in patients treated with SLNB followed by immediate lymphadenectomy (as compared to controls)[139]. As to the utility of SLNB for identifying patients for adjuvant therapy with interferon, additional trials are needed to ascertain the relative utility of this approach[140].

In conclusion, intraoperative lymphatic mapping and SLNB followed by selective complete lymphadenectomy has revolutionized the management of the regional lymph node basin in patients with melanoma. The sentinel node procedure has been validated by a multicenter clinical trial showing that SLNB in melanoma can be accurately performed in a uniform manner by multidisciplinary teams. Although the diagnostic and prognostic accuracy as well as usefulness of SLNB has been established, its therapeutic use has not been demonstrated.

Adjuvant therapy

The goal of adjuvant therapy is the elimination of clinically inapparent micrometastases. The major target population for adjuvant therapy is patients with resected high-risk stage II and III melanoma. Some trials have also targeted resected stage IV patients. A number of postsurgical adjuvant approaches have been tested, including systemic chemotherapy and immunotherapy using microbial agents such as bacille Calmette–Guérin (BCG) or *Corynebacterium parvum*[141–143]. None of these approaches were successful in randomized controlled trials[144].

The current recommendation is to include appropriate patients in well-controlled clinical studies to obtain valid data leading to recommendations about future adjuvant therapy. Currently, the major candidates for adjuvant therapy in patients with melanoma are recombinant biological response modifiers, in particular the intensively studied IFN-α. IFN-α is a type I member of the interferon family of proteins and has pleiotropic functions. These include complex immunoregulatory functions such as induction of MHC class I expression as well as an impact on immune effector cells such as the activation of natural killer (NK) cells and the maturation of dendritic cells. Some of its activities may have direct or indirect antitumor effects[145]. Limited antitumor activity has been demonstrated in metastatic stage IV melanoma, with overall response rates of 10–15%. IFN-α has been most widely studied in the adjuvant setting for stage II and III disease. It is important to distinguish high-dose IFN-α therapy with the aim of reaching maximally tolerated dosage (20 MU/m^2 intravenously during the induction phase, followed by 10 MU/m^2 subcutaneously three times per week) from low-dose IFN-α therapy which is much better tolerated in terms of side effects (typically 3 MU subcutaneously three times per week) (Table 113.12).

High-dose IFN-α has demonstrated an improvement in relapse-free and overall survival compared to controls in two studies (ECOG 1684 as well as ECOG 1694) (see Table 113.12). However, a beneficial effect

SELECTED TRIALS FOR ADJUVANT INTERFERON-α_2 THERAPY IN MELANOMA

	Trial	TNM	N	Agent	Treatment	RFS	OS
Low-dose	EORTC 18871	T3–4, N1	800	IFN-α_{2b} IFN-γ	1 MU sc, qod, 52 wk versus 0.2 mg sc, qod, 52 wk versus Iscador versus Observation	–	–
	WHO 16[146]	N1–2	444	IFN-α_{2a}	3 MU sc, t.i.w, 36 mo versus Observation	–	–
	Austrian trial[147]	T3–4, N0	311	IFN-α_{2a}	3 MU sc, daily, 3 wk, followed by 3 MU, t.i.w., 48 wk versus Observation	+	–
	French trial[148]	T3, N0	499	IFN-α_{2a}	3 MU sc, t.i.w., 18 mo versus Observation	+	–
Intermediate-dose	EORTC 18952	T4, N1–2	1388	IFN-α_{2b}	10 MU sc, daily x 5/7 d/wk, 4 wk followed by either 10 MU sc, t.i.w., 52 wk or 5 MU, t.i.w., 104 wk versus Observation	–	–
High-dose	NCCTG 837052[149]	T3–4, N1	262	IFN-α_{2a}	20 MU/m^2 im, t.i.w., 12 wk	–	–
	ECOG 1684[150]	T4, N1	287	IFN-α_{2b}	20 MU/m^2 iv, daily × 5/7 d/wk, 4 wk followed by 10 MU/m^2 sc, t.i.w., 48 wk	+	+
High-dose versus low-dose	ECOG 1690[151]	T4, N1	642	IFN-α_{2b}	20 MU/m^2 iv, daily × 5/7 d/wk, 4 wk followed by 10 MU/m^2 sc, t.i.w., 48 wk (HDI) versus 3 MU sc, t.i.w, 24 mo (LDI)	+	–
High-dose versus ganglioside	ECOG 1694[152]	T4, N1	880	IFN-α_{2b} versus GMK	20 MU/m^2 iv, daily × 5/7 d/wk, 4wk followed by 10 MU/m^2 sc, t.i.w., 48 wk (HDI) versus GMK sc, weekly, 3 mo	+	+

Table 113.12 Selected trials for adjuvant interferon (IFN)-α_2 therapy in melanoma. +, statistically significant improvement with IFN; –, statistically insignificant impact; ECOG, Eastern Cooperative Oncology Group; GMK, GM2 ganglioside, keyhole limpet hemocyanin plus OS21 adjuvant; HDI, high-dose interferon; im, intramuscular; iv, intravenous; LDI, low-dose interferon; mo, months; MU, million units; NCCTG, North Central Cancer Treatment Group; OS, overall survival; qod, every other day; RFS, relapse-free survival; sc, subcutaneous; t.i.w., three times per week; wk, weeks.

on overall survival was not seen in another high-dose IFN-α study (ECOG 1690). A recent study showed the association of the appearance of autoantibodies or clinical manifestations of autoimmunity during treatment with IFN-α_{2b} with significant improvements in relapse-free survival and overall survival in patients with melanoma[153].

Toxicities from high-dose IFN-α include constitutional (flu-like) symptoms and neuropsychiatric (depression, suicidal intention), hematologic and hepatic side effects, as well as cases of fatal rhabdomyolysis[154,155]. These toxicities have a major impact on the patient's quality of life and lead to dose modifications in two-thirds of patients in the first month of high-dose IFN-α therapy. IFN-α is the only FDA-approved adjuvant therapy for melanoma in the US. The use of high-dose IFN-α adjuvant therapy has been questioned, especially in Europe, due to the inconsistent reports of its impact on overall survival and the considerable dose-dependent toxicity[156,157]. It has, however, been suggested that patients view recurrence of metastases as having a greater impact on quality of life than high-dose IFN-α-associated toxicity[158,159]. For low-dose IFN-α, randomized studies have consistently reported a benefit with regard to relapse-free but not overall survival compared to untreated controls[147,148]. Ongoing trials have been designed to address the utility of long-term maintenance low-dose IFN-α therapy.

A meta-analysis has been performed of all available IFN-α trial results, largely based on published reports. The endpoints evaluated were disease-free survival and overall survival in approximately 3700 patients included in ten trials[160]. For disease-free survival, there was clear benefit for IFN-α, but the advantage was less clear for overall survival. There was no statistically significant evidence that the benefit of IFN-α was greater in higher- than in lower-dose trials. The authors concluded that 'decisions on the use of IFN-α for melanoma will need to be based on considerations such as the relative importance of benefits on disease-free survival compared to overall survival, patient quality of life and financial costs.'

Management of Distant Metastases (Stage IV)

Despite new treatment options, the prognosis for patients with distant metastatic melanoma has not changed significantly over recent decades, with survival rates of 6% and median survival of 7.5 months[88]. The initial site of metastasis determines prognosis. For example, non-regional nodal metastases and gastrointestinal metastases (median survival of 12.5 months; estimated 5-year survival rate, 14%) have a better prognosis than pulmonary metastases (median survival of 8.3 months; estimated 5-year survival rate, 4%). The worst prognosis is associated with metastases to the liver, brain or bone (median survival of 4.4 months; estimated 5-year survival rate, 3%)[88]. Thus, the focus is often on palliative therapy with special emphasis on quality of life. In the absence of proven highly effective therapies, a discussion of the option of participation in clinical trials is appropriate in the management of most stage IV melanoma patients. There is evidence that patients included in clinical trials may have a better outcome[161]. Recent developments with a favorable benefit:side effect profile include oral chemotherapeutic agents and innovative approaches to therapeutic cancer vaccination. It should also be noted that surgery plays a limited but important role in the management of stage IV patients. Randomized trials have demonstrated that the value of surgery for local metastatic disease is probably underestimated, while the value of extensive surgery and prophylactic surgical procedures is overestimated[157].

Evaluation of the patient with suspected metastatic disease

It is essential to get an accurate picture of the metastatic burden before considering therapy. Evaluation should be guided by an in-depth medical history and physical examination. Further staging investigations include a CT scan of the chest, abdomen and pelvis, as well as an MRI of the brain. FDG-PET provides an additional method with a high sensitivity for detection of metastases (see above). Measuring soluble

SYMPTOMS AND DIAGNOSTIC TESTS FOR METASTATIC MELANOMA

Metastatic site (TNM)	Symptoms	Diagnostic tests*
Skin, soft tissue metastasis (TxNxM1a), in-transit metastasis (TxN2cM0)	Papules or nodules that vary in color from skin-toned to pink–red to blue, brown or black; secondary ulceration or bleeding	Histologic examination
Brain metastasis (TxNxM1c)	Headache, nausea, seizures, focal weakness, visual disturbance, paresthesias	CT, PET-CT or MRI
Lung metastasis† (TxNxM1b)	Chest pain, dyspnea, cough, hemoptysis	Chest radiograph, CT or PET-CT
Gastrointestinal (including liver) metastasis (TxNxM1c)	• GI: abdominal pain, signs of anemia (e.g. fatigue, chest pain), vomiting, constipation, melena • Liver: abdominal pain, jaundice	• CBC, fecal occult blood test, CT with oral contrast or PET-CT; colonoscopy, endoscopy or video capsule endoscopy • Liver function tests, LDH; ultrasound, CT, PET-CT or MRI
Bone metastasis (TxNxM1c)	Pain, spontaneous fractures	Bone scan or PET-CT

*Always include a thorough medical history and physical examination as well as complete blood count (CBC) and blood chemistry including lactate dehydrogenase (LDH). Special procedures such as detection of soluble melanoma markers (e.g. S100, melanoma inhibitory activity [MIA] protein) are performed at selected melanoma referral centers for increased sensitivity of metastasis detection as part of controlled studies.
† Often asymptomatic.

Table 113.13 Symptoms and diagnostic tests for metastatic melanoma. CT, computed tomography; MRI, magnetic resonance imaging; PET, positron emission tomography.

melanoma serum markers such as S100 and MIA may give an early indication of metastatic disease as well as treatment response in some stage IV patients[162,163]. Further specialized diagnostic tests are performed according to individual symptoms of the patient (Table 113.13).

Surgery

Despite the well-known behavior of melanoma to disseminate to multiple organs, resection of metastases may provide excellent palliation and, in selected patients, long-term survival (Table 113.14). Factors that positively influence prognosis are isolated non-visceral metastasis and complete resection with free surgical margins. In certain cases, median 5-year survival can approach 35% after surgical treatment.

TREATMENT OPTIONS FOR METASTATIC MELANOMA

Metastatic site (TNM)	Treatment choice
In-transit metastasis (TxN2cM0)	1st: <5 – surgery; >5 – extremity perfusion* 2nd: radiotherapy, CO2 laser ablation, intralesional IL-2, topical imiquimod, topical miltefosine 3rd: systemic therapy
Brain metastasis (TxNxM1c) Single Multiple	1st: surgery, stereotactic radiosurgery 1st: radiotherapy 2nd: systemic therapy
Lung metastasis (TxNxM1b) Single Multiple	1st: surgery 1st: systemic therapy
Gastrointestinal metastasis (TxNxM1c) Single Multiple	1st: surgery 1st: systemic therapy; for liver metastases, isolated liver perfusion
Skin, soft tissue metastasis (TxNxM1a) Single Multiple	1st: surgery 1st: surgery, systemic therapy, topical imiquimod, topical miltefosine
Painful bone metastasis (TxNx1c)	1st: radiotherapy
Disseminated metastasis (TxNxM1c)	1st: systemic therapy ± surgery, radiotherapy of symptomatic metastasis

*Should be performed as part of controlled studies.

Table 113.14 Treatment options for metastatic melanoma. IL-2, interleukin-2.

Complete resection of lung metastases can lead to a median survival of 19 months and a 5-year survival of 25%. Patients rarely survive long term after brain or gastrointestinal metastases, but surgical resection extends median survival to about 10 months in this group, with a significant improvement in quality of life[164]. The combination of cytoreductive surgery, with the goal of resecting clinically evident disease, and immunotherapy has been tried as an approach to management of stage IV patients[165].

Radiation therapy

The efficacy of radiotherapy for melanoma is often understated due to unfavorable clinical results observed in early studies. Recent evidence indicates that melanoma is not only highly variable in its radiosensitivity but that radioresistance might be overcome using large individual dose fractions[166]. Radiation therapy has been useful in some extensive lentigo malignas (see Ch. 139). Radiotherapy also provides effective palliation in symptomatic advanced melanoma (Table 113.14)[167]. Specific indications include pain associated with bone metastases, spinal cord compression, brain metastases and local control of cutaneous disease. Studies do not support the administration of adjuvant radiotherapy following resection of regional lymph node metastases[168].

Whole brain radiotherapy combined with surgical resection has been the mainstay of the treatment of cerebral metastases. This approach results in a median survival of about 10 months[169]. A recent development producing at least similar results is stereotactic radiosurgery using either the so-called 'Gamma Knife' or linear accelerator radiosurgical techniques. Radiosurgery has been shown to be effective for metastatic tumors in surgically inaccessible sites such as the brainstem. A benefit of radiosurgery is the virtual absence of perioperative complications, with a reduced adverse impact on quality of life compared to surgery or whole brain radiotherapy. Long-term complications of radiosurgery are infrequent and primarily relate to short-term failure of local tumor control (10%) and radiation-induced edema or necrosis[169].

Systemic therapy

The mainstay of therapy in patients with distant metastases is systemic therapy. The systemic agents that have been used include chemotherapy, immunotherapy, and combination biochemotherapy. A recent development has been the introduction of molecularly targeted therapy for melanoma[170]. The overall results with these therapies have been sufficiently disappointing that participation in clinical trials should be considered, if not encouraged, for this patient population.

Chemotherapy

Over the past four decades, cytotoxic chemotherapy has had a low but reproducible level of activity against metastatic melanoma (Table 113.14). Drugs employed include dacarbazine (DTIC)/temozolomide, cisplatin, vindesine/vinblastine, BCNU/fotemustine and taxol/taxotere[171]. Chemotherapeutic treatment of stage IV melanoma has been disappointing. Advances in chemotherapy have not had a significant impact on melanoma survival over the last 20 years despite the identification of multiple chemotherapeutic agents with activity against melanoma as demonstrated *in vitro* and in phase I/II clinical trials[88]. A promising area of research is the selection of melanoma chemotherapy according to *in vitro* chemosensitivity assays[172]. Recent developments include oral delivery of the prodrug of dacarbazine (temozolomide), combination chemotherapy, and combinations of chemotherapy and immunotherapy[173].

The most widely used single chemotherapeutic agent remains dacarbazine (DTIC). It has shown the greatest effectiveness as a single agent in most trials and was equally effective when combined with IFN-α or tamoxifen[174]. With DTIC as a single agent, an approximately 20% response rate can be achieved with a median response duration of 5 to 6 months and complete response rates of 5%[175]. The oral alkylating agent temozolomide (a prodrug of MTIC, the active metabolite of DTIC) has some efficacy in CNS metastasis and equal efficacy to DTIC[176,177]. Fotemustine is a member of the nitrosourea family and has some efficacy in melanoma including brain metastases[178].

Combination chemotherapy regimens like CVD (cisplatin, vinblastine, DTIC) and BOLD (bleomycin, vincristine, lomustine, DTIC) have induced responses in metastatic lesions typically unresponsive to DTIC alone, including in the liver, bone and brain, but have failed to improve overall patient survival. Another approach is chemohormonal therapy using tamoxifen in addition to chemotherapy. The CBDT (cisplatin, carmustine, DTIC and tamoxifen) or 'Dartmouth regimen' achieved high response rates in earlier trials (up to 55%), but a phase III trial did not show a statistical survival benefit compared to DTIC alone[179]. Therefore, DTIC remains the reference standard for chemotherapy in stage IV melanoma.

Immunotherapy

Immunotherapy builds on the concept that the immune system is able to fight cancer[180]. Melanoma is one of the prototypic immunogenic cancers[21]. Therefore, therapeutic effect might be achieved by infusing effectors of the immune system such as cytokines, killer cells or antibodies. Immunization seeks to stimulate the patient's immune effector cells in response to an injected vaccine (antigen plus adjuvant).

Treatment of advanced melanoma with single cytokines such as IFN-α or IL-2 has been disappointing, even though high-dose IL-2 might lead to long-term remissions[181]. Antibody-based therapies, including the use of anti-ganglioside antibody or anti-high-molecular-weight melanoma-associated antigen (MAA) antibody, which might be coupled to a toxin (e.g. ricin) or radioactive isotope have yet to demonstrate marked activity in melanoma comparable to the activity of anti-CD20 antibody in B-cell lymphoma[182]. Adoptive immunotherapy using *in vitro* expansion of tumor-infiltrating killer cells targeting melanoma epitopes is an interesting concept but has failed to translate into practical use due to low response rates and technical difficulties. Combined adoptive immunotherapy and lymphodepleting chemotherapy is undergoing trials[183].

There has been considerable interest in the use of active immunization/vaccination for the treatment of advanced melanoma. In the past, most vaccines under study were whole cell preparations or lysates of melanoma in combination with a variety of adjuvants. Examples are: (1) polyvalent allogeneic melanoma cell lines ± BCG (CancerVax™, Canvaxin™)[184]; (2) allogeneic melanoma lysates plus 'detox' (a 'detoxified' bacterial endotoxin) (Melacine®)[185]; (3) autologous melanoma cells modified with the hapten dinitrophenol (M-VAX™)[186]; and (4) shed antigen vaccine[187]. These showed some effects in phase II trials in advanced melanoma patients but were for the most part disappointing in randomized controlled trials[188]. Gene-modified whole cell vaccines have so far failed to demonstrate a significant clinical effect[189]. An antigen-based ganglioside vaccine (GM2-KLH/QS21) induced antibody responses but was less effective than high-dose IFN-α in a randomized trial[152].

Progress in the field of melanoma immunology has allowed the identification of new melanoma antigens. Based on this knowledge, the new field of antigen-specific *peptide vaccination* is rapidly expanding. These peptides are defined stretches of amino acids corresponding to a known melanoma epitope. An advantage of the peptide approach is the ability to exactly follow the melanoma-specific immune response during vaccination. Rosenberg et al.[190] have demonstrated clinical responses in patients injected with melanoma peptides, incomplete Freund's adjuvant and IL-2. In other trials, tumor regression as well as immunologic responses were observed[191,192]. An alternative approach is the use of dendritic cells to boost a melanoma-specific immune response. Early clinical trials using dendritic cells pulsed with melanoma peptides have demonstrated immune responses as well as clinical responses in selected patients[193,194]. However, the first multicenter phase II/III trial demonstrated low therapeutic efficacy which was not statistically different from that of systemic DTIC[195].

An innovative approach represents the interference with the immunosuppressive environment of melanoma by blocking downregulatory signals (i.e. releasing the brake) of the immune system using anti-CTLA-4 antibodies[196].

Biochemotherapy

A combination of biological response modifiers and chemotherapy has been termed chemo-immunotherapy, also referred to as 'biochemotherapy'. The most promising combinations have involved the use of high doses of IFN-α or IL-2 with cisplatin-based chemotherapy regimens[197]. Initial phase II trials of biochemotherapy demonstrated favorable response rates of 40–60%, complete response rates of 10–20%, and a median survival of 11–12 months[198]. These clinical benefits were associated with very significant toxicity[199,200]. Unfortunately, phase III clinical trials failed to confirm the response rates that had been previously observed and did not demonstrate superiority of biochemotherapy to single-agent IL-2 therapy[199]. There have been many modifications of the doses and the relative timing of the administration of the components of these regimens, making interpretation of the data difficult. There have also been significant improvements in the prevention of life-threatening toxicities through the use of growth factor support. In light of the limitations of the phase III studies that have been conducted to date, some authors have concluded that biochemotherapy remains an important treatment modality in young patients with no CNS metastases[170].

Molecularly targeted therapy

As described above, ongoing molecular studies are identifying the genetic pathways, genes and gene products involved in melanoma progression. These studies are providing molecular targets for melanoma therapy[201]. Examples of successful molecularly targeted therapy for other malignancies include tretinoin in acute promyelocytic leukemia and imatinib for chronic myelocytic leukemia and gastrointestinal stromal tumor[202]. Despite the complexity of the genetic alterations observed in melanoma, there is evidence to suggest that the inhibition of a single critical pathway in tumor cells may lead to cell death and an associated clinical response[203]. Antibody- and small molecule-based therapies are being successfully developed to target kinases, extracellular ligands, and cell surface receptors critical to these pathways. Initial therapeutic trials have focused on the use of a not very specific Raf kinase inhibitor, as up to 70% of melanomas have been demonstrated to harbor a specific activating somatic mutation of the *BRAF* proto-oncogene[204].

In addition to direct molecular targeting of the cancer cell, insights into tumor/host biology are providing additional therapeutic targets within the tumor microenvironment. One important class of agents is that targeting angiogenesis. Melanomas are associated with robust angiogenesis and the overexpression of vascular endothelial growth factor (VEGF) is associated with poor prognosis. Thalidomide, which has many potential mechanisms of action, is under study as a potential antiangiogenic agent for melanoma. Bevacizumab, a humanized anti-VEGF mouse monoclonal antibody, is being investigated as well[201].

1. Lens MB, Dawes M. Global perspectives of contemporary epidemiological trends of cutaneous malignant melanoma. Br J Dermatol. 2004; 150:179–85.

2. Jemal A, Murray T, Ward E, et al. Cancer statistics, 2005. CA Cancer J Clin. 2005;55:10–29.

3. Elder DE, Clark WH Jr, Elenitsas R, Guerry D, Halpern AC. The early and intermediate precursor lesions of tumor progression in the melanocytic system: common acquired nevi and atypical (dysplastic) nevi. Semin Diagn Pathol. 1993;10:18–35.

4. Clark WH Jr. A classification of malignant melanoma in man correlated with histogenesis and biological behaviour. In: Advances in Biology of the Skin. Oxford: Pergamon Press, 1967:621–47.

5. Curtin JA, Fridlyand J, Kageshita T, et al. Distinct sets of genetic alterations in melanoma. N Engl J Med. 2005;353:2135–47.

6. Hayward NK. Genetics of melanoma predisposition. Oncogene. 2003;22:3053–62.

7. Sharpless E, Chin L. The INK4a/ARF locus and melanoma. Oncogene. 2003;22:3092–8.

8. Yang G, Rajadurai A, Tsao H. Recurrent patterns of dual RB and p53 pathway inactivation in melanoma. J Invest Dermatol. 2005;125:1242–51.

9. Bataille V. Genetic epidemiology of melanoma. Eur J Cancer. 2003;39:1341–7.

10. Hansen CB, Wadge LM, Lowstuter K, Boucher K, Leachman SA. Clinical germline genetic testing for melanoma. Lancet Oncol. 2004;5:314–19.

11. Kefford R, Bishop JN, Tucker M, et al. Genetic testing for melanoma. Lancet Onco1. 2002;3:653–4.

12. Wachsmuth RC, Turner F, Barrett JH, et al. The effect of sun exposure in determining nevus density in UK adolescent twins. J Invest Dermatol. 2005;124:56–62.

13. Landi MT, Kanetsky PA, Tsang S, et al. MC1R, ASIP, and DNA repair in sporadic and familial melanoma in a Mediterranean population. J Natl Cancer Inst. 2005;97:998–1007.

14. Rivers JK. Is there more than one road to melanoma? Lancet. 2004;363:728–30.

15. Steingrimsson E, Copeland NG, Jenkins NA. Melanocyte stem cell maintenance and hair graying. Cell. 2005;121:9–12.

16. Widlund HR, Fisher DE. Microphthalamia-associated transcription factor: a critical regulator of pigment cell development and survival. Oncogene. 2003;22:3035–41.

17. Gupta PB, Kuperwasser C, Brunet JP, et al. The melanocyte differentiation program predisposes to metastasis after neoplastic transformation. Nat Genet. 2005;37:1047–54.

18. Chudnovsky Y, Adams AE, Robbins PB, Lin Q, Khavari PA. Use of human tissue to assess the oncogenic activity of melanoma-associated mutations. Nat Genet. 2005;37:745–9.

19. Chin L. The genetics of malignant melanoma: lessons from mouse and man. Nat Rev Cancer. 2003;3:559–70.

20. De Fabo EC, Noonan FP, Fears T, Merlino G. Ultraviolet B but not ultraviolet A radiation initiates melanoma. Cancer Res. 2004;64:6372–6.

21. Nestle FO, Burg G, Dummer R. New perspectives on immunobiology and immunotherapy of melanoma. Immunol Today. 1999;20:5–7.

22. Boon T, Coulie PG, Van den Eynde BJ, Van der Bruggen P. Human T cell responses against melanoma. Annu Rev Immunol. 2005;24:175–208.

23. Rosenberg SA. Progress in human tumour immunology and immunotherapy. Nature. 2001;411:380–4.

24. Hofbauer GF, Schaefer C, Noppen C, et al. MAGE-3 immunoreactivity in formalin-fixed, paraffin-embedded primary and metastatic melanoma: frequency and distribution. Am J Pathol. 1997;151:1549–53.

25. Marincola FM, Jaffee EM, Hicklin DJ, Ferrone S. Escape of human solid tumors from T-cell recognition: molecular mechanisms and functional significance. Adv Immunol. 2000;74:181–273.

26. Antony PA, Restifo NP. CD4+CD25+ T regulatory cells, immunotherapy of cancer, and interleukin-2. J Immunother. 2005;28:120–8.

27. Beddingfield FC 3rd. The melanoma epidemic: res ipsa loquitur.[see comment]. Oncologist. 2003;8:459–65.

28. Welch HG, Woloshin S, Schwartz LM. Skin biopsy rates and incidence of melanoma: population based ecological study. BMJ. 2005;331:481.

29. Marks R. The changing incidence and mortality of melanoma in Australia. Recent Results Cancer Res. 2002;160:113–21.

30. MacKie RM, Bray CA, Hole DJ, et al; Scottish Melanoma Group. Incidence of and survival from malignant melanoma in Scotland: an epidemiological study. Lancet. 2002;360:587–91.

31. Clegg LX, Feuer EJ, Midthune DN, Fay MP, Hankey BF. Impact of reporting delay and reporting error on cancer incidence rates and trends. J Natl Cancer Inst. 2002;94:1537–45.

32. Weinstock MA. Epidemiology, etiology, and control of melanoma. Med Health R I. 2001;84:234–6.

33. Gandini S, Sera F, Cattaruzza MS, et al. Meta-analysis of risk factors for cutaneous melanoma: II. Sun exposure. Eur J Cancer. 2005;41:45–60.

34. Whiteman DC, Watt P, Purdie DM, Hughes MC, Hayward NK, Green AC. Melanocytic nevi, solar keratoses, and divergent pathways to cutaneous melanoma [see comment]. J Natl Cancer Inst. 2003;95:806–12.

35. Autier P. Perspectives in melanoma prevention: the case of sunbeds. Eur J Cancer. 2004;40:2367–76.

36. Gandini S, Sera F, Cattaruzza MS, et al. Meta-analysis of risk factors for cutaneous melanoma: I. Common and atypical naevi. Eur J Cancer. 2005;41:28–44.

37. Goldstein AM, Fraser MC, Clark WH Jr, Tucker MA. Age at diagnosis and transmission of invasive melanoma in 23 families with cutaneous malignant melanoma/dysplastic nevi. J Natl Cancer Inst. 1994;86:1385–90.

38. Evans RD, Kopf AW, Lew RA, et al. Risk factors for the development of malignant melanoma – I: Review of case-control studies. J Dermatol Surg Oncol. 1988;14:393–408.

39. Noonan FP, Recio JA, Takayama H, et al. Neonatal sunburn and melanoma in mice. Nature. 2001;413:271–2.

40. Atillasoy ES, Seykora JT, Soballe PW, et al. UVB induces atypical melanocytic lesions and melanoma in human skin. Am J Pathol. 1998;152:1179–86.

41. Donawho C, Wolf P. Sunburn, sunscreen, and melanoma. Curr Opin Oncol. 1996;8:159–66.

42. Ley RD. Dose response for ultraviolet radiation A-induced focal melanocytic hyperplasia and nonmelanoma skin tumors in Monodelphis domestica. Photochem Photobiol. 2001;73:20–3.

43. Westerdahl J, Ingvar C, Masback A, Olsson H. Sunscreen use and malignant melanoma. Int J Cancer. 2000;87:145–50.

44. Dennis LK, Beane Freeman, LE, VanBeek MJ. Sunscreen use and the risk for melanoma: a quantitative review [see comment]. Ann Intern Med. 2003;139:966–78.

45. Thieden E, Philipsen PA, Sandby-Moller J, Wulf HC. Sunburn related to UV radiation exposure, age, sex, occupation, and sun bed use based on time-stamped personal dosimetry and sun behavior diaries. Arch Dermatol. 2005;141:482–8.

46. Lee TK, Rivers JK, Gallagher RP. Site-specific protective effect of broad-spectrum sunscreen on nevus development among white schoolchildren in a randomized trial. J Am Acad Dermatol. 2005;52:786–92.

47. Clark WH Jr, From L, Bernardino EA, Mihm MC. The histogenesis and biologic behavior of primary human malignant melanomas of the skin. Cancer Res. 1969;29:705–27.

48. Skender-Kalnenas TM, English DR, Heenan PJ. Benign melanocytic lesions: risk markers or precursors of cutaneous melanoma? [see comment]. J Am Acad Dermatol. 1995;33:1000–7.

49. Demierre MF, Chung C, Miller DR, Geller AC. Early detection of thick melanomas in the United States: beware of the nodular subtype. Arch Dermatol. 2005;141:745–50.

50. Weinstock MA, Sober AJ. The risk of progression of lentigo maligna to lentigo maligna melanoma. Br J Dermatol. 1987;116:303–10.

51. Tannous ZS, Lerner LH, Duncan LM, Mihm MC Jr, Flotte TJ. Progression to invasive melanoma from malignant melanoma in situ, lentigo maligna type. Hum Pathol. 2000;31:705–8.

52. Cress RD, Holly EA. Incidence of cutaneous melanoma among non-Hispanic whites, Hispanics, Asians, and blacks: an analysis of California Cancer Registry data, 1988-93. Cancer Causes Control. 1997;8:246–52.

53. Leyden JJ, Spott DA, Goldschmidt H. Diffuse and banded melanin pigmentation in nails. Arch Dermatol. 1972;105:548–50.

54. McNutt NS. "Triggered trap": nevoid malignant melanoma. Semin Diagn Pathol. 1998;15:203–9.

55. Bastian BC. Molecular cytogenetics as a diagnostic tool for typing melanocytic tumors. Recent Results Cancer Res. 2002;160:92–9.

56. Koch H, Zelger B, Cerroni L. Malignant blue nevus: malignant melanoma in association with blue nevus. Eur J Dermatol. 1996;6:335–8.

57. Zettersten E, Sagebiel RW, Miller JR 3rd, Tallapureddy S, Leong SP, Kashani-Sabet M. Prognostic factors in patients with thick cutaneous melanoma (> 4 mm). Cancer. 2002;94:1049–56.

58. Segal NH, Pavlidis P, Noble WS, et al. Classification of clear-cell sarcoma as a subtype of melanoma by genomic profiling. J Clin Oncol. 2003;21:1775–81.

59. Crowson AN, Magro CM, Mihm MC Jr. Malignant melanoma with prominent pigment synthesis: "animal type" melanoma – a clinical and histological study of six cases with a consideration of other melanocytic neoplasms with prominent pigment synthesis. Hum Pathol. 1999;30:543–50.

60. Richtig E, Langmann G, Mullner K, Smolle J. Ocular melanoma: epidemiology, clinical presentation and relationship with dysplastic nevi. Ophthalmologica. 2004;218:111–14.

61. Char DH. Ocular melanoma. Surg Clin North Am. 2003;83:253–74.

62. Tomicic J, Wanebo HJ. Mucosal melanomas. Surg Clin North Am. 2003;83:237–52.

63. Sanchez JL, Figueroa LD, Rodriguez E. Behavior of melanocytic nevi during pregnancy. Am J Dermatopathol. 1984;6(suppl.):89–91.

64. MacKie RM. Pregnancy and exogenous hormones in patients with cutaneous malignant melanoma. Curr Opin Oncol. 1999;11:129–31.

65. Lens MB, Rosdahl I, Ahlbom A, et al. Effect of pregnancy on survival in women with cutaneous malignant melanoma. J Clin Oncol. 2004; 22:4369–75.

66. Grin CM, Driscoll MS, Grant-Kels JM. The relationship of pregnancy, hormones, and melanoma. Semin Cutan Med Surg.1998;17:167–71.

67. Pappo AS. Melanoma in children and adolescents. Eur J Cancer. 2003;39:2651–61.

68. Barnhill RL. Childhood melanoma. Semin Diagn Pathol. 1998;15:189–94.

69. Saenz NC, Saenz-Badillos J, Busam K, LaQuaglia MP, Corbally M, Brady MS. Childhood melanoma survival. Cancer. 1999;85:750–4.

70. Abbasi NR, Shaw HM, Rigel DS, et al. Early diagnosis of cutaneous melanoma: revisiting the ABCD criteria. JAMA. 2004;292:2771–6.

71. Cerroni L, Kerl H. Simulators of malignant melanoma of the skin. Eur J Dermatol. 1998;8:388–96.

72. Massone C, Di Stefani A, Soyer HP. Dermoscopy for skin cancer detection. Curr Opin Oncol. 2005;17:147–53.

73. Argenziano G, Soyer HP, Chimenti S, et al. Dermoscopy of pigmented skin lesions: results of a consensus meeting via the Internet. J Am Acad Dermatol. 2003;48:679–93.

74. Halpern AC. Total body skin imaging as an aid to melanoma detection. Semin Cutan Med Surg. 2003;22:2–8.

75. Feit NE, Dusza SW, Marghoob AA. Melanomas detected with the aid of total cutaneous photography. Br J Dermatol. 2004;150:706–14.

76. Ackerman A, Cerroni L, Kerl H. Pitfalls in Histopathologic Diagnosis of Malignant Melanoma. Philadelphia: Lea & Febiger, 1994.

77. Anonymous. A nationwide survey of observer variation in the diagnosis of thin cutaneous malignant melanoma including the MIN terminology. CRC Melanoma Pathology Panel [see comment]. J Clin Pathol. 1997;50:202–5.

78. Clemente C, Cook M, Ruiter D, Mihm M. Histopathologic diagnosis of melanoma. In: World Health Organization Melanoma Programme Publications, Number 5. Milan: Trezzano SN; 2001.

79. Clark WH Jr, Elder DE, Guerry D, et al. Model predicting survival in stage I melanoma based on tumor progression. J Natl Cancer Inst. 1989; 81:1893–904.

80. Cochran AJ, Bailly C, Cook M, et al. Recommendations for the reporting of tissues removed as part of the surgical treatment of cutaneous melanoma. The Association of Directors of Anatomic and Surgical Pathology. Am J Clin Pathol. 1998;110:719–22.

81. de Wit NJ, van Muijen GN, Ruiter DJ. Immunohistochemistry in melanocytic proliferative lesions. Histopathology. 2004;44:517–41.

82. Balch CM, Soong SJ, Gershenwald JE, et al. Prognostic factors analysis of 17,600 melanoma patients: validation of the American Joint Committee on Cancer melanoma staging system. J Clin Oncol. 2001;19:3622–34.

83. Balch CM, Buzaid AC, Soong SJ, et al. Final version of the American Joint Committee on Cancer staging system for cutaneous melanoma. J Clin Oncol. 2001;19:3635–48.

84. Ruiter DJ, Testori A, Eggermont AM, Punt CJ. The AJCC staging proposal for cutaneous melanoma: comments by the EORTC Melanoma Group. Ann Oncol. 2001;12:9–11.

85. Garbe C, Buttner P, Bertz J, et al. Primary cutaneous melanoma. Identification of prognostic groups and estimation of individual prognosis for 5093 patients. Cancer. 1995;75:2484–91.

86. Levi F, Randimbison L, La Vecchia C, Te VC, Franceschi S. Prognostic factors for cutaneous malignant melanoma in Vaud, Switzerland. Int J Cancer. 1998;78:315–19.

87. Schuchter L, Schultz DJ, Synnestvedt M, et al. A prognostic model for predicting 10-year survival in patients with primary melanoma. The Pigmented Lesion Group [see comment]. Ann Intern Med. 1996;125:369–75.

88. Barth A, Wanek LA, Morton DL. Prognostic factors in 1,521 melanoma patients with distant metastases. J Am Coll Surg. 1995;181:193–201.

89. Seiter S, Rappl G, Tilgen W, Ugurel S, Reinhold U. Facts and pitfalls in the detection of tyrosinase mRNA in the blood of melanoma patients by RT-PCR. Recent Results Cancer Res. 2001;158:105–12.

90. Brochez L, Naeyaert JM. Serological markers for melanoma. Br J Dermatol. 2000;143:256–68.

91. Deichmann M, Benner A, Bock M, et al. S100-Beta, melanoma-inhibiting activity, and lactate dehydrogenase discriminate progressive from nonprogressive American Joint Committee on Cancer stage IV melanoma. J Clin Oncol. 1999;17:1891–6.

92. Johnson TM, Chang A, Redman B, et al. Management of melanoma with a multidisciplinary melanoma clinic model. J Am Acad Dermatol. 2000;42:820–6.

93. McGovern TW, Litaker MS. Clinical predictors of malignant pigmented lesions. A comparison of the Glasgow seven-point checklist and the American Cancer Society's ABCDs of pigmented lesions. J Dermatol Surg Oncol. 1992;18:22–6.

94. Grob JJ, Bonerandi JJ. The 'ugly duckling' sign: identification of the common characteristics of nevi in an individual as a basis for melanoma screening. Arch Dermatol. 1998;134:103–4.

95. Kopf AW, Mintzis M, Bart RS. Diagnostic accuracy in malignant melanoma. Arch Dermatol. 1975;111:1291–2.

96. Binder M, Puespoeck-Schwarz M, Steiner A, et al. Epiluminescence microscopy of small pigmented skin lesions: short-term formal training improves the diagnostic performance of dermatologists. J Am Acad Dermatol. 1997;36:197–202.

97. Wang TS, Johnson TM, Cascade PN, Redman BG, Sondak VK, Schwartz JL. Evaluation of staging chest radiographs and serum lactate dehydrogenase for localized melanoma. J Am Acad Dermatol. 2004;51:399–405.

98. Sober AJ, Chuang TY, Duvic M, et al. Guidelines of care for primary cutaneous melanoma. J Am Acad Dermatol. 2001;45:579–86.

99. Kumar R, Alavi A. Clinical applications of fluorodeoxyglucose – positron emission tomography in the management of malignant melanoma. Curr Opin Oncol. 2005;17:154–9.

100. Strauss LG. Sensitivity and specificity of positron emission tomography (PET) for the diagnosis of lymph node metastases. Recent Results Cancer Res. 2000;157:12–19.

101. Schwimmer J, Essner R, Patel A, et al. A review of the literature for whole-body FDG PET in the management of patients with melanoma. Q J Nucl Med. 2000;44:153–67.

102. Krug B, Dietlein M, Groth W, et al. Fluor-18-fluorodeoxyglucose positron emission tomography (FDG-PET) in malignant melanoma. Diagnostic comparison with conventional imaging methods. Acta Radiol. 2000;41:446–52.

103. Collins BT, Lowe VJ, Dunphy FR. Correlation of CT-guided fine-needle aspiration biopsy of the liver with fluoride-18 fluorodeoxyglucose positron emission tomography in the assessment of metastatic hepatic abnormalities. Diagn Cytopathol. 1999;21:39–42.

104. Voit C, Mayer T, Proebstle TM, et al. Ultrasound-guided fine-needle aspiration cytology in the early detection of melanoma metastases. Cancer. 2000; 90:186–93.

105. Lederman JS, Sober AJ. Does biopsy type influence survival in clinical stage I cutaneous melanoma? J Am Acad Dermatol. 1985;13:983–7.

106. Veronesi U, Cascinelli N, Adamus J, et al. Thin stage I primary cutaneous malignant melanoma. Comparison of excision with margins of 1 or 3 cm. N Engl J Med. 1988;318:1159–62.

107. Veronesi U, Cascinelli N. Narrow excision (1-cm margin). A safe procedure for thin cutaneous melanoma. Arch Surg. 1991;126:438–41.

108. Bono A, Bartoli C, Clemente C, et al. Ambulatory narrow excision for thin melanoma (< or = 2 mm): results of a prospective study. Eur J Cancer. 1997;33:1330–2.

109. Cascinelli N. Margin of resection in the management of primary melanoma. Semin Surg Oncol.1998;14:272–5.

110. Balch CM, Soong SJ, Smith T, et al. Long-term results of a prospective surgical trial comparing 2 cm vs. 4 cm excision margins for 740 patients with 1–4 mm melanomas. Ann Surg Oncol. 2001;8:101–8.

111. Johnson TM, Sondak VK. A centimeter here, a centimeter there: does it matter? J Am Acad Dermatol. 1995;33:532–4.

112. Ross MI, Balch C. Surgical treatment of primary melanoma. In: Balch CM, Houghton AN, Sober AJ, Soong S-J (eds). Cutaneous Melanoma. St Louis: Quality Medical Publishing, 1998:141–53.

113. Kanzler MH, Mraz-Gernhard S. Primary cutaneous malignant melanoma and its precursor lesions: diagnostic and therapeutic overview. J Am Acad Dermatol. 2001;45:260–76.

114. Landthaler M, Braun-Falco O, Leitl A, Konz B, Holzel D. Excisional biopsy as the first therapeutic procedure versus primary wide excision of malignant melanoma. Cancer. 1989;64:1612–16.

115. Gershenwald JE, Thompson W, Mansfield PF, et al. Multi-institutional melanoma lymphatic mapping experience: the prognostic value of sentinel lymph node status in 612 stage I or II melanoma patients. J Clin Oncol. 1999;17:976–83.

116. DiFronzo LA, Wanek LA, Elashoff R, Morton DL. Increased incidence of second primary melanoma in patients with a previous cutaneous melanoma. Ann Surg Oncol. 1999;6:705–11.

117. Brobeil A, Rapaport D, Wells K, et al. Multiple primary melanomas: implications for screening and follow-up programs for melanoma. Ann Surg Oncol. 1997;4:19–23.

118. Karakousis CP, Bartolucci AA, Balch C. Local recurrence and its managment. In: Balch CM, Houghton AN, Sober AJ, Soong S-J (eds). Cutaneous Melanoma. St Louis: Quality Medical Publishing, 1998:155–62.

119. Tsao H, Cosimi AB, Sober AJ. Ultra-late recurrence (15 years or longer) of cutaneous melanoma. Cancer. 1997;79:2361–70.

120. Buzaid AC, Ross MI, Soong SJ. Classification and staging. In: Balch CM, Houghton AN, Sober AJ, Soong S-J (eds). Cutaneous Melanoma. St Louis: Quality Medical Publishing, 1998:37–49.

121. Ng AK, Jones WO, Shaw JH. Analysis of local recurrence and optimizing excision margins for cutaneous melanoma. Br J Surg. 2001;88:137–42.

122. Cohn-Cedermark G, Mansson-Brahme E, Rutqvist LE, Larsson O, Singnomklao T, Ringborg U. Outcomes of patients with local recurrence of cutaneous malignant melanoma: a population-based study. Cancer. 1997;80:1418–25.

123. Dong XD, Tyler D, Johnson JL, DeMatos P, Seigler HF. Analysis of prognosis and disease progression after local recurrence of melanoma. Cancer. 2000;88:1063–71.

124. Lienard D, Eggermont AM, Kroon BB, Schraffordt Koops H, Lejeune FJ. Isolated limb perfusion in primary and recurrent melanoma: indications and results. Semin Surg Oncol. 1998;14:202–9.

125. Mraz-Gernhard S, Sagebiel RW, Kashani-Sabet M, Miller JR 3rd, Leong SP. Prediction of sentinel lymph node micrometastasis by histological features in primary cutaneous malignant melanoma. Arch Dermatol. 1998;134:983–7.

126. Zinkernagel RM. Immunity against solid tumors? Int J Cancer. 2001;93:1–5.

127. Cole DJ, Baron PL. Surgical management of patients with intermediate thickness melanoma: current role of elective lymph node dissection. Semin Oncol. 1996;23:719–24.

128. Veronesi U, Adamus J, Bandiera DC, et al. Delayed regional lymph node dissection in stage I melanoma of the skin of the lower extremities. Cancer. 1982;49:2420–30.

129. Veronesi U, Adamus J, Bandiera DC, et al. Inefficacy of immediate node dissection in stage 1 melanoma of the limbs. N Engl J Med. 1977;297:627–30.

130. Sim FH, Taylor WF, Pritchard DJ, Soule EH. Lymphadenectomy in the management of stage I malignant melanoma: a prospective randomized study. Mayo Clin Proc. 1986;61:697–705.

131. Balch CM, Soong SJ, Bartolucci AA, et al. Efficacy of an elective regional lymph node dissection of 1 to 4 mm thick melanomas for patients 60 years of age and younger. Ann Surg. 1996;224:255–63; discussion 263–6.

132. Cascinelli N, Morabito A, Santinami M, MacKie RM, Belli F. Immediate or delayed dissection of regional nodes in patients with melanoma of the trunk: a randomised trial. WHO Melanoma Programme. Lancet. 1998;351:793–6.

133. Morton DL, Chan AD. The concept of sentinel node localization: how it started. Semin Nucl Med. 2000;30:4–10.

134. Morton DL, Thompson JF, Essner R, et al. Validation of the accuracy of intraoperative lymphatic mapping and sentinel lymphadenectomy for early-stage melanoma: a multicenter trial. Multicenter Selective Lymphadenectomy Trial Group. Ann Surg. 1999;230:453–63; discussion 463–5.

135. Gershenwald JE, Colome MI, Lee JE, et al. Patterns of recurrence following a negative sentinel lymph node biopsy in 243 patients with stage I or II melanoma. J Clin Oncol. 1998;16:2253–60.

136. Blaheta HJ, Schittek B, Breuninger H, Garbe C. Detection of micrometastasis in sentinel lymph nodes of patients with primary cutaneous melanoma. Recent Results Cancer Res. 2001;158:137–46.

137. McMasters KM, Reintgen DS, Ross MI, et al. Sentinel lymph node biopsy for melanoma: how many radioactive nodes should be removed? Ann Surg Oncol. 2001;8:192–7.

138. McMasters KM. The Sunbelt Melanoma Trial. Ann Surg Oncol. 2001;8(suppl.):41S–43S.

139. Morton DL, Thompson JF, Cochran AJ, et al.; MSLT Group. Sentinel-node biopsy or nodal observation in melanoma. N Engl J Med. 2006;355:1307–17.

140. Reintgen D, Pendas S, Jakub J, et al. National trials involving lymphatic mapping for melanoma: the Multicenter Selective Lymphadenectomy Trial, the Sunbelt Melanoma Trial, and the Florida Melanoma Trial. Semin Oncol. 2004;31:363–73.

141. Cascinelli N, Rumke P, MacKie R, Morabito A, Bufalino R. The significance of conversion of skin reactivity to efficacy of bacillus Calmette-Guerin (BCG) vaccinations given immediately after radical surgery in stage II melanoma patients. Cancer Immunol Immunother. 1989;28:282–6.

142. Wallack MK, McNally K, Michaelides M, et al. A phase I/II SECSG (Southeastern Cancer Study Group) pilot study of surgical adjuvant immunotherapy with vaccinia melanoma oncolysates (VMO). Am Surg. 1986;52:148–51.

143. Balch CM, Smalley RV, Bartolucci AA, Burns D, Presant CA, Durant JR. A randomized prospective clinical trial of adjuvant C. parvum immunotherapy in 260 patients with clinically localized melanoma (Stage I): prognostic factors analysis and preliminary results of immunotherapy. Cancer. 1982;49:1079–84.

144. Lotze MT, Dallal RM, Kirkwood JM, Flickinger JC. Cutaneous melanoma. In: de Vita VT, Rosenberg SA (eds). Cancer: Principles and Practice of Oncology. Philadelphia: Lippincott Williams & Wilkins, 2001:2012–68.

145. Kirkwood JM. Adjuvant interferon in the treatment of melanoma. Br J Cancer. 2000;82:1755–6.

146. Cascinelli N, Bufalino R, Morabito A, Mackie R. Results of adjuvant interferon study in WHO melanoma programme. Lancet. 1994;343: 913–14.

147. Pehamberger H, Soyer HP, Steiner A, et al. Adjuvant interferon alfa-2a treatment in resected primary stage II cutaneous melanoma. Austrian Malignant Melanoma Cooperative Group. J Clin Oncol. 1998; 16:1425–9.

148. Grob JJ, Dreno B, De La Salmoniere P, et al. Randomised trial of interferon alpha-2a as adjuvant therapy in resected primary melanoma thicker than 1.5 mm without clinically detectable node metastases. Lancet. 1998;351:105–10.

149. Creagan ET, Dalton RJ, Ahmann DL, et al. Randomized, surgical adjuvant clinical trial of recombinant interferon alfa-2a in selected patients with malignant melanoma. J Clin Oncol. 1995; 13:2776–83.

150. Kirkwood JM, Strawderman MH, Ernstoff MS, et al. Interferon alfa-2b adjuvant therapy of high-risk resected cutaneous melanoma: the Eastern Cooperative Oncology Group Trial EST 1684. J Clin Oncol. 1996;14:7–17.

151. Kirkwood JM, Ibrahim JG, Sondak VK, et al. High- and low-dose interferon alfa-2b in high-risk melanoma: first analysis of intergroup trial E1690/S9111/C9190. J Clin Oncol. 2000;18:2444–58.

152. Kirkwood JM, Ibrahim JG, Sosman JA, et al. High-dose interferon alfa-2b significantly prolongs relapse-free and overall survival compared with the GM2-KLH/ QS-21 vaccine in patients with resected stage IIB-III melanoma: results of intergroup trial E1694/S9512/ C509801. J Clin Oncol. 2001;19:2370–80.

153. Gogas H, Ioannovich J, Dafni U, et al. Prognostic significance of autoimmunity during treatment of melanoma with interferon. N Engl J Med. 2006;354:709–18.

154. Weiss K. Safety profile of interferon-alpha therapy. Semin Oncol. 1998;25:9–13.

155. Reinhold U, Hartl C, Hering R, Hoeft A, Kreysel HW. Fatal rhabdomyolysis and multiple organ failure associated with adjuvant high-dose interferon alfa in malignant melanoma. Lancet. 1997;349:540–1.

156. Hauschild A, Volkenandt M. [Adjuvant therapy of malignant melanoma]. Ther Umsch. 1999;56:324–9.

157. Eggermont AM. Surgical management of primary and metastatic melanoma: what we have learned from randomized trials [Abstract]. Melanoma Res. 2001;11(suppl. 1):61.

158. Kilbridge KL, Weeks JC, Sober AJ, et al. Patient preferences for adjuvant interferon alfa-2b treatment. J Clin Oncol. 2001;19:812–23.

159. Kirkwood JM. Interferon (IFN) is the standard therapy of high-risk resectable cutaneous melanoma. Melanoma Res. 2001;11(suppl. 1):7.

160. Wheatley K, Hancock B, Gore M, et al. Interferon-α as adjuvant therapy for melanoma: a meta-analysis of the randomised trials. Proc Am Soc Clin Oncol. 2001;20:349a (Abstr. 1394).

161. Stiller CA. Centralised treatment, entry to trials and survival. Br J Cancer. 1994;70:352–62.

162. Schmitz C, Brenner W, Henze E, Christophers E, Hauschild A. Comparative study on the clinical use of protein S-100B and MIA (melanoma inhibitory activity) in melanoma patients. Anticancer Res. 2000;20:5059–63.

163. Juergensen A, Holzapfel U, Hein R, Stolz W, Buettner R, Bosserhoff A. Comparison of two prognostic markers for malignant melanoma: MIA and S100 beta. Tumour Biol. 2001;22:54–8.

164. Sharpless SM, Das Gupta TK. Surgery for metastatic melanoma. Semin Surg Oncol. 1998;14:311–18.

165. Morton DL, Ollila DW, Hsueh EC, Essner R, Gupta RK. Cytoreductive surgery and adjuvant immunotherapy: a new management paradigm for metastatic melanoma. CA Cancer J Clin. 1999;49:101–116, 165.

166. Ang KK, Geara FB, Byers RM, Peters LJ. Radiotherapy for melanoma. In: Balch CM, Houghton AN, Sober AJ, Soong S-J (eds). Cutaneous Melanoma. St Louis: Quality Medical Publishing, 1998:389–403.

167. Seegenschmiedt MH, Keilholz L, Altendorf-Hofmann A, et al. Palliative radiotherapy for recurrent and metastatic malignant melanoma: prognostic factors for tumor response and long-term outcome: a 20-year experience. Int J Radiat Oncol Biol Phys. 1999; 44:607–18.

168. Fuhrmann D, Lippold A, Borrosch F, Ellwanger U, Garbe C, Suter L. Should adjuvant radiotherapy be recommended following resection of regional lymph node metastases of malignant melanomas? Br J Dermatol. 2001;144:66–70.

169. Young RF. Radiosurgery for the treatment of brain metastases. Semin Surg Oncol. 1998;14:70–8.

170. Buzaid AC. Management of metastatic cutaneous melanoma. Oncology (Williston Park). 2004;18:1443–50; discussion 1457–9.

171. Legha S. Treatment of advanced melanoma with cytotoxic drugs. Melanoma Res. 2001;11(suppl. 1):13.

172. Cree IA, Neale MH, Myatt NE, et al. Heterogeneity of chemosensitivity of metastatic cutaneous melanoma. Anticancer Drugs. 1999;10:437–44.

173. Dummer R, Nestle FO, Hofbauer G, Burg G. [Systemic therapy of metastatic melanoma]. Ther Umsch. 1999; 56:330–3.

174. Falkson CI, Ibrahim J, Kirkwood JM, Coates AS, Atkins MB, Blum RH. Phase III trial of dacarbazine versus dacarbazine with interferon alpha-2b versus dacarbazine with tamoxifen versus dacarbazine with interferon alpha-2b and tamoxifen in patients with metastatic malignant melanoma: an Eastern Cooperative Oncology Group study. J Clin Oncol. 1998;16:1743–51.

175. Serrone L, Zeuli M, Sega FM, Cognetti F. Dacarbazine-based chemotherapy for metastatic melanoma: thirty-year experience overview. J Exp Clin Cancer Res. 2000;19:21–34.

176. Middleton MR, Grob JJ, Aaronson N, et al. Randomized phase III study of temozolomide versus dacarbazine in the treatment of patients with advanced metastatic malignant melanoma. J Clin Oncol. 2000;18:158–66.

177. Agarwala SS, Kirkwood JM. Temozolomide, a novel alkylating agent with activity in the central nervous system, may improve the treatment of advanced metastatic melanoma. Oncologist. 2000;5:144–51.

178. Ulrich J, Gademann G, Gollnick H. Management of cerebral metastases from malignant melanoma: results of a combined, simultaneous treatment with fotemustine and irradiation. J Neurooncol. 1999;43:173–8.

179. Chapman PB, Einhorn LH, Meyers ML, et al. Phase III multicenter randomized trial of the Dartmouth regimen versus dacarbazine in patients with metastatic melanoma. J Clin Oncol. 1999;17:2745–51.

180. Shankaran V, Ikeda H, Bruce AT, et al. IFNgamma and lymphocytes prevent primary tumour development and shape tumour immunogenicity. Nature. 2001;410:1107–11.

181. Atkins MB, Kunkel L, Sznol M, Rosenberg SA. High-dose recombinant interleukin-2 therapy in patients with metastatic melanoma: long-term survival update. Cancer J Sci Am. 2000;6(suppl. 1):S11–14.

182. Chapman PB, Parkinson DR, Kirkwood JM. Biologic therapy. In: Balch CM, Houghton AN, Sober AJ, Soong S-J (eds). Cutaneous Melanoma. St. Louis: Quality Medical Publishing, 1998:419–36.

183. Dudley ME, Wunderlich JR, Yang JC, et al. Adoptive cell transfer therapy following non-myeloablative but lymphodepleting chemotherapy for the treatment of patients with refractory metastatic melanoma. J Clin Oncol. 2005;23:2346–57.

184. Chan AD, Morton DL. Active immunotherapy with allogeneic tumor cell vaccines: present status. Semin Oncol. 1998;25:611–22.

185. Mitchell MS. Perspective on allogeneic melanoma lysates in active specific immunotherapy. Semin Oncol. 1998;25:623–35.

186. Berd D. Autologous, hapten-modified vaccine as a treatment for human cancers. Vaccine. 2001;19:2565–70.

187. Bystryn JC, Zeleniuch-Jacquotte A, Oratz R, Shapiro RL, Harris MN, Roses DF. Double-blind trial of a polyvalent, shed-antigen, melanoma vaccine. Clin Cancer Res. 2001;7:1882–7.

188. Livingston P. The unfulfilled promise of melanoma vaccines. Clin Cancer Res. 2001;7:1837–8.

189. Sun Y, Paschen A, Schadendorf D. Cell-based vaccination against melanoma – background, preliminary results, and perspective. J Mol Med. 1999;77:593–608.

190. Rosenberg SA, Yang JC, Schwartzentruber DJ, et al. Immunologic and therapeutic evaluation of a synthetic peptide vaccine for the treatment of patients with metastatic melanoma. Nat Med. 1998;4:321–7.

191. Marchand M, van Baren N, Weynants P, et al. Tumor regressions observed in patients with metastatic melanoma treated with an antigenic peptide encoded by gene MAGE-3 and presented by HLA-A1. Int J Cancer. 1999;80:219–30.

192. Jager D, Jager E, Knuth A. Vaccination for malignant melanoma: recent developments. Oncology. 2001;60:1–7.

193. Nestle FO, Alijagic S, Gilliet M, et al. Vaccination of melanoma patients with peptide- or tumor lysate-pulsed dendritic cells. Nat Med. 1998;4:328–32.

194. Thurner B, Haendle I, Roder C, et al. Vaccination with mage-3A1 peptide-pulsed mature, monocyte-derived dendritic cells expands specific cytotoxic T cells and induces regression of some metastases in advanced stage IV melanoma. J Exp Med. 1999;190:1669–78.

195. Schadendorf D, Ugurel S, Schuler-Thurner B, et alDacarbazine (DTIC) versus vaccination with autologous peptide-pulsed dendritic cells (DC) in first-line treatment of patients with metastatic melanoma: a randomized phase III trial of the DC study group of the DeCOG. Ann Oncol. 2006;17:563–70.

196. Attia P, Phan GQ, Maker AV, et al. Autoimmunity correlates with tumor regression in patients with metastatic melanoma treated with anti-cytotoxic T-lymphocyte antigen-4. J Clin Oncol. 2005;23:6043–53.

197. Ross PJ, Gore ME. Scientific evidence and expert clinical opinion for the investigation and management of stage IV malignant melanoma. In: MacKie RM, Murray D, Roisin RD, Hancock B, Miles A (eds). The Effective Management of Malignant Melanoma. London: Aesculapius Medical, 2001:83–104.

198. O'Day SJ, Kim CJ, Reintgen DS. Metastatic melanoma: chemotherapy to biochemotherapy. Cancer Control. 2002;9:31–8.

199. Margolin KA. Biochemotherapy for melanoma: rational therapeutics in the search for weapons of melanoma destruction. Cancer. 2004;101:435–8.

200. Flaherty LE, Gadgeel SM. Biochemotherapy of melanoma. Semin Oncol. 2002;29:446–55.

201. Flaherty KT. New molecular targets in melanoma. Curr Opin Oncol. 2004;16:150–4.

202. Tallman MS. Acute promyelocytic leukemia as a paradigm for targeted therapy. Semin Hematol. 2004;41:27–32.

203. Tuveson DA, Weber BL, Herlyn M. BRAF as a potential therapeutic target in melanoma and other malignancies. Cancer Cell. 2003;4:95–8.

204. Karasarides M, Chiloeches A, Hayward R, et al. B-RAF is a therapeutic target in melanoma. Oncogene. 2004;23:6292–8.

Vascular Neoplasms and Neoplastic-like Proliferations

Paula E North and Jay Kincannon

114

INTRODUCTION

In this chapter, we use the term *neoplasm* synonymously with *tumor* in a general, albeit imperfect[1], sense, consistent with its common usage: *an abnormal proliferation ('new growth') of cells that appears to be relatively autonomous (i.e. not reactive).* Common infantile hemangiomas, although arguably neoplastic in nature, especially in light of recent demonstrations of clonality in these lesions[2,3], are discussed separately in Chapter 103. Some entities with established or suspected features of reactive processes that mimic neoplasms are included in this chapter (Table 114.1). Angiokeratomas and telangiectatic lesions are discussed in Chapter 106. Kaposi's sarcoma, a virus-associated and possibly virus-induced process of as-yet-uncertain position on the hyperplasia–neoplasia spectrum (but with the potential to kill), is covered here, while two benign vascular proliferations of more seemingly straightforward infectious etiology (bacillary angiomatosis and verruga peruana) are covered elsewhere (see Ch. 73). Vascular malformations, which may be associated, in some cases, with a number of the cellular vascular proliferations discussed here, are discussed formally in Chapter 104. With these caveats in mind, a broad working classification of vascular neoplasms and neoplastic-like conditions is presented in Table 114.1. Vascular neoplasms with classic associations with syndromes or laboratory findings appear in Figure 114.1.

BENIGN VASCULAR NEOPLASMS AND REACTIVE HYPERPLASIAS

Papillary Endothelial Hyperplasia

> **Synonyms:** ■ Masson's lesion ■ Masson's tumor ■ Masson's hemangio-endotheliome vegetant intravasculaire ■ Masson's pseudoangiosarcoma ■ Intravascular or extravascular papillary endothelial hyperplasia

Key features

- Not a specific disease entity, but rather a distinct histopathologic pattern that can be confused with angiosarcoma
- The primary or 'pure' form is not associated with a pre-existing vascular anomaly and appears as a solitary, slowly growing, often painful nodule located within a dilated dermal or subcutaneous vein
- Secondary forms are associated with venous malformations and other vascular anomalies prone to thrombosis
- Rare forms are extravascular, probably arising in hematomas
- Thought to represent an unusual, exuberant response of endothelial cells to organizing thrombus

Introduction

Masson first described this process in 1923 in hemorrhoidal veins, terming it *hemangio-endotheliome vegetant intravasculaire*, and interpreted it as a neoplastic process mimicking angiosarcoma. In 1932, Henschen re-interpreted the process as reactive, and in 1971 Kauffman & Stout noted its occurrence not only in thrombosed vessels but also

A WORKING CLASSIFICATION OF VASCULAR TUMORS AND ANOMALIES
Reactive conditions
• Papillary endothelial hyperplasia*
• Reactive angioendotheliomatosis*
• Glomeruloid hemangioma*
• Microvenular hemangioma*
• Angiolymphoid hyperplasia with eosinophilia*
• Spindle cell hemangioma*
• Pyogenic granuloma*
Vascular and lymphatic malformations (see Chs 104 & 106)
• Capillary malformation (port-wine stain)
• Venous malformation
• Lymphatic malformation (microcystic and macrocystic)
• Mixed capillary/venous/lymphatic malformation
• Arteriovenous malformation
• Angiokeratoma
• Verrucous 'hemangioma'
• Angioma serpiginosum
Telangiectasias (see Ch. 106)
• Generalized essential telangiectasia
• Unilateral nevoid telangiectasia
• Hereditary hemorrhagic telangiectasia[†]
• Spider angioma
• Venous lake
Benign vascular neoplasms
• Infantile hemangioma (see Ch. 103)
• Congenital hemangioma (see Ch. 103)
• Cherry angioma*
• Sinusoidal hemangioma*
• Hobnail hemangioma*
• Tufted angioma*
• Multifocal lymphangioendotheliomatosis with thrombocytopenia*
Borderline and low-grade malignant vascular neoplasms
• Kaposiform hemangioendothelioma*
• Dabska-type hemangioendothelioma*
• Retiform hemangioendothelioma*
• Epithelioid hemangioendothelioma*
• Kaposi's sarcoma*
Malignant vascular neoplasms
• Angiosarcoma*
Perivascular neoplasms and neoplastic-like conditions
• Glomus tumor (proper)*
• Glomuvenous malformation ('glomangioma')*
• Infantile-type hemangiopericytoma/myofibromatosis* (also see Ch. 116)
• Adult-type hemangiopericytoma
• Glomangiopericytoma
• Myopericytoma

*Covered in this chapter.
[†]*Represent arteriovenous malformations.*

Table 114.1 A working classification of vascular tumors and anomalies.

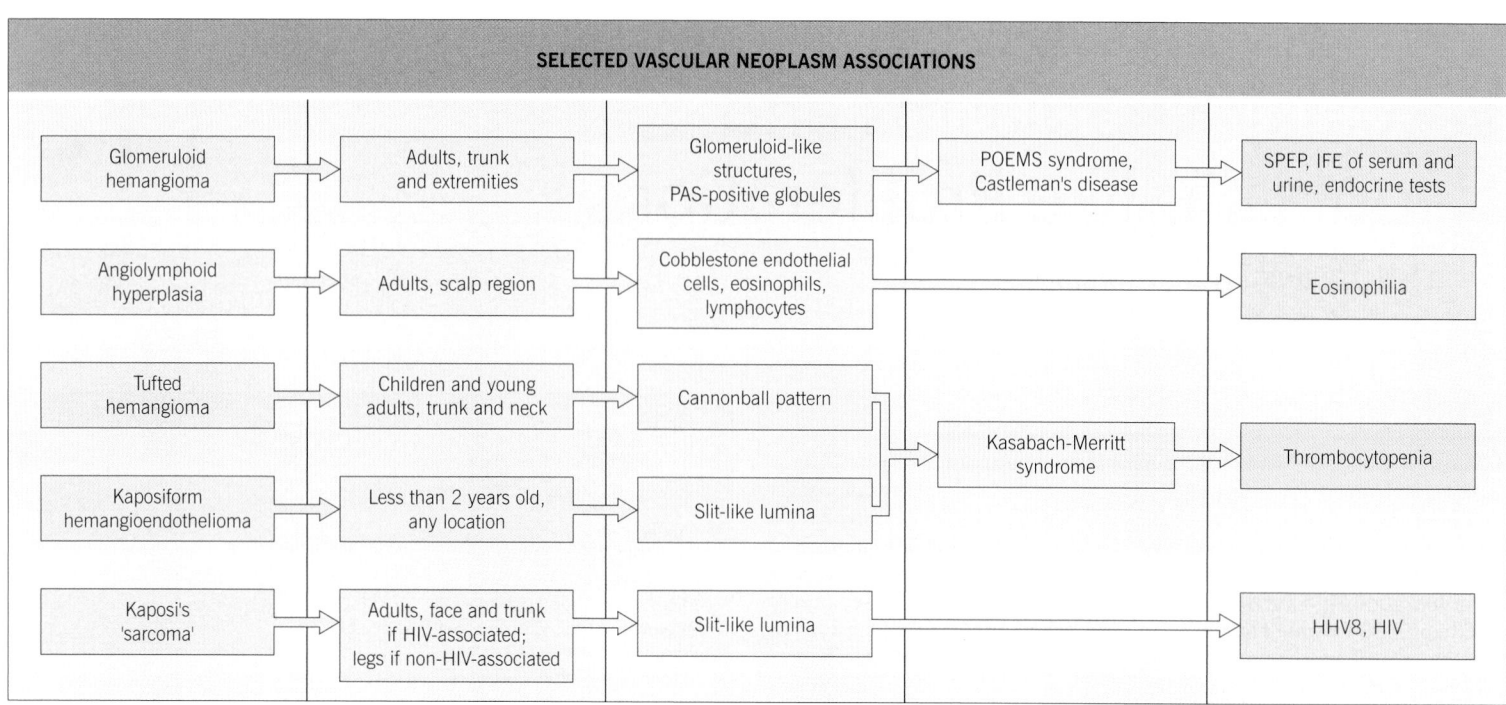

SELECTED VASCULAR NEOPLASM ASSOCIATIONS

Glomeruloid hemangioma	Adults, trunk and extremities	Glomeruloid-like structures, PAS-positive globules	POEMS syndrome, Castleman's disease	SPEP, IFE of serum and urine, endocrine tests
Angiolymphoid hyperplasia	Adults, scalp region	Cobblestone endothelial cells, eosinophils, lymphocytes		Eosinophilia
Tufted hemangioma	Children and young adults, trunk and neck	Cannonball pattern	Kasabach-Merritt syndrome	Thrombocytopenia
Kaposiform hemangioendothelioma	Less than 2 years old, any location	Slit-like lumina		
Kaposi's 'sarcoma'	Adults, face and trunk if HIV-associated; legs if non-HIV-associated	Slit-like lumina		HHV8, HIV

Fig. 114.1 Selected vascular neoplasm associations. IFE, immunofixation electrophoresis; SPEP, serum protein electrophoresis.

in a hematoma, further demonstrating the potential for confusion with soft tissue angiosarcoma. In 1976, the name *Masson's pseudoangiosarcoma* was proposed by Kuo et al.[4] to emphasize this fact. A lymphatic vessel counterpart of Masson's lesion was reported in 1979 in a cystic lymphatic malformation[5].

Epidemiology

Papillary endothelial hyperplasia has a slight female predominance, most pronounced for the rare extravascular forms[6]. Although lesions can occur at any age, most are in adults, with an average age of 34 years. A history of trauma was elicited in only 4% of patients[6].

Pathogenesis

Areas of papillary endothelial hyperplasia can in most cases be seen to merge with definitive thrombus material, in support of the notion that they represent an unusual form of thrombus organization.

Clinical features

Primary lesions within superficial tissues appear as solitary, firm masses, often with red or blue discoloration of the overlying skin. The history is typically one of slow growth over a period of several months or years. These lesions occur most commonly within veins of the head and neck and, interestingly, the fingers, but they may also arise elsewhere[6]. In a study of 314 cases, 56% were of the primary form, 40% were associated with other vascular lesions, and 4% appeared extravascular[6]. Clinical features of the secondary forms are those of the underlying vascular anomaly.

Pathology

Intravascular examples may be limited to the confines of a single thin-walled vein or may arise, often multifocally, within pre-existing vascular lesions such as venous malformations, glomuvenous malformations (glomangiomas) and pyogenic granulomas (Fig. 114.2). Foci of intravascular papillary endothelial hyperplasia are extremely common in venous malformations and serve to distinguish these low-flow lesions from high-flow arteriovenous malformations. Rarely, the involved vessel wall is ruptured, allowing the proliferative vascular process to spill out into the adjacent stroma. Extravascular examples that on serial sectioning show no evidence of a surrounding blood vessel wall may have arisen within an organizing hematoma[6].

Early lesions show growth of endothelial sprouts into fibrinous thrombus material, dividing it into papillary fronds lined by a single layer of plump endothelial cells with minimal mitotic activity and no significant cytologic atypia (Fig. 114.2 inset). The early fibrin cores of the papillae become collagenized and hyalinized with time, and the

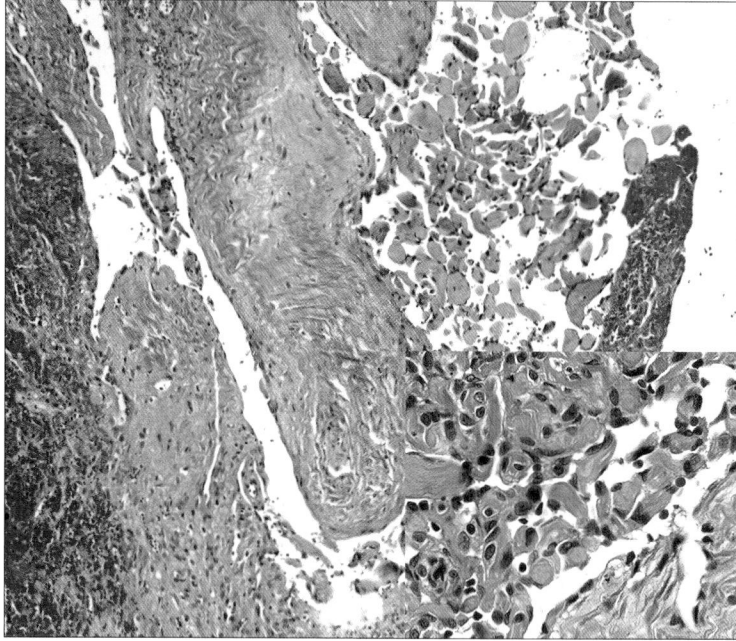

Fig. 114.2 Histology of papillary endothelial hyperplasia. Hyperplastic endothelial cells line stromal papillae formed within organizing thrombus material. Complex networks of recanalizing thrombus may mimic angiosarcoma (inset).

endothelial lining becomes thin and attenuated. Lesional papillae may fuse to form an anastomosing meshwork of vessels separated by connective tissue stroma that mimics angiosarcoma. However, the relatively high mitotic rate, striking pleomorphism and necrosis that characterize angiosarcoma are lacking[7].

Differential diagnosis

The clinical appearance of these lesions is non-specific, and diagnosis relies on microscopic examination. The most important differential diagnostic consideration for the pathologist is well-differentiated angiosarcoma.

Treatment

Surgical excision is usually curative. Local recurrences may occur when the lesion is superimposed on a vascular malformation that may generate new foci of endothelial hyperplasia.

Reactive Angioendotheliomatosis

Key features

- Rare, self-limited process occurring exclusively in the skin, characterized histologically by a dense proliferation of small capillaries
- The most common form is predominantly intravascular, resulting in luminal obliteration of pre-existing dermal vessels; many of these patients have cryoglobulinemia or systemic infections
- Should be distinguished from *intravascular lymphomatosis*, an angiotropic lymphoma erroneously termed *malignant angioendotheliomatosis* prior to the advent of discriminating immunohistochemistry

Introduction

Angioendotheliomatosis has historically been considered to be a single disease entity, divided into benign and malignant variants. As such, the large pleomorphic cells found within blood vessels in malignant angio-endotheliomatosis were thought to be transformed endothelial cells. More recently, immunohistochemical studies have convincingly demonstrated that these cells are neoplastic lymphocytes. Accordingly, malignant angioendotheliomatosis has been renamed *intralymphatic lymphomatosis* (see Ch. 119). The benign form is a true angioendotheliomatosis and is considered reactive.

Epidemiology

Reactive angioendotheliomatosis is rare and may occur at any age without gender discrimination. Although most cases are idiopathic, the condition may be associated with systemic disorders such as bacterial endocarditis, cryoglobulinemia, hepatic disease, monoclonal gammopathies, rheumatoid arthritis, antiphospholipid syndrome and atherosclerotic disease.

Pathogenesis

Reactive angioendotheliomatosis is a benign self-limited process. Its frequent association with various systemic conditions has led some investigators to propose that the capillary proliferation may be caused by a circulating angiogenic factor[8]. However, the fact that many of the disorders associated with this process cause vascular occlusion or tissue ischemia suggests that a local, hypoxia-induced increase in vascular endothelial growth factor may be instrumental.

Clinical features

Lesions appear as erythematous nodules or plaques, often associated with petechiae or ecchymoses. Focal ulceration may be evident.

Pathology

This exclusively cutaneous, largely dermal process shows a proliferation of closely packed capillaries lined by plump endothelial cells rimmed by small numbers of pericytes. Immunohistochemical positivity for endothelial markers such as von Willebrand factor, and focally for pericyte/smooth muscle-associated actins, confirms the cellular composition. Cytologic atypia and mitotic figures are not present. The capillary lumina are small and may be occluded by fibrin thrombi and bulging endothelial cells. In many cases, the proliferating capillaries appear to be contained within a larger, pre-existing vessel, obliterating its lumen. Cases associated with cryoglobulinemia show intraluminal and intracellular eosinophilic globules.

Differential diagnosis

Diagnostic considerations include other forms of intravascular endothelial proliferation, including intravascular pyogenic granuloma, Dabska tumor, intravascular papillary endothelial hyperplasia, and glomeruloid hemangioma.

Treatment

Lesions associated with systemic disease may regress upon resolution of the underlying condition.

Glomeruloid Hemangioma

Key features

- Reactive, histologically distinctive vascular proliferation that occurs in patients with POEMS syndrome
- Presents as multiple, firm angiomatous papules scattered mainly on the trunk and proximal extremities
- Characterized histologically by glomeruloid nests of capillaries within dilated dermal vessels
- May be induced by increased circulating levels of vascular endothelial growth factor

Introduction and history

The term glomeruloid hemangioma was coined by Chan et al.[9] in 1990 to describe a distinctive vascular proliferation that occurs in patients with POEMS syndrome (*p*olyneuropathy, *o*rganomegaly, *e*ndocrinopathy, *m*onoclonal gammopathy and *s*kin lesions), sometimes in association with multicentric Castleman's disease.

Clinical features

The reported incidences of angiomas in patients with POEMS syndrome range from 25% to 45%. These appear as multiple, firm, dome-shaped, red-to-purple papules up to several millimeters in diameter, scattered predominantly over the trunk and proximal extremities (see Ch. 52). Other cutaneous manifestations of POEMS syndrome include hyperpigmentation, hypertrichosis, hyperhidrosis, sclerodermoid features, digital clubbing, acquired ichthyosis, multiple seborrheic keratoses, livedo reticularis and purpura[10]. Glomeruloid hemangiomas appear to be specific for POEMS syndrome.

Pathogenesis

Although specific pathogenic mechanisms in glomeruloid hemangioma remain speculative, it is generally perceived to be reactive, rather than neoplastic. It is arguably a peculiar variant of reactive angioendotheliomatosis in which the glomeruloid architecture is pronounced, perhaps as the result of endothelial stimulation by deposited immunoglobulins[9] or in response to the increased levels of vascular endothelial growth factor (VEGF) that have been consistently observed in patients with POEMS syndrome. Approximately 85% of patients with POEMS syndrome in association with multicentric Castleman's disease have evidence of HHV-8 infection by PCR; viral IL-6 produced by HHV-8 may indirectly promote angiogenesis by inducing VEGF expression.

Pathology

Most of the angiomas seen in patients with POEMS syndrome are found, upon histologic examination, to be consistent with common cherry angiomas, with numerous dilated dermal capillaries lined by flattened endothelial cells. Only a few demonstrate the distinctive features of glomeruloid hemangioma. These consist of dilated dermal vessels filled by congeries of small capillaries, forming structures reminiscent of renal glomeruli (Fig. 114.3). The capillaries comprising these glomeruloid formations are lined by flat endothelial cells surrounded by an outer layer of pericytes and they are separated by a scant stroma containing large cells with lightly eosinophilic cytoplasm and multiple eosinophilic globules. The latter are PAS-positive, diastase-resistant, and immunopositive for polytypic immunoglobulin, presumably derived from the serum of these patients with paraproteinemia[9]. The interstitial, immunoglobulin-containing cells are of endothelial derivation. Some patients have both cherry angiomas and glomeruloid hemangiomas, and the cherry angiomas may display focal glomeruloid formation[9]. This suggests that these two histologic subsets may reflect different stages of the same process.

Differential diagnosis

The differential diagnosis of glomeruloid hemangioma is essentially that described above for reactive angioendotheliomatosis and includes several entities characterized by intravascular vascular proliferation, including intravascular pyogenic granuloma, Dabska tumor, tufted angioma, and intravascular papillary endothelial hyperplasia.

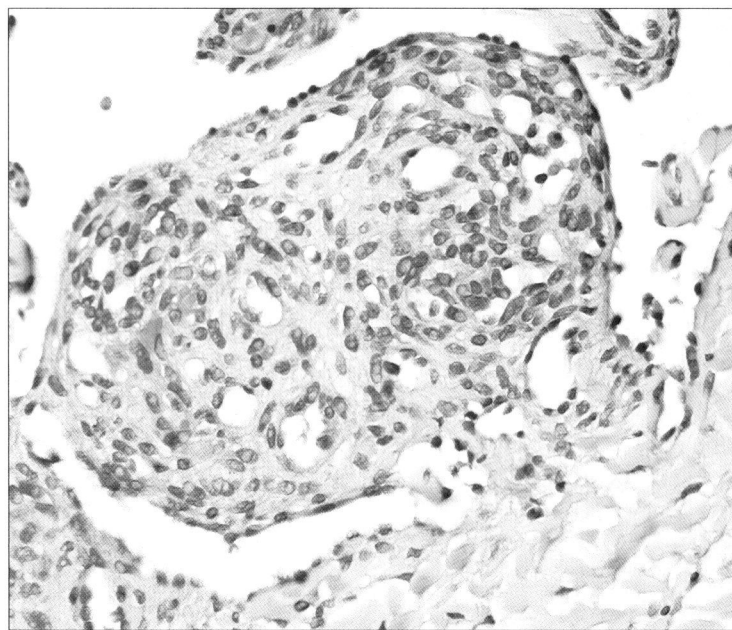

Fig. 114.3 **Histology of a glomeruloid hemangioma from a patient with POEMS syndrome.** Dilated dermal vessels are filled with congeries of small capillaries reminiscent of renal glomeruli.

Treatment

Treatment is not required, although shave excision, cryosurgery, electrodesiccation or pulsed dye laser surgery will remove the vascular tumors.

Microvenular Hemangioma

Synonym: ■ Microcapillary hemangioma

Key features

- An uncommon acquired vascular tumor of young to middle-aged adults of both genders
- Presents as a small, usually solitary, red papule on the trunk or extremities, with a predilection for the forearms
- Consists of small branching capillaries and venules with collapsed lumina and conspicuous pericytes infiltrating the full thickness of the reticular dermis
- May be subject to hormonal influences in some women

Introduction and history

Microvenular hemangioma was first described by that name in 1991 by Hunt, Santa Cruz & Barr[11], although cases reported as microcapillary hemangiomas are probably identical.

Epidemiology

Reported cases have been in young and middle-aged adults of both sexes. Some lesions in women have been temporally related to pregnancy or oral contraceptive use.

Pathogenesis

Microvenular hemangiomas have been reported in patients with POEMS syndrome[10], suggesting that these lesions, like glomeruloid hemangiomas, may be of reactive etiology. Observations that some microvenular hemangiomas affecting women present in association with pregnancy or oral contraceptive use arguably suggest a hormonal influence.

Clinical features

Microvenular hemangioma typically presents as a solitary, purple to red, slowly enlarging papule, plaque or small nodule on the trunk, arms or legs (rarely the face). There appears to be a particular predilection for the forearms, and most lesions are less than 2 cm in diameter[10]. In general, they are asymptomatic, although mild erythema and tenderness have been reported.

Pathology

Histologically, lesions are poorly circumscribed proliferations of small, relatively monomorphous, branching capillaries and venules involving the full thickness of the reticular dermis. Unlike port-wine stains, in which vascular ectasia is prominent, the vascular lumina of this tumor are inconspicuous and often collapsed. Cells lining the vessels show no atypia and are strongly positive for endothelial markers and are associated with smooth muscle actin-positive pericytes. The vessels are not as delicate or angulated as the lymphatic-like vessels of Kaposi's sarcoma or benign lymphangiomatosis, and they often contain red blood cells. The pericytic component is obvious even in routine H&E-stained sections.

Differential diagnosis

The major differential diagnostic consideration for these acquired lesions of adulthood is macular (patch-stage) Kaposi's sarcoma. Kaposi's sarcoma differs by the presence of delicate lymphatic-like vessels, plasma cell infiltrates, eosinophilic globules and more spindle cells.

Treatment

Surgical excision has been effective in reported cases.

Angiolymphoid Hyperplasia with Eosinophilia (AHE)

Synonyms: ■ Epithelioid hemangioma ■ Pseudopyogenic granuloma ■ Inflammatory angiomatous nodule ■ Papular angioplasia ■ Inflammatory arteriovenous hemangioma ■ Intravenous atypical vascular proliferation ■ Histiocytoid hemangioma[12]

Key features

- Benign angiomatous nodules or plaques, often multiple and grouped, located in the head and neck region, especially around the ears
- May be painful, pruritic or pulsatile, and often recur after excision
- Characterized histologically by proliferations of capillary-sized vessels with epithelioid endothelial cells surrounding larger, thick-walled vessels, accompanied by eosinophils and lymphocytes
- In many cases, associated with arteriovenous shunts
- Kimura's disease now thought to be a separate clinicopathologic entity

Introduction and history

Angiolymphoid hyperplasia with eosinophilia (AHE) was first described in 1969 by Wells & Whimster[13]. They considered AHE to be a late stage of Kimura's disease, described in the Japanese literature in 1948. It is now generally accepted that these are two separate entities[14].

Epidemiology

AHE occurs in young to middle-aged adults, with a female preponderance. Superficial lesions around the ear may have a greater female preponderance than lesions of deeper tissues. A history of trauma can be elicited in some cases[15].

Pathogenesis

The frequent presence of mural damage or rupture in intralesional large vessels of AHE has suggested a role of trauma or arteriovenous shunting in its pathogenesis[15]. Cases have been reported in association with arteriovenous fistulae and malformations. These findings suggest that at least many lesions of this histologic type may be reactive, rather than neoplastic.

Clinical features

AHE typically presents as papules or nodules, tan, brown, pink or dull red in color, located predominantly in the head and neck region, especially around the ears and on the forehead and scalp (Fig. 114.4). Lesions have less commonly been described in the mouth or on the trunk, arms, vulva and penis. Most are dermal in location, but some are subcutaneous. Occasional cases involve deep soft tissues or arise from vessels[7]. About half of the patients have multiple lesions, generally grouped in the same area[7]. AHE can be asymptomatic or it can be painful, pruritic or pulsatile[15]. Some patients have regional lymph node enlargement and peripheral eosinophilia. Lesions tend to recur after excision.

Pathology

Typical lesions involving the dermis and subcutaneous tissue are well circumscribed and show vaguely lobular proliferations of capillary-sized vessels around larger central vessels, with a variably dense perivascular inflammatory infiltrate rich in lymphocytes and eosinophils (Fig. 114.5). Mast cells and plasma cells are usually also present, and nodular lymphoid aggregates, with or without germinal centers, may be prominent in subcutaneous lesions. The stroma is fibrous, and the larger vessels have thick walls with prominent myxoid degeneration. Many of the vessels, particularly the larger ones, are lined by enlarged endothelial cells that protrude into the lumen, producing a scalloped or 'cobblestone' appearance. These epithelioid endothelial cells are responsible for the synonym

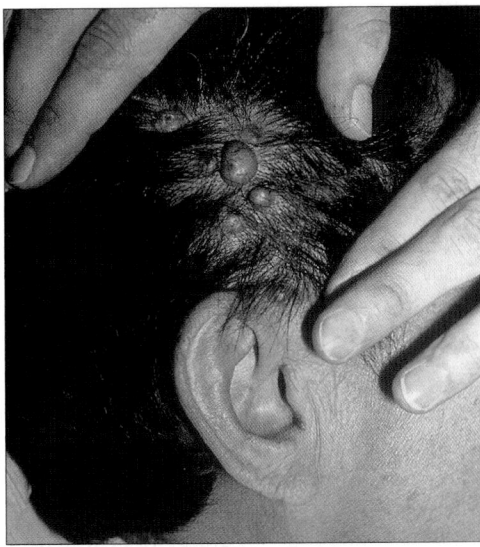

Fig. 114.4 **Angiolymphoid hyperplasia with eosinophilia.** Multiple pink papulonodules are often seen on the scalp.

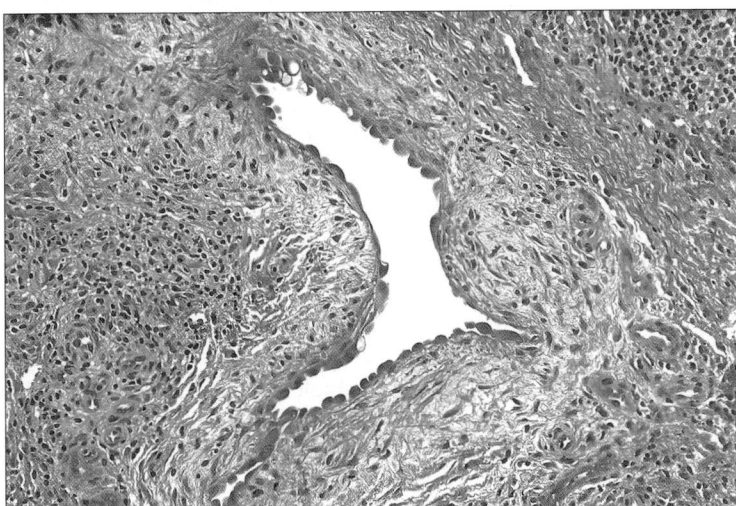

Fig. 114.5 **Histology of angiolymphoid hyperplasia with eosinophilia.** Cobblestone or hobnail endothelial cells prominently bulge into the lumen of the larger-sized vessel, surrounded by lymphocytes and eosinophils. Courtesy of Ronald P Rapini MD.

epithelioid hemangioma. Inflammatory infiltration of medium- to large-sized arteries, with variable luminal occlusion, damage to elastic laminae, and even mural rupture, is common.

Differential diagnosis

AHE may resemble benign lymphoid hyperplasia, lymphoma cutis, sarcoidosis and richly vascularized metastatic tumors. Kimura's disease has much larger lymphoid follicles and is usually located on the posterior neck. Angiosarcoma lacks the eosinophils and is usually cytologically more atypical and hemorrhagic.

Treatment

Although rare instances of spontaneous regression have been reported, surgical excision is generally required. About one-third of lesions recur after excision[7]. Intraoperative bleeding can be problematic. Carbon dioxide laser therapy or electrosection may be helpful[16].

Spindle Cell Hemangioma

Synonym: ■ Spindle cell hemangioendothelioma

Key features

- Blue–red nodules that typically appear in the dermal and subcutaneous tissue of the distal extremities of young adults and children and tend to multiply locally
- Composed of thin-walled cavernous veins containing organizing thrombi, interspersed with fascicles of spindle cells resembling Kaposi's sarcoma
- Originally interpreted as a low-grade angiosarcoma (*spindle cell hemangioendothelioma*), but now viewed as a benign lesion without metastatic potential (*spindle cell hemangioma*)
- Currently viewed by many as a vascular malformation complicated by thrombosis and irregular vascular collapse
- Tends to recur following resection

Introduction and history

This entity was first described by Weiss & Enzinger in 1986[17] as *spindle cell hemangioendothelioma* in order to recognize its spindle cell morphology and the fact that one case from their series of 26 had metastasized to a regional lymph node. Results of larger studies with extended follow-up have led to the current view that this tumor has no inherent malignant potential[7,18]. Based on these observations, Perkins & Weiss suggested in 1996[18] that the entity be renamed *spindle cell hemangioma*.

Epidemiology

Spindle cell hemangiomas usually occur in children and young adults, although in a recent series of 78 cases compiled by Perkins & Weiss[18], patient ages ranged from 8 to 78 years, with a median age of 32 years. Males and females are affected equally. Spindle cell hemangiomas are occasionally associated with Maffucci's syndrome[17–19], Klippel–Trenaunay syndrome[19], congenital lymphedema[17,19] and, rarely, epithelioid hemangioendothelioma.

Pathogenesis

This lesion is widely considered to be non-neoplastic[19–21], possibly a vascular malformation dominated by the effects of thrombosis and irregular vascular collapse[7,18]. The typical development of multiple nodules over time within a given anatomic region may represent intravascular propagation[18].

Clinical features

Most spindle cell hemangiomas begin as a solitary, firm, red–blue nodule in the subcutaneous tissue and dermis of the distal upper or lower extremity, then develop multifocally in the same general anatomic area (Fig. 114.6). They are largely asymptomatic. Approximately 60%

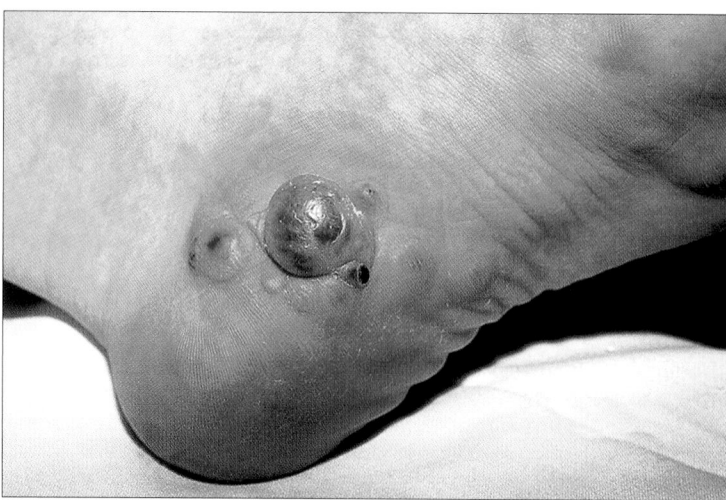

Fig. 114.6 Spindle cell hemangioma. Clustered blue–red multifocal nodules are typical.

recur following resection[18]. Rare cases have been reported in skeletal muscle.

Pathology

These lesions present as hemorrhagic, often multiple, nodules in the dermis and subcutaneous tissue and are composed of two basic histologic elements: thin-walled, cavernous spaces containing organizing thrombi, and more cellular areas containing spindle cells and occasional aggregates of vacuolated epithelioid cells (Fig. 114.7). The spindled areas stain focally for actin, form slit-like vascular spaces, and appear to consist of fibroblastic cells, pericytes and collapsed vessels[7]. The epithelioid interstitial cells, as well as the flattened cells lining the cavernous spaces, immunoreact positively for endothelial markers[19]. Cavernous vessels may show foci of intravascular papillary endothelial hyperplasia (Masson's lesion) consistent with the presence of organizing thrombus material.

Differential diagnosis

These tumors may resemble nodular lesions of Kaposi's sarcoma, but the latter lack cavernous vascular spaces and vacuolated epithelioid endothelial cells. The frequent presence of foci of intravascular papillary endothelial hyperplasia (Masson's lesion) in spindle cell hemangioma may lead to misdiagnosis. Primary Masson's lesion is solitary and lacks epithelioid endothelial cells.

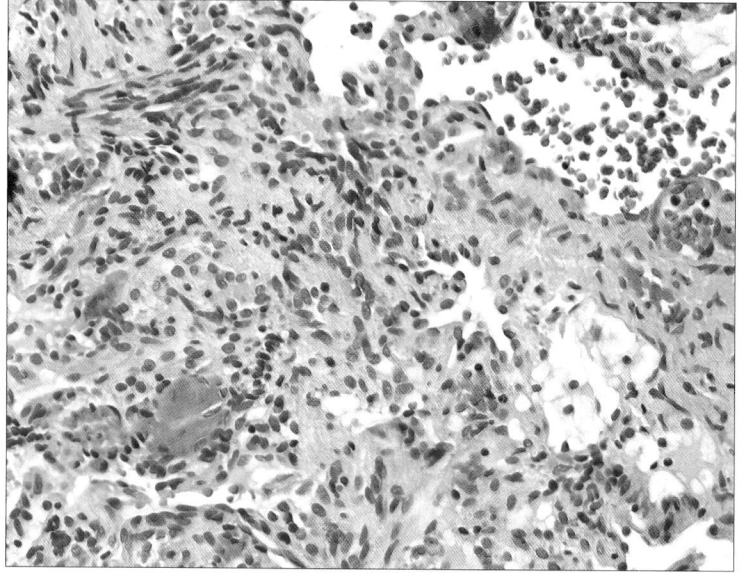

Fig. 114.7 Histology of spindle cell hemangioma. Collapsed veins containing organizing thrombi alternate with more cellular spindled areas and occasional vacuolated epithelioid cells.

Treatment

There is one report of successful intralesional and intra-arterial treatment of spindle cell hemangioma with recombinant interleukin-2, with no signs of recurrence at 24 months[22]. Based on the large series of Perkins & Weiss, simple surgical excision is successful in many patients (approximately 40%)[18]. The frequent local recurrences may reflect the inherent multifocality of these lesions, with growth via vessels to discontinuous regional sites[18].

Pyogenic Granuloma

Synonyms: ■ Lobular capillary hemangioma ■ Granuloma pyogenicum ■ Tumor of pregnancy ■ Eruptive hemangioma ■ Granulation tissue-type hemangioma

Key features

- Rapidly growing, friable, red papule or polyp of skin or mucosa that frequently ulcerates; most common in children and young adults
- Examples arising on the gingiva of pregnant women (*granuloma gravidarum*) are considered a separate subgroup, but are histologically indistinguishable
- Consist of lobules of small capillaries set in a fibromyxoid matrix, often distinctly exophytic and bounded by collarettes of hyperplastic epithelium
- Occasionally found in subcutaneous or intravascular locations
- Neither infectious in etiology nor granulomatous in histology; considered a benign neoplasm by some, a reactive process by others

Introduction and history

Poncet & Dor are credited with the first description of these lesions in 1897, which they believed were caused by *Botryomyces* infection. The term *granuloma pyogenicum* was coined in 1904 by Hartzell to describe four similar cases that he believed represented a non-specific granulation tissue-type response to any type of pyogenic agent[23]. Although the etiology of these common lesions remains uncertain today, the term *pyogenic granuloma* is clearly a misnomer. There is no evidence to implicate any infectious agent, and the histologic appearance is not granulomatous.

Epidemiology

Pyogenic granulomas may occur at any age, but are more common in children and young adults. They are equally prevalent in males and females and show no racial or familial predisposition. Gingival lesions are relatively common in pregnancy.

Pathogenesis

Pyogenic granulomas exhibit a number of clinical features suggestive of reactive neovascularization, including common association with a pre-existing injury or irritation, limited capacity for growth, and a propensity for multiple eruptions that may be localized or disseminated. The occasional eruption of pyogenic granulomas within pre-existent port-wine stains[24] suggests that abnormalities in blood flow may be etiologically important in some cases.

Clinical features

The lesion presents as a solitary red papule or polyp that grows rapidly over the course of several weeks or months, then stabilizes (Fig. 114.8). Its final size is rarely greater than 1 cm, and it may persist indefinitely if not removed. Approximately one-third develop following minor trauma. In one series of 289 cases, the most common sites, in decreasing order of frequency, were the gingiva, fingers, lips, face and tongue[25]. They are extremely friable, frequently ulcerate, and may bleed profusely with minor trauma. Multiple satellite lesions occasionally develop near a primary pyogenic granuloma, usually after destruction of that lesion[26].

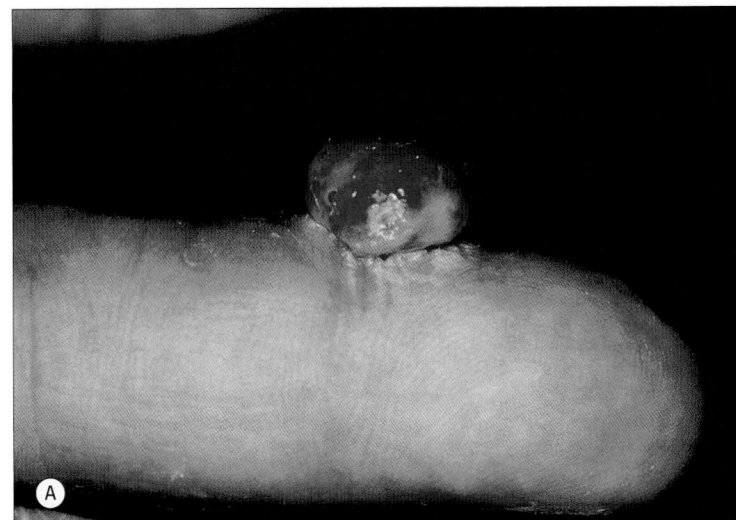

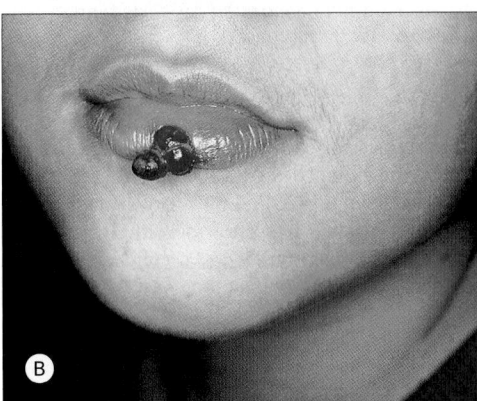

Fig. 114.8 Pyogenic granuloma. **A** Pedunculated papule on the finger. **B** Grouped red papules on the lip. Both are common sites.

variable, and a scant infiltrate of lymphocytes, plasma cells and mast cells may be present. Capillary lumina within the lobules vary from small and angular to branching and ectatic, and foci of intravascular papillary endothelial hyperplasia may be present. A few larger vessels with smooth muscle walls, usually venous, are often present at the base of the lesion. Thick, intervening bands of dense fibrous tissue sharply define the lobularity and help distinguish pyogenic granuloma from other lobular forms of capillary proliferation such as infantile hemangioma.

Lateral margins are often defined by prominent epithelial 'collarettes' resulting from peripheral adnexal hyperplasia or, in some cases, from downward growth of rete ridges, bridged by flattened epidermis. The histology of many early lesions is altered by ulceration and secondary inflammatory change, lending a similarity in appearance to granulation tissue, with radially oriented capillaries, fibrin deposition, and loss of lobularity. Intravascular and subcutaneous forms demonstrate features similar to superficial lesions, without the inflammatory complications. Late-stage lesions are characterized by intralobular as well as interlobular fibrosis, and quiescent, flattened capillary endothelia.

Differential diagnosis

The diagnosis of pyogenic granuloma can be made clinically if the red, bleeding papule is coupled with the characteristic location and history. Otherwise they can be easily confused with amelanotic melanoma and, in the immunosuppressed patient, bacillary angiomatosis or Kaposi's sarcoma. Glomus tumors, hemangiomas, irritated melanocytic nevi and warts can all mimic pyogenic granulomas. Histologic conformation is always helpful in cases where the diagnosis is in question.

Treatment

Shave excision followed by electrosurgery of the base under local anesthesia is sufficient for most lesions. Patients and parents should be alerted to the possibility of recurrence after removal. Excision with suturing may result in less postoperative bleeding and a lower recurrence rate.

Pulsed dye laser has also been shown to be a safe and effective treatment for small pyogenic granulomas and may be particularly useful in pediatric patients[29]. There is a recent report of successful sclerotherapy of pyogenic granulomas in nine patients using monoethanolamine oleate, with inconspicuous scar formation and no recurrence[30].

Rare instances of disseminated, eruptive forms have occurred[27]. Pyogenic granulomas have been reported in association with systemic retinoids[28], indinavir and anti-EGFR antibodies, but in some cases this may represent excessive granulation tissue.

Pathology

The quintessential lesion is a well-circumscribed, exophytic, sometimes pedunculated, proliferation of small capillaries, often arranged in a lobular pattern (Fig. 114.9). Lesional capillaries are lined by flattened to slightly plump endothelial cells rimmed by pericytes and surrounded by a variably edematous fibromyxoid interstitial stroma containing fibroblasts. Endothelial and stromal cell mitotic activity is highly

Cherry Angioma

Synonyms: ■ Cherry hemangioma ■ Senile angioma ■ Campbell–De Morgan spot

Key features

- Bright red, dome-shaped to polypoid papules up to a few millimeters in diameter that begin appearing in adult life, most commonly on the trunk and upper extremities
- A common, benign lesion found in most individuals by the age of 60 years, often in large numbers
- Consist of dilated, congested capillaries and postcapillary venules in the papillary dermis

Introduction and history

Cherry angiomas are the most common of the acquired cutaneous vascular proliferations. They can be unattractive, and may in rare instances of eruptive onset herald an underlying systemic abnormality.

Epidemiology

These lesions affect both sexes. Although some angiomas may appear during adolescence, they usually first appear in individuals in at least their third decade of life or later, and increase in number over time. Most people over 60 years of age have one or more of these lesions.

Pathogenesis

Cherry angiomas often appear in increased numbers during pregnancy and may involute in the postpartum period, suggesting that hormonal

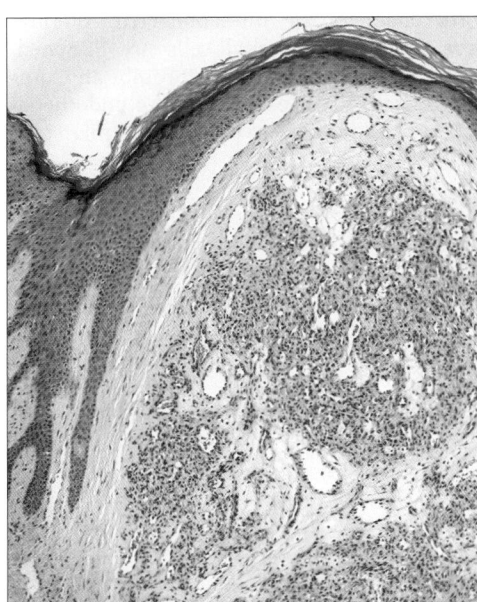

Fig. 114.9 Histology of pyogenic granuloma. Proliferating capillaries are often grouped into lobules by dense fibrous bands, hence the synonym lobular capillary hemangioma. The lesion is often clutched by an epithelial collarette.

factors may be important in their pathogenesis. Two women with hundreds of eruptive cherry hemangiomas, both with increased serum levels of prolactin, have also been reported[10]. Most angiomas that appear in the setting of POEMS syndrome are cherry angiomas, often in association with glomeruloid hemangiomas.

Clinical features

Cherry angiomas are round to oval, bright red, dome-shaped papules ranging in size from barely visible to several millimeters in diameter (Fig. 114.10). Well-developed lesions may be polypoid. They most commonly occur on the trunk and proximal extremities and are rare on the hands, feet and face. It is not unusual for elderly adults to have 50 to 100 cherry angiomas on their trunk. Patients are usually aware of the benign nature of these extremely common lesions and bring them to a physician's attention only when concerned about their appearance. They are generally asymptomatic, but may bleed when traumatized.

Pathology

Histologically, these lesions consist of congested, ectatic capillaries and postcapillary venules in the papillary dermis (Fig. 114.10 inset). Early lesions are characterized by small lumina and plump endothelial cells. With maturation, the vessels dilate and endothelial cells flatten. The epidermis shows central loss of rete ridges with peripherally placed adnexal epithelial collarettes.

Differential diagnosis

The distinctive appearance and characteristic distribution of cherry angiomas limit other diagnostic considerations. Glomeruloid hemangiomas, although similar in clinical appearance, can be distinguished histologically. Tiny cherry angiomas may resemble petechiae.

Treatment

Patients may request removal of cosmetically undesirable or chronically traumatized cherry angiomas. This can be accomplished by shave excision, electrodesiccation or laser ablation.

Sinusoidal Hemangioma

> **Synonyms:** ■ Variant sinusoidal hemangioma ■ Sinusoidal venous malformation

Key features

- Relatively rare, small, well-demarcated acquired lesion most commonly seen in the subcutis of middle-aged women and traditionally described as a variant of 'cavernous hemangioma' (venous malformation)
- Histologically distinguished by dilated, interconnecting venous channels exhibiting a prominent sieve-like or sinusoidal pattern
- May be confused with well-differentiated angiosarcoma, although distinguished from the latter by lack of significant cytologic atypia, lack of infiltrative growth, and lack of endothelial multilayering
- Probably malformative, rather than neoplastic or reactive in etiology, with delayed presentation
- Similar sinusoidal patterns are seen focally in many venous malformations, presumably due to thrombosis and recanalization, raising doubt as to whether the sinusoidal variant should be considered a singular entity

Introduction and history

Sinusoidal hemangioma was described as a distinctive subset of so-called cavernous hemangioma by Calonje & Fletcher in 1991[31]. In contrast to typical venous malformations (so-called 'cavernous hemangiomas') of childhood, sinusoidal hemangiomas have been singled out by their acquired presentation and by an unusually prominent sinusoidal or sieve-like histologic pattern.

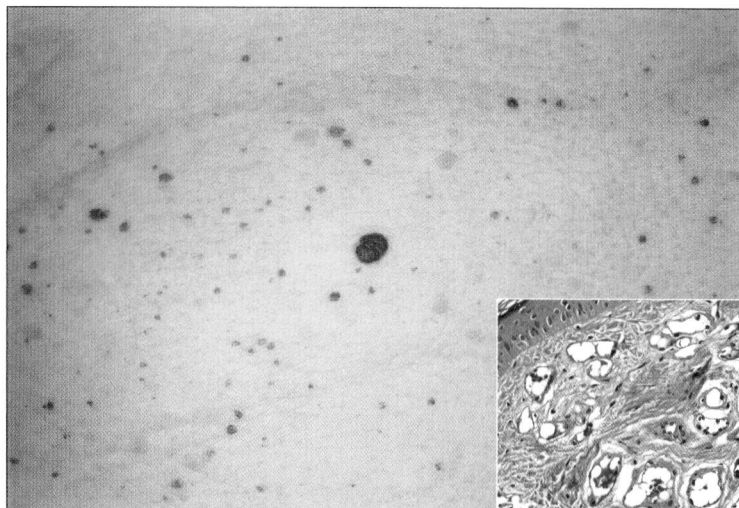

Fig. 114.10 Cherry hemangiomas. Multiple compressible red papules. Courtesy of Jean L Bolognia MD. Histologically, congested capillaries and postcapillary venules expand the papillary dermis (inset).

Epidemiology

Acquired lesions with the characteristic sinusoidal histology have most commonly been identified in middle-aged women and are relatively rare (fewer than two dozen cases reported). Their not uncommon occurrence in breast subcutaneous tissue has emphasized the need to differentiate these lesions from angiosarcoma.

Pathogenesis

Typical presentation in adulthood has suggested a neoplastic or reactive etiology for sinusoidal hemangioma. Nevertheless, the strong histologic parallels with venous malformations of childhood suggest that these mitotically quiescent vascular lesions are probably congenital developmental disorders that become evident later in life due to remodeling, thrombosis and progressive vascular dilation. Focal sinusoidal patterns have also been described in congenital venous malformations.

Clinical features

Sinusoidal hemangiomas, as traditionally defined, are relatively well-demarcated, solitary lesions that present in adults, usually women, most commonly presenting on the arms and torso (including the breast) as freely mobile deep dermal or subcutaneous papules or nodules. Color varies from red in superficial lesions to bluish or colorless in subcutaneous lesions. Follow-up studies have revealed no evidence of metastasis or of local recurrence following resection.

Pathology

Generally well-defined lobules of dilated, thin-walled veins with scant mural smooth muscle form characteristic interconnected, 'emphysematous', sieve-like spaces. Lining endothelial cells are flattened, single-layered, and mitotically inactive. Organizing thrombi are common, with occasional superimposed changes of papillary endothelial hyperplasia. There is no significant cytologic atypia. Central infarction and necrosis have been reported.

Differential diagnosis

Given the typical presentation in adulthood and anastomosing vascular pattern, the most clinically significant simulator is well-differentiated angiosarcoma. The latter is distinguished by a more infiltrative pattern, endothelial multilayering, and cytologic atypia.

Treatment

Complete surgical resection, which is facilitated by the typical well demarcation, is curative.

Hobnail Hemangioma

> **Synonyms:** ■ Targetoid hemosiderotic hemangioma

Key features

- Uncommon, benign tumor that usually presents as a red–blue or brown papule on the trunk or extremities of children and young to middle-aged adults
- The papule is sometimes surrounded by a pale ring and ecchymotic halo
- Biphasic pattern of dilated vessels with hobnail endothelial cells and slit-like vessels
- Can be confused with patch-stage Kaposi's sarcoma

Introduction and history

Santa Cruz & Aronberg described lesions of this histologic type in 1988 using the term *targetoid hemosiderotic hemangioma* to emphasize the targetoid clinical appearance and hemosiderin deposition seen in their series of eight cases. Since then, it has become apparent that only a minority of these lesions demonstrate the ecchymotic halo, and hemosiderin deposition is variable. The term *hobnail hemangioma* has been proposed to encompass lesions with the characteristic biphasic growth pattern and marked hobnail endothelial morphology, with or without a targetoid clinical appearance and/or marked hemosiderin deposition[32,33]. More than 60 cases have now been reported[33,34]. All have had a benign clinical course.

Epidemiology

There is an equal male–female distribution[33]. In the largest series to date (62 cases), patients ranged in age from 6 to 72 years (median of 32 years)[34].

Pathogenesis

The presence of vascular endothelial growth factor receptor-3 (VEGFR-3) immunoreactivity suggests the possibility of lymphatic derivation. It has been proposed that this tumor represents the benign end of a spectrum of vascular tumors with hobnail endothelial cells that also includes Dabska tumor and retiform hemangioendothelioma[32].

Clinical features

Most lesions are solitary, well-circumscribed, red–blue to brown papules, 2 to 3 mm in diameter. In some patients, the papule is surrounded by a thin, pale area and an ecchymotic ring (Fig. 114.11). The halo may fade and disappear with time, and some lesions have been reported to undergo cycles of spontaneous regression and recurrence[33]. Sites, in decreasing order of frequency, are the lower extremities, upper extremities, back, buttock and hip, and chest wall. Lesions have also been reported on the tongue and gingiva[33].

Pathology

A biphasic growth pattern is observed, consisting of a superficial dermal complement of dilated, thin-walled vessels containing small numbers of red blood cells and lined by prominent hobnail endothelial cells, merging with smaller, more slit-like vessels that dissect between collagen bundles in deeper areas of the dermis (Fig. 114.12). Extravasated red blood cells and hemosiderin deposits are common, but may be absent. Although the superficial vessels occasionally show delicate intraluminal papillary fronds, the more complex, multilayered endothelial tufts of Dabska tumor are lacking.

Differential diagnosis

Hobnail hemangiomas are benign in clinical appearance and may resemble melanocytic nevi or a sclerosing hemangioma as well as other benign vascular proliferations[33]. The histopathologic differential diagnosis is much more complex and includes patch-stage and lymphangioma-like variants of Kaposi's sarcoma, well-differentiated angiosarcoma, retiform hemangioendothelioma, Dabska tumor and benign lymphangiomatosis.

Treatment

Hobnail hemangioma is successfully treated by simple excision. Follow-up information in a study of 35 patients, ranging from 1 to 4 years, revealed no local recurrence or systemic metastasis[34].

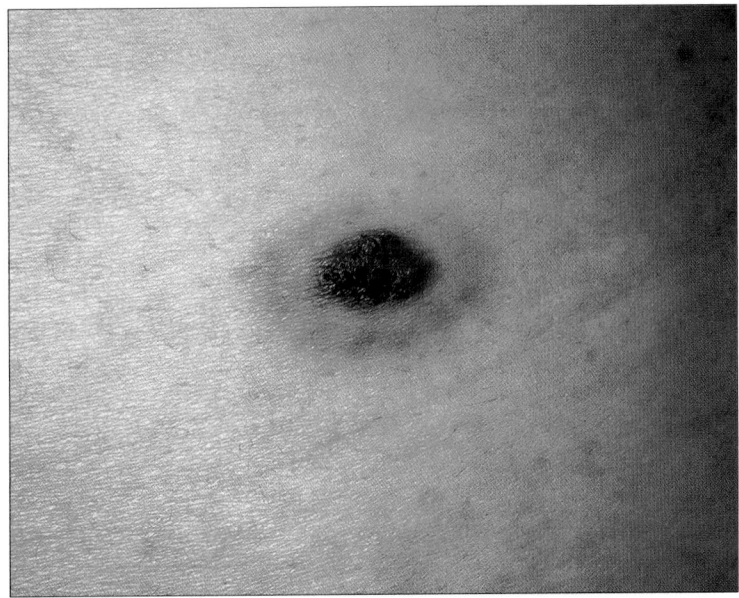

Fig. 114.11 Hobnail hemangioma (targetoid hemosiderotic hemangioma). Note the target-like appearance. Courtesy of Ronald P Rapini M.D.

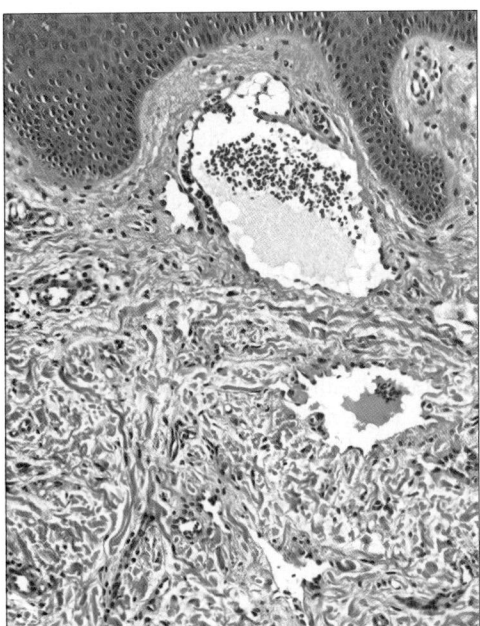

Fig. 114.12 Histology of hobnail hemangioma. Dilated superficial dermal vessels lined by hobnail endothelial cells, merging with smaller slit-like vessels in the lower dermis.

Tufted Angioma

Synonyms: ■ Acquired tufted angioma ■ Angioblastoma of Nakagawa ■ Tufted hemangioma ■ Hypertrophic hemangioma ■ Progressive capillary hemangioma

Key features

- Inhomogeneous pink-to-red macules and plaques with superimposed papules that spread slowly, often to involve large areas, then stabilize; rarely may regress
- Most commonly located on the neck or trunk
- Usually presents as an acquired lesion in children and young adults, but may be congenital or appear late in life
- May be associated with Kasabach–Merritt phenomenon in congenital cases
- Characterized histologically by tightly packed tufts of tiny capillaries distributed within the dermis and subcutis in a 'cannonball' pattern

Introduction

Tufted angioma has often been lumped erroneously with infantile hemangioma under the generic term 'capillary hemangioma'. It is important to recognize it as a separate entity, due to its association with Kasabach–Merritt syndrome in some infants. In older children and adults, it may clinically mimic Kaposi's sarcoma. Current opinion is that it represents a mild, superficial form of kaposiform hemangioendothelioma.

History

Tufted angioma was first described in 1989 by Wilson-Jones & Orkin[35]. Apparently identical lesions had been described many years previously as angioblastoma[36] and progressive capillary hemangioma[37]. The association of tufted angioma with Kasabach–Merritt phenomenon, shared by kaposiform hemangioendothelioma, has only recently been recognized[38].

Epidemiology

Most lesions occur in young adults and children, many in the first year of life. Over 50% present before 5 years of age[35]. Approximately 15% are congenital[35], and rare lesions may occur late in life[39]. Although one family with several affected family members has been reported[40], the vast majority of cases are sporadic.

Pathogenesis

Tufted angioma and kaposiform hemangioendothelioma show a significant degree of overlap in histologic features, with resection specimens of kaposiform hemangioendothelioma often demonstrating dermal changes that would have been interpreted in small biopsy specimens as tufted angioma. In light of the virtually exclusive association of these two entities with Kasabach–Merritt phenomenon, this histologic overlap suggests that tufted angioma may be a milder form of kaposiform hemangioendothelioma[38,41,42].

Clinical features

Tufted angiomas appear as mottled red macules or plaques with superimposed angiomatous papules on the neck, trunk or shoulders that grow slowly by lateral extension over a period of 5 months to 10 years[35] (Fig. 114.13). A platelet-trapping syndrome (Kasabach–Merritt phenomenon) may develop in congenital cases, although less commonly than in kaposiform hemangioendothelioma. Lesions eventually stabilize in size, then may shrink and leave a fibrotic residuum or persist unchanged. Rare complete spontaneous regression has been reported[43]. Occasional lesions are painful, and this may be exacerbated during periods of uncontrolled platelet trapping[44].

Pathology

Tufted angiomas are characterized by multiple discrete lobules of capillaries set within the dermis and often the subcutis in what has been termed a 'cannonball' pattern (Fig. 114.14). Borders of the area of tissue involvement are poorly defined. Dermal collagen and subcutis separating capillary lobules may be histologically normal, but are often fibrotic. The lobules themselves, unlike those of pyogenic granuloma, are composed of tiny capillaries with pinpoint lumina, occasionally containing fibrin microthrombi, tightly packed together without intervening stroma and frequently bulging into peripherally placed thin-walled vessels suggestive of lymphatics. Collections of angular, slightly ectatic lymphatic vessels are also common between lobules and in adjacent tissue, and are consistently seen in large resection specimens, suggesting the possibility that the capillary proliferations arise from a field of aberrant lymphatics. The endothelial cells of tufted angioma do not immunoreact for the infantile hemangioma-associated antigens glucose transporter isoform 1 (GLUT1) and Lewis Y antigen[45]. Ultrastructural studies have demonstrated classic Weibel–Palade bodies. Platelet trapping in cases associated with Kasabach–Merritt phenomenon has been confirmed with CD61 immunoreaction[46].

Differential diagnosis

Congenital tufted angiomas must be differentiated from infantile hemangiomas, the most common tumors of infancy (see Ch. 103). The latter show more rapid growth without lateral extension, and usually extend more deeply. Other entities that may mimic the clinical appearance of tufted angioma include pyogenic granulomas arising within a

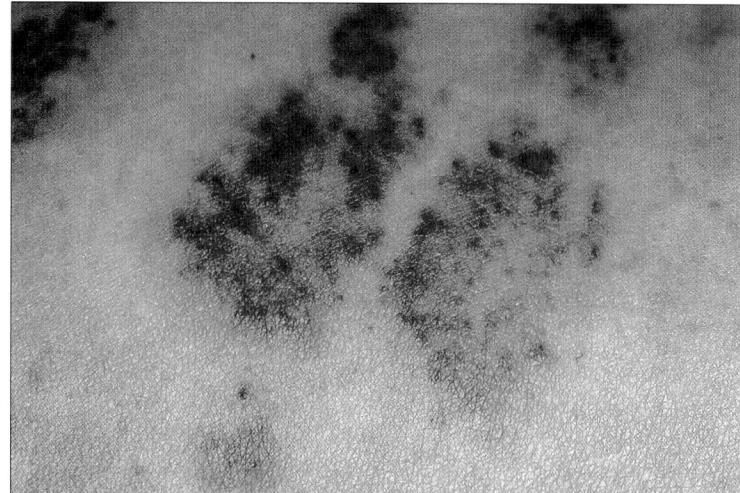

Fig. 114.13 Tufted angioma. Mottled red macules and superimposed papules are typical.

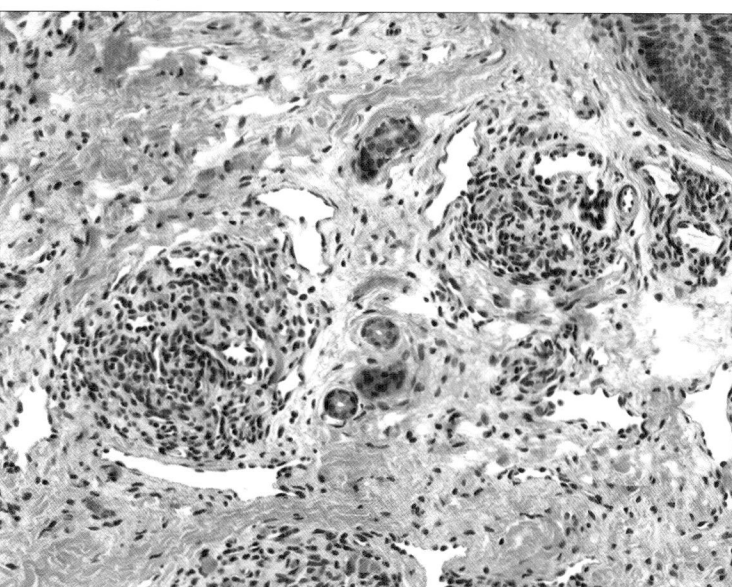

Fig. 114.14 Histology of tufted angioma. A cannonball distribution of dense capillary lobules in the dermis is classic.

vascular malformation and Kaposi's sarcoma. Pyogenic granuloma can be distinguished histologically by its characteristic edematous stroma, granulation tissue-type changes, lack of association with lymphatic vessels, and generally larger, more loosely packed lesional vessels. Kaposi's sarcoma differs in its lack of tufting, presence of a plasma cell infiltrate, and prominent fascicles of spindle cells forming slit-like spaces. Kaposiform hemangioendothelioma, although overlapping in histology with tufted angioma, is typically a more bulky, deeply seated lesion, infiltrating across multiple tissue planes.

Treatment

Complete surgical excision is the treatment of choice for small tufted angiomas, although recurrence is common. Use of a pulsed dye laser has been ineffective[44,47], although the argon tunable dye laser has been successfully used. High-dose systemic corticosteroids may also be useful[48], and interferon-α has produced partial regression[47]. Aspirin may help control the platelet interaction, pain and growth of tufted angiomas that are associated with Kasabach–Merritt syndrome[44].

Multifocal Lymphangioendotheliomatosis with Thrombocytopenia

Synonym: ■ Congenital cutaneovisceral angiomatosis with thrombocytopenia

Key features

- A newly recognized disorder, characterized by multiple congenital and progressive vascular lesions involving skin and viscera and, in some cases, synovium or muscle, complicated by chronic mild-to-moderate thrombocytopenia

- Clinically significant gastrointestinal bleeding appears universal and may be life-threatening

- Distinctive histopathologic features, including intraluminal papillary proliferations, resemble benign lymphangioendothelioma, with variable expression of lymphatic-associated immunohistochemical markers, including LYVE-1 and podoplanin

- Cutaneous lesions are red–brown to burgundy plaques, up to hundreds in number and measuring up to a few centimeters in diameter

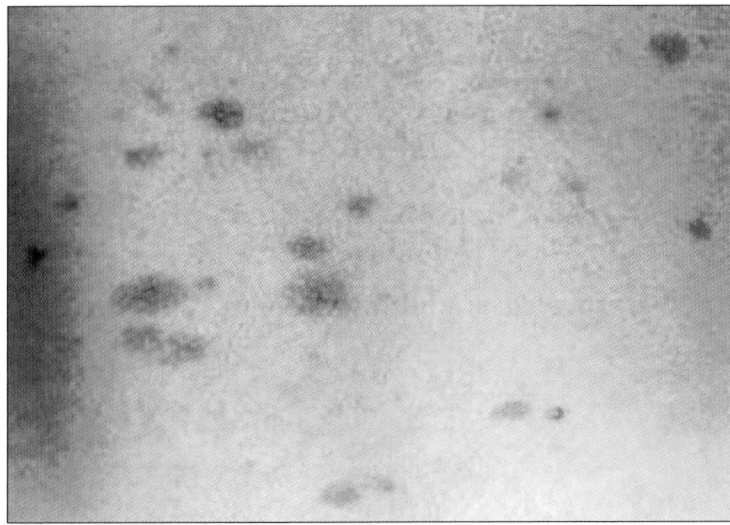

Fig. 114.15 **Multifocal lymphangioendotheliomatosis with thrombocytopenia.** Multiple red–brown plaques or papules that may slowly enlarge and increase in number; associated with similar visceral lesions and mild to moderate thrombocytopenia.

Introduction and history

This distinctive, but only recently recognized, clinicopathologic entity was first described in 2004 by North et al.[49] as *multifocal lymphangio-endotheliomatosis with thrombocytopenia* (MLT), based upon the highly characteristic histology, multifocal tissue involvement, and consistent expression of the lymphatic-associated marker LYVE-1. A clinically and histologically equivalent series of cases was independently recognized by the vascular anomalies teams at the Children's Hospital in Boston and Hôpital Sainte-Justine, Montreal, and reported by Prasad et al.[50] in 2005 using the term *congenital cutaneovisceral angiomatosis with thrombocytopenia* (CCAT).

Epidemiology

Most cases are evident at birth, although many lesions are slowly progressive and increase in number with time. No clear racial or sexual predilections have emerged.

Pathogenesis

Reported cases are sporadic and it is not yet clear if the lesions are best considered tumors or malformations. Lesional endothelial cells coexpress CD34 and LYVE-1 and may focally express podoplanin, making blood-vascular versus lymphatic-vascular differentiation ambiguous. The association with selective thrombocytopenia draws parallels with kaposiform hemangioendothelioma and tufted angioma – two vascular entities uniquely linked to severe platelet trapping (Kasabach–Merritt phenomenon) that also express mixed blood vascular and lymphatic endothelial markers[38,42,49].

Clinical features

Cutaneous lesions, often numbering in the hundreds at birth, are flat or indurated, red–brown to burgundy plaques or papules, often with central pallor and, occasionally, central scar-like areas (Fig. 114.15). Slow progression of pre-existing lesions and progressive appearance of new lesions is typical, without evidence of regression. Similar lesions in the gastrointestinal tract cause severe gastrointestinal bleeding beginning in infancy. Some patients have extensive pulmonary involvement complicated by hemoptysis[50]. Rare reported cases have involved the liver, spleen, muscle and/or synovium[49,50]. Thrombocytopenia is mild to moderate, chronic, and fluctuating, with essentially normal prothrombin time (PT), partial thromboplastin time (PTT) and serum fibrinogen levels.

Pathology

Lesions are composed of thin-walled vessels scattered throughout the dermis and subcutis and lined by a monolayer of slightly hobnailed endothelial cells that focally form papillary projections (Fig. 114.16). Some of the papillary formations are complex and appear to float in the luminal plane of section (Fig. 114.16 inset). Many vessel lumens, especially the smaller ones, are largely devoid of red blood cells. Endothelial cells show strong immunopositivity for CD31, CD34 and LYVE-1, light-to-absent positivity for D2-40 (podoplanin), and negativity for GLUT1[49]. Mitotic figures are rare or absent, although increased

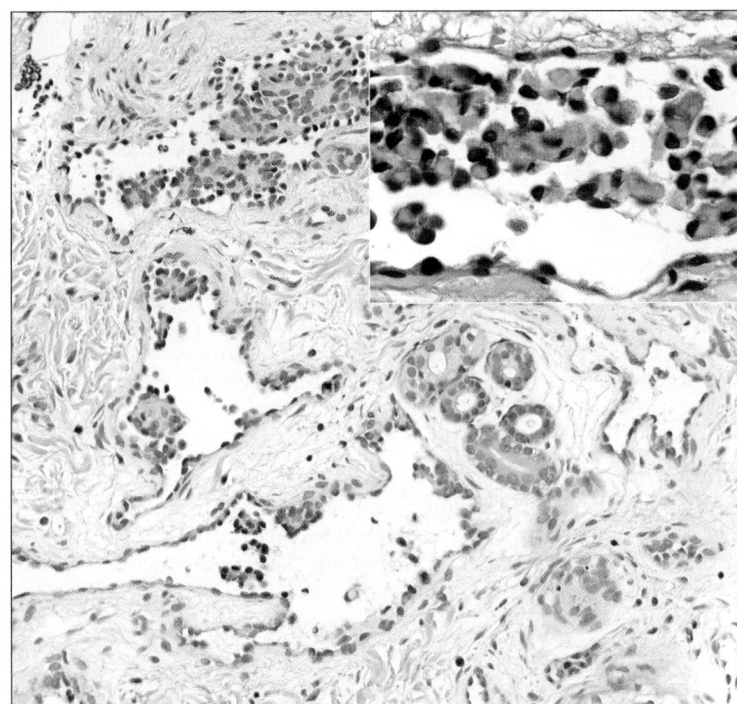

Fig. 114.16 **Histology of multifocal lymphangioendotheliomatosis with thrombocytopenia.** Thin-walled vessels focally forming intraluminal papillary projections scattered throughout the dermis and subcutis. Complex papillary projections lined by endothelium may appear to float in the lumen (inset).

endothelial expression of Ki-67 (approximately 15% of cells) correlates with the clinically observed progressive behavior[49].

Differential diagnosis

This entity must be differentiated from other multifocal vascular skin disorders presenting in infancy or childhood, including diffuse neonatal hemangiomatosis, blue rubber bleb nevus syndrome, glomuvenous malformations (glomangiomas), and Maffucci's syndrome. The clinical differential diagnosis also includes other causes of a 'blueberry muffin baby', such as extramedullary hematopoiesis, leukemia cutis, cutaneous metastases and infantile myofibromatosis (see Table 121.2). The skin lesions of MLT, however, are unique in their clinical plus histologic appearance, and are far more numerous than would be typical for any of the other vascular conditions except diffuse neonatal hemangiomatosis. Biopsy and histologic evaluation, supplemented by GLUT1 and LYVE-1 immunohistochemistry, is diagnostic.

Treatment

Gastrointestinal bleeding may spontaneously stabilize or require colectomy for effective control. Corticosteroids, interferon-α and thalidomide have been reported to be of possible value in some, but not all, cases[49,50].

BORDERLINE AND LOW-GRADE MALIGNANT VASCULAR NEOPLASMS

Kaposiform Hemangioendothelioma

Synonyms: ■ Infantile kaposiform hemangioendothelioma ■ Kaposi-like infantile hemangioendothelioma

Key features

- A rare vascular tumor of childhood associated with lymphangiomatosis and, in some cases, with a life-threatening platelet-trapping syndrome (Kasabach–Merritt phenomenon)
- Locally aggressive, but thought not to metastasize
- Cutaneous tumors present as ill-defined violaceous plaques; many tumors are more deeply seated
- Unlike common infantile hemangioma, does not spontaneously involute
- Some have responded well to therapy with corticosteroids, interferon-α-2a or vincristine, although surgical excision is best, where feasible

Introduction and history

Kaposiform hemangioendothelioma was described as such by Zukerberg et al.[41] in 1993, although equivalent lesions had been previously reported as 'hemangioma with Kaposi's sarcoma-like features'[51] and 'Kaposi-like infantile hemangioendothelioma'[52]. Many lesions of this type were previously diagnosed as infantile hemangioma.

Epidemiology

Most lesions present in children younger than 2 years of age, and some are congenital. Three cases have been reported in adults, all without evidence of Kasabach–Merritt syndrome[53]. The incidence is approximately equal in males and females.

Pathogenesis

Recent studies have demonstrated immunoreactivity for the lymphatic endothelium-associated antigen VEGFR-3 in kaposiform hemangioendotheliomas, supporting the concept that these tumors, like Kaposi's sarcoma and a subset of angiosarcomas, have a lymphatic endothelial phenotype[54]. Histologic and immunohistochemical similarities between Kaposi's sarcoma and kaposiform hemangioendothelioma have suggested that these entities might be etiologically related. Human herpesvirus-8 sequences have not been identified in kaposiform hemangioendothelioma[55], and children with coincident kaposiform hemangioendothelioma and HIV infection have not been reported. The more striking histologic overlap between kaposiform hemangioendothelioma and tufted angioma, and the shared, possibly unique, association of these two lesions with Kasabach–Merritt phenomenon, has been noted above. The life-threatening thrombocytopenia that characterizes Kasabach–Merritt phenomenon has been attributed to platelet trapping within these tumors[38,46]. Although platelet transfusions may be necessary, they have in some cases paradoxically worsened the coagulopathy[38,56]. Based on these incidents and on observations of rapid tumor shrinkage following pharmacologic control of platelet trapping, it has been suggested that intratumoral platelet activation may 'add fuel to the fire' by stimulating vascular proliferation[38], presumably by release of angiogenic agonists such as platelet-derived growth factor. A self-sustaining cycle of platelet trapping and tumor growth may thus be important for development of the full-blown Kasabach–Merritt phenomenon.

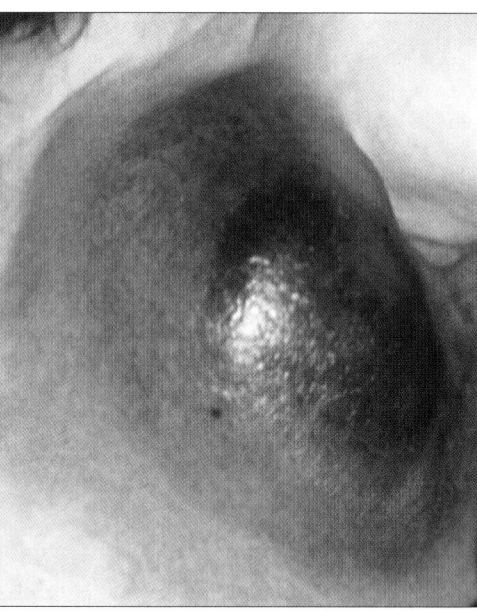

Fig. 114.17 Kaposiform hemangioendothelioma. An infiltrative indurated mass on the trunk of a child.

Clinical features

Cutaneous forms present as locally infiltrative vascular macules or plaques that may develop nodules. Deeper soft tissue lesions may present as bulging, indurated masses (Fig. 114.17) or be undetected on physical examination. Untreated lesions do not appear to regress, and patients with tumors complicated by Kasabach–Merritt phenomenon often have purpura and ecchymoses. In a compilation of reported cases with skin involvement[55], the initial age at presentation averaged 43 months, which is later than that of classical infantile hemangioma. More deeply seated tumors, particularly those in the retroperitoneum, are more likely to cause Kasabach–Merritt phenomenon[55].

The two most common causes of death from kaposiform hemangioendothelioma are complications of thrombocytopenia and direct tumor infiltration[55]. No distant metastases have been reported to date, although one case spread to regional lymph nodes[57]. Clinical evaluation of suspected cases – for instance, new-onset vascular tumors in children more than 3 months old[55] – should include MRI, a complete blood cell count, coagulation studies to detect coexistent Kasabach–Merritt phenomenon, and, if not prohibited by severe thrombocytopenia, biopsy for histopathologic diagnosis. MRI typically shows ill-defined tumor margins with the involvement of multiple tissue layers.

Pathology

Kaposiform hemangioendotheliomas are characterized by ill-defined, frequently coalescing nodules composed of fascicles of moderately plump spindle cells with eosinophilic-to-clear cytoplasm and bland nuclei that form elongated, slit-like lumina containing erythrocytes, reminiscent of Kaposi's sarcoma (Fig. 114.18A). These lumina may also contain platelet-rich microthrombi. At the margin of the lesion, the spindle cells may infiltrate freely into the surrounding adipose tissue and between collagen bundles, or may be encased by dense fibrosis. The spindle cells are immunoreactive for both the pan-endothelial marker CD31 and the lymphatic endothelial marker podoplanin (Fig. 114.18B). Mitotic activity is variable, but generally low. Focally, lobules of small, rounded capillaries lined by flat endothelia merge with the spindled areas, and nests of epithelioid cells with eosinophilic cytoplasm are occasionally observed. Extravasated erythrocytes and hemosiderin granules are typically present, and tumor cells may contain intracytoplasmic erythrocyte fragments and hyaline globules. Many cases display a prominent component of dilated lymphatic vessels that intermingle with the tumor lobules, but are often most obvious in the marginal soft tissues. 'Involuted' kaposiform hemangioendotheliomas remaining after successful treatment of platelet trapping represent dormant, often sclerotic, versions of the original disease process.

Differential diagnosis

The most important differential considerations are common infantile hemangioma, Kaposi's sarcoma and tufted angioma. Infantile

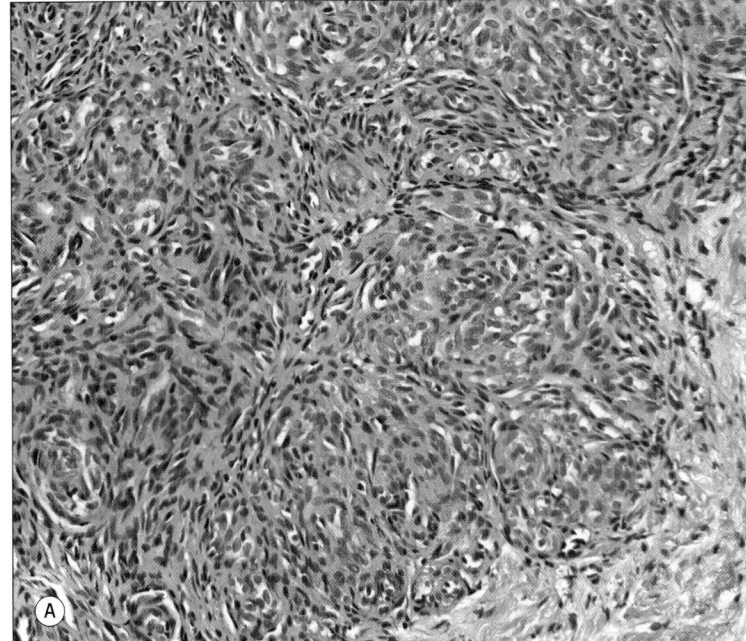

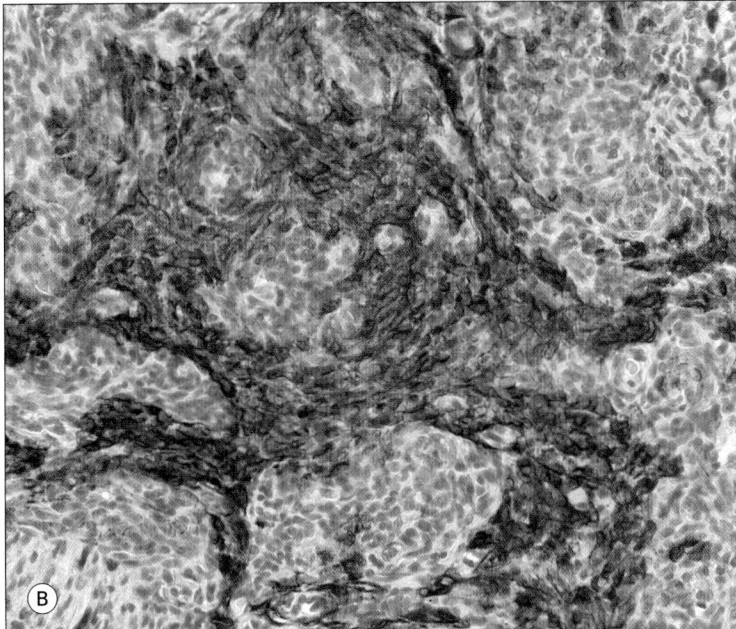

Fig. 114.18 Histology of kaposiform hemangioendothelioma. A. Fascicles of spindled endothelial cells forming slit-like lumina surround nests of more epithelioid areas rich in pericytes. **B.** The endothelial cells show evidence of lymphatic differentiation, here evidenced by positivity for podoplanin.

hemangiomas, unlike kaposiform hemangioendotheliomas, express a number of unusual vascular markers such as GLUT1[45,58] and do not contain fascicles of spindle cells. Kaposi's sarcoma, which is rare in children (outside of Africa), lacks the lobularity of kaposiform hemangioendothelioma and characteristically may show a few plasma cells. Tufted angioma is probably a milder relative of kaposiform hemangioendothelioma, characterized histologically by a 'cannonball' distribution of small, non-coalescent vascular tufts or nodules, without prominent cellular spindling.

Treatment
Tumors that are localized and superficial can be cured by wide local excision. Tumors in the mediastinum or retroperitoneum are often large and unresectable. Standard treatment regimens for unresectable cases with associated Kasabach–Merritt syndrome have not been well established because of their rarity, and responses to available therapies have been inconsistent. Current therapeutic options with a history of success in some patients include interferon-α-2a[59], vincristine[60], radiation therapy, aspirin plus ticlopidine, multimodal therapy[61], and a chemotherapeutic regimen consisting of cyclophosphamide, vincristine and actinomycin D[62]. Corticosteroids alone do not appear to be effective[55].

Dabska-type Hemangioendothelioma

Synonyms: ■ Papillary intralymphatic angioendothelioma (PILA) ■ Endovascular papillary angioendothelioma ■ Malignant endovascular papillary angioendothelioma ■ Dabska tumor ■ Hobnail hemangioendothelioma

Key features
- Rare neoplasm of lymphatic differentiation and very low metastatic potential that occurs primarily in children
- Enlarging dermal or subcutaneous mass or plaque, mostly in children, often on distal extremities
- Histologically defined by prominent papillary intralymphatic growth and peculiar rosette-like clusters of hobnail, columnar endothelial cells
- Thought to be closely related to retiform hemangioendothelioma, a similar tumor occurring mainly in adults

Introduction and history
Dabska first described tumors of this type as 'malignant endovascular papillary angioendothelioma' in 1969 based on a series of six cases, all in children. Two patients in this original series had lymph node metastases, and one of them later developed distant metastases and died[63]. Cases reported subsequently have behaved in a benign fashion, although follow-up for some has been limited[64]. Based on these observations and on the defining presence of papillary intravascular proliferation in these tumors, Fanburg-Smith et al.[64] have proposed designating these tumors as *papillary intralymphatic angioendotheliomas* (PILA), reflecting both their consistent lymphatic phenotype and their tentative potential for malignant or borderline clinical behavior. Weiss & Goldblum[7] have recently proposed that the term *hobnail hemangioendothelioma* be used to embrace both Dabska-type hemangioendothelioma and retiform hemangioendothelioma, recognizing their shared hobnail endothelial morphology, lymphatic differentiation and similar biologic behavior.

Epidemiology
Compilations of reported cases have shown no clear sex predilection, with approximately 75% of patients being children. Many cases have been congenital. A recent series of 12 patients where the mean age was 30 years suggests a wider age range for Dabska-like hemangioendotheliomas[64].

Clinical features
Lesions may appear as enlarging, diffuse, firm swellings of skin and subcutaneous tissue, or as soft intradermal plaques, sometimes with pink or blue skin discoloration. The size range is wide, with one reported mass, involving the buttock of a 16-year-old girl, measuring 40 cm[64]. A number of cases appear to have arisen in pre-existing lymphatic malformations or 'lymphangiomas'. Sites involving superficial tissues have included the head and neck, trunk, and extremities. Local recurrences are relatively common (about 40%). As noted above, only two cases of lymph node metastasis and one case of distant metastasis[63] have been reported.

Pathology
The unifying microscopic feature is the presence within the dermis and/or subcutis of intercommunicating, thin-walled vessels lined by hobnail endothelial cells forming characteristic intraluminal papillary projections that focally assume a rosetting or matchstick-like pattern (Fig. 114.19). Lesional vessels are variable in size. Hyaline papillary stromal cores are immunoreactive for collagen type IV, and focal actin-positive pericytes may be present within the papillary projections in some cases[64]. Lymphocytes may cluster along the endothelial lining of

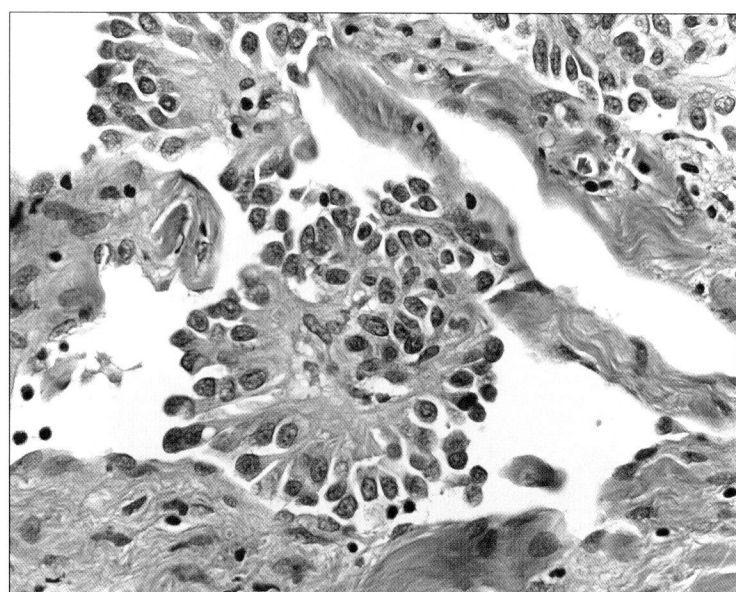

Fig. 114.19 Histology of Dabska-type hemangioendothelioma. Rosette-like intravascular clusters of hobnail, columnar endothelial cells.

the vessels and infiltrate into the surrounding stroma. Recent studies have shown strong endothelial immunopositivity for VEGFR-3 in these tumors[54,64], consistent with lymphatic differentiation.

Differential diagnosis

Dabska-type hemangioendotheliomas must be differentiated histologically from retiform hemangioendothelioma, hobnail hemangioma and well-differentiated angiosarcoma. In retiform hemangioendothelioma, intravascular papillary tufts, so prominent in the Dabska-type tumors, are infrequent and poorly developed. Hobnail hemangioma is a more superficial dermal process, again without the exuberant papillary tufts of Dabska-type hemangioendothelioma. Conventional angiosarcoma, even when well differentiated, usually presents on the head of the elderly or in areas of lymphedema, lacks hobnail endothelial cells, and demonstrates significant cytologic atypia not seen in Dabska-type hemangioendothelioma.

Treatment

The optimal therapy is conservative surgical excision with close follow-up. Recurrences are common.

Retiform Hemangioendothelioma

Synonym: ▪ Hobnail hemangioendothelioma

Key features

- Rare neoplasm of lymphatic differentiation and very low metastatic potential that occurs primarily in adults
- Presents as a slow-growing exophytic tumor or plaque on the trunk or extremities, especially the distal lower extremities
- Histologically characterized by a diffuse infiltration of the dermis and/or subcutis by elongated vessels with hobnail endothelial cells arborizing in a pattern similar to that of the normal rete testis
- Local recurrence following excision occurs in about 60% of patients; two cases with lymph node metastasis have been reported
- Thought to be closely related to Dabska-type hemangioendothelioma, a similar tumor occurring mainly in children

Introduction and history

Retiform hemangioendothelioma was first described as an entity in 1994 by Calonje et al.[32] based on a series of 15 cases, and was inter-

preted as a low-grade angiosarcoma. Six additional cases have subsequently been reported. Similarities in histology and clinical behavior to Dabska-like hemangioendothelioma, a tumor mainly affecting children, have led to a proposal that these two entities be jointly described by the term *hobnail hemangioendothelioma*[7], not to be confused with hobnail hemangioma discussed previously.

Epidemiology

Men and women are equally affected. The patient age range for reported cases is 9 to 78 years.

Clinical features

The clinical appearance of retiform hemangioendothelioma is not specific. Lesions present as solitary, slowly growing exophytic masses, plaques, or dermal and subcutaneous nodules. The site most commonly involved has been the extremities. In the series of Calonje et al.[32], nearly 60% of tumors recurred locally, and 1 of 14 patients followed developed a lymph node metastasis. There have been no tumor-related deaths.

Pathology

Retiform hemangioendothelioma is one of a small group of vascular tumors, also including hobnail hemangioma and Dabska tumor, that are characterized by endothelial cells with so-called hobnail appearance. Low-power views reveal diffuse infiltration of the reticular dermis and/or subcutis by an arborizing network of elongated, thin-walled vessels forming a pattern reminiscent of normal rete testis. The margins are ill defined. High-power views of the lesional vessels reveal a lining of bland endothelial cells with prominent apical nuclei that protrude into the lumina in a hobnail or 'matchstick' fashion. Mitotic figures are rare, and cytologic atypia is minimal. Solid foci of spindle cells expressing endothelial markers are often present, as are occasional intravascular papillae. The cavernous lymphatic-like vessels and prominent intravascular proliferations characteristic of Dabska-type hemangioendothelioma are absent. The endothelial cells of retiform hemangioendothelioma, like those of hobnail hemangioma and Dabska-type hemangioendothelioma, strongly express the lymphatic endothelium-associated marker VEGFR-3[54,64].

Differential diagnosis

The most clinically important differential for retiform hemangioendothelioma, as for Dabska-type hemangioendothelioma, is well-differentiated angiosarcoma, which is distinguished by cytologic atypia and lack of hobnail endothelial cells.

Treatment

Wide excisional biopsy with follow-up is appropriate.

Epithelioid Hemangioendothelioma

Key features

- Vascular tumor of adults with intermediate malignant potential
- Skin involvement is uncommon and is usually associated with more deeply seated disease, often associated with a vein
- Characterized histologically by cords and nests of epithelioid endothelial cells in a myxoid or hyalinized background
- Approximately 30% develop metastases in regional lymph nodes, lung, liver or bone
- Less than 50% of patients with metastases die of their disease

Introduction and history

Epithelioid hemangioendothelioma is a low-grade angiosarcoma (hemangioendothelioma) first described by Weiss & Enzinger in 1982. It has more metastatic potential than other lesions classified as hemangioendotheliomas[65]. Most arise in deep soft tissues, but lesions can occur in skin, viscera and bone. Since its original description, 19 cutaneous cases have been reported in the literature[65,66].

Epidemiology

Epithelioid hemangioendothelioma typically occurs in adults. Males and females are affected in an approximately equal ratio.

Pathogenesis

Epithelioid hemangioendotheliomas are clonal neoplastic proliferations of endothelial cells with low to intermediate potential to metastasize. Chromosomal translocation has been reported[67].

Clinical features

Most epithelioid hemangioendotheliomas present as a solitary, slightly painful, soft tissue mass. Skin involvement is often associated with an underlying soft tissue or bone tumor, but purely cutaneous examples do occur[65]. The most frequent sites of cutaneous involvement that have been reported are the extremities. Many tumors are closely associated with or arise from a vessel, usually a vein[68]. Occlusion of that vessel in some cases may cause secondary symptoms, such as edema or thrombophlebitis. Overall, approximately 30% of patients develop metastatic disease in regional lymph nodes, lung, liver or bone, and fewer than 50% of these patients with metastases have died of their disease[68]. One study of 30 cases suggests that dermal tumors may have a better prognosis than more deeply seated lesions[64].

Pathology

Like their more common counterparts involving soft tissue and bone, epithelioid hemangioendotheliomas involving the skin show an infiltrative growth pattern of epithelioid tumor cells with eosinophilic cytoplasm forming poorly canalized nests and cords within a distinctive myxohyaline stroma. An important clue to their endothelial origin is the presence of small intracytoplasmic vacuoles containing red blood cells (Fig. 114.20). Nuclei are vesicular with little or no atypia and contain small, inconspicuous nucleoli. Unlike in epithelioid hemangioma (angiolymphoid hyperplasia with eosinophilia), inflammation is sparse. Mitotic rate is variable and only weakly correlated with clinical outcome[65].

Differential diagnosis

The differential diagnosis is wide and includes epithelioid sarcoma, metastatic carcinoma, melanoma and epithelioid angiosarcoma. An essential criterion for diagnosis of epithelioid hemangioendothelioma is immunohistochemical evidence of endothelial differentiation[65]. Differentiation from epithelioid angiosarcomas may be problematic and relies upon recognition of the typical architectural pattern of epithelioid hemangioendothelioma throughout the lesion.

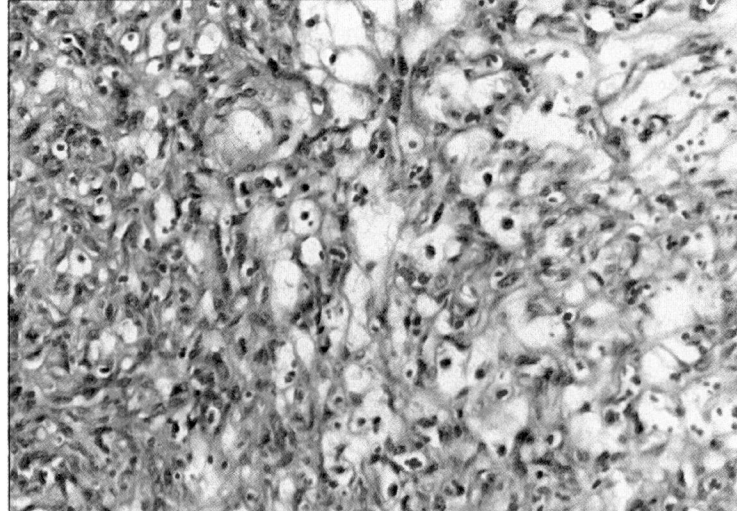

Fig. 114.20 Histology of epithelioid hemangioendothelioma. Poorly canalized cords and nests of endothelial cells in a myxoid background which form small intracytoplasmic vacuoles containing red blood cells.

Treatment

Appropriate therapy involves wide local excision without adjuvant chemotherapy or radiotherapy, given the low-grade nature of these tumors. Regional lymph nodes should be evaluated since these represent a common metastatic site.

Kaposi's Sarcoma

Key features

- It is controversial whether Kaposi's sarcoma (KS) represents neoplasia or hyperplasia; all clinical variants are viewed as a virally induced disease – human herpesvirus-8 (HHV-8) is the implicated agent
- KS is a multifocal systemic disease with four principal clinical variants: (1) chronic or classic KS; (2) African endemic KS, including a fulminant lymphadenopathic type; (3) KS in iatrogenically immunocompromised patients; and (4) AIDS-related epidemic KS
- Cutaneous lesions present as variably distributed pink patches, blue–violet to black nodules or plaques, and polyps, depending on the clinical variant and stage
- The histologic appearance of KS does not vary significantly between clinical subtypes, but does vary with stage of the lesion
- Most cases in childhood, with or without HIV infection, are of the lymphadenopathic type and are rapidly fatal due to visceral dissemination
- Because of multifocality, treatment with chemotherapy and/or radiation is favored over surgery

Introduction and history

In 1872, Moritz Kaposi described five men with an unusual multifocal sarcoma of the skin in Hungary which he termed 'idiopathic multiple pigmented sarcoma of the skin'. This disease entity became known as *Kaposi's sarcoma* and has been historically considered a chronic, protracted disease primarily affecting elderly men, generally Jewish or of Mediterranean/Eastern European descent. Despite occasional reports regarding its occurrence in organ transplant patients and its endemic form in Africa, KS received little attention until it became epidemic among men who have sex with men and was recognized as a sign of AIDS. A new human herpesvirus (HHV-8) was recognized as the probable inductive agent of all clinical variants of KS. The mechanisms that control the clinical variability of KS are likely to involve a number of interrelated factors modulated by the patient's immune status and have yet to be fully defined.

Epidemiology
Classic KS

The annual incidence of classic KS in the US is estimated to be 0.02% to 0.06% of all malignant tumors. People of Jewish Ashkenazi descent and/or of Mediterranean descent are predominantly afflicted. Clustered occurrences have been reported on Sardinia and in the Peloponnesus[69], although familial occurrence is rare. The male-to-female incidence ratio has varied in different studies, from 15 to 1 in the older literature to 3 to 1 and 1 to 1 in more recent literature[70]. Two-thirds of patients with classic KS develop disease after the age of 50 years.

African endemic KS

The incidence of KS among black Africans is high, ranging from 1.3% to 10% according to locality, with an increased incidence first noted in the 1950s before the AIDS pandemic. Presentations equivalent to classic KS account for up to 9% of all reported cancers in the equatorial region of Africa[71]. Another form of KS endemic in Africa is the lymphadenopathic variant (see below), which mainly affects children. There is a clear male predominance in African KS, mainly in adults, but also in children.

KS in iatrogenically immunosuppressed patients

This form of KS has been increasing in incidence among individuals with organ transplants, cancer or autoimmune diseases, due to the increased use of various immunosuppressive and cytotoxic agents. KS has been observed in organ transplant recipients receiving traditional immunosuppressive agents such as azathioprine and corticosteroids, as well as in individuals receiving cyclosporine therapy. Cyclosporine therapy is associated with a higher incidence and more rapid onset of disease. The estimated incidence of post-transplantation KS in Western countries is estimated to be less than 1%, although it is nearly 4% in the Near East[7]. As in classic KS, men are more commonly affected than women.

AIDS-related epidemic KS

This form of KS occurs almost exclusively in men who have sex with men and, to a lesser degree, in female partners of the latter and in women from certain regions of Africa and the Caribbean who have acquired HIV by heterosexual contact. In the pre-HAART era, about 40% of men who had sex with men and who had AIDS developed KS, compared with less than 5% in other risk groups. In children with AIDS, the incidence of KS was 4%[72].

Pathogenesis

Immunohistochemical and ultrastructural studies have firmly established the endothelial nature of KS, but it remains controversial whether this endothelial phenotype is vascular, lymphatic, or perhaps a composite of both. Moreover, many, if not most, cells forming the substance of a plaque or nodule of KS are spindled cells distinctly unlike endothelial cells in morphology, although expressing pan-endothelial markers like CD31 as well as markers of lymphatic differentiation such as VEGFR-3[54,73], podoplanin[74] and LYVE-1, and in vitro, HHV-8 can infect both lymphatic and blood vascular endothelial cells and induce transcriptional reprogramming, leading to expression of lymph-angiogenic molecules[74a]. It also remains unclear whether KS is essentially hyperplastic or neoplastic in nature. Studies employing X-chromosome inactivation (methylation) patterns have supported clonality[75,76]. Interestingly, studies of sets of multiple lesions from single patients by this method have in some cases shown singular, presumably disseminated clones[75], and in other cases have indicated dissimilar, presumably independently developing clones[76].

Despite these uncertainties, these is currently a large body of evidence indicating that infection with HHV-8 causes, or at least strongly influences, the development of KS[77] (see Ch. 79). This virus was first identified in KS cells of a patient with AIDS and now is known to be present in most patients with all clinical types of KS. Seroreactivity to HHV-8 is not present to a significant degree in the normal population. The HHV-8 genome, when detected in the blood of HIV-positive men, strongly predicts their subsequent development of KS. HHV-8 contains homologues of cellular genes that can stimulate cell proliferation, inflammation and angiogenesis and perhaps inhibit apoptosis[78]. The host immune response and cytokines (particularly fibroblast growth factor) released by the virally infected cells may further support tumor growth in an autocrine and paracrine manner[79,80].

Clinical features

Classic KS typically presents as slowly growing, blue–red to violet macules on the distal lower extremities that may coalesce to form large plaques (Fig. 114.21), or develop into nodules or polypoid tumors. Initially unilateral lesions progress to a more widely disseminated multifocal pattern. Early lesions may regress, while others evolve, leading to lesions at different stages. Patients with longstanding KS may have lesions in the mouth and gastrointestinal tract that are usually asymptomatic.

African endemic KS can be classified into four subgroups: nodular, florid, infiltrative and lymphadenopathic. The nodular variant resembles classic KS in course and appearance, whereas the florid and infiltrative types are more biologically aggressive. The lymphadenopathic type is notably different in several regards: it predominantly affects children, the primary tumors involve the lymph nodes (although skin and mucosal lesions may also be present), and its course is fulminant and fatal.

Immunosuppressive drug-induced KS (transplantation-associated KS) is generally clinically similar to classic KS. It may resolve completely upon removal of immunosuppressive therapy. KS associated with prolonged high-dose immunosuppression may behave in a more

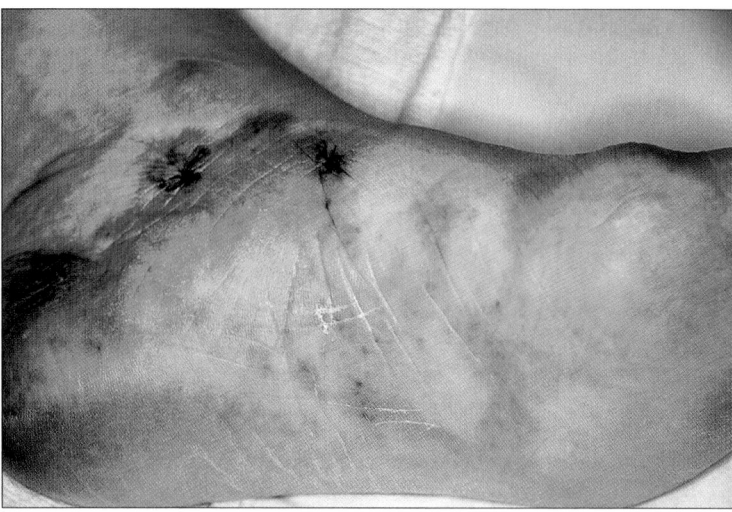

Fig. 114.21 Classic Kaposi's sarcoma. Red macules and patches on the plantar surface of the foot, with violaceous plaques on the ankle.

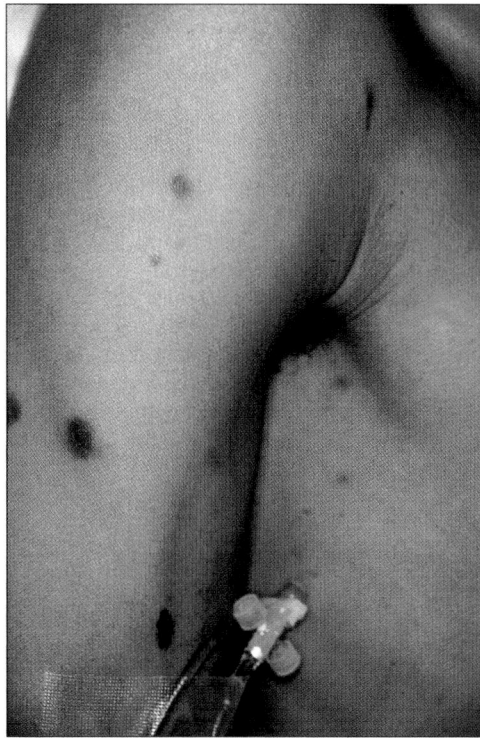

Fig. 114.22 Kaposi's sarcoma in a patient with AIDS. Violet–brown papules or nodules are often oval to lanceolate and are usually more widely distributed than in classic KS.

aggressive fashion, causing death in patients who develop internal involvement.

AIDS-related epidemic KS most commonly affects HIV-infected patients with advanced immune impairment and CD4+ T cell counts of less than 500 cells per cubic millimeter[81]. Clinical features of KS in the HIV-infected patient are protean. While some patients experience only a single lesion, others have disseminated cutaneous disease. Individual lesions range from faint erythematous macules, papules and plaques to purple–black tumors and nodules. Macules and plaques are frequently oval to lanceolate and may array along lines of cleavage of the skin (Fig. 114.22). Coalescing papules and plaques occasionally form extensive armor-like constricting plaques that may impair the function of extremities and cause lymphedema. While any skin surface may be involved, the trunk and midface (particularly the nose) are common sites, causing significant cosmetic disfigurement (see Ch. 77). Bluish to violaceous macules, plaques and tumors may arise on the oral mucosa. Plaques and tumors at any site may ulcerate and become secondarily infected.

KS frequently involves the viscera, including the gastrointestinal tract, lymph nodes and lungs. The prognosis of pulmonary disease is grave.

Pathology

The histologic appearance of KS does not vary significantly between the different clinical subtypes, but does vary with the stage of the lesion. The *patch* stage is characterized by a superficial dermal proliferation of small, angulated vessels lined by inconspicuous endothelial cells, suggestive of lymphatics (Fig. 114.23). These delicate but 'jagged' vessels tend to separate collagen bundles and are accompanied by a sparse infiltrate of lymphocytes and plasma cells. In the more advanced *plaque* stage, the vascular proliferation extends to include the deeper dermis and may involve the subcutis. A spindle cell population expressing endothelial markers appears among the ramifying small vessels during the *plaque* stage and expands, replacing dermal collagen and producing the *nodular* stage of KS. Pleomorphism and significant numbers of mitotic figures are absent. The spindle cells form intersecting fascicles and are separated by characteristic slit-like spaces containing erythrocytes (Fig. 114.24). The resulting sieve-like pattern of vascular spaces is highly characteristic of KS. Intracellular and extracellular hyaline globules are thought to represent degenerated erythrocytes[7]. The tumor nodules are often rimmed by ectatic or crescentic vessels, hemosiderin deposits, lymphocytes and plasma cells and may be compartmentalized by fibrous bands. Some tumors contain prominent ectatic meshworks of vessels and have been referred to as 'lymphangioma-like' KS. Tumors with a frankly sarcomatous appearance, nuclear pleomorphism and brisk mitotic activity may occur either as a late stage within previously indolent lesions or as an initial presentation, the latter most commonly in African endemic cases.

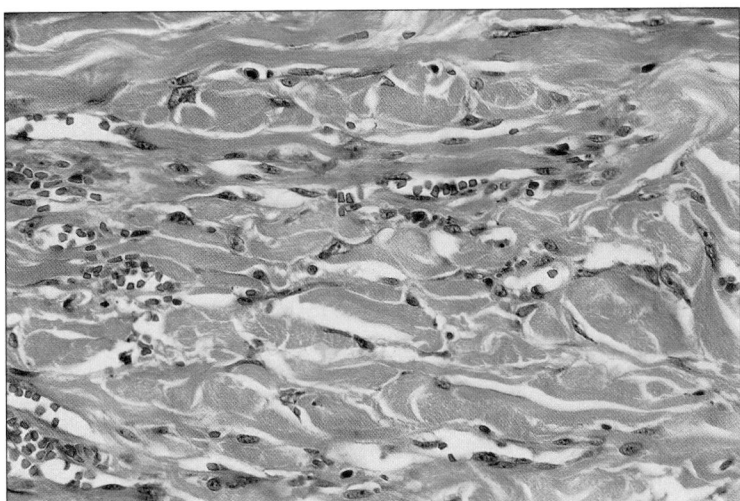

Fig. 114.23 Histology of Kaposi's sarcoma – patch stage. Slit-like vascular spaces are present. Courtesy of Ronald P Rapini MD.

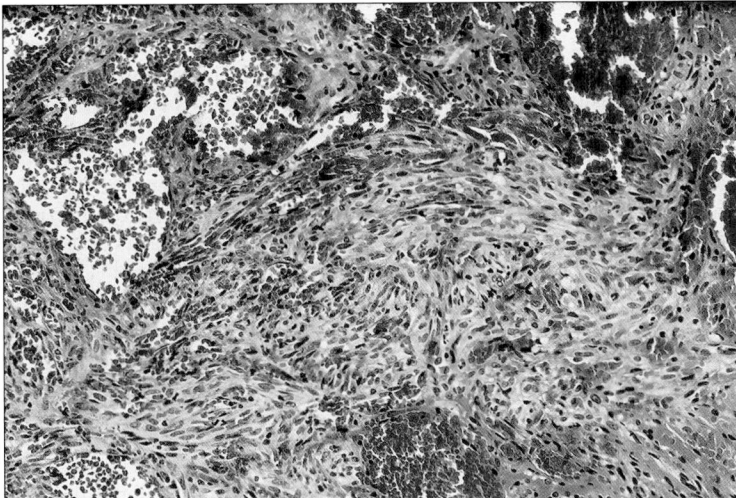

Fig. 114.24 Histology of Kaposi's sarcoma – tumor/nodular stage. Dilated blood vessels and solid areas of bland spindle cells, slit-like spaces, and hemorrhage. Courtesy of Ronald P Rapini MD.

Demonstration of expression of the latency-associated nuclear antigen (LNA-1) of HHV-8 has proved in a number of studies to be a highly sensitive and specific marker of KS (see Fig. 79.22) and other HHV-8-associated disorders such as multicentric Castleman's disease and primary effusion lymphoma in both HIV-positive and HIV-negative patients[81a,81b]. Immunohistochemical detection of this antigen in vascular tumors is more diagnostically useful than detection of the HHV-8 genome by PCR, since a few non-KS vascular tumors in both immunocompromised and immunocompetent patients have been found to be positive for HHV-8 by PCR, but not by LNA immunohistochemistry, presumably due to detection of HHV-8 within blood cells circulating through the tumors[81a].

Differential diagnosis

Lesions of KS may resemble a number of other diseases in clinical and histologic appearance, especially the early- and late-stage lesions. The clinical differential for macular-stage KS includes well-differentiated angiosarcoma, benign lymphangiomatosis, microvenular hemangioma and hobnail hemangioma. These can be distinguished histologically, with the plasma cell-rich infiltrate of KS being an important discriminating factor.

The most important differential diagnostic considerations in nodular-stage KS are kaposiform hemangioendothelioma, spindle cell hemangioma and moderately differentiated angiosarcoma. Although KS and spindle cell hemangioma both are characterized by proliferations of spindle cells, KS lacks the cavernous spaces of the latter. Kaposiform hemangioendothelioma is almost exclusively a disease of infancy and childhood and is distinguished from KS by a strongly lobular architecture and lack of plasma cell infiltrates. Angiosarcoma is characterized by endothelial atypia and mitotic activity, both absent in KS.

Late-stage KS may both clinically and histologically resemble acro-angiodermatitis of chronic venous insufficiency and Stewart–Bluefarb syndrome (pseudo-Kaposi's sarcoma). These reactive, hyperplastic entities differ from KS in that the hyperplasia can be seen to derive from pre-existing vasculature. Late-stage KS lesions can also be confused histologically with a number of non-vascular spindle cell sarcomas such as fibrosarcoma and leiomyosarcoma. In these cases, demonstration of CD31 immunoreactivity helps confirm the vascular differentiation of KS.

Other entities that can mimic KS clinically, but can be easily distinguished on the basis of histologic features include cutaneous metastases, leukemia or lymphoma cutis, venous and lymphatic malformations, and the cutaneous manifestations of polyarteritis nodosa and erythema elevatum diutinum.

Treatment

In many patients with KS, obtaining a complete cure may be an unrealistic expectation, since recurrence rates are high. Treatment of visible lesions, even in HIV-positive patients with widely disseminated disease, improves appearance, heightens self-esteem and provides patients with a sense of control in an otherwise difficult situation. In older immunocompetent patients with static disease, observation and close follow-up is an option. Surgery is only useful for tissue diagnosis and removal of solitary lesions. Cryotherapy, laser surgery, photodynamic therapy and topical alitretinoin gel have been used to treat superficial macules and plaques. Freezing must usually be sufficiently vigorous to cause epidermal ulceration. The resulting scar seems to replace the vascular proliferation of KS. Extensive, multifocal disease requires irradiation and chemotherapy.

Radiation therapy is a treatment option for the patient presenting with multifocal but relatively localized KS. Regimens reported to be successful include single-dose radiation (8 to 12 Gy) delivered to an extended field and total body electron beam therapy (4 Gy) once a week for 6 to 8 weeks. Radiation therapy clearly plays a role in the treatment of localized cutaneous and oral KS, but may have a briefer effect in AIDS-related KS than in classic KS[82].

Rapidly progressive KS (defined by development of 10 or more new cutaneous lesions per month), pulmonary KS, symptomatic visceral involvement, and lymphedema are indications for systemic chemotherapy. Vincristine, doxorubicin and bleomycin have been commonly employed singly and in combination[83]. Nowadays, liposomal preparations of the anthracyclines doxorubicin and daunorubicin are being used in the hope of reducing side effects. Bone marrow toxicity remains the major limiting factor in these therapies[84]. The taxanes paclitaxel and docetaxel are used for the treatment of disseminated KS not responsive to anthracyclines and depending upon co-morbities, may be used initially.

For treatment of individual lesions, intratumoral vinblastine (0.1 mg/ml) causes a slow fading of erythema and thickness. High concentrations or volumes of injection may cause ulceration of the overlying epidermis, but lesions still resolve with adequate cosmesis.

Interferon-α is a biological response modifier that has been proven effective as a systemic therapy for KS. It is administered either intravenously or with daily subcutaneous injections, with the dose required to achieve success in the treatment of disseminated KS approaching 30 million units per day. However, interferon has a number of undesirable side effects (see Ch. 128).

A number of new topical and systemic therapies are emerging. Etoposide, at higher doses, has resulted in response rates >75% in patients with AIDS-associated KS[85]. Systemic therapies specifically designed for AIDS-related KS are being developed, including angiogenesis inhibitors and drugs targeting HHV-8. Angiogenesis inhibitors that currently show promise include thalidomide, the matrix metalloproteinase inhibitor COL-3, bevacizumab (anti-VEGF), and TNP-470 (fumagillin analog)[85,86]. Additional agents under investigation as adjuvants in the treatment of AIDS-related KS include imatinib, sorafenib, gefitinib, pentosan polysulfate, and interleukin-12[85,86]. Highly active antiretroviral therapy (HAART) has been profoundly helpful in alleviating AIDS-related KS, probably indirectly by decreasing viral load and increasing the CD4 count. The exact mechanism of this effect is unclear. Of note, there are reports of flares of KS as a manifestation of the immune recovery syndrome (see Ch. 77), but this does not necessarily translate into a poor prognosis.

Organ transplant patients with KS pose a particular therapeutic challenge, that of balancing the risk of graft rejection with the benefit of improvement in KS. Reduction of immunosuppression dosage by 50% in one study showed a 100% response rate in reduction of KS lesions[87]. Substitution of sirolimus (rapamycin) for cyclosporine can lead to complete resolution of the lesions of KS. These patients will also respond to conventional local and systemic therapies used in other forms of KS. There are few published studies on the treatment of African endemic KS.

MALIGNANT VASCULAR NEOPLASMS

Angiosarcoma

Synonyms: ■ Malignant hemangioendothelioma
■ Hemangiosarcoma ■ Lymphangiosarcoma

Key features

- Uncommon malignant neoplasm of endothelium, accounting for less than 1% of all sarcomas

- Unlike most sarcomas, has a predilection for skin and superficial soft tissue

- Most commonly affects the scalp and face of the elderly and areas of chronic lymphedema or radiodermatitis; rare in children

- Cutaneous forms are usually well to moderately differentiated lesions composed of anastomosing vessels that dissect between bundles of collagen

- Approximately 50% of cases express markers of lymphatic differentiation

- Prognosis is extremely poor, with fewer than 15% of patients surviving 5 years

- Most long-term survivors received early radical ablative surgery

Introduction and history

The term *angiosarcoma* is traditionally used to denote all biologically high-grade malignant neoplasms of endothelial derivation, regardless of the evidence of lymphatic or vascular differentiation. Endothelial tumors of low or intermediate malignant potential are designated *hemangioendotheliomas*, although in the past these borderline tumors were often referred to as *low-grade angiosarcomas*. An exception to this rule is Kaposi's sarcoma, a virus-associated disease of highly variable behavior that maintains a controversial place in the spectrum between neoplasia and hyperplasia. Angiosarcomas were first described systematically by Caro & Stubenrauch in 1945. Only 3 years later, Stewart & Treves described the association between angiosarcoma and post-mastectomy lymphedema[88]. The cutaneous form of angiosarcoma that primarily affects the face and scalp of the elderly was characterized by Wilson-Jones in 1964[89].

Epidemiology

Angiosarcomas are rare neoplasms that usually occur in adults. Rare examples that occur in childhood or adolescence are more likely to arise in viscera or in association with other disease states, including chronic or congenital lymphedema, chronic radiodermatitis and immunosuppression. Among elderly patients with angiosarcomas of the face and scalp, there is a strong predilection for Caucasians compared to individuals of African or Asian descent, and approximately a 2:1 predilection for males[90].

Pathogenesis

Angiosarcomas are clonal proliferations of malignantly transformed cells expressing endothelial differentiation. Mechanisms of the association between chronic lymphedema and angiosarcoma remain uncertain. Theories include induction of neoplastic change by unknown carcinogens in accumulated lymphatic fluid[88] and the idea that areas with chronic lymphedema are 'immunologically privileged sites' due to loss of afferent lymphatic connections. The latter idea is supported by observations that skin grafts transferred to lymphedematous areas show prolonged survival. Although angiosarcomas arising in the setting of chronic lymphedema have often been presumed to originate from lymphatics, this has not been definitively proven. Expression of the lymphatic endothelium-associated antigen VEGFR-3 was observed in 8 of 16 angiosarcomas in one series in which cases associated with lymphedema and prior irradiation were excluded[71]. Another series found VEGFR-3 positivity in only one of two spindled angiosarcomas and in none of four epithelioid angiosarcomas[64]. Most angiosarcomas in another series were found to coexpress podoplanin and podocalyxin, thought to be markers of lymphatic and vascular endothelium, respectively[74]. This suggests that many angiosarcomas are of mixed lineage. Until this issue is further clarified, use of the more generic term *angiosarcoma*, rather than *lymphangiosarcoma* or *hemangiosarcoma*, seems prudent. HHV-8, strongly linked to Kaposi's sarcoma, appears not to be associated with angiosarcoma. Cumulative sun exposure has also not been shown to be a predisposing factor.

Clinical features

The most common form of angiosarcoma is cutaneous angiosarcoma without lymphedema in the elderly. Approximately 70% of these tumors occur in patients greater than 40 years of age, with the highest incidence in those over 70 years of age. About 50% involve the head and neck. Lesions typically present as a deceptively benign-appearing bruise-like patch on the central face, forehead or scalp. Facial swelling and edema may be present. More advanced lesions are violaceous, elevated nodules (Fig. 114.25) that bleed easily. Ulceration may be present. The area of involvement spreads centrifugally, eventually covering large portions of the head and neck. The prognosis is invariably poor, with a less than 15% survival rate over a 5-year period[90].

Angiosarcomas that arise in the setting of chronic lymphedema present as firm, coalescing violaceous nodules or an indurated plaque on a background of brawny, non-pitting edema. Greater than 90% of all angiosarcomas associated with lymphedema arise after mastectomy and lymph node dissection (Stewart–Treves syndrome). In these cases, the inner aspect of the upper arm is the most common site of involvement. Other forms of chronic lymphedema are associated with angiosarcoma, including congenital, filarial, traumatic and idiopathic. The duration of lymphedema prior to the appearance of angiosarcoma ranges from 4 to 27 years. Rare post-irradiation angiosarcomas have been documented[91], usually as abdominal or chest wall tumors

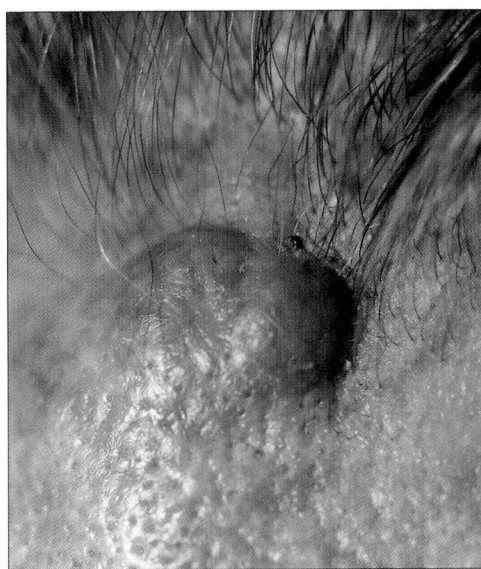

Fig. 114.25 Angiosarcoma. Violet-colored nodule on the scalp, a common site for this malignancy. Courtesy of Kenneth Greer MD.

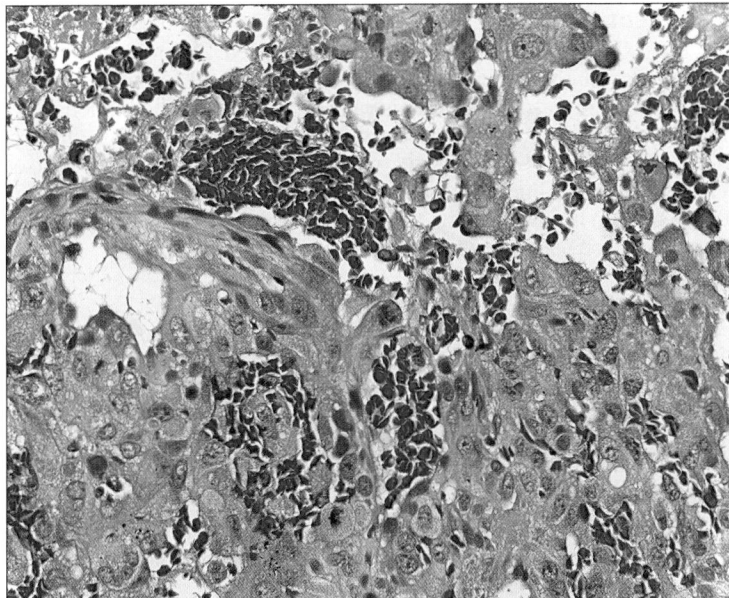

Fig. 114.26 Histology of angiosarcoma. Infiltration of the dermis by ill-defined vascular spaces lined by atypical, piled-up endothelial cells.

following radiation for gynecologic malignancies or breast carcinoma. Recently, with increased use of breast-sparing surgery paired with irradiation for breast carcinoma, more post-irradiation sarcomas have arisen in breast parenchyma and overlying skin, with an average post-treatment duration of 6 years. However, the incidence of angiosarcoma among women treated conservatively for breast cancer is still very low (less than 0.05% in a recent survey[92]). Post-irradiation angiosarcomas appear as infiltrative plaques or nodules in or near the area of tissue irradiated and share the poor prognosis of all forms of angiosarcoma. These are aggressive, infiltrative, multicentric tumors that enlarge incessantly. Local recurrence and metastasis to regional lymph nodes and lung are common. Angiosarcomas of skin and soft tissue have been reported in association with benign and malignant nerve sheath tumors[93], defunctionalized arteriovenous shunts in renal transplant patients[94], long-term exposure to various foreign materials[95], xeroderma pigmentosum[96] and bilateral retinoblastoma[97]. MRI, which shows a non-specific decreased or variable signal intensity in T1, an increased signal in T2, and enhancement with gadolinium, is more useful than CT in accurately delineating the extent of local disease, including involvement of neurovascular structures and joints. It is also the imaging modality of choice for evaluating tumor response to preoperative radiation or chemotherapy.

Pathology

Angiosarcomas involving the skin, although highly variable in degree of endothelial differentiation both between and within individual tumors, do not vary in histology as a class between those of the 'usual type' not associated with lymphedema, those associated with chronic lymphedema, and those associated with chronic radiodermatitis. Well-differentiated areas display an anastomosing network of sinusoidal vessels, often bloodless, lined by a single layer of endothelial cells of slight to moderate nuclear atypia. These exhibit a highly infiltrative pattern, splitting apart collagen bundles and groups of adipose cells. In less well-differentiated areas, the endothelial cells with more pronounced nuclear pleomorphism and mitotic activity pile up (Fig. 114.26) and form papillary projections. In poorly differentiated areas, luminal formation may be non-apparent and mitotic activity may be high, mimicking other high-grade sarcomas, carcinoma or melanoma. Hemorrhage and blood-filled cavities may be present.

In tumors associated with chronic lymphedema, networks of small lymphatics lined by endothelial cells with hyperchromatic nuclei may ramify through adjacent soft tissues and have been interpreted as premalignant change. Angiosarcomas developing in this setting may retain lymphatic characteristics (Fig. 114.27). Most angiosarcomas immunoreact positively for CD31 and CD34, with CD31 being the more sensitive and endothelium-specific of the two. Immunohistochemical detection of factor VIII-related antigen, although highly specific for endothelial cells, lacks sensitivity for vascular neoplasms and is negative or very weak even in well-differentiated angiosarcomas.

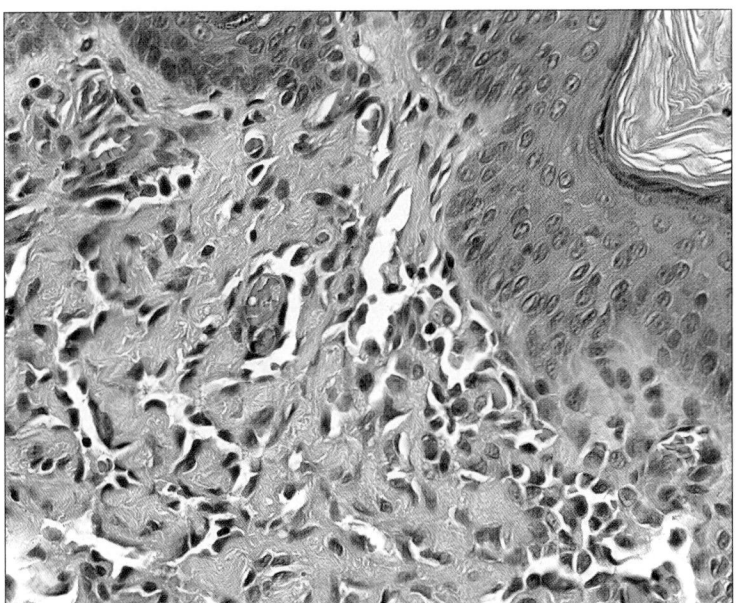

Fig. 114.27 Histology of angiosarcoma with lymphatic characteristics ('lymphangiosarcoma'). Some of the vascular channels are angular and lack erythrocytes.

Angiosarcomas with an epithelioid appearance occasionally occur in the skin, although this variant is more common in deep soft tissues. These so-called 'epithelioid angiosarcomas' consist of large rounded cells with prominent eosinophilic nucleoli in which the only morphologic evidence of vascular differentiation may be the presence of occasional intracytoplasmic vacuoles. Cytokeratin positivity is present in about one-third of epithelioid angiosarcomas[98,99], making distinction from carcinoma problematic. Fortunately, this distinction can be accomplished by demonstration of coexistent CD31 expression.

Differential diagnosis

Early recognition and histologic diagnosis are crucial in the treatment of angiosarcoma. Well-differentiated angiosarcomas, which display only slight cytologic atypia despite their high-grade biologic behavior, may closely resemble benign lymphangiomatosis. Other vascular neoplasms that must be distinguished from angiosarcoma histologically include Dabska-like and retiform hemangioendothelioma, epithelioid hemangioendothelioma and tufted angioma. Intravascular proliferation of atypical endothelial cells is not a feature of Kaposi's sarcoma.

Treatment

Surgical excision with wide margins is indicated. Even with negative margins by histologic examination, the recurrence rate and chance of metastatic disease is high. This may in part reflect the tendency for multifocality. In a recent retrospective review, 10 of 13 patients showed a response to weekly paclitaxel versus 14 of 27 for non-paclitaxel regimens, but the difference was not statistically significant (p=0.18)[99a]. There are also isolated reports of successful thalidomide therapy. Radiotherapy may be palliative, but does not improve survival.

PERIVASCULAR NEOPLASMS AND NEOPLASTIC-LIKE PROLIFERATIONS

Glomus Tumors and Glomuvenous Malformations (Glomangiomas)

Synonyms: ■ Glomus tumor: solitary glomus tumor, solid glomus tumor ■ Glomuvenous malformation: glomangioma, infiltrating glomus tumor, multiple glomus tumors

Key features

- A heterogeneous group of benign tumors characterized by presence of glomus cells
- The two major subgroups are *glomus tumor* and *glomuvenous malformation (glomangioma)*
- The glomus tumor typically presents in young adults, is a *solitary*, *painful* papule or nodule on the extremities with a predilection for subungual sites, and consists of a relatively solid proliferation of glomus cells associated with *small* vessels
- The less common glomuvenous malformation (glomangioma) typically presents in infancy or childhood, is often *multiple*, *asymptomatic* and histologically resembles a venous malformation in which *dilated* vessels are rimmed by a *few glomus cells*
- Histologic variants in which glomus cells merge with well-differentiated smooth muscle cells are referred to as *glomangiomyomas*
- Extremely rare atypical and malignant forms have been described

Introduction

Tumors distinguished by the presence of benign glomus cells have been subclassified in the past into a number of descriptive types, such as solid type, solitary type, multiple type, adult type, pediatric type and diffuse type. Current evidence supports division of these tumors into two major disparate categories: (1) the glomus tumor proper, a cellular lesion that tends to be well circumscribed, solitary and subungual; and (2) the glomangioma, a frequently multifocal tumor, more properly termed glomuvenous malformation, that most commonly presents in infants or children and histologically resembles a venous malformation in which lesional vessels are rimmed by glomus cells.

Epidemiology

Solitary glomus tumors can occur at any age, but are most common in young adults. Although these tumors in general show no gender predilection, subungual lesions are more common in women. Glomangiomas are less common (accounting for 10–20% of all glomus cell lesions) and typically present in children; many are congenitally evident.

Pathogenesis

The fact that the most common site of occurrence of glomus tumors (the subungual region of the finger) corresponds to one of the densest areas of distribution of the normal glomus body suggests that many glomus tumors represent neoplastic proliferations originating from pre-existing normal glomus cell populations. However, the occasional occurrence of glomus tumors at sites where normal glomus bodies may not be found, including bone, gastrointestinal tract, trachea and nerve, suggests that some glomus tumors may arise from pluripotent mesenchymal cells or even ordinary smooth muscle cells.

Despite their shared complement of benign glomus cells, glomus tumors and glomangiomas differ widely in clinical and histopathologic features and are unlikely to be closely related in pathogenesis. The resemblance to venous malformations and the early presentation of glomangiomas strongly supports a malformative etiology, thus the recent preference for the term *glomuvenous malformation*. Although most glomuvenous malformations are sporadic, some cases are familial and have demonstrated an autosomal dominant pattern of inheritance[100,101]. Based on linkage disequilibrium studies with 12 of these families, a locus for glomuvenous malformations (termed VMGLOM) has been mapped to chromosome 1p21–p22[102], and loss of function of a cytoplasmic protein termed *glomulin* has been credited with causation of familial forms of these lesions[103]. Interestingly, a familial form of venous malformation has been linked to a different locus on chromosome 9p[104].

Clinical features

The glomus tumor is a benign lesion that usually presents in young adults (20–40 years of age) as a small (less than 2 cm), blue–red papule or nodule in the deep dermis or subcutis of the distal upper or lower extremities. They are tender to touch, and may be associated with severe paroxysmal pain in response to temperature changes and pressure. The hand, especially the nail beds and palm, is most commonly affected (Fig. 114.28), but lesions can also occur at other cutaneous locations. Unusual extracutaneous glomus tumors have been reported in the gastrointestinal tract, bone, mediastinum, trachea, mesentery, cervix and vagina. Extremely rare instances of malignant transformation within glomus tumors, with documented metastasis, have been described[105]. Radiographs are of limited usefulness in diagnosis, but in subungual tumors often show bony erosion and may show increased distance between the nail and the dorsum of the phalanx. MRI is frequently the primary diagnostic imaging modality of choice (Fig. 114.29), followed by contrast-enhanced CT. Glomus tumors are strongly enhancing masses by both CT and MRI.

Glomuvenous malformations arise in children and adolescents and tend to be multiple. They are generally asymptomatic lesions covering a large cutaneous area that appear either as multiple, soft, red-to-blue nodules that may be widely distributed or confluent (Figs 114.30 & 114.31), or as pink to deep blue plaque-like lesions, also multifocal. Although they clinically resemble venous malformations, glomuvenous malformations differ in appearance from the latter in a number of aspects, as recently described by Mounayer et al.[106]: they tend to be more nodular or cobblestone-like in appearance, more blue and less compressible, and they do not swell with exercise or dependency. Lesions typically thicken and become more blue in color with time. Although

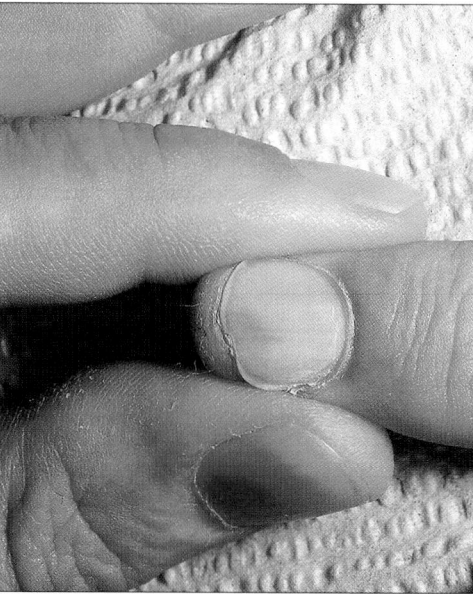

Fig. 114.28 Glomus tumor. The lesion presented with pain and ill-defined subungual erythema. Courtesy of Ronald P Rapini MD.

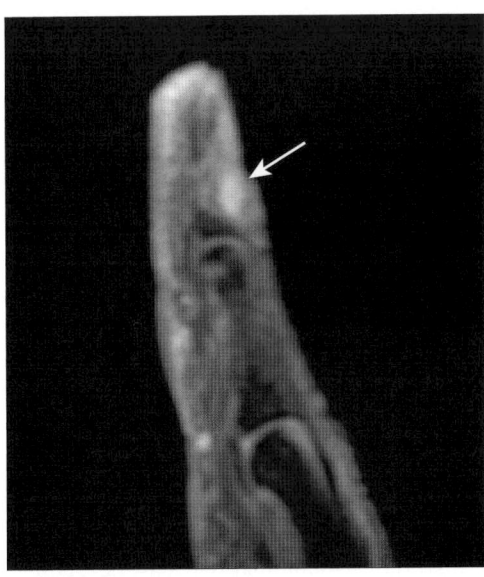

Fig. 114.29 MRI of a glomus tumor located in the proximal portion of the nail bed and matrix. While there was a low signal lesion noted in T1-weighted images of the left index finger, the lesion was very bright in T2-weighted images with diffuse homogeneous enhancement with gadolinium (arrow). Courtesy of Kalman Watsky MD.

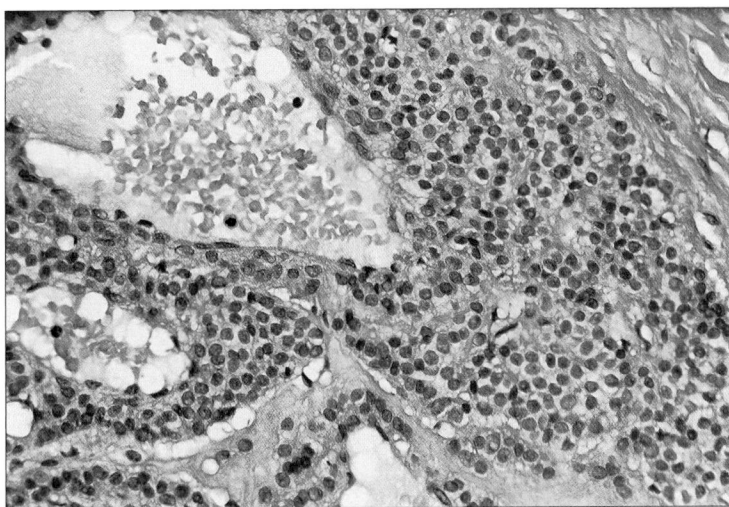

Fig. 114.32 Histology of glomus tumor. Glomus cells are monotonously rounded and sometimes arranged in a single-file manner. Courtesy of Ronald P Rapini MD.

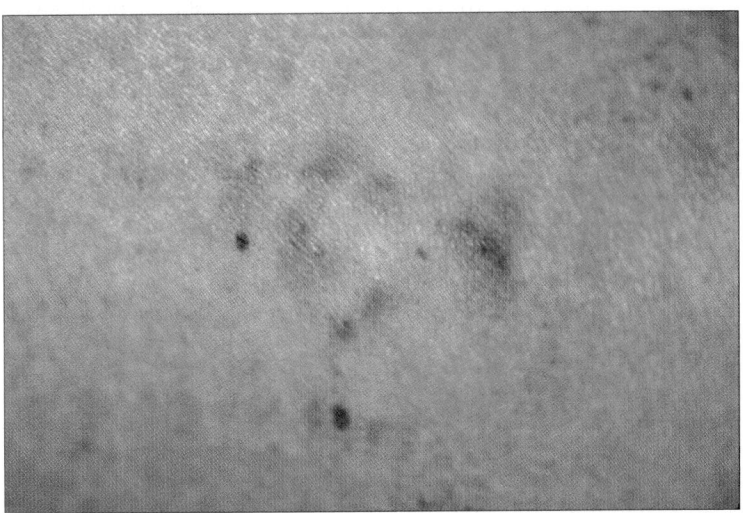

Fig. 114.30 Glomuvenous malformation ('glomangioma'). Note the cluster of slightly compressible blue papules.

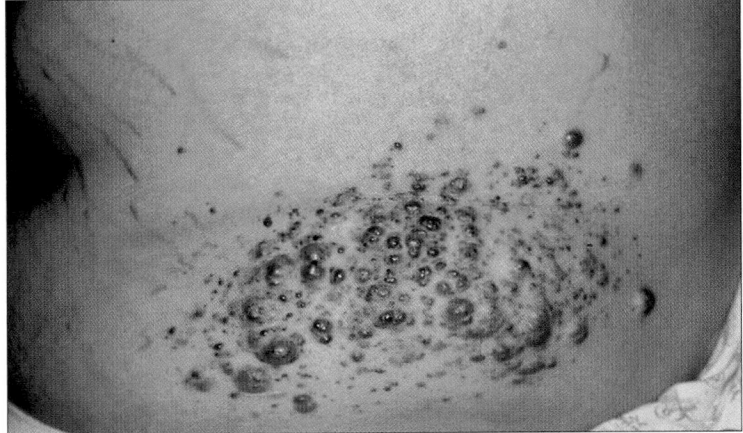

Fig. 114.31 Glomuvenous malformation ('glomangioma'). Large cluster of blue papulonodules becoming confluent centrally.

less painful than the glomus tumor, glomuvenous malformations may be tender to palpation, and attacks of pain may occur in association with menstruation and pregnancy. All reported cases have behaved in a benign fashion.

Pathology

The common glomus tumor is a generally well-circumscribed proliferation of solid sheets and clusters of uniform glomus cells focally clustering around a variable complement of capillary-sized, endothelium-lined vessels (Fig. 114.32). The stroma is typically myxoid or hyalinized and may contain numerous small nerve twigs. A dense fibrous pseudo-capsule may be present. The glomus cells are distinctive in their uniformly rounded or polygonal shape, centrally placed, rounded nuclei, and pale eosinophilic cytoplasm. PAS staining reveals basement membrane material around individual tumor cells. Mitotic figures may be present, but are normally configured. The ultrastructural features of these cells are consistent with modified smooth muscle cells, replete with relatively abundant myofilaments (that focally condense to form dense bodies) and pinocytotic vesicles[107]. Immunohistochemical studies reveal consistent expression of vimentin and muscle actin isoforms, and variably reported expression of desmin. Examples demonstrating gradual transition from rounded glomus cells to elongated, well-differentiated smooth muscle cells have been termed glomangiomyomas[108]. Although the great majority of glomus tumors display no significant cytologic atypia, some have atypical or frankly malignant features. Based on an analysis of 53 atypical and malignant glomus tumors, Folpe et al.[109] have recently proposed a histopathologic classification of glomus tumors with unusual features, with malignant glomus tumors defined as those of large size (>2 cm) and deep location, or those with marked atypia and high mitotic rate (≥5/50 HPF), or those with atypical mitotic figures. Malignant examples show a compressed rim of benign glomus tumor around the malignant areas in about one-half of cases, consistent with malignant transformation from a pre-existing benign tumor.

Glomuvenous malformations consist of large, dilated, thin-walled veins in the dermis and subcutaneous tissue histologically equivalent to those comprising venous malformations, but surrounded by one or more layers of uniform, cuboidal glomus cells (Fig. 114.33). Some microscopic fields may lack the glomus cells and be indistinguishable from common venous malformations. They are less circumscribed than solitary glomus tumors and may be distributed as separate nodules in the same anatomic area. Like venous malformations without glomus cells, many glomuvenous malformations contain organizing thrombi or phleboliths.

Differential diagnosis

Solitary glomus tumors may clinically be confused with other painful nodules (see the Introductory chapter) such as eccrine spiradenomas and leiomyomas that can readily be distinguished from glomus tumors histologically and immunohistochemically. From a histologic point of view, solid forms of hidradenoma may closely resemble glomus tumors, especially when sweat ducts acquire erythrocytes, but can be distinguished by their keratin expression. Cellular glomus tumors are occasionally mistaken for pseudoangiomatous intradermal nevi, but the latter are positive for S100.

Glomuvenous malformations must be distinguished from ordinary venous malformations that lack glomus cells by histologic examination,

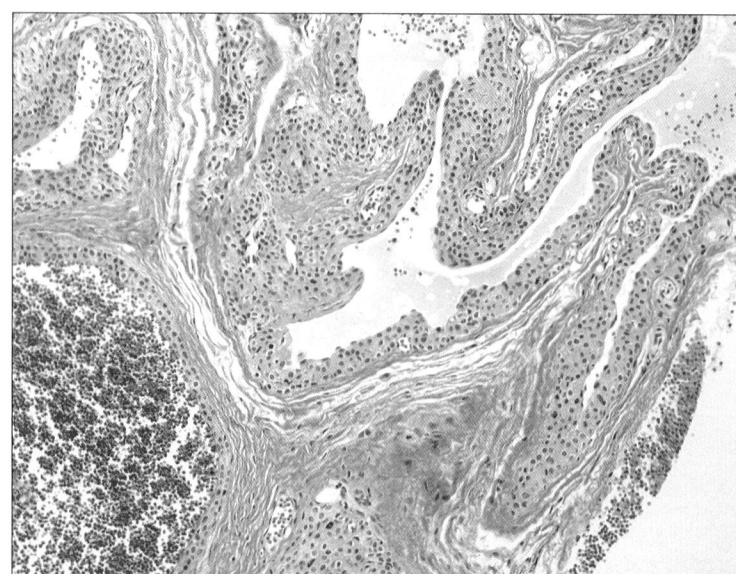

Fig. 114.33 Histology of glomuvenous malformation ('glomangioma'). One or more, often incomplete, layers of glomus cells rim abnormal venous channels that are otherwise histologically consistent with venous malformation.

although several clinical features of these lesions help make this distinction (see section above). It is likely that many cases of the so-called blue rubber bleb nevus syndrome, a familial disorder characterized by multiple venous malformations, actually represent examples of multiple glomuvenous malformations (glomangiomatosis).

Treatment

Solitary glomus tumors can be treated successfully by local surgical excision. Other options include electrodesiccation and sclerotherapy.

Glomuvenous malformations are less amenable to surgery than common glomus tumors, due to their more extensive and multifocal nature. In a recent series of large facial glomangiomas[108], MRI was the best modality for definition of the extent of the lesions and their relationship to other anatomic structures. In this same series, surgical resection reduced the area of discoloration and improved facial contour, while sclerotherapy was less effective than for venous malformations[108]. Laser surgery employing CO_2, argon and pulsed dye lasers may also be helpful. Residual lesions following subtotal resections may slowly re-expand[108].

Infantile Hemangiopericytoma

Synonym: ■ Congenital hemangiopericytoma

Key features

- Benign neoplasm of perivascular myoid differentiation that usually presents at birth or in the first years of life
- Clinical appearance is that of single or multiple dermal and subcutaneous nodules that may be alarmingly large at birth or grow rapidly
- Differs in both histology and clinical behavior from adult-type hemangiopericytoma, which rarely involves the skin
- Multilobulated tumor with cellular areas of spindle cells and antler-like branching blood vessels, merging with less cellular areas containing plump myofibroblasts
- Closely related to infantile myofibromatosis
- Behaves in a benign fashion, despite frequent focal necrosis and increased mitotic activity

Introduction and history

The concept of hemangiopericytoma as an entity has been controversial since these tumors were described in 1942 by Stout & Murray, who considered them to be composed mainly of pericytes. Congenital or infantile hemangiopericytoma was recognized as a separate entity from adult-type hemangiopericytoma in 1976 by Enzinger & Smith[110] in consideration of its distinguishing clinical and histologic features. Classical adult-type hemangiopericytomas will not be discussed here because of their extreme rarity in superficial tissues.

Epidemiology

Infantile hemangiopericytomas are uncommon tumors that typically appear in the first year of life and are usually congenital. There is a male predominance by approximately 2:1. Tumors in older children have occasionally been reported.

Pathogenesis

The frequent zonal pattern of myofibroblastic differentiation in infantile hemangiopericytomas has led to the proposal that infantile hemangiopericytoma and infantile myofibromatosis may lie upon a continuous spectrum of myofibroblastic lesions[111]. A family of adult tumors with perivascular myoid differentiation has recently been described that overlaps in histologic appearance with infantile myofibromatosis and includes two new entities termed *glomangiopericytoma* and *myopericytoma*. Granter et al.[112], in support of similar observations by Requena and colleagues[113], have proposed that this widening spectrum of tumors and their distinctive cellular components might be better explained by derivation from a pluripotent periendothelial cell capable of differentiating along smooth muscle, pericytic and glomus cell lines, rather than from myofibroblasts.

Clinical features

Infantile hemangiopericytomas are nodules that primarily occur in the subcutaneous and dermal tissues of the head and neck. Congenital examples may be alarming in size at birth or grow rapidly thereafter. Multicentric cases have been reported and have in some instances been misinterpreted as examples of distant metastasis. Although benign behavior appears to be the rule, large tumors may be problematic if they hemorrhage or threaten vital structures. Lesions in deeply seated sites, such as the tongue, mediastinum and abdomen, have been reported. Rare multisystemic forms in neonates may be lethal. Local recurrence after excision is common, although spontaneous tumor regression has also been documented.

Pathology

Infantile-type hemangiopericytomas, unlike the adult type, are usually dermal or subcutaneous in location and are often multilobulated. They typically show a biphasic growth pattern in which primitive hemangiopericytomatous areas resembling the adult tumors (short spindle cells arranged around thin-walled, branching vessels) blend with less cellular areas containing plump, myofibroblast-like cells set within a collagenous matrix. Focal necrosis and significant mitotic activity may be present, but are not indicative of poor prognosis.

Differential diagnosis

Infantile hemangiopericytomas demonstrate non-specific clinical and radiologic features and require histologic examination for definitive diagnosis. They may be confused clinically with infantile hemangiomas owing to rapid postnatal growth, and large congenital lesions may suggest rapidly involuting congenital hemangioma or infantile fibrosarcoma. Further diagnostic considerations include infantile myofibromatosis and subcutaneous pyogenic granuloma.

Treatment

Conservative treatment following establishment of the diagnosis of infantile hemangiopericytoma by biopsy is generally recommended, given the potential for spontaneous regression. Complete surgical resection is a good option in some cases, although there appears to be a conflicting tendency of these tumors to both locally recur and spontaneously regress.

REFERENCES

1. Ackerman AB. Resolving Quandaries in Dermatology, Pathology, and Dermatopathology. New York: Ardor Scribendi, 2001.
2. Boye E, Yu Y, Paranya G, et al. Clonality and altered behavior of endothelial cells from hemangiomas. J Clin Invest. 2001;107:745–52.
3. Walter JW, North PE, Waner M, et al. Somatic mutation of vascular endothelial growth factor receptors in juvenile hemangioma. Genes Chromosomes Cancer. 2002;33:295–303.
4. Kuo T, Sayers CP, Rosai J. Masson's "vegetant intravascular hemangioendothelioma:" a lesion often mistaken for angiosarcoma: study of seventeen cases located in the skin and soft tissues. Cancer. 1976;38:1227–36.
5. Kuo T, Gomez LG. Papillary endothelial proliferation in cystic lymphangiomas. A lymphatic vessel counterpart of Masson's vegetant intravascular hemangioendothelioma. Arch Pathol Lab Med. 1979;103:306–8.
6. Pins MR, Rosenthal DI, Springfield DS, Rosenberg AE. Florid extravascular papillary endothelial hyperplasia (Masson's pseudoangiosarcoma) presenting as a soft-tissue sarcoma. Arch Pathol Lab Med. 1993;117:259–63.
7. Weiss SW, Goldblum JR. Enzinger and Weiss's Soft Tissue Tumors, 4th edn. St. Louis: Mosby, 2001.
8. Pasyk K, Depowski M. Proliferating systematized angioendotheliomatosis of a 5-month-old infant. Arch Dermatol. 1978;114:1512–15.
9. Chan JK, Fletcher CD, Hicklin GA, Rosai J. Glomeruloid hemangioma. A distinctive cutaneous lesion of multicentric Castleman's disease associated with POEMS syndrome. Am J Surg Pathol. 1990; 14:1036–46.
10. Requena L, Sangueza OP. Cutaneous vascular proliferation. Part II. Hyperplasias and benign neoplasms. J Am Acad Dermatol. 1997;37:887–919; quiz 920–2.
11. Hunt SJ, Santa Cruz DJ, Barr RJ. Microvenular hemangioma. J Cutan Pathol. 1991;18:235–40.
12. Allen PW, Ramakrishna B, MacCormac LB. The histiocytoid hemangiomas and other controversies. Pathol Ann. 1992;27:51–87.
13. Wells GC, Whimster IW. Subcutaneous angiolymphoid hyperplasia with eosinophilia. Br J Dermatol. 1969;81:1–14.
14. Googe PB, Harris NL, Mihm MC Jr. Kimura's disease and angiolymphoid hyperplasia with eosinophilia: two distinct histopathological entities. J Cutan Pathol. 1987;14:263–71.
15. Olsen TG, Helwig EB. Angiolymphoid hyperplasia with eosinophilia. A clinicopathologic study of 116 patients. J Am Acad Dermatol. 1985;12:781–96.
16. Hobbs ER, Bailin PL, Ratz JL, Yarbrough CL. Treatment of angiolymphoid hyperplasia of the external ear with carbon dioxide laser. J Am Acad Dermatol. 1988;19:345–9.
17. Weiss SW, Enzinger FM. Spindle cell hemangioendothelioma. A low-grade angiosarcoma resembling a cavernous hemangioma and Kaposi's sarcoma. Am J Surg Pathol. 1986;10:521–30.
18. Perkins P, Weiss SW. Spindle cell hemangioendothelioma. An analysis of 78 cases with reassessment of its pathogenesis and biologic behavior. Am J Surg Pathol. 1996;20:1196–204.
19. Fletcher CD, Beham A, Schmid C. Spindle cell haemangioendothelioma: a clinicopathological and immunohistochemical study indicative of a non-neoplastic lesion. Histopathology. 1991;18:291–301.
20. Imayama S, Murakamai Y, Hashimoto H, Hori Y. Spindle cell hemangioendothelioma exhibits the ultrastructural features of reactive vascular proliferation rather than of angiosarcoma. Am J Clin Pathol. 1992;97:279–87.
21. Battocchio S, Facchetti F, Brisigotti M. Spindle cell haemangioendothelioma: further evidence against its proposed neoplastic nature. Histopathology. 1993;22:296–8.
22. Setoyama M, Shimada H, Miyazono N, et al. Spindle cell hemangioendothelioma: successful treatment with recombinant interleukin-2. Br J Dermatol. 2000;142:1238–9.
23. Hartzell MB. Granuloma pyogenicum (botryomycosis of French authors). J Cutan Dis. 1904;22:520–3.
24. Katta R, Bickle K, Hwang L. Pyogenic granuloma arising in port-wine stain during pregnancy. Br J Dermatol. 2001;144:644–5.
25. Kerr DA. Granuloma pyogenicum. Oral Surg Oral Med Oral Pathol. 1951;4:158.
26. Warner J, Jones EW. Pyogenic granuloma recurring with multiple satellites. A report of 11 cases. Br J Dermatol. 1968;80:218–27.
27. Wilson BB, Greer KE, Cooper PH. Eruptive disseminated lobular capillary hemangioma (pyogenic granuloma). J Am Acad Dermatol. 1989;21:391–4.
28. Campbell JP, Grekin RC, Ellis CN, et al. Retinoid therapy is associated with excess granulation tissue responses. J Am Acad Dermatol. 1983;9:708–13.
29. Tay YK, Weston WL, Morelli JG. Treatment of pyogenic granuloma in children with the flashlamp-pumped pulsed dye laser. Pediatrics. 1997;99:368–70.
30. Matsumoto K, Nakanishi H, Seike T, et al. Treatment of pyogenic granuloma with a sclerosing agent. Dermatol Surg. 2001;27:521–3.
31. Calonje E, Fletcher CD. Sinusoidal hemangioma. A distinctive benign vascular neoplasm within the group of cavernous hemangiomas. Am J Surg Pathol. 1991;15:1130–5.
32. Calonje E, Fletcher CD, Wilson-Jones E, Rosai J. Retiform hemangioendothelioma. A distinctive form of low-grade angiosarcoma delineated in a series of 15 cases. Am J Surg Pathol. 1994;18:115–25.
33. Guillou L, Calonje E, Speight P, et al. Hobnail hemangioma: a pseudomalignant vascular lesion with a reappraisal of targetoid hemosiderotic hemangioma. Am J Surg Pathol. 1999;23:97–105.
34. Mentzel T, Partanen TA, Kutzner H. Hobnail hemangioma ('targetoid hemosiderotic hemangioma'): clinicopathologic and immunohistochemical analysis of 62 cases. J Cutan Pathol. 1999;26:279–86.
35. Wilson-Jones E, Orkin M. Tufted angioma (angioblastoma). A benign progressive angioma, not to be confused with Kaposi's sarcoma or low-grade angiosarcoma. J Am Acad Dermatol. 1989;20:214–25.
36. Nakagawa K. Case report of angioblastoma of the skin. Nippon Hifuka Gakkai Zasshi. 1949;59:92–4.
37. Macmillan A, Champion RH. Progressive capillary haemangioma. Br J Dermatol. 1971;85:492–3.
38. Enjolras O, Wassef M, Mazoyer E, et al. Infants with Kasabach-Merritt syndrome do not have 'true' hemangiomas. J Pediatr. 1997;130:631–40.
39. Hebeda CL, Scheffer E, Starink TM. Tufted angioma of late onset. Histopathology. 1993;23:191–3.
40. Heagerty AH, Rubin A, Robinson TW. Familial tufted angioma. Clin Exp Dermatol. 1992;17:344–5.
41. Zukerberg LR, Nickoloff BJ, Weiss SW. Kaposiform hemangioendothelioma of infancy and childhood. An aggressive neoplasm associated with Kasabach-Merritt syndrome and lymphangiomatosis. Am J Surg Pathol. 1993;17:321–8.
42. Sarkar M, Mulliken JB, Kozakewich HP, et al. Thrombocytopenic coagulopathy (Kasabach-Merritt phenomenon) is associated with Kaposiform hemangioendothelioma and not with common infantile hemangioma. Plast Reconstr Surg. 1997;100:1377–86.
43. Lam WY, Mac-Moune Lai F, Look CN, et al. Tufted angioma with complete regression. J Cutan Pathol. 1994;21:461–6.
44. Leaute-Labreze C, Bioulac-Sage P, Labbe L, et al. Tufted angioma associated with platelet trapping syndrome: response to aspirin. Arch Dermatol. 1997;133:1077–9.
45. North PE, Waner M, Mizeracki A, et al. A unique microvascular phenotype shared by juvenile hemangiomas and human placenta. Arch Dermatol. 2001;137:559–70.
46. Seo SK, Suh JC, Na GY, et al. Kasabach-Merritt syndrome: identification of platelet trapping in a tufted angioma by immunohistochemistry technique using monoclonal antibody to CD61. Pediatr Dermatol. 1999;16:392–4.
47. Suarez SM, Pensler JM, Paller AS. Response of deep tufted angioma to interferon alfa. J Am Acad Dermatol. 1995;33:124–6.
48. Munn SE, Jackson JE, Jones RR. Tufted haemangioma responding to high-dose systemic steroids: a case report and review of the literature. Clin Exp Dermatol. 1994;19:511–14.
49. North PE, Kahn T, Cordisco MR, et al. Multifocal lymphangioendotheliomatosis with thrombocytopenia: a newly recognized clinicopathological entity. Arch Dermatol. 2004;140:599–606.
50. Prasad V, Fishman SJ, Mulliken JB, et al. Cutaneovisceral angiomatosis with thrombocytopenia. Pediatr Dev Pathol. 2005;8:407–19.
51. Niedt GW, Greco MA, Wieczorek R, et al. Hemangioma with Kaposi's sarcoma-like features: report of two cases. Pediatr Pathol. 1989;9:567–75.
52. Tsang WY, Chan JK. Kaposi-like infantile hemangioendothelioma. A distinctive vascular neoplasm of the retroperitoneum. Am J Surg Pathol. 1991;15:982–9.
53. Mentzel T, Mazzoleni G, Dei Tos AP, Fletcher CD. Kaposiform hemangioendothelioma in adults. Clinicopathologic and immunohistochemical analysis of three cases. Am J Clin Pathol. 1997;108:450–5.
54. Folpe AL, Veikkola T, Valtola R, Weiss SW. Vascular endothelial growth factor receptor-3 (VEGFR-3): a marker of vascular tumors with presumed lymphatic differentiation, including Kaposi's sarcoma, kaposiform and Dabska-type hemangioendotheliomas, and a subset of angiosarcomas. Mod Pathol. 2000;13:180–5.
55. Vin-Christian K, McCalmont TH, Frieden IJ. Kaposiform hemangioendothelioma. An aggressive, locally invasive vascular tumor that can mimic hemangioma of infancy. Arch Dermatol. 1997;133:1573–8.
56. Phillips WG, Marsden JR. Kasabach-Merritt syndrome exacerbated by platelet transfusion. J R Soc Med. 1993;86:231–2.
57. Lai FM, Allen PW, Yuen PM, Leung PC. Locally metastasizing vascular tumor. Spindle cell, epithelioid, or unclassified hemangioendothelioma? Am J Clin Pathol. 1991;96:660–3.
58. North PE, Waner M, Mizeracki A, Mihm MC Jr. GLUT1: a newly discovered immunohistochemical marker for juvenile hemangioma. Hum Pathol. 2000;31:11–22.
59. Deb G, Jenkner A, De Sio L, et al. Spindle cell (Kaposiform) hemangioendothelioma with Kasabach-Merritt syndrome in an infant: successful treatment with alpha-2A interferon. Med Pediatr Oncol. 1997;28:358–61.
60. Enjolras O, Wassef M, Dosquet C, et al. Kasabach-Merritt syndrome on a congenital tufted angioma. Ann Dermatol Venereol. 1998;125:257–60.
61. Blei F, Karp N, Rofsky N, et al. Successful multimodal therapy for kaposiform hemangioendothelioma complicated by Kasabach-Merritt phenomenon: case report and review of the literature. Pediatr Hematol Oncol. 1998;15:295–305.
62. Hu B, Lachman R, Phillips J, et al. Kasabach-Merritt syndrome-associated kaposiform hemangioendothelioma successfully treated with cyclophosphamide, vincristine, and actinomycin D. J Pediatr Hematol Oncol. 1998;20:567–9.
63. Argani P, Athanasian E. Malignant endovascular papillary angioendothelioma (Dabska tumor) arising within a deep intramuscular hemangioma. Arch Pathol Lab Med. 1997;121:992–5.
64. Fanburg-Smith JC, Michal M, Partanen TA, et al. Papillary intralymphatic angioendothelioma (PILA): a report of twelve cases of a distinctive vascular tumor with phenotypic features of lymphatic vessels. Am J Surg Pathol. 1999;23:1004–10.
65. Mentzel T, Beham A, Calonje E, et al. Epithelioid hemangioendothelioma of skin and soft tissues: clinicopathologic and immunohistochemical study of 30 cases. Am J Surg Pathol. 1997;21:363–74.
66. Quante M, Patel NK, Hill S, et al. Epithelioid hemangioendothelioma presenting in the skin: a clinicopathologic study of eight cases. Am J Dermatopathol. 1998;20:541–6.
67. Mendlick MR, Nelson M, Pickering D, et al. Translocation t(1;3)(p36.3;q25) is a nonrandom aberration in epithelioid hemangioendothelioma. Am J Surg Pathol. 2001;25:684–7.
68. Weiss SW, Ishak KG, Dail DH, et al. Epithelioid hemangioendothelioma and related lesions. Semin Diagn Pathol. 1986;3:259–87.
69. Rappersberger K, Tschachler E, Zonzits E, et al. Endemic Kaposi's sarcoma in human immunodeficiency virus type 1-seronegative persons: demonstration of retrovirus-like particles in cutaneous lesions. J Invest Dermatol. 1990;95:371-81.
70. Friedman-Birnbaum R, Weltfriend S, Katz I. Kaposi's sarcoma: retrospective study of 67 cases with the classical form. Dermatologica. 1990;180:13–17.
71. Bluefarb SM. Kaposi's Sarcoma. Springfield, IL: Charles C Thomas, 1966.
72. Rogers MF, Thomas PA, Starcher ET, et al. Acquired immunodeficiency syndrome in children: report of

the Centers for Disease Control National Surveillance, 1982 to 1985. Pediatrics. 1987;79:1008–14.

73. Jussila L, Valtola R, Partanen TA, et al. Lymphatic endothelium and Kaposi's sarcoma spindle cells detected by antibodies against the vascular endothelial growth factor receptor-3. Cancer Res. 1998;58:1599–604.

74. Weninger W, Partanen TA, Breiteneder-Geleff S, et al. Expression of vascular endothelial growth factor receptor-3 and podoplanin suggests a lymphatic endothelial cell origin of Kaposi's sarcoma tumor cells. Lab Invest. 1999;79:243–51.\

74a. Wang H-W, Trotter MWB, Lagos D, et al. Kaposi sarcoma herpesvirus-induced cellular reprogramming contributes to the lymphatic gene expression in Kaposi sarcoma. Nat Genet. 2004;36:687–93.

75. Rabkin CS, Janz S, Lash A, et al. Monoclonal origin of multicentric Kaposi's sarcoma lesions. N Engl J Med. 1997;336:988–93.

76. Gill PS, Tsai YC, Rao AP, et al. Evidence for multiclonality in multicentric Kaposi's sarcoma. Proc Natl Acad Sci USA. 1998;95:8257–61.

77. Weiss RA, Whitby D, Talbot S, et al. Human herpesvirus type 8 and Kaposi's sarcoma. J Natl Cancer Inst Monogr. 1998;(23):51–4.

78. Moore PS, Chang Y. Kaposi's sarcoma-associated herpesvirus-encoded oncogenes and oncogenesis. J Natl Cancer Inst Monogr. 1998;(23):65–71.

79. Sciacca FL, Sturzl M, Bussolino F, et al. Expression of adhesion molecules, platelet-activating factor, and chemokines by Kaposi's sarcoma cells. J Immunol. 1994;153:4816–25.

80. Masood R, Cai J, Tulpule A, et al. Interleukin 8 is an autocrine growth factor and a surrogate marker for Kaposi's sarcoma. Clin Cancer Res. 2001;7:2693–702.

81. Tappero JW, Conant MA, Wolfe SF, Berger TG. Kaposi's sarcoma. Epidemiology, pathogenesis, histology, clinical spectrum, staging criteria and therapy. J Am Acad Dermatol. 1993;28:371–95.

81a. Hammock L, Reisenauer A, Wang W, et al. Latency-associated nuclear antigen expression and human herpesvirus-8 polymerase chain reaction in the evaluation of Kaposi sarcoma and other vascular tumors in HIV-positive patients. Mod Pathol. 2005;18:463–8.

81b. Dupin N, Fisher C, Kellam P, et al. Distribution of human herpesvirus-8 latently infected cells in Kaposi's sarcoma, multicentric Castleman's disease, and primary effusion lymphoma. Proc Natl Acad Sci USA 1999;96:4546–51.

82. Antman K, Chang Y. Kaposi's sarcoma. N Engl J Med. 2000;342:1027–38.

83. Krown SE. Acquired immunodeficiency syndrome-associated Kaposi's sarcoma. Biology and management. Med Clin North Am. 1997;81:471–94.

84. Gascon P, Schwartz RA. Kaposi's sarcoma. New treatment modalities. Dermatol Clin. 2000;18:169–75.

85. Vanni T, Sprinz E, Machado MW, et al. Systemic treatment of AIDS-related Kaposi sarcoma: current status and perspectives. Cancer Treatment Rev. 2006;32:445–55.

86. Di Lorenzo G, Konstantinopoulos PA, Pantanowitz L, et al. Management of AIDS-related Kaposi's sarcoma. Lancet Oncol. 2007;8:167–76.

87. Qunibi WY, Barri Y, Alfurayh O, et al. Kaposi's sarcoma in renal transplant recipients: a report on 26 cases from a single institution. Transplant Proc. 1993;25:1402–5.

88. Stewart FW, Treves N. Lymphangiosarcoma in postmastectomy lymphedema. Cancer. 1948;1:64–81.

89. Wilson-Jones E. Malignant angioendothelioma of the skin. Br J Dermatol. 1964;76:21–39.

90. Holden CA, Spittle MF, Jones EW. Angiosarcoma of the face and scalp, prognosis and treatment. Cancer. 1987;59:1046–57.

91. Cafiero F, Gipponi M, Peressini A, et al. Radiation-associated angiosarcoma: diagnostic and therapeutic implications – two case reports and a review of the literature. Cancer. 1996;77:2496–502.

92. Marchal C, Weber B, de Lafontan B, et al. Nine breast angiosarcomas after conservative treatment for breast carcinoma: a survey from French comprehensive Cancer Centers. Int J Radiat Oncol Biol Phys.1999;44:113–19.

93. Brown RW, Tornos C, Evans HL. Angiosarcoma arising from malignant schwannoma in a patient with neurofibromatosis. Cancer. 1992;70:1141–4.

94. Bessis D, Sotto A, Roubert P, et al. Endothelin-secreting angiosarcoma occurring at the site of an arteriovenous fistula for haemodialysis in a renal transplant recipient. Br J Dermatol. 1998;138:361–3.

95. Jennings TA, Peterson L, Axiotis CA, et al. Angiosarcoma associated with foreign body material. A report of three cases. Cancer. 1988;62:2436–44.

96. Leake J, Sheehan MP, Rampling D, et al. Angiosarcoma complicating xeroderma pigmentosum. Histopathology. 1992;21:179–81.

97. Dunkel IJ, Gerald WL, Rosenfield NS, et al. Outcome of patients with a history of bilateral retinoblastoma treated for a second malignancy: the Memorial Sloan-Kettering experience. Med Pediatr Oncol. 1998;30:59–62.

98. Gray MH, Rosenberg AE, Dickersin GR, Bhan AK. Cytokeratin expression in epithelioid vascular neoplasms. Hum Pathol. 1990;21:212–17.

99. Meis-Kindblom JM, Kindblom LG. Angiosarcoma of soft tissue: a study of 80 cases. Am J Surg Pathol. 1998;22:683–97.

99a. Saroha S, Litwin S, von Mehren M. Retrospective review of treatment for angiosarcoma at Fox Chase Cancer Center over the past 15 years. J Clin Oncol . 2007;25(18S):10034.

100. Rycroft RJ, Menter MA, Sharvill DE, et al. Hereditary multiple glomus tumours. Report of four families and a review of literature. Trans St Johns Hosp Dermatol Soc. 1975;61:70–81.

101. Wood WS, Dimmick JE. Multiple infiltrating glomus tumors in children. Cancer. 1977;40:1680–5.

102. Irrthum A, Brouillard P, Enjolras O, et al. Linkage disequilibrium narrows locus for venous malformation with glomus cells (VMGLOM) to a single 1.48 Mbp YAC. Eur J Hum Genet. 2001;9:34–8.

103. Brouillard P, Boon LM, Mulliken JB, et al. Mutations in a novel factor, glomulin, are responsible for glomuvenous malformations ("glomangiomas"). Am J Hum Genet. 2002;70:866–74.

104. Gallione CJ, Pasyk KA, Boon LM, et al. A gene for familial venous malformations maps to chromosome 9p in a second large kindred. J Med Genet. 1995;32:197–9.

105. Brathwaite CD, Poppiti RJ Jr. Malignant glomus tumor. A case report of widespread metastases in a patient with multiple glomus body hamartomas. Am J Surg Pathol. 1996;20:233–8.

106. Mounayer C, Wassef M, Enjolras O, Boukobza M, Mulliken JB. Facial 'glomangiomas': large facial venous malformations with glomus cells. J Am Acad Dermatol. 2001;45:239–45.

107. Gould EW, Manivel JC, Albores-Saavedra J, Monforte H. Locally infiltrative glomus tumors and glomangiosarcomas. A clinical, ultrastructural, and immunohistochemical study. Cancer. 1990;65:310–18.

108. Yang JS, Ko JW, Suh KS, Kim ST. Congenital multiple plaque-like glomangiomyoma. Am J Dermatopathol. 1999;21:454–7.

109. Folpe AL, Fanburg-Smith JC, Miettinen M, Weiss SW. Atypical and malignant glomus tumors: analysis of 52 cases, with a proposal for the reclassification of glomus tumors. Am J Surg Pathol. 2001;25:1–12.

110. Enzinger FM, Smith BH. Hemangiopericytoma. An analysis of 106 cases. Hum Pathol. 1976;7:61–82.

111. Mentzel T, Calonje E, Nascimento AG, Fletcher CD. Infantile hemangiopericytoma versus infantile myofibromatosis. Study of a series suggesting a continuous spectrum of infantile myofibroblastic lesions. Am J Surg Pathol. 1994;18:922–30.

112. Granter SR, Badizadegan K, Fletcher CD. Myofibromatosis in adults, glomangiopericytoma, and myopericytoma: a spectrum of tumors showing perivascular myoid differentiation. Am J Surg Pathol. 1998;22:513–25.

113. Requena L, Kutzner H, Hugel H, et al. Cutaneous adult myofibroma: a vascular neoplasm. J Cutan Pathol. 1996;23:445–57.

Neural and Neuroendocrine Neoplasms (Other than Neurofibromatosis)

Zsolt B Argenyi

Chapter Contents

For decades, neural tumors were often misdiagnosed histopathologically because of confusing classifications; as a result, their clinical relevance was poorly understood. Clinically, cutaneous neural tumors often look alike and most of them are benign. However, their correct diagnosis can be helpful in recognizing important clinical syndromes and can contribute to better patient management. Moreover, with the advancement of immunohistochemistry, new variants of cutaneous neural neoplasms have been described[1].

CLASSIFICATION, TERMINOLOGY AND HISTOGENESIS

Cutaneous neural tumors can be classified into two major groups: those derived from peripheral nerves and those derived from ectopic or heterotopic neural tissue (Table 115.1). The former group is often subdivided into true nerve sheath neoplasms and hamartomatous tumors, although this classification may not be universally accepted[2].

Cutaneous neural tumors either arise from or differentiate toward one or more elements of the nervous system. During their differentiation, neural neoplasms often recapitulate to varying degrees the morphogenesis of normal peripheral nerves. Therefore, knowledge of the organization of the normal peripheral nerve is crucial to understanding the histogenesis of tumors that arise from it[3]. The peripheral nerve can be compared to a conventional telephone cable, in which each axon and its surrounding Schwann cell layer correspond to a telephone wire and its insulation, respectively (Fig. 115.1).

The basic units of a peripheral nerve are nerve fibers, composed of axons and the surrounding Schwann cells. These fibers form nerve fascicles and are held together by a sheath of specialized cells, which is called the perineurium. The space between the individual nerve fibers is called the endoneurium. As in a telephone cable system where the smaller cable units are separated, protected and held together by an outer wrapping, bundles of nerve fascicles are also encased in a supportive fibrous sheath that is called the epineurium. To variable extent,

CLASSIFICATION OF CUTANEOUS NEURAL TUMORS

Peripheral nerve sheath tumors	Neural heterotopias
Hamartomas	**Meningothelial**
• Neuromas	• Meningocele
• Traumatic	• Rudimentary meningocele
• Spontaneous	• Meningioma
• Solitary, encapsulated	**Neuroglial**
• Multiple, non-encapsulated	• Nasal glioma
• Variants	**Neuroblastic/ganglionic**
• Neurofibromas	• Metastatic neuroblastoma
• Superficial, solitary	• Primary primitive neuroectodermal
• Deep	tumor
• Diffuse	• Ganglioneuroma
• Pigmented	**Miscellaneous**
• Plexiform	• Pigmented neuroectodermal tumor
• Variants	of infancy
True nerve sheath neoplasms	
• Schwannomas	
• Common, solitary	
• Ancient	
• Cellular	
• Plexiform	
• Variants	
• Malignant peripheral nerve sheath tumor	
Miscellaneous	
• Nerve sheath myxoma/ neurothekeoma	
• Classic	
• Cellular	
• Granular cell tumor	
• Neuroendocrine carcinoma of the skin (Merkel cell carcinoma)	
• Perineurioma	

Table 115.1 Classification of cutaneous neural tumors.

this architectural arrangement is recognizable in many cutaneous neural neoplasms.

The most important constituent cells are the Schwann cell, the perineurial cell, and the various non-specific mesenchymal cells, such as fibroblasts and mast cells. These cells are capable of proliferation and malignant transformation. Other elements of the peripheral nerve, which are cell parts or products (i.e. axons and myelin), cannot duplicate. Schwann cells are derived from the neural crest, and there is evidence that perineurial cells are modified fibroblasts of mesodermal origin. This difference in histogenesis is also reflected in the distinct antigenic expression of these cells. Schwann cells express S100 protein but not epithelial membrane antigen, whereas perineurial cells stain for epithelial membrane antigen but not for S100 protein. Axons contain a specific type of intermediate filament called neurofilament, and myelinated axons contain myelin basic protein, both of which can be detected by immunohistochemistry. These and other immunohistochemical markers often can help to establish the correct diagnosis.

In the following sections, each clinically relevant neural neoplasm is discussed (Tables 115.2–115.4; Fig. 115.2).

THE STRUCTURE OF THE PERIPHERAL NERVE

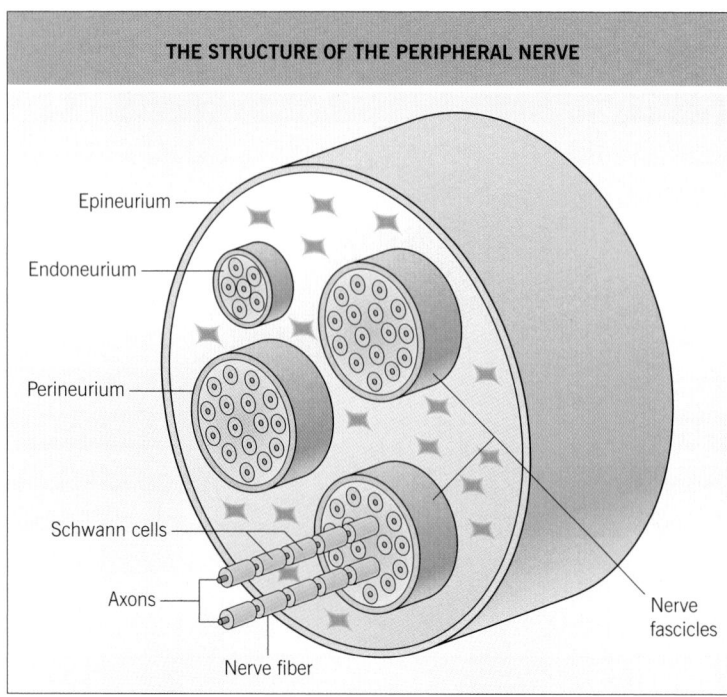

Epineurium

Endoneurium

Perineurium

Schwann cells

Axons

Nerve fiber

Nerve fascicles

Fig. 115.1 The structure and components of the peripheral nerve.

NEUROMAS

Key features

Traumatic neuroma
- At the site of previous trauma
- Skin-colored papules or nodules
- Often painful or sensitive
- Circumscribed, but not encapsulated
- Regenerative proliferation of axons and Schwann cells with fibrous tissue

Palisaded encapsulated neuroma
- Usually on the face of adults
- Solitary
- Skin-colored papule or nodule
- Circumscribed, partly or completely encapsulated
- Compactly arranged fascicles of spindle cells with vague palisading of nuclei

	CLINICAL FEATURES OF BENIGN NEURAL NEOPLASMS						
	Traumatic neuroma	Palisaded encapsulated neuroma	Schwannoma (neurilemmoma)	Neurofibroma	Nerve sheath myxoma	Cellular neurothekeoma	Granular cell tumor
Incidence	Uncommon	Rare	Uncommon	Very common	Rare	Rare	Rare
Age	Any	Adults (mean age, 45.5 years)	Adults (20–50 years)	Adults (20–60 years)	Adults (mean age, 48 years)	Early adulthood (mean age, 24 years)	Adults (30–50 years)
Gender	Any	M:F = 1:1	F > M	M:F = 1:1	M:F = 1:2	F > M	M:F =1:3
Number	Usually solitary	Usually solitary	Usually solitary	Usually solitary	Usually solitary	Usually solitary	Usually solitary
Location	At sites of trauma, surgical scars, amputations	90% face, 10% elsewhere	Flexor aspects of extremities, head	Trunk, head (solitary type)	Head and upper extremities	Predominantly on head, but also anywhere	30% tongue, 70% elsewhere, mainly head and neck
Size	0.5–2.0 cm	0.2–0.6 cm	0.3–3.0 cm	0.2–2.0 cm	0.5–1.0 cm	0.5–3.0 cm	0.5–3.0 cm
Clinical appearance	Skin-colored, firm papules or nodules	Skin-colored or pink, rubbery, firm papules or nodules	Soft, pink or yellow, smooth-surfaced nodules or tumors	Skin-colored, soft or rubbery papules or nodules, sometimes pedunculated	Soft, skin-colored papules and nodules	Pink, red or brown firm papules and nodules	Skin-colored or brownish red, raised, firm nodules; may have ulceration and verrucous surface
Symptoms	Variable, tingling, itching, lancinating pain	Asymptomatic	Asymptomatic; rarely painful, tender or paresthetic; occasionally freely movable	Asymptomatic; 'buttonhole' sign may be present	Asymptomatic	Usually asymptomatic, rarely sore or itchy	Asymptomatic or occasionally tender or pruritic
Association	NA	Multiple mucosal neuromas are seen in MEN 2B	Rarely with neurofibromatosis (primarily type 2) or CNS tumors	If multiple, may be sign of one of the various forms of neurofibromatosis (see Ch. 60)	NA	NA	10% multiple; predilection for blacks; rare in children
Clinical differential diagnosis	Hypertrophic scar, dermatofibroma, granuloma	Dermal melanocytic nevi, basal cell carcinoma, neurofibroma	Lipoma, angiolipoma, adnexal tumors, dermoid or pilar cysts, leiomyoma, ganglion cyst	Dermal nevi, neuroma, soft fibroma, dermatofibroma	Myxoid cysts, ganglion cyst, dermal melanocytic nevi, fibrolipoma	Dermatofibroma, keloid, hemangioma, dermal melanocytic nevi	Dermatofibroma, neurofibroma, adnexal tumor, compound melanocytic nevi
Other	'Rudimentary supernumerary digit' is considered as variant	May be induced by minor trauma	May be multiple; 'schwannomatosis'	Plexiform variant is pathognomonic for neuro-fibromatosis type 1			Visceral forms occur; malignant transformation may occur (3%)

Table 115.2 Clinical features of benign neural neoplasms. NA, not applicable; MEN 2B, multiple endocrine neoplasia, type 2B.

HISTOLOGIC DIFFERENTIAL DIAGNOSTIC FEATURES OF COMMON CUTANEOUS NEURAL NEOPLASMS				
	Traumatic neuroma	**Palisaded encapsulated neuroma**	**Schwannoma**	**Neurofibroma**
Location in the skin	Any level of dermis or subcutis	Upper or mid dermis	Deep dermis or subcutis	Any location in the dermis
Growth pattern	Usually well circumscribed but may be irregular at the distal end	Well circumscribed, nodular, rarely plexiform	Well circumscribed, nodular or ovoid	Poorly to well circumscribed
Encapsulation	Usually encased by fibrous sheath	Yes, by perineurium	Yes, by perineurium	Not encapsulated in the dermis
Architecture	Chaotic, poorly organized tangle of fascicles of various sizes and shapes	Compactly arranged fascicles; frequent clefts between fascicles	Hypercellular areas (Antoni-A), fascicles in various patterns, hypocellular areas (Antoni-B), edematous, myxoid	Fine fibrillary lattice of haphazardly arranged spindle cells in variably dense matrix
Constituent cell types	Schwann cells, fibroblasts, perineurial cells, inflammatory cells, macrophages	Schwann cells (99%), perineurial cells (in capsule only)	Schwann cells (99%), perineurial cells (in capsule only)	Schwann cells, perineurial cells, fibroblasts, mast cells
Cytologic features	Spindle cells with indistinct cytoplasmic membrane and tapered slender nuclei	Spindle cells with indistinct cytoplasmic membrane and tapered slender nuclei	Spindle cells with indistinct cytoplasmic membrane and slender nuclei	Spindle cells with slender nuclei, plump fibroblasts
Nuclear palisading	None	Usually present, but indistinct	Yes, prominent in Antoni-A areas	Rarely
Verocay bodies	None	None	Often	None
Nerve fibers (axons)	Yes, abundant irregular pattern	Yes, abundant often in parallel arrangement	None or only at the site of the connecting nerve	Yes, rare, scattered
Other important features	Nerve of origin frequently present, extensive fibrosis	Nerve of origin frequently present, no fibrosis	Mast cells; may have extensive degenerative changes (hyalinization, hemorrhage, etc.) in Antoni-B areas ('ancient changes')	Variable fibrosis and myxoid changes, occasional blood vessels, mast cells
Histopathologic differential diagnosis	Hypertrophic scar, neurofibroma, schwannoma	Traumatic neuroma, schwannoma, angioleiomyoma, myofibroma	Palisaded encapsulated neuroma, angiomyoma, fibrous histiocytoma	Dermatofibroma, hypertrophic scar, dermatofibrosarcoma protuberans, traumatic neuroma, neural nevus

Table 115.3 Histologic differential diagnostic features of common cutaneous neural neoplasms.

TUMORS AND TUMOR-LIKE CONDITIONS OF ECTOPIC AND HETEROTOPIC NEURAL TISSUE INVOLVING THE SKIN				
	Nasal glioma*	**Rudimentary meningocele**	**Cutaneous meningioma (Types II and III)**	**Peripheral neuroblastoma**
Incidence	Rare	Rare	Extremely rare	Extremely rare
Age	Neonates	Neonates or infants	Usually adults	Late adulthood
Location	Most common near the root of the nose but can be intranasal	Scalp, forehead, paravertebral areas	Scalp	Head and trunk
Size	0.5–3.0 cm	0.5–3.0 cm	0.5–4.0 cm	0.5–5.0 cm
Clinical appearance	Firm, smooth, red–purple nodule or tumor	Soft to firm nodules, often with alopecia or the 'hair collar' sign; occasionally cystic; blue–red hue common	Soft to firm nodules, often with alopecia	Soft, skin-colored or red, often ulcerated nodules
Clinical differential diagnosis	Infantile hemangioma, nasal polyp, juvenile xanthogranuloma, dermoid cyst	Membranous aplasia cutis, heterotopic brain tissue, dermoid cyst, infantile hemangioma	Epidermoid or trichilemmal cyst, adnexal neoplasm, cutaneous metastasis	Lipoma, dermatofibroma, cutaneous metastasis
Associations	Intracranial connection in ~20% ('atretic' encephalocele)	An intracranial connection may be present ('atretic' meningocele)	May be associated with von Recklinghausen disease and acoustic neuromas	NA
Other	NA	NA	Metastasis of CNS meningioma must be excluded	Metastasis of ganglionic or adrenal neuroblastoma and extension of olfactory neuroblastoma must be excluded, especially in children
Histopathologic features	Lobulated neural tissue (glial cells, astrocytes, rarely true neurons)	Cystic or cavernous spaces, scattered meningothelial cells, pseudovascular pattern, psammoma bodies	Solid nests and strands, whorls of epithelioid or spindle cells, psammoma bodies	Rosette-like (Homer Wright type) structures of small, round, blue cells, extensive infiltration and necrosis
Biologic course	Benign	Benign	Locally aggressive and destructive	Extremely malignant with widespread metastases

*Heterotopic brain tissue can also be located in the midline scalp, orbit, lip and oropharynx.

Table 115.4 Tumors and tumor-like conditions of ectopic and heterotopic neural tissue involving the skin. NA, not applicable.

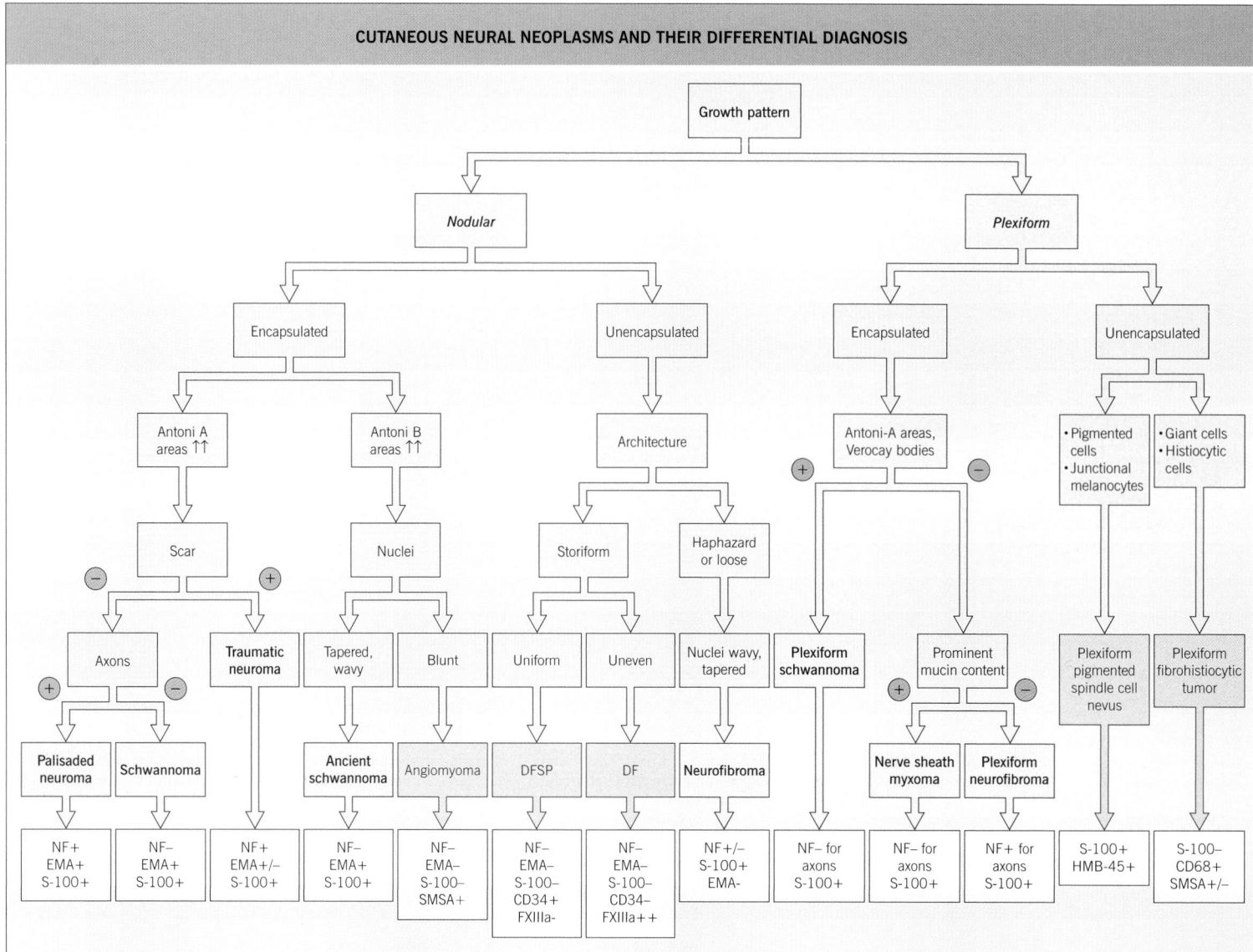

Fig. 115.2 Cutaneous neural neoplasms and their differential diagnosis. DF, dermatofibroma; DFSP, dermatofibrosarcoma protuberans; EMA, epithelial membrane antigen; FXIIIa, Factor XIII antigen; HMB45, melanocyte-related antibody; NF, neurofilament; S100, S100 protein; SMSA, smooth muscle-specific actin; +, positive; –, negative.

Introduction

Neuromas are proliferations of neural tissue in which Schwann cells and axon components are found in roughly equal numbers. There are two major subtypes: *traumatic* or *amputation neuroma* and *palisaded encapsulated neuroma* (PEN). Traumatic or amputation neuromas are complex regenerative proliferations of nerve fibers secondary to injury. Palisaded encapsulated or solitary circumscribed neuromas are complex hamartomatous proliferations of nerve fibers without apparent previous tissue injury.

History

The current view of traumatic neuroma was introduced by Huber & Lewis based on the concept of Wallerian degeneration[4]. PEN was described by Reed and co-workers in 1972[5].

Epidemiology

Traumatic neuromas are relatively uncommon but can occur at any age and in either sex. They are more prevalent in professions with a high probability for physical injuries. The solitary form of PEN develops spontaneously and gradually, without evidence of obvious previous trauma. These tumors appear during adulthood (mean age, 45.5 years) with about equal occurrence in men and women[5]. With the solitary form, there is no specific association with neurofibromatosis or the mucosal neuroma syndrome (MEN 2B).

Pathogenesis

Any extrinsic damage to nerve fibers can cause a traumatic neuroma. Amputation neuroma is considered the most common form and represents an attempted but failed regeneration of nerve fibers after transection. Following transection, the distal segments of the nerve fibers degenerate, whereas the proximal segments regenerate in an attempt to reunite with the distal portion of the transected nerve fibers[6]. In cases of severe trauma, this regenerative process is unsuccessful and the growing nerve fibers form a tangle of fascicles within fibrotic tissue. Despite marked variations in arrangement, size and shape of the regenerating fascicles, in traumatic neuromas the constituent fibers have a Schwann cell to axon ratio close to normal (1:1), which helps to distinguish true neuromas from other nerve sheath neoplasms[7].

In PEN there is an overgrowth of axons and their sheath cells within the confinement of the perineurium. This benign tumor most likely represents a hamartomatous growth in which there is a close reduplication of the normal axon to Schwann cell ratio[5]. The cause of the overgrowth of neurites is unknown. Although minor tissue injury such as inflammation induced by acne was suggested as a cause, a definite traumatic origin cannot be established[7].

Clinical Features

Traumatic neuromas are usually solitary, skin-colored or reddish purple, firm papules or nodules at sites of wounds, surgical scars and amputations[8–10] (Fig. 115.3). On the lower extremities they tend to be multiple[9].

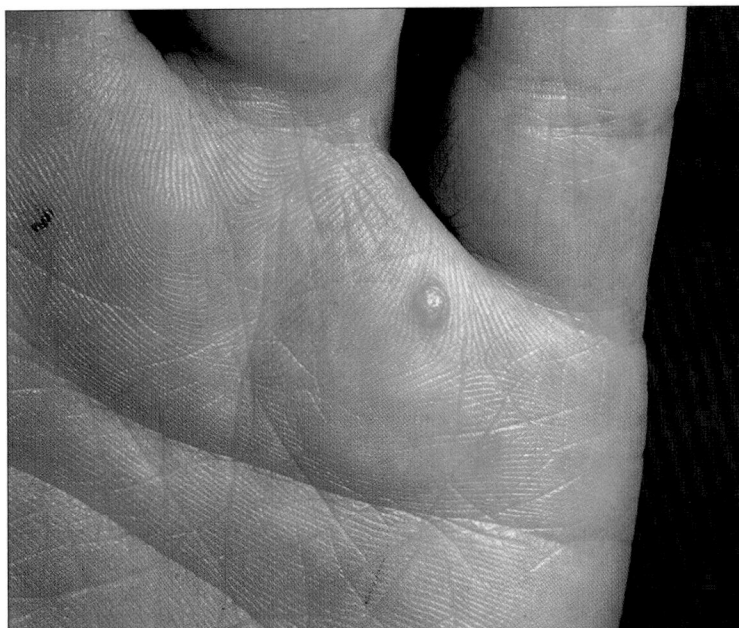

Fig. 115.3 **Traumatic neuroma.** Presenting as a painful, firm papule after a deep puncture injury.

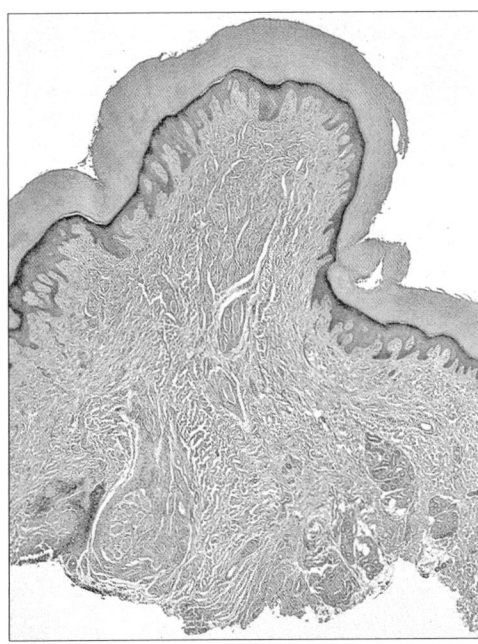

Fig. 115.4 **Amputation neuroma.** A polypoid lesion. Note the proliferation of nerve fascicles in the fibrotic stroma, and the lack of bony structures.

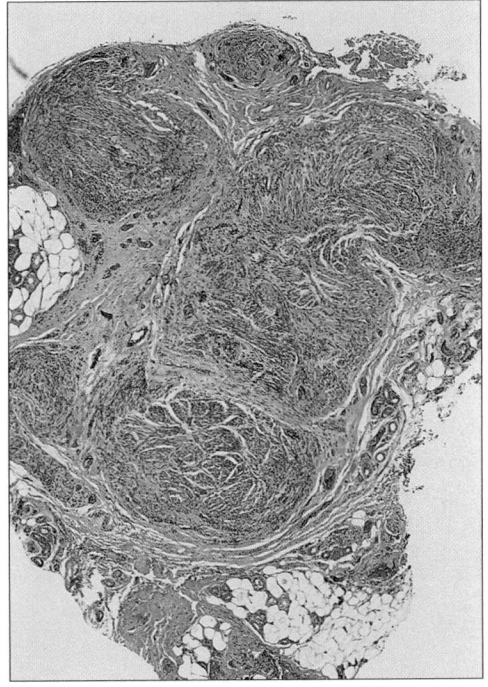

Fig. 115.5 **Traumatic neuroma.** The chaotic proliferation of nerve fascicles is embedded in a fibrous stroma.

Early lesions are asymptomatic, but after a few months they gradually become painful, frequently with a lancinating character. Variable tingling and itching can be associated with the pain.

In neonates and small infants, lesions may be located at the lateral-volar aspect of the hands, in which case they represent amputation neuromas secondary to amputation *in utero* of supernumerary digits[11] (see Ch. 63). These tumors are occasionally referred to as 'rudimentary supernumerary digits'; however, on histologic examination, they do not contain either normal or rudimentary elements of a digit.

In the solitary form of PEN, the individual lesions are asymptomatic, rubbery, firm, skin-colored to pink papules or nodules ranging in size from 0.2 to 0.6 cm in diameter[5]. Approximately 90% are located on the face, primarily around the nose, but they also occur on the cheek, chin and lips[12]. The remaining 10% occur elsewhere, including the trunk and extremities. In the multiple mucosal neuroma syndrome, numerous soft, skin- or mucosa-colored papules and nodules occur on the lips, tongue and conjunctivae, as well as in the nasal and laryngeal mucosa. Multiple mucosal neuromas are uncommon and represent a key feature of the multiple endocrine neoplasia syndrome (type 2B; see Ch. 62, Table 62.2), in which pheochromocytoma, medullary carcinoma of the thyroid, and gastrointestinal ganglioneuromas also occur; therefore, its early recognition can be life-saving. Multiple mucocutaneous neuromas with a predilection for the face and distal extremities can also represent a manifestation of the PTEN hamartoma-tumor syndrome, which includes Cowden and Bannayan–Riley–Ruvalcaba syndromes (see Ch. 62).

Pathology

Traumatic or amputation neuromas are usually well-circumscribed nodules located at any level of the dermis or the subcutis (Fig. 115.4). They are encased by a fibrous sheath, although the distal end can be poorly defined. The proliferation is composed of a chaotic, poorly organized tangle of fascicles of various sizes and shapes[8] (Fig. 115.5). Between the fibers are variable amounts of fibrous tissue with or without inflammatory cells or mucin[7]. The constituent cells are Schwann cells and perineurial cells with spindle-shaped nuclei and cytoplasm. Special stains show many axons in an irregular, haphazard pattern[1,5].

Solitary PENs are well-circumscribed, ovoid or round tumors located in the mid dermis, although some lesions may extend into the subcutis. The tumor appears encapsulated by a thick condensation of collagen fibers that surround it, and there is often some clefting from the adjacent dermis[5] (Fig. 115.6). The parenchyma is composed of interwoven fascicles of spindled cells. The fascicles are compactly and relatively uniformly arranged, separated only by clefts. There is no evidence of

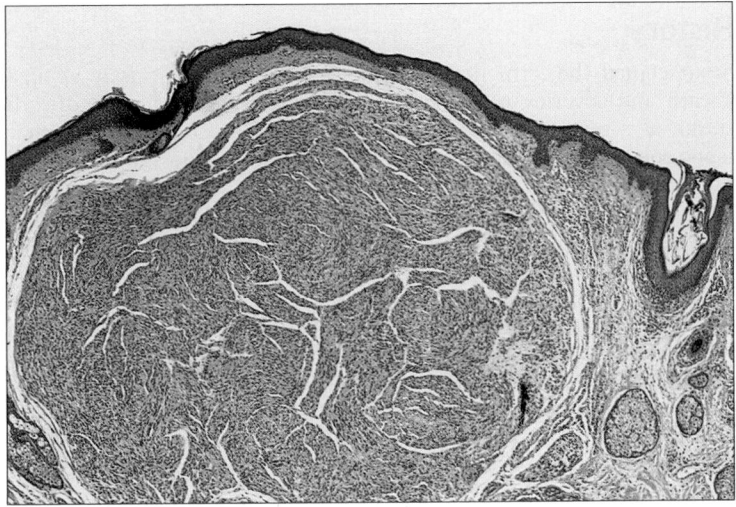

Fig. 115.6 **Palisaded encapsulated neuroma.** The well-circumscribed dermal nodule appears encapsulated.

extensive fibrosis, inflammation, granulation tissue, degenerative changes or foreign bodies, in contrast to traumatic neuromas[7].

The nuclei of the spindle-shaped tumor cells are elongated and wavy with tapered ends, and have an evenly basophilic chromatin pattern. Occasionally, a parallel arrangement of the nuclei is present, but, despite its name, distinct palisading or Verocay body formation is rare[13–15]. There is no appreciable nuclear pleomorphism, and mitotic figures are scant or absent. Special stains show abundant axons in a variable pattern[13]. The tumors of the mucosal neuroma syndrome may be considered to be a variant of PEN but are not encapsulated and are multiple.

Differential Diagnosis

The diagnosis of traumatic neuroma is usually suspected by the history of a painful or symptomatic papulonodule at a site of injury and is confirmed by pathologic examination.

PENs resemble intradermal nevi, basal cell carcinomas, adnexal tumors, and neurofibromas (Table 115.2). The diagnosis is seldom made clinically, and depends upon histologic examination (Table 115.3).

Treatment

Surgical excision of traumatic neuromas is indicated, with an attempt to reposition the proximal nerve stump into a scar-free area[9].

PENs are easily excised, and some can be enucleated from the surrounding dermis or subcutaneous tissue[5].

SCHWANNOMA

Synonyms: ■ Neurilemmoma ■ Neurolemmoma ■ Neurinoma ■ Schwann cell tumors ■ Acoustic neuroma

Key features

- Solitary papulonodule that usually appears on the flexural aspects of extremities along a peripheral nerve
- Occasionally painful or tender
- Deep dermal or subcutaneous location
- Histologically, there is an encapsulated spindle cell proliferation with biphasic Antoni A and B areas, palisading of nuclei, and Verocay bodies; axons are usually absent

Introduction

Schwannomas are benign true nerve sheath neoplasms composed entirely of Schwann cell proliferation.

History

Stout coined the term neurilemoma, referring to the closely applied sheath and covering of the tumor[16]. Verocay suggested nerve sheath tumor as a general classification[17]. Based on almost the entire tumor being composed of Schwann cells, the designation schwannoma is now preferred.

Epidemiology

Schwannomas are relatively uncommon tumors that can occur at any age, but are seen most often in adults and are slightly more frequent in women than in men. Approximately 90% of schwannomas are solitary without an association with any specific syndromes[2]. Occasionally, solitary schwannomas are seen in patients with neurofibromatosis (primarily type 2) and can be associated with various CNS tumors, usually meningiomas[2]. Rare cases of multiple schwannomas have been described under the term neurilemmomatosis or schwannomatosis, sometimes with a familial occurrence[18,19] or features shared with neuro-fibromatosis type 2 (NF2)[20–22].

Pathogenesis

Schwannomas are derived from the proliferation of periaxonal or endoneurial Schwann cells. As a result of the Schwann cell proliferation, the remaining normal nerve fibers are displaced to the periphery of tumor, creating an absence of the other components of a peripheral nerve[2]. Only after careful dissection can the attached nerve trunk be demonstrated. Since only the Schwann cells proliferate, the neoplasm remains within the confine of the perineurium, forming an encapsulated tumor. The cause of the exclusive Schwann cell proliferation is unknown, although an alteration or loss of the NF2 gene product on chromosome 22 has been implicated[23].

Clinical Features

Schwannomas present as a solitary, soft, pink to yellow, smooth-surfaced, dermal or subcutaneous nodule or tumor (Fig. 115.7). In general, their size ranges between 0.5 and 3.0 cm in diameter[24]. They are most commonly found on the flexor aspects of the extremities along the larger nerve trunks, followed by the head and neck[25,26]. The tumors are usually asymptomatic, but rarely pain and tenderness occur, especially if the tumor is forcefully moved and the attached nerve is placed under tension. Motor disturbances and paresthesias are extremely rare[27].

Pathology

Schwannomas are well-circumscribed, nodular or ovoid tumors located in the deep dermis or subcutis. They are almost always encapsulated. The tumors are composed of hypercellular (also called Antoni A-type tissue) and hypocellular (Antoni B-type tissue) areas[2]. The hypercellular areas show proliferation of spindle cells with indistinct cytoplasmic membranes and uniform nuclei[28]. Nuclear palisading and arrangement of palisaded nuclei in double rows, the so-called Verocay bodies, are characteristic features of these tumors[16,29] (Fig. 115.8). Mitotic figures are absent or rare.

The hypocellular areas show variable degrees of degeneration, including cystic, edematous, mucinous, fibrotic and vascular changes. Degenerative changes are often associated with some degree of cytologic atypia. These so-called *ancient schwannomas* should not be confused with the more specific entity of cellular schwannomas, which may display similar degenerative changes but rarely occur in the skin[30]. As a general rule, schwannomas are devoid of axons or they can be detected only at the site at which they are attached to a nerve[2]. There are additional less common subtypes of schwannomas, i.e. plexiform (no association with neurofibromatosis), cellular, pigmented, epithelioid and glandular[2,31–35].

Differential Diagnosis

The clinical differential diagnosis includes lipoma, angiolipoma, adnexal tumors, dermoid cyst, leiomyoma, nevi and ganglion cysts. The diagnosis is made by histopathologic examination.

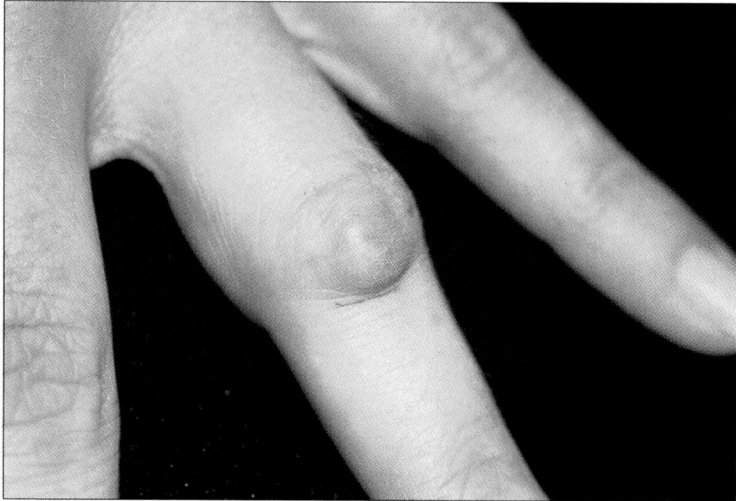

Fig. 115.7 Solitary schwannoma. Subcutaneous skin-colored nodule on the finger.

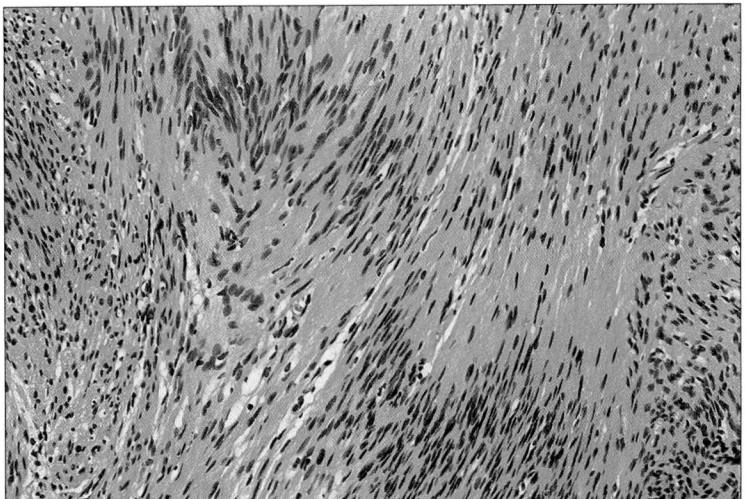

Fig. 115.8 Solitary cutaneous schwannoma. Hypercellular areas often show nuclear palisading and Verocay bodies.

Treatment

The tumor is benign and a simple excision is curative. If the clinical diagnosis is suspected, the lesion should be removed by enucleation, preserving normal nerve function.

NEUROFIBROMA

Synonyms: ■ Solitary or sporadic neurofibroma ■ Solitary nerve sheath tumor ■ Plexiform neurofibroma ■ Multiple neurofibromatosis

Key features
Solitary type
- Skin-colored to tan–violet papules or nodules
- May be pedunculated or have 'buttonhole' sign
- Predilection for trunk and head
- Spindle cell proliferation with variable mixture of the components of the peripheral nerve, including residual axons
- Fibrosis and mucinous changes are common

Plexiform type
- Pathognomonic of NF1
- Large, occasionally pigmented, bag-like masses
- Favor trunk and proximal extremities
- The plexiform variant has similar cytologic constituents as the solitary or sporadic type

Introduction

Neurofibromas are benign tumors composed of a complex proliferation of neuromesenchymal tissue (Schwann cells, perineurial cells, fibroblasts and mast cells), with residual nerve fibers (axons)[2]. Neurofibromas are common, especially as solitary lesions. The presence of multiple neurofibromas raises the possibility of one of the several types of neurofibromatosis (including the mosaic form; see Ch. 60). Plexiform neurofibromas are seen in patients with neurofibromatosis type 1 (NF1).

History

Neurofibromas were originally described as fibrous tumors by von Recklinghausen. Subsequently, a neuroectodermal origin was suggested by Verocay[36], which was eventually confirmed by immunohistochemical and ultrastructural studies.

Epidemiology

Solitary cutaneous neurofibromas are relatively common, especially in young adults, and have no gender preferences. Plexiform neurofibromas almost always indicate that the patient has NF1.

Pathogenesis

Neurofibromas differ from schwannomas in that several cell types are involved in their histogenesis. Regardless of the various histologic subtypes of neurofibromas (e.g. solitary, diffuse, combined, plexiform), the basic process is proliferation of the entire 'neuromesenchyme', which includes the Schwann cells, endoneurial fibroblasts, perineurial cells, mast cells, and cell types with intermediate features[2]. Since the extent of proliferation of each cell line is often different, the resulting histologic composition and architecture are variable. As stated earlier, the axons do not duplicate; therefore, their relative ratio to the Schwann cells will be less than 1:1. Genetic studies indicate that mutations in the *NF1* gene predict inactivation of the neurofibromin protein (i.e. haploinsufficiency); however, tumorigenesis may be the result of loss of heterozygosity (see Chs 53 and 60). The pathogenesis of isolated solitary neurofibromas is unclear.

Clinical Features

Neurofibromas are usually solitary, skin-colored, soft or rubbery papulonodules. They range in size from 0.2 to 2.0 cm and may become pedunculated[2]. They grow slowly and are asymptomatic. The 'buttonhole' sign is often present[2], i.e. the tumor is easily invaginated. Approximately 10% of patients with common neurofibromas have multiple lesions, and some of these patients have one of the several types of neurofibromatosis (see Ch. 60). There are several clinical and pathologic subtypes of neurofibroma, such as the diffuse, pigmented and plexiform variants. The diffuse and pigmented types may present as elevated, indurated or soft nodules and plaques with or without hyperpigmentation. Except for the plexiform variant, these types of neurofibromas rarely undergo malignant changes.

The plexiform neurofibroma is especially important because it is considered pathognomonic of von Recklinghausen disease and carries a higher probability of malignant transformation[2]. Typically, these tumors are baggy or pedunculated rope-like dermal and subcutaneous masses that, on occasion, are covered by hyperpigmented skin (Fig. 115.9). Recognition and correct patient management is crucial in these cases, especially in subtle forms of NF1, when the other cutaneous stigmata

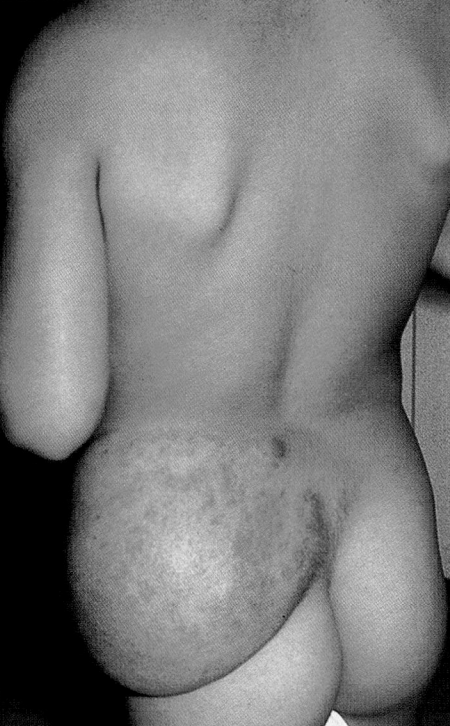

Fig. 115.9 Plexiform neurofibroma in a child with neurofibromatosis. Bag-like mass with overlying patches of hyperpigmentation.

may not be obvious[37]. The exact incidence of malignant transformation of plexiform neurofibroma is not known; it ranges from 2% to 13% (the lower percentage cited more recently).

Pathology

Neurofibromas are poor- to well-circumscribed, usually unencapsulated, nodular or oblong tumors that can be located anywhere in the dermis and subcutis[2,38]. The common solitary variant is usually present in the superficial dermis, creating a dome-shaped or polypoid elevation of its surface. The tumor is composed of a fine fibrillary lattice of haphazardly arranged slender spindle cells[39] (Fig. 115.10). The stroma can be variably vascular, fibrotic, edematous or myxomatous. Besides the Schwann cells and perineurial cells, plump fibroblasts and mast cells are present. Palisading of nuclei can occur, but true Verocay body formation is rare[38,39]. Mitotic figures are absent or rare. The diffuse form has essentially similar cytology, but without a well-defined growth pattern infiltrating the adjacent structures. Atypical forms of neurofibromas have been described[40].

As opposed to the superficial, solitary and diffuse forms, neurofibromas which are seated in the deep dermis, subcutis and other deep soft tissues are usually encapsulated by the perineurium or the epineurium and may show a plexiform growth pattern (Fig. 115.11)[2]. Variants with a combined diffuse and plexiform growth pattern usually occur in NF1. By utilizing special stains, rare scattered axons can be demonstrated in both the superficial and the deep variants of neurofibromas.

Differential Diagnosis

The clinical differential diagnosis of solitary neurofibromas includes dermal melanocytic nevi, neuromas, soft fibromas and dermatofibromas (Table 115.2). The majority of solitary or sporadic neurofibromas have similar clinical and histologic features as the multiple papular neurofibromas in patients with NF1. Plexiform neurofibromas with overlying hyperpigmentation and hypertrichosis can resemble congenital melanocytic nevi. Histologically, plexiform neurofibroma must be differentiated from other plexiform tumors, including plexiform schwannoma.

Treatment

Neurofibromas are usually treated by simple excision. The evaluation and management of plexiform neurofibromas and neurofibromatosis is discussed in Chapter 60.

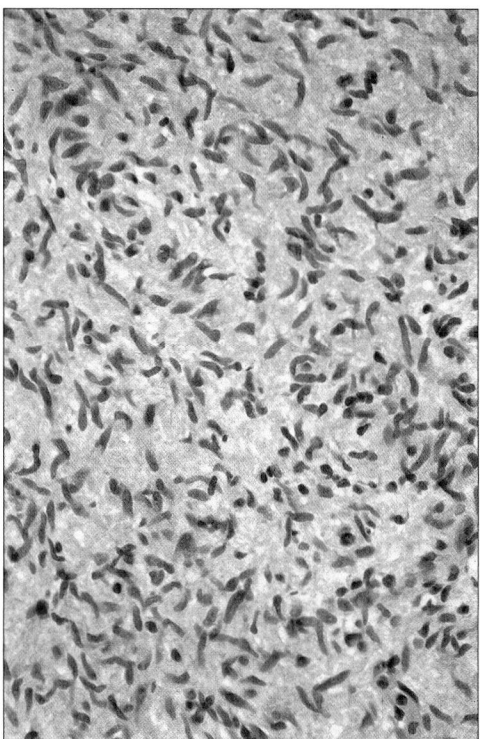

Fig. 115.10 **Neurofibroma.** The tumor contains diffuse proliferation of spindle cells with slender, ovoid nuclei in a fibrillary matrix.

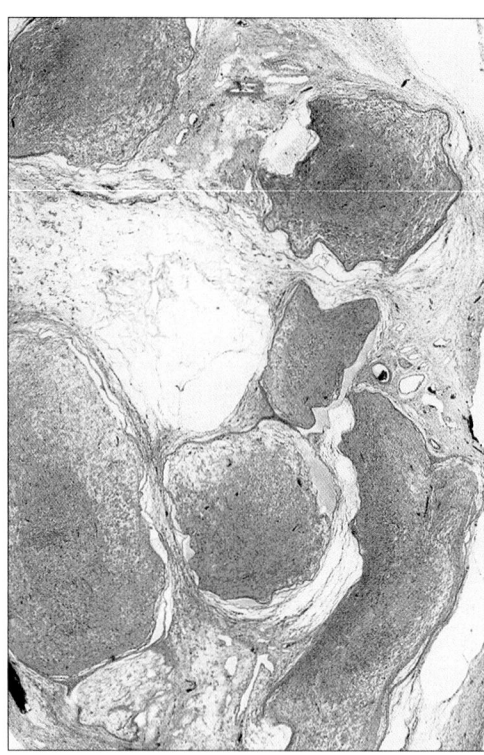

Fig. 115.11 **Plexiform neurofibroma showing irregularly expanded, twisted nerve fascicles.**

NERVE SHEATH MYXOMA AND CELLULAR NEUROTHEKEOMA

Synonyms: ■ Neurothekeoma ■ Cutaneous lobular neuromyxoma ■ Myxomatous perineurioma ■ Bizarre cutaneous neurofibroma ■ Myxoma of the nerve sheath

Key features

- Occurs most commonly in young and middle-aged women
- Skin-colored papules and nodules with a predilection for the head and neck region
- Histologically, lobular and fascicular pattern with a lack of axons
- There is a hypocellular myxomatous pattern and a cellular type with scant mucin
- Benign behavior, but local recurrences may occur

Introduction

Nerve sheath myxoma refers to a spectrum of neuromesenchymal tumors that are characterized by the proliferation of nerve sheath cells in a variably myxomatous stroma. Nerve sheath myxomas can be classified into a *classic myxoid type* and a *cellular type* (cellular neurothekeoma)[41,42], based on the degree of cytologic differentiation and the relative amount of myxomatous stroma.

History

Nerve sheath myxoma was first described as a specific entity by Harkin & Reed in 1969[43]. The term 'cellular neurothekeoma' was coined by Rosati et al. in 1986[44].

Epidemiology

The classic or myxoid type of nerve sheath myxoma occurs commonly in middle-aged adults (mean age, 48 years) with an approximate 1:2 male-to-female ratio[45,46].

The cellular form of nerve sheath myxoma (cellular neurothekeoma) is also a tumor of adulthood, but it usually affects younger adults (mean age, 24 years) and is also more common in women[47,48].

Pathogenesis

Nerve sheath myxoma has a controversial histogenesis. Both Schwann cells and perineurial cells are present in classic nerve sheath myxoma[41,42]. The reason for extreme mucin production is unknown, although mucin is part of the normal endoneurium. Some authors speculate that nerve sheath myxoma could represent a variant of neurofibroma with extreme myxoid degeneration[45]. This degeneration may explain the virtual lack of axons in these tumors.

Although the available immunohistochemical and ultrastructural data support nerve sheath differentiation in the classic myxoid variant, there is no uniformly accepted view regarding the histogenesis of the cellular variant[41,42,47,48]. Cellular neurothekeomas usually do not express S100 protein (as do Schwann cells) or epithelial membrane antigen (as perineurial cells do), but can be partially positive for smooth muscle-specific antigen and for a melanocyte marker, NKI/C3 antigen[49,50]. A recent study suggests that protein gene product 9.5 (PGP 9.5) is a good marker for this tumor[51].

Clinical Features

Classic nerve sheath myxomas are soft, skin-colored papules or nodules, generally 0.5 to 1.0 cm in diameter, and are typically located on the head and upper extremities[45].

Although cellular neurothekeomas tend to occur predominantly on the head, cases from a variety of anatomic sites have been reported. The tumors are characterized by firm, pink, red or brown papulo-nodules ranging in size from 0.5 to 3.0 cm (Fig. 115.12). Symptoms are non-specific and seem to relate to the size and firmness of the tumor[47,48].

Pathology

The classic myxoid type of nerve sheath myxoma is a well-defined, lobular or plexiform neoplasm that is usually located in the reticular dermis (Fig. 115.13). It often appears encapsulated by a compression of the surrounding fibrous tissue[41]. There is hypocellular myxoid stroma with rare, scattered, spindled, stellate or dendritic cells. The cells usually have scant, pale cytoplasm with indistinct cytoplasmic contours and hyperchromatic, ovoid or angulated nuclei[41,45]. Nucleoli are small and mitotic figures are rare or absent. On occasion, multinucleated giant cells with eosinophilic cytoplasm can be identified. Histochemically, the myxoid stroma stains strongly positive for acidic mucopolysaccharides (see Ch. 46)[45]. While entrapped nerves in and around the tumor can be identified, the presence of scattered axons or direct continuity of axons with tumor cells has not been established[41,42].

Cellular neurothekeoma is composed of ill-defined multilobular masses or fascicles in the reticular dermis[41] (Fig. 115.14A). In some cases, the growth pattern can be frankly infiltrative or dissecting without any hint of a residual capsule, and there may be involvement of the superficial subcutis[7]. Cytologically, the predominant cell types are epithelioid or polygonal cells with ample eosinophilic cytoplasm and round nuclei with an open chromatin pattern[48,49] (see Fig. 115.14B). Many cells have prominent nucleoli. Less often, the constituent cells are spindle-shaped with hyperchromatic nuclei, as seen in the classic

form of nerve sheath myxoma. Mitotic figures are often present but are usually normal morphologically. Rare cases with increased mitotic figures and cytologic atypia have been reported[52]. The stroma can be markedly fibrotic or even hyalinized. An obvious direct connection with the peripheral nerves has not been established, but branches of pre-existing nerve fibers can be demonstrated by special stains.

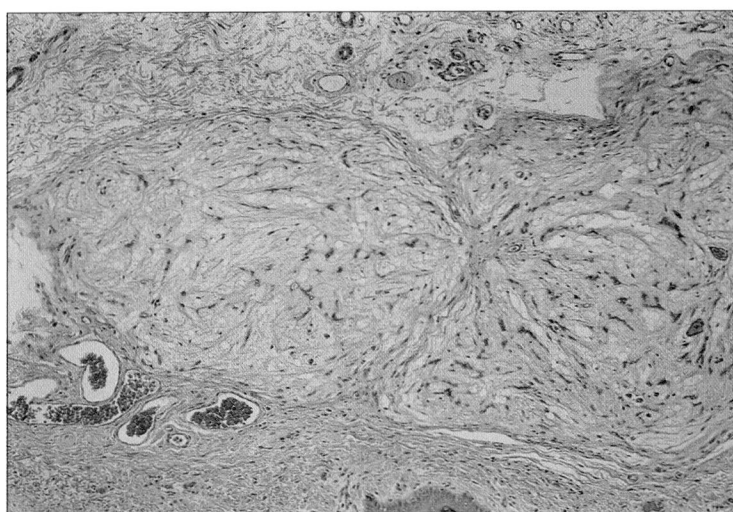

Fig. 115.13 Nerve sheath myxoma, classic type. Well-defined fascicles with myxoid stroma.

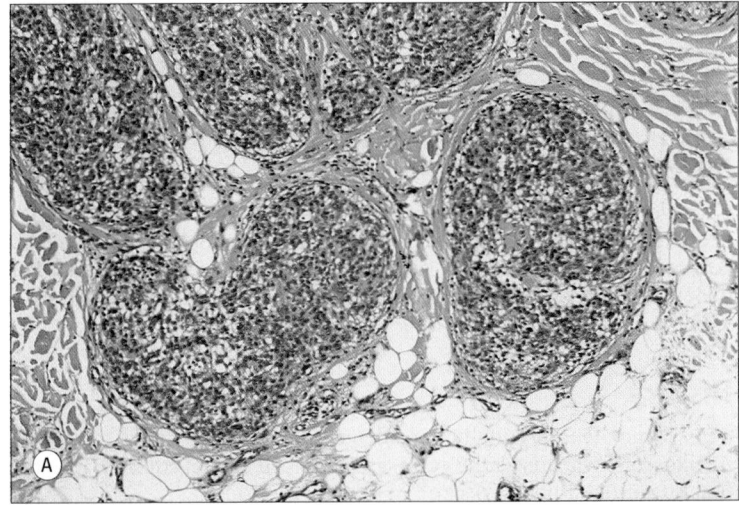

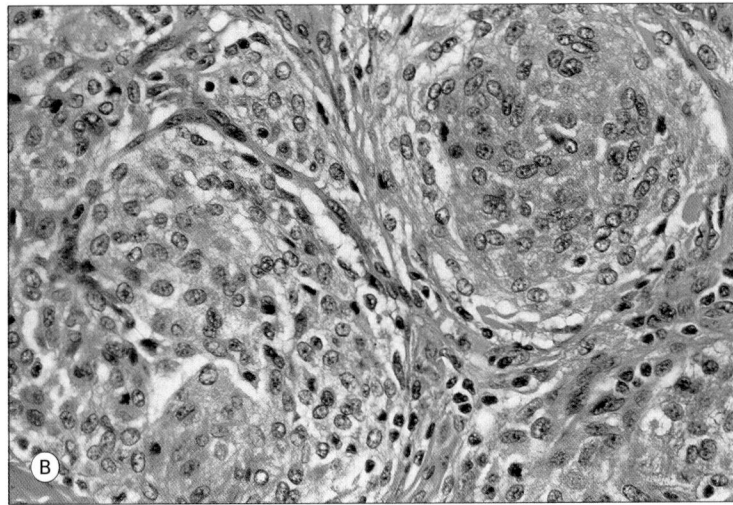

Fig. 115.14 Nerve sheath myxoma, cellular type or cellular neurothekeoma. A Epithelioid nests are dispersed in a hyalinized stroma. **B** Whorl-like arrangement of epithelioid cells showing nuclear pleomorphism and rare mitotic figures.

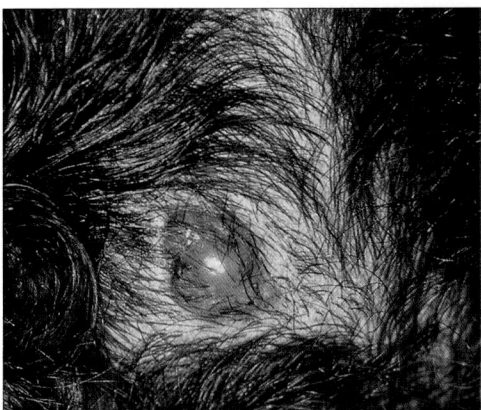

Fig. 115.12 Cellular neurothekeoma of the scalp, presenting as an erythematous, firm papule.

Differential Diagnosis

Nerve sheath myxomas are usually asymptomatic and clinically are mistaken for myxoid or ganglion cysts, dermal melanocytic nevi, fibrolipomas and adnexal neoplasms. The clinical impression of cellular neurothekeoma is usually that of a dermatofibroma, keloid, hemangioma, dermal melanocytic nevus or pyogenic granuloma.

Treatment

These lesions are usually treated by simple excision; however, in case of incomplete removal, nerve sheath myxoma may recur. A few case reports have described atypical variants of cellular neurothekeomas with postulated uncertain behavior in which case complete excision becomes important.

GRANULAR CELL TUMOR

Synonyms: ■ Granular cell nerve sheath tumor ■ Granular cell myoblastoma ■ Granular cell schwannoma ■ Abrikossoff's tumor

Key features

- Seen more commonly in adults, women and darkly pigmented races
- Predilection for the tongue, but can occur anywhere, including the viscera
- Malignant transformation is rare and usually occurs with deep-seated lesions
- Histologically, an ill-defined, infiltrative tumor with associated pseudoepitheliomatous hyperplasia is common
- Large polygonal cells with finely granular eosinophilic cytoplasm; the granules are PAS-positive, diastase-resistant

Introduction

Granular cell tumor is a descriptive term for a heterogeneous group of neoplasms composed of cells with granular cytoplasm due to the accumulation of lysosomal granules. Most cutaneous granular cell neoplasms are of neural origin, but granular cell change occurs in a variety of neoplasms.

History

This tumor was originally considered to be derived from muscle by Abrikossoff, who used the term granular cell myoblastoma[53]. Feyrter first suggested a neural origin[54].

Epidemiology

Granular cell tumor is a relatively rare tumor that occurs mainly in adults (age 30–50 years) with a 1:3 male-to-female ratio. The tumor is characteristically solitary, and 70% of them are located in the head and neck region, including 30% of these on the tongue[53]. Other common locations are the breast (5–15%) and the proximal extremities. Rare visceral lesions have also been reported. In approximately 10% of patients, the lesions are multiple, especially in African-Americans.

Pathogenesis

The neural origin of this tumor has been a subject of controversy, and was originally based on the observation that granular cells are sometimes intimately associated with nerves and other neural tumors[55–57]. In addition, granular cells express S100 protein and CD57, as do many Schwann cell tumors[58]. However, the classic form of this tumor does not resemble any other type of peripheral nerve sheath tumor. Recent immunohistochemical studies suggest a neural crest-derived peripheral nerve-related cell differentiation[59]. Despite the controversy regarding its histogenesis, the tumor is histologically distinct and rarely presents a diagnostic problem.

Clinical Features

A granular cell tumor presents as an asymptomatic or occasionally tender or pruritic, skin-colored or brownish red, firm dermal or subcutaneous papulonodule, ranging in size from 0.5 to 3.0 cm in diameter. Occasionally, the surface can show ulceration or verrucous changes. Granular cell tumors are slowly growing and in general have benign behavior. In approximately 3% of cases, malignant behavior may ensue (local infiltration or metastasis), usually when the tumor arises from a visceral or deep location.

Pathology

The dermis contains a poorly circumscribed nodule composed of polygonal, pale-stained cells that may infiltrate into the adjacent dermis. The cells have abundant, granular, faintly eosinophilic cytoplasm with round, dark nuclei (Fig. 115.15)[60]. Characteristic larger cytoplasmic granules are called pustulo-ovoid bodies. With PAS reaction the granules are positive, but diastase-resistant. Occasionally, a perineurial growth pattern is present; however, the tumor is devoid of axons. Increased numbers of mast cells are present in some lesions[55]. The overlying epidermis is frequently acanthotic. Rarely, a plexiform growth pattern has been described[61]. The histologic criteria to prospectively identify the rare aggressive tumors are not well established[62]. The presence of necrosis, increased mitotic rate, and spindling of the cells have been suggested as predictive of aggressive behavior[63].

Differential Diagnosis

The clinical differential diagnosis includes dermatofibroma, adnexal tumors, compound melanocytic nevi and seborrheic keratoses. Granular cell tumors can induce considerable pseudocarcinomatous hyperplasia of the overlying epithelium, and superficial biopsy samples have been mistaken for squamous cell carcinoma, especially on the tongue[64]. A variety of epithelial and mesenchymal neoplasms can show granular cell change, including basal cell carcinomas, leiomyomas and leiomyosarcomas[60,65].

Treatment

The treatment is complete excision. If incompletely excised, this tumor has a high local recurrence rate, due to the plexiform or perineurial growth pattern.

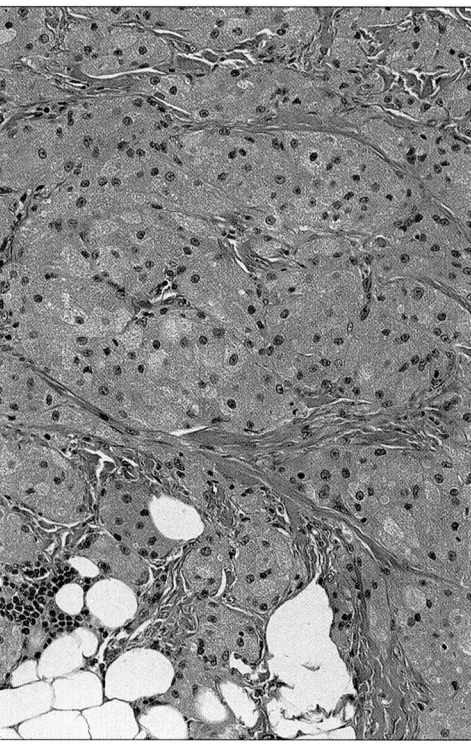

Fig. 115.15 Granular cell tumor. The tumor may show a nodular or infiltrative growth pattern. The large polygonal cells have finely granular cytoplasm and round nuclei.

MALIGNANT PERIPHERAL NERVE SHEATH TUMOR

Synonyms: ■ Neurosarcoma ■ Neurofibrosarcoma ■ Malignant schwannoma

The term malignant peripheral nerve sheath tumor is preferable to the widely used but confusing synonyms above. This is because any cellular component of the peripheral nerve could give rise to these tumors. In the majority of cases, perineural or endoneurial fibroblasts rather than Schwann cells form the bulk of the tumor[66–68].

Malignant peripheral nerve sheath tumor is a tumor of deep soft tissues and rarely involves the skin. A definitive diagnosis requires a biopsy usually with immunohistochemistry, electron microscopy, and molecular biologic analysis. Histologically, in the most common form, there is a proliferation of atypical spindle cells, often arranged in a 'herring-bone' pattern. There is variable cytologic atypia, numerous abnormal mitotic figures, areas of necrosis and hemorrhage (Fig. 115.16)[67–69]. Despite its rarity, malignant peripheral nerve sheath tumor has clinical relevance for the dermatologist, because 2–13% of plexiform neurofibromas, associated with neurofibromatosis, develop into this malignancy[69] (Ch. 60).

MERKEL CELL CARCINOMA

Synonyms: ■ Primary neuroendocrine carcinoma of the skin ■ Trabecular carcinoma of the skin ■ Primary small cell carcinoma of the skin ■ Cutaneous apudoma

Key features

- Predilection for the head and neck region of older adults
- Solitary, rapidly growing nodule
- Histologically, small, round, blue cell tumor, often with a nested or trabecular growth pattern
- High mitotic rate, frequent single-cell necrosis, and often zonal necrosis
- Aggressive, malignant behavior

Introduction

Merkel cell carcinoma is a malignant proliferation of highly anaplastic cells which share structural and immunohistochemical features with various neuroectodermally derived cells, including cutaneous Merkel cells. These tumors display non-specific clinical features and highly aggressive behavior. Early recognition and adequate therapy are therefore critical.

History

This tumor was originally described by Toker and given the name 'trabecular carcinoma' based on its lattice-like and infiltrative growth pattern[70]. Subsequently, the neuroendocrine nature of this tumor was recognized with similarities to the normal Merkel cell of the skin[71].

Epidemiology

Merkel cell carcinoma most commonly occurs in the elderly, and it is slightly more prevalent in women[72].

Pathogenesis

Although the cells of this tumor and the normal Merkel cell, which is a specialized receptor cell of touch located in the basal layer of the epidermis, share several morphologic, immunohistochemical and ultrastructural features, there is little evidence for a direct histogenetic relationship between the two[71]. Furthermore, extracutaneous neuroendocrine tumors display similar features. Therefore, the conceptually more unifying term primary neuroendocrine carcinoma of the skin (PNECS) is preferred by pathologists over Merkel cell carcinoma[4], as it indicates the tumor's relationship with neuroendocrine tumors of other origins. Clinicians seem to prefer the shorter term Merkel cell carcinoma, which seems entrenched in the lexicon.

Clinical Features

The tumor favors the head and neck region, followed by the extremities and the buttocks. The usual appearance is a pink–red or violaceous, firm, dome-shaped solitary nodule that grows rapidly (Fig. 115.17)[72]. Ulceration can occur. The behavior is that of an aggressively growing tumor, with frequent recurrences after excision. Distant metastases develop in approximately 40% of the patients, and about 30% will die of their disease within 5 years[72].

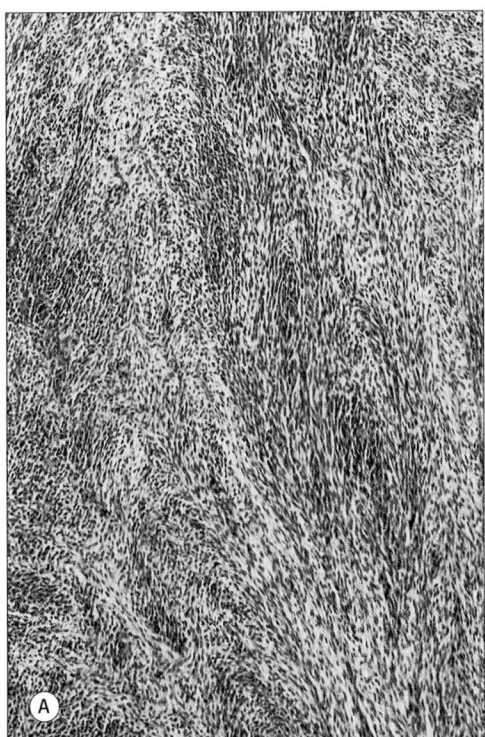

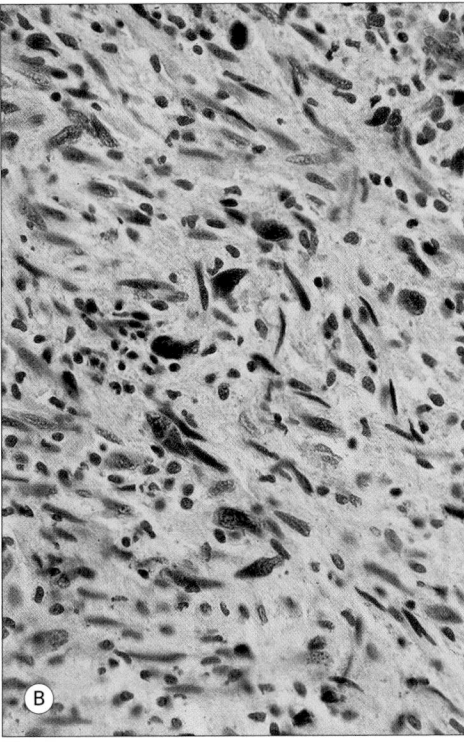

Fig. 115.16 Malignant peripheral nerve sheath tumor. A The tumor is composed of intersecting fascicles creating a 'herring-bone' pattern. **B** Marked cellular pleomorphism with cytologic atypia and mitotic activity.

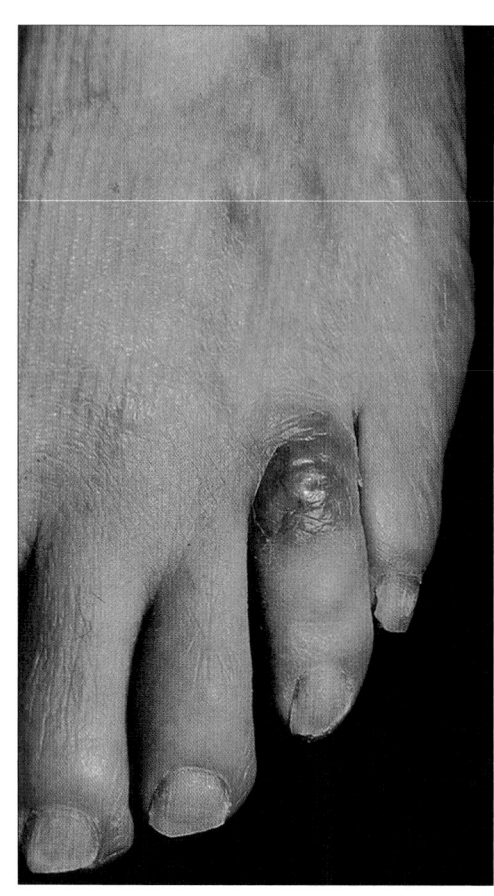

Fig. 115.17 Merkel cell carcinoma (primary neuroendocrine carcinoma) presenting as a rapidly growing, violaceous nodule on the toe.

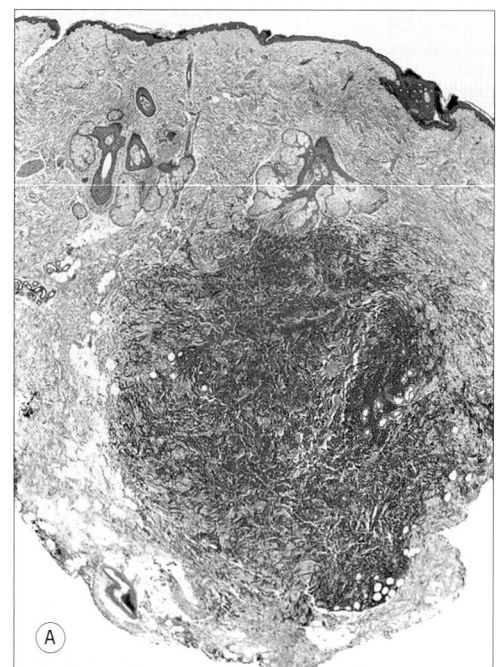

Fig. 115.18 Primary neuroendocrine carcinoma of the skin (Merkel cell carcinoma). **A** Dermal nodule with infiltrating borders. **B** Anaplastic tumor cells with round to ovoid shape, scant nuclei, and fine chromatin pattern. **C** Immunohistochemical stain for cytokeratin 20 demonstrates a characteristic perinuclear dot pattern. C Courtesy of Ronald P Rapini MD.

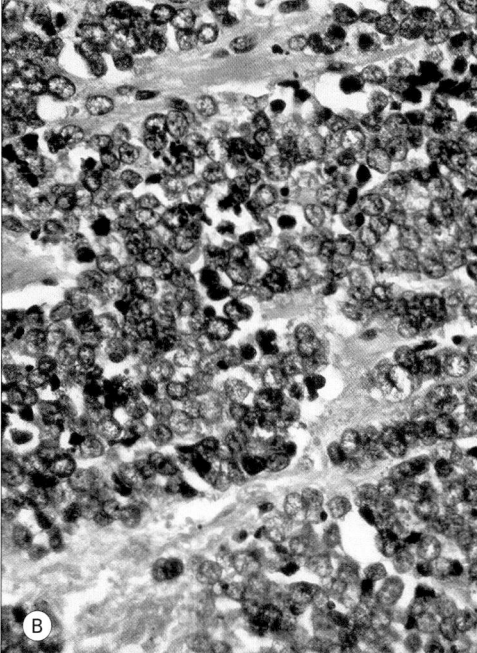

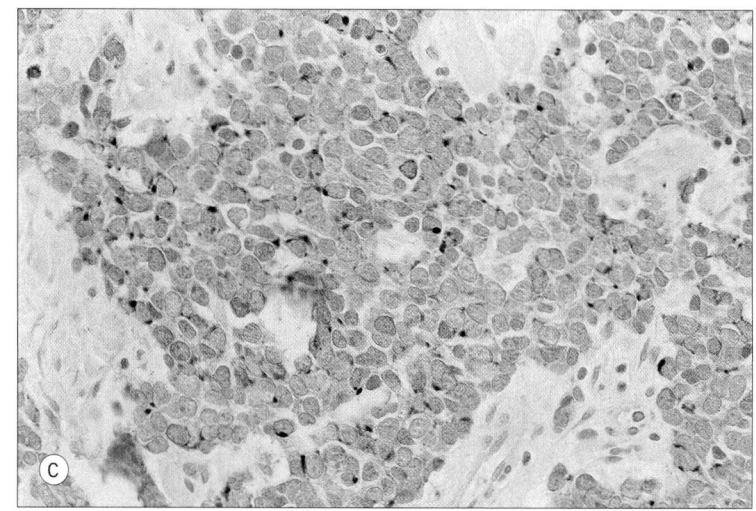

Pathology

The tumor appears as a poorly defined dermal mass frequently infiltrating the subcutaneous fat, fascia and muscle. While it may show various growth patterns, a sheet-like growth is the most common, followed by the nested and trabecular types (Fig. 115.18A)[73]. Characteristically, the edge of the tumor shows a trabecular infiltrating pattern[70]. The tumor is composed of monotonously uniform, small, round to oval cells that are about two to three times larger than mature lymphocytes[70,71]. The nuclei of these cells are ovoid with a finely dispersed chromatin pattern and distinct nuclear membranes (Fig. 115.18B). Nucleoli are usually not prominent. Mitotic figures are abundant. The cytoplasm is scant and faintly amphophilic. Extensive areas of necrosis, individual cell necrosis and characteristic crush artifact are common[73].

Various types of differentiation have been described in Merkel cell carcinoma, including rosette-like structures resembling Homer Wright rosettes of neuroblastoma, epidermotropic involvement with pagetoid spread, and eccrine and squamoid differentiation[74,75]. Immuno-histochemically, there is a characteristic perinuclear globule upon staining for low-molecular-weight cytokeratins (CK) such as CK20 and CK8/18/19 (CAM 5.2). This corresponds to the ultrastructural distri-bution of paranuclear whorls of intermediate filaments[73,74]. In addition, there is a reaction with various neuroendocrine markers, including chromogranin, synaptophysin, somatostatin, calcitonin, vasoactive intestinal peptides and others[74]. These peptides are associated with the ultrastructurally demonstrable membrane-bound dense-core secretory granules. The tumor also expresses neuron-specific enolase and, occasionally, neural filaments, but immunostaining for S100 protein is characteristically negative[74]. Likewise, a negative reaction for thyroid transcription factor 1 (TTF-1) helps to differentiate between Merkel cell carcinoma and cutaneous metastasis from other small cell carcinomas (pulmonary and extrapulmonary); the latter is characteristically positive for this marker[74].

Differential Diagnosis

Due to the violaceous, sometimes hemorrhagic appearance of the tumor, the differential diagnosis includes hemangioma, abscess, angio-sarcoma and lymphoma. Other common clinical diagnoses are non-melanoma skin cancer and cyst. There is a broad spectrum of small, round, blue cell tumors of diverse histogenesis that can be confused with PNECS[74]. These include metastatic neuroendocrine carcinoma of the lung (small cell or oat cell carcinoma), poorly differentiated eccrine carcinoma, lymphoma, metastatic neuroblastoma, primary peripheral primitive neuroectodermal tumor, Ewing's sarcoma, melanoma and poorly differentiated squamous cell carcinoma[73,74] (see introductory chapter).

Treatment

Surgery is the primary approach; however, adjuvant chemotherapy, immunotherapy and radiation therapy are often simultaneously administered owing to the aggressive course of the disease[76]. Sentinel lymph node mapping has also been recommended[77,77a] (Fig. 115.19).

TUMORS AND TUMOR-LIKE CONDITIONS OF ECTOPIC AND HETEROTOPIC NEURAL TISSUE OF THE SKIN

These rare lesions develop from embryologically misplaced neural tissue within the skin. They range from benign malformations to cellular proliferations with potential for metastasis. There are three major clinicopathologic manifestations of neural heterotopias in the skin: (1) neuroglial; (2) meningeal; and (3) neuroblastic/ganglionic abnormalities.

HETEROTOPIC NEUROGLIAL TISSUE

Synonyms: ■ Nasal glioma ■ Brain-like heterotopia ■ Glial hamartoma

Key features

- Rare, benign, congenital lesion
- Most common near the root of the nose, but can be intranasal
- Solitary, firm, smooth, red–purple papule or nodule
- May be associated with an encephalocele
- Microscopically, lobulated neuroglial tissue

History

The term 'nasal glioma' was introduced by Schmidt in 1900[78].

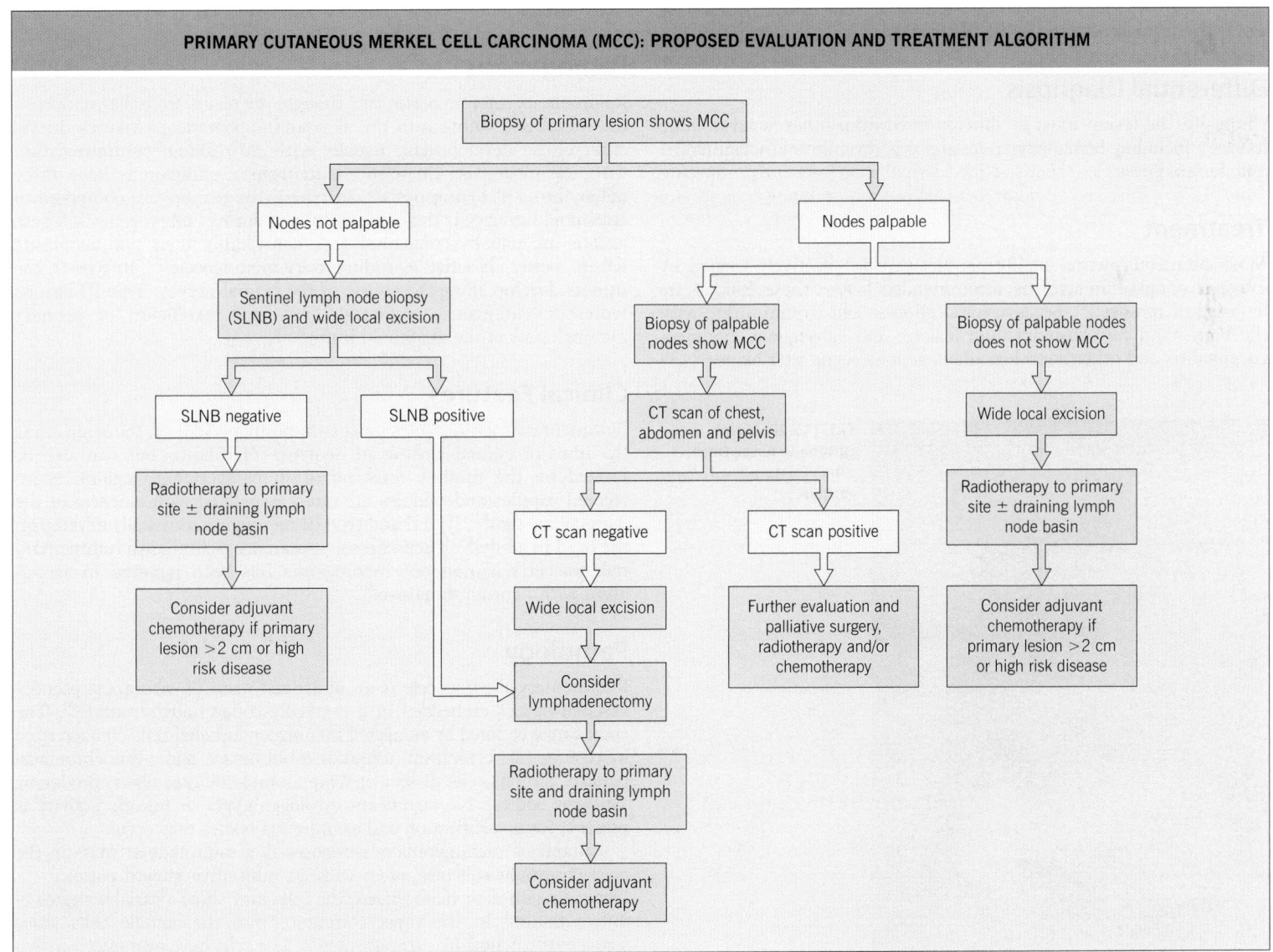

Fig. 115.19 Primary cutaneous Merkel cell carcinoma (MCC): proposed evaluation and treatment algorithm. Courtesy of Paul Nghiem MD PhD. Based upon: Gupta SG, Wang LC, Penas PF, et al. Sentinel lymph node biopsy for evaluation and treatment of patients with Merkel cell carcinoma: The Dana-Farber experience and meta-analysis of the literature. Arch Dermatol. 2006;142:685–90.

Epidemiology

These tumors are rare and usually manifest at the time of birth.

Pathogenesis

A nasal glioma is the result of embryologic displacement of brain tissue usually along the cranial closure lines without apparent communication with the underlying structures[79]. It has a predilection for the perinasal areas; therefore, it is commonly referred to as a nasal glioma. As this is not a true neoplasm, the term is misleading[80].

Clinical Features

Nasal gliomas are firm, smooth-surfaced, skin-colored or pink, sometimes slightly vascularized nodules ranging in size from 1 to 3 cm (Fig. 115.20). Approximately 60% are located on the bridge of the nose, with the remainder often located intranasally or in both locations[80,81].

Pathology

In a nasal glioma, an ill-defined, unencapsulated neuropil-like mass is seen in the dermis and subcutis. The neuropil-like tissue is composed of nests and strands of pale-staining, finely vacuolated or fibrillary matrix in which various types of astrocytes can be found[79]. Gemistocytic astrocytes, with polygonal, eosinophilic cytoplasm and eccentric nuclei, as well as multinucleated giant cells, are relatively common. Mature neurons are present in variable numbers[80]. Occasionally, residual meningoendothelial cells, ependymal cells, choroid plexus-like structures and pigmented cells can be identified[81]. No mitotic activity or aggressive growth pattern has been described.

Differential Diagnosis

Clinically, the lesion must be differentiated from other facial midline lesions[82] including hemangioma, nasal polyp, juvenile xanthogranuloma and dermoid cyst.

Treatment

Most cutaneous neural malformations can be effectively treated by excision. Cranial imaging is recommended before these lesions are biopsied or removed[83], because nasal gliomas can communicate with the brain, and cerebrospinal fluid leakage and subsequent meningoencephalitis and other neurologic damage may occur after biopsy[80].

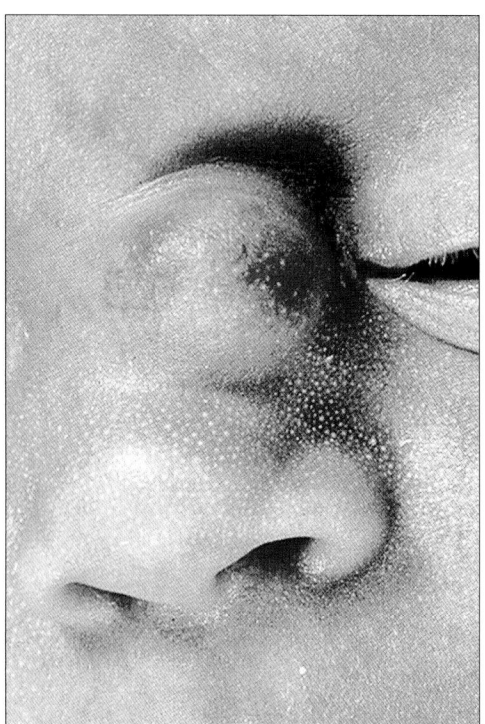

Fig. 115.20 Nasal glioma in a newborn. Pink violaceous soft nodule.

HETEROTOPIC MENINGEAL TISSUE

Synonyms: ■ Cutaneous meningioma ■ Rudimentary meningocele

Key features

- Rare disorder that usually presents in neonates and infants and favors the scalp, forehead and paravertebral region
- Soft to firm, skin-colored nodules often with partial alopecia or the 'hair collar' sign
- Can be associated with neurofibromatosis or other developmental anomalies
- Histologically, solid nests and strands, whorls of epithelioid or spindle cells and psammoma bodies

History

The rare cutaneous presentation of meningioma was first reported by Winkler[84] in 1904, and the concept of rudimentary meningocele was introduced by Lopez et al.[85].

Epidemiology

Meningeal heterotopias are rare lesions, usually present at or shortly after birth[85].

Pathogenesis

Rudimentary meningoceles are thought to result from herniation of the meningeal lining into the skin and subcutaneous tissues during embryologic development, usually with no residual communication with the CNS (see Ch. 63)[86]. Cutaneous meningiomas have three major forms of histogenesis[85]. In type I, the tumors are composed of arachnoid lining cells that were misplaced during embryogenesis. These lesions are usually congenital and, considering their non-neoplastic nature, better classified as rudimentary meningoceles[86]. In type II, the tumors develop along the course of the cranial nerves. Type III lesions represent cutaneous 'metastasis' or direct extension of primary meningiomas of the arachnoid lining[87,88].

Clinical Features

Rudimentary meningoceles most commonly present on the scalp along the lines of cranial closure in neonates or infants, but can also be located on the midline forehead or in paravertebral regions. Skin-colored papules and nodules are often associated with alopecia or the 'hair collar' sign[87]. Type II and type III meningiomas usually develop on the head in adults[85]. Their clinical appearance is similar to rudimentary meningoceles. Cutaneous meningioma has been reported in association with neurofibromatosis[89].

Pathology

Rudimentary meningocele is an ill-defined mass of cavernous, pseudo-vascular spaces embedded in a markedly collagenous stroma[86,90]. The spaces may be lined by elongated meningoendothelial cells characterized by eosinophilic cytoplasm, round or ovoid nuclei, and a fine chromatin pattern. Similar cells dissect or wrap around collagen fibers, producing 'collagen bodies'. No significant cytologic atypia or mitotic activity is present. Focal calcification and psammoma bodies may occur.

Cutaneous meningioma is composed of a multinodular mass in the deep dermis or subcutis, often with an infiltrative growth pattern[91-93]. Depending on their histogenesis, the cells may show a variable degree of differentiation. In the most common form, the spindle cells show a concentric, whorl-like arrangement[91]. The cells have oval nuclei with a vesicular chromatin pattern. Mitotic figures are rare in type II and variably increased in type III. Psammoma bodies (eosinophilic laminated and whorled structures with variable calcification) are often present[91-93].

Differential Diagnosis

Rudimentary meningoceles must be distinguished from 'atretic' meningoceles (an intermediate form with an intracranial connection), membranous aplasia cutis congenita, heterotopic brain tissue, dermoid cysts and infantile hemangiomas. Clinically, cutaneous meningiomas may resemble cysts and other adnexal neoplasms as well as metastatic tumors.

Treatment

As with heterotopic neuroglial tissue (nasal glioma), imaging studies are required prior to biopsy or excision. The latter is usually performed by neurosurgeons.

HETEROTOPIC NEUROBLASTIC TISSUE AND THEIR TUMORS

Synonyms: ■ Neuroblastoma (primary or metastatic) ■ Primitive neuroectodermal tumor ■ Neuroepithelioma

Key features

- The third most common malignant neoplasm in children
- Cutaneous metastases (children) seen more frequently than primary cutaneous tumors (adults)
- Cutaneous metastases present as multiple, purple–blue dermal nodules in association with elevated serum and urine catecholamines
- Histologically, small, round, blue cells in a nested or infiltrative growth pattern, with formation of Homer Wright rosettes
- Prognosis depends on the patient's age, clinical stage and tumor suppressor gene expression

Introduction

Neuroblastic-ganglionic tumors are derived from the germinal neuroepithelium and/or from the neural crest. They display a wide spectrum of clinicopathologic features based on their relative degree of differentiation, ranging from very primitive neuroectodermal tumors to more mature forms such as neuroblastomas.

History

The concept of neuroectodermal tumors was introduced by Stout in 1918[94]. Since then, different terms have been used for tumors with cytologically similar features, reflecting the controversy regarding this entity. Dehner performed a comprehensive review of the nosology of this diverse group of lesions, suggesting the term primitive neuroectodermal tumors (PNET)[95].

Epidemiology

Neuroblastoma is the third most commonly occurring childhood neoplasm, and cutaneous metastases are frequent[3]. Most neuroblastomas develop as sporadic tumors, although rare familial cases have been reported. Primary cutaneous PNETs are tumors of adulthood (mean age is 40 years) and are exceedingly rare[3].

Pathogenesis

PNETs of the skin either represent metastases from a PNET of the adrenals and/or the ganglionic chain (traditionally designated as neuroblastomas) or develop *de novo* from heterotopic neural crest cells[3]. In the latter case, they are referred to as peripheral PNETs or as peripheral neuroblastomas. Recent studies have shown loss of heterozygosity involving chromosome bands 1p36 and 11q23, abnormal amplification of N-*myc*, and abnormal nerve growth factor/nerve growth factor receptor pathways[3,96].

Clinical Features

The cutaneous metastases of neuroblastoma in children often manifest as multiple blue or purple dermal papules or nodules (Fig. 115.21), resembling the 'blueberry muffin' lesions seen with congenital infectious or hematologic disorders[5] (see Ch. 121). These nodules may blanch on stroking[97,98]. Serum and urine catecholamine levels are typically elevated. Spontaneous regression has been described in stage IV-S[7] but rarely can occur in other stages.

PNETs in adults are rapidly growing dermal or subcutaneous nodules that favor the trunk or head. Ulceration is common. These highly aggressive neoplasms have an almost invariably fatal outcome[99].

Pathology

Metastatic neuroblastoma is an ill-defined or infiltrative mass in the dermis and/or the subcutis. However, smaller, more superficial deposits are more well defined. The mass is composed of atypical, small, dark cells with scant cytoplasm[3,95]. The cells have larger nuclei than mature lymphocytes, with a coarse chromatin pattern. The cells form irregular nests, cords or poorly cohesive sheets. Rosette formation, by concentrically arranged tumor cells in double or multiple circles, is common. The center of the rosettes contains converging fine fibrillary material characteristic of Homer Wright-type rosettes[3] (Fig. 115.22). Mitotic activity is high, and abnormal mitoses are abundant. Extensive areas of necrosis and hemorrhage are common.

As the tumor differentiates, the relative proportion of neuroblastoma components decreases, and the ganglioneuromatous elements increase. Eventually, the tumor may become a ganglioneuroma[99]. Immunohistochemically, the cells react variably with neural and neuroendocrine markers, depending on their state of differentiation. These markers

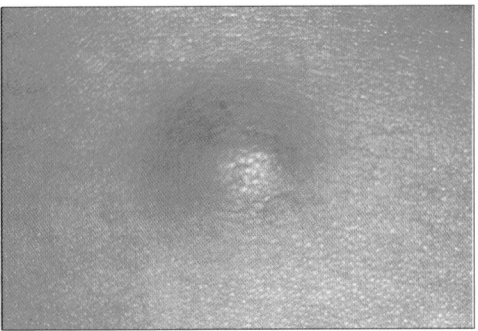

Fig. 115.21 Neuroblastoma. A cutaneous metastasis of neuroblastoma in a child presenting as a violaceous, blanchable, dermal nodule on the abdomen.

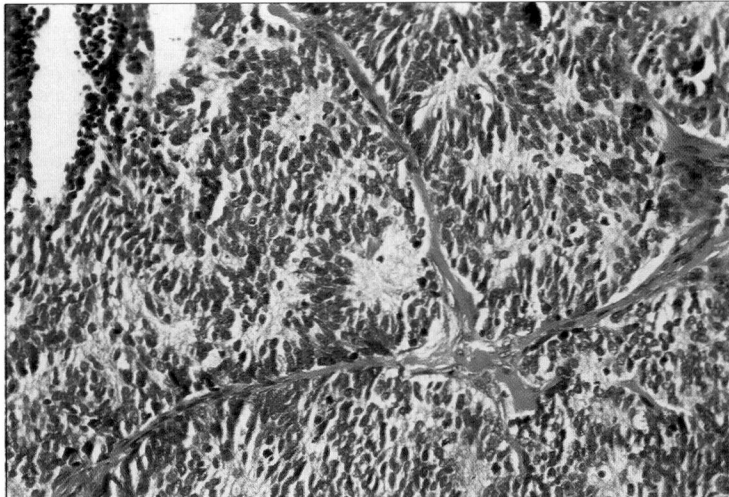

Fig. 115.22 Cutaneous neuroblastoma. The tumor is composed of small cells with small, round to ovoid nuclei that can be arranged in rosettes. The fibrillary material in the center of Homer Wright-type rosettes is characteristic.

include neuron-specific enolase, S100 protein, neurofilaments, synaptophysin, chromogranin and CD99[96].

Primary PNETs have similar histopathologic features to those of the classic neuroblastoma, but ganglionic or neuromatous differentiation is not characteristic. PNET also shares the main immunohistochemical features with classic neuroblastoma. However, Mic-2(013) is commonly expressed by PNETs, but not by neuroblastoma, facilitating their distinction[96,101–104].

Differential Diagnosis

The clinical differential diagnosis includes other types of cutaneous metastasis, mastocytomas, angiolipomas, adnexal tumors, cutaneous lymphoma and melanoma. Histologically, both metastatic neuro-

blastoma and primary cutaneous neuroectodermal tumor must be differentiated from other rosette-forming small, round, blue cell tumors that may involve the skin[102–104] (see introductory chapter).

Treatment

The effective treatment of neuroblastoma requires an interdisciplinary team that includes oncologists, surgeons and radiation therapists. The overall prognosis of localized tumor involvement has recently improved with combined multiagent chemotherapy, radiation therapy and surgical excision. Important prognostic factors include the presence of metastasis, tumor size, histologic parameters, type of tumor suppressor gene expression and response to initial chemotherapy[3].

REFERENCES

1. Argenyi ZB. Recent developments in cutaneous neural neoplasms. J Cutan Pathol. 1993;20:97–108.
2. Scheithauer BW, Woodruff JM, Erlandson RA. Tumors of the peripheral nervous system. In: Atlas of Tumor Pathology, 3rd series, Fascicle 24. Washington, DC: Armed Forces Institute of Pathology, 1999:1–415.
3. Enzinger FM, Weiss SW. Benign tumors of peripheral nerves. In: Soft Tissue Tumors, 4th edn. St. Louis: Mosby, 2001:1111–207.
4. Huber CC, Lewis LD. Amputation neuroma: their development and prevention. Arch Surg. 1920; 1:85–9.
5. Reed RJ, Fine RM, Meltzer HD. Palisaded, encapsulated neuromas of the skin. Arch Dermatol. 1972; 106:865–70.
6. Lundborg G. Nerve regeneration and repair: a review. Acta Orthop Scand. 1987;58:145–69.
7. Argenyi ZB, Santa Cruz D, Bromley C. Comparative light-microscopic and immunohistochemical study of traumatic and palisaded, encapsulated neuromas of the skin. Am J Dermatopathol. 1992;14:504–10.
8. Das Gupta TW, Brasfield RD. Amputation neuromas in cancer patients. NY J Med. 1969;69:2129–32.
9. Matthews GJ, Osterholm JL. Painful traumatic neuromas. Surg Clin North Am. 1972;51:1313–24.
10. Burtner DD, Goodman M. Traumatic neuroma of the nose. Arch Otolaryngol. 1972;103:108–9.
11. Shapiro L, Juklin EA, Brownstein HM. Rudimentary polydactyly. Arch Dermatol. 1973;108:223–5.
12. Dakin MC, Leppard B, Theaker JM. The palisaded, encapsulated neuroma (solitary circumscribed neuroma). Histopathology. 1992;20:405–10.
13. Argenyi ZB. Immunohistochemical characterization of palisaded encapsulated neuroma. J Cutan Pathol. 1990;17:329–35.
14. Argenyi ZB, Cooper PH, Santa Cuz D. Plexiform and other unusual variants of palisaded encapsulated neuroma. J Cutan Pathol. 1993;20:34–9.
15. Argenyi ZB. Newly recognized neural neoplasms relevant to the dermatopathologist. Dermatol Clin. 1992;10:219–34.
16. Stout AP. The peripheral manifestations of specific nerve sheath tumor (neurilemoma). Am J Cancer. 1935;24:751–96.
17. Verocay J. Multiple Geschwülste als Systemerkrankung am nervösen Apparate. Festschrift Hans Chiari aus Anlasz Seines 25 Jèhrigen Professoren-Jubilaüms Gewidmet. W. Braumüller, Wein and Leipzig, 1908:378–415.
18. Izumi AK, Rosato FE, Wood MG. Von Recklinghausen's disease associated with multiple neurilemomas. Arch Dermatol. 1971;104:172–6.
19. Shishiba T, Niimura M, Ohtsuka F, et al. Multiple cutaneous neurilemomas as a skin manifestation of neurilemmomatosis. J Am Acad Dermatol. 1984;10:744–54.
20. Purcell SM, Dixon SL. Schwannomatosis: an unusual variant of neurofibromatosis or a distinct clinical entity? Arch Dermatol. 1989;125:390–3.
21. MacCollin M, Woodfin W, Kronn D, Short MP. Schwannomatosis: a clinical and pathologic study. Neurology. 1996;46:1072–9.
22. Reith JD, Goldblum JR. Multiple cutaneous plexiform schwannomas: report of a case and review of the literature with particular reference to the association with types 1 and 2 neurofibromatosis and

schwannomatosis. Arch Pathol Lab Med. 1996;120:399–401.
23. Sainz J, Huynh PD, Figueroa K, et al. Mutations of the neurofibromatosis type 2 gene and lack of the gene product in vestibular schwannomas. Hum Mol Genet. 1994;3:885–91.
24. Das Gupta TK, Brasfield RD, Strong EW, et al. Benign solitary schwannomas (neurilemomas). Cancer. 1969;24:355–66.
25. White NB. Neurilemomas of the extremities. J Bone Joint Surg Am. 1967;49:1605–10.
26. Whitaker WG, Droulias C. Benign encapsulated neurilemoma: a report of 76 cases. Am Surg. 1976;42:675–8.
27. Jacobs RL, Barmada R. Neurilemoma: a review of the literature with six case reports. Arch Surg. 1971;102:181–6.
28. Vilanova JR, Burgos-Bretones JJ, Alvarez JA, et al. Benign schwannomas: a histopathological and morphometric study. Pathology. 1982;137:281–6.
29. Dahl I, Hagmar B, Idvall I. Benign solitary neurilemoma (schwannoma): a correlative cytological and histological study of 28 cases. Acta Pathol Microbiol Immunol Scand. 1984;92:91–101.
30. Argenyi ZB, Balogh K, Abraham AA. Degenerative ('ancient') changes in benign cutaneous schwannoma: a light microscopic, histochemical and immunohistochemical study. J Cutan Pathol. 1993;20:148–53.
31. Woodruff JM, Marshall ML, Gowin TA, et al. Plexiform (multinodular) schwannoma: a tumor simulating the plexiform neurofibroma. Am J Surg Pathol. 1983; 7:691–7.
32. Kao GF, Laskin WB, Olsen TG. Solitary cutaneous plexiform neurilemmoma (schwannoma): a clinicopathologic, immunohistochemical and ultrastructural study of 11 cases. Mod Pathol. 1986;2:20–6.
33. Argenyi ZB, Goodenberger ME, Strauss JS. Congenital neural hamartoma ('fascicular schwannoma'): a light microscopic, immunohistochemical, and ultrastructural study. Am J Dermatopathol. 1990;12:283–93.
34. Woodruff JM, Susin M, Godwin TA, et al. Cellular schwannoma: a variety of schwannoma sometimes mistaken for a malignant tumor. Am J Surg Pathol. 1981;5:733–44.
35. Hajdu SI. Schwannomas. Mod Pathol. 1995;8:109–14.
36. Verocay J. Zur kenntnis der Neurofibrome. Beitr Pathol Annat Allg Pathol. 1910;48:1–69.
37. Riccardi VM. Neurofibromatosis: the importance of localized or otherwise atypical forms. Arch Dermatol. 1987;123:882–9.
38. Lassmann H, Jurecka W, Lassmann W, et al. Different types of benign nerve sheath tumors: light microscopy, electron microscopy, and autoradiography. Virchows Arch A Pathol Anat Histol. 1977;375:197–210.
39. Megahed M. Histopathological variants of neurofibroma. A study of 114 lesions. Am J Dermatopathol. 1994;16:486–95.
40. Lin BT, Weiss LM, Medeiros LJ. Neurofibroma and cellular neurofibroma with atypia: a report of 14 tumors. Am J Surg Pathol. 1997;21:1443–9.
41. Argenyi ZB, LeBoit PE, Santa Cruz D, Swanson PE, Kutzner H. Nerve sheath myxoma (neurothekeoma) of the skin: light microscopic and immunohistochemical

reappraisal of the cellular variant. J Cutan Pathol. 1993;20:294–303.
42. Argenyi ZB, Kutzner H, Seaba MM. Ultrastructural spectrum of cutaneous nerve sheath myxoma/cellular neurothekeoma. J Cutan Pathol. 1995;22:137–45.
43. Harkin JC, Reed RJ. Tumors of the peripheral nervous system. In: Atlas of Tumor Pathology, 2nd series, Fascicle 3. Washington, DC: Armed Forces Institute of Pathology, 1969:60–4.
44. Rosati LA, Fratamico FCM, Eusebi V. Cellular neurothekeoma. Appl Pathol. 1986;4:186–91.
45. Angervall L, Kindblom LG, Haglid K. Dermal nerve sheath myxoma. A light and electron microscopic, histochemical and immunohistochemical study. Cancer 1984;53:1752–9.
46. Aronson PJ, Fretzin DF, Potter BS. Neurothekeoma of Gallagher and Helwig (dermal nerve sheath myxoma variant): report of a case with electron microscopic and immunohistochemical studies. J Cutan Pathol. 1985;12:506–19.
47. Barnhill RL, Mihm MC Jr. Cellular neurothekeoma. A distinctive variant of neurothekeoma mimicking nevomelanocytic tumors. Am J Surg Pathol. 1990;14:113–20.
48. Barnhill RL, Dickersin GR, Nickeleit V, et al. Studies on the cellular origin of neurothekeoma: clinical, light microscopic, immunohistochemical and ultrastructural observations. J Am Acad Dermatol. 1991;25:80–8.
49. Fletcher CD, Chan JK, McKee PH. Dermal nerve sheath myxoma: a study of three cases. Histopathology. 1986;10:135–45.
50. Calonje E, Wilson-Jones E, Smith NP, Fletcher CD. Cellular neurothekeoma: an epithelioid variant of pilar leiomyoma? Morphological and immunohistochemical analysis of a series. Histopathology. 1992;20:397–404.
51. Wang AR, May D, Bourne P, Scott G. PGP9.5: a marker for cellular neurothekeoma. Am J Surg Pathol. 1999;23:1401–7.
52. Busam KJ, Mentzel T, Colpaert C, et al. Atypical or worrisome features in cellular neurothekeoma. A study of 10 cases. Am J Surg Pathol. 1998;22:1067–72.
53. Abrikossoff A. Myomas originating from transversely striated voluntary musculature. Virchow Arch. 1926;260:215–33.
54. Feyrter F. Uber die granularen neurogenen Gewachse. Beitr Pathol Anat. 1949;110:181–208.
55. Abenoza P, Sibley RK. Granular cell myoma and schwannoma: fine structural and immunohistochemical study. Ultrastruct Pathol. 1987;11:19–28.
56. Bedetti CD, Martinez AJ, Beckford NS, May M. Granular cell tumor arising in myelinated peripheral nerves. Light and electron microscopy and immunoperoxidase study. Virchows Arch. 1983;402:175–83.
57. Fisher ER, Wechsler H. Granular cell myoblastoma – a misnomer. Electron-microscopic and histochemical evidence concerning its Schwann cell derivation and nature (granular cell schwannoma). Cancer. 1962;15:936–54.
58. Armin A, Connelly EM, Rowden G. An immunoperoxidase investigation of S-100 protein in granular cell myoblastomas: evidence for Schwann cell derivation. Am J Clin Pathol. 1983;79:37–44.
59. Filie AC, Lage JM, Azumi N. Immunoreactivity of S-100 protein, alpha-1 antitrypsin, and CD68 in adult and congenital granular cell tumors. Mod Pathol. 1996;9:888–92.

115

60. Mentzel T, Wadden C, Fletcher CD. Granular cell change in smooth muscle tumors of skin and soft tissue. Histopathology. 1994;24:223–31.

61. Lee J, Bhawan J, Wax F, Farber J. Plexiform granular cell tumor. A report of two cases. Am J Dermatopathol. 1994;16:537–41.

62. Simsir A, Osborne BM, Greenebaum E. Malignant granular cell tumor: a case report and review of the recent literature. Hum Pathol. 1996;27:853–8.

63. Fanburg-Smith JC, Meis-Kindblom JM, Fante R, Kindblom LG. Malignant granular cell tumor of soft tissue. Diagnostic criteria and clinicopathologic correlation. Am J Surg Pathol. 1998;22:779–94.

64. Apisarnthanarax P. Granular cell tumor. An analysis of 16 cases and review of the literature. J Am Acad Dermatol. 1981;5:171–82.

65. Suster S, Rosen LB, Sanchez JL. Granular cell leiomyosarcoma of the skin. Am J Dermatopathol. 1988;10:234–9.

66. Erlandson RA, Woodruff JM. Peripheral nerve sheath tumors: an electron microscopic study of 43 cases. Cancer. 1982;49:273–87.

67. Wanebo JE, Malik JM, Vandenberg SE, et al. Malignant peripheral nerve sheath tumors: a clinicopathologic study of 28 cases. Cancer. 1993; 71:1247–53.

68. Hirose T, Hasegawa T, Kudo E. Malignant peripheral nerve sheath tumors: an immunohistochemical study in relation to ultrastructural features. Hum Pathol. 1992;23:865–70.

69. Wick MR, Swanson PE, Scheithauer BW, et al. Malignant peripheral nerve sheath tumor: an immunohistochemical study of cases. Am J Clin Pathol. 1987;87:425–33.

70. Toker C. Trabecular carcinoma of the skin. Arch Dermatol. 1972;105:107–10.

71. Sibley RK, Dehner LP, Rosai J. Primary neuroendocrine (Merkel cell?) carcinoma of the skin. I. Am J Surg Pathol. 1985;9:95–108.

72. Ratner D, Nelson BR, Brown MD, et al. Merkel cell carcinoma. J Am Acad Dermatol. 1993;29:143–56.

73. Wick MR, Scheithauer BW. Primary neuroendocrine carcinoma of the skin. In: Wick MR (ed.). Pathology of Unusual Malignant Cutaneous Tumors. New York: Marcel Dekker, 1985;107–72.

74. Cheuk W, Kwan MY, Suster S, Chan JK. Immunostaining for thyroid transcription factor 1 and cytokeratin 20 aids the distinction of small cell carcinoma from Merkel cell carcinoma, but not pulmonary from extrapulmonary small cell carcinomas. Arch Pathol Lab Med. 2001;125:228–31.

75. LeBoit PE, Crutcher WA, Shapiro PE. Pagetoid intraepidermal spread in Merkel cell (primary neuroendocrine) carcinoma of the skin. Am J Surg Pathol. 1992;16:584–92.

76. Medina-Franco H, Urist MM, Fiveash J, Heslin MJ, Bland KI, Beenken SW. Multimodality treatment of Merkel cell carcinoma: case series and literature review of 1024 cases. Ann Surg Oncol. 2001;8:204–8.

77. Duker I, Starz H, Bachter D, Balda BR. Prognostic and therapeutic implications of sentinel lymphonodectomy and S-staging in Merkel cell carcinoma. Dermatology. 2001;202:225–9.

77a. Gupta SG, Wang LC, Penas LC, et al. Sentinel lymph node biopsy for evaluation and treatment of patients with Merkel cell carcinoma: The Dana-Farber experience and meta-analysis of the literature. Arch Dermatol. 2006;142:771–4.

78. Schmidt MB. Über seltene Spaltbildungen im Bereiche des mittleren Stirnfortsatzes. Virchow Arch Pathol Anat. 1900;162:340–70.

79. Patterson K, Kapur S, Chandra RS. 'Nasal gliomas' and related brain heterotopias: a pathologist's perspective. Pediatr Pathol. 1986;5:353–62.

80. Yeoh GPS, Bale PM, DeSilva M. Nasal cerebral heterotopia: the so-called nasal glioma or sequestered encephalocele and its variants. Pediatr Pathol. 1989;9:531–49.

81. Orkin M, Fisher I. Heterotopic brain tissue (heterotopic neural rest): case report with review of related anomalies. Arch Dermatol. 1966;94:699–708.

82. Fletcher CDM, Carpenter G, McKee PH. Nasal glioma: a rarity. Am J Dermatopathol. 1986;8:341–6.

83. Kennard CD, Rasmussen JE. Congenital midline nasal masses: diagnosis and management. J Dermatol Surg Oncol. 1990;16:1025–36.

84. Winkler M. Ueber Psammome der Haut und des Unterhautgewebes. Arch Pathol Anat. 1904;178:323–50.

85. Lopez DA, Silvers DN, Helwig EB. Cutaneous meningiomas: a clinicopathologic study. Cancer. 1974;34:728–44.

86. Sibley DA, Cooper PH. Rudimentary meningocele: a variant of 'primary cutaneous meningioma'. J Cutan Pathol. 1989;16:72–80.

87. Berry AD III, Patterson W. Meningoceles, meningomyeloceles, and encephaloceles: a neuro-dermatopathologic study of 132 cases. J Cutan Pathol. 1991;18:164–77.

88. Argenyi ZB. Cutaneous neural heterotopias and related tumors relevant for the dermatopathologist. Semin Diagn Pathol. 1996;13:60–71.

89. Argenyi ZB, Thielberg MD, Hayes CM, Whitaker DC. Primary cutaneous meningioma associated with von Recklinghausen disease. Cutan Pathol. 1994;21:549–56.

90. Marrogi AJ, Swanson PE, Kyriakos M, et al. Rudimentary meningocele of the skin: clinicopathologic features and differential diagnosis. J Cutan Pathol. 1991;18:178–88.

91. Nochomovitz LE, Jannotta F, Orenstein JM. Meningioma of the scalp: light and electron microscopic observations. Arch Pathol Lab Med. 1985;109:92–5.

92. Theaker JM, Fleming KA. Meningioma of the scalp: a case report with immunohistological features. J Cutan Pathol. 1987;14:49–53.

93. Gelli MC, Pasquinelli G, Martinelli G, et al. Cutaneous meningioma: histochemical, immunohistochemical and ultrastructural investigation. Histopathology. 1993;23:576–8.

94. Stout AP. A tumor of the ulnar nerve. Proc NY Pathol Soc. 1918;18:2–12.

95. Dehner LP. Peripheral and central primitive neuroectodermal tumors: a nosologic concept seeking a consensus. Arch Pathol Lab Med. 1986;110:997–1005.

96. Stevenson AJ, Chatten J, Bertoni F, et al. CD99 (p30/32 MIC2) neuroectodermal/Ewing's sarcoma antigen as an immunohistochemical marker: review of more than 600 tumors and the literature experience. Appl Immunohistochem. 1994;2:231–40.

97. Shown TE, Durfee MF. Blueberry muffin baby: neonatal neuroblastoma with subcutaneous metastases. J Urol. 1970;104:193–5.

98. Hawthorne HC, Nelson JS, Witzelben CL, et al. Blanching subcutaneous nodules in neonatal neuroblastoma. J Pediatr. 1970;77:297–300.

99. Evans AE, Chatten J, D'Angio GD, et al. A review of 17 IV-S neuroblastoma patients at the Children's Hospital of Philadelphia. Cancer. 1980;45:833–9.

100. Aleshire DL, Glick AD, Cruz VE, et al. Neuroblastoma in adults: pathologic findings and clinical outcome. Arch Pathol Lab Med. 1985;109:352–6.

101. Argenyi ZB, Bergfeld WF, McMahon JT, et al. Primitive neuroectodermal tumor in the skin with features of neuroblastoma in an adult patient. J Cutan Pathol. 1986;13:420–30.

102. Nguyen AV, Argenyi ZB. Cutaneous neuroblastoma: peripheral neuroblastoma. Am J Dermatopathol. 1993;15:7–14.

103. Joshi VV, Silverman JF. Pathology of neuroblastic tumors. Semin Diagn Pathol. 1994;11:107–17.

104. Banerjee SS, Agbamu DA, Eyden BP, Harris M. Clinicopathological characteristics of peripheral primitive neuroectodermal tumour of skin and subcutaneous tissue. Histopathology. 1997;31:355–66.

Fibrous and Fibrohistiocytic Proliferations of the Skin and Tendons

116

Hideko Kamino, Shane A Meehan and John Pui

Chapter Contents

Key features

- Fibrous and fibrohistiocytic proliferations of the skin and tendons are common lesions that include both neoplastic and 'reactive' processes

- Common benign fibrous and fibrohistiocytic proliferations, some of their atypical variants that could be misdiagnosed as malignant tumors, and corresponding malignant neoplasms are reviewed

- These tumors are composed of fibroblasts, myofibroblasts, histiocytes, dermal dendritic cells, collagen fibers, elastic fibers, and connective tissue mucin, and they are present in variable proportions, depending upon the particular lesion

- Immunohistochemical stains for vimentin for non-specific mesenchymal components; factor XIIIa and CD34 for dermal dendritic cells; KP-1, HAM 56, MAC 387 and α_1-antichymotrypsin for histiocytes; and muscle-specific actin for myofibroblasts are helpful in evaluating these lesions

SKIN TAG

Synonyms: ■ Acrochordon ■ Fibroepithelial polyp ■ Soft fibroma

Clinical Features

This is the most common fibrous lesion of the skin and presents as a soft skin-colored to slightly hyperpigmented pedunculated papule, predominantly on the neck and in the axilla and groin, as well as scattered elsewhere. They may be single or multiple and range in size from 1–2 mm papules on the eyelids to 1–2 cm baggy polyps on the trunk. They are usually asymptomatic, but on occasion can become painful secondary to irritation or torsion and infarction, with an accompanying change in color to a darker red–brown hue (Fig. 116.1).

Epidemiology

Skin tags are very common, and their incidence increases with age. Men and women are equally affected, and close to 50% of all individuals have at least one skin tag[1]. Clinically, skin tags can resemble intra-dermal melanocytic nevi, seborrheic keratoses and, less commonly, a pedunculated neurofibroma.

Although skin tags were initially thought to be associated with colonic polyps[2] and diabetes mellitus[3], later studies have not confirmed this finding[4,5]. The skin tags associated with Birt–Hogg–Dubé syndrome and Cowden disease are hamartomatous in origin and histologically different from conventional skin tags[6,7]. The skin tags in Birt–Hogg–Dubé syndrome are fibrofolliculomas, trichodiscomas and perifollicular fibromas, whereas in Cowden disease the skin tags are sclerotic fibromas.

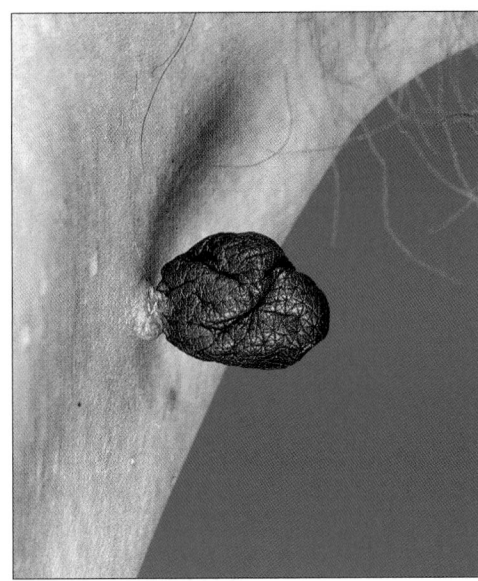

Fig. 116.1 Infarcted skin tag. A pedunculated dark-red papule in the axilla. Courtesy of the Ronald O. Perelman Department of Dermatology, New York University.

Pathology

Histologically, skin tags are polypoid with variably loose to dense collagenous stroma with thin-walled, dilated blood vessels in the center. The overlying epidermis may have increased pigment within the basal keratinocytes, but is not hyperplastic unless the lesion has been rubbed. Adipocytes are sometimes seen admixed within the core of larger skin tags (sometimes called lipofibroma or fibroma molle). The histopathologic differential diagnosis includes seborrheic keratosis, nevus lipomatosus superficialis, angiofibroma and intradermal melanocytic nevus.

Treatment

Unless irritated or infarcted, skin tags are more of a cosmetic issue than a clinical concern and can be easily removed by simple scissor excision, electrodesiccation or cryosurgery.

CUTANEOUS ANGIOFIBROMA

Synonyms: ■ Fibrous papule ■ Pearly penile papule ■ Periungual fibroma

Cutaneous angiofibroma is a descriptive term for a group of lesions with different clinical presentations and implications, but similar histologic findings.

Clinical Features

Fibrous papules are solitary, skin-colored, shiny, dome-shaped papules located on the face of adults, most commonly on the nose (Fig. 116.2)[8]. Clinically, they can mimic small intradermal melanocytic nevi, basal cell carcinomas or appendageal tumors. Although benign, they are commonly sampled to exclude basal cell carcinoma. Shave excision and electrodesiccation have been used to remove them completely.

Pearly penile papules are pearly, white, dome-shaped, closely aggregated small papules located on the glans penis, commonly in a multi-layered and circumferential manner on the corona (Fig. 116.3). They are found in up to 30% of young postpubertal adults, and are more common in uncircumcised men[9]. They can be mistaken for condyloma acuminata or hypertrophied sebaceous glands. They are benign but sometimes of significant cosmetic concern to the patient. No treatment is needed, only reassurance.

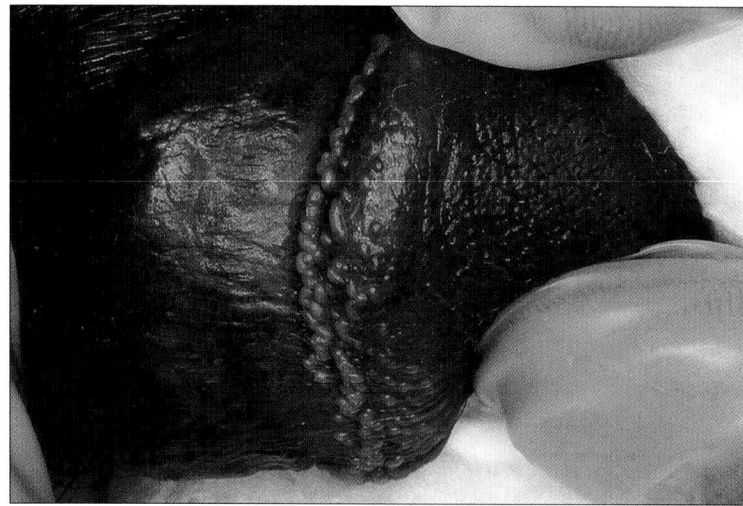

Fig. 116.3 Pearly penile papules. Multiple small white papules along the corona of the glans penis. Note the multilayered distribution. Courtesy of Kalman Watsky MD.

Multiple facial angiofibromas are associated with tuberous sclerosis (Fig. 116.4; see Ch. 60). Once known as *adenoma sebaceum* (a misnomer, as they are not adenomas, nor are they sebaceous), facial angiofibromas are usually distributed bilaterally on the cheeks, nasolabial folds and chin as well as the nose. Patients with tuberous sclerosis can also have multiple periungual fibromas, which are also angiofibromas and may have significant epidermal hyperplasia and orthokeratosis, depending on their location in relationship to the nail unit. The onset of facial angiofibromas in tuberous sclerosis is usually during early to mid childhood, with 75% of individuals with tuberous sclerosis developing these lesions. Periungual fibromas are less common in childhood but increase in incidence with age to 40% in adulthood. Both of these skin lesions are considered to be primary diagnostic features of tuberous sclerosis (see Table 60.6).

Pathology

All angiofibromas, including the facial angiofibromas associated with tuberous sclerosis, are dome-shaped lesions composed of a dermal proliferation of fibroblasts in a collagenous stroma with an increase in the number of thin-walled, dilated blood vessels. The collagen bundles tend to be arranged perpendicularly to the epidermis or in a concentric fashion around hair follicles and blood vessels (a variant known as perifollicular fibroma). Elastic fibers are decreased in number. Some fibroblasts are stellate in shape and can be multinucleated (Fig. 116.5). By immunohistochemistry, these cells are positive for factor XIIIa and negative for S100 protein, consistent with a dermal dendrocyte origin.

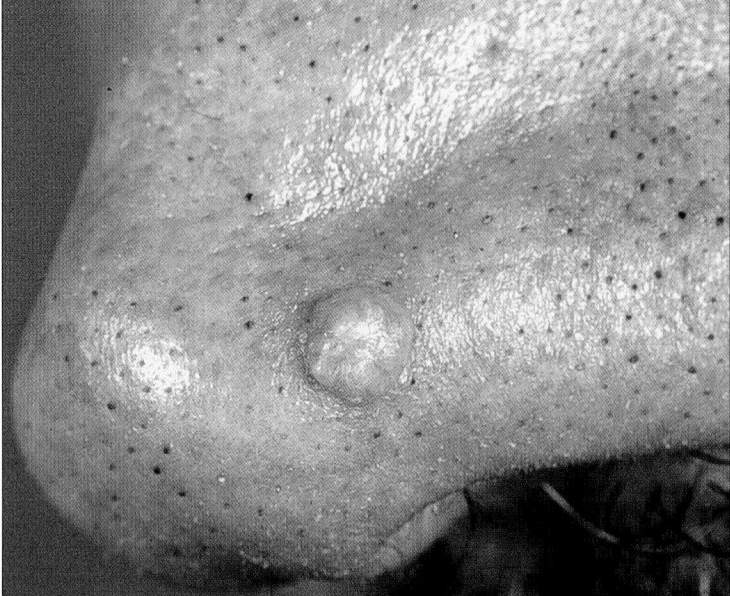

Fig. 116.2 Fibrous papule of the nose. A smooth, dome-shaped, skin-colored papule on the nose. Courtesy of the Ronald O. Perelman Department of Dermatology, New York University.

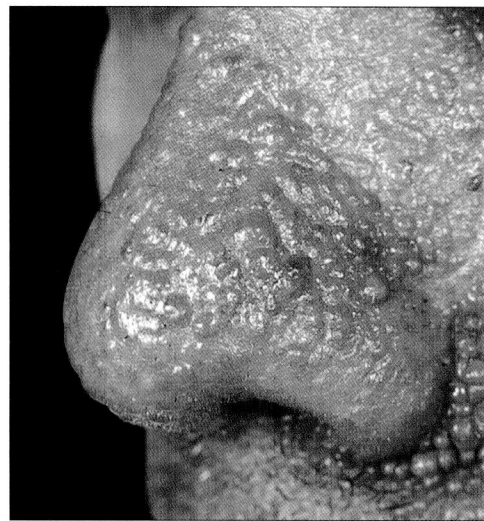

Fig. 116.4 Facial angiofibromas of tuberous sclerosis. There are multiple firm papules of the nose and cheek. Courtesy of the Ronald O. Perelman Department of Dermatology, New York University.

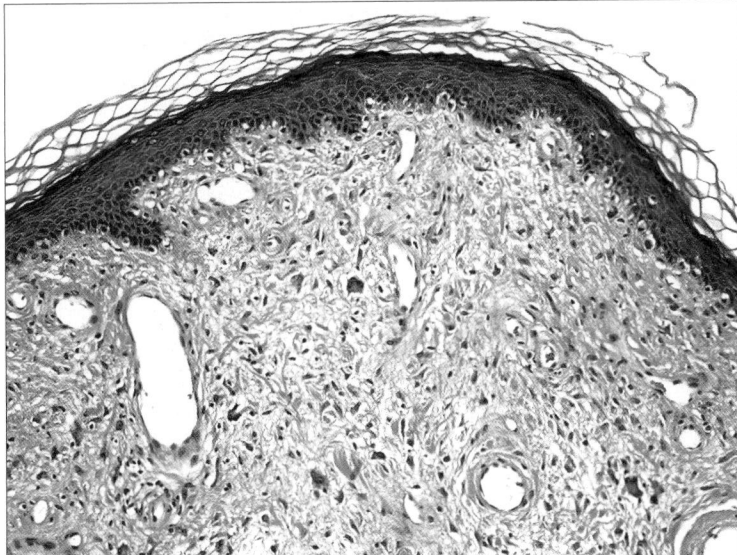

Fig. 116.5 Angiofibroma. Dermal fibroplasia with dilated, thin-walled vessels and large stellate fibroblasts is seen.

The overlying epidermis is sometimes slightly atrophic. The histopathologic differential diagnosis includes skin tags and intradermal melanocytic nevi.

DERMATOFIBROMA

Synonyms: ■ Fibroma simplex ■ Benign fibrous histiocytoma ■ Nodular subepidermal fibrosis ■ Histiocytoma ■ Sclerosing hemangioma ■ Dermal dendrocytoma

Clinical Features

Dermatofibromas are the second most common fibrohistiocytic tumor of the skin. They are seen primarily in adults and favor the lower extremities (Fig. 116.6) but may arise in any location. They are firm, minimally elevated to dome-shaped papules that usually measure from a few millimeters to 1 cm in diameter, but occasionally are up to 2 cm in size. The lesions are commonly hyperpigmented, but in patients with lightly pigmented skin may appear tan to pink in color. On palpation, they may seem attached to the subcutaneous tissue; pinching the lesion gently usually results in apparent downward movement of the tumor, also known as the dimple sign.

Although some dermatofibromas are thought to arise at sites of trauma or arthropod bites, their precise etiology is not known. Multiple

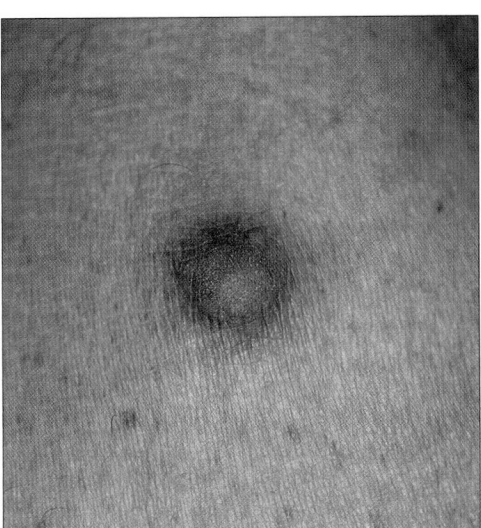

Fig. 116.6 Dermatofibroma. Hyperpigmented firm papule on the lower extremity. Courtesy of Jean L Bolognia MD.

eruptive dermatofibromas have been observed in patients with autoimmune disorders (e.g. lupus erythematosus), atopic dermatitis and in the setting of immunosuppression (e.g. HIV infection)[10]. Clinically, dermatofibromas can be confused with cysts or melanocytic nevi, especially those with fibrosis. In the case of larger lesions, the possibility of dermatofibrosarcoma protuberans (DFSP), which is less well defined and multilobulated, can be considered.

Pathology

Dermatofibromas are characterized by a nodular dermal proliferation, predominantly of spindle-shaped fibroblasts and myofibroblasts arranged as short intersecting fascicles (Fig. 116.7). The fibroblasts and myofibroblasts have plump oval nuclei with small nucleoli. Mitoses may be present. There may be a component of mono- or multinucleated histiocytes with vacuolated foamy (xanthomatous) cytoplasm (hence the synonym benign fibrous histiocytoma). Thick hyalinized collagen bundles are seen at the periphery ('keloidal' collagen), which are refractile with polarized light (Fig. 116.8)[11]. An increased number of small blood vessels and a perivascular infiltrate of lymphocytes and plasma cells may be present. Hemorrhage into a dermatofibroma (sclerosing hemangioma) is, at times, quite striking and explains the common finding of hemosiderin.

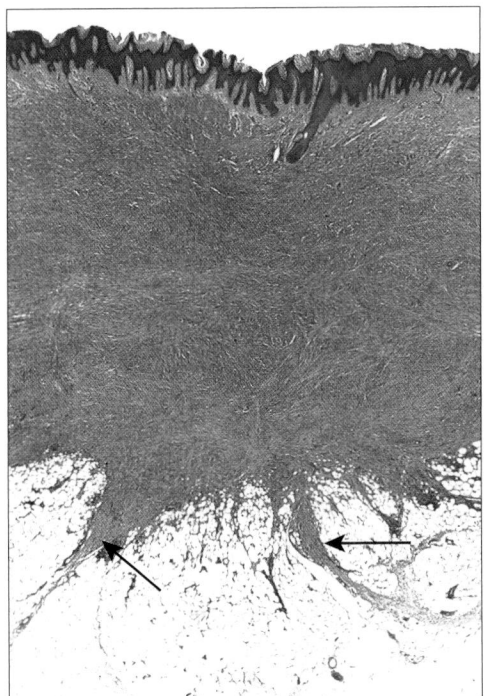

Fig. 116.7 Dermatofibroma. There is a nodular proliferation of spindled fibroblasts and histiocytes in the reticular dermis, with hyperplasia and hyperpigmentation of the overlying epidermis. Extension into the subcutaneous tissue occurs in a radial pattern (arrows).

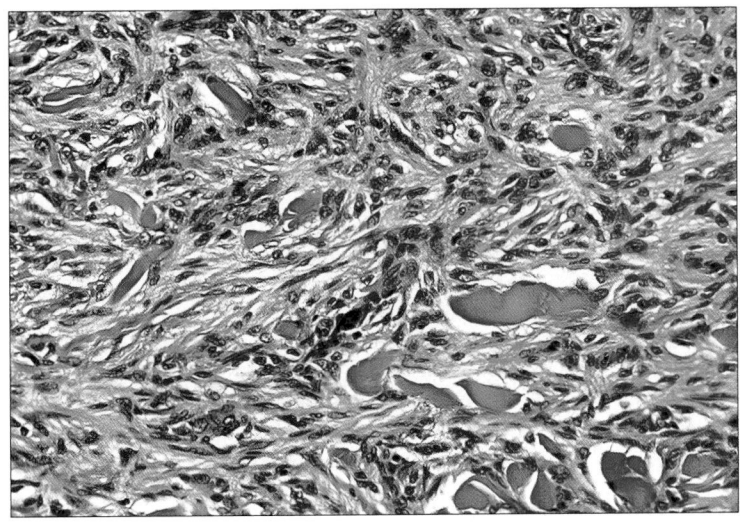

Fig. 116.8 Dermatofibroma. The fibroblasts are arranged in broad intersecting fascicles with entrapment of thick collagen bundles.

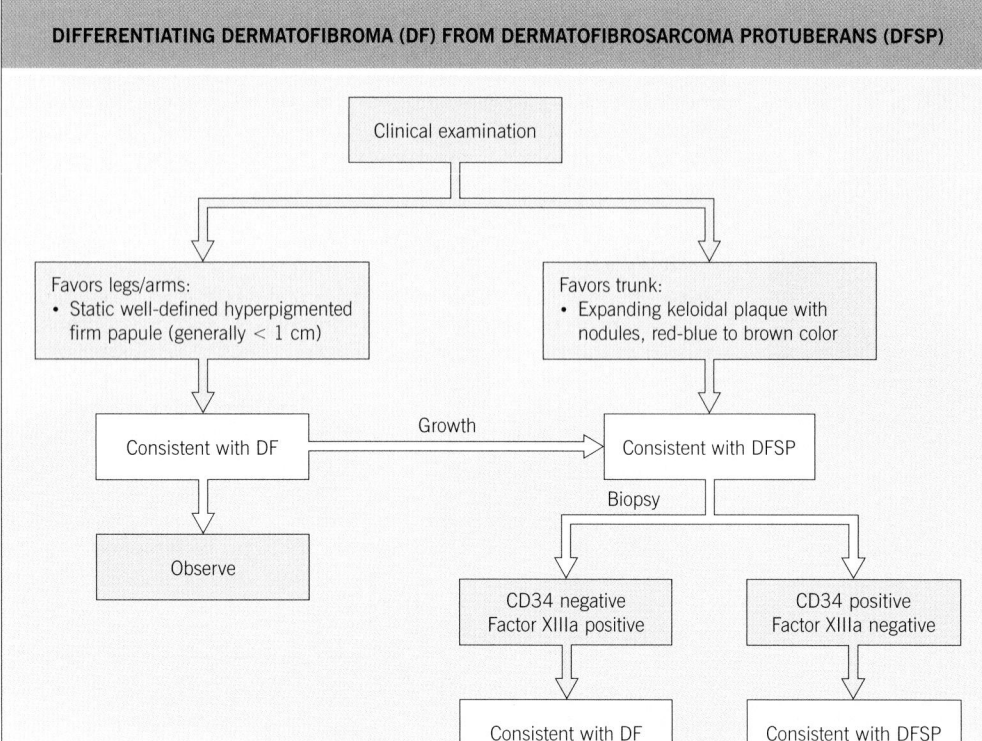

Fig. 116.9 Differentiating dermatofibroma (DF) from dermatofibrosarcoma protuberans (DFSP).

The overlying epidermis is usually hyperplastic with flat confluent rete ridges and hyperpigmentation of the basal layer (so-called 'dirty fingers'). Adnexal structures are usually absent at the center of the lesion; however, very often, small follicular or sebaceous structures are connected to the epidermis. Sometimes there are aggregates of basaloid cells with follicular differentiation emanating from the epidermis, which may be confused with a superficial basal cell carcinoma. There are, however, a few reported cases of true basal cell carcinomas evolving within longstanding dermatofibromas[12]. Histologic variants of dermatofibroma are listed in Table 116.1 (see below).

Positive immunohistochemical reactions for vimentin, factor XIIIa[13–16], muscle-specific actin, and histiocytic markers such as KP-1 and HAM 56, as well as a negative reaction for CD34, support a diagnosis of dermatofibroma (Fig. 116.9)[13,17]. Sometimes, however, at the periphery of dermatofibromas there is a relatively increased number of CD34-positive dermal dendritic cells, which appear to be the pre-existing dendritic cells that have been displaced by the expanding constituent cells of the dermatofibroma. The histologic differential diagnosis includes keloid, scar, dermatomyofibroma, DFSP (CD34+) and nodular Kaposi's sarcoma. Whether dermatofibromas are reactive or neoplastic has been an area of controversy. Recent studies have reported evidence of clonality in dermatofibromas, which supports the neoplastic nature of this tumor[18,19].

Treatment

Dermatofibromas may be biopsied or excised to exclude a melanocytic proliferation, a fibrosed cyst or other mesenchymal neoplasm. Excision for cosmetic purposes is of questionable value, as the resultant scar is often quite evident and sometimes more noticeable than the original lesion, especially on the legs. However, some patients prefer a scar rather than the nodular appearance of a dermatofibroma, and they may also wish to have histologic confirmation of the diagnosis. Undisturbed dermatofibromas usually persist, but with time may undergo partial regression, especially centrally.

Histologic Variants of Dermatofibroma (Table 116.1)
Dermatofibroma with atypical cells
- Pseudosarcomatous dermatofibroma[20]
- Atypical ('pseudosarcomatous') cutaneous histiocytoma[21]

HISTOLOGIC VARIANTS OF DERMATOFIBROMA

With atypical cells
Atrophic
Extending into the subcutaneous tissue (deep dermatofibroma)
Palisading
Aneurysmal (angiomatoid, hemosiderotic sclerosing hemangioma)
With osteoclast-like cells
Ossifying
Clear cell
Xanthomatous*
With granular cells

*May be yellow in color.

Table 116.1 Histologic variants of dermatofibroma.

- Atypical cutaneous fibrous histiocytoma[22]
- Dermatofibroma with monster cells[23].

The clinical presentation of dermatofibromas with atypical cells is similar to that of common dermatofibromas, except that the former are usually in middle-aged adults and are slightly larger than 1 cm in diameter. Clinical follow-up in three studies showed no evidence of recurrence after simple excision[21–23].

Dermatofibromas with atypical cells have the architectural pattern and components of common dermatofibromas. In addition, they have large atypical mono- and multinucleated cells with large pleomorphic and hyperchromatic nuclei, some of which have prominent nucleoli (Fig. 116.10). The atypical cells have abundant vacuolated cytoplasm, very often with hemosiderin deposits. Mitotic figures are rare, and atypical mitoses are not seen. The histopathologic differential diagnosis includes atypical fibroxanthoma (superficial malignant fibrous histiocytoma) and pleomorphic fibroma.

Deep dermatofibroma extending into the subcutaneous tissue
The deep variant of dermatofibroma can be confused clinically and histopathologically with DFSP. Deep dermatofibromas are usually seen on the trunk and proximal extremities of young to middle-aged patients and tend to be larger than the common variety, measuring 1–2 cm in diameter. The skin surface may be depressed, flat or dome-shaped, and

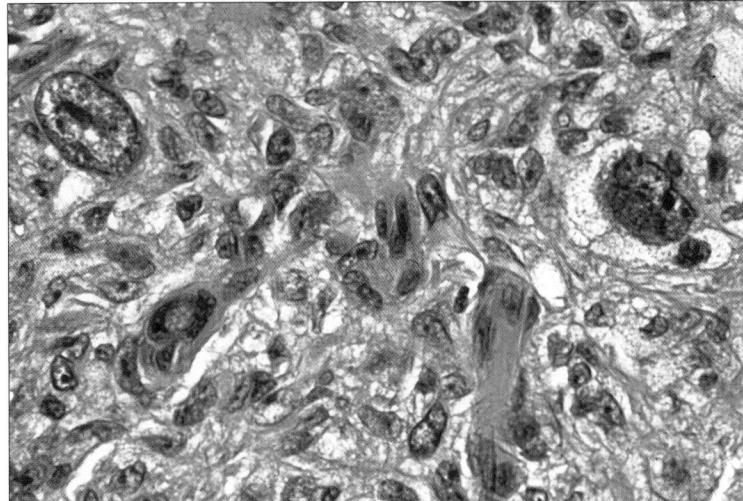

Fig. 116.10 **Dermatofibroma with atypical cells.** There are histiocyte-like cells with large hyperchromatic nuclei as well as scattered fibroblasts.

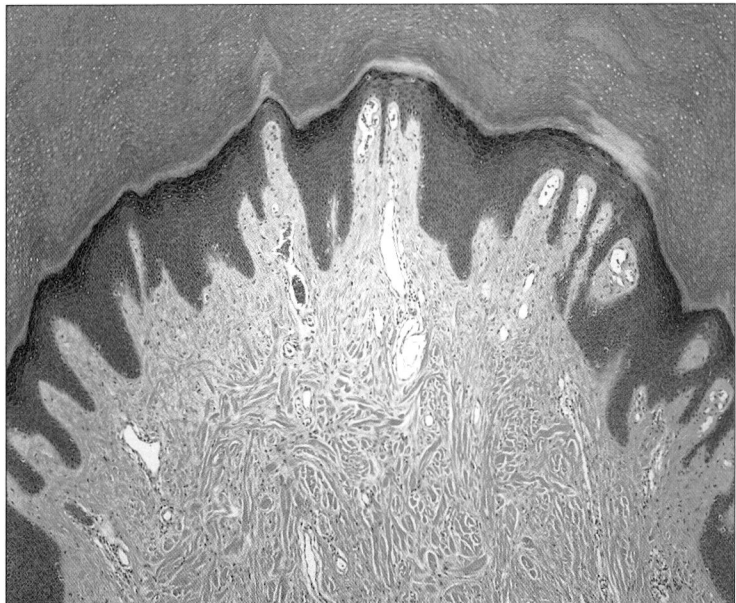

Fig. 116.12 **Acral fibrokeratoma.** There is a digitated fibrovascular core with vertically arranged collagen bundles lined by epidermal hyperplasia. Note the thick stratum corneum.

on palpation the tumor is attached to the underlying subcutaneous tissue. The clinical differential diagnosis includes a cyst, lipoma and DFSP.

The deep variant has histopathologic features similar to those of the common dermal dermatofibroma, but with extensions into the subcutaneous tissue in two main patterns[24]. In approximately 70% of cases, the dermatofibroma extends in a vertical or radial fashion, predominantly along the septae, which have a wedge-shaped appearance (see Fig. 116.7). In approximately 30% of cases, the base is well circumscribed, with a smooth deep margin. All the components present in the dermis extend into the subcutaneous tissue: fibroblasts, histiocytes, thick collagen bundles, and the lymphoplasmacytic inflammatory infiltrate. These patterns are different from the multilayered and 'honeycomb' patterns characteristic of DFSP. The histologic differential diagnosis includes DFSP, malignant fibrous histiocytoma and fibromatosis.

ACRAL FIBROKERATOMA

Synonym: ■ Acquired digital fibrokeratoma

Clinical Features

These uncommon lesions typically present as a solitary, skin-colored to pink, slightly keratotic exophytic papulonodule with a collarette of elevated skin. The most common site is the fingers (Fig. 116.11), but

they may appear elsewhere on acral skin. Acquired fibrokeratomas usually occur in middle-aged adults, and there is an unclear relationship to prior trauma[25]. Clinically, they can resemble a supernumerary digit (see Ch. 63), periungual fibroma, verruca, eccrine poroma, pyogenic granuloma or fibroma, and, less often, a cutaneous horn or dermatofibroma. Fibrokeratomas are benign and can be removed by shave excision.

Pathology

Acral fibrokeratomas are composed of thick collagen bundles surrounded by blood vessels, oriented perpendicularly to the epidermis. There is orthokeratosis with variable epidermal hyperplasia, and elastic fibers in the dermis are decreased (Fig. 116.12)[26]. The histopathologic differential diagnosis includes dermatofibroma, angiofibroma and supernumerary digit. The latter is congenital, almost always appears on the ulnar aspect of the hand, usually contains many nerves, and sometimes has central cartilage or bone. Periungual fibroma should also be considered, and some authors believe that the two entities are the same[8,27].

SUPERFICIAL ACRAL FIBROMYXOMA

Superficial acral fibromyxoma is a rare mesenchymal neoplasm that typically occurs on the digits of middle-age adults.

Clinical Features

In the original description by Fetsch et al.[28], there was a male predominance with patients ranging from 14 to 72 years of age (mean, 43 years; median, 46 years). The lesions are usually slow growing and seldom painful; some are preceded by trauma. These tumors most often appear in the ungual region, occasionally in association with deformity of the underlying bone. Less common sites are the finger or palm. If incompletely excised, lesions may persist or recur, but have not recurred if removed completely. There have been no reports to date of malignant transformation. The clinical differential diagnosis includes periungual fibroma, verruca, acquired fibrokeratoma, pyogenic granuloma and foreign body reaction.

Pathology

Superficial acral fibromyxomas are located within the dermis or subcutis and are non-encapsulated, moderately cellular and comprised of spindle- and stellate-shaped cells. The cells are arranged in a storiform

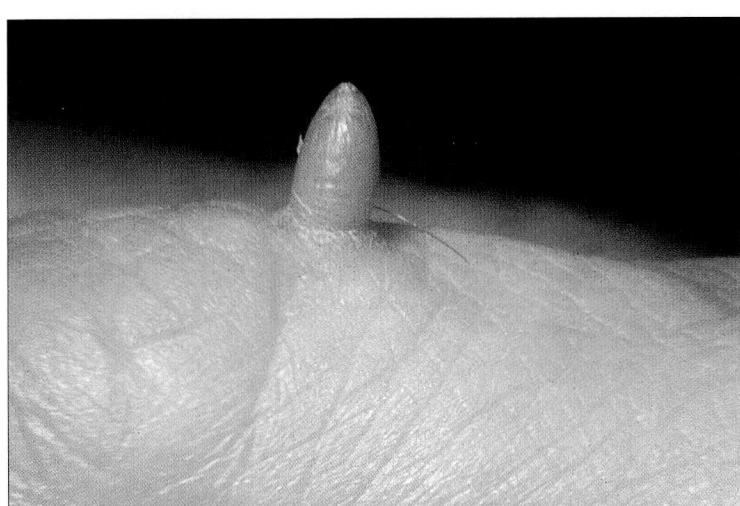

Fig. 116.11 **Acral fibrokeratoma.** A light-pink exophytic papule arising from the dorsal surface of the finger. Courtesy of the Ronald O. Perelman Department of Dermatology, New York University.

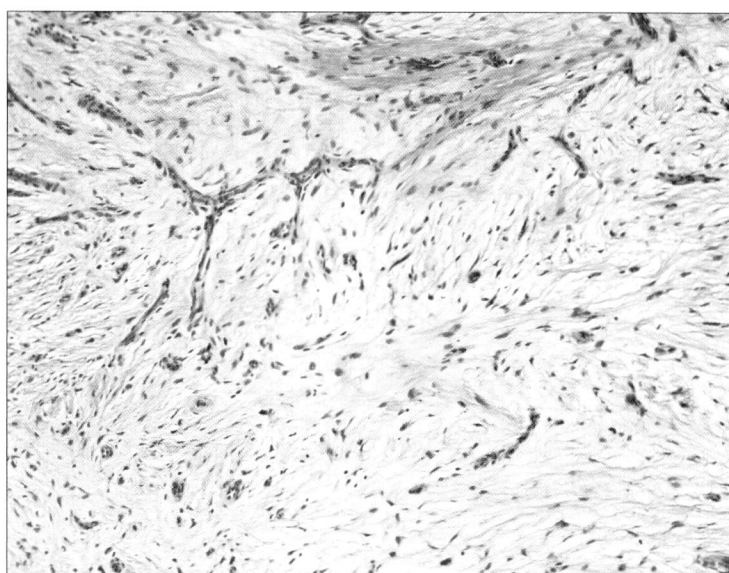

Fig. 116.13 Superficial acral fibromyxoma. The lesion is composed of spindle and stellate cells arranged in a loose storiform pattern with a myxoid collagenous matrix.

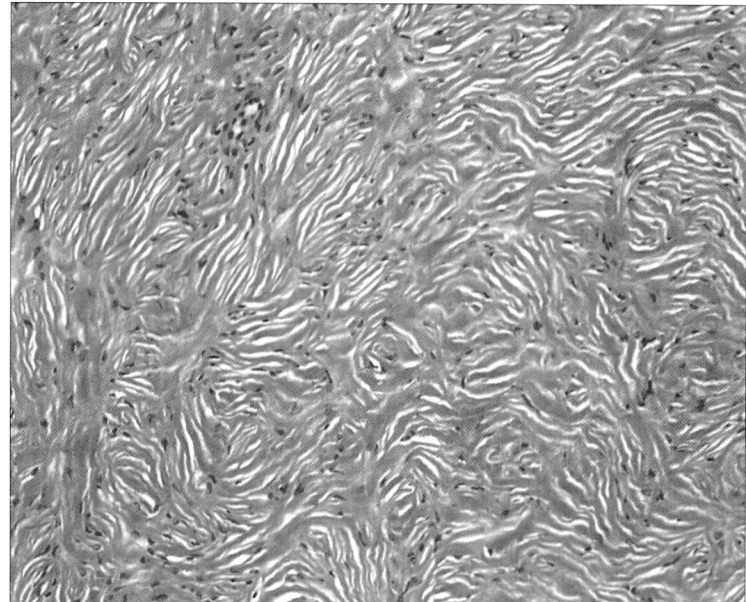

Fig. 116.14 Sclerotic fibroma. The collagen bundles in this hypocellular tumor are arranged in short parallel bundles, leading to a laminated or 'plywood' appearance.

or fascicular pattern within a myxoid or collagenous stroma that may have an increased number of blood vessels and mast cells (Fig. 116.13). CD34 is expressed in almost all tumors, with focal expression of epithelial membrane antigen in the majority of cases[29]. The differential diagnosis includes myxoid neurofibroma, sclerosing perineurioma, superficial angiomyxoma, acquired fibrokeratoma, dermatofibroma, DFSP and acral myxoinflammatory fibroblastic sarcoma.

SCLEROTIC FIBROMA OF THE SKIN

Clinical Features

This distinct, very collagenous variant of fibroma was originally reported as a component of the multiple hamartoma syndrome or Cowden disease[7]. However, a sporadic solitary form without association with other hamartomas has been more recently described[30].

In Cowden disease, the sclerotic fibromas can be solitary or multiple, and present on the skin and/or mucous membranes as pearly papules or nodules that measure from a few to up to 10 mm in diameter. The lesion usually appears during adulthood, and there is no gender predominance. In the sporadic form, there is no predilection for any particular anatomic site.

Pathology

Sclerotic fibromas are well-circumscribed, dome-shaped, dermal hypocellular nodules composed predominantly of sclerotic thick collagen bundles arranged as short intersecting stacks in a parallel arrangement and separated by spaces containing connective tissue mucin (plywood-like or whorl-like pattern; Fig. 116.14). Between the collagen bundles, there are thin fibroblasts with scanty cytoplasm and small nuclei. The blood vessels are small and inconspicuous, and the overlying epidermis is usually thin. The spindle cells react positively for vimentin and muscle-specific actin (and to a lesser degree for CD34), which highlights the spindle cells between thick collagen bundles[31,32]. Positivity for CD34 may result in the misdiagnosis of early DFSP. The matrix of sclerotic fibroma shows variable staining for collagen IV, procollagen and laminin[33]. The differential diagnosis includes pleomorphic fibroma of the skin, keloid and early DFSP.

PLEOMORPHIC FIBROMA OF THE SKIN

Clinical Features

This unusual variant of a fibroma was described by Kamino et al.[34] in 1989. Pleomorphic fibromas of the skin usually present in adults, with

a slight preponderance in women. They favor the extremities and present as asymptomatic, solitary, skin-colored, dome-shaped or polypoid papules which measure from a few millimeters to nearly 2 cm in diameter. Clinically, they resemble skin tags, neurofibromas or intradermal melanocytic nevi. Treatment is simple excision, and to date there have been no reports of recurrence.

Pathology

Pleomorphic fibromas are polypoid or dome-shaped, well-circumscribed dermal lesions characterized by low cellularity with a predominance of thick collagen bundles in a haphazard array. There are scattered spindle and irregularly shaped cells with scanty cytoplasm, indistinct cellular borders, and large pleomorphic and hyperchromatic nuclei. There are multinucleated giant cells, some of which show multilobed nuclei (Fig. 116.15). Mitotic figures are rare. In some cases, moderate amounts of connective tissue mucin and scattered adipocytes are present. The overlying epidermis is thinned. The spindle-shaped cells and the irregularly shaped, multinucleated giant cells are positive for vimentin. The larger multinucleated cells are also positive for CD34[35] and the spindle-shaped cells react positively for muscle-specific actin[31]. The

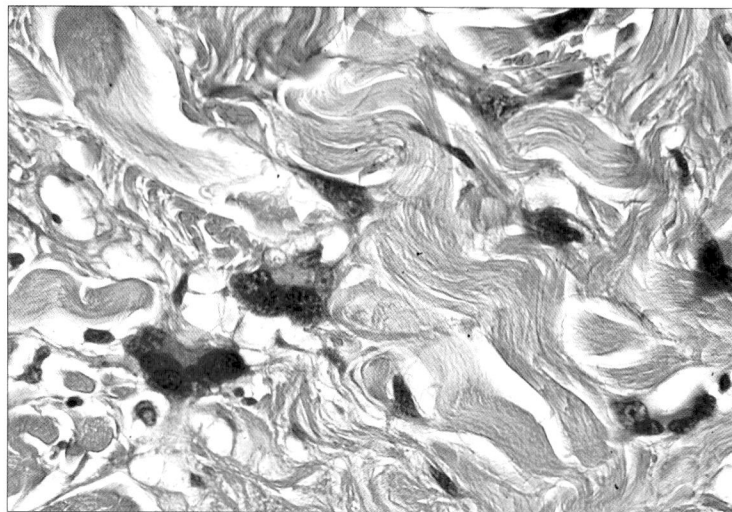

Fig. 116.15 Pleomorphic fibroma. There are interwoven coarse collagen bundles with a few interspersed large mono- and multinucleated atypical fibroblasts.

differential diagnosis includes dermatofibroma with atypical cells, atypical fibroxanthoma, and neurofibroma with atypical cells.

EPITHELIOID CELL HISTIOCYTOMA

This benign epithelioid cell mesenchymal neoplasm was first described in 1989 by Wilson Jones and co-workers[36].

Clinical Features

Epithelioid cell histiocytomas are more commonly present in adults during the fifth decade of life, with a slight predominance in women. They favor the extremities, and the thigh is the most frequent location. They are firm, sessile or polypoid papules or nodules measuring 0.5–1.5 cm in diameter. Because this neoplasm is highly vascular, common clinical diagnoses are pyogenic granuloma and dermatofibroma (sclerosing hemangioma). The treatment consists of simple excision.

Pathology

Epithelioid cell histiocytomas are dome-shaped or polypoid dermal nodules with a well-demarcated base and a collarette of epithelium at their periphery. It is a cellular lesion comprised of a monomorphous population of large, epithelioid stellate and triangular cells with angulated borders. The cells have oval nuclei with small nucleoli; some cells have two or more nuclei. Mitotic figures are rarely seen. The cells are separated by delicate collagen fibers and variable amounts of connective tissue mucin, and there is no evidence of nesting. Adnexal structures are not present at the center of the lesion.

The neoplastic cells react positively for vimentin and most of the cells are also positive for factor XIIIa, indicating differentiation toward dermal dendrocytes[36,37]. Most of the epithelioid cells are negative for histiocytic markers such as HAM 56, KP-1, MAC 387, lysozyme, α_1-antitrypsin and α_1-antichymotrypsin. The differential diagnosis includes intradermal Spitz nevus and cellular neurothekeoma.

MULTINUCLEATE CELL ANGIOHISTOCYTOMA

Clinical Features

The typical clinical presentation of multinucleate cell angiohistocytomas is that of slowly growing, multiple, discrete but grouped, red to violaceous papules, usually on the lower extremities (Fig. 116.16) or the dorsal aspect of the hands. The lesions may be unilateral or bilateral, and typically affect women over 40 years of age[38]. A generalized form has also been described in a young man[39]. Clinically, lesions may resemble Kaposi's sarcoma, granuloma annulare or sarcoidosis.

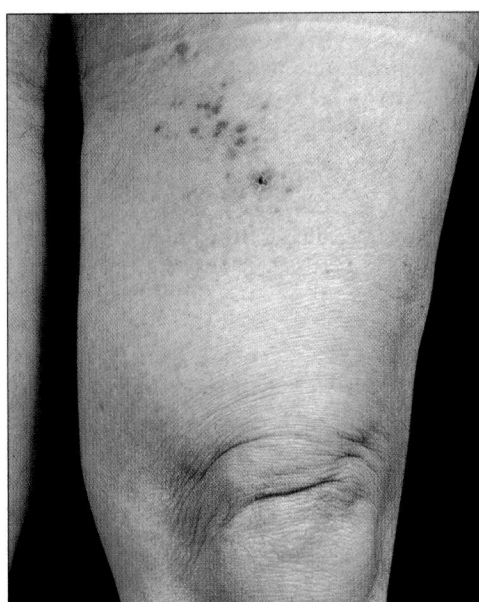

Fig. 116.16 Multinucleate cell angiohistocytoma. Grouped erythematous macules and papules on the thigh. Hemorrhagic crust represents biopsy site. Courtesy of the Ronald O. Perelman Department of Dermatology, New York University.

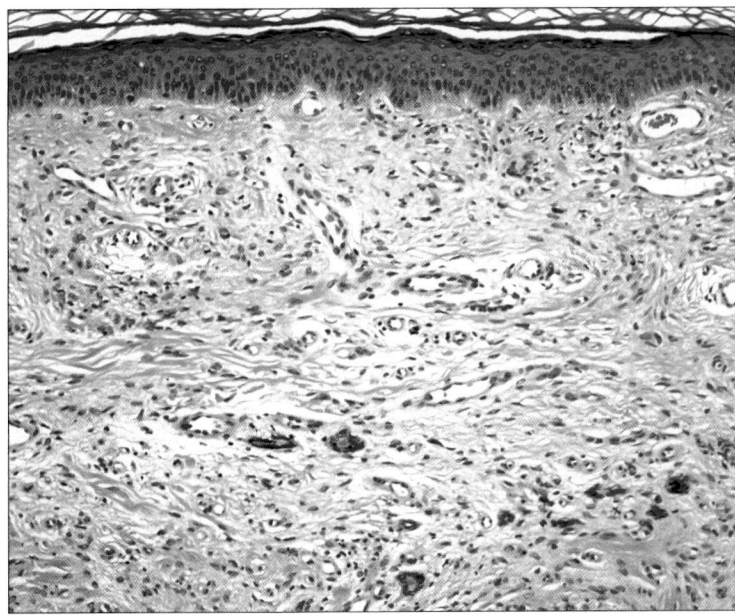

Fig. 116.17 Multinucleate cell angiohistocytoma. There is a proliferation of thin-walled, dilated blood vessels and multinucleated giant cells. The fibrous stroma is more delicate than that seen in angiofibromas.

Pathology

These lesions are composed of a proliferation of dilated capillaries and small venules in the superficial to mid dermis within thickened collagen bundles. The characteristic cell is a multinucleated giant cell, sometimes with peripheral palisading of the nuclei within eosinophilic cytoplasm, located within the collagenous stroma (Fig. 116.17). By immunohistochemistry, these cells are positive for vimentin and negative for S100 protein and factor XIIIa. A mixed inflammatory cell infiltrate can also be seen. The overlying epidermis may be hyperplastic, with hyperpigmentation and orthokeratosis. The histopathologic differential diagnosis includes dermatofibroma, angiofibroma, hemangioma and interstitial granuloma annulare.

Treatment

These lesions are benign and can be removed by simple excision. If left untreated, most cases progress slowly without evidence of spontaneous resolution.

DERMATOMYOFIBROMA

This tumor was described as plaque-like dermal fibromatosis in 1991 by Hugel[40] and as dermatomyofibroma by Kamino et al.[41] the following year.

Clinical Features

Dermatomyofibromas are lesions predominantly of young women and usually involve the shoulder area, axilla, upper arm, and neck. They are asymptomatic, well-circumscribed, oval or annular, skin-colored to red-brown plaques measuring 1–2 cm in greatest diameter, with a smooth skin surface. The clinical differential diagnosis includes dermatofibroma, cyst, granuloma annulare and pseudolymphoma.

Pathology

Dermatomyofibromas present as well-circumscribed plaques involving the reticular dermis and the upper portion of the subcutaneous septae; they are composed of well-defined, long intersecting fascicles of spindle-shaped cells parallel to the skin surface. The cells have a very uniform appearance, with elongated nuclei having rounded or pointed ends and one or two small nucleoli (Fig. 116.18). There is no evidence of nuclear atypia, and mitotic figures are rare. The cells are separated by thin collagen fibers and the elastic fibers are preserved; the adnexal structures are spared. The fascicles, spindle-shaped cells, collagen fibers and elastic fibers may have a wavy appearance.

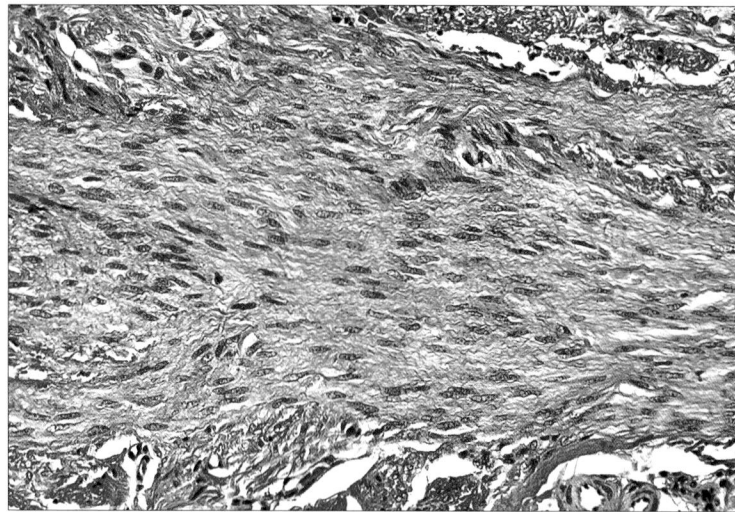

Fig. 116.18 Dermatomyofibroma. The myofibroblasts are arranged in long intersecting fascicles that are parallel to the skin surface.

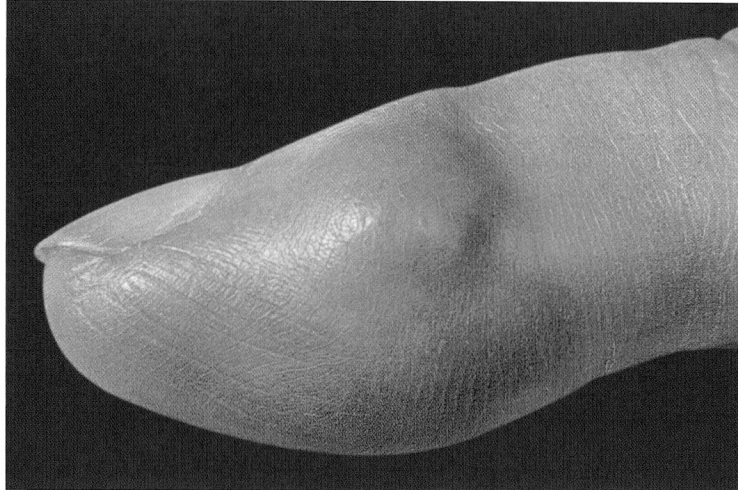

Fig. 116.19 Giant cell tumor of tendon sheath. A skin-colored nodule on the lateral aspect of the index finger. Courtesy of the Ronald O. Perelman Department of Dermatology, New York University.

Masson's trichrome stain highlights the presence of thin collagen fibers between the spindle cells. With Verhoeff van Gieson's stain, the elastic fibers appear slightly increased in number compared with the surrounding uninvolved dermis. The spindle-shaped cells react positively for vimentin and muscle-specific actin. They are variably positive for smooth muscle actin and negative for desmin, factor XIIIa and CD34. These results support a fibroblastic-myofibroblastic differentiation rather than smooth muscle differentiation[40,41]. On electron microscopy, the myofibroblasts contain prominent rough endoplasmic reticulum and intracytoplasmic myofilaments[41]. The histologic differential diagnosis includes dermatofibroma, leiomyoma and neurofibroma.

Treatment

The treatment is simple excision. Incompletely excised dermatomyofibromas may persist or recur.

GIANT CELL TUMOR OF TENDON SHEATH

Synonyms: ■ Localized nodular tenosynovitis ■ Giant cell synovioma ■ Pigmented villonodular synovitis

Clinical Features

This tumor usually presents as a firm nodule on the hands or fingers (Fig. 116.19), but can also occur on the toes and other periarticular sites. It is typically slow growing and fixed to subcutaneous structures without attachment to the overlying skin, except on the distal fingers and toes. Although usually asymptomatic, there can be pain, numbness or stiffness of the affected digit.

Giant cell tumor of tendon sheath is the most common tumor of the hand and can present at any age, but usually appears in adults 30 to 50 years of age, and is more common in women than in men[42]. The clinical differential diagnosis is broad and includes rheumatoid nodule, myxoid or ganglion cyst, subcutaneous granuloma annulare and the rare entities epithelioid sarcoma and clear cell sarcoma (melanoma of soft parts).

Pathology

These tumors have a lobular outline and are attached to the tendon sheath. They have a biphasic appearance, with moderately cellular areas of rounded to polygonal cells blending into hypocellular collagenized areas with spindle cells. The characteristic multinucleated giant cells are scattered throughout the tumor in variable densities. These cells have eosinophilic cytoplasm and from a few to 50 nuclei (Fig. 116.20). There are also mononucleated histiocytes with abundant pale foamy or vacuolated cytoplasm having variable amounts of hemo-

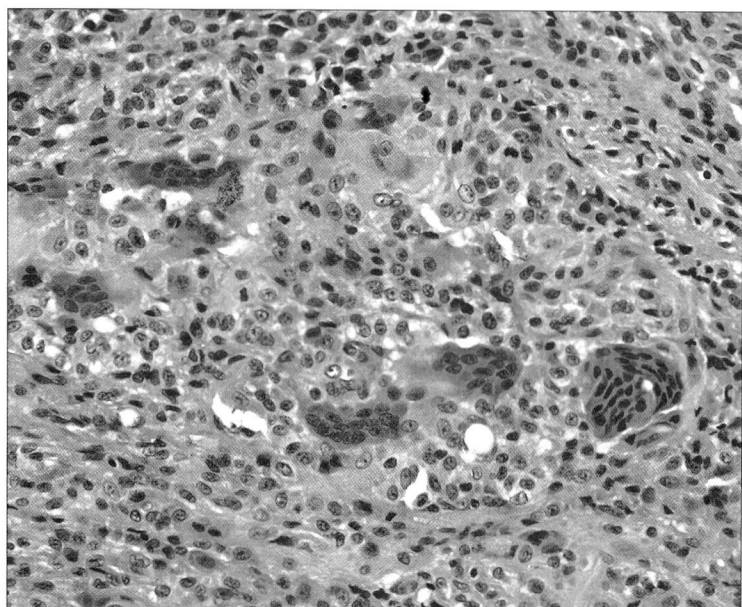

Fig. 116.20 Giant cell tumor of tendon sheath. The tumor is composed of sheets of epithelioid histiocytes with a variable number of the characteristic multinucleated osteoclast-like giant cells. Some of the histiocytes may have pale foamy cytoplasm. Courtesy of Jacqueline M Wharton MD.

siderin deposits. Stromal clefts or spaces, mitotic figures and, rarely, vascular involvement may be observed. The histologic differential diagnosis includes subcutaneous granuloma annulare, necrobiosis lipoidica, rheumatoid nodule, epithelioid sarcoma, synovial sarcoma, deep dermatofibroma, fibroma of tendon sheath, and foreign body granuloma.

Treatment

Despite the hypercellularity and large cells in this tumor, it is benign, with a local recurrence rate of 30%. It can be treated by a simple excision that includes a small margin of normal tissue[42]. It remains controversial as to whether this tumor is reactive or neoplastic in nature. Although karyotypic abnormalities have been reported by some, others have found that the tumors are polyclonal[43,44].

FIBROMA OF TENDON SHEATH

Clinical Features

This benign tumor presents as a small subcutaneous nodule that slowly increases in size. It is most frequently found on the hands and feet, with the thumb being the most common site of involvement.

They are usually asymptomatic, but there can be mild tenderness and limitation in the range of motion of involved joints[45].

The usual age of presentation is between 20 and 50 years. Men develop these tumors three times more often than women. The clinical differential diagnosis includes giant cell tumor of tendon sheath, neuroma, myxoid or ganglion cyst, rheumatoid nodule and subcutaneous granuloma annulare.

Pathology

The tumor has a well-circumscribed lobular appearance and is attached to a tendon sheath. It is composed of dense hyalinized collagen with scattered spindle-shaped fibroblasts and stromal clefts. There are occasional foci of myxoid change, with stellate fibroblasts. Rare giant cells are noted in occasional tumors, but there are no associated vacuolated histiocytes. The histopathologic differential diagnosis includes giant cell tumor of tendon sheath, fibromatosis, angioleiomyoma, nodular fasciitis, benign fibrous histiocytoma, synovial sarcoma and fibrosarcoma.

Treatment

Like giant cell tumor of tendon sheath, this tumor is benign, with a recurrence rate of about 25%. Treatment is usually a simple excision that includes a small margin of normal tissue[46]. Some authors believe that this tumor may represent a sclerotic end-stage variant of giant cell tumor of tendon sheath[47].

NODULAR FASCIITIS

Clinical Features

Nodular fasciitis is a benign reactive process seen in young to middle-aged adults. The upper extremity is the most common site. In children, the head and neck region is the most frequent location[48]. There is no gender predominance. Nodular fasciitis presents as a rapidly growing (but self-limited) subcutaneous nodule measuring from 1 to 5 cm in diameter, which may be tender. Some lesions are triggered by trauma.

Pathology

There is a well-circumscribed subcutaneous, fascial or intramuscular nodule with a stellate appearance. Dermal and intravascular variants have been reported[49]. Present are plump spindle and stellate fibroblasts and myofibroblasts with oval nuclei that have a fine chromatin pattern and prominent nucleoli. Mitoses are frequent. In early lesions, the fibroblasts and myofibroblasts are loosely arranged in an edematous, myxomatous stroma imparting a 'feathered' appearance (Fig. 116.21), with a proliferation of small blood vessels, scattered lymphocytes and extravasated erythrocytes. Occasionally, clusters of siderophages may be present. Older lesions show hyalinized collagen bundles. The fibroblasts and myofibroblasts react positively for vimentin and muscle-specific actin and, to a lesser degree, for smooth muscle actin. Some cells are positive for the histiocytic marker KP-1[50]. The histologic differential diagnosis includes fibrosarcoma and malignant fibrous histiocytoma.

Treatment

Nodular fasciitis is treated with a conservative excision and rarely recurs. The rate of recurrence is approximately 1%[51].

CONNECTIVE TISSUE NEVUS

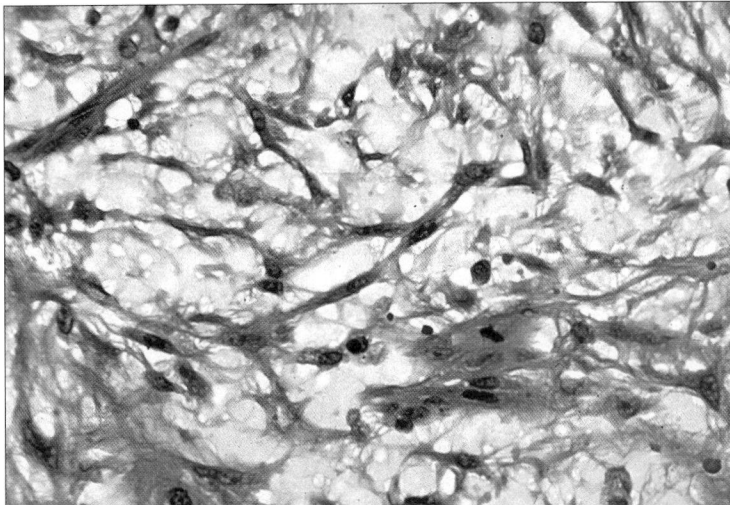

Fig. 116.21 Nodular fasciitis. Spindle-shaped and stellate fibroblasts are loosely arranged in a myxomatous stroma, with some cells in mitosis.

Clinical Features

Connective tissue nevi are firm, solitary or multiple, skin-colored papules, nodules or plaques that usually present at birth or arise during childhood (Fig. 116.22). They may represent hamartomas rather than neoplasms. Clinically and histologically, they may be subtle and even resemble normal skin. There are several variants, including the shagreen patch of tuberous sclerosis (see Ch. 60), which most commonly presents as a pebbly plaque with a 'pigskin' appearance on the lower back.

In the Buschke–Ollendorf syndrome, multiple skin-colored or slightly yellowish papules are seen and are referred to as dermatofibrosis lenticularis disseminata. The disease is due to loss-of-function mutations in the *LEMD3* gene which then lead to loss of antagonism of the TGF-β and bone morphogenic protein signaling pathways. The disorder is inherited in an autosomal dominant pattern and the papules begin at an early age. In radiograms, a characteristic stippled appearance to the bone is seen, called osteopoikilosis, and it represents islands of increased bone density (Fig. 116.23). This abnormality is asymptomatic.

Pathology

There is usually a poorly demarcated area of increased dermal collagen bundles in a haphazard array, without an apparent increase in fibroblasts. These lesions are designated collagenomas. A variant with increased elastic fibers has been called elastoma. Many of the cutaneous lesions in Buschke–Ollendorf syndrome tend to have increased elastic

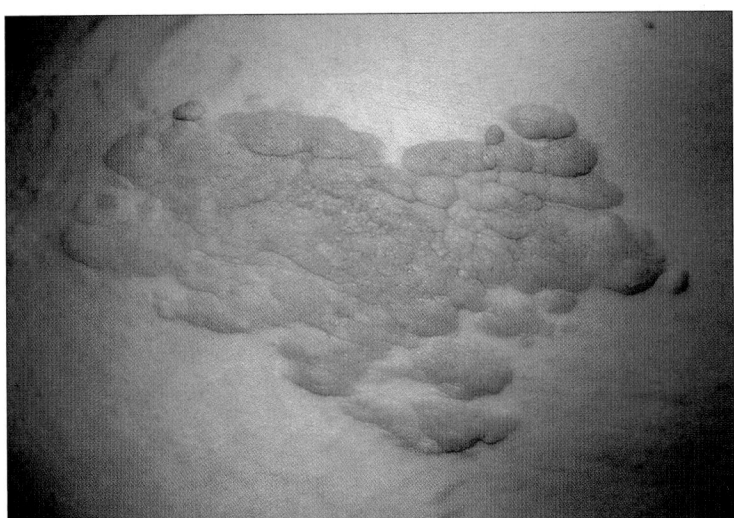

Fig. 116.22 Connective tissue nevus. Coalescence of multiple tan papules and plaques on the lower back. The lesion was firm to palpation and histologically had increased collagen.

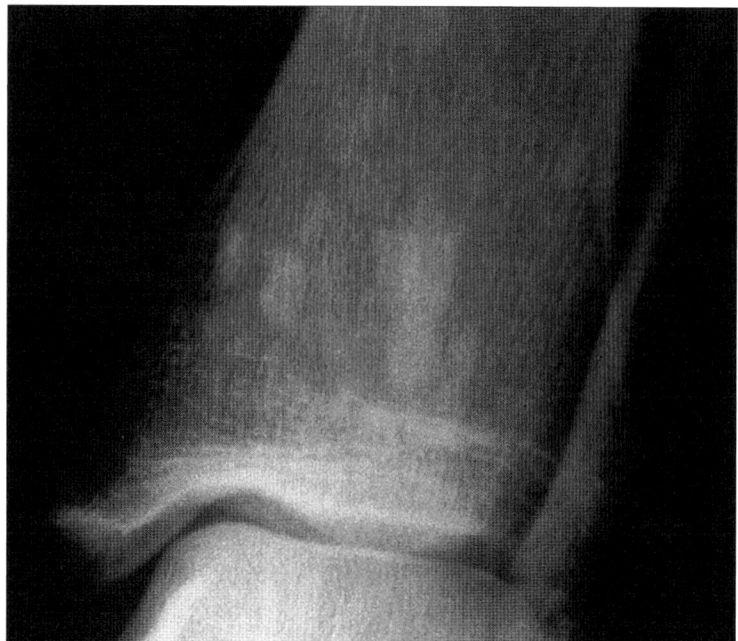

Fig. 116.23 **Osteopoikilosis.** In this radiograph, multiple asymptomatic round to oval areas of increased bone density are seen in the tibia. Courtesy of Jean L Bolognia MD.

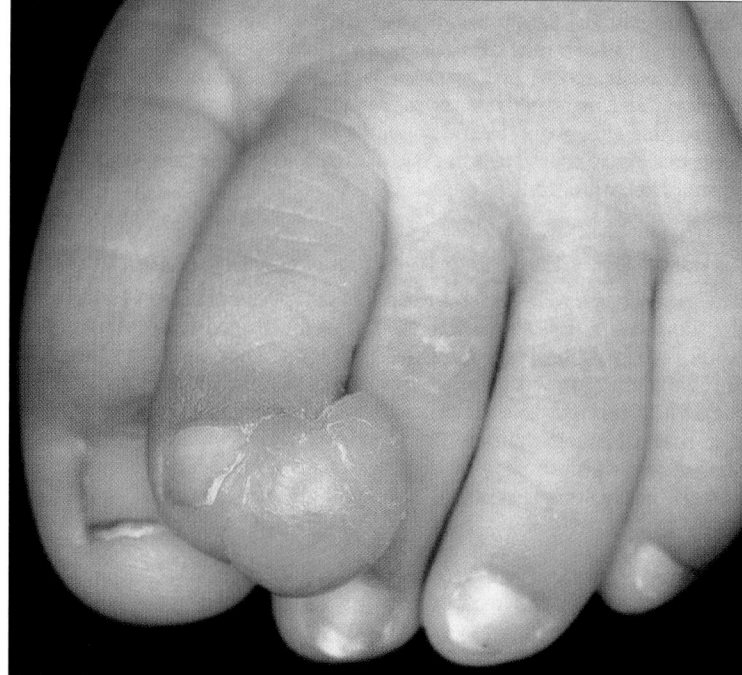

Fig. 116.24 **Infantile digital fibroma.** Firm skin-colored nodule on the dorsolateral aspect of the second toe in a young child.

fibers, but some appear to be primarily collagenous. Elastoma should not be confused with elastofibroma, which is a large mass in the deep subcutaneous tissue or fascia of the infrascapular area that is rarely treated by dermatologists. In many examples of connective tissue nevi, the connective tissue alterations may not be readily apparent unless the surrounding normal skin is examined histologically for comparison. A thin elliptical excision oriented with normal skin at one end and lesional skin at the other can be sectioned longitudinally for an optimal demonstration of the lesion.

Differential Diagnosis

Although the differential diagnosis includes fibromatoses, fibrous hamartoma of infancy, infantile myofibromatosis and dermatofibromas, clinicopathologic correlation usually establishes the diagnosis fairly easily.

INFANTILE DIGITAL FIBROMA

Synonyms: ■ Recurring digital fibrous tumor of childhood ■ Inclusion body fibromatosis

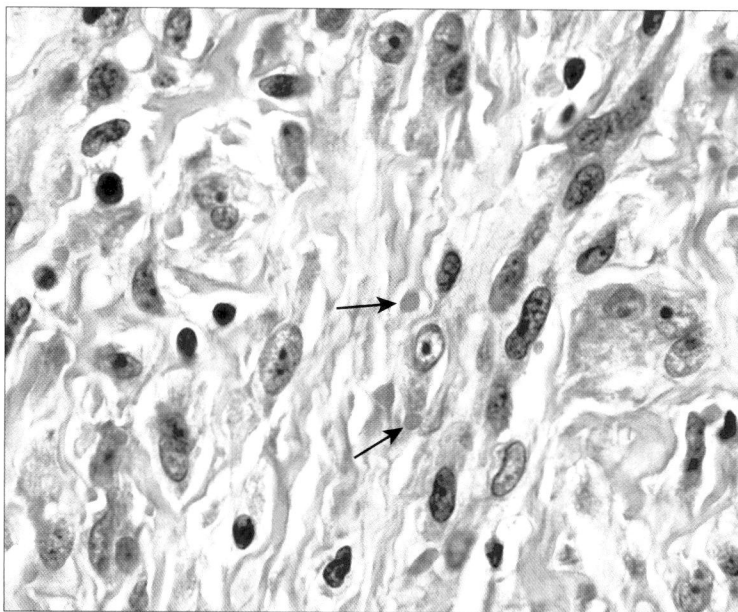

Fig. 116.25 **Infantile digital fibroma.** Myofibroblasts have pathognomonic cytoplasmic eosinophilic hyalin globules (arrows).

Clinical Features

Infantile digital fibromas commonly present as multiple, firm, smooth, skin-colored, dome-shaped nodules on the dorsolateral aspects of the fingers and toes (Fig. 116.24). They can be up to several centimeters in diameter, and tend to spare the thumb and great toe.

Almost all cases occur in infants under 1 year of age, and boys and girls are equally affected[52]. Rare adult cases of a histologically similar tumor have been reported at extradigital sites[53]. The smaller tumors can resemble acral fibrokeratomas, periungual fibromas and supernumerary digits.

Pathology

Infantile digital fibromas are poorly circumscribed proliferations of spindle-shaped myofibroblasts, arranged as interwoven fascicles with a collagenous stroma within the dermis or subcutaneous tissue. The cells have uniform spindle-shaped wavy nuclei without nuclear atypia or mitoses. The pathognomic feature is the presence of eosinophilic intra-cytoplasmic inclusions within the spindle cells (Fig. 116.25); the inclusions are often perinuclear. These inclusions stain red with Masson's trichrome and purple with phosphotungsten acid–hematoxylin (PTAH). Ultrastructurally, the inclusions are composed of bundles of actin-like filaments. Although this tumor is histologically very characteristic, the histopathologic differential diagnosis includes a dermal scar, dermatofibroma, angiofibroma, neurofibroma and angiofibromatous verruca vulgaris.

Treatment

In general, there is a benign clinical course, although functional impairment is possible. Spontaneous regression within 2–3 years is the usual natural history[54]. Contractures can be problematic. Recommendations for therapy range from conservative observation to wide local excision and possible amputation because of high local recurrence rates[55,56]. In the absence of special circumstances, conservative therapy seems prudent.

INFANTILE MYOFIBROMATOSIS

Synonyms: ■ Congenital multicentric fibromatosis ■ Congenital generalized fibromatosis

Clinical Features

Although this entity is rare, it is the most common of the juvenile fibromatoses. Clinically, it presents as one or more, firm to rubbery, skin-colored to purple, dermal or subcutaneous nodules, commonly located in the head and neck region (Fig. 116.26) or on the trunk. Skeletal involvement in the form of lytic metaphyseal lesions occurs in half of the patients, and the tumors can involve multiple internal organs, including the gastrointestinal tract, kidneys, lungs and heart.

Half of all patients have lesions present at birth, with more appearing during the first 2 years of life. Familial cases have been reported, but with an unclear inheritance pattern, and female infants tend to have visceral involvement more often[57]. The clinical differential diagnosis includes other infantile tumors such as neurofibromas, hemangiomas, cutaneous metastases (e.g. neuroblastoma, leukemia) and sarcomas (e.g. rhabdomyosarcoma), as well as juvenile xanthogranulomas; when the lesion is solitary, it may resemble a mastocytoma, solitary histiocytoma or infantile digital fibroma. Similar tumors appearing in older children or adults are usually solitary and have a good prognosis. They are termed solitary myofibromas[58].

Pathology

These tumors are composed of circumscribed nodules with a biphasic appearance. Areas of plump spindle-shaped myofibroblasts, with abundant cytoplasm arranged in fascicles within a collagenous stroma, blend with more cellular areas of smaller, rounder cells having less cytoplasm and an associated stag-horn pattern of dilated branching blood vessels. Mitotic figures, necrosis, intravascular growth and stromal hyalinization can be present. Immunohistochemically, the spindle and rounded cells are positive for vimentin and actin, with negative staining for desmin, as is seen in myofibroblasts. Infantile hemangiopericytomas (see Ch. 114) have similar histologic features, typically with more prominent immature rounded cells and associated vascularity, and it has been suggested that the two disorders exist on a continuum. The histologic differential diagnosis also includes fibrosarcoma, leiomyosarcoma, leiomyoma, juvenile fibromatosis, nodular fasciitis and fibrous hamartoma of infancy.

Treatment

Patients with only soft tissue and bony involvement have a good prognosis, as the tumors regress spontaneously within months via massive apoptosis[59]. Patients with visceral involvement have a high mortality rate within the first 4 months owing to the compromise of vital organ function. However, if patients survive beyond this period to when the tumors begin to regress, the prognosis is much improved[60]. Because the tumors tend to regress, debulking surgery is recommended only for symptomatic lesions. Combination chemotherapy has been used in severe cases[57].

CALCIFYING APONEUROTIC FIBROMA

Synonyms: ■ Juvenile aponeurotic fibroma ■ Calcifying fibroma ■ Cartilage analogue of fibromatosis

Clinical Features

This is a very rare entity that presents as a slowly growing, asymptomatic, solitary, firm, subcutaneous nodule that is usually fixed to underlying structures. It occurs primarily on the hands, and sometimes on the feet. A characteristic radiologic finding is the presence of stippled calcifications. Most cases occur in young children and adolescents and

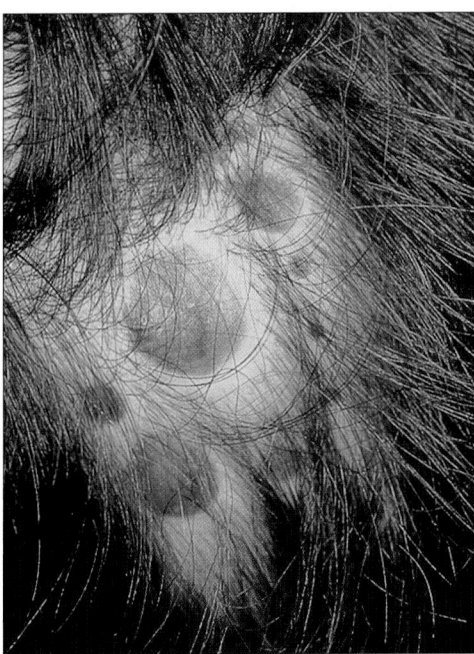

Fig. 116.26 Infantile myofibromatosis. Multiple firm violaceous papulonodules on the scalp.

there is a tendency for boys to be affected more frequently than girls[61]. The clinical differential diagnosis includes other tumors of the hands and feet, such as giant cell tumor of tendon sheath, fibroma of tendon sheath and neuroma, as well as rheumatoid nodules.

Pathology

The tumor is poorly circumscribed with an infiltrating border. It is composed of sheets of spindled and epithelioid fibroblasts with parallel nuclei in a collagenous stroma. There are characteristic islands of calcifications surrounded by palisaded epithelioid fibroblasts (Fig. 116.27). In older lesions, these areas of calcification can undergo chondroid and osseous metaplasia. Occasional multinucleated giant cells may also be present. The histopathologic differential diagnosis includes other forms of juvenile fibromatosis, palmar and plantar fibromatosis, chondroma and pseudogout.

Treatment

These tumors are benign, with a local recurrence rate of 50%[61]. Treatment consists of local excision, with re-excision as necessary for recurrences[62].

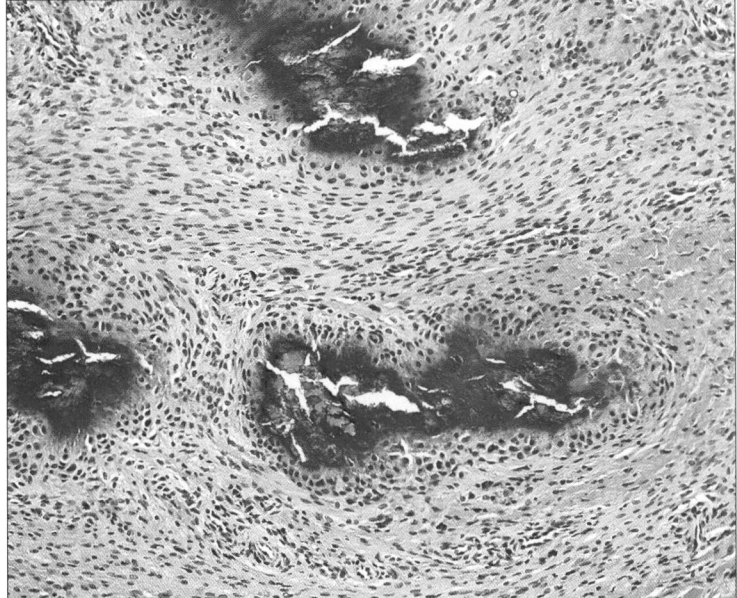

Fig. 116.27 Calcifying aponeurotic fibroma. Islands of calcification are surrounded by palisaded and osteoclast-like fibroblasts. In between these areas are sheets of spindled and epithelioid fibroblasts in a collagenous stroma.

FIBROUS HAMARTOMA OF INFANCY

Synonym: ■ Subdermal fibromatous tumor in infancy

Clinical Features

The typical clinical presentation for this tumor is a painless, solitary, skin-colored subcutaneous nodule. It favors the axilla, shoulder and upper arm, although it can appear in other sites such as the groin[63,64]. There is a variable rate of growth, and this tumor can become quite large. Fixation to underlying structures may be observed. Occasionally, overlying changes such as hypertrichosis are present[65].

Most of these tumors appear within the first year of life, but some are congenital. Boys are affected three times as often as girls[63,66]. These tumors mimic other subcutaneous malignancies of infancy such as rhabdomyosarcoma and cutaneous metastases (e.g. neuroblastoma, leukemia) as well as other fibromatoses, subcutaneous fat necrosis and mucinosis of infancy.

Pathology

This tumor is not well circumscribed, and it is composed of three distinctive elements in variable proportions: (1) a proliferation of spindle-shaped myofibroblasts arranged as broad fascicles within a collagenous stroma; (2) nests and aggregates of smaller, round to plump, spindle-shaped, immature mesenchymal cells within a myxoid matrix; and (3) mature adipocytes (Fig. 116.28). The histopathologic differential diagnosis includes infantile myofibromatosis, embryonal rhabdomyosarcoma, neurofibroma, early calcifying aponeurotic fibroma, fibrolipoma and lipoblastoma.

Treatment

Fibrous hamartoma is benign and the usual treatment is local excision, with recurrence being fairly uncommon[66]. If left untreated, the tumor continues to grow and stabilizes in size by mid-childhood[67].

FIBROMATOSES

Synonym:
■ Superficial fascial fibromatosis:
  – palmar fibromatosis (Dupuytren's disease)
  – plantar fibromatosis (Ledderhose's disease)
  – penile fibromatosis (Peyronie's disease)
  – knuckle pads (holoderma)
■ Deep musculoaponeurotic fibromatosis:
  – desmoid tumor (extra-abdominal)

Clinical Features

Fibromatoses are slowly growing tumors. The superficial variants may reach up to several centimeters in greatest diameter[68]. They appear as firm nodules, plaques or cord-like tumors along the flexor tendons, in particular the fourth finger (see Ch. 98).

Palmar and plantar fibromatoses usually appear during adulthood and the incidence increases with age. Flexion contractures, especially of the fourth and fifth fingers, can result. Penile fibromatosis is more common in middle-aged to elderly men; pain and erectile dysfunction are common. Knuckle pads affect the extensor surfaces of the interphalangeal and metacarpophalangeal joints (Fig. 116.29) and may be associated with palmar and plantar fibromatosis. They can be a reflection of chronic trauma.

Deep musculoaponeurotic fibromatoses or desmoid tumors are usually rather large – up to 25 cm in diameter. There are both abdominal and extra-abdominal variants. They may present after pregnancy in the abdominal wall, in postsurgical scars, and as mesenteric fibromatosis in Gardner syndrome (see Ch. 62). Trauma[69] and cytogenetic abnormalities, including trisomies of chromosomes 8 and 14 (in plantar fibromatosis), may play a role in the pathogenesis of these tumors[70].

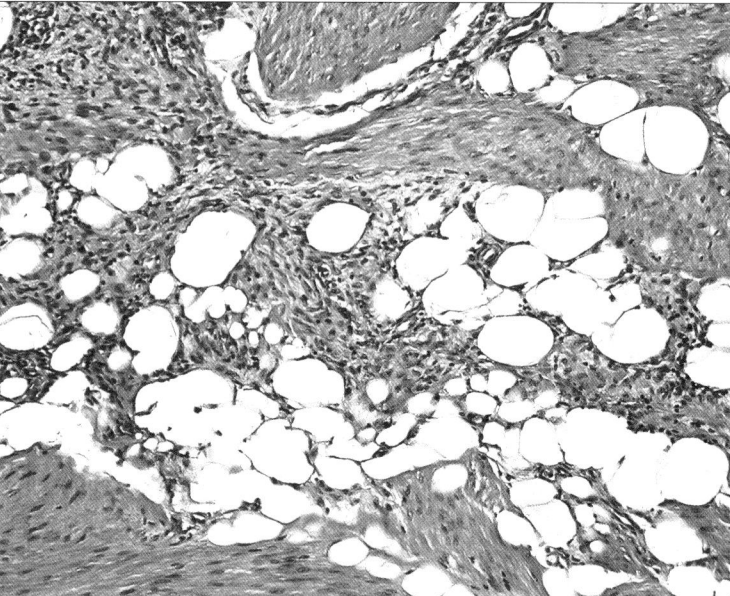

Fig. 116.28 Fibrous hamartoma of infancy. It is composed of a mixture of elongated bundles of spindle-shaped myofibroblasts, clusters of smaller immature mesenchymal cells in a myxoid stroma, and mature adipocytes.

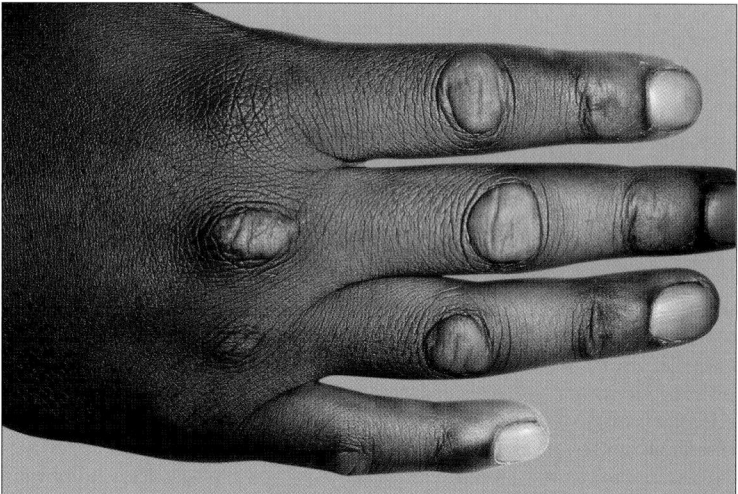

Fig. 116.29 Knuckle pads. Note the localization to the skin overlying the knuckles. Courtesy of Ronald P Rapini MD.

Pathology

Fibromatoses consist of large dermal and subcutaneous plaques and nodules that are poorly circumscribed. They are composed of long fascicles of monomorphous fibroblasts and myofibroblasts with elongated nuclei that have a fine chromatin pattern and small nucleoli (Fig. 116.30). Mitotic figures are rare. There are cellular foci in which the cells are scattered between thin collagen fibers. In hypocellular areas, the cells are separated by thick collagen fibers. The neoplastic cells usually infiltrate the adjacent aponeurosis, fascia and skeletal muscle. The histopathologic differential diagnosis includes fibrosarcoma, dermatomyofibroma, DFSP and keloid.

Cytogenetic abnormalities have been identified less frequently in superficial fibromatoses as compared to their deep counterparts, and, in the former, usually exhibit simple numerical changes, especially gains of chromosome 8[71].

Treatment

Surgical excision with fasciectomy is the treatment for palmar and plantar fibromatosis[72,73], with the goal of reduction of functional impairment rather than complete disease removal. Penile fibromatoses may resolve spontaneously in approximately a third of patients[74]. Therefore,

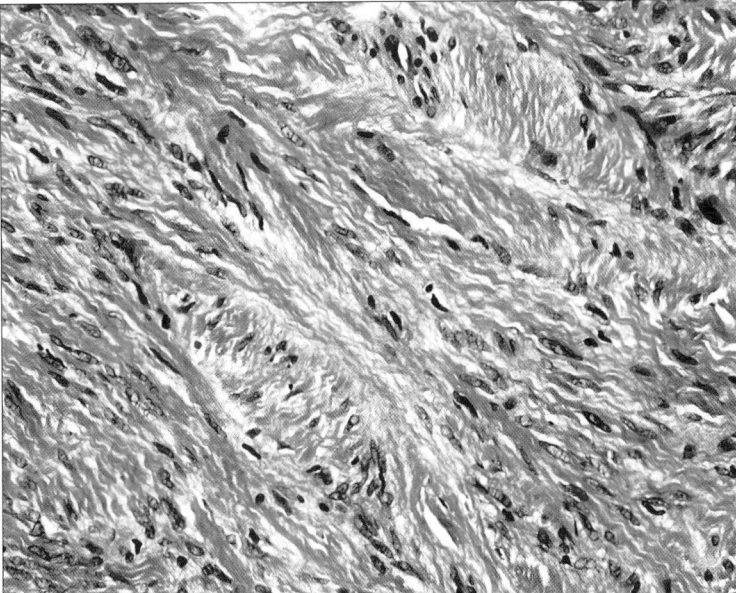

Fig. 116.30 **Fibromatosis.** Slender spindle-shaped fibroblasts and collagen strands are arranged in broad sweeping fascicles.

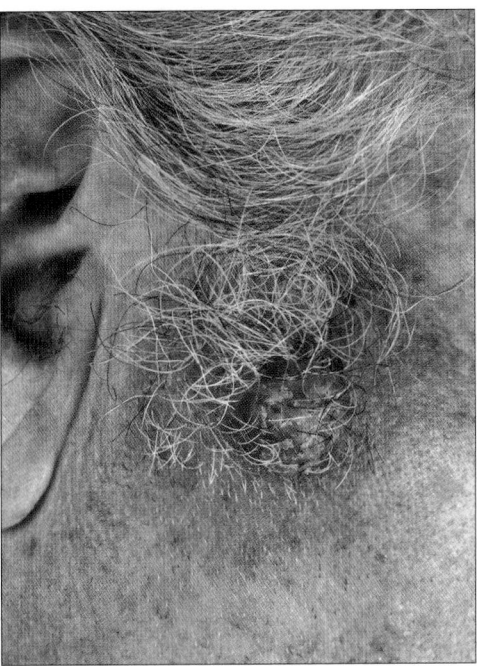

116

Fig. 116.31 **Atypical fibroxanthoma.** A purplish exophytic nodule on the lateral cheek of an elderly man.

a waiting period is recommended before surgical excision or laser treatment. The deep musculoaponeurotic fibromatoses have a higher recurrence rate and appropriate treatment of these is beyond the scope of this book.

ATYPICAL FIBROXANTHOMA

Synonym: ■ Superficial variant of malignant fibrous histiocytoma

Clinical Features

Atypical fibroxanthoma is a low-grade sarcoma that occurs in the sun-damaged skin of the head and neck in elderly patients. They usually measure from 1 to 2 cm in diameter and present as a rapidly growing nodule (Fig. 116.31). Secondary changes include serosanguineous crusts and ulceration[75]. There is a rare variant that appears in non-sun-damaged skin of the trunk or extremities in younger patients. A few cases have been reported in children with xeroderma pigmentosum[76]. The clinical differential diagnosis includes basal cell carcinoma, squamous cell carcinoma, amelanotic melanoma, Merkel cell carcinoma and cutaneous metastasis.

Pathology

Atypical fibroxanthoma is a dome-shaped nodule covered by a thin epidermis and is composed of a proliferation of both atypical spindle-shaped cells with moderate amounts of cytoplasm and large atypical cells with abundant pale-staining vacuolated cytoplasm. The cells have large pleomorphic and hyperchromatic nuclei and some of them are multinucleated. There are numerous typical and atypical mitotic figures (Fig. 116.32). For those tumors that arise in sun-damaged skin, there is solar elastosis at the periphery and base of the neoplasm. A rare variant with scattered osteoclast-like multinucleated giant cells has been reported[77].

Both the spindle-shaped cells and the histiocyte-like cells react positively for vimentin. The spindle-shaped cells are positive for muscle-specific actin, while the large histiocyte-like cells react positively for α_1-antichymotrypsin[78]. Both populations of cells are negative for CD34. The differential diagnosis includes spindle cell squamous cell carcinoma, spindle cell melanoma, dermatofibroma with atypical cells, and pleomorphic fibroma. Atypical fibroxanthoma is considered to be a superficial form of malignant fibrous histiocytoma. The latter presents as a deep subcutaneous or visceral mass which regularly metastasizes, unlike atypical fibroxanthoma.

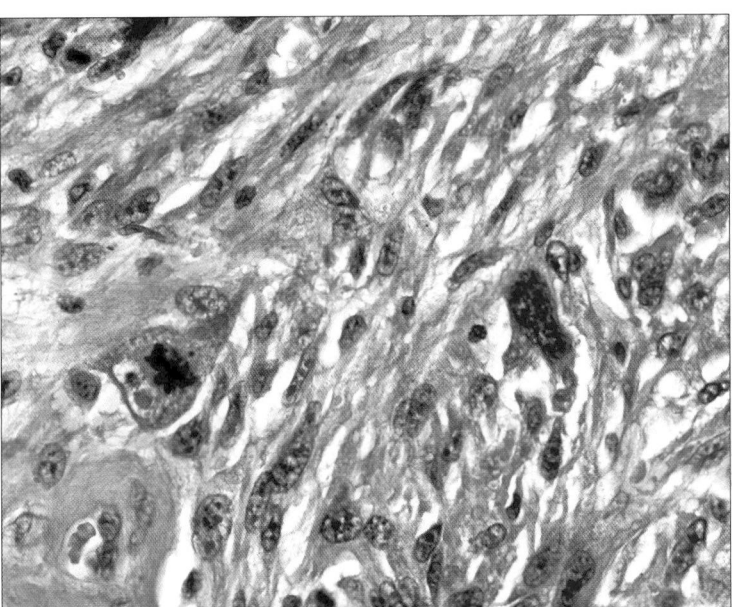

Fig. 116.32 **Atypical fibroxanthoma.** The spindle cells have pale foamy cytoplasm and hyperchromatic nuclei with small nucleoli. There is also a large atypical giant cell with darker nuclear chromatin as well as a cell in atypical mitosis.

Treatment

Atypical fibroxanthoma is a low-grade sarcoma that usually is cured by complete excision. It has a very low incidence of local recurrence, and only rare cases have metastasized[79].

DERMATOFIBROSARCOMA PROTUBERANS

Clinical Features

Dermatofibrosarcoma protuberans (DFSP) is a locally aggressive sarcoma of intermediate malignancy that favors young to middle-aged adults. Lesions that are present at birth or with an onset during childhood have also been reported. DFSP occurs on the trunk in 50–60% of patients, the proximal extremities in 20–30%, and the head and neck in 10–15%. There is a predilection for the tumor to involve the shoulder or pelvic areas. Initially, it presents as a slowly growing, asymptomatic, skin-colored indurated plaque that eventually develops violaceous to red–brown nodules measuring from one to several centimeters in diameter (Fig. 116.33)[80,81]. On palpation, the lesion is

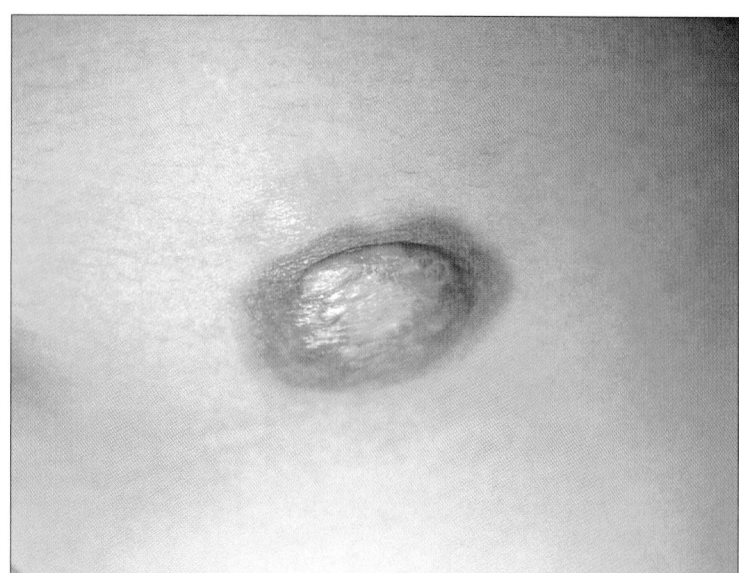

Fig. 116.33 Dermatofibrosarcoma protuberans. A broad red–brown plaque on the abdomen, with superimposed nodules.

firm and attached to the subcutaneous tissue. The early plaque stage may be misdiagnosed as a benign tumor and incompletely excised. Moreover, superficial samples may not yield diagnostic material. There are cases reported of accelerated growth during pregnancy[82]. The clinical differential diagnosis includes keloid, large dermatofibroma, dermatomyofibroma and morphea. Congenital and childhood-onset DFSP (and occasionally early lesions in adults) may have an atrophic appearance and/or hypopigmented to blue-red color, with the latter potentially leading to misdiagnosis as a vascular malformation or tumor.

Pathology

Early plaque lesions are characterized by a flat surface and low cellularity and are comprised of a proliferation of slender spindle-shaped cells arranged as long fascicles parallel to the skin surface. The cells are scattered between thin collagen fibers and infiltrate thick collagen bundles which appear cellular and wavy. In this stage, the slender cells show minimal nuclear atypia and rare mitotic figures. The adnexal structures are infiltrated and obliterated. In the plaque stage, the spindle cells infiltrate into the subcutaneous tissue, very often in a multilayered pattern (Fig. 116.34)[24].

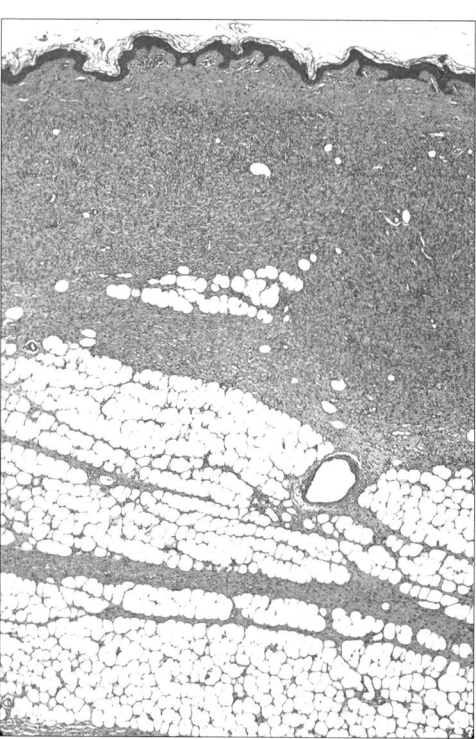

Fig. 116.34 Dermatofibrosarcoma protuberans, plaque stage. Characteristic multilayered pattern of infiltration into the subcutaneous tissue.

As the tumor develops into its nodular stage, it becomes more cellular, with the cells arranged as short fascicles in a 'storiform' or mat-like arrangement (Fig. 116.35). The cells infiltrate the subcutaneous tissue in a 'honeycomb' pattern (Fig. 116.36). In the nodular stage, the cells have hyperchromatic nuclei, and mitotic figures are easily identified. The nodules may develop myxomatous areas, characterized by more rounded to stellate cells in a highly vascular myxomatous stroma. The less differentiated fibrosarcomatous foci have a more cellular appearance, with intersecting fascicles in a 'herringbone' pattern, with increased cytologic atypia and frequent mitoses. In less than 5% of cases, a DFSP may contain melanin-producing cells with schwannian differentiation, and this is termed a Bednar tumor[83].

In the plaque stage, the spindle-shaped cells are strongly positive by anti-CD34 antibody immunostaining[13,17,84,85] (see Fig. 116.9). The reaction is stronger in the plaque areas than in the nodular foci[86]. Plaque and nodular areas are negative for factor XIIIa[13,17]. The general immunostaining pattern of DFSP – CD34-positive, factor XIIIa-negative – serves to distinguish it from large and/or highly cellular dermatofibromas, which are CD34-negative and factor XIIIa-positive.

Unique cytogenetic abnormalities have been reported, such as reciprocal t(17;22) translocations (see below) and supernumerary ring

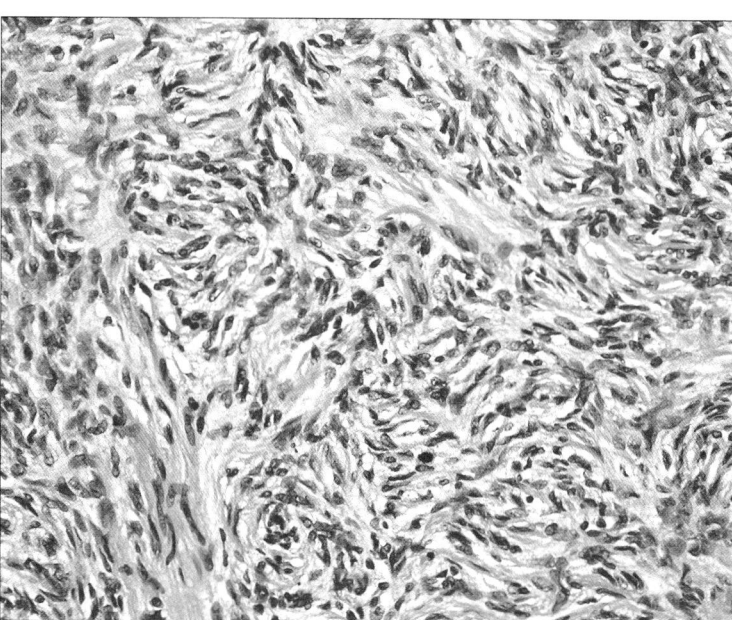

Fig. 116.35 Dermatofibrosarcoma protuberans. The spindle-shaped cells are arranged in a 'storiform' pattern.

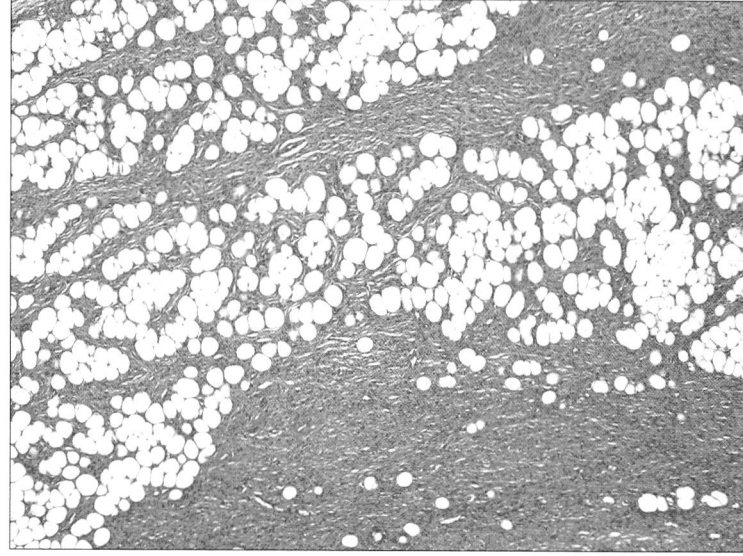

Fig. 116.36 Dermatofibrosarcoma protuberans, nodular stage. At the base of the tumor, the neoplastic cells infiltrate the subcutaneous tissue to produce a honeycomb pattern.

chromosomes containing sequences from chromosomes 17 and 22[87]. Overexpression of *p53* has been found in the fibrosarcomatous foci of DFSP with higher proliferative activity and aneuploidy[88].

The pathologic differential diagnosis of the plaque stage of DFSP includes atrophic dermatofibroma, dermatomyofibroma and neurofibroma. For the nodular stage, it includes deep dermatofibroma extending to the subcutaneous tissue, fibrosarcoma and malignant peripheral nerve sheath tumor. Incisional biopsy specimens, including ample subcutaneous tissue, are optimal for diagnosis.

Treatment

Complete surgical excision, including Mohs micrographic surgery, is the treatment for DFSP[89]. This tumor is characterized by its local invasion and tendency to recur. However, in rare cases, recurrent tumors with fibrosarcomatous areas have metastasized to the lungs[90]. Because the translocation places the platelet-derived growth factor (PDGF) B-chain gene under the control of the collagen 1A1 promoter, imatinib mesylate (Gleevec®), which targets the PDGF receptor (as well as other tyrosine kinase receptors, e.g. KIT and BCR-ABL), has been tried in patients with DFSP. In one series of eight patients with locally advanced disease, there was a complete response in 50% of the patients[90a].

GIANT CELL FIBROBLASTOMA

Clinical Features

This is a rare, solitary, slow-growing, asymptomatic, skin-colored, dermal or subcutaneous nodule involving the neck, trunk or groin. The lesion usually occurs during early childhood, with a strong predilection for boys[91]. Clinically, these tumors can appear to be cystic hygromas, lipomas or other juvenile subcutaneous tumors (see fibrous hamartoma of infancy section).

Pathology

This lesion is composed of diffusely infiltrating sheets of spindle-shaped fibroblasts and multinucleated cells with hyperchromatic nuclei within a slightly myxoid matrix. Irregular 'angiectoid' or pseudovascular spaces lined by multinucleated giant cells are present throughout the tumor (Fig. 116.37). These giant cells do not react with markers for endothelial differentiation, but do react with anti-CD34 antibodies[92,93]. Similar-appearing giant cells can be seen in the solid portions of the tumor as well. On occasion, some tumors have hypercellular spindle

cell areas with a storiform pattern similar to that seen in DFSP[93], and some authors consider giant cell fibroblastoma to be the juvenile form of DFSP[94]. More recent molecular studies have revealed that giant cell fibroblastomas and DFSP share the same t(17;22) chromosomal translocation which fuses the PDGF B-chain gene to the collagen type I α_1 gene[95].

Treatment

Giant cell fibroblastoma is a low-grade sarcoma with occasional recurrences following local excision[91].

FIBROSARCOMA

Clinical Features

Fibrosarcoma usually affects young to middle-aged adults. The most common location is the lower extremities, followed by the upper extremities, trunk, and then the head and neck region. This is a neoplasm predominantly of the deep soft tissues, with secondary involvement of the overlying subcutis and skin. A fibrosarcoma is a slowly growing tumor that measures from 1 to 10 cm in diameter and is usually diagnosed when it becomes a palpable painful nodule[96]. It may appear in old burn scars and in areas of prior radiation[97].

Pathology

When a fibrosarcoma involves the dermis and subcutaneous tissue, it usually represents an extension from a fibrosarcoma arising in the underlying soft tissues. The tumor is composed of a proliferation of atypical spindle-shaped cells arranged as intersecting fascicles in a 'herringbone' pattern (Fig. 116.38). There are thin collagen bundles between the cells. The cells have scanty cytoplasm and elongated hyperchromatic nuclei. Mitotic figures are easily identified and myxomatous foci may be present. A sclerosing epithelioid variant that simulates an infiltrating carcinoma has been described[98]. High-grade or poorly differentiated fibrosarcomas are characterized by increased cellularity with more atypical nuclei, a higher mitotic rate, foci of necrosis, and a less distinct 'herringbone' pattern. In most cases, the constituent cells only react positively for vimentin (non-specific) and, to a lesser degree, for muscle-specific actin.

The histopathologic differential diagnosis includes nodular fasciitis, fibromatosis, DFSP, malignant fibrous histiocytoma, and malignant peripheral nerve sheath tumor (see Ch. 115).

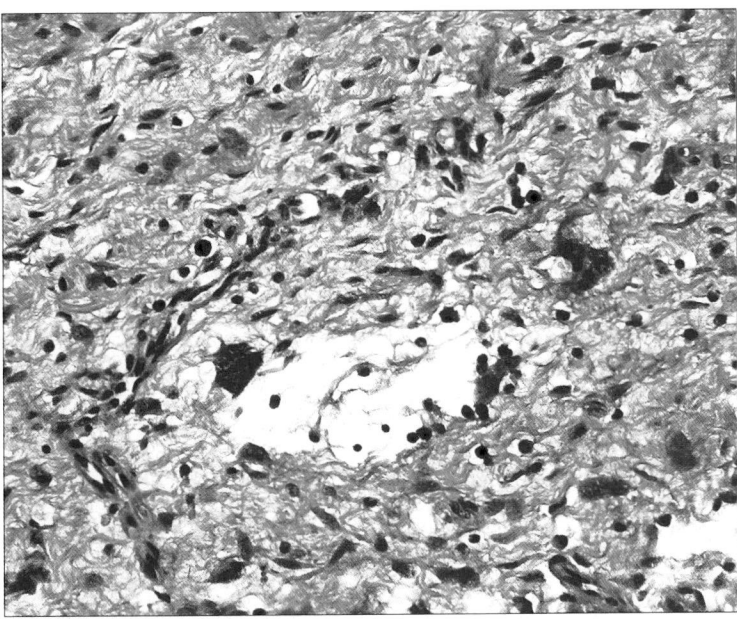

Fig. 116.37 Giant cell fibroblastoma. This pseudovascular or 'angiectoid' space lined by giant cells with hyperchromatic nuclei is characteristic of this tumor.

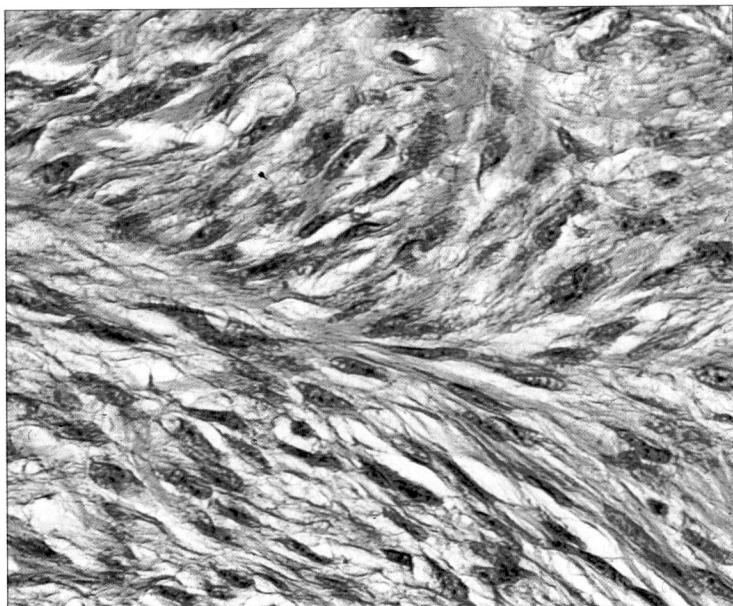

Fig. 116.38 Fibrosarcoma. Cellular fascicles of atypical spindle-shaped fibroblasts with coarse nuclear chromatin are arranged in a 'herringbone' pattern.[95]

Treatment

The treatment for fibrosarcoma is wide excision. When wide free margins cannot be achieved, adjuvant radiation therapy and amputation are additional options. In high-grade fibrosarcomas, adjuvant systemic chemotherapy is given. Hematogenous metastases to the lung, and less often to the bones, develop in patients with high-grade or poorly differentiated fibrosarcomas. The overall 5-year survival rate is approximately 40%.[96] There are rare cases of congenital or infantile fibrosarcomas that tend to be less aggressive[99].

EPITHELIOID SARCOMA

Synonym: ■ Epithelioid cell sarcoma

Clinical Features

This rare tumor presents as a slow-growing, firm to hard, subcutaneous nodule of the distal extremities, usually the hands and fingers. There may be associated ulceration if the tumor involves the dermis. Advanced disease can present as a linear arrangement of ulcerated nodules extending from distal to proximal sites on affected extremities. If there is involvement of a large nerve, associated pain, paresthesias and muscle wasting can occur[100].

The majority of patients are between 20 and 40 years of age, and men are affected twice as often as women. Hand and finger lesions may resemble giant cell tumor of tendon sheath, fibroma of tendon sheath, nodular fasciitis, granuloma annulare, rheumatoid nodule, or myxoid or ganglion cyst. Penile lesions can mimic Peyronie's disease[100].

Pathology

The tumor is composed of a nodular proliferation of spindle-shaped to round or polygonal cells with abundant eosinophilic cytoplasm and small uniform nuclei without prominent nucleoli. The tumor is frequently associated with fascia, periosteum, tendons and nerves. The larger tumor nodules have zones of central necrosis surrounded by palisaded tumor cells and a mixed chronic inflammatory cell infiltrate (Fig. 116.39). Distinction from other tumors usually requires immunohistochemical analysis. The tumor cells of epithelioid sarcoma are positive for both keratins (hence 'epithelioid') and vimentin (hence 'sarcoma'). They are also positive for epithelial membrane antigen and

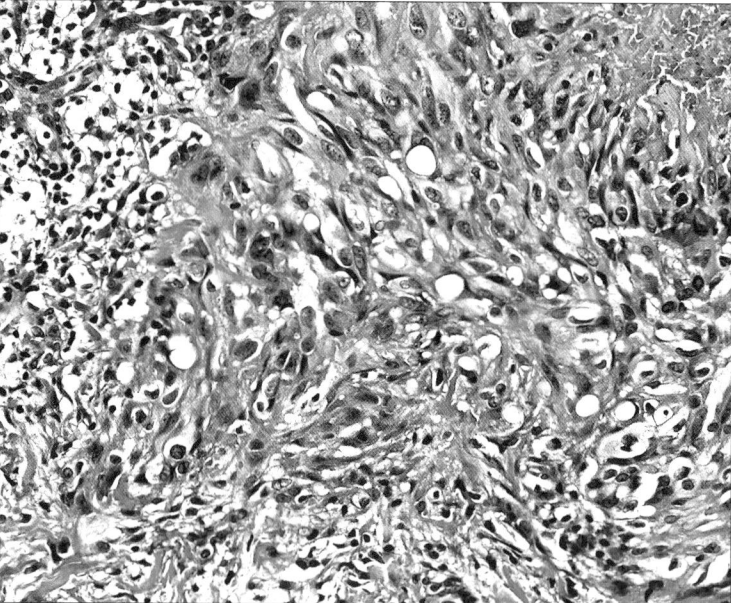

Fig. 116.39 Epithelioid sarcoma. The atypical epithelioid cells are palisaded around an area of necrosis. Courtesy of Jacqueline M Wharton MD.

negative for S100, HMB45 and CD31. The histopathologic differential diagnosis includes granuloma annulare, necrobiosis lipoidica, rheumatoid nodule, infectious granuloma, giant cell tumor of tendon sheath, squamous cell carcinoma, fibrosarcoma, melanoma, synovial sarcoma, epithelioid angiosarcoma, epithelioid hemangioendothelioma, and malignant fibrous histiocytoma.

Treatment

This sarcoma tends to be multifocal, with an infiltrating growth pattern along tendons, nerves and fascia. Although earlier therapeutic approaches involved radical surgery, including amputation, there has been a movement toward more conservative surgery with adjuvant radiation therapy[101]. Local recurrences are frequent, as are pleuropulmonary metastases (seen in 50% of patients)[100]. The 5-year survival rate is 50%, and metastases can present as late as two decades after the initial diagnosis[100,102].

REFERENCES

1. Banik R, Lubach D. Skin tags: localization and frequencies according to sex and age. Dermatologica. 1987;174:180–3.
2. Beitler M, Eng A, Kilgour M, Lebwohl M. Association between acrochordons and colonic polyps. J Am Acad Dermatol. 1986;14:1042–4.
3. Kahana M, Grossman E, Feinstein A, et al. Skin tags: a cutaneous marker for diabetes mellitus. Acta Derm Venereol. 1987;67:175–7.
4. Gould BE, Ellison RC, Greene HL, Bernhard JD. Lack of association between skin tags and colon polyps in a primary care setting. Arch Intern Med. 1988;148:1799–800.
5. Mathur SK, Bhargava P. Insulin resistance and skin tags. Dermatology. 1997;195:184.
6. De la Torre C, Ocampo C, Doval IG, et al. Acrochordons are not a component of the Birt-Hogg-Dube syndrome: does this syndrome exist? Case reports and review of the literature. Am J Dermatopathol. 1999;21:369–74.
7. Starink TM, Meijer CJ, Brownstein MH. The cutaneous pathology of Cowden's disease: new findings. J Cutan Pathol. 1985;12:83–93.
8. Meigel WN, Ackerman AB. Fibrous papule of the face. Am J Dermatopathol. 1979;1:329–40.
9. Rehbein HM. Pearly penile papules: incidence. Cutis 1977;19:54–7.
10. Yazici AC, Baz K, Ikizoglu G, et al. Familial eruptive dermatofibromas in atopic dermatitis. J Eur Acad Dermatol Venereol. 2006;20:90–2.

11. Barr RJ, Young EM Jr, King DF. Non-polarizable collagen in dermatofibrosarcoma protuberans: a useful diagnostic aid. J Cutan Pathol. 1986;13:339–46.
12. Goette DK, Helwig EB. Basal cell carcinomas and basal cell carcinoma-like changes overlying dermatofibromas. Arch Dermatol. 1975;111:589–92.
13. Abenoza P, Lillemoe T. CD34 and factor XIIIa in the differential diagnosis of dermatofibroma and dermatofibrosarcoma protuberans. Am J Dermatopathol. 1993;15:429–34.
14. Cerio R, Spaull J, Wilson Jones E. Histiocytoma cutis: a tumour of dermal dendrocytes (dermal dendrocytoma). Br J Dermatol. 1989;120:197–206.
15. Cerio R, Spaull J, Oliver GF, Wilson Jones E. A study of factor XIIIa and MAC 387 immunolabeling in normal and pathological skin. Am J Dermatopathol. 1990;12:221–33.
16. Reid MB, Gray C, Fear JD, Bird CC. Immunohistological demonstration of factors XIIIa and XIIIs in reactive and neoplastic fibroblastic and fibrohistiocytic lesions. Histopathology. 1986;10:1171–8.
17. Zelger BW, Ofner D, Zelger BG. Atrophic variants of dermatofibroma and dermatofibrosarcoma protuberans. Histopathology. 1995;26:519–27.
18. Vanni R, Marras S, Faa G, et al. Cellular fibrous histiocytoma of the skin: evidence of a clonal process with different karyotype from dermatofibrosarcoma. Genes Chromosomes Cancer. 1997;18:314–17.
19. Chen TC, Kuo T, Chan HL. Dermatofibroma is a clonal proliferative disease. J Cutan Pathol. 2000;27:36–9.

20. Levan NE, Hirsch P, Kwong MQ. Pseudosarcomatous dermatofibroma. Arch Dermatol. 1963;88:908–12.
21. Fukamizu H, Oku T, Inoue K, et al. Atypical ('pseudosarcomatous') cutaneous histiocytoma. J Cutan Pathol. 1983;10:327–33.
22. Leyva WH, Santa Cruz DJ. Atypical cutaneous fibrous histiocytoma. Am J Dermatopathol. 1986;8:467–71.
23. Tamada S, Ackerman AB. Dermatofibroma with monster cells. Am J Dermatopathol. 1987;9:380–7.
24. Kamino H, Jacobson M. Dermatofibroma extending into the subcutaneous tissue. Differential diagnosis from dermatofibrosarcoma protuberans. Am J Surg Pathol. 1990;14:1156–64.
25. Cooper PH, Mackel SE. Acquired fibrokeratoma of the heel. Arch Dermatol. 1985;121:386–8.
26. Kint A, Baran R, De Keyser H. Acquired (digital) fibrokeratoma. J Am Acad Dermatol. 1985;12:816–21.
27. Kint A, Baran R. Histopathologic study of Koenen tumors. Are they different from acquired digital fibrokeratoma? J Am Acad Dermatol. 1988; 18:369–72.
28. Fetsch JF, Laskin WB, Miettinen M. Superficial acral fibromyxoma: a clinicopathologic and immunohistochemical analysis of 37 cases of a distinctive soft tissue tumor with a predilection for the fingers and toes. Hum Pathol. 2001;32:704–14.
29. Andre J, Theunis A, Richert B, de Saint-Aubain N. Superficial acral fibromyxoma: clinical and pathological features. Am J Dermatopathol. 2004;26:472–4.

30. Rapini RP, Golitz LE. Sclerotic fibromas of the skin. J Am Acad Dermatol. 1989;20:266–71.

31. Garcia-Doval I, Casas L, Toribio J. Pleomorphic fibroma of the skin, a form of sclerotic fibroma: an immunohistochemical study. Clin Exp Dermatol. 1998;23:22–4.

32. Wilk M, Kaiser HW, Steen KH, Kreysel HW. Sclerotic fibroma. Hautarzt. 1995;46:413–16.

33. Shitabata PK, Crouch EC, Fitzgibbon JF, et al. Cutaneous sclerotic fibroma. Immunohistochemical evidence of a fibroblastic neoplasm with ongoing type I collagen synthesis. Am J Dermatopathol. 1995;17:339–43.

34. Kamino H, Lee JY, Berke A. Pleomorphic fibroma of the skin: a benign neoplasm with cytologic atypia. A clinicopathologic study of eight cases. Am J Surg Pathol. 1989;13:107–13.

35. Rudolph P, Schubert C, Zelger BG, et al. Differential expression of CD34 and Ki-M1p in pleomorphic fibroma and dermatofibroma with monster cells. Am J Dermatopathol. 1999;21:414–19.

36. Wilson Jones E, Cerio R, Smith NP. Epithelioid cell histiocytoma: a new entity. Br J Dermatol. 1989;120:185–95.

37. Dezfoulian B, Nikkels AF, Pierard-Franchimont C, Pierard GE. Epithelioid cell histiocytoma: a report of two cases. Dermatology. 1995;190:349–50.

38. Wilson Jones E, Cerio R, Smith NP. Multinucleate cell angiohistiocytoma: an acquired vascular anomaly to be distinguished from Kaposi's sarcoma. Br J Dermatol. 1990;122:651–63.

39. Chang SN, Kim HS, Kim SC, Yang WI. Generalized multinucleate cell angiohistiocytoma. J Am Acad Dermatol. 1996;35:320–2.

40. Hugel H. Plaque-like dermal fibromatosis/dermatomyofibroma. Hautzart. 1991;42:223–6.

41. Kamino H, Reddy VB, Gero M, Greco MA. Dermatomyofibroma. A benign cutaneous, plaque-like proliferation of fibroblasts and myofibroblasts in young adults. J Cutan Pathol. 1992;19:85–93.

42. Rao AS, Vigorita VJ. Pigmented villonodular synovitis (giant-cell tumor of the tendon sheath and synovial membrane). A review of eighty-one cases. J Bone Joint Surg Am. 1984;66:76–94.

43. Ray RA, Morton CC, Lipinski KK, et al. Cytogenetic evidence of clonality in a case of pigmented villonodular synovitis. Cancer. 1991;67:121–5.

44. Vogrincic GS, O'Connell JX, Gilks CB. Giant cell tumor of tendon sheath is a polyclonal cellular proliferation. Hum Pathol. 1997;28:815–19.

45. Chung EB, Enzinger FM. Fibroma of tendon sheath. Cancer. 1979;44:1945–54.

46. Smith RD, O'Leary ST, McCullough CJ. Trigger wrist and flexor tenosynovitis. J Hand Surg [Br]. 1998;23:813–14.

47. Satti MB. Tendon sheath tumours: a pathological study of the relationship between giant cell tumour and fibroma of the tendon sheath. Histopathology. 1992;20:213–20.

48. Sarangarajan R, Dehner LP. Cranial and extracranial fasciitis of childhood: a clinicopathologic and immunohistochemical study. Hum Pathol. 1999;30:87–92.

49. Price SK, Kahn LB, Saxe N. Dermal and intravascular fasciitis. Unusual variants of nodular fasciitis. Am J Dermatopathol. 1993;15:539–43.

50. Montgomery EA, Meis JM. Nodular fasciitis. Its morphologic spectrum and immunohistochemical profile. Am J Surg Pathol. 1991;15:942–8.

51. Bernstein KE, Lattes R. Nodular (pseudosarcomatous) fasciitis, a nonrecurrent lesion: clinicopathologic study of 134 cases. Cancer. 1982;49:1668–78.

52. Beckett JH, Jacobs AH. Recurring digital fibrous tumors of childhood: a review. Pediatrics. 1977;59:401–6.

53. Viale G, Doglioni C, Iuzzolino P, et al. Infantile digital fibromatosis-like tumour (inclusion body fibromatosis) of adulthood: report of two cases with ultrastructural and immunocytochemical findings. Histopathology. 1988;12:415–24.

54. Kawaguchi M, Mitsuhashi Y, Hozumi Y, Kondo S. A case of infantile digital fibromatosis with spontaneous regression. J Dermatol. 1998;25:523–6.

55. Azam SH, Nicholas JL. Recurring infantile digital fibromatosis: report of two cases. J Pediatr Surg. 1995;30:89–90.

56. Dabney KW, MacEwen GD, Davis NE. Recurring digital fibrous tumor of childhood: case report with long-term follow-up and review of the literature. J Pediatr Orthop. 1986;6:612–17.

57. Stanford D, Rogers M. Dermatological presentations of infantile myofibromatosis: a review of 27 cases. Australas J Dermatol. 2000;41:156–61.

58. Beham A, Badve S, Suster S, Fletcher CD. Solitary myofibroma in adults: clinicopathological analysis of a series. Histopathology. 1993;22:335–41.

59. Fukasawa Y, Ishikura H, Takada A, et al. Massive apoptosis in infantile myofibromatosis. A putative mechanism of tumor regression. Am J Pathol. 1994;144:480–5.

60. Zeller B, Storm-Mathisen I, Smevik B, et al. Cure of infantile myofibromatosis with severe respiratory complications without antitumour therapy. Eur J Pediatr. 1997;156:841–4.

61. Fetsch JF, Miettinen M. Calcifying aponeurotic fibroma: a clinicopathologic study of 22 cases arising in uncommon sites. Hum Pathol. 1998;29:1504–10.

62. DeSimone RS, Zielinski CJ. Calcifying aponeurotic fibroma of the hand. A case report. J Bone Joint Surg Am. 2001;83-A:586–8.

63. Paller AS, Gonzalez-Crussi F, Sherman JO. Fibrous hamartoma of infancy. Eight additional cases and a review of the literature. Arch Dermatol. 1989;125:88–91.

64. Popek EJ, Montgomery EA, Fourcroy JL. Fibrous hamartoma of infancy in the genital region: findings in 15 cases. J Urol. 1994;152:990–3.

65. Yoon TY, Kim JW. Fibrous hamartoma of infancy manifesting as multiple nodules with hypertrichosis. J Dermatol. 2006;33:427–9.

66. Sotelo-Avila C, Bale PM. Subdermal fibrous hamartoma of infancy: pathology of 40 cases and differential diagnosis. Pediatr Pathol. 1994;14:39–52.

67. Efem SE, Ekpo MD. Clinicopathological features of untreated fibrous hamartoma of infancy. J Clin Pathol. 1993;46:522–4.

68. Allen PW. The fibromatoses: a clinicopathologic classification based on 140 cases. Am J Surg Pathol. 1977;1:255–70.

69. Devine CJ Jr, Somers KD, Jordan SG, Schlossberg SM. Proposal: trauma as the cause of the Peyronie's lesion. J Urol. 1997;157:285–90.

70. Breiner JA, Nelson M, Bredthauer BD, et al. Trisomy 8 and trisomy 14 in plantar fibromatosis. Cancer Genet Cytogenet. 1999;108:176–7.

71. De Wever I, Dal Cin P, Fletcher CDM, et al. Cytogenetic, clinical and morphological correlations in 78 cases of fibromatosis: a report from the CHAMP study group. Mod Pathol. 2000;13:1080–5.

72. Brotherson TM, Balakrishnan C, Milner RH, Brown HG. Long term follow-up of dermofasciectomy for Dupuytren's contracture. Br J Plast Surg. 1994;47:440–3.

73. Aluisio FV, Mair SD, Hall RL. Plantar fibromatosis: treatment of primary and recurrent lesions and factors associated with recurrence. Foot Ankle Int. 1996;17:672–8.

74. Gelbard MK, Dorey F, James K. The natural history of Peyronie's disease. J Urol. 1990;144:1376–9.

75. Fretzin DF, Helwig EB. Atypical fibroxanthoma of the skin. A clinicopathologic study of 140 cases. Cancer. 1973;31:1541–52.

76. Dilek FH, Akpolat N, Metin A, Ugras S. Atypical fibroxanthoma of the skin and the lower lip in xeroderma pigmentosum. Br J Dermatol. 2000;143:618–20.

77. Ferrara N, Baldi G, Di Marino MP, et al. Atypical fibroxanthoma with osteoclast-like multinucleated giant cells. In Vivo. 2000;14:105–7.

78. Leong AS, Milios J. Atypical fibroxanthoma of the skin: a clinicopathological and immunohistochemical study and a discussion of its histogenesis. Histopathology. 1987;11:463–75.

79. Helwig EB, May D. Atypical fibroxanthoma of the skin with metastasis. Cancer. 1986;57:368–76.

80. Taylor HB, Helwig EB. Dermatofibrosarcoma protuberans: a study of 115 cases. Cancer. 1962;15:717–25.

81. Gloster HM Jr. Dermatofibrosarcoma protuberans. J Am Acad Dermatol. 1996;35:355–74.

82. Parlette LE, Smith CK, Germain LM, et al. Accelerated growth of dermatofibrosarcoma protuberans during pregnancy. J Am Acad Dermatol. 1999;41:778–83.

83. Ding JA, Hashimoto H, Sugimoto T, et al. Bednar tumor (pigmented dermatofibrosarcoma protuberans). An analysis of six cases. Acta Pathol Jpn. 1990;40:744–54.

84. Aiba S, Tabata N, Ishii H, Ootani H, Tagami H. Dermatofibrosarcoma protuberans is a unique fibrohistiocytic tumour expressing CD34. Br J Dermatol. 1992;127:79–84.

85. Kutzner H. Expression of the human progenitor cell antigen CD34 (HPCA-1) distinguishes dermatofibrosarcoma protuberans from fibrous histiocytoma in formalin-fixed, paraffin-embedded tissue. J Am Acad Dermatol. 1993;28:613–17.

86. Kamino H, Burchette J, Garcia J. Immunostaining for CD34 in plaque and nodular areas of dermatofibrosarcoma protuberans. J Cutan Pathol. 1992;19:530.

87. Pedeutour F, Simon MP, Minoletti F, et al. Translocation, t(17;22)(q22;q13), in dermatofibrosarcoma protuberans: a new tumor-associated chromosome rearrangement. Cytogenet Cell Genet. 1996;72:171–4.

88. Hisaoka M, Okamoto S, Morimitsu Y, et al. Dermatofibrosarcoma protuberans with fibrosarcomatous areas. Molecular abnormalities of the p53 pathway in fibrosarcomatous transformation of dermatofibrosarcoma protuberans. Virchows Arch. 1998;433:323–9.

89. Gloster HM Jr, Harris KR, Roenigk RK. A comparison between Mohs micrographic surgery and wide surgical excision for the treatment of dermatofibrosarcoma protuberans. J Am Acad Dermatol. 1996;35:82–7.

90. Mentzel T, Beham A, Katenkamp D, Dei Tos AP, Fletcher CD. Fibrosarcomatous ('high-grade') dermatofibrosarcoma protuberans: clinicopathologic and immunohistochemical study of a series of 41 cases with emphasis on prognostic significance. Am J Surg Pathol. 1998;22:576–87.

90a. McArthur GA, Demetri GD, van Oosterom A, et al. Molecular and clinical analysis of locally advanced dermatofibrosarcoma protuberans treated with imatinib: Imatinib Target Exploration Consortium Study B2225. J Clin Oncol. 2005;23:866–73.

91. Dymock RB, Allen PW, Stirling JW, et al. Giant cell fibroblastoma. A distinctive, recurrent tumor of childhood. Am J Surg Pathol. 1987;11:263–71.

92. Fletcher CD. Giant cell fibroblastoma of soft tissue: a clinicopathological and immunohistochemical study. Histopathology. 1988;13:499–508.

93. Harvell JD, Kilpatrick SE, White WL. Histogenetic relations between giant cell fibroblastoma and dermatofibrosarcoma protuberans. CD34 staining showing the spectrum and a simulator. Am J Dermatopathol. 1998;20:339–45.

94. Shmookler BM, Enzinger FM, Weiss SW. Giant cell fibroblastoma. A juvenile form of dermatofibrosarcoma protuberans. Cancer. 1989;64:2154–61.

95. Simon MP, Pedeutour F, Sirvent N, et al. Deregulation of the platelet-derived growth factor B-chain gene via fusion with collagen gene COL1A1 in dermatofibrosarcoma protuberans and giant-cell fibroblastoma. Nat Genet. 1997;15:95–8.

96. Scott SM, Reiman HM, Pritchard DJ, Ilstrup DM. Soft tissue fibrosarcoma. A clinicopathologic study of 132 cases. Cancer. 1989;64:925–31.

97. Wiklund TA, Blomqvist CP, Raty J, et al. Postirradiation sarcoma. Analysis of a nationwide cancer registry material. Cancer. 1991;68:524–31.

98. Meis-Kindblom JM, Kindblom LG, Enzinger FM. Sclerosing epithelioid fibrosarcoma. A variant of fibrosarcoma simulating carcinoma. Am J Surg Pathol. 1995;19:979–93.

99. Soule EH, Pritchard DJ. Fibrosarcoma in infants and children: a review of 110 cases. Cancer. 1977;40:1711–21.

100. Chase DR, Enzinger FM. Epithelioid sarcoma. Diagnosis, prognostic indicators, and treatment. Am J Surg Pathol. 1985;9:241–63.

101. Callister MD, Ballo MT, Pisters PW, et al. Epithelioid sarcoma: results of conservative surgery and radiotherapy. Int J Radiat Oncol Biol Phys. 2001;51:384–91.

102. Evans HL, Baer SC. Epithelioid sarcoma: a clinicopathologic and prognostic study of 26 cases. Semin Diagn Pathol. 1993;10:286–91.

Muscle, Adipose and Cartilage Neoplasms

117

Sabine Kohler

In this chapter, benign and malignant neoplasms of muscle, adipose tissue and cartilage will be reviewed (Fig. 117.1). The entities include:

- leiomyoma
- leiomyosarcoma
- smooth muscle hamartoma
- lipoma
- angiolipoma
- spindle cell lipoma
- hibernoma
- nevus lipomatosus superficialis
- lipoblastoma/lipoblastomatosis
- liposarcoma/atypical lipomatous tumor
- extraskeletal chondroma.

TUMORS OF SMOOTH MUSCLE

Leiomyoma

Synonyms: ■ Superficial leiomyoma ■ Leiomyoma cutis
■ Superficial benign smooth muscle tumor

Key features

- Three distinct variants: piloleiomyoma, genital leiomyoma and angioleiomyoma
- Usually presents as a solitary or multiple clustered (piloleiomyomas) papules or nodules in a young adult
- Piloleiomyoma and angioleiomyoma may be painful
- Most patients with multiple piloleiomyomas have multiple cutaneous and uterine leiomyomatosis syndrome with a germline mutation in the fumarate hydratase gene
- Myocytes are fusiform with centrally located, cigar-shaped nuclei

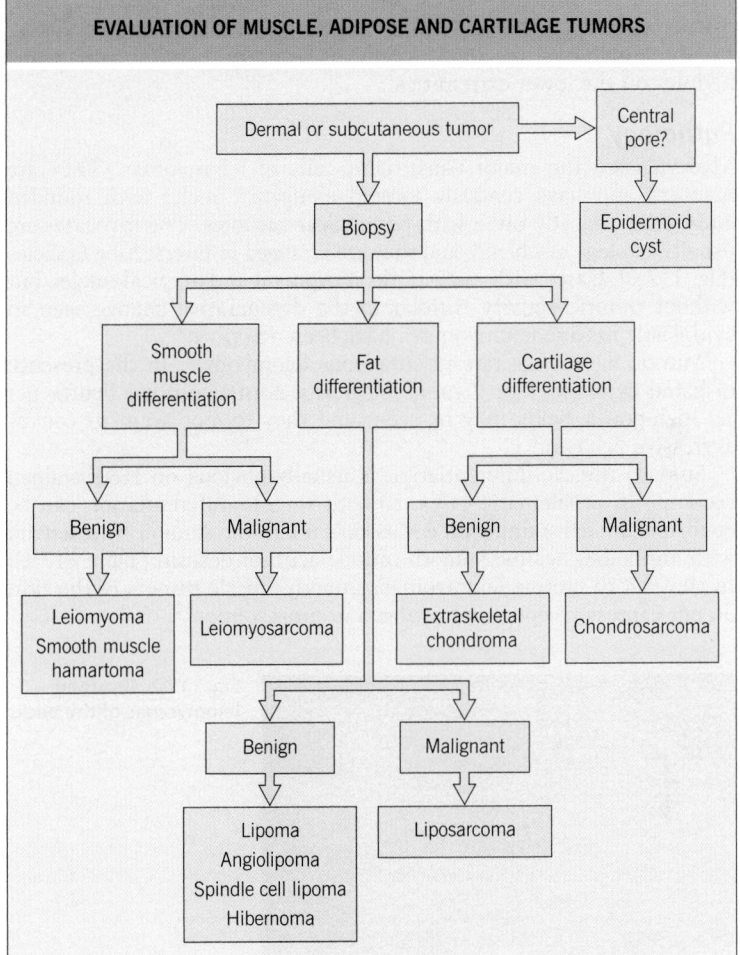

Fig. 117.1 Evaluation of muscle, adipose and cartilage tumors.

Introduction

Leiomyomas are benign dermal tumors, arising from the arrector pili muscles, the dartoic, vulvar or mammary smooth muscles, or the muscles enveloping dermal blood vessels. Accordingly, they are subclassified into piloleiomyomas, solitary genital leiomyomas and angioleiomyomas.

History

In an early review article, Arthur Purdy Stout[1] cites an 1854 publication of Rudolf Virchow as the first case report of multiple leiomyomas involving the skin near the areola in a 32-year-old man.

Epidemiology

Cutaneous leiomyomas are uncommon neoplasms, but exact figures of their incidence are not available. Of 85 349 pathology specimens in a general surgical pathology practice, 34 (0.04%) represented cutaneous leiomyomas[2]. The reported incidence of the various leiomyoma subtypes differs. Piloleiomyomas outnumbered genital leiomyomas in a study from El Salvador[2], while the reverse incidence was found in a series of patients from Japan[3]. It is more common for an individual patient to have multiple cutaneous piloleiomyomas than solitary tumors.

Pathogenesis

Piloleiomyomas arise from smooth muscle cells in the arrectores pilorum. Genital leiomyomas derive from the network of smooth muscle in the deep dermis of the genital area and the areola, including the erectile muscles of the nipple and areola, the scrotal dartos muscle, and the dartos labialis within the labia majora. Smooth muscle cells within vessel walls give rise to angioleiomyomas.

Most patients with multiple cutaneous leiomyomas have a germline mutation of the fumarate hydratase gene, located on chromosome 1q42.3–43. Germline mutations in the fumarate hydratase gene underlie the multiple cutaneous and uterine leiomyomatosis syndrome (multiple leiomyomatosis; Reed's syndrome; leiomyomatosis cutis et uteri). Fumarate hydratase is an enzyme of the mitochondrial Krebs cycle. A high percentage of affected women develop symptomatic uterine leiomyomas requiring treatment. A small number of patients with multiple cutaneous and uterine leiomyomatosis develop early-onset papillary renal cell carcinoma[4,5].

Clinical features

Piloleiomyomas present as dermal reddish-brown, pink or skin-colored papules or nodules that can be solitary or multiple. They typically develop during adolescence or early adulthood, and they have an approximately equal sex distribution[6]. Rare congenital or pediatric cases are described. When multiple, the distribution is most commonly clustered, linear, or along Blaschko's lines, but widespread lesions are observed. Most tumors measure 1–2 cm in diameter, and the most common sites of involvement are the extremities and trunk (especially the shoulder), with solitary lesions favoring the limbs and multiple lesions the trunk[6] (Fig. 117.2). Piloleiomyomas are often associated with spontaneous or induced pain, especially in cool weather. The mechanism of the pain is unclear. Contraction of smooth muscle, compression of nearby nerves, or an increased number of nerve bundles have been proposed as possible etiologies[6].

Genital leiomyomas are most often solitary, and they are usually painless. They can appear on the vulva, penis, scrotum, nipple and areola, usually measure less than 2 cm in diameter, and may be pedunculated. **Angioleiomyomas** usually present as solitary firm subcutaneous nodules on the lower extremities[7].

Pathology

Myocytes are the major constituent cells of leiomyomas. They are fusiform and have centrally located elongated nuclei with rounded ends (cigar-shaped), often with perinuclear vacuoles. The myocytes are usually cytologically bland, and they are arranged in intersecting fascicles (Fig. 117.3). Cases with nuclear pleomorphism and atypical nuclei, but without mitotic activity (similar to the degenerative change seen in symplastic uterine leiomyomas), have been described[8,9].

Mitotic figures are rare in cutaneous leiomyomas. In the presence of bland cytology, 1 or 2 morphologically normal mitotic figures per 10 high-power fields may be seen, and they do not seem to convey aggressive behavior[6].

Smooth muscle differentiation is usually obvious on H&E-stained sections. In problematic cases, smooth muscle differentiation can be confirmed by red staining on a Masson's trichrome stain or by reactivity with antibodies against smooth muscle actin or desmin (Table 117.1). In contrast to uterine leiomyomas, smooth muscle tumors of the skin do not express receptors for estrogen or progesterone[10].

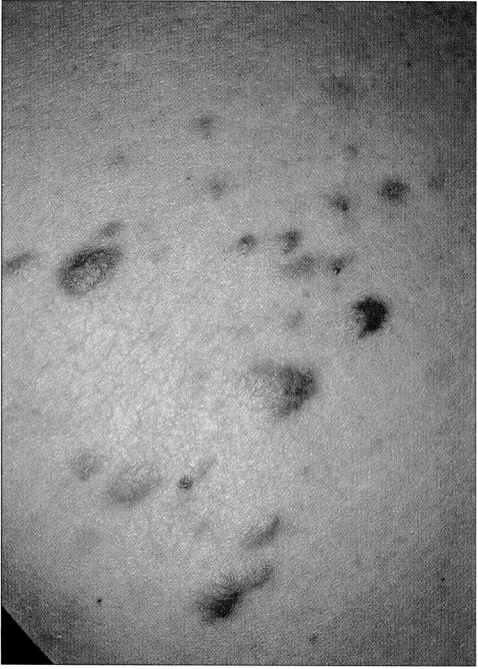

Fig. 117.2 Grouped leiomyomas of the back.

Table 117.1 Special stains to confirm smooth muscle differentiation.

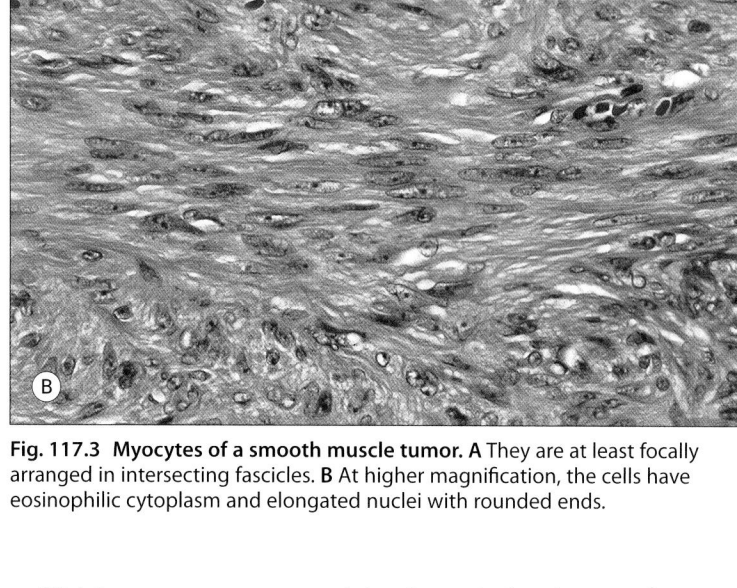

Fig. 117.3 Myocytes of a smooth muscle tumor. A They are at least focally arranged in intersecting fascicles. **B** At higher magnification, the cells have eosinophilic cytoplasm and elongated nuclei with rounded ends.

Piloleiomyomas are centered in the reticular dermis; they may extend into the fat and maintain a grenz zone beneath the overlying epidermis; the latter may be effaced, hyperplastic, or normal[5]. The center of these neoplasms is formed by interdigitating fascicles. The periphery is infiltrative, with fascicles of myocytes extending between collagen bundles (Fig. 117.4).

Genital leiomyomas of the scrotum or vulva tend to be larger and better circumscribed than piloleiomyomas. Scrotal leiomyomas are usually homogeneous spindle cell tumors, while vulvar lesions can show epithelioid cytology, myxoid change, or hyalinization[11]. Leiomyomas of the nipple closely resemble piloleiomyomas.

Angioleiomyomas are well-circumscribed tumors in the lower reticular dermis and subcutis (Fig. 117.5). Smooth muscle bundles surround patent thick-walled vascular channels. Collections of fat or foci of calcification may be present.

Differential diagnosis

The clinical appearance of cutaneous leiomyomas is varied, and includes solitary, clustered, and widespread lesions. Accordingly, the clinical differential diagnosis comprises a wide spectrum of dermal neoplasms, including dermatofibromas, schwannomas, neurofibromas, adnexal tumors, and metastases. The association with pain, or a pseudo-Darier's sign due to muscle fiber contraction, may be suggestive, but ultimately the definitive diagnosis depends upon a biopsy.

Spindle cell tumors with fibrohistiocytic or peripheral nerve sheath differentiation are in the histopathologic differential diagnosis. Usually, the cytologic features are sufficiently distinct to allow for morphologic diagnosis. The differential diagnosis with leiomyosarcoma is discussed below.

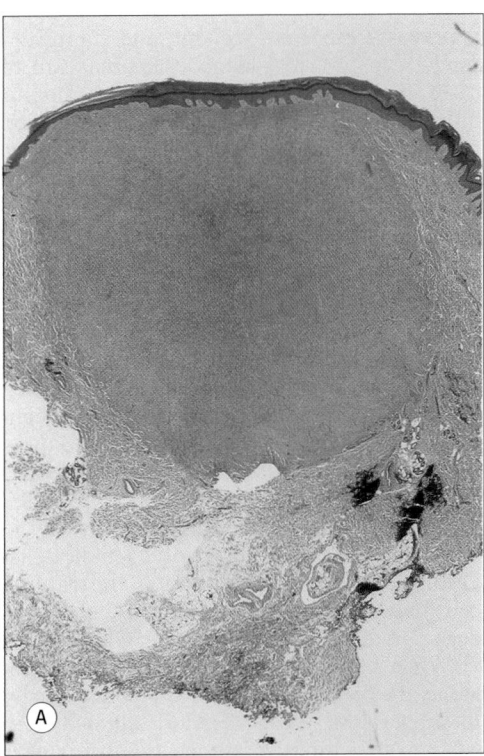

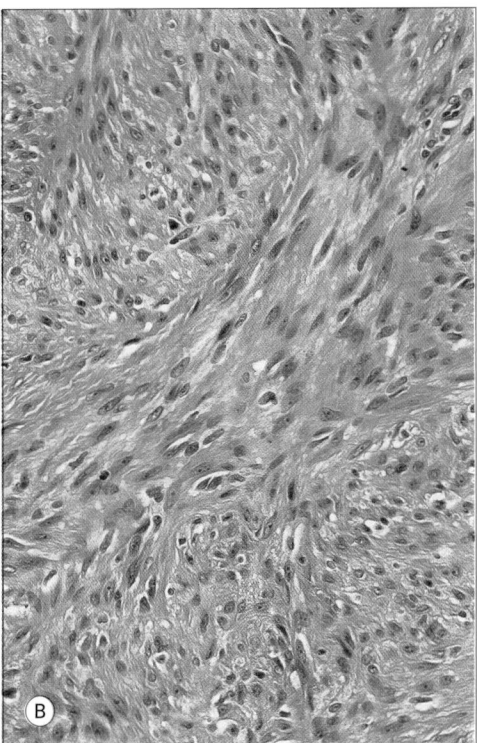

Fig. 117.4 Piloleiomyoma. A Piloleiomyoma centered in the reticular dermis forming a nodule with fascicles of myocytes interdigitating between collagen bundles at its periphery. **B** The center of the lesion shows intersecting fascicles of smooth muscle cells.

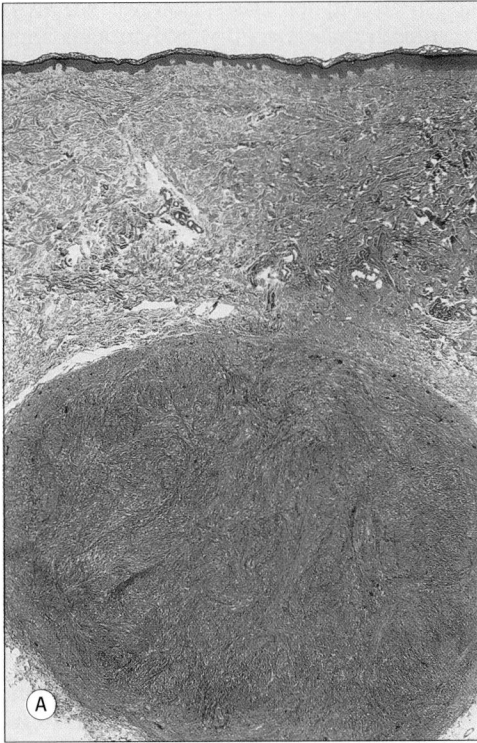

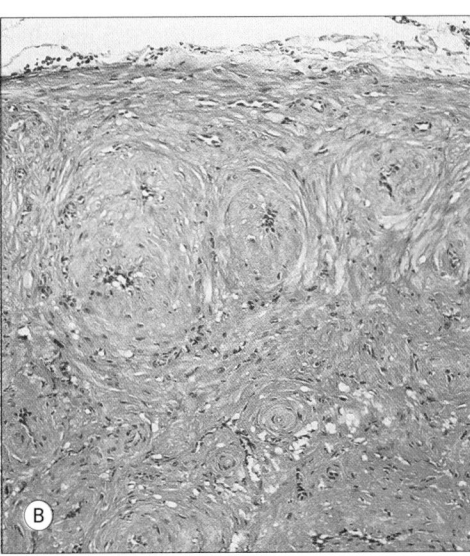

Fig. 117.5 Angioleiomyoma. A Angioleiomyomas are well circumscribed and often located in the deep dermis, extending into the subcutis. **B** At higher magnification, thick-walled vessels are surrounded by bundles of smooth muscle cells.

Treatment

The degree of symptoms and extent of lesions determine therapy. Simple excision is curative for solitary or limited tumors. For those tumors that are not amenable to surgery because of their number or location, treatment with nitroglycerine, nifedipine, or CO_2 laser ablation may provide relief from pain[12,13]. To the best of our knowledge, cutaneous leiomyomas do not undergo malignant transformation, allowing for a conservative approach to treatment. The experience with mitotically active leiomyomas (see above) is very limited. There are no definite criteria used to distinguish mitotically active leiomyomas from leiomyo-sarcomas and, accordingly, there is significant overlap between these two entities. It would, therefore, appear prudent to completely excise mitotically active leiomyomas.

Leiomyosarcoma

Synonyms: ▪ Superficial leiomyosarcoma ▪ Superficial malignant smooth muscle tumor

Key features

- Malignant neoplasm with smooth muscle differentiation, affecting patients beyond the fifth decade of life
- Most commonly located on the extensor surfaces of the extremities
- Management and prognosis depend on location: *dermal* leiomyosarcomas can be cured by simple excision, and they rarely recur and rarely metastasize; *subcutaneous* leiomyosarcomas carry a 30–40% risk of metastasis and require wide excision

Introduction

For management and prognostic reasons, it is important to differentiate between 'superficial leiomyosarcomas' that are limited to the dermis, and lesions that primarily arise in or extensively involve the subcutis. The former have a favorable prognosis, can recur, but very rarely metastasize. Subcutaneous leiomyosarcomas, in contrast, metastasize in approximately 25–40% of cases[13a].

Epidemiology

Cutaneous and subcutaneous leiomyosarcomas are rare neoplasms, comprising only 4.0–6.5% of soft tissue sarcomas[14]. Approximately 400 cases have been reported in the English language literature[13a,15].

Pathogenesis

Dermal leiomyosarcomas are thought to arise from either the arrector pili or genital smooth muscle. Subcutaneous leiomyosarcomas probably originate from vascular smooth muscle. A subset of either variant may derive from undifferentiated mesenchymal cells that, in the course of malignant transformation, acquire smooth muscle features. The etiology is largely unknown. Anecdotal reports describe an association with trauma and radiation[15]. However, a leiomyosarcoma arising in a radiation field is exceptionally rare, and it is much less common than radiation-induced fibrosarcoma, osteosarcoma, or malignant fibrous histiocytoma[16].

Clinical features

Cutaneous and subcutaneous leiomyosarcomas predominantly affect individuals in the fifth to seventh decades of life, but they can occur at any age[16]. They can arise anywhere on the body, but have a predilection for the extensor surfaces of the extremities and (for dermal lesions) the head and neck. The clinical appearance is not distinctive, and the tumors often come to attention because of rapid enlargement or ulceration (Fig. 117.6). Leiomyosarcomas are typically solitary, deeply seated, firm nodules, with variable associated erythema and hyperpigmentation. If multiple tumors are encountered, the possibility of metastases from a retroperitoneal or visceral location should be considered[17].

Most dermal tumors measure less than 2 cm in diameter, while subcutaneous lesions are often larger. The prognosis of dermal leiomyosarcomas is excellent, and complete excision is curative; they rarely recur. Dermal leiomyosarcomas can metastasize in exceptional cases, mainly because the recurrent tumors are often deeper and more difficult to treat. Subcutaneous leiomyosarcomas metastasize in 30–40% of cases. The risk of metastasis seems to be related to size, as metastasis is unlikely in lesions measuring less than 5 cm in diameter. Metastatic spread occurs hematogenously to the lung and, less often, other visceral organs, or via the lymphatics to regional lymph nodes[16,18].

Pathology

The histopathologic features of leiomyosarcoma span a morphologic continuum that, at the well-differentiated end, demonstrate overlap with leiomyoma, while the poorly differentiated lesions can closely resemble atypical fibroxanthoma and malignant fibrous histiocytoma. A leiomyosarcoma of moderate differentiation will be comprised of cells that cytologically resemble normal smooth muscle cells. Compared with leiomyomas, malignant smooth muscle tumors are more cellular, exhibit cytologic atypia, and contain easily identifiable mitotic figures (Fig. 117.7). At least focally, the spindle cells are arranged in fascicles. During neoplastic transformation, the cytologic features change and the cells may come to resemble myofibroblasts or fibrohistiocytic cells. The degree of differentiation may vary throughout the tumor.

While a leiomyoma can usually be diagnosed on morphologic grounds alone, the diagnosis of leiomyosarcoma usually requires adjuvant studies to support the lineage. Historically, red staining of the cytoplasm on Masson's trichrome stain was used to support smooth muscle differentiation. Nowadays, immunophenotypic studies with antibodies to smooth muscle actin and desmin represent the standard of care. Of the two markers, actin is more sensitive and desmin is somewhat more specific. Unfortunately, neither marker is entirely specific for smooth muscle differentiation, and reactivity can also be observed in myofibroblasts and fibroblasts. However, negative staining with an antibody to smooth muscle actin would strongly argue against smooth muscle differentiation. Usually a combination of morphology and immunophenotype will prove most helpful.

Rarely, leiomyosarcomas can show epithelioid cytology[19]. These neoplasms are usually actin-positive and desmin-negative, but clinically they seem to behave similarly to ordinary leiomyosarcomas.

In dermal leiomyosarcomas, at least 90% of the neoplasm should be confined to the dermis[18]. Dermal tumors are poorly circumscribed and infiltrate between adjacent collagen bundles, while subcutaneous lesions are better circumscribed and are surrounded by a pseudocapsule formed by compressed tissue.

Differential diagnosis

The clinical differential diagnosis comprises all lesions presenting as solitary nodules, including cysts, dermatofibromas, dermatofibrosarcoma protuberans and appendageal tumors. Definitive diagnosis is not possible based on clinical appearance alone; it requires histopathologic confirmation. Adequate sampling is imperative.

The histopathologic differential diagnosis raises two problems: the differentiation of leiomyosarcoma from leiomyoma and its delineation from other spindle cell neoplasms. The diagnostic criteria at the well-differentiated end are imprecise and not clearly defined. Anaplasia, high mitotic activity, necrosis and angiolymphatic invasion will easily establish a smooth muscle neoplasm as malignant.

Traditionally, the number of mitotic figures is used as the most reliable diagnostic criterion when trying to predict clinical behavior[16]. In the presence of cytologic atypia, a mitotic rate of one or more mitotic figures per high-power field is generally considered to be indicative of malignancy[14]. It is important to remember, however, that the prognosis seems to depend more on the location (dermal vs subcutaneous), and that the extent of mitotic activity is probably more important in subcutaneous lesions. A cytologically bland dermal smooth muscle tumor with 1 to 2 mitotic figures per 10 high-power fields should not be classified as leiomyosarcoma based on the presence of mitoses alone[6].

The differential diagnosis of leiomyosarcoma from other dermal spindle cell neoplasms nearly always requires immunophenotyping. This is best approached by using a panel of antibodies that examine the neoplasm for its line of differentiation (Table 117.2). A standard panel

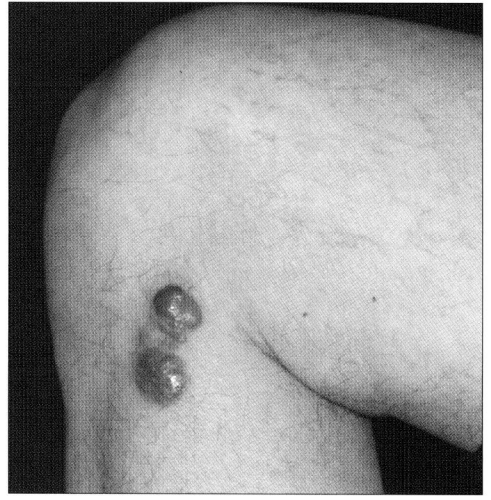

Fig. 117.6 Leiomyosarcoma. Two hyperpigmented tumor nodules on the lower extremity. Courtesy of Lorenzo Cerroni MD.

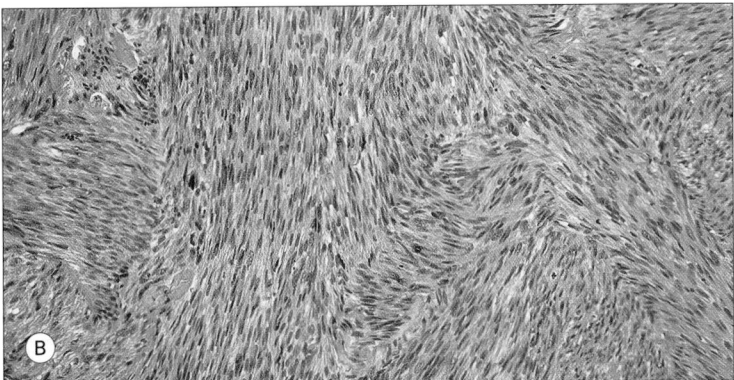

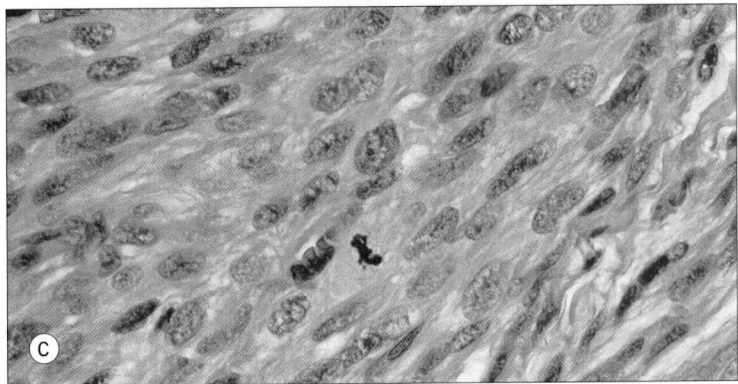

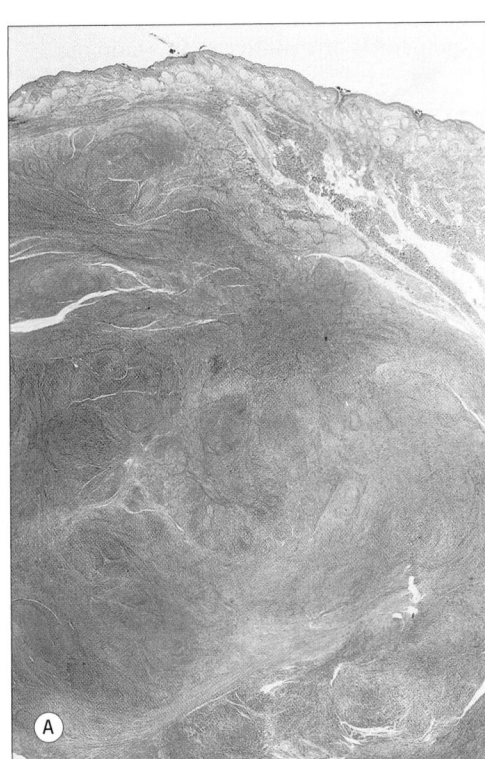

Fig. 117.7 Leiomyosarcoma. A A large tumor extending from upper reticular dermis deep into the subcutis. **B** At higher magnification, this neoplasm is more cellular than a leiomyoma. The nuclei are pleomorphic, more hyperchromatic, and have coarse chromatin. **C** Mitotic figures are numerous and are easily identified.

IMMUNOHISTOCHEMICAL FINDINGS IN LEIOMYOSARCOMA RELATIVE TO OTHER SPINDLE CELL TUMORS					
	Leiomyosarcoma	SCC	Melanoma	Nerve sheath tumors	AFX/ MFH
Actin	+	–	–	–	±
Desmin	±	–	–	–	–
Cytokeratin	–	+	–	–	–
S100 protein	–	–	+	+	–
CD68	–	–	±	–	±

Table 117.2 Immunohistochemical findings in leiomyosarcoma relative to other spindle cell tumors. AFX, atypical fibroxanthoma; MFH, malignant fibrous histiocytoma; SCC, spindle cell squamous carcinoma. CD68 is a glycoprotein expressed by monocytes and macrophages.

consists of antibodies to actin, desmin, keratin, S100 protein and CD68. Leiomyosarcoma will be actin-positive, mostly desmin-positive and negative for keratin, S100 protein and CD68. Other dermal and subcutaneous spindle cell neoplasms that figure in the differential diagnosis include spindle cell squamous carcinoma (keratin-positive), spindle cell and desmoplastic melanoma (S100-positive), nerve sheath tumors (S100-positive), atypical fibroxanthoma (AFX)/malignant fibrous histiocytoma (MFH) and nodular fasciitis. AFX/MFH can show some overlap in the immunohistochemical profile with leiomyosarcoma. Actin and CD68 are positive in about 30% of AFX/MFH but desmin, S100 and keratin are negative. The diagnosis of nodular fasciitis depends mainly on morphologic criteria. This neoplasm is composed of loose bundles of spindle cells, arranged in S- and C-shaped sweeping fascicles, in contrast to the tightly cellular fascicles of leiomyosarcoma.

Treatment

Wide excision with meticulous examination of all surgical margins is crucial in order to prevent recurrence. Recurrent tumors tend to infil-

trate more deeply, and they are often less well differentiated. They are more difficult to treat and carry a higher risk of metastasis. Several authors report successful treatment with Mohs micrographic surgery[15,20], allowing for complete margin control.

Smooth Muscle Hamartoma

Key features

- Congenital or acquired skin-colored to hyperpigmented plaque on the trunk or proximal extremities
- Common follicular prominence and hypertrichosis
- Clinical and histopathologic overlap with Becker's nevus (melanosis)

Introduction

Hamartoma is derived from the Greek word *hamartanein*, which means 'to err' or 'to fail'. Hamartomas are defined as lesions that are: (1) most commonly present at birth, but can also be acquired; and (2) are composed of aberrant mature or nearly mature structures. The term hamartoma is synonymous with 'nevus'; for example, nevus sebaceus, apocrine nevus, eccrine nevus. Smooth muscle hamartoma may be congenital or acquired and associated with a Becker's nevus (melanosis).

History

The first description of a smooth muscle hamartoma is attributed to Stokes in 1923[21].

Epidemiology

The estimated incidence ranges from 1:1000 to 1:27 000 live births.

Clinical features

Smooth muscle hamartomas not associated with a Becker's nevus present as firm skin-colored or hyperpigmented plaques, most commonly located on the trunk, buttocks or proximal extremities (Fig. 117.8). Surface changes may be present in the form of small follicular papules

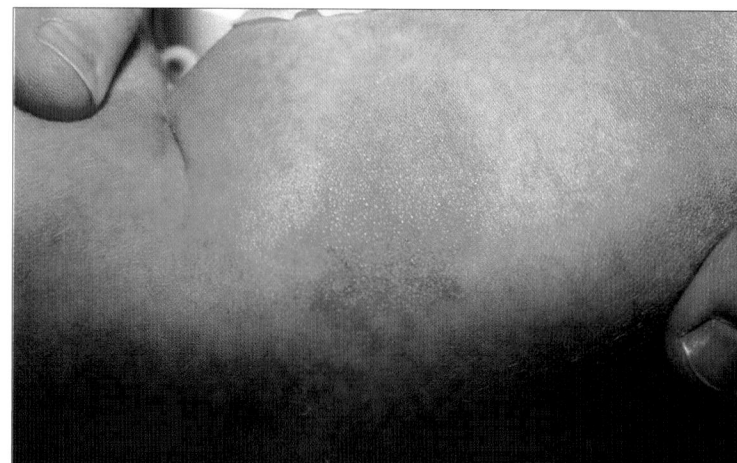

Fig. 117.8 Smooth muscle hamartoma. This infant presented with a firm plaque on the thigh. Courtesy of Ronald P Rapini MD.

or hypertrichosis. If hypertrichosis and hyperpigmentation are present, then the lesion shows significant overlap with a Becker's nevus (see Ch. 112). The lesions are most often solitary, but may be multiple. A generalized variant produces hypertrichosis and folding of the skin; it is another cause of a 'Michelin tire baby'[22]. Rubbing of the plaque may result in a pseudo-Darier's sign, consisting of transient induration of the affected area. There is no known case of malignant transformation in a smooth muscle hamartoma.

Pathology
Well-defined and thickened bundles of smooth muscle are haphazardly distributed throughout the dermis. Connections with hair follicles may be present. The epidermis is often acanthotic and has hyperpigmentation of the basal layer.

Differential diagnosis
Clinically and histologically, smooth muscle hamartomas demonstrate overlap with Becker's nevus, and the two lesions possibly represent a spectrum of phenotypic expression of the same process. Leiomyomas usually present as papulonodules rather than plaques. Additional entities in the clinical differential diagnosis are congenital melanocytic nevus and neurofibroma. Histologically, the smooth muscle fibers in a piloleiomyoma aggregate to dermal tumors with irregular margins, but they are not haphazardly scattered throughout the dermis as in smooth muscle hamartoma.

Treatment
Therapy may be indicated for cosmetic reasons. A small lesion may be amenable to excision. A recent report describes treatment of a Becker's nevus with the ruby laser[23].

TUMORS OF FAT

Lipoma

Key features
- Benign tumor of mature fat
- One of the most common neoplasms in humans
- Asymptomatic soft subcutaneous nodule of any site
- Multiple lipomas are seen in diffuse lipomatosis, Madelung's disease, adiposis dolorosa, familial multiple lipomatosis, Gardner syndrome, Bannayan–Riley–Ruvalcaba syndrome and Proteus syndrome

Introduction
Lipomas are benign tumors composed of mature lipocytes. They are among the most common neoplasms in humans, and they represent

the most common mesenchymal neoplasm[24]. Lipomas are more often solitary than multiple. In some patients, multiple lipomas are a manifestation of a lipomatosis or a multisystem syndrome.

Epidemiology
Lipomas can occur at any age, but most commonly become evident beyond the fourth decade of life. Most, but not all, statistical studies report the incidence in men to be higher than in women[24]. The incidence seems to be approximately equal in all races.

Pathogenesis
The vast majority of lipomas are incidental, and little is known about their pathogenesis. Occasionally, in the setting of familial multiple lipomatosis, there is a hereditary component. The incidence of lipomas is increased in overweight individuals, diabetics, and patients with elevated serum cholesterol[24]. Some lesions appear to be related to preceding trauma, and they may evolve from large hematomas[24].

Clonal chromosomal aberrations are found within lipomas in approximately two-thirds of patients. The abnormalities are heterogeneous, and the most common abnormalities are translocations between 12q13–15 and various other chromosomes. The *HMBA2* gene is located in the 12q13–15 region, and it may play a role in lipoma development. *HMBA2* encodes a high mobility group protein involved in the regulation of transcription[25].

Clinical features
Lipomas can occur in any fatty tissue of the body. The subcutis is the most commonly affected tissue. Sites of predilection are the neck, trunk, arms, proximal lower extremities, and buttocks. The face, hands and distal lower extremities are unusual locations[24,26,27]. Most lipomas are a few centimeters in diameter, but they can range in size from a few millimeters to 10 cm. Rare lesions attain a much larger size.

Lipomas are round to oval, soft, mobile subcutaneous nodules with a normal overlying epidermis. They may feel multilobular. Lipomas are asymptomatic, unless they encroach upon and compress nerves, in which case they may be painful. They are more common in overweight individuals, and they are characterized by slow growth. Once they achieve a certain size, they tend to remain stable and show no tendency to involute. Interestingly, the rate of growth may accelerate during periods of weight gain, but weight loss, even when extreme, does not seem to affect the size.

Multiple lipomas may be seen in patients with one of the lipomatoses or in the setting of a multisystem syndrome, such as Proteus syndrome.

Infiltrating or diffuse lipomatosis is characterized by non-encapsulated mature fat infiltrating subcutaneous tissue, muscle, skin, and, at times, even fascia and bone. This entity usually occurs before 30 years of age and, rarely, it may be congenital. Diffuse lipomatosis has been described in association with tuberous sclerosis (see Ch. 60) and paralytic poliomyelitis[28–30]. The lower extremities are most commonly affected, but involvement of the head, neck, face and upper extremities have all been reported. Pelvic involvement may lead to urinary tract, intestinal, and even vena caval obstruction[31].

Familial multiple lipomatosis is also known as familial multiple lipomas, multiple circumscribed lipomas, hereditary multiple lipomas, and discrete lipomatosis (Fig. 117.9). The disorder is defined as multiple lipomas occurring in several members of one kindred. In contrast to benign symmetric lipomatosis (Madelung's disease), the tumors are discrete, mobile, and surrounded by a capsule, as opposed to the diffuse and infiltrative tumor growth observed in Madelung's disease[32]. Favored sites include, but are not limited to, forearms and thighs. The neck and shoulders are generally spared.

Proteus syndrome is a complex disorder characterized by asymmetric, disproportionate (i.e. progressive and distorting) overgrowth of multiple tissues and multiple hamartomatous malformations (see Ch. 61). Because of its wide variability in phenotypic expression, the disease is named after Proteus, who, in Greek mythology, was a wise old man of the sea. Despite knowing everything, he was very reluctant to share his knowledge. Those who wanted to consult him had to surprise him during his midday nap and tie him down. He would try to

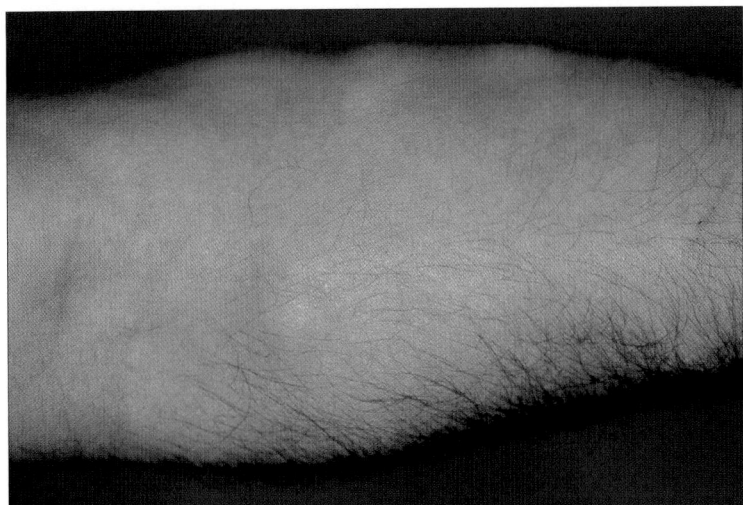

Fig. 117.9 Familial multiple lipomatosis. Several discrete lipomas are present on the forearm.

escape his captors by assuming a variety of shapes. Those who managed to hold him down long enough were rewarded with their desired answer when he returned to his original shape. Proteus syndrome received public attention through the book, play and movie describing the life of John Carey Merrick as *The Elephant Man*.

In patients with Proteus syndrome, congenital lipomatosis may be associated with overgrowth of multiple tissues in a mosaic pattern, leading to partial gigantism of the head or limbs, organomegaly, skeletal deformities, benign and malignant tumors, vascular malformations, areas of lipoatrophy, and deep venous thromboses[33]. Connective tissue nevi (particularly cerebriform lesions on the palms and soles) and epidermal nevi are commonly observed. Since the syndrome is highly variable, workshops have been conducted to try to establish diagnostic guidelines[34]. Mandatory diagnostic criteria include mosaic distribution of lesions, progressive course, and sporadic occurrence. The tissue overgrowth is progressive until after adolescence, but then seems to plateau. A subset of patients with Proteus-like phenotypes have germline mutations in the *PTEN* tumor suppressor gene (the susceptibility gene for Cowden disease and Bannayan–Riley–Ruvalcaba syndrome, see below)[35], and whether such cases represent true Proteus syndrome has been debated in the literature. **Hemihyperplasia–multiple lipomatosis syndrome** is a related but distinct condition characterized by multiple lipomas in association with asymmetric (but non-progressive and non-distorting) overgrowth, cutaneous capillary malformations, and thickened plantar skin with prominent creases.

Benign symmetric lipomatosis is also known as Madelung's disease in the American literature[36] and as benign symmetric lipomatosis of Launois-Bensaude in the European literature[37]. It consists of extensive symmetric fat deposits in the head, neck, and shoulder girdle area. When the mediastinum is involved, complications related to a space-occupying mass may ensue. Most patients are men, and a high percentage suffer from alcoholism; this may account for several disorders reported in association with benign symmetric lipomatosis, such as peripheral neuropathy, malignant tumors of the upper airways, and macrocytic anemia. Mutations in the mitochondrial tRNA lysine gene (which also result in neuropathy) have been described in a subset of patients with benign symmetric lipomatosis.

Multiple painful lipomas are present primarily on the arms, trunk, and in the periarticular soft tissue in **adiposis dolorosa (Dercum's disease)**. This disease most commonly affects postmenopausal women, and it is associated with weakness and psychiatric symptoms such as depression[38]. Pain is intermittent, but it may be debilitating, necessitating sophisticated pain management.

Lipomas may be part of **Gardner syndrome**. This syndrome consists of polyposis of the colon (eventuating in colonic carcinoma in about 50% of cases), odontomas, multiple epidermoid cysts, osteomas, leiomyomas and desmoid fibromatosis. Congenital hypertrophy of the retinal pigment epithelium is the characteristic ocular finding in Gardner syndrome. Mutations in the *APC* gene are responsible for this syndrome as well as familial adenomatous polyposis.

Multiple lipomas are also seen in **Bannayan–Riley–Ruvalcaba syndrome**, an autosomal dominantly inherited hamartoma syndrome. The characteristic constellation of findings has been described under at least five different eponyms, including Riley–Smith syndrome (1960), Bannayan–Zonana syndrome (1971), Ruvalcaba–Myre syndrome (1980) and Bannayan–Riley–Ruvalcaba syndrome (1980). While macrocephaly is the most consistent finding, other symptoms include pigmented macules on the penis and hamartomas, such as multiple lipomas, intestinal polyposis, and 'hemangiomas'[39,40].

Bannayan–Riley–Ruvalcaba syndrome and Cowden disease share the same genetic basis. Both diseases have mutations in the *PTEN* gene (phosphatase and tensin homolog deleted from chromosome 10), a tumor suppressor gene located on 10q23. Patients with Cowden disease have hamartomas in multiple organ systems, including skin, breast, thyroid, gastrointestinal tract, endometrium and brain. Cutaneous manifestations consist of trichilemmomas, acral and palmoplantar keratoses, and oral papillomatosis. Cowden disease and Bannayan–Riley–Ruvalcaba syndrome show partial clinical overlap, including lipomas, macrocephaly and intestinal polyps. Given that both syndromes share the same genetic basis, and families with both phenotypes have been described[29], the two disorders probably represent a spectrum of phenotypic expressions of the same disease.

Pathology

Lipomas are composed of a uniform population of mature fat cells with small, uniform and eccentric nuclei (Fig. 117.10). The fat cells are arranged in lobules with capillaries scattered throughout the lesion. Mitotic figures are absent. Microscopically, lipomas are indistinguishable from mature adipose tissue. If fibrous tissue or myxoid stroma are focally admixed, the terms fibrolipoma or myxolipoma are used, respectively. Cartilaginous or osseous metaplasia may occur. Intramuscular lipomas lack the circumscription of ordinary subcutaneous lipomas and infiltrate between muscle fibers.

Differential diagnosis

Clinically, lipomas may be mistaken for epidermoid cysts, hibernomas, and other special variants of benign fatty tumors. Lipomas lack the patulous follicular orifice of epidermoid cysts. As lipomas are histologically indistinguishable from normal fat, a definitive diagnosis cannot be made based on tissue examination.

Treatment

Small solitary lipomas of the subcutis can be easily excised, because they tend to be sharply circumscribed and can be shelled out. Local recurrence after excision is more common with larger-sized lipomas. Larger lesions, or systemic lipomatoses, may be amenable to liposuction.

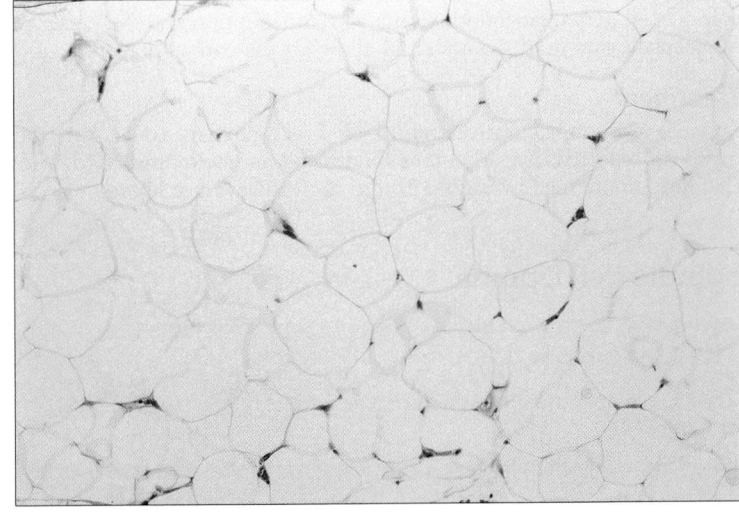

Fig. 117.10 Lipomas. They are composed of a uniform population of mature fat cells with small and eccentric nuclei.

Angiolipoma

Key features

- Soft subcutaneous nodules, usually less than 2 cm in diameter
- Typically located on the forearms of young adults
- More often painful than ordinary lipomas
- Small vessels occasionally contain fibrin thrombi

Introduction

An angiolipoma is a benign subcutaneous tumor composed of mature fat and a vascular component.

Epidemiology

Patients with angiolipomas are typically young adults in their late teens or early twenties. About 5% of cases are familial.

Pathogenesis

The pathogenesis of angiolipomas is not known. A small number of cases are familial, thus suggesting a genetic component. Unlike lipomas, hibernomas and many other fatty tumors, angiolipomas have a normal karyotype.

Clinical features

Angiolipomas are clinically similar to lipomas, but they measure less than 2 cm in diameter and may be painful. In approximately two-thirds of patients, the tumors are found on the forearms. Other, less common, sites include the trunk and upper arms. An estimated two-thirds of patients have multiple tumors[24].

Pathology

On cut section, angiolipomas are well-circumscribed or encapsulated yellow tumors with a reddish tinge. Histologic sections show mature adipose tissue admixed with a variable number of small vessels (Fig. 117.11). The degree of vascularity varies among different lesions and within different areas of the same tumor. Occasional vessels are occluded by fibrin thrombi. Tumors with a predominantly vascular component may be difficult to distinguish from a vascular neoplasm. Mast cells are more numerous than in lipomas, and older lesions may contain areas of fibrosis.

Differential diagnoses

Clinically, angiolipomas cannot be reliably distinguished from other benign fatty tumors, although the presence of pain may hint towards a diagnosis of angiolipoma. The histopathologic differential diagnosis includes ordinary lipoma, and no lower threshold exists for the minimal number of vessels required to warrant the diagnosis of angiolipoma. The identification of thrombosed vessels may be helpful in this situation, as they are usually not seen in lipomas. Highly vascular angiolipomas may be difficult to distinguish from Kaposi's sarcoma and spindle cell hemangioendothelioma. Circumscription and the presence of a capsule and mature fat should allow for the correct diagnosis.

Treatment

Surgical excision is curative and, to date, no malignant transformation has been reported. Angiolipomas tend to be more circumscribed, and, therefore, more readily excised *in toto* than the average lipoma.

Spindle Cell Lipoma

Key features

- Subcutaneous nodule on the upper back of middle-aged to older men
- Clinically indistinguishable from a lipoma
- Histologic triad of spindle cells, mature fat cells, and strands of dense collagen

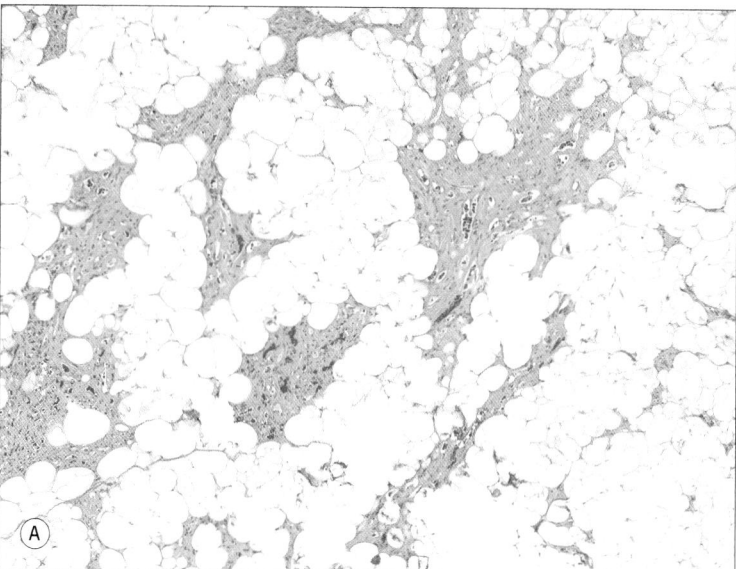

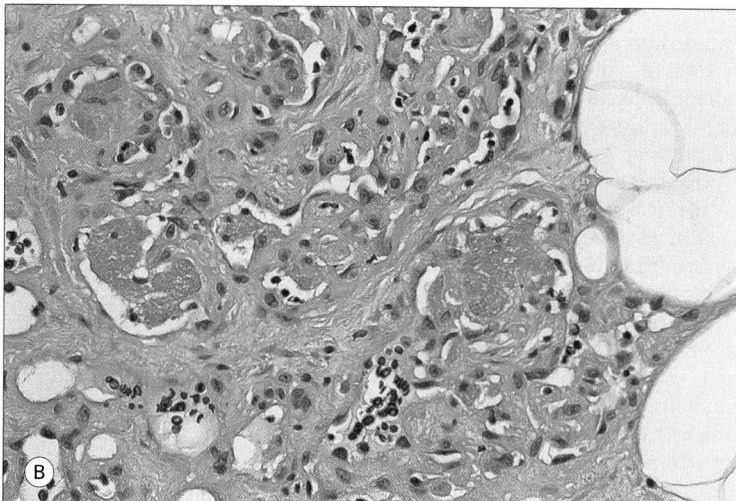

Fig. 117.11 Angiolipoma. A In angiolipomas, mature fat is admixed with a variable number of small vessels. **B** Occasional vessels are occluded by fibrin thrombi.

Introduction

Spindle cell lipoma is a histologically distinct tumor composed of mature fat cells, a population of spindle cells, and strands of dense collagen. The tumor occurs almost exclusively on the upper back and posterior neck of middle-aged and older men. However, it has no clinical characteristics that would allow it to be distinguished from other fatty tumors.

History

Spindle cell lipoma was first described by Enzinger & Harvey in 1975[41].

Epidemiology

Although cases involving women and young men have been reported, almost all patients with spindle cell lipoma are middle-aged to older men. In the original series of 114 patients, 91% were men[41].

Pathogenesis

The pathogenesis of spindle cell lipoma is unknown. Only a small fraction of cases occur in a familial setting.

Clinical features

Spindle cell lipoma presents in a similar fashion to an ordinary lipoma, as a solitary, slow-growing, mobile and painless subcutaneous mass without epidermal changes. The most common locations are the posterior neck, upper back, and shoulders, but other sites, including the breast, upper aerodigestive tract, and orbit have been described[24]. Multiple spindle cell lipomas and familial cases are rare.

Pathology

The histopathologic diagnosis of spindle cell lipoma requires the presence of three components, admixed in varying proportions: (1) mature fat cells; (2) small, uniform spindle cells; and (3) strands of dense, eosinophilic ('ropey') collagen[42] (Fig. 117.12). The spindle cell component is often set in a mucoid matrix. The vascularity is usually inconspicuous, but cleft-like spaces are occasionally prominent. The tumors are well circumscribed. The spindle cells are CD34-positive, actin-negative and S100-negative, and probably represent undifferentiated mesenchymal cells.

Differential diagnosis

Clinically, spindle cell lipoma is indistinguishable from other benign lipomatous tumors, with location being the most characteristic finding. The histopathologic appearance is characteristic, and diagnostic problems should arise only when the spindle cell population is predominant. In the latter situation, immunophenotyping may be helpful. Nodular fasciitis is actin-positive and CD34-negative. Neurofibroma and schwannoma are also in the differential diagnosis, but these are S100-positive.

Treatment

Surgical excision is curative for this benign tumor. It is rare for spindle cell lipoma to recur after complete excision.

Hibernoma

Synonyms: ■ Lipoma of immature adipose tissue ■ Lipoma of embryonic fat ■ Fetal lipoma

Key features

- Rare benign fatty tumor derived from brown fat, which is clinically indistinguishable from lipoma
- Patients with a hibernoma tend to be younger than those with lipomas and are typically in their thirties
- The most common locations are in the interscapular area, thighs, neck and chest
- The average size is approximately 10 cm

Introduction

A hibernoma is a rare benign tumor that is derived from brown fat. Brown fat is prominent in hibernating animals, but it is also found in humans. Brown fat first appears in the human fetus and persists into childhood. In children, brown fat is most prominent in the interscapular area, neck, mediastinum, anterior abdominal wall, and around some of the intraperitoneal and retroperitoneal organs. Brown fat gradually disappears with increasing age, and, in adults, it only persists around the kidneys, adrenal glands, aorta and in the neck. The main function of brown fat is heat production.

History

This neoplasm was first described in 1906 by Merkel[43] as a pseudo-lipoma of the breast. The term hibernoma was first introduced by Gery in 1914[44].

Epidemiology

Hibernomas occur primarily in adults. Individuals who develop these tumors are younger than patients with lipomas, and are typically in their thirties. A recent series of 170 hibernomas found an age range from 2 to 75 years, with a mean age of 38 years. The series included nine children[44].

Pathogenesis

Little is known about the pathogenesis of hibernoma. Characteristic clonal chromosomal abnormalities consist of structural rearrangements of 11q13 and 11q21.

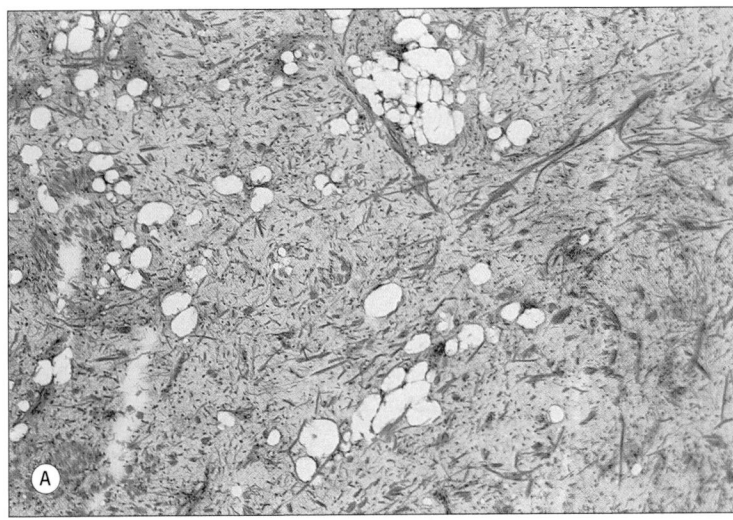

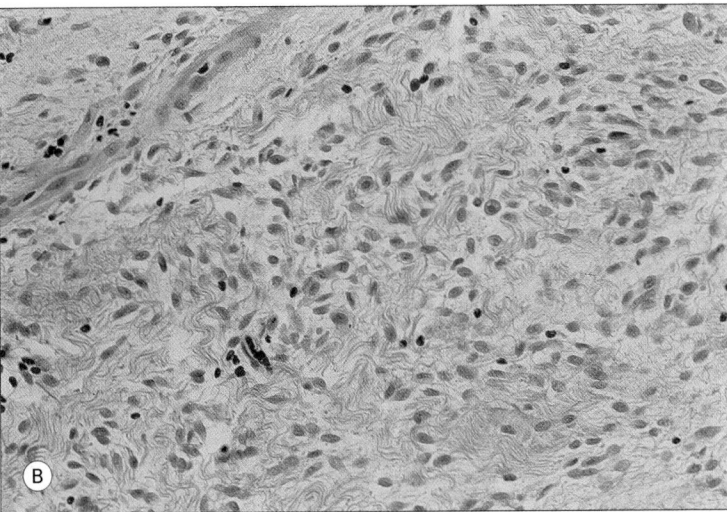

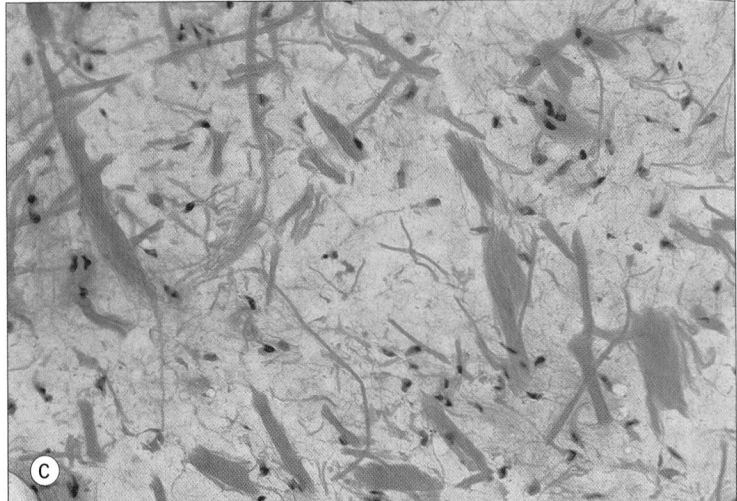

Fig. 117.12 Spindle cell lipoma. A This low-power photomicrograph shows all three components of a spindle cell lipoma – spindle cells, mature fat cells and 'ropey' collagen. **B** The spindle cells are small, uniform, bland, and have inconspicuous cytoplasm. **C** High magnification of thick, 'ropey' collagen.

Clinical features

Hibernomas are slow-growing tumors located in the subcutis or, occasionally, within skeletal muscle. On examination, they are indistinguishable from a lipoma, and they consist of soft, mobile, round to oval subcutaneous nodules. The most common anatomic locations are the interscapular area, thighs, shoulder, neck, chest, arms and abdominal cavity/retroperitoneum. They can measure up to 25 cm in diameter, with an average size of 10 cm[45].

Pathology

On cut section, hibernomas have a characteristic tan to deep red–brown color. Histologic examination shows pronounced lobulation. Highly vascular interlobular septa surround individual lobules (Fig. 117.13). Common to hibernomas are the characteristic brown fat cells with a small central nucleus and multivacuolated to granular eosinophilic cytoplasm. The cell membrane is distinct. These typical hibernoma cells are admixed with variable numbers of mature fat cells and pale multivacuolated cells. Rare cases have a myxoid stroma or have features of both spindle cell lipoma and hibernoma[45].

Differential diagnosis

Hibernomas are clinically indistinguishable from lipomas. The histopathologic appearance is characteristic, and confusion with other entities is unlikely.

Treatment

Surgical excision is curative. None of the 66 cases in a recent clinicopathologic study recurred after complete excision[45].

Nevus Lipomatosus Superficialis

Synonym: ■ Nevus lipomatosis of Hoffman and Zurhelle

Key features

■ Grouped soft papulonodules on the hips and upper thighs

■ Hamartomatous lesion with onset during the first two decades of life

■ Mature fat cells in the dermis are the defining histopathologic feature

Introduction

Nevus lipomatosus superficialis of Hoffman and Zurhelle is a connective tissue nevus or hamartoma, characterized by grouped soft papulonodules, most commonly located on the buttocks or upper thighs.

History

Nevus lipomatosus was first described by Hoffman & Zurhelle in 1921[46].

Epidemiology

This rare hamartoma develops shortly after birth or during the first two decades of life, and it does not seem to exhibit a gender preference.

Pathogenesis

The pathogenesis of nevus lipomatosus superficialis is unknown. There is speculation that precursor cells around dermal blood vessels give rise to the mature fat cells in the dermis that characterize this lesion.

Clinical features

Nevus lipomatosus superficialis consists of soft clustered papulonodules that are usually present at birth, or appear during childhood or adolescence. Initial presentation in adults has been described. The lesions consist of soft, yellow to skin-colored papules or nodules that are clustered, do not cross the midline, and may follow Blaschko's lines (Fig. 117.14A). Individual lesions may be sessile or pedunculated, and they have a smooth or cerebriform surface. The pelvic girdle area and upper thighs are the most common locations.

For large lesions that form linear masses along skin folds, the term 'Michelin tire baby' has been applied[47]. Michelin tire syndrome only describes the phenotypic appearance of affected individuals, and it does not define the underlying histopathologic abnormality, as patients with large smooth muscle hamartomas can have a similar clinical appearance[22].

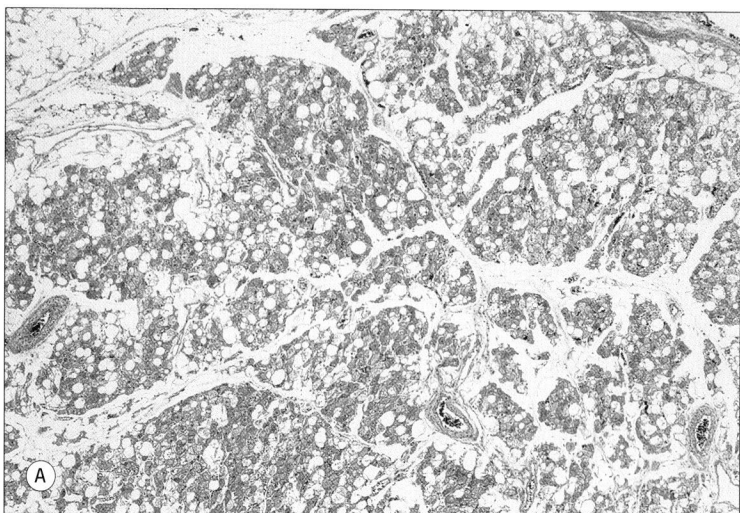

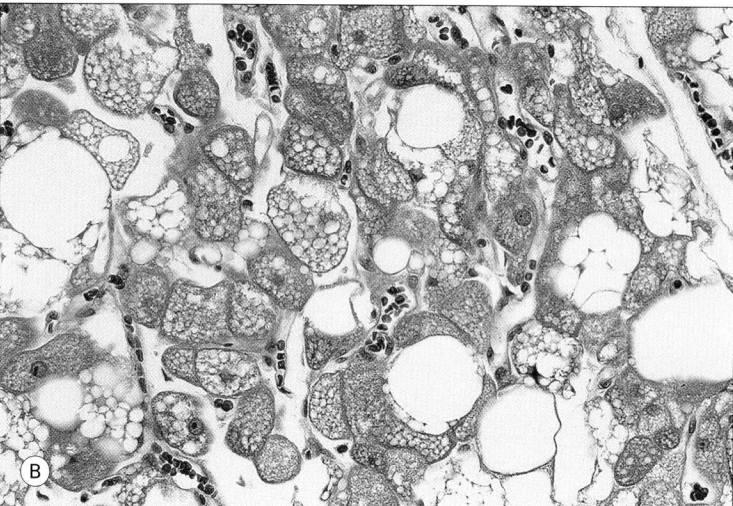

Fig. 117.13 Hibernoma. A Hibernoma with characteristic lobulation. **B** The cytoplasm of hibernoma cells ranges from multivacuolated to granular.

Pathology

The defining histopathologic feature consists of mature fat cells in the dermis (Fig. 117.14B). Skin appendages are not displaced.

Differential diagnosis

A solitary acquired papilloma that contains fat cells but no skin appendages in the dermis is a variant of skin tag known as lipofibroma, not a nevus lipomatosus superficialis. In focal dermal hypoplasia (Goltz syndrome), the dermis is either absent and completely replaced by fat cells, or significantly thinned. Skin appendages are missing. Clinically, agminated neurofibromas may be mistaken for nevus lipomatosus.

Treatment

Most lesions are amenable to excision.

Lipoblastoma/Lipoblastomatosis

Synonym: ■ Embryonic lipoma

Key features

■ Benign neoplasm of immature fat cells seen primarily in children less than 3 years of age

■ The circumscribed form is termed lipoblastoma, and the diffuse form is termed lipoblastomatosis

■ Extremities represent the site of predilection

■ It can be histopathologically indistinguishable from myxoid liposarcoma, which almost always occurs in adults

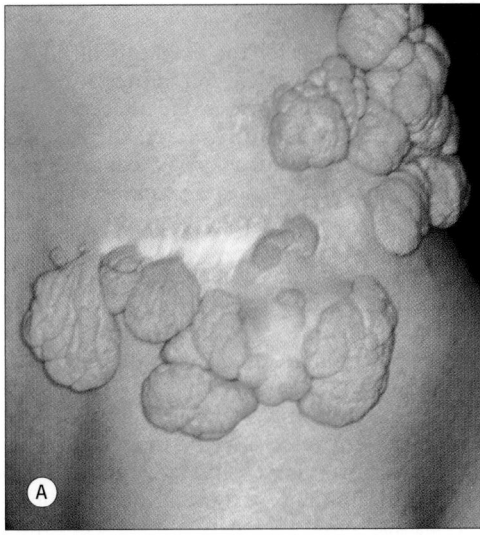

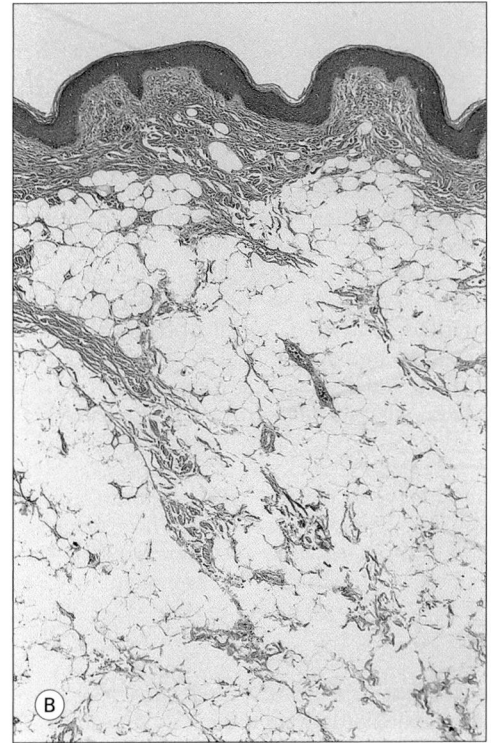

Fig. 117.14 Nevus lipomatosus superficialis.
A This hamartoma is characterized by grouped soft, pedunculated, skin-colored tumors; a partial resection had been performed. With permission from Kopf AW and Bart RS. J Dermatol Surg Oncol 9:279–281, 1983. **B** Histopathologically, mature fat cells seen in the dermis are pathognomonic.

Introduction

This is a rare variant of lipoma, and it represents a benign tumor of immature fat cells that occurs almost exclusively in children. When circumscribed, this neoplasm is termed lipoblastoma, and, when diffuse, it is known as lipoblastomatosis.

History

The term lipoblastoma was coined by Vellios et al.[48] in 1958, when they reported a case of lipoblastomatosis.

Epidemiology

Lipoblastoma and lipoblastomatosis are tumors of infancy. Occasionally, these neoplasms are described in older children, or even teenagers, but the majority occur before the age of 3 years. Congenital tumors have been observed. Boys are affected twice as often as girls.

Pathogenesis

Lipoblastomas are neoplasms of immature white fat, and they may represent residual areas of immature fat. The latter is suggested by sequential biopsies showing maturation to mature fat and by the almost exclusive occurrence in infancy and childhood. On the other hand, the presence of chromosomal rearrangements affecting chromosome 8q argues for a clonal neoplasm.

Clinical features

Most lipoblastomas occur before the age of 3 years, and they are twice as common in boys as in girls. The upper and lower extremities are the sites of predilection. Most tumors are limited to the subcutis and circumscribed, and hence represent lipoblastomas. In addition to the extremities, lipoblastomas may be found in the head and neck region and on the trunk. These superficial lesions clinically simulate lipomas, and they present as slow-growing, soft, mobile, painless nodules, measuring 3–5 cm in diameter.

Lipoblastomatosis affects the deeper soft tissue, and often diffusely infiltrates adjacent skeletal muscle. This process can occur in the mediastinum, mesentery and retroperitoneum. Rare tumors weigh up to 1 kg. Depending on the location, the tumor may result in symptoms of local obstruction or compression.

Pathology

Grossly, lipoblastomas are paler than ordinary lipomas, and they have a myxoid quality. Histologically, it is a lobulated neoplasm. The stroma is often myxoid, contains a plexiform vascular network, and is divided into lobules by connective tissue septa. Deep-seated tumors often lack the lobulation, and they may grow in a diffuse pattern. The tumors are composed of fat cells spanning the range of maturation from immature stellate and spindled mesenchymal cells, to lipoblasts with a single cytoplasmic vacuole that indents a peripherally located nucleus, to small and mature adipocytes. Lipoblastomas are paucicellular, cytologically bland, and lack mitotic activity. Serial biopsies of a lipoblastoma may show gradual maturation to a mature fatty tumor.

Differential diagnosis

Histopathologically, lipoblastoma and myxoid liposarcoma can be indistinguishable. Clinical parameters that aid in the differential diagnosis are the age of the patient and the location of the tumor. Myxoid liposarcomas almost always develop in individuals older than 20 years of age, and they are located in the deep soft tissue, rather than the subcutis. Nevertheless, in a child, an immature fat tumor that contains areas of marked cellularity, loss of lobulation, and mitotic figures should raise concern for a myxoid liposarcoma.

Treatment

Lipoblastoma, if treated with complete excision, rarely recurs. Unusual cases of spontaneous resolution without treatment exist[49]. In a series of 14 patients with lipoblastomas/lipoblastomatosis[50] 22% recurred after excision. Recurrences are usually restricted to cases of lipoblastomatosis, particularly if the excision was incomplete. Wide excision is the therapy of choice for the diffuse form of the disease.

Liposarcoma/Atypical Lipomatous Tumor

Synonym: ■ Atypical lipoma

Key features

- Sarcoma of deep soft tissue that is only rarely limited to the skin
- There are five histologic subtypes, ranging in biologic behavior from locally aggressive neoplasms without metastatic potential to malignant tumors with a significant risk of metastatic dissemination
- If the skin is involved, extension from a more deeply situated tumor needs to be excluded

Introduction

Liposarcoma is the second most common soft tissue sarcoma after malignant fibrous histiocytoma. Five histopathologic subtypes are recognized by the World Health Organization (WHO), with important prognostic, cytogenetic, molecular and epidemiologic differences. The biologic behavior of the subtypes ranges from locally aggressive tumors without metastatic potential to highly malignant neoplasms with a significant risk of systemic spread. There is considerable controversy among soft tissue pathologists regarding the nomenclature of this tumor. Some experts prefer the term atypical lipomatous tumor for all liposarcomas in the subcutis, because these tumors recur but have virtually no metastatic potential[51,52]. Others prefer to retain the term liposarcoma because histologically and cytogenetically these tumors are the same, regardless of location, and also because these tumors carry a small risk for dedifferentiation, which confers metastatic potential[53].

Epidemiology

The annual incidence of all types of soft tissue liposarcoma is estimated at 2.5 per million, based on a Swedish study. The average age at presentation is 50 years. Rare cases arise in children older than 10 years of age, but virtually never in children younger than 10 years of age.

Pathogenesis

It appears that liposarcomas arise de novo, rather than from pre-existing lipomas. A reciprocal translocation between chromosomes 12 and 16 is consistently present in myxoid and round cell liposarcomas, and this results in the expression of fusion transcripts; the latter play an important role in oncogenesis. Well-differentiated liposarcomas have giant and ring chromosomes that are derived from chromosome 12 and result in gene amplification. Unlike other soft tissue sarcomas, radiation does not appear to play a role in their pathogenesis.

Clinical features

Liposarcoma is a tumor primarily of the deep soft tissue of the extremities and retroperitoneum. Legs and buttocks are more frequently affected than the upper extremities (Fig. 117.15). It originates in, and is limited to, the dermis or subcutis only in exceptional circumstances[54,55]. Primary cutaneous liposarcomas are described as dome-shaped or polypoid, and they measure between 1 and 19.5 cm[55]. If a liposarcoma presents in the subcutis, this will often be due to direct extension from an underlying sarcoma of the deep soft tissue.

Tumors limited to the dermis or subcutis can recur, but they do not metastasize or cause patient death. Liposarcomas of the deep soft tissue and retroperitoneum are malignant neoplasms, capable of recurrence, metastasis, and causing patient death. The prognosis depends on the location, degree of differentiation, and the histopathologic subtype.

Pathology

The sine qua non for the diagnosis of liposarcoma is the presence of lipoblasts. Lipoblasts are immature fat cells, characterized by a hyperchromatic nucleus that is indented or scalloped by cytoplasmic fat vacuoles (Fig. 117.16). However, the lipoblasts need to be present in the appropriate histopathologic context, as they are not specific for liposarcomas, but can also be found in lipoblastomas and pleomorphic lipomas, or can closely resemble histiocytes found in fat necrosis or fat atrophy.

The histopathologic appearance is highly variable and depends on the particular subtype (Fig. 117.17). A **well-differentiated** liposarcoma consists of mature fat with a variable number of lipoblasts and cells with hyperchromatic nuclei. **Myxoid** liposarcoma resembles immature fat and can be histologically indistinguishable from a lipoblastoma. Small and uniformly bland spindle cells are set in a myxoid matrix with plexiform vessels. In the more cellular areas, myxoid liposarcoma merges with **round cell** liposarcoma, which is characterized by sheets of primitive round cells. Several classification schemes recognize round cell liposarcoma as a part of the spectrum of myxoid liposarcoma. **Pleomorphic** liposarcoma is the least common subtype; it exhibits an extreme degree of nuclear pleomorphism and resembles a malignant fibrous histiocytoma. **Dedifferentiated** liposarcoma is a biphasic tumor comprised of areas of well-differentiated liposarcoma/atypical lipomatous tumor and areas of a non-lipogenic sarcoma.

Differential diagnosis

Liposarcomas of the subcutaneous tissue are exceedingly rare, and they should only be diagnosed after histopathologic mimics, metastases, and direct extension from a deep soft tissue sarcoma have been excluded. Pleomorphic lipoma, a subcutaneous tumor usually found on the posterior neck in the same location as spindle cell lipoma, can closely resemble liposarcoma. It is found in elderly men, and there are hyperchromatic atypical lipocytes, often with floret-type giant cells. Liposarcomas are more infiltrating, more cellular, and more atypical in most cases.

Myxoid liposarcoma can be histologically indistinguishable from lipoblastoma and lipoblastomatosis. This differential diagnosis relies on clinical parameters and is discussed above under lipoblastoma.

Treatment

Wide excision is the treatment of choice. Tumors limited to the dermis and subcutis may be treated by dermatologists. The treatment of most liposarcomas, however, will require an oncologic soft-tissue surgeon. It is not uncommon for liposarcomas to have a multinodular growth pattern and extend into muscle and fascial planes. Excision needs to be carefully planned using MRI and radiographic information.

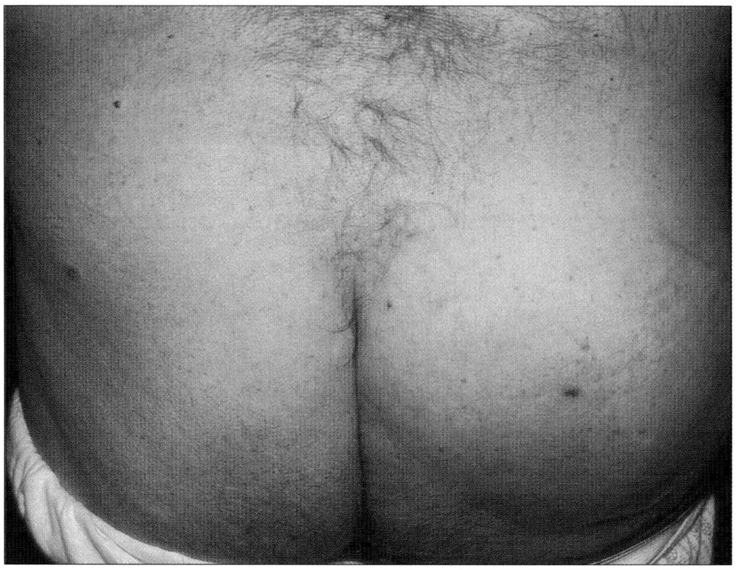

Fig. 117.15 Liposarcoma. Note the large mass in the right buttock. Courtesy of Ronald P Rapini MD.

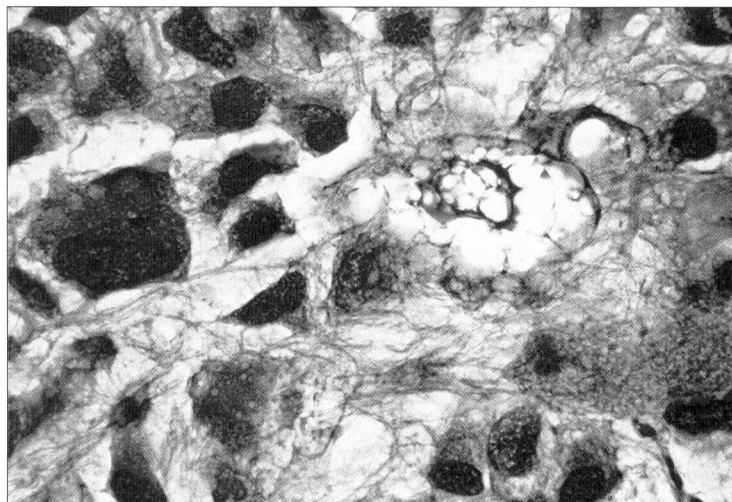

Fig. 117.16 Liposarcoma. Lipoblasts are immature fat cells, with a hyperchromatic nucleus that is scalloped by cytoplasmic fat vacuoles. Their presence is mandatory for a diagnosis of liposarcoma. Courtesy of Richard Kempson MD.

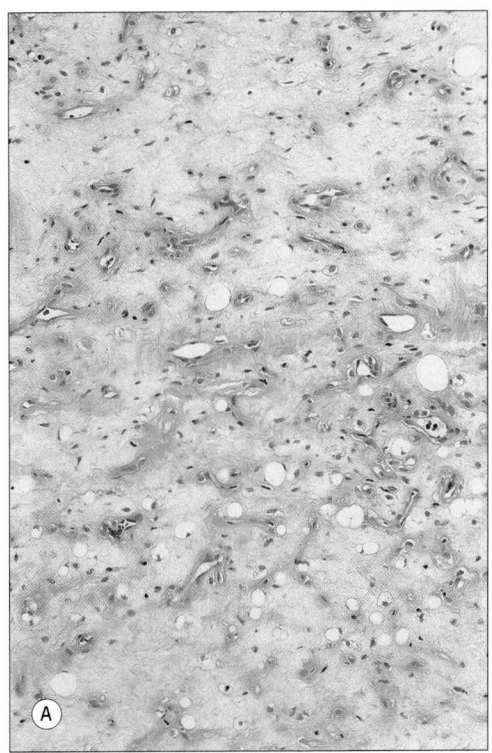

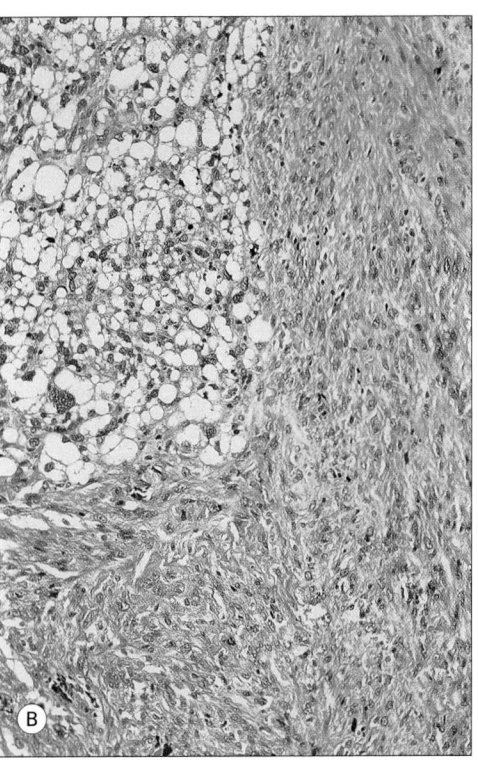

Fig. 117.17 The varied histopathologic features of liposarcoma. A Myxoid liposarcoma – without the clinical context, this tumor can be indistinguishable from lipoblastoma. Bland spindle cells occur in a myxoid matrix with plexiform vessels. **B** Pleomorphic liposarcoma – anaplastic and cellular neoplasm. Lipoblasts may be difficult to find.

TUMORS OF CARTILAGE

Extraskeletal Chondroma

Synonym: ▪ Chondroma of soft parts

Key features

- Rare benign tumor of mature cartilage
- Most commonly located near the small joints of the hands and feet

Introduction

Cartilage can be found in the skin as a result of metaplasia, as a component of chondroid syringomas, and as the exclusive component of extraskeletal chondromas. By definition, extraskeletal chondromas are not attached to bone and occur outside the synovial space. With the exception of two clinical series[56,57], most of the experience with extraskeletal chondromas is in the form of case reports.

Epidemiology

Extraskeletal chondromas are rare tumors that occur in children as well as adults, but most patients are beyond their third decade.

Clinical features

Extraskeletal chondromas present as solitary painless nodules on the hands and feet and, most frequently, on the fingers. They grow slowly and are often associated with tendons. Other rare locations include the trunk, head, neck, oral cavity, larynx and pharynx.

Pathology

On gross examination, chondromas are sharply circumscribed and often lobulated. Most measure less than 2 cm, but larger lesions can occur. Histopathologically, they consist of hyaline cartilage that may be admixed with variable amounts of fibrous tissue or myxoid stroma. The cartilage may comprise only a small portion of the tumor. Mature hyaline cartilage displays a dense basophilic matrix with nuclei in lacunae. Calcification is common, preferentially affects the center of the tumor, and may be extensive. Like normal chondrocytes, the lesional cells of chondroma are reactive for S100 protein.

Differential diagnosis

Synovial chondromatosis consists of multiple discrete osteocartilaginous nodules and favors the large joints, such as the knee, hip and elbow. Histologic differentiation from grade I chondrosarcoma or myxoid chondrosarcoma may be difficult, but chondrosarcomas rarely affect hands and feet, and they are in continuity with bone and cartilage.

Treatment

Local excision is usually curative. Up to 20% of extraskeletal chondromas may recur. To the best of our knowledge, malignant transformation to chondrosarcoma does not occur.

REFERENCES

1. Stout AP. Solitary cutaneous and subcutaneous leiomyoma. Am J Cancer. 1937;29:435–69.
2. Orellana-Diaz O, Hernandez-Perez E. Leiomyoma cutis and leiomyosarcoma: a 10-year study and a short review. J Dermatol Surg Oncol. 1983;9:283–7.
3. Yokoyama R, Hashimoto H, Daimaru Y, Enjoji M. Superficial leiomyomata. A clinicopathologic study of 34 cases. Acta Pathol Jpn. 1987;37:1415–22.
4. The Multiple Leiomyoma Consortium. Germline mutations in *FH* predispose to dominantly inherited uterine fibroids, skin leiomyomata and papillary renal cell cancer. Nat Genet. 2002;30:406–10.
5. Alam NA, Barclay E, Rowan AJ, et al. Clinical features of multiple cutaneous and uterine leiomyomatosis. Arch Dermatol. 2005;141:199–206.
6. Raj S, Calonje E, Kraus M, et al. Cutaneous pilar leiomyoma: clinicopathologic analysis of 53 lesions in 45 patients. Am J Dermatopathol. 1997;19:2–9.
7. Hachisuga T, Hashimoto H, Enjoji M. Angioleiomyoma. A clinicopathologic reappraisal of 562 cases. Cancer. 1984;54:126–30.
8. Kawagishi N, Kashiwagi T, Ibe M, et al. Pleomorphic angioleiomyoma. Am J Dermatopathol. 2000; 22:268–71.
9. Slone S, O'Connor D. Scrotal leiomyomata with bizarre nuclei: a report of three cases. Mod Pathol. 1998;11:282–7.
10. McGinley KM, Bryant S, Kattine AA, et al. Cutaneous leiomyomata lack estrogen and progesterone receptor immunoreactivity. J Cutan Pathol. 1997; 24:241–5.
11. Newman PL, Fletcher CD. Smooth muscle tumours of the external genitalia: clinicopathological analysis of a series. Histopathology. 1991;18:523–9.
12. Thompson JA Jr. Therapy for painful cutaneous leiomyomata. J Am Acad Dermatol. 1985;13:865–7.

18

NEOPLASMS OF THE SKIN

13. Christenson LJ, Smith K, Arpey CJ. Treatment of multiple cutaneous leiomyomata with CO$_2$ laser ablation. Dermatol Surg. 2000;26:319–22.

13a. Svarvar C, Bohling T, Berlin O, et al. Clinical course of nonvisceral soft tissue leiomyosarcoma in 225 patients from the Scandinavian Sarcoma Group. Cancer. 2007;109:282–91.

14. Fields JP, Helwig EB. Leiomyosarcoma of the skin and subcutaneous tissue. Cancer. 1981;47:156–69.

15. Bernstein SC, Roenigk RK. Leiomyosarcoma of the skin. Treatment of 34 cases. Dermatol Surg. 1996;22:631–5.

16. Weiss SW, Goldblum JR. Leiomyosarcoma. In: Weiss SW (ed.). Soft Tissue Tumors, 4th edn. St Louis: Mosby, 2001:727–48.

17. Dahl I, Angervall L. Cutaneous and subcutaneous leiomyosarcoma. A clinicopathologic study of 47 patients. Pathol Eur. 1974;9:307–15.

18. Kempson RL, Fletcher CDM, Evans HL, et al. Smooth muscle tumors. In: Rosai J, Sobin LH (eds). Tumors of Soft Tissues, 3rd Series. Washington, DC: Armed Forces Institute of Pathology, 2001:239–56.

19. Suster S. Epithelioid leiomyosarcoma of the skin and subcutaneous tissue. Clinicopathologic, immunohistochemical, and ultrastructural study of five cases. Am J Surg Pathol. 1994;18:232–40.

20. Huether MJ, Zitelli JA, Brodland DG. Mohs micrographic surgery for the treatment of spindle cell tumors of the skin. J Am Acad Dermatol. 2001;44:656–9.

21. Stokes JH. Nevus pilaris with hyperplasia of non-striated muscle. Arch Dermatol Syph. 1923;7:479–81.

22. Glover MT, Malone M, Atherton DJ. Michelin-tire baby syndrome resulting from diffuse smooth muscle hamartoma. Pediatr Dermatol. 1989;6:329–31.

23. Nanni CA, Alster TS. Treatment of a Becker's nevus using a 694-nm long-pulsed ruby laser. Dermatol Surg. 1998;24:1032–4.

24. Weiss SW, Goldblum JR. Benign lipomatous tumors. In: Weiss SW (ed.). Soft Tissue Tumors, 4th edn. St Louis: Mosby, 2001:571–639.

25. Rubin BP, Fletcher CD. The cytogenetics of lipomatous tumours. Histopathology. 1997;30:507–11.

26. Rydholm A, Berg NO. Size, site and clinical incidence of lipoma. Factors in the differential diagnosis of lipoma and sarcoma. Acta Orthop Scand. 1983;54:929–34.

27. Myhre-Jensen O. A consecutive 7-year series of 1331 benign soft tissue tumours. Clinicopathologic data. Comparison with sarcomas. Acta Orthop Scand. 1981;52:287–93.

28. Karademir M, Kocak M, Usal A, et al. A case of infiltrating lipomatosis with diffuse, symmetrical distribution. Br J Clin Pract. 1990;44:728–30.

29. Klein JA, Barr RJ. Diffuse lipomatosis and tuberous sclerosis. Arch Dermatol. 1986;122:1298–302.

30. Kindblom LG, Moller-Nielsen J. Diffuse lipomatosis in the leg after poliomyelitis. Acta Pathol Microbiol Scand [A]. 1975;83:339–44.

31. Klein FA, Smith MJ, Kasenetz I. Pelvic lipomatosis: 35-year experience. J Urol. 1988;139:998–1001.

32. Leffell DJ, Braverman IM. Familial multiple lipomatosis. Report of a case and a review of the literature. J Am Acad Dermatol. 1986;15:275–9.

33. Biesecker LG. The multifaceted challenges of Proteus syndrome. JAMA. 2001;285:2240–3.

34. Biesecker LG, Happle R, Mulliken JB, et al. Proteus syndrome: diagnostic criteria, differential diagnosis, and patient evaluation. Am J Med Genet. 1999; 84:389–95.

35. Zhou X, Hampel H, Thiele H, et al. Association of germline mutation in the PTEN tumour suppressor gene and Proteus and Proteus-like syndromes. Lancet. 2001;358:210–11.

36. Enzi G. Multiple symmetric lipomatosis: an updated clinical report. Medicine (Baltimore). 1984;63:56–64.

37. Ruzicka T, Vieluf D, Landthaler M, Braun-Falco O. Benign symmetric lipomatosis Launois-Bensaude. Report of ten cases and review of the literature. J Am Acad Dermatol. 1987;17:663–74.

38. Reece PH, Wyatt M, O'Flynn P. Dercum's disease (adiposis dolorosa). J Laryngol Otol. 1999;113:174–6.

39. Bannayan GA. Lipomatosis, angiomatosis, and macrencephalia. A previously undescribed congenital syndrome. Arch Pathol. 1971;92:1–5.

40. Wanner M, Celebi JT, Peacocke M. Identification of a PTEN mutation in a family with Cowden syndrome and Bannayan-Zonana syndrome. J Am Acad Dermatol. 2001;44:183–7.

41. Enzinger FM, Harvey DA. Spindle cell lipoma. Cancer. 1975;36:1852–9.

42. Kempson RL, Fletcher CDM, Evans HL, et al. Lipomatous tumors. In: Rosai J, Sobin LH (eds). Tumors of Soft Tissues. 3rd Series. Washington, DC: Armed Forces Institute of Pathology, 2001:187–238.

43. Merkel H. On a pseudolipoma of the breast (peculiar fat tumor). Beitr Pathol Anat. 1906;39:152–7.

44. Gery L. Discussions. Bull Mem Soc Anat (Paris). 1914;89:111–12.

45. Furlong MA, Fanburg-Smith JC, Miettinen M. The morphologic spectrum of hibernoma: a clinicopathologic study of 170 cases. Am J Surg Pathol. 2001;25:809–14.

46. Hoffman E, Zurhelle E. Über einen Nävus lipomatosus cutaneus superficialis der linken Glutealgegend. Arch Dermatol. 1921;130:327.

47. Ross CM. Generalized folded skin with an underlying lipomatous nevus. "The Michelin Tire baby". Arch Dermatol. 1969;100:320–3.

48. Vellios F, Baez JM, Shumacker HB. Lipoblastomatosis: a tumor of fetal fat different from hibernoma: report of a case, with observations on the embryogenesis of human adipose tissue. Am J Pathol. 1958;34:1149.

49. Mognato G, Cecchetto G, Carli M, et al. Is surgical treatment of lipoblastoma always necessary? J Pediatr Surg. 2000;35:1511–13.

50. Mentzel T, Calonje E, Fletcher CD. Lipoblastoma and lipoblastomatosis: a clinicopathological study of 14 cases. Histopathology. 1993;23:527–33.

51. Azumi N, Curtis J, Kempson RL, et al. Atypical and malignant neoplasms showing lipomatous differentiation. A study of 111 cases. Am J Surg Pathol. 1987;11:161–83.

52. Evans HL, Soule EH, Winkelmann RK. Atypical lipoma, atypical intramuscular lipoma, and well differentiated retroperitoneal lipoma: a reappraisal of 30 cases formerly classified as well differentiated liposarcoma. Cancer. 1979;43:574–84.

53. Weiss SW, Rao VK. Well-differentiated liposarcoma (atypical lipoma) of deep soft tissue of the extremities, retroperitoneum, and miscellaneous sites. A follow-up study of 92 cases with analysis of the incidence of 'dedifferentiation'. Am J Surg Pathol. 1992; 16:1051–8.

54. Yoshikawa H, Ueda T, Mori S, et al. Dedifferentiated liposarcoma of the subcutis. Am J Surg Pathol. 1996;20:1525–30.

55. Dei Tos AP, Mentzel T, Fletcher CD. Primary liposarcoma of the skin: a rare neoplasm with unusual high grade features. Am J Dermatopathol. 1998;20:332–8.

56. Dahlin DC, Salvador AH. Cartilaginous tumors of the soft tissues of the hands and feet. Mayo Clin Proc. 1974;49:721–6.

57. Chung EB, Enzinger FM. Benign chondromas of soft parts. Cancer. 1978;41:1414–24.

Mastocytosis

Michael D Tharp

Key features

- The onset of mastocytosis can occur from birth to adulthood and may involve only the skin (most children) or multiple organs such as the bone marrow, liver, spleen and/or lymph nodes (some adults)

- Childhood disease is more common and often presents with one or more tan to brown papules or plaques (*urticaria pigmentosa*) that frequently resolve in late adolescence

- *Mastocytomas* are thicker plaques or nodules that occur mostly in children

- Adults with mastocytosis may or may not have cutaneous lesions; when present, they appear as 2–5 mm red–brown macules or papules. Adult disease persists throughout life

- *Telangiectasia macularis eruptiva perstans* is a variation that occurs mostly in adults

- Stroking of lesions of mastocytosis often causes urtication (*Darier's sign*), which is more common in children due to a higher density of mast cells

- Blisters may occur and are most common during early childhood

- Patients may be asymptomatic or have accompanying symptoms of mast cell mediator release such as pruritus, flushing, abdominal pain, diarrhea, hypotension and syncope

INTRODUCTION

Mastocytosis represents a spectrum of clinical disorders with a common phenotype of tissue mast cell hyperplasia. Patients with this disorder were initially thought to have only cutaneous disease; however, it was then discovered that mastocytosis patients could have involvement of multiple organs. Although the clinical aspects of the disorder have been well documented for decades, the pathogenesis of mastocytosis became better defined during the early 1990s. It now appears that the mechanism responsible for most cases of childhood mastocytosis differs from that of adult-onset disease, thus helping to explain differences in the clinical presentations and courses between these two patient groups (Fig. 118.1). While therapy for mastocytosis currently centers on inhibiting the effects of mast cell mediators released into tissues, it is expected that an improved understanding of the pathogenesis of this disorder should lead to more directed and effective treatments in the future.

HISTORY

The original description of mastocytosis was by Nettleship & Tay, who reported on a 2-year-old girl with hyperpigmented papules that spontaneously urticated[1]. It was not until 8 years later in 1877 that Paul Ehrlich formally discovered the mast cell. The next year, Sangster described a patient with pruritus, urticaria and pigmentation; he labeled this peculiar eruption urticaria pigmentosa[2]. Unna was the first to demonstrate that mast cells were responsible for the cutaneous eruption in mastocytosis patients, and over 60 years later, Ellis reported the first patient with systemic disease[3]. While a number of descriptive terms have been applied to patients with mast cell disease, mastocytosis is now the accepted term for this disorder.

EPIDEMIOLOGY

Mastocytosis can present at the time of birth or develop any time thereafter into late adulthood. Childhood mastocytosis is defined as

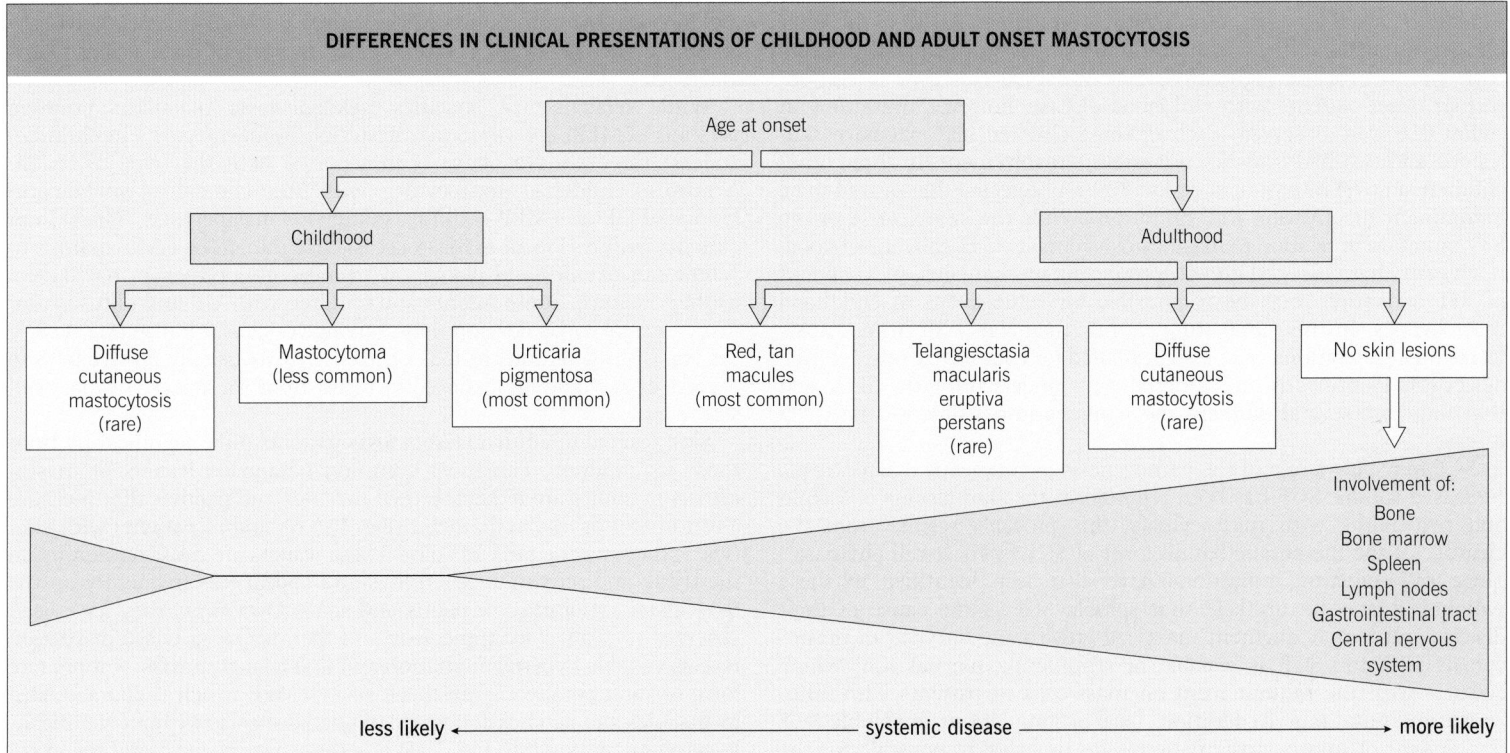

Fig. 118.1 Differences in clinical presentations of childhood and adult-onset mastocytosis. The mechanism responsible for most cases of childhood mastocytosis differs from that of adult-onset disease.

that with an onset before puberty. Approximately 55% of mastocytosis patients develop their disease by 2 years of age, and another 10% experience disease onset between the ages of 2 and 15 years. This disorder has no gender preference, and it has been reported in all races[4]. While most patients with mastocytosis have no family history of the disorder, to date there have been approximately 70 familial cases of mastocytosis reported, including at least 15 sets of monozygotic twins (although several monozygotic twin pairs discordant for mastocytosis have also been described). Familial mastocytosis has been documented in three generations of a single kindred[5].

PATHOGENESIS

Mast cells are derived from pluripotent CD34$^+$ precursors in the bone marrow and circulate in the peripheral blood as agranular, monocytic-appearing cells. After migrating into tissues, these immature mast cells assume their typical granular morphology. Circulating mast cell precursors express CD34, the tyrosine kinase KIT (CD117), and IgG receptors (FcγRII), but not high-affinity IgE receptors (FcεRI)[6]. KIT is the protein product of the proto-oncogene c-kit located on chromosome 4q12, and it belongs to the type III receptor tyrosine kinase subfamily. KIT is expressed on mast cells, melanocytes, primitive hematopoietic stem cells, primordial germ cells, and interstitial cells of Cajal. Activation of KIT induces cellular growth and extends cell survival by preventing apoptosis. The ligand for KIT is stem cell factor (SCF), which is an important growth factor for mast cells. The gene for SCF is located on chromosome 12, and encodes a protein that localizes to the cell membrane. A membrane-bound and a soluble form of SCF exist, and both induce KIT activation; the latter is thought to arise via enzymatic cleavage of the former. SCF is produced by bone marrow stromal cells, fibroblasts, keratinocytes, endothelial cells, and reproductive Sertoli and granulosa cells. Peripheral blood mast cell precursors cultured in the presence of SCF and other cytokines become KIT$^+$/CD34$^-$/FcγRII$^-$/FcεRI$^+$ and develop characteristic cytoplasmic mast cell granules[6,7].

Alterations in KIT structure and activity are central to the pathogenesis of some forms of mastocytosis. Somatic point mutations in codon 816 of the c-kit proto-oncogene have been identified in adult mastocytosis patients without familial disease[5]. This mutation causes constitutive activation of KIT, thereby leading to continued mast cell development. Other mutations in c-kit, at codons 560 and 820, have also been reported in patients with systemic mastocytosis, but these appear to be rare and are less well characterized as a direct cause of the disease. In one study, 22 children and adults with sporadic mastocytosis were investigated for c-kit autoactivating mutations[5]. All 11 of the adult patients studied had the 816 mutation, whereas four pediatric patients with typical urticaria pigmentosa lesions lacked this gene alteration. In four other patients with childhood disease, however, mutations in codon 816 were observed. Each of these children had extensive skin lesions and two had evidence of systemic involvement. In three other children, a novel mutation at codon 839 was detected that proved to be a dominant inactivating KIT mutation. While the significance of the 839 mutation in relation to mastocytosis remains to be fully understood, it suggests that mast cell growth-promoting mechanisms, independent of KIT activation, may be responsible for some forms of childhood mastocytosis. In this same study, family members with mastocytosis from three generations were also evaluated for c-kit mutations. No KIT defect was identified in this kindred, thus underscoring the likelihood that there are several different mechanisms responsible for mast cell disease.

SCF may play a role in the pathogenesis of cutaneous mastocytosis. Increased soluble SCF has been reported in the skin lesions of a child and two adults with mastocytosis; this probably results from the cleavage of the membrane-bound form of SCF by mast cell chymase[8]. Since KIT-activating mutations have also been identified in these patients, it appears unlikely that soluble SCF is the cause of their disease, but it may augment mast cell growth and survival in mastocytosis patients. SCF is capable of stimulating normal KIT, which coexists with the mutant form on mast cells in patients with auto-activating mutations. In addition, local accumulations of soluble SCF in the skin of mastocytosis patients are probably responsible for the hyperpigmentation seen in cutaneous mastocytosis lesions, since stimulation of KIT on melanocytes leads to melanin production.

Recently, a transgenic mouse model of mastocytosis was developed[9]. Specifically within their mast cells, these mice express a human kit gene with an activating mutation at codon 816, and as a result, the human KIT receptor is 'turned on' (as in patients with adult mastocytosis). The clinical findings ranged from indolent mast cell hyperplasia to an invasive mast cell tumor. A second mouse model, based upon the injection of cells from a murine mastocytoma that contain an activating mutation homologous to D816V, has also been described[10]. The hope is to utilize these models to understand the pathogenesis of mastocytosis, including its clinical heterogeneity, as well as to examine the effects of new therapeutic agents.

CLINICAL FEATURES

Signs and Symptoms

Many children and adults have few, if any, symptoms. When symptoms do occur, they are due to the diverse physiologic effects of secreted mast cell mediators, such as histamine, eicosanoids and cytokines (Fig. 118.2). These complaints and findings may range from pruritus and flushing to abdominal pain and diarrhea to palpitations, dizziness and syncope. Of interest is the relative absence of pulmonary symptoms in mastocytosis. Complaints of fever, night sweats, malaise, weight loss, bone pain, epigastric distress, and problems with mentation (cognitive disorganization) often signal the presence of extracutaneous disease. Deaths associated with extensive mast cell mediator release also are rare, but have been reported in both children and adults. Symptoms of mastocytosis can be exacerbated by exercise, heat or local trauma to skin lesions. In addition, alcohol, narcotics, salicylates and other non-steroidal anti-inflammatory drugs (NSAIDs), polymyxin B, and anti-cholinergic medications have been implicated in precipitating symptoms of mastocytosis. Some systemic anesthetic agents may precipitate anaphylaxis (see Treatment).

Cutaneous Lesions

Skin lesions of **childhood mastocytosis** patients include a solitary tan or yellow–tan plaque or nodule (mastocytoma; Fig. 118.3) or variable numbers of tan to brown macules or papules (urticaria pigmentosa, UP; Fig. 118.4). Mastocytomas may be present at birth or they may arise during infancy; they represent approximately 15–20% of all childhood mastocytosis lesions. These lesions often appear on the distal extremities, but can occur in any anatomic location. UP usually presents early in childhood, most commonly on the trunk although it can involve any anatomic site. However, it often spares the central face, scalp, palms and soles.

While telangiectatic macules (telangiectasia macularis eruptiva perstans, TMEP) are a rare manifestation of mastocytosis in children, at least three children have been reported with this type of lesion. A form of childhood mastocytosis with little clinical resemblance to lesions of UP or TMEP is diffuse cutaneous mastocytosis. The skin of patients with this form of mastocytosis has numerous erythematous to yellow–tan papules and plaques with areas of confluence that have a leathery texture. Some infants and children with UP and diffuse cutaneous mastocytosis develop non-scarring vesicles or bullae (Fig. 118.5; see Fig. 35.14). Bullous lesions of mastocytosis usually resolve by 3 to 5 years of age, and are believed to result from the release of mast cell serine proteases.

Skin lesions in **adult mastocytosis** patients differ significantly from those in children. The most common cutaneous lesions of mastocytosis in adults are reddish-brown macules and papules that measure a centimeter or less in diameter (Fig. 118.6), and in patients with skin type I, they may be pink in color. These lesions are most numerous on the trunk and proximal extremities and appear less frequently on the face, distal extremities or palms and soles. Over time, they have been observed to resolve spontaneously and then reappear. Close inspection reveals variable hyperpigmentation and fine telangiectasias. A more rare form of adult cutaneous mastocytosis is TMEP, which is characterized by macules and patches composed of telangiectasias without significant hyperpigmentation (Fig.118.7). While there have been several reports of mastocytomas in adults, these are extremely rare. Diffuse cutaneous mastocytosis has also been documented in adults. The skin of these

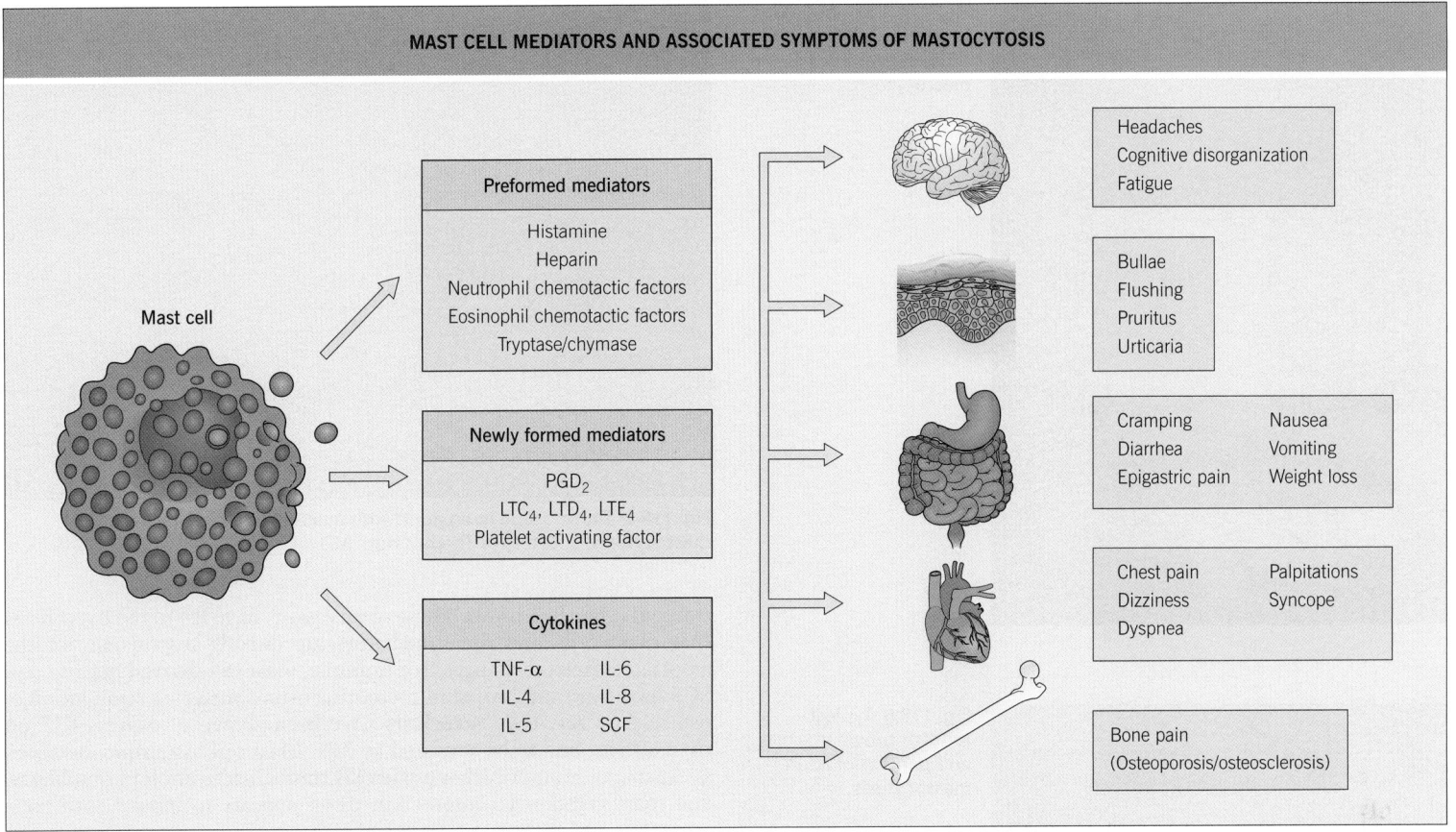

Fig. 118.2 Mast cell mediators and associated symptoms of mastocytosis. IL, interleukins; LT, leukotrienes; PGD$_2$, prostaglandin D$_2$; SCF, stem cell factor; TNF, tumor necrosis factor.

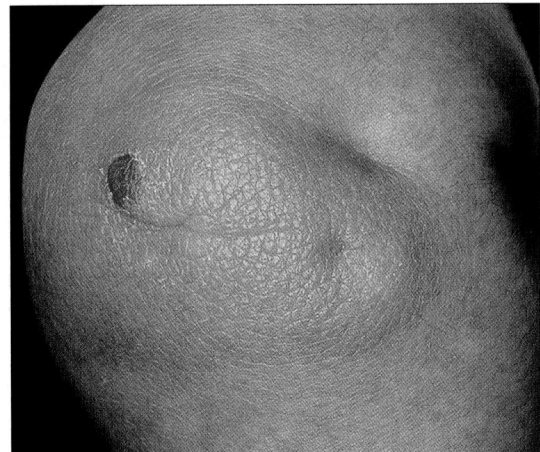

Fig. 118.3 A mastocytoma on the knee of an infant.

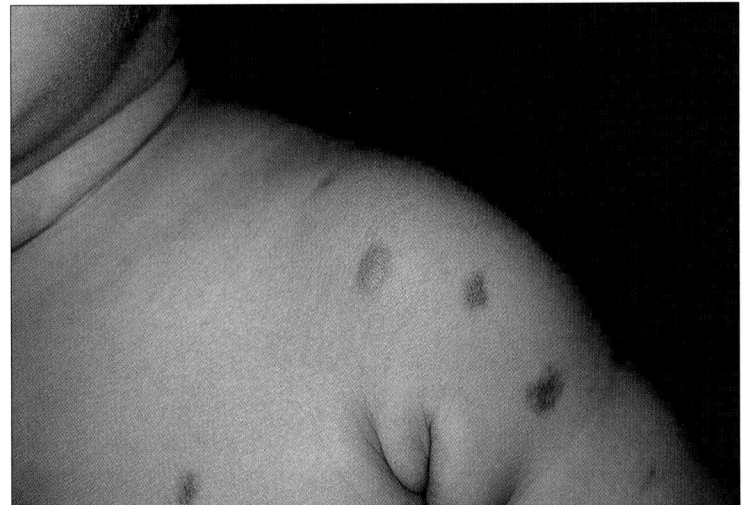

Fig. 118.4 Typical lesions of urticaria pigmentosa in a child.

patients has a doughy consistency, and the presence of numerous, confluent, yellow–tan papules has led to the descriptive term xanthelasmoidal mastocytosis. In more advanced stages, skin folds of patients with diffuse disease become markedly thickened and distort facial features.

The presence of mast cell hyperplasia in the skin of mastocytosis patients can be confirmed clinically by firmly rubbing a characteristic lesion. The formation of an urticarial wheal (Darier's sign; Fig. 118.8) at the lesion site is indicative of mast cell mediator release. Darier's sign is readily demonstrated in mastocytomas and childhood UP lesions, whereas it may be less apparent in common adult mastocytosis lesions and barely detectable in TMEP. This can be explained from studies quantifying mast cells in the skin of children and adults with mastocytosis. Mast cell concentrations in mastocytomas and childhood UP have been reported to be 150-fold and 40-fold greater than normal skin,

respectively, whereas the mast cell content of lesional skin in adult mastocytosis patients was only 8-fold greater than normal skin[11].

Systemic Manifestations

Skeletal lesions commonly occur in adult patients with mastocytosis, but they are rarely seen in children. They may appear as radio-opacities, radiolucencies, or a mixture of the two. The skull, spine and pelvis are most commonly involved. In one large study of 58 adult systemic mastocytosis patients, 57% had diffuse bone involvement, whereas only 2% had focal lesions. Demineralization was the most common change in patients with diffuse skeletal disease, followed by osteosclerosis and mixed lesions of osteosclerosis and osteoporosis[12]. Undecalcified iliac crest biopsies from adult mastocytosis patients have demonstrated increased numbers of mast cells and evidence of enhanced cortical and

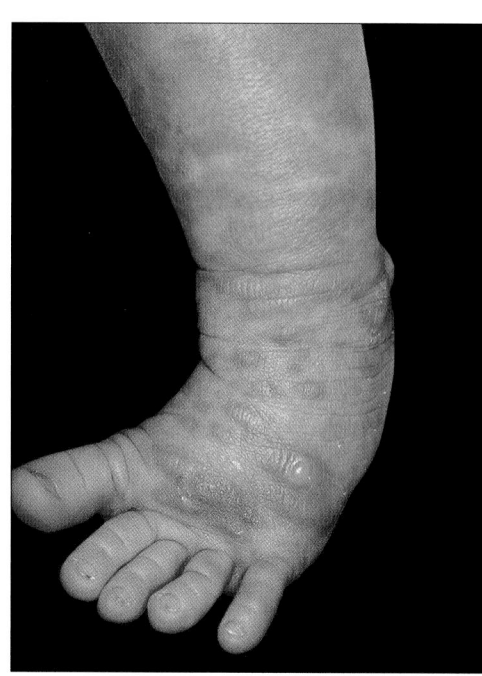

Fig. 118.5 Spontaneous blister in an infant with diffuse cutaneous mastocytosis.

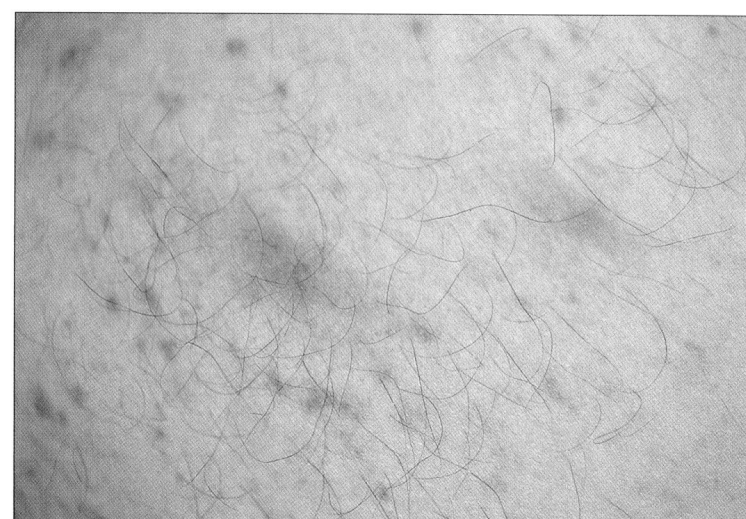

Fig. 118.8 Darier's sign in an adult with macular and papular lesions of mastocytosis. Courtesy of Thomas Horn MD.

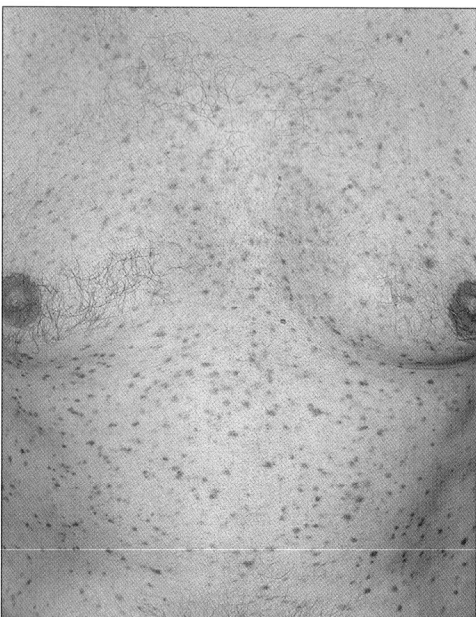

Fig. 118.6 Typical reddish-brown macules and papules of adult mastocytosis.

trabecular bone turnover. These observations have led to the hypothesis that mast cells and their mediators are directly responsible for the associated skeletal changes. For example, mast cell-derived heparin and SCF have been implicated in promoting osteoporosis via stimulation of osteoclastic activity. Osteoclasts have been shown to express KIT on their surface and to be activated by SCF. Mast cell histamine, however, is capable of promoting bone sclerosis through activation of fibroblasts, and mast cell-derived interleukin (IL)-6 appears to induce both bone resorptive and fibrotic activities[13,14].

The bone marrow is commonly involved in adult patients with mastocytosis. In a report of 71 adults with mastocytosis, 90% had increased numbers of spindle-shaped bone marrow mast cells with focal perivascular, peritrabecular and/or intertrabecular accumulations[15]. Scattered lymphocytes and eosinophils have been associated with these mast cell aggregates, leading to the term mast cell, eosinophil, lymphocyte (MEL) lesion. The identification of MEL lesions in the bone marrow is often useful in differentiating mastocytosis from other hematologic disorders with increased bone marrow mast cells, such as myeloproliferative and myelodysplastic diseases. Bone marrow biopsies were performed in one study of 19 children with mastocytosis. In 10 of these patients, only focal perivascular mast cell aggregates were observed. Eight of the remaining nine children had normal marrow cellularity, and the ninth child had hypocellular changes[16]. These and similar observations have led to the recommendation that bone marrow biopsies should not be routinely performed in children with mastocytosis. Also, in healthy adults with cutaneous mastocytosis and normal hematologic parameters, bone marrow biopsies are not required.

Splenomegaly, detected either clinically or by CT scan, has been reported in 50% to 60% of adult mastocytosis patients[15,16]. Increased numbers of mast cells and eosinophils are frequently observed in the spleen, as are various degrees of fibrosis and hematopoiesis. Lymph node enlargement is uncommon in most mastocytosis patients, but occurs in patients with more advanced systemic disease. Among 58 systemic mastocytosis patients, 26% had peripheral lymphadenopathy, whereas 19% had central nodal disease[17]. Histologically, early involvement of lymph nodes often consists of just clusters of mast cells, while in more advanced disease, mast cell infiltrates involve the paracortex, and are often accompanied by eosinophils.

Gastrointestinal (GI) symptoms, such as abdominal pain, diarrhea, nausea and vomiting, may occur in mastocytosis patients[12,15]. Pain is often exacerbated by alcohol, certain foods, stress, and increased mast cell mediator release. Diarrhea in patients with mastocytosis is usually episodic; it can result from malabsorption, increased motility and acid hypersecretion, probably as a result of the release of mast cell histamine and prostaglandins. GI hemorrhage has been reported in some patients with systemic mastocytosis and is often secondary to gastritis or peptic ulcers. A number of radiographic changes in the GI tract have been described in patients with systemic mastocytosis and they include urticaria-like lesions, thickened gastric, duodenal and jejunal folds, as well as mucosal nodules and/or peptic ulcers. Biopsies of mucosal

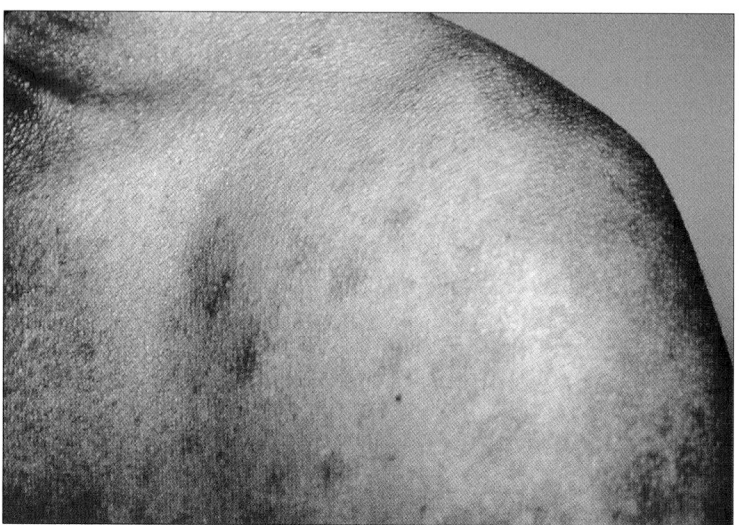

Fig. 118.7 Telangiectasia macularis eruptiva perstans. Multiple lesions composed of telangiectasias are present.

nodules have demonstrated numerous mast cells with varying numbers of eosinophils. Hepatomegaly has also been documented in some systemic mastocytosis patients. In a report of 58 patients with systemic mastocytosis, 41% had detectable hepatomegaly; however, only 12% had abnormal liver function tests[12].

A mixed organic brain syndrome with a constellation of symptoms – including irritability, fatigue, headache, poor attention span and motivation, limited short-term memory, inability to work effectively, and difficulty in interacting with other people – has been described in patients with mastocytosis[18]. It has been hypothesized that these symptoms may be secondary to released mast cell mediators. Electroencephalographic studies in these patients range from normal to changes consistent with a toxic or metabolic process.

Classification of Mastocytosis

A classification scheme for mastocytosis has been proposed, to include four patient types: types I–IV (Table 118.1). Patients with indolent mastocytosis (type I) represent the largest group and include most children and many adults with this disease. Most of these patients have cutaneous lesions, but they may also have systemic involvement. Patients with indolent mastocytosis have one or more of the following clinical signs and symptoms:

- increased numbers of cutaneous mast cells
- gastric and/or duodenal ulcers
- malabsorption secondary to intestinal mast cell infiltration and mediator release
- skeletal changes resulting from increased mast cells and their mediators
- hemodynamic instability manifested by repeated episodes of flushing and possibly syncope
- evidence of mast cell infiltration of the bone marrow, liver, spleen and/or lymph nodes.

In contrast to children, adults are more likely to have systemic symptoms and evidence of extracutaneous involvement. Most children with indolent mastocytosis have a limited course, with approximately 50% experiencing resolution of their disease by adolescence and the remainder noting a marked reduction in lesion number[4]. Activating c-*kit* mutations have been reported in a few children with mastocytosis, and it has been postulated that this patient group may represent the 10–15% of children whose disease persists into adulthood[5]. It is believed that children with activating c-*kit* mutations have the same prognosis as adult-onset mastocytosis patients, including an increased potential for systemic involvement and more aggressive disease.

Type II mastocytosis patients have an associated hematologic disease, and they may or may not have cutaneous lesions. Often, however, these patients have liver, spleen and/or lymph node involvement. Among five mastocytosis patients with type II disease, studied by CT scan, all had hepatic enlargement and/or ascites, and one had Budd–Chiari syndrome. Splenomegaly was noted in all patients in whom a splenectomy had not been performed, and abdominal lymphadenopathy was present in all but one[19]. Type II mastocytosis patients are often older adults, and they may have other symptoms such as fever, anorexia, weight loss, generalized malaise, GI complaints, pruritus, dermographism and flushing. Hematologic disorders associated with type II mastocytosis include: myeloproliferative and myelodysplastic disorders (e.g. polycythemia rubra vera, chronic myeloid leukemia, chronic myelomonocytic leukemia, idiopathic myelofibrosis), hypereosinophilic syndrome, lymphocytic leukemia (acute and chronic), and lymphoma (non-Hodgkin and Hodgkin disease). Secondary acute myeloblastic or myelomonocytic leukemias have also developed in this patient group. Bone marrow biopsies are indicated in patients with type II mastocytosis and usually demonstrate increased numbers of mast cells accompanying the hematologic changes. The overall prognosis of type II mastocytosis patients appears directly dependent upon the severity of the hematologic disease.

Type III mastocytosis is rare. Frequently, these patients do not have cutaneous lesions, but they often have mast cell infiltrates involving the bone marrow, GI tract, liver, spleen and lymph nodes[20]. Most patients have an expected survival of between 2 and 4 years.

Mast cell leukemia (type IV mastocytosis) is also rare. The diagnosis of mast cell leukemia requires the peripheral blood nucleated cell

CLASSIFICATION OF MASTOCYTOSIS

Classification based on clinical criteria		WHO classification
Type Ia	Indolent mastocytosis without systemic disease	Cutaneous mastocytosis
Type Ib	Indolent mastocytosis with systemic disease	Indolent systemic mastocytosis
Type II*	Mastocytosis associated with a myeloproliferative or myelodysplastic disease	Systemic mastocytosis with *associated clonal hematological non-mast cell-lineage disease* (AHNMD)
Type III[†]	Lymphadenopathic mastocytosis (with eosinophilia)	Aggressive systemic mastocytosis
Type IV[†]	Mast cell leukemia	Mast cell leukemia

WHO criteria for the diagnosis of systemic mastocytosis

Requires either the major criterion plus one minor criterion *or* three minor criteria

Major criterion
- Multifocal dense infiltrates of mast cells (aggregates of >15 mast cells) in bone marrow or extracutaneous tissues

Minor criteria
- >25% of mast cells in bone marrow samples or extracutaneous tissues are spindle-shaped or otherwise atypical
- Extracutaneous mast cells (CD117⁺) express CD2, CD25 or both (determined via flow cytometry)
- Presence of c-*kit* codon 816 mutation in blood, bone marrow or extracutaneous tissues
- Serum total tryptase level is persistently >20 ng/ml (except in AHNMD)

Classification based on c-*kit* mutations detected to date

Childhood disease
No activating mutation (most)
816 activating mutation (few)[‡]
Inactivating mutation (e.g. E839K) (few)

Adult disease
816 activating mutation (most)[‡]
Other activating mutations (e.g. F522C[§], V560G, D820G) (few)

Familial disease
No activating or inactivating mutation (most)
Activating mutations (e.g. K509I[§], A533D) (few)

Familial gastrointestinal stromal tumors (GISTs) plus hyperpigmentation or mast cell disease
Activating mutations (e.g. deletion of V559 & V560; V559A; L576_P577insQL; deletion of D419)

*Includes patients with the FIP1L1-PDGFRA mutation in association with hypereosinophilic syndrome/chronic eosinophilic leukemia.
[†] Patients often do not have cutaneous lesions.
[‡] For example, when it leads to an Asp/Val substitution, the abbreviation is D816V, and when it leads to an Asp/Phe substitution, D816F.
[§] Disease responsive to imatinib; an F522C germline mutation was described in a woman with adult-onset systemic mastocytosis and a history of childhood urticaria pigmentosa that resolved by adolescence.

Table 118.1 Classification of mastocytosis. WHO classification from Valent P, Horny HP, Escribano L, et al. Diagnostic criteria and classification of mastocytosis: a consensus proposal. Leuk Res. 2001;25:603–25.

population to be composed of at least 10% mast cells[12,17]. However, because mature mast cells are rarely observed in the peripheral blood of normal individuals, their presence should raise the suspicion of mast cell leukemia. Most patients with type IV mastocytosis do not have cutaneous lesions, but frequently experience recurrent fever, weight loss, abdominal pain, diarrhea, nausea and vomiting. The prognosis for mast cell leukemia is extremely poor, with an expected survival of a year or less from the time of diagnosis.

With the detection of c-*kit* mutations, an alternative classification for childhood, adult-onset, and familial mastocytosis may be more clinically relevant (see Table 118.1). It appears that most children and patients with familial disease lack c-*kit* mutations. A small number of children with mastocytosis, however, have either the 816 autoactivating mutation or the 839 inactivating mutation. All sporadic adult-onset mastocytosis patients have c-*kit* activating mutations. Patients who

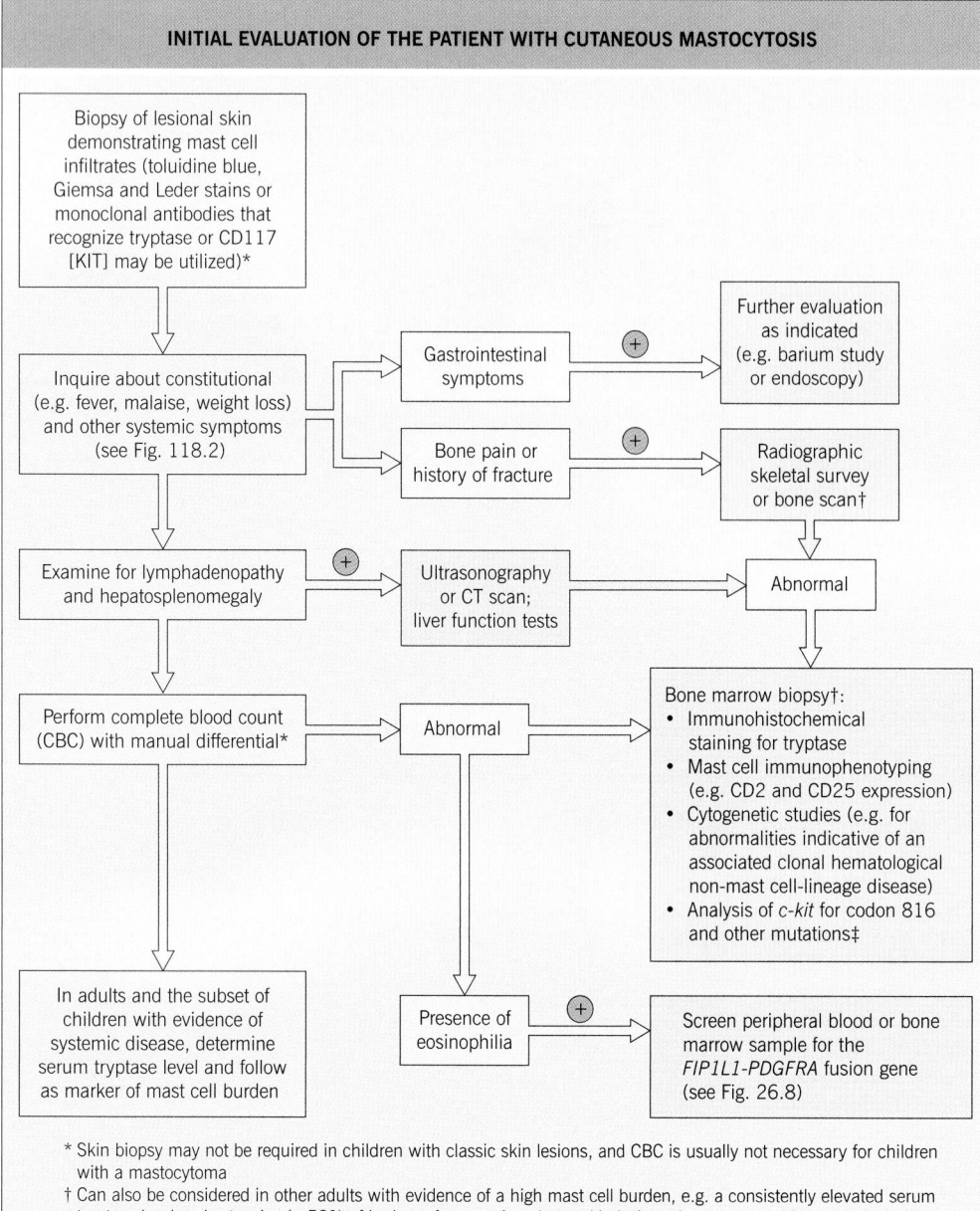

Fig. 118.9 Initial evaluation of the patient with cutaneous mastocytosis.

INITIAL EVALUATION OF THE PATIENT WITH CUTANEOUS MASTOCYTOSIS

Biopsy of lesional skin demonstrating mast cell infiltrates (toluidine blue, Giemsa and Leder stains or monoclonal antibodies that recognize tryptase or CD117 [KIT] may be utilized)*

Inquire about constitutional (e.g. fever, malaise, weight loss) and other systemic symptoms (see Fig. 118.2)

Gastrointestinal symptoms → (+) → Further evaluation as indicated (e.g. barium study or endoscopy)

Bone pain or history of fracture → (+) → Radiographic skeletal survey or bone scan†

Examine for lymphadenopathy and hepatosplenomegaly → (+) → Ultrasonography or CT scan; liver function tests → Abnormal

Perform complete blood count (CBC) with manual differential* → Abnormal →

Bone marrow biopsy†:
• Immunohistochemical staining for tryptase
• Mast cell immunophenotyping (e.g. CD2 and CD25 expression)
• Cytogenetic studies (e.g. for abnormalities indicative of an associated clonal hematological non-mast cell-lineage disease)
• Analysis of c-kit for codon 816 and other mutations‡

In adults and the subset of children with evidence of systemic disease, determine serum tryptase level and follow as marker of mast cell burden

Presence of eosinophilia → (+) → Screen peripheral blood or bone marrow sample for the FIP1L1-PDGFRA fusion gene (see Fig. 26.8)

* Skin biopsy may not be required in children with classic skin lesions, and CBC is usually not necessary for children with a mastocytoma
† Can also be considered in other adults with evidence of a high mast cell burden, e.g. a consistently elevated serum tryptase level and extensive (>50% of body surface area) or dense skin lesions; bone marrow biopsy rarely needed in children.
‡ It is also possible to analyze paraffin-embedded lesional skin biopsy specimens for c-kit mutations

express activating mutations, regardless of the age of onset, appear likely to have adult-type disease that persists throughout life, and which may be associated with systemic involvement. In contrast, children without activating mutations appear to have mild disease that resolves by adulthood. The clinical course and overall prognosis of familial disease appears good, but is less well defined.

An approach to the initial evaluation of a patient with cutaneous mastocytosis is presented in Figure 118.9.

PATHOLOGY

Direct Studies

The diagnosis of mastocytosis is established by demonstrating characteristic mast cells in one or more organs. For patients with cutaneous lesions, mast cell infiltrates can be demonstrated in a biopsy of lesional skin (Fig. 118.10). Special stains, such as toluidine blue, Giemsa and Leder (Fig. 118.11A), or monoclonal antibodies that recognize tryptase or CD117 (KIT; Fig. 118.11B) are helpful for identifying tissue mast cells. Mast cells in nodular, papular and macular lesions (including TMEP) of mastocytosis have been quantified using a morphometric technique and shown to contain mean mast cell densities of 63.2%

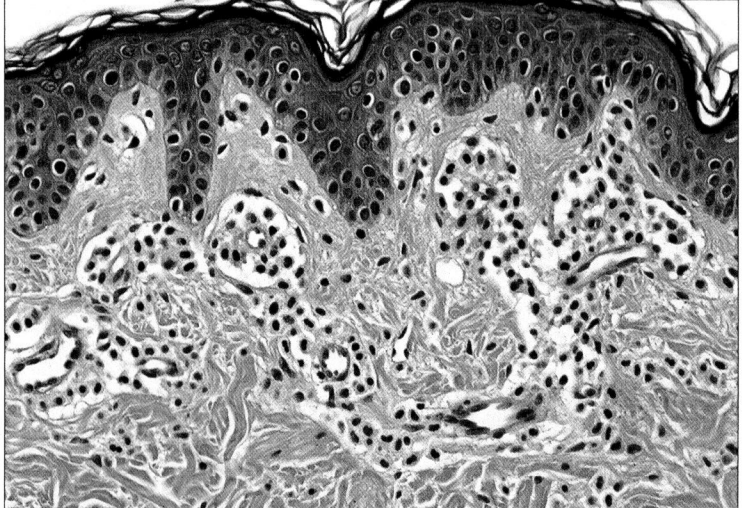

Fig. 118.10 Histologic features of cutaneous mastocytosis. Mast cells, seen here within the dermis, have a 'fried egg' appearance with granules in the amphophilic cytoplasm.

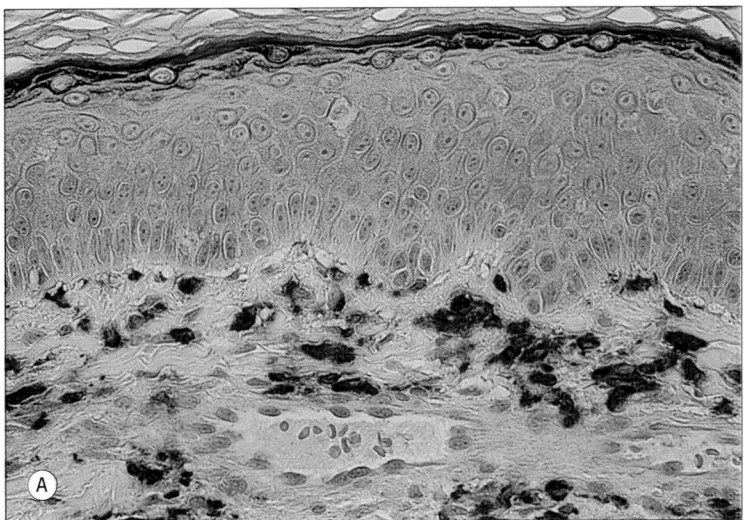

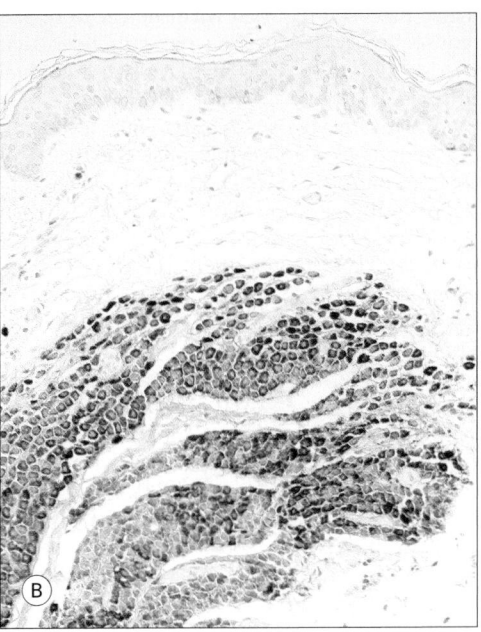

Fig. 118.11 Special stains to detect dermal mast cells. A The Leder method utilizes naphthol AS-D chloroacetate esterase and the mast cell granules appear red. **B** Tryptase immunohistochemical stain.

serum tryptase levels have been correlated with the extent of mast cell disease. Fifty percent of patients with total serum tryptase levels between 20 and 75 ng/ml had evidence of systemic mastocytosis, whereas all patients with levels >75 ng/ml had proven systemic involvement.

Urinary histamine and its metabolites have also been measured in mastocytosis patients. In many instances, unmetabolized urinary histamine levels may be normal in asymptomatic systemic mastocytosis patients, whereas the major metabolite of histamine, 1,4-methylimidazole acetic acid (MeImAA) is often persistently elevated. When urinary MeImAA levels were correlated with the extent of mast cell disease, patients with widespread systemic involvement had the highest concentrations, and patients with only cutaneous disease had normal or only slightly elevated MeImAA[24]. It is important to note that certain foods with high histamine content, such as spinach, eggplant, cheeses (Parmesan, Roquefort and blue) and red wines, can artificially elevate the levels of urinary histamine and its metabolites.

The urinary excretion of the major urinary metabolite of prostaglandin D_2 (PGD_2), 9α,11β-dihydroxy-15-oxo-2,3,18,19-tetranorprost-5-ene-1,20-diolic acid (PGD_2M), has also been reported to be increased in some systemic mastocytosis patients[25]. In one study of 17 patients with mastocytosis, the levels of PGD_2M were compared to urinary methylhistamine concentrations. In all patients, urinary PGD_2M levels were increased to a greater extent than those of methylhistamine, and markedly elevated PGD_2M levels were detected in four patients with a normal concentration of urinary methylhistamine. Urinary PGD_2M levels have not been compared to urinary MeImAA or serum α-tryptase determinations, and as a result it is unclear whether measuring PGD_2M offers any advantage over obtaining commercially available urinary MeImAA or serum tryptase levels. Most recently, plasma levels of IL-6 have been shown to be elevated in patients with mastocytosis, correlating with severity of bone marrow pathology, organomegaly and extent of skin involvement.

DIFFERENTIAL DIAGNOSIS

The lesions of childhood and adult mastocytosis are so characteristic that they are rarely confused with other skin disorders. Childhood lesions of UP may spontaneously urticate and thus may be mistaken for urticaria. However, lesions of urticaria last only a few hours and do not have the associated hyperpigmentation seen in UP. Some childhood mastocytosis patients may develop bullae. Therefore, the differential diagnosis for blisters in these children includes bullous arthropod bites, bullous impetigo, herpes simplex viral infection, linear IgA bullous dermatosis and, less often, other autoimmune bullous dermatoses. In addition, children with diffuse cutaneous mastocytosis may develop widespread blisters early in their course, which may be mistaken for epidermolysis bullosa or toxic epidermal necrolysis. Demonstration of increased mast cells in either the blister fluid or skin biopsy of the mastocytosis patient helps to establish the correct diagnosis. Occasionally, nodular scabies has been misdiagnosed as mastocytosis. Lastly, a variant of mastocytosis has been described that mimics a histiocytic disorder clinically (red–yellow–brown lesions), but, histologically, eosinophils, neutrophils and nuclear debris mask the infiltrate of mast cells[26].

Skin lesions of adult mastocytosis patients may at first glance appear as lentigines or melanocytic nevi, but mastocytosis lesions usually have an associated erythema. Mastocytomas in children may be confused with café-au-lait macules, arthropod bites, Spitz nevi, pseudolymphomas and juvenile xanthogranulomas.

TREATMENT

Treatment of patients with mastocytosis is directed primarily at alleviating symptoms, since there is no cure for this disorder. Many indolent mastocytosis patients have few, if any, symptoms, and therefore require little or no therapy. Mastocytosis patients should be cautioned to avoid potential mast cell degranulating agents such as ingested alcohol, anticholinergic preparations, aspirin and other NSAIDs, narcotics and polymyxin B sulfate. In addition, heat and friction can induce local or systemic symptoms and should be avoided whenever possible (Table 118.2). A number of systemic anesthetic agents, including lidocaine, d-tubocurarine, metocurine, etomidate, thiopental, succinylcholine

(± 8.2% SEM), 16.1% (± 4.8% SEM) and 3.5% (± 1.8% SEM), respectively[21]. In contrast, the mast cell content of normal skin was reported to be 0.4% (± 0.1% SEM). In cases of adult mastocytosis with cutaneous lesions that contain only borderline numbers of mast cells, molecular diagnostic studies for c-*kit* mutations may help confirm or establish a diagnosis. However, these studies are time consuming and not routinely available. Recently, immunohistochemical staining for CD117 (KIT) proved helpful in establishing the diagnosis of TMEP[22].

Biopsy specimens of normal-appearing skin from patients with mastocytosis have normal concentrations of mast cells, and thus are not helpful in establishing the diagnosis. A biopsy of the bone marrow or GI tract may be indicated for patients in whom the diagnosis of mastocytosis is a possibility, but who lack skin lesions. Increased mast cell numbers in association with variable numbers of eosinophils are observed in these tissue specimens. In addition, the combination of monoclonal antibodies against CD117 (KIT) and tryptase may be particularly useful for identifying atypical mast cells in various tissues.

Indirect Studies

Detection of circulating mast cell mediators and/or their metabolites can offer indirect evidence of mastocytosis. Two forms (α and β) of mast cell tryptase have been identified[23]. Alpha-tryptase is elevated in patients with systemic mastocytosis, regardless of whether or not they are experiencing acute symptoms, and therefore may be useful in assessing total body mast cell burden. Beta-tryptase, however, is often detected both in mastocytosis patients and in patients without mastocytosis who are experiencing anaphylactic symptoms. Total (α and β)

THERAPEUTIC LADDER FOR MASTOCYTOSIS

Avoidance of potential mast cell stimuli

Alcohol
Anticholinergic medications
Aspirin
Non-steroidal anti-inflammatory drugs
Heat
Friction
Narcotics (e.g. morphine, codeine)
Polymyxin B sulfate
Systemic anesthetics (see text)

Local therapy for symptom control

Potent and superpotent topical corticosteroids, including under occlusion (2)
Intralesional corticosteroids (3)

Systemic therapy for symptom control

Oral H_1 and H_2 receptor antagonists (2)
Oral cromolyn sodium (1)
Oral corticosteroids (3)
Oral PUVA (2)

Systemic therapy for aggressive/severe mastocytosis

Interferon-α-2b (2)
Cladribine (2)
Imatinib mesylate, depending upon type of c-kit mutation (3)

Table 118.2 Therapeutic ladder for mastocytosis. Key to evidence-based support: (1) prospective controlled trial; (2) retrospective study or large case series; (3) small case series or individual case reports.

hydrochloride (suxamethonium chloride), enflurane and isoflurane, have been directly or indirectly implicated in precipitating anaphylactoid reactions in mastocytosis patients. In contrast to systemic anesthetics, local injections of lidocaine can be used safely in these patients, and a recent report indicates that propofol, vecuronium bromide and fentanyl are safe alternative systemic anesthetics for patients with mastocytosis[27].

Histamine type 1 (H_1) receptor antagonists, or combined H_1 and H_2 receptor antagonists, are often helpful in controlling many of the symptoms associated with mastocytosis. The second-generation antihistamines cetirizine, loratadine and fexofenadine have distinct advantages over first-generation antihistamines because they have longer half-lives and are more specific H_1 antagonists. In some instances, the addition of an H_2 antagonist (cimetidine, ranitidine, famotidine or nizatidine) may prove beneficial, especially in patients with gastric acid hypersecretion. Ketotifen fumarate, which has both antihistamine and mast cell stabilizing properties, has been effective in combination with ranitidine in controlling symptoms of mastocytosis, as has the tricyclic antidepressant doxepin, which, on a molar basis, is nearly 800-fold more active at the H_1 receptor *in vitro* than diphenhydramine. Oral cromolyn sodium (disodium cromoglycate; 400–800 mg/day) may alleviate GI, cutaneous and CNS symptoms associated with mastocytosis. At doses ranging from 100 to 600 mg/day, oral cromolyn has proven effective in controlling pruritus and blister formation in some patients.

Psoralen plus UVA (PUVA) therapy given four times a week can help to control the pruritus and cutaneous whealing in patients with mastocytosis. This treatment, however, does not alter other symptoms associated with this disorder[28,29]. While PUVA is capable of reducing skin mast cell histamine content, it does not permanently eliminate cutaneous mast cell infiltrates. In contrast to oral PUVA, bath PUVA is not beneficial for symptomatic mastocytosis patients[29].

Potent topical corticosteroids under occlusion for 6 weeks or more eliminates pruritus, cutaneous whealing, histamine levels, and the number of lesional skin mast cells. Patients may remain clinically improved for up to 12 months after therapy[30]. Intralesional injections of triamcinolone acetonide have also been successful in clearing mast cell infiltrates in the skin of mastocytosis patients. The use of systemic corticosteroids in mastocytosis patients has been anecdotal, but relief of both cutaneous and GI symptoms has been reported using prednisone doses ranging from 40 to 60 mg/day. Systemic corticosteroids in combination with cyclosporine were used in a patient with aggressive mastocytosis. This combined therapy resulted in a reduction in symptoms that paralleled a decline in serum tryptase and urinary histamine metabolite levels[31].

Interferon-α-2b (IFN-α-2b) has also been used with some success in patients with more aggressive forms of mastocytosis. In a prospective study, six patients with indolent systemic mastocytosis were treated with IFN-α-2b (0.5×10^6 U/day)[32]. Five of the six patients completed 12 months of treatment, and in each of these patients the number of bone marrow mast cells declined by 5–10%. A modest decline in urinary MeImAA levels was also noted, but there was no change in serum tryptase levels. Side effects of the IFN therapy included hypothyroidism, thrombocytopenia and depression. Although not observed in this study, anaphylaxis also has been reported with the use of higher doses of IFN-α-2b, and, consequently, it has been recommended that the initial dose of IFN-α-2b should be 0.5×10^6 U/day with a gradual increase over weeks to months.

Some patients with systemic mastocytosis may experience recurrent, life-threatening episodes of hypotension following mast cell mediator release. Patients who experience such episodes should be instructed to have a premeasured epinephrine preparation (EpiPen®) with them at all times for emergency use. In some instances, these patients may experience recurrent similar attacks within hours of the initial event; when this occurs, prednisone (20–40 mg/day for 2–4 days) should be initiated, since it often suppresses these recurrent reactions.

Chemotherapeutic agents have been used with limited success in the treatment of severe mastocytosis; however, intravenous cladribine (2-chlorodeoxyadenosine) was reportedly effective in eliminating skin lesions and markedly reducing the number of bone marrow mast cells in a patient with advanced systemic disease[33]. For patients with type II disease, chemotherapy may be effective and should be directed at treating the associated hematologic disorder, since this is the primary determining factor for overall prognosis. Local radiation therapy (approximately 2000 to 30 000 cGy over a 7- to 14-day period) may benefit patients with bone pain. In some instances, pain relief can be achieved during treatment (or shortly thereafter), thus decreasing the frequency and amount of oral analgesics required for pain control. Splenectomy may be indicated for mastocytosis patients with hypersplenism who experience significant cytopenia, and it appears to improve survival in patients with more aggressive disease. Non-myeloablative allogeneic hematopoietic stem cell transplantation for life-threatening disease is still under investigation.

Imatinib mesylate (Gleevec®) is an oral tyrosine kinase inhibitor that was developed for the treatment of chronic myelogenous leukemia in which the translocation that results in the Philadelphia chromosome also results in an activated fusion tyrosine kinase receptor. In addition, imatinib is very effective in treating KIT-related gastrointestinal stromal tumors (GIST). With regard to mastocytosis, mutational analysis should be performed prior to considering the use of 'KIT-targeting' tyrosine kinase inhibitors, because adult patients with the common D816V mutation usually have little response to imatinib[34], although some efficacy was noted in a recent study. However, patients with systemic mastocytosis plus hypereosinophilic syndrome and expression of *FIPL1/PDGFRA* fusion gene (see Fig. 26.8) do respond. Also, an individual with mastocytosis whose mutation (F522C) was in exon 10, i.e. outside exon 17 (the location of the 816 codon), was treated successfully with imatinib, as was a patient with familial mastocytosis whose mutation was K509I (exon 9)[35]. Identification of agents that are capable of inhibiting the more common form of mutated KIT will undoubtedly be the focus of future research efforts.

1. Nettleship E, Tay W. Rare forms of urticaria. Br Med J. 1869;2:323–4.
2. Sangster A. An anomalous mottled rash accompanied by pruritus, factitious urticaria and pigmentation. Urticaria pigmentosa? Trans Clin Svc, London. 1878;11:161–3.
3. Ellis JM. Urticaria pigmentosa – report of a case with autopsy. Arch Pathol. 1949;48:435–8.
4. Caplan RM. The natural course of urticaria pigmentosa. Arch Dermatol. 1963;87:146–57.
5. Longley BJ, Metcalfe DD, Tharp MD, et al. Activating and dominant inactivating c-kit catalytic domain mutations in distinct clinical forms of human mastocytosis. Proc Natl Acad Sci USA. 1999;96:1609–14.
6. Rottem M, Okada T, Goff JP, et al. Mast cells cultured from the peripheral blood of normal donors and patients with mastocytosis originate from a CD34+/FcεRI– cell population. Blood. 1994;84:2489–96.
7. Anderson DM, Lyman SD, Baird A, et al. Molecular cloning of mast cell growth factor, a hematopoietin that is active in both membrane bound and soluble forms. Cell. 1990;63:235–43.
8. Longley BJ, Tyrrell L, Ma Y, et al. Chymase cleavage of stem cell factor yields a bioactive, soluble product. Proc Natl Acad Sci USA. 1998;94:9017–21.
9. Zappulla JP, Dubreuil P, Desbois S, et al. Mastocytosis in mice expressing human Kit receptor with the activating Asp816Val mutation. J Exp Med. 2005;202:1635–41.
10. Demehri S, Corbin A, Loriaux M, et al. Establishment of a murine model of aggressive systemic mastocytosis/mast cell leukemia. Exp Hematol. 2006;34:284–8.
11. Kasper CS, Tharp MD. Quantification of cutaneous mast cells using morphometric point counting and a conjugated avidin stain. J Am Acad Dermatol. 1987;16:326–31.
12. Travis W, Li C-Y, Bergstrahl E, et al. Systemic mast cell disease. Medicine (Baltimore). 1988;67:345–68.
13. Andrew SM, Freemont AJ. Skeletal mastocytosis. J Clin Pathol. 1993;46:1033–5.
14. Linkhart TA, Linkhart SG, MacCharles DC, et al. Interleukin-6 messenger RNA expression and interleukin-6 protein secretion in cells isolated from normal human bone: regulation by interleukin-1. J Bone Miner Res. 1991;6:1285–94.
15. Sagher F, Even-Paz Z. Mastocytosis and the mast cell. Chicago: Yearbook Medical, 1967:10–291.
16. Metcalfe DD. The liver, spleen, and lymph nodes in mastocytosis. J Invest Dermatol. 1991;96:45S–46S.
17. Travis WD, Li C-Y. Pathology of the lymph node and spleen in systemic mast cell disease. Mod Pathol. 1986;1:4–14.
18. Rogers M, Bloomingdale K, Murawski B, et al. Mixed organic brain syndrome as a manifestation of systemic mastocytosis. Psychosomatic Med. 1986;48:437–47.
19. Avila NA, Ling A, Worobec AS, et al. Systemic mastocytosis: CT and US features of abdominal manifestations. Radiology. 1997;202:367–72.
20. Meggs WJ, Friedman MM, Kramer N, et al. Lymphadenopathic mastocytosis with eosinophilia. 1985;33:162A (abstract).
21. Kasper C, Freeman RG, Tharp MD. Diagnosis of mastocytosis subsets using a morphometric point counting technique. Arch Dermatol. 1987;123:1017–21.
22. Lee HW, Jeong YI, Choi JC, et al. Two cases of telangiectasia macularis eruptiva perstans demonstrated by immunohistochemistry for c-kit (CD117). J Dermatol. 2005;32:817–20.
23. Schwartz LB, Sakai K, Bradford TR, et al. The α form of human tryptase is the predominant type present in blood at baseline in normal subjects and is elevated in those with systemic mastocytosis. J Clin Invest. 1995;96:2702–10.
24. Keyzer JL, DeMonchy JGR, van Doormaal JJ, et al. Improved diagnosis of mastocytosis by measurement of urinary histamine metabolites. N Engl J Med. 1983;309:1603–5.
25. Morrow J, Guzo C, Lazarus G, et al. Improved diagnosis of mastocytosis by measurement of the major urinary metabolite of prostaglandin D2. J Invest Dermatol. 1995;104:937–40.
26. Dunst KM, Huemer GM, Zelger BG, et al. A new variant of mastocytosis: report of three cases clinicopathologically mimicking histiocytic and vasculitic disorders. Br J Dermatol. 2005;153:642–6.
27. Borgeat A, Ruetsch YA. Anesthesia in a patient with malignant systemic mastocytosis using a total intravenous anesthetic technique. Anesth Analg. 1998;86:442–4.
28. Kolde G, Frosch P, Czarnetzki B. Response of cutaneous mast cells to PUVA in patients with urticaria pigmentosa: histomorphometric, ultrastructural, and biochemical investigations. J Invest Dermatol. 1984;83:175–8.
29. Godt O, Proksch E, Streit V, et al. Short- and long-term effectiveness of oral and bath PUVA therapy in urticaria pigmentosa and systemic mastocytosis. Dermatology. 1997;195:35–9.
30. Barton J, Lavker RM, Schechter NM, et al. Treatment of urticaria pigmentosa with corticosteroids. Arch Dermatol. 1985;121:1516–23.
31. Kurosawa M, Amano H, Kanbe N, et al. Response to cyclosporin and low dose methylprednisone in aggressive systemic mastocytosis. J Allergy Clin Immunol. 1999;103:S412–20.
32. Butterfield JH. Response of severe systemic mastocytosis to interferon-alpha. Br J Dermatol. 1998;138:489–95.
33. Teferi A, Li CY, Butterfield, JH, Hoagland HC. Treatment of systemic mast cell disease with cladribine. N Engl J Med. 2001;344:307–8.
34. Metcalfe DD. Mastocytosis. Novartis Found Symp. 2005;271:232–42.
35. Zhang LY, Smith ML, Schultheis B, et al. A novel K509I mutation of KIT identified in familial mastocytosis – in vitro and in vivo responsiveness to imatinib therapy. Leuk Res. 2006;30:373–8.

B-Cell Lymphomas of the Skin

Lorenzo Cerroni

Synonyms: ■ Cutaneous B-cell lymphomas ■ Skin-associated lymphoid tissue (SALT)-related B-cell lymphomas

Key features

- Cutaneous B-cell lymphomas represent a group of lymphomas whose primary site is the skin; they are derived from B lymphocytes in different stages of differentiation. The skin can also be the site of secondary involvement by extracutaneous (usually nodal) B-cell lymphomas

- Most cutaneous B-cell lymphomas are low-grade malignancies, and they are characterized by indolent behavior and a good prognosis

- The widespread use of immunohistochemical and molecular genetic techniques has shown that many of the cases previously classified as cutaneous B-cell pseudolymphomas actually represent low-grade malignant B-cell lymphomas of the skin

- Precise classification can be achieved only after a complete synthesis of clinical, histopathologic, immunophenotypic and molecular features. The new WHO–EORTC classification provides the basis for a consistent classification of patients

- In many patients, treatment consists primarily of local radiotherapy; when one to two lesions are present, surgical excision is an option. Systemic or intralesional anti-CD20 antibody may be used in some patients, while systemic chemotherapy is necessary in only a small proportion of patients

INTRODUCTION

The majority of cutaneous lymphomas are examples of mycosis fungoides, a malignant cutaneous T-cell lymphoma. Although B-cell lymphomas represent the majority of non-Hodgkin lymphomas arising within lymph nodes, they represent only a minority of the non-Hodgkin lymphomas whose primary site is the skin. In the classification of cutaneous lymphomas published recently by the World Health Organization (WHO) and the European Organization for Research and Treatment of Cancer (EORTC) Cutaneous Lymphoma Project Group (Table 119.1), B-cell lymphomas represented 22.5% of all cutaneous lymphomas (data were based on the Dutch and Austrian registries for cutaneous lymphomas)[1]. A similar figure was derived from a large series of patients observed in Graz between 1960 and 1999, in which B-cell lymphomas represented 26.4% of all cases of primary cutaneous lymphoma[2].

WHO–EORTC CLASSIFICATION OF CUTANEOUS B-CELL LYPHOMAS WITH PRIMARY CUTANEOUS MANIFESTATIONS

- Primary cutaneous marginal zone B-cell lymphoma*
- Primary cutaneous follicle center lymphoma
- Primary cutaneous diffuse large B-cell lymphoma, leg type
- Primary cutaneous diffuse large B-cell lymphoma, other
- Intravascular large B-cell lymphoma

Includes cases previously designated as primary cutaneous immunocytoma and primary cutaneous plasmacytoma.

Table 119.1 WHO–EORTC classification of cutaneous B-cell lymphomas with primary cutaneous manifestations.

In the new WHO–EORTC classification, primary cutaneous lymphomas are defined as *malignant lymphomas confined to the skin at presentation after complete staging procedures*[1]. In general, most patients with primary cutaneous B-cell lymphoma are diagnosed by dermatologists, as extracutaneous symptoms and signs are observed only very rarely at the onset of the disease. Consequently, dermatologists should be conversant with the clinicopathologic features of this group of diseases, in order to be able to establish the diagnosis in its early stages. Additionally, as aggressive treatment modalities are needed only in selected cases, these patients should be managed primarily in dermatology departments with special expertise in cutaneous lymphomas.

HISTORY

In the past, cutaneous B-cell lymphomas were thought to be invariably secondary, that is, due to dissemination of extracutaneous (usually nodal) B-cell lymphomas to the skin. In recent years, it was recognized that B-cell lymphomas whose primary site is the skin represent a distinct and very important group of extranodal lymphomas[3]. They occur far more frequently than was generally appreciated. The widespread use of immunohistochemical and molecular genetic techniques has shown that many of the cases previously classified as cutaneous B-cell pseudolymphomas actually represent low-grade malignant B-cell lymphomas of the skin[3,4]. Cases reported in the past as examples of 'transformation' of B-cell pseudolymphomas into overt cutaneous B-cell lymphomas are, most likely, examples of true primary cutaneous B-cell lymphomas from the onset.

Some authors have suggested that all cases of primary cutaneous B-cell lymphoma represent both a distinct and a unique type of extra-nodal B-cell lymphoma, and they have proposed use of the term 'skin-associated lymphoid tissue (SALT)-related B-cell lymphomas'[5], but this view has not gained widespread acceptance. The new WHO–EORTC classification provides a valid basis for a uniform classification, and it should be used consistently, in order to allow comparison of data amongst different centers.

EPIDEMIOLOGY

Although reports of single cases or small series of primary cutaneous B-cell lymphoma have been published from around the world, there are only a few studies of large series of patients. Consequently, epidemiologic data are still fragmentary and are based primarily on the experience of three major centers in the Netherlands, Italy and Austria[1,2,5].

Primary cutaneous B-cell lymphomas may occur more frequently in particular regions of the world. In fact, analysis of data from four academic centers in the US showed that primary cutaneous B-cell lymphoma represented only 4.5% of all the cases of primary cutaneous lymphoma registered in those centers[6]. In contrast, as already mentioned, primary cutaneous B-cell lymphoma represented 22.5% of all the cases of primary cutaneous lymphoma in the Dutch and Austrian registries for cutaneous lymphomas[1].

Regional variations have also been observed with regard to the incidence of specific types of primary cutaneous B-cell lymphoma. In the two largest series published to date, the relative frequencies of follicle center cell lymphoma and marginal zone lymphoma/immunocytoma varied considerably. For example, follicle center cell lymphoma represented 71.1% of all primary cutaneous B-cell lymphomas in the Netherlands, but only 40.8% in Graz; conversely, marginal zone lymphoma/immunocytoma represented 42.4% of all cases of primary cutaneous B-cell lymphoma in Graz, but only 10.1% in the Netherlands. On the other hand, the relative frequency of the third most common type of primary cutaneous B-cell lymphoma, the so-called large B-cell lymphoma of the leg, was similar in the two series (Netherlands: 15.3%; Austria: 15.6%), indicating that, in these two series, differences in the relative frequencies were confined to B-cell lymphomas characterized by an indolent behavior. This suggests that these variations may be due, at least in part, to a different classification of patients in different centers.

Although variations in the relative frequency of primary cutaneous B-cell lymphomas, and of specific subtypes, may be explained by differences in diagnostic and classification standards, true regional variations in the incidence of special types of primary cutaneous B-cell lymphoma may be due to the presence of different etiologic factors. For example, the association between primary cutaneous B-cell lymphoma and infection with specific *Borrelia* species in endemic areas has been known for many years (see Ch. 73). This association may explain, in part, regional differences in the incidence of primary cutaneous B-cell lymphomas, but the relatively low percentage of such cases (even in countries with endemic *Borrelia* infections) suggests that other etiologies are also involved in regional variations.

Primary cutaneous B-cell lymphoma affects adults of both sexes. In a study of 147 patients, there was a slight predominance of men (male:female = 1.1:1)[2]. With the exception of B-cell lymphoblastic lymphoma (which almost never represents an example of true primary cutaneous B-cell lymphoma), only a few cases have been observed in patients less than 20 years of age.

ETIOLOGY AND PATHOGENESIS

The pathogenesis of primary cutaneous B-cell lymphoma is unknown. In contrast to the many nodal B-cell lymphomas that have been linked to specific genetic alterations (e.g. nodal follicular lymphomas and interchromosomal 14;18 translocations), there are no data on the specific genetic features of primary cutaneous B-cell lymphoma. Extensive studies have failed thus far to detect the presence of genetic alterations common to specific subtypes of primary cutaneous B-cell lymphoma.

Some similarities to the clinicopathologic features observed in B-cell lymphomas arising in the gastric mucosa (so-called mucosa-associated lymphoid tissue or MALT lymphomas) led to the hypothesis that primary cutaneous B-cell lymphomas are caused by longstanding antigenic stimulation, possibly due to chronic infection with specific microorganisms. In fact, it has been long established that MALT lymphomas originating in the stomach are linked to chronic antigenic stimulation due to infection with *Helicobacter pylori*. As previously mentioned, *Borrelia* species are thought to play a role in the etiology of a minority of cases of primary cutaneous B-cell lymphoma. Recently, in patients from a region in Austria with endemic *Borrelia* infections, specific DNA sequences of *Borrelia* were detected in 18% of all cases of primary cutaneous B-cell lymphoma[7]; similar findings have been reported from Scotland[8].

At present, no other microorganism has been convincingly linked to the development of primary cutaneous B-cell lymphoma. Studies of lymphotropic viruses such as Epstein-Barr virus and human herpesvirus types 7 and 8 have failed to demonstrate clearcut evidence of an etiologic association[9,10]. Finally, it should also be noted that primary cutaneous B-cell lymphomas have been described in patients with AIDS, and that reversible primary cutaneous B-cell lymphomas have been observed in patients undergoing therapy with methotrexate, thus suggesting that immune dysregulation may play a role in the development of this disease[11,12].

CLINICAL FEATURES

In the WHO–EORTC classification (see Table 119.1), primary cutaneous B-cell lymphomas have been divided into four major types[1]. Follicle center lymphoma and marginal zone B-cell lymphoma are in a group characterized by an indolent clinical behavior, whereas diffuse large B-cell lymphoma, leg type, and diffuse large B-cell lymphoma, other (the latter including rare variants such as intravascular large B-cell lymphoma) are in a group with intermediate clinical behavior.

It must be emphasized that, in addition to primary cutaneous B-cell lymphomas, the skin can be a site of secondary involvement for practically all types of extracutaneous (usually nodal) B-cell lymphomas and leukemias. Consequently, complete staging must be performed in all patients with a confirmed diagnosis of B-cell lymphoma involving the skin. This includes a complete blood examination, flow cytometry of peripheral blood, and CT examination of the chest, abdomen and pelvis. Bone marrow biopsy and flow cytometry of the bone marrow are optional studies that can prove useful in low-grade lymphomas. Gallium scans have been replaced by positron emission tomography (PET).

In the following two sections, the clinicopathologic features of each type of primary cutaneous B-cell lymphoma listed in Table 119.1 will be discussed. In addition, the characteristics of cutaneous B-cell lymphoblastic lymphoma will be presented.

Primary Cutaneous Follicle Center Lymphoma

Primary cutaneous follicle center lymphoma (PCFCL) is defined as a neoplastic proliferation of germinal center cells confined to the skin. It represents a common subtype of primary cutaneous B-cell lymphoma.

Clinically, patients present with solitary or grouped, pink- to plum-colored papules, plaques or tumors, which, especially on the trunk, can be surrounded by patches of erythema (Figs 119.1 & 119.2). Ulceration is uncommon. Preferential locations are the scalp and forehead or the back. In the past, lesions located on the back were referred to as Crosti's lymphoma or reticulohistiocytoma of the dorsum[13]. The skin lesions are usually asymptomatic, and, as a rule, symptoms are rare. The serum level of lactate dehydrogenase (LDH), which is a powerful prognostic factor in systemic lymphomas, is within normal limits.

The prognosis is favorable[1,14,15]. Recurrences are observed in up to 50% of patients, but dissemination to lymph nodes or internal organs is rare.

Primary Cutaneous Marginal Zone B-Cell Lymphoma

Primary cutaneous marginal zone B-cell lymphoma (PCMZL) has been recognized as a distinct variant of low-grade malignant primary cutaneous B-cell lymphoma[4,16]. It is closely related to MALT lymphomas. Because of the inconsistent use of terminology in the past, cases classified as PCMZL in some centers were variously diagnosed as immunocytoma, plasmacytoma, MALT-type cutaneous B-cell

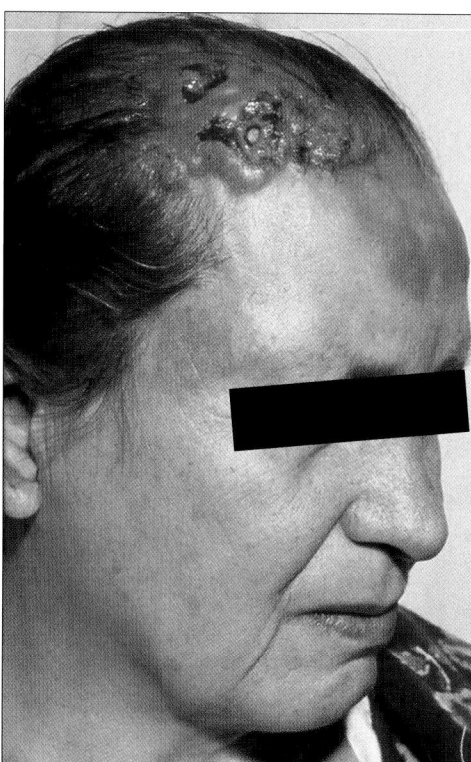

Fig. 119.1 Cutaneous follicle center lymphoma. Large ulcerated tumors on the scalp surrounded by infiltrated erythematous nodules and plaques.

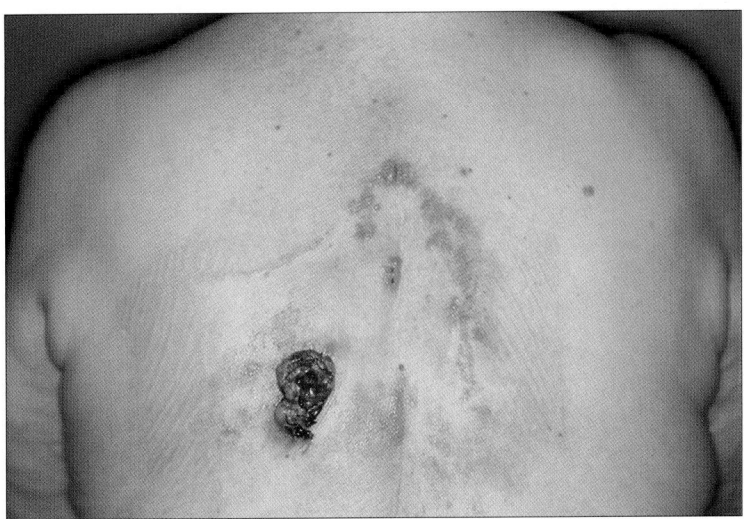

Fig. 119.2 Cutaneous follicle center lymphoma. Large ulcerated tumor on the back. Note surrounding erythematous papules, patches and plaques (Crosti's lymphoma).

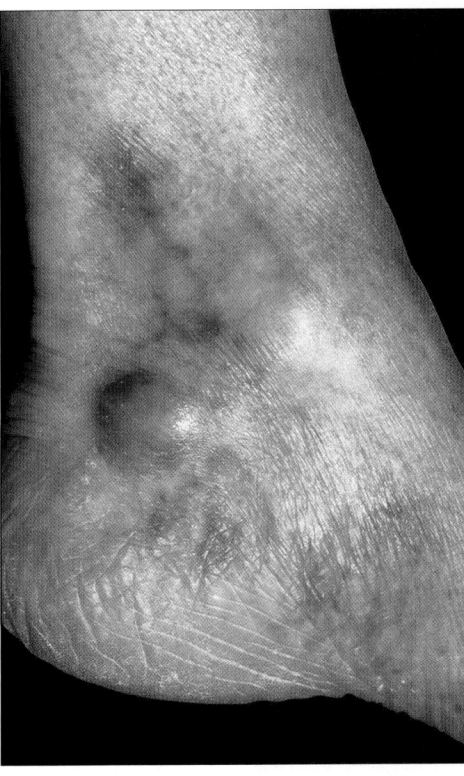

Fig. 119.4 Cutaneous marginal zone B-cell lymphoma. Dome-shaped erythematous nodule with smooth surface. The surrounding area shows features of acrodermatitis chronica atrophicans. This tumor, which demonstrated prominent lymphoplasmacytic differentiation histologically, was classified as cutaneous immunocytoma in the past.

lymphoma or SALT-related B-cell lymphoma in other centers. Of note, cases classified in the past as *primary cutaneous immunocytoma* or *primary cutaneous plasmacytoma* most likely represented examples of PCMZL with prominent lymphoplasmacytic or plasmacytic differentiation, respectively, and the terms cutaneous immunocytoma and cutaneous plasmacytoma are not used in the new WHO–EORTC classification[1]. In addition, lesions previously designated as *cutaneous atypical lymphoid hyperplasia with monotypic plasma cells* probably represent examples of PCMZL as well.

Clinically, patients present with recurrent red to red–brown papules, plaques and nodules localized preferentially on the extremities (upper more so than lower) (Figs 119.3 & 119.4) or trunk. Generalized lesions can be observed in a small number of patients. Ulceration rarely, if ever, occurs; skin lesions are usually asymptomatic, and systemic signs and symptoms, such as fever, night sweats, weight loss and malaise (B-symptoms), are generally not present. The serum level of LDH is within normal limits. In some instances, resolution of lesions may be accompanied by secondary anetoderma due to loss of elastic fibers in the area of the tumor infiltrate[17].

The prognosis of PCMZL is excellent. In a study of 32 patients with PCMZL, none of them developed lymph node or internal involvement during a mean follow-up of more than 4 years[4].

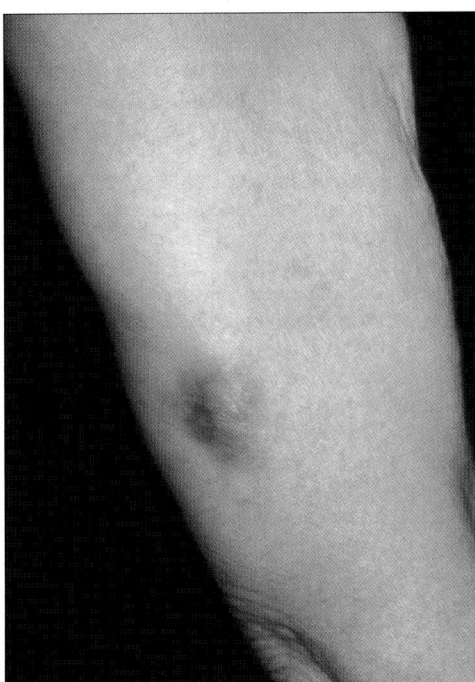

Fig. 119.3 Cutaneous marginal zone B-cell lymphoma. Solitary, large, erythematous nodule on the upper arm.

Of note, PCMZL can arise in areas affected by acrodermatitis chronica atrophicans (see Fig. 119.4), and it may be linked to infection by *Borrelia* species more frequently than are other types of primary cutaneous B-cell lymphoma. In fact, *Borrelia* DNA sequences have been demonstrated by PCR analysis in cutaneous lesions[7].

Primary Cutaneous Diffuse Large B-Cell Lymphoma, Leg Type

Primary cutaneous *diffuse large B-cell lymphoma, leg type* (DLBCLLT) represents a form of primary cutaneous B-cell lymphoma that is characterized by a predominance of large round cells (centroblasts, immunoblasts) positive for Bcl-2[1]. It has an intermediate prognosis and occurs almost exclusively in elderly patients, predominantly women[18].

Clinically, patients present with solitary or clustered erythematous to red–brown nodules, located primarily on the distal aspect of one leg (Fig. 119.5). In some patients, lesions may arise on both lower extremities contemporaneously or within a short interval of time. Ulceration is common. Small erythematous papules can be seen adjacent to larger nodules. It must be emphasized that tumors with similar morphologic and phenotypic features can arise in *areas other than the lower extremities*[4].

The prognosis of DLBCLLT is less favorable than that of other types of primary cutaneous B-cell lymphoma, with a 5-year survival rate of approximately 50%[1,2]. In the past, the prognosis of cutaneous diffuse large B-cell lymphomas had been linked to several factors, including Bcl-2 expression, morphology of the cells, number of lesions at presentation, and location on the legs[19,20]. A recent study, however, demonstrated that accurate classification based upon the new WHO–EORTC categories is the single most important prognostic criterion, and other features are of little or no relevance when patients are stratified into these specific categories[21].

It must be stressed that some patients with nodal large B-cell lymphoma can present with secondary cutaneous lesions located exclusively on the legs. We have observed a number of patients who presented with clinicopathologic features otherwise indistinguishable from those of primary cutaneous DLBCLLT, underlying the need for complete staging investigations before a diagnosis of DLBCLLT can be established. The addition of PET scans to CT studies is a useful way of discovering evidence of systemic disease.

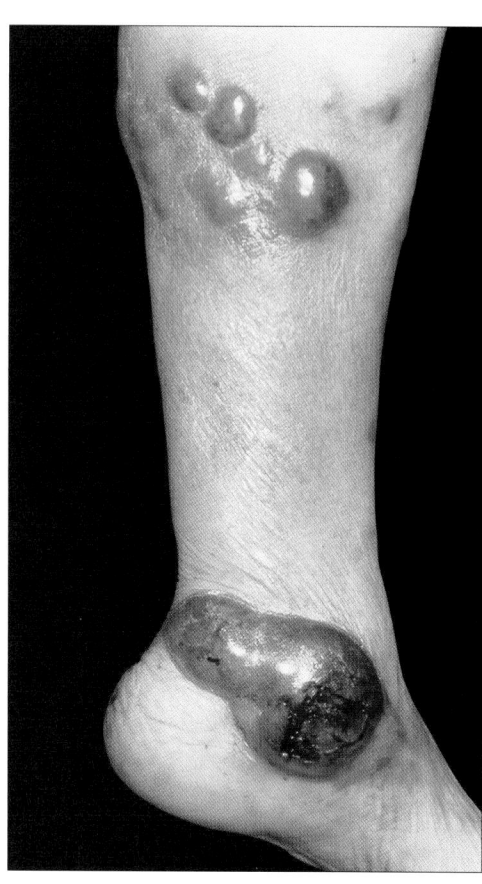

Fig. 119.5 Cutaneous diffuse large B-cell lymphoma, leg type. Multiple red–brown tumors on the lower leg.

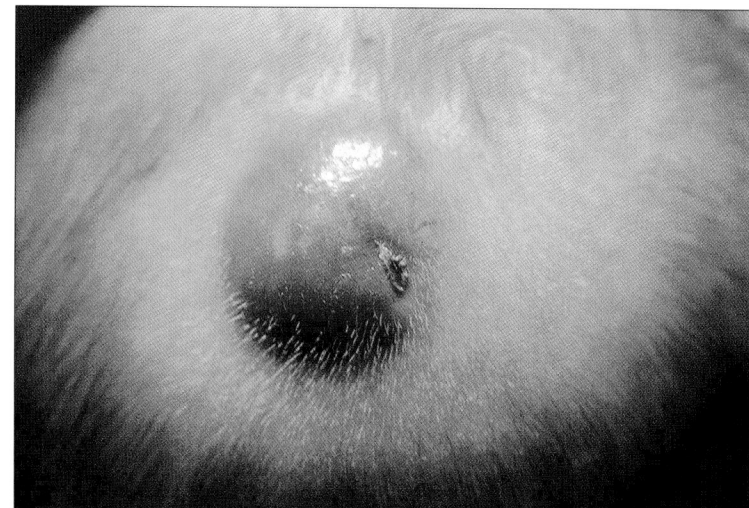

Fig. 119.6 Cutaneous B-cell lymphoblastic lymphoma. Large erythematous tumor on the scalp of an 11-month-old child.

Primary Cutaneous Diffuse Large B-Cell Lymphoma, Other

This group consists of rare patients who do not fit into one of the other categories of primary cutaneous B-cell lymphoma, including those with diffuse large B-cell lymphoma with a round cell morphology but without Bcl-2 expression (clinicopathologic features intermediate between PCFCL, diffuse type, and DLBCLLT); intravascular large B-cell lymphoma; and the rare large B-cell lymphomas arising in the setting of immune suppression (e.g. plasmablastic lymphoma)[1].

Intravascular large B-cell lymphoma is a malignant proliferation of large B lymphocytes within blood vessels[22]. Most patients have a B-cell phenotype, but a T-cell variant has been reported. In rare patients, the skin may be the only affected site, although more often there is systemic involvement (including the CNS) from the onset. Clinically, patients present with indurated, erythematous or violaceous patches and plaques, preferentially located on the trunk and thighs. The clinical appearance is not typical of cutaneous lymphoma, and it may sometimes suggest a diagnosis of panniculitis or vascular tumors. Interestingly, intravascular large B-cell lymphoma has been observed to be confined to cherry angioma lesions[23]. The prognosis of intravascular large B-cell lymphoma limited to the skin has been reported to be better than that of the systemic (disseminated) form, but only a limited number of cases have been studied.

Plasmablastic lymphoma is a rare lymphoma that usually arises within the oral cavity in patients with severe immunosuppression, especially HIV-related. It is often associated with infection by human herpesvirus-8 (HHV-8).

B-Cell Lymphoblastic Lymphoma

B-cell lymphoblastic lymphomas are malignant proliferations of precursor B lymphocytes. Reports of patients whose primary site is the skin have been rare. It should be emphasized, however, that all patients should be assumed to have, and treated for, systemic disease, even in the absence of documented systemic involvement at the time of presentation.

In contrast to the other cutaneous B-cell lymphomas, this disease shows a clearcut predilection for children and young adults[24,25].

Clinically, patients present with solitary large erythematous tumors, commonly located on the head (Fig. 119.6) and neck. Patients with primary skin disease often have asymptomatic lesions of a few weeks duration. Those with secondary skin lesions may have systemic symptoms (e.g. weight loss, fever, fatigue, malaise, night sweats). The serum level of LDH is often elevated, reflecting the aggressive and often systemic nature of the disease.

The disease is highly aggressive, and the prognosis of untreated patients is poor. It has been suggested that expression of CD34, an antigen known to be present on the surface of normal hematopoietic stem cells as well as in a subset of immature thymocytes, is associated with a longer disease-free survival in patients with acute lymphoblastic lymphoma/leukemia compared with those who do not express CD34, thus implying a prognostic significance for this antigen.

PATHOLOGY

Primary Cutaneous Follicle Center Lymphoma

In PCFCL, nodular or diffuse infiltrates are seen within the entire dermis, often extending into the subcutaneous fat (Fig. 119.7A)[3]. The epidermis is usually spared. A clearcut follicular pattern with formation of neoplastic germinal centers was observed in a minority of cases (25%) in the series from Graz[2,14]. However, a higher percentage of cases may show at least some follicular architecture. In the cases with a follicular pattern, the neoplastic follicles show morphologic features of malignancy, including the presence of a reduced or absent mantle zone, the lack of tingible body macrophages, and a monomorphism of the follicles – so-called 'dark' and 'clear' areas are no longer recognizable (Fig. 119.8)[14].

In both the follicular and diffuse variants, centroblasts (large, non-cleaved follicle center cells with prominent nucleoli) and centrocytes (small to large, cleaved follicle center cells) predominate within the neoplastic infiltrate, admixed with a variable number of immunoblasts, small lymphocytes, histiocytes, and, in some cases, eosinophils and plasma cells (Fig. 119.7B). On a cytomorphologic basis, some cases of PCFCL with a diffuse pattern of growth have the appearance of a large cell lymphoma, but the prognosis of these cases is similar to that of lesions without the large cell morphology[1,21,26]. An accompanying infiltrate of small T lymphocytes and histiocytes/macrophages is usually present, and, in some instances, these cells can be predominant.

In addition to cases characterized by numerous large cells, other morphologic variants of PCFCL include those with a predominant spindle cell morphology, which can simulate sarcomas or other spindle cell tumors histopathologically, thus representing a diagnostic pitfall[27]. Cases in which a few B-cell blasts are admixed with numerous T lymphocytes have been classified as 'T-cell-rich B-cell lymphomas', and in the skin probably represent another rare morphologic variant of PCFCL[3].

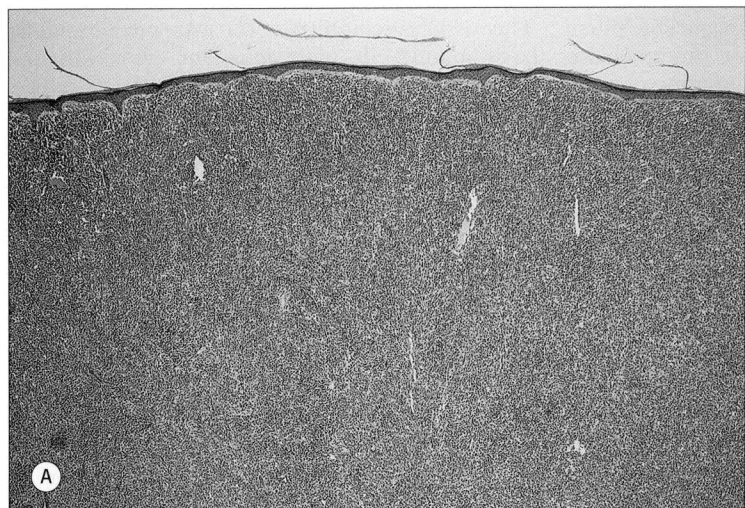

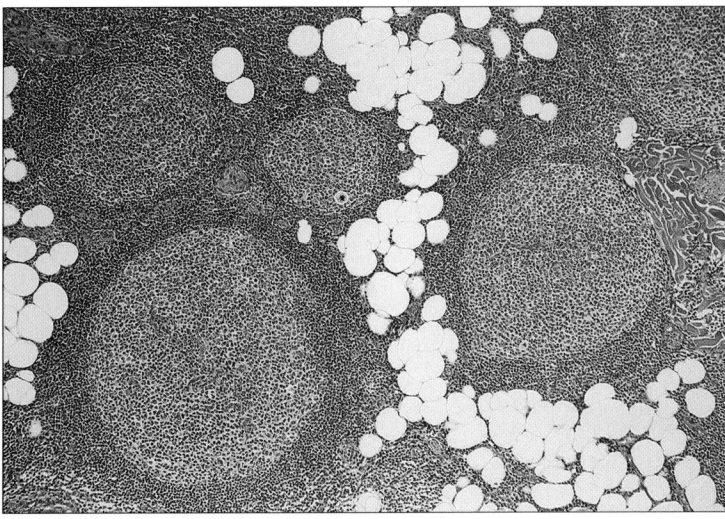

Fig. 119.8 Cutaneous follicle center lymphoma, follicular type. Neoplastic follicles with monomorphous morphology.

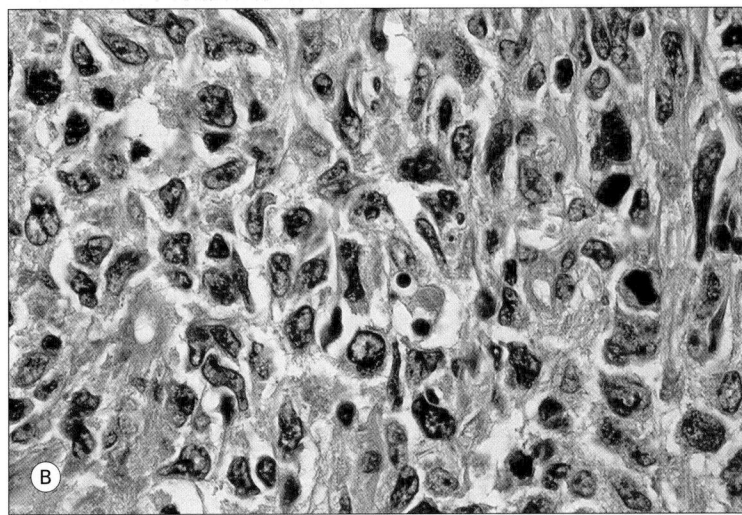

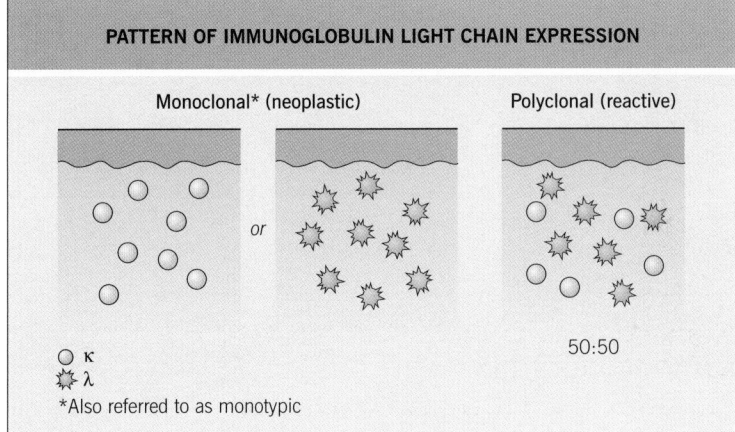

Fig. 119.7 Cutaneous follicle center lymphoma, diffuse type. A Diffuse infiltrate without follicular pattern. **B** Centroblasts and medium- and large-sized centrocytes (cleaved cells) predominate.

Fig. 119.9 Pattern of immunoglobulin light chain expression.

The tumor cells express monotypic surface immunoglobulins (e.g. all the neoplastic cells stain positively for either κ or λ light chains; Fig. 119.9) as well as B-cell-associated antigens (CD20, CD79a); they are CD5⁻ and CD43⁻ (see Table I.7 for the specificities of CD markers). When follicles are present, they are characterized by an irregular network of CD21⁺ follicular dendritic cells. Bcl-6 (a marker of germinal center cells and other blastic cells) is positive in virtually all cases, irrespective of the pattern of growth. In all cases with a follicular growth pattern, and in a minority of those with a diffuse growth pattern, neoplastic cells also stain positively for CD10. The presence of small clusters of Bcl-6⁺ cells outside the follicles is considered strongly suggestive of a diagnosis of follicular lymphoma[14].

In the overwhelming majority of cases, staining for the protein product of *bcl-2* (Bcl-2) yields negative results, representing a major difference from follicular lymphomas arising within lymph nodes[28]. A useful, though somewhat counterintuitive, immunohistochemical feature (for differential diagnosis) is the lower degree of proliferative activity within malignant follicles as detected by the MIB-1 antibody (which detects the Ki-67 antigen expressed by proliferating cells), contrasting with the strong MIB-1-positivity in reactive follicles[14,29]. In cases with large cell morphology (predominance of large cleaved cells), immunohistochemical staining for MUM-1 (multiple myeloma oncogene 1 or interferon regulatory factor 4; expressed by germinal center B cells and plasma cells) is usually either negative or is positive in a minority of neoplastic cells (in contrast to strong expression of MUM-1 by DLBCLLT; see below)[1,21].

The interchromosomal 14;18 translocation, typically found in nodal follicular lymphomas, is present in up to 40% of PCFCLs[30]. However, the presence of the 14;18 translocation, and especially expression of Bcl-2, should still raise suspicion that the patient has a systemic lymphoma involving the skin. Analysis of the genes that encode the joining segment (J_H) and other regions of the immunoglobulin heavy chain (IGH) reveals the presence of a monoclonal rearrangement in the majority of patients (60–70%). In cases with a follicular growth pattern, monoclonality of the follicular structures has been proven by PCR analysis of J_H gene rearrangements after microdissection of the follicular cells[14].

Analysis of morphologic, immunohistochemical and molecular data suggests that follicular lymphomas originating in the lymph nodes and the skin, although characterized by a similar morphologic pattern, have different pathogenic mechanisms.

Primary Cutaneous Marginal Zone B-Cell Lymphoma

Histology of PCMZL shows a patchy, nodular or diffuse infiltrate involving the dermis and subcutaneous fat. The epidermis is spared. A characteristic pattern can be observed at scanning magnification: nodular infiltrates, sometimes containing reactive germinal centers, are surrounded by a pale-staining population of small- to medium-sized cells with indented nuclei, inconspicuous nucleoli and abundant pale cytoplasm – variously described as marginal zone cells, centrocyte-like cells or monocytoid B cells (Fig. 119.10A)[3,4]. In addition, plasma cells (at the margins of the infiltrate), lymphoplasmacytoid cells, small lymphocytes and occasional large blasts are observed. Eosinophils are also a common finding. In some patients, there may be a granulomatous reaction with epithelioid and giant cells. Cases with a predominance of lymphoplasmacytoid lymphocytes were once classified as cutaneous immunocytoma[31]; PAS-positive intranuclear inclusions (Dutcher bodies) are sometimes observed and represent a valuable

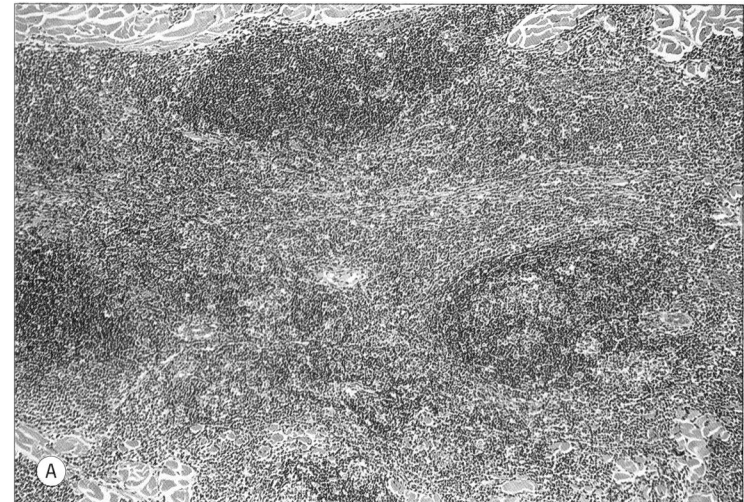

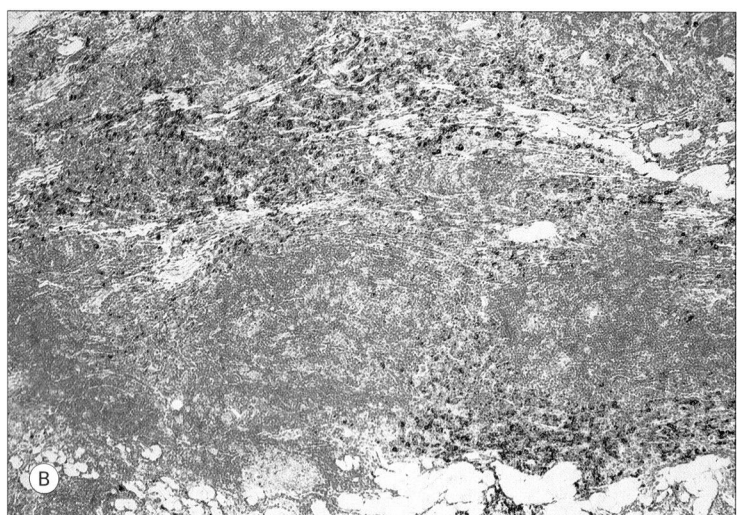

Fig. 119.10 Cutaneous marginal zone B-cell lymphoma. A Small nodules of reactive lymphocytes (dark areas) surrounded by neoplastic marginal zone cells, lymphoplasmacytoid cells and plasma cells (clear areas). **B** Monotypic expression of λ immunoglobulin light chain within the neoplastic population of cells.

diagnostic clue. Occasionally, the predominant cell type is a plasma cell, and although such cases used to be classified as primary cutaneous plasmacytomas, they (and cutaneous immunocytomas) are now considered to be variants of PCMZL[1].

The centrocyte-like cells stain positively for CD20, CD79a and Bcl-2, and they are negative for CD5, CD10 and Bcl-6. In the overwhelming majority of cases, intracytoplasmic monotypic expression of immunoglobulin light chains (either κ or λ, but not both) can be observed (see Fig. 119.9). The monoclonal population of B lymphocytes is often characteristically arranged at the periphery of the cellular aggregates (Fig. 119.10B). Monoclonal rearrangement of the *IGH* genes can be observed in the majority of cases (60–80%).

A particular translocation, t(14;18)(q32;q21), that involves the *IGH* and *MALT1* genes has been detected recently in a subset of PCMZL as well as MALT lymphomas arising in organs other than the skin. Other genetic aberrations include trisomy 3 and rarely an 11;18 translocation. However, in more than 50% of patients, no molecular abnormalities have been found.

Primary Cutaneous Diffuse Large B-Cell Lymphoma, Leg Type

In DLBCLLT, a dense diffuse infiltrate is seen within the dermis and subcutis. The infiltrate usually involves the entire papillary dermis extending to the dermal–epidermal junction. Involvement of the epidermis by clusters of large atypical cells, simulating the Pautrier's microabscesses found in cutaneous T-cell lymphoma, can be observed in some cases (B-cell epidermotropism), representing a potential

diagnostic pitfall[3]. The neoplastic infiltrate consists predominantly of immunoblasts (large round cells with abundant cytoplasm and prominent nucleoli) and centroblasts (Fig. 119.11). Cases of diffuse large B-cell lymphoma with a predominance of large cleaved cells are classified among the PCFCLs[1]. Reactive small lymphocytes are few or absent, and mitoses are frequent. Based on the common finding of immunoglobulin gene hypermutations, it has been proposed that most cases of DLBCLLT represent large cell lymphomas originating from lymphocytes of the germinal center[32].

Neoplastic cells express monoclonal surface immunoglobulins and/or cytoplasmic immunoglobulins. They are positive for B-cell markers (CD20, CD79a), but there can be (partial) loss of antigen expression. MUM-1 (see above) is strongly expressed by neoplastic cells in most patients[1,21]. This marker is useful in the differential diagnosis of DLBCLLT from PCFCL, diffuse type (in the latter, MUM-1 is usually either negative or expressed by a small minority of cells) (Fig. 119.12). The tumors demonstrate monoclonal rearrangement of the *IGH* genes. The interchromosomal 14;18 translocation is not present.

Staining for Bcl-2 is positive in all patients with primary cutaneous DLBCLLT. In fact, cases of cutaneous diffuse large B-cell lymphoma with a predominance of large round cells and an absence of Bcl-2 expression are categorized as primary cutaneous diffuse large B-cell lymphoma, other, according to the WHO–EORTC classification[1]. An algorithmic approach to the diagnosis of cutaneous diffuse large B-cell lymphomas is provided in Figure 119.13.

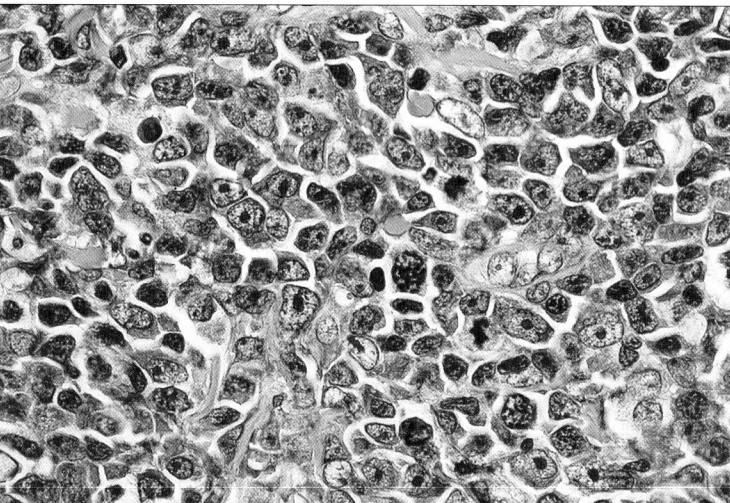

Fig. 119.11 Cutaneous diffuse large B-cell lymphoma, leg type. Large cells with a round morphology (mainly immunoblasts) predominate.

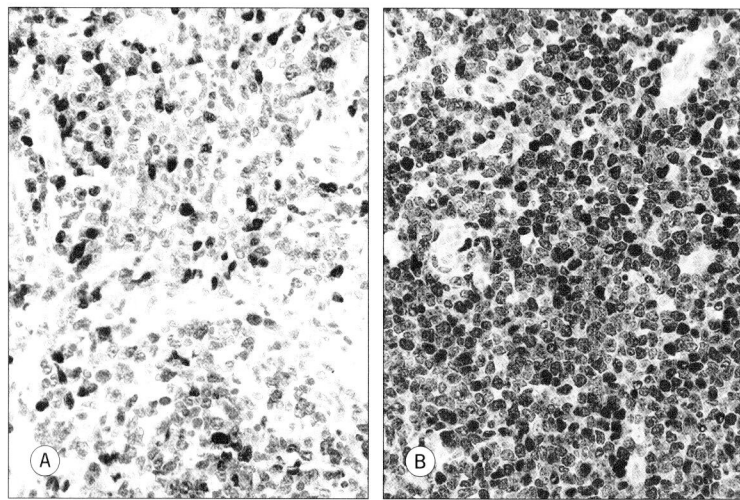

Fig. 119.12 Immunohistochemical staining with the anti-MUM-1 antibody. A Only a minority of cells are positive in primary cutaneous follicle center lymphoma, diffuse type. **B** Virtually all tumor cells are positive in primary cutaneous diffuse large B-cell lymphoma, leg type.

APPROACH TO THE DIAGNOSIS OF CUTANEOUS LARGE B-CELL LYMPHOMAS

```
                    Predominant cell type
                    /                \
          Large round cells      Large cleaved cells
                |                        |
          Location of cells      Primary cutaneous
            /        \           follicle center lymphoma,
    Intravascular   In the dermis    diffuse type
        |           and/or subcutis
Intravascular large      |
B-cell lymphoma      Immunophenotype
                      /         \
                   Bcl-2+      Bcl-2–
                     |           |
            Diffuse large B-cell    Diffuse large B-cell
            lymphoma, leg type      lymphoma, other
```

Fig. 119.13 Approach to the diagnosis of cutaneous large B-cell lymphomas.

Rare cases of otherwise typical cutaneous DLBCLLT show expression of CD30 by neoplastic cells[21]. These cases should not be mistakenly classified as cutaneous CD30+ anaplastic large cell lymphomas, but must be considered as a rare phenotypic variant of DLBCLLT. In contrast to cutaneous T-cell lymphomas, prognosis in large B-cell lymphomas (both cutaneous and extracutaneous) is not related to CD30 expression.

Genetic data obtained by fluorescence *in situ* hybridization (FISH) or microarray chip technologies have confirmed that DLBCLLTs show clear molecular differences from PCFCL, diffuse type, confirming the need of classifying these cases separately[33,34]. Some of the aberrations found in DLBCLLT are similar to those observed in diffuse large B-cell lymphomas of the lymph nodes.

Primary Cutaneous Diffuse Large B-Cell Lymphoma, Other

Cases of primary cutaneous B-cell lymphoma with a predominance of large round cells, but lacking Bcl-2 expression, are classified in this group. Other histopathologic and immunohistochemical features are similar to those of either DLBCLLT or PCFCL, diffuse type, suggesting that these lymphomas represent a morphologic or phenotypic variant of the latter groups[21].

Intravascular large B-cell lymphoma is characterized by a proliferation of large atypical lymphocytes that fills dilated blood vessels within the dermis and subcutaneous tissues (Fig. 119.14). In some patients, a variable number of atypical cells may also be observed around blood vessels. The malignant cells are large with scanty cytoplasm and often have prominent nucleoli. They are positive for B-cell-associated markers and express monoclonal surface immunoglobulins. Staining with endothelial cell-related antibodies (e.g. CD31, CD34) highlights the characteristic intravascular location of the cells. Molecular analysis shows monoclonal rearrangement of the *IGH* genes.

Plasmablastic lymphoma is characterized by a proliferation of plasmablasts (large eccentric nuclei, abundant cytoplasm, prominent nucleoli). The neoplastic cells are positive for CD38 and CD138, and they express monotypic immunoglobulin light chains.

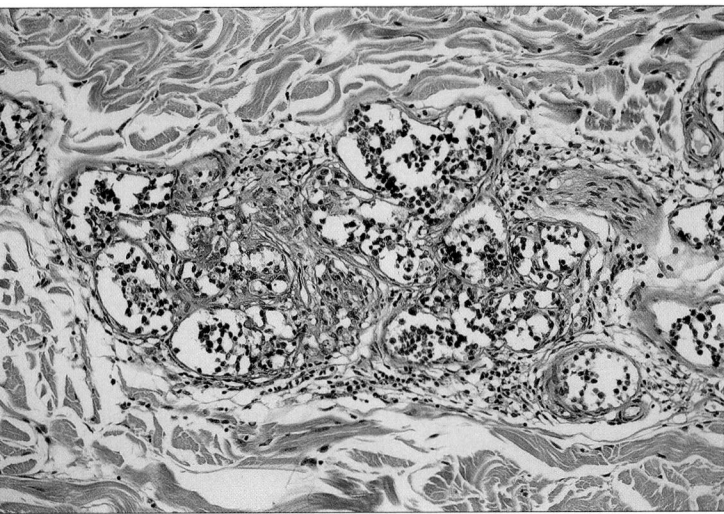

Fig. 119.14 Cutaneous intravascular large B-cell lymphoma. Intravascular proliferation of medium- to large-sized atypical lymphocytes.

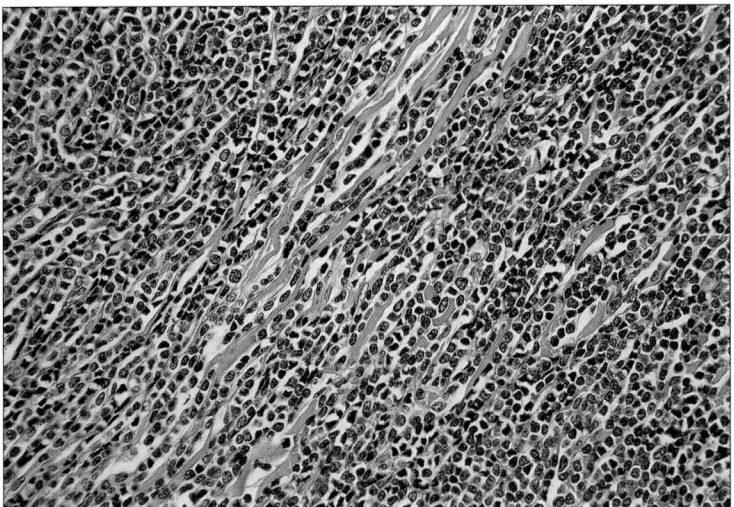

Fig. 119.15 Cutaneous B-cell lymphoblastic lymphoma. Medium-sized blasts with the characteristic 'mosaic-stone' linear arrangement.

B-Cell Lymphoblastic Lymphoma

Histologically, B-cell lymphoblastic lymphoma shows a monomorphous proliferation of medium-sized cells with scanty cytoplasm and round or convoluted nuclei with fine chromatin (Fig. 119.15). A 'starry sky' pattern is commonly seen at low power, due to the presence of macrophages with inclusion bodies ('tingible bodies'). Another characteristic feature is the arrangement of neoplastic cells in a 'mosaic-stone' pattern. Mitoses and necrotic cells are abundant. It must be stressed that histologic features alone do not allow differentiation of lymphoblastic lymphomas of B-cell phenotype from those of T-cell lineage. Immunohistology demonstrates positive staining for TdT (terminal deoxynucleotidyl transferase; present on precursor T and B cells), CD10 and the cytoplasmic μ-chain of immunoglobulins and, in most cases, CD20 and CD79a. CD20 is negative in the pre-pre-B-cell variant, which is CD34+. Lesions in most patients also express CD99, and some are positive for CD43. Molecular analyses usually show a monoclonal rearrangement of the *IGH* genes and a polyclonal pattern for the T-cell receptor (*TCR*) genes, but a lack of rearrangement of the *IGH* genes or monoclonal rearrangement of both the *TCR* and *IGH* genes may be observed.

DIFFERENTIAL DIAGNOSIS

Differential diagnoses of primary cutaneous B-cell lymphomas vary according to the type of lymphoma and include primarily inflammatory processes that may simulate malignant lymphomas either clinically, histopathologically, or both (so-called cutaneous pseudolymphomas; see Ch. 121). It must be emphasized that a definitive diagnosis of primary cutaneous B-cell lymphoma can be reached only after careful examination of the clinical, histopathologic, immunophenotypic and molecular features; in some cases, only repeated examination of the patient and sequential biopsy specimens will allow the correct classification[3,35–37].

Patients for whom no definitive diagnosis can be established at the time of presentation should provisionally be classified as having 'cutaneous atypical lymphoid proliferation of B-cell lineage', and they should be re-examined at regular intervals. A complete staging investigation does not belong in the diagnostic evaluation of these patients; that is, patients without a definitive diagnosis of cutaneous B-cell lymphoma should not be screened for extracutaneous disease until the diagnosis is established with certainty. In contrast, once the diagnosis of cutaneous B-cell lymphoma has been established, complete staging is mandatory, as clinicopathologic features alone do not allow the differentiation of primary from secondary cutaneous B-cell lymphomas. A diagnostic algorithm for evaluation of patients at first presentation is provided in Figure 119.16. In the following section, the major differential diagnoses of each of the main types of primary cutaneous B-cell lymphoma are outlined separately, as they differ according to the lymphoma type.

As already mentioned, before the recent establishment of the WHO–EORTC classification system, distinguishing between the different forms of low-grade primary cutaneous B-cell lymphoma

(PCFCL and PCMZL) was complicated by the lack of consistency in the categorization of these diseases among different centers and by the lack of homogeneity of data reported in the literature. In fact, patients presenting with similar clinicopathologic features were classified into different categories in different studies, thus contributing to the difficulties in distinguishing among the various types of primary cutaneous B-cell lymphomas of low-grade malignancy.

PCFCL with a follicular pattern of growth should be differentiated from B-cell pseudolymphomas with prominent germinal centers, such as *Borrelia*-induced lymphocytoma cutis (cutaneous lymphoid hyperplasia)[14,38]. Lymphocytoma cutis often occurs in children, and it shows a predilection for particular body sites such as the earlobes, nipples and scrotum[38]. Clinically, lesions are usually solitary and relatively small. Although histologically a follicular pattern is almost always observed, germinal centers in lymphocytoma cutis are reactive, and they are accompanied by inflammatory infiltrates with small lymphocytes, plasma cells and often eosinophils[3,38]. The germinal centers in *Borrelia*-induced lymphocytoma cutis are often devoid of a clearcut mantle, but they are characterized by the presence of: many tingible body macrophages, 'clear' and 'dark' areas, and a normal (high) proliferation rate[38].

Rare cases of cutaneous PCMZL can have a prominent presence of reactive germinal centers, and they should be differentiated from the follicular type of PCFCL. In these cases, so-called follicular colonization by neoplastic marginal zone cells can indeed cause significant problems in histopathologic differential diagnosis, similar to what happens in

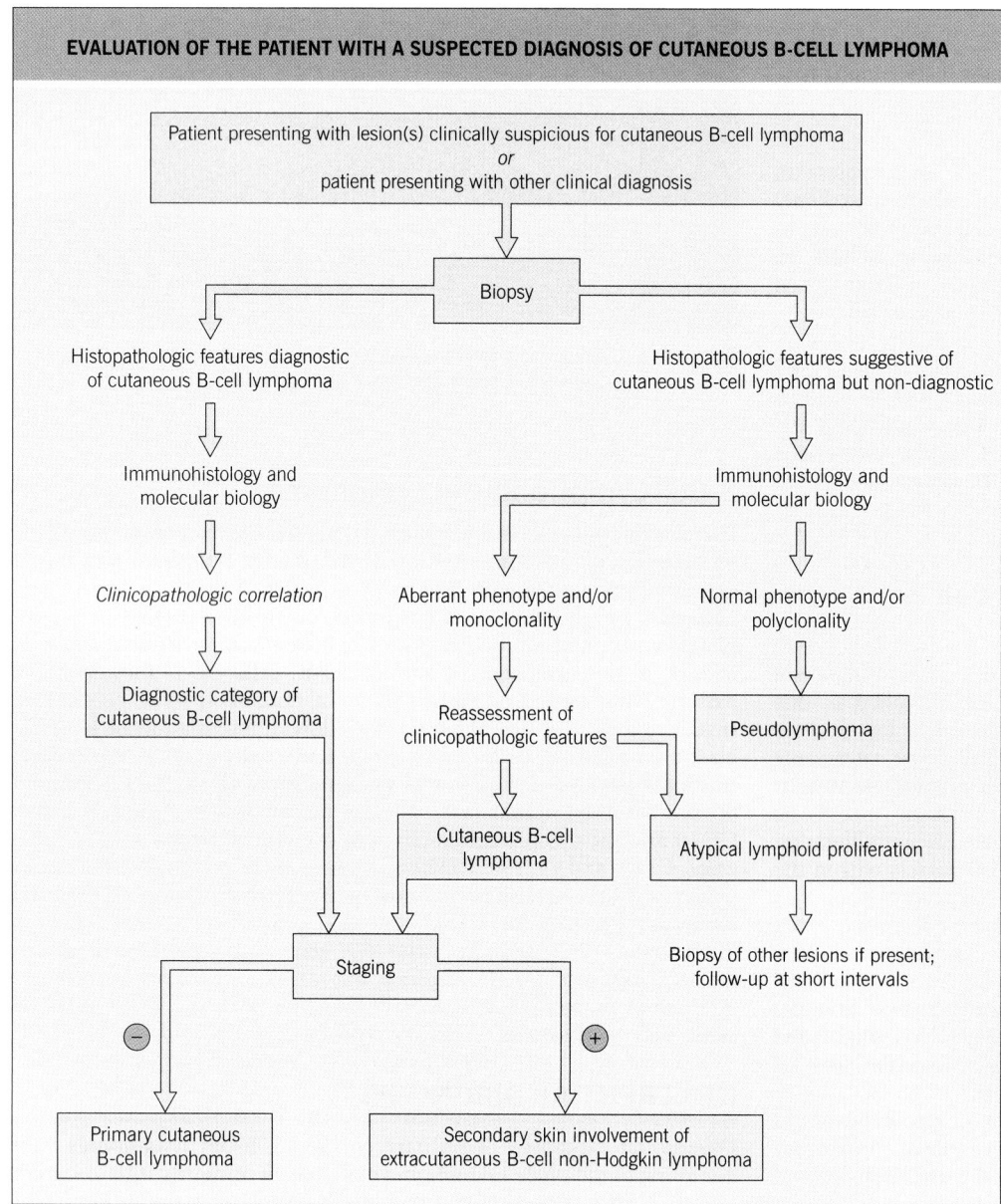

Fig. 119.16 Evaluation of the patient with a suspected diagnosis of cutaneous B-cell lymphoma.

EVALUATION OF THE PATIENT WITH A SUSPECTED DIAGNOSIS OF CUTANEOUS B-CELL LYMPHOMA

B-cell lymphomas of the MALT type. However, the overall architecture of the infiltrate, the presence of a population of monoclonal plasma cells belonging to the neoplastic clone, and the negativity of neoplastic cells for CD10 and Bcl-6 usually allow the diagnosis of cutaneous PCMZL to be established.

As mentioned previously, secondary cutaneous involvement by primary extracutaneous follicular lymphomas has morphologic and phenotypic features similar or identical to those observed in primary cutaneous B-cell lymphoma, except for the usual positivity of neoplastic cells for Bcl-2 in secondary cutaneous lesions. Consequently, the occurrence of a cutaneous follicular lymphoma with clearcut positivity for Bcl-2 within neoplastic follicles should be considered as a strong hint (although exceptions have been reported) for the diagnosis of secondary skin lesions of nodal lymphoma.

The differential diagnosis of PCMZL consists primarily of reactive processes and other types of low-grade primary cutaneous B-cell lymphoma. Benign, reactive processes do not have monotypic restriction of immunoglobulin light chain expression, in contrast to what is observed in the great majority of cases of PCMZL. Lymphocytic infiltration of Jessner-Kanof can present with clinicopathologic features similar to those observed in some cases of PCMZL, but the infiltrates in the former are composed predominantly of T lymphocytes and monoclonality is not present.

PCFCL, diffuse type, can be differentiated from PCMZL by the architectural pattern and cytomorphology, the former being characterized by a diffuse infiltrate of B lymphocytes with a predominance of centrocytes and centroblasts. Moreover, in contrast to in PCMZL, neoplastic cells in PCFCL express Bcl-6. PCMZL with germinal centers must also be differentiated from cases of PCFCL, follicular type. As already pointed out, germinal centers in PCMZL are reactive, whereas they display a variety of atypical features in PCFCL, follicular type. Care should be taken to avoid misinterpretation of follicular colonization by marginal zone cells as neoplastic germinal centers.

PCMZL should also be distinguished from secondary cutaneous lesions of B-cell chronic lymphocytic leukemia (B-CLL), a condition in which neoplastic B lymphocytes display positivity for CD20 and CD43, and usually positivity for CD5. Helpful diagnostic features are: (1) the absence, in B-CLL, of plasma cells belonging to the neoplastic clone; and (2) the positivity for CD5 observed in most cases of cutaneous B-CLL, but practically never in PCMZL. Finally, it seems likely that cases classified in the past as 'cutaneous lymphoid hyperplasia with monotypic plasma cells' represent, in fact, examples of PCMZL with prominent plasma cell differentiation.

PCMZL with prominent plasma cell differentiation must be differentiated from reactive plasma cell proliferations and inflammatory pseudotumors (plasma cell granulomas). In reactive conditions, plasma cells are not atypical, and they display a polyclonal pattern of immunoglobulin light chain expression. Besides inflammatory pseudotumors, reactive skin diseases with a predominance of plasma cells are very rare, with the exception of lesions arising on mucosal surfaces and syphilis. A silver stain (e.g. Warthin-Starry) or immunohistochemical staining for *Treponema pallidum* can help to highlight the microorganisms in cases of syphilis (see Ch. 81).

DLBCLLT must be differentiated from a number of entities, including cutaneous involvement from systemic lymphomas as well as specific infiltrates of acute myelogenous leukemia and non-lymphoid tumors (e.g. solid organ metastases). The clinicopathologic pattern together with phenotypic and molecular features allow correct classification of these lesions in most instances. In order to avoid diagnostic errors, detailed immunophenotyping is mandatory in all cases of cutaneous lymphoma, especially in those showing medium- to large-cell morphology.

The differential diagnosis of cutaneous intravascular large B-cell lymphoma is not a problem in typical cases. The large number of atypical cells within blood vessels is pathognomonic of this condition. Distinction between T- and B-cell types cannot be achieved on morphologic grounds alone, but it does not seem to be relevant for prognosis and treatment. Intravascular large B-cell lymphoma should be distinguished from so-called intravascular histiocytosis, a condition in which the vessels in the dermis show intraluminal collections of histiocytes. Morphologic, immunophenotypic and molecular features allow one to distinguish these entities with confidence. Intravascular

histiocytosis has been observed in different clinical settings, including chronic erysipelas.

Cases of B-cell lymphoblastic lymphoma should be differentiated from other cutaneous lymphomas and from non-lymphoid tumors such as Ewing's sarcoma and small cell lung carcinoma. Positivity for TdT represents the most important immunohistochemical feature for the diagnosis of cutaneous lymphoblastic lymphoma. It has been suggested that CD99, TdT and CD34, alone or in combination, strongly support the diagnosis of lymphoblastic lymphoma/leukemia and allow distinction of these neoplasms from small non-cleaved cell lymphomas (e.g. Burkitt's lymphoma). Histologic features of cutaneous lesions do not allow the differentiation of T-cell from B-cell lymphoblastic lymphomas, thus emphasizing the importance of complete immunophenotypic and genotypic analyses.

TREATMENT

The most appropriate treatment modality for patients with a primary cutaneous B-cell lymphoma is selected after exact classification of the lymphoma, analysis of results of staging investigations, and consideration of the overall condition of the patient. Those patients with secondary cutaneous lesions of extracutaneous B-cell lymphoma should be treated in a hemato-oncologic, not dermatologic, setting, and they will not be discussed in this chapter[3,39–41].

Before reviewing the major therapeutic strategies, it must be emphasized that many patients with low-grade primary cutaneous B-cell lymphoma can be managed conservatively with a so-called watchful–waiting strategy, similar to what is often adopted for indolent B-cell lymphomas and leukemias at extracutaneous sites[40]. Follow-up examinations in these patients should be performed at least every 6 months or at the onset of new lesions and/or new symptoms, in order to treat the patient as soon as it is necessary. Many patients treated conservatively with a watchful–waiting strategy experience a prolonged course and long survival, and they do not need aggressive treatment.

Most patients with primary cutaneous B-cell lymphomas that are low grade (PCFCL, PCMZL) and who have a solitary or few lesions can be treated by local radiotherapy, simple surgical excision, or surgical excision followed by radiotherapy of the surgical field[39]. It has been reported that recurrences are less frequently seen in patients treated by radiotherapy with wide margins (about 10–20 cm beyond clinically apparent lesions); this approach seems to be justified for so-called Crosti's lymphoma, a type of PCFCL arising on the back, in which erythematous nodules, papules and patches surrounding the tumor represent specific infiltrates that can extend far beyond the main bulk of the lesion[42]. Radiotherapy with wide margins, however, does not seem to be justified for lesions other than Crosti's lymphoma, as margins of about 3–5 cm usually suffice (depending on the size of the lesion). Surgical excision with narrow margins is a valuable therapeutic modality for patients with solitary well-circumscribed lesions. In these patients, relapse rates do not seem to be higher than in patients treated with more time-intensive modalities such as local radiotherapy.

In recent years, a few reports have appeared in which low-grade primary cutaneous B-cell lymphomas were treated with systemic antibiotics, achieving a complete resolution in at least a percentage of the patients[40,43,44]. This type of treatment is conceptually analogous to that adopted for *Helicobacter pylori*-associated MALT lymphomas of the stomach, which in their early stages can be cured by eradication of *H. pylori* infection. Complete response to antibiotic therapy has been observed recently in some patients with *Borrelia*-associated primary cutaneous B-cell lymphoma. Although not yet corroborated by adequate data, antibiotic treatment of patients with primary cutaneous B-cell lymphomas should be considered before more aggressive therapeutic options are employed, particularly in European countries endemic for *Borrelia* infections. It is important to treat patients at the onset of the disease, because, in later stages, lesions may no longer be sensitive to systemic antibiotics. PCR analysis of *Borrelia* DNA is a rapid test that should be performed in all patients with primary cutaneous B-cell lymphoma from endemic areas, in order to identify those who would more likely benefit from antibiotic treatment.

Another treatment modality for low-grade primary cutaneous B-cell lymphoma is subcutaneous or intralesional interferon, particularly interferon-α-2a[40,45]. Although some favorable results have been reported, it seems that treatment with interferon is associated with a complete response in about 50% of patients. Therapy with interferon should be considered for patients presenting with multiple lesions at different body sites, such that local radiotherapy becomes difficult to administer.

Intralesional or systemic injection of anti-CD20 monoclonal antibody (rituximab) has been recently used to induce tumor reduction in patients with indolent primary cutaneous B-cell lymphomas[46–48]. Intralesional administration should be considered in patients presenting with a few, localized lesions. Therapy with intravenous rituximab represents a valid alternative to established treatments, especially in patients who present with disseminated skin lesions or relapse after radiotherapy. Anti-CD20 monoclonal antibody can also be administered in combination with other treatment modalities for cutaneous B-cell lymphomas with more aggressive behavior (e.g. DLBCLLT).

Patients with disseminated lesions of PCFCL, diffuse type, or particularly DLBCLLT need more aggressive treatment modalities (e.g. systemic chemotherapy plus rituximab). This treatment, however, is usually necessary in only a small proportion of patients with PCFCL[40,49,50]. The regimen used most frequently is cyclophosphamide, doxorubicin, vincristine and prednisone (CHOP) plus rituximab. In the absence of signs of transformation into high-grade lymphoma, aggressive treatment is not indicated in patients with PCMZL. For patients with DLBCLLT, either local radiotherapy or systemic chemotherapy plus rituximab is the standard therapy. However, in the setting of significant comorbidities, rituximab alone may be administered.

Systemic chemotherapy plus rituximab is the treatment of choice for patients with intravascular large B-cell lymphoma, regardless of results of staging investigations. Finally, patients with B-cell lymphoblastic lymphoma should be treated in a hematologic setting; even in those with negative staging at presentation, aggressive chemotherapy plus rituximab should be administered. The option of hematopoietic stem cell transplantation should be discussed.

MULTIPLE MYELOMA

Multiple myeloma is a malignant proliferation of plasma cells that rarely involves the skin. However, there are a number of cutaneous manifestations of monoclonal gammopathies (Table 119.2), which can occur in the setting of multiple myeloma. The possibility of underlying multiple myeloma needs to be considered in any patient with a monoclonal gammopathy detected by serum electrophoresis. A bone marrow aspirate and biopsy is performed, especially when the monoclonal protein is >1 g/dl. The evaluation also includes immunofixation electrophoresis of the serum, in order to identify the class of immunoglobulin that is being produced (IgG > IgA > IgD), as well as of the urine, to determine the presence of Bence-Jones light chains. Skeletal radiographs of the spine and long bones are done to look for osteolytic lesions (sclerotic lesions are seen in POEMS syndrome; see below).

Histopathology

In specific lesions, diffuse infiltration of the dermis by atypical plasma cells or lymphoplasmacytoid cells is present, usually with prevalent mitoses. Multinucleated plasma cells may be found. The infiltrating cells can be difficult to recognize as plasma cells, and CD45 and CD20 are negative as a rule. Neoplastic plasma cells can be stained with CD38 and CD138, and they express monotypic immunoglobulins. Intracytoplasmic eosinophilic inclusions (Russell bodies) are often present; the cells are called Mott cells when these bodies form grape-like clusters. Eosinophilic inclusions in the nucleus (Dutcher bodies) can also be observed. These are thought to be immunoglobulin or glycoprotein accumulations, and can be found in other conditions in which plasma cells are prevalent (see introductory chapter of this text for a list of plasma cell-rich conditions).

CUTANEOUS CONDITIONS ASSOCIATED WITH MONOCLONAL GAMMOPATHY

Proliferation of lymphoplasmacytic cells in the skin
- Extramedullary cutaneous plasmacytoma
- Cutaneous Waldenström's macroglobulinemia*

Deposition of the monoclonal protein in the skin, by definition
- Primary systemic amyloidosis
- Cryoglobulinemic occlusive vasculopathy (type I cryoglobulins†)
- Hyperkeratotic spicules (follicular > non-follicular)
- IgM storage papules (cutaneous macroglobulinosis)*
- Subepidermal bullous dermatosis associated with IgM gammopathy*

Deposition of the monoclonal protein in the skin frequently observed
- Plasma cell dyscrasia-associated acquired cutis laxa, acral or generalized (amyloid or IgG)
- Plasma cell dyscrasia-associated reactive angioendotheliomatosis (type I cryoglobulins or amyloid)

Almost always associated with monoclonal gammopathy
- Scleromyxedema
- POEMS syndrome
- Schnitzler's syndrome*
- Necrobiotic xanthogranuloma

Frequently associated with monoclonal gammopathy
- Normolipemic plane xanthoma
- Scleredema (type 2; see Ch. 46)
- Angioedema secondary to acquired C1 esterase inhibitor deficiency

Significant association with monoclonal gammopathy (at least 15% of cases)
- Erythema elevatum diutinum
- Subcorneal pustular dermatosis (SPD) and SPD-type IgA pemphigus
- Pyoderma gangrenosum

Occasionally associated with monoclonal gammopathy
- Sweet's syndrome
- Cutaneous small vessel vasculitis†,‡
- Xanthoma disseminatum
- Epidermolysis bullosa acquisita
- Paraneoplastic pemphigus
- Atypical scleroderma§

*IgM monoclonal gammopathy is present by definition; in Schnitzler's syndrome, IgG gammopathy has occasionally been observed.
† Cryoglobulinemic vasculitis can occur secondary to type II cryoglobulins.
‡ Henoch–Schönlein purpura in adults is occasionally associated with an IgA monoclonal gammopathy.
§ Possible association; sclerodermoid changes can also occur in the setting of primary systemic amyloidosis.

Table 119.2 Cutaneous conditions associated with monoclonal gammopathy.

Differential Diagnosis

The diagnosis of PCMZL with prominent plasma cell differentiation (formerly called cutaneous plasmacytoma) rests upon a lack of involvement of the bone marrow. Waldenström's macroglobulinemia has histology similar to PCMZL with prominent lymphoplasmacytic differentiation (formerly called cutaneous immunocytoma), except that direct immunofluorescence demonstrates monoclonal IgM within and around the infiltrating cells. Immunofixation electrophoresis of the serum detects the circulating monoclonal protein as IgM.

POEMS syndrome (Takatsuki syndrome, Crow–Fukase syndrome), is characterized by *p*olyneuropathy, *o*rganomegaly, *e*ndocrinopathies, *m*onoclonal gammopathy, and *s*kin changes such as diffuse hyperpigmentation, edema and glomeruloid hemangiomas (see Ch. 114).

REFERENCES

1. Willemze R, Jaffe ES, Burg G, et al. WHO-EORTC classification for cutaneous lymphomas. Blood 2005;105:3768–85.
2. Fink-Puches R, Zenahlik P, Bäck B, et al. Primary cutaneous lymphomas: applicability of current classification schemes (EORTC, WHO) based on clinicopathologic features observed in a large group of patients. Blood. 2002;99:800–5.
3. Cerroni L, Gatter K, Kerl H. An Illustrated Guide to Skin Lymphoma, 2nd edn. Malden: Blackwell, 2004.
4. Cerroni L, Signoretti S, Höfler G, et al. Primary cutaneous marginal zone B-cell lymphoma: a recently described entity of low-grade malignant cutaneous B-cell lymphoma. Am J Surg Pathol. 1997;21:1307–15.
5. Santucci M, Pimpinelli N, Arganini L. Primary cutaneous B-cell lymphoma: a unique type of low-grade lymphoma – clinicopathologic and immunologic study of 83 cases. Cancer. 1991;67:2311–26.
6. Zackheim HS, Vonderheid EC, Ramsay DL, et al. Relative frequency of various forms of primary cutaneous lymphomas. J Am Acad Dermatol. 2000;43:793–6.
7. Cerroni L, Zöchling N, Pütz B, Kerl H. Infection by Borrelia burgdorferi and cutaneous B-cell lymphoma. J Cutan Pathol. 1997;24:457–61.
8. Goodlad JR, Davidson MM, Hollowood K, et al. Primary cutaneous B-cell lymphoma and Borrelia burgdorferi infection in patients from the highlands of Scotland. Am J Surg Pathol. 2000;24:1279–85.
9. Zöchling N, Pütz B, Wolf P, et al. Human herpesvirus 8-specific DNA sequences in primary cutaneous B-cell lymphomas. Arch Dermatol. 1998;134:246–7.
10. Nagore E, Ledesma E, Collado C, et al. Detection of Epstein-Barr virus and human herpesvirus 7 and 8 genomes in primary cutaneous T- and B-cell lymphomas. Br J Dermatol. 2000;143:320–3.
11. Viraben R, Brousse P, Lamant L. Reversible cutaneous lymphoma occurring during methotrexate therapy. Br J Dermatol. 1996;135:116–18.
12. Beylot-Barry M, Vergier B, Masquelier B, et al. The spectrum of cutaneous lymphomas in HIV infection. A study of 21 cases. Am J Surg Pathol. 1999;23:1208–16.
13. Berti E, Alessi E, Caputo R, et al. Reticulohistiocytoma of the dorsum. J Am Acad Dermatol. 1988;19:259–72.
14. Cerroni L, Arzberger E, Pütz B, et al. Primary cutaneous follicle center cell lymphoma with follicular growth pattern. Blood. 2000;95:3922–8.
15. Pimpinelli N, Santucci M, Bosi A, et al. Primary cutaneous follicular centre-cell lymphoma: a lymphoproliferative disease with favourable prognosis. Clin Exp Dermatol. 1989;14:12–19.
16. Bailey EM, Ferry JA, Harris NL, et al. Marginal zone lymphoma (low-grade B-cell lymphoma of mucosa-associated lymphoid tissue type) of skin and subcutaneous tissue. A study of 15 patients. Am J Surg Pathol. 1996;20:1011–23.
17. Child FJ, Woollons A, Price ML, et al. Multiple cutaneous immunocytoma with secondary anetoderma: a report of two cases. Br J Dermatol. 2000;143:165–70.
18. Vermeer MH, Geelen FAMJ, van Haselen CW, et al. Primary cutaneous large B-cell lymphomas of the legs. A distinct type of cutaneous B-cell lymphoma with an intermediate prognosis. Arch Dermatol. 1996;132:1304–8.

19. Grange F, Bekkenk MW, Wechsler J, et al. Prognostic factors in primary cutaneous large B-cell lymphomas: a European multicenter study of 145 cases. J Clin Oncol. 2001;19:3602–10.
20. Grange F, Petrella T, Beylot-Barry M, et al. Bcl-2 protein expression is the strongest independent prognostic factor of survival in primary cutaneous large B-cell lymphomas. Blood. 2004;103:3662–8.
21. Kodama K, Massone C, Chott A, et al. Primary cutaneous large B-cell lymphomas: clinicopathologic features, classification, and prognostic factors in a large series of patients. Blood. 2005;106:2491–7.
22. Perniciaro C, Winkelmann RK, Daoud MS, et al. Malignant angioendotheliomatosis is an angiotropic intravascular lymphoma. Immunohistochemical, ultrastructural, and molecular genetics studies. Am J Dermatopathol. 1995;17:242–8.
23. Cerroni L, Zalaudek I, Kerl H. Intravascular large B-cell lymphoma colonizing cutaneous hemangiomas. Dermatology. 2004;209:132–4.
24. Chimenti S, Fink-Puches R, Peris K, et al. Cutaneous involvement in lymphoblastic lymphoma. J Cutan Pathol. 1999;26:379–85.
25. Sander CA, Medeiros LJ, Abruzzo LV, et al. Lymphoblastic lymphoma presenting in cutaneous sites: a clinicopathologic analysis of six cases. J Am Acad Dermatol. 1991;25:1023–31.
26. Willemze R, Meijer CJLM, Sentis HJ, et al. Primary cutaneous large cell lymphomas of follicular center cell origin: a clinical follow-up study of nineteen patients. J Am Acad Dermatol. 1987;16:518–26.
27. Cerroni L, El-Shabrawi-Caelen L, Fink-Puches R, LeBoit PE, Kerl H. Cutaneous spindle-cell B-cell lymphoma. A morphologic variant of cutaneous large B-cell lymphoma. Am J Dermatopathol. 2000;22:299–304.
28. Cerroni L, Volkenandt M, Rieger E, et al. bcl-2 protein expression and correlation with the interchromosomal 14;18 translocation in cutaneous lymphomas and pseudolymphomas. J Invest Dermatol. 1994;102:231–5.
29. Cerroni L, Kerl H. Primary cutaneous follicle center cell lymphoma. Leuk Lymphoma. 2001;42:891–900.
30. Streubel B, Scheucher B, Valencak J, et al. Molecular cytogenetic evidence of t(14;18)(IGH;BCL2) in a substantial proportion of primary cutaneous follicle center lymphomas. Am J Surg Pathol. 2006;30:529–36.
31. Rijlaarsdam JU, van der Putte SCJ, Berti E, et al. Cutaneous immunocytomas: a clinicopathologic study of 26 cases. Histopathology. 1993;23:117–25.
32. Gellrich S, Rutz S, Golembowski S, et al. Primary cutaneous follicle center cell lymphomas and large B cell lymphomas of the leg descend from germinal center cells. A single cell polymerase chain reaction analysis. J Invest Dermatol. 2001;117:1512–20.
33. Hoefnagel JJ, Dijkman R, Basso K, et al. Distinct types of primary cutaneous large B-cell lymphoma identified by gene expression profiling. Blood. 2005;105:3671–8.
34. Wiesner T, Streubel B, Huber D, et al. Genetic aberrations in primary cutaneous large B-cell lymphoma. A fluorescence in situ hybridization study of 25 cases. Am J Surg Pathol. 2005;29:666–73.
35. Cerroni L, Goteri G. Differential diagnosis between cutaneous lymphoma and pseudolymphoma. Anal Quant Cytol Histol. 2003;25:191–8.

36. Yang B, Tubbs RR, Finn W, et al. Clinicopathologic reassessment of primary cutaneous B-cell lymphomas with immunophenotypic and molecular genetic characterization. Am J Surg Pathol. 2000;24:694–702.
37. Leinweber B, Colli C, Chott A, et al. Differential diagnosis of cutaneous infiltrates of B lymphocytes with follicular growth pattern. Am J Dermatopathol. 2004;26:4–13.
38. Colli C, Leinweber B, Müllegger R, et al. Borrelia burgdorferi-associated lymphocytoma cutis: clinicopathologic, immunophenotypic, and molecular study of 106 cases. J Cutan Pathol. 2004;31:232–40.
39. Parry EJ, Stevens SR, Gilliam AC, et al. Management of cutaneous lymphomas using a multidisciplinary approach. Arch Dermatol. 1999;135:907–11.
40. Zenahlik P, Fink-Puches R, Kapp KS, et al. Therapy of primary cutaneous B-cell lymphomas. Hautarzt. 2000;51:19–24.
41. Kerl H, Kodama K, Cerroni L. Diagnostic principles and new developments in primary cutaneous B-cell lymphomas. J Dermatol Sci. 2004;34:167–75.
42. Piccinno R, Caccialanza M, Berti E, Baldini L. Radiotherapy of cutaneous B cell lymphomas: our experience in 31 cases. Int J Radiat Oncol Biol Phys. 1993;27:385–9.
43. Kütting B, Bonsmann G, Metze D, et al. Borrelia burgdorferi-associated primary cutaneous B cell lymphoma: complete clearing of skin lesions after antibiotic pulse therapy or intralesional injection of interferon α-2a. J Am Acad Dermatol. 1997;36:311–14.
44. Roggero E, Zucca E, Mainetti C, et al. Eradication of Borrelia burgdorferi infection in primary marginal zone B-cell lymphoma of the skin. Hum Pathol. 2000;31:263–8.
45. Parodi A, Micalizzi C, Rebora A. Intralesional natural interferon alpha in the treatment of Crosti's lymphoma (primary cutaneous B follicular centre-cell lymphoma): report of four cases. J Dermatol Treat. 1996;7:105–7.
46. Heinzerling LM, Urbanek M, Funk JO, et al. Reduction of tumor burden and stabilization of disease by systemic therapy with anti-CD20 antibody (rituximab) in patients with primary cutaneous B-cell lymphoma. Cancer. 2000;89:1835–44.
47. Sabroe RA, Child FJ, Woolford AJ, et al. Rituximab in cutaneous B-cell lymphoma: a report of two cases. Br J Dermatol. 2000;143:157–61.
48. Fink-Puches R, Wolf IH, Zalaudek I, et al. Treatment of primary cutaneous B-cell lymphoma with rituximab. J Am Acad Dermatol. 2005;52:847–53.
49. Bekkenk MW, Vermeer MH, Geerts ML, et al. Treatment of multifocal primary cutaneous B-cell lymphoma: a clinical follow-up study of 29 patients. J Clin Oncol. 1999;17:2471–8.
50. Rijlaarsdam JU, Toonstra J, Meijer CJLM, et al. Treatment of primary cutaneous B-cell lymphomas of follicle center cell origin: a clinical follow-up study of 55 patients treated with radiotherapy or polychemotherapy. J Clin Oncol. 1996;14:549–55.

Cutaneous T-Cell Lymphoma

Rein Willemze

Chapter contents

Introduction

The term cutaneous T-cell lymphoma (CTCL) describes a heterogeneous group of neoplasms of skin-homing T cells that show considerable variation in clinical presentation, histologic appearance, immunophenotype and prognosis. CTCLs represent approximately 75–80% of all primary cutaneous lymphomas, whereas primary cutaneous B-cell lymphomas (CBCLs) account for approximately 20–25%[1]. For many years, mycosis fungoides (MF) and Sézary syndrome (SS) were the only known types of CTCL. In the last decade, based on a combination of clinical, histologic and immunophenotypic criteria, new types of CTCL and CBCL have been defined and new classification schemes for the group of primary cutaneous lymphomas have been formulated[1-3]. A major advantage of these primary cutaneous lymphomas over malignant lymphomas arising at other sites is that they can be seen and can be biopsied easily, giving the dermatologist the unique opportunity to correlate the clinical appearance and clinical behavior with histologic, immunophenotypic and genetic aspects of these conditions. Hence, the dermatologist can play a key role in the diagnosis, the classification and the treatment of these diseases.

History

In 1806, a French physician, Jean Louis Alibert, was the first to describe a patient with MF. This case was designated *pian fungoïde* in his atlas, but, in 1835, was renamed *mycosis fungoïde*, because of the resemblance of some skin tumors to mushrooms. In 1870, Bazin described the natural progression from a non-specific premycotic phase to plaque lesions and finally to tumors, which probably represents one of the first descriptions of the 'multistep model' in the development of a malignancy. In 1885, Vidal & Brocq described MF d'emblée, in which patients presented with skin tumors not preceded by patches or plaques. It has now become clear that such cases represent another type of CTCL or a CBCL. The erythrodermic form of MF was described in 1892 by Besnier & Hallopeau. These early descriptions of the main clinical forms of MF were followed by descriptions of Sézary syndrome by Sézary & Bouvrain in 1938, pagetoid reticulosis by Woringer & Kolopp in 1939, and lymphomatoid papulosis (LyP) by Macaulay in 1968.

Thus, in the early 1970s, MF and some related conditions were the only types of cutaneous lymphoma that had been rather well described. Reports on cutaneous lymphomas other than MF/SS, commonly designated in the past as malignant reticulosis or reticulum cell sarcoma, were few. Moreover, they were firmly believed to represent skin manifestations of a systemic lymphoma, and treated as such.

The CTCL concept

In 1968, Lutzner & Jordan described the ultrastructural features of the circulating atypical cells in SS. Characteristically, the nuclei of these cells had deep and narrow indentations, giving them a cerebriform appearance. In 1971, similar cells were found in the skin and lymph nodes of patients with MF. In 1975, based on the observation that the neoplastic cells in MF, SS and related conditions had not only the same morphology but also a common T-cell phenotype, Edelson suggested the term CTCL for this group of diseases[4,5]. Within a short time, this term gained wide acceptance, particularly in the US. The introduction of the CTCL concept can be considered as a landmark in the history of this group of diseases. However, a major disadvantage has been that in many subsequent studies, distinction was no longer made between MF or SS versus other T-cell neoplasms, entities which may vary considerably in their clinical presentation and clinical behavior.

The concept of primary cutaneous lymphomas

At about the same time that the CTCL concept was introduced, several European groups started to classify cutaneous lymphomas according to the criteria of the Kiel classification, a classification system used by hematopathologists for the classification of nodal lymphomas. It was then determined that many types of CBCL and CTCL (other than classical MF and SS) can present in the skin without any evidence of extracutaneous disease at the time of diagnosis. It appeared that these primary cutaneous lymphomas often have a completely different clinical behavior and prognosis when compared to morphologically similar lymphomas arising in lymph nodes, and therefore require different types of treatment[1]. In addition, differences in the presence of specific translocations and in the expression of oncogenes, viral sequences or antigens (e.g. EBV), and adhesion receptors involved in tissue-related lymphocyte homing were found[1].

Such differences underscored that these primary cutaneous lymphomas represent a distinct group, and may explain, at least in part, their different clinical behavior. For instance, the observation that the neoplastic T cells in most CTCLs express cutaneous lymphocyte antigen (CLA) and the CC-chemokine receptor 4 (CCR4) indicates that they are the neoplastic counterparts of normal skin-homing T cells, and this explains why these CTCLs present in the skin. Perhaps most important, it appeared that different types of CTCL and CBCL with different clinical behaviors and different therapeutic requirements may have an identical histologic appearance. This implies that histologic features should always be combined with clinical and immunophenotypic data, before a definite diagnosis (classification) can be made.

In the last decade, such an approach resulted in the delineation of several new types of CTCL and CBCL, and it formed the basis of the European Organization for Research and Treatment of Cancer (EORTC) classification for primary cutaneous lymphomas.

EORTC, WHO and WHO–EORTC classification schemes

In recent years, awareness has grown that: (a) malignant lymphomas should be viewed as a group of disease entities, defined by a constellation of morphologic, immunologic, genetic and clinical criteria; (b) extranodal lymphomas are not identical to their nodal counterparts; and (c) the site of presentation is important. These novel insights resulted in new classification schemes, such as the EORTC

WHO–EORTC CLASSIFICATION FOR CUTANEOUS T-CELL LYMPHOMAS

WHO-EORTC Classification	Frequency (%)*	5-year survival rate (%)*
Indolent clinical behavior		
Mycosis fungoides	54	88
Mycosis fungoides variants and subtypes		
• Folliculotropic MF	6	80
• Pagetoid reticulosis	1	100
• Granulomatous slack skin	<1	100
Primary cutaneous CD30+ lymphoproliferative disorders		
• Primary cutaneous anaplastic large cell lymphoma	10	95
• Lymphomatoid papulosis	16	100
Subcutaneous panniculitis-like T-cell lymphoma§	1	82
Primary cutaneous CD4+ small/medium-sized pleomorphic T-cell lymphoma‡	3	75
Aggressive clinical behavior		
Sézary syndrome	4	24
Adult T-cell leukemia/lymphoma	NDA	NDA
Extranodal NK/T-cell lymphoma, nasal type	1	<5
Primary cutaneous aggressive epidermotropic CD8+ cytotoxic T-cell lymphoma‡	<1	18
Cutaneous γ/δ T-cell lymphoma‡	1	<5
Primary cutaneous peripheral T-cell lymphoma, unspecified†	3	16

*Data are based on 1476 CTCL patients registered by the Dutch and Austrian Cutaneous Lymphoma Groups[3].
†Primary cutaneous T-cell lymphoma, unspecified, excluding the three provisional entities indicated by ‡.
§α/β T-cell phenotype.

Table 120.1 WHO–EORTC classification for cutaneous T-cell lymphomas[3]. NDA, no data available.

classification[1] and the World Health Organization (WHO) classification[2]. In 2004, representatives from both classification systems reached an agreement on a new classification scheme for the group of cutaneous lymphomas: the WHO–EORTC classification[3]. The frequency and survival of patients with the different types of CTCL recognized in the WHO–EORTC classification are presented in Table 120.1. Following a description of practical guidelines for the diagnosis, classification and staging, relevant features of the different types of CTCL included in this classification are presented.

Practical Guidelines for Diagnosis, Classification and Staging of CTCL

Diagnosis

The first step in the evaluation of a patient suspected of having a CTCL is to decide if it represents a lymphoma or a benign condition. Skin biopsies – preferably deep punch biopsies 4–6 mm wide or an excisional or incisional biopsy from the most representative skin lesions – should be performed.

Since prior treatment with topical corticosteroids or PUVA may profoundly change the original histology, biopsies from untreated skin lesions are preferred. Even if an adequate biopsy specimen is obtained, a definite diagnosis is not always possible. First, several types of CTCL, such as MF, are often preceded for years by skin lesions that are neither clinically nor histologically diagnostic. The gradual progression from this prediagnostic phase to overt lymphoma explains why it has always

been so difficult to reach a consensus on the minimal histologic criteria needed for an unequivocal diagnosis of MF[6]. Because of the indolent clinical behavior of the disease in such patients, a conservative approach is justified. In most cases, repeated biopsies, when appropriate, will ultimately result in the correct diagnosis.

Secondly, atypical T-cell infiltrates are found not only in CTCL, but also in reactive conditions, for example, lymphomatoid drug eruptions (pseudo-T-cell lymphomas)[7]. Therefore, a definite diagnosis should always be based on a combination of clinical, histologic and, in most cases, immunophenotypic criteria, and it may be supplemented with the results of gene rearrangement analysis.

Immunophenotyping

Immunohistochemical studies on paraffin or frozen sections using antibodies reactive with cell surface or cytoplasmic molecules are extremely important in the diagnosis and classification of cutaneous lymphomas. Using a panel of such antibodies, distinction can be made between neoplasms of T-cell, B-cell, NK-cell and myeloid or monocytic origin. Within the group of CTCLs, such studies have contributed to the delineation of new subtypes and provided important diagnostic and prognostic criteria (see Table 120.1).

With respect to the diagnosis of CTCL, demonstration of an aberrant phenotype, i.e. loss of one or more T-cell-associated antigens (such as CD2, CD3, CD4 or CD5) by the neoplastic T cells, can be considered as an important additional criterion in establishing a definite diagnosis of CTCL[8]. However, loss of CD7 expression, which may be caused by chronic T-cell stimulation, and is commonly observed in benign dermatoses as well, is not a reliable marker[9]. Recently, new antibodies have become available, which, in combination with antigen retrieval techniques, now also allow demonstration of 'marker loss' on paraffin sections.

T-cell receptor gene rearrangement analysis

In the last decade, T-cell receptor (TCR) gene rearrangement analysis, either by Southern blot analysis or by more sensitive PCR-based techniques, has increasingly been used in the diagnosis and staging of malignant lymphomas[10]. However, caution is warranted in interpreting the results of such analyses. Clonal T-cell populations have been detected not only in skin lesions, lymph nodes and peripheral blood of patients with CTCL, and in cases of chronic dermatitis preceding MF ('clonal dermatitis'), but also in skin lesions of patients with apparently benign conditions, such as pityriasis lichenoides et varioliformis acuta, lichen planus, chronic pigmented purpura, lichen sclerosus and some pseudolymphomas[10–12].

Therefore, demonstration of clonal T-cell populations cannot be used as an absolute criterion of malignancy, but should always be considered in conjunction with clinical and histologic features, which together remain the 'gold standard'. If the clinical and histologic findings are not consistent, and an aberrant phenotype is not detected, a definite diagnosis of CTCL should not be made.

Classification

Once a diagnosis of CTCL has been made, the type of CTCL should be determined. As noted before, the histologic diagnosis is not the final diagnosis, which means that CTCL cannot be classified on the basis of histologic criteria alone. For instance, in the case of a skin biopsy showing a dermal infiltrate which is composed predominantly of CD30+ large anaplastic or pleomorphic T cells, the *histologic diagnosis* will be (CD30+) anaplastic large cell lymphoma (ALCL). However, depending on the clinical presentation, the *definite diagnosis* may be a primary cutaneous ALCL, skin involvement from a systemic ALCL, MF with transformation into a CD30+ diffuse large T-cell lymphoma, or LyP (in cases of recurrent self-healing papules). Obviously, each of these conditions requires a different approach in terms of staging and treatment.

In Table 120.2, the differential diagnosis of four histologic categories has been elaborated. This histologic subdivision into epidermotropic CTCL, CTCL with diffuse pleomorphic infiltrates, CD30+ CTCL, and subcutaneous CTCL is neither complete nor meant as an alternative classification. It is only presented as an illustration of how histology should be combined with clinical and immunophenotypic data to arrive at a definite diagnosis.

DIFFERENTIAL DIAGNOSIS OF COMMON HISTOLOGIC PATTERNS IN CTCL

Histologic category	Differential diagnosis	Diagnostic criteria/clues
Epidermotropic CTCL (simulating or consistent with plaque stage MF)	Mycosis fungoides (MF)	• Characteristic patches and plaques • Most atypical cells within the epidermis (basal layer)
	Pagetoid reticulosis	• Solitary plaque, commonly on distal extremities • Neoplastic cells confined to an often acanthotic epidermis • Often CD8+ phenotype; CD30 expression common
	Lymphomatoid papulosis (LyP), type B	• Recurrent, self-healing papular eruption • Sometimes extension of infiltrate into lower dermis • In some cases admixture with large atypical cells as in type A LyP (mixed type A and B)
	Aggressive epidermotropic CD8+	• Infiltrated plaques, but often eruptive nodules and tumors with ulceration • Intraepidermal accumulation of medium-sized pleomorphic T cells or small blast cells; no typical cerebriform appearance • Phenotype: CD8+, TIA-1+, granzyme B+, CD45RA+, CD7−/+
	Sézary syndrome	• Often more monotonous infiltrate histologically • Erythroderma • Peripheral blood involvement
	Adult T-cell leukemia/lymphoma	• Sometimes clinically and histologically identical to MF • Check HTLV-1 status in patients from endemic areas
CTCL with diffuse pleomorphic infiltrates (CD30−) (simulation or consistent with tumor stage MF; few CD30+ tumor cells may be present)	Tumor stage MF	• Concurrent patches and plaques • Variable numbers of small, medium-sized and/or large cerebriform T-cells and/or blast cells and variable admixture with inflammatory cells
	Peripheral T-cell lymphoma, unspecified	• Histologically, often indistinguishable from MF with blastic transformation • No prior or concurrent patches and plaques
	CD4+ small/medium-sized pleomorphic CTCL	• Less than 30% large neoplastic T cells • Histologically, sometimes indistinguishable from tumor stage MF • No prior or concurrent patches and plaques
	Pseudo-T-cell lymphoma	• Presentation with solitary plaque or tumor (2–3 cm) • Scattered medium-sized to large pleomorphic T cells (no clusters) • Many admixed CD8+ T cells, B cells and histiocytes • No aberrant phenotype ('marker loss') • No clonal T-cell population
CD30-positive CTCL	Lymphomatoid papulosis, type A/C	• Recurrent self-healing papules and nodules • Histologic spectrum (from typical LyP to C-ALCL)
	Primary cutaneous anaplastic large cell lymphoma (C-ALCL)	• Generally, solitary or localized nodules or tumors • No evidence of prior or concurrent MF, LyP or another type of CTCL • No extracutaneous disease (staging negative) • Histologic spectrum (from typical C-ALCL to LyP) • Phenotype: CLA+, EMA−, ALK−
	Systemic ALCL with secondary skin involvement	• Prior or concurrent extracutaneous involvement (exception: involvement of one regional lymph node basin) • Often generalized skin lesions • Phenotype: CLA−, EMA+, ALK+ (mainly in pediatric subgroup)
	MF with blastic transformation	• Histologically, an admixture with typical cerebriform cells, but sometimes indistinguishable from C-ALCL • Prior or concurrent patches and plaques
CTCL with subcutaneous involvement	Subcutaneous panniculitis-like T-cell lymphoma	• Infiltrates confined to subcutis • Characteristic rimming of individual fat cells by neoplastic T cells • Deeply seated nodules and plaques, mainly involving the legs and trunk • Characteristic CD3+, CD4−, CD8+, CD56−, βF1+ T-cell phenotype
	Other types of CTCL	• Subcutaneous infiltrates represent extension from dermal infiltrates • For specific features: see text

Table 120.2 Differential diagnosis of common histologic patterns in cutaneous T-cell lymphoma (CTCL). ALK, anaplastic lymphoma kinase; CLA, cutaneous lymphocyte antigen; C-ALCL, cutaneous anaplastic large cell lymphoma; EMA, epithelial membrane antigen; TIA, T-cell restricted intracellular antigen; βF1, positivity reflects α/β T-cell origin.

Practical guidelines

For those not regularly involved in the diagnosis and classification of CTCL and perhaps overwhelmed by the many new types of CTCL introduced within recent years, a stepwise approach, as presented in Figure 120.1, may serve as a practical guide[13].

Step one: Based on a combination of clinical, histologic and immunophenotypic criteria, distinction is first made between classical MF, MF variants and SS on the one hand versus CTCL other than these conditions on the other. The rationale for this first step is that dermatologists are familiar with the former set of conditions, which comprise approximately 65% of CTCLs, and these lymphomas require a different clinical approach in terms of staging and therapy compared to the other forms of CTCL. Cases of unequivocal LyP can be included in this first step.

Step two: The second category to be considered is the group of primary cutaneous CD30+ lymphoproliferative disorders. It implies that evaluation of skin biopsies from patients with (suspected) CTCL should always include staining for CD30. This group includes cases of cutaneous ALCL (C-ALCL) and LyP, which together represent the second most common group of CTCL (see Table 120.1). Patients within this spectrum of disease generally have an excellent prognosis, and, in most instances, can be easily managed by dermatologists.

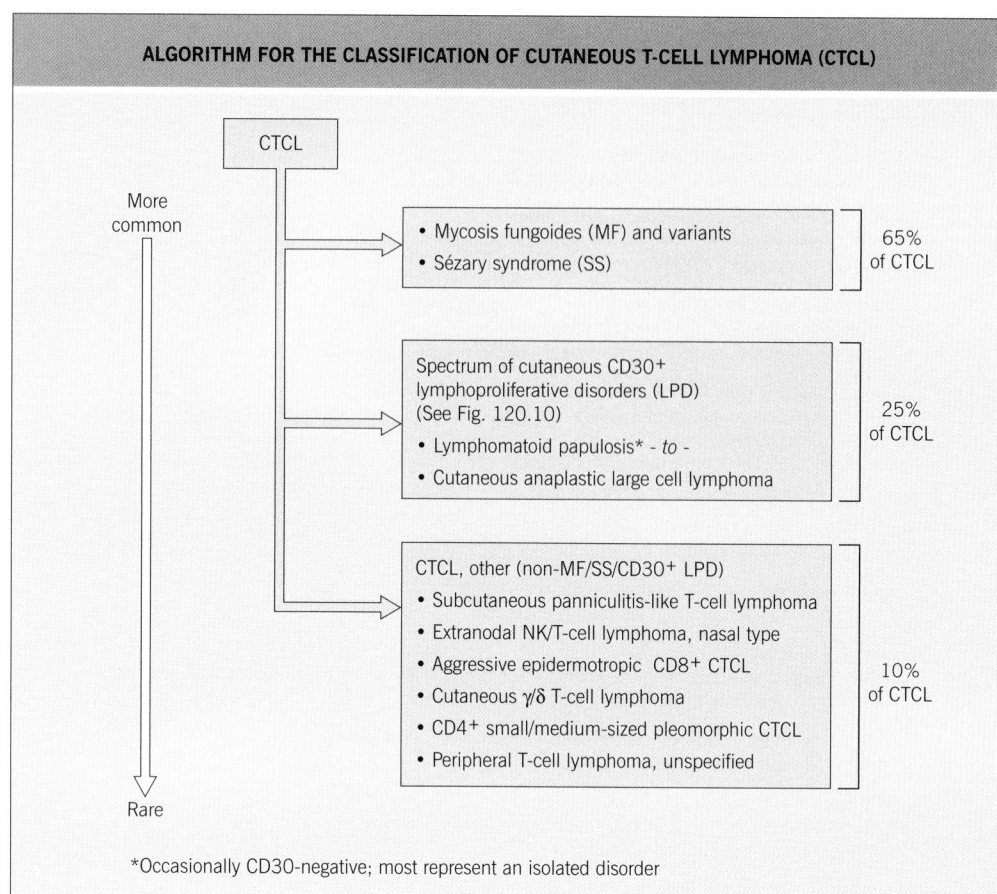

ALGORITHM FOR THE CLASSIFICATION OF CUTANEOUS T-CELL LYMPHOMA (CTCL)

*Occasionally CD30-negative; most represent an isolated disorder

Fig. 120.1 Algorithm for the classification of cutaneous T-cell lymphoma (CTCL). Adapted from Willemze R, Beljaards RC, Meijer CJLM. Classification of primary cutaneous T-cell lymphoma. Histopathology. 1994;24:405–15.

Step three: With the first two steps, approximately 90% of CTCLs will have been classified correctly. The remaining 10% represents rare types of CTCL, including subcutaneous panniculitis-like T-cell lymphoma (SPTL), extranodal NK/T-cell lymphoma, nasal type, and the broad group of primary cutaneous peripheral T-cell lymphoma, unspecified. From this latter group, aggressive epidermotropic CD8+ cytotoxic T-cell lymphoma, cutaneous γ/δ T-cell lymphoma and primary cutaneous CD4+ small/medium-sized pleomorphic T-cell lymphoma have been separated out as provisional entities[3]. In the WHO–EORTC classification scheme, the term peripheral T-cell lymphoma, unspecified, is maintained for remaining cases that do not fit into one of these three provisional entity categories. In the EORTC classification, all these lymphomas, except for SPTL, were classified as either primary cutaneous CD30− large T-cell lymphoma or primary cutaneous CD30− small/medium-sized pleomorphic T-cell lymphoma[1].

Apart from SPTL and primary cutaneous CD4+ small/medium-sized pleomorphic T-cell lymphomas (see Table 120.1), lymphomas included in this third category have an aggressive clinical course, and should be treated by, or in close collaboration with, a hemato-oncologist. It should be emphasized that distinction between these different types of aggressive CTCLs is sometimes very difficult, because of overlapping clinicopathologic features and highly aberrant phenotypes. Distinction between primary and secondary cutaneous involvement is less important than in other types of cutaneous lymphoma. Patients presenting with only skin lesions generally develop extracutaneous disease within a short period of time and have a poor prognosis as well.

Staging

Apart from CTCL, a term preferably used only for *primary* CTCL, systemic T-cell lymphomas frequently present or relapse in the skin. Adequate staging procedures are required to differentiate between CTCL and these systemic lymphomas secondarily involving the skin. The extent of staging procedures is dependent on the type of (suspected) CTCL, and, in the case of classical MF, on the clinical stage of the disease. In cases of early patch/plaque stage MF, and unequivocal cases of LyP and probably pagetoid reticulosis as well, staging procedures are generally not worthwhile. In cases of suspected SS, adequate staging with special emphasis on assessment of peripheral blood involvement by cytology, immunophenotyping and TCR gene rearrangement analysis is essential. In all other types of CTCL, routine hematologic staging, including complete and differential blood cell counts, a blood chemistry panel, CT scans of the chest and abdomen, and bone marrow biopsy, is required.

MYCOSIS FUNGOIDES

Definition

Mycosis fungoides (MF) represents the most common type of CTCL and accounts for approximately 50% of all primary cutaneous lymphomas (see Table 120.1). The term MF should be restricted to the classical 'Alibert–Bazin' type characterized by the typical evolution of patches, plaques and tumors, or for clinicopathologic variants showing a similar clinical course.

Epidemiology

MF is a rare disorder, with an incidence of about 0.3 per 100 000 inhabitants per year[14]. MF typically affects older adults (median age at diagnosis: 55–60 years), but may occur in children and adolescents as well. Men are affected more often than women, with a male-to-female ratio of 1.6–2.0:1.

Pathogenesis

The etiology and the pathogenetic mechanisms involved in the development and stepwise progression of MF are largely unknown. Genetic, environmental and immunologic factors have all been considered.

Genetic factors

Lymphomagenesis is considered to be a multifactorial process, in which a stepwise accumulation of genetic abnormalities may result in clonal proliferation, malignant transformation and, ultimately, progressive and widely disseminated disease. Although the successive clinical steps of tumor progression were described more than a century ago, the molecular events underlying the different steps of tumor progression have not been identified. Many genetic abnormalities have been reported in patients with MF, but a consistent pattern has not emerged[15]. Chromosomal loss at 10q and genetic alterations in *p53* and *CDKN2A* genes have been reported in the advanced, but not in the early, stages of MF[16,17].

Environmental factors

Persistent antigenic stimulation has been demonstrated to play a crucial role in the development of various malignant lymphomas, including MALT lymphomas (*Helicobacter pylori* infection), CBCL (*Borrelia burgdorferi* infection) and enteropathy-type T-cell lymphoma (celiac disease). Also in MF, persistent antigenic stimulation has been proposed as an initial event, but the nature of the antigen(s) involved is unknown. Large case–control studies do not support a relationship between industrial or environmental exposure and the development of MF[14]. Whereas the etiologic role of human T-cell leukemia virus 1 (HTLV-1) in adult T-cell leukemia/lymphoma, and of EBV in extranodal NK/T-cell lymphoma, nasal type has been firmly established, conclusive evidence for a primary etiologic role of these viruses in MF is lacking[18].

Immunologic factors

Recent studies suggest that CD8+ cytotoxic T cells (CTL) play a crucial role in the antitumor response in MF. A relationship between high percentages of CD8+ CTL in the dermal infiltrates and a better survival has been described[19,20]. These CD8+ T cells exert their antitumor effect both by a direct cytotoxic effect and by the production of cytokines, particularly interferon (IFN)-γ. They can mediate tumor cell lysis by exocytosis of cytotoxic granules containing perforin, granzymes and T-cell-restricted intracellular antigen (TIA-1), and by expression of Fas ligand (FasL), which interacts with Fas (CD95; APO-1) on the neoplastic T cells[20]. Both pathways ultimately lead to activation of caspase 3 and tumor cell death via apoptosis. Loss of Fas expression or function by the neoplastic T cells is one of the many mechanisms by which tumor cells can evade an effective antitumor response[21].

Recent studies suggest that the neoplastic T cells in Sézary syndrome (SS) and tumor stage MF are derived from CD4+ T cells with a Th2 cytokine profile (production of IL-4, IL-5 and IL-10), whereas the cytotoxic T cells are the main producers of IFN-γ, which plays an important role in augmenting T-cell- and NK-cell-mediated killing. In accordance with this concept, a gradual shift from a predominantly type 1 cytokine profile in MF plaques to a predominantly type 2 cytokine profile in MF tumors has been suggested[22]. Increased levels of Th2 cytokines may impair the Th1 cell-mediated antitumor response and contribute to the immunosuppression seen in patients with advanced MF.

Clinical features

Characteristically, patients with classical MF progress from patch stage to plaque stage and finally to tumor stage disease, and they have a protracted clinical course over years or even decades. Before a definite diagnosis is made, patients generally have many years of non-specific eczematous or psoriasiform skin lesions and non-diagnostic biopsies. The median duration from onset of skin lesions to the diagnosis of MF is 4–6 years, but may vary from several months to more than five decades[23,24].

Early patch stage MF is characterized by the presence of variably sized erythematous, finely scaling lesions, which may be mildly pruritic (Fig. 120.2A). These early lesions may show variable degrees of atrophy, and a poikilodermatous variant consisting of patches with mottled hyper- and hypopigmentation, atrophy and telangiectasia has been described (formerly called poikiloderma vasculare atrophicans or PVA). The initial skin lesions have a predilection for the buttocks and other covered sites of the trunk and limbs. With progression, more infiltrated reddish-brown, scaling plaques may develop, which gradually enlarge, and which may have an annular, polycyclic or typical horseshoe-shaped configuration (Fig. 120.3A). It should be stressed that many patients never progress beyond the plaque stage of the disease. However, a number of patients may develop nodules or tumors. These patients with tumor stage MF characteristically show a combination of patches, plaques and tumors (Fig. 120.4A); the latter often show ulceration.

If only skin tumors are present without preceding or concurrent patches or plaques, a diagnosis of MF is highly unlikely and another type of CTCL should be considered. The risk of developing extracutaneous disease correlates with the extent and type of skin lesions. It is exceedingly rare in patients with limited patch/plaque stage disease, relatively uncommon in patients with generalized plaques, and most likely in patients with skin tumors or erythroderma[23,24]. Extracutaneous dissemination almost without exception first involves the regional lymph nodes draining areas of extensive skin involvement. Visceral involvement may develop subsequently, and may involve any organ. The bone marrow is only rarely involved.

Pathology

Early patch lesions in MF show superficial band-like or lichenoid infiltrates, mainly composed of lymphocytes. Atypical lymphocytes with small to medium-sized, highly convoluted (cerebriform) and sometimes hyperchromatic nuclei are few, and they are mostly confined to the epidermis (epidermotropism). These lymphocytes characteristically colonize the basal layer of the epidermis as single cells surrounded by vacuolated halos, often in a linear configuration (Fig. 120.2B)[25]. In typical plaques epidermotropism is generally more pronounced (Fig. 120.3B). The presence of intraepidermal nests of atypical cells (Pautrier's microabscesses) is a highly characteristic feature, but is observed in only a minority of cases. The epidermis may

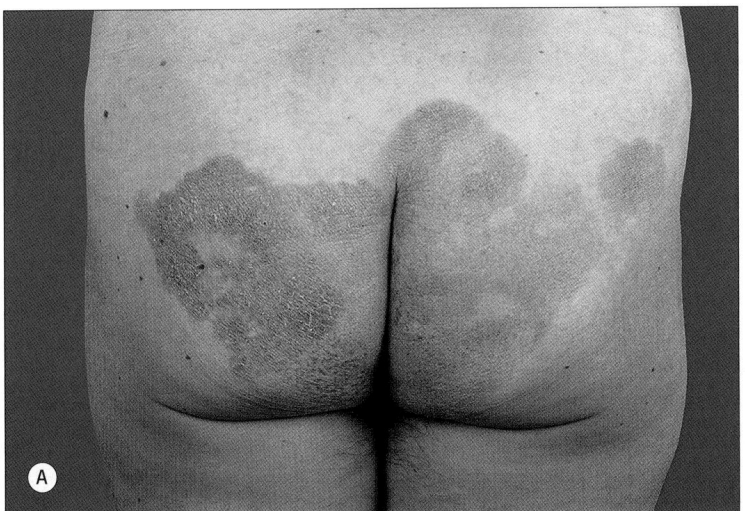

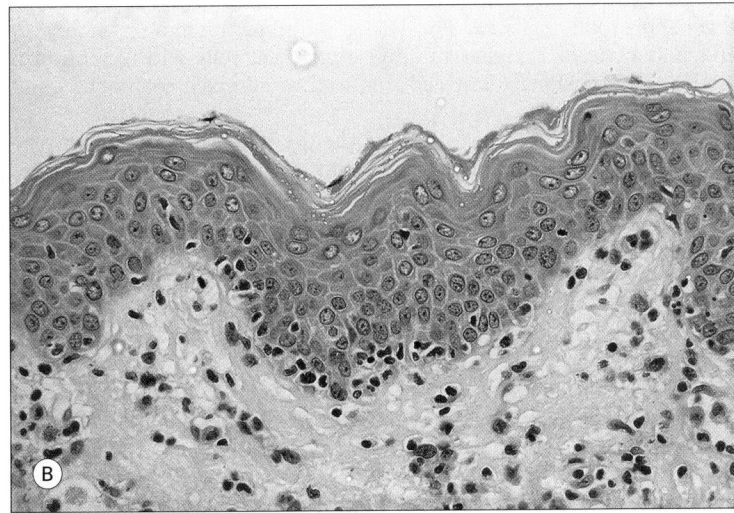

Fig. 120.2 Mycosis fungoides, limited patch/plaque stage disease (stage 1A). A Patches on the buttocks, involving less than 10% of the skin surface. **B** Atypical lymphocytes in a typical linear configuration along the epidermal basal layer.

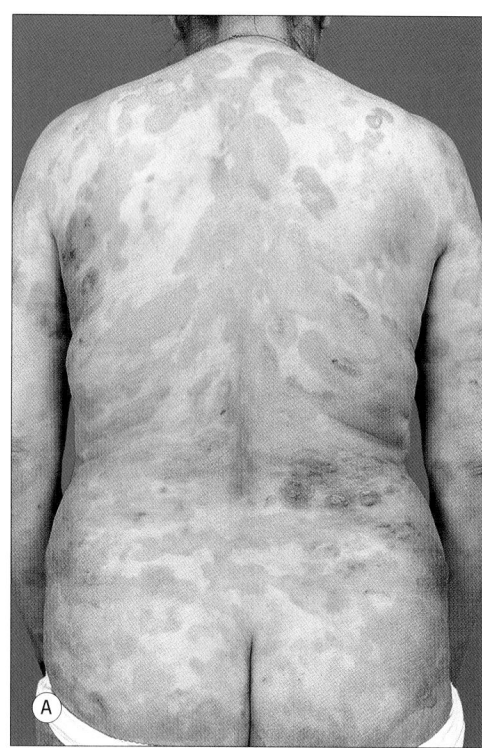

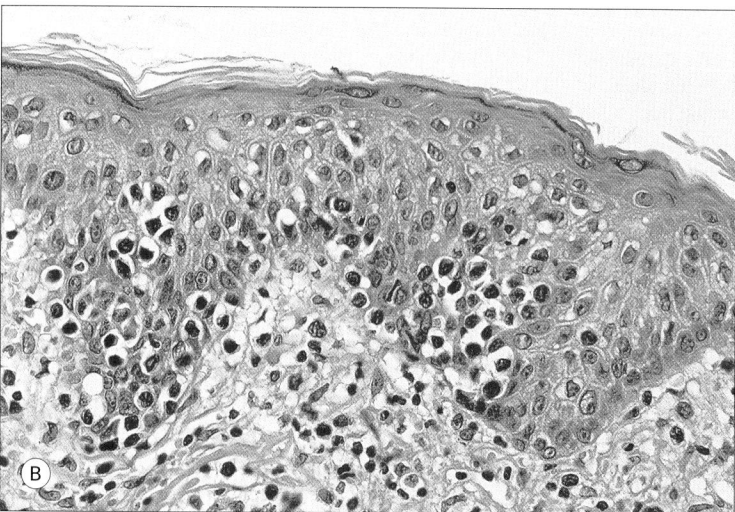

Fig. 120.3 Mycosis fungoides, generalized patch/plaque stage disease (stage 1B). A Extensive patches and plaques involving more than 10% of the skin surface. **B** Pronounced epidermotropism with the formation of small nests of atypical cells (Pautrier's microabscesses).

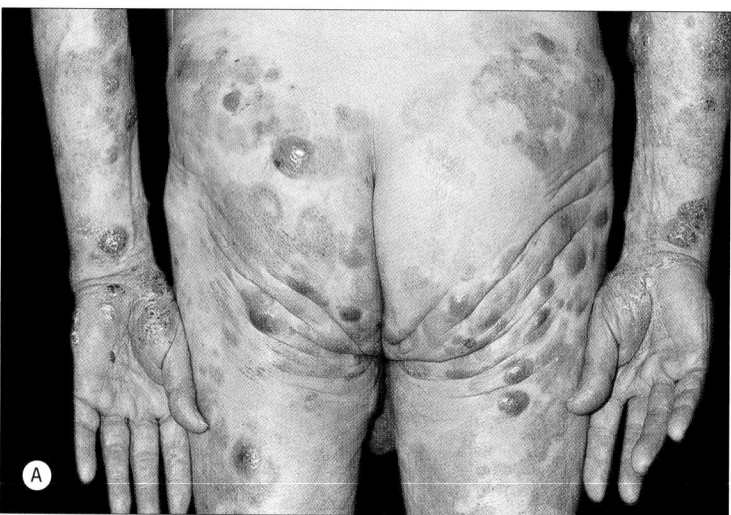

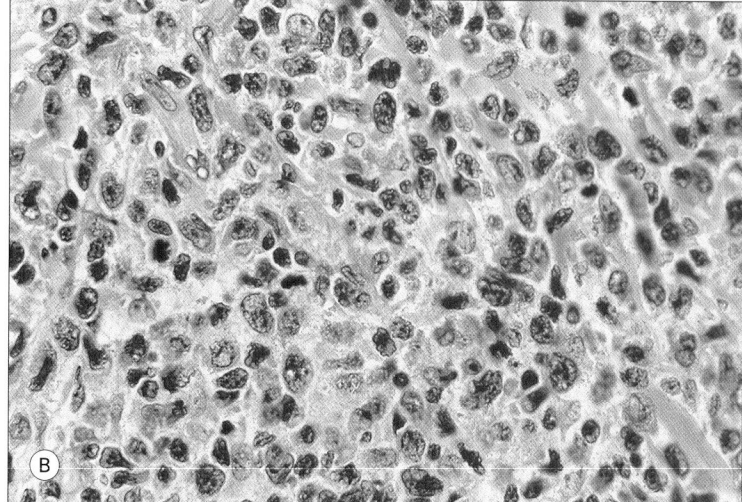

Fig. 120.4 Mycosis fungoides, tumor stage. A Multiple skin tumors in combination with typical patches and plaques. **B** Diffuse dermal infiltrate of medium-sized to large neoplastic T cells.

show acanthosis and elongated psoriasiform rete ridges, but spongiosis is generally mild or absent. The dermal infiltrates are more pronounced, and may contain a higher number of atypical cells with cerebriform nuclei and occasional blast cells, as well as admixed eosinophils and plasma cells.

With progression to tumor stage, the dermal infiltrates can involve the entire dermis and extend into the subcutaneous tissue. Epidermotropism may no longer be present. The tumor cells increase in number and size, showing variable proportions of small, medium-sized or large cells with cerebriform nuclei, blast cells with prominent nuclei, and intermediate forms (Fig. 120.4B). Transformation to a CD30[−] or CD30[+] diffuse large T-cell lymphoma may occur, and this is often associated with a poor prognosis[26].

Immunophenotype

The neoplastic cells in MF have a mature CD3[+], CD4[+], CD45RO[+], CD8[−] memory T-cell phenotype. In rare cases of otherwise classical MF, a CD3[+], CD4[−], CD8[+] mature T-cell phenotype may be seen. Immunophenotyping may demonstrate an aberrant phenotype in plaque or tumor stage MF, but rarely in early patch lesions, and is therefore of little help in early diagnosis[8].

Differential diagnosis

Regarding the differential diagnosis of MF, three categories should be considered. The first category contains a diverse group of benign dermatoses, which early MF may resemble clinically, and it includes several types of eczema, psoriasis, superficial fungal infections, and drug reactions. These specific diagnoses can generally be excluded by histologic and other standard dermatologic examinations. This category may also include patients with *large plaque parapsoriasis* (parapsoriasis en plaque) who show slightly scaly, sometimes atrophic, erythematous patches or plaques which are commonly located on the trunk and buttocks (see Ch. 10). Whereas large plaque parapsoriasis cannot be distinguished clinically from early patch or plaque stage MF, the histologic features are often not consistent with MF. Long-term follow-up studies have documented progression of large plaque parapsoriasis to overt MF in approximately 10% of cases[27]. One prevailing opinion is that large plaque parapsoriasis should be considered a form of MF, rather than a potential precursor of MF, but the author feels there is no consensus. There is even less consensus about whether small plaque parapsoriasis represents MF.

A second category includes several benign conditions with histologic features highly suggestive of MF. Examples of these are lymphomatoid contact dermatitis, lymphomatoid drug reactions and actinic reticuloid. Apart from subtle histologic differences (e.g. the predominance of atypical T cells in the dermal infiltrate rather than in the epidermis), careful evaluation of the clinical features, which are generally not consistent with MF, often results in a correct diagnosis[7].

The third category includes other types of (epidermotropic) CTCL, which may resemble MF histologically. Diagnostic features of these entities are presented in Table 120.2.

Staging systems and staging procedures

In 1979 the Mycosis Fungoides Cooperative Group developed a staging system for CTCL based on the TNM (tumor-node-metastasis) classification scheme[28]. This staging system has been used for many decades, but proved not particularly helpful for CTCL other than MF and SS. Recently, revisions of the original TNMB and clinical staging system have been published (Tables 120.3 & 120.4)[28a]. This revised classification and staging system pertains specifically to MF and SS. In addition, a separate staging system for primary cutaneous (T-cell) lymphomas other than MF and SS has recently been proposed[29].

Evaluation of patients suspected of having MF should include a thorough physical examination with special attention to the type and extent of skin lesions and the presence of palpable lymph nodes, as well as skin biopsies, complete blood counts and serum chemistries. Enlarged lymph nodes should be biopsied. Histologically, a distinction can be made between lymph nodes showing dermatopathic lymph-adenopathy without involvement by MF (category I), dermatopathic lymphadenopathy with early MF involvement (category II), and lymph nodes showing partial or complete effacement of the normal lymph node architecture by neoplastic T cells (category III)[2]. The prognostic significance of such a subdivision has been well established.

In patients with stage IA–B disease, no further examinations are indicated. CT scans of the abdomen and chest are useful in patients in whom extracutaneous disease may be suspected, but they have not been shown to be useful on a routine basis. Examination of other organs, including bone marrow, should only be performed if clinically indicated. TCR gene rearrangement analysis of the peripheral blood has shown conflicting results, depending on the sensitivity of the technique employed, and is not advised as a standard diagnostic procedure.

Treatment

The choice of an initial treatment in MF depends upon the stage of the disease and the general condition and age of the patient[22,30]. In general, therapies are effective in controlling disease, but they have not been shown to prolong life. Three different types of treatment can be considered: skin-targeted therapies (including topical application of corticosteroids or cytotoxic agents, phototherapy and radiotherapy) systemic chemotherapy, and biological response modifiers. Combination therapies, which may have synergistic effects and may reduce the toxicity of the single agents, are increasingly being used.

It should be kept in mind that, unlike with other cancers, the choice of treatment in MF is not based on the results of controlled clinical trials. Prospective randomized trials that compare therapies have rarely been performed in MF, which may relate to the rarity of the disease, and this is further impeded by the lack of a staging system which clearly defines homogeneous patient groups.

Following the traditional dermatologic approach, skin-directed therapies are preferred in the early stages of MF, whereas systemic chemotherapy is used in the advanced stages with nodal or visceral involvement (Table 120.5). In a randomized study it was demonstrated that in the early stages of CTCL, systemic multiagent chemotherapy as

TNMB CLASSIFICATION OF MYCOSIS FUNGOIDES AND SÉZARY SYNDROME

T (skin)

T_1	Limited patch/plaque (involving <10% of total skin surface)
T_2	Generalized patch/plaque (involving ≥10% of total skin surface)
T_3	Tumor(s)
T_4	Erythroderma

N (lymph node)

N_0	No enlarged lymph nodes
N_1	Enlarged lymph nodes, histologically uninvolved
N_2	Enlarged lymph nodes, histologically involved (nodal architecture uneffaced)
N_3	Enlarged lymph nodes, histologically involved (nodal architecture (partially) effaced)

M (viscera)

M_0	No visceral involvement
M_1	Visceral involvement

B (blood)

B_0	No circulating atypical (Sézary) cells (or <5% of lymphocytes)
B_1	Low blood tumor burden (≥5% of lymphocytes are Sézary cells, but not B_2)
B_2	High blood tumor burden (≥1000/µL Sézary cells + positive clone)

Table 120.3 TNMB classification of mycosis fungoides and Sézary syndrome.

CLINICAL STAGING SYSTEM FOR MYCOSIS FUNGOIDES AND SÉZARY SYNDROME

Clinical stage				
IA	T_1	N_0	M_0	B_{0-1}
IB	T_2	N_0	M_0	B_{0-1}
IIA	T_{1-2}	N_{1-2}	M_0	B_{0-1}
IIB	T_3	N_{0-2}	M_0	B_{0-1}
III	T_4	N_{0-2}	M_0	B_{0-1}
IVA_1	T_{1-4}	N_{0-2}	M_0	B_2
IVA_2	T_{1-4}	N_3	M_0	B_{0-2}
IVB	T_{1-4}	N_{0-3}	M_1	B_{0-2}

Table 120.4 Clinical staging system for mycosis fungoides and Sézary syndrome.

TREATMENT OF MYCOSIS FUNGOIDES

Premycotic phase

- Topical corticosteroids; UVB
- If not effective, PUVA

Stage IA–IIA (patches/plaques)

- PUVA; HN2; topical BCNU
- UVB (if only patches)
- Topical corticosteroids or topical bexarotene (if only limited patches/thin plaques)
- RT (if single lesion)
- TSEB (if generalized thick plaques)

Stage IIB (skin tumors)

- PUVA or HN2 + RT (if only a few tumors)
- TSEB (followed by skin-targeted therapies)
- Relapse: PUVA + IFN-α; PUVA + retinoids (acitretin; oral bexarotene*); denileukin diftitox*
- Add RT (if persistent tumors); consider second TSEB (10–20 Gy)

Stage III (erythroderma)

- ECP; if not effective, add IFN-α
- Low-dose chlorambucil and prednisone; low-dose methotrexate
- Add skin-targeted therapies (PUVA; HN2; RT), if necessary
- Oral bexarotene*

Stage IV (nodal, visceral involvement)

- Multiagent chemotherapy (e.g. CHOP)
- Biological response modifiers (denileukin diftitox*; IL-12*, etc.)
- Add skin-targeted therapies (PUVA; HN2), if necessary

Efficacy compared to traditional treatments yet to be determined.

Table 120.5 Treatment of mycosis fungoides. ECP, extracorporeal photopheresis; HN2, topical nitrogen mustard; IFN, interferon; RT, local radiotherapy; TSEB, total skin electron beam.

initial therapy did not result in improved survival as compared to traditional treatment with skin-targeted therapies, and the former was associated with considerable morbidity[31]. The efficacy of the skin-targeted therapies in MF is explained by the preferential localization of the neoplastic skin-homing T cells to the epidermis and superficial dermis.

Skin-targeted therapies

Topical corticosteroids

In many MF patients with only patches and thin plaques, application of topical corticosteroids is effective in controlling disease activity. In patients with limited patch/plaque stage disease (mainly patches), complete remissions in up to 60% of patients have been reported[32]. In the more advanced stages, they continue to be an important adjuvant therapy.

Topical chemotherapy

Topical application of the chemotherapeutic agents mechlorethamine (nitrogen mustard) and carmustine (BCNU) has proven to be an effective treatment for early stage MF. Nitrogen mustard, either dissolved in water or used as an ointment-based preparation, results in complete remissions in approximately 60–80% of patients with stage IA–B disease[33]. Most patients with early MF remain clear on maintenance therapy. Side effects include skin irritation, allergic contact dermatitis and an increased risk for the development of skin cancer related to long-term use. The complete remission rate with BCNU is similar to that of nitrogen mustard[34]. Side effects of BCNU include telangiectasia and myelosuppression, which requires careful monitoring of the complete blood count.

Radiotherapy

Total skin electron beam irradiation (TSEB) with an energy of 4–6 MeV is a highly effective treatment in patients with skin-limited MF (see Ch. 139)[23,35]. The total dose is generally 36 Gy administered in fractions of 1.5–2 Gy over an 8–10-week period. TSEB is most effective in patients with stage IA–B disease, leading to complete response rates of more than 80%. However, in most centers, such patients are treated with PUVA or topical chemotherapy. TSEB is particularly useful in patients with tumor stage MF, where complete response rates of approximately 40% have been reported. Side effects are generally mild, and include erythema, scaling, and temporary loss of hair, nails and sweat gland function.

Local radiotherapy with X-ray or preferably electron beam may be considered for single tumors in patients with plaque stage disease, either in combination with other modalities (e.g. PUVA) as an alternative for TSEB, or for new tumors following TSEB. A dose of 10–20 Gy suffices. In patients with unilesional MF, local radiotherapy may be curative.

Phototherapy

Several types of phototherapy can be used in the treatment of MF (see Ch. 134). These include UVA irradiation following photosensitization with 8-methoxypsoralen (PUVA therapy), broadband and narrowband UVB therapy, and, more recently, UVA1 therapy. Extracorporeal photopheresis (ECP) may be effective in patients with erythrodermic MF (see the section on Sézary syndrome).

PUVA treatment has become a standard therapy for the early stages of MF[36]. In patients with stage IA–IIA disease, complete response rates of 80–90% have been reported. In many centers, maintenance PUVA therapy (every 2 to 4 weeks) is given to prolong remission. Although sustained complete remissions have been reported, most patients will relapse after cessation of PUVA therapy or during maintenance treatment. Recurrent or persistent lesions particularly favor UV-shielded areas, such as the inner thighs and the gluteal cleft. In tumor stage MF, PUVA therapy alone is unlikely to result in complete responses, but favorable results may be achieved when combined with radiotherapy or biological response modifiers.

In patients with only patches, broadband UVB therapy has been reported as a safe and effective alternative, with complete response rates of up to 75%[37]. More recent studies reported favorable results with narrowband UVB (311 nm) and UVA1 therapy in the early stages of MF, but it remains to be determined how these new therapies compare to the established forms of phototherapy[38].

Systemic chemotherapy

Systemic multiagent chemotherapy should only be used in patients with unequivocal lymph node or visceral involvement, or in patients with progressive skin tumors, which cannot be controlled with skin-targeted therapies. In many centers, the standard treatment in such cases is the administration of six cycles of CHOP. CHOP stands for cyclophosphamide, hydroxydaunomycin (doxorubicin), Oncovin® (vincristine) and prednisone. With this and other combination regimens, high response rates can be achieved for extracutaneous disease, but the responses are generally short-lived. Moreover, concurrent patches and plaques are often less responsive, and may require additional treatment with PUVA or topical nitrogen mustard. In recent years, purine analogues (2-deoxycoformycin, fludarabine and 2-chlorodeoxyadenosine), gemcitabine and liposomal doxorubicin have demonstrated activity in patients with advanced MF, but controlled studies are still lacking[39].

Experience with autologous and allogeneic bone marrow transplantation in the management of MF is limited[39].

Biological response modifiers

Biological response modifiers are aimed at potentiating the host's immune response to the neoplastic T cells. This category includes cytokines, retinoids, immunotoxins and vaccination therapy. Current evidence suggests that biological response modifiers are most effective when combined with (or preceded by) traditional therapies aimed at tumor cell eradication.

Interferons

The most commonly used biological response modifier is IFN-α. In most centers, IFN-α is administered subcutaneously in doses of 3 to 9 million units three times a week. Side effects are generally mild and reversible, and include flu-like symptoms, hair loss, nausea, depression and bone marrow suppression. The overall response rate of IFN-α, when used as a single agent, is approximately 50%, with 17% representing complete remissions[40]. The combination of PUVA and IFN-α appears to produce higher response rates than PUVA alone, and may also be considered in patients with early tumor stage disease when PUVA therapy alone is insufficient. The suggestion that maintenance treatment with low-dose IFN-α following PUVA therapy may prolong complete remissions needs to be confirmed by controlled studies.

Retinoids

The overall and complete response rates of established oral retinoids (isotretinoin, etretinate and acitretin) and a novel RXR-selective retinoid (bexarotene), used as a single oral agent, are roughly similar to those of IFN-α[40]. A combination of retinoids and PUVA (RePUVA) shows response rates similar to that of PUVA alone, although patients treated with RePUVA require fewer treatments and a significantly lower cumulative UVA dose. In patients with patches or thin plaques, topical bexarotene may be considered.

Miscellaneous

Newer immunomodulatory therapies in MF include the usage of receptor-targeted cytotoxic fusion proteins (DAB$_{389}$IL2; denileukin diftitox), cytokines (e.g. IL-12), monoclonal antibodies (e.g. anti-CD4 and anti-CD52 [alemtuzumab]) and various vaccination strategies[39]. DAB$_{389}$IL2 is a fusion protein, in which diphtheria toxin is linked to IL-2. It binds to the high-affinity IL-2 receptor expressed by the neoplastic T cells in MF; this results in inhibition of protein synthesis and cell death and in overall and complete clinical response rates of approximately 30% and 10%, respectively. It remains to be determined which patients are most likely to benefit from this therapy.

Vaccination with peptides or peptide-loaded dendritic cells is currently under investigation. However, unlike in melanoma, useful CTCL-associated antigens have not yet been identified.

Prognosis

The prognosis of patients with MF is dependent upon the stage, and in particular the type and extent of skin lesions and the presence of extracutaneous disease[24,41]. Patients with limited patch/plaque stage MF have a similar long-term life expectancy as an age-, sex- and race-matched control population. In a study of 309 Dutch MF patients, the disease-related 10-year survival rate of patients with limited patch/

plaque disease, generalized patch/plaque disease, and tumor stage disease without concurrent lymph node involvement was 97%, 83% and 42%, respectively, but was only 20% for patients with histologically documented lymph node involvement[24]. An aggressive clinical course is seen in patients with effaced lymph nodes, visceral involvement, and transformation into a large T-cell lymphoma. Patients usually die of systemic involvement or infections.

VARIANTS OF MYCOSIS FUNGOIDES

Apart from the classical Alibert–Bazin type of mycosis fungoides (MF), many clinical and/or histologic variants have been reported. Clinical variants, such as bullous and hyper- or hypopigmented MF, have a clinical behavior similar to that of classical MF, and are therefore not considered separately. In contrast, folliculotropic MF (MF-associated follicular mucinosis), pagetoid reticulosis and granulomatous slack skin have distinctive clinicopathologic features, and therefore have been included as distinct variants or subtypes of MF in the WHO–EORTC classification scheme.

Folliculotropic MF

Synonyms: ■ MF-associated follicular mucinosis ■ Folliculocentric or pilotropic MF

Definition

Folliculotropic MF is a distinct variant of MF characterized by the presence of folliculotropic infiltrates, often with sparing of the epidermis and preferential involvement of the head and neck region. Most cases show mucinous degeneration of the hair follicles (follicular mucinosis; see Ch. 46) and are traditionally designated as MF-associated follicular mucinosis. Similar cases, but without follicular mucinosis, have been reported as folliculocentric or pilotropic MF. From a biologic point of view, the most relevant feature (in cases both with and without associated follicular mucinosis) is the deep, follicular and perifollicular localization of the neoplastic infiltrates, which makes them less accessible to skin-targeted therapies. For both groups, the term folliculotropic MF is therefore preferred[3].

Epidemiology

This variant is found in approximately 10% of MF patients[24]. It occurs mostly in adults, but may occasionally affect children and adolescents. Men are more often affected than women.

Clinical features

Patients may present with (grouped) follicular papules, acneiform lesions, indurated plaques and sometimes tumors, which preferentially involve and are most pronounced in the head and neck area. The skin lesions are often associated with alopecia, and sometimes with mucinorrhea. Infiltrated plaques in the eyebrow region with concurrent alopecia are a common and highly characteristic finding (Fig. 120.5A). Pruritus is often more severe than in classical MF, and may represent a reliable parameter of disease activity. Secondary bacterial infections are frequently observed.

It should be stressed that the clinical staging systems for MF are not very helpful in patients with folliculotropic MF. Because of the perifollicular localization of the neoplastic infiltrates, patients presenting with one or a few plaques on the face do not have stage IA disease, but should always be considered as having tumor stage disease. Consistently, the survival of patients with folliculotropic MF is similar to that of classical tumor stage MF[42,43].

Pathology

Characteristic findings include the primarily perivascular and periadnexal localization of the dermal infiltrates, with variable infiltration of the follicular epithelium by small, medium-sized or sometimes large T cells with hyperchromatic and cerebriform nuclei, and sparing of the epidermis (folliculotropism instead of epidermotropism) (Fig. 120.5B). Most cases show mucinous degeneration of the follicular epithelium (follicular mucinosis), as assessed with Alcian blue or colloidal iron staining. There is often a considerable admixture with eosinophils and sometimes plasma cells. In the perifollicular infiltrates, the neoplastic T cells may be blast cells rather than cerebriform cells, and therefore may be easily mistaken for histiocytes. In most cases, the neoplastic T cells have a CD3+, CD4+, CD8– phenotype as in classical MF. Admixture with CD30+ blast cells is common.

Differential diagnosis

The distinctive clinical and histologic features should facilitate an early and correct diagnosis. However, because of the preferential involvement

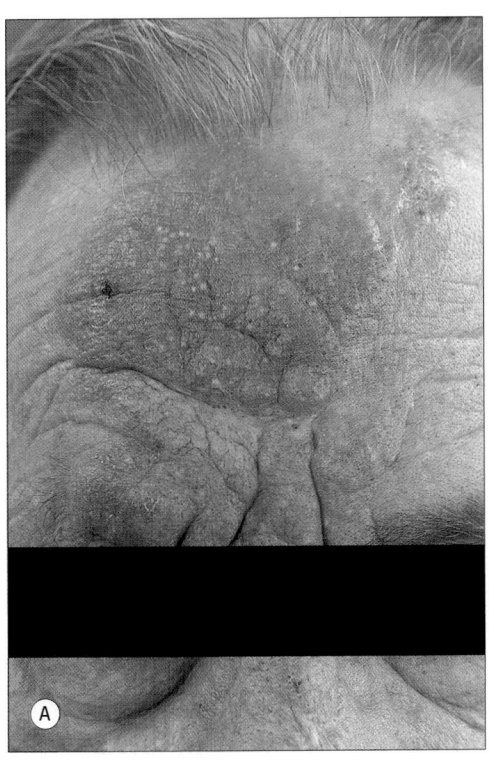
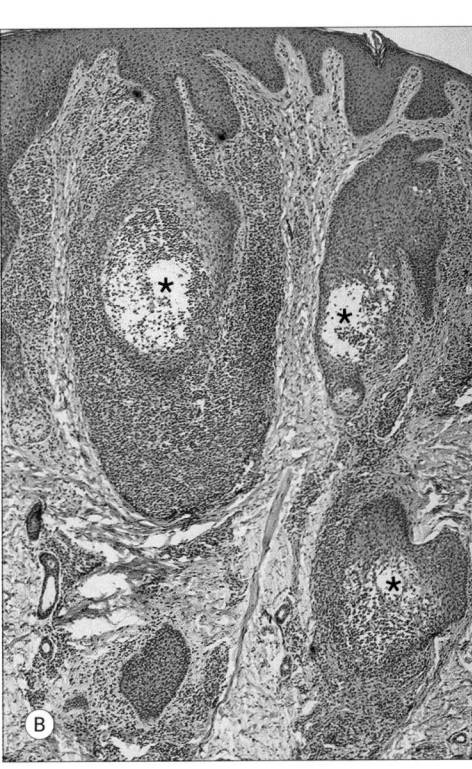

Fig. 120.5 Folliculotropic mycosis fungoides.
A Infiltrated plaques of the forehead and eyebrow with concurrent hair loss. **B** Characteristic perifollicular infiltrates with extensive follicular mucinosis (asterisks). Note absence of epidermotropism.

of the head and neck area, the absence of patches and plaques on the trunk and buttocks, and particularly because of the absence of epidermotropic atypical T cells, the diagnosis of MF or CTCL is often not considered and is misinterpreted as seborrheic dermatitis or atopic dermatitis. Clinicopathologic correlation is also required to differentiate folliculotropic MF from other types of CTCL[42]. The relationship between folliculotropic MF and the so-called benign or idiopathic form of folliculotropic mucinosis (alopecia mucinosa) resembles the relationship between classical MF and 'parapsoriasis'. In the case of persistent lesions, patients should be monitored regularly, since progression into overt folliculotropic MF has been frequently reported.

Treatment
Because of the perifollicular localization of the dermal infiltrates, folliculotropic MF is often less responsive to skin-targeted therapies, such as PUVA and topical nitrogen mustard, than is classical plaque stage MF. If not successful, local radiotherapy or total skin electron beam irradiation is the preferred mode of treatment, although sustained complete remissions are rarely achieved[42].

Pagetoid Reticulosis

> **Synonyms:** ■ Woringer–Kolopp disease ■ Unilesional MF

Definition
This is a rare variant of MF, characterized by the presence of localized patches or plaques with an intraepidermal proliferation of neoplastic T cells. The term pagetoid reticulosis should be used only for the localized type (Woringer–Kolopp type) and not for the disseminated type (Ketron–Goodman type), which is a manifestation of an aggressive epidermotropic CD8[+] CTCL or of classical tumor stage MF[1].

Epidemiology
Pagetoid reticulosis is extremely rare, and accounts for less than 1% of CTCL cases. It mostly affects adults.

Clinical features
Patients present with a solitary psoriasiform or hyperkeratotic patch or plaque, which is usually localized on an extremity, and is slowly progressive (Fig. 120.6A). In contrast to classical MF, extracutaneous dissemination or disease-related deaths have never been reported.

Pathology
The typical histologic picture consists of a hyperplastic epidermis with marked infiltration by large atypical pagetoid cells, arranged singly or in nests or clusters (Fig. 120.6B). The atypical cells have medium-sized or large, sometimes hyperchromatic and cerebriform nuclei and abundant, vacuolated cytoplasm. The superficial dermis may have an infiltrate of mostly small lymphocytes, but rarely contains neoplastic T cells.

Immunophenotype
The neoplastic T cells may show either a CD3[+], CD4[+], CD8[−] or a CD3[+], CD4[−], CD8[+] phenotype. CD30 is often expressed[44,45].

Differential diagnosis
Pagetoid reticulosis should be differentiated from other types of epidermotropic CTCL, such as MF, lymphomatoid papulosis type B and aggressive epidermotropic CD8[+] CTCL with a cytotoxic phenotype (see Table 120.2). Useful criteria for pagetoid reticulosis include the characteristic clinical presentation and the often strictly epidermal localization of the neoplastic T cells.

Treatment
The preferred mode of treatment is radiotherapy or surgical excision.

Granulomatous Slack Skin

Definition
This is an extraordinarily rare type of CTCL, characterized by the slow development of folds of lax skin and a granulomatous infiltrate with clonal T cells[46].

Epidemiology
This is an extremely rare type of CTCL, with less than 30 cases reported. It may affect adolescents and adults, and mostly occurs in men.

Clinical features
This condition is characterized by circumscribed areas of pendulous lax skin with a predilection for the axillae and groin (Fig. 120.7A). In approximately one-third of the reported patients, an association with Hodgkin disease was observed[46]. An association with classical MF has also been described. Most patients have an indolent clinical course.

Pathology
Fully developed lesions show dense granulomatous dermal infiltrates containing atypical T cells with cerebriform nuclei, macrophages, and often many multinucleated giant cells, as well as destruction of elastic tissue and elastophagocytosis by the multinucleated cells (Fig. 120.7B). The epidermis is infiltrated by often small atypical T cells with cerebriform nuclei, as in classical MF. The atypical T cells have a CD3[+], CD4[+], CD8[−] phenotype.

Treatment
Radiotherapy may be effective, but experience is still limited. Rapid recurrences after surgical excision have been reported.

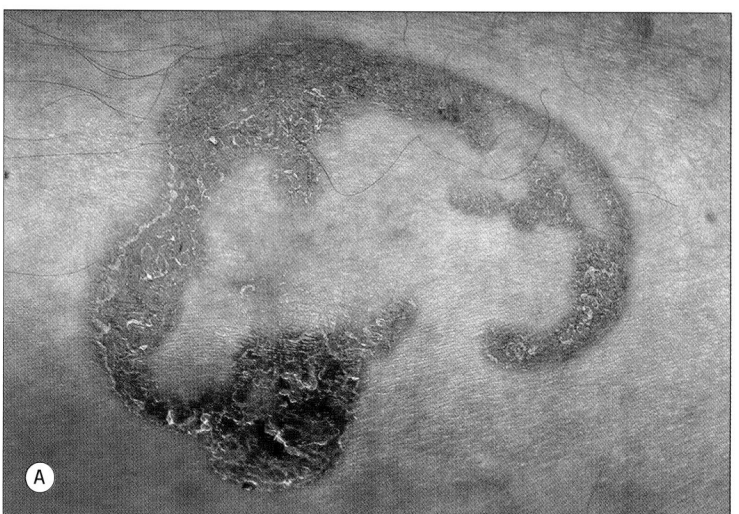

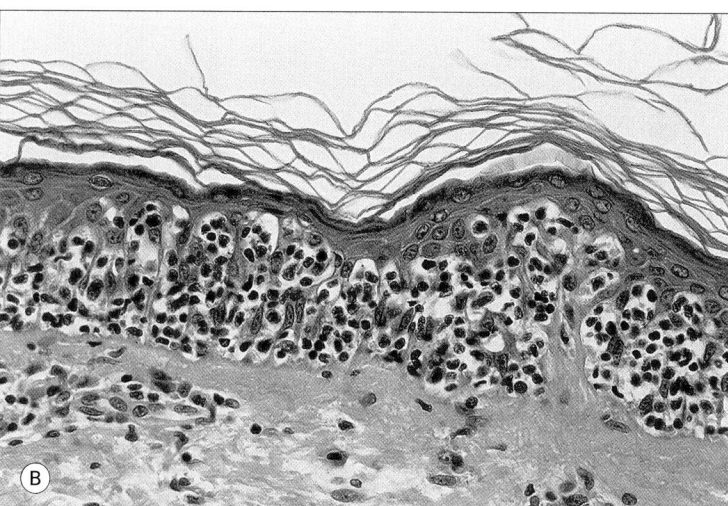

Fig. 120.6 Pagetoid reticulosis. A Solitary plaque on the left upper leg. **B** Purely intraepidermal proliferation of atypical T cells.

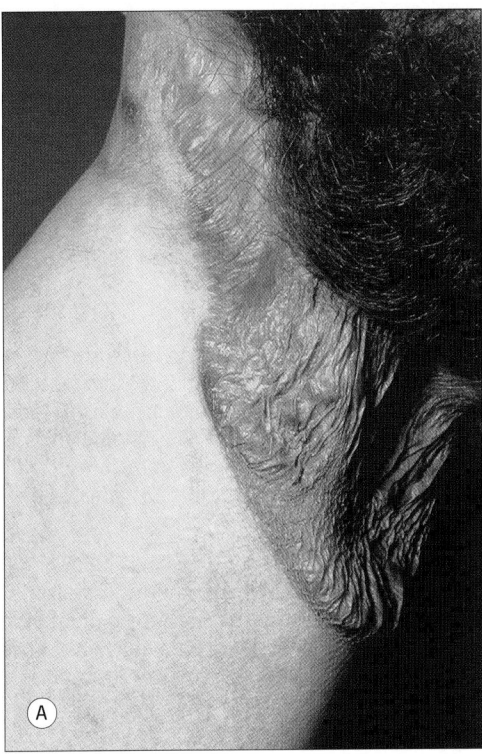

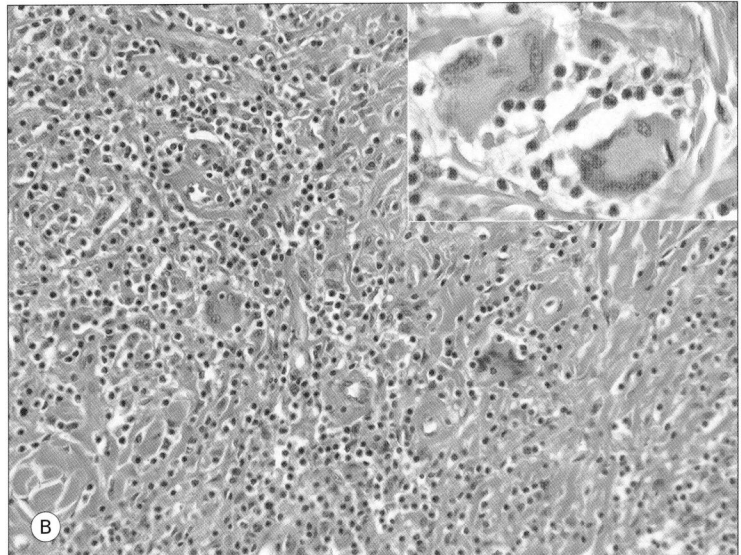

Fig. 120.7 Granulomatous slack skin. A Pendulous fold of atrophic lax skin in the right inguinal area. **B** Multinucleated giant cells with intracellular leukocytes (emperipolesis), surrounded by a dense leukocytic infiltrate. Inset: Elastic tissue stain showing a multinucleated giant cell containing an elastic fiber (elastophagocytosis).

SÉZARY SYNDROME

Definition

Sézary syndrome (SS) is defined historically by the triad of erythroderma, generalized lymphadenopathy, and the presence of neoplastic T cells (Sézary cells) in the skin, lymph nodes and peripheral blood (Fig. 120.8). Criteria recommended for the diagnosis of SS include demonstration of a T-cell clone in the peripheral blood by molecular or cytogenetic methods, demonstration of immunophenotypic abnormalities (an expanded CD4$^+$ T-cell population resulting in a CD4:CD8 ratio >10 and/or aberrant expression of pan-T-cell antigens), and an absolute Sézary cell count of least 1000 cells per μl[47]. In the WHO–EORTC classification, demonstration of a T-cell clone (preferably the same T-cell clone in the skin and peripheral blood) in combination with one of the above-mentioned cytomorphologic or immunophenotypic criteria are suggested as minimal criteria for the diagnosis of SS in order to exclude patients with benign inflammatory condition simulating SS.

Epidemiology

SS is a rare disease, accounting for less than 5% of all CTCLs (see Table 120.1). It occurs exclusively in adults.

Clinical features

SS is characterized by an erythroderma, which may be associated with marked exfoliation, edema and lichenification; it is intensely pruritic (Fig. 120.9). Lymphadenopathy, alopecia, onychodystrophy and palmoplantar hyperkeratosis are common findings[48]. The overt clinical picture may be preceded by a non-diagnostic dermatitis. The bone marrow may contain neoplastic cells, but real replacement of bone marrow tissue is rare. The prognosis is generally poor, with an overall

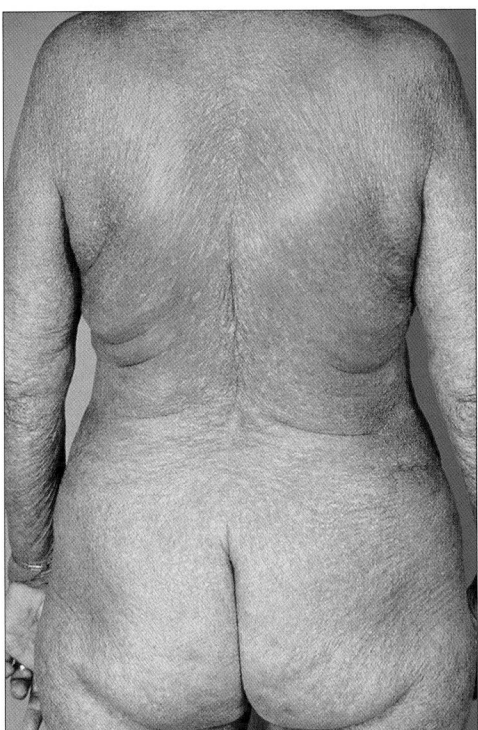

Fig. 120.9 Sézary syndrome. Diffuse erythroderma is present.

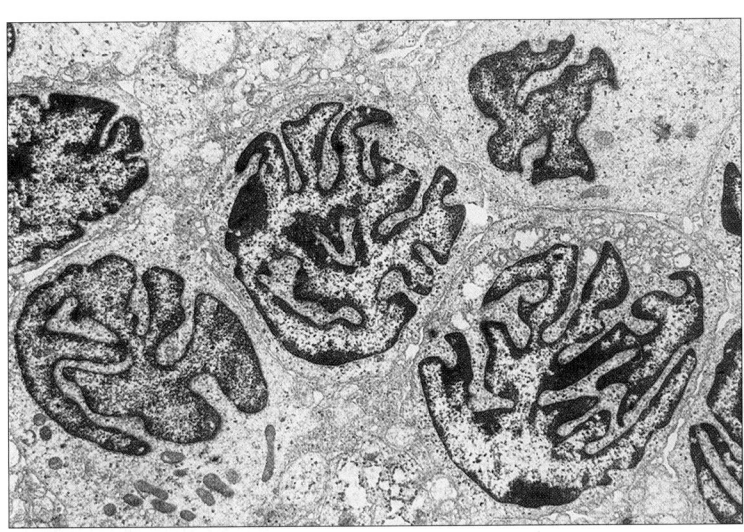

Fig. 120.8 Sézary syndrome. Electron photomicrograph of a skin biopsy showing characteristic Sézary cells.

5-year survival of approximately 25%. Most patients die of opportunistic infections due to immunosuppression.

Pathology

The histologic features in SS may be similar to those in mycosis fungoides (MF). However, the cellular infiltrates in SS are more often monotonous, and epidermotropism may sometimes be absent. Involved lymph nodes characteristically show a dense, monotonous infiltrate of Sézary cells with effacement of the normal lymph node architecture. The neoplastic T cells have a CD3+, CD4+, CD8− phenotype.

Pathogenesis

The pathogenesis of SS is unknown. Conclusive evidence of an etiological role for HTLV-1 is lacking. Recurrent chromosomal translocations have not been detected in SS, but complex karyotypes are common. Several studies have identified a consistent pattern of identical chromosomal abnormalities in SS, which was almost identical to that in MF, suggesting that both conditions represent entities within the same spectrum of disease with a similar pathogenesis[17,49,50].

Differential diagnosis

Differentiation between SS and non-neoplastic forms of erythroderma may be extremely difficult. The differential diagnosis includes erythroderma on the basis of psoriasis, atopic dermatitis or other form of eczema, drug reactions, and idiopathic erythroderma (see Ch. 11). Demonstration of clonal T cells in the peripheral blood is considered an important diagnostic criterion favoring a diagnosis of SS. Demonstration of a predominant CD3+, CD4−, CD8+ T-cell population in the skin and peripheral blood is highly suggestive of actinic reticuloid[51].

Treatment

Being a systemic disease (leukemia) by definition, systemic treatment is required. Skin-directed therapies like PUVA or potent topical corticosteroids may be used as adjuvant therapy. Extracorporeal photopheresis (ECP), either alone or in combination with other treatment modalities, has been suggested as the treatment of choice in SS and erythrodermic MF, with overall response rates of 30–80%, and complete response rates of 14–25%[52,53]. This great variation in response rates may reflect differences in patient selection and/or concurrent therapies. The suggested superiority of ECP over the traditional low-dose chemotherapy regimens has not yet been substantiated by randomized controlled trials[53]. Beneficial effects have also been reported with IFN-α (either alone or in combination with PUVA therapy), prolonged treatment with a combination of low-dose chlorambucil and prednisone, or with methotrexate, but complete responses are uncommon. CHOP or CHOP-like regimens may produce higher response rates, but these responses are generally short-lived. Recent studies demonstrated activity with bexarotene and alemtuzumab (anti-CD52), but the long-term effects of these therapies remain to be established[30,39].

ADULT T-CELL LEUKEMIA/LYMPHOMA

Definition

Adult T-cell leukemia/lymphoma (ATLL) is a type of T-cell neoplasm etiologically associated with HTLV-1. Skin lesions are generally a manifestation of widely disseminated disease. However, a slowly progressive form that sometimes has only skin lesions has been described (smoldering variant)[54].

Epidemiology

ATLL is endemic in areas with a high prevalence of HTLV-1 in the population, such as southwestern Japan, the Caribbean Islands and parts of Central Africa. In addition, a high prevalence is seen in Jewish people whose ancestors were from Mashad, Iran. However, only a minor proportion of seropositive patients eventually develop ATLL. The disease occurs in adults, and men are affected more frequently than women. HTLV-1 is generally transmitted from infected mother to infant via breast milk (vertical transmission). Less commonly, infected cells are transmitted by sexual contacts, blood transfusions or intravenous drug usage (horizontal transmission).

Clinical features

Most patients present with acute ATLL characterized by the presence of leukemia, lymphadenopathy, organomegaly, hypercalcemia and, frequently, skin lesions; it has a poor prognosis. Chronic and smoldering variants often present with patches, plaques and papular skin lesions which may closely resemble mycosis fungoides (MF), while circulating neoplastic T cells are few or absent. Such cases have a more protracted clinical course, but progression to a high-grade malignant disseminated form of the disease may occur.

Pathology

Skin lesions demonstrate a superficial or more diffuse infiltration of small, medium-sized or large pleomorphic T cells, which often display marked epidermotropism. The histologic picture may be indistinguishable from MF. Skin lesions in the smoldering type may have sparse dermal infiltrates with only slightly atypical cells. The neoplastic T cells express a CD3+, CD4+, CD8−, CD25+ phenotype.

Differential diagnosis

Differentiation between chronic or smoldering variants of ATLL and MF may be extremely difficult, particularly in endemic areas. In such cases, a definite diagnosis of ATLL requires demonstration of clonally integrated HTLV-1. By flow cytometry or immunohistochemistry, the presence of an abnormal population of T lymphocytes expressing CD25 is suggestive of ATLL.

Treatment

In most cases, systemic chemotherapy is required[55]. In chronic and smoldering cases mainly affecting the skin, skin-targeted therapies as in MF are preferred.

PRIMARY CUTANEOUS CD30+ LYMPHOPROLIFERATIVE DISORDERS

Primary cutaneous CD30+ lymphoproliferative disorders represent the second most common group of CTCL, accounting for approximately 25% of CTCLs (see Table 120.1). This group includes primary cutaneous anaplastic large cell lymphoma (C-ALCL), lymphomatoid papulosis (LyP), and borderline cases. C-ALCL and LyP have overlapping clinical, histologic and immunophenotypic features and form a spectrum of disease[56]. Thus, histologic criteria alone are often insufficient to distinguish between the two ends of the spectrum. In the end, the clinical appearance and course are used as decisive criteria for the definite diagnosis and choice of treatment. The term 'borderline case' refers to patients in whom, despite careful clinicopathologic correlation, a definite distinction between C-ALCL and LyP cannot be established. Longitudinal clinical evaluation will generally disclose whether the patient has C-ALCL or LyP[57]. Cases previously designated as *regressing atypical histiocytosis*, as well as rare cases of primary cutaneous Hodgkin disease with an indolent clinical course, also belong to this spectrum[57].

These primary cutaneous CD30+ lymphoproliferative disorders should be differentiated from: (1) skin involvement by systemic ALCL; (2) cases of mycosis fungoides (MF) with transformation into a CD30+ large cell lymphoma; and (3) other well-defined types of CTCL which may sometimes express the CD30 antigen (see Table 120.2). Guidelines for the diagnosis and treatment of these cutaneous CD30+ lymphoproliferations are provided in Figure 120.10.

Primary Cutaneous Anaplastic Large Cell Lymphoma

Definition

Primary C-ALCL is characterized by large cells with an anaplastic, pleomorphic or immunoblastic cytomorphology and expression of the CD30 antigen by the majority (>75%) of the tumor cells. There is no clinical evidence or history of LyP, MF or another type of CTCL. In the EORTC classification, these lymphomas were designated as primary cutaneous CD30+ large T-cell lymphoma[1].

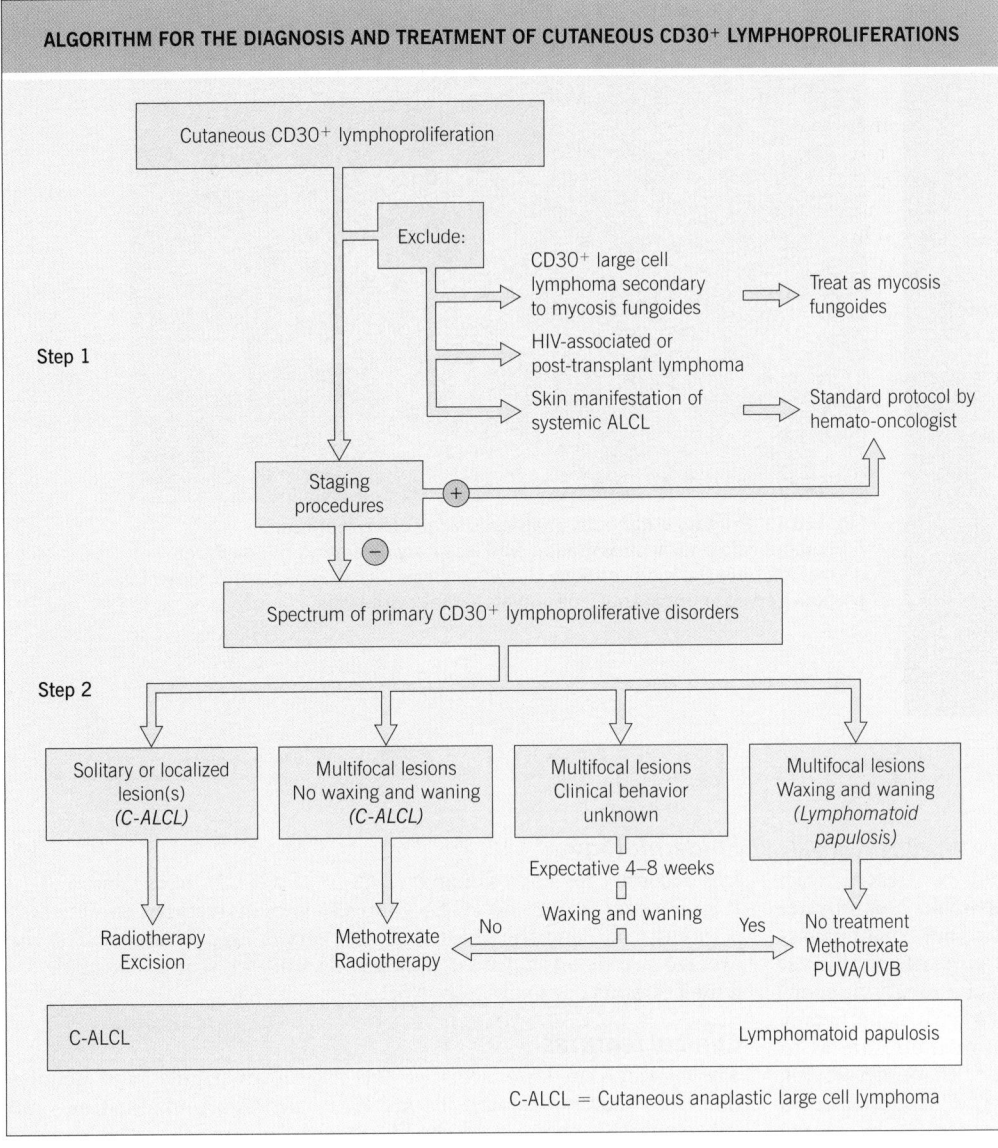

Fig. 120.10 Algorithm for the diagnosis and treatment of primary cutaneous CD30[+] lymphoproliferations[57].

ALGORITHM FOR THE DIAGNOSIS AND TREATMENT OF CUTANEOUS CD30[+] LYMPHOPROLIFERATIONS

Step 1

Cutaneous CD30[+] lymphoproliferation

Exclude:
- CD30[+] large cell lymphoma secondary to mycosis fungoides → Treat as mycosis fungoides
- HIV-associated or post-transplant lymphoma
- Skin manifestation of systemic ALCL → Standard protocol by hemato-oncologist

Staging procedures
(+) Standard protocol by hemato-oncologist
(−) Spectrum of primary CD30[+] lymphoproliferative disorders

Step 2

- Solitary or localized lesion(s) (C-ALCL) → Radiotherapy Excision
- Multifocal lesions No waxing and waning (C-ALCL) → Methotrexate Radiotherapy
- Multifocal lesions Clinical behavior unknown → Expectative 4–8 weeks → Waxing and waning — No / Yes
- Multifocal lesions Waxing and waning (Lymphomatoid papulosis) → No treatment Methotrexate PUVA/UVB

C-ALCL   Lymphomatoid papulosis

C-ALCL = Cutaneous anaplastic large cell lymphoma

Epidemiology

These lymphomas account for approximately 10% of all CTCLs (see Table 120.1). They predominantly affect adults, and are rare in children or adolescents. The male-to-female ratio is approximately 2:1.

Clinical features

Most patients present with solitary or localized nodules or tumors (sometimes papules) that often develop ulceration (Fig. 120.11A). Multifocal lesions are seen in about 20% of the patients. The skin lesions may show partial or complete spontaneous regression, as in LyP. These lymphomas frequently relapse in the skin. Extracutaneous dissemination occurs in approximately 10% of the patients, and primarily involves the regional lymph nodes. The prognosis is usually favorable, with a 10-year disease-related survival rate exceeding 85%[57,58].

Pathology

These lymphomas have diffuse non-epidermotropic infiltrates with cohesive sheets of large CD30[+] tumor cells (Fig. 120.11B). In most cases, the tumor cells have the characteristic morphology of anaplastic cells, with round, oval or irregularly shaped nuclei, prominent (eosinophilic) nucleoli and abundant cytoplasm. Less commonly (20–25% of patients), the tumor cells have a pleomorphic, immunoblastic or Reed–Sternberg cell-like appearance. The mitotic index is generally high. Reactive lymphocytes are often present at the periphery of the tumor. Ulcerating lesions may show an LyP-like histology with an abundant inflammatory infiltrate of reactive T cells, histiocytes,

eosinophils, neutrophils, and relatively few CD30[+] cells. In such cases, epidermal hyperplasia may be prominent.

Immunophenotype

The neoplastic cells often express a CD4[+] T-cell phenotype with variable loss of CD2, CD5 and/or CD3. Some patients (<5%) have a CD8[+] T-cell phenotype. CD30 must be expressed by the majority of neoplastic cells[59]. Expression of cytotoxic proteins (granzyme B, TIA-1, perforin) is noted in approximately 70% of the cases. Unlike systemic CD30[+] lymphomas, most primary C-ALCLs express the cutaneous lymphocyte antigen (CLA), but do not express epithelial membrane antigen (EMA) or anaplastic lymphoma kinase (ALK); the latter is indicative of the t(2;5) chromosomal translocation[57,60]. Unlike with Hodgkin and Reed–Sternberg cells in Hodgkin disease, staining for CD15 is generally negative. Coexpression of CD56 is observed in rare cases, but does not appear to be associated with an unfavorable prognosis[61].

Genetic features

The t(2;5) translocation, which is predominantly found in systemic ALCL in children, is not or rarely found in C-ALCL[60].

Treatment

Radiotherapy is the initial choice of treatment in patients presenting with a solitary or a few localized nodules or tumors. However, if a solitary lesion has been excised completely, or has disappeared

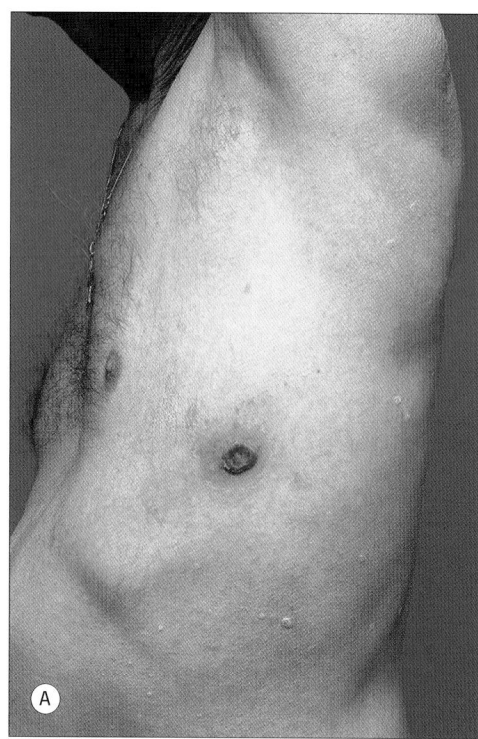

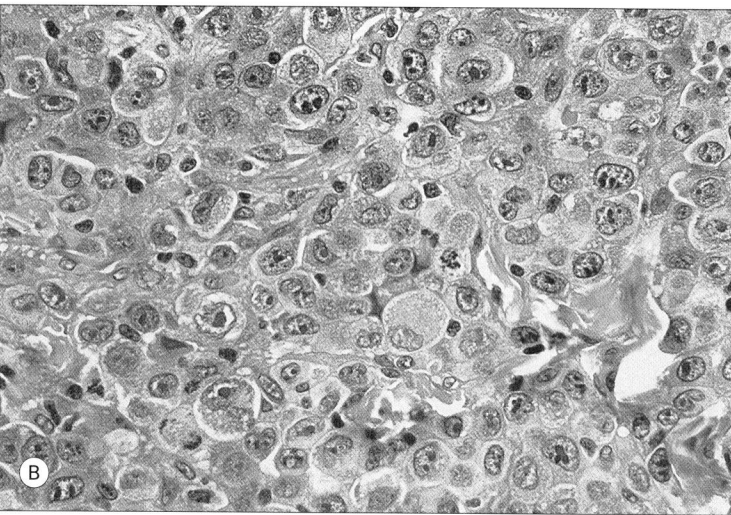

Fig. 120.11 Primary cutaneous anaplastic large cell lymphoma.
A Characteristic clinical presentation with a solitary ulcerating tumor. **B** Detail of dermal infiltrate showing cohesive clusters of large (CD30⁺) anaplastic cells with pronounced eosinophilic nucleoli and abundant cytoplasm.

spontaneously, no further therapy is required. Whether patients presenting with multifocal skin lesions should be treated with doxorubicin-based multiagent chemotherapy is debatable. Not only are skin relapses following CHOP therapy common, but spontaneous regression of all skin lesions has been noted in patients with multifocal skin disease. Current evidence suggests that patients in whom spontaneous regression does not occur are best treated with radiotherapy (if there are only a few lesions) or with low-dose methotrexate as in LyP[57,62] (see Fig 120.10). In patients presenting with or developing extracutaneous disease, multiagent chemotherapy is still considered the safest option.

Lymphomatoid Papulosis

Definition

Lymphomatoid papulosis (LyP) is defined as a chronic, recurrent, self-healing papulonecrotic or papulonodular skin disease with histologic features suggestive of a (CD30⁺) malignant lymphoma. Since the introduction of the term LyP in 1968 by Macaulay[63], there has been continued discussion as to whether LyP is a malignant, a premalignant or a benign condition. Because of the overlapping clinical and histologic features between LyP and C-ALCL, including the presence of an aberrant T-cell phenotype, the presence of clonally rearranged TCR genes in 60–70% of the patients, and the presence of identical T-cell clones in LyP lesions and associated lymphoma lesions, LyP is best regarded as a low-grade malignant CTCL[56,64].

Pathogenesis

The initiating event in LyP is unknown. Several authors have suggested a viral etiology. However, studies searching for an etiologic role for HTLV-1, EBV or other herpes viruses (e.g. herpes simplex virus types 1 and type 2, human herpesvirus-6) have been consistently negative. The mechanisms involved in the spontaneous disappearance of skin lesions, or in tumor progression, as observed in some patients with LyP, have not yet been identified. It has been suggested that interactions between CD30 and its ligand (CD30L) may contribute to apoptosis of the neoplastic T cells and the subsequent regression of the skin lesions, but the exact mechanism is as yet unknown[65]. Unresponsiveness to the growth inhibitory effect of transforming growth factor-β (TGF-β) due to a mutation in the TGF-β type I receptor on the CD30⁺ tumor cells has been suggested as one of the possible mechanisms in tumor progression[66].

Epidemiology

LyP accounts for approximately 15% of all CTCLs (see Table 120.1). It may occur at any age. The youngest patient reported to date was 8 months old, and the oldest was 84 years of age. In large series, the average age of onset varied between 35 and 45 years. The male-to-female ratio is approximately 1.5:1.

Clinical features

The typical skin lesions in LyP are red–brown papules and nodules that may develop central hemorrhage, necrosis and crusting, and subsequently spontaneously disappear within 3 to 8 weeks. Characteristically, skin lesions in different stages of evolution coexist (Fig. 120.12A). The papulonodules may leave transient hypopigmented or hyperpigmented macules and, occasionally, superficial atrophic (varioliform) scars, or disappear without apparent necrosis and ulceration. The number of lesions may vary from several to more than 100. Lesions may be localized, sometimes clustered within rather well-defined areas, or generalized. The predominant sites of involvement are the trunk and limbs. The eruption is generally asymptomatic.

The duration of the disease may vary from several months to more than 40 years. In up to 20% of patients, LyP may be preceded by, associated with, or followed by another type of malignant (cutaneous) lymphoma, generally MF, C-ALCL or Hodgkin disease[67]. However, the prognosis is usually excellent. In a recent study of 118 patients with LyP, only five patients (4%) developed a systemic lymphoma, and only two patients (2%) died of systemic disease over a median follow-up period of 77 months[57]. Risk factors for the development of a systemic lymphoma are unknown.

Pathology

The histologic picture of LyP is extremely variable, but in part correlates with the age of the sampled skin lesion. In addition, three histologic types of LyP have been described: types A, B and C.

LyP type A lesions show a wedge-shaped, initially non-epidermotropic, infiltrate with scattered or small clusters of large atypical, sometimes multinucleated or Reed–Sternberg-like, CD30⁺ T cells, interspersed in an extensive inflammatory infiltrate composed of small lymphocytes, neutrophils and/or eosinophils (Fig. 120.12B,C). The large atypical cells, which have the morphologic and immunophenotypic characteristics of the neoplastic cells in C-ALCL, are relatively few in early lesions and more numerous in fully developed

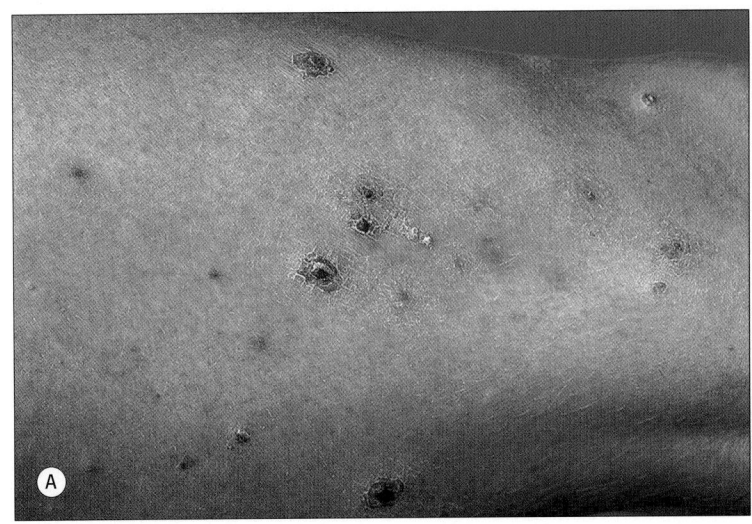

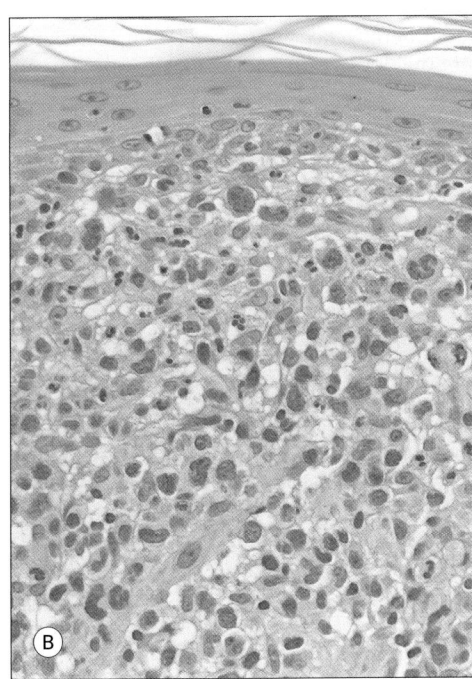

Fig. 120.12
Lymphomatoid papulosis (LyP). **A** Clinical presentation with papulonecrotic skin lesions at different stages of evolution. **B** Diffuse infiltrate with many large atypical lymphocytes. Scattered neutrophils both in the epidermis and dermis. **C** Detail of dermal infiltrate showing a mixed inflammatory infiltrate with scattered (CD30+) large anaplastic T cells (LyP, type A).

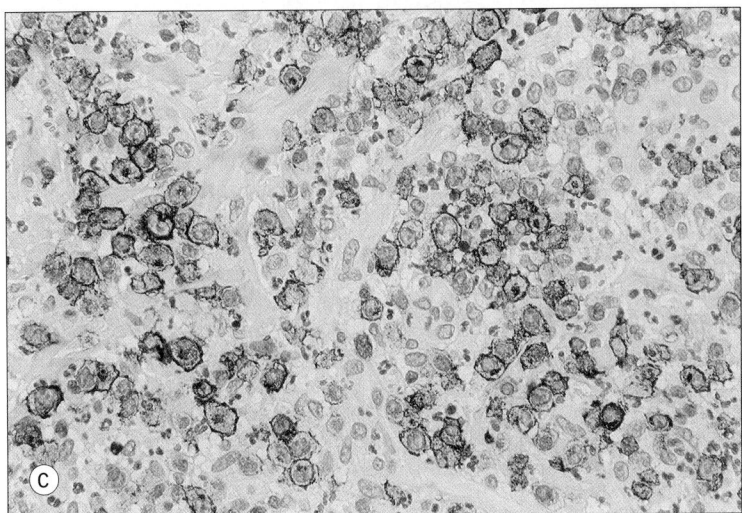

lesions, but may be completely absent in resolving lesions. The presence of scattered neutrophils within a moderately acanthotic and parakeratotic, but otherwise unaffected, epidermis is a characteristic finding.

LyP type B lesions are relatively uncommon (<10%) and are characterized by superficial perivascular to band-like lymphocytic infiltrates, which show early infiltration of the basal and parabasal layers of the epidermis. Occasionally, these perivascular infiltrates can also be found in the deeper dermis. The infiltrates are composed predominantly of small to medium-sized atypical cells with cerebriform nuclei and the phenotype of CD3+, CD4+, but CD30-, T cells, similar to those observed in MF.

Features of LyP type A and type B may occur in different but concurrent lesions, and some LyP lesions may show histologic findings characteristic of both type A and type B[57].

LyP type C lesions demonstrate a monotonous population or large clusters of large CD30+ T cells with relatively few admixed inflammatory cells, a histologic appearance typically found in C-ALCL.

Recognition of these three histologic types has contributed to our understanding of the relationship between LyP and other types of CTCL and to the definition of the spectrum of primary cutaneous CD30+ lymphoproliferations. However, from a practical point of view, histologic subtyping is not necessary, since the three histologic subtypes do not differ clinically.

Differential diagnosis

Small recurrent LyP lesions on the trunk are commonly misinterpreted as folliculitis or arthropod bites for years. Because of the presence of multifocal skin lesions with the histologic features of CD30+ large cell lymphoma, LyP patients are sometimes treated unnecessarily with multiagent chemotherapy by physicians not familiar with this condition. When the clinical features are taken into account along with the histologic findings, differentiation between LyP and the malignant lymphomas is not difficult.

Because of the clinical similarities between LyP and pityriasis lichenoides, a relationship between the two conditions was initially suggested. Clonal T-cell populations have been demonstrated in skin biopsies of both conditions. Pityriasis lichenoides occurs more often in younger patients, is generally short-lived, does not develop nodular lesions, and progression to a malignant lymphoma is exceedingly rare, if it occurs at all. CD30+ blast cells are generally not seen in pityriasis lichenoides[68,69].

Treatment

The treatment of patients with LyP is unsatisfactory. Topical or systemic corticosteroids or antibiotics are not effective. Aggressive treatment modalities such as systemic chemotherapy or total skin electron beam irradiation may produce complete remissions, but, after discontinuation of therapy, the LyP lesions generally reappear within weeks or months, and the disease follows its natural course. Since a curative therapy is not available and none of the available treatment modalities affects the natural course of the disease, the short-term benefits of active treatment should be balanced carefully against the potential side effects[57]. In patients with relatively few non-scarring lesions, active treatment is not necessary. In the case of cosmetically disturbing lesions (e.g. scarring or many papulonodules), low-dose oral methotrexate (5–20 mg/week) is the most effective therapy for reducing the number of skin lesions[62]. Beneficial effects have been reported with PUVA, topical nitrogen mustard or BCNU, and low-dose etoposide. When larger skin tumors develop in the course of LyP, they can be observed for a period of 4 to 12 weeks for the possibility of spontaneous remission. If spontaneous resolution does not occur, such lesions can be excised or treated with radiotherapy. Because of the potential risk for developing a systemic lymphoma, long-term follow-up is required in all patients with LyP.

SUBCUTANEOUS PANNICULITIS-LIKE T-CELL LYMPHOMA

Definition

In both the EORTC and WHO classification schemes, subcutaneous panniculitis-like T-cell lymphoma (SPTL) was defined as a cytotoxic T-cell lymphoma characterized by the presence of primarily subcutaneous infiltrates of small, medium-sized or large pleomorphic T cells in addition to many macrophages, predominantly affecting the legs and often complicated by a hemophagocytic syndrome[1,2]. The disorder included cases with an α/β T-cell phenotype (75%) as well as cases with a γ/δ T-cell phenotype (25%). Recent studies have shown clinical, histologic and immunophenotypic differences between cases of SPTL with an α/β T-cell phenotype versus those with a γ/δ T-cell phenotype, suggesting that they may represent different entities. Whereas SPTLs with an α/β T-cell phenotype are homogeneous with a rather indolent clinical behavior in many patients, SPTLs with a γ/δ T-cell phenotype overlap with other types of γ/δ-positive T-cell lymphoma and invariably run a very aggressive clinical course (Table 120.6)[70–74]. In the WHO–EORTC classification scheme, the term SPTL is only used for cases with an α/β+ T-cell phenotype, whereas cases with a γ/δ+ T-cell phenotype are included in the category of cutaneous γ/δ T-cell lymphoma (see Table 120.1).

Epidemiology

SPTL is a rare condition, accounting for less than 1% of all CTCLs. It may occur in adults as well as in young children, and both sexes are equally affected.

Clinical features

In general, patients present with subcutaneous nodules and plaques, primarily involving the extremities and less often the trunk; ulceration is uncommon. Systemic symptoms such as fever, fatigue and weight loss may be present. A hemophagocytic syndrome, which is generally associated with a rapidly progressive course, may occur, but is much less common than in cutaneous γ/δ+ T-cell lymphomas with panniculitis-like lesions. Dissemination to extracutaneous sites is rare. Many patients with SPTL have a protracted clinical course with recurrent subcutaneous lesions but without extracutaneous dissemination or the development of a hemophagocytic syndrome[72,74]. This

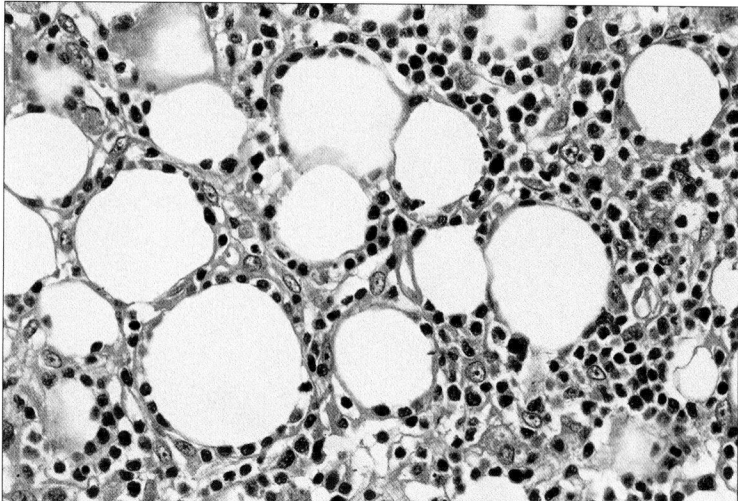

Fig. 120.13 Subcutaneous panniculitis-like T-cell lymphoma. Subcutaneous infiltrate with characteristic rimming of individual fat cells by the neoplastic T cells.

entity may include cases previously referred to as *cytophagocytic histiocytic panniculitis* (see Ch. 100)[75]. Recent studies suggest that the 5-year survival rate for patients with SPTL is approximately 80%[74].

Pathology

Subcutaneous infiltrates simulate a panniculitis, with a mixture of neoplastic pleomorphic T cells of various sizes and often numerous macrophages. The overlying epidermis and dermis are typically uninvolved. Rimming of individual fat cells by neoplastic T cells is a helpful (though not entirely specific) diagnostic feature (Fig. 120.13). Necrosis, karyorrhexis and cytophagocytosis are common findings. In the early stages, the neoplastic infiltrates may lack significant atypia, and a heavy inflammatory infiltrate may predominate[74,75].

Immunophenotype

These lymphomas have a TCR-α/β+, CD3+, CD4−, CD8+ T-cell phenotype, with expression of cytotoxic proteins. CD30 and CD56 are rarely expressed.

Treatment

Patients have generally been treated with systemic chemotherapy or radiotherapy. However, recent studies suggest that many patients can be controlled for long periods of time with systemic corticosteroids[72,74].

EXTRANODAL NK/T-CELL LYMPHOMA, NASAL TYPE

Definition

Extranodal NK/T-cell lymphoma, nasal type is nearly always an EBV-positive lymphoma with an NK-cell, or more rarely a cytotoxic T-cell, phenotype. The skin is the second most common site of involvement after the nasal cavity/nasopharynx, and skin involvement may be a primary or secondary manifestation of the disease.

Epidemiology

Extranodal NK/T-cell lymphoma is a rare disease, particularly in Europe and the US. It is more common in Asia, Central America and South America. Patients are adults, with a predominance of males.

Clinical features

Patients generally present with multiple plaques or tumors, preferentially on the trunk and extremities. In the case of NK/T-cell lymphoma, nasal type, the clinical presentation is a midfacial destructive tumor; the latter was previously referred to as lethal midline granuloma[74,76,77] (Fig. 120.14). Ulceration is common. Although patients presenting with only skin lesions have a somewhat better prognosis than patients presenting with both cutaneous and extracutaneous disease, both groups experience a very aggressive clinical course and require the same type of treatment[78].

TWO TYPES OF SUBCUTANEOUS PANNICULITIS-LIKE T-CELL LYMPHOMA (SPTL)		
	SPTL α/β T-cell phenotype	SPTL γ/δ T-cell phenotype
Phenotype – T-cell receptor – T-cell phenotype – Coexpression of CD56	βF1+, TCRδ1− CD3+, CD4−, CD8+ Absent	βF1−, TCRδ1+ CD3+, CD4−, CD8− Common
Architecture	Subcutaneous	Subcutaneous and epidermal/dermal
Clinical features	Nodules and plaques Rarely ulceration	Nodules and plaques Ulceration common
Hemaphagocytic syndrome	Uncommon	Common
Survival rate (5-year)	>80%	<10%
Treatment	Systemic corticosteroids	Systemic chemotherapy
WHO-EORTC classification[3]	Subcutaneous panniculitis-like T-cell lymphoma	Cutaneous γ/δ T-cell lymphoma

Table 120.6 Two types of subcutaneous panniculitis-like T-cell lymphoma (SPTL)[1,2]. βF1, positivity reflects α/β T-cell origin; TCR, T-cell receptor.

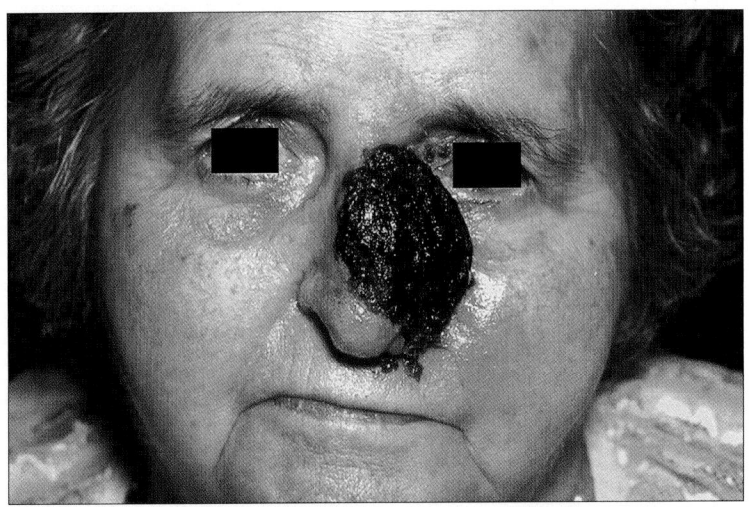

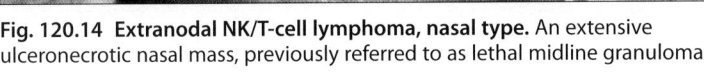

Fig. 120.14 **Extranodal NK/T-cell lymphoma, nasal type.** An extensive ulceronecrotic nasal mass, previously referred to as lethal midline granuloma.

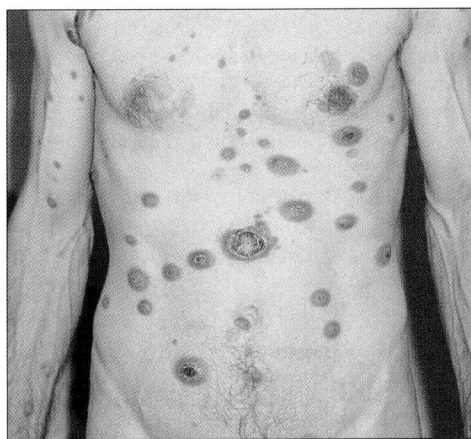

Fig. 120.15 **Aggressive epidermotropic CD8+ cutaneous T-cell lymphoma.** Generalized skin tumors with central ulceration. Previously, such cases were designated as disseminated pagetoid reticulosis (Ketron–Goodman type).

Pathology

These lymphomas are characterized by dense infiltrates involving the dermis and often the fat and deeper tissues. Prominent angiocentricity and angiodestruction are frequently accompanied by extensive necrosis[76,77]. NK/T-cell lymphoma has a broad cytologic spectrum ranging from small to large cells, with most cases consisting of medium-sized cells with irregular or oval nuclei, moderately dense chromatin and pale cytoplasm. In some cases, a heavy inflammatory infiltrate of small lymphocytes, histiocytes, plasma cells and eosinophils can be seen.

Immunophenotype

The neoplastic cells express CD2, CD56, cytoplasmic CD3ε and cytotoxic proteins (TIA-1, granzyme B, perforin), but lack surface CD3. In rare CD56− cases, detection of EBV by *in situ* hybridization and expression of cytotoxic proteins is required for diagnosis[79].

Treatment

Systemic chemotherapy is the recommended treatment, but the results are disappointing[76,77].

PRIMARY CUTANEOUS AGGRESSIVE EPIDERMOTROPIC CD8+ CYTOTOXIC T-CELL LYMPHOMA

These tumors are characterized by a proliferation of epidermotropic CD8+ cytotoxic T cells and an aggressive clinical behavior[80,81]. Differentiation from other types of CTCL expressing a CD8+ cytotoxic T-cell phenotype (i.e. >50% of patients with pagetoid reticulosis as well as rare cases of mycosis fungoides, lymphomatoid papulosis and C-ALCL) is based on the clinical presentation and clinical behavior. In these latter conditions, no differences in clinical presentation or prognosis are observed between CD4+ and CD8+ cases.

Clinically, aggressive epidermotropic CD8+ cytotoxic T-cell lymphomas are characterized either by the presence of localized or disseminated eruptive papules, nodules and tumors with central ulceration and necrosis or by superficial, hyperkeratotic patches and plaques (Fig. 120.15). The lymphoma may disseminate to other visceral sites (lung, testis, CNS, oral mucosa), but lymph nodes are often spared[80].

Histologically, these lymphomas show strongly epidermotropic, band-like to diffuse infiltrates of small, medium-sized or large pleomorphic T cells with a CD3+, CD4−, CD8+, CD7−/+, CD45RA+, granzyme B+, perforin+, TIA-1+ phenotype[71,80]. The epidermis may be acanthotic or atrophic, and it may have necrotic keratinocytes, ulceration and variable spongiosis, sometimes with blister formation. Invasion and destruction of adnexal structures are commonly seen. Angiocentricity and angioinvasion may be present.

These epidermotropic CD8+ cytotoxic T-cell lymphomas run an aggressive clinical course and should be treated with systemic chemotherapy[80].

CUTANEOUS γ/δ T-CELL LYMPHOMA

Cutaneous γ/δ T-cell lymphoma is characterized by a clonal proliferation of mature, activated γ/δ T cells with a cytotoxic phenotype. This group includes cases previously known as subcutaneous panniculitis-like T-cell lymphoma with a γ/δ phenotype (see Table 120.6).

Cutaneous γ/δ T-cell lymphomas generally present with disseminated plaques and/or ulceronecrotic nodules or tumors, particularly on the extremities[71,73]. Involvement of mucosal and other extranodal sites is frequently observed, but involvement of the lymph nodes, spleen or bone marrow is uncommon. In patients with panniculitis-like tumors, a hemophagocytic syndrome may occur[75].

Histologically, these lymphomas often show marked epidermotropism as well as involvement of the subcutaneous tissues[79]. The neoplastic cells are generally medium to large in size with coarsely clumped chromatin, and have a βF1−, CD3+, CD2+, CD4−, CD5−, CD7+/−, CD8−, CD56+ phenotype with strong expression of cytotoxic proteins. In frozen sections, the cells are strongly positive for TCR-δ. Angiocentricity and angiodestruction are commonly seen. The subcutaneous cases may show rimming of fat cells, similar to subcutaneous panniculitis-like T-cell lymphoma of α/β origin.

Most patients have an aggressive, often rapidly fatal, disease, which is resistant to multiagent chemotherapy. Patients with subcutaneous fat involvement may have a worse prognosis compared to patients with epidermal or dermal disease only[73].

PRIMARY CUTANEOUS CD4+ SMALL/MEDIUM-SIZED PLEOMORPHIC T-CELL LYMPHOMA

These lymphomas are defined as CTCL with a predominance of small to medium-sized CD4+ pleomorphic T cells without (a history of) patches and plaques typical of mycosis fungoides and in most cases a favorable clinical course[82]. In contrast to in the EORTC classification, in the WHO–EORTC classification scheme the term small/medium-sized pleomorphic CTCL is restricted to cases with a CD4+ T-cell phenotype. Cases with a CD3+, CD4−, CD8+ phenotype usually have a more aggressive clinical course similar to that of aggressive epidermotropic CD8+ cytotoxic T-cell lymphoma[83].

Characteristically, CD4+ small/medium-sized pleomorphic T-cell lymphomas present with a solitary plaque or tumor, generally on the face, the neck or the upper trunk. Less commonly, they present with one or several papules, nodules or tumors. These lymphomas have a rather favorable prognosis, especially those presenting with a solitary tumor or localized skin lesions[83–85].

Histologically, these lymphomas are characterized by dense, diffuse or nodular infiltrates within the dermis, with a tendency to infiltrate the subcutis. Epidermotropism may be present focally. There is a predominance of small/medium-sized CD3+, CD4+, CD8−, CD30− pleomorphic T cells. A small proportion (<30%) of large pleomorphic cells may be present[82]. In some cases, a considerable admixture with small reactive lymphocytes and histiocytes may be observed. Demonstration of an aberrant T-cell phenotype and clonality represent useful criteria for differentiating these small/medium-sized pleomorphic CTCLs from pseudo-T-cell lymphomas, which may also present with a solitary plaque or nodule[86].

In patients with solitary localized skin lesions, surgical excision or radiotherapy is the preferred mode of treatment. Cyclophosphamide (as single-agent therapy) and IFN-α have been reported as effective in patients with more generalized skin disease[87]. However, the optimal treatment for this group is still to be defined.

PRIMARY CUTANEOUS PERIPHERAL T-CELL LYMPHOMA, UNSPECIFIED

The designation peripheral T-cell lymphoma, unspecified is retained for cutaneous T-cell lymphomas that do not fit into any of the better-defined subtypes of CTCL, including the three provisional entities just described (see Table 120.1). Most cases in this category would have been classified as a primary cutaneous CD30⁻ large T-cell lymphoma in the EORTC classification, particularly those with a CD4⁺ T-cell phenotype. Clinically, these patients present with solitary or localized, but more frequently generalized, nodules or tumors[83] (Fig. 120.16).

Histologically, nodular or diffuse infiltrates with variable numbers of medium-sized to large pleomorphic or immunoblast-like T cells are observed. Epidermotropism is generally mild or absent. Most cases are characterized by an aberrant CD4⁺ T-cell phenotype with variable loss of pan-T-cell antigens. CD30 staining is negative or restricted to a few scattered tumor cells. Rare cases may show coexpression of CD56.

Patients should be treated with systemic chemotherapy, but the prognosis is generally poor, with a 5-year survival rate of less than 20%[3,83,85].

CD4⁺/CD56⁺ HEMATODERMIC NEOPLASM (BLASTIC NK-CELL LYMPHOMA)

In the WHO classification, blastic NK-cell lymphoma was included as a clinically aggressive neoplasm commonly involving the skin and probably derived from NK-cell precursors. However, more recent studies suggest derivation from a plasmacytoid dendritic cell precursor. *CD4⁺/CD56⁺ hematodermic neoplasm* and *early plasmacytoid dendritic cell leukemia/lymphoma* have been proposed as more appropriate terms for this condition[87,88]. In the WHO–EORTC classification, the term CD4⁺/CD56⁺ hematodermic neoplasm is preferred.

These neoplasms commonly present in the skin as solitary or multiple nodules or tumors with or without concurrent extracutaneous involvement. However, most patients who present with only cutaneous lesions rapidly develop involvement of the bone marrow, peripheral blood, lymph nodes and extranodal sites.

Histologically, these neoplasms are composed of non-epidermotropic, monotonous infiltrates of medium-sized cells with finely dispersed chromatin and absent or indistinct nucleoli. The cells resemble lymphoblasts or myeloblasts and usually have a CD4⁺, CD56⁺, CD8⁻, CD7⁺/⁻, CD2⁻/⁺, CD45RA⁺ phenotype, but do not express surface and cytoplasmic CD3 or cytotoxic proteins (Fig. 120.17). Staining for terminal deoxynucleotidyl transferase (TdT) and CD68 may be positive. Since lymphoblastic and myelomonocytic neoplasms can also be positive for CD56, stains for CD3 and myeloid markers should

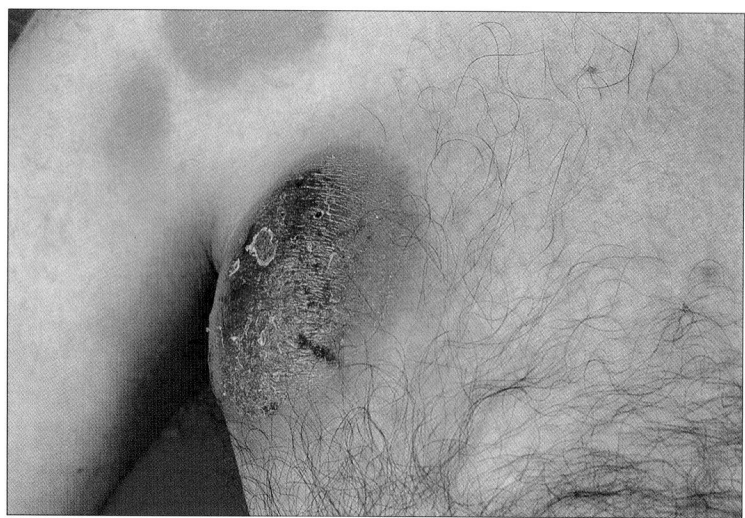

Fig. 120.16 Primary cutaneous peripheral T-cell lymphoma, unspecified. Rapidly growing nodules and tumors. Note: the skin lesions in the left upper corner do not represent patches, but rather deep plaques present for 2 weeks.

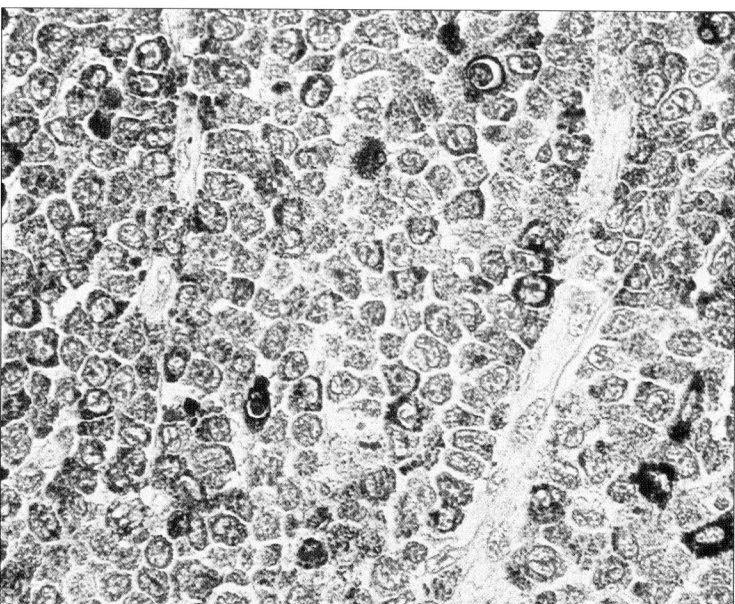

Fig. 120.17 CD4⁺/CD56⁺ hematodermic neoplasm (blastic NK-cell lymphoma). Monotonous proliferation of medium-sized to large CD3⁻, CD4⁺, CD8⁻ tumor cells, here showing strong expression of CD56.

always be performed in order to exclude these entities. The tumor cells also express CD123 (IL-3 receptor α-chain) and T-cell leukemia 1 (TCL1) antigen, both of which support a relationship to plasmacytoid dendritic cells[87,88]. Expression of TCL1 may be a useful additional marker to differentiate these CD4⁺/CD56⁺ hematodermic neoplasms from cutaneous lesions of acute myelogenous leukemia[88,89].

CD4⁺/CD56⁺ hematodermic neoplasm is an aggressive disease with a poor prognosis (median survival, 14 months)[78,88]. Systemic chemotherapy usually results in a complete remission, but quick relapses unresponsive to further chemotherapy are the rule. Recent studies suggest that allogeneic stem cell transplantation may be a better option in these patients[78].

REFERENCES

1. Willemze R, Kerl H, Sterry W, et al. EORTC classification for primary cutaneous lymphomas. A proposal from the Cutaneous Lymphoma Study Group of the European Organization for Research and Treatment of Cancer (EORTC). Blood. 1997;90:354–71.

2. Jaffe ES, Harris NL, Stein H, Vardiman JW (eds). World Health Organization Classification of Tumours. Pathology and Genetics of Tumours of Haematopoietic and Lymphoid Tissues. Lyon: IARC Press, 2001.

3. Willemze R, Jaffe ES, Burg G, et al. WHO-EORTC classification for cutaneous lymphomas. Blood 2005;105:3768–85.

4. Lutzner MA, Edelson RL, Schein P, et al. Cutaneous T-cell lymphomas: the Sézary syndrome, mycosis fungoides, and related disorders. Ann Intern Med. 1975;83:534–52.

5. Edelson RL. Cutaneous T cell lymphoma: mycosis fungoides, Sézary syndrome, and other variants. J Am Acad Dermatol. 1980;2:89–106.

6. Santucci M, Burg G, Feller AC. Interrater and intrarater reliability of histologic criteria in early cutaneous T-cell lymphoma: an EORTC Cutaneous Lymphoma Project Study Group. Dermatol Clin. 1994;12:323–7.

7. Rijlaarsdam JU, Scheffer E, Meijer CJLM, Willemze R. Cutaneous pseudo-T-cell lymphomas. A clinicopathologic study of 20 patients. Cancer. 1992;69:717–24.

8. Ralfkiaer E. Controversies and discussion on early diagnosis of cutaneous T-cell lymphoma: phenotyping. Dermatol Clin. 1994;12:329–34.

9. Moll M, Reinhold U, Kukel S, et al. CD7-negative helper T cells accumulate in inflammatory skin lesions. J Invest Dermatol. 1994;102:328–32.

10. Wood GS. T-cell receptor and immunoglobulin gene rearrangements in diagnosing skin disease. Arch Dermatol. 2001;137:1503–6.

11. Flaig MJ, Schumann K, Sander CA. Impact of molecular analysis in the diagnosis of cutaneous lymphoid infiltrates. Semin Cutan Med Surg. 2000;19:87–90.

12. Lukowski A, Muche JM, Sterry W, Audring H. Detection of expanded T-cell clones in skin biopsy samples of patients with lichen sclerosus et atrophicus by T-cell receptor-gamma polymerase chain reaction assays. J Invest Dermatol. 2000;115:254–9.

13. Willemze R, Beljaards RC, Meijer CJLM. Classification of primary cutaneous T-cell lymphoma. Histopathology. 1994;24:405–15.

14. Weinstock MA. Epidemiology of mycosis fungoides. Semin Dermatol 1994;13:154–9.

15. Karenko L, Hytinen E, Sarna S, Ranki A. Chromosomal abnormalities in cutaneous T-cell lymphoma and its premalignant conditions as detected by G-banding and interphase cytogenetic methods. J Invest Dermatol. 1997;108:22–9.

16. Navas JC, Ortiz-Romero PL, Villuendas R, et al. P16(INK4a) gene alterations are frequent in lesions of mycosis fungoides. Am J Pathol. 2000;156:1565–72.

17. Smoller BR, Santucci M, Wood GS, Whittaker SJ. Histopathology and genetics of cutaneous T-cell lymphoma. Hematol Oncol Clin North Am. 2003;17:1277–311.

18. Li G, Vowels BR, Benoit BM, et al. Failure to detect human T-lymphotropic virus type I (HTLV-I) proviral DNA in cell lines and tissues from patients with cutaneous T-cell lymphoma. J Invest Dermatol. 1996;7:308–13.

19. Hoppe RT, Medeiros LJ, Warnke R, et al. CD8-positive tumor-infiltrating lymphocytes influence the long-term survival of patients with mycosis fungoides. J Am Acad Dermatol. 1995;32:448–53.

20. Vermeer MH, van Doorn R, Dukers D, et al. CD8+ T-cells in cutaneous T-cell lymphoma: expression of cytotoxic proteins, FAS ligand and killing inhibitory receptors and relationship with clinical behaviour. J Clin Oncol. 2001;19:4322–9.

21. van Doorn R, Dijkman R, Vermeer MH, et al. A novel splice variant of the fas gene in patients with cutaneous T-cell lymphoma. Cancer Res. 2002;62:5389–92.

22. Kim EJ, Hess S, Richardson SK, et al. Immunopathogenesis and therapy of cutaneous T-cell lymphoma. J Clin Invest. 2005;115:798–812.

23. Hoppe RT, Wood GS, Abel EA. Mycosis fungoides and the Sézary syndrome: pathology, staging and treatment. Curr Probl Cancer. 1990;14:295–371.

24. van Doorn R, van Haselen CW, van Voorst PC, et al. Mycosis fungoides: disease evolution and prognosis of 309 Dutch patients. Arch Dermatol. 2000;136:504–10.

25. Smoller BR, Bishop K, Glusac E, Warnke R. Reassessment of histologic parameters in the diagnosis of mycosis fungoides. Am J Surg Pathol. 1995;19:1423–30.

26. Diamandidou E, Colome-Grimmer M, Fayad L, et al. Transformation of mycosis fungoides/Sézary syndrome: clinical characteristics and prognosis. Blood. 1998; 92:1150–9.

27. Lambert WC, Everett MA. The nosology of parapsoriasis. J Am Acad Dermatol. 1981;5:373–95.

28. Bunn P, Lamberg S. Report of the Committee on Staging and Classification of Cutaneous T-cell Lymphoma. Cancer Treat Rep. 1979;63:725–8.

28a. Olsen E, Vonderheid E, Pimpinelli N, et al. Revisions to the staging and classification of mycosis fungoides and Sézary syndrome: a proposal of the International Society for Cutaneous Lymphomas (ISCL) and the Cutaneous Lymphoma Task Force of the European Organization of Research and Treatment of Cancer (EORTC). Blood. 2007 May 31; [Epub ahead of print].

29. Kim YH, Willemze R, Pimpinelli N, et al. TNM classification system for primary cutaneous lymphomas other than mycosis fungoides and Sézary syndrome: a proposal of the International Society for Cutaneous Lymphomas (ISCL) and the cutaneous lymphoma task force of the European Organization of Research and Treatment of Cancer (EORTC). Blood. 2007;110:479–84.

30. Whittaker SJ, Marsden JR, Spittle M, Russell Jones R. Joint British Association of Dermatologists and U.K. Cutaneous Lymphoma Group guidelines for the management of primary cutaneous T-cell lymphomas. Br J Dermatol. 2003;149:1095–107.

31. Kaye FJ, Bunn PA, Steinberg SM, et al. A randomized trial comparing combination electron beam radiation and chemotherapy with topical therapy in the initial treatment of mycosis fungoides. N Engl J Med. 1989;321:784–90.

32. Zackheim HS, Kashani-Sabet M, Amin S. Topical corticosteroids for mycosis fungoides. Experience in 79 patients. Arch Dermatol. 1998;134:949–54.

33. Vonderheid EC, Tan E, Kantor AF, et al. Long-term efficacy, curative potential and carcinogenicity of topical mechlorethamine chemotherapy in cutaneous T-cell lymphoma. J Am Acad Dermatol. 1989;20:416–28.

34. Zackheim HS, Epstein EH, Crain WR. Topical carmustine (BCNU) for cutaneous T-cell lymphoma: a 15-year experience in 143 patients. J Am Acad Dermatol. 1990;22:802–10.

35. Jones GW, Kacinski BM, Wilson LD, et al. Total skin electron radiation in the management of mycosis fungoides: Consensus of the European Organization for Research and Treatment of Cancer (EORTC) Cutaneous Lymphoma Project Group. J Am Acad Dermatol. 2002; 47:364–70.

36. Querfield C, Rosen ST, Kuzel TM, et al. Long-term follow-up of patients with early-stage cutaneous T-cell lymphoma who achieved complete remission with psoralen plus UV-A monotherapy. Arch Dermatol. 2005;141:305–11.

37. Ramsey D, Lish K, Yalowitz C, et al. Ultraviolet-B phototherapy for early stage cutaneous T-cell lymphoma. Arch Dermatol. 1992;128:931–3.

38. Clark C, Dawe RS, Evans AT, et al. Narrowband TL-01 phototherapy for patch stage mycosis fungoides. Arch Dermatol. 2000;136:748–52.

39. Foss F. Mycosis fungoides and Sézary syndrome. Curr Opin Oncol. 2004;16:421–8

40. Olsen EA, Bunn PA. Interferon in the treatment of cutaneous T-cell lymphoma. Hematol Oncol Clin North Am. 1995;9:1089–97.

41. Kim YH, Hoppe RT. Mycosis fungoides and the Sézary syndrome. Semin Oncol. 1999;26:276–89.

42. van Doorn R, Scheffer E, Willemze R. Follicular mycosis fungoides: a distinct disease entity with or without associated follicular mucinosis. Arch Dermatol. 2002;138:191–8.

43. Bonta MD, Tannous ZS, Demierre MF, et al. Rapidly progressing mycosis fungoides presenting as follicular mucinosis. J Am Acad Dermatol. 2000;43:635–40.

44. Burns MK, Chan LS, Cooper KD. Woringer-Kolopp disease (localized pagetoid reticulosis) or unlesional mycosis fungoides? Arch Dermatol. 1995;131:325–9.

45. Haghighi B, Smoller BR, LeBoit PE, et al. Pagetoid reticulosis (Woringer-Kolopp disease): an immunophenotypic, molecular and clinicopathologic study. Mod Pathol. 2000;13:502–10.

46. LeBoit PE. Granulomatous slack skin. Dermatol Clin. 1994;12:375–89.

47. Vonderheid EC, Bernengo MG, Burg G, et al. Update on erythrodermic cutaneous T-cell lymphoma: report of the International Society for Cutaneous Lymphomas. J Am Acad Dermatol. 2002;46:95–106.

48. Wieselthier JS, Koh HK. Sézary syndrome: diagnosis, prognosis and critical review of treatment options. J Am Acad Dermatol. 1990;22:381–401.

49. Karenko L, Kahkonen M, Hyytinen ER, Lindlof M, Ranki A. Notable losses at specific regions of chromosomes 10q and 13q in the Sezary syndrome detected by comparative genomic hybridization. J Invest Dermatol. 1999;112:392–5.

50. Mao X, Lillington D, Scarisbrick JJ, et al. Molecular cytogenetic analysis of cutaneous T-cell lymphomas: identification of common genetic alterations in Sezary syndrome and mycosis fungoides. Br J Dermatol. 2002;147:464–75.

51. Toonstra J, Henquet CJM, van Weelden H, et al. Actinic reticuloid: a clinical, photobiologic, histopathologic and follow-up study of 16 cases. J Am Acad Dermatol. 1989;21:205–14.

52. Edelson R, Berger C, Gasparro F, et al. Treatment of cutaneous T-cell lymphoma by extracorporeal photochemotherapy. N Engl J Med. 1987;316:297–303.

53. Russell-Jones R. Extracorporeal photopheresis in cutaneous T-cell lymphoma. Inconsistent data underline the need for randomized studies. Br J Dermatol. 2000;142:16–21.

54. Shimoyama M. Diagnostic criteria and classification of clinical subtypes of adult T-cell leukemia-lymphoma: a report from the Lymphoma Study Group (1984-1987). Br J Haematol. 1991;79:428–37.

55. Yamada Y, Tomonaga M. The current status of therapy for adult T-cell leukemia-lymphoma in Japan. Leuk Lymphoma. 2003;44:611–18.

56. Willemze R, Beljaards RC. Spectrum of primary cutaneous CD30+ lymphoproliferative disorders. A proposal for classification and guidelines for management and treatment. J Am Acad Dermatol. 1993;28:973–80.

57. Bekkenk M, Geelen FAMJ, van Voorst Vader PC, et al. Primary and secondary cutaneous CD30-positive lymphoproliferative disorders: long term follow-up data of 219 patients and guidelines for diagnosis and treatment. A report from the Dutch Cutaneous Lymphoma Group. Blood. 2000;95:3653–61.

58. Liu HL, Hoppe RT, Kohler S, Harvell JD, Reddy S, Kim YH. CD30+ cutaneous lymphoproliferative disorders: the Stanford experience in lymphomatoid papulosis and primary cutaneous anaplastic large cell lymphoma. J Am Acad Dermatol. 2003;49:1049–58.

59. Beljaards RC, Meijer CJ, Scheffer E, et al. Prognostic significance of CD30 (Ki-1/Ber-H2) expression in primary cutaneous large-cell lymphomas of T-cell origin. A clinicopathologic and immunohistochemical study in 20 patients. Am J Pathol. 1989;135:1169–78.

60. DeCouteau JF, Butmarc JR, Kinney MC, Kadin ME. The t(2;5) chromosomal translocation is not a common feature of primary cutaneous CD30+ lymphoproliferative disorders: comparison with anaplastic large cell lymphoma of nodal origin. Blood. 1996;87:3437–41.

61. Natkunam Y, Warnke RA, Haghighi B, et al. Co-expression of CD56 and CD30 in lymphomas with primary presentation in the skin: clinicopathologic, immunohistochemical and molecular analyses of seven cases. J Cutan Pathol. 2000;27:392–9.

62. Vonderheid EC, Sajjadian A, Kadin ME. Methotrexate is effective therapy for lymphomatoid papulosis and other primary cutaneous CD30-positive lymphoproliferative disorders. J Am Acad Dermatol. 1996;34:470–80.

63. Macaulay WL. Lymphomatoid papulosis. A continuing self-healing eruption, clinically benign: histologically malignant. Arch Dermatol. 1968;97:23–30.

64. Davis TM, Morton CC, Miller-Cassman R, et al. Hodgkin's disease, lymphomatoid papulosis, and cutaneous T-cell lymphoma derived from a common T-cell clone. N Engl J Med. 1992;326:1115–22.

65. Mori M, Manuelli C, Pimpinelli N, et al. CD30-CD30L interaction in primary cutaneous CD30+ T-cell lymphomas: a clue to the pathophysiology of clinical regression. Blood. 1999;94:3077–83.

66. Schieman WP, Pfeifer WM, Levi E, et al. A deletion in the gene for transforming growth factor beta type I receptor abolishes growth regulation by transforming growth factor beta in cutaneous T-cell lymphoma. Blood. 1999;94:2854–61.

67. Beljaards RC, Willemze R. The prognosis of patients with lymphomatoid papulosis associated with malignant lymphomas. Br J Dermatol. 1992;126:596–602.

68. Willemze R, Scheffer E. Clinical and histological differentiation between lymphomatoid papulosis and

pityriasis lichenoides. J Am Acad Dermatol. 1985;133:418–28.

69. Varga FJ, Vonderheid EC, Olbricht SM, et al. Immunohistochemical distinction of lymphomatoid papulosis and pityriasis lichenoides et varioliformis acuta. Am J Pathol. 1990;136:979–87.

70. Salhany KE, Macon WR, Choi JK, et al. Subcutaneous panniculitis-like T-cell lymphoma: clinicopathologic, immunophenotypic, and genotypic analysis of alpha/beta and gamma/delta subtypes. Am J Surg Pathol. 1998;22:881–93.

71. Santucci M, Pimpinelli N, Massi D, et al. Cytotoxic/natural killer cell cutaneous lymphomas. Report of EORTC Cutaneous Lymphoma Task Force Workshop. Cancer. 2003;97:610–27.

72. Hoque SR, Child FJ, Whittaker SJ, et al. Subcutaneous panniculitis-like T-cell lymphoma: a clinicopathological, immunophenotypic and molecular analysis of six patients. Br J Dermatol. 2003;148:516–25.

73. Toro JR, Liewehr DJ, Pabby N, et al. Gamma-delta-T-cell phenotype is associated with significantly decreased survival in cutaneous T-cell lymphoma. Blood. 2003;101:3407–12.

74. Massone C, Chott A, Metze D, et al. Subcutaneous, blastic natural killer (NK), NK/T-cell and other cytotoxic lymphomas of the skin: a morphologic, immunophenotypic and molecular study of 50 patients. Am J Surg Pathol. 2004;28:719–35.

75. Marzano AV, Berti E, Paulli M, Caputo R. Cytophagocytic histiocytic panniculitis and subcutaneous panniculitis-like T-cell lymphoma. Arch Dermatol. 2000;136:889–96.

76. Cheung MMC, Chan JKC, Lau WH, et al. Primary non-Hodgkin lymphoma of the nose and nasopharynx: clinical features, tumor immunophenotype, and treatment outcome in 113 patients. J Clin Oncol. 1998;16:70–7.

77. Chan JK, Sin VC, Wong KF, et al. Nonnasal lymphoma expressing the natural killer cell marker CD56: a clinicopathologic study of 49 cases of an uncommon aggressive neoplasm. Blood. 1997;89:4501–13.

78. Bekkenk MW, Jansen PM, Meijer CJLM, Willemze R. CD56+ hematological neoplasms presenting in the skin: a retrospective analysis of 23 new cases and 130 cases from the literature. Ann Oncol. 2004;15:1097–108.

79. Jaffe ES, Krenacs L, Raffeld M. Classification of cytotoxic T-cell and natural killer cell lymphomas. Semin Hematol. 2003;40:175–84.

80. Berti E, Tomasini D, Vermeer MH, et al. Primary cutaneous CD8-positive epidermotropic cytotoxic T-cell lymphoma: a distinct clinicopathologic entity with an aggressive clinical behavior. Am J Pathol. 1999;155:483–92.

81. Agnarsson BA, Vonderheid EC, Kadin ME. Cutaneous T-cell lymphoma with suppressor/cytotoxic (CD8) phenotype: identification of rapidly progressive and chronic subtypes. J Am Acad Dermatol. 1990;22:569–77.

82. Beljaards RC, Meijer CJLM, van der Putte SCJ, et al. Primary cutaneous T-cell lymphomas. Clinicopathologic features and prognostic parameters of 35 cases other than mycosis fungoides and CD30-positive large cell lymphoma. J Pathol. 1994;172:53–60.

83. Bekkenk MW, Vermeer MH, Jansen PM, et al. Peripheral T-cell lymphomas unspecified presenting in the skin: analysis of prognostic factors in a group of 82 patients. Blood. 2003;102:2213–19.

84. Friedmann D, Wechsler J, Delfau MH, et al. Primary cutaneous pleomorphic small T-cell lymphoma. Arch Dermatol. 1995;31:1009–15.

85. Fink-Puches R, Zenahlik P, Bäck B, Smolle J, Kerl H, Cerrone L. Primary cutaneous lymphomas: applicability of current classification schemes (EORTC, WHO) based on clinicopathologic features observed in a large group of patients. Blood. 2002;99:800–5.

86. Bakels V, van Oostveen JW, van der Putte CJ, et al. Immunophenotyping and gene rearrangement analysis provide additional criteria to differentiate between cutaneous T-cell lymphomas and pseudo-T-cell lymphomas. Am J Pathol. 1997;150:1941–9.

87. Jacob MC, Chaperot C, Mossuz P, et al. CD4+ CD56+ lineage negative malignancies: a new entity developed from malignant early plasmacytoid dendritic cells. Haematologica. 2003;88:941–55.

88. Petrella T, Bagot M, Willemze R, et al. Blastic NK-cell lymphomas (agranular CD4+CD56+ hematodermic neoplasms). Am J Clin Pathol 2005;123:662–75.

89. Dijkman R, van Doorn R, Szuhai K, et al. Gene-expression profiling and array-based CGH classify CD4+CD56+ hematodermic neoplasm and cutaneous myelomonocytic leukemia as distinct disease entities. Blood. 2007;109:1720–7.

Other Lymphoproliferative and Myeloproliferative Diseases

121

Bruce R Smoller and Harry L Winfield

BENIGN LYMPHOCYTIC INFILTRATES

LYMPHOCYTIC INFILTRATE OF JESSNER

Synonyms: ■ Benign lymphocytic infiltration of the skin ■ Jessner's lymphocytic infiltration of the skin ■ Jessner's lymphocytic infiltrate of the skin ■ Jessner–Kanof lymphocytic infiltration of the skin

Key features

- Erythematous papules, plaques and, less commonly, nodules
- Most common on the head, neck and back
- Dermal infiltrate of lymphocytes without epidermal involvement

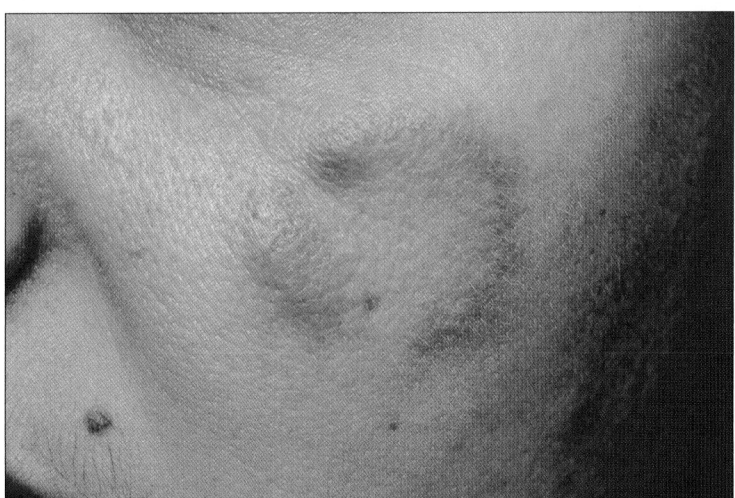

Fig. 121.1 Lymphocytic infiltrate of Jessner. Annular erythematous plaque on the face.

History

Lymphocytic infiltrate of Jessner was initially described in 1953 by Jessner & Kanof[1] as circinate papules on the face, surrounding a central area of clearing.

Epidemiology

Lymphocytic infiltrate of Jessner occurs with equal incidence in men and women, and it is a disease primarily of middle-aged adults. It is very rare in children. There does not appear to be any regional or seasonal variation in incidence.

Pathogenesis

Lymphocytic infiltrate of Jessner is an entity whose existence remains controversial. Various authors believe it is a variant of either lupus erythematosus, cutaneous lymphoid hyperplasia or polymorphous light eruption[2]. Others believe it to represent an infectious process (possibly related to *Borrelia burgdorferi* infection), while some have raised the possibility that lymphocytic infiltrate of Jessner is an early, evolving cutaneous T-cell lymphoma. There are cases of co-occurrence with lupus erythematosus and with polymorphous light eruption in the literature, further raising the possibility that these entities are related. Rare cases of drug-induced lymphocytic infiltrate of Jessner have been described. Incriminated drugs include glatiramer acetate, a polypeptide that shares amino acids with myelin used to treat multiple sclerosis, and angiotensin-converting enzyme (ACE) inhibitors[3,4].

Clinical features

Lymphocytic infiltrate of Jessner most commonly appears on the head, neck and upper back as one or several asymptomatic erythematous papules, plaques and, less commonly, nodules (Fig. 121.1). There are no secondary changes, such as scale, and annular plaques with central clearing are commonly observed. Individual lesions last several weeks to months. There are no systemic manifestations associated with lymphocytic infiltrate of Jessner. Emotional stress has been associated with exacerbation of the eruption in a minority of patients. The eruption resolves spontaneously and without sequelae in most patients.

Pathology

The epidermis is relatively unremarkable, with little evidence of lymphocytic exocytosis or interface dermatitis. There is a superficial and deep, primarily perivascular, lymphocytic infiltrate that may surround

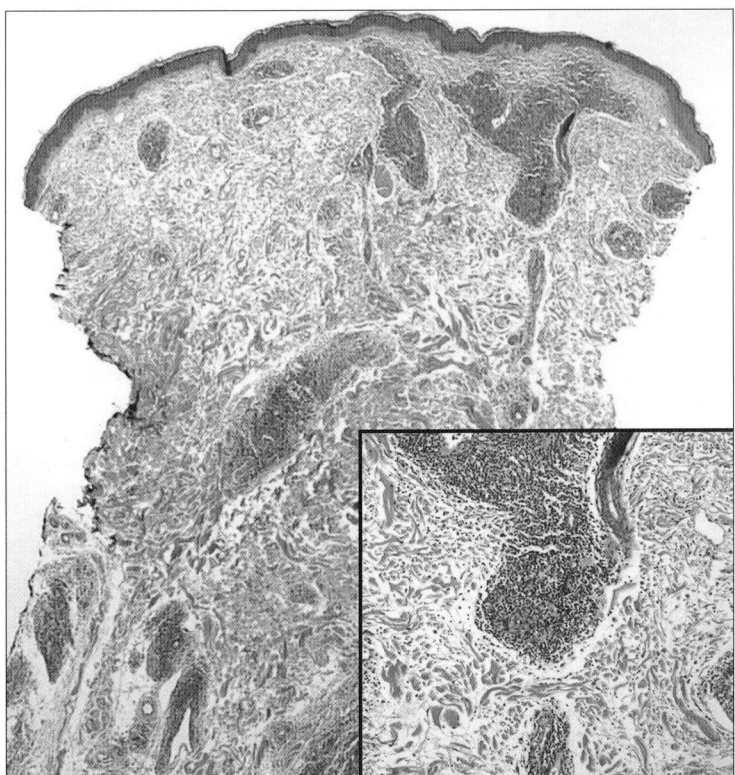

Fig. 121.2 Lymphocytic infiltrate of Jessner. A superficial and deep perivascular infiltrate without an interface component is characteristic.

hair follicles in some cases (Fig. 121.2). The majority of infiltrating lymphocytes express CD4 (T helper lymphocyte marker). Plasmacytoid monocytes may be present in small clusters or as single cells surrounding dermal venules, and their presence may be helpful in arriving at the diagnosis[5]. Slightly increased amounts of dermal mucin may be seen in the reticular dermis.

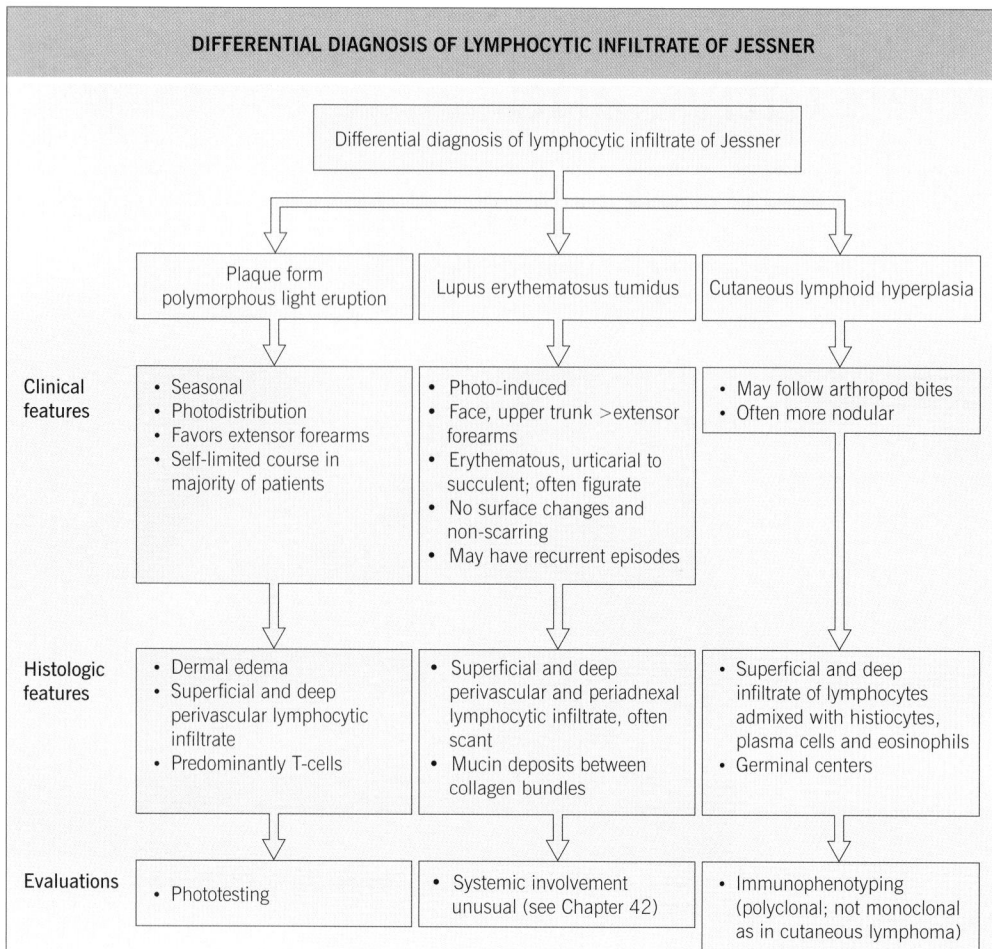

Fig. 121.3 Differential diagnosis of lymphocytic infiltrate of Jessner.

Differential diagnosis

The differential diagnosis includes the plaque form of polymorphous light eruption, cutaneous lymphoid hyperplasia (see below), cutaneous lymphoma, palpable migratory arciform erythema, and lupus erythematosus (Fig. 121.3). In contrast to lymphocytic infiltrate of Jessner, lesions of subacute and chronic lupus erythematosus have secondary changes, including scale, follicular plugging and central hypopigmentation. Histologically, interface changes with basal vacuolopathy and necrotic keratinocytes are seen, which are also features distinct from lymphocytic infiltrate of Jessner. However, in lupus erythematosus tumidus, interface changes are sparse, if present at all, and distinction is more difficult. Phototesting may prove helpful in establishing the diagnosis.

Polymorphous light eruption can be distinguished based upon its relationship to sun exposure and its usually self-limited clinical course. In addition, polymorphous light eruption frequently demonstrates abundant papillary dermal edema, a feature not present in lymphocytic infiltrate of Jessner. For some patients, however, it may be difficult (if not impossible) to distinguish between these entities. Phototesting may be of benefit (see Fig. 121.3).

Cutaneous lymphomas can have significant overlap with lymphocytic infiltrate of Jessner, both clinically and histologically. If the dermal lymphocytic infiltrate is extensive, immunophenotypic and genotypic analyses may help to distinguish the mixed cellular infiltrate seen in lymphocytic infiltrate of Jessner from a more uniform population characteristic of cutaneous lymphomas (see Chs 119 & 120; Fig. 119.9). Palpable migratory arciform erythema is a rare eruption, characterized histologically by dermal lymphoid infiltrates and clinically by irregularly shaped, enlarging plaques on the trunk, arms and thighs. The lesions tend to arise and resolve over a period of days to weeks, as opposed to weeks to months for lymphocytic infiltrate of Jessner. Histologically, palpable migratory arciform erythema lacks the mucin occasionally seen in lymphocytic infiltrate of Jessner and it has a distinct absence of any plasma cells[6].

Treatment

The cutaneous manifestations of lymphocytic infiltrate of Jessner resolve spontaneously within months to years, and they do not result in scarring. Oral antibiotics and topical or intralesional corticosteroids have been used with limited success. Up to 50% of patients may improve with hydroxychloroquine. Lymphocytic infiltrate of Jessner is generally resistant to radiation therapy. A crossover study of oral thalidomide (100 mg/day) versus placebo in 25 patients resulted in a clinical response of 76% for thalidomide and 16% for placebo.

CUTANEOUS LYMPHOID HYPERPLASIA (LYMPHOCYTOMA CUTIS)

Synonyms: ■ Lymphocytoma cutis ■ Lymphadenosis benigna cutis (LABC) ■ Spiegler–Fendt sarcoid

Key features

- Erythematous to violaceous nodule or plaque
- Most common on the face and upper trunk
- Mixed dermal infiltrate of lymphocytes, plasma cells and eosinophils
- Follicular centers are common
- Polyclonal inflammatory infiltrate

History

Cutaneous lymphoid hyperplasia (CLH) was first reported by Spiegler in 1894. He described patients who presented with clinical features of a sarcoma but experienced a benign clinical course. Subsequent investigators recognized the reactive lymphocytic nature of the process.

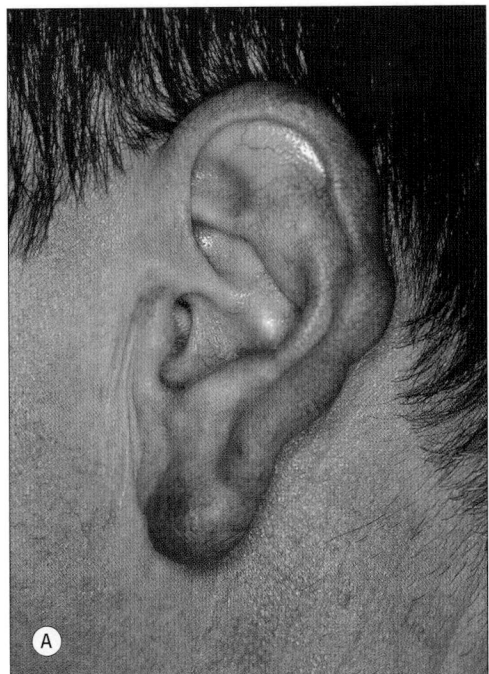 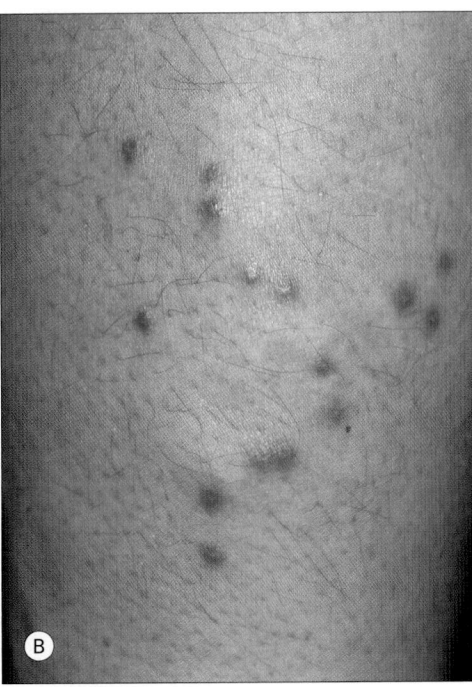

Fig. 121.4 Cutaneous lymphoid hyperplasia (lymphocytoma cutis). A Violet papulonodules on the helix and lobe of the ear (unknown etiology). **B** Multiple red–brown to violet papules at the sites of *Hirudo medicinalis* (medicinal leech) application. B, Courtesy of Josef Smolle MD.

Epidemiology

CLH is seen most often in adults, and it may be slightly more common in women than in men. The disorder has been reported in children.

Pathogenesis

CLH almost certainly does not represent a single disease state, but rather reflects an exaggerated local immunologic reaction to a stimulus, often unrecognized. Inciting agents include arthropod bites, tattoos, vaccinations and medications, including antihistamines, antidepressants and angiotensin II receptor blockers[7-9]. In Europe, *Borrelia burgdorferi* infection has been associated with CLH[10].

Clinical features

A firm, erythematous to violaceous papule, plaque or nodule is most commonly located on the head and neck or upper extremities (Fig. 121.4). Clusters of papules are also seen. The majority of lesions have no surface changes. Rarely, slight scale or follicular accentuation has been described.

Pathology

A superficial and deep nodular or diffuse infiltrate of lymphocytes, admixed with histiocytes and occasional plasma cells and eosinophils, characterizes CLH. The dermal infiltrate is quite dense and recapitulates nodal architecture. In florid cases, germinal centers with prominent tingible-body macrophages are apparent (Fig. 121.5). A mantle zone may be present surrounding the lymphoid follicles. Differentiation from cutaneous lymphoma may be difficult; however, in most cases, the distinction can be made on routine histologic sections or with the addition of immunostains.

Although immunophenotypic analysis may reveal either a T- or B-cell-predominant pattern, the overall appearance is that of a mixed infiltrate. Typically, B-cell-predominant infiltrates express a mixture of both kappa and lambda light chains (see Fig. 119.10). In T-cell-predominant infiltrates, the most common cell type is a CD4+ T helper lymphocyte with a significant minority population of CD8+ cytotoxic/suppressor T cells. Expression of CD68 demonstrates the presence of histiocytes, occasionally containing tingible bodies. A subpopulation of cases, 61% in one study, may possess clonal populations of either T or B cells, and CLH may rarely eventuate into overt cutaneous lymphoma. Whether the presence of clonal populations is a marker for progression to lymphoma, or reflects a lymphoma at the outset, remains uncertain[11,12].

Differential diagnosis

The clinical differential diagnosis includes lymphoma cutis, non-lymphoid metastatic disease, lymphocytic infiltrate of Jessner, and, occasionally, adnexal tumors. The histologic differential diagnosis of CLH includes cutaneous lymphoma (usually of the B cell type; Table 121.1),

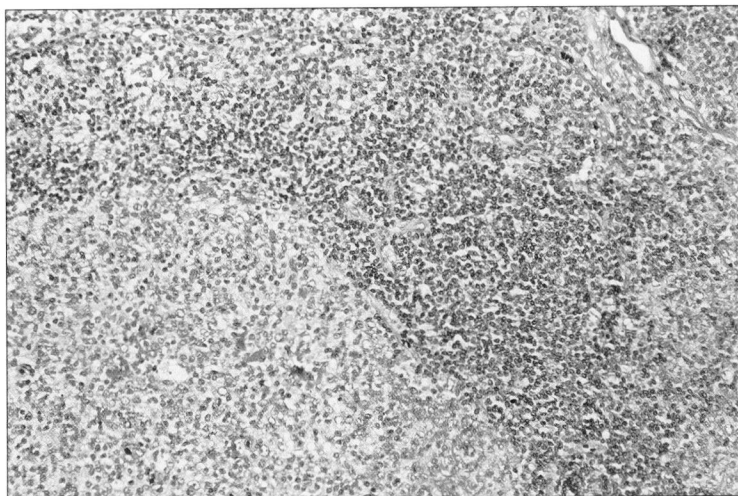

Fig. 121.5 Cutaneous lymphoid hyperplasia (lymphocytoma cutis). Germinal center formation, tingible-body macrophages, and a mantle zone are present.

MICROSCOPIC DIFFERENCES BETWEEN CUTANEOUS LYMPHOID HYPERPLASIA AND CUTANEOUS LYMPHOMA	
Cutaneous lymphoid hyperplasia	**Cutaneous B-cell lymphoma**
Histologic features	
Mixed cellular infiltrate	Lymphocytic infiltrate
Mixed population of lymphocytes	Uniform-appearing lymphocytes
Germinal follicles	No germinal follicles
Mantle zone	No mantle zone
Tingible-body macrophages	No tingible-body macrophages
No destruction of appendages	Appendageal infiltration and destruction
Patterned infiltrate	Diffuse infiltrate
Immunophenotypic features	
T and B lymphocytes	Uniform B lymphocytes
Mixed CD4+ and CD8+ lymphocytes	Rare CD4+ or CD8+ cells*
Mixed kappa and lambda expression	Restricted kappa or lambda expression
Bcl-2 only on T lymphocytes	Bcl-2 on neoplastic B cells (some cases)
Exception is T-cell-rich B-cell lymphoma.	

Table 121.1 Microscopic differences between cutaneous lymphoid hyperplasia and cutaneous lymphoma.

lymphocytic infiltrate of Jessner, the plaque form of polymorphous light eruption, and, occasionally, tumid lesions of lupus erythematosus. Cutaneous lymphoid hyperplasia can be differentiated from lymphoma based upon the presence of reactive germinal centers, a polymorphous infiltrate of lymphocytes and histiocytes, and the presence of eosinophils and/or plasma cells. If these distinctions cannot be made on routine histologic sections, immunophenotyping of the lymphocytes can distinguish between the two, with reactive states demonstrating a mixed population of cells and neoplastic ones a more restricted population.

Lymphocytic infiltrate of Jessner is difficult to characterize precisely (see above), but it is thought to be a predominantly T cell infiltrate, whereas, in most cases, CLH demonstrates a brisk B lymphocytic component. The distinguishing features of polymorphous light eruption and lupus erythematosus tumidus are outlined in Figure 121.3. The inflammatory infiltrates of polymorphous light eruption display a more perivascular distribution than do those of CLH, and eosinophils and plasma cells are uncommon.

Acral pseudolymphomatous angiokeratoma of children (APACHE) was originally thought to represent a vascular nevus, but is now categorized as a pseudolymphoma. In contrast to CLH, it favors the extremities of children between the ages of 2 and 16 years, usually presenting with a unilateral grouping of small, red to violet, 'angiomatous' papules. Histologically, a dermal infiltrate of lymphocytes, histiocytes and plasma cells is often accompanied by prominent thickened capillaries.

Treatment

Cutaneous lymphoid hyperplasia is a benign, reactive condition, and it should be treated conservatively. Often, there is spontaneous resolution without scarring. In persistent or florid cases, topical and/or intralesional corticosteroids have been used with some efficacy. Simple excision, cryosurgery, laser ablation and radiation therapy are other options. Thalidomide has also been utilized with success in recalcitrant cases[13].

EXTRAMEDULLARY HEMATOPOIESIS

Key features

- Evidence of bone marrow dysfunction
- Most commonly associated with TORCH (*t*oxoplasmosis, *r*ubella, *c*ytomegalovirus and *h*erpes virus) infections in neonates and myelofibrosis in adults
- Widely disseminated erythematous to violaceous papules and nodules, with neonatal form referred to as 'blueberry muffin baby'
- Diffuse dermal infiltrate of immature erythrocytes, leukocytes and, sometimes, megakaryocytes

Epidemiology

Extramedullary hematopoiesis is most commonly seen in neonates secondary to underlying bone marrow dysfunction. It may occur in adults secondary to myelofibrosis or other myeloproliferative disorders or after splenectomy.

Pathogenesis

Extramedullary hematopoiesis within the skin can occur normally during early embryogenesis but abates prior to birth. Thereafter, it occurs only as a secondary phenomenon in response to altered bone marrow function. Rarely, primary cutaneous neoplasms such as pilomatricomas, nevus sebaceus, hemangiomas and pyogenic granulomas may be associated with localized extramedullary hematopoiesis[14].

Clinical features

The clinical presentation is usually one of erythematous to violaceous papules and nodules, with occasional plaques, ulcers or nasal polyps[15]. When widely disseminated, as is seen most frequently in neonates, it leads to the classic 'blueberry muffin baby' (Fig. 121.6). This can be seen as a consequence of congenital viral infections or severe and chronic prenatal anemias (Table 121.2). Serologic titers for the TORCH

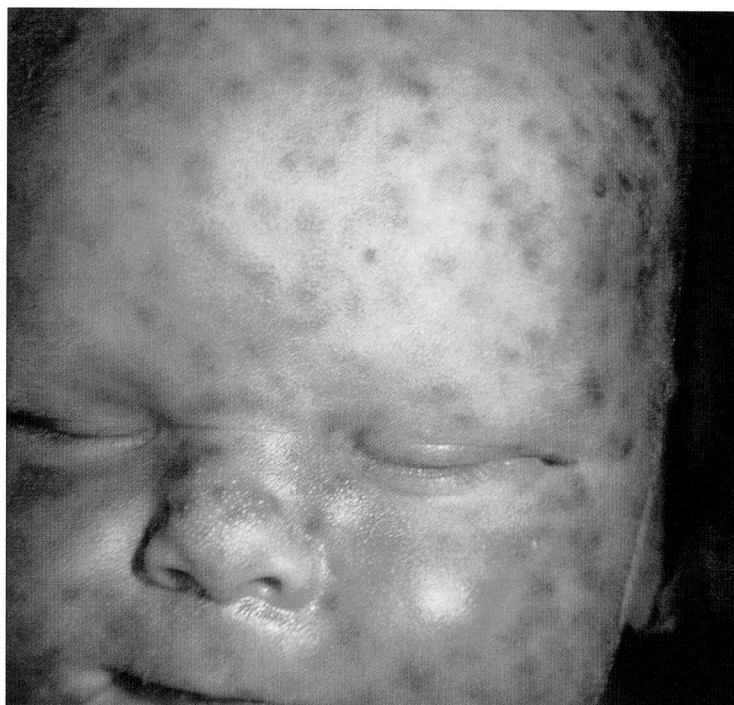

Fig. 121.6 Extramedullary hematopoiesis. 'Blueberry muffin baby' secondary to congenital rubella. Courtesy of James Graham MD.

DIFFERENTIAL DIAGNOSIS OF 'BLUEBERRY MUFFIN BABY'

Disseminated extramedullary hematopoiesis
- Prenatal infections
  - TORCH
    - Congenital rubella
    - Cytomegalovirus
    - Toxoplasmosis
  - Coxsackievirus
  - Parvovirus
- Severe and chronic prenatal anemias
  - Severe hemolytic anemias
    - Congenital spherocytosis
    - Rhesus hemolytic disease
    - ABO incompatibility
  - Twin–twin transfusion
  - Chronic fetomaternal hemorrhage
  - Severe internal bleeding (e.g. intracranial)
  - Myelodysplasia, congenital leukemia
Congenital leukemia cutis
Neonatal neuroblastoma
Congenital Langerhans cell histiocytosis
Congenital alveolar cell rhabdomyosarcoma
Hemangiomatosis, other vascular lesions (e.g. multifocal lymphangioendotheliomatosis, glomuvenous malformations)

Table 121.2 Differential diagnosis of 'blueberry muffin baby'.

---

infections are useful in evaluating neonates. Biopsy-proven dermal hematopoiesis is most often seen with rubella and cytomegalovirus.

Pathology

Extramedullary hematopoiesis is characterized by a dermal infiltrate of immature red and white blood cell precursors and megakaryocytes. It is usually centered around vessels of the superficial vascular plexus, but it may also involve the deeper reticular dermis extending into the interstitial collagen, becoming diffuse and dense in more florid cases. Precursors of all three hematopoietic cell lines are present in varying ratios, depending upon the underlying disease process.

Differential diagnosis

Histologically, the differential diagnosis of extramedullary hematopoiesis is relatively limited. The most important distinctions are with disseminated congenital leukemia cutis and neonatal neuroblastoma.

In extramedullary hematopoiesis, all three hematopoietic cell lines (erythrocytes, leukocytes and megakaryocytes) are represented, whereas in leukemias, the cutaneous infiltrate is comprised predominantly of immature leukocytes, many of which are cytologically atypical. In patients with overwhelming marrow involvement by leukemia, extramedullary hematopoiesis can occur simultaneously with the leukemic involvement of the skin, further complicating the differential diagnosis.

Treatment

Treatment of the cause of the underlying bone marrow dysfunction results in reversal of the cutaneous process. Spontaneous resolution can occur with some viral infections.

MALIGNANT HEMATOPOIETIC INFILTRATES

LEUKEMIA CUTIS

Key features

- Red to purple papules and nodules; hemorrhagic ulcers
- Diffuse dermal infiltrate of neoplastic leukocytes
- Immature precursor cells in some types

Epidemiology

There are multiple types of leukemia, each of which has its own epidemiologic characteristics. Acute lymphoblastic leukemia (ALL) tends to be a neoplasm of childhood. Acute myelogenous leukemia (AML) and chronic myelogenous leukemia (CML) occur primarily in adults, and chronic lymphocytic leukemia (CLL) and hairy cell leukemia are most common in elderly patients.

Pathogenesis

Certain types of leukemia have been associated with specific chromosomal abnormalities. For example, the Philadelphia chromosome, the primary diagnostic feature of CML, represents a translocation between chromosomes 9 and 22 [t(9;22)]. This translocation results in a fusion of the two genes BCR and ABL, with constitutive activation of the tyrosine kinase activity of Abl. It is this kinase activity that is selectively inhibited by imatinib mesylate (Gleevec®). In addition, 95% of patients with promyelocytic leukemia have a t(15;17) anomaly, which leads to abnormal expression of a fusion retinoic acid receptor that is the target of all-trans retinoic acid therapy. In ALL and AML, there is a variety of non-random chromosomal abnormalities, and Table 121.3 demonstrates the relationship between specific abnormalities and prognosis in ALL. Detection and analysis of these chromosomal abnormalities are leading to a greater understanding of the pathogenesis of leukemias, more accurate prognostic information, and more effective directed therapies.

RELATIONSHIP BETWEEN SPECIFIC CHROMOSOMAL ABNORMALITIES AND PROGNOSIS IN ACUTE LYMPHOCYTIC LEUKEMIA	
Chromosomal abnormalities	**Prognosis**
t(9;22)(q34;q11.2)	Unfavorable
t(4;11)(q21;q23)	Unfavorable
t(1;19)(q23;p13.3)	Unfavorable
t(12;21)(p13;q22)	Favorable
Hyperdiploid >50	Favorable
Trisomy 4, 10, 17	Favorable
Hypodiploidy	Unfavorable

Table 121.3 **Relationship between specific chromosomal abnormalities and prognosis in acute lymphocytic leukemia (precursor B lymphoblastic leukemia/lymphoblastic lymphoma type).**

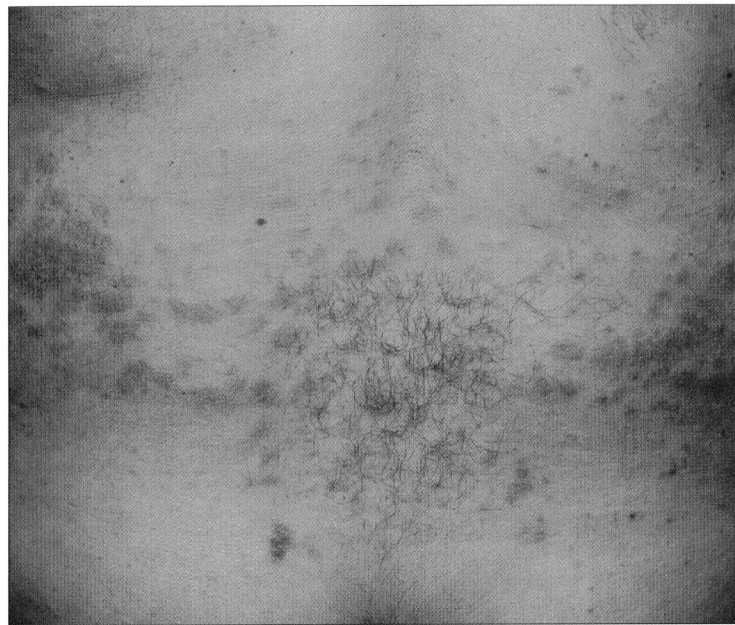

Fig. 121.7 **Leukemia cutis.** Multiple red–brown papules and plaques in a patient with hairy cell leukemia.

Clinical features

Leukemia can cause non-specific reactive skin lesions (Table 121.4) or specific infiltrates of leukemia cutis. In the latter, firm papules and nodules (Fig. 121.7), often hemorrhagic, are frequently seen; thrombocytopenia probably plays a role in the associated hemorrhage. Purpura, ulcers and, rarely, blisters have been described. While lesions of leukemia cutis can appear in any location, the head, neck and trunk are most commonly involved. Leukemic infiltrates can also arise at sites of trauma or scars. Rarely, myelogenous leukemias may present with dermal nodules known as chloromas or granulocytic sarcomas. Upon sectioning and exposure to air, these nodules assume a blue–green color due to the myeloperoxidase granules within the neoplastic leukocytes. Granulocytic sarcomas may precede the development of systemic leukemia by months. Gingival hyperplasia secondary to leukemic infiltrates is seen in some patients with acute monocytic and acute myelomonocytic leukemias.

In one series, cutaneous eruptions of leukemia accounted for 30% of all skin biopsy specimens in patients with leukemia[16]; although >60% of the patients with leukemia cutis had AML, cutaneous leukemic infiltrates accounted for a smaller proportion of total skin biopsies from patients with AML and ALL compared to patients with CLL and CML. Other common cutaneous findings in this group of patients were GVHD, drug eruptions, infectious processes, purpura and small vessel vasculitis. In most patients with acute leukemia, cutaneous lesions are present at the time of diagnosis or recurrence. On occasion, skin involvement precedes the appearance of leukemia in the peripheral smear. This situation is referred to as 'aleukemic' leukemia cutis. Rarely, leukemia cutis predates apparent bone marrow involvement by months. Recurrence of AML can lead to leukemic infiltrates in extramedullary sites, including the skin. These are sometimes designated extramedullary myeloid cell tumors[17].

Table 121.4 summarizes the 'inflammatory' disorders associated with acute and chronic leukemias.

Pathology

The histologic features of leukemia cutis vary with the type of leukemia. Typically, there is an infiltrate of leukemic cells throughout the dermis, which may be perivascular or form tumor nodules with diffuse spread of single cells through the interstitial collagen. There is frequently a dense peri-eccrine infiltrate of neoplastic hematopoietic cells[22].

AML is characterized by an infiltrate of immature myeloid cells. These cells recapitulate myeloid precursor cells at the most immature stages of development. In many cases, cytoplasmic granules can be found. A chloroacetate esterase stain may be helpful in detecting myeloid differentiation but, in very immature precursor cells, myeloid granules may not be present. There is often abundant hemorrhage within skin biopsy specimens of AML. ALL is characterized by an infiltrate of

'INFLAMMATORY' DISORDERS ASSOCIATED WITH ACUTE AND CHRONIC LEUKEMIAS	
Disorder	**Associated leukemias**
Neutrophilic dermatoses	
Sweet's syndrome	AML > CML, hairy cell leukemia, CNL > ALL, CLL
Pyoderma gangrenosum*	AML, CML, hairy cell leukemia > ALL, CLL
Neutrophilic eccrine hidradenitis	AML >> ALL, CML, CLL
Reactive erythemas	
Exaggerated arthropod reactions	CLL
Erythroderma	CLL[†]
Vasculitis	
Polyarteritis nodosa	Hairy cell leukemia >> CMML
Vasculitis (small vessel/ leukocytoclastic)	Hairy cell leukemia, CLL > AMML, ALL
Erythema elevatum diutinum	Hairy cell leukemia, CLL
Panniculitis	
Erythema nodosum[‡]	AML, CML, CMML
Other panniculitides[§]	Hairy cell leukemia, AML, CMML
Other	
Erythema multiforme[#]	CLL
Urticaria	CLL, hairy cell leukemia
Paraneoplastic pemphigus	CLL
Recalcitrant adult-onset eczema	CLL (T cell)
Acral ischemia with lividity	CML[¶]

*Especially bullous.
[†]Many probably represented Sézary syndrome.
[‡]Isolated case reports; may occur concomitantly with Sweet's syndrome.
[§]Sweet's syndrome may have a subcutaneous component.
[#]May have represented paraneoplastic pemphigus.
[¶]Leukostasis/hyperleukocytosis syndrome.

Table 121.4 'Inflammatory' disorders associated with acute and chronic leukemias[18–22]**.** ALL, acute lymphoblastic leukemia; AML, acute myelogenous leukemia; AMML, acute myelomonocytic leukemia; CLL, chronic lymphocytic leukemia; CML, chronic myelogenous leukemia; CMML, chronic myelomonocytic leukemia; CNL, chronic neutrophilic leukemia.

immature-appearing lymphoid cells. Cytoplasmic granularity is not present. These cells may be difficult to identify in skin biopsy specimens, and immunostaining for terminal deoxytransferase (tdt) is helpful in identifying these cells.

CML demonstrates a range of myeloid precursors, including promyelocytes, metamyelocytes, bands and mature neutrophils. All but the most immature cells will stain with a chloroacetate stain. CLL is characterized by a dense infiltrate of remarkably uniform-appearing small round lymphocytes (Fig. 121.8). The infiltrating cells appear mature, but the monomorphous nature and paucity of other cell types within the infiltrate are evidence in favor of a leukemic infiltrate.

Differential diagnosis

The clinical presentations of leukemia cutis are so protean that there is a lengthy clinical differential diagnosis, including lymphoma cutis, infectious emboli, vasculitis and drug eruptions. The histologic differential diagnosis of leukemia cutis depends upon the type of leukemia present. For lymphoid leukemias, the differential diagnosis includes lymphoma. In most cases, this distinction is made on the basis of bone marrow and lymph node involvement. Histologically, it can be very difficult, if not impossible, to distinguish some cases of leukemia cutis from lymphomas involving the skin. For myeloid leukemias, the differential diagnosis includes extramedullary hematopoiesis (see above), Sweet's syndrome, cutaneous small vessel vasculitis and other neutrophilic dermatoses. Recognizing immature and atypical leukocytic precursors in leukemic infiltrates allows the distinction from reactive neutrophilic infiltrates. A question yet to be addressed is whether immature leukocytes can appear in the skin with various 'reactive rashes' (as opposed to 'leukemia cutis') just because they are a prominent component of a patient's circulating cells.

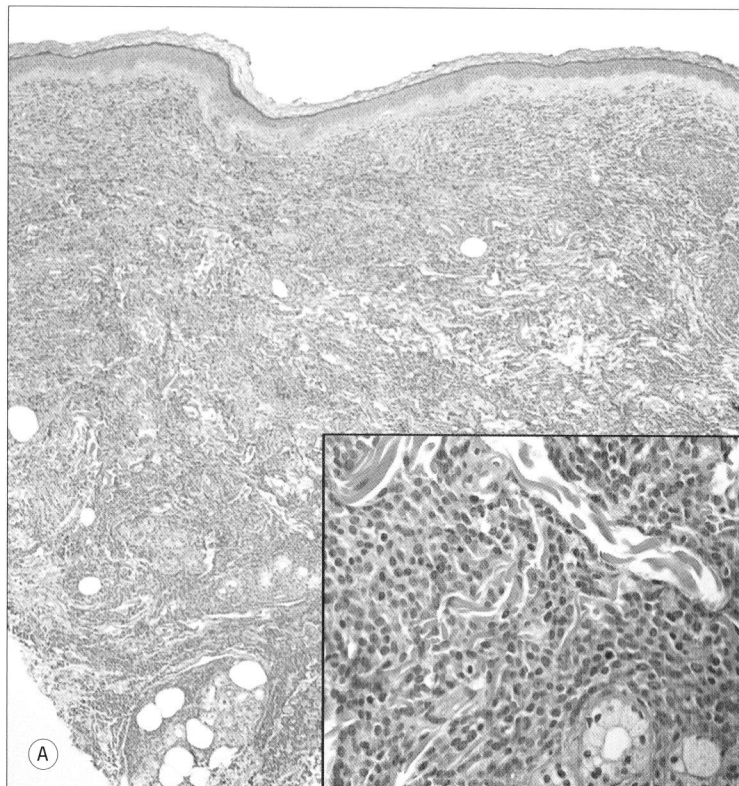

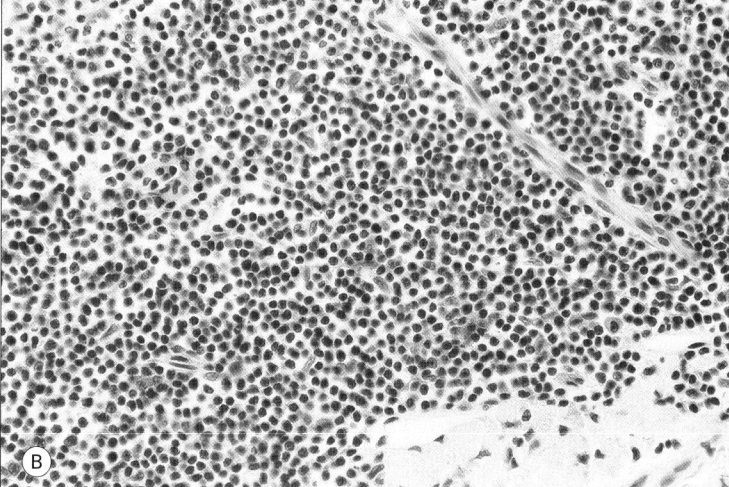

Fig. 121.8 Chronic lymphocytic leukemia (CLL). A CLL infiltrates the skin in a dense and diffuse manner. **B** The cells in CLL are strikingly monomorphous and lack significant cytologic atypia.

Treatment

There is no specific treatment for leukemia cutis. The cutaneous eruptions typically resolve in the setting of successful treatment of the leukemia.

NON-B-CELL, NON-T-CELL LYMPHOMAS

Hodgkin Disease

Synonym: ■ Hodgkin lymphoma

Key features

- Advanced stage in most patients with skin involvement
- Dermal nodules and plaques, sometimes ulcerated
- Dense dermal infiltrate with lymphocytes and eosinophils
- Atypical cells (lacunar cells, Reed–Sternberg cells)

History

In 1832, Thomas Hodgkin described a series of patients with lymphadenopathy, splenomegaly and weight loss, all of whom died of their disease. Wilks reported a subsequent series of patients in 1885, and designated the illness Hodgkin's disease.

Epidemiology

Isolated cutaneous involvement by Hodgkin disease (HD) is very unusual. In the vast majority of cases, cutaneous involvement occurs in patients with advanced disease. In one large study, 0.5% of patients with HD had cutaneous involvement, and the skin manifestations preceded apparent nodal disease in only one patient[23]. These rare isolated cutaneous cases may follow a more indolent course than their systemic counterparts, even with the subsequent development of nodal involvement. Isolated cutaneous cases, some with an aggressive course, have been reported in patients with advanced HIV infection[24]. There is no known gender preference. The incidence of HD peaks in young adults, with a second smaller peak in people in their fifties.

Pathogenesis

The pathogenesis of HD remains unknown, although Epstein–Barr virus (EBV) has been implicated in a minority of cases[25]. Recent evidence suggests that in the majority of cases of classic HD, the Reed–Sternberg cell represents a malignant B lymphocyte[26]; however, in isolated cutaneous cases, there is evidence that the malignant cells are of a T-cell lineage[27].

Clinical features

Isolated cutaneous HD presents as one or several ulcerated nodules with no apparent site predilection. Constitutional symptoms such as fevers, chills and night sweats may not be present, and there may be no evidence of hepatosplenomegaly or lymphadenopathy. Spontaneous regression of primary lesions has been reported.

The more common presentation is that of multiple disseminated papulonodules and plaques appearing rapidly in a patient with known, advanced disease. Cutaneous lesions often occur at sites distal to affected lymph nodes. The trunk is the most common site of involvement (Fig. 121.9).

Pathology

The histologic features of cutaneous HD (primary or secondary) are similar to affected lymph nodes. A dense dermal infiltrate consisting of lymphocytes with occasional eosinophils and plasma cells is present. Epidermotropism is usually not seen. Depending upon the histologic subtype, Reed–Sternberg cells (or mononuclear variants) may be present (Fig. 121.10). Lacunar cells may also be present. The latter, most common in the nodular sclerosing subtype of HD, are large cells with abundant eosinophilic cytoplasm. The retraction of this cytoplasm from adjacent cells during fixation gives rise to a giant cell residing within a clear space. Areas of dermal sclerosis may be seen, and extension into the subcutaneous fat is common.

Reed–Sternberg cells express CD30 (Ki-1), fascin and CD15, but fail to express CD45RB (leukocyte common antigen). The background infiltrate of lymphocytes is composed predominantly of T cells[28]. In lymphocytic-predominant HD, the malignant cell stains positively for CD20.

Differential diagnosis

The histologic differential diagnosis of HD includes large cell anaplastic lymphoma and lymphomatoid papulosis (see Ch. 120). The clinical presentation is important in differentiating between these entities. Lymphomatoid papulosis and large cell anaplastic lymphoma each present with scattered nodules and papules. In the patients with lymphomatoid papulosis, there is no evidence of systemic involvement (unless there is a concomitant lymphoma) and crops of lesions appear and spontaneously resolve. In patients with large cell anaplastic lymphoma, nodal involvement may be seen. In contrast, primary cutaneous HD is very rare, and virtually all patients with cutaneous involvement have advanced disease.

Histologically, each of these entities demonstrates a mixed infiltrate with varying numbers of large, atypical cells. These cells may be CD30-positive in all three diseases. In HD, unlike the other two, the cells will

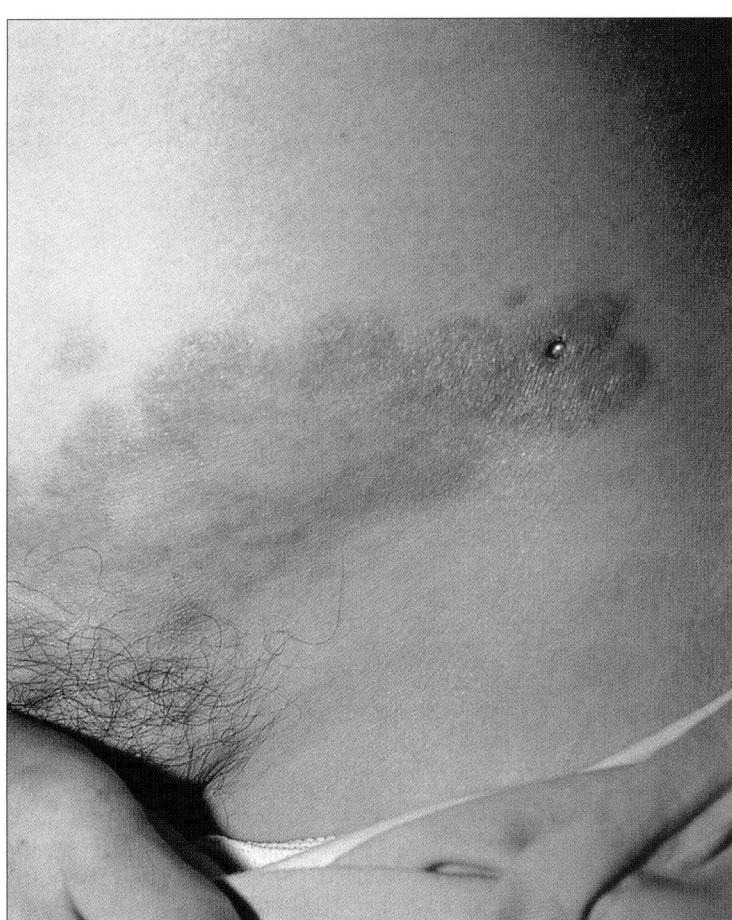

Fig. 121.9 Cutaneous Hodgkin disease. A large pink plaque with central clearing is noted on the lower abdomen.

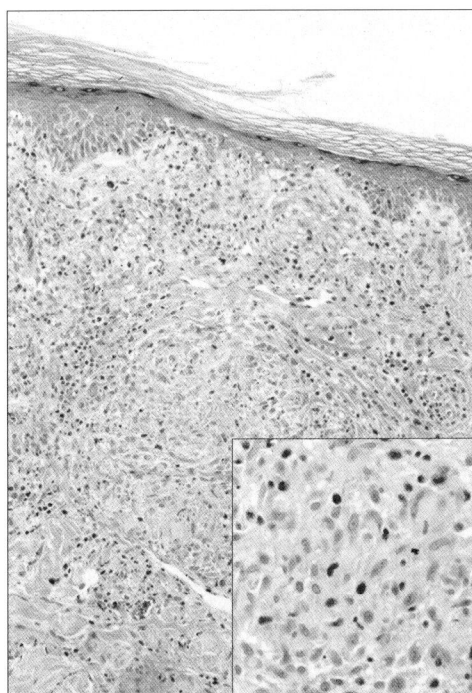

Fig 121.10 Cutaneous Hodgkin disease. Characteristic Reed–Sternberg cells may be seen amidst a mixed lymphocytic background.

also express CD15. In large cell anaplastic lymphoma, the majority of the infiltrate is composed of malignant cells, with a relatively small number of reactive inflammatory cells. In lymphomatoid papulosis, the infiltrate is more heterogeneous, with fewer large, atypical cells.

Treatment

Though the number of cases reported is small, the prognosis for patients with primary cutaneous HD appears to be similar to that of other patients with early stage disease. Many patients do not develop systemic disease. Currently, patients with stage IV HD have a cure rate of approximately 60% following combination chemotherapy[29].

Extranodal Natural Killer Cell Lymphoma

Synonyms: ■ NK/T-cell lymphoma ■ Nasal-type NK lymphoma ■ Angiocentric lymphoma ■ Polymorphic/malignant midline reticulosis

Key features

- Nodules, often with ulceration
- Extranodal sites of involvement are common
- Dense perivascular infiltrate of atypical lymphocytes
- Vascular destruction and thrombosis
- CD56 expression by neoplastic cells

History

The concept of the natural killer (NK) cell lymphoma is still developing. The entity may be closely related, if not identical, to entities previously known as lethal midline granuloma and midline malignant reticulosis. It seems likely that NK cell lymphoma does not represent a single entity, but rather is a group of lymphomas with overlapping clinical, histologic and immunologic properties.

Epidemiology

NK cell lymphoma is an uncommon disease that affects middle-aged to older adults of Asian, Central American and South American heritage. There is no gender predilection. In a large series, NK cell lymphomas accounted for less than 3% of cutaneous lymphomas[30].

Pathogenesis

NK cell lymphomas appear to be related to latent EBV infection in some, but not all, variants of this disease.

Clinical features

Patients with NK cell lymphoma usually present with nodules or plaques (Fig 121.11), some of which may be ulcerated. Less commonly, purpura may be the predominant cutaneous manifestation. In addition to the skin, the upper aerodigestive tract, CNS and skeletal muscle are frequently involved, and may be the site of initial involvement[30]. Hepatosplenomegaly and lymphadenopathy can appear with disease progression.

Pathology

NK cell lymphomas are characterized by a dense perivascular infiltrate of pleomorphic medium-sized lymphocytes. The cells invade dermal

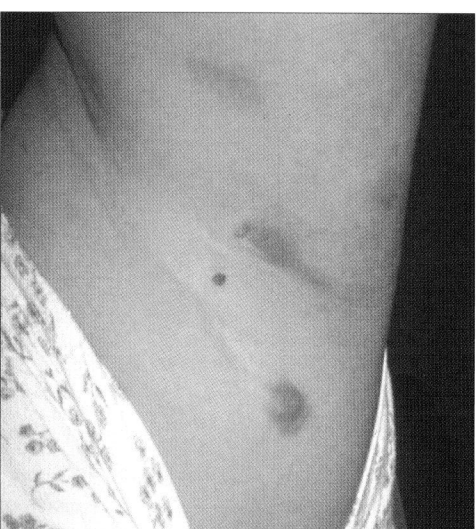

Fig. 121.11 Natural killer (NK) cell lymphoma. Multiple erythematous nodules and plaques in the axilla. Courtesy of Jeffrey E Frederic MD.

vessels, causing vascular destruction, thrombosis and extravasation of erythrocytes. The vascular occlusion frequently results in dermal and epidermal necrosis and ulceration – a common histologic change in this type of lymphoma. The infiltrate is almost always rather dense and extends into the subcutaneous fat. Epidermotropism is not a usual feature. Plasma cells and eosinophils are not abundant in most cases[31].

The neoplastic cell labels with CD56, a neural adhesion molecule expressed by NK cells. They are often CD2-, granzyme B-, TIA-1- and perforin-positive. Although membrane expression of CD3 is often negative, the cytoplasmic epsilon fragment of CD3 is frequently positive. Evidence for a clonal T-cell gene rearrangement is usually lacking[30].

Differential diagnosis

The histopathologic differential diagnosis of NK cell lymphoma includes other types of lymphomas. Many cutaneous T-cell lymphomas display epidermotropism and adnexotropism that are not characteristic of NK cell lymphomas. In addition, NK cell lymphomas are much more likely to invade and destroy vessels, causing thrombosis and necrosis, than are cutaneous T-cell lymphomas. Subcutaneous panniculitis-like T-cell lymphomas can be angiocentric, but are distinguished from NK cell lymphomas by different immunostaining profiles of the neoplastic cells as well as by the presence of a clonally arranged T-cell receptor that is usually not detected in NK cell lymphomas.

B-cell lymphomas are also in the differential diagnosis, but these do not ordinarily invade and destroy blood vessels. Immunolabeling studies serve to make the distinction relatively straightforward in most cases.

Treatment

These tumors frequently follow an aggressive course resulting in the death of the patient[30]. The mean survival time in one study was 12.2 months from the time of diagnosis[32].

ANGIOIMMUNOBLASTIC LYMPHADENOPATHY

Synonyms: ■ Angioimmunoblastic lymphadenopathy with dysproteinemia ■ Immunoblastic lymphadenopathy ■ Angioimmunoblastic T-cell lymphoma ■ Lymphogranulomatosis X

Key features

- Constitutional symptoms (fever, sweats, weight loss)
- Morbilliform erythema
- Polyclonal gammopathy, autoantibodies, hemolytic anemia, thrombocytopenia, eosinophilia and pleural effusions
- Generalized lymphadenopathy and hepatosplenomegaly
- Dermal infiltrate with immunoblasts and increased vascularity

History

Several groups in the mid-1970s described the syndrome of generalized lymphadenopathy, hepatosplenomegaly and systemic symptoms[33].

Epidemiology

Angioimmunoblastic lymphadenopathy (AILD) is a rare disease of adults, with up to 80% of cases occurring in individuals over the age of 50 years.

Pathogenesis

Angioimmunoblastic lymphadenopathy is a lymphoproliferative disorder whose exact pathogenesis remains unknown. One theory is that it represents an exaggerated response to (super)antigens. It has been associated with exposure to various drugs, including antibiotics and anticonvulsants. Others have implicated EBV infection in the pathogenesis, but this is an inconstant finding[34]. Chromosomal abnormalities are found in those patients who have progressed to peripheral T-cell lymphoma (e.g. trisomy 3, trisomy 5, an additional X chromosome).

Clinical features

Patients with AILD present with fever, weight loss, night sweats, generalized lymphadenopathy, and hepatosplenomegaly[34]. Approximately half of patients with AILD have cutaneous manifestations. The most common presentation is a widespread morbilliform erythema that resembles a viral exanthem[35]. Other cutaneous findings include petechiae (often associated with thrombocytopenia), urticaria, purpura and, rarely, erythroderma. Generalized pruritus may be a presenting symptom. The majority of patients with AILD progress to a high-grade T-cell lymphoma[34].

Pathology

A mixed infiltrate of lymphocytes, plasma cells, histiocytes and immunoblasts coursing along blood vessels is seen. When seen in the context of increased dermal vascularity, the diagnosis can be suspected or confirmed. T-cell gene rearrangements are detected in most patients.

Differential diagnosis

The morbilliform nature of the eruption belies its malignant nature. Consequently, confusion with a drug eruption or viral exanthem is common. As histologic changes are often subtle, a specific diagnosis often cannot be rendered.

Treatment

Treatment with systemic corticosteroids and multidrug chemotherapeutic regimens has been advocated. Response to treatment varies widely. The prognosis for patients with AILD is generally quite poor, with a 50–75% mortality rate and a mean survival of 1 to 2 years from time of presentation[36]. Most patients die of infectious complications rather than tumor burden, leading to the suggestion that a significant contributing factor to mortality is an underlying immunodeficiency.

LYMPHOMATOID GRANULOMATOSIS

> ## Key features
>
> - EBV-driven angiocentric/destructive lymphoproliferative disorder
> - Presents with cough, dyspnea, chest pain and constitutional symptoms
> - Cavitary pulmonary nodules on chest radiograph
> - Nodular to ulcerative cutaneous lesions in 25–50% of patients

History

Lymphomatoid granulomatosis was initially described in 1972 as a pulmonary angiitis/granulomatosis closely mimicking Wegener's granulomatosis. Although initially thought to represent a reactive process, subsequent studies demonstrated a malignant clonal B-cell population admixed with an abundant polyclonal reactive T-cell population.

Epidemiology

Lymphomatoid granulomatosis is a rare disease of adults, usually presenting in the fifth to sixth decade of life. The male-to-female ratio is approximately 2:1. The disease can affect children, most commonly in the setting of immunodeficiency syndromes.

Pathogenesis

The pathogenesis of lymphomatoid granulomatosis is often related to EBV infection, occasionally in combination with immunosuppression. Based upon case reports, immunosuppressive factors associated with lymphomatoid granulomatosis include renal transplantation, Wiskott–Aldrich syndrome, HIV infection and X-linked lymphoproliferative syndrome[37].

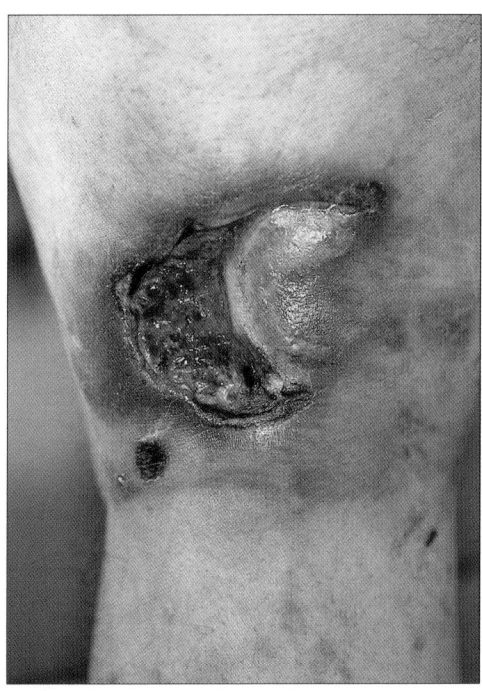

Fig. 121.12 Lymphomatoid granulomatosis. Ulcerated violaceous plaque in the popliteal fossa. Courtesy of Jean L Bolognia MD.

Clinical features

Patients with lymphomatoid granulomatosis typically present with symptoms related to respiratory tract involvement, such as cough, dyspnea and chest pain. Additional constitutional symptoms include fever, weight loss, malaise, arthralgias and myalgias. Cutaneous lesions are present in 25–50% of patients and usually range from nodules to ulcerated plaques (Fig. 121.12). Rarely, lymphomatoid granulomatosis may present as an exanthem of macules and papules. The kidney, brain and gastrointestinal tract may be affected. In contrast to angioimmunoblastic lymphadenopathy, the lymph nodes and spleen are rarely involved.

Pathology

Lesions of lymphomatoid granulomatosis show nodular lymphoid infiltrates composed of lymphocytes, plasma cells and large atypical mononuclear cells surrounding and invading arteries and veins. Granulomatosis, as defined by necrosis within lymphoid aggregates in the absence of granuloma formation, is a distinct and prominent feature. The atypical cells stain with B-cell markers and EBV DNA can be detected via *in situ* hybridization.

Differential diagnosis

The clinical differential diagnosis includes various forms of cutaneous lymphoma as well as infectious and inflammatory disorders (e.g. medium vessel vasculitis, pyoderma gangrenosum). The histologic differential diagnosis is broad and encompasses most of the lymphoproliferative disorders mentioned above, including B-cell and T-cell lymphomas. Other disorders with histologic evidence of granulomatosis (as defined above) include Wegener's granulomatosis, sarcoidosis and infectious processes. Diagnosis is based upon histopathologic findings plus immunophenotypic and genotypic analyses.

Treatment

Lymphomatoid granulomatosis generally follows an aggressive course, with 5-year mortality ranging from 60% to 90%. Treatment commonly involves anti-CD20 antibody, multidrug chemotherapy and, for milder cases, interferon-α.

REFERENCES

1. Jessner M, Kanof NB. Lymphocytic infiltration of the skin. Arch Dermatol. 1953;68:447–9.

2. Toonstra J, Wildschut A, Boer J, et al. Jessner's lymphocytic infiltration of the skin. A clinical study of 100 patients. Arch Dermatol. 1989;125:1525–30.

3. Nolden S, Casper C, Kuhn A, Petereit HF. Jessner-Kanof lymphocytic infiltration of the skin associated with glatiramer acetate. Mult Scler. 2005;11:245–8.

4. Schepis C, Lentini M, Siragusa M, Batolo D. ACE-inhibitor-induced drug eruption resembling lymphocytic infiltration (of Jessner-Kanof) and lupus erythematosus tumidus. Dermatology. 2004;208:354–5.

5. Toonstra J, van der Putte SC. Plasmacytoid monocytes in Jessner's lymphocytic infiltration of the skin. A valuable clue for the diagnosis. Am J Dermatopathol. 1991;13:321–8.

6. Abeck D, Ollert MW, Eckert F, et al. Palpable migratory arciform erythema. Clinical morphology, histopathology, immunohistochemistry and response to treatment. Arch Dermatol. 1997;133:763–6.

7. Crowson AN, Magro CM. Antidepressant therapy. A possible cause of atypical cutaneous lymphoid hyperplasia. Arch Dermatol. 1995;131:925–9.

8. Magro CM, Crowson AN. Drugs with antihistaminic properties as a cause of atypical cutaneous lymphoid hyperplasia. J Am Acad Dermatol. 1995;32:419–28.

9. Viraben R, Lamant L, Brousset P. Losartan-associated atypical cutaneous lymphoid hyperplasia. Lancet. 1997;350:1366.

10. Albrecht S, Hofstadter S, Artsob H, et al. Lymphadenosis benigna cutis resulting from *Borrelia* infection (*Borrelia* lymphocytoma). J Am Acad Dermatol. 1991;24:621–5.

11. Gilliam AC, Wood GS. Cutaneous lymphoid hyperplasias. Semin Cutan Med Surg. 2000;19:133–41.

12. Nihal M, Mikkola D, Horvath N, et al. Cutaneous lymphoid hyperplasia: a lymphoproliferative continuum with lymphomatous potential. Hum Pathol. 2003;34:617–22.

13. Benchikhi H, Bodemer C, Fraitag S, et al. Treatment of cutaneous lymphoid hyperplasia with thalidomide: report of two cases. J Am Acad Dermatol. 1999;40:1005–7.

14. Vega Harring SM, Niyaz M, Okada S, Kudo M. Extramedullary hematopoiesis in a pyogenic granuloma: a case report and review. J Cutan Pathol. 2004;31:555–7.

15. Brennan LV, Mayer T, Devitt J. Extramedullary hematopoiesis occurring as a nasal polyp in a man with a myeloproliferative disorder. Ear Nose Throat J. 2004;83:258–9.

16. Desch JK, Smoller BR. The spectrum of cutaneous disease in leukemias. J Cutan Pathol. 1993;20:407–10.

17. Traweek ST, Arber DA, Rappaport H, Brynes RK. Extramedullary myeloid cell tumors. An immunohistochemical and morphologic study of 28 cases. Am J Surg Pathol. 1993;17:1011–19.

18. Arai E, Ikeda S, Itoh S, Katayama I. Specific skin lesions as the presenting symptom of hairy cell leukemia. Am J Clin Pathol. 1988;90:459–64.

19. Carsuzaa F, Pierre C, Jaubert D, Viala JJ. Cutaneous findings in hairy cell leukemia. Review of 84 cases. Nouv Rev Fr Hematol. 1994;35:541–3.

20. Spann CR, Callen JP, Yam LT, Apgar JT. Cutaneous leukocytoclastic vasculitis complicating hairy cell leukemia (leukemic reticuloendotheliosis). Arch Dermatol. 1986;122:1057–9.

21. Fischer G, Commens C, Bradstock K. Sweet's syndrome in hairy cell leukemia. J Am Acad Dermatol. 1989;21:573–4.

22. Longacre TA, Smoller BR. Leukemia cutis. Analysis of 50 biopsy-proven cases with an emphasis on occurrence in myelodysplastic syndromes. Am J Clin Pathol. 1993;100:276–84.

23. Smith JL Jr, Butler JJ. Skin involvement in Hodgkin's disease. Cancer. 1980;45:354–61.

24. Jurisic V, Bogunovic M, Colovic N, Colovic M. Indolent course of the cutaneous Hodgkin's disease. J Cutan Pathol. 2005;32:176–8.

25. Vasef MA, Kamel OW, Chen Y-Y, et al. Detection of Epstein-Barr virus in multiple sites involved by Hodgkin's disease. Am J Pathol. 1995;147:1408–15.

26. Chan WC. The Reed-Sternberg cell in classical Hodgkin's disease. Hematol Oncol. 2001;19:1–17.

27. Kadin ME, Drews R, Samel A, et al. Hodgkin's lymphoma of T cell type: clonal association with a CD30+ cutaneous lymphoma. Hum Pathol. 2001;32:1269–72.

28. Cerroni L, Beham-Schmid C, Kerl H. Cutaneous Hodgkin's disease. J Cutan Pathol. 1995;22:229–35.

29. Tesch H, Diehl V, Lathan B, et al. Moderate dose escalation for advanced stage Hodgkin's disease using the bleomycin, etoposide, adriamycin, cyclophosphamide, vincristine, procarbazine, and prednisone scheme and adjuvant radiotherapy: a study of the German Hodgkin's Lymphoma Study Group. Blood. 1998;92:4560–7.

30. Savoia P, Fierro MT, Novelli M, et al. CD56 positive cutaneous lymphoma: a poorly recognized entity in the spectrum of primary cutaneous disease. Br J Dermatol. 1997;137:966–71.

31. Petrella T, Dalac S, Maynadie M, et al. CD4+ CD56+ cutaneous neoplasms: a distinct hematological entity. Am J Surg Pathol. 1999;23:137–46.

32. Nagatani T, Okazawa H, Kambara T, et al. Cutaneous monomorphous CD4- and CD56-positive large-cell lymphoma. Dermatology. 2000;200:202–8.

33. Frizzera G, Moran EM, Rappaport H. Angio-immunoblastic lymphadenopathy with dysproteinemia. Lancet. 1974;1:1070–3.

34. Martel P, Laroche L, Courville P, et al. Cutaneous involvement in patients with angioimmunoblastic lymphadenopathy with dysproteinemia: a clinical, immunohistological, and molecular analysis. Arch Dermatol. 2000;136:881–6.

35. Gross AS, Kagan SA, Hargreaves HK, et al. Fever, maculopapular eruption, and lymphadenopathy: angioimmunoblastic lymphadenopathy (AILD). Arch Dermatol. 1994;130:1551, 1554.

36. Pangalis GA, Moran EM, Nathwani BN, et al. Angioimmunoblastic lymphadenopathy: long-term follow-up study. Cancer. 1983;52:318–21.

37. Jaffe ES, Wilson WH. Lymphomatoid granulomatosis: pathogenesis, pathology and clinical implications. Cancer Surv. 1997;30:233–48.

Cutaneous Metastases

Daniel Davis and Donna Pellowski

Key features

- Cutaneous metastasis is rare, may be the presenting sign of a malignancy, and has historically had a bad prognosis
- In women, breast carcinoma and melanoma are the most common malignancies metastatic to the skin
- In men, melanoma and head and neck, lung and colon carcinoma are the most common malignancies metastatic to the skin
- Of the common malignancies, breast carcinoma is the most likely and prostate carcinoma is the least likely to metastasize to the skin
- The typical morphology of a cutaneous metastasis is a firm, painless, mobile, erythematous dermal papule that grows to a nodule which may ulcerate
- Cutaneous metastases are generally in the anatomic vicinity of the primary cancer
- Cutaneous metastases often have histologic features similar to, but not identical to, those of the primary malignancy
- Treatment options include chemotherapy, radiotherapy, immunotherapy, excision and observation
- The therapeutic response of cutaneous metastases may mirror the systemic response

THE PERCENTAGES OF PATIENTS WITH METASTATIC CANCER WHO HAD CUTANEOUS METASTASES		
Primary malignancy	Patients with metastatic cancer (n = 4020)	Patients with cutaneous metastases (n = 420; 10%)
Melanoma	172	77 (45%)
Breast	707	212 (30%)
SCC of the head & neck (e.g. laryngeal, oral)	221	29 (13%)
Endocrine glands	24	3 (12.5%)
Esophagus	35	3 (8.5%)
Urinary bladder	85	7 (8%)
Unknown	271	20 (7.5%)
Gallbladder/bile ducts	38	2 (5.5%)
Liver	21	1 (5%)
Kidney	130	6 (4.5%)
Colon/rectum	413	18 (4.5%)
Ovary	249	10 (4%)
Lung	802	21 (2.5%)
Endometrium	183	4 (2%)
Stomach	147	3 (2%)
Pancreas	107	2 (2%)
Uterine cervix	195	2 (1%)
Prostate	207	0
Testes	13	0

Table 122.1 **The percentages of patients with metastatic cancer who had cutaneous metastases.** SCC, squamous cell carcinoma. Adapted from Lookingbill DP, Spangler N, Helm KF. Cutaneous metastases in patients with metastatic carcinoma: a retrospective study of 4020 patients. J Am Acad Dermatol. 1993;29:228–36.

INTRODUCTION

Cancer metastatic to the skin requires a pre-existing cancer at another site. Cutaneous metastasis is rare, may be the presenting sign of a malignancy, and has historically signified a bad prognosis. Cancer may spread to the skin via vascular transit, lymphatic transit, contiguous growth, or iatrogenic implantation.

EPIDEMIOLOGY

The literature regarding cutaneous metastasis is limited because it is retrospective and based significantly on autopsy series, referral patterns, and biased demographics[1–7]. Frequently cited statistics of metastatic rates are from a retrospective study published in 1993[7]. Table 122.1 ranks the percentage of cutaneous metastases as a subset of systemic metastasis. For example, lung cancer has the highest incidence of total metastasis, but ranks very low with regard to percentage of cutaneous metastases. Table 122.1 does not indicate those patients who had exclusively cutaneous metastasis. Table 122.2 ranks the overall percent likelihood of particular primary malignancies in patients with cutaneous metastases, according to gender. In comparison to Table 122.1, a cancer such as lung carcinoma is ranked highly even though it rarely metastasizes to skin, simply because it is so common.

It is doctrine that the most common cutaneous metastases are from breast carcinoma in women and melanoma in both sexes. It is likely not a coincidence that the breast is a modified skin appendage and that melanocytes largely reside in the skin, and this may explain these observations. In adult men, metastases from the oropharynx and from lung and colon carcinoma also rank highly. Cutaneous metastasis is most common from the fifth to seventh decade. Metastasis in children is uncommon and is not included in Tables 122.1 or 122.2. In children, the highest ranking malignancies are leukemia, neuroblastoma, and rhabdomyosarcoma[8].

PATHOGENESIS

Cancer results after a number of successive stages in a process known as tumorigenesis. A cancer is the clonal product of somatic and hereditary genetic alterations that have been selected to have a phenotypic advantage. Although a tumorigenic phenotype is a prerequisite for metastasis, metastasis does not always follow tumorigenicity, as exemplified by basal cell carcinoma[9].

Metastasis is a complex, dynamic, and relatively inefficient process. Few cancers complete the metastatic sequence[10]. It occurs only after the cancer has acquired the positive attributes that allow it to survive in the host's environment and after the cancer has lost the negative regulators that impeded its spread. Early in the metastatic sequence, cancer cells begin to function autonomously. Some cells produce autocrine motility factors that stimulate their own tissue movement. Invasion is enhanced by loss of normal cell–cell adhesion, which is largely mediated by cadherins. Experimental increases of E-cadherin production resulted in cancer cells with a less invasive phenotype, implicating E-cadherin as a metastasis suppressor[10]. Integrin-mediated cell migration and adhesion between cells and extracellular matrix components is also altered. The increased expression of some integrins correlates with the ability of a

A RANKING OF THE UNDERLYING PRIMARY MALIGNANCIES IN PATIENTS WITH CUTANEOUS METASTASES			
Men		**Women**	
Primary malignancy	Patients with cutaneous metastases (n = 127)	Primary malignancy	Patients with cutaneous metastases (n = 300)
Melanoma	41 (32%)	Breast	212 (70%)
SCC of the head & neck	21 (16.5%)	Melanoma	36 (12%)
Lung	15 (12%)	Ovary	10 (3.5%)
Colon/rectum	14 (11%)	Unknown	9 (3%)
Unknown	11 (8.5%)	SCC of the head & neck	7 (2.5%)
Kidney	6 (4.5%)	Lung	6 (2%)
Upper GI	5 (4%)	Colon/rectum	4 (1.5%)
Breast	3 (2.5%)	Endometrium	4 (1.5%)
Urinary bladder	3 (2.5%)	Urinary bladder	4 (1.5%)
Esophagus	3 (2.5%)	Uterine cervix	2 (0.7%)
Endocrine glands	2 (1.5%)	Stomach	2 (0.7%)
Stomach	1 (1%)	Bile ducts	2 (0.7%)
Pancreas	1 (1%)	Pancreas	1 (0.3%)
Liver	1 (1%)	Endocrine glands	1 (0.3%)
Total	127 (100%)	Total	300 (100%)

Table 122.2 **A ranking of the underlying primary malignancies in patients with cutaneous metastases.** GI, gastrointestinal; SCC, squamous cell carcinoma. Adapted from Lookingbill DP, Spangler N, Helm KF. Cutaneous metastases in patients with metastatic carcinoma: a retrospective study of 4020 patients. J Am Acad Dermatol. 1993;29:228–36.

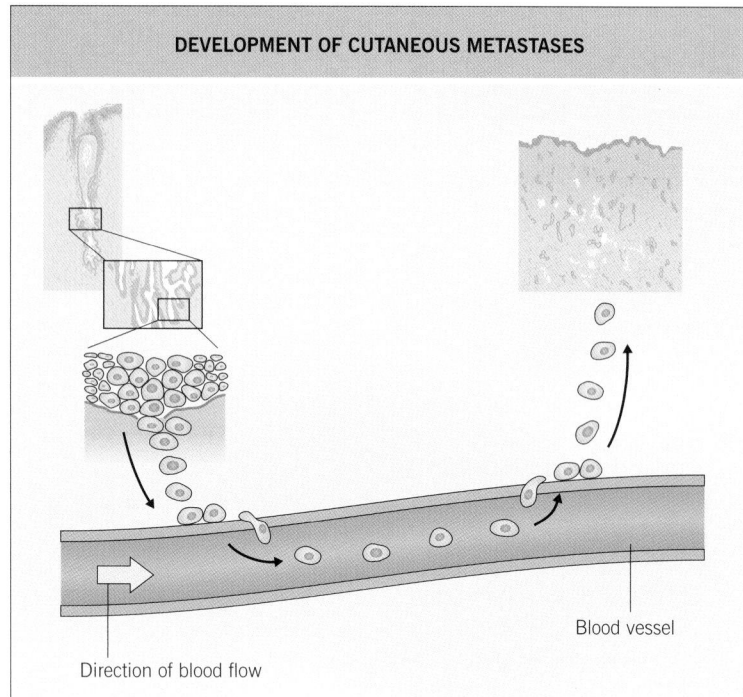

DEVELOPMENT OF CUTANEOUS METASTASES

Fig. 122.1 **Development of cutaneous metastases.** A prototypic breast cancer cell is successively selected to have a phenotypic advantage that allows it to proliferate, migrate, implant, and survive at a distant site.

variety of cancers to invade, while decreased expression of others may be associated with enhanced tumorigenicity and invasion. For example, cutaneous melanomas show enhanced expression of $\alpha_4\beta_1$ and $\alpha_V\beta_3$, and a loss of $\alpha_6\beta_1$, when compared to benign melanocytic lesions[11]. Changes in expression of these integrins correlate with prognosis. In human breast cancer, loss of $\alpha_2\beta_1$ expression correlates with loss of differentiation and tumorigenicity, while re-expression of this integrin abolishes the malignant phenotype and restores differentiation[12].

The release of proteases such as urokinase plasminogen activator (uPA), cathepsins and matrix metalloproteases (MMPs) leads to degradation and remodeling of the extracellular matrix, which is essential for tumor cell invasion. High uPa levels have been shown to be a poor prognostic marker in a variety of cancers, particularly breast cancer[13]. MMPs participate in many normal and abnormal functions; for example, they can activate growth factors and influence angiogenesis and cell migration, but because of their complex interactions, the various roles of MMPs in metastasis is still an area of active investigation. High levels of MMP-1, MMP-2, MMP-9, and membrane type-1 MMP (MT1-MMP) have been associated with progression of head and neck squamous cell carcinoma[14]. Trials with MMP inhibitors have been disappointing, although more selective targeting may prove of therapeutic benefit in the future.

Once cancer cells become autonomous, their highway to metastasis is the vasculature. Angiogenesis, the production and recruitment of new capillaries, is required for both cancer growth and metastasis[15]. Cancer must make an 'angiogenic switch' by tipping the local balance in favor of proangiogenic factors such as vascular endothelial growth factor (VEGF) or by downregulating antiangiogenic factors such as angiostatin and endostatin[15]. It seems counterintuitive that, in addition to angiogenic factors, cancers also produce such antiangiogenic factors. However, this may be the reason why removal of a primary cancer that secretes antiangiogenic factors has been associated with an increased risk of subsequently successful metastases. Angiostatin and endostatin inhibit human epidermal growth factor receptor-2 (HER2), and HER2

stimulates VEGF expression[15]. Thus, inhibiting HER2 indirectly results in decreased endothelial proliferation and diminished angiogenesis.

A number of potential cancer treatments have burgeoned from this newly discovered role of angiogenic factors. Inhibitors that both directly and indirectly block VEGF are in various phases of development, including anti-VEGF antibodies, anti-VEGF receptor-2 antibodies, and endogenous angiogenesis inhibitor proteins. Trastuzumab, an anti-HER2 antibody, is used as an immunotherapy for breast cancer.

Intravasation, or movement of cancer into the vasculature, requires penetration of basement membrane and endothelium. Once in circulation, relatively few tumor cells can bypass both mechanical and immune host defenses in order to invade an organ. The century-old 'seed and soil' theory of site-specific metastasis remains conceptually pertinent today[16]. The cancer 'seed' must be genetically successful enough to survive the metastatic sequence. Yet, implantation still depends on the fertile 'soil' of a permissive and biologically unique microenvironment in specific organs. Once it has implanted, cancer distribution within an end organ is again determined by its altered genetic ability and constitution. Figure 122.1 demonstrates the successive stages of cancer development and successful metastasis.

Other mechanisms of cancer spread are well known. In addition to direct cancer extension typified by squamous cell carcinoma of the oropharynx and subtypes of breast carcinoma, mechanisms such as 'extravascular migratory metastasis' have been proposed. Extravascular migratory metastasis, where cancer migrates *outside* of vessels, has been suspected in select melanomas where metastasis occurred, but there was no sign of intravasation and the melanoma was seen investing the vascular pericytes[17]. Iatrogenic implantation following biopsy or incomplete excision of solid organ malignancies has been described. It does not seem to play an important role in skin cancer and there are currently no data to support its occurrence with cutaneous melanoma. Lymphatic spread is obviously one of the many routes by which cancer can metastasize. As typified by melanoma, hematogenous and lymphatic spread is often concurrent. In-transit metastases are examples of the latter (see Ch. 113).

CLINICAL FEATURES

While cutaneous metastasis from one organ may be indistinguishable from that from another, the appearance, distribution and timing of cutaneous metastasis can provide clues to the discerning clinician. The clinical appearance of cutaneous metastasis is frequently dismissed by the patient because it can be a commonplace, painless, freely mobile, erythematous papule that grows to an inflammatory nodule[5]. Furthermore, malignancies from many organ systems can appear identical once they have metastasized to the skin. The very firm, even hard, nature of a dermal nodule can lead to a high clinical index of suspicion that a lesion represents a metastasis, especially in a patient with a history of a previous malignancy. However, some metastases do have a distinct clinical appearance.

Breast carcinoma metastatic to the chest wall may have several distinctive clinical appearances. Carcinoma erysipeloides is manifested by a sharply demarcated, elevated, red plaque reminiscent of erysipelas (Fig. 122.2); carcinoma telangiectoides is manifested by red papules and telangiectasias; and carcinoma *en cuirasse* is manifested by dusky, translucent skin with an orange peel appearance which mimics morphea due to the associated induration (Fig. 122.3).

Metastasis from lung cancer is typically to the chest wall or mediastinal or supraclavicular lymph nodes. Unlike the more common breast cancer metastases, there are no special clinical subtypes and lesions are usually pink to red nodules. Lung cancer can metastasize to the posterior thorax, which is a more unusual site for breast carcinoma. Colon carcinoma usually metastasizes to the abdominal wall, liver, and mesenteric lymph nodes. A Sister (Mary) Joseph nodule is a pink to red–brown, umbilical or periumbilical metastasis. Although many abdominal visceral malignancies can present as a Sister (Mary) Joseph nodule (Table 122.3), it was originally described as a cutaneous manifestation of metastatic gastric carcinoma. Metastases from head and neck carcinoma are erythematous nodules that are often located adjacent to surgical sites or in overlying skin, and may be accompanied by metastases to cervical lymph nodes.

Alopecia neoplastica may present as a scarring alopecia, appearing anywhere on the scalp, and it has been described with cutaneous metastasis from breast, gastric, lung, renal and pancreatic carcinomas (Fig. 122.4)[5]. When visceral carcinomas spread to the skin in

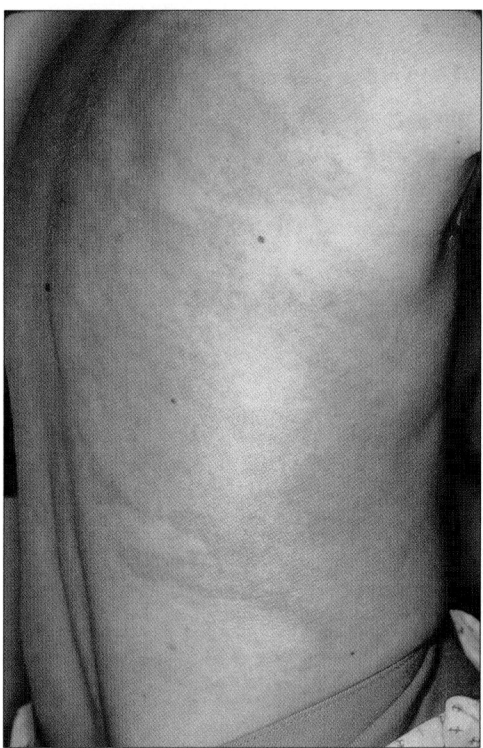

Fig. 122.2 Inflammatory breast carcinoma (carcinoma erysipeloides). Such lesions may initially be misdiagnosed as infectious cellulitis.

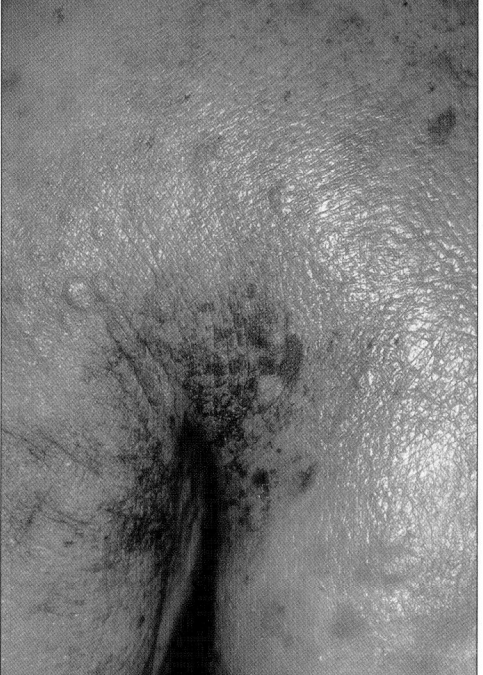

Fig. 122.3 Metastatic breast cancer involving the chest and upper arm. The skin is indurated due to fibrosis and has an orange peel appearance, referred to as carcinoma *en cuirasse*.

SITES OF METASTASES RELATIVE TO THE PRIMARY MALIGNANCY		
Sites of metastases	Sites of primary tumors	Primary malignancies
Metastases localized to the excision site		
Variable	Variable	Oral, lung, kidney, endometrium, ovary, colorectal
Metastases in the vicinity of the primary tumor		
Head & neck	Head & neck	SCC of the head & neck (e.g. laryngeal, oral)
Anterior chest wall	Chest	Breast, lung
Anterior abdominal wall	Abdomen, chest	Gastrocolic, breast
Umbilical*	Abdomen, pelvis	Gastrocolic, pancreas, ovary, endometrium
Perineum	Pelvis	Ovary, endometrium, cervix, prostate
Distant metastases		
Scalp	Variable	Breast, lung, stomach, pancreas, kidney

*Sister Mary Joseph nodule.

Table 122.3 Sites of metastases relative to the primary malignancy. SCC, squamous cell carcinoma.

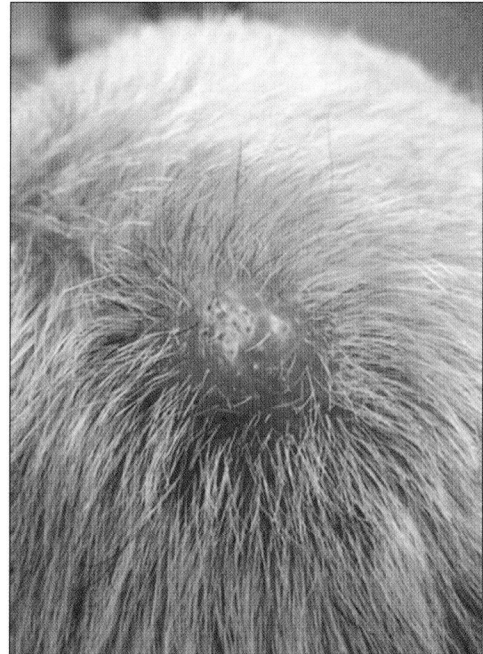

Fig. 122.4 An erythematous scalp nodule representing a metastasis from a primary lung squamous cell carcinoma. Notice the alopecia.

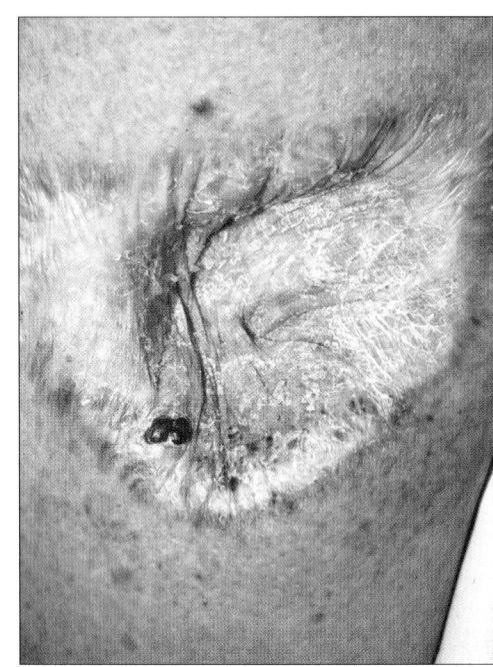

Fig. 122.5 Localized melanoma metastases. Discrete black papules are present within and at the periphery of the skin graft placed at the excision site. Courtesy of Ronald P Rapini MD.

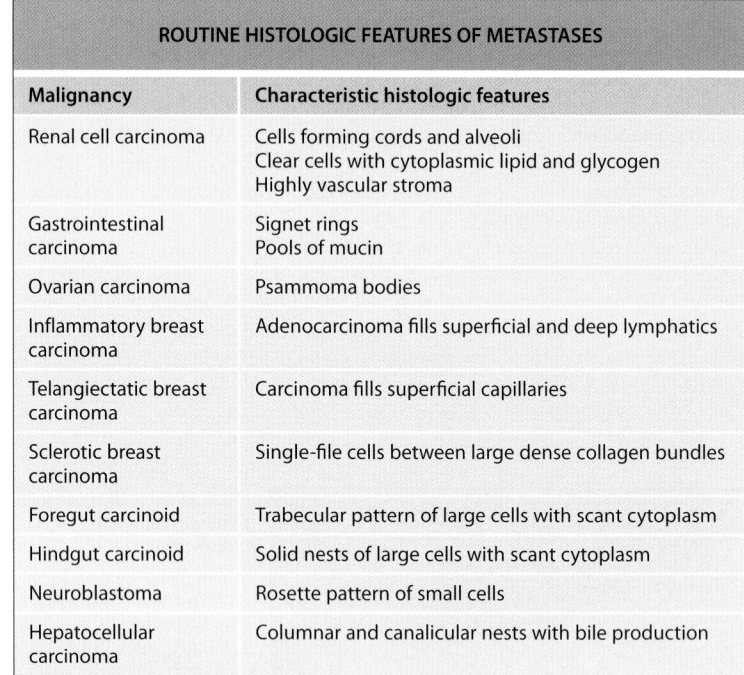

ROUTINE HISTOLOGIC FEATURES OF METASTASES	
Malignancy	**Characteristic histologic features**
Renal cell carcinoma	Cells forming cords and alveoli Clear cells with cytoplasmic lipid and glycogen Highly vascular stroma
Gastrointestinal carcinoma	Signet rings Pools of mucin
Ovarian carcinoma	Psammoma bodies
Inflammatory breast carcinoma	Adenocarcinoma fills superficial and deep lymphatics
Telangiectatic breast carcinoma	Carcinoma fills superficial capillaries
Sclerotic breast carcinoma	Single-file cells between large dense collagen bundles
Foregut carcinoid	Trabecular pattern of large cells with scant cytoplasm
Hindgut carcinoid	Solid nests of large cells with scant cytoplasm
Neuroblastoma	Rosette pattern of small cells
Hepatocellular carcinoma	Columnar and canalicular nests with bile production

Table 122.4 Routine histologic features of metastases.

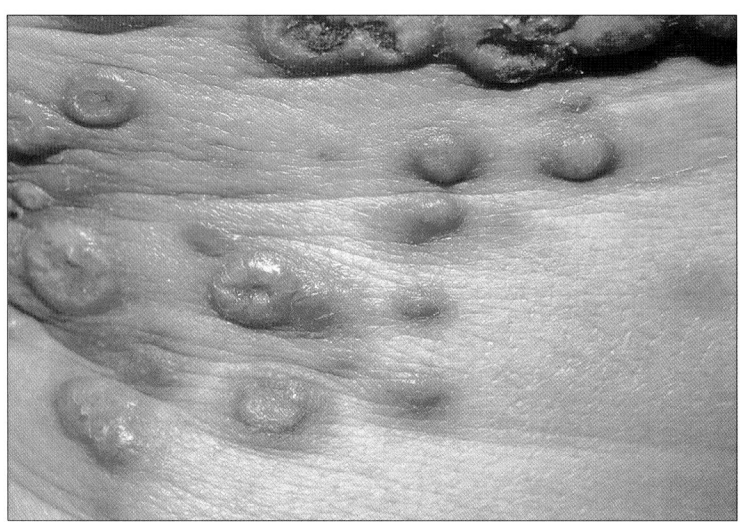

Fig. 122.6 Ulcerated erythematous nodules on the anterior trunk due to metastases of adenocarcinoma of the lung.

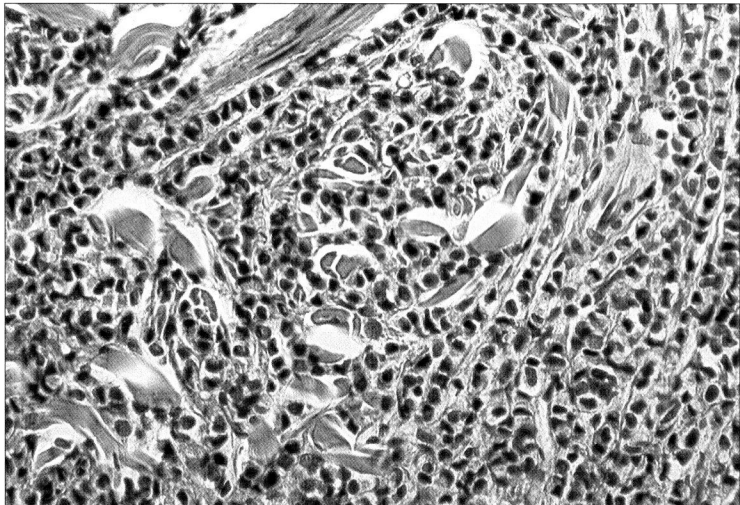

Fig. 122.7 Photomicrograph of a cutaneous metastasis of breast carcinoma. Note the single-file pattern of the tumor cells.

dermatomal crops of succulent nodules, this is known as zosteriform metastasis[5]. Finally, melanoma metastatic to skin can be brown to black to blue, indicative of melanin production (Fig. 122.5). A prominent vascular appearance has been described for cutaneous metastases from renal cell carcinoma.

Cutaneous metastases are generally in the anatomic vicinity of the primary cancer (Fig. 122.6), but the distribution of metastases can also be distinctive (see Table 122.3). When melanoma, breast carcinoma and lung carcinoma metastasize to skin, they often concurrently metastasize to other sites such as the lungs, liver, lymph nodes and brain[7].

PATHOLOGY

Organ-specific diagnosis of the cutaneous metastasis can be a daunting task. Such diagnosis routinely involves numerous phone calls, histologic sections, and application of new technologies to ferret out the answer. There is never too much clinical information or too much submitted tissue. Patient gender, race, age, cancer history, cancer location(s), and a biopsy specimen are a mandatory beginning.

The histologic appearance of the cutaneous metastasis may be identical to the primary cancer. More commonly, however, the metastasis is dedifferentiated. There are three degrees of dedifferentiation as compared to the primary. First, the metastasis may be slightly dedifferentiated, but visually resembles the primary cancer enough to make the diagnosis. This is the most common situation[18,19]. Distinct light microscopic features of particular malignancies are listed in Table 122.4. Second, the metastasis may be phenotypically dedifferentiated, but the organ of origin can be elucidated via immunohistochemistry and, less commonly, electron microscopy (Table 122.5). Finally, the metastasis may be dedifferentiated to the point that it is impossible to ascertain the organ of origin by any technology.

A commonsense approach to the histologic diagnosis of the dedifferentiated metastasis deserves mention. Identified by their oncologic pattern, by far the most common metastases to skin are adenocarcinoma, squamous carcinoma, and melanoma. Cutaneous metastatic adenocarcinoma is especially common from the breast (Fig. 122.7), but also from the colon and lung. Cutaneous metastatic squamous carcinoma is typically from the oropharynx and lung. Cutaneous metastatic melanoma is typically from the skin. A panel of three immunohistochemical stains, anti-cytokeratin -5/6, -7, -20 and anti-S100, may be useful in classifying the primary organ in most patients, but may be less useful for breast carcinoma[20]. Immunohistochemical staining for estrogen receptors, progesterone receptors and epidermal growth factor (anti-HER2/neu) can have diagnostic and prognostic significance in breast carcinoma patients[21]. Immunohistochemical staining for anti-epithelial membrane antigen (EMA), also known as

Malignancy	Feature
IMMUNOHISTOCHEMICAL STAINS AND ULTRASTRUCTURAL FEATURES USED TO DIFFERENTIATE AMONG METASTASES AND LYMPHOMA CUTIS	
Immunohistochemical staining	
Breast	Estrogen & progesterone receptors, HER2/neu*, gross cystic disease fluid protein-15, epithelial membrane antigen (EMA)
Colon	CK 7, carcinoembryonic antigen (CEA)
Lung (small cell, adenocarcinoma)	CK 20*, thyroid transcription factor (TTF)
Prostate	Prostate-specific antigen (PSA)
Follicular thyroid	Thyroglobulin

Lymphoma
  B cell
  T cell
	CD20, CD22
	CD3, CD4, CD8

Medullary thyroid	Calcitonin
Renal	Renal tubular antigen
Choriocarcinoma	Human chorionic gonadotropin (hCG)
Ovarian	CA-125
Neuroendocrine, including Merkel cell carcinoma	CK 20, neuron-specific enolase, chromogranin A, synaptophysin
Melanoma	S100, HMB45, Melan-A/MART-1, Mel-5
Squamous cell carcinoma	CK 5/6
Carcinoma (general)	Cytokeratin (e.g. pankeratin, AE1/AE3)
Ultrastructural features	
Melanoma	Melanosomes
Carcinoma (general)	Keratin intermediate filaments Desmosomes
Neuroendocrine carcinoma	Neurosecretory granules
Adenocarcinoma	Cytoplasmic mucin
Positive in a minority of cases.	

Table 122.5 Immunohistochemical stains and ultrastructural features used to differentiate among metastases and lymphoma cutis. CK, cytokeratin; HER2, human epidermal growth factor receptor-2.

MUC1, may be found in many carcinomas such as cutaneous squamous cell carcinoma, ductal breast carcinoma, and colon carcinoma.

DIFFERENTIAL DIAGNOSIS

Ironically, the lack of distinctive clinical features may be a clue to the diagnosis of cutaneous metastases. Anatomic location, the primary morphology, and lesional color can sometimes be helpful. When distinct clinical features are not present, the primary morphology of most metastases is a papule or especially a nodule. Most sources cite the usual morphologic differential diagnosis of a dermal/subcutaneous nodule, i.e. a cyst, lipoma, appendageal tumor or fibroma[5]. Since the pathogenesis of metastasis intimately involves angiogenesis, the primary color is often some shade of red. As a result, metastatic carcinoma can simulate a number of benign and malignant vascular lesions. The differential diagnosis of metastatic breast cancer, as discussed above, includes morphea, erysipelas and radiation dermatitis, and a range of scarring alopecias as well as benign and malignant appendageal tumors must be considered with scalp metastases.

TREATMENT AND PROGNOSIS

Therapy can be tailored to treat any combination of primary cancer and cutaneous metastasis. Treatment of the latter includes chemotherapy, immunotherapy, radiotherapy, excision, heat and observation. Occasionally intralesional and topical (e.g. imiquimod) agents are employed. Tumor burden, maintaining daily function, cosmesis, and the possibility of pain, bleeding and infection are factored into the treatment algorithm. Although the disease course depends on the underlying malignancy and its therapeutic response, cutaneous metastasis is a marker of advanced disease and, historically, life expectancy has been short[4]. That the skin is accessible particularly facilitates the observation of systemic therapeutic response.

SUMMARY

Metastasis is an inefficient, dynamic process whereby carcinoma cells are successively selected to have a phenotypic advantage that allows them to proliferate, migrate, implant, and survive at a distant site. Considering the myriad malignancies that can metastasize, the clinical and histologic appearance of cutaneous metastases is often surprisingly nondescript. However, there are a finite number of clinical presentations that deserve attention. History and immunohistochemistry may be useful diagnostic tools. Despite the travail, an organ-specific diagnosis is not a fruitless exercise. Metastasis may be the presenting sign of malignancy and may have prognostic significance.

REFERENCES

1. McWhorter JE, Cloud AW. Malignant tumors and their metastases: a summary of the necropsies on eight hundred and sixty-five cases performed at the Bellevue Hospital of New York. Ann Surg. 1930; 92:434–43.
2. Abrams HL, Spiro R, Goldstein N. Metastases in carcinoma: analysis of 1000 autopsied cases. Cancer. 1950;3:74–85.
3. Enticknap JB. An analysis of 1000 cases of cancer with special reference to metastasis. Guy's Hosp Rep. 1952;101:273–9.
4. Reingold IM. Cutaneous metastases from internal carcinoma. Cancer. 1966;19:162–8.
5. Brownstein MH, Helwig EB. Spread of tumors to the skin. Arch Dermatol. 1973;107:80–6.
6. Lookingbill DP, Spangler N, Sexton FM. Skin involvement as the presenting sign of internal carcinoma. A retrospective study of 7316 cancer patients. J Am Acad Dermatol. 1990:22;19–26.
7. Lookingbill DP, Spangler N, Helm KF. Cutaneous metastases in patients with metastatic carcinoma: a retrospective study of 4020 patients. J Am Acad Dermatol. 1993;29:228–36.
8. Wesche WA, Khare VK, Chesney TM, Jenkins JJ. Non-hematopoietic cutaneous metastases in children and adolescents: thirty years experience at St Jude Children's Research Hospital. J Cutan Pathol. 2000;27:485–92.
9. Brodland DG, Zitelli JA. Mechanisms of metastasis. J Am Acad Dermatol. 1992;27:1–8.
10. Stetler-Stevenson WG. Invasion and metastases. In: Devita, VT, Hellman, S, Rosenber, SA (eds). Cancer: Principles and Practice of Oncology, 7th edn. Philadelphia: Lippincott Williams & Wilkins, 2005:113–27.
11. Johnson JP. Cell adhesion molecules in the development and progression of malignant melanoma. Cancer Metastasis Rev. 1999;18:345–57.
12. Zutter MM, Santoro SA, Staatz WD, Tsung YL. Re-expression of the alpha2beta1 integrin abrogates the malignant phenotype of breast carcinoma cells. Proc Natl Acad Sci USA. 1995;92:7411–15.
13. Duffy MJ, Duggan C. The urokinase plasminogen activator system: a rich source of tumour markers for the individualized management of patients with cancer. Clin Biochem. 2004;37:541–8.
14. Rosenthal EL, Matrisian LM. Matrix metalloproteases in head and neck cancer. Head Neck 2006;28:639–48.
15. Folkman, J. Role of angiogenesis in tumor growth and metastasis. Semin Oncol. 2002;29(suppl. 16):15–18.
16. Hart IR. 'Seed and soil' revisited: mechanisms of site-specific metastasis. Cancer Metastasis Rev. 1982;1:5–16.
17. Barnhill RL, Lugassy C. Angiotropic malignant melanoma and extravascular migratory metastasis: description of 36 cases with emphasis on a new mechanism of tumour spread. Pathology 2004;36:485–90.
18. Schwartz RA. Histopathologic aspects of cutaneous metastatic disease. J Am Acad Dermatol. 1995;33:649–57.
19. Schwartz RA. Cutaneous metastatic disease. J Am Acad Dermatol. 1995;33:161–82.
20. Saeed S, Keehn CA, Morgan MB. Cutaneous metastasis: a clinical pathological, and immunohistochemical appraisal. J Cutan Pathol. 2004;31:419–30.
21. Cobleigh MA, Tabesh B, Bitterman P, et al. Tumor gene expression and prognosis in breast cancer patients with 10 or more positive lymph nodes. Clin Cancer Res. 2005;11:8623–31.

Public Health Science in Dermatology

123

Thomas L Diepgen and Suephy Chen

INTRODUCTION

Skin diseases are very common, affecting approximately 20–33% of the population at any one time[1,2]. In addition, skin cancers are the most common malignancies that occur in the Caucasian population each year[3]. The majority of skin diseases are not life threatening, but the psychological effects of relatively minor skin abnormalities can often cause more distress to the patients than other more serious medical disorders[4]. The skin is very important in many ways: it is a sensitive dynamic boundary between the body and the outside world; it is essential for controlling water and heat loss; and it has defensive functions against infections and infestations, as well as protective properties against irritants, allergens and UV radiation.

The skin is the largest organ in the body and not a simple 'inert' barrier. It is an important sensory organ that is able to distinguish pain, touch, itch, heat and cold. The skin is an important organ for social and sexual contact, and contains other important structures, including hair, blood vessels, nerves, sweat and sebaceous glands. In addition, vitamin D is synthesized in the skin. Thus, skin failure can be as worthy of medical attention as cardiac or renal failure as it affects all of the functions just described[4].

Chronic suffering rather than mortality is the characteristic of most skin diseases. In addition to physical symptoms, perhaps the most significant way in which skin disease affects people is the effect it has on psychological well-being[4]. Disfiguring skin disease in visible sites such as the face (e.g. acne) can result in loss of self-esteem, depression and poorer job prospects. Indeed, quality-of-life scores for people with skin disease are often worse than for people with more traditional 'medical' disorders such as angina and hypertension. The skin is therefore a sensitive and dynamic organ that has a crucial and frequently underestimated social function. The study of the magnitude of skin diseases and their impacts on patient lives is captured with disciplines such as epidemiology and health services research. Further, these research arenas depend on standardized case definitions and an understanding of the limitations of diagnostic tests and potential biases.

WHY IS EPIDEMIOLOGY IMPORTANT FOR DERMATOLOGY?

Epidemiology refers to the study of the distribution and causes of disease in human populations[5]. Epidemiology, as applied to dermatology, explores issues such as how *many* people suffer from skin disease in a given community. By comparing affected people to those without disease with respect to a range of plausible causes, epidemiology offers one of the simplest and most direct ways of evaluating the *causes* of skin diseases in various populations. One of the first epidemiologic discoveries in dermatology can be traced to 1746, when James Lind concluded that scurvy in sailors was related to dietary factors[6]. He then showed by means of a controlled study that the disease readily responded to the addition of fresh oranges and lemons to the sailors' diet. Therefore, knowledge of cause opens up the possibility for prevention of cutaneous and venereal disease – a powerful and perhaps more appropriate way of approaching the problem of skin disease at a population level than is investment into expensive drugs and therapies, which may often only modify established disease[7].

Epidemiologic studies can be categorized as observational descriptive, analytical and intervention studies (Table 123.1). Observational descriptive studies demonstrate the public health importance, characterize the demographics of a population, describe the natural history of particular skin diseases, and suggest possible disease-related hazards and risks. Analytical studies examine risk factors for new disease and prognostic factors for established disease. Intervention studies evaluate the effectiveness of measures to prevent or reduce the impact of a skin disease[8]. Information from epidemiologic studies may provide answers to the following questions:

- What are the prevalence and incidence rates?
- What is the public health importance and impact of a skin disease?
- Who gets the skin disease of interest, who is at risk?
- When and where does the skin disease of interest occur? What exposures are associated with a higher risk?
- What is the natural history and prognosis of the skin disease?
- What preventive measures and interventions are effective?

Whereas most clinical research is involved in describing individual cases, epidemiology is concerned with relating individuals with a particular skin disease to entire *populations*, so that effective healthcare strategies that benefit *all* can be developed. The term dermato-epidemiology refers to the study of the epidemiology of dermatologic disorders. Some examples of the relevance of epidemiology in dermatology are given in Table 123.2.

WHY IS HEALTH SERVICES RESEARCH IMPORTANT FOR DERMATOLOGY?

Health services research refers to the study of healthcare services and interventions in the real life setting. Information from health services research helps patients and policymakers to make informed decisions and improve the quality of healthcare services. Unlike traditional clinical trials, health services research does not focus on physiologic endpoints

---

DESCRIPTIVE, ANALYTIC AND INTERVENTION DERMATO-EPIDEMIOLOGY

Descriptive epidemiology

- How *many* people suffer from skin disease in a given community
- In which ways such skin diseases affect people (e.g. adverse quality-of-life, loss of employment, economic burden)

Analytic epidemiology

- By contrasting affected people versus those without disease with respect to a range of plausible causes, it offers one of the simplest and most direct ways of evaluating the *causes* of skin diseases in populations (cross-sectional, case–control or cohort studies)

Intervention epidemiology

- Knowledge of causes opens up the possibility for prevention
- A powerful and perhaps more appropriate way of approaching the problem of skin disease at a population level than is investment into expensive treatments, which may often only modify established disease

Table123.1 **Descriptive, analytic and intervention dermato-epidemiology.**

THE RELEVANCE OF EPIDEMIOLOGY FOR DERMATOLOGY

- To quantify the volume of skin disease in the community
- To identify the causes or risk factors for skin diseases
- To describe the natural history, prognosis and disease associations of skin diseases
- To evaluate the effectiveness of dermatologic health services and prevention programs
- To provide a methodologic framework for designing and interpreting clinical dermatologic research

Table 123.2 **The relevance of epidemiology for dermatology.**

THE RELEVANCE OF HEALTH SERVICES RESEARCH FOR DERMATOLOGY

- To quantify the quality-of-life burden of skin disease
- To quantify the economic burden of skin disease
- To determine the relative cost-effectiveness of new therapies
- To determine the usage of and access barriers to dermatologic services
- To quantitatively determine the level of patient satisfaction with dermatologic services

Table 123.3 **The relevance of health services research for dermatology.**

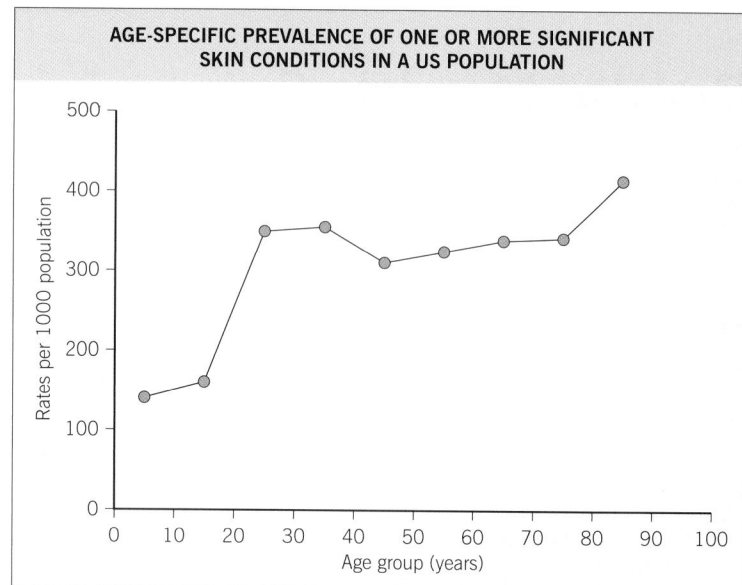

Fig. 123.1 **Age-specific prevalence of one or more significant skin conditions in a US population.** According to Johnson, 1978[2].

(e.g. PASI scores). Instead, parameters include clinical outcomes, quality-of-life outcomes, quality of care, cost, patient satisfaction, usage of healthcare services, and access to such services. Health services research also informs decision-makers about the best ways to deliver appropriate care with societal constraints. Specifically, with limited healthcare resources, the most cost-effective treatments for skin disease must be elucidated. Information from health services research may provide answers to the following questions:

- What is the quality-of-life impact?
- What subpopulations utilize dermatologists?
- What barriers exist to healthcare access?
- Is this new therapy cost-effective relative to existing ones?
- Are patients satisfied with their healthcare delivery?
- What standards exist, and what evidence supports such standards, for delivering specific health care?
- Are most dermatologists complying with existing standards of care?

Some examples of the relevance of health services research in dermatology are given in Table 123.3.

THE PUBLIC HEALTH IMPORTANCE OF SKIN DISEASES

Although it is true that skin disease is rarely life threatening, its moderate morbidity rate multiplied by its high prevalence rate places skin disease among the top four chronic disease groups when entire communities are considered[9]. In addition, several important skin diseases such as skin cancer, atopic dermatitis, venous stasis ulcers and psoriasis are becoming more common. Unlike most other medical specialities, dermatology as a specialty has between 1000 and 2000 diseases. However, fewer than ten categories of skin disorders account for over 70% of dermatologic consultations: skin cancer, acne, atopic dermatitis, psoriasis, viral warts, infective skin disorders, benign tumors and vascular lesions, leg ulceration, and contact dermatitis (and other eczema)[9].

The economic implications of the magnitude of skin disorders are not trivial. Various studies have assessed the economic impact of specific skin diseases and these have shown that direct costs are as high as for many other diseases, with much of that cost being carried by patients as well as by the state or by third-party payers. Small changes in the way this balance functions can have a profound effect on a country's healthcare budget because skin disease affects so many people[9].

Other costs such as unemployment and losing an economically viable sector of a country's workforce are also important when considered at a population level. Indirect costs (e.g. the time lost from work to take care of skin problems) and the opportunity costs (i.e. costs that could be gained by doing something other than taking care of skin problems) also need to be considered in such economic evaluations.

HOW COMMON ARE SKIN DISEASES?

A survey of 20 000 randomly chosen residents between the ages of 20 and 65 years in Gothenburg, Sweden, found that 27% of women and 25% of men reported symptoms of skin diseases in the preceding 12 months[10]. Surveys in the UK and US suggest that skin conditions as a whole represent a large and important problem: one study of adults in London suggested that 22.5% of those surveyed had a skin disease that could benefit from medical care, yet only 24% of such individuals with moderate to severe skin disease had utilized medical services in the last 6 months[1]. The overall proportion of the population found to have any form of skin disease was 55% (95% confidence intervals,

49.6–61.3%). Another detailed cross-sectional study of skin diseases was conducted by the first US Health and Nutrition Examination Survey[2] on a representative population sample of 20 749 persons between 1 and 74 years of age. Nearly one-third (312 per 1000 population) had one or more significant skin conditions that were considered by a dermatologist to justify evaluation by a physician at least once. The prevalence of significant skin pathology increases steadily with age, reflecting the increase in chronic diseases such as psoriasis, vitiligo, malignant and benign tumors, and actinic and seborrheic keratoses (Fig. 123.1).

Both surveys, along with a trend towards an increase in consultation rates for skin disease as a whole, suggest that there is a large hidden iceberg of unmet dermatologic needs[7]. This iceberg of dermatologic need is likely to surface over the next 20 years as consumers of health care become more aware of their rights, and some of the common skin diseases such as skin cancer and venous leg ulcers become more common due to an aging population[9]. Frequent travel between countries and continents, migrant populations in search of work, and widening socioeconomic divides are factors that could contribute to increases in infectious skin diseases and an increase in venereal diseases.

Inflammatory skin diseases such as atopic dermatitis, contact dermatitis, psoriasis, hand eczema and acne are very common in the population. Infectious skin diseases account for a large portion of skin disorders presenting to both primary care physicians and dermatologists, and skin cancer represents the most common form of human cancer, although many cancer registries probably underestimate its true incidence. Chronic venous insufficiency is a major (although generally underestimated) health problem which affects approximately 15% of the adult population in European countries, with 1% suffering from active venous leg ulcers[7].

People with skin complaints obtain help from various sources, including self-help, advice from pharmacists, treatment from primary care physicians, and services from other specialists. For example, of 291 individuals complaining of acne/spots/greasy skin, 47% took no action, 34% used or bought an over-the-counter preparation, and 12% used medicines prescribed by a doctor; the remaining 7% used home remedies[11]. The estimated number of people utilizing dermatologic health services in the UK at various entry points for a population of 100 000 over a 1-year period is shown in Table 123.4[9,12–15].

In a consumer study from Great Britain, skin complaints in the preceding 2 weeks were reported by 25% of adults and 36% of children[11]. According to the Lambeth study[1], approximately 30% of adults with a skin complaint decided to self-medicate; this proportion was similar for trivial as well as for moderate to severe skin disease. Approximately 15% of the UK population consulted their general practitioner (GP) because of a skin condition (excluding benign and malignant skin tumors and some skin infections)[12]. These visits represented 19% of all

SKIN DISEASES IN A UK POPULATION OF 100 000 PEOPLE (1-YEAR PERIOD)	
Skin complaints	25 000 (25%)
Self-treatment	7500 (30% of 25 000)
Seek advice from GP	14 500* (15%)
Referred to dermatologist	1162 (1.2%)
Admitted to hospital	24–31 (2–3% of referrals)
Deaths	5 (0.4% of referrals)
Excludes cutaneous neoplasms, viral warts, herpes simplex and scabies.	

Table 123.4 Skin diseases in a UK population of 100 000 people over a 1-year period[9,12–15]. GP, general practitioner.

CLINICAL DIAGNOSIS AND DIAGNOSTIC TESTS

Clinical Diagnosis

The accuracy of the diagnosis in dermatology depends on the experience, knowledge and skill level of the physician who makes the diagnosis, and on the degree of difficulty in confirming the relationship between the diagnosis and a positive diagnostic test or an exposure (e.g. for exogenous dermatoses). For example, detailed patch testing or provocation testing may be necessary to determine whether sensitization to certain agents has occurred, but even then it is sometimes not certain whether the contact dermatitis is irritant or allergic. Patch testing and provocation testing are helpful in assessing patients with suspected allergic contact dermatitis, but are often not used by general dermatologists because of the high false-positive rates, irritant reactions or difficulties in interpretation.

Diagnostic Tests

To ascertain the validity of a diagnostic test (e.g. laboratory test, patch tests, etc.), the terms 'sensitivity', 'specificity' and 'predictive value' are used. Sensitivity indicates the *probability* that the skin disease of interest is correctly diagnosed, while the specificity requires that non-diseased cases are correctly excluded. From a clinical perspective, it is more appropriate to calculate the positive predictive value (PPV), which is the proportion of individuals who actually have the disease of interest among those diagnosed as such by the diagnostic test that was used[16].

The PPV is a function of the prevalence of the disease in the population, and of the sensitivity and specificity of the diagnostic test. In Figure 123.2, the PPV is shown as a function of the prevalence,

THE NUMBER OF CORRECT AND FALSE-POSITIVE PATCH TEST RESULTS ACCORDING TO DIFFERENT PREVALENCE RATES OF SENSITIZATION, ASSUMING A SENSITIVITY AND SPECIFICITY OF 90%					
	Prevalence of allergic contact dermatitis (ACD)				
	1%	5%	10%	20%	50%
Patients with ACD	10	50	100	200	500
Patients without ACD	990	950	900	800	500
Total no. of patients	1000	1000	1000	1000	1000
No. of true positives	9	45	90	180	450
No. of false positives	99	95	90	80	50

Table 123.5 The number of correct and false-positive patch test results according to different prevalence rates of sensitization, assuming a sensitivity and specificity of 90%. Numbers are given with the assumption that 1000 patients have been patch tested.

assuming a fixed sensitivity of 90% and four different specificities: 99%, 97.5%, 95% and 90%, respectively. If, for example, the prevalence of allergic contact dermatitis due to an allergen (e.g. nickel) is 10% and the sensitivity is 90%, then the PPV would be 91% if the specificity is 99%. The PPV will decrease to 80% if the specificity is 97.5%, 67% if the specificity is 95%, and 50% if the specificity is 90%.

Example: Patch Testing

If we assume that the prevalence of being sensitized to nickel is 10%, and the sensitivity and specificity of patch testing are 90%, then from a statistical point of view, a positive reaction results in only 50% of the cases being diagnosed correctly. Therefore, individuals are frequently missed who are sensitized, while others are wrongly diagnosed as being sensitized. Table 123.5 illustrates the magnitude of this problem assuming that the sensitivity and specificity of patch testing are 90% and the prevalence of sensitization to different allergens ranges from 1% to 50% in a sample of 1000 patients tested in a specific time period. The resulting false-positive patch test results would misdiagnose between 99 and 50 patients. If the true prevalence was 1% (not uncommon for many contact allergies), then of 10 truly sensitized patients, the test would correctly diagnose 9 patients, but of 990 individuals in the truly not sensitized group, 99 would have false-positive patch test results. Even if we assume a true prevalence of 50%, the expected number of false-positives would be 50 out of 500 non-sensitized patients.

This example demonstrates how important it is to achieve a high prevalence rate of truly sensitized patients in the clinical setting in order to reduce the number of false-positive patch test results. Thus, also from a statistical point of view, it is crucial to explore the patient's history carefully and exactly before performing patch testing: indiscriminate testing of many patients with a doubtful allergic origin of their

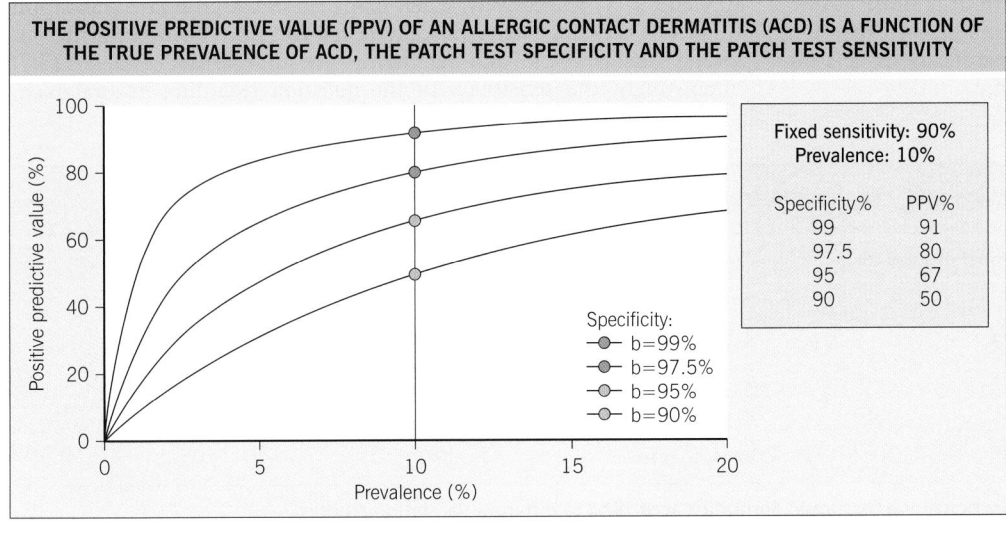

Fig. 123.2 The positive predictive value (PPV) of an allergic contact dermatitis (ACD) is a function of the true prevalence of ACD, the patch test specificity and the patch test sensitivity.

STATISTICAL SIGNIFICANCE CAN BE INFLUENCED BY SENSITIVITY AND SPECIFICITY			
	Dyshidrotic hand eczema		
	Yes	No	Total
Nickel allergy yes	11	9	20
Nickel allergy no	19	61	80
Total	30	70	100
Chi-square test:	$\chi^2 = 7.44$; $p = 0.006$		

Sensitivity and specificity for patch testing 90% and worst-case scenario			
	Dyshidrotic hand eczema		
	Yes	No	Total
Nickel allergy yes	2	10	12
Nickel allergy no	28	60	88
Total	30	70	100
Chi-square test:	$\chi^2 = 1.15$; $p = 0.28$, indicating no significant association		

Table 123.6 **Statistical significance can be influenced by sensitivity and specificity.** The upper table shows a statistically significant association between hand eczema and nickel allergy. The lower table shows the effects of misclassification, assuming a sensitivity and specificity of 90% for patch testing (worst-case scenario).

skin problem (i.e. a low prevalence of true allergies) will lead to many cases of incorrectly diagnosed contact dermatitis.

The Effect of Sensitivity and Specificity on *p*-Values

A second example demonstrates other possible pitfalls associated with sensitivity and specificity. Suppose one would like to study whether there is a statistically significant association between dyshidrotic hand eczema and a sensitization to nickel. Assuming that patch tests were performed in the next 100 patients with hand eczema in an outpatient clinic, and if 30% of those patients were diagnosed as having dyshidrotic hand eczema, and if a positive patch test was found in 20% of patients, then the results (shown in Table 123.6) demonstrate a statistically highly significant association between dyshidrotic hand eczema and nickel allergy. But, if it is assumed that the sensitivity and specificity of patch testing is 90%, then one would expect 10% false negative results among patients with nickel allergy and 10% false positive results among patients without nickel allergy. Based on these statistics, it can be calculated that approximately 9 out of the 20 patients with a positive patch test for nickel were in reality not sensitized (PPV = 55%), and 1 out of the 80 patients with negative patch test results would in fact have nickel allergy (negative predictive value = 99%). In the worst-case scenario, if the 9 false-positive patients have dyshidrotic hand eczema and the 1 false-negative patient does not have dyshidrotic hand eczema, the result would actually switch to a higher frequency of nickel allergy in patients without dyshidrosis than in those with dyshidrosis. However, with a chi-square test statistic of 1.15 and a corresponding *p*-value of 0.28, this would mean no statistically significant association between dyshidrotic hand eczema and nickel allergy.

The example described above represents a common measurement error of categorical data that is well known in the statistical literature as a phenomenon of misclassification[17]. The occurrence of this phenomenon is unfortunately the rule more often than the exception in the dermatologic literature. The example shows the consequences when representing our contact dermatitis data in a 2×2 table. The possible consequences are widely discussed in the statistical literature[18]. Various techniques to deal with this problem, other than just increasing the sample size, have been developed in recent decades.

CASE DEFINITION, CASE ASCERTAINMENT, MISCLASSIFICATION AND BIAS

Case Definition

It is crucial that clinical trials and epidemiologic studies have accurate criteria for disease definition; such criteria are referred to as case definitions. Although most dermatologists have little difficulty in making a firm diagnosis in most patients, there are very few case definitions that lend themselves to research such that the diagnosis of the disease is without uncertainty. Specific issues include clinical variants of a disease (e.g. pustular psoriasis vs. inverse psoriasis vs. plaque-type psoriasis), different levels of disease severity, and difficulties in differentiating between similar dermatologic conditions. The lack of a standard case definition for many skin diseases leads to difficulties in obtaining accurate epidemiologic data because a precise case definition is a prerequisite for the gathering of epidemiologic data. Consequently, in many dermatoses, the case definition can vary from one data source to another. For example, atopic dermatitis (AD) can be a difficult disease to define because of variable distribution and morphology, variable time course, and the lack of a pathognomonic diagnostic test. In addition, every country has several synonyms that are commonly used by physicians and patients for the disease which is here named atopic dermatitis. Given these difficulties, it is not surprising that a range of different methods and definitions for AD have been used in studies, ranging from questionnaire recall of 'eczema during childhood' or parental recall, to health visitor and physician recall.

Clinical diagnostic features of AD have been based largely on patients admitted to hospitals and visiting outpatient clinics[19]. These criteria are very helpful in describing the various aspects of the clinical syndrome of AD, but they are less useful for epidemiologic studies because of their complexity and because of their unknown validity. Various other diagnostic tools have been suggested based on clinical examination[20,21] or questionnaires[22]. Williams et al.[23] have proposed and validated a minimum set of diagnostic criteria for AD that are recommended to serve as a 1-year period prevalence measure in epidemiologic studies. These UK criteria were shown to have a sensitivity and specificity of 80% and 96%, respectively, in children attending hospital-based dermatology outpatient clinics, when compared to a dermatologist's diagnosis[23]. In a community survey of London children 3 to 11 years of age from mixed ethnic and socio-economic groups, the sensitivity and specificity for AD prevalence were 80% and 97%, respectively, when using these UK criteria[24]. Validation studies of the UK diagnostic criteria for AD have been performed in several other countries and the findings are summarized in Table 123.7. Interestingly, the sensitivity of the question regarding flexural rash,

SENSITIVITY AND SPECIFICITY OF THE UK DIAGNOSTIC CRITERIA FOR ATOPIC DERMATITIS ACCORDING TO DIFFERENT VALIDATION STUDIES					
Author	Country	Number of subjects	Age of subjects (years)	Sensitivity (%)	Specificity (%)
Williams et al. 1996[24]	UK	695	3–11	80	97
Popescu et al. 1998[25]	Romania	1114	6–12	74	99
Kramer et al. 1998[26]	Germany	1511	6	51	93.6
Marks et al. 1999[27]	Australia	2491	4–18	43	95
Firooz et al. 1999[28]	Iran	416	<4, 4–10, >10	10	98.3

Table 123.7 **Sensitivity and specificity of the UK diagnostic criteria for atopic dermatitis according to different validation studies.**

a hallmark of AD, was only 76% in the UK study[24], 74% in the Romanian study[25], and 49% in the Hong Kong study[29].

None of the definitions of the outcome variables for AD are 100% valid. Individuals are nearly always missed who do carry an atopic disposition, while others are wrongly designated as cases of AD. Theoretically, from a statistical point of view, an observed increase in the prevalence of AD can be explained by a decrease in specificity over time because of an increased awareness of allergic diseases in the population (resulting in more false positives). Assuming a true prevalence of 10%, a sensitivity of 95% and a specificity of 95%, the percentage of individuals diagnosed as cases of AD would be 13.5%. If the specificity were to decrease over time to 90%, then 18.5% would be diagnosed as AD cases (Table 123.8). This example also demonstrates that an overestimation of the true prevalence must be assumed in most studies, and comparing studies using different instruments (even with seemingly minor differences regarding sensitivity and specificity) can lead to false conclusions[30].

Case Ascertainment

Case ascertainment is a surveillance technique that seeks to capture eligible cases of a particular disease. Case ascertainment depends not only on a rigorous case definition, but also largely on the sources of data that are used, e.g. morbidity statistics or observational studies. Mortality statistics are not helpful because skin diseases generally are not fatal. In morbidity statistics, case ascertainment usually involves registration of persons with dermatoses who fulfill additional criteria for registration, e.g. hospital admission, sickness leave or referral to a specialist physician. This restriction in the definition of a case will probably result in selective inclusion of the more severe cases, since a large proportion of individuals suffering from skin diseases do not come to medical attention or are seen in other settings (Fig. 123.3).

Systematic Errors and Bias

Further possibilities for systematic errors in samples of patients with skin diseases exist (Table 123.9). Biases are defined as sources of variation that distort the findings in one direction[31].

The important question 'how do we know who has the disease and who does not?' can cause ***selection bias***. Ideally, the sample of cases would be a random sample of everyone who has the disease. Especially in case–control studies, cases are usually sampled from patients in whom contact dermatitis, for example, has already been diagnosed and who are available for the study. This sample is not representative of all patients with the disease, because those who are undiagnosed, misdiagnosed or lost to follow-up are less likely to be included.

To avoid bias resulting from the method of case ascertainment, it is usually not enough to restrict case ascertainment within a defined study population to reviewing the files of dermatologists or general practitioners. In general, it requires some effort to bring all cases in the study population to the attention of the investigator. Screening of the complete study population according to standardized criteria by one or more trained dermatologist(s) is the most reliable, and therefore preferred, method.

In observational studies of skin diseases, the ascertainment of cases varies from intensive efforts by a medical examination of the complete study population to the relatively easy-to-apply method of self-administered questionnaires, or a combination of both. The advantage of observational studies is that case ascertainment can be performed utilizing uniform criteria for the definition of cases. However, the frequency of cases ascertained by questionnaire may be quite different from those ascertained by clinical examination. The size of the difference in prevalence estimates that may arise as a result of differences in the definition and method of diagnosing hand eczema (***information bias***) has been investigated by Smit et al.[32]. Two types of questionnaire-based diagnoses, a 'symptom-based' and a 'self-reported' diagnostic approach, were compared with the medical diagnosis of hand eczema. The prevalence of hand eczema according to the medical diagnosis was 18%, but according to the symptom-based diagnostic questionnaire it was 48%, and for the self-reported diagnostic questionnaire was 17%. The sensitivity and specificity of the symptom-based

A HYPOTHETICAL EXAMPLE WHERE AN INCREASE IN THE PREVALENCE OF ATOPIC DERMATITIS (AD) CAN BE EXPLAINED BY A DECREASE IN SPECIFICITY	1st study	2nd study
True prevalence of AD	10%	10%
Sensitivity	95%	95%
Specificity	95%	90%
Sample size	1000	1000
Estimated number of cases with AD	135	185
Study estimate of AD prevalence	13.5%	18.5%

Table 123.8 A hypothetical example where an increase in the prevalence of atopic dermatitis (AD) can be explained by a decrease in specificity.

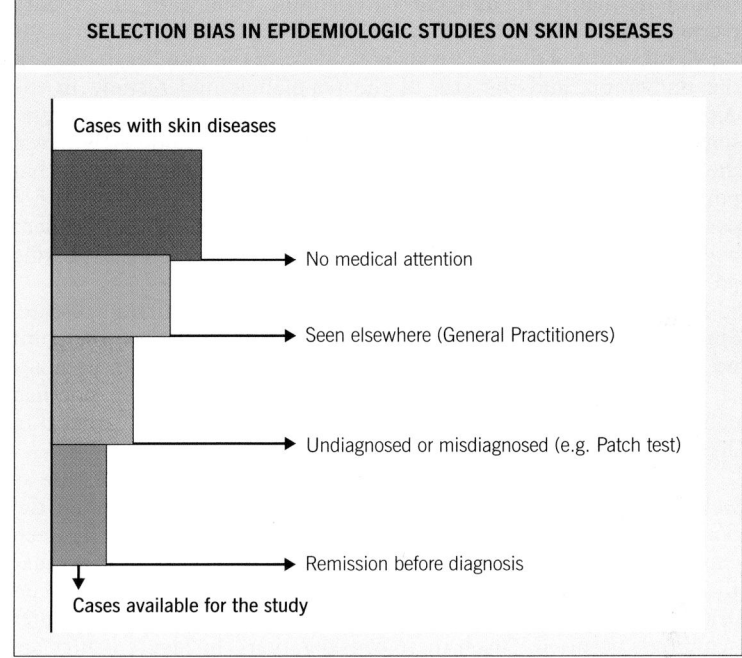

SELECTION BIAS IN EPIDEMIOLOGIC STUDIES ON SKIN DISEASES

Cases with skin diseases

No medical attention

Seen elsewhere (General Practitioners)

Undiagnosed or misdiagnosed (e.g. Patch test)

Remission before diagnosis

Cases available for the study

Fig. 123.3 Selection bias in epidemiologic studies on skin diseases.

REASONS FOR SYSTEMATIC ERRORS IN SAMPLES OF PATIENTS WITH SKIN DISEASES	
Type of errors	**Reasons**
Misclassification	• Overlap between skin disease and 'cosmetic' skin problem • Sensitivity and specificity of diagnostic tests are often not very high • Lack of standard case definition
Information bias	• Ascertainment of cases varies from dermatologic examination to self-administered questionnaires • Instruments are neither standardized nor evaluated (over- or underestimation)
Selection bias	• Samples of skin diseases are not selected randomly • Samples are not population-based • Only less than one-third of patients with skin complaints result in medical attention

Table 123.9 Reasons for systematic errors in samples of patients with skin diseases.

diagnostic questionnaire were 100% and 64%, respectively, and for the self-reported questionnaire, they were 65% and 93%, respectively. That means that the symptom-based diagnosis overestimated the incidence of hand eczema, and the self-reported diagnosis underestimated the prevalence of hand eczema according to the medical diagnosis.

INCIDENCE AND PREVALENCE

Measures of disease frequencies include 'prevalence', which is the amount of disease that is already present in a population, 'incidence', which refers to the number of new cases of skin diseases during a defined period in a specified population, and 'incidence rate', which is the number of non-diseased persons who become diseased within a certain period of time, divided by the number of person-years in the population. Prevalence of a disease is a cross-sectional 'snap-shot' of the total number of diseased subjects (new and old) within a defined population at a point in time (point prevalence) or in a defined period (period prevalence) and should not be confused with incidence, which gives the number of new cases in a defined period.

Data on the incidence and prevalence of skin diseases are scarce and population-based studies are lacking. There is a huge amount of data from case series of patients visiting dermatology clinics, but a limited number of cross-sectional studies in different samples of subgroups of the population (e.g. atopic dermatitis in schoolchildren, occupational contact dermatitis in different occupations, viral warts in military recruits, etc.).

All measures of disease frequency consist of the number of cases in the numerator, and the size of the population under study in the denominator. As mentioned above, in case series the sample represented by the numerator is often biased. With few exceptions, however, the size of the denominator is unknown in many publications that purport to discuss the frequencies of skin diseases. Therefore it is not possible to calculate rates. This is the reason why studies among patient populations from dermatology clinics are not adequate for estimating prevalence or incidence rates.

Point prevalence includes only subjects with actual skin disease. Since skin diseases are often chronically relapsing diseases, the point prevalence is less informative than the period prevalence. The accuracy of recall decreases with time, because persons who have not had complaints recently are more likely to forget to report their earlier skin disease.

Period prevalence includes subjects with long-lasting skin disease as well as relatively recent cases, and thus is characterized by all the possible interpretational difficulties. No inference can be made between exposure and the dermatosis of interest (e.g. contact dermatitis) because the exposure may have changed over time, past exposure may be over- or underestimated, and preventive measures may have been taken after symptoms occurred. Given these considerations, incidence figures are mostly preferred for analyzing risk factors for skin diseases.

Prevalence is in fact a measure of the product of incidence and duration of disease. Despite the appearance of an increased prevalence of a disease, it is possible that the incidence has remained steady if disease chronicity has increased. Therefore, in examining the changes in the biology of a disease, incidence data are preferable.

Example: Non-melanoma Skin Cancer

Cancer registries exist in many countries and can be very helpful when used to estimate the annual incidence rate of a disease. However, skin cancer registration data are of variable completeness and accuracy[33], and incidence data of high epidemiologic quality on non-melanoma skin cancer (NMSC) are sparse because traditional cancer registries often exclude NMSC data or are incomplete[3]. Table 123.10 shows the age-standardized rates of NMSC in Caucasians per 100 000 population from Australia, the US and Europe. This figure is based on selected studies reported after 1990 and an analysis of the data demonstrates the uncertainty of the real incidence rate of NMSC in populations from different parts of the world.

For example, the reported incidence varies according to the method of case ascertainment. Population-based epidemiologic surveys, surveying random sample of residents, indicate that the incidence in Australia is 1% to 2% per year (1000 to 2000 per 100 000 population per year). In contrast, estimates based on cancer registries were much lower (see Table 123.10). Systematic and complete recording of NMSCs is difficult or even unlikely to be achieved because of the large numbers involved, the rarity with which these lesions require hospital treatment, and the large proportion of clinically recognized skin cancers that may be treated destructively without histologic confirmation of the diagnosis.

Country	Year of report	BCC		SCC	
		Men	*Women*	*Men*	*Women*
AUSTRALIA					
Townsville[34]	1998	2055	1195	1332	755
Nambour[35]	1996	2074	1579	1035	472
Tasmania[36]	1993	145	83	64	20
UNITED STATES					
Various[37]	1994	407	212	81	26
New Hampshire[38]	1991	159	87	32	8
Rochester[39]	1997	175	124	155	71
EUROPE					
Wales, UK[40]	2000	128	105	25	9
Hull, UK[41]	1994	116	103	29	21
Scotland[42]	1998	50	37	18	8
Finland[43]	1999	49	45	7	4
The Netherlands[44]	1991	46	32	11	3

AGE-STANDARDIZED RATES OF NMSC IN CAUCASIANS PER 100 000 POPULATION FROM AUSTRALIA, US AND EUROPE

Table 123.10 Age-standardized rates of NMSC in Caucasians per 100 000 population from Australia, US and Europe. Selected studies after 1990, according to Diepgen & Mahler[3].

Therefore, few cancer registries in the world routinely collect notifications of NMSCs, thus necessitating special surveys. Such surveys are still missing for Europe.

The incidence of NMSC is increasing rapidly. In Caucasian populations in Europe, the US, Canada and Australia, the average increase in NMSC has been 3–8% per year since the 1960s[45]. The rising incidence rates of NMSC are probably due to a combination of increased sun exposure or exposure to UV light, increased outdoor activities, changes in clothing style, increased longevity, and ozone depletion[1]. The incidence of NMSC in Caucasians increases proportionally with proximity of residence to the equator, with the incidence of squamous cell carcinoma (SCC) doubling for each 8–10 degree decline in latitude[46]. UV dosage per unit time at the equator in the Pacific is very high, about 200% that of Europe or the northern US, and 30% higher than that of the southern US[47]. The incidence of NMSC is elevated in individuals with a high cumulative exposure to UV light, but the paradox of the lack of quantitative evidence of a causal link between sun exposure and skin cancer was found in outdoor workers[38]. The incidence also increases with age. According to Holme et al.[40], in 1998 the incidence of basal cell carcinoma (BCC) in individuals over 75 years old was approximately five times higher than in individuals between 50 and 55 years of age, and for SCC it was approximately 35 times higher. The incidence of SCC increases more rapidly with age than does BCC. Therefore there is a need for more analytic epidemiologic studies assessing the risk factors for NMSC.

ECONOMIC EVALUATION OF SKIN DISEASES

The economics of skin diseases can serve two main purposes: to measure the financial burden of skin diseases as well as to determine whether new therapies and technologies are worth providing.

Estimating the financial burden of skin disease requires consideration of the perspective of the study. These perspectives include those from society, payer, or patient. The costs of skin disease are divided into 'direct' and 'indirect' costs. Direct costs refer to those directly related to the treatment of the skin disease (e.g. cost of dressings and antibiotics for leg ulcers). Indirect costs refer to costs not directly related to the care of the skin disease, and may include those patient or caretaker's days lost from work, and travel costs. The Panel of Cost-Effectiveness in Health and Medicine, convened by the US Public Health Service, has standardized methods to estimate these costs[48]. Recently, a joint project between the American Academy of Dermatology Association and the Society for Investigative Dermatology estimated the annual cost of skin disease in the US in 2004 to be $39.3 billion, including $29.1 billion in direct medical costs and $10.2 billion in lost productivity costs (defined as costs related to consumption of medical care, costs associated with impaired ability to work, and lost future earning potential because of premature death)[48a].

Since the effect of the intervention is as important as the cost, economic analyses also consider the outcome produced for the resources consumed. The choice of outcome measure in the analysis determines whether the analysis is classified as a cost-effectiveness, a cost–utility or a cost–benefit evaluation. Each type of analysis differs in the type of information it provides. Cost-effectiveness analyses use disease-specific clinical measures as the endpoint, for example, ulcer healed or number of nails cleared. Because the outcome measure is disease-specific, cost-effectiveness analysis is useful to compare alternative therapies *within* a specific skin disorder. Cost-effectiveness analysis is not useful, however, for making comparisons between different diseases because the unit of clinical effect in these cases would not be comparable: one cannot meaningfully compare, for example, the cost-effectiveness of '$100 per ulcer healed' to '$200 per patient nails cleared'[49]. Cost–utility studies circumvent this limitation by using the QALY (quality-adjusted life-year) as the outcome measure. QALYs summarize quality-of-life impact and mortality into a summary score that is applicable to all disease states. The quality-of-life impact is measured with a metric called utilities (see below). QALYs may thus be used as a common metric to compare the 'cost per QALY gained' across different conditions. Cost–benefit analyses use the dollar as the metric to compare among healthcare interventions or with other economic sectors[50]. In cost–benefit analysis, a surplus in benefits relative to costs implies that the therapy is worth providing, whereas a negative result suggest that costs would exceed benefits. The requirement to put a monetary value on health, however, is ethically problematic for some health providers, and represents an obstacle to widespread use of cost–benefit analysis[50]. Economic analyses such as cost-effectiveness, cost–utility and cost–benefit represent an additional application piece of information to inform policymakers in their quest for rational resource allocation.

QUALITY-OF-LIFE IMPACT OF SKIN DISEASES

The importance of the quality of patients' lives with their disease has gained increasing recognition as new therapies and technologies extend life. In fields where mortality is not a prominent feature, such as dermatology, quality-of-life improvement has particular relevance.

The WHO definition of quality of life (QOL) includes 'impairment', 'disability', and 'handicap', which represent symptoms, functional impact, and broad psychological, social and emotional impact, respectively. Two distinct but related ways to measure QOL are health status measures and utilities (Table 123.11). Health status measures address QOL in a detailed comprehensive manner such that the three constructs defined above are represented. Health status measures can also address QOL

from general health, skin-specific or disease-specific perspectives. The more general the measure, the more applicable the instrument is across different diseases and populations. However, in contrast to disease-specific measures, the general measures are less sensitive to issues specific to the disease. The health status measures can be targeted towards children as well as adults. However, the children-oriented instruments must take into account the age of the patient. Also, the issues that affect adults may differ from those that affect children. Lastly, health status instruments can address the impact on the family. The health status approach, which has its roots in psychometric scaling methods, can result in a single summary score, reflecting the overall impact of skin disease on QOL, separate scores for various sub-domains, or both.

By far the most dominant skin-specific QOL instrument is the 'Dermatology Life Quality Index (DLQI)'[51]. This 10-item scale taps into symptoms/feelings, daily activities, leisure, work/school, personal relationships, and treatment. The instrument produces a single score ranging from 0 to 30, with higher scores reflecting greater QOL impact. The results can also be expressed as a % of the total score obtained (i.e. a score of 10 would translate to 33.3%). Since its publication in 1994, the DLQI has been used in over 100 studies with a wide variety of skin diagnoses; its reliability, validity and responsiveness have been well established and it has been translated into over 20 languages. While the DLQI has certainly shown good to excellent psychometric properties, its brevity can also be seen as a weakness. With only 10 items, there is little chance for detailed assessment, and the instrument has only one item directly examining the emotional or psychological impact of skin disease. Further, a single item asks 'How itchy, sore, painful, or stinging has your skin been?', mixing multiple symptoms.

The primary alternative to the DLQI is the 'Skindex'[52], a 61-item instrument that has been shortened to 29-item[53] and 16-item versions[54]. The 29-item version – which taps the three dimensions of symptoms, functioning and emotions – has been the most widely adopted, having been used in nearly 20 studies with a variety of skin diagnoses, translated into five languages, and had its psychometric properties fairly well established. The Skindex instrument focuses more on the social and emotional aspects of skin disease than does the DLQI. The remaining skin-specific QOL instruments for adults have been used much less frequently and for fewer skin diagnoses, despite fairly well established psychometric properties.

A variety of disease-specific health status measures have also been developed, but these have been used much less frequently than the skin-specific instruments. Similarly, a few children-specific and family-specific instruments have been developed with limited applications.

Utilities are the other means of addressing QOL. They are health economic measures that involve eliciting patient preferences for particular health states. These preferences are usually in the form of trading life to have perfect health or taking a certain risk of death to

QUALITY-OF-LIFE (QOL) MEASURES			
Type of QOL measure	Advantages	Disadvantages	Examples/Methods
Health status measures			
Generic health	Applicable and thus comparable across all diseases, both cutaneous and non-cutaneous	May not be sensitive to issues related to specific skin disorders	Medical Outcome Survey, Short Form 36 (SF-36)
Skin-specific	Applicable and thus comparable across all skin diseases	May not be sensitive to issues related to specific skin disorders	Dermatology Life Quality Index (DLQI) Skindex
Disease-specific	Sensitive to specific issues related to a particular disease; may be more sensitive to responsiveness	Not comparable to other measures	Scalpdex Melasma Quality of Life Scale (MELASQOL)
Health economic measures			
Utilities	Reflects patients' preferences; metric to incorporate QOL into cost-effectiveness analyses	Takes a long time to elicit from patients	Standard gamble, time trade-off
Willlingness-to-pay	Reflects patients' preferences; metric to incorporate QOL into cost–benefit analyses	Health professionals often uncomfortable in assigning dollar value to QOL	Revealed preferences

Table 123.11 Quality-of-life measures.

have perfect health. The advantage of the utility approach is that it results in a single, standardized score, allowing comparison of patients with a variety of medical conditions. Utilities are the QOL metric used in cost-effectiveness analyses to account for QOL outcomes. A related measure is the willingness-to-pay, which quantifies patient preferences into a dollar amount.

EVIDENCE-BASED DERMATOLOGY AND SYSTEMATIC REVIEWS

All clinical practice and clinically oriented research benefits from acknowledgement of the level of evidence that underlies the assumptions made in the course of either a therapeutic decision or designing a research question. According to Sackett et al.[55], evidence-based medicine (EBM) is the conscientious, explicit and judicious use of the best current evidence in making decisions about the care of individual patients. Practicing evidence-based dermatology may be defined as integrating clinical expertise with the best external evidence from systematic research in the field of skin diseases. It is not 'cook-book' medicine, because it integrates the best external evidence with individual clinical expertise and patient choice. External clinical evidence can inform, but it can never replace individual clinical expertise. Clinical expertise and discussion of patient preferences determine whether the external evidence applies to the individual patient and, if so, how it should be integrated into a clinical decision. The patient's unique situation, values, and expectations have to be considered. EBM is not an excuse to cut costs or a restriction on clinical freedom.

The process of evidence-based dermatology can be broken down into four separate steps:
- asking a patient-driven structured question
- searching for relevant information
- critically appraising the information, and
- applying it back to the patient.

Asking a Patient-Driven Structured Question

A structured evidence-based question should address the four key elements[56]: (1) the patient or problem being addressed; (2) the intervention, whether by nature or by clinical design (e.g. a cause, prognostic factor or treatment) being considered; (3) a comparison intervention, when relevant; and (4) the clinical outcome or outcomes of interest.

Searching for Relevant Information

Searching for relevant information is difficult, since general physicians who want to keep up to date with articles relevant to their practice face the task of examining 19 articles a day, 365 days a year[56]. With over 200 specialty journals, the situation in dermatology is no different. A quick search for dermatologic trials in the Medline database by restricting the search to publication type 'clinical trials' will retrieve only about half of those on the database[57]. A far more efficient database to search for treatment efficacy is the Cochrane Controlled Clinical Trial Register, part of the Cochrane Library.

Critically Appraising the Information

Once we find potentially useful evidence, we need to critically appraise it to determine if it is valid and useful. At the top of the evidence hierarchy is the systematic review (Table 123.12). The Cochrane

THE SIX STEPS INVOLVED IN CONDUCTING A SYSTEMATIC REVIEW	
Step 1	Framing an important and answerable question
Step 2	Defining the outcome measures
Step 3	Systematically retrieving all relevant study reports
Step 4	Abstracting and critically appraising the quantitative information
Step 5	Synthesis of quantitative data, quality rating of studies, appropriate sensitivity analyses
Step 6	Interpreting the results

Table 123.13 The six steps involved in conducting a systematic review.

Collaboration, of which there is the Cochrane Skin Group, was formed to prepare, maintain and disseminate unbiased external systematic reviews of the effects of health care based on randomized controlled clinical trials (RCTs)[58].

Unlike traditional reviews, systematic reviews have an explicit structure and methodology that another researcher could replicate if necessary. Systematic reviews of RCTs, such as those developed by the Cochrane Collaboration, are a summary of accurate, up-to-date, high-quality external evidence of the effectiveness of interventions for treating or preventing human disease. They are done systematically along a series of well-defined steps (Table 123.13) that are outlined in a protocol. However, like any study design, systematic reviews can be good or bad[56]. Sometimes, combining data quantitatively is inappropriate, and other techniques, such as best-evidence synthesis or a search for the reasons for conflicting findings or studies, are more informative[59]. Systematic reviews are needed in dermatology because it has become increasingly difficult or impossible to keep up with the over 200 journals currently being published. Second, they can reduce the uncertainty produced by the conflicting results of several small inconclusive studies by combining their results – provided they are sufficiently similar. Another reason for systematic reviews is to reduce bias. The protocol provides an opportunity to state which participants should ideally be studied, which comparisons are appropriate, and which outcomes make a difference clinically. However, the main reason why systematic reviews are needed in dermatology is that such reviews provide an excellent opportunity to identify and promote further research, and to help change the RCT agenda which is often driven by the pharmaceutical industry.

RCTs are one of the strongest designs in modern medicine for assessing treatment efficacy because of the potential to minimize bias. According to Juni et al.[60] the four most important elements that have been shown to inflate treatment effects in RCTs are: (1) unclear method of generation of the randomization sequence; (2) unclear concealment of the allocation sequence; (3) non-blinding of the intervention from participants and assessors; and (4) failure to perform an analysis of all those originally randomized (an intention-to-treat analysis).

Applying it Back to the Patient

The last, but perhaps one of the most difficult steps is applying the results of our critical appraisal back to the patient. The external evidence has to be integrated with the clinical expertise of the physician, along with the knowledge of the unique features of the individual patients and their situations, rights and expectations. The five key questions that should be asked are shown in Table 123.14.

THE HIERARCHY OF EVIDENCE
Systematic reviews
Randomized controlled trials
Non-randomized trials
Uncontrolled trials (case series)
Case report
Anecdotal

Table 123.12 The hierarchy of evidence.

QUESTIONS TO ASK WHEN APPLYING THE RESULTS OF A CRITICAL APPRAISAL BACK TO THE PATIENT
Are my patient's characteristics similar to those of the patients in these trials?
Are the outcomes of clinical sense to me?
Is the magnitude of benefit likely to be worthwhile to my patient?
What are the adverse effects?
Does the treatment fit with my patient's values and beliefs?

Table 123.14 Questions to ask when applying the results of a critical appraisal back to the patient. Modified according to Williams HC. Dowling Oration 2001: Evidence-based dermatology – a bridge too far? Clin Exp Dermatol. 2001;26:714–24.

Knowing how to read a clinical trial reporting a new treatment for a skin disease is arguably a core competency and lifelong skill for any dermatologist[61].

Websites

European Dermato-Epidemiology Network (EDEN):
   http://www.dermis.net/org/eden
Cochrane Skin Group: http://www.nottingham.ac.uk/~muzd

REFERENCES

1. Rea JN, Nehouse ML, Halil T. Skin disease in Lambeth: a community study of prevalence and use of medical care. Br J Prev Soc Med. 1976;30:107–14.
2. Johnson M-LT. Skin conditions and related need for medical care among persons aged 1–74 years, United States, 1971-74. Vital and Health Statistics: Series 11, No. 212. DHEW publication No. (PHS) 79-1660. National Center for Health Statistics 1978:1–72.
3. Diepgen TL, Mahler V. The epidemiology of skin cancer, Br J Dermatol. 2002;146(suppl.):1–6.
4. Ryan TJ. Disability in dermatology. Br J Hosp Med. 1991;46:33–6.
5. Williams HC, Strachan DP (eds). The Challenge of Dermato-Epidemiology. Boca Raton: CRC Press Inc., 1997.
6. Williams HC. Epidemiology of skin diseases. In: Champion RH, Burton JL, Burns DA, Breathnach SM (eds). Textbook of Dermatology, 6th edn. Oxford: Blackwell Science, 1998:139–57.
7. Williams HC, Naldi L, Diepgen TL, et al. Epidemiology of skin disease in Europe. In: Fritsch P (ed.). White Book Dermatology and Venereology in Europe. Bern: European Dermatology Forum, 2001.
8. Diepgen TL, Coenraads PJ. Inflammatory skin disease II: contact dermatitis. In: Williams HC, Strachan DP (eds). The Challange of Dermato-Epidemiology. Boca Raton: CRC Press, 1997:141–57.
9. Williams HC. Dermatology. In: Stevens A, Raftery J (eds). Health Care Needs Assessment, second series. Oxford: Radcliffe Medical Press, 1997.
10. Meding B. Normal standards of dermatological health screening at places at work. Contact Dermatitis. 1992;27:269–70.
11. Everyday Health Care: A Consumer Study of Self-medication in Great Britain. London: British Market Research Bureau, 1987.
12. Royal College of General Practitioners. Morbidity statistics from General Practice. Fourth National Study 1991-92. London: HMSO, 1995.
13. Carmichael AJ. Achieving an accessible dermatology service. Dermatol Pract. 1995;3:13–16.
14. Ferguson JA, Goldacre MJ, Newton JN, Dawber RPR. An epidemiological profile of inpatient workload in dermatology. Clin Exp Dermatol. 1992;17:407–12.
15. Office of Population Censuses and Surveys. 1992 Mortality Statistics. London: HMSO, 1994.
16. Diepgen TL, Coenraads PJ. The impact of sensitivity, specificity and positive predictive value of patch testing: the more you test, the more you get? Contact Dermatitis. 2000;42:315–17.
17. Agresti A. Categorical Data Analysis. New York: Wiley, 1990.
18. Greenland S. Statistical uncertainty due to misclassification: implications for validation substudies. J Clin Epidemiol. 1988;41:1167–74.
19. Hanifin JM, Rajka G. Diagnostic features of atopic dermatitis. Acta Derm Venereol (Stockh). 1980;92:44–7.
20. Diepgen TL, Sauerbrei W, Fartasch M. Development and validation of diagnostic scores for atopic dermatitis incorporating criteria of data quality and practical usefulness. J Clin Epidemiol. 1996;49:1031–8.
21. Svenson A, Edman B, Möller H. A diagnostic tool for atopic dermatitis based on clinical criteria. Acta Dermatol Venereol (Stockh). 1985;114:33–40.
22. Schultz Larsen F, Diepgen TL, Svensson A. The occurrence of atopic dermatitis in North Europe. An international questionnaire study. J Am Acad Dermatol. 1996;34:760–4.

23. Williams HC, Burney P, Pembroke A, Hay RJ. The U.K. Working Party's Diagnostic Criteria for Atopic Dermatitis. III: Independent hospital validation. Br J Dermatol. 1994;131:406–16.
24. Williams HC, Burney P, Pembroke A, Hay RJ. Validation of the UK diagnostic criteria for atopic dermatitis in a population setting. Br J Dermatol. 1996;135:12–17.
25. Popescu CM, Popescu R, Williams H, Forsea D. Community validation of the United Kingdom diagnostic criteria for atopic dermatitis in Romanian schoolchildren. Br J Dermatol. 1998;138:436–42.
26. Kramer U, Schafer T, Behrendt H, Ring J. The influence of cultural and educational factors on the validity of symptom and diagnosis questions for atopic eczema. Br J Dermatol. 1998;139:1040–6.
27. Marks R, Kilkenny M, Plunkett A, Merlin K. The prevalence of common skin conditions in Australian school students: 2. Atopic dermatitis. Br J Dermatol. 1999;140:468–73.
28. Firooz A, Davoudi SM, Farahmand AN, et al. Validation of the diagnostic criteria for atopic dermatitis. Arch Dermatol. 1999;135:514–16.
29. Chan HH, Pei A, van Krevel C, et al. Validation of the Chinese translated version of ISAAC core questions for atopic eczema. Clin Exp Allergy. 2001;31:903–7.
30. Diepgen TL. Is the prevalence of atopic dermatitis increasing? In: Williams HC (ed.). Epidemiology of Atopic Eczema. Cambridge: Cambridge University Press, 2000:96–109.
31. Hulley S, Cummings S, Browner W, et al. Designing Clinical Research: An Epidemiologic Approach, 2nd edn. Philadelphia: Lippincott Williams & Wilkins, 2001.
32. Smit HA, Coenraads PJ, Lavrijsen APM, Nater JP. Evaluation of a self-administered questionnaire on hand dermatitis. Contact Dermatitis. 1992;26:11–16.
33. Richards C, Richards H, Pheby D. Skin cancer: how accurate are local data? Br Med J. 1995;310:503.
34. Buettner PG, Raasch BA. Incidence rates of skin cancer in Townsville, Australia. Int J Cancer. 1998;78:587–93.
35. Green A, Battistutta D, Hart V, et al. Skin cancer in a subtropical Australian population: incidence and lack of association with occupation. Am J Epidemiol. 1996;144:1034–40.
36. Kaldor J, Shugg D, Young B, et al. Non-melanoma skin cancer: ten years of cancer-registry-based surveillance. Int J Cancer. 1993;53:886–91.
37. Miller DL, Weinstock MA. Nonmelanoma skin cancer in the United States: incidence. J Am Acad Dermatol. 1994;30:774–8.
38. Serrano H, Scotto J, Shornick G, et al. Incidence of nonmelanoma skin cancer in New Hampshire and Vermont. J Am Acad Dermatol. 1991;24:574–9.
39. Gray DT, Suman VJ, Su WPD, et al. Trends in the population-based incidence of squamous cell carcinoma of the skin first diagnosed between 1984 and 1992. Arch Dermatol. 1997;133:735–40.
40. Holme SA, Malinovszky K, Roberts DL. Changing trends in non-melanoma skin cancer in South Wales, 1988-98. Br J Dermatol. 2000;143:1224–9.
41. Ko CB, Walton S, Keczkes HPR, et al. The emerging epidemic of skin cancer. Br J Dermatol. 1994;130:269–72.
42. Scottish Cancer Intelligence Unit, ISD, National Health Service in Scotland. Cancer Registration Statistic. Scotland 1990-95. Edinburgh: Scottish Executive, 1998.
43. Hannuksela-Svahn A, Pukkala E, Karvonen J. Basal cell skin carcinoma and other nonmelanoma skin cancers in

Finland from 1956 through 1995. Arch Dermatol. 1999;135:781–6.
44. Coebergh JW, Neumann HA, Vrints LW, et al. Trends in the incidence of non-melanoma skin cancer in the SE Netherlands 1975-88: a registry based study. Br J Dermatol. 1991;125:353–9.
45. Green A. Changing patterns in incidence of nonmelanoma skin cancer. Epithelial Cell Biol. 1992;1:47–51.
46. Giles G, Marks R, Foley P. Incidence of nonmelanocytic skin cancer treated in Australia. Br Med J. 1988;269:13–17.
47. Fears TR. Estimating increase in skin cancer morbidity due to increase in ultraviolet radiation exposure. Cancer Invest. 1983;1:119–26.
48. Russel L, Gold M, Siegel J, et al. The role of cost-effectiveness analysis in health and medicine. JAMA. 1996;276:1172–7.
48a. Bickers DR, Lim HW, Margolis D, et al. American Academy of Dermatology Association. Society for Investigative Dermatology. The burden of skin diseases: 2004 a joint project of the American Academy of Dermatology Association and the Society for Investigative Dermatology. J Am Acad Dermatol. 2006;55:490–500.
49. Detsky A, Naglie I. A clinician's guide to cost-effectiveness analysis. Ann Int Med. 1990;113:147–54.
50. Ellis C, Reiter K, Wheeler J, Fendrick A. Economic analysis in dermatology. J Am Acad Dermatol. 2002;46:271–83.
51. Finlay AY, Khan GK. Dermatology Life Quality Index (DLQI) – a simple practical measure for routine clinical use. Clin Exp Dermatol. 1994;19:210–16.
52. Chren MM, Lasek RJ, Quinn LM, et al. Skindex, a quality-of-life measure for patients with skin disease: reliability, validity, and responsiveness. J Invest Dermatol. 1996;107:707–13.
53. Chren MM, Lasek RJ, Flocke SA, Zyzanski SJ. Improved discriminative and evaluative capability of a refined version of Skindex, a quality-of-life instrument for patients with skin diseases. Arch Dermatol 1997;133:1433–40.
54. Chren MM, Lasek RJ, Sahay AP, Sands LP. Measurement properties of Skindex-16: a brief quality-of-life measure for patients with skin diseases. J Cutan Med Surg 2001;5:105–10.
55. Sackett DL, Richardson WS, Rosenberg WMC, Haynes RB. Evidence-Based Medicine: How to Practice and Teach EBM. New York: Churchill Livingstone, 1997.
56. Davidoff F, Haynes RB, Sackett DL, Smith R. Evidence based medicine: a new journal to help doctors identify the information they need. Br Med J. 1995;310:1085–6.
57. Adetugbo K, Williams HC. How well are randomised controlled trials reported in the dermatology literature? Arch Dermatol. 2001;137:332–5.
58. Williams HC, Adetugbo K, Wan Po AL, et al. The Cochrane Skin Group: preparing, maintaining and disseminating systematic reviews of clinical interventions in dermatology. Arch Dermatol. 1998;134:1620–6.
59. Chalmers I, Altman DG (eds). Systematic Reviews. London: BMJ Publishing Group, 1995.
60. Juni P, Altman DG, Egger M. Assessing the quality of controlled clinical trials. Br Med J. 2001;323:42–6.
61. Williams HC. Dowling Oration 2001: Evidence-based dermatology – a bridge too far? Clin Exp Dermatol. 2001;26:714–24.

Skin Barrier and Percutaneous Drug Delivery

124

SKIN BARRIER AND PERCUTANEOUS DRUG DELIVERY

Peter M Elias, Jui-Chen Tsai, Gopinathan K Menon, Walter M Holleran and Kenneth R Feingold

Stratum Corneum Structure and Organization

The paper-thin stratum corneum is a composite material made of proteins and lipids that is crucial for life in a terrestrial environment. In the traditional view, the stratum corneum is regarded as impermeable, but inert and highly resilient, analogous to a sheet of plastic wrap (Table 124.1). According to this model, transepidermal permeation is governed solely by the physico-chemical properties of this supposedly homogeneous tissue[1], and barrier properties can be assessed readily *in vitro*, in either devitalized or fresh epidermal sheets. Anatomic site-related variations in the number of stratum corneum cell layers, which govern the diffusion path length, can also be integrated into the kinetics predicted by the plastic-wrap model.

The first development to cast doubt upon both the plastic-wrap model and its suppositions was the discovery of the unique structural heterogeneity of the stratum corneum, i.e. its 'bricks and mortar' organization (Fig. 124.1)[2]. Rather than being uniformly dispersed, the highly hydrophobic lipids in normal stratum corneum are sequestered within the extracellular spaces, where this lipid-enriched matrix is organized into lamellar membranes that surround the corneocytes[2,3]. Hence, instead of stratum corneum thickness, variations in number of lamellar membranes (= lipid weight %), membrane structure, and/or lipid composition provide the structural and biochemical basis for site-related variations in permeability[4]. It follows, then, that the extracellular,

lipid-enriched matrix of the stratum corneum comprises not only the structure that limits transdermal delivery of hydrophilic drugs, but also the so-called stratum corneum 'reservoir'[5], within which lipid-soluble drugs, such as topical corticosteroids, can accumulate and be slowly released.

Human stratum corneum typically comprises about 20 corneocyte cell layers, which differ in their thickness, packing of keratin filaments, filaggrin content, and number of corneodesmosomes, depending on

EVOLVING CONCEPTS OF THE STRATUM CORNEUM

Outdated

1. Disorganized and no functional significance: 'basket-weave'
2. Homogeneous film: 'Saran Wrap'

Current

3. Two-compartment organization: 'bricks and mortar'
4. Microheterogeneity within extracellular spaces: 'There's more to the mortar than lipid'
5. Persistent metabolic activity: dynamic changes in cytosol, cornified envelope, and interstices from inner to outer stratum corneum
6. Homeostatic links to the nucleated cell layers: barrier function regulates epidermal DNA and lipid synthesis
7. Pathophysiologic links to deeper skin layers: barrier abrogation and/or epidermal injury initiates epidermal hyperplasia and inflammation
8. Stratum corneum as a biosensor: changes in external humidity alone regulate proteolysis of filaggrin, epidermal DNA/lipid synthesis, and initiation of inflammation

Table 124.1 Evolving concepts of the stratum corneum.

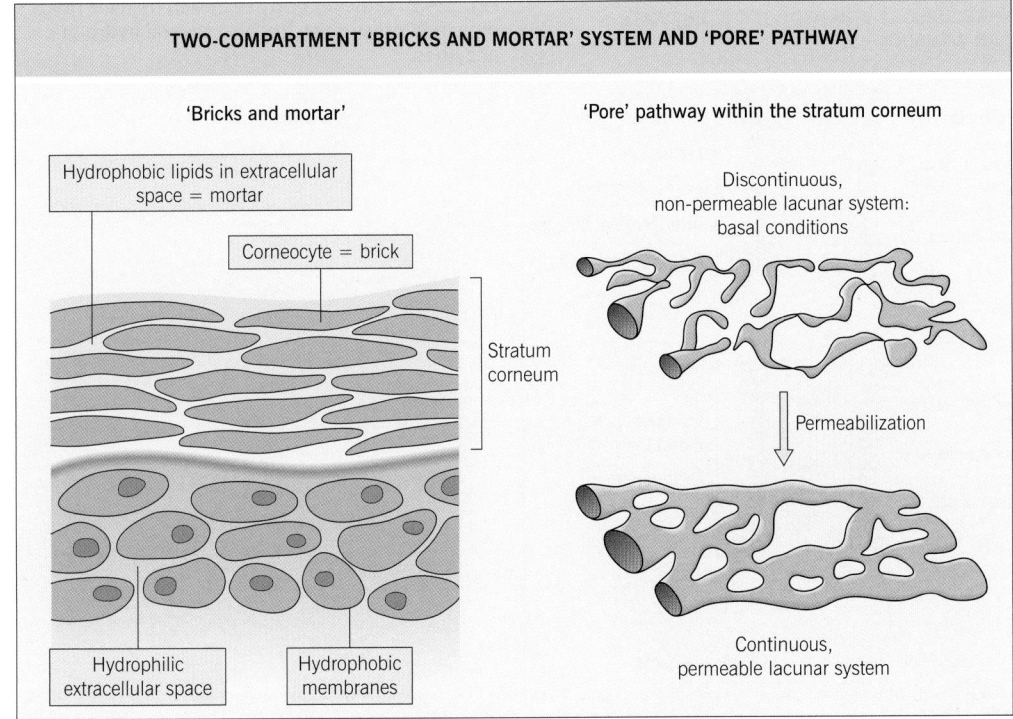

TWO-COMPARTMENT 'BRICKS AND MORTAR' SYSTEM AND 'PORE' PATHWAY

'Bricks and mortar'

Hydrophobic lipids in extracellular space = mortar

Corneocyte = brick

Hydrophilic extracellular space

Hydrophobic membranes

Stratum corneum

'Pore' pathway within the stratum corneum

Discontinuous, non-permeable lacunar system: basal conditions

Permeabilization

Continuous, permeable lacunar system

Fig. 124.1 Two-compartment 'bricks and mortar' system and 'pore' pathway. A The stratum corneum is a unique two-compartment system, analogous to a brick wall. Whereas lipids are sequestered extracellularly within the stratum corneum, the corneocyte is lipid-depleted, but protein-enriched. **B** The degradation of corneodesmosomes results in discontinuous lacunar domains, which represent the likely aqueous 'pore' pathway. These lacunae can enlarge and extend, forming a continuous, but collapsible network under certain conditions, e.g. occlusion, prolonged hydration, sonophoresis.

body site. Corneocytes are surrounded by a highly cross-linked, resilient sheath, the cornified envelope, while the cell interior is packed with keratin filaments embedded in a matrix composed mainly of filaggrin and its breakdown products (= 'natural moisturizing factor'). As noted above, individual corneocytes, in turn, are surrounded by a lipid-enriched extracellular matrix, organized largely into lamellar membranes, which derive from secreted lamellar body precursor lipids (Fig. 124.2). Following secretion, lamellar body contents fuse end-to-end, forming progressively elongated membrane sheets[3], a sequence requiring the action of a battery of lipolytic 'processing' enzymes (see below). Yet, despite the clear importance of corneocytes both as spacers and as a scaffold for the extracellular matrix, transdermal drug development has focused primarily on manipulations of the extracellular lipid milieu[6,7]. The existence of aqueous pores within the extracellular matrix[8] not only adds further complexity to the extracellular pathway (see Fig. 124.1), but also provides additional opportunities for novel delivery strategies.

The exceptionally low permeability of normal stratum corneum to water-soluble drugs is the consequence of several characteristics of the lipid-enriched, extracellular matrix (Table 124.2), including its organization into a highly convoluted and tortuous extracellular pathway imposed by geometrically arrayed corneocyte 'spacers'[9]. Moreover, not only the paired-bilayer arrangement of extracellular lipids, but also their extreme hydrophobicity and the composition and distribution of the three key species (ceramides, cholesterol and free fatty acids) in a critical (1:1:1) molar ratio are further characteristics that provide for barrier function.

Ceramides account for approximately 50% of the total stratum corneum lipid mass[10,11], and are crucial for the lamellar organization of the stratum corneum barrier[12]. Of the nine ceramide classes, acylceramides or ceramides 1, 4 and 7 (which contain ω-hydroxy-linked, essential fatty acids in an ester linkage) are epidermis-unique compounds, known to be important for the barrier[13]. Cholesterol, the second most abundant lipid by weight in the stratum corneum, promotes the intermixing of different lipid species, and regulates its 'phase' behavior[14]. Free fatty acids, which account for 10–15% of stratum corneum lipids, consist predominantly of very-long-chain, saturated species with ≥18 carbon atoms[10]. A decrease in the concentrations of any of these critical lipid species compromises barrier integrity, by altering the molar ratio of the membranes that mediate normal barrier function.

The 'domain-mosaic model' advocates a meandering, polar (pore) pathway for water transport through lamellar boundaries within the lipid mosaic[15], adding potential complexity to the already tortuous, extracellular pathway. An alternative model relates to the presence of lacunar domains embedded within the lipid bilayers[8] (see Fig. 124.1). These lacunae correspond to sites of subjacent corneodesmosome degradation (see Fig. 124.2), and presumably they contain the hydrophobic degradation products of corneodesmosomes[16]. Whereas these lacunae are scattered and discontinuous under basal conditions, following certain types of permeabilization (e.g. occlusion, prolonged hydration, sonophoresis, iontophoresis), they expand until they interconnect, forming a continuous 'pore pathway' (see Fig. 124.1). The pore pathway reverts back to its original, discontinuous state once the permeabilizing stimulus disappears. Such a lacunar system, then, does not correspond to the grain boundaries of the 'domain mosaic model', but instead it forms an 'extended mosaic macrodomain' within the stratum corneum interstices[17].

Epidermal Lipid Metabolism and the Skin Barrier
Biosynthetic activities

Epidermal differentiation is a vectorial process that is accompanied by dramatic changes in lipid composition, including loss of phospholipids with the emergence of ceramides, cholesterol and free fatty acids in the stratum corneum[11,13] (see Fig. 124.2). Although epidermal lipid synthesis is both highly active and largely autonomous from systemic influences, it can be regulated by external influences, i.e. changes in the status of the permeability barrier[18]. Acute perturbations of the permeability barrier stimulate a characteristic recovery sequence that leads to restoration of normal function over about 72 hours in young skin (the cutaneous stress test). This sequence includes an increase in cholesterol, free fatty acid and ceramide synthesis that is restricted to the underlying epidermis,

---

HOW STRATUM CORNEUM LIPIDS MEDIATE BARRIER FUNCTION

- Extracellular localization: only intercellular lipids play a role
- Amount of lipid (lipid weight %)
- Elongated, tortuous pathway: increases diffusion length
- Organization into lamellar membrane structures
- Hydrophobic composition: absence of polar lipids and presence of very-long-chain, saturated fatty acids
- Correct molar ratio: approximately 1:1:1 of three key lipids: ceramides, cholesterol and free fatty acids
- Unique molecular structures (e.g. acylceramides)

Table 124.2 How stratum corneum lipids mediate barrier function.

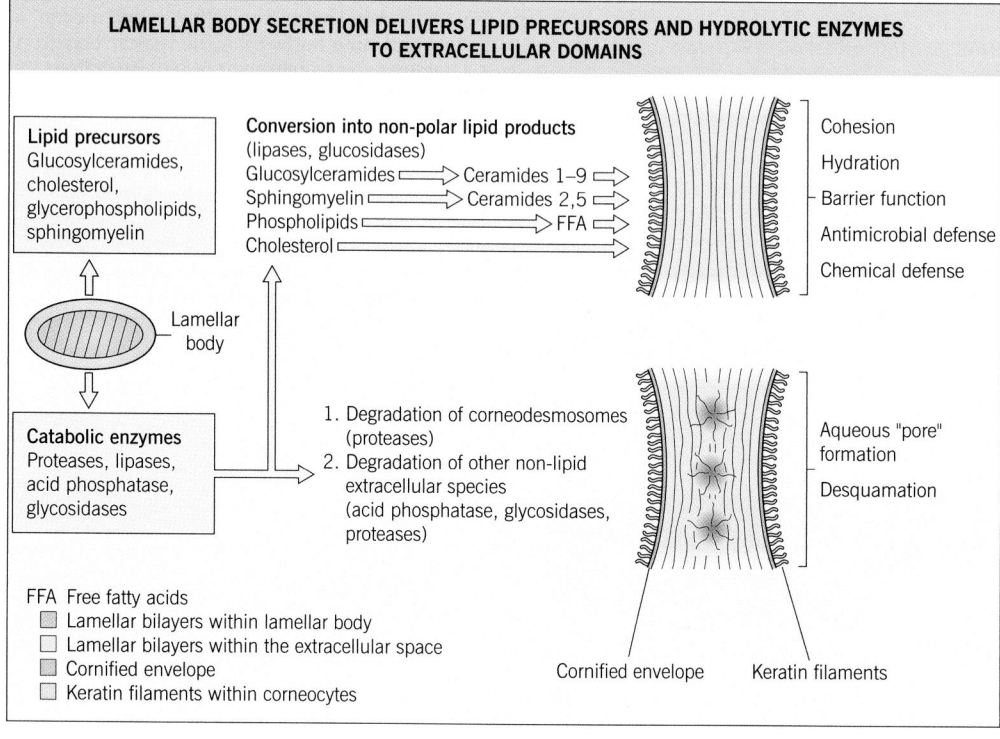

Fig. 124.2 Lamellar body secretion delivers not only lipid precursors, but also several hydrolytic enzymes.

LAMELLAR BODY SECRETION DELIVERS LIPID PRECURSORS AND HYDROLYTIC ENZYMES TO EXTRACELLULAR DOMAINS

Lipid precursors
Glucosylceramides, cholesterol, glycerophospholipids, sphingomyelin

Lamellar body

Catabolic enzymes
Proteases, lipases, acid phosphatase, glycosidases

Conversion into non-polar lipid products
(lipases, glucosidases)
Glucosylceramides ⟹ Ceramides 1–9 ⟹
Sphingomyelin ⟹ Ceramides 2,5 ⟹
Phospholipids ⟹ FFA ⟹
Cholesterol ⟹

1. Degradation of corneodesmosomes (proteases)
2. Degradation of other non-lipid extracellular species (acid phosphatase, glycosidases, proteases)

Cohesion
Hydration
Barrier function
Antimicrobial defense
Chemical defense

Aqueous "pore" formation
Desquamation

Cornified envelope   Keratin filaments

FFA Free fatty acids
☐ Lamellar bilayers within lamellar body
☐ Lamellar bilayers within the extracellular space
☐ Cornified envelope
☐ Keratin filaments within corneocytes

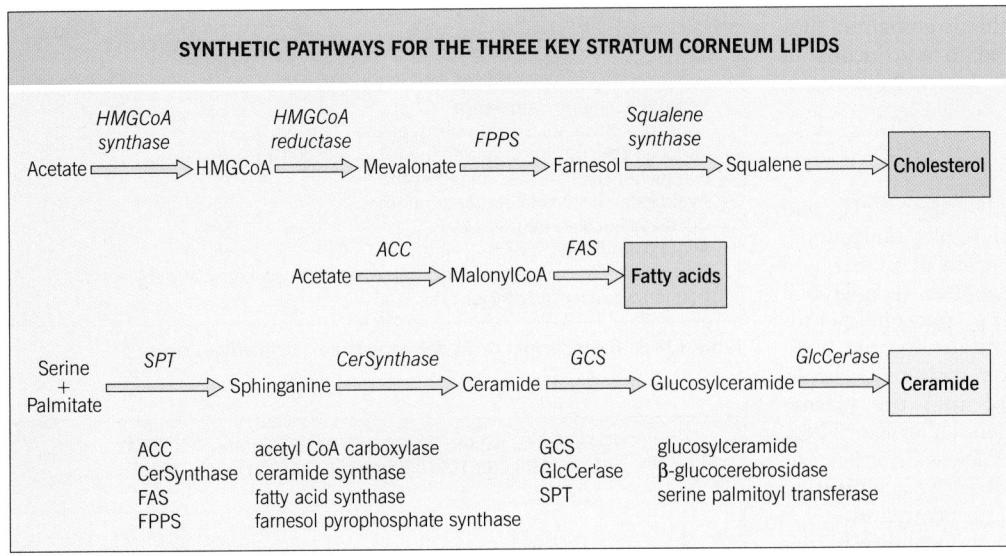

Fig. 124.3 The major synthetic pathways that lead to the generation of the three key barrier lipids of the stratum corneum. The rate-limiting enzymes in each pathway are shown. Each enzyme, in turn, represents a potential target for a metabolic intervention to enhance drug delivery (see Fig. 124.8). Applications of specific, conduritol-type inhibitors of β-glucocerebrosidase to intact skin lead to a progressive abnormality in barrier function. In both a transgenic murine model of Gaucher disease (GD) (produced by targeted disruption of the β-glucocerebrosidase gene) and in the severe, type 2 neuronopathic form of GD, infants present with a barrier abnormality. This was attributable to accumulation of glucosylceramides, depletion of ceramides, and persistence of immature lamellar bodies within the interstices of the stratum corneum.

and attributable to a prior increase in mRNA and enzyme activity/mass for each of the key synthetic enzymes (Fig. 124.3). Furthermore, synthesis of each of the three key lipids is required for normal barrier homeostasis, i.e. topically applied inhibitors of the key enzymes in each pathway produce abnormalities in permeability barrier homeostasis[18]. These experiments provided the seminal observations, as well as the model ('stress test'), that led to development of a biochemical strategy to enhance drug delivery (see below).

Lamellar body secretion

The unique two-compartment organization of the stratum corneum is attributable to the secretion of lamellar body-derived lipids and co-localized hydrolases at the stratum granulosum–stratum corneum interface[3]. Under basal conditions, lamellar body secretion is slow, but sufficient to provide for barrier integrity. Following acute barrier disruption, calcium is lost from the outer epidermis, and much of the preformed pool of lamellar bodies in the outermost cells of the stratum granulosum is quickly secreted[19–21]. Calcium is an important regulator of lamellar body secretion, with the high levels of Ca^{2+} in the stratum granulosum restricting lamellar body secretion to low, maintenance levels[22]. Finally, barrier homeostasis and lamellar body secretion are regulated not only by changes in Ca^{2+}, but also by agents that block organellogenesis and secretion, e.g. monensin and brefeldin A (see below).

Extracellular processing

Extrusion of the polar lipid contents of lamellar bodies at the stratum granulosum–stratum corneum interface is followed by the processing of those lipids into more hydrophobic species that form mature, lamellar membranes[8] (Fig. 124.4). The extracellular processing of glucosylceramides, phospholipids and cholesterol sulfate with accumulation of ceramides, free fatty acids and cholesterol in the stratum corneum is attributable to the co-secretion of a set of hydrolytic enzymes[3] (see Fig 124.2).

Extracellular processing of glucosylceramides plays a key role in barrier homeostasis (see legend to Fig. 124.3). In addition, phospholipid hydrolysis, catalyzed by one or more, still uncharacterized, 14 kDa secretory phospholipases ($sPLA_2$), generates a family of non-essential free fatty acids, which are required for barrier homeostasis[23–25]. Since applications of either bromphenacylbromide or MJ33 (chemically unrelated $sPLA_2$ inhibitors) modulate barrier function in intact skin, $sPLA_2$ appears to play a critical role in barrier homeostasis[23–25]. Moreover, applications of either inhibitor to perturbed skin sites delays barrier recovery.

Sphingomyelin hydrolysis by acidic sphingomyelinase generates two of the nine ceramides required for normal barrier homeostasis (see Fig 124.2). Moreover, patients with mutations in the gene encoding acidic sphingomyelinase (Niemann-Pick, Type A) that lead to low enzyme activity display an ichthyosiform dermatosis, and transgenic mice with an absence of acidic sphingomyelinase also demonstrate a barrier abnormality. Finally, applications of non-specific inhibitors of acidic sphingomyelinase to perturbed skin sites lead to a delay in barrier recovery[26].

Just as with glucosylceramides and sphingomyelin, cholesterol sulfate content increases during epidermal differentiation, and then decreases progressively as the latter is desulfated during passage from the inner to the outer stratum corneum[27]. Both cholesterol sulfate and its processing enzyme, steroid sulfatase, are concentrated in membrane domains of the stratum corneum. Conversely, the content of cholesterol sulfate in these sites increases by approximately tenfold[27] in recessive X-linked ichthyosis (see Ch. 56). Not only is recessive X-linked ichthyosis characterized by a barrier defect[28], but also repeated applications of cholesterol sulfate to intact skin produce a barrier abnormality[29]. In both cases, the barrier abnormality is attributable to cholesterol

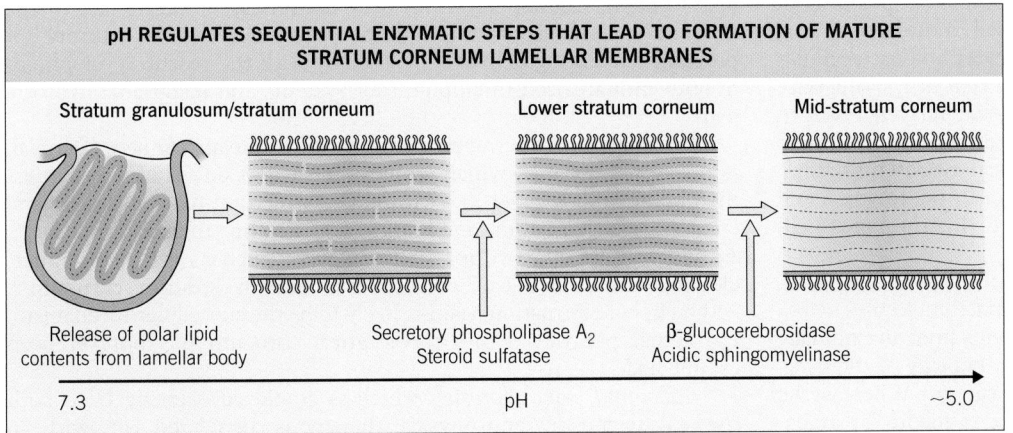

Fig. 124.4 pH regulates sequential enzymatic steps that lead to formation of mature stratum corneum lamellar membranes. The process begins at the stratum granulosum–stratum corneum interface.

sulfate-induced phase separation in lamellar membrane domains[28]. But the barrier defect may also be, in part, attributed to a reduction in cholesterol content, since cholesterol sulfate is a potent inhibitor of HMGCoA reductase (see Fig. 124.3).

Acidification

The fact that the stratum corneum displays an acidic external pH ('acid mantle') is well documented, but its origin is not fully understood. Extraepidermal mechanisms (including surface deposits of eccrine- and sebaceous gland-derived products as well as metabolites of microbial metabolism), endogenous catabolic processes (e.g. phospholipid-to-free fatty acid hydrolysis, deamination of histidine to urocanic acid), and local generation of protons within the lower stratum corneum (by sodium-proton antiporters [NHE_1] inserted into the plasma membrane[30,31]) could actively acidify the extracellular space. These mechanisms would explain not only the pH gradient across the interstices of the stratum corneum (see Fig. 124.4), but also selective acidification of membrane microdomains within the lower stratum corneum.

The concept that acidification is required for permeability barrier homeostasis is supported by the observation that barrier recovery is delayed when acutely perturbed skin sites are immersed in neutral pH buffers[32], or when either the sodium-proton exchanger/antiporter or $sPLA_2$-mediated phospholipid catabolism to free fatty acids is blocked[30]. Acidification appears to impact barrier homeostasis through regulation of enzymes involved in extracellular processing, such as β-glucocerebrosidase and acidic sphingomyelinase, which exhibit acidic pH optima (see Fig. 124.4).

Strategies to Enhance Transdermal Drug Delivery

Because of its theoretical advantages (Table 124.3; Fig. 124.5), enormous efforts have been expended on the development of new approaches to enhance transdermal drug delivery. Yet, despite these efforts, the current list of drugs that have been delivered transdermally for systemic applications is still small, and largely limited to lipophilic compounds of both low molecular weight and low total absorbed dose (e.g. nitroglycerin, clonidine, sex steroids, scopolamine and nicotinic acid) (Table 124.4). The strategies that have been devised to enhance transdermal drug delivery can be classified as either physical, chemical, mechanical or biochemical approaches. Combinations of these strategies can also be employed to increase efficacy[33–35], or for extending the time available for transdermal delivery (see below). Physical techniques vary from straightforward approaches, such as occlusion or tape stripping, to highly sophisticated instrumentation and miniaturization (e.g. iontophoresis, electroporation).

The most straightforward physical method is prolonged *occlusion*, which alters the barrier properties of the stratum corneum[36,37]. Following 24–48 hours of occlusion with resultant hydration, corneocytes swell, the intercellular spaces become distended, and the lacunar network becomes dilated. Distention of lacunae eventually leads to connections within an otherwise discontinuous system, creating 'pores' in the stratum corneum interstices through which polar and non-polar substances can penetrate more readily (see Fig. 124.1).

Stripping consists of another straightforward physical method to abrogate the barrier. Sequential stripping, with either adhesive tapes or cyanoacrylate glue, increases transepidermal water loss, an indicator of a barrier defect, which correlates with enhanced transdermal drug delivery[34,38]. Tape stripping removes both corneocytes and extracellular lipids, thereby reducing the elongated path length that drugs otherwise need to traverse, and mechanically disrupts lamellar bilayers, even in retained, lower stratum corneum layers. Barrier disruption of human skin requires multiple strippings, which can lead to inflammation. More strippings are required to disrupt the barrier in phototype 5 and 6 (darkly pigmented) than in phototype 1 and 2 (lightly pigmented) subjects[39].

Iontophoresis and *electroporation* represent electrically assisted, physical approaches to enhance delivery of drugs/macromolecules across the stratum corneum[40]. Iontophoresis uses low currents from an externally placed electrode, with the same charge as the net polarity of the drug, to drive these molecules across the stratum corneum. Whereas the predominant pathway of iontophoretic transport is reportedly trans-

Table 124.3 Transdermal drug delivery: theoretical advantages.

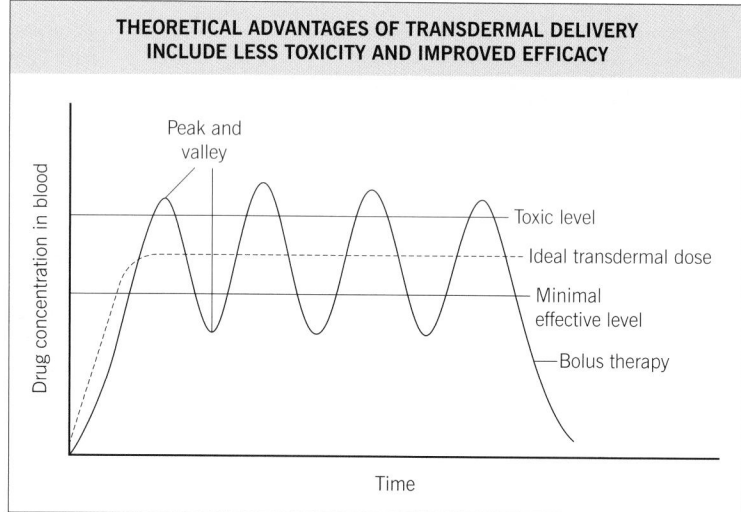

Fig. 124.5 **Theoretical advantages of transdermal delivery include less toxicity and improved efficacy.** This is due to a reduction in the 'peaks' and 'valleys' associated with bolus therapy.

TRANSDERMAL DRUG DELIVERY: ISSUES WITH CURRENT APPROACHES

- Device- or patch-dependent
- Reliance on *in vitro* models alone: limits relevance
- Limitations:
  - Dose (<10 mg/day)
  - Polarity (1° lipophilic)
  - Drug class (peptides excluded)

Therefore, relatively few successful examples: nitroglycerin, scopolamine, clonidine, estrogen, progestins, testosterone, nicotinic acid, fentanyl, lidocaine, oxybutynin, selegiline, ritigotine, methyphenidate

Table 124.4 Transdermal drug delivery: issues with current approaches.

appendageal (hair follicles, sweat glands), extracellular routes across the stratum corneum are also traversed[41]. Iontophoretic delivery through the interstices of the stratum corneum occurs via aqueous pores (see Fig. 124.1); thus, it operates at both a macro- (appendageal) and micro- (extracellular, lacunar) level. As drug delivery is proportionate to the amount of applied current, iontophoresis offers an opportunity for programmable drug delivery[42], especially with the recent development of both miniaturized microprocessor systems and disposable hydrogel pads.

Electroporation (electropermeabilization) is a relatively new electrical, non-thermal method, which employs ultrashort pulses of large, transmembrane voltages (~100 V) to induce structural rearrangement and conductance changes in membranes, again leading to pore formation[40]. Although most effective for single bilayers, such as cell membranes, electroporation also can permeabilize human stratum corneum[43]. Although pore formation again is likely to be the subcellular mechanism, the actual pathway across the stratum corneum has not yet been established.

Ultrasound (sonophoresis), which is employed extensively in both medical diagnostics and physical therapy, is considered safe, with no known short- or long-term side effects. Upon encountering the stratum corneum, ultrasound waves generate defects in its structure[44], leading to permeabilization. Although frequencies in the range of 1–3 MHz are minimally effective, higher frequencies (10–20 MHz) significantly enhance drug delivery[45]. During sonophoresis, electron-dense tracers, such as lanthanum and FITC-conjugated dextrans, penetrate across the stratum corneum into the epidermis and dermis within 5 minutes with no apparent damage to the keratinocytes[46]. Moreover, tracer movement again occurs through lacunae, which become dilated and transiently continuous, followed by collapse of the pore pathway with cessation of applied energy[8,45] (see Fig. 124.1).

A recently developed technique utilizes pulsed laser beams to generate *photomechanical (stress) waves* that interact directly with the stratum corneum in ways that are different from ultrasound. These waves are generated by ablation of a target material (polystyrene) that covers the drug-containing solution that is to be delivered. The target first absorbs the laser radiation, and the solution then serves as a coupling medium for stress waves to propagate across the stratum corneum. As with sonophoresis and iontophoresis, the pathway of permeation is thought to be extracellular, but morphologic studies are lacking. In murine models, both dextran and latex particles were delivered across the stratum corneum by a single photomechanical wave, generated by using a Q-switched ruby laser. As with sonophoresis and iontophoresis, single photomechanical compression waves modulate the permeability of human stratum corneum only transiently, and barrier function recovers almost immediately. Recently, this method has been used to deliver small molecules (e.g. 5-aminolevulenic acid) into human skin both without discomfort and without adverse effects on skin structure or viability[46].

Solvents, such as ethanol, methanol, chloroform and acetone, as well as *detergents* can extract barrier lipids and permeabilize the stratum corneum. Morphologic changes in human stratum corneum following exposure to solvents[17] include phase separation and disruption of lamellar bilayers in addition to the creation of defects in corneocyte membranes (with detergents). Moreover, surfactants, such as sodium dodecyl (lauryl) sulfate, and vehicles (e.g. propylene glycol) extract lipids and create extensive expansion of pre-existing lacunar domains. Furthermore, solvent-based penetration enhancers, such as azone, sulfoxides, urea and free fatty acids, not only extract extracellular lipids, but they also alter stratum corneum lipid organization (phase behavior), thereby increasing transdermal delivery and expanding intercellular domains[5] (Fig. 124.6).

Finally, *liposomes* represent yet another 'chemical' method, frequently employed to enhance drug delivery. However, liposomes appear to enhance transdermal delivery solely via the appendageal pathway[47,48], i.e. as yet, there is no convincing evidence that they penetrate intact stratum corneum[49,50].

Metabolic Approaches to Enhance Transdermal Drug Delivery

As noted above, although a wide variety of methods have been deployed to enhance transdermal drug delivery, they have been minimally effective (see Table 124.4). *In vitro* assessments of efficacy are limited by the lack of a normal metabolic response, while *in vivo* repair responses inevitably restrict the efficacy of any enhancing method. Thus, an alternative, metabolically based approach aims to enhance the efficacy of standard enhancers by inhibiting the repair (metabolic) response *in vivo*[34] (Fig. 124.7). Moreover, this metabolic approach can be used in conjunction with physical methods (see above) to further increase their efficacy[35].

The concept of a biochemical approach to enhance transdermal drug delivery came from pharmacologic studies aimed at inhibiting key metabolic sequences that restore and maintain barrier function, i.e. epidermal lipid synthesis (see Fig. 124.3), lamellar body secretion, extracellular processing (see Fig. 124.4), and maintenance of lamellar bilayers (Fig. 124.8). These methods all either alter the critical molar ratio of the three key stratum corneum lipids or induce discontinuities in the lamellar bilayer system. Pharmacologic 'knockout' studies support the concept that interference with the biosynthesis of any of the key stratum corneum lipids can lead to a temporary increase in trans-

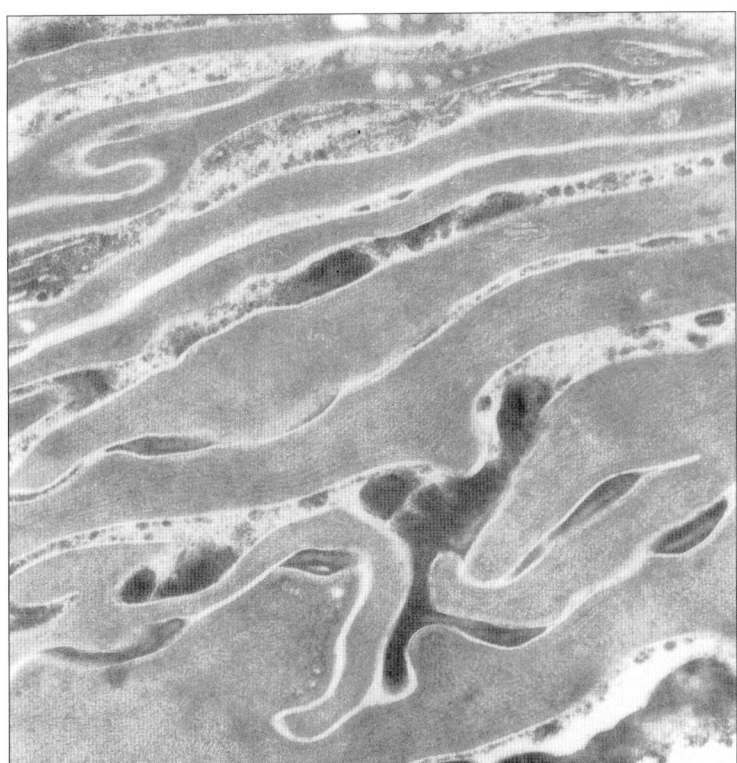

Fig. 124.6 Lipophilic agents (e.g. *n*-butanol) penetrate across the stratum corneum (SC) via the intercellular spaces. Note huge volume expansion of extracellular domains in this electron photomicrograph, representing the putative SC reservoir. *Method*: *n*-butanol precipitation *in situ* with osmium vapors.

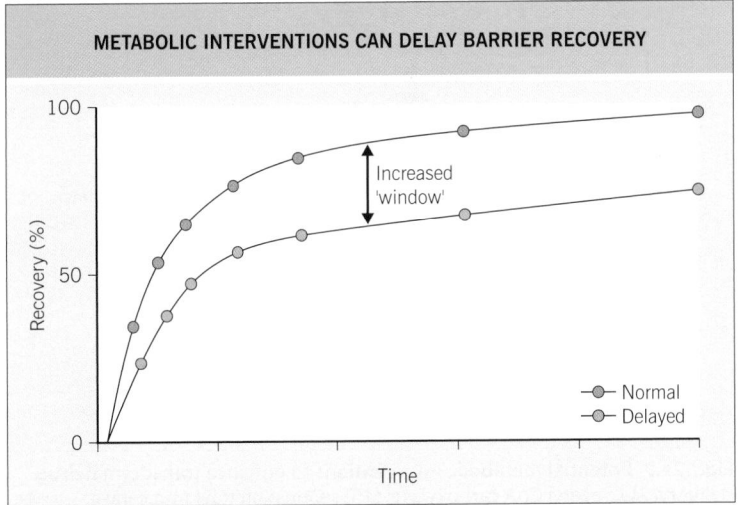

Fig. 124.7 After initial barrier perturbations, metabolic interventions can delay barrier recovery. This creates an increased potential, i.e. a 'window', for transdermal drug delivery.

epidermal water loss, with obvious implications for transdermal drug delivery. In addition to lipid synthesis inhibitors (see Fig. 124.8), agents that interfere with assembly, secretion or extracellular processing of lamellar bodies delay barrier recovery after acute perturbations, and, in some cases, create defects in intact skin. Examples include: (1) brefeldin A, which blocks lamellar body assembly by disorganizing preformed Golgi structures; (2) monensin and chloroquine, which inhibit the apical translocation and secretion of lamellar bodies; (3) exposure to high Ca^{2+}/K^+ levels, which inhibits lamellar body secretion; (4) inhibitors of β-glucocerebrosidase, acidic sphingomyelinase and $sPLA_2$, which are required for normal extracellular processing; and (5) neutral pH buffers, which impede barrier recovery after acute perturbations, presumably by inactivating pH-dependent, extracellular processing enzymes.

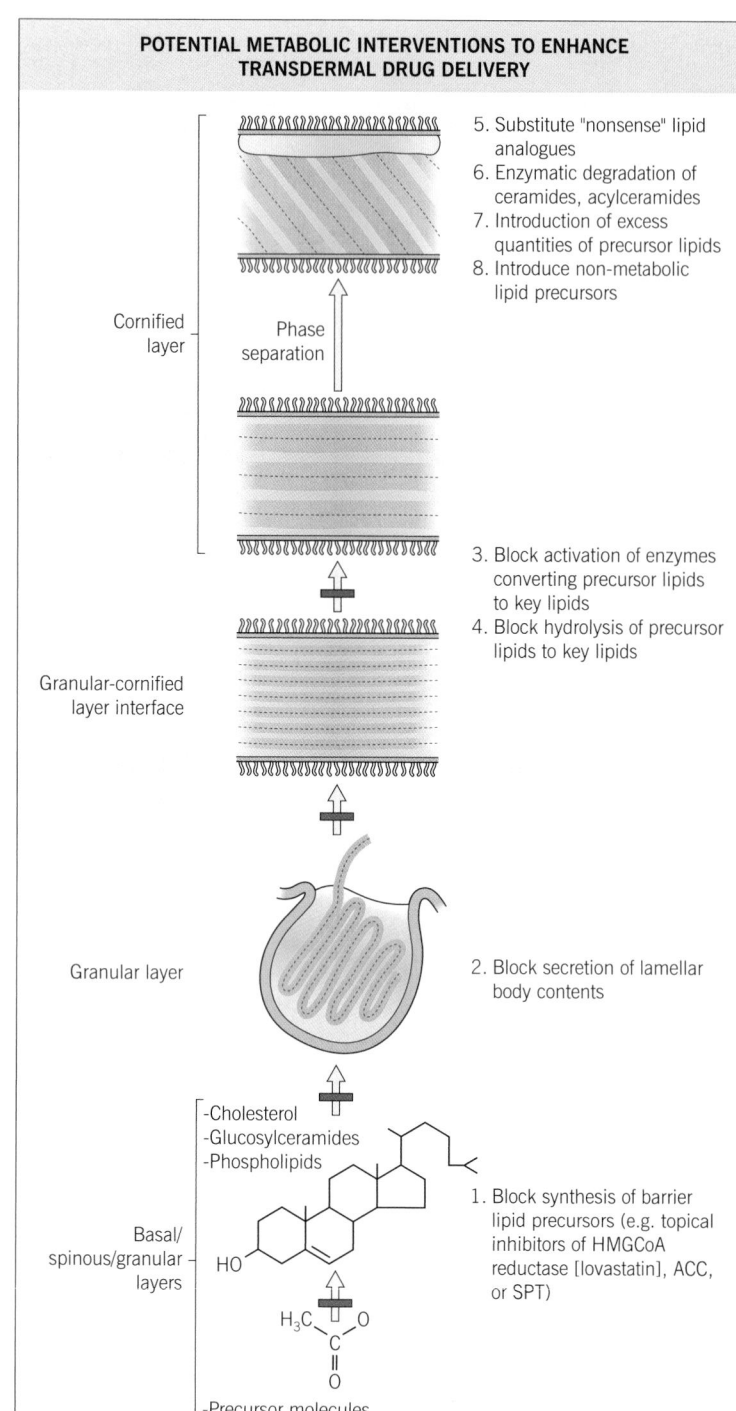

POTENTIAL METABOLIC INTERVENTIONS TO ENHANCE TRANSDERMAL DRUG DELIVERY

Cornified layer

Phase separation

5. Substitute "nonsense" lipid analogues
6. Enzymatic degradation of ceramides, acylceramides
7. Introduction of excess quantities of precursor lipids
8. Introduce non-metabolic lipid precursors

Granular-cornified layer interface

3. Block activation of enzymes converting precursor lipids to key lipids
4. Block hydrolysis of precursor lipids to key lipids

Granular layer

2. Block secretion of lamellar body contents

Basal/ spinous/granular layers

-Cholesterol
-Glucosylceramides
-Phospholipids

HO

1. Block synthesis of barrier lipid precursors (e.g. topical inhibitors of HMGCoA reductase [lovastatin], ACC, or SPT)

H_3C

-Precursor molecules

Fig. 124.8 Potential metabolic interventions to enhance transdermal drug delivery. ACC, acetyl CoA carboxylase; SPT, serine palmitoyl transferase.

An additional category of biochemical enhancers utilizes approaches that alter the supramolecular organization of preformed lamellar bilayers. These include: (1) synthetic analogues of cholesterol, ceramides and free fatty acids, such as *trans*-vaccenic acid and epicholesterol, which induce abnormalities in lamellar membrane organization; (2) complex precursors of cholesterol, ceramides and free fatty acids, such as sterol esters, which are not metabolized efficiently to their respective products in the stratum corneum, thereby providing non-lamellar phase separation; (3) supraphysiologic concentrations of physiologic lipids, such as cholesterol sulfate, which also can induce phase separation in preformed membrane bilayers; and (4) hydrolytic enzymes, such as acid ceramidase, which degrade one or more of the three key stratum corneum species. Finally, it should be noted that any single- or double-component mixture of the three key lipids, or any mixture of all three species, which includes a greater than threefold excess of one of the three key lipid species, will delay barrier repair after acute perturbations.

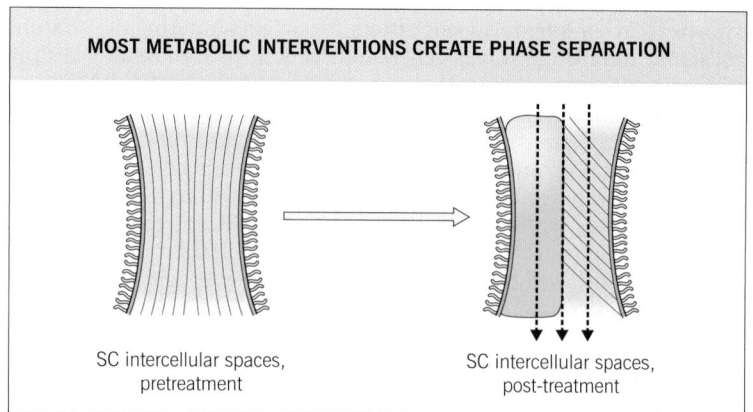

MOST METABOLIC INTERVENTIONS CREATE PHASE SEPARATION

SC intercellular spaces, pretreatment

SC intercellular spaces, post-treatment

Fig. 124.9 Most metabolic interventions create phase separation. The formation of non-lamellar domains leads to additional potential pathways for transdermal drug delivery. SC, stratum corneum.

Together, these strategies induce the formation of separate lamellar and non-lamellar domains within the interstices of the stratum corneum (Fig. 124.9). In most cases, the basis for such domain separation relates to changes in the critical mole ratio, i.e. with deletion or excess of any one of the three key lipids, a portion of the excess species no longer can remain in a well-organized lamellar phase. For example, a 50% reduction in cholesterol would result in an excess of both ceramides and free fatty acids, with a portion of the excess forming a non-lamellar phase. The result of phase separation is more permeable stratum corneum interstices, due not only to deletion of a key hydrophobic lipid, but also to the creation of additional penetration pathways, distinct from the primary lamellar membrane route (see Fig. 124.9).

In theory, then, strategies that interfere with the synthesis, assembly, secretion, activation, processing, or assembly/disassembly of the extracellular lamellar membranes can increase drug delivery by interfering with permeability barrier homeostasis. These biochemical/metabolic approaches can also be viewed vectorially, i.e. as operative within different layers of the epidermis (see Fig. 124.8). For example, most lipid synthesis occurs within the basal layer, while lamellar body formation, acidification and secretion occur in suprabasal, nucleated cell layers. Finally, extracellular processing and membrane assembly occur even more distally, i.e. within the interstices of the stratum corneum. Ultimately, strategies could be deployed that not only target specific biochemical mechanisms, but also take advantage of the localization and relative importance of the steps leading to the generation and maintenance of functional extracellular lamellae within the stratum corneum.

PRINCIPLES OF PERCUTANEOUS DRUG DELIVERY

Thomas J Franz

Parameters Controlling Absorption

Percutaneous drug delivery is a passive process governed by Fick's law, that is, the rate of absorption or flux (J) of any substance across a barrier is proportional to its concentration difference across that barrier. For topically applied drugs, the concentration difference is simply the concentration of drug in the vehicle, C_v, and the proportionality constant relating flux to concentration is the permeability coefficient, K_p (equation 1). K_p is composed of factors that relate to both drug and barrier as well as the interaction between the two. These factors are K_m, the partition coefficient; D, the diffusion coefficient; and L, the length of the diffusion pathway (equation 2). Thus, four factors control the kinetics of percutaneous drug absorption (equation 2); however, it is of great practical importance that two of the four (C_v, K_m) are highly dependent on one additional factor, the vehicle[51].

$$J = K_p C_v \qquad (1)$$

$$J = \left(\frac{DK_m}{L}\right)C_v \qquad (2)$$

Role of Vehicle

The vehicle is the link between drug potency and therapeutic effectiveness, since extensive pharmaceutical research has shown that the composition of the vehicle can profoundly influence the rate and extent of absorption (bioavailability). Innate potency is only expressed when a drug reaches its site of action within the skin at an effective dose. As illustrated by the potency ranking scale for glucocorticoids[52], the same drug appears in different potency classes when formulated in different vehicles (Table 124.5). It was once axiomatic that ointments were more potent than creams. Though true for the early glucocorticoid products, it is no longer generally applicable. Greater understanding of the science underlying topical formulations has allowed creams, gels and solutions to be specifically formulated equipotent to ointments (see Table 124.5). The profound effect careful vehicle design can have on enhancing drug delivery and subsequently on efficacy is clearly seen with the newest of the vehicle types, the low residue foam (Fig 124.10)[54].

In the rational design of dermatologic vehicles that maximize bioavailability, two factors are of critical importance: (1) solubilizing the drug in the vehicle (C_v); and (2) maximizing movement (partitioning) of drug from vehicle to stratum corneum (K_m). The partition coefficient describes the ability of a drug to escape from the vehicle and move into the outermost layer of the stratum corneum. It is defined as the equilibrium solubility of drug in the stratum corneum relative to its solubility in the vehicle ($K_m=C_{sc}/C_v$).

Drug Concentration

The driving force for percutaneous absorption is the concentration of *soluble* drug in the vehicle. Many older topical drug products were marketed with the expectation that higher concentrations were more potent. Although true for some products, e.g. tretinoin gels and creams (0.01–0.1%) in which the drug is completely solubilized at all concentrations, for others it is not. Hydrocortisone 1% and 2.5% in a cream formulation have been shown to be of equal potency, as have triamcinolone acetonide 0.025%, 0.1% and 0.5% creams[52]. One of the major advances

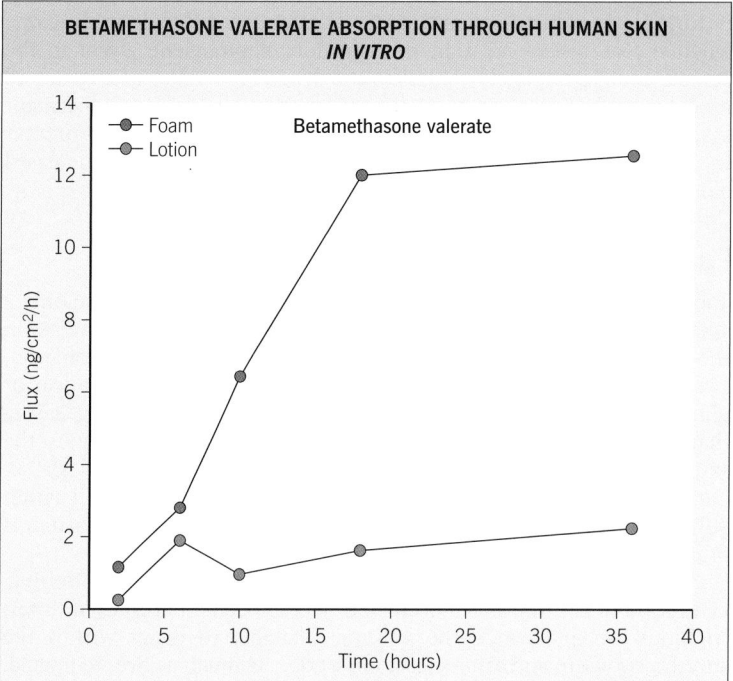

Fig. 124.10 **Betamethasone valerate absorption through human skin *in vitro*.** The same two products (foam and lotion) were also evaluated clinically. A sixfold increase in absorption from a foam product versus a lotion product (as shown here) resulted in a 50% increase in efficacy in the treatment of scalp psoriasis. Reproduced from Franz TJ, et al. Betamethasone valerate foam 0.12%: a novel vehicle with enhanced delivery and efficacy. Int J Dermatol. 1999;38:628–32.

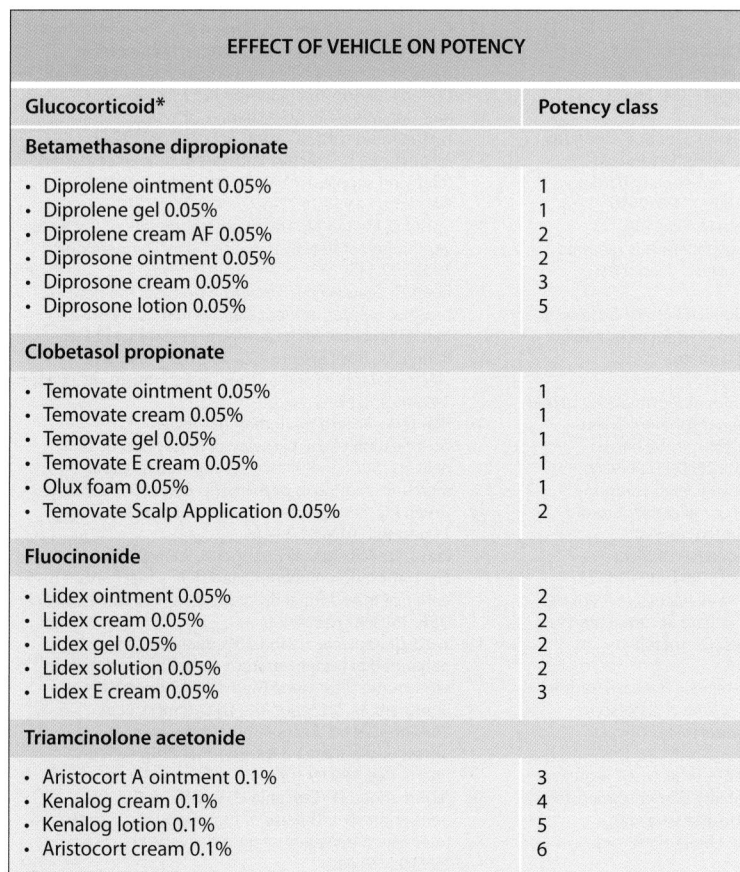

EFFECT OF VEHICLE ON POTENCY	
Glucocorticoid*	**Potency class**
Betamethasone dipropionate	
• Diprolene ointment 0.05%	1
• Diprolene gel 0.05%	1
• Diprolene cream AF 0.05%	2
• Diprosone ointment 0.05%	2
• Diprosone cream 0.05%	3
• Diprosone lotion 0.05%	5
Clobetasol propionate	
• Temovate ointment 0.05%	1
• Temovate cream 0.05%	1
• Temovate gel 0.05%	1
• Temovate E cream 0.05%	1
• Olux foam 0.05%	1
• Temovate Scalp Application 0.05%	2
Fluocinonide	
• Lidex ointment 0.05%	2
• Lidex cream 0.05%	2
• Lidex gel 0.05%	2
• Lidex solution 0.05%	2
• Lidex E cream 0.05%	3
Triamcinolone acetonide	
• Aristocort A ointment 0.1%	3
• Kenalog cream 0.1%	4
• Kenalog lotion 0.1%	5
• Aristocort cream 0.1%	6

Table 124.5 **Effect of vehicle on potency**[52,53]. *Generic name in header followed by trade names.

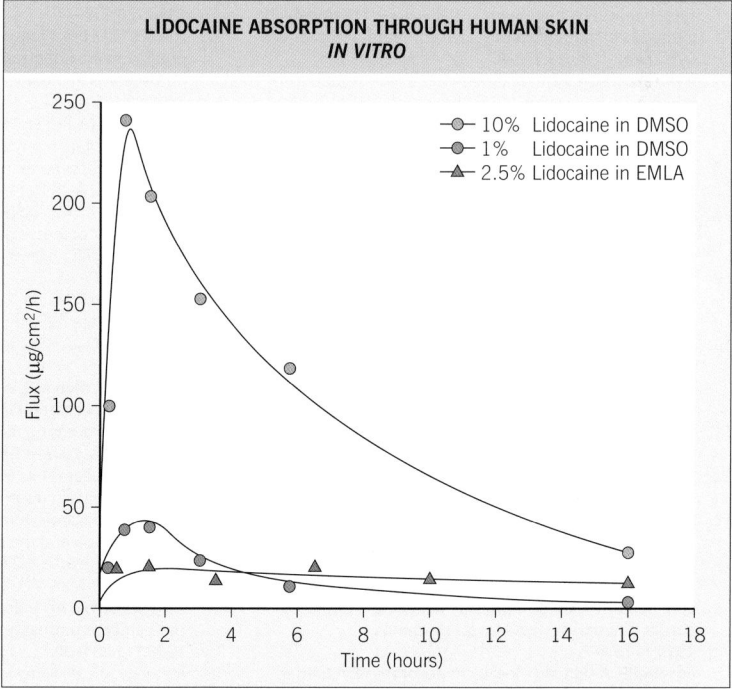

Fig. 124.11 **Lidocaine absorption through human skin *in vitro*.** Incorporation of DMSO as a co-solvent with ethanol results in both increased drug solubility (C_v) and partitioning (K_m). At 10% drug concentration, the maximum flux is 10-fold greater than that achieved in an emulsion formulation (eutectic mixture of lidocaine 2.5% and prilocaine 2.5% [EMLA]). At 1% drug concentration in DMSO the maximum flux is twofold greater than 2.5% drug in EMLA. Reproduced from Mallory SB, et al. Topical lidocaine for anesthesia in patients undergoing pulsed dye laser treatment for vascular malformations. Pediatr Dermatol. 1993;10:370–5.

in formulating glucocorticoids, as first shown with fluocinonide, came when it was discovered that the addition of propylene glycol to the vehicle could completely solubilize the drug. This led to corticosteroid products with greater potency, as demonstrated in the vasoconstrictor assay. Newer products are now tested during the development process to insure that increased drug concentration results in increased bioavailability.

Partition Coefficient

Topically applied drugs are poorly absorbed, in general, because only a small fraction partitions into the stratum corneum. Most remains on the skin surface, subject to loss from a multitude of factors (exfoliation, sweating, wash-off, rub-off, adsorption to clothing, and chemical or photochemical degradation). Even 10–12 hours following dosing, a drug that has not been lost by exfoliation or rub-off remains largely on the skin surface, and is easily removed by a simple soap and water wash[55,56]. One of several positive effects on drug delivery achieved with either polyethylene occlusion or drug contained within a transdermal patch is protection from loss to external factors.

A number of physical and chemical factors can improve partitioning. Hydration of the skin from occlusion, which occurs naturally in intertriginous sites, expands the volume available to drugs within the stratum corneum and can increase absorption as much as five- to tenfold. Common excipients such as ethanol and propylene glycol can also alter

barrier structure to increase partitioning. In addition, they have good solvent properties and, therefore, positively affect C_v as well as K_m. The use of high concentrations of propylene glycol to maximize bioavailability has become pervasive among the super- and high-potency glucocorticoid products, but at a price. Adverse events such as burning and stinging are common when applied to fissured or eroded skin, and contact dermatitis may occur.

Many other compounds have been identified as enhancers. Dimethylsulfoxide (DMSO), the archetypical enhancer, exemplifies the effects that can be achieved (Fig. 124.11). Like with ethanol and propylene glycol, both C_v and K_m are affected. It is a superb solvent, thus, higher drug concentrations can be achieved than with other solvents, but it also expands the barrier to permit increased drug uptake and, possibly, an increased rate of diffusion (D) through the barrier. Expansion of the stratum corneum by DMSO, water and other solvents, to enhance drug uptake, is often referred to as establishing a skin 'reservoir' (see Fig. 124.6).

Regional Variation

All body sites are not equally permeable[57]. Variations in stratum corneum thickness, number of sebaceous glands, and hydration status can all affect absorption. Current data and clinical experience suggest that one can crudely rank regional permeability as follows: nail << palm/sole < trunk/extremities < face/scalp << scrotum.

REFERENCES

1. Scheuplein RJ, Blank IH. Permeability of the skin. Physiol Rev. 1971;51:702–47.
2. Elias PM. Epidermal lipids, barrier function, and desquamation. J Invest Dermatol. 1983;80(suppl.):44S–49S.
3. Elias PM, Menon GK. Structural and lipid biochemical correlates of the epidermal permeability barrier. Adv Lipid Res. 1991;24:1–26.
4. Lampe MA, Burlingame AL, Whitney J, et al. Human stratum corneum lipids: characterization and regional variations. J Lipid Res. 1983;24:120–30.
5. Nemanic MK, Elias PM. In situ precipitation: a novel cytochemical technique for visualization of permeability pathways in mammalian stratum corneum. J Histochem Cytochem. 1980;28:573–8.
6. Flynn GL. Mechanism of percutaneous absorption from physicochemical evidence. In: Bronaugh RL, Maibach HI (eds). Percutaneous Absorption. New York: Marcel Dekker, 1989:27–51.
7. Schaefer H, Redelmeier TE. Skin barrier. In: Principles of Percutaneous Absorption. Basel: Karger, 1996.
8. Menon GK, Elias PM. Morphologic basis for a pore-pathway in mammalian stratum corneum. Skin Pharmacol. 1997;10:235–46.
9. Potts RO, Francoeur ML. The influence of stratum corneum morphology on water permeability. J Invest Dermatol. 1991;96:495–9.
10. Wertz PH, Downing DL. Epidermal lipids. In: Goldsmith LA (ed). Physiology, Biochemistry and Molecular Biology of the Skin. New York: Oxford University Press, 1991:205–36.
11. Schurer NY, Elias PM. The biochemistry and function of stratum corneum lipids. Adv Lipid Res. 1991;24:27–56.
12. Bouwstra JA, Gooris GS, Cheng K, et al. Phase behavior of isolated skin lipids. J Lipid Res. 1996;37:999–1011.
13. Wertz PW, Downing DT. Ceramides of pig epidermis: structure determination. J Lipid Res. 1983;24:759–65.
14. Norlen L, Nicander I, Lundh Rozell B, et al. Inter- and intra-individual differences in human stratum corneum lipid content related to physical parameters of skin barrier function in vivo. J Invest Dermatol. 1999;112:72–7.
15. Forslind B. A domain mosaic model of the skin barrier. Acta Derm Venereol. 1994;74:1–6.
16. Haftek M, Teillon MH, Schmitt D. Stratum corneum, corneodesmosomes and ex vivo percutaneous penetration. Microsc Res Tech. 1998;43:242–9.
17. Menon GK, Lee SH, Roberts MS. Ultrastructural effects of some solvents and vehicles on the stratum corneum and other skin components: evidence for an 'extended mosaic-partitioning model of the skin barrier'. In: Robert MS, Walters KA (eds). Dermal Absorption and Toxicity Assessment. New York: Marcel Dekker, 1998:727–51.
18. Feingold KR. The regulation and role of epidermal lipid synthesis. Adv Lipid Res. 1991;24:57–82.
19. Menon GK, Elias PM, Lee SH, Feingold KR. Localization of calcium in murine epidermis following disruption and repair of the permeability barrier. Cell Tissue Res. 1992;270:503–12.
20. Menon GK, Feingold KR, Elias PM. Lamellar body secretory response to barrier disruption. J Invest Dermatol. 1992;98:279–89.
21. Menon GK, Elias PM, Feingold KR. Integrity of the permeability barrier is crucial for maintenance of the epidermal calcium gradient. Br J Dermatol. 1994;130:139–47.
22. Lee SH, Elias PM, Proksch E, et al. Calcium and potassium are important regulators of barrier homeostasis in murine epidermis. J Clin Invest. 1992;89:530–8.
23. Mao-Qiang M, Brown BE, Wu-Pong S, et al. Exogenous nonphysiologic vs physiologic lipids. Divergent mechanisms for correction of permeability barrier dysfunction. Arch Dermatol. 1995;131:809–16.
24. Mao-Qiang M, Feingold KR, Jain M, Elias PM. Extracellular processing of phospholipids is required for permeability barrier homeostasis. J Lipid Res. 1995;36:1925–35.
25. Mao-Qiang M, Jain M, Feingold KR, Elias PM. Secretory phospholipase A2 activity is required for permeability barrier homeostasis. J Invest Dermatol. 1996;106:57–63.
26. Schmuth M, Man MQ, Weber F, et al. Permeability barrier disorder in Niemann-Pick disease: sphingomyelin-ceramide processing required for normal barrier homeostasis. J Invest Dermatol. 2000;115:459–66.
27. Elias PM, Williams ML, Maloney ME, et al. Stratum corneum lipids in disorders of cornification. Steroid sulfatase and cholesterol sulfate in normal desquamation and the pathogenesis of recessive X-linked ichthyosis. J Clin Invest. 1984;74:1414–21.
28. Zettersten E, Man MQ, Sato J, et al. Recessive X-linked ichthyosis: role of cholesterol-sulfate accumulation in the barrier abnormality. J Invest Dermatol. 1998;111:784–90.
29. Maloney ME, Williams ML, Epstein EH Jr, et al. Lipids in the pathogenesis of ichthyosis: topical cholesterol sulfate-induced scaling in hairless mice. J Invest Dermatol. 1984;83:252–6.
30. Behne MJ, Meyer JW, Hanson KM, et al. NHE1 regulates the stratum corneum permeability barrier homeostasis. Microenvironment acidification assessed with fluorescence lifetime imaging. J Biol Chem. 2002;277:47399–406.
31. Chapman SJ, Walsh A. Membrane-coating granules are acidic organelles which possess proton pumps. J Invest Dermatol. 1989;93:466–70.
32. Mauro T, Holleran WM, Grayson S, et al. Barrier recovery is impeded at neutral pH, independent of ionic effects: implications for extracellular lipid processing. Arch Dermatol Res. 1998;290:215–22.
33. Johnson ME, Mitragotri S, Patel A, et al. Synergistic effects of chemical enhancers and therapeutic ultrasound on transdermal drug delivery. J Pharm Sci. 1996;85:670–9.
34. Tsai JC, Guy RH, Thornfeldt CR, et al. Metabolic approaches to enhance transdermal drug delivery. 1. Effect of lipid synthesis inhibitors. J Pharm Sci. 1996;85:643–8.
35. Choi EH, Lee SH, Ahn SK, Hwang SM. The pretreatment effect of chemical skin penetration enhancers in transdermal drug delivery using iontophoresis. Skin Pharmacol Appl Skin Physiol. 1999;12:326–35.
36. Van Den Merwe E, Ackermann C. Physical changes in hydrated skin. Int J Cosmet Sci. 1987;9:237–47.
37. Mikulowska A. Reactive changes in human epidermis following simple occlusion with water. Contact Dermatitis. 1992;26:224–7.
38. Spruit D, Malten KE. The regeneration rate of the water vapour loss of heavily damaged skin. Dermatologica. 1966;132:115–23.
39. Reed JT, Ghadially R, Elias PM. Skin type, but neither race nor gender, influence epidermal permeability barrier function. Arch Dermatol. 1995;131:1134–8.
40. Banga AK, Bose S, Ghosh TK. Iontophoresis and electroporation: comparisons and contrasts. Int J Pharm. 1999;179:1–19.
41. Monteiro-Riviere NA, Inman AO, Riviere JE. Identification of the pathway of iontophoretic drug delivery: light and ultrastructural studies using mercuric chloride in pigs. Pharm Res. 1994;11:251–6.
42. Green PG. Iontophoretic delivery of peptide drugs. J Contr Rel. 1996;41:33–48.
43. Prausnitz MR, Bose VG, Langer R, Weaver JC. Electroporation of mammalian skin: a mechanism to enhance transdermal drug delivery. Proc Natl Acad Sci USA. 1993;90:10504–8.
44. Wu J, Chappelow J, Yang J, Weimann L. Defects generated in human stratum corneum specimens by ultrasound. Ultrasound Med Biol. 1998;24:705–10.
45. Bommannan D, Menon GK, Okuyama H, et al. Sonophoresis. II. Examination of the mechanism(s) of ultrasound-enhanced transdermal drug delivery. Pharm Res. 1992;9:1043–7.
46. Bommannan D, Okuyama H, Stauffer P, Guy RH. Sonophoresis. I. The use of high-frequency ultrasound to enhance transdermal drug delivery. Pharm Res. 1992;9:559–64.
47. Yarosh D, Bucana C, Cox P, et al. Localization of liposomes containing a DNA repair enzyme in murine skin. J Invest Dermatol. 1994;103:461–8.

48. Domashenko A, Cotsarelis G. Transfection of human hair follicles using topical liposomes is optimal at the onset of anagen. J Invest Dermatol. 1999;112:552.

49. Lasch J, Laub R, Wohlrab W. How deep do intact liposomes penetrate into human skin? J Contr Rel. 1992;18:55–8.

50. Korting HC, Stolz W, Schmid MH, Maierhofer G. Interaction of liposomes with human epidermis reconstructed in vitro. Br J Dermatol. 1995;132:571–9.

51. Franz TJ. Kinetics of cutaneous drug penetration. Int J Dermatol. 1983;22:499–505.

52. Stoughton RB. Vasoconstrictor assay: specific applications. In: Maibach HI, Surber C (eds). Topical corticosteroids. Basel: Karger, 1992:42–53.

53. Franz TJ, Parsell DA, Myers JA, et al. Clobetasol propionate foam 0.05%: a novel vehicle with enhanced delivery. Int J Dermatol. 2000;39:535–8.

54. Franz TJ, Parsell DA, Halualani M, et al. Betamethasone valerate foam 0.12%: a novel vehicle with enhanced delivery and efficacy. Int J Dermatol. 1999;38:628–32.

55. Franz TJ, Lehman PA. Percutaneous absorption of sulconazole nitrate in man. J Pharm Sci. 1988;77:489–91.

56. Franz TJ, Lehman PA. Systemic absorption of retinoic acid. J Toxicol Cutaneous Ocul Toxicol. 1989;8:517–24.

57. Wester RC, Maibach HI. Regional variation in percutaneous absorption. In: Bronaugh RL, Maibach HI (eds). Percutaneous Absorption: Drugs, Cosmetics, Mechanisms, Methodology. New York: Marcel Dekker, 1999:107–16.

Glucocorticosteroids

Lee T Nesbitt Jr

Key features

- Glucocorticosteroids continue to be among the most commonly prescribed anti-inflammatory agents in dermatology and all of medicine, with a large number of disorders responding to these drugs
- Proper systemic use of glucocorticosteroids requires a working knowledge of the hypothalamic–pituitary–adrenal (HPA) axis
- Proper local (topical and intralesional) use of glucocorticosteroids requires a thorough knowledge of their various formulations, potencies, and local duration of effect
- Awareness of the various adverse effects of these agents is extremely important, with many methods utilized to minimize the associated side effects
- Clinical usage guidelines are important in proper dosing and administration of glucocorticosteroids for both short-term and long-term therapy

INTRODUCTION AND PHARMACOLOGY

The Nobel Prize in Medicine was awarded in 1950 to Hench and associates[1] for their initial work on the effects and toxicities of glucocorticosteroids, especially in rheumatic disorders. In 1951, Sulzberger and colleagues[2] first reported on the use of systemic cortisone and adrenocorticotropic hormone (ACTH) in inflammatory skin diseases. One year later, Sulzberger & Witten successfully used topical hydrocortisone to treat eczematous eruptions. In 1961, Reichling & Kligman[3] first employed oral alternate-day glucocorticosteroids for treating certain skin conditions. Another method of high-dose glucocorticosteroid therapy was introduced to dermatology in 1982 by Johnson & Lazarus[4], when they first used pulse intravenous therapy for pyoderma gangrenosum. During the past 30–40 years, numerous non-steroidal drugs have been introduced which allow for a 'steroid-sparing' effect and minimization of risks from long-term therapy with systemic glucocorticosteroids.

Structure/Metabolism

All steroids, including glucocorticosteroids, have the basic four-ring structure of cholesterol, with three hexane rings and one pentane ring. Figure 125.1 shows the chemical structure of hydrocortisone (cortisol). Modifications in the basic four-ring structure of glucocorticosteroids result in systemic agents which have varying potency, mineralocorticoid effect, duration of action (biologic half-life), and metabolism[5]. Table 125.1 lists the key pharmacologic properties of the major oral agents used today. Similar changes in the basic structure of the glucocorticosteroid molecule have resulted in various topical agents with differing solubility, lipophilic properties, percutaneous absorption, and glucocorticoid receptor-binding activity.

When examining the chemical structure of glucocorticosteroids, it is important to recognize that active agents, such as hydrocortisone in Figure 125.1, have a hydroxyl group at the 11 position. The corresponding inactive drug, cortisone, has a ketone group at the 11 position and must undergo hepatic conversion to hydrocortisone for biologic activity. The same is true for prednisone, which must undergo the identical 11-hydroxylation by the liver to produce the active agent, prednisolone. Since patients who have severe hepatic disease will have impaired conversion of the inactive drug to its active analogue, it is best to use an active agent such as prednisolone in such situations[6].

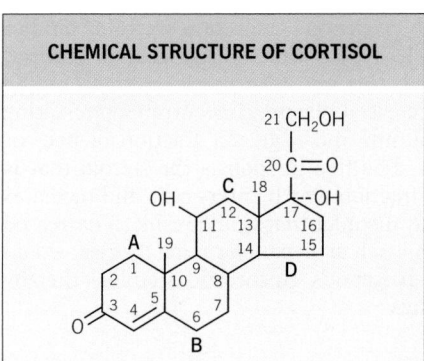

CHEMICAL STRUCTURE OF CORTISOL

Fig. 125.1 Chemical structure of cortisol (hydrocortisone). Note the hydroxyl group at the 11 position.

PHARMACOLOGY OF GLUCOCORTICOSTEROIDS				
	Equivalent GCS dose (mg)	Mineralocorticoid potency (relative)	Duration of action (hours)	Plasma half-life (minutes)
Short-acting				
Cortisone	25	1.0	8–12	60
Hydrocortisone	20	0.8	8–12	90
Intermediate-acting				
Prednisone	5	0.25	24–36	60
Prednisolone	5	0.25	24–36	200
Methylprednisolone	4	0	24–36	180
Triamcinolone	4	0	24–36	300
Long-acting				
Dexamethasone	0.75	0	36–54	200
Betamethasone	0.6	0	36–54	200

Table 125.1 Pharmacology of glucocorticosteroids (GCS).

In addition to showing the equivalent glucocorticosteroid potency in milligrams, Table 125.1 also shows that these agents differ in their relative mineralocorticoid potency. The older drugs, cortisone and hydrocortisone, have fairly significant mineralocorticoid potency, but it should be noted that prednisone and prednisolone both have slight mineralocorticoid effects. A drug such as methylprednisolone has no mineralocorticoid potency, and would be an excellent choice in situations in which one needs to eliminate all mineralocorticoid effects[7].

Plasma half-lives of the various glucocorticosteroid agents vary from about 1 to 5 hours, as seen in Table 125.1. However, it is noteworthy that the plasma half-life is a poor indicator of the duration of action (biologic activity) of each glucocorticosteroid. Duration of biologic effect is best assessed by the period of suppression of ACTH secretion by the pituitary gland after the administration of a single dose of the particular glucocorticosteroid. As seen in Table 125.1, short-acting glucocorticosteroids have an effect for 8–12 hours, intermediate-acting agents for 24–36 hours, and long-acting agents for more than 48 hours. Duration of biologic activity is the property of glucocorticosteroids that is of utmost importance in choosing an agent for alternate-day therapy. Intermediate-acting agents should be used for this purpose, with long-acting agents avoided because there would be no period for recovery of the hypothalamic–pituitary–adrenal (HPA) axis[6].

Absorption/Distribution

Oral glucocorticosteroids are absorbed in the jejunum, with peak plasma levels occurring in 30–90 minutes[8]. Administration of these drugs with food does not decrease absorption, but it may be delayed. Once glucocorticosteroids reach the plasma, the primary carrier protein is corticosteroid-binding globulin, also known as transcortin. Most endogenous cortisol is bound to this protein, and low doses of exogenous glucocorticosteroids are initially primarily bound by this high-affinity, but low-capacity, carrier system. With larger glucocorticosteroid doses, some binding also occurs to albumin in a low-affinity fashion, but with a greater capacity because of the larger amounts of albumin in the serum. The avidity with which exogenous glucocorticosteroids bind to these two carrier proteins is less than that of endogenous cortisol. Exogenous glucocorticosteroid therapy fills corticosteroid-binding globulin binding sites, with increased plasma concentrations resulting in low-affinity binding to albumin and a greater fraction of free, or unbound, glucocorticosteroids. The free fraction is the steroid that is biologically active, and is that fraction which enters cells and mediates glucocorticosteroid effects[5]. Any disorder that would result in decreased binding proteins in the plasma, such as hepatic or renal disease, would increase the free fraction of exogenous glucocorticosteroids, thereby increasing toxicity of these drugs.

MECHANISM OF ACTION

HPA Axis Function

A working knowledge of the normal function of the HPA axis is invaluable in understanding glucocorticosteroid physiology, and it leads to an understanding of the molecular mechanisms of action of these agents[9]. The hypothalamus produces corticotropin-releasing hormone, which is released in small pulses into the pituitary circulation. The anterior pituitary responds to corticotropin-releasing hormone with synthesis of ACTH and its subsequent pulsatile secretion into the peripheral circulation. ACTH is the hormone that stimulates the inner adrenal cortex to generate and release cortisol. In an individual with a normal sleep cycle, the greatest amount of cortisol is released during the early morning hours prior to waking. Under basal conditions, the adrenals produce approximately 20–30 mg of cortisol per day, but this may increase up to tenfold under times of maximal stress. ACTH also has some role in stimulating adrenal androgen production, but is not significantly involved in the production of the major mineralocorticoid, aldosterone. The major mineralocorticoid control mechanisms are the renin–angiotensin system and serum potassium levels.

There are three main control mechanisms for endogenous cortisol secretion[10]. The first is the negative feedback effect by plasma cortisol levels, which inhibit the secretion of corticotropin-releasing hormone and ACTH by the hypothalamus and pituitary, respectively. The second control is the pulsatile secretion of ACTH, which is based on a circadian cycle, with increasing pulses several hours after the onset of sleep, reaching a maximum shortly before waking. From these ACTH pulses, the peak release of cortisol in a normal sleep cycle is about 6–8 a.m. With abnormal sleep cycles, this circadian pattern will adjust so that peak cortisol levels occur just prior to waking. The third form of control of endogenous cortisol production comes from neural effects on the HPA axis in response to various emotional or physical stresses. These neural stimuli include catecholamine production from the brainstem, corticotropin-releasing hormone from sites other than the hypothalamus, and vasopressin.

Molecular Mechanisms

The glucocorticosteroid free (i.e. unbound) fraction enters cells and exerts its effect by binding to glucocorticoid receptors[11]. Binding of glucocorticosteroids to these receptors results in both beneficial and adverse effects. The receptor is located in the cytoplasm of almost all cells of the body, and, upon binding by glucocorticosteroids, the release of 90 kDa heat shock protein occurs, exposing two nuclear localization signals which facilitate the nuclear translocation of the glucocorticoid receptor complex.

In the nucleus, the glucocorticoid receptor forms a dimer that binds to the glucocorticoid response element of the promoter region of steroid-responsive genes. Approximately 10–100 genes are regulated directly by glucocorticosteroids. This binding affects the rate of transcription, repressing or inducing messenger RNA production and protein synthesis.

The glucocorticoid receptor also interacts with other transcription factors that have a central role in the inflammatory response as well as their coactivator molecules, such as cAMP response element binding protein (CREB)-binding protein[12]. Nuclear factor-κB is an important transcription factor that induces transcription of many genes that play a significant role in chronic inflammation, including genes for various cytokines, adhesion molecules, inflammatory enzymes, and growth factors. By indirectly and directly inhibiting nuclear factor-κB, the glucocorticoid receptor can dramatically reduce the inflammatory process. The glucocorticoid receptor also interacts with activating protein 1 (AP-1) (a collective term for the heterodimeric transcription factor composed of c-jun, c-fos and activating transcription factor), which controls transcription of growth factor and cytokine genes. In much the same way as described previously for nuclear factor-κB, glucocorticosteroids inhibit TNF-α, granulocyte–macrophage colony-stimulating factor, and several interleukins (e.g. IL-1, IL-2, IL-6, IL-8). Adhesion molecules such as intercellular adhesion molecule-1 and E-selectin are also inhibited, as is cyclooxygenase.

Inflammatory Cell Effects

Glucocorticosteroids produce accelerated release of neutrophils from the bone marrow, thereby producing a neutrophilia, with an increase in the circulating pool of these cells but not the body's total number of neutrophils[13]. Although neutrophils move from the bone marrow to the circulation, they are inhibited from moving to inflammatory sites in tissue. There is also decreased apoptosis of these cells. The reduction of neutrophils at inflammatory sites is likely due to inhibition of endothelial adhesion molecule expression and chemoattractants. Neutrophil phagocytosis and bactericidal function are relatively unaffected by glucocorticosteroids in pharmacologic doses.

A transient lymphopenia is also produced during glucocorticosteroid therapy, as a result of redistribution of all T-lymphocyte subpopulations to lymphoid depots, likely through a change in adhesion molecule expression[14]. T-cell activation is also inhibited by decreased IL-2 production and IL-2 gene transcription. Although the subpopulations of helper, suppressor and cytotoxic T lymphocytes all have inhibition of proliferation and function after administration of glucocorticosteroids, helper cells are affected more than suppressor cells. Inhibition of B-cell function requires very high doses of glucocorticosteroids. Pulse therapy is a way of delivering high-dose glucocorticosteroids as a means of decreasing antibody production by B lymphocytes.

The number of circulating eosinophils is reduced directly by glucocorticosteroids through decreased release of these cells from the bone marrow and increased apoptosis[15]. Glucocorticosteroids also decrease the production and differentiation of monocyte-macrophage cell lines. Antigen presentation to T lymphocytes by dendritic cells is also inhibited. Finally, reduced destruction of erythrocytes from glucocorticosteroid therapy is related to both decreased autohemolysis and decreased erythrophagocytosis.

INDICATIONS, DOSAGES AND CONTRAINDICATIONS (CLINICAL USE)

Table 125.2 lists most of the broad categories of diseases in which systemic glucocorticosteroids are used in dermatology[7]. There are many more disorders in which topical and intralesional glucocorticosteroids can be useful, such as the papulosquamous disorders and other localized inflammatory processes.

Oral Therapy

Dermatologists use glucocorticosteroids for short periods to treat acute conditions such as extensive allergic contact dermatitis and other acute eczematous disorders[11]. Short-term therapy is usually defined as treatment that occurs for approximately 3 weeks or less. An oral agent with an intermediate duration of action, such as prednisone, is usually given in a single early-morning dose to achieve the least HPA axis suppression[16]. In some severe acute dermatoses, the dose can be divided and administered from two to four times per day for better initial control, but conversion to a single early-morning dose should occur as soon as possible. The clinician should realize that split-dose therapy has a parallel increase in both efficacy and toxicity. The split dose can simply be considered to represent the equivalent of a slightly higher simple morning dose despite the same total number of milligrams. The daily dose of prednisone can vary depending on the severity of the dermatosis, but for most moderate, self-limited conditions in average-weight adults, a common initial dose is 40–60 mg/day.

Long-term therapy is usually defined as therapy lasting 4 weeks or longer[6]. Often, long-term therapy refers to treatment lasting for months to years. In these situations, corticosteroid-sparing agents are usually added in an attempt to reduce the glucocorticosteroid dose required to control the disease process, or to eliminate the corticosteroid altogether.

Prednisone is often the intermediate-acting glucocorticosteroid of choice for both short-term and long-term therapy. It is both inexpensive and available in many dosage forms[10].

Methylprednisolone can be used if there is a need to reduce all mineralocorticoid effects. Intermediate-acting drugs such as prednisone and methylprednisolone are also utilized for alternate-morning therapy, which allows the HPA axis to recover in the last 12 hours of the off-day of therapy. In tapering the glucocorticosteroid dosage, eventual alternate-morning therapy is often utilized to promote HPA axis recovery. Two important side effects of long-term glucocorticosteroid therapy that are not minimized by alternate-morning dosing are osteoporosis and cataracts, both discussed later in the side effects section.

Tapering of the glucocorticosteroid dose may not be necessary from the adrenal recovery standpoint in very short-term therapy, but has great importance when treatment is for longer than a few weeks. Symptoms of corticosteroid withdrawal syndrome include arthralgias, myalgias, mood changes, fatigue, headache, and gastrointestinal symptoms[17]. To counteract this syndrome, a return to the previous dose of glucocorticosteroid with more gradual tapering is recommended. The rate of prednisone tapering depends on both the type and severity of the dermatosis and adrenal recovery issues. Tapering the prednisone dose can usually be accomplished even by 20 mg tapers at doses greater than 60 mg/day, 10 mg tapers between 30 and 60 mg/day, and 5 mg tapers between 30 mg and the physiologic dose range. Once the physiologic dose range of 5–7.5 mg/day of prednisone is reached, a more gradual reduction of 1 mg per taper may be necessary due to adrenal recovery issues.

Another method of glucocorticosteroid dosage tapering is to convert from daily to alternate-day therapy once the prednisone dose is about 20–30 mg/day[6]. The simplest way to convert is to multiply the previous daily dose by 2–2.5 times for the on-day dose, and taper therapy rapidly on the off-day. An alternate way is to increase the on-day dose by 5 mg increments and decrease the off-day dose by a similar amount, until therapy is eventually doubled on the on-day and stopped on the off-day. Finally, simultaneous tapering and alternate-morning conversion can be accomplished by decreasing the dose by 5 mg on the alternate morning, with the patient eventually taking the same dose every other morning as they were taking daily.

Intramuscular Therapy

Dermatologists occasionally use intramuscular administration of glucocorticosteroids for control of acute dermatoses[18]. Although acute dermatoses respond very well to intramuscular glucocorticosteroid therapy, serious conditions such as pemphigus vulgaris or severe drug reactions are best treated by other routes of administration because of the initial need for higher daily dose levels and the need for more control of dosage changes. Advantages of intramuscular administration of glucocorticosteroids include physician administration of therapy, guaranteed compliance, and an assured steady release of glucocorticosteroids achieved by depot preparations. Opponents of intramuscular therapy stress that oral morning doses are more physiologic, are more predictably absorbed, can be more precisely tapered, and can be administered on alternate-morning schedules to decrease HPA axis suppression even further. There also is the possibility of lipoatrophy or a sterile abscess at an injection site, especially with triamcinolone if the

MAJOR INDICATIONS FOR THE POSSIBLE USE OF SYSTEMIC GLUCOCORTICOSTEROIDS IN DERMATOLOGY
Severe dermatitis
• Contact dermatitis (various forms)
• Atopic dermatitis
• Photodermatitis
• Exfoliative erythrodermas
Bullous dermatoses
• Pemphigus (all forms)
• Bullous pemphigoid
• Cicatricial pemphigoid
• Linear IgA bullous dermatosis
• Epidermolysis bullosa acquisita
• Gestational pemphigoid
• Erythema multiforme (major)
Vasculitis
• Cutaneous (various types)
• Systemic (various types)
Autoimmune connective tissue diseases
• Lupus erythematosus
• Dermatomyositis
• Systemic sclerosis
• Eosinophilic fasciitis
• Mixed connective tissue disease
• Relapsing polychondritis
Neutrophilic dermatoses
• Pyoderma gangrenosum
• Sweet's syndrome (acute febrile neutrophilic dermatosis)
• Behçet's disease
Miscellaneous dermatoses
• Sarcoidosis
• Lichen planus
• Panniculitis (some types)
• Urticaria/angioedema – acutely
• Arthropod bites/stings
• Infantile hemangiomas

Table 125.2 Major indications for the possible use of systemic glucocorticosteroids in dermatology.

injection is not given deeply enough into the muscle. Intramuscular agents such as betamethasone and dexamethasone, which have a duration of action of less than 1 week, may be preferred in self-limited dermatoses. Long-acting intramuscular agents which produce effects for about 3 weeks, such as triamcinolone acetonide, should not be given more than about four to six times per year[7]. The physician might be lulled into thinking that therapy is intermittent and relatively safe, while in fact therapy is continuous for 3 weeks per injection, necessitating time for HPA axis recovery.

Intravenous and Pulse Therapy

Intravenous doses of glucocorticosteroids may be necessary in life-threatening dermatologic conditions. A total daily dose of 2 mg/kg or more of methylprednisolone is given initially in divided doses every 6–8 hours in these acute and critical situations. Another method of dosing glucocorticosteroids in severe dermatologic disease is intravenous pulse therapy[19]. With this method, methylprednisolone is given intravenously in doses of 0.5–1 g over 2 hours daily for 1–5 days. This therapy was formerly given in an inpatient setting with appropriate cardiac monitoring because arrhythmias and rare cases of sudden death were possible with this treatment if it was given too quickly. Acute electrolyte shifts are a possible cause for these cardiac effects, so infusion of potassium during the methylprednisolone administration may prevent this problem[20]. In addition, slow infusion of the methylprednisolone over 2 hours usually prevents cardiac effects and has allowed use of this therapy in an outpatient setting. Most commonly, oral doses are continued on a maintenance basis after pulse therapy is given. Pulse therapy allows for a dramatic acute effect in severe dermatoses, but hopes that it would greatly reduce the need or dose of maintenance therapy have not been realized.

Topical Therapy

For topical glucocorticosteroid therapy, there are large numbers of medications[21] available in a wide range of potency. Seven classes have been suggested based on potency. They range from the superpotent topical glucocorticosteroids in class 1 to the very low-potency topical glucocorticosteroids in class 7. These classes have been developed based on vasoconstrictor assays and double-blind clinical studies[22]. A partial list of these topical preparations is shown in Table 125.3. For some agents, brand-name preparations may have greater potency than generics. It is also clear that the vehicle can greatly influence the percutaneous absorption and therapeutic efficacy of the particular glucocorticosteroid. As a result, in the era of generic substitutions, the clinician needs to consider this point, as well as noncompliance, as an explanation for reduced efficacy.

In general, a glucocorticosteroid molecule in an ointment vehicle is more potent than the same molecule in a cream, lotion or other vehicle, because occlusive vehicles enhance percutaneous absorption through increased hydration of the stratum corneum. Gel preparations also tend to be readily absorbed. In choosing a topical glucocorticosteroid preparation for clinical use, one must first choose the desired potency based on the severity, location and extent of lesions. Next, one must select the proper vehicle based on the type of lesions to be treated, need for hydration or drying effect, location on the body, and potential for irritation or sensitization by components of the vehicle. Lotions are elegant for the face, creams rub in well, ointments are beneficial for dry lesions, and gels are more useful in hairy areas or for a drying effect. For the face and body folds, the more potent and superpotent glucocorticosteroid preparations are to be avoided due to the risks of epidermal atrophy in both locations and steroid rosacea/perioral dermatitis on the face. There is anecdotal evidence that pulse dosing (i.e. twice daily weekend dosing only) may reduce the risk of epidermal atrophy with more potent corticosteroids. It is not certain that any modification reduces the risk of cutaneous atrophy or perioral dermatitis/steroid rosacea independent of potency.

An innovative topical corticosteroid is mometasone furoate, which has a low percutaneous absorption and is rapidly metabolized in the liver[23]. Fluticasone is another innovation, as it is highly lipophilic and binds specifically to the glucocorticoid receptor without significant binding to androgen-, progestogen-, estrogen- or mineralocorticoid receptors[24].

POTENCY RANKING OF SOME COMMONLY USED TOPICAL GLUCOCORTICOSTEROIDS

Class 1 (Superpotent)

- Clobetasol propionate gel, ointment, cream and foam 0.05%
- Betamethasone dipropionate gel* and ointment* 0.05%
- Diflorasone diacetate ointment* 0.05%
- Fluocinonide cream 0.1%
- Flurandrenolide tape 4 μg/cm²
- Halobetasol propionate ointment and cream 0.05%

Class 2 (High Potency)

- Amcinonide ointment 0.1%
- Betamethasone dipropionate cream* and ointment 0.05%
- Clobetasol propionate solution ('scalp application') 0.05%
- Desoximetasone ointment and cream 0.25% and gel 0.05%
- Diflorasone diacetate ointment and cream* 0.05%
- Fluocinonide gel, ointment, cream and solution 0.05%
- Halcinonide ointment and cream 0.1%
- Mometasone furoate ointment 0.1%

Class 3 (High Potency)

- Amcinonide cream and lotion 0.1%
- Betamethasone dipropionate cream and lotion 0.05%
- Betamethasone valerate ointment 0.1%
- Desoximetasone cream 0.05%
- Diflorasone diacetate cream 0.05%
- Fluticasone propionate ointment 0.005%
- Triamcinolone acetonide ointment 0.1% and cream 0.5%

Class 4 (Medium Potency)

- Betamethasone valerate foam 0.12%
- Fluocinolone acetonide ointment 0.025%
- Flurandrenolide ointment 0.05%
- Hydrocortisone valerate ointment 0.2%
- Mometasone furoate cream and lotion 0.1%
- Triamcinolone acetonide ointment (Kenalog®) and cream 0.1%

Class 5 (Medium Potency)

- Betamethasone dipropionate lotion 0.05%
- Betamethasone valerate cream and lotion 0.1%
- Clocortolone pivalate cream 0.1%
- Fluocinolone acetonide cream 0.025% and oil 0.01%
- Fluticasone propionate cream and lotion 0.05%
- Flurandrenolide cream and lotion 0.05%
- Hydrocortisone butyrate ointment, cream and lotion 0.1%
- Hydrocortisone probutate cream 0.1%
- Hydrocortisone valerate cream 0.2%
- Prednicarbate ointment and cream 0.1%
- Triamcinolone acetonide lotion 0.1%

Class 6 (Low Potency)

- Aclometasone dipropionate ointment and cream 0.05%
- Triamcinolone acetonide cream 0.1% (Aristocort®)
- Betamethasone valerate lotion 0.1%
- Desonide gel, ointment, cream, lotion and foam 0.05%
- Fluocinolone acetonide cream 0.01% and solution 0.05%
- Triamcinolone acetonide cream and lotion 0.025%

Class 7 (Low Potency)

- Topicals with hydrocortisone, dexamethasone and prednisolone

*Optimized vehicle.

Table 125.3 Potency ranking of some commonly used topical glucocorticosteroids.

Intralesional Therapy

For many localized disorders, when topical therapy does not produce a significant effect and systemic therapy is best avoided, intralesional glucocorticosteroid therapy can be very effective. With this method, triamcinolone acetonide is diluted to the desired concentration depending on the lesion to be treated and is injected in small amounts into the lesion, usually with a 30-gauge needle. With thick dermal lesions such as keloids, concentrations as high as 20–40 mg/ml of triamcinolone can be injected, as the desired result is to decrease the connective tissue present in the lesion. However, with other lesions where atrophy of the dermis or fat can occur, a dilute concentration as low as 2 mg/ml of triamcinolone should be used. The concentration can vary greatly, depending on the lesion and location to be treated. This method of administration allows the clinician to bypass the barrier of a thickened stratum corneum and/or to treat the dermal inflammatory process (e.g. sarcoidosis, granuloma annulare) without epidermal atrophy and with higher concentrations of corticosteroid at the site of the pathology.

Contraindications

Finally, one must always consider contraindications to glucocorticosteroid therapy, whether it be systemic or local[10]. Herpes simplex keratitis is considered a contraindication to local glucocorticosteroid therapy of the eye. Also, active tuberculosis or systemic fungal infections are usually considered a contraindication to systemic glucocorticosteroid therapy. Previous history of hypersensitivity to an intravenous preparation, which is rare, should preclude further use of that particular intravenous drug. Many other situations, such as active peptic ulcer disease, severe depression or psychosis, and extensive chronic dermatoses (e.g. psoriasis) likely to flare with a rebound after rapid corticosteroid taper, should be relative contraindications to systemic glucocorticosteroid therapy, with these agents used only when necessary.

MAJOR SIDE EFFECTS

Short-term glucocorticosteroid therapy is usually extremely safe for treatment of self-limited and acute dermatoses[7]. When side effects do occur with short courses of therapy, those listed in Table 125.4 are seen most commonly. With long-term glucocorticosteroid therapy at supraphysiologic doses, there is an increased incidence of more serious effects. Table 125.5 lists the major categories of complications, with the more common adverse effects in each category. For most of these adverse effects, side effects are dose-related.

As shown in Table 125.6, some patients have a higher risk of side effects from glucocorticosteroids[6]. Women have greater risks than men, due to slower metabolism and clearance of glucocorticosteroids secondary to estrogen, lower bone density, and dosages that are often not adjusted based on weight. Postmenopausal women are much more prone to osteoporosis, as are all elderly patients with decreased physical activity. Children and adolescents also have a significant incidence of osteoporosis from exogenous glucocorticosteroids, and along with possible temporary retardation of growth, they may develop striae distensae. Patients with systemic lupus erythematosus (SLE) have a higher incidence of aseptic necrosis of bone, rheumatoid arthritis patients have a greater incidence of osteoporosis, and patients with myositis have a tendency to muscle atrophy when treated with long-term glucocorticosteroids. Those with liver disease and alcoholism have difficulty metabolizing glucocorticosteroids and abnormal metabolism of lipids, which together often result in high serum triglyceride levels. Those with hypoalbuminemia have an increased free fraction of exogenous glucocorticosteroids, and, therefore, may have much greater side effects. Smoking and increased alcohol intake greatly increase the risks of osteoporosis, peptic ulcer disease, and certain other major side effects.

The following discussion highlights selected toxicities of glucocorticosteroid therapy.

Osteoporosis

Osteoporosis is one of the most prevalent side effects that occur in patients receiving long-term systemic glucocorticosteroids. Osteoporosis occurs in 30–50% of all patients treated chronically with glucocorticosteroids without proper preventive measures[25]. The most significant demineralization occurs during the first 6–12 months of therapy, with slowing after this time. Postmenopausal women are most at risk for complications such as fractures, because they have the lowest bone mass before beginning therapy. The greatest amount of bone loss is usually observed in young men, because they have the highest pretreatment bone mass. Osteoporosis is not minimized by alternate-morning treatment schedules.

SIDE EFFECTS OF SHORT-TERM SYSTEMIC GLUCOCORTICOSTEROID THERAPY	
• Mood changes, nervousness, insomnia	• Acneiform eruptions
• Gastrointestinal intolerance	• Increased infections
• Hyperglycemia	• Amenorrhea
• Fluid/sodium retention	• Muscular weakness, muscle effects
• Increased appetite, weight gain	• Wound healing effects

Table 125.4 Side effects of short-term systemic glucocorticosteroid therapy.

MAJOR SIDE EFFECTS OF LONG-TERM SYSTEMIC GLUCOCORTICOSTEROID THERAPY	
Musculoskeletal	**Gynecologic, obstetric**
Osteoporosis	Amenorrhea
Osteonecrosis (e.g. hip)	Fetal effects
Growth retardation	
Muscle atrophy	
Myopathy	
Ophthalmologic	**Hematologic, cellular**
Cataracts	Leukocytosis
Glaucoma	Lymphopenia
Infection	Eosinopenia
Hemorrhage	Immunosuppression
Exophthalmos	Impaired fibroplasia
	Decreased mitotic rate
	Infections
Gastrointestinal	**Nervous system**
Nausea, vomiting	Mood, personality changes
Peptic ulcer disease	Psychiatric problems, psychosis
Intestinal perforation	Seizures
Pancreatitis	Pseudotumor cerebri
Esophagitis	Peripheral neuropathy
Metabolic	**Cutaneous**
Hyperglycemia	Atrophy
Hyperlipidemia	Vascular fragility, purpura
Obesity	Acne, acneiform eruptions
Hypocalcemia	Hirsutism
Hypokalemic alkalosis	Infections
	Hyperpigmentation
Cardiovascular	**Hypothalamic-pituitary-adrenal (HPA) axis**
Hypertension	Suppression
Peripheral edema	Withdrawal syndrome
Atherosclerosis	Adrenal crisis

Table 125.5 Major side effects of long-term systemic glucocorticosteroid therapy.

PATIENTS AT HIGHER RISK FOR TOXICITY FROM GLUCOCORTICOSTEROID THERAPY
• Female patients
• Postmenopausal women, elderly patients
• Young children
• Patients with SLE, myositis or rheumatoid arthritis
• Patients with hepatic disease
• Alcoholics
• Patients with hypoalbuminemia

Table 125.6 Patients at higher risks for toxicity from glucocorticosteroid therapy. SLE, systemic lupus erythematosus.

Trabecular bone, present in the axial skeleton (vertebrae, ribs), has a metabolic turnover rate eight times that of cortical bone (long bones), so that trabecular bone is much more prone to demineralization[26]. Although there are no symptoms from osteoporosis in many patients, more advanced disease can produce bone pain, fractures and vertebral collapse. The mechanism of glucocorticosteroid-induced bone loss includes both reduced intestinal absorption of calcium and decreased renal tubular resorption of calcium. A diet high in sodium may increase calcium loss even further. Decreased calcium results in parathyroid hormone release and produces a form of secondary hyperparathyroidism, stimulating osteoclast activity in bone and producing bone resorption. There is also inhibition of osteoblasts in bone and inhibition of collagen matrix synthesis through several mechanisms.

Although routine radiographs can detect vertebral compression fractures, these plain X-ray studies are not sensitive enough to detect osteoporosis until 20–60% of bone mass is lost[27] (Fig. 125.2). The best measurement of osteoporosis available today is quantification of bone mineral density with dual-energy X-ray absorptiometry (DEXA), now the preferred method because of its sensitivity, reproducibility, and low radiation exposure. Ideally, patients on long-term glucocorticosteroids should have a baseline DEXA examination at the hip and lumbar spine, with a repeat study performed at least annually at the same bone sites because there is variability in density among different sites[28]. In densitometry reports, T scores are used to connote a standard deviation from the mean of a healthy control standard. Osteopenia is defined as a T score between –1 and –2.5 standard deviations below the mean, with a T score less than –2.5 defining osteoporosis[25].

Certain other risk factors for osteoporosis from glucocorticosteroids are pre-existing osteoporosis, immobilization, menopause, low-calcium or high-sodium diet, increased tobacco or alcohol use, high caffeine intake, rheumatoid arthritis, renal failure, and hyperparathyroidism or hyperthyroidism.

For patients beginning long-term glucocorticosteroid therapy, guidelines should be followed (Fig. 125.3)[29]. Abstinence from tobacco should be recommended and both alcohol and caffeine intake should be restricted. Exercise against gravity should be encouraged to stimulate osteoblast function, and patients should have a calcium intake of 1.5 g/day along with a vitamin D intake of 800 IU/day, if there are no contraindications, such as nephrolithiasis. It is suggested that if there is greater than 300 mg of calcium in a 24-hour urine collection (performed every 3–6 months, particularly in patients with a history of hypercalciuria or nephrolithiasis), a thiazide diuretic be added to decrease urinary calcium excretion.

In general, experts agree that postmenopausal women, men over 65 years of age, and patients with a T score below –1 or –1.5 on DEXA examination should begin concomitant bisphosphonate therapy when started on long-term glucocorticosteroids. Since the largest reduction in bone mass occurs in the first 6 months of glucocorticosteroid therapy, the American College of Rheumatology recommends that all patients who begin long-term glucocorticosteroid therapy be started concomitantly on a bisphosphonate[29]. Alendronate 70 mg or risedronate 35 mg orally once per week are first-line agents. They should be taken on an empty stomach, only with water, upon arising in the morning and patients should not lie flat for 1 hour after taking them. Although generally well tolerated, gastrointestinal side effects can occur and may necessitate change to alternative agents, if severe. Intravenous bisphosphonates such as pamidronate 30 mg iv every 3 months or zolendronate 4–5 mg iv once yearly are alternatives. All bisphosphonates, especially those with long half-lives, should be avoided in premenopausal women who might become pregnant, as these agents cross the placenta and produce teratogenicity, including fetal skeletal abnormalities. Although not as effective as bisphosphonates, intranasal calcitonin 200 IU daily is a second-line agent when bisphosphonates are not tolerated or are contraindicated.

Hormonal therapy in women was once considered a treatment of choice for management of postmenopausal osteoporosis, and it is effective, as demonstrated by the Women's Health Initiative (WHI) study[30]. Unfortunately, the WHI also revealed increased breast cancer, stroke, thromboembolism and myocardial infarction in women on estrogen–progesterone hormonal therapy, with these risks outweighing the osteoporosis benefits. It is as yet unclear if low-dose estrogen without progesterone has the same risk profile. Raloxifene, a selective estrogen receptor modulator (SERM), is not as effective as estrogen in preventing osteoporosis, but has beneficial effects in breast cancer prevention and treatment, making it a consideration in preventing bone loss in some women on long-term glucocorticosteroids. Men on long-term glucocorticosteroids, who are found to have low testosterone levels, can be considered for treatment with 250 mg testosterone replacement intramuscularly each month, if there is no risk of prostate cancer or prostate hypertrophy.

Finally, patients who have failed bisphosphonates and other osteoporosis management, with T scores less than –3.0 to –3.5, or with osteoporotic fractures, should be considered for teriparatide, a fragmented portion of human parathyroid hormone (PTH). The cost of teriparatide is a limiting factor in its use, and it should not be used in combination with bisphosphonates, as they may inhibit the effectiveness of teriparatide. Endocrinologic consultation should always be utilized in patients who develop significant osteopenia or osteoporosis. For guidelines on osteoporosis prevention and treatment for patients on long-term glucocorticosteroids, see Fig. 125.3.

Osteonecrosis

Also known as aseptic necrosis or avascular necrosis, osteonecrosis has numerous causes, one of which is as a complication of glucocorticosteroid treatment[31]. Co-risk factors include physical trauma, alcohol abuse, cigarette smoking, and elevated serum triglycerides. The incidence of glucocorticosteroid-related osteonecrosis is higher in renal transplant recipients and patients with SLE, altered lipid metabolism, and fatty degeneration of the liver or alcoholism.

Localized bone pain during activity is the usual initial symptom of osteonecrosis, with the pain eventually occurring at rest and requiring analgesics for relief. The proximal femur is the most common site affected, although the distal femur or humeral head may be affected. Most patients who develop osteonecrosis while on glucocorticosteroids will have been treated for at least 6–12 months, paralleling the time needed to induce changes in bone marrow fat deposition and clinical cushingoid features.

The mechanism of this condition is not completely understood, although intraosseous hypertension secondary to fat cell enlargement may compromise terminal arterioles at certain sites. Some investigators believe that fat emboli can originate from fatty deposits in the liver or from serum triglycerides, whereas others believe that only bone-derived fat emboli produce arterial occlusion with subsequent infarction[31].

Radiographic signs of osteonecrosis may not occur for as long as 6 months after bone pain begins (Fig. 125.4). Therefore, early MRI, the most specific and sensitive radiologic examination, is recommended for confirmation of diagnosis (Fig. 125.5). Early medical treatment is conservative and consists of trauma prevention, rest, and modified weight bearing with the use of crutches[32]. More advanced cases in young patients may require hip salvaging procedures such as core

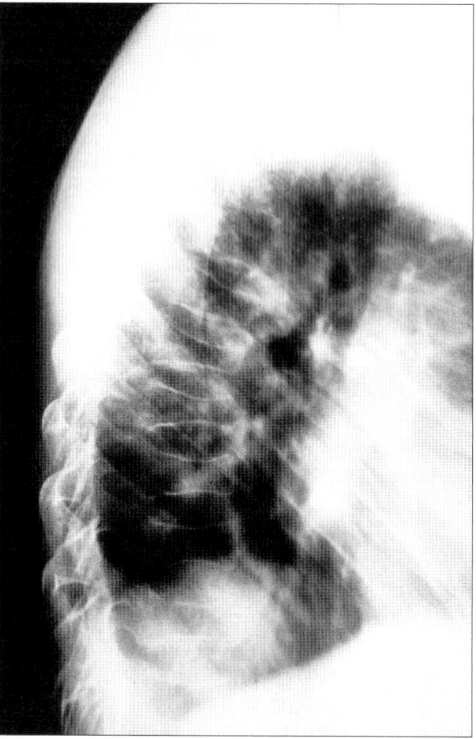

Fig. 125.2 Radiograph of the spine showing severe demineralization. This is indicative of advanced osteoporosis.

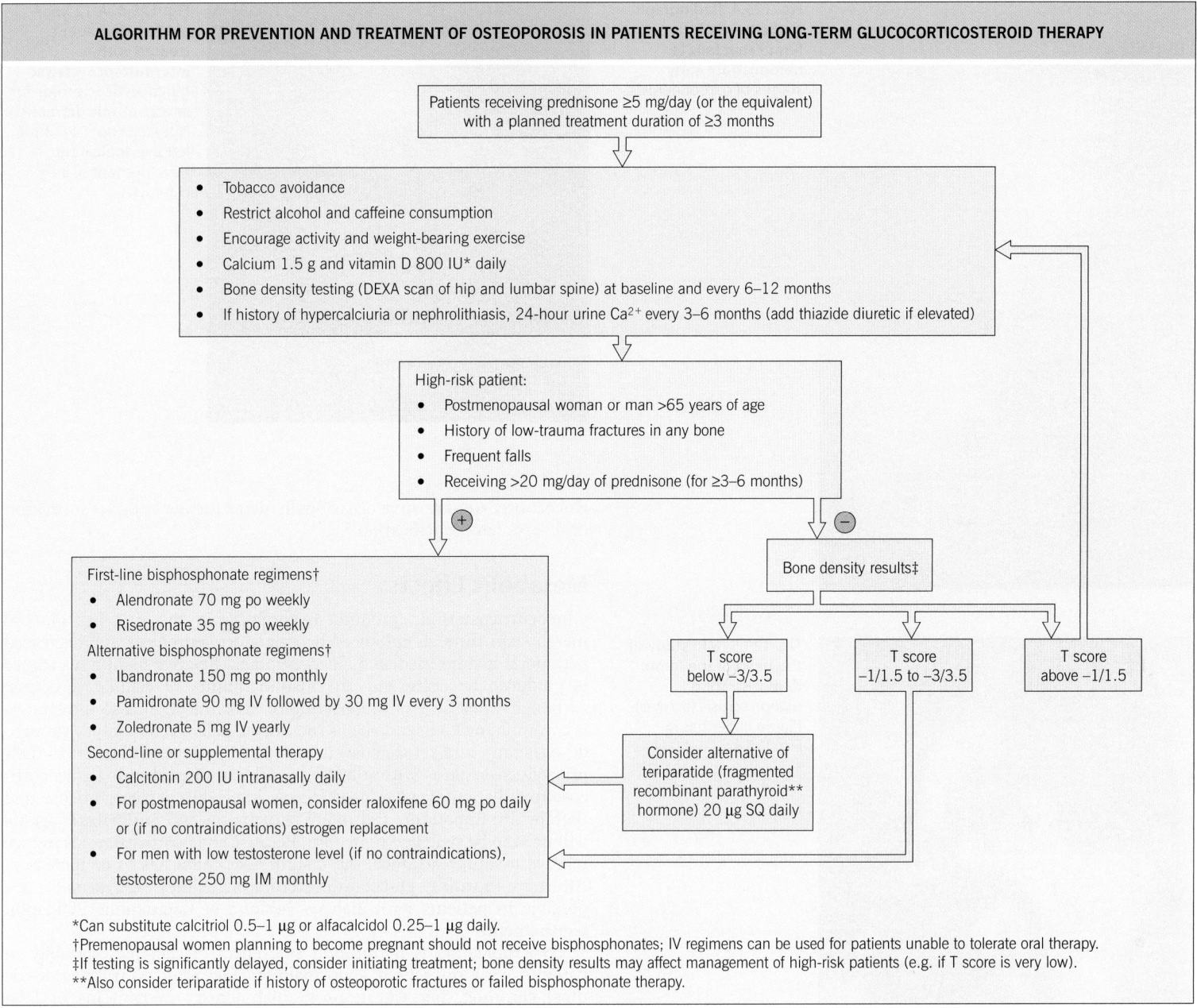

ALGORITHM FOR PREVENTION AND TREATMENT OF OSTEOPOROSIS IN PATIENTS RECEIVING LONG-TERM GLUCOCORTICOSTEROID THERAPY

Patients receiving prednisone ≥5 mg/day (or the equivalent) with a planned treatment duration of ≥3 months

- Tobacco avoidance
- Restrict alcohol and caffeine consumption
- Encourage activity and weight-bearing exercise
- Calcium 1.5 g and vitamin D 800 IU* daily
- Bone density testing (DEXA scan of hip and lumbar spine) at baseline and every 6–12 months
- If history of hypercalciuria or nephrolithiasis, 24-hour urine Ca^{2+} every 3–6 months (add thiazide diuretic if elevated)

High-risk patient:
- Postmenopausal woman or man >65 years of age
- History of low-trauma fractures in any bone
- Frequent falls
- Receiving >20 mg/day of prednisone (for ≥3–6 months)

Bone density results‡

First-line bisphosphonate regimens†
- Alendronate 70 mg po weekly
- Risedronate 35 mg po weekly

Alternative bisphosphonate regimens†
- Ibandronate 150 mg po monthly
- Pamidronate 90 mg IV followed by 30 mg IV every 3 months
- Zoledronate 5 mg IV yearly

Second-line or supplemental therapy
- Calcitonin 200 IU intranasally daily
- For postmenopausal women, consider raloxifene 60 mg po daily or (if no contraindications) estrogen replacement
- For men with low testosterone level (if no contraindications), testosterone 250 mg IM monthly

T score below –3/3.5

T score –1/1.5 to –3/3.5

T score above –1/1.5

Consider alternative of teriparatide (fragmented recombinant parathyroid** hormone) 20 µg SQ daily

*Can substitute calcitriol 0.5–1 µg or alfacalcidol 0.25–1 µg daily.
†Premenopausal women planning to become pregnant should not receive bisphosphonates; IV regimens can be used for patients unable to tolerate oral therapy.
‡If testing is significantly delayed, consider initiating treatment; bone density results may affect management of high-risk patients (e.g. if T score is very low).
**Also consider teriparatide if history of osteoporotic fractures or failed bisphosphonate therapy.

Fig. 125.3 Algorithm for prevention and treatment of osteoporosis in patients receiving long-term glucocorticosteroid therapy.

decompression to reduce intraosseous pressure, vascularized fibular grafting, or electric stimulation. Eventual total joint arthroplasty is often unavoidable[33].

Growth Retardation

The doses of systemic glucocorticosteroids required to produce growth suppression are not much larger than physiologic doses. Alternate-morning therapy can minimize this effect, but does not eliminate it completely[34]. Glucocorticosteroid therapy via inhalants or extensive and chronic use of topical agents may also rarely produce growth suppression. Once the glucocorticosteroid therapy is discontinued, there is often a compensatory growth spurt with normal development of height, except if glucocorticosteroids are given during the two major spurts of childhood – prior to age 2 years and at puberty. If glucocorticosteroids are given just before puberty, the usual compensatory growth may be negated by epiphyseal closure.

Glucocorticosteroids produce growth retardation by many mechanisms, including interference with nitrogen and mineral retention, inhibition of collagen and protein matrix synthesis, and a decreased growth hormone effect[34]. Growth suppression monitoring should be done every 3–6 months, and growth hormone therapy might be considered in certain situations to restore linear growth and reverse certain other catabolic effects.

Myopathy

The form of glucocorticosteroid-related myopathy relevant to dermatology is uncommon, but, when it occurs, it is a painless, symmetrical, proximal muscle weakness, usually of the lower extremities. It typically begins many weeks to months after therapy is initiated and usually at doses greater than 40 mg/day of prednisone equivalent. Although possibly more common with fluorinated glucocorticosteroids, the condition can occur with any agent[35]. Alternate-morning therapy may decrease its incidence. Diagnosis of myopathy may be difficult, as muscle enzymes, muscle biopsy, and electromyographic studies will usually be normal. Elevation of urinary creatine may be helpful in the diagnosis. Gradual reduction of the glucocorticosteroid dose along with physical therapy is useful in managing this complication, although muscle function may not return to normal for many months or up to 1 year.

When treating inflammatory muscle diseases, such as dermatomyositis, glucocorticosteroids are vital for controlling the disorder but they may actually increase the tendency for muscle atrophy. Therefore,

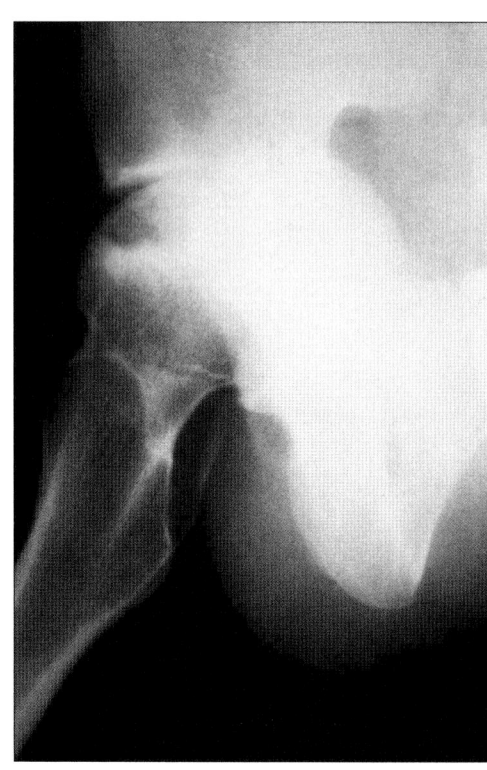

Fig. 125.4 Radiograph of the head of the femur that fails to demonstrate early stages of osteonecrosis.

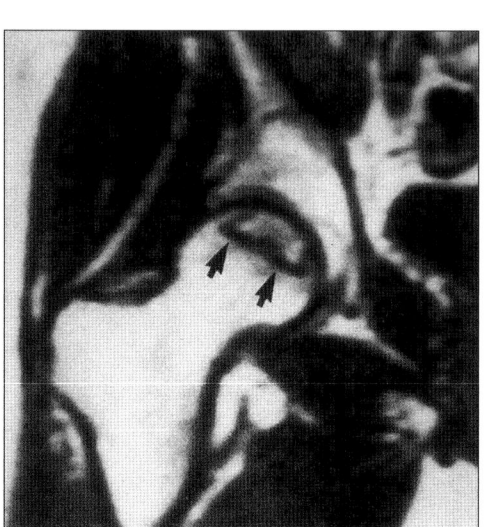

Fig. 125.5 MRI study of the head of the femur demonstrating osteonecrosis (arrows). (Same patient as in Fig. 125.4.)

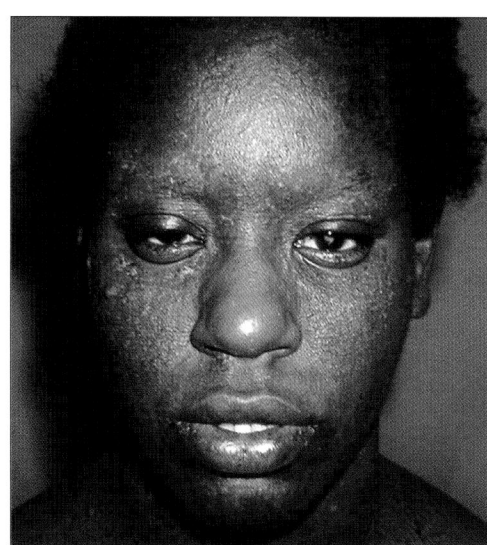

Fig. 125.6 A 12-year-old female patient treated with intermittent systemic glucocorticosteroids for severe atopic dermatitis. Note lens opacity of the left eye, indicating development of a cataract.

glucocorticosteroids may occasionally deter further cataract formation or reverse lens opacification[36].

Metabolic Effects

Glucocorticosteroids produce hyperglycemia by affecting glucose metabolism through enhanced hepatic gluconeogenesis and decreased peripheral insulin-mediated glucose uptake. Relative insulin resistance is produced by decreasing the insulin affinity of cellular receptors. Although worsening of pre-existing or subclinical glucose intolerance is common, new-onset diabetes mellitus usually occurs only with high-dose therapy, and ketoacidosis is rare. Most patients will revert to their prior glucose status within a few months of discontinuing glucocorticosteroid therapy. Regular blood glucose levels during glucocorticosteroid therapy are important, and many patients on oral antidiabetic agents will need to be switched to insulin. Because glucocorticosteroids induce relative insulin resistance, the insulin dose often has to be increased. Alternate-morning glucocorticosteroid schedules are usually not possible in patients with diabetes because of fluctuations in insulin requirements[37].

Hyperlipidemia is a common side effect of therapy, especially in patients with prior lipid abnormalities. Elevation of triglycerides is most common, but elevations of high-density lipoproteins or low-density lipoproteins occur in some patients. The mechanism of hypertriglyceridemia is likely related to relative insulin insufficiency. A diet low in saturated fat and calories should be instituted in all patients on long-term glucocorticosteroids[38].

Other metabolic effects from glucocorticosteroids include weight gain with redistribution of fat (including the classic 'buffalo hump'), hypokalemic alkalosis associated with high-dose therapy, and the uncommon development of hypocalcemia, which can rarely cause tetany in children on high-dose therapy. Potassium supplementation is often necessary, and adequate calcium intake is mandatory.

Cardiovascular Effects

Although the majority of patients with endogenous glucocorticosteroid excess (Cushing's syndrome) have hypertension, exogenous glucocorticosteroid therapy produces hypertension in only about 20% of patients, because of the lower mineralocorticoid effect of exogenous agents. When glucocorticosteroid-associated hypertension does occur, it is more common in patients with pre-existing hypertension or with decreased renal function, in the elderly, or when glucocorticosteroids with greater mineralocorticoid activity are used[39]. Because glucocorticosteroids rarely affect blood pressure during the first 2 weeks of therapy, short courses of glucocorticosteroids in hypertensive patients almost never produce problems. In patients receiving long-term therapy, sodium restriction is important along with the possible institution of a thiazide diuretic. Alternate-morning therapy may produce some reduced effect on the blood pressure. The pathogenesis of glucocorticosteroid-induced

corticosteroid-sparing agents may be utilized in treating these disorders after initial control with glucocorticosteroids, if glucocorticosteroid tapering is not occurring at an acceptable rate[6] (see Ch. 43).

Cataracts

The overall total dosage and duration of therapy are the most important factors in the development of posterior subcapsular cataracts in patients on glucocorticosteroids. This effect has been noted in patients receiving as little as 10 mg/day of prednisone for 1 year. Cataract development is not minimized by alternate-morning schedules, and patients on continuous therapy are at higher risk than patients on intermittent therapy. Although there may be some individual susceptibility, children are at greatest risk because they can develop cataracts with lower doses and shorter treatment duration than do adults. Cataracts that occur as a manifestation of the disease process in atopic dermatitis are usually anterior plaques in the papillary zone, but cataracts may occur in a posterior location and be indistinguishable from those associated with glucocorticosteroids (Fig. 125.6).

Ophthalmologic examinations are recommended every 6–12 months for patients on long-term systemic glucocorticosteroid therapy. Progression of the cataract may still occur despite decreasing or discontinuing glucocorticosteroid therapy, but discontinuing the hypertension is not totally understood, but is likely related to vaso-constriction (from potentiation of catecholamines and inhibition of vasodilators), sodium retention, and intravascular volume expansion.

Certain patients, including patients with SLE, rheumatoid arthritis, and renal transplants, have demonstrated accelerated atherosclerosis with long-term glucocorticosteroid use[40]. Young children treated with glucocorticosteroids may also show this effect, and it has long been noted in patients with Cushing's syndrome from chronic endogenous glucocorticosteroid excess. Instances of thromboembolic complications and atrioventricular conduction problems have also been reported with glucocorticosteroid therapy.

Gastrointestinal Effects

Association of glucocorticosteroid therapy with peptic ulcer disease is controversial, with varying results in different published case series. There does seem to be an increased incidence in patients treated concomitantly with non-steroidal anti-inflammatory drugs or with aspirin, such as those with rheumatoid arthritis[41]. Other additive risk factors include smoking, alcohol use, and past history of peptic ulcer disease. When ulcer disease does occur in patients on glucocorti-costeroids, it is more likely to be gastric than duodenal, with milder pain symptoms and greater chance of a major complication such as hemorrhage or perforation. This is related to the tendency of gluco-corticosteroids to mask signs and symptoms of inflammation and to inhibit wound healing. A possible mechanism of ulceration in these situations is decreased mucus production and mucosal cell renewal. The administration of oral glucocorticosteroids with food, as well as the use of H_2 receptor antagonists or proton pump inhibitors, minimize the chance for peptic ulcer disease in patients on glucocorticosteroids. Other gastrointestinal side effects that may occur in patients receiving glucocorticosteroids are nausea and vomiting (minimized by a dyspepsia prophylactic regimen and dosing the glucocorticosteroids with food), reflux or candidal esophagitis (the latter is a particular problem in patients with erosive oral mucosal disease, such as pemphigus vulgaris, which requires treatment with oral antifungals, e.g. fluconazole), pan-creatitis in patients with hypertriglyceridemia, intestinal perforation, and fatty liver changes.

Infection

Patients receiving glucocorticosteroids have an increased susceptibility to many bacterial, viral, fungal and parasitic infections. Cutaneous staphylococcal and superficial fungal infections are extremely common. Fever and the usual signs of inflammation may be masked; therefore, the early diagnosis of infection in patients on glucocorticosteroids may be difficult. Alternate-morning therapy and doses of less than 10 mg/day of prednisone equivalent may significantly reduce the chance of oppor-tunistic infection[42].

Reactivation of tuberculosis has long been a concern in patients on long-term glucocorticosteroids, but this risk may be less than previously believed. A tuberculosis history should be taken and, if negative or uncertain, a tuberculin skin test performed prior to beginning therapy. A baseline chest radiograph should be obtained for patients with a positive tuberculin reaction (defined as ≥5 mm of induration in indi-viduals receiving the equivalent of ≥15 mg/day of prednisone for a month or more), a history of tuberculosis or other risk factors (e.g. pre-existing immunosuppression), and a 9-month course of isoniazid is recommended for those with an untreated latent tuberculosis infection[43].

Some physicians have noted an increased risk of *Pneumocystis jiroveci* pulmonary infection in certain patient groups receiving systemic glucocorticosteroid therapy for longer than 2 months[44]. These patient groups include those with HIV infection, Wegener's granulomatosis or SLE, as well as those receiving additional immunosuppressives. Trimethoprim–sulfamethoxazole or dapsone can be used for prophylaxis in certain of these situations.

Normal antibody responses to immunizations are seen in patients who receive less than about 20 mg/day of prednisone. However, any live virus vaccine should not be given to children being treated with glucocorticosteroids. An increase in significant complications associated with naturally acquired varicella has also been reported.

Obstetric and Gynecologic Effects

A higher incidence than normal of cleft palate has been noted in rodents given very large doses of glucocorticosteroids early in gestation; therefore, the safety of glucocorticosteroids during the first trimester of pregnancy has been debated. However, clinical experience and several clinical trials have shown minimal human effects[45]. Only small amounts of prednisone reach the fetus of a pregnant patient in an active form, because a placental enzyme, 11-hydroxysteroid dehydro-genase type 2, inactivates most prednisolone crossing into the fetal circulation. This enzyme has limited metabolism for fluorinated gluco-corticosteroids, such as betamethasone and dexamethasone, so that greater amounts reach the fetus if these agents are utilized[46]. Pregnant patients on glucocorticosteroids do have a slightly increased risk of hypertension, which might account indirectly for smaller fetal gestational size, and gestational glucose intolerance, which is relatively common on moderate to high glucocorticosteroid doses. When large glucocorticosteroid doses are used near the time of delivery, fetal HPA axis suppression may occasionally occur, producing a pseudo-Addisonian neonate. Even though there is excretion of glucocorticosteroids into maternal breast milk, the American Academy of Pediatrics has deter-mined that prednisone therapy is compatible with breastfeeding, although it is best delayed for approximately 4 hours after dosing[47].

In non-pregnant women, amenorrhea may occur from therapy with glucocorticosteroids, most frequently with intramuscular injections[18]. Premenopausal women receiving glucocorticosteroids should be alerted to this possibility, to prevent unnecessary alarm. Impairment of fertility does not appear to be a risk in women, although decreased sperm counts have been reported in men on glucocorticosteroids.

Nervous System Effects

Mood changes, nervousness and insomnia are common dose-related side effects of glucocorticosteroid use. Patients with a prior history of personality pattern disorders are at a greater risk for increased neuro-psychiatric symptoms[35]. Depression and fatigue are not uncommon during the tapering phase of glucocorticosteroid therapy.

Psychosis is an uncommon side effect, but it is dose-related and is seen more commonly in patients with a previous history of major psychiatric disease. When psychosis develops in patients with SLE on glucocorticosteroids, it may be difficult to determine if the psychosis is due to the underlying disease or the glucocorticosteroid. If glucocorti-costeroid doses are reduced, steroid psychosis should improve, whereas it should worsen or remain the same with lupus encephalopathy[35].

Pseudotumor cerebri is a possible complication of high-dose or long-term glucocorticosteroid therapy, in which the patient presents with headache, nausea, vomiting, visual changes and papilledema. Most often, this problem develops after rapid tapering or discontinuation of the glucocorticosteroid, so that a return to previous doses with more gradual tapering is recommended[35]. Although the condition is rever-sible, there is potential for visual loss.

Seizures occur uncommonly, primarily in seizure-prone patients on high glucocorticosteroid doses. Other uncommon neurologic compli-cations include EEG changes, enhancement of tremor, and peripheral neuropathy[35]. In treating neuropsychiatric complications, consultation with a psychiatrist or neurologist may be necessary in some instances and pharmacologic therapy with neuroleptics may be needed. Tricyclic antidepressants may even worsen symptoms and are best used under the recommendation of a specialist. Alternate-morning therapy may be beneficial, but bipolar behavior has sometimes been noted to worsen with these schedules.

Cutaneous Effects

A host of cutaneous effects can occur in patients on systemic and topical glucocorticosteroids, most of which are similar to those of the hyperadrenal state associated with Cushing's syndrome. These include purpura, telangiectasias, atrophy, striae (Fig. 125.7), pseudoscars, acnei-form or rosacea-like eruptions, and facial plethora[48].

Systemic glucocorticosteroid-induced acne or folliculitis character-istically presents with uniform papulopustules on the chest and back. Acne vulgaris itself is also usually worsened by continuous gluco-corticosteroid therapy, although inflammatory and cystic acne lesions

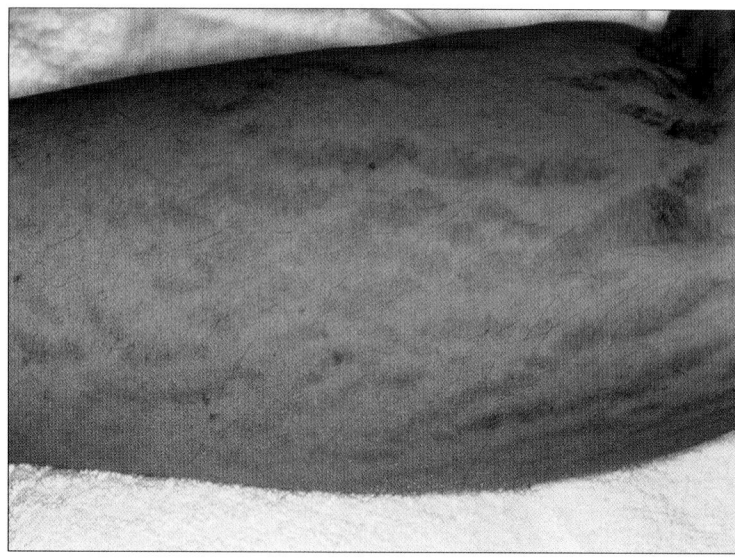

Fig. 125.7 Striae in a patient on chronic oral prednisone therapy.

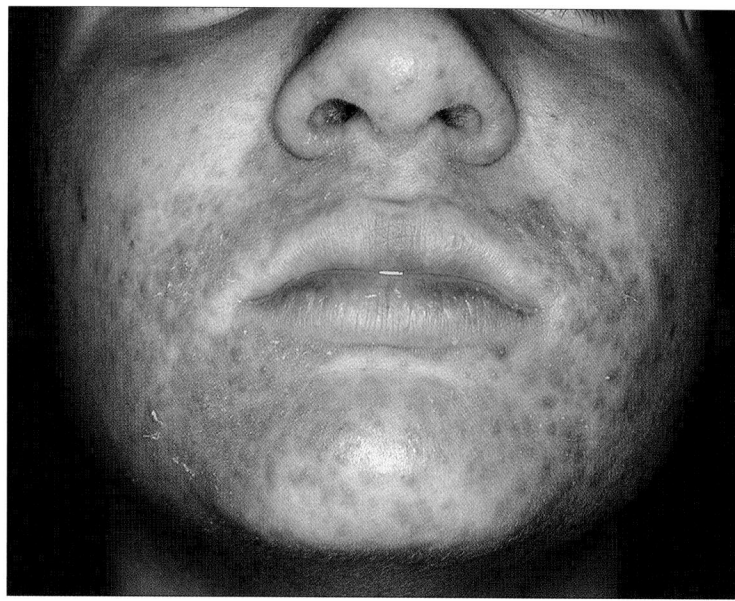

Fig. 125.9 Steroid rosacea due to application of mid-potency glucocorticosteroids to the face. Courtesy of Kalman Watsky MD.

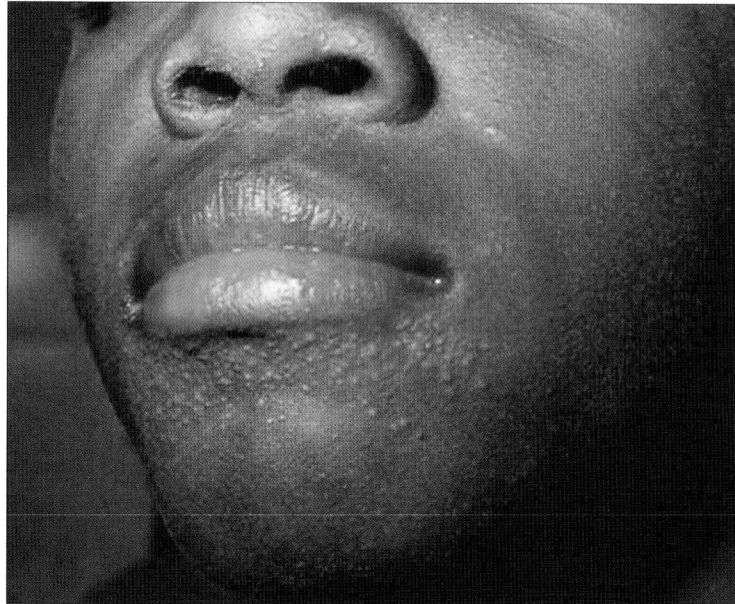

Fig. 125.8 Papular perioral eruption from fluorinated topical glucocorticosteroids in a young male patient.

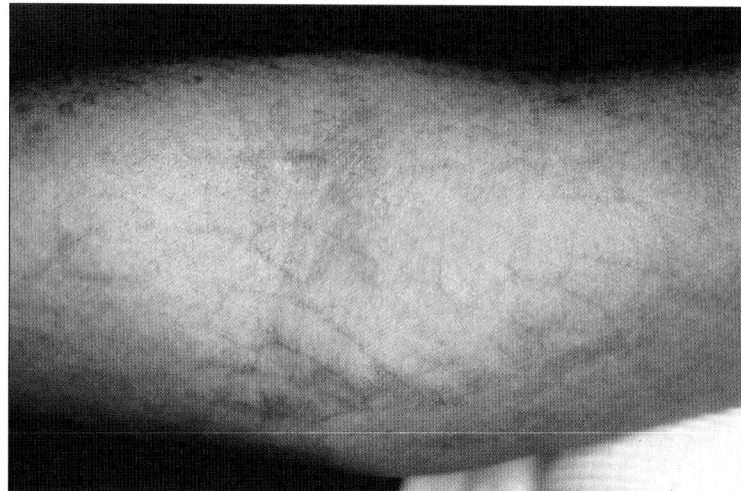

Fig. 125.10 Cutaneous atrophy due to topical corticosteroids. Note the prominent vascular pattern.

may be temporarily improved by very short intermittent courses of systemic glucocorticosteroids, or by intralesional injections of cysts (see Ch. 37). An acneiform or rosacea-like perioral or periorbital eruption also occurs with significant use of inhalant glucocorticosteroids or application of potent topical glucocorticosteroids from classes 1–5 to the face (Figs 125.8 & 125.9). Topical tacrolimus or pimecrolimus may be helpful in treating perioral dermatitis/steroid rosacea (see Ch. 38), although these agents have also been reported to exacerbate rosacea.

Other cutaneous effects from systemic glucocorticosteroids include hirsutism, alopecia, hyperpigmentation, and acanthosis nigricans[48]. A telogen effluvium type of transient hair loss on the scalp may occur with systemic glucocorticosteroid therapy. Hirsutism and increased vellus hair growth on other areas of the body can develop. Topical and intralesional glucocorticosteroids can produce local effects, including telangiectasias, atrophy (Figs 125.10 & 125.11) and hypopigmentation (see Ch. 65).

Topical and systemic glucocorticosteroid therapy may impair wound healing by inhibiting fibroblast function and collagen production. Angiogenesis, production of ground substance, and re-epithelialization of wounds are also inhibited[7]. Some authors have advocated using vitamin C to improve wound healing in glucocorticosteroid-treated patients.

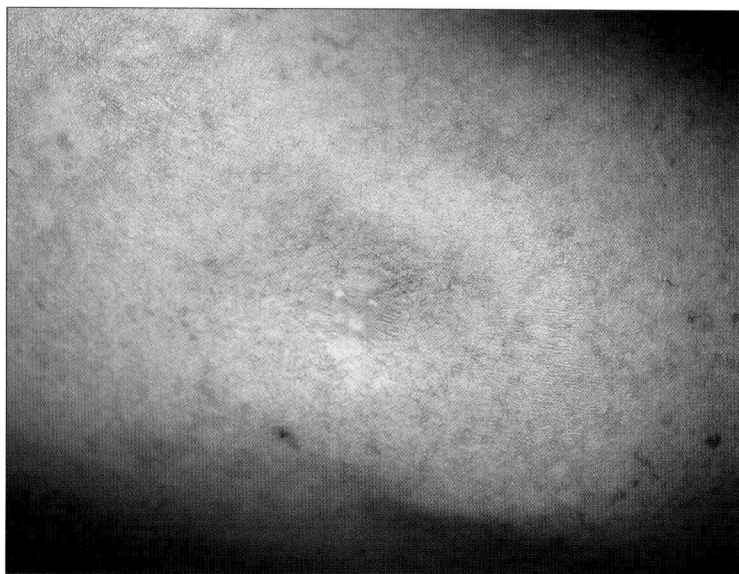

Fig. 125.11 Local side effects of intralesional glucocorticosteroids. Telangiectasias, dermal and subcutaneous atrophy, and yellow–white deposits of triaminolone acetonide. Courtesy of Jean L Bolognia MD.

HPA Axis Suppression

Exogenous glucocorticosteroids can produce a secondary type of adrenal insufficiency which is related to both dose and duration of treatment, with adrenal suppression occurring at doses just above physiologic levels at 4 weeks, and earlier with higher doses. This effect is minimized by using single morning doses, and even more so by using an intermediate-acting agent on alternate mornings[16].

The entire HPA axis is affected by exogenous glucocorticosteroid doses. The hypothalamus is the first to be suppressed and the quickest to recover. The adrenals are the last of the three glands to be suppressed and the slowest to recover. After high-dose therapy for many months to years, ACTH levels may not return to normal for several months. Full recovery of the adrenal glands with normal serum cortisol levels may take even longer, sometimes up to 1 year[10]. There can be altered stress responsiveness in situations such as infection or surgery. Symptoms of weakness, fatigue, anorexia, nausea and fever may occur, and the patient may even rarely develop hypotension or shock. Small doses of intravenous glucocorticosteroids may be needed prior to physically stressful situations such as major surgical procedures[49]. Minor surgical procedures under local anesthesia do not require replacement therapy. Endocrinologic consultation should always be obtained if the rare Addisonian crisis occurs.

A more common problem than adrenal crisis is the corticosteroid withdrawal syndrome. In this situation, the patient develops arthralgias, headache, mood swings, lethargy and nausea upon rapid tapering of long-term glucocorticosteroid therapy. Low intracellular corticosteroid levels are thought to be the cause. A return to previous doses with slower tapering alleviates this syndrome[19].

With regard to HPA axis suppression, the primary test for basal function of the entire axis is the morning serum cortisol level. Any morning glucocorticosteroid dose should be omitted on the day the cortisol level is checked. Impaired basal HPA axis function is suggested by serum cortisol levels below $10\,\mu g/100\,dl$. Adrenal function alone can be tested by using the ACTH stimulation test, in which basal, 30-minute and 60-minute serum cortisol levels are measured after $250\,\mu g$ of parenteral ACTH[10]. If it is necessary to test stress responsiveness of the HPA axis or the adrenal glands in greater detail, endocrinologic consultation should be obtained for the ACTH stimulation test or for other evaluations including the corticotropin-releasing factor test, the insulin hypoglycemia test, or the metyrapone test.

INTERACTIONS AND DOSE ALTERATIONS

The pharmacokinetics of glucocorticosteroids may be altered by certain medications[7] (see Ch. 131). Inducers of the P450 hepatic microsomal enzyme system, such as phenytoin, phenobarbital and rifampin, may greatly increase the clearance of glucocorticosteroids, and thereby increase the prednisone requirement of patients on these drugs. When prednisone is given concurrently with hepatic enzyme inhibitors, such as ketoconazole, a decrease in the prednisone requirement should apply. One study showed that coadministration of prednisolone and ketoconazole resulted in 50% higher prednisolone levels than when the former was administered alone. In patients on concomitant oral contraceptives or estrogens, the estrogen increases the glucocorticosteroid effect because the two drugs have similar protein-binding characteristics and are metabolized similarly. This effect may allow for a lowered glucocorticosteroid requirement in patients taking estrogens.

Glucocorticosteroids may also alter the kinetics of certain other medications[7]. In patients on concomitant salicylates, the renal salicylate clearance is increased by glucocorticosteroids, requiring higher doses; highly elevated salicylate levels have been reported after tapering or discontinuing glucocorticosteroids. Glucocorticosteroids may also impair conversion of carotene to vitamin A, with carotenemia occurring in patients on β-carotene and concomitant glucocorticosteroids.

As mentioned previously, certain medical conditions may require glucocorticosteroid dose alteration[7]. With hypoalbuminemia, a larger unbound fraction of the glucocorticosteroid dose can lead to a greater incidence of side effects. In patients with reduced renal function and chronic active hepatitis, decreased renal clearance will require a reduction in glucocorticosteroid doses. In patients with hyperthyroidism, a higher glucocorticosteroid dose may be required because these patients have reduced biologic effects from prednisolone.

Most of the above interactions and dose-alteration requirements have been assessed using short-term studies evaluating pharmacologic results rather than biologic effects. Therefore, the clinician should always keep these interactions in mind, but make treatment decisions based on individual patients and their responses to treatment.

REFERENCES

1. Hench PS, Kendall EC, Slocumb CH, et al. Effects of cortisone acetate and pituitary ACTH on rheumatoid arthritis, rheumatic fever, and certain other conditions. Study in clinical physiology. Arch Intern Med. 1950;85:545–666.
2. Sulzberger MB, Witten VH, Yaffe SN. Cortisone acetate administered orally in dematologic therapy. Arch Dermatol Syphilol. 1951;64:573–8.
3. Reichling GH, Kligman AM. Alternate-day corticosteroid therapy. Arch Dermatol. 1961;83:980–3.
4. Johnson RB, Lazarus GS. Pulse therapy: therapeutic efficacy in the treatment of pyoderma gangrenosum. Arch Dermatol. 1982;118:76–84.
5. Schimmer BP, Parker KL. Adrenocorticotropic hormone: adrenocortical steroids and their synthetic analogs; inhibitors of the synthesis and actions of adrenocortical hormones. In: Hardman JG, Limbird LE, Molinoff PB, et al. (eds). The Pharmacological Basis of Therapeutics, 9th edn. New York: McGraw-Hill, 1996:1459–85.
6. Nesbitt LT. Minimizing complications from systemic glucocorticoid use. Dermatol Clin. 1995;13:925–39.
7. Williams LC, Nesbitt LT. Update on systemic glucocorticosteroids in dermatology. Dermatol Clin. 2001;19:63–77.
8. Lester RS. Corticosteroids. Clin Dermatol. 1989;7:80–97.
9. Orth DN, Kovacs WJ. The adrenal cortex. In: Wilson JD, Foster DW, Kronenberg HM, et al. (eds). Williams Textbook of Endocrinology, 9th edn. Philadelphia: WB Saunders, 1998:517–47.
10. Wolverton SE. Systemic corticosteroids. In: Wolverton SE (ed.). Comprehensive Dermatologic Drug Therapy. Philadelphia: WB Saunders, 2001:109–46.
11. Feldman SR. The biology and clinical application of systemic corticosteroids. In: Callan JP (ed.). Current Problems in Dermatology. St Louis: Mosby Year Book, 1992:211–35.
12. Werth VP. Management and treatment with systemic glucocorticoids. Adv Dermatol. 1993; 8:81–101.
13. Fauci AS, Dale DC, Balow JE. Glucocorticoid therapy: mechanisms of action and clinical considerations. Ann Intern Med. 1976;84:304–15.
14. Boumpas DT, Chrousos GP, Wilder RL, et al. Glucocorticoid therapy for immune-mediated diseases: basic and clinical correlates. Ann Intern Med. 1993;119:1198–208.
15. Barnes PJ, Pedersen S, Busse WM. Efficacy and safety of inhaled corticosteroids. Am J Respir Crit Care Med. 1998;157:S1–S53.
16. Myles AB. Single daily dose corticosteroid treatment. Ann Rheum Dis. 1971;30:149–53.
17. Dixon RB, Christy NP. On the various forms of corticosteroid withdrawal syndrome. Am J Med. 1980;68:224–30.
18. Storrs FJ. Intramuscular corticosteroids: a second point of view. J Am Acad Dermatol. 1981;5:600–2.
19. Baethge BA, Lidsky MD, Goldberg JW. A study of adverse effects of high-dose intravenous (pulse) methylprednisolone therapy in patients with rheumatic disease. Ann Pharmacother. 1992;26:316–20.
20. Bonnotte B, Chauffert B, Martin F, et al. Side-effects of high-dose intravenous (pulse) methylprednisolone therapy cured by potassium infusion. Br J Rheumatol. 1998;37:109.
21. Yohn JJ, Weston WL. Topical glucocorticoids. Curr Probl Dermatol. 1990;2:38–63.
22. Cornell RC, Stoughton RB. Correlation of the vasoconstrictor assay and clinical activity. Arch Dermatol. 1985;121:63–7.
23. Degreef H, Dooms-Goossens A. The new corticosteroids: are they effective and safe? Dermatol Clin. 1993;11:155–60.
24. Chu AC, Munn S. Fluticasone propionate in the treatment of inflammatory dermatoses. Br J Clin Pract. 1995;49:131–3.
25. Iqbal MM. Osteoporosis: epidemiology, diagnosis and treatment. South Med J. 2000;93:2–18.
26. Lane NE, Lukert B. The science and therapy of glucocorticoid-induced bone loss. Endocrinol Metab Clin North Am. 1998;27:465–83.
27. Gulko PS, Mulloy AL. Glucocorticoid-induced osteoporosis: pathogenesis, prevention and treatment. Clin Exp Rheumatol. 1996;14:199–206.
28. Werth VP. Systemic glucocorticoids and the skin: dermatologists can prevent steroid-induced osteoporosis. Med Surg Dermatol. 1996;3:343–6.
29. American College of Rheumatology Ad Hoc Committee on Glucocorticoid Induced Osteoporosis. Recommendations for the prevention and treatment of glucocorticoid-induced osteoporosis. Arthritis Rheum. 2001;44:1496–503.
30. Cauley JA, Robbins J, Chen Z, et al. Effects of estrogen plus progestin on risk of fracture and bone mineral density: Women's Health Initiative randomized trial. JAMA. 2003;290:1729–38.
31. Lester RS, Knowles SR, Shear NH. The risks of systemic corticosteroid use. Dermatol Clin. 1998;16:277–86.
32. Mankin HJ. Nontraumatic necrosis of bone (osteonecrosis). N Engl J Med. 1992;326:1473–9.
33. Scully SP, Aaron RK, Urbaniak JR. Survival analysis of hips treated with core decompression or vascularized fibular grafting because of avascular necrosis. J Bone Joint Surg Am. 1998;80:1270–5.

34. Allen DB. Growth suppression by glucocorticoid therapy. Endocrinol Metab Clin North Am. 1996; 25:699–717.

35. Lacomis D, Samuels MA. Adverse neurologic effects of glucocorticosteroids. J Gen Intern Med. 1991; 6:367–77.

36. Renfro L, Snow JS. Ocular effects of topical and systemic steroids. Dermatol Clin. 1992;10:505–12.

37. Braithwaite SS, Barr WG, Rahman A, Quddusi S. Managing diabetes during glucocorticoid therapy. Postgrad Med. 1998;104:163–75.

38. Ariza-Andraca CR, Barile-Fabris LA, Frati-Munari AC, Baltazar-Montufar A. Risk factors for steroid diabetes in rheumatic patients. Arch Med Res. 1998;29:259–62.

39. Whitworth JA. Mechanisms of glucocorticoid-induced hypertension. Kidney Int. 1987;31:1213–24.

40. Nashel DJ. Is atherosclerosis a complication of long-term corticosteroid treatment? Am J Med. 1986;80:925–9.

41. Piper JM, Ray WA, Daugherty JR, Griffin MR. Corticosteroid use and peptic ulcer disease: role of nonsteroidal anti-inflammatory drugs. Ann Intern Med. 1991;114:735–40.

42. Stuck AE, Minder CE, Frey FJ. Risk of infectious complications in patients taking glucocorticosteroids. Rev Infect Dis. 1989;11:954–63.

43. American Thoracic Society (ATS) and Centers for Disease Control and Prevention (CDC). Targeted tuberculin testing and treatment of latent tuberculosis infection. Am J Respir Crit Care Med. 2000;161:S221–47.

44. Yale SH, Limper AH. *Pneumocystis carinii* pneumonia in patients without acquired immunodeficiency syndrome: associated illnesses and prior corticosteroid therapy. Mayo Clin Proc. 1996;71:5–13.

45. Esplin MS, Branch DW. Immunosuppressive drugs and pregnancy. Obstet Gynecol Clin North Am. 1997;24:601–16.

46. Parish DC. How safe is long-term prenatal glucocorticoid treatment? JAMA. 1997;277:1077–80.

47. Reed BR. Pregnancy, drugs, and the dermatologist. Curr Probl Dermatol. 1994;6:33–54.

48. Trahan AP, Ahmed AR. Corticosteroids: a review with emphasis on complications of prolonged systemic therapy. Ann Allergy. 1989;62:375–90.

49. Salem M, Tainsh RE, Bromberg J, et al. Perioperative glucocorticoid coverage. Ann Surg. 1994;219:416–25.

Retinoids

Stéphane Kuenzli and Jean-Hilaire Saurat

126

Key features

- Retinoids are structural and functional analogues of vitamin A that exert multiple effects on cellular differentiation and proliferation, the immune system, and embryonic development, primarily by regulating gene transcription via intracellular nuclear receptors

- The nuclear receptors – retinoic acid receptors (RARs) and retinoid X receptors (RXRs) – are both ligand-dependent transcriptional factors belonging to the steroid-thyroid hormone family

- Topical retinoids are used to treat acne, photoaging, and limited psoriasis, as well as a number of other conditions; the limiting factor is dose-related but temporary skin irritation. Teratogenicity risk is very low to non-existent

- Oral retinoids are the single most effective class of drugs available for severe acne (isotretinoin) and many disorders of cornification (isotretinoin; acitretin). They are also helpful tools in the management of psoriasis vulgaris, especially pustular and erythrodermic forms (acitretin > isotretinoin), pityriasis rubra pilaris, and cutaneous T-cell lymphoma

- Systemic toxicity, such as laboratory abnormalities (e.g. hypertriglyceridemia, transaminitis), ocular, musculoskeletal, endocrinologic or hematologic (bexarotene) adverse effects, and particularly teratogenicity, make careful thorough patient selection and ongoing laboratory monitoring critical when using systemic retinoid therapy

INTRODUCTION

Vitamin A (retinol) and related compounds with either structural (retinol derivative) or functional (vitamin A activity) analogy are known as retinoids (Fig. 126.1). The importance of retinoids in cutaneous biology was first appreciated early in the 20th century by Wolbach, who observed that vitamin A-deficient animals manifested altered keratinization, such as epidermal hyperkeratosis and squamous metaplasia of mucous membranes as well as certain precancerous conditions[1]. The 'antikeratinizing properties' of vitamin A led pioneers von Stuettgen and Bollag to administer topical and systemic retinoids to treat disorders of keratinization. In initial clinical trials with oral vitamin A, it was either ineffective at tolerable doses or too toxic at higher dosage levels. Because of this narrow therapeutic window, a large program was launched to engineer synthetic retinoids that would have the highest therapeutic activity with the lowest level of toxicity. Although retinoids may be produced naturally during vitamin A metabolism, most prescribed retinoids are synthetic. Parallel to these efforts, a growing interest in topical retinoids emerged.

All-*trans*-retinoic acid (tretinoin, *at*-RA), a naturally occurring metabolite of retinol (see Fig. 126.1), was the first retinoid to be synthesized. Orally, it did not have significant advantages over vitamin A and, as a result, the primary focus became its topical use for a number of conditions, including acne vulgaris and photoaging. The ability of tretinoin to promote cellular differentiation has been exploited for the systemic treatment of patients with acute promyelocytic leukemia, but resistance has been shown to eventually occur in those who receive tretinoin as a sole agent.

13-*cis*-retinoic acid (isotretinoin, 13-*cis*-RA) was first synthesized in 1955, but was tested years later in clinical trials. Its initial use was hampered by concerns regarding its teratogenicity and memories of the thalidomide tragedy. Initially, Orfanos and co-workers obtained equivocal results when they used isotretinoin to treat psoriasis, but etretinate

(used either alone or as combination therapy) was subsequently found to be very effective for treating psoriasis. These latter findings led to the temporary abandonment of studies of isotretinoin. Interest in isotretinoin was rekindled by the discovery of its effectiveness in the treatment of lamellar ichthyosis and other cutaneous disorders of keratinization[2], as well as its ability to produce complete responses with prolonged remissions in patients with previously treatment-resistant cystic acne and acne conglobata[3]. Isotretinoin is also available for topical use, where it matches tretinoin in its efficacy for moderate acne. In the US, 9-*cis*-retinoic acid (alitretinoin, 9-*cis*-RA) 0.1% gel is approved for the topical treatment of cutaneous Kaposi's sarcoma.

In 1972, Bollag, within the framework of his research program aimed at discovering retinoids with better therapeutic margins, developed two aromatic retinoids: etretinate and acitretin. These compounds demonstrated a therapeutic index ten times more favorable than that for tretinoin in the chemically induced rodent papilloma test model. Etretinate and its free acid metabolite, acitretin, are considered second-generation retinoids, and their identification constituted a real breakthrough in the systemic treatment of psoriasis and of many disorders of keratinization.

A major advance in understanding the molecular pharmacologic features and mechanisms of action of retinoids came with the discovery of nuclear receptors known as retinoic acid receptors (RARs) and retinoid X receptors (RXRs). New retinoids are being developed as a result of basic research that focuses on their binding properties to specific retinoid receptors. The third-generation retinoids include topical adapalene (acne), topical tazarotene (psoriasis and acne) and oral as well as topical bexarotene (cutaneous T-cell lymphoma). Lastly, topical retinol and retinaldehyde, the precursors of retinoic acid, are now being included in 'cosmeceutical products' since they induce much less irritation than topical tretinoin.

MECHANISM OF ACTION

Retinoids are involved in the regulation of diverse biologic functions (Table 126.1). They affect cellular growth, differentiation and morphogenesis, inhibit tumor promotion and malignant cell growth, exert immunomodulatory actions, and alter cellular cohesiveness.

BIOLOGIC FUNCTIONS OF RETINOIDS

Functions of vitamin A (retinol)*

- Embryonic growth
- Morphogenesis
- Differentiation and maintenance of epithelial tissues
- Reproduction (retinol)
- Visual function (retinaldehyde)

Biologic effects of retinoids

- Modulation of proliferation and differentiation
- Antikeratinization
- Alteration of cellular cohesiveness
- Antiacne and antiseborrheic effects
- Immunologic and anti-inflammatory effects
- Tumor prevention and therapy
- Induction of apoptosis
- Effects on extracellular matrix components

Retinoic acid can substitute for retinol with regard to growth, morphogenesis and epithelial differentiation; it cannot substitute completely for retinol in reproductive function, nor can it replace retinaldehyde in the visual cycle.

Table 126.1 **Biologic functions of retinoids.**

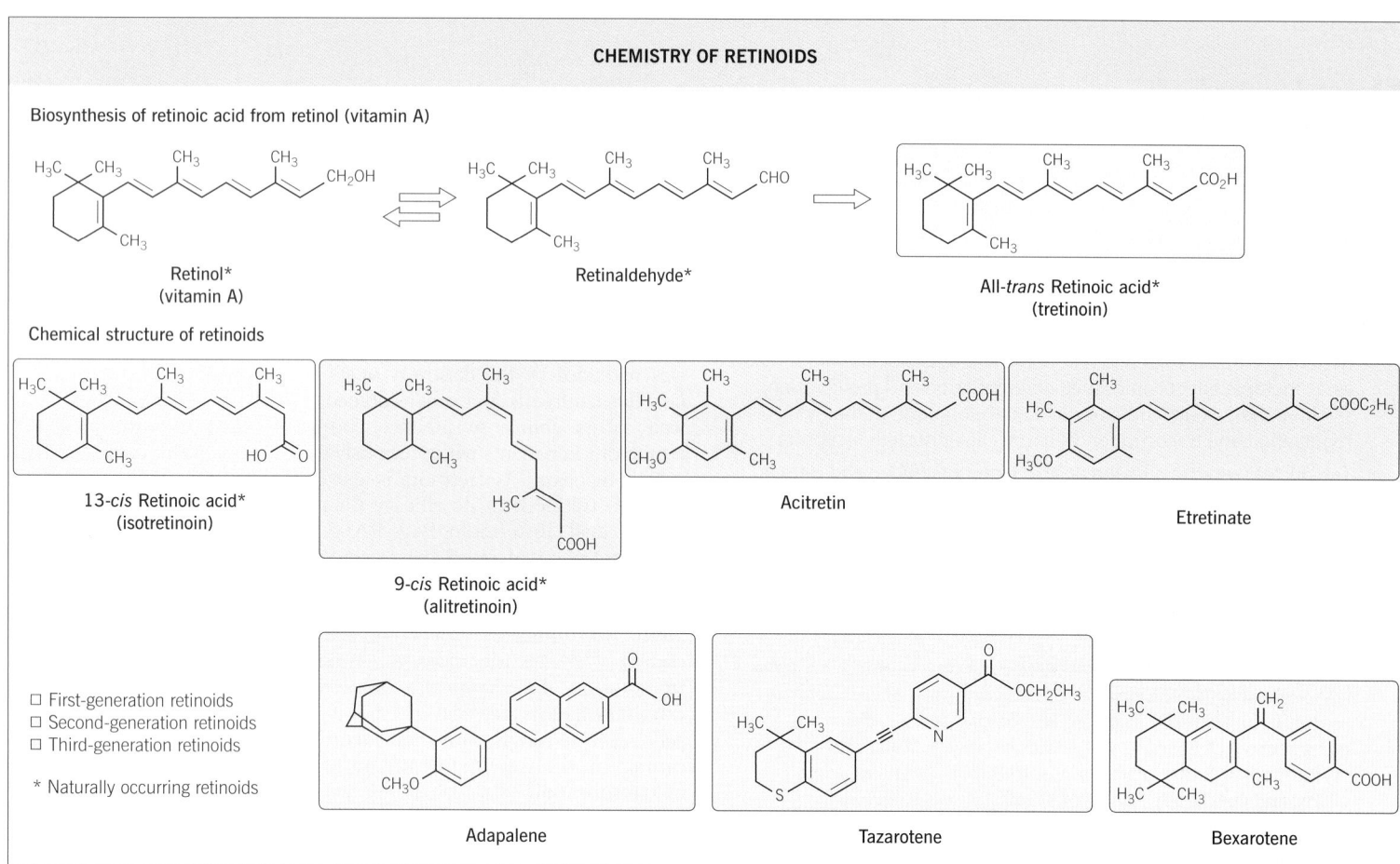

Fig. 126.1 **Chemistry of retinoids.**

Vitamin A Metabolism

Vitamin A (retinol) must be acquired through the diet and is ingested as retinyl esters and as provitamin A carotenoids; of the latter, β-carotene is particularly efficient in its ability to be converted to vitamin A. Within the intestinal lumen, retinyl esters are hydrolyzed to retinol, which is then absorbed and stored in the liver in the ester form (especially retinol palmitate; Fig. 126.2). Retinol represents the main dietary source, as well as transport and storage form of vitamin A. Once inside the bloodstream, after release of the retinol ester/storage form from the liver, retinol is transported bound to a complex of retinol binding protein (RBP) and transthyretin.

The basic cellular pathway leading to conversion of retinol to *at*-RA, the biologically active ligand that binds to nuclear receptors, consists of a two-step process (see Figs 126.1 & 126.2). In a reversible process, retinol (vitamin A alcohol) is oxidized to retinaldehyde (vitamin A aldehyde), which is then irreversibly converted to retinoic acid (vitamin A acid). A binding protein, called cytosolic RBP (CRBP-I), facilitates these enzymatic reactions by delivering retinol to appropriate enzymes.

Two additional intracellular carriers, cytosolic retinoic acid binding proteins (CRABP-I and CRABP-II), are thought to function in transporting retinoic acid to the nucleus as well as buffering the level of free *at*-RA in the cell. The latter is accomplished by sequestering *at*-RA and by promoting metabolism of *at*-RA by cytochrome P450 enzymes belonging to the CYP 2D6 family. CRABP-I regulates the metabolic fate of its ligands by directly affecting the activities of RA-metabolizing enzymes (cytochrome P450), while CRABP-II markedly stimulates the RA-induced transcriptional activity of RAR through protein–protein interactions[4].

Intracellularly, retinoic acid is found in both all-*trans* and 9-*cis* configurations (see Fig. 126.2). Physiologically, *at*-RA is the predominant retinoic acid form; only a small fraction is isomerized into 13-*cis*-RA. *at*-RA is the active ligand that binds to the three known nuclear RARs, which mediate, at least in part, the molecular and cellular effects of retinoic acid.

Retinoid Receptors

A major breakthrough in the understanding of retinoid action came from the discovery of nuclear receptors for retinoids. Retinoids exert their physiologic effects on DNA transcription through the binding to two distinct families of nuclear receptors: RAR (retinoic acid receptors) and RXR (retinoid X receptors). RAR and RXR belong to a superfamily of nuclear receptors that act as ligand-activated transcription factors and include the steroid, vitamin D3 and thyroid hormone receptors, as well as peroxisome proliferator-activated receptors (PPAR). The RAR receptor family contains three receptor isotypes (α, β and γ) encoded by different genes. In addition, the various retinoids have different binding properties; for example, *at*-RA binds only to RAR, whereas 9-*cis*-RA binds both to RAR and RXR (see Table 126.2).

RAR functions as a heterodimer with RXR, whereas RXR may act as a homodimer or participate in the formation of heterodimers with a variety of other nuclear receptors, including vitamin D3, thyroid hormone and peroxisome proliferator-activated receptors. Such heterodimers can provide a mechanism for cross-talk between nuclear hormone signaling pathways. Dimers of retinoid receptors (RAR/RXR or RXR/RXR) are localized to the nucleus and bind even in the unliganded state to specific DNA regulatory sequences (called hormone response elements) in the promoter regions of retinoid-responsive genes (see Fig. 126.2). The unliganded receptors bind to co-repressor molecules and repress transcription. However, when the receptor binds its ligand, it undergoes a conformational change resulting in the release of co-repressors and recruitment of co-activators. These molecules include histone acetylases that change the conformation of the chromatin and allow access to the DNA by transcriptional machinery. Finally, the retinoid–receptor complex modulates the transcription of specific sets of genes.

Retinoids can induce both direct and indirect effects on gene transcription. Their direct effects are mediated through binding to their hormone response element (retinoid hormone response element; RARE) in the promotor region of target genes whose transcription is activated. It is probable that many of the differentiation-inducing actions are mediated by this mechanism. In contrast, the indirect effects of retinoids result from the downregulation of genes that do not contain RARE in their promoter region. The retinoid–receptor complex probably antagonizes various transcription factors such as AP1 or NF-IL6 by competing for commonly required co-activator proteins, thereby downregulating expression of AP1 or NF-IL6-responsive genes. The antiproliferative and anti-inflammatory actions of retinoids are believed to be mediated by this type of negative, indirect gene regulatory mechanism. AP1 and NF-IL6 are key transcription factors in proliferative and inflammatory responses, and 'dissociating retinoids' have been synthesized that possess indirect anti-AP1 function but not direct gene transactivation function. Recently, the anti-inflammatory effects of at-RA have been associated, at least in part, with the ability to regulate the expression and activation of Toll-like receptors[5]. The biologic relevance of non-genomic effects of retinoids (e.g. phosphorylation, membrane effects) is still a matter of investigation.

The existence of several types and varied distributions of receptors, dimers, hormone response elements, mechanisms of action, and regulatory proteins means that retinoid action is mediated via multiple pathways and results in the complex activation or inhibition of a large set of coordinately regulated genes. However, the mechanism of retinoid action in many dermatologic conditions is still unknown, and, so far, the nuclear receptor concept does not satisfactorily explain the biologic diversity of retinoid effects.

Synthetic Retinoids

Three generations of synthetic retinoids have been developed (see Fig. 126.1). The first-generation monoaromatic retinoids (tretinoin, isotretinoin) are produced by chemically modifying the polar end group and the polyene side chain of vitamin A. Second-generation monoaromatic retinoids (etretinate, acitretin) are formed by replacing the cyclic end group of vitamin A with different substituted and unsubstituted ring systems. The third-generation polyaromatic retinoids, also called arotinoids, are produced by cyclization of the polyene side chain, and these include adapalene, bexarotene and tazarotene.

Commercially available retinoids differ not only in their spectrum of clinical efficacy but also in their observed toxicity and pharmacokinetics. Consequently, each retinoid should be investigated as a unique drug, and the lack of disease response to one retinoid does not necessarily signify unresponsiveness to the others.

The oral bioavailability of all retinoids is considerably enhanced when administered with food, especially with fatty meals, due to their lipophilic properties. The metabolism of retinoids occurs mainly in the liver. It involves oxidation and chain shortening to biologically inactive and polar metabolites, facilitating biliary and/or renal elimination. The oxidative metabolism is induced mainly by retinoids themselves and possibly also by other agents known to induce hepatic cytochrome P450 isoforms. Table 126.2 summarizes the key pharmacologic features and nuclear binding profile of retinoids used in dermatology.

Adapalene

Adapalene is a light-stable, rigid, and highly lipophilic synthetic retinoid with higher affinity for RAR-β/γ than for RAR-α. Since RAR-β is not expressed in keratinocytes, RAR-γ is the primary retinoid target receptor for adapalene in the epidermis. It does not bind to CRABPs but does induce expression of CRABP-II. Due to its lipophilic properties, there is selective uptake into the pilosebaceous unit, which may contribute to its low systemic absorption (due to dissolution within the sebum) and its activity in acne. Systemically absorbed adapalene is excreted through the hepatobiliary route and, given its negligible transdermal absorption, teratogenic risks appear minimal. Adapalene affects cellular differentiation, keratinization, and inflammatory processes that are abnormal in acne. However, it has no sebostatic effect.

Tazarotene

Tazarotene is a prodrug that is rapidly converted by skin esterases to its free carboxylic acid (tazarotenic acid), which is the active metabolite. It has a higher affinity for RAR-β/γ than for RAR-α and no affinity for RXR. Because of its rapid metabolism, systemic exposure is low.

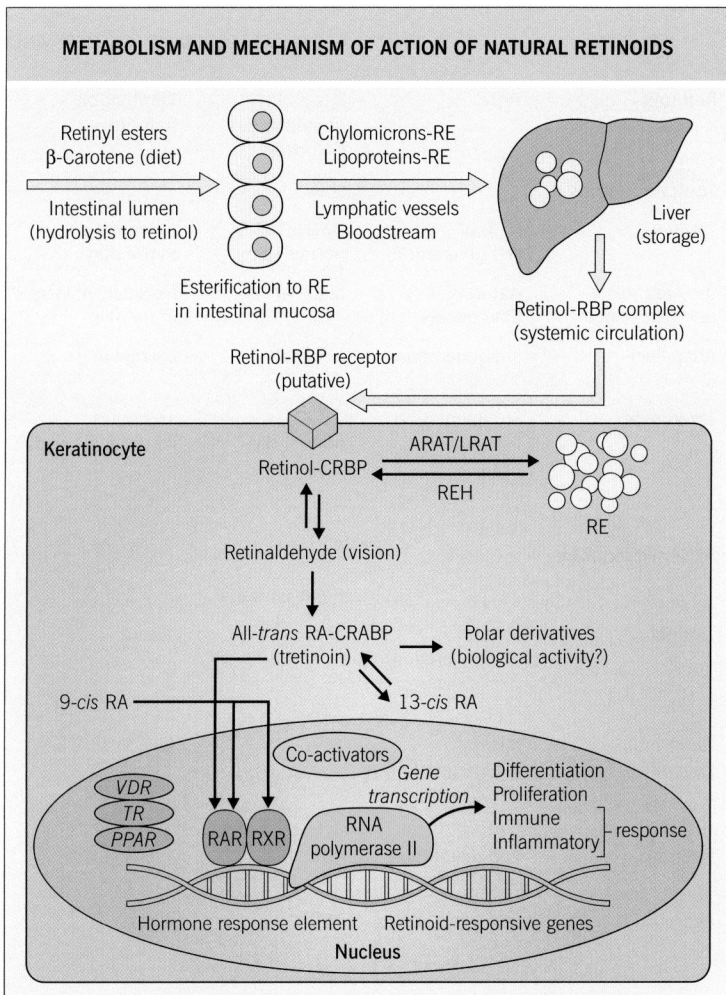

Fig. 126.2 Metabolism and mechanism of action of natural retinoids.
RE, retinyl esters; RBP, retinol binding protein; CRBP, cytosolic retinol binding protein; LRAT, lecithin:retinol acyl transferase; ARAT, acyl-CoA:retinol acyl transferase; REH, retinyl ester hydrolase; RA, retinoic acid; CRABP, cytosolic retinoic acid binding protein; RAR, retinoic acid receptor; RXR, retinoid X receptor; VDR, vitamin D3 receptor; TR, thyroid receptor; PPAR, peroxisome proliferator-activated receptor.

Tazarotene appears to modulate the pathogenesis of psoriasis by regulating expression of retinoid responsive genes, including those involved in: (1) cell proliferation (leading to downregulation of various proliferation-associated proteins, including ornithine decarboxylase, hyperproliferative keratins [i.e. K6, K16] and epidermal growth factor receptor); (2) cell differentiation; and (3) inflammation (downregulation of proinflammatory cytokine interleukin-6 and migration inhibition factor-related protein 8). In addition, tazarotenic acid upregulates tazarotene-inducible genes (TIG-1,2,3) and has antiproliferative properties that were demonstrated in patients with psoriasis[6]. Subsequently, an oral form was developed and phase III clinical trials completed that showed beneficial effects in psoriatic patients, but oral tazarotene is currently not approved by the US Food and Drug Administration (FDA). Interestingly, preliminary clinical studies suggested that topical tazarotene may cause regression of human sporadic basal cell carcinoma[7].

Acitretin

Acitretin is the major metabolite and the pharmacologically active compound of etretinate. Although acitretin and etretinate are equally effective, acitretin has a profound pharmacokinetic advantage because of its more rapid elimination compared with etretinate. Etretinate is approximately 50 times more lipophilic than acitretin and it binds strongly to plasma proteins, particularly lipoproteins and albumin. These properties have a marked influence on the respective pharmacokinetic properties of the two drugs.

The major serious adverse effect associated with synthetic retinoids is teratogenicity, and, therefore, the length of time that these drugs

KEY PHARMACOLOGIC FEATURES AND NUCLEAR BINDING PROFILE OF RETINOIDS

Retinoid	Type	Systemic absorption (% dose):	Elimination half-life	Metabolism	Excretion	Nuclear receptor and binding protein profile
Topical retinoids		Low*				
Tretinoin	Natural (1st generation)	<2% in normal skin	Normally present in the skin	Isomerization to 13-cis-RA (epidermis)	Desquamation, hepatobiliary	RAR; CRABP; no RXR
9-cis-retinoic acid (alitretinoin)	Natural (2nd generation)	Minimal	Normally present in the skin	Main metabolite: 4-oxo-9-cis-RA	Desquamation, hepatobiliary	RXR and RAR
Adapalene	3rd generation	Minimal	Unknown	Minimal biotransformation due to chemical rigidity	Desquamation, hepatobiliary	RAR-β, -γ > -α; no RXR
Tazarotene	3rd generation	<1–6% in normal skin	16 hours (tazarotenic acid)	Rapid skin ester hydrolysis to form its active metabolite, tazarotenic acid (within 20 min); excreted metabolites: sulfoxides, sulfones	Desquamation, urine (within 3 days), feces (within 7 days)	RAR-β, -γ > -α; no RXR
Systemic retinoids						
		Bioavailability†				
Tretinoin	Natural (1st generation)	50%	1 hour	Hepatic; main metabolites: cis- and trans-4-oxo derivatives	Biliary, renal	RAR; CRABP; no RXR (9-cis binds both RXR and RAR)
Isotretinoin (13-cis-RA)	Natural (1st generation)	25%	20 hours	Hepatic, endogenous concentration reached within 2 weeks; main metabolite: 4-oxo-isotretinoin	Biliary, renal	–‡
Etretinate	2nd generation	40%	120 days	Hepatic, hydrolysis to acitretin	Biliary, renal (accumulation in fat)	–‡
Acitretin	2nd generation	60%	2 days	Hepatic, re-esterification to etretinate indirectly increased by alcohol consumption; main metabolite: cis-acitretin	Biliary, renal	–‡
Bexarotene	3rd generation	Unknown	7–9 hours	Hepatic	Hepatobiliary	RXR

*Limited propensity for distribution to systemic tissues.
†Increased with food intake, highly variable.
‡No clearly identified affinity for any retinoid receptor.

Table 126.2 The key pharmacologic features and nuclear binding profile of retinoids. CRABP, cellular retinoic acid binding protein; RA, retinoic acid; RAR, retinoic acid receptor; RXR, retinoid X receptor.

are present in the body is of great importance. Etretinate is stored in adipose tissue, including subcutaneous fat, from which it is released slowly. Therefore, it has a long terminal half-life of up to 120 days. In contrast, under identical conditions, acitretin carries a negatively charged group and, not being nearly as lipophilic as etretinate, it does not accumulate in adipose tissue and so is eliminated from the body more rapidly. Acitretin has an elimination half-life of 2 days[8]. Paradoxically, acitretin activates all three RAR subtypes, but binds poorly to them.

Re-esterification of acitretin to etretinate may occur when acitretin is taken simultaneously with alcohol. This finding prompted the manufacturer to extend the time of compulsory contraception in patients taking acitretin to 2 years after discontinuation, as it is for etretinate. Indeed, the FDA advises a therapeutic contraceptive period of at least 3 years for acitretin, based on the pharmacokinetics of acitretin and etretinate observed in clinical trials and on previous safety experience with etretinate. The pharmacokinetic advantage of acitretin over etretinate still holds true, however, for all women who strictly avoid alcohol during treatment and for 2 months thereafter[8].

The mechanism of action of acitretin is still not clearly understood. Evidence supports a normalization of differentiation and proliferation as well as a modification of inflammatory responses and neutrophil function.

For all of these reasons, acitretin represents a therapeutic alternative with greater clinical potential than etretinate; in June 1997, acitretin was approved by the FDA as a substitute for etretinate with similar indications[8]. The latter is no longer commercially available.

Isotretinoin (13-cis-retinoic acid)

Isotretinoin is a naturally occurring physiologic compound resulting from the metabolism of vitamin A (see Fig. 126.2). 13-cis-RA and at-RA are two interconvertible isomers that differ in their elimination half-lives: approximately 20 hours for isotretinoin and 1 hour for retinoic acid. Isotretinoin undergoes first pass metabolism in the liver and subsequent enterohepatic recycling. In plasma, isotretinoin is greater than 99% bound to plasma protein, mainly albumin. There is neither liver storage nor adipose tissue storage, in sharp contrast to vitamin A. The major metabolite of isotretinoin (4-oxo-isotretinoin) is produced by oxidation. Isotretinoin and its major metabolites are excreted in the urine and feces.

After discontinuation of isotretinoin, natural concentrations of 13-cis-RA and its major metabolites are reached within 2 weeks, ranging from 2 days for at-RA to 10 days for 4-oxo-isotretinoin. Therefore, 1 month of post-therapy contraception provides an adequate safety margin. Among natural and synthetic retinoids, only oral isotretinoin significantly suppresses sebum production and considerably improves acne. Since no clear affinity with isotretinoin has been identified for any retinoid receptor, other mechanisms of action must be considered[9]. It may even be that isotretinoin is a prodrug that targets the sebaceous gland with sebo-suppressive metabolites.

Bexarotene

Bexarotene, a specific RXR-selective retinoid (rexinoid), was approved in 1999 in the US for treatment of cutaneous T-cell lymphoma (CTCL).

This compound is about 100-fold more potent at binding to RXR than to RAR. In plasma, bexarotene is highly bound (>99%) to various proteins that have yet to be characterized. Both the ability of bexarotene to displace other drugs bound to plasma proteins and the ability of other drugs to displace bexarotene are unknown. Bexarotene probably has a clearance profile similar to that of isotretinoin, with a terminal half-life of between 7 and 9 hours[10]. Bexarotene is metabolized by cytochrome P450 3A4 (see Ch. 131) and generates its own oxidative metabolites via hepatic CYP 3A4 induction. Neither bexarotene nor its metabolites are excreted in urine; their elimination is thought to occur primarily via the hepatobiliary system[10]. The exact mechanism of action of bexarotene in CTCL is still unknown, but bexarotene probably acts through regulation of cellular differentiation and proliferation and induction of apoptosis.

INDICATIONS (Table 126.3)

Topical Retinoids

Regardless of the preparation or indication, the most important element in topical therapy with retinoids is education of the patient. Local skin irritation characterized by erythema and peeling can be expected, and noticeable beneficial effects may take weeks or months to appear. Administration of topical retinoids should be titrated depending on cutaneous irritant reactions, which may mean decreasing the concentration or the frequency of application. It is generally wise to begin with the lowest strength formulation, then increase the concentration as tolerance builds. Another tactic is to start by applying a given concentration every other day. Daytime moisturizers with sunscreen are important components of any topical retinoid regimen.

CLINICAL INDICATIONS FOR RETINOIDS			
Topical retinoids	FDA-approved indications	Acne vulgaris Photoaging (wrinkling, mottled pigmentation, facial roughness) Psoriasis (<20% of body surface area) Cutaneous T-cell lymphoma (bexarotene) Kaposi's sarcoma (alitretinoin)	
	Selected non-approved indications	Limited disorders of keratinization (Darier disease, ichthyoses, pityriasis rubra pilaris) Rosacea Pigmentary disorders (melasma, lentigines, postinflammatory hyperpigmentation) Actinic keratoses Striae Wound healing Lichen planus (oral and cutaneous) Verrucae planae (flat warts) Corticosteroid-induced atrophy Therapy and prevention of skin cancer (basal cell carcinoma; xeroderma pigmentosum)	
Systemic retinoids	FDA-approved indications	Psoriasis (acitretin)	Pustular psoriasis (localized and von Zumbusch) Erythrodermic psoriasis Severe and recalcitrant psoriasis
		Acne (isotretinoin)	Nodulocystic acne Recalcitrant acne with tendency for scarring
		Cutaneous T-cell lymphoma (bexarotene)	Resistant to at least one systemic therapy
	Selected non-FDA-approved indications	Rosacea and acne-related disorders	Hidradenitis suppurativa Eosinophilic pustular folliculitis (Ofuji's disease) AIDS-associated eosinophilic folliculitis Pyoderma faciale (rosacea fulminans) Acne with solid facial edema Dissecting cellulitis of the scalp
		Disorders of keratinization	Ichthyosis, various forms (see Ch. 56) Darier disease Pityriasis rubra pilaris Keratoderma Papillon–Lefèvre syndrome
		Chemoprophylaxis of neoplastic processes	Xeroderma pigmentosum Nevoid basal cell carcinoma syndrome Skin cancer in solid-organ transplant patients
		Treatment of neoplastic processes	Epithelial precancerous conditions Basal cell carcinoma Advanced squamous cell carcinoma Keratoacanthoma Kaposi's sarcoma Sebaceous hyperplasia Muir–Torre syndrome Leukoplakia Langerhans cell histiocytosis
		Miscellaneous conditions	Atrophoderma vermiculatum Ulerythema ophryogenes Confluent and reticulated papillomatosis of Gougerot and Carteaud Bazex paraneoplastic acrokeratosis Follicular mucinosis Lupus erythematosus Sarcoidosis Granuloma annulare Lichen planus Lichen sclerosus Subcorneal pustular dermatosis

Table 126.3 Clinical indications for retinoids.

Acne

Topical retinoids, of which tretinoin (at-RA) is the prototype, are mainstays in the treatment of comedonal and inflammatory acne. The primary mode of action in acne is normalization of abnormal differentiation and proliferation of the follicular epithelium (see Ch. 37), which leads to the loosening and unseating of microcomedones, thereby allowing sebum to reach the surface of the skin and preventing obstruction of the pilosebaceous unit. In addition, topical retinoids may have anti-inflammatory activity. The mechanism of action of topical isotretinoin, used therapeutically only in Europe, is similar to that of topical tretinoin because of intraepithelial isomerization of isotretinoin to tretinoin. In contrast to oral isotretinoin, topical isotretinoin fails to suppress sebum production to the same extent. Isotretinoin is less irritating, but it is probably somewhat less effective than tretinoin. Because of the birth defects induced by the oral formulation, topical isotretinoin has not received FDA approval in the US.

The newer synthetic derivatives, adapalene and tazarotene, are intended to improve tolerability while at least maintaining similar efficacy when compared to topical tretinoin. In company-sponsored studies of patients with acne, adapalene 0.1% gel was as effective as tretinoin 0.025% gel against open and closed comedones and more effective against inflammatory lesions, and with less irritation[11]. Tazarotene 0.05% and 0.1% topical gels significantly decreased acne lesions compared with control patients, with tolerability clinically comparable to tretinoin (again in company-sponsored trials).

Topical retinoids should be applied to the entire face, once a day (if tolerated) and in the evening to minimize photodestruction (i.e. inactivation of the retinoid by UV). The medication should be applied on dry skin to minimize dermal absorption, which correlates with skin irritation. Patients should be advised that the therapeutic response is slow, and beneficial effects do not become evident for weeks to months. An apparent exacerbation may occur during the first month of therapy, representing the externalization of deeper-seated acne lesions as the follicular epithelium is loosening. Topical retinoids, except in very mild acne, should be used concomitantly with antibiotics (oral or topical) or benzoyl peroxides, which have modes of action that differ from those of topical retinoids and target primarily inflammatory lesions.

Psoriasis

Topical application of tretinoin or isotretinoin has limited efficacy in psoriasis. Tazarotene is the first topical retinoid proven effective in treating mild to moderate plaque-type psoriasis not exceeding 20% of the body surface area. When compared with twice-daily fluocinonide cream, tazarotene 0.05% and 0.1% gels applied once daily were shown to produce similar reductions in plaque elevation (in company-sponsored trials). Nevertheless, tazarotene 0.1% gel carries a significantly lower risk of relapse than does fluocinonide cream after 12 weeks off therapy[12]. A combination of tazarotene and a mid-potency corticosteroid improved efficacy (possibly by taking advantage of the rapid onset of action of the topical corticosteroid) and reduced the incidence of local adverse effects; this combination may also reduce the risk of corticosteroid-induced atrophy[13].

Photoaging

Photodamaged skin is characterized by fine and coarse wrinkling, rough texture, sallow color, and irregular pigmentation. Several controlled studies have clearly demonstrated that topical retinoids, particularly tretinoin, and more recently tazarotene cream, improve fine wrinkling and lighten uneven pigmentation. It generally takes 3–6 months of daily applications to see significant clinical improvement. Cutaneous irritation is usually the limiting factor. Retinaldehyde was demonstrated to be as effective as tretinoin in treating photodamage in less extensive trials, but has a better tolerance profile[14]. It has been hypothesized that the reduction in side effects seen with retinaldehyde (compared with retinoic acid) may be due to a more controlled delivery of retinoic acid to target cells, thus limiting an 'overload' of retinoic acid in the skin, which may be responsible, in part, for producing the cutaneous irritation.

Photoaging is the consequence of UV-induced damage to the skin, and it is characterized by decreased expression of RXR-α and RAR-γ (the two major nuclear receptors in keratinocytes) in the acute setting, and by upregulation of AP1-driven matrix metalloproteinases. Topical retinoids promote cellular dedifferentiation and extracellular matrix synthesis, including an increase in hyaluronate acid via a CD44-mediated mechanism[14a]. Histologic findings after repeated topical application of tretinoin include: compaction of the stratum corneum, epidermal hyperplasia (acanthosis), correction of atypia (e.g. actinic keratoses), dispersion of melanin granules, increased dermal collagen synthesis, and angiogenesis. These findings explain the reported smoother skin, rosy glow, decrease in blotchy pigmentation, and diminished fine lines and wrinkles.

Other indications

Alitretinoin (9-cis-RA) 0.1% gel, a pan-receptor agonist (RAR and RXR), is FDA-approved for the topical treatment of cutaneous Kaposi's sarcoma. The oral formulation is under investigation for HIV-associated Kaposi's sarcoma, psoriasis and chronic hand eczema. Topical bexarotene is FDA-approved for the treatment of CTCL. In one study, 67 patients with early-stage (IA–IIA) CTCL achieved an overall response rate of 63% and a clinical complete response rate of 21% after using topical bexarotene for a median of 20 weeks[15]. Although non-FDA-approved indications, topical retinoids have also been used to treat pigmentary irregularities (melasma, postinflammatory hyperpigmentation, lentigines), actinic keratoses, corticosteroid-induced atrophy, verrucae planae (flat warts), actinic cheilitis and striae, as well as a number of other disorders (see Table 126.3).

Systemic Retinoids

Psoriasis

Several randomized multicenter trials have been performed to ascertain the efficacy of acitretin in plaque-type[16] and pustular psoriasis, and to compare its effectiveness with that of etretinate. Acitretin appears to be as effective as etretinate, and it can be used in the same combination regimens. Adverse effects appear to be similar in quality and incidence. The best results have been obtained in acral or generalized (von Zumbusch) pustular psoriasis, in which etretinate and acitretin are considered to be first-line therapies. The lesions of both localized and generalized pustular psoriasis, as well as those of erythrodermic psoriasis, cleared more rapidly with etretinate or acitretin monotherapy than with most other therapies[17]. Rebound does not usually occur after stopping acitretin or etretinate treatment[18], and reintroduction of the drug when it does occur produces a beneficial response[18].

The most common form of psoriasis, plaque-type psoriasis, responds variably to both drugs. Although complete clearance of plaques is achieved in only about 30% of treated patients, a significant improvement is obtained in an additional 50%[19]. The decrease in the Psoriasis Area and Severity Index (PASI) score is approximately 60–70%, depending on the dosage and duration of treatment. Many of the plaques may remain, but they are thinner with less scale and erythema. Approximately 20% of patients may be considered treatment failures[19,20].

One of the main reasons for treatment interruption is an initial worsening of the disease with an increase in erythema and/or extent of the involvement. This may occur within a few days of starting therapy at a dosage of 0.5–1 mg/kg/day (i.e. 30–70 mg/day in adults). A therapeutic dosage scheme utilizing a low dosage (10 mg/day) of etretinate or acitretin initially, followed by progressively increasing the dosage, seems to avoid this complication. In order to define the efficacy of acitretin as monotherapy for psoriasis, different dosages (10–75 mg/day) were compared with placebo in a double-blind fashion. At the end of an 8-week treatment period in two studies, acitretin at doses of 25 and 50 mg/day[21] or 50 and 75 mg/day[22] was superior to placebo. The efficacy of low-dose acitretin at 10 mg/day was not significantly different from that of placebo in either study.

Total clearance of psoriatic lesions usually requires a combination of therapies, such as retinoids plus topical corticosteroids, topical vitamin D derivatives, anthralin (dithranol) or photochemotherapy (PUVA). The main advantage of the Re–PUVA combination, in which retinoids are given for 14 days before starting PUVA, is the acceleration of the response rate of psoriatic lesions and the clearance of lesions that otherwise could not be cleared with retinoid or PUVA alone (Fig. 126.3). A further advantage is that the cumulative radiation exposure required to produce a remission is significantly lower with Re–PUVA. The lower radiation dosage is likely to diminish the risk of PUVA-induced

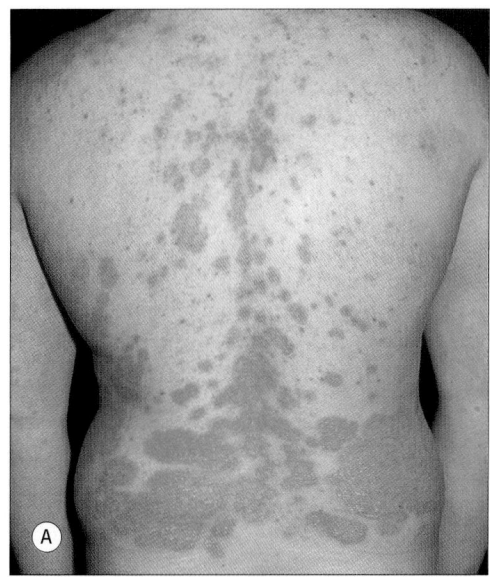
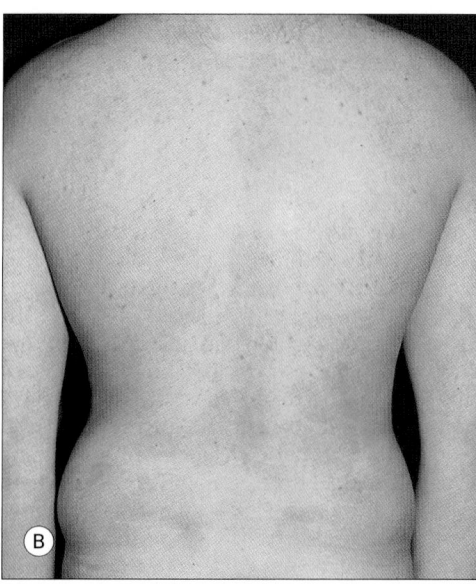

Fig. 126.3 Chronic plaque-type psoriasis. Before (**A**) and after (**B**) treatment with a combination of acitretin and PUVA.

carcinogenesis, which is clearly UVA dose-dependent. Oral retinoids can also be combined with bath PUVA, a combination that also allows a reduction in the cumulative dose of UVA. Lastly, the combination of etretinate or acitretin with UVB phototherapy has been shown to be more effective in patients with psoriasis than is retinoid or UVB phototherapy alone[23,24].

Isotretinoin has a lesser effect on psoriasis than has acitretin or etretinate, although some efficacy has been shown in combination with PUVA[25]. Nevertheless, some dermatologists continue to use isotretinoin in women of childbearing age with psoriasis who need systemic retinoids, to avoid the long post-acitretin contraception period. As with acne, isotretinoin prescriptions are currently limited to 1 month of medication in the US.

Acne

The introduction of isotretinoin was a key advance in the history of dermatologic therapy. Isotretinoin is still the only compound that has been shown to induce long-term remissions and even 'cure' acne, because it is the only one that affects, albeit not to the same degree or permanently, all the etiologic factors implicated in acne: sebum production, comedogenesis, and colonization with *Propionibacterium acnes* (Fig. 126.4).

Among natural and synthetic retinoids tried in humans, only isotretinoin was found to suppress sebum excretion and to significantly improve acne. It is still a matter of conjecture why only isotretinoin has sebo-suppressive effects. The 'sebo-specificity' of oral isotretinoin cannot be explained on the basis of the molecular biology of retinoid nuclear receptors because isotretinoin has no special affinity to any of the identified retinoid nuclear receptors. Attempts have been made to relate the sebo-suppressive effect to a metabolite, and 4-oxo-isotretinoin has been considered a possible candidate, but little supporting evidence has been forthcoming.

In the early 1980s, isotretinoin use was restricted to patients suffering from severe nodulocystic acne. With increasing experience, however, its use has been extended to patients with less severe disease who have responded unsatisfactorily to conventional therapies such as long-term antibiotics. Patients with moderate acne that may induce scars have also been treated.

Acne morbidity is now generally considered to extend beyond the mere aesthetics of physical appearance. Significant psychosocial consequences of acne range from depression and anxiety to interpersonal and work-related difficulties. Studies with quality-of-life instruments have shown that isotretinoin treatment significantly improves sociability and self-esteem.

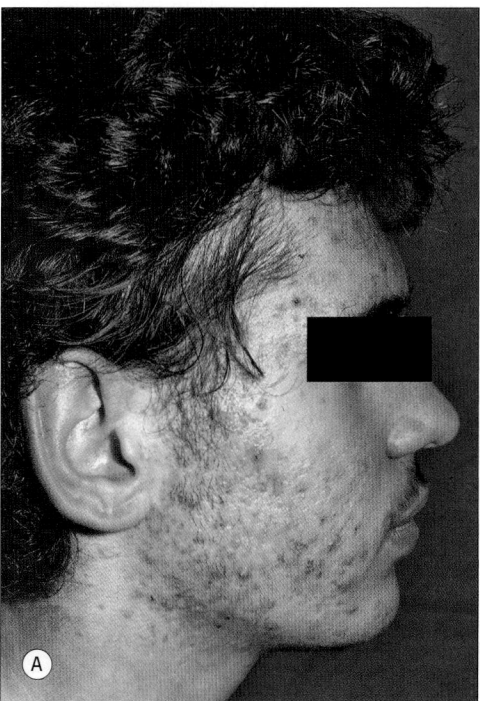
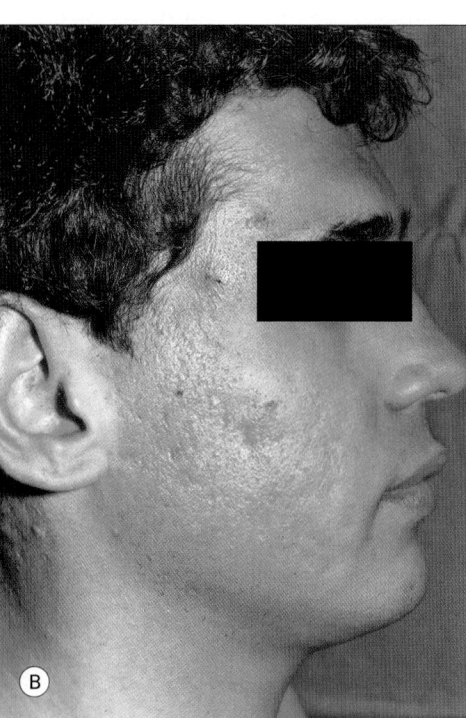

Fig. 126.4 Severe acne vulgaris. Before (**A**) and after (**B**) treatment with oral isotretinoin.

It was initially considered that optimal benefit would be achieved with a high daily dose of approximately 1 mg/kg/day[26]. However, this high dose can induce undesirable effects, and similar short-term therapeutic results were obtained with doses below 0.5 mg/kg/day. In order to avoid the higher incidence of relapses associated with low-dose isotretinoin, the latter approach required that the treatment be maintained over a longer period of time in order to reach a critical cumulative dose threshold. The concept of cumulative dose (mg/kg body weight), introduced by Harms in 1989[27], is the total amount of oral isotretinoin taken by the patient over the entire duration, divided by his or her body weight. Thus, a patient weighing 50 kg and receiving 25 mg/day of isotretinoin for 100 days would have received a cumulative dose of 50 mg/kg (25 mg × 100 = 2500 mg, divided by 50 kg = 50 mg/kg). Data from several centers indicated that post-therapy relapse was minimized by a treatment course amounting to a total of at least 120 mg/kg[28], with no further therapeutic gain beyond about 150 mg/kg[29]. Some dermatologists have suggested that generic isotretinoin preparations may not be absorbed as well as the original trade drug, leading to the need for higher daily doses and/or longer courses of therapy. However, this has not been proven in controlled trials and more pharmacokinetic details are needed on the generic products.

A lag period of 1–3 months may exist before the onset of the therapeutic effect. Continued healing after the discontinuation of therapy is regularly observed. Consequently, it is not necessary to maintain treatment until total clearance is achieved. Approximately one-third of patients with acne require a second course of therapy, either for persistent disease or for relapse. The only predictive factor of resistance to isotretinoin treatment is closed comedonal acne and microcystic acne[30]. Women with a history of acne that is refractory to isotretinoin or with repeated relapses should be examined for hirsutism, questioned regarding abnormal menstruation, and referred for an endocrinologic evaluation to exclude ovarian or adrenal dysfunction[31] (see Ch. 37).

A flare of disease during the first few weeks of treatment, and subsequent evolution of acne cysts into lesions resembling pyogenic granulomas, may be observed with isotretinoin treatment. Retinoids may alter directly or indirectly the expression of pro- or anti-angiogenic growth factors such as vascular endothelial growth factor/vascular permeability factor (VEGF/VPF). The incidence of this side effect may be reduced by using lower doses of isotretinoin during the first 3–4 weeks of therapy.

Women of childbearing potential must have a (in the US, two) negative pregnancy test(s) and practice effective contraception for 1 month prior to therapy, during therapy, and for 1 month after completing therapy. To afford a sufficient safety margin, a 1-month post-therapy contraceptive period is mandatory because plasma concentrations of isotretinoin return to physiologic levels within 10 days of completing therapy[32].

Isotretinoin has a more limited effect on hidradenitis suppurativa and dissecting cellulitis of the scalp. These disorders may occur together as part of the follicular occlusion tetrad (see Ch. 39). Some investigators recommend oral isotretinoin during the weeks or months preceding surgery for hidradenitis suppurativa, and sometimes also during the postoperative period[33].

Cutaneous T-cell lymphoma

Isotretinoin and etretinate are somewhat effective and are considered to be of equal potency in the treatment of mycosis fungoides (MF). Retinoids can be used in combination with PUVA, interferon or systemic chemotherapy. Despite initial improvement of the various stages of MF, it is often impossible to maintain remissions with these retinoids as monotherapy.

Both oral and topical bexarotene have produced responses in CTCL. Two multicenter clinical trials of oral bexarotene were conducted in patients with stage I–IIA disease (n=58)[34] and with stage IIB–IVB disease (n=94)[35]. Patients in the early-stage study who were randomly assigned to the low-dose arm of 6.5 mg/m^2/day had a 20% response rate, in contrast to 54% and 67% for patients receiving a starting dose of 300 mg/m^2/day versus 650 mg/m^2/day (then decreased to 500 mg/m^2/day), respectively[34]. However, dose-dependent toxicity was a significant problem at the higher doses. Responses rates were approximately 50% for the patients with advanced CTCL[35].

The FDA approved bexarotene in December 1999 as oral therapy for the treatment of CTCL that is refractory to at least one systemic therapy, and in June 2000 as a gel formulation for cutaneous manifestations of early-stage refractory or persistent CTCL[35]. The recommended initial oral dose is 300 mg/m^2/day, administrated as a single daily dose with a meal. Based on the severity of adverse effects (see below), the dosage may be decreased to 100 or 200 mg/m^2/day, or temporarily suspended. If there is no tumor response after 8 weeks of therapy, the dose may be increased to 400 mg/m^2/day with careful monitoring.

Other 'off label' clinical uses

The pleomorphic effects of retinoids, as well as their relative selective targeting of skin structures, explain the broad potential benefit they could provide to patients with skin disease. Many other skin disorders respond to retinoids (see Table 126.3), but for only a few has the benefit been established in controlled studies[36].

Ichthyosis

Among the different types of ichthyoses (see Ch. 56), the best results can be obtained by using acitretin for non-bullous congenital ichthyosiform erythroderma and lamellar ichthyosis (Fig. 126.5). Treatment of bullous congenital ichthyosiform erythroderma may result in an initial increase in bulla formation. Good results have also been observed in patients with recessive X-linked ichthyosis and ichthyosis vulgaris; however, in contrast to lamellar ichthyosis, the more limited severity of these diseases does not usually require systemic retinoid therapy. Given the lifelong duration of these disorders, intermittent courses are sometimes prescribed.

Darier disease

Severe forms of Darier disease are often treated with systemic retinoids, but special care should be taken to initiate therapy with a very low dose (e.g. acitretin 10 mg/day) in order to prevent an initial exacerbation of the disease; usually 20 mg/day is sufficient for significant improvement.

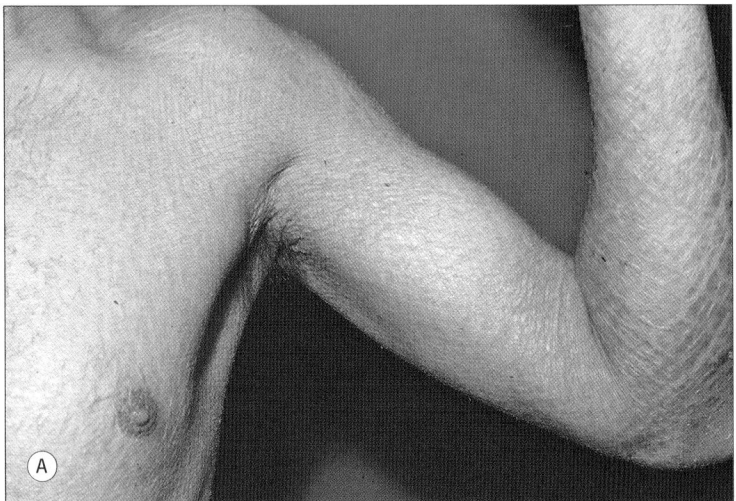 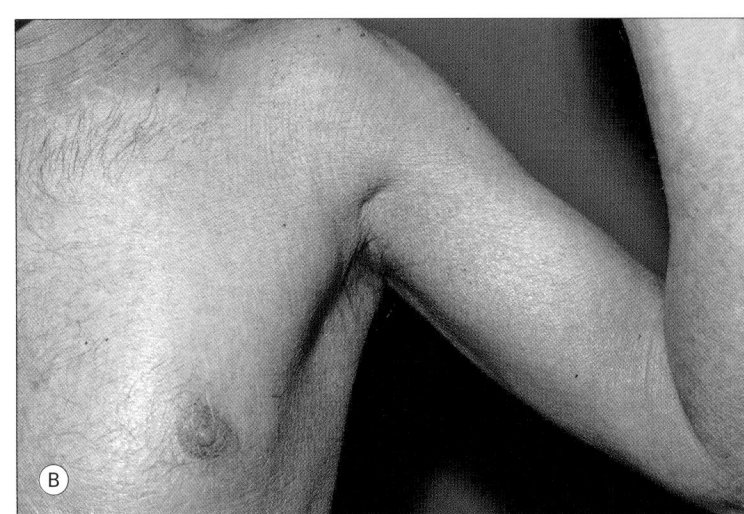

Fig. 126.5 Lamellar ichthyosis. Before (**A**) and after (**B**) treatment with acitretin.

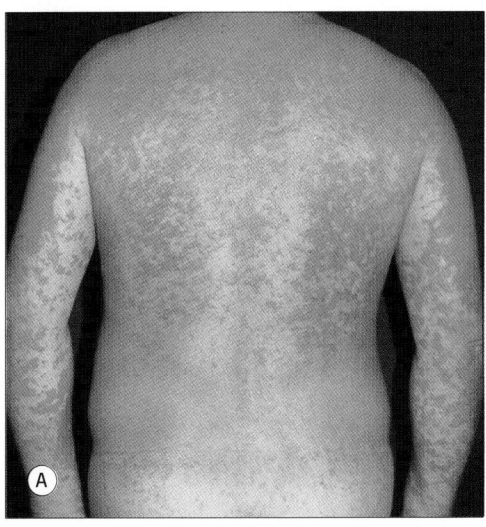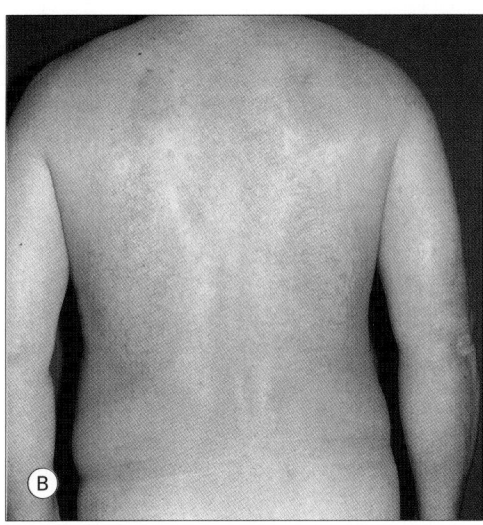

Fig. 126.6 Pityriasis rubra pilaris. Before (**A**) and after (**B**) treatment with acitretin.

Pityriasis rubra pilaris

Early treatment with retinoids appears to offer the best chance for clearing pityriasis rubra pilaris (PRP) (Fig. 126.6). In extensive cases, concomitant use of methotrexate may be advantageous. Etretinate (now acitretin) is considered to be superior to isotretinoin for the treatment of adult-onset PRP[37].

Rosacea

In severe forms or treatment-resistant rosacea, isotretinoin often has a greater effect on inflammatory lesions than on vascular lesions[38]. A low daily dose (10 mg) is often sufficient, although acne vulgaris regimens are sometimes used in severe disease.

Premalignant and malignant skin lesions

Etretinate and acitretin were both shown to be effective in the treatment of premalignant skin lesions, including HPV-induced tumors and actinic keratoses. In the nevoid basal cell carcinoma syndrome and in xeroderma pigmentosum, these drugs are able to dramatically reduce the incidence of malignant evolution of cutaneous lesions. A double-blind study demonstrated that acitretin (30 mg/day for 6 months) prevented the development of premalignant and malignant cutaneous neoplasms in renal transplant recipients[39].

Graft-versus-host disease

In an open study, 3 months of etretinate therapy produced encouraging responses among patients with refractory sclerodermatous chronic GVHD resulting from allogeneic bone marrow transplantation[40].

Lichen sclerosus

The use of acitretin is an effective treatment for patients with severe vulvar (and, occasionally, non-genital) lichen sclerosus. It may be used intermittently in patients who are intolerant of or resistant to topical therapies.

Lupus erythematosus

Both isotretinoin and acitretin have been used successfully in patients with various forms of lupus erythematosus (LE). However, recurrence of the lesions after completion of the treatment is a limiting factor. Comparable therapeutic efficacy has been observed for acitretin and hydroxychloroquine in chronic cutaneous (i.e. 'discoid') LE and in subacute cutaneous LE[41].

DOSAGE

The different formulations, strengths and standard dosage ranges of topical retinoids and systemic retinoids currently available for use in dermatology are outlined in Table 126.4.

CONTRAINDICATIONS

Topical Retinoids

Topical retinoids should be avoided during pregnancy and nursing, due primarily to medicolegal issues raised by the teratogenicity of oral isotretinoin. Due to the irritant effects of topical retinoids, concomitant use of irritating topical products (e.g. abrasive soaps, astringents, cosmetics, toners, scrubs, exfoliants, buff puffs, and other potentially irritating agents) should be avoided.

Systemic Retinoids

The absolute contraindications are pregnancy or women contemplating becoming pregnant, non-compliance with contraception, breastfeeding, and hypersensitivity to preservatives present in acitretin's capsule (parabens). Relative contraindications are leukopenia, moderate to severe hypercholesterolemia or hypertriglyceridemia, significant hepatic (especially bexarotene) or renal dysfunction, hypothyroidism (especially bexarotene), young children, suicidal ideation and pseudotumor cerebri. Furthermore, patients should be advised not to take vitamin A supplements in excess. In the US, recent FDA requirements for use of isotretinoin have progressed from voluntary patient entry into a treatment registry and registration of prescribing physicians to a full mandatory registration (ipledge) program.

MAJOR SIDE EFFECTS (Table 126.5)

Topical Retinoids

By far the most common side effect of topical retinoids is skin irritation characterized by erythema, scaling, pruritus, burning, stinging and dryness. This 'retinoid dermatitis' occurs within the first month of treatment and tends to recede thereafter. It responds to a temporary reduction in the frequency or amount of retinoid application and to application of moisturizers. Although pharmaceutical companies focus on differences between the products regarding irritation, the clinically observed differences are often greater between patients using the same product than between products[42]. Desquamation and peeling correspond to the hyperproliferative response of the epidermis to tretinoin mediated by RARs, but the erythema does not seem to be receptor-mediated[43]. The perioral area of the face is most sensitive to peeling and use in this area can be limited or avoided.

Although no photoallergic or phototoxic reactions have been proven for topical retinoids, many patients note a decreased tolerance to UV radiation shortly after sun exposure. This reaction is often accentuated by a sensation of heat, raising the question of involvement of infrared irradiation. Potential teratogenicity from long-term use of topical retinoids is very low: systemic absorption of topically applied retinoids is inconsequential in both animal and human studies[44], and there is no evidence that application of tretinoin causes congenital disorders.

VARIOUS FORMULATIONS OF TOPICAL AND SYSTEMIC RETINOIDS				
Retinoid	Route (Pregnancy category)	Formulations	Standard dosage range	Major indications
Retinol	Topical	Various (0.15%; 0.3%)		Cosmeceutical products
Retinaldehyde	Topical	Various (0.05–0.1%)		
Tretinoin	Topical (C)	Gel, cream, solution (0.1, 0.05, 0.04, 0.025, 0.02, 0.01%)		Acne vulgaris Photoaging
	Systemic (X)	10 mg	45 mg/m²/day	Acute promyelocytic leukemia
Tazarotene	Topical (X)	Cream, gel (0.05%; 0.1%)		Acne vulgaris Plaque-type psoriasis Facial photodamage
Adapalene	Topical (C)	Gel, cream, solution (0.1%; 0.3%)		Acne vulgaris
Isotretinoin	Topical (C)	Gel (0.05%)		Acne vulgaris*
	Systemic (X)	10, 20, 40 mg capsules	0.5–2 mg/kg/day	Severe, recalcitrant acne; related dermatoses*
Acitretin	Systemic (X)	10, 25 mg capsules	25–50 mg/day	Psoriasis Severe disorders of keratinization*
Bexarotene	Topical (C)	Gel (0.1%)		Cutaneous T-cell lymphoma
	Systemic (X)	75 mg	300 mg/m²/day	
Alitretinoin	Topical (D) Systemic†	Gel (0.1%)		Kaposi's sarcoma Kaposi's sarcoma*; psoriasis*; chronic hand eczema*
Motretinide (etretinate derivative)	Topical (C)	Cream, solution (0.1%)		Acne vulgaris*

*Not an FDA-approved indication.
†Under clinical investigation.

Table 126.4 Various formulations of topical and systemic retinoids. C, pregnancy category C; D, pregnancy category D; X, Pregnancy category X.

Temporary worsening of acne may occur within the first weeks of therapy. Uncommon side effects include transitory hypo- or hyper-pigmentation, koebnerization of psoriasis (especially tazarotene), allergic contact dermatitis, and ectropion.

Systemic Retinoids

Teratogenicity is the most troublesome adverse effect of oral retinoids. The side-effect profile of systemic retinoids (see Table 126.5) qualitatively resembles that of the toxic effects of vitamin A or hyper-vitaminosis A syndrome. Acute expressions of retinoid toxicity include mucocutaneous (most cases) and laboratory abnormalities (less common but may be severe), while chronic retinoid toxicity can involve bony changes (unusual).

Teratogenicity

Systemic retinoids are potent teratogens, and fetal deformities are the major concern in treating fertile women with oral retinoids. So far, with regard to teratogenicity, no safe minimal dose during pregnancy has been established. The range of defects seen in retinoid embryopathy includes abnormalities of the CNS (hydrocephalus, microcephaly), ear (anotia, small or absent external auditory canals), cardiovascular system (cardiac septal defects, complex malformations), eye (microphthalmia) and acral skeleton, as well as craniofacial and thymus gland anomalies (Table 126.6)[45]. In some instances, the abnormalities may lead to pre-mature birth, spontaneous abortion or fetal death. The putative mech-anism involves toxic effects on neural crest cells, particularly in the case of exposure during the fourth week of gestation[46].

So far, no typical retinoid embryopathy malformations have been reported in pregnancies where the male partner had been the one taking acitretin or isotretinoin at the time of conception. However, it is usually recommended that men who are actively trying to father children avoid systemic retinoid therapy. The mandatory registry in the US applies equally to men, in part because there have been pregnancies in women who 'shared' a prescription with a male patient.

Skin and mucous membrane adverse effects

Dose-dependent mucocutaneous toxicity is the most commonly observed side effect with oral retinoids, and it mainly reflects a decreased production of sebum, reduced stratum corneum thickness, and altered skin barrier function. Dry lips or cheilitis is the earliest and the most frequent sign that appears after starting therapy (Fig. 126.7). Dryness of the mouth accompanied by thirst, and dryness and fragility of the nasal mucosa leading to epistaxis are also frequently observed.

Xerosis of the skin, associated with pruritus and peeling, especially of the palms and soles, is a frequent side effect. Skin fragility and fissuring of the fingertips may create a specific problem for those who must perform manual labor. Photosensitivity may be observed, in particular with isotretinoin, and probably reflects a reduction in the thickness of the stratum corneum. *Staphylococcus aureus* colonization correlates with the isotretinoin-induced reduction in sebum production and may lead to overt cutaneous infections[47]. In atopic patients, eczema and pruritus may be exacerbated by oral retinoids.

Xerophthalmia due to decreased meibomian gland secretion may prohibit the use of contact lenses and can lead to blepharoconjunctivitis, with varying degrees of severity. Corneal ulceration can occur as a complication in up to one-third of patients. If artificial tears and topical ophthalmologic antibiotic ointment fail to alleviate the conjunctivitis, ophthalmologic consultation should be sought. Diffuse or localized hair loss (telogen effluvium) is a common complaint, although objective alopecia tends to occur only at high dosage levels. Systemic retinoid therapy can induce a variety of undesirable effects on the nail apparatus, including nail thinning, fragility and shedding, paronychia-like changes, and periungual granulation tissue.

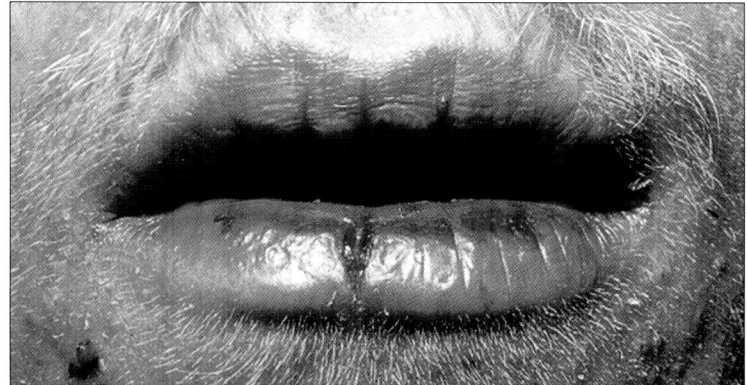

Fig. 126.7 Cheilitis in an isotretinoin-treated patient.

			ADVERSE EFFECTS OF RETINOIDS	
Topical retinoids	Adverse effects	Skin irritation (retinoid dermatitis)	Erythema Peeling, desquamation Dryness Burning Pruritus Photosensitivity	
		Uncommon	Hypo- or hyperpigmentation Ectropion Allergic contact dermatitis	
Systemic retinoids	Acute adverse effects	Mucocutaneous	Xerosis with pruritus* Cheilitis* Dry mucosa* (mouth, eyes, nose; epistaxis) Skin fragility* Retinoid dermatitis* Palmoplantar peeling* Photosensitivity Blepharoconjunctivitis, corneal ulceration Stickiness sensation (palms, soles) Granulation tissue and pyogenic granuloma-like lesions Telogen effluvium, hair thinning Nail fragility with softening, paronychia, onycholysis *Staphylococcus aureus* infection	
		Systemic	Myalgias Arthralgias Anorexia, nausea, diarrhea, abdominal pain Headache, pseudotumor cerebri (rare) Fatigue, lethargy, irritability Reduced night vision Blurred vision, photophobia, keratitis Depression, suicidal ideation (rare and controversial) Toxic hepatitis (rare) Hypothyroidism (bexarotene)* Pancreatitis secondary to hypertriglyceridemia (rare) Hyperuricemia with gout (rare)	
		Laboratory	Elevated liver function tests (usually transient, minor): AST, ALT, alkaline phosphatase, LDH, bilirubin Hyperlipidemia: hypertriglyceridemia; increased cholesterol, VLDL and LDL; decreased HDL Elevated creatine kinase Leukopenia (bexarotene) Agranulocytosis (bexarotene) Thrombocytosis, thrombocytopenia Hypercalcemia (rare)	
	Chronic adverse effects	Mucocutaneous	Alopecia (rare) Dry eyes (rare)	

		Systemic	DISH syndrome-like bone changes:
			   Osteophyte and bony bridge formation, especially of vertebrae (rarely clinically significant at dosages for acne)
			   Anterior and posterior spinal ligament calcification
			Extraspinal tendon and ligament calcification
			Osteoporotic change in long bones
			Premature epiphyseal closure
			Periosteal thickening
			Myopathy	

Common adverse effects.

Table 126.5 Adverse effects of retinoids. See Table 126.6 for teratogenicity. DISH, diffuse idiopathic skeletal hyperostosis.

Systemic retinoids do have different mucocutaneous side effect profiles. For example, isotretinoin causes more mucosal dryness, and acitretin has been associated with higher incidences of alopecia and palmoplantar peeling, whereas bexarotene induces milder mucocutaneous and ocular side effects than do other classes of retinoids.

Systemic toxic effects
Bone toxicity
Bone pain can be observed in retinoid-treated patients, although without objective evidence of any abnormalities and without sequelae. While these minor complaints appear to have no long-term pathologic effects on the skeleton, several reports have implicated synthetic retinoids, including etretinate and isotretinoin, in the formation of diffuse hyperostoses of the spine (diffuse idiopathic skeletal hyperostosis [DISH] syndrome-like bone changes), as well as calcification of tendons and ligaments, particularly in the ankles[48]. Specific findings

include anterior spinal ligament calcification, osteophyte formation, extraspinal calcifications, and bony bridges, but without a narrowing of the disk space (Fig. 126.8). More rarely, ossification of the spinal posterior longitudinal ligament has been reported; this change, which can be progressive, may lead to spinal cord compression with signs of partial spastic paraplegia[49].

Based on data from retrospective studies, it was concluded that although many of the bone changes observed could not be positively attributed to etretinate or acitretin therapy, spurs and interosseous membrane and tendon calcifications were probably treatment-related[50]. Of note, prospective studies have shown that the effect of retinoids on bone, if present at all, is likely to involve worsening of pre-existing skeletal overgrowth rather than induction of *de novo* changes[51]. Even long-term use of isotretinoin in acne patients rarely causes clinically significant radiologic abnormalities, as most hyperostoses are asymptomatic and clinically insignificant[52].

RETINOID EMBRYOPATHY

Craniofacial

- Atresia of the ear canal, microtia, anotia
- Microphthalmia
- Microcephaly
- Asymmetry of the face
- Cleft palate
- Micrognathia
- Anomalies of the thymus and parathyroid glands, e.g. hypoplasia

Cardiovascular – conotruncal

- Transposition of the great vessels
- Tetralogy of Fallot
- Truncus arteriosus communis
- Supracristal ventricular septal defect

Cardiovascular – branchial arch mesenchyme

- Interrupted aortic arch
- Retroesophageal right subclavian artery
- Hypoplastic aorta

Central nervous system

- Hydrocephalus
- Cortical agenesis
- Cerebellar hypoplasia
- Mental retardation
- Difficulty with visual-motor integration

Other

- Limb anomalies
- Anal and vaginal atresia

Table 126.6 Retinoid embryopathy.

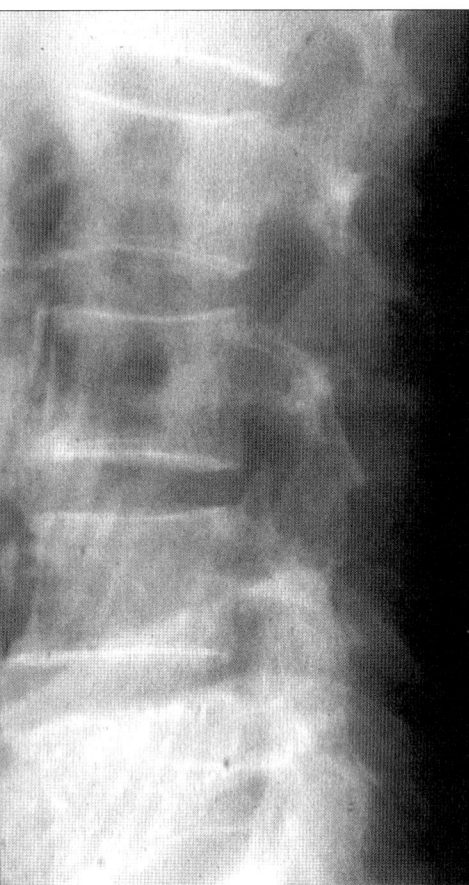

Fig. 126.8 Osteophytes and bony ridges without narrowing of the disk spaces in an acne patient treated with a prolonged (several-year) course of isotretinoin.

Osteoporosis has been observed with hypervitaminosis A and after long-term therapy with etretinate but not with isotretinoin[53]. However, more recently, a loss of bone density of 4.4% was observed in 18 young men (without measurable alterations of calcium metabolism) after 6 months of isotretinoin use (1 mg/kg), compared with controls[54]. A subsequent open-label trial in 217 adolescents receiving a similar regimen showed no significant change in bone mineral density[55]. In children, only a few cases of skeletal abnormalities, including osteoporosis, periosteal thickening, slender long bone, and premature epiphyseal closure[56,57], have been reported. No baseline X-rays are required, although monitoring high-risk patients who require prolonged high-dose retinoid therapy may be useful.

Muscle effects

Muscular pain and cramps can be observed in patients taking etretinate or acitretin; however, these symptoms are associated primarily with isotretinoin, especially in individuals involved in vigorous physical activity. Occasionally, elevated creatine kinase levels may be observed. Increased muscle tone as well as axial muscle rigidity and myopathy were reported to be related to etretinate and acitretin therapy, respectively[58].

Central nervous system and psychiatric effects

CNS side effects are rare. Although individual signs of increased intracranial pressure, such as headache, nausea and vomiting, are occasionally observed, the complete syndrome with papilledema (pseudotumor cerebri) and blurred vision is considered very rare[59]. Concomitant use of other drugs associated with intracranial hypertension (e.g. tetracycline, doxycycline or minocycline) is considered a major risk factor for developing pseudotumor cerebri and should therefore be avoided[60]. Examination for papilledema should be performed immediately when a patient receiving retinoid therapy complains of persistent headache, especially if it is accompanied by visual changes, nausea or vomiting, or when pseudotumor cerebri is otherwise suspected.

There have been anecdotal reports suggesting a causal association between isotretinoin therapy in acne patients and severe depression, psychosis and suicide attempts[61]. However, a systematic review of studies comparing depression before and after treatment with isotretinoin did not find a statistically significant increase in depression

diagnoses or depressive symptoms[62], and a large population-based cohort study provided no evidence for a causal link between isotretinoin exposure and an increased risk of newly diagnosed depression, suicidal behavior, psychosis or other psychiatric disorders[63]. Nevertheless, patients with depressive symptoms or suicidal ideation should be carefully monitored.

Ophthalmologic side effects

The most common ocular retinoid effects are dryness and irritation. Alterations in visual function, mainly nyctalopia (night blindness), excessive glare sensitivity, and changes in color perception have also been reported[64]. Competitive inhibition of ocular retinol dehydrogenase by retinoids, resulting in decreased rhodopsin formation, may be the cause of nyctalopia.

Other systemic effects
Hypothyroidism

Clinical and biochemical central hypothyroidism occurred in 40% of patients in the CTCL trials with bexarotene and it was rapidly and completely reversible with cessation of therapy without any clinical sequelae[34,65]. This effect is probably mediated through suppression of thyrotropin β-subunit (TSH-β) secretion by the thyrotrope cells of the anterior pituitary, which express RXR-γ.

Gastrointestinal side effects

Uncommon non-specific gastrointestinal complaints (e.g. abdominal pain, nausea, diarrhea) have been reported in association with retinoid therapy. Synthetic retinoids have been temporally linked with other toxicities, such as inflammatory bowel disease, on rare occasions; however, no cause-and-effect relationship has been established.

Renal effects

Renal toxicity is not characteristic of retinoid therapy. Isotretinoin has been safely administered to patients with end-stage kidney disease who were undergoing hemodialysis. However, case reports of reversible renal dysfunction (with elevated creatinine levels) during etretinate therapy have been described. Therefore, renal function should be monitored during retinoid therapy in patients with a history of renal disorders[66].

Laboratory abnormalities
Dyslipidemia

Hypertriglyceridemia is the most frequently observed systemic effect of retinoid therapy. Isotretinoin and etretinate/acitretin elevate triglycerides in 50% and cholesterol in 30% of treated patients[67], whereas bexarotene induces elevated triglycerides and cholesterol in approximately 79% and 48% of patients, respectively[34]. In addition, a concomitant increase in total and low-density lipoprotein (LDL) cholesterol is frequently observed. In cases of severe retinoid-induced hypertriglyceridemia, eruptive xanthomas and acute hemorrhagic pancreatitis may occur. A higher incidence of acute hemorrhagic pancreatitis has been encountered in patients taking bexarotene, as compared to first- or second-generation retinoids.

These observations have led to the suggestion that baseline serum lipids be obtained before initiating bexarotene therapy, as well as every 1 to 2 weeks during therapy until levels become stable (generally in 4 to 8 weeks). For other oral retinoids, monitoring levels monthly for the first 2 months and then at 2- to 3-month intervals (if there are no increases in dosage) is adequate in cases of normal baseline lipid levels and an absence of risk factors (obesity, high alcohol intake, diabetes). Discontinuation of therapy is suggested if fasting triglycerides reach 800 mg/dl (8 g/l). Less severe increases may be treated by dose reduction, withdrawing therapy until normalization of serum lipids occurs, and dietary (reduction in alcohol and tobacco consumption) or physical management. In some instances, lipid-lowering agents may be indicated[68]. Co-administration of atorvastatin or fenofibrate (or both) with bexarotene is recommended to treat the retinoid-induced hyperlipidemia and to lower the risk of pancreatitis[8,69].

The effect of retinoid-induced hyperlipidemia, and its management during long-term therapy, on the development of atherosclerotic cardiovascular disease is unknown. Retinoids probably cause hyperlipidemia by interfering with lipid clearance. Bexarotene increases the expression of apolipoprotein C-III, which prevents the uptake of lipids from very-low-density lipoproteins (VLDL) into cells[70]. Of note, in a cross-sectional comparison study, individuals who developed hypertriglyceridemia during isotretinoin therapy for acne were found to be at increased risk for future hyperlipidemia and the metabolic syndrome[70a].

Liver toxicity

Transitory abnormal elevations in serum transaminases have been reported in approximately 20% of patients treated with either etretinate or acitretin, occurring much less frequently with isotretinoin or bexarotene therapy. Circulating levels of alkaline phosphatase, lactic dehydrogenase and bilirubin may also become elevated during retinoid therapy. Liver function abnormalities, mostly mild, usually occur between 2 and 8 weeks of starting therapy, and they return to normal within another 2–4 weeks, despite continued therapy. Severe or persistent hepatotoxic reactions have been seen in less than 1% of patients. Acitretin therapy elicited no biopsy-proven hepatotoxicity in a 2-year prospective study, thus suggesting that periodic liver biopsy is not necessary[71]. No specific studies have evaluated the use of retinoids in patients with hepatic insufficiency. However, since retinoids are metabolized by hepatic cytochrome P450 isoenzymes (CYP 3A4) and undergo partial biliary elimination, significant hepatic insufficiency may be expected to interfere with drug elimination. Transaminase elevations to greater than three times the upper limit of normal should lead to discontinuation of retinoid therapy. With two- to three-fold transaminase elevations, therapy should be withdrawn until normalization of tests of liver function occurs[8]. Other causes of these elevations should simultaneously be excluded.

Hematologic toxicities

A high incidence (28%) of dose-related leukopenia was reported in the studies of bexarotene in CTCL, occurring as early as 2–4 weeks, with a decrease in neutrophils rather than lymphocytes[34]. Hematologic abnormalities are much less common with other retinoids, but careful hematologic monitoring in HIV-infected patients is warranted.

Summary

Most adverse effects associated with retinoids are preventable and manageable through proper patient selection, dose adjustments or discontinuation of treatment, and routine monitoring for potential toxicity.

INTERACTIONS

Concurrent use of retinoids with alcohol or other medications having similar side effects may increase their incidence. The following should be avoided or used with caution:

- tetracycline, doxycycline, minocycline (may increase intracranial pressure)
- alcohol (associated with increased conversion of acitretin to etretinate and hepatotoxicity)
- methotrexate (displays synergistic liver toxicity with retinoids; however, combination used with caution in patients with PRP or severe psoriasis)
- vitamin A supplements (carries the risk of hypervitaminosis A)[72].

Retinoid drug levels and resultant potential for toxicity may increase with CYP 3A4 inhibitors such as azoles and macrolides. In contrast, antituberculosis drugs (rifampin) and anticonvulsants (phenytoin and carbamazepine) may decrease the drug levels of retinoids via CYP 3A4 induction. Retinoids may also increase the drug levels of cyclosporine via competition for CYP 3A4 metabolism[8]. Concomitant administration of bexarotene and gemfibrozil results in a substantial increase in plasma concentrations of bexarotene, at least partially because of cytochrome P450 CYP 3A4 inhibition that is induced by gemfibrozil. Concomitant atorvastatin or fenofibrate administration does not affect bexarotene plasma levels and is, therefore, the recommended concomitant antilipemic therapy.

In rare instances, patients with diabetes mellitus may have more difficult glucose control while taking a retinoid; however, the causal relationship remains uncertain. In addition, acitretin has been shown to possibly reduce the efficacy of progestin-only contraceptives[73]. Also, unprotected UV radiation exposure or photosensitizing medications should be avoided because of increased photosensitivity caused by retinoid therapy. Since retinoids act through nuclear receptor dimers, cross-talk with other nuclear receptors may provide synergistic effects: for example, interactions between RXR and VDR positively influence the action of vitamin D3[74]; however, cross-talk with PPAR and its ligands is still under investigation.

USE IN PREGNANCY AND LACTATION

All systemic retinoids are teratogenic, and they are, therefore, absolutely contraindicated during pregnancy and lactation (FDA category X), which should be excluded by a pregnancy test before considering retinoid therapy and then at regular intervals (e.g. monthly in the case of isotretinoin) during its administration. In the US, two pregnancy tests are recommended before instituting isotretinoin therapy. Pregnancy is not only an absolute contraindication to starting therapy; it must also be avoided throughout therapy and for an appropriate interval after completion of therapy. Adequate contraception for at least 1 month before therapy is required for all systemic retinoid therapy. Acitretin requires contraception for 3 years (USA) or 2 years (Europe) after cessation of therapy, whereas isotretinoin and bexarotene require contraception for just 1 month after cessation of therapy. The recommended duration of contraception after discontinuation of oral retinoid therapy varies for the different retinoid compounds, based mainly on their pharmacologic profiles (half-life, deposit in adipose tissue; see Table 126.2).

Although no evidence exists for teratogenicity of topical retinoids in humans, they are nevertheless not recommended for use during pregnancy. Since no dermatologic condition that is known to be responsive to topical retinoids, and which may be observed during pregnancy, is life threatening to the mother or fetus, it is wiser to postpone treatment until after delivery (primarily due to medicolegal rather than scientific data in the opinion of these authors). The same recommendations are also valid for lactating women, as it is not known whether topical retinoids (tretinoin, isotretinoin, adapalene, tazarotene and bexarotene) pass into the breast milk. Consequently, topical retinoid use is not recommended during breastfeeding; it may cause unwanted effects in the nursing baby.

REFERENCES

1. Wolbach SB, Howe PR. Tissue changes following deprivation of fat-soluble A vitamin. J Exp Med. 1925;42:753–78.

2. Peck GL, Yoder FW. Treatment of lamellar ichthyosis and other keratinising dermatoses with an oral synthetic retinoid. Lancet. 1976;ii:1172–4.

3. Peck GL, Olsen TG, Yoder FW, et al. Prolonged remissions of cystic and conglobata acne with 13-cis-retinoic acid. N Engl J Med. 1979;300:329–33.

4. Dong D, Ruuska SE, Levinthal DJ, et al. Distinct roles for cellular retinoic acid-binding proteins I and II in regulating signaling by retinoic acid. J Biol Chem. 1999;274:23695–8.

5. Liu PT, Krutzik SR, Kim J, Modlin RL. Cutting edge: all-trans retinoic acid down-regulates TLR2 expression and function. J Immunol. 2005;174:2467–70.

6. Duvic M, Nagpal S, Asano AT, et al. Molecular mechanisms of tazarotene action in psoriasis. J Am Acad Dermatol. 1997;37:S18–24.

7. Bianchi L, Orlandi A, Campione E, et al. Topical treatment of basal cell carcinoma with tazarotene: a clinicopathological study on a large series of cases. Br J Dermatol. 2004;151:148–56.

8. Wiegand UW, Chou RC. Pharmacokinetics of acitretin and etretinate. J Am Acad Dermatol. 1998;39:S25–33.

9. Torma H. Interaction of isotretinoin with endogenous retinoids. J Am Acad Dermatol. 2001;45:S143–9.

10. Ethan-Quan HN, Wolverton S. Systemic retinoids. In: Wolverton SE (ed.). Comprehensive Dermatologic Drug Therapy. Philadelphia: WB Saunders, 2001:269–310.

11. Cunliffe WJ, Caputo R, Dreno B, et al. Clinical efficacy and safety comparison of adapalene gel and tretinoin gel in the treatment of acne vulgaris: Europe and US multicenter trials.J Am Acad Dermatol. 1997;36:S126–34.

12. Lebwohl M, Ast E, Callen JP, et al. Once-daily tazarotene gel versus twice-daily fluocinonide cream in the treatment of plaque psoriasis. J Am Acad Dermatol. 1998;38:705–11.

13. Thacher SM, Standeven AM, Athaniker J, et al. Receptor specificity of retinoid-induced epidermal hyperplasia: effect of RXR-selective agonists and correlation with topical irritation. J Pharmacol Exp Ther. 1997;282:528–34.

14. Creidi P, Vienne M-P, Ochonisky S, et al. Profilometric evaluation of photodamage after topical retinaldehyde and retinoic acid treatment. J Am Acad Dermatol. 1998;39:960–5.

14a. Calikoglu E, Sorg O, Tran C, et al. UVA and UVB decrease the expression of CD44 and hyaluronate in mouse epidermis, which is counteracted by topical retinoids. Photochem Photobiol. 2006;82:1342–7.

15. Breneman D, Duvic M, Kuzel T, et al. Phase 1 and 2 trial with bexarotene gel for skin-directed treatment of patients with cutaneous T cell lymphoma. Arch Dermatol. 2002;138:325–32.

16. Arechalde A, Saurat J-H. Management of psoriasis: the position of retinoid drugs. Bio Drugs. 2000;13:327–33.

17. White SI, Marks JM, Shuster S. Etretinate in pustular psoriasis of palms and soles. Br J Dermatol. 1985;113:581–5.

18. Dubertret L, Chastang C, Beylot C, et al. Maintenance treatment of psoriasis by Tigason: a double-blind randomized clinical trial. Br J Dermatol. 1985;113:323–30.

19. Lowe NL. When systemic retinoids fail to work in psoriasis. In: Saurat JH (ed.). Retinoids: 10 Years On. Basel: Karger, 1991:341–9.

20. Geiger JM, Czarnetzki BM. Acitretin (Ro 10-1670, etretin): overall evaluation of clinical studies. Dermatologica. 1988;176:182–90.

21. Lassus A, Geiger JM, Nyblom M, et al. Treatment of severe psoriasis with etretin (Ro 10-1670). Br J Dermatol. 1987;117:333–41.

22. Goldfarb MT, Ellis CN, Gupta AK, et al. Acitretin improves psoriasis in a dose-dependent fashion. J Am Acad Dermatol. 1988;18:655–62.

23. Saurat JH, Geiger JM, Amblard P, et al. Randomized double-blind multicenter study comparing acitretin-PUVA, etretinate-PUVA and placebo-PUVA in the treatment of severe psoriasis. Dermatologica. 1988;177:218–24.

24. Lebwohl M. Acitretin in combination with UVB or PUVA. J Am Acad Dermatol. 1999;41:S22–4.

25. Saurat JH. Systemic retinoids. What's new? Dermatol Clin. 1998;16:331–40.

26. Layton AM, Knaggs H, Taylor J, et al. Isotretinoin for acne vulgaris – 10 years later: a safe and successful treatment. Br J Dermatol. 1993;129:292–6.

27. Harms M, Duvanel T, Williamson C, et al. Isotretinoin for acne: should we consider the total cumulative dose? In: Marks R, Plewig G (eds). Acne and Related Disorders. London: Martin Dunitz, 1989:203–6.

28. Lehucher-Ceyrac D, Weber-Buisset MJ. Isotretinoin and acne: a prospective analysis of 188 cases over 9 years. Dermatology. 1993;186:123–8.

29. Cunliffe WJ, van de Kerkhof PCM, Caputo R, et al. Roaccutane treatment guidelines: results of an international survey. Dermatology. 1997;194:351–7.

30. Lehucher-Ceyrac D, de La Salmoniere P, Chastang C, et al. Predictive factors for failure of isotretinoin treatment in acne patients: results from a cohort of 237 patients. Dermatology. 1999;198:278–83.

31. Chaspoux C, Lehucher-Ceyrac D, Morel P, et al. [Acne in the male resistant to isotretinoin and responsibility of androgens: 9 cases, therapeutic implications]. Ann Dermatol Venereol. 1999;126:17–19.

32. Wiegand UW CW, Wyss R, et al. Treatment of female patients with isotretinoin: what is the safe post-therapy contraceptive period? In: Clinical Dermatology 2000 meeting, Vancouver, 1996.

33. Boer J, van Gemert MJ. Long-term results of isotretinoin in the treatment of 68 patients with hidradenitis suppurativa. J Am Acad Dermatol. 1999;40:73–6.

34. Duvic M, Martin AG, Kim Y, et al. Phase 2 and 3 clinical trial of oral bexarotene (Targretin capsules) for the treatment of refractory or persistent early-stage cutaneous T-cell lymphoma. Arch Dermatol. 2001;137:581–93.

35. Duvic M, Hymes K, Heald P, et al. Bexarotene is effective and safe for treatment of refractory advanced-stage cutaneous T-cell lymphoma: multinational phase II-III trial results. J Clin Oncol. 2001;19:2456–71.

36. Arechalde A, Saurat JH. Retinoids: unapproved uses or indications. Clin Dermatol. 2000;18:63–76.

37. Clayton BD, Jorizzo JL, Hitchcock MG, et al. Adult pityriasis rubra pilaris: a 10-year case series. J Am Acad Dermatol. 1997;36:959–64.

38. Erdogan FG, Yurtsever P, Aksoy D, et al. Efficacy of low-dose isotretinoin in patients with treatment-resistant rosacea. Arch Dermatol. 1998;134:884–5.

39. Bavinck JNB, Tieben LM, Vanderwoude FJ, et al. Prevention of skin cancer and reduction of keratotic skin lesions during acitretin therapy in renal transplant recipients: a double-blind, placebo-controlled study. J Clin Oncol. 1995;13:1933–8.

40. Marcellus DC, Altomonte VL, Farmer ER, et al. Etretinate therapy for refractory sclerodermatous chronic graft-versus-host disease. Blood. 1999;93:66–70.

41. Ruzicka T, Sommerburg C, Goerz G, et al. Treatment of cutaneous lupus erythematosus with acitretin and hydroxychloroquine. Br J Dermatol. 1992;127:513–18.

42. Prystowsky J. Topical retinoids. In: Wolverton SE (ed.). Comprehensive Dermatologic Drug Therapy. Philadelphia: WB Saunders, 2001.

43. Kang S, Duell EA, Fisher GJ, et al. Application of retinol to human skin in vivo induces epidermal hyperplasia and cellular retinoid binding proteins characteristic of retinoic acid but without measurable retinoic acid levels or irritation. J Invest Dermatol. 1995;105:549–56.

44. Jick H. Retinoids and teratogenicity. J Am Acad Dermatol. 1998;39:S118–22.

45. Lammer EJ, Chen DT, Hoar RM, et al. Retinoic acid embryopathy. N Engl J Med. 1985;313:837–41.

46. Sulik KK. Teratogenicity of the retinoids. In: Saurat JH (ed.). Retinoids: 10 Years On. Basel: Karger, 1991:282–95.

47. Williams RE, Doherty VR, Perkins W, et al. Staphylococcus aureus and intra-nasal mupirocin in patients receiving isotretinoin for acne. Br J Dermatol. 1992;126:362–6.

48. Carey BM, Parkin GJ, Cunliffe WJ, et al. Skeletal toxicity with isotretinoin therapy: a clinico-radiological evaluation. Br J Dermatol. 1988;119:609–14.

49. Tfelt-Hansen P, Knudsen B, Petersen E, et al. Spinal cord compression after long-term etretinate. Lancet. 1989;2:325–6.

50. Kilcoyne RF. Effects of retinoids in bone. J Am Acad Dermatol. 1988;19:212–16.

51. van Dooren-Greebe R, Lemmens J, De Boo T, et al. Prolonged treatment with oral retinoids in adults: no influence on the frequency and severity of spinal abnormalities. Br J Dermatol. 1996;134:71–6.

52. Ling TC, Parkin G, Islam J, et al. What is the cumulative effect of long-term, low-dose isotretinoin on the development of DISH? Br J Dermatol. 2001;144:630–2.

53. DiGiovanna JJ, Sollitto RB, Abangan DL, et al. Osteoporosis is a toxic effect of long-term etretinate therapy. Arch Dermatol. 1995;131:1263–7.

54. Leachman SA, Insogna KL, Katz L, et al. Bone densities in patients receiving isotretinoin for cystic acne. Arch Dermatol. 1999;135:961–5.

55. DiGiovanna JJ, Langman CB, Tschen EH, et al. Effect of a single course of isotretinoin therapy on bone mineral density in adolescent patients with severe, recalcitrant, nodular acne. J Am Acad Dermatol. 2004;51:709–17.

56. Halkier-Sörensen L, Laurberg G, Andersen J. Bone changes in children on long-term treatment with etretinate. J Am Acad Dermatol. 1987;16:999–1006.

57. Nishimura G, Mugishima H, Hirao J, et al. Generalized metaphyseal modification with cone-shaped epiphyses following long-term administration of 13-cis-retinoic acid. Eur J Pediatr. 1997;156:432–5.

58. Lister RK, Lecky BRF, Lewis-Jones MS, et al. Acitretin-induced myopathy. Br J Dermatol. 1996;134:989–90.

59. Bonnetblanc JM, Hugon J, Dumas M. Intracranial hypertension with etretinate. Lancet. 1983;2:974.

60. Lee AG. Pseudomotor cerebri after treatment with tetracycline and isotretinoin for acne. Cutis. 1995;55:165–8.

61. Chu A, Cunliffe WJ. The inter-relationship between isotretinoin/acne and depression. J Eur Acad Dermatol Venereol. 1999;12:263.

62. Marqueling AL, Zane LT. Depression and suicidal behavior in acne patients treated with isotretinoin: a systematic review. Sem Cutan Med Surg. 2005;24:92–102.

63. Jick SS, Kremers HM, Vasilakis-Scaramozza C. Isotretinoin use and risk of depression, psychotic symptoms, suicide, and attempted suicide. Arch Dermatol. 2000;136:1231–6.

64. Safran AB, Haliaoua B, Roth A, et al. Ocular side-effects of oral treatment with retinoids. In: Saurat JH (ed.). Retinoids: 10 Years On. Basel: Karger, 1991:315–26.

65. Sherman SI, Gopal J, Haugen BR, et al. Central hypothyroidism associated with retinoid X receptor-selective ligands. N Engl J Med. 1999;340:1075–9.

66. Cribier B, Welsch M, Heid E. Renal impairment probably induced by etretinate. Dermatology. 1992;185:266–8.

67. Koo J, Nguyen Q, Gambla C. Advances in psoriasis therapy. Adv Dermatol. 1997;12:47–72.

68. Vahlquist C, Olsson A, Lindholm A, et al. Effects of gemfibrozil (Lopid®) on hyperlipidemia in acitretin-treated patients. Acta Dermato-Venereol. 1995;75:377–80.

69. Talpur R, Ward S, Apisarnthanarax N, Breuer-Mcham J, Duvic M. Optimizing bexarotene therapy for cutaneous T-cell lymphoma. J Am Acad Dermatol. 2002;47:672–84.

70. Vu Dac N, Gervois P, Torra IP, et al. Retinoids increase human apo C-III expression at the transcriptional level via the retinoid X receptor – contribution to the hypertriglyceridemic action of retinoids. J Clin Invest. 1998;102:625–32.

70a. Rodondi N, Darioli R, Ramelet AA, et al. High risk for hyperlipidemia and the metabolic syndrome after an episode of hypertriglyceridemia during 13-cis retinoic acid therapy for acne: a pharmacogenetic study. Ann Intern Med. 2002;136:582–9.

71. Roenigk HH Jr, Callen JP, Guzzo CA, et al. Effects of acitretin on the liver. J Am Acad Dermatol. 1999;41:584–8.

72. Katz HI, Waalen J, Leach EE. Acitretin in psoriasis: an overview of adverse effects. J Am Acad Dermatol. 1999;41:S7–12.

73. Berbis P, Bun H, Geiger JM, et al. Acitretin (RO10-1670) and oral contraceptives: interaction study. Arch Dermatol Res. 1988;280:388–9.

74. Kang S, Li XY, Duell EA, et al. The retinoid X receptor agonist 9-cis-retinoic acid and the 24-hydroxylase inhibitor ketoconazole increase activity of 1,25-dihydroxyvitamin D3 in human skin in vivo. J Invest Dermatol. 1997;108:513–18.

Antimicrobial Drugs

Jack Lesher and Carol McConnell Woody

Key features

- Bacterial, fungal and viral infections of the skin and soft tissue are very common
- Selection of the appropriate treatment depends on the infecting microbe, the medication and the patient
- Physicians must be aware of the drug interactions and potential adverse effects of antimicrobial medications

ANTIBACTERIAL AGENTS

Introduction

The development of antibiotics has provided physicians with a formidable armamentarium against bacterial diseases. Literally hundreds of antibiotics are now available. While physicians have gained abundant therapeutic options, some find the vast number of antibacterial medications confusing and overwhelming. Selection of the most appropriate antibiotic depends on identification of the infecting organism and its sensitivity to antimicrobial agents. Often a patient will present with a clinical picture strongly suggestive of a particular organism. Ideally, culture of the organism should be obtained prior to starting therapy. However, a microbiologic diagnosis may not always be possible or practical.

In acutely ill patients, empiric therapy with broad-spectrum antibiotics may be necessary initially. Knowledge of local bacterial resistance patterns should guide antibiotic selection. Once the microbe is identified, preferably along with antibiotic sensitivities, medication should be adjusted accordingly. Indiscriminate use of broad-spectrum antibiotics leads to the development of resistant bacteria[1,2]. The site and extent of the infection, the safety, side effects and cost of the medication, and patient characteristics, including renal and hepatic function as well as pregnancy and lactation, also influence drug selection.

Antibacterial drugs are characterized as being either bacteriostatic or bactericidal. Bacteriostatic drugs stop growth and replication of bacteria and limit spread of infection, allowing the immune system to eliminate the pathogen. Bactericidal agents kill bacteria directly. Table 127.1 outlines into which category commonly used antibiotics are classified.

Topical Antibacterial Agents

Introduction

Topical antibacterials are used to treat acne vulgaris, rosacea and superficial bacterial infections and to prevent infection after surgery or injuries. Topical antibacterials have several advantages over oral and parenteral antibiotics. They can be applied easily directly to the affected area and thus deliver a high concentration of the medication locally with relatively little chance of adverse systemic effects. However, their utility is limited to those conditions that are superficial and localized.

Topical antibacterial agents used to treat acne vulgaris and rosacea

Table 127.2 lists topical antibiotics commonly used to treat acne vulgaris and rosacea. Topical antibiotics are used in these conditions for their anti-inflammatory effects as well as for their antibacterial effect. They have relatively little effect on non-inflammatory, comedonal acne.

BACTERIOSTATIC VERSUS BACTERICIDAL DRUGS	
Bacteriostatic	**Bactericidal**
Chloramphenicol	Aminoglycosides
Clindamycin	Bacitracin
Erythromycin	Carbapenems
Sulfonamides	Monobactams
Tetracyclines	Penicillins
Trimethoprim	Polymyxin B
	Quinolones
	Vancomycin

Table 127.1 Bacteriostatic versus bactericidal drugs. Clindamycin may be either bacteriostatic or bactericidal depending on the susceptibility of the infecting organism and the concentration achieved at the site of infection.

Mechanisms of action

Table 127.3 lists the mechanisms of action of the topical antibacterials used to treat acne vulgaris and rosacea.

Azelaic acid is a dicarboxylic acid derivative found in whole grain cereals and animal products and is normally present in human plasma. The exact mechanism of action of azelaic acid is unknown. *In vitro*, it has activity against *Propionibacterium acnes* and *Staphylococcus epidermidis*. It is usually bacteriostatic, but may be bactericidal in high concentrations. Its activity may be due to an inhibition of microbial cellular protein synthesis. Azelaic acid also normalizes keratinization and is anticomedonal. It thins the stratum corneum, decreases the number and size of keratohyaline granules, and reduces the amount and distribution of filaggrin in the epidermis. Azelaic acid has antiproliferative effects against hyperactive and abnormal melanocytes without causing depigmentation of normally pigmented skin except in rare cases (see Table 127.4).

Benzoyl peroxide is bacteriostatic against *P. acnes*. Once absorbed by the skin, it is converted to benzoic acid. Its effects are believed to be due to oxidation of bacterial proteins by active oxygen, which is released when the drug is decomposed by cysteine in the skin. Two weeks of daily 10% benzoyl peroxide decreases free fatty acids by 50% and *P. acnes* by 98%, which is comparable to results obtained after 4 weeks of antibiotics[3]. It is also keratolytic and desquamative.

Clindamycin is a semisynthetic lincosamide antibiotic that suppresses protein synthesis by binding to the bacterial 50S ribosomal subunit. It is active against Gram-positive cocci and anaerobes including staphylococci, streptococci, *P. acnes*, *Corynebacterium*, *Clostridium* and *Gardnerella vaginalis*. Clindamycin may be either bacteriostatic or bactericidal depending on the susceptibility of the infecting organism and the concentration achieved at the site of infection.

Erythromycin is a macrolide antibiotic, made as a fermentation product by *Streptomyces erythreus*. It inhibits protein synthesis by binding to the 50S ribosomal subunit. Erythromycin is active against Gram-positive cocci including group A β-hemolytic streptococci, α-hemolytic streptococci and *Staphylococcus aureus*; it is also active against some Gram-negative bacilli. Erythromycin also has anti-inflammatory properties.

Studies have shown that the combination of erythromycin and benzoyl peroxide is more effective than erythromycin alone both *in vivo* and *in vitro*[4–8]. This combination may be synergistic and may slow the development of antibiotic resistance. The topical erythromycin and benzoyl peroxide formulation may be prescribed separately or as a combination product.

A 5% benzoyl peroxide/1% clindamycin gel has also recently become available for the topical treatment of acne. Randomized, double-blind,

TOPICAL ANTIBACTERIALS USED FOR ACNE VULGARIS AND ROSACEA				
Generic name	**Trade name(s)®**	**Formulations**	**Dosing frequency**	**FDA pregnancy category**
Azelaic acid	Azalea, Azelex, Cutacelan, Skinkoren, Skinoderm, Skinorem, Skinoren	20% cream	bid	B
Benzoyl peroxide	Acetoxyl, Acne-Aid, Acnomel, Ambi, Benoxyl, Benzac, Benzagel, BenzaShave, Brevoxyl, Clearasil, Clearplex, Del-Aqua, Dermoxyl, Desquam-E, Desquam-X, Fostex, Loroxide, Oxy, Oxyderm, PanOxyl, Solugel, Triaz	2.5–10% lotion, cream, gel, stick, cleansing bar, cleansing lotion, mask, shaving cream	qd–tid; mask qwk	C
Clindamycin	Basocin, Cindala, Cleocin T, Clicinin, Clinac, Clinda-Derm, Clindets, Cutaclin, Dalacin, Dalacin T, Dalacine, Dalagis, Euroclin, Evoclin	1% gel, lotion, solution, pledgets; 2% vaginal cream	bid	B
Erythromycin	Akne-Mycin, A/T/S, Emgel, Erycette, Eryderm, Erygel, Erymax, Ery-Sol, Erythra-Derm, ETS, Ilotycin, Sans-Acne, Staticin, Theramycin Z, T-Stat	1.5% or 2% solution, 2% pledgets; gel, ointment	bid	B
Sodium sulfacetamide	Klaron, Novacet, Plexion, Sulfacet-R, Fostex, Acnederm, Rosac, Rosanil, Rosula, Zetacet	10% lotion	bid	C
Metronidazole	MetroGel, MetroCream, MetroLotion, Noritate	0.75% or 1% gel, cream, lotion	qd–bid	B
Benzoyl peroxide/ erythromycin	Benzamycin	5%/3% gel	bid	C
Benzoyl peroxide/ clindamycin	Benzaclin, Duac	5%/1% gel	bid	C
Clindamycin phosphate/ tretinoin	Ziana	1.2/0.025% gel	qd	C

Table 127.2 Topical antibacterials used for acne vulgaris and rosacea.

MECHANISMS OF ACTION OF TOPICAL ANTIBACTERIAL AGENTS USED TO TREAT ACNE VULGARIS AND ROSACEA		
Generic name	**Class**	**Mechanism of action**
Azelaic acid	Dicarboxylic acid derivative	Unknown
Benzoyl peroxide	Active oxygen releaser	Oxidation of bacterial proteins by active oxygen
Clindamycin	Lincosamide	Inhibits protein synthesis by binding to the bacterial 50S ribosomal subunit
Erythromycin	Macrolide	Inhibits protein synthesis by binding to the bacterial 50S ribosomal subunit
Sodium sulfacetamide	Sulfonamide	Inhibits nucleic acid and protein synthesis and cell growth by impeding bacterial synthesis of dihydrofolic acid. Competitive inhibition of dihydropteroate synthetase prevents condensation of pteridine precursors with PABA (see Fig. 127.4)
Metronidazole	Nitroimidazole	May cause DNA strand breaking. Also has antioxidant and anti-inflammatory effects

Table 127.3 Mechanisms of action of topical antibacterial agents used to treat acne vulgaris and rosacea. PABA, para-aminobenzoic acid.

competitive inhibition of the enzyme dihydropteroate synthetase (see Table 127.3). It thereby inhibits nucleic acid and protein synthesis and cell growth. It is active against some Gram-positive and Gram-negative organisms.

Metronidazole is a nitroimidazole. How this medication exerts its bactericidal effect is not fully understood. It may cause DNA strand breaking. Topical metronidazole also has antioxidant and anti-inflammatory effects.

Indications

Azelaic acid, benzoyl peroxide, clindamycin, erythromycin and sodium sulfacetamide are often used for mild to moderate inflammatory acne vulgaris. Several of these medications have additional indications. For instance, azelaic acid may also be useful for melasma and other forms of hyperpigmentation. Benzoyl peroxide has been used for decubitus and stasis ulcers. Either topical clindamycin or erythromycin may be used for superficial bacterial infections of the skin. Topical clindamycin and metronidazole are both indicated for bacterial vaginosis. Sodium sulfacetamide and topical metronidazole are indicated for the treatment of rosacea.

Dosages

Topical antibacterial agents are usually applied once or twice a day (see Table 127.2). A small amount of medication is applied in a thin layer and massaged gently into clean, dry skin. Benzoyl peroxide bar and wash are used as cleansers one to three times a day. Benzoyl peroxide shave cream is used like any other shaving cream. The mask is applied in a thin layer once a week, left on for 15 to 25 minutes, and then rinsed off.

Contraindications

As is the case with all topical medicines, the chief contraindication for these medications is a history of hypersensitivity to any component of the formulations. Azelaic acid contains propylene glycol, which may be a potent sensitizer. Topical clindamycin is contraindicated in patients with a history of regional enteritis, ulcerative colitis or antibiotic-associated colitis. These conditions may increase the chance of gastrointestinal side effects.

Major side effects

Adverse reactions to the topical antibacterial agents used to treat acne vulgaris and rosacea are usually mild and transient. The most commonly occurring side effects are burning, stinging, tingling, pruritus, erythema, xerosis, peeling, irritant contact dermatitis and allergic

controlled trials demonstrated that patients treated with the combination product had a greater reduction in the number of inflammatory papules and pustules than did those treated with benzoyl peroxide alone, clindamycin alone or vehicle alone[9,10]. The initial disadvantage of these combination products was their need to be refrigerated to prevent degradation. There is also a new combination product with clindamycin and tretinoin for the treatment of acne.

Erythromycin (4%) has been combined with 1.2% zinc acetate, as has benzoyl peroxide 3–10% with zinc lactate. The former product is not available in the US. Zinc has antiandrogen activity *in vitro* and suppresses sebum secretion[11]. Studies have shown erythromycin combined with zinc to be superior to placebo *in vivo*[12–15] and effective *in vitro* against erythromycin-resistant *P. acnes*[16]. However, it may be inferior to benzoyl peroxide combined with erythromycin[17].

Sodium sulfacetamide is bacteriostatic. Sulfonamides inhibit bacterial synthesis of dihydrofolic acid by preventing the condensation of pteridine precursors with para-aminobenzoic acid (PABA) through

SIDE EFFECTS OF TOPICAL ANTIBACTERIAL AGENTS USED FOR ACNE VULGARIS AND ROSACEA	
Generic name	Side effects
Azelaic acid	Pruritus, burning, stinging, tingling, erythema, xerosis, peeling, irritant contact dermatitis, allergic contact dermatitis Rarely reported: worsening of asthma, hypopigmentation, depigmentation, hypertrichosis, keratosis pilaris, exacerbation of recurrent herpes labialis
Benzoyl peroxide	Painful irritation, blistering, crusting, severe erythema, and edema Bleaches hair and colored fabrics
Clindamycin	Gram-negative folliculitis Rare cases of pseudomembranous colitis (the suggested risk of pseudomembranous colitis from topical use appears not to be clinically significant[18])
Erythromycin	Eye irritation, skin tenderness, Gram-negative folliculitis, rarely generalized urticarial reactions Bacterial resistance
Sodium sulfacetamide	Xerosis, pruritus; may cross-react in patients allergic to the oral form
Metronidazole	Watery eyes, metallic taste in the mouth, nausea, numbness and paresthesias have been reported with topical use[19]; may cross-react in patients allergic to the oral form

Table 127.4 Side effects of topical antibacterial agents used for acne vulgaris and rosacea.

contact dermatitis. Stinging is especially common with the alcohol-containing solutions and pledgets. Table 127.4 shows additional side effects of individual drugs.

Interactions
Application of more than one topical medication simultaneously may increase or decrease the effect of one or both of the medications. Benzoyl peroxide, topical clindamycin and topical erythromycin may have additive irritant effects when used with other topical acne medications. Topically applied clindamycin may interact with other drugs as a result of systemic absorption. Clindamycin has neuromuscular blocking properties that may enhance the effects of similar agents. It should be used with caution in patients receiving neuromuscular blocking agents. Clindamycin, erythromycin and chloramphenicol may antagonize each other due to their similar mechanisms of action. Oral metronidazole may potentiate the anticoagulant effect of warfarin, resulting in a prolonged prothrombin time. It is not known whether topical preparations have the same effect.

Pregnancy and lactation
Table 127.2 lists the FDA pregnancy categories of the topical antibacterial agents used to treat acne vulgaris and rosacea.

Azelaic acid has not been adequately studied in pregnant women. There is a small amount of systemic absorption of azelaic acid through topical application. Passage of azelaic acid into maternal milk may occur. There have been no reported problems due to azelaic acid in nursing infants.

Studies on the effects of benzoyl peroxide in pregnancy have not been done in either humans or animals. There may be systemic absorption of topically applied benzoyl peroxide. It is not known whether benzoyl peroxide is excreted in breast milk. It has not been reported to cause problems in nursing infants.

There are no adequate studies of topical clindamycin in pregnant or lactating women. It is not known whether topically applied clindamycin passes into breast milk. No serious adverse effects have been reported in nursing infants. Clindamycin vaginal cream is not recommended during pregnancy, except for women who are at high risk for a bad outcome due to bacterial vaginosis or in women who are at low risk of adverse pregnancy outcomes who also have symptomatic bacterial vaginosis.

Studies on the effect of topical erythromycin in pregnancy have not been done in humans or animals. Animal reproduction studies have not been done. Systemically administered erythromycin is excreted in breast milk. However, it is not known whether topical erythromycin is excreted in breast milk. Erythromycin topical preparations have not been reported to cause problems in nursing infants. However, the safety of this medication in children has not been established via controlled trials.

Sulfonamides may increase the chance of kernicterus in newborns and should not be used late in pregnancy. Systemic sulfonamides are excreted in breast milk and may cause kernicterus, anemia and other adverse effects in nursing infants, especially those with glucose-6-phosphate dehydrogenase deficiency.

Topical metronidazole has not been studied in pregnant women. Systemic metronidazole does cross the placental barrier and enters the fetal circulation. It has not been shown to cause birth defects or other problems in animal studies. Topical metronidazole results in blood levels much lower than those achieved with systemically administered metronidazole. The small amounts of this medication that are absorbed are unlikely to cause serious problems in nursing infants.

Topical antibacterial agents used to treat superficial infections
Table 127.5 lists antibacterial agents commonly used to prevent and treat superficial wound infections.

Mechanisms of action
The mechanisms of action of the topical antibacterial agents used to treat superficial infections are listed in Table 127.6.

Mupirocin (pseudomonic acid A) is derived from Pseudomonas fluorescens. It inhibits protein synthesis by reversibly binding to bacterial isoleucyl transfer RNA synthetase. It is clinically active against staphylococci, groups A, B, C and G streptococci, and some Gram-negative aerobic bacteria. It is usually bacteriostatic, but may be bactericidal at high concentrations.

Retapamulin is the first drug in the new pleuromutilin class, derived from fermentation of a mushroom, Clitopilus passeckerianus. It works

TOPICAL ANTIBACTERIAL AGENTS USED FOR SUPERFICIAL INFECTIONS				
Generic name	Trade name(s)®	Formulations	Dosing frequency	FDA pregnancy category
Mupirocin	Bactoderm, Bactroban, Centany, Bactroban Nasal, Eismycin	2% ointment or cream	tid	B
Retapamulin	Altabax	1% ointment	bid	B
Neomycin	Myciguent, Framycetin	0.5% ointment or cream	qd–tid	C
Gentamicin	Garamycin, Gentamar, G-Myticin	0.1% ointment or cream	tid–qid	C
Bacitracin	Baciguent	400–500 units per gram ointment	tid	C
Polymyxin B	Polysporin ointment = bacitracin + polymyxin B Neosporin ointment = bacitracin, polymyxin B + neomycin Neosporin cream = polymyxin B + neomycin only	5000–10 000 units per gram ointment	qd–tid	C

Table 127.5 Topical antibacterial agents used for superficial infections.

MECHANISMS OF ACTION OF TOPICAL ANTIBACTERIAL AGENTS USED FOR SUPERFICIAL INFECTIONS		
Generic name	**Class**	**Mechanism of action**
Mupirocin	Unique	Inhibits protein synthesis by reversibly binding to bacterial isoleucyl transfer RNA synthetase
Retapamulin	Pleuromutilin	Selectively inhibits bacterial protein synthesis by interacting with the ribosomal protein L3 on the 50S ribosomal subunit
Neomycin	Aminoglycoside	Binds to the 30S subunit of the bacterial ribosome and causes misreading of the mRNA and inhibition of bacterial protein synthesis. May also inhibit bacterial DNA polymerase
Gentamicin	Aminoglycoside	Binds to the 30S subunit of the bacterial ribosome and causes misreading of the mRNA and inhibition of bacterial protein synthesis
Bacitracin	Cyclic polypeptide	Forms a complex with C55-phenol pyrophosphate, a component of the bacterial cell wall, impeding bacterial cell wall synthesis
Polymyxin B	Cyclic lipopeptide	Interacts with the phospholipids of bacterial cell membranes, increasing their cellular permeability

Table 127.6 Mechanisms of action of topical antibacterial agents used for superficial infections.

by selectively inhibiting bacterial protein synthesis by interacting with the ribosomal protein L3 on the 50S ribosomal subunit[19a].

Neomycin and *gentamicin* are aminoglycoside antibiotics isolated from cultures of *Streptomyces fradiae* and *Micromonospora purpurea*, respectively. They bind to the 30S subunit of the bacterial ribosome and cause misreading of mRNA and inhibition of bacterial protein synthesis. Neomycin may also inhibit bacterial DNA polymerase. Neomycin is bactericidal against Gram-positive and Gram-negative bacteria, including *S. aureus, Escherichia coli, Haemophilus influenzae, Proteus* species and *Serratia* species. It is generally not effective against *Pseudomonas aeruginosa*. Gentamicin is effective against sensitive strains of group A β-hemolytic and α-hemolytic streptococci, *S. aureus* (coagulase-positive, coagulase-negative and some penicillinase-producing strains) and Gram-negative bacteria, including *P. aeruginosa*, *Aerobacter aerogenes*, *E. coli*, *P. vulgaris* and *Klebsiella pneumoniae*.

Bacitracin is a cyclic polypeptide antibiotic produced by the Tracey I strain of *Bacillus subtilis*. It has a thiazolidine ring and peptide side chains. *In vivo* it forms a complex with C55-phenol pyrophosphate, a component of the bacterial cell wall, impeding bacterial cell wall synthesis. Bacitracin is active against Gram-positive organisms such as staphylococci, streptococci, corynebacteria and clostridia.

Polymyxin B is a cyclic lipopeptide antibiotic isolated from the aerobic Gram-positive rod *Bacillus polymyxa*, a soil organism. It interacts with the phospholipids of bacterial cell membranes, increasing their cellular permeability. It is rapidly bactericidal for various Gram-negative organisms, including *P. aeruginosa*, *E. coli*, *K. pneumoniae*, *Enterobacter aerogenes*, *H. influenzae*, *Proteus mirabilis* and *Serratia marcescens*. It is not active against Gram-positive organisms.

Indications
Mupirocin, neomycin, gentamicin, bacitracin and polymyxin B are all indicated for the treatment and prevention of superficial bacterial skin infections. The intranasal preparation made with the calcium salt of mupirocin is indicated for the eradication of nasopharyngeal carriage of *S. aureus*. Recent studies implicating nasal staphylococci as a potential source for wound infections and bacteremia suggest mupirocin intranasally may have an effect in decreasing the incidence of these bacterial infections[20]. Mupirocin has been shown to be as effective as systemic antibiotics for limited impetigo[21,22]. Retapamulin is indicated for the topical treatment of impetigo due to *Streptococcus pyogenes* and methicillin-susceptible *S. aureus* in patients as young as 9 months.

Dosages
Table 127.5 outlines the formulations and dosing frequency for the antibacterial agents used for the treatment of superficial skin infections. Intranasal mupirocin is applied into the nares two to four times a day for 5 to 14 days.

Contraindications
As with all topical medications, the main contraindication is a history of hypersensitivity to any component of the formulations.

Major side effects
Side effects of mupirocin include burning, stinging, tenderness, pain and pruritus, as well as erythema, edema, increased exudate, allergic contact dermatitis, cellulitis, headache and nausea. Nasal mupirocin can occasionally cause headaches, rhinitis, respiratory tract congestion, pharyngitis, taste perversion, burning, stinging and cough. Use of mupirocin on generalized areas has been reported to cause systemic absorption of polyethylene glycol leading to renal toxicity. Retapamulin can cause application site irritation or pruritus.

Side effects of neomycin include allergic contact dermatitis in 5% to 15% of patients[19], in particular when neomycin is applied to cutaneous ulcerations. The most common symptoms are pruritus, erythema and edema. The risk of potential side effects increases if the patient has impaired renal function; for example, patients with decreased renal function may develop irreversible ototoxicity manifested by hearing loss. Caution should be exercised if the medication is used over extensive areas where rapid absorption may occur. Nephrotoxicity, neuromuscular blockade and death have been reported after application of neomycin[19]. It may also cause mast cell degranulation and histamine release[3].

Possible side effects of gentamicin are erythema, pruritus, edema and photosensitization. There is a risk of producing gentamicin-resistant strains of *Pseudomonas* when this topical agent is applied to heavily colonized skin (e.g. leg ulcers).

Adverse effects of bacitracin include irritant and allergic contact dermatitis. Chronic stasis dermatitis predisposes to the latter. Anaphylaxis has been reported in patients with a history of multiple previous exposures when bacitracin was applied to open wounds.

There are very few side effects from polymyxin B. Contact sensitization has been reported. Of note, some cross-reactivity exists between bacitracin and polymyxin B because they are both derived from *Bacillus* species.

Interactions
In studies utilizing *E. coli*, chloramphenicol interferes with the effect of mupirocin on bacterial RNA synthesis. Otherwise, there are no known significant drug interactions with regard to the topical antibiotics used for superficial skin infections.

Pregnancy and lactation
Table 127.5 lists the FDA pregnancy categories of the topical antibacterials used to treat superficial infections.

Neither topical nor nasal mupirocin has been adequately studied in pregnant women. It has not been shown to cause birth defects or other problems in animal studies using rats and rabbits. It is not known whether topical or nasal mupirocin is excreted in breast milk. There is very little systemic absorption of topically applied mupirocin. Topical neomycin has not been shown to cause birth defects in humans and has not been reported to cause problems in nursing infants. Animal studies have not been conducted with polymyxin B, and it is not known whether polymyxin B is excreted in breast milk.

Other topical antibacterial agents
Fusidic acid is a unique fusidane antibiotic isolated from the fungus *Fusidum coccineum*[23]. It is not approved in the US but is used in Europe and Canada for mild to moderately severe cutaneous infections, external eye infections, and for eradication of nasopharyngeal carriage of *S. aureus*. It is available as a 2% cream, ointment and impregnated gauze that is applied three times a day. It may also be given orally or intravenously. It has a steroid-like structure, but does not have any steroid effects[23,24]. Fusidic acid inhibits bacterial protein synthesis by interfering with elongation factor G. It is active against Gram-positive

bacteria. Specifically, it is highly effective against *S. aureus*. This medication has a bacteriologic efficacy comparable to that of mupirocin for impetigo and may be more cost-effective[25–27]. When combined with topical corticosteroids, it is useful in treating atopic dermatitis with superimposed staphylococcal infection[24]; it is also effective in erythrasma[28,29]. Fusidic acid has few adverse effects, although allergic contact dermatitis has been reported.

Iodoquinol (1%) combined with 1% hydrocortisone has been commercially available for many years. Iodoquinol is a halogenated oxyquinoline with antibacterial and antifungal activity. Its mechanism of action is unknown. The combination product is applied three to four times a day for superficial bacterial and fungal skin infections. It is in FDA pregnancy category C and its safety during pregnancy is unknown. Topical iodoquinol (1%) preparations have a high iodine content. There is a systemic form of iodoquinol used for amebiasis, which is contra-indicated in patients with iodine intolerance, may interfere with thyroid function tests, and may cause iododerma[30]. A related medica-tion, topical *clioquinol* (iodochlorhydroxyquin), is used primarily for the treatment of superficial fungal infections (see below).

Mafenide acetate cream is a sulfonamide used for thermal burns and is available as a cream applied once or twice daily. It has antibacterial and antifungal activity. The most common side effect is burning, and, less often, urticaria or facial edema can occur. Rarely, mafenide acetate may cause bone marrow suppression or lead to hemolytic anemia in patients with glucose-6-phosphate dehydrogenase (G6PD) deficiency. It should be used with caution in patients with renal or pulmonary disease owing to its potential to cause metabolic acidosis. Furthermore, mafenide acetate may cause intense pain upon application and may be associated with *Candida* superinfection.

Nitrofurazone is used for thermal burns and skin grafting. It is available as a 0.2% cream, ointment and solution. Nitrofurazone is used once a day. It works by inhibiting bacterial metabolic enzymes and is effective against staphylococci, streptococci, *E. coli*, *Clostridium perfringens*, *Aerobacter enterogenes* and *Proteus* species.

Silver sulfadiazine is a 1% cream applied once to twice a day for thermal burns. In addition to its sulfonamide properties, the silver interacts with bacterial cell walls and membranes. When used in conjunction with cimetidine, there is an increased risk of leukopenia. Silver sulfadiazine may interfere with collagenase (Santyl®), papain (Panafil®) and sutilains (Travase®). It is contraindicated in patients with a history of hypersensitivity to sulfonamides and should be used with caution in patients with G6PD deficiency, renal or hepatic disease, and porphyria. Sulfonamides can generate oxidants and induce an acute hemolytic anemia in patients with G6PD deficiency. They may pre-cipitate an attack of pseudoporphyria or unmask a case of true porphyria. The mechanism for this is unclear, but may be direct hepatocellular damage, increased cytochrome P450 activity, or inhibition of liver enzymes leading to increased production of porphyrins. Localized argyria due to deposits of silver in the dermis can also occur.

Topical tetracyclines

Tetracycline hydrochloride is available as a 3% solution and as an ointment. It is applied twice a day for acne vulgaris and is also indicated for superficial skin infections. Meclocycline sulfosalicylate solution and cream are indicated for acne but are not available in the US. Chlortetracycline ointment is indicated for superficial skin infections. Topical tetracyclines may be less effective than topical clindamycin or erythromycin. They work by inhibition of protein synthesis and are bacteriostatic against a wide range of Gram-negative and Gram-positive bacteria. These products have been reformulated to reduce the yellow color associated with topical tetracyclines. Side effects include stinging, burning and an unpleasant odor. It is not known whether topically applied tetracyclines are excreted in breast milk. However, because tetracyclines can cause permanent yellow, gray or brown discoloration of the teeth, they should not be used in pregnant women, nursing mothers, or children under 8 years of age. Topical tetracycline contains sodium bisulfite which may cause anaphylaxis in susceptible people.

Systemic Antibacterial Agents

Systemic antibacterial agents have the potential to cause wide-ranging adverse side effects and significant interactions with other systemic

medications. For example, systemic antibacterials such as rifampin may reduce the efficacy of oral contraceptives. Furthermore, bacterio-static antibacterial agents may decrease the efficacy of bactericidal antibacterial agents, because the latter drugs target actively dividing cells. Additionally, there is a greater potential risk for the development of bacterial resistance with the use of systemic antibacterials. The mechanisms of action of the major classes of antibacterial drugs are listed in Table 127.7 and illustrated in Figure 127.1. Systemic antibiotics are used perioperatively by dermatologic surgeons for the prophylaxis of postoperative wound infections, endocarditis and contamination of prostheses. Prophylaxis against endocarditis after cutaneous surgery is indicated in patients with prosthetic heart valves and in patients with high-risk cardiac lesions who have surgery involving infected tissue[31].

SITES OF ACTION OF DIFFERENT CLASSES OF SYSTEMIC ANTIBACTERIAL DRUGS

Site of action	Drug class(es)
Cell wall	Penicillins Cephalosporins Carbapenems Monobactams Vancomycin β-lactamase inhibitors
Inhibit nucleic acid synthesis	Sulfonamides Trimethoprim
DNA gyrase	Quinolones
DNA strand breakage	Metronidazole
Ribosomal subunit	Aminoglycosides – 30S Tetracyclines – 30S Chloramphenicol – 50S Clindamycin – 50S Macrolides – 50S

Table 127.7 Sites of action of different classes of systemic antibacterial drugs.

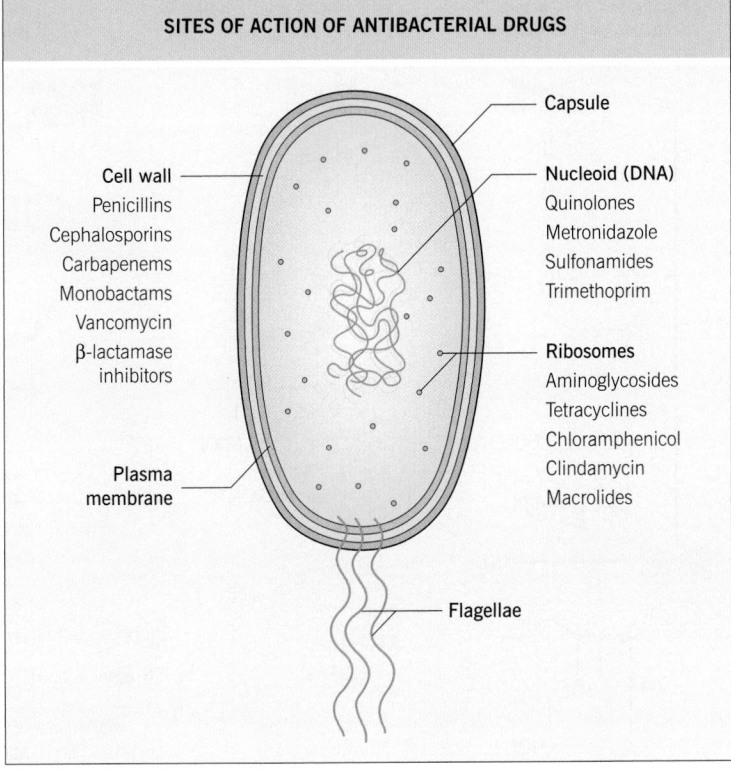

SITES OF ACTION OF ANTIBACTERIAL DRUGS

Capsule

Cell wall
Penicillins
Cephalosporins
Carbapenems
Monobactams
Vancomycin
β-lactamase inhibitors

Nucleoid (DNA)
Quinolones
Metronidazole
Sulfonamides
Trimethoprim

Ribosomes
Aminoglycosides
Tetracyclines
Chloramphenicol
Clindamycin
Macrolides

Plasma membrane

Flagellae

Fig. 127.1 Sites of action of antibacterial drugs. This figure illustrates a prototypical bacterial cell. Each class of antibacterial drug exerts its effect on a particular component of the cell.

Penicillins

Mechanism of action

Penicillins are β-lactam antibiotics that exert a bactericidal effect by binding to and inactivating penicillin-binding proteins in the bacterial cell wall. Their exact mechanism of action is not known, but they somehow inhibit the synthesis of the bacterial cell wall. One possibility is that penicillins inhibit the transpeptidase cross-linking of peptidoglycan chains, resulting in an unstable bacterial cell wall (Fig. 127.2).

The natural penicillins (penicillin G and penicillin V) are active against Gram-positive and Gram-negative cocci, most Gram-positive bacilli, and spirochetes. The penicillinase-resistant penicillins or anti-staphylococcal penicillins (methicillin, nafcillin and dicloxacillin) have greater efficacy against *S. aureus*. The aminopenicillins (ampicillin, amoxicillin) have an extended spectrum to include *H. influenzae*, *E. coli*, *Salmonella* and *Shigella* and some other Gram-negative bacteria, but not *Pseudomonas*. The antipseudomonal penicillins (carbenicillin, ticarcillin and piperacillin) cover *P. aeruginosa* and *B. fragilis*. Carbenicillin and ticarcillin have no activity against *Klebsiella*, whereas mezlocillin, azlocillin and piperacillin do. Addition of the β-lactamase inhibitors clavulanic acid, sulbactam and tazobactam extends the spectrum of penicillins to include staphylococci and other β-lactamase-producing bacteria (Fig. 127.3).

Indications

Penicillins are used for streptococcal skin infections such as blistering distal dactylitis and perianal dermatitis as well as erysipeloid and anthrax[32]. Amoxicillin with clavulanic acid is the drug of choice for cat, dog and human bites. It is useful also for acute paronychia. The penicillinase-resistant penicillins, e.g. dicloxacillin, are used for staphylococcal skin infections including impetigo, folliculitis and furunculosis, although the incidence of methicillin-resistant *Staphylococcus aureus* (MRSA) is rising and sensitivity testing should be obtained when MRSA is a clinical concern. Amoxicillin may be used for Lyme disease when tetracyclines are contraindicated. Penicillins are also used to treat non-cutaneous infections caused by susceptible bacteria,

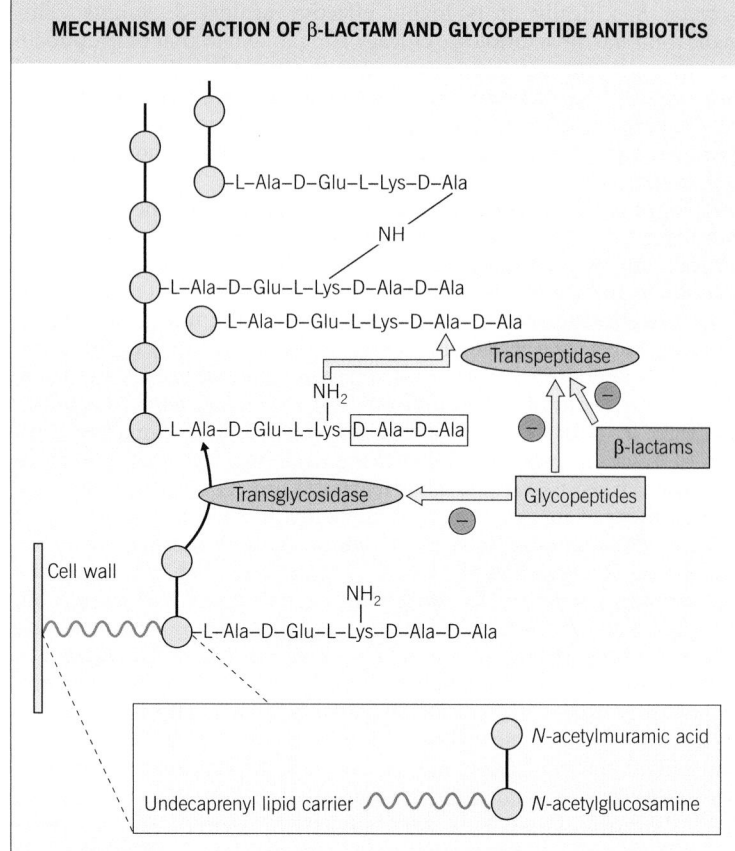

MECHANISM OF ACTION OF β-LACTAM AND GLYCOPEPTIDE ANTIBIOTICS

Fig. 127.2 Mechanism of action of β-lactam and glycopeptide antibiotics. Simplified schematic of probable mechanism of action of β-lactam antibiotics (penicillins, cephalosporins) and glycopeptides (e.g. vancomycin, dalbavancin) in interfering with enzymatic steps in bacterial cell wall (peptidoglycan) synthesis.

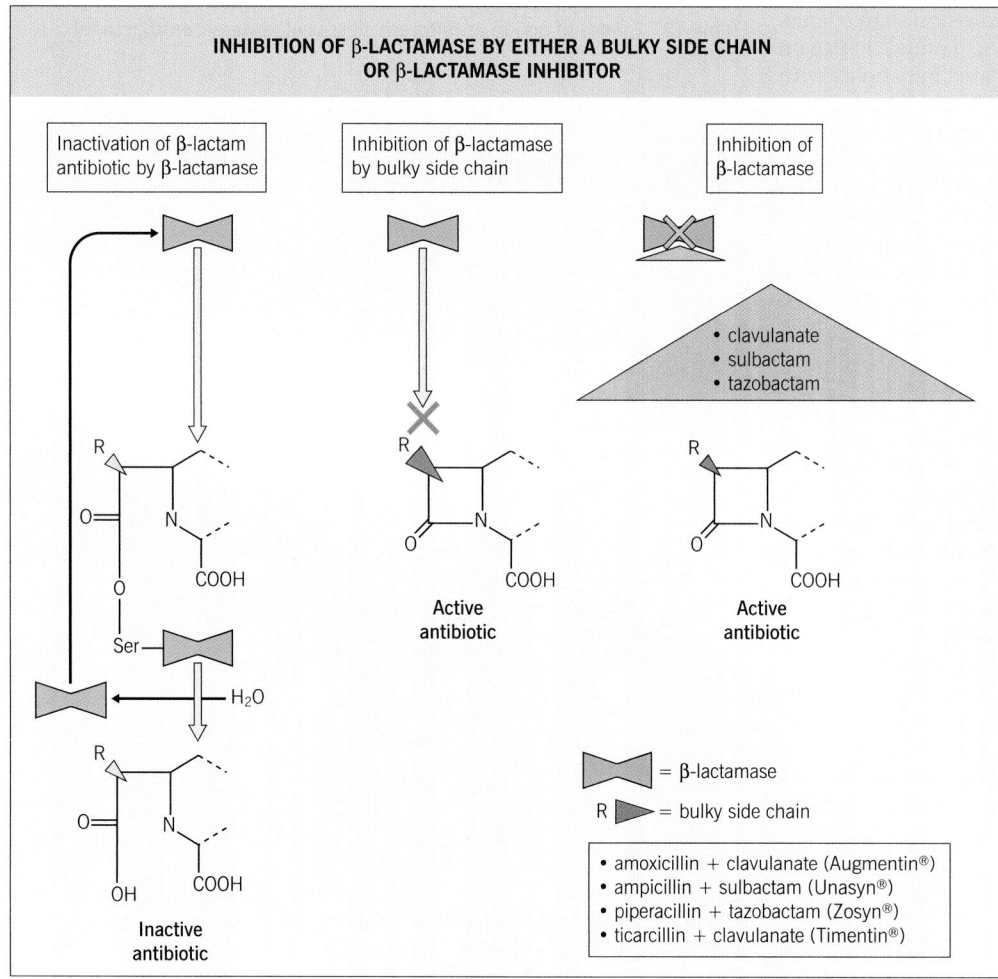

INHIBITION OF β-LACTAMASE BY EITHER A BULKY SIDE CHAIN OR β-LACTAMASE INHIBITOR

- amoxicillin + clavulanate (Augmentin®)
- ampicillin + sulbactam (Unasyn®)
- piperacillin + tazobactam (Zosyn®)
- ticarcillin + clavulanate (Timentin®)

Fig. 127.3 Inhibition of β-lactamase by either a bulky side chain or β-lactamase inhibitor. Placement of a bulky side chain (R▶) on the penicillin molecule (e.g. methicillin, nafcillin and dicloxacillin) can result in inhibition of bacterial β-lactamase, as can the combination of a penicillin with a β-lactamase inhibitor (e.g. clavulanic acid, sulbactam and tazobactam). The latter group of drugs has no inherent antibacterial activity. Inhibition of β-lactamase then allows the antibiotic to be active and inhibit bacterial transpeptidase.

including pneumonia, gonorrhea, syphilis, urinary tract infections, otitis media and sinusitis.

Dosages
The pediatric and adult dosages of commonly used penicillins are listed in Table 127.8. Amoxicillin and amoxicillin with clavulanic acid should be taken with food. Other penicillins should be taken on an empty stomach.

Contraindications
Penicillins are contraindicated in patients with a known hypersensitivity to any penicillin or other β-lactam antibiotic, in particular a history of urticaria, angioedema or anaphylaxis. A recent study found, however, that only 10% to 20% of patients reporting a history of allergy to penicillins had a true allergy proven by skin testing[33]. Benzylpenicilloyl polylysine, benzylpenicillin G, benzylpenicilloate and penicilloyl propylamine, as well as negative (saline) and positive (histamine) controls, are used to test for penicillin allergy. Antihistamines should be avoided prior to testing. Patients who have had a life-threatening reaction to penicillin should be tested with 100-fold dilutions of the allergens before being tested with full-strength allergens in a monitored setting where treatment for anaphylaxis is available. Epicutaneous (prick) testing may be performed by placing drops of antigen solutions on the volar forearm and using a 26-gauge needle to pierce the epidermis without drawing blood. An epicutaneous test is positive if, within 15 minutes, the average wheal diameter is 4 mm larger than the wheal of negative controls. For intradermal testing, antigen solutions and controls are injected in the volar forearm. An intradermal test is positive if, 15 minutes after injection, the average wheal diameter is at least 2 mm greater than the initial wheal size and is also at least 2 mm greater than the negative controls. Patients who report a history of penicillin allergy but are skin-test-negative to the entire battery of major (benzylpenicilloyl polylysine), minor (benzylpenicillin G and benzylpenicilloate and penicilloyl propylamine) allergens can use penicillin in a monitored setting. Skin-test-positive patients may be desensitized orally or intravenously in a hospital setting in about 4 hours. Rarely, serious IgE-mediated allergic reactions can occur. A radioallergosorbent test (RAST) may also be performed on a patient's blood to determine penicillin allergy. In general, RASTs are less sensitive and give less information than skin tests.

Major side effects
Drugs in the penicillin group cause hypersensitivity reactions characterized by urticaria, flushing and pruritus in 7% to 15% of patients. In severe cases, they may give rise to anaphylaxis, shock and death. Penicillins may also cause delayed hypersensitivity reactions with drug fever, eosinophilia and serum sickness-like reaction. Stevens–Johnson syndrome, toxic epidermal necrolysis, and pustular eruptions such as acute generalized exanthematous pustulosis are also potential side effects. These drugs sometimes lead to autoimmune phenomena, including hemolytic anemia or vasculitis. Ampicillin and amoxicillin almost invariably cause a diffuse morbilliform eruption when used in patients with infectious mononucleosis; this type of reaction is also

more likely in patients with lymphocytic leukemia or those who are taking concomitant allopurinol. When administered in high doses to patients with renal insufficiency, penicillins may lead to neurotoxicity with hyperirritability, confusion, seizures and coma. Rapid infusion, high blood levels or intrathecal injection may cause convulsions.

Penicillins can induce an acute interstitial nephritis characterized by proteinuria, hematuria, renal casts, eosinophilia, eosinophiluria, fever, arthralgias and declining renal function. Prolonged use of penicillins may lead to reversible neutropenia, anemia, agranulocytosis and platelet dysfunction. Penicillins can cause diarrhea, pseudomembranous colitis and hepatic dysfunction. For example, oxacillin and carbenicillin are associated with 'oxacillin hepatitis', an anicteric liver dysfunction with eosinophilia that may occur in as many as 15% of patients. Treatment with penicillins can lead to oral or vaginal overgrowth of *Candida* in over 10% of patients[34].

Interactions
Because probenecid blocks the secretion of penicillins in the distal renal tubules, concomitant administration of these two drugs increases the serum levels and duration of action of the penicillins. When amoxicillin or ampicillin is used with allopurinol, there is an increased risk of morbilliform drug eruption, and when tetracyclines are used with penicillins, the bactericidal effect of penicillins is decreased.

Pregnancy and lactation
Penicillins are grouped in pregnancy category B and are considered to be safe for use in nursing mothers.

Cephalosporins
Mechanism of action
Like the penicillins, the cephalosporins (Table 127.9) are bactericidal β-lactam antibiotics that bind to penicillin-binding proteins and interfere with bacterial cell wall synthesis. First-generation cephalosporins are very effective against Gram-positive organisms (staphylococci and streptococci) and less effective against Gram-negative organisms; however, they are active against *E. coli*, *Klebsiella* and *Proteus*. Second-generation cephalosporins are equally effective against Gram-positive and Gram-negative bacteria. Their spectrum includes all of the organisms covered by first-generation cephalosporins plus *Enterobacter*, *Neisseria gonorrhea* and *H. influenzae*. Third-generation cephalosporins are more effective against Gram-negative bacteria than Gram-positive bacteria. Fourth-generation cephalosporins have an extended spectrum for Gram-negative and Gram-positive organisms, but have minimal resistance to β-lactamase. They are active against *Enterobacter* and *Klebsiella*. Cephamycins are resistant to β-lactamase and have a broad spectrum, including *E. coli*, *Klebsiella*, *Proteus*, *Serratia* and *Bacteroides*.

Indications
Cephalosporins are useful in staphylococcal and streptococcal skin and soft tissue infections. Cephalexin is the cephalosporin of choice in uncomplicated skin infections[32]. These drugs are very useful for uncomplicated impetigo, cellulitis, furunculosis, erysipelas and ecthyma; however, strains of MRSA are resistant to cephalosporins as well.

Dosages
See Table 127.10 for dosages of the more commonly used cephalosporins.

Contraindications
Cephalosporins are contraindicated in patients with a history of hypersensitivity to this class of drugs. Approximately 15% of patients allergic to penicillins have cross-reactivity to cephalosporins (2% in pediatric patients)[35].

Major side effects
Cephalosporins may cause morbilliform eruptions, urticaria, anaphylaxis, drug fever, eosinophilia, and acute generalized exanthematous pustulosis. Cutaneous reactions are similar to those seen with the penicillins. Approximately 2% of patients allergic to cephalosporins cross-react with penicillins. Cefaclor has been reported to have a significantly higher rate of drug eruptions in children compared to other cephalosporins and other antibiotic classes[36]. Cephalosporins may also

DOSAGES OF COMMONLY USED PENICILLINS

Generic name	Pediatric dosage	Adult dosage
Penicillin V potassium	25–50 mg/kg/day divided q6–8 h	250–500 mg qid
Dicloxacillin	12.5–50 mg/kg/day divided q6 h	125–500 mg qid
Ampicillin	50–100 mg/kg/day divided q6 h	250–500 mg qid
Amoxicillin	20–40 mg/kg/day divided q8 h	250–500 mg bid
Amoxicillin/ clavulanate	20–40 mg/kg/day (of amoxicillin) divided q8 h or q12 h*	500–875 mg bid

Table 127.8 Dosages of commonly used penicillins. *Do not double the dose of clavulanate if you double the amoxicillin dose, as this causes excessive clavulanate dosage and increased risk of GI side effects like diarrhea.

DIFFERENT CLASSES OF CEPHALOSPORINS AND ROUTES OF ADMINISTRATION

Generic name	Trade name(s)®	Route(s) of administration
First generation		
Cefadroxil	Duracef, Ultracef	po
Cefazolin	Ancef, Kefzol, Zolicef	im, iv
Cephalexin	Keflex, Keftab, Biocef	po
Cephalothin	Keflin, Seffin	im, iv
Cephapirin	Cefadyl	im, iv
Cephradine	Velosef, Anspor	po, im, iv
Second generation		
Cefaclor	Ceclor, Ceclor CD	po
Cefamandole	Mandol	im, iv
Cefmetazole	Zefazone	iv
Cefonicid	Monocid	im, iv
Cefprozil	Cefzil	po
Cefuroxime sodium	Zinacef, Kefurox	im, iv
Cefuroxime axetil	Ceftin	po
Loracarbef (a carbacephem)	Lorabid	po
Third generation		
Cefdinir	Omnicef	po
Cefixime	Suprax	po
Cefoperazone	Cefobid	im, iv
Cefotaxime	Claforan	im, iv
Cefpodoxime proxetil	Vantin	po
Ceftazidime	Ceptaz, Fortaz, Tazidime, Tazicef	im, iv
Ceftibuten	Cedax	po
Ceftizoxime	Cefizox	im, iv
Ceftriaxone	Rocephin	im, iv
Fourth generation		
Cefepime	Maxipime	im, iv
Cephamycins		
Cefoxitin	Mefoxin	im, iv
Cefotetan	Cefotan	im, iv

Table 127.9 Different classes of cephalosporins and routes of administration.

DOSAGES OF COMMONLY PRESCRIBED CEPHALOSPORINS

Generic name	Pediatric dosage	Adult dosage
Cephalexin	25–100 mg/kg/day divided q6 h or q12 h	250–500 mg qid
Cefadroxil	30 mg/kg/day divided q12 h	1–2 g qd
Cefaclor	40 mg/kg/day divided q8 h or q12 h	250–500 mg tid
Loracarbef	15–30 mg/kg/day divided q12 h	200–400 mg bid
Cefprozil	30 mg/kg/day divided q12 h	250–500 mg qd
Cefuroxime axetil	20–30 mg/kg/day divided q12 h	250–500 mg bid
Cefpodoxime proxetil	10 mg/kg/day divided q12 h	100–400 mg bid
Ceftibuten	9 mg/kg/day divided q24 h	400 mg qd
Cefixime	8 mg/kg/day divided q12 h or q24 h	200 mg bid or 400 mg qd
Ceftriaxone	50 mg/kg im × 1 (max. 1 g)	1–4 g im qd; 250 mg im × 1 for uncomplicated gonorrhea
Cefdinir	14 mg/kg/day divided q12 h or q24 h	300 mg bid or 600 mg qd

Table 127.10 Dosages of commonly prescribed cephalosporins.

safety has not been definitively established. Cephalosporins are excreted in breast milk.

Sulfonamides and co-trimoxazole
Mechanism of action
Sulfamethoxazole, sulfasalazine and sulfisoxazole are sulfonamides which compete with para-aminobenzoic acid (PABA) to be the substrate for the enzyme dihydropteroate synthetase (Fig. 127.4). Dihydropteroate synthetase catalyzes the reaction that combines pteridine precursors

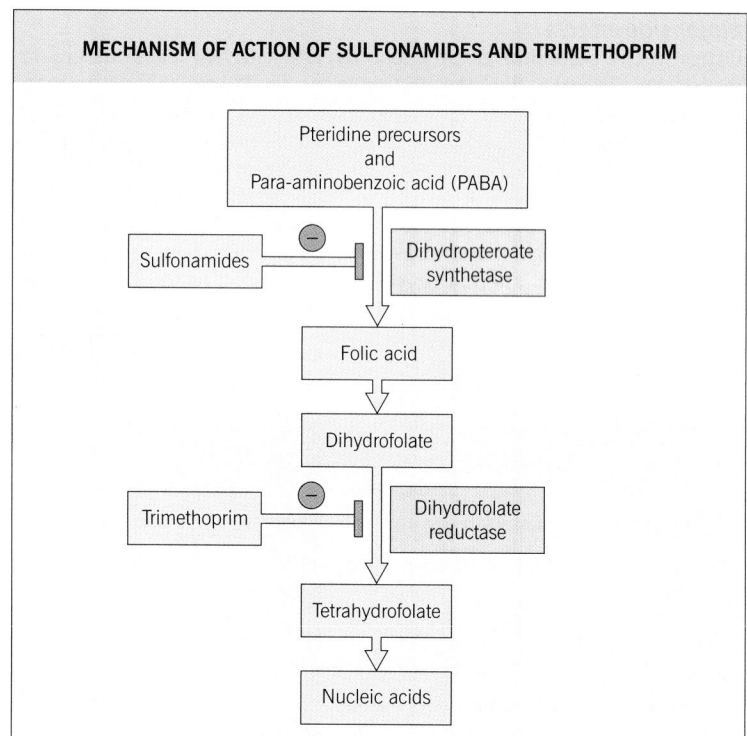

MECHANISM OF ACTION OF SULFONAMIDES AND TRIMETHOPRIM

Fig. 127.4 Mechanism of action of sulfonamides and trimethoprim. Sulfonamides inhibit the conversion of pteridine precursors and PABA to folic acid by dihydropteroate synthetase. Trimethoprim inhibits the conversion of dihydrofolate to tetrahydrofolate by dihydrofolate reductase. The end result of both actions is inhibition of bacterial nucleic acid synthesis.

lead to neutropenia, thrombocytopenia, hemolytic anemia and a positive direct Coombs test, especially in the setting of renal insufficiency. When given orally, they can also cause diarrhea, nausea and pseudomembranous colitis. Certain cephalosporins with a methylthiotetrazoleside group can cause a disulfiram-like effect when alcohol is ingested concomitantly and have antivitamin K effects leading to an enhanced risk of bleeding (e.g. cefotetan, cefoperazone, cefamandole).

Interactions
Oral cephalosporins administered in conjunction with aminoglycosides can lead to increased nephrotoxicity. Probenecid may decrease renal clearance of cephalosporin. Antacids, didanosine and proton pump inhibitors may decrease absorption of some oral cephalosporins, e.g. cefuroxime.

Pregnancy and lactation
Cephalosporins are in FDA pregnancy category B. They have not shown any adverse effects during pregnancy or lactation. However, their

with PABA to make folic acid. Thus, sulfonamides prevent the synthesis of bacterial folic acid, an essential cofactor for bacterial nucleic acid synthesis. They have a bacteriostatic effect against Gram-positive bacteria (including *S. aureus* and *S. pyogenes*), Gram-negative bacteria, *Chlamydia* and *Nocardia*.

Co-trimoxazole is a synergistic combination of sulfamethoxazole and trimethoprim. It blocks two consecutive steps in the biosynthesis of bacterial nucleic acids (see Fig. 127.4). The sulfonamide inhibits dihydropteroate synthetase and trimethoprim blocks the action of dihydrofolate reductase, which normally converts dihydrofolate to tetrahydrofolate (the active form of folic acid). This combination may be bactericidal or bacteriostatic depending on the concentration of the drug and the susceptibility of the infecting organism. It is active against most Gram-positive organisms and Gram-negative organisms.

Indications

Systemic sulfonamides are indicated for uncomplicated urinary tract infections. They are also used for *Chlamydia* conjunctivitis and *Nocardia* infections. Sulfasalazine is commonly prescribed for ulcerative colitis. Co-trimoxazole is used to treat respiratory tract, prostate, urinary tract and gastrointestinal infections, as well as to treat, and as prophylaxis against, *Pneumocystis jiroveci* pneumonia. The latter indication is for patients who are immunosuppressed, e.g. as a result of HIV infection or systemic medications. Co-trimoxazole is also used for superficial skin infections, inflammatory acne vulgaris recalcitrant to other antibacterial agents, cat scratch disease, and granuloma inguinale.

Dosages

In pediatric patients, sulfadiazine and sulfisoxazole are given as 120–150 mg/kg/day divided every 4 to every 6 hours. One double-strength capsule of co-trimoxazole contains 160 mg of trimethoprim and 800 mg of sulfamethoxazole, and in adults is given twice a day. In children, the dose is 6–12 mg/kg of trimethoprim and 30–60 mg/kg of sulfamethoxazole every 12 hours.

Contraindications

The sulfonamides and co-trimoxazole are contraindicated in patients with a history of hypersensitivity to this class of medications. Sulfonamides are contraindicated in the third trimester of pregnancy and in lactating patients (see below). They are also contraindicated in patients with porphyria. Sulfonamides may precipitate an acute attack of pseudoporphyria or true porphyria. The mechanism by which they do this is unclear. They may cause hepatocellular damage or increase cytochrome P450 activity or inhibit liver enzymes, thereby increasing the production of porphyrins. Co-trimoxazole is contraindicated in patients with megaloblastic anemia, folate deficiency or G6PD deficiency. It should be used cautiously in patients with impaired hepatic or renal function and in patients with bone marrow suppression.

Major side effects

The sulfonamides and co-trimoxazole may cause fixed drug or morbilliform eruptions, urticaria, angioedema, photosensitivity, Stevens–Johnson syndrome, toxic epidermal necrolysis, exfoliative erythroderma and vasculitis. Additional cutaneous side effects include acute generalized exanthematous pustulosis, Sweet's syndrome, linear IgA bullous dermatosis, erythema nodosum and radiation recall. In HIV-infected patients, these drugs are common causes of cutaneous eruptions. Non-cutaneous side effects include hemolytic anemia in the setting of G6PD deficiency, agranulocytosis, thrombocytopenia, eosinophilia, methemoglobinemia, nephrotoxicity, hepatotoxicity, neurotoxicity, and kernicterus in newborns. Co-trimoxazole may also cause nausea, vomiting, glossitis and stomatitis, as well as dizziness and headaches. Trimethoprim (alone or in combination with sulfamethoxazole) can induce a folate deficiency with megaloblastic anemia, leukopenia and granulocytopenia. It can also cause thrombocytopenia. Giving folinic acid, which does not impair antibacterial activity because it does not enter bacteria, can reverse all of the effects of folate deficiency.

Interactions

The sulfonamides and co-trimoxazole can potentiate the effects of oral hypoglycemics and the anticoagulant effect of warfarin. They should not be used in patients on methenamine for urinary tract infections. Sulfonamides decrease protein binding and renal clearance of methotrexate, leading to potentially life-threatening methotrexate myelosuppression toxicity. Monoamine oxidase (MAO) inhibitors and probenecid may increase sulfonamide adverse effects through altered hepatic metabolism and renal clearance, respectively.

Pregnancy and lactation

Co-trimoxazole must be avoided during pregnancy and lactation and for the first 2 months of life. The sulfonamides and co-trimoxazole are in pregnancy category C during the first two trimesters owing to their inhibition of folic acid, but they are in category D during the third trimester owing to the increased risk of kernicterus. Systemic sulfonamides are excreted in breast milk, and may cause hepatic toxicity, anemia and other adverse effects in nursing infants.

Macrolides
Mechanism of action

Macrolides are bacteriostatic and inhibit bacterial protein synthesis by binding to the 50S ribosomal subunit. Erythromycin is effective against Gram-positive and Gram-negative cocci, most Gram-positive bacilli, and spirochetes. Clarithromycin has an expanded spectrum that includes *H. influenzae* and *Moraxella catarrhalis*. Azithromycin also covers *H. influenzae*. Clarithromycin and azithromycin are both effective against atypical mycobacteria, *Toxoplasma gondii*, *Treponema pallidum* and *Borrelia burgdorferi*.

Indications

Macrolides are commonly used for staphylococcal and streptococcal skin infections as they often represent a suitable treatment alternative for patients allergic to penicillin. However, there are regions where a significant percentage of *S. aureus* isolates are erythromycin-resistant. Erythromycin may be used for inflammatory acne, erythrasma, pitted keratolysis, bacillary angiomatosis and cat scratch disease. For several venereal diseases, e.g. chancroid, lymphogranuloma venereum, chlamydia and granuloma inguinale, it represents an alternative therapy.

Erythromycin has been used for both the acute and chronic forms of pityriasis lichenoides. Macrolides are also indicated for pharyngitis, bacterial respiratory infections (including *Mycoplasma* pneumonia and Legionnaire's disease), diphtheria, pertussis and disseminated *Mycobacterium avium-intracellulare* complex treatment and prophylaxis.

Dosages

Table 127.11 outlines the dosages for commonly prescribed macrolides. Erythromycin base should be taken on an empty stomach, while the other formulations should be taken with food.

DOSAGES OF COMMONLY USED MACROLIDES		
Generic name	**Oral pediatric dosage**	**Oral adult dosage**
Azithromycin	20 mg/kg once or 5 mg/kg/day Maximum 1 g/day	Bacterial infections: 500 mg on day 1, then 250 mg qd on days 2–5 Chancroid: 1 g once
Clarithromycin	15 mg/kg qd divided q12 h Maximum 1 g/day Adjust for decreased renal function	500 mg qd Adjust for decreased renal function
Erythromycin base	30–50 mg/kg qd divided q6–8 h Maximum 2 g/day	250–500 mg qid or 333 mg tid or 500 mg bid
Erythromycin estolate	20–50 mg/kg qd divided q6–12 h Maximum 2 g/day	250–500 mg q6–12 h
Erythromycin ethyl succinate	20–50 mg/kg qd divided q8–12 h	400 mg qid
Erythromycin stearate	20–50 mg/kg qd divided q6 h	250–500 mg q6–12 h

Table 127.11 Dosages of commonly used macrolides.

Contraindications

Macrolides are contraindicated in patients with hepatic dysfunction, renal dysfunction (clarithromycin) and in patients with hypersensitivity to the drug. Macrolides are contraindicated in patients taking terfenadine, astemizole or cisapride (three drugs which have been removed from the US market and are either banned or severely restricted in many other countries).

Major side effects

Erythromycin is one of the least toxic antibiotics. However, gastrointestinal intolerance characterized by nausea, vomiting and abdominal cramping may limit its use. Hypersensitivity reactions are unusual. Erythromycin estolate may cause intrahepatic cholestasis in adults, and this risk increases during pregnancy. Less common side effects include stomatitis, jaundice, transient deafness and cardiac arrhythmias. Pustular eruptions such as generalized exanthematous pustulosis may occur with the macrolides, as well as Stevens–Johnson syndrome, toxic epidermal necrolysis, urticaria and vasculitis.

Interactions

Macrolides have numerous significant drug interactions. Due to CYP3A4 inhibition (see Ch.131), macrolides increase the risk of *torsades de pointes* when used with grepafloxacin, sparfloxacin, terfenadine, astemizole or cisapride. By the same mechanism, macrolides increase serum levels and potential toxicity of anticonvulsants, benzodiazepines, buspirone, corticosteroids, warfarin, HMG-CoA reductase inhibitors, oral contraceptives, cyclosporine, tacrolimus, disopyramide, felodipine and ergot alkaloids. Macrolides may increase serum levels of theophylline by inhibiting CYP1A2, leading to cardiac arrhythmias. Macrolides may also increase digoxin levels by altering gut flora, which metabolize digoxin.

Clarithromycin administered in conjunction with calcium channel blockers carries an increased risk for bradycardia and hypotension. Erythromycin used concomitantly with lovastatin has been reported to cause rhabdomyolysis. Macrolides may interfere with the effectiveness of chloramphenicol or clindamycin (see below), and antacids can decrease the absorption of azithromycin. Clarithromycin levels may be increased when this drug is administered with fluconazole, hexobarbital, alfentanil, disopyramide or bromocriptine. Of note, azithromycin has improved gastrointestinal tolerance and little potential for significant metabolism-based drug interactions[37].

Pregnancy and lactation

Erythromycin and azithromycin are in FDA pregnancy category B; clarithromycin is category C. The macrolides are generally considered safe during pregnancy, except for erythromycin estolate. This drug is contraindicated in pregnancy owing to the risk of maternal cholestatic hepatitis. The latter may represent a hypersensitivity reaction to the estolate component and it may be accompanied by fever, leukocytosis and eosinophilia in addition to findings related to liver disease (nausea, vomiting, abdominal pain, jaundice, liver enzyme abnormalities); occasionally, a cutaneous eruption is seen.

Tetracyclines
Mechanism of action

Tetracyclines (Table 127.12) inhibit bacterial protein synthesis by binding to the 30S ribosomal subunit. They are mainly bacteriostatic, but may be bactericidal at high concentrations. Tetracyclines are active against most bacteria, *Rickettsia*, *Chlamydia* and *Mycoplasma*. However, they are not active against *Proteus* species or *P. aeruginosa*.

Indications

Tetracyclines are indicated for acne vulgaris, rosacea and perioral dermatitis, as well as rickettsial infections (Rocky Mountain spotted fever, rickettsialpox, typhus, Q fever and trench fever), Lyme disease and ehrlichiosis. They are used in syphilis (in penicillin-allergic patients), granuloma inguinale, chlamydial infections (lymphogranuloma venereum, psittacosis), non-gonococcal urethritis and actinomycosis, in addition to brucellosis, pulmonary infections (e.g. *Mycoplasma* pneumonia) and cholera. Tetracyclines are also useful for treating infections due to *Vibrio vulnificus* or *Mycobacterium marinum*. High-dose tetracycline is used in conjunction with nicotinamide for bullous pemphigoid.

DOSAGES AND ROUTES OF ADMINISTRATION OF THE TETRACYCLINES			
Generic name	**Trade name(s)®**	**Routes of administration**	**Adult dosage**
Demeclocycline	Declomycin	po	300 mg q12 h
Doxycycline hydrate	Vibramycin, Doryx, Vibra-Tabs, Periostat	po	50 mg qd–100 mg q12 h
Doxycycline monohydrate	Monodox, Oracea*, Adoxa	po	50 mg qd–100 mg q12 h
Minocycline	Minocin, Dynacin, Vectrin, Solodyn	po	50 mg qd–100 mg q12 h
Oxytetracycline	Terramycin	po, im	500 mg q6 h
Tetracycline	Sumycin, Achromycin, Robitet, Panmycin	po, iv	250–1500 mg/day in divided doses

Table 127.12 Dosages and routes of administration of the tetracyclines. *40 mg qd.

Dosages

Tetracycline should be taken 1 hour before or 2 hours after meals. Doxycycline and minocycline may be taken with or without food. To try to avoid esophagitis, the pills should not be 'dry swallowed' and should be taken at least half an hour prior to bedtime. Table 127.12 lists the dosages of more commonly prescribed tetracyclines.

Contraindications

Tetracyclines should not be used in patients under 8 years of age (to avoid tooth discoloration) or in pregnant women. All tetracyclines except doxycycline should be avoided in patients with renal impairment, because they can accumulate; doxycycline has a compensatory gastrointestinal secretion.

Major side effects

Common side effects of tetracyclines include gastrointestinal upset, phototoxicity (especially doxycycline) and vaginal candidiasis. Minocycline may cause dizziness and bluish discoloration of scars (including those due to acne) and normal skin (in particular the lower extremities)[32]. Gray to blue–gray discoloration of the oral mucosa, sclerae, nails and teeth can also occur, as can black pigmentation of the thyroid gland. Deposition of tetracyclines in the teeth and bones occurs in children, causing discoloration and hypoplasia of the teeth and occasionally temporarily stunting growth.

Tetracyclines (especially minocycline) may cause hypersensitivity reactions, including urticaria, which can be accompanied by pneumonitis[38]; perhaps these reactions are seen more frequently in black patients[39]. Tetracyclines may also cause serum sickness-like reactions, esophageal ulcerations, infectious enterocolitis, blood dyscrasias, a pseudotumor cerebri-like syndrome (especially when given with retinoids or vitamin A), nephrotoxicity, nephrogenic diabetes insipidus and even fatal hepatotoxicity. Of all the tetracyclines, minocycline has been associated more often with more serious adverse events, including drug-induced lupus[40] and polyarteritis nodosa. These latter drug reactions may be seen after months or years of therapy.

Interactions

Food decreases the absorption of tetracycline by about 50%. Therefore, tetracycline should be taken 1 hour before or 2 hours after a meal. Minocycline and doxycycline may be taken with food to diminish gastrointestinal upset caused by these medications. Absorption of tetracyclines is impaired by polyvalent cations such as calcium, aluminum, magnesium, iron, zinc and bismuth. Thus, antacids, some laxatives, medications containing magnesium (e.g. quinapril), dietary supplements and dairy products may inhibit absorption of tetracyclines. Antacids, H_2 blockers and proton pump inhibitors increase stomach pH and thereby decrease tetracycline absorption. Tetracyclines increase the serum levels and potential toxicity of digoxin, lithium and warfarin, whereas they can reduce insulin requirements. Barbiturates, hydantoins and carbamazepine will decrease the half-life of doxycycline. Bacteriostatic tetracyclines may interfere with the effectiveness of bactericidal penicillins.

Pregnancy and lactation
Systemic tetracyclines should not be used during pregnancy or lactation because they cross the placenta and are excreted in breast milk. They cause staining of the deciduous teeth and enamel hypoplasia and may impair skeletal growth in developing fetuses and in nursing infants[41]. They are designated pregnancy category D.

Clindamycin
Mechanism of action
Clindamycin is a lincosamide that suppresses bacterial protein synthesis by binding to the bacterial 50S ribosomal subunit. It is active against Gram-positive cocci including *S. aureus*, *Streptococcus pneumoniae*, *Str. pyogenes*, *Str. viridans* and anaerobic streptococci. It is not active against enterococci. Clindamycin is active against anaerobes including peptostreptococci, peptococci, *Bacteroides* species and fusobacteria.

Indications
Clindamycin is indicated in infections caused by susceptible bacteria, including anaerobic abscesses, chlamydial infections and bacterial vaginosis. Clindamycin is also used for skin infections including impetigo, cellulitis, folliculitis, furunculosis and ecthyma. It may also be useful in necrotizing fasciitis.

Dosages
Clindamycin is formulated for oral, intravenous and intramuscular administration. It is typically dosed from 150 to 450 mg four times a day.

Contraindications
Clindamycin is contraindicated in patients with hypersensitivity to the drug and in patients with colitis.

Major side effects
Clindamycin carries a relatively high risk of pseudomembranous colitis. Studies have reported rates from 0.1% to 10%[42–44]. It occasionally increases serum levels of liver enzymes. Clindamycin may also cause hypersensitivity reactions, especially in HIV-positive patients. It may cause transient neutropenia or thrombocytopenia and eosinophilia and possible neuromuscular blockade. Stevens–Johnson syndrome rarely occurs.

Interactions
Clindamycin binds at or near the sites of binding of erythromycin and chloramphenicol. These drugs should not be used concomitantly. It may potentiate the neuromuscular effect of botulinum toxin or neuromuscular blockers.

Pregnancy and lactation
Clindamycin is in pregnancy category B. There are no known adverse effects of systemic clindamycin on the developing fetus. In rat and mouse studies, oral and subcutaneous clindamycin have not been shown to cause birth defects or other problems. Clindamycin may modify the bowel flora of nursing infants and may interfere with the interpretation of bacterial culture results obtained during a fever evaluation of a nursing infant.

Quinolones
Mechanism of action
Quinolones are rapidly bactericidal by inhibiting DNA gyrase (topoisomerase II). They are active against Gram-negative aerobes, staphylococci and streptococci, but are not active against anaerobes.

Table 127.13 lists the drugs in this class.

Indications
Quinolones are indicated for sinusitis, acute exacerbations of chronic bronchitis, community acquired pneumonia, urinary tract infections, gastrointestinal infections, chlamydia, osteomyelitis, and skin and soft tissue infections. Second-generation quinolones (ciprofloxacin, ofloxacin,

QUINOLONES		
Generic name	**Trade name(s)®**	**Routes of administration**
Alatrofloxacin	Trovan IV	iv, im
Ciprofloxacin	Cipro	po, iv
Enoxacin	Penetrex	po
Gatifloxacin*	Tequin	po, iv
Levofloxacin	Levaquin	po, iv
Lomefloxacin	Maxaquin	po
Moxifloxacin	Avelox	po
Norfloxacin	Chibroxin, Noroxin	po
Ofloxacin	Floxin	po, iv
Sparfloxacin	Zagam	po
Trovafloxacin*	Trovan	po, iv
Withdrawn from US market.		

Table 127.13 Quinolones.

enoxacin, lomefloxacin and norfloxacin) have good coverage of Gram-negative rods and some Gram-positive coverage. They are the most potent antipseudomonal quinolones. Third-generation quinolones (levofloxacin, gatifloxacin and sparfloxacin) are broad spectrum, with coverage of Gram-negative rods and greater Gram-positive cocci coverage, especially of *Pneumococcus*. Fourth-generation quinolones (alatrofloxacin, moxifloxacin and trovafloxacin) are very broad spectrum, with coverage of Gram-negative rods, Gram-positive cocci, anaerobes and atypical bacteria. They cover streptococcus and methicillin-susceptible *S. aureus*. They have minimal antipseudomonal activity.

Dosages
Ciprofloxacin and levofloxacin are dosed at 250 to 750 mg twice a day. Quinolones must be adjusted for renal impairment. The safety of quinolones in pediatric patients has not been established. However, ciprofloxacin has been given to children at doses of 20–30 mg/kg per day in divided doses (q12h).

Contraindications
Quinolones are contraindicated in pregnancy and in patients with QT prolongation or hypokalemia. Historically, quinolones have been contraindicated in patients under 18 years of age because of a potential risk for producing arthropathy. However, quinolones have been used to treat pediatric cystic fibrosis patients, with only mild and reversible joint changes observed[45].

Major side effects
In studies involving juvenile animals, quinolones can damage cartilage in weight-bearing joints[46]. Quinolones may cause gastrointestinal upset, changes in taste, abnormal liver function tests, nephrotoxicity, headache, dizziness, lightheadedness, drowsiness and, rarely, increased intracranial pressure and seizures. Rupture of tendons, in particular the Achilles tendon, has been rarely observed.

Interactions
Cations (e.g. calcium, aluminum, magnesium, iron and zinc salts) as well as antacids and sucralfate prevent absorption of quinolones and thereby reduce serum levels. Quinolones increase serum levels and potential toxicities of caffeine, theophylline and aminophylline due to CYP1A2 inhibition. They may also increase serum levels of warfarin, increasing the INR. Quinolones used in combination with cyclosporine may increase serum creatinine levels in transplant patients. Quinolones can also increase circulating levels of procainamide by decreasing renal clearance of this drug.

Quinolones should be used with caution in patients who are taking antiarrhythmics, erythromycin, antipsychotics, tricyclic antidepressants or other drugs that cause QT prolongation or lower seizure threshold.

NEW ANTIBACTERIAL AGENTS				
Generic name	Trade name(s)®	Formulations	Indications and dosing	FDA pregnancy category
Daptomycin	Cubicin	iv	Complicated skin infections: 4 mg/kg iv q24 h × 7–14 days Adjust dose for renal or hepatic impairment	B
Linezolid	Zyvox	600 mg tablet 100 mg/5 ml oral suspension iv	Uncomplicated skin infections: 400 mg po q12 h × 10–14 days MRSA or complicated skin infections: 600 mg iv or po q12 h × 10–28 days Adjust dose for renal impairment	C
Quinupristin/dalfopristin	Synercid	iv	Serious skin infections due to *S. aureus* or *S. pyogenes*: 7.5 mg/kg iv q12 h	B
Tigecycline	Tygacil	iv	Complicated skin infections: 50 mg iv q12 h × 5–14 days Adjust dose for hepatic impairment	D

Table 127.14 New antibacterial agents. MRSA, methicillin-resistant *Staphylococcus aureus*.

They may increase seizure risk if administered with non-steroidal anti-inflammatory drugs. Gatifloxacin may cause hypoglycemia when used with sulfonylureas.

Pregnancy and lactation
Quinolones are designated pregnancy category C. They should not be used during pregnancy or nursing because of the arthropathy found in animal studies.

Metronidazole
Mechanism of action
Metronidazole is an imidazole. Its mechanism of action is not completely understood, but may be due to DNA strand breaking.

Indications
In addition to its antiprotozoal actions, metronidazole has activity against anaerobic cocci (including *Peptococcus* and *Peptostreptococcus*), anaerobic Gram-negative bacilli (including *Bacteroides* and *Fusobacterium* species) and anaerobic Gram-positive bacilli (including *Clostridium*). It is indicated for trichomoniasis, amebiasis and anaerobic bacterial infections. Metronidazole has been used for skin and soft tissue infections, oral and dental infections, intra-abdominal, pelvic and brain abscesses, anaerobic pulmonary infections and osteomyelitis. It can be used in combination with a broad-spectrum β-lactamase inhibitor–penicillin combination to treat Fournier's gangrene. Metronidazole is also used to treat giardiasis, New World mucocutaneous leishmaniasis and bacterial vaginosis.

Dosages
Metronidazole is available for oral and intravenous administration. For bacterial infections, it is given as 500 mg orally every 6 to 8 hours for 7 to 14 days. For bacterial vaginosis or trichomoniasis, a single 2 g dose is given or 500 mg may be taken twice a day for 7 days. The pediatric dose is 30 mg/kg/day in divided doses every 6 hours.

Contraindications
Metronidazole is contraindicated in patients with prior hypersensitivity to the drug and also during the first trimester of pregnancy. It should be used with caution in patients with impaired liver function.

Major side effects
Metronidazole may cause a morbilliform eruption, pruritus, fever, gastrointestinal disturbances, a metallic taste and xerostomia, in addition to thrombophlebitis, transient leukopenia, dark urine and neurologic symptoms (e.g. headache, confusion, syncope, seizures, sensory neuropathy).

Interactions
Metronidazole increases circulating levels of cyclosporine, tacrolimus and phenytoin; it may increase the anticoagulant effect of warfarin. Metronidazole can cause a disulfiram-like reaction when combined with ethanol or with protease inhibitors, and administration of metronidazole with disulfiram may precipitate psychosis. Metronidazole may increase the risk of neuropathy due to reverse transcriptase inhibitors.

Pregnancy and lactation
Metronidazole is pregnancy category B. It has been shown to be teratogenic in rodents, but there are no known adverse effects of systemic metronidazole on the developing fetus. It is contraindicated during the first trimester of pregnancy based on reported cases of fetal malformation in women exposed to metronidazole, despite the fact that there has never been a reported increase in the overall risk of birth defects. Metronidazole should be used with caution in nursing women because of reports of mutagenesis and carcinogenesis in some species.

New Antibacterial Agents
Linezolid and quinupristin/dalfopristin are useful in serious staphylococcal and streptococcal skin infections, including MRSA. Both inhibit bacterial protein synthesis. Daptomycin is a cyclic lipopeptide used for complicated skin infections. It kills bacteria by binding to and depolarizing bacterial cell membranes, inhibiting protein and nucleic acid synthesis. Tigecycline interferes with protein synthesis by binding to the 30S ribosomal subunit and is also used in complicated skin infections. Table 127.14 lists these newer antibacterials and their dosages and indications.

ANTIFUNGAL AGENTS

Superficial dermatophytoses usually respond to topical therapy. Topical antifungal agents are outlined in Table 127.15. With topical medications, there is less potential for major side effects, and many of these products are available without a prescription. Fungal infections of the hair and nails as well as systemic mycoses generally necessitate treatment with systemic antifungal medications. Furthermore, patients who are immunocompromised or who have extensive skin involvement will likely require systemic treatment. Sometimes even in immunocompetent patients, systemic antifungal therapy is necessary for superficial infections resistant to topical treatments[47].

Mechanisms of action
The mechanisms of action of the antifungal agents are outlined in Table 127.16 and illustrated in Figures 127.5 and 127.6.

Imidazole and triazole antifungal drugs inhibit C-14-α-demethylation of lanosterol to 14-demethyl-lanosterol by 14-α-demethylase. This reaction is normally catalyzed by and dependent on cytochrome P450. Imidazoles bind to a heme iron on cytochrome P450, blocking the binding of oxygen necessary for activation of the molecule. This results in the accumulation of 14-α-methyl sterols and prohibits the synthesis of ergosterol, a fungal cell membrane steroid needed for normal permeability and structural integrity. Most azoles are fungistatic, although some are fungicidal at very high concentrations. Additionally, miconazole affects triglyceride and fatty acid synthesis and inhibits fungal oxidative and peroxidase enzymes[48].

Allylamines and benzylamines are fungistatic by inhibiting squalene epoxidase, thereby inhibiting ergosterol biosynthesis and disrupting fungal cell membrane synthesis. Moreover, the resultant accumulation of intracellular squalene is fungicidal. Unlike imidazoles, the activity of allylamines is not dependent on cytochrome P450.

	TOPICAL ANTIFUNGAL AGENTS			
Generic name	Trade name(s)®	Formulation(s)	FDA pregnancy category	OTC/Rx
Imidazoles				
Butoconazole	Femstat-3, Gynazole-1, Mycelex-3	2% vaginal cream	C	OTC
Clotrimazole	Canesten, Clotrimaderm, Cruex, Desenex AF, FemCare, Gyne-Lotrimin, Lotrimin, Lotrimin AF, Mycelex, Mycelex Troches, Myclo, Myclo-Gyne, Neo-Zol	1% lotion, solution, cream, aerosol solution, lozenges, troches, powder	B	OTC, Rx
Econazole	Spectazole, Ecostatin	1% cream	C	Rx
Ketoconazole	Nizoral, Nizoral AD	1% and 2% cream, shampoo	C	OTC, Rx
Miconazole	Femizole-M, Micatin, Micozole, Monistat, Monistat-Derm, Zeasorb AF	2% cream, lotion, powder, aerosol powder, aerosol solution	C	OTC
Oxiconazole	Derimine, Myfungar, Oceral, Oceral GB, Okinazole, Oxistat, Oxizole	1% cream, lotion	B	Rx
Sertaconazole	Ertaczo	2% cream	C	Rx
Sulconazole	Exelderm, Sulcosyn	1% cream, solution	C	Rx
Terconazole	Fungistat, Fungistat 3, Fungistat 5, Byno-Terazol, Cyno-Terazol 3, Terazol, Terazol 3, Terazol 7, Tercospor	0.4% and 0.8% vaginal cream, 80 mg vaginal suppositories	C	Rx
Tioconazole	GyneCure, Monistat 1, Trosyd AF, Trosyd J, Vagistat 1	20% nail lacquer, 6.5% vaginal cream, ointment	C	OTC
Allylamines				
Naftifine	Naftin	1% cream, gel	B	Rx
Terbinafine	Lamisil, Lamifen	1% cream, solution, aerosol solution	B	OTC
Benzylamine				
Butenafine	Mentax, Lotrimin Ultra	1% cream	B	OTC, Rx
Polyenes				
Nystatin	Acronistina, Barstatin, Bio-Statin, Candacin, Candex, Candida-Lokalicid, Candio, Candio-Hermal, Canstat, Conio, Fongistat, Kandistatin, Korostatin, Lystin, Micostatin, Moronal, Mycastatin, Mycocide, Mycostatin, Mycostatine, Mykinac, Mytrex, Nadostine, Nilstat, Nyaderm, Nysert, Nystacid, Nystan, Nystaina, Nystex, Nystop, O-V Statin, Oranyst, Pedi-Dry, Scanytin, Statin, Vagistat	100 000 USP units/g cream, ointment, powder, oral suspension, lozenges (pastilles), vaginal tablets	C, Pastilles A	Rx
Amphotericin B	Fungizone	3% cream, ointment, lotion	B	Rx
Others				
Ciclopirox olamine	Batrafen, Batrafen Nail Lacquer, Brumixol, Ciclochem, Fungowas, Loprox, Loprox Laca, Miclast, Micoxolamina, Mycoster, Nail Batrafen, Penlac, Primax	0.77% and 1% cream, gel, lotion, solution, 8% nail lacquer	B	Rx
Tolnaftate	Aftate, Equate, Genaspore, NP-27, Pitrex, Tinactin, Ting, Zeasorb-AF	1% cream, gel, powder, solution, aerosol liquid, aerosol powder	–	OTC
Undecylenic acid	Caldesene, Cruex, Decylenes, Gordochom	20% cream, 25% ointment, solution, 15% powder, aerosol foam, aerosol powder	–	OTC
Clioquinol	Vioform MC, Lococorten-Vioform	3% cream, ointment	C	–
Iodoquinol	Alcortin	1% iodoquinol with 2% hydrocortisone gel	C	Rx

Table 127.15 Topical antifungal agents. Other topical agents with antifungal activity not listed in this table include Whitfield's ointment (benzoic acid and salicylic acid), selenium sulfide, sodium thiosulfate, salicylic acid and sulfur, zinc pyrithione, haloprogin, mafenide, amorolfine, propylene glycol and benzoyl peroxide.

The polyene antifungal agents – nystatin and amphotericin B – have a macrolide ring of carbon atoms with double bonds. They work by binding irreversibly to fungal cell membrane sterols and increasing permeability. They have a higher affinity for fungal sterols, including ergosterol, than they do for human cell cholesterol. Polyenes are fungistatic at low concentrations and fungicidal at high concentrations. Amphotericin is available in three lipid-complexed forms that are less nephrotoxic and much more expensive.

Ciclopirox olamine is a hydroxypyridine, broad-spectrum, fungicidal and fungistatic antifungal. It interferes with the uptake of precursors required for cell membrane synthesis, alters cellular permeability, and inhibits fungal respiratory activity, i.e. it interferes with iron-dependent systems including cytochromes, catalases and peroxidases[49]. At lower concentrations, the drug blocks the transport of amino acids into the cell. At higher concentrations, it alters fungal cell membranes so that intracellular material leaks out of the cell.

The aforementioned classes of antifungal agents all have anti-inflammatory effects. Allylamine and benzylamine antifungal drugs have a greater anti-inflammatory action than azole antifungal drugs. For example, naftifine inhibits chemotaxis and the production of reactive oxygen intermediates by neutrophils[50]. Azoles inhibit neutrophil chemotaxis, calmodulin activity, synthesis of leukotrienes and prostaglandins, and histamine release from mast cells[51–53]. Ketoconazole has anti-inflammatory activity comparable to that of hydrocortisone[54]. Ciclopirox olamine is also anti-inflammatory due to its inhibition of prostaglandin and leukotriene synthesis[52,55].

Tolnaftate is a thiocarbamate antifungal that inhibits squalene epoxidase and thus fungal cell membrane sterol synthesis. As with the

Table 127.16 Mechanism of action of antifungal drugs.

MECHANISM OF ACTION OF ANTIFUNGAL DRUGS	
Site of action	Drug class(es)
Binds cell membrane sterols	Polyenes
Interferes with cell wall synthesis via inhibition of β-(1,3)-D-glucan synthesis	Echinocandins
Interferes with cell membrane synthesis via inhibition of 14-α-demethylase	Imidazoles Triazoles
Interferes with cell membrane synthesis via inhibition of squalene epoxidase	Allylamines Benzylamines
Blocks DNA synthesis	Flucytosine
Disrupts mitotic spindle	Griseofulvin
Inhibits respiration, blocks transport of amino acids, and alters cell membrane permeability	Ciclopirox olamine

Table 127.16 Mechanism of action of antifungal drugs.

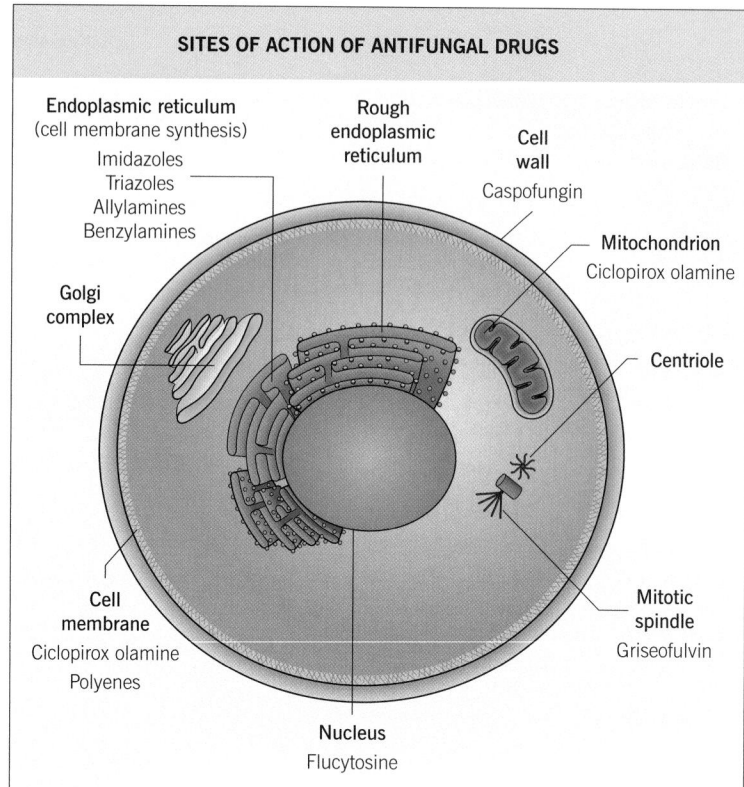

Fig. 127.5 Sites of action of antifungal drugs. The different classes of antifungal drugs exert their effects at different sites in the fungal cell. Notably, ciclopirox olamine and polyenes have more than one site of action.

allylamine antifungal drugs, this results in the accumulation of squalene. The mechanism of action of undecylenic acid is not fully understood. Selenium sulfide is antimitotic and reduces cellular adhesion in the stratum corneum, allowing for shedding of fungi. Clioquinol (iodochlorhydroxyquin) is a synthetic hydroxyquinoline and has both antifungal and antibacterial effects. Its mechanism of action is unknown.

Griseofulvin inhibits the mitosis of dermatophytes by interacting with microtubules and disrupting the mitotic spindle. It is fungistatic against *Trichophyton*, *Microsporum* and *Epidermophyton*. It is not active against yeast (including *Malassezia*), dimorphic fungi, *Cryptococcus* or the fungi that cause chromomycosis. Flucytosine is an analogue of cytosine, and it may interfere with DNA synthesis. However, its exact mechanism of action is not known.

Caspofungin acetate is a new antifungal agent in a unique class, the echinocandins. It inhibits the synthesis of β-(1,3)-D-glucan, an essential fungal cell wall component. This leads to alterations in fungal cell wall permeability[56].

Indications

Topical azoles are indicated for tinea corporis, tinea pedis, tinea cruris, pityriasis versicolor and mucocutaneous candidiasis. Of this group, oxiconazole and sulconazole have relatively weak activity against *Candida*. Butoconazole, clotrimazole, econazole, miconazole, terconazole and tioconazole are available in vaginal preparations to treat *Candida* vaginitis. Ketoconazole is additionally indicated for seborrheic dermatitis.

Topical allylamines and benzylamines are indicated for tinea pedis, tinea cruris and tinea corporis. Butenafine has been shown, *in vitro*, to be 10 to 100 times more effective against common dermatophytes than azole antifungals[57]. Terbinafine is 2 to 30 times more potent than azole antifungal agents against common dermatophytes *in vitro*[58]. Clinical trials have shown that terbinafine, butenafine and naftifine are superior to azole antifungals for tinea pedis[59,60]. The mycologic cure rates are significantly higher a month after treatment has stopped[61]. Post-

treatment relapse rates are also lower for allylamines and benzylamines than for azole antifungal drugs[59,62,63]. For example, butenafine 1% cream applied once a day for 2 weeks for tinea cruris resulted in an 81% mycologic cure rate 4 weeks after the end of treatment[64]. In addition, topical terbinafine and butenafine are indicated for *Candida* infections, though they have relatively weak anti-*Candida* action compared to the topical azoles.

Of the two topical polyenes, only nystatin is commonly used. It is indicated for mucocutaneous *Candida* infections. Polyenes are not effective against dermatophytes[65,66]. Nystatin is not well absorbed when taken orally. However, this fact may be used to an advantage in treating anogenital candidiasis and candidal diaper dermatitis[66,67].

Ciclopirox olamine is active against dermatophytes, *Malassezia* species, *Candida*, actinomycetes, molds, and Gram-positive and Gram-negative bacteria. It is indicated for tinea corporis, tinea pedis, tinea cruris, pityriasis versicolor and mucocutaneous candidiasis. *In vitro*, it is less potent against dermatophytes than the allylamine and benzylamine antifungals, but more potent than the azole antifungals. However, it is more effective against *Candida* than the azoles, allylamines or benzylamines.

Tolnaftate, undecylenic acid and clioquinol are indicated for dermatophyte infections, but are less efficacious than the aforementioned topical agents; tolnaftate is also effective for *Malassezia* infections.

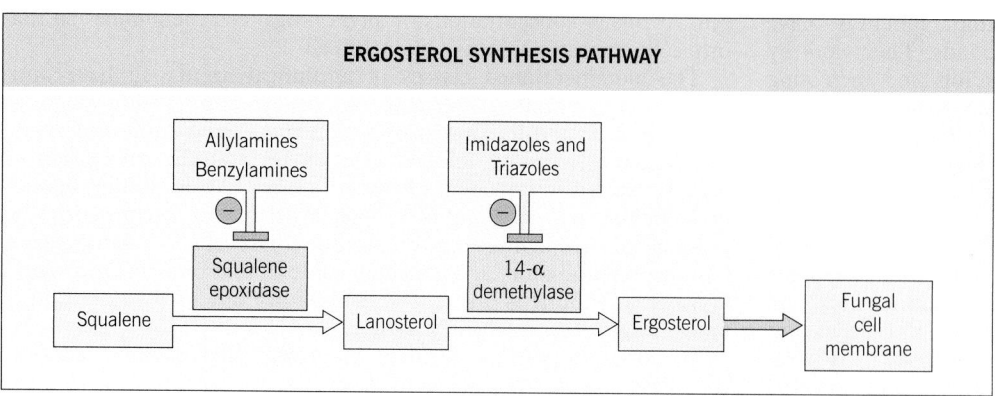

Fig. 127.6 Ergosterol synthesis pathway. Squalene is converted to lanosterol by squalene epoxidase. This enzyme is inhibited by the allylamine and benzylamine antifungals. 14-α demethylase converts lanosterol to ergosterol. Imidazole and triazole antifungals inhibit this conversion.

	INDICATIONS FOR SYSTEMIC ANTIFUNGAL AGENTS		
Generic name	**Antifungal spectra**	**Indications**	**FDA pregnancy category**
Terbinafine	*Epidermophyton floccosum, Trichophyton mentagrophytes, T. rubrum, T. tonsurans*	Onychomycosis Superficial fungal infections: widespread, severe or resistant to topical antifungals*	B
Ketoconazole	Most dermatophytes, *Candida* spp.	Systemic fungal infections: histoplasmosis, non-meningeal cryptococcosis, blastomycosis, mucocutaneous candidiasis, oropharyngeal and esophageal candidiasis, vaginal candidiasis and nail candidiasis Superficial fungal infections: widespread, severe or resistant to topical antifungals*	C
Itraconazole	Dermatophytes, yeasts (*Candida, Pityrosporum*), some molds	Blastomycosis, histoplasmosis and aspergillosis (oral and intravenous), onychomycosis (oral), oropharyngeal and esophageal candidiasis (solution) Superficial fungal infections: widespread, severe or resistant to topical antifungals*	C
Fluconazole	*Candida* spp., *T. tonsurans, T. rubrum, Microsporum canis*	Oropharyngeal, esophageal, vaginal and systemic candidiasis Cryptococcal meningitis Superficial fungal infections resistant to topical antifungals*	C
Voriconazole	*Aspergillus, Candida, Fusarium, Scedosporium*	Invasive aspergillosis (superior to amphotericin B), esophageal candidiasis, serious infections caused by *Fusarium* and *Scedosporium apiospermum*	D
Posaconazole	*Candida, Aspergillus, Cryptococcus, Fusarium,* Zygomycetes	Prevention of invasive aspergillosis and *Candida* infections in immunosuppressed hosts	C
Griseofulvin	*Trichophyton, Microsporum, Epidermophyton* spp. (no activity against *Candida* or *Malassezia*)	Tinea capitis and onychomycosis Superficial fungal infections: widespread, severe or resistant to topical antifungals	C
Amphotericin B	*Candida, Cryptococcus neoformans,* dimorphic fungi (*Histoplasma capsulatum, Coccidioides immitis* and *Blastomyces dermatitidis*), *Aspergillus*	Severe fungal infections including disseminated systemic candidiasis, cryptococcal meningitis, blastomycosis, disseminated histoplasmosis, extracutaneous sporotrichosis, coccidiodomycosis, paracoccidiodomycosis, mucormycosis and aspergillosis	B
Flucytosine	*Candida, Cryptococcus, Aspergillus,* agents of chromomycosis	Second-line therapy for severe fungal infections including candidiasis, cryptococcosis, aspergillosis and chromomycosis	C
Caspofungin acetate	*Aspergillus fumigatus, A. flavus, A. terrus, Candida*	Invasive aspergillosis in patients refractory to or intolerant of other antifungals, candidemia, esophageal candidiasis	C
Micafungin	*Candida, Aspergillus*	Prophylaxis for *Candida* infections in hematopoietic stem cell transplant patients, esophageal candidiasis	C
Anidulafungin	*Candida, Aspergillus*	Candidemia, esophageal candidiasis, intra-abdominal *Candida* infections and peritonitis	C

*Resistant superficial fungal infections treated by systemic terbinafine and azole antifungals include tinea corporis, tinea cruris and tinea pedis. The azoles are also used for pityriasis versicolor. Certain of these indications may not be available in some countries.

Table 127.17 Indications for systemic antifungal agents. The use of flucytosine is declining, but it is still used in certain situations.

Indications for the systemic antifungal agents are outlined in Table 127.17. Superficial fungal skin infections usually respond to topical agents. However, systemic therapy is sometimes required. Griseofulvin is generally the drug of choice for treating dermatophyte infections resistant to topical therapy in children. Mycologic cure rates are usually 80% to 95%. Terbinafine, itraconazole and fluconazole have also been successful in treating superficial dermatophyte infections of the skin, hair and nails in adults and children[47,68]. Terbinafine at standard doses results in a mycologic cure rate of approximately 70% for onychomycosis of the toenails and 80% for fingernails. Itraconazole, used continuously or as a pulse regimen, produces similar mycologic cure rates. Terbinafine has been shown to have a higher combined clinical and mycologic cure rate than itraconazole (37.7% versus 23.2%, $p = 0.004$) after 12 weeks of continuous oral therapy for toenail onychomycosis[69]. Fluconazole is generally the drug of choice for systemic candidiasis. However, cases of fungemia due to azole-resistant *Candida* have been reported[70]; amphotericin B is then the next best alternative. Fluconazole is relatively hydrophilic compared to other systemic azole antifungal drugs and thus is distributed to the cerebro-spinal fluid and can be used to treat fungal meningitis. Flucytosine is generally used concomitantly with amphotericin B for synergistic effect and to decrease the likelihood of resistance.

Dosages

Topical antifungal agents are generally applied twice a day until clinical signs and symptoms are improved, usually for 1 to 4 weeks. Occlusion should not be used. Shampoos are used every 3 to 4 days and are left in place for 5 minutes before rinsing. Nystatin oral suspension is held in the mouth for as long as possible before swallowing or expectorating, four times a day. There is essentially no systemic absorption. The pastilles are allowed to dissolve slowly in the mouth four to five times a day for up to 14 days. Ciclopirox olamine nail lacquer is applied daily for 1 week and then removed with alcohol; this cycle is then repeated.

A typical treatment course of systemic terbinafine is 12 weeks for toenail onychomycosis or 6 weeks for fingernail onychomycosis, and 2 weeks for superficial tinea infections resistant to topical antifungal agents. Dosages are based on age and weight and are shown in Table 127.18. In adults, for example, terbinafine 250 mg daily for 1 to 2 weeks is effective for tinea corporis and tinea cruris; a 2-week course is effective for tinea pedis[47]. For tinea capitis in children, terbinafine is given continuously for 2 to 4 weeks.

Ketoconazole is available in 200 mg tablets. Adults take one or two tablets daily. Children over 2 years of age take 6.6 mg/kg orally once for

DOSAGES OF TERBINAFINE	
Adults	250 mg qd
Children over 2 years old and under 20 kg	62.5 mg qd
Children over 2 years old and 20–40 kg	125 mg qd
Children over 2 years old and over 40 kg	250 mg qd

Table 127.18 Dosages of terbinafine. Oral granules of terbinafine, which can be sprinkled on food, have recently been approved by the FDA for use in children.

pityriasis versicolor. For other tinea infections and cutaneous candidiasis, children over 2 years of age take 3.3 to 6.6 mg/kg/day orally for 2 to 4 weeks. For mucocutaneous candidiasis in children, the dose is 5 to 10 mg/kg/day divided into two doses; the maximum dose is 400 mg a day. Absorption is improved with an acidic stomach pH. The manufacturer suggests ketoconazole should be taken with food. However, some clinicians suggest plasma levels are higher when the drug is taken on an empty stomach.

Itraconazole is available as 100 mg capsules and a 10 mg/ml cherry-caramel-flavored solution. The solution should be taken on an empty stomach, and the capsules should be taken with a full meal to enhance absorption. Pediatric dosing is 3 to 5 mg/kg daily[68,71]. Doses over 200 mg should be divided into two doses per day. For tinea capitis in children, itraconazole may be given continuously for 2 to 4 weeks or given as 1- to 3-week-long pulses (with 3 weeks without drug in between each pulse). Adult oral dosages for various indications are outlined in Table 127.19. Itraconazole is also available for intravenous infusion, given 200 mg intravenously twice a day for four doses and then 200 mg every day. Patients should be switched from intravenous to oral itraconazole when appropriate. The maximum length of intravenous treatment is usually 14 days. Treatment of oropharyngeal and esophageal candidiasis is for at least 3 weeks and should be continued for at least 2 weeks after symptoms resolve. Itraconazole solution is swished in the mouth, 10 mg at a time, for several seconds and then swallowed.

Fluconazole is available as 50 mg, 100 mg and 200 mg tablets and as an orange-flavored suspension in 10 mg/ml and 40 mg/ml strengths. Table 127.20 outlines the dosages of fluconazole for its various indications. Unlike ketoconazole and itraconazole, fluconazole is not dependent on a low gastric pH for absorption.

Voriconazole is used for invasive aspergillosis at 4 mg/kg intravenously every 12 hours or 100 to 200 mg orally every 12 hours. A loading dose of 6 mg/kg intravenously, given twice, 12 hours apart, is administered prior to the intravenous or oral regimen. Dose adjustments must be made in patients with renal or hepatic dysfunction.

ADULT DOSING OF ORAL ITRACONAZOLE	
Indication	Adult dosage
Pityriasis versicolor	200 mg po qd for 5–7 days
Tinea corporis, tinea cruris	100 mg po qd for 2 weeks *or* 200 mg po qd for 1 week
Tinea pedis	100 mg po qd for 2 weeks *or* 200 mg po qd for 1 week
Blastomycosis, histoplasmosis	200 mg po qd. May increase by 100 mg increments to a maximum of 400 mg po qd for at least 3 months
Aspergillosis	200–400 mg po qd for at least 3 months. May give loading dose of 200 mg tid for first 3 days in life-threatening conditions
Onychomycosis of toenails	200 mg po qd for 12 weeks or 200 mg po bid for 1 week, then 3 weeks without treatment, repeated twice more for a total of three pulses of therapy
Onychomycosis of fingernails	200 mg po bid for 1 week, then 3 weeks without treatment, then 200 mg po bid for 1 week
Oropharyngeal candidiasis	Swish and swallow 200 mg qd for 1–2 weeks
Oropharyngeal candidiasis refractory to fluconazole	Swish and swallow 100 mg bid
Esophageal candidiasis	Swish and swallow 100–200 mg qd

Table 127.19 **Adult dosing of oral itraconazole.** The safety of itraconazole in children has not been established. Some children 3 to 16 years old have been treated for systemic fungal infection with itraconazole capsules at a dose of 100 mg po qd and suffered no ill effects. Additionally, children have taken itraconazole solution at a dose of 5 mg/kg/day without any problems. Animal studies showed bone defects caused by itraconazole.

DOSING OF ORAL FLUCONAZOLE		
Indication	Pediatric dosage	Adult dosage
Pityriasis versicolor		400 mg po once or 300 mg po once, with possible second dose in 1 week, depending on clinical response
Tinea corporis, tinea cruris		50–100 mg po qd or 150 mg po qwk for 2–4 weeks
Tinea pedis		Pulse doses of 150 mg po qwk for 2–6 weeks
Tinea capitis		6 mg/kg/day for 2–3 weeks
Oropharyngeal candidiasis	6 mg/kg on day 1 then 3 mg/kg q24–72 h for 14 days*	200 mg on day 1 then 100 mg qd for at least 2 weeks
Vaginal candidiasis		150 mg po once
Esophageal candidiasis	6 mg/kg on day 1 then 3–12 mg/kg q24–72 h for 21 days*	200 mg on day 1 then 100 mg qd for at least 3 weeks. Treat for at least 2 weeks after symptoms resolve
Systemic candidiasis	6–12 mg/kg q24–72 h for 28 days*	Up to 400 mg qd
Prophylaxis of candidiasis in bone marrow transplantation	10–12 mg/kg q24 h (maximum 600 mg/day)	400 mg qd
Cryptococcal meningitis	12 mg/kg iv on day 1 then 6–12 mg/kg q24–72 h* (maximum 600 mg/kg iv qd; continue until 10–12 weeks after culture is negative)	400 mg on day 1 then 200–400 mg qd. Continue until 10–12 weeks after spinal fluid is negative
Prevention of relapse of cryptococcal meningitis in HIV patients		200 mg po qd

*If the patient is less than 14 days old, dosing is every 24–72 h. If the patient is over 14 days old, dosing is every 24 h.

Table 127.20 **Dosing of oral fluconazole.**

Posaconazole is a 40 mg/ml suspension, given with food. It is indicated for prophylaxis of invasive fungal infections in immunocompromised patients. The dosage is 200 mg orally three times daily in patients over 13 years of age. For oropharyngeal candidiasis, it may be given as 100 mg orally twice daily (on the first day) and then 100 mg daily for 12 days. In cases refractory to fluconazole or itraconazole, the dose is increased to 400 mg orally twice daily. Duration of treatment varies according to patient response[71a].

Dosages for griseofulvin are shown in Table 127.21. In the US, increasing doses have been required for the treatment of tinea capitis, due to changes in the most common causative organism to *Trichophyton tonsurans*. The long duration of therapy required with griseofulvin is a significant disadvantage and leads to non-compliance. Absorption of griseofulvin is significantly improved by dietary fat intake. Drug particle size reduction through micronization and ultramicronization has significantly enhanced oral absorption.

Dosing of intravenous amphotericin B varies depending upon the formulation of the medication (e.g. 0.75–1 mg/kg/day of amphotericin B versus 3–5 mg/kg/day of lipid-complexed amphotericins). In adults, flucytosine is given at a dose of 150 mg/kg orally daily, divided every 6 hours. Taking the medicine over 15 minutes decreases the nausea. Doses of both drugs should be adjusted in patients with renal insufficiency.

Caspofungin acetate is given as a slow intravenous infusion over 1 hour. For treatment of *Aspergillus* infections, the loading dose on the first day is 70 mg. The dose is 50 mg intravenously per day thereafter. Patients who do not respond to this dose may respond to 70 mg intravenously per day. Caspofungin must not be mixed with solutions containing dextrose, and patients with moderate hepatic insufficiency should receive 35 mg per day after the 70 mg loading dose. This drug has not been adequately studied in children[56].

Micafungin is only available in an IV form. For esophageal candidiasis, it is administered as 150 mg IV daily. In hematopoietic stem cell transplant patients, as prophylaxis for *Candida* infections, it may be given at a dose of 50 mg IV daily. Anidulafungin is also available in an IV form for *Candida* infections[71b]. In candidemia, the dose is 100 mg IV daily after a loading dose of 200 mg; treatment should continue until two weeks after the most recent positive blood culture. For esophageal candidiasis, the dose is 50 mg daily.

Contraindications

Topical and systemic antifungals are contraindicated in patients with hypersensitivity to any of the formulation components. Systemic antifungals are contraindicated in patients who are taking other drugs that may cause potentially serious interactions (see below). Itraconazole is contraindicated in patients with left-sided heart disease and should be avoided in pregnant or lactating patients. Ketoconazole and itraconazole may not be absorbed in patients with achlorhydria. Fluconazole, however, is not dependent on a low gastric pH[72]. Griseo-

fulvin is contraindicated in patients with acute intermittent porphyria, variegate porphyria, porphyria cutanea tarda or liver failure. All systemic antifungal agents should be used with caution in patients with liver or kidney disease. Flucytosine should be used with caution in patients with bone marrow suppression.

Major side effects

The most common side effect of topical antifungal drugs is local skin irritation, which may be more severe with occlusion. Clinical manifestations include burning, stinging, pruritus, erythema, edema, peeling, blistering, allergic contact dermatitis and urticaria. Clioquinol can cause discoloration of clothes, skin, hair and nails.

Oral terbinafine may cause a morbilliform eruption and, less commonly, urticaria, pruritus, alopecia or dermatitis. Severe cutaneous reactions that have been caused by systemic terbinafine include Stevens–Johnson syndrome and toxic epidermal necrolysis, as well as acute generalized exanthematous pustulosis, pustular psoriasis, flares of psoriasis and subacute cutaneous lupus erythematosus[73–77]. Noncutaneous side effects of terbinafine include gastrointestinal disturbances, elevated liver enzymes, headaches, taste and visual disturbances, transient decreases in absolute lymphocyte count, and rare neutropenia in immunosuppressed patients. This drug should be used with caution in patients with liver or kidney disease. Liver enzyme tests should be monitored before and during treatment. The side effects of the systemic azole antifungals are listed in Table 127.22.

Griseofulvin has been used for over 40 years with infrequent side effects and is considered a very safe medication. Its most common side effects are headache and gastrointestinal disturbances. It also may cause a fixed drug eruption, photosensitivity, petechiae, pruritus, exfoliative dermatitis or urticaria, and may precipitate or exacerbate lupus or porphyria. It has occasionally been associated with enuresis, proteinuria and urinary frequency, arthralgias, fever, hypersensitivity reactions (including angioedema and serum sickness-like reaction), neurologic side effects (e.g. confusion, blurred vision, vertigo, depression, nightmares, insomnia, ataxia and paresthesias), syncope, epistaxis, estrogen-like effects, sore throat, hepatotoxicity and leukopenia.

Amphotericin B commonly causes fever, chills, nausea and vomiting. These side effects may be minimized by pretreatment with aspirin or acetaminophen, diphenhydramine and/or intravenous hydrocortisone. Less commonly, it may also cause anorexia, diarrhea, orthostatic hypotension or hypertension, tachycardia, dyspnea, headache and skin eruptions, including exanthems, exfoliative dermatitis, fixed drug eruption, flushing, urticaria and infusion-site reactions. Amphotericin B can produce hypokalemia, thrombocytopenia and renal toxicity characterized by increased BUN and creatinine. Damage to the kidney may be mediated directly or through vasoconstriction and can be severe and irreversible after high doses. Less commonly, amphotericin B can cause seizures, arrhythmias, agranulocytosis, liver failure or anaphylaxis.

	ORAL DOSING OF GRISEOFULVIN		
Generic name	**Adult**		**Pediatric (over 2 years old)**
	Tinea corporis, capitis, cruris	Tinea pedis, unguium	
Griseofulvin microsize*	500–1000 mg qd *or* 250–500 mg bid	750–1000 mg qd	10–20 mg/kg/day (maximum 1 g/day); use higher range (15–20 mg/kg/day) for tinea capitis 2–4 weeks for tinea corporis 6–12 weeks for tinea capitis 4–8 weeks for tinea pedis 3–6 months or more for onychomycosis
Griseofulvin ultramicrosize	330–375 mg qd	660–750 mg qd	5–10 mg/kg/day (maximum 750 mg/day) 2–4 weeks for tinea corporis 6–12 weeks for tinea capitis 4–8 weeks for tinea pedis 4 months for fingernail onychomycosis 6 months for toenail onychomycosis†

*To increase absorption, griseofulvin microsize should be taken with a fatty meal.
†Use declining.

Table 127.21 Oral dosing of griseofulvin.

SIDE EFFECTS OF SYSTEMIC AZOLE ANTIFUNGAL AGENTS	
Generic name	**Side effects**
Ketoconazole	• Nausea, vomiting, abdominal pain, idiosyncratic hepatotoxicity • Anaphylaxis, urticaria, pruritus • At higher doses, suppresses testosterone and cortisol synthesis
Itraconazole	• Morbilliform eruption, pruritus, urticaria, alopecia; rarely, Stevens–Johnson syndrome; parenteral administration may result in injection-site reactions • Anorexia, nausea, vomiting, abdominal pain, hepatic dysfunction • Fatigue, headaches, dizziness • Fever, edema, hypokalemia, neutropenia (rarely) • Rarely causes congestive heart failure, pulmonary edema, anaphylaxis, peripheral neuropathy
Fluconazole	• Morbilliform eruption and, rarely, exfoliative dermatitis • Nausea, vomiting, abdominal pain, diarrhea, hepatotoxicity • Headache
Voriconazole	• Visual disturbances, headache • Nausea, vomiting, diarrhea, abdominal pain • Fever, peripheral edema

Table 127.22 Side effects of systemic azole antifungal agents.

Flucytosine can cause a number of neurologic side effects, including headaches, fatigue, vertigo, ataxia, paresthesias, confusion and hallucinations. In addition to gastrointestinal disturbances (e.g. nausea, vomiting, abdominal pain and diarrhea), hypokalemia and hypoglycemia may occur with use of this drug. Flucytosine can also cause more serious side effects, including cardiac and respiratory arrest, renal failure, aplastic anemia, agranulocytosis, thrombocytopenia, gastrointestinal bleeding and colitis.

Caspofungin acetate may cause headaches, fever, infusion-site reactions, phlebitis, flushing, erythema, induration, facial swelling, pruritus and warmth, as well as nausea and vomiting. To date, one case of anaphylaxis has been reported. Laboratory abnormalities encountered include increased alkaline phosphatase, hypokalemia, eosinophilia, proteinuria and hematuria. Micafungin may uncommonly cause anaphylaxis, liver or kidney dysfunction, thrombophlebitis or hemolytic anemia. It can cause headache, nausea, rigors and leukopenia. Skin reactions include 'rash' and injection site reactions. Anidulafungin may cause liver toxicity, diarrhea, hypokalemia and infusion reactions.

Interactions
Topical antifungals have no significant drug interactions.

Systemic terbinafine inhibits the cytochrome P450 isoform CYP2D6. As such, it may increase serum levels and toxic effects of other drugs metabolized by this pathway, including β-blockers, tricyclic antidepressants, selective serotonin reuptake inhibitors (SSRIs), MAO inhibitors, and type B and class IC antiarrhythmics. Terbinafine increases cyclosporine clearance by 15% and decreases caffeine clearance by 19%. It also decreases the efficacy of codeine. Terbinafine used with thioridazine may cause prolonged QT intervals and arrhythmias. Whereas cimetidine increases terbinafine levels, rifampin decreases terbinafine levels by doubling its rate of clearance[69].

Azole antifungal drugs exert their therapeutic effect by inhibiting cytochrome P450 enzymes (see above). Cytochrome P450 enzymes play a major role in transforming lipophilic drugs to more easily excreted metabolites[72]. Inhibition of this enzyme family is the cause of many of the azole antifungals' drug–drug interactions. These interactions have resulted in black-box warnings in the package insert by the FDA in the US. The interactions are listed in Table 127.23.

Griseofulvin may decrease the levels and efficacy of warfarin and salicylates. Barbiturates may decrease griseofulvin efficacy by decreasing its absorption. Griseofulvin potentiates the effect of alcohol or may induce a disulfiram-like reaction[72]. It also increases estrogen-metabolizing liver enzymes, which may make oral contraceptives less effective or cause menstrual irregularities.

DRUG INTERACTIONS OF SYSTEMIC AZOLE ANTIFUNGAL AGENTS		
Interacting drug	**Result**	**Azoles involved**
Astemizole, terfenadine, cisapride (banned or restricted)	Arrhythmia, torsade de pointes	K, I, F, V
Warfarin	Increased warfarin levels	K, I, F, V
Cyclosporine, tacrolimus	Increased cyclosporine or tacrolimus levels, nephrotoxicity, neurotoxicity, hypertension	K, I, F, V
Rifampin, rifamycin	Decreased plasma levels of azole antifungals (ketoconazole also decreases absorption of rifamycin)	K, I, F, V
Phenytoin	Phenytoin causes decreased levels of itraconazole, ketoconazole Fluconazole causes increased levels of phenytoin	K, I, F, V
Sildenafil (Viagra®)	Increased sildenafil	K, I, F, V
Oral hypoglycemics	Hypoglycemia	K, I, F, V
Oral contraceptives	Decreased levels, contraceptive failure	K, I, F, V
Antacids, H₂ antihistamines, proton pump inhibitors, anticholinergics, didanosine	Decreased GI absorption of azole antifungals Omeprazole and voriconazole causes increased levels of both drugs	K, I, V
Benzodiazepines	Excessive sedation	K, I, F, V
Indinavir	Increased indinavir levels	K
Corticosteroids	Increased corticosteroid levels	K
Digoxin	Increased digoxin levels	I, F, V
HMG-CoA reductase inhibitors (e.g. atorvastatin, simvastatin)	Rhabdomyolysis, myopathy	I, V
Dihydropyridine calcium channel blockers	Edema	I, V
Phenobarbital, carbamazepine, isoniazid, revirapine	Decreased serum levels of itraconazole	I, V
Pimozide, buspirone, quinidine, vincristine	Increased drug levels	I, V
Thiazide diuretics (e.g. HCTZ)	Increased serum levels of fluconazole	F
Theophylline, nucleoside analogs	Increased drug levels	F, V

Table 127.23 Drug interactions of systemic azole antifungal agents. K, ketoconazole; I, itraconazole; F, fluconazole; V, voriconazole.

Systemic corticosteroids, loop diuretics and thiazide diuretics increase the risk of developing hypokalemia due to amphotericin B. Antipsychotics used concomitantly with amphotericin B may cause QT prolongation and cardiac arrhythmias. Nephrotoxic drugs such as cisplatin, flucytosine, gentamicin and vancomycin may compound the nephrotoxicity of amphotericin B. Amphotericin may increase digoxin levels. Cisplatin used in conjunction with flucytosine increases the risk for nephrotoxicity and bone marrow suppression.

Caspofungin acetate does not affect the cytochrome P450 system. It does decrease tacrolimus levels, and cyclosporine increases caspofungin levels. Phenytoin, rifampin, dexamethasone, carbamazepine and several antiretroviral drugs (efavirenz, nelfinavir, nevirapine) can decrease caspofungin levels.

Pregnancy and lactation
Topical imidazoles have not been shown to cause any problems during pregnancy. Clotrimazole used intravaginally during the second and

third trimesters has not been shown to cause birth defects or other problems in humans. Topical imidazoles have not been shown to cause any problems during breastfeeding. Topical oxiconazole is excreted in breast milk. It is not known whether the other topical imidazoles are excreted in breast milk. Topical nystatin has not been shown to cause birth defects or other problems in humans; it is not known whether topically applied nystatin is excreted in breast milk. There are not adequate studies of ciclopirox olamine in pregnant women. A small amount of drug is absorbed through the skin. Animal studies involving mice, rats, rabbits and monkeys showed no impairment of fertility or harm to the fetus at doses ten times higher than the topical human dose. It is not known whether ciclopirox olamine is secreted in breast milk. Tolnaftate and undecylenic acid have not been reported to cause problems during pregnancy or with breastfeeding.

The FDA pregnancy categories of the systemic antifungal drugs are listed in Table 127.17. These drugs should not be used to treat onychomycosis if the patient is pregnant or contemplating pregnancy. During pregnancy, they should be reserved for systemic fungal infections only if the benefit outweighs the risk. Although animal studies of oral terbinafine have shown no adverse effects during pregnancy, there are no adequate studies in pregnant women. Orally administered terbinafine is secreted in breast milk and is not recommended for use in nursing mothers.

There are no adequate human studies of the effects of azole antifungals during pregnancy or nursing. Itraconazole is contraindicated in lactating patients because it is excreted in human milk. Fluconazole is excreted in breast milk. Griseofulvin has been associated with fetal abnormalities in rats and dogs. Rare cases of conjoined twins have been reported in women taking griseofulvin in the first trimester of pregnancy. Patients should avoid pregnancy for at least 1 month after discontinuing griseofulvin[78]. There are no adequate studies of amphotericin B or flucytosine in pregnant or lactating women. Flucytosine has been teratogenic in rat and mouse studies. Caspofungin acetate is toxic to rat and rabbit embryos and is excreted in breast milk in rats.

ANTIVIRAL AGENTS

This section reviews antiviral agents used for herpes simplex virus (HSV) and varicella zoster virus (VZV) infections. Table 127.24 lists the topical antiherpetic antiviral medications. Antiretroviral medications (see Ch. 77) and immunomodulating medications (see Ch. 128) are addressed elsewhere in the text.

Mechanisms of action

Figure 127.7 illustrates the mechanism of action of the major antiherpetic drugs.

Acyclovir is a synthetic purine nucleoside analogue similar in chemical structure to deoxyguanosine but with an acyclic side chain. It has a high affinity for HSV-1, HSV-2 and VZV thymidine kinase, which phosphorylates and activates the drug. Human cellular guanylate kinase then phosphorylates acyclovir twice more to transform it into acyclovir triphosphate. This substance blocks viral DNA synthesis by competitively inhibiting and inactivating viral DNA polymerase and by becoming irreversibly incorporated into the viral DNA chain, causing DNA chain termination.

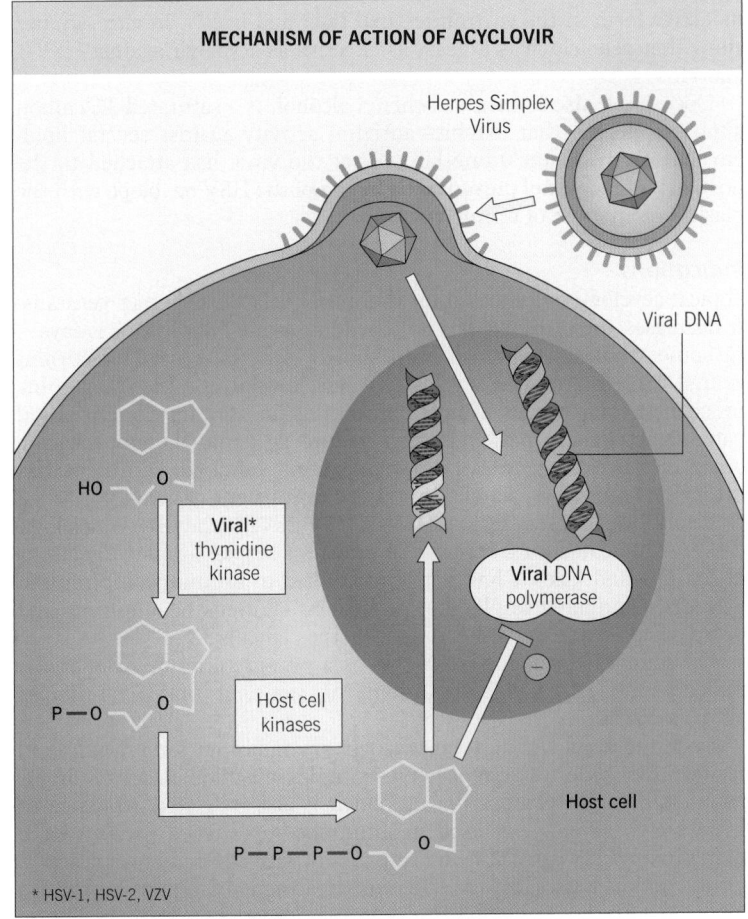

Fig. 127.7 **Mechanism of action of acyclovir.** Acyclovir, a purine analogue, has a high affinity for HSV-1, HSV-2 and VZV thymidine kinase, which phosphorylates and activates the drug. Human cellular guanylate kinase then phosphorylates acyclovir twice, to transform it into acyclovir triphosphate, which blocks viral DNA synthesis by competitively inhibiting and inactivating viral DNA polymerase and by becoming irreversibly incorporated into the viral DNA chain, causing DNA chain termination. Valacyclovir, penciclovir and famciclovir have mechanisms of action similar to acyclovir.

Valacyclovir is the prodrug of acyclovir. It is almost completely converted to acyclovir by valacyclovir hydrolase while passing through the gastrointestinal tract and liver. It has an oral bioavailability approximately three times greater than that of acyclovir (55% versus 15–30%, respectively) and is also more conveniently dosed than acyclovir.

Penciclovir is an acyclic guanosine analogue with a mechanism of action similar to acyclovir. It reaches higher intracellular concentrations and has a longer intracellular half-life than acyclovir (2.3–3 hours versus 1.3–1.5 hours, respectively). However, it is less potent because it does not cause chain termination of viral DNA, and it has a poor oral bioavailability. For these reasons, this medication is only available in topical form[79]. Famciclovir is the prodrug of penciclovir. The bioavailability of famciclovir is about 77%. Like valacyclovir, it is converted to

	TOPICAL ANTIHERPETIC ANTIVIRAL AGENTS			
Generic name	Trade name(s)®	Formulations	FDA pregnancy category	OTC/Rx
Acyclovir	Acic, Acicloftal, Aciclor, Aciclosina, Acivir, Acivir Eye, Aclovir, Acyclo-V, Acyvir, Avirax, Avorax, Azovir, Cicloferon, Cicloviral, Clinovir, Clovicin, Clovix, Cusiviral, Cyclivex, Cyclovir, Deherp, Eduvir, Entir, Herpefug, Herpex, Herpoviric Rp, Hexidol, Inmerax, Lisovyr, Lovir, Lovire, Maynor, Norum, Oppvir, Poviral, Quavir, Supra-Vir, Supraviran, Vacrovir, Vicorax, Virogon, Virex, Virless, Virobis, Zevin, Zoter, Zovir, Zovirax, Zyclir	5% ointment, cream	B	Rx
Penciclovir	Denavir, Vectavir	1% cream	B	Rx
Docosanol	Abreva	10% cream	B	OTC

Table 127.24 Topical antiherpetic antiviral agents.

its active form in the gastrointestinal tract and liver[80]. *In vitro* studies show that penciclovir is at least as effective as acyclovir against HSV-1 and HSV-2[81].

Docosanol, also known as behenyl alcohol, is a saturated 22-carbon aliphatic alcohol that exhibits antiviral activity against several lipid-enveloped viruses including HSV. After the virus has attached to the host cell, n-docosanol prevents the fusion of the HSV envelope with the plasma membrane of uninfected cells[82].

Indications

Topical acyclovir is indicated for the initial episode of herpes genitalis. It decreases the duration of viral shedding from 7 days to 4.1 days[83]. In some studies it has also been shown to be effective in recurrent genital herpes[84]. Topical acyclovir is indicated for non-life-threatening mucocutaneous herpes simplex infections in immunocompromised patients, but these patients often require systemic therapy. Despite being effective for genital herpes infections, acyclovir ointment has little effect on herpes labialis in immunocompetent patients[79].

Penciclovir is active against HSV-1, HSV-2, VZV and EBV. Penciclovir cream is indicated for treatment of recurrent herpes simplex infections of the lips and face. It has not been studied in immunocompromised patients. Compared to placebo, penciclovir shortens healing time and decreases pain and viral shedding in herpes labialis[79].

Docosanol is available in the US as a non-prescription drug and is indicated for the topical treatment of recurrent oral-facial herpes simplex infections.

Systemic acyclovir and valacyclovir are indicated for primary and recurrent episodes of genital herpes simplex infection, herpes simplex suppression and herpes zoster. Acyclovir is also indicated for varicella. Intravenous acyclovir is used in immunocompromised patients with disseminated HSV or VZV and in patients with severe herpes zoster[85]. Other off-label uses of acyclovir are treatment of recurrent herpes-associated erythema multiforme, eczema herpeticum, primary herpes gingivostomatitis, herpetic whitlow and neonatal herpes. Famciclovir is indicated for herpes zoster, primary or recurrent genital herpes, herpes suppression in immunocompetent patients and recurrent herpes simplex in HIV-infected patients. Valacyclovir and famciclovir are used off-label for varicella and oral valganciclovir and valacyclovir are used for CMV prophylaxis in solid-organ transplant patients.

Acyclovir, valacyclovir and famciclovir are considered equivalent in safety and efficacy (time to healing, duration of pain, and viral shedding) for initial episodes of genital herpes. Famciclovir and valacyclovir have the advantage of greater oral bioavailability and more convenient dosing. Famciclovir 250 mg three times a day for 5 to 10 days is comparable to acyclovir in the treatment of initial episodes of genital herpes simplex[86]. Valacyclovir is at least as effective as acyclovir in decreasing the duration of pain in herpes zoster[87,88]. Table 127.25 lists the relative susceptibilities of herpes viruses to the antiviral drugs.

Dosages

Antivirals (topical or systemic) should be started as soon as possible after the onset of signs and symptoms. A glove or applicator should be used to apply topical antivirals to prevent autoinoculation of the finger. Table 127.26 details the dosing regimens of the topical antiviral drugs. Table 127.27 lists the available formulations of systemic antiviral medications. Table 127.28 outlines the dosages of the systemic anti-herpetic medications for their various indications. Intravenous, rather than oral, treatment may be required in severely immunosuppressed patients, patients who cannot take medications orally, and those who cannot be relied upon to take the medication correctly[89].

Although the majority of people who are seropositive for HSV-2 are asymptomatic[90,91], it is thought that asymptomatic viral shedding leads to most transmission of genital herpes. The physician must decide whether to treat on an episodic basis or in a continuous suppressive fashion. Factors that influence this decision are the number of outbreaks per year, the severity of outbreaks, the lack of prodromal symptoms, and an HSV-seronegative sexual partner[89]. Suppression with acyclovir 400 mg twice daily decreased recurrences by 80–90% and decreased asymptomatic shedding by 95%[92]. A year-long, double-blind, placebo-controlled study demonstrated 1 g of valacyclovir taken daily reduced recurrence rates by 78%[93]. In addition, a multicenter, randomized, placebo-controlled study showed that daily valacyclovir significantly

COMPARATIVE SUSCEPTIBILITY OF HERPESVIRUSES TO ANTIVIRAL DRUGS					
Antiviral drug	**Viral susceptibility**				
	HSV-1	**HSV-2**	**VZV**	**CMV**	**Main target organisms**
Acyclovir, valacyclovir	+++	+++	++	–	HSV-1, HSV-2, VZV
Cidofovir	+	+	++	+++	CMV, resistant HSV
Famciclovir	+++	+++	++	–	HSV-1, HSV-2, VZV
Foscarnet	++	++	+	++	CMV, resistant HSV, VZV
Ganciclovir, valganciclovir	+	+	+	+++	CMV

Table 127.25 Comparative susceptibility of herpesviruses to antiviral drugs.

DOSING OF TOPICAL ANTIVIRAL DRUGS		
Antiviral drug	**Dosage**	**Side effects**
Acyclovir	q3 h, 6 times/day for 7 days In Canada: 4–6 times/day for up to 10 days	Burning, stinging, discomfort and mild pain at the application site. Less commonly: pruritus, erythema, edema or mucosal irritation when applied to genital lesions
Penciclovir	q2 h while awake (at least 6 times/day) for 4 days	Burning, stinging, discomfort and mild pain at the application site, headache, dysgeusia, decreased cutaneous sensation (particularly to touch), and erythema
Docosanol	5 times/day until episode is resolved	Burning, pruritus, xerosis, acne, erythema and edema

Table 127.26 Dosing of topical antiviral drugs.

FORMULATIONS OF SYSTEMIC ANTIVIRAL DRUGS	
Antiviral drug	**Available formulations**
Acyclovir	200 mg capsules; 400 mg and 800 mg tablets; iv solution; 200 mg/5 ml banana-flavored suspension
Valacyclovir	500 mg and 1000 mg tablets
Famciclovir	125 mg, 250 mg and 500 mg tablets
Valganciclovir	450 mg tablets

Table 127.27 Formulations of systemic antiviral drugs.

lowered the risk of transmission of genital herpes in heterosexual, immunocompetent, monogamous, HSV-2 discordant couples[94].

Acyclovir, valacyclovir and famciclovir are all effective against herpes labialis when used intermittently or suppressively, and they are all effective in treating herpes zoster. Treatment of varicella in children is controversial, but does not alter antibody production at 28 days and at 1 year[95]. It is recommended for children over 13 years of age, as well as those patients with chronic skin or lung disease, on long-term salicylates, receiving corticosteroids or immunocompromised from malignancy[96].

Contraindications

As with all medications, antiviral agents are contraindicated in patients with hypersensitivity to the drug, prodrug or any components of the formulation. Systemic antivirals need to be dose-adjusted for patients with impaired renal function, and, in patients taking nephrotoxic medications, renal function needs to be monitored. There have been reports of thrombotic thrombocytopenic purpura and hemolytic uremic syndrome in immunocompromised patients receiving valacyclovir[97].

INDICATIONS AND DOSAGES OF SYSTEMIC ANTIHERPETIC DRUGS

Indication	Dosage
Primary genital herpes	Acyclovir 200 mg po q4 h while awake (5 times a day) for 10 days Valacyclovir 1 g po bid for 10 days Famciclovir 250 mg po tid for 7–10 days
Recurrent genital herpes	Acyclovir 200 mg po q4 h while awake (5 times a day) for 5 days Valacyclovir 500 mg po q12 h for 3 days -or- 1 g po qd for 5 days Famciclovir 125 mg po q12 h for 5 days -or- 1 g po bid × 1 day
Chronic suppression of genital herpes	Acyclovir 400 mg po bid or 200 mg po 3–5 times a day, reassess after 12 months Valacyclovir 500 mg–1 g po qd for patients with 10 or fewer recurrences per year Valacyclovir 1 g po qd for patients with over 10 recurrences per year Famciclovir 250 mg po q12 h
Herpes zoster	Acyclovir 800 mg po q4 h while awake (5 times a day) for 7–10 days Valacyclovir 1 g po q8 h for 7 days Famciclovir 500 mg po q8 h for 7 days
Varicella	Patients over 2 years of age, over 40 kg: Acyclovir 800 mg po qid for 5 days Patients over 2 years of age, under 40 kg: Acyclovir 20 mg/kg po qid for 5 days (maximum 800 mg per dose)
Recurrent mucocutaneous herpes simplex in immunocompromised patients, including HIV-infected	Acyclovir 5 mg/kg iv q8 h for 7 days* Acyclovir 400 mg po 5 times a day for 14–21 days* Valacyclovir 1 g po tid for 7 days* Famciclovir 500 mg po q12 h for 5–10 days*
HSV encephalitis	Acyclovir 10 mg/kg iv q8 h for 10 days
Disseminated herpes zoster	Acyclovir 5–10 mg/kg iv q8 h for 7–10 days
Orolabial herpes	Famciclovir 1500 mg once Valacyclovir 2 g po q12 h twice

*Or until healed.

Table 127.28 Indications and dosages of systemic antiherpetic drugs. Dosage frequency and amount must be adjusted for renal failure and dialysis.

SIDE EFFECTS OF SYSTEMIC ANTIVIRAL AGENTS

Acyclovir and valacyclovir	• Cutaneous: morbilliform eruption, Stevens-Johnson syndrome, injection-site reaction, urticaria, angioedema • Gastrointestinal: nausea, vomiting, diarrhea, abdominal pain • Hematologic: aplastic anemia, leukopenia, thrombocytopenia • Neurologic: headaches, vertigo, lethargy, confusion, hallucinations, depression, seizures, encephalopathy, coma (CNS disturbances more likely in elderly) • Cardiovascular: hypertension, tachycardia, anaphylaxis • Other: malaise, arthralgia, myalgia, dyspnea, dysmenorrhea • Reversible crystalluria-induced nephropathy with intravenous acyclovir • Thrombotic thrombocytopenic purpura or hemolytic uremic syndrome in immunocompromised patients with valacyclovir
Famciclovir	• Pruritus, paresthesias, headache, fatigue, nausea, vomiting, diarrhea, and flatulence

Table 127.29 Side effects of systemic antiviral agents.

DRUG INTERACTIONS OF SYSTEMIC ANTIVIRAL AGENTS

Interacting drug	Result
Amphotericin	Increases serum acyclovir level
Cimetidine	Decreases rate of conversion of valacyclovir to acyclovir Increases serum levels of acyclovir and valacyclovir
Digoxin	Famciclovir increases digoxin levels
Glyburide with metformin (Glucovance®)	Acyclovir or valacyclovir may cause lactic acidosis in patients with decreased renal function
Interferon	May worsen potential neurotoxicity of acyclovir
Intrathecal methotrexate	May worsen potential neurotoxicity of acyclovir
Nephrotoxic drugs (i.e. cisplatin)	Acyclovir increases risk of nephrotoxicity
Probenecid	Decreases rate of conversion of valacyclovir to acyclovir Increases serum levels of acyclovir and valacyclovir
Theophylline	Acyclovir causes decreased metabolism and increased serum levels of theophylline Theophylline increases serum levels of acyclovir and valacyclovir
Zidovudine	Increases serum levels of acyclovir and valacyclovir

Table 127.30 Drug interactions of systemic antiviral agents.

Major side effects

Table 127.26 lists the side effects of the topical antiviral agents. Absorption of topical antivirals is limited.

Table 127.29 lists the side effects of systemic antiherpetic medications. The crystalline nephropathy caused by intravenous acyclovir is more likely to occur in patients with pre-existing renal dysfunction or in dehydrated patients.

Interactions

No clinically important drug interactions with topical antivirals have been identified. Table 127.30 lists the interactions of the systemic antiviral agents with other medications.

Pregnancy and lactation

There are no adequate studies of topical antiviral agents in pregnant or lactating women. Small amounts of topical acyclovir are absorbed through the skin and mucous membranes. However, it is not known if topically applied antivirals are excreted in breast milk. Topical docosanol has not been shown to cause birth defects or other problems in animal studies using rats or rabbits. It is unknown whether docosanol passes into breast milk. To date, no problems in nursing infants due to topical antiviral agents have been reported.

Systemic antiviral drugs should not be used during pregnancy unless potential benefit justifies the potential risk to the fetus. Systemic acyclovir is FDA pregnancy category C. At high doses in vitro, acyclovir is mutagenic[98]. It has not been shown to be teratogenic in standard animal studies. However, acyclovir does cross the placenta and could theoretically cause renal dysfunction in the fetus[99]. A prospective registry of 756 pregnant patients who took acyclovir showed an incidence of birth defects similar to that of the general population[99]. Acyclovir is the drug of choice for primary genital herpes in pregnant women, because it has been used safely more often than other antivirals. Recurrent herpes simplex is not an indication for acyclovir. Varicella in pregnant women should be treated with acyclovir due to the high risk of maternal mortality from varicella pneumonia as well as fetal death or premature delivery[100]. It is not known, however, whether acyclovir prevents congenital varicella syndrome. Acyclovir is excreted in breast milk, but no data are available regarding the risk to nursing infants. There are no adequate human studies of valacyclovir (pregnancy category B) in pregnancy or lactation.

Systemic famciclovir (pregnancy category B) and penciclovir have not been shown to be teratogenic in animal studies. Very high doses of penciclovir are mutagenic, and prolonged exposure to high-dose famciclovir is associated with benign mammary tumors in rats[98]. There is an ongoing registry maintained by the manufacturer to monitor pregnant patients exposed to famciclovir[19]. Penciclovir does pass into the milk in animals when given orally. The safety of famciclovir and penciclovir use during lactation has not been established.

Other antiviral agents

Herpes infection resistant to commonly used drugs is a problem in immunocompromised patients. Foscarnet and cidofovir are two alternative treatments in this situation (see Table 127.25).

Foscarnet is an intravenous antiviral used for CMV retinitis or CMV skin infection in HIV-infected patients and for acyclovir-resistant herpes simplex infections. Foscarnet is an inorganic pyrophosphate analogue that selectively inhibits viral DNA polymerase. It blocks the pyrophosphate binding sites on viral polymerases. This prevents the cleavage of pyrophosphate from deoxyadenosine triphosphate. It does not require phosphorylation to be activated, and thus it circumvents the commonest mode of viral resistance involving viral thymidine kinase. Foscarnet is active against all herpesviruses. Side effects of the intravenous form include nephrotoxicity, anemia, changes in serum calcium, magnesium and phosphate, erosive penile lesions, thrombophlebitis, seizures and gastrointestinal disturbances[101,102]. Topical formulations of the drug are being studied.

Cidofovir is an acyclic nucleoside phosphate analogue of deoxycytosine monophosphate. It inhibits viral DNA polymerase and causes DNA chain termination. It differs from acyclovir and penciclovir in that it does not require viral thymidine kinase to become activated[102]. It is also used for CMV retinitis in HIV-infected patients. Cidofovir is currently available in intravenous form only, and side effects include nephrotoxicity, iritis, neutropenia, metabolic acidosis and gastrointestinal disturbances. However, a topical form for acyclovir-resistant herpes simplex infections is being studied. It has been used with some success for herpes simplex resistant to acyclovir, molluscum contagiosum, condyloma acuminata and verruca vulgaris[103,104]. *In vitro*, it is active against DNA viruses including monkeypox, variola and vaccinia.

New compounds with a novel antiherpetic mechanism have recently been reported. These antiviral agents target the helicase–primase complex (three HSV proteins which unravel DNA) and have been shown to be effective *in vitro* as well as in animal models[105–107]. Also, resiquimod, a topical immune-response modifier, has been shown to reduce the number of recurrences of genital herpes.

REFERENCES

1. Espersen F. Resistance to antibiotics used in dermatological practice. Br J Dermatol. 1998;139(suppl. 53):4–8.
2. Veien NK. The clinician's choice of antibiotics in the treatment of bacterial skin infection. Br J Dermatol. 1998;139(suppl. 53):30–6.
3. Tunkel AR. Topical antibacterials. In: Mandell GL, Bennett JE, Dolin R (eds). Mandell, Douglas, and Bennett's Principles and Practice of Infectious Disease, 5th edn. Philadelphia: Churchill Livingstone, 2000;428–35.
4. Eady EA, Bojar RA, Jones CE, et al. The effects of acne treatment with a combination of benzoyl peroxide and erythromycin on skin carriage of erythromycin-resistant propionibacteria. Br J Dermatol. 1996;134:107–13.
5. Eady EA, Cove JH, Holland KT, Cunliffe WJ. Erythromycin resistant propionibacteria in antibiotic treated acne patients: association with therapeutic failure. Br J Dermatol. 1989;121:51–7.
6. Eady EA, Farmery MR, Ross JI, Cove JH, Cunliffe WJ. Effects of benzoyl peroxide and erythromycin alone and in combination against antibiotic-sensitive and -resistant skin bacteria from acne patients. Br J Dermatol. 1994;131:331–6.
7. Harkaway KS, McGinley KJ, Foglia AN, et al. Antibiotic resistance patterns in coagulase-negative staphylococci after treatment with topical erythromycin, benzoyl peroxide, and combination therapy. Br J Dermatol. 1992;126:586–90.
8. Chalker DK, Shalita A, Smith JG Jr, Swann RW. A double-blind study of the effectiveness of a 3% erythromycin and 5% benzoyl peroxide combination in the treatment of acne vulgaris. J Am Acad Dermatol. 1983;9:933–6.
9. BenzaClin® topical gel (clindamycin – benzoyl peroxide gel). [Prescribing Information]. Bridgewater, NJ: Dermik Laboratories; 2006.
10. Lookingbill DP, Chalker DK, Lindholm JS, et al. Treatment of acne with a combination clindamycin/benzoyl peroxide gel compared with clindamycin gel, benzoyl peroxide gel and vehicle gel: combined results of two double-blind investigations. J Am Acad Dermatol. 1997;37:590–5.
11. Pierard GE, Pierard-Franchimont C. Effect of topical erythromycin-zinc formulation on sebum output. Evaluation by combined photometric-multi-step samplings with Sebutape. Clin Exp Dermatol. 1993;18:410–13.
12. Feucht CL, Allen BS, Chalker DK, Smith JG Jr. Topical erythromycin with zinc in acne. A double-blind controlled study. J Am Acad Dermatol. 1980;3:483–91.
13. Pierard-Franchimont C, Goffin V, Visser JN, et al. A double-blind controlled evaluation of the sebosuppressive activity of topical erythromycin-zinc complex. Eur J Clin Pharmacol. 1995;49:57–60.
14. Schachner L, Eaglstein W, Kittles C, Mertz P. Topical erythromycin and zinc therapy for acne. J Am Acad Dermatol. 1990;22:253–60.
15. Strauss JS, Stanieri AM. Acne treatment with topical erythromycin and zinc: effect of Propionibacterium

16. Holland KT, Bojar RA, Cunliffe WJ, et al. The effect of zinc and erythromycin on the growth of erythromycin-resistant and erythromycin-sensitive isolates of Propionibacterium acnes: an in-vitro study. Br J Dermatol. 1992;126:505–9.
17. Chu A, Huber FL, Plott RT. The comparative efficacy of benzoyl peroxide 5%/erythromycin 3% gel and erythromycin 4%/zinc 1.2% solution in the treatment of acne vulgaris. Br J Dermatol. 1997;136:235–8.
18. van Hoogdalem EJ. Transdermal absorption of topical anti-acne agents in man; review of clinical pharmacokinetic data. J Eur Acad Dermatol Venerol. 1998;11:S13–19.
19. McEvoy GK (ed). American Hospital Formulary Service (AHFS) Drug Information. Bethesda: American Society of Health-System Pharmacists, 2001;539–41,3322–4.
19a. Altabax ointment (retapamulin ointment), 1% [package insert]. Research Triangle Park, NC: GlaxoSmithKline; 2007.
20. von Eiff C, Becker K, Machka K, et al. Nasal carriage as a source of Staphylococcus aureus bacteremia. N Engl J Med. 2001;344:11–16.
21. Leyden JJ. Review of mupirocin ointment in the treatment of impetigo. Clin Pediatr. 1992;31:549–53.
22. Rice TD, Duggan AK, DeAngelis C. Cost-effectiveness of erythromycin versus mupirocin for the treatment of impetigo in children. Pediatrics. 1992;89:210–14.
23. Mandell LA. Fusidic acid. In: Mandell GL, Bennett JE, Dolin R (eds). Mandell, Douglas, and Bennett's Principles and Practice of Infectious Disease, 5th edn. Philadelphia: Churchill Livingstone, 2000;306–7.
24. Wilkinson JD. Fusidic acid in dermatology. Br J Dermatol. 1998;139(suppl. 53):37–40.
25. Sutton JB, Lagdon CG. An analysis of the cost effectiveness of fusidic acid cream and mupirocin ointment in the treatment of superficial skin sepsis in general practice. Br J Med Econ. 1993;6:367–43.
26. Sutton JB. Efficacy and acceptability of fusidic acid cream and mupirocin ointment in facial impetigo. Curr Ther Res. 1992;51:673–8.
27. Morley PAR, Munot LD. A comparison of sodium fusidate ointment and mupirocin ointment in superficial skin sepsis. Curr Med Res Opin. 1988;11:142–8.
28. Macmillan AL, Sarkany I. Specific topical therapy for erythrasma. Br J Dermatol. 1970;82:507–9.
29. Hamann K, Thorn P. Systemic or local treatment of erythrasma? A comparison between erythromycin tablets and fucidin cream in general practice. Scand J Prim Health Care. 1991;9:35–9.
30. Pearson RD. Agents active against parasites and Pneumocystis carinii. In: Mandell GL, Bennett JE, Dolin R (eds). Mandell, Douglas, and Bennett's Principles and Practice of Infectious Disease, 5th edn. Philadelphia: Churchill Livingstone, 2000;505–9.
31. Rabb DC, Lesher JL Jr. Antibiotic prophylaxis in cutaneous surgery. Dermatol Surg. 1995;21:550–4.
32. Darmstadt GL. Antibiotics in the management of pediatric skin disease. Dermatol Clin. 1998;16:509–25.

33. Salkind AR, Cuddy PG, Foxworth JW. Is this patient allergic to penicillin? An evidence-based analysis of the likelihood of penicillin allergy. JAMA. 2001;285:2498–505.
34. Litt JZ. Drug Eruption Reference Manual. New York: Parthenon, 2001:263.
35. Anderson JA. Antibiotic drug allergy in children. Curr Opin Pediatr. 1994;6:656–60.
36. Ibia EO, Schwartz RH, Wiedermann BL. Antibiotic rashes in children. A survey in a private practice setting. Arch Dermatol. 2000;136:849–54.
37. Raimer SS. New and emerging therapies in pediatric dermatology. Dermatol Clin. 2000;18:73–8.
38. Sullivan JR, Shear NH. The drug hypersensitivity syndrome. What is the pathogenesis? Arch Dermatol. 2001;137:357–64.
39. Le Cleach L, Bocquet H, Roujeau JC. Reactions and interactions of some commonly used systemic drugs in dermatology. Dermatol Clin. 1998;16:421–9.
40. Shapiro LE, Knowles SR, Shear NH. Comparative safety of tetracycline, minocycline, and doxycycline. Arch Dermatol. 1997;133:1224–30.
41. Cohan S, Bevelander G, Tiamisc T. Growth inhibition of prematures receiving tetracycline. Am J Dis Child. 1963;105:1008.
42. Bartlett JG. Antimicrobial agents implicated in Clostridium difficile toxin-associated diarrhea or colitis. Johns Hopkins Med J. 1981;149:6–9.
43. Bartlett JG. Anti-anaerobic antibacterial agents. Lancet. 1982;2:478–81.
44. Tedesco FJ. Clindamycin and colitis: a review. J Infect Dis. 1977;135:S95–8.
45. Burkhardt JE, Walterspiel JN, Schaad UB. Quinolone arthropathy in animals versus children. Clin Infect Dis. 1997;25:1196–204.
46. Hooper DC. Quinolones. In: Mandell GL, Bennett JE, Dolin R (eds). Mandell, Douglas, and Bennett's Principles and Practice of Infectious Disease, 5th edn. Philadelphia: Churchill Livingstone, 2000;306–7.
47. Lesher JL Jr. Oral therapy of common superficial fungal infections of the skin. J Am Acad Dermatol. 1999;40:S31–4.
48. Mosby's GenRx, 11th edn. St Louis: Mosby, 2001:1655–9.
49. Wortzman MS. Ciclopirox Clinical Data Review. Medicis Pharmaceutical Corporation, 2001.
50. Evans EG, James IG, Seaman RA, Richardson MD. Does naftifine have anti-inflammatory properties? A double-blind comparative study with 1% clotrimazole/1% hydrocortisone in clinically diagnosed fungal infection of the skin. Br J Dermatol. 1993;129:437–42.
51. Hegemann L, Toso SM, Lahijani KI, et al. Direct interaction of antifungal azole-derivatives with calmodulin: a possible mechanism for their therapeutic activity. J Invest Dermatol. 1993;100:343–6.
52. Rosen T, Schell BJ, Orengo I. Anti-inflammatory activity of antifungal preparations. Int J Dermatol. 1997;36:788–92.
53. Bremm KD, Plempel M. Modulation of leukotriene metabolism from human polymorphonuclear granulocytes by bifonazole. Mycoses. 1991;34:41–5.

54. van Cutsem J, van Gerven F, Cauwenbergh G, et al. The anti-inflammatory effects of ketoconazole. A comparative study with hydrocortisone acetate in a model using living and killed *Staphylococcus aureus* on the skin of guinea-pigs. J Am Acad Dermatol. 1991;25:257–61.
55. Abrams BB, Hanel H, Hoehler T. Ciclopirox olamine: a hydroxypyridine antifungal agent. Clin Dermatol. 1991;9:471–7.
56. Cancidas® product information. Merck & Co Inc., Whitehouse Station, NJ, 2001.
57. Arika T, Yokoo M, Yamaguchi H. Topical treatment with butenafine significantly lowers relapse rate in an interdigital tinea pedis model in guinea pigs. Antimicrob Agents Chemother. 1992:36:2523–5.
58. Shadomy S, Wang H, Shadomy HJ. Further *in vitro* studies with oxiconazole nitrate. Diagn Microbiol Infect Dis. 1988;9:231–7.
59. Evans EG. A comparison of terbinafine (Lamisil) 1% cream given for one week with clotrimazole (Canesten) 1% cream given for four weeks, in the treatment of tinea pedis. Br J Dermatol. 1994;130(suppl. 43):12–14.
60. Bergstresser PR, Elewski B, Hanifin J, et al. Topical terbinafine and clotrimazole in interdigital tinea pedis: a multicenter comparison of cure and relapse rates with 1- and 4-week treatment regimens. J Am Acad Dermatol. 1993;28:648–51.
61. Ablon G, Rosen T, Spedale J. Comparative efficacy of naftifine, oxiconazole, and terbinafine in short-term treatment of tinea pedis. Int J Dermatol. 1996; 35:591–3.
62. Smith EB, Breneman DL, Griffith RF, et al. Double-blind comparison of naftifine cream and clotrimazole/betamethasone dipropionate cream in the treatment of tinea pedis. J Am Acad Dermatol. 1992;26:125–7.
63. Elewski B, Bergstresser P, Hanifin J, et al. Long-term outcome of patients with interdigital tinea pedis treated with terbinafine or clotrimazole. J Am Acad Dermatol. 1995;32:290–2.
64. Lesher JL Jr, Babel DE, Stewart DM, et al. Butenafine 1% cream in the treatment of tinea cruris: a multicenter, vehicle-controlled, double-blind trial. J Am Acad Dermatol. 1997;36:S20–4.
65. Brennan B, Leyden JJ. Overview of topical therapy for common superficial fungal infections and the role of new topical agents. J Am Acad Dermatol. 1997;36:S3–8.
66. Lesher JL Jr, Smith JG Jr. Antifungal agents in dermatology. J Am Acad Dermatol. 1987;17:383–94.
67. Lynch PJ, Minkin W, Smith EB. Ecology of *Candida albicans* in candidiasis of the groin. Arch Dermatol. 1969;99:154–60.
68. Friedlander SF, Suarez S. Pediatric antifungal therapy. Dermatol Clin. 1998;16:527–37.
69. De Backer M, De Vroey C, Lesaffre E, et al. Twelve weeks of continuous oral therapy for toenail onychomycosis caused by dermatophytes: double-blind comparative trial of terbinafine 250 mg/day versus itraconazole 200 mg/day. J Am Acad Dermatol. 1998;38:S57–63.
70. Jandourek A, Brown P, Vazquez JA. Community-acquired fungemia due to a multiple-azole-resistant strain of *Candida tropicalis*. Clin Infect Dis. 1999;29:1583–4.

71. Elewski BE. Tinea capitis: a current perspective. J Am Acad Dermatol. 2000;42:1–20.
71a. Cornely OA, Maertens J, Winston DJ, et al. Posaconazole vs. fluconazole or itraconazole prophylaxis in patients with neutropenia. N Eng J Med. 2007;356:348–59.
71b. Vazquez JA, Sobel JD. Anidulafungin: a novel Echinocandin. Clin Inf Dis. 2006;43:215–22.
72. Katz HI. Systemic antifungal agents used to treat onychomycosis. J Am Acad Dermatol. 1998; 38:S48–52.
73. Gupta AK, Lynde CW, Lauzon GJ, et al. Cutaneous adverse effects associated with terbinafine therapy: 10 case reports and a review of the literature. Br J Dermatol. 1998;138:529–32.
74. Brooke R, Coulson IH, al-Dawoud A. Terbinafine-induced subacute cutaneous lupus erythematosus. Br J Dermatol. 1998;139:1132–3.
75. Holmes S, Kemmett D. Exacerbation of systemic lupus erythematosus induced by terbinafine. Br J Dermatol. 1998;139:1133.
76. Murphy M, Barnes L. Terbinafine-induced lupus erythematosus. Br J Dermatol. 1998;138:708–9.
77. Bonsmann G, Schiller M, Luger TA, Stander S. Terbinafine-induced subacute cutaneous lupus erythematosus. J Am Acad Dermatol. 2001;44:925–31.
78. Smith EB. The treatment of dermatophytosis: safety considerations. J Am Acad Dermatol. 2000; 43:S113–19.
79. Spruance SL, Rea TL, Thoming C, et al. Penciclovir cream for the treatment of herpes simplex labialis. JAMA. 1997;277:1374–9.
80. Vere Hodge RA. Review: antiviral portraits series, number 3. Famciclovir and penciclovir: the mode of action of famciclovir including its conversion to penciclovir. Antiviral Chem Chemother. 1993; 4:67–84.
81. Bacon TH, Howard BA, Spender LC, Boyd MR. Activity of penciclovir in antiviral assays against herpes simplex virus. J Antimicrob Chemother. 1996;37:303–13.
82. Pope LE, Marcelletti JF, Katz LR, et al. The anti-herpes simplex virus activity of n-docosanol includes inhibition of the viral entry process. Antiviral Res. 1998;40:85–94.
83. Corey L, Nahmias AJ, Guinan ME, et al. A trial of topical acyclovir in genital herpes simplex virus infections. N Engl J Med. 1982;306:1313–19.
84. Fiddian AP, Kinghorn GR, Goldmeier D, et al. Topical acyclovir in the treatment of genital herpes: a comparison with systemic therapy. J Antimicrob Chemother. 1983;12:67–77.
85. Evans TY, Tyring SK. Advances in antiviral therapy in dermatology. Dermatol Clin. 1998;16:409–20.
86. Loveless M, Sacks SL, Harris JRW. Famciclovir in the management of first-episode genital herpes. Infect Dis Clin Pract. 1997;6:S12–16.
87. Tyring S, Barbarash RA, Nahlik JE, et al. Famciclovir for the treatment of acute herpes zoster: effects on acute disease and postherpetic neuralgia. A randomized, double-blind, placebo-controlled trial. Collaborative Famciclovir Herpes Zoster Study Group. Ann Intern Med. 1995;123:89–96.
88. Herne K, Cirelli R, Lee P, Tyring SK. Antiviral therapy of acute herpes zoster in older patients. Drugs Aging. 1996;8:97–112.

89. Evans TY, Vander Straten M, Carrasco DA, et al. Systemic antiviral agents. In: Wolverton SE (ed.). Comprehensive Dermatologic Drug Therapy. Philadelphia: Saunders, 2001:85–106.
90. Fleming DT, McQuillan GM, Johnson RE, et al. Herpes simplex virus type 2 in the United States, 1976 to 1994. N Engl J Med. 1997;337:1105–11.
91. Johnson RE, Nahmias AJ, Magder LS, et al. A seroepidemiologic survey of the prevalence of herpes simplex virus type 2 infection in the United States. N Engl J Med. 1989;321:7–12.
92. Wald A, Zeh J, Barnum G, Davis LG, Corey L. Suppression of subclinical shedding of herpes simplex virus type 2 with acyclovir. Ann Intern Med 1996; 124(1 Pt 1):8–15.
93. Reitano M, Tyring S, Lang W, et al. Valacyclovir for the suppression of recurrent genital herpes simplex virus infection: a large-scale dose range-finding study. J Infect Dis. 1998;178:603–10.
94. Corey L, Wald A, Patel R, et al. Once-daily valacyclovir to reduce the risk of transmission of genital herpes. N Engl J Med. 2004;350:11–20.
95. Englund JA, Arvin AM, Balfour HH Jr. Acyclovir treatment for varicella does not lower gpI and IE-62 (p170) antibody responses to varicella-zoster virus in normal children. J Clin Microbiol. 1990;28:2327–30.
96. Chapel KL, Rasmussen JE. Pediatric dermatology: advances in therapy. J Am Acad Dermatol. 1997;36:513–26.
97. Valtrex® product information. Glaxo Wellcome Inc., Research Triangle Park, NC, October 2000.
98. Hayden FG. Antiviral drugs (other than antiretrovirals). In: Mandell GL, Bennett JE, Dolin R (eds). Mandell, Douglas, and Bennett's Principles and Practice of Infectious Disease, 5th edn. Phildadelphia: Churchill Livingstone, 2000:460–90.
99. Zovirax® product information. Glaxo Wellcome Inc., Research Triangle Park, NC, March 2000.
100. Mutalik S, Gupte A, Gupte S. Oral acyclovir therapy for varicella in pregnancy. Int J Dermatol. 1997; 36:49–51.
101. Sasadeusz JJ, Sacks SL. Systemic antivirals in herpesvirus infections. Dermatol Clin. 1993;11:171–85.
102. Leung DT, Sacks SL. Current recommendations for the treatment of genital herpes. Drugs. 2000;60:1329–52.
103. Calista D. Topical cidofovir for severe cutaneous human papillomavirus and molluscum contagiosum infections in patients with HIV/AIDS. A pilot study. J Eur Acad Dermatol Venereol. 2000;14:484–8.
104. Zabawski EJ Jr, Cockerell CJ. Topical and intralesional cidofovir: a review of pharmacology and therapeutic effects. J Am Acad Dermatol. 1998;39:741–5.
105. Crumpacker CS, Schaffer PA. New anti-HSV therapeutics target helicase-primase complex. Nat Med. 2002;8:327–8.
106. Crutte JJ, Grygon CA, Hargrave KD. Herpes simplex virus helicase-primase inhibitors are active in animal models of human disease. Nat Med. 2002;8:386–91.
107. Kleymann G, Fischer R, Betz UAK, et al. New helicase-primase inhibitors as drug candidates for the treatment of herpes simplex disease. Nat Med. 2002;8:392–8.

Immunomodulators

Jeffrey P Callen

INTERFERONS

Key features

- Human cells produce three antigenically distinct forms of interferon (IFN), originally described as leukocyte (α), fibroblast (β) and immune (γ)
- Recombinant DNA technology can produce large quantities of highly purified human IFN
- IFNs have antiviral, antiproliferative and immunoregulatory properties
- Dermatologic FDA-approved indications for IFNs include condyloma acuminata (IFN-α₂ᵦ), melanoma (IFN-α₂ᵦ), and AIDS-associated Kaposi's sarcoma (IFN-α₂ₐ and IFN-α₂ᵦ)
- Side effects include flu-like symptoms, leukopenia, nausea, vomiting and hepatitis

INTRODUCTION

Interferons (IFNs) are a family of secretory glycoproteins produced by most eukaryotic cells in response to a variety of viral and non-viral inducers. All IFNs display antiviral activity, but also modulate other cellular functions. IFN does not inactivate viruses directly, but rather renders cells resistant to viruses.

There are three antigenically distinct IFNs, originally described as leukocyte (α), fibroblast (β) and immune (γ)[1] (Table 128.1). Utilization of recombinant DNA technology has led to the production of large quantities of highly purified human IFN by *Escherichia coli*. This chapter will focus primarily on IFN-α₂ₐ and IFN-α₂ᵦ, which are the most frequently used IFNs for patients with dermatologic diseases.

PHARMACOLOGY AND MECHANISM OF ACTION

There are over 30 species of IFN-α, with a molecular weight of approximately 20 kDa, composed of 165–172 amino acids and with very similar amino acid sequences. IFN-α₂ₐ and IFN-α₂ᵦ differ in just a single amino acid. IFN-β has 29% structural homology to IFN-α, but IFN-γ has no statistically significant structural homology to either IFN-α or IFN-β[2].

IFNs must be injected intralesionally or be given parenterally. Systemic absorption via the intramuscular or subcutaneous route is greater than 80% for IFN-α. The peak effect of IFN-α₂ᵦ (administered intramuscularly or subcutaneously) is reached between 3 and 12 hours after injection, and IFN becomes undetectable after 24 hours[1].

IFNs undergo renal catabolism. Proteolytic degradation of IFN during renal tubular absorption is the likely mechanism and the primary site of inactivation is probably the kidney. Human IFN does not appear to cross the placental barrier, but IFN-α is FDA pregnancy category C. The safety of IFN-α during lactation is unknown.

IFN activity is dependent upon its ability to bind to specific receptors on the surface of target cells. IFN-α and IFN-β share the same receptor encoded on chromosome 21, whereas IFN-γ binds to an unrelated receptor encoded on chromosome 6. The intracellular events following receptor binding leading to gene expression are still under investigation. The antiviral activity of various IFNs can be explained in part by their ability to induce the expression of oligo-adenylate synthetase (2'–5'A synthetase) (Table 128.2). The antiproliferative effects of the various IFNs may involve the induction of 2'–5'A synthetase (with its products inhibiting mitosis), the inhibition of several growth factors, and the downregulation of c-*myc*, c-*fos* and certain c-*ras* oncogenes, as well as the ability of IFN to induce expression of *p53*, the tumor suppressor gene, and enhance apoptosis.

MECHANISMS OF ACTION FOR INTERFERONS

Cellular mechanisms	Clinical effect
Induction of 2'–5'A synthetase Induction of ribonuclease Induction of protein kinase P1	Antiviral
Induction of 2'–5'A synthetase Inhibition of various growth factors Enhanced *p53* tumor suppressor gene expression Downregulation of c-*myc*, c-*fos* and certain c-*ras* oncogenes	Antiproliferative
Induction of class I & II MHC antigens Increased number of natural killer (NK) cells Inhibits production of Th2 cytokines such as IL-4 and IL-5	Immunoregulatory

Table 128.2 **Mechanisms of action for interferons.** IL, interleukin; MHC, major histocompatibilty complex. Courtesy of Brian Berman MD, Tami De Araujo MD, and Mark Lebwohl MD.

Table 128.1 **The interferons.** il, intralesional; im, intramuscular; iv, intravenous; sc, subcutaneous.

THE INTERFERONS

Generic name	Trade name®	Manufacturer	Route	Half-life	Peak effect
Interferon-α₂ₐ	Roferon	Roche	sc	5.1 h	3.8–7.3 h
Interferon-α₂ᵦ	Intron A Rebetron when combined with ribavirin	Schering	iv, il, im, sc	2–3 h	30 min (iv) 3–12 h (im, sc)
Interferon-αN3	Alferon N	Hemispherx	il	2–3 h	3–12 h
Interferon-β₁ₐ	Avonex Rebif	Biogen-Idec Serono	im sc	10 h 69 h	3–15 h 16 h
Interferon-β₁ᵦ	Betaseron	Berlex	sc	4.3 h	1–8 h
Interferon-γ₁ᵦ	Actimmune	Intermune	sc	5.9	4.7
Interferon alphacon-1	Infergen	Valeant	sc	-	24–36 h

IFN-α therapy can induce the formation of neutralizing antibodies. However, the clinical significance of neutralizing antibodies remains to be elucidated[3].

INDICATIONS AND DOSAGES (Table 128.3)

Condylomata Acuminata (Genital Warts)

Intralesional IFN-α_{2b} was found to be safe and effective in the treatment of condylomata acuminata on the external surfaces of genital and perianal areas[4]. The dose used for condyloma is 1 million IU per wart three times weekly for 3 weeks, with a maximal dose of 5 million IU per session. It is not clear whether IFN therapy for condyloma acuminata is superior to other therapies available[5], because studies have focused on IFN use in patients who have previously failed other therapies. However, IFN should be reserved for highly motivated patients who have failed other simpler and less costly modes of therapy.

Cutaneous T-Cell Lymphoma

The use of IFN for cutaneous T-cell lymphoma dates back to the early 1980s. Interferon-α_{2a} is the most frequently used preparation. Although IFN may be used as a monotherapy, its use in combination with PUVA, total skin electron beam therapy, oral retinoids, and other chemotherapeutic agents seems to enhance the effectiveness of the other agents (see Ch. 120) and in many instances results in a complete response rate of between 70% and 80%[6].

Hemangiomas

IFN-α_{2a} has been used to treat severe, life-threatening and/or corticosteroid-unresponsive hemangiomas[7] (see Ch. 103). However, this therapy has been associated with spastic diplegia and other neurologic dysfunction; consequently, its use as a therapy for hemangiomas has declined[8].

AIDS-Associated Kaposi's Sarcoma

Both IFN-α_{2a} and IFN-α_{2b} are used to treat Kaposi's sarcoma associated with AIDS (see Ch. 77). The overall objective response rates with IFN-α_{2a} and IFN-α_{2b} have equaled or surpassed those achieved with conventional cytotoxic chemotherapy. The recommended dosages of IFN-α_{2a} and IFN-α_{2b} are 36 and 30 million IU, respectively, administered subcutaneously daily. As a single agent, a high dose of IFN-α_{2a} has been reported to induce a response rate of 7% among asymptomatic patients with fewer than 200 CD4$^+$ cells/mm^3. Response rates of 27% and 45% were seen in those with 200–400 and over 400 cells/mm^3, respectively[9].

Currently, the optimal duration of IFN treatment for Kaposi's sarcoma is not known. In many patients, tumor recurrence occurs within 6 months in complete responders and the response to the second course of treatment is less reliable. These facts have led to a recommendation for maintenance therapy for as long as adverse effects are tolerated[9]. Unlike highly active antiretroviral therapy (see Ch. 77), IFN does not reverse the underlying immunodeficiency. In addition to its immune-enhancing and antiproliferative effects, the response of Kaposi's sarcoma to IFN could be explained by an antiviral effect on human herpesvirus-8 (see Ch. 77).

Basal Cell Carcinoma

Intralesional injection of IFN-α_{2b} into nodular or superficial basal cell carcinoma (BCC) can be regarded as an alternative to surgery in highly selected patients[10]. Although studies demonstrated significant cure rates (compared to placebo), the highest rates were roughly 85% for such lesions, which is far below what might be expected for traditional surgical approaches.

Squamous Cell Carcinoma and Keratoacanthoma

As with BCC, IFN-α_{2b} therapy can be considered for patients with actinically induced or human papillomavirus (HPV)-associated squamous

---

CLINICAL DISEASES TREATED WITH INTERFERONS

FDA-approved indications

Condyloma acuminata (α)
AIDS-associated Kaposi's sarcoma (α)
Melanoma (adjuvant) (α)
Chronic granulomatous disease (γ)

Some off-label dermatologic uses

Basal cell carcinoma (α)
Actinic keratoses (α)
Squamous cell carcinoma (α)
Giant condyloma of Buschke–Lowenstein (α)
Cutaneous T-cell lymphoma (α, β, γ)
Granulomatous slack skin (α, γ)
Keloids (α, γ)
Hemangioma (α)

Tufted angioma (α)
Verruca vulgaris (α, β, γ)
Epidermodysplasia verruciformis (α)
Herpes zoster (α)
Herpes simplex (α)
Necrolytic acral erythema (with hepatitis C) (α)
Leishmaniasis (γ)
Leprosy (γ)
Mycobacterium avium complex (γ)
Atopic dermatitis (γ)
Chronic cutaneous lupus erythematosus (α)
Behçet's disease (α)
Progressive systemic sclerosis (γ)
Scleromyxedema (α)

Table 128.3 Clinical diseases treated with interferons. Adapted from Wolverton SE, Comprehensive Dermatologic Drug Therapy, 2nd edition. Philadelphia: WB Saunders, 2007.

---

cell carcinoma (SCC) or keratoacanthoma who are not candidates for surgical excision or who are not amenable to surgery[11,12].

Melanoma

The results of several trials of adjuvant interferon therapy for cutaneous melanoma are outlined in Table 113.12.

Keloids

In 1989, Berman & Duncan[13] reported a 41% reduction in the area of a keloid, following intralesional injections of 1.5 million IU of IFN-α_{2b} twice over 4 days (the effect was seen by day 9 after the injection, by which time a biopsy specimen of the keloid was obtained).

Granstein et al.[14] performed a placebo-controlled, double-blind trial of intralesional recombinant IFN-γ for the treatment of keloids in 10 patients. Eight of the patients completed the course of treatment with injections of either diluent or 0.1 or 0.01 mg IFN-γ three times per week for 3 weeks. The average percentage reduction in keloidal height 22 days after the initial injection was 30.4% for the IFN-γ-treated keloids and only 1.1% for the diluent-treated keloids ($P<0.002$). No statistically significant difference was found between the effects of the lower versus the higher dose of IFN-γ. In another study of 10 scars, interferon-γ at doses of 0.5 mg (intralesionally) once weekly for 10 weeks decreased the linear dimension by at least 50% in 5 of 10 scars, with minimal adverse effects being reported[15].

In the postoperative setting, Berman & Flores[16] demonstrated that intralesional IFN-α_{2b} was superior to triamcinolone acetonide injections in preventing recurrences of excised keloids. However, in a report by Davison et al.[17], triamcinolone was more effective than IFN-α_{2b}.

Verruca Vulgaris

In the early 1980s, Nimura et al.[18] reported a 'good response' in 81% of common warts treated with intralesional non-recombinant IFN-β, compared to a 17% response rate in controls. Berman and co-workers[19] then reported a mean reduction of 86% in the lesional area of common warts treated with 0.1 million IU IFN-α_{2b}, compared to a 38% improvement in the placebo-injected group.

Atopic Dermatitis

Evidence of reduced production of IFN-γ *in vitro* by mononuclear cells of patients with atopic dermatitis, and the suppression of interleukin (IL)-4-mediated IgE stimulation by IFN-γ, prompted evaluation of the use of IFN for atopic dermatitis. A randomized, placebo-controlled, double-blind, multicenter trial studied the effects of daily subcutaneous injection (50 μg/m²) of recombinant IFN-γ versus placebo for 12 weeks in 78 patients. Altogether, 45% of the recombinant IFN-γ-treated group and 21% of the placebo-treated patients achieved a significant response (>50% improvement) by physicians' evaluations[20]. The results with other dosages have varied from 57% clinical improvement (open trial of 14 patients)[20] to no differences compared with controls[21].

Therapy with IFN-α has also been investigated in patients with atopic dermatitis, again with varied and contradictory results. Torrelo et al.[22] reported a satisfactory response (investigator and patient global assessment) in five of 13 patients treated with IFN-α_{2a} (3 million IU subcutaneously three times weekly for 4 weeks). However, Mackie[23] reported no benefit from the same regimen administered for a total duration of 12–14 weeks. Further clinical trials are obviously necessary in order to determine the clinical effectiveness of this expensive treatment.

Behçet's Disease

Fourteen patients with Behçet's disease who had oral ulcers, genital ulcers, pustular vasculitis, erythema nodosum and/or thrombophlebitis were treated with IFN-α_{2a} (3 million IU subcutaneously three times per week, escalating to 12 million IU, for a 2-month period). All patients were symptom-free at 2 months and had fewer recurrences in the post-treatment period[24]. Similar response rates with recombinant IFN-γ injected subcutaneously have been reported[25]. Maintenance doses once or twice weekly, however, were required to prevent early relapses.

Systemic Sclerosis

The ability of IFN to inhibit *in vitro* activated functions of dermal fibroblasts derived from the involved skin of patients with scleroderma, morphea or keloids (see above) has been demonstrated[26]. The elevated collagen production by scleroderma, morphea and keloid fibroblasts can be inhibited by IFN-α, -β and -γ. The latter also inhibited the proliferation of scleroderma fibroblasts, although the inhibition did not persist[26]. Kahan et al.[27] reported benefit of therapy with recombinant IFN-γ in a small group of patients with systemic sclerosis.

CONTRAINDICATIONS

Absolute contraindications are hypersensitivity to mouse immunoglobulin and to IFN-α and -γ formulations. The relative contraindications are cardiac arrhythmias, depression or other psychiatric disorders, leukopenia, coagulopathies, pregnancy (category C) and previous organ transplantation.

MAJOR SIDE EFFECTS

The adverse effects of IFN are dose-dependent and generally improve or remit during continued therapy or following dose reduction. In addition, the adverse effects are usually rapidly reversible upon cessation of therapy.

Cutaneous Reactions

Approximately 5% of patients treated with IFN-β_{1b} for multiple sclerosis have developed skin necrosis at the site of injection secondary to a localized vasculopathy[28] (Fig. 128.1). Plaques of psoriasis can also develop at the sites of injection of IFN, as can flares of psoriasis in patients receiving IFN (Fig. 128.2).

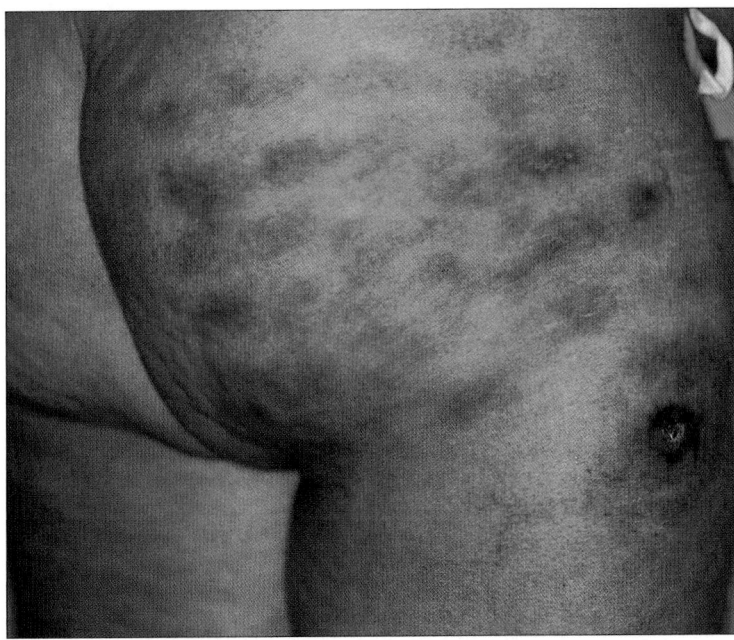

Fig. 128.1 Postinflammatory hyperpigmentation and ulceration at sites of interferon-β_{1b} injection in a woman with multiple sclerosis. Courtesy of Jean L Bolognia MD.

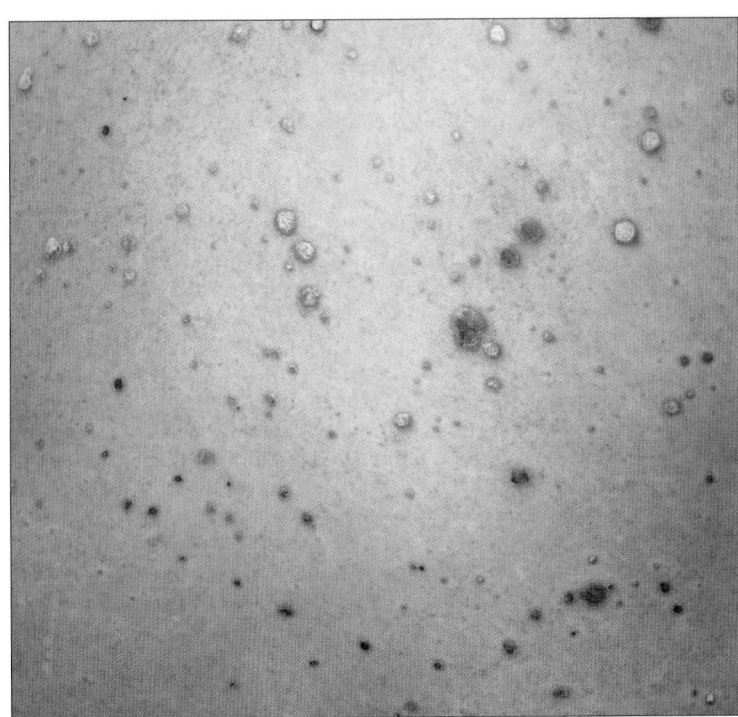

Fig. 128.2 Interferon-induced flare of psoriasis.

Flu-like Symptoms

The most commonly associated adverse effects are flu-like symptoms of fever, chills, fatigue, myalgias, headache and arthralgias. Generally, in healthy individuals, subcutaneous administration of IFN-α in doses of ≤3 million IU every other day induces nominal and tolerable flu-like symptoms, or no adverse effects at all. Prophylactic (1–2 hours prior to injection) administration of acetaminophen (650 mg), aspirin (650 mg) or non-steroidal anti-inflammatory drugs (e.g. ibuprofen 400 mg) helps to prevent these effects.

Neurologic and Psychiatric Effects

Spastic diplegia was reported in five of 26 patients with hemangiomas treated with 1.02–3.60 million IU/day of IFN-α_{2a}[8]. Preservatives such as benzyl and phenol alcohol in the commercially available injectable solution may have been playing a role and a preservative-free saline solution was recommended by the authors. An additional explanation is the immaturity of the infant's central nervous system. Depression and suicidal behavior, including suicidal ideation, attempts and completed suicides, have been reported in association with IFN-α therapy[29].

Cardiovascular Effects

Significant hypotension, arrhythmias or tachycardia (heart rate ≥150 beats/minute) can be seen in association with IFN therapy[30]. Although these side effects are usually managed by modifying the dosages of IFN or by discontinuing treatment, they may require specific additional therapy. Patients with a recent history of a myocardial infarction or a history of arrhythmias require close monitoring.

Rhabdomyolysis

Rhabdomyolysis is occasionally seen, and proved fatal in at least one patient treated with high-dose IFN-α_{2b} (20 million IU intravenously twice daily for 5 days)[31]. Elevated serum creatine kinase levels should lead to a reduction in dose or cessation of therapy, depending on the severity of the elevation.

Gastrointestinal Effects and Bone Marrow Suppression

Gastrointestinal disturbances such as nausea, vomiting and diarrhea can occur, as can anorexia and hepatitis. Fatal cases of hepatitis have been reported in patients receiving high-dose IFN. Bone marrow suppression is another side effect of IFN, and it is a particular problem in patients receiving high-dose therapy or who have other reasons for bone marrow suppression (e.g. concomitant medications). Serial evaluation of liver function tests and complete blood counts is recommended.

Other Adverse Effects

Neutralizing antibodies can develop in patients receiving IFN-α_{2a} or IFN-α_{2b}, and they appear to be specific to the recombinant IFN and not to natural IFN[32].

INTERACTIONS

In one study of nine patients, a single intramuscular injection of IFN-α_{2a} and a single injection of aminophylline led to a variable effect on the clearance of aminophylline[33]; a 50% reduction in median clearance of aminophylline was observed, probably due to inhibition of the cytochrome P450 enzyme system. Caution must be used when IFN is administered in conjunction with other myelosuppressive drugs, as well as potentially neurotoxic vinca alkaloids. The concomitant use of IFN and IL-2 may increase the risk of renal failure. The concomitant use of IFN-α_{2a} with zidovudine may increase the risk of myelosuppression.

USE IN PREGNANCY

Interferons are rated as pregnancy category C, and although it is unknown whether IFN is excreted into human milk, it is excreted into mouse milk.

IMIQUIMOD

Key features

- Commercially available as a 5% cream
- Initially used for anogenital warts, it is now FDA-approved for actinic keratoses on the head and neck and superficial BCCs
- It has also been used off-label in individual patients or small case series for common warts, molluscum contagiosum, keloids, lentigo maligna, SCC *in situ* and extramammary Paget's disease
- An immune response modifier that stimulates an innate immune response via induction of IFN-α and TNF-α and stimulates cell-mediated immunity as well

INTRODUCTION

Imiquimod (1-(2 methylpropyl)-1 H-imidazo [4, 5c] quinolin-4 amine) is an immune response modifier that stimulates innate and adaptive immune pathways, resulting in antiviral, antitumor and immunoregulatory properties. Imiquimod is a stimulator of the innate immune response via the induction, synthesis and release of cytokines, such as IFN-α, IL-6 and TNF-α[34] (Fig. 128.3). In addition, imiquimod acts to stimulate other elements of innate immunity, such as natural killer cell activity and secretion of nitric oxide from macrophages[35]. Imiquimod's effects on the cell-mediated arm of the adaptive immune system include indirect stimulation of the Th1 cytokine IFN-γ (Fig. 128.3). Imiquimod also activates and enhances the migration of Langerhans cells, the major antigen-presenting cell type within the epidermis, to the regional lymph nodes, resulting in antigen presentation to T-lymphocytes[36].

MECHANISM OF ACTION

In vitro, imiquimod induces cytokine production, most likely via activation of Toll-like receptor 7 (TLR7). Upon TLR7 stimulation, nuclear factor-κB activation stimulates production of IFN-α and cytokines such as interleukin(IL)-12 and IL-18 (see Fig. 128.3). The stimulation of IL-12 production and the stimulation of CD4$^+$ T cells to produce the IL-12 β_2 receptor (by IFN-α) lead to the production of IFN-γ and the enhancement of cell-mediated immunity.

After topical application of imiquimod to hairless mice, increased IFN-α and TNF-α were seen in treated (but not control) mouse skin[34]. Imiquimod's antiviral and antitumor activity in animal models is explained at least in part by the actions of IFN-α (see Table 128.2). In addition, IFN-γ stimulates cytotoxic T lymphocytes, which kill virally infected cells as well as tumors and provide the immune memory needed for future protection. Long-term protection following imiquimod treatment was observed in the guinea pig model for herpes simplex and in a murine tumor model. In the latter, imiquimod-treated mice became free of tumor at the end of a 30-day experiment and remained resistant to challenge with the same tumor cells 8 months later without further drug treatment. In summary, imiquimod has effects in both the innate and the adaptive arms of the immune system.

Metabolism

Percutaneous absorption of imiquimod from the 5% cream is minimal, with less than 0.9% of a radiolabeled 5 mg dose being recovered in the urine and feces. The site of potential metabolism is unknown, as is the degree of protein binding, if any.

INDICATIONS

Human Papillomavirus Infection

HPV is not easily recognized by the immune system. The various subtypes associated with anogenital and non-genital warts, as well as the 'oncogenic' subtypes, are reviewed in Chapter 78. The importance of treating HPV infection is highlighted by the association of the latter subtypes with anogenital SCCs as well as the discomfort and psychological effects of HPV-associated conditions such as genital warts.

External genital and perianal warts[37]

In randomized vehicle-controlled clinical trials, the topical application of imiquimod 5% cream three times a week for up to 16 weeks completely clears lesions in roughly 50% of patients. There is a difference in the clearance rates between women and men, which is thought to be due to the location of the warts, with a lower degree of keratinization of the vulva compared with the shaft of the penis, the most common locations of warts, respectively. The topical imiquimod is well tolerated by the patients. The exact place for this therapy in the therapeutic armamentarium remains unclear, but it is believed to be among first-line topical therapies.

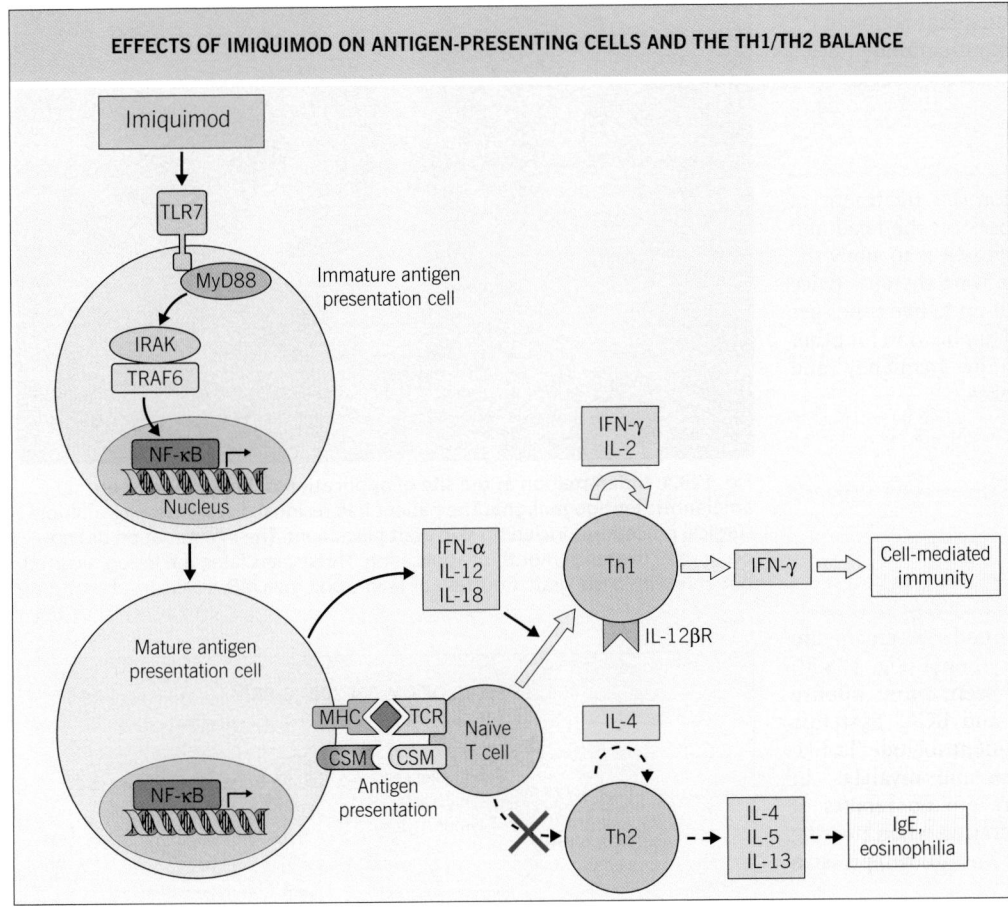

EFFECTS OF IMIQUIMOD ON ANTIGEN-PRESENTING CELLS AND THE TH1/TH2 BALANCE

Fig. 128.3 Effects of imiquimod on antigen-presenting cells and the Th1/Th2 balance. Binding of imiquimod to Toll-like receptor 7 (TLR7) on antigen-presenting cells (e.g. Langerhans cells, other dendritic cells, macrophages) leads to interaction of the cytoplasmic portion of the receptor with MyD88. This facilitates association of MyD88 with IL-1 receptor-associated kinase (IRAK), which in turn activates TNF receptor-activated 6 (TRAF6) and ultimately results in stimulation of nuclear factor-κB-mediated signaling. Imiquimod thereby promotes antigen-presenting cell maturation and secretion of IL-12 and other cytokines, which induce IFN-γ production by naive T cells and result in a Th1-type immune response. CSM, costimulatory molecule; MHC, major histocompatibility complex; TCR, T-cell receptor.

Common warts

The efficacy of topical imiquimod in the treatment of common warts (verrucae vulgaris), periungual warts and plantar warts appears to be quite a bit lower than its efficacy for genital and perianal warts. It is possible that imiquimod might be used as an adjuvant therapy or might be combined with sequential application of acid preparations that might enhance its penetration and effectiveness.

Several case studies have reported the successful treatment of common warts in immunocompromised patients[38]. There are also reports of the successful treatment of recalcitrant facial flat warts with imiquimod 5% cream.

Molluscum Contagiosum

Molluscum contagiosum, a cutaneous infection caused by a large double-stranded DNA virus of the Poxviridae family, has been successfully treated with imiquimod 5% cream. Molluscum contagiosum tends to occur in young children, sexually active adults, and HIV-infected patients (up to 20% of the latter group). Open-label trials and some case reports have suggested that imiquimod might be beneficial for molluscum contagiosum. One double-blind, placebo-controlled trial involving 23 children found a significant decrease in the number of molluscum lesions within 12 weeks of imiquimod applied three times per week compared to placebo[39]. As with verrucae, patients may try sequential application of a keratolytic.

Keloids

A pilot study was undertaken to evaluate the recurrence rate of keloids following surgical excision and subsequent localized topical application of imiquimod 5% cream[40]. Thirteen keloids (12 earlobe, 1 mid-back) in 12 patients were surgically excised and closed primarily. Nightly application of imiquimod 5% cream directly to the suture line and to the surrounding area was initiated on the day of surgery for a total of 8 weeks. None of the 11 (0%) keloids recurred in the 10 patients who completed both the treatment period and at least 6 months of post-

operative follow-up[40]. In a subsequent small study, comparing post-surgical application of imiquimod to intralesional corticosteroid therapy, Martin-Garcia & Busquets found the imiquimod to be beneficial[41].

Basal Cell Carcinoma[42]

Imiquimod is approved for the treatment of superficial BCCs. Studies of both superficial and nodular BCCs have been performed using imiquimod 5% cream. Applications either 5 days per week or 7 days per week for 6–12 weeks were employed in various studies. The rate of clinical and histologic clearance was roughly 70–75%, which was highly statistically significant compared to placebo. This rate is substantially lower than rates for destructive and surgical methods.

Actinic Keratoses

Imiquimod is FDA-approved for treatment of actinic keratoses of the head and neck. Its efficacy and toxicity have been recently reviewed in a systematic review and meta-analysis. The authors concluded that application of imiquimod 5% cream three times per week for 12–16 weeks resulted in complete clearing of 50% versus 5% for those patients treated with placebo[43]. Toxicity was common, but was primarily limited to local irritant reactions that are often managed with a drug holiday.

Bowen's Disease

Imiquimod has been studied in a double-blind, placebo-controlled study in patients with Bowen's disease[44]. This relatively small study demonstrated a highly significant level of efficacy compared to placebo (73% vs 0%). Follow-up periods averaging 9 months failed to demonstrate any recurrence among the complete responders.

Other Dermatologic Diseases[45,46]

Imiquimod 5% cream has been reported in non-controlled case reports and series to be effective in the treatment of nevoid basal cell carcinoma syndrome[47], SCC including in patients who are transplant recipients[48], SCC of the penis[49], cutaneous T-cell lymphoma[50], extramammary Paget's disease[51], lentigo maligna[52] and cutaneous melanoma metastases[53].

DOSAGES

Imiquimod 5% cream is approved in the US for the treatment of external genital and perianal warts, actinic keratoses on the head and neck, and superficial BCCs. The recommended regimen is to apply the cream three times weekly for up to 16 weeks for wart therapy, twice weekly for up to 16 weeks for actinic keratoses, and up to five times per week for up to 6 weeks for BCCs. The frequency of application for other 'off-label' indications varies and optimal therapy frequency and duration are still being determined in most instances.

CONTRAINDICATIONS

None are known.

MAJOR SIDE EFFECTS

The most common adverse reactions to imiquimod 5% cream are restricted to the site of application and include erythema (Fig. 128.4), ulceration, edema and scaling. These reactions seem more intense and frequent in patients with actinic keratoses and BCC. Systemic adverse effects possibly or probably related to treatment include flu-like symptoms, i.e. fatigue, fever, headache, diarrhea and myalgias, in approximately 1–2% of patients. Thus far, there are no reports of systemic immune alteration, an important consideration when treating patients with solid organ transplants who are on immunosuppressive therapies.

INTERACTIONS

There are no known drug interactions with imiquimod 5% cream.

USE IN PREGNANCY

Imiquimod 5% cream is classified pregnancy category B. It is not known whether topically applied imiquimod 5% cream is excreted in breast milk.

GRANULOCYTE–MACROPHAGE AND GRANULOCYTE COLONY-STIMULATING FACTOR (GM-CSF AND G-CSF)

Key features

- Used primarily to treat neutropenia
- Cutaneous side effects include neutrophilic dermatoses and vasculitis

INTRODUCTION

Colony-stimulating factors are glycoproteins that regulate the survival, proliferation, differentiation and functional activation of hematopoietic cells. They include erythropoietin, granulocyte–macrophage colony-stimulating factor (GM-CSF), granulocyte colony-stimulating factor (G-CSF), macrophage colony-stimulating factor (M-CSF), IL-3 and IL-II. Erythropoietin (erythroid precursors), GM-CSF, G-CSF and IL-II (megakaryocytes) are currently commercially available.

MECHANISM OF ACTION

The mechanism of action of GM-CSF and G-CSF is illustrated in Figure 128.5.

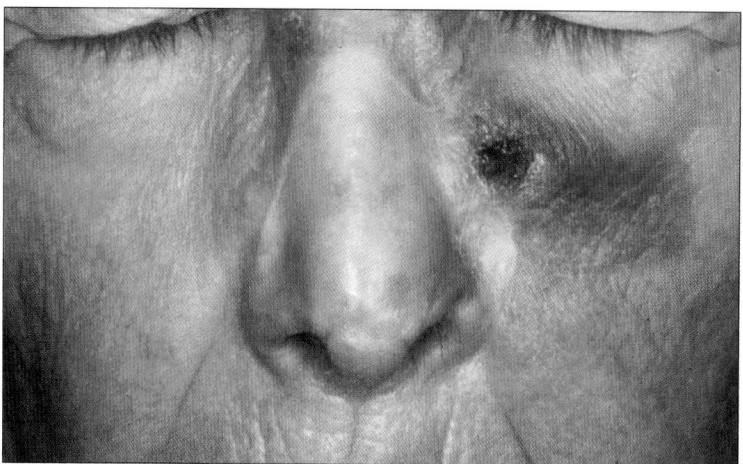

Fig. 128.4 Inflammation at the site of application of imiquimod to an amelanotic lentigo maligna. The patient had residual disease despite multiple surgical procedures including skin graft placement. The inflammation did not occur until the tenth month of application. Three years later, the lesion recurred, but only within the graft. Courtesy of Jean L Bolognia MD.

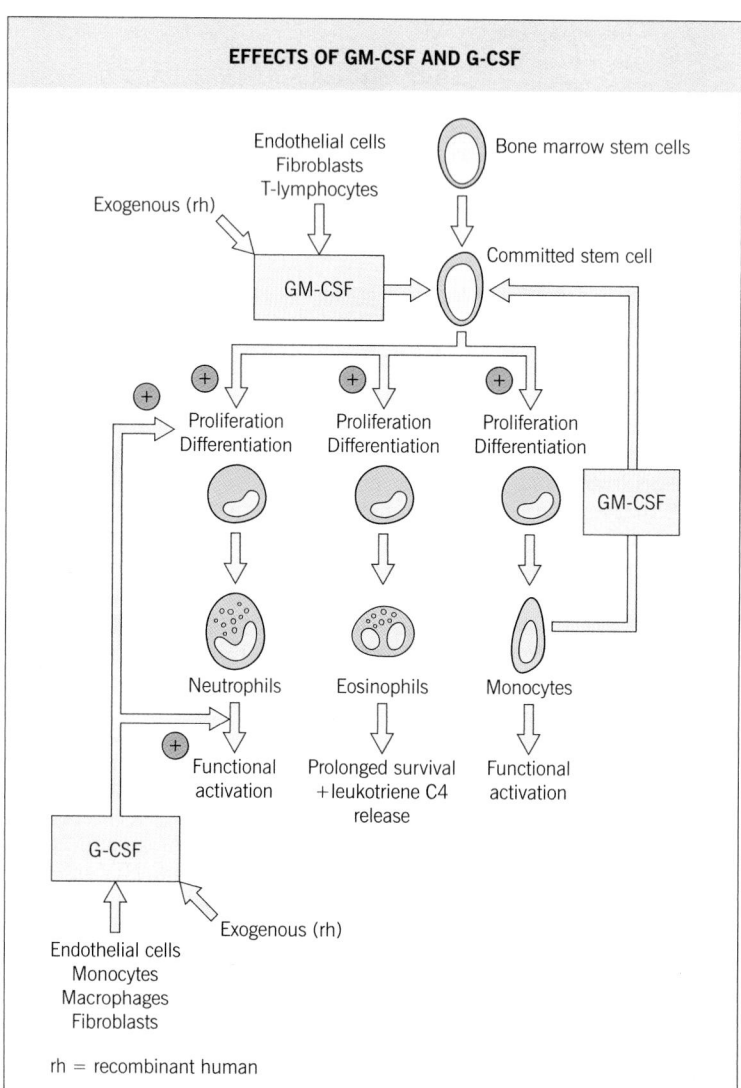

Fig. 128.5 The effects of GM-CSF and G-CSF. rh, recombinant human. Courtesy of Brian Berman MD and Tami De Araujo MD.

INDICATIONS

Both recombinant human GM-CSF and G-CSF are used primarily to treat neutropenia in the setting of marrow-suppressive chemotherapy, bone marrow transplantation and peripheral blood stem cell transplantation, as well as for mobilization of peripheral blood progenitor cells. Additional uses include aplastic anemia, AIDS-related neutropenia, severe chronic neutropenia and the neutropenia associated with dyskeratosis congenita[54]. In dermatology, both have been investigated as promoters of wound healing and GM-CSF has been studied as a possible therapy for melanoma.

MAJOR SIDE EFFECTS

GM-CSF

Commonly reported systemic side effects of GM-CSF administration include fever, myalgias, bone pain, and occasionally flares of autoimmune disease. Horn et al.[55] reported a morbilliform cutaneous eruption as a side effect of GM-CSF administration. The widespread eruption usually presents within 24–48 hours of GM-CSF administration; histologic findings include spongiosis, lymphocytic exocytosis, and an upper dermal inflammatory cell infiltrate composed of eosinophils, neutrophils, mononuclear cells and an increased number of macrophages. The eruption typically resolves with a decrease in the dosage or with discontinuation of the drug. Other cutaneous side effects of GM-CSF (some of which are anticipated, given its mechanism of action) include local urticarial (Fig. 128.6) or pustular reactions at the site of injection, urticarial plaques with tense bullae, epidermolysis bullosa acquisita, exacerbation of psoriasis, leukocytoclastic vasculitis and Sweet's syndrome[56].

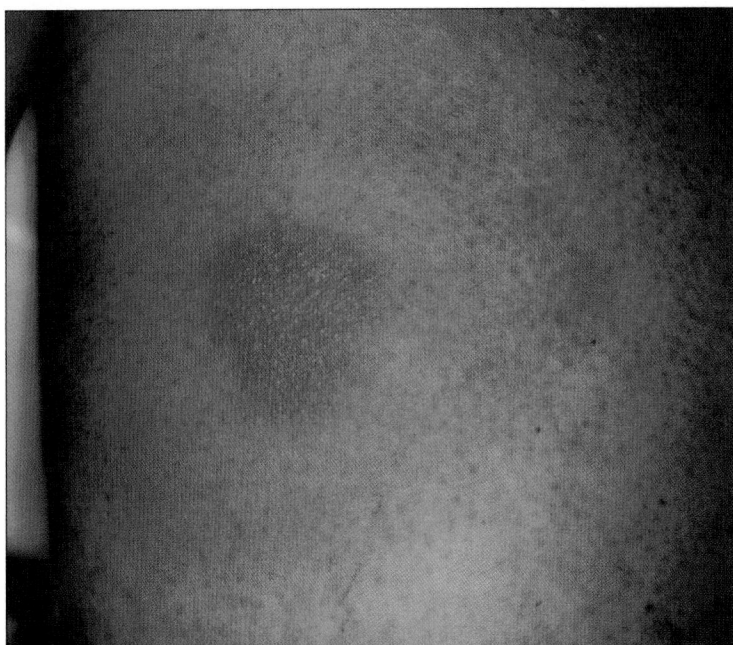

Fig. 128.6 Urticarial plaque at the site of GM-CSF injection.

G-CSF

G-CSF is generally well tolerated. The most common side effect is bone pain, which is characterized by a transient mild, dull ache that occurs in up to 20% of recipients. Rarely, reversible elevations in serum levels of uric acid, lactic dehydrogenase or alkaline phosphatase, seizures, anaphylactic reactions and transient decreases in blood pressure occur.

Recently, there have been several reports of Sweet's syndrome induced by G-CSF within 1–2 weeks after administration. Other cutaneous side effects include injection site reactions, pyoderma gangrenosum, cutaneous vasculitis and widespread folliculitis[57]. Histopathologically, a perivascular and interstitial infiltrate composed of neutrophils, eosinophils and large, plump histiocytes with cytologic atypia and numerous mitotic figures are seen.

INTERACTIONS

Additive effects can be seen between G-CSF or GM-CSF and other drugs that can cause neutrophilia, e.g. corticosteroids and lithium. A proliferation of blasts can be seen in patients with neutropenia in the setting of myelodysplasia (with excess blasts) treated with these growth factors.

USE IN PREGNANCY

GM-CSF and G-CSF have been classified as pregnancy risk category C. It is unknown whether either is excreted in human milk.

TOPICAL CALCINEURIN INHIBITORS: TACROLIMUS AND PIMECROLIMUS

Key features

- Topical calcineurin inhibitors are effective anti-inflammatory agents that allow treatment of inflammatory dermatoses without the side effects of topical corticosteroids
- Topical tacrolimus and pimecrolimus are approved for the treatment of moderate to severe and mild to moderate atopic dermatitis, respectively. They are also effective in treating a number of other corticosteroid-responsive dermatoses

INTRODUCTION

Topical corticosteroids have been the mainstay of therapy for eczematous dermatoses and other inflammatory disorders since their introduction decades ago. Unfortunately, they are associated with local disease rebound and tachyphylaxis and with well-described side effects, such as the development of cutaneous atrophy, telangiectasias, striae, perioral dermatitis (when used on the face), and cataracts and glaucoma (when used around the eyes). Systemic absorption can also occur.

Oral tacrolimus has been used in transplant patients for many years. Tacrolimus ointment (Protopic®) and pimecrolimus cream (Elidel®) are approved for the treatment of atopic dermatitis, and they have been used for other eczematous dermatoses and steroid-responsive dermatoses.

MECHANISM OF ACTION

Tacrolimus and pimecrolimus are inhibitors of the phosphatase calcineurin[58]. T-lymphocyte activation begins when costimulatory ligands on antigen-presenting cells interact with T-cell receptors. This increases the levels of free calcium within the cell, which binds to calmodulin, which in turn activates calcineurin (Fig. 128.7). Calcineurin dephosphorylates the cytoplasmic subunit of the nuclear factor of activated T cells (NFAT) – a step that is essential, since the dephosphorylated subunit is then able to translocate to the nucleus, where it forms a complex that assists in transcription of numerous cytokines. Tacrolimus and pimecrolimus bind to FK506-binding protein, forming complexes that inhibit calcineurin, thus preventing the dephosphorylation activity of this important phosphatase.

INDICATIONS

Tacrolimus ointment 0.1% and 0.03% are indicated for the treatment of moderate to severe atopic dermatitis in adults and in children over the age of 2 years, respectively. Pimecrolimus cream is indicated for the treatment of mild to moderate atopic dermatitis in individuals over the age of 2 years. There are a number of anecdotal reports and case series in which these agents have been used to treat other inflammatory dermatoses, including oral and/or genital lichen planus, chronic GVHD, eyelid and intertriginous dermatitis, facial and intertriginous psoriasis, periocular vitiligo, pyoderma gangrenosum, cutaneous Crohn's disease, seborrheic dermatitis, hand dermatitis, granulomatous rosacea, cutaneous lesions of dermatomyositis, cutaneous lupus erythematosus and lichen sclerosus[59].

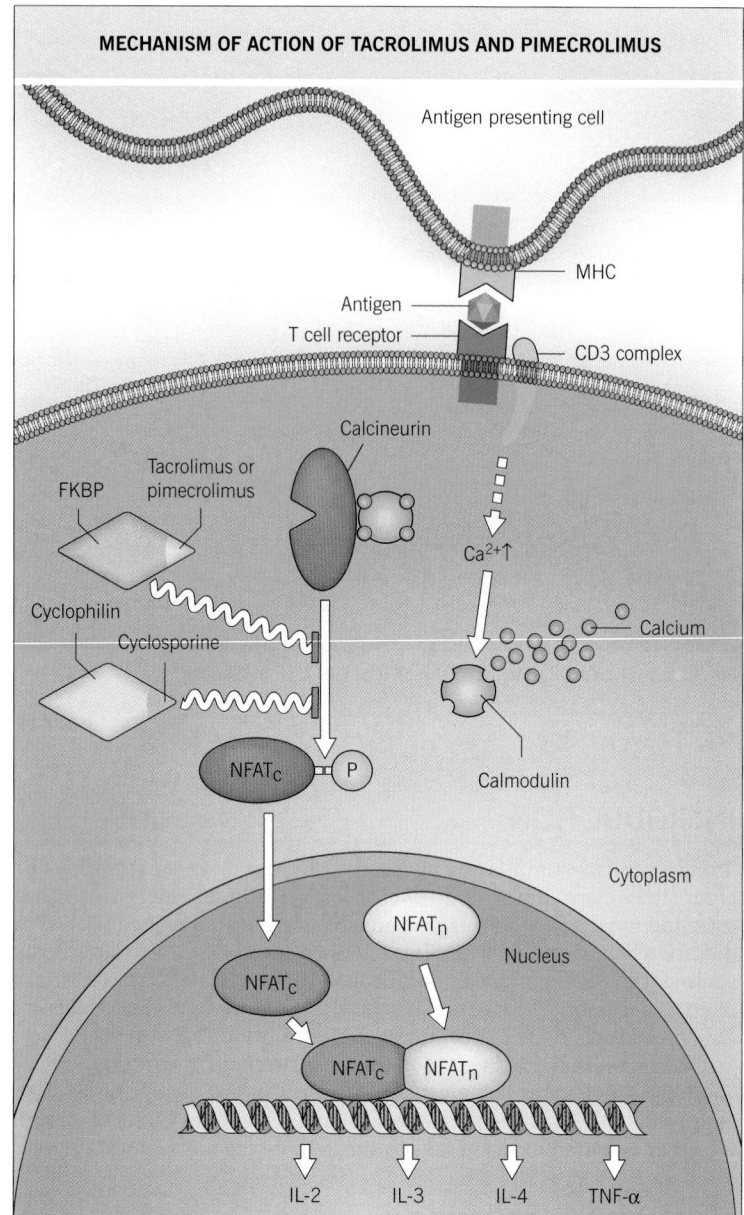

MECHANISM OF ACTION OF TACROLIMUS AND PIMECROLIMUS

Fig. 128.7 Mechanism of action of tacrolimus and pimecrolimus. FKBP, FK506-binding protein. NFAT, nuclear factor of activated T cells. With permission from Nghiem P, Pearson G, Langley RG. Tacrolimus and pimecrolimus: from clever prokaryotes to inhibiting calcineurin and treating atopic dermatitis. J Am Acad Dermatol. 2002;46:228–41.

DOSAGES

Topical tacrolimus is commercially available in 0.1% and 0.03% concentrations. The 0.1% formulation is somewhat more effective than the 0.03% formulation, but the 0.03% formulation is FDA-approved for use in children with atopic dermatitis. Pimecrolimus cream is available in a 1% concentration.

CONTRAINDICATIONS

The package inserts recommend that the benefits and risks of tacrolimus ointment and pimecrolimus cream be evaluated when prescribing them in the presence of varicella, active herpes simplex virus infection or eczema herpeticum. In addition, both labels were revised to include warnings about the potential for future malignancy and other effects of immune suppression due to absorption of the active agent. A systematic review failed to identify an increased level of risk from the use of these agents in humans; however, risks associated with long-term use of either of these agents remain unknown[60].

Because tacrolimus and pimecrolimus shorten the time to skin tumor formation in animal photocarcinogenicity studies, patients are asked to minimize or avoid natural or artificial sunlight exposure. Because of the increased absorption of tacrolimus ointment in patients with Netherton syndrome, its use and the use of pimecrolimus cream in this condition are not recommended[61].

MAJOR SIDE EFFECTS

Application site reactions (e.g. burning, stinging) are among the most common side effects of tacrolimus ointment and pimecrolimus cream. There are scattered reports of allergic contact dermatitis and a rosacea-like granulomatous reaction on the face due to tacrolimus. Regarding skin infections, it is interesting that *Staphylococcus aureus* colonization is reduced in the skin of atopic dermatitis patients treated with tacrolimus ointment.

INTERACTIONS

Formal clinical studies have not been conducted using tacrolimus ointment with other topical or systemic medications, but anecdotal use of tacrolimus in conjunction with topical corticosteroids suggests that the combination reduces burning and enhances efficacy. Compatibility studies of tacrolimus ointment applied in combination with desoximetasone ointment or clobetasol ointment indicate that both agents remain stable in the setting of concomitant use.

USE IN PREGNANCY

Because there are no adequate studies of topically administered tacrolimus or pimecrolimus in pregnant women, both are rated as category C. Animal studies with systemically administered tacrolimus indicate harmful fetal affects only at doses that are toxic to the mother.

BIOENGINEERED IMMUNOMODULATORS

Key features

- Agents that interfere with T-cell activation (alefacept, efalizumab) or T-cell trafficking in the skin (efalizumab) are effective in the treatment of psoriasis

- Agents that block TNF-α (etanercept, infliximab, adalimumab) are also effective as treatments for psoriasis, psoriatic arthritis, and other dermatoses with elevated levels of TNF-α

- Anakinra is an agent that binds to IL-1 receptors and downregulates the inflammatory effects of IL-1, which is important in patients with rheumatoid arthritis, but also has benefit for a few rare cutaneous diseases

- An agent that blocks CD20 on B cells (rituximab) is approved for treatment of B-cell lymphoma and rheumatoid arthritis, but is also useful in B-cell-mediated skin diseases

- There are multiple bioengineered agents that are being developed to attack other parts of the immune/inflammatory system and might have therapeutic implications for dermatologic disease. In addition, each new therapy has the potential for adverse cutaneous reactions

INTRODUCTION

New developments in genetic engineering and biotechnology have allowed the creation of bioengineered molecules that target specific steps in the pathogenesis of several immune-mediated disorders, including Crohn's disease, juvenile idiopathic arthritis, rheumatoid arthritis, psoriasis and psoriatic arthritis, ankylosing spondylitis, pemphigus and B-cell lymphoma. These drugs work by eliminating pathogenic T cells, blocking T-cell activation, inhibiting the trafficking of T cells, changing the immune profile from Th1 to Th2, blocking cytokines or eliminating pathogenic B cells.

ALEFACEPT

Introduction

Alefacept (Amevive®) is a fusion protein in which the extracellular domain of lymphocyte function-associated antigen (LFA)-3 is fused with the Fc portion of human IgG$_1$[62].

Mechanism of Action

Two costimulatory signals must be delivered between antigen-presenting cells and T cells for activation to occur. The first signal occurs when molecules of the major histocompatibility complex on the antigen-presenting cells interact with receptors on the surface of resting T cells (see Fig. 5.8). The second costimulatory signal can be one of a number of interactions between antigen-presenting cells and T cells, as shown in Figure 128.8A. Alefacept binds to CD2, preventing its normal interaction with LFA-3 and T-cell activation (Fig. 128.8B). Moreover, CD2 is maximally expressed in activated CD45RO$^+$ T cells. The LFA-3 portion of alefacept binds to CD2 and the Fc portion fixes natural killer cells, which reduces the number of CD45RO$^+$ cells in the circulation.

Indications

Alefacept was the first biologic agent approved for the treatment of moderate to severe plaque type psoriasis, but it might have a role in the treatment of other T-cell-dependent diseases such as lichen planus[63], lupus erythematosus, chronic GVHD[64], and alopecia areata[65]. Although alefacept was studied in both intravenous and intramuscular forms, shortly after its approval the intravenous preparation was withdrawn from the market. Studies demonstrated that alefacept was significantly more effective than placebo in achieving a 75% reduction in the Psoriasis Area and Severity Index (PASI) score. However, a minority of patients achieve this level of improvement, which has affected its use in psoriasis.

Dosages

In clinical trials that have been published or presented, alefacept has been administered either intramuscularly or intravenously at weekly intervals for 12 weeks[62]. Following a 12-week period of observation, a second course of 12 weekly injections results in additional improvement. Doses of 7.5 and 15 mg (per week) have been used intravenously or intramuscularly, respectively. Additional courses seem to result in more prolonged remissions.

Contraindications

Alefacept should not be administered to patients with active infections or malignancies.

Major Side Effects

The most frequent side effect is local injection site reactions. Although the label suggests that malignancy risk is increased, there have not been excessive numbers of malignancies noted during or following therapy with alefacept. However, patients with an active malignancy should probably not be treated with this drug. Primary and secondary immune responses are unaffected by treatment with alefacept, as demonstrated by a normal immune response to either new antigens (phix174) or recall antigens (tetanus and diphtheria toxoids). Although a significant decrease in circulating T cell counts can occur, there does not appear to

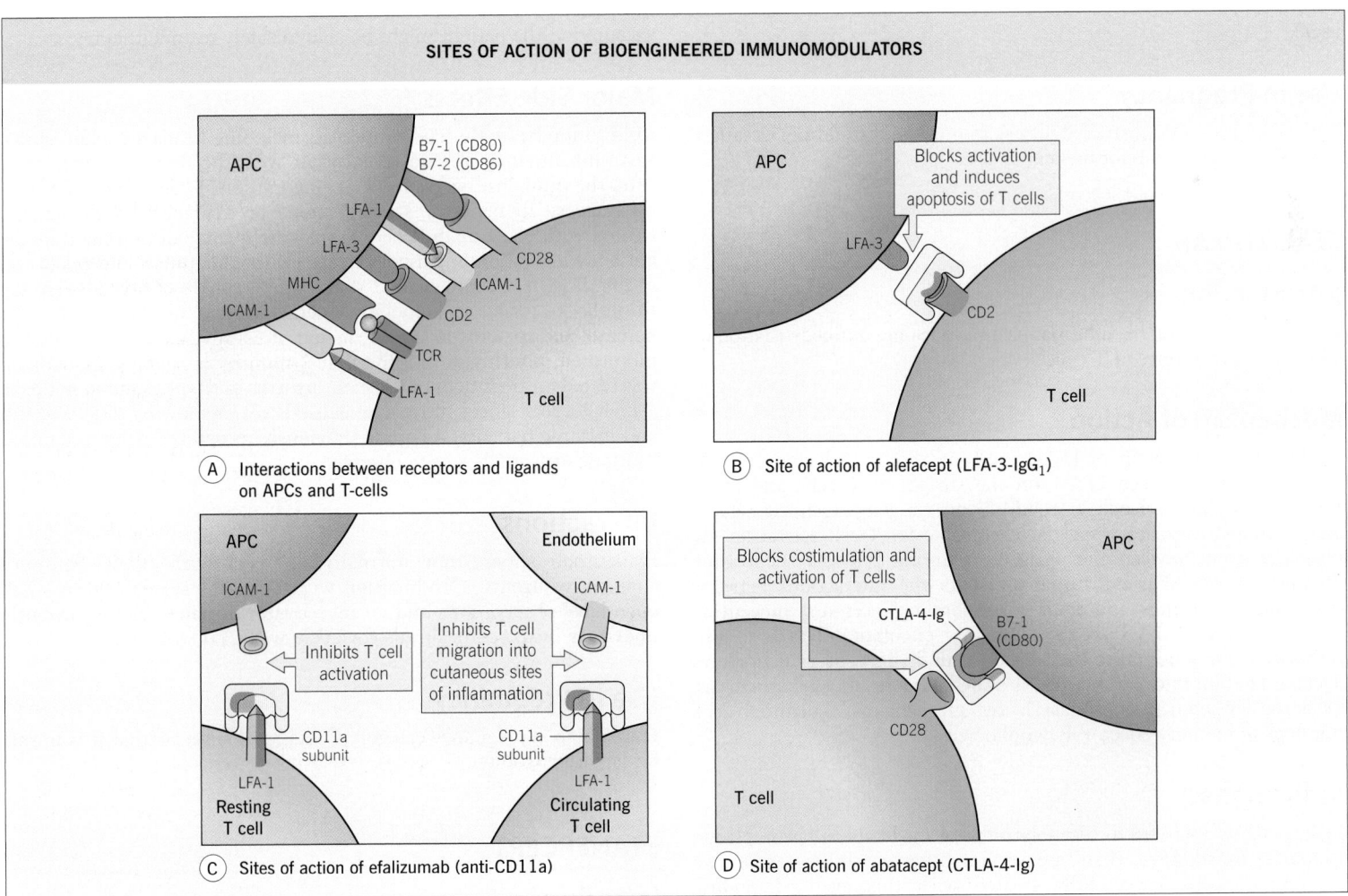

SITES OF ACTION OF BIOENGINEERED IMMUNOMODULATORS

(A) Interactions between receptors and ligands on APCs and T-cells

(B) Site of action of alefacept (LFA-3-IgG$_1$)

(C) Sites of action of efalizumab (anti-CD11a)

(D) Site of action of abatacept (CTLA-4-Ig)

Fig. 128.8 Sites of action of bioengineered immunomodulators. A Activation of T cells requires two signals. The first occurs when the major histocompatibility complex antigen interacts with the T-cell receptor. A second costimulatory signal is required for T-cell activation to occur. **B** Sites of action of alefacept. **C** Sites of action of efalizumab. **D** Site of action of abatacept.

RECOMMENDED LABORATORY EVALUATION FOR PATIENTS RECEIVING BIOENGINEERED IMMUNOMODULATORS FOR PSORIASIS AND/OR PSORIATIC ARTHRITIS		
Drug	Prior to treatment	During treatment
Adalimumab	PPD Chest x-ray (optional)	Annual PPD and/or chest x-ray*
Alefacept	CBC with differential T cell count	T cell (CD4+) count weekly or every other week
Efalizumab	CBC with differential	Monthly CBC with differential ×3 Thereafter, perhaps quarterly*
Etanercept	PPD* Chest x-ray (optional)	Annual PPD*
Infliximab	PPD Chest x-ray (optional)	Annual PPD and/or chest x-ray*

*Routinely performed, but not FDA-required.

Table 128.4 Recommended laboratory evaluation for patients receiving bioengineered immunomodulators for psoriasis and/or psoriatic arthritis.

be any increase in the risk of infections in patients treated with this agent[66]. Recommended laboratory tests are outlined in Table 128.4.

Interactions

Alefacept has been tested in combination with other psoriasis treatments in only a limited number of patients. It might be safe to combine with UV light therapies, retinoids and perhaps methotrexate[67,68]. It is unlikely that there will be adverse interactions with topical treatments. The combination with other biologic agents, either sequentially or simultaneously, has not been studied and concern over potentiation of immunosuppression suggests that studies are needed to clarify this issue.

Use in Pregnancy

Alefacept has not been studied for use in pregnancy or during lactation. It is labeled category B for pregnancy use.

EFALIZUMAB

Introduction

Efalizumab (Raptiva®) is a humanized monoclonal antibody that binds CD11a on the surface of T cells[69–72].

Mechanism of Action

CD11a is a component of LFA-1, and, as shown in Figure 128.8A, the interaction between LFA-1 on the surface of T cells and intercellular adhesion molecule-1 (ICAM-1) on antigen-presenting cells is one of the costimulatory signals responsible for T-cell activation. By inserting itself between the antigen-presenting cell and the resting T cell (Fig. 128.8C), efalizumab prevents the interactions between costimulatory ligands and their corresponding receptors, preventing T-cell activation. LFA-1 on the surface of circulating T cells is also responsible for adhesion to ICAM-1 on endothelial cells, which allows T-cell migration into the skin (Fig. 128.8C). As a result, efalizumab can block the development of psoriasis by two mechanisms. Efalizumab does not deplete memory effector T lymphocytes.

Indications

Efalizumab is approved for the treatment of moderate to severe plaque psoriasis. In addition, there are several other conditions that have presumably been successfully treated with this agent, including generalized granuloma annulare, cutaneous lupus erythematosus, cutaneous dermatomyositis, atopic dermatitis and alopecia areata[72–74]. Somewhere between 25% (at 12 weeks) and 40% of patients treated

with efalizumab will achieve a 75% improvement in their PASI score, depending on the timing of the analysis. Cessation of the drug is associated with worsening of the psoriasis, which in most instances is gradual. In occasional patients, the psoriasis and/or psoriatic arthritis rebounds following tapering or cessation of therapy, and in another subset of patients the disease seems to change character, e.g. development of intertriginous disease or even pustular disease[75]. In at least one report, the development of pustular disease or a rebound did not predict the same occurrence with future use of the efalizumab[76]. Plans for management of flares or a change in character of the disease should be made at the onset of therapy. Physicians unwilling to use other systemic agents such as methotrexate, acitretin or cyclosporine for patients whose disease flares with efalizumab should reconsider the use of this agent.

Dosages

Efalizumab is administered subcutaneously by the patient at a dose of 1 mg/kg once weekly. A lower initial dose (0.7 mg/kg) lessens the possibility of flu-like symptoms that may accompany use of this agent. In several studies of psoriasis, higher doses were not more efficacious. It is not known whether tachyphylaxis might develop with long-term use of this agent. In addition, longer intervals between drug administration have not proved to maintain efficacy.

Contraindications

Efalizumab is an immunosuppressant and it could have additive effects if used in conjunction with other immunosuppressive medications. It is contraindicated in patients with infections and malignancy. Live vaccines should be avoided in patients on efalizumab and the use of attenuated vaccines might be associated with a poor immune response to the vaccine. It is not known how long before administering a vaccine the patient should stop therapy, nor is it known how long after the vaccination the patient might be able to safely resume therapy.

Major Side Effects[77]

Mild to moderate flu-like symptoms, including headache, pain, chills, gastrointestinal upset and fever, occur with the first few treatments. After the third dose, side effects are uncommon. To date, there has been no increase in opportunistic infections or malignancies in patients treated with efalizumab. There is a low frequency of non-neutralizing antibody formation in patients treated with efalizumab. After approval of the drug, it became evident that a small subset of patients develop thrombocytopenia or hemolytic anemia[77]. The mechanism for the hematologic toxicity is not clear, but it is advised that patients be monitored monthly during the first 3 months of therapy. Efalizumab was tested for treatment of psoriatic arthritis and was found to not have a high level of effect (http://clinicaltrials.gov/ct/show/NCT00051662), and in some patients, a flare of previously recognized or unrecognized psoriatic arthritis has been observed.

Interactions

Efalizumab should not normally be used with other immunosuppressive agents. Combination with UV light seems safe in small open-label observations and an investigator-initiated trial is currently underway (http://clinicaltrials.gov/ct/show/NCT00302445).

Use in Pregnancy

Efalizumab is pregnancy category C. Its label suggests that it is unsafe for lactating women.

ETANERCEPT

Introduction

Etanercept (Enbrel®) is a fusion protein consisting of the extracellular domain of the TNF-α receptor fused with the Fc portion human IgG$_1$[78].

Mechanism of Action

Etanercept binds to TNF-α, inhibiting its activity (Fig. 128.9). Etanercept has two p75 binding sites, which gives it greater affinity for TNF-α as compared to the naturally occurring monomeric receptor. TNF appears to be involved in more than just inflammation, and may have an impact on the neuroendocrine system[79].

Indications

Etanercept is approved for the treatment of rheumatoid arthritis, psoriatic arthritis, moderate to severe plaque psoriasis, ankylosing spondylitis, and juvenile idiopathic arthritis (children 4 to 17 years of age). In addition, it has been used to treat a variety of mucocutaneous disorders, including dermatomyositis, neutrophilic dermatoses, cutaneous lupus erythematosus, autoimmune bullous diseases, lichen planus, pyoderma gangrenosum, hidradenitis suppurativa, sarcoidosis, multicentric reticulohistiocytosis, relapsing polychondritis, and GVHD[80–82]. Only individual case reports or small case series have been reported, and, in randomized trials, etanercept failed to demonstrate improvement for several systemic manifestations of sarcoidosis[83]. Presumably all of the disorders for which it might be effective are characterized by elevated levels of TNF-α in the circulation or tissue or both. Some patients with psoriasis or rheumatoid arthritis have coexistent hepatitis C infection and etanercept appears not to have an adverse effect on viral load or hepatitis in such patients[84].

Dosages

For most of its indications, etanercept was initially approved to be administered subcutaneously at a dose of 25 mg twice weekly. Shortly after its approval for psoriatic arthritis, it was demonstrated that 50 mg weekly gave equivalent results to 25 mg twice weekly. The approved dose for moderate to severe plaque psoriasis is 50 mg twice weekly for the first 3 months, followed by 50 mg weekly. Some physicians have chosen to initiate therapy at a dose of 50 mg weekly and only escalate the dose if the patient fails to respond after 6 to 12 months. Etanercept is available in a 25 mg dose that must be reconstituted by the patient, and 50 mg prefilled syringes and pens.

Upon initiating therapy with etanercept, patients often report a feeling of well-being that seems to occur prior to the onset of clinically measurable responses. This effect might be due to a reduction in depression that may accompany psoriasis and psoriatic arthritis[85].

Contraindications

Etanercept is contraindicated in patients with sepsis or with known hypersensitivity to the medication. It should also be avoided in patients with a history of multiple sclerosis or a significant active infection or malignancy.

Major Side Effects

Injection site reactions are the most common side effect, but in general they are of little clinical significance. All are mild to moderate and diminish in frequency after the first month of treatment. Erythema, pruritus, pain and swelling have been described.

In open and double-blind placebo-controlled trials, there has been a slight increase in the incidence of upper respiratory tract infections in patients treated with etanercept, but no increase in the incidence of serious infections. Serious infections have been reported in patients receiving etanercept, but the rate of occurrence is not clear and may vary from one population to the next. Opportunistic infections such as histoplasmosis, coccidioidomycosis and *Pneumocystis jiroveci* (*carinii*) pneumonia may occur and, therefore, a new onset of fever or cough should not be overlooked. Reactivation of latent tuberculosis has been reported and, although skin testing for tuberculosis is not mandated by the package insert, many insurers mandate screening.

The oncogenic potential of etanercept, particularly for lymphoma, is a much debated issue. It may be dependent upon the disease state that is being treated. Recent reports have suggested a slight (perhaps up to threefold) increase in the risk of lymphoma, particularly in patients with rheumatoid arthritis[86] (a group known to have an increased susceptibility to lymphoma). Whether this translates into an increase for patients with psoriasis or other diseases is unknown. Most studies have not demonstrated an increase in solid malignancies, including non-melanoma skin cancer[87]. However, patients with psoriasis have not been fully studied and the risk of non-melanoma skin cancer remains unknown. In a study of patients with Wegener's granulomatosis, there appeared to be an increase in solid malignancies[88]. Therefore, choosing to use a TNF antagonist in patients with a history of malignancy should be carefully considered.

There is also an increase in the development of antinuclear antibodies, as well as one small case series of patients who developed signs and symptoms of systemic lupus erythematosus (SLE), while receiving etanercept[89]. Conversely, there are several small case series in which the use of etanercept was associated with disappearance of subacute cutaneous lupus erythematosus[82,90]. The lupus-like disease that has been linked to etanercept is readily reversible. It is not necessary to evaluate patients for antinuclear antibodies before or during therapy.

While etanercept was originally used as treatment for multiple sclerosis, several patients treated with etanercept or other TNF antagonists have developed multiple sclerosis[91]. Others with multiple sclerosis have had exacerbations of their disease when treated with etanercept. In some patients, the symptoms of multiple sclerosis have

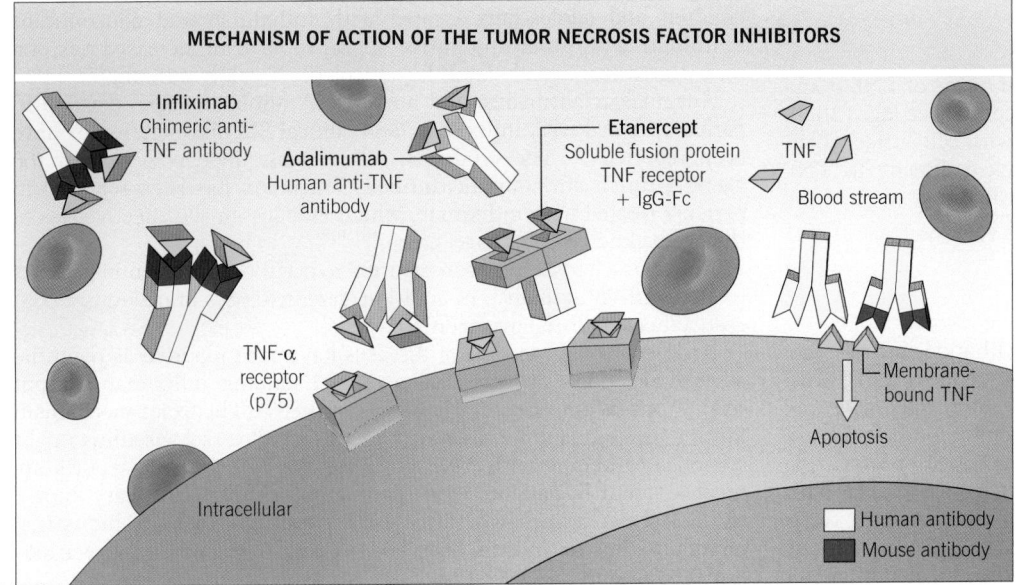

Fig. 128.9 Mechanism of action of the tumor necrosis factor (TNF) inhibitors.

abated despite continued therapy. It seems reasonable to avoid using etanercept or other TNF antagonists in patients with a history of multiple sclerosis, unless there is no other alternative.

Etanercept was tested for the treatment of congestive heart failure and did not confer any benefit[92]. In addition, there have been reports of etanercept-induced congestive heart failure. This event appears to be very rare, but therapy with etanercept for patients with unstable cardiac disease is best avoided.

A variety of skin lesions or diseases have been reported as potential adverse reactions to anti-TNF agents. Recent reports of new-onset psoriasis have appeared[93]. The exact mechanism for this reaction is not known and the possibility exists that these patients with presumed rheumatoid arthritis actually suffered from psoriatic arthritis. Cutaneous small vessel vasculitis might complicate therapy with TNF agents[94], but the reports are most frequent in patients with rheumatoid arthritis, a disease known to be associated with vasculitis. Lastly, multiple cases of interstitial granulomatous dermatitis have been reported in patients on various anti-TNF agents[95].

Interactions

Etanercept has been used successfully in combination with methotrexate and is approved for concomitant use in patients with rheumatoid arthritis and psoriatic arthritis. The combination of etanercept with other biologic agents should be avoided until well-designed studies demonstrate efficacy and safety. A specific example was a study of anakinra plus etanercept for patients with rheumatoid arthritis. In this study, there was no increase in efficacy, but there was a substantial increase in the frequency of infection[96].

Use in Pregnancy

Etanercept is pregnancy category B, with no evidence of harm to the fetus in animal studies. Studies in pregnant women have not been conducted. In a recent editorial, Salmon & Alpert suggest that etanercept and other TNF antagonists might be best avoided after the first trimester[97]. It is not known whether etanercept is secreted in breast milk and therefore it is suggested that its use in nursing mothers be avoided. However, at least in adults, this drug is metabolized and not absorbed via an oral route; consequently, the suggestion to avoid nursing is perhaps not scientifically sound.

INFLIXIMAB

Introduction

Infliximab (Remicade®) is a chimeric (human–mouse) monoclonal antibody and its target is human TNF-α[98].

Mechanism of Action

Infliximab binds to soluble and membrane-bound forms of TNF-α and blocks the interaction of TNF-α with TNF-α receptors (see Fig. 128.9). In addition, infliximab causes apoptosis of cells with cell-surface TNF. Although the effectiveness is believed to be linked directly to TNF blockade on cells and in the circulation, it is possible that some of the effects are mediated through effects on hormonal axes[79].

Indications

Infliximab is approved for the treatment of adults with moderate to severe psoriasis, psoriatic arthritis, Crohn's disease, fistulae associated with Crohn's disease, rheumatoid arthritis, ulcerative colitis and ankylosing spondylitis. Infliximab is approved for the treatment of Crohn's disease in children above the age of 6 years. Infliximab also appears to be useful for pyoderma gangrenosum, whether it is associated with inflammatory bowel disease or not[99]. It has been effective as a treatment for sarcoidosis, granulomatous cheilitis, Behçet's disease, various vasculitides, pityriasis rubra pilaris, reactive arthritis (formerly Reiter's

disease), subcorneal pustular dermatosis, GVHD, Sjögren's syndrome, multicentric reticulohistiocytosis and hidradenitis suppurativa[100]. Like etanercept, infliximab appears to have positive effects without excessive toxicity in patients with psoriasis, psoriatic arthritis and rheumatoid arthritis who have a concomitant infection with hepatitis C virus.

Dosages

Infliximab has been used at doses of 5 or 10 mg/kg administered by slow intravenous infusion approximately every 8 weeks. The frequency of administration is increased when the response is less than adequate. For Crohn's disease, rheumatoid arthritis and psoriatic arthritis, it is approved for concomitant administration with methotrexate, azathioprine or low-dose prednisone.

Contraindications

Infliximab is contraindicated in patients with known sensitivity to murine proteins or to the drug itself. It should be avoided in patients with serious active infections or malignancies. Patients with multiple sclerosis or congestive heart failure should avoid infliximab[91,92].

Major Side Effects

Infusion-related reactions are the most commonly reported side effect, occurring in 16% of infliximab-treated patients compared to 6% of placebo-treated patients. Symptoms consist of fever, chills, pruritus, urticaria, chest pain, hypotension, hypertension and shortness of breath. Infusion reaction risk has also been linked to the presence of human antichimeric antibodies. This risk may be lessened by concomitant use of methotrexate, azathioprine or corticosteroids[101].

Serious infections such as pneumonia, cellulitis or sepsis were reported in 3% of infliximab-treated patients compared to 2% of placebo-treated patients, but many of these patients were also treated with other immunosuppressive agents, such as methotrexate or corticosteroids. There is concern regarding the frequency with which mycobacterial infections have emerged in patients treated with infliximab compared to disease control patients. Therefore, a purified protein derivative (PPD) skin test is mandated in the labeling of this agent. In addition, most clinicians will also obtain a chest X-ray prior to infliximab therapy. Patients with a positive PPD test can be treated with antituberculous therapy prior to initiating infliximab, or an alternative agent may be selected. Opportunistic infections such as histoplasmosis, coccidioidomycosis, listeriosis and *Pneumocystis jiroveci* (*carinii*) pneumonia may occur more frequently in patients on infliximab than in matched patients with Crohn's disease and rheumatoid arthritis who are not on infliximab[102]. Careful monitoring and early evaluation for these types of infections are necessary.

A recent meta-analysis involving infliximab and adalimumab demonstrated an increased risk of lymphoproliferative diseases and malignancies in patients treated with these agents[103]. In addition, children and adolescents treated with infliximab and concomitant azathioprine or 6-mercaptopurine appear to have an increased risk of a rare, aggressive, usually fatal, hepatosplenic T-cell lymphoma[104].

Antinuclear antibodies and anti-nDNA antibodies also develop in patients treated with infliximab, and clinical SLE-like syndromes have been reported[105]. The syndrome is reversible upon cessation of the agent. Human antichimeric antibody formation has been reported in patients treated with infliximab, which may lessen the effectiveness of the agent (known as 'dosage' creep)[101,106].

Multiple sclerosis has been reported to occur or to worsen in patients treated with infliximab[91]. In addition, rare instances of new-onset congestive heart failure have been reported[92].

A variety of skin lesions or diseases have been reported as potential adverse reactions to anti-TNF agents, including infliximab. Recent reports of new-onset psoriasis have appeared[93]. The exact mechanism for this reaction is not known. Cutaneous small vessel vasculitis might complicate therapy with TNF blocking agents[94], but the reports are most frequent in patients with rheumatoid arthritis, a disease known to be associated with vasculitis. Lastly, multiple cases of interstitial granulomatous dermatitis have been observed in patients on various anti-TNF agents[95].

Interactions

Infliximab has been used in combination with methotrexate, azathioprine, 6-mercaptopurine and systemic corticosteroids. The main concern has been additive immunosuppression. Infliximab should not be administered with other biologic agents until adequate studies have examined the safety and effectiveness of such combinations. Live vaccines are contraindicated in patients on infliximab. The effectiveness of attenuated vaccines is unknown, but a recent report has suggested that immunity was conferred after influenza vaccination[107].

Use in Pregnancy

Infliximab is rated pregnancy category B. Its use in pregnancy should probably be avoided until long-term studies demonstrate a lack of adverse effect. It is not known whether infliximab is secreted in breast milk; thus, its use probably should be avoided in nursing mothers.

ADALIMUMAB

Introduction

Adalimumab (Humira®) is a 'fully' human recombinant IgG$_1$ monoclonal antibody with specificity for human TNF-α[108].

Mechanism of Action

Adalimumab binds to soluble and membrane-bound TNF-α (see Fig. 128.9), leading to a blockade of activity of TNF. Apoptosis of cells with membrane-bound TNF occurs. Adalimumab does not bind to TNF-β (lymphotoxin). Adalimumab may have similar effects on the endocrine axes as other TNF antagonists[79].

Indications

Adalimumab was initially approved for the treatment of rheumatoid arthritis and then it was subsequently approved for treatment of psoriatic arthritis, ankylosing spondylitis and Crohn's disease. Currently, it is under study for moderate to severe plaque type psoriasis. It might be useful for hidradenitis suppurativa, pustular psoriasis[109], sarcoidosis, pyoderma gangrenosum, neutrophilic dermatoses, dermatomyositis and Behçet's disease[79]. Like etanercept, adalimumab appears to have positive effects without excessive toxicity in patients with psoriasis, psoriatic arthritis and rheumatoid arthritis who have a concomitant infection with hepatitis C virus.

Dosages

Adalimumab is supplied in a 40 mg prefilled syringe or pen. It may be administered 40 mg every other week, or weekly. Its approved dose for psoriatic arthritis, rheumatoid arthritis and ankylosing spondylitis is 40 mg every other week. An initial loading dose of 80 mg might increase the rapidity of the response.

Contraindications

Adalimumab is contraindicated in patients with known sensitivity. It should be avoided in patients with serious active infections or malignancies. Patients with multiple sclerosis or congestive heart failure should avoid adalimumab.

Major Side Effects

There is concern regarding the mycobacterial infections that have emerged in patients treated with adalimumab. Therefore, a PPD test is mandated in the labeling of this agent. In addition, most clinicians will also obtain a chest X-ray prior to therapy. Patients with a positive PPD test can be treated with antituberculous therapy prior to initiating adalimumab, or an alternative agent may be selected. Opportunistic infections such as histoplasmosis, coccidioidomycosis, listeriosis and *Pneumocystis jiroveci* (*carinii*) pneumonia probably occur more frequently in patients on adalimumab.

A recent meta-analysis involving infliximab and adalimumab demonstrated an increased risk of lymphoproliferative diseases and malignancies in patients treated with these agents[103].

Antinuclear antibodies appear to be increased in patients treated with adalimumab, and clinical SLE-like syndromes have been reported. The syndrome is reversible upon cessation of the agent.

Multiple sclerosis has been reported to occur or to worsen in patients treated with adalimumab. In addition, rare instances of new-onset congestive heart failure have been reported.

A variety of skin lesions or diseases have been reported as potential adverse reactions to anti-TNF agents, including adalimumab. Recent reports of new-onset psoriasis have appeared[93]. The exact mechanism for this reaction is not known. Cutaneous small vessel vasculitis might complicate therapy with TNF blocking agents[94], but the reports are most frequent in patients with rheumatoid arthritis, a disease known to be associated with vasculitis. Lastly, multiple cases of interstitial granulomatous dermatitis have been observed in patients on various anti-TNF agents[95].

Interactions

Live vaccines should be avoided. The response to attenuated vaccines may be muted. Other biologic agents should not be combined with adalimumab. The concomitant administration of other immunosuppressive agents might increase the risk of infection.

Use in Pregnancy

Adalimumab is pregnancy category B. Its safety during lactation is unknown.

ANAKINRA

Introduction

Anakinra (Kineret®) is an IL-1 antagonist[110].

Mechanism of Action

Anakinra binds to IL-1 type 1 receptors and downregulates the inflammatory effects of IL-1.

Indications

Anakinra is approved for rheumatoid arthritis[110]. It has recently been demonstrated to be effective for neonatal-onset multisystem inflammatory disease (NOMID), also known as chronic infantile neurologic cutaneous articular (CINCA) syndrome[111]. This disorder is characterized by fever, CNS disease and a deforming arthropathy with an accompanying urticarial eruption (see Table 45.2). Treatment with corticosteroids or TNF antagonists are often imperfect in their ability to control this disease. This disorder has been linked to mutations in the cold-induced autoinflammatory syndrome 1 (*CIAS1*) gene, which encodes cryopyrin, a protein that regulates inflammation in NOMID and other cold-induced inflammatory diseases, including Muckle–Wells syndrome, another disease with urticarial papules and plaques (see Table 45.2).

Dosages

Anakinra is administered at a dose of 100 mg daily via a subcutaneous route in adults. Children are treated with 2 mg/kg/day.

Contraindications

Anakinra should not be given to patients with active infections, severe renal impairment, or hypersensitivity to the drug.

Major Side Effects

Infection, neutropenia and thrombocytopenia are the most serious reactions that can occur. Monitoring patients with complete blood counts is indicated. Injection site reactions are usually mild and seem to abate with continued therapy. Flu-like symptoms may also occur with anakinra. Long-term safety is not known.

Interactions

Other immunosuppressive agents, particularly biologic agents, should be avoided in patients taking anakinra (see Etanercept, Interactions)[96]. Live vaccines should also be avoided, but it is unknown whether attenuated vaccines have a full effect.

Use in Pregnancy

Anakinra is pregnancy category B. It is not known if it can be given to lactating women.

RITUXIMAB

Introduction

Rituximab (Rituxan®) is a chimeric monoclonal antibody directed against the CD20 antigen present on the surface of mature B cells[112].

Mechanism of Action

Rituximab binds to CD20 on the cell surface of mature B cells and causes apoptosis of the cells. Rituximab is a therapeutic antibody that targets and selectively depletes CD20+ B cells without targeting stem cells or existing plasma cells. Possible mechanisms of cell lysis include complement-dependent cytotoxicity and antibody-dependent cell-mediated cytotoxicity.

Indications

Rituximab was first approved for non-Hodgkin B-cell lymphoma. It has been recently approved for patients with rheumatoid arthritis[113]. In addition to its approved indications, rituximab has been used successfully to treat patients with autoimmune bullous dermatoses (including pemphigus vulgaris[114], bullous pemphigoid and paraneoplastic pemphigus), SLE and cutaneous lupus erythematosus[115], chronic GVHD[116], ANCA-associated vasculitis, small vessel vasculitis[117], cutaneous B-cell lymphoma[118] and dermatomyositis[119].

Dosages

Rituximab is approved at a dose of 375 mg/m^2 intravenously weekly for 4–8 weeks for lymphoma. For rheumatoid arthritis, it is given as a 1000 mg infusion on each of two consecutive weeks. It is usually administered with methylprednisolone 100 mg intravenously 30 minutes prior to each infusion. Repeat dosing for maintenance therapy is often required, but the exact timing and frequency of the dosing is still under study. It is approved for concomitant use with methotrexate in patients with rheumatoid arthritis, and with chemotherapy in patients with B-cell lymphoma.

Contraindications

Rituximab is contraindicated in patients allergic to the drug or its components, hepatitis B carriers, and patients with cardiac arrhythmias, angina pectoris, high tumor burden or active infections.

Major Side Effects

Deaths within 24 hours of rituximab infusion have been reported. These fatal reactions followed an infusion reaction complex which included hypoxia, pulmonary infiltrates, acute respiratory distress syndrome, myocardial infarction, ventricular fibrillation and cardiogenic shock. Approximately 80% of fatal infusion reactions occurred in association with the first infusion. Acute renal failure, requiring dialysis with instances of fatal outcome, has been reported in the setting of tumor lysis syndrome following treatment with rituximab. Severe mucocutaneous reactions, including Stevens–Johnson syndrome/toxic

epidermal necrolysis, have been rarely observed in patients given rituximab. Rare patients have had the onset of paraneoplastic pemphigus during infusion, but it is not clear whether this phenomenon is drug-related or disease-related.

The safety profile of rituximab has been established primarily in patients with lymphoproliferative diseases and includes more than 730 000 patient exposures over a period of 8 years. In general, the adverse events observed in patients with rheumatoid arthritis were similar in type to those seen in patients with non-Hodgkin lymphoma. The most common adverse events observed in clinical trials were infusion reactions and infections. No significant change in average immunoglobulin levels was observed in treated patients within clinical trials.

There was no increase in hematologic malignancies, demyelinating events, or risk of opportunistic infections (including tuberculosis) in rituximab-treated patients over 24 weeks of treatment. Although 5% of rituximab-treated patients developed human antichimeric antibodies, this was not associated with loss of clinical response or additional safety observations.

Interactions

Hepatitis B reactivation is possible in patients treated with rituximab. Live vaccines are contraindicated and the response to attenuated vaccines may be muted. Combination with other biologic agents, particularly natalizumab, may increase the risk of infection. Combination with cisplatin increases the risk of nephrotoxicity.

Use in Pregnancy

Rituximab is pregnancy category C and is possibly unsafe during lactation.

OTHER BIOENGINEERED AGENTS UNDER INVESTIGATION

Development of many other bioengineered agents for use in dermatology continues. Table 128.5, derived from the National Psoriasis Foundation website (accessed in October 2007), is a partial listing of the drugs that are currently under investigation for psoriasis. There are drugs that are being developed for non-cutaneous inflammatory diseases which might be effective for skin disease, or might be associated with adverse cutaneous effects. For example, it is possible that omalizumab, a drug approved for the treatment of steroid-resistant asthma, will be useful for some patients with atopic dermatitis and/or urticaria[120].

Recent investigations into the pathogenesis of psoriasis have pointed to a role for Th17 cells, which produce IL-17. In addition to the latter, these cells also release IL-22 when stimulated by IL-23 (produced by dendritic cells). The IL-22 then leads to proliferation of keratinocytes and dermal inflammation, and circulating levels of IL-22 correlate with disease activity (see Ch. 9). Human monoclonal antibodies against the

SOME OF THE BIOLOGIC AGENTS THAT ARE UNDER DEVELOPMENT				
Name	Company	Delivery mechanism	Mechanism of action	Phase
ABT874	Abbott Immunology	Injectable	IL-12/IL-23 inhibitor	II
CC-10004	Celgene	Oral	TNF-α inhibitor	II
Ustekinumab (CNTO 1275)	Centocor, Inc.	Injectable	IL-12/IL-23 inhibitor	III
Certolizumab pegol	UCB	Injectable	TNF-α inhibitor	II
Golimumab (CNTO 148)	Centocor, Inc.	Injectable	TNF-α inhibitor	III

Table 128.5 Some of the biologic agents that are under development. IL, interleukin; LFA, lymphocyte function-associated antigen. Adapted from the National Psoriasis Foundation website – accessed October 15, 2007.

p40 subunit of IL-23 (IL-12 has the same p40 subunit) block the interactions of these two cytokines with their cognate cell-surface receptors (see Table 128.5). In a recently published clinical trial, ustekinumab (CNTO 1275) was shown to be highly effective in patients with psoriasis[120a]. It is administered via weekly subcutaneous injection and was given in this study in doses of 45 or 90 mg/week for four weeks.

IMMUNE GLOBULIN

Key features

- IVIg is useful for inflammatory disorders, including some cutaneous diseases
- Doses for inflammatory disorders are empiric, but have generally been 2 g/kg/month for chronic diseases, and 3 g/kg total for acute disorders
- There are only a few disorders for which there is a high level of evidence indicating effectiveness

INTRODUCTION

IVIg is currently used in the treatment of immunodeficiency syndromes, inflammatory disorders and infectious diseases[121]. Clinical studies, most of which are uncontrolled, and anecdotal reports suggest that IVIg is useful for some cutaneous conditions (Table 128.6), but randomized clinical trials, barring those for dermatomyositis, are lacking. IVIg offers new hope for the treatment of many severe dermatologic conditions, including toxic epidermal necrolysis/Stevens–Johnson syndrome[122], dermatomyositis[123] and chronic autoimmune blistering diseases[124].

MECHANISM OF ACTION

The exact mechanism of action for IVIg is unknown. The immunomodulatory effects of IVIg may be exerted through one or more of the following: 1) functional blockade of Fc receptors; 2) inhibition of complement-mediated damage; 3) alteration of cytokine and cytokine antagonist profiles; 4) reduction of circulating antibodies via anti-idiotype antibodies; and 5) neutralization of toxins which trigger auto-antibody production[121,125]. In toxic epidermal necrolysis, IVIg is believed to block Fas (CD95)-mediated keratinocyte death by inhibiting Fas–Fas ligand interactions.

INDICATIONS

IVIg is approved for treatment of primary and secondary immunodeficiency diseases. Table 128.6 details the reported dermatologic disorders for which IVIg has been used.

DOSAGES

At least nine different preparations of IVIg are available in the US[126]. The products differ in their sugar content, sodium content, osmolality, pH and IgA levels (Table 128.7). The doses recommended vary depending upon the disease state being treated (see Table 128.6).

CONTRAINDICATIONS

Preparations containing IgA are contraindicated in patients with IgA deficiency. In such patients, there is a risk of anaphylaxis and sudden death should IgA-containing preparations be administered.

MAJOR SIDE EFFECTS

Major toxicity includes the potential for anaphylaxis, renal failure, thromboembolic events, hyperviscosity syndromes, cardiac collapse, pulmonary edema and aseptic meningitis. These risks vary with the preparation selected and the patient being treated. Pretreatment with acetaminophen and diphenhydramine may lessen infusion reactions, and decreasing the rapidity of the infusion lessens the risk of thromboembolic events, aseptic meningitis, and renal and cardiovascular events.

GUIDELINES FOR USE OF IVIg IN DERMATOLOGY			
Indication	Summary of evidence	Dosing	Comments
Dermatomyositis	Benefit established	2 g/kg (over 2 days) Initially given every month, maintenance schedule individualized	Resistant or intolerant to prednisone or immunosuppressives
Kawasaki's disease	Benefit established	2 g/kg (over 6–12 hours)	
Toxic epidermal necrolysis	Case series, anecdotal evidence	1 g/kg/day for 3 days	
Pemphigus variants	Case series, anecdotal evidence	2 g/kg (over 2–3 days) Initially given every month, maintenance schedule individualized	Adjunctive or second-line therapy
Bullous pemphigoid	Case series, anecdotal evidence	2 g/kg (over 2–3 days) Initially given every month, maintenance schedule individualized	Adjunctive or second-line therapy
Mucous membrane (cicatricial) pemphigoid	Case series, anecdotal evidence	2–3 g/kg (over 3 days) Initially given every 2–6 weeks, maintenance schedule individualized	Adjunctive or second-line therapy
Epidermolysis bullosa acquisita	Anecdotal evidence	2 g/kg (over 2–3 days) Initially given every month, maintenance schedule individualized	Adjunctive or second-line therapy
Necrotizing fasciitis	Uncertain benefit	2 g/kg (over 6–12 hours); repeat 1–2 g/kg in 2–5 days if disease progresses	Adjunctive for progressive disease
Pyoderma gangrenosum	Uncertain benefit	2 g/kg (over 2 days) Initially given every month, maintenance schedule individualized	May be considered

Table 128.6 Guidelines for use of IVIg in dermatology. From Mydlarski PR, Mittman N, Shear NH: Intravenous immunoglobulin: use in dermatology. Skin Therapy Lett. 2004;9:1–6, with permission.

SOME PREPARATIONS OF IVIg THAT ARE AVAILABLE IN THE US				
	Gammagard	**Iveegam**	**Gamunex**	**Carimune NF**
Manufacturer	Baxter	Baxter	Bayer	ZLB Bioplasma
Form	Lyophilized	Lyophilized	Liquid	Lyophilized
Concentration	5%	10%	10%	3–12%
Infusion rate	4.0 ml/kg/h	2.0 ml/kg/h	8.4 ml/kg/h	2.5 ml/kg/h
Time to infuse 70 g	5.3 h	12 h	<2 h	<6.6 h
Storage	Room temperature	2–8°C	2–8°C, room temperature	Room temperature
Shelf-life	24 months	24 months	36 months	24 months
pH	6.8	6.4–7.2	4.25	6.4–6.8
Osmolarity (mOsm/l)	636 at 5%	>240	260	192–1074
Sugar content	2% glucose	5% glucose	No sugar (glycine)	1.67 g sucrose/g of protein
Sodium content	0.85%	0.3%	Traces	<20 mg/g of protein
IgA (mg/ml)	<3.7	<10	46	720 µg/ml

Table 128.7 Some preparations of IVIg that are available in the US.

INTERACTIONS

There are no interactions that appear to be clinically significant with IVIg.

USE IN PREGNANCY

There does not appear to be an excessive risk in pregnancy or lactation associated with the use of IVIg.

OTHER AGENTS

Many other agents that are immunomodulators are used in other areas of medicine (Table 128.8). There are frequent cutaneous adverse reactions with some of these agents (e.g. the epidermal growth factor inhibitors used to treat solid tumors). Additionally, some of these agents might have some benefit for dermatologic conditions (e.g. imatinib for fibrosing conditions including scleroderma)[127].

OTHER 'BIOLOGIC AGENTS' CURRENTLY USED IN MEDICINE		
Drug (Trade name®)	**Target**	**FDA-approved indications/non-approved dermatologically relevant uses**
Abatacept (Orencia)	B7-1 (CD80)	Rheumatoid arthritis/melanoma, psoriasis (historical) (see Fig. 128.8D)
Bevacizumab (Avastin) Ranibizumab (Lucentis; intravitreal agent)	VEGF	Colorectal cancer Age-related macular degeneration
Cetuximab (Erbitux; IgG1)*,** Panitumumab (Vectibix; IgG2)*	EGFR	Head and neck SCC, colorectal cancer Metastatic colorectal cancer
Trastuzumab (Herceptin)	HER2/neu	Breast cancer
Daclizumab (Zenapax) Basiliximab (Simulect)	IL2Rα (CD25)	Solid organ transplantation/GVHD
Gemtuzumab (Mylotarg)	CD33	AML
Alemtuzumab (Campath)	CD52	B-cell CLL/mycosis fungoides, ATLL
Tyrosine kinase inhibitors		
Erlotinib (Tarceva)*,**	EGFR	Non-small cell lung and pancreatic cancer
Gefitinib (Iressa)*,**	EGFR	Non-small cell lung cancer
Lapatinib (Tykerb, Tycerb)*	EGFR, HER2/neu	Metastatic breast cancer
Imatinib (Gleevec, Glivec)**	c-KIT, c-Abl, PDGFR	CML, GIST, DFSP, systemic mastocytosis (see Ch. 118), hypereosinophilic syndrome (see Fig. 26.8)
Dasatinib (Sprycel)	c-KIT, c-Abl	CML, Philadelphia chromosome-positive ALL
Sorafenib (Nexavar)**	VEGFR1&2, PDGFR, BRAF	Renal cell carcinoma/melanoma
Sunitinib (Sutent)**	VEGFR1&2, PDGFR, c-KIT, FLT3	Renal cell carcinoma, GIST

Table 128.8 Other 'biologic agents' currently used in medicine. *See Ch. 37. **See Table 22.9. ALL, acute lymphoblastic leukemia; AML, acute myelogenous leukemia; ATLL, adult T-cell leukemia-lymphoma; CLL, chronic lymphocytic leukemia; CML, chronic myelogenous leukemia; DFSP, dermatofibrosarcoma protuberans; EGFR, epidermal growth factor receptor; FLT3, FMS-like tyrosine kinase 3; GIST, gastrointestinal stromal tumors; GVHD, graft-versus-host disease; IL2Rα, interleukin-2 receptor α; PDGFR, platelet-derived growth factor receptor; SCC, squamous cell carcinoma; VEGF, vascular endothelial growth factor; VEGFR, VEGF receptor.

REFERENCES

1. Havell EA, Berman B, Ogburn CA, et al. Two antigenically distinct species of human interferon. Proc Natl Acad Sci USA. 1975;72:2185–7.
2. Wills RJ. Clinical pharmacokinetics of interferons. Clin Pharmacokinet. 1990;19:390–9.
3. Rajan GP, Seifert B, Prummer O, et al. Incidence and in-vivo relevance of anti-interferon antibodies during treatment of low-grade cutaneous T-cell lymphomas with interferon alpha-2a combined with acitretin or PUVA. Arch Dermatol Res. 1996; 288:543–8.
4. Vance JC, Bart BJ, Hansen RC, et al. Intralesional recombinant alpha-2 interferon for the treatment of patients with condyloma acuminatum or verruca plantaris. Arch Dermatol. 1986;122:272–7.
5. Ling M. Therapy of genital papillomavirus infections. Part II: Methods of treatment. Int J Dermatol. 1992;32:769–76.
6. Knobler E. Current management strategies for cutaneous T-cell lymphoma. Clin Dermatol. 2004;22:197–208.
7. Ezekowitz RA, Mulliken JB, Folkman J. Interferon-alfa-2a therapy for life-threatening hemangiomas of infancy. N Engl J Med. 1992;326:1456–63.

8. Barlow CF, Priebe CJ, Mulliken JB, et al: Spastic diplegia as a complication of interferon alfa-2a treatment of hemangiomas of infancy. J Pediatr. 1998;132:527–30.
9. Krown SE. Interferon and other biological agents for the treatment of Kaposi's sarcoma. Hematol Oncol Clin North Am. 1991;5:311–22.
10. Cornell RC, Greenway HT, Tucker SB, et al. Intralesional interferon therapy for basal cell carcinoma. J Am Acad Dermatol. 1990;23:694–700.
11. Edwards L, Berman B, Rapini RP, et al. Treatment of cutaneous squamous cell carcinoma by intralesional interferon alfa-2b therapy. Arch Dermatol. 1992;128:1486–9.
12. Grob JJ, Suzini F, Richard A, et al. Large keratoacanthomas treated with intralesional interferon alfa-2a. J Am Acad Dermatol. 1993;29:237–41.
13. Berman B, Duncan MR. Short-term keloid treatment *in vivo* with human interferon-α_{2b} results in a selective and persistent normalization of keloidal fibroblast collagen, glycosaminoglycan and collagenase production *in vitro*. J Am Acad Dermatol. 1989;21:694–702.
14. Granstein RD, Rook A, Flotte TJ, et al. A controlled trial of intralesional recombinant interferon-γ in the treatment of keloidal scarring. Arch Dermatol. 1990;126:1295–302.
15. Larrabee WF Jr, East CA, Jaffe HS, et al. Intralesional interferon gamma treatment for keloids and hypertrophic scars. Arch Otolaryngol Head Neck Surg. 1990;116:1159–62.
16. Berman B, Flores F. Recurrence rates of excised keloids treated with postoperative triamcinolone acetonide injections or interferon-α_{2b} injections. J Am Acad Dermatol. 1997;37:755–7.
17. Davison SP, Mess S, Kauffman LC, Al-Attar A. Ineffective treatment of keloids with interferon alpha-2b. Plast Reconstr Surg. 2006;117:247–52.
18. Nimura M. Intralesional human fibroblast interferon in common warts. J Dermatol. 1983;10:217–20.
19. Berman B, Davis-Reed L, Silverstein L, et al. Treatment of verruca vulgaris with α-2 interferon. J Infect Dis. 1986;154:328–30.
20. Hanifin SM, Schneider LC, Leung DY, et al. Recombinant interferon gamma therapy for atopic dermatitis. J Am Acad Dermatol. 1993;28:189–97.
21. Nishioka K, Matsunaga T, Katayama I. Gamma-interferon therapy for severe cases of atopic dermatitis of the adult type. J Dermatol. 1995;22:181–5.
22. Torrelo A, Harto A, Sendagorta E, et al. Interferon-α therapy in atopic dermatitis. Acta Derm Venereol. 1992;72:370–2.
23. Mackie RM. Interferon-α for atopic dermatitis. Lancet. 1990;335:1282–3.
24. Alpsoy E, Yilmaz E, Basaran E. Interferon therapy for Behcet's disease. J Am Acad Dermatol. 1994;31:617–19.
25. Mahrle G, Schulze HJ. Recombinant interferon-gamma (rIFN-gamma) in dermatology. J Invest Dermatol. 1990;95:132S–7S.
26. Rosenbloom J, Feldman G, Freundlich B, Jimenez SA. Inhibition of excessive scleroderma fibroblast collagen synthesis by recombinant gamma interferon. Arthritis Rheum. 1966;29:851–6.
27. Kahan A, Amor B, Menkes CJ, Strauch G. Recombinant interferon-γ in the treatment of systemic sclerosis. Am J Med. 1989;87:273–7.
28. Elgart GW, Sheremata W, Ahn YS. Cutaneous reactions to recombinant human interferon beta-1b: the clinical and histologic spectrum. J Am Acad Dermatol. 1997;37:553–8.
29. Interferon-β1a, -β1b, α_{2a}, α_{2b}, α n3. In: Physicians' Desk Reference, 52nd edn. Montvale: Medical Economics Company, 1998:305–7,1290–2, 2489–4, 2637–44.
30. Deyton LR, Walker RE, Kovac JA, et al. Reversible cardiac dysfunction associated with interferon-alfa therapy in AIDS patients with Kaposi's sarcoma. N Engl J Med 1989;321:1246–9.
31. Reinhold U, Hartl C, Hering R, et al. Fatal rhabdomyolysis and multiple organ failure associated with adjuvant high dose interferon alfa in malignant melanoma. Lancet. 1997;349:540–1.
32. Steis RG, Smith JW, Urba WJ, et al. Resistance to recombinant interferon-alfa$_{2a}$ in hairy-cell leukemia associated with neutralizing anti-interferon antibodies. N Engl J Med. 1988;318:1409–13.
33. Williams SJ, Baird-Lambert JA, Farrell GC. Inhibition of theophylline metabolism by interferon. Lancet. 1987;2:939–41.
34. Imbertson LM, Bearurline JM, Couture AM, et al. Cytokine induction in hairless mouse and rat skin after topical application on the immune response modification. J Invest Dermatol. 1998;110:734–9.
35. Miller RL, Gerster JF, Owens ML, et al. Imiquimod applied topically: a novel immune response modifier and new class of drug. Int J Immunopharmacol. 1999;21:1–14.
36. Suzuki H, Wang B, Shivji GM, et al. Imiquimod, a topical immune response modifier, induces migration of Langerhans cells. J Invest Dermatol. 2000; 114:135–41.
37. Workowski KA, Berman SM; Centers for Disease Control and Prevention. Sexually transmitted diseases treatment guidelines, 2006. MMWR Recomm Rep. 2006;55:1–94.
38. Weisshaar E, Gollnick H. Potentiating effect of imiquimod in the treatment of verrucae vulgares in immunocompromised patients. Acta Derm Venereol. 2000;80:306–7.
39. Theos AM, Cummings R, Silverberg NB, Paller AS. Effectiveness of imiquimod cream 5% for treating childhood molluscum contagiosum in a double-blind, randomized pilot trial. Cutis. 2004;74:141–2.
40. Berman B, Kaufman J. Pilot study of the effect of postoperative imiquimod 5% cream on the recurrence rate of excised keloids. J Am Acad Dermatol. 2002;47(suppl.):S209–11.
41. Martin-Garcia RF, Busquets AC. Postsurgical use of imiquimod 5% cream in the prevention of earlobe keloid recurrences: results of an open-label, pilot study. Dermatol Surg. 2005;31:1394–8.
42. Ceilley RI, Del Rosso JQ. Current modalities and new advances in the treatment of basal cell carcinoma. Int J Dermatol. 2006;45:489–98.
43. Hadley G, Derry S, Moore RA. Imiquimod for actinic keratosis: systematic review and meta-analysis. J Invest Dermatol. 2006;126:1251–5.
44. Patel GK, Goodwin R, Chawla M, et al: Imiquimod 5% cream monotherapy for cutaneous squamous cell carcinoma in situ (Bowen's disease): a randomized, double-blind, placebo-controlled trial. J Am Acad Dermatol. 2006;54:1025–32.
45. Berman B, Poochareon VN, Villa AM. Novel dermatologic uses of the immune response modifier imiquimod 5% cream. Skin Therapy Lett. 2002;7:1–6.
46. Berman B, Perez OA, Zell D. Immunological strategies to fight skin cancer. Skin Therapy Lett 2006;11:1–7.
47. Kagy MK, Amonette R. The use of imiquimod 5% cream for the treatment of superficial basal cell carcinomas in a basal cell nevus syndrome patient. Dermatol Surg. 2000;26:577–9.
48. Pehoushek J, Smith KJ. Imiquimod and 5% fluorouracil therapy for anal and perianal squamous cell carcinoma *in situ* in an HIV-1-positive man. Arch Dermatol. 2001;137:14–17.
49. Orengo I, Rosen T, Guill CK. Treatment of squamous cell carcinoma *in situ* of the penis with 5% imiquimod cream. J Am Acad Dermatol. 2002;47(suppl.):S225–8.
50. Suchin KR, Junkins-Hopkins JM, Rook AH. Treatment of stage IA cutaneous T-cell lymphoma with topical application of the immune response modifier imiquimod. Arch Dermatol. 2002;138:1137–9.
51. Cohen PR, Schulze KE, Tschen JA, Hetherington GW, Nelson BR. Treatment of extramammary Paget disease with topical imiquimod cream: case report and literature review. South Med J. 2006; 99:396–402.
52. Ahmed I, Berth-Jones J. Imiquimod: a novel treatment for lentigo maligna. Br J Dermatol. 2000; 143:843–5.
53. Wolf IH, Smolle J, Binder B, Cerroni L, Richtig E, Kerl H. Topical imiquimod in the treatment of metastatic melanoma to skin. Arch Dermatol. 2003;139:273–6.
54. Root RK, Dale DC. Granulocyte colony-stimulating factor and granulocyte-macrophage colony-stimulating factor: comparisons and potential for use in the treatment of infections in neutropenic patients. J Infect Dis. 1999;179:S342–52.
55. Horn TD, Burke PJ, Karp JE, Hood AF. Intravenous administration of recombinant granulocyte-macrophage colony-stimulating factor causes a cutaneous eruption. Arch Dermatol. 1991;127:49–52.
56. Scott GA. Report of three cases of cutaneous reactions to granulocyte-macrophage colony-stimulating factor and a review of the literature. Am J Dermatopathol. 1995;17:107–14.
57. Johnson ML, Grimwood RE. Leukocyte colony-stimulating factors. A review of associated neutrophilic dermatosis and vasculitides. Arch Dermatol. 1994;130:77–81.
58. Stuetz A, Baumann K, Grassberger M, et al. Discovery of topical calcineurin inhibitors and pharmacological profile of pimecrolimus. Int Arch Allergy Immunol. 2006;141:199–212.
59. Carroll CL, Fleischer AB Jr. Tacrolimus ointment: treatment of atopic dermatitis and other inflammatory cutaneous disease. Expert Opin Pharmacother. 2004;5:2127–37.
60. Callen JP, Chamlin S, Eichenfield LF, et al. A systematic review of the safety of topical therapies for atopic dermatitis. Br J Dermatol. 2007;156:203–21.
61. Allen A, Siegfried E, Silverman R, et al. Significant absorption of topical tacrolimus in 3 patients with Netherton syndrome. Arch Dermatol. 2001;137:747–50.
62. Ellis CN, Krueger GG. Treatment of chronic plaque psoriasis by selective targeting of memory effector T lymphocytes. N Engl J Med. 2001;345:248–55.
63. Fivenson DP, Mathes B. Treatment of generalized lichen planus with alefacept. Arch Dermatol 2006;142:151–2.
64. Shapira MY, Resnick IB, Bitan M, et al. Rapid response to alefacept given to patients with steroid resistant or steroid dependent acute graft-versus-host disease: a preliminary report. Bone Marrow Transplant. 2005;36:1097–101.
65. Heffrenan M, Hurley MY, Martin KS, et al: Alefacept for alopecia areata. Arch Dermatol. 2005;141:1513–16.
66. Goffe B, Papp K, Gratton D, et al. An integrated analysis of thirteen trials summarizing the long-term safety of alefacept in psoriasis patients who have received up to nine courses of therapy. Clin Ther. 2005;27:1912–21.
67. Mease PJ, Gladman DD, Keystone EC; Alefacept in Psoriatic Arthritis Study Group. Alefacept in combination with methotrexate for the treatment of psoriatic arthritis: results of a randomized, double-blind, placebo-controlled study. Arthritis Rheum. 2006;54:1638–45.
68. Ortonne JP, Khemis A, Koo JY, Choi J. An open-label study of alefacept plus ultraviolet B light as combination therapy for chronic plaque psoriasis. J Eur Acad Dermatol Venereol. 2005;19:556–63.
69. Gottlieb AB, Krueger JG, Wittkowski K, et al. Psoriasis as a model for T-cell mediated disease: immunobiologic and clinical effects of treatment with multiple doses of efalizumab and anti-CDIIa antibody. Arch Dermatol. 2002;138:591–60.
70. Gordon KB, Papp KA, Hamilton TK, et al. Efalizumab for patients with moderate to severe plaque psoriasis: a randomized controlled trial. JAMA. 2003;290:3073–80.
71. Lebwohl M, Tyring SK, Hamilton TK, et al. A novel targeted T-cell modulator, efalizumab, for plaque psoriasis. N Engl J Med. 2003;349:2004–13.
72. Wellington K, Perry CM. Efalizumab.Am J Clin Dermatol. 2005;6:113–18.
73. Weinberg JM, Siegfried EC. Successful treatment of severe atopic dermatitis in a child and an adult with the T-cell modulator efalizumab. Arch Dermatol. 2006;142:555–8.
74. Kaelin U, Hassan AS, Braathen LR, Yawalkar N. Treatment of alopecia areata partim universalis with efalizumab. J Am Acad Dermatol. 2006;55:529–32.
75. Golda N, Benham SM, Koo J. Rebound of psoriasis during treatment with efalizumab. J Drugs Dermatol. 2006;5:63–5.
76. Lowes MA, Turton JA, Krueger JG, Barneston RS. Psoriasis vulgaris flare during therapy does not preclude future use: a case series. BMC Dermatol. 2005;5:9.
77. Sheinfeld N. Efalizumab: a review of events reported during clinical trials and side effects. Expert Opin Drug Saf. 2006;5:197–209.
78. Mease PJ, Goffe BS, Metz J, VanderStoep A, Finck B, Burge DJ. Etanercept in the treatment of psoriatic arthritis and psoriasis: a randomized trial. Lancet. 2000;356:385–90.
79. Straub RH, Härle P, Sarzi-Puttini P, Cutolo M. Tumor necrosis factor-neutralizing therapies improve altered hormone axes. An alternative mode of anti-inflammatory action. Arthritis Rheum. 2006;54:2039–46.
80. Alexis AF, Strober BE. Off-label dermatologic uses of anti-TNF-α therapies. J Cutan Med Surg. 2005;9:296–302.
81. Keystone EC, Thorne C, Haraoui B. The utility of biologics in orphan diseases. New Developments in Rheumatic Diseases. 2005;3:9–28.
82. Norman R, Greenberg RG, Jackson JM. Case reports of etanercept in inflammatory dermatoses. J Am Acad Dermatol. 2006;54(suppl. 2):S139–42.

83. Baughman RP, Lower EE, Bradley DA, et al. Etanercept for refractory ocular sarcoidosis: results of a double-blind randomized trial. Chest. 2005;128:1062–7.

84. Peterson JR, Hsu FC, Simkin PA, Wener MH. Effect of tumour necrosis factor alpha antagonists on serum transaminases and viraemia in patients with rheumatoid arthritis and chronic hepatitis C infection. Ann Rheum Dis. 2003;62:1078–82.

85. Tyring S, Gottlieb A, Papp K, et al. Etanercept and clinical outcomes, fatigue, and depression in psoriasis: double-blind placebo-controlled randomized phase III trial. Lancet. 2006;367:29–35.

86. Wolfe F, Michaud K. Lymphoma in rheumatoid arthritis: the effect of methotrexate and anti-tumor necrosis factor therapy in 18,572 patients. Arthritis Rheum. 2004;50:1740–51.

87. Lebwohl M, Blum R, Berkowitz E, et al. No evidence for increased risk of cutaneous squamous cell carcinoma in patients with rheumatoid arthritis receiving etanercept for up to 5 years. Arch Dermatol. 2005;141:861–4.

88. Wegener's Granulomatosis Etanercept Trial (WGET) Research Group. Etanercept plus standard therapy for Wegener's granulomatosis. N Engl J Med. 2005;352:351–61.

89. Shakoor N, Michalska M, Harris CA, Block JA. Drug-induced systemic lupus erythematosus associated with etanercept. Lancet. 2002;359:579–80.

90. Fautrel B, Foltz B, Frances C, et al. Regression of subacute cutaneous lupus erythematosus in a patient with rheumatoid arthritis treated with a biologic tumor necrosis factor alpha-blocking agent: comment on the article by Pisetsky and the letter from Aringer et al. Arthritis Rheum. 2002;46:1408–9.

91. Mohan N, Edwards ET, Cupps TR, et al. Demyelination occurring during anti-tumor necrosis factor alpha therapy for inflammatory arthritides. Arthritis Rheum. 2001;44:2862–9.

92. Behnam SM, Behnam SE, Koo JY. TNF-alpha inhibitors and congestive heart failure. Skinmed. 2005;4:363–8.

93. Kary S, Worm M, Audring H, et al. New onset or exacerbation of psoriatic skin lesions in patients with definite rheumatoid arthritis receiving tumour necrosis factor alpha antagonists. Ann Rheum Dis. 2006;65:405–7.

94. Mohan N, Edwards ET, Cupps TR, et al. Leukocytoclastic vasculitis associated with tumor necrosis factor-alpha blocking agents. J Rheumatol. 2004;31:1955–8.

95. Deng A, Harvey V, Sina B, et al. Interstitial granulomatous dermatitis associated with the use of tumor necrosis factor alpha inhibitors. Arch Dermatol. 2006;142:198–202.

96. Genovese MC, Cohen S, Moreland L, et al. Combination therapy with etanercept and anakinra in the treatment of patients with rheumatoid arthritis

97. who have been treated successfully with methotrexate. Arthritis Rheum. 2004;50: 412–19.

97. Salmon JE, Alpert D. Are we coming to terms with tumor necrosis factor inhibition in pregnancy? Arthritis Rheum. 2006;54:2353–5.

98. Chaudhari U, Romano P, Mulcahy LD, et al. Efficacy and safety of infliximab monotherapy for plaque-type psoriasis: a randomized trial. Lancet. 2001;357:1842–6.

99. Brooklyn TN, Dunnill MG, Shetty A, et al. Infliximab for the treatment of pyoderma gangrenosum: a randomized, double-blind, placebo controlled trial. Gut. 2006;55:505–9.

100. Scheinfeld N. Off-label uses and side effects of infliximab. J Drugs Dermatol. 2004;3:273–84.

101. Baert F, Noman M, Vermeire S, et al. Influence of immunogenicity on the long-term efficacy of infliximab in Crohn's disease. N Engl J Med. 2003;348:601–8.

102. Bergstrom L, Yocum DE, Ampel NM, et al. Increased risk of coccidioidomycosis in patients treated with tumor necrosis factor alpha antagonists. Arthritis Rheum 2004;50:1959–66.

103. Bongartz T, Sutton AJ, Sweeting MJ, et al. Anti-TNF antibody therapy in rheumatoid arthritis and the risk of serious infections and malignancies: systematic review and meta-analysis of rare harmful effects in randomized controlled trials. JAMA. 2006;295:2275–85.

104. Thayu M, Markowitz JE, Mamula P, et al. Hepatosplenic T-cell lymphoma in an adolescent patient after immunomodulator and biologic therapy for Crohn disease. J Pediatr Gastroenterol Nutr. 2005;40:220–2.

105. Comby E, Tanaff P, Mariotte D, et al. Evolution of antinuclear antibodies and clinical patterns in patients with active rheumatoid arthritis with longterm infliximab therapy. J Rheumatol. 2006;33:24–30.

106. Miele E, Markowitz JE, Mamula P, Baldassano RN. Human antichimeric antibody in children and young adults with inflammatory bowel disease receiving infliximab. J Pediatr Gastroenterol Nutr. 2004; 38:502–8.

107. Fomin I , Caspi D, Levy V, et al. Vaccination against influenza in rheumatoid arthritis: the effect of disease modifying drugs, including TNF alpha blockers. Ann Rheum Dis. 2006;65:191–4.

108. Mease PJ. Adalimumab: an anti-TNF agent for the treatment of psoriatic arthritis. Expert Opin Biol Ther. 2005;5:1491–504.

109. Callen JP, Jackson JH. Adalimumab effectively controlled recalcitrant generalized pustular psoriasis in an adolescent. J Dermatol Treat. 2005;16:350–2.

110. Furst DE. Anakinra: review of recombinant human interleukin-1-receptor antagonist in the treatment of rheumatoid arthritis. Clin Ther. 2004;26:1960–75.

111. Goldbach-Mansky R, Dailey NJ, Canna SW, et al. Neonatal-onset multisystem inflammatory disease responsive to interleukin-1beta inhibition. N Eng J Med. 2006;355:581–92.

112. Scheinfeld N. A review of rituximab in cutaneous medicine. Dermatol Online J. 2006;12:3.

113. Anonymous. Rituximab (Rituxan) for rheumatoid arthritis. Med Lett Drugs Ther. 2006;48:34–5.

114. El Tal AK, Posner MR, Spigelman Z, Ahmed AR. Rituximab: a monoclonal antibody to CD20 used in the treatment of pemphigus vulgaris. J Am Acad Dermatol. 2006;55:449–59.

115. Anolik JH, Aringer M. New treatments for SLE: cell-depleting and anti-cytokine therapies. Best Pract Res Clin Rheumatol. 2005;19:859–78.

116. Cutler C, Miklos D, Haesook T, et al. Rituximab for steroid-refractory chronic graft-versus-host disease. Blood. 2006;108:756–62.

117. Chung L, Funke AA, Chakravarty EF, et al. Successful use of rituximab for cutaneous vasculitis. Arch Dermatol 2006;142:1407–10.

118. Bonnekoh B, Schulz M, Franke I, Gollnick H. Complete remission of primary cutaneous B-cell lymphoma of the lower leg by first-line monotherapy with the CD20-antibody rituximab. J Cancer Res Clin Oncol. 2002;128:161–6.

119. Levine TD. Rituximab in the treatment of dermatomyositis: an open-label pilot study. Arthritis Rheum. 2005;52:601–7.

120. Beck LA, Saini S. Wanted: a study with omalizumab to determine the role of IgE-mediated pathways in atopic dermatitis. J Am Acad Dermatol. 2006;55:540–1.

120a. Krueger GG, Langley RG, Leonardi C, et al. CNTO 1275 Psoriasis Study Group. A human interleukin-12/23 monoclonal antibody for the treatment of psoriasis. N Engl J Med 2007;356:580–92.

121. Mydlarski PR, Mittman N, Shear NH. Intravenous immunoglobulin: use in dermatology. Skin Therapy Lett. 2004;9:1–6.

122. French LT, Trent JT, Kerdel FA. Use of intravenous immunoglobulin in toxic epidermal necrolysis and Stevens-Johnson syndrome: our current understanding. Int Immunopharmacol. 2006;6:543–9.

123. Dalakas MC. The role of high-dose immune globulin in the treatment of dermatomyositis. Int Immunopharmacol. 2006;6:550–6.

124. Ahmed AR. Use of intravenous immunoglobulin therapy in autoimmune blistering diseases. Int Immunopharmacol. 2006;6:557–78.

125. Bayary J, Dasgupta S, Misra N, et al. Intravenous immunoglobulin in autoimmune disorders: an insight into the immunoregulatory mechanisms. Int Immunopharmacol. 2006;6:528–34.

126. Siegel J. Safety considerations in IGIV utilization. Int Immunopharmacol. 2006;6:523–7.

127. Distler JH, Jungel A, Huber LC, et al. Imatinib mesylate reduces production of extracellular matrix and prevents development of experimental dermal fibrosis. Arthritis Rheum. 2007;56:311–22.

Other Topical Medications

Annemarie Uliasz and Mark Lebwohl

Key features

- Absorption of topical medications depends upon several factors, including cutaneous barrier function, anatomic site, the active agent, characteristics of the vehicle, and patient factors such as quality of application
- Combination topical therapy may result in increased efficacy with a reduction in side effects
- In neonates, there is a greater risk of systemic toxicity due to topical medications

FACTORS THAT AFFECT PERCUTANEOUS ABSORPTION

Barrier function/disruption (e.g. Netherton syndrome)
Molecular size of the drug or prodrug
Lipophilicity of the drug
Active drug concentration
Drug metabolism
Composition of the vehicle
Anatomic location
Thickness of the stratum corneum
Skin hydration
Occlusion
Patient age

Table 129.1 Factors that affect percutaneous absorption.

GENERAL PRINCIPLES OF TOPICAL THERAPY

Topical therapy is advantageous in that medications may be applied directly to the target organ. As a result, systemic side effects and toxicities may be reduced, while maximizing cutaneous effects. Unfortunately, application of topical therapies may be more time consuming than the ingestion or injection of systemic medications; they also require detailed patient instruction and can leave messy residues or stains. Furthermore, it is not always practical to apply topical medications to large areas of the body. Despite these potential shortcomings, topical medications represent a key component of dermatologic treatment strategies.

Topical formulations consist of an active ingredient in a non-active base (vehicle). To be effective, topical medications must gain entry into the skin, travel through its layers, and reach the desired site of action in adequate concentrations. The site of action is often the epidermis (beneath the stratum corneum) or the dermis. Successful topical therapy depends on effective percutaneous absorption. Several variables affect percutaneous absorption, including the active agent, its concentration, the vehicle, skin hydration, and anatomic site (Table 129.1).

Given that it functions to protect the skin against desiccation and environmental insult, the stratum corneum acts as the primary barrier to percutaneous absorption (see Ch. 124). The semipermeable stratum corneum is often described as a 'brick and mortar' structure with keratinocytes acting as the bricks and intercellular lipid domains acting as the mortar. Agents move across the stratum corneum by way of passive diffusion, often via the intercellular lipid domains. Alternatively, agents may be transported via pores within a continuous lacunar system or via a transappendageal route (e.g. along hair follicles or sweat glands).

Cutaneous absorption is proportional to the concentration of the active agent in the topical medication, i.e. given the same vehicle, higher concentrations increase absorption. Concentration may also be altered based upon properties of the vehicle. For example, volatile components of vehicles may evaporate, rapidly reducing the volume of the vehicle and thus increasing the concentration of the medication.

Skin hydration has also been shown to affect percutaneous absorption, with increased skin hydration resulting in higher degrees of absorption. Occlusion (in the form of an ointment, physical dressing or skin fold) may increase hydration by a factor of 10 by preventing epidermal water loss. In addition, it prevents removal of the topical agent by evaporation, friction or exfoliation.

Anatomic location is another factor that influences percutaneous absorption. Both occlusion (e.g. in intertriginous zones) and the thickness of the stratum corneum play a role. Feldman & Maibach[1] were the first to describe such regional variations, based upon their studies on the absorption of topical corticosteroids and pesticides in various anatomic sites (Table 129.2). In areas where the stratum corneum was thicker, such as the palms and soles, absorption was lower. Conversely,

PERCUTANEOUS ABSORPTION BY ANATOMIC REGION

Site of application	Absorption
Forearm (ventral) – control site	1
Forearm (dorsal)	1.1
Plantar surface	0.14
Ankle	0.42
Palm	0.83
Back	1.7
Scalp	3.5
Axilla	3.6
Forehead	6.0
Jaw	13
Scrotum	42

Table 129.2 Percutaneous absorption by anatomic region[1]. Ratio consisting of total absorption for each anatomic site compared to the forearm (estimated by amount of ^{14}C-hydrocortisone excreted in urine).

absorption was higher in areas where the stratum corneum was thin (e.g. the scrotum and face).

Furthermore, chemicals, diseases or physical injury that disrupt barrier function can result in increased absorption. The markedly enhanced absorption of topical tacrolimus in patients with Netherton syndrome is a prime example of this phenomenon. Although there appears to be no difference between adults and full-term neonates (see below), the cutaneous barrier function in premature babies is markedly impaired.

Another factor that influences cutaneous absorption is molecular size of the drug. Molecules must traverse a tortuous path through the intercellular lipid domains. Hence, the diffusion of a compound is inversely proportional to its frictional coefficient, which is a function of the molecular size of the compound.

Lastly, in the stratum corneum, a unique mixture of lipids that includes ceramides, cholesterol and fatty acids prevents desiccation and acts as a barrier to the diffusion of substances into the skin. As a result, lipophilic agents are more likely to permeate the skin than are hydrophilic agents.

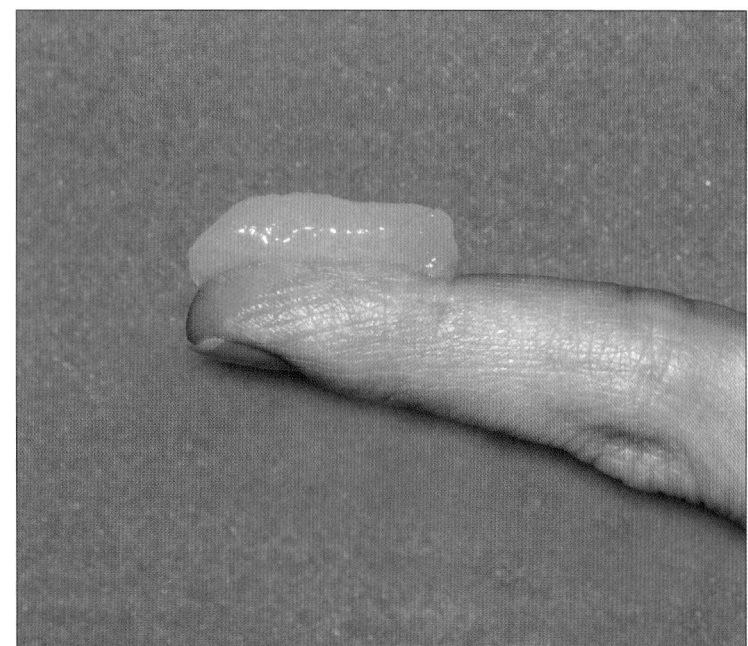

Fig. 129.1 An adult fingertip unit.

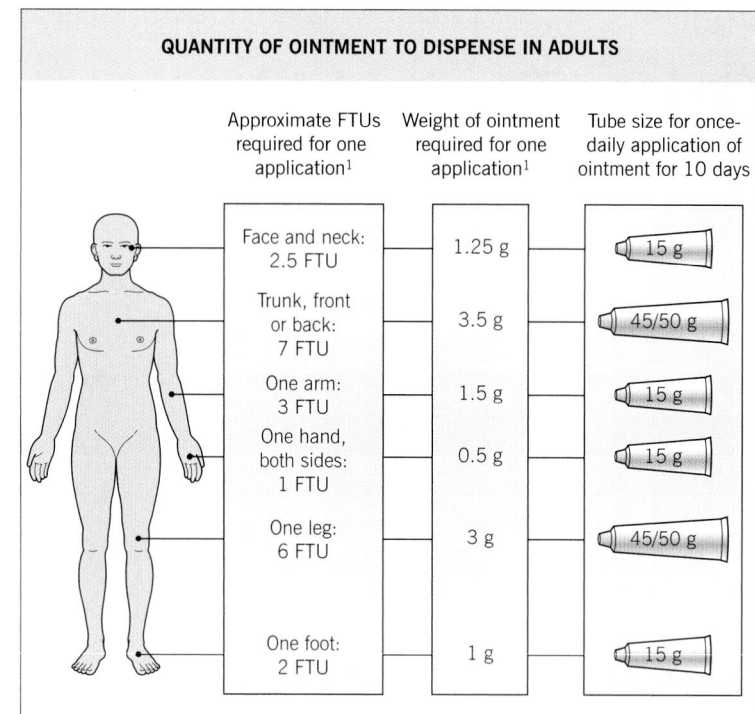

QUANTITY OF OINTMENT TO DISPENSE IN ADULTS		
Approximate FTUs required for one application[1]	Weight of ointment required for one application[1]	Tube size for once-daily application of ointment for 10 days
Face and neck: 2.5 FTU	1.25 g	15 g
Trunk, front or back: 7 FTU	3.5 g	45/50 g
One arm: 3 FTU	1.5 g	15 g
One hand, both sides: 1 FTU	0.5 g	15 g
One leg: 6 FTU	3 g	45/50 g
One foot: 2 FTU	1 g	15 g

Fig. 129.2 Quantity of ointment to dispense in adults. FTU, fingertip unit. Redrawn from Long CC, Finlay AY. The finger-tip unit – a new practical measure. Clin Exp Dermatol. 1991;16:444–7.

Quantity of Application

Topical medications should be applied to the skin as a thin layer measuring approximately 0.1 mm. A thicker layer of medication does not result in enhanced penetration or a better therapeutic effect (due to the medication itself). According to Arndt & Bowers[2], 1 g of cream covers a 10 cm × 10 cm area of skin; 1 g of ointment spreads approximately 10% further than the same amount of cream.

A practical guide to quantifying the amount of ointment necessary to treat different areas of the body was developed by Long & Finlay[3]. They described the fingertip unit (FTU) as the amount of ointment dispensed from a 5 mm diameter nozzle that is applied to the distal third of the index finger, from the crease under the distal interphalangeal joint to the fingertip (Fig. 129.1). One FTU is equal to approximately 0.5 g. In their study, the number of FTUs required to treat different areas of the body was determined (Fig. 129.2). They found that approximately 20 g were needed to treat the entire body of an adult man, or roughly 280 g per week if the medication were applied twice daily for 1 week.

Long & Finlay[4] subsequently devised the 'rule of hand' method for determining the amount of topical medication to apply to a given area. They determined that the area of one side of an extended, flat hand requires approximately 0.5 FTU. In turn, four hand areas require 2 FTUs or 1 g of ointment. In this way, the number of 'flat hand' areas of affected skin can be estimated, and the number of FTUs required for treatment calculated. The fingertip unit and 'rule of hand' methods were subsequently used to devise guidelines for pediatric patients (Fig. 129.3)[5].

Combination Therapy

Advantages of using a single therapeutic agent for disease control include lower cost and improved compliance. However, combination therapy is often employed because monotherapy has proven inadequate or associated side effects are unacceptable. Combination therapy can allow for a reduction in the dosage of one or both agents, potentially decreasing side effects (especially if there are different adverse-effect profiles)[6–9]. In addition, by combining medications with different mechanisms of action, additive or even synergistic therapeutic effects can occur.

As an example, in a study by Lebwohl et al.[10], a combination of calcipotriene applied daily in the morning in conjunction with halobetasol in the evening for 2 weeks was found to be more effective than either component alone in the treatment of psoriasis. Additionally, patients treated with this combination had fewer cutaneous adverse effects than patients treated with either halobetasol or calcipotriene alone. Enhanced efficacy is also seen when mid-potency topical corti-

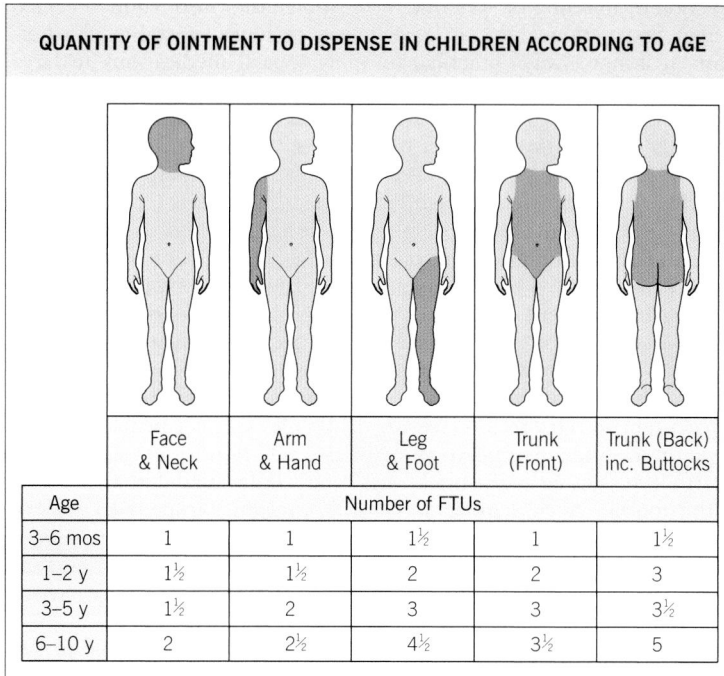

QUANTITY OF OINTMENT TO DISPENSE IN CHILDREN ACCORDING TO AGE				
Face & Neck	Arm & Hand	Leg & Foot	Trunk (Front)	Trunk (Back) inc. Buttocks
Age	Number of FTUs			
3–6 mos	1	1	1½	1	1½
1–2 y	1½	1½	2	2	3
3–5 y	1½	2	3	3	3½
6–10 y	2	2½	4½	3½	5

Fig. 129.3 Quantity of ointment to dispense in children, according to age. FTU, fingertip unit. Redrawn from Long CC, Mills CM, Finlay AY. A practical guide to topical therapy in children. Br J Dermatol. 1998; 138:293–6.

costeroids are combined with topical calcineurin inhibitors in the treatment of atopic dermatitis and psoriasis[11]. Sometimes, combination therapy results in similar endpoint results but more rapid improvement (e.g. daily calcipotriene plus betamethasone dipropionate for 8 weeks followed by daily calcipotriene for 4 weeks versus calcipotriene twice daily for 12 weeks[12]).

Longer remission times can also be observed, in addition to enhanced efficacy and reduced side effects. For example, when tazarotene gel is combined with topical corticosteroids for the treatment of psoriasis, enhanced efficacy, longer remission times, and a decrease in tazarotene-associated irritation have all been observed[13,14]. Yet another clinical approach is to use high-potency topical corticosteroids 2 days per week (weekends) and a second agent (e.g. calcipotriene or calcineurin inhibitors) 5 days per week (weekdays) as a means of decreasing side effects and prolonging remission times[15].

Combination therapy is commonly employed in the treatment of acne. As the pathogenesis of acne is multifactorial, the combination of agents with different mechanisms of action often provides faster, more effective results. In the treatment of mild papulopustular acne, a combination of topical retinoids and topical antibiotics is first-line therapy. Moreover, because topical retinoids normalize desquamation and comedogenesis, they allow increased penetration of other topical agents. A study of the combination of clindamycin 1% gel and tretinoin 0.025% gel demonstrated superior efficacy compared to either agent alone. Furthermore, the combination was better tolerated than tretinoin monotherapy[16]. Additionally, the combination of adapalene 0.1% gel and clindamycin 1% was found to be more effective than clindamycin plus vehicle[17]. The combination of topical tretinoin 0.05% and topical erythromycin 2% has demonstrated synergistic results and was found to be well tolerated[18].

One concern in the treatment of acne is the increasing incidence of resistant strains of *Propionibacterium acnes*. However, to date, there have not been reports of resistance when topical antibiotics were used in combination with benzoyl peroxide. Benzoyl peroxide is bactericidal, and when used in conjunction with topical antibiotics, it is effective in the long-term treatment of acne and in those patients who have previously developed resistant *P. acnes*[19].

In addition to using two agents concurrently, sequential therapy is another strategy for combining topical (as well as systemic) treatments[20]. In this approach, a more powerful agent is used during the clearance phase. Thereafter, the frequency of use is gradually reduced in order to prolong remission time and minimize adverse effects. Other less powerful but safer agents are then used on the remaining days to reduce recurrence of disease. Eventually, the latter often serve as the sole agent during the maintenance phase. This method is commonly used in 'pulse therapy' with superpotent topical corticosteroids.

Although combination therapy may provide greater efficacy and decreased adverse effects, it should be noted that not all medications are compatible. The combination of certain agents may, in fact, compromise the effects of one another. For example, the addition of tar to anthralin was observed to decrease the cutaneous irritation associated with anthralin. However, it was found that coal tar caused anthralin to oxidize, suggesting that tar minimizes anthralin-induced irritation by inactivating the anthralin[21]. Similarly, calcipotriene has been demonstrated to be unstable when combined with hydrocortisone-17-valerate 0.2% ointment, 12% ammonium lactate lotion and 6% salicylic acid[22].

Topical Therapy and Neonates

The neonatal period is defined as the first 30 days of life. At birth, neonatal skin is functionally mature. The stratum corneum, the main barrier to percutaneous absorption, is fully developed and similar in thickness to that of adults[23]. Despite these findings, the neonate is at risk for systemic toxicity from topically applied medications. Studies have reported toxicity in infants exposed to topical corticosteroids, salicylic acid, lindane, hexachlorophene and chlorhexidine, as well as to topical phenol, mercury, boric acid, epinephrine, estrogens and propylene glycol (Table 129.3)[24,25].

There are several factors that contribute to this increased risk (Table 129.4). First, at birth, full-term infants have a surface area to body weight ratio four times that of adults. This allows infants to absorb percutaneously proportionately greater quantities of topical medication than adults. Although the stratum corneum is fully formed at birth, optimal barrier function may be delayed until the transition from neutral to acidic pH that occurs over the first few weeks of life is complete. Furthermore, several organ systems in the neonate, including the hepatic, renal and central nervous system, are not yet fully developed, neither structurally nor functionally. This may result in altered drug distribution, metabolism and excretion.

Decreased plasma protein binding in neonates may lead to drug toxicity at lower blood levels. Additionally, drug distribution may be altered by the lower blood pressure and variable blood flow patterns seen in neonates. The immature hepatic system can lead to longer half-

POTENTIAL SYSTEMIC SIDE EFFECTS OF TOPICAL MEDICATIONS	
Medication	**Systemic side effect**
Androgens	Virilization in women
Boric acid	Generalized erythema, fever, vomiting, mental status change
Calcipotriene	Hypercalcemia
Carmustine (BCNU)	Bone marrow toxicity
Chlorhexidine	Nausea, signs of ethanol intoxication
Clindamycin	Diarrhea, pseudomembranous colitis (controversial)
Corticosteroids	Iatrogenic Cushing's syndrome, inhibition of hypothalamic–pituitary axis
Dimethylsulfoxide	Nausea, abdominal pain
Epinephrine	Tachycardia
Estrogens	Pseudoprecocious puberty, gynecomastia, hypogonadism in men
Gentamicin	Ototoxicity
Hexachlorophene	Neurotoxicity, coma, death
Iodine	Hypothyroidism
Lindane	CNS toxicity
Malathion	CNS toxicity, hyperglycemia
Mechlorethamine	Myelosuppression
Mercury	CNS and renal toxicity, acrodynia
Minoxidil	Cardiac toxicity, death
Neomycin	Ototoxicity, nephrotoxicity
Phenol	Cardiac arrhythmia, death
Podophyllin	Polyneuropathy, coma
Prilocaine–lidocaine (EMLA®)	Methemoglobinemia
Propylene glycol	Hyperosmolality, with or without lactic acidosis
Salicylic acid	Tinnitus, CNS and gastrointestinal toxicity, coma, death
Silver (silver nitrate, silver sulfadiazine)	Leukopenia, argyria

Table 129.3 Potential systemic side effects of topical medications. For most, the risk of these side effects is either theoretical or exists only in instances where the medication is applied to neonates or in quantities greatly exceeding normal exposure.

FACTORS THAT INCREASE THE RISK OF SYSTEMIC TOXICITY FROM TOPICAL MEDICATIONS IN NEONATES
Increased ratio of surface area to body weight
Suboptimal epidermal barrier function due to the higher pH of neonatal stratum corneum
Decreased hepatic metabolism
Decreased renal excretion
Increased distribution of drug, including the CNS
Decreased plasma protein binding

Table 129.4 Factors that increase the risk of systemic toxicity from topical medications in neonates.

lives of drugs that are metabolized into inactive or excretable metabolites by the liver.

In addition, the neonatal glomerular filtration rate is half that of adults and does not reach adult levels until approximately 1 year of age. As the renal system is not fully developed, drug excretion may be affected.

Lastly, myelination within the CNS is completed slowly during infancy, and the blood–brain barrier of the neonate is more permeable than that of adults. This may increase the likelihood of drug-induced seizures.

In sum, when prescribing topical medications for neonates, the increased risk of systemic toxicity must be kept in mind.

Topical Therapy during Pregnancy and Lactation

When treating any woman of childbearing age, it is important to be aware of available recommendations regarding the use of specific drugs during pregnancy and lactation. Unfortunately, a pregnant or lactating woman may not always notify her physician of her status. Additionally, a woman's pregnancy status may be unknown.

The decision to use topical medications during pregnancy should be based on the potential risk of the medication and the extent to which the condition affects the health of the woman. Although not a comprehensive list, use of the following topical medications during pregnancy is either contraindicated or at least controversial: podophyllin (teratogenic), anthralin, phenol (neurotoxicity), lindane (potentially neurotoxic), chemotherapeutics including carmustine, mechlorethamine hydrochloride and 5-fluorouracil (teratogenic), and salicylic acid (premature closure of the ductus arteriosus and consequent pulmonary hypertension in the newborn when used in late pregnancy). Table 129.5 details the Food and Drug Administration (FDA) classification system of pharmaceutical pregnancy categories. Table 129.6 provides lists of topical medications with minimal risk during pregnancy and lactation.

Dermatologists should realize that both patients and our obstetrical colleagues may carry preconceived notions about the use of specific medications during pregnancy. Open lines of communication can avoid misunderstandings.

Formulations and Vehicles

A classification of the various formulations for external preparations is provided in Table 129.7 and their clinical applications in Table 129.8. A discussion of vehicles is found in Chapter 124, and this section will focus on the most recently developed vehicle, foam.

Foam vehicles are pressurized collections of gaseous bubbles in a matrix of liquid film. Dispensed in an aluminum can with a hydrocarbon propellant, the foam matrix is thermolabile. It is stable at room temperature, but readily breaks down and melts at body temperature. The matrix is comprised of several components. Once applied to the skin, volatile ingredients, including alcohol and water, evaporate. Lipid and polar components interact with skin-surface lipids, resulting in supersaturated solutions on the stratum corneum. Supersaturated solutions at the vehicle–skin interface enable maximum drug transfer into the skin and increased bioavailability. Furthermore, components of the foam, particularly alcohol, may reversibly alter the stratum corneum's barrier properties, resulting in enhanced penetration. The presence of

---

FDA CLASSIFICATION SYSTEM OF PHARMACEUTICAL PREGNANCY CATEGORIES

Category	Description
A	Controlled studies show no risk. Adequate well-controlled studies in pregnant women have failed to demonstrate risk to the fetus.
B	No evidence of risk in humans. Either animal studies show risk, but human studies do not; or, if no adequate human studies have been done, animal findings are negative.
C	Risk cannot be ruled out. Human studies are lacking, and animal studies are either positive for fetal risk or lacking as well. However, potential benefits may justify the potential risk.
D	Positive evidence for risk. Human studies, or investigational or post-marketing data, show risk to fetus. Nevertheless, potential benefits may outweigh potential risk.
X	Contraindicated in pregnancy. Studies in animals or humans, or investigational or post-marketing reports, have shown fetal risk, which clearly outweighs any possible benefit to the patient.

Table 129.5 **FDA classification system of pharmaceutical pregnancy categories**[26]. FDA, Food and Drug Administration.

TOPICAL MEDICATIONS WITH MINIMAL RISK DURING PREGNANCY AND LACTATION

Pregnancy	FDA category (see Table 129.5)	Lactation
Azelaic acid	B	Acyclovir
Ciclopirox	B	Bacitracin
Clindamycin	B	Benzoyl peroxide
Clotrimazole	B	Butoconazole
Erythromycin	B	Calcipotriene
Metronidazole*	B	Ciclopirox
Mupirocin	B	Clotrimazole
Naftifine	B	Erythromycin
Nystatin†	A (pastilles)	Hydroquinone
Oxiconazole	B	Ketoconazole
Permethrin	B	Metronidazole
Terbinafine	B	Mupirocin
		Nystatin
		Oxiconazole
		Terbinafine
		Tretinoin

*Contraindicated in the first trimester.
† Intravaginal topical application not advised close to term because of risk of contamination if membranes have ruptured.

Table 129.6 **Topical medications with minimal risk during pregnancy and lactation**[27,28]. Minimal risk defined here as FDA pregnancy category B.

CLASSIFICATION OF EXTERNAL PREPARATIONS

Liquid

- Monophasic solutions
  - Pure aqueous: lotions, gels
  - Alcoholic, alcoholic-aqueous: paints
  - Oily: oils
- Emulsions
  - Oil in water (O/W)
  - Water in oil (W/O)
- Suspensions
- Aerosols (solutions with pressurized gaseous propellants)
  - Foam
  - Spray

Semisolid

- Water-free: ointments
- Water-containing
  - Monophasic: hydrogels
  - Multiphasic: emulsions, creams (O/W or W/O)
- Highly concentrated suspensions: pastes

Solid

- Powders (e.g. zinc oxide, titanium dioxide, talc)

Table 129.7 **Classification of external preparations.** Vehicles can also contain preservatives, emulsifiers, absorption promoters, and fragrances.

FACTORS IN THE CHOICE OF FORMULATION AND VEHICLE FOR TOPICAL MEDICATIONS

Nature of the dermatosis

- Wet dermatoses (e.g. oozing) – water-based formulations, drying paste
- Dry dermatoses (e.g. scaling) – oil-based formulations
- Highly inflamed or crusted dermatoses – ointment or cream following or combined with wet compresses (e.g. open wet dressings, wet wraps) or soaks
- Fissured or eroded skin – avoid formulations containing alcohol or salicylates, which can lead to stinging and burning

Location of the dermatosis

- Glabrous skin – ointment, cream or emulsion
- Skin folds – lotion or O/W cream; avoid occlusive ointments and W/O formulations
- Hairy areas – lotion, gel, foam or oil

Table 129.8 **Factors in the choice of formulation and vehicle for topical medications.** O/W, oil in water; W/O, water in oil.

alcohol also explains the stinging and burning seen with foams, especially when there are fissures or erosions.

In addition to enhanced penetration, foams may be more cosmetically appealing than traditional vehicles. They are quick-drying, fragrance-free, stain-free, and leave little to no residue. This makes them better suited for application to hair-bearing areas. As foams are lighter than other vehicles, they also produce less shearing forces when applied to inflamed skin. These characteristics may lead to improved compliance.

In vitro studies have shown increased absorption, rates of delivery, and permeation of active agents in foams as compared to other vehicles[29]. With regard to combination therapy, calcipotriene solution, tacrolimus ointment and pimecrolimus cream are stable in the presence of betamethasone valerate and clobetasol propionate foams[29].

SPECIFIC TOPICAL MEDICATIONS

In the remainder of the chapter, topical medications not discussed elsewhere in this textbook (Table 129.9) will be reviewed. Table 129.10 outlines the agents commonly used to treat ulcers and burns.

ANESTHETICS

Eutectic Mixture of Lidocaine and Prilocaine

Introduction
EMLA® (eutectic mixture of lidocaine and prilocaine) cream is comprised of 2.5% prilocaine and 2.5% lidocaine. With occlusion, these agents can penetrate the keratinized stratum corneum to deliver adequate anesthesia to the skin. The combination mixture offers greater penetration than either drug alone.

Mechanism of action
Lidocaine and prilocaine block nerve impulses and conduction by decreasing the entry of sodium into nerve cells (see Ch. 143).

Dosages
EMLA® is available as a cream and in the form of a disc (which itself provides occlusion). In adults, approximately 5–10 g is applied 1 to 2 hours prior to a procedure under occlusion. The duration of anesthesia is approximately 1 to 2 hours. In children, the dose and area of application should be reduced to avoid methemoglobinemia (Table 129.11).

Side effects
Side effects are generally mild and most commonly consist of application-site blanching (vasoconstriction) or erythema. Less often, urticaria, contact dermatitis (irritant or allergic), petechiae and purpura are observed. Methemoglobinemia may occur when the product is applied in greater than recommended amounts, especially in neonates or infants (see Table 129.3).

Indications
EMLA® is used for pain relief associated with procedures such as venipuncture, debridement, curettage, epilation, circumcision[30], and superficial surgeries (including with lasers). It is also utilized for postherpetic neuralgia and painful ulcers.

Contraindications
Patients at risk for methemoglobinemia should not use EMLA®. This includes children with congenital or idiopathic methemoglobinemia; neonates with a gestational age <37 weeks; and children <12 months of age receiving methemoglobinemia-inducing agents.

Interactions
EMLA® should not be used in children receiving medications associated with drug-induced methemoglobinemia, including acetaminophen, benzocaine, chloroquine, dapsone, nitrofurantoin, nitroglycerin, nitroprusside, phenazopyridine, phenelzine, phenytoin, quinine and sulfonamides. Topical benzoyl peroxide may reduce the efficacy of topical anesthetics, including lidocaine and prilocaine.

TOPICAL MEDICATIONS DISCUSSED IN OTHER CHAPTERS	
Topical medications	**Chapter(s)**
Aluminum chloride	40
Antimicrobials (antibacterials, antifungals, antivirals)	127
Glucocorticosteroids	125
Immunomodulators (e.g. calcineurin inhibitors, imiquimod)	128
Keratolytic agents	56, 57
Retinoids	126
Hydroquinone	65, 66
Monobenzyl ether of hydroquinone	65
Lindane, malathion, pyrethrins, thiabendazole	83
Minoxidil	68
Sensitizers (e.g. squaric acid)	68
Eflornithine	69
Cantharidin	80, 84

Table 129.9 Topical medications discussed in other chapters.

APPLICATION OF EMLA® TO INTACT SKIN IN CHILDREN			
Age and body weight	**Maximum dose (g)**	**Maximum application area (cm²)**	**Maximum application time (h)**
0–3 months or <5 kg	1	10	1
3–12 months and >5 kg	2	20	4
1–6 years and >10 kg	10	100	4
7–12 years and >20 kg	20	200	4

Table 129.11 Application of EMLA® to intact skin in children. EMLA, eutectic mixture of lidocaine and prilocaine.

AGENTS COMMONLY USED FOR EROSIONS, ULCERS AND BURNS		
Topical agent	**Indication**	**Action**
Aqueous silver nitrate	Cauterization of oozing ulcers, reduction of granulation tissue, antiseptic prophylaxis in burns	Coagulation of cellular proteins to form an eschar; bactericidal against Gram-positive and Gram-negative bacteria (including *Pseudomonas aeruginosa* and *Staphylococcus aureus*) and *Candidia albicans*
Silver sulfadiazine	Prevention of infection in second- and third-degree burns	Bactericidal against Gram-positive and Gram-negative bacteria (including *P. aeruginosa* and *S. aureus*) and *C. albicans*
Enzymatic debriding agents (collagenase, papain, fibrinolysin and deoxyribonuclease)	Debridement of burns and ulcers	Selective digestion of necrotic matter

Table 129.10 Agents commonly used for erosions, ulcers and burns. This is in addition to topical antibiotics (Ch. 127) and growth factors (e.g. PDGF; Chs 103 & 105).

Use in pregnancy

EMLA® is pregnancy category B.

Other Anesthetics

Topical lidocaine is available in a liposomal delivery system as LMX™ in concentrations of 4% and 5%; the latter formulation is for anorectal use and both are available over-the-counter (OTC). This preparation does not require occlusion and the recommended application time is 30 minutes. It is comparable in efficacy to EMLA®[31]. Additional topical anesthetics are discussed in Chapter 143.

ANTIMITOTIC AGENTS

Anthralin (Dithranol)

Introduction

Anthralin is a topical antiproliferative agent used in the treatment of psoriasis and alopecia areata. An effective alternative or adjunct to topical corticosteroids, it has largely fallen out of favor secondary to its odor, staining properties and irritant effects, as well as the availability nowadays of other better-tolerated medications. However, anthralin is still used in the inpatient setting and in psoriasis daycare treatment centers as a component of the Ingram regimen, especially outside of the US.

Mechanism of action

The exact mechanism of action is unknown. Anthralin is cytotoxic and inhibits a variety of cellular functions, including mitochondrial respiration and cell growth. In addition, it has been reported to inhibit glycolic enzymes *in vitro*. These effects lead to a reduction in keratinocyte proliferation[32].

Dosages

This topical medication is available as an ointment, paste, cream or stick, with concentrations ranging from 0.1% to 1%. While low concentrations of anthralin can be administered overnight, concentrations of 0.5% or greater are applied once daily for short periods of time ('short contact' therapy). Sequentially, the concentration and duration of application are slowly increased as tolerated, based upon irritation. For example, the first application may consist of 0.5% anthralin applied for 10 minutes, with further advancements in 10-minute increments until 1 hour is reached. A sample protocol for the treatment of alopecia areata is outlined in Table 129.12.

Following treatment, anthralin should be promptly washed off with an acid soap and an emollient should be applied. Anthralin is quite irritating to normal skin. Combination therapy with topical corticosteroids has been reported to reduce irritation without decreasing efficacy[33]. Additionally, application of triethanolamine following short-contact anthralin therapy has been found to inhibit anthralin-induced irritation without altering the therapeutic effect[34].

Side effects

Anthralin use is limited by irritant contact dermatitis (more so of non-involved skin) and non-permanent staining.

Indications

The principal use of anthralin is for the treatment of chronic psoriasis. However, it has also been used to stimulate an inflammatory response and hair regrowth in alopecia areata (see Table 129.12) as well as to treat cutaneous warts.

Contraindications

Anthralin should not be used on irritated or excoriated skin, on mucosa, or in patients with known hypersensitivity to the medication.

Use in pregnancy

Anthralin is pregnancy category C.

Alternatives

Alternative treatments for psoriasis include topical corticosteroids, vitamin D analogues, coal tar, tazarotene, and calcineurin inhibitors (the latter in locations where efficacious, e.g. face, groin).

Coal Tar

Introduction

Coal tar, a crude distillate of heated coal, has long been used for the treatment of dermatologic disorders[35]. There are four types of tar: wood tar, bituminous tar, petroleum tar, and coal tar. Of these, coal tar is most widely used for the treatment of inflammatory dermatoses, in particular psoriasis and less often dermatitis. Despite the availability of newer topical agents, coal tar continues to be a useful treatment for psoriasis in many parts of the world due to its wide availability, low cost, and efficacy.

Mechanism of action

Although the exact mechanism remains elusive, coal tar appears to possess antimicrobial, anti-inflammatory and antipruritic effects. Additionally, it is thought to suppress DNA synthesis, imparting an antiproliferative effect, as evidenced by decreased plaque thickness when applied to psoriatic lesions. Coal tar has also been shown to be photosensitizing, with its effects enhanced by exposure to UV light.

Dosages

Coal tar is available in many forms, including shampoo, solution, gel, lotion, oil, ointment and soap, in concentrations ranging from 0.5% to 10%. Liquor carbons detergens (LCD) is a distillate of crude coal tar and concentrations of 3–10% are usually prescribed. Coal tar preparations are used in conjunction with UVB irradiation in the Goeckerman regimen.

Side effects

Drawbacks of tar include its offensive odor, messiness, and staining properties. Additionally, tar may cause erythema, irritant contact dermatitis, tar folliculitis, pustules within plaques of psoriasis, and 'tar smarts' (following UVA irradiation). Crude coal tar preparations are generally not used in flexural areas, in order to avoid irritation, but LCD (e.g. 5% cream) is usually well tolerated. An increased risk of cutaneous carcinomas related to tar use has not been observed in studies in which coal tar was used to treat psoriasis[36,37]. Oftentimes, salicylic acid is added to coal tar preparations, and when the combination is applied to large surface areas, the same precautions apply as for salicylic acid alone.

Indications

Coal tar preparations are indicated for the treatment of psoriasis, seborrheic dermatitis, dandruff, pruritus, and various forms of dermatitis.

SAMPLE PROTOCOL FOR SHORT-CONTACT ANTHRALIN THERAPY FOR ALOPECIA AREATA

- Anthralin 0.5% cream is applied sparingly to all affected areas of the scalp daily, followed by washing with shampoo/acid soap and water
- An initial application time of 10 minutes is increased in 10-minute increments every 4–5 days until slight irritation (e.g. erythema, scaling, pruritus) occurs
- If excessive irritation develops, treatment is withheld for several days and resumed at the last tolerated application time
- If there is no irritation with a 60-minute contact time, 1% anthralin is applied for 10 minutes and application times increased as above
- If there is no irritation with 1% anthralin applied for 60 minutes, contact the doctor's office regarding the possibility of overnight application
- Initial responses are typically seen within 12 weeks; cosmetically acceptable responses require a mean of 24 weeks

Additional information

- Brownish staining of treated areas of the scalp and hair is expected
- To prevent staining of clothing, bedding and furniture, patients should wash their hands thoroughly after applying anthralin and avoid touching fabrics with their scalp until it has been washed off (see above)
- Avoid getting anthralin into the eyes; do not apply to eyelids or eyelashes
- Special care should be taken in sensitive areas (areas of scalp near the ears, eyebrows)

Table 129.12 Sample protocol for the use of anthralin to treat alopecia areata. Courtesy of Julie V Schaffer MD and Jean L Bolognia MD.

Use in pregnancy

Coal tar is pregnancy category C.

Alternatives

Alternative treatments for psoriasis include topical corticosteroids, vitamin D analogues, tazarotene, anthralin, and calcineurin inhibitors (the latter in locations where efficacious, e.g. face, groin).

Azelaic Acid

Introduction

Azelaic acid, a naturally occurring dicarboxylic acid, is used in the treatment of rosacea and acne vulgaris (the latter represents an off-label indication). Despite scattered reports of its use in lentigo maligna[38], azelaic acid is more commonly used off-label for postinflammatory hyperpigmentation and melasma.

Mechanism of action

Azelaic acid has been reported to inhibit the production of free radical oxygen by neutrophils[39]. This results in a reduction of oxidative tissue injury at sites of inflammation as well as decreased melanin formation. Studies have also demonstrated selective cytotoxic and antiproliferative effects on hyperactive and abnormally proliferating melanocytes, with little effect on normal melanocytes[38,40]. Azelaic acid 20% cream has been shown to be equally efficacious as hydroquinone 4% in the treatment of melasma.

Furthermore, azelaic acid demonstrates antimicrobial activity against *P. acnes* and *Staphylococcus epidermidis*. To date, there have been no reports of bacterial resistance. Additionally, this medication possesses moderate anti-comedogenic properties via modification of epidermal keratinization. Azelaic acid is often used in combination with other topical agents such as benzoyl peroxide, clindamycin, erythromycin, or a topical retinoid. Azelaic acid 15% gel has been shown to be more effective than metronidazole 0.75% cream in the treatment of rosacea[41].

Dosages

Azelaic acid, available in a 20% cream and 15% gel, is applied twice daily.

Side effects

Azelaic acid may cause mild (i.e. peeling, dryness, erythema) to moderate irritant contact dermatitis, and seborrhea; side effects may subside after 2 to 4 weeks of treatment.

Indications

Azelaic acid is used to treat rosacea, mild to moderate acne, melasma and postinflammatory hyperpigmentation.

Use in pregnancy

Azelaic acid is pregnancy category B.

Alternatives

Alternative treatments for rosacea and acne include topical metronidazole, antibiotics (including sodium sulfacetamide), benzoyl peroxide, sulfur, retinoids and salicylic acid, and for postinflammatory hyperpigmentation and melasma, hydroquinone.

Fluorouracil

Introduction

Topical 5-fluorouracil (5-FU) is a chemotherapeutic agent that has been used successfully in the treatment of actinic keratoses (AKs). In comparison to ablative treatments, 5-FU may reduce the risk of pain, scarring and infection. This medication is advantageous in treating large-sized AKs, numerous AKs within a circumscribed area, and areas of severe actinic damage without clinically detectable lesions. In patients with background facial erythema or pigment, topical 5-FU does not result in the circular hypopigmented macules that are often seen following liquid nitrogen therapy. Also, if the cream is applied beyond the obvious clinical margin of the AKs, there is less of a chance of lateral residual disease.

Mechanism of action

5-FU is a pyrimidine antimetabolite that inhibits thymidylate synthetase, a critical enzyme in DNA synthesis. This prevents cellular proliferation and results in cell death. The effects are most pronounced in rapidly dividing cells.

Indications

5-FU is used in the treatment of AKs. It is much less effective in treating hypertrophic AKs, due to decreased percutaneous absorption resulting from the thickened stratum corneum. In addition, it is sometimes used in the treatment of psoriasis (e.g. involving the nails) and condyloma acuminata, as well as Bowen's disease and extramammary Paget's disease limited to the epidermis[42].

Dosages

This medication is available as a cream (0.5–5%) and solution (2–5%). It is applied once or twice daily for 2 to 3 weeks, depending upon the formulation. Application of 5-FU results in inflammation and subsequent destruction of lesions. During treatment, the skin progresses through escalating stages of erythema then crusting (Fig. 129.4) prior to re-epithelialization, which may take 2 to 4 weeks. While early studies found that inflammation could be suppressed without loss of efficacy, it has recently been suggested that this inflammation is likely required to achieve a therapeutic effect[43]. Topical corticosteroids may be applied subsequent to 5-FU application (once peak inflammation has been reached) in order to reduce inflammation more rapidly. Investigations involving prolonged courses of less frequent application are currently underway, as are studies assessing the effect of suppressing inflammation.

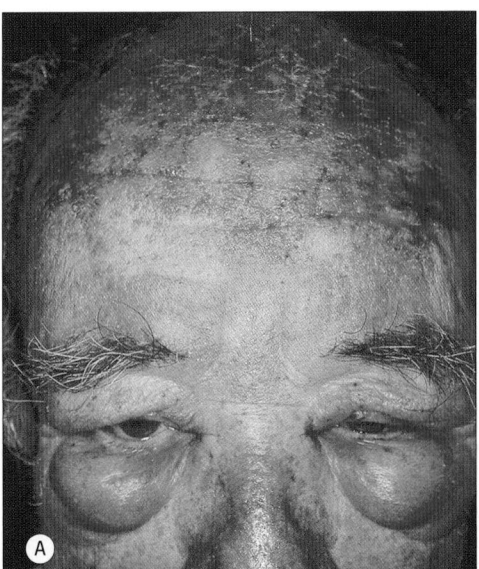

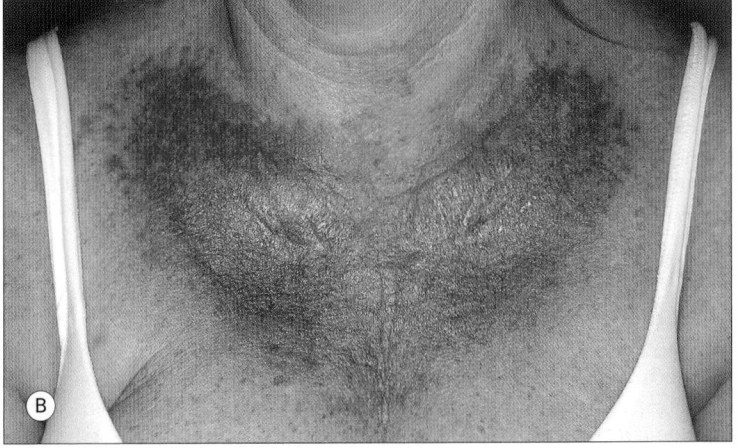

Fig. 129.4 Reactions to topical 5-fluorouracil.
A Note the erythema and crusting in areas of solar damage, as well as periorbital edema.
B Large red–purple patches at sites of application in a patient with severe photodamage.
B, Courtesy of Jean L Bolognia MD.

Side effects

Side effects include application-site pain, burning and swelling, which may interfere with compliance. Patients should be warned to discontinue therapy once significant erythema has occurred. On the dorsal hands, extensor forearms and shins, pretreatment with a topical retinoid for several weeks prior to 5-FU application can improve efficacy.

Contraindications

Use is contraindicated in those with hypersensitivity to 5-FU or dihydropyrimidine dehydrogenase deficiency, as well as during pregnancy and lactation.

Use in pregnancy

5-FU is potentially teratogenic and therefore contraindicated during pregnancy and lactation. It is pregnancy category X.

Alternatives

Other therapies for AKs include imiquimod, diclofenac, cryosurgery, curettage, and other destructive modalities such as photodynamic therapy (e.g. topical aminolevulinic acid plus blue light illumination).

Mechlorethamine Hydrochloride

Introduction

Mechlorethamine HCl (topical nitrogen mustard) is one of the primary treatments for patients with limited or generalized patch- and/or plaque-stage mycosis fungoides.

Mechanism of action

The mechanism of action of topical nitrogen mustard remains speculative. Systemically, mechlorethamine acts as an alkylating agent with a cytotoxic effect on rapidly dividing cells. The therapeutic effects of topical nitrogen mustard have also been postulated to be the result of immune mechanisms.

Dosages

Mechlorethamine HCl is available as an aqueous solution or an anhydrous ointment-based preparation in concentrations of 0.01–0.04%. It is applied daily to the total skin surface (excluding genitals and sparingly to intertriginous areas) until clearance is achieved. Once remission is reached, maintenance therapy may continue for 6 months or longer.

Side effects

Mechlorethamine HCl may cause allergic or irritant contact dermatitis in approximately 50% of patients and urticarial or anaphylactoid reactions in 5–10%. Irritant reactions may improve with continued use or with concurrent administration of topical corticosteroids. The ointment preparation is associated with a lower incidence of hypersensitivity reactions compared to the aqueous formulation.

Indications

Mechlorethamine HCl is used for the treatment of limited or generalized patch- and/or plaque-stage mycosis fungoides.

Use in pregnancy

Mechlorethamine HCl is contraindicated during pregnancy (category D) and lactation.

Alternatives

Other therapies for limited or generalized patch- and/or plaque-stage mycosis fungoides include topical corticosteroids, carmustine and bexarotene, narrowband UVB, PUVA, total skin electron beam therapy, oral bexarotene, and systemic interferon.

Carmustine

Introduction

Carmustine – 1,3-bis(2-chloroethyl)-1-nitrosurea (BCNU) – is a topical chemotherapeutic agent used to treat patch- or plaque-stage mycosis fungoides. It may be used as an alternative therapy in those who develop contact dermatitis to topical mechlorethamine HCl. However, because of the potential for hematologic complications due to systemic absorption, it is prescribed less often than topical nitrogen mustard.

Mechanism of action

Carmustine is a nitrosourea alkylating agent with cytotoxic effects.

Dosages

Carmustine may be formulated as an aqueous solution or an ointment. A 0.2% alcoholic solution is made by injecting 5 ml of 95% ethanol into a vial containing 100 mg of BCNU; the 5 ml are then withdrawn and diluted to 50 ml with 95% ethanol[43a]. An ointment may be prepared by mixing the alcohol solution with white petrolatum to a desired concentration of 10 mg/100 g petrolatum. Plastic gloves, gauze pads or a soft brush should be used for daily application to involved areas only. Alternatively, in patients with very limited disease, the undiluted alcohol solution may be applied directly to lesions with a cotton-tipped applicator. This may result in an erythematous reaction which generally subsides in a few weeks.

Side effects

Carmustine may cause erythema, bullae, irritant or allergic contact dermatitis, and permanent telangiectasia in sites of application. Although bone marrow suppression is an uncommon side effect, complete blood counts should be monitored during carmustine treatment.

Indications

Topical carmustine is used in the treatment of limited or generalized patch- and/or plaque-stage mycosis fungoides.

Use in pregnancy

Carmustine is contraindicated during pregnancy (category D) and lactation.

Alternatives

Other therapies for limited or generalized patch- and/or plaque-stage mycosis fungoides include topical mechlorethamine HCl as well as therapies listed above (see Mechlorethamine, Alternatives).

Podophyllin and Podophyllotoxin

Introduction

Podophyllin is a plant resin derived from *Podophyllum peltatum* or *P. emodi*. Podophyllin resin is not standardized and therefore varies in composition by batch. It is recommended that podophyllin administration be performed under medical supervision, given its potential for systemic side effects as well as its variability in composition.

Podophyllotoxin is a standardized compound containing one of the active ingredients of podophyllin. In comparison to podophyllin, it lacks mutagenic potential, is effective in lower concentrations, and has lower potential for systemic toxicity. Furthermore, podophyllotoxin may be safely administered by the patient.

Mechanism of action

Podophyllin and podophyllotoxin are antiproliferative agents that arrest epithelial cell mitosis during metaphase and lead to tissue necrosis.

Dosages

Podophyllin is available as a 10–25% solution that is applied sparingly by the physician to lesions once a week; a common vehicle is tincture benzoin. At 1 to 4 hours after application, the lesion should be washed with soap and water. Duration of treatment usually ranges from 4 to 6 weeks.

Podophyllotoxin is available as a 0.5% solution, 0.5% gel, and 0.15% cream. It may be applied by the patient to lesions twice daily for three consecutive days alternating with four days without therapy. Lesions should not be rinsed after application. Duration of therapy is 4 to 6 weeks.

Side effects

Side effects of both podophyllin and podophyllotoxin include local irritation and pruritus. Application of petrolatum to normal surrounding skin can reduce this side effect. Because of the high percutaneous absorption of podophyllin, the potential for systemic toxicity exists when large amounts are applied, manifesting as nausea, vomiting, mental status changes, peripheral neuropathy, thrombocytopenia, leukopenia and renal failure.

Indications
Podophyllin and podophyllotoxin are indicated in the treatment of anogenital condyloma acuminata[44].

Contraindications
Podophyllin is teratogenic and therefore contraindicated in pregnancy. It also has mutagenic potential, which has been implicated in carcinogenesis. In general, podophyllin should not be applied to cervical, urethral or oral warts, and it should not be used in either pregnant or lactating women or children.

Use in pregnancy
Podophyllin and podophyllotoxin are pregnancy category X, and are therefore contraindicated in pregnancy.

Alternatives
Other therapies for condyloma acuminata include cryosurgery and other destructive modalities, imiquimod, topical 5-fluorouracil, and trichloroacetic acid.

ANTIPRURITIC THERAPY

Doxepin

Introduction
Doxepin is a topical tricyclic antidepressant used for the relief of pruritus and pain.

Mechanism of action
Doxepin is a topical antihistamine with anticholinergic properties. The exact mechanism of its antipruritic and analgesic activity is unknown. However, doxepin is known to antagonize both H_1 and H_2 histamine receptors.

Indications
Doxepin is indicated for the management of moderate pruritus in patients with atopic dermatitis or lichen simplex chronicus[45]. It is also used to treat the pruritus associated with other forms of dermatitis as well as neuropathic pain (sometimes in combination with topical capsaicin). In a large case series, doxepin oral rinse was reported to reduce oral mucosal pain due to cancer or its treatment.

Dosages
A 5% doxepin hydrochloride cream is commercially available. It may be applied as a thin film four times a day and is used for short-term (less than 8 days) relief of pruritus.

Side effects
Topical doxepin can cause localized burning, irritation, and allergic contact dermatitis. In patients with allergic contact dermatitis, subsequent administration of oral doxepin can lead to systemic contact dermatitis. Topical doxepin may cause drowsiness (>20% of patients) and even marked sedation due to systemic absorption of the active drug.

Contraindications
Topical doxepin is contraindicated in patients with untreated narrow angle glaucoma, a tendency to urinary retention, and a known sensitivity to any of its components, in addition to those receiving monoamine oxidase (MAO) inhibitors.

Use in pregnancy
Doxepin is pregnancy category B. It is not recommended for use during lactation.

Capsaicin

Introduction
Capsaicin, a natural constituent of red chili peppers, acts as an antipruritic and analgesic by desensitizing nerve endings.

Mechanism of action
Capsaicin exerts its pharmacologic effects on the peripheral sensory nervous system by depleting substance P from C fibers (via the release of substance P; see Ch. 6). Substance P mediates pain impulses from peripheral sensory neurons to the CNS. With repeated capsaicin use, transmission of sensations of heat, pain and itch is prevented. The therapeutic effect is observed approximately 1 week after initiation of treatment.

Indications
The dermatologic uses of capsaicin include treatment of intractable localized pruritus (e.g. prurigo nodularis, brachioradial pruritus), uremic pruritus, and superficial pain secondary to postherpetic neuralgia and diabetic neuropathy[46,47]. In double-blind vehicle/placebo-controlled studies, capsaicin was shown to be effective in the treatment of notalgia paresthetica, pruritic psoriasis and pruritus ani.

Dosages
Capsaicin is available as a cream, gel, lotion, patch and stick, with concentrations ranging from 0.025% to 0.75%. It is applied in a consistent manner to the affected area three to four times per day.

Side effects
Common side effects of capsaicin include transient application-site itching, burning and erythema, which may diminish with frequent use.

Use in pregnancy
Capsaicin is pregnancy category C.

Other Antipruritic Agents

Pramoxine (1%) is a topical anesthetic that is used in the treatment of pruritus ani and cutaneous disorders associated with burning and pruritus (e.g. notalgia paresthetica). Within a few minutes of application, partial anesthesia is attained. Duration of the therapeutic effect is approximately 2–4 hours[2]. Pramoxine is available as a gel, or in combination with 0.5% to 2.5% hydrocortisone as a lotion, cream or ointment. A foam preparation with 1% hydrocortisone is also available. Pramoxine has very low sensitizing potential, which offers an advantage over other topical anesthetics.

Camphor (0.25–0.5%) is a ketone with a local anesthetic effect that may relieve milder degrees of pruritus or burning. *Phenol*, an ingredient found in throat sprays and lozenges, imparts its antipruritic effects as a result of its anesthetic action. It should not be used in pregnant women or infants less than 6 months of age. Another agent that may provide some relief is *menthol* (0.25–0.5%), an alcohol compound derived from mint, which imparts a cooling effect as a result of its low boiling point (see Ch. 6). These agents may serve as counter irritants.

Emollients are agents that also help to relieve pruritus, especially if the latter is related to xerosis or asteatotic eczema. It is recommended that emollients be applied after bathing. The most effective emollients are water-free ointments and water-in-oil emulsions and creams (see Table 129.7). Preparations containing urea (10–20%) and lactic acid (5–12%) are also used to reduce the pruritus associated with xerosis, but burning is a potential side effect with topical lactic acid products, especially if any fissures or erosions are present.

SULFUR

Introduction
Sulfur, a yellow, non-metallic element, has long been employed (alone or in combination with sodium sulfacetamide or salicylic acid) as a safe and effective alternative in the treatment of a number of dermatologic conditions. An offensive odor that resembles rotten eggs (due to H_2S) has limited its use in the absence of masking fragrances.

Mechanism of action

Sulfur has antibacterial, antifungal and keratolytic properties. Its exact mechanism of action is unknown. It reduces itching and scaling of seborrheic dermatitis and dandruff. In addition, it acts as an antifungal against *Malassezia* yeasts.

Dosages

Sulfur can be compounded in a range of concentrations from 2% to 10%. In commercially available products, sulfur is usually combined with a second agent, e.g. 2% sulfur plus 2% salicylic acid in shampoos or 5% sulfur plus 10% sodium sulfacetamide in a cream, suspension or gel formulation. The former is used to treat dandruff and seborrheic dermatitis, while the latter is used for rosacea, acne and seborrheic dermatitis. A 20% sodium thiosulfate solution may be applied to treat pityriasis versicolor[48].

Side effects

Side effects are generally mild and include dryness and itching. Approximately 1% of topically applied sulfur is systemically absorbed and a fatal outcome has been reported in infants after extensive application for scabies.

Indications

Sulfur is used in the treatment of seborrheic dermatitis, rosacea, acne, tinea versicolor and scabies.

Contraindications

Topical sulfur is contraindicated in patients with a sensitivity to sulfur.

Use in pregnancy

Topical sulfur (5–10%) has been used to treat scabies in pregnant and lactating women but precise safety data are lacking.

Alternatives

For seborrheic dermatitis, topical corticosteroids and imidazoles are alternative medications, and for rosacea, topical azelaic acid and all the alternatives listed in the section on azelaic acid (see above).

SALICYLIC ACID

Introduction

Salicylic acid is a keratolytic agent with a slight anti-inflammatory effect, used in the treatment of acne, warts, psoriasis and seborrheic dermatitis. Lower concentrations (1–5%) are often used for scaling dermatoses of glabrous skin, while higher concentration may be used for scalp or palmoplantar skin. In concentrations of 10–40%, salicylic acid is used for the treatment of corns, calluses, warts and local hyperkeratosis.

Mechanism of action

The keratolytic effect of salicylic acid is a result of its inhibition of cholesterol sulfotransferase, which leads to a decrease in cholesterol sulfate formation within keratinocytes. The solubilization of intracellular 'cement' and subsequent decreased cell-to-cell adhesion enhances the shedding of corneocytes. Of note, this solubilizing effect may increase the penetration of other topical agents. Additionally, as a competitive inhibitor of pantothenic acid, salicylic acid is bacteriostatic and fungistatic. Furthermore, it has a slight anti-inflammatory effect.

Dosages

Commercially, salicylic acid is available in concentrations ranging from 0.5% to 40%; the various formulations include liquids, gels, creams, ointments, shampoos, soaps, patches, pads, foams and plasters. When compounding a topical preparation, the clinician can choose a specific concentration.

Side effects

Depending upon the site and concentration, salicylic acid can cause irritation, peeling and even erosions. Systemic intoxication may result from extensive application, particularly in newborns and infants, resulting in neurologic and gastrointestinal toxicity.

Indications

Salicylic acid is used for the treatment of seborrheic dermatitis, superficial fungal infections, psoriasis, acne, warts, ichthyoses, keratodermas and other scaling dermatoses. It is also used as a peeling agent for disorders such as melasma (see Ch. 153).

Use in pregnancy

Salicylic acid is pregnancy category C and premature closure of the ductus arteriosus in the fetus (with subsequent pulmonary hypertension in newborns) has been reported when used in late in pregnancy.

Alternatives

Depending upon the disorder, alternatives include topical corticosteroids, tar or vitamin D derivatives (inflammatory dermatoses), lactic or glycolic acid or urea (hyperkeratosis), retinoids or topical antibiotics (acne), and antifungals.

VITAMIN D ANALOGUES

Key features

- Vitamin D analogues inhibit proliferation and promote differentiation of keratinocytes
- They are as efficacious as mid-potency topical corticosteroids for the treatment of psoriasis and may be safely used on a long-term basis
- They are efficacious as monotherapy as well as in combination with other treatments for psoriasis (e.g. topical corticosteroids, phototherapy, acitretin)

Introduction

The therapeutic potential of vitamin D as a treatment for psoriasis was first discovered when a patient receiving systemic vitamin D for osteoporosis was observed to have improvement of severe psoriasis[49]. Calcitriol, the active form of vitamin D_3 (1,25-dihydroxyvitamin D_3 [1,25(OH)$_2$D$_3$]; Fig. 129.5), was found to inhibit proliferation and promote differentiation of keratinocytes[50], in addition to regulating calcium absorption and bone mineralization.

The therapeutic use of calcitriol is limited, however, by its effects on calcium homeostasis. In order to reduce the risk of hypercalcemia and hypercalciuria, vitamin D_3 analogues were developed for clinical use. Table 129.13 lists the generic and trade names of commercially available vitamin D_3 analogues.

Mechanism of action

Vitamin D exerts its effects via interaction with vitamin D receptors on target cells, including keratinocytes, Langerhans cells, melanocytes, fibroblasts, endothelial cells, monocytes and T cells. In the setting of psoriasis, vitamin D has an antiproliferative effect on hyperplastic psoriatic keratinocytes.

CALCITRIOL (1,25-DIHYDROXYVITAMIN D$_3$) THE ACTIVE FORM OF VITAMIN D$_3$

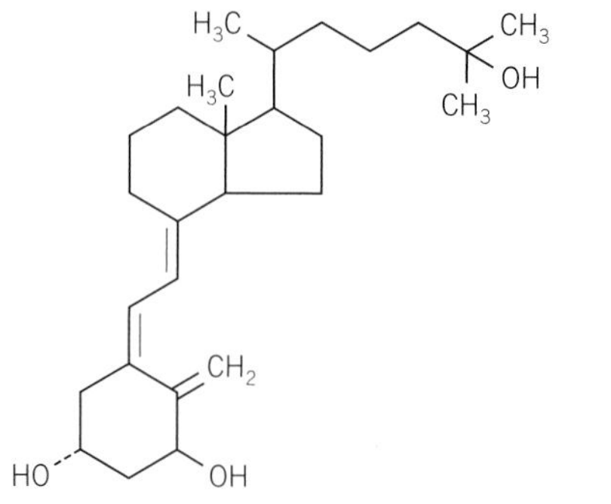

Fig. 129.5 Calcitriol (1,25-dihydroxyvitamin D$_3$), the active form of vitamin D$_3$.

RECOMMENDED MAXIMUM DOSE PER WEEK OF VITAMIN D₃ AND ITS ANALOGUES		
Generic name	Trade names®	Maximum dose per week
Calcipotriene (calcipotriol)	Dovonex Daivonex Psorcutan	100 g of 50 µg/g
Calcipotriene/betamethasone dipropionate	Daivobet Dovobet Taclonex	Same as above
Calcitriol [1,25(OH)₂D₃]	Silkis	30 g
Maxacalcitol	Oxarol	70 g
Tacalcitol [1,24(OH)₂D₃]	Bonalfa Apsor Vellutan Curatoderm	35 g

Table 129.13 **Recommended maximum dose per week of topical vitamin D₃ and its analogues.** Calcipotriene is the US Adopted Name (USAN) and calcipotriol is the International Nonproprietary Name (INN).

Additionally, vitamin D possesses immunomodulatory activities. Studies have shown increased levels of interleukin (IL)-10 (an anti-inflammatory and immunosuppressive cytokine) and decreased levels of IL-8 (a proinflammatory chemokine) in calcipotriene-treated psoriatic plaques[51]. IL-8 promotes proliferation of keratinocytes and is found in high levels in lesions of psoriasis. Its reduction by calcipotriene may be another explanation for the therapeutic action of calcipotriene in psoriasis.

Calcitriol

Calcitriol [1,25(OH)₂D₃], the active form of vitamin D₃, inhibits proliferation and induces terminal differentiation of keratinocytes. Additionally, it has immunomodulatory effects via the inhibition of specific interleukins (see above). Calcitriol affects calcium metabolism by releasing calcium from bone, decreasing parathyroid hormone, increasing tubular resorption of calcium in the kidney, and stimulating calcium transport in the intestines. Its actions may result in hypercalcemia and hypercalciuria if excessive amounts are applied.

Calcipotriene (calcipotriol)

Calcipotriene is the only vitamin D analogue available in the US. It is a synthetic vitamin D₃ derivative with similar affinity for vitamin D receptors[52] and similar therapeutic effects as 1,25(OH)₂D₃[50]. Its molecular structure differs from 1,25(OH)₂D₃ in that it contains a double bond and a ring structure in its side chain (Fig. 129.6). This difference enables it to be metabolized much more rapidly, and as a result, calcipotriene was shown in animal studies to be approximately 100 to 200 times less potent than 1,25(OH)₂D₃ in producing hypercalcemia and hypercalciuria[52]. Nevertheless, over-application can result in hypercalcemia and hypercalciuria.

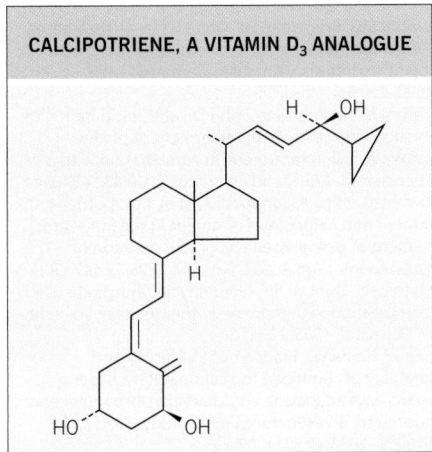

CALCIPOTRIENE, A VITAMIN D₃ ANALOGUE

Fig. 129.6 **Calcipotriene (calcipotriol), a vitamin D₃ analogue.**

Tacalcitol

Tacalcitol [1,24(OH)₂D₃] is similar to 1,25(OH)₂D₃ with regard to its affinity for vitamin D receptors and therapeutic effects. This analogue has been shown to induce hypercalcemia at comparable doses to 1,25(OH)₂D₃, demonstrating less selectivity than calcipotriene in its effect on calcium metabolism. Immunomodulatory actions include inhibition of chemokine production by epidermal keratinocytes[53].

Maxacalcitol

Maxacalcitol (1α,25-dihydroxy-22-oxacalcitriol) has been shown to be approximately 10 times more potent than calcitriol in inhibiting keratinocyte proliferation and exhibits a similar log difference in promoting differentiation when compared to calcipotriene and tacalcitol[54]. Additionally, maxacalcitol is approximately 60 times less calcemic than calcipotriene.

Clinical effects
Calcipotriene (calcipotriol)

Calcipotriene is available as a cream, ointment and solution for the treatment of mild to moderate psoriasis. Studies have revealed that the optimal concentration is 50 µg/g applied twice daily[55,56]. Although less efficacious than twice-daily therapy, once-daily treatment was shown to be more efficacious than placebo[57,58]. This option may increase compliance in patients who experience skin irritation with calcipotriene application. Depending upon the study and the formulation, topical calcipotriene has been found to be more, equally, or less effective (ointment, cream, or solution, respectively) than topical betamethasone 17-valerate.

Although studies have demonstrated the safety and efficacy of twice-daily calcipotriene ointment in the treatment of intertriginous psoriasis[59], irritation can be a problem. Consideration should be given to once-daily application or the use of the cream formulation in these areas.

As maintenance therapy, calcipotriene has been shown to be safe and effective for the long-term treatment of psoriasis. Sustained disease improvement was observed with the use of calcipotriene ointment (50 µg/g) twice daily for 1 year, without an increase in mean serum calcium levels[60].

For very thick plaques, occlusion may increase the therapeutic response to calcipotriene[61]. However, occlusion should be limited to small areas of psoriasis to avoid systemic absorption.

Tacalcitol and maxacalcitol

The other vitamin D analogues, tacalcitol and maxacalcitol, have not yet been studied in great detail. In a double-blind study (n = 63), tacalcitol ointment (4 µg/g) was determined to be as effective as 0.1% betamethasone valerate ointment[62]. Other studies have demonstrated that tacalcitol ointment (2 µg/g) twice daily is as effective as hydrocortisone butyrate and slightly less effective than betamethasone valerate. In a study examining long-term usage, daily application of tacalcitol ointment (4 µg/g) was found to be safe and effective in the treatment of psoriasis, for up to 18 months.

In a comparison of various concentrations of once-daily maxacalcitol ointment (6, 12.5, 25 and 50 µg/g) with placebo, as well as with once-daily calcipotriene ointment (50 µg/g), for a period of 8 weeks, all concentrations of maxacalcitol were more effective than placebo, with the greatest effect reported for maxacalcitol 25 µg/g[54]. Additionally, 55% of patients treated with maxacalcitol ointment (25 µg/g) showed marked improvement or clearance of psoriasis, compared with 46% of patients treated with calcipotriene.

Side effects, tolerability and safety

The main side effect is application-site burning, stinging and irritation. Irritation may be a greater problem in facial and intertriginous regions. However, unlike topical corticosteroids, calcipotriene use does not result in atrophic changes.

Studies have shown that application of up to 100 g per week of calcipotriol ointment (50 µg/g) had no effect on calcium and bone metabolism[63]. It is therefore recommended that the weekly amount of topical calcipotriene (50 µg/g) be kept below 100 g[64]. If weekly amounts exceed 100 g, serum parathyroid hormone levels should be monitored. Of note, patients with renal disease may be at risk for developing hypercalcemia when applying less than 100 g per week.

Calcipotriene (50 µg/g) ointment applied twice daily has been shown to be safe and effective for the treatment of psoriasis in children[65,66].

Use in pregnancy

Calcipotriene is pregnancy category C.

Combination therapy

Corticosteroids and calcipotriene

When calcipotriene is used in conjunction with topical corticosteroids, increased clinical response and tolerance has been demonstrated (Table 129.14). That is, the combination of calcipotriene and corticosteroids reduced the risks associated with long-term use of topical corticosteroids, including atrophy and rebound, as well as the irritation associated with calcipotriene.

In a study by Lebwohl et al.[10], a regimen of calcipotriene ointment applied in the morning with halobetasol applied at night was found to be more efficacious and produced fewer cutaneous side effects than either agent alone; similar results have been observed with calcipotriene cream[67]. Ruzicka & Lorenz[73] demonstrated that following 2 weeks of calcipotriene monotherapy, combination therapy consisting of calcipotriene plus betamethasone valerate led to an additive clinical effect with reduction in both psoriatic lesions and local irritation (when compared to continuation of calcipotriene alone).

The combination of corticosteroids with calcipotriene has also resulted in an increase in remission time. When weekday calcipotriene was added to weekend-only superpotent topical corticosteroids (sometimes referred to as pulse therapy), 76% of the patients maintained a remission for 6 months, compared to 40% receiving weekend corticosteroids and placebo during the week[74].

Formulations containing a fixed combination of calcipotriene (50µg/g) and betamethasone 17-valerate 0.1% ointment have demonstrated greater efficacy and a more rapid onset of action (compared to either medication alone) in a short-term (4-week) study[75]. Skin irritation associated with calcipotriene appeared to be minimized by the anti-inflammatory effects of the corticosteroid. However, caution should be exercised with prolonged use or with use in intertriginous zones, given the potential for corticosteroid-related side effects.

Phototherapy and calcipotriene

The combination of calcipotriene and phototherapy has been shown to be beneficial in the treatment of psoriasis. Molin[68] demonstrated that the addition of calcipotriene twice daily to UVB phototherapy three times a week enhanced therapeutic effects without affecting safety or tolerability (see Table 129.14). Studies combining calcipotriene with PUVA also demonstrated increased efficacy when compared to PUVA alone[69]. This may serve to decrease total cumulative UVA exposure required for clearance of psoriasis, thereby reducing the risk of developing cutaneous malignancies. It should be noted that when employing these combination regimens, calcipotriene should be applied after phototherapy. Lebwohl et al.[76] demonstrated that more than 90% of calcitriol

COMBINATION STUDIES WITH CALCIPOTRIENE (CALCIPOTRIOL)		
Calcipotriene	**Comparison**	**Outcome**
Ointment 50 µg/g[10]	Ointment 50 µg/g + halobetasol	Calcipotriene + corticosteroid equal to or better than monotherapy with either agent
Cream 50 µg/g[67]	Cream 50 µg/g + clobetasone 17-butyrate cream 0.5 mg/g	Calcipotriol + corticosteroid equal to or better than calcipotriol monotherapy
Ointment 50 µg/g[68]	Ointment 50 µg/g + UVB phototherapy	Calcipotriol + UVB better than calcipotriol monotherapy
Ointment 50 µg/g + PUVA[69]	PUVA	Reduction in PUVA dose with combination therapy
Ointment 50 µg/g + cyclosporine (CSA) 2 mg/kg/day[70] Ointment 50 µg/g + CSA 4.5 mg/kg/day[71]	Placebo + CSA (2 mg/kg/day; 4.5 mg/kg/day)	Calcipotriol + CSA better than placebo + CSA
Ointment 50 µg/g + acitretin 10–20 mg/day[72]	Placebo + acitretin (similar dosages)	Calcipotriol + acitretin better than placebo + acitretin and an acitretin-sparing effect

Table 129.14 Combination studies with calcipotriene (calcipotriol). Calcipotriene is the US Adopted Name (USAN) and calcipotriol is the International Nonproprietary Name (INN).

3 µg/g ointment is degraded upon exposure to UVA, broadband UVB or narrowband UVB. Additionally, UVA light has been shown to degrade calcipotriene[77].

Systemic agents and calcipotriene

The combination of topical calcipotriene and oral acitretin has been shown to enhance the clinical response in patients with psoriasis, as compared to acitretin alone (see Table 129.14)[72]. Furthermore, clearance or improvement was attained with a significantly lower cumulative dose of acitretin, offering a reduction in the dose-dependent side effects of acitretin.

Cyclosporine is another systemic agent successfully used in combination with calcipotriene in the treatment of psoriasis. The combination of oral cyclosporine plus topical calcipotriene has been studied in an attempt to reduce the effective dose of cyclosporine and, consequently, the associated side effects. Studies using a combination of low-dose cyclosporine (2 mg/kg/day) and twice-daily calcipotriene showed enhanced efficacy when compared to cyclosporine and placebo[70]. Furthermore, the combination of cyclosporine (4.5 mg/kg/day) and calcipotriene ointment twice daily was more effective than cyclosporine alone[71].

REFERENCES

1. Feldman RJ, Maibach HI. Regional variation in percutaneous penetration of ^{14}C cortisol in man. J Invest Dermatol. 1967;48:181–3.
2. Arndt KA, Bowers KE. Manual of Dermatologic Therapeutics, 6th edn. Philadelphia: Lippincott Williams & Wilkins, 2002:279.
3. Long CC, Finlay AY. The finger-tip unit – a new practical measure. Clin Exp Dermatol. 1991;16:444–7.
4. Long CC, Finlay AY, Averill RW. The rule of hand: 4 hand areas + 2 FTU + 1g. Arch Dermatol. 1992;128:1129–30.
5. Long CC, Mills CM, Finlay AY. A practical guide to topical therapy in children. Br J Dermatol. 1998; 138:293–6.
6. Menter MA, See JA, Amend WJ, et al. Proceedings of the Psoriasis Combination and Rotation Therapy Conference. Deer Valley, Utah, Oct. 7-9, 1994. J Am Acad Dermatol. 1996;34:315–21.
7. Lebwohl M, Menter A, Koo J, et al. Combination therapy to treat moderate to severe psoriasis. J Am Acad Dermatol. 2004;50:416–30.

8. Norris DA. Mechanisms of action of topical therapies and the rationale for combination therapy. J Am Acad Dermatol. 2005;53:S17–25.
9. Del Rosso J, Friedlander SF. Corticosteroids: options in the era of steroid-sparing therapy. J Am Acad Dermatol. 2005;53:S50–8.
10. Lebwohl M, Siskin S, Epinette W, et al. A multicenter trial of calcipotriene ointment and halobetasol ointment compared with either agent alone for the treatment of psoriasis. J Am Acad Dermatol. 1996;35:268–9.
11. Torok HM, Maas-Irsinger R, Slayton RM. Clocortolone pivalate cream 0.1% used concomitantly with tacrolimus ointment 0.1% in atopic dermatitis. Cutis. 2003;72:161–6.
12. Kragballe K, Noerrelund KL, Lui H, et al. Efficacy of once-daily treatment regimens with calcipotriol/betamethasone dipropionate ointment and calcipotriol ointment in psoriasis vulgaris. Br J Dermatol. 2004;150:1167–73.

13. Lebwohl MG, Breneman DL, Goffe BS, et al. Tazarotene 0.1% gel plus corticosteroid cream in the treatment of plaque psoriasis. J Am Acad Dermatol. 1998; 39:590–6.
14. Lebwohl M. Strategies to optimize efficacy, duration of remission, and safety in the treatment of plaque psoriasis by using tazarotene in combination with a corticosteroid. J Am Acad Dermatol. 2000;43:S43–6.
15. Lebwohl M, Yoles A, Lombardi K, et al. Calcipotriene ointment and halobetasol ointment in the long-term treatment of psoriasis: effects on the duration of improvement. J Am Acad Dermatol. 1998;39:447–50.
16. Rietschel RL, Duncan SH. Clindamycin phosphate used in combination with tretinoin in the treatment of acne. Int J Dermatol. 1983;22:41–3.
17. Wolfe JE, Kaplan D, Kraus SJ, et al. Efficacy and tolerability of combined topical treatment of acne vulgaris with adapalene and clindamycin: a multicenter, randomized, investigator-blinded study. J Am Acad Dermatol. 2003;49:S211–17.

18. Mills OH, Kligman AM. Treatment of acne vulgaris with topically applied erythromycin and tretinoin. Acta Derm Venereol. 1978;58:555–7.
19. Toyoda M, Morohashi M. An overview of topical antibiotics for acne treatment. Dermatology. 1998;196:130–4.
20. Koo J. Systemic sequential therapy of psoriasis: a new paradigm for improved therapeutic results. J Am Acad Dermatol. 1999;41:S25–8.
21. Muller R, Naumann E, Detmar M, et al. Stability of cignolin (dithranol) in ointments containing tar with and without the addition of salicylic acid. Oxidation to danthron and dithranol dimer. Hausarzt. 1987;38:107–111.
22. Patel B, Siskin S, Krazmien R, et al. Compatibility of calcipotriene with other topical medications. J Am Acad Dermatol. 1998;38:1010–11.
23. Fairley JA, Rasmussen JE. Comparison of stratum corneum thickness in children and adults. J Am Acad Dermatol. 1983;8:652–4.
24. West DP, Worobec S, Solomon LM. Pharmacology and toxicology of infant skin. J Invest Dermatol. 1981;76:147–50.
25. Darmstadt GL, Dinulos JG. Neonatal skin care. Pediatr Clin North Am. 2000;47:757–82.
26. Code of Federal Regulations: 21 (part 120.57): 21–27, 2005.
27. Hale EK, Pomeranz MK. Dermatologic agents during pregnancy and lactation and clinical review. Int J Dermatol. 2002;14:197–203.
28. Reed BR. Dermatologic drugs, pregnancy, and lactation. Arch Dermatol. 1997;133:894–8.
29. Huang X, Tanojo H, Lenn J, et al. A novel foam vehicle for delivery of topical steroids. J Am Acad Dermatol. 2005;53:S26–38.
30. Taddio A, Ohlsson A, Einarson TR, et al. A systematic review of lidocaine-prilocaine cream (EMLA) in the treatment of acute pain in neonates. Pediatrics. 1998;101:299.
31. Koh JL, Harrison D, Myers R, et al. A randomized, double-blind comparison study of EMLA cream and ELA-Max for topical anesthesia in children undergoing intravenous insertion. Paediatr Anaesth. 2004;14:977–82.
32. Mahrle G. Dithranol. Clin Dermatol. 1997;15:723–37.
33. Swinkels OQ, Prins M, Tosserams EF, et al. The influence of a topical corticosteroid on short-contact high-dose dithranol therapy. Br J Dermatol. 2001;145:63–9.
34. Ramsay B, Lawrence CM, Bruce JM, et al. The effect of triethanolamine application on anthralin-induced inflammation and therapeutic effect in psoriasis. J Am Acad Dermatol. 1990;23:73–6.
35. Thami GP, Sarkar R. Coal tar: past, present and future. Clin Exp Dermatol. 2002;27:99–103.
36. Pittelkow MR, Perry HO, Muller SA, et al. Skin cancer in patients with psoriasis treated with coal tar. A 25-year follow-up study. Arch Dermatol. 1981;117:465–8.
37. Arnold WP. Tar. Clin Dermatol. 1997;15:739–44.
38. Breathnach AS. Azelaic acid: potential as a general antitumoural agent. Med Hypotheses. 1999;52:221–6.
39. Akamatsu H, Komura J, Asada Y, et al. Inhibitory effect of azelaic acid on neutrophil functions: a possible cause for its efficacy in treating pathogenetically unrelated diseases. Arch Dermatol. 1991;283:162–6.
40. Fitton A, Goa KL. Azelaic acid: a review of its pharmacologic properties and therapeutic efficacy in acne and hyperpigmentary skin disorders. Drugs. 1991;41:780–98.

41. Elewski BE, Fleischer AB, Pariser DM. A comparison of 15% azelaic acid gel and 0.75% metronidazole gel in the topical treatment of papulopustular rosacea. Arch Dermatol. 2003;139:1444–50.
42. Krebs HB. The use of topical 5-fluorouracil in the treatment of genital condylomas. Obstet Gynecol Clin North Am. 1987;14:559–68.
43. Jury CS, Ramraka-Jones V, Gudi V, et al. A randomized trial of topical 5% 5-fluorouracil (Efudex cream) in the treatment of actinic keratoses comparing daily with weekly treatment. Br J Dermatol. 2005;153:808–10.
43a. Zackheim HS. Topical carmustine (BCNU) in the treatment of mycosis fungoides. Dermatol Ther. 2003;16:299–302.
44. Bonnez W, Elswick RK, Bailey-Farchione A, et al. Efficacy and safety of 0.5% podofilox solution in the treatment and suppression of anogenital warts. Am J Med. 1994;96:420–5.
45. Drake LA, Millikin LE. The antipruritic effect of 5% doxepin cream in patients with eczematous dermatitis. Doxepin Study Group. Arch Dermatol. 1995;131:1403–8.
46. Markovits E, Gilhar A. Capsaicin – an effective topical treatment in pain. Int J Dermatol. 1997;36:401–4.
47. Choy L, Liu HN, Huang TP, et al. Uremic pruritus: roles of parathyroid hormone and substance P. J Am Acad Dermatol. 1997;36:538–43.
48. Bamford JTM. Treatment of tinea versicolor with sulfur-salicylic shampoo. J Am Acad Dermatol. 1983;8:211–13.
49. Morimoto S, Kumahara Y. A patient with psoriasis cured by 1 alpha-hydroxyvitamin D_3. Med Osaka Univ. 1985;35:51–4.
50. Kragballe K, Wildfang IL. Calcipotriol (MC 903), a novel vitamin D_3 analogue, stimulates terminal differentiation and inhibits proliferation of cultured human keratinocytes. Arch Dermatol Res. 1990;282:164–7.
51. Kang S, Yi S, Griffiths CE, et al. Calcipotriene-induced improvement in psoriasis is associated with reduced interleukin-8 levels and increased interleukin-10 levels within lesions. Br J Dermatol. 1998;138:77–83.
52. Binderup L, Bramm E. Effects of a novel vitamin D analogue MC 903 on cell proliferation and differentiation in vitro and on calcium metabolism in vivo. Biochem Pharmacol. 1988;37:889–95.
53. Fukuoka M, Ogino Y, Sato H, et al. RANTES expression in psoriatic skin, and regulation of RANTES and IL-8 production in cultured epidermal keratinocytes by active vitamin D_3 (tacalcitol). Br J Dermatol. 1998;138:63–70.
54. Barker JNWN, Ashton RE, Marks R, et al. Topical maxacalcitol for the treatment of psoriasis vulgaris: a placebo-controlled, double-blind, dose-finding study with active comparator. Br J Dermatol. 1999;141:274–8.
55. Dubertret L, Wallach D, Souteyrand P, et al. Efficacy and safety of calcipotriol (MC 903) ointment in psoriasis vulgaris. J Am Acad Dermatol. 1992;27:983–8.
56. Kragballe K. Treatment of psoriasis by the topical application of the novel cholecalciferol analogue calcipotriol (MC903). Arch Dermatol. 1989;125;1647–52.
57. Pariser DM, Pariser RJ, Breneman D, et al. Calcitriene ointment applied once a day for psoriasis: a double-blind, multicenter, placebo-controlled study. Arch Dermatol. 1996;132:1527.
58. Kragballe K, Barnes L, Hamberg KJ, et al. Calcipotriol cream with or without concurrent topical corticosteroid in psoriasis: tolerability and efficacy. Br J Dermatol. 1998;139:649–54.

59. Keinbaum S, Lehmann P, Ruzicka T. Topical calcipotriol in the treatment of intertriginous psoriasis. Br J Dermatol. 1996;135:647–50.
60. Ramsay CA, Berth-Jones J, Brundin G, et al. Long-term use of topical calcipotriol in chronic plaque psoriasis. Dermatology. 1994;189:260–4.
61. Bourke JF, Berth-Jones J, Hutchinson PE. Occlusion enhances the efficacy of topical calcipotriol in the treatment of psoriasis vulgaris. Clin Exp Dermatol. 1993;18:504–6.
62. Scarpa C. Tacalcitol ointment is an efficacious and well tolerated treatment for psoriasis. J Eur Acad Dermatol Venereol. 1996;6:142–6.
63. Mortensen L, Kragballe K, Wegman E, et al. Treatment of psoriasis vulgaris with topical calcipotriol has no short-term effect on calcium or bone metabolism. Acta Derm Venereol. 1993;73:300–4.
64. Fogh K, Kragballe K. Vitamin D3 analogues. Clin Dermatol. 1997;15:705–13.
65. Darley CR, Cunliffe WJ, Green CM, et al. Safety and efficacy of calcipotriol ointment (Dovonex) in treating children with psoriasis vulgaris. Br J Dermatol. 1996;135:390–3.
66. Oranje A, Marcoux D, Svensson A, et al. Topical calcipotriol in childhood psoriasis. J Am Acad Dermatol. 1997;36:203–8.
67. Kragballe K, Barnes L, Hamberg KJ, et al. Calcipotriol cream with or without concurrent topical corticosteroid in psoriasis: tolerability and efficacy. Br J Dermatol. 1998;139:649–54.
68. Molin L. Topical calcipotriol combined with phototherapy for psoriasis. Dermatology. 1999;198:375–81.
69. Speight EL, Farr PM. Calcipotriol improves the response of psoriasis to PUVA. Br J Dermatol. 1994;130:79–82.
70. Grossman RM, Thivolet J, Claudy A, et al. A novel therapeutic approach to psoriasis with combination calcipotriol ointment and very low-dose cyclosporine: results of a multicenter placebo-controlled study. J Am Acad Dermatol. 1994;31:68–74.
71. Kokelj F, Torsello P, Plozzer C. Calcipotriol improves the efficacy of cyclosporine in the treatment of psoriasis vulgaris. J Eur Acad Dermatol. 1998;10:143–6.
72. Van de Kerkhof PCM, Cambazard F, Hutchinson PE, et al. The effect of addition of calcipotriol ointment (50 μg/g) to acitretin therapy in psoriasis. Br J Dermatol. 1998;138:84–9.
73. Ruzicka T, Lorenz B. Comparison of calcipotriol monotherapy and a combination of calcipotriol and betamethasone valerate after 2 weeks' treatment with calcipotriol in the topical therapy of psoriasis vulgaris: a multicentre, double-blind, randomized study. Br J Dermatol. 1998;138:254–8.
74. Lebwohl M. Topical application of calcipotriene and corticosteroids: combination regimens. J Am Acad Dermatol. 1997;37:S55–8.
75. Papp KA, Guenther L, Boyden B, et al. Early onset of action and efficacy of a combination of calcipotriene and betamethasone dipropionate in the treatment of psoriasis. J Am Acad Dermatol. 2003;48:48–54.
76. Lebwohl M, Quijije J, Gillard J, et al. Topical calcitriol is degraded by ultraviolet light. J Invest Dermatol. 2003;121:594–5.
77. Lebwohl M, Hecker D, Martinez J, et al. Interactions between calcipotriene and ultraviolet light. J Am Acad Dermatol. 1997;37:93–5.

Systemic Drugs

Julia R Nunley, Stephen Wolverton and Marc Darst

INTRODUCTION

This chapter is designed to be a broad overview of a variety of systemic therapies for dermatologic diseases. It provides an historical perspective for each drug, a discussion of its mechanism of action and side effects, and then touches briefly on indications and clinical use. This information should serve as a starting point, allowing the reader to readily compare and contrast various treatment options. It is not a substitute for the in-depth knowledge and experience necessary to implement these systemic therapies, nor is it a complete library of systemic drugs used in dermatology. A number of systemic medications have been reviewed in other chapters (Table 130.1) and therefore will not be discussed here.

Systemic drugs used in dermatology may be subdivided into broad categories, such as immunosuppressive, cytotoxic and antiproliferative (Table 130.2), as a means of organization when approaching this exten-sive topic. Drugs in a single category act in a relatively similar fashion and generally have similar important side effects. For example, immuno-suppressive drugs suppress the body's ability to recognize or eliminate infections and neoplastic cells. Patients may be at increased risk for opportunistic infections and selected lymphoproliferative malignancies as well as squamous cell carcinomas. Given this increased risk for opportunistic infections, patients with either an active infection or one that may reactivate (such as tuberculosis) should be given these drugs with tremendous caution.

Among the drugs discussed are several older drugs which have been reformulated either into a prodrug that is more tolerable from a side-effect standpoint (e.g. mycophenolate mofetil) or into a more readily absorbed formulation such as Neoral® (cyclosporine). Others represent older drugs that have found new uses in dermatology. Most lack Food and Drug Administration (FDA) approval for the diseases for which dermatologists use them. This is not an incrimination of the practice, but is rather due to a lack of pharmaceutical company enthusiasm for putting drugs through lengthy, expensive approval processes for diseases that are relatively uncommon. This is why familiarity with each drug and the recent literature is important.

When choosing therapy for an individual patient, certain broad general principles always apply. First, the physician should be aware of all the common therapeutic modalities available and become very familiar with the drugs most frequently used and most likely to yield optimal results. Certain systemic medications will not be utilized frequently enough for a given clinician to become comfortable with their use; therefore, patients requiring more specialized drugs should be referred to colleagues more experienced with their use. Patients should be advised of all the reasonable therapeutic choices as well as the risk–benefit profile of each modality. Non-compliance is a relative contraindication for all of the medications discussed in this chapter.

Part of every initial prescription should be a complete history and physical examination, with specific emphasis on the organ systems that may be affected by the particular drug. Tuberculin skin testing should be performed prior to using some of the immunosuppressive medications, specifically corticosteroids and tumor necrosis factor inhibitors (for a few, it is FDA-required). Consultation with appropriate generalists or specialists in selected situations may be required prior to initiating therapy as well as for periodic screening for complications of therapy. Table 130.3 outlines suggested monitoring guidelines for the systemic medications discussed in this chapter. However, these tests may need to be performed more frequently in high-risk patients or in patients with abnormal results. Furthermore, each outpatient visit should include an appropriate review of systems and physical examination.

The use of each drug during pregnancy and lactation is reviewed. Wherever possible, this has been referenced with the seventh edition of *Drugs in Pregnancy and Lactation* by Briggs and colleagues. In general, one should be very circumspect in prescribing systemic medications to women of childbearing potential. It is not adequate to merely ask the patient if she is utilizing birth control before prescribing most of the medications discussed in this chapter; the patient must be made acutely aware of the risks associated with using the medication during pregnancy and the prudence of continuing therapy if pregnancy does occur. The prescribing physician also needs to keep in mind that birth defects have sometimes been ascribed to systemic medications despite the lack of scientific evidence. Family planning consultation and open communication with the patient's obstetrician or primary care physician can prove particularly helpful.

Several drugs discussed herein have parenteral formulations. Clinicians who administer parenteral medications in the office setting should be current in their Advanced Cardiac Life Support (ACLS) training and keep emergency resuscitation supplies readily available.

SYSTEMIC MEDICATIONS COVERED IN OTHER CHAPTERS	
Antihistamines	Ch. 19
Antimicrobials	Ch. 127
Bioengineered immunomodulators • Adalimumab • Alefacept • Anakinra • Efalizumab • Etanercept • Infliximab • Rituximab	Ch. 128
Cytokines • GM-CSF and G-CSF • Interferons	Ch. 128
Glucocorticosteroids	Ch. 125
Ivermectin	Ch. 83
Psoralens	Ch. 134
Psychotropic agents • Pimozide • Atypical antipsychotic agents	Ch. 8
Retinoids • Acitretin • Bexarotene • Isotretinoin	Chs 9 & 126 Ch. 126 Chs 37 & 126
Spironolactone	Ch. 37

Table 130.1 Systemic medications covered in other chapters.

CATEGORIES OF SYSTEMIC DRUGS USED IN DERMATOLOGY BASED UPON MECHANISM OF ACTION			
Immunosuppressive/ Anti-inflammatory	Cytotoxic	Antiproliferative	Miscellaneous
Azathioprine Mycophenolate mofetil Cyclosporine Tacrolimus (FK506) Thalidomide	Cyclophosphamide Bleomycin	Methotrexate Hydroxyurea	Dapsone Antimalarials Saturated solution of potassium iodide (SSKI)

Table 130.2 Categories of systemic drugs used in dermatology based upon mechanism of action.

MONITORING GUIDELINES FOR SYSTEMIC MEDICATIONS

Drug	Initial screening	Follow-up monitoring	Special considerations
Antimalarials	Ocular: Slit lamp and fundoscopic examination: assessment of visual acuity and visual field testing	Ocular: Repeat testing every 6 months for 1 year and then yearly	G6PD testing before antimalarial therapy is controversial and is probably most important with the use of primaquine
	Laboratory: CBC CMP G6PD (selected cases)	Laboratory: CBC monthly for 3 months, then every 4–6 months CMP after 1 and 3 months, then every 4–6 months	Urine or serum porphyrins should be measured when porphyria is clinically suspected Retinopathy risk is greatest for those on treatment for at least 5 years (especially with chloroquine) and if maximum daily safe dose has been exceeded
Azathioprine	CBC with plt count CMP UA	CBC with plt count every 2 weeks for 2 months, then every 2–3 months if stable	25% dose reduction is necessary if GFR 10–50 ml/min; 50% dose reduction if GFR <10 ml/min
	Consider pregnancy test for women of childbearing potential	AST/ALT every 2 weeks for 2 months, then every 2–3 months if stable	Frequency of laboratory studies is based on baseline TPMT determination; if TPMT is not known, hematologic parameters should be more closely monitored
	TPMT level, if available		Discontinue therapy if WBC declines to <4000–4500 cells/mm^3 or if hemoglobin <10 g/dl
	Tuberculin skin testing (should be considered depending on clinical situation)		Yearly skin examination and age-appropriate cancer screening, including yearly gynecologic examination in women
Cyclophosphamide	CBC with plt count CMP UA	CBC with plt count every week for 2–3 months, then every 2 weeks if stable. After 3–6 months, may decrease to every 3 months if stable	Discontinue or lower dose if WBC declines to <4000–4500 cells/mm^3 or plt count to <100 000 cells/mm^3
	Pregnancy test for women of childbearing potential	UA every week for 2–3 months, then every 2 weeks if stable. After 3–6 months, may decrease to every 3 months if stable	Stop treatment if red blood cells appear in urine; refer to urologist if hematuria persists Urine cytology after a cumulative dose of 50 g or after an episode of hemorrhagic cystitis; consider repeating yearly and/or after each 50 g
		CMP monthly for 3–6 months, then every 3 months if stable	Yearly physical examination and CBC as well as age-appropriate cancer screening
Cyclosporine	At least 2 baseline blood pressure readings	CBC with plt count at 1 month, then every 2–4 months	Blood pressure must be monitored every 2 weeks for first 3 months and then monthly if stable
	At least 2 baseline serum creatinine levels	CMP (must include BUN, creatinine, uric acid, potassium, magnesium) every 2 weeks for 1–2 months, then monthly	Lower dose by 25–50% if serum creatinine remains elevated (over 2 weeks) by >25% of baseline
	CMP (must include BUN, magnesium, potassium and uric acid)	UA with microscopic examination every month if abnormal; otherwise yearly	Lower dose by 25–50%, or discontinue, if at any time serum creatinine is elevated by ≥50% of baseline
	CBC with plt count		
	UA with microscopic examination	Fasting lipid panel every 2–4 weeks for 1–2 months, then monthly	Consider creatinine clearance if >6 months of therapy
	Fasting lipid profile (TG, cholesterol, HDL)		Skin examination at least yearly and age-appropriate cancer screening Consider trough whole drug cyclosporine level if response is inadequate or if drug interactions are suspected
Dapsone	CBC with plt count CMP UA G6PD level	CBC with plt count every week for 1 month, then every 2 weeks for 2 months, then every 3–4 months	Each visit should include an assessment of peripheral motor function and an assessment for the signs and symptoms of methemoglobinemia and peripheral neuropathy
		Reticulocyte count if anemia develops	Methemoglobin level if clinically indicated
		CMP every 3–4 months	Increase monitoring frequency when dose is increased
		UA every 3–4 months	

Table 130.3 Monitoring guidelines for systemic medications, as recommended by the authors (i.e. not standards of care).*,† ALT, alanine aminotransferase; AST, aspartate aminotransferase; BUN, blood urea nitrogen; CBC, complete blood count with differential; CMP, comprehensive metabolic panel (includes liver function tests); G6PD, glucose-6-phosphate dehydrogenase; GFR, glomerular filtration rate; HDL, high-density lipoproteins; IM, intramuscular; plt, platelet; TG, trigycerides; TPMT, thiopurine methyltransferase; TSH, thyroid-stimulating hormone; UA, urinalysis; WBC, white blood count. *Continued*

MONITORING GUIDELINES FOR SYSTEMIC MEDICATIONS

Drug	Initial screening	Follow-up monitoring	Special considerations
Gold	CBC with plt count CMP (must include creatinine and transaminases) UA	IM: CBC with plt count and UA prior to each injection; CMP (must include creatinine and transaminases) every 1–2 months until stable, then every 6 months Oral: CBC with plt count and UA monthly; CMP every 1–2 months until stable, then every 6 months	Hold dose or discontinue therapy if WBC declines to <4000–4500 cells/m^3 or plt count <100 000 cells/m^3
Hydroxyurea	CBC with plt count CMP UA Pregnancy test for women of childbearing potential	CBC with plt count weekly for at least 1 month until stable, then monthly CMP and UA monthly until stable, then every 3–6 months	A drop in hemoglobin of 1–2 g should be expected. Discontinue or decrease dose if the hemoglobin declines by more than 3 g or the WBC to <4000–4500 cells/mm^3 or the plt count to <100 000/mm^3
Methotrexate	CBC with plt count CMP Pregnancy test for women of childbearing potential Serologic tests for hepatitis A, B, C HIV testing if indicated	CBC with plt and AST/ALT after initial 5–10 mg test dose CBC with plt and AST/ALT every week for 2–4 weeks and after each dose escalation, then monthly for 2–4 months, and then every 3–4 months, if stable BUN and serum creatinine every 6–12 months	Consider periodic liver biopsies: Baseline and then after every 1.5–2 g in low-risk patients, after every 1 g in high-risk patients, and every 6 months in patients with grade IIIA liver biopsy changes Consider creatinine clearance, especially in elderly patients
Mycophenolate mofetil	CBC with plt count CMP Pregnancy test for women of childbearing potential	CBC with plt count every 2 weeks for 2–3 months, then monthly for first year CMP after 1 month and then every 3–4 months	Discontinue or decrease dose if WBC declines to <3500–4000 cells/mm^3
Saturated solution of potassium iodide (SSKI)	Thyroid function testing, including TSH, T$_4$ Pregnancy test for women of childbearing potential	TSH after 1 month of therapy	Consider antithyroglobulin and antimicrosomal antibodies in those with a history of thyroid disease
Tacrolimus	At least 2 baseline blood pressure readings At least 2 baseline serum creatinine levels CMP (must include BUN, magnesium, potassium and uric acid) CBC with plt count UA with microscopic examination Fasting lipid profile (TG, cholesterol, HDL)	CBC with plt count at 1 month, then every 2–4 months CMP (must include BUN, creatinine, uric acid, potassium, magnesium) every 2 weeks for 1–2 months, then monthly UA with microscopic examination every month if abnormal; otherwise yearly Fasting lipid panel every 2–4 weeks for 1–2 months, then monthly	The risk of diabetes mellitus post-transplant is higher with tacrolimus than with cyclosporine Blood pressure must be monitored every visit Lower dose or discontinue treatment if serum creatinine rises by >30% of baseline Consider creatinine clearance if >6 months of therapy Skin examination at least yearly and age-appropriate cancer screening Consider trough whole drug tacrolimus level if response is inadequate or if drug interactions are suspected
Thalidomide	CBC with plt count CMP Pregnancy test in women of childbearing potential Subjective review of sensory and motor neurologic function and neurologic examination	Consider CBC with plt count and AST/ALT every 2–3 months Pregnancy test every week for 4 weeks, then monthly for women of childbearing potential with regular menses, or every 2 weeks for those with irregular menses and as clinically indicated Neurologic examination monthly for 3 months, then every 1–6 months	Measurements of sensory nerve action potential amplitudes (SNAP) if indicated by history prior to therapy Consider SNAP measurements every 6 months, or as indicated

*Before using any of these medications, the risk–benefit profiles and adverse effects should be thoroughly discussed with each patient.
†More frequent monitoring is needed in high-risk patients, when results are abnormal or when increasing doses.

Table 130.3, cont'd Monitoring guidelines for systemic medications, as recommended by the authors (i.e. not standards of care).*,† ALT, alanine aminotransferase; AST, aspartate aminotransferase; BUN, blood urea nitrogen; CBC, complete blood count with differential; CMP, comprehensive metabolic panel (includes liver function tests); G6PD, glucose-6-phosphate dehydrogenase; GFR, glomerular filtration rate; HDL, high-density lipoproteins; IM, intramuscular; plt, platelet; TG, trigycerides; TPMT, thiopurine methyltransferase; TSH, thyroid-stimulating hormone; UA, urinalysis; WBC, white blood count.

ANTIMALARIALS

Quinine and its derivatives have been used since the 1600s for the treatment of malaria. Quinine is derived from the bark of the cinchona tree in South America and was first used in dermatology by Payne in 1894 to treat discoid lesions in patients with lupus erythematosus (LE). The most common antimalarials are hydroxychloroquine (Plaquenil®), chloroquine (Aralen®) and quinacrine; the latter, which can lead to yellow discoloration of the skin, is only available via compounding pharmacies in the US and it will not be covered in detail here.

The antimalarials are absorbed extensively into tissues and slowly released, leading to a half-life of 40–50 days. A steady state is achieved slowly and it may take 3–4 months to see an adequate clinical effect. Hydroxychloroquine is catabolized into two metabolites, desethylhydroxychloroquine and desethylchloroquine. Chloroquine is metabolized only into the latter. The initial metabolites undergo further change into the primary amine form. Overall, 50% of each drug undergoes renal excretion[1].

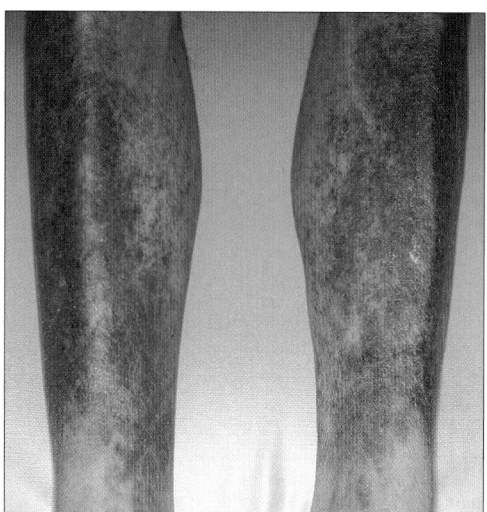

Fig. 130.1 Dark blue discoloration of the shins due to chloroquine.

Mechanism of Action

The mechanism of action of the antimalarials is not well known. These drugs can inhibit interleukin-2 (IL-2) release from T-helper (CD4+) cells and may inhibit macrophage expression of major histocompatibility complex (MHC) antigens. Antimalarials also exert various anti-inflammatory effects and they decrease platelet aggregation. The speculation that antimalarials may affect UV absorption in the skin remains unproven[2].

Dosages

Most conditions will respond to dosages between 200 and 400 mg per day of hydroxychloroquine or 250 mg per day of chloroquine, with a maximum safe dose (from an ocular standpoint) being 6.5 mg/kg/day and 4.0 mg/kg/day, respectively. After a suitable therapeutic response has been achieved, the response may be maintained with hydroxychloroquine 100–200 mg daily. If available, quinacrine 100 mg/day can be added to 200 mg twice daily of hydroxychloroquine, to maximize the clinical benefit without an increased risk of ocular toxicity. Lower doses of chloroquine (125 mg twice weekly) or hydroxychloroquine (100 mg three times weekly) must be used in patients with porphyria cutanea tarda, in order to minimize the risk of a toxic reaction (e.g. hepatotoxicity) in addition to a marked increase in urinary uroporphyrin output.

If no response is noted after 3–4 months, the specific antimalarial has failed and should be discontinued; however, a different antimalarial can be tried. In patients with porphyria cutanea tarda, the antimalarial can slowly be increased to daily dosing, if necessary.

Monitoring guidelines are outlined in Table 130.3. Because of the risk of dose-related ocular toxicity, a referral to an ophthalmologist is necessary for examination at baseline and then every 6 to 12 months[3].

Major Side Effects

Antimalarials are highly concentrated in the iris and choroid, reaching levels 480 000 times that of plasma[2]. Irreversible retinopathy may rarely occur and patients must be monitored by an ophthalmologist experienced with the ocular effects of antimalarials (Table 130.4). Of note, the risk of retinopathy is much less with hydroxychloroquine as compared with chloroquine.

Up to one-third of patients who receive antimalarials for over 4 months will develop a blue–gray to black hyperpigmentation on their shins (Fig. 130.1), face, palate and/or nail beds. The discoloration fades after cessation of therapy, but may take months to resolve completely. Reversible bleaching of the hair roots (achromotrichia) occurs in up to 10% of patients, presumably due to interference with melanosomal function. Another 10–20% may develop an exanthem ranging from urticaria to lichenoid reactions to exfoliative erythroderma. Of interest, morbilliform and urticarial exanthems have been observed with greater frequency in individuals with dermatomyositis as compared to those with LE.

Antimalarials have been reported to worsen psoriasis in some patients, even though in the past they were commonly used to treat psoriatic arthritis. Psoriatic patients traveling to malaria-endemic areas may take these drugs prophylactically.

Laboratory abnormalities do not commonly occur, but it is the practice of the authors to monitor patients as outlined in Table 130.3. An overdose of antimalarials can be fatal, and although pediatric usage is safe and effective, patients should be warned to keep the drug out of the reach of small children.

Indications

The most common dermatologic use of antimalarials is as second-line therapy for cutaneous LE, after topical or intralesional corticosteroids. Antimalarials are especially useful in patients with widespread discoid lesions and in those with the annular or papulosquamous lesions of subacute cutaneous LE (SCLE).

Other diseases that may respond to antimalarial therapy include photodermatoses, especially polymorphous light eruption. Small case series of patients with dermatomyositis, sarcoidosis, granuloma annulare, lymphocytic dermal infiltrates (including LE tumidus), chronic GVHD, panniculitis, porphyria cutanea tarda (see above) and lichen planus indicate that antimalarials may be of use in these diseases as well[4].

Contraindications

The only true contraindication is hypersensitivity to the drug. Caution should be used in patients with severe blood dyscrasias or hepatic disorders, because hepatitis and bone marrow suppression can occasionally occur. Ophthalmologic changes of premaculopathy call for discontinuation of the drug. Ocular changes at this stage are potentially reversible, but could progress if the drug were continued.

Use in Pregnancy and Lactation

Chloroquine is thought to be safe for treatment and prophylaxis of malaria during pregnancy; however, there have been anecdotal reports of an increase in birth defects in pregnant women being treated for systemic LE (SLE). Hydroxychloroquine is thought to be safer during pregnancy, even with its much longer half-life.

Although excreted into breast milk, standard doses of either drug are not harmful to breastfed infants and are approved by the American Academy of Pediatrics for use during lactation[5].

Drug Interactions

Cimetidine may increase circulating levels of antimalarials, and antimalarials may increase digoxin levels. Kaolin and magnesium trisilicate, over-the-counter gastrointestinal drugs, decrease absorption of antimalarials. The most significant potential interaction is the additive risk of retinal toxicity when chloroquine and hydroxychloroquine are used concomitantly. Combined therapy consisting of chloroquine or hydroxychloroquine plus quinacrine is acceptable.

SIDE EFFECTS OF SYSTEMIC DRUGS USED IN DERMATOLOGY

Drug	Common	Uncommon	Rare
Antimalarials	Derm: blue–gray to black discoloration; yellowing from quinacrine	Derm: bleaching of hair roots, exanthem GI: nausea, vomiting, elevated liver enzymes Neuro: irritability, nervousness	Ophtho: reversible (early) and irreversible retinopathy, vision changes Heme: pancytopenia, hemolysis (G6PD-deficient, primarily with non-dermatologic antimalarials)
Azathioprine	Heme: leukopenia, thrombocytopenia, immunosuppression	GI: nausea, vomiting ID: opportunistic infections	Heme: pancytopenia GI: pancreatitis, hepatitis Malignancy: lymphoma, cutaneous and gynecologic SCC Hypersensitivity syndrome
Cyclophosphamide	GI: nausea, vomiting Heme: leukopenia GU: sterility (higher doses or long-term administration)	Heme: anemia, thrombocytopenia GU: dysuria, hemorrhagic cystitis, amenorrhea, azoospermia, sterility (lower doses) ID: opportunistic infections Derm: diffuse hyperpigmentation, alopecia	GI: hemorrhagic colitis, hepatotoxicity Heme: aplastic anemia Malignancy: bladder, lymphoma, acute leukemia Pulmonary: pneumonitis, interstitial fibrosis Anaphylaxis
Cyclosporine	Cardiac: hypertension GU: renal dysfunction* Neuro: headache, tremor Metabolic: hyperlipidemias	ID: infections GI: nausea, diarrhea Neuro: paresthesia, hyperesthesia Derm: hypertrichosis, gingival hyperplasia, sebaceous hyperplasia Metabolic: hyperkalemia, hypomagnesemia, hyperuricemia	Musculoskeletal: myalgias, myositis GI: hepatotoxicity Pulmonary: dyspnea, bronchospasm ID: infections
Dapsone	Heme: hemolysis, methemoglobinemia	GI: dyspepsia, anorexia	Heme: agranulocytosis Neuro: peripheral neuropathy Sulfone syndrome
Hydroxyurea	Heme: anemia, megaloblastic changes	Heme: leukopenia Derm: dermatomyositis-like lesions	Heme: thrombocytopenia GI: hepatitis Malignancies: acute leukemia GU: renal dysfunction Derm: hyperpigmentation, leg ulcers
Methotrexate	Heme: leukopenia	GI: elevated liver enzymes, nausea, vomiting, anorexia, cirrhosis Derm: photosensitivity, alopecia, oral ulcers Heme: thrombocytopenia	Heme: pancytopenia Pulmonary: pneumonitis, fibrosis Derm: necrosis of psoriasis plaques, accelerated reversible cutaneous nodulosis ID: infections
Mycophenolate mofetil	GI: diarrhea, cramps, nausea, vomiting	Heme: anemia, leukopenia, thrombocytopenia ID: opportunistic infections	GU: dysuria, sterile pyuria Neuro: insomnia, dizziness, tinnitus
Saturated solution of potassium iodide (SSKI)	GI: nausea, vomiting, diarrhea, abdominal pain Derm: acneiform eruption	Metabolic: hyperkalemia Derm: iododerma	Metabolic: hypothyroidism, hyperthyroidism, goiter, 'iodism' GI: salivary gland enlargement, Derm: flair of dermatitis herpetiformis Cardiac: heart failure, pulmonary edema Hypersensitivity reactions
Tacrolimus	Derm: localized burning sensation GU: renal dysfunction* Cardiac: hypertension	ID: infections	Metabolic: diabetes mellitus
Thalidomide	Fetal abnormalities Neuro: peripheral neuropathy, sedation GI: constipation Gyn: amenorrhea Derm: xerosis, pruritus	Psych: headache, mood changes GI: xerostomia, increased appetite Heme: thromboses Peripheral edema Gyn: primary ovarian failure	Heme: leukopenia Derm: exfoliative erythroderma, TEN Hypersensitivity reaction (in HIV+)

*Not permanent during short-term treatment if guidelines are followed.

Table 130.4 Side effects of systemic drugs used in dermatology. Derm, dermatologic; G6PD, glucose-6-phosphate dehydrogenase; GI, gastrointestinal; GU, genitourinary; Gyn, gynecologic; Heme, hematologic; ID, infectious diseases; Neuro, neurologic; Optho, ophthalmologic; Psych, psychiatric; SCC, squamous cell carcinoma; TEN, toxic epidermal necrolysis.

In patients with LE, cigarette smoking has been associated with decreased efficacy of antimalarials. Whether this represents a 'drug–drug' interaction or decreased compliance (as a manifestation of high-risk behavior) is not known.

AZATHIOPRINE

Azathioprine was developed in 1959 from its parent drug 6-mercaptopurine (6-MP). After its anti-inflammatory and immuno-suppressive effects were noted, dermatologists began to utilize azathioprine for the treatment of inflammatory diseases. With its moderately potent immunosuppressive and anti-inflammatory effects, azathioprine has a reasonable risk–benefit profile. However, it should be reserved for more serious, life-threatening or recalcitrant dermatoses after other therapies have failed.

Azathioprine (Imuran®, Azasan®) has an 88% bioavailability. Immediately after absorption, it is converted to 6-MP and subsequently processed through three different and competing pathways. When

6-MP is catabolized via two of these metabolic pathways, by either xanthine oxidase or thiopurine methyltransferase (TPMT), inactive metabolites result. Active metabolites, such as the purine analogue thioguanine monophosphate and others, are produced from the third and only anabolic pathway via hypoxanthine-guanine phosphoribosyltransferase (HGPRT)[6]. Should either the xanthine oxidase or TPMT catabolic pathway be blocked, more 6-MP will be shunted through the anabolic HGPRT pathway, leading to more active metabolites; excessive immunosuppression and pancytopenia may result[7].

The TPMT pathway is interesting because it can have variable activity (polymorphism) on a genetic basis. Three distinct phenotypes exist and ethnicity may be a factor in the frequency of certain alleles. Encoded at the 6p22.3 locus, the TPMT activity trait is inherited in an autosomal codominant manner. Overall, 89% of Caucasians are homozygous for the high-activity allele and have relatively elevated levels, 11% are heterozygotes and have moderate activity, and 1/300 is homozygous for one of the seven low-activity alleles and has low TPMT activity. Red blood cell (RBC) TPMT activity mirrors systemic activity and a test for RBC TPMT activity has been developed. Although TPMT activity may vary somewhat between different laboratories and within different batches of the same test kit, knowledge of the baseline TPMT activity is clinically useful in the majority of patients who will receive azathioprine. However, vigilance in monitoring for pancytopenia will also identify those with low TMPT activity who will require dose reduction. Likewise, patients with high TMPT activity may need higher doses.

Decreased xanthine oxidase activity is rarely genetic in nature, but this enzyme is inhibited by allopurinol. Azathioprine dosage should be decreased by 75% in patients receiving allopurinol.

Mechanism of Action

6-Thioguanine, the active metabolite of azathioprine, is a purine analogue similar in structure to both adenine and guanine. Instead of an amino or hydroxyl group, it contains a thiol moiety. Incorporation of 6-thioguanine into DNA and RNA inhibits purine metabolism and cell division. 6-Thioguanine has other activities which are not well understood, such as suppression of T-cell function and B-cell antibody production. It also decreases the number of Langerhans cells in the skin and inhibits their ability to present antigens[6].

Dosages

Available in 25, 50, 75 and 100 mg tablets, empiric dosing is generally started at 50 mg/day and increased to a maximum of 2.5 mg/kg/day according to clinical efficacy and careful monitoring. Maximum doses based on baseline TPMT determination are as follows: TPMT <5 U, azathioprine contraindicated; 5–13.7 U, up to 0.5 mg/kg/day; 13.7–19 U, up to 1.5 mg/kg/day; and >19 U, up to 2.5 mg/kg/day. Doses must be reduced in the setting of renal insufficiency (see Table 130.3). Baseline evaluation should include a complete medication history because of adverse effects when azathioprine is used concomitantly with allopurinol, captopril or warfarin (see below). Monitoring guidelines are outlined in Table 130.3.

Major Side Effects

Major side effects are related to the immunosuppressive effects of azathioprine (see Table 130.4). Pancytopenia occurs rarely, particularly when doses are based on TPMT activity. Patients may be at increased risk for malignancies, especially lymphoproliferative disorders and squamous cell carcinomas of the skin and female genitourinary tract, and patients should be monitored accordingly. Factors influencing a patient's malignancy risk include degree and duration of immunosuppression, ethnicity, and existing comorbid diseases.

Azathioprine may rarely cause a life-threatening hypersensitivity reaction, which most commonly develops during the first month of therapy and when the drug is used in combination with cyclosporine or methotrexate. The cutaneous eruption is typically morbilliform with areas of confluence (Fig. 130.2). Other components of the syndrome include fever, respiratory and gastrointestinal distress, hepatotoxicity, and the possibility of cardiovascular collapse.

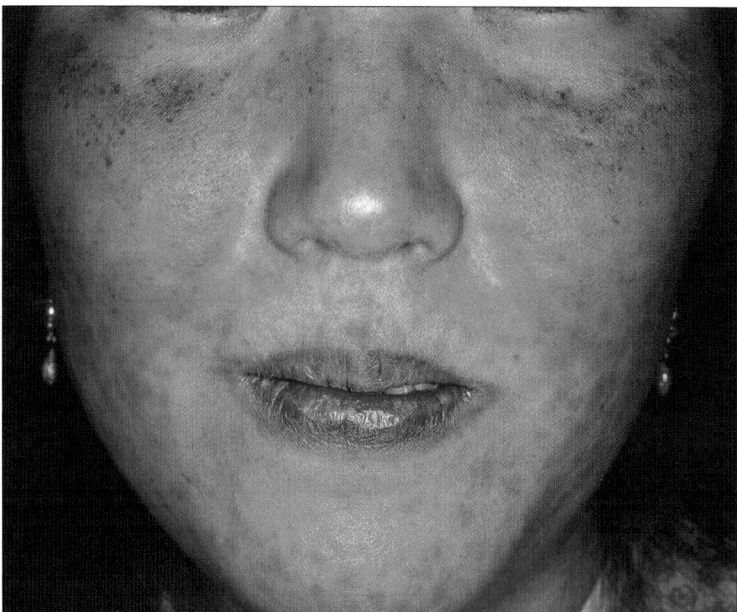

Fig. 130.2 Azathioprine hypersensitivity reaction. Pink to red macules, papules and areas of confluence are seen. Courtesy of Kalman Watsky MD.

Indications

Although azathioprine has FDA approval for non-dermatologic uses only, dermatologists have been using this drug for over 35 years to treat severe dermatologic conditions as dictated by risk–benefit considerations. It is inexpensive and has moderate immunosuppressive and anti-inflammatory effects.

Azathioprine is most often used as a corticosteroid-sparing agent in the treatment of immunobullous diseases such as pemphigus vulgaris, bullous pemphigoid and cicatricial pemphigoid. Various subsets of cutaneous vasculitis and Wegener's granulomatosis also respond well to azathioprine[8]. There may be a delay of 4–6 weeks in the onset of full clinical benefits.

Although azathioprine is more effective in improving the systemic features of autoimmune connective tissue diseases such as SLE and dermatomyositis, it may improve the cutaneous manifestations as well. Azathioprine may be selectively utilized for severe, recalcitrant atopic dermatitis and chronic actinic dermatitis in adults.

Contraindications

Absolute contraindications to azathioprine therapy include the history of a hypersensitivity reaction, as rechallenge may be fatal. Active serious infection and pregnancy are relative contraindications. Concomitant use of allopurinol requires dose reduction of azathioprine (see above).

Use in Pregnancy and Lactation

Azathioprine is pregnancy prescribing category D. Even though it is considered relatively safe for use in transplant patients who become pregnant, for dermatologic purposes it should not be prescribed during pregnancy[5]. No information is available regarding the risk to breastfed infants.

Drug Interactions

Allopurinol inhibition of xanthine oxidase (see above) increases the risk of pancytopenia in azathioprine-treated patients. Captopril may increase the risk of leukopenia. Azathioprine can decrease the effectiveness of warfarin and pancuronium, necessitating larger doses of these drugs. Since azathioprine may decrease the effectiveness of intrauterine contraceptive devices, alternative birth control methods should be employed.

BLEOMYCIN

The dosage, indications and side effects are outlined in Table 130.5.

<table>
<tr><td colspan="1">BLEOMYCIN</td></tr>
</table>

Source: *Streptomyces verticillus*

Mechanism of action: inhibits DNA synthesis in infected keratinocytes, but no direct effect on the human papilloma virus

Dermatologic indication: intralesional treatment of therapy-resistant verrucae vulgaris; 65–80% of lesions clear after 1 to 2 injections

Dosage: 0.1 to 0.3 ml of 1 U/ml (of saline) injected into targeted lesions, with maximum total dose per treatment = 2 ml; repeated every 3 to 6 weeks until resolution; given its rapid degradation and expense, newly constituted solution should be divided into glass vials and stored at 20°C

Side effects: injection is extremely painful (local or regional anesthesia may be required); pain and burning postinjection; Raynaud's phenomenon occasionally; nail dystrophy; no systemic toxicity with recommended total dose

Contraindications: pregnancy, immunosuppression, vascular compromise

Pregnancy and lactation: not recommended; pregnancy prescribing category D

Table 130.5 Bleomycin.

CLOFAZAMINE

The dosage, indications and side effects are outlined in Table 130.6.

COLCHICINE

The dosage, indications and side effects are outlined in Table 130.7.

CYCLOPHOSPHAMIDE

Cyclophosphamide (Cytoxan®) was derived from nitrogen mustard in 1958; the latter was combined with phosphoric acid in an effort to make an inert drug capable of entering and releasing active nitrogen mustard within target cells[9]. It has approximately 75% oral bioavailability, peaks in the plasma at about 1 hour, and crosses the blood–brain barrier. Cyclophosphamide itself is inactive, but it is metabolized by cytochrome P-450 (CYP) enzymes into the active metabolite 4-hydroxy-cyclophosphamide (nornitrogen mustard, $t_{1/2}$ 3.3 hours), which may then be converted into the other active metabolite phosphoramide mustard ($t_{1/2}$ 9 hours). Metabolites are excreted primarily via the kidney (50%). The inactive metabolite acrolein is believed to cause hemorrhagic cystitis and associated transitional cell carcinoma of the bladder[10].

Mechanism of Action

Cyclophosphamide functions in a cell cycle-independent fashion. Although its major effect is suppression of B-cell function, it also suppresses that of T cells (especially regulatory T cells). Clearly, the T-cell effects are greatest if the drug is given prior to antigen presentation. Cyclophosphamide crosses the nuclear membrane, covalently binds with DNA, and inhibits the synthesis of guanine, cytosine and adenine. Cytotoxicity occurs by several mechanisms: (1) DNA cross-linking with various proteins or other DNA strands; (2) G–C → A–T substitution; and (3) depurination resulting in chain scission. These mechanisms can overwhelm the DNA repair mechanisms, inducing cell death[9].

Dosages

Cyclophosphamide is available in 25 and 50 mg tablets. Doses range from 1 to 3 mg/kg/day, either as a single morning dose or in equally divided doses. Dermatologic diseases seldom require more than 2 to 2.5 mg/kg/day of cyclophosphamide. Dose reduction is necessary in patients with hepatic or renal dysfunction. Because of the risk of cystitis, patients should be advised to consume plenty of fluids on a daily basis. A monthly intravenous infusion (pulse) of 500 to 1000 mg has been used to treat a number of rheumatologic disorders, including severe SLE.

Prior to prescribing cyclophosphamide, patients should have documentation of a white blood count (WBC) of >4500/mm[3] and a

<table>
<tr><td>CLOFAZIMINE</td></tr>
</table>

Drug properties: riminophenazine dye (red color)

Mechanism of action: disrupts cell membranes (activation of phospholipase A_2 leads to generation of membrane-destabilizing lysophospholipids); enhances superoxide production; inhibits neutrophil motility and lymphocyte proliferation

Dermatologic indications: treatment of multibacillary leprosy, other infections (mycobacterial, malacoplakia, rhinoscleroma) and inflammatory skin diseases including neutrophilic dermatoses (pyoderma gangrenosum, Sweet's syndrome), granuloma faciale, orofacial granulomatosis, erythema dyschromicum perstans and discoid LE

Dosage: 50–400 mg orally daily*; avoid long-term administration of >200 mg daily; see Table 74.4 for leprosy regimens

Side effects: discoloration of skin (red to red–brown diffusely, bluish to violet–brown in lesional sites), cornea/conjunctiva and body fluids (urine, sweat, tears); xerosis/ichthyosis; gastrointestinal symptoms (abdominal pain, nausea, vomiting, diarrhea); ocular irritation; elevated hepatic enzymes; crystal deposition-related enteropathy (rarely); cardiac arrhythmias (rarely; associated with electrolyte disturbances)

Contraindications: prior hypersensitivity reaction

Pregnancy and lactation: for dermatologic disorders, should be avoided during pregnancy (category C) and lactation (concentrated in breast milk)

Larger doses are usually divided two to four times daily.

Table 130.6 Clofazimine. LE, lupus erythematosus.

<table>
<tr><td>COLCHICINE</td></tr>
</table>

Source: alkaloid from *Colchicum autumnale* (autumn crocus)

Mechanism of action: prevents microtubule assembly, resulting in mitotic arrest at metaphase and inhibiting cellular motility; decreases neutrophil chemotaxis, adhesion and degranulation

Dermatologic indications: treatment of neutrophilic dermatoses (Behçet's disease, Sweet's syndrome), small vessel vasculitis, neutrophil-rich autoimmune bullous diseases (EBA, linear IgA bullous dermatosis) and aphthous stomatitis

Dosage: 0.5 or 0.6 mg orally two to three times daily; drug must be shielded from light (degraded by UVR)

Side effects: commonly, gastrointestinal symptoms (diarrhea, abdominal pain, nausea, vomiting; dose-related); occasionally, alopecia, peripheral neuropathy, myopathy and bone marrow suppression (with prolonged therapy*); multiorgan failure with acute overdose†

Contraindications: prior hypersensitivity reaction; severe renal, hepatic, gastrointestinal or cardiac disease; blood dyscrasias

Pregnancy and lactation: for dermatologic disorders, should be avoided during pregnancy (category C); excreted in breast milk, but use during lactation allowed per AAP recommendations

Particularly in patients with renal insufficiency.
†*A toxic epidermal necrolysis-like reaction has been described.*

Table 130.7 Colchicine. AAP, American Academy of Pediatrics; EBA, epidermolysis bullosa acquisita; UVR, ultraviolet radiation.

granulocyte count of >1500/mm[3]. Laboratory monitoring guidelines are outlined in Table 130.3. Of note, it is not necessary to induce significant myelosuppression in order to achieve immunosuppression[11].

Major Side Effects

The most common side effects from cyclophosphamide treatment are hematologic and gastrointestinal (see Table 130.4). Dermatologic side effects include anagen effluvium (5–30%, which is typically reversible), pigmented bands of the teeth (irreversible), diffuse hyperpigmentation, transverse ridging of nails, acral erythema and, rarely, Stevens–Johnson syndrome. Up to 40% of patients have hemorrhagic cystitis, presumably from the acrolein metabolite, which is associated with a 10-fold increase in the risk for transitional cell carcinoma of the bladder. This risk is greater in patients who receive chronic 'low-dose' cyclophosphamide (as given for dermatologic diseases) than in those exposed to brief courses of high-dose pulse therapy (as given for systemic lymphomas and SLE). Immunosuppression is significant, especially in patients concomitantly receiving systemic corticosteroid therapy. Infection and malignancy risks are real, and appropriate monitoring is suggested. Long-term or high-dose therapy may be associated with infertility in either sex.

Indications

Although cyclophosphamide is only FDA-approved for use in advanced mycosis fungoides and hematopoietic malignancies, it can be extremely useful in treating a number of severe cutaneous diseases as well. Cyclophosphamide is a major component of treatment regimens for systemic vasculitides, especially Wegener's granulomatosis and allergic granulomatosis. It can also be used as a prednisone-sparing agent in a variety of cutaneous diseases or as monotherapy after prednisone is discontinued.

Contraindications

Absolute contraindications are pregnancy, lactation, depressed bone marrow function, and hypersensitivity to the drug. Cyclophosphamide-allergic patients may have cross-reactions with chlorambucil or mechlorethamine. Relative contraindications include active infections and significantly impaired hepatic or renal function.

Use in Pregnancy and Lactation

Cyclophosphamide is a first-trimester teratogen and is immuno-suppressive in breastfed infants. It is pregnancy prescribing category D and should not be used during pregnancy or lactation.

Drug Interactions

Allopurinol, cimetidine and chloramphenicol may elevate cyclophos-phamide drug levels and produce toxicity (via CYP450 interactions), whereas barbiturates may enhance conversion to inactive metabolites. Digoxin absorption may be decreased. Cyclophosphamide may enhance the effect of succinylcholine, increase cardiotoxicity of doxorubicin, and cause additive immunosuppressive and carcinogenic effects with other immunosuppressive drugs. Unpredictable effects can be seen when used with the inhalation anesthetics halothane and nitrous oxide.

CYCLOSPORINE

Cyclosporine, a cyclic peptide of 11 amino acids, was isolated from the soil fungus *Tolypocladium inflatum Gams* in 1970 and was found to have clinical immunosuppressive effects in 1976. In 1979, during a rheumatoid arthritis trial, it was discovered that cyclosporine improved cutaneous psoriasis in patients with psoriatic arthritis. Two forms are available, the original preparation (Sandimmune®) and a predigested microemulsion (Neoral®) that is more completely and consistently absorbed. The latter is available as capsules (25 mg, 100 mg) or as an oral solution (100 mg/ml)[12]. The solution can be mixed in orange juice or apple juice, but grapefruit juice should be avoided because it alters cyclosporine's metabolism (see Ch. 131).

Bioavailability of the microemulsion is not known, but it yields 40–106% higher peak blood levels than the original formulation. Cyclosporine is metabolized by the CYP 3A4 pathway, and primary excretion is via bile and feces. Only 6% of cyclosporine is excreted unchanged in the urine. Monitoring blood levels of cyclosporine is not routinely necessary since levels correlate poorly with efficacy or toxicity; determination of drug levels (11-hour trough) is primarily of value when drug–drug interactions are a concern.

Mechanism of Action

T-cell receptor activation causes release of intracellular calcium that in turn binds to calmodulin and activates calcineurin (see Ch. 128). This calcineurin complex dephosphorylates the cytoplasmic portion of the nuclear factor of activated T cells ($NFAT_c$), allowing it to migrate into the nucleus and bind with its intranuclear counterpart $NFAT_n$. This complex is a transcription factor for inflammatory cytokines such as IL-2. IL-2 receptors are also upregulated as a result of this process. IL-2 receptor stimulation in turn triggers a cascade of enzymes that affects mRNAs crucial for the cell to progress from G1 to S phase.

Cyclosporine binds to cyclophilin, a member of the family of intra-cytoplasmic proteins called immunophilins. This complex blocks the dephosphorylation of $NFAT_c$ and the subsequent upregulation of IL-2 and IL-2 receptors, resulting in a decrease in the number of $CD4^+$ and $CD8^+$ (cytotoxic) T cells in the epidermis.

Dosages

Cyclosporine is best used on a short-term basis (<6–12 months) to control flares of psoriasis and to provide an alternative to the patient's current regimen (see Ch. 9). However, safety has been documented in psoriasis patients receiving therapy for up to 2 years[13]. It is reasonable to use cyclosporine as sequential therapy with acitretin, methotrexate or other systemic therapies. After psoriasis clearance has been initiated by cyclosporine, the alternative medicine may be started and advanced to the therapeutic dose. At the same time, cyclosporine may be weaned by 1 mg/kg/day each month until the patient is receiving acitretin or methotrexate alone. Historically, the maximum dermatologic dose for cyclosporine is 5 mg/kg/day, although a maximum dose of 4 mg/kg/day of the microemulsion formulation should be considered, given the greater bioavailability of this formulation. The dose for obese patients is based on ideal body weight.

For psoriasis patients with a severe flare or recalcitrant disease, cyclosporine may be initiated at the maximum dosage until significant disease resolution occurs. The dose is then tapered by 1 mg/kg/day every 2 weeks until the minimum effective maintenance dose is deter-mined. For most patients with more moderate disease, therapy should be initiated at 2.5 mg/kg/day and increased by 0.5 to 1 mg/kg/day every other week until clinical improvement is seen or the maximum dose of 4–5 mg/kg/day (depending upon the formulation) is reached. If no improvement is observed after 3 months at the maximum dose, therapy has failed and should be discontinued[14].

Patients must be adequately monitored for the development of hypertension and laboratory abnormalities as outlined in Table 130.3. If the serum creatinine rises by >25% over baseline, the value should be rechecked within 2 weeks. If it returns to <25% over baseline, therapy can be continued at the current dose. However, if the elevation persists at that level, the dose should be decreased by 25–50% for 1 month and then the serum creatinine rechecked. If it is still >25% above baseline, therapy should be discontinued until the serum creatinine is within 10% of the baseline value. At that time, restarting therapy may be considered, but at a lower dose.

Major Side Effects

Cyclosporine is associated with a wide variety of adverse effects, including hypertension, hepatotoxicity, myositis, hyperlipidemia, hyper-trichosis, gingival hyperplasia and renal failure (see Table 130.4). Most of the side effects associated with short-term therapy are reversible upon discontinuation of the drug. A quarter of all psoriasis patients on cyclosporine will develop hypertension, which is usually mild and manageable. Direct vasoconstrictive effect of cyclosporine on the kidney vasculature is responsible for the development of hypertension short-term[15]. Hypertension due to cyclosporine is both time- and dose-related.

Modern, conservative dosing guidelines have prevented significant kidney damage in the vast majority of patients on short-term therapy. However, renal interstitial fibrosis has been demonstrated histologically even in the absence of abnormal laboratory tests in patients on appropriate dosing and monitoring regimens. Renal biopsy specimens from patients on long-term treatment demonstrate irreversible changes including renal tubular atrophy, arteriolar hyalinosis, glomerular obsolescence and interstitial fibrosis[16,17]. In fact, all patients on cyclosporine for >2 years were shown to have some of these abnormalities.

Although transplant recipients on high doses and prolonged courses of cyclosporine have an increased risk of certain malignancies (e.g.

cutaneous squamous cell carcinoma and lymphomas), patients with skin diseases on cyclosporine for less than 2 years and on lower 'dermatologic' doses have not been observed to have a similar risk.

Indications

Cyclosporine can be beneficial for patients with psoriasis who have failed or cannot tolerate other therapies and for those with widespread, inflammatory disease (see Ch. 9). In fact, cyclosporine has FDA approval for three 'types' of psoriasis: (1) severe; (2) recalcitrant; and (3) disabling. Patients with plaque-type psoriasis may also benefit from cyclosporine in rotating or sequential regimens with other modalities.

The use of cyclosporine in atopic dermatitis has been examined and a high percentage of patients improve with therapy; unfortunately, atopic dermatitis is a chronic disease and most patients relapse within 4 weeks of its discontinuation. Cyclosporine efficacy has been established in patients with severe pyoderma gangrenosum, but the disease may take several months to clear, depending on the size of the ulcer. Some clinicians prefer cyclosporine for idiopathic pyoderma gangrenosum, arguing that when there is a known underlying cause, therapy is best aimed at the latter (e.g. inflammatory bowel disease, myelodysplasia). Most other uses of cyclosporine are based upon anecdotal evidence[17a].

Contraindications

Absolute contraindications include significant renal impairment, uncontrolled hypertension, and hypersensitivity to cyclosporine. Relative contraindications include age <18 years or >64 years, controlled hypertension, and medication usage that may interfere with cyclosporine metabolism or worsen renal function. Tremendous caution is necessary if used in patients with significant infections, recent live virus vaccinations, immunodeficiency syndromes, or in combination with methotrexate, phototherapy or other immunosuppressive drugs.

Use in Pregnancy and Lactation

Cyclosporine is not teratogenic, and it is classified as a pregnancy prescribing category C drug. Use during pregnancy should be considered only in exceptional patients for whom the potential benefits of cyclosporine therapy dramatically outweigh the risks. Cyclosporine is excreted into breast milk and should not be used during lactation, due to risks of immunosuppression and possible carcinogenesis in the breastfed infant[5].

Drug Interactions

Drugs that interact with cyclosporine are discussed in Chapter 131. The clinician should review the patient's medication list for potential interactions using the following guidelines. In general, drugs that inhibit the CYP 3A4 pathway will increase cyclosporine levels, while inducers of the 3A4 pathway will decrease the effectiveness of cyclosporine, due to lower serum levels. Some drugs will potentiate renal toxicity, such as non-steroidal anti-inflammatory drugs (NSAIDs), aminoglycosides, amphotericin B and miscellaneous antibiotics (vancomycin, trimethoprim/sulfamethoxazole). Cyclosporine will reduce the renal clearance of digoxin, lovastatin and prednisolone. Increased risk of hyperkalemia occurs with concurrent use of angiotensin-converting enzyme (ACE) inhibitors, potassium supplements and potassium-sparing diuretics.

DAPSONE

Dapsone is a sulfone drug, and sulfones are related to the sulfonamide family (see Ch. 22). Sulfonamides were initially derived from coal tar in the early 1900s for use as fabric dyes. Medically, they were first demonstrated to be effective against streptococcal infections. Synthesized in 1908, dapsone was shown to be effective against tuberculosis and leprosy. During the first half of the 20th century, the related drugs sulfapyridine and sulfoxone were used to treat dermatitis herpetiformis (DH). However, since 1953, dapsone (the parent compound of sulfoxone) has been the mainstay of treatment for DH. Due to its activity in neutrophil-mediated dermatoses, dapsone has also proven useful in

the treatment of several forms of autoimmune bullous diseases and vasculitis syndromes.

Dapsone is 80% orally bioavailable, peaks in the serum between 2 and 6 hours post-administration, and has a half-life of 24–30 hours. Being highly lipophilic, it has excellent cell penetration. Dapsone and its major metabolite monoacetyldapsone are strongly protein-bound and undergo enterohepatic recirculation. Thus, dapsone may be found in the bloodstream up to 1 month following a single dose.

Dapsone is metabolized by N-acetylation and N-hydroxylation in the liver. Acetylation yields monoacetyldapsone, which is then de-acetylated to dapsone, yielding an equilibrium between dapsone and monoacetyldapsone. Hydroxylation via CYP enzymes produces N-hydroxy-dapsone, the metabolite which is believed to be responsible for the majority of dapsone side effects. Both dapsone and N-hydroxy-dapsone undergo glucuronidation in the liver, which results in more water-soluble compounds that are rapidly excreted in the urine[18].

Mechanism of Action

Dapsone is clinically most useful in the treatment of dermatologic diseases involving neutrophilic infiltrates. Researchers have demonstrated that dapsone inhibits neutrophil myeloperoxidase, thus reducing damage from the neutrophil respiratory burst mediated by this enzyme. Furthermore, dapsone has been shown to inhibit neutrophil chemotaxis to N-formyl-methionyl-leucyl-phenylalanine and to interfere with the CD11b/CD18-mediated neutrophil binding that induces chemoattractant signal transduction. IgA adherence is also inhibited. It is of clinical interest that dapsone also inhibits eosinophil myeloperoxidase activity, and thus may be efficacious in diseases in which eosinophils have a central role in pathogenesis, such as eosinophilic cellulitis[19].

Dosages

Dapsone is available in 25 mg and 100 mg tablets. The initial dose is often 50 mg/day in a single dose. Most conditions require 50–200 mg/day for adequate control of symptoms; rarely are dosages up to 300 mg/day required. In those with DH who respond to dapsone, rapid resolution of symptoms (within 48 hours) is usually noted; conversely, symptoms flare relatively rapidly after discontinuing therapy. Patients must be strictly warned against self-adjustment of the dosage, due to the various side effects that are dose-dependent.

Because of potential adverse effects, any cardiopulmonary or neurologic symptoms should be assessed prior to therapy. Documentation of peripheral motor nerve function may occasionally be necessary before or during therapy. Table 130.3 outlines monitoring guidelines for therapy. The clinician must be aware of all signs and symptoms associated with methemoglobinemia and the peripheral neuropathy to ensure proper monitoring.

Major Side Effects

Serious systemic side effects of dapsone may be idiosyncratic or pharmacologic. The pharmacologic and dose-dependent adverse effects include methemoglobinemia and hemolytic anemia (see Table 130.4). Agranulocytosis, peripheral neuropathy and dapsone hypersensitivity are idiosyncratic reactions; however, patients on higher daily doses or long-term therapy may be more likely to develop a peripheral neuropathy. Although rare, dapsone hypersensitivity syndrome may be fatal. Patients present with fever, hepatitis and a generalized cutaneous eruption. Cutaneous reactions range from a maculopapular eruption to toxic epidermal necrolysis (TEN). Liver failure has occurred in patients with the dapsone hypersensitivity syndrome[20].

Indications

Dapsone works well in a number of neutrophilic dermatoses. Although only FDA-approved for DH, dapsone is very useful in diseases such as linear IgA bullous dermatosis, bullous eruption of SLE and erythema elevatum diutinum. It is also a key component of combination therapy for leprosy.

Dapsone has variable efficacy in the treatment of other autoimmune bullous diseases (e.g. pemphigus foliaceus, bullous pemphigoid), neutrophilic dermatoses (e.g. Sweet's syndrome, pyoderma gangrenosum) and selected vasculitic syndromes.

Contraindications

The absolute contraindication to dapsone therapy is prior hypersensitivity to dapsone. Relative contraindications include a low glucose-6-phosphate dehydrogenase (G6PD) level, significant cardiopulmonary disease, and an allergy to sulfonamide antibiotics (because of the possibility of cross-reactivity). Patients with low G6PD levels are at an increased risk of the oxidative stress of the dapsone metabolites on RBCs. Those with significant cardiopulmonary disease may not tolerate the methemoglobinemia and hemolysis induced by dapsone.

Use in Pregnancy and Lactation

Dapsone does not appear to present a major risk to the fetus; however, it remains a pregnancy prescribing category C drug and should only be used during pregnancy if the benefits clearly outweigh the risks. There have been published papers reporting its use in pregnant patients with leprosy. Dapsone is found in breast milk and can cause hemolytic anemia in breastfed infants; however, it is approved by the American Academy of Pediatrics for use during lactation when required, as in patients with leprosy[5].

Drug Interactions

Drugs that may increase dapsone levels (and side effects) are probenecid (via decreased renal clearance), trimethoprim and other folate antagonists. Sulfonamides and hydroxychloroquine increase the oxidative stress on RBCs and may worsen hemolysis. Dapsone levels may be reduced by activated charcoal, para-aminobenzoic acid (PABA) and rifampin. Although cimetidine can increase absolute levels of dapsone, the former leads to a reduction in the more toxic hydroxylamine metabolite and thus the end result is a lower level of methemoglobin.

GOLD

The dosage, indications and side effects are outlined in Table 130.8.

HYDROXYUREA

Although hydroxyurea (Hydrea®) was first synthesized in 1869, its beneficial effect in psoriasis was not discovered until 100 years later. Being 100% bioavailable, hydroxyurea is very well absorbed. Peak levels are seen in 2 hours, its half-life is 5.5 hours, and 80% is excreted via the kidneys. Hydroxyurea is not highly protein-bound and can cross the blood–brain barrier. Metabolic mechanisms are poorly understood, but hydroxyurea is noted to accumulate in greater concentrations in leukocytes than erythrocytes. With about 60% of patients noticing no side effects, hydroxyurea is typically well tolerated[21]. The macrocytic anemia that commonly occurs is the primary factor limiting hydroxyurea therapy.

Mechanism of Action

Hydroxyurea inhibits the M_2 subunit of ribonucleotide reductase, thus blocking DNA synthesis. Accumulation of DNA precursors may lead to DNA damage and strand scission. Cells are arrested in the G_2 phase and thus are unable to repair UV- and ionizing radiation-induced damage. Hydroxyurea also causes hypomethylation of genes, inducing differentiation and normalization of psoriatic skin. Resistance may arise via increased levels of ribonucleotide reductase or by alteration of the enzyme leading to decreased susceptibility[11].

Dosages

The usual dosage is 20–30 mg/kg/day in divided doses, with a maximum of 2 g/day. Doses ranging from 1 to 2 g/day are commonly used[10]. Hydroxyurea is available in 200, 250, 300, 400 and 500 mg tablets. Monitoring guidelines are outlined in Table 130.3. A decrease in dosage

---

GOLD THERAPY (CHRYSOTHERAPY)

Formulations:
Parental (IM): aurothioglucose (Solganal®); aurothiomalate (Myochrysine®, Myocrisin®) with 70% renal excretion and half-life of 6 days
Oral: auranofin (Ridaura®) with primarily hepatobiliary elimination, 25% bioavailability, and half-life of 21 days

Mechanism of action: inhibits chemotactic and phagocytic responses of neutrophils and macrophages *in vitro*; inhibits lysosomal enzymes and interferes with prostaglandin synthesis

Dermatologic indications: treatment of autoimmune bullous diseases (pemphigus vulgaris, cicatricial pemphigoid, EBA) and connective tissue diseases (discoid LE, systemic LE)

Dosage:
IM: 10 mg, followed in 1 week by 25 mg, then 50 mg biweekly in adults*; for maintenance, taper dose or increase interval
Oral: 3 mg two to three times daily with maintenance dose of 3 mg daily; because of delayed onset, should be continued for up to 6 months

Side effects:
- Mucocutaneous (40% IM; 30% oral) – lichenoid and pityriasis rosea-like eruptions (Fig. 130.3), erythroderma, cheilitis, stomatitis; may persist for weeks after discontinuing drug
- Diarrhea (35–40%)
- Hematologic (1–2%) – leukopenia[†], thrombocytopenia, eosinophilia
- Proteinuria (2–10%)
- Nitroid reaction (IM) – dizziness, metallic taste, hypotension, syncope
- Pulmonary fibrosis (rarely)
- Anaphylaxis

Contraindications: prior significant reactions to gold (e.g. anaphylaxis, erythroderma, severe hematologic abnormalities, necrotizing enterocolitis, pulmonary fibrosis)

Pregnancy and lactation: for dermatologic disorders, should be avoided during pregnancy (category C); experts disagree regarding lactation (excreted in breast milk) but allowed per AAP recommendations

*In children, eventual dose is 1 mg/kg/week.
†Rarely, aplastic anemia with auranofin.

Table 130.8 Gold therapy (chrysotherapy). AAP, American Academy of Pediatrics; EBA, epidermolysis bullosa acquisita; IM, intramuscular; LE, lupus erythematosus.

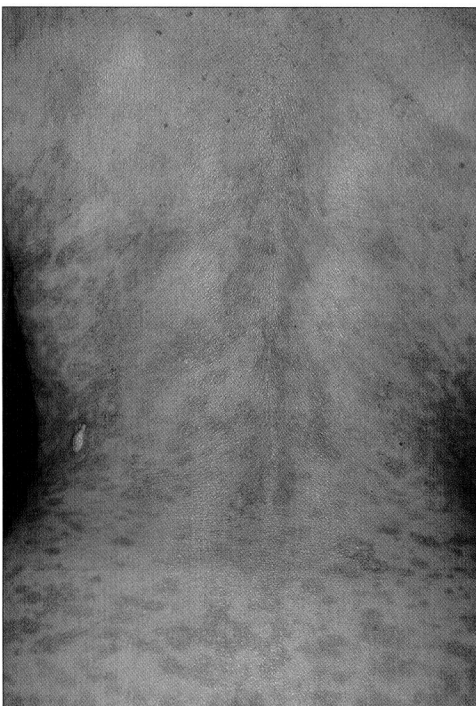

Fig. 130.3 Postinflammatory hyperpigmentation secondary to gold eruption. There were features of both a lichenoid drug eruption and a pityriasis rosea-like drug eruption.

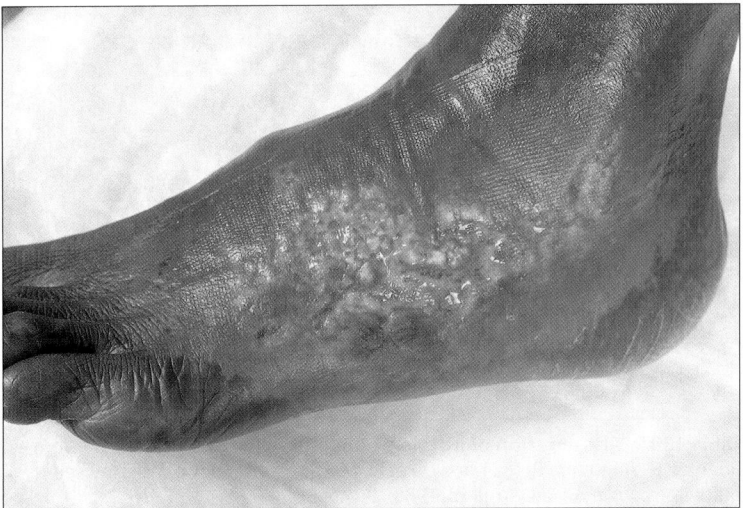

Fig. 130.4 Hydroxyurea-induced lower extremity ulcers.

(or discontinuation of therapy) is warranted if evidence develops of any type of significant cytopenia, concomitant infection, or other organ system involvement (see Table 130.4).

Major Side Effects

All patients on hydroxyurea develop megaloblastosis; however, only 10–35% develop anemia (see Table 130.4). Leukopenia is seen in 7% and thrombocytopenia in 2–3%. These changes may occur as soon as 48 hours after initiation of therapy, but typically resolve promptly with discontinuation of the drug. Transient, reversible hepatitis occurs occasionally and is associated with an acute 'flu-like' syndrome. Sporadic elevations of blood urea nitrogen (BUN) and serum creatinine have been reported, but frank renal failure is rare.

Rare cutaneous side effects include diffuse hyperpigmentation (including the buccal mucosa and tongue) and leg ulcers that resolve on discontinuation of the drug (Fig. 130.4). A characteristic dermatomyositis-like eruption on the dorsum of the hands has been reported. A wide variety of relatively minor side effects are well documented in the package insert.

Indications

Hydroxyurea is typically ineffective as monotherapy for clearing psoriasis, but it is quite effective as maintenance therapy following control of the disease by another modality, either phototherapy or a systemic medication. More commonly used throughout the 1970s, it is rarely prescribed in the current era of immunomodulating agents. Hydroxyurea is ineffective in psoriatic arthritis. Other uses include lymphocytic hypereosinophilic syndrome unresponsive to corticosteroids and chronic myeloproliferative disorders. Current FDA-approved indications include squamous cell carcinoma of the head and neck, prophylaxis against sickle cell anemia crises, resistant chronic myelogenous leukemia, metastatic melanoma and ovarian cancer.

Contraindications

Absolute contraindications include pregnancy, lactation and hypersensitivity to hydroxyurea. Relative contraindications include concomitant use of cytarabine, blood dyscrasias, infection, cardiac, renal or pulmonary disease, and unstable or fulminant psoriasis.

Use in Pregnancy and Lactation

Hydroxyurea is a teratogen and should not be used in pregnancy or lactation. It is pregnancy prescribing category D[5].

Drug Interactions

Hydroxyurea has no significant drug interactions.

INTRAVENOUS IMMUNOGLOBULIN (IVIg)

Mechanism of Action

IVIg has historically been used to provide passive immunity to selected individuals. It is a sterile solution of globulins extracted from pooled plasma donated by 10 000–20 000 individuals per production cycle. Processing results in a product that is predominantly IgG, having eliminated all but trace amounts of IgA and other soluble immunologically active particles. Administered intravenously, IVIg peaks almost immediately and has a half-life between 3 and 5 weeks.

A variety of immunoregulatory properties have been attributed to IVIg, including the blockade of reticuloendothelial fragment crystallizable (Fc) receptors, prevention of complement-mediated damage, reduction of circulating pathogens and antibodies, and alteration of cytokine-to-cytokine antagonist ratios[22]. Its recent success in treating TEN is believed to be a function of its ability to inhibit apoptosis. Theoretically, IVIg acts as a Fas (CD95)-blocking antibody, inhibiting Fas:Fas ligand-induced keratinocyte death[23].

Dosages

Since a number of different IVIg preparations are commercially available, each package insert should be consulted before use. Low doses are generally used in immunodeficiency disorders. Higher doses are utilized for the inflammatory and autoimmune blistering disorders[23]. 'High dose' ranges from 1 to 2 g/kg/cycle, given either as a single dose or in divided doses over a number of days. The rate of response to IVIg varies from days to months, with the duration of effect being unknown. Although generally administered every 2–4 weeks then tapered to every 2–4 months, there is no standard schedule for maintenance dosing in chronic diseases.

Major Side Effects

IVIg is generally well tolerated. Most side effects are mild and self-limited. Under most circumstances, decreasing the rate of infusion can improve the general side effects as well as the risk of hyperviscosity and thrombosis. Acute renal failure, stroke and myocardial infarction have been described on rare occasion, primarily in patients with predisposing medical conditions. Renal failure is most common after use of sucrose-containing products which can cause an 'osmotic nephrosis.'

Indications

IVIg is approved for use in a variety of immunodeficiency syndromes and hematologic conditions. Although utilized for a variety of dermatologic conditions, IVIg is currently FDA-approved for GVHD only. Off-label uses include the primary autoimmune blistering diseases (pemphigus vulgaris, bullous pemphigoid, EBA, dermatomyositis, Kawasaki disease, toxic shock syndrome, recalcitrant atopic dermatitis, pyoderma gangrenosum and TEN[22–24b]. Adequate data now exist supporting the use of IVIg in patients with dermatomyositis who have failed conventional therapy, and studies are ongoing to evaluate its effectiveness in blistering diseases. Although the current cost of IVIg prohibits its use as first-line treatment in any cutaneous diseases, it may be effective in inducing remission or at least gaining control of recalcitrant and difficult-to-treat cases[24], which can then be transitioned to other therapies.

Contraindications

Absolute contraindications include a history of hypersensitivity to IVIg, the presence of IgA antibodies, IgA deficiency and sensitivity to thimerosal. Relative contraindications include renal dysfunction and pregnancy.

Use in Pregnancy and Lactation

IVIg is pregnancy prescribing category C.

Drug Interactions

Live virus vaccination induces a suboptimal result in those receiving IVIg.

METHOTREXATE

The effectiveness of the folic acid analogue methotrexate (MTX) in psoriasis was noted in the early 1950s, but remained without FDA approval until the 1960s. MTX is not difficult to use and oral administration achieves reliable blood levels unaffected by food intake. MTX is widely distributed throughout the body, but penetrates the blood–brain barrier poorly.

Within 1 hour of ingestion, distribution and active cellular uptake is complete. Plasma MTX is 50% protein-bound, and irreversibly bound to dihydrofolate reductase, the enzyme it inhibits. By 4 hours, the kidneys have excreted the plasma portion of the drug. Over the next 10–27 hours, the drug is slowly released from body tissues.

Mechanism of Action

Dihydrofolate reductase (DHFR) converts dihydrofolate to tetrahydrofolate (fully reduced folic acid; see Ch. 127), which is a necessary cofactor in the synthesis of thymidylate and purine nucleotides, which, in turn, are required for DNA/RNA synthesis. MTX competitively inhibits DHFR, although this inhibition can be at least partially reduced by concomitant folic acid administration. MTX also exerts partially reversible inhibition downstream on thymidylate synthetase, inhibiting cell division in the S phase.

Although originally believed to suppress keratinocyte proliferation, it is more likely that MTX inhibits DNA synthesis in immunologically active cells. MTX decreases inflammation through other mechanisms as well. By inhibiting aminoimidocarboxyamido-ribonucleotide transformylase, MTX increases local tissue concentrations of the potent anti-inflammatory mediator adenosine. By inhibiting methionine synthase, MTX reduces production of the proinflammatory mediator S-adenyl methionine[25].

Dosages

MTX is administered as a once-weekly dose of up to 30 mg for dermatologic and rheumatologic diseases. Oncologists may prescribe 20–40 mg/m^2 every 1 to 4 weeks with folinic acid rescue. Historically, MTX was administered in three doses over 24 hours (8 a.m. and 8 p.m. day 1, and 8 a.m. day 2). There were theoretical advantages for the divided dosing regimen from a cell-cycle kinetics standpoint. However, since the clinical result is the same, a single dose, which is easier and less confusing (for the patient and the pharmacist), is currently recommended. The patient should be admonished to adhere to the dosing schedule religiously, as more frequent dosing invariably causes major hematologic complications and potentially an increased risk of liver fibrosis. Parenteral administration (intramuscular or subcutaneous) is available for patients who cannot tolerate oral MTX and has also been advocated by some clinicians for use in erythrodermic patients who may have decreased gastrointestinal absorption or when compliance is an issue.

Available in 2.5 mg tablets, therapy should begin with a test dose of 5–10 mg followed 5–6 days later with a complete blood count with differential (CBC), platelet count and hepatic profile. The dose may be gradually increased by 2.5 to 5 mg every 2–4 weeks until satisfactory results are obtained with minimal toxicity. Once disease control has been attained for at least 1–2 months, the MTX can be tapered by 2.5 mg every 1–2 weeks to the lowest dose that still maintains disease control. The usual weekly dose for psoriasis is 10–15 mg, although doses up to 25 mg per week are not uncommonly used, except in patients with renal insufficiency. Rheumatologic and dermatologic monitoring regimens do differ (i.e. liver biopsies are not routinely recommended by rheumatologists); monitoring guidelines that are utilized by the authors for those with psoriasis are in Table 130.3. In general, dosing and duration of therapy may be higher and longer for psoriasis patients than for those with rheumatologic diseases.

Major Side Effects

The most important side effects of MTX include pancytopenia and hepatotoxicity (see Table 130.4). Pancytopenia typically develops early,

Grade	Histologic findings	Methotrexate
	CLASSIFICATION OF HISTOLOGIC FINDINGS IN LIVER BIOPSIES	
I	Essentially normal liver	Continue
II	Moderate to severe fatty infiltration, nuclear variability, portal tract expansion, portal tract inflammation and necrosis	Continue; repeat biopsy after additional 1.5 g
IIIA	Mild fibrosis; fibrotic septae which extend into the lobules	Repeat biopsy in 6 months
IIIB	Moderate to severe fibrosis	Discontinue
IV	Cirrhosis	Discontinue

Table 130.9 Classification of histologic findings in liver biopsies. Data from Roenigk H, Auerbach R, Maibach HI, et al. Methotrexate in psoriasis: revised guidelines. J Am Acad Dermatol. 1988;19:145–56.

compared to hepatic fibrosis and cirrhosis, which take years to develop. There is considerable debate over the risk of hepatotoxicity in psoriasis patients on long-term MTX. Suffice it to say that the higher the cumulative dose of MTX, the greater the risk of significant liver damage (Table 130.9). Compounding risk factors for hepatic impairment include: previous or current excessive alcohol intake, persistent abnormal liver chemistries, a history of liver disease (including hepatitis B and C viral infections), family history of inheritable liver disease, diabetes mellitus, obesity, and a history of significant exposure to hepatotoxic drugs or chemicals. References discussing this issue in detail[26–28] should be consulted before prescribing MTX. In limited studies, elevated levels of procollagen III amino peptide were observed to be a serologic marker of fibrosis, and, in the future, this (or a similar) assay may help to determine which patients should be sent for liver biopsy.

Photosensitivity may occur and patients should take appropriate sun precautions[26,27]. Gastrointestinal intolerance is often abated with concomitant folic acid therapy (1–5 mg orally daily, based on symptoms). When used in very high doses, MTX may cause reversible oligospermia.

Drug Indications

MTX has FDA approval for use in psoriasis (see Ch. 9); however, it is used for those individuals with severe, debilitating or recalcitrant disease. Clinical improvement is striking and occurs within 2–3 months in up to 80% of patients.

Other disorders such as pityriasis rubra pilaris (PRP), pityriasis lichenoides et varioliformis acuta (PLEVA), lymphomatoid papulosis and reactive arthritis (formerly Reiter's disease) may also respond to MTX. PRP commonly requires up to twice the typical psoriasis dose, whereas PLEVA often responds to small MTX doses (2.5–5 mg/week).

Several inflammatory diseases may also improve with MTX, most notably dermatomyositis and sarcoidosis. Significant improvement can be seen within 2 months of initiating MTX, allowing corticosteroid doses to be reduced. MTX demonstrates corticosteroid-sparing effects in other immunologic diseases such as certain types of vasculitic, neutrophilic and immunobullous dermatoses[28], in particular bullous pemphigoid. In the elderly, monotherapy with weekly MTX is an option for the treatment of bullous pemphigoid.

Contraindications

Absolute contraindications to MTX use are pregnancy and lactation. Relative contraindications include significant liver disease or elevated liver enzymes and excessive alcohol intake. The presence of active infection or immunodeficiency, and the desire for imminent pregnancy are relative contraindications to MTX therapy. Caution is indicated and a dose reduction necessary if used in the setting of decreased renal function. In the elderly, serum creatinine levels may be deceptively low and may not reflect true renal function.

Use in Pregnancy and Lactation

MTX is an abortifacient and teratogen and should not be used during pregnancy. The American Academy of Pediatrics considers MTX to be contraindicated in breastfeeding owing to concerns of immune suppression, growth retardation and carcinogenesis[5].

Drug Interactions

Drugs that elevate MTX blood levels include NSAIDs, salicylates, sulfonamides, chloramphenicol, phenothiazines, phenytoin and tetracyclines. Dipyridamole and probenecid increase intracellular accumulation of MTX. Trimethoprim, sulfonamides and dapsone also inhibit the folate metabolic pathway (see Ch. 127) and markedly increase the risk for pancytopenia with concomitant use. Systemic retinoids and alcohol may cause synergistic liver damage in combination with MTX.

MYCOPHENOLATE MOFETIL

Mycophenolic acid (MPA) has been used in various forms for the treatment of psoriasis since the 1970s. Its use declined until the early 1990s, when a more bioavailable and safer formulation, mycophenolate mofetil (Cellcept®), became commercially available. Initially inactivated during first-pass glucuronidation in the liver (into the phenolic glucuronide of MPA, MPAG), MPA is then reactivated in the epidermis and gastrointestinal tract by β-glucuronidase. Mycophenolate mofetil has greater bioavailability than MPA, undergoes complete presystemic conversion to MPA after ingestion, and then follows the same inactivation/activation cycle[29]. Mycophenolate mofetil is 94% bioavailable. MPA is 97% and MPAG 82% albumin-bound. Over 90% of the drug is excreted in the urine, mainly as MPAG. Renal insufficiency can increase plasma concentrations up to sixfold[10].

Mechanism of Action

MPA selectively and non-competitively inhibits the enzyme inosine monophosphate dehydrogenase (IMPDH), preventing conversion of inosine- and xanthine-5-phosphate to guanosine-5-phosphate. This blocks de novo synthesis of guanine nucleotides and their subsequent incorporation into DNA. DNA synthesis in T and B lymphocytes is preferentially inhibited because these cells lack the purine salvage pathway and are dependent on de novo purine synthesis. MPA decreases immunoglobulin levels and delayed-type hypersensitivity responses by inhibiting proliferative responses to mitogenic and allospecific stimulation; MPA also suppresses antibody formation by B lymphocytes.

Dosages

Mycophenolate mofetil is available in 250 mg capsules and 500 mg tablets. For dermatologic diseases, the best results are obtained with doses of 2000 mg daily. Selected patients may require doses carefully titrated up to 3000 mg daily.

Major Side Effects

The most common side effects of mycophenolate mofetil are gastrointestinal and include nausea, vomiting, diarrhea, abdominal cramps and tenderness (see Table 130.4). Significant hematologic and hepatic toxicity occur uncommonly. Monitoring guidelines are outlined in Table 130.3. The dosage should be reduced or therapy discontinued for a WBC <3500–4000 cells/mm[3].

Indications

Mycophenolate mofetil is currently FDA-approved for renal allograft rejection only. However, it is quite useful in the treatment of autoimmune bullous diseases (e.g. different types of pemphigus and pemphigoid) owing to its unique metabolism noted above[30]. Occasionally, it is used for patients with severe forms of atopic dermatitis, cutaneous lupus or psoriasis or refractory pyoderma gangrenosum. Mycophenolate mofetil is generally used in conjunction with other immunosuppressive agents, most commonly corticosteroids.

Contraindications

Absolute contraindications to mycophenolate mofetil use are pregnancy and allergy to MPA. Relative contraindications include lactation, as MPA is partially excreted in breast milk. Peptic ulcer disease and hepatic, renal or cardiopulmonary disease are also relative contraindications. As noted previously, renal insufficiency can increase plasma concentrations up to sixfold[10].

Use in Pregnancy and Lactation

Due to the paucity of human data, mycophenolate mofetil is currently rated as a pregnancy prescribing category D medication. However, animal data suggest a significant risk for fetal structural malformations, and effective contraception is recommended[5]. Mycophenolate mofetil is contraindicated during lactation, due to potential immunosuppression.

Drug Interactions

Drugs that alter the enterohepatic recirculation or gastrointestinal absorption of mycophenolate mofetil, such as cholestyramine, iron or aluminum and magnesium hydroxides, decrease the effectiveness of mycophenolate mofetil (see Ch. 131). Plasma levels of acyclovir and mycophenolate mofetil are both elevated when used concomitantly.

SATURATED SOLUTION OF POTASSIUM IODIDE (SSKI)

Mechanism of Action

First discovered in seaweed in the 1800s, iodine was soon used medically for a variety of conditions, such as thyroid disease, syphilis, psoriasis and atopic dermatitis[31]. To this day, it remains an important tool in the treatment of sporotrichosis and a variety of inflammatory conditions, especially panniculitis. Most conveniently administered as a saturated solution of potassium iodide (SSKI), it is rapidly absorbed, widely distributed into the thyroid and salivary glands, choroid plexus and placenta, and then excreted primarily through the kidneys. Although its mechanism of action with regard to inflammatory diseases is speculative, it is thought to exert its effects via immune modulation. Similar to dapsone, SSKI appears to be effective in suppressing neutrophil migration and toxicity. The mechanism through which it eradicates sporotrichosis is unknown[31].

Dosages

SSKI is most commonly available in a solution with a concentration of 1000 mg/ml. The accompanying dropper has markings at 0.3 ml (300 mg) and 0.6 ml (600 mg); when lower doses are prescribed, drops (gt) are counted. The initial dose to treat inflammatory skin conditions is generally 150–300 mg three times daily, increased weekly as tolerated[32]. Improvement is generally seen within days to weeks. The dose for sporotrichosis is usually higher, beginning at 600 mg three times daily, with a maximum dose of 6 g, if tolerated[33]. The course of treatment for sporotrichosis is approximately 6–10 weeks.

Major Side Effects

Gastrointestinal side effects are common and may be ameliorated by slow dose escalation (see Table 130.4). Long-term use can be associated with the development of 'iodism', manifested by a burning mouth, a metallic taste, soreness of the teeth and gums, and a severe headache. Acneiform eruptions and iododerma can also occur, especially at higher dosages. Fortunately, symptoms abate quickly with cessation of therapy. SSKI may also alter thyroid metabolism, resulting in either hypo- or hyperthyroidism, with reversible hypothyroidism being relatively common. While hyperkalemia can occur, other side effects are rare.

Indications

Although SSKI is not FDA-approved for any cutaneous disease, it is a highly effective treatment for cutaneous and lymphocutaneous sporotrichosis. However, for systemic sporotrichosis, other drugs should be prescribed (see Ch. 76). SSKI has also been used successfully for a variety of neutrophilic disorders (Sweet's syndrome, pyoderma gangrenosum), granulomatous disorders (Wegener's granulomatosis, granuloma annulare), and several types of panniculitis (erythema nodosum, nodular vasculitis, subacute nodular migratory panniculitis; see Ch. 100).

Contraindications

The only absolute contraindication is a hypersensitivity reaction to iodides. Relative contraindications include thyroid or cardiac disease, renal insufficiency and Addison's disease[34].

Use in Pregnancy and Lactation

Iodide crosses the placenta and is considered pregnancy prescribing category D; fetal defects have been described. Although it is present in breast milk, the American Academy of Pediatrics considers its use to be compatible with breastfeeding[5].

Drug Interactions

Concurrent use with other medications such as ACE inhibitors, potassium-sparing diuretics and potassium-containing medications may result in significant hyperkalemia. Hypothyroidism may result when used in combination with amiodarone, lithium, phenazone and, possibly, sulfones[31].

TACROLIMUS

Tacrolimus (Prograf®; previously known as FK 506) is a macrolide lactone that is most commonly used to prevent rejection after organ transplantation and to treat acute and chronic forms of GVHD. Despite promising results in clinical trials, side effects have limited its systemic use in other dermatologic diseases. However, a topical form is FDA-approved for the treatment of atopic dermatitis (see Ch. 128). The molecular weight of 822.05 allows it to penetrate intact human skin, in contrast to cyclosporine, a significantly larger molecule.

Mechanism of Action

Tacrolimus has a mechanism of action similar to cyclosporine (see above), but is 10–100 times more potent per milligram administered. In addition, tacrolimus inhibits production of other cytokines such as IL-8, which appears to promote neutrophil and T-cell accumulation in psoriatic dermis and epidermis[12].

Dosages

Although trials of systemic tacrolimus have demonstrated effectiveness in psoriasis, renal toxicity and hypertension limit its usefulness[35]. Available in 0.5, 1 and 5 mg capsules, the usual dose for GVHD is approximately 1–2 mg daily, but dose adjustments are necessary to achieve a blood level of 5–15 ng/ml.

Major Side Effects

Systemic use can result in significant elevations of BUN and serum creatinine, which is less acceptable in dermatologic practice than in transplant medicine (but can be minimized by following blood levels closely). Significant adverse cardiovascular effects include hypertension and concentric left ventricular hypertrophy. The incidence of hypertrichosis is significantly less than with cyclosporine, while the incidence of diabetes mellitus is increased.

Contraindications

Absolute contraindications include allergy to tacrolimus or to HCO-60 (polyoxyl 60 hydrogenated castor oil). The castor oil allergy is important only with parenteral administration, as intravenous infusions can cause anaphylaxis in sensitive patients.

Use in Pregnancy and Lactation

Tacrolimus is pregnancy prescribing category C. Fetal abnormalities and spontaneous abortions have been observed in pregnant rabbits and rats. Systemic tacrolimus is excreted into breast milk and should be avoided during lactation.

Drug Interactions

Formal drug interaction studies have not been performed with systemic tacrolimus. Caution is necessary if drugs with potential renal toxicity are used concomitantly. Drugs that affect the hepatic CYP 3A4 enzyme system and alter cyclosporine levels may similarly affect tacrolimus levels (see Ch. 131).

THALIDOMIDE

Few drugs have garnered such notoriety as has thalidomide. Originally introduced in Europe during the 1950s as a sedative/hypnotic, it was commonly used to control morning sickness during pregnancy. Thus, it was prescribed to thousands of pregnant women, with tragic results. By 1961, thalidomide was withdrawn from the market worldwide after being linked to thousands of babies born with phocomelia (severe underdevelopment of the extremities)[36]. At the time of worldwide withdrawal, thalidomide had never received FDA approval for use in the US. Renewed interest in the drug ensued in the mid-1960s with reports that thalidomide provided significant relief from the symptoms of erythema nodosum leprosum (ENL). Thalidomide received FDA approval for treatment of ENL in 1997.

In the US, both the prescribing physician and the dispensing pharmacist must be enrolled in the system for thalidomide education and prescribing safety (STEPS) program administered by the FDA and the Celgene Corporation (1-888-4-CELGENE to enroll). Standardized informed consent forms, patient education packets, and monitoring requirements are included in the program.

Thalidomide (Thalomid®) is a lipophilic, non-polar piperidine-dione that is poorly absorbed and highly protein-bound. Peak plasma levels are attained 2–6 hours post-ingestion and absorption is not affected by food intake. The half-life of thalidomide is 9 hours. Although the major degradative pathway is non-enzymatic hydrolysis, the drug is also metabolized by the CYP enzymes. The precise method of excretion is not known, but it is non-renal[22].

Mechanism of Action

The precise mechanisms of action of thalidomide are unknown. However, its anti-inflammatory and immunomodulatory effects on dermatologic diseases are thought to be largely through inhibition of TNF-α release and activity.

Dosages

A major emphasis of the STEPS program is pregnancy prevention. Prior to therapy, women of childbearing potential must be on birth control for 1 month and have a negative serum pregnancy test within 24 hours of the first dose. If the initial history or physical examination indicates peripheral nervous system disease, neurologic consultation should be sought. Monitoring guidelines are listed in Table 130.3. Thalidomide is available in 50, 100 and 200 mg capsules. Dosing regimens will vary according to the particular disease and its severity. Used in combination with antileprosy chemotherapy, the dose for ENL ranges from 100 to 400 mg per day (see package insert). Dosages for HIV-associated oral aphthae and neutrophilic dermatoses are generally 100 mg per day. The most common dose-limiting side effect is sedation.

Patients with recalcitrant discoid or SCLE lesions (Fig. 130.5) have 75–90% clearance rates with thalidomide. The initial dose of 50–100 mg/day is subsequently tapered to 25–50 mg/day after a clinical effect is seen, usually within 2 weeks. Acute cutaneous lesions of SLE have a 90% resolution rate, but require higher doses and a longer treatment period before results are noted. For some patients, intermittent courses of thalidomide (for 2–3 months) can be used to clear lesions, with antimalarials given concomitantly and as maintenance therapy.

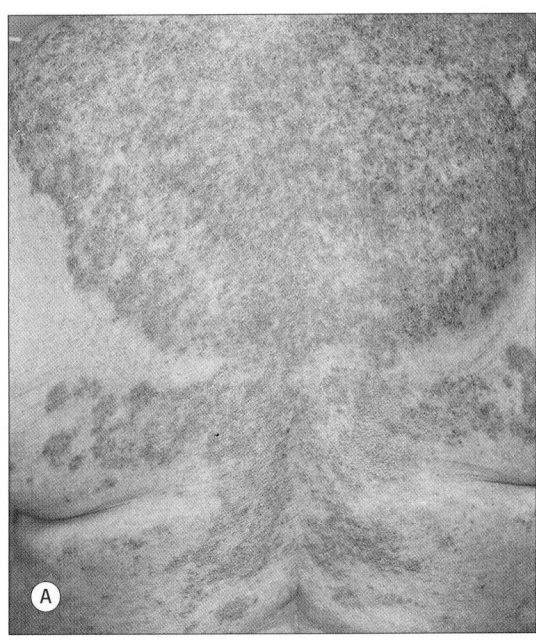

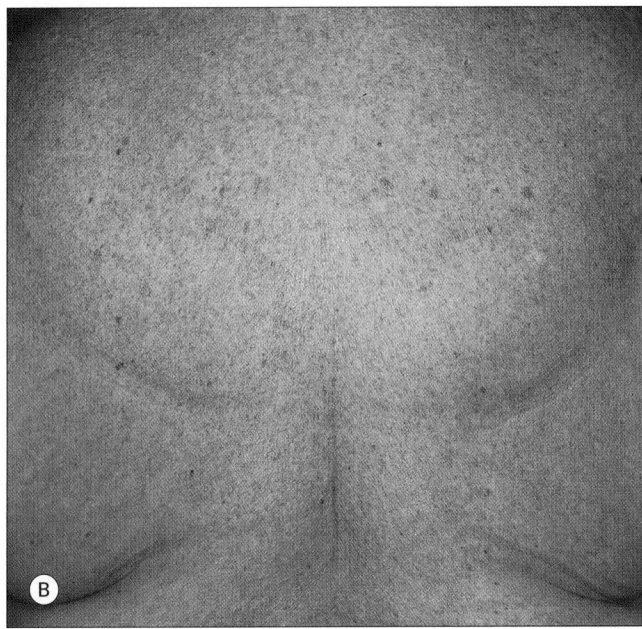

Fig. 130.5 Effect of thalidomide on subacute cutaneous lupus erythematosus. The patient's disease was not controlled despite prednisone (60 mg/day), hydroxychloroquine (600 mg/day!) and isotretinoin (60 mg/day), all for at least 2 months (**A**). Thalidomide (50–100 mg/day) was begun and the lesions resolved over 6 to 8 weeks (**B**). Courtesy of Jean L Bolognia MD.

Major Side Effects

A single dose of thalidomide during the first 21–36 days of gestation yields a 100% incidence of birth defects (see Table 130.4). Sedation is by far the most common adverse side effect and may necessitate night-time dosing and a gradual titration of the thalidomide dose. Constipation is also relatively common. Permanent nerve damage (primarily sensory neuropathy) can develop and is more common with long-term therapy. Measurements of sensory nerve action potential amplitudes (SNAP) may be indicated before and/or during therapy. Amenorrhea and primary ovarian failure may occur.

Severe leukopenia, exfoliative erythroderma and TEN are rare, but severe, consequences of thalidomide treatment. A hypersensitivity reaction specific to HIV-positive patients has been described. Common dermatologic side effects include brittle fingernails, xerosis, pruritus and red palms. Peripheral edema can develop occasionally. Vascular thromboses are unusual unless the patient is receiving concomitant corticosteroids or chemotherapy.

Indications

Thalidomide is FDA-approved and 99% effective for ENL (type II leprosy reaction). It has no effect on type I leprosy reactions. A variety of off-label uses of thalidomide have emerged over the years[37]. The beneficial effects for cutaneous lupus are discussed above. HIV-associated mucosal ulceration and aphthae associated with neutrophilic dermatoses (including Behçet's disease) respond rapidly to thalidomide, but also relapse quickly when it is discontinued. Patients with either GVHD or unusually severe treatment-resistant prurigo nodularis may also experience significant improvement with thalidomide. However, the highest rate of peripheral neuropathy has been observed in prurigo nodularis patients[37]. Thalidomide can also be an effective treatment for multiple myeloma and scleromyxedema.

Contraindications

Absolute contraindications to thalidomide therapy include sensitivity to thalidomide, pregnancy and a pre-existing peripheral neuropathy. Women of childbearing potential must agree to use highly effective methods of birth control (e.g. two reliable forms of contraception simultaneously). Men taking thalidomide who have female partners of childbearing potential must wear condoms (even if they have had a vasectomy) while their partners use an additional form of birth control (either oral or barrier). *Relative* contraindications include significant hepatic or renal disease, a history of neurologic disease, congestive heart failure, hypertension, constipation and hypothyroidism. In patients with a predisposing condition (e.g. antiphospholipid antibodies, myeloma), there can be an increased risk of thromboses. Individuals receiving antimalarials should continue to do so, because these drugs have been reported to inhibit platelet aggregation and adhesion.

Use in Pregnancy and Lactation

Thalidomide is pregnancy prescribing category X and should not be used in pregnant women. It is wise to avoid thalidomide in nursing mothers.

Drug Interactions

Thalidomide may amplify the sedative effects of alcohol, barbiturates, chlorpromazine and reserpine. Any drug that significantly induces the CYP 3A4 enzymes may decrease the effectiveness of hormonal contraception, increasing the potential of pregnancy and, thus, teratogenicity.

REFERENCES

1. Callen JP, Camisa C. Antimalarial agents. In: Wolverton SE (ed.). Comprehensive Dermatologic Drug Therapy. Philadelphia: WB Saunders, 2001:251–68.
2. Weiss JS. Antimalarial medications in dermatology. Dermatol Clin. 1991;9:377–85.
3. Willoughby JS, Shear NH. Antimalarials. Clin Dermatol. 1989;7:60–8.
4. Isaacson D, Elgart M, Turner ML. Anti-malarials in dermatology. Int J Dermatol. 1982;21:379–95.
5. Briggs GG, Freeman RK, Yaffe SJ. Drugs in Pregnancy and Lactation, 7th edn. Baltimore: Lippincott Williams & Wilkins, 2005.
6. Nashel DJ. Mechanisms of action and clinical applications of cytotoxic drugs in rheumatic disorders. Med Clin North Am. 1985;69:817–40.
7. Badalamenti S, Kerdel FA. Azathioprine. In: Wolverton SE (ed.). Comprehensive Dermatologic Drug Therapy. Philadelphia: WB Saunders, 2001:165–79.
8. Rapini RP. Cytotoxic drugs in the treatment of skin disease. Int J Dermatol. 1991;30:313–22.
9. Ahmed AR, Hombal SM. Cyclophosphamide, a review on relevant pharmacology and clinical uses. J Am Acad Dermatol. 1984;11:1115–26.
10. Pan TD, McDonald CJ. Cytotoxic agents. In: Wolverton SE (ed.). Comprehensive Dermatologic Drug Therapy. Philadelphia: WB Saunders, 2001:180–204.
11. McDonald CJ. Cytotoxic agents for use in dermatology. J Am Acad Dermatol. 1985;12:753–75.
12. Koo JYM, Lee CS, Maloney JE. Cyclosporine and related drugs. In: Wolverton SE (ed.). Comprehensive Dermatologic Drug Therapy. Philadelphia: WB Saunders, 2001:205–29.
13. Dutz JP, Ho VC. Immunosuppressive agents in dermatology, an update. Dermatol Ther. 1998; 16:235–51.

14. Koo J, Lee J. Cyclosporine, what clinicians need to know. Psoriasis. 1995;13:897–907.

15. Grossman RM, Chevret S, Abi-Rached J, et al. Long-term safety of cyclosporin in the treatment of psoriasis. Arch Dermatol. 1996;132:623–9.

16. Zachariae H. Renal toxicity of long-term cyclosporin. Scand J Rheumatol. 1999;28:65–8.

17. Luke RG. Mechanism of cyclosporine-induced hypertension. Am J Hypertension. 1991;4:468–71.

17a. Griffiths CEM, Katsambas A, Dijkmans BAC, et al. Update on the use of ciclosporin in immune-mediated dermatoses. Br J Dermatol. 2006;155(Suppl 2):1–16.

18. Zuidema J, Hilbers-Modderman ESM, Merkus FWHM. Clinical pharmacokinetics of dapsone. Clin Pharmacokinet. 1986;11:299–315.

19. Hall RP. Dapsone. In: Wolverton SE (ed.). Comprehensive Dermatologic Drug Therapy. Philadelphia: WB Saunders, 2001:230–50.

20. Coleman MD. Dapsone: modes of action, toxicity and possible strategies for increasing patient tolerance. Br J Dermatol. 1993;129:507–13.

21. Boyd AS, Neldner KH. Hydroxyurea therapy. J Am Acad Dermatol. 1991;25:518–24.

22. Knable AL. Miscellaneous systemic drugs. In: Wolverton SE (ed.). Comprehensive Dermatologic Drug Therapy. Philadelphia: WB Saunders, 2001:445–70.

23. Viard I, Wehrli P, Bullani R, et al. Inhibition of toxic epidermal necrolysis by blockade of CD95 with human intravenous immunoglobulin. Science. 1998;282:490–3.

24. Ahmed AR, Dahl MV. Consensus statement on the use of intravenous immunoglobulin therapy in the treatment of autoimmune mucocutaneous blistering diseases. Arch Dermatol. 2003;139:1051–9.

24a. Segura S, Iranzo P, Martinez-dePablo I, et al. High-dose intravenous immunoglobulins for the treatment of autoimmune mucocutaneous blistering diseases: Evaluation of its use in 19 cases. J Am Acad Dermatol. 2007;56:960–7.

24b. Pereira FA, Mudgil AV, Rosmarin DM. Toxic epidermal necrolysis. J Am Acad Dermatol. 2007;56:181–200.

25. Olsen EA. The mechanism of action of methotrexate. Rheum Dis Clin North Am. 1997;23:739–55.

26. Roenigk HH Jr, Auerbach R, Maibach HI, et al. Methotrexate in psoriasis: consensus conference. J Am Acad Dermatol. 1998;25:478–85.

27. Zachariae H. Liver biopsies and methotrexate: a time for reconsideration. J Am Acad Dermatol. 2000; 42:531–4.

28. Callen JP, Kulp-Shorten CL, Wolverton SE. Methotrexate. In: Wolverton SE (ed). Comprehensive Dermatologic Drug Therapy. Philadelphia: WB Saunders, 2001:147–64.

29. Kitchin JES, Pomeranz MK, Pak G, et al. Rediscovering mycophenolic acid: a review of its mechanism, side effects, and potential uses. J Am Acad Dermatol. 1997;37:445–9.

30. Grundmann-Kollmann M, Korting HC, Behrens S, et al. Mycophenolate mofetil: a new therapeutic option in the treatment of blistering autoimmune diseases. J Am Acad Dermatol. 1999;40:957–60.

31. Sterling JB, Heymann WR. Potassium iodide in dermatology: a 19th century drug for the 21st century – uses, pharmacology, adverse effects, and contraindications. J Am Acad Dermatol. 2000;43:691–7.

32. Horio T, Danno K, Okamoto H, et al. Potassium iodide in erythema nodosum and other erythematous dermatoses. J Am Acad Dermatol. 1983;9:77–91.

33. Restrepo A. Treatment of tropical mycoses. J Am Acad Dermatol. 1994;31:S91–102.

34. Davis LS. Newer uses of older drugs – an update. In: Wolverton SE (ed.). Comprehensive Dermatologic Drug Therapy. Philadelphia: WB Saunders, 2001:426–44.

35. Lin AN. Topical immunotherapy. In: Wolverton SE (ed.). Comprehensive Dermatologic Drug Therapy. Philadelphia: WB Saunders, 2001:607–29.

36. Powell RJ, Gardner-Medwin JMM. Guideline for the clinical use and dispensing of thalidomide. Postgrad Med J. 1994;70:901–4.

37. Faver IR, Guerra SG, Su WP, el-Azhary R. Thalidomide for dermatology: a review of clinical uses and adverse effects. Int J Dermatol. 2005;44:61–7.

Drug Interactions

Lori E Shapiro, Sandra R Knowles and Neil H Shear

131

INTRODUCTION

There are two concerns in drug safety: drug reactions and drug interactions. When multiple drug therapies are prescribed, drug interactions become an important safety and efficacy consideration for patients and physicians alike[1]. Non-prescription drugs, and herbal or alternative medicines and foods (such as grapefruit juice), may also be implicated in interactions with drug therapy.

It is difficult to obtain precise rates of incidence and prevalence, as specific diagnostic codes for drug interactions are lacking[2]. Drug interactions are responsible for up to 2.8% of hospital admissions[3,4]. It has been estimated that adverse drug outcomes occur about once every 100 patient days[3,5]. Although it is impossible to remember all potential drug interactions, knowledge of the interactive properties of drugs can help reduce the risk of serious adverse outcomes. Moreover, it is the responsibility of physicians to counsel patients regarding drug interactions[6]. Unfortunately, even when serious new drug interactions are recognized and reported, physicians, pharmacists and patients are often unaware that there is a risk[7].

PUTTING INTERACTIONS INTO PERSPECTIVE

Prescribing drugs with the potential for a deleterious interaction increases the risk of, but need not lead to, an adverse outcome. Many drug interactions are susceptible to control by dose adjustment. Some are even beneficial and are exploited to therapeutic advantage. In a cross-sectional study, all prescriptions involving two or more drugs dispensed to the Swedish population from all Swedish pharmacies in January 1999 were analyzed[8]. This paper was reassuring in that potential interactions that could have had serious clinical consequences occurred in 1.4% each of prescriptions for men and women. Of note, over half (52%) of these potential interactions were between ipratropium and β-adrenergic agonists, with an increased risk of acute angle closure glaucoma only when the drugs were used in nebulized form, an uncommon method of delivery.

Most drugs are associated with interactions, but many do not produce significant outcomes[9]. Not all listed or reported drug interactions are clinically significant. Some have little clinical relevance, whereas others are clearly defined as contraindications on the basis of substantiation of risk, potential severity and frequency of cases. Others can be successfully managed by dosage adjustment and monitoring. One recent study looked at the occurrence of drug interactions from the adverse events reported during mega clinical trials[10]. The authors concluded that serious adverse drug reactions (ADRs) secondary to drug–drug interactions are infrequent; however, drug–drug interactions that involved selected drugs with a narrow therapeutic index (which elicited life-threatening undesired effects) did occur. Serious ADRs secondary to drug–drug interactions were most frequent in elderly patients, in the presence of polypharmacy, in the psychiatric patient population, and in the presence of inappropriate prescriptions or multiple prescribers. Again, the vast majority of reported drug interactions result in adverse outcomes in a minority of patients who receive the interacting combination. Thus, for most drug interactions, it is necessary to assess each patient situation individually.

ASSESSMENT OF RISK IN THE CLINICAL OUTCOME OF DRUG INTERACTIONS

The clinical importance of specific drug interactions is often either over- or underestimated, as these assessments are largely based on clinical experience in using a particular drug combination[11]. The clinical outcome of most drug interactions is highly situational, as most patients who receive drugs with the potential for interactions do not develop adverse effects. Emphasis should be placed on those factors that increase or decrease the risk to a given patient.

To prevent or detect drug interactions, the physician needs to identify risk factors in the individual patient. Some patient groups are more likely than others to develop adverse events caused by drug interactions (Table 131.1). Risk factors are listed and grouped by category in this table[12].

The elderly frequently experience drug interactions because of the physiologic changes that accompany the aging process and the types of drugs that older patients tend to receive[13]. Polypharmacy, which is common in the elderly, makes them particularly susceptible. Various medications may impair pathways of drug elimination by interfering with drug metabolism, thereby increasing the likelihood of adverse drug reactions. Alterations due to advanced age, including changes in drug–protein binding and drug distribution in tissue, may promote drug interactions. Most adverse metabolic drug interactions occur when an inhibitor or inducer is begun in a patient who previously had stable levels of a substrate drug.

Patients with AIDS also have a high rate of adverse drug reactions[14]. In some instances, this may relate to phenotypic changes in drug metabolism, which can vary with HIV progression[15]. HIV can alter enzyme function, with resultant changes in drug metabolism and a higher rate of adverse reactions in these patients.

A major source of interindividual differences in drug metabolism is genetic polymorphisms, which are inherited significant variations in the activity of drug metabolizing enzymes. These polymorphisms exist for various cytochrome P450 (CYP) isoforms and N-acetyltransferase. There are also interethnic differences in drug metabolism, with differences in the expression of cytochrome P450 isoforms and glucuronyl transferase as well as different frequencies of genetic polymorphisms. Several genetic polymorphisms have been well studied at the epidemiologic, protein and DNA level. In some cases, it is possible to determine an individual's genotype[16]. Further details on genetic polymorphisms are discussed later in the chapter.

Interactions with other drugs can predispose a patient to the development of certain types of ADR. For example, systemic corticosteroids

PATIENT RISK FACTORS FOR DRUG INTERACTIONS
• Multiple medications – polypharmacy
• Demographic risk factors
– Female gender
– Extremes of age (very young and elderly)
• Major organ dysfunction (especially multiple medical problems)
– Liver dysfunction
– Renal dysfunction*
– Congestive heart failure
• Metabolic and endocrine risk factors
– Obesity
– Hypothyroidism
– Hypoproteinemia
• Pharmacogenetic risk factors
– Slow acetylator phenotype
– Other genetic polymorphisms (see text)
• Other medical issues
– Hypothermia
– Hypotension
– Dehydration

May be underestimated in elderly patients.

Table 131.1 Patient risk factors for drug interactions[13].

may increase the background risk of Stevens–Johnson syndrome or toxic epidermal necrolysis due to other drugs[17]. Valproic acid increases the risk of severe cutaneous adverse reactions to lamotrigine[18], and allopurinol increases the risk of exanthematous eruptions to antibiotics. A disease state itself may directly affect the likelihood of an ADR. For example, active infection with EBV or CMV increases the risk of exanthematous eruptions to amoxicillin. The basis of these interactions is unknown but may represent a combination of factors, including alterations in drug metabolism, drug detoxification, antioxidant defenses and immune reactivity[19]. The disease state may dictate the way in which a drug is used, and this will subsequently affect the outcome. When a drug has more than one therapeutic action, an interacting drug may affect the action of another drug when it is used to treat one disease but not when it is used to treat another disease. This is known as pharmacologic selectivity.

An example of intrinsic effects of disease states would be when epinephrine is given to patients receiving non-cardioselective β-adrenergic blockers (but who do not have anaphylaxis) and this results in hypertension. In contrast, the same β-blockers inhibit the pressor response to epinephrine[20] when the latter is given to patients with anaphylaxis.

An example of a disease-dependent drug interaction is the concomitant use of non-steroidal anti-inflammatory drugs (NSAIDs) and methotrexate. Available evidence indicates that the risk of this combination is considerably greater in patients receiving high-dose methotrexate for cancer than it is in patients receiving lower weekly dosages for psoriasis[21]. This is because the distribution of the drug is not very important mechanistically in determining drug interactions, but changes in drug elimination are. When larger doses of methotrexate (as are used in cancer therapy) are given in combination with an NSAID, drug elimination becomes an important issue, increasing the risk of methotrexate toxicity.

Gender-related differences in pharmacokinetics may cause variations in drug absorption, gastric emptying and distribution based on percentage of adipose tissue[22]. Gender-related differences in receptor density and sensitivity, enzyme activity (CYP2D6) and underlying disease activities also contribute to pharmacokinetic variation. The effect of obesity on metabolism is cytochrome-specific. For example, obesity decreases the activity of CYP3A4 and increases the activity of CYP2E1[17].

That certain medications are most likely to be involved in drug interactions must also be borne in mind. Clinically significant interactions occur more frequently with drugs that have a narrow margin of safety, i.e. a narrow therapeutic window. Drugs with the potential for such serious interactions include warfarin, monoamine oxidase inhibitors, and cyclosporine.

Medication-related factors that contribute to the clinical risk include the dose, route of administration and duration of administration of the precipitant drug (the drug that causes the interaction) and the sequence of administration of the interacting drugs. Most metabolic drug interactions are dose-related. That is, as the dose of the precipitant drug is increased, the magnitude of its effect on the object drug tends to increase. Thus, the dose of the precipitant drug is often an important determinant of risk to the patient. The dose of the object drug may also affect the risk of an adverse drug interaction. For example, a patient who takes small doses of an object drug with serum concentrations at the lower end of the target range is at a lesser risk when an enzyme-inhibiting precipitant drug is added than would be a patient taking large doses of the same object drug.

The route of administration is an important risk factor for some non-metabolic drug interactions, such as when one drug binds another in the gastrointestinal (GI) tract. However, the route of administration can also be important for metabolic drug interactions, especially when the drug undergoes extensive first-pass metabolism in the gut wall and liver by CYP3A4 or P-glycoprotein. Most drug interactions have a typical time course over which the effects develop. Therefore, giving rifampin, a typical inducer of CYP3A4, for only a few days is unlikely to have much effect on substrates of CYP3A4, as induction of an enzyme takes weeks to occur.

In summary, there is pharmacodynamic and pharmacokinetic variability between people, as well as host variability in terms of disease state. Overall, this variability contributes to confusion, as tables and lists that outline potentially interacting medications vary between different sources. One reason is that various levels of evidence exist for many drugs in terms of their ability to contribute to/cause drug interactions. This is outlined in more detail below.

LEVELS OF EVIDENCE

Drug interaction literature is often confusing due to poorly substantiated claims[23]. This confusion occurs as a result of inaccurate or cursory evaluations of published cases or inappropriate extrapolations from the literature. Metabolic drug interactions are a major source of potential clinical problems, but their investigation during drug development is often incomplete. *In vitro* studies give very accurate data on the interactions of drugs with selective CYP isozymes, but their interpretation in the clinical context is difficult. Although *in vitro* systems have been developed to test the effects of certain drugs on the metabolism of other drugs, these systems may not accurately predict the effect in patients receiving drugs with complex metabolism. Also, problems with the detection of adverse events after a drug has been released arise mainly because such events are rare. It takes a surveillance system with a high degree of sensitivity to detect such problems[24].

Furthermore, most *in vivo* and *in vitro* studies of drug interactions evaluate two-drug regimens, and the results may not apply to the multidrug regimens used clinically. This is especially true for a regimen consisting of three or more drugs with opposing effects on CYP3A4 metabolism. The lack of studies of multiple drug interactions provides little assistance to the prescribing physician, who is left to rely on adverse events or treatment failure to demonstrate whether an interaction has occurred. In addition, the design of *in vivo* studies is sometimes poor (choice of prototype substrate, doses, schedule of administration, number of volunteers), with the risk of minimizing the real potential for interaction. To link *in vitro* and *in vivo* studies, several authors have suggested using extrapolation techniques, based on the comparison of *in vitro* inhibition data with the active *in vivo* concentrations of the inhibitor. However, the lack of knowledge with regard to one or several important parameters, such as the role of metabolites and intrahepatocyte accumulation, often limits the ability to make safe and accurate predictions. The uncertainty and inaccuracy of predicting the extent and duration of *in vivo* drug interactions currently stems from a lack of definitive models by which to assess likely substrate and inhibitor concentrations at the active site of metabolism. Additional issues contributing to the uncertainty of predicting drug interactions include assumptions of the contribution of presystemic drug extraction and the effect of inhibitors on the processes involved. As a consequence, these methods are useful for complementing *in vitro* studies and helping to design clinically relevant *in vivo* studies, but in the foreseeable future they will not totally replace *in vivo* investigations. One group has developed a computerized application, the quantitative drug interactions prediction system (Q-DIPS), to make both qualitative deductions and quantitative predictions on the basis of a database containing updated information on CYP substrates, inhibitors and inducers, as well as pharmacokinetic parameters[25].

ABSORPTION

Interactions that alter the absorption of drugs often lead to dramatic changes in plasma drug concentrations. Drug interactions within the GI tract can result in decreased absorption. This reduces the bioavailability or the amount of drug available to the systemic circulation and results in subtherapeutic serum concentrations. The underlying mechanisms of most drug interactions that alter GI absorption involve: (1) the formation of drug complexes that reduce absorption; (2) alterations in the gastric pH; and/or (3) changes in GI motility that alter transit time[26].

Common drugs that form complexes with other drugs include antacids, sucralfate, and cholesterol-binding resins. A significant interaction occurs between multivalent cations – such as calcium, aluminum, iron and magnesium – and tetracyclines and fluoroquinolone antibiotics. For example, there is an 85% reduction in the absorption of ciprofloxacin when ingested 5–10 minutes after a dose of an aluminum hydroxide/magnesium hydroxide antacid[27]. These interactions can be easily avoided by administering the fluoroquinolone at least 2 hours

MYCOPHENOLATE METABOLISM

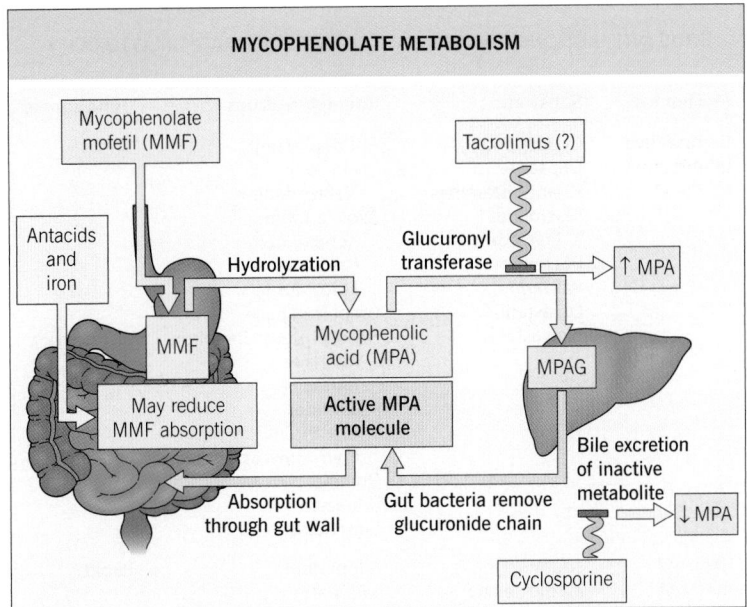

Fig. 131.1 Mycophenolate metabolism. Mycophenolate is hydrolyzed to mycophenolic acid (MPA). Following glucuronidation in the liver, inactive MPA glucuronide (MPAG) is excreted into the gut via bile acid secretion. In the gut, bacteria remove the glucuronide chain to produce MPA, the active molecule, which is then reabsorbed through the gut wall. Cyclosporine impairs MPA enterohepatic recirculation by inhibiting biliary excretion of MPAG (thereby *decreasing* MPA levels), whereas tacrolimus may inhibit UDP-glucuronyl transferase (thereby *increasing* MPA levels).

before or 6 hours after the antacid. Alendronate, as well as other bisphosphonates prescribed for the prevention and treatment of osteoporosis, form complexes with cations and many other drugs, thereby further decreasing their already low oral absorption. When mycophenolate mofetil and iron preparations were administered concomitantly, a remarkable decrease in mycophenolate mofetil absorption was observed (Fig. 131.1)[28]. When mycophenolate mofetil and iron ion preparations were administered concomitantly, a decrease in mycophenolate mofetil absorption was observed in some studies.

Drugs that increase gastric pH, such as proton pump inhibitors, antacids and H_2 antihistamines, may reduce the absorption of drugs such as ketoconazole and itraconazole, which are best absorbed in an acidic environment[29]. Although itraconazole is best absorbed when the gastric pH is low, its administration with food is more important for achieving high plasma concentrations[30]. The absorption of fluconazole is unaffected by variations in gastric pH[31]. Drugs that affect GI motility, such as anticholinergic agents, may decrease the rate of absorption but not the extent of absorption. An overall reduction in drug absorption has more clinical significance[32].

Some drugs may interfere with the enterohepatic recirculation of a substrate drug. When the substrate is excreted into the GI tract, a second drug can bind to it and prevent its reabsorption back into the systemic circulation. The bound substrate drug is excreted in the feces, thereby effectively shortening its half-life. An example of this is the concurrent administration of warfarin and cholestyramine, in which the half-life of warfarin is shortened by oral cholestyramine.

P-glycoprotein (PGP)

Membrane-bound transport systems may also determine drug disposition[33]. PGP is an ATP-dependent plasma membrane glycoprotein (Fig. 131.2) belonging to the superfamily of ATP-binding cassette transporters[34]. In humans, the multidrug resistance (MDR) genes, including *MDR1*, encode membrane glycoproteins that function as drug transporters and hence affect both drug absorption and elimination. High levels of PGP are found in superficial columnar epithelial cells of the small intestine, apical surface epithelial cells of the proximal tubules of the kidney, and in the biliary canalicular membrane of hepatocytes. PGP is also detected in high concentrations in the endothelial cells of the capillaries of the blood–brain barrier, testes, uterus and placenta. An understanding of the physiologic regulation of these transporter

P-GLYCOPROTEIN

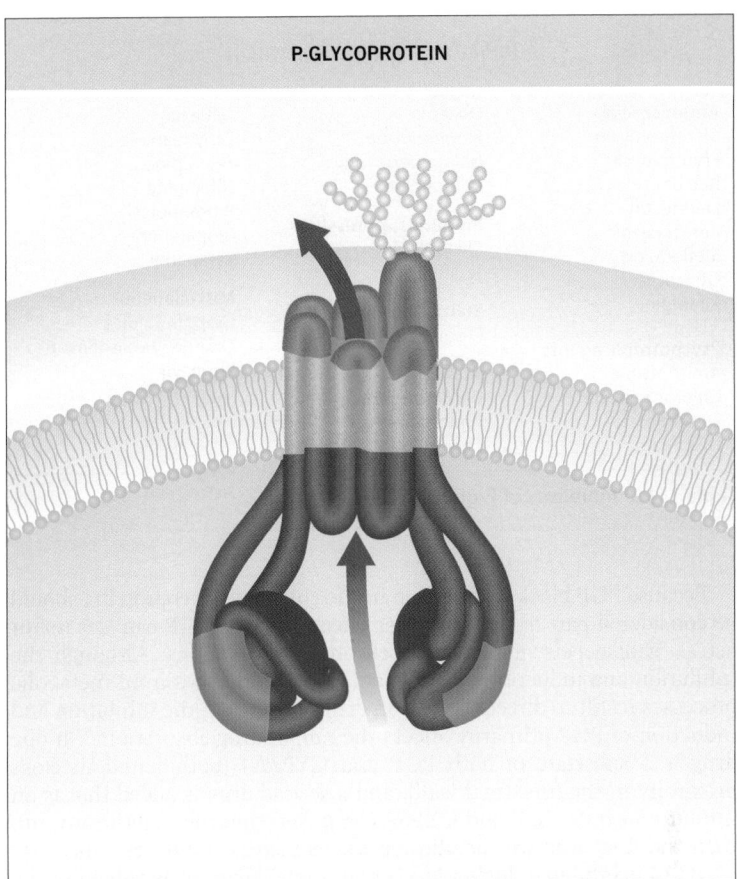

Fig. 131.2 P-Glycoprotein. This is an ATP-dependent plasma membrane glycoprotein that functions as a drug transporter and hence affects both drug absorption and elimination. Adapted from Kartner N, Ling V. Scientific American 1989;260:44–51.

P-GLYCOPROTEIN SUBSTRATES

Antimicrobials	Mitomycin C	**Cardiac agents**
Ciprofloxacin	Paclitaxel	Amiodarone
Erythromycin	Taxol	Atorvastatin
Ivermectin	Vinblastine	Diltiazem
Other quinolones	Vincristine	Digoxin
Rifampin		Lovastatin
	Antiemetics	Nadolol
HIV protease inhibitors	Domperidone	Pravastatin
Indinavir	Ondansetron	Propranolol
Nelfinavir		Timolol
Ritonavir	**Rheumatologic agents**	Quinidine
Saquinavir	Colchicine	Verapamil
	Methotrexate	
Anticancer agents	Quinine	**Miscellaneous**
Actinomycin D		Cimetidine
Daunorubicin	**Immunosuppressives**	Lidocaine
Doxorubicin	Cyclosporine	Loperamide
Etoposide	Tacrolimus	Terfenadine*

*Historical

Table 131.2 P-Glycoprotein substrates.

proteins is key to designing strategies for improving the therapeutic efficacy of drugs that serve as their substrates (Table 131.2).

These membrane-bound transport systems appear to have developed as a mechanism for protecting the body from harmful substances. It appears that PGP acts as a pump whereby the efflux of drugs from the cell membrane or cytoplasm is powered by the energy from ATP hydrolysis. For example, the aminoglycoside antibiotics amikacin and tobramycin are not effectively delivered orally, perhaps because of active efflux from the brush border cells of the small intestine by the PGP pump. The most remarkable property of PGP is its ability to transport a diverse array of compounds that do not appear to share obvious structural characteristics. The range of substrates, inhibitors and inducers of PGP is vast and expanding (Tables 131.2 & 131.3).

INHIBITORS OF P-GLYCOPROTEIN		
Antimicrobials Clarithromycin Erythromycin Itraconazole Ivermectin Ketoconazole Mefloquine Ofloxacin Rifampin **Psychotropic agents** Amitriptyline Chlorpromazine Desipramine Disulfiram	Doxepin Fluphenazine Haloperidol Imipramine **Immunosuppressives** Cyclosporine Tacrolimus **Steroid hormones** Progesterone Testosterone **Cardiac agents** Amiodarone Carvedilol	Diltiazem Dipyridamole Felodipine Nifedipine Propranolol Propafenone Verapamil **Miscellaneous** Grapefruit juice Orange juice isoflavones Ritonavir

Table 131.3 Inhibitors of P-glycoprotein.

Because PGP blocks absorption in the gut, these glycoproteins should be considered part of the 'first-pass effect'. In fact, PGP can 'set up' or act as 'gatekeepers' for later cytochrome P450 actions. Although the inhibition and induction of intestinal CYP3A enzymes from metabolic processes result in direct changes in drug absorption, the inhibition and induction of PGP primarily affects the rate of drug absorption[35]. If one drug is a substrate of both PGP and CYP3A4 (both found in close proximity in the intestinal wall), and a second drug is added that is an inhibitor of both PGP and CYP3A4 (e.g. ketoconazole, erythromycin), then the first drug will be allowed in, in increased amounts. Because CYP3A4 is inhibited, higher levels of unmetabolized drug will enter the blood. The effect of PGP blockade is to 'open the gates' so that the later actions of CYP3A4 inhibition will be increased.

Evidence suggests that intestinal PGP plays a significant role in the first-pass elimination of cyclosporine, probably by being a rate-limiting step in absorption. Intestinal CYP3A4 is thought to play a lesser role[36]. However, the overlap of tissue distribution and substrate specificity of CYP3A4 and PGP in the intestinal wall makes it difficult to define the precise mechanisms of some drug interactions and to predict the plasma concentrations of certain drug combinations. Moreover, the involvement of CYP3A4 and PGP in drug interactions is not always complementary.

PGP also plays a role in the development of resistance to medications. One pertinent dermatologic example is that resistance to ivermectin has been documented in animals to occur through PGP[37].

DISTRIBUTION

Drugs that are highly protein bound (>90%) may cause interactions based on alterations in distribution. When one drug displaces another from plasma protein-binding sites, the free serum concentration of the displaced drug is increased and its pharmacologic effect increases. However, the unbound fraction of the drug is not only more available to sites of action but is also more readily eliminated. Any enhanced pharmacologic effect occurs only transiently because of a compensatory increase in elimination, and the *effect of displacement interactions is then negligible*. Therefore, interactions involving drug displacement from binding proteins tend to be self-limiting[38]. Typically, the pharmacologic activity of the displaced drug is increased for a few days. This is followed by a return of the pharmacologic response back to the previous unbound serum concentration, even if the concomitant therapy is continued. Therefore, it is safe to say that if a patient does not manifest an adverse event from the combination therapy in the first week or so of administration, an adverse event probably will not occur. In practice, protein-binding displacement interactions do not produce clinically important changes in drug response unless the drug also has a limited distribution in the body, is slowly eliminated, or has a low therapeutic index[32]. For this reason, protein-binding displacement interactions may assume greater importance when the displacing drug also reduces the elimination of the substrate drug. A good example of this principle involves interactions between NSAIDs and methotrexate (Table 131.4).

DRUG INTERACTIONS THAT INCREASE RISK OF SUBSTRATE DRUG TOXICITY			
Mechanism	**Substrate**	**Interactive drugs**	**Time course**

Competitive inhibition of CYP3A4*	Cyclosporine
	Dapsone
	H_1 antihistamines
	Macrolides
	  Erythromycin
	Phenytoin
	Warfarin
	Lovastatin
	Simvastatin
		Antidepressants
		  Fluoxetine
		  Nefazodone
		Azole antifungals
		  Ketoconazole
		  Itraconazole
		  Fluconazole
		Grapefruit juice
		HIV-1 protease inhibitors
		  Indinavir
		  Ritonavir
		Macrolides
		  Clarithromycin
		  Erythromycin
		Quinine
		Diltiazem
		Cimetidine
			Rapid

Reduced metabolic clearance	Azathioprine Methotrexate	Allopurinol Salicylates	Rapid
Displacement from plasma proteins	Methotrexate	NSAIDs Salicylates Sulfonamides	Rapid
Reduced renal elimination	Methotrexate	NSAIDs Penicillins Probenecid Salicylates Sulfonamides	Rapid
Synergy	Methotrexate Retinoids Acitretin Serotonin reuptake inhibitors	Retinoids Sulfonamides Tetracyclines Alcohol Monoamine oxidase inhibitors	Variable Variable Variable

Also A5 and A7.

Table 131.4 Drug interactions that increase risk of substrate drug toxicity[2,3].

Medications that are most susceptible to interactions based on changes in drug distribution involving displacement from binding proteins include warfarin, sulfonamides and phenytoin[13].

PGP is an important component of the blood–brain barrier. Active PGP will prevent drugs from entering the brain. It has been suggested that the reason newer antihistamines do not cause sedation is due to PGP activity acting as a barrier to central penetration. This would suggest that PGP inhibitors (see Table 131.3) could interact with and allow increased cerebral concentrations of these antihistamines, with an attendant increase in sedation[39].

DRUG BIOTRANSFORMATION

Cytochrome P450 Enzymes

After their administration, drugs are metabolized through a series of reactions to enhance their hydrophilicity and to facilitate excretion. These drug biotransformation reactions are broadly grouped into two phases, I and II. Phase I reactions involve intramolecular changes such as oxidation, reduction and hydrolysis that make the drug more polar and therefore more readily eliminated. Phase II reactions are conjugation reactions in which an endogenous substance combines with the functional group derived from phase I reactions to produce a highly polar drug conjugate that can be even more readily eliminated. These reactions involve glucuronidation and sulfation.

The cytochrome P450 enzymes (Fig. 131.3) are the major drug-metabolizing enzymes. They are present in the endoplasmic reticulum of many cells but are at their highest concentration in hepatocytes[40]. In the GI tract, P450 enzymes are present in the crypt cells, but the highest concentration is found in the enterocytes at the tips of the villi;

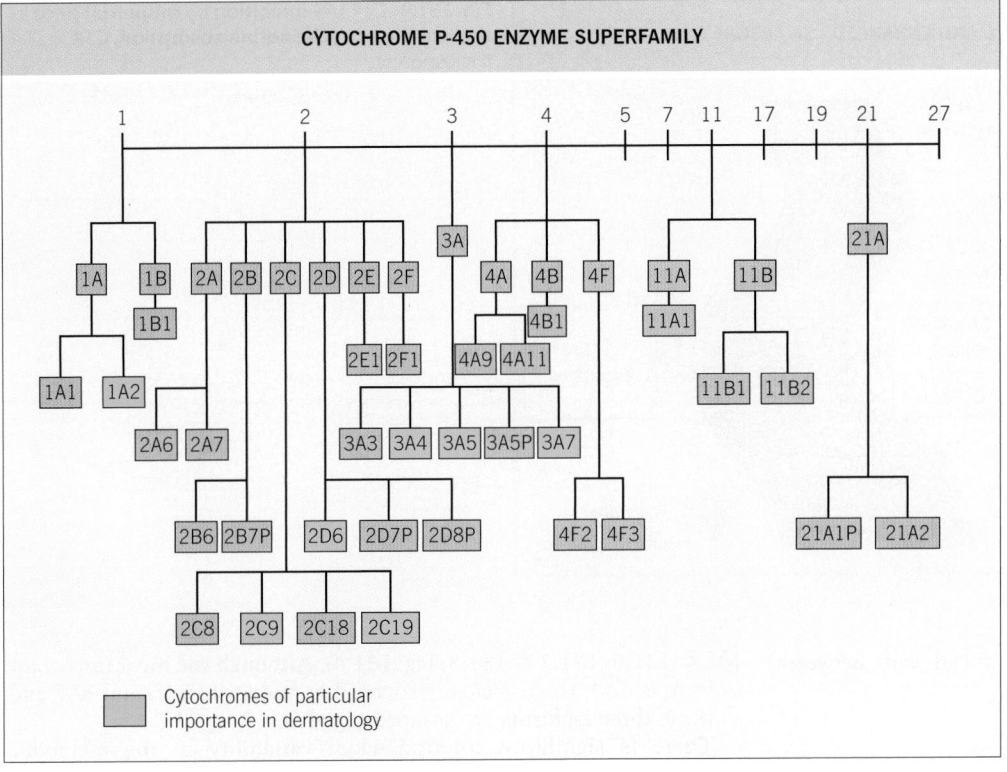

Fig. 131.3 Cytochrome P-450 enzyme superfamily.

their presence accounts for the first-pass metabolism of many drugs. These heme-containing proteins are encoded by a gene superfamily, with the encoded isoforms exhibiting distinct but overlapping substrate specificities and isoform-specific regulatory and pharmacogenetic properties[41]. The nomenclature employs a three-tier classification consisting of the family (40% homology in amino acid sequence), the subfamily (77% homology) and the individual protein (e.g. CYP2D6).

An increased understanding of drug metabolism has solved much of the mystery behind drug interactions. Over 90% of drug oxidation can be attributed to six main cytochromes: CYP1A2, 2C9, 2C19, 2D6, 2E1 and 3A4. The metabolism of a drug by a specific isoenzyme indicates that it is a substrate for that enzyme. Whether enzyme inhibition or induction occurs is an entirely separate issue. Many drugs serve only as substrates and produce no significant enzyme inhibition or induction. It is entirely possible for a drug to be a substrate for one enzyme and inhibit or induce another enzyme that is not involved with its own metabolism. Therefore, drug interactions are more aptly termed drug–protein–drug (food) interactions. These are affected by genetics (polymorphic genes cause particular enzymes to be less effective, 2D6 being an example), drugs (a drug may inhibit or induce a cytochrome, or interfere in the chemical pathway of another drug, e.g. ketoconazole inhibits cyclosporine metabolism), chemicals (dioxin is an inducer of CYP3A4, and a food such as grapefruit juice is an inhibitor of CYP3A4 metabolism) and the environment (cigarette smoke is an inducer of CYP1A2). Deciding what is clinically relevant is a challenging, relatively new field of investigation.

Drug metabolism is investigated even before human exposure. With recombinant human cytochrome P450 enzymes, it is possible to determine the metabolic pathways, potential genetic polymorphisms, ability to induce or inhibit drug metabolism, and possible drug interactions. Although there are limitations to the information gleaned from *in vitro* studies, nonetheless this information can be used to guide more expensive *in vivo* studies.

Using *in vitro* tests that focus on cytochrome enzymes alone to predict clinical interactions may not always be reliable for a variety of reasons. First, it is not always possible to know the therapeutic concentration of a new drug and its primary metabolites in specific tissues[33]. Second, there are a large number of pathways and interactions, and it is impossible to test them all even in an *in vitro* system. Third, the demonstration of an *in vitro* effect does not tell physicians whether that effect is likely to occur in clinical practice, i.e. the clinical significance of an *in vitro* interaction is unknown. Fourth, there may be a contribution of the underlying disease state to the development of a drug interaction that is unaccounted for by *in vitro* studies alone. Until clinical data demonstrate the presence or absence of a clinically significant interaction, dosage adjustments are premature[42].

THE CONFUSING WORLD OF DRUG INTERACTIONS

Why does it take so long to learn about interactions? Some drugs come to market and their various interactions are not realized for several years. Drugs are prescribed on the basis of indications that may have their own adverse effects on patient outcome. Studies in healthy volunteers are not sufficient to determine the contribution of underlying diseases to the development of interactions. The latter are affected by genetics, drugs, chemicals, the underlying health status of the patient, the therapeutic index of the drug affected by the interaction, dose-related factors, the duration of coadministration, the time course of the interaction, whether active metabolites are involved, and the environment (Table 131.5).

The multiple metabolic pathways of some drugs make it difficult to predict the outcome of drug interactions. Gender-related differences in pharmacokinetics might cause variations in drug absorption, gastric emptying and distribution based on percentage of adipose tissue[22]. Gender-related differences in receptor density and sensitivity, enzyme activity (2D6) and underlying disease activities also contribute to pharmacokinetic variation. This variability causes confusion, as tables

INFLUENCES ON CYTOCHROME P450 ACTIVITY					
	Cytochrome P450				
	1A2	2C	2D6	2E1	3A4
Nutrition	↑			↑ (obesity ↑)	↓ (obesity ↓)
Smoking	↑				
Alcohol				↑	
Drugs	↑ or ↓	↑ or ↓	↑ or ↓		↑ or ↓
Environmental factors	↑			↑	↑
Genetics		↑ or ↓	+		

Table 131.5 Influences on cytochrome P450 activity.

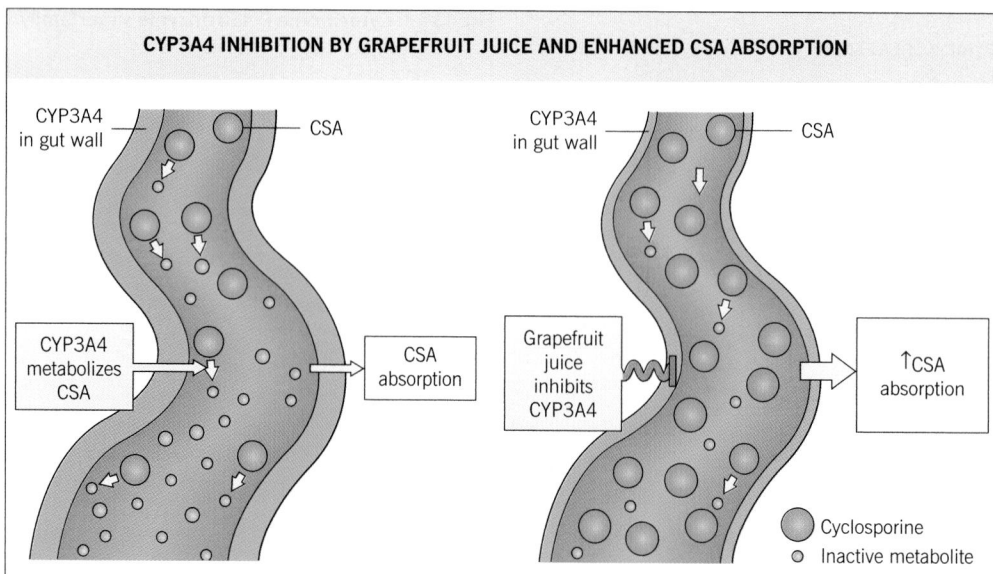

CYP3A4 INHIBITION BY GRAPEFRUIT JUICE AND ENHANCED CSA ABSORPTION

CYP3A4 in gut wall

CSA

CYP3A4 metabolizes CSA

CSA absorption

CYP3A4 in gut wall

CSA

Grapefruit juice inhibits CYP3A4

↑CSA absorption

○ Cyclosporine
· Inactive metabolite

Fig. 131.4 CYP3A4 inhibition by grapefruit juice and enhanced cyclosporine absorption. CSA, cyclosporine.

and lists outlining potentially interacting agents can vary between different sources[43].

Metabolism

The most clinically relevant drug interactions are caused by alterations in drug metabolism.

Members of the cytochrome P450 3A subfamily are the most abundant of the human hepatic cytochromes and account for up to 70% of GI cytochromes. CYP3A4 is also located in the placenta, uterus, kidney, lung and fetus. This subfamily is the major metabolizing isoform for many of the drugs prescribed by dermatologists (Tables 131.4, 131.6, 131.7 & 131.8; Fig. 131.4). Although the most important isoform is 3A4, there is close structural homology to 3A5 and 3A7 and so these three isoforms are grouped together.

There is significant interindividual variability in the metabolic activity of CYP3A. The extent of variability may be as much as 20-fold and the individual level of CYP3A4 activity probably has clinical relevance. Obesity also plays a role in drug metabolism in an enzyme-specific way[44]. Obesity decreases isoform 3A4 metabolism, and 33% of Americans are obese.

The successful application of information regarding cytochrome P450 to prevent drug interactions and improve the therapeutic risk:benefit ratio can occur only if we know which enzyme is responsible for the metabolism of a particular drug. Drug interactions should also be more predictable based on the knowledge of which compounds induce and inhibit specific P450 enzymes. Knowing all of the major enzyme substrates, inhibitors and inducers is a formidable task. Tables 131.7 to 131.10 are intended to summarize large amounts of this information.

DRUG INTERACTIONS THAT REDUCE THE EFFICACY OF SUBSTRATES

Mechanism	Substrate/ parent drug	Concomitant drugs	Time course
Reduced GI absorption	Itraconazole Ketoconazole	Antacids Didanosine H₂ antihistamines Proton pump inhibitors Sucralfate	Rapid
	Fluoroquinolones	Antacids Iron Sucralfate	
	Tetracycline	Divalent cations Calcium Magnesium Iron	
	Dapsone	Didanosine	
	Mycophenolate mofetil	Iron	
Induction of CYP3A4*	Calcineurin inhibitors Cyclosporine Tacrolimus Oral contraceptives Prednisone Warfarin	Anticonvulsants Carbamazepine Phenytoin Phenobarbital Antituberculous agents Isoniazid Rifampin Dexamethasone Griseofulvin	1–2 weeks
Antagonistic effects	Epinephrine Cyproheptadine	β-Blockers SSRI antidepressants Fluoxetine Paroxetine	

*Also A5, A7.

Table 131.6 Drug interactions that reduce the efficacy of substrates.

SUBSTRATES OF CYP3A4,5,7

Antiarrhythmics
Amiodarone
Digoxin
Lidocaine
Propafenone
Quinidine

Anticonvulsants
Carbamazepine
Ethosuximide
Phenytoin

Antidepressants
Amitriptyline
Doxepin
Imipramine
Sertraline

Antihistamines
Fexofenadine
Loratadine

Benzodiazepines
Alprazolam
Diazepam
Midazolam
Triazolam

Calcium channel blockers
Amlodipine

Diltiazem
Felodipine
Isradipine
Nifedipine
Verapamil

Cancer chemotherapy
Busulfan
Cyclophosphamide
Docetaxel
Doxorubicin
Etoposide
Ifosfamide
Paclitaxel
Tamoxifen
Vinblastine
Vincristine

HMG-CoA reductase inhibitors
Atorvastatin
Cerivastatin
Lovastatin
Simvastatin

Immunosuppressive drugs
Corticosteroids
Cyclophosphamide
Cyclosporine

Dapsone
Tacrolimus

Protease inhibitors
Indinavir
Nelfinavir
Ritonavir
Saquinavir

Miscellaneous
Acetaminophen
Cisapride*
Clarithromycin
Codeine
Enalapril
Erythromycin
Estrogens
Flutamide
Losartan
Montelukast
Omeprazole
Oral contraceptives
Pimozide
Retinoic acid
Rifampin
Sildenafil
Terazosin
Theophylline
Warfarin
Zileuton

Table 131.7 Substrates of CYP3A4,5,7[45]. *Historical.

CYP3A4 INHIBITORS AND INDUCERS

Inhibitors	Inducers
Antibiotics	**Anticonvulsants**
Clarithromycin	Carbamazepine
Ciprofloxacin	Ethosuximide
Erythromycin	Phenobarbital
Metronidazole	Phenytoin
Norfloxacin	Primidone
Troleandomycin	
	Antituberculous agents
Azole antifungals	Isoniazid
Fluconazole	Rifampin
Itraconazole	
Ketoconazole	**HIV antivirals**
	Efavirenz
HIV antivirals	Nevirapine
Amprenavir	Ritonavir
Delavirdine	
Indinavir	**Miscellaneous**
Nelfinavir	Dexamethasone
Ritonavir	Griseofulvin
Saquinavir	St John's wort
	Ticlopidine
Calcium channel blockers	Troglitazone
Diltiazem	
Nifedipine	
Verapamil	
SSRIs	
Fluoxetine	
Fluvoxamine	
Nefazodone	
Paroxetine	
Sertraline	
Others	
Amiodarone	
Antiprogestins	
Cannabinoids	
Cimetidine	
Grapefruit juice	
Interferon-gamma	
Quinine	
Tacrolimus	
Zafirlukast	

Table 131.8 CYP3A4 inhibitors and inducers[45]. Drugs in italics are particularly potent inhibitors.

DRUG METABOLIZING ENZYMES CYP1A2, 2C9 AND 2C19: SELECTED SUBSTRATES, INHIBITORS AND INDUCERS

Isozyme	Substrate	Inhibitors	Inducers
CYP1A2	Amitriptyline	*Cimetidine*	Barbiturates
	Caffeine	*Ciprofloxacin*	Brussel sprouts
	Clomipramine	Clarithromycin	Cabbage
	Clozapine	*Erythromycin*	Carbamazepine
	Desipramine	*Fluvoxamine*	Charbroiled foods
	Fluvoxamine	Ketoconazole	Cigarette smoking
	Haloperidol	*Norfloxacin*	Omeprazole
	Imipramine	*Paroxetine*	Phenobarbital
	Propranolol	Terbinafine	Phenytoin
	Tacrine	Ticlopidine	Rifampin
	Theophylline		Ritonavir
	Warfarin		
	Zileuton		
	Zolmitriptan		
CYP2C9	Diclofenac	*Amiodarone*	Barbiturates
	Fluvastatin	*Cimetidine*	Carbamazepine
	Ibuprofen	Fluconazole	Ethanol
	Losartan	Fluvoxamine	Rifampin
	Montelukast	Ketoconazole	
	Phenytoin	Omeprazole	
	Piroxicam	Ritonavir	
	Sulfonamides	Sulfonamides	
	Tricyclic antidepressants	Trimethoprim	
	Valproic acid	Zafirlukast	
	Warfarin		
	Zafirlukast		
CYP2C19	Citalopram	Cimetidine	Norethindrone
	Cyclophosphamide	Felbamate	Prednisone
	Diazepam	Fluconazole	Rifampin
	Hexobarbital	Fluoxetine	
	Imipramine	Fluvoxamine	
	Indomethacin	Indomethacin	
	Lansoprazole	Ketoconazole	
	Nelfinavir	Lansoprazole	
	Nilutamide	Modafinil	
	Omeprazole	Omeprazole	
	Pantoprazole	Paroxetine	
	Progesterone	Ticlopidine	
	Proguanil	Topiramate	
	Teniposide		
	Warfarin		

Table 131.9 Drug metabolizing enzymes CYP1A2, 2C9 and 2C19: selected substrate inhibitors and inducers[45,46]. Drugs in italics are particularly potent inhibitors.

Cytochrome induction

Many enzymes involved in drug biotransformation are able to increase in amount and activity in response to substances known as inducers. The onset and offset of enzyme induction is gradual because the induction phase depends on the accumulation of the particular inducing agent and the subsequent synthesis of new enzyme. The offset depends on elimination of the inducer and decay of the increased enzyme levels.

Inducers may enhance parent drug metabolism, so that therapeutic efficacy is actually reduced if the parent drug is the active moiety (Fig. 131.5). Alternatively, inducers may enhance the metabolism of a substrate to active metabolites, with the potential for exaggerated toxicity. The alkylating agent cyclophosphamide is a prodrug that requires metabolic activation to phosphoramide mustards for its therapeutic effect. Unfortunately, metabolic activation also leads to the formation of acrolein, which causes the bladder toxicity seen with this medication[47].

Cytochrome inhibition

The inhibition of drug metabolism is the most important mechanism for drug interactions because it can lead to an increase in plasma drug concentration, enhanced drug response, and toxicity. In contrast to the time course seen with enzyme induction, inhibition of drug metabolism begins within the first one or two doses of the inhibitor and is maximal when a steady-state concentration of the inhibitor is achieved. Therefore, the time course for inhibitory actions is usually in terms of days not weeks.

Inhibitory interactions can be either competitive or non-competitive. An example of competitive inhibition involves the tight binding of inhibitors such as ketoconazole, cimetidine and macrolides to the heme moiety of the cytochrome P450 isozyme. As long as the inhibitor occupies this specific site of the P450 cytochrome, the substrate cannot be biotransformed[48]. As the concentration of the inhibiting drug increases, the degree of saturation of the isoenzyme increases. When the enzyme system is saturated, further metabolic activity by that enzyme system is limited. At that point, a patient becomes the equivalent of a poor metabolizer and concentrations of co-prescribed medications begin to rise. The extent of inhibition of one drug by another depends on the affinity each compound has for the P450 isoform. Competitive inhibition depends on the affinity of the substrate for the enzyme being inhibited, the concentration of substrate required to saturate the system, and the half-life of the inhibitor drug. The onset and offset of enzyme inhibition are dependent on the half-life and time to steady state of the inhibitor.

The significance of an elevated plasma level of a particular drug is determined largely by the therapeutic margin of the drug. Therefore, when considering the potential clinical relevance of an interaction, one must exercise more caution with drugs that have a narrow therapeutic range. Non-competitive inhibition is less common and occurs when the enzyme is destroyed, inactivated, or changed by the inhibitor such that it can no longer metabolize the original substrate. Spironolactone forms suicidal reactive intermediate metabolites that inactivate cytochromes.

The antiprogestins mefepristone, lilopristone and onapristone are oxidized to reactive species capable of inactivating their metabolizing enzyme[49]. These drugs are a relatively new class of agents with promise in the treatment of some forms of breast and prostate cancer, meningioma, uterine leiomyoma and endometriosis, and as contraceptive agents.

HOW TO MINIMIZE THE RISK OF DRUG–DRUG INTERACTIONS

One commonly perpetuated myth is that all drugs in a given class are equally susceptible or contributory to drug interactions. Understanding the differences between drugs in a particular class with regard to potential for drug interactions is clinically relevant. Specific drugs, from a given class of drugs associated with interactions, may have little or no clinical potential for drug interactions and are therefore safer choices (Table 131.11).

SUBSTRATES AND INHIBITORS OF CYP2D6

Substrates of CYP2D6		Inhibitors of CYP2D6
Antiarrhythmics	**Antidepressants**	*Amiodarone*
Amiodarone	Amitriptyline	Amitriptyline
Encainide	Clomipramine	Celecoxib
Flecainide	*N*-desmethyl-	Chlorpheniramine
Mexiletine	clomipramine	Cimetidine
Propafenone	Desipramine	Clomipramine
	Fluoxetine	Desipramine
Antipsychotics	Imipramine	Donepezil
Clozapine	Maprotiline	Doxepin
Haloperidol	Mianserin	*Fluoxetine*
Perphenazine	Norfluoxetine	Fluphenazine
Remoxipride	Nortriptyline	Haloperidol
Risperidone	Paroxetine	Imipramine
Thioridazine	Trazodone*	Indinavir
Zuclopenthixol	Trimipramine	Moclobemide
	Venlafaxine	Nortriptyline
β-Blockers		*Paroxetine*
Alprenolol	**Miscellaneous**	Pimozide
Bufuralol	Captopril	Propafenone
Metoprolol	Codeine	*Quinidine*
Propranolol	Dextromethorphan	Ranitidine
Timolol	Diphenhydramine	*Ritonavir*
	Domperidone	Sertraline (weak)
	Donepezil	Terbinafine
	Ethylmorphine	Thioridazine
	4-hydroamphetamine	Ticlopidine
	Oxycodone	Venlafaxine (weak)
	Phenformin	
	Terfenadine**	

*Applies to metabolite rather than the parent drug.
**Historical.

Table 131.10 Substrates and inhibitors of CYP2D6[45,46]. Drugs in italics are particularly potent inhibitors.

DRUGS AND FOODS WITH DIFFERING POTENTIAL FOR DRUG–DRUG INTERACTIONS BASED ON METABOLISM

Drug/food class	Agents with more potential	Agents with less potential
Macrolides	Clarithromycin Erythromycin	Azithromycin
Quinolones	Ciprofloxacin Enoxacin	Levofloxacin Lomefloxacin Ofloxacin
H2 blockers	Cimetidine	Famotidine Nizatidine Ranitidine
Protease inhibitors	Ritonavir Indinavir	Saquinavir Nelfinavir
HMG-CoA reductase inhibitors	Simvastatin Lovastatin Atorvastatin Cerivastatin	Pravastatin Fluvastatin
Citrus fruit juice	Grapefruit juice	Orange juice

Table 131.11 Drugs and foods with differing potential for drug–drug interactions based on metabolism.

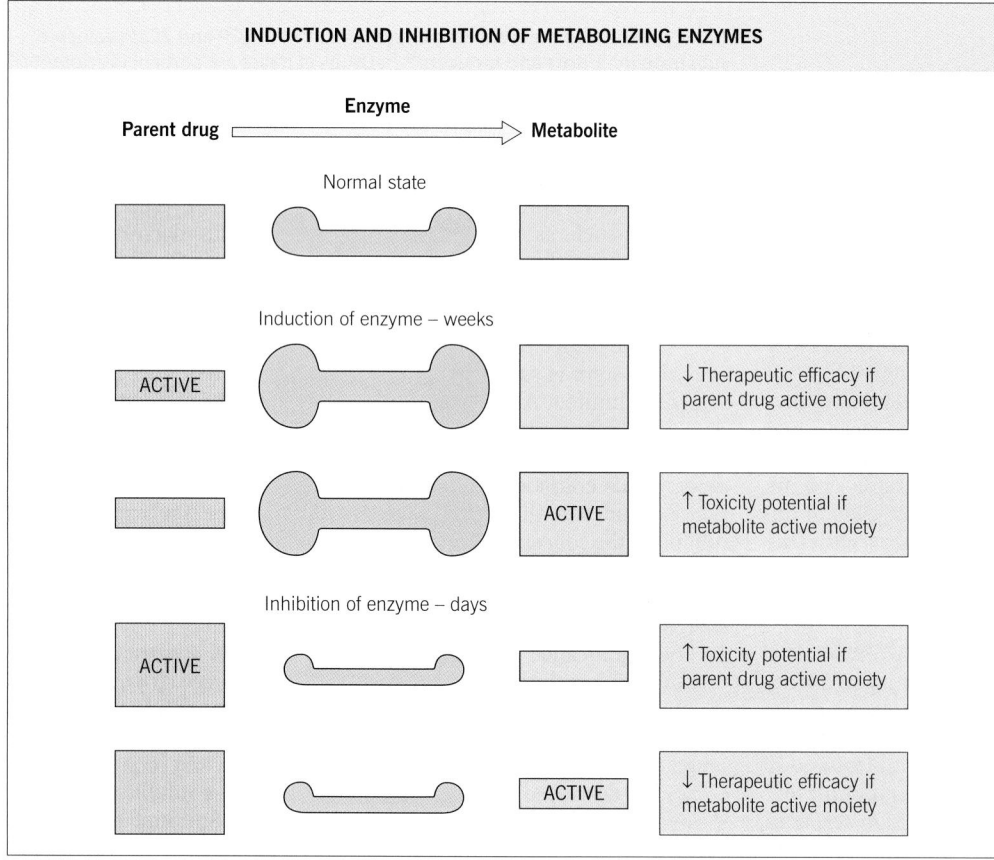

INDUCTION AND INHIBITION OF METABOLIZING ENZYMES

Parent drug → Enzyme → Metabolite

Normal state

Induction of enzyme – weeks

↓ Therapeutic efficacy if parent drug active moiety

ACTIVE — ↑ Toxicity potential if metabolite active moiety

Inhibition of enzyme – days

ACTIVE — ↑ Toxicity potential if parent drug active moiety

↓ Therapeutic efficacy if metabolite active moiety — ACTIVE

Fig. 131.5 Induction and inhibition of metabolizing enzymes.

Various drug classes commonly encountered by dermatologists will be discussed, with emphasis on important interactions and ways to minimize risks by appropriate drug choices within a given drug class.

Allylamine Antifungals

Terbinafine is an orally active allylamine antifungal used in the treatment of dermatophytoses. Reports suggest some degree of significant inhibition of CYP2D6 and CYP1A2 by terbinafine[50]. There are three levels of activity of CYP2D6 in the population: poor metabolizers (PM), extensive metabolizers (EM) and ultrarapid metabolizers. The EM status is by far the most common and is considered 'normal'. Approximately 7.5% of Caucasians and less than 2% of Asian and African-Americans are poor metabolizers. Inhibition of CYP2D6 by terbinafine would make individuals who have active enzyme (extensive metabolizers) into poor metabolizers, and this effect could possibly last for weeks after discontinuing terbinafine. This can cause two problems. First, there may be an accumulation of the parent drug (substrate), and this can result in dose-dependent drug toxicity, or there can be reduced formation of active metabolites, and this can result in loss of efficacy (see Fig. 131.5)[51]. To date, over 17 different CYP2D6 mutations have been described and the commonest allele is designated CYP2D6*1A (PM); drug effects may differ, depending on the different alleles.

For now, terbinafine appears to be a potent inhibitor of CYP2D6, and so clinicians should be aware of potential interactions (see Table 131.10). The area of greatest concern, because of possible severity and common use, would be bradycardia from excess β-blockade (e.g. propanolol) or from the accumulation of donepezil (used to treat Alzheimer's disease)[52]. Codeine could lose its analgesic effect, as the active metabolite morphine is not formed when CYP2D6 activity is low[53]. The clinical impact of this interaction remains unknown. It should, however, change the information that patients are given when this drug is prescribed.

Azole Antifungals

The imidazole ketoconazole and the triazole itraconazole require an acid milieu for absorption; therefore, concomitant antacids, H₂ blockers, proton pump inhibitors, sucralfate and didanosine significantly reduce absorption (see Table 131.6). Decreased GI absorption has been demonstrated with antacids, cyclosporine and omeprazole.

Among the systemic azole antifungals, ketoconazole has been shown *in vitro* to be the strongest inhibitor of CYP3A4. Many substrates are metabolized via these enzymes (see Tables 131.4, 131.6, 131.7), and those that can lead to moderate to severe drug interactions include phenytoin, warfarin and cyclosporine. Itraconazole is contraindicated when the patient is also receiving the following CYP3A substrate drugs: triazolam, oral midazolam, lovastatin, simvastatin, astemizole, quinidine or pimozide. Caution has been suggested with warfarin, cyclosporine, digoxin and atorvastatin. Significant effects on the metabolism of fluvastatin or pravastatin by itraconazole do not appear to occur[54] (see Table 131.11).

More specifically, when the azole antifungals are administered with cyclosporine, the concentrations of the latter are increased, requiring careful monitoring of cyclosporine levels. Similarly, frequent monitoring of the international normalized ratio (INR) is required for patients on warfarin who require therapy with an azole antifungal. The azole antifungals reportedly increase the anticoagulant effects of warfarin by two- to threefold. In one study, phenytoin concentrations were significantly increased 48 hours after fluconazole administration, owing to a 33% decrease in the clearance of phenytoin[55].

Azole antifungals interfere with the metabolism of benzodiazepines such as triazolam and midazolam, leading to increased levels and sedation. There is also decreased metabolism of some HMG-CoA reductase inhibitors, e.g. lovastatin and simvastatin, leading to increased levels, as well as to rhabdomyolysis. Additional drugs whose metabolism is decreased by azoles include tacrolimus and indinavir. Peripheral edema due to an interaction between nifedipine and itraconazole has been reported. It was suspected that itraconazole inhibited the metabolism of this calcium channel blocker, resulting in an increased serum nifedipine concentration and leg edema. This hypothesis was confirmed by obtaining serum levels of nifedipine, itraconazole and hydroxy-

itraconazole (the active metabolite of itraconazole) before and after the administration of itraconazole[56]. The authors recommended that patients receiving both azole or triazole antifungals and calcium channel blockers be monitored for side effects such as leg edema and, more importantly, hypotension, because of the increased serum concentration of the calcium channel blocker.

Fluconazole, but not itraconazole, interacts with losartan, an angiotensin II receptor antagonist antihypertensive. Fluconazole inhibits losartan's metabolism to the active metabolite E-3174[57]. The clinical significance of this interaction remains unclear, but the possibility of a reduced therapeutic effect of losartan should be borne in mind. Phenytoin is a CYP2C9 substrate, and concurrent fluconazole use at bedtime has resulted in several cases of phenytoin toxicity[58].

In contrast to the azole antifungals, terbinafine is an allylamine that does not inhibit CYP3A4[59]. This antifungal may be a viable therapeutic option in patients on concomitant therapy with a high likelihood of drug interactions with the azoles.

Cimetidine

Cimetidine can produce significant inhibition of CYP1A2, 2C, 2C19, 2D6 and 3A4. This is a concern, as this medication is available without prescription in the US. It is used by dermatologists as a therapy for urticaria and verrucae vulgares. Examples of clinically relevant interactions exist between cimetidine and theophylline, aminophylline, metoprolol, propranolol, nifedipine and quinidine. The interaction involving the β-blockers metoprolol and propranolol can result in clinically relevant sinus bradycardia and hypotension. Therefore, the dose of the β-blocker may need to be reduced if these agents are administered together. Atenolol and nadolol have been shown not to interact with cimetidine.

Azathioprine

Azathioprine is metabolized to 6-mercaptopurine (6-MP). There are then three subsequent pathways for the metabolism of this metabolite. Thiopurine methyltransferase (TPMT) metabolizes 6-MP to inactive products (see below) and xanthine oxidase metabolizes 6-MP to inactive metabolites. The third pathway involves hypoxanthine guanine phosphorobosyltransferase (HGPRT) and the end products are active purine analogues, in particular 6-thioguanine. Allopurinol inhibits the metabolism of 6-MP via xanthine oxidase. The resultant effect is increased antimetabolite effect and toxicity of azathioprine and 6-MP. Combining either of these drugs with allopurinol should be avoided. If allopurinol must be used, an alternate immunosuppressant should be selected.

Cyclosporine

Numerous drug interactions with cyclosporine have surfaced that are associated with its metabolism and presystemic metabolism (both by the CYP3A4 enzyme and by PGP), in the liver and intestine, respectively. It is thought that this GI tract metabolism may explain its erratic absorption. In fact, 3A4 inhibitors have been administered intentionally to improve cyclosporine's bioavailability, thereby reducing dosing requirements and lowering overall drug costs. Ketoconazole 200–400 mg/day can decrease the required daily dose of cyclosporine by 60–80%[60].

Diltiazem can decrease cyclosporine dosing by as much as 30%[61], but effects with grapefruit juice have been variable. Other drugs that alter cyclosporine concentrations via cytochrome 3A4 inhibition include verapamil, nifedipine, fluconazole, itraconazole, ketoconazole, erythromycin, clarithromycin and tacrolimus. Conversely, isoform 3A4 inducers, such as rifampin, phenytoin, carbamazepine and phenobarbital, decrease cyclosporine concentrations. Newer reports include decreased cyclosporine levels occurring with coadministration of troglitazone or ticlopidine[62]. Cyclosporine trough levels, as well as signs of toxicity versus adequate immunosuppressive response, should be monitored when any of these drugs are combined with cyclosporine.

Grapefruit Juice

Grapefruit juice interactions are of potential clinical relevance in the individual patient for a wide range of drugs. The mechanisms of grapefruit juice interactions are exclusively pharmacokinetic in nature. The effect is mediated mainly by the suppression of CYP3A4 and PGP in the small intestinal wall by either fresh or frozen grapefruit juice[63] (see Fig. 131.4). This results in a diminished first-pass metabolism, with higher bioavailability and increased maximal plasma concentrations of substrates of this transporter and/or enzyme. The effect is most pronounced in drugs with high first-pass degradation, such as felodipine, nifedipine, saquinavir, cyclosporine, midazolam, triazolam, terazosin, ethinylestradiol, 17β-estradiol, prednisone, and the HMG-CoA reductase inhibitors lovastatin and simvastatin[64,65].

It is not yet clear which component in grapefruit juice is to blame. Psoralen, mainly a bergamottin compound, is thought to be the major inhibitor, with a minor role attributable to flavonoids such as naringenin and quercetin[66]. These furocoumarins are strong candidates as causative agents of grapefruit juice-mediated drug interactions because they have an inhibition potential that is equal to or stronger than that of the prototypical CYP3A4 inhibitor, ketoconazole[67].

Even a change in the brand or batch of grapefruit juice may influence the grapefruit juice/drug interaction to an unpredictable degree, as grapefruit juice is a natural product that is not standardized in composition. Similar interactions have not been seen with other citrus fruit juices, such as orange juice. Lack of 6,7-dihydroxybergamottin in orange juice probably accounts for the absence of inhibitory effects[68]. However, isoflavones in orange juice may mediate this food's inhibitory effect on PGP.

The idea of using grapefruit juice as a cost-cutting measure has been used in patients on concomitant cyclosporine therapy[69]. It was thought that because grapefruit juice can inhibit the metabolism of cyclosporine, combining the two would lower the required daily dose of cyclosporine, thereby reducing drug costs. More recent studies have also demonstrated that grapefruit juice increases the bioavailability of saquinavir without affecting its clearance, suggesting that inhibition of intestinal CYP3A4 may represent a way to enhance effectiveness without increasing the dose[70].

However, in general, it is recommended that patients refrain from ingesting grapefruit juice when taking a drug that is extensively metabolized, unless a lack of interaction has been documented. Many hospital cafeterias now place warnings of the potential for drug interactions in areas where grapefruit juice is sold. Orange juice is a good alternative (see Table 131.11).

Herbal Remedies

Herbal medicines (see Ch. 133) have become a popular form of therapy. They are perceived to be 'natural' by the public and thus harmless. Although many current therapeutic agents (including digitalis, atropine, vincristine, and narcotic derivatives) have been derived from plants, little is known about the relative safety of current herbal therapies compared with prescription drugs, and even less is known when the two are co-consumed. Because of under-reporting, our present knowledge represents the tip of the iceberg. It is estimated that 80% of the world's population relies primarily on traditional medicines utilizing plant extracts or their active ingredients.

The interactions of phytomedicines with prescription medications are under-researched[71]. Because herbs are not sold as drugs, no proof of efficacy or warnings about side effects are required. When a drug is prescribed, the dosage and quality of the substance are assured. No such standardization or quality control exists for herbal preparations. Contamination, mislabeling and misidentification of herbs are also problems. Some patients do not know what they are taking, as they may purchase a product whose ingredients are listed in a foreign language only.

A study in 12 healthy volunteers examined the effect of the ingestion of St John's wort on cytochrome activity[72]. Short-term administration (less than 2 weeks) of St John's wort had no effect on CYP activity, whereas long-term St John's wort administration resulted in a significant and selective induction of CYP3A activity in the intestinal wall. St John's wort did not alter the activity of CYP2C9, CYP1A2 or CYP2D6. Reduced therapeutic efficacy of drugs metabolized by CYP3A should be anticipated during long-term administration of St John's wort.

When taking a history regarding medications, it is important to ask specifically about prescription, non-prescription and herbal therapies.

HERBAL REMEDIES/PRESCRIPTION DRUG INTERACTIONS		
Herbal remedy	**Side effects**	**Drug interaction**
Zemaphyte (Chinese herbal therapy)	Diarrhea, increased liver function tests, reversible dilated cardiomyopathy, reversible acute hepatic illness, fatal hepatic necrosis, worsening of atopic dermatitis, acute urticaria	Methotrexate
Coenzyme Q10[3]	Reduced efficacy of warfarin	Warfarin
Ginseng[73]	Can reduce the anticoagulant response of warfarin	Warfarin
Licorice (*Glycyrrhiza glabra* or *uralensis*)	Contraindicated in hypertension, diabetes mellitus, hypokalemia, liver/kidney disorders	Cyclosporine, digoxin, prednisone, thiazides
Purple coneflower (*Echinacea angustifolia* or *purpurea*)	Recurrent erythema nodosum Caution in patients with HIV, autoimmune CTD, TB, MS, or ragweed, sunflower allergies	Immunomodulators and cyclosporine, methotrexate, corticosteroids
Ginkgo (*Ginkgo biloba*) Garlic, ginger, ginseng (*Panax ginseng*)[74]	Can cause spontaneous bleeding	Can potentiate aspirin, NSAIDs, warfarin, heparin
St. John's wort[3] (oral)	Photosensitivity Erectile dysfunction	Cyclosporine Oral contraceptive

Table 131.12 Herbal remedies/prescription drug interactions. CTD, connective tissue disease; MS, multiple sclerosis; TB, tuberculosis.

Patients should tell their physician if they are using herbal remedies, to improve monitoring of side effects and potential interactions. See Table 131.12 for some important drug interactions between herbal medicines and dermatologic therapies.

HMG-CoA Reductase Inhibitors

Although dermatologists may not prescribe these lipid-lowering agents, their use by family physicians and specialists is so widespread that it is fairly common to encounter patients who are taking this class of drugs. To date, all reports of significantly increased rates of myalgias from combination therapy with a 'statin' plus certain other drugs involve simvastatin or lovastatin. These are the statins with the highest known metabolic dependency on the CYP3A4 pathway for elimination[75]. Fluvastatin is metabolized via CYP2C9 and therefore is not expected to interact with CYP3A4 inhibitors, but may interact with 2C9 inhibitors. Pravastatin is not metabolized by CYP3A4, nor is it cleared by PGP to a clinically significant degree[76].

Leukotriene Receptor Antagonists

Montelukast is metabolized by cytochrome P450 3A4 and 2C9 isoforms. Inducers of these CYP enzymes may reduce concentrations of montelukast. Zafirlukast is metabolized by CYP2C9 and it inhibits 3A4 and 2C9. Coadministration of warfarin with zafirlukast produces clinically significant increases in prothrombin time. Serum theophylline levels have reportedly increased to toxic levels after the addition of zafirlukast to the regimen[77].

Macrolide Antibiotics

When a macrolide is required in a patient who is receiving systemic tacrolimus, azithromycin should be used (rather than erythromycin or clarithromycin) because this does not produce significant inhibition of CYP3A4[78]. When erythromycin is prescribed to a patient on long-term warfarin, there is a risk of increased plasma warfarin levels, with increased anticoagulation and hemorrhage. This occurs because tacrolimus and warfarin are CYP3A4 substrates and erythromycin is a potent inhibitor. As with azole antifungals, historically the coadministration of erythromycin and astemizole or terfenadine was associated with a risk of cardiotoxicity.

Erythromycin also inhibits the metabolism of sildenafil, resulting in a significant increase in serum levels of sildenafil[79]. If concurrent administration is unavoidable, reduced doses of sildenafil are recommended. In addition, an interaction between erythromycin and carbamazepine has been well established[80]. Erythromycin significantly inhibits hepatic metabolism of carbamazepine; the interaction is highly predictable, develops with rapid onset, and may also occur with clarithromycin or troleandomycin[80]. Concurrent use should therefore be avoided.

Quinolone Antibiotics

In the GI tract, all fluoroquinolones interact with multivalent cation-containing products, and the bioavailability of the quinolone can be reduced by up to 50% when coadministered with iron compounds (ciprofloxacin and moxifloxacin are more affected than levofloxacin or gemifloxacin). There is also a significant decrease in the bioavailability of quinolones when given with sucralfate[80], and antibiotic treatment failure has been documented. If sucralfate cannot be discontinued, the quinolone should be taken 2–6 hours before the sucralfate. Similar decreases in bioavailability occur when a quinolone is given concurrently with an antacid[80]. The antacid should therefore be taken 6 hours prior to or 2 hours after the antibiotic.

The interaction between theophylline and fluoroquinolones is most marked with enoxacin, pefloxacin and ciprofloxacin, with no such interaction reported for levofloxacin. Sparfloxacin is associated with cardiac manifestations in the form of QTc prolongation and has a high phototoxicity potential. Moxifloxacin is currently under observation because of concern regarding QTc effects. While moxifloxacin can prolong the QT interval, it does not alter the QT dispersion (QT dispersion is thought to be a more sensitive predictor of the risk of torsades de pointes). As such, the increased risk of torsades de pointes attributable to moxifloxacin is questionable[81]. Levofloxacin has no QT prolongation and a very low phototoxic potential, making it one of the safest newer fluoroquinolones[82]. An enhanced anticoagulant effect of warfarin has been reported after coadministration with norfloxacin, ciprofloxacin, ofloxacin or enoxacin[62].

Pimozide

Pimozide is a neuroleptic that may be used for psychogenic dermatologic problems such as delusions of parasitosis (see Ch. 8). Hopefully, in the future, newer antipsychotics with fewer side effects may replace pimozide. However, as long as it is still being prescribed, dermatologists must be aware of its drug–drug interactions. Case reports suggest that pimozide prolongs the cardiac QT interval and may lead to arrhythmias. Pimozide is oxidized by two CYP450 isoforms, CYP3A4 and CYP1A2, with the former being the responsible isoform at therapeutically relevant pimozide concentrations[83]. Pimozide is also an inhibitor of CYP2D6 without being a substrate of this isoform. Therefore, a greater risk of adverse effects is expected when pimozide is co-prescribed with metabolic inhibitors.

The risk of concomitant administration of CYP3A inhibitors with pimozide is highlighted by a recent report of fatal cardiac arrhythmias in patients taking pimozide plus clarithromycin[84]. To examine the latter interaction, investigators gave a single oral dose of pimozide with and without clarithromycin to 12 healthy subjects who were documented as either extensive or poor metabolizers of CYP2D6[85]. Pimozide itself was capable of prolonging QT intervals, and pimozide concentrations were increased in the presence of clarithromycin; the average QT prolongation was longer when both drugs were taken. CYP2D6 activity, however, was not a factor.

In summary, patients who are at risk of ventricular arrhythmias because of prolonged QT intervals or electrolyte disturbances, or who take other drugs that affect QT intervals, should use pimozide with caution. Adding a CYP3A4 inhibitor such as clarithromycin, erythromycin or an azole antifungal may increase the risk of toxicity. A baseline assessment of the QT interval and reassessment 6 hours after a pimozide dose may be helpful in patients at risk who require pimozide.

Protease Inhibitors

HIV protease inhibitors are associated with numerous drug interactions, many of which are clinically important. Ritonavir, indinavir, saquinavir and nelfinavir are all substrates and inhibitors of CYP3A4, and ritonavir also inhibits CYP2D6[86]. Ritonavir and indinavir are significant 3A4 inhibitors, whereas saquinavir and nelfinavir are less potent. Ritonavir is the most potent inhibitor, having inhibitory potency slightly less than that of ketoconazole. Consequently, ritonavir is the most likely to interact with other drugs. Indinavir, amprenavir and nelfinavir have a moderate probability of causing interactions, and saquinavir has the lowest probability[14].

Ritonavir may also induce CYP3A4 and 1A2, leading to auto-induction of its own metabolism in a dose-dependent manner during the first 14 days of therapy. Since it induces its own metabolism, one would expect a higher dose requirement after 14 days. By inducing CYP1A2, ritonavir decreases the plasma concentration of theophylline. Ritonavir and nelfinavir also increase glucuronyl transferase activity, which may partly explain the substantial decreases in plasma ethinylestradiol concentration during concurrent therapy with these protease inhibitors. Therefore, alternative or additional methods of contraception are recommended in women taking ritonavir or nelfinavir[87].

Protease inhibitors should be prescribed cautiously with drugs metabolized primarily by the CYP3A4 system and those metabolized by the CYP2D6 system (ritonavir only). Concurrent administration should be accompanied by clinical monitoring for enhanced side effects that may require dosage adjustments in some patients.

Genetic Polymorphisms

Each of the isoenzymes of the P450 system is under genetic control. Because of genetic polymorphisms, different individuals have different levels of activity of different P450 isoforms. Genetic polymorphism means that within a general population individuals have different levels of enzyme activity due to the presence of variant alleles. People with genetically determined low levels of activity are referred to as poor metabolizers. People who have a functional enzyme are known as extensive metabolizers. There are yet others who have more than the usual complement of functional genes and more than the usual amounts of certain enzymes, who are referred to as ultrarapid metabolizers. Still others have partially functional enzymes and are slower metabolizers than normal. Poor metabolizers may have a larger response and be at greater risk of toxicity than extensive metabolizers for drugs that are highly dependent on clearance to an inactive metabolite by the particular isoform[88]. On the other hand, ultrarapid metabolizers might not reach therapeutically active plasma concentrations of certain drugs, thereby not achieving the anticipated desired effect.

P450 enzymes that exhibit genetic polymorphisms include CYP1A2, CYP2C19, CYP2D6 and CYP2E1. Ethnic differences exist with regard to the percentage of a population who are extensive, ultrarapid or poor metabolizers. As discussed in the section on allylamine antifungals, approximately 7.5% of Caucasians and less than 2% of Asians and African-Americans are poor metabolizers and have minimal CYP2D6 activity[51]. Cytochrome 2C19 also exhibits genetic polymorphism, with 20% of Asians and African-Americans and 3–5% of Caucasians reported to be poor metabolizers. Lastly, in one study, 12% of subjects were found to be slow 1A2 metabolizers and approximately 40% were found to be fast metabolizers[89].

Poor metabolizers can be identified through a drug challenge test using debrisoquine sulfate for the 2D6 system, mephenytoin for the 2C19 system, and caffeine for the 1A2 system[89]. However, these tests are not routinely used in clinical practice and unfortunately there are no clinical parameters that are useful in predicting the metabolizing status of a given individual.

Pharmacogenetic Variation

Pharmacogenetic variation can also occur in other drug-metabolizing enzymes. Pertinent to dermatologists, the enzyme thiopurine S-methyltransferase (TPMT) is important in the metabolism of azathioprine and 6-mercaptopurine to non-toxic metabolites. There is a 0.3% rate of homozygous deficiency of this enzyme, putting these patients at great risk for toxicity, especially myelosuppression[90]. Conversely, 88% of the population is homozygous for the active TPMT enzyme and may therefore require doses greater than the recommended daily dose of azathioprine (1–2 mg/kg/day) to achieve therapeutic success. Determination of the patient's TPMT level provides *a priori* information that allows the individualization of azathioprine dosing, thereby minimizing toxicity and maximizing efficacy.

Drug–Cytokine Interactions

Cytochrome P450 drug metabolism can be altered by certain proinflammatory cytokines, such as interleukin (IL)-6, IL-1 and TNF-α[91]. These cytokines can cause reduced P450 3A function and they are released during periods of stress, trauma or infection, as well as following the administration of immunomodulators such as IL-2[92].

Drug–HIV Interactions

New information about drug interactions in patients with HIV infection becomes available nearly weekly. A recent review presents current information[15].

CONCLUSION

Dealing with drug interactions is a challenge in clinical practice. Although no one can be expected to know all drug interactions, good resources are available, e.g. the Medical Letter's *Handbook of Adverse Drug Interactions*, or a hospital drug information service. In addition, computer programs now exist that can flag potential interactions, and their use will increase as electronic records become more common. However, such sources are limited, as are most desk references, by class-related statements. Broad statements may falsely and unnecessarily restrict therapeutic options.

More research during the early stages of drug development is required to identify new interactions, define mechanisms of older interactions, and examine the safety of new drugs from classes that are known to cause interactions. We also need more sensitive post-marketing surveillance tools to identify important drug interactions that become evident over time in diseased hosts and that were not seen in pre-marketing studies of healthy volunteers. Physicians need better tools, but, in the meantime, understanding the nuances of the cytochrome P450s will help take the fright out of prescribing.

Because the best evidence for clinically relevant drug interactions comes from case reports, prescribing physicians can have a major impact. Observations of drug interactions should be confirmed, if possible, by serum drug concentrations. Then they should be reported to regulatory bodies and submitted to journals. By understanding the mechanisms behind drug interactions and staying alert for toxicities, we can help make drug therapy safer and reduce the fear of drug interactions.

REFERENCES

1. Shapiro LE, Shear NH. Drug-drug interactions – how scared should we be? CMAJ. 1999;161:1266–7.
2. Weideman RA, McKinney WP, Bernstein IH. Predictors of potential drug interactions. Hosp Pharm. 1998;33:835–40.
3. Hansten P, Horn J. The Top 100 Drug Interactions: A Guide to Patient Management, Year 2005. Edmonds, WA: H&H Publications, 2007.
4. Schneitman-McIntire O, Farnen TA, Gordon N, et al. Medication misadventures resulting in emergency department visits at an HMO medical center. Am J Health Syst Pharm. 1996;53:1416–22.
5. Hamilton RA, Briceland LL, Andritz MH. Frequency of hospitalization after exposure to known drug-drug interactions in a Medicaid population. Pharmacotherapy. 1998;18:1112–20.
6. Hoey J. Drug interactions: who warns the patients? [editorial]. CMAJ. 1999;161:117.
7. Smalley W, Shatin D, Wysowski DK, et al. Contraindicated use of cisapride: impact of Food and Drug Administration regulatory action. JAMA. 2000;284:3036–9.
8. Merlo J, Liedholm H, Lindblad U, et al. Prescription with potential drug interactions dispensed at Swedish pharmacies in January 1999: cross sectional study. BMJ. 2001;323:427–8.
9. Shapiro LE, Shear NH. Drug interactions/P450. Curr Probl Dermatol. 2001;13:141–52.
10. du Souich P. In human therapy, is the drug-drug interaction or the adverse drug reaction the issue? Can J Clin Pharmacol. 2001;8:153–61.
11. Hansten PD, Horn JR. Drug Interactions Analysis and Management. St Louis, MO: Facts & Comparisons (Wolters Kluwer Health); 2007.
12. Andersen W, Feingold D. Adverse drug interactions clinically important for the dermatologist. Arch Dermatol. 1995;131:468–73.
13. Montamat SC, Cusack BJ, Vestal RE. Management of drug therapy in the elderly. N Engl J Med. 1989;321:303–9.
14. Piscitelli S, Gallicano K. Interactions among drugs for HIV and opportunistic infections. N Engl J Med. 2001;344:984–96.
15. www.hiv-druginteractions.org; University of Liverpool.
16. Brly F, Marez D, Sabbagh N, et al. An efficient strategy for detection of known and new mutations of the CYP 2D6 gene using single stand conformation polymorphism analysis. Pharmacogenetics. 1995;5:373–84.
17. Roujeau JC, Kelly JP, Naldi L, et al. Medication use and the risk of Stevens-Johnson syndrome or toxic epidermal necrolysis. N Engl J Med. 1995;333:1600–7.

18. Sullivan JR, Watson A. Lamotrigine-induced toxic epidermal necrolysis treated with intravenous cyclosporine: a discussion of pathogenesis and immunosuppressive management. Australas J Dermatol. 1996;37:208–12.
19. Sullivan JR, Shear NH. The drug hypersensitivity syndrome: what is the pathogenesis? Arch Dermatol. 2001;137:357–64.
20. Toogood J. Beta blocker therapy and the risk of anaphylaxis. CMAJ. 1987;136:929–33.
21. Tugwell P, Bennett K, Bell M, Gent M. Methotrexate in rheumatoid arthritis: indications, contraindications, efficacy and safety. Ann Intern Med. 1987;107:358–66.
22. Thurmann PA, Hompesch BC. Influence of gender on the pharmacokinetics and pharmacodynamics of drugs. Int J Clin Pharmacol Ther. 1998;36:586–90.
23. Del Rosso JQ. Clinically significant drug interactions: recognition and understanding of common mechanisms. Curr Pract Med. 1998;1:62–4.
24. Hoey J. Postmarketing drug surveillance: what it would take to make it work. CMAJ. 2001;165:1293.
25. Bonnabry P, Sievering J, Leemann T, Dayer P. Quantitative drug interactions prediction system (Q-DIPS): a dynamic computer-based method to assist in the choice of clinically relevant in vivo studies. Clin Pharmacokinet. 2001;40:631–40.
26. Anastasio G, Cornell K, Menscer D. Drug interactions: keeping it straight. Am Fam Phys. 1997;56:883–94.
27. Marchbanks C. Drug-drug interactions with fluoroquinolones. Pharmacotherapy. 1993;13:23–5.
28. Morii M, Ueno K, Ogawa A, et al. Impairment of mycophenolate mofetil absorption by iron ion. Clin Pharmacol Ther. 2000;68:613–16.
29. Bodey GP. Azole antifungal drugs. Clin Infect Dis. 1992;14:5161–9.
30. Zimmermann T, Yeates RA, Laufen H, et al. Influence of concomitant food intake on the oral absorption of two triazole antifungal agents, itraconazole and fluconazole. Eur J Clin Pharmacol. 1994;46:147–50.
31. Blum RA, D'Andrea DT, Florentino BM. Increased gastric pH and the bioavailability of fluconazole and ketoconazole. Ann Intern Med. 1991;114:755–7.
32. Hansten PD. Drug interactions. Drug Interactions Newsletter. 1996:893–906.
33. Drug interactions. Med Lett Drugs Ther. 1999; 41:61–2.
34. Preiss R. P-glycoprotein and related transporters. Int J Clin Pharmacol Ther. 1998;36:3–8.
35. Benet LZ, Izumi T, Zhang Y, et al. Intestinal MDR transport proteins and P-450 enzymes as barriers to oral delivery. J Control Release. 1999;62:25–31.

36. Lown KS, Mao RR, Leichtman AB, et al. Role of intestinal p-glycoprotein (mdr1) in interpatient variation in the oral bioavailability of cyclosporine. Clin Pharmacol Ther. 1997;62:248–60.
37. Burkhart CN. Ivermectin: an assessment of its pharmacology, microbiology and safety. J Bet Toxicol. 2000;13:292–6.
38. Shapiro LE, Singer MI, Shear NH. Pharmacokinetic mechanisms of drug-drug and drug-food interactions in dermatology. Curr Opin Dermatol. 1997;4:25–31.
39. Chishty M, Reichel A, Siva J, Abbott NJ, Begley DJ. Affinity for the P-glycoprotein efflux pump at the blood-brain barrier may explain the lack of CNS side-effects of modern antihistamines. J Drug Target. 2001;9:223–8.
40. Watkins PB. Drug metabolism by cytochromes P450 in the liver and small bowel. Gastroenterol Clin North Am. 1992;21:511–26.
41. Birkett DJ, Mackenqie PI, Veronese ME, et al. In vitro approaches can predict human drug metabolism. Trends Pharmacol Sci. 1993;14:292–4.
42. Ford N, Sonnichsen D. Clinically significant cytochrome P-450 drug interactions – a comment. Pharmacotherapy. 1998;18:890–1.
43. Singer MI, Shapiro LE, Shear NH. Cytochrome P450 3A: interactions with dermatologic therapies. J Am Acad Dermatol. 1997;37:765–71.
44. Kotlyar M, Carson SW. Effects of obesity on the cytochrome P450 enzyme system. Int J Clin Pharmacol Ther. 1999;39:8–19.
45. Michalets E. Update: Clinically significant cytochrome P450 drug interactions. Pharmacotherapy. 1998;18:84–112.
46. Rendic S, Di Carlo FJ. Human cytochrome P450 enzymes. Drug Metab Rev. 1997;29:413–580.
47. Park BK, Pirmohamed M, Kitteringham N. The role of cytochrome P450 enzymes in hepatic and extrahepatic human drug toxicity. Pharmacol Ther. 1995;68:385–424.
48. Virani A, Mailis A, Shapiro LE, Shear NH. Drug interactions in human neuropathic pain pharmacotherapy. Pain. 1997;73:3–13.
49. Jang GR, Benet LZ. Antiprogestin-mediated inactivation of cytochrome P450 3A4. Pharmacology. 1998;56:150–7.
50. Abdel Rahman SM, Gotschall RR, Kaufmann RE, et al. Investigation of terbinafine as a CP2D6 inhibitor in vivo. Clin Pharmacol Ther. 1999;65:465–72.
51. Wormhoudt LW, Commandeur JN, Vermeulen NP. Genetic polymorphism of human N-acetyltransferase, cytochrome P450, glutathione-S-transferase, and epoxide hydrolase enzymes: relevance to xenobiotic metabolism and toxicity. Crit Rev Toxicol. 1999;29:59–124.

52. Barner EL, Gray SL. Donepezil use in Alzheimer disease. Ann Pharmacother. 1999;32:70–7.

53. Tseng CY, Wang SL, Lai MD, Lai ML, Huang JD. Formation of morphine from codeine in Chinese subjects of different CYP2D6 genotypes. Clin Pharmacol Ther. 1996;60:177–82.

54. Neuvonen PJ, Kantola T, Kivisto KT. Simvastatin but not pravastatin is very susceptible to interaction with the CYP3A4 inhibitor itraconazole. Clin Pharmacol Ther. 1998;64:332–41.

55. Touchette MA, Chandrasekar PH, Milad MA, Edwards DJ. Contrasting effects of fluconazole and ketoconazole on phenytoin and testosterone disposition in man. Br J Clin Pharmacol. 1992;34:75–8.

56. Tailor S, Gupta A, Walder S, Shear N. Peripheral edema due to nifedipine-itraconazole interaction: a case report. Arch Dermatol. 1996;132:350–2.

57. Kaukonen KM, Olkkola KT, Neuvonen PJ. Fluconazole but not itraconazole decreased the metabolism of losartan to E-3174. Eur J Clin Pharmacol. 1998;53:445–9.

58. Cadle RM, Zenon GJ III, Rodriguez-Bvarradas MC, et al. Fluconazole induced symptomatic phenytoin toxicity. Ann Pharmacother. 1994;28:292–5.

59. Gupta AK, Katz HI, Shear NH. Drug interactions with itraconazole, fluconazole and terbinafine and their management. J Am Acad Dermatol. 1999;41:237–48.

60. Gomez D, Wacher VJ, Tomlanovich SJ, et al. The effects of ketoconazole on the intestinal metabolism and bioavailability of cyclosporine. Clin Pharmacol Ther. 1995;58:15–19.

61. Shennib H, Auger JL. Diltiazem improves cyclosporine dosage in cystic fibrosis lung transplant recipients. J Heart Lung Transplant. 1994;10:292–6.

62. Tatro DS (ed.). Drug Interaction Facts (with quarterly updates). St Louis: Facts & Comparisons, 1999:xxi–xxvii, 39–40, 2406–42, 720a–b.

63. Fuhr U. Drug interactions with grapefruit juice. Drug Safety. 1998;18:251–72.

64. Roller L. Drugs and grapefruit juice [letter]. Clin Pharmacol Ther. 1998;63:87–8.

65. Kantola T, Kivisto KT, Neuvonen PJ. Grapefruit juice greatly increases serum concentrations of lovastatin and lovastatin acid. Clin Pharmacol Ther. 1998;63:397–402.

66. Schmiedlin-Ren P, Edwards DJ, Fitzsimmons ME, et al. Mechanisms of enhanced oral availability of CYP3A4 substrates by grapefruit juice constituents. Decreased enterocyte CYP3A4 concentration and mechanism-based inactivation by furanocoumarins. Drug Metab Dispos. 1997;25:1228–33.

67. Fukuda K, Ohta T, Oshima Y, et al. Specific CYP3A4 inhibitors in grapefruit juice: furocoumarin dimers as components of drug interaction. Pharmacogenetics. 1997;7:391–6.

68. Edwards DJ, Bellevue FH, Woster PM. Identification of 6,7-dihydroxybergamottin, a cytochrome P450 inhibitor, in grapefruit juice. Drug Metab Dispos. 1996;24:1287–90.

69. Hollander AA, van der Woude FJ, Cohen AF. Effect of grapefruit juice on blood cyclosporin concentration [letter]. Lancet. 1995;346:123.

70. Kupferchmidt HH, Fattinger KE, Ha HR, et al. Grapefruit juice enhances the bioavailability of the HIV protease inhibitor saquinavir in man. Br J Clin Pharmacol. 1998;45:355–9.

71. Ernst E. Harmless herbs? A review of the recent literature. Am J Med. 1998;104:170–8.

72. Wang Z, Gorski JC, Hamman MA, Huang SM, Lesko LJ, Hall SD. The effects of St John's wort (Hypericum perforatum) on human cytochrome P450 activity. Clin Pharmacol Ther. 2001;70:317–26.

73. Yuan CS, Wei G, Dey L, et al. Brief communication: American ginseng reduces warfarin's effect in healthy patients. A randomized controlled trial. Ann Intern Med. 2004;141:23–7.

74. Matthews MK Jr. Association of ginkgo biloba with intracerebral hemorrhage. Neurology. 1998;50:1933–4.

75. Bottorf MB. Distinct drug-interaction profiles for statins. Am J Health Syst Pharm. 1999;56:1019–20.

76. Ford NE, Sonnichsen DS. Clinically significant cytochrome P450 drug interactions – a comment. Pharmacotherapy. 1998;18:890–1.

77. Katial RK, Stelzle RC, Bonner MW, et al. A drug interaction between zafirlukast and theophylline. Arch Intern Med. 1998;158:1713–15.

78. McKindley D, Dufresne R. Current knowledge of the cytochrome p-450 isozyme system: can we predict clinically important drug interactions? Med Health. 1998;81:38–42.

79. Hansten PD, Horn JR. Drug Interactions Newsletter (with quarterly updates): a clinical perspective and analysis of current developments. Vancouver: Applied Therapeutics, 1998.

80. Tatro DS (ed.). Drug Interaction Facts (with quarterly updates). St Louis: Facts & Comparisons, 1998:91–92, 609a–10, 685d–g, 714a–b.

81. Tsikouris JP, Peeters MJ, Cox CD, Meyerrose GE, Seifert CF. Effects of three fluoroquinolones on QT analysis after standard treatment courses. Ann Noninvasive Electrocardiol. 2006;11:52–6.

82. Lode H. Evidence of different profiles of side effects and drug-drug interactions among the quinolones – the pharmacokinetic standpoint. Chemotherapy. 2001;47(suppl. 3):24–31, 44–8.

83. Desta Z, Kerbusch T, Soukhova N, et al. Identification and characterization of human cytochrome P450 isoforms interacting with pimozide. J Pharmacol Exp Ther. 1998;285:428–37.

84. Flockhart DA, Richard E, Woosley RL, et al. Metabolic interaction between clarithromycin and pimozide may result in cardiac toxicity. Clin Pharmacol Ther. 1996;59:189A.

85. Desta Z, Kerbusch T, Flockhart DA. Effect of clarithromycin on the pharmacokinetics and pharmacodynamics of pimozide in healthy poor and extensive metabolizers of cytochrome P450 2D6 (CYP2D6). Clin Pharmacol Ther. 1999;65:10–20.

86. Deeks SG, Smith M, Holodniy M, Kahn JO. HIV-1 protease inhibitors. JAMA. 1997;277:145–53.

87. Ouellet D, Hsu A, Qian J, et al. Effect of ritonavir on the pharmacokinetics of ethinyl estradiol in healthy female volunteers. Br J Clin Pharmacol. 1998;46:111–16.

88. Daly AK. Molecular basis of polymorphic drug metabolism. J Mol Med. 1995;73:539–53.

89. Butler M, Lang N, Young J, et al. Determination of CYP1A2 and NAT2 phenotypes in human populations by analysis of caffeine urinary metabolites. Pharmacogenetics. 1992;2:116–27.

90. Snow J, Gibson L. A pharmacogenetic basis for the safe and effective use of azathioprine and other thiopurine drugs in dermatologic patients. J Am Acad Dermatol. 1995;32:114–16.

91. Prandota J. Important role of proinflammatory cytokines/other endogenous substances in drug-induced hepatotoxicity: depression of drug metabolism during infections/inflammation states, and genetic polymorphisms of drug-metabolizing enzymes/cytokines may markedly contribute to this pathology. Am J Ther. 2005;12:254–61.

92. Schwartz DH, Merigan TC. Interleukin-2 in the treatment of HIV disease. Biotherapy. 1990;2:119–36.

Sunscreens

Vincent A DeLeo

132

Key features

- Modern sunscreens were first developed during the 1940s with the primary aim of preventing sunburn: today, sunscreens are also used to prevent other aspects of photodamage, including carcinogenesis and photoaging

- The active ingredients in sunscreens include inorganic agents (i.e. physical blockers) and organic compounds (i.e. chemical absorbers). The latter are further classified as UVB and/or UVA absorbers

- The ability of sunscreens to prevent cutaneous squamous cell carcinoma has been demonstrated in human studies. Their ability to prevent basal cell carcinoma and cutaneous melanoma remains controversial, although evidence supports efficacy in this regard

- Side effects from sunscreens include irritation (which is common) and allergy (which is rare)

- Sunscreen usage and sun avoidance may lead to a decrease in vitamin D levels in some individuals. The medical significance of this effect remains controversial, although optimum vitamin D levels can be achieved with a healthy diet and supplements

INTRODUCTION AND HISTORY

Sun Exposure

Evidence exists that even ancient civilizations sought protection from the damaging effects of the sun. The concept of excessive sun exposure as unhealthy or at least cosmetically unacceptable eventually spread to Northern Europe, especially among the aristocracy, and continued into the 19th century, until the period of the Industrial Revolution. In 1890, Palm noted that children in urban slums of England had rickets whereas those in similar housing conditions in sunny India did not, and linked the lack of sun to the development of rickets[1]. Physicians then began to treat such children with artificial UV radiation. At the same time, Finsen began to treat a number of other diseases, including tuberculosis and, interestingly, lupus erythematosus, with artificial light. He was awarded the Nobel Prize for his work in 1903. At the turn of the 20th century, the image of tanned skin as aesthetically pleasing began to emerge. The French fashion designer Coco Chanel is often credited with developing the concept of tanned skin as beautiful that still persists today. However, the 20th century also saw the recognition of sunburn as an effect of UVB, the discovery of UVC- and UVB-induced DNA mutations, and establishment of UVB as a complete carcinogen.

During the 1990s, dermatologists and other healthcare professionals made serious efforts to educate consumers regarding the damaging effects of excessive sun exposure as well as exposure to artificial tanning devices. Despite these efforts, recent studies show that while understanding of the adverse effects of exposure has increased, there has been very little positive change in behavior. This is especially true for adolescents, who continue to suffer sunburns in alarming numbers and who continue to seek a tan through natural and artificial exposure. Over 20 million Americans go to tanning salons every year and sunscreen usage has actually been declining in some studies[2,3,3a]. Achieving better compliance with sun protection will depend on a better understanding of behavior modification and techniques of disseminating the right message to consumers in an effective manner.

Sunscreens

Sunscreens are pharmaceutical preparations that attenuate UV wavelengths that would otherwise interact with molecules in the skin (chromophores) to generate photochemical reactions, leading to photobiologic change. These preparations are usually combinations of active agents or ingredients which absorb or scatter incident radiation, and they are dispersed in a variety of bases. The active ingredients are not absorbed in any large quantity into the living epidermis or dermis or the general circulation.

The first modern sunscreen was a product containing benzyl salicylate and benzyl cinnamate, which was introduced in the US in 1928. However, widespread use of sunscreens did not occur until World War II, when the US Military provided preparations containing red petrolatum to prevent sunburn in troops stationed in sunny areas. After the war, there was an increased interest in UV-absorbing chemicals, and para-aminobenzoic acid (PABA), patented in 1943, was the first of these to gain widespread usage. It was not until the mid-1970s that sunscreens gained a degree of consumer acceptance and sales of such products have continued to grow.

The initial sunscreens were produced primarily to prevent sunburn and therefore contained primarily UVB-absorbing agents. As scientific evidence grew documenting the deleterious effects of longer-wavelength UVA radiation and as manufacturers strove to develop higher levels of protection against burning, agents with absorption in the longer wavelengths (e.g. benzophenones) were combined with UVB absorbers. The physical blocking sunscreens (e.g. titanium dioxide) were used from the early days of sunscreen manufacturing, but, because of large particle size, were not cosmetically acceptable in high concentrations. Newer technology allowed for micronization of such particles, with an increase in transparency and therefore greater cosmetic acceptability. More recently, chemical agents with greater UVA absorption have been introduced (see below) and are gaining in popularity.

In addition to sunscreens for 'beach' use, manufacturers also began to develop various cosmetics for daily use which contained sunscreen agents. Today, a wide array of sunscreen-containing preparations, including foundations, moisturizers and lipsticks, are commercially available. Another improvement in sunscreen products has been the development of agents with increased substantivity. Such agents, usually marketed as 'sports' products, have bases which persist on the stratum corneum for longer than do the usual bases, allowing for vigorous outdoor activity and even swimming with retained photoprotection.

SUNSCREEN REGULATION

Since sunscreens alter the structure or function of skin, they are considered over-the-counter drugs in the US and are regulated by the Food and Drug Administration (FDA). Regulations include the maximum concentration of active ingredients, safety labeling, and the method for determining the sun protection factor (SPF).

Sun Protection Factor

The measure of efficacy of sunscreens is designated the sun protection factor (SPF), and the SPF is determined as outlined in Table 132.1. If properly tested and applied, a product with an SPF of 10 would allow 10 times as much time in the sun with the same resultant level of erythema as without the product in a given individual. An SPF 20 similarly would allow 20 times as much exposure with the same result. As shown in Table 132.2, this does not mean that the SPF 20 product absorbs twice as much radiation as the SPF 10 product.

Table 132.1 Determination of the sun protection factor (SPF). Based upon the 2007 FDA proposed regulations for sunscreen labeling, the SPF would still be measured in the same manner but would be renamed the *sunburn* protection factor and a rating system for UVA protection would consist of 1 to 4 stars (low, medium, high, highest). The UVA protection rating would be based upon an *in vivo* and an *in vitro* assay and would consist of the lower of the two results; the *in vitro* assay for assessing UVA protection would be based upon the breadth of reduction of UVA penetrance and the *in vivo* assay would measure the effect of the sunscreen on prevention of delayed pigment darkening.

RELATIONSHIP OF THE SUN PROTECTION FACTOR (SPF) TO BLOCKAGE OF ERYTHEMAL RADIATION

SPF	Blockage of erythemal radiation (%)
10	90
15	92.5
20	95
40	97.5

Table 132.2 Relationship of the sun protection factor (SPF) to blockage of erythemal radiation.

Testing for UVA Protection

Since scientists have become aware of the damage that can be caused by photons of wavelengths longer than 320 nm, many attempts have been made to develop a standard method of testing for protection against long-wave or UVA radiation. Since there is no easily reproducible and biologically relevant endpoint for UVA radiation (like erythema for the UVB range), investigators have suggested a number of assays, including both *in vitro* and *in vivo* methodology. Some researchers have suggested that erythema produced by UVA sources could be utilized, but the irradiation times for such wavelengths are too long to make such an assay practical. Others have utilized psoralen-sensitized human skin plus UVA, with delayed erythema as the endpoint. Such an assay, however, has the shortcoming of measuring protection from only the photons responsible for psoralen photosensitivity.

The most commonly utilized assays developed in human skin include immediate pigment darkening and delayed or persistent pigment darkening, both with endpoints that measure the skin's overall tanning response to UVA radiation. The former, as discussed elsewhere in this text, is dependent upon radiation-induced darkening of pre-formed melanin, while the latter is a more complex response which includes increased production and transfer of melanin as well as proliferation of melanocytes. Both endpoints can be produced with relatively small amounts of UVA radiation, making them reasonable for human assays. The assay for persistent pigment darkening is utilized in Japan[4].

The most commonly accepted *in vitro* method for assaying UVA protection is the critical wavelength determination, which is utilized in some countries in the European Union and in Australia. This is a relatively simple assay in which the sunscreen is dissolved in solvent and the absorption spectrum is determined in a spectrophotometer. The critical wavelength for the product is determined as the wavelength at which 90% of solar-simulated radiation above 320 nm is absorbed[5].

In 1999, the most current FDA regulations regarding sunscreens were published. They included a labeling cap of 30+ for the SPF and the term *waterproof* was changed to *very water resistant*. However, methods for testing and labeling for long-wave range protection were not addressed and manufacturers had to limit claims of efficacy (in labeling or marketing) to protection from sunburn. In response to the 1999 regulations, a consensus conference was held[6]. One recommendation was that there be no cap on the SPF; it was thought that such a cap would discourage manufacturers from producing more protective sunscreens, since without labeling there would be no way for clinicians and consumers to identify such products. A second recommendation was to standardize testing and labeling for long-wave range protection; both critical wavelength determination (see above) and an *in vivo* human assay such as delayed pigment darkening could be utilized and the level of UVA protection of a product should be included on the label (along with the standard SPF value). A third recommendation was for the UVA protection afforded by a product be proportional to its level of UVB protection, so that products that were highly protective in the UVB range would have comparable protection in the UVA range. Lastly, assessments of sunscreen efficacy should go beyond protection against sunburn, since additional benefits would increase consumer awareness of other harmful effects of sun exposure and hopefully lead to greater usage of sunscreens.

In August 2007, the FDA released proposed regulations for sunscreen labelling (The Final Rule) that included several changes: (1) the SPF claim could be increased from 30+ to 50+; (2) the SPF would still be measured in the same manner but would be renamed the *sunburn* protection factor; (3) a rating system for UVA protection would consist of 1 to 4 stars (low, medium, high, highest); (4) the UVA protection rating would be based upon an *in vivo* and an *in vitro* assay and would consist of the lower of the two results; and (5) a warning label that UV exposure from the sun 'increases the risk of skin cancer, premature aging and other skin damage' as well as a recommendation that it is important to reduce UV exposure 'by limiting time in the sun, wearing protective clothing, and using a sunscreen' would be placed on the sunscreen label. The *in vitro* assay for assessing UVA protection would be based upon the breadth of reduction of UVA penetrance and the *in vivo* assay would measure the effect of the sunscreen on prevention of delayed pigment darkening in a manner similar to the way in which SPF is determined based on prevention of sunburn.

MECHANISMS OF SUNSCREEN ACTION

Sunscreens, when applied properly, form a film or coating on the surface of the stratum corneum and attenuate radiation that would otherwise reach the living epidermis and dermis. The active agents in sunscreen products do this by either absorbing or scattering the photons reaching the skin (Fig. 132.1). Agents which scatter radiation are opaque particles of inorganic materials and are referred to as physical agents or sunblockers. Agents which absorb radiation are organic compounds, referred to as chemical agents or sunscreens. Scattering of radiation by inorganics is based on particle size, while chemical absorption is related to chemical structure. The photons scattered by the inorganic screens are reflected back out of the skin, whereas the energy absorbed by the organic agents is converted to non-damaging energy and dissipated primarily as heat. Many sunscreen products today contain combinations of both types of agents.

Because of the large particle size of the original preparations of inorganic agents, they were not deemed cosmetically acceptable, owing to their opaque appearance on the skin. Nowadays, these agents are formulated as micronized particles, resulting in products that are more cosmetically acceptable. However, such micronized inorganics actually act more like organic sunscreens, scattering as well as absorbing radiation to some extent.

Currently, most sunscreens contain a combination of two or more agents created to offer high levels of protection against both UVB and longer-wavelength radiation.

ACTIVE INGREDIENTS IN SUNSCREENS

Figure 132.2 lists, according to type of activity and spectrum of protection, the active agents currently used in sunscreens[7].

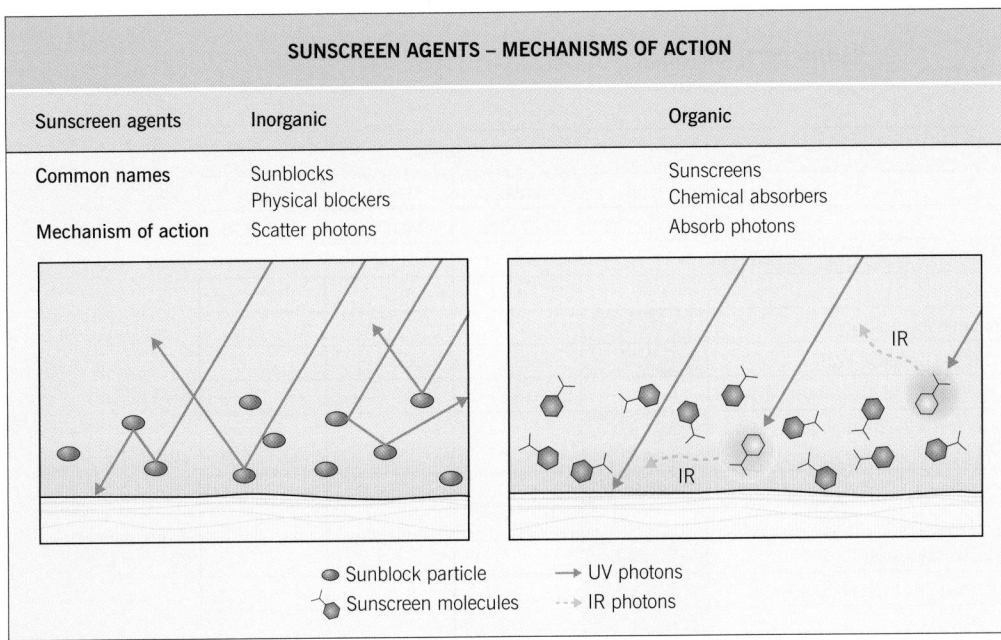

Fig. 132.1 Sunscreen agents – mechanisms of action. IR, infrared. Schematics courtesy of Mark Naylor MD.

Organic Screens

Para-aminobenzoic acid and derivatives

Padimate O (or octyl dimethyl PABA) is a PABA ester and one of the most common UVB absorbers found in sunscreens today. Both padimate O and its parent compound, PABA, are highly effective UVB absorbers. However, the latter causes staining of clothing and today is utilized infrequently.

Cinnamates

Octyl methoxycinnamate is a good UVB absorber but is not as potent as PABA and its esters. Presently, it is the most common sunscreen ingredient in the US. Although an approved agent, cinoxate is currently not used in any sunscreens in the US.

Salicylates

The salicylates are relatively weak UVB absorbers but do have the ability to stabilize other agents, thereby preventing photodegradation. Consequently, they are used in combination with other organics. This group includes octisalate, homosalate and trolamine salicylate.

Benzophenones

Benzophenones are good UVA absorbers, although their effectiveness is primarily in the UVA2 range. Oxybenzone is the most commonly used agent in this group and actually affords both UVB and UVA protection. Sulisobenzone and dioxybenzone have similar protective spectra but are infrequently utilized.

Other organic screens

Octocrylene is a commonly used UVB filter which is primarily employed to stabilize photolabile agents. Ensulizole is likewise a photostable UVB absorber. Avobenzone is an excellent UVA filter with absorption well into the UVA1 range, but is very photolabile. It is combined with other agents which assist in stabilizing its protective ability. Meradimate is a UVA filter with a maximum absorption in the UVA2 range, but its efficacy is relatively weak.

Mexoryl™ SX is a camphor derivative with an absorption maximum at 345 nm, well into the UVA1 range. Mexoryl™ XL is a benzotriazole with both UVB and UVA absorption, with a maximum absorption at 344 nm. Lastly, Tinosorb® M is a combination agent with both UVB and UVA absorption (maximum at 358 nm) and Tinosorb® S is a UVA filter with absorption into the UVA1 range.

Inorganic Screens

The two major inorganic screens are titanium dioxide and zinc oxide. There are a few so-called 'chemical-free' products that contain only inorganics, but usually these agents are combined with organic screens. The activity of the inorganic agents depends upon particle size. Agents with large particle size like those on the market in the 1970s offered protection well into the UVA1 and even visible ranges, but because of their opaque appearance they were not acceptable to many consumers. More cosmetically acceptable agents were developed with smaller particle size (i.e. micronized), but at the expense of shifting the protection toward the shorter UVA2 range. Micronized zinc oxide appears to have better activity in the UVA1 range than does titanium dioxide at comparable concentrations[8].

Other Agents

Dihydroxyacetone is the compound most commonly used in sunless tanners. This agent, which when applied is colorless, binds to the stratum corneum and colors the skin to produce a tanned appearance. Although it has a very low SPF, it does offer protection from long-wave radiation (even into the visible range). Iron oxide offers protection across the UV spectrum and into the visible range, and is used a colorant in some products[9].

Other 'active' ingredients have been added to sunscreens, with claims of increasing efficacy of the finished products[7]. The most popular of these are antioxidants, including vitamins E and C and green tea polyphenols, some of which have decreased UV-induced damage in *in vitro* and *in vivo* assays. However, factors including chemical structure, concentration and stability in a finished product cannot be determined from package labels, so at this point it is impossible for the clinician and the consumer to judge efficacy.

SUNSCREEN EFFICACY

A good modern sunscreen should protect against sunburn, carcinogenesis, photoaging, photoimmune suppression and photosensitivity. Efficacy of a given sunscreen product is usually assumed if the combined absorption spectra of the agents in a product match the action spectrum of a given adverse event.

The action spectra for the adverse effects of sun exposure are listed in Table 132.3. There is abundant evidence that sunburn, non-melanoma skin cancer induction, photoimmune suppression and photoaging are all most efficiently produced by UVB radiation. However, studies have shown that for some of these events, UVA also plays a greater or lesser role. For example, UVB is about 1000 times as effective at inducing erythema in human skin as is UVA. On the other hand, photoaging was originally thought to be primarily due to UVB radiation, but UVA penetrates more deeply into the dermis and is likely to have an important role in this process. Similarly, although most studies (in a number of model systems) show that the maximal effective radiation

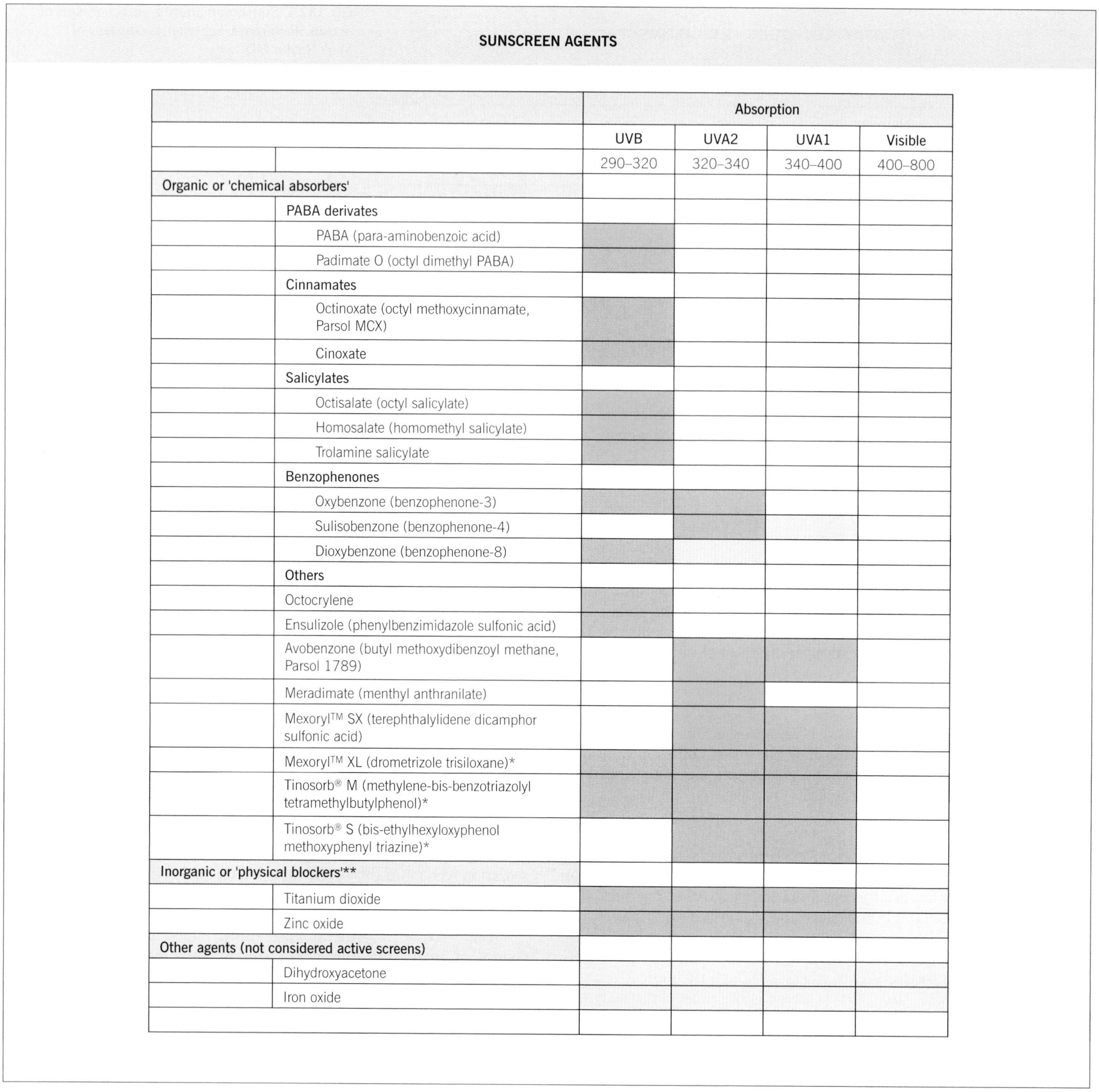

		Absorption			
		UVB	UVA2	UVA1	Visible
		290–320	320–340	340–400	400–800
Organic or 'chemical absorbers'					
	PABA derivates				
	PABA (para-aminobenzoic acid)	▓			
	Padimate O (octyl dimethyl PABA)	▓			
	Cinnamates				
	Octinoxate (octyl methoxycinnamate, Parsol MCX)	▓			
	Cinoxate	▓			
	Salicylates				
	Octisalate (octyl salicylate)	▓			
	Homosalate (homomethyl salicylate)	▓			
	Trolamine salicylate	▓			
	Benzophenones				
	Oxybenzone (benzophenone-3)	▓	▓		
	Sulisobenzone (benzophenone-4)	▓	▓		
	Dioxybenzone (benzophenone-8)	▓	▓		
	Others				
	Octocrylene	▓			
	Ensulizole (phenylbenzimidazole sulfonic acid)	▓			
	Avobenzone (butyl methoxydibenzoyl methane, Parsol 1789)		▓	▓	
	Meradimate (menthyl anthranilate)		▓		
	Mexoryl™ SX (terephthalylidene dicamphor sulfonic acid)		▓		
	Mexoryl™ XL (drometrizole trisiloxane)*	▓	▓	▓	
	Tinosorb® M (methylene-bis-benzotriazolyl tetramethylbutylphenol)*	▓	▓	▓	
	Tinosorb® S (bis-ethylhexyloxyphenol methoxyphenyl triazine)*	▓	▓	▓	
Inorganic or 'physical blockers'					
	Titanium dioxide	▓	▓	▓	
	Zinc oxide	▓	▓	▓	
Other agents (not considered active screens)					
	Dihydroxyacetone				
	Iron oxide				

Fig. 132.2 Sunscreen agents. * Currently not FDA-approved. ** Depending on particle size. Lighter colored bars represent variable efficacy (based upon particle size).

for producing photoimmune suppression is in the UVB range, sunscreens with only UVB protective agents are not totally effective in blocking this effect[10].

With regard to cutaneous squamous cell carcinoma (SCC), epidemiologic and animal studies combined with the identification of UVB and UVA 'signature' mutations in human SCCs strongly support causation primarily by UVB, but UVA may also play a role[11]. Most evidence also supports the role of UVB in basal cell carcinoma (BCC) induction, but a great deal of controversy exists as to the action spectrum for melanoma. Still, UVB seems the most likely culprit. New models for melanoma are currently under investigation and may prove enlightening in this debate in the near future.

It must also be remembered that even though UVA may be less effective at inducing a given event in the skin when compared to UVB, there is 10 to 20 times as much UVA as UVB in sunlight (Fig. 132.3).

This ratio is even higher in the skin of an individual wearing a UVB-protective sunscreen (especially if the SPF is ≤8) which might allow him or her to stay in the sun longer and get larger amounts of UVA radiation[12]. Therefore, the use of broad-spectrum sunscreens should be a goal of any photoprotection strategy.

Although the effectiveness of the protection of a given product might be predicted from a comparison of the action spectrum (see Table 132.3) versus the absorption spectrum (see Fig. 132.2), the most valid measures of efficacy are prospective studies in human subjects. However, in the case of skin cancer and photoaging, these studies are difficult to conduct because the photobiologic processes have such a long latency period. Animal models can be utilized, and this has often been done for photoaging and SCC induction, but has been quite limited for BCC (e.g. mice with only one normal allele for *Ptch*) and melanoma (e.g. opossums). Another approach has been to employ assays that measure

Effect	Spectrum of light			Type of evidence
	UVB	**UVA**	**Visible**	
Sunburn	++++	+		1
Photoaging	++++	++	?	3,4
Squamous cell carcinoma	++++	+		2,3,4
Basal cell carcinoma	+++	?		2,4
Cutaneous melanoma	++	+		3,4
Photoimmune suppression	++++	++		1,3,4
Photosensitivity	+	+++	+	1 (varies with disease)

ACTION SPECTRA FOR PHOTODAMAGE

Relative values.

Table 132.3 Action spectra for photodamage*. 1, human studies; 2, epidemiologic studies; 3, animal studies; 4, *in vitro* studies of associated biologic endpoints.

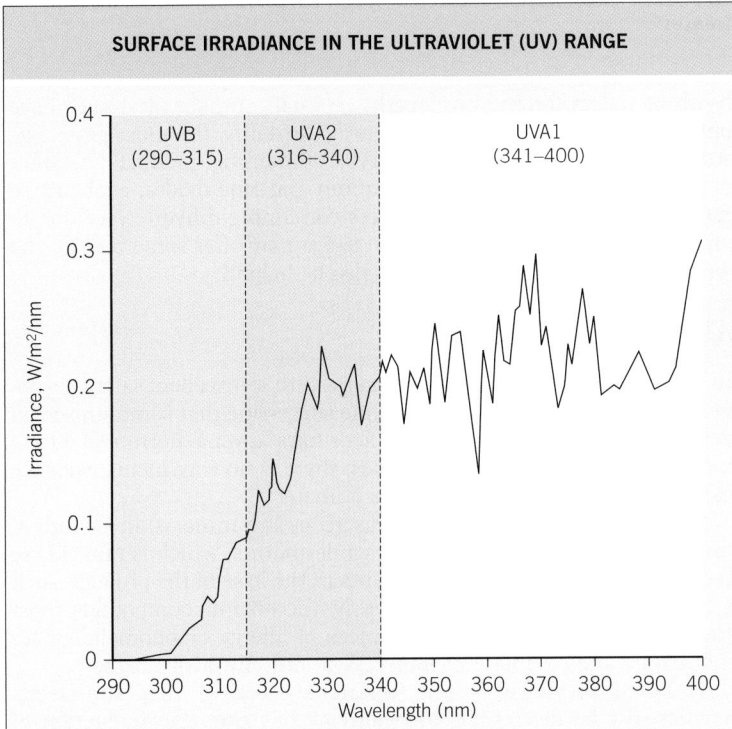

Fig. 132.3 Surface irradiance in the UV range. Courtesy of Mark Naylor MD.

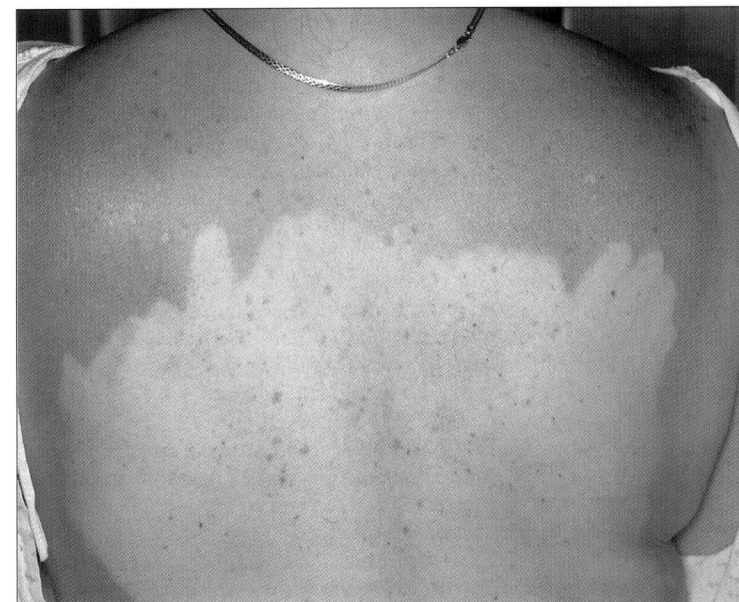

Fig. 132.4 Lack of sunburn in areas of sunscreen application. Peripheral edge represents outline of fingers. Courtesy of Kalman Watsky MD.

the effect of sunscreens on biologic endpoints known to be important precursors in a pathologic process (but before the development of a recognizable lesion). Examples would be studying the effects of sunscreens on the development of actinic keratoses or assaying for DNA damage or mutated genes in human skin[12].

Much of the information on sunscreen efficacy is based on retrospective case-controlled studies. Because of the lower level of validity of such studies and because of variability of study design and especially the inherent recall bias, many such studies arrive at conflicting results. In addition, prospective trials are limited by the ability to blind subjects (to control vehicle vs active ingredients) in the setting of sun exposure.

Sunburn

Literally tens of thousands of unpublished SPF studies performed in the pre-marketing testing of sunscreens attest to their ability to prevent sunburn. Controlled human studies in 'real world' settings have found, however, that sunscreen usage does not always prevent sunburn[13]. The major reason for this dichotomy is that individuals do not apply

sunscreens at the same concentrations as are utilized in controlled SPF testing – that is, 2 mg/cm^2. Some studies have shown that most sunscreen users apply only 25–75% of that quantity[14]. This means that the SPF is similarly reduced, i.e. applying only one-half of the standard amount of an SPF 15 product will result in protection comparable to a product with an SPF of 7.5. The proper quantity of sunscreen to cover the skin of an adult is approximately 30 cm^3 or two tablespoons. Strategies to improve compliance include applying the product twice to gain the proper concentration which also cuts down on skip areas (Fig. 132.4) or to use a product with twice the SPF as desired[15,16].

Photoaging

There are numerous animal studies demonstrating that sunscreen usage prevents clinical and histologic changes of photoaging and such usage can actually help reduce some of the damage that has already occurred. In addition, Boyd et al.[17] noted a significant reduction in dermal elastosis with daily sunscreen use over a 2-year period during an actinic keratosis study. A shorter-term study found that sunscreens with broad spectral coverage (extending significantly into the UVA spectrum) prevented many biochemical measures of sun damage (from solar-simulated radiation) in human volunteers[18].

Photoimmune Suppression

Immune suppression by UV radiation was first reported in animal studies that showed that mice could no longer reject UV-induced skin tumors if they had been irradiated with non-tumorigenic doses of UV before transplantation of the tumors. This immunosuppressive effect of UV has been shown to affect delayed-type hypersensitivity and contact sensitivity as well as tumor rejection and has been shown to be active in humans as well as animals[19,19a]. While the responsible action spectrum has been shown to be predominantly in the UVB range, in experimental studies UVB sunscreens have not always afforded protection against immune suppression[20]. In an elegantly designed study in a large number of human volunteers, Kelly and colleagues[21] reported that sunscreen did offer some protection against suppression but the level of protection was not as great as its protection against sunburn. The researchers utilized a measure of photoprotection against suppression, designated the immune protective factor (IPF), and compared it with the erythema protection factor (EPF), a measure similar to SPF. The IPF was only 4.9, while the EPF was 14.2. The authors postulated that this difference was due to UVA radiation not blocked by the applied sunscreen[21]. Some investigators concerned about the effect of photoimmune suppression on various aspects of human health have suggested that sunscreens should be tested and labeled for IPF as well as SPF.

Non-melanoma Skin Cancer

Because of the long latency period for the development of SCC and BCC, the first two prospective studies in humans examining the effect of sunscreen on cancer prevention used actinic keratoses, precursors of SCC, as surrogates for the cancer. Naylor et al.[22] studied the daily application of an SPF 29 sunscreen applied over a 2-year period in a group of 53 individuals with a previous history of actinic keratoses. The sunscreen-treated group had significantly fewer actinic keratoses over the 2-year period compared with the placebo group. The difference between the two groups with regard to skin cancers was not significant, probably due to the relatively short duration of the trial.

Thompson et al.[23] studied the effects of an SPF 17 sunscreen applied daily in 588 individuals over 40 years of age during a single Australian summer. This study also found a significant reduction in the number of actinic keratoses in the sunscreen-treated group.

Later, Green et al.[24] undertook a prospective study of the daily use of an SPF 17 sunscreen in individuals in Australia. This study compared an active intervention group, in which sunscreen was supplied and its use encouraged, against the background rate of sunscreen use in the general population. SCCs were found to be significantly less in the sunscreen-treated group, but there was no difference in the number of BCCs between the two groups. From clinical observations regarding anatomic distribution, the relationship between UV radiation and BCC is known to be more complex than with SCC.

Cutaneous Melanoma

Developing sunscreen efficacy studies for decreasing the risk of melanoma would be very difficult and might not be considered ethical. As with SCC and actinic keratoses, a number of researchers have used the development of melanocytic nevi in children as a marker for melanoma risk. The number of nevi has been related to sun exposure in children and the former has also been linked to risk for melanoma[25]. In several retrospective epidemiologic studies, researchers have actually reported that children who used sunscreens had an increased number of nevi[26]. However, in the single published prospective controlled study to date, Gallagher et al.[27] demonstrated that sunscreens could suppress the development of nevi. The study was conducted over a 3-year period with an SPF 30 sunscreen in a total of 485 schoolchildren 6 to 9 years of age.

Currently, there is no direct experimental evidence in humans to support the use of sunscreens as a means to prevent melanoma, although it is likely that they can, if used appropriately. However, this view is not held by all investigators. The results from case-controlled retrospective studies of melanoma patients are conflicting with regard to sunscreen usage and the risk of developing melanoma. Some of these studies show a decreased risk, while others actually show an increased risk. Meta-analyses of the published studies by two different groups concluded that sunscreen usage did not increase the risk of developing melanoma, but the analyses could not confirm a protective effect from using sunscreen[28,29].

This dichotomy of results has led to the most important controversy concerning the use of sunscreens. The controversy is based on two different but related lines of reasoning. The first relates to the action spectrum for induction of melanoma. If in fact the action spectrum for melanoma is in the UVA range (as suggested by studies in fish), then wearing sunscreens with UVB protection will allow individuals to stay in the sun longer and receive larger doses of UVA, thereby increasing their risk of developing melanoma. However, several animal models suggest that the action spectrum is probably predominantly in the UVB range. The second theory is based on the concept that sunscreen usage decreases vitamin D levels in humans and that vitamin D has been shown to reduce proliferation and increase differentiation of various normal and tumor cells; as a result, low vitamin D levels may increase the risk of developing some cancers, including melanoma[30].

Photosensitivity Disorders (see Ch. 86)

The action spectra of the more common photosensitivity disorders are listed in Table 132.4. Some of these reactions are caused by UVB radiation, but the majority of affected individuals react to UVA and/or visible light. Therefore they require photoprotection with agents that

Disease	Spectrum of light		
	UVB	UVA	Visible
Polymorphous light eruption	+	++	
Hydroa vacciniforme	+	++	
Solar urticaria	+	++	++
Chronic actinic dermatitis	+++	++	+
Actinic prurigo	++	++	
Photoallergic contact dermatitis		+++	
Photoirritant contact dermatitis		+++	
Photodrug reactions	+	+++	+
Porphyria			+++
Lupus erythematosus	+++	++	

CLASSIFICATION AND ACTION SPECTRA OF PHOTOSENSITIVE SKIN DISEASES

*Relative values.

Table 132.4 Classification and action spectra of photosensitive skin diseases*.

absorb or reflect longer wavelengths; a small number of studies have confirmed the efficacy of such agents[30]. Currently, the most protective formulations appear to be Mexoryl™-containing products[31]. Other useful agents include inorganic titanium and zinc oxides, avobenzone and benzophenones. The self-tanners containing dihydroxyacetone in combination with regular sunscreen usage may offer some benefit and iron oxide-containing products can also be helpful.

SUNSCREEN SAFETY

Sunscreens have been utilized for decades with an excellent safety record. While studies appear from time to time suggesting that some sunscreen agents are mutagenic or carcinogenic or have adverse hormonal effects in various *in vitro* and animal studies, there is no convincing evidence that such studies have relevance for humans[32].

The major adverse effects of sunscreens are minor skin irritation, which is common, and allergic contact dermatitis, which is rare. These reactions are usually due to ingredients in the base of the product, such as fragrance or preservatives. Presently, the organic compounds most often responsible for the rare instances of allergy or photoallergy are oxybenzone and padimate O, and, less commonly, avobenzone[33].

As noted previously, some researchers believe that sunscreens may actually be deleterious to health by blocking the production of vitamin D. The first step in the production of this important nutrient is the conversion within the epidermis of 7-dehydroxycholesterol to pro-vitamin D_3 by UVB radiation (see Ch. 51). Sunscreens that are effective at blocking UVB photons would therefore be expected to decrease levels of vitamin D, and studies have shown that this does in fact occur. However, the majority of human studies that measured serum vitamin D levels in sunscreen users (as compared to non-users) found that the levels, though reduced, were within the normal range[34]. In addition, studies have shown that dark-skinned individuals, women, and, during the wintertime, individuals who live in northerly climes all have reduced levels[35].

Recently, scientists in the fields of nutrition and bone metabolism have presented data suggesting that individuals who have serum vitamin D levels in the low normal range may actually have insufficient vitamin D for optimum health. Some of these studies suggest that not only do these low normal or 'insufficient' levels of vitamin D adversely affect good musculoskeletal health, but that they may also increase the risk of other adverse events like cancer and decreased immune function[36]. One recent publication linked lower levels of sun exposure to decreased survival in melanoma patients and suggested that this was related to insufficient vitamin D[36,37].

A controversy has arisen because scientists cannot agree on what constitutes the 'normal' range for serum 25-OH vitamin D levels and similarly cannot agree on the minimum suggested daily intake for the vitamin. Although vitamin D can be obtained from foods such as fish oils, in developed countries the more common sources are vitamin D-fortified milk and milk products, as well as vitamin supplements. At the time of writing, 400–600 IU is considered the daily minimum for adults. Unfortunately, the tanning salon industry has 'fanned the flames' by suggesting that UV light exposure and tanning represent the optimum way to assure healthy vitamin D metabolism. This prompted a multidisciplinary conference on 'Sunlight, Tanning Booths, and Vitamin D' to be convened in 2004[38].

This area of medicine is evolving and, as specialists in skin health and disease, we should not simply deny any merit to this controversy. We should await solid science from our colleagues in other fields to guide us as to what constitutes normal laboratory values for circulating levels of vitamin D and what the adequate daily intake of this vitamin should be. However, this does not mean that we should change our message about sun avoidance and sunscreen usage; we simply have to suggest that all individuals maintain adequate vitamin D intake through diet and supplements.

SUNSCREEN RECOMMENDATIONS

There is ever-increasing evidence that although the public is aware of the damaging effects of sun exposure, there does not seem to be a significant degree of alteration in behavior. In an effort to re-energize the medical community's need to try to change behavior, the American Academy of Dermatology has reformulated its message concerning protection (www.aad.org). While the importance of sunscreen is stressed, the recommendations are broader and more positive, and hopefully this and other improvements in consumer education will eventually lead to a decrease in photodamage in the world's population.

REFERENCES

1. Giacomoni PU. Sunprotection: historical perspective. In: Shaath NA (ed.). Sunscreens: Regulations and Commercial Development, 3rd edn. Boca Raton, FL: Taylor & Francis, 2005:71–81.
2. Geller AC, Colditz G, Oliveria S, et al. Use of sunscreen, sunburning rates, and tanning bed use among more than 10,000 US school children and adolescents. Pediatrics. 2002;109:1009–14.
3. Davis KJ, Cokkinides VE, Weinstock MA, et al. Summer sunburn and sun exposure among US youths ages 11–18: national prevalence and associated factors. Pediatrics. 2002;110:27–35.
3a. El Sayed F, Ammoury A, Nakhle F, et al. Photoprotection in teenagers. Photodermatol Photoimmunol Photomed. 2006; 22:18–21.
4. Moyal D, Chardon A, Kollias N. UVA protection efficacy of sunscreens can be determined by the persistent pigment darkening (PPD) method (part 1): calibration of the method. Photodermatol Photoimmunol Photomed. 2000;16:245–9.
5. Diffey BL, Tanner PR, Matts PJ, et al. In vitro assessment of the broad spectrum ultraviolet protection of sunscreen products. J Am Acad Dermatol. 2000; 43:1024–35.
6. Lim HW, Naylor M, Honigsmann H, et al. American Academy of Dermatology consensus conference on UVA protection of sunscreens: summary and recommendations. Washington, DC: Feb 4, 2000. J Am Acad Dermatol. 2001;44:505–8.
7. Kullavanijaya P, Lim HW. Photoprotection. J Am Acad Dermatol. 2005;52:938–58.
8. Pinnell SR, Fairhurst D, Gillies R, et al. Microfine zinc oxide is a superior sunscreen ingredient to microfine titanium dioxide. Dermatol Surg 2000;26:309–14.
9. Murphy GM. Sunblocks: mechanism of action. Photodermatol Photoimmunol Photomed. 1999;15:34–6.
10. Young AR. Are broad-spectrum sunscreens necessary for immunoprotection? J Invest Dermatol. 2003;121:ix–x.
11. Agar NS, Halliday GM, Barnetson, RS, et al. The basal layer in human squamous tumors harbors more UVA than UVB fingerprint mutations: a role for UVA in human skin carcinogenesis. Proc Natl Acad Sci USA. 2004;101:4954–9.
12. Fourtanier A. Mexoryl SX protects against solar-simulated photocarcinogenesis in mice. Photodermatol Photoimmunol Photomed. 1996;64:688–93.

13. Wright MW, Wright ST, Wagner RF. Mechanisms of sunscreen failure. J Am Acad Dermatol. 2001;44:781–4.
14. Azuridia RM, Pagliaro JA, Diffey BL, et al. Sunscreen application by photosensitive patients is inadequate for protection. Br J Dermatol.1999;140:255–8.
15. Diffey BL. When should sunscreens be reapplied? J Am Acad Dermatol. 2001;45:882–5.
16. Pruim B, Green A. Photobiological aspects of sunscreen re-application. Australas J Dermatol. 1999; 40:14–18.
17. Boyd AS, Naylor M, Cameron GS, et al. The effects of chronic sunscreen use on the histologic changes of dermatoheliosis. J Am Acad Dermatol. 1995;33:941–6.
18. Stenberg C, Larko O. Sunscreen application and its importance for the sun protection factor. Arch Dermatol. 1985;121:1400–2.
19. Ullrich SE. Photoimmune suppression and photocarcinogenesis. Front Biosci. 2002;17:d684–703.
19a. Hanneman KK, Cooper KD, Baron ED. Ultraviolet immunosuppression: mechanisms and consequences. Dermatol Clin. 2006;24:19–25.
20. Baron ED, Fourtanier A, Compan D, et al. High ultraviolet A protection affords greater immune protection confirming that ultraviolet A contributes to photoimmunosuppression in humans. J Invest Dermatol. 2003;121:869–75.
21. Kelly DA, Seed PT, Young AR, et al. A commercial sunscreen's protection against ultraviolet radiation-induced immunosuppression is more than 50% lower than protection against sunburn in humans. J Invest Dermatol. 2003;120:65–71.
22. Naylor MF, Boyd A, Smith DW, et al. High sun protection factor (SPF) sunscreens in the suppression of actinic neoplasia. Arch Dermatol. 1995;131:170–5.
23. Thompson SC, Jolley D, Marks R. Reduction of solar keratoses by regular sunscreen use. N Engl J Med. 1993;329:1147–51.
24. Green A, Williams G, Neale R, et al. Daily sunscreen application and betacarotene supplementation in prevention of basal-cell and squamous-cell carcinomas of the skin: a randomised controlled trial. Lancet.1999;354:723–9.
25. Azizi E, Iscovich J, Pavlotsky F, et al. Use of sunscreen is linked with elevated naevi counts in Israeli school children and adolescents. Melanoma Res. 2000;10:491–8.
26. Autier P, Dor JF, Severi G. More about sunscreen use, wearing clothes, and number of nevi in 6 to 7 year

old European children. J Natl Cancer Inst. 1999; 91:1165–6.
27. Gallagher RP, Rivers JK, Lee TK, et al. Broad-spectrum sunscreen use and the development of new nevi in white children: a randomized controlled trial. JAMA. 2000;283:2955–60.
28. Bastuji-Garin S, Diepgen TL. Cutaneous malignant melanoma, sun exposure, and sunscreen use: epidemiological evidence. Br J Dermatol. 2002;146(suppl. 61):24–30.
29. Huncharek M, Kupelnick B. Use of topical sunscreens and the risk of malignant melanoma: a meta-analysis of 9067 patients from 11 case control studies. Am J Public Health. 2003;93:11–12.
30. Eide MJ, Weinstock MA. Public health challenges in sun protection. Dermatol Clin. 2006;24:119–24.
31. DeLeo V. Sunscreen use in photodermatoses. Dermatol Clin. 2006;24:27–33.
32. Gasparro FP, Mitchnick M, Nash JF. A review of sunscreen safety and efficacy. Photochem Photobiol. 1998;68:243–56.
33. DeLeo VA. Photocontact dermatitis. Dermatol Ther. 2004;17;279–88.
34. Sollitto RB, Kraemer KH, DiGiovanna JJ. Normal vitamin D levels can be maintained despite rigorous photoprotection: six years' experience with xeroderma pigmentosum J Am Acad Dermatol. 1997;37:942–7.
35. Nesby-O'Dell S, Scanlon KS, Cogswell ME, et al. Hypovitaminosis D prevalence and determinants among African American and white women of reproductive age: third National Health and Nutrition Examination Survey, 1988–1994. Am J Clin Nutr. 2002;76:187–92.
36. Egan KM, Sosman JA, Blot WJ. Sunlight and reduced risk of cancer: is the real story vitamin D? J Natl Cancer Inst. 2005;97:161–3.
37. Berwick M, Armstrong BK, Ben-Porat L, et al. Sun exposure and mortality from melanoma. J Natl Cancer Inst. 2005;97:195–8.
38. Lim, HW, Gilchrest BA, Cooper KD, et al. Sunlight, tanning booths, and vitamin D. J Am Acad Dermatol. 2005;52:868–76.

Complementary and Alternative Medicine

Amy Geng and Raymond G Dufresne Jr

Key features

- Complementary and alternative medicine (CAM) is being used by many patients, and is rising in popularity
- CAM consists of a large set of unrelated methods
- Amongst dermatology patients, the most popular forms of CAM include herbals, dietary supplements, and homeopathy
- Scientific research into CAM treatments is growing

INTRODUCTION

Complementary and alternative medicine (CAM) is also known as integrative, unconventional, or traditional medicine. CAM represents a diverse set of healthcare systems, practices and treatment modalities, which are grouped together because they are not considered part of conventional medicine. Various classifications of CAM have been suggested, including one summarized in Table 133.1[1].

An estimated 65% to 80% of the world's population uses CAM as their initial and perhaps only type of medical care[1]. The prevalence of CAM usage is higher in developing countries, but is significant and rising in developed countries. In the US, use of alternative therapies rose from 33.8% in 1990 to 42.1% in 1997[2]. Fifty percent of the US population takes supplements[3], and 18.4% of all prescription users also take herbals or high-dose vitamins[1]. Out-of-pocket expenditures on alternative medicine totaled US$27.0 billion in 1997, a figure comparable to out-of-pocket costs for all US physician services[2]. In Europe and Australia, CAM usage is also significant, with estimates from 20% to 70% of the general population.

Patients who use CAM tend to be female, middle-aged, middle-class, better-educated, and express a high degree of satisfaction with their care. However, CAM usage is likely underestimated in children, the elderly, and lower-income populations.

The few existing studies regarding dermatology and CAM usage suggest that patients use CAM to complement conventional medicine in the treatment of most dermatologic conditions. An estimated 35% to 70% of dermatology patients use CAM during their lifetimes, most frequently herbals, dietary supplements, and homeopathy[4].

This chapter provides a survey of CAM used for dermatologic conditions, with preference given to those modalities with more supportive evidence in the literature.

BOTANICALS AND OTHER BIOLOGICALLY BASED PRACTICES

Introduction

Biologically based practices include botanicals, animal-derived products, vitamins, minerals, fatty acids, amino acids, proteins, prebiotics, probiotics (substances that promote growth of microorganisms), diets, and functional foods. Consumption of these products represents the most commonly used CAM in dermatology. Between 40% and 46% of the US population uses supplements regularly; usage may be more frequent among those who have one or more health problems, consume high amounts of alcohol, or are obese[1].

Modern medicine has its roots in natural substances; however, biologically based practices and conventional medicine differ funda-

mentally. Conventional medicine takes a reductionist view of the body's functions, emphasizing a belief in science's ability to isolate the active molecules needed to treat specific diseases. In contrast, biologically based practices would ideally take a holistic approach to health and emphasize disease prevention and health promotion by strengthening the body's own healing mechanisms.

Dermatologic Applications

Conventional dermatology uses many products of herbal origins, including podophyllin, psoralens, oatmeal and pyrethrins. This chapter limits its discussion to herbals that are less well known to dermatologists but are commonly used; additional herbals are listed in Table 133.2.

Witch hazel and other astringents

Witch hazel (*Hamamelis virginiana*) and other astringent herbs such as white oak bark (*Quercus*) and English walnut leaf (*Juglans regia*) are used for treating acne. Witch hazel can also be used to treat eczema and oral ulcers; its vasoconstrictive effects may be beneficial in treating varicose veins and hemorrhoids. Astringent herbs contain tannins, which coagulate cell-surface proteins to form a protective barrier. Other tannin-containing herbs include St. John's wort, agrimony, Labrador tea, goldenrod, lady's mantle, lavender, rhubarb and yellow dock[5,6].

Aloe vera

The gel from *Aloe vera* leaves is used topically on wounds and burns. Aloe reduces burning and itching as well as scarring from radiation burns; it also aids in the healing of chronic leg ulcers, postsurgical wounds, and frostbite. Double-blind placebo-controlled studies of aloe have shown statistically significant improvement for psoriasis (83% vs. 7%) and seborrheic dermatitis (62% vs. 25%). Aloe has multiple active components: salicylic acid decreases vasoconstriction and platelet aggregation by decreasing thromboxane A_2, thromboxane B_2 and prostaglandin 2α, and thus improves dermal perfusion. A carboxypeptidase inactivates bradykinin and may act to decrease pain. Polysaccharides such as acemannon have anti-inflammatory, antimicrobial (bactericidal, antifungal) and immune-stimulating actions. Other components include magnesium sulfate, amino acids, vitamin E, vitamin C, zinc and essential fatty acids. Aloe can cause allergic contact dermatitis[5].

Honey

Honey is traditionally used for wound healing, and it can be applied directly to burns, decubitus ulcers, and infected wounds. In a study of nine infants with culture-positive, postoperative wound infections that had failed appropriate treatment (>14 days of chlorhexidine and intravenous antibiotics), the wounds were treated with unprocessed honey twice a day. The wounds cleared clinically by day 5 and were culture-negative at day 21. In a randomized, controlled trial, burns treated with honey healed earlier than those treated with polyurethane film. Honey contains catalase, which is thought to encourage debridement. Honey also promotes granulation and re-epithelialization and treats edema. *In vitro*, it is antibacterial and antifungal. Honey contact dermatitis has been reported rarely[5].

Calendula

Marigold (*Calendula officionalis*) is an antiseptic and is commonly used for diaper dermatitis. *Calendula* preparations have been recommended for wounds, ulcers, burns (especially radiation-induced), furuncles,

CLASSIFICATION OF COMPLEMENTARY AND ALTERNATIVE MEDICINE (CAM) BY THE NATIONAL CENTER FOR COMPLEMENTARY AND ALTERNATIVE MEDICINE AT THE NATIONAL INSTITUTES OF HEALTH, UNITED STATES		
Biologically based practices	Botanicals Animal-derived extracts Vitamins Minerals Fatty acids Amino acids Proteins Prebiotics, probiotics Whole diets Functional foods	
Whole medical systems	Traditional Chinese medicine Ayurvedic medicine Homeopathy Naturopathy Curanderismo Others: Native American, African, Middle Eastern, Tibetan, Central and South American	
Mind–body medicine	Relaxation Hypnosis Visual imagery Meditation Yoga Biofeedback Tai-chi Qi-gong Cognitive-behavioral therapies Group support Autogenic training Spirituality Prayer	
Manipulative and body-based practices	Alexander technique Bowen technique Chiropractic manipulation Craniosacral therapy Feldenkrais method Massage therapy Osteopathic manipulation Reflexology Rolfing Trager bodywork Tui-na	
Energy medicine	**Energy types**	**Energy therapies**
	Veritable energy: Mechanical vibrations Electromagnetic energy (light, magnetic fields, monochromatic radiation [laser beams], infrared)	Sound therapy Light therapy Magnetic therapy Millimeter wave therapy Infrared therapy
	Putative energy, 'biofields': Qi (Chinese) Ki (Japanese)	Traditional Chinese Medicine (acupuncture, qi-gong) Reiki Johrei
	Dosha Prana Homeopathic resonance	Ayurvedic medicine Pranayama, yoga Homeopathy
	Other energy types: Ether (Greek) Fohat (Tibetan) Mana (Polynesian) Orgone, Odic force (European)	*Other energy therapies:* Therapeutic touch Vortex healing Polarity therapy Distant healing Intercessory prayer

Table 133.1 Classification of complementary and alternative medicine (CAM) by the National Center for Complementary and Alternative Medicine at the National Institutes of Health, United States[1].

'rashes', dermatitis, herpes zoster, varicose veins, and mouth and throat inflammation. Marigold contains flavonoids, triterpene saponins and carotenoids, which have anti-inflammatory properties and may be antimicrobial as well as immunomodulating. Animal studies have demonstrated increased glycoproteins and collagen at wound sites treated with marigold. There are rare reports of contact dermatitis to *Calendula*[5].

Capsaicin

Capsaicin is found in cayenne pepper (*Capsicum frutescens*). Topical capsaicin is used for treating pain, especially postherpetic neuralgia. Capsaicin stimulates the release and subsequent depletion of substance P, a neurotransmitter. In clinical trials, capsaicin decreased scaling, thickness, erythema and pruritus in patients with psoriasis. A common side effect is temporary burning[5].

Arnica

Arnica (*Arnica montana*) is approved by the German Commission E for its anti-inflammatory effects. It has been used for centuries in the treatment of myalgia, arthralgia, bruises, insect bites, furuncles, inflamed gums, acne, hemorrhoids, seborrheic dermatitis, and psoriasis. Arnica is toxic when ingested and should only be used topically. Although it has been recommended for postsurgical pain and wound healing, arnica should not be applied to open wounds[5]. Active components include sesquiterpene lactones, which reduce inflammation by inhibiting nuclear factor-κB, an important transcription factor which regulates the production of cytokines and other proinflammatory molecules. Contact dermatitis is a possible adverse effect[5]. A single case report of Sweet's syndrome with pathergy to arnica occurred in a patient with leukemia[7].

Chamomile

Chamomile (*Matricaria recutita*) is used for inflammatory conditions of the skin and mucous membranes and to promote wound healing. It is traditionally used for dermatitis. Chamomile may be ingested as a tea or applied topically. Studies have demonstrated that the anti-inflammatory effects of topical chamomile are 60% to 100% that of topical hydrocortisone 0.25%. One double-blind trial showed decreased wound surface area and healing time with chamomile. *In vitro*, chamomile has antimicrobial effects, while animal studies demonstrated anti-inflammatory and antispasmodic effects. Active components include α-bisabolol, α-bisabolol oxides A and B, matricin, chamazulene, and the flavonoids apigenin, luteolin and quercetin. These substances inhibit cyclooxygenase and lipoxygenase, inhibit histamine release, and promote granulation tissue formation. There are rare reports of allergic reactions to chamomile, including contact dermatitis and anaphylaxis[5,8].

Horse chestnut seed extract and others

Horse chestnut seed extract (HCSE) (*Aesculus hippocastanum*) has anti-inflammatory and astringent properties, and it is used in treating chronic venous insufficiency. HCSE contains aescin (a type of triterpene glycoside) and saponin, which inhibits leukocyte activation and decreases vascular leakage by inhibiting elastase and hyaluronidase. Oral HCSE is prescribed for chronic venous insufficiency; topical HCSE formulations can be used for varicose veins, phlebitis and hemorrhoids. There have been multiple studies regarding the efficacy of oral HCSE in the treatment of chronic venous insufficiency. HCSE decreases leg volume in addition to calf and ankle circumference. Studies comparing HCSE with grade II compression stockings demonstrated equivalent efficacies. HCSE is well-tolerated; adverse effects are similar to those of placebo. Natural horse chestnut seeds are poisonous and need to be processed to remove toxic components. To date, there has been one case report of drug-induced lupus from a German HCSE-containing medication. Contact dermatitis has also been reported[5].

Butcher's broom (*Ruscus aculeatus*) and sweet clover (*Melilotus officinalis*) are two other herbs approved by the German Commission E for the treatment of symptoms of chronic venous insufficiency such as pain, heaviness, pruritus and swelling. Butcher's broom has diuretic properties, and sweet clover increases venous return. Plant-derived polyphenols, or bioflavonoids, have antioxidant effects that can be used to strengthen capillaries. For example, citrus pulp, grape seed, grape skin and Pacific maritime pine bark (*Pinus maritima*) extracts can be

BOTANICALS AND OTHER BIOLOGICALLY ACTIVE SUBSTANCES USED FOR DERMATOLOGIC CONDITIONS

Common name	Latin name	Active components	Description	Known side effects
Pineapple extract	*Ananas comosus*	Bromelain (a protease)	• Aids in wound healing and hematoma resorption • Ingestion 1 to 2 hours prior to meals enhances uptake by WBCs	Hypersensitivity; anaphylaxis
Chaparral	*Larrea tridentata*	Nordihydroguaiaretic acid	• Native American remedy used to treat actinic keratoses • Antioxidant; antibiotic	Contact dermatitis; abnormal renal and hepatic function tests
Oregon grape root	*Mahonia aquifolium* (syn. *Berberis aquifolium*)	Berberine	• Used for chronic pustular eruptions • Antimicrobial; anti-inflammatory; antihistamine; increases bile production; inhibits sebaceous gland lipogenesis	Reports of jaundice in infants; caution during pregnancy and breastfeeding
Gotu kola, luei gong gen	*Centella asiatica*	Triterpenoids	• Used for burns, scars, varicose veins, psoriatic arthritis • Stimulates collagen and fibronectin production; inhibits keratinocyte growth • Used for scleroderma to increase finger mobility and decrease skin hardening	Absolute contraindication in pregnancy and breastfeeding
Sarsaparilla	*Smilax* spp.	Saponins, sarsaponin, β-sitosterol	• Anti-inflammatory • Used for psoriasis, eczema, scleroderma	Gastrointestinal symptoms; abnormal renal function
Echinacea	*Echinacea purpurea, Echinacea angustifolia, Echinacea pallida*	Inulin	• Stimulates neutrophils and macrophages; affects cytokine secretion • Antimicrobial; antihyaluronidase • Used for eczema, burns, herpes simplex, wound healing	Hypersensitivity eruption; contraindicated in autoimmune diseases
Fruit acids	From grapes, apples, sugar cane, sugar maple trees, pineapple, papaya, lemons, limes, sour milk, blackberries, yogurt and cider	Lactic, citric, glycolic, malic and tartaric acids	• As effective as 5% benzoyl peroxide in clearing inflamed acne lesions and comedones	Irritant contact dermatitis
Vitex	*Vitex agnuscastus*	Flavonoids, iridoid glycosides, terpenoids	• For acne related to menstrual cycle • Acts on pituitary to increase progesterone and decrease estrogen	Contraindicated in pregnancy and breastfeeding
Garlic	*Allium sativum*	Allicin, allyl sulfides, ajoene, vinyldithiins	• Antibacterial; antiviral; antifungal; lowers cholesterol and triglycerides • Inhibits platelet aggregation; increases fibrinolysis • Usually used for atherosclerosis and hypercholesterolemia • May be used for warts, tinea pedis	Excessive anticoagulation; contact dermatitis
Bittersweet nightshade	*Solanum dulcamara*		• Condylomata, verrucae	Contraindicated in pregnancy and breastfeeding
Wild oats (straw)	*Avena sativa*	Straw contains silica	• Condylomata, verrucae	
Calotropis	*Calotropis procera*		• Condylomata, verrucae	Contraindicated in pregnancy and breastfeeding
Greater celandine	*Chelidonium majus*		• Condylomata, verrucae	Contraindicated in pregnancy and breastfeeding
Chrysanthemums	*Asteraceae family*	Pyrethrins	• Antimicrobial • Used for scabies	Contact dermatitis; photosensitivity
Anise seeds	*Pimpinella anisum*	Terpenoid anethole, phytoestrogens	• Antibacterial; anti-insecticidal • Used for infestations	Contraindicated in pregnancy and breastfeeding
Neem	*Azadirachta indica*	Azadirachtin (tetranortriterpenoid)	• Used for infestations	Contraindicated in pregnancy, breastfeeding, and children
Pansy flower	*Viola tricolor*	Salicylic acid, saponins, mucilage	• For seborrheic dermatitis in infants	None reported, but salicylate toxicity is a theoretical risk
Jewelweed	*Impatiens biflora, Impatiens capensis*	Tannins	• Used for poison ivy and other forms of allergic contact dermatitis, but studies have shown conflicting evidence	
Rosemary	*Rosmarinus officinalis*	Cineole, rosmarinic acid, carnosol	• Antibacterial; antioxidant; inhibits tumorigenesis	Contraindicated in pregnancy
Ginseng	*Panax ginseng*	Ginsenosides, panaxans, polysaccharides	• Used to strength immune system • May lower risk of some cancers	Not recommended in pregnancy and breastfeeding
Propolis	Resinous substance collected by bees, especially from poplars and conifers	Flavonoids, phenolic acids, clerodane diterpenoid	• Antimicrobial; anti-inflammatory; antioxidant; antitumorigenic/tumoricidal; analgesic • Used for aphthous ulcers, herpes simplex • One study showed decreased healing time of genital herpes with propolis compared to topical antivirals	Hypersensitivity reactions (Fig. 133.1); contraindicated in people with allergies to honey, bee products, conifers or poplars
Zinc chloride	Not applicable	Zinc chloride	• Strong escharotic • Used for skin cancers • Can debride leg ulcers, sites of osteomyelitis	Pain, burns, scarring
Bloodroot	*Sanguinaria canadensis*	Sanguinarine	• Strong escharotic • Used for skin and other cancers • Induces apoptosis; may inhibit NF-κB; may block cell cycle; antimicrobial	Pain, burns, scarring; contraindicated in pregnancy, breastfeeding, and children
Goldenseal	*Hydrastis canadensis*	Berberine, hydrastine (isoquinoline alkaloids)	• Mild escharotic • Used for skin and other cancers • Anticarcinogenic; inhibits glucose uptake by cancer cells; antimicrobial	Not recommended in pregnancy and breastfeeding

Table 133.2 Botanicals and other biologically active substances used for dermatologic conditions. The most commonly used herbals are discussed in the text.

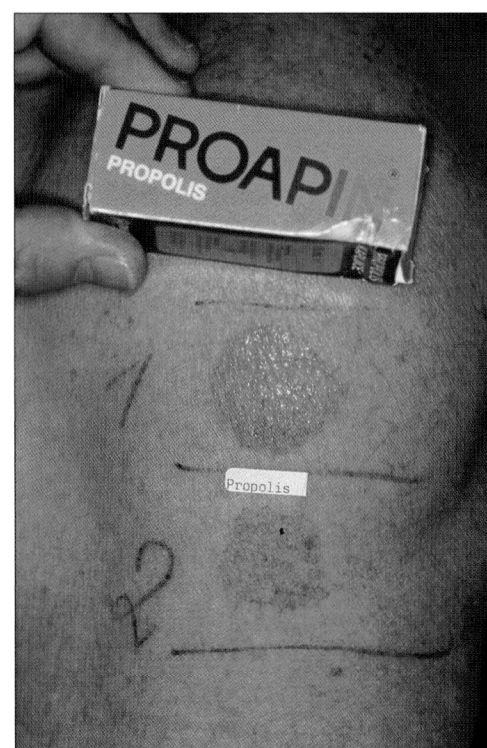

Fig. 133.1 Contact allergy to propolis. This is a frequently used topical agent in central Europe. Courtesy of Josef Smolle MD.

DIETARY SUPPLEMENTS AND EFFECTS ON COAGULATION		
Name	**Medicinal uses**	**Effects on coagulation**
Alfalfa	Prothrombinemic purpura	Contains coumarins
Bilberry	Diabetes, retinopathy, diarrhea	Contains coumarins
Capsicum	Dyspepsia, arthritis	Contains coumarins, inhibits platelet aggregation
Celery	Arthritis, urinary infection	Contains coumarins
Chamomile	Dyspepsia, anxiety	Contains coumarins
Dan shen	Cardiovascular disease	Inhibits platelet aggregation, decreases elimination of warfarin in rats
Dang gui	Menopausal complaints, menstrual disorders	Contains coumarins
Fenugreek	Dyspepsia, gastritis	Contains coumarins
Feverfew	Migraines, arthritis, fever	Inhibits platelet aggregation
Fish oils	Hypercholesterolemia	Decreases platelet aggregation and platelet adhesion
Garlic	Atherosclerosis, hypertension, hypercholesterolemia, infection	Decreases plasma viscosity, increases clotting time, inhibits platelet aggregation
Ginger	Nausea, arthritis	Inhibits platelet function
Ginkgo biloba	Cardiovascular disease	Inhibits platelet aggregation and function, decreases plasma viscosity
Ginseng	Stress reduction, improves vitality	Inhibits platelet aggregation, contains coumarins
Goldenseal	Infection, inflammation	Contains coumarins
Green tea	Cancer prevention, gastrointestinal disorders, cognition enhancement	Inhibits platelet aggregation
Horseradish	Infection, inflammation	Contains coumarins
Huang qi	Immunostimulant	Inhibits platelet aggregation and fibrinolysis
Kava kava	Anxiety, stress, muscle pain	Decreases platelet aggregation
Licorice	Cough, inflammation	Contains coumarins
Passionflower	Anxiety, insomnia	Contains coumarins
Red clover	Infections, psoriasis	Contains coumarins
Vitamin E	Antioxidant	Decreases platelet adhesion and aggregation

Table 133.3 Dietary supplements and effects on coagulation. Based on Collins SC, Dufresne RG. Dietary supplements in the setting of Mohs surgery. Dermatol Surg. 2002;28:447–452 with permission.

used for solar purpura. Rutin, a bioflavonoid found in buckwheat, has been shown to decrease leg volume[5].

Tea

There are numerous studies of tea (*Camellia sinensis*) and its antioxidant, anti-inflammatory, anticarcinogenic, wound-healing and antiaging effects. Tea contains flavonoid compounds with polyphenolic structures which serve as scavengers for reactive oxygen species[9]. Green tea polyphenols, especially epigallocatechin gallate (EGCG), also modulate gene transcription and signaling pathways. Both topical and oral green tea can protect against inflammation, chemical carcinogenesis, photocarcinogenesis and UVA-induced photodamage. White and green teas have higher amounts of polyphenols than black teas. Black tea is fermented and oxidized, which destroys polyphenols, converting them into theaflavins and thearubigins. Black tea can decrease UVB-induced damage and inhibit tumor proliferation. Caffeine, which is present in teas, appears to have an independent protective effect against photocarcinogenesis[5].

Licorice root

Licorice root (*Glycyrrhiza glabra*, *Glycyrrhiza uralensis*) is used for its anti-inflammatory properties by both European and Chinese herbalists. Licorice root contains glycyrrhizin and carbenoxolone and it can produce mineralocorticoid-like effects. Excessive use may lead to hypertension, edema, congestive heart failure and hypokalemia (i.e. syndrome of apparent mineralocorticoid excess). Licorice also contains potent flavonoids and chalcones (which are antioxidants) and liquiritin. Liquiritin cream has been used for treating melasma, with enhanced efficacy compared to placebo (70% vs. 20%)[5].

Escharotics

Escharotics are used topically for treating skin cancer; these agents are caustic, producing necrotic crusts and possible scarring. Escharotics include zinc chloride, bloodroot (*Sanguinaria canadensis*) and goldenseal (*Hydrastis canadensis*) (see Table 133.2)[10].

Side Effects

Herbs are composed of organic and inorganic components that are biologically active and, as with any medication, may have serious side effects or interact with other medications. Several herbal and dietary supplements potentiate anticoagulation (Table 133.3). Because patients often do not report the use of CAM, it is recommended that preoperative assessments include specific questioning regarding dietary supplements (see Ch. 151).

A common misperception exists that herbs are 'natural' and 'safer' than prescription medications. Hematologic, nephrotoxic, cardiotoxic and hepatotoxic effects have been observed, as well as phototoxicity (Fig. 133.2) and hypersensitivity reactions, including Stevens–Johnson syndrome. Additionally, in most countries, herbal medicine is not subject to the same regulation as prescription medications. Herbal supplements have been found to be contaminated with metals, prescription drugs such as non-steroidal anti-inflammatory drugs (NSAIDs) or corticosteroids, microorganisms, and other substances.

Several challenges stem from the use of plants as therapeutics. These considerations include differences in: climate and soil; cultivars and species; growing, harvesting and storage conditions; methods of extraction; chemical standardization of products; and bioavailability of formulations[1].

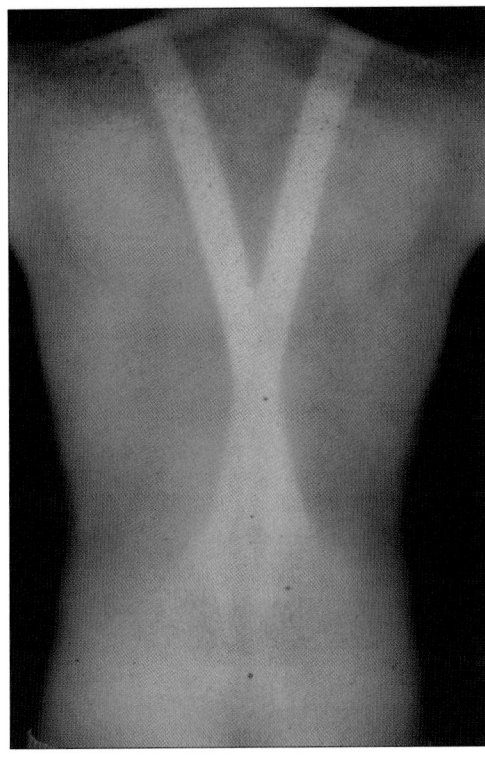

Fig. 133.2 Phototoxic reaction due to herbal tea. Courtesy of Josef Smolle MD.

TRADITIONAL CHINESE MEDICINE

Introduction

Traditional Chinese Medicine (TCM) is a complete system of healing that began prior to 2000BC. TCM originated in China, but unique versions developed in Japan, Korea and other countries. TCM encompasses a myriad of treatment modalities, including herbal medicine, acupuncture, massage, exercise, and dietary and lifestyle modifications (Table 133.4). Herbal medicine comprises approximately two-thirds of the TCM armamentarium, and acupuncture the remaining third.

TCM takes a holistic attitude towards health. For health to occur, balance and harmony must be achieved between two opposing and complementary forces, Yin and Yang. Central to Yin–Yang theory is the concept that no single part can be understood except in relation to the whole. Yin–Yang theory takes a dialectical view of health, and thus TCM differs fundamentally from conventional medicine, which is based on a reductionist view of disease[11].

In TCM, normal flow patterns of Qi, or life-force (which is Yang), and Blood (which is Yin) are essential for health. Disruptions of Qi and Blood flow can cause pain and disease, and regulation of flow is the goal of therapy. For example, it is believed that stimulation of precise points on the body using acupuncture, moxibustion or massage can correct the flow of Qi and Blood.

Given its roots as a complete system of healing, TCM has been employed for most dermatologic conditions, and a complete discussion is beyond the scope of this chapter. This chapter focuses on the use of TCM for atopic dermatitis and psoriasis.

TCM Herbal Medicine

Dermatologic applications

A Cochrane systematic review of the literature analyzed a number of studies involving the use of Chinese herbal preparations in the treatment of atopic dermatitis, including three double-blind, randomized, controlled, crossover trials, all investigating a standardized mixture of raw herbs[12]. The herbal preparation was composed of ten herbs: *Ledebouriella seseloides, Potentilla chinensis, Anebia clematidis, Rehmannia glutinosa, Paeonia lactiflora, Lophatherum gracile, Dictamnus dasycarpus, Tribulus terrestris, Glycyrrhiza uralensis* and *Schizonepeta tenuifolia.*

Two of the three trials demonstrated greater improvement with the ten-herb decoction (an extraction of water-soluble components via boiling) as compared with placebo, both by Sheehan and colleagues[13,14]. The first study involved 40 adult patients with refractory atopic dermatitis, randomized to receive 8 weeks of study herbs versus placebo, followed by a crossover after a 4-week washout period[13]. A similar study was also conducted in 47 children with extensive atopic dermatitis[14]. In both the adults and the children, the TCM ten-herb decoction led to greater reductions in erythema, surface area of involvement, and pruritus, as well as improved sleep quality, when compared with placebo.

The third trial reviewed by the Cochrane Collaboration failed to demonstrate any difference between the ten-herb decoction and placebo. Hematologic cell counts, renal function, and liver function studies were performed in all three studies, and no changes were observed.

Sheehan et al.[15] also performed 1-year follow-up observational studies in which patients could choose to continue the TCM herbal decoction. Those who continued the preparation showed significant benefit compared with patients who chose not to take the preparation. Of note, during this 1-year study, 2 of 37 children experienced asymptomatic elevations in serum levels of aspartate aminotransferase which normalized after discontinuing the herbs. No adult patients experienced laboratory abnormalities.

Several herbs with anti-inflammatory and immunosuppressive effects have been used to treat psoriasis, including *Indigo natualis, Tripterygium wilfordii* Hook and *Camptotheca acuminata* Decne. Herbs that contain furocoumarins, such as *Radix angelicae dahuricae* and *Radix angelicae pubescentis,* can be used instead of psoralens with UVA phototherapy. In a study of 801 psoriatic patients, 50% to 85% of patients responded to a decoction of *Rhizoma sparganii, Rhizoma zedoariae, Herba serissae, Resnia boswelliae* and *Myrrha*[16].

Mechanism of action and clinical evidence

Numerous studies have been performed regarding the pharmacologic properties and clinical efficacies of herbs, primarily in the non-English language literature. With regard to the above-mentioned ten-herb combination used for atopic dermatitis, multiple studies have sought to characterize the mechanisms of action. The studies have focused on the role of CD23, a low-affinity IgE receptor found on monocytes/macrophages in the peripheral blood and skin, which is overexpressed in patients with atopic dermatitis. These herbs may lead to a dose-dependent reduction in CD23 expression and may also reduce HLA-DR expression. Additionally, these herbs have antioxidant properties.

Tripterygium wilfordii Hook is anti-inflammatory and immunosuppressive. A randomized, placebo-controlled trial showed a significant dose-dependent response to *T. wilfordii* Hook in patients with rheumatoid arthritis[17]. Two Japanese remedies, Sho-seiryu-to and Moku-boi-to, have significant antihistamine effects estimated to equal that of diphenhydramine.

TRADITIONAL CHINESE MEDICINE (TCM) TREATMENT MODALITIES	
Modality	**Delivery methods/Related modalities**
Herbal medicine	Decoctions – water is used to simmer herbs, then the decanted fluid is taken in divided doses Topical poultices Essential oils Lotions, creams, ointments Tablets, capsules
Acupuncture	Needles – stainless steel (most common), gold, silver Moxibustion Cupping, coining, rubbing Acupressure Electroacupuncture Auricular acupuncture Laser acupuncture Medicamentous acupuncture Magnet therapy
Therapeutic exercise	Tai-ji (tai-chi), qi-gong (chi-gong)
Massage therapy	Tui-na, acupressure
Dietary modification	
Meditation	

Table 133.4 Traditional Chinese Medicine (TCM) treatment modalities.

Side effects

As discussed in the previous section on botanicals, herbs have biologically active components, and may have serious side effects. TCM herbs should only be used under the supervision of a licensed practitioner.

Acupuncture

Dermatologic applications

In TCM, acupuncture is considered less useful than herbal medicine for dermatologic conditions. A review of the literature revealed one controlled trial of acupuncture for psoriasis, which failed to demonstrate any efficacy over placebo[18].

There have been multiple studies supporting the use of acupuncture for pain, pruritus, and emotional states such as stress, anxiety and depression, which may be associated with dermatologic conditions. Acupuncture has been reportedly used for atopic dermatitis, neurodermatitis, lichen planus, psoriasis, scleroderma, alopecia areata, warts, acne, herpes viral infection, postherpetic neuralgia, and urticaria[19,20].

Mechanism of action and clinical efficacy

Numerous studies have been performed to try to elucidate the mechanisms of action of acupuncture. Proposed mechanisms for acupuncture analgesia include: gate control, diffuse noxious inhibitory control, and stimulating the release of neuroactive substances including endorphins and enkephalins[21].

In addition, acupuncture may have anti-inflammatory and immunomodulatory effects by altering the release of neurotransmitters. Acupuncture has been shown to increase adrenal production of corticosterone and cortisol as well as production of β-endorphin and corticotropin by the pituitary.

Proposed mechanisms of action of acupuncture for depression and anxiety are not well characterized, but incorporate the monoamine hypothesis for affective disorders. Cerebral serotonin release is stimulated by specific acupuncture points. Additionally, intracephalic blood flow may be altered by acupuncture[22].

Side effects

The most common side effects associated with acupuncture are: tiredness (8.2%), drowsiness (2.8%), aggravation of pre-existing symptoms (2.8%), pruritus (1.0%), dizziness/vertigo (0.8%), faintness/nausea (0.8%), headache (0.5%) and chest pain (0.3%). Local reactions include: minor bleeding on needle withdrawal (2.6%), pain on needle insertion (0.7%), petechiae/ecchymosis (0.3%), pain/ache after the treatment (0.1%), subcutaneous hematoma (0.1%) and pain/discomfort during needle retention (0.03%)[23]. Infection, hematomas and pneumothorax have been reported. Infectious risks are minimized by utilizing single-use needles. The risk of pneumothorax is avoided by using traditional angles of insertion. Localized argyria has been rarely reported from using subcutaneous permanent needles made of silver instead of stainless steel.

Moxibustion, Cupping and Other TCM Treatment Modalities

Moxibustion is the practice of burning dried moxa (*Artemisia vulgaris*) placed in small cone-shaped piles over acupuncture points. Moxibustion may be either direct, in which the moxa-cones are allowed to burn completely down to the skin surface, or indirect, in which the moxa-cones are removed prior to the burning fibers touching the skin. Side effects include first- and second-degree burns.

Cupping is another method used to stimulate acupuncture points. It is accomplished by igniting alcohol-soaked cotton, placing the burning cotton in a jar, and placing the jar on the skin. A vacuum is created, and circular areas of erythema and ecchymosis may result.

Skin scraping, also known as coining or spooning, is more commonly practiced in Southeast Asia, and is used to improve circulation. Skin scraping is performed by rubbing a tool in streaks on skin treated with oil. Symmetric linear ecchymoses may result (Fig. 133.3).

Any Asian patient with cutaneous lesions in patterns suggestive of external causes should be asked about traditional medicine before accusations of abuse arise. Ethiopians have similar practices of moxibustion and cupping.

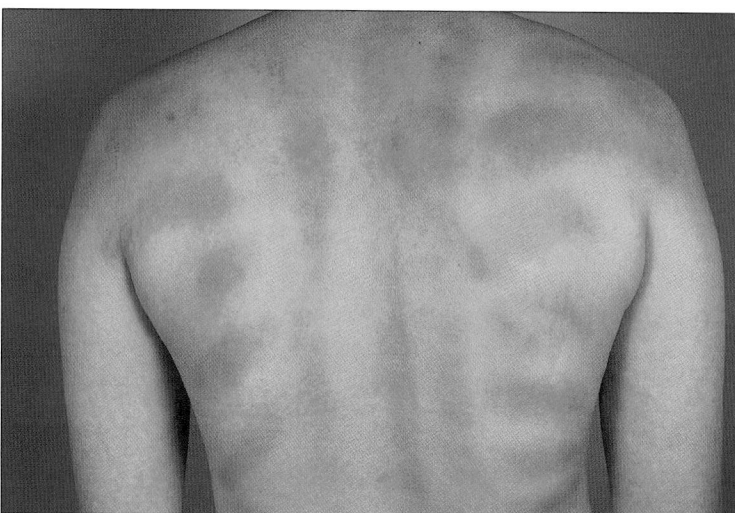

Fig. 133.3 Linear ecchymoses on the back due to coining.

HOMEOPATHY

Introduction

Homeopathy is a system of healing founded by Samuel Hahnemann (1755–1843), a German physician. He hypothesized that one can select treatments based on the 'principle of similars', which states that symptoms may be cured by giving a therapy that induces the same symptoms. A homeopathic therapy provides the additional stimulus needed for the body to recognize and fight an illness. Hahnemann studied remedies by giving repeated doses to healthy volunteers and then observing their physical symptoms, emotions, and mental states[24].

Homeopathic remedies are given in dilutions; a second assumption of homeopathy, the 'principle of infinitesimals', hypothesizes that the higher the dilution, the greater the effect. Some remedies are so highly diluted (one part in 10^{24} or higher) that not a single molecule of the substance remains according to the laws of chemistry using Avogadro's number (6.023×10^{23}). In homeopathy, however, it is believed that the dilutant, usually water, carries an 'essence' of the original substance, and can be used to treat disease.

Dermatologic Applications

Homeopathy may be used for multiple dermatologic conditions, including: atopic dermatitis, seborrheic dermatitis, psoriasis, acne, rosacea, actinic keratoses, verrucae and infections. At a British homeopathic hospital, eczema and psoriasis accounted for 13% of referrals[25]. Seborrheic dermatitis reportedly responds to a homeopathic tobacco preparation.

Mechanism of Action and Clinical Evidence

The literature regarding the use of homeopathy for dermatologic conditions consists mostly of anecdotal case reports. A few studies have tried to demonstrate the 'essence' of water dilutant. A study published in *Nature* demonstrated degranulation of human basophils using very dilute antiserum against IgE[26]; this has not been replicated.

Meta-analyses of the literature have found conflicting evidence regarding the efficacy of homeopathy. Randomized, controlled trials of homeopathic treatment of warts have not found any efficacy beyond that of placebo[24].

Side Effects

Homeopathic remedies are usually highly diluted, therefore side effects are rare and may include headache, fatigue, myalgia, arthralgia and diarrhea[25]. There have also been reports of contact dermatitis. Homeopathy should only be used with the supervision of a licensed practitioner.

AROMATHERAPY

Introduction

Aromatherapy is the therapeutic use of aromatic essential oils. Considered a subset of botanical medicine, aromatherapy may use any plant part, including leaves, stems, flowers, fruits, roots and wood resins. Essential oils are extracted using steam distillation, cold-pressing or other methods.

The term 'aromathérapie' was coined in 1927 by René-Maurice Gattefossé, a French chemist, whose interest began after a personal incident. After burning his hand in the laboratory, Gattefossé dipped it into a nearby vat of lavender oil. His hand healed rapidly, and he subsequently studied essential oils at military hospitals during World War I. Today, France is a leader in aromatherapy research.

Aromatherapy is used to treat a wide range of physical, mental and emotional states. Oils may be used externally or internally. External methods are more common and include massage, compresses, gels/creams/pastes, sprays, baths and inhalation. Internal routes include oral, otic, intrarectal and intravaginal[27].

Dermatologic Applications

Aromatherapy may be used directly to treat dermatologic conditions, or indirectly to treat symptoms (e.g. emotional) associated with dermatologic disease (Table 133.5). Indications for aromatherapy include: acne, alopecia areata, pruritus, psoriasis, burns, ulcers, herpes viral infections, radiation dermatitis, xerosis, contact dermatitis, scars and analgesia. It is also used for wound-healing, antimicrobial, anti-inflammatory and antispasmodic properties. In the treatment of psoriasis, for example, lemon balm is used to reduce xerosis and pruritus, chamomile to reduce stress, and lavender to promote relaxation[27].

Mechanism of Action and Clinical Evidence

Essential oils are mixtures of organic compounds including acids, alcohols, aldehydes, coumarins, esters, ethers, ketones, lactones, oxides, phenols and terpenes. Therapeutic properties vary with the concentrations of specific compounds. Essential oils high in ketones are used for wound healing. Acids, aldehydes and alcohols have antimicrobial and immunostimulatory properties. Phenols, ethers and terpenes are antimicrobial. Terpenes also have antihistamine and cortisone-like effects.

There are very few studies on the use of aromatherapy in dermatology. A single-blind trial in acne patients found similar efficacies for tea tree oil 5% gel and benzoyl peroxide 5% lotion; tea tree oil had a slower onset of action but fewer side effects. The efficacy profile of tea tree oil 100% for onychomycosis is similar to that of clotrimazole 1% solution. For tinea pedis, tea tree oil 10% cream helps ameliorate symptoms, but is no more effective than placebo in achieving mycologic cure[27].

A randomized, controlled, double-blind trial in alopecia areata patients showed significantly more improvement with aromatherapy versus placebo (44% vs. 15%). Thyme, rosemary, lavender and cedarwood oils were used[28].

Lemon balm (Melissa officinalis) may be used for herpes labialis. In a double-blind, randomized, controlled trial, balm decreased the size and healing time of lesions[29]. Studies suggest that the active components are tannins, polyphenols, terpenes and sesquiterpenes, including citronella, citral-A and citral-B.

Other areas of research regarding essential oils in dermatology have included antimicrobial properties, antitumor effects, enhancing transdermal drug absorption, and promoting cutaneous blood flow.

Side Effects

Like all botanicals, essential oils have biologically active components and may be toxic. Cutaneous side effects include contact dermatitis and phytophotodermatitis. Ketones have neurotoxic effects, especially in patients with seizure disorders, pregnant women, and children. Some compounds are potentially carcinogenic, including safrole in sassafras oil and beta-asarone in calamus oil[27].

AROMATHERAPY: ESSENTIAL OILS USEFUL IN DERMATOLOGIC CONDITIONS

Latin name	Common name	Actions/Indications
Boswellia carterii	Frankincense	Immunostimulant; wound healing
Citrus aurantium var. amara	Petitgrain	Infected acne
Citrus bergamia	Bergamot	Pruritus, psoriasis, HSV-1 infection, wound disinfection
Citrus senesis	Sweet orange	Wound disinfection
Cymbopogen citrates	Lemongrass	Anti-inflammatory
Eucalyptus citriodora	Eucalyptus (lemon-scented)	Anti-inflammatory, analgesic; herpes zoster, candidiasis
Eucalyptus radiata	Australian eucalyptus	Acne
Jasminum officinalis	Jasmine	Antiseptic, anti-inflammatory
Juniperus communis	Juniper berry	Anti-inflammatory, analgesic; skin 'problems'
Juniperus communis	Juniper twig	Acne
Lavandula angustifolia	True lavender	Burns, wound healing, analgesic
Lavandula latifolia	Spike lavender (French)	Severe first-degree burns, neuralgia
Lavandula stoechas	Stoechas lavender	Dermatitis
Melaleuca alternifolia	Tea tree	Antifungal, antiviral, antibacterial; acne, warts, radiation burn prevention
Melaleuca leucodendron	Cajeput	Genital herpes viral infection, radiation burn prevention
Melaleuca quinquenervia/ viridifolia	Nialouli	Dermatitis
Melissa officinalis	Lemon balm	Viral skin infections
Mentha x piperita	Peppermint	Dermatitis, herpes viral infections
Ocimum basilicum	Basil	'Dry' dermatitis
Pelargonium x asperum	Geranium	Acne, impetiginized dermatitis
Pinus sylvestrus	Scotch pine	Allergy, inflammation
Piper nigrum	Black pepper	Analgesic
Pogostemon cablin	Patchouli	Anti-inflammatory, antiseptic, antimicrobial; acne, seborrhea, dermatitis (including weeping forms), scars, tinea pedis
Ravensara aromatica	Ravensara	Herpes zoster
Rosa damascena	Rose	Dermatitis
Rosamarinus officinalis	Rosemary (verbenone) CT verbenone	Antispasmodic
Satureja montana	Winter savory	Oil used for its antibacterial, antiparasitic, antiviral and antifungal properties; psoriasis, analgesia
Styrax benzoe	Benzoin	Skin infections, acne, dermatitis, psoriasis, ulcers

Table 133.5 Aromatherapy: essential oils useful in dermatologic conditions. Reproduced with permission from Stevensen CJ. Aromatherapy in dermatology. Clin Dermatol. 1998;16:689–694.

MIND–BODY MEDICINE

Introduction

Mind–body medicine comprises a wide range of therapeutic interventions which emphasize the complex interactions involving the brain, mind, behavior, spirit and body.

Mind–body interventions include meditation, relaxation, hypnosis, imagery, yoga, tai-chi, qi-gong, biofeedback, cognitive-behavioral therapies, group therapy, breathing techniques, autogenic training, dance therapy, music therapy, spirituality, and prayer. Excluding prayer, approximately 30% of the US population has used mind–body therapy, most commonly meditation, guided imagery, and yoga. Prayer was used by more than 50%[1].

The belief that the mind plays an important role in health and healing is integral to many systems of traditional medicine, including Western medicine. Scientific and technologic development subsequently led to an emphasis on the physical aspects of medicine and a separation from the less tangible facets to healing. The medical community is more accepting of mind–body relationships that can be 'scientifically' demonstrated, such as the placebo effect, which accounts for 35% of the therapeutic response to any treatment[1]. The mental and spiritual aspects of health are challenging to study scientifically, but the evidence for mind–body medicine continues to grow.

Dermatologic Applications

Hypnosis may be used for treating warts, with response rates of 27% to 55%. Hypnosis is also used for atopic dermatitis. Children respond to hypnosis better than adults for both conditions[30].

Mind–body interventions have been found to be useful in treating problems indirectly associated with dermatologic conditions. Nociception is readily altered by meditation and behavioral techniques[31]. Mind–body relationships can influence immunity, positively or negatively. Finally, there are potential uses of mind–body medicine in dermatologic surgery for improved wound healing and pain reduction.

Certain dermatologic conditions, including acne or psoriasis, are associated with psycho-emotional factors (Table 133.6) and may be good candidates for mind–body interventions.

Mechanism of Action and Clinical Evidence

Mind–body medicine is an active area of research, and there is good evidence for biofeedback, cognitive-behavioral interventions, and hypnosis. One of the first scientific demonstrations of the mind–body relationship was termed the 'relaxation response' by Benson, who observed that, after 20 minutes of meditation, study participants experienced decreased heart rate, breathing rate, blood pressure, oxygen consumption, carbon dioxide production and serum lactic acid production, while skin resistance increased and blood flow was altered. Since then, researchers have demonstrated numerous physiologic changes following mind–body interventions.

One model that synthesizes these changes is the 'neuro-immuno-cutaneous-endocrine (NICE)' network, in which four physiologic systems interact through a complex amalgamation of neurotrophic substances, cytokines, hormones including glucocorticoids, and other molecules. For example, physical stimulation of the skin induces the release of neuropeptides, which influence the CNS as well as having local effects. In particular, α-melanocyte stimulating hormone (α-MSH), which is produced by the skin and the pituitary gland, may

DERMATOLOGIC CONDITIONS ASSOCIATED WITH PSYCHO-EMOTIONAL FACTORS	
Dermatologic conditions associated with psycho-emotional factors	
Hyperhidrosis	Telogen effluvium
Dyshidrosis	Alopecia areata
Pruritus sine materia	Psoriasis
Urticaria	Seborrheic dermatitis
Lichen simplex chronicus	Nummular dermatitis
Atopic dermatitis	Lichen planus
Herpes simplex	Warts
Acne vulgaris	Rosacea
Perioral dermatitis	Vitiligo
Median nail dystrophy	
Psychiatric syndromes associated with dermatologic conditions	
Dermatitis artefacta	Dermatologic phobias:
Neurotic excoriations	Venereophobia
Trichotillomania	Oncophobia
Onychotillomania	Dysmorphophobia
Delusions of parasitosis	(dermatologic non-disease)
(Ekbom's syndrome)	Bromidrosiphobia
Body dysmorphic syndrome	Glossodynia/glossopyrosis
Hypochondriasis	Vulvodynia/vulvopyrosis

Table 133.6 Dermatologic conditions associated with psycho-emotional factors. Based on Panconesi E, Gallassi F, Sarti MG, Bellini MA. Biofeedback, cognitive-behavioral methods, hypnosis: 'alternative psychotherapy'? Clin Dermatol. 1998:16:709–710 with permission.

play a key role. α-MSH inhibits experimentally induced cutaneous inflammation[33]. Langerhans cells have neuropeptide receptors and secrete neurotrophic factors, and may form part of the NICE network. Through this network, the mind can exert a myriad of physiologic effects on nociception, wound healing, immunity and other aspects of health.

The mind–body effect on wound healing has been studied using the blister chamber wound model in human skin. Cytokines, matrix metalloproteinases (MMPs) and tissue inhibitors of metalloproteinases (TIMPs) can affect wound healing. Stress or different moods change the expression of MMPs and TIMPs and slow wound healing, partially through activation of the hypothalamic–pituitary–adrenal axis[1].

Side Effects

Mind–body interventions have minimal side effects because physical agents are not used. Potential side effects include autonomic responses such as lightheadedness, nausea, vomiting or syncope.

CONCLUSION

CAM is increasing in popularity globally for all diseases, including many dermatologic conditions. It is important for dermatologists to recognize and acknowledge the use of CAM in their patients, both to better empathize with their patients as well as to recognize potential side effects. There are a few studies supporting the role of CAM modalities in dermatology, including herbal medicine, traditional Chinese medicine, homeopathy, aromatherapy and mind–body medicine. However, many of these studies are case series, or animal or *in vitro* studies, and there is a need for additional and better-designed studies.

REFERENCES

1. National Center for Complementary and Alternative Medicine. *www.nccam.nih.gov.* 2004.
2. Eisenberg DM, Davis RB, Ettner SL, et al. Trends in alternative medicine use in the United States, 1990-1997. JAMA. 1998;280:1569–75.
3. Collins SC, Dufresne RG. Dietary supplements in the setting of Mohs surgery. Dermatol Surg. 2002;28:447–52.
4. Ernst E. The usage of complementary therapies by dermatological patients: a systematic review. Br J Dermatol. 2000;142:857–61.
5. Bedi MK, Shenefelt PD. Herbal therapy in dermatology. Arch Dermatol. 2002;138:232–42
6. Dattner AM. From medical herbalism to phytotherapy in dermatology: back to the future. Dermatol Ther. 2003;16:106–13.
7. Delmonte S, Brusati C, Parodi A, Rebora A. Leukemia-related Sweet's syndrome elicited by pathergy to arnica. Dermatology. 1998;197:195–7.
8. Brown DJ, Dattner AM. Phytotherapeutic approaches to common dermatologic conditions. Arch Dermatol. 2002;134:1401–4.
9. Hsu S. Green tea and the skin. J Am Acad Dermatol. 2005;52:1049–59.
10. Jellinek N, Maloney ME. Escharotic and other botanical agents for the treatment of skin cancer: a review. J Am Acad Dermatol. 2005;53:487–95.
11. Kaptchuk TJ. The Web That Has No Weaver: Understanding Chinese Medicine, 2nd edn. Chicago: Contemporary, 2000.
12. Zhang W, Leonard T, Bath-Hextall F, et al. Chinese herbal medicine for atopic eczema. Cochrane Database Syst Rev. 2005;(2):CD002291.

13. Sheehan MP, Rustin MHA, Atherton DJ, et al. Efficacy of traditional Chinese herbal therapy in adult atopic dermatitis. Lancet 1992;340:13–17.

14. Sheehan MP, Ahterton DJ. A controlled trial of traditional Chinese medicinal plants in widespread non-exudative atopic eczema. Br J Dermatol. 1992;126:179–84.

15. Sheehan MP, Atherton DJ. One-year follow up of children treated with Chinese medicinal herbs for atopic eczema. Br J Dermatol. 1994;130:488–93.

16. Koo J, Desai R. Traditional Chinese medicine in dermatology. Dermatol Ther. 2003;16:98–105.

17. Tao X, Younger J, Fan FZ, et al. Benefit of an extract of *Tripterygium wilfordii* Hook F in patients with rheumatoid arthritis: a double-blind, placebo-controlled study. Arthritis Rheum. 2002;46:1735–43.

18. Koo J, Arain S. Traditional Chinese Medicine for the treatment of dermatologic disorders. Arch Dermatol. 1998;134:1388–93.

19. Iliev E. Acupuncture in dermatology. Clin Dermatol. 1998;16:659–88.

20. Chen CJ, Yu HS. Acupuncture, electrostimulation, and reflex therapy in dermatology. Dermatol Ther. 2003;16:87–92.

21. National Institutes of Health. Acupuncture: NIH Consensus Statement. 1997;15:1–34.

22. Geng A, Geng J. Acupuncture Primer. *http://www.geocities.com/koaika*. 2002.

23. Yamashita H, Tsukayama H, Hori N, Kimura T, Tanno Y. Incidence of adverse reactions associated with acupuncture. J Altern Complement Med. 2000; 6:345–50.

24. Smolle J. Homeopathy in dermatology. Dermatol Ther. 2003;16:93–7.

25. Thompson E, Barron S, Spence D. A preliminary audit investigating remedy reactions including adverse events in routine homeopathic practice. Homeopathy. 2004;93:203–9.

26. Davenas E, Beauvais F, Amara J, et al. Human basophil degranulation triggered by very dilute antiserum against IgE. Nature. 1988;333:816–18.

27. Stevensen CJ. Aromatherapy in dermatology. Clin Dermatol. 1998;16:689–94.

28. Hay IC, Jamieson M, Ormerod AD. Randomized trial of aromatherapy: successful treatment for alopecia areata. Arch Dermatol. 1998;134:1349–52.

29. Wobling RH, Leonardt K. Local therapy of herpes simplex with dried extract of *Melissa officinalis*. Phytomedicine. 1994;1:25–31.

30. Bellini MA. Hypnosis in dermatology. Clin Dermatol. 1998;16:725–6.

31. Mundy EA, DuHamel KN, Montgomery GH. The efficacy of behavioral interventions for cancer treatment-related side effects. Semin Clin Neuropsychiatry. 2003;8:253–75.

32. Panconesi E, Gallassi F, Sarti MG, Bellini MA. Biofeedback, cognitive-behavioral methods, hypnosis: "alternative psychotherapy"? Clin Dermatol. 1998;16:709–10.

33. Brazzini B, Ghersetich I, Hercogova J, Lotti T. The neuro-immuno-cutaneous-endocrine network: relationship between mind and skin. Dermatol Ther. 2003;16:123–31.

Ultraviolet Therapy

Herbert Hönigsmann and Thomas Schwarz

Key features

- Phototherapy denotes the use of UV light in the treatment of skin disease
- Currently, phototherapy encompasses irradiations with broadband UVB (290–320 nm), narrowband UVB (311–313 nm), 308 nm excimer laser, UVA1 (340–400 nm), UVA plus psoralens (PUVA), and extracorporeal photochemotherapy (photopheresis)
- Therapeutic success depends upon proper selection of the phototherapy modality for a given disease
- Proper dosimetry is required to avoid acute side effects such as sunburn reaction, blistering and burning sensations
- The risk of skin carcinogenesis represents the major long-term side effect of phototherapy. Except for PUVA, the magnitude of this risk is yet not clearly delineated

INTRODUCTION

Over the past 25 years, phototherapy has greatly influenced treatment concepts in dermatology. Studies focusing on the effects of electromagnetic radiation (Fig. 134.1) on the skin have induced fruitful collaborations between basic scientists and clinicians.

Although UV radiation had been used for decades in the management of common skin diseases such as psoriasis and atopic dermatitis, the introduction of PUVA in the mid-1970s sparked a whole new series of discoveries, including high-intensity UV sources and selective spectra in the UVB and UVA range, e.g. narrowband UVB (311–313 nm) and UVA1 (340–400 nm).

PHOTOTHERAPY WITH UVB

Historical Aspects

Phototherapy using artificial light sources has a tradition dating back more than 75 years. The combination of topical crude coal tar and subsequent UV irradiation for the treatment of psoriasis was introduced by Goeckerman in 1925 and became a standard therapy for psoriasis for half a century, particularly in the US. In the 1970s, it was observed that broadband UVB radiation alone, if given in doses that produce a slight erythema, could clear the milder forms of psoriasis, particularly the seborrheic and guttate types. A major advance was the development of fluorescent bulbs that emitted narrowband UVB radiation at 311–313 nm in the mid-1980s. This narrow spectrum is superior in clearing psoriasis and thus represents the most effective and most frequently used UVB phototherapy for psoriasis; it is also beneficial for a variety of other dermatoses that were previously treated with PUVA (see below).

Principles and Mechanisms

UVB phototherapy refers to the use of artificial UVB radiation without the addition of exogenous photosensitizers. The radiation is absorbed by endogenous chromophores, and photochemical reactions involving these UV-absorbing biomolecules mediate a variety of biologic effects, ultimately leading to the therapeutic effects. The most important chromophore for UVB is nuclear DNA. Absorption of UV by nucleotides causes the formation of DNA photoproducts, primarily pyrimidine dimers[1].

UVB exposure reduces DNA synthesis and thus is used to suppress the accelerated DNA synthesis found in psoriatic epidermal cells. UVB also induces the expression of the tumor suppressor gene *p53*, and this can lead to either cell cycle arrest (allowing time for DNA repair) or apoptosis of keratinocytes ('sunburn cells') if the DNA damage is too severe to be repaired. Through these mechanisms, *p53* prevents photocarcinogenesis.

In addition to its effect on the cell cycle, UV induces the release of prostaglandins and cytokines. Interleukin (IL)-6 and IL-1, for example, seem to play important roles in producing the systemic symptoms of UV phototoxicity (sunburn) and immune suppression, respectively[1]. These responses may, however, prove to be equally important for therapeutic effectiveness.

There is also increasing evidence that UV radiation can affect, in addition to DNA, extranuclear molecular targets located in the cytoplasm and cell membrane. These targets include cell surface receptors, kinases, phosphatases and transcription factors. It was recently shown that nuclear and cytoplasmic/membrane effects are not mutually exclusive, rather they independently contribute to the various biologic effects of UVB.

Fig. 134.1 Electromagnetic spectrum with expanded UV region.

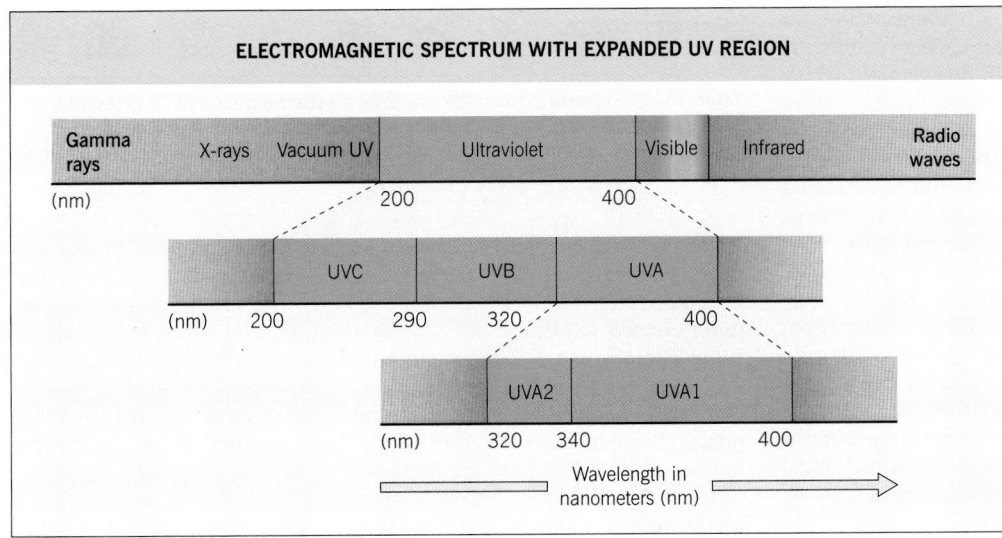

ELECTROMAGNETIC SPECTRUM WITH EXPANDED UV REGION

Many of the therapeutic effects of UVB may be due to its immuno-suppressive properties that have been linked to the formation of pyrimidine dimers. UV radiation suppresses contact allergy, delayed-type hypersensitivity, and immune surveillance against UV-induced non-melanoma skin cancers in mice. Of note, Langerhans cells are very sensitive to UVB, which alters their antigen-presenting function. Keratinocytes also secrete soluble mediators such as IL-1 and IL-6, prostaglandin E_2 and TNF-α, which by themselves can alter the immune response. Therapeutic UVB suppresses the type 1 (proinflammatory) axis as defined by IL-12, interferon-γ and IL-8, and can selectively reduce proinflammatory cytokine production by individual T cells[1].

The interplay of the various photobiologic pathways is far from being completely understood. In psoriasis, both epidermal keratinocytes and cutaneous lymphocytes may be targeted by UVB. Immune suppression, alteration of cytokine expression, and cell cycle arrest may all contribute to the suppression of disease activity in psoriatic plaques[2].

Action Spectrum and Radiation Sources

A comparison of therapeutic spectra by Fischer indicated that the highest antipsoriatic efficacy was in the range of 313 nm. This was confirmed by Parrish & Jaenicke[3], who demonstrated that 304 and 313 nm were optimally effective (Fig. 134.2), even at suberythemogenic doses. Erythemogenic UVA doses are also therapeutically effective, but 1000 times higher fluences are needed (as compared with UVB), and, on a practical level, this is not feasible. The addition of UVA also does not enhance the therapeutic efficacy of UVB in psoriasis (unlike atopic dermatitis). The Philips TL01 fluorescent lamp that emits narrowband UVB (311–313 nm) was introduced to optimally meet the requirements for antipsoriatic activity (Fig. 134.3).

Treatment Protocols

Before starting phototherapy, determination of the patient's UV sensitivity via phototesting is recommended, since skin typing alone does not always reflect the actual sensitivity of a particular individual. However, phototesting is not mandatory for the experienced therapist and, for practical reasons, is often not done. Testing is performed by exposing six small template areas (e.g. 1 cm diameter circles) of usually non-sun-exposed skin (lower back, buttocks) to an incremental series of UVB irradiations. Increases are made by fixed values (e.g. 10 mJ/cm²) or by a fraction of the last dose (e.g. 40%). An example is given in Table 134.1. Note that these doses strongly depend on the photometer used. Narrowband UVB is much less erythemogenic with regard to physical units (mJ/cm²) than broadband UVB.

The minimal erythema dose (MED) is defined as the lowest dose that causes a minimally perceptible erythema reaction at 24 hours after irradiation. Sunbathing or exposure to 'sunlamps' should be avoided before phototesting. It is crucial to document the type of lamp used for the MED determination, since the values obtained with broadband and narrowband sources differ tremendously (see Table 134.1).

Despite controversial discussion as to whether visual assessment of the MED is the optimal method for establishing a reference value for dosimetry, it is an easily performed procedure that does not require any specialized equipment. An initial therapeutic UVB dose equal to 70% of the MED is recommended. Treatments are given two to five times weekly. Since UVB erythema peaks within 24 hours after exposure, doses may be increased with each successive treatment. However, if treatments are given five times weekly, the doses should be increased every other treatment. The rate of increase depends on treatment frequency and the outcome of the preceding UVB exposure. The objective of the dose increments is to achieve a minimally perceptible erythema as a clinical indicator of optimal dosimetry. For example, with thrice-weekly exposures, doses are increased by 40% if no erythema appears, and by 20% upon development of slight erythema. If mild erythema persists, the dose should be maintained. With daily exposures, these rates are no more than 30%, 15% and 0%, respectively. If more intensive or painful erythema develops, irradiations are stopped until the symptoms disappear. Treatment is then continued until complete remission is achieved or no further improvement can be obtained with continued phototherapy (Fig. 134.4).

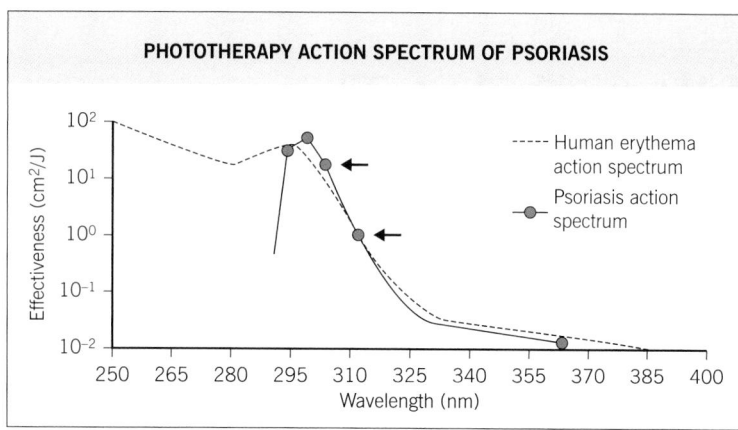

Fig. 134.2 Phototherapy action spectrum of psoriasis. The phototherapy action spectrum of psoriasis is plotted as the reciprocal of the lowest effective daily dose to clearing versus wavelength. The dashed line shows human erythema action spectrum. The solid line is the action spectrum of psoriasis. Circles represent the reciprocal of the lowest effective daily dose for wavelengths that cleared psoriasis (295, 300, 304, 313, 365 nm); the arrows point to the wavelengths that were optimally effective (304, 313 nm). Presently, narrowband UVB sources that emit wavelengths between 311 and 313 nm are available. Adapted from Parrish JA, Jaenicke KF. Action spectrum for phototherapy of psoriasis. J Invest Dermatol. 1981;76:359–62.

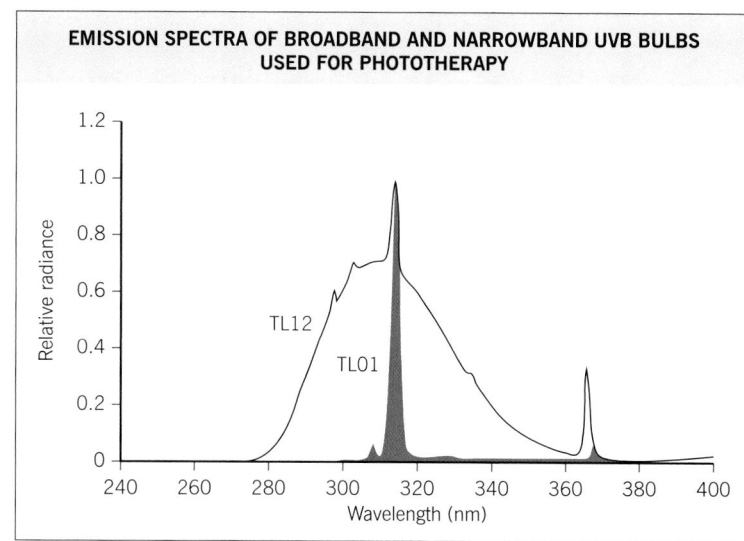

Fig. 134.3 Emission spectra of broadband and narrowband UVB bulbs used for phototherapy. Philips TL12, broadband UVB bulb; Philips TL01, narrowband UVB bulb.

EXPOSURE DOSES FOR MED ASSESSMENT WITH BROADBAND AND NARROWBAND UVB SOURCES (mJ/cm²)						
Broadband UVB	20	40	60	80	100	120
Narrowband UVB	200	400	600	800	1000	1200

Table 134.1 Exposure doses for minimal erythema dose (MED) assessment with broadband and narrowband UVB sources (mJ/cm²). Physical doses as measured with an integrated UV meter (Waldmann, Schwenningen, Germany).

Whether maintenance treatment leads to a more prolonged remission time is still a matter of debate, since no precise data are available. In cutaneous T-cell lymphoma (CTCL), most therapists perform maintenance treatment for several months to a year. For psoriasis, some centers use a 2-month maintenance phase with twice-weekly exposures for 1 month and once-weekly exposures for another month. The last effective UVB dose is given throughout the maintenance phase. If relapses occur during the maintenance phase, treatment frequency and UVB dose are increased again until clearing.

Excellent guidelines for use of narrowband UVB have been prepared by the British Photodermatology Group. They present evidence-based

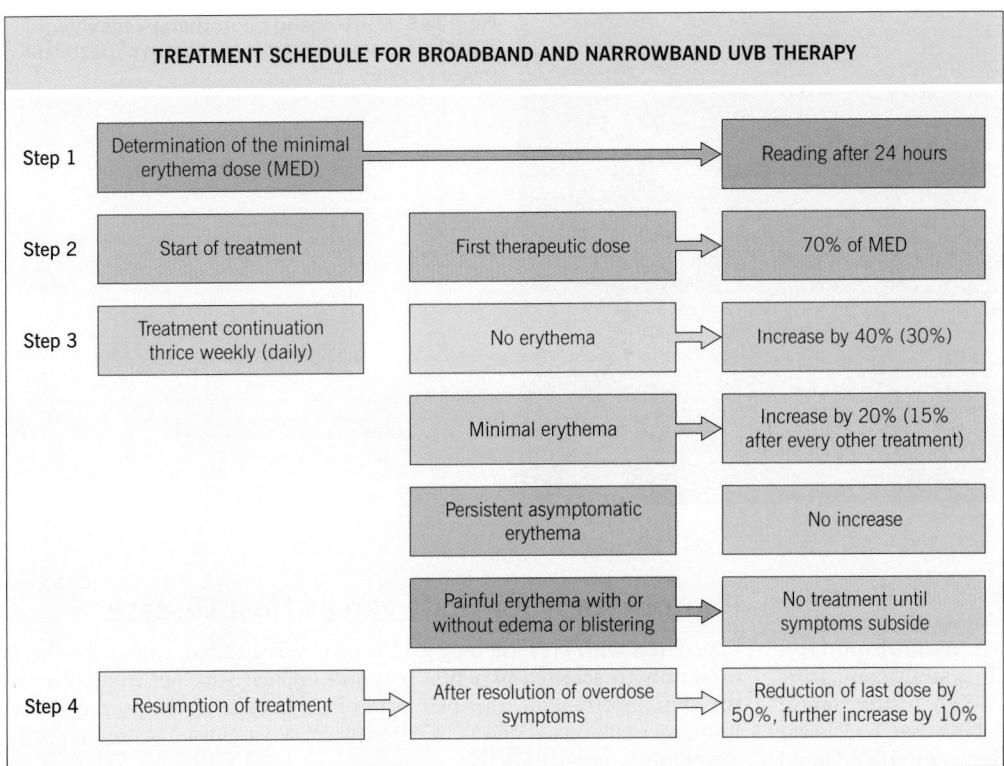

Fig. 134.4 Treatment schedule for broadband and narrowband UVB therapy.

guidance for treatment of patients with a variety of dermatoses and photodermatoses, with identification of the strength of evidence available at the time of preparation[4].

Phototherapy for Psoriasis

Guttate and seborrheic (minimally elevated) forms of psoriasis respond most favorably and rapidly to broadband UVB, while chronic, plaque-type psoriasis is more resistant. Despite its proven efficacy, UVB is certainly inferior to PUVA, both in terms of clearing efficiency and duration of remission.

However, narrowband UVB phototherapy is superior to conventional broadband UVB with respect to both clearing and remission times. In many countries, narrowband UVB has mostly replaced conventional UVB phototherapy. Based on our own studies and other publications, we regard narrowband UVB phototherapy to be nearly as effective as PUVA[5].

In addition to the protocols mentioned above, other regimens may be used. Some schedules utilize skin type-dependent starting doses and fixed increments regardless of skin reaction. Sometimes, the patient's extremities (in particular the lower extremities) are exposed to higher doses than the trunk.

Adjunctive topical agents and combination therapies are often tried in order to improve efficacy and to reduce the cumulative UVB dose, with the ultimate aim of minimizing the risk of long-term side effects. Narrowband UVB has been successfully combined with therapies such as anthralin and calcipotriol. The use of bland emollients before UVB treatment is laborious and time-consuming. In our experience, it does not dramatically increase treatment efficacy. The concurrent use of topical corticosteroids may reduce remission times and thus is discouraged[6].

Systemic drugs such as retinoids increase efficacy, particularly in patients with chronic plaque-type psoriasis[7,8]. In addition, retinoids may reduce the carcinogenic potential of UVB phototherapy.

Phototherapy for Cutaneous T-Cell Lymphoma (Mycosis Fungoides)

In early stages (IA, IB and IIA) of CTCL, conventional treatment strategies consist of topical therapies with an increasing stage-dependent aggressiveness. Options include topical corticosteroids, UV radiation, and topical cytotoxic agents such as nitrogen mustard. More

advanced stages are treated with total body electron beam radiation therapy (see Ch. 139), X-irradiation, and systemic polychemotherapy, but none of these regimens has been demonstrated to induce permanent remission.

Mycosis fungoides (MF) lesions frequently occur in non-sun-exposed areas of the body, and patients with early-stage MF can benefit from exposure to natural sunlight. In a long-term follow-up report, 74% patients treated with broadband UVB remained in complete remission after a median treatment period of 5 months[9]. Response to phototherapy was determined by the type (i.e. patch-stage MF did better than the plaque type) but not the extent of skin involvement. Using a similar protocol, Ramsay et al.[10] observed complete clearing in 83% of patients with early-stage CTCL after a median period of 5 months. With prolonged maintenance therapy, the median duration of remission within the observational period was 22 months. Twenty percent of patients with complete responses had recurrence of their disease; the four patients with plaques did not respond to UVB treatment. In a further study, prolonged maintenance therapy (up to 30 months) resulted in a relapse-free period of 26 ± 10 months[11].

The proposed mechanisms for UVB phototherapy of CTCL include impairment of epidermal Langerhans cell function and alterations in cytokine production and adhesion molecule expression by keratinocytes[12]. More recently, it was noted that narrowband UVB induces apoptosis of T lymphocytes, which may contribute particularly to the beneficial effect of this light source[13].

UVB phototherapy is clearly less efficient than PUVA, and the duration of treatment in the clearing and maintenance phases is longer and thus requires higher patient compliance. Whether patients would benefit from adding UVA as is sometimes recommended remains questionable. Likewise, narrowband UVB and broadband UVB therapy have not been compared in MF. Recently, a pilot study documented the efficacy of medium- to high-dose UVA1 therapy in patients with stage IA and IB MF (see below).

Phototherapy for Vitiligo

Many patients observe follicular repigmentation in areas of vitiligo following sun exposure. Because of seasonal and weather-dependent variations in sunlight intensity in moderate climates, exposure to natural sunlight is often not a practical option for inducing complete repigmentation. In the past, PUVA was most frequently used for the treatment of vitiligo, but exposure to artificial UVB irradiation, in

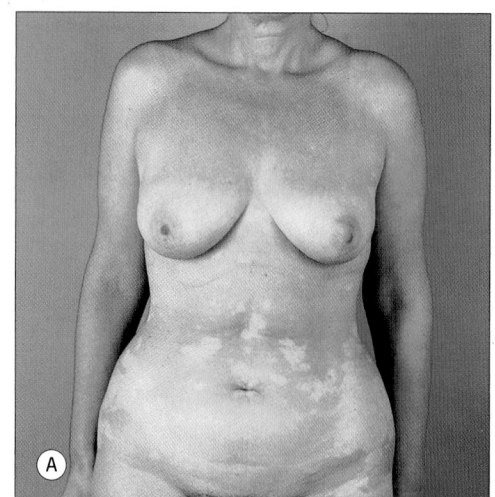 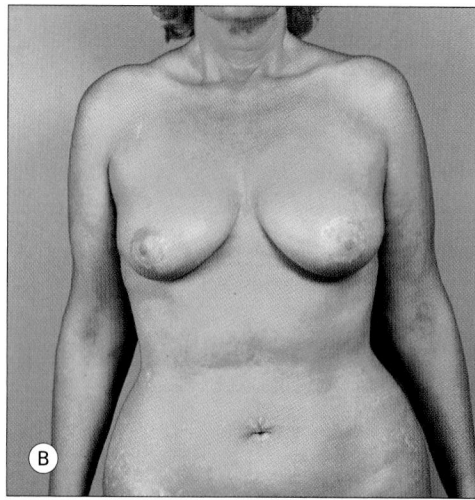

Fig. 134.5 Narrowband phototherapy for vitiligo.
A Before treatment. **B** After 10 months of treatment (twice weekly).

particular narrowband UVB, can also provide an acceptable therapeutic effect, if given for a sufficiently long period. Although the action spectrum for phototherapy of vitiligo is not known, narrowband UVB has clearly become quite popular in recent years. In a study comparing whole-body narrowband UVB irradiations with PUVA (using topical psoralen), narrowband UVB was as effective as PUVA but had fewer side effects[14] (Fig. 134.5). Also, in a recent randomized double-blind trial of nonsegmental vitiligo, NB-UVB therapy was superior to oral PUVA therapy[14a]. UVA alone is of limited benefit.

Since intense erythema may induce the Koebner phenomenon and worsening of the disease, it is necessary to stay within a dose range that induces minimally perceptible erythema. Therefore, initial assessment of the MED in a vitiliginous area that is normally not sun-exposed (e.g. buttocks, lower back or abdomen) is recommended. The UVB doses have to be increased more carefully than in other disorders, because of the increased photosensitivity.

The initial exposure is 70% of the MED in lesional skin, and subsequent doses are chosen according to the response in vitiligo areas, i.e. the goal is to induce a barely perceptible erythema. This minimal erythema is the only useful parameter for determining dosage increments. The dose should not be increased more than once weekly by 10–20% of the preceding dose. Despite the lack of pigment, vitiliginous skin does develop some tolerance, probably as a result of epidermal hyperplasia and thickening of the stratum corneum. Usually, a maximum dose will be reached during the first couple of months that is used throughout the entire treatment period. Most commonly, two to three treatments per week are given. However, too few controlled studies are available for any particular phototherapy regimen to be preferred over another.

Phototherapy for Atopic Dermatitis
Broadband UVB phototherapy
Based on the empirical experience that sun exposure was beneficial for patients with atopic dermatitis, broadband UVB has been used to treat atopic dermatitis since the end of the 1970s.

UVA/UVB phototherapy
Recent studies suggest that a combination of UVB plus UVA irradiation (UVA/UVB therapy) is superior to conventional broadband UVB, conventional UVA, and low-dose UVA1 therapy in the management of chronic, moderate atopic dermatitis. A paired-comparison study demonstrated statistically significant differences in favor of UVA/UVB therapy, compared with broadband UVB therapy[15].

Narrowband UVB phototherapy
George et al.[16] first used an air-conditioned narrowband UVB irradiation unit to treat atopic dermatitis. It not only improved the total clinical score, but also substantially reduced the need for potent corticosteroids. These beneficial effects were still present in the majority of patients 6 months after cessation of phototherapy. Other trials have shown similar results[17]. Narrowband UVB therapy has been used successfully in conjunction with UVA1 therapy.

Phototherapy for Graft-versus-Host Disease
Experience with UVB therapy of GVHD is very limited, since it has been used only in selected patients. It is still unclear whether irradiation of the skin shortly after transplantation is of benefit in the prevention of human cutaneous GVHD[18]. Currently, PUVA represents the mainstay for phototherapy of GVHD.

Phototherapy for Pityriasis Lichenoides and Lymphomatoid Papulosis
Both pityriasis lichenoides acuta and chronica can have a prolonged course and be rather resistant to therapy. As sunlight may lead to some improvement, UVB phototherapy has also been associated with some success. However, PUVA seems to be more effective (see below), especially in the acute form of the disease (perhaps because of the deeper extension of the dermal inflammatory infiltrate). Although Honig et al.[19] have recommended PUVA as the treatment of choice for the acute form, PUVA may be reserved for cases of pityriasis lichenoides chronica that are UVB-resistant.

Phototherapy for Seborrheic Dermatitis
Seborrheic dermatitis generally improves during the summer and 'sunny' vacations. Accordingly, UV radiation also seems to have a beneficial effect on this condition. However, flares of dermatitis may occasionally occur. Recently, narrowband UVB was found to be an effective treatment in severe cases[20].

Phototherapy for Pruritus
Both narrowband and broadband UVB therapy can be beneficial in various forms of pruritus, particularly those associated with diabetes and hepatic disorders or those that are idiopathic in nature. Remissions in hepatic disease, however, are relatively short-lived. Controlled studies have clearly demonstrated its efficacy in uremic pruritus[21].

Side Effects of Phototherapy with UVB
Short-term side effects include erythema (Fig. 134.6), xerosis accompanied by pruritus, occasional blistering, and an increased frequency of recurrent herpes simplex viral infections. Painful erythema resulting from overexposure is treated with topical corticosteroids. Systemic non-steroidal anti-inflammatory drugs and corticosteroids can prove useful in severe cases, if administered early.

Long-term side effects include photoaging and carcinogenesis. Although UVB is a known carcinogen, its carcinogenic potential seems to be lower than that of PUVA. A 16-center study conducted by Stern & Laird[22] did not detect a relationship between UVB phototherapy and non-melanoma skin cancer. In a British study comprised of 1908 patients treated with narrowband UVB, a small but significant increase of basal cell carcinomas, but not squamous cell carcinomas, was detected.

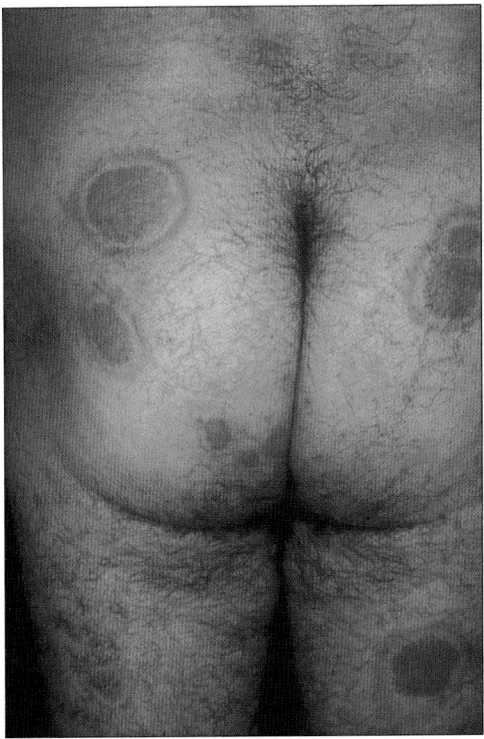

Fig. 134.6 Target-like appearance of psoriatic lesions secondary to phototoxicity due to UVB. Annular erythema is separated from the psoriatic plaques by Woronoff's ring.

According to the authors, this could be explained by a number of factors, including ascertainment bias. To determine the true carcinogenic risk of narrowband UVB phototherapy, further follow-up studies are essential[23].

Because narrowband UVB has been in use for just the last two decades, its long-term side effects are not yet known. Compared with broadband UVB, up to tenfold higher physical doses of narrowband UVB are required to produce erythema, edema and sunburn cell formation. Using single-cell gel electrophoresis (the comet assay), therapeutically equivalent doses from these two radiation sources produced minimal differences in the amount of DNA damage[24]. As narrowband UVB is clinically more effective than broadband UVB, the former requires less MED-equivalents to achieve a therapeutic response, implying that narrowband UVB is less carcinogenic than broadband UVB[25].

PHOTOTHERAPY WITH THE 308 NM EXCIMER LASER

The use of the 308 nm excimer laser represents an enhancement of narrowband UVB delivery. The clinical use of this laser for plaque-type psoriasis was first reported in 1997[26]. Subsequent reports[27] showed that high multiples of the MED, such as 4 and 6 MEDs, could induce a longer duration of remission than achieved with conventional narrowband therapy in some patients. Other advantages of the use of the excimer laser for psoriasis is the lower number of treatments that may be necessary to induce clearing and the ability to treat exclusively the affected skin and with a reduced cumulative dose, thus perhaps reducing the long-term risk of carcinogenicity[28,29]. However, widespread psoriasis generally cannot be treated with this modality because the spot size is less than 2 cm². Clearly, the excimer laser will be most suitable for patients with stubborn plaques unresponsive to other treatment and/or those having difficult-to-treat localized areas such as the palms, soles, knees and elbows. The excimer laser is now approved by the Food and Drug Administration (FDA) for the treatment of psoriasis. Whether it really represents a therapeutic advancement still remains to be determined by larger and longer-term studies, particularly in view of the high costs of the laser treatment.

Targeted phototherapy with the excimer laser may also serve as a new treatment modality for the management of stable vitiligo and for a variety of other chronic inflammatory localized dermatoses such as granuloma annulare, lichen planus, lichen simplex chronicus and alopecia areata[30,31].

PHOTOTHERAPY WITH UVA1

The UVA spectrum (320–400 nm) has been arbitrarily subdivided into two parts: UVA1 (340–400 nm) and UVA2 (320–340 nm) (see Fig. 134.1). The main reason for this subdivision was the observation that UVA2 resembled UVB in its ability to cause erythema as well as immuno-modulation and photocarcinogenesis. Because of its longer mean wave-length, UVA1 radiation penetrates more deeply into the skin than UVA2 (see Ch. 86), and thus affects not only epidermal structures, but also mid and deep dermal components, especially blood vessels. Since the skin is a large organ, exposure of circulating immune cells to UVA1 irradiation may have significant systemic ramifications. In particular, its ability to induce T-lymphocyte apoptosis is likely to be relevant in the treatment of atopic dermatitis and possibly of mycosis fungoides. It may reduce the number of Langerhans cells and mast cells in the dermis in atopic dermatitis, and in cutaneous mastocytosis. In addition, it has been shown that increased collagenase expression in treated lesions of localized scleroderma accompanies improvement with UVA1 irradiation. Perhaps the efficacy of UVA1 in localized scleroderma, and in other sclerosing conditions, is in part due to this action.

UVA1 phototherapy is currently being investigated as a safer alternative to PUVA for treating chronic conditions. To date, most of the UVA1 studies have been performed in Europe, where efficient sources of UVA1 radiation are more widely available (Fig. 134.7).

UVA1 has some limited effects on atopic dermatitis[32–34] (Fig. 134.8). It seems to be more effective than UVA/UVB therapy, at least for severe exacerbations of atopic dermatitis. When used as a monotherapy, medium and high daily doses are better than low doses. However, UVA1 has not yet been compared directly with the standard phototherapies for atopic dermatitis (narrowband UVB or PUVA). Moreover, the published studies do not tell us whether or not adding UVA1 to treatment with potent topical steroids is beneficial[35].

UVA1 therapy was reported to be beneficial in several other dermatoses, including localized scleroderma[36,37], chronic sclerodermoid GVHD[38], urticaria pigmentosa[39] and CTCL[40]. However, the latter indication in particular requires confirmation in larger patient series. Clearly, this area of phototherapy is still under evaluation.

Side Effects of Phototherapy with UVA1

The adverse effects of UVA1 are less severe than those of UVB and UVA2. Until more is known about UVA1 therapy, its use (especially with high doses such as 130 J/cm²) should be limited to treating

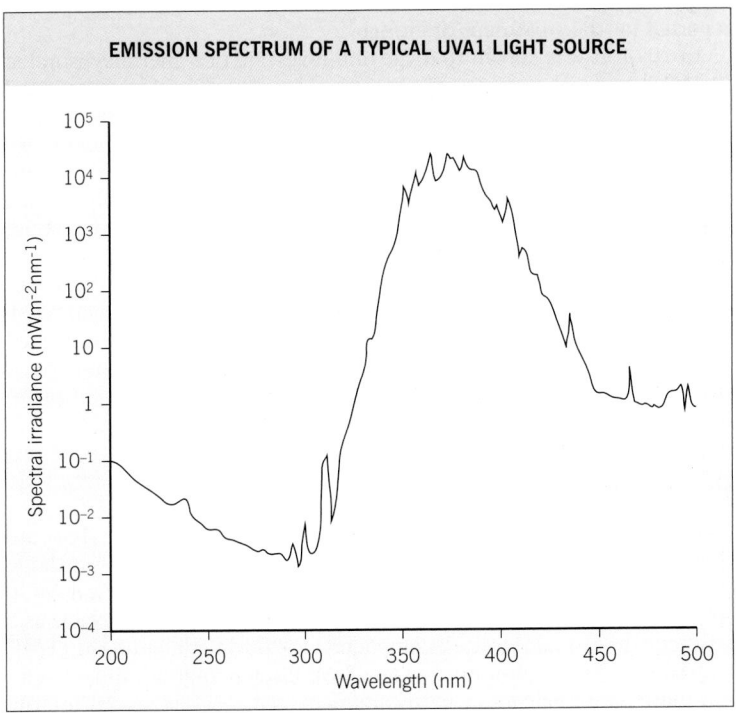

Fig. 134.7 Emission spectrum of a typical UVA1 light source (filtered metal halide lamp).

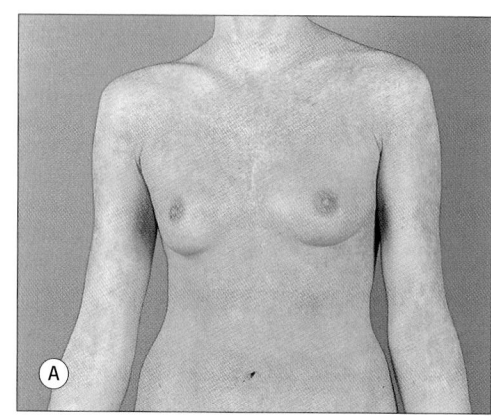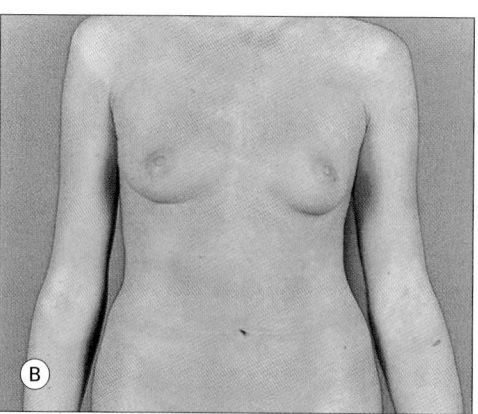

Fig. 134.8 UVA1 phototherapy of atopic dermatitis. High-dose (130 J/cm², left side) versus medium-dose (65 J/cm², right side) UVA1 phototherapy of atopic dermatitis. **A** Before treatment. **B** After treatment (15 exposures). Note that there is no difference in the therapeutic result. From Tzaneva et al.[34] From Tzaneva S, Seeber A, Schwaiger M, et al. High-dose versus medium-dose UVA1 phototherapy for patients with severe, generalized atopic dermatitis. J Am Acad Dermatol. 2001;45:503–7.

diseases with periods of severe, acute exacerbations, and, in general, one treatment cycle should not exceed 10–15 successively administered exposures and should not be repeated more than once a year. A European prospective longitudinal study has been initiated to monitor patients treated with UVA1 phototherapy for the development of skin cancer and photoaging. An increased expression of *p53* and a slight increase in Bcl-2 protein expression in keratinocytes have been recently found in human skin after UVA1 irradiation (even with suberythemogenic doses), suggesting that UVA1 may cause DNA damage[41]. Of note, in the years since the widespread use of UVA1 phototherapy in Europe began in 1992, no serious negative side effects in humans have been reported.

PHOTOCHEMOTHERAPY WITH PSORALENS (PUVA)

Psoralen photochemotherapy (PUVA) combines the use of psoralens (P) and long-wave UV radiation (UVA). This combination results in a therapeutically beneficial phototoxic effect, which is not produced by either of the components alone. Psoralens can be administered orally or applied topically in the form of solutions, creams or baths, with subsequent UVA exposure.

Historical Aspects

Topical exposure to extracts, seeds or parts of plants (e.g. *Ammi majus*, *Psoralea corylifolia*) that contain natural psoralens, followed by exposure to sunlight, was used as a remedy for vitiligo for thousands of years in ancient Egypt and India. Encouraging results with topical or oral psoralens and exposure to sunlight or UV radiation were initially reported for the treatment of vitiligo[42].

In 1974, it was shown that the oral ingestion of 8-methoxypsoralen (8-MOP) and subsequent exposure to a new, high-intensity, artificial UVA radiation source was highly effective in the treatment of psoriasis[43]. This new therapeutic concept was called photochemotherapy or acronymously PUVA. However, even before the development of high-intensity UVA sources, it had already been shown that topically applied psoralens plus irradiation with low-intensity UVA (black light) could clear psoriatic lesions[42].

Subsequently, the use of psoralen baths and subsequent UVA exposure (bath PUVA), which originated in Scandinavia[44], has been used. The effectiveness of all variants of PUVA has been widely documented and has profoundly influenced dermatologic therapy in general, given the responsiveness of a number of different disorders in addition to psoriasis (Table 134.2)[19].

Psoralens

Psoralens are naturally occurring linear furocoumarins that are found in a large number of plants, and there are several synthetic psoralen compounds. For oral and topical (bath, cream) PUVA, 8-MOP (methoxsalen) is used primarily; it is of plant origin but also available as a synthetic drug. The synthetic compound, 4,5',8-trimethylpsoralen (TMP, trioxsalen), is less phototoxic than 8-MOP after oral administration, but more phototoxic when bathwater-delivered. TMP is used primarily in Scandinavia for bath PUVA. 5-Methoxypsoralen (5-MOP, bergapten) is also therapeutically effective when given orally; it is less

erythemogenic and is not associated with gastrointestinal intolerance (Fig. 134.9). In Europe (where available) it is now used for routine PUVA. Oral preparations of 8-MOP and 5-MOP contain either crystals, micronized crystals or solubilized psoralens in a gel matrix. The liquid preparation induces earlier, higher and more reproducible peak plasma levels than the crystalline preparations.

The steps between the ingestion of a psoralen and its arrival in the skin include disintegration and dissolution of the drug, absorption, first-pass effect, blood transportation, and tissue distribution. The absorption rate of a psoralen from the gut depends on the physicochemical properties

PUVA-RESPONSIVE DISEASES

Therapy of disease	Prevention of disease
Psoriasis	Polymorphous light eruption[†]
Palmoplantar pustulosis	Solar urticaria[†]
Atopic dermatitis	Chronic actinic dermatitis[*,†]
Mycosis fungoides (stages IA, IB, IIA)	Hydroa vacciniforme[*,†]
Vitiligo	Erythropoietic protoporphyria[*,†]
Generalized lichen planus	
Urticaria pigmentosa	
Cutaneous GVHD	
Generalized granuloma annulare	
Prurigo nodularis	
Pityriasis lichenoides (acute and chronic)[*]	
Lymphomatoid papulosis[*]	
Pityriasis rubra pilaris[*,†]	
Purpura pigmentosa chronica[*]	
Langerhans cell histiocytosis[*]	
Localized scleroderma[*]	

Experience is limited to a small number of patients.
[†]*May flare.*

Table 134.2 PUVA-responsive diseases.

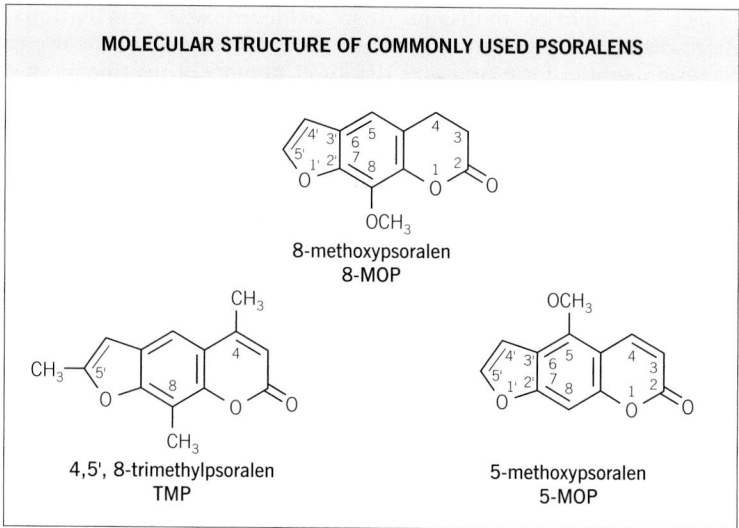

MOLECULAR STRUCTURE OF COMMONLY USED PSORALENS

8-methoxypsoralen
8-MOP

4,5', 8-trimethylpsoralen
TMP

5-methoxypsoralen
5-MOP

Fig. 134.9 Molecular structure of commonly used psoralens.

of the molecule, the rate of dissolution, the galenic characteristics of the preparation, and the fat content of concomitantly ingested food. 5-MOP is less water-soluble than 8-MOP and its absorption rate is approximately 25% of that of 8-MOP. Like 8-MOP, liquid preparations of 5-MOP give higher and earlier peak serum levels than do crystalline formulations. In addition, peak serum levels are achieved by liquid preparations after a relatively reproducible time interval, whereas wide time variability occurs with crystalline formulations. Before reaching the skin via the circulation, psoralens are metabolized during their passage through the liver. Plasma levels of 8-MOP administered orally at different doses show a strong non-linearity indicating a saturable first-pass effect. Thus, small differences in the ingested doses and absorption rates of psoralens lead to large differences in plasma levels. As a practical consequence, small amounts of the drug are almost completely metabolized by the liver during the first pass and therefore may be therapeutically inactive.

8-MOP and 5-MOP serum levels show a wide range of inter-individual differences. Even on different occasions in the same patient, serum levels may differ; however, the levels are usually sufficiently constant to provide for relatively reproducible therapeutic results. This unpredictable pharmacokinetic behavior is probably due to inter- and intra-individual variations in intestinal absorption, first-pass effect, blood distribution in the body, and metabolism and elimination of the drug.

In a particular individual, serum levels of 8-MOP correspond fairly well with skin reactivity, with the peak of skin phototoxicity coinciding with peak serum levels. A correlation between 8-MOP and 5-MOP serum levels and epidermal concentrations does exist. Whether there is a significant correlation between maximum psoralen blood concentrations and the minimal phototoxicity dose remains equivocal.

The pharmacokinetics of topical 8-MOP depend on the mode of application. 8-MOP administered topically as a 0.15% emulsion or solution has been shown to result in plasma levels comparable to those obtained by oral delivery, if large areas of the body are treated. In contrast, due to the much lower concentrations that are used, plasma levels following bath-PUVA treatment of almost the entire body surface are very low. Bathwater-delivered psoralens are readily absorbed into the skin, but are promptly eliminated without cutaneous accumulation[2].

Psoralen photochemistry

Psoralens react with DNA in three steps. First, in the absence of UV radiation, the psoralen intercalates into the DNA double strand. Absorption of photons in the UVA range results in the formation of a 3,4- or 4',5'-cyclobutane monoadduct with pyrimidine bases of native DNA. The 4',5' monoadducts can absorb a second photon and this reaction leads to the formation of an interstrand cross-link of the double helix with the 5,6 double bond of the pyrimidine base of the opposite strand (Fig. 134.10).

Excited psoralens can also react with molecular oxygen. The reactive oxygen species formed by this reaction cause cell membrane damage by lipid peroxidation and may activate the cyclooxygenase and arachidonic acid metabolic pathways (for references, see refs 45 & 46).

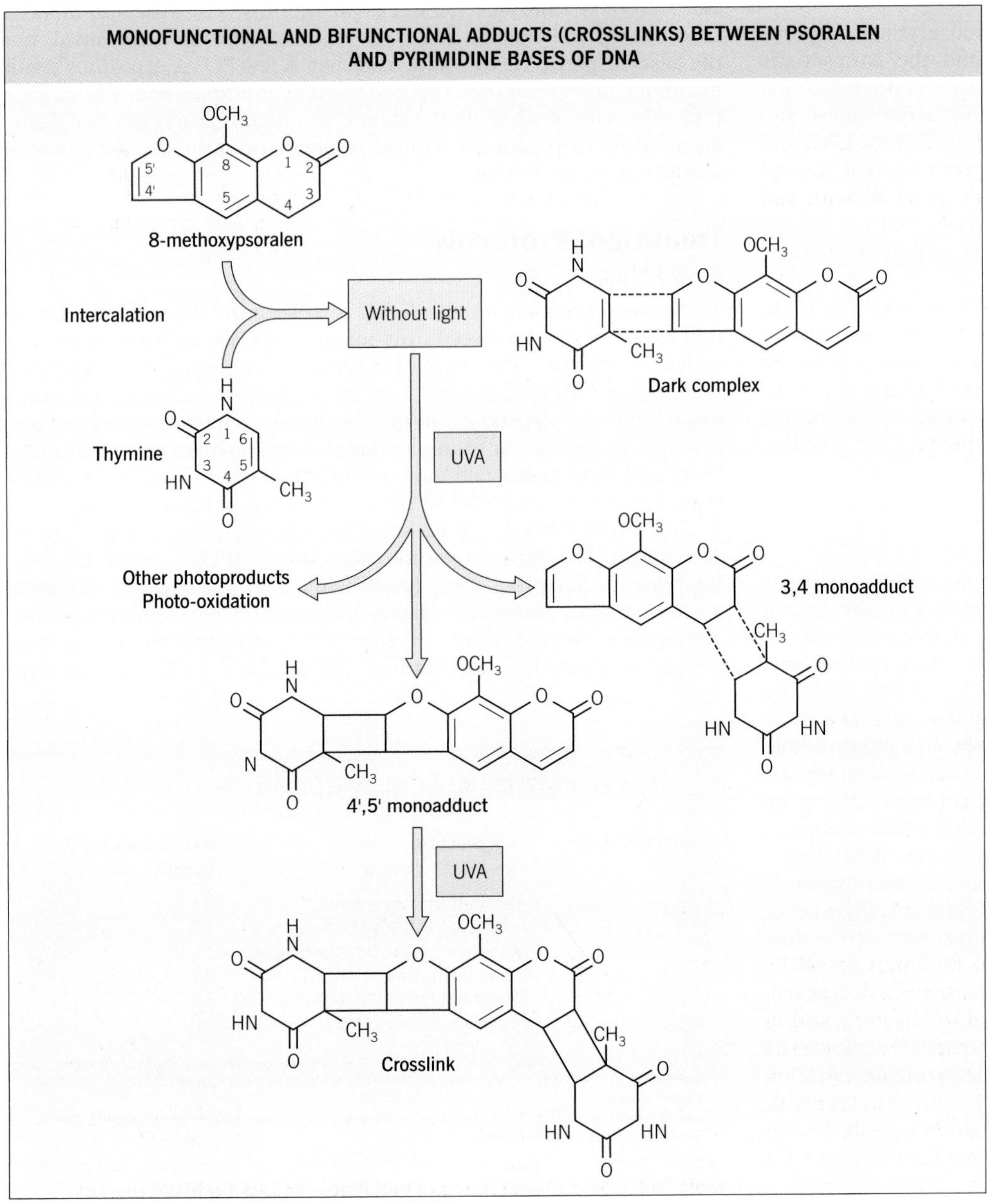

MONOFUNCTIONAL AND BIFUNCTIONAL ADDUCTS (CROSSLINKS) BETWEEN PSORALEN AND PYRIMIDINE BASES OF DNA

Fig. 134.10 Monofunctional and bifunctional adducts (cross-links) between psoralen and pyrimidine bases of DNA.

The conjunction of psoralens with epidermal DNA inhibits DNA replication and causes cell cycle arrest. Although not proven, it is generally assumed that this effect may be the therapeutic mechanism in psoriasis. Psoralen photosensitization also causes an alteration in the expression of cytokines and cytokine receptors. However, DNA cross-linking does not appear to be a prerequisite for all the therapeutic effects of PUVA, and the successful treatment of other skin diseases is unlikely to be due directly to this molecular reaction. Psoralens also interact with RNA, proteins and other cellular components and indirectly modify proteins and lipids via singlet oxygen-mediated reactions or by generating free radicals[46].

PUVA can reverse the pathologically altered patterns of keratinocyte differentiation markers and reduce the number of proliferating epidermal cells. Infiltrating lymphocytes are strongly suppressed by PUVA, with variable effects on different T-cell subsets. PUVA is far more potent in inducing apoptosis in lymphocytes than in keratinocytes[1], which may explain its efficacy in CTCL as well as in inflammatory skin diseases. Although much is known about pathways and mechanisms in psoralen photosensitization, the interactions and relative contributions to the clearing of a specific disease are not well understood.

Psoralens also stimulate melanogenesis. This involves the photoconjugation of psoralens to DNA in melanocytes, followed by mitosis and subsequent proliferation of melanocytes, increased formation and melanization of melanosomes, enhanced transfer of melanosomes to keratinocytes, and increased synthesis of tyrosinase via stimulation of cAMP activity.

Action Spectrum and Light Sources

The action spectrum for 8-MOP-induced delayed erythema has its maximum activity in the 330–335 nm range and the antipsoriatic activity of 8-MOP (plus UVA) appears to parallel its erythema action spectrum[47]. Conventional therapeutic UVA fluorescent tubes and broad-spectrum metal halide lamps, which are filtered in the UVB and UVC range, cover well the psoralen action spectrum. The typical fluorescent UVA lamp used for PUVA therapy peaks at 352 nm and emits approximately 0.5% in the UVB range (Fig. 134.11). Major advantages of mercury halide units are the stability of output and their high irradiance, enabling short treatment times.

UVA doses are given in J/cm², instead of mJ/cm² used for UVB, usually measured with a photometer with a maximum sensitivity at 350–360 nm. Within the treatment system, the irradiance must be relatively uniform so that the dose does not vary at different anatomic sites. UVB emission should be kept low enough to avoid erythemogenic UVB doses before sufficient UVA is absorbed to produce the psoralen photosensitivity reaction.

Photosensitivity Effects of PUVA

PUVA treatment produces an inflammatory response that manifests as delayed phototoxic erythema. The reaction depends on the dose of drug, the dose of UVA, and the individual's sensitivity (skin type). Recently, it was shown that changes in 8-MOP dose had no detectable effect on the maximum slope of the PUVA erythema dose–response curve. Thus, 8-MOP dose changes within individuals, over a narrow but clinically relevant range, appear to significantly alter the threshold response to PUVA erythema but not the rate of increase in erythema with increasing UVA dose[48]. PUVA erythema differs remarkably from the sunburn or UVB erythema that appears after 4–6 hours and peaks 12–24 hours after exposure. PUVA erythema does not occur before 24–36 hours and it peaks at 72–96 hours or even later after exposure. It has a shallower dose–response curve than UVB erythema (by a factor of approximately 2) and this difference is maintained even at the time of maximum erythema[49]. PUVA erythema persists for longer periods of time (lasting up to more than 1 week) and it consists of a deeper red, even a violaceous, hue. Severe reactions may lead to blistering and to superficial skin necrosis. Overdoses of PUVA are frequently followed by edema, intense pruritus and sometimes by a peculiar stinging sensation in the affected skin area. At this time, erythema is the only available parameter that allows an assessment of the magnitude of the PUVA reaction and thus represents an important factor for determining UVA dose adjustments[2].

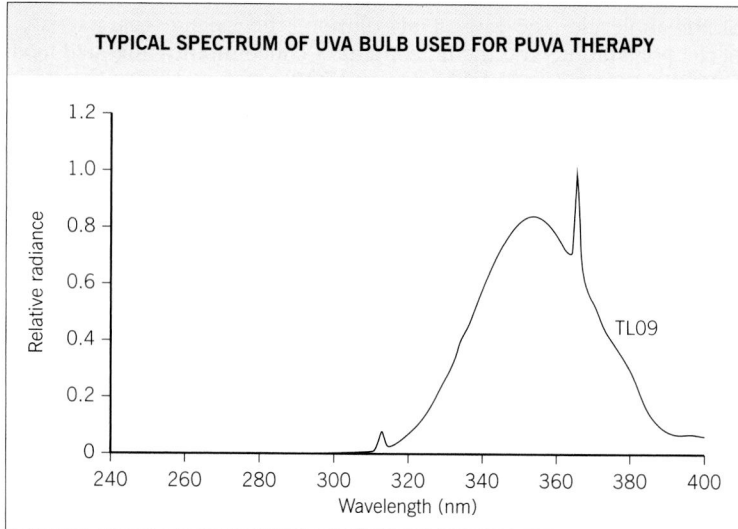

Fig. 134.11 Typical spectrum of a UVA bulb (Philips TL09) used for PUVA therapy.

Pigmentation, the second important effect of PUVA, may develop without clinically evident erythema, especially when oral 5-MOP or TMP is used; this is of particular importance in the treatment of vitiligo and for the preventive treatment of some photodermatoses. In normal skin, PUVA pigmentation peaks about 7 days after exposure and may last from several weeks to months. As with sun-induced tanning, the individual's ability to tan is genetically determined, but the dose–response curve is much steeper. A few PUVA exposures result in a much deeper tan than that produced by multiple exposures to solar radiation. One goal of phototherapy of inflammatory and neoplastic disorders is to produce a clinical response prior to the induction of significant pigmentation.

Treatment Protocols

Oral PUVA

The general principle of oral PUVA is to keep the dose of psoralen, as well as the interval between drug intake and UVA exposure, constant, and to vary the UVA dose according to the patient's sensitivity. A dosage of 8-MOP of 0.6 to 0.8 mg/kg is administered orally 1–3 hours before exposure, depending on the absorption characteristics of the particular drug brand. For example, liquid drug preparations are absorbed faster and yield higher and more reproducible serum levels than microcrystalline forms. For 5-MOP, the usual dosage is 1.2–1.8 mg/kg.

The initial UVA doses are selected either by skin typing[50,51] or by determining the minimal phototoxicity dose (MPD)[52]. In the US, skin reactivity to solar radiation is evaluated and patients are classified based on a skin phototype scheme according to their sunburn history. Therapeutic doses of UVA are then given according to an empirical scheme based on this classification[50] (Table 134.3). In Europe, the most

SKIN PHOTOTYPES AND INITIAL DOSE OF UVA FOR PUVA THERAPY		
Skin phototype*	Skin reaction	Recommended dose (J/cm²)
I[†]	Always burn, never tan	0.5
II	Always burn, but sometimes tan	1.0
III	Sometimes burn, but always tan	1.5
IV	Never burn, always tan	2.0
V[‡]	Moderately pigmented skin	2.5
VI	Darkly pigmented skin	3.0

*Types I–IV are determined by history; types V and VI by physical examination (racial descent).
[†] Patients with erythrodermic psoriasis are to be classified as skin phototype I for determination of UVA dosage.
[‡] Patients with this phototype should be classified into a lower skin phototype category if the sunburning history so indicates.

Table 134.3 Skin phototypes and initial dose of UVA for PUVA therapy.

widely used approach consists of MPD determination analogous to MED determination. The MPD is defined as the minimal dose of UVA (following psoralen ingestion) that produces a barely perceptible, but well-defined, erythema. The doses range from 0.5 to 5 J/cm^2 if 8-MOP is used and 1 to 10 J/cm^2 if 5-MOP is used. Erythema readings are performed 72 (not later than 96) hours after irradiation, when the phototoxicity reaction usually peaks. As with the MED, the MPD should be determined on previously non-sun-exposed skin (lower back or buttocks). This will yield lower values than on previously exposed skin and thus contributes to a safer initial dosimetry. Although performing an MPD is more time-consuming than phototyping, it should be done whenever possible, since it allows far more accurate and higher UVA doses during the initial treatment phase. As with UVB therapy, some experienced therapists do not consider phototesting to be mandatory.

Oral PUVA should not be used in patients with hepatitis, because slower metabolization of psoralens may prolong photosensitivity. Also, impaired renal function may slow down psoralen excretion.

Bath PUVA

Bath-water delivery of psoralens is becoming increasingly popular because it provides a uniform drug distribution over the skin surface, very low psoralen plasma levels, and a quick elimination of free psoralens from the skin, thereby reducing the period of photosensitivity. Due to the absence of systemic photosensitization, bath-water delivery of 8-MOP circumvents gastrointestinal side effects and potential ocular effects. Skin psoralen levels are highly reproducible and photosensitivity lasts no more than 2 hours. The higher incidence of unwanted phototoxicity can be prevented by a lower starting dose (30% of the initial MPD) and more cautious dosimetry during the initial treatment phase. Originally, bath PUVA was performed with TMP, but 8-MOP and 5-MOP are now being used as well. Bath PUVA consists of 15–20 minutes of whole-body (or hand and foot) immersion in solutions of 0.5–5.0 mg of 8-MOP per liter of bath water. Irradiation has to be performed immediately thereafter, as photosensitivity decreases rather rapidly. TMP is more phototoxic after topical application and thus is used at lower concentrations than 8-MOP. MPD testing for bath PUVA must take into account that, unlike with oral PUVA, the phototoxic threshold declines during the early treatment phase. In our experience, when the MPD is determined on a consecutive daily basis, the fourth MPD is approximately 50% of the first MPD (this may be due to persistent psoralen adducts)[2].

Topical PUVA

Application of 8-MOP (0.1–0.01%) in creams, ointments or lotions, followed by UVA irradiation, is effective but has several disadvantages. The non-uniform distribution on the skin surface may produce unpredictable phototoxic erythema reactions, and inadvertent application to surrounding uninvolved skin can lead to cosmetically unacceptable hyperpigmentation; this is a particular problem in patients with vitiligo. Furthermore, if numerous lesions are present, the application is laborious and time-consuming, and the treatment does not prevent the development of new active lesions in previously unaffected, untreated areas. Finally, extensive application ('paint' PUVA) of a 0.15% 8-MOP emulsion was found to cause plasma levels comparable to those detected with oral ingestion. Therefore, topical PUVA utilizing psoralen creams, ointments or lotions is now reserved primarily for psoriasis of the palms and soles and limited stable vitiligo.

Guidelines for bath, local immersion and other forms of topical PUVA were recently published by the British Photodermatology Group. These recommendations are based, where possible, on the results of controlled studies; otherwise they represent a consensus view on current practice[53].

Initial Treatment (Clearing) Phase

The initial treatment phase is defined as the treatment period until clearing of the disease is achieved; repeated exposures are required, with gradual dose increments as pigmentation develops. Doses that are too low frequently result in failure of treatment, except in those diseases in which induction of pigmentation is the desired objective. In most dermatoses amenable to PUVA, the frequency of treatments should be reduced after satisfactory control of the disease.

Treatment should not be started until the end of the 72-hour period after MPD testing. A safe initial therapeutic dose for oral PUVA is 70% of the MPD (recent studies have shown that 50% is often sufficient for the effective treatment of psoriasis). For bath PUVA, it is advisable to start at only 30% of the MPD, because photosensitivity is up to 10 times higher than with oral PUVA (Fig. 134.12).

Irradiations are given two to four times weekly. Dose increments are performed no more often than twice a week (at least 72 hours apart) and never during the first week of treatment (if initial dose is based on MPD), in order to avoid accumulation of delayed cutaneous phototoxicity. Although not necessary for therapeutic success, a minimally perceptible erythema is considered a clinical indicator of adequate dosimetry. There exists no rigid scheme for dose increments; the major parameter for dose adjustments should be the clinical response of the disease. It is essential to note that with bath PUVA, the MPD can even decrease during the first days after initiation of treatment by up to 50%, but then increases at later stages. This may be due to persistent psoralen adducts which are converted into cross-links upon subsequent exposures.

In the absence of erythema, the UVA dose can be increased safely by 30% in both oral PUVA and bath PUVA (see Fig. 134.12). However, some patients will not need dose adjustments over prolonged periods of time, because of erythema formation (e.g. vitiligo) and/or adequate treatment response.

Maintenance Phase

The purpose of maintenance therapy is to achieve a longer remission. In the European regimen, maintenance therapy consists of one month of twice-weekly treatments utilizing the final UVA dose administered during the clearing phase, followed by another month of once-weekly exposures. According to the recommendations of the British Photodermatology Group[54], maintenance treatment should be considered only in the setting of rapid relapses. Although PUVA has now been in use for more than three decades, the question remains whether maintenance therapy can prevent early relapses, particularly in psoriasis. For CTCL, many institutions recommend some form of permanent maintenance therapy. However, due to the lack of prospective studies, no valid recommendation can be given. Perhaps a once-monthly treatment would be a feasible compromise.

Mild relapses during the maintenance phase are handled by temporarily increasing the frequency of treatments; in the case of a severe relapse, the original clearing phase schedule must be resumed until clearing is once again achieved. A disadvantage of maintenance therapy for patients with a remission is the potential to overtreat the patient and to increase the potential for long-term toxicity that is related to the total cumulative dose of the PUVA.

PUVA for Psoriasis

Basically, all types of psoriasis respond to PUVA, although the management of erythrodermic or generalized pustular psoriasis is more difficult[2]. Both the US and the European regimens proved to be highly efficient and have therefore remained in use, although with the advent of biologic therapies (see Ch. 128), phototherapy of all types has lessened. Table 134.4 lists the differences between these two methods of administering oral 8-MOP PUVA[50,52].

Three studies have compared bath-water delivery of 8-MOP with oral administration[55–57]. In two reports, initial doses were determined by skin typing and treatments were given two to three times weekly. Dosage increments were done with every treatment in the first study[55], whereas smaller increments were performed every third treatment in the second[56]. Patients in the third study were treated according to the guidelines of the standard European regimen for oral PUVA; this group had the lowest incidence of treatment failures and overdose episodes[57]. Relative to the results obtained with oral PUVA, bath PUVA showed equal clearing rates with lower numbers of exposures. The greater therapeutic efficacy could be due to a higher penetration of psoralens through the abnormal stratum corneum overlying psoriatic plaques as compared with healthy perilesional skin where phototoxicity is monitored during the therapy. The incidence of erythema and pruritus

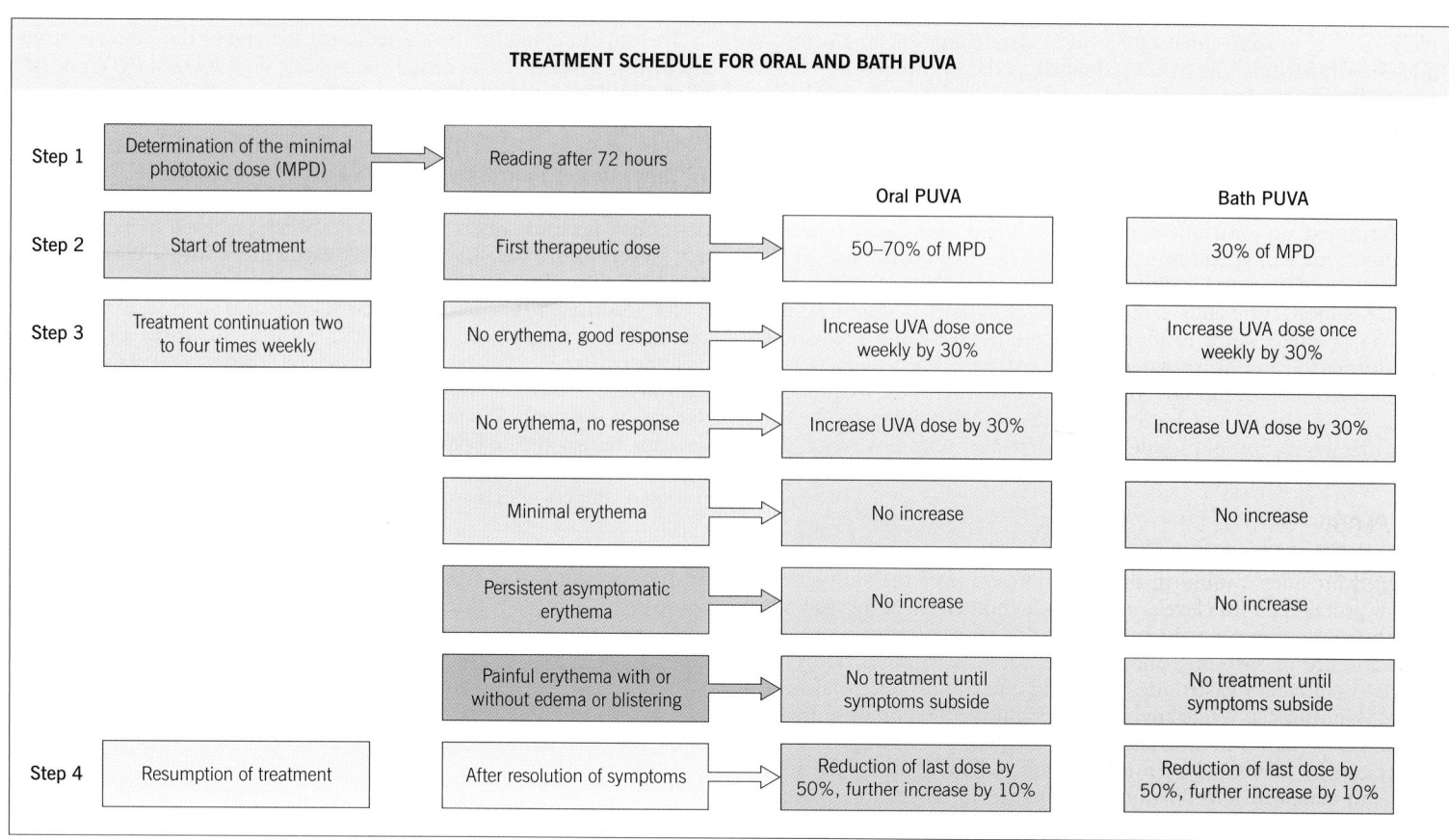

TREATMENT SCHEDULE FOR ORAL AND BATH PUVA

			Oral PUVA	Bath PUVA
Step 1	Determination of the minimal phototoxic dose (MPD)	Reading after 72 hours		
Step 2	Start of treatment	First therapeutic dose	50–70% of MPD	30% of MPD
Step 3	Treatment continuation two to four times weekly	No erythema, good response	Increase UVA dose once weekly by 30%	Increase UVA dose once weekly by 30%
		No erythema, no response	Increase UVA dose by 30%	Increase UVA dose by 30%
		Minimal erythema	No increase	No increase
		Persistent asymptomatic erythema	No increase	No increase
		Painful erythema with or without edema or blistering	No treatment until symptoms subside	No treatment until symptoms subside
Step 4	Resumption of treatment	After resolution of symptoms	Reduction of last dose by 50%, further increase by 10%	Reduction of last dose by 50%, further increase by 10%

Fig. 134.12 Treatment schedule for oral and bath PUVA.

DIFFERENCES BETWEEN THE US AND EUROPEAN PROTOCOLS FOR PUVA THERAPY

	US	Europe
UVA dosimetry	Predetermined dose according to skin phototype	Individualized dose according to MPD determination
Frequency of treatment	Two to three times/week	Four times/week
Dose increments	Predetermined	Individualized
Principle of approach	Rigid, cautious	Flexible, aggressive
Goal	To clear without ponderous testing and acute side effects	To clear rapidly before maximum pigmentation develops

Table 134.4 Differences between the US and European protocols for PUVA therapy. MPD, minimal phototoxicity dose.

was similar or lower with bath PUVA as compared to oral therapy. In all the investigations, episodes of systemic intolerance such as nausea and vomiting were recorded only with oral PUVA[2].

Oral 5-MOP PUVA represents another alternative to 8-MOP PUVA. Psoriatic lesions clear with a comparable number of exposures, but 5-MOP requires significantly higher cumulative UVA doses (Fig. 134.13). This is due to the lower phototoxic potential of 5-MOP and to its greater tanning activity. Nevertheless, 5-MOP PUVA therapy seems particularly valuable because of the absence of nausea and vomiting, and the lower incidence of pruritus and severe phototoxic skin reactions.

PUVA alone can produce a definite remission in many cases of psoriasis, but a considerable number of patients require additional therapies for clearing. Such combination therapy (see below) can help to clear the majority of patients.

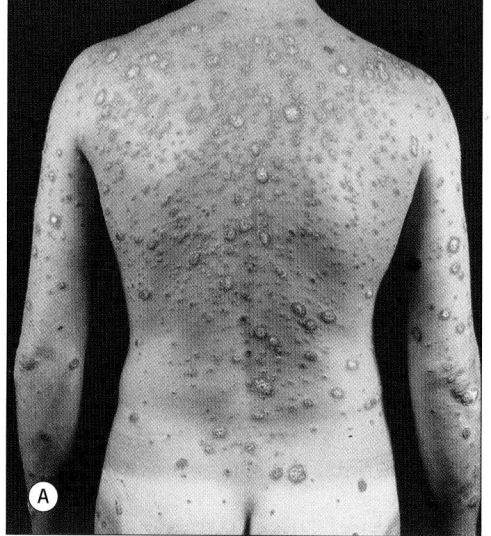

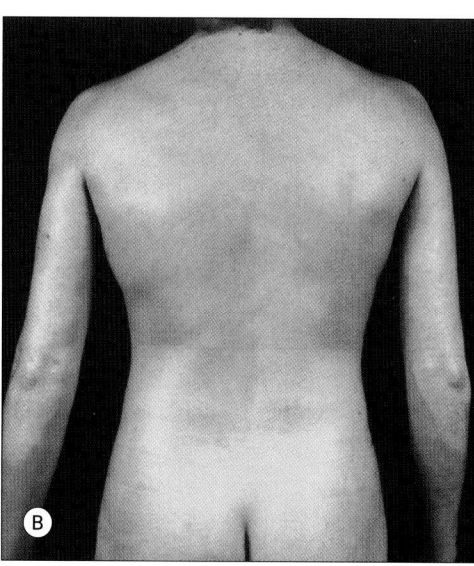

Fig. 134.13 PUVA treatment for psoriasis (5-MOP; four times weekly). A Before treatment. **B** After 6 weeks of treatment.

Combination Treatments

Topical combination

As with UVB phototherapy, PUVA can be combined with other treatment modalities to improve efficacy and to reduce potential side effects[2]. Topical adjuvant therapies include corticosteroids, anthralin and tar, and, more recently, calcipotriol and tazarotene (see Chs 125, 126 & 129). However, some patients are reluctant to 'retry' topical agents that previously proved unsuccessful when used alone.

Methotrexate (see Ch. 131)

The combination of PUVA and methotrexate (MTX) during the clearing phase reduces the duration of treatment, number of exposures, and cumulative UVA dose, and is also effective in clearing patients unresponsive to PUVA or UVB alone[58]. If used for long-term treatment, this combination could be potentially hazardous because PUVA and MTX may act synergistically in the development of skin cancers[22]. However, to date, no increased risk of non-melanoma skin cancer has been reported for this combination. In contrast, cyclosporine plus PUVA has been clearly shown to dramatically enhance skin carcinogenesis. Thus, this combination should be categorically discouraged[60,61].

Retinoids

The combination of PUVA with systemic retinoids (RePUVA) is one of the most potent therapeutic regimens for psoriasis. The therapeutic efficacy of PUVA therapy is significantly enhanced upon daily combination with oral retinoids (etretinate, acitretin, isotretinoin) (0.75–1 mg/kg for etretinate and isotretinoin, 0.5–0.75 mg/kg for acitretin) administered for 5–10 days before PUVA is started, with the combination continued throughout the clearing phase[51]. RePUVA reportedly can reduce the number of exposures by one-third and the total cumulative UVA dose by more than one-half. RePUVA can also clear 'poor PUVA responders'[62].

The underlying mechanism of the synergistic action of retinoids plus PUVA may be a reduction in the inflammatory infiltrate and an accelerated desquamation of the psoriatic plaques, thereby optimizing the optical properties of the skin. In theory, retinoids may also reduce the long-term carcinogenic risk of PUVA by reducing the number of exposures and providing chemoprevention against skin cancers. Some evidence for this was presented in a recent study where patients with psoriasis treated with PUVA in combination with systemic retinoids showed a reduced risk of squamous cell carcinoma but not a significantly altered incidence of basal cell carcinoma[63].

Short-term side effects of retinoids are completely reversible upon discontinuation, and long-term toxicity is not relevant because of the limited duration of their use (until clear). The potential teratogenicity of retinoids represents a serious concern. For women of childbearing age, the use of isotretinoin is an option, because contraception is only necessary for 1–2 months after discontinuation of therapy, as opposed to etretinate and acitretin, which require at least 2 years of contraception[2].

PUVA for Cutaneous T-Cell Lymphoma (Mycosis Fungoides)

Based on the empirical beneficial effect of natural sunlight on early-stage MF, Gilchrest et al.[64] first reported the successful use of PUVA for CTCL. Patients with unsatisfactory responses to other therapies and histologically confirmed plaque- or tumor-stage MF or the erythrodermic form of CTCL were subjected to PUVA. Complete clearing was observed, except in those areas that were shielded from UVA exposures, thus excluding the possibility of spontaneous remission. This also indicated that the therapeutic effect of PUVA was local rather than systemic.

Numerous studies followed which addressed the rates of initial response and average duration of remission in relation to the stage of CTCL, the efficacy of PUVA compared with other established treatment options, the efficacy of combination treatments, the mechanisms responsible for the therapeutic effects, and the risk of short- and long-term side effects[2].

Treatment schedules and dosimetry in the photochemotherapy of CTCL are essentially the same as for psoriasis, consisting of three phases – clearing, maintenance and follow-up. Some authors suggest that remission should be confirmed by histologic examination of previously involved areas. In some institutions, maintenance therapy includes two exposures per week for one month and one exposure per week for another month. If still in remission, therapy is discontinued and the patient is monitored monthly and then bimonthly. If a relapse occurs, the patient is again treated with three or four PUVA exposures per week until complete clearing. However, some investigators advocate permanent maintenance treatment consisting of treatments once monthly or every other month, as it appears that PUVA treatment is not curative. Since the course of CTCL varies considerably from patient to patient, the final answer remains to be determined. Clinical experience indicates that patients benefit most from individualized schedules.

Several studies involving large patient cohorts have provided information on the initial response rates of PUVA treatment in relation to disease stage. However, the use of different treatment protocols, psoralen preparations and light sources may have contributed to some heterogeneity in results.

The percentage of patients who experienced a complete remission during their first course of PUVA treatment was reported to be 75–100% for stage IA, 47–100% for stage IB, 67–83% for stage IIA, 40–100% for stage IIB, and 33–100% for stage III. Only a few patients with stage IV disease have been treated with PUVA monotherapy, because, in this stage, PUVA is generally considered to be only a palliative or adjunctive therapy. An analysis of the outcome of five of these studies (comprising a total of 244 patients) provided the following average complete initial response rates: stage IA, 90%; stage IB, 76%; stage IIA, 78%; stage IIB, 59%; and stage III, 61%.

The long-term outcome is strictly dependent on the relapse rates and the mean disease-free intervals. In the first follow-up study of 44 PUVA-treated patients, 56% (5/9) with stage IA disease and 39% (10/26) with stage IB disease remained in remission during a mean follow-up period of 44 months[65]. Patients who experienced relapses had mean disease-free intervals of 20 months for stage IA and 17 months for stage IB. All patients (7/7) with stage IIB disease had multiple recurrences, and of the two patients with stage III disease (both of whom were initially brought into remission), one relapsed during maintenance therapy and one was lost to follow-up. In a more recent study of 82 patients with a median follow-up period of 43 months, 53% in stage IA, 37% in stage IB, 50% in stage IIA, and the only one in stage IVA did not develop recurrences after complete clearing. One stage IIB patient and two of six stage III patients initially cleared, but they all eventually relapsed[66].

Relapses usually respond to PUVA in the same manner as the initial response. Clinical remissions appear to be directly related to phototoxic destruction of the malignant infiltrate. Thus, complete clearing may be induced when the cells are confined to the epidermis and the superficial dermis and do not exceed the depth of UVA penetration into the skin. Patients with tumor-stage CTCL exhibit a high rate of early recurrences, which require permanent maintenance treatment; often only the combination of PUVA with local radiotherapy and/or systemic chemo-immunotherapy can result in complete tumor resolution[65].

In summary, the data thus far indicate that PUVA is an excellent treatment option for early stage (IA–IIA) CTCL (Fig. 134.14). High rates of complete clearing can be achieved and a substantial percentage of patients remain free of disease for many years. In advanced stages (IIB–IVB), PUVA is not sufficient as monotherapy, but as adjunctive treatment it can reduce the tumor burden in the skin and can improve the quality of life for patients. Presently, no therapeutic regimen is known to arrest eventual progression of advanced stages of CTCL to tumor formation, dissemination and fatal outcome. Prolonged remissions have been observed with combinations of PUVA with either conventional retinoids, or bexarotene[67–69] or interferon-α_{2a}[70]. Possible long-term side effects related to frequent PUVA treatments are probably meaningless for patients with CTCL compared with patients with benign conditions.

While PUVA therapy is very effective in inducing remission as long as the lymphoma is confined to the skin, the impact of this therapy on the natural course of CTCL and on patient survival is not yet determined. However, data from Sweden have shown a significant drop in the death rates of CTCL patients since the introduction of PUVA[71].

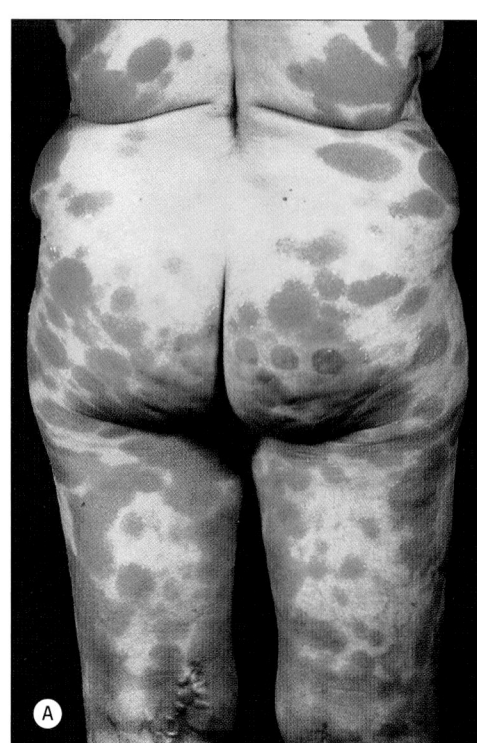
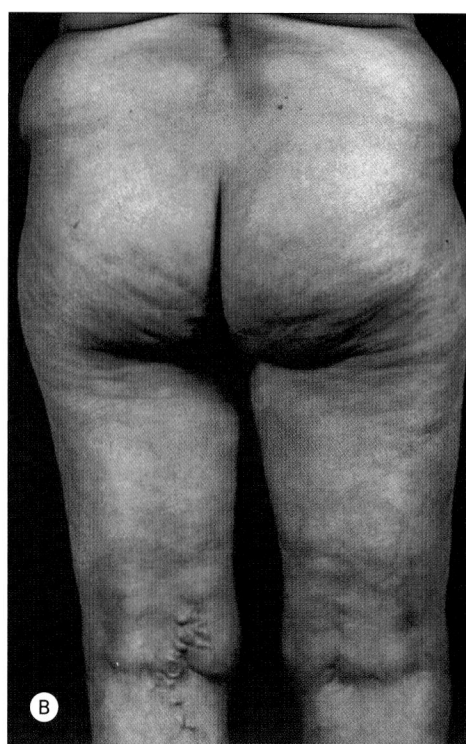

Fig. 134.14 PUVA treatment for cutaneous T-cell lymphoma (mycosis fungoides) (8-MOP; four times weekly). A Before treatment. **B** After 12 weeks of treatment.

PUVA for Vitiligo

As mentioned above, vitiligo was the first disease treated with an ancient form of psoralen photochemotherapy in India and Egypt. PUVA in its modern form stimulates melanogenesis, melanocyte proliferation and migration, and reconstitutes the normal skin color in more than 50% of vitiligo patients.

Treatment Protocols and Results

Oral 8-MOP or TMP are the photosensitizers most frequently used, followed by exposure to sunlight or artificial UVA radiation. A large, controlled clinical trial by the Harvard group provided detailed information regarding different treatment schedules. Also, 5-MOP was in a large trial in India and is used in Europe, where available, with good success (for references, see ref. 1). To induce repigmentation, patients need constant long-term therapy. It is crucial that the patient understands that PUVA, like other vitiligo therapies, may require months or even years to achieve a satisfactory result. All too optimistic prognoses regarding therapeutic efficacy and length of time to produce adequate repigmentation should be avoided. The patients must also be aware that the treatments stimulate the pigmentation of normal skin, which will intensify the contrast between normal and vitiliginous skin.

Because of weaker phototoxicity, oral TMP is preferred to 8-MOP for treatment with sunlight as the radiation source. Treatments should be given at least twice a week, but not more than three times, with at least one day between treatments. If there is no response after 4–5 months or approximately 30–40 treatments, PUVA should be terminated. Responsiveness is defined as development of multiple perifollicular macules of repigmentation, or, in the case of small (<2 cm) lesions, contraction in size. If treatment is discontinued, reversal of acquired repigmentation may occur unless the lesion has completely repigmented. Completely repigmented areas can be stable for a decade or more without relapse[72].

Another photochemotherapeutic regimen for vitiligo consists of khellin (a furanochromone) as the photosensitizer and UVA irradiation (KUVA). Khellin is not phototoxic and exhibits substantially lower mutagenic activity than psoralens. Its efficacy and failure rate in vitiligo are comparable with PUVA[73]. The major advantage of khellin is that, given its lack of phototoxicity, it can be considered safe for home treatment or treatment with natural sunlight. The treatment schedule is the same as for PUVA; khellin is administered orally at a dose of 100 mg 2 hours before treatment or applied topically as a 5% cream. Khellin is not available in the US. With oral khellin, approximately 30% of vitiligo patients develop reversible increases in liver transaminases that

remain to be explained[73]. Under special circumstances, KUVA may be considered an alternative to conventional photochemotherapy. However, the efficacy of topical KUVA in comparison with oral PUVA or other therapeutic modalities has not been established.

Photochemotherapy with topical 8-MOP can be used in patients with small lesions (less than 5% total body surface area) or in children in whom one may hesitate to use systemic PUVA. The therapy must be done in an office setting, since home treatment involves a high risk of severe phototoxic side effects. Topical 8-MOP preparations (0.01 or 0.1% 8-MOP in a cream or ointment base) are applied evenly on the treatment area 30 minutes prior to irradiation. Exposure times (beginning at ≤0.25 J/cm²) are increased weekly in increments of 0.25 J/cm² unless marked erythema occurs. Once- to twice-weekly treatments are recommended. TMP and 5-MOP can also be used for topical PUVA but are more phototoxic than 8-MOP. For topical application, the vehicle plays a major role in delivery and resulting cutaneous psoralen levels[14]. Solutions should be avoided as they can 'run', producing hyperpigmented streaks. Application of sunscreen to the surrounding uninvolved skin prior to application of the topical psoralen can reduce hyperpigmented rims.

Patient selection appears to be critically important in vitiligo treatment. For oral PUVA, the patients should be ages 10–12 years or older, and for all forms, they must be available for 12–24 months of continuous therapy. Lips, distal dorsal hands, fingers and toes, palms, soles and nipples are very refractory to treatment, as are large areas with only white hairs. Patients need to be made aware of this fact.

Stable disease, e.g. segmental vitiligo present for at least a year, is usually easier to treat. On average, a complete treatment course consists of at least 150 exposures. However, because of the different response rates in different body areas, total repigmentation is only rarely achieved, and approximately 30% of patients do not respond at all, despite months of therapy.

The mechanisms by which PUVA induces repigmentation in vitiligo remain mostly speculative. Bearing in mind the immunomodulating effect of UV radiation, one might postulate a hypothetical suppressor cell population generated by PUVA that suppresses the stimulus for melanocyte destruction.

PUVA for Atopic Dermatitis (see Ch. 13)

Many patients with moderate, severe and even erythrodermic forms of atopic eczema can benefit from PUVA therapy[58]. The treatment guidelines are essentially the same as for psoriasis. However, as compared to psoriasis, atopic dermatitis is more difficult to treat; quite often, a higher number of treatments is required. Although atopic eczema may be cleared by PUVA, recurrence rates are high and rapid, requiring frequent maintenance exposures. Due to the average patient's young age, long-term maintenance therapy should be avoided. A combination of PUVA with topical corticosteroids appears to be superior to PUVA alone in maintaining remissions. The mechanism of action of photochemotherapy in atopic dermatitis is unclear; current concepts support an alteration of lymphocyte function in the dermal infiltrate.

PUVA for Lichen Planus (see Ch. 12)

The beneficial effect of PUVA in lichen planus was first reported shortly after its introduction. In generalized lichen planus, PUVA can provide an effective alternative to systemic corticosteroids. Later studies pointed to an overall response rate between 50% and 90%, suggesting that lichen planus was less responsive to PUVA than psoriasis. In addition, more treatment sessions and higher cumulative UVA doses were generally necessary for complete remission and not all patients responded satisfactorily. Marked postinflammatory hyperpigmentation may impair the final cosmetic result. An exacerbation during PUVA treatment has been reported in a few patients[22,74].

Bath PUVA also works in lichen planus and in one study appeared to be even better than oral PUVA. However, early relapses occurred with both regimens[74]. A combined RePUVA regimen (as is used for psoriasis) may accelerate clearing in disseminated and particularly keratotic forms of lichen planus. Thus, overall, PUVA is an effective therapeutic option for extensive lichen planus; however, this disease is usually more resistant than psoriasis.

PUVA for Chronic Graft-versus-Host Disease

An indication of increasing importance may be acute and chronic cutaneous GVHD. Due to clinical and histologic similarities between idiopathic lichen planus and lichenoid GVHD, PUVA treatment was evaluated for the latter[75]. Beneficial effects were observed in patients who had not responded to conventional immunosuppressive therapy alone. PUVA can also improve acute GVHD[76]. Results of the PUVA therapy of scleroderma-like variants of cutaneous GVHD are controversial. In our experience, the more localized and circumscribed morpheaform lesions appear to respond to PUVA fairly rapidly, concomitantly with softening of the associated sclerosis. However, the more advanced and widespread sclerodermoid form hardly responds to PUVA.

As opposed to other conditions, PUVA may exert not only local, but also systemic, effects, since improvement of mucosal erosions was observed during treatment of chronic lichenoid GVHD with PUVA, but this could also be mere coincidence. Apparently, there is no improvement of GVHD of other organs, e.g. liver and gut. Of note, deterioration of liver GVHD has not been reported thus far. This is important, since psoralens are metabolized by the liver.

The therapeutic regimen used for the treatment of chronic GVHD is basically the same as for psoriasis. UVA doses should not be increased too aggressively, in order to avoid erythema and possible (re)activation of GVHD. The UVA dosage is increased by no more than 0.5 J/cm^2 every second to fourth exposure, and patients are treated three to four times weekly. After clearing of skin lesions, exposures are reduced according to the maintenance schedule outlined for psoriasis.

There may be a slight overall increased risk of cutaneous malignancies in all hematopoietic stem cell recipients, but much less than in solid organ transplant patients who receive long-term immunosuppression. Serial cutaneous examinations are recommended, especially in those who have received PUVA and are fair complexioned.

PUVA for Urticaria Pigmentosa (see Ch. 19)

PUVA causes a temporary involution of cutaneous mastocytosis[77,78]. The treatment results in loss of Darier's sign, relief of itching, and flattening and sometimes even complete disappearance of cutaneous papules and macules. Surprisingly, even systemic symptoms such as histamine-induced migraines and flushing fade gradually as treatment is continued[77]. In most patients, the manifestations of the disease

recurred several months after discontinuation of PUVA. The recurrences respond as well as the original lesions and complete clearing of signs and symptoms can again be achieved. In children, PUVA is also often helpful, and appears to be justified in widespread, disabling mastocytosis. To avoid sudden mediator release from mast cells, a PUVA regimen of gradually increasing doses, especially during the initial phase, seems advisable, although the therapy should otherwise be undertaken according to the usual guidelines.

PUVA for Miscellaneous Dermatoses

Both acute and chronic *pityriasis lichenoides*[19] respond to photochemotherapy and favorable results have been reported for *lymphomatoid papulosis*[19,79]. Nevertheless, the experience with these conditions is limited to a few anecdotal cases. In *pityriasis rubra pilaris*, the results are quite inconsistent. Some patients seem to respond well[19], while others may flare and some require combination treatment with retinoids or methotrexate. Generalized *granuloma annulare* has been reported to clear completely, but long-term maintenance treatment was required to maintain remissions[80]. Regrowth of hair was noted in *alopecia areata* with either topical or systemic PUVA in which exposures were localized to the alopecia areas. There was a great variation in the number of treatments required for regrowth, and circumscribed lesions responded better than did total alopecia. However, follow-up studies of larger patient groups concluded that PUVA is generally not effective in alopecia areata[81,82], which is in accordance with our own experience. *Localized scleroderma* and *pansclerotic morphea* have been successfully treated with bath PUVA and oral PUVA[83,84].

PUVA for Photodermatoses

Tolerance to sunlight can be induced in several photodermatoses with PUVA. In *polymorphous light eruption* (PMLE), the most common photodermatosis, PUVA is a very effective preventive treatment (via hardening)[85]. In approximately 70% of patients with this condition, a 3- to 4-week course of PUVA suffices to suppress the disease upon subsequent exposure to sunlight. The initial exposure and dose increments should be performed according to the guidelines outlined for psoriasis. PUVA induces pigmentation rapidly and intensively at relatively low (suberythemogenic) UVA doses that usually remain well below the threshold doses for eliciting the PMLE. About 10% of the patients develop typical lesions during the initial phase of PUVA. Interruption of treatment or reduction in the UVA dose is rarely required in such cases. Usually, brief symptomatic treatment with topical corticosteroids suffices.

PUVA hardening is indicated in selected patients with severe PMLE whose disease cannot be prevented with the use of sunscreens or UVB phototherapy. Treatment is given three times weekly over a period of 4 weeks in the early spring. Both 8-MOP and 5-MOP can be used as photosensitizers; however, 5-MOP is preferable because of better tolerability and higher pigment potential. The PUVA therapy protects only temporarily, and regularly repeated sun exposures are subsequently required to maintain protection. However, a considerable number of patients remain protected for 2 to 3 months, even after pigmentation has faded.

The mechanisms by which phototherapy induces tolerance to sunlight are not clear. Hyperpigmentation and thickening of the stratum corneum may be important factors for this protective effect. However, other mechanisms may also be involved, since PMLE does occur in darkly pigmented individuals and even patients with skin type I who do not tan profit from hardening. Modulation of cutaneous immune functions is a possible explanation.

The therapeutic value of preventive photochemotherapy for PMLE has to be balanced against its potential long-term side effects. Given the fact that very few treatments and low cumulative UVA doses (ranging from 15 to 40 J/cm^2 per treatment course, depending on skin type and photosensitizer) are required for photoprotection and that PMLE can severely impair patients in their outdoor activities, PUVA treatment of PLE is justified when other preventive measures (e.g. antimalarials) fail[85].

There is also some experience with PUVA prophylaxis of other photodermatoses. In *solar urticaria*, PUVA therapy appears to the most effective preventive treatment available and it is certainly better than antihistamines. Tolerance to sunlight can be increased tenfold or more after a single treatment course[86–88]. The suppressive effect may last throughout the summer, depending on regularly repeated sunlight exposures. Problems may occur during the first several PUVA exposures, since in some patients the urticaria threshold dose appears to be lower than their MPD. In these cases, stepwise UVA irradiation of single quadrants of the body a few hours before each PUVA treatment has proved useful. PUVA is then administered during the refractory period.

Successful photochemotherapy has also been reported in occasional patients with *chronic actinic dermatitis*[86–88] and *hydroa vacciniforme*[89]. Limited experience in patients with *erythropoietic protoporphyria* indicates that, with a very cautious approach and in combination with β-carotene, PUVA may increase light tolerance considerably[90].

Side Effects and Long-Term Hazards of PUVA

As discussed above, oral 8-MOP has a high incidence of nausea (30% of patients) and vomiting (10% of patients), and this may occasionally require discontinuation of the treatment. These side effects are more common with liquid than with crystalline preparations, probably because of higher psoralen serum levels. With 5-MOP, nausea is nearly absent, even with doses up to 1.8 mg/kg, and this is the major reason for increased usage of this compound.

The short-term side effects of the combined action of psoralens plus UVA radiation consist of redness, swelling, and occasionally blister formation as can be seen with excessive sunburns. Generalized pruritus or tingling sensations may herald phototoxic side effects. When large areas of skin are affected, systemic symptoms of excess phototoxicity such as fever and general malaise may occur. Non-steroidal anti-inflammatory drugs and topical and systemic corticosteroids may be required to alleviate the symptoms, but have to be given early. Such overdosage phenomena are more common after topical psoralen application, because of high epidermal psoralen concentrations. Cumulation of phototoxic effects after several consecutive UVA exposures is also more common with topical PUVA.

Some patients experience persistent pruritus during PUVA treatment, particularly after slight UVA overdosage, and, in rare cases, a stinging pain may develop in circumscribed areas. PUVA-induced skin pain unrelated to actual phototoxic burns occurs rarely, but it may necessitate discontinuation of treatment. The mechanism is unknown and the symptoms are unresponsive to antihistamines. Usually, these complaints subside slowly upon continuation of treatment.

Ophthalmologic effects

Eye protection is mandatory during UVA exposure, and UVA-opaque glasses are required for ambient exposure until the evening of the treatment day. UVA penetrates into the ocular lens and potentially could induce cataracts by forming psoralen-protein photoproducts. The higher permeability of the ocular lens at a younger age led to the relative contraindication of oral PUVA in children younger than 12 years of age. Despite the experimental data indicating a risk of premature cataract formation, clinical evaluation has shown no increase in lens opacities even in patients who neglected careful eye protection[91,91a]. Obviously, there is no risk with topical or bath PUVA.

Laboratory data

Because psoralens can cause liver damage in laboratory animals when given in excessive doses, concern was expressed in the past regarding possible hepatotoxic effects in humans. Several large-scale studies demonstrated no significant abnormal laboratory findings in patients receiving PUVA over prolonged periods of time[50,52,92]. In particular, serial laboratory examinations performed over a period of several years have not revealed any substantial evidence for an impairment of hepatic function. Liver biopsies after 1 year of therapy did not show signs of hepatotoxicity. Anecdotal case reports of hepatitis during PUVA treatment were most likely unrelated to therapy. Several large-scale studies have negated a possible relation between PUVA therapy and the occurrence of antinuclear antibodies[93].

Potential long-term risks of PUVA

Repeated phototoxic injury to the skin can be expected to result in cumulative actinic damage regardless of whether it is induced by sunlight, artificial UV radiation or PUVA. Although the precise action spectrum of actinic damage has not been determined, epidermal changes are attributed to UVB and dermal changes more to UVA, because the latter penetrates more deeply into the skin. Thus, chronic exposure to PUVA may produce changes in the skin that generally resemble those known as dermatoheliosis and may add to the injury induced by sunlight. High cumulative doses of whole-body UVB or PUVA result in pigmentary changes, xerosis, loss of elasticity, wrinkle formation and actinic keratoses. Additionally, PUVA may induce profuse formation of dark lentigines, termed PUVA lentiginosis[52]. These result from repeated and prolonged treatment and are commonly associated with high cumulative doses of UVA and a high number of treatments. So far, no increased risk of cutaneous melanoma associated with these lentigines has been recorded, but the cosmetic effect may be quite disturbing.

The major concern with prolonged and repeated phototherapeutic regimens is photocarcinogenesis. Therefore, from the onset, PUVA-treated patients were carefully monitored for the development of precursors and malignant skin tumors. Almost all data were obtained from psoriatics, since they represent the largest group of patients receiving PUVA.

The risk is certainly related to DNA damage, but PUVA-induced immunosuppression may play a role as well. In PUVA patients, the risk of squamous cell carcinoma, but not of basal cell carcinoma, is significantly increased in comparison with matched controls, and the magnitude of the increase appears to be dose-dependent[22,94]. However, there is uncertainty regarding PUVA being the sole factor; many of the affected patients had previous exposure to excessive sunlight and to treatments with carcinogenic potential, including arsenic, UVB and antimetabolite therapy[95]. Particularly, high levels of UVB exposure appear to increase the risk of non-melanoma skin cancer in PUVA-treated patients[96].

According to a single study, the genitalia of male patients previously treated with tar and UVB appeared to be particularly susceptible to the carcinogenic stimuli of PUVA[97], but the risk seemed not to be increased if only PUVA was used[98]. In a retrospective study from France comprised of 5400 patients treated between 1978 and 1998, no case of genital skin cancer was found, despite the fact that the genital area had not been protected during UVA exposure, and this raises the question whether genital shielding is absolutely necessary[99]. Interestingly, no increased risk of skin carcinoma has so far been reported for patients treated with PUVA for vitiligo.

The carcinogenicity of 5-MOP PUVA is unknown, but in *in vitro* photomutagenicity and photocarcinogenicity studies in mice, the activity of 5-MOP was similar to that of 8-MOP.

Only a few anecdotal cases of cutaneous melanoma have been described in long-term PUVA-treated psoriatics, and, with one exception, no increased risk of melanoma has been observed in any large-scale study reported thus far. However, Stern et al.[100] recently reported on the cohort of 1380 patients enrolled in the PUVA Follow-up Study (16-center study), and, since 1975, 23 patients had developed 26 invasive or *in situ* cutaneous melanomas. Beginning 15 years after the initial exposure to PUVA, an increased risk of melanoma was observed in their cohort of PUVA-treated patients.

The authors concluded that perhaps PUVA has been treated unfairly. Its long-term risks have been subject to much greater scrutiny than the risks of other therapies utilized for severe psoriasis, such as methotrexate and particularly immunosuppressive therapies such as cyclosporine (CSA). An increased risk of cutaneous squamous cell carcinoma has been observed in patients with solid organ transplants who have received long-term CSA and in patients who have received CSA subsequent to PUVA therapy[101]. UVA-sparing, aggressive regimens without prolonged maintenance therapy may be safer than continuous non-aggressive regimens[102] (see Table 134.4).

In a recent study in 944 Swedish and Finnish patients[103], bath PUVA with TMP appeared to have no relevant risk of carcinogenesis. In addition, no association between cutaneous carcinoma and 8-MOP bath PUVA was found in 158 Finnish psoriatic patients[104]. Perhaps related to lower cumulative UVA doses, these data on the long-term safety of bath PUVA are encouraging, but no premature conclusions should be drawn. The risk/benefit ratio still seems very favorable for PUVA[105], and, so far, no single therapy, except perhaps narrowband UVB, has been accepted as equally safe and efficient.

UVB and PUVA in HIV-Infected Patients

With oral PUVA, treatment of psoriasis did not induce progression of HIV disease nor was there an increase in side effects[106,107]. It was concluded from these studies that PUVA may be safe for HIV-infected patients with psoriasis. Theoretical modeling of UVB- and PUVA-induced HIV promoter activation in human skin indicated that UVB is more likely than PUVA to activate viral transcription *in vivo*[108]. Data from long-term observations are currently awaited. Thus, it is presently impossible to advocate the use of PUVA in (HIV-) immunosuppressed individuals in general, but major hazards are unlikely. The available data and theoretical considerations indicate that UVB is more likely to be a hazard than PUVA in an HIV-infected population[108,109].

EXTRACORPOREAL PHOTOCHEMOTHERAPY (PHOTOPHERESIS)

Extracorporeal photochemotherapy (photopheresis, ECP) was introduced in the early 1980s for the palliative treatment of erythrodermic CTCL[110]. Its efficacy was confirmed later by several uncontrolled clinical trials and approved as a device in 1988 by the FDA for the treatment of this disease. In 1994, at the International Consensus Conference on Staging and Treatment Recommendations for CTCL, ECP was recommended as the first-line of treatment for patients with erythrodermic CTCL[111]. However, not all authorities agree (see Ch. 120).

Attempts to better characterize those CTCL patients who are more likely to respond to ECP revealed the following:

- There seems to be a significant linear association between response and CD4:CD8 ratio. Patients with a ratio <10 are more likely to respond than are patients with a ratio >10.
- There is a marginally significant linear association between response and LDH level. Patients whose LDH is not elevated at the start of treatment tend to have a better response to ECP compared to patients with an elevated LDH[112].

Treatment Protocols

The ECP procedure involves the oral administration of 8-MOP followed by passage of blood fractions from one arm vein through a photopheresis machine and then back. A discontinuous flow cell separator harvests mononuclear cells (PBMC) within a buffy coat collection. The red cell fraction is returned to the patient without further treatment. 8-MOP can also be administered directly into the collection of the PBMC, thereby avoiding 8-MOP-induced nausea. The collection of PBMC is then exposed to $2\,J/cm^2$ of UVA and reinfused into the patient. This treatment is typically repeated on two successive days with 2- to 4-week intervals.

Mechanism of Action

Despite the fact that ECP has been in use for almost 20 years, the mode of action still remains enigmatic. It was postulated that the response of CTCL to ECP is due to the induction of an immune response against the malignant cells. Recent experimental results suggest that infusion of autologous haptenated cells, in which apoptosis was induced by 8-MOP/UVA, induces immunologic tolerance. The nature of this tolerance is due primarily to regulatory T cells, because transfer in an animal model conferred similar protection. The demonstration of the induction of regulatory T cells may explain why, in humans, ECP exerts a beneficial effect in a wide variety of diseases which would be amenable to such activity. The generation of antigen-specific regulatory T cells may explain why generalized immunosuppression has not been noted with ECP[113].

Side Effects

Side effects of ECP are uncommon and consist of transient nausea after oral ingestion of 8-MOP and episodes of hypotension and vasovagal reflex due to volume shifts during treatments; the latter usually do not interfere with the treatment.

Other Indications

A number of studies have been performed in order to evaluate the efficacy of ECP in inflammatory diseases other than CTCL where autoreactive T cells play a key role. Uncontrolled clinical trials have revealed variable success in selected entities such as atopic dermatitis, systemic sclerosis, pemphigus vulgaris, and systemic lupus erythematosus.

ECP may also play a role in the treatment of acute and chronic GVHD after allogeneic bone marrow transplantation[114,115].

Lastly, ECP has been used to treat acute allograft rejection among cardiac, lung and renal transplant recipients[116,117].

REFERENCES

1. Weichenthal M, Schwarz T. Phototherapy. How does UV work? Photodermatol Photoimmunol Photomed. 2005;21:260–6.
2. Hönigsmann H. Phototherapy for psoriasis. Clin Exp Dermatol. 2001;6:343–50.
3. Parrish JA, Jaenicke KF. Action spectrum for phototherapy of psoriasis. J Invest Dermatol. 1981;76:359–62.
4. Ibbotson SH, Bilsland D, Cox NH, et al. An update and guidance on narrowband ultraviolet B phototherapy: a British Photodermatology Group Workshop Report. Br J Dermatol. 2004;151:283–97.
5. Tanew A, Radakovic-Fijan S, Schemper M, Hönigsmann H. Narrow UV-B phototherapy vs photochemotherapy in the treatment of chronic plaque-type psoriasis: a paired comparison study. Arch Dermatol. 1999;135:519–24.
6. Meola T Jr, Soter NA, Lim HW. Are topical corticosteroids useful adjunctive therapy for the treatment of psoriasis with ultraviolet radiation? A review of the literature. Arch Dermatol. 1991;127:1708–13.
7. Iest J, Boer J. Combined treatment of psoriasis with acitretin and UVB phototherapy compared with acitretin alone and UVB alone. Br J Dermatol. 1989;120:665–70.
8. Green C, Lakshmipathi T, Johnson BE, Ferguson J. A comparison of the efficacy and relapse rates of narrowband UVB (TL-01) monotherapy vs. etretinate (re-TL-01) vs. etretinate-PUVA (re-PUVA) in the treatment of psoriasis patients. Br J Dermatol. 1992;127:5–9.
9. Resnik KS, Vonderheid EC. Home UV phototherapy of early mycosis fungoides: long-term follow-up observations in thirty-one patients. J Am Acad Dermatol. 1993;29:73–7.
10. Ramsay DL, Lish KM, Yalowitz CB, Soter NA. Ultraviolet-B phototherapy for early-stage cutaneous T-cell lymphoma. Arch Dermatol. 1992;128:931–3.
11. Boztepe G, Sahin S, Ayhan M, et al. Narrowband ultraviolet B phototherapy to clear and maintain clearance in patients with mycosis fungoides. J Am Acad Dermatol. 2005;53:242–6.
12. Volc-Platzer B, Hönigsmann H. Photoimmunology of PUVA and UVB therapy. In: Krutmann J, Elmets CA (eds). Photoimmunology. Oxford: Blackwell Science, 1995:265–73.
13. Ozawa M, Ferenczi K, Kikuchi T, et al. 312-nanometer ultraviolet B light (narrow-band UVB) induces apoptosis of T cells within psoriatic lesions. J Exp Med. 1999;189:711–18.
14. Westerhof W, Nieuweboer-Krobotova L. Treatment of vitiligo with UV-B radiation vs topical psoralen plus UV-A. Arch Dermatol. 1997;133:1525–8.
14a. Yones SS, Palmer RA, Garibaldinos TM, Hawk JLM. Randomized double-blind trial of treatment of vitiligo. Arch Dermatol. 2007;143:578–84.
15. Jekler J, Larkö O. Phototherapy for atopic dermatitis with ultraviolet A (UVA), low-dose UVB and combined UVA and UVB: two paired comparison studies. Photodermatol Photoimmunol Photomed. 1991;8:151–6.
16. George SA, Bilsland DJ, Johnson BE, Ferguson J. Narrow-band (TL-01) UVB air-conditioned phototherapy for chronic severe adult atopic dermatitis. Br J Dermatol. 1993;128:49–56.
17. Reynolds NJ, Franklin V, Gray JC, et al. Narrow-band ultraviolet B and broad-band ultraviolet A phototherapy in adult atopic eczema: a randomised controlled trial. Lancet. 2001;357:2012–16.
18. Torinuki W, Mauduit G, Guyotat D, et al. Effect of UVB radiation on the skin after allogeneic bone-marrow transplantation in man. Arch Dermatol Res. 1987;279:424–6.
19. Honig B, Morison WL, Karp D. Photochemotherapy beyond psoriasis. J Am Acad Dermatol. 1994;31:775–90.
20. Pirkhammer D, Seeber A, Hönigsmann H, Tanew A. Narrow-band ultraviolet B (TL-01) phototherapy is an effective and safe treatment option for patients with severe seborrhoeic dermatitis. Br J Dermatol. 2000;143:964–8.
21. Gilchrest BA. Ultraviolet phototherapy of uremic pruritus. Int J Dermatol. 1979;18:741–8.
22. Stern RS, Laird N. The carcinogenic risk of treatments for severe psoriasis. Cancer. 1994;73:2759–64.

23. Man I, Crombie IK, Dawe RS, Ibbotson SH, Ferguson J. The photocarcinogenic risk of narrowband UVB (TL-01) phototherapy: early follow-up data. Br J Dermatol. 2005;152:755–7.
24. Tzung TY, Rünger TM. Assessment of DNA damage induced by broadband and narrowband UVB in cultured lymphoblasts and keratinocytes using the comet assay. Photochem Photobiol. 1998;67:647–50.
25. Young AR. Carcinogenicity of UVB phototherapy assessed. Lancet. 1995;345:1431–2.
26. Bónis B, Kemeny L, Dobozy A, et al. 308-nm UVB excimer laser for psoriasis. Lancet. 1997;350:1522.
27. Asawanonda P, Anderson RR, Chang Y, Taylor CR. 308 nm excimer laser for the treatment of psoriasis: a dose-response study. Arch Dermatol. 2000;136:619–24.
28. Feldman SR, Mellen BG, Housman TS, et al. Efficacy of the 308 nm excimer laser for treatment of psoriasis: results of a multicenter study. J Am Acad Dermatol. 2002;46:900–6.
29. Köllner K, Wimmershoff MB, Hintz C, Landthaler M, Hohenleutner U. Comparison of the 308-nm excimer laser and a 308-nm excimer lamp with 311-nm narrowband ultraviolet B in the treatment of psoriasis. Br J Dermatol. 2005;152:750–4.
30. Spencer JM, Nossa R, Ajmeri J. Treatment of vitiligo with the 308-nm excimer laser: a pilot study. J Am Acad Dermatol. 2002;46:727–31.
31. Aubin F, Vigan M, Puzenat E, et al. Evaluation of a novel 308-nm monochromatic excimer light delivery system in dermatology: a pilot study in different chronic localized dermatoses. Br J Dermatol. 2005;152:99–103.
32. Krutmann J, Diepgen TL, Luger TA, et al. High-dose UVA1 therapy for atopic dermatitis: results of a multicenter trial. J Am Acad Dermatol. 1998; 38:589–93.
33. Abeck D, Schmidt T, Fesq H, et al. Long-term efficacy of medium-dose UVA1 phototherapy in atopic dermatitis. J Am Acad Dermatol. 2000;42:254–7.
34. Tzaneva S, Seeber A, Schwaiger M, et al. High-dose versus medium-dose UVA1 phototherapy for patients with severe, generalized atopic dermatitis. J Am Acad Dermatol. 2001;45:503–7.
35. Dawe RS. Ultraviolet A1 phototherapy. Br J Dermatol. 2003;148:626–37.
36. Kerscher M, Volkenandt M, Gruss C, et al. Low-dose UVA phototherapy for treatment of localized scleroderma. J Am Acad Dermatol. 1998;38:21–6.
37. Stege H, Berneburg M, Humke S, et al. High-dose UVA1 radiation therapy for localized scleroderma. J Am Acad Dermatol. 1997;36:938–44.
38. Ständer H, Schiller M, Schwarz T. UVA1-therapy for treatment of sclerodermic graft-versus-host-disease of the skin. J Am Acad Dermatol. 2002;46:799–800.
39. Stege H, Schöpf E, Ruzicka T, Krutmann J. High-dose UVA1 for urticaria pigmentosa [letter]. Lancet. 1996;347:64.
40. Zane C, Leali C, Airo P, et al. 'High-dose' UVA1 therapy of widespread plaque-type, nodular, and erythrodermic mycosis fungoides. J Am Acad Dermatol. 2001;44:629–33.
41. Edström DW, Porwit A, Ros A-M. Effects on human skin of repetitive ultraviolet-A1 (UVA1) irradiation and visible light. Photodermatol Photoimmunol Photomed. 2001;17:66–70.
42. Pathak MA Fitzpatrick TB. The evolution of photochemotherapy with psoralens and UVA (PUVA): 2000 BC to 1992 AD. J Photochem Photobiol B. 1992;14:3–22.
43. Parrish JA, Fitzpatrick TB, Tanenbaum L, Pathak MA. Photochemotherapy of psoriasis with oral methoxsalen and long wave ultraviolet light. N Engl J Med. 1974;291:1207–11.
44. Fischer T, Alsins J. Treatment of psoriasis with trioxsalen baths and dysprosium lamps. Acta Derm Venereol. 1976;56:383–90.
45. Dall'Acqua F, Vedaldi D, Caffieri S, et al. Principles of psoralen photosensitization. In: Hönigsmann H, Jori G, Young AR (eds). The Fundamental Bases of Phototherapy. Milan: OEMF SpA, 1996:1–16.
46. Averbeck D. Recent advances in psoralen phototoxicity mechanism. Photochem Photobiol. 1989;50:859–82.
47. Brücke J, Tanew A, Ortel B, Hönigsmann H. Relative efficacy of 335 and 365 nm radiation in photochemotherapy of psoriasis. Br J Dermatol. 1991;124:372–4.
48. Ibbotson SH, Dawe RS, Farr PM. The effect of methoxsalen dose on ultraviolet-A-induced erythema. J Invest Dermatol. 2001;116:813–15.
49. Ibbotson SH, Farr PM. The time-course of psoralen ultraviolet A (PUVA) erythema. J Invest Dermatol. 1999;113:346–50.
50. Melski JW, Tanenbaum L, Parrish JA, et al. Oral methoxsalen photochemotherapy for the treatment of psoriasis: a cooperative clinical trial. J Invest Dermatol. 1977;68:328–35.
51. Anonymous. Guidelines of care for phototherapy and photochemotherapy, American Academy of Dermatology Committee on Guidelines of Care. J Am Acad Dermatol. 1994;31:643–8.
52. Henseler T, Wolff K, Hönigsmann H, et al. Oral 8-methoxypsoralen photochemotherapy of psoriasis. The European PUVA study: a cooperative study among 18 European centres. Lancet. 1981;i:853–7.
53. Halpern SM, Anstey AV, Dawe RS, et al. Guidelines for topical PUVA: a report of a workshop of the British photodermatology group. Br J Dermatol. 2000;142:22–31.
54. Anonymous. British Photodermatology Group guidelines for PUVA. Br J Dermatol. 1994;130:246–55.
55. Lowe NJ, Weingarten D, Bourget T, et al. PUVA therapy for psoriasis: comparison of oral and bath-water delivery of 8-methoxypsoralen. J Am Acad Dermatol. 1986;14:754–60.
56. Collins P, Rogers S. Bath-water compared with oral delivery of 8-methoxypsoralen PUVA therapy for chronic plaque psoriasis. Br J Dermatol. 1992;127:392–5.
57. Calzavara-Pinton PG, Ortel B, Hönigsmann H, et al. Safety and effectiveness of an aggressive and individualized bath-PUVA regimen in the treatment of psoriasis. Dermatology. 1994;189:256–9.
58. Morison WL. Phototherapy and photochemotherapy. Adv Dermatol. 1992;7:255–70.
60. Molin L, Larkö O. Cancer induction by immunosuppression in psoriasis after heavy PUVA treatment [letter]. Acta Derm Venereol. 1997;77:402.
61. van de Kerkhof PC, De Rooij MJ. Multiple squamous cell carcinomas in a psoriatic patient following high-dose photochemotherapy and cyclosporin treatment: response to long-term acitretin maintenance. Br J Dermatol. 1997;136:275–8.
62. Hönigsmann H, Wolff K. Results of therapy for psoriasis using retinoid and photochemotherapy (RePUVA). Pharmacol Ther. 1989;40:67–73.
63. Nijsten TEC, Stern RS. Oral retinoid use reduces cutaneous squamous cell carcinoma risk in patients with psoriasis treated with psoralen-UVA: a nested cohort study. J Am Acad Dermatol. 2003;49:644–50.
64. Gilchrest BA, Parrish JA, Tanenbaum L, et al. Oral methoxsalen photochemotherapy of mycosis fungoides. Cancer. 1976;38:683–9.
65. Tanew A, Hönigsmann H. Ultraviolet B and psoralen plus UVA phototherapy for cutaneous T-cell lymphoma. Dermatol. Ther. 1997;4:38–46.
66. Herrmann JJ, Roenigk HH Jr, Hurria A, et al. Treatment of mycosis fungoides with photochemotherapy (PUVA): long-term follow-up. J Am Acad Dermatol. 1995;33:234–42.
67. Thomsen K, Hammar H, Molin L, et al. Retinoids plus PUVA (RePUVA) and PUVA in mycosis fungoides, plaque stage. A report from the Scandinavian Mycosis Fungoides Group. Acta Derm Venereol. 1989; 69:536–8.
68. Zhang C, Duvic M. Retinoids: therapeutic applications and mechanisms of action in cutaneous T-cell lymphoma. Dermatol Ther. 2003;16:322–30.
69. Singh F, Lebwohl MG. Cutaneous T-cell lymphoma treatment using bexarotene and PUVA: a case series. J Am Acad Dermatol. 2004;51:570–3.
70. Stadler R, Otte HG, Luger T, et al. Prospective randomized multicenter clinical trial on the use of interferon-α-2a plus acitretin versus interferon-α-2a plus PUVA in patients with cutaneous T-cell lymphoma stages I and II. Blood. 1998;92:3578–81.
71. Swanbeck G, Roupe G, Sandström MH. Indications of a considerable decrease in the death rate in mycosis fungoides by PUVA treatment. Acta Derm Venereol. 1994;74:465–6.
72. Ortel B, Tanew A, Hönigsmann H. Vitiligo treatment. Curr Probl Dermatol. 1986;15:265–71.
73. Ortel B, Tanew A, Hönigsmann H. Treatment of vitiligo with khellin and ultraviolet A. J Am Acad Dermatol. 1988;18:693–701.
74. Helander I, Jansén CT, Meurman L. Long-term efficacy of PUVA treatment in lichen planus: comparison of oral and external methoxsalen regimens. Photodermatology. 1987;4:265–8.
75. Volc-Platzer B, Hönigsmann H, Hinterberger W, Wolff K. Photochemotherapy improves chronic cutaneous graft-versus-host disease. J Am Acad Dermatol. 1990;23:220–8.
76. Kunz M, Wilhelm S, Freund M, et al. Treatment of severe erythrodermic acute graft-versus-host disease with photochemotherapy. Br J Dermatol. 2001;144:901–2.
77. Christophers E, Hönigsmann H, Wolff K, Langner A. PUVA-treatment of urticaria pigmentosa. Br J Dermatol. 1978;98:701–2.
78. Kolde G, Frosch PJ, Czarnetzki BM. Response of cutaneous mast cells to PUVA in patients with urticaria pigmentosa: histomorphometric, ultrastructural, and biochemical investigations. J Invest Dermatol. 1984;83:175–8.
79. Wantzin GL, Thomsen K. PUVA-treatment in lymphomatoid papulosis. Br J Dermatol. 1982;107:687–90.
80. Kerker BJ, Huang CP, Morison WL. Photochemotherapy of generalized granuloma annulare. Arch Dermatol. 1990;126:359–61.
81. Healy E, Rogers S. PUVA treatment for alopecia areata – does it work? A retrospective review of 102 cases. Br J Dermatol. 1993;129:42–4.
82. Taylor CR, Hawk JLM. PUVA treatment of alopecia areata partialis, totalis and universalis: audit of 10 years' experience at St. John's Institute of Dermatology. Br J Dermatol. 1995;133:914–18.
83. Kerscher M, Volkenandt M, Meurer M, et al. Treatment of localised scleroderma with PUVA bath photochemotherapy. Lancet. 1994;343:1233.
84. Scharfetter-Kochanek K, Goldermann R, Lehmann P, et al. PUVA therapy in disabling pansclerotic morphoea of children. Br J Dermatol. 1995; 132:830–1.
85. Hönigsmann H. Polymorphous light eruption. In: Lim HW, Soter NA (eds). Clinical Photomedicine. New York: Marcel Dekker, 1993:167–79.
86. Hölzle E, Hofmann C, Plewig G. PUVA-treatment for solar urticaria and persistent light reaction. Arch Dermatol Res. 1980;269:87–91.
87. Parrish JA, Jaenicke KF, Morison WL, et al. Solar urticaria: treatment with PUVA and mediator inhibitors. Br J Dermatol. 1982;106:575–80.
88. Hindson C, Spiro J, Downey A. PUVA therapy of chronic actinic dermatitis. Br J Dermatol. 1985;113:157–60.
89. Jaschke E, Hönigsmann H. Hydroa vacciniforme – action spectrum. UV-tolerance following photochemotherapy. Hautarzt. 1981;32:350–3.
90. Roelandts R. Photo(chemo)therapy and general management of erythropoietic protoporphyria. Dermatology. 1995;190:330–1.
91. Cox NH., Jones SK, Downey DJ, et al. Cutaneous and ocular side-effects of oral photochemotherapy: results of an 8-year follow-up study. Br J Dermatol. 1987;116:145–52.
91a. Malanos D, Stern RS. Psoralen plus ultraviolet A does not increase the risk of cataracts: A 25-year prospective study. J Am Acad Dermatol. 2007;57:231–7.
92. Hönigsmann H. Psoralen photochemotherapy – mechanisms, drugs, toxicity. Curr Probl Dermatol. 1986;15:52–66.
93. Calzavara-Pinton PG, Franceschini F, Rastrelli M, et al. Antinuclear antibodies are not induced by PUVA treatment with uncomplicated psoriasis. J Am Acad Dermatol. 1994;30:955–8.
94. Henseler T, Christophers E, Hönigsmann H, Wolff K. Skin tumors in the European PUVA study. Eight year follow-up of 1643 patients treated with PUVA for psoriasis. J Am Acad Dermatol. 1987;16:108–16.
95. Stern RS, Liebman EJ, Vakeva L. Oral psoralen and ultraviolet-A light (PUVA) treatment of psoriasis and persistent risk of nonmelanoma skin cancer. PUVA Follow-up Study. J Natl Cancer Inst. 1998;90:1278–84.
96. Lim JL, Stern RS. High levels of ultraviolet B exposure increase the risk of non-melanoma skin cancer in psoralen and ultraviolet A-treated patients. J Invest Dermatol. 2005;124:505–13.
97. Stern RS. Genital tumors among men with psoriasis exposed to psoralens and ultraviolet A radiation (PUVA) and ultraviolet B radiation. N Engl Med J. 1990;322:1093–7.
98. Wolff K, Hönigsmann H. Genital carcinomas in psoriasis patients treated with photochemotherapy. Lancet. 1991;337:439.
99. Aubin F, Puzenat E, Arveux P, et al. Genital squamous cell carcinoma in men treated by photochemotherapy. A cancer registry-based study from 1978 to 1998. Br J Dermatol. 2001;144:1204–6.

100. Stern RS; PUVA Follow up Study. The risk of melanoma in association with long-term exposure to PUVA. J Am Acad Dermatol. 2001;44:755–61.

101. Marcil I, Stern RS. Squamous-cell cancer of the skin in patients given PUVA and ciclosporin: nested cohort crossover study. Lancet. 2001;358:1042–5.

102. Young AR. Photochemotherapy and skin carcinogenesis: a critical review. In: Hönigsmann H, Jori G, Young AR (eds). The Fundamental Bases of Phototherapy. Milan: OEMF, 1996:77–87.

103. Hannuksela-Svahn A, Sigurgeirsson B, Pukkala E, et al. Trioxsalen bath PUVA did not increase the risk of squamous cell skin carcinoma and cutaneous malignant melanoma in a joint analysis of 944 Swedish and Finnish patients with psoriasis. Br J Dermatol. 1999;141:497–501.

104. Hannuksela-Svahn A, Pukkala E, Koulu L, et al. Cancer incidence among Finnish psoriasis patients treated with 8-methoxypsoralen bath PUVA. J Am Acad Dermatol. 1999;40:694–6.

105. Morison WL, Baughman RD, Day RM, et al. Consensus workshop on the toxic effects of long-term PUVA therapy. Arch Dermatol. 1998;134:595–8.

106. Ranki A, Puska P, Mattinen S, et al. Effect of PUVA on immunologic and virologic findings in HIV-infected patients. J Am Acad Dermatol. 1991;24:404–10.

107. Horn TD, Morison WL, Farzadegan H, et al. Effects of psoralen plus UVA radiation (PUVA) on HIV-1 in human beings: a pilot study. J Am Acad Dermatol. 1994;31:735–40.

108. Zmudzka BZ, Miller SA, Jacobs ME, et al. Medical UV exposures and HIV activation. Photochem Photobiol. 1996;64:246–53.

109. Morison WL. PUVA therapy is preferable to UVB phototherapy in the management of HIV-associated dermatoses. Photochem Photobiol. 1996;64:267–8.

110. Edelson R, Berger C, Gasparro F, et al. Treatment of cutaneous T-cell lymphoma by extracorporeal photochemotherapy. Preliminary results. N Engl J Med. 1987;316:297–303.

111. Demierre MF, Foss F, Koh H. Proceedings of the International Consensus Conference on Cutaneous T-Cell Lymphoma (CTCL) Treatment Recommendations. J Am Acad Dermatol. 1997;36:460–6.

112. Knobler E, Warmuth I, Cocco C, et al. Extracorporeal photochemotherapy – the Columbia Presbyterian experience. Photodermatol Photoimmunol Photomed. 2002;18:232–7.

113. Maeda A, Schwarz A, Kernebeck K, et al. Intravenous infusion of syngeneic apoptotic cells by photopheresis induces antigen-specific regulatory T cells. J Immunol. 2005;174:5968–76.

114. Greinix HT, Volc-Platzer B, Rabitsch W, et al. Successful use of extracorporeal photochemotherapy in the treatment of severe acute and chronic graft-versus-host disease. Blood. 1998;92:3098–104.

115. Foss FM, DiVenuti GM, Chin K, et al. Prospective study of extracorporeal photopheresis in steroid-refractory or steroid-resistant extensive chronic graft-versus-host disease: analysis of response and survival incorporating prognostic factors. Bone Marrow Transplant. 2005;35:1187–93.

116. Dall'Amico R, Murer L. Extracorporeal photochemotherapy: a new therapeutic approach for allograft rejection. Transfus Apher Sci. 2002;26:197–204.

117. Kumlien G, Genberg H, Shanwell A, Tyden G. Photopheresis for the treatment of refractory renal graft rejection. Transplantation 2005;79:123–5.

Photodynamic Therapy

Whitney D Tope and Sachin S Bhardwaj

135

Synonym: ■ Photoradiation therapy

Key features

- The use of photodynamic therapy by dermatologists has expanded over the past two decades, beginning with actinic keratoses and basal cell carcinomas and now including a wide range of disorders, from acne and photoaging to mycosis fungoides and psoriasis

- The photodynamic effect is a photochemical reaction which requires the presence of a photosensitizing molecule, photoactivating wavelengths of light, and tissue oxygen

- Photosensitizers may be administered systemically as intact macrocycles or topically as pro-photosensitizers, which are metabolized to photoactive macrocycles

- A time period is required after drug administration to allow photosensitizer production and partitioning into targeted tissue and cellular compartments

- Visible light from coherent (laser) or non-coherent sources is used to illuminate the skin and the light can be low power, non-thermal and continuous wave, or high power, photothermal and pulsed; the latter introduces varying degrees of photothermal injury via biologic chromophores, augmenting overall clinical injury

- Across the visible and near infrared spectrum, the depth of photon penetration into skin correlates positively with increased wavelength

- Target cells may undergo either apoptosis due to membrane-bound photosensitizers or ischemic necrosis due to vascular injury from photosensitizers concentrated in endothelial cells, or both

- Systemic photosensitizers cause variable degrees of pain, erythema and edema in treated skin and generalized photosensitivity may occur due to retention of photosensitizers; topical photosensitizers result in brief local photosensitivity

HISTORY AND DEVELOPMENT

Although cutaneous photodynamic therapy was described almost a century ago, directed clinical and basic research did not begin until the 1960s[1–3]. In 1900, medical student Oscar Raab reported that killing of paramecia required both acridine orange and light and he correctly correlated the effect with the fluorescence of acridine. Von Tappeiner, Raab's mentor, continued this work and, with Jesionek, reported 3 years later on the use of topical or intralesional eosin plus light (sunlight or arc lamp) to treat skin cancer, cutaneous lupus and condylomata. Von Tappeiner also reported the requirement for oxygen and coined the term 'photodynamic therapy' (PDT) for this method of photosensitization.

Meyer-Betz[4] himself demonstrated the generalized photosensitizing effects of systemic hematoporphyrin (Fig. 135.1), an iron-free preparation of blood with which Hausmann, in 1908, had demonstrated photodynamic killing of paramecia and photosensitization of mice. Policard subsequently observed tumor localization of porphyrins in 1924. Auler & Banzer confirmed this finding using hematoporphyrin and correlated tissue fluorescence with the presence of tumor necrosis in animal models in 1942. In attempting to purify hematoporphyrin's more active compounds, Schwartz created an esterified porphyrin which localized to tumor tissue even more strongly than hematoporphyrin. Schwartz convinced Richard Lipson, a resident performing research at

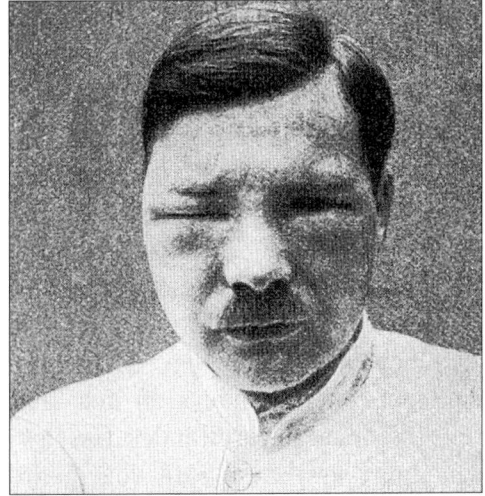

Fig. 135.1 Acute photosensitivity due to hematoporphyrin. Meyer-Betz, who noted pain and swelling of exposed skin within minutes of injection of 200 mg of hematoporphyrin. Generalized photosensitivity lasted more than 2 months. Photograph taken from Dtsch Arch Klin Med. 1913;112:476.

the University of Minnesota, to employ this new compound, hematoporphyrin derivative (HPD). In 1960, Lipson[5] reported his characterization of the photodynamic action of HPD and white light on normal murine skin, and later (1961) the successful fluorescent detection of murine and rat tumors after systemic injection of HPD.

Thomas Dougherty initiated human trials of HPD in 1976, treating primarily cutaneous cancer metastases. Subsequent studies utilized optical fiber-delivered laser light for PDT of esophageal, lung and intracranial malignancies. HPD eventually became known as porfimer sodium, or Photofrin®. In 1995, nearly 100 years after Raab's initial observations, porfimer sodium plus red light was approved by the Food and Drug Administration (FDA) for the palliative treatment of esophageal carcinoma.

Many recognized that the significant prolonged photosensitivity induced by HPD stood in the way of its potential clinical applications. In the search for photosensitizers with less prolonged tissue retention, protoporphyrin IX (PpIX), a highly hydrophobic compound (suggesting greater tissue retention) synthesized within the liver and the blood, was originally viewed as a poor candidate. The challenge then was to allow cells to produce PpIX themselves (by administration of a pro-photosensitizer rather than providing PpIX directly), and, in 1986, Kennedy & Pottier successfully demonstrated the use of 5δ-aminolevulinic acid HCl (ALA) to induce tissue production of photoactivating PpIX. Beginning in 1987, patients with basal cell carcinoma (BCC), actinic keratoses (AKs), and squamous cell carcinoma (SCC) were successfully treated with topical ALA plus red light[6,7]. In 1999, topical ALA and blue light were FDA-approved for the treatment of AKs.

PHOTOCHEMISTRY OF PDT

PDT may be briefly defined as the use of cytotoxic oxygen radicals (primarily singlet oxygen, $^1O_2$) generated from photoactivated molecular species to achieve a therapeutic response. The necessary components are photoactivating light, an exogenous photosensitizer, tissue oxygen, and a target cell (Fig. 135.2). The processes that convert photon energy to singlet oxygen are best explained using the modified Jablonski energy state diagram shown in Figure 135.3. Within any molecule, outer ring electrons exist in a ground state orbital or region. Absorption of an appropriately energetic photon $(E = h\nu_1)$ allows an electron to jump to an excited state orbital further from the nucleus. All such absorption events lead first to the excited singlet state. The term singlet denotes a specific pattern of electron spin in paired electrons and associated energy levels occupied by the electrons. Excited state electrons, which tend to seek the more stable ground state, may deactivate by several paths. The additional molecular energy may be dissipated as heat through vibration or through a jump back to a lower energy state. When radiative decay occurs from singlet states, a photon ($E = h\nu_2$) is emitted during the process of fluorescence. Because energy transfer is imperfectly conserved, this emitted photon carries less energy and necessarily a longer or redder wavelength (Stokes shift). Singlet states are unstable and extremely short-lived (nanosecond time domain). Certain molecules possess potential singlet states whose vibrational energy levels correspond with those of triplet states (different electron spin pairing). This radiationless conversion from singlet to triplet states occurs through a process termed intersystem crossing. Porphyrins and similar molecules produce triplet states very efficiently. Triplet states may deactivate through heat loss or by emitting a photon ($E = h\nu_3$) through phosphorescence. Triplet states possess a significantly longer lifetime (microsecond time domain), making them more available for molecular interaction. In oxygenated biologic tissues, excited triplet state electrons tend to interact with tissue oxygen (O_2) to create singlet oxygen ($^1O_2$). This absolute requirement for oxygen is characteristic of the photodynamic effect and defines type II photochemical reactions in biologic systems[8]. The ground state photosensitizer molecule is regenerated and may again participate

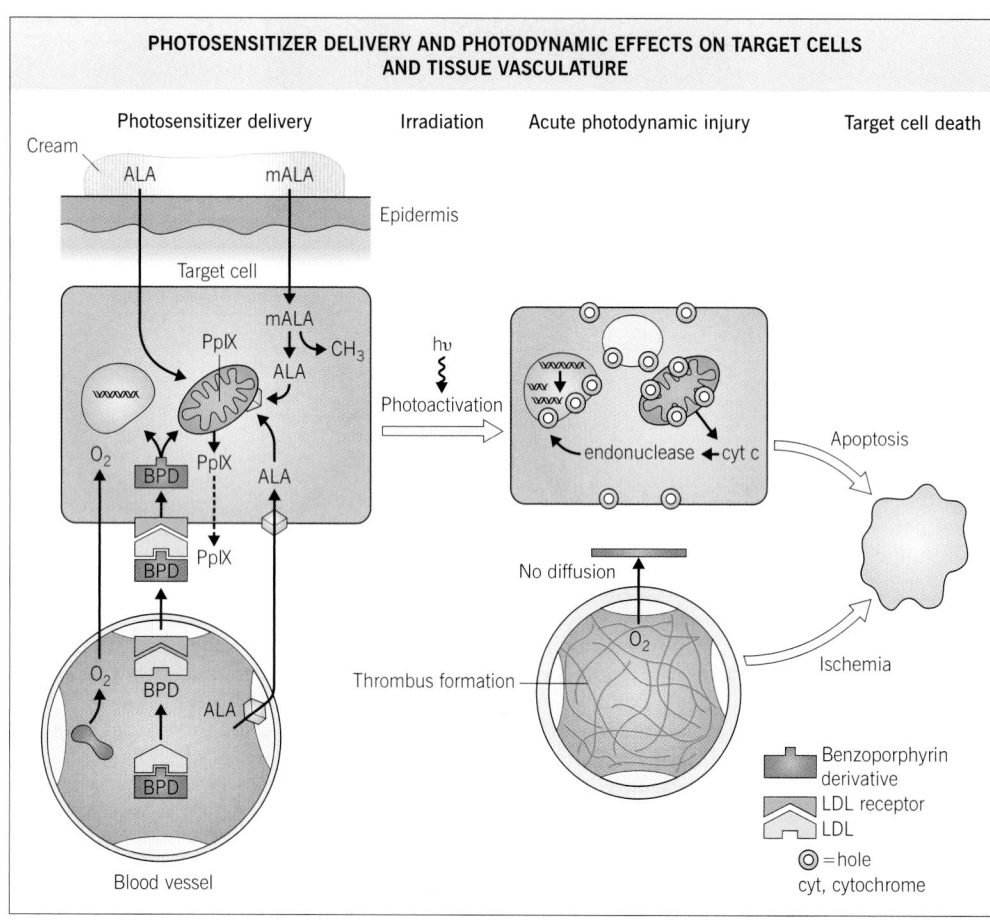

Fig. 135.2 Photosensitizer delivery and photodynamic effects on target cells and tissue vasculature. Topical photosensitizers 5-aminolevulinic acid (ALA) and methyl-esterified ALA (mALA) diffuse through the stratum corneum into target epithelial cells. Systemic photosensitizers arrive through the serum (ALA) or bound to low-density lipoproteins (LDL; e.g. benzoporphyrin derivative monoacid ring A [BPD], porfimer, temoporfin). Oxygen is delivered via erythrocyte circulation. Systemically delivered photosensitizers concentrate in endothelial cells and diffuse through the interstitium to target cells. ALA derived from any source is converted to protoporphyrin IX (PpIX) within mitochondria. PpIX then leaks from the mitochondria to other cellular structures, and eventually to the vasculature for removal. After sufficient time for photosensitizer partitioning to subcellular structures, target tissue is irradiated with photoactivating light. During acute photodynamic injury, mitochondria leak cytochrome c, initiating endonuclease activity, and plasma and nuclear membranes lose integrity. Acute injury in endothelial cells leads to thrombus formation and vascular collapse. Target cell and tissue oxygen delivery cease. Both apoptosis and ischemic necrosis contribute to irreversible target cell injury and death.

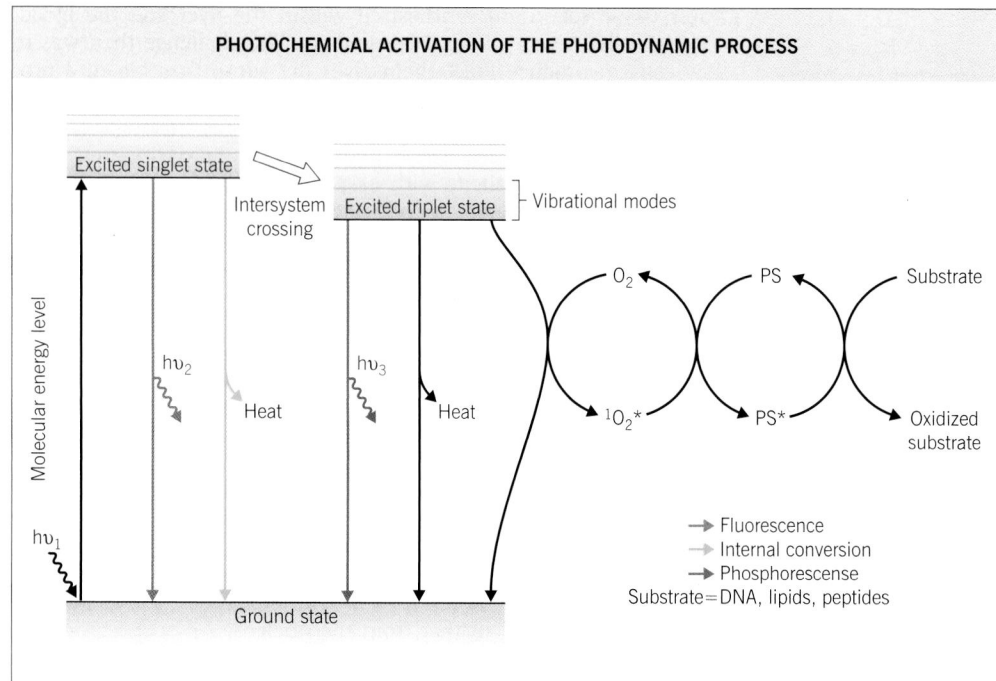

Fig. 135.3 Photochemical activation of the photodynamic process: the Jablonski energy state diagram. See Photochemistry section for explanation. PS, photosensitizer. *Excited state.

in photon absorption. Singlet oxygen, one of the most potent oxidant species known, may then oxidize critical cellular components (lipid, peptides, nucleic acids) with sufficient oxidative damage to lead to cell death. How this cellular effect leads to tissue responses will be discussed below. It is important to note that singlet oxygen, or its downstream oxidation products, may also attack and disable the photosensitizer itself, a process termed photobleaching. With continued light application to a given amount of photosensitizer present in oxygenated tissue, photobleaching may eventually limit and terminate PDT.

LIGHT DOSIMETRY AND INSTRUMENTATION

Historically, photochemical processes such as PDT typically employed continuous wave (non-pulsed) light. These light sources deliver low-power, low-irradiance light, which does not create photothermal or photomechanical effects. The light source's spectral output must be selected to match an absorption peak of the photosensitizer and the location of the target at depth. Across the visible and near infrared spectrum, the depth of the photon penetration into skin correlates positively with increased wavelength. For epidermal lesions, blue light gives adequate penetration and photosensitizer absorption; dermal processes typically require deeply penetrating red light which needs to correspond with one of the photosensitizer's absorption peaks (Fig. 135.4).

Functionally, the potential treatment wavelength for PDT must be longer than the wavelengths that comprise the UV spectrum (i.e. >400 nm) so that there is limited tissue penetration of UV light and consequent risk of cancer induction. The wavelength must also have sufficient photon energy to initiate photochemical processes (<800 nm). Thus, the therapeutic wavelength window for PDT lies between 400 and 800 nm. As an example, blue light was chosen because the largest porphyrin absorption peak is near 400 nm (the Soret band). The 'light dose' (number of photons per unit area) used in PDT is given as the total *fluence* delivered in joules per square centimeter (J/cm^2). *Power*, the photons delivered per unit time, is given in watts (W). One watt equals one joule delivered in one second. The *irradiance*, or power per unit area, is given as $J/cm^2 \cdot s$ or W/cm^2. The exposure time (t, seconds) required to deliver the total light dose may be derived from fluence (F, J/cm^2) and the irradiance (I, W/cm^2) using the relationship: $t = F/I$. Within this light dosing schema exists time:intensity reciprocity; that is, doubling the irradiance requires half the exposure time to deliver the same light dose.

Light sources now used in PDT have evolved nearly full circle over a century, from broadband light sources to monochromatic coherent sources (lasers) and to more efficient broadband sources. Early sources were non-coherent, white light sources, such as xenon arc lamps. These sources were filtered to obtain broadband light more appro-

priately matched to the absorption peaks of specific photosensitizers. The development of laser light sources, particularly the argon-pumped tunable dye laser (630 nm), presented an opportunity to utilize very specific wavelengths of light produced at high irradiance in order to: drastically shorten treatment times, provide sufficient light through optical fibers to treat internal organs, and, through beam splitting, allow the treatment of multiple tumors simultaneously. Newer photosensitizers activated by even longer wavelengths (650–755 nm) have enabled the use of less costly diode lasers and light-emitting diode (LED) sources. Although very small, individual diodes can easily be constructed in arrays to provide uniform fields of light covering hundreds of square centimeters. Recently, filtered broadband lamp sources have again been designed for dermatologic applications of PDT.

Nowadays, both high-power pulsed lasers (595 nm) and filtered (~500–1200 nm) light sources are being used for PDT. These sources produce wavelengths absorbed by porphyrins, but deliver light in short intense pulses sufficient to produce photothermal injury via skin chromophores (e.g. melanosomes, blood vessels). A comparison of PDT using pulsed light sources versus continuous wave sources found that the clinical photodynamic effects of the latter were dramatically less than with pulsed light[9]. Thus, the overall clinical effect of treatments that utilize such pulsed sources is the sum of photodynamic plus photothermal effects; the contribution of each effect is as yet undefined.

DRUG DELIVERY AND TISSUE LOCALIZATION

The characteristics of photosensitizers and pro-photosensitizers currently approved or under investigation for dermatologic applications are found in Figure 135.5 and Table 135.1. Topical, oral, intralesional and intravenous routes have all been explored as photosensitizer delivery systems. Target tissue localization of the photosensitizer depends upon whether the photosensitizer is delivered as an intact molecule or as a pro-photosensitizer subject to target cellular metabolic processes that lead to photosensitizer production.

Intact photosensitizers are often large, lipophilic, macrocyclic molecules (e.g. PpIX MW = 562). Because of their immiscibility in typical dermatologic bases and/or inability to penetrate the stratum corneum, intact macrocycles typically require intravenous administration as aqueous solutions (porfimer sodium) or lipid emulsions (benzoporphyrin derivative monoacid ring A; BPD-MA). These molecules then bind chiefly to serum lipoproteins within the circulation (see Fig. 135.2)[10]. Low-density lipoproteins (LDLs) play a major role in the delivery of amphiphilic and hydrophobic photosensitizers to tumor tissue. Both endothelial cells of tumor neovasculature and rapidly dividing cells demonstrate high expression of LDL receptors as well as significant photosensitizer uptake via LDL receptor-mediated endocytosis. The photosensitizer is then transported intracellularly to the lysosomal, endoplasmic reticular, mitochondrial and nuclear membranes. High-density lipoproteins (HDLs) may play a lesser role in the delivery of photosensitizers to target tissue, and perhaps a greater role in clearance from the liver and spleen for elimination via the bile. Of note, tissue macrophages, in both normal and tumor interstitium, also consume and retain macrocyclic photosensitizers. The presence of photosensitizers within cutaneous macrophages accounts for the long-term photosensitivity observed after their use.

In contrast, the low-molecular-weight and hydrophilic pro-photosensitizers, ALA and methyl-esterified ALA (mALA), are administered as topical preparations to the diseased skin surface (see Fig. 135.2). mALA is often applied after 'skin preparation' or light curettage to remove the stratum corneum and superficial tumor tissue. Once absorbed into tissue, esterases cleave and demethylate mALA to ALA. ALA, an amino acid, is readily taken up through the cellular membrane. In all nucleated cells, ALA is normally produced from glycine and succinyl CoA by ALA synthetase, a rate-limiting step in porphyrin and heme biosynthesis. The presence of exogenous ALA circumvents this rate-limiting step and subsequent enzymatic reactions proceed to convert ALA to protoporphyrin IX (PpIX). The addition of iron to PpIX by ferrochelatase to create heme constitutes the final rate-limiting step of the porphyrin biosynthetic pathway (see Ch. 49). By virtue of tight regulation by both heme levels and strictly controlled iron availability, nucleated cells exposed to exogenous ALA produce large intracellular quantities of PpIX. As observed in patients with inherited

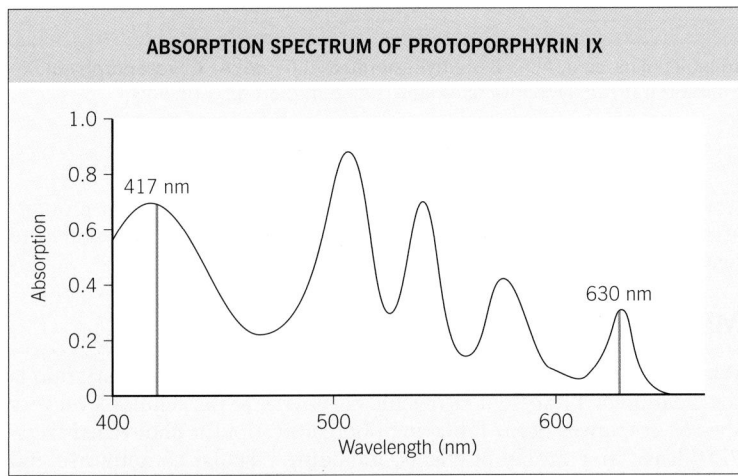

ABSORPTION SPECTRUM OF PROTOPORPHYRIN IX

Fig. 135.4 Absorption spectrum of protoporphyrin IX (PpIX). The absorption spectrum demonstrates the probability of absorption for each wavelength of light. It reveals the major absorption (photoactivation) peaks of PpIX. The blue (417 nm) and red (630 nm) wavelengths typically used to activate PpIX in photodynamic therapy are designated (spectrum for PpIX dissolved in pyridine).

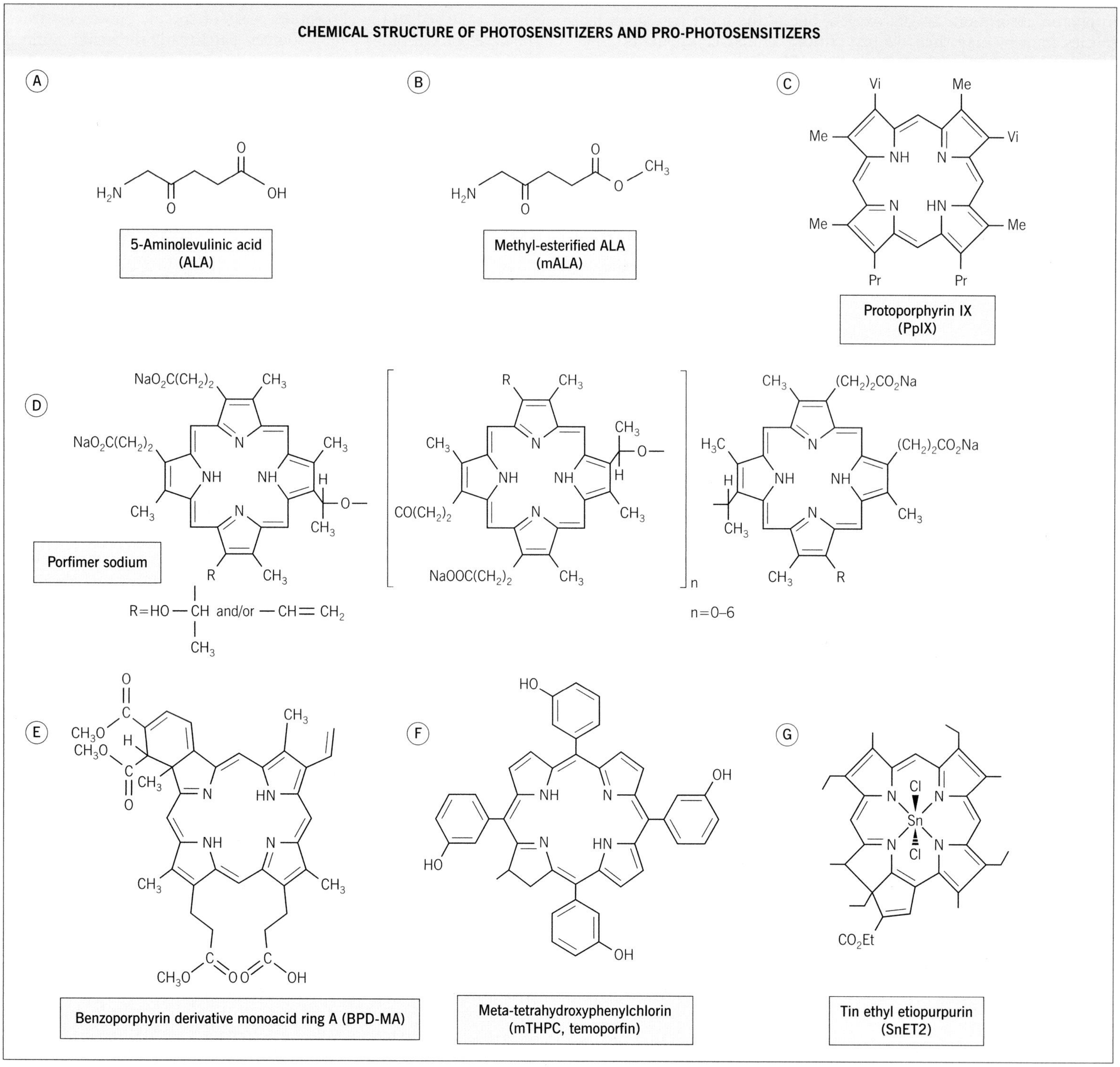

CHEMICAL STRUCTURE OF PHOTOSENSITIZERS AND PRO-PHOTOSENSITIZERS

A 5-Aminolevulinic acid (ALA)

B Methyl-esterified ALA (mALA)

C Protoporphyrin IX (PpIX)

D Porfimer sodium

R=HO—CH and/or —CH=CH₂

n=0–6

E Benzoporphyrin derivative monoacid ring A (BPD-MA)

F Meta-tetrahydroxyphenylchlorin (mTHPC, temoporfin)

G Tin ethyl etiopurpurin (SnET2)

Fig. 135.5 Chemical structures of photosensitizers and pro-photosensitizers. A 5-aminolevulinic acid (ALA); **B** Methyl-esterified ALA (mALA); **C** Protoporphyrin IX (PpIX); **D** Porfimer sodium; **E** Benzoporphyrin derivative monoacid ring A (BPD-MA); **F** Meta-tetrahydroxyphenylchlorin (mTHPC, temoporfin); **G** Tin ethyl etiopurpurin (SnET2).

deficiency of ferrochelatase (erythropoietic protoporphyria), PpIX is a potent and immediate photosensitizer.

Once delivered intact to, or produced within, tissue, photosensitizers will leak or be transported from both normal and target tissues. The differential chronologies of photosensitizer delivery and removal from various tissues directly affect the timing of light delivery. To enhance target tissue destruction (yet minimize normal tissue destruction), photoactivation should occur when target:normal tissue photosensitizer ratios are maximized. Membrane localization and pH changes within different subcellular compartments act to retain hydrophobic photosensitizers within cells. The relative dearth of organized lymphatic drainage from neoplastic tissues creates a stromal sink for the accumulation and slow release of photosensitizers from malignant tissues. These effects tend to enhance the target versus normal tissue localization of photosensitizers and the therapeutic ratio for PDT. Retention of photosensitizers in inflammatory conditions such as psoriasis is less

well understood, but probably depends upon enhanced cellular proliferation, the presence of activated lymphocytes, and the vasculature necessary to support these processes.

MECHANISM OF ACTION

Whereas the outward clinical effect of photosensitizer administration is the creation of a transient iatrogenic porphyria, at the cellular level very specific responses occur following photoactivation of photosensitizers. PDT leads to a variety of effects, including vascular compromise and direct cell kill (see Fig. 135.2), as well as inflammatory and immunologic responses. The subcellular distance-of-action of $^1O_2$ confers a precise specificity such that photodynamic injury occurs within the immediate vicinity of the photosensitizer molecule. Singlet oxygen may oxidize specific amino acids (cysteine, histidine, tryptophan, tyrosine and methionine), guanine moieties in nucleic acids, and unsaturated

PHOTOSENSITIZERS AND PRO-PHOTOSENSITIZERS USED FOR DERMATOLOGIC PHOTODYNAMIC THERAPY

Drug (generic)	5-aminolevulinic acid HCl (ALA)	Methyl-esterified ALA (mALA)	Porfimer Na	Benzoporphyrin derivative monoacid ring A (BPD-MA)	Meta-tetrahydroxyphenylchlorin (mTHPC; temoporfin)	Tin ethyl etiopurpurin (SnET2)
Drug (trade)®	Levulan	Metvix	Photofrin	Verteporfin	Foscan	Purlytin
Photosensitizer produced	PpIX	PpIX	–	–	–	–
Treatment λ (nm)	417, 630	630	630	690	652	660
Delivery routes	Topical (T), oral (O)	Topical	Intravenous (iv)	iv	iv	iv
Time period between administration and irradiation	24 h (T)*, 2–4 h (O)	3–4 h	48–72 h	1–3 h	48–96 h	24 h
Light source**	Dye laser (630) Filtered broadband	Dye laser (630) Filtered broadband	Dye laser (630)	Diode	Dye laser (652)	Diode
Cutaneous FDA-approved indications†	AK	AK	None	None	None	None
Experimental indications	BCC, SCC *in situ*, mycosis fungoides, photoaging, acne, hirsutism, HPV	BCC, AK, SCC *in situ*	BCC, SCC, SCC *in situ*	BCC, SCC *in situ*, psoriasis	BCC, SCC, SCC *in situ*	BCC, psoriasis
Duration of generalized cutaneous photosensitivity	0 h (T), 24 h (O)	0 h	1–4 months	3–5 days	1–2 weeks	1–3 weeks

*Often reduced to 1–3 h to reduce pain and clinical efficacy.
**Dye laser = argon- or KTP-pumped dye laser.
†At the time of writing.

Table 135.1 Photosensitizers and pro-photosensitizers utilized for dermatologic photodynamic therapy. AK, actinic keratosis; BCC, basal cell carcinoma; FDA, Food and Drug Administration; HPV, human papillomavirus infections; PpIX, protoporphyrin IX; SCC, squamous cell carcinoma.

bonds of lipids. Photo-oxidation may in turn create altered molecular conformation and molecular cross-linking, preventing performance of normal functional and structural roles or enhancing susceptibility to degradation[11]. The photodynamic effect due to photosensitizers localizing to plasma, lysosomal and mitochondrial membranes leads to increased plasma membrane permeability, intracellular release of lysosomal enzymes, and the induction of apoptosis, respectively (see Fig. 135.2). When cytochrome c enters the cytosol from the mitochondria, endonuclease activity increases and caspase-3 is activated, triggering the apoptosis cascade[12].

Assuming sufficient tissue oxygen and light levels, observed PDT responses depend upon the pattern of tissue localization of photosensitizers. Activation of photosensitizers delivered in large amounts via LDL receptors to tissue vasculature induces endothelial cell damage, local vascular collapse, and ischemic tissue necrosis[13]. This group includes porfimer, BPD-MA, meta-tetrahydroxyphenylchlorin (mTHPC, temoporfin), and tin ethyl etiopurpurin (SnET2; see Table 135.1). In contrast, photosensitizers gaining ready access to target cells or produced intracellularly produce a preponderance of direct cell death over vascular injury. This group includes PpIX generated from either ALA or mALA. In gross terms, vascular injury predominates when large macrocyclic photosensitizers are used for PDT, whereas direct cell injury predominates when pro-photosensitizers are employed for PDT.

A host of factors influence the clinical specificity of PDT. For successful treatment of precancers and cutaneous malignancies, one must achieve a degree of injury that surpasses inherent repair mechanisms, i.e. sufficient to produce clinical tissue necrosis. This concept of a threshold of injury defines the minimum 'photodynamic dose' (PDD). The photodynamic threshold dose incorporates the tissue concentration of photosensitizer as well as the wavelength (absorption coefficient) and local tissue fluence of photoactivating light. Assuming an adequate PDD is delivered, the clinical specificity of PDT for a particular target tissue depends upon: preferential tissue localization of the chosen photosensitizer; the timing and intensity (irradiance) of the applied light dose; the tissue penetration of the chosen wavelength; shielding of adjacent normal tissue; local oxygen concentration during irradiation; and the sensitivity of the photosensitizer to photobleaching. The majority of photosensitizers currently available demonstrate sub-

stantial absorption of both blue–green and red wavelengths. As noted previously, across the visible and near infrared spectrum, the depth of tissue penetration correlates positively with increasing wavelength. Thus, one may enhance selectivity for superficial conditions (e.g. psoriasis, actinic keratoses) by employing photoactivating blue wavelengths, and for deeper conditions (e.g. BCC, mycosis fungoides) by employing red wavelengths. High irradiances (as observed with brief, high fluence, pulsed light) may cause more rapid tissue oxygen depletion and photobleaching, both acting to limit the photodynamic effect.

A complete analysis of the immune and inflammatory effects of PDT is the subject of intense investigation. A variety of studies have documented modulation of photodynamic effects in immunosuppressed animals (e.g. SCID mice) or by the use of adjuvants. PDT alters the expression of cell surface proteins (e.g. adhesion molecules) and patterns of cytokine expression[14]. Porfimer PDT induces an immunosuppression which is adoptively transferable and antigen-specific, suggesting the generation of T suppressor cells, but without altered delayed-type hypersensitivity (DTH)[15]. Except for intact DTH, this pattern is similar to that induced by UVB irradiation. Also, ALA PDT appears to selectively target activated and malignant T lymphocytes based on their high levels of transferrin receptor (CD71) expression[16]. There is also evidence that PDT may act as a biological response modifier[17]. In summary, PDT is a broadly inflammatory event, and cytokines, chemokines and other immunogenic proteins released by injured and dying cells create an inflammatory and immunologically active milieu. Information gleaned from these and future studies should enable a better understanding and implementation of PDT for inflammatory and immunologic dermatoses.

INDICATIONS/CONTRAINDICATIONS

The skin lends itself to PDT, given that the condition to be treated is easily exposed to an external light source and the drug may be applied topically. Consequently, investigators have tried using PDT as a potential therapeutic modality for many conditions. Common cutaneous neoplasms represent well-studied targets for PDT. Only more recently has significant attention been paid to the use of PDT for inflammatory dermatoses and photodamage. Accurate assessment of the PDT literature is challenging. As there are no set protocols for many diseases, significant variation exists with regard to the histology, the photosensitizers used, wavelengths employed, and dosimetry. Many early PDT tumor studies relied heavily upon clinical, rather than histopathologic, assessment of tumor response and initial reports of high response rates were then followed by less sanguine data. In addition, few early studies attempted direct comparison of PDT with established treatments. Fortunately, better-designed, recent studies clearly support the efficacy and safety of PDT. The following section provides data from selected studies emphasizing large study populations, prospective design, appropriate controls, histopathologic outcomes assessment, appropriate follow-up duration, and direct comparisons with standard therapies, where available. More extensive reviews of PDT should be consulted for information on the use of PDT in cutaneous diseases not discussed below[18-20].

NEOPLASIA

Actinic Keratoses/Actinic Cheilitis

Initial investigation into the possibility of ALA-based photodynamic treatment of actinic keratoses (AKs) was first reported in 1990[6]. Since then, numerous studies have reported lesion cure rates for AKs in the range of 70–100% (Table 135.2). The concentration of ALA varied from 10% to 30%, with 20% being the most commonly employed. Incubation times ranged from 4 hours under occlusion to 18 hours without occlusion, and light sources included the argon-pumped dye laser (630 nm)[21], intense pulsed light[25], red light[22,24,26] and blue light[23]. The latter non-laser light sources provided adequate fluence, but at a lower cost. In one study, only weak PpIX fluorescence was observed in hypertrophic AKs after ALA application and this correlated with a poorer clinical response[21]. The authors concluded that hyperkeratosis was a limiting factor for ALA tissue penetration. In addition, certain sites (e.g. face, scalp) had better response rates than others (e.g. hands, forearms, trunk). Overall, PDT provided excellent cosmetic results and no generalized and only rare local photosensitivity was noted.

Because cutaneous malignancies, particularly SCCs, are such a problem in recipients of solid organ transplants, PDT has been tried in this patient population. However, response rates for AKs and SCC in situ were significantly lower than in immunocompetent controls (see Table 135.2)[24]. One possible explanation was provided by an in vitro study in which cyclosporine was shown to inhibit apoptosis in a SCC cell line subjected to phthalocyanine PDT[27]. More recent studies have investigated the role of PDT in the prevention of SCC in the transplant population. In a prospective, paired study (n = 40 patients) comparing prophylactic topical ALA PDT (plus violet light) versus no treatment, assigned in a random fashion to either the right or the left hand and forearm, the occurrence of new SCCs was not significantly different between the PDT-treated arms and the control arms[28]. Specifically, 15 SCCs were diagnosed in nine PDT-treated arms and 10 SCCs were diagnosed in nine control arms during a 2-year evaluation period. In addition, whether the patient received one versus two PDT treatments was of no consequence. Several explanations have been offered for the lack of efficacy observed in this study: reduced response rates for PDT of SCCs in situ (and AKs) on the hands and forearms[24] (compared to other sites such as the face; see Table 135.2); the superficial penetration of the violet light (compared to red light); and the low total dose of light (5.5–6 J/cm^2) being suboptimal (traditional protocols use 10 J/cm^2). In addition, given the immunosuppression, more frequent and a higher total number of treatments may be necessary to achieve a killing response (mediated by inflammatory cell activation) against atypical or malignant keratinocytes. Given the propensity of transplant recipients to develop numerous and aggressive skin cancers, and the lack of

---

SELECTED STUDIES OF PHOTODYNAMIC THERAPY OF ACTINIC KERATOSES

Type of study (ref)	No. of patients	Topical photosensitizer (concentration)	Incubation time	Light source	Response rate	Comments
Prospective, vehicle-controlled, varying doses of drug (21)	40 (240 AKs)	ALA (10%, 20%, 30%)	Overnight	Argon-pumped dye laser (630 nm); maximum effect at 10 J/cm^2	With 30% ALA and in non-hypertrophic (grade 1 or 2) AKs of the face and scalp, 91% Truncal lesions, 45%	• All three ALA concentrations better than placebo vehicle • Grade 1 (mild, palpable) and grade 2 (moderately thick) AKs responded better than hypertrophic (grade 3) AKs
Prospective, paired comparison to topical 5-FU (22)	14 (hand AKs)	ALA (20%) under occlusion	4 h	Red light (580–740 nm) at 150 J/cm^2 and mean irradiance of 86 mW/cm^2	Total surface area of AKs reduced by 70% (73% for 5-FU)	• 5% 5-FU cream was applied bid for 3 weeks • Assessed over 6 months • Pain and erythema similar in two groups*
Prospective, vehicle-controlled (23)	36	ALA (20%)	14–18 h	Blue light (417 nm) at 10 J/cm^2	88% at 8 weeks (6% for vehicle alone)	• Less potential for deeper damage, compared to red light • The ALA solution was applied three times prior to one irradiation
Prospective, immuno-suppressed transplant patients versus immunocompetent patients as the control group (24)	20 (20 controls)	ALA (20%) under occlusion	5 h	Red light at 75 J/cm^2	86% at 1 month & 48% at 1 year (94% & 72% for controls)	• Both AKs and SCC in situ were treated • Better results for lesions of the scalp, face and neck than for hands and forearms
Prospective single arm (25)	17 (38 AKs)	ALA (20%) under occlusion	4 h	Intense pulsed light (615–1200 nm) at 40 J/cm^2	91% at 3 months	• Two PDT treatments, 1 month apart • A single pass of 4 ms pulse/ 20 ms delay/4 ms pulse
Prospective, randomized, comparison with cryotherapy (26)	193 (95 cryo-therapy controls)	mALA under occlusion	3 h	Red light (570–670 nm) at 75 J/cm^2	69% (75% for cryotherapy)	• Prior to PDT or cryotherapy, superficial curettage was performed • Two cycles of cryotherapy • Excellent or good cosmetic outcome: PDT, 98%; cryotherapy, 91%

Pain and erythema was maximal at the start of therapy for PDT and at the end of therapy for 5-FU.

Table 135.2 Selected studies of photodynamic therapy (PDT) of actinic keratoses (AKs). Unless noted otherwise, each patient received a single PDT treatment. ALA, 5-aminolevulinic acid; 5-FU, 5-fluorouracil; mALA, methyl-esterified ALA. Adapted from Anderson, R. Laser–tissue interactions. In: Goldman M, Fitzpatrick R (eds). Cutaneous Laser Surgery, 2nd ed. St. Louis: Mosby; 1999:5.

effective treatments for wide 'fields' of photodamaged skin, PDT warrants further investigation as a potential tool in this population.

In the case of actinic cheilitis, the absence of a stratum corneum should facilitate topical PDT of this mucosal surface. In one small series, one to three topical ALA PDT sessions (using filtered red light doses of 55 J/cm^2) successfully cleared three patients with actinic cheilitis recalcitrant to conventional treatments[29]; the clearance was maintained at 12 months' follow-up. Desquamative peeling lasted for months, but the eventual cosmetic result was reported as excellent. On a cautionary note, one might well expect that poorer treatment responses would result from the greater challenge to establish accurate dosimetry in the setting of *en face* illumination and three-dimensionally complex sites.

In Situ and Invasive Squamous Cell Carcinoma

SCC *in situ*, including erythroplasia of Queyrat, is also quite responsive to PDT. High cure rates have been observed with both systemic photosensitizers and topical pro-photosensitizers in conjunction with lasers (630 nm) and non-coherent red light (Table 135.3)[6,30-33]. More deeply penetrating red light should be used to treat SCC *in situ* in order to ensure adequate treatment of adnexal extensions and to compensate for three-dimensionally complex cutaneous and mucosal sites. PDT may be a particularly attractive alternative for large lesions, those sites associated with significant morbidity after surgical excision, and for those patients unwilling or unable to undergo other treatment modalities.

Few reports detail the photodynamic treatment of invasive cutaneous SCC and thus far the results have been unsatisfactory compared to surgical excision (including microscopically controlled; see Table 135.3)[34-36]. Not surprisingly, a higher response rate was observed with superficially invasive SCCs as compared to nodular SCCs[6]. The results obtained to date suggest that PDT for invasive cutaneous SCC has not yet been optimized. Primary treatment of SCC with PDT should be reserved for early invasive disease (<1 mm) and must take advantage of multiple treatments and high doses of deeply penetrating red light. In advanced head and neck SCC, PDT should be considered an adjunctive treatment modality[35].

Basal Cell Carcinoma

The most common, and perhaps most sought-after, oncologic indication for PDT remains BCC. Studies comparing its efficacy against standard therapies, such as cryosurgery, surgical excision or Mohs micrographic surgery, are limited or absent. Early studies of systemic porphyrin-based PDT clearly showed that BCCs do respond (80–100% complete response), but these studies relied upon short-term follow-up and clinical responses. In retrospect, the data may have been overly optimistic and are difficult to interpret accurately[18-20]. The desire to have a successful therapeutic modality as well as the problem of prolonged generalized photosensitivity with systemic photosensitizers has fueled intensive development of more rapidly cleared systemic (e.g. BPD-MA) and topical (ALA, mALA) photosensitizers (see Table 135.1). The latter are highly desirable because of their ease of use and limited adverse effects. Only in recent years have results from larger study groups, with adequate clinical and/or histopathologic follow-up, been published, providing a seasoned view of PDT for BCC.

Table 135.4 outlines the results of selected studies where either systemic or topical photosensitizers were used to treat BCCs. The systemic agents included porfimer sodium, BPD-MA and mTHPC[37-40]

SELECTED STUDIES OF PHOTODYNAMIC THERAPY OF SQUAMOUS CELL CARCINOMA						
Type of study (ref)	No. of patients or lesions	Topical or iv photosensitizer (concentration)	Incubation time	Light source	Response rate	Comments
In situ SCC						
Case series (30)	8 lesions	Porfimer sodium (iv)	48 h	630 nm argon-dye laser at 185–250 J/cm^2	100% at 12 months	• Lesions were either large in size or in difficult-to-treat sites
Case series (6)	6 lesions	ALA (20%)	3–6 h	Filtered red light (600+ nm)	100%	
Prospective single arm (31)	36 lesions	ALA (20%)	3–6 h	Copper vapor laser (630 nm) at 125 or 150 J/cm^2	89% at 18 months	
Prospective single arm (32)	40 large (>2 cm) lesions and 45 'multiple' lesions	ALA (20%)	4 h	Red light (615–645 nm) at 100 J/cm^2	78% (large lesions); 89% (multiple lesions) at 1 year	• Small lesions required 1–2 treatments at 6-week intervals and large lesions 2–3 treatments
Prospective, randomized, comparison with cryo (33)	40 lesions (<2 cm)	ALA (20%)	4 h	Red light (615–645 nm) at 125 J/cm^2 and 70 mW/cm^2	75% [15/20] vs 50% [10/20]	• Cryo was a 20-s freeze–thaw cycle • For complete clearance of non-responding tumors, cryo group required 2–3 more cryo treatments (2 recurrences at 1 year) and PDT-treated group required 1 more PDT treatment (0 recurrences)
Invasive SCC						
Pilot clinical study (34)	32 lesions	Porfimer sodium (iv)	72 h	Red light (630 nm) at 30 J/cm^2	81% at 6 months	• 50% had recurred by 1 year
Case reports (35)	20 lesions in 2 patients	Temoporfin (iv)	96 h	Red laser light (652 nm)	50% at 6 and 14 months	• Immunosuppressed patients
Prospective single arm (36)	12 superficial (<1 mm depth or elevation) 6 nodular (>1 mm) 4 KAs	ALA (20%)	6–8 h	630 nm argon-pumped dye laser at 60–80 J/cm^2	100% KAs 83% superficial 33% nodular at a mean of 29 months	• Treatment was repeated every other day until clinical destruction of tumor • Treatments required: superficial, 1–3; KAs, 2; nodular, 2–6

Table 135.3 Selected studies of photodynamic therapy (PDT) of squamous cell carcinoma (SCC). Unless noted otherwise, each patient received a single PDT treatment. ALA, 5-aminolevulinic acid; cryo, cryotherapy; iv, intravenous; KA, keratoacanthoma.

SELECTED STUDIES OF PHOTODYNAMIC THERAPY OF BASAL CELL CARCINOMA

Type of study (ref)	No. of patients or lesions	Photosensitizer (concentration)	Incubation time	Light source	Response rate	Comments
Systemic photosensitizer						
Prospective, single arm (37)	37 patients (151 lesions: 125 primary; 26 recurrent)	Porfimer sodium (1 mg/kg iv)	48–72 h	Red light (630 nm) at 78–288 J/cm² and 150 mW/cm²	88% at 29 months	• BCCs of the nose and morpheaform BCCs more likely to recur – 36% and 89%, respectively • Moderate local pain
Prospective, randomized (for light dose), multicenter (38)	421 lesions of NMSC (92% BCCs)	BPD-MA (14 mg/m² iv)	1–3 h	Red light (678–698 nm; LED source) at 60, 120 or 180 J/cm²	78% at 6 months based on histology: 69% for 60 J/cm²; 79% for 120 J/cm²; 93% for 180 J/cm²	• Clinical response at 2 years also correlated with fluence – 51% for 60 J/cm²; 79% for 120 J/cm²; 95% for 180 J/cm² • 17% had intolerable pain during irradiation • 72% had post-treatment pain
Prospective, varying light and drug doses (39)	18 patients with 97 lesions	mTHPC (0.1–0.15 mg/kg iv)	96 h	652 nm laser at 5–20 J/cm²	92% at a mean of 14 months	• Lower drug and light doses associated with poorer clinical response
Prospective, varying light and drug doses (40)	5 patients with 187 lesions	mTHPC (0.1 mg/kg iv – maximal response)	48 h	Red light (652 nm) at 15 J/cm² – maximal response	86% at 1 year (with 15 J/cm²)	• Shorter illumination times are needed with mTHPC
Topical photosensitizers						
Prospective single arm (41)	80 lesions (55 superficial, 25 nodular)	ALA (20%)	3–6 h	630 nm laser at 60 J/cm²	100% for superficial, 64% for nodular	• Non-responding nodular BCCs given a second treatment
Prospective, randomized comparison with cryosurgery (42)	83 lesions (44 PDT; 39 cryosurgery)	ALA (20%)	6 h	635 nm laser at 60 J/cm² and 60–100 mW/cm²	70% for PDT at 1 year (74% for cryosurgery)	• Response rate based on both clinical and histologic evaluation • Prior to PDT, crusts, stratum corneum and lipids removed • Cryosurgery consisted of two 25–30-s freeze–thaw cycles with a 2–4-min interval
Prospective, randomized, comparison to excisional surgery with ≥5 mm margins (43)	52 patients (nodular lesions)	mALA under occlusion	3 h	Red light (570–670 nm) at 75 J/cm²	• 91% at 3 months after last PDT treatment (98% for surgical excision) • 83% at 1 year (96% for surgical excision)	• Two PDT treatments 7 days apart • If incomplete response at 3 months, second course of PDT given • Prior to PDT, superficial curettage was performed
Prospective, with varying light doses depending upon histologic subtype (44)	350 lesions (54% were nodular)	mALA (160 mg/g)	4 h (mean)	Filtered red light (570–670 nm) at 64 (superficial), 78 (nodular), 88 (morpheaform) or 100 J/cm² (mixed)	87.5% at 3–6 months (see text for additional details)	• 6% of the tumors had a second PDT treatment • Gentle curettage was performed prior to mALA application
Nevoid basal cell carcinoma syndrome						
Case reports (45)	2 patients (9 superficial; 16 nodular)	ALA (20%; face)	1–5 h	Blue light (417 nm) at 10 J/cm²	89% for superficial, 31% for nodular	• Two courses of treatment, 2–4 months apart • Decrease in new BCCs over 8 months
Case reports (46)	3 children (up to 22% BSA)	ALA (20%) under occlusion	24 h	Red light (633 nm) from an argon-pumped dye laser & filtered tungsten-halogen lamp (590–700 nm)	85–98% clearance at 1.8–6 years	• Large areas were treated over 3 to 6 h, requiring general anesthesia • Individual areas were retreated once or twice • No new BCCs were observed in the follow-up period

Table 135.4 Selected studies of photodynamic therapy (PDT) of basal cell carcinoma (BCC). Unless noted otherwise, each patient received a single PDT treatment. ALA, 5-aminolevulinic acid; BPD-MA, benzporphyrin derivative monoacid ring A; BSA, body surface area; iv, intravenous; LED; light-emitting diode; mALA, methyl-esterified ALA; mTHPC, meta-tetrahydroxyphenylchlorin; NMSC, non-melanoma skin cancer.

(see Table 135.1), while ALA and mALA were the primary topical agents[41,42,43,45]; with one exception, red light (either from coherent or non-coherent sources) was used exclusively. Although response rates were very encouraging with systemic PDT (Fig. 135.6), there were several expected drawbacks, including generalized photosensitivity, facial edema, pain during irradiation (requiring its discontinuation), and post-treatment pain, sometimes necessitating opioid analgesics.

In more than one study, higher doses of the photosensitizer and higher fluences of light were associated with better response rates; use of mTHPC was associated with significantly shorter illumination times.

As noted previously, topical approaches to the photodynamic treatment of BCC have been based almost entirely upon ALA and, more recently, mALA[41–44]. Topical photosensitization for PDT offers the significant clinical advantages of ease of drug delivery and photosensitivity

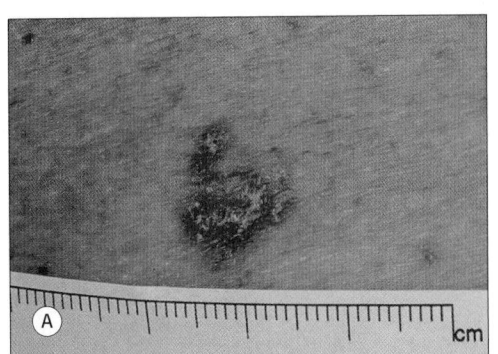
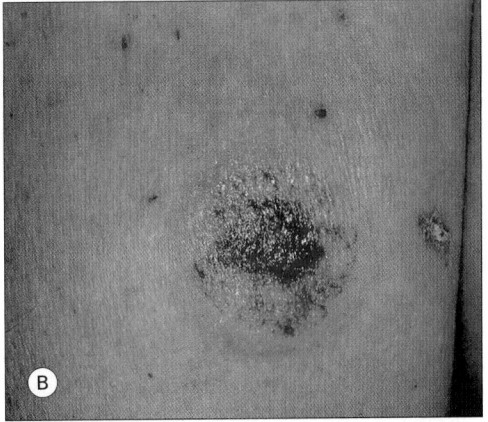
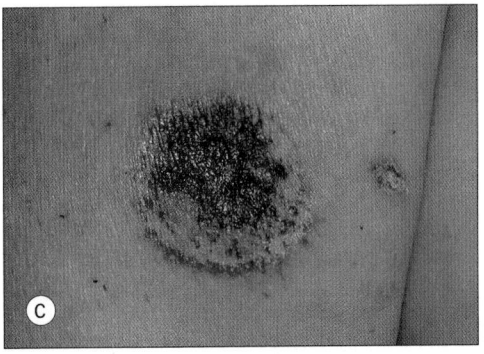
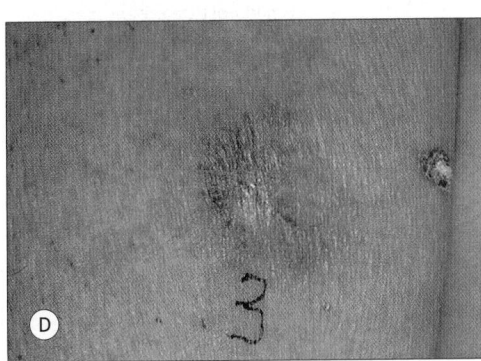
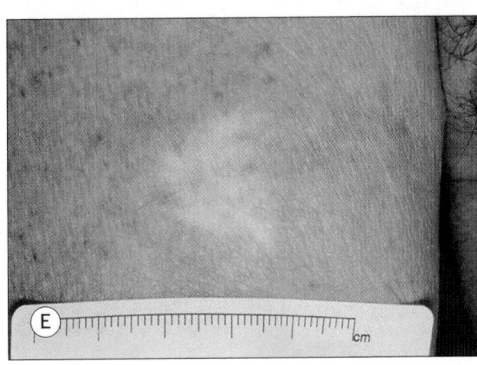

Fig. 135.6 Photodynamic therapy of a nodular basal cell carcinoma (BCC) using intravenous benzoporphyrin derivative monoacid ring A (BPD-MA) plus red light. A Nodular BCC prior to treatment. **B** At 48 hours, early tissue necrosis correlates with pretreatment tumor, with a lesser response in normal surrounding skin. **C** At 9 days, tissue necrosis affects the tumor and some adjacent irradiated skin. Necrotic tissue went on to slough and the resulting superficial ulcer healed. **D** At 3 months, the treatment site shows an erythematous scar. **E** At 2 years, the treatment site has been replaced with a pale soft scar with no evidence of recurrent tumor.

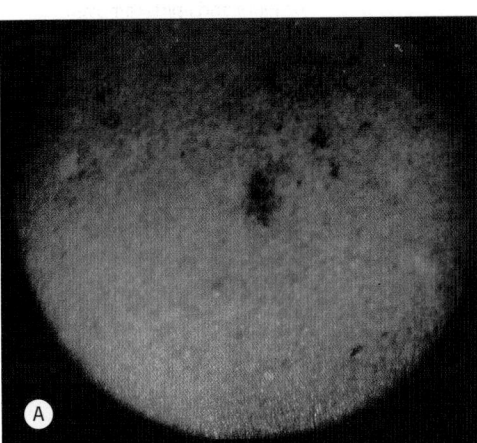
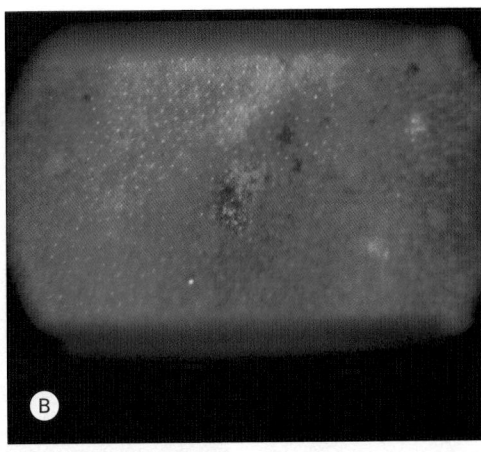
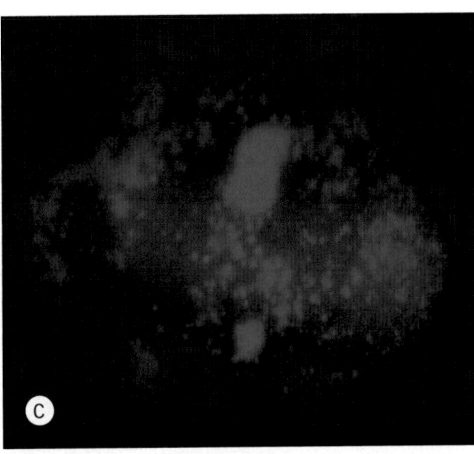

Fig. 135.7 Topical 5-aminolevulinic acid (ALA) photosensitization of a nodular basal cell carcinoma (BCC). A White light image of a nodular BCC after topical ALA application. **B** The same tumor viewed under blue excitation light, revealing pink protoporphyrin IX (PpIX) fluorescence within the BCC and lighter signal in adjacent photodamaged skin. **C** The same tumor viewed using blue excitation light and a red (635 ± 10 nm) filter to reveal only PpIX fluorescence, now seen in the tumor, nearby actinic keratoses and normal hair follicles.

confined to the application site (Fig. 135.7). No generalized photosensitivity occurs because of the limited systemic absorption of ALA or PpIX from the treatment site. Kennedy & Pottier in the late 1980s discovered the rapid uptake of ALA, its conversion to PpIX, and the subsequent catabolism of PpIX, all of which leads to very limited cutaneous photosensitivity. In their early studies, they reported a 79% complete response rate at 3 months for 300 superficial BCCs treated with 20% ALA (applied for 3–6 hours) and then irradiated with filtered red (600+ nm) light[6,7]. Additional clinical trials utilizing *topical* photosensitizers to treat BCCs are outlined in Table 135.4. Response rates for superficial tumors were better than for nodular BCCs. In comparison studies, the cosmetic results from PDT were judged to be superior to either cryosurgery or standard surgical excisions with margins >5 mm.

An attractive feature of topical PDT is the ability to treat relatively large body surface areas with a single intervention, often with a minimal amount of scarring. This is particularly important for patients with familial cancer syndromes, including Gorlin syndrome (nevoid basal cell carcinoma syndrome). Such patients often suffer from multi-tudinous BCCs, which require numerous surgical procedures that over time may result in disfiguring scarring. Both a traditional approach where individual lesions are treated[45] as well as treatment of large surface areas (up to 22% BSA) over 3 to 6 hours (requiring general anesthesia)[46] have been tried in patients with nevoid basal cell carcinoma syndrome (see Table 135.4).

Assuming adequate tissue oxygenation, topical PDT of BCCs may suffer from two potential pitfalls: inadequate drug delivery at depth or inadequate light delivery at depth. In order to examine the two potential problems, a rigorous histologic assessment of topical ALA PDT for non-melanoma skin cancers (eight BCCs, three SCCs *in situ*, two invasive SCCs) was performed[47]. ALA cream 20% was applied for 3 hours to tumors, which were then irradiated with filtered red light (570 nm; 100 J/cm^2; 19–44 mW/cm^2). Tumor responses were judged clinically and then at 3 months, each treatment site was excised and examined histologically for residual tumor. Although 69% (9/13) of the tumors were judged to be clinical cures, only 46% (6/13) of the treated tumors were clear by histopathologic examination. Persistent tumor typically subtended a layer of normal-appearing skin. Because red light penetrates well into the deep dermis, this study strongly suggested that inadequate penetration of topically applied ALA might account for the clinical recurrences of non-melanoma skin cancer following PDT. Using a similar ALA application protocol, tumor-associated PpIX fluorescence was measured spectroscopically and then the tumors were excised just after peak fluorescence[48]. In 6 of 16 tumors, fluorescent microscopic examination clearly showed either a depth-limited pattern of PpIX production or no evident PpIX production. The depth limitation of topical ALA penetration prevented uniform PpIX production to the depth of a significant number of BCCs examined. Drug penetration would be expected to be the least for aggressive-growth (sclerosing, morpheaform, micronodular) BCCs, because these tumors often maintain an intact overlying stratum corneum.

Measures that have been attempted in order to improve the cure rate of BCCs with topical ALA PDT include: curettage to debulk tumor tissue from thick (>2 mm) nodular BCCs just prior to ALA application; pretreatment or admixture with dimethylsulfoxide (DMSO) to enhance penetration of ALA; admixture of ALA with ethylenediaminetetraacetic acid (EDTA) or desferrioxamine to enhance PpIX formation through iron chelation; more prolonged ALA application (up to 48 hours); intralesional infiltration of ALA; and routine use of multiple treatment protocols. All of these manipulations have provided increased long-term cure rates.

Manipulations of administration route and novel topical photosensitizers may well circumvent the drug penetration problem of topical ALA, yet maintain efficacy while minimizing the risk of generalized photosensitivity. In a non-irradiation protocol, we showed complete tumor PpIX fluorescence, even in a morpheaform BCC (Fig. 135.8), after administration of a single *oral* dose of ALA (40 mg/kg)[49]. However, subjects receiving this dose of oral ALA did manifest generalized photo-

sensitivity and nausea lasting more than 24 hours as well as transient elevation of liver enzyme levels for 1–3 weeks. A subsequent pilot treatment trial demonstrated a complete response for BCCs treated with fractionated oral ALA (60 mg/kg delivered in 20 mg/kg increments) and fractionated red light (600–650 nm; 50 or 100 J/cm²) (Fig. 135.9). Although 1 day's photosensitivity still occurred in 1 of 6 subjects, ALA dose fractionation completely prevented the transient liver enzyme elevations seen in the previous study (Tope WD and Cronk JS, unpublished data).

In a different approach, topical delivery of mALA proved effective in treating non-melanoma skin cancer[44]. Methylation removes a negative charge, enhances lipophilicity and, in turn, confers increased penetration. Absorbed within viable cells, mALA is demethylated, allowing the conversion of ALA to PpIX (see Fig. 135.2). Three to 6 months after the initial PDT session, 87.5% (310/350) of the BCCs had responded completely (see Table 135.4 for protocol)[44]. Ninety-three percent of the BCCs received a single treatment session, 6% a second session. In a retrospective review years later (mean 35 months), the initial complete response was confirmed in 277 (89%) treatment sites, with 11% recurring. Of note, both of the morpheaform BCCs recurred after treatment. In this review, mALA performed well, particularly in treating nodular BCCs which might have responded less well to ALA (see above). An added benefit of mALA may be found in reduced treatment pain. ALA may be taken up into peripheral nerve cells via GABA receptors, whereas mALA is not[50].

Mycosis Fungoides/Cutaneous T-Cell Lymphoma

Both systemic porfimer sodium and topical ALA PDT have produced beneficial responses in tumors, plaques and patches of mycosis fungoides

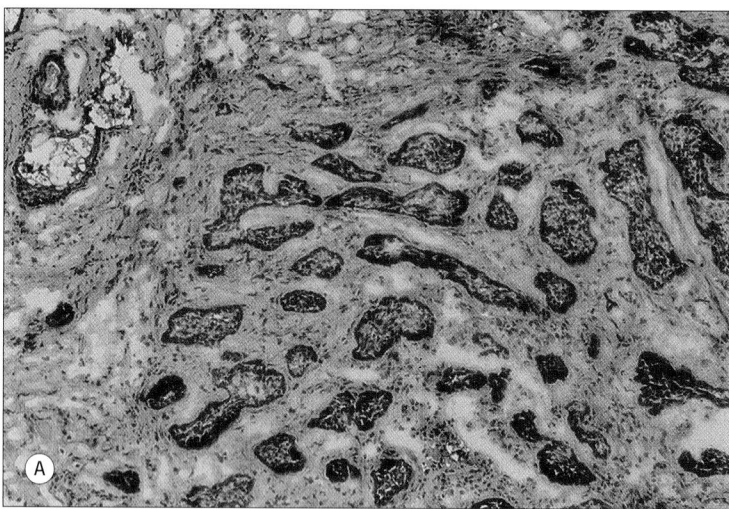
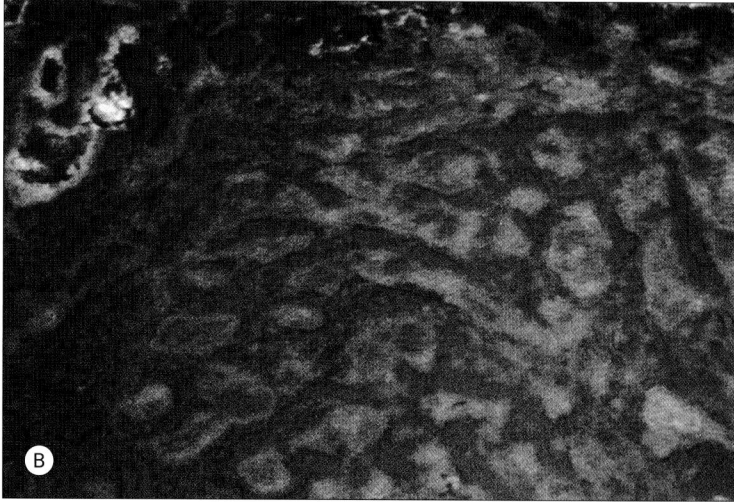

Fig. 135.8 Oral 5-aminolevulinic acid (ALA) photosensitization of basal cell carcinoma (BCC). A Routine light microscopy of an H&E-stained frozen section demonstrates a morpheaform-pattern BCC. **B** The same frozen section examined by fluorescence microscopy shows protoporphyrin IX (PpIX) fluorescence in every tumor island several hours after oral ALA (40 mg/kg).

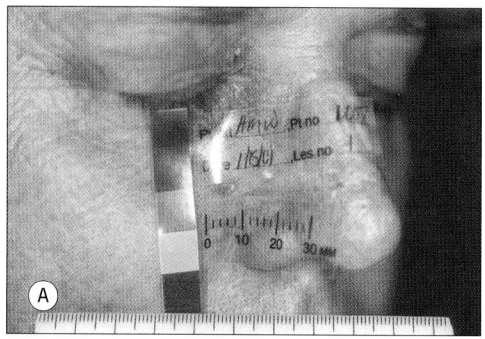
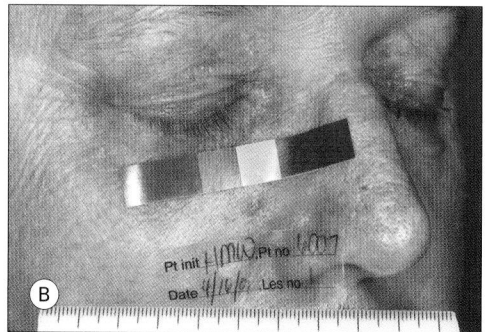
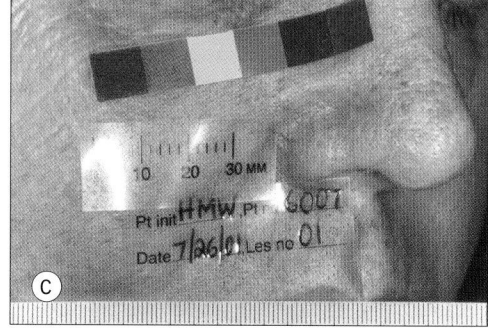

Fig. 135.9 Photodynamic therapy of a superficial basal cell carcinoma (BCC) using oral 5-aminolevulinic acid (ALA) plus red light. BCC prior to treatment (**A**) and then 3 months (**B**) and 6 months (**C**) following photodynamic therapy.

(MF)[18–20]. Topical ALA PDT would seem particularly attractive for MF because activated and malignant T lymphocytes express the transferrin receptor (CD71) at high levels in order to maximize iron absorption. High CD71 expression correlates with low intracellular iron levels, which would facilitate PpIX production; thus, CD71$^+$ status may predict selectivity of ALA PDT for dermatoses associated with activated and malignant T lymphocytes[16]. In one study involving two patients, prolonged remission (8 and 14 months) of MF plaques was observed after multiple (four to five) treatments using topical 20% ALA and filtered red light[51]. Also, lasting complete remissions (6 and 14 months) were noted in two of four cutaneous T-cell lymphoma lesions subjected to multiple ALA PDT sessions[41]. Although these patients appeared to do well, based on the currently limited data, PDT cannot be recommended as first-line therapy for MF; however, PDT might be considered as alternative therapy for resistant lesions. Larger controlled prospective studies should establish the role of PDT for MF.

Melanoma

The responses of cutaneous melanoma have not been sufficiently beneficial to consider PDT a viable option at the present time. Although common sense dictates that melanized cells would be relatively resistant to light-based therapies, lutetium texaphyrin, a photosensitizer activated by very deeply penetrating 752 nm red light, did demonstrate the destruction of subcutaneous melanoma metastases in phase I trials[20]. At present, PDT might only be considered as a final-option, palliative treatment for small cutaneous and subcutaneous metastases of advanced melanoma.

Other Cutaneous Malignancies

At present, only anecdotal evidence is available regarding PDT of uncommon skin tumors, but as the technology develops, broader applications will likely be further investigated. In three HIV-infected patients, Kaposi's sarcoma (KS) was reported to respond to systemic PDT consisting of intravenous indocyanin green (two boluses 30 minutes apart) plus irradiation with an 805 nm diode laser[52]. The lesions irradiated (100 J/cm^2) 10–30 minutes after the last dose of indocyanin green demonstrated complete clearance; those treated at longer time intervals between injection and irradiation showed only a partial response.

In a study of 16 cases of extramammary Paget's disease, 11 of which had received previous treatments (including Mohs micrographic surgery, laser ablation and excision), 8 (50%) showed a complete response at 6 months[53]. However, 3 of these 8 recurred within 1 year, for a durable complete response of 5/16 (31%). In this protocol, topical ALA 20% was applied to axillary and anogenital lesions and occluded for 18–24 hours. Each lesion received red argon pumped dye laser light (632 nm; 200–300 J/cm^2), followed in some cases by further filtered red light (590–700 nm) irradiation.

Port-Wine Stains (Capillary Vascular Malformations)

As noted previously, given the appropriate photosensitizer, PDT has the ability (via LDL receptor-mediated endocytosis) to induce endothelial cell damage and local vascular collapse (see Fig. 135.2). This potential for vascular destruction has led to examination of the use of PDT for the treatment of port-wine stain (PWS) vascular malformations.

In an *in vivo* chick chorioallantoic membrane model, the combined use of PDT plus photothermal pulsed dye laser (PDL) was evaluated as a means of inducing selective vascular damage[54]. Following administration of BPD-MA intraperitoneally into the chick embryos, they were irradiated with a continuous wave argon pumped-dye laser (576 nm), a PDL (585 nm), or both. When compared to control groups (e.g. no intervention, photosensitizer alone) or photosensitizer plus single-source irradiation, PDT plus PDL resulted in significantly more severe vascular damage than any other group, notably 127% more damage than PDT alone and 47% more than PDL alone. This experimental technique, which employed subtherapeutic PDT, followed immediately by PDL irradiation, achieved an improved yet selective vascular injury. In addition, the use of yellow light for both PDT and PDL confined the

therapeutic effects to the upper 1000 µm of the dermis, thus reducing the risk of skin infarction by avoiding destruction of the lower vascular plexus.

Initial clinical studies of PDT alone demonstrated reasonable blanching of PWSs, but the treatment was complicated by the development of skin necrosis when both blue and red light sources were employed[54]. In a series of 118 patients with PWSs[55], one intravenous injection of a purified mixture of six types of porphyrin molecules, followed within 30 minutes by irradiation with a copper vapor laser (578 nm), led to good to excellent clearing in 74% of patients. The highest rate of success was seen in macular PWSs (91.5%). Patients did experience approximately 1 week of severe edema in the treated areas, as well as temporary relative hyperpigmentation, which resolved within 2–6 months. Avoidance of direct sunlight was advised for 2 weeks following PDT, as the photosensitizers used in this study cause photosensitivity for this period of time. Notably, no hypertrophic scarring or permanent pigmentary alteration was reported in this study group.

In one small series[56], PDT, consisting of oral ALA plus PDL, was investigated as a possible treatment for PWSs. Eight patients with non-facial PWSs were administered oral ALA (30 mg/kg), followed by PDL irradiation 1 hour later to one portion of the PWS and 2 hours later to another portion of the PWS. In addition, a portion of each PWS was also treated with PDL alone (7 mm, 6.5 J/cm^2), prior to the administration of ALA. Patients received a total of four treatments given at 4-week intervals. The investigators noted no consistent difference between either of the PDT-treated portions and the PDL-only-treated portion. This lack of efficacy may have been due to one or more of several factors, including the laser pulse duration, the fluence, ALA dose, poor localization of ALA to endothelial cells, or a genuine lack of an additive effect of ALA PDT in combination with PDL (in areas treated with both).

Investigations are ongoing, as PDT has shown to be the only significant alternative to photothermal treatments alone as a means of enhancing the rapidity and degree of PWS improvement.

INFLAMMATORY AND INFECTIOUS DERMATOSES

Psoriasis

In 1937, psoriasis was first reported to respond to PDT consisting of HPD (i.e. porfimer sodium) plus UV light, with seven patients noting a marked improvement[20]. Since then, both systemic (e.g. porfimer, BPD-MA) and topical (ALA) photosensitizers, in combination with visible light, have produced partial or complete clearance of psoriatic plaques. PDT poses an attractive alternative because of the potential for: more rapid clearance of lesions; reduced cumulative exposure to UV irradiation (by using photoactivating doses); and the use of visible light. The latter two factors could reduce the carcinogenic risk, when compared to traditional UV irradiation therapies.

A number of studies have demonstrated the accumulation of PpIX within psoriatic plaques (as well as clinical responses) after the application of *topical* ALA, although the amount and distribution of PpIX within and among plaques have not been consistent[57]. As with ALA photosensitization of BCCs, more uniform production of PpIX within psoriatic plaques may be induced by using *oral* ALA[58]. Currently, oral ALA and BPD-MA appear to be the most attractive *systemic* photosensitizers, based on their rapid clearance and limited photosensitivity, but precise treatment regimens for psoriasis have yet to be established. In addition, while novel *topical* photosensitizers probably offer the safest therapeutic option for limited disease, there is also no reliable topical PDT protocol at this time due to the lack of consistent results.

Acne

Both porphyrin expression by naturally occurring *Propionibacterium acnes* as well as PpIX production occurring primarily within sebaceous glands and hair follicles after topical ALA application have suggested the potential of PDT for diseases of the pilosebaceous unit. Several studies have pointed to the effectiveness of PDT for acne (Table 135.5).

In addition to broadband red light and red light from a diode laser, numerous devices, including pulsed dye (595 nm) lasers, intense pulsed

SELECTED STUDIES OF PHOTODYNAMIC THERAPY FOR THE TREATMENT OF ACNE						
Type of study (ref)	No. of patients	Topical photosensitizer (concentration)	Incubation time	Light source	Response	Comments
Prospective, controlled (59)	22 (posterior trunk acne)	ALA (20%) under occlusion	3 h	Red light (550–700 nm) at 150 J/cm^2	• Only sites treated at least once with PDT showed significant improvement (reduced acne score, sebum production, *P. acnes* porphyrin production) • Multiple treatments enhanced response up to three treatments	• Control groups consisted of red light alone, ALA alone, and no therapy • Half of the patients were treated once and half four times at weekly intervals • Sebaceous glands showed immediate acute damage and were smaller than non-PDT-treated glands for 20 weeks • All PDT-treated sites developed a transient inflammatory folliculitis, beginning at 3–4 days and lasting 1–3 weeks • Adverse effects included erythema, crusting, pain, hyperpigmentation
Prospective single arm (60)	10 (posterior trunk acne)	ALA (20%) under occlusion	3 h	Red light diode laser (635 nm) at 15 J/cm^2 and 25 mW/cm^2	• Reduction in lesion count • No effect on numbers of *P. acnes* or sebum excretion	• Weekly for 3 weeks
Prospective single arm (61)	10 (posterior trunk acne)	Indocyanine green* under occlusion	24 h	Diode laser (810 nm; 4 mm spot size; 50 ms pulses) at 40 J/cm^2	• Short-term improvement and 'encouraging' long-term results at 10 months	• Selective histologic damage to enlarged sebaceous glands
Prospective, varying lasers and incubation times (62)	22 (inflammatory acne of the face and back)	Indocyanine green* under occlusion	5–15 min	Diode laser (803 nm or 809 nm)	• Less inflammation, lesion flattening, and reduction in *P. acnes* and sebum production up to 2 months	• No adverse reactions • Hypothesized to cause both photodynamic and photothermal effects within the pilosebaceous unit

*Peak absorption at 805 nm and preferentially accumulated by sebaceous glands.

Table 135.5 Selected studies of photodynamic therapy (PDT) for the treatment of acne. ALA, 5-aminolevulinic acid.

light (560–1200 nm), BLU-U® (417 nm) and LED sources have been shown to be effective in the treatment of acne, with ALA application times as brief as 15–60 minutes. Success with multiple light sources and delivery modes is testimony to the multiple absorption peaks of PpIX. PDT utilizing topical ALA and mALA (as well as indocyanine green) may well have an increasing role in the treatment of acne, particularly in patients unable or unwilling to undergo isotretinoin therapy. Significant restriction of access to isotretinoin, especially in the US, should fuel the interest in using PDT for papulocystic acne.

Human Papillomavirus Infections

The efficacy of PDT in the treatment of superficial malignancies led investigators to try this modality for treating cutaneous human papillomavirus (HPV) infections[18–20]. Verrucae and condylomata often affect multiple sites, are superficial in nature and difficult to treat, particularly in immunosuppressed individuals. Systemic and topical PDT have led to lesion regression in rabbit models. In addition, some in-vitro studies have pointed to a direct antiviral effect of PDT. As with any cutaneous tumor, *topical* PDT would be preferred for its lesion specificity and limited photosensitivity. In one study, a maximal condylomata:normal skin PpIX fluorescence ratio was detected at 2 hours[63], suggesting that virally infected cells could be preferentially targeted by PDT at this same time point. Lastly, because mucosal lesions (i.e. condylomata) typically do not have associated hyperkeratotic scale (which inhibits drug penetration) and cutaneous lesions (i.e. verrucae) are characteristically keratotic, more variable responses to topical PDT would be anticipated with verrucae.

In a prospective, randomized, double-blind trial, 232 recalcitrant hand and foot warts were treated with six sessions of either ALA PDT or placebo PDT[64]. Both groups also received standard treatment with paring followed by a topical keratolytic. At 18 weeks, both the number of warts cleared and the mean wart area reduction (100% for ALA and

71% for placebo PDT) were significantly superior in the ALA PDT group. The overall high level of improvement in the placebo group testifies to the power of placebo therapy as well as paring and keratolysis, emphasizing the need for carefully designed prospective controlled comparisons in order to determine the proper place for PDT in treating HPV infections. It is also noteworthy that most studies, because they are experimental, select patients whose warts have been recalcitrant to multiple therapies, and the possibility that PDT might perform well as a therapy for uncomplicated or untreated warts could go unconfirmed.

Other Infectious Diseases

A number of studies, utilizing several different photosensitizers and light sources, have demonstrated the antimicrobial activity of PDT. Among the susceptible organisms are bacteria commonly responsible for primary and secondary cutaneous infections, including *Staphylococccus aureus* and *Streptococcus pyogenes*[65].

PDT has also been investigated for the treatment of cutaneous leishmaniasis[66]. In one patient with cutaneous leishmaniasis due to *Leishmania donovani* (diagnosed by clinical and histologic criteria as well as serologic assays), five lesions, recalcitrant to treatment with repeated courses of systemic sodium stibogluconate, were treated with topical mALA PDT. Following application of mALA ointment (20%) under occlusion for 5 hours, the lesions were illuminated with red light (570–670 nm; 75 J/cm^2); this treatment regimen was repeated twice weekly for 12 weeks, and then once weekly for an additional 4 weeks. All treated sites demonstrated clinical clearance with an excellent cosmetic result. Furthermore, three additional lesions in the same patient, previously recalcitrant to treatment with topical paromomycin sulfate, were also successfully treated utilizing the same PDT protocol.

With concerns regarding emerging antibiotic resistance in a variety of organisms, PDT may prove to be a viable alternative for patients

SELECTED STUDIES OF PHOTODYNAMIC THERAPY FOR THE TREATMENT OF PHOTOAGING						
Type of study (ref)	No. of patients	Topical photosensitizer (concentration)	Incubation time	Light source	Response	Comments
Prospective, randomized, varying incubation times (67)	18	ALA (20%) solution	1, 2 or 3 h	Blue light (417 nm) at 10 J/cm²	Improvement in skin quality, fine wrinkling and sallowness of facial skin	• 90% of treated hypertrophic AKs also responded
Prospective, randomized, split-face, with comparison to intense pulsed light (IPL) alone (68)	20	ALA (20%) solution applied twice	30–60 min after an acetone scrub	IPL (515–1200 nm) at 23–28 J/cm² (single pass; 2.4 ms pulse/ 15 ms delay/ 4 ms pulse)	4 weeks after the last treatment, in the ALA IPL PDT group, global photodamage and mottled pigmentation were improved*; fine lines and pigmentation were successfully treated†	• Three treatments at 3-week intervals • All patients received two additional full-face IPL treatments • Contact cooling was used • Blinded observer • ALA IPL PDT vs IPL – similar effects on tactile roughness and sallowness
Case series, varying incubation times and light doses (69)	3 (phototypes I–III)	ALA (20%)	30 or 60 min	IPL (28 J/cm² and 26 J/cm² for skin types I/II and III, respectively)	Possible synergistic photo-rejuvenation due to potentiation of PDT by concomitant hyperthermia, but there were no PDT-alone or radiofrequency-alone controls	• IPL PDT was combined with radiofrequency (20 J/cm²) • Erythema seen with 60-min incubation times but not with 30-min incubation times

*Improved defined as a decrease in score by 1 point (5-point scale).
†Successful treatment defined as a decrease in score to 0 or 1.

Table 135.6 Selected studies of photodynamic therapy (PDT) for the treatment of photoaging. ALA, 5-aminolevulinic acid; AKs, actinic keratoses.

unwilling or unable to undergo conventional antibiotic treatment or who are unresponsive to such therapies.

Photodamage

Recently, the use of topical PDT for the treatment of photodamage has been investigated. Results from several selected studies are outlined in Table 135.6. Depending upon the study, improvements in fine lines, sallowness and mottled pigmentation have been reported. However, assessing subtle improvements in the cutaneous changes associated with photoaging can be difficult and readers often rely on an overall impression based upon clinical photographs; however, the latter have not always been included in the publications[68]. The duration of improvements has yet to be determined and, while the tissue targets responsible for photoaging alterations (e.g. melanocytes, telangiectatic vasculature, elastosis, dyskeratinization) may be known, to date the independent response of each of these targets to photothermal, photodynamic and radiofrequency injury has been only variably described. Further investigations are clearly needed.

PREOPERATIVE CONSIDERATIONS

Before undertaking PDT, the physician must consider various aspects, in particular those related to the condition and the patient being treated. First, the condition to be treated should be one that is likely to respond to PDT. The specific histopathology must be analyzed, taking into account tissue optics, desired photosensitizer localization within the diseased skin, the logistics of light delivery and dosimetry, and PDT responses previously demonstrated in the literature. In the opinion of the authors, a punch biopsy specimen to fat should be obtained in the case of cutaneous tumors in order to determine the associated histologic features. Tumors that are infiltrating, sclerotic, hyperkeratotic or multifocal may not respond well to topical PDT, or they may require multiple treatment sessions. If PDT is an experimental modality for the condition, such as psoriasis or acne, then the clinician should have adequately considered, discussed and utilized other first-line therapies before initiating PDT.

Each subject should be evaluated with clinical exclusion criteria in mind. The preoperative evaluation must seek to discern a history of porphyria or other relevant photosensitivity disorders; documented

allergy to the photosensitizer, similar chemical structures or trace manufacturing agents; the potential impact of sunlight exposure during the expected period of photosensitivity; a history of hepatic disease or concurrent medications subject to hepatic metabolism; and a prior or current herpes simplex virus (HSV) infection in or near the treatment site, especially if there is a history of HSV flares with UV light exposure. Appropriate patients should receive antiviral therapy. Medications known to cause phototoxicity reactions in combination with UV light should not be activated by the visible wavelengths used in PDT. Baseline liver function tests should be obtained prior to systemic photosensitizer administration, particularly in those patients with a history of or suspected hepatic disease.

A general assessment should be made as to whether the patient will be able to tolerate the procedure. Most PDT systems can create painful stimuli, described by patients as ranging from 'warmth' to 'needle pricks' to intense 'burning pain'. Pain reduction during irradiation may be accomplished with local ice packs, cool air, or local anesthetic injection. Local anesthetics should be administered without epinephrine in order to maintain tissue oxygen delivery during irradiation. Every effort should be made to complete the planned irradiation schedule, but pain can be dramatically curtailed by turning off the light source. Currently approved ALA PDT, which utilizes blue light for the treatment of AKs, requires the use of opaque protective goggles as well as placing the face within a relatively confined space illuminated by bright blue light. Some patients may feel 'claustrophobic' or find this a stimulus for a panic attack. The potential patient or caregivers should be evaluated for their ability to provide daily care for the treatment sites. Patients should be carefully advised regarding the risk and duration of local or generalized photosensitivity. Of particular note, UVA/B sunscreens will not protect against photodynamic burns caused by visible wavelengths. Although physical sunscreens (ZnO_2, TiO_2, Fe_2O_3) should provide greater protection into the visible spectrum, patients must be advised to cover up with appropriate clothing, wear protective goggles, and simply avoid bright light from any source.

TECHNIQUE

Before any PDT is undertaken, adequate documentation of the lesions to be treated, a full history and informed consent should be obtained. Preoperative photographs are helpful to adequately assess the result of treatment and to monitor long-term responses in those with multiple lesions. PDT should be carried out in an appropriate clinical setting; it should provide for low light levels (preferably no windows and a dimmer switch or lamp), cooling and ventilating for the heat generated by the light source, and a room whose size is adequate for the necessary equipment. In a large room, floor-to-ceiling opaque black curtains function well to cordon off an area free of unwanted photons. Like any similar situation, the uncomfortable sensations caused by PDT can evoke vasovagal responses. These are largely preventable by instructing patients to eat a moderate meal before therapy, and by prone or supine positioning during intravenous infusions and irradiation.

Topical PDT

This section describes the technique for topical ALA or mALA PDT. The current FDA-approved PDT system for the treatment of AKs incorporates a single-use 20% ALA solution applicator (Levulan® Kerastick®) and a blue (417 nm) non-coherent light source (BLU-U®). The area to be treated may initially be cleansed with acetone to remove sebum and facilitate ALA absorption or subjected to microdermabrasion to remove the stratum corneum. A glass capsule containing the alcoholic diluent is crushed to allow dissolution of the ALA into solution. Care must be taken to achieve a thorough mixture, or an inadequate ALA concentration and consequent PDT effect may result. The sponge applicator is applied thrice to the desired lesions and allowed to dry after each application. The manufacturer estimates that one applicator is adequate for treating up to 250 lesions. Initial incubation times of 18 to 24 hours were previously the norm; however, to reduce associated pain, most practitioners now perform irradiations within 1 to 3 hours after ALA application. The patient wears protective goggles and is positioned within the blue light unit. Irradiation occurs for 16 minutes and 40 seconds. The intensity of pain typically becomes maximal towards the end of the treatment. Distraction using a radio or television and skin cooling using a fan should make the patient more comfortable. If the patient complains of too much discomfort, the therapy can be stopped and continued after a short break. Patients must be able to contact a staff member if they feel discomfort or have a question, and a nurse or the physician should check on the patient occasionally during irradiation. Of note, pulsed light sources complete irradiation more quickly, irradiate small areas, allow inherent rest periods during treatment, and cause less discomfort for patients, but recent work has shown that pulsed light may be less effective than continuous wave sources[9].

Administration of mALA (Metvix®) PDT is similar, except for tumor preparation. Without anesthesia, tumors are gently curetted to remove crusts and the superficial tissue of any bulky lesion. The mALA cream (160 mg/g) is then immediately applied under occlusion for 3 hours. After gently removing the cream with cotton gauze, the patient is positioned an appropriate distance from the light source (CureLight®). This therapy is FDA-approved for non-hyperkeratotic AKs of the face and scalp. The calculated light dose is then delivered using shields to define the treatment area and prevent unnecessary phototoxic reactions in adjacent normal skin. Discomfort during irradiation is handled as discussed above. In a recent study involving 20 patients, topical mALA was shown to be associated with less pain than topical ALA when each was applied to tape-stripped normal forearm skin (for 3 hours under occlusion) and then the sites irradiated with red light (570–670 nm; 70 J/cm²)[50]. Significantly less pain was noted both during and 2 hours after treatment at the mALA-treated site. After PDT with either agent, patients are given post-treatment skin care instructions and released from the clinic.

Systemic PDT

Systemic PDT involves oral or intravenous administration of the drug or prodrug. Porfimer, BPD-MA, SnET2 or mTHPC (see Table 135.1) can be given by a slow, fixed-rate infusion; the time until light application is typically determined with reference to the initiation of the intravenous infusion. When given orally, ALA powder is mixed with orange juice and given either as a single oral bolus or fractionated into 20 mg/kg doses, imbibed hourly. The time until light application is determined with reference to the last oral dose.

The patient should be kept in a low-light room to prevent both acute phototoxicity and photobleaching. Because of their rapid and broad distribution, systemic photosensitizers do require more attention to normal skin shielding during irradiation. Disposable, adhesive-backed foil reflecting paper can be used to define the lesion and perilesional treatment margin; thick opaque card stock also works well. Regional photoprotection can be easily achieved using opaque cloths. Patients are given goggles for ocular protection and instructed to avoid bright light exposure (see below).

Postoperative Care

Immediately after PDT, the treatment sites develop erythema and edema, often leading to a *peau d'orange* appearance. Pain typically reduces dramatically with cessation of irradiation. Postoperative pain is usually easily controlled with acetaminophen or non-steroidal anti-inflammatory drugs, but some individuals may require opioid analgesics. The patients should again be advised how to avoid photosensitivity reactions by covering themselves with clothing. Those receiving systemic agents should use eyewear that blocks the appropriate wavelengths faithfully until the risk of photosensitivity is minimal. It should be noted that a position near a window on a sunny day will cause photo-activation of most photosensitizers.

Wound care requirements depend upon the photosensitizer used and the consequent nature of the photodynamic injury. More superficial epithelial conditions (e.g. AKs, psoriasis, SCCs *in situ*) may crust and then peel, with newly healed skin appearing within 1–2 weeks. With deeper dermal conditions and photosensitizers that cause more vascular injury, treated sites first blister or turn gray, then deeper ulcerative wounds develop requiring more prolonged healing times (weeks to months). Over the next few days, the pain is variable while blistering, crusting, ulceration and eschar formation begin to occur. The pain gradually subsides and unoccluded wounds form eschars, which persist in relation to the depth of photodynamic injury and anatomic site. Patients should keep the wounds moist by applying a topical antibiotic or white petrolatum two to three times a day. Autolytic eschar debridement may be hastened by occlusion with hydrocolloid or film dressings. The frequency of postoperative visits should be based on symptoms and the need to assess wound healing. A 1-week postoperative visit should allow full declaration of wounding and discernment of optimal wound healing requirements. Wound infections may occur, but at no greater frequency than with other wounds healing by second intention. Therefore, unless there is a strong propensity to wound infections, patients should only receive antibiotics for identified infections. Patients with a history of HSV infection should receive antiviral prophylaxis if PDT will be administered to the site of a prior infection or an adjacent area.

ADVERSE EFFECTS AND COMPLICATIONS

The expected and adverse effects of PDT vary with the photosensitizer and light source that are used. With the exception of photosensitivity, most effects related to the therapy itself are common to any destructive therapeutic modality with a similar depth of wounding.

Cutaneous Photosensitivity and Photophobia

The main concern and limitation of systemic administration is prolonged generalized cutaneous photosensitivity, lasting up to 2 or 3 months for porfimer sodium, but as short as several days for BPD-MA or 1 day for oral ALA (Fig. 135.10). The action spectrum for the associated phototoxicity lies within the visible (blue–green and red) portion of the electromagnetic spectrum. Patients must clearly understand that sunscreens that block UV light are ineffective protection. Physical sunscreens (ZnO_2, Fe_2O_3 or TiO_2) and dihydroxyacetone (DHA)-induced 'tans' may provide some protection, but the best option is to cover all skin surfaces with tightly woven dark clothing. This extreme photosensitivity necessitates a lifestyle of sunlight avoidance during the at-risk time period; if this is ignored, the result is a severe cutaneous phototoxic reaction characterized by significant edema, erythema and, occasionally, bullae. Such phototoxic reactions in those

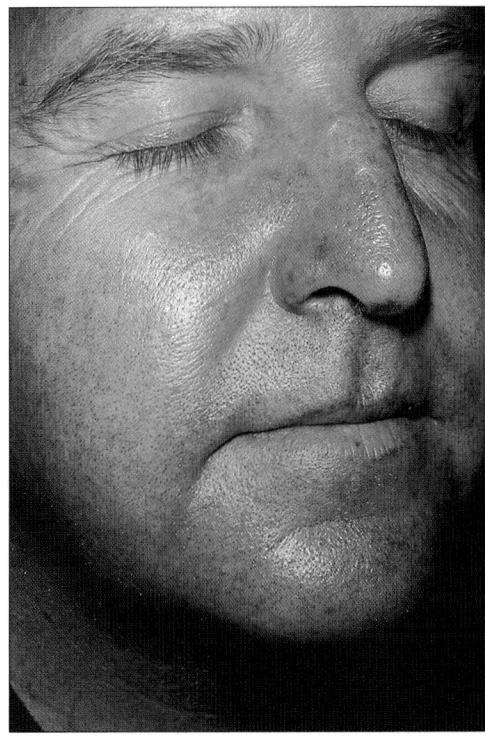

Fig. 135.10 Photosensitivity after oral 5-aminolevulinic acid (ALA). This patient sustained a phototoxic reaction 24 hours earlier by walking in bright sunlight several hours after oral ALA administration. The reaction resolved several days later.

Constitutional Symptoms

Other adverse effects reported during or after systemic PDT include nausea, emesis, headache and flu-like symptoms. Virtually all macrocyclic photosensitizers are subject to hepatic metabolism, and liver toxicity has occurred with HPD (porfimer sodium)[20]. Large (30–40 mg/kg) oral doses of ALA may cause a transient (1–3 weeks), dose-dependent elevation of hepatic enzyme and bilirubin levels[49,58,70]. However, to date there has been no evidence of permanent liver damage or changes in neurologic function or hematologic indices after oral ALA administration at these doses. More recent experience suggests that ALA dose fractionation (20 mg/kg given at hourly intervals) circumvents the elevation of hepatic enzymes.

Local Site Reactions

Immediately after illumination, edema typically develops and may last for several days or longer when facial sites are treated. Significant edema may abate earlier with systemic corticosteroid therapy, if felt to be necessary. With topical PDT, crusting and occasional blistering then occur, followed by slough and healing within a week or so. For systemic PDT, crusting and blistering also occur, but this is followed by necrosis, ulceration and eschar formation. Ulcers heal within 2–8 weeks, depending upon wounding depth, anatomic site and wound care methods. Treatment site pruritus commonly follows both topical and systemic PDT. The frequency of postinflammatory hyperpigmentation depends largely upon Fitzpatrick skin phototype. Treatment sites that develop ulceration typically heal with hypopigmentation and some degree of scarring. In prone anatomic sites, hypertrophic scarring may occur and should be appropriately managed as soon as it is identified. Permanent alopecia may also occur in treated areas.

Allergic Contact Dermatitis

To date, a single case of allergic contact dermatitis has been reported with topical ALA, but not with other topical photosensitizers, and one case of transient urticaria was observed during an HPD infusion[20].

Mutagenic Potential

Although visible light carries no risk of cutaneous carcinogenesis, concern has been raised about the potential genotoxicity of PDT-induced oxygen free radicals. There is one report of melanoma developing within the treatment site after multiple PDT sessions for keratinocytic neoplasia[71]. Although the authors proposed that the immunosuppression caused by PDT might act as a tumor promoter, the location of the treatment site within a heavily sun-exposed area makes the association more likely fortuitous. An *in vitro* sister chromatid exchange assay was used to evaluate the effects of zinc phthalocyanine PDT and no differences were found as compared with untreated controls, suggesting that PDT did not produce cell death through chromosomal damage[72]. The current data suggest that there is no increased risk of secondary tumors[73], thus offering the advantage of repeated treatments.

FUTURE DIRECTIONS

PDT brings biotechnology companies together with a broad range of basic and clinical scientists. The future of this highly promising diagnostic and therapeutic technique will depend upon the intricate relationship between technology and clinical medicine. Clinicians should expect advances in light delivery (automated sources with real-time monitoring of dosimetry), photosensitizer development (e.g. indium methyl pyropheophorbide, a chlorin derivative capable of topical delivery), basic research to elucidate in detail the mechanism of photodynamic action *in vivo*, and clinical research to establish the safety and efficacy of new photosensitizers as well as to compare proven photosensitizers against standard therapies. In addition to the indications previously discussed, there will be ongoing evaluation of the role of PDT in the treatment of pilosebaceous tumors, lichen planus, morphea, port-wine stain vascular malformations and hirsutism ('photodynamic tricholysis'), to name just a few.

with Fitzpatrick phototypes III–VI may resolve as a 'photodynamic tan' which is deep and persistent. Patients should also avoid any intense visible light source, such as phototherapy units, tanning beds, bright medical examination lamps, operating theater lights or pulse oximeters. Low indoor lighting is usually not sufficient to trigger a reaction. Ocular protection is particularly important after systemic photosensitizer administration. A few patients may report photophobia after receiving systemic photosensitizers, but the duration is usually less than for the cutaneous photosensitivity.

Phototoxic reactions to systemic ALA are characterized by mild to moderate erythema and edema followed by desquamation 48–72 hours later. Phototoxic reactions secondary to BPD-MA or porfimer begin as rapidly, but resolve more slowly. Topical photosensitizer delivery will usually not lead to sufficient systemic absorption to cause a generalized photosensitivity reaction. Even local photosensitivity due to topical photosensitizer application is rare, but can occur and should be prevented by opaque clothing or dressings. PDT has been reported to reactivate photosensitive conditions such as lupus, and the Koebner phenomenon was described after PDT treatment of a superficial SCC in a patient with psoriasis[18–20].

Pain

This is the most commonly reported side effect of PDT and it can vary from a slight ache to severe pain. The degree of pain experienced will vary from patient to patient and depends on the size and anatomic site of the lesion being treated as well as the particular photosensitizer. For example, a comparative study of mALA versus ALA found that the associated pain was less severe with mALA, and the explanation was greater absorption of ALA by cutaneous nerves[50]. Uniform application of topical photosensitizers (and light) to large treatment fields usually results in significant (7–10/10) pain. However, this pain has been dramatically reduced with the current practice of using 1- to 3-hour incubation times for topical PDT. During the irradiation, discomfort can be alleviated by cool air fans, ice packs placed around the treatment field, pretreatment narcotic analgesics, intradermal anesthetic injections, or cessation of light application; in general, topical anesthetics are not sufficient. More specific measures may become available in the future as the mediators of the associated pain become known. Post-treatment pain should be managed with appropriate levels of analgesia.

REFERENCES

1. Daniell MD, Hill JS. A history of photodynamic therapy. Aust NZ J Surg. 1991;61:340–8.
2. Dougherty TJ. A brief history of clinical photodynamic therapy development at Roswell Park Cancer Institute. J Clin Laser Med Surg. 1996;14:219–22.
3. Ackroyd R, Kelty C, Brown N, Reed M. The history of photodetection and photodynamic therapy. Photochem Photobiol. 2001;74;656–69.
4. Meyer-Betz F. Untersuchungen uber die biologische (photodynamische) Wirkung des Hamatoporphyrins und anderer Derivate des Blut- und Gallenfarbstoffs. Dtsch Arch Klin Med. 1913;112:476–503.
5. Lipson RL, Baldes EJ. The photodynamic properties of a particular hematoporphyrin derivative. Arch Dermatol. 1960;82:508–16.
6. Kennedy JS, Pottier RH, Pross DC. Photodynamic therapy with endogenous protoporphyrin IX: basic principles and present clinical experience. J Photochem Photobiol B. 1990;6:143–8.
7. Kennedy JS, Pottier RH. Endogenous protoporphyrin IX, a clinically useful photosensitizer for photodynamic therapy. J Photochem Photobiol B. 1992;14:275–92.
8. Fuchs J, Thiele J. The role of oxygen in cutaneous photodynamic therapy. Free Radic Biol Med. 1998;24:835–47.
9. Strasswimmer J, Grande DJ. Do pulsed lasers produce an effective photodynamic therapy response? Lasers Surg Med. 2006;38:22–5.
10. Jori G. Low-density lipoproteins-liposome delivery systems for tumor photosensitizers *in vivo*. In: Henderson BW, Dougherty TJ (eds). Photodynamic Therapy: Basic Principles and Clinical Applications. New York: Marcel Dekker, 1992:173–86.
11. Dubbelmann TMAR, Prinsze C, Penning LC, van Steveninck J. Photodynamic therapy: membrane and enzyme physiology. In: Henderson BW, Dougherty TJ (eds). Photodynamic Therapy: Basic Principles and Clinical Applications. New York: Marcel Dekker, 1992:37–46.
12. Kessel D, Castelli M. Evidence that bcl-2 is the target of three photosensitizers that induce a rapid apoptotic response. Photochem Photobiol. 2001;74:318–22.
13. Zhou CN. Mechanisms of tumor necrosis induced by photodynamic therapy. J Photochem Photobiol B. 1989;3:299–318.
14. Simkin GO, Tao JS, Levy JG, Hunt DW. IL-10 contributes to the inhibition of contact hypersensitivity in mice treated with photodynamic therapy. J Immunol. 2000;164:2457–62.
15. Musser DA, Oseroff AR. Characteristics of the immunosuppression induced by cutaneous photodynamic therapy: persistence, antigen specificity and cell type involved. Photochem Photobiol. 2001;73:518–24.
16. Rittenhouse-Diakun K, Van Leengoed H, Morgan J, et al. The role of transferring receptor (CD71) in photodynamic therapy of activated and malignant lymphocytes using the heme precursor delta-aminolevulinic acid (ALA). Photochem Photobiol. 1995;61:523–8.
17. Oseroff A. PDT as a cytotoxic agent and biological response modifier: implications for cancer prevention and treatment in immunosuppressed and immunocompetent patients. J Invest Dermatol. 2006;126:542–4.
18. Fritsch C, Goerz G, Ruzicka T. Photodynamic therapy in dermatology. Arch Dermatol. 1998;134:207–14.
19. Lui H, Bissonnette R. Photodynamic therapy. In: Goldman MP, Fitzpatrick RE (eds). Cutaneous Laser Surgery: the Art and Science of Selective Photothermolysis. St Louis: Mosby, 1999:437–58.
20. Kalka K, Merk H, Mukhtar H. Photodynamic therapy in dermatology. J Am Acad Dermatol. 2000;42:389–413.
21. Jeffes EW, McCullough JL, Weinstein GD, et al. Photodynamic therapy of actinic keratosis with topical 5-aminolevulinic acid. A pilot dose-ranging study. Arch Dermatol. 1997;133:727–32.
22. Kurwa HA, Yong-Gee SA, Seed PT, Markey AC, Barlow RJ. A randomized paired comparison of photodynamic therapy and topical 5-fluorouracil in the treatment of actinic keratoses. J Am Acad Dermatol. 1999;41:414–18.
23. Jeffes EW, McCullough JL, Weinstein GD, et al. Photodynamic therapy of actinic keratoses with topical aminolevulinic acid hydrochloride and fluorescent blue light. J Am Acad Dermatol. 2001;45:96–104.
24. Dragieva G, Hafner J, Dummer R, et al. Topical photodynamic therapy in the treatment of actinic keratoses and Bowen's disease in transplant recipients. Transplantation. 2004;77:115–21.
25. Ruiz-Rodriguez R, Sanz-Sanchez T, Cordoba S. Photodynamic photorejuvenation. Dermatol Surg. 2002;28:742–4.
26. Szeimies RM, Karrer S, Radakovic-Fijan S, et al. Photodynamic therapy using topical methyl 5-aminolevulinate compared with cryotherapy for actinic keratoses: a prospective, randomized study. J Am Acad Dermatol. 2002;47:258–62.
27. Lam M, Oleinick NL, Nieminen AL. Photodynamic therapy-induced apoptosis in epidermoid carcinoma cells. Reactive oxygen species and mitochondrial inner membrane permeabilization. J Biol Chem. 2001;276:47379–86.
28. de Graff YGL, Kennedy C, Wolterbeek R, et al. Photodynamic therapy does not prevent cutaneous squamous cell carcinoma in organ transplant recipients: results of a randomized-controlled trial. J Invest Dermatol. 2006;126:569–74.
29. Stender IM, Wulf HC. Photodynamic therapy with 5-aminolevulinic acid in the treatment of actinic cheilitis. Br J Dermatol. 1996;135:454–6.
30. Jones CM, Mang T, Cooper M, et al. Photodynamic therapy in the treatment of Bowen's disease. J Am Acad Dermatol. 1992;27:979–82.
31. Cairnduff F, Stringer MR, Hudson EJ, et al. Superficial photodynamic therapy with topical 5-aminolaevulenic acid for superficial primary and secondary skin cancer. Br J Cancer. 1994;69:605–8.
32. Morton CA, Whitehurst C, McColl JH, et al. Photodynamic therapy for large or multiple patches of Bowen disease and basal cell carcinoma. Arch Dermatol. 2001;137:319–24.
33. Morton CA, Whitehurst C, Moseley H, et al. Comparison of photodynamic therapy with cryotherapy in the treatment of Bowen's disease. Br J Dermatol. 1996;135:766–71.
34. Pennington DG, Waner M, Knox A. Photodynamic therapy for multiple skin cancers. Plast Reconstr Surg. 1988;82:1067–71.
35. Dilkes MG, DeJode ML, Rowntree-Taylor A, et al. m-THPC photodynamic therapy for head and neck cancer. Lasers Med Sci. 1996;11:23–9.
36. Calzavara-Pinton PG. Repetitive photodynamic therapy with topical d-aminolevulinic acid as an approach to the routine treatment of superficial non-melanoma skin tumors. J Photochem Photobiol B. 1995;29:53–7.
37. Wilson BD, Mang TS, Stoll H, et al. Photodynamic therapy for the treatment of basal cell carcinoma. Arch Dermatol. 1996;128:1597–601.
38. Lui H, Hobbs L, Tope WD, et al. Photodynamic therapy of non-melanoma skin cancers with verteporfin and red light. Lasers Surg Med. 2001;29(S13):9.
39. Kubler AC, Haase T, Staff C, et al. Photodynamic therapy of primary nonmelanomatous skin tumours of the head and neck. Lasers Surg Med. 1999;25:60–8.
40. Baas P, Saarnak AE, Oppelaar H, et al. Photodynamic therapy with meta-tetrahydroxyphenylchlorin for basal cell carcinoma: a phase I/II study. Br J Dermatol. 2001;145:1–2.
41. Svanberg K, Andersson T, Killander D, et al. Photodynamic therapy of non-melanoma malignant tumors of the skin using topical d-amino levulinic acid sensitization and laser irradiation. Br J Dermatol. 1994;130:743–51.
42. Wang I, Bendsoe N, Klinteberg CAF, et al. Photodynamic therapy vs. cryosurgery of basal cell carcinomas: results of a phase III clinical trial. Br J Dermatol. 2001;144:832–40.
43. Rhodes LE, de Rie M, Enstrom Y, et al. Photodynamic therapy using topical methyl aminolevulinate vs surgery for nodular basal cell carcinoma. Arch Dermatol. 2004;140:17–23.
44. Soler AM, Warloe T, Berner A, Giercksky KE. A follow-up study of recurrence and cosmesis in completely responding superficial and nodular basal cell carcinomas treated with methyl 5-aminolevulinate-based photodynamic therapy alone and with prior curettage. Br J Dermatol. 2001;145:467–71.
45. Itkin A, Gilchrest BA. Delta-aminolevulinic acid and blue light photodynamic therapy for treatment of multiple basal cell carcinomas in two patients with nevoid basal cell carcinoma syndrome. Dermatol Surg. 2004;30:1054–61.
46. Oseroff AR, Shieh S, Frawley NP, et al. Treatment of diffuse basal cell carcinomas and basaloid follicular hamartomas in nevoid basal cell carcinoma syndrome by wide-area 5-aminolevulinic acid photodynamic therapy. Arch Dermatol. 2005;141:60–7.
47. Lui H, Salasche S, Kollias N, et al. Photodynamic therapy of nonmelanoma skin cancer with topical aminolevulinic acid: a clinical and histologic study. Arch Dermatol. 1995;131:737–8.
48. Martin A, Tope WD, Grevelink JM, et al. Lack of selectivity of protoporphyrin IX fluorescence for basal cell carcinoma after topical application of 5-aminolevulinic acid: implications for photodynamic treatment. Arch Dermatol Res. 1995;287:665–74.
49. Tope WD, Ross EV, Kollias N, et al. Protoporphyrin IX fluorescence induced in basal cell carcinoma by oral delta-aminolevulinic acid. Photochem Photobiol. 1998;67:249–55.
50. Wiegell SR, Stender IM, Na R, Wulf HC. Pain associated with photodynamic therapy using 5-aminolevulinic acid or 5-aminolevulinic acid methylester on tape-stripped normal skin. Arch Dermatol. 2003;139:1173–7.
51. Wolf P, Fink-Puches R, Kerl H. Photodynamic therapy for mycosis fungoides after topical photosensitization with 5-aminolevulinic acid. J Am Acad Dermatol. 1995;33:541 (letter).
52. Abels C, Karrer S, Baumler W, et al. Indocyanine green and laser light for the treatment of AIDS-associated cutaneous Kaposi's sarcoma. Br J Cancer. 1998;77:1021–4.
53. Shieh S, Dee AS, Cheney RT, et al. Photodynamic therapy for the treatment of extramammary Paget's disease. Br J Dermatol. 2002;146:1000–5.
54. Kelly KM, Kimel S, Smith T, et al. Combined photodynamic and photothermal induced injury enhances damage to in vivo model blood vessels. Lasers Surg Med. 2004;34:407–13.
55. Xiao-xi L, Wei W, Shuo-fan W, et al. Treatment of capillary vascular malformation (port wine stains) with photochemotherapy. Plast Reconstr Surg. 1997;99:1826–30.
56. Evans AV, Robson A, Barlow J, Kurwa H. Treatment of port wine stains with photodynamic therapy using pulsed dye laser as a light source, compared with pulse dye laser alone: a pilot study. Lasers Surg Med. 2005;36:266–9.
57. Robinson DJ, Collins P, Stringer MR, et al. Improved response of plaque psoriasis after multiple treatments with topical 5-aminolaevulinic acid photodynamic therapy. Acta Dermatol Venereol. 1999;79;451–5.
58. Bissonnette R, Zeng H, McLean DI, et al. Oral aminolevulinic acid induces protoporphyrin IX fluorescence in psoriatic plaques and peripheral blood cells. Photochem Photobiol. 2001;74:339–45.
59. Hongcharu W, Taylor CR, Chang Y, et al. Topical ALA-photodynamic therapy for the treatment of acne vulgaris. J Invest Dermatol. 2000;115:183–92.
60. Pollock B, Turner D, Stringer MR, et al. Topical aminolevulinic acid-photodynamic therapy for the treatment of acne vulgaris: a study of clinical efficacy and mechanism of action. Br J Dermatol. 2004;151:616–22.
61. Lloyd JR, Mirkov M. Selective photothermolysis of the sebaceous glands for acne treatment. Lasers Surg Med. 2002;31:115–20.
62. Tuchin VV, Genina EA, Bashkatov AN, et al. A pilot study of ICG laser therapy of acne vulgaris: photodynamic and photothermolysis treatment. Lasers Surg Med. 2003;33:296–310.
63. Ross EV, Romero R, Kollias N, et al. Selectivity of protoporphyrin IX fluorescence for condylomata after topical application of 5-aminolaevulinic acid: implications for photodynamic treatment. Br J Dermatol. 1997;137:736–42.
64. Stender IM, Na R, Fogh H, et al. Photodynamic therapy with 5-aminolaevulinic acid or placebo for recalcitrant hand and foot warts: randomized double-blind trial. Lancet. 2000;355:963–6.
65. Maisch T, Szeimies RM, Jori G, Abels C. Antibacterial photodynamic therapy in dermatology. Photochem Photobiol Sci. 2004;3:907–17.
66. Gardlo K, Horska Z, Enk CD, et al. Treatment of cutaneous leishmaniasis by photodynamic therapy. J Am Acad Dermatol. 2003;48:893–6.
67. Touma DJ, Gilchrest BA. Topical photodynamic therapy: a new tool in cosmetic dermatology. Semin Cutan Med Surg. 2003;22:124–30.
68. Dover JS, Bhatia AC, Stewart B, Arndt KA. Topical 5-aminolevulinic acid combined with intense pulsed light

in the treatment of photoaging. Arch Dermatol. 2005;141:1247–52.

69. Hall JA. Keller PJ, Keller GS. Dose response of combination photorejuvenation using intense pulsed light-activated photodynamic therapy and radiofrequency energy. Arch Facial Plast Surg. 2004;6:374–8.

70. Webber J, Kessel D, Fromm D. Side effects and photosensitization of human tissues after aminolevulinic acid. J Surg Res. 1997;68:31–7.

71. Wolf P, Fink-Puches R, Reimann-Weber A, Kerl H. Development of malignant melanoma after repeated topical photodynamic therapy with 5-aminolevulinic acid at the exposed site. Dermatology. 1997;194:53–4.

72. Halkiotis K, Yova D, Pantelias G. *In vitro* evaluation of the genotoxic and clastogenic potential of photodynamic therapy. Mutagenesis. 1999;14:193–8.

73. Fuchs J, Weber S, Kaufmann R. Genotoxic potential of porphyrin type photosensitizers with particular emphasis on 5-aminolevulinic acid: implications for clinical photodynamic therapy. Free Radic Biol Med. 2000;28:537–48.

Principles of Laser–Skin Interactions

Ranella J Hirsch, Tomi L Wall, Mathew M Avram and R Rox Anderson

PHYSICAL TREATMENT MODALITIES

Synonym: ■ LASER – light amplification by stimulated emission of radiation

Key features

- Laser surgery works by precise tissue heating, which occurs when optical energy is absorbed within the skin
- Heat is created within skin where light is absorbed by molecules called chromophores
- The major skin chromophores for visible and near-infrared light are melanin and hemoglobins. Water is the major chromophore for the far-infrared spectrum
- Red and near-infrared wavelengths are deeply penetrating, due to reduced absorption and scattering
- Wavelength(s) of lasers or intense pulsed light (IPL) sources are often matched for absorption by chromophores in skin targets such as blood vessels, hair follicles, melanin-containing cells, tattoo ink or tissue layers
- Selective heating and damage of targets can occur when a pulse of selectively absorbed light is delivered faster than the targets can cool by heat conduction
- The time for a tissue target to cool is its thermal relaxation time, equal in seconds to approximately the square of the target size in millimeters
- Very short (nanosecond) laser pulses, produced by Q-switched lasers, can precisely damage small targets such as individual melanocytes
- Millisecond lasers and IPLs selectively affect multicellular targets such as blood vessels, hair follicles and tissue layers
- Fractional laser treatments use precise microscopic patterns of thermal injury for skin treatment
- Laser microscopy of live, intact skin is an emerging diagnostic tool for dermatology

INTRODUCTION

Modern dermatology is inextricably linked to photomedicine, which includes all diagnostic and therapeutic uses of light. The last century took us from Einstein's insight into the quantum nature of light, to the invention of the ruby laser in 1960, to the wide spectrum of lasers available today. In particular, the principle of selective photothermolysis guided the development of pulsed lasers that target specific skin structures such as blood vessels, melanosomes and hair follicles. Laser dermatology is a dynamic field and a steady source of therapeutic innovation. Its applications are broad and include soft tissue ablation as well as the treatment of vascular lesions, tattoos, pigmented lesions, hirsutism, and photoaged skin. Lasers are also the preferred treatment for a variety of medical conditions affecting other organs such as the eyes. Recent advances in light-activated drug therapy and laser-based diagnostics are promising.

LASERS

LASER is an acronym for *light amplification by stimulated emission of radiation*, which describes the physical process by which a laser produces light[1]. Lasers are unique light sources rooted in the process of stimulated emission. A discussion of laser principles begins with Einstein's formulation of principles of electromagnetic radiation[2]. Electromagnetic radiation is a basic form of energy that can exhibit both wave and particle properties. A quantum of electromagnetic energy called a photon can stimulate an excited atom to emit another photon with the same energy. The resultant photons have equal energy and wavelength and are in phase (temporal and spatial). In 1960, Maiman observed stimulated emission of red light in a flashlamp-excited ruby crystal[3]. Later that decade, Leon Goldman became the first physician to utilize a laser on humans, initiating dermatologic application of laser technology.

All laser systems are composed of four essential components (Figs 136.1 & 136.2):
- a gas, liquid or solid medium (Table 136.1) that can be excited to generate laser light by stimulated emission
- a source of energy to excite the medium ('pumping system')
- mirrors at the ends of the laser, forming the 'optical cavity' that surrounds the medium and confines the amplification process
- a delivery system.

Population inversion occurs when greater than half of the atoms within the laser medium are excited by the energy source; this is a prerequisite for a laser to function. With population inversion, photons traveling in the laser medium are more likely to encounter an excited atom (leading to stimulated emission) than a resting atom that can simply absorb the light. As light travels back and forth between the laser's mirrors, very high intensity can be achieved.

Laser light possesses several properties (monochromicity, coherence, collimation and high intensity) that differentiate it from other light

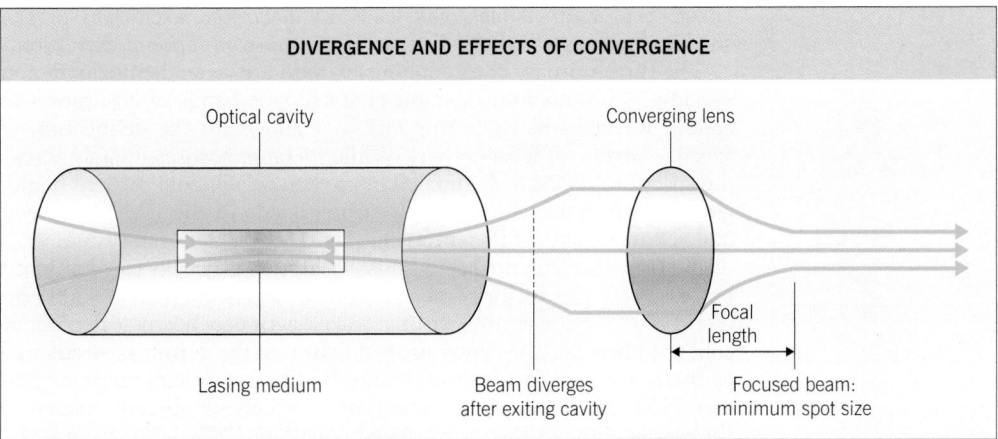

DIVERGENCE AND EFFECTS OF CONVERGENCE

Optical cavity

Converging lens

Lasing medium

Beam diverges after exiting cavity

Focal length

Focused beam: minimum spot size

Fig. 136.1 Divergence and effects of convergence. Lasers produce beams of light with low divergence (spread) as the beam travels. Low divergence allows the beam to be tightly focused by a converging lens or mirror. Laser focusing is used in dermatology for confocal microscopy and for 'fractional' treatments (which stimulate responses to an array of small thermal injury zones).

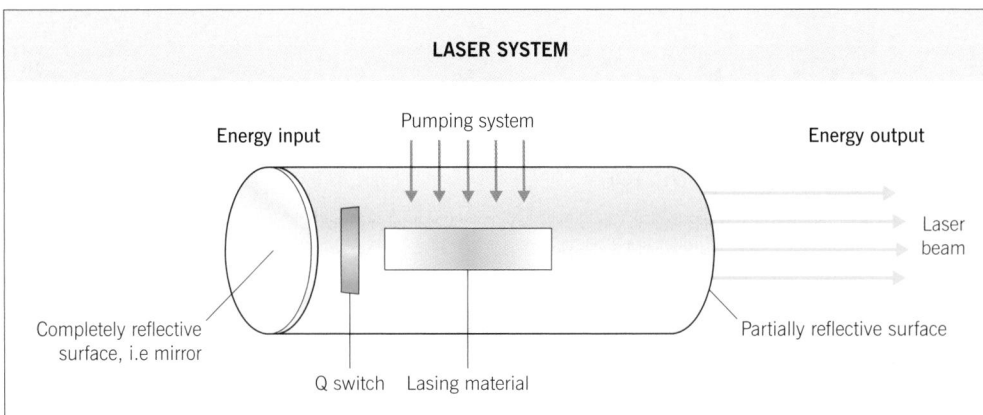

LASER SYSTEM

Fig. 136.2 Laser system. The pumping system stimulates the lasing medium to emit photons. The mirrors at the ends of the cavity reflect this light back and forth along one axis, leading to amplification of the stimulated emission process. One of the mirrors is only partially reflective, allowing the laser light to exit.

Gas	Liquid	Solid
Argon	Rhodamine dye	Crystal
Carbon dioxide	dissolved in	• Alexandrite
Copper vapor	organic solvent[†]	• Erbium-doped yttrium aluminum garnet (YAG)
Helium–neon		• Holmium-doped YAG
Krypton		• Neodymium-doped YAG
Xenon chloride*		• Potassium titanyl phosphate
		• Ruby
		Semiconductor
		• Diode (e.g. aluminium gallium arsenide)

TYPES OF LASER MEDIA

*In excimer lasers.
[†]In pulsed dye lasers.

Table 137.1 Types of laser media. Lasers are often named for the medium contained within their optical cavity.

sources[4]. Monochromicity refers to the emission of only one wavelength or a very narrow band of wavelengths. Coherence describes light waves that travel in phase, both in time and space, similar to a column of soldiers marching in step (Fig. 136.3). Coherence allows lasers to be focused to spot sizes as narrow as the wavelength itself. Collimation refers to the parallel nature and lack of divergence of the coherent light

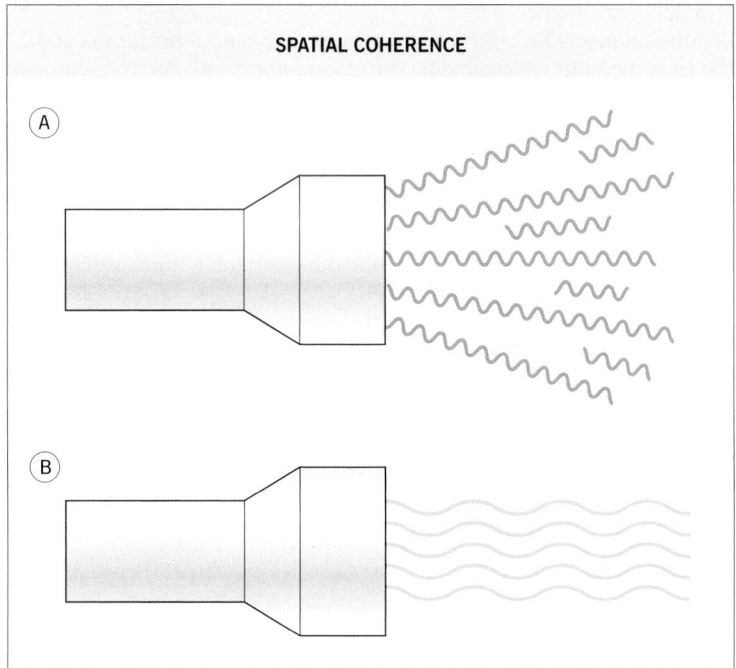

SPATIAL COHERENCE

Ⓐ

Ⓑ

Fig. 136.3 Spatial coherence. A Portable flashlight emitting non-coherent light. **B** Laser emitting coherent light, with waves that are in phase and parallel (collimated).

waves. Laser beams can travel over long distances without significant loss of intensity.

Laser light can be delivered in continuous and pulsed waves. In continuous-wave mode, lasers produce a constant beam of light. Argon lasers are an example of this type of laser. These lasers usually have a limited peak power, whereas high peak powers can be achieved by pulsing a laser over a short time period[5]. Q-switched lasers produce very short pulses at very high peak power. 'Q' refers to a quality factor of energy storage in the lasing medium, which is changed suddenly to produce a short, intense burst of light. The repetition rate for pulsed lasers is expressed in hertz (Hz). Some lasers emit a rapid train of low-energy pulses that behave surgically like continuous-wave lasers and are called quasicontinuous.

Dermatologic Q-switched lasers are designed to produce pulses of 10–100 ns, with fluence (energy density) typically in the 2–10 joules $(J)/cm^2$ range. These short, high-power pulses are particularly useful for selective removal of tattoos and pigmented lesions[6].

SKIN OPTICS

Laser light interacts with the skin in four principal ways: reflection, scattering, transmission and absorption (Fig. 136.4). As a beam of light strikes the skin surface, 4–7% is reflected because of the difference in the refractive indices of air ($n = 0$) and stratum corneum ($n = 1.45$)[7]. This is termed the Fresnel reflectance because it follows Fresnel's equations relating reflectance to the angle of incidence (least reflectance with perpendicular incident light) and plane of polarization as well as refractive index[8]. The remaining 93–96% of incident light enters the skin, where it is scattered, transmitted or absorbed. Scattering occurs when particles within the skin spread the incoming beam of light in all directions, limiting its depth of penetration. Light is transmitted when it passes through the tissue unaltered.

In general, tissue effects occur only when light is absorbed. The absorption coefficient is defined as the probability per unit path length that a photon at a particular wavelength will be absorbed, and it depends on the concentration of chromophores (absorbing molecules) present. When absorption occurs, the photon surrenders its energy to the chromophore. Once absorbed by the chromophore, the photon ceases to exist and the chromophore becomes excited. Absorption of ultraviolet (UV) and visible light leads to *electronic* excitation of the chromophore. Infrared (IR) light tends to cause *vibrational* excitation.

The three primary chromophores in skin are water, hemoglobin and melanin. Chromophores exhibit characteristic bands of absorption at certain wavelengths. It is this fact that allows for the delineation of specific targets for laser activity. While melanin absorbs broadly across the spectrum, blood is dominated by oxyhemoglobin and reduced hemoglobin absorption, which exhibit strong bands in the UV, blue, green and yellow regions of the spectrum (Fig. 136.5).

In normally pigmented epidermis, absorption is usually the dominant process over the majority of the optical spectrum (200–10 000 nm) (Fig. 136.6). In the dermis, strong, wavelength-dependent scattering by collagen fibers occurs. Penetration of light into the dermis is attenuated by this scattering, which varies inversely with wavelength. Between 280 and 1300 nm, the depth of penetration is generally directly related to the wavelength; in this broad region covering UVB, UVA, visible and

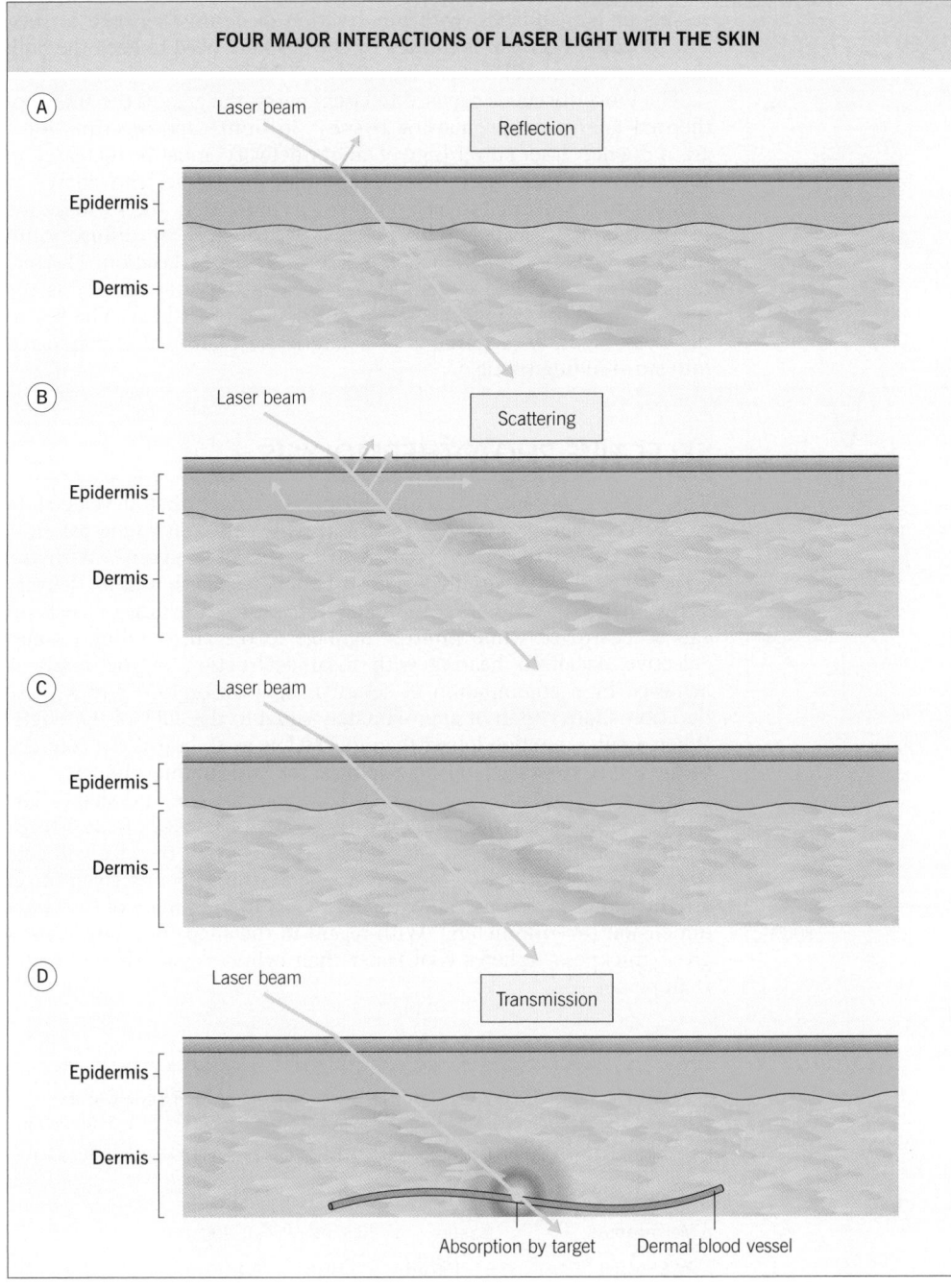

FOUR MAJOR INTERACTIONS OF LASER LIGHT WITH THE SKIN

A
Laser beam
Reflection
Epidermis
Dermis

B
Laser beam
Scattering
Epidermis
Dermis

C
Laser beam
Epidermis
Dermis

D
Laser beam
Transmission
Epidermis
Dermis
Absorption by target   Dermal blood vessel

Fig. 136.4 Four major interactions of laser light with the skin. These are reflection, scattering, transmission and absorption.

near-IR light, longer wavelengths have deeper penetration. At wavelengths below 300 nm there is strong absorption by protein, urocanic acid and DNA. Above 1300 nm, penetration decreases due to the absorption of light by water. The most deeply penetrating wavelengths are in the 650–1200 nm red and near-IR region of the spectrum. The least penetrating wavelengths are in the far-UV and far-IR regions.

THERMAL INTERACTIONS

In dermatologic applications, the majority of laser interactions produce heat. As temperature is raised, many of the essential structures within cells are denatured; these include DNA, RNA and cell membranes. Denaturation results in loss of function via unfolding and coagulation of macromolecules. Thermal coagulation yields cell necrosis and, if widespread, a burn. Laser skin surgery requires precise control over the placement and amount of heat-induced injury.

Most human cells can easily withstand temperatures of up to 40°C (104°F). Whether a given cell population can survive higher temperatures is dependent upon both exposure time and temperature. This is because the rate of thermal denaturation depends on temperature: heat increases the rate at which molecules denature. Exposure to elevated temperatures in most organisms and cells induces a physiologic reaction

called the heat shock response. This response is characterized by the inhibition of normal protein synthesis and the induction of synthesis of a particular set of proteins termed heat shock proteins (HSPs), which confer some resistance to thermal injury[9]. A fascinating example found in nature is some thermophilic bacteria that can survive at 80–90°C (175–195°F). These organisms have thermally stable membranes that are protected by the production of HSPs.

Laser-induced thermal injury is well described by an Arrhenius model[10], which states that the rate of denaturation is exponentially related to temperature. Thus, the accumulation of denatured material rises exponentially with temperature and proportionally with time[11]. Near a critical temperature (which is different for different tissues), rapid coagulation occurs; this is what accounts for the well-defined histologic boundaries of dermal coagulation in laser and other burn injuries. In the dermis, the extracellular matrix structural protein collagen plays a primary role in coagulation, whereas elastin is extremely thermally stable and can survive boiling without apparent injury. Type I collagen, the predominant collagen subtype in the dermis, has a sharp melting transition to the fibrillar form between 60°C and 70°C (140–160°F). At or above this temperature range, collagen denaturation typically occurs and scarring becomes likely. Selective photothermolysis permits selected heating of targets within the dermis, such as blood

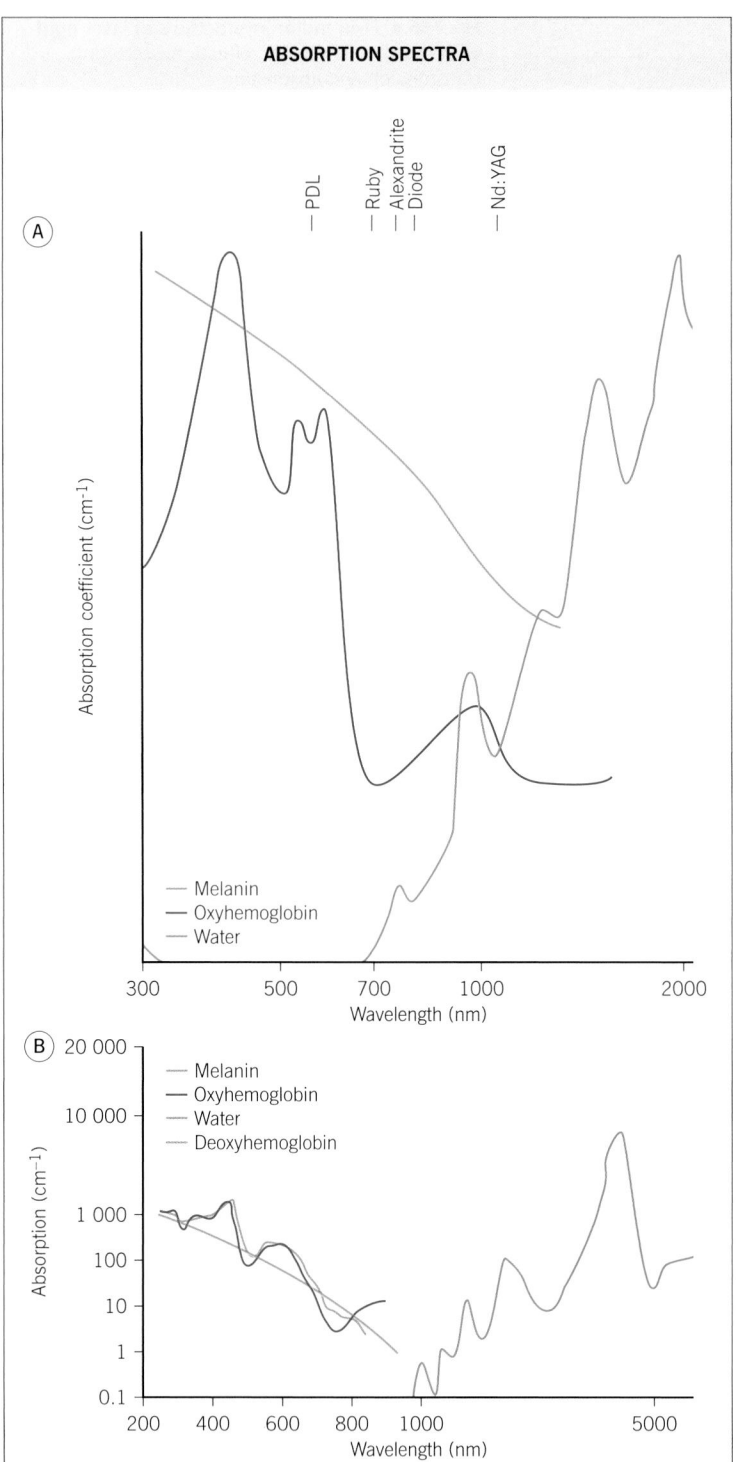

Fig. 136.5 Absorption spectra. The heterogeneous absorption spectra of chromophores allow selective photothermolysis to work.

vessels or hair follicles, with preservation of dermis between targets. The process in general is limited by the absolute need to keep the bulk skin temperature below approximately 60–70°C.

The longer tissue is exposed to laser energy, the greater the spread of thermal energy to neighboring tissues. To limit exposure time for a given fluence, laser power (rate of energy delivery) must be increased to compensate. Once laser light is absorbed by tissue, the energy is immediately converted to heat energy. Via conduction, the surrounding tissue becomes heated. The process by which heat diffuses into neighboring tissues by conduction is termed thermal relaxation. Thermal relaxation time (TRT) is defined, for a given tissue structure, as the time required for the heated tissue to lose half of its heat. The key to the clean ablation of tissue is to ablate faster than heat is conducted into surrounding tissue[12].

SELECTIVE PHOTOTHERMOLYSIS

The concept of selective photothermolysis[13] was first developed to guide the design of a laser to treat port-wine stains in young patients, and it initiated the use of pulsed dye lasers in medicine. With the selection of a preferentially absorbed laser wavelength and its delivery at the appropriate pulse duration and fluence, specific target structures can be destroyed while limiting damage to the surrounding tissues. Selective, localized heating with focal destruction of the target is achieved by a combination of selective light absorption and a pulse duration shorter than or approximately equal to the TRT of the target. When a pulse duration longer than the TRT is used, heat is not confined to the target structure and may damage the surrounding tissues.

A target structure's TRT is related to both its size and shape. The TRT of a target is proportional to the square of its size (Table 136.2). Thus, for a given material and shape, an object half the size will cool in one-quarter of the time. For most tissues, the TRT of a given target structure (in seconds) is approximately equal to the square of the target dimension (in millimeters). With regard to the shape of a target, for a given thickness, spheres cool faster than cylinders, which cool faster than planes.

PULSE DURATIONS AND TARGETS OF SELECTIVE PHOTOTHERMOLYSIS			
Chromophore	**Diameter**	**TRT**	**Typical laser pulse duration**
Tattoo ink particle	0.1 μm	10 ns	10 ns
Melanosome	0.5 μm	250 ns	10–100 ns
PWS vessels	30–100 μm	1–10 ms	0.4–20 ms
Terminal hair follicle	300 μm	100 ms	3–100 ms
Leg vein	1 mm	1 s	0.1 s

Table 136.2 Pulse durations and targets of selective photothermolysis. PWS, port-wine stain; TRT, thermal relaxation time.

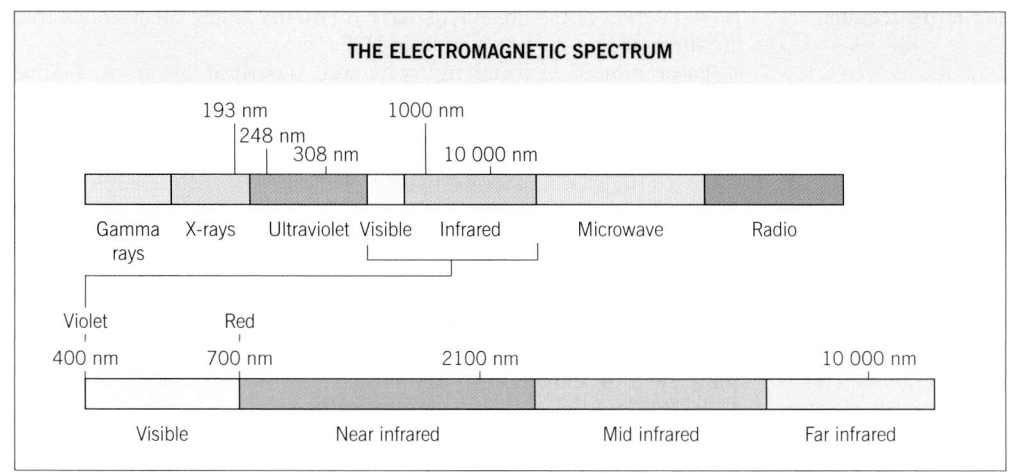

Fig. 136.6 The electromagnetic spectrum. The visible portion is only a small range of the spectrum.

In general, the optimal pulse duration for selective photothermolysis is approximately equal to the TRT. Selective photothermolysis of various skin lesions is best achieved using pulsed rather than continuous laser technology because of the relatively short TRTs of cutaneous targets such as blood vessels and melanosomes[14]. Blood vessels represent a broad category with a wide range of TRTs, including capillaries (tens of microseconds), large venules of adult port-wine stains (up to tens of milliseconds) and leg veins (hundreds of milliseconds). Small pigmented targets (e.g. melanosomes within pigmented melanocytes in a nevus of Ota) are best treated with short (sub-microsecond) pulses, while larger pigmented targets (e.g. hair follicles) have longer TRTs and are best treated with longer (millisecond) pulses[15].

PHOTOMECHANICAL EFFECTS

Pulsed lasers can also cause photomechanical effects[16]. Sudden heating causes sudden thermal expansion that produces stress waves, including acoustic and/or shock waves. The stress waves can rupture or increase permeability of cell membranes. Photomechanical disruption is also achieved through cavitation. This occurs when the combination of temperature and pressure is such that evaporation of water leads to the appearance, expansion and violent collapse of vapor bubbles. Cavitation is the dominant mechanism of vessel rupture achieved by pulsed dye lasers emitting pulses less than ~20 ms[17].

LASER–TISSUE INTERACTIONS

A number of parameters control laser–tissue effects, including wavelength, fluence, irradiance, spot size, and pulse duration (Table 136.3). With smaller spot sizes, a greater fraction of the light is removed from the beam path by scattering of photons in its outer portion (Fig. 136.7). To achieve the greatest effective penetration depth into skin, a combination of a penetrating wavelength (600–1300 nm) and a large spot size is used (Fig. 136.8).

SKIN COOLING

Epidermal melanin is often an undesired chromophore when lasers are used to treat vascular lesions and to remove hair. Epidermal damage can be minimized through the use of skin cooling directed at the superficial portion of the skin (but sparing deeper target tissues). This is especially important in the treatment of darkly pigmented skin, in which pigmentary side effects are more common.

Most of the cooling methods involve the extraction of heat by conduction at the skin surface. The cooling agent (gas, liquid or solid) may flow or move along the skin surface. For spray cooling, the cooling agent is a *liquid* whose temperature is lower than the skin surface temperature. In this case, cooling occurs via evaporation of the coolant layer, which evolves from liquid to gas during the process. In *solid* contact cooling, the agent (typically a solid with high thermal capacity and conductivity) is kept at a constant temperature via active cooling mechanisms. With cold *gel*, passive cooling occurs; because there is no removal of heat from the cooling agent, its temperature eventually rises. A combination of the temperature, quality of contact and thermal conductivity of the cold medium determines how quickly heat can be extracted from the skin.

There are three basic types of skin cooling: precooling, parallel cooling and postcooling, which correspond to extracting heat from the skin before, during and after the laser exposure, respectively[18]. For pulse durations shorter than 5 ms (e.g. with a Q-switched laser), the period of time during which the epidermis needs to remain cool is minimized, and *precooling* provides the requisite protection. Dynamic cooling devices, such as cryogen liquid spray, provide the most aggressive and superficial (epidermal) precooling.

Parallel cooling is the most effective method for pulses longer than 5–10 ms. Spray cooling physically interferes with the laser pulse and is therefore not suited for parallel cooling. Solid contact cooling with cold sapphire pressed to the skin just before and during a long laser pulse enables the safe delivery of very large fluences even in darkly pigmented skin[19]. *Postcooling* (e.g. with ice) is useful to minimize pain and erythema[15].

LASER AND LASER DERMATOLOGY TERMS		
Terms	Definitions	Units
Energy	Fundamental unit of work	Joules (J)
Power	Rate at which energy is delivered	Watts (W)
Fluence	Amount of energy delivered per unit area	J/cm^2
Irradiance	Power delivered per unit area	W/cm^2
Pulse duration (pulse width)	Laser exposure duration	Seconds (s)
Spot size	Diameter of the laser beam on the skin surface	mm
Chromophore	Medium that absorbs light	
Thermal relaxation time	Time required for heated tissue to lose 50% of its heat through diffusion	Seconds (s)

Table 136.3 Laser and laser dermatology terms.

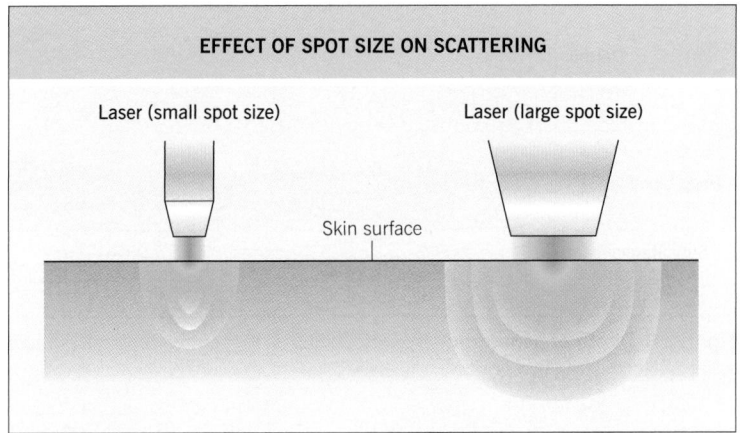

EFFECT OF SPOT SIZE ON SCATTERING

Laser (small spot size)   Laser (large spot size)

Skin surface

Fig. 136.7 The effects of spot size on scattering. The larger spot size allows more photons to remain within a beam's diameter, whereas with a smaller spot size a greater fraction of photons scatters outside the beam and is ineffective. Thus, a beam of a given wavelength penetrates to a deeper level with a larger spot size.

APPLICATIONS OF LASER PRINCIPLES

Lasers are utilized in the treatment of a wide variety of cutaneous and extracutaneous medical conditions and represent a component of several non-invasive medical imaging systems. Properties of lasers that are used in medicine and their specific applications are summarized in Table 136.4.

Ablative Skin Resurfacing

The ablative lasers in dermatology are far-infrared CO_2 (10 600 nm) or Er:YAG (2940 nm) devices which emit wavelengths that are strongly absorbed by water. These lasers emit pulsed and/or scanned focused beams that precisely ablate superficial tissue, causing a 'plume' of material leaving the skin. Most of the heat is removed during vaporization, but a thin layer of residual thermal damage remains that is useful for hemostasis. Laser resurfacing is very useful for treating photoaging, scars and lesions such as epidermal nevi and seborrheic keratoses. Resurfacing removes the old epidermis and stimulates contraction and remodeling of the dermis for many months after treatment. Being a controlled partial-thickness burn, meticulous perioperative technique and wound care are important in order to avoid infection and other complications. Scarring, transient hyperpigmentation, delayed-onset permanent hypopigmentation, prolonged erythema, and bacterial, viral and fungal infections have been reported after laser resurfacing[20].

Treatment of Vascular Lesions

Argon lasers were the original treatment of choice for vascular lesions until the advent of pulsed dye laser (PDL) technology. The argon laser

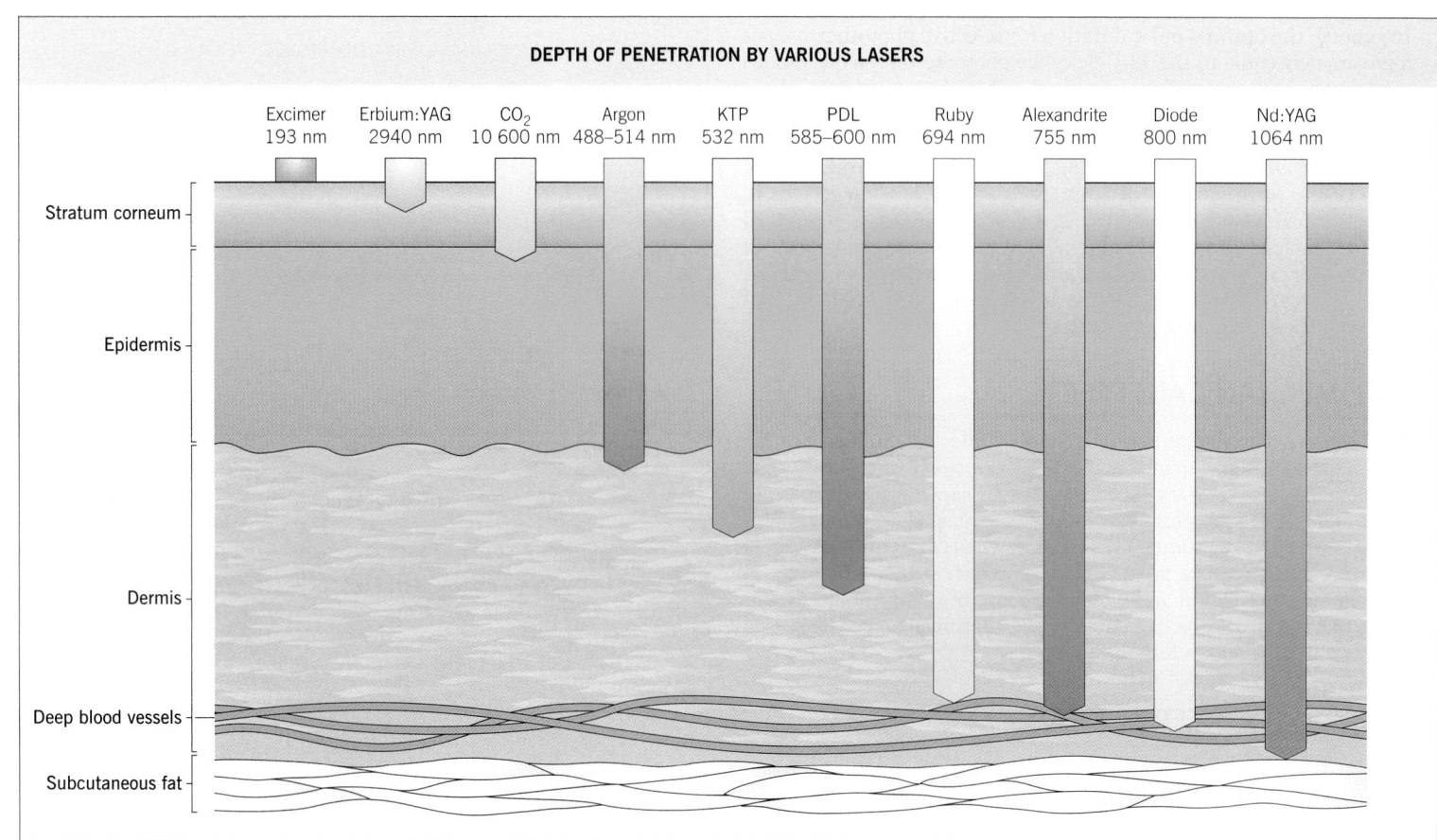

DEPTH OF PENETRATION BY VARIOUS LASERS

Excimer 193 nm · Erbium:YAG 2940 nm · CO₂ 10 600 nm · Argon 488–514 nm · KTP 532 nm · PDL 585–600 nm · Ruby 694 nm · Alexandrite 755 nm · Diode 800 nm · Nd:YAG 1064 nm

Stratum corneum · Epidermis · Dermis · Deep blood vessels · Subcutaneous fat

Fig. 136.8 Depth of penetration by various lasers. KTP, potassium titanyl phosphate; Nd, neodymium; PDL, pulsed dye laser; YAG, yttrium aluminum garnet.

wavelengths of 488 and 514 nm do not correlate well with hemoglobin's absorption spectrum and are strongly absorbed by melanin. This, and the fact that they are continuous-wave lasers, yields non-specific heating of the surrounding tissue. The result is a high risk of scarring with treatment. Argon lasers are no longer commonly used in clinical practice.

A peak of absorption by oxyhemoglobin occurs in the yellow spectrum (see Fig. 136.5). The principle of selective photothermolysis suggests that a pulse duration of approximately 1 ms would be ideal for targeting the small-caliber vessels in port-wine stains and effecting blood coagulation. The flashlamp-pumped PDL was initially designed with a wavelength of 577 nm, the yellow absorption peak of oxyhemoglobin, and a pulse duration of 0.45 ms. Subsequent modifications included increasing the wavelength to 585–600 nm (improving the depth of penetration to approximately 1.2 mm but requiring higher fluences due to decreased absorption by oxyhemoglobin) and increasing the pulse duration to 1.5 ms or longer. Dynamic cooling with cryogen spray can be utilized to minimize epidermal damage, allowing the use of these higher fluences. Still, the majority of port-wine stains require six or more treatments, and some lesions fail to respond to therapy. This resistance appears to be attributable to the presence of vessels that are deeper than 1.5 mm. Of note, high-fluence, long-pulsed neodymium: YAG (Nd:YAG) lasers may offer an improvement over PDLs in the treatment of port-wine stains with a deeper component; while there is similar selectivity for blood vessels at 1064 nm and 585 nm, the Nd:YAG laser wavelength penetrates far more deeply (see Fig. 136.8). Other lasers with wavelengths in the near-IR range (e.g. long-pulsed alexandrite, diode) have also been utilized to target larger, deeper vessels (e.g. leg veins).

Currently, the 585 nm flashlamp PDL is the standard treatment for vascular lesions, including port-wine stains, hemangiomas and telangiectasias. Since epidermal melanin also absorbs 585 nm PDL pulses, fluence is decreased for more deeply pigmented skin. The principal side effect is purpura, which is dependent on fluence and spot size[21]. Purpura is the result of immediate microvascular hemorrhage, subsequent thrombosis and delayed appearance of vasculitis. Spot sizes range from 5 to 10 mm and fluences from 4 to 15 J/cm². With increasing spot size, deeper tissue penetration can be observed. If a smaller spot size is used,

a higher fluence is required to produce comparable clinical results. In general, therefore, the largest practical spot size should be used.

Immediate post-treatment purpura after PDL exposure poses a cosmetic problem for some patients. When the pulse duration (or dwell time) exceeds approximately 20 ms, there is little or no immediate purpura because cavitation and vessel rupture are avoided. Instead, the vessels collapse and tend to disappear immediately after treatment. A stuttered PDL, with pulse train up to 20 ms, has also been developed to reduce the side effect of immediate purpura. It should be noted, however, that delayed purpura can still occur due to a phase of vasculitis several days after treatment, even when no immediate purpura is observed. Continuous- and quasicontinuous-wave green and yellow lasers have less vascular specificity than PDLs, but they offer the advantage of markedly less post-treatment purpura because of longer pulse duration or dwell time. Patients with discrete telangiectasias rather than areas of confluent telangiectasias are excellent candidates for this class of laser.

Copper vapor or copper bromide lasers emit either green light at 511 nm or yellow light at 578 nm. With a repetition rate of 15 000 pulses per second, tissue effects comparable to a continuous-wave laser are seen, and this laser is categorized as quasicontinuous. Minimal swelling and crusting can occur, with resolution within 1 week[22].

Potassium titanyl phosphate (KTP) lasers, at a wavelength of 532 nm, have been introduced for treating telangiectasias, with less resultant purpura than with PDLs. The specificity for vessels is nearly as good at 532 nm as at 585 nm. The most common side effects are crusting and, less frequently, vesiculation. Variable pulse width 532 nm lasers have been created by intracavity frequency doubling of Nd:YAG lasers. In combination with skin cooling, these lasers are versatile for vascular lesion treatment.

Treatment of Pigmented Lesions and Removal of Tattoos

Several types of lasers have been developed specifically for the treatment of pigmented skin lesions. These lasers are utilized for the removal of exogenous tattoo pigment as well as treatment of skin lesions

Laser	Wavelength (nm)	Mode	Average power (W)	Average energy per pulse (J)	Pulse duration (sec)	Pulse rep. rate (Hz)	Typical uses
				LASERS IN MEDICINE			
Excimer (ArF)	193	Pulsed	10	0.1	10^{-8}	100	Corneal surgery
Excimer (XeCl)	308	Pulsed	10	0.1	10^{-7}	100	Angioplasty, psoriasis, vitiligo
Argon	488, 514	CW	1–10				Vascular lesions
Copper vapor	511, 578	Quasi-CW	1–10	10^{-3}	10^{-8}	2×10^3	Skin lesions
KTP	532	Quasi-CW	1–10	10^{-4}	10^{-8}	10^4	Skin lesions
Q-switched, frequency-doubled Nd:YAG	532	Pulsed (ns)	1–3	0.2^{-1}	10^{-8}	5–10	Epidermal pigment, tattoos (red)
Pulsed dye	585–600	Pulsed	10	5	$(1.5–40) \times 10^{-3}$	2	Vascular lesions
Argon dye	630	CW	0.5–2				Photodynamic therapy
Ruby	694	Pulsed	30	30	10^{-3}	1	Hair removal, tattoos, pigmented lesions
Q-switched ruby	694	Pulsed (ns)	2	2	3×10^{-8}	1	Hair removal, tattoos, pigmented lesions
Alexandrite	755	Pulsed	30	30	10^{-3}	1	Hair removal, tattoos, pigmented lesions
Q-switched alexandrite	755	Pulsed	5	0.5–5	10^{-7}	1–10	Hair removal, tattoos, pigmented lesions
Diode (AlGaAs)	800	CW/pulsed	5–3000	5–100	$(5–400) \times 10^{-3}$	1–2	Hair removal, leg veins
Nd:YAG	1064	CW	10–100				Endoscopic surgery
Q-switched Nd:YAG	1064	Pulsed (ns)	5–10	1	10^{-8}	5–10	Tattoos (black)
Long-pulsed Nd:YAG	1064	Pulsed	1–50	1–50	$(1–200) \times 10^{-3}$	0–10	Hair removal, leg veins
Long-pulsed Nd:YAG	1320	Pulsed	1–50	1–50	$(1–200) \times 10^{-3}$	0–10	Skin rejuvenation
Diode	1450	Pulsed	10–15	10–15	0.15–0.25	1	Skin rejuvenation
Erbium:glass	1540	Pulsed	10	5	1×10^{-3}	2	Skin rejuvenation
Holmium:YAG	2000	Pulsed	5–100	0.2–5	10^{-3}	10–20	Orthopedics, lithotripsy
Erbium:YAG	2940	Pulsed	10–20	0.1–3	$(3–100) \times 10^{-4}$	5–100	Skin resurfacing
Carbon dioxide	10 600	CW/pulsed	1–500	0.05–0.5	$10^{-5}–10^{-3}$	$10^2–10^4$	Vaporization/coagulation, skin resurfacing

Table 136.4 Lasers in medicine. AlGaAs, aluminium gallium arsenide; ArF, argon fluoride; CW, continuous wave; KTP, potassium titanyl phosphate; ns, nanosecond; Nd, neodymium; XeCl, xenon chloride; YAG, yttrium aluminum garnet.

containing endogenous melanin pigment. Melanin is located within melanosomes, organelles that range from 0.5 to 1.0 μm in size. The latter have been shown to represent the primary target structure during laser treatment of pigmented lesions[23]. Melanin has an absorption spectrum that ranges from UV to near-IR (see Fig. 136.5), which lends itself to possible treatment with a wide variety of lasers[24]. The selection of treatment wavelength is based, in part, on avoidance of the absorption peaks of other chromophores. Based on the theoretical TRT of melanosomes, the optimal pulse duration is 70–250 ns[13]. Q-switched lasers are, therefore, excellent for targeting melanosomes. When the fluence threshold for melanosome disruption is reached, the pigmented cell dies.

Treatment of tattoos with short-pulsed lasers leads to fragmentation of the ink particles and selective death of pigment-containing cells, with resultant pigment release. There are several speculated mechanisms for removal of the pigment particles. Some ink is lost in an epidermal crust, some is lost via the lymphatics, and some is rephagocytosed by dermal cells[25].

Different lasers are required to manage different pigments. Q-switched ruby lasers can be used at fluences of up to approximately 10 J/cm², and they emit a 694 nm deep red light that is well absorbed by melanin. At a 20–40 ns pulse duration, this laser can also effectively treat most tattoo colors except bright shades such as red and yellow (see Table 137.5 and Fig. 137.5). Q-switched ruby lasers are particularly useful in the treatment of dermal melanocytoses such as nevus of Ota. The literature also contains multiple reports of the successful use of the ruby laser for the treatment of solar lentigines and ephelides. Café-au-lait macules and melanocytic nevi may respond to treatment with Q-switched ruby lasers (or, for nevi, long-pulsed ruby lasers that target nests of melanocytes), but recurrences are common (and, considering the residual dermal melanocytes in laser-treated nevi, not surprising)[26,27]. Treatment of acquired melanocytic nevi is controversial, given the lack of

histologic evaluation. Of note, postinflammatory hyperpigmentation and melasma are poorly responsive to treatment with ruby or other lasers[28]. The Q-switched alexandrite laser emits deep red light at 755 nm with 50–100 ns pulse durations, and it has nearly equivalent uses to Q-switched ruby lasers.

The Q-switched Nd:YAG laser emits energy in the near-IR range at 1064 nm, with typical pulse durations of 10 ns. Its primary use is in the treatment of dermal melanocytoses, such as nevus of Ota, and removal of blue–black tattoo pigment. The 1064 nm energy can be frequency doubled to produce 532 nm visible green light by passing it through a KTP crystal. This frequency-doubled Nd:YAG laser can effectively remove epidermal melanin pigment as well as red and yellow tattoo ink, but not green ink. Complications include hypopigmentation or hyperpigmentation, and transient textural changes at higher fluences.

Hair Removal

Permanent hair removal probably requires damage to follicular stem cells in the bulge region of the outer root sheath and/or the dermal papilla at the base of the hair follicle. These are non-pigmented targets, located at a distance from melanin chromophores within pigmented hair shafts. In order to damage the non-pigmented targets, heat must diffuse from the pigmented portion. This has been achieved with high-energy, millisecond-domain pulses of wavelengths in the red to near-IR region of the spectrum, which penetrate into the deep dermis and are preferentially absorbed by melanin. Ruby, alexandrite, diode and Nd:YAG lasers are currently used for hair removal. None of these sources works well for blond or white hair due to the paucity of melanin chromophores.

Since melanin in the epidermis and in the hair follicle have nearly identical absorption spectra, laser hair removal poses a risk of epidermal injury. Light must first travel through the pigmented epidermis to reach hair follicles. Skin cooling is essential to safe removal of hair, especially in individuals with darkly pigmented skin. The mechanism for temporary hair loss is primarily induction of catagen. Permanent hair loss, in contrast, appears to occur via two separate pathways: (1) miniaturization of terminal hair follicles to produce vellus-like hairs; and (2) complete degeneration with fibrosis, particularly with pulses of 20 ms or longer. Of note, temporary hair loss can be achieved with lower fluences and longer pulse durations than those needed for permanent hair reduction. For example, an 810 nm diode laser source intended for home use by consumers was recently reported to reliably induce temporary reduction of pigmented terminal hair[29].

Non-ablative Skin Rejuvenation

Non-ablative facial rejuvenation is a non-invasive approach for the treatment of fine lines and non-movement-associated rhytides that eliminates the prolonged side effects and extended recovery period characteristic of traditional resurfacing techniques. Study results vary, but indicate that non-ablative treatments are far less effective than resurfacing. However, patient satisfaction is high because the treatment is nearly devoid of side effects.

Non-ablative lasers (e.g. 1320 nm Nd:YAG, 1450 nm diode and 1540 nm erbium:glass lasers) and intense pulsed light sources (see below) work by subtle thermal effects on the dermis, but they leave the epidermis intact. The mechanisms are unknown, but presumably involve stimulating a wound healing response in the dermis. Non-ablative therapy may also help fade irregular pigmentation of the skin. Unlike a facelift or conventional laser resurfacing, the results from non-ablative rejuvenation are gradual and subtle. Well-controlled studies are lacking. The present commercial marketing for non-ablative rejuvenation probably overstates its value.

Fractional Photothermolysis

Fractional photothermolysis, a newer resurfacing technique in which microscopic zones of thermal injury are created, stimulates turnover of both epidermis and dermis[30]. Focused mid-IR laser microbeams are used to create a pixilated pattern of multiple columns of thermal damage, referred to as microthermal treatment zones (MTZs). Typically, about 1 million MTZs are placed per full-face treatment. Pattern density and depth of thermal damage are separately controlled. Density affects coverage, while energy per MTZ is used to control the depth of dermal treatment (up to about 1.2 mm). Tissue spared around each MTZ initiates rapid repair and stimulates remodeling. Desquamation of the epidermal portion of each MTZ removes some basal layer pigment and a small amount of papillary dermal debris. With the loss and replacement of damaged tissue, fractional resurfacing occurs.

Laser-Based Diagnostics

In addition to its therapeutic applications, laser technology has contributed to the development of diagnostic techniques. Optical coherence tomography (OCT) uses IR light for high-resolution cross-sectional imaging of body tissues. An example of an OCT application is in the imaging of atherosclerotic plaques in the coronary arteries[31]. Plaques that are vulnerable to rupture (and therefore prone to cause myocardial infarction) are composed largely of lipid and have a thin, fibrous surface layer. Since these features can be identified in OCT images, OCT is being developed to differentiate stable from unstable coronary plaques, an important criterion in determining the most appropriate therapy. OCT uses a low-coherence laser or diode source and may have applications in dermatology[32]. For example, a Doppler version has been shown to be capable of imaging blood flow before and after laser treatment of vascular lesions[33].

IR-laser confocal microscopy captures scattered light from a thin plane 'section' inside skin. Real-time confocal microscopy is able to view the skin in vivo with histology-like resolution down to a depth of approximately 0.3 mm. By using this technique, the epidermis and upper dermis can be examined rapidly in vivo. The resolution is approximately 1 μm, similar to conventional microscopy. Confocal microscopy of human skin tumors reveals features different from those of conventional histology. For example, microvascular blood flow and trafficking of lymphocytes can be observed. However, the absence of stains for in vivo confocal microscopy and OCT is a limitation. In a preliminary study, the sensitivity and specificity of in vivo confocal microscopy for differentiating benign (melanocytic nevi [n = 90] and seborrheic keratoses [n = 30]) and malignant (melanoma [n = 27] and basal cell carcinoma [n = 15]) skin lesions was 94% and 98%, respectively[34].

NON-LASER LIGHT SOURCES

Filtered xenon flashlamps, called intense pulsed light (IPL) sources, have also been utilized for non-ablative skin rejuvenation, hair removal and the treatment of vascular and pigmented lesions. Unlike lasers, IPL devices emit polychromatic, non-coherent light. The wavelengths are in the visible to near-IR range (480–1200 nm), and different filters (480–755 nm) that exclude shorter wavelengths can be selected in order to target particular chromophores.

Additional IR and radiofrequency devices that have been utilized for skin rejuvenation are described in Chapter 137.

PRINCIPLES OF LASER SAFETY

Laser safety standards are legal requirements for practice, adopted in the US from the American National Standards Institute (ANSI; designation code Z136.3). With increased use of lasers, there has been an alarming increase in eye injuries in both patients and dermatologists. Near-infrared Q-switched dermatological lasers (e.g. Q-switched alexandrite and Nd:YAG lasers) are the most eye-hazardous tools in medical use. *Blindness occurs rapidly and painlessly*, even when only 1% of the beam is reflected into the eye from glossy metal, glass or plastic surfaces. Even laser-experienced dermatologists have suffered blindness by inadvertent lack of appropriate eyewear.

All lasers and IPL sources used for hair removal are designed to damage deep, pigmented structures and the retina and uveal tract are highly pigmented. Anterior eye injury from lasers or IPL sources usually involves inexperienced personnel attempting to remove the lower eyebrow or vascular lesions near the eye, without an eye shield in place[35]. Even an opaque laser eye shield covering the patient's cornea will not prevent damage if the laser or IPL directly impacts exposed sclera. The risk of trans-scleral eye injury may in practice be somewhat greater with IPL sources because of imprecise placement of these bulky devices.

Laser-protective eyewear consists of wrap-around glasses and goggles, rated by optical density (OD) at various wavelengths (corresponding to various lasers). OD = log (1/T), where T is the transmittance of light through the eyewear. By law, OD and wavelength ranges of protection are printed directly on the eyewear. For dermatological lasers, proper protection is considered to be an OD of 4 or greater at the wavelength of the laser being used. The color of the goggles is *not* an indication of protection, especially when using an infrared (invisible) laser. To ensure that the patient, the dermatologist and others in attendance are protected, the following are recommended: (1) know the wavelength of the laser being used; (2) check that the glasses or goggles have an OD of at least 4 for that wavelength; and (3) use both the laser and the eyewear properly.

Fire hazard is greatest with the CO_2 and erbium lasers used for skin resurfacing. There have been many injury cases after drapes, clothing, hair or plastic materials were ignited by CO_2 lasers. The most common cause is failure to place the laser in STANDBY mode when not actually treating the patient, followed by inadvertently activating the laser footswitch. Some patients have died from laser-ignited plastic endotracheal tube fires, which release toxic fumes directly into the patient's airway; reducing the oxygen concentration to less than 40% reduces this risk. Hair can be ignited by several different lasers, and it should be moistened near the treatment field. A fire extinguisher should also be nearby. Inhalation of laser-generated 'plume' materials is a biohazard, especially during resurfacing. Of note, many of the hair removal lasers vaporize hair shafts, which release irritating sulfur and other oxides. Submicrometer surgical filter masks provide some protection when worn properly, but a smoke evacuator and good ventilation are more effective measures.

REFERENCES

1. Goldman L, Blaney DJ, Kindel DJ, et al. Effect of the laser beam on the skin: preliminary report. J Invest Dermatol. 1963;40:121.

2. Einstein A. Zur quantentheorie der strahlung. Physiol Z. 1917;18:121–8.

3. Maiman TH. Stimulated optical radiation in ruby. Nature. 1960;187:493–4.

4. Carroll L, Humphreys TR. LASER-tissue interactions. Clin Dermatol. 2006;24:2–7.

5. Herd RM, Dover JS, Arndt KA. Basic laser principles. Dermatol Clin. 1997;15:355–72.

6. Raulin C, Schonermark MP, Greve B, et al. Q-switched ruby laser treatment of tattoos and benign pigmented skin lesions: a critical review. Ann Plast Surg. 1998;41:555–65.

7. Anderson RR, Parrish JA. The optics of human skin. J Invest Dermatol. 1981;77:13–19.

8. Anderson RR. Polarized light examination and photography of the skin. Arch Dermatol. 1991;127:1000–5.

9. Polla BS, Anderson RR. Thermal injury by laser pulse: protection by heat shock despite failure to induce heat shock response. Lasers Surg Med. 1987;7:398–404.

10. Henriques FC. Studies of thermal injury. Arch Pathol. 1947;43:489.

11. Welch AJ. The thermal response to laser irradiated tissue. IEEE J Quant Electron. 1984;20:1471.

12. Hruza GJ, Geronemus RG, Dover JS, et al. Lasers in dermatology. Arch Dermatol. 1993;129:1026–33.

13. Anderson RR, Parrish JA. Selective photothermolysis: precise microsurgery by selective absorption of pulse radiation. Science. 1983;220:524–7.

14. Anderson RR. Laser-tissue interactions. In: Goldman MP, Fitzpatrick RE (eds). Cutaneous Laser Surgery. St Louis: Mosby, 1994:1–17.

15. Anderson RR. Lasers in dermatology – a critical update. J Dermatol. 2000;27:700–5.

16. Watanabe S, Flotte TJ, McAuliffe DJ, et al. Putative photoacoustic damage in skin induced by pulsed ArF excimer laser. J Invest Dermatol. 1988;90:761–6.

17. Garden JM, Tan OT, Kerschmann R, et al. Effect of dye laser pulse duration on selective cutaneous vascular injury. J Invest Dermatol. 1986;87:653–7.

18. Zenzie HH, Altshuler GB, Smirnov MZ, et al. Evaluation of cooling methods for laser dermatology. Lasers Surg Med. 2000;26:130–44.

19. Battle EF, Suthamjariya K, Alora MB, et al. Very long-pulsed (20-200 ms) diode laser for hair removal on all skin types. Lasers Surg Med. 2000;12(suppl.):85.

20. Nanni CA, Alster TS. Complications of CO_2 laser resurfacing: an evaluation of 500 patients. Dermatol Surg. 1998;24:1–6.

21. Lanigan SW. Patient reported morbidity following flashlamp-pumped pulsed tunable dye laser treatment of port wine stains. Br J Dermatol. 1995;133:423–5.

22. Dinehart SM, Waner M. Comparison of the copper vapor and flashlamp-pulsed dye laser in the treatment of facial telangiectasia. J Am Acad Dermatol. 1991;24:116.

23. Polla LL, Margolis RJ, Dover JS, et al. Melanosomes are a primary target of Q-switched ruby laser irradiation in guinea pig skin. J Invest Dermatol. 1987;89:281–6.

24. Murphy GF, Shepard RS, Paul BS, et al. Organelle specific injury to melanin containing cells in human skin by pulsed laser irradiation. Lab Invest. 1983;49:680–5.

25. Taylor CR, Anderson RR, Gange RW, et al. Light and electron microscope analysis of tattoos treated by Q-switched ruby laser. J Invest Dermatol. 1991;97:131–6.

26. Goldberg DJ. Benign pigmented lesions of the skin and treatment with the Q-switched ruby laser. J Dermatol Surg Oncol. 1993;19:376–9.

27. Grossman MC, Anderson RR, Farinelli W, et al. Treatment of café au lait macules with lasers. Arch Dermatol. 1985;131:1416–20.

28. Taylor CR, Anderson RR. Ineffective treatment of mzelasma and postinflammatory hyperpigmentation by Q switched ruby laser. J Dermatol Surg Oncol. 1994;20:592–7.

29. Wheeland RG. Simulated consumer use of a battery-powered, hand-held portable diode laser (810 nm) for hair removal: a safety, efficacy and ease-of use study. Lasers Surg Med. 2007;39:476–93.

30. Manstein D, Herron GS, Sink RK, et al. Fractional photothermolysis: a new concept for cutaneous remodeling using microscopic patterns of thermal injury. Lasers Surg Med. 2004;34:426–38.

31. Tearney GJ, Jang IK, Kang DH, et al. Porcine coronary imaging in vivo by optical coherence tomography. Acta Cardiol. 2000;55:233–7.

32. Gambichler T, Moussa G, Sand M, et al. Applications of optical coherence tomography in dermatology. J Dermatol Sci. 2005;40:85–94.

33. Nelson JS, Kelly KM, Zhao Y, et al. Imaging blood flow in human port-wine stain in situ and in real time using optical Doppler tomography. Arch Dermatol. 2001;137:741–4.

34. Gerger A, Koller S, Weger W, et al. Sensitivity and specificity of confocal laser-scanning microscopy for in vivo diagnosis of malignant skin tumors. Cancer. 2006;107:193–200.

35. Hammes S, Augustin A, Raulin C, et al. Pupil damage after periorbital laser treatment of a port-wine stain. Arch Dermatol. 2007;143:392–4.

Laser Therapy

Macrene R Alexiades-Armenakas, Jeffrey S Dover and Kenneth A Arndt

Key features

- The selectivity and efficacy of lasers are continually being improved, targeting specific structures in a variety of locations within the skin (e.g. blood vessels of different sizes and depths; pigment contained in the epidermis, dermis and hair follicles)

- Improved understanding of laser–tissue interactions and protection of the epidermis with active cooling systems during laser treatment of dermal targets reduce the risk of side effects, increase patient tolerability and permit the use of higher fluences for enhanced efficacy

- Laser treatment of vascular lesions has been optimized through the use of different wavelengths, variable pulse durations and higher fluences in conjunction with active epidermal cooling

- Laser treatment of pigmented lesions employs very short pulse durations, with short wavelengths for epidermal targets and longer wavelengths for dermal targets

- Laser hair removal targets pigment within the hair shaft; it has become safe and effective for individuals of all skin types through the use of longer wavelengths and pulse durations to bypass epidermal melanosomes and allow higher fluences to be employed

- Laser resurfacing includes non-ablative, fractional and ablative techniques

- Non-ablative laser skin rejuvenation using near-infrared-wavelength lasers, intense pulsed light or radiofrequency energy targets the dermis and produces mild improvement in rhytides and laxity

- Fractional laser resurfacing ablates microscopic columns of epidermal and upper dermal tissue, resulting in improvement of rhytides and dyspigmentation with a short recovery time

- Ablative laser resurfacing, which employs erbium:YAG and pulsed or scanned carbon dioxide lasers, requires the longest recovery period but yields the highest level of efficacy in treating rhytides and photodamage

- Lasers can be used in conjunction with aminolevulinic acid photodynamic therapy for the treatment of actinic keratoses, actinic cheilitis, photodamage and acne

INTRODUCTION AND BACKGROUND

Laser technology has continually evolved over the past half century, and it now provides an important therapeutic modality that is widely used in dermatology and many other medical and surgical specialties. The concept of laser radiation has its roots in Einstein's *The Quantum Theory of Radiation*, which was published in 1917. A method for *M*icrowave *A*mplification by *S*timulated *E*mission of *R*adiation (MASER) was invented by Townes & Schalow in 1958[1], and the first laser was developed in 1960 by Maiman, who observed stimulated emission of radiation utilizing visible light and ruby crystals and modified the term to *L*ight *A*mplification by *S*timulated *E*mission of *R*adiation (LASER). In the 1960s and 70s, argon and continuous-wave carbon dioxide (CO_2) lasers that created non-specific tissue damage were used for cutting or coagulating superficial skin lesions. The *principle of selective photothermolysis*, proposed by Anderson and Parrish in 1983[2], led to the development of high-energy pulsed lasers that were capable of selectively destroying cells, organelles and other microscopic targets within the skin. Since then, the specificity and efficacy of lasers have been honed, producing a generation of lasers with excellent safety profiles and the ability to precisely target skin structures.

TYPES OF LASERS

Basic principles such as the 'anatomy' of lasers, the process of stimulated emission of radiation and types of laser media (gas, liquid and solid) are discussed in Chapter 136. Lasers can be categorized according to the wavelengths of the photons they emit (Fig. 137.1). Lasers used in dermatology emit specific wavelengths within the UV (10–400 nm), visible (400–720 nm) and IR (720–1 000 000 nm) portions of the electromagnetic spectrum. Intense pulsed light (IPL) devices emit broadband visible and near-IR light (400–1200 nm), whereas radiofrequency devices emit broadband radiofrequency energy. The wavelengths and skin targets of the lasers that are most commonly used by dermatologists are shown in Table 137.1.

A molecule that selectively absorbs light of certain wavelengths is termed a *chromophore*, from the Greek word for 'color absorber'. Each chromophore within the skin has a characteristic *absorption spectrum*, i.e. a curve of *absorption coefficients* (probability per unit path length that a photon at a particular wavelength will be absorbed by the chromophore) plotted for different wavelengths. This curve is dependent

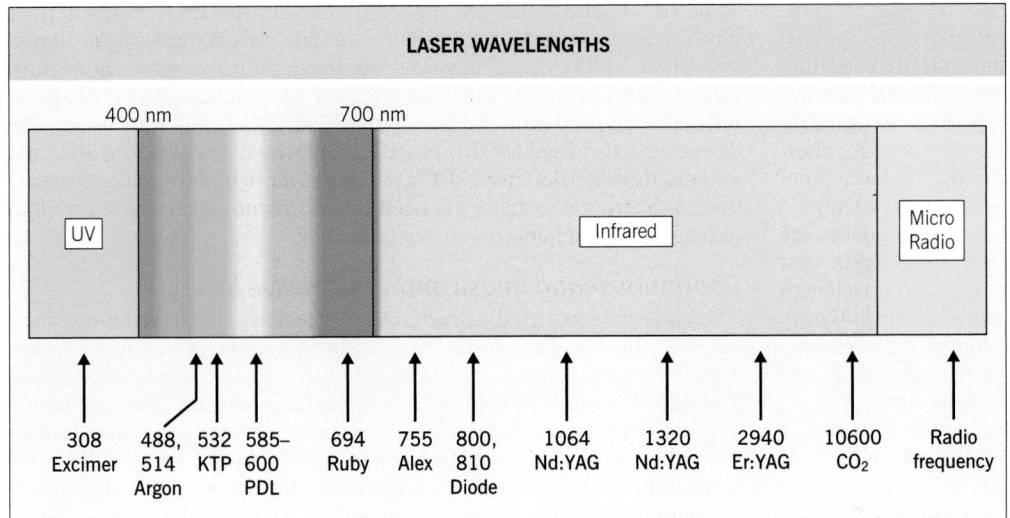

LASER WAVELENGTHS

| 308 Excimer | 488, 514 Argon | 532 KTP | 585–600 PDL | 694 Ruby | 755 Alex | 800, 810 Diode | 1064 Nd:YAG | 1320 Nd:YAG | 2940 Er:YAG | 10600 CO_2 | Radio frequency |

Fig. 137.1 Laser wavelengths. Laser wavelengths lie predominantly within the ultraviolet (10–400 nm), visible (400–720 nm) and infrared (720–1 000 000 nm) portions of the spectrum. Broad bands of visible and radiofrequency wavelengths are emitted by intense pulsed light and radiofrequency devices, respectively.

WAVELENGTHS AND TARGETS OF LASERS COMMONLY USED IN DERMATOLOGY

Laser	Wavelength	Target chromophore
Argon	488, 514 nm	Melanin, hemoglobin
Frequency-doubled Nd:YAG/KTP	532 nm	Vascular (LP); melanin/tattoo pigment (QS)
Pulsed dye	585–600 nm	Vascular
Ruby	694 nm	Melanin/tattoo pigment
Alexandrite	755 nm	Melanin/tattoo pigment
Diode	800 nm	Melanin, hemoglobin
Nd:YAG	1064 nm	Hemoglobin (LP), melanin/tattoo pigment (QS)
Erbium:YAG	2940 nm	Water
Carbon dioxide	10 600 nm	Water

Table 137.1 Wavelengths and targets of lasers commonly used in dermatology. KTP, potassium titanyl phosphate; LP, long pulsed; Nd, neodymium; QS, Q-switched; YAG, yttrium aluminum garnet.

OPTICAL PENETRATION DEPTHS OF LASERS IN CAUCASIAN SKIN

Laser	Wavelength (nm)	Penetration depth reached by 50% of the incident beam (μm)
Excimer (argon fluoride)	193	0.5
Argon	488	200
Argon	514	300
Q-switched Nd:YAG (frequency-doubled)	532	400
Pulsed dye	577	400
Pulsed dye	585	600
Q-switched ruby	694	1200
Q-switched alexandrite	755	1300
Q-switched Nd:YAG	1064	1600
Erbium:YAG	2940	1
Carbon dioxide	10 600	20

Table 137.2 Optical penetration depths of lasers in Caucasian skin. Penetration decreases when the beam radius is less than the penetration depth or when the concentration of chromophores, such as pigment or vascular structures, is increased. Adapted from Anderson R. Laser-tissue interactions. In: Goldman M, Fitzpatrick R (eds) Cutaneous Laser Surgery, 2nd edn. St Louis: Mosby, 1999: 5.

upon the relative concentration of the chromophore in skin structures, interference via absorption by surrounding chromophores, and depth of penetration of each wavelength.

The absorption spectra of water, hemoglobin and melanin, the most important chromophores in the skin, are plotted in Figure 136.5. Ablative lasers typically emit wavelengths in the IR range of the spectrum and their primary chromophore is water, which results in thermal damage to all skin cells to a certain depth. Vascular and pigment lasers emit wavelengths in the visible to near-IR region that are highly absorbed by hemoglobin and melanin, respectively.

LASER SPECIFICITY

The *principle of selective photothermolysis* allows specific target structures in the skin to be destroyed with limited damage to surrounding tissues via utilization of: (1) a wavelength of light that is preferentially absorbed by the target; (2) a pulse duration shorter than or approximately equal to the target's *thermal relaxation time* (TRT; time it takes for a structure to dissipate half of its thermal energy to surrounding tissues); and (3) an appropriate fluence (energy density) (see Chapter 136)[2]. For most target structures, the TRT (in seconds) is approximately equal to the square of its diameter (in mm). For example, the estimated TRT for a melanosome measuring $0.5\,\mu m$ ($5 \times 10^{-4}\,mm$) in diameter is 250 ns ($25 \times 10^{-8}\,s$), and that for a capillary with a 0.1 mm diameter is 10 ms ($1 \times 10^{-2}\,s$)[3]. Thus, very short pulses (in the nanosecond range) are used to target very small structures such as melanosomes and tattoo pigment particles, while much longer pulses (in the millisecond range) are used to heat larger structures such as capillaries and hair follicles.

When lasers are used to target dermal structures (e.g. blood vessels) or to remove hair, epidermal melanin represents an undesired chromophore. Skin-surface cooling can be used to minimize epidermal damage, allowing the safe delivery of large fluences even in patients with darkly pigmented skin. *Precooling* (before laser exposure) is beneficial for short pulse durations (e.g. <5 ms), while *parallel cooling* (during laser exposure) is more effective for longer pulse durations (see Chapter 136).

The *penetration depth* of the laser determines which targets are reached by the laser beam, and it is dependent upon wavelength, spot size and fluence. Penetration depth is directly proportional to wavelength for light in the UVB, UVA, visible and near-IR regions (280–1300 nm); this is due to decreased dermal scattering of longer wavelengths. However, light in the far-UV and far-IR regions penetrates less deeply because of increased protein and water absorption, respectively.

The influence of spot size on penetration depth is related to optical scattering and progressive dissipation of photons in the outer portion of a laser beam; larger spot sizes allow more photons to reach a greater depth. If the radius of the beam is less than or equal to the wavelength's

usual penetration depth into the dermis, penetration and beam intensity decrease. Thus, the spot size for a laser of a particular wavelength should be at least twice the penetration depth reached by 50% of the incident beam (Table 137.2).

LASER TREATMENT OF VASCULAR LESIONS

Through application of the aforementioned principles, laser treatment of congenital and acquired vascular lesions has become increasingly selective and effective. In the past, treatment of vascular lesions with continuous wave lasers (e.g. the argon laser) was often complicated by scarring due to non-specific thermal damage. Subsequent development of pulsed lasers and employment of the theory of selective photothermolysis have enabled excellent targeting of vascular structures while avoiding dissipation of heat into surrounding tissues. In addition, the use of longer pulse durations and skin-surface cooling devices can minimize or eliminate post-treatment purpura and pigmentary alterations.

Types of Vascular Lasers

The wavelengths, targets and applications of the vascular lasers most commonly used in current dermatologic practice are presented in Table 137.3. Those that are applied to the skin surface to target dermal blood vessels include pulsed dye, variable-pulsed potassium titanyl phosphate (KTP; frequency-doubled neodymium:yttrium aluminum garnet [Nd:YAG]; 532 nm), long-pulsed alexandrite (755 nm), long-pulsed diode (800 nm) and long-pulsed Nd:YAG (1064 nm) lasers; IPL devices are also used for this purpose. Endovascular lasers (e.g. 810 and 940 nm diodes, 1320 nm Nd:YAG) that deliver light within blood vessels using a fiberoptic catheter are used to treat incompetent varicosities in patients with saphenous vein insufficiency.

Continuous- and quasicontinuous-wave lasers

The earliest lasers used to treat vascular lesions were continuous- and quasicontinuous-wave lasers, including the argon (488 nm, 514 nm), argon pumped tunable dye (488–638 nm), copper vapor and copper bromide (511 nm, 578 nm), KTP (532 nm) and krypton (568 nm) lasers. The argon laser was the treatment of choice for many vascular lesions from the 1970s to 1980s. It was particularly useful for nodular port-wine stains (PWSs)[4], facial telangiectasias[5], high-flow spider angiomas[6], pyogenic granulomas and venous lakes. However, despite selective

Laser/device	Wavelength (nm)	Fluence (J/cm²)	Pulse duration (ms)	Target structure	Applications
Skin-surface application					
Variable-pulsed KTP laser	532	Up to 240	1–100	Telangiectasia, venulectasia	Facial telangiectasias, erythematotelangiectatic rosacea, leg telangiectasias, venous malformations, cherry angiomas
Pulsed dye laser	585, 590, 595, 600	Up to 40	0.45–40	Telangiectasia	Port-wine stains, erythematotelangiectatic rosacea, facial and leg telangiectasias, infantile hemangiomas, hypertrophic scars, striae rubra, verrucae
Long-pulsed alexandrite laser	755	Up to 100	3–100	Venulectasia, telangiectasia	Spider leg telangiectasias
Diode laser	800	10–100	5–400	Venulectasia, telangiectasia	Spider leg venulectasias and telangiectasias, blue reticular veins
Long-pulsed Nd:YAG laser	1064	5–900	0.25–500	Venulectasia, telangiectasia	Spider leg venulectasias and telangiectasias, blue reticular veins, facial telangiectasias
Intense pulsed light	400–1200	10–80	2–200	Telangiectasia, venulectasia	Erythematotelangiectatic rosacea, spider leg telangiectasias
Endovascular application					
Diode lasers	810, 940			Varicose veins	Saphenous vein insufficiency
Nd:YAG laser	1320			Varicose veins	Saphenous vein insufficiency
Radiofrequency energy source	Radiofrequency			Varicose veins	Saphenous vein insufficiency

Table 137.3 Lasers and other devices used for the treatment of vascular lesions.

absorption of the argon laser's wavelengths by hemoglobin in blood vessels, the continuous nature of the beam produced non-specific thermal injury in adjacent tissue, increasing the risk of scarring. In addition, concomitant absorption by melanin frequently resulted in permanent hypopigmentation.

The quasicontinuous-wave lasers (copper bromide, krypton and KTP) were used for a variety of vascular lesions[7,8]. Because of the short interval between pulses, the vessels did not cool adequately and thermal injury to surrounding tissues was identical to that of a continuous-wave laser. In an effort to optimize treatment and limit non-specific tissue damage, automated scanning hand pieces were attached to continuous-wave and quasicontinuous-wave lasers, delivering small, non-adjacent spots in a predetermined treatment area. However, the pulse duration remained too long for selective photothermolysis to be achieved, and collateral thermal damage still occurred.

Pulsed lasers

The advent of pulsed lasers allowed adequate energy to be delivered to the vascular target while minimizing heat dissipation to surrounding structures[2,9]. This has greatly improved the efficacy and decreased the side effects of vascular lasers. These lasers are categorized into three main groups: (1) pulsed dye lasers (PDLs); (2) pulsed KTP lasers; and (3) pulsed IR lasers (see Table 137.3).

Pulsed dye lasers

The flashlamp-pumped PDL was the first laser developed based on the principle of selective photothermolysis, and it was designed specifically to treat vessels within PWSs in children. It uses a high-power flashlamp to energize an organic dye (rhodamine) and produce a true pulse of yellow light. The original PDL emitted at a wavelength of 577 nm, coinciding with the last absorption peak of oxyhemoglobin. The dye was then modified to produce light at 585 nm to allow for deeper tissue penetration, despite slightly less selective vascular injury[10].

The pulse duration of the traditional PDL (450 μs) is shorter than the calculated thermal relaxation time of cutaneous vasculature (1–10 ms for vessel diameters of 30–100 μm) and allows sufficient energy absorption by oxyhemoglobin to cause red blood cell coagulation. Histologic examination of PWSs after PDL treatment demonstrates an intact epidermis and superficial dermal blood vessels containing agglutinated erythrocytes, fibrin and thrombi. These histologic findings correlate with the purpura seen clinically immediately after PDL irradiation. One month after treatment, the destroyed ectatic vessels are replaced by normal-appearing vessels without evidence of dermal scarring[11].

The classic PDL is considered to be the treatment of choice for many vascular lesions, including PWSs (Fig. 137.2), facial telangiectasias (including spider angiomas and telangiectatic erythema associated with rosacea; Fig. 137.3), and some superficial infantile hemangiomas[10,12,13]. Its applications have also been expanded to include benign cutaneous neoplasms (e.g. angiofibromas) and other skin conditions (e.g. verrucae, hypertrophic scars, striae distensae and psoriasis) with a prominent vascular component. Modifications to PDLs have included the addition of active cooling systems, such as cryogen-spray cooling that delivers millisecond spurts of cryogen to the skin's surface prior to laser pulsing (e.g. Dynamic Cooling Device™) and an air cooling system with a continuous flow of chilled air onto the skin during laser treatment (e.g. SmartCool™, Zimmer Cooler™). By protecting the epidermis, these cooling methods permit the use of higher fluences for the treatment of resistant vascular lesions and reduce discomfort.

Disadvantages of classic PDLs include post-treatment purpura, which lasts 2–3 weeks, and limited penetration depth of the 585 nm wavelength, which minimizes efficacy when treating deep lesions with larger blood vessels (e.g. leg telangiectasias and some PWSs). In addition, the optimal pulse duration for treatment of vessels 30–100 μm in diameter is in the 1–10 ms range, longer than the 450 μs pulses delivered by the classic PDL[14]. These factors led to the development of PDLs with deeper-penetrating wavelengths (590–600 nm) and slightly longer pulse durations (1.5 ms) that heated vessels more slowly, producing less profound and shorter-lasting purpura than classic PDLs. Combined with cryogen-spray coolant and very high fluences, this generation of PDLs achieved faster clearance of PWSs and some infantile hemangiomas in fewer treatment sessions. Facial telangiectasias and deeper, blue vessels that were unresponsive to treatment with classic PDLs showed significant improvement following treatment with long-pulsed PDLs[15]. However, although somewhat effective for the treatment of leg veins less than 0.4 mm in diameter, the 1.5 ms PDL was unable to target larger-caliber leg vessels[16].

Ultralong- or variable-pulsed PDLs (e.g. V-Beam™, V-Star™) represent a more recent advance in the vascular laser field. Collectively referred to as long-pulsed PDLs, they offer pulse durations of up to 40 ms. By delivering equivalent fluences over variable pulse durations (1.5–40 ms), these versatile lasers are capable of treating vessels of different sizes.

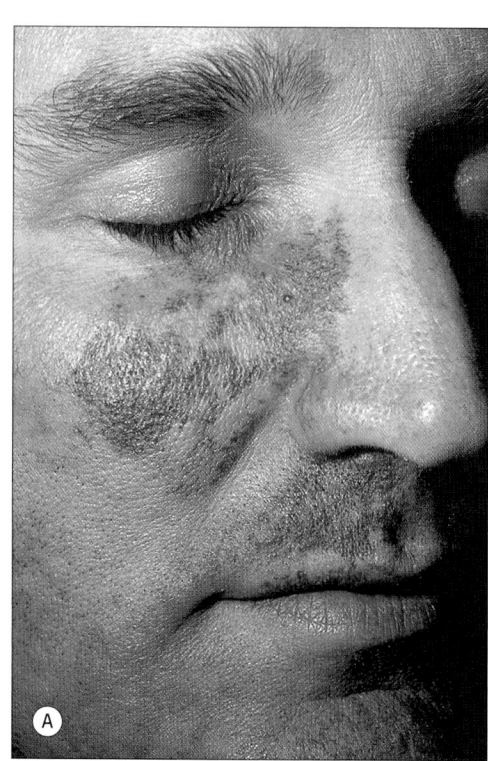
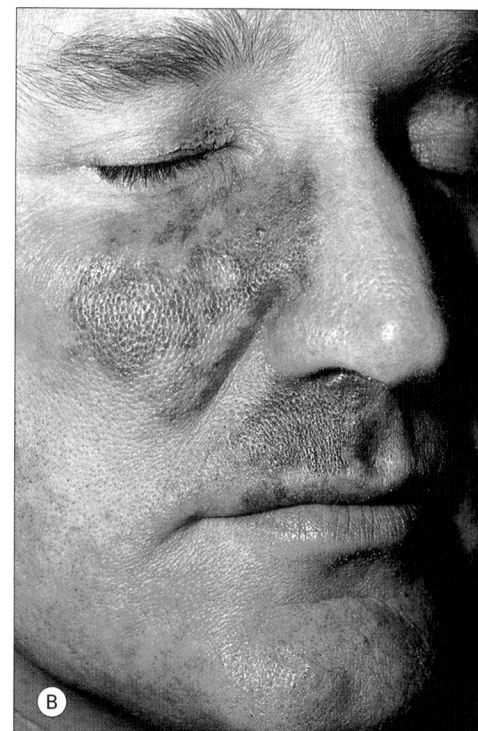
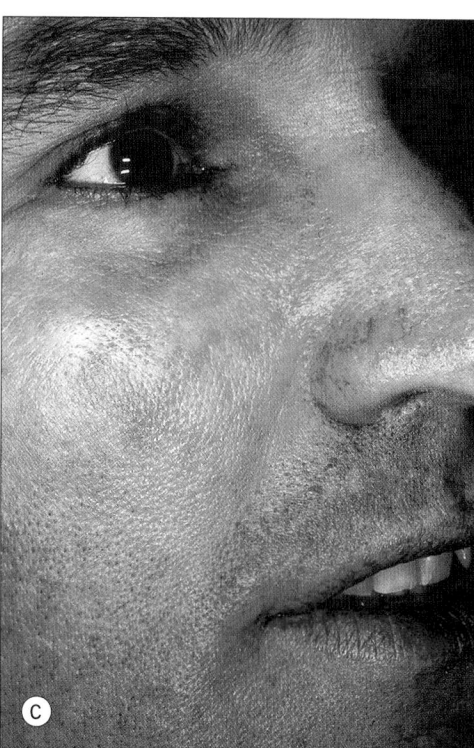

Fig. 137.2 Port-wine stain. A Before treatment. **B** Purpuric response immediately after treatment with the 585 nm, 450 ms pulsed dye laser. **C** Six weeks after the fourth pulsed dye laser treatment.

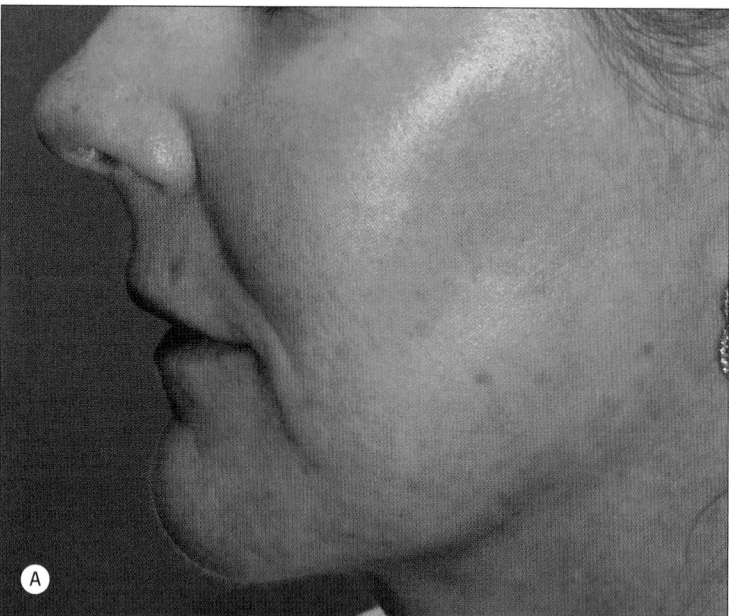
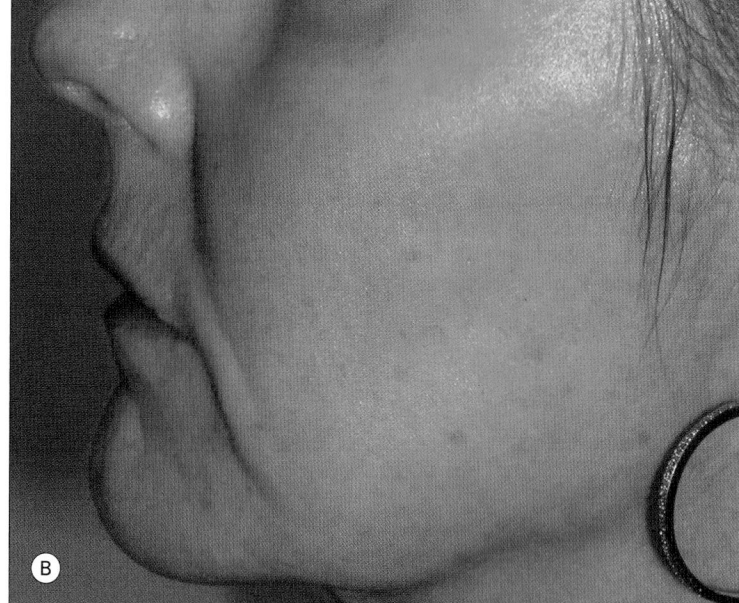

Fig. 137.3 Erythematotelangiectatic rosacea. A Before treatment. **B** After a series of long-pulsed pulsed dye laser treatments.

In addition, their longer pulse durations allow for slower and uniform heating of the targeted vessels, resulting in reduced or absent post-treatment purpura.

Long-pulsed PDLs are highly effective for the treatment of facial erythema (with no visible vessels) in patients with conditions such as rosacea. Longer pulse durations (approximately 6 ms) allow clearance to be achieved at relatively high fluences (6–8 J/cm^2) that remain below the purpura threshold. Large spot sizes of 10 mm and firing speeds of 1 Hz allow for rapid treatment, while epidermal cooling devices minimize discomfort and increase safety in darker skin types. Clearance of visible facial telangiectasias (including spider angiomas) and PWSs can be also achieved, but this typically requires fluences immediately above the threshold for purpura induction. The application of multiple long pulses on top of one another during a treatment session, termed *pulse stack-*

ing, improves efficacy without producing purpura[17]. Alternatively, a treatment session with a long-pulsed PDL using *multiple passes* at non-purpuragenic settings (e.g. 6 ms and 6 J/cm^2) results in a decrease in facial telangiectasias comparable to treatment with a single pass at purpuragenic settings (e.g. 6 ms and 12 J/cm^2)[18].

The mechanism of action of PDL in the treatment of vascular lesions has been elucidated, and *in vivo* findings are in agreement with mathematical models. The initial physical effects of PDL are followed by additional biological processes. The use of a PDL (585 nm and 0.45 ms) on the dorsal skin of hamsters resulted in the following histologic findings: (1) restriction of tissue injury to the irradiated area 1 hour after treatment, with aggregated erythrocytes within blood vessels; (2) extension of tissue injury to surrounding areas 24 hours after treatment, with thrombus formation. These results demonstrated that delayed biological processes can result in further reduction of blood vessel perfusion after initial photocoagulation. Small blood vessels measuring 2–16 μm in diameter were incompletely photocoagulated, which corresponds to the incomplete blanching of a PWS that is observed clinically[19].

Pulsed KTP lasers

Long-pulsed or variable-pulsed KTP lasers, which represent frequency-doubled Nd:YAG lasers that emit green light at 532 nm, were also developed in an effort to treat vascular anomalies without purpura and have become the optimal treatment modality for discrete facial telangiectasias (see Table 137.3). Several pulsed KTP lasers are currently in clinical use, with pulse durations ranging from 1 ms to as long as 100 ms delivered to tissue through a fiberoptic hand piece. Studies have shown these lasers to be effective in the treatment of a variety of vascular lesions, including spider leg telangiectasias and venous malformations as well as facial telangiectasias.

The distinct advantages of this group of lasers are the strong absorption of their 532 nm wavelength by hemoglobin and the absence of purpura. The latter results from the slow heating of blood vessels that occurs at longer pulse durations, which avoids rupture of the vessel wall or red blood cell extravasation into the interstitial space. The major disadvantage of pulsed KTP lasers is the limited depth of skin penetration due their short wavelength. In addition, 532 nm light competes for absorption with epidermal melanin more than longer wavelengths, resulting in potential pigmentary changes (particularly in suntanned or darkly pigmented patients).

Long-pulsed infrared lasers

The absorption spectra of oxyhemoglobin and reduced hemoglobin have useful bands in the near-IR region (720–1200 nm; see Fig. 136.5). Several pulsed lasers emitting near-IR wavelengths have been used for the treatment of leg veins, including the alexandrite (755 nm), diode (800 nm) and Nd:YAG (1064 nm) lasers (see Table 137.3). Their longer wavelengths are absorbed less by melanin and penetrate deeper into the skin, but their absorption by hemoglobin is far less than with other vascular lasers. Nonetheless, long-pulsed IR lasers can effectively photocoagulate superficial and deeper vessels up to 3 mm in diameter. These lasers are primarily used to target venulectasias in the reticular dermis, such as spider leg venulectasias, and blue reticular veins. Owing to their longer wavelengths, the diode and long-pulsed Nd:YAG lasers are particularly safe for darkly pigmented skin.

Intense pulsed light sources

IPL devices use a flashlamp to produce non-coherent, pulsed, broadband light. Wavelengths are in the visible to near-IR range (400–1200 nm), and pulse durations and intervals are variable (see Table 137.3). Although IPL is not considered to be a first-line treatment for vascular lesions, a series of cut-off filters (including 515, 550, 570, 595, 610, 645, 695 and 755 nm) can be used to shift the short end of the spectrum in order to target hemoglobin. Versatility is a major advantage of IPL sources, given the wide range of wavelengths and pulse durations that allow treatment of both superficial and deeper vascular lesions. They can generate a variety of fluences (up to 80 J/cm²) in single-, double- or triple-pulse modes in the 2–10 ms domain. The light is delivered by a fiber to an 8 × 15 mm or 8 × 35 mm aperture, allowing treatment of large areas. In an effort to decrease epidermal damage and increase depth of targeting, a cooling gel is applied on the skin. Post-treatment purpura is not produced in most instances, but it may occur with the use of high fluences and short pulse durations.

Disadvantages of IPL include longer and more numerous treatment sessions as compared to PDLs; a higher learning curve for the practitioner; and a greater risk of pigmentary alteration, blistering and scarring (particularly in dark-skinned patients). However, recent software upgrades have helped reduce adverse events and lower the learning curve. IPL can effectively treat facial telangiectasias, leg telangiectasias and port-wine stains[20–22]. It has also been used in non-ablative photorejuvenation and laser hair removal (see sections below).

Endovascular lasers

The use of lasers for the treatment of varicose veins in the setting of saphenous vein insufficiency has revolutionized therapy for this disorder, which was formerly treated primarily by surgical vein stripping (see Chapter 155). Light from 810 nm diode, 940 nm diode or 1320 nm Nd:YAG lasers or radiofrequency energy is delivered by a fiberoptic catheter, which is inserted into the incompetent saphenous vein; this results in thermal closure of the affected vessel. Complete closure rates of >90% after a single treatment have been reported for this modality[23,24]. Endovascular laser obliteration (in contrast to surgical approaches) has the advantages of rapid recovery and a lack of scarring.

Clinical Applications of Vascular Lasers

Port-wine stains

PWSs are capillary malformations that are found in 0.3–0.5% of newborns. Initially composed of small ectatic vessels in the papillary and reticular dermis, the lesions tend to become thickened over time due to a progressive increase in the diameter of the vessels and involvement of the deeper dermis and subcutis. In 65% of patients, PWSs are hypertrophic and nodular by the fifth decade of life.

PDL is the treatment of choice for PWS, and substantial lightening with few side effects can be achieved at a 585 nm wavelength and 450 μs or 1.5 ms pulse duration. More advanced, nodular or hypertrophic forms are best treated with 595–600 nm long-pulsed (1.5–40 ms) PDLs at high fluences (15–20 J/cm²) with cryogen cooling spray. The addition of cooling systems to PDLs has allowed for higher fluences to be used with minimal epidermal damage and less discomfort, resulting in faster clearance rates, reduced healing time and better patient tolerance[25]. A series of 4–12 treatment sessions with PDL are required to clear most PWSs, but in approximately 50% of patients portions of the lesion remain resistant to treatment[13]. In addition, a recent study of 51 patients with classic PDL-treated PWSs found that the lesions had darkened significantly after a median follow-up period of 10 years, although they were still lighter than prior to treatment[26].

Laser treatment of PWSs (especially those located on the face) is typically initiated early in life in order to decrease the potential psychological impact of the birthmark and avoid the development of hypertrophy. The results of some studies have suggested that PWSs in very young patients (e.g. <1 year old) tend to respond better to PDL therapy, but a large clinical study showed that treating PWSs during early childhood versus later childhood or early adulthood had similar results[27]. Although one study of 3- to 5-year-old children with PWSs found no association with problems in psychosocial development, studies of adolescents and adults with facial PWSs have demonstrated significant negative psychosocial consequences.

The rate of PWS clearance is inversely proportional to *lesion size* and also depends on *anatomic location*, with lesions on the distal extremities responding less favorably than those on the head and neck[28]. Among facial PWSs, lesions in the periorbital area and on the forehead, lateral cheeks and chin clear faster than those on the medial cheeks, upper cutaneous lip and nose[29]. In addition, red PWSs (which have relatively superficial ectatic vessels) tend to clear faster than pink PWSs (which have more deeply situated ectatic vessels). The degree of lightening is often not uniform due to various calibers and depths of the vessels within a particular PWS.

Comparative studies between different PDLs suggest that the 585 nm wavelength is more efficacious for some types of PWS than the 595 nm wavelength. In one prospective, randomized study of 15 patients, PDL treatment at a wavelength of 585 nm and pulse duration of 0.5 ms was found to be most efficacious (although it was associated with more adverse events); this was followed by 595 nm and 20 ms, then 595 nm and 0.5 ms[30]. Purple PWSs fared better than red, which responded better than pink lesions. Of note, pink PWSs (with larger, deeper vessels) responded best to the longer wavelength (595 nm) and pulse duration (20 ms). Clearance directly correlated with the degree of post-treatment purpura.

Recently, a study was conducted on 89 patients with PWSs treated with a variable-pulsed 532 nm KTP laser (at fluences of 9.5–20.0 J/cm², spot sizes of 2–6 mm and pulse durations of 15–20 ms) for 1–12 treatment sessions[31]. More than 50% improvement was observed in the majority of patients, with a low incidence of pigmentary alteration or scarring. In a different study, portions of resistant PWSs treated with a variable-pulsed 532 nm KTP laser and portions treated with a long-pulsed 595 nm PDL improved to a similar degree.

Infantile hemangiomas

Infantile hemangiomas are the most common tumor of infancy, with a 3% incidence among newborns (see Chapter 103). Lasers can effectively treat some superficial infantile hemangiomas and promote healing of ulcerated hemangiomas. PDL therapy (e.g. 595 nm, 6–7 J/cm^2 with epidermal cooling) is most beneficial for treatment of the early 'macular stain' precursor stage of infantile hemangiomas. However, lesions are usually well into the proliferative phase by the time patients present to a dermatologist[13]. The use of PDLs to treat hemangiomas in the proliferative phase (which occurs during the first 6–12 months of life) is controversial, although one report suggested that PDL therapy may accelerate involution[32]. On the other hand, laser treatment is not currently recommended for proliferating infantile hemangiomas with a deep component[13]. Finally, PDL remains the treatment of choice for residual telangiectasias present after involution of infantile hemangiomas, although multiple treatments are often needed[33].

Rosacea/telangiectasias

Rosacea is a common disease, and the erythematotelangiectatic subtype is characterized by flushing, persistent central facial erythema and telangiectasias (see Chapter 38). In general, telangiectasias may be classified into four types: linear, arborizing, spider and punctiform or papular[34]. Linear and arborizing telangiectasias measuring 0.1–1.0 mm in diameter frequently occur on the face, particularly the nose, cheeks and chin. Telangiectasias may also result from factors such as chronic sun exposure, hormones (in particular estrogen), pregnancy, physical stress and (rarely) genetic disorders.

PDLs and pulsed KTP lasers are the most rigorously studied lasers for the treatment of rosacea and telangiectasias, although the use of IPL for this purpose has been increasing in recent years. The traditional PDL had the disadvantage of postoperative purpura and has been largely replaced by the long-pulsed PDL (up to 40 ms), which is currently the treatment of choice for diffuse erythema and confluent telangiectasias due to rosacea and other conditions. The long-pulsed PDL provides purpura-free treatment with excellent efficacy for all types of telangiectasias and telangiectatic erythema using relatively high fluences (6–8 J/cm^2) and longer pulse durations (6–10 ms) (see above). Pulsed KTP lasers also clear facial telangiectasias without purpura and are the treatment of choice for linear and arborizing, discrete telangiectasias. Both lasers result in minimal postoperative erythema that resolves within a few hours (with rare crusting in the case of pulsed KTP) and high patient acceptance. Several treatment sessions are often required for patients with numerous telangiectasias or telangiectatic erythema, usually 3–5 sessions for the long-pulsed PDL and 2–3 for pulsed KTP lasers. The use of IPL also results in non-purpuric treatment of rosacea and telangiectasias with excellent patient acceptance, but it requires more (>5) treatment sessions[35]. The long-pulsed Nd:YAG laser (1064 nm, 1–100 ms) is effective in clearing deeper and larger facial vessels and is safer for dark-skinned patients.

Spider leg veins

Sclerotherapy remains the gold standard for spider leg veins (see Chapter 155). Although lasers have become highly effective, they require more treatment sessions. The 585 nm PDL is effective for leg veins less than 0.2 mm in diameter but not larger-caliber vessels[36], and almost half of patients develop post-treatment hypo- or hyperpigmentation. The long-pulsed (≥1.5 ms) 595 or 600 nm PDL at high fluences clears leg telangiectasias with infrequent complications; in one study, three treatment sessions with the 595 nm PDL (elliptical spot of 2–7 mm) at fluences of 15–20 J/cm^2 resulted in ~80% clearance of leg telangiectasias 0.4–1.5 mm in diameter[37]. The addition of a cryogen-spray cooling system to the PDL has allowed these high fluences (which are necessary to cause irreversible vascular damage) to be used safely with minimal epidermal injury. The disadvantages of the PDL include post-treatment purpura, which takes 1–2 weeks to resolve, and limited penetration depth.

Pulsed, visible lasers and other light sources are the preferred treatments for isolated, non-arborizing, superficial telangiectasias of the legs that are less than 0.3 mm in diameter, as well as for postsclerotherapy telangiectatic matting[38]. The pulsed KTP (532 nm) is an excellent therapeutic modality for superficial leg telangiectasias and venulectasias when used at high fluences (15–20 J/cm^2) and pulse durations of 15–20 ms,

requiring at least 3–5 treatment sessions at 3–4 week intervals. The advantages include high efficacy and rapid healing time, with resolution of minimal to moderate erythema within 1–2 weeks. The disadvantages of pulsed KTP are its time- and labor-intensiveness, as each vessel must be individually traced, and the poor targeting of deeper vessels. In addition, it is not an option in suntanned or darker-skinned patients due to absorption of the 532 nm wavelength by epidermal melanin, which leads to crusting and potential dyspigmentation.

IPL has been used for the treatment of leg veins with sizes ranging from 0.3 to 1 mm in diameter. In one study, treatment consisted of a sequence of pulses at fluences ranging from 25 to 70 J/cm^2, with cut-off wavelengths of 515, 550, 570 or 590 nm (depending on the diameter of the vessel)[20]. After 1–5 treatments at 2- to 4-week intervals, 94% of the patients had >50% clearance of vessels, with a low risk of scarring and hyperpigmentation.

Lasers with deeper-penetrating, near-IR wavelengths and higher fluences, in conjunction with various epidermal cooling methods, have demonstrated good clearance of larger-diameter (up to 2–3 mm) and more deeply situated leg telangiectasias and reticular veins. Long-pulsed alexandrite lasers (755 nm, 3 ms) with a cryogen-spray cooling system achieved 75% clearance in 65% of the treated vessels (up to 2 mm in diameter) 12 weeks after 1–3 laser passes[39]. Transient hyperpigmentation was seen in 35% of treatment sites. The 810 nm diode laser (30–40 ms) was used to treat leg telangiectasias 0.4–1.0 mm in diameter in conjunction with a contact-cooling sapphire hand piece[40]. At fluences of 40 J/cm^2 there was 50% clearance after two treatments and 75% clearance after three treatments. Similar results have been achieved with a long-pulsed Nd:YAG laser (1064 nm, 10–16 ms) at fluences of 80–130 J/cm^2. Approximately 75% of veins 0.5–3.0 mm in diameter cleared 3 months after a single treatment. As observed with sclerotherapy, improved treatment outcomes are achieved when incompetent perforator and reticular feeding veins are treated first using appropriate surgical approaches or large-vessel sclerotherapy.

Other vascular lesions

A great variety of vascular lesions can be treated effectively with currently available laser devices. Cherry angiomas and low-flow spider angiomas clear within 1–2 treatment sessions using almost any of the vascular lasers, but results are best with the pulsed KTP. High-flow spider angiomas require more aggressive treatment with PDL, using cooling to protect the overlying epidermis. Venous lakes, venous malformations, angiokeratomas and Kaposi sarcoma have all been successfully treated with vascular lasers.

Laser Treatment Methodologies for Vascular Lesions

Anesthesia

PDL therapy is relatively well tolerated by adults, although treatment of particularly sensitive sites (e.g. the infranasal and periorbital skin, digits and anogenital region) is best performed with the use of a topical or local anesthetic (see Chapter 143). In infants and children, treatment is often traumatic and typically requires topical anesthesia; in certain cases, local, regional or general anesthesia may be necessary. Discomfort during PDL treatment is described as akin to a rubber band snapped against the skin. With 532 nm pulsed KTP laser therapy, patients experience a transient stinging or burning sensation that is usually well tolerated without any local anesthesia. IPL therapy is associated with minimal discomfort and does not require topical anesthesia. Although treatment with older near-IR lasers resulted in significant discomfort, improvements in newer near-IR lasers have minimized the discomfort and eliminated the need for topical anesthesia.

Technique

With PDL therapy, individual laser pulses can be delivered at a repetitive rate of up to 2 Hz with spot sizes ranging from 2 to 12 mm. The pulses are placed adjacent to one another with approximately 20% overlap to avoid missing areas in between the circular spots, thus preventing a reticular or honeycombed appearance of the treated site. The therapeutic endpoint is either appearance of light gray discoloration (purpuric mode) or transient purpura that lasts no longer than 1–2 seconds (non-purpuric mode).

With pulsed KTP lasers, the hand piece is held perpendicular to the skin surface at a predetermined distance and the vessels are traced individually at the speed necessary to heat and seal them without producing overlying epidermal damage. Disappearance of the vessels and a subtle blanching effect within the treated area are the treatment endpoints. For IPL therapy, aqueous gel is applied and 1–3 passes of non-overlapping pulses are administered, increasing the fluence in subsequent treatment sessions. Treatment with near-IR lasers differs depending on the device that it utilized, but it also typically involves non-overlapping pulses administered in 1–3 passes, with subsequent application of cool packs to minimize side effects such as erythema and edema.

LASER TREATMENT FOR PIGMENTED LESIONS AND TATTOO REMOVAL

The first use of lasers to treat pigmented lesions or remove tattoos was with the normal-mode ruby laser in the 1960s[41]. Continuous-wave lasers (e.g. CO_2, Nd:YAG and argon lasers) were also utilized to remove pigmentation but often caused scarring. The development of short-pulsed, pigment-specific lasers (Q-switched lasers) over the past two decades has enabled the targeting of subcellular pigment with high selectivity and a low risk of complications. These lasers emit high-powered pulses with extremely short durations that selectively target exogenous or endogenous pigment with minimal damage to adjacent tissues.

Experimental studies have shown that Q-switched lasers can target and destroy the melanosome[42]. The thermomechanical action on melanosomes and the generation of acoustic waves result in dispersion of the pigment within keratinocytes and melanocytes to the periphery of the cell, which appears as a 'ring-cell' formation histologically[43]. This is thought to correlate with the whitening phenomenon observed clinically immediately after Q-switched laser therapy of pigmented lesions.

Types of Pigment Lasers

The lasers that are currently used to treat pigmented lesions are grouped into three categories: (1) highly selective Q-switched lasers; (2) the less pigment-selective, longer-pulsed lasers; and (3) non-pigment-specific ablative lasers (Table 137.4). The highly selective Q-switched lasers include the Q-switched frequency-doubled Nd:YAG (532 nm), Q-switched ruby (694 nm), Q-switched alexandrite (755 nm) and Q-switched Nd:YAG (1064 nm) lasers. The 532 nm wavelength targets epidermal pigment, the 694 and 755 nm wavelengths target epidermal and dermal pigment, and the 1064 nm wavelength targets deeper dermal pigment.

The less-selective lasers that are currently used for pigment removal include the long-pulsed ruby (694 nm), variable-pulsed diode (800 nm) and long-pulsed Nd:YAG, which through manipulation of fluence and pulse duration may be used to target pigment in the epidermis and dermis, although less effectively than with the Q-switched lasers. Given their ability to target larger pigmented structures, these long-pulsed lasers have been employed for the treatment of certain melanocytic nevi (e.g. congenital), presumably by destroying nests of melanocytes and (in hypertrichotic nevi) hair follicles. Pigment removal can also be achieved with an IPL source, which can generate polychromatic light in the visible to IR region at variable pulse widths and intervals. Lastly, pigment non-selective ablative lasers, such as CO_2 (10 600 nm) and erbium:YAG (Er:YAG; 2940 nm) lasers, may remove superficial pigmented lesions via non-specific destruction.

The approach to the treatment of pigmented lesions and tattoo removal with lasers depends on the anatomic location of the pigment (epidermal, dermal or mixed), the type of pigment (melanin, tattoo ink) and its distribution in tissue (extracellular, intracellular). In most cases the chromophore is melanin, although other exogenous and endogenous pigments can be targeted. Epidermal pigmented lesions respond well to lasers with shorter wavelengths (up to 755 nm), whereas for deeper lesions the longer-wavelength, pigment-specific lasers (694 nm and beyond, preferably 1064 nm) are more suitable. The Q-switched Nd:YAG at 1064 nm is best for treating darkly pigmented skin because of the lower risk of inducing pigmentary changes. In general, laser-treated lentigines,

LASERS AND OTHER LIGHT-BASED DEVICES USED FOR THE TREATMENT OF PIGMENTED LESIONS				
Laser/device	Wavelength (nm)	Fluence (J/cm²)	Pulse duration	Applications
Q-switched lasers (highly pigment-specific)				
Q-switched Nd:YAG, frequency-doubled	532	0.4–6	5–10 ns	Lentigines
Q-switched ruby	694	3–12	20–40 ns	Lentigines, nevi*
Q-switched alexandrite	755	0.85–12	50–100 ns	Lentigines, nevi*
Q-switched Nd:YAG	1064	0.75–12	5–10 ns	Nevi*
Long-pulsed lasers and intense pulsed light (less pigment-specific)				
Long-pulsed ruby†	694	Up to 100	0.2–25 ms	Nevi*
Diode	800	Up to 100	5–400 ms	Lentigines, nevi*
Nd:YAG	1064	Up to 600	0.25–300 ms	Nevi*
Intense pulsed light source	500–1200	Up to 80	10–150 ms	Lentigines, nevi*

Treatment of melanocytic nevi (especially acquired lesions) is controversial.
† *No longer being manufactured.*

Table 137.4 Lasers and other light-based devices used for the treatment of pigmented lesions. Q-switched lasers are most effective for treating pigmented lesions due to their very short pulse durations, which effectively target the melanosome. In addition to the lasers listed below, pigment non-selective ablative lasers, such as CO_2 (10 600 nm) and erbium:YAG (Er:YAG; 2940 nm), can remove superficial pigmented lesions via non-specific destruction.

ephelides and dermal melanocytoses improve markedly or clear completely, while café-au-lait macules (CALMs), postinflammatory hyperpigmentation and melasma exhibit variable responses and higher recurrence rates after laser treatment.

Clinical Applications of Pigment Lasers
Epidermal pigmented lesions
Superficial pigmented lesions, such as ephelides, solar (Fig. 137.4) and labial lentigines, and flat pigmented seborrheic keratoses, can be effectively treated with most of the pigment-specific pulsed lasers (see Table 137.4)[44]. The healing time and the side effect profile among these lasers are similar, but infrequent purpura after treatment with Q-switched ruby (694 nm) and alexandrite (755 nm) lasers makes them slightly preferable over green-light, Q-switched Nd:YAG (532 nm) lasers, especially when treating facial lesions. One or two laser treatment sessions are usually sufficient to clear most lentigines, although further treatments are occasionally required for larger and more resistant lesions. Post-treatment pigmentary changes (in particular hyperpigmentation) are most frequently observed in individuals with skin types III–IV or suntanned skin. The risk of hypopigmentation is higher with the Q-switched ruby laser than with the Q-switched alexandrite laser.

In contrast, clinical experience with Q-switched lasers for the treatment of CALMs has yielded variable responses. Short-term lightening or complete clearing is frequently achieved after repeated laser treatments over a period of several weeks or months. Despite initial improvement, however, recurrences are frequent, occurring in as many as 50% of patients. There are a few reports of complete lightening of CALMs treated with the 510 nm pigmented lesion dye laser or Er:YAG laser resurfacing, with no evidence of recurrence 1–1½ years later[45,46]. The frequent recurrences of CALMs after laser therapy may be due to relatively rapid resumption of melanosome production, melanization and transfer from melanocytes to keratinocytes and/or replenishment with 'overactive' melanocytes that presumably harbor a somatic mutation.

In Becker's melanosis, where hypertrichosis as well as hyperpigmentation are often present, multiple Q-switched laser treatments typically result in incomplete removal, hypopigmentation and recurrences.

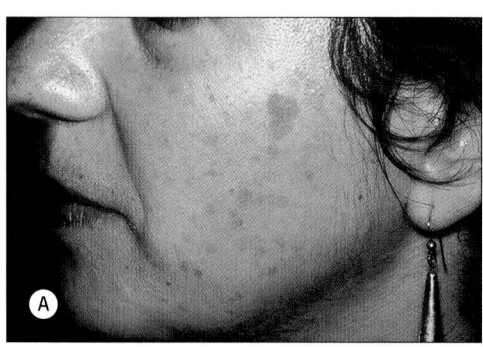

Fig. 137.4 Lentigines. Before (**A**) and 6 weeks after (**B**) a single Q-switched ruby laser treatment. There is lightening of the treated lesions, but an additional treatment is required to achieve full improvement.

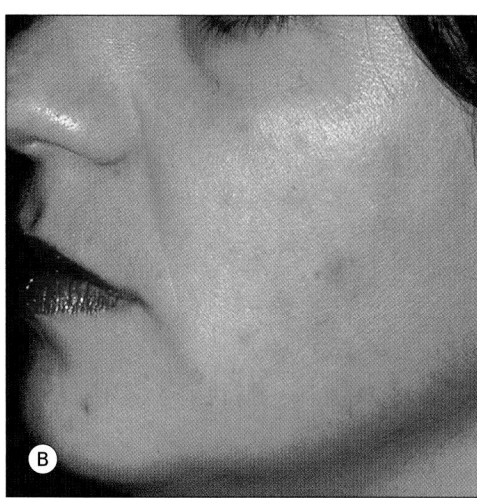

Although superficial pigment is eliminated after Q-switched ruby laser irradiation, a significant amount of pigment persists in the adnexal structures[47]. The complex hamartomatous nature of Becker's melanosis and its hormone dependency, demonstrated by enhanced lesional androgen receptor activity, may play a role in the resistance to treatment. The best approach for Becker's melanosis is a combination of a Q-switched laser to remove the epidermal pigment and a long-pulsed alexandrite, diode or Nd:YAG laser to remove the hypertrichosis.

Laser therapy of epidermal nevi is a useful alternative in cases where other surgical methods cannot be employed. In the past, continuous-wave argon lasers (488 nm, 514 nm) were used for soft, velvety lesions, whereas the continuous-wave CO_2 laser (10 600 nm) was applied for thicker, hyperkeratotic nevi. Pulsed CO_2 and Er:YAG resurfacing lasers are now preferable, circumventing the risk of scarring from continuous-wave lasers. Epidermal nevi have also been successfully treated with the long-pulsed ruby laser (694 nm, pulse duration of <0.2 ms, fluences of 18–25 J/cm^2), with occasional post-treatment hypopigmentation but no scarring[48].

Dermal and mixed epidermal/dermal pigmentary disorders (other than melanocytic nevi)

Despite repeated attempts to treat melasma with lasers, longstanding clearing has rarely been achieved and recurrence is the rule. Epidermal melasma shows a moderate response to laser treatment, similar to bleaching agents or chemical peels, while the dermal and mixed types of melasma are generally resistant to laser therapy[49]. In addition, darkly pigmented melasma patients have a significant risk of darkening following laser treatment. Treatment of the more refractory, dermal-type melasma with resurfacing lasers (pulsed/scanned CO_2 or Er:YAG) to ablate the superficial portion of the skin (including melanocytes) has been attempted. Despite the marked improvement noted immediately after treatment with the Er:YAG laser, in one study all the patients developed postinflammatory hyperpigmentation that required frequent glycolic acid peels, with ultimate sustained improvement 6 months later[50]. Complete clearance of dermal-type melasma has been achieved with pulsed CO_2 laser resurfacing followed by Q-switched alexandrite laser treatment to selectively target dermal melanin[51].

Until the development of short-pulsed lasers, there was no effective treatment for dermal melanocytoses such as nevus of Ota, nevus of Ito

and persistent Mongolian spots. Q-switched laser therapy has become the treatment of choice for these disorders[52]. The Q-switched ruby, alexandrite and Nd:YAG (1064 nm) lasers are all highly effective in targeting the pigmented, dendritic dermal melanocytes, producing significant (>75%) or complete lesional clearing after an average of 4–8 laser treatments with fluences ranging from 5 to 12 J/cm^2 [53–55]. The number of treatments required is determined by the degree of pigmentation and the depth of the dermal melanocytes[56,57]. Aside from temporary postinflammatory hyperpigmentation, no significant complications have been reported after laser treatment, and once the nevus has fully cleared the results are usually permanent.

Laser treatment of postinflammatory hyperpigmentation may result in initial improvement, but recurrences or even worsening of the pigmentation often occur in susceptible individuals due to additional epidermal trauma from the laser's impact. In addition, individual treatment spots may develop central lightening together with peripheral postinflammatory hyperpigmentation.

Dark infraorbital circles are caused by dermal pigmentation, shadowing from excess lid laxity and prominent cutaneous vasculature. When dermal pigmentation is the main cause, dark circles respond favorably to several treatments with the Q-switched ruby laser, in spite of the frequent incidence of postinflammatory hyperpigmentation[58]. Significant reduction of infraorbital pigmentation has also been achieved with CO_2 laser resurfacing[59].

Certain forms of drug-induced hyperpigmentation have improved with the use of short-pulsed lasers. The blue-black hyperpigmentation caused by minocycline has been reported to clear after treatment with Q-switched ruby, alexandrite and Nd:YAG (1064 nm) lasers[60]. Similar results have been reported for amiodarone-induced discoloration treated with the Q-switched ruby laser[61]. However, laser treatment should be deferred until the drug has been discontinued and a reasonable time has been allowed for spontaneous resolution.

Melanocytic nevi and lentigo maligna

Controversy remains regarding laser treatment of congenital and acquired melanocytic nevi; for the latter lesions, the lack of histologic evaluation is especially problematic. Laser therapy is most often considered for facial congenital melanocytic nevi when surgical excision would be difficult to perform or would leave a cosmetically unacceptable scar. Q-switched ruby, alexandrite and Nd:YAG (1064 nm) laser treatments of small- to medium-sized congenital nevi have led to clinical improvement after several sessions[62–64]. Histologic examination following laser treatment has demonstrated a reduction of nevus cells in the papillary and upper reticular dermis, with residual nevomelanocytes in the deeper dermis. This explains the partial responses and frequent recurrences that have been observed[63,64].

Long-pulsed lasers have also been utilized to treat melanocytic nevi, offering the theoretical advantage of eliminating larger and deeper pigmented structures within the skin, i.e. nests of cells rather than subcellular organelles. The use of a normal-mode, long-pulsed (0.3–1 ms) ruby laser at fluences of 10–20 J/cm^2 produced almost complete clearance of two giant congenital nevi and a medium-sized congenital nevus of the eyelid after four treatment sessions, with minimal side effects[65]. In a study of 13 patients with medium- or large-sized congenital melanocytic nevi, long-pulsed ruby laser treatment (with or without use of a Q-switched ruby laser) showed efficacy despite residual nevus cells only 1 mm below the skin surface[66]. Fibroplasia above the remaining nevomelanocytes was seen histologically, which may have accounted for the marked clinical lightening of the nevi (as is also seen with dermabrasion or curettage performed during the neonatal period). The patients had no clinical or histologic evidence of malignant degeneration during follow-up periods of up to 8 years[66].

In one study, only partial clearing of acquired banal and dysplastic melanocytic nevi was noted after treatment with a Q-switched ruby laser (40–60 ns, 7.5–8.0 J/cm^2), a normal-mode ruby laser (3 ms, 40 J/cm^2) or both[67]. No lesion had a complete histologic response and no malignant or atypical changes were observed microscopically. In other studies, treatment of acquired banal melanocytic nevi with a Q-switched (± normal mode) ruby laser resulted in persistence or recurrence of nevi with a dermal component, but histologically confirmed complete removal of a subset of purely junctional nevi (with no recurrence after a follow-up period of up to 1 year)[68].

Although longer follow-up studies are needed, to date there have been several reports of melanoma arising in laser-treated lesions presumed to represent melanocytic nevi, including a superficial spreading melanoma at the periphery of a large congenital melanocytic nevus on the back that had been treated with an argon laser 10 years earlier as well as melanoma developing within lesions initially diagnosed clinically or via partial biopsy as acquired melanocytic nevi and treated with a Q-switched ruby or CO_2 laser. In addition, there have been descriptions of lentigo maligna melanoma arising within lesions initially diagnosed clinically as atypical-appearing solar lentigines and treated with a Q-switched ruby or alexandrite laser[69]. Patients with a personal or family history of melanoma or dysplastic nevi should not be considered candidates for laser treatment of their nevi. Individuals who have had a nevus removed by laser should be followed closely and any signs of recurrence require a biopsy or total excision of the lesion. Because early melanomas can have a subtle clinical appearance, the major concern is their misdiagnosis as banal nevi and subsequent laser treatment.

Laser treatment of a speckled lentiginous nevus (nevus spilus) typically improves the darker superimposed 'spots' (lentigines and melanocytic nevi of various types) more so than the macular CALM-like background. Multiple Q-switched ruby laser treatments result in variable clearing with frequent recurrences, particularly of the macular background[70]. Melanomas have been reported to arise within speckled lentiginous nevi, so (as for other types of congenital melanocytic nevi) patients who undergo laser therapy should be followed closely.

Lentigo maligna, a form of melanoma *in situ* that develops in sites of chronic sun exposure, has been treated with a variety of lasers as a palliative modality. Early studies employing the argon and CO_2 lasers were associated with a 50% recurrence rate on long-term follow-up[71]. Patients with an unresectable lentigo maligna have been treated with the Q-switched ruby laser (10 J/cm^2) with significant clearance, but in one case the lesion recurred as an amelanotic melanoma. In general, laser treatment for lentigo maligna is not recommended.

Tattoos

Tattoos are classified as cosmetic, medical or traumatic, with the last resulting from accidental penetration of a foreign, pigmented material such as carbon, lead, asphalt or gunpowder into the skin. In the past, a number of different modalities were employed for tattoo removal, including surgical excision, dermabrasion, salabrasion, cryosurgery and destruction with caustic chemicals, yielding variable responses and frequently causing scarring. The use of Q-switched lasers has revolutionized the field of tattoo removal by selectively targeting and clearing tattoo pigment with a minimal risk of textural changes.

For effective tattoo removal, laser light must be absorbed by the tattoo pigment and the pulse duration must be shorter than the thermal relaxation time of the pigmented particles. Q-switched lasers meet these criteria by delivering high-energy, ultrashort (nanosecond range) pulses of a wavelength that is preferentially absorbed by the tattoo pigment. This leads to fragmentation of the tattoo particles and selective death of pigment-containing cells, which is followed by re-phagocytosis and lymphatic elimination[72,73]. Lamellated pigment material that is left behind in the dermis is also less visibly apparent.

Removal of Different Colors and Types of Tattoos

Black tattoo pigment absorbs all laser wavelengths, making it the most susceptible to treatment, while colored tattoos selectively absorb laser light and can therefore be effectively treated by only some of the available laser devices (Table 137.5). *Blue* tattoo pigment can be removed by Q-switched ruby, alexandrite and Nd:YAG lasers. *Green* tattoo pigment absorbs maximally in the 630–740 nm wavelength range and is best treated with the Q-switched ruby (694 nm) and alexandrite (755 nm) lasers. *Yellow* and *red* tattoo pigments have maximal absorption in the 505–560 nm range, making the ruby and alexandrite lasers ineffective for treating these tattoos. The frequency-doubled Q-switched Nd:YAG laser (532 nm) and pigmented lesion dye laser (510 nm flashlamp-pumped PDL) emit more suitable wavelengths and are also useful for other bright tattoo colors such as *orange* and *violet*[74]. Thus, multicolored tattoos often require more than one laser wavelength for complete removal (Fig. 137.5).

Amateur tattoos require fewer laser treatments (3–6 sessions) because they usually consist of a single carbon-based pigment that is more easily disrupted by pulses of laser light. Professional tattoos are typically more resistant to laser treatment because they are more densely pigmented and may contain multiple and less responsive pigments,

TATTOO PIGMENTS, LASERS USED FOR THEIR REMOVAL AND POTENTIAL COMPLICATIONS			
Color/etiology	Pigment	Lasers	Complications
Traumatic	Lead, dirt, gunpowder, other	QS ruby, QS alexandrite, QS Nd:YAG (1064)	Hypopigmentation, microexplosions (gunpowder)
Amateur black	India ink, carbon	QS ruby, QS alexandrite, QS Nd:YAG (1064)	Hypopigmentation
Professional black	Carbon, iron oxide, logwood extract	QS ruby, QS alexandrite, QS Nd:YAG (1064)	Hypopigmentation
Blue	Cobalt aluminate (azure blue)	QS ruby, QS alexandrite, QS Nd:YAG (1064)	Hypopigmentation
Green	Chromium oxide (casalis green), hydrated chromium sesquioxide (guignet green), malachite green, lead chromate, ferro-ferric cyanide, curcumin green, phthalocyanine dyes (copper salts with yellow coal tar dyes)	QS ruby, QS alexandrite	Hypopigmentation, allergic reactions (chromium)
Red	Mercury sulfide (cinnabar), cadmium selenide (cadmium red), sienna (red ochre; ferric hydrate and ferric sulfate), azo dyes	QS Nd:YAG (532), pigmented lesion dye (510)	Hypopigmentation, tattoo ink darkening, allergic reactions (mercury sulfide, cadmium, azo dyes)
Yellow	Cadmium sulfide (cadmium yellow), ochre, curcumin yellow	QS Nd:YAG (532), pigmented lesion dye (510)	Hypopigmentation, tattoo ink darkening, allergic reactions (cadmium)
Brown	Ochre	Tan/light brown: QS Nd:YAG (532), pigmented lesion dye (510) Dark brown: QS ruby, QS alexandrite, QS Nd:YAG (1064)	Hypopigmentation, tattoo ink darkening
Violet	Manganese violet	QS Nd:YAG (532), pigmented lesion dye (510)	Hypopigmentation, tattoo ink darkening
White	Titanium dioxide, zinc oxide	QS Nd:YAG (532), pigmented lesion dye (510)	Hypopigmentation, tattoo ink darkening
Flesh	Iron oxides	QS Nd:YAG (532), pigmented lesion dye (510)	Hypopigmentation, tattoo ink darkening

Table 137.5 Tattoo pigments, lasers used for their removal and potential complications. Hyperpigmentation and textural changes also occasionally occur as complications. Hypo- and hyperpigmentation are more common in individuals with darkly pigmented skin, and they are best treated with the Q-switched (QS) Nd:YAG (1064) laser to reduce this risk.

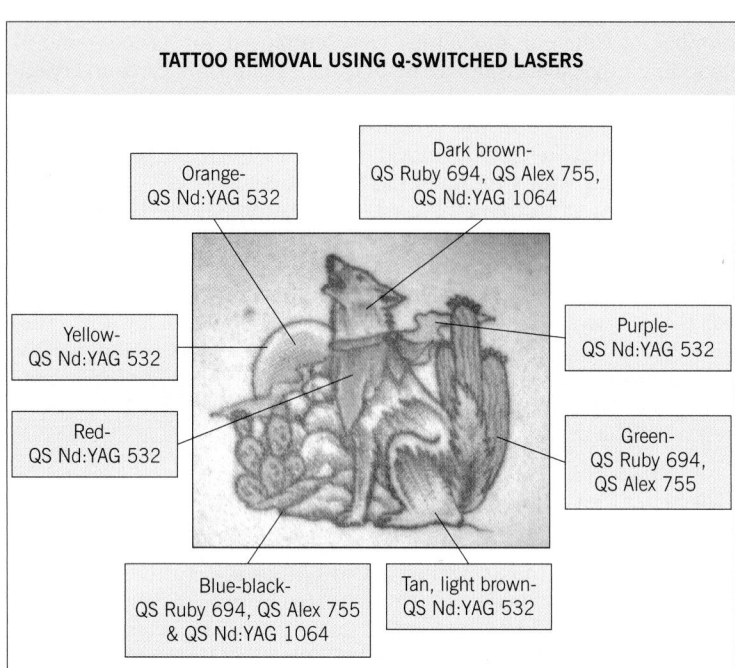

TATTOO REMOVAL USING Q-SWITCHED LASERS

Orange- QS Nd:YAG 532

Dark brown- QS Ruby 694, QS Alex 755, QS Nd:YAG 1064

Yellow- QS Nd:YAG 532

Purple- QS Nd:YAG 532

Red- QS Nd:YAG 532

Green- QS Ruby 694, QS Alex 755

Blue-black- QS Ruby 694, QS Alex 755 & QS Nd:YAG 1064

Tan, light brown- QS Nd:YAG 532

Fig. 137.5 Tattoo removal using Q-switched lasers. The Q-switched (QS) Nd:YAG (532 nm) and pigmented lesion dye (510 nm) lasers can be used to remove red, orange, yellow, purple and tan/light brown pigments. The QS alexandrite (Alex; 755 nm) and QS ruby (694 nm) lasers can be employed to remove green tattoo ink, while the QS Alex, QS ruby and Q-switched Nd:YAG (1064 nm) lasers can remove blue-black and dark brown tattoo ink. Courtesy of Jean L Bolognia MD.

particularly yellow and dark green colors. At least 6–10 treatments are necessary to markedly improve professional tattoos, and it is often not possible to totally clear the tattoo pigment. In one study of blue-black tattoos treated with the Q-switched ruby laser, 85% of amateur tattoos were completely removed in an average of three treatment sessions, whereas only 10% of professional tattoos completely resolved and 70% were partially removed after an average of six treatment sessions[75].

Older tattoos tend to have less dense pigment deposits and may be easier to remove than fresh tattoos. Traumatic tattoos typically respond well to Q-switched lasers because of their predominately superficial location and carbon-based pigment. The Q-switched Nd:YAG laser (1064 nm), which penetrates deeper into the skin, may be more effective than the ruby laser for deeper tattoos. Because its longer wavelength is less likely to be absorbed by epidermal melanin, the Q-switched Nd:YAG laser is also advantageous for patients with darkly pigmented skin.

Laser treatment of tattoos can be remarkably effective, but approximately one-third of patients have residual laser-altered tattoos despite multiple treatments. Current research efforts are focusing on the use of lasers with shorter pulse durations (subnanosecond range) for more effective treatment of tattoos[76]. The use of picosecond pulses is theoretically attractive because the thermal relaxation time of most tattoo pigment particles is less than 10 ns[77]. In addition, technical advances may allow the future development of either lasers with wavelength tunability (in order to match the absorption spectra of different tattoo pigments) or tattoo materials that are more easily dispersed with laser therapy.

Adverse Effects of Laser Tattoo Removal

Common adverse effects of laser tattoo removal include pigmentary and textural changes. Transient and rarely long-term hypopigmentation may develop, particularly with the Q-switched ruby and alexandrite lasers. Hyperpigmentation develops in up to 15% of cases, occurring most frequently in patients with darkly pigmented skin. Transient textural changes are occasionally seen after Q-switched laser therapy, especially with the Q-switched Nd:YAG (1064 nm), but scarring occurs in less than 5% of patients.

Local allergic reactions to various tattoo pigments (e.g. cadmium sulfide, chromium) have been reported, and systemic allergic reactions to mobilized tattoo antigens have been precipitated by Q-switched laser

treatment[78,79]. Local cutaneous reactions to tattoo pigments can include eczematous, granulomatous (sarcoidal or foreign body), lichenoid and pseudolymphomatous inflammatory responses as well as pseudo-epitheliomatous hyperplasia of the overlying epidermis (see Chapter 93). In patients with a history of allergic reactions to tattoo ink, laser treatment is generally not recommended, although the concomitant use of oral antihistamines and topical or systemic corticosteroids as a preventive measure has been successful in some patients.

A well-established complication of treatment with Q-switched lasers is paradoxical darkening of cosmetic tattoos containing beige, red, white or light brown tattoo pigments[80]. This phenomenon has been attributed to reduction of ferric oxide pigment (Fe^{3+}) to ferrous oxide (Fe^{2+}). It leads to the immediate appearance of gray-black color that is difficult to remove, although it may improve with further Q-switched Nd:YAG (1064 nm) laser therapy. Hence, the treatment of cosmetic tattoos (e.g. lip tattoos) should be approached cautiously by performing a test site with a single pulse and following up 2 weeks later to assess the clinical outcome. In selected cases, the use of high-powered continuous-wave or pulsed CO_2 and Er:YAG lasers may remove these tattoos effectively and bypass the ink-darkening effect.

Occasionally, Q-switched lasers may cause hyperpigmentation in patients receiving certain drugs. Localized chrysiasis was induced in a patient receiving parenteral gold therapy who underwent treatment with a Q-switched ruby laser for postinflammatory hyperpigmentation[81]. This effect was probably due to a physicochemical alteration of the dermal gold deposits by the laser, similar to the darkening effect of Q-switched lasers on cosmetic tattoos.

Q-switched Laser Treatment Methodologies

Anesthesia

Anesthesia is rarely required for the treatment of small pigmented lesions and tattoos. When treating larger areas or lesions on sensitive sites, topical or intralesional anesthetics may be necessary. In the treatment of nevus of Ota, a regional nerve block utilizing a 1–2% lidocaine solution with 1:100 000 or 1:200 000 epinephrine followed by supplementary local infiltration of the treated area usually provides adequate anesthesia.

Technique

The parameters of laser treatment vary and depend on the type of laser, the type of pigmented lesion or tattoo and the patient's skin type. In general, higher fluences are necessary for dermal lesions compared to those used for epidermal lesions. A uniform whitening immediately after treatment is considered an adequate therapeutic response. Excessive fluences that disrupt the epidermis should be avoided as they may result in tissue sloughing, prolonged healing time and an increased risk of pigmentary alterations. Patients with skin types IV–VI should be treated cautiously with lower fluences because their threshold response is likely to occur at a lower energy than patients with lightly pigmented skin.

The whitening that develops immediately after treatment with Q-switched lasers usually fades within 30 minutes. An urticarial reaction may also develop in and around the treated area, causing some itching or stinging that typically resolves within a few hours, rarely requiring oral antihistamines. After the whitening fades, the treated lesion appears darker in color and forms a superficial crust that usually falls off in 7–14 days, depending on the site and the aggressiveness of treatment. Following treatment with the frequency-doubled Q-switched Nd:YAG laser (532 nm), purpura usually appears after the whitening fades because of concomitant absorption of hemoglobin at this wavelength and consequent rupture of blood vessels. The purpura usually lasts for 5–7 days.

LASER HAIR REMOVAL

Laser hair removal is one of the most frequently performed laser procedures. It has supplanted electrolysis as the preferred mode of long-term hair removal, because laser treatment is more effective, faster (requiring less time per session and fewer sessions) and less painful. Laser hair removal targets the pigment present in hair follicles (e.g. within the hair shaft). Long wavelengths (which penetrate into the deep dermis and are preferentially absorbed by melanin) and high fluences are delivered in long (millisecond domain) pulse durations, allowing diffusion of heat from the pigmented chromophores in an amount sufficient to damage stem cells in the bulge region of the follicle (which does not contain substantial amounts of melanin).

The first laser hair removal technique approved by the US Food and Drug Administration (FDA) involved application of a carbon particle suspension to the skin followed by exposure to Q-switched Nd:YAG (1064 nm) laser pulses[82]. The carbon particles were postulated to penetrate into the hair follicle, allowing selective absorption of laser energy. Although temporary hair removal was achieved with this method in patients with light and dark hair colors, long-lasting results were not achieved, presumably because of the limited spatial injury that was caused by the carbon–Q-switched Nd:YAG laser combination.

Current laser hair removal systems use follicular melanin as a chromophore and are therefore most effective and safe for patients with lightly pigmented skin and dark hair. In 1996, high fluences from a long-pulsed or normal-mode ruby laser (694 nm) were shown to effectively remove pigmented human terminal hair, based on the principle of selective photothermolysis[83]. This was followed by the development of several laser systems and light sources that specifically targeted hair follicles. The first laser hair removal system employed was the normal-mode ruby laser, but the pulse duration of 0.3 ms was not efficacious; longer pulse durations of 0.7–0.8 ms subsequently increased its usefulness. When the pulse duration of the ruby laser was lengthened to 3 ms, permanent hair removal was demonstrated; however, there was a significant risk of dyspigmentation. Longer-wavelength lasers such as the alexandrite (755 nm), diode (800 nm) and Nd:YAG (1064 nm) were subsequently employed at long pulse durations, resulting in safe, effective, long-lasting hair removal. The decreased absorption of these longer wavelengths by melanin, together with the use of epidermal cooling devices and longer pulse durations, has enabled patients with darkly pigmented skin to be safely treated with the latter group of lasers (particularly the Nd:YAG).

Two follicular responses can be observed after laser treatment: (1) temporary hair growth arrest (primarily via induction of catagen); and (2) longstanding or permanent hair removal[84]. The latter can occur by miniaturization of terminal hair follicles (producing vellus-like hairs) or via degeneration and fibrosis of the follicle. Clinically, regrowing hairs are often thinner and lighter than the original hairs as well as reduced in number. The overall cosmetic outcome is determined not only by the absolute number of hairs, but also by the diameter, length and color of hairs in the treated area. Histologically, selective thermal injury to the superficial and deep follicular epithelium has been observed immediately after treatment with the long-pulsed ruby, alexandrite, diode and Nd:YAG lasers. Biopsies performed a year or more later show replacement of terminal hairs by vellus-like hairs and/or the presence of fibrosis.

Types of Hair Removal Lasers

The hair removal systems most commonly used in current clinical practice are near-IR lasers (alexandrite, diode and Nd:YAG) and IPL sources (400–1200 nm) (Table 137.6)[85,86]. The majority of patients with brown or black, coarse terminal hair treated with high fluences (>30 J/cm²) using the ruby, alexandrite or diode laser experience long-term hair reduction. The long-pulsed Nd:YAG laser, although less effective, can also result in long-term hair reduction. Controlled studies utilizing hair counts have demonstrated an average of 15–35% long-term hair loss after each laser treatment when appropriate fluences were used[87].

Long-pulsed ruby laser

The permanence of hair reduction appears to require that a critical fluence threshold be reached regardless of the laser used. The long-pulsed ruby (694 nm) was the first laser studied, with as much as 20–60% hair reduction reported after a single treatment[86]. In an initial study, a single treatment with the long-pulsed ruby laser (0.3 ms pulse duration, fluences ranging from 30 to 60 J/cm²) induced temporary hair growth arrest for 1–3 months (compared to unexposed control sites), with a greater degree of hair loss at 6 months in sites treated with higher fluences[83]. A subset of these patients was followed for 2 years,

LASERS AND OTHER LIGHT-BASED DEVICES USED FOR HAIR REMOVAL					
Laser/device	Wavelength (nm)	Pulse duration (ms)	Fluence (J/cm²)	Skin types treated	Efficacy
Long-pulsed lasers					
Ruby*	694	0.2–25	10–60	I–III	Moderate
Alexandrite	755	2–20	10–100	I–III	Moderate
Diode	800	5–400	10–100	I–VI	High
Nd:YAG	1064	0.25–300	0–600	I–VI	Moderate
Intense pulsed light					
Intense pulsed light source	400–1200	2.5–100	10–150	I–III	Low
*No longer being manufactured.					

Table 137.6 Lasers and other light-based devices used for hair removal.

and the majority (4 of 7 individuals) still demonstrated partial hair loss (30–60%) in the irradiated sites[84]. In a multicenter study using a long-pulsed (3 ms) ruby laser with sapphire skin cooling in 183 patients, most of whom had dark hair, the majority had hair loss of >75% and about 1 in 10 had complete laser-induced hair loss 6 months after a mean of 4 treatments[88]. In general, use of the ruby laser for hair removal is limited to patients with skin types I–III, since absorption of 694 nm light by epidermal melanin results in a higher risk of complications (e.g. blistering, pigmentary changes) in individuals with darkly pigmented skin.

Long-pulsed alexandrite laser

Multiple studies have demonstrated effective hair removal with the long-pulsed alexandrite laser at fluences of 10–40 J/cm² and pulse durations of 2–20 ms[86]. At fluences of 20–40 J/cm², several investigators have reported hair reductions of 70–80% after multiple (at least 3–5) treatments[89–91]. Use of the long-pulsed alexandrite in patients with darkly pigmented skin has been reported, but side effects such as blistering and pigmentary alteration can occur; in general, this laser is best suited for hair removal in patients with skin types I–III[92].

Long-pulsed diode laser

The long-pulsed diode (800 nm; 5–400 ms) laser has also been studied extensively and shown to result in long-term hair removal, with the advantage of safety for patients with darkly pigmented skin[86]. High fluences can be safely employed using long pulse durations, thus yielding high efficacy of hair destruction per treatment session. In a comparative study with the long-pulsed ruby laser, the diode laser was found to be more effective for removal of coarse terminal hair. Permanent hair loss on the order of 20–35% per treatment has been reported with the diode laser[93,94]. A 40% long-term (20-month follow-up) hair reduction after two treatments was reported in one study[95], and an 84% hair reduction after four treatments was observed in another[89]. In dark-skinned patients, 75–90% hair reduction was reported after 8–10 treatments at 10 J/cm² and a 30 ms pulse duration[96]. Longer pulse durations (100–400 ms) may allow for higher fluences (20–30 J/cm²) to be employed safely and with improved efficacy. Figure 137.6 shows a patient with effective long-term hair removal two years after three treatments with the diode laser.

Long-pulsed Nd:YAG laser

The long-pulsed Nd:YAG laser (1064 nm) is considered to be the safest for hair removal in darkly pigmented patients; however, it is also less efficacious[86]. Several reports have shown its safety in skin types IV–VI, but with slightly lower efficacy than other types of lasers[97,98]. Mean hair reductions of 44% on the face and 50% on the body were reported following three treatments at 30–60 J/cm² and a 10–30 ms pulse duration[99]. Both the long-pulsed diode and Nd:YAG lasers have been used to treat pseudofolliculitis barbae, given their improved safety profiles in darkly pigmented skin[86].

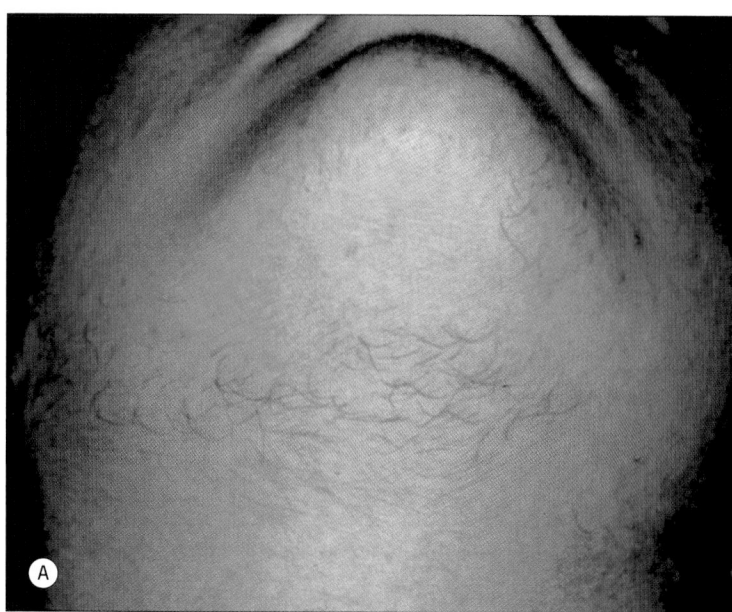 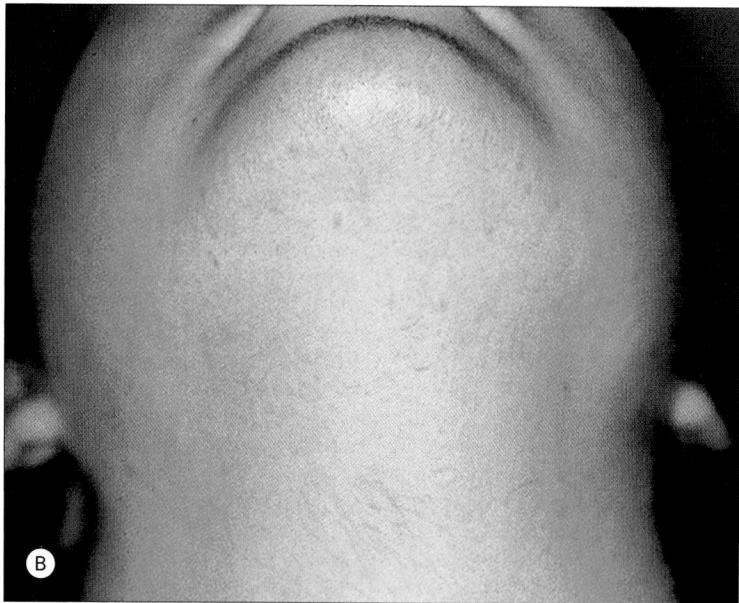

Fig. 137.6 Laser hair removal. A Before treatment. **B** Two years after three long-pulsed diode laser treatments; there is almost complete and permanent hair growth reduction.

Intense pulsed light

IPL sources (400–1200 nm) are versatile devices with a wide range of applications that includes hair removal. Cut-off filters are placed to delete short wavebands, thereby limiting damage to pigmented skin. Reports have suggested variable efficacy for hair removal, likely due to differences in wavelength output and irradiances among different IPL devices[100–102]. It remains to be determined whether IPL is as effective as long-pulsed lasers for hair removal, and it does carry an increased risk of pigmentary alteration.

Clinical Applications of Hair Removal Lasers
Patients with light hair colors

The efficiency of hair removal is affected by hair color: dark, coarse hair is the most responsive, followed by less pigmented hair. Blonde-, red- and gray-haired patients will experience temporary hair loss that can be maintained by treatments at regular intervals (every 1–3 months). Blonde and red hairs do contain low levels of melanin, and permanent reduction may occur after many treatments with the long-pulsed lasers discussed above. A study of combined radiofrequency and IPL showed 44% and 52% clearance of white and blonde hair, respectively, after four treatments[103], but these results await replication. In a small pilot study of photodynamic therapy with topical 5-aminolevulinic acid (ALA), 40% hair loss was reported at 6 months; however, waxing prior to the therapy was included in the protocol and larger studies need to be performed to confirm the effectiveness of this therapeutic modality[103].

Patient selection – preoperative considerations

Any individual with hypertrichosis or hirsutism should be thoroughly investigated for potential hormonal imbalances, family history of excess hair, medication use and the presence of androgen-secreting tumors (see Chapter 69). Because suntanned skin is less responsive to laser treatment and has a higher risk of adverse effects such as blistering and scarring, it is best to postpone the laser treatment until the tan has completely faded. Patients with active cutaneous infections should not be treated, and those with a history of recurrent HSV (particularly in perioral or pubic areas undergoing laser treatment) or staphylococcal infections should receive appropriate prophylactic antibiotics starting 1 day prior to the procedure to diminish the likelihood of an outbreak.

Although not considered an absolute contraindication, a history of keloidal or hypertrophic scarring should be taken into consideration and individuals with such conditions should be treated less aggressively. In individuals who have taken isotretinoin within the past 6 months, there is a risk for atypical scarring after a laser procedure and many experts suggest postponing the treatment until a sufficient period of time (6–12 months) has elapsed following discontinuation of the medication. Patients with skin diseases such as psoriasis or vitiligo should be warned about the risk of koebnerization following laser surgery. The use of Q-switched lasers should be avoided in hair-bearing areas that overlie cosmetically applied white, beige, tan or pink tattoos due to the risk of paradoxical darkening.

Waxing, plucking of hair and electrolysis should not be performed for at least 6 weeks prior to laser treatment. One day prior to laser treatment, or even on the same day, the areas should be shaved or epilated with a depilatory cream. Between treatments, the use of broad-spectrum sunscreens is essential and suntanning should be avoided.

Side effects and complications

Complications are uncommon provided that patients have been carefully selected and appropriate guidelines have been followed. Virtually all patients will experience pain, erythema and swelling that usually last 1–3 days after laser treatment, depending on the hair color and density and the fluences used. Epidermal damage may occur when excessive energy fluences are used and is more common in patients with a suntan or skin types IV–VI. The most common adverse effects are pigmentary changes, which are usually temporary. Postinflammatory hyperpigmentation has been reported in 5% of patients, particularly suntanned patients or individuals with skin types IV–VI. In patients who develop postinflammatory hyperpigmentation, topical hydroquinone and tretinoin can be initiated and sun exposure should be avoided. Hypopigmentation has also been reported after laser hair removal and is usually due to excessive epidermal injury. Scarring has not been reported but remains a possible adverse event if high fluences are used or postoperative infections occur.

Laser Treatment Methodologies for Hair Removal
Anesthesia

Laser treatments for hair removal are generally well tolerated by patients and do not usually require anesthesia. However, because the hair follicle is surrounded by nerve endings, topical anesthesia is necessary when treating large surfaces of the body or sensitive areas such as the upper lip and bikini area. Local infiltration of anesthetic or nerve blocks using 2% lidocaine can also be useful in selected patients.

Technique

The ideal treatment parameters are individualized for each patient, based on hair color and skin type (see Table 137.6). Pulses are delivered in a slightly overlapping mode with a predetermined spot size. The ideal immediate response is vaporization of the hair shaft, followed a few minutes later by the appearance of perifollicular edema and erythema. It is generally recommended that the highest tolerable

		LASERS AND OTHER DEVICES USED FOR REJUVENATION AND RESURFACING	
Laser/device	Target	Advantages	Disadvantages
Non-ablative			
Vascular lasers (532 nm pulsed KTP, 585 and 595 nm pulsed dye)	Dermal vasculature	Excellent safety, no recovery time, improvement in telangiectasias	Minimal efficacy, multiple treatments necessary
Near-infrared lasers (1310 nm diode, 1320 nm long-pulsed Nd:YAG, 1450 nm diode, 1540 nm Er:glass) and light devices (1100–1800 nm)	Dermal collagen and water	Excellent safety, no recovery time, greater efficacy for rhytides	Modest efficacy, multiple treatments necessary
Intense pulsed light source	Dermal vasculature, pigment, collagen and water	Moderate safety, no recovery time, improvement in telangiectasias and dyspigmentation	Minimal to modest efficacy, multiple treatments necessary
Radiofrequency energy source	Dermal collagen; dermal and subcutaneous charged particles and water	Excellent safety, no recovery time, greater efficacy for rhytides and laxity	Modest efficacy, multiple treatments necessary
Fractional			
Fractionated lasers (1320/1440 nm Nd:YAG; 1410, 1540 and 1550 nm erbium-doped fiber; 2940 nm erbium:YAG; 10 600 nm carbon dioxide) and light devices (825–1350 nm)	Water	Greater efficacy than non-ablative modalities for rhytides, also improves dyspigmentation	Moderate efficacy, 2–3-day recovery time, multiple treatments necessary (but fewer than non-ablative modalities)
Ablative			
Carbon dioxide (10 600 nm) laser	Water	Excellent efficacy for rhytides and photoaging	3-week recovery time, higher risk profile
Erbium:YAG (2940 nm) laser	Water	Excellent efficacy for rhytides and photoaging	3-week recovery time, higher risk profile
Nitrogen plasma	Cell membranes	Moderate to excellent efficacy for rhytides and photoaging	3-day to 3-week recovery time

Table 137.7 Lasers and other devices used for rejuvenation and resurfacing.

fluence and the largest spot size be used in order to obtain the best results. However, excessive fluences that cause epidermal separation or blistering should be avoided. If the device is not equipped with a cooling mechanism, a thick layer of cool gel is applied before the delivery of laser pulses.

The plume that is produced during laser vaporization of hair shafts has a characteristic sulfurous smell that can irritate the respiratory tract. Laser vacuums and good ventilation are recommended in order to eliminate such unpleasant odors. Some laser systems have self-contained vacuums and therefore do not require additional vacuums.

LASER SKIN RESURFACING

The desire for cosmetic enhancement of facial skin with minimal risk and rapid recovery has inspired laser-mediated means of wrinkle and photodamage reduction (Table 137.7)[104,105]. In the 1980s and early 1990s, continuous-wave CO_2 lasers were used to resurface photo-damaged skin in a procedure called 'thermabrasion'; however, this ablative procedure was associated with an unacceptably high risk of scarring. The advent of short-pulsed, high-peak-power and rapidly scanned, focused-beam CO_2 lasers and normal-mode Er:YAG lasers, which remove photodamaged skin layers in a precisely controlled manner, revolutionized skin rejuvenation and scar treatment[104].

The prolonged recovery time and complication risk of ablative laser resurfacing prompted the development of non-ablative and, more recently, fractional resurfacing in an effort to further minimize risk and recovery. Non-ablative laser resurfacing induces dermal thermal injury to improve rhytides and photodamage without epidermal damage. Fractional resurfacing thermally ablates microscopic columns of epidermal and dermal tissue in a regularly spaced array comprising a fraction of the skin surface. This intermediate approach increases efficacy as compared to non-ablative resurfacing and speeds recovery as compared to ablative resurfacing. Neither non-ablative nor fractional resurfacing produces results comparable to ablative laser skin resurfacing, but both have become much more popular than the latter because of minimal risks and acceptable improvement (see Table 137.7)[104].

Non-Ablative Resurfacing

Non-ablative laser and light systems can be classified into three main groups: (1) vascular lasers such as the PDL and pulsed KTP laser; (2) mid-IR lasers targeting the dermis; and (3) IPL (Table 137.8)[105,106]. Initially, the Q-switched Nd:YAG laser (1064 nm) was shown to induce dermal remodeling[107]. Subsequently, vascular lasers such as the PDL and pulsed 532 nm lasers were employed but with minimal efficacy. Longer-wavelength IR lasers, which more effectively target the mid dermis, have since become the most prominent non-ablative lasers, resulting in more consistent mild improvement in rhytides. IPL improves dyspigmentation and vascularity while at the same time emitting near-IR wavelengths that target the dermis, thereby resulting in global improvement in photodamage. More recently, radiofrequency systems have been developed, delivering electrical energy (with or without concomitant laser or light) that results in more pronounced reduction of skin laxity and rhytides. The mechanisms for non-ablative rejuvenation involve photothermal and other effects resulting in collagen contracture and neocollagenesis.

Vascular lasers

A role for PDLs in treating photodamage had been suggested based upon the clinical and histologic collagen changes observed in PDL-treated hypertrophic scars, striae distensae and acne scars[108–112]. One of the first lasers of this type to be utilized for wrinkle reduction was a 585 nm PDL at a 350 µs pulse duration and subpurpuric fluences (N-lite™) (see Table 137.8). In an initial study with this laser, a single treatment session resulted in a significant reduction in mild to severe rhytides[113]. Another early study showed that a single PDL treatment session at a 450 µs pulse duration led to a clinical improvement in 75–90% of mild to moderate rhytides and 40% of moderate to severe rhytides[114]. However, further studies with PDLs were unable to reproduce these findings and demonstrated only minimal effects. For example, in one study a long-pulsed PDL (595 nm) only demonstrated 18% improvement in clinical grading of photodamage[115]. This was largely due to the laser's ability to target facial telangiectasias associated with photodamage[116]. In spite of FDA approval of the long-pulsed PDL for treating

NON-ABLATIVE LASER RESURFACING SYSTEMS				
Laser	Wavelength (nm)	Fluence (J/cm²)	Pulse duration	Spot size (mm)
Vascular lasers				
Pulsed KTP	532	15	20 ms	10
Pulsed dye (PDL)	585	3	350–450 µs	5
Long-pulsed PDL	595	6–8	6 ms	10
Infrared (IR) lasers				
Nd:YAG	1064	50	50 ms	12
Nd:YAG	1320	18	200 µs	6
Diode	1450	8–14	250 ms	6
Er:glass	1540	10	3.5 ms	4
Intense pulsed light (IPL)				
	400–1200	Variable	Variable	
Radiofrequency (RF)				
RF, monopolar	RF current	58–144	NA	0.25–3 cm² tip
RF, unipolar	RF electro-magnetic radiation	2–220	NA	1 cm tip
RF, bipolar	RF current	2–110	NA	8 mm interelectrode distance
Combined modalities				
RF, bipolar + diode laser + IPL or IR light	RF current; 900; 500–2000	5–100; 20–50; 6–45	NA	8 mm interelectrode distance

Table 137.8 Non-ablative laser resurfacing systems.

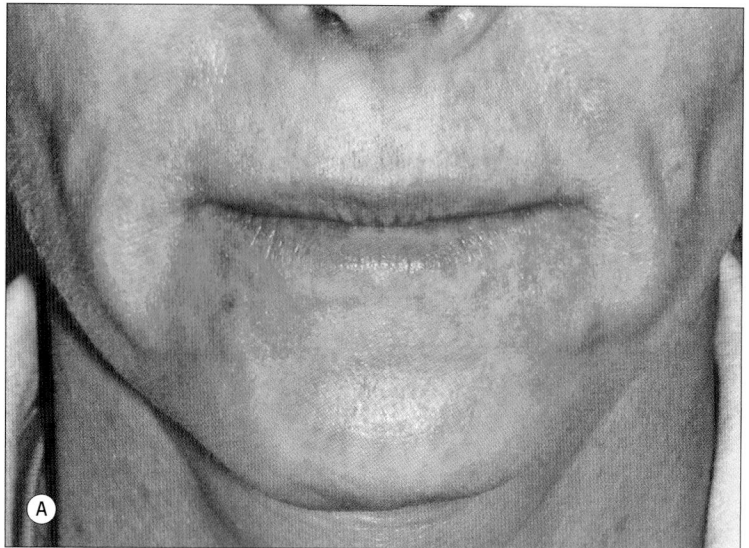

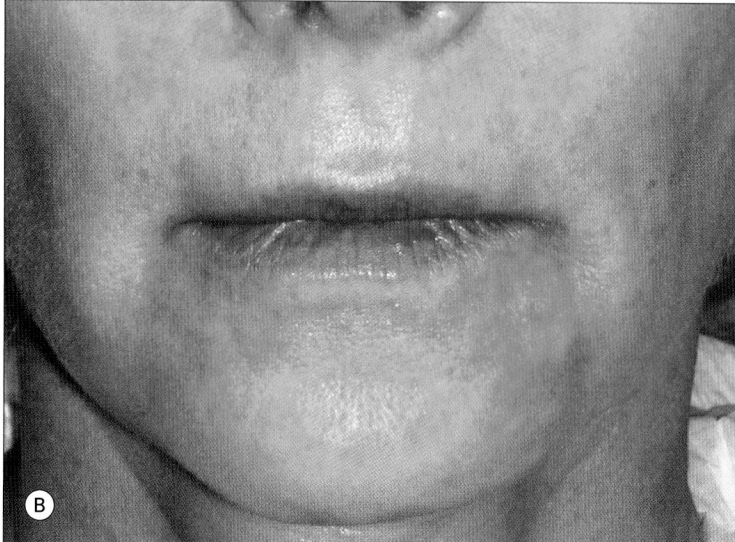

Fig. 137.7 Non-ablative laser resurfacing. A Before treatment. **B** One year after a single treatment with combination of diode laser (900 nm), intense pulsed light and bipolar radiofrequency.

photodamage, only modest results have been observed, presumably due to predominantly vascular targeting and only superficial penetration (to the papillary dermis) of the short wavelengths.

Recently, topical application of the precursor photosensitizer ALA in combination with long-pulsed PDL (595 nm) irradiation was found to enhance the ability of this laser to treat photodamage[117]. Photodynamic therapy (PDT) mediated by the long-pulsed PDL is effective in the removal of actinic keratoses, actinic cheilitis, lentigines, fine rhytides and textural changes due to photodamage[117–119]. The mechanism of these effects is activation by the 595 nm light of the photosensitizer proto-porphyrin IX (derived from ALA), which preferentially accumulates in photodamaged cells and results in their destruction by apoptosis or an immune-mediated response. Thus, the effects of PDL on photodamaged skin have been significantly augmented by ALA application.

Infrared lasers

The prototype of non-ablative rejuvenation is the Nd:YAG (1320 nm) laser with a 200 µs pulse duration (e.g. CoolTouch™)[120], which has been followed by the diode (1450 nm) laser (e.g. Smoothbeam®) and the erbium-doped phosphate glass (Er:glass; 1540 nm) laser[121] (see Table 137.8). Multiple clinical studies employing these lasers showed mild but reproducible improvement in rhytides and scars, with histo-logic evidence of neocollagenesis 6 months after treatment[122]. In studies of the 1320 nm Nd:YAG laser, the majority of the patients who were treated demonstrated minimal to mild and a minority moderate improvement[123]; similar results have been obtained with the 1450 nm diode laser. Treatment with the 1540 nm Er:glass laser also results in mild to moderate improvement in rhytides, with histologic evidence of an increase in dermal collagen months after treatment[124]. For example, a study of 60 patients with periorbital and perioral rhytides treated with the Er:glass laser demonstrated a mean increase in dermal thickness of 17% and a patient satisfaction rate of 62%[125]. The Nd:YAG (1320 nm) laser can also be effective in the treatment of acne scarring, but in a comparative study of the 1450 nm diode and 1320 nm Nd:YAG lasers

in treating atrophic facial scars, the diode was superior[126]. In summary, the drawback of non-ablative skin rejuvenation with IR lasers is that it only induces dermal changes and, therefore, has limited benefit for patients with epidermal photodamage. It is best suited for the treatment of wrinkles and acne scarring.

Histologic analysis of the skin following non-ablative resurfacing has found predominantly dermal, with some epidermal, changes. Three passes with the 1320 nm Nd:YAG laser resulted in epidermal edema (especially of the basal layer) 1 hour after treatment and microthrombi, sclerosis of blood vessels and neutrophilic infiltration in the dermis at 3 days. These findings correlated with clinical improvement, suggesting that epidermal and vascular injury may be mechanisms of action[127]. The 1450 nm diode laser results in fibrosis of the upper dermis and the 1540 nm Er:glass laser produces an increase in dermal thickness[124,126].

A newer IR device emitting wavelengths from 1100 to 1800 nm (Titan™) was recently introduced for treating skin laxity. This technology is purported to induce volumetric heating of the dermis, followed by tissue contraction. Early data suggest its safety and a moderate degree of efficacy in treating rhytides and skin laxity. A preliminary study of 25 patients showed that fluences of 20–30 J/cm² produced immediate changes and moderate improvement in facial rhytides. A preliminary split-face design study comparing this modality to radio-frequency reported milder improvement using the IR device. In an additional study, mild improvements were reported in the majority and dramatic findings in a minority of patients treated[128].

Most recently, a 1310 nm diode laser with a wide variety of pulse durations in the multisecond range (allowing a variable depth of penetration) has been shown in preliminary studies to produce moderate improvements in rhytides and laxity of the face and neck.

Intense pulsed light

The advantage of IPL (400–1200 nm) is its ability to target both melanin and hemoglobin, resulting in global improvement in dyspigmentation and vascularity, termed 'photorejuvenation' (see Table 137.7). Cut-off filters are placed to exclude shorter wavelengths, thereby preferentially targeting various chromophores. IPL results in a modest clinical improvement in rhytides, although pigmentary and vascular abnormalities of photodamaged skin show more dramatic improvement[120]. Histologic evaluation of the skin after IPL illumination for wrinkle reduction demonstrated neocollagenesis 6 months after treatment in one study[129] and an increase in extracellular matrix proteins and collagen in another study. Patient perception of improvement is enhanced by the concomitant diminution of dyspigmentation and vascularity, which are more easily detectable than the mild changes in rhytides. This has led to the widespread use of IPL for non-ablative resurfacing. With the addition of topical ALA before each of a series of IPL treatments, greater pigmentary and vascular improvement can be achieved while increasing the degree of improvement of fine wrinkles[130].

Radiofrequency

In an effort to increase penetration depth, collagen contracture and skin tightening, devices with radiofrequency wavelengths have been developed (see Table 137.8). Non-ablative radiofrequency devices produce electrical energy that heats the dermis at relatively low temperatures without plume, resulting in mild tissue contracture. The first was a monopolar radiofrequency device (ThermaCool™) that delivers a uniform volumetric heating effect into the deep dermis, generated by the tissue's resistance to the current flow. The electric field polarity is changed 6 million times per second, causing charged particles within the electric field to change orientation at that rate and to generate heat due to the resistance of the tissue. The minimal erythema and lack of significant side effects are advantageous. However, substantial improvement occurs in a minority of patients, with minimal changes in the majority, and patients often experience discomfort during treatment[131]. In one study using a monopolar radiofrequency device to treat the lower face, only 5 of 15 patients rated the results satisfactory and photographic analysis did not yield statistically significant results[132]. Recent technologic and protocol modifications (e.g. using a larger tip to deliver an increased number of passes at lower energy settings) may result in a more consistent benefit. In addition, newer radiofrequency devices with both unipolar (penetrating to the deep dermis and subcutaneous junction) and bipolar (targeting the superficial and mid dermis) modes (Accent™) or vacuum-assisted positioning of bipolar electrodes (Aluma™) were found to improve rhytides and skin laxity in initial studies.

The combination of electrical and optical energy (*electro-optical synergy*; ELOS™) can potentially augment the non-ablative effects achieved by either modality alone. Various combinations of bipolar radiofrequency with pulsed diode (900 nm) laser, IPL (500–1000 nm) and/or IR light (700–2000 nm) treatments have been shown to reduce photodamage, rhytides and skin laxity[133,134] (Fig. 137.7). This combination technology has also been assessed for the treatment of striae and cellulite[135]. Further studies, including control groups treated with the diode laser, IPL or IR light alone, will be important to evaluate whether or not there is a synergistic effect (when combined with radiofrequency).

Fractional Resurfacing

Fractional resurfacing or fractional photothermolysis is a resurfacing technique recently developed by Anderson[136] (Table 137.9). This approach thermally ablates a fraction of the skin, leaving intervening regions of normal skin that serve to rapidly repopulate the ablated columns of tissue. A 1550 nm (mid-IR) erbium-doped fiber laser (Fraxel® SR, Mosaic™) causes cylindrical areas of thermal damage to the epidermis and upper dermis, which are spaced at a density of approximately 1000–3000 microscopic treatment zones of photothermolysis per cm^2. Each column or 'microthermal zone' is approximately 70–150 μm in width with a vertical thermal injury depth of 400–700 μm into the dermis. Approximately 15–25% of the skin surface area is ablated per

FRACTIONAL RESURFACING				
Indication	Energy/ MTZ (mJ)	Density (MTZ/cm²)	Number of passes	Total treatment density (MTZ/cm²)
Melasma				
Skin types I–II	6	250	12	3000
Skin types III–VI	6	250	8	2000
Rhytides				
Mild	12	125	12	1500
Moderate	15	125	8	1000
Severe	20	125	8	1000
	12	125	16	2000
Acne scarring				
Skin types I–II	15–20	125	8–12	1500–1000
Skin types III–VI	15	125	8	1000
Photoaging				
Skin types I–II	10	250	8	2000
Skin types III–VI	8	250	8	2000

Table 137.9 **Fractional resurfacing.** MTZ, microscopic treatment zone. Note that the total treatment density is obtained by multiplying the density by the number of passes.

treatment session. The original fractional resurfacing laser (maximum fluence, 40 J/cm^2) was approved by the FDA for soft tissue coagulation in 2003; periorbital rhytides and pigmented lesions in 2004; and skin resurfacing, melasma and scars (acne, surgical) in 2006. More recently, a version with a penetration depth of up to 1.4 mm (maximum fluence, 70 mJ/cm^2; Fraxel® SR1500/re:store™) has been utilized for the treatment of deeper rhytides and scars. Fractionated 1410-nm erbium-doped fiber (Fraxel® re:fine™), 2940-nm erbium:YAG (Er:YAG; e.g. Lux2940™, Pixel™, Profractional™) and 10 600-nm CO_2 (e.g. ActiveFX™, Fraxel® AFR/re:pair™, Slim MiXto SX™) lasers have also been developed.

As in ablative laser resurfacing, the areas of thermally ablated tissue are repopulated by fibroblast neocollagenesis and epidermal proliferation. In contrast to ablative resurfacing, fractional resurfacing provides faster recovery and fewer side effects, with resolution of erythema and edema within a few days in most patients. However, the improvement in rhytides and photodamage is not as impressive as with ablative resurfacing. Mild to moderate improvement requires multiple (5–6) treatment sessions at 1- to 4-week intervals. Dyspigmentation improves quickly, whereas wrinkles and scars require more treatments for significant improvement. Pigmentary improvement is comparable to that seen with pigment-specific Q-switched lasers and IPL, but acne scars and wrinkles appear to improve faster and to a greater extent than with the non-ablative devices.

Additional devices for fractional resurfacing include IR (825–1350 nm), 1540 nm and 2940 nm (LuxIR™, Lux1540™ and Lux2940™) hand pieces that divide pulsed light (StarLux™) into an array of microbeams, creating a periodic lattice of hyperthermic columns. The 1540 nm device produces 100–320 microbeams per cm^2, with a penetration depth of up to 1 mm. Another fractional resurfacing device (Affirm™) sequentially emits 1320 nm and 1440 nm wavelengths at fixed intervals. A microlens array is employed to diffuse the laser light into a lattice of microbeams, with deeper and more superficial penetration depths of the two wavelengths, respectively. Peer-reviewed publications are pending for these newer fractional resurfacing modalities.

Ablative Laser Resurfacing

Ablative laser systems

Continuous-wave CO_2 lasers were used in the 1980s and 1990s to resurface photodamaged skin. While very effective, the risk of thermal damage and scarring was unacceptably high. To improve the safety of laser skin resurfacing, which uses water as a chromophore, the

ABLATIVE RESURFACING LASERS							
Type	Wavelength (nm)	Beam delivery	Power (W)	Pulse duration	Energy per pulse	Fluence	Spot size
Carbon dioxide lasers							
Pulsed	10 600	Individual pulses	500 (peak)	<950 µs	50–500 mJ	5–7 J/cm²	3 mm collimated or computer pattern generator
Scanned continuous-wave	10 600	Spiral or rasterized scan	7–100 (average)	0.03–0.52 s scan duration, 300–1000 µs dwell time	N/A	5–15 J/cm²	0.6–15 mm scan size with 0.1–0.25 mm focused beam
Erbium:YAG laser							
	2940	Individual pulses	10–20 (average)	250 µs–50 ms	0.1–3.0 J	1–50 mJ/cm²	2–7 mm collimated or focused; pattern generator

Table 137.10 Ablative resurfacing lasers.

principle of selective photothermolysis has been utilized[2]. In order to limit the depth of thermal damage to 100–150 µm, the pulse duration needs to be less than 1 ms, and in order to achieve tissue vaporization, sufficient energy needed to be delivered within this time. Short-pulsed, high-peak-power CO_2 lasers, rapidly scanned continuous-wave CO_2 lasers and normal-mode Er:YAG lasers adhering to these principles have been developed to precisely control the depth of thermal ablation (Table 137.10).

Carbon dioxide laser

The CO_2 laser emits a 10 600 nm wavelength, which is strongly absorbed by tissue water (absorption coefficient of 800 cm^{-1}). The penetration depth is dependent upon a tissue's water content, but not the melanin or hemoglobin content. With a pulse duration of less than 1 ms, CO_2 laser light penetrates approximately 20–30 µm into the skin, and residual thermal damage can be confined to a 100–150 µm layer of tissue, although thermal coagulation up to 1 mm has been reported[137].

The vaporization or boiling point of water at 1 atmosphere is 100°C (212°F). The fluence required to achieve pulsed-laser ablation of skin tissue is 5 J/cm², with less energy producing diffuse tissue heating without vaporization[138]. At these parameters, the skin temperature reaches approximately 120–200°C. The diameter of the beam plays a role, with small beams (100–300 µm in diameter) achieving high fluences and rapid tissue vaporization; however, the beam must be moved rapidly across the skin surface to avert desiccation, charring and heat diffusion. Beam diameters of greater than 2 mm induce non-vaporization heating and increase the risk of deep thermal damage due to the need to apply low fluences for longer periods of time in order for visible vaporization to occur. Based on these findings, the pulsed or scanned CO_2 lasers were designed to combine high peak powers with short pulses and/or rapid movement across the skin surface.

Two basic CO_2 laser systems have been utilized in cutaneous resurfacing (see Table 137.10). The first type is the high-powered pulsed CO_2 laser system, which delivers energy in individual pulses of about 1 ms or less (e.g. UltraPulse™). This laser produces up to 500 mJ of energy in each individual 600 µs^{-1} ms pulse. Vaporization can be performed either with a 3 mm spot size or by a computer pattern generator, which can deliver various patterns of up to 80 pulses, each pulse measuring 2.25 mm in diameter.

The second type of CO_2 resurfacing laser achieves well-controlled tissue ablation by rapidly scanning the focal spot of a focused continuous-wave CO_2 laser over the skin (e.g. FeatherTouch™ and SilkTouch™ flash scanners). Computer-driven mechanical devices can scan a 0.2 mm spot in a spiral manner, ranging in diameter from 8 to 16 mm in several shapes at a constant velocity. No individual spot is irradiated more than once and the dwell time on any individual spot is less than 1 ms, while achieving fluences above the ablation threshold.

Despite these technical differences, the two laser systems accomplish similar clinical results[139]. In general, two passes with the SilkTouch™ are approximately equal to three pulses with the UltraPulse™ and four passes with the FeatherTouch™ in terms of the amount of tissue removed and the depth of residual thermal damage. Other CO_2 laser systems using varied parameters have been developed (e.g. TruPulse™, UltraPulse Encore™, UniPulse™), with clinical results similar to those

of the prototype CO_2 lasers[140]. The main differences are in the specific parameters used with each laser system.

All of the recently developed CO_2 laser systems result in significant improvement of photoaged skin. Most patients with wrinkles attain a 50–90% improvement (Fig. 137.8)[141,142]. Optical profilometry has been utilized to objectively quantify wrinkle improvement[143]. The improvement is usually more marked for fine wrinkles, especially those around the eyes or mouth, and less pronounced for deeper rhytides and creases.

CO_2 laser treatment of acne scars is moderately effective. Severe acne scars are less responsive than mild to moderate acne scars. One investigator reported 81% improvement in moderate atrophic scars[144], whereas another found adequate improvement in only two of four patients with severe acne scarring[145].

Erbium:YAG laser

The Er:YAG laser was the next ablative laser developed for skin resurfacing. It emits IR light with a wavelength of 2940 nm, which is close to the absorption peak of water and yields an absorption coefficient 16 times that of the CO_2 laser. The Er:YAG laser's penetration depth is limited to about 1–3 µm of tissue per J/cm² versus the 20–30 µm observed with the CO_2 laser[146]. This provides more precise ablation of skin with minimal thermal damage to the surrounding tissues; the residual thermal damage is estimated to be 10–40 µm. Operating the Er:YAG laser at a fluence of 5 J/cm² vaporizes the epidermis in four passes, 8–12 J/cm² achieves this after two passes.

Overall efficacy of the Er:YAG is rather similar to the CO_2 laser, although the CO_2 laser has been found to be superior in most comparative studies. The Er:YAG laser has been associated with less tissue tightening or contraction as compared to the CO_2 laser, which may impact the long-term outcome in photoaged skin[147]. The variable-pulsed Er:YAG laser (pulse durations of 10–50 ms) demonstrates immediate tissue contraction and a healing rate that is intermediate between the short-pulsed Er:YAG (pulse durations of 250–350 µs) and CO_2 lasers[148]. In comparative studies, the variable-pulsed Er:YAG laser was very effective in the removal of rhytides, although the CO_2 laser was still found to be slightly more efficacious[149,150].

The Er:YAG laser results in less severe side effects of discomfort, erythema and edema, and overall healing times are faster than with the CO_2 laser[151]. When compared according to the depth of ablation performed, healing times for the two lasers have been similar[152]. In contrast to the bloodless nature of CO_2 laser treatment (due to photocoagulation of blood vessels less than 0.5 mm in diameter), bleeding increases with successive passes with the Er:YAG laser.

Ablative resurfacing with the CO_2 and Er:YAG lasers results in histologic evidence of neocollagenesis approximately 6 weeks postoperatively. Early on, however, the inflammatory cell infiltrates differ, with a band-like infiltrate of neutrophils following CO_2 treatment as opposed to a mild perivascular infiltrate of neutrophils and eosinophils following Er:YAG treatment. Recently, changes in expression of extracellular matrix proteins and cytokines following CO_2 laser resurfacing have been evaluated. Reverse transcriptase polymerase chain reaction (RT-PCR) and immunohistochemical staining of facial skin biopsies from 28 patients following resurfacing demonstrated upregulation of procollagens I and II, interleukin-1β, tumor necrosis factor-α,

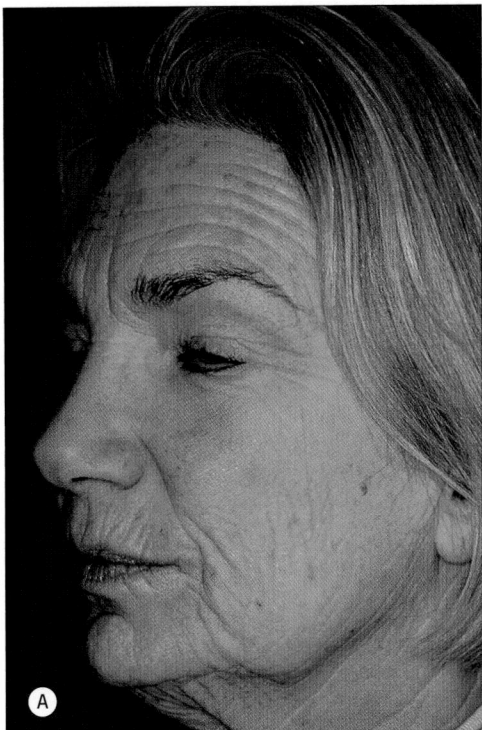
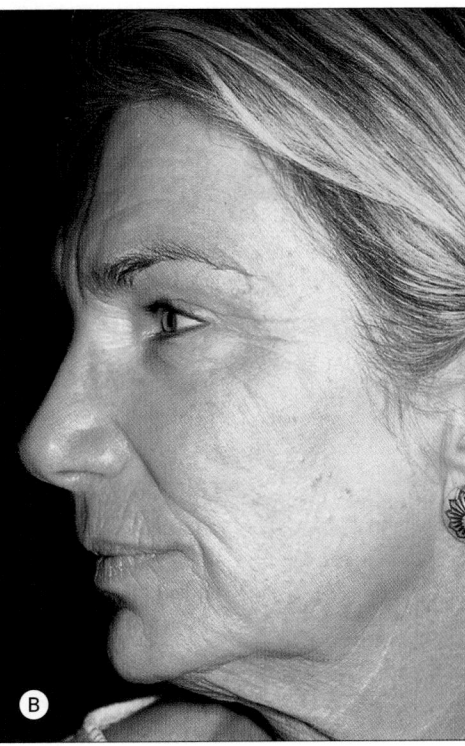

Fig. 137.8 Ablative laser resurfacing. A Before treatment. **B** One year after carbon dioxide laser resurfacing.

transforming growth factor-β1 and matrix metalloproteinases (MMPs)-1, -3, -9 and -13[153].

Plasma skin resurfacing

This novel device for ablative resurfacing works by passing radiofrequency energy into nitrogen gas. The 'nitrogen plasma' causes rapid heating of the skin with limited tissue ablation and minimal collateral thermal damage. Preliminary reports indicate improvement in facial rhytides and scars following treatment. Epidermal regeneration occurs by 7 days postoperatively, with neocollagenesis visible on histologic analysis at 90 days. Comparative studies are needed to evaluate the safety and efficacy of this device as compared to CO_2 and Er:YAG laser resurfacing.

Indications for ablative laser resurfacing

Laser skin resurfacing has been employed to treat a large number of skin conditions, but the two most common indications are photoaging and scarring. Photoaging, which may defined based on criteria of rhytides, lentigines, telangiectasias, elastosis and actinic keratoses, is highly responsive to laser resurfacing. Perioral and periorbital rhytides, which are resistant to facelift procedures, are highly amenable to laser resurfacing. Fine rhytides (particularly in the periorbital, perioral and cheek areas) may be completely eradicated with laser resurfacing; deeper creases are also improved, probably secondary to a general tightening effect. Rhytides and creases that appear with active movement and facial expression, such as glabellar and nasolabial folds, tend to be more resistant to laser resurfacing.

The ideal laser resurfacing candidate is a healthy, lightly pigmented patient with realistic expectations. Patients with a history of keloids, radiation therapy to the area or scleroderma are not candidates. Diseases that exhibit koebnerization, such as psoriasis and vitiligo, are relative contraindications. Prior isotretinoin therapy has been associated with atypical scarring after dermabrasion or chemical peeling, even if the procedure were performed more than 1 year after isotretinoin treatment[154]. Therefore, it is generally recommended that patients wait for at least 1–2 years before undergoing this procedure. Resurfacing performed at the same time or soon after facelifting or blepharoplasty increases the risk of skin necrosis and scarring due to the altered blood circulation of the undermined skin following these procedures[155]. Hence, laser resurfacing of undermined skin should be deferred for at least 6 months after the original surgical procedure. Laser resurfacing is not used on the hands, neck and chest due to the unacceptably high risk of scarring.

Ablative laser resurfacing is effective for scars, including those caused by acne, trauma and surgery. It is most effective for elevated or deep, distensible acne scars, in which the fibrotic tissue can be removed or the shoulders of the scars ablated, respectively. Ice-pick or bound-down scars are less responsive, requiring a combined approach of subcision and punch excision/grafting, followed by laser resurfacing 6–8 weeks later[156]. Varicella scars may be improved with spot laser resurfacing, with fresh scars (6–10 weeks after varicella) responding more completely than older scars. Postsurgical and traumatic scars may achieve dramatic improvement, especially if resurfaced 6–10 weeks after the surgery or injury. Resurfacing well-vascularized wound edges immediately after surgery, prior to suture placement, may also improve cosmetic outcome[157].

Since laser resurfacing is relatively bloodless and allows for controlled tissue removal with a low risk of scarring, it has also been used to treat rhinophyma[158], diffuse actinic cheilitis[159], actinic keratoses, benign neoplasms/hamartomas (e.g. angiofibromas, appendageal tumors) and verrucae.

Side effects and complications of ablative laser resurfacing

While side effects following ablative laser resurfacing are frequent and predictable, serious complications are uncommon and preventable with proper technique and postoperative management.

Erythema: Postoperative erythema will persist for an average of 1–4 months due to increased blood flow, an inflammatory response, reduced melanin and decreased dermal optical scattering. It often lasts 1 month for Er:YAG and 2 months for CO_2 laser resurfacing, but may persist for up to 12 months. Flushing within the treated site upon physical exertion or emotional stress may occur for up to 1 year after resurfacing.

Dyspigmentation: The risk of pigmentary alteration correlates with the depth of laser damage. Injury into the papillary dermis is more likely to cause postinflammatory hyperpigmentation, whereas deeper passes may lead to hypopigmentation. Postinflammatory hyperpigmentation is the most common adverse event, occurring in up to a third of patients[160]. It is observed more often in individuals with skin types III–VI, during the summer months and in sunny regions. At the first sign of hyperpigmentation, hydroquinone and tretinoin are prescribed and sun exposure is avoided; it usually resolves within a few months. Rates of hyperpigmentation as low as 3% have been reported among patients pretreated with bleaching creams and tretinoin[161].

Two types of hypopigmentation secondary to ablative laser resurfacing have been reported. One is a relative hypopigmentation compared to the background untreated skin[151]. This can be avoided by resurfacing the entire face (or at least entire cosmetic units) and feathering the treatment into the surrounding areas. The other type is delayed hypopigmentation that develops 6–12 months after resurfacing, reported in 15% of patients.

Acneiform eruptions: Milia may occur during the healing process due to follicular re-epithelialization or the use of occlusive moisturizers. Acne occurs frequently in the first few weeks post-resurfacing, especially in acne-prone patients, and responds to standard acne treatments. Isotretinoin is avoided postoperatively due to the possibility of hypertrophic scarring.

Dermatitis: Irritant contact dermatitis may be observed following application of topical anesthetics; it does not correlate with patch test findings but resolves with appropriate treatment (e.g. topical corticosteroids). This occurrence increases the likelihood of postoperative erythema and hyperpigmentation. Irritant or allergic contact dermatitis due to other etiologies (e.g. wound dressings, topical antibiotics) may also develop during the first 4 weeks after treatment and also responds to mid- to high-potency topical corticosteroids. Perioral dermatitis is infrequently observed 1–3 months after resurfacing of the perioral region, and responds to oral doxycycline.

Infections: Prophylactic systemic antibiotics (e.g. dicloxacillin or cephalexin for a minimum of 5 days) and appropriate topical care (e.g. saline or tap water soaks followed by application of petrolatum) are used to minimize the risk of bacterial infection. *Staphylococcus aureus* or *Pseudomonas aeruginosa* infections may occur despite prophylactic antibiotics, presenting as pustules, yellow crusting, patchy erythema or delayed healing. Broad-spectrum antibiotic coverage should be instituted while awaiting the culture results. Antiviral chemoprophylaxis for 10–14 days is standard practice in all patients, because even individuals with no history of 'cold sores' frequently develop herpes simplex viral infections in treated areas[162]. Candidiasis may also occur and responds well to treatment with systemic antifungal agents. Some laser surgeons administer antifungal prophylaxis (e.g. fluconazole) in all patients.

Scarring: The risk of scarring from ablative laser resurfacing is small. It can be minimized by proper patient selection, conservative technique and careful wound care. Scarring can occur following a large number of passes, excessive energy fluences or pulse stacking (overlap of laser pulses)[163]. Scars should be promptly treated with topical or intralesional corticosteroids, silicone gel sheeting and PDL therapy.

LASER-MEDIATED PHOTODYNAMIC THERAPY

Over the past two decades, lasers have been used in conjunction with photosensitizers for the treatment of skin neoplasia and other conditions (Table 137.11)[119]. PDT is discussed in detail in Chapter 135. Systemic porphyrins, such as hematoporphyrin, were the first photosensitizers to be employed, mostly to treat tumors. The first light sources used were broadband, non-coherent lights, such as quartz, xenon, tungsten or halogen lamps. The wavelengths of light chosen were based upon the absorption spectrum of porphyrins: blue because the largest porphyrin absorption peak is at ~400 nm (Soret band) and red because of its greater penetration depth and the smaller porphyrin absorption peak (Q band) at 650 nm. Systemic photosensitizers caused prolonged photosensitivity and broadband light sources had limitations and side effects. The development of topical photosensitizers such as ALA and advances in laser technology have led to the emergence of laser-mediated PDT as a treatment option for a variety of skin conditions[119].

In the 1990s, red lasers were used for PDT due to their increased skin penetration (see above)[119]. In addition, broadband blue light and red light were studied extensively, the former achieving FDA approval in combination with topical ALA for the treatment of actinic keratoses in 1997. However, these lasers and light sources caused side effects, such as discomfort during illumination, erythema, crusting, blistering and dyspigmentation. The use of the long-pulsed PDL (595 nm) following topical ALA has minimized these side effects without compromising efficacy[117]. Long-pulsed PDL-mediated PDT has since been shown to be effective for the treatment of actinic keratoses, actinic cheilitis, sebaceous hyperplasia, extragenital lichen sclerosus and acne vulgaris[117–119,164,165]. Finally, IPL sources have been introduced for PDT

of photodamage and acne, offering advantages of versatility in wavelengths and applications[119].

The lasers and light sources used for PDT are presented in Table 137.11. Currently, blue light (e.g. Blu-U®), long-pulsed PDL and IPL are most often utilized for PDT. Prior to irradiation with blue light, topical ALA is applied for 14–18 hours. A shorter incubation period (3 hours) was found to be as effective for the treatment of actinic keratoses as longer application times when the ALA was combined with long-pulsed PDL[117]. Even shorter incubations of 1 hour have been used with success[118,119].

When blue light is used for PDT, illumination times are typically 16–17 minutes. In the case of the long-pulsed PDL (595 nm), a fluence of 7–7.5 J/cm² and pulse duration of 10 ms (with dynamic cooling spray) are employed following ALA application for 1–3 hours[117,118]. With the latter method, efficacy rates are 88% lesional clearance following a single treatment for actinic keratoses at 8 months' follow-up and 68% complete clearance following 1–3 treatments for actinic cheilitis, with a mean follow-up of 4 months[118,119]. Recently, long-pulsed PDL-mediated PDT combined with topical therapy (e.g. benzoyl peroxide, antibiotics and retinoids) for the treatment of mild to severe comedonal, inflammatory and cystic acne resulted in complete clearance in 14 of 14 patients following a mean of 3 (range 1–6) treatments and 6 months of follow-up[164].

Given the modest efficacy of IPL therapy alone for photodamage, IPL-mediated PDT (with ALA) has been used in patients with actinic keratoses and photodamage. The cosmetic outcome has been favorable and ALA has been added to photorejuvenation protocols that utilize IPL[119,130]. To date, reports of IPL-mediated PDT for acne have demonstrated efficacy rates that are lower than those for PDL-mediated PDT[119,164].

LASERS USED IN CONJUNCTION WITH PHOTODYNAMIC THERAPY			
Laser/light source	Wavelength (nm)	Photosensitizer	Disorders treated
Blue–green			
Argon	488, 514	HPD, porfimer sodium	
Yellow			
Pulsed dye	585, 595	ALA	AKs, AC, SCC, BCC, acne, photodamage
Red			
Gold vapor	628	HPD, porfimer sodium	SCC, BCC
Tunable dye	630	HPD, porfimer sodium	SCC, BCC
Copper vapor-dye	630	ALA	AK, SCC, BCC
Nd:YAG	630	ALA	AK, SCC, BCC
Argon ion-dye	630	ALA	AK, SCC, BCC
Red diode	635	ALA	Acne
Argon pumped-dye	638	ALA	BCC
Diode	688	Verteporfin	SCC, BCC
Broadband light			
Broadband 'blue' light	405–440	ALA	AKs, acne, photodamage
Intense pulsed light	400–1200	ALA	AKs, acne, photodamage

Table 137.11 Lasers used in conjunction with photodynamic therapy. 5-aminolevulinic acid (ALA) can be applied topically, whereas the remainder of the photosensitizers are administered systemically. AC, actinic cheilitis; AKs, actinic keratoses; BCC, basal cell carcinoma; HPD, hematoporphyrin derivative; SCC, squamous cell carcinoma.

LASERS FOR OTHER SKIN CONDITIONS

Clinical applications of laser therapy have expanded greatly, with lasers being used for conditions that are unresponsive to conventional therapies and as adjuncts to surgical procedures. Such indications include scars, keloids, striae, warts, hair transplantation, appendageal tumors, sebaceous hyperplasia, hair transplantation and incisional surgery.

Hypertrophic Scars and Keloids

Continuous-wave lasers (e.g. CO_2, argon and Nd:YAG lasers) were the first to be used for treating hypertrophic scars and keloids[166,167], but their non-selective tissue ablation led to recurrences or worsening of the scars within a few years of treatment. Since then, PDL has become the laser of choice for treatment of hypertrophic scars and keloids. In the first published study, hypertrophic and atrophic scars (induced by argon laser treatment of PWSs) treated with five PDL sessions over a 10-month period improved in erythema, texture and pliability[108]. Subsequently, there have been multiple reports of successful PDL treatment of hypertrophic scars and keloids resulting from sternotomy[109], surgical excisions, trauma[168], burns and acne[110]. Clinical response rates have ranged from 55% to 85% after multiple laser treatments, with hypertrophic scars responding better than keloids. However, these findings have been disputed by a prospective comparative study of PDL treatment versus silicone gel sheeting for hypertrophic scars, which showed no differences in clinical appearance, symptoms or histologic response[112].

The mechanisms underlying the possible effects of PDL on scars and keloids are unclear. The targeted destruction of blood vessels may result in tissue ischemia, leading to regression of the keloid. Other possibilities include alteration of collagen metabolism and immune-mediated mechanisms, as suggested by the increased number of mast cells in PDL-treated scars. Histologic assessment of scars following PDL has shown the disappearance of dilated vascular channels, a normal number of dermal fibroblasts, and looser, less coarse collagen fibers. A study of PDL treatment of hypertrophic scar tissue implanted in athymic mice showed that the extent of inhibition of growth of the scar tissue correlated with the extent of vascular damage, which was maximal at the highest fluence used (10 J/cm^2)[169].

The ideal time to initiate laser treatment, as well as the ideal number and frequency of laser treatments, are currently being defined; complete remodeling of scars usually takes 12 months to occur. In keloid-prone individuals, it is possible that early treatment may prevent their formation, but this awaits the results of clinical trials. A combination of intralesional corticosteroids with PDL at relatively high fluences (above the purpura threshold) may improve efficacy, particularly in the treatment of keloids.

Striae Distensae

Although a cosmetic concern, there has been considerable demand for the treatment of striae. In anecdotal reports, some benefit has been observed from topical tretinoin, α-hydroxy acids and topical vitamin C. PDL (450 μs, 585 nm) was the first laser treatment utilized for striae[170]. Improvement was seen clinically and by means of optical profilometry, while histologic analysis showed an increase in the elastin content of laser-treated lesions. Further research has shown that smaller striae respond better than large striae, and that the location and age of the striae did not affect the response rate. PDL is most efficacious for striae rubra, ostensibly by eliminating the erythema and potentially by inhibiting the progression of the striae (which are akin to superficial atrophic scars).

Striae alba, which have a hypopigmented appearance, have been notoriously more difficult to treat. The 308 nm xenon chloride excimer laser was shown to be efficacious in improving striae alba; however, maintenance treatments were required to preserve the cosmetic correction[171]. During the course of that study, reflectance spectroscopy revealed that the hypopigmented appearance was not due to decreased pigmentation, but rather resulted from increased reflectance by the superficial array of collagen fibers in the striae[171]. A combination of radiofrequency, diode laser (900 nm) and IPL may also be efficacious in reversing the textural atrophy associated with striae and restoring normal skin texture and appearance. The optimal approach is to target the superficial dermis and increase collagen production in this area.

Warts

The CO_2 laser in the continuous-wave mode has been used for treating periungual and plantar warts and condyloma acuminata. It has the advantages of well-controlled tissue destruction and hemostasis. Although the CO_2 laser is capable of vaporizing periungual warts without nail avulsion, permanent onychodystrophy frequently develops. For plantar warts, the lesions need to be pared down followed by successive laser passes, debridement and curettage. Response rates for CO_2 laser treatment of warts range from 30% to 80%[172,173]. This moderate response may be related to the presence of viral particles in normal-appearing epidermis 5–10 mm from the clinical lesion[174]. Thus a treatment margin of at least 1 cm of normal skin is essential to achieve a cure. A risk of this procedure is the presence of viable human papilloma virus particles in the laser plume of vaporized warts[175]. Appropriate precautions should be taken to minimize the risk of inhalation of these viral particles.

The dermal papillae beneath verrucae contain dilated and congested vasculature adjacent to the elongated rete ridges. The PDL, which selectively destroys superficial dermal capillaries, has been shown to effectively treat verrucae[138]. In one study of 39 patients treated with a 5 mm spot size at a fluence of 6.25–7.5 J/cm^2, 72% were cleared of their warts after an average of 1.7 treatments[176]. However, there have also been reports of disappointing results with PDL treatment for verrucae[177]. In order to achieve clearance, stacking of 8–10 pulses at high fluences and multiple treatments are needed, suggesting that thermal ablation is the mechanism.

Psoriasis

A number of different lasers have been used for the treatment of localized plaques of psoriasis. The PDL (585 nm, 450 μs) has been shown to partially improve psoriatic lesions, presumably through its ability to target the superficial dermal vessels[178]. In addition, a CO_2 laser was used to resurface isolated psoriatic plaques, but despite clinical and histologic evidence of complete ablation of the epidermis and the papillary dermis, psoriasis recurred in most patients within 8 weeks[179]. The 308 nm excimer laser, emitting at a wavelength within the effective narrowband UVB spectrum (305–311 nm), was found to clear psoriatic plaques in a shorter time and with fewer treatments than standard UVB phototherapy[180]. The advantages of the former therapy are the lack of exposure of unaffected skin to UV radiation and the ability to use higher fluences of UV on individual psoriatic plaques. In a multicenter study of 124 patients, 72% of treated subjects achieved at least 75% clearing in an average of six treatment sessions, while 84% responded with more than 75% improvement after 10 or more treatment sessions[181]. The major disadvantage of this approach is that it is time- and labor-intensive, thereby limiting it to patients with <10% body surface area involvement. Other UVB-responsive diseases such as vitiligo, mycosis fungoides and atopic dermatitis also appear to benefit from laser phototherapy.

LASER SAFETY

Laser hazards are divided in two categories: beam hazards, which are related to direct or incidental impact, and non-beam hazards.

Beam hazards such as fire, thermal burns and ocular damage can occur whenever the laser is activated. Flammability accidents occur when the laser is used in the presence of oxygen; fires induced by the PDL during general anesthesia have been reported[182]. Flammable items such as drapes, towels and sponges can be ignited by a direct or reflected laser beam. To avoid this risk, wet or non-flammable material should be placed in the surgical field, all excess draping should be removed from the site, and a laryngeal mask should be used if oxygen is administered. Surgical instruments with a bright reflective surface should be either ebonized or covered with wet sponges to prevent inadvertent irradiation. Alcohol is extremely hazardous when exposed to the intense heat generated by the lasers. Thus solutions containing alcohol may easily ignite and should be avoided in the laser impact site. Exposure to the solvents and organic dyes in dye laser systems is also potentially hazardous.

Ocular risks are the most serious safety hazard encountered in laser use. The eye may be exposed directly in the laser beam's path or indirectly by a reflected beam. Each wavelength interacts differently with tissue and therefore can produce different types of ocular damage. CO_2 laser radiation (10 600 nm) is absorbed by water. When light of this wavelength impacts the eye, it gets absorbed by the cornea, leading to extensive corneal damage. Laser light in the visible (400–720 nm) and near-IR (720–1400 nm) portions of the electromagnetic spectrum are transmitted through the transparent cornea and lens and are focused on a retinal spot of 10–20 µm, resulting in a retinal burn and visual damage. To protect the eyes from laser damage, adequate wraparound glasses must be worn by all present in the treatment room. There are many manufacturers who produce goggles in several designs for use with any of the lasers.

Non-beam hazards include plume hazards and are currently the subject of widespread concern. Research has shown that harmful particulates such as intact virions and viral DNA are present in the plume during CO_2 laser radiation. Intact human papilloma virus DNA has been found in continuous-wave CO_2 laser vapor (as discussed above). Transmission and infection by hepatitis B virus and HIV through laser plume or smoke represent a serious potential hazard. Molecular studies have detected HIV and simian immunodeficiency virus (SIV) DNA in laser smoke from irradiation of infected cultured cells by a continuous-wave CO_2 laser[183]. However, the infectivity is unknown since both viruses appeared to be damaged by the laser.

More concern exists regarding the aerosolization of tissue particles during the microexplosions of tissue that occur when it is treated by ultrashort pulses, such as those from the Q-switched ruby laser or the Q-switched Nd:YAG laser. The debris contains viable cells, micro-organisms and blood. The velocity of microexplosions and the spread of tissue fragments exceed the speed of sound and may escape collection by smoke evacuators. This problem has been addressed by some manufacturers by the use of a splatter shield for the laser hand piece. However, additional protective measures such as the use of gloves and gowns must be implemented during treatment with Q-switched lasers.

Lasers are high-voltage electrical devices and carry a risk of inadvertent discharge. Today most laser systems have safety controls built into them that shield the operator and the patient from high voltage, minimizing the possibility of electrical accidents. Other appropriate safety precautions include the use of proper gloves and gowns by all personnel throughout all laser procedures. The wearing of properly filtered and tied laser masks can greatly reduce the respiratory exposure to viral and other infectious agents. Laser surgery should be presumed to contain liberated viable infectious particles in the plume of smoke. The risk of infection in laser operators can be minimized through the use of a high-efficiency smoke filtration system.

Future Directions

Lasers are continually being optimized to effectively treat specific cutaneous disorders, while at the same time increasing their versatility to target different conditions. Combination laser systems are being developed, which will allow practitioners to minimize the number of devices required and maximize the number of skin conditions which can be safely and effectively treated. Lasers are becoming an essential part of the repertoire of technologies available to dermatologists, providing treatment options for skin neoplasia, inflammatory conditions, acne, hypertrichosis and scars as well as vascular and pigmented lesions, tattoos and photoaging.

REFERENCES

1. Dover JS, Arndt KA, Geronemus RG, Alora MBT (eds). Illustrated Cutaneous and Aesthetic Laser Surgery. 2nd edn. Stamford, CT: Appleton and Lange, 2000.

2. Anderson RR, Parrish JA. Selective photothermolysis: precise microsurgery by selective absorption of pulsed radiation. Science. 1983;220:524–7.

3. Anderson RR. In: Arndt KA, Dover JS, Olbricht SM (eds). Lasers in cutaneous and aesthetic surgery. Philadelphia: Lippincott-Raven, 1997:25–51.

4. Arndt KA. Treatment techniques in argon laser therapy: comparison of pulsed and continuous exposures. J Am Acad Dermatol. 1984;11:90–7.

5. Achauer BM, Vander Kam VM. Argon laser treatment of telangiectasia of the face and neck: 5 years' experience. Laser Surg Med. 1987;7:495–8.

6. Arndt KA. Argon laser therapy of small cutaneous vascular lesions. Arch Dermatol. 1982;118:220–4.

7. Pickering JW, Walker EB, Butler PH, et al. Copper vapour laser treatment of port-wine stains and other vascular malformations. Br J Plast Surg. 1990;43:273–82.

8. Keller GS. Use of KTP in cosmetic surgery. Am J Cosmetic Surg. 1992;9:177–80.

9. Anderson RR, Parrish JA. Microvasculature can be selectively damaged using dye lasers: a basic theory and experimental evidence in human skin. Lasers Surg Med. 1981;1:263–76.

10. Tan OT, Morrison P, Kurban AK. 585 nm for the treatment of port-wine stains. Plast Reconstr Surg. 1990;86:1112–17.

11. Tan OT, Carney M, Margolis R, et al. Histologic responses of port-wine stains treated by argon, carbon dioxide and tunable dye lasers. Arch Dermatol. 1986;122:1016–22.

12 Lowe NJ, Behr KL, Fitzpatrick R, et al. Flash lamp-pumped dye laser for rosacea-associated telangiectasia and erythema. J Dermatol Surg Oncol. 1991;17:522–5.

13. Astner S, Anderson RR. Treating vascular lesions. Dermatol Ther. 2005;18:267–81.

14. Dierickx CC, Casparian JM, Venugopalan V, et al. Thermal relaxation time of port wine stain vessels probed in vitro: the need for 1–10 millisecond laser pulse treatment. J Invest Dermatol. 1995;105:709–14.

15. West TB, Alster TS. Comparison of the long-pulsed dye and KTP lasers in the treatment of facial and leg telangiectasia. Dermatol Surg. 1998;24:221–6.

16. Bernstein EF, Lee J, Lowery J, et al. Treatment of spider veins with the 595 nm pulsed dye laser. J Am Acad Dermatol. 1998;39:746–50.

17. Rohrer TE, Chatrath V, Iyengar V. Does pulse stacking improve the results of treatment with variable pulsed-dye lasers? Dermatol Surg. 2004;30:163–7.

18. Iyer S, Fitzpatrick RE. Long-pulsed dye laser treatment for facial telangiectasias and erythema. Dermatol Surg. 2005;31:898–903.

19. Babiles P, Shaferstein G, Baumler W, et al. Selective photothermolysis of blood vessels following flashlamp-pumped pulsed dye laser irradiation in vivo results and mathematical modelling are in agreement. J Invest Dermatol. 2005;125:343–52.

20. Goldman MP, Eckhouse S. Photothermal sclerosis of leg veins. Dermatol Surg. 1996;22:323–30.

21. Raulin C, Hellwig S, Schonermark MP, et al. Treatment of a non-responding port-wine stain with a new pulsed source (Photoderm VL). Lasers Surg Med. 1997;21:203–8.

22. Schroeter C, Wilder D, Reineke T, et al. Clinical significance of an intense, pulsed light source on leg telangiectasias of up to 1 mm diameter. Eur J Dermatol. 1997;7:38–42.

23. Goldman MP. Intravascular lasers in the treatment of varicose veins. J Cosmet Dermatol. 2004;3:162–6.

24. Proebstle TM, Moehler T, Gul D, Herdemann S. Endovenous treatment of the great saphenous vein using a 1320 nm Nd:YAG laser causes fewer side effects than using a 940 nm diode laser. Dermatol Surg. 2005;31:1678–83.

25. Kauvar ANB, Lou WW, Zelickson B. Effect of cryogen spray on 595 nm, 1.5 msec pulsed dye laser treatment of port wine stains. Lasers Surg Med. 1999;22:19.

26. Huikeshoven M, Koster PH, de Borgie CA, et al. Redarkening of port-wine stains 10 years after pulsed-dye-laser treatment. N Engl J Med. 2007;356:1235–40.

27. van der Horst CM, Koster PH, De Borgie CA, et al. Effect of timing of treatment of port-wine stains with the flashlamp-pumped pulsed dye laser. N Engl J Med. 1998;338:1028–33.

28. Goldman MP, Fitzpatrick RE. Laser treatment of cutaneous vascular lesions. In: Goldman MP, Fitzpatrick RE (eds). Cutaneous Laser Surgery: The Art and Science of Selective Photothermolysis, 2nd edn. St Louis: Mosby, 1999:19–178.

29. Renfro L, Geronemus RG. Anatomical differences of port-wine stains in response to treatment with the pulsed dye laser. Arch Dermatol. 1993;129:182–8.

30. Greve B, Raulin C. Prospective study of port wine stain treatment with dye laser: comparison of two wavelengths (585 nm vs. 595 nm) and two pulse durations (0.5 milliseconds vs. 20 milliseconds). Laser Surg Med. 2004;34:168–73.

31. Pence B, Aybey B, Ergenekon G. Outcomes of 532 nm frequency-doubled Nd:YAG laser use in the treatment of port-wine stains. Dermatol Surg. 2005;31:509–17.

32. Batta K, Goodyear HM, Moss C, et al. Randomised controlled study of early pulsed dye laser treatment of uncomplicated childhood haemangiomas: results of a 1-year analysis. Lancet. 2002;360:521–7.

33. Ashinoff R, Geronemus RG. Capillary hemangioma and treatment with the flashlamp-pumped pulsed dye laser. Arch Dermatol. 1991;127:202–5.

34. Goldman MP, Weiss RA, Brody HJ, et al. Treatment of facial telangiectasia with sclerotherapy, laser surgery, and/or electrodessication: a review. J Dermatol Surg Oncol. 1993;19:899–906.

35. Schroeter CA, Neumann HAM. An intense light source. The photoderm VL-flashlamp as a new treatment possibility for vascular lesions. Dermatol Surg. 1998;24:743–8.

36. Goldman MP, Fitzpatrick RE. Pulsed-dye laser treatment of telangiectasia: with and without simultaneous sclerotherapy. J Dermatol Surg Oncol. 1990;16:338–44.

37. Bernstein EF, Lee J, Lowery J, et al. Treatment of spider veins with the 595 nm pulsed dye laser. J Am Acad Dermatol. 1998;39:746–50.

38. Kauvar ANB. The role of lasers in the treatment of leg veins. Semin Cutan Med Surg. 2000;19:245–52.

39. Kauvar ANB, Lou WW. Pulsed alexandrite laser for the treatment of leg telangiectasia. Arch Dermatol. 2000;136:1371–5.

40. Dierickx CC, Duque V, Anderson RR. Treatment of leg telangiectasia. Lasers Surg Med. 1998;21(suppl):40.

41. Goldman L, Wilson RG, Hornby P, et al. Radiation from a Q-switched ruby laser. J Invest Dermatol. 1965;44:69–71.

42. Polla LL, Margolis RJ, Dover JS, et al. Melanosomes are a primary target of Q-switched ruby laser irradiation in guinea pig skin. J Invest Dermatol. 1987;89:281–6.

43. Dover JS, Margolis RJ, Polla LL. Pigmented guinea pig skin irradiated with Q-switched ruby lasers. Arch Dermatol. 1989;125:43–9.

44. Kilmer SL, Wheeland RG, Goldberg DJ, et al. Treatment of epidermal pigmented lesions with the frequency doubled Q-switched Nd:YAG laser. A controlled, single impact, dose-response, multicenter trial. Arch Dermatol. 1994;130:1515–19.

45. Grossman MC, Anderson RR, Farinelli W, et al. Treatment of café-au-lait macules with lasers. A clinicopathological correlation. Arch Dermatol. 1995;131:1416–20.

46. Alora MB, Arndt KA. Treatment of a café-au-lait macule with the erbium:YAG laser. J Am Acad Dermatol. 2001;45:566–8.

47. Kopera D, Hohenleutner U, Landthaler M. Quality-switched ruby laser treatment of solar lentigines and Becker's nevus: a histopathological and immunochemical study. Dermatology. 1997;194:338–43.

48. Baba T, Narumi H, Hanada K, et al. Successful treatment of dark-colored epidermal nevus with ruby laser. J Dermatol. 1995;22:567–70.

49. Taylor CR, Anderson RR. Ineffective treatment of refractory melasma and post-inflammatory hyperpigmentation by Q-switched laser. J Dermatol Surg Oncol. 1994;20:592–7.

50. Manaloto RM, Alster T. Erbium:YAG laser resurfacing for refractory melasma. Dermatol Surg. 1999;25:121–3.

51. Nouri K, Bowes L, Chartier T, et al. Combination treatment of melasma with pulsed CO_2 laser followed by Q-switched alexandrite laser: a pilot study. Dermatol Surg. 1999;25:494–7.

52. Watanabe S, Takahashi H. Treatment of nevus of Ota with the Q-switched ruby laser. N Engl J Med. 1994;331:1745–50.

53. Apfelberg DB. Argon and Q-switched yttrium-aluminum-garnet laser treatment of nevus of Ota. Ann Plastic Surg. 1995;35:150–3.

54. Alster TS, Williams CM. Treatment of nevus of Ota by the Q-switched alexandrite laser. Dermatol Surg. 1995;21:592–6.

55. Geronemus RG. Q-switched laser therapy of nevus of Ota. Arch Dermatol. 1992;128:1618–22.

56. Ueda S, Isoda M, Imayama S. Response of naevus of Ota to Q-switched ruby laser treatment according to lesion colour. Br J Dermatol. 2000;142:77–83.

57. Kang W, Lee E, Choi GS. Treatment of Ota's nevus by Q-switched alexandrite laser: therapeutic outcome in relation to clinical and histopathologic findings. Eur J Dermatol. 1999;9:639–43.

58. Lowe NJ, Wieder JM, Shorr N, et al. Infraorbital pigmented skin. Preliminary observations of laser therapy. Dermatol Surg. 1995;21:767–70.

59. West TB, Alster TS. Improvement of infraorbital hyperpigmentation following carbon dioxide laser resurfacing. Dermatol Surg. 1998;24:615–16.

60. Tsao H, Busam K, Barnhill RL, et al. Treatment of minocycline-induced hyperpigmentation with the Q-switched ruby laser. Arch Dermatol. 1996;132:1250–1.

61. Karrer S, Hohenleutner U, Szeimies RM, et al. Amiodarone-induced pigmentation resolves after treatment with the Q-switched ruby laser. Arch Dermatol. 1999;135:251–3.

62. Waldorf HA, Kauvar AN, Geronemus RG. Treatment of small and medium congenital nevi with the Q-switched ruby laser. Arch Dermatol. 1996;132:301–4.

63. Grevelink JM, van Leeuwen RL, Anderson RR, et al. Clinical and histological responses of congenital melanocytic nevi after single treatment with Q-switched lasers. Arch Dermatol. 1997;133:349–53.

64. Rosenbach A, Williams CM, Alster TS. Comparison of the Q-switched alexandrite (755 nm) and Q-switched Nd:YAG (1064 nm) lasers in the treatment of benign melanocytic nevi. Dermatol Surg. 1997;23:239–44.

65. Ueda S, Imayama S. Normal-mode ruby laser for treating congenital nevi. Arch Dermatol. 1997;133:355–9.

66. Imayama S, Ueda S. Long- and short-term histological observations of congenital nevi treated with the normal-mode ruby laser. Arch Dermatol. 1999;135:1211–18.

67. Duke D, Byers R, Sober A, et al. Treatment of benign and atypical nevi with the normal mode ruby laser and the Q-switched ruby laser. Arch Dermatol. 1999;135:290–6.

68. Westerhof W, Gamei M. Treatment of acquired junctional melanocytic naevi by Q-switched and normal mode ruby laser. Br J Dermatol. 2003;148:80–5.

69. Lee PK, Rosenberg CN, Tsao H, et al. Failure of Q-switched laser to eradicate atypical-appearing solar lentigo: report of two cases. J Am Acad Dermatol. 1998;38:314–17.

70. Grevelink JM, Gonzalez S, Bonoan R, et al. Treatment of nevus spilus with the Q-switched ruby laser. Dermatol Surg. 1997;23:365–9.

71. Arndt KA. Argon treatment of lentigo maligna. J Am Acad Dermatol. 1984;10:953–7.

72. Taylor CR, Anderson RR, Gange W, et al. Light and electron microscopic analysis of tattoos treated with the Q-switched ruby laser. J Invest Dermatol. 1991;97:131–6.

73. Kilmer SL, Anderson RR. Clinical use of the Q-switched ruby and the Q-switched Nd:YAG (1064 and 532 nm) lasers for the treatment of tattoos. J Dermatol Surg Oncol. 1993;19:330–8.

74. Grekin RC, Shelton RM, Geisse JK, et al. 510-nm pigmented lesion dye laser: its characteristics and clinical uses. J Dermatol Surg Oncol. 1993;19:380–7.

75. Taylor CR, Gange W, Dover JS, et al. Treatment of tattoos by the Q-switched ruby laser: a dose–response study. Arch Dermatol. 1990;126:893–7.

76. Roosee EV, Naseef GS, Lin C, et al. Comparison of responses of tattoos to picosecond and nanosecond Q-switched neodymium:YAG lasers. Arch Dermatol. 1998;134:167–71.

77. Herd RM, Alora MB, Smoller B, et al. A clinical and histological prospective controlled study of the picosecond titanium:sapphire (795 nm) laser versus the Q-switched alexandrite (752 nm) laser for removing tattoo pigment. J Am Acad Dermatol. 1999;40:603–6.

78. Ashinoff R, Levine VJ, Soter NA. Allergic reactions to tattoo pigment after laser treatment. Dermatol Surg. 1995;21:291–4.

79. Bjornberg A. Reactions to light in yellow tattoos from cadmium sulfide. Arch Dermatol. 1963;88:267.

80. Anderson RR, Geronemus R, Kilmer SL, et al. Cosmetic tattoo ink darkening: a complication of Q-switched and pulsed-laser treatment. Arch Dermatol. 1993;129:1010–14.

81. Trotter MJ, Tron VA, Hollingdale J, et al. Localized chrysiasis induced by laser therapy. Arch Dermatol. 1995;131:1411–14.

82. Goldberg DJ, Littler CT, Wheeland RG. Topical suspension-assisted Q-switched Nd:YAG laser hair removal. Dermatol Surg. 1997;23:741–5.

83. Grossman MC, Dierickx C, Farinelli W, et al. Damage to hair follicles by normal-mode ruby laser pulses. J Am Acad Dermatol. 1996;35:889–94.

84. Dierickx CC, Grossman MC, Farinelli WA, et al. Permanent hair removal by normal-mode ruby laser. Arch Dermatol. 1998;134:837–44.

85. Finkel B, Eliezri YD, Waldman A, et al. Pulsed alexandrite laser technology for non-invasive hair removal. J Clin Laser Med Surg. 1997;15:225–9.

86. Wanner M. Laser hair removal. Dermatol Ther. 2005;18:209–16.

87. Grossman MC, Lou WW, Geronemus RG, et al. Long term comparison of different lasers and light sources for hair removal. Lasers Surg Med. 2000;12(suppl):89.

88. Anderson RR, Burns AJ, Garden J, et al. Multicenter study of long-pulse ruby laser hair removal. Lasers Surg Med. 1999;11(suppl):14.

89. Eremia S, Li C, Newman N. Laser hair removal with alexandrite versus diode laser using four treatment sessions: 1-year results. Dermatol Surg. 2001; 27:925–9.

90. Finkel B, Eliezri YD, Waldman A, Slatkine M. Pulsed alexandrite laser technology for noninvasive hair removal. J Clin Laser Med Surg. 1997;15:225–9.

91. Gorgu M, Aslan G, Akoz T, Erdogan B. Comparison of alexandrite laser and electrolysis for hair removal. Dermatol Surg. 2000;26:37–41.

92. Garcia C, Alamoudi H, Nakib M, Zimmo S. Alexandrite laser hair removal is safe for Fitzpatrick skin types IV–VI. Dermatol Surg. 2000;26:130–4.

93. Baugh WP, Trafeli JP, Barnette DJ Jr, Ross EV. Hair reduction using a scanning 800 nm diode laser. Dermatol Surg. 2001;27:358–64.

94. Bouzari N, Tabatabai H, Abbasi Z, Firooz A, Dowlati Y. Hair removal using an 800-nm diode laser: comparison at different treatment intervals of 45, 60, and 90 days. Int J Dermatol. 2005;44:50–3.

95. Lou WW, Quintana AT, Geronemus RG, Grossman MC. Prospective study of hair reduction by diode laser (800 nm) with long-term follow-up. Dermatol Surg. 2000;26:428–32.

96. Greppi I. Diode laser hair removal of the black patient. Lasers Surg Med. 2001;28:150–5.

97. Alster TS, Bryan H, Williams CM. Long-pulsed Nd:YAG laser-assisted hair removal in pigmented skin: a clinical and histological evaluation. Arch Dermatol. 2001;137:885–9.

98. Goldberg DJ, Silapunt S. Hair removal using a long-pulsed Nd:YAG laser: comparison at fluences of 50, 80, and 100 J/cm^2. Dermatol Surg. 2001;27:434–6.

99. Tanzi EL, Alster TS. Long-pulsed 1064-nm Nd:YAG laser-assisted hair removal in all skin types. Dermatol Surg. 2004;30:13–17.

100. Weiss RA, Weiss MA, Marwaha S, Harrington AC. Hair removal with a noncoherent filtered flashlamp intense pulsed light source. Lasers Surg Med. 1999;24:128–32.

101. Sadick NS, Shea CR, Burchette JL Jr, Prieto VG. High-intensity flashlamp photoepilation: a clinical, histological, and mechanistic study in human skin. Arch Dermatol. 1999;135:668–76.

102. Gold MH, Bell MW, Foster TD, Street S. Long-term epilation using the EpiLight broadband, intense pulsed light hair removal system. Dermatol Surg. 1997;23:909–13.

103. Sadick NS, Shaoul J. Hair removal using a combination of conducted radiofrequency and optical energies – an 18-month follow-up. J Cosmet Laser Ther. 2004;6:21–6.

104. Alexiades-Armenakas MR, Dover JS, Arndt KA. The spectrum of laser skin resurfacing: nonablative, fractional and ablative laser resurfacing. J Am Acad Dermatol. 2007, in press.

105. Herne KB, Zachary CB. New facial rejuvenation techniques. Semin Cutan Med Surg. 2000;19:221–31.

106. Alam M, Dover JS, Arndt KA. Energy delivery devices for cutaneous remodeling: lasers, lights, and radio waves. Arch Dermatol. 2003;139:1351–60.

107. Goldberg DJ, Whitworth J. Laser skin resurfacing with the Q-switched Nd:YAG laser. Dermatol Surg. 1997;23:903–7.

108. Alster TS, Kurban AK, Grove GL, et al. Alteration of argon laser-induced scars by the pulsed dye laser. Lasers Surg Med. 1993;13:368–73.

109. Alster TS, Williams CM. Improvement of hypertrophic and keloidal median sternotomy scars by the 585 nm flashlamp-pumped pulsed dye laser: a controlled study. Lancet. 1995;345:1198–200.

110. Alster TS, McMeekin TO. Improvement of facial acne scars by the 585 nm flashlamp-pumped pulsed dye laser. J Am Acad Dermatol. 1996;35:79–81.

111. McDaniel DH, Ask K, Zubowski M. Treatment of stretch marks with the 585 nm flashlamp pumped pulsed dye laser. Dermatol Surg. 1996;22:332–7.

112. Wittenberg GP, Fabian BG, Bogomilsky JL, et al. Prospective, single-blind, randomized, controlled study to assess the efficacy of the 585-nm flashlamp-pumped pulsed-dye laser and silicone gel sheeting in hypertrophic scar treatment. Arch Dermatol. 1999;135:1049–55.

113. Bjerring P, Clement M, Heickendroff L, et al. Selective non-ablative laser reduction by laser. J Cutan Laser Ther. 2000;2:9–15.

114. Zelickson BD, Kilmer SL, Bernstein E, at al. Pulsed dye therapy for sundamaged skin. Lasers Surg Med. 1999;25:229–36.

115. Rostan E, Bowes LE, Iyer S, Fitzpatrick RE. A double-blind, side-by-side comparison study of low fluence long pulsed dye laser to coolant treatment of wrinkling of the cheeks. J Cosmet Laser Ther. 2001;3:129–36.

116. Goldberg D, Tan M, Dale Sarradet M, Gordon M. Nonablative dermal remodeling with a 585-nm, 350-microsec, flashlamp pulsed dye laser: clinical and ultrastructural analysis. Dermatol Surg. 2003;29:161–4.

117. Alexiades-Armenakas MR, Geronemus RG. Laser-mediated photodynamic therapy of actinic keratoses. Arch Dermatol. 2003;139:1313–20.

118. Alexiades-Armenakas MR, Geronemus RG. Laser-mediated photodynamic therapy of actinic cheilitis. J Drugs Dermatol. 2004;3:548–52.

119. Alexiades-Armenakas M. Laser-mediated photodynamic therapy. Clin Dermatol. 2006:24:16–25.

120. Bitter P, Campbell CA, Goldman M. Nonablative skin rejuvenation using intense pulsed light. Lasers Surg Med. 2000;12:16.

121. Ross EV, Sajben FP, Hsia J, et al. Nonablative skin remodeling: selective dermal heating with a mid-infrared laser and contact cooling combination. Lasers Surg Med. 2000;26:186–95.

122. Kelly KM, Nelson JS, Lask GP, et al. Cryogen spray cooling with nonablative laser treatment of facial rhytides. Arch Dermatol. 1999;135:691–4.

123. Goldberg DJ. Non-ablative subsurface remodeling: clinical and histological evaluations of a 1320-nm Nd:YAG laser. J Cutan Laser Ther. 1999;1:153–7.

124. Lupton JR, Williams CM, Alster TS. Nonablative laser skin resurfacing using a 1540 nm erbium glass laser: a clinical and histologic analysis. Dermatol Surg. 2002;28:833–5.

125. Fournier N, Dahan S, Barneon G, et al. Non-ablative remodeling: clinical histologic ultrasound imaging, and profilometric evaluation of a 1540-nm Er:glass laser. Dermatol Surg. 2001;27:799–806.

126. Tanzi EL, Alster TS. Comparison of a 1450-nm diode laser and a 1320-nm Nd:YAG laser in the treatment of atrophic facial scars: a prospective clinical and histologic study. Dermatol Surg. 2004;30:152–7.

127. Fatemi A, Weiss MA, Weiss RA. Short-term histologic effects of nonablative resurfacing: results with a dynamically cooled millisecond-domain 1320 nm Nd:YAG laser. Dermatol Surg. 2002;28:172–6.

128. Goldberg DJ, Hussain M, Fazeli A, Berlin AL. Treatment of skin laxity of the lower face and neck in older individuals with a broad-spectrum infrared light source. J Cosmet Laser Ther. 2007;9:35–40.

129. Goldberg D. New collagen formation after dermal remodeling with an intense pulsed light source. J Cutan Laser Ther. 2000;2:59–61.

130. Dover JS, Bhatia AC, Stewart B, Arndt KA. Topical 5-aminolevulinic acid combined with intense pulsed light in the treatment of photoaging. Arch Dermatol. 2005;141:1247–54.

131. Jacobson LG, Alexiades-Armenakas MR, Bernstein L, Geronemus, RG. Treatment of nasolabial folds and jowls with a non-invasive radiofrequency device. Arch Dermatol. 2003;139:1313–20.

132. Hsu TS, Kaminer MS. The use of nonablative radiofrequency technology to tighten the lower face and neck. Semin Cutan Med Surg. 2003;22:115–23.

133. Sadick N, Alexiades-Armenakas M, Bitter P, et al. Enhanced full-face skin rejuvenation using synchronous intense pulsed optical and conducted, bipolar radiofrequency energy (ELOS): introducing selective radiophotothermolysis. J Drugs Dermatol. 2005;4:181–6.

134. Doshi SN, Alster TS. Combination radiofrequency and diode laser for treatment of facial rhytides and skin laxity. J Cosmet Laser Ther. 2005;7:11–15.

135. Sadick NS, Mullholland RS. A prospective clinical study to evaluate the efficacy and safety of cellulite treatment using the combination of optical and RF energies for subcutaneous tissue heating. J Cosmet Laser Ther. 2004;6:187–90.

136. Manstein D, Herron GS, Sink RK, et al. Fractional photothermolysis: a new concept for cutaneous remodeling using microscopic patterns of thermal injury. Lasers Surg Med. 2004;34:426–38.

137. Walsh JT, Flotte TJ, Anderson RR, et al. Pulsed CO_2 laser tissue ablation: effect of tissue type and pulse duration on thermal damage. Lasers Surg Med. 1988;8:108–18.

138. Walsh JT, Deutsch TF. Pulsed CO_2 laser tissue ablation: measurement of the ablation rate. Lasers Surg Med. 1988;8:264–75.

139. Alster TS, Nanni C, Williams CM. Comparison of four carbon dioxide resurfacing lasers. A clinical and histopathologic evaluation. Dermatol Surg. 1999;25:3:153–9.

140. Duke D, Khatri K, Grevelink J, et al. The comparison of a 60 µsec pulse duration to a 1 ms pulse duration CO_2 laser system in laser resurfacing. Lasers Surg Med. 1997;20:30–1.

141. Fitzpatrick RE, Goldman MP, Satur NM, et al. Pulsed carbon dioxide laser resurfacing of photoaged facial skin. Arch Dermatol. 1996;132:395–402.

142. Alster TS, Garg S. Treatment of facial rhytides with a high-energy pulsed carbon dioxide laser. Plast Reconstr Surg. 1996;98:791–4.

143. Grover R, Grobbelaar AO, Morgan BD, et al. A quantitative method for the assessment of facial rejuvenation. Br J Plast Surg. 1998;51:8–13.

144. Alster TS, West TB. Resurfacing of atrophic facial acne scars with a high-energy, pulsed carbon dioxide laser. Dermatol Surg. 1996;22:151–5.

145. Apfelberg DB. A critical appraisal of high-energy pulsed carbon dioxide laser facial resurfacing for acne scars. Ann Plast Surg. 1997;38:95–100.

146. Miller ID. The erbium laser gains a role in cosmetic surgery. Biophotonics Int. 1997;May/June:38–42.

147. Ross VE, McKinlay JR, Anderson RR. Why does carbon dioxide resurfacing work? Arch Dermatol. 1999;135:444–54.

148. Adrian MA. Pulsed carbon dioxide and long pulse 10-ms erbium-YAG laser resurfacing. A comparative clinical and histological study. J Cutan Laser Ther. 1999;1:197–202.

149. Newman JB, Lord JL, Ash K, et al. Variable pulse erbium:YAG laser skin resurfacing of perioral rhytides and side-by-side comparison with carbon dioxide laser. Lasers Surg Med. 2000;26:208–14.

150. Rostan EF, Fitzpatrick RE, Goldman MP. Laser resurfacing with a long pulse erbium:YAG laser compared to the 950 ms CO_2 laser. Lasers Surg Med. 2001;29:136–41.

151. Manuskiatti W, Fitzpatrick RE, Goldman MP. Long-term effectiveness and side effects of carbon dioxide laser resurfacing for resurfacing of photoaged facial skin. J Am Acad Dermatol. 1999;40:401–11.

152. Khatri KA, Ross V, Grevelink JM, et al. Comparison of erbium:YAG and carbon dioxide lasers in resurfacing of facial rhytides. Arch Dermatol. 1999;135:1416–17.

153. Orringer J, Kang S, Johnson TM, et al. Connective tissue remodeling induced by carbon dioxide laser resurfacing of photodamaged human skin. Arch Dermatol. 2004;140:1326–32.

154. Rubenstein R, Roenigk HH Jr, Stegman SJ, et al. Atypical keloids after dermabrasion of patients taking isotretinoin. J Am Acad Dermatol. 1986;15:280–5.

155. Hayes DK, Berkland ME, Stambaugh KI. Dermal healing after local skin flaps and chemical peels. Arch Otolaryngol Head Neck Surg. 1990;116:794–7.

156. Jacob CI, Dover JS, Kaminer MS. Acne scarring: a classification system and review of treatment options. J Am Acad Dermatol. 2001;45:109–17.

157. Greenbaum SS, Rubim MG. Surgical pearl: the high energy pulsed carbon dioxide laser for immediate scar resurfacing. J Am Acad Dermatol. 1999;40:988–90.

158. Gjuric M, Rettinger G. Comparison of carbon dioxide laser and electrosurgery in the treatment of rhinophyma. Rhinology. 1993;31:37–9.

159. Johnson TM, Sebastien TS, Lowe L, et al. Carbon dioxide laser treatment of actinic cheilitis: clinicopathologic correlation to determine the optimal depth of destruction. J Am Acad Dermatol. 1992;27:737–40.

160. Ho C, Nguyen Q, Lowe NJ, et al. Laser resurfacing in pigmented skin. Dermatol Surg. 1995;21:1035–7.

161. Bernstein LJ, Kauvar ANB, Grossman MC. The short- and long-term side effects of carbon dioxide laser resurfacing. Dermatol Surg. 1997;23:519–25.

162. Sriprachya-Anunt S, Fitzpatrick RE, Goldman MP, et al. Infections complicating pulsed carbon dioxide laser resurfacing for photoaged facial skin. Dermatol Surg. 1997;23:527–35.

163. Fitzpatrick RE, Smith SR, Sriprachya-Anunt S. Depth of vaporization and the effect of pulse stacking with a high energy, pulsed carbon dioxide laser. J Am Acad Dermatol. 1999;40:615–22.

164. Alexiades-Armenakas MR. Long pulsed dye laser-mediated photodynamic therapy combined with topical therapy for the treatment of mild to severe, comedonal, inflammatory and cystic acne. J Drugs Dermatol. 2006;5:1–11.

165. Alexiades-Armenakas MR. Laser-mediated photodynamic therapy of lichen sclerosus. J Drugs Dermatol. 2004;3:S25–7.

166. Apfelberg DB, Maser MR, Lash H, et al. Preliminary results of argon and carbon dioxide laser treatment of keloid scars. Lasers Surg Med. 1984;4:283–90.

167. Sherman R, Rosenfeld H. Experience with the Nd:YAG laser in the treatment of keloid scars. Ann Plast Surg. 1988;21:231–5.

168. Dierickx C, Goldman MP, Fitzpatrick R. Laser treatment of erythematous/hypertrophic and pigmented scars in 26 patients. Plast Reconstr Surg. 1995;95:84–90.

169. Reiken SR, Wolfort SF, Berthiaume F, et al. Control of hypertrophic scar growth using selective photothermolysis. Lasers Surg Med. 1997;21:7–12.

170. McDaniel DH, Ask K, Zubowski M. Treatment of stretch marks with the 585 nm flashlamp pumped pulsed dye laser. Dermatol Surg. 1996;22:332–7.

171. Alexiades-Armenakas MR, Bernstein LJ, Friedman PM, Geronemus RG. The safety and efficacy of the 308 nm excimer laser for pigment correction of hypopigmented scars and striae alba. Arch Dermatol. 2004;140:955–60.

172. Lim JT, Goh CL. Carbon dioxide laser treatment of periungual and subungual viral warts. Australas J Dermatol. 1992;33:87–91.

173. Street ML, Roenigk RK. Recalcitrant periungual verrucae: the role of carbon dioxide laser vaporization. J Am Acad Dermatol. 1991;25:730–1.

174. Ferenczy A, Mitao M, Nagai N, et al. Latent papillomavirus and recurring genital warts. N Engl J Med. 1985;313:784–8.

175. Sawchuk WS, Weber PJ, Lowy DR, et al. Infectious papillomavirus in the vapor of warts treated with carbon dioxide laser or electrocoagulation: detection and protection. J Am Acad Dermatol. 1989;21:41–9.

176. Tan OT, Hurwitz RM, Stafford TJ. Pulsed dye laser treatment of recalcitrant verrucae: a preliminary report. Lasers Surg Med. 1993;13:127–37.

177. Huilgol SC, Barlow RJ, Markey AC. Failure of pulsed dye laser therapy for resistant verrucae. Clin Exp Dermatol. 1996;21:93–5.

178. Zelickson BD, Mehregan DA, Wendelschfer-Crabb G, et al. Clinical and histologic evaluation of psoriatic plaques treated with a flashlamp pumped pulsed dye laser. J Am Acad Dermatol. 1996;35:64–8.

179. Alora MB, Anderson RR, Quinn TT, et al. CO_2 laser resurfacing of psoriatic plaques: a pilot study. Lasers Surg Med. 1998;22:165–70.

180. Asawanonda P, Anderson RR, Chang Y, et al. 308-nm excimer laser for the treatment of psoriasis. A dose–response study. Arch Dermatol. 2000; 136:619–24.

181. Feldman SR, Mellen BG, Salam TN, et al. Efficacy of 308 nm excimer laser for treatment of psoriasis: results of a multicenter study. J Am Acad Dermatol. 2002;46:900–6.

182. Fretklin S, Beeson WH, Hanke CW. Ignition potential of the 585 nm pulsed-dye laser. J Dermatol Surg Oncol. 1996;22:699–702.

183. Baggish MS, Poiesz B, Jorot D, et al. Presence of immunodeficiency virus DNA in laser smoke. Lasers Surg Med. 1991;4:197–203.

Cryosurgery

Emanuel G Kuflik

Synonyms: ■ Cryotherapy ■ Contact therapy ■ Freezing

Key features

- Versatile modality for benign, premalignant and malignant lesions on all areas of the body
- Entails fast freezing and slow thawing, with a single freeze–thaw cycle for benign lesions and a double freeze–thaw cycle for malignant ones
- A tissue temperature of –50°C to –60°C is needed for destruction of malignant lesions, while lesser degrees of freezing are needed for benign lesions
- Because of its lower boiling point (–196°C), liquid nitrogen is preferred as the cryogen over nitrous oxide, carbon dioxide and fluorinated hydrocarbons
- Depth dose is determined by observation, palpation, freeze time, thaw time, lateral spread of freeze, and measurement of the tissue temperature. Cancer depth dose is achieved when these factors have reached the desired endpoint
- The tissue reactions are predictable, including crust or bulla formation after treatment of a benign lesion, and exudation, edema and sloughing after treatment of a malignant one
- Melanocytes are more sensitive to freezing than are keratinocytes, thus cryosurgery can lead to depigmentation

INTRODUCTION AND BACKGROUND

Cryosurgery is a treatment modality that is used frequently, to one degree or another, by all dermatologists. For several reasons, it is useful as a primary or as an alternate form of treatment (Table 138.1). The word cryotherapy is often used interchangeably with cryosurgery, although the latter is a more accurate description of the destruction that is now attainable with this modality.

The objective of cryosurgery is to cause selective necrosis of tissue, the extent of which depends on the type of lesion and the volume of freezing needed. Tissue alterations are caused by reduction of the skin temperature with consequent freezing of cells[1]. The rate of heat transfer

ADVANTAGES IN THE USE OF CRYOSURGERY
• Versatility for treatment of diverse conditions
• Treatment of any area of body
• Palliative therapy for inoperable tumors
• Excellent cosmetic results
• Suitable for office, nursing home, or outpatient facility
• Low cost
• No general anesthesia; local anesthesia optional
• Operative suite not required
• Safe and relatively simple procedure
• No restriction of work or sports
• Useful in pregnancy
• For patients who are fearful of undergoing surgery
• For poor surgical risk patients
• No age limitations – excellent for the very elderly
• Suitable for wheelchair and stretcher patients

Table 138.1 Advantages in the use of cryosurgery.

is a function of the temperature difference between the skin and the heat sink, or liquid nitrogen. Because the difference between the skin temperature and the temperature of liquid nitrogen is great, rapid heat transfer away from the skin results.

The tissue response ranges from an inflammatory reaction, as in the treatment of acne, to mild destruction for benign lentigo, or even more destruction as for actinic keratosis. A greater amount of necrosis is needed for eradication of malignant lesions[2–4]. The mechanisms of injury in cryosurgery can be attributed to the direct effects of freezing tissue and to vascular stasis. Freezing tissue results in intracellular and extracellular ice crystal formation, disruption of cell membrane integrity, pH changes, impairment of multiple homeostatic functions, and thermal shock. This damage is enhanced during subsequent thawing of the tissue by the development of vascular stasis, which leads to failure of the local microcirculation. Slow cooling produces extracellular ice, but this is not as damaging as rapid cooling, which produces intracellular ice formation. Therefore, rapid cooling of the target tissue is desirable. On the other hand, the rate of rewarming, or thawing, should proceed slowly. With repeated freeze–thaw cycles, maximum destructive effects are produced. The tissue reactions that ensue after either light or deep freezing are predictable, and the underlying stroma provides a structural framework for wound repair.

Liquid nitrogen is the coldest cryogenic agent (–196°C boiling point) with the greatest freezing capability. It can be used for cutaneous malignancies as well as for small benign lesions. Although other cryogenic agents are available, including nitrous oxide, carbon dioxide and fluorinated hydrocarbons, they are not recommended for skin cancer but rather for lesions that require lesser degrees of freezing. Modern cryosurgery uses an apparatus that employs liquid nitrogen in a closed system that permits continuous and rapid extraction of heat from tissue. The dominant apparatus for dermatologic use is a hand-held unit that can be used either with a spray-tip accessory or with a closed cryoprobe (also known as contact therapy). Although the same equipment is used for a wide variety of conditions, the volume of liquid nitrogen, the technique of treatment, the duration of cooling and the amount of tissue being destroyed varies. Other techniques still in use include a cotton-tipped applicator and crushed carbon dioxide.

INDICATIONS AND CONTRAINDICATIONS

Cryosurgery is a versatile modality that is used for many benign, premalignant and malignant lesions. The indications are related to the nature of the lesion and to the type of patient.

More than 50 benign conditions are amenable to cryosurgical management (Table 138.2). This is in addition to premalignant lesions and *in situ* malignancies including actinic keratoses, actinic cheilitis, lentigo maligna, Bowen's disease and erythroplasia of Queyrat.

Various subtypes of basal and squamous cell carcinomas can be treated, including papulonodular, cystic, superficial, ulcerative, keratotic and exophytic tumors[5]. Lesions most amenable to treatment have well-delineated borders, but they can be of any size. Cryosurgery is suitable for single or multiple tumors, or difficult tumors, especially for those patients who are elderly, debilitated, or with limited mobility. It is useful for patients with pacemakers or coagulopathies, for lesions located within psoriatic plaques, or when other methods of treatment are impractical or undesirable. Any area of the body can be treated, including the eyelids.

While not the usual initial therapeutic approach, cryosurgery has been used for selected recurrent tumors and ones that are fixed to cartilage or bone[6]. Reviewers of this chapter feel that cryosurgery is not a good choice for treating most recurrent tumors. It can be used for inoperable tumors or where the goal of therapy is palliation, e.g. to relieve pain, reduce tumor bulk or to facilitate nursing care.

BENIGN CONDITIONS AMENABLE TO CRYOSURGERY	
• Acne cysts	• Lichen sclerosus (of vulva)
• Acne keloidalis	• Lymphangioma
• Acne vulgaris	• Lymphocytoma cutis
• Acquired perforating disorder (Kyrle's disease)	• Molluscum contagiosum
• Angiofibroma	• Mucocele
• Angiokeratomas, including of Fordyce	• Myxoid cyst
• Cherry angioma	• Nevoid hyperkeratosis of the nipple
• Chondrodermatitis nodularis helicis	• Orf
• Chromoblastomycosis	• Pearly penile papules
• Clear cell acanthoma	• Porokeratosis
• Condyloma acuminatum	• Prurigo nodularis
• Dermatofibroma	• Pyogenic granuloma
• Discoid lupus erythematosus	• Rhinophyma
• Eccrine poroma	• Rosacea
• Elastosis perforans serpiginosa	• Sarcoidosis
• Epidermal nevus	• Sebaceous hyperplasia
• Erosive adenomatosis of the nipple	• Seborrheic keratosis
• Folliculitis keloidalis	• Syringocystadenoma papilliferum
• Granuloma annulare	• Syringoma
• Granuloma faciale	• Trichiasis
• Hemangioma	• Trichoepithelioma
• Herpes simplex	• Venous lake
• Keloid	• Verruca vulgaris
• Leishmaniasis	• Xanthoma
• Lentigo	

Table 138.2 Benign conditions amenable to cryosurgery.

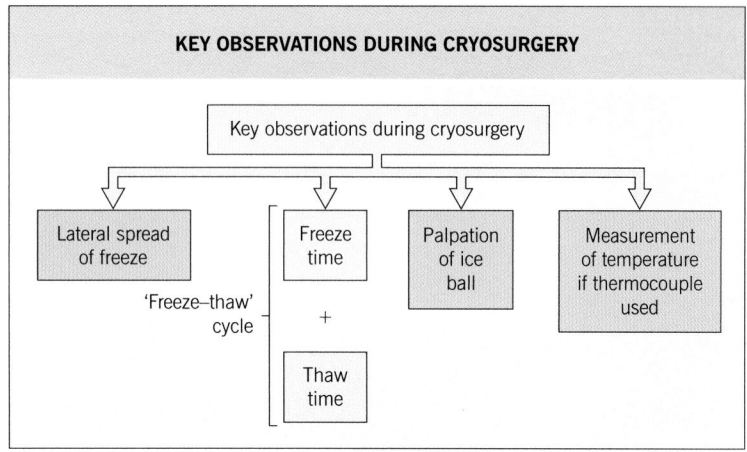

Fig. 138.1 Key observations during cryosurgery.

There are some contraindications for cryosurgery. Patients who have cold urticaria, cold intolerance, cryofibrinogenemia or cryoglobulinemia are best treated by other means. Tumors with indistinct or ill-defined borders (e.g. morpheaform or infiltrative histologic subtypes), as well as deeply penetrating and very aggressive lesions, are best treated by other modalities. Cryosurgery is not considered to be a standard treatment for invasive melanoma.

Caution should be observed when confronted with patients who have darkly pigmented skin, since freezing of skin can result in hypopigmentation. Overfreezing should be avoided in the case of benign and premalignant lesions. On the other hand, undertreatment of malignancies can lead to inadequate destruction or recurrence. Also, lesions that overlie superficial nerves, such as on the fingers or ulnar fossa, should be carefully treated. Some anatomic areas where cryosurgery should be undertaken cautiously include the corners of the mouth, the vermilion margin of the lips, eyebrows, inner canthi, the free margin of the ala nasi, and the auditory canal, since scarring or retraction of the tissue can occur. As mentioned previously, lesions that are not sharply defined may not be good candidates for cryosurgery. Also, lesions in which treatment might lead to functional alterations or an unsightly cosmetic appearance are best treated by other means. Patients may opt for another form of treatment when faced with the prospect of a long healing period.

PREOPERATIVE HISTORY AND CONSIDERATIONS

In planning treatment, consideration should be given to the characteristics of the lesion, which technique of cryosurgery to employ, and the expected results. An explanation of the procedure and the anticipated response of the tissue to freezing, e.g. exudation, crusting, re-epithelialization and healing time, should be discussed with the patient.

TREATMENT FACTORS

When tissue is frozen, the surface freezing and extension of the ice ball is visible, yet the depth of freeze cannot be seen. Therefore, the amount of freezing and the temperature reached beneath and surrounding the lesion must be determined by the surgeon. This is referred to as the depth of freeze (depth dose) and consists of measuring certain clinical factors (observation, palpation, freeze time, thaw time and lateral spread of freeze) as well as the tissue temperature. The proper

depth dose estimation is achieved when clinical observations and the tissue temperature, if measured, have reached the desired endpoint (Fig. 138.1)[7].

Freeze Time

The freeze time refers to the duration of cooling. It is shorter for a benign lesion than it is for a malignancy. For example, about 10 seconds with the open-spray technique will cure 80% of actinic keratoses[8], whereas 45 seconds may be required for a small basal cell carcinoma. For large tumors, a proportionately longer freeze time is needed. The freeze time can be altered by the thickness of the lesion and by the amount of liquid nitrogen being emitted from the spray tip. When the cryoprobe technique is used, the freeze time is approximately two to three times longer than with the open-spray technique. After freezing with either technique, the tissue is permitted to thaw spontaneously and the thaw time is usually two to three times longer than the freeze time.

Lateral Spread of Freeze

The lateral spread of freeze refers to the freezing of the tissue beyond the margins of the lesion. For some benign lesions, such as verrucae or dermatofibromas, it should reach 2 to 3 mm for the treatment to be successful. For basal cell and squamous cell carcinomas, the lateral spread of freeze should extend at least 3 to 5 mm or more around the tumor.

Freeze–Thaw Cycle

A freeze–thaw cycle refers to the actual freezing and thawing of the lesion. A single cycle is usually sufficient for benign and premalignant conditions, while a double cycle is recommended for malignant lesions. This is done to ensure greater lethality to cancerous cells.

Temperature at the Base of the Tissue

To supplement the clinical estimations, one can measure the temperature at the base of a malignancy with the use of a thermocouple that is mounted in the tip of a 25- to 30-gauge needle. It is inserted into the skin at a 25° to 30° angle, from a point lateral to the lesion, with the tip coming to lie beneath the lesion (Fig. 138.2). This is useful for those lesions that lie more than 3 mm below the skin surface and for medicolegal reasons. Since the temperature recorded is very localized, more than one thermocouple may need to be inserted for a large lesion. The recommended temperature for malignancies is between –50°C and –60°C.

DESCRIPTION OF TECHNIQUES

There are six techniques of cryosurgical treatment, and the choice of which to use depends on the lesion and preference of the operator.

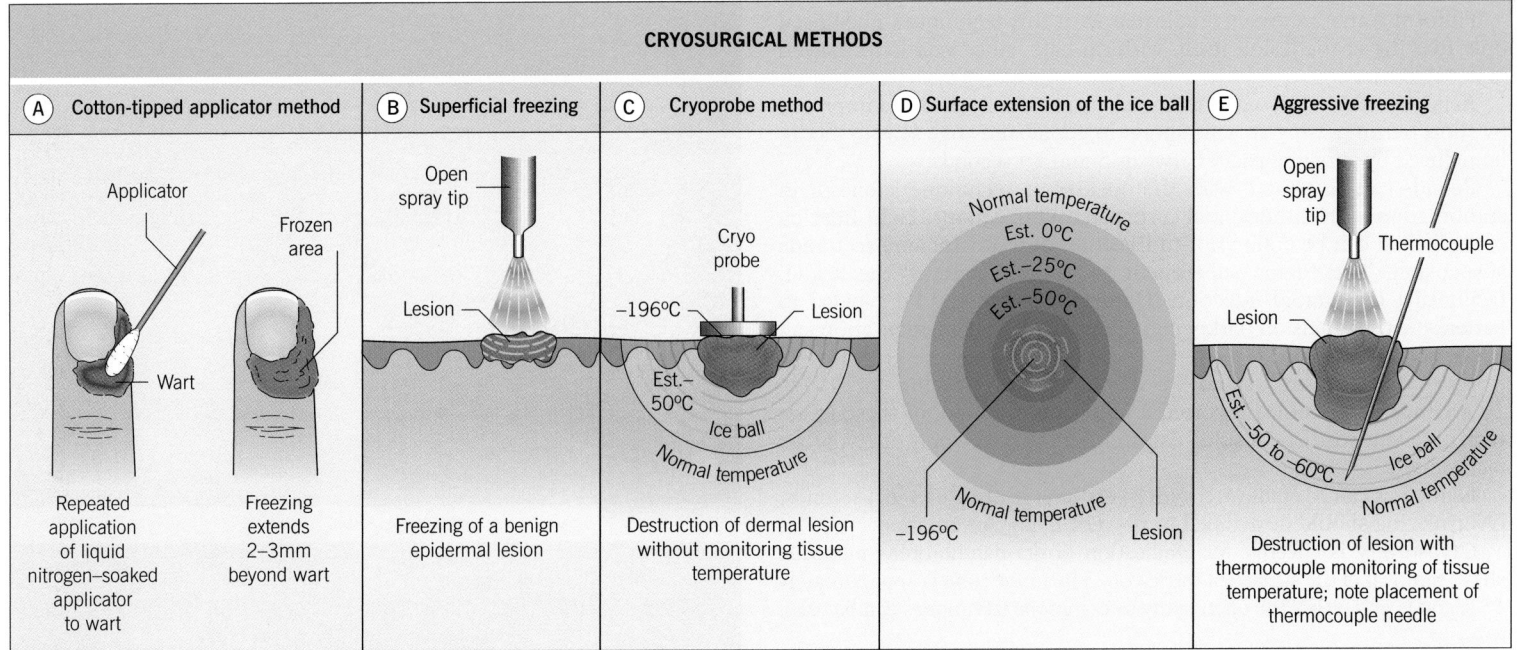

CRYOSURGICAL METHODS

| Ⓐ Cotton-tipped applicator method | Ⓑ Superficial freezing | Ⓒ Cryoprobe method | Ⓓ Surface extension of the ice ball | Ⓔ Aggressive freezing |

Applicator

Frozen area

Wart

Repeated application of liquid nitrogen–soaked applicator to wart

Freezing extends 2–3mm beyond wart

Open spray tip

Lesion

Freezing of a benign epidermal lesion

Cryo probe

−196°C

Lesion

Est.−50°C

Ice ball

Normal temperature

Destruction of dermal lesion without monitoring tissue temperature

Normal temperature

Est. 0°C

Est.−25°C

Est.−50°C

Normal temperature

−196°C

Lesion

Open spray tip

Thermocouple

Lesion

Est. −50 to −60°C

Ice ball

Normal temperature

Destruction of lesion with thermocouple monitoring of tissue temperature; note placement of thermocouple needle

Fig. 138.2 Cryosurgical methods. A The cotton-tipped applicator method used in the treatment of verrucae vulgares, including periungual warts. **B** Superficial freezing used for treating benign lesions and actinic keratoses. **C** Cryoprobe method which is useful for round lesions and those on flat surfaces. **D** Surface extension of the ice ball: note the diminution of the temperature as the ice ball progresses outwards; this can be determined with palpation. **E** Aggressive freezing is deeper and employs thermocouple monitoring of tissue temperature.

Dipstick Technique

The dipstick technique is the oldest method that employs liquid nitrogen. It consists of application of a saturated, cotton-tipped applicator onto the lesion (Fig. 138.2A). It is a method preferred by the author for verrucae.

Solidified Carbon Dioxide

An old and less commonly performed method is crushed solidified carbon dioxide, contained in a disposable towel, and secured around a pestle. It is dipped in acetone and applied lightly onto the skin for mild freezing and exfoliation. This is known as slush therapy and can be used for acne vulgaris, acne cysts, rosacea and flat warts.

Open Spray

The open-spray method is the most frequently used technique, employing a cryosurgical unit, liquid nitrogen, and spray-tip attachments. It is suitable for diverse conditions, including seborrheic keratoses, acne cysts, lentigines, verrucae, dermatofibromas, condyloma acuminata, actinic keratoses, actinic cheilitis, keratoacanthoma, lentigo maligna, basal cell carcinoma and squamous cell carcinoma. A fine spray of liquid nitrogen is directed at the lesion from a distance of approximately 1 to 2 cm. It is particularly useful for superficial, irregular, and multiple lesions and for those on a curved surface. An intermittent spray of liquid nitrogen of 60 seconds or more is used for malignant lesions, to allow a deeper freeze (Fig. 138.2B&E).

Cryoprobe

The cryoprobe technique, also known as contact therapy, employs a cryosurgical unit and consists of application of a flat, pre-cooled metal tip that is placed firmly onto the lesion. It is useful for round lesions and those on flat surfaces (Fig. 138.2C). Venous lakes, hemangiomas, dermatofibromas, myxoid cysts, sebaceous hyperplasia, condyloma acuminata, and basal cell and squamous cell carcinomas are examples of lesions that can be managed with this technique[9]. The freeze time can range between 15 and 20 seconds for the benign lesions and up to several minutes for malignancies.

Confined Spray

The confined-spray technique is a variation of the open-spray in which the liquid nitrogen spray is confined within a cone that is held against the skin. Plastic otoscope cones have been used to precisely localize the spray, for example. The freeze time is the same as for the open-spray technique.

Closed Cone

The closed-cone technique also confines the spray, but the freeze time is half that of the open-spray since the liquid nitrogen is concentrated to a very focal area of skin. This accessory is attached directly to the cryosurgical unit at one end, allowing the nitrogen to enter the cone. It is held against the skin, enabling it to rapidly freeze the lesion.

TREATMENT

Benign Lesions

Freezing is carried out after determination of the type of lesion and selection of the technique of treatment. For benign lesions, one may choose between the cotton-tipped applicator method, a spray technique or the cryoprobe.

For verrucae vulgares and periungual warts, the dipstick or open-spray techniques can be used[10]. The author prefers the former because of greater control, exactness of the freeze and for its predictability. The cotton-tipped applicator is repeatedly dipped into a cup of liquid nitrogen and applied directly onto the wart until a 2 to 3 mm halo forms around it (see Fig. 138.2A). Large lesions that encircle the nail are also treatable. The freeze time ranges between 20 and 60 seconds. A local anesthetic can be used to alleviate the stinging associated with this type of treatment. A bulla develops after several hours that should extend beyond the wart for treatment to be successful. The blister is caused by separation at the dermal-epidermal junction. The author recommends puncture of the bulla (approximately 12 hours following freezing) and washing of the site. Healing occurs within 3 weeks, without scarring or damage to the nail plate, and the cosmetic results are excellent. If a lesion recurs, it can be retreated in a similar manner.

Filiform warts are easily eradicated with this technique. They need only freezing of the lesion itself, with no halo, since vesicle formation is not necessary.

Acne comedones, closed or inflamed, can be diminished and improved by short freezing using an acne spray-tip. Small and large acne cysts can be reduced by spraying them between 5 and 15 seconds.

Keloids can be treated with the open-spray technique, alone or in combination with intralesional corticosteroid injections. Light freezing of the keloid can be done prior to injection of triamcinolone acetonide suspension. The edema subsequent to freezing 'softens' the keloid, facilitating the steroid injection. Hard freezing should be avoided in patients with keloids on darkly pigmented skin, as depigmentation can occur.

Myxoid cysts are treated by deroofing and freezing for 15 to 20 seconds. The author reported a cure rate of 76.7% of these cysts, with excellent cosmetic results, using either the open-spray or cryoprobe technique[11].

Lentigines can be eradicated with a very brief freezing of 3 to 4 seconds. Overfreezing should be avoided to prevent hypopigmentation.

Cryosurgery is effective for eradication of dermatofibromas following shave removal of the surface of the lesion. The freeze time is approximately 15 seconds and either the open-spray or cryoprobe techniques can be used.

Premalignant Lesions

Premalignant lesions are treated with one of the spray techniques or a cryoprobe. A local anesthetic and dressings are optional. The prototype lesion for the open-spray technique is actinic keratosis (see Fig. 138.2B). A shallow crust forms and falls off within 2 weeks. Multiple lesions can be easily treated at one visit[12]. The freeze time for actinic cheilitis ranges between 10 and 20 seconds. Bowen's disease can be treated with a single freeze–thaw cycle and a freeze time of approximately 20 seconds for a small lesion.

Cryosurgery is useful as an alternative modality for lentigo maligna (Fig. 138.3). Aggressive treatment using the open-spray technique is recommended, including freezing to –40°C to –50°C and a 1 cm lateral spread of freeze. With this technique, a recurrence rate of 6.6% was observed[13].

Malignant Lesions

In the treatment of malignant lesions, the same volume of tissue must be destroyed by freezing that would have been removed by conservative local excision if that had been the chosen procedure. Complete destruction is possible with cryosurgery. Lesions are treated aggressively using one of the spray techniques or the cryoprobe. Several preoperative biopsy specimens can be obtained to delineate the margins of a tumor. The target site is cleansed and a local anesthetic can be injected. Thermocouple needles can be implanted at this time. The entire tumor is generally frozen in one session using a double freeze–thaw cycle. The aforementioned clinical factors are observed, and through palpation one can ascertain the extent of the ice ball (Fig. 138.2D). The recommended temperature is between –50°C and –60°C at the base of the tumor, and the freeze time is approximately 45 seconds for a 1 cm lesion. During the past two decades, there has been an increased use of colder temperatures, greater use of debulking techniques, and a trend toward more aggressive treatment for basal and squamous cell carcinomas. At the conclusion of treatment, a dry gauze dressing is applied and instructions given to the patient for postoperative care.

The author reported a 5-year cure rate of 99% for 522 new cancers[14]. The overall 30-year cure rate was 98.6% for 4406 basal cell, squamous cell and basosquamous cell carcinomas. Other investigators have obtained similar results[14a,14b]. Graham[15] had a combined cure rate of 98% for 3593 new basal cell carcinomas using mostly the open-spray technique. Holt[16] reported a 5-year cure rate of 97% in 395 non-melanoma skin cancers. Zacarian[17] reported an 18-year cure rate of 97.4% in the treatment of 4228 carcinomas. A 5-year follow-up study by Nordin et al.[18] of 50 patients with large primary basal cell carcinomas on the nose resulted in only one recurrence. The cure rate for recurrent basal cell carcinomas was found to be lower (88.4%)[19].

After treatment of a malignancy, the tissue responds in a predictable manner that leads to healing of the wound by second intention. The

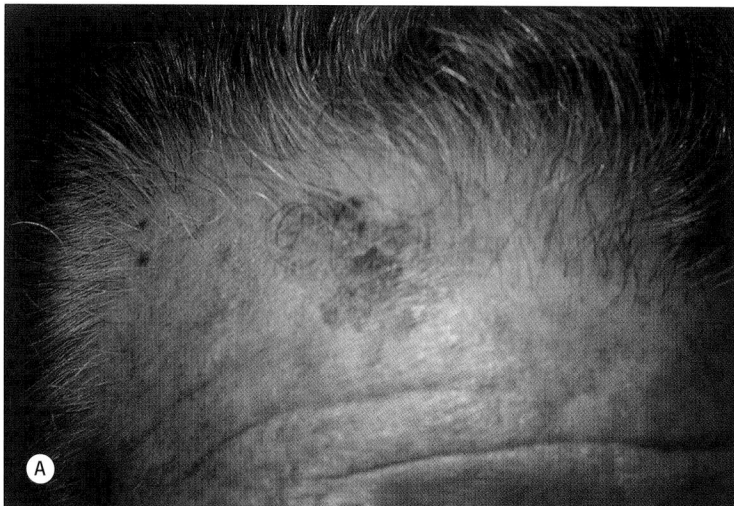

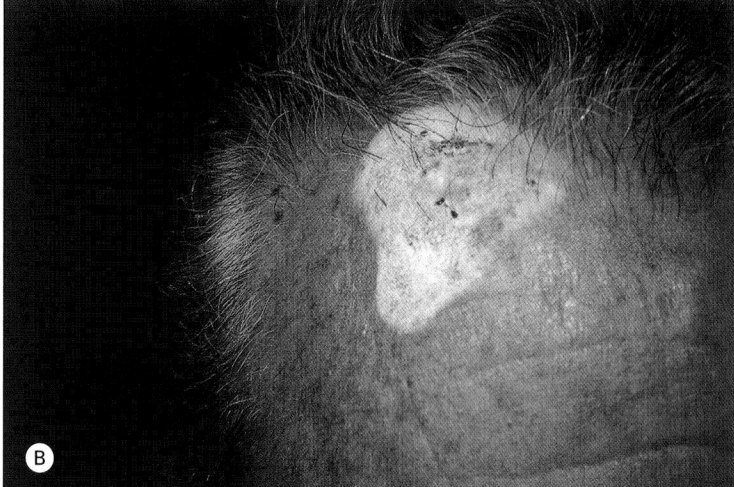

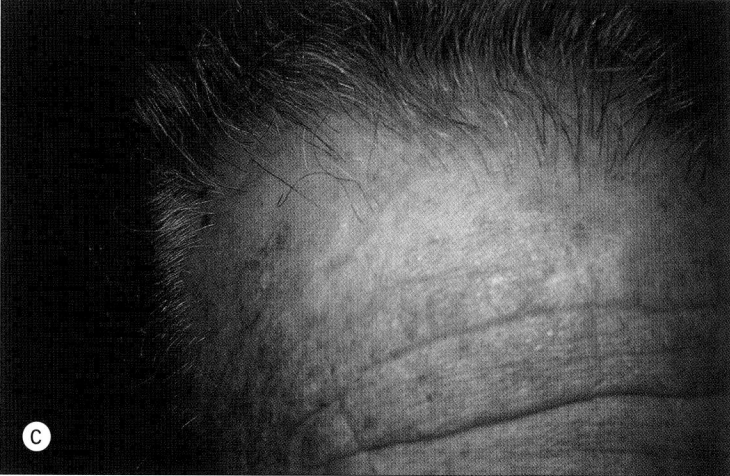

Fig. 138.3 A lentigo maligna on the forehead of a 72-year-old man. A The lesion measures 3.1 cm × 2.5 cm. **B** Cryosurgery to the entire lesion. Note the wide lateral spread of freeze. **C** The healed cryosurgical site 5 months after treatment.

reactions that ensue after freezing include erythema, vesiculation, edema, exudation and sloughing (Fig. 138.4). Benign and premalignant lesions usually heal between 2 and 4 weeks. Malignant lesions on the face, eyelids, nose, ears and neck generally heal between 4 and 6 weeks. Large tumors and those on the trunk and extremities take longer to heal, sometimes up to 14 weeks. The cosmetic results after cryosurgery are often equal or superior to those achieved by other modalities. Wounds reproduce natural skin contours and keloid formation typically does not occur. Cryosurgery is advantageous for tumors on the ears and nose because cartilage is relatively resistant to freezing damage and the architecture of the structure is preserved. Lesions on the eyelids and in the vicinity of the lacrimal duct are good candidates for cryosurgery as

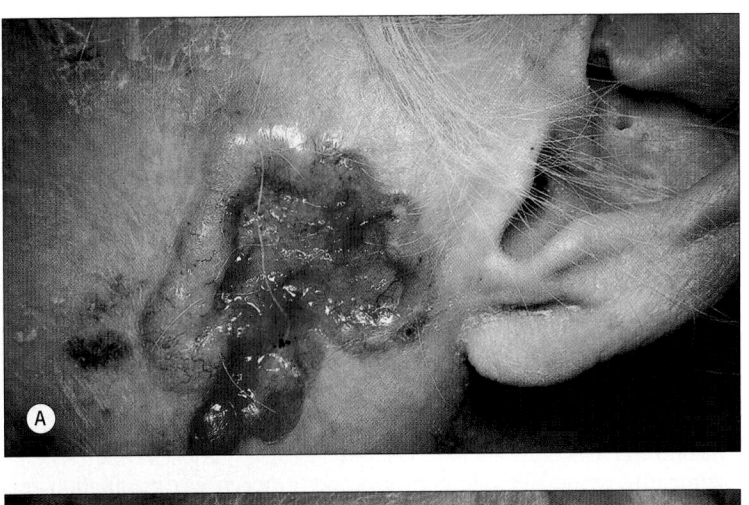

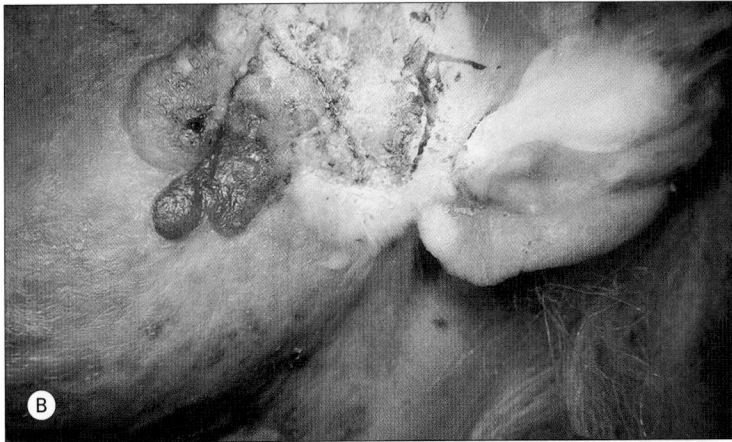

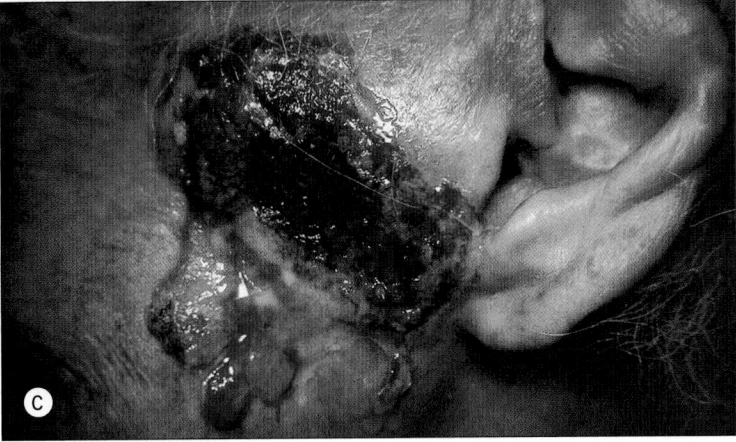

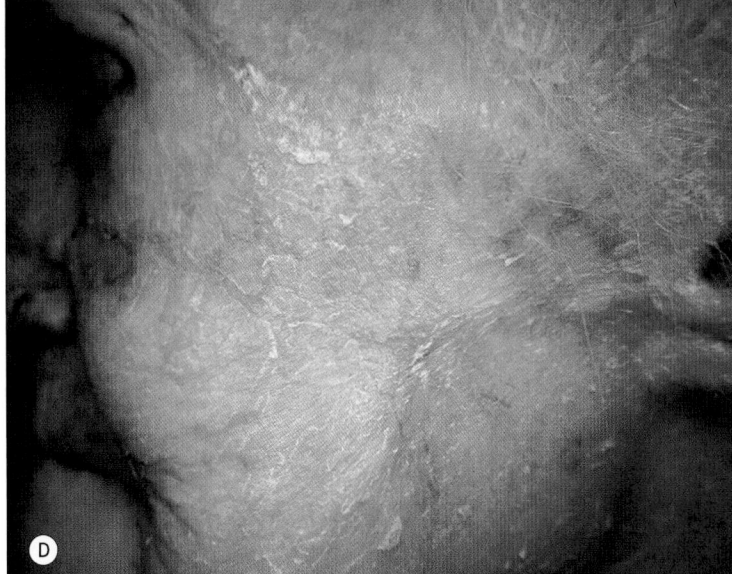

Fig. 138.4 A squamous cell carcinoma on the cheek in a 95-year-old woman.
A The lesion measures 4.5 cm × 3 cm. **B** Cryosurgery to upper half of the lesion. Segmental treatment was used to reduce the morbidity. Note lateral spread of freeze and protection of ear canal with cotton. **C** Tissue response after cryosurgery: exudation and sloughing 1 week after treatment. **D** The completely healed site shows an excellent cosmetic result 4 months after second section of tumor was treated.

the likelihood of ectropion is small and damage to the lacrimal outflow system is rare (Fig. 138.5)[20].

VARIATIONS AND UNUSUAL SITUATIONS

If a lesion is thick or bulky, it is beneficial to reduce it to a shallow one by debulking with a curette, scissors or electrosurgery. This is done because the mass is detrimental to proper treatment, either by hindering the advancement of the ice ball, misjudging the placement of thermocouple needles or by prevention of proper assessment of the lateral margins and base of the lesion. After debulking, hemostasis must be obtained before proceeding with cryosurgery.

It is sometimes beneficial to inject lidocaine for the purpose of lifting a lesion away from underlying tissue or superficial nerves. Examples include the treatment of warts or actinic keratoses on the fingers and hands, and malignancies on the head, neck and scalp.

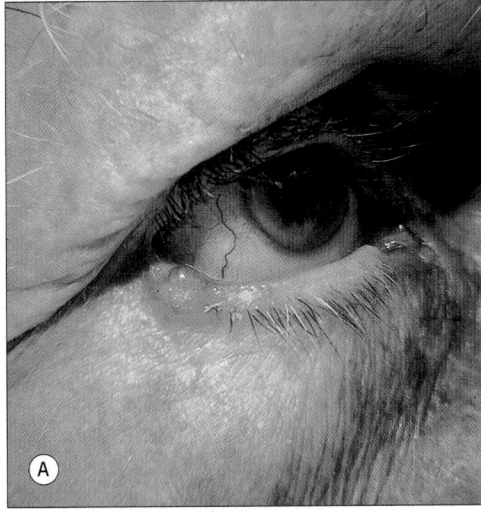

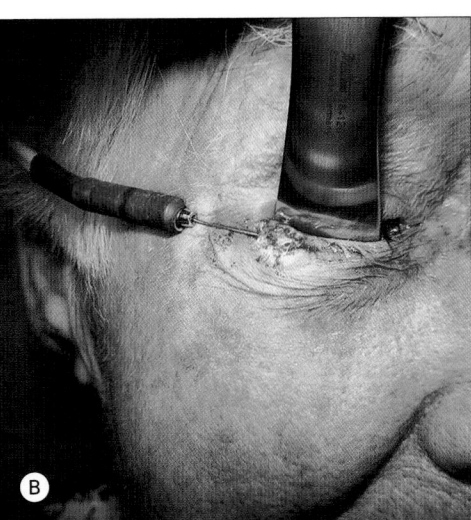

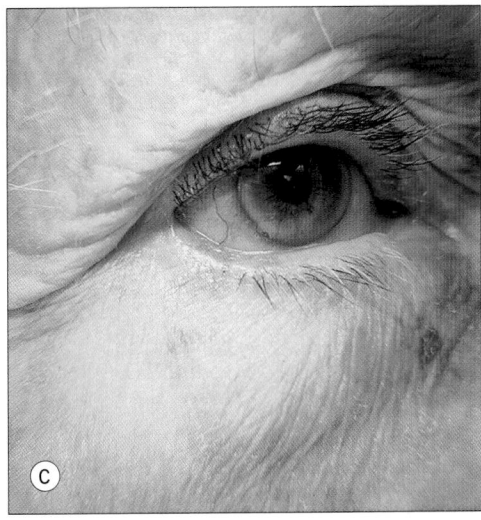

Fig. 138.5 Basal cell carcinoma on the right lower eyelid. A Papular lesion at margin of lid in an 82-year-old woman. **B** Cryosurgery to lesion: note placement of thermocouple needle and protection of eye. **C** The healed cryosurgical site 6 months after treatment. Excellent cosmetic result; note loss of cilia.

Selected large basal or squamous cell carcinomas are amenable to cryosurgery using segmental treatment (see Fig. 138.4)[21]. A lesion is treated in stages after being divided and can be treated either on the same day or at subsequent visits. Each section is treated according to its characteristics and depth. Wound healing is not hindered by overlapping treatment at the margins.

POSTOPERATIVE CARE

Postoperative care varies according to the lesion, location and depth of freeze. Most benign lesions require little or no aftercare except for ordinary washing. A shallow eschar develops that falls off spontaneously. In some instances, a watery exudate may develop beneath an eschar or excessive granulation tissue may develop. This can be treated by debridement with a curette or simply cleansed with soap and water. An antibiotic ointment can be applied.

In the case of malignancies, extensive exudation begins within 24 hours and diminishes in an orderly manner as the wound heals and re-epithelializes. The author recommends washing with soap and water four times daily in the exudative stage and less often during the granulating period. A dry gauze dressing is initially applied, and, as the wound begins to heal, an antibiotic ointment is used. In some instances, oral antibiotics are beneficial, such as for lesions on the legs and ears, or where otherwise indicated. Bullae may form at the periphery of a large lesion and is not a complication. The bullae are drained and healing is not affected.

COMPLICATIONS

The incidence of complications after cryosurgery is low. It is important to distinguish between expected sequelae and untoward results. A complication may arise in several ways: (1) as an unexpected event (e.g.

infection); (2) as an unsatisfactory cosmetic result (e.g. hypertrophic scarring); and (3) as a more pronounced response of the tissue to freezing than had been anticipated (e.g. residual hypopigmentation).

Temporary complications may develop during the healing stage or after completion of treatment and generally resolve spontaneously. Commonly described examples include edema of the eyelids or ears and hypertrophic scarring. Edema, particularly periorbital, can be minimized or ameliorated with open wet compresses, corticosteroid cream or a short course of systemic corticosteroids. The author reported using an intramuscular injection of 4 mg betamethasone sodium phosphate, 1 ml 30 minutes before treatment, followed by an adult dose of oral prednisone, 20 mg/day for 3 days[22]. Occasionally, hypertrophic scarring may develop, particularly after treatment of a large lesion, but this always improves and resolves with time, usually within months. If desired, intralesional injection of a corticosteroid suspension can hasten resolution. Uncommon reactions include delayed bleeding, headache, paresthesia, neuropathy, secondary infection, syncope, nitrogen gas insufflation (gas bubbles in skin), milia, hyperpigmentation and pyogenic granuloma.

Permanent complications include retraction of tissue, (e.g. lips, eyebrows, ala nasi), tissue defect, depigmentation, notching, ectropion, alopecia and contour defects. Improvement in some can occur, often in an elderly patient, as a result of skin laxity.

FUTURE TRENDS

Cryosurgery is an old technique that will remain very popular for the treatment of actinic keratoses and warts. The technique has remained relatively unchanged for several decades. It is far less commonly performed than excision and Mohs surgery for cutaneous malignancies, and the expert use of cryoprobes has become an art performed mainly by a limited number of dermatologists. The author feels that new instrumentation and techniques may be forthcoming.

REFERENCES

1. Kuflik EG, Gage AA. Cryobiology. In: Cryosurgical Treatment for Skin Cancer. New York: Igaku-Shoin, 1990:35–51.
2. Kuflik EG. Cryosurgery updated. J Am Acad Dermatol. 1994;31:925–44.
3. Yamada S, Tsubouchi S. Rapid cell death and cell population recovery in mouse skin epidermis after freezing. Cryobiology. 1976;13:317–27.
4. von Sebastian G, Scholz A. Histopathologie der Basaliom-Kryolasion. Dermatol Monatasschrift. 1983;169:9–17.
5. Kuflik EG, Gage AA. Cryosurgical Treatment for Skin Cancer. New York: Igaku-Shoin, 1990.
6. Kuflik EG, Gage AA. Recurrent basal cell carcinoma treated with cryosurgery. J Am Acad Dermatol. 1997;37:82–4.
7. Torre D. Depth dose in cryosurgery. J Dermatol Surg Oncol. 1983;9:219–25.
8. Thai K-E, Fergin P, Freeman M, et al. A prospective study of the use of cryosurgery for the treatment of actinic keratosis. Int J Dermatol. 2004;43:686–91.
9. Suhonen R, Kuflik EG. Venous lakes treated by liquid nitrogen cryosurgery. Br J Dermatol. 1997;137:1018–19.

10. Kuflik EG. Cryosurgical treatment of periungual warts. J Dermatol Surg Oncol. 1984;10:673–6.
11. Kuflik EG. Specific indications for cryosurgery of the nail unit. Myxoid cysts and periungual verrucae. J Dermatol Surg Oncol. 1992;18:702–6.
12. Lubritz RR, Smolewski SA. Cryosurgery cure rate of actinic keratoses. J Am Acad Dermatol. 1982;7:631–2.
13. Kuflik EG, Gage AA. Cryosurgery for lentigo maligna. J Am Acad Dermatol. 1994;31:75–8.
14. Kuflik EG. Cryosurgery for skin cancer: 30-year experience and cures rates. Dermatol Surg. 2004; 24:297–300.
14a. Bernardeau K, Derancourt C, Cambie M, et al. Cryosurgery of basal cell carcinoma: a study of 358 patients. Ann Dermatol Venereol. 2000;127:175–9.
14b. Kokoszka A, Scheinfeld N. Evidence-based review of the use of cryosurgery in treatment of basal cell carcinoma. Dermatol Surg. 2003;29:566–71.
15. Graham GF. Cryosurgery. Clin Plast Surg. 1993;20:131–47.
16. Holt P. Cryotherapy for skin cancer: results over a 5-year period using liquid nitrogen spray cryotherapy. Br J Dermatol. 1998;119:231–40.

17. Zacarian SA. Cryosurgery of cutaneous carcinomas: an 18-year study of 3022 patients with 4228 carcinomas. J Am Acad Dermatol. 1983;9:947–56.
18. Nordin P, Larko O, Stenquist B. Five-year results of curettage-cryosurgery of selected large basal cell carcinomas on the nose: an alternative treatment in a geographical area underserved by Mohs' surgery. Br J Dermatol. 1997;136:180–3.
19. Kuflik EG, Gage AA. Results. In: Cryosurgical Treatment for Skin Cancer. New York: Igaku-Shoin. 1990:243–54.
20. Kuflik EG. Cryosurgery for carcinomas of the eyelids: a 12-year experience. J Dermatol Surg Oncol. 1985; 11:243–6.
21. Kuflik EG. Cryosurgical treatment of large basal cell carcinomas on the trunk. J Dermatol Surg Oncol. 1983;9:226–30.
22. Kuflik EG, Webb W. Effects of systemic corticosteroids on post-cryosurgical edema and other manifestations of the inflammatory response. J Dermatol Surg Oncol. 1985;11:464–8.

Radiotherapy

Michael Veness and Shawn Richards

Synonyms: ■ Radiation treatment ■ Radiation therapy ■ X-ray therapy

Key features

- Radiotherapy is an important modality in the treatment of patients with skin malignancies
- Radiotherapy may reduce morbidity (as compared to surgery), decrease the risk of recurrent disease, and even be life-saving
- Although most patients with skin cancer are adequately treated by modalities other than radiotherapy, there are factors that may favor its recommendation (e.g. comorbidities, location)
- Modern radiotherapy has an established role as a definitive, adjuvant or palliative treatment
- Treating benign skin disease with radiotherapy must always be carefully considered in light of the risk of radiation-induced malignancy, especially in younger patients

BASICS OF RADIOTHERAPY

Indications

In dermatology, the primary role of radiotherapy is to treat basal cell carcinoma (BCC) and cutaneous squamous cell carcinoma (SCC; see Ch. 108)[1]. It is also used to treat less common, but potentially aggressive, cutaneous malignancies and, occasionally, benign diseases. The former include Merkel cell carcinoma, Kaposi's sarcoma (AIDS- and non-AIDS-related), angiosarcoma, adnexal carcinoma, lymphoma and melanoma (especially lentigo maligna).

While the majority of skin cancers are amenable to excision (see Chs 146–148) or other treatment modalities (e.g. electrodessication and curettage; see Chs 135, 138, 140, 150) which are often more cost-effective, there are clinical settings where radiotherapy is favored. For example, *definitive* radiotherapy is often recommended when the outcome (functional and/or cosmetic) is likely to be better with radiotherapy than with surgery, especially in the situation where the clinician is constrained by the site or size of the tumor. Likewise, elderly patients with advanced lesions for whom complex surgery is best avoided are also excellent candidates for radiotherapy. The aim of *adjuvant* radiotherapy is to reduce the risk of recurrence, whereas *palliative* radiotherapy plays an important role in patients with advanced and/or incurable disease.

Mechanism of action

X-rays are a powerful form of ionizing electromagnetic radiation and the lethal damage they produce within double-stranded DNA represents the basis for radiation therapy[2]. When X-rays (often referred to as photons) are absorbed by biological matter, an electron may be ejected from an atom with the local release of large amounts of energy. The result is that replicating, i.e. more rapidly dividing, malignant cells undergo a mitotic death. Although normal adjacent tissues maintain mechanisms for repair following sublethal damage, there are limitations as to the dose of ionizing radiation normal tissue can tolerate, beyond which late reactions arise (see below). Enhancement of the difference in the response of malignant cells versus normal tissue is accomplished via delivery of the radiation in small divided doses (referred to as fractions).

Treatment machines

In the modern era of radiation oncology, high-energy megavoltage (mV) photons (6–25 mV) are generated by a linear accelerator (LINAC) located within a heavily shielded concrete bunker. One of the advantages of megavoltage radiotherapy is its ability to treat deep-seated internal malignancies with relative skin sparing. However, when treating cutaneous lesions, deep beam penetration and skin sparing are usually not desirable. The delivery of *low-energy* kilovoltage (kV) photons (50–300 kVp) by a *superficial/orthovoltage* machine is preferable, as it avoids both skin sparing and the irradiation of deeper tissues. With low-energy photons, tissue penetration is measured in millimeters to centimeters. Shielding is achieved by applying 3–4 mm of lead either directly onto the skin or by using an internal (e.g. eye or mouth) shield.

Terminology

The International Unit of radiotherapy is a Gray (Gy)[3]. One Gy is equivalent to 100 cGy or 100 rads (in the older terminology). A fraction of radiotherapy refers to the dose delivered in one treatment. A typical course of radiotherapy for a cutaneous malignancy in an otherwise healthy patient is 50 Gy delivered in 20 daily (Monday through Friday) fractions (2.5 Gy/fraction). Historically, patients were often administered only two or three fractions per week. At the very least, this latter schedule simply protracted the overall treatment period, but in some cases may have resulted in decreased local control. The daily outpatient irradiations are only minutes in duration and treatment regimens usually consist of 10 to 30 weekday visits.

Radiotherapy doses

Hypofractionation refers to the delivery of larger doses per fraction (4–7 Gy). However, when the dose per fraction is increased, the total dose delivered is then decreased. For example, commonly prescribed dose fractionation schedules are 45 Gy in 15 (3 Gy) fractions, 40 Gy in 10 (4 Gy) fractions, and 35 Gy in 5 (7 Gy) fractions. Using a 2 Gy per fraction equivalent, this variation in the total dose results when the biological effective dose (BED) needed for eradicating a tumor is calculated[4]. Despite this, the data suggest that, at least for small (≤2 cm) SCCs and BCCs, there is not a marked dose-response, and local control is similar whether a patient receives 40 Gy in 10 fractions (47 Gy BED) or 50 Gy in 20 fractions (52 Gy BED). However, when the tumors are larger or more infiltrative, better local control is achieved with a BED of around 60 Gy. Of note, late effects increase as the total dose and dose per fraction increase and it is these late effects that will impact on cosmesis and late tissue damage (necrosis).

Radiation physics

The qualities and 'hardness' of a superficial/orthovoltage photon beam are determined by the placement of filters within the radiation beam[5]. In radiation physics, a standard term is the 'half value layer' (HVL) which refers to the thickness of a material (often copper [Cu] or aluminum [Al]) that is required to reduce the beam intensity by 50%. The filter serves to remove the softer photon component and improve the penetration quality of the beam. A second concept is half value depth ($D^{1}/_{2}$) and here filters are used to achieve radiation with a $D^{1}/_{2}$ that corresponds to tumor depth. For each superficial and orthovoltage beam, at least one to two filters should be available.

Low-energy photons (superficial/orthovoltage) and common cutaneous protocols

A typical 100 kVp superficial photon beam with an HVL of 7 mm of aluminium will deliver 100% of prescribed dose to the surface, 85% at 5 mm, and 70% at 10 mm. A 250 kVp orthovoltage beam with an HVL of 2.5 mm of copper will deliver 95% of prescribed dose at 5 mm and 90% at 10 mm. Most superficial lesions (<5 mm depth) will be adequately treated by a 100 kVp beam with an HVL of 6–8 mm aluminum (or similar). Deeper, more invasive lesions (5–10 mm in depth) are adequately encompassed by a 250 kVp orthovoltage beam with an HVL of 2–4 mm copper.

Some clinicians estimate tumor thickness and then choose an appropriate beam energy and HVL that will achieve 90–95% of the prescribed dose at the depth of the tumor. However, this latter approach requires an accurate estimate of tumor thickness.

The photoelectric effect is a phenomenon whereby underlying bone or cartilage receives a higher dose of radiation when low-energy photons are used. This is not the case with electrons (see below) and is used by some clinicians as a justification for the use of electrons when treating lesions in close proximity to bone or cartilage. However, there are no convincing data that the late effects in these tissues are markedly increased when low-energy photons are used instead of electrons[6].

Grenz ray treatment

Grenz rays are very-low-energy (5–15 kVp) photons that penetrate only superficially (0.5–1 mm)[7]. Nowadays, the use of this modality is very limited, but, in the past, several inflammatory dermatoses (e.g. chronic hand dermatitis) were treated with grenz rays. The latter are reported to be relatively safe in lifetime doses of up to 50 Gy to treated areas. Nevertheless, grenz rays should *never* be viewed as first-line therapy. Worldwide, the machines used to generate these very soft X-rays are rare and are not utilized in modern departments of radiation oncology.

Electrons

A linear accelerator can also generate electrons and they are utilized in a variety of treatment settings. Unlike X-rays, electrons are a particulate radiation that carries a negative charge. Low-energy electrons (6–8 MeV [million electron volts]) offer an alternative to low-energy photons when treating cutaneous tumors, but the former do have some disadvantages[8]. For example, electron beams are relatively skin sparing (Fig. 139.1), and, as a result, a tissue equivalent bolus needs to be placed on the skin surface (Fig. 139.2); small treatment fields (<4 cm²) may result in tumor underdosing at the deepest extent of the tumor.

Electrons offer the advantage of a rapid linear decline in dose beyond a well-defined tissue depth that is a function of the selected beam energy (see Fig. 139.1). For example, a 6 MeV electron beam provides some of its dose (~87%) at the surface, but deposits 100% of the specified dose at a depth of approximately 1 cm. Using a higher-energy beam will result in deposition of a higher percentage of the dose at the skin surface, but with a higher dose to subcutaneous tissues. On the other hand, if a tissue equivalent bolus of 1 cm is applied in conjunction with a 6 MeV beam, close to 100% of the desired dose will be obtained at the skin surface (see Fig. 139.2). All of the deposition of dose will be brought 1 cm closer to the skin surface, further minimizing the dose to underlying structures.

In addition, tumors treated with electrons require 10–20 mm margins as a consequence of a wider penumbra (dose drop off at the field edge). Electrons also have a lower relative biological effectiveness (RBE) in comparison to photons, leading some clinicians to recommend a 10–15% increase in total dose to compensate.

In summary, there are data to suggest that local control of skin tumors may not be as good with electrons when compared to low-energy photons. However, this may reflect an under-appreciation by some clinicians of the intricacies of using small field electrons to treat skin cancers.

Brachytherapy

Brachytherapy is a type of radiotherapy that is delivered by the direct application of a radioactive source to involved tissues. In the vast majority of clinical settings, radioactive molds and implants offer little advantage over the range of energies of external beam photons and electrons currently available. As a result, they are rarely used nowadays to treat BCCs and SCCs. Nonetheless, some clinicians have advocated using radioactive molds for areas with poor vascularity and slow rates of healing (e.g. the anterior lower limb or dorsum of the hand)[9]. However, suitable lesions need to be superficial (<3–4 mm depth) and there are radiation safety issues if this approach is utilized.

Office-based radiotherapy

Office-based superficial radiotherapy was once the standard modality by which dermatologists treated skin cancer[10]. Typical machines delivered photons of 70–100 kVp with a depth dose suitable for most patients with cutaneous malignancies. However, in the past two decades, the rising cost of radiotherapy machines combined with increased enthusiasm and training in dermatologic surgery have led to a significant decline in office-based radiotherapy. Nowadays, radiotherapy for skin cancer is performed almost exclusively by radiation oncologists. However, this does not diminish the need for dermatologists to understand the role of radiotherapy and to become familiar with its indications and treatment regimens, since dermatologists frequently diagnose skin cancer and outline therapeutic options.

Advantages of radiotherapy

Radiotherapy offers the advantage of a non-surgical approach, thereby avoiding surgical morbidity, scarring and the need for reconstruction. In situations where reconstruction with grafts or flaps is required, improved cosmesis may result from radiotherapy[11]. Radiotherapy fields can also be tailored with generous margins in order to encompass 'at-risk' areas (e.g. possible sites of clinically inapparent tumor extensions) that, if surgically approached, would require involved and complex surgery. In addition, standard oncologic excision margins in certain sites are often difficult to achieve without causing surgical morbidity; such sites include the midface triangle, i.e. the periorbital region (especially the medial canthus), the lower eyelid, nose (especially the ala nasi and nasal tip), nasolabial fold, lip and chin.

Disadvantages of radiotherapy

Radiotherapy does have its disadvantages; in particular, most patients require a protracted course of treatment compared to what is often a simple outpatient excision. Patients should also be informed that because of the risk of serious late effects such as soft tissue and cartilage necrosis, a second course of definitive radiotherapy cannot be delivered to the same site. In addition, the reduced 'quality' of irradiated skin

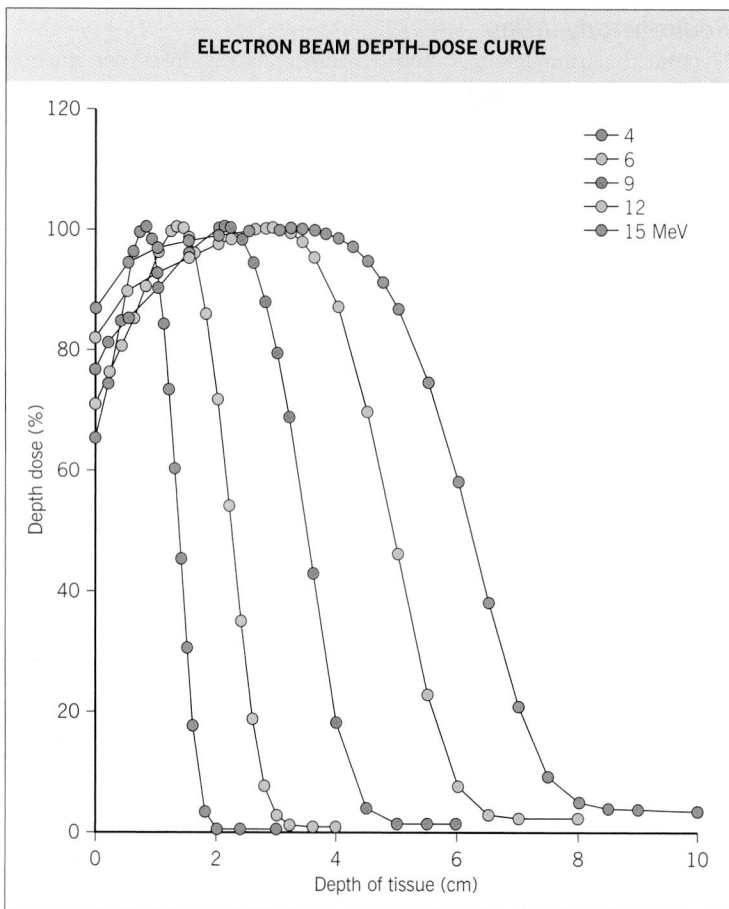

ELECTRON BEAM DEPTH–DOSE CURVE

Legend: 4, 6, 9, 12, 15 MeV

Depth dose (%) vs *Depth of tissue (cm)*

Fig. 139.1 Electron beam depth–dose curve. Electrons offer the advantage of a rapid linear decline in dose beyond a well-defined tissue depth that is a function of the selected beam energy. Courtesy of Lynn Wilson MD.

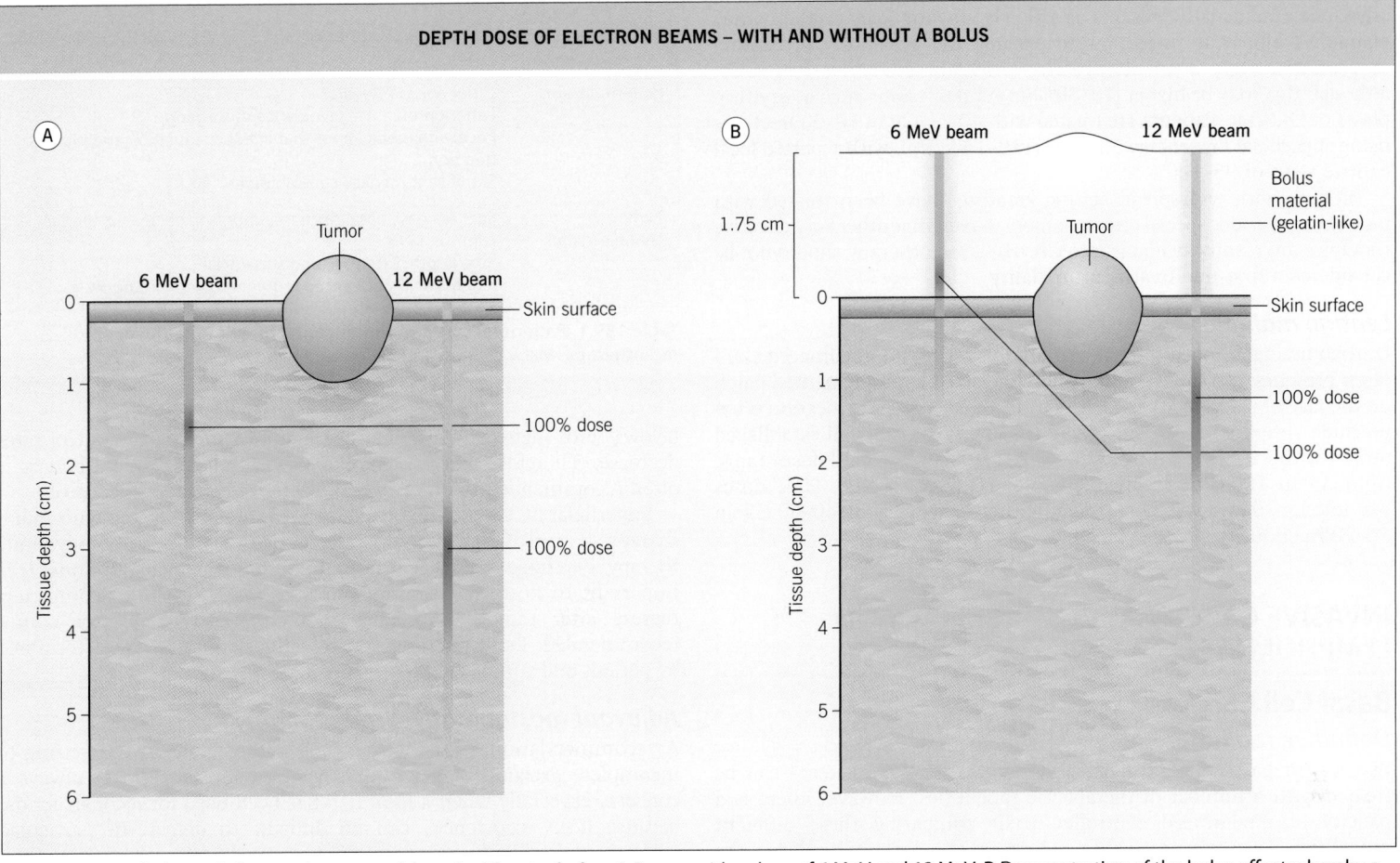

Fig. 139.2 Depth dose of electron beams – with and without a bolus. A Beams with a dose of 6 MeV and 12 MeV. **B** Demonstration of the bolus effect whereby a more appropriate dose of radiation is obtained at the skin surface. Courtesy of Lynn Wilson MD.

makes subsequent surgery difficult if the tumor recurs or persists following radiation therapy. Lastly, individuals with xeroderma pigmentosum or nevoid basal cell carcinoma syndrome should not be irradiated owing to their marked predisposition for developing multiple and recurrent skin cancers, often at a young age.

Lesions that have deeply invaded cartilage or bone often do better with a combination of excision plus adjuvant radiotherapy, although definitive radiotherapy still remains an option (local control 60–70%). Radiotherapy of lesions located on the foot, anterior lower leg or dorsum of the hand, although not contraindicated, should be avoided if possible; lesions in such sites are best treated with excision. Unfortunately, radiotherapy to poorly vascularized, edematous tissues is often associated with poor healing. Skin cancers arising in sites of chronic ulceration, trauma or burns should not be irradiated if at all possible. These sites often have poor vascularity and consequently poor healing. Patients with scleroderma and other causes of cutaneous fibrosis are also best treated by surgical means, as radiotherapy may enhance the fibrosis and lead to poor healing.

Radiotherapy has a very small (~1 in 1000) risk of causing a radiation-induced malignancy (often soft tissue/bone sarcoma) 10–15 years after exposure[12]. However, these data were obtained from studies involving many different malignancies treated by various techniques and dosing schedules. It is likely that with modern radiotherapeutic techniques as well as the smaller volumes being irradiated when treating skin cancers, a figure of 1 in 1000 represents an overestimate of the real risk. Despite this, in younger patients (<50 years of age) this is an important issue and patients must be informed of the risk.

RADIOTHERAPY OF BENIGN SKIN DISORDERS

Background
The role of radiotherapy in treating benign disorders has markedly diminished over the past several decades. It is no longer ethically acceptable to offer radiotherapy as a treatment for acne, warts, hirsutism or tinea capitis. The role of radiotherapy in treating inflammatory skin conditions (e.g. dermatitis, psoriasis, lichen planus) is primarily historical due to efficacious alternative treatments (e.g. corticosteroids, phototherapy) and the risk of exposing patients to ionizing radiation. Previous studies suggested that low-dose (8–12 Gy) soft X-rays often resulted in satisfactory resolution of symptoms, especially in eczematous conditions, but clinicians must carefully weigh the risks versus the benefits before recommending radiotherapy. Specific guidelines have been published regarding the risk/benefit ratio and obtaining informed consent when radiotherapy for benign disorders is being considered[13].

Keloids
Recurrent keloids, often refractory to re-excision and intralesional corticosteroid injections, can have significant cosmetic and psychologic sequelae for patients, many of whom are young women. The addition of low-dose (12–16 Gy) adjuvant radiotherapy delivered in three to four fractions, beginning within 24–48 hours following surgery, can markedly and safely reduce the incidence of recurrence[14]. A common site is the earlobe and patients can be treated with low-energy photons plus lead shielding of surrounding tissues. Young patients with keloids of the lower anterior neck (in close proximity to the thyroid gland) should not be irradiated.

Pseudolymphomas
Cutaneous pseudolymphoma (cutaneous lymphoid hyperplasia) often arises on the face (see Ch. 121). When lesions fail to respond to intralesional corticosteroids, low-dose fractionated radiotherapy (10–15 Gy in five fractions) utilizing low-energy photons is an efficacious treatment option with minimal, if any, side effects.

RADIOTHERAPY OF CUTANEOUS MALIGNANCIES

In Situ Malignancies
Squamous cell carcinoma in situ (Bowen's disease)
Radiotherapy can be used, albeit infrequently, to treat SCC *in situ*. The malignancy is limited to the epidermis and its appendages, can arise

anywhere, and usually presents as a slowly growing scaly erythematous plaque. A biopsy is important to exclude the possibility of eczema or psoriasis. Only a small minority (<5%) become invasive SCCs, although this may be higher (10–30%) in genital lesions such as erythroplasia of Queyrat. Patients are treated with 40–50 Gy in 10–20 fractions using superficial low-energy photons (110–150 kVp), with reported local control rates of 98–100%[15].

Patients with widespread actinic keratoses have been treated with radiotherapy under special circumstances. Given that other very effective therapies are readily available (see Ch. 108), radiotherapy should not be considered a first-line treatment modality.

Lentigo maligna

Lentigo maligna (melanoma *in situ* arising within photodamaged skin) often presents as a longstanding and large-sized hyperpigmented patch on the face of elderly patients (see Ch. 113). The size and location often preclude simple excision, and radiotherapy remains a well-established option with excellent control rates (Fig. 139.3)[16]. Reported doses range from 35 to 100 Gy administered in 5–10 fractions, i.e. large doses per fraction. However, dose fractionation schedules of 40–50 Gy in 10–20 fractions would also be efficacious[17].

INVASIVE CARCINOMAS, SARCOMAS AND LYMPHOMAS

Basal Cell Carcinoma

Definitive radiotherapy

BCCs – in particular, primary tumors <2 cm in diameter – can be treated with a number of therapeutic modalities. However, there is a paucity of randomized controlled trials comparing these different modalities. In a recent Cochrane Review, the authors analyzed the published results of seven different treatment categories[18]. Although they suggested the need for further research, surgery and radiotherapy appeared to be the two most efficacious modalities, with surgery probably leading to the lowest recurrence rates[18]. Of note, Mohs micrographic surgery is said to result in some of the highest cure rates.

While local control rates (90–95%) for either excision or radiotherapy are probably similar, management decisions are often based on other factors (Table 139.1). For example, radiotherapy would be favored in an elderly patient with a BCC located on the nasal tip or nasal alae (Fig. 139.4). In the locations outlined in Table 139.1, excision followed by primary closure is often difficult to accomplish and grafts or flaps are frequently required if surgical excision is chosen. Although larger lesions (>20 mm) can still be eradicated via definitive radiotherapy (see

PATIENT FACTORS AND TUMOR CHARACTERISTICS THAT FAVOR RADIOTHERAPY	
Patient factors	Older age (>70 years) Patient preference (avoidance of surgery) Receiving medications that affect coagulation and platelet function Significant medical comorbidities
Tumor characteristics	Site: Ala nasi, nasal tip, nasal bridge, lower eyelid, medial canthus, helix Size/depth: Extensive and superficial Stage: Locally advanced requiring complex surgery

Table 139.1 Patient factors and tumor characteristics that favor radiotherapy. Many of these indications are relative.

below), with increasing size and depth of invasion, local control rates decrease. Therefore, surgery combined with adjuvant radiotherapy is often recommended in order to try to achieve better local control.

Superficial BCCs that involve large areas are also treated with radiotherapy (Fig. 139.5), although alternatives such as photodynamic therapy, curettage and topical imiquimod are reasonable options. It is important to note that tumors can take many weeks to completely regress after radiotherapy and, therefore, early re-biopsy is not recommended. Dose fractionation schedules vary and are determined by patient and tumor factors (see below).

Adjuvant (postoperative) radiotherapy

A recommendation for radiotherapy is often made in the setting of incomplete excision of a BCC. A positive deep margin is always a concern, especially when a local flap has been used for reconstruction, because deep recurrences can be difficult to detect. In particular, undetected deep recurrences of tumors located within the midface and periorbital region may be associated with significant local morbidity. It is accepted that at least 20–30% of incompletely excised BCCs will recur[19] and re-excision is often recommended in order to achieve a negative margin[20]. In one study, for example, residual BCC was found in 45% of the re-excised specimens[19]. However, in some circumstances, the involved margin precludes simple re-excision (e.g. the periosteum of the nose). In these situations, radiotherapy is an option. The aim of adjuvant radiotherapy is to reduce the incidence of local recurrence by eradicating residual microscopic BCC[20]. In a Canadian trial, the addition of adjuvant radiotherapy improved the 5-year local control rate from 61% to 91%[21]. Not surprisingly, the 10-year local control rates were similar (92% vs 90%), as the majority of recurrences were successfully salvaged via surgery.

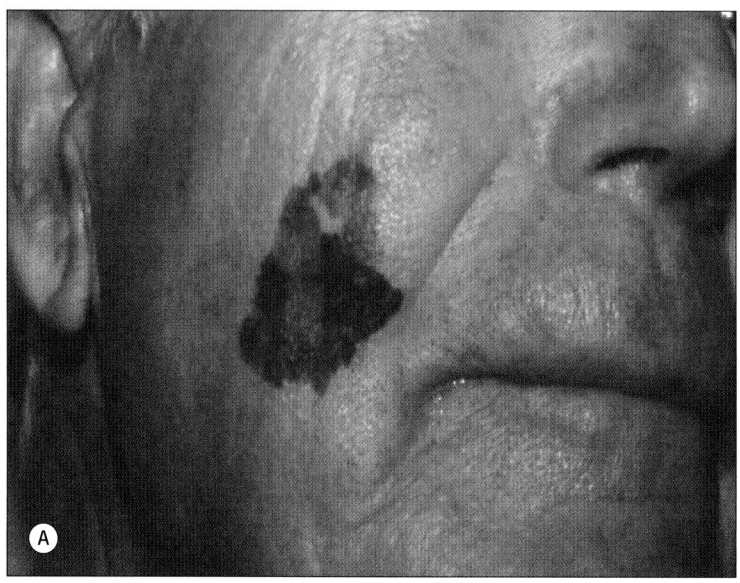
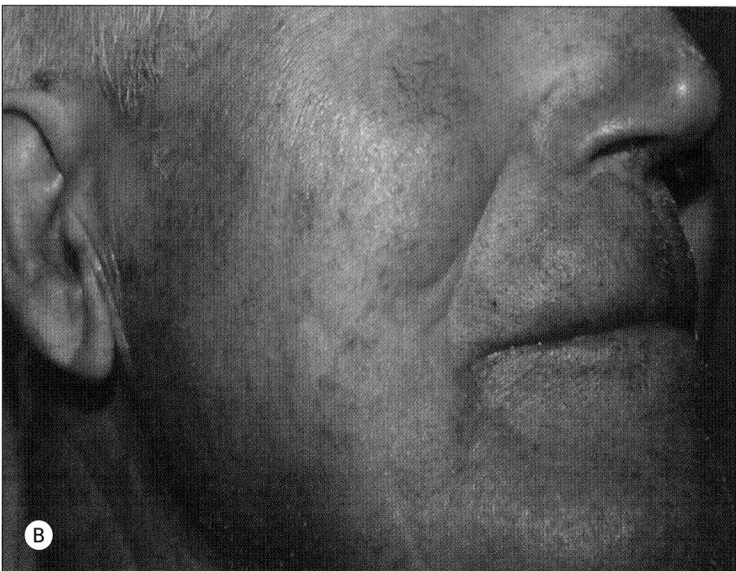

Fig. 139.3 Lentigo maligna (melanoma *in situ*). A An 82-year-old man with a lentigo maligna on his right cheek. **B** Three months after superficial radiotherapy (45 Gy in 15 daily fractions, 120 kVp, HVL 4.2 mm Al).

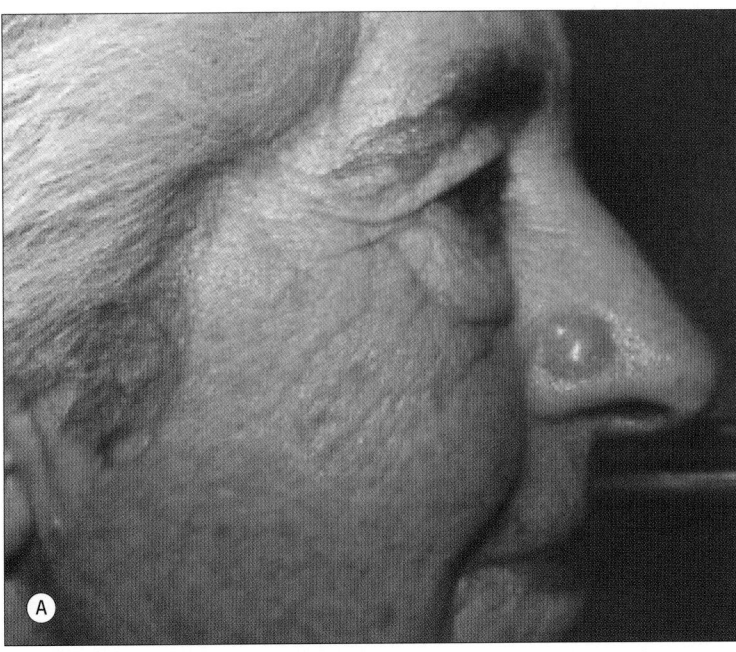
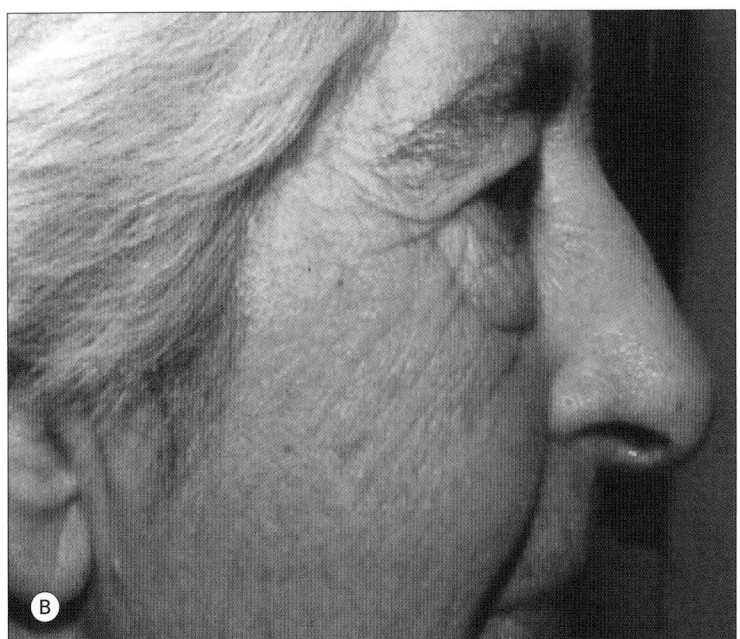

Fig. 139.4 Nodular basal cell carcinoma. A A 72-year-old woman with a 1 cm nodular basal cell carcinoma on the right ala nasi. **B** Four months after superficial radiotherapy (45 Gy in 15 daily fractions, 100 kVp, HVL 7 mm Al).

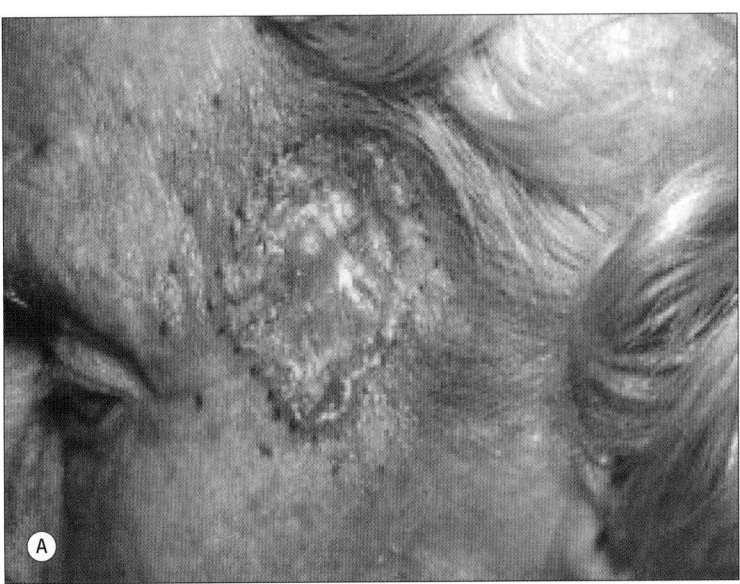
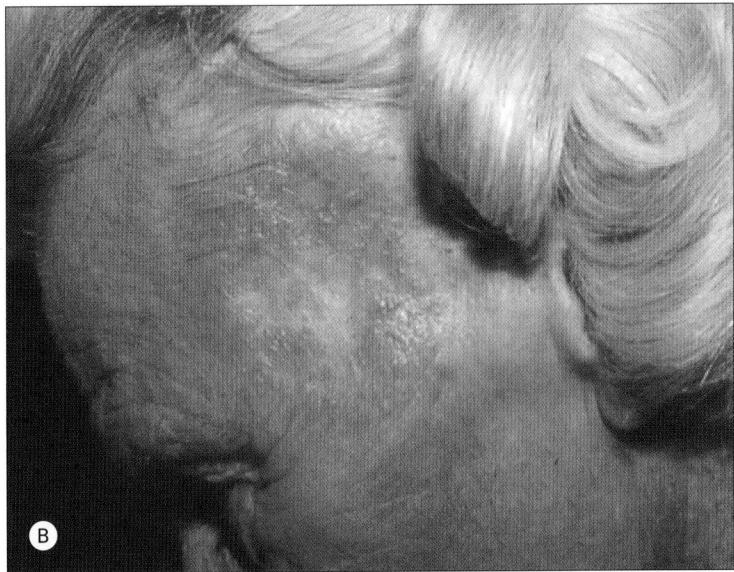

Fig. 139.5 Extensive basal cell carcinoma. A An elderly woman with a large basal cell carcinoma occupying much of the left temple region. **B** Three months after 40 Gy in 10 daily fractions using superficial energy photons (100 kVp, HVL 7 mm Al).

Squamous Cell Carcinoma

Definitive radiotherapy

The approach to treating patients with cutaneous SCC is influenced by the small risk (<5%[22] to <1%) of metastatic spread to regional lymph nodes and the need to achieve local control. Of note, some patients can be considered as having high-risk SCC when certain unfavorable features are present; these include thickness >4–5 mm, diameter >2 cm, recurrent tumor, high-grade (i.e. poorly differentiated) histology, neurotropism, location on or around the ear or lower lip, and immunosuppressed host. These SCCs have a greater risk of developing recurrences and metastatic nodal disease[23,23a].

In general, high-risk patients should have lesions excised with wider margins (see below) and be followed closely for at least 5 years[24]. However, depending upon the circumstances (see Table 139.1), some patients are treated with definitive (or adjuvant) radiotherapy. To date, there is no consensus as to which high-risk patients should be offered elective treatment (e.g. surgical, radiotherapy) of regional lymph nodes, but future sentinel lymph node biopsy studies may help resolve this issue.

The aim in excising any SCC is to achieve adequate margins, taking into consideration cosmesis and function. Surgical excision of SCC is often more extensive than for BCC, with wider margins (>5 mm) usually recommended[25], and it may entail the Mohs micrographic surgical technique or wide local excision under general anesthesia with flap/graft reconstruction. In a study of cutaneous SCCs <2 cm in diameter, the investigators reported that with a 4 mm excision margin, 95% of the tumors were removed with negative margins. For SCCs >2 cm, a 6 mm excision margin led to negative margins in 95% of the cases[26]. Of note, the local control rate for SCCs is, on average, 10–15% lower than for equivalent-sized BCCs[1,4,27].

It is generally not appropriate to merely observe an incompletely excised SCC. Recurrent SCC is associated with a higher incidence of regional metastases (compared to the initial presentation), with rates of up to 25–45%, depending on the tumor location[22]. Both recurrent BCC and recurrent SCC are associated with a control rate that is lower by at least 10% (compared to untreated lesions of equivalent size), again emphasizing the need to reduce the risk of local relapse[4,26].

Definitive radiotherapy of cutaneous SCC is an excellent treatment option, especially in the clinical settings outlined in Table 139.1. For

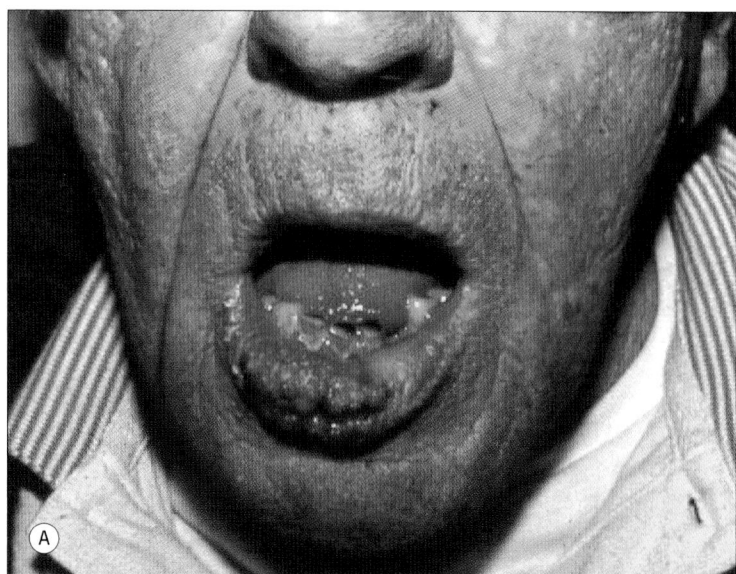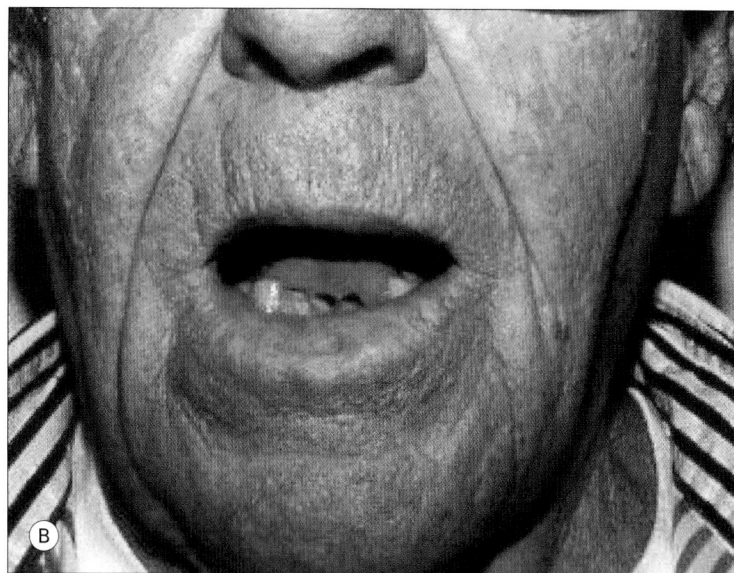

Fig. 139.6 Squamous cell carcinoma. A A 67-year-old man with a squamous cell carcinoma occupying much of the lower lip. The patient received 50 Gy in 20 daily fractions using orthovoltage energy photons (250 kVp, HVL 2.5 mm Cu) and oral cavity lead shielding to protect the teeth and mandible. **B** An excellent cosmetic and functional outcome has been achieved.

example, multiple medical comorbidities may preclude patients from having extensive surgery. In addition, in sites such as the lower lip, radiotherapy can result in excellent maintenance of function (even with more extensive tumors; Fig. 139.6) as well as cure rates comparable to surgery (see section on lip SCC)[28].

Keratoacanthomas

A keratoacanthoma (KA) typically presents as a rapidly enlarging papulonodule with a central keratin plug. Difficulty often arises in distinguishing these tumors histologically from well-differentiated SCCs, and many authorities consider most KAs to be a well-differentiated variant of SCC. Although KAs often regress spontaneously, a significant number become large and unsightly. Radiotherapy is an efficacious treatment option if excision is not contemplated. Regimens consisting of 25 Gy in five fractions have been reported to lead to a durable regression. Despite this, if the diagnosis of KA versus well-differentiated SCC is uncertain, a dose fractionation schedule appropriate for a SCC should be prescribed (40–50 Gy in 10–20 fractions; see section below on dose fractionation schedules).

Adjuvant (postoperative) radiotherapy

Adjuvant radiotherapy is an option when excision of an SCC is incomplete and re-excision is not considered possible. It is imperative that every pathology report document and quantify margin status, and a patient with an incompletely excised SCC, i.e. positive or close margin, remains at risk of local recurrence. While there is no consensus with regard to the most appropriate surgical margin for cutaneous SCCs, published recommendations range from 3 to 10 mm[29], often depending upon size (see above). In one series of patients with SCC of the lip, a 37% local recurrence rate was observed in patients who underwent excision alone (27% close/positive margins) versus a 6% local recurrence rate in patients treated with surgery plus adjuvant radiotherapy (94% close/positive margins)[30].

Special clinical situations
SCC of the lip

In regions of the world that have a high incidence of non-melanoma skin cancer (e.g. Australia), SCC of the lip is considered a skin cancer, not an oral cancer[28]. Compared to oral SCC, there is a lower propensity for spread to regional nodes. Nearly all lesions arise on the lower lip, usually as a consequence of chronic sun exposure.

As with small- to moderate-sized SCCs of the skin, the outcome with surgery versus radiotherapy is similar. The laxity of the lip means that wedge excision (± vermilionectomy) is the procedure of choice, with primary closure often possible. When >30–50% of the lip is involved, excision with appropriate margins is usually not achievable without

risking function (e.g. oral competency). Complex reconstruction is an option, but insensate tissue may be needed for reconstruction, again with an impact on function. Radiotherapy is therefore an excellent treatment option for SCC of the lip. The lower lip lends itself very well to treatment with orthovoltage photons following insertion of a 3 mm intraoral lead shield to protect the mandible and teeth (see Fig. 139.6). Doses are similar to those for any other equivalent-sized SCC, with a recommended total dose of 50–55 Gy in 20–25 fractions[30].

Lymph node metastases of SCC

Patients with metastatic SCC involving regional lymph nodes (usually of the head and neck) are best referred to a multidisciplinary cancer service[30a]. Metastases within the cervical lymph nodes can be due to a silent SCC of the oropharynx or a previously treated cutaneous SCC. Parotid lymph nodes represent a common site for metastases from a previously treated scalp, forehead or ear SCC; in such cases, surgery (parotidectomy ± neck dissection) is required.

Adjuvant radiotherapy is nearly always recommended in patients with nodal metastases in order to improve locoregional control, as the risk of nodal relapse remains high despite surgery[31]. Even patients with multiple unfavorable features (e.g. involvement of multiple nodes, extranodal spread, close margins) can still expect a 5-year disease-free survival of 70–75% with the combination of surgery and adjuvant radiotherapy[31].

Perineural invasion of SCC

Perineural invasion is an uncommon but serious consequence of SCC[32]. Up to 5% of excised SCCs are noted to have incidental perineural invasion and a minority (30–40%) will actually present with, or eventually develop, neurologic signs (e.g. motor deficit) or symptoms. Formication (sensation of ants crawling) may herald the diagnosis of perineural invasion, but dysesthesias, paresthesias, numbness and pain are all suggestive symptoms. The diagnosis is frequently delayed because perineural invasion is often not suspected.

A consensus is lacking regarding the most appropriate treatment following the diagnosis of perineural invasion. Patients with limited disease usually undergo surgery plus adjuvant radiotherapy, while radiotherapy alone is often recommended for those with advanced disease extending into the cranial cavity. Prognosis is poor once signs (e.g. craniopathies) or symptoms develop, with 5-year survival rates reported to be around 50%. When periorbital SCCs, especially those in the supraorbital area, are associated with perineural invasion, further treatment should definitely be considered[33]. Retrograde spread of SCC along the first division of the trigeminal nerve towards the orbital apex can occur. In addition, both the second division of this nerve and the facial nerve are potential conduits for spread back to the CNS.

In some circumstances, additional surgery, often extensive, may be undertaken to explore and dissect out potentially involved nerves. Alternatively, radiotherapy, often requiring multi-field megavoltage photons to treat neural pathways to the brainstem as well as first echelon lymph nodes, can be recommended[32–34]. While radiotherapy has the advantage of avoiding surgery, there is some risk of late radiation damage to orbital and CNS structures. Doses of 50–70 Gy (2 Gy/fraction) are often utilized, although late complications (10–35% of patients) can occur. Hyperfractionated radiotherapy (i.e. delivery of smaller-than-usual doses per fraction) and concomitant chemotherapy may improve outcome and decrease late reactions[34].

Immunosuppressed hosts

Immunosuppression in the setting of solid-organ transplantation (usually renal or cardiac) may be associated with significant morbidity due to the development of malignancies, especially lymphomas and skin cancers[35]. In some transplant populations, the risk of developing a cutaneous SCC exceeds 50%, and there is a greater risk of metastatic spread (compared to the general population). An interesting phenomenon is the higher incidence of SCCs compared to BCCs. Transplant patients also have an increased incidence of cutaneous melanoma, Merkel cell carcinoma and Kaposi's sarcoma. Additional patients at increased risk for developing aggressive cutaneous SCCs are individuals infected with HIV and those with chronic lymphocytic leukemia, especially when undergoing therapy (e.g. fludarabine, alemtuzumab). A subset of the SCCs that arise in immunosuppressed patients are clearly aggressive, with rapid growth and the development of regional and distant metastases[36]. There is some evidence that reducing the level of immunosuppression may be beneficial, although this potentially puts the patient at risk of organ rejection. The role of chemoprophylaxis (retinoids) in reducing the future development of skin cancers is unclear, although there is recent evidence to suggest a possible benefit. However, tolerability of dose-related side effects remains an issue.

The basic tenets of obtaining adequate surgical margins and examining for perineural invasion are of particular importance in this group of patients. Whilst prophylactic treatment to regional lymph nodes cannot be recommended, adjuvant radiotherapy to incompletely excised tumors or those with perineural invasion should be strongly considered. Transplant patients usually tolerate radiotherapy quite well, with no greater degree of acute toxicity.

Dose fractionation schedules and fields

An appropriate dose fractionation schedule depends upon both patient and tumor factors. However, decisions should not be based on age alone, as the presence or absence of relevant comorbidities must also be considered. As a generalization, smaller lesions (2–3 cm) in older patients (>70 years of age) are adequately treated by using 40–45 Gy in 10–15 daily fractions, resulting in acceptable local control and cosmesis (Table 139.2). Elderly or infirm patients may be best served by prescribing single large fractions (see palliation below) or even three to five fractions of 6–7 Gy. For larger invasive lesions (>3–4 cm) and/or

younger patients, a lower fraction size (2–2.5 Gy) and a 'hotter' total dose of 50–60 Gy are recommended in order to optimize local control and produce acceptable late effects. Some clinicians administer a higher dose for cutaneous SCCs than for equivalent-sized BCCs. However, the data to support this practice are conflicting, and, in the opinion of the authors, this is not required. Also, the dose for different subtypes or grades of BCC or SCC does not need to vary nor does the dose prescribed in the adjuvant setting.

A field margin of 5–10 mm beyond macroscopic disease or a surgical site is usually adequate. For a small, well-defined BCC, a 5 mm field margin is adequate if superficial photons are used. For SCCs and infiltrative BCCs, a wider margin of 10–15 mm is required in order to encompass surrounding subclinical spread. Ideally, adjuvant treatment should start within 6–7 weeks of excision. Whilst some clinicians are reticent to administer radiotherapy to a grafted site, it is uncommon for a healed skin graft to be lost because of radiotherapy[37]. Occasionally, poorly vascularized or infected grafts, especially on the scalp, do not tolerate radiotherapy.

Merkel Cell Carcinoma

Merkel cell carcinoma is a primary cutaneous neuroendocrine (small cell) carcinoma that most often arises in the head and neck region (see Ch. 115)[38]. These tumors often lack diagnostic clinical features. Merkel cell carcinomas are aggressive, having a high propensity for locoregional relapse and distant spread, and patients need to be appropriately evaluated prior to instituting therapy. Merkel cell carcinoma is both a radio- and chemo-responsive carcinoma. Currently, wide local excision of the primary lesion with margins of at least 10–20 mm or Mohs micrographic surgery is recommended. Some clinicians also advocate sentinel lymph node biopsy, and treatment of the regional lymph nodes must always be considered. When adjuvant locoregional radiotherapy is administered, there is evidence that extensive local surgery may not necessarily lead to a better outcome[39].

Although there are proponents of surgery alone for selected cases of Merkel cell carcinoma, adjuvant locoregional radiotherapy should nearly always be considered and represents 'best practice' in the opinion of the authors[40,40a]. Treatment should include the excision site, in-transit tissue (because of the risk of in-transit metastases), and regional lymph nodes. In an attempt to reduce the risk of locoregional relapse (which occurs in 40–50% of patients treated with surgery alone), a typical dose fractionation schedule would be 50 Gy in 20–25 daily fractions, usually requiring megavoltage photons or moderate-energy (9–12 MeV) electrons plus bolus. The role of adjuvant chemotherapy is currently unresolved, though recent trials may ultimately lead to the incorporation of carboplatin/etoposide-based chemotherapy[41]. In advanced or metastatic disease, both palliative radiotherapy and chemotherapy can offer effective symptom improvement.

Angiosarcoma

Most angiosarcomas present as violaceous plaques on the scalp and face of older adults (see Ch. 114). These tumors often extend well beyond the clinically evident/apparent margins[42] and locally extensive disease is usually present at the time of diagnosis. Unfortunately, excision alone is usually followed by local recurrences because of the multicentric and insidious nature of this tumor. Relapses can occur at the periphery of treated sites as well as regionally.

Angiosarcomas tend to be radio-responsive and therefore can be treated with radiotherapy. Patients with limited and operable disease may undergo excision followed by *adjuvant* radiotherapy. Alternatively, *definitive* radiotherapy is also an option, with a reasonable likelihood of obtaining in-field control[43]. In the case of scalp involvement, a technique can be used that encompasses the entire scalp and combines matching photon and electron fields[42]. Other options include multiple static electron fields or electron arcs. Lastly, single-agent chemotherapy with paclitaxel may be helpful in patients with recurrent disease.

Kaposi's Sarcoma

Kaposi's sarcoma (KS) is a type of spindle cell malignancy that arises from the vascular endothelium, usually presenting violaceous papules

SUGGESTED DOSE FRACTIONATION SCHEDULES FOR BASAL CELL CARCINOMAS (BCCs) AND SQUAMOUS CELL CARCINOMAS (SCCs)		
Dose fractionation schedule	**Indication**	**Biological effective dose***
Single 12–20 Gy fraction	Elderly, infirm (palliation)	
35 Gy in 7 fractions of 5 Gy	Elderly, medical comorbidity	44 Gy
40 Gy in 10 fractions of 4 Gy	Older, otherwise well	47 Gy
45 Gy in 15 fractions of 3 Gy	Older, otherwise well	49 Gy
50 Gy in 20 fractions of 2.5 Gy	Younger and/or lesion <2–3 cm	52 Gy
60 Gy in 30 fractions of 2 Gy	Younger and/or large lesion	60 Gy

*Calculated by converting to 2 Gy/fraction using the linear quadratic equation.

Table 139.2 Suggested dose fractionation schedules for basal cell carcinomas (BCCs) and squamous cell carcinomas (SCCs).

and plaques (see Ch. 114). Classic KS favors the legs of elderly men of Mediterranean or Jewish origin[44], whereas AIDS-associated KS has a more widespread distribution pattern, including the oral cavity (see Ch. 77).

While the role of radiotherapy for AIDS-related KS has markedly diminished with the advent of highly active antiretroviral therapies (HAART), it is a radio-responsive tumor and various dose fractionation schedules have been used to effectively treat cutaneous lesions. Regimens range from a single 8 Gy irradiation to 30–40 Gy in 10–20 daily fractions[45]. Because patients often develop acute painful reactions from radiotherapy to the oral cavity and the plantar surface, they should undergo radiotherapy to only one foot at a time.

Classic KS usually has a long and indolent clinical course. Patients with localized resectable tumors that are symptomatic may undergo excision, but the multifocal nature of the disease must be kept in mind. Radiotherapy is also an effective modality for palliating areas of symptomatic disease. Single small doses of 8–12 Gy are reported to result in symptom relief and tumor reduction in most patients, but in some circumstances, higher more fractionated doses may be considered to sites of limited disease. Occasionally, there is a sense of chasing the disease as lesions gradually appear at the periphery of irradiated sites. For patients with widespread disease, total skin electron beam therapy (see below) has been utilized.

Cutaneous Lymphomas

Cutaneous lymphomas are exquisitely radio-sensitive. However, with the exception of primary cutaneous B-cell lymphoma (see Ch. 119) and selected patients with cutaneous T-cell lymphoma (CTCL; see Ch. 120), the role of radiotherapy is essentially palliative. Patients with sites of symptomatic local disease (lymph nodes, dermal nodules and plaques, ulcers) can be palliated with doses of 20–30 Gy, often requiring orthovoltage or megavoltage energy photons. In cutaneous B-cell lymphoma, a form of indolent extranodal non-Hodgkin lymphoma, local radiotherapy with doses of 36–40 Gy may be curative[46].

Total skin electron beam therapy

Selected patients with mycosis fungoides and Sézary syndrome may be treated with total skin electron beam therapy (TSEBT) to a dose of 36 Gy over 9 weeks[47]. This treatment, which is complex and usually delivered by specialized centers of radiation oncology, has particular advantages:

- comprehensive coverage of the entire skin surface
- can be repeated should other modalities fail to control the CTCL
- an acceptable toxicity profile when given over a 6–9-week period.

While TSEBT can be offered to patients with all stages of disease, it is usually reserved for more advanced stages (IIB, III, IV) and/or disease that has failed to respond to less aggressive therapies (e.g. phototherapy, topical alkylating agents).

Treatment consists of a 4–6 MeV beam (see Fig 139.1), with patients often treated in the standing position at a distance of 7 m from the linear accelerator. Irradiation is administered 4 days per week for 9 weeks (i.e. 36 fractions). To some degree, X-ray contamination is always a feature of electron beam therapy. Typically, if using a 4–6 MeV electron beam, X-ray contamination is less than 2% of the dose. Each week, the entire skin surface receives two cycles of treatment and a total of 2 Gy is given to the entire skin surface each cycle. The perineum, plantar surface and scalp receive supplemental 'boosts', as these areas are not adequately treated with the patient in the standing position. Lead contact lenses are used to shield the eyes during the initial 18 fractions of TSEBT, and external shielding of the eyelids is done during the second portion of the treatment; hands and feet are also shielded 50% of the time during TSEBT. Patients with tumor stage disease often receive supplemental boosts via orthovoltage or electrons at the completion of the TSEBT.

As there is no significant dose of radiation to the bone marrow or viscera[48], patients receiving TSEBT should not have systemic sequelae (e.g. cytopenias, nausea, vomiting, diarrhea). However, alopecia, dyspigmentation and hypohidrosis often occur and in many patients are permanent side effects. A repeat course of TSEBT may be given months to years later for those who develop recurrent treatment-resistant disease. The most suitable candidates for repeat TSEBT are

individuals with longer intervals between courses (> 6 months) and those who had a longer disease-free interval following the first course.

Adnexal Carcinomas

Adnexal (appendageal) carcinomas, such as microcystic adnexal carcinomas and sebaceous, eccrine or apocrine carcinomas, are rare and therefore any treatment approach needs to be individualized (Ch. 112). Many of these tumors are aggressive in nature, with a propensity to develop regional and distant metastases. While patients with operable cancers should have them excised with appropriate margins, inoperable lesions may respond to radiotherapy. Adjuvant radiotherapy may also be recommended in the setting of incomplete excision. Doses similar to those for equivalent non-melanoma skin cancers should be administered (see Table 139.2).

PALLIATION

Locally Advanced Tumors

Occasionally, elderly, debilitated or mentally ill patients present with advanced and neglected skin cancers, which, though not curable, can be palliated. Such tumors are often painful, bleeding and infected, causing problems for both the patient and the caregiver. With the addition of a bolus (see Fig. 139.2), single large fractions of 12–20 Gy can be given quickly (within minutes) using megavoltage photons. Uncooperative patients may require mild sedation prior to treatment. These large single fractions are well tolerated with minimal toxicity. Alternative regimens include multiple medium-sized fractions given once or twice a week (e.g. 8 Gy × 3). In elderly patients who are otherwise well, higher total dose fractionation schedules such as 35 Gy in 5–7 fractions or 40 Gy in 10 fractions may be more appropriate and can be considered more radical in intent. These are often given as two or three fractions per week.

Metastases

Dermal-based metastases occur most frequently in patients with lung and breast cancer, and, in general, are associated with a poor prognosis (see Ch. 122). Both in-transit metastases and distant dermal metastases can develop in patients with cutaneous SCC, Merkel cell carcinoma, and melanoma. Cutaneous metastases may also present as rapidly enlarging subcutaneous masses with intact overlying skin.

Ulceration and bleeding are complications of cutaneous metastases that respond to palliative radiotherapy. Orthovoltage photons or mega-voltage photons (with a bolus) administered as a single 8 Gy fraction or 20 Gy in five fractions are effective regimens. Metastatic deposits elsewhere (e.g. skeletal) are also palliated with a similar dose fractionation schedule.

REACTIONS AND COMPLICATIONS

Acute Reactions

Acute morbidity from radiotherapy is usually minimal (in-field cutaneous erythema and desquamation) and limited to a small area (Table 139.3). Systemic side effects such as fatigue, nausea and vomiting do not occur. The daily application of a bland emollient, aloe vera or vitamin E cream is recommended while receiving radiotherapy. Most patients can expect to have local discomfort and moist desquamation by the conclusion of the radiation therapy (Fig. 139.7), which then lasts for a few weeks. Hemorrhagic crusting can also develop and re-epithelization usually occurs by week 3 or 4 following completion of radiotherapy. During the healing phase, patients are advised to keep the irradiated tissue clean and dry (after washing). Delayed healing (beyond 6–8 weeks) is uncommon, as is associated soft tissue infection.

Late Reactions

The late effects of radiotherapy (e.g. telangiectasia, epidermal atrophy, dyspigmentation; see Table 139.3 & Fig. 139.7) often appear months to

Table 139.3 RADIOTHERAPY REACTIONS AND COMPLICATIONS

	Reaction or complication
Acute	Dry desquamation, moderate erythema Moist desquamation and mild bleeding
Late*	Hypo- or hyperpigmentation[†] Telangiectasia[†] Epidermal atrophy[†] and fragility Permanent epilation/alopecia, sweat gland atrophy Necrosis of soft tissue, cartilage and/or bone Subdermal fibrosis Radiation-induced malignancy

*Many late effects are uncommon.
[†]Components of poikiloderma.

Table 139.3 Radiotherapy reactions and complications.

years later. They are more likely to appear with continued unprotected sun exposure, when a large dose per fraction (>3–4 Gy) was delivered, if the total dose was >55 Gy, and when large fields were irradiated.

In a review of over 400 patients treated with radiotherapy, 92% were considered to have a good or excellent cosmetic result[1]. However, 36% of those receiving >60 Gy in ≤2 Gy fractions had only a fair (16%) or poor (20%) cosmetic result. Smaller treatment fields (2–3 cm) tolerate hypofractionation better than do larger areas, but, even so, if cosmesis is an important consideration, larger fractions should be avoided. Patients should also be warned of the small risk (<5%) of late soft tissue and cartilage necrosis, which are related to larger tumor size and larger doses per fraction.

Younger Patients

When irradiating younger patients, better long-term cosmetic results are more likely if a low dose per fraction (2 Gy/fraction) is administered. A typical dose for a small BCC would be 50–54 Gy delivered in 25–27 daily fractions[49]. However, even with this dose fractionation schedule, patients can still expect some degree of in-field hypopigmentation and telangiectasia. Other options, therefore, should be considered prior to recommending radiotherapy to younger patients.

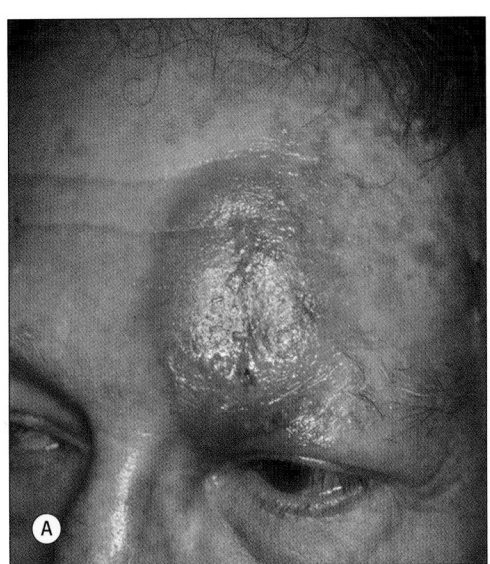

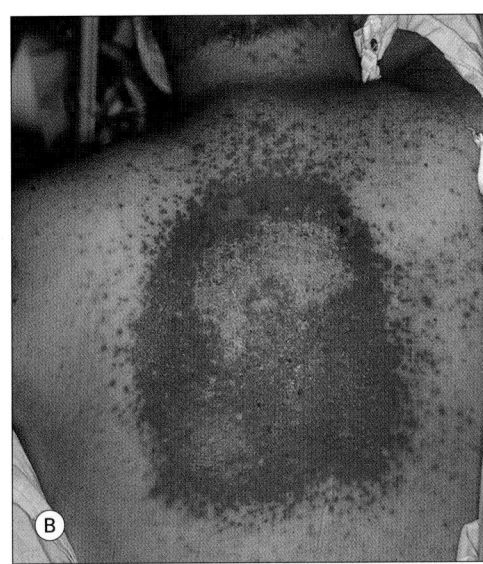

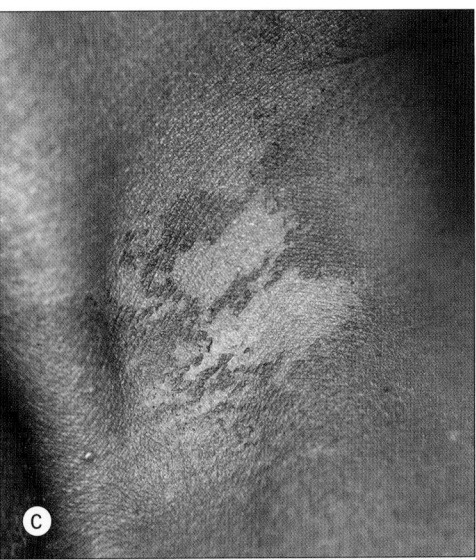

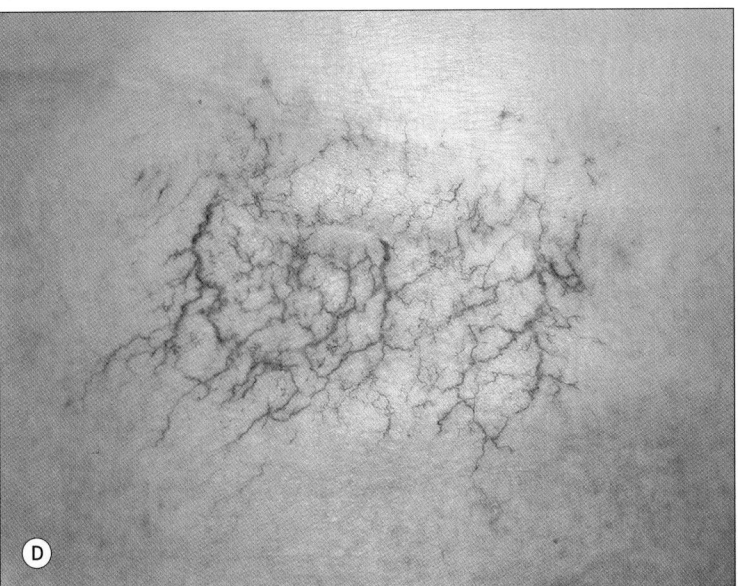

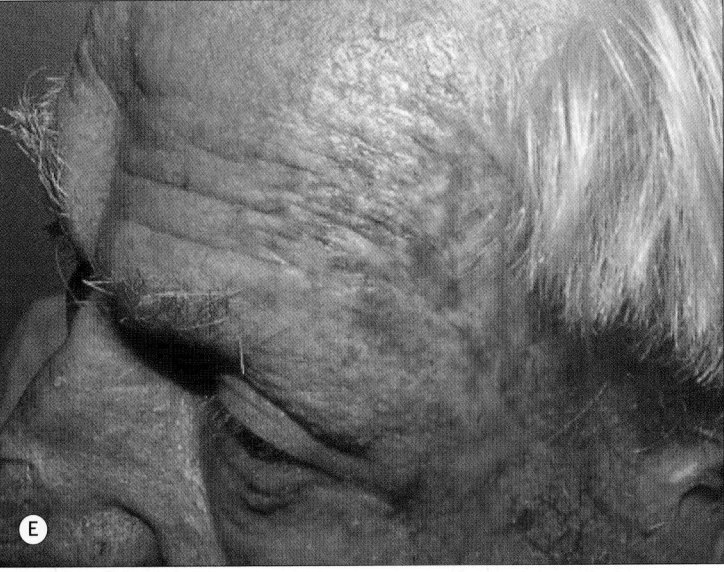

Fig. 139.7 Acute and chronic cutaneous side effects of radiation therapy. A Confluent moist desquamation and marked edema in a patient near completion of radiation therapy for a squamous cell carcinoma with neurotropism. **B** Stevens–Johnson syndrome localized to multiple radiation ports in a patient receiving phenobarbital. **C** Dry desquamation of the neck several weeks following radiation therapy for a pharyngeal squamous cell carcinoma. **D** In-field telangiectasias; note the square distribution pattern. **E** In-field hypo- and hyperpigmentation 10 years after radiotherapy for a basal cell carcinoma. *Continued*

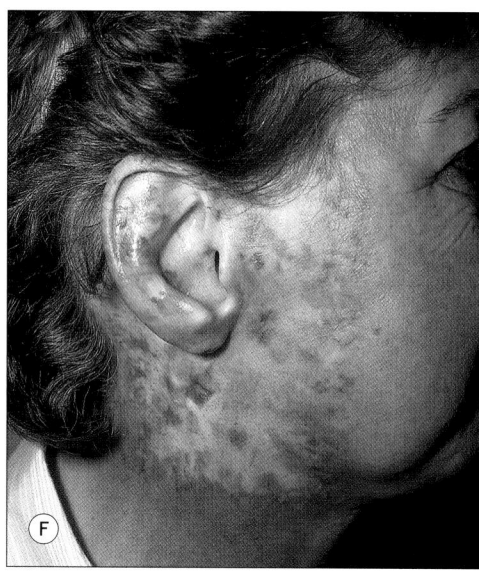
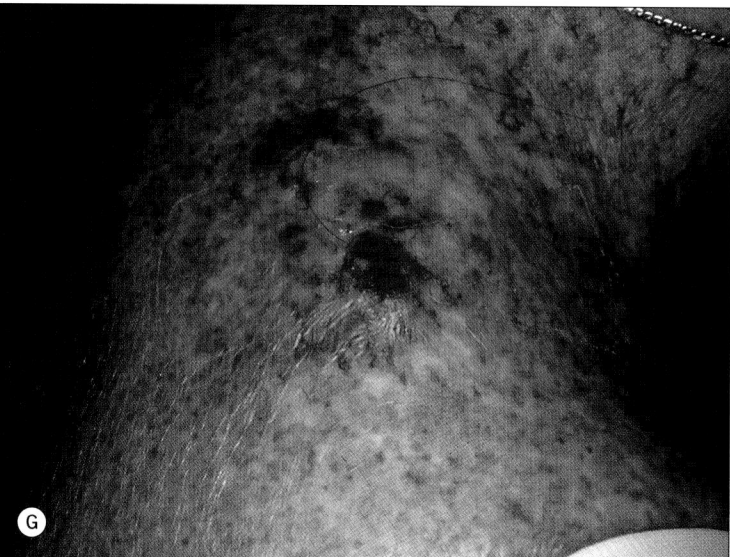

Fig. 139.7, cont'd Acute and chronic cutaneous side effects of radiation therapy. F In-field poikiloderma, fibrosis and ulceration; nowadays, this is seen much less often. **G** Spindle cell carcinoma within a radiation port. Note the background poikiloderma. A, C, D, Courtesy of Jean L Bolognia MD. B, Reprinted with permission from Duncan KO, Tigelaar RE, Bolognia JL. J Am Acad Dermatol 1999;40:493–6. G, Courtesy of Robert Hartman MD.

Cutaneous Diseases Induced by Radiation Therapy

Table 139.4 outlines the cutaneous disorders that are induced by radiotherapy, with some occurring outside the field of radiation and others limited to the site of irradiation.

FUTURE TRENDS

Modern radiotherapy has entered a new and exciting era[50]. Accurate conformal radiotherapy is being delivered via sophisticated three-dimensional CT-based planning and treatment systems. Intensity-modulated radiotherapy (IMRT) is allowing tumor doses to escalate and normal tissue doses to decrease. The integration of MRI and functional imaging such as positron emission tomography (PET) into planning systems will further enhance the accurate delivery of radiotherapy.

DISEASES INDUCED BY RADIATION THERAPY
Disease not confined to the sites of radiation
• Erythema multiforme
• Bullous pemphigoid
• Pemphigus foliaceus, pemphigus vulgaris
• Brunsting–Perry cicatricial pemphigoid
• Paraneoplastic pemphigus
• Herpes zoster
Disease limited to sites of radiation
• Bullous pemphigoid
• Erythema multiforme
• Comedonal acne, folliculitis
• Graft-versus-host disease
• Lichen planus
• Lichen sclerosus
• Morphea (localized scleroderma)
• Pseudosclerodermatous panniculitis
Lesions spare radiation site
• Exanthematous drug eruption

Table 139.4 Diseases induced by radiation therapy. This list does not include neoplasms.

REFERENCES

1. Locke J, Karimpour S, Young G, Lockett MA, Perez CA. Radiotherapy for epithelial skin cancers. Int J Radiat Oncol Biol Phys. 2001;51:748–55.

2. Withers HR. Biological basis of radiation therapy for cancer. Lancet. 1992;339:156–63.

3. Goldschmidt H, Breneman JC, Breneman DL. Ionizing radiation therapy in dermatology. J Am Acad Dermatol. 1994;30:157–82.

4. Silva JJ, Tsang RW, Panzarella T, Levin W, Wells W. Results of radiotherapy for epithelial skin cancer of the pinna: the Princess Margaret Hospital experience, 1982-1993. Int J Radiat Oncol Biol Phys. 2000; 47:451–9.

5. Khan FM. Quality of x-ray beams. In: Khan FM (ed.). The Physics of Radiation Therapy, 1st edn. Baltimore: Williams & Wilkins, 1984:110–20.

6. Tsao MN, Tsang RW, Liu FF, Panzella T, Rotstein L. Radiotherapy management for squamous cell carcinoma of the nasal skin: the Princess Margaret Hospital experience. Int J Radiat Oncol Biol Phys. 2002;52:973–9.

7. Goldschmidt H. FDA recommendations on radiotherapy of benign diseases. J Dermatol Surg Oncol. 1978;4:619–20.

8. Miller RA, Spittle MF. Electron beam therapy for difficult cutaneous basal and squamous cell carcinoma. Br J Dermatol. 1982;106:429–30.

9. Svoboda VHJ, Kovarik J, Morris F. High dose-rate microselection molds in the treatment of skin tumors. Int J Radiat Oncol Biol Phys. 1995;31:967–72.

10. de Launey JW, MacKenzie-Wood AR. Office radiotherapy in dermatology: a contemporary perspective. Australas J Dermatol. 1996;37:71–9.

11. Poulsen M, Burmeister B, Kennedy D. Preservation of form and function in the management of head and neck skin cancer. World J Surg. 2003; 27:868–74.

12. Feigen M. Should cancer survivors fear radiation induced sarcomas? Sarcoma. 1997;1:5–15.

13. Order SE, Donaldson SS. Radiation Therapy of Benign Diseases: A Clinical Guide, 2nd edn. New York: Springer, 1998:7.

14. Huang Q, Veness M, Richards S. The role of adjuvant radiotherapy in recurrent keloids. Austral J Dermatol. 2004;45:162–6.

15. Dupree MT, Kitely RA, Weismantle K, Panos R, Johnstone PAS. Radiation therapy for Bowen's disease: lessons for lesions of the lower extremity. J Am Acad Dermatol. 2001;45:401–4.

16. Schmid-Wendtner MH, Brunner B, Konz B, et al. Fractionated radiotherapy of lentigo maligna and lentigo maligna melanoma in 64 patients. J Am Acad Dermatol. 2000;43:477–82.

17. Huynh NT, Veness MJ. Radiotherapy for lentigo maligna. Arch Dermatol. 2002;138:981–2.

18. Bath FJ, Bong J, Perkins W, Williams HC. Interventions for basal cell carcinoma of the skin (Cochrane Review). In: The Cochrane Library, Issue 2, 2004. Chichester, UK: John Wiley & Sons.

19. Wilson AW, Howsam G, Santhanam V, et al. Surgical management of incompletely excised basal cell carcinomas of the head and neck. Br J Oral Maxillofac Surg. 2004;42:311–14.

20. Dieu T, Macleod AM. Incomplete excision of basal cell carcinomas: a retrospective audit. ANZ J Surg. 2002;72:219–21.
21. Liu FF, Maki E, Warde P, Payne D, Fitzpatrick P. A management approach to incompletely excised basal cell carcinomas of the skin. Int J Radiat Oncol Biol Phys. 1991;20:423–8.
22. Rowe DE, Carroll RJ, Day CD. Prognostic factors for local recurrence, metastasis, and survival rates in squamous cell carcinoma of the skin, ear and lip. J Am Acad Dermatol. 1992;26:976–90.
23. Cherpelis BS, Marcusen C, Lang PG. Prognostic factors for metastasis in squamous cell carcinoma of the skin. Dermatol Surg. 2002;28:268–73.
23a. Veness MJ, Palme CE, Morgan GJ. High-risk cutaneous squamous cell carcinoma of the head and neck: Results from 266 patients treated with metastatic nodal disease. Cancer. 2006;106:2389–96.
24. Motley R, Kersey P, Lawrence C. Multiprofessional guidelines for the management of the patient with primary cutaneous squamous cell carcinoma. Br J Dermatol. 2002;146:18–25.
25. Griffiths RW, Feeley K, Suvarna SK. Audit of clinical and histological prognostic factors in primary invasive squamous cell carcinoma of the skin: assessment in a minimum 5 year follow-up study after conventional excisional surgery. Br J Plast Surg. 2002;55:287–92.
26. Brodland DG, Zitelli JA. Surgical margins for excision of primary cutaneous squamous cell carcinoma. J Am Acad Dermatol. 1992;27:241–8.
27. Kwan W, Wilson D, Moravan V. Radiotherapy for locally advanced basal cell and squamous cell carcinomas of the skin. Int J Radiat Oncol Biol Phys. 2004;60:406–11.
28. Veness MJ, Ong C, Cakir B, Morgan G. Squamous cell carcinoma of the lip. Patterns of relapse and outcome: reporting the Westmead Hospital experience, 1980–1997. Australas Radiol. 2001;45:195–9.
29. de Visscher JG, Gooris PJJ, Vermey A, Roodenburg JLN. Surgical margins for resection of squamous cell carcinoma of the lower lip. Int J Oral Maxillofac Surg. 2002;31:154–7.
30. Babington S, Veness MJ, Cakir B, Gebski VJ, Morgan GJ. Squamous cell carcinoma of the lip: is there a role for adjuvant radiotherapy in improving local control following incomplete or inadequate excision? ANZ J Surg. 2003;73:621–5.
30a. Veness MJ, Porceddu S, Palme CE, Morgan GJ. Cutaneous head and neck squamous cell carcinoma metastatic to parotid and cervical lymph nodes. Head Neck. 2007;29:621–31.
31. Veness MJ, Morgan GJ, Palme CE, Gebski V. Surgery and adjuvant radiotherapy in patients with cutaneous head and neck squamous cell carcinoma metastatic to lymph nodes: combined treatment should be considered best practice. Laryngoscope. 2005; 115:870–5.
32. Garcia-Serra A, Hinerman RW, Mendenhall WM, et al. Carcinoma of the skin with perineural invasion. Head Neck. 2003;25:1027–33.
33. Veness MJ, Biankin S. Perineural spread leading to orbital invasion from skin cancer. Australas Radiol. 2000;44:296–302.
34. Galloway TJ, Morris CG, Mancuso AA, Amdur RJ, Mendenhall WM. Impact of radiographic findings on prognosis for skin carcinoma with clinical perineural invasion. Cancer. 2005;103:1254–7.
35. Preciado DA, Matas A, Adams GL. Squamous cell carcinoma of the head and neck in solid organ transplant recipients. Head Neck. 2002;24:319–25.
36. Veness MJ, Quinn DI, Ong CS, et al. Aggressive cutaneous malignancies following cardiothoracic transplantation: the Australian experience. Cancer. 1999;85:1758–64.
37. Bui DT, Chunilal A, Mehrara BJ, Disa JJ, Alektiar KM, Cordeiro PG. Outcome of split-thickness skin grafts after external beam radiotherapy. Ann Plast Surg. 2004;52:551–7.
38. Goessling W, McKee PH, Mayer RJ. Merkel cell carcinoma. J Clin Oncol. 2002;20:588–98.
39. Poulsen M, Harvey J. Is there a diminishing role for surgery for Merkel cell carcinoma of the skin? A review of current management. ANZ J Surg. 2002;72:142–6.
40. Veness MJ, Perera L, McCourt J, et al. Merkel cell carcinoma: improved outcome with adjuvant radiotherapy. ANZ J Surg. 2005;75:275–81.
40a. Clark JC, Veness MJ, Gilbert R, O'Brien CJ, Gullane PJ. Merkel cell carcinoma of the head and neck: Is adjuvant radiotherapy necessary? Head Neck 2007; 29: 249–57.
41. Poulsen M, Rischin D, Walpole E, et al. Analysis of toxicity of Merkel cell carcinoma of the skin treated with synchronous carboplatin/etoposide and radiation: a Trans-Tasman Radiation Oncology Group study. Int J Radiat Oncol Biol Phys. 2001;51:156–63.
42. Veness M, Cooper S. Treatment of cutaneous angiosarcomas of the head and neck. Australas Radiol. 1995;39:277–81.
43. Sasaki R, Soejima T, Kishi K, et al. Angiosarcoma treated with radiotherapy: impact of tumor type and size on outcome. Int J Radiat Oncol Biol Phys. 2002;52:1032–40.
44. Antman K, Chang Y. Kaposi's sarcoma. N Engl J Med. 2000;342:1027–37.
45. Lukawska J, Cottrill C, Bower M. The changing role of radiotherapy in AIDS-related malignancies. Clin Oncol. 2003;15:2–6.
46. Smith BD, Glusac EJ, McNiff JM, et al. Primary cutaneous B-cell lymphoma treated with radiotherapy: a comparison of the European Organization for Research and Treatment of Cancer and the WHO classification systems. J Clin Oncol. 2004;22:634–9.
47. Jones GW, Kacinski BM, Wilson LD, et al. Total skin electron radiation in the management of mycosis fungoides: Consensus of the European Organisation for Research and Treatment of Cancer (EORTC) Cutaneous Lymphoma Project Group. J Am Acad Dermatol. 2002;47:364–70.
48. Wilson LD. Delivery and sequelae of total skin electron beam therapy. Arch Dermatol. 2003;139:812–13.
49. Huynh NT, Veness MJ. Basal cell carcinoma of the lip treated with radiotherapy. Australas J Dermatol. 2002;43:15–19.
50. Moran JM, Elshaikh MA, Lawrence TS. Radiotherapy: what can be achieved by technical improvements in dose delivery? Lancet Oncol. 2005;6:51–8.

Electrosurgery

Sheldon V Pollack

140

Synonym: ■ Radiosurgery

Key features

- Electrosurgery encompasses a group of procedures by which tissue is removed or destroyed through the application of electrical energy

- True electrocautery uses direct current to create a red-hot tip, which can be safer for patients with pacemakers and implantable cardioverter-defibrillators

- In modern electrosurgery, high-frequency alternating current is converted to heat within the treated tissues as a result of resistance to its passage

- Electrodesiccation is superficial ablation by touching the tissue with a monoterminal device

- Electrofulguration is superficial ablation by use of a monoterminal device whose electrode is held at a slight distance from the tissue, allowing a spark to jump to the tissue

- Electrocoagulation uses a biterminal device for deeper ablation

- Electrosection uses a biterminal device to cut while achieving hemostasis by mild lateral heat spread

- In order to minimize adverse sequelae, lateral heat spread should be kept to a minimum by using the appropriate waveform, power setting and electrode size

INTRODUCTION AND BACKGROUND

Definition

Modern electrosurgery is a group of techniques by which high-frequency alternating electrical current is applied to living tissues in order to achieve superficial ablation, deep ablation or cutting of the skin. Since living tissue is a poor conductor of electricity, the flow of electrical current is hampered and builds up at the site of application. This resistance to the flow of electricity results in its conversion to heat. The use of different varieties of electrosurgical current, each characterized by a distinctive waveform, results in unique biologic outcomes, including desiccation, coagulation or section of treated skin.

Electrocautery

The forerunner of modern electrosurgery was electrocautery (from Greek *kauterion*, branding iron)[1]. In electrocautery, invented in 1875, a metal wire is heated by resistance to the flow of direct current electricity. The principle is the same as that used in an electric toaster or range in which an element is heated 'red-hot' by the application of an electric current. Hemostasis (even in a wet field) can be obtained with electrocautery, but the resulting third-degree burn may result in prolonged healing times and may cause inferior cosmetic outcomes.

It is important to understand that electrocautery, with its hot element, is different from modern electrosurgery, in which high-frequency alternating current is applied via an unheated electrode. Some doctors use the term electrocautery incorrectly to cover all forms of electrosurgery in this chapter. Electrocautery units are of value for providing hemostasis for surgical patients with pacemakers and implantable cardioverter-defibrillators (ICDs). External electromagnetic fields may compromise the function of these devices. A number of electrocautery units are

currently produced, among them the Thermal Cautery Unit by Geiger Medical Technologies Inc. (Monarch Beach, CA).

Historical Aspects

Although used by most dermatologists on a daily basis, high-frequency electrosurgery (often referred to as 'radiosurgery') could not have been developed if several major advances in the knowledge of electricity had not occurred. In order for alternating current electricity to be utilized for medical purposes, it was necessary for high-frequency currents to be produced. A generator that could provide such current was developed in 1889 by Thompson, who noted heat in his wrists when current was passed through his hands when immersed in saline solution[2]. Experiments conducted by Jacques Arsene d'Arsonval in 1891 established that the application, in human subjects, of electric currents with frequencies greater than 10 000 cycles per second (10 000 hertz [Hz]) failed to cause neuromuscular stimulation and the associated tetanic response[3,4]. Also in the 1890s, Oudin, following some modifications to d'Arsonval's equipment, was able to generate a spray of sparks that caused superficial tissue destruction.

During the next few years, the major forms of high-frequency electrosurgery were elucidated and described. Rivière, at the turn of the 20th century, conceived the notion of using very small treatment electrodes in order to concentrate the current density. This would enable one to treat a skin lesion with an electric spark[5]. Walter de Keating-Hart and Pozzi[6] in 1907 introduced the term fulguration (from Latin *fulgur*, lightning), referring to the superficial carbonization that resulted when the spark from the Oudin coil was used to treat skin. They claimed that this modality was ideal for treating skin cancer and that the spark could selectively destroy tumor cells by interfering with their source of nutrition.

In 1909, Doyen[7] introduced the term 'electro-coagulation' (from Latin *coagulare*, to curdle) to describe a different form of electrosurgery in which tissue was touched directly with the treatment electrode and an indifferent electrode was added to the circuit. The indifferent electrode allowed for direct removal of the electricity entering the patient and caused the latter to flow back into the electrosurgical device. By removing this static energy build-up, shocks were avoided in surgeons and other bystanders. The amperage was effectively increased while the 'recycling' of electrical current allowed for lower voltages to be utilized. The current produced with this biterminal arrangement penetrated more deeply than fulguration and directly coagulated tissues rather than causing only surface carbonization. Doyen claimed that this more deeply penetrating current was more likely to be effective in the destruction of tumor cells.

William Clark, in 1911, reported on the use of an electrosurgical output that caused dehydration of tissue without carbonization at the surface[8]. He substituted a multiple spark gap for the usual single one in a monoterminal Oudin current generator. This provided a smoother current that resulted in the production of fine sparks as opposed to the long, thick sparks seen with electrofulguration. Clark used the term desiccation (from Latin *desiccare*, to dry out) to describe this action.

The next major event in the development of electrosurgery came in 1923 when Dr George A Wyeth, a noted tumor surgeon, used electrosurgery for cutting tissues[9]. His apparatus, which he termed an 'endotherm knife' (Greek *endo*, within; *thermē*, heat), used a thermionic vacuum tube instead of a spark gap[10]. Wyeth called the technique 'electrothermic endothermy'. He believed that the technique was particularly applicable to tumor surgery since it sealed off not only the smaller blood vessels but also the lymphatics that might otherwise provide for dissemination of metastatic disease.

A Harvard physicist, William Bovie PhD, probably made the most important contribution to the development of electrosurgery. With financial assistance from the Liebel-Flarsheim Company of Cincinnati, he built an operating room electrosurgical device that offered both coagulation and cutting currents[11]. Dr Harvey Cushing, a distinguished neurosurgeon, became quite interested in these techniques and, with Bovie at the controls, began using electrosurgery for controlling bleeding and cutting through tissues during surgical procedures at Peter Bent Brigham Hospital in 1926. Dr Cushing's favorable impressions of electrosurgery assured acceptance of this technique by the surgical world. The subsequent impact of Bovie's machine upon medicine was so great that the word 'bovie' is still often used generically as a noun to refer to an electrosurgical apparatus or even as a verb to describe the act of performing electrosurgery[12].

Electrosurgical Devices and Outputs

Over the years, electrosurgical devices have become increasingly sophisticated. A variety of electrical outputs, each with a characteristic waveform and use, can be generated by a single apparatus. Clinical application of the appropriate output results in selective incision, excision, ablation, or coagulation of tissue. To optimize the use of an electrosurgical device, the clinician should have some understanding of how such equipment functions.

The circuitries of all electrosurgical instruments share certain design features necessary for production of suitable electrical outputs for electrosurgery. Standard household current first passes through a transformer which alters the voltage, providing the levels and characteristics required for the instrument's various circuit functions. The current next travels through an oscillating circuit that may employ a spark gap, a thermionic vacuum tube, or solid state transistors to increase electrical frequency. Finally, this altered electrical energy is delivered to the treatment electrode.

Each electrosurgical current produces its own unique wavy pattern of current flow, or *waveform*. The waveforms thus produced can be visualized on the screen of an oscilloscope or traced on an oscillograph. These may be either *damped* or *undamped*, depending on the type of oscillating circuit used. In general, damped waveforms provide electrodesiccation and electrofulguration, whereas the application of undamped currents results in electrocoagulation and cutting currents (Fig. 140.1). The spark gap generator produces a damped wave, consisting of bursts of energy in which successive wave amplitudes gradually return to zero. This occurs due to the resistance to energy flow presented by the gap.

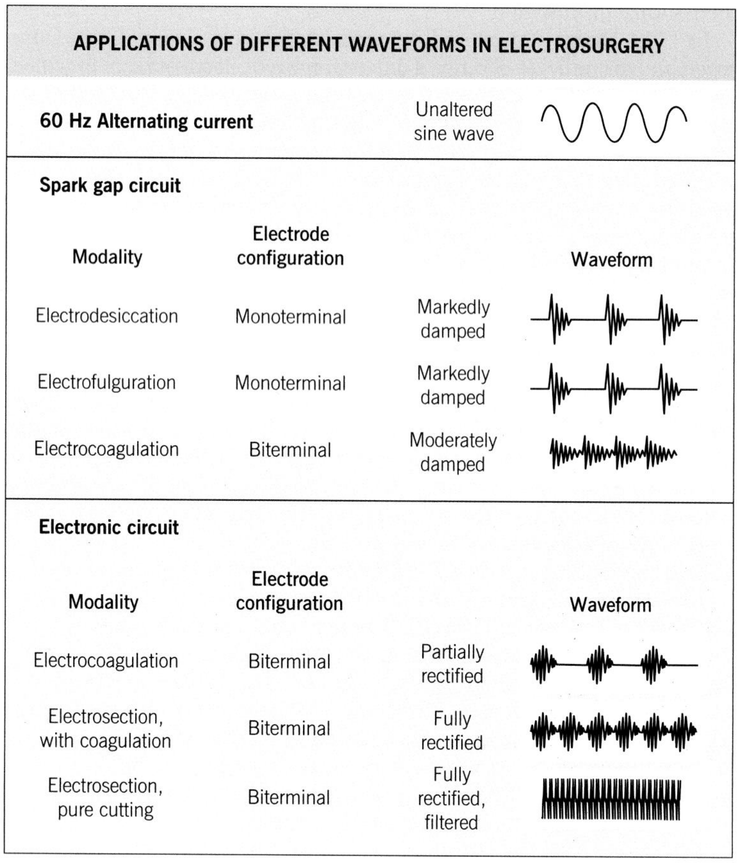

Use of a thermionic tube results in a more uniform output. The valve tube circuit is able to neutralize the internal resistance responsible for the damping effect seen in the spark gap circuit, and the amplitude of output therefore remains unchanged. Depending on the circuitry used, the output can be moderately damped (partially rectified) or slightly damped (fully rectified). A filtered, fully rectified output is essentially continuous and uniform, similar to an undamped wave. The different types of waveforms each result in different biologic outcomes and are, therefore, used for different electrosurgical procedures.

Terminology: Monopolar, Bipolar, Monoterminal and Biterminal

Prior to exploring the individual electrosurgical currents in detail, it is appropriate to first clarify four common electrosurgical terms that have been used inconsistently by various authors, causing much confusion. The terms *monopolar* and *bipolar* denote the number of tissue contacting tips at the end of the surgical electrode. When the surgical electrode has only one tip projecting from its end, it is a monopolar electrode. If it has two tips, it is a bipolar electrode.

Simply put, monoterminal refers to the use of a treatment electrode without an indifferent or dispersive electrode ('ground plate'). Biterminal denotes that both treatment and indifferent electrodes are used. Such is the case with electrocoagulation and electrosection, in which use of the indifferent plate, although not *technically* necessary for the machine to work, will definitely enhance the efficiency of the electrosurgical apparatus. Electrodesiccation and its variant, electrofulguration, are monoterminal procedures in which the indifferent electrode serves no purpose.

When a ball electrode is used to electrocoagulate a bleeding vessel, one is using biterminal, monopolar electrosurgery. In the case of bipolar forceps in which the electrode is connected to both the active and the dispersive electrode termini, we are using a biterminal, bipolar modality.

INDICATIONS/CONTRAINDICATIONS

The simplest way to think of electrosurgical applications in the clinical setting is to consider the three major capabilities of electrosurgery units. These include superficial tissue destruction (electrodesiccation), deep tissue destruction (electrocoagulation) and cutting (electrosection)[13,14]. Destruction or excision of skin lesions by electrosurgery should be accomplished with the smallest possible amount of damage to normal tissues. Whether electrosurgery, cryosurgery or CO_2 laser surgery is used, the greater the penetration of the destructive modality into the skin, the greater the likelihood that unacceptable scarring will result. Because the destructive effects of electrocoagulation extend more deeply than those of electrodesiccation, the clinician must consider the histologic characteristics of the lesion to be treated when selecting the appropriate current. A partial list of dermatologic conditions that are commonly treated by each electrosurgical modality is found in Table 140.1.

There are no absolute contraindications to the use of electrosurgery, but precautions should be taken during the treatment of patients with pacemakers or ICDs (see Variations/unusual situations, below).

PREOPERATIVE HISTORY AND CONSIDERATIONS

The preoperative assessment of patients undergoing electrosurgery should concentrate on potential hazards to either the patient or the treatment team. A patient history of previous allergic reactions to skin cleansers, anesthetics, or postoperative topicals and dressings should be sought. Electrosurgery should be used with care in patients with cardiac pacemakers and ICDs.

Smoke evacuation equipment should always be available to safely remove the smoke plume when extensive electrosurgery, particularly electrosection, is performed. In such procedures, the operator and assistants should wear masks and use eye protection to prevent exposure to smoke-borne microbes. Gloves should always be worn when electrosurgical procedures are performed.

APPLICATIONS OF DIFFERENT WAVEFORMS IN ELECTROSURGERY

60 Hz Alternating current		Unaltered sine wave	

Spark gap circuit

Modality	Electrode configuration		Waveform
Electrodesiccation	Monoterminal	Markedly damped	
Electrofulguration	Monoterminal	Markedly damped	
Electrocoagulation	Biterminal	Moderately damped	

Electronic circuit

Modality	Electrode configuration		Waveform
Electrocoagulation	Biterminal	Partially rectified	
Electrosection, with coagulation	Biterminal	Fully rectified	
Electrosection, pure cutting	Biterminal	Fully rectified, filtered	

Fig.140.1 Applications of different waveforms in electrosurgery.

COMMON DERMATOLOGIC INDICATIONS FOR ELECTROSURGERY
Electrofulguration/electrodesiccation (superficial skin ablation)
Acrochordon
Actinic keratosis
Angioma (small)
Epidermal nevus
Hemostasis (capillary bleeding)
Lentigo
Seborrheic keratosis
Verruca plana
Electrocoagulation (deep skin ablation)
Angiofibroma
Angioma (large)
Basal cell carcinoma
Bowen's disease
Hemostasis (arterial bleeding)
Hirsutism
Ingrown toenail matrixectomy
Banal melanocytic nevi
Sebaceous hyperplasia
Squamous cell carcinoma
Syringoma
Telangiectasia
Trichoepithelioma
Verruca vulgaris (all locations)
Electrosection (skin incision/excision)
Acne keloidalis nuchae
Blepharoplasty incision
Debulking procedures
Hair transplant strip harvesting
Rhinophyma repair
Rhytidectomy incisions and undermining
Scar revision
Shave removal of benign skin lesions (fibromas, nevi, etc.)
Skin flap incisions and undermining
Skin resurfacing (under investigation)
Surgical excision of malignant or benign skin lesions

Table 140.1 **Common dermatologic indications for electrosurgery.**

Preparatory to electrosurgery, the lesion and surrounding skin should be cleansed with a non-alcoholic skin cleanser such as chlorhexidine or povidone iodine. There is a potential for alcohol to ignite with electrosurgery, so it should be avoided or allowed to thoroughly dry prior to therapy.

Local anesthesia, usually via 1% lidocaine with epinephrine, is almost always used when performing electrosurgery. The usual exception is in the treatment of small facial telangiectases, in which anesthesia is omitted. Local infiltration is most often used for anesthetizing localized surface lesions, whereas field blocks and/or nerve blocks should be considered when performing larger electrosurgical procedures such as rhinophyma repair. When a local anesthetic is used prior to treatment of a dome-shaped lesion, such as a large angioma, it is helpful to massage the swollen anesthetized treatment site prior to electrosurgery in order to flatten it. This prevents the development of a depressed scar subsequent to the procedure.

Electrosurgical procedures are most often undertaken with patients lying on a treatment or operating table. This positioning of patients also tends to lessen their risk of fainting and suffering resultant bodily injury. If possible, the table should be adjusted to a height which allows the operator to perform the procedure most comfortably. Prior to activating the electrosurgery unit, the operator should determine that the appropriate current and power settings for the particular procedure have been selected, that the dispersive electrode has been properly placed and that the correct treatment electrode has been chosen. Sterile sleeves that slip over the handle of the wand and disposable electrode tips are often utilized. Nowadays it is unacceptable to use the same electrode tip on multiple patients without sterilization, erroneously assuming that heat will destroy pathogens.

DESCRIPTION OF TECHNIQUES

Electrodesiccation

For very superficial lesions, such as those involving only the epidermis, electrosurgical destruction by *electrodesiccation* can be achieved with little, if any, scarring. The markedly damped, high-voltage current generated by spark gap electrosurgical units causes superficial tissue damage by dehydration of the treatment site. It is delivered in a monoterminal (concentrative) fashion. If the electrode is held at a slight distance from the tissue, a spark is formed between the electrode and the tissue. This technique, termed *electrofulguration*, achieves very superficial destruction because the surface carbonization it produces insulates the underlying tissues from thermal heat spread.

Electrodesiccation is the method of choice when the most superficial type of tissue destruction is desired. For example, it is ideal for treatment of epidermal lesions such as seborrheic or actinic keratoses (Fig. 140.2), acrochordons, verruca plana or small epidermal nevi. Hemostasis of mild capillary bleeding can also be achieved by use of electrodesiccation. A standard technique for treating keratoses by this method is to move the electrode slowly across the surface of the lesion (for small lesions) or to insert it directly into the lesion (for larger lesions), while applying current at a low power setting. After a few seconds, the lesion bubbles as the epidermis separates from the underlying dermis. It can then be easily removed with a curette or simply by rubbing a piece of gauze across the treatment site. The clinical endpoint in treating epidermal lesions is punctate bleeding, which is controlled with pressure, by spot electrocoagulation, or by topical hemostatic agents such as aluminum chloride. More profuse bleeding indicates probable damage to the dermis, with a greater likelihood of subsequent scarring. Extremely small superficial lesions can be treated by electrofulguration, which causes the least amount of damage to adjacent tissues.

Electrocoagulation

In electrocoagulation, a moderately damped current is applied in a *biterminal* manner (both concentrative and dispersive electrodes are used). This current is of higher amperage and lower voltage than that utilized for electrodesiccation. Because this type of current penetrates more deeply, it has the potential for greater tissue destruction.

Electrocoagulation is particularly useful for deep tissue destruction and surgical hemostasis. It is our preferred modality for treating small and uncomplicated primary basal cell and squamous cell carcinomas, as well as other lesions such as trichoepitheliomas, which extend into the dermis. The electrode is brought into direct contact with the tissue to be treated and is moved slowly across the lesion, which eventually becomes charred. A curette may then be used to gently remove the charred tissue. For treatment of skin cancers, this procedure is repeated two more times in an attempt to remove any small tumor extensions. During the last curettage, a small curette is often used to remove the final tiny 'roots' of the tumor. Scarring must be expected with this procedure, as with any other tissue-destroying therapy, and must therefore be discussed with the patient when therapeutic alternatives are considered.

Electrocoagulation is also effective for treatment of superficial telangiectasias (Fig. 140.3), unwanted hair (electroepilation) and ingrown toenails (electrosurgical matrixectomy). Hemostasis using electrocoagulation can be achieved by either monopolar or bipolar means. Because the electrosurgical energy may be transmitted for several millimeters along the vessel wall, it is important to use the minimum effective exposure time and power setting in order to prevent delayed bleeding from damaged vessels. We often use monopolar electrocoagulation, in which the electrode is touched directly to the bleeding vessel. Coagulation can also be achieved by touching the electrode to a hemostat that has been clamped on the severed vessel. In bipolar electrocoagulation (Fig. 140.4), a bipolar forceps is used to provide more directed pinpoint hemostasis. Electrocoagulation current delivered in this manner causes less adjacent tissue damage but requires a dry operative field to be effective.

Electrosection (cutting)

Electrosection involves the biterminal application of a slightly damped current. The current, of low voltage and high amperage, causes

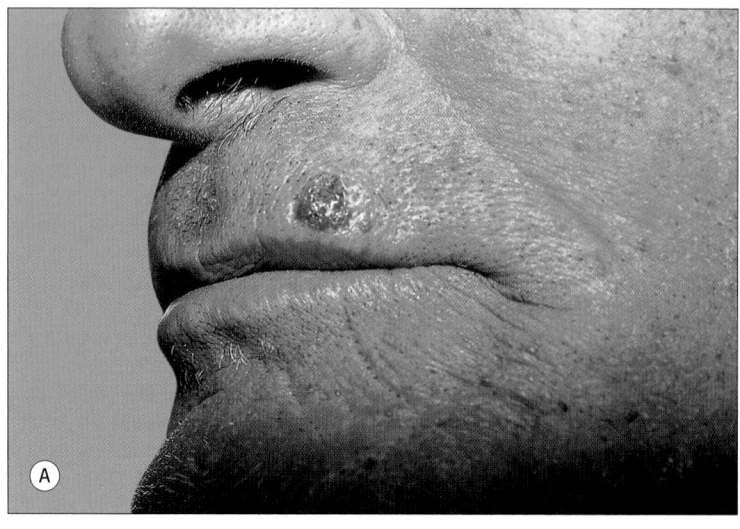
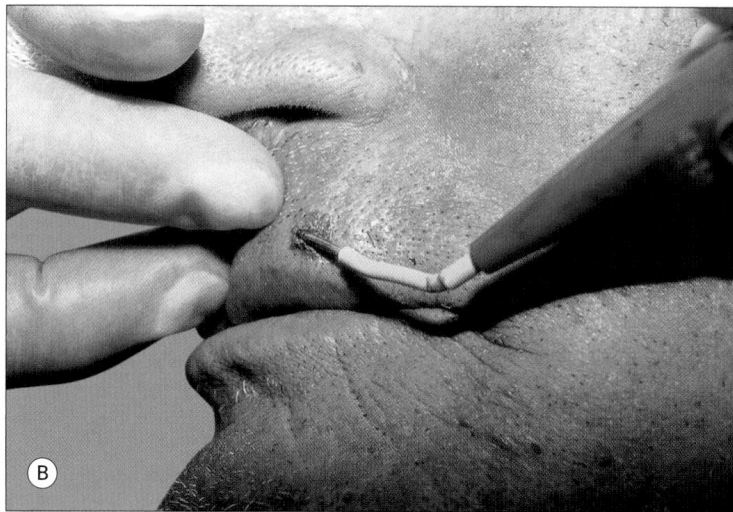
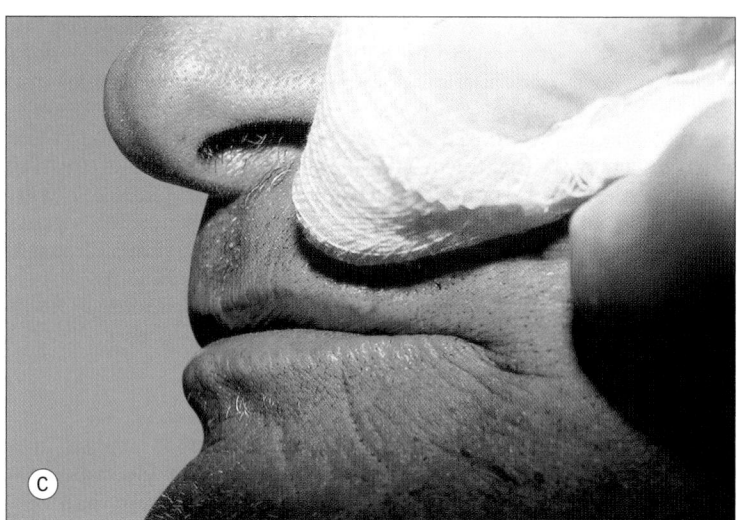
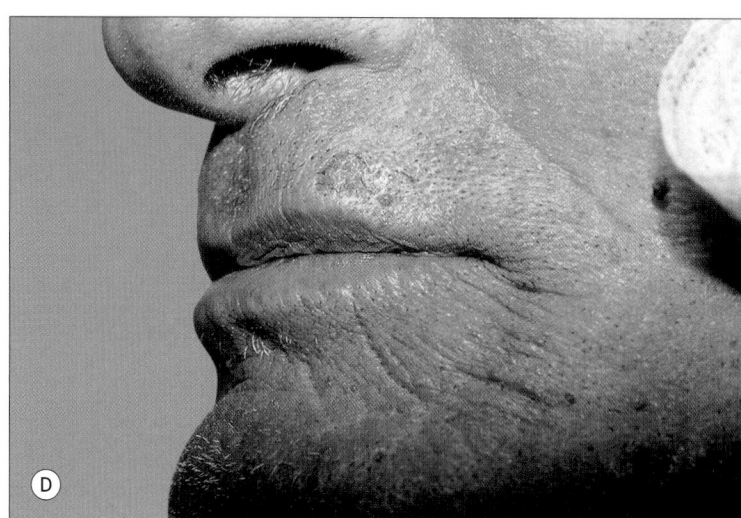

Fig. 140.2 Seborrheic keratosis on the upper lip. A Given its epidermal location, electrosurgical destruction should employ a current that provides the most superficial type of tissue damage. **B** Under local anesthesia, the lesion is treated by electrodesiccation. Delivery of current is stopped when the lesion begins to 'bubble'. **C** In lieu of a curette, a gauze pad is useful for removing charred tissue after desiccation of superficial lesions. **D** There is minimal bleeding, indicating that damage did not penetrate deeply into the dermis.

minimal lateral heat spread and tissue damage, and has the additional advantage of simultaneously achieving hemostasis and cutting. 'Pure' cutting can be obtained using a true undamped tube current, which provides the least amount of lateral heat spread and causes vaporization of tissue without hemostasis. Such current has been suggested by Chiarello[15] to be useful in debulking large skin cancers, contouring surrounding skin following shave excisions, scar revision following skin flaps and grafts, and rhinophyma repair. When electrosection is performed using a filtered, fully rectified current, subsequent spot electrocoagulation can be achieved by changing to the electrocoagulation current.

Electrosection can be used to perform rapid and effortless excisions or incisions. Virtually no manual pressure by the operator is required. Electrodes configured as loops, triangles or diamonds can be used for quick removal of skin tags, papillomas, intradermal nevi and other exophytic skin lesions. A straight, narrow electrode is most often used to incise the skin and is applied to the tissue in brisk, continuous paintbrush-like strokes. The difference between electrosection and scalpel excision is immediately apparent to the first-time user of electrosection. At the appropriate power setting, the electrode passes smoothly through the tissue like a 'hot knife through butter'. If perceptible sparking occurs during incision, the power setting is too high; if the electrode 'drags', the power setting is too low.

Slightly damped currents cause some charring at the margins of the excised tissue. Therefore, when a specimen suitable for histopathologic analysis is required, the filtered current should be used because it does not create significant electrosurgical artifact. It is recommended that the new initiate to electrosection develop technical skills and concepts

by practicing on beefsteak before utilizing these techniques in the clinical arena.

The major advantage of electrosection over scalpel surgery is that when a blended cutting and coagulating current is utilized, hemostasis is achieved immediately as the incision is made. However, larger blood vessels (more than 2 mm in diameter) require additional spot electrocoagulation at the completion of the excision. Another drawback is that vaporization of the tissue generates a smoke plume, which can be unpleasant for both the patient and the operator and may contain potentially infectious viral particles (see below). Consequently, effective smoke evacuation equipment should be available during such procedures.

Electrosection is extremely useful for achieving relatively bloodless excision of large, bulky lesions, such as acne keloidalis nuchae and rhinophyma (Fig. 140.5), in which the surgical defect is allowed to heal by second intention. Electrosurgical excision followed by primary closure can also be undertaken with no impairment of wound healing, as compared with conventional scalpel surgery. This modality has been used, without complication, to create skin flaps and perform cosmetic facial surgery, including blepharoplasty and rhytidectomy, with excellent outcomes.

VARIATIONS/UNUSUAL SITUATIONS

Cardiac Pacemakers and ICDs

The use of electrosurgery in patients with cardiac pacemakers or ICDs raises the question of whether the flow of electrical energy during

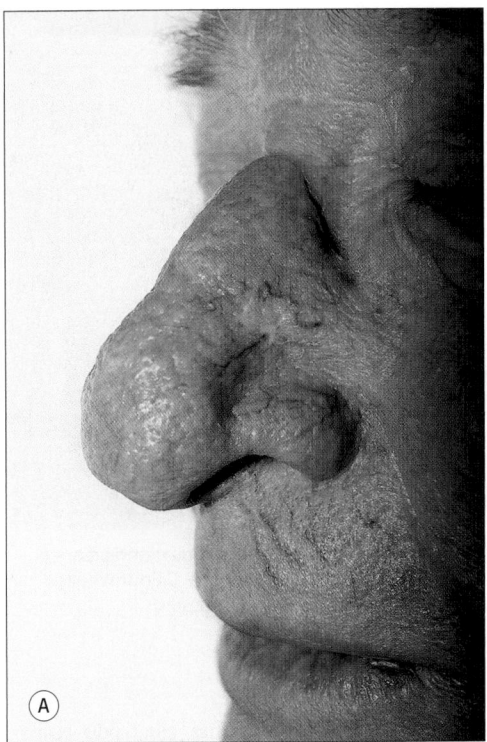
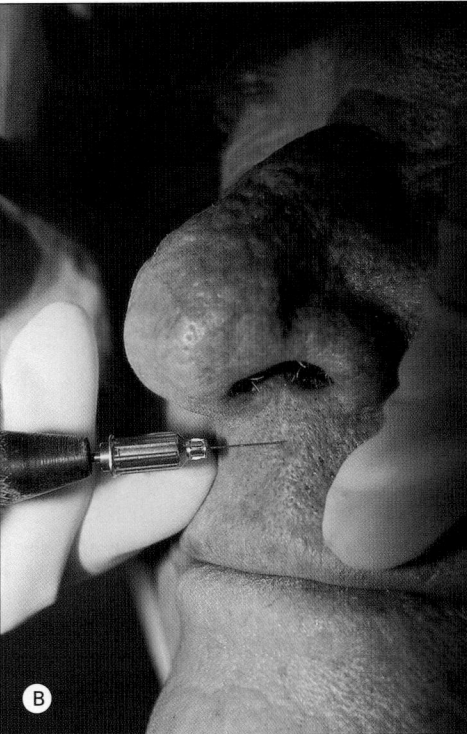
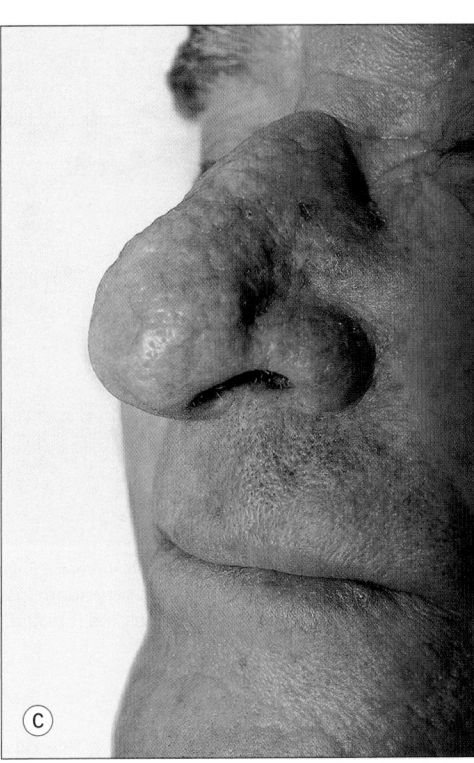

Fig. 140.3 Telangiectasias on nose and upper lip being treated by fine-needle electrocoagulation. A Preoperative photograph shows linear telangiectasias on the nose and upper lip. **B** The electrode consists of a hub adapter with a 30-gauge metal-hubbed needle attached. The machine is energized at a low power setting and the electrode momentarily touches the skin surface, along the length of the vessel being treated, at 3 to 4 mm intervals. The patient experiences some discomfort during the procedure, but this is usually tolerable. **C** The same patient immediately after treatment. This technique is usually performed quickly without anesthesia.

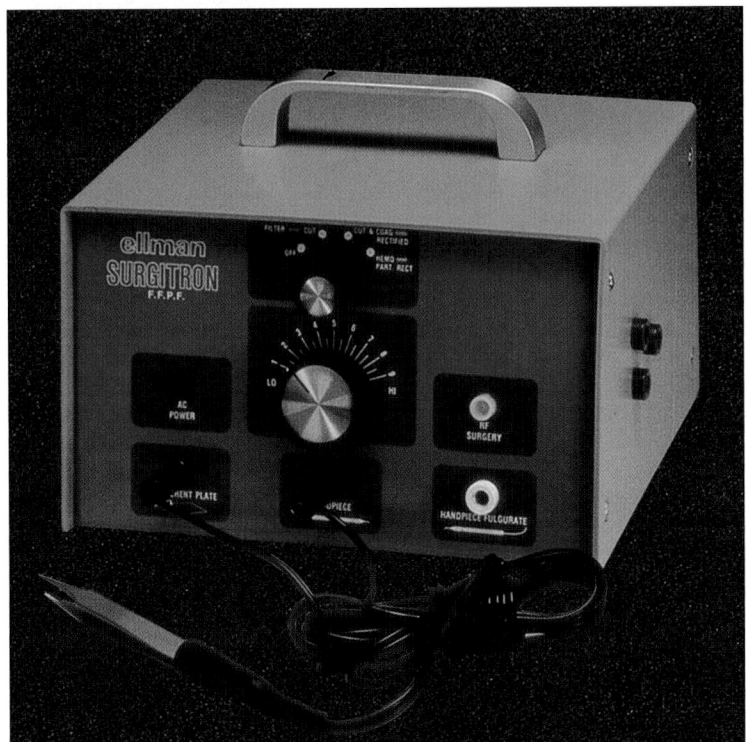

Fig. 140.4 Bipolar forceps attached to an electrosurgical apparatus. These are useful for providing pinpoint electrocoagulation in hemostasis. Bipolar electrocoagulation is also recommended for use in patients with cardiac pacemakers or implantable cardioverter-defibrillators (ICDs).

electrosurgery might interfere with the function of these devices[16]. Although modern pacemakers and ICDs have improved shielding technology to guard them from the influence of external electromagnetic currents, prudence requires that a modicum of precaution be taken. If used indiscriminately in these patients, electrosurgery can occasionally trigger skipped beats, reprogramming of a pacemaker, firing of an ICD, asystole or bradycardia.

Routine precautions recommended when using electrosurgery in patients with pacemakers and ICDs include: (i) utilize short bursts of energy that are less than 5 seconds in duration; (ii) keep power settings as low as possible; (iii) avoid the use of cutting current; and (iv) avoid use on the skin around the pacemaker or ICD. Although recommended in the literature, most dermatologists do not follow specific precautions such as intraoperative monitoring, preoperative cardiology consultation, or postoperative evaluation of the cardiac device by a cardiologist. This may be due to the fact that to date there have been no reported cases of interference to a pacemaker or ICD in a dermatologic setting. Also, at least one article suggests that practical experience of complications due to electrosurgical interference is rare among dermatologic surgeons[17].

There is less risk of potential side effects when the electrosurgical current is confined to a very small area, as is the case when bipolar forceps are used as electrodes. A way to virtually eliminate such risk in very unstable cardiac patients or those with ICDs is to use true electrocautery, rather than other forms of electrosurgery[18]. Although the use of this modality may cause more of a burn injury than does true electrosurgery, there is no flow of current to cause electrical interference. In a survey of Mohs surgeons, 34% used electrocautery and 19% used bipolar forceps in patients with pacemakers or ICDs. Among this group, there was only one reported case of interference in one of the electrocautery patients. However, since there is no current flow in true electrocautery, this was likely an error in reporting.

It is the author's belief that the use of either electrocautery or bipolar forceps as electrodes in pacemaker and ICD patients will eliminate the need for intraoperative monitoring, preoperative cardiology consultation or postoperative evaluation by a cardiologist in the majority of patients.

POSTOPERATIVE CARE

Standard postoperative wound management, incorporating antibiotic ointments and/or semiocclusive dressings, is followed. For superficial skin ablations, such as those following electrodesiccation or electrofulguration, twice-daily application of an antibiotic ointment is generally all that is required. An adhesive plaster may be used if the area is prone

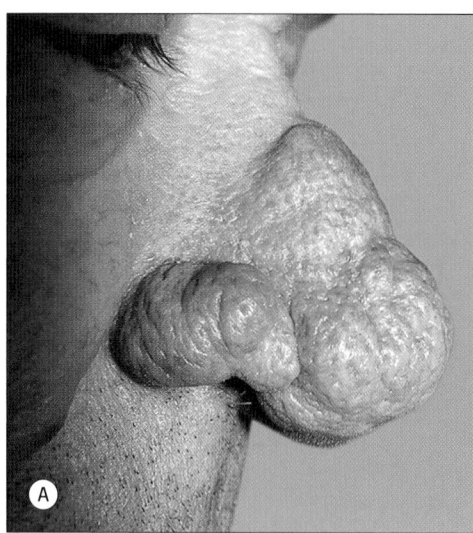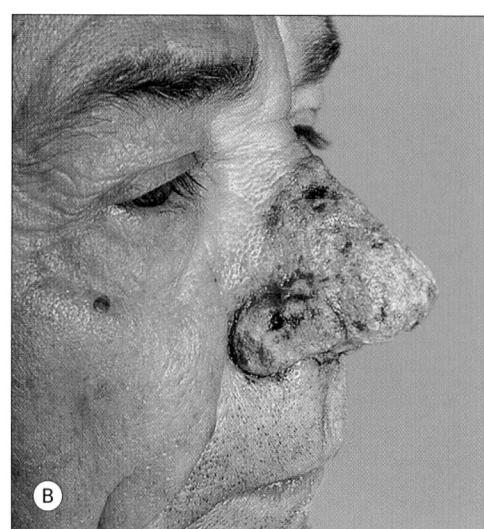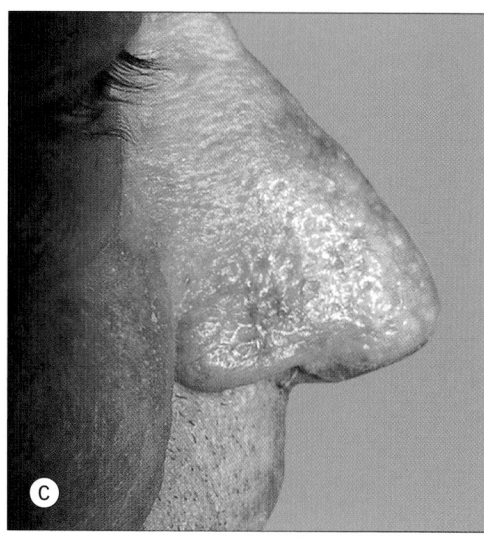

Fig. 140.5 Rhinophyma. A Moderately severe rhinophyma in a middle-aged man. **B** Immediately after electrosurgical planing of excess sebaceous glands. Care is taken to perform subtotal removal as very aggressive therapy can result in significant scarring and possible deformity caused by scar contracture. **C** Four weeks later, healing with good cosmetic outcome is noted. During healing, the wound is kept moist with an antibiotic ointment and semiocclusive dressings.

to rubbing. An eschar forms within a few days and separates in about 10 days. For deeper wounds, in which healing can take 2–4 weeks (or longer on the lower extremities), once- or twice-daily application of an antibiotic ointment followed by an adhesive plaster is recommended. For larger wounds, such as those following rhinophyma repair, Telfa™ sheets are cut to size to cover the defect and kept in place with semiocclusive paper tape (e.g. Micropore®, 3M Corporation, MN).

COMPLICATIONS

Patients should be warned of the possibility of delayed bleeding and should be reassured that it can, in the vast majority of cases, be controlled by 20–30 minutes of constant direct pressure over the wound. Trips to the local emergency room to stop postoperative bleeding are unusual but can occur. Patients should also be advised that for ablative procedures, scarring, in the form of a hypopigmented area, may occur.

Other potential hazards of electrosurgery are briefly discussed below.

Fire

There is a risk of fire or explosion if electrosurgical procedures are conducted in the presence of alcohol, oxygen or bowel gases (methane). Care should be taken to be certain that the operative site is free of alcohol residue. Oxygen is usually not a problem except in the operating room setting. Bowel gases are highly inflammable! Use care in the perianal region.

Thermoelectric Burns

Although modern generators are isolated from earth, and are often equipped with sophisticated monitor systems, current can still be diverted away from the return electrode and cause an accidental burn at the point at which it leaves the patient's body. Alternative pathways occur when the current is diverted from the return electrode and finds an alternative path to return to the generator. When the point of contact between the patient and the earthed object is small, even a relatively low-power current can generate sufficient current density to cause a burn. Earthed objects may include metal parts of the operating table, table accessories, or ECG electrodes.

This problem is reduced, but not eliminated, by the use of isolated electrosurgical units, which have little or no connection to the common earth.

Microorganism Transmission

The potential exists for transmission of microorganisms either via the electrode[19,20] or via smoke plume inhalation. Neither possibility has been investigated in sufficient depth to yield conclusive results.

Practitioners should minimize the risk of possible electrode transmission by using disposable or sterilized electrodes. Adapters are available that allow disposable metal hypodermic needles to be used as electrodes.

Surgical Smoke

During surgical procedures using a laser or electrosurgical unit, the thermal destruction of tissue creates a smoke byproduct. Research studies have confirmed that this smoke plume can contain toxic gases and vapors such as benzene, hydrogen cyanide and formaldehyde, bioaerosols, dead and live cellular material (including blood fragments)[21], and viruses[22]. At high concentrations, the smoke causes ocular and upper respiratory tract irritation in healthcare personnel and creates visual problems for the surgeon. The smoke has unpleasant odors and has been shown to have mutagenic potential[23].

Research by the National Institute for Occupational Safety and Health (NIOSH) has shown that airborne contaminants generated by these surgical devices can be effectively controlled by appropriate ventilation using a portable smoke evacuation system. Smoke evacuators contain a suction unit (vacuum pump), filter, hose, and an inlet nozzle. The smoke evacuator should have high efficiency in airborne particle reduction and should be used in accordance with the manufacturer's recommendations to achieve maximum efficiency. A capture velocity of approximately 100–150 feet per minute at the inlet nozzle is generally recommended. It is also important to choose a filter that is effective in collecting the contaminants. A high-efficiency particulate air (HEPA) filter or equivalent is recommended for trapping particulates. Various filtering and cleaning processes also exist which remove or inactivate airborne gases and vapors. The different filters and absorbers used in smoke evacuators require monitoring and replacement on a regular basis and are considered a possible biohazard requiring proper disposal.

The smoke evacuator hose inlet nozzle must be kept within 2 inches of the surgical site to effectively capture airborne contaminants generated by these surgical devices. The smoke evacuator should be activated at all times when airborne particles are produced during all surgical or other procedures. At the completion of the procedure, all tubing, filters and absorbers must be considered infectious waste and be disposed of appropriately. New filters and tubing should be installed on the smoke evacuator for each procedure.

FUTURE TRENDS

It is interesting to note that interest and innovation in electrosurgery have increased in the past two decades, since continuous wave CO_2 laser systems were introduced. Practitioners came to realize that superficial ablation, deep ablation and tissue incision with immediate hemostasis were available through electrosurgery without the need for expensive laser systems. The role of electrosurgery in dermatologic care has continued to expand. For example, specially adapted electrosurgery equipment that utilizes electricity to remove the epidermis and upper dermis for facial skin resurfacing has been introduced, providing an alternative treatment to deep chemical peeling, dermabrasion or CO_2 laser resurfacing[24]. In a like manner, at a recent meeting of the American Academy of Dermatology, Dr Stephen Chiarello described the use of electrosurgical cutting current, using the Ellman Surgitron® (Ellman International Manufacturing, Hewlett, NY), to resurface surgical scars and improve cosmetic outcomes (personal communication, February 2001). A myriad of articles describing new electrosurgical techniques continue to appear in the medical literature. The latest such development involves the use of non-ablative tightening of skin laxity, using a standard Radiosurgery device (Surgitron Dual Frequency RF,

Ellman International). Radiofrequency current produces heat through resistance in the dermis and subcutaneous tissue. When heated, collagen fibrils will denature and contract, presumably leading to the observed tissue tightening. This new indication for the Surgitron Dual Frequency RF was approved by the US Food and Drug Administration in 2007, and preliminary reports suggest patient satisfaction with little or no down time[25].

Many developments in recent years have also served to make electrosurgery safer and more user-friendly. The availability of a variety of disposable electrodes, smoke evacuation systems, and more fully functional electrosurgery equipment at reasonable prices suggest that this modality will continue to be of import to all dermatologists in the future. The current emphasis on cosmetic dermatology will also serve to keep electrosurgery at the forefront of dermatology as the cosmetic applications of this modality continue to evolve.

REFERENCES

1. Blankenship ML. Physical modalities. Electrosurgery, electrocautery and electrolysis. Int J Dermatol. 1979;18:443–52.
2. Mitchell JP, Lumb GN. Principles of surgical diathermy and its limitations. Br J Surg. 1962;50:314–20.
3. d'Arsonval A. Action physiologique des courants alternatifs. Soc Biol. 1891;43:283–6.
4. d'Arsonval A. Action physiologique des courants alternatifs à grande fréquence. Arch Physiol Norm Path. 1893;5:401–8.
5. Rivière AJ. Action des courants de haute fréquence et des effleuves du résonateur Oudin sur certaines tumeurs malignes. J Méd Intern. 1900;4:776-7.
6. Pozzi M. Remarques sur la fulguration. Bull Assoc Franc Cancer. 1909;2:64–9.
7. Doyen D. Sur la destruction des tumeurs cancéreuses accessibles par la méthode de la voltaisation bipolaire et de l'électro-coagulation thermique. Arch Elec Med Exp Clin. 1909;17:791–5.
8. Clark WL. Oscillatory desiccation in the treatment of accessible malignant growths and minor surgical conditions: a new electrical effect. J Adv Therap. 1911;29:169–83.
9. Wyeth GA. Endothermy, surgical adjunct in accessible malignancy and precancerous conditions. Surg Gynec Obstet. 1923;36:711–14.

10. Wyeth GA. The endotherm. Am J Electrotherapeut Radiol. 1924;42:186–7.
11. Cushing H. Electro-surgery as an aid to the removal of intracranial tumors, with a preliminary note on a new surgical-current generator by WT Bovie, Ph.D. Surg Gynec Obstet.1928;47:751–2.
12. Goldwyn RM. Bovie: the man and the machine. Ann Plast Surg. 1979;2:135–53.
13. Pollack SV. Electrosurgery of the Skin. New York: Churchill Livingstone, 1991.
14. Sebben JE. Cutaneous Electrosurgery. Chicago: Year Book Medical Publishers, 1989.
15. Chiarello S. Controlled vaporization of tumor tissue utilizing radio frequency cutting current through a blunt hockey stick scalpel or radio frequency knife. Dermatol Surg. 1998;24:158–60.
16. Riordan AT, Gamache C, Fosko SW. Electrosurgery and cardiac devices. J Am Acad Dermatol. 1997;37:250–5.
17. El-Gamal HM, Dufresne RG Jr, Saddler K. Electrosurgery, pacemakers and ICDs: a survey of precautions and complications experienced by cutaneous surgeons. Dermatol Surg. 2001;27:385–90.
18. Wilson JH, Lattner S, Jacob R, Stewart R. Electrocautery does not interfere with the function of the automatic implantable cardioverter defibrillator. Ann Thorac Surg. 1991;51:225–6.

19. Sherertz EF, Davis GL, Rice RW, et al. Transfer of hepatitis B virus by contaminated reusable needle electrodes after electrodesiccation in simulated use. J Am Acad Dermatol. 1986;15:1242–6.
20. Bennett RG, Kraffert CA. Bacterial transference during electrodesiccation and electrocoagulation. Arch Dermatol. 1990;126:751–5.
21. Berberian BJ, Burnett JW. The potential role of common dermatologic practice techniques in transmitting disease. J Am Acad Dermatol. 1986;15:1057–8.
22. Sawchuck WS, Weber PJ, Lowy DR, et al. Infectious papillomavirus in the vapor of warts treated with carbon dioxide laser or electrocoagulation: detection and protection. J Am Acad Dermatol. 1989;21:41–9.
23. Tomita Y, Mihashi S, Nagata K, et al. Mutagenicity of smoke condensates induced by CO_2-laser irradiation and electrocauterization. Mutat Res. 1981;89:145–9.
24. Grekin RC, Tope WD, Yarborough JM Jr, et al. Electrosurgical facial resurfacing: a prospective multicenter study of efficacy and safety. Arch Dermatol. 2000;136:1309–16.
25. Rusciani A, Curinga G, Menichini G, et al. Nonsurgical tightening of skin laxity: A new radiofrequency approach. J Drugs Dermatol. 2007;6:381–6.

Wound Healing

Robert S Kirsner

Key features

- Wound healing occurs in three overlapping phases: the inflammatory phase, the proliferative phase, and the remodeling phase

- The depth of the wound determines the degree of contraction and the source of keratinocytes for re-epithelialization

- Platelets, the first cells to appear in the healing process, and macrophages, the most important cells in the healing process, mediate most of their actions via cytokines or growth factors

- Endothelial cells, previously thought to be bystanders in wound healing, play an active role in facilitating leukocyte migration

- The cell that is the most important in the production of the dermal matrix is the fibroblast

- Wound healing can be enhanced by a variety of interventions, e.g. avoiding the application of toxic substances, keeping the wound free of necrotic tissue, and the appropriate use of occlusive dressings

INTRODUCTION

Cutaneous wound healing involves the complex interaction of several types of cells, the cytokines or mediators they produce, and the extracellular matrix. Vascular responses, cellular and chemotactic activity, and the release of chemical mediators within wounded tissues combine to form the inherent, interrelated components of healing. For dermatologists, an understanding of wound healing is critical, as many skin disorders involve a break in the cutaneous barrier. In addition, wounds and ulcers represent the most expensive skin condition[1]. Dermatologists, perhaps to a greater degree than other physicians, also create wounds for diagnostic and therapeutic purposes.

Appreciation of the normal is a prerequisite to addressing the pathologic. Understanding the processes involved in wound repair is also vitally important for a specialty that devotes a significant amount of its time to creating wounds. At the onset, however, a disclaimer needs to be made. Although wound healing is traditionally divided into three phases – the inflammatory phase, the proliferative phase, and the remodeling phase (Fig. 141.1) – the process is a continuous one and the phases actually overlap. In addition, it has been suggested that a 'coagulation phase', which would precede the inflammatory phase, may

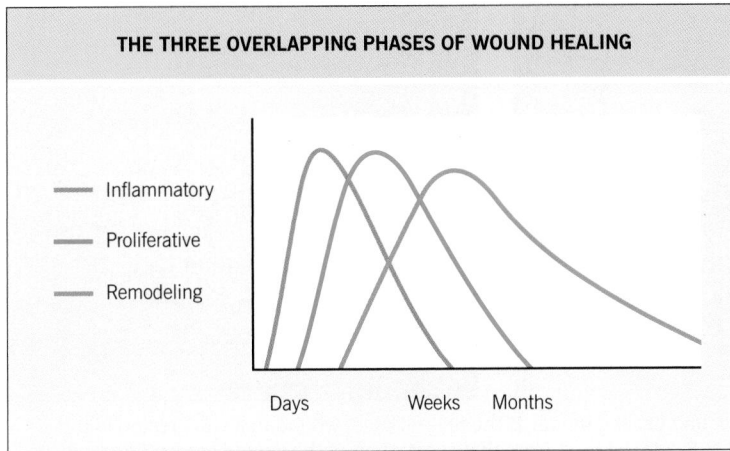

Fig. 141.1 The three overlapping phases of wound healing.

also exist. Therefore, the conceptual distinction between phases serves only as an outline for discussing events that occur during wound repair.

Historically, fundamental definitions of events during wound healing have been chosen arbitrarily, albeit logically. Defining the point at which wound healing begins and ends has often been based on macroscopic examination. As a result, injury and repair of the skin that occurs at a microscopic or a molecular level may not be appreciated. Although they are not yet known, understanding the events occurring at early and/or unrealized times may be invaluable to enhancing our knowledge of the dynamic process of wound healing.

The process of healing may proceed in a timely or an untimely (slow) fashion, and the two processes are conveniently called acute and chronic wounds, respectively. Determination of the exact healing time and the designation of a wound as acute or chronic remain arbitrary and are based on variables including location and cause of the wound as well as the age and physical condition of the patient. An elliptical wound on the face of a healthy child will heal faster than a circular burn wound on an elderly infirm person, even though both might heal in a timely fashion given the circumstances. The Wound Healing Society has, somewhat arbitrarily, defined chronic wounds as '… wounds (that) have failed to proceed through an orderly and timely process to produce an anatomic and functional integrity, or proceed through the repair process without establishing a sustained and functional result'.

TYPES OF WOUNDS

PARTIAL-THICKNESS VERSUS FULL-THICKNESS WOUNDS

Injury to just the epidermis differs from injury involving the underlying dermis. After an injury limited to the epidermis, the epidermis restores itself to a structure similar to the preinjury state. This is in contrast to injury to deeper structures such as the dermis, where regeneration does not normally occur, but rather repair occurs. In certain situations, regeneration does occur after dermal injury. For example, regeneration occurs *in utero*, where higher concentrations of type III collagens and glycosaminoglycans in addition to decreased levels of transforming growth factor-β (TGF-β) likely play a role in mediating regeneration as opposed to repair. Also, reduced inflammation *in utero* may play a role in the 'scarless' healing observed during the first 20 weeks of gestation[1a].

Wounds can be categorized depending on their depth. If only the epidermis (or a portion of the epidermis) is lost, this is referred to as an erosion. When the wound involves structures deep to the epidermis, it is termed an ulceration. Wounds that involve the epidermis and varying parts of the dermis are termed partial thickness (Fig. 141.2A), while those involving the epidermis, all of the dermis, and deeper structures are called full-thickness wounds (Fig. 141.2B). Chronic wounds are also categorized by the thickness of the wound; for example, pressure ulcer staging depends upon wound depth (see Fig. 105.22)[1b].

For acute wounds, there is an additional reason to differentiate partial-thickness from full-thickness wounds, in that partial-thickness wounds epithelialize by a different mechanism than do full-thickness wounds[2]. In partial-thickness wounds, since the deep dermis has not been lost or destroyed, adnexal structures are present. These structures serve as a reservoir of epithelial cells for repopulating the epidermis. Epithelia from these structures, as well as from the ulcer edge, migrate across the wound surface to provide coverage (Fig. 141.3). In full-thickness wounds, on the other hand, adnexal structures are no longer present; therefore epithelium can only migrate from the ulcer edge.

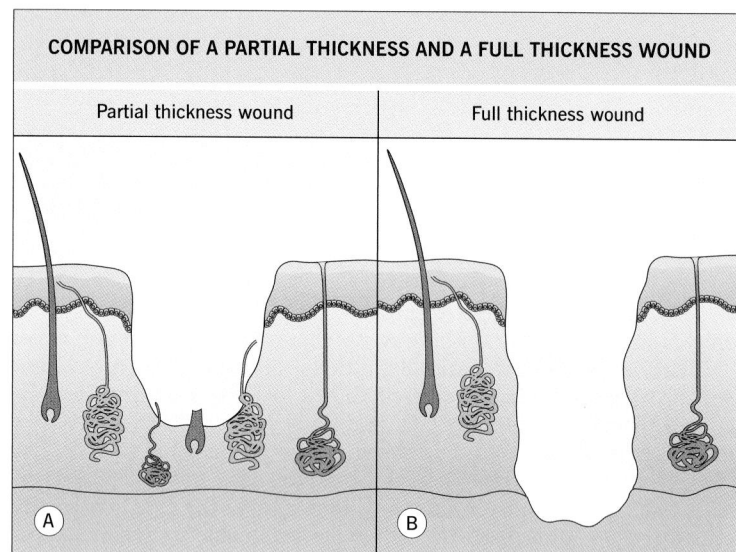

Fig. 141.2 **Comparison of a partial-thickness and a full-thickness wound.**
A The partial-thickness wound is one in which the epidermis and part of the dermis are missing but the adnexal structures remain. **B** A full-thickness wound is one in which all of the epidermis and dermis are missing as well as the adnexal structures.

Full-thickness wounds heal to some extent by contraction (Fig. 141.4), while there is minimal contraction in partial-thickness wounds[3]. The reason for this is not clear and the contraction may be mediated by mechanical or biologic factors (or both). During contraction, the area of the wound decreases and this involves movement of pre-existing tissue centripetally, not the formation of new tissue. Usually, contraction does not go to completion, except occasionally in small wounds. Clinically,

contraction of the wound may result in cosmetically disfiguring contractures. Because the contraction of wounds occurs in predictable directions (via so-called 'skin tension lines'), surgeons often place incisions in the direction of the skin tension lines in order to direct the contracture. They may also utilize full-thickness skin grafts to prevent wound contraction and subsequent contracture (see Ch. 148).

PRIMARY VERSUS SECONDARY INTENTION HEALING

When an acute wound, such as one created by a surgical excision, is left to heal on its own, it is termed secondary (second) intention healing. Primary intention healing occurs when a surgeon directs closure of the wound by approximating the wound edges; the latter includes side-to-side closures, flaps and grafts. Even if the wound edges are approximated using a primary intention method, the wound still needs to proceed through the three phases of healing. In secondary intention healing, the time until re-epithelialization is complete is dependent on several factors. These include wound depth (superficial wounds heal faster), wound location (facial wounds heal faster than acral wounds) and geometric shape (given a particular area, the smallest diameter wound heals faster). For smaller wounds, primary versus secondary intention healing may produce similar cosmetic results, but as the wound becomes larger (≥8 mm), preferred cosmetic results occur with primary intention healing[3a]. Tertiary intention healing refers to when a wound is closed via a primary intention method, but then dehisces and is left to heal by secondary intention (Fig. 141.5).

The decision to close a wound primarily or not depends on a number of variables, including patient factors, concerns regarding cosmetic outcome, and the location, depth and size of the wound. Examples of patient factors are a patient's age, the presence of comorbid conditions such as venous hypertension and arteriosclerosis, the patient's risk for developing infection (which may be increased by leaving wounds open),

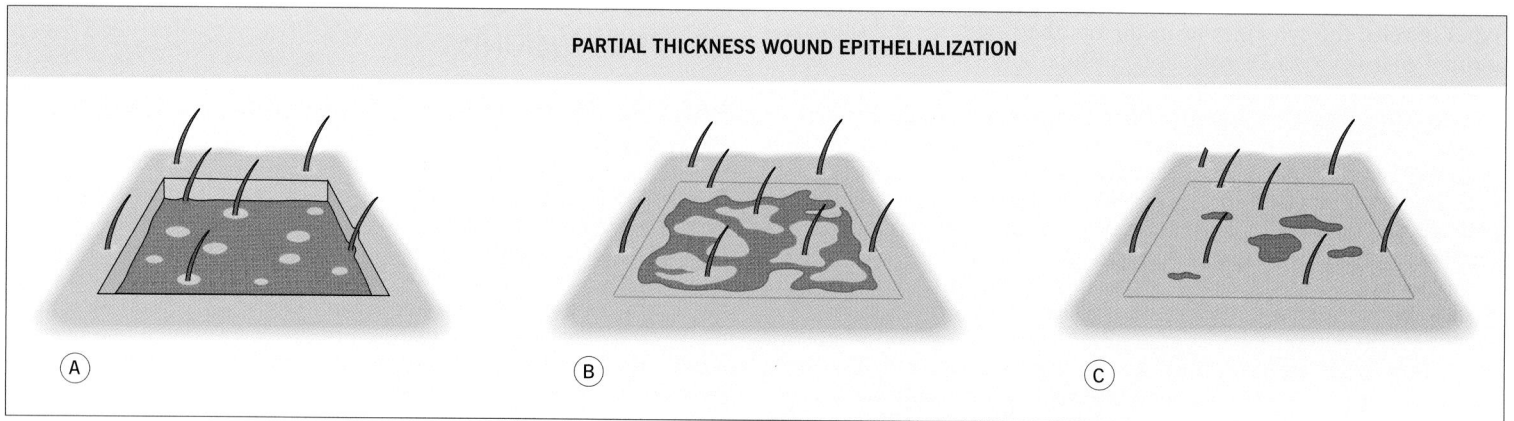

Fig. 141.3 **Partial-thickness wound epithelialization. A** The red is the wound bed and the pink areas within the wound bed represent the remaining adnexal structures. After partial-thickness wounding, microscopic adnexal structures remain as a source of keratinocytes. **B** During the first few days after wounding, cells migrate from both the wound edges and the adnexal structures and eventuate in epithelialization (**C**).

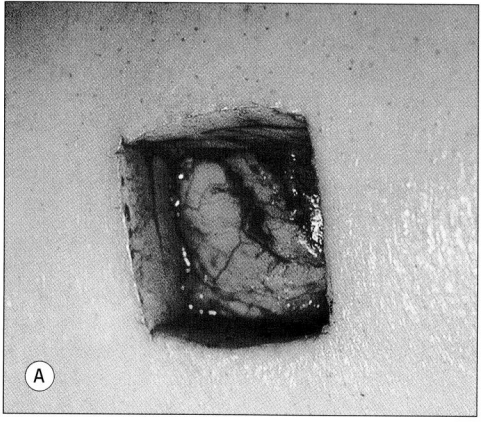
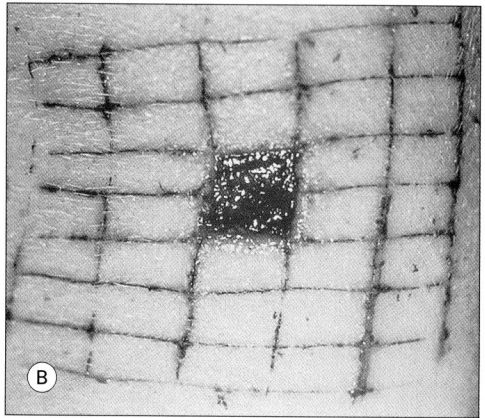
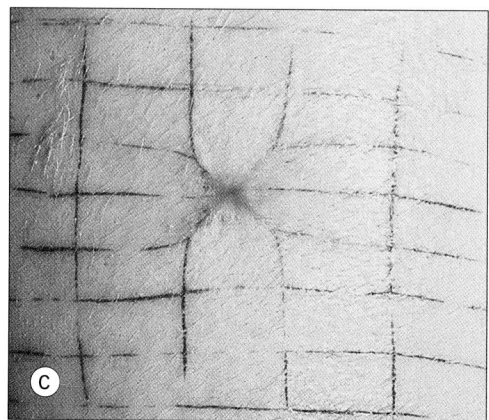

Fig. 141.4 **A full-thickness wound. A** A full-thickness wound is created in a porcine wound healing model. **B** The full-thickness wound that was created in the center of a tattoo grid has been allowed to granulate for several days. **C** Same wound as B, after healing. Note that contraction of the wound has occurred, which results in a distorted grid.

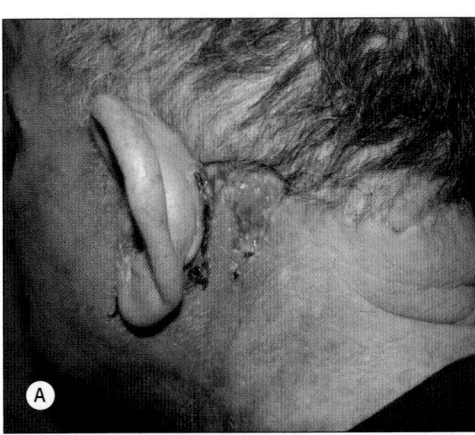

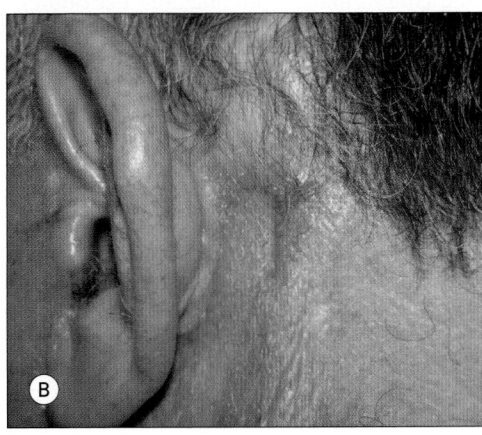

Fig 141.5 Tertiary intention healing. A Dehiscence of a primarily closed skin cancer excision site posterior to the left ear. **B** Same wound as A, 1 month later.

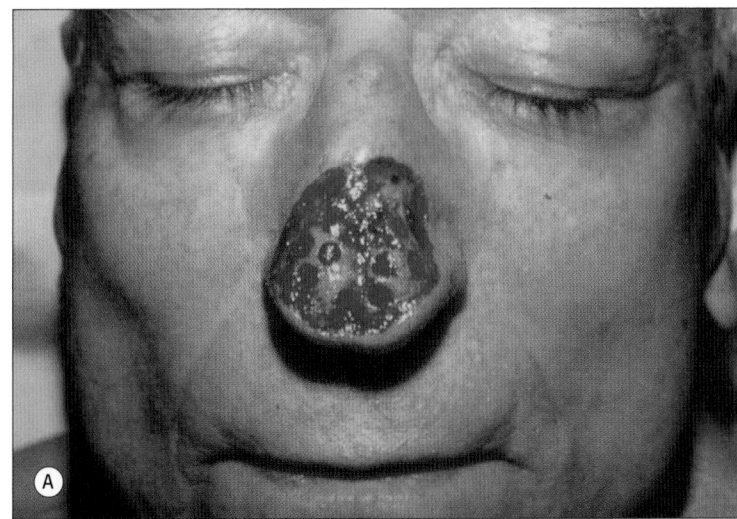

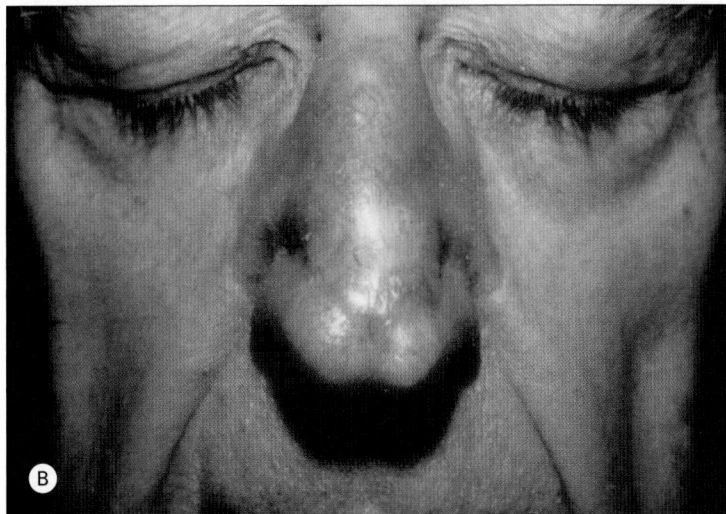

Fig 141.6 Second intention healing over cartilage. A Defect after excision of a skin cancer on the nose. The holes were created in the cartilage to allow granulation tissue formation. **B** Same wound as A, after healing by secondary intention. The presence of cartilage limited wound contracture.

and the ability of the individual to tolerate a surgical repair. In the case of secondary intention healing, wounds located in concavities and over fixed structures (Fig. 141.6) heal cosmetically better than those in other locations.

METHODS OF CREATING ACUTE WOUNDS

The method by which wounds are created may also influence their healing. Acute wounds can be created in a variety of ways. For example, a surgeon may utilize a scalpel (steel), a laser (heat), liquid nitrogen (cold) or chemicals (acid) to create a wound. Alternatively, a patient may develop an acute wound by a variety of methods such as burns or traumatic accidents. Depending upon how the wound was created, wounds heal differently and at different rates. In general, wounds created by steel heal faster than other methods of wounding. For example, surgical incisions heal faster than burn wounds, primarily because burns have a lag period prior to healing[4]. This is the rationale for debridement of burn wounds to speed their healing. Healing of traumatic wounds may be slowed due to foreign substances having been inoculated into the wound, leading to a prolongation of the inflammatory phase (discussed below).

PHASES OF WOUND HEALING

INFLAMMATORY PHASE

Overview and the Vascular Response

The initial reaction to wounding can be subdivided into cellular and vascular responses, and *in toto* they produce the inflammatory response. Platelets, the first cells to appear after wounding, not only aid in hemostasis but also initiate the healing cascade via the release of important growth factors such as platelet-derived growth factor (PDGF)[5]. Early in the wounding process, local vasodilation, fluid leakage into the extravascular space, and blocking of lymphatic drainage can produce the cardinal signs of inflammation, including rubor (redness), tumor (swelling) and calor (heat). This acute inflammatory reaction that is seen following the creation of a new wound usually lasts 24–48 hours and may be misinterpreted as an infectious process, since infection can

have a similar appearance. Although usually lasting 1–2 days, the inflammation may persist for up to 2 weeks in some patients. Should the inflammation persist, then it is referred to as chronic inflammation.

The most common acute wound, a surgical wound, serves as a good conceptual model. One can easily envision with an incisional wound that there is concomitant bleeding secondary to disruption of blood vessels and extravasation of red blood cells. Therefore, the first step in wound healing is hemostasis[2]. Hemostasis can be divided into two parts: development of a fibrin plug and coagulation (via the coagulation cascade).

With damage to endothelial cells and blood vessels, collagen is exposed. Platelets are stimulated at the wound site by locally generated thrombin as well as exposed fibrillar collagen; they then undergo activation, adhesion and aggregation. The amino acids proline and hydroxyproline that are found in collagen serve as important determinants in the initiation of platelet activation. Upon activation, platelets release a number of mediators found within their granules, including serotonin, adenosine diphosphate (ADP), thromboxane A_2, fibrinogen, fibronectin and thrombospondin. Induced by these chemicals and proteins, other passing platelets adhere to the exposed connective tissue at the site of injury in the endothelial wall and this leads to a relatively unstable platelet plug that may temporarily occlude small vessels sufficiently to slow or stop bleeding. Concomitantly, endothelial cells produce prostacyclin, which inhibits platelet aggregation and thus limits the extent of platelet aggregation to the site of injury.

Platelet-derived fibrinogen is converted to fibrin, which acts as a matrix for the influx of monocytes and fibroblasts[6]. Of note, platelets also produce PDGF, which is chemotactic and mitogenic for fibroblasts

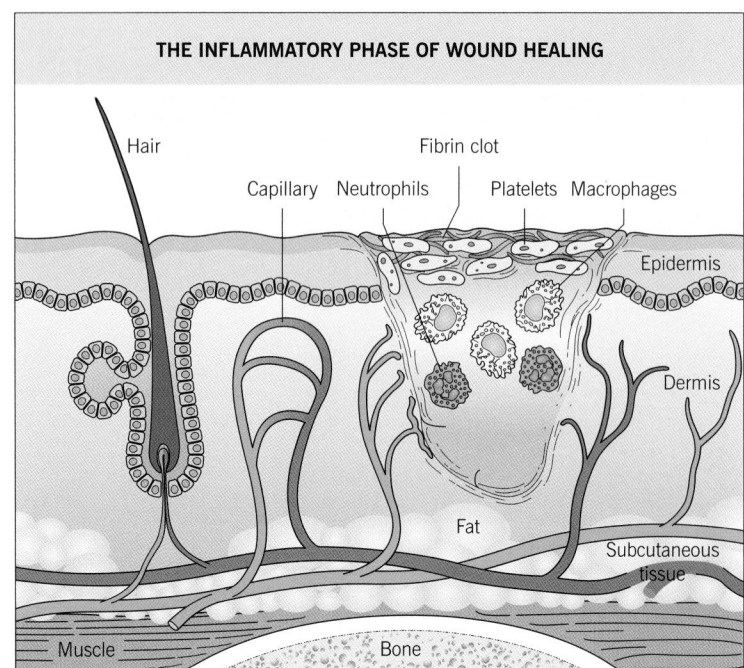

THE INFLAMMATORY PHASE OF WOUND HEALING

Hair

Fibrin clot

Capillary Neutrophils Platelets Macrophages

Epidermis

Dermis

Fat

Subcutaneous tissue

Muscle Bone

Fig. 141.7 The inflammatory phase of wound healing. Cells are recruited to the wound site and initiate a healing cascade mediated primarily by cytokines, including platelet-derived and macrophage-derived factors.

and smooth muscle cells *in vitro*[5]. In addition, PDGF is chemotactic for macrophages[7], monocytes and neutrophils[8], and thrombin-activated platelets possess angiogenic activity[9]. Through these functions, platelets clearly not only are important in hemostasis, but also significantly contribute to the regulation of fibrin deposition, fibroplasia and angiogenesis (Fig. 141.7).

As noted previously, platelet aggregation temporarily occludes small vessels enough to slow or stop bleeding. Whether or not prolonged vasoconstriction occurs, this process triggers the circulating enzyme Hageman factor XII to initiate clotting by converting prothrombin to thrombin, which in turn converts fibrinogen to fibrin (see Ch. 23). In addition to coagulation, thrombin has multiple effects on platelets, macrophages, fibroblasts and endothelial cells. However, deficiency of the thrombin receptor (protease-activated receptor 1), which mediates many of the effects of thrombin, does not alter normal wound healing[10].

Initial vasoconstriction leads damaged, small vessels to be pressed together, which induces a stickiness within the endothelial lining that is capable of occluding vessels even after active vasoconstriction has begun to relax. Almost immediately after injury, neutrophils begin to adhere to the sticky endothelium of venules. Within 1 hour after the onset of inflammation, the entire endothelial margin of the venules may be covered with neutrophils. Soon after this margination occurs, the neutrophils begin an amoeboid behavior by inserting narrow projections into the junctions between endothelial cells and releasing chemotactic factors. In the early inflammatory state, neutrophils (which have a survival time in the circulation of only a few hours) and monocytes are the predominant cells at the site of injury. Later in the inflammatory phase, the number of neutrophils declines and macrophages (tissue-derived monocytes) predominate.

Shortly after margination, histamine is released into the area from mast cells, basophils and platelets. This causes vasodilation and an increase in the endothelial wall permeability of venules to low-molecular-weight plasma proteins. Although the action of histamine action is very short-lived (probably lasting no longer than 30 minutes), its effects tend to last longer due to this increase in vascular wall permeability.

The Cellular Response

Leukocytes

The inflammatory phase of wound healing derives its name from the influx of white blood cells into the site of injury. Neutrophils, the first white blood cells to arrive, and monocytes are induced to migrate to the

wound by chemotactic factors produced by the coagulation cascade. These chemotactic factors, such as kallikrein, fibrinopeptides released from fibrinogen, and fibrin degradation products, also serve to upregulate the expression of important adhesion molecules that mediate cell–cell binding.

Upregulation of adhesion molecules allows leukocyte–endothelial cell interactions (see Ch. 102), which facilitate diapedesis of neutrophils. Endothelial cells, previously thought of as bystanders in inflammatory processes and wound healing, are now believed to play an active role in facilitating leukocyte migration. Neutrophils release elastase and collagenase, which likely enhance their passage through the blood vessel basement membrane. Once in the wound site, integrins found on the surface of neutrophils enhance cell–matrix interactions. This allows neutrophils to perform their functions of killing and phagocytosing bacteria as well as degrading matrix proteins within the wound bed. The presence of wound contamination prolongs the neutrophilic presence within the wound. Normally this lasts only a few days. However, the presence of neutrophils in the wound environment is not critical, as neutropenia does not interfere with wound healing in the absence of infection[11].

The eosinophil may also be involved in phagocytosis to some degree, but the basophil is not a phagocytic cell. Basophils contain histamine, which is released locally following injury and contributes to the early increased vascular permeability. When monocytes emigrate from the bloodstream into the tissue spaces, they are transformed into macrophages. Monocytes and their tissue counterparts, macrophages, soon become the dominant figures in the inflammatory phase. Monocytes are initially attracted to the wound site by some of the same chemoattractants that attract neutrophils, and their recruitment continues as a result of monocyte-specific chemoattractants. The latter include extracellular degradation products, thrombin and TGF-β[12].

Macrophages are critical to repair and are considered the most important regulatory cell in the inflammatory reaction as far as tissue healing is concerned. Along with other leukocytes, macrophages digest, phagocytose and kill pathogenic organisms, scavenge tissue debris and destroy any remaining neutrophils. After binding to the cellular membrane and subsequent phagocytosis, bacterial, cellular and tissue destruction is accomplished through release of biologically active oxygen intermediates and proteases. These all-important processes performed by the monocyte/macrophage allow for induction of angiogenesis and formation of granulation tissue.

Macrophages tolerate severe hypoxia well. This may explain why they are usually present within sites of chronic inflammation. In addition, macrophages release chemotactic factors (e.g. fibronectin) that attract fibroblasts to the wound and play a role in localizing inflammation; they also aid in the adhesion of fibroblasts to fibrin during the transition between the inflammatory and proliferative phases of wound repair. In this regard, macrophages may enhance collagen deposition, as their depletion markedly decreases the deposition of collagen within the wound[13]. In the absence of macrophages, fibroblasts migrate to the site of injury in considerably reduced numbers, and, when found, are somewhat immature.

The angiogenic potential of macrophages has also been demonstrated by the ability of macrophage-derived growth factor to induce neovascularization in the rat cornea model. New blood vessel growth follows the gradient of angiogenic factor produced by hypoxic macrophages (fully oxygenated or anoxic macrophages do not produce this angiogenic factor). If macrophages are removed from the tissue spaces, angiogenesis and wound debridement may be temporarily or permanently inhibited[11]. *In toto*, macrophages can be considered factories for growth factor production, synthesizing and secreting PDGF, fibroblast growth factor (FGF), vascular endothelial growth factor (VEGF), TGF-β and TGF-α[14]. These cytokines are important in inducing cell migration and proliferation as well as matrix production.

Chemical Mediators of Inflammation

A number of chemical mediators are involved in the initiation and control of inflammation (Table 141.1). These mediators work in concert, as some are protagonists and others antagonists of inflammation. While the actions of some of these substances may be synergistic, for others their precise role has not been clearly elucidated.

CHEMICAL MEDIATORS OF INFLAMMATION THAT PLAY A ROLE IN WOUND HEALING	
Chemical mediator	**Action**
Histamine	Increased vascular permeability
Serotonin	Stimulation of fibroblast proliferation Cross-linking of collagen molecules
Kinins	Increased vascular permeability
Prostaglandins	Increased vascular permeability Sensitize pain receptors Increased synthesis of GAGs
Complement	Increased vascular permeability Increased phagocytosis Enhanced bacterial lysis Mast cell and basophil activation

Table 141.1 Chemical mediators of inflammation that play a role in wound healing. GAGs, glycosaminoglycans.

Histamine

One of many products of the mast cell is histamine. In addition to histamine, mast cell granules, whose contents are released at the time of injury, contain a number of active compounds, including heparin and serotonin. Release of histamine leads in part to the initial short-lived increase in the permeability of venules – when mast cells are depleted of histamine or histamine receptors are blocked, the early increase in vascular permeability is prevented. Heparin, an anticoagulant, serves to temporarily prevent coagulation of the excess tissue fluid and blood components during the early phase of the inflammatory response.

Serotonin

Serotonin, or 5-hydroxytryptamine, is a potent vasoconstrictor, but it is unlikely that it has a significant effect on vascular permeability in humans. However, serotonin appears to be involved in other activities related to later phases of wound healing, such as fibroblast proliferation and the cross-linking of collagen molecules (see Ch. 94). Cross-linking of collagen molecules not only affects the tensile strength of newly formed desirable scar tissue, but also accounts for certain negative effects of scarring, such as the toughness and lack of resilience of unwanted fibrous tissue.

Kinins

The kinins are a family of biologically active and nearly indistinguishable peptides that are found in areas of tissue destruction. The most familiar kinin, bradykinin, is a potent inflammatory mediator released from plasma proteins in injured tissue by the plasma enzyme, kallikrein. The action of the kinins on the microvasculature is similar to that of histamine, i.e. potent vasodilation. Kinins are rapidly destroyed by tissue proteases, suggesting that their importance is limited to the early inflammatory stage of wound healing.

Prostaglandins

Prostaglandins (PGs) are produced by nearly all cells of the body in response to cell membrane injury. When cellular membranes are altered, their phospholipid content is degraded by the enzyme phospholipase A2 and this results in the formation of arachidonic acid. The oxidation of arachidonic acid by 5-lipoxygenase initiates the formation of a series of potent compounds, the leukotrienes. Several different types of leukotrienes combine to form what was previously referred to as 'the slow-reacting substance of anaphylaxis', which alters capillary permeability during the inflammatory reaction.

Arachidonic acid can also be oxidized by cyclooxygenase and this initiates the formation of PGs, prostacyclin and thromboxane (see Ch. 6). PGs are extremely potent biologic substances that exert marked effects in very low concentrations. Specific classes of PGs appear to control or perpetuate the local inflammatory response. For example, PGE_2 may increase vascular permeability by antagonizing vasoconstriction, and its chemotactic activity may attract leukocytes to the locally inflamed area. The PGs that are proinflammatory (e.g. PGE_2) act

synergistically with other inflammatory substances such as bradykinin. Proinflammatory PGs are thought to be responsible for sensitizing pain receptors, causing the state of hyperalgesia associated with the inflammatory reaction, while other classes of PGs act as inhibitors. Together, these opposing effects of various PGs lead to a tightly controlled response. PGs may also regulate repair processes during the early phases of healing by contributing to the synthesis of glycosaminoglycans (GAGs).

One action of corticosteroids (e.g. prednisone) and non-steroidal anti-inflammatory drugs (NSAIDs) is inhibition of PG synthesis via inhibition of cyclooxygenase activity. Suppressing the inflammatory response and its associated pain may be appropriate treatment for chronic inflammation but is usually not indicated for the normal acute inflammatory response.

Complement system

The complement system collectively represents a cascade of multiple proteins, many of which are enzyme precursors (see Ch. 59). All of these proteins may be present among the plasma proteins that leak from capillaries into the tissue spaces of a wound. Whether the cascade is triggered by the classical pathway (via antibody–antigen complexes) or the alternative pathway (via membranes of microorganisms), sequential reactions produce multiple end-products that help prevent damage by an invading organism or toxin. With regard to wound healing, some of the end-products activate phagocytosis by both neutrophils and macrophages, whereas others enhance lysis and agglutination of invading organisms (e.g. C5b–9). Still others activate mast cells and basophils to release histamine (e.g. C5a).

Growth factors

Numerous terms are used to designate growth factors, including cytokines, interleukins and colony-stimulating factors (see Ch. 5)[14]. This, coupled with the fact that the name of a growth factor does not necessarily identify its only or its primary biologic role, has made the nomenclature for growth factors quite confusing. For instance, PDGF is found in platelets, but is also found in keratinocytes and other cells[5]. These growth factors work through cell surface receptors and may bind to a single or multiple receptors. Growth factors can have an effect on the original cell of origin (autocrine mode), on neighboring cells (paracrine mode), or on distant cells (exocrine mode).

Chronic Inflammation

Most of the symptoms associated with the acute inflammatory response last approximately 2 weeks. After a subacute phase, inflammation persisting for months or years is referred to as chronic inflammation. Chronic inflammation associated with wounds often occurs when a wound is habitually sealed by necrotic tissue, is contaminated with pathogens, or contains foreign material that cannot be phagocytosed or solubilized by granulocytes during the acute inflammatory phase. Granulocytes disappear (through lysis and migration) with the resolution of the acute inflammatory phase, while mononuclear cells (specifically, lymphocytes, monocytes and macrophages), which are more resistant to lysis, increase in number and persist at the site of inflammation. Prolonged persistence and proliferation of mononuclear cells in chronically inflamed wounds may indicate the presence of foreign material. In particular, macrophages that have ingested foreign particulate material will remain in inflamed tissue if they are unable to solubilize the material. Macrophages attract fibroblasts, and over time the latter may produce increased quantities of collagen, leading to a slowly forming encapsulated granuloma (see Ch. 93). This is considered the body's last defense against a foreign material that cannot be phagocytosed or solubilized.

PROLIFERATIVE PHASE

The initial responses to injury provide the necessary framework for the production of a new functional barrier. In the proliferative phase of healing, cellular activity predominates. This phase involves the creation of a permeability barrier (re-epithelialization) as well as the establishment of an appropriate blood supply (neovascularization) and reinforcement of the injured tissue (fibroplasia; Figs 141.8 & 141.9).

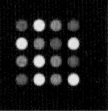

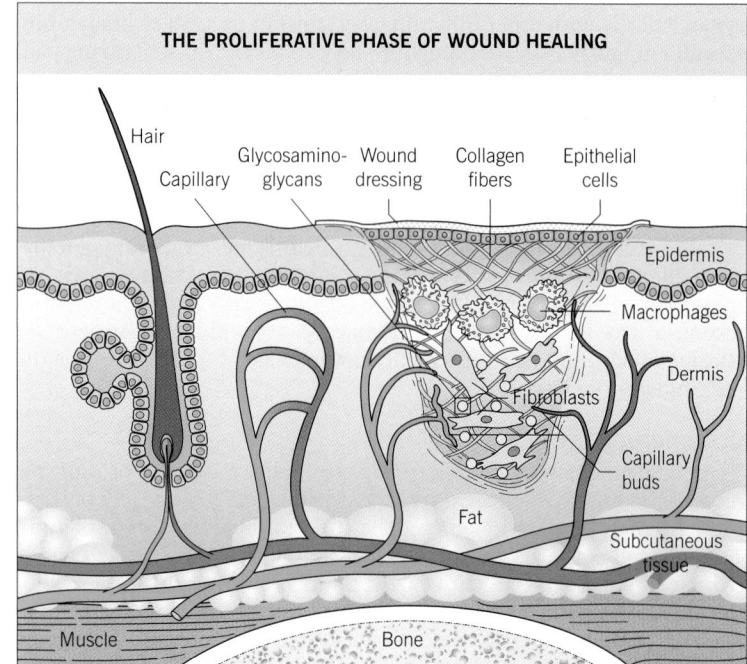

Fig. 141.8 **The proliferative phase of wound healing.** Deposition of matrix materials allows cells to proliferate, leading to the development of granulation tissue and re-epithelialization.

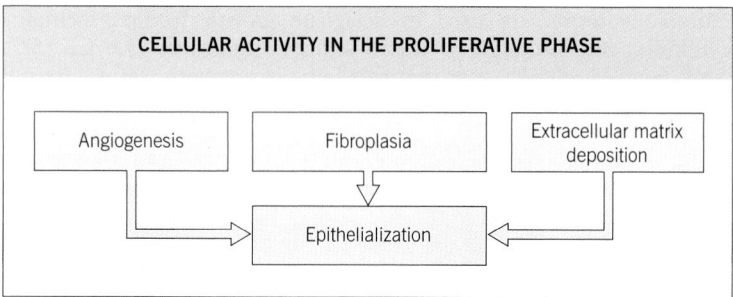

Fig. 141.9 **Cellular activity in the proliferative phase.**

Epidermis

Re-epithelialization

The epidermis reacts to the defect caused by injury within 24 hours. Keratinocytes initially respond to an epidermal defect by migrating from the free edge of the wound. Epidermal cell migration in partial-thickness wounds, which have remaining adnexal structures, occurs from both the wound edges and from skin appendages, in particular the hair follicles. Epidermal stem cells from the hair follicle are now thought to originate from the hair bulge, which is believed to be the germinative portion of the hair (see Ch. 67)[15,16].

Approximately 12 hours after wounding, epidermal cells become somewhat flattened, develop pseudopod-like projections and lose their desmosomal intercellular attachments, retract their intracellular tonofilaments, and form actin filaments at the edge of the cell cytoplasm. While epidermal cells are migrating, their proliferative potential is inhibited. The migrating keratinocytes from the basal layer are thought to differ from normal resting basal cells and may express selective cell surface markers such as CD44 as well as some markers usually expressed by keratinocytes above the basal layer[16].

Re-epithelialization of the wound surface may occur in several ways[3]. The classic mechanism of epithelial cell migration over the wound surface is the 'leap frog' model[3,17] (Fig. 141.10), where epidermal cells migrate two or three cell-lengths from their initial position and slide or roll over epidermal cells previously implanted in the wound. The migrating cell becomes fixed, and other epidermal cells successively migrate over these cells. The epidermal layer progressively advances and closes the epithelial defect. A single layer of epidermal cells can

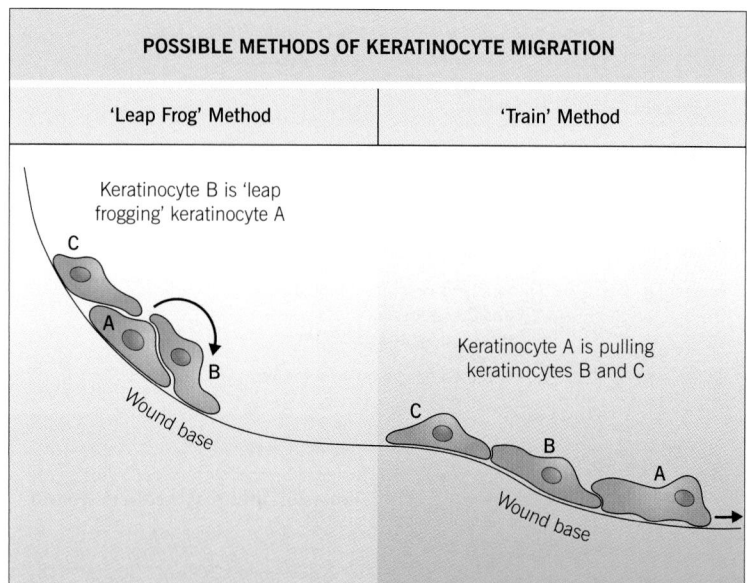

Fig. 141.10 **Possible methods of keratinocyte migration.**

resurface a wound during the first week of healing if frictional trauma to the site is prevented.

A second proposed method of re-epithelialization is where epidermal cells migrate across a wound surface as a 'train' of epidermal cells, with each cell maintaining its original position in the chain. Characteristic of this migrating epidermal tongue is the loss of tight binding between epidermal cells and the basement membrane and underlying dermis. Fibronectin appears to be instrumental in allowing continual epidermal migration. An early provisional matrix formed by fibrin, fibronectin and type V collagen enables keratinocytes to migrate and dissect under eschar and debris covering the wound[18]. Keratinocytes dissect under eschar because a moist environment is necessary for their migration and may be one reason for the success of occlusive dressings in speeding wound healing. Fibronectin is produced from plasma initially, and from plasma and fibroblasts later, and may also be derived from the migrating keratinocytes themselves. This suggests that the migrating tongue of epithelial cells may provide its own lattice for continued migration. Among the stimuli for re-epithelialization thought to be important are TGF-β, keratinocyte growth factor (KGF) and epidermal growth factor (EGF).

Another example of the active role of basal keratinocytes in cell migration is their secretion of collagenase-1 when in contact with fibrillar collagen but not while on intact basement membrane[19]. This production of collagenase-1 by basal keratinocytes disrupts any attachment to fibrillar collagen and allows for continued migration of keratinocytes. Once the wound is epithelialized, keratinocytes bind to $\alpha_2\beta_1$ integrin and production of collagenase-1 ceases. This specificity with regard to collagenase-1 impacts not only on the outcome of epithelial migration, but also on the maintenance of the directionality of the migrating tongue of epithelium.

Just proximal to these migrating cells are actively proliferating cells, which lie between the migrating tongue of epithelium and the normal cells at the wound edge. Once the wound is covered with at least a single layer of keratinocytes, all of the keratinocytes enter the proliferative mode. Among the growth factors important in this rapid proliferation are EGF and its homologue TGF-α. Wounding also induces expression of keratins 6, 16 and 17 by epidermal keratinocytes, and mouse embryos lacking keratin 17 show a striking delay in wound closure[20]. Recently, this cytoskeleton protein was shown to be able to regulate the cell growth of keratinocytes by influencing protein synthesis[21].

The basement membrane zone changes in several ways after wounding. Two important basement membrane proteins, laminin and type IV collagen, which normally mediate epidermal–dermal adhesion, disappear. In fact, the presence of these proteins appears to retard epidermal cell migration *in vitro*. Within 7–9 days after the reformation of the functional barrier of the skin, the basement membrane zone returns to normal. Bullous pemphigoid antigen is the first detected component of the basement membrane, followed by laminin and then type IV collagen. Synthesis of these last two components begins only after the epidermal cells have ceased migrating.

Factors affecting wound epithelialization

Local factors that adversely affect wound healing include: (1) poor surgical techniques, e.g. excessive tension or excess devitalized tissue; (2) vascular disorders, e.g. arteriosclerosis or venous insufficiency; (3) tissue ischemia; (4) infectious processes[22]; (5) certain topically applied medications[23–26], e.g. potent corticosteroids, iodine; (6) hemostatic agents such as aluminum chloride or ferric subsulfate[27]; (7) foreign body reactions; and (8) an adverse wound microenvironment, e.g. the use of dry as opposed to occlusive dressings. In addition, pressure, neuropathy and chronic radiation injury all adversely affect wound healing.

Systemic factors that may be detrimental to wound healing include malnutrition, insufficient protein intake[28], and vitamin A or C deficiency. Systemic medications such as corticosteroids, penicillamine, nicotine, NSAIDs and antineoplastic agents may interfere with the wound healing process at various stages and often arrest progress, resulting in a poorly healing or non-healing wound[29]. Chronic debilitating illnesses (e.g. hepatic, renal, hematopoietic, cardiovascular, autoimmune, oncologic), endocrine disorders (e.g. diabetes mellitus, Cushing's syndrome), systemic vascular disorders (e.g. vasculitis, atherosclerosis), and connective tissue disease (e.g. Ehlers–Danlos syndrome) often have adverse effects on wound healing. Finally, advancing age contributes to poor wound healing, possibly through impaired expression of metalloproteinases[30].

The Dermis

Angiogenesis

Angiogenesis refers to new vessel growth or neovascularization. There are at least three ways angiogenesis occurs in wounds: the generation of a *de novo* vascular network in the wound space; anastomosis to pre-existing vessels (i.e. naturally occurring grafts); and the coupling or recoupling of vessels throughout the wound space. From existing blood vessels adjacent to the wound, new capillary buds extend into the wound itself. Neovascularization involves a phenotypic alteration of endothelial cells, directed migration, and various mitogenic stimuli.

Similar to the migrating tongue of epithelium, endothelial cells at the tip of capillaries migrate into the wound but do not undergo active proliferation[31]. This early aspect of neovascularization depends upon chemotactic factors supplied by neighboring cells and matrix. A pre-existing extracellular matrix and the 'free edge effect' (absence of neighboring endothelial cells) are essential for formation of new vessels[32]. On day 2 post wounding, cytoplasmic pseudopodia extend from the endothelial cells, collagenase is secreted, and migration into the perivascular space occurs[33]. Proliferation of endothelial cells, on the other hand, has been postulated to be a secondary effect of cell migration. As a result, fibronectin, heparin and platelet factors that are known to stimulate endothelial cell migration into the wound also directly or indirectly stimulate endothelial cell proliferation.

Endothelial cells have a critical role during the wound healing process, including formation of new blood vessels, allowing for leukocyte migration, providing for transport of oxygen and nutrients into the wound, and secretion of biologically active substances. Cytokines released by cells such as macrophages stimulate angiogenesis during wound healing, as does low oxygen tension, lactic acid and biogenic amines[34]. The presence of low oxygen tension or hypoxia in wounds may also be a potent stimulus for TGF-β and collagen synthesis and may be the cause of excess fibrosis observed in certain chronic wounds[35].

The family of fibroblast growth factors (FGFs) and vascular endothelial growth factor (VEGF) are also potent stimuli for angiogenesis during healing[15]. Two forms of FGF exist, acidic FGF and basic FGF. Basic FGF, the more potent of the two (after injury takes place), interacts with heparin and enhances new vessel growth. The family of FGFs is secreted by macrophages and fibroblasts during cutaneous wound healing. In the presence of VEGF, activated vascular endothelial cells undergo the consecutive steps of angiogenesis, whereas in the absence of VEGF, vascular endothelial cells undergo apoptosis (see Ch. 102 for details). Thrombospondins are endogenous inhibitors of skin angiogenesis, and while overexpression may result in impaired

granulation tissue formation and wound vascularization, decreased expression may lead to enhanced skin vascularization.

Fibroplasia

Granulation tissue, a sign that healing is progressing, consists of new vessels that migrate into the wound as well as the accumulation of fibroblasts and ground substances (Fig. 141.11). The cell that is most important in the production of the dermal matrix is the fibroblast. Fibroblasts migrate into the wound between 48 and 72 hours. Chemotactic factors for fibroblasts are complex, but are, in part, derived from macrophages already present in the wound. Fibroblasts perform several functions and may undergo phenotypic changes over a period of time in order to accomplish these different functions[15]. However, it is possible that certain subpopulations of these cells exist (similar to lymphocytes) and these individual subpopulations may perform different roles during wound healing.

Fibroblasts initially undergo a phenotypic change whereby cellular organelles retract within the cell and the myofibroblast, a spindle-shaped cell, proliferates and migrates into the wound[36]. Having electron microscopic characteristics of both smooth muscle cells and fibroblasts, these cells contain abundant rough endoplasmic reticulum needed for the production of large amounts of matrix proteins. Myofibroblasts participate in wound contraction, with actin filaments aligning along the cell periphery to allow movement and contractile strength[36]. Fibroblast growth factors and chemoattractants are likely inducing factors for fibroblasts to undergo their change in shape and to synthesize matrix, with fibroblast proliferation and migration being modulated by PDGF, EGF and FGF, among others[37,38]. Fibroblast proliferation is stimulated by a low oxygen environment found in the center of the wound. As angiogenesis proceeds with the formation of new vessels and increased oxygen-carrying capacity, this stimulus diminishes.

The myofibroblast provides structure and synthesizes fibronectin, collagen, GAGs, thrombospondin and various enzymes[39]. Fibronectin, a glycoprotein, is initially secreted and provides for enhanced myofibroblast activity. Thrombin and EGF stimulate fibronectin synthesis and secretion. Fibronectin allows fibroblasts to bind to the extracellular matrix and provides an adherent base for cell migration, allowing fibroblasts to attach to collagen, fibrin and hyaluronic acid[40]. The fibronectin matrix also provides a scaffolding for collagen fibrils and mediates wound contraction. The vectors of fibroblast migration into the wound are directed by fibronectin's molecular and gross fibrillar structure and therefore it plays a critical role in the speed and direction of dermal repair. Fibroblasts migrate by pulling themselves along a fibronectin matrix, which occurs by contraction of intracellular microfilaments such as actin.

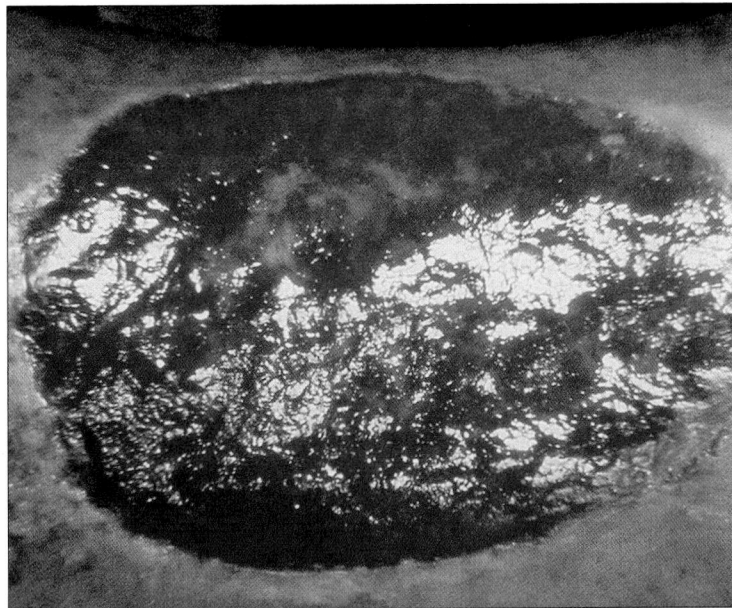

Fig. 141.11 Granulation tissue characterizes the proliferative phase with angiogenesis and fibroplasia.

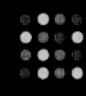

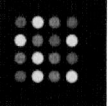
Phenotypic changes that occur in the fibroblast correlate with the cell's various roles in wound healing. First fibroblasts migrate and then later they produce large amounts of matrix materials, including collagen, proteoglycans and elastin[41]. As was the case for fibroblast proliferation, optimal conditions for fibroblasts to produce matrix proteins consist of an acidic, low-oxygen environment. However, wound environments that are anoxic inhibit collagen cross-linking, as oxygen is a necessary cofactor. Vitamin C is also a cofactor for collagen cross-linking[42], and individuals with vitamin C deficiency suffer from poor wound healing.

Several different types of collagen exist, sharing in common a triple-helical structure (see Ch. 94). While type I collagen is the major collagen in normal adult dermis, type III collagen, present in large quantities in fetal dermis, is a minority component of normal adult dermis. However, during early wound healing, type III collagen is the predominant type of collagen synthesized. It first appears after 48–72 hours and is maximally secreted between 5 and 7 days. TGF-β stimulates both types I and III collagen *in vitro*, and likely serves as a potent stimulus for collagen production *in vivo*. Excess TGF-β has been found in the dermis of chronic venous ulcers and may play a role in the fibrosis associated with that and other diseases (e.g. scleroderma)[43].

Extracellular matrix

Connective tissues are composed of three elements: cells, fibers and amorphous ground substance. Fibers and ground substance collectively are referred to as extracellular matrix (see Ch. 94), and GAGs and proteoglycans (GAGs covalently linked to proteins) are major components of the ground substance. The latter is an amorphous viscous gel secreted by fibroblasts, which occupies the spaces between the cells and fibers of connective tissue. Ground substance helps determine compliance, flexibility and integrity of the dermis as well as providing strength, support and density to the tissue; it reduces friction between connective tissue fibers during tissue stress or strain and protects against tissue invasion by microorganisms. Ground substance allows tissue fluid, which contains nutrients for the cells as well as waste products, to diffuse among cells and capillaries. It also transports many soluble substances and stores electrolytes and water, the other two primary components of ground substance (in addition to GAGs and proteoglycans).

Hyaluronic acid is the primary non-sulfated GAG found within the extracellular matrix of the wound[8] (see Table 46.1). It is found in the highest amounts during the first 4–5 days of healing. Hyaluronic acid serves as a stimulus for fibroblast proliferation and migration[44] and can absorb large amounts of water, producing tissue edema. This swelling provides additional space for the migration of fibroblasts into the wound. Hyaluronidase enzymatically degrades hyaluronic acid once the need for hyaluronic acid diminishes.

Sulfated GAGs, e.g. chondroitin sulfate, dermatan sulfate, are attached to a protein core and are therefore proteoglycans (see Ch. 94). They provide a stable and resilient matrix that inhibits cell migration and proliferation. Chondroitin-4-sulfate and dermatan sulfate eventually replace hyaluronic acid as the major GAGs on days 5–7. Saccharide chains in the chondroitin sulfate–protein complex cross-link to collagenous fibers. These sulfated GAGs promote collagen synthesis and maturation (i.e. polymerization). Of note, levels of GAGs, especially chondroitin sulfate, are increased in pathologic states such as Dupuytren's contracture or hypertrophic scarring. Lastly, heparan sulfate (another proteoglycan), absent initially after wounding, controls cell division and inhibits the growth of smooth muscle cells.

The mechanism of wound contraction

For full-thickness wounds, contraction begins soon after wounding and peaks at 2 weeks. In these wounds, the defect is deeper than the adnexa, and contraction is an important component of wound healing, accounting for up to a 40% decrease in the size of the wound. In contrast, in partial-thickness wounds, portions of the adnexa remain and allow epithelialization to occur from within the wound. Therefore, partial-thickness wounds contract less than full-thickness wounds and in direct proportion to their depth. As a result, superficial wounds contract little, if at all. Wound contraction also varies from species to species, generally being less in humans than in many animals.

Because of their ability to extend and retract, myofibroblasts are the predominant mediator of this contractile process. Myofibroblasts

contain one of the highest concentrations of actinomyosin of any cell type. The cells within the wound align along the lines of contraction and differ from the other cellular components, including leukocytes and endothelial cells, which do not exhibit such organized orientation. This muscle-like contraction of myofibroblasts is mediated by PGF₁, 5-hydroxytryptamine, angiotensin, vasopressin, bradykinins, epinephrine and norepinephrine. The contraction is unified and requires cell–cell and cell–matrix communication.

The rate of wound contraction is proportional to the cell number and inversely proportional to the lattice collagen concentration[45]. Cytoplasmic pseudopodia extend, attach to collagen fibers and then retract, drawing the collagen fibers to the cell, thereby producing wound contraction. Fibronectin not only provides the multiple functions described previously but also assists in wound contraction. *In vitro*, fibronectin has been localized to the matrix surrounding myofibroblasts in monolayers of healing human and hamster fibroblasts. Fibroblasts within wounds express fibronectin receptors, and fibronectin contains an actin-binding site. Lastly, wound contraction can be inhibited by smooth muscle relaxants, but thus far this has proved impractical.

REMODELING PHASE

Remodeling, the third phase of wound repair, consists of the deposition of matrix materials and their subsequent change over time (Fig. 141.12). Dermal macromolecules such as fibronectin, hyaluronic acid, proteoglycans and collagen are deposited during repair and serve as a scaffold for cellular migration and tissue support. Deposition and remodeling of the extracellular matrix proteins are dynamic processes and differences in amounts of matrix proteins occur even between the center and periphery of the wound.

Long after the skin's functional barrier is restored, events continue to occur that are related to wound injury and repair. The total amount of collagen increases early in repair, reaching a maximum between 2 and 3 weeks after injury. Tensile strength, a functional assessment of collagen, increases to 40% of preinjury strength at 1 month post injury and may continue to increase for up to a year. Even at its peak, tensile strength of the healed wound is never greater than 80% of its preinjury strength[46].

During the remodeling phase, there are changes in the types of collagen present and synthesized. While type III collagen is the major

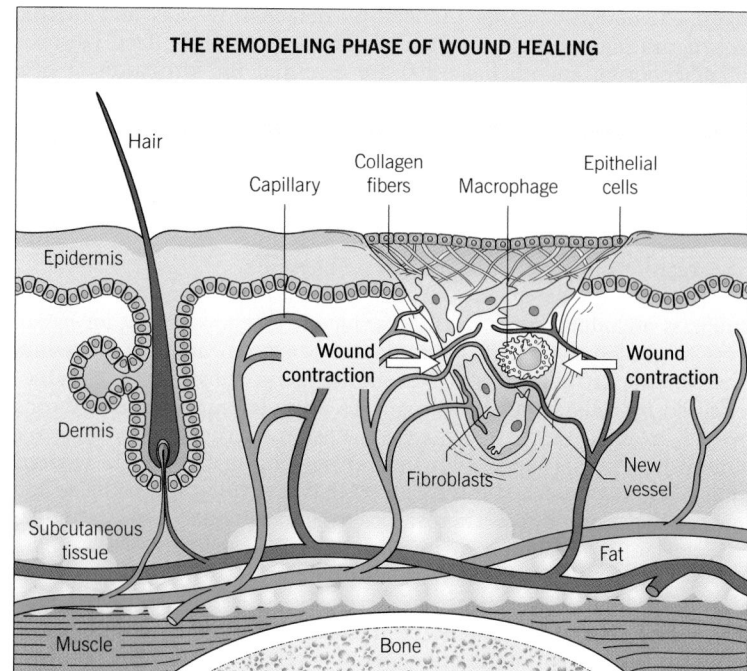

Fig. 141.12 The remodeling phase of wound healing. During the remodeling phase of wound healing, deposition of matrix materials and their subsequent change over time occurs. The process includes converting a dermis of predominantly type III collagen to one of predominantly type I collagen, which is accomplished via a tightly controlled synthesis of new and lysis of old collagen.

type of collagen synthesized by fibroblasts during wound repair, over the period of a year or more, the remodeling dermis must return to the stable, preinjury phenotype, consisting largely of type I collagen. In addition, the composition of other matrix material within the wound changes as the amount of water content and GAGs decreases. The process of converting a dermis of predominantly type III collagen to one of predominantly type I collagen is accomplished via a tightly controlled synthesis of new and lysis of old collagen, the latter being accomplished through the actions of collagenases. This leads to a change in the orientation of scar tissue. The collagen that escapes the action of collagenases is that which was initially laid down parallel to the lines of tension.

Collagen

Collagen is the principal protein providing structure, strength and stiffness to dermal tissue. Collagenous fibers constitute approximately 70% of the skin's dry weight and have a high tensile strength; because these bundles are relatively inextensible and non-elastic, they resist stretching, mechanical forces and deformation[47]. The collagenous fibers do, however, form a loose interlacing network that is deformable. The fibers align in directions that accommodate applied stress, thereby allowing skin to stretch[47].

Collagen varies genetically and structurally. Type I collagen, the most prevalent form, accounts for approximately 90% of the collagen in the body. It is found in dermis, tendons, fascia, bone and teeth. Type III collagen is found in embryonic connective tissue and, in adults, in reticular networks of the deep dermis, blood vessels and wounds. All collagens possess triple-helical structures but differ in the primary structure of their polypeptide chains (see Ch. 94).

The first collagen to be produced during wound repair is highly disorganized and gel-like, yielding poor wound strength. Initially, the collagen is structurally similar to type III collagen. With wound closure, a gradual turnover of collagen occurs. As type III collagen undergoes degradation, type I collagen is synthesized. The stimulus for conversion from type III collagen to type I collagen may be the biomechanical stress and strain placed across a closed wound. Stress and strain also may direct realignment of connective tissue fibers; as noted previously, collagenous fibers under tension appear to be resistant to the action of collagenase, whereas random fibers not under tension are susceptible to lysis by collagenase. The amount of stress on the wound is responsible for how much scar tissue forms. For example, more scar tissue is necessary in wounds that are on mobile extremities than in a less mobile area such as the abdomen.

The diameters of collagenous fibers also vary within the dermis. Type I collagenous fibrils range in diameter from 100 to 500 nm, whereas type III collagenous fibrils range from 40 to 60 nm. In addition to the amount of total collagen and collagen cross-linkages, the ratio of larger-diameter fibrils to smaller-diameter fibrils ultimately determines the tissue tensile strength.

Biosynthesis of collagen

Collagen biosynthesis is reviewed in detail in Chapter 94. Both magnesium and zinc (trace minerals) are needed for translation to occur, whereas hydroxylation of proline and lysine requires oxygen, ferrous iron and ascorbic acid (vitamin C).

Collagenase

Three main types of enzymes have the ability to degrade and digest collagen: (1) bacterial collagenase; (2) lysosomal proteases; and (3) tissue collagenase. However, before these enzymes can work, other enzymes (e.g. hyaluronidase, other proteases) must expose the collagen fibrils by removing non-collagen substances. Then, these three groups of enzymes are able to function to restore the postinjury dermis towards normalcy. The first two groups work upon fragmented collagen that has been previously digested and phagocytosed. The third group, the tissue collagenases, is the most important of the set of enzymes that can digest collagen. Epithelial cells, fibroblasts, macrophages and leukocytes all secrete tissue collagenases under appropriate stimulation[48]. All of the tissue collagenases are similar in that they require calcium to function and are inhibited by chelating agents such as EDTA.

The collagenases, along with stromelysins and gelatinases, belong to a family of proteinases known as matrix metalloproteinases (MMPs; Table 141.2). With a few exceptions (matrilysin produced in eccrine glands, gelatinase A stored but not produced in healthy tissue), MMPs are not expressed in healthy resting tissue but rather expressed in physiologic (repair, remodeling, proliferation) or pathologic states (inflammation, tumor growth). MMPs have the ability to degrade extracellular matrix, and substrate specificity is an important issue with regard to the action of MMPs. Collagenase-1 and collagenase-2 specifically cleave fibrillar collagen (types I, II, III) in a site-specific fashion[19]. Thus, the actions of these enzymes are the rate-limiting step in the turnover of the major protein component of the extracellular matrix, collagen. After this site-specific cleavage, at body temperature, collagen will denature (turn into gelatin) and be susceptible to further degradation by the gelatinases.

Elastic fibers

Elastic fibers are long, thin, wavy and highly retractile, and they are entwined amongst the collagenous fibers. Elastin, a highly hydrophobic structural protein, provides elasticity and extensibility to the dermis and assists in recovery from deformation; however, it comprises only 2% of the total protein within the dermis[49]. The structure and function of elastic fibers are discussed in Chapter 94. Elastin, lipids and glycoproteins bind to form microfibrils that serve as the scaffolding or foundation for fiber orientation.

Reticular fibers

Reticular fibers are very fine, thin fibrils. Functionally, reticular fibers form a supporting framework for many organs and glands and reticular fibers form a framework upon which collagenous fibers are laid down. As the least prevalent fiber in the connective tissue substrate, reticulin is found in small numbers in normal skin. However, in early phases of healing, reticulin does increase in amount.

Factors Affecting Connective Tissue Repair

Connective tissue repair is affected by several factors, including blood supply, available proteins, minerals, amino acids and enzymes, circulating hormones, mechanical stress and infection. Lack of cellular oxygen impedes wound healing and leads to a decrease in the strength of the resultant tissue. Hypoxia that occurs without neovascularization

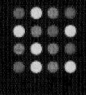

DIFFERENT TYPES OF METALLOPROTEINASES INVOLVED IN WOUND REPAIR	
Enzyme	**MMP number**
Collagenase-1	MMP-1
Collagenase-2	MMP-8
Collagenase-3	MMP-13
Collagenase-4	MMP-18
Stromelysin-1	MMP-3
Stromelysin-2	MMP-10
Stromelysin-3	MMP-11
Gelatinase-A	MMP-2
Gelatinase-B	MMP-9
Matrilysin	MMP-7
Macrophage metalloproteinase (elastase)	MMP-12
MT1-MMP	MMP-14
MT2-MMP	MMP-15
MT3-MMP	MMP-16
MT4-MMP	MMP-17

Table 141.2 Different types of metalloproteinases (MMPs) involved in wound repair. MT1, membrane-type 1.

reduces energy production. In addition, tissue oxygen tension is important in collagen synthesis and, therefore, tensile strength of wounds[50].

Other factors that may hinder wound healing include medications such as antineoplastic agents and antibiotics. Penicillin, for example, decreases cross-linking of collagen and, therefore, impairs the strength of the wound. This does not appear, however, to be of clinical importance. Radiation and exposure to cold also have a detrimental effect on healing. Malnutrition, in which inadequate protein intake impairs healing, may result in decreased wound strength owing to a reduction in collagen synthesis[51].

Whether collagen biosynthesis is retarded or potentiated depends on available minerals and vitamins. Lack of available ascorbic acid (vitamin C) impedes the hydroxylation of amino acids needed during collagen synthesis. Without ascorbic acid, underhydroxylated collagen is produced and, consequently, the collagen fails to aggregate into fibers. In persons with vitamin C deficiency, reopening of old wounds has actually occurred.

Vitamin A also potentiates epithelial repair and collagen synthesis by enhancing inflammatory reactions, particularly macrophage availability[52]. Therefore, its absence slows repair. Minerals also may affect healing. Zinc depletion reduces the rate of epithelialization and retards cellular proliferation, and dietary zinc deficiency has been shown to decrease wound strength[53].

A direct relationship exists between available macrophages and fibroblast production. In fact, if the initial inflammatory process is blocked by the use of systemic corticosteroids during the first 3 days after wounding, healing time is retarded, with a resultant loss of skin turgor. Furthermore, the mitotic activity of fibroblasts is suppressed by corticosteroids. The suppression of wound healing caused by corticosteroids has been shown to be ameliorated with administration of local and systemic vitamin A[52], and a single injection of TGF-β[54].

Ways to Speed Healing of Acute Wounds

In acute wounds, wound edges may be brought together in direct apposition to one another with the use of sutures or Steri-Strips™. Performed in a clean wound using aseptic technique, the apposition of the wound edges decreases or eliminates the distance that cells need to migrate. Aseptic surgical technique minimizes the risk of bacterial contamination, which can prolong healing. Prevention of hematoma formation through proper hemostasis and elimination of necrotic tissue also decreases the chance for infection.

Surgical techniques involving steel instruments, as opposed to electrosurgery or cryosurgery, decrease the risk for infection because less necrotic tissue is produced and healing is faster. Elimination of dead space through the appropriate use of buried deep sutures also lessens the risk for hematoma formation and subsequent infection. However, wounds closed too tightly with sutures may become ischemic and subsequently necrotic at the edges, and healing is then delayed. For large wounds (e.g. burns, trauma, abdominal or cardiac surgeries), vacuum-assisted closure (VAC) can be used to reduce infection and enhance healing. This procedure entails placing a sponge into the wound, applying an occlusive dressing, and attaching a suction device that removes fluid from the wound.

The intelligent use of occlusive dressings can be very effective in speeding wound healing (see Ch. 145). Stemming from observations that blisters that remained roofed healed faster than those that had their roof removed, it was found that wounds covered with an occlusive dressing healed up to 40% faster than those left air-exposed[55]. Why occlusive dressings work is not entirely understood. Among the ways occlusive dressings might function include enhancement of keratinocyte migration by maintenance of a moist environment, prevention of infection, establishment of an electromagnetic current, or containment of wound fluid and the growth factors present within it. In addition to speeding the rate of healing, occlusive dressings also decrease pain and improve the cosmetic outcome of wounds healed by both primary and secondary intention[55].

The use of autologous and allogeneic grafts can also speed healing of acute wounds (Fig. 141.13), and there have been recent attempts via bioengineering to include viable blood vessels within these grafts. Several growth factors, including PDGF, growth hormone, EGF and FGF, have been shown to speed healing of acute wounds in various settings, and although recombinant PDGF (becaplermin) is commercially available, currently it is only Food and Drug Administration (FDA)-approved for the treatment of diabetic ulcers (see Ch. 105). The details of several of the studies utilizing growth factors for wounds are outlined in Table 141.3.

Future Directions (Table 141.4)

In addition to the potential role of cytoskeleton proteins, e.g. keratin 17 (see above), recent studies have also examined the impact of the innate immune system on wound healing[56]. Manipulation of several of its components may lead to improved wound repair. While the effects of

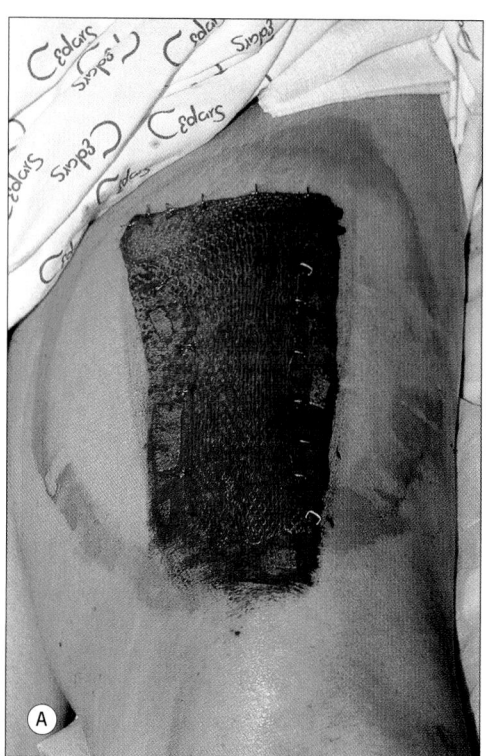

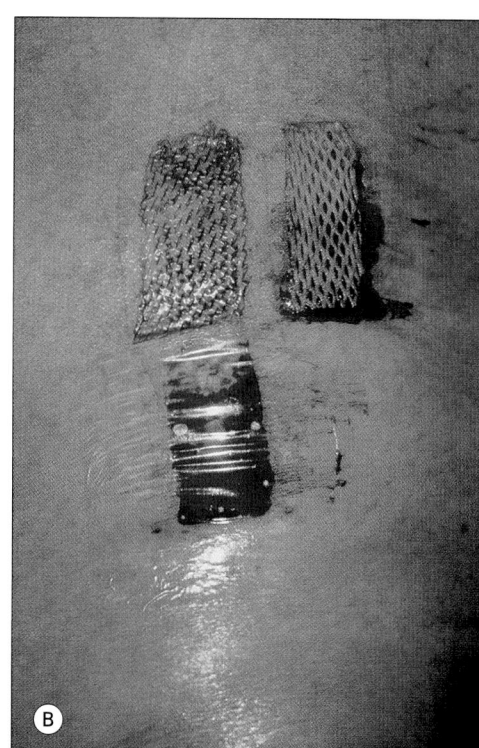

Fig. 141.13 Split-thickness skin graft donor sites regrafted to speed healing. A Donor site regrafted with meshed and pinch autografts to speed healing. **B** Comparison of donor sites treated with meshed bilayered allogeneic living skin equivalent (top left), meshed autograft (top right), and polyurethane film dressing (bottom left). The meshed bilayered allogeneic living skin equivalent and the meshed autograft both sped healing compared to the film dressing.

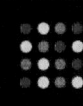

Table 141.3 — GROWTH FACTORS FOUND TO SPEED HEALING OF ACUTE WOUNDS IN HUMANS

Growth factor	Wound type	Reference
Platelet-derived growth factor (PDGF)	Full-thickness punch biopsy sites Surgical wound separation	J Am Acad Dermatol. 2001; 145:857–62 Am J Obstet Gynecol. 2002; 186:701–4
Epidermal growth factor (EGF)	Donor site wounds	N Engl J Med. 1989;321:76–9
Fibroblast growth factor (FGF)	Burn wounds	Lancet. 1998;352;1661–4
Growth hormone	Donor sites in burned children	Ann Surg. 1990;212:430–1

Table 141.3 Growth factors found to speed healing of acute wounds in humans.

FUTURE DIRECTIONS IN WOUND HEALING

Gene therapy (e.g. PDGF)
Stem cell therapy (bone marrow-derived)
Microarray analysis of healing and nonhealing wounds
Novel anti-inflammatory agents (e.g. adenosine agonists, lactoferrin)
Stimulation of angiogenesis (e.g. nicotinic receptor agonists)
Growth factor therapy (e.g. VEGF)
Antimicrobial agents (e.g. anti-biofilm agents)

Table 141.4 Future directions in wound healing.

electromagnetic currents on wounds have been investigated for decades, insights into the underlying mechanisms (e.g. phosphatidylinositol-3-OH kinase-γ, PTEN) have provided potential avenues for exploring ways to improve wound healing[57]. Also, stress has been found to inhibit healing via elevated cortisol levels, suggesting a role for stress reduction to speed healing[57a]. In the future, investigators will focus not only on the speed of healing[58], but also on the quality (strength and cosmetic appearance) of the resultant scar.

REFERENCES

1. Bickers DR, Lim HW, Margolis D, et al. The burden of skin diseases: 2004 a joint project of the American Academy of Dermatology Association and the Society for Investigative Dermatology. J Am Acad Dermatol. 2006;55:490–500.
1a. Naik-Mathuria B, Gay AN, Zhu X, et al. Age-dependent recruitment of neutrophils by fetal endothelial cells: implications in scarless wound healing. J Pediatr Surg 2007;42:166–171.
1b. Kanj, LF, Wilkins SV, Phillips TJ, et al. Pressure ulcers. J Am Acad Dermatol. 1998;38:517–36.
2. Li J, Chen J, Kirsner RS. Pathophysiology of acute wound healing. Clin Dermatol. 2007;25:9–18.
3. Krawczyk WS. A pattern of epidermal cell migration during wound healing. J Cell Biol. 1971;49:247–63.
3a. Christenson LJ, Phillips PK, Weaver AL, Otley CC. Primary closure vs second-intention treatment of skin punch biopsy sites: a randomized trial. Arch Derm 2005; 141;1093–1099.
4. Hell E, Lawrence JC. The initiation of epidermal wound healing in cuts and burns. Br J Exp Pathol. 1979; 60:171–9.
5. Katz MH, Alvarez AF, Kirsner RS, et al. Human wound fluid from acute wounds stimulates fibroblast and endothelial cell growth. J Am Acad Dermatol. 1991;25:1054–8.
6. Grinnell F, Billingham RE, Burgess L. Distribution of fibronectin during wound healing in vivo. J Invest Dermatol. 1981;76:181–9.
7. Uutela M, Wirzenius M, Paavonen K, et al. PDGF-D induces macrophage recruitment, increased interstitial pressure, and blood vessel maturation during angiogenesis. Blood. 2004;104:3198–204.
8. Deuel TF, Senior RM, Huang JS, et al. Chemotaxis of monocytes and neutrophils to platelet-derived growth factor. J Clin Invest. 1982;69:1046–9.
9. Knighton DR, Hunt TK, Thakral KK, et al. Role of platelets and fibrin in the healing sequence: an in vivo study of angiogenesis and collagen synthesis. Ann Surg. 1982;196:379–88.
10. Connolly AJ, Suh DY, Hunt TK, et al. Mice lacking the thrombin receptor, PAR1, have normal skin wound healing. Am J Pathol. 1997;151:1199–204.
11. Simpson DM, Ross R. The neutrophilic leukocyte in wound repair. A study with antineutrophil serum. J Clin Invest. 1972;51:2009–23.
12. Postlethwaite AE, Kang AH. Collagen- and collagen peptide-induced chemotaxis of human blood monocytes. J Exp Med. 1976;143:1299–307.
13. Olsen CE. Macrophage factors affecting wound healing. In: Hunt TK, Heppenstall RB, Pines E, Rovee D (eds). Soft and Hard Tissue Repair. Biological and Clinical Aspects. New York: Praeger, 1984:343.
14. Falanga V. Growth factors and wound healing. J Dermatol Surg Oncol. 1993;19:711–14.
15. Clark RAF. Cutaneous wound repair: molecular and cellular controls. Prog Dermatol. 1988;22:1–12.

16. Sun TT, Cotsarelis G, Lavker RM. Hair follicular stem cells: the bulge-activation hypothesis. J Invest Dermatol. 1991;96:77S–78S.
17. Winter GD. Epidermal regeneration studied in the domestic pig. In: Maibach HI, Rovee DT (eds). Epidermal Wound Healing. Chicago: Year Book Medical, 1972.
18. Grove GL. Age-related differences in healing of superficial skin wounds in humans. Arch Dermatol Res. 1982;272:381–5.
19. Parks WC. Matrix metalloproteinases in repair. Wound Repair Regen. 1999;7:423–32.
20. Bishr Omary M, Nam-On K. Skin care by keratins. Nature. 2006;441:296–7.
21. Kim S, Wong P, Coulombe PA. A keratin cytoskeletal protein regulates protein synthesis and epithelial cell growth. Nature. 2006;441:362–5.
22. Leyden JJ. Effect of bacteria on healing of superficial wounds. Clin Dermatol. 1984;2:81–5.
23. Corball M, O'Dwyer P, Brady MP. The interaction of vitamin A and corticosteroids on wound healing. Ir J Med Sci. 1985;154:306–10.
24. Geronemus RG, Mertz PM, Eaglstein WH. Wound healing. The effects of topical antimicrobial agents. Arch Dermatol. 1979;115:1311–14.
25. Eaglstein WH, Mertz PM. 'Inert' vehicles do affect wound healing. J Invest Dermatol. 1980;74:90–1.
26. Marks JG Jr, Cano C, Leitzel K, et al. Inhibition of wound healing by topical steroids. J Dermatol Surg Oncol. 1983;9:819–21.
27. Armstrong RB, Nichols J, Pachance J. Punch biopsy wounds treated with Monsel's solution or a collagen matrix. A comparison of healing. Arch Dermatol. 1986;122:546–9.
28. Langemo D, Anderson J, Hanson D, et al. Nutritional considerations in wound care. Adv Skin Wound Care. 2006;19:297–303.
29. Stadelmann WK, Digenis AG, Tobin GR. Impediments to wound healing. Am J Surg. 1998;176:39S–47S.
30. Ashcroft GS, Herrick SE, Tarnuzzer RW, et al. Human ageing impairs injury-induced in vivo expression of tissue inhibitor of matrix metalloproteinases (TIMP)-1 and -2 protein and mRNA. J Pathol. 1997;183:169–76.
31. Folkman J. Angiogenesis: initiation and control. Ann NY Acad Sci. 1982;401:212–27.
32. Arnold F, West D, Kumar S. Wound healing: the effect of macrophage and tumour derived angiogenesis factors on skin graft vascularization. Br J Exp Pathol. 1987;68:569–74.
33. Kalebic T, Garbisa S, Glaser B, Liotta LA. Basement membrane collagen: degradation by migrating endothelial cells. Science. 1983;221:281–3.
34. Remensnyder JP, Majno G. Oxygen gradients in healing wounds. Am J Pathol. 1968;52:301–23.
35. Falanga V, Martin TA, Takagi H, et al. Low oxygen tension increases mRNA levels of alpha 1 (I) procollagen in human dermal fibroblasts. J Cell Physiol. 1993;157:408–12.

36. Majno G. The story of the myofibroblasts. Am J Surg Pathol. 1979;3:535–42.
37. Ross R, Bowen-Pope DF, Raines EW. Platelet-derived growth factor: its potential roles in wound healing, atherosclerosis, neoplasia, and growth and development. Ciba Found Symp. 1985;116:98–112.
38. Roberts AB, Sporn MB. Transforming growth factor-beta: potential common mechanisms mediating its effects on embryogenesis, inflammation-repair, and carcinogenesis. Int J Rad Appl Instrum B. 1987; 14:435–9.
39. Kurkinen M, Vaheri A, Roberts PJ, Stenman S. Sequential appearance of fibronectin and collagen in experimental granulation tissue. Lab Invest. 1980;43:47–51.
40. Pearlstein E. Plasma membrane glycoprotein which mediates adhesion of fibroblasts to collagen. Nature. 1976;262:497–500.
41. Woodley DT, O'Keefe EJ, Prunieras M. Cutaneous wound healing: a model for cell-matrix interactions. J Am Acad Dermatol. 1985;12:420–33.
42. Gessin JC, Darr D, Kaufman R, et al. Ascorbic acid specifically increases type I and type III procollagen messenger RNA levels in human skin fibroblasts. J Invest Dermatol. 1988;90:420–4.
43. Higley HR, Ksander GA, Gerhardt CO, Falanga V: Extravasation of macromolecules and possible trapping of transforming growth factor-beta in venous ulceration. Br J Dermatol. 1995;132:79–85.
44. Toole BP, Gross J. The extracellular matrix of the regenerating newt limb: synthesis and removal of hyaluronate prior to differentiation. Dev Biol. 1971;25:57–77.
45. Bell E, Ehrlich HP, Buttle DJ, et al. Living tissue formed in vitro and accepted as skin-equivalent tissue of full thickness. Science. 1981;211:1052–4.
46. Abercrombie M, Flint MH, James DW. Wound contraction in relation to collagen formation in scorbutic guinea-pigs. J Embryol Exp Morphol. 1956;4:167–75.
47. Booth BA, Polak KL, Uitto J. Collagen biosynthesis by human skin fibroblasts. Biochem Biophys Acta. 1980;607:145–60.
48. McDonald JA, Baum BJ, Rosenburg DM, et al. Destruction of a major extracellular adhesive glycoprotein (fibronectin) of human fibroblasts by neutral proteases from polymorphonuclear leukocyte granules. Lab Invest. 1979;40:350–7.
49. Braverman IM, Fonferko E. Studies in cutaneous aging: I. The elastic fiber network. J Invest Dermatol. 1982;78:434–43.
50. Jonsson K, Jensen JA, Goodson WH, et al. Tissue oxygenation, anemia, and perfusion in relation to wound healing in surgical patients. Ann Surg. 1991;214:605–13.
51. Modolin M, Bevilacqua RG, Margarido NF, Lima-Goncalves E. Effects of protein depletion and repletion on experimental open wound contraction. Ann Plast Surg. 1985;15:123–6.

52. Hunt TK. Vitamin A and wound healing. J Am Acad Dermatol. 1986;15:817–21.

53. Agren MS, Franzen L. Influence of zinc deficiency on breaking strength of 3-week-old skin incisions in the rat. Acta Chir Scand. 1990;156:667–70.

54. Beck LS, De Guzman L, Lee WP, et al. One systemic administration of transforming growth factor-beta 1 reverses age- or glucocorticoid-impaired wound healing. J Clin Invest. 1993;92:2841–9.

55. Eaglstein WH. Experiences with biosynthetic dressings. J Am Acad Dermatol. 1985;12:434–40.

56. Sorensen OE, Thapa DR, Roupe KM, et al. Injury-induced innate immune response in human skin mediated by transactivation of the epidermal growth factor receptor. J Clin Invest. 2006;116:1878–85.

57. Zhao M, Song B, Pu J, et al. Electrical signals control wound healing through phosphatidylinositol-3-OH kinase-gamma and PTEN. Nature. 2006;442:457–60.

57a. Vileikyte L. Stress and wound healing. Clin Dermatol. 2007;25:49–55.

58. Coulombe PA. Wound epithelialization: accelerating the pace of discovery. J Invest Dermatol. 2003;121:219–30.

Surgical Anatomy of the Head and Neck

Franklin P Flowers and Jennifer C Zampogna

Key features

- The muscles of facial expression all arise from the second branchial arch, are concentrated in the central facial region, and receive their motor innervation from the facial (7th cranial) nerve

- The superficial musculoaponeurotic system (SMAS) is a fibromuscular layer that ensheathes and connects the facial muscles and plays an intricate role in coordinating facial expressions

- The SMAS can be utilized as a guide to dissection, tissue mobilization and closure, minimizing trauma to neurovascular tissues

- The three branches of the trigeminal (5th cranial) nerve provide sensory innervation to the face, while various branches of the cervical plexus provide sensory innervation to the neck, parts of the ear, and posterior scalp

- Familiarity with the muscular and neurovascular structures of the head and neck region allow the surgeon to properly approach the 'danger zones', e.g. Erb's point in the neck, the temporal nerve as it crosses the zygomatic arch, and the marginal mandibular nerve at the jawline just anterior to the masseter muscle

- The rich and anastomosing vascular supply of the face and scalp, derived from both the external and internal carotid arteries, explains the excellent healing potential and viability of local flaps and grafts in this region

- Cosmetic subunits and the junction lines separating them should be considered when planning excisions, repairs and cosmetic procedures of the head and neck

The dermatologic surgeon must have a comprehensive knowledge of regional anatomy in order to obtain acceptable operative results. Tissue movement on the face and neck must be considered in order to obtain closure under minimal tension without cosmetic distortion or functional loss of vital structures. Preservation of tissue viability, sensory and motor innervation, and prevention of postoperative morbidity can be achieved with a fundamental appreciation for the macromechanics of the head and neck[1,2]. The fascial planes, vascular supply, innervation, and aesthetic subunits of the face must be considered when planning a surgical or cosmetic procedure. In order to accurately and thoroughly counsel patients regarding procedural risks and benefits, the surgeon must have a thorough appreciation of head and neck anatomy.

TOPOGRAPHIC ANATOMY OF THE HEAD AND NECK

It is possible to pinpoint underlying anatomic structures of the head and neck by observing surface anatomy. The bony structure of the face serves as a simple anatomic framework (Fig. 142.1). The supraorbital ridges are formed by the frontal bone and are more prominent in men. The supraorbital foramen transmits the sensory supraorbital nerve (from the ophthalmic division of the trigeminal nerve), artery and vein. It is palpable on the bony supraorbital ridge at the vertical midpupillary line. This line lies approximately one finger-breadth lateral to the lateral nasal root or 2.5 cm lateral of the midline on the face (Fig. 142.2). Other important foramina lie in this midpupillary line and transmit important neurovascular bundles. The infraorbital foramen is located 1 cm below the infraorbital rim in the midpupillary line. It transmits the sensory infraorbital nerve (from the maxillary division of the

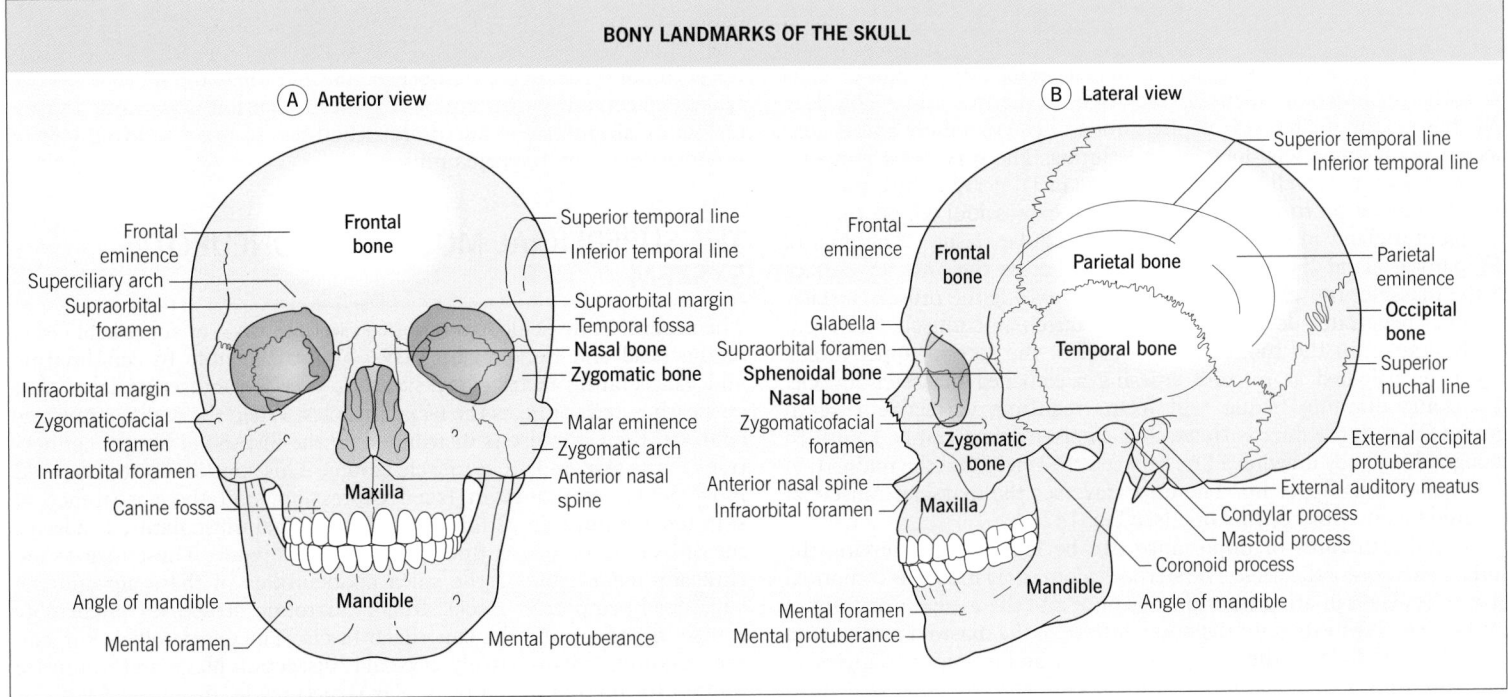

BONY LANDMARKS OF THE SKULL

Ⓐ Anterior view

Frontal eminence
Superciliary arch
Supraorbital foramen
Frontal bone
Superior temporal line
Inferior temporal line
Supraorbital margin
Temporal fossa
Nasal bone
Zygomatic bone
Infraorbital margin
Zygomaticofacial foramen
Infraorbital foramen
Malar eminence
Zygomatic arch
Maxilla
Anterior nasal spine
Canine fossa
Angle of mandible
Mandible
Mental foramen
Mental protuberance

Ⓑ Lateral view

Frontal eminence
Frontal bone
Parietal bone
Superior temporal line
Inferior temporal line
Parietal eminence
Occipital bone
Glabella
Supraorbital foramen
Sphenoidal bone
Nasal bone
Zygomaticofacial foramen
Temporal bone
Superior nuchal line
Zygomatic bone
Anterior nasal spine
Infraorbital foramen
Maxilla
External occipital protuberance
External auditory meatus
Condylar process
Mastoid process
Coronoid process
Mandible
Angle of mandible
Mental foramen
Mental protuberance

Fig. 142.1 Bony landmarks of the skull. A Anterior view. **B** Lateral view.

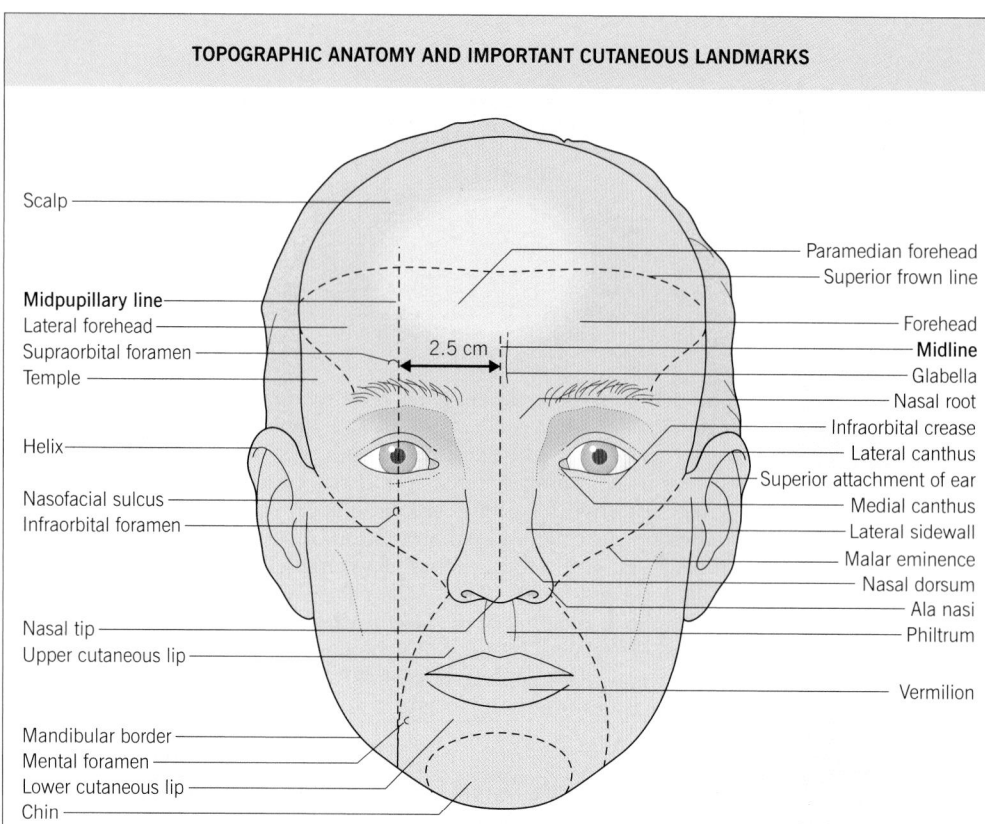

TOPOGRAPHIC ANATOMY AND IMPORTANT CUTANEOUS LANDMARKS

Scalp

Midpupillary line
Lateral forehead
Supraorbital foramen
Temple

2.5 cm

Helix

Nasofacial sulcus
Infraorbital foramen

Nasal tip
Upper cutaneous lip

Mandibular border
Mental foramen
Lower cutaneous lip
Chin

Paramedian forehead
Superior frown line

Forehead
Midline
Glabella
Nasal root
Infraorbital crease
Lateral canthus
Superior attachment of ear
Medial canthus
Lateral sidewall
Malar eminence
Nasal dorsum
Ala nasi
Philtrum

Vermilion

Fig. 142.2 Topographic anatomy and important cutaneous landmarks.

trigeminal nerve) and its associated artery and vein. The mental foramen lies in the same vertical line in the midportion of the mandible. The mental neurovascular bundle emerges here as a terminal sensory branch of the mandibular division of the trigeminal nerve.

The anterior border of the temporalis muscle can be palpated in the temporal fossa above the zygomatic bone. The latter bone forms the malar eminence of the cheek. The buccal fat pad provides fullness to the cheek; elderly or cachectic patients often have very prominent zygomatic arches. These arches form the widest points on the face and serve as the point of attachment for several muscles of facial expression and for a muscle of mastication called the masseter. The masseter muscle spans the zygomatic arch and mandibular ramus, serving as a muscle of mastication innervated by a motor branch of the trigeminal nerve. This muscle is easily palpated by clenching the jaw.

The parotid gland lies beneath the subcutaneous fat of the lateral cheek and is invested by parotid fascia. The superficial lobe of the parotid covers the posterior half of the masseter muscle and extends from the preauricular sulcus to the angle of the mandible. The deep lobe lies on the medial side of the ramus of the mandible and is connected to the superficial lobe by an isthmus. The superficial temporal artery and vein, as well as branches of the facial nerve (which provides motor innervation to the muscles of facial expression) course through the parotid gland in channels between glandular tissue[3]. The duct of the parotid gland (Stensen's duct) travels across the anterior surface of the masseter muscle (Fig. 142.3). After crossing the muscle surface, the duct penetrates deeper to pierce the buccinator muscle and eventually drain into the mouth at the level of the second upper molar. It can be palpated as a 'cord' crossing a clenched masseter muscle. A chronic draining fistula will form, requiring corrective surgical intervention, if the duct is transected. Stensen's duct can be identified topographically by drawing a line between the tragus and the midportion of the cutaneous upper lip. The duct traverses the masseter muscle at the middle one-third of this line (see Fig. 142.3).

Several structures of importance can be located by observing the surface anatomy of the neck. The sternocleidomastoid muscle is comprised of two heads originating from the sternum and the medial one-third of the clavicle. It inserts onto the outer surface of the mastoid process and nuchal ridge, dividing the neck into anterior and posterior triangles. A dermatologic surgeon should be familiar with the anatomic structures that lie within each of these topographic triangles (Fig. 142.4). Although

the sternocleidomastoid muscle covers and protects most of the major anatomic structures in the neck, the external jugular vein traverses its surface with many cutaneous sensory nerves of the cervical plexus. In addition, the posterior triangle of the neck contains trunks of the brachial and cervical plexus as well as the spinal accessory nerve (cranial nerve XI). Cranial nerve XI innervates the trapezius muscle of the back. It may be damaged when operating in this posterior triangle. This may result in chronic shoulder and neck pain, shoulder drop and trapezius atrophy, arm paresthesias, and the inability to abduct the arm greater than 80°.

Erb's point designates the area where the cervical plexus emerges from the posterior margin of the sternocleidomastoid muscle. The spinal accessory nerve courses through this area on its way to the trapezius muscle. This surgical danger zone can be visualized by drawing a line connecting the angle of the jaw to the mastoid process. A perpendicular line dropped 6 cm from the midpoint of this connector will intersect the posterior border of the sternocleidomastoid where the spinal accessory nerve and cervical plexus emerge[4]. Extreme caution is warranted when dissecting around these anatomic structures, in order to avoid loss of innervation to the trapezius muscle.

THE SUPERFICIAL MUSCULOAPONEUROTIC SYSTEM

The superficial musculoaponeurotic system (SMAS) or superficial fascia of the head and neck region plays an intricate role in coordinating and exaggerating facial expressions. It is a fibromuscular layer that ensheathes and connects the facial muscles. When the regional muscles contract, their impulse is distributed by the SMAS via fibrous connections to the skin and other muscle groups. This contributes to organized movements, symmetry in facial expression, and the appearance of skin tension lines. In certain areas where facial musculature is absent, the SMAS layers form a thick, inelastic membrane. These regions are clinically identifiable as the galea aponeurotica of the scalp and the superficial temporalis fascia. Major anatomic structures predictably course in and around the superficial fascia. The dermatologic surgeon can maximize this relatively avascular dissection plane and minimize trauma to important neurovascular structures by using the SMAS as a guide to dissection, tissue mobilization, and closure. Rejuvenation

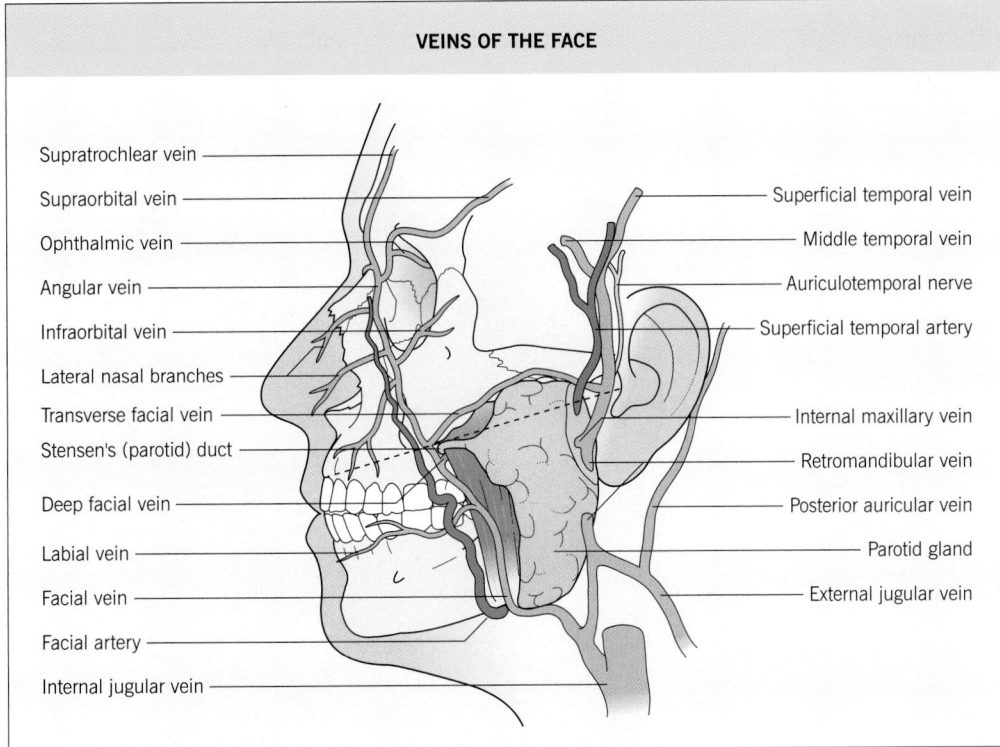

VEINS OF THE FACE

Supratrochlear vein
Supraorbital vein
Ophthalmic vein
Angular vein
Infraorbital vein
Lateral nasal branches
Transverse facial vein
Stensen's (parotid) duct
Deep facial vein
Labial vein
Facial vein
Facial artery
Internal jugular vein

Superficial temporal vein
Middle temporal vein
Auriculotemporal nerve
Superficial temporal artery
Internal maxillary vein
Retromandibular vein
Posterior auricular vein
Parotid gland
External jugular vein

Fig. 142.3 Veins of the face. Stensen's duct can be identified topographically by drawing a line between the tragus and mid portion of the cutaneous upper lip (dotted line). It can be palpated as a cord at the middle third of this line.

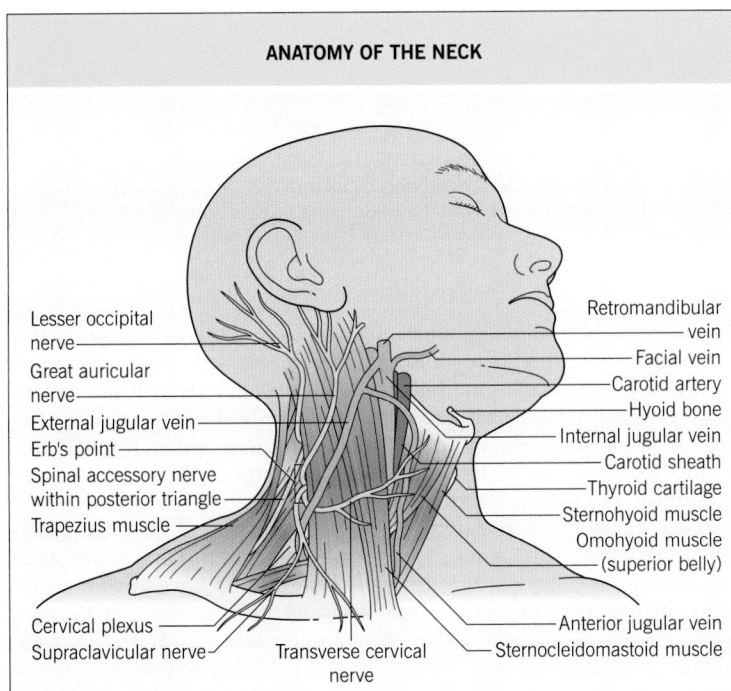

ANATOMY OF THE NECK

Lesser occipital nerve
Great auricular nerve
External jugular vein
Erb's point
Spinal accessory nerve within posterior triangle
Trapezius muscle
Cervical plexus
Supraclavicular nerve
Transverse cervical nerve

Retromandibular vein
Facial vein
Carotid artery
Hyoid bone
Internal jugular vein
Carotid sheath
Thyroid cartilage
Sternohyoid muscle
Omohyoid muscle (superior belly)
Anterior jugular vein
Sternocleidomastoid muscle

Fig. 142.4 Anatomy of the neck.

procedures such as facelifts rely on the redistribution and manipulation or plication of the head and neck SMAS.

The deep fascia of the face covers bone, cartilage, muscles of mastication, and visceral structures. It is a continuous sheath, forming periosteum, perichondrium, temporalis muscle fascia, and the parotid-masseteric fascia[1]. This fascia is resistant to stretch and particularly impedes tissue movement on the scalp. Plication or suspension sutures are often used to 'tack' overlying structures to the deeper fascia in order to secure tissue and redirect tension vectors.

The SMAS of the cheek is located between the skin and the deeper muscles of mastication. By mobilizing the preauricular SMAS plane, the anterolateral neck and lower cheek below the zygomatic arch can be repositioned as a whole. The SMAS of the cheek is continuous with the orbicularis oculi muscle of the lower eyelid and has several bony attachments in the periocular region[5]. Note that the SMAS of the upper face is discontinuous with the SMAS below the zygoma. Different embryologic development patterns of the upper and lower facial muscle groups account for this separation. The galea aponeurotica of the scalp and the fascia of the superficial temporalis muscle split to envelop the frontalis muscle of the forehead and the occipitalis muscle of the posterior scalp. This superior SMAS terminates 1 cm below the zygomatic arch.

The parotid gland, Stensen's duct, and emerging branches of the facial nerve lie on the deep masseteric fascia. They are covered by thin fibrotic platysma remnants called the parotid fascia, which is covered by the SMAS. The aponeurotic investiture of the central face is thin and often indistinct. The intrinsic nasal muscles and lip elevators and depressors are essentially devoid of superficial fascial interconnections. This makes dissection in this area challenging, because the planes are often difficult to establish and many important anatomic structures are under threat of compromise.

Large sensory nerves and axial blood vessels that supply the face ascend to lie within the SMAS or between the SMAS and subcutaneous fat (Fig. 142.5). Motor nerves run deep to the SMAS and penetrate the muscles of facial expression from their undersurface. Knowledge of these anatomic relationships assists the surgeon in establishing a relatively avascular and safe plane of dissection. Blunt dissection of the scalp SMAS separates the galea aponeurotica from the skull periosteum, the superficial temporalis fascia from the deep temporalis fascia, and the subfrontalis SMAS from the forehead periosteum. This is called the subgaleal plane, and it is the ideal avascular dissection plane for scalp surgery. Beware of the supraorbital/supratrochlear neurovascular bundles above the eyebrows when dissecting to the deep galea, as these can be damaged as they exit the inferior frontalis muscle origin. In the SMAS-parotid fascial plane of the cheek, the buccal and zygomatic branches of the facial nerve are endangered due to thin protective aponeurotic tissue in this area. The superficial temporal vessels and auriculotemporal nerve course within the superficial temporalis fascia above the zygomatic arch, then assume a superficial plane in the subcutaneous fat.

Surgical undermining and dissection should maximize the horizontal planes provided by the superficial fascial network of the head and neck. Undermining in the subcutaneous fat of the face below the subdermal plexus minimizes the risk to motor nerves, but remember that sensory branches and blood vessels do course through this area. There is sparse subcutaneous fat on the dorsal nose, forehead, upper lip, and eyelid. The ideal dissection plane in these regions lies just superficial to the thin investing fascia (SMAS) covering the regional muscles of facial expression[6].

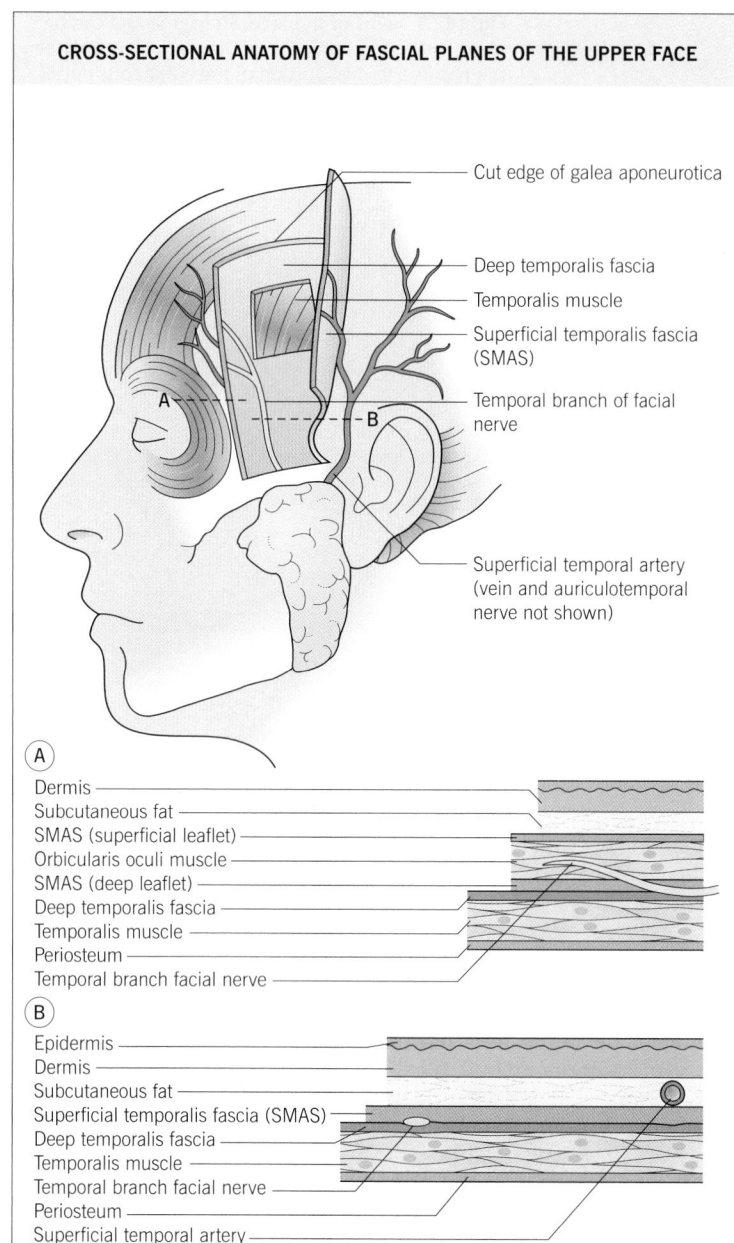

CROSS-SECTIONAL ANATOMY OF FASCIAL PLANES OF THE UPPER FACE

Cut edge of galea aponeurotica

Deep temporalis fascia

Temporalis muscle

Superficial temporalis fascia (SMAS)

Temporal branch of facial nerve

Superficial temporal artery (vein and auriculotemporal nerve not shown)

A

Dermis
Subcutaneous fat
SMAS (superficial leaflet)
Orbicularis oculi muscle
SMAS (deep leaflet)
Deep temporalis fascia
Temporalis muscle
Periosteum
Temporal branch facial nerve

B

Epidermis
Dermis
Subcutaneous fat
Superficial temporalis fascia (SMAS)
Deep temporalis fascia
Temporalis muscle
Temporal branch facial nerve
Periosteum
Superficial temporal artery

Fig. 142.5 Cross-sectional anatomy of fascial planes of the upper face. SMAS, superficial musculoaponeurotic system.

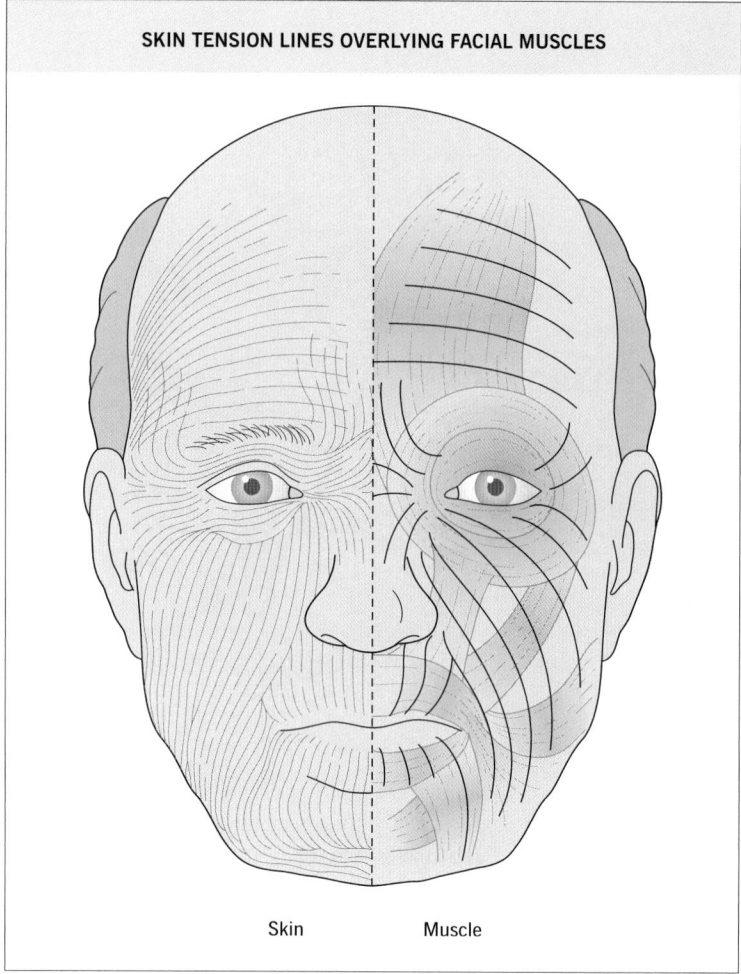

SKIN TENSION LINES OVERLYING FACIAL MUSCLES

Skin   Muscle

Fig. 142.6 Skin tension lines overlying facial muscles. Note that wrinkles are often directed perpendicularly to the underlying muscle fibers of facial expression.

In short, the SMAS acts as a unifying infrastructure to the head and neck that creates an anatomic plane for identification and protection of key structures. Knowledge of neurovascular anatomy with respect to the superficial investing fascia will promote effective surgical dissection and closures that minimize functional compromise and maximize cosmesis.

SKIN TENSION LINES

Collagen and elastin afford flexibility and extensibility to the skin, and derangements of their architecture or abundance contribute to the aging process. Wrinkles (rhytides) develop over time in predictable areas on the face. The fine wrinkles seen on an aged face may be referred to as the skin tension lines (Fig. 142.6). Many environmental and intrinsic factors, such as ultraviolet exposure, smoking, underlying facial muscles, etc., contribute to the appearance of the expressive human face. A thorough understanding of the derivation and implications of skin tension lines is essential to successful dermatologic surgery.

Continuous tension is exerted on the skin of the head and neck by the muscles of facial expression. A complicated network composed of muscles, fibrous septae of collagen, elastin and fascial planes contributes to this stress, which eventually results in sagging, wrinkling and redundant skin. Collagen is flexible but much less extensible than elastic fibers.

The resistance to tensile forces by collagen promotes a 'youthful' appearance. Over time, the prolonged tension exerted on the skin from many factors forces collagen fibrils to accommodate by way of elongation. Eventually, aged skin manifests the consequences of persistent skin tension. The collagenous tissue becomes increasingly intertwined, diminished in volume, and permanently elongated. This causes the accentuation of skin tension lines[4].

Elastic fibers promote extensibility (i.e. the ability of skin to stretch) and elasticity (i.e. the skin's capacity to restore its original shape after physical stress). They contribute to the skin tension lines by promoting vector distribution of tension along fascial planes. The elastic properties of the skin explain the phenomenon whereby round surgical wounds relax into an axis parallel to the patient's wrinkles. Tension vectors are increased parallel to the skin tension lines and are diminished perpendicular to them; therefore, the linear appearance of wrinkles is often directed perpendicularly to the underlying muscle fibers of facial expression. The continuous tension exerted on the overlying skin by these muscles challenges the competency of elastic tissue and collagen. They induce this geometric linearity via fibrous connections to the dermis via the SMAS. For example, the forehead undergoes transverse wrinkling due to contractions of the frontalis muscle, whose fibers run in a cephalo-caudad direction. Periocular rhytides are often radially oriented due to underlying contraction of the orbicularis oculi. Similarly, perioral wrinkling occurs under the influence of the concentric orbicularis oris muscle, which induces a radial arrangement of skin tension lines as well. The procerus muscle causes transverse nasal root lines, and vertical glabellar lines are determined by the corrugator supercilii muscles (Fig. 142.7).

Knowledge of these functional anatomic principles is necessary in surgical and cosmetic dermatology. For example, the successful use of botulinum toxin for the diminution of rhytides requires an understanding of the anatomic relationships between various muscle groups

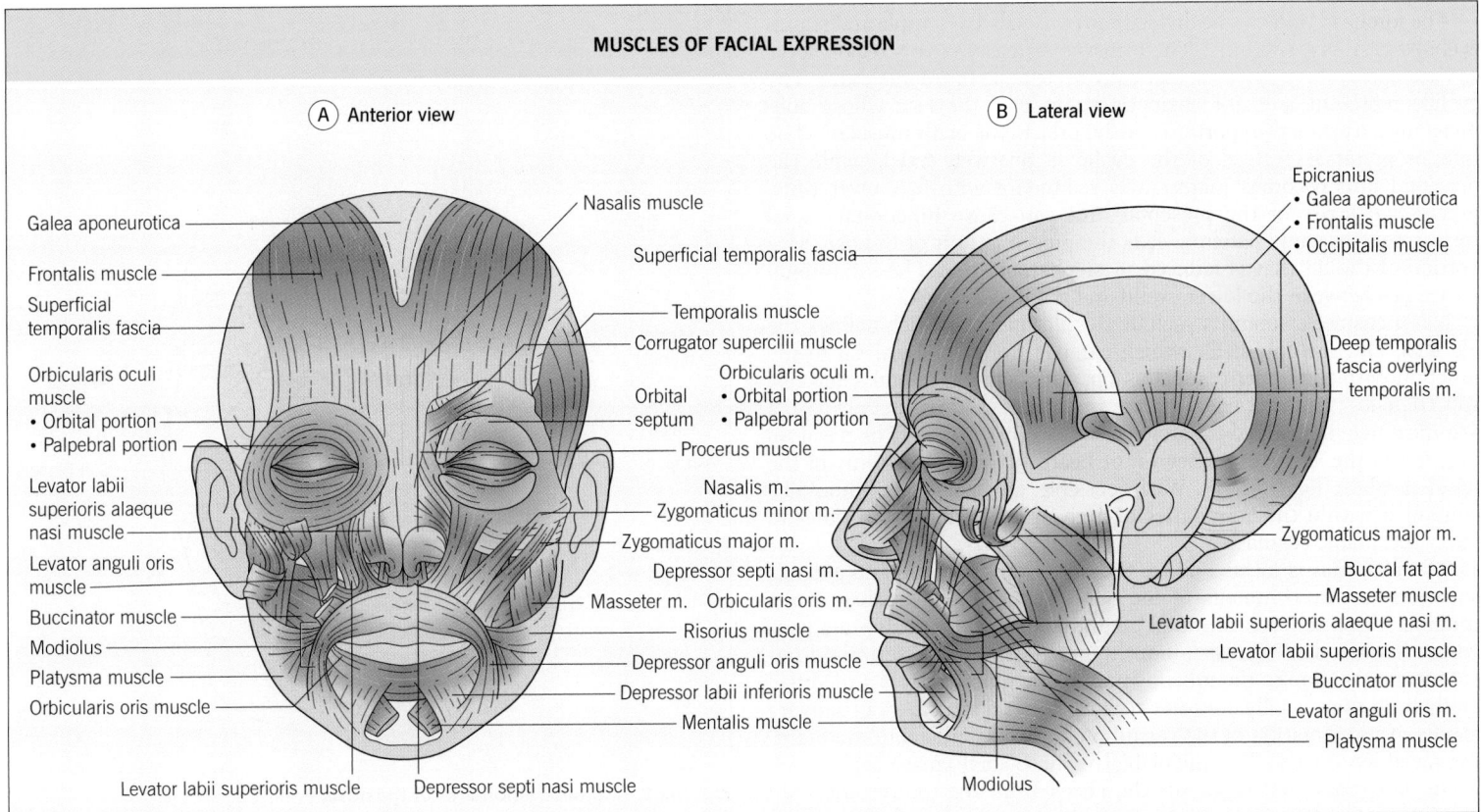

MUSCLES OF FACIAL EXPRESSION

A Anterior view

Galea aponeurotica
Frontalis muscle
Superficial temporalis fascia
Orbicularis oculi muscle
• Orbital portion
• Palpebral portion
Levator labii superioris alaeque nasi muscle
Levator anguli oris muscle
Buccinator muscle
Modiolus
Platysma muscle
Orbicularis oris muscle

Nasalis muscle

Levator labii superioris muscle   Depressor septi nasi muscle

B Lateral view

Superficial temporalis fascia
Temporalis muscle
Corrugator supercilii muscle
Orbicularis oculi m.
Orbital   • Orbital portion
septum   • Palpebral portion
Procerus muscle
Nasalis m.
Zygomaticus minor m.
Zygomaticus major m.
Depressor septi nasi m.
Masseter m.   Orbicularis oris m.
Risorius muscle
Depressor anguli oris muscle
Depressor labii inferioris muscle
Mentalis muscle

Modiolus

Epicranius
• Galea aponeurotica
• Frontalis muscle
• Occipitalis muscle

Deep temporalis fascia overlying temporalis m.

Zygomaticus major m.
Buccal fat pad
Masseter muscle
Levator labii superioris alaeque nasi m.
Levator labii superioris muscle
Buccinator muscle
Levator anguli oris m.
Platysma muscle

Fig. 142.7 Muscles of facial expression. A Anterior view. **B** Lateral view.

and their influence on the skin tension lines. Proper surgical technique entails placement of incisional lines parallel to the skin tension lines in order to achieve excellent cosmesis. It is helpful to determine and even sketch the patient's skin tension lines with a Gentian violet pen. This will help orient the axis of incision and guide the closure parallel to and preferably 'buried' within individual lines of tension.

There is often a significant amount of recruitable or 'redundant' skin within the skin tension lines. In addition, 'extra' skin may also be found in the preauricular folds, glabella, nasolabial folds, and the 'jowls' or lower cheeks[7]. These tissue reservoirs can be used as donor sites for flaps (see Ch. 147) and grafts (see Ch. 148) in order to achieve surgical closure under minimal tension.

COSMETIC SUBUNITS

Cosmetic units (i.e. aesthetic, topographic or regional units) represent the major structural areas of the face that are separated by contour or junctional lines or boundaries (Fig. 142.8). Units are designated based upon their similarity in topographic anatomy, texture and color, solar exposure, hair density, and sebaceous features. The forehead, temples, eyelids, nose, cheeks, upper and lower lips, chin, and ears represent the major cosmetic subunits of the face. Within each division, smaller units are designated that further guide surgical closures. The junctional or contour lines between cosmetic units serve as excellent locations to place incisions and hide surgical scars. They include the hairline, alar and nasolabial creases, eyebrows, the philtrum, the labiomental crease, and the upper and lower vermilion-cutaneous interfaces (see Fig. 142.2).

In general, defects should be repaired with tissue from within the same cosmetic unit in order to preserve topographic consistency. If this cannot be achieved, it is reasonable to utilize tissue from an adjacent aesthetic unit, which will most closely 'match' the skin of the recipient cosmetic unit. The goal is to optimize the match in skin texture, color, actinic damage and thickness. Scars that cross aesthetic units and boundary lines are obvious and often cosmetically unacceptable. A primary goal of cutaneous surgery is to 'respect' the cosmetic subunits.

An appreciation for cosmetic units and contour lines also helps the surgeon determine areas of 'recruitable' tissue for closures. Redundant or freely mobile skin can be mobilized from the preauricular folds, neck, nasolabial folds, temple, glabella, the lower and lateral cheeks,

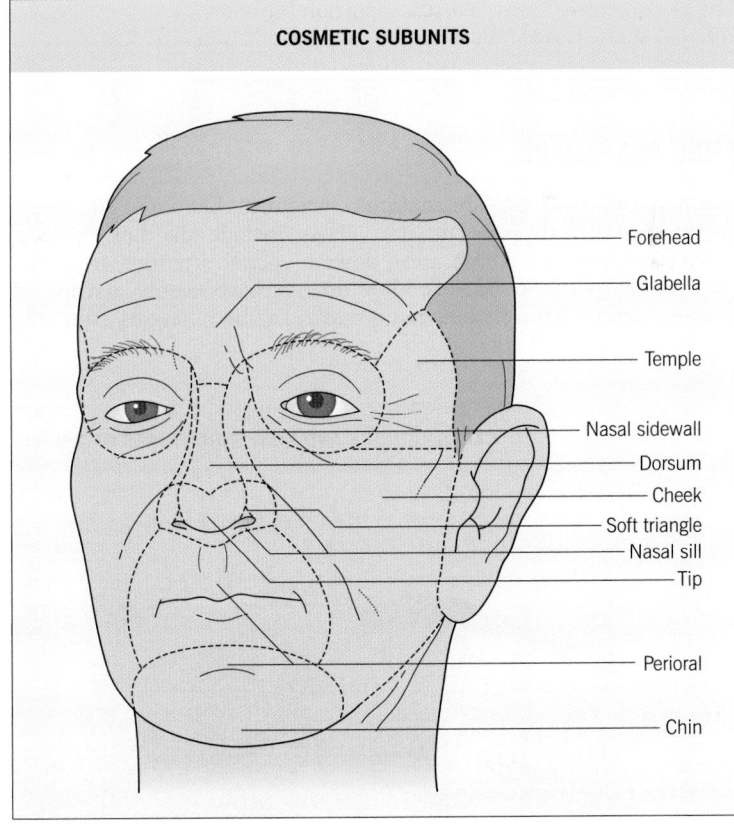

COSMETIC SUBUNITS

Forehead
Glabella
Temple
Nasal sidewall
Dorsum
Cheek
Soft triangle
Nasal sill
Tip
Perioral
Chin

Fig. 142.8 Cosmetic subunits.

and the 'jowls'. The potential for such tissue recruitment depends on the patient's age, degree of actinic damage and skin elasticity, which varies from patient to patient. Areas of redundancy or high elasticity may serve as excellent donor sites within or adjacent to the cosmetic subunit which contains a given surgical defect. For example, cheek advancement flaps and temple to lateral forehead advancement and rotation flaps are frequently used for defect repairs.

The forehead unit can be divided into the glabella, temple and supra-eyebrow aesthetic subunits. The transverse creases of this region serve as excellent sites to place cosmetically acceptable incisional scars. The eyelids represent a major cosmetic subunit of the face whose subdivisions correspond to portions of the orbicularis oculi muscles[8]. The inferior pretarsal portion of the eyelid is relatively fixed, while the preseptal unit becomes increasingly redundant with age. Over time, progressive laxity of the preseptal unit can cause functional visual impairment in some patients. It is the preseptal unit of the palpebral portion of the lid that is reduced in blepharoplasties. The infraorbital crease lies between the lower eyelid and the upper cheek.

Nasal cosmetic subunits include the alar groove (which defines the ala nasi) and the columella, which extends from the nasal tip to the junction with the upper cutaneous lip. The dorsum, lateral sidewalls, soft triangles, root and nasal tip are important landmarks that pose a significant challenge in dermatologic surgery (Fig. 142.9). The nasal tip unit forms the shape of a chevron or heart due to the anatomy of the nasal cartilage (Fig. 142.10). When possible, surgical defects should be contained within the boundaries of a given nasal subunit in order to effect acceptable cosmesis[9].

The philtrum is located above the upper vermilion lip and extends superiorly to the columella of the nose (Fig. 142.11). Because it is a midline structure, even minimal anatomic distortion results in a poor cosmetic outcome. The vermilion lip extends from the vermilion lip-cutaneous junction to the mucous membrane junction. It is a modified epithelium that usually does not contain adnexal structures or salivary glands. Approximation of the vermilion borders is crucial to maintaining facial symmetry. The melolabial or nasolabial crease serves as a useful landmark that separates the cheek from the mouth and chin aesthetic units. It is an ideal place to hide suture lines and often serves as a generous donor site for repairs.

The external ear (auricle or pinna) consists of a single cartilaginous plate that results in the complex curves and folds of the ear (Fig. 142.12). The skin is loose on the posterior portion but tightly adherent on the anterior surface. Awareness of the anatomic landmarks of the ear is important in planning reconstruction and in demarcation of the precise location of neoplasias.

FREE MARGINS

Free margins of the face are anatomic structures that are in some way discontinuous with adjacent skin. They include the lips, helices, eyelids and nostrils. These areas deserve special attention from the dermatologic surgeon because they do not have evenly distributed tension vectors. This characteristic makes the free margins especially

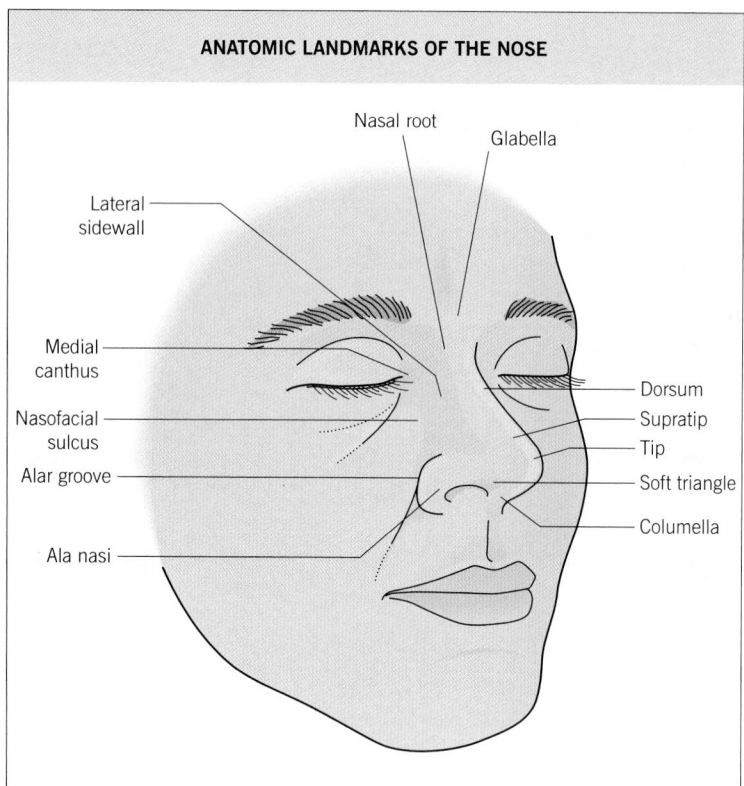

Fig. 142.9 Anatomic landmarks of the nose.

vulnerable to any iatrogenic directional pull. Surgical closures, wound healing and scar contraction can cause these free margins to lose their cosmetic or functional integrity. Ectropion (eyelid eversion) or eclabium (lip eversion) may ensue. Primary elliptical closures that are strictly parallel to a free margin and second intention healing are not frequently used in these areas.

The opposing force inflicted upon a free margin depends on closure axis orientation, flap or graft design, and the tensile strength and elasticity of the skin. Aged skin is often less able to resist directional vectors. The lower eyelid often becomes especially lax with cumulative actinic damage and age. The 'pinch' or 'snap' test can be used in free margin evaluation by gently pulling the lower lid away from the eye. Upon release, a competent lower lid should assume its original shape against the globe, while a lax lid will regain its configuration slowly[4].

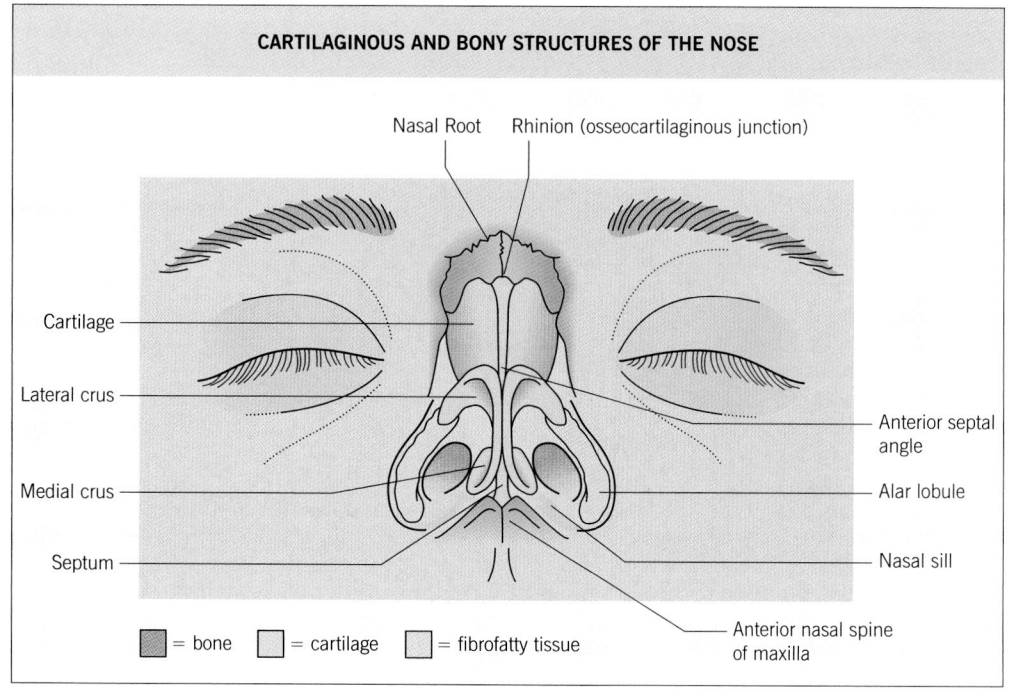

Fig. 142.10 Cartilaginous and bony structures of the nose.

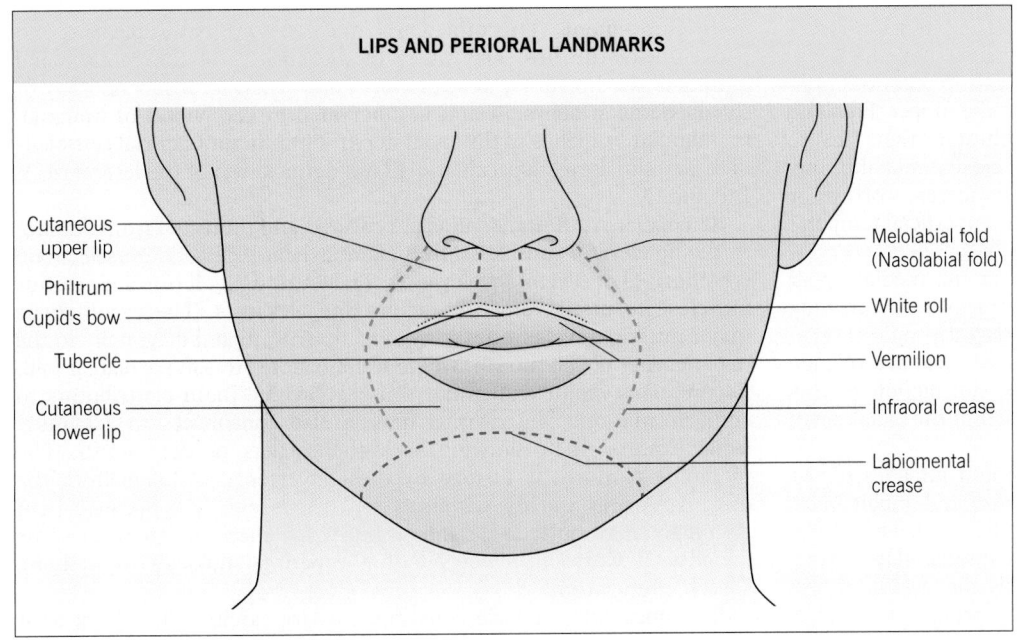

LIPS AND PERIORAL LANDMARKS

Cutaneous upper lip

Philtrum

Cupid's bow

Tubercle

Cutaneous lower lip

Melolabial fold (Nasolabial fold)

White roll

Vermilion

Infraoral crease

Labiomental crease

Fig. 142.11 Lips and perioral landmarks.

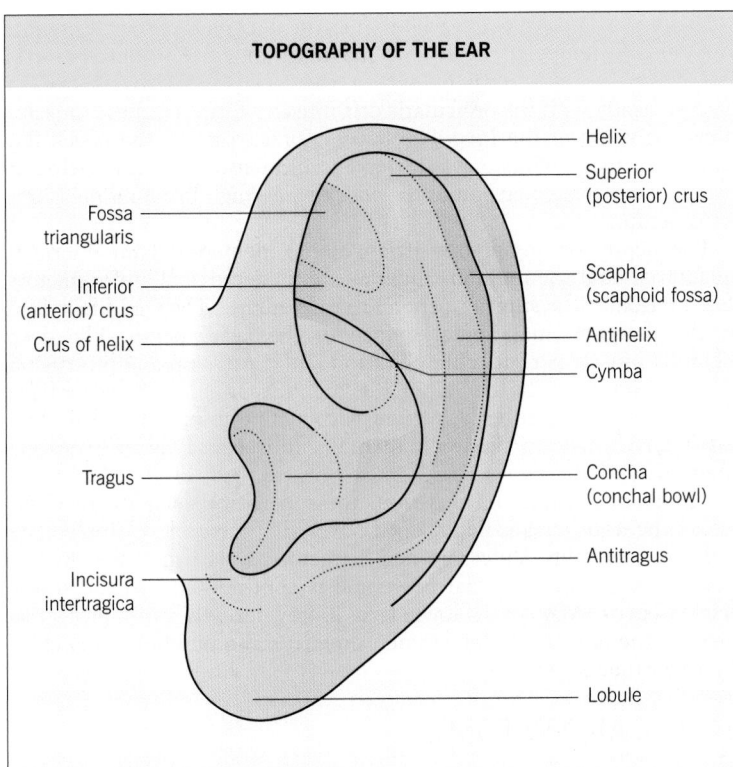

TOPOGRAPHY OF THE EAR

Fossa triangularis

Inferior (anterior) crus

Crus of helix

Tragus

Incisura intertragica

Helix

Superior (posterior) crus

Scapha (scaphoid fossa)

Antihelix

Cymba

Concha (conchal bowl)

Antitragus

Lobule

Fig. 142.12 Topography of the ear.

Instruct the patient to open his or her mouth and gaze upwards while simulating closure options under the eye. This generates the maximum intraoperative tension on the lower eyelid and can help to estimate the risk for distortion of this free margin. No more than 2 mm of inferior pull or 'drag' on the lower eyelid can generally be tolerated during cutaneous surgical repairs. Any additional inferior tension puts the patient at high risk for ectropion[10].

Maintenance of cosmesis and function of the lip vermilion is of utmost importance. Elliptical closures often create drag on these free margins, but careful redirection of tension vectors may allow simple closures here as well. A-T closures may help in this area, as a way to maintain cosmetic boundaries. Full-thickness skin grafts are not commonly employed on the lips, but may serve as useful closures at other free margin areas like the lower eyelids and the nasal tip and alae. Full-thickness skin grafts prevent distortion at these sites by minimizing the possibility of scar contraction (see Ch. 128).

Although the helical rims are free margins, they are far more 'forgiving' than the aforementioned sites. Second intention healing and axial elliptical closures can achieve excellent results on the ear. The tissue is easily dissected and the posterior auricular skin provides excellent mobility. Most patients have some ear asymmetry at baseline, thus making this free margin less cosmetically sensitive.

The nasal tip, alae and adjacent lateral sidewall require special consideration due to their classification as 'free margins' and the underlying cartilage framework that prevents significant tissue mobility. Elevation and distortion of the nasal rim may occur if second intention healing or simple primary closure is attempted. Full-thickness skin grafts and transposition or rotation flaps from adjacent areas are particularly appealing repairs in this cosmetically sensitive area[11].

MUSCLES OF FACIAL EXPRESSION

The muscles of facial expression arise from the second branchial arch, are innervated by the seventh cranial nerve (i.e. the facial nerve, cranial nerve VII), and are concentrated in the central facial region. They insert into overlying skin and other local muscle groups and contribute to the relaxed skin tension lines of this region. Fluidity of facial movements is orchestrated by their interaction with the SMAS. A surgeon must have detailed knowledge of these muscles and the potential consequences of disrupting their innervation.

The epicranius or occipitofrontalis muscle of the scalp has an anterior and posterior region connected by the galea aponeurotica (see Fig. 142.7). Contraction of these muscles allows the skin to slide over the scalp. Humans no longer have voluntary control of the posterior muscle group, which is innervated by the posterior auricular branch of the facial nerve. The frontalis muscle is a member of the epicranius complex that begins at the anterior hairline and inserts into the forehead and eyebrow skin. It also connects with the procerus, orbicularis oculi and corrugator supercilii muscles. Midline vertical forehead skin tension lines occur due to variation in distance between the left and right frontalis bellies. Horizontal skin tension lines occur perpendicular to the frontalis contractile orientation. Loss of frontalis function results in flattening of forehead skin tension lines and a drooping eyebrow. This occurs when the temporal branch of the facial nerve is disrupted. Patients with compromised frontalis function may be unable to open their eyes widely, due to the synergistic effect this muscle has with the orbicularis oculi muscle.

The small periauricular muscles or the temporoparietalis group arise from the superficial temporalis SMAS and the lateral galea. They help draw back the temporal skin and are innervated by the posterior ramus of the temporal branch of the facial nerve. The orbicularis oculi muscle complex is the major group that acts on the eyelid and periorbital skin. It inserts into the medial and lateral canthal tendons and encircles the eye region. Its palpebral portion has a preseptal component overlying the orbital septum and a pretarsal portion overlying the tarsal plate of the eyelid. The palpebral orbicularis oculi muscle aids in tear excretion. Upper pretarsal and preseptal muscles depress the upper lid. The orbital component of this muscle group allows voluntary tight closure of the eye. The palpebral portion allows gentle eye closure and blinking. The orbicularis oculi is intertwined with the procerus, corrugator supercilii, and frontalis muscles and attaches to the superficial temporal fascia at its lateral border.

The corrugator supercilii muscle is located over the medial upper orbital rim. It contributes to a 'scowling' facial expression by drawing the eyebrows medially and downward. It interdigitates with and is covered by the frontalis and orbicularis oculi muscles. The vertical and oblique skin tension lines of the glabella are caused by contraction of this muscle, which is innervated by the temporal branch of the facial nerve (Table 142.1).

The procerus muscle overlies the nasal bone and attaches to the nasal root skin. It causes foreshortening of the nose and 'rabbit lines' (i.e. skin tension lines exaggerated by wrinkling up the nose). The nasalis muscle courses across the nasal dorsum and facilitates alar 'flaring' and compression. These muscles are innervated by the zygomatic and buccal branches of the facial nerve. The depressor septi nasi muscle lies deep to the orbicularis oris and can form a transverse skin tension line across the philtrum. It plays a minor role in facial expression by pulling the columella down toward the lip.

An intricate network of interdigitating agonist and antagonist muscle groups contributes to lip movements and oral expression. Lip elevators, depressors and retractors assist the sphincteric orbicularis oris muscle

INNERVATION OF THE MUSCLES OF FACIAL EXPRESSION VIA CRANIAL NERVE VII (THE FACIAL NERVE)

Temporal branch
- Frontalis muscle (m.)
- Corrugator supercilii m.
- Orbicularis oculi m. (upper portion)
- Auricular m. (anterior and superior; also known as the temporoparietalis m.)

Posterior auricular branch
- Occipitalis m.
- Auricular m. (posterior)

Zygomatic branch
- Orbicularis oculi m. (lower portion)
- Nasalis m. (alar portion)
- Procerus m.
- Upper lip muscles
  - Levator anguli oris m.
  - Zygomaticus major m.

Buccal branch
- Buccinator m. (muscle of mastication)
- Depressor septi nasi m.
- Nasalis m. (transverse portion)
- Upper lip muscles
  - Zygomaticus major and minor m.
  - Levator labii superioris m.
  - Orbicularis oris m.
  - Levator anguli oris m.
- Lower lip muscles (orbicularis oris m.)

Marginal mandibular branch
- Lower lip muscles
  - Orbicularis oris m.
  - Depressor anguli oris m.
  - Depressor labii inferioris m.
  - Mentalis m.
- Risorius m.
- Platysma m. (upper portion)

Cervical branch
- Platysma m.

Table 142.1 Innervation of the muscles of facial expression via cranial nerve VII (the facial nerve)[4,12].

in lip movement. The orbicularis oris muscle allows pursing and puckering of the lips, apposition of the corners of the mouth, and pulling of the lips up against the teeth and gingivae. It has no bony or cartilaginous attachment and is innervated by the buccal or marginal mandibular branches of the facial nerve. This circumferential muscle is necessary for correct speech and allows enunciation of the letters M, V, F, P and O[4].

The facial arteries and veins are covered and protected from damage by the lip elevator muscles. The quadratus labii superioris muscle group is comprised of several lip elevators. The levator anguli oris and risorius muscles are mouth angle retractors and elevators. The zygomaticus major muscle travels from the zygoma downward and diagonally to the upper corner of the mouth, where it contributes to the nasolabial fold. Zygomaticus major and minor muscles are the main contributors to smile formation. The risorius muscle also contributes to a smiling facial expression by drawing back the corners of the mouth. The modiolus platform is formed by the convergence of fibers from the orbicularis oris and lip elevators and depressors. It is located 1 cm lateral to the mouth angle and accounts for cheek 'dimples' in some patients. It works in synergy with the perioral muscles to facilitate speech enunciation.

The buccinator muscle constitutes a large area of the cheek as it courses from the posterior maxillary area to the upper medial surface of the mandible, where it interdigitates with the orbicularis oris. The facial vascular bundle crosses its surface. The parotid duct and transverse facial artery run parallel to each other as the duct pierces the buccinator to enter the mouth at the second maxillary molar. The buccinator is innervated by the buccal branch of the facial nerve and contracts synergistically with the orbicularis oris muscle. Together, these muscles allow whistling of the lips. The buccinator also keeps the cheek flat against the teeth, which prevents food accumulation during chewing. It also prevents overextension of the cheek when high intraoral pressures are generated.

The depressor anguli oris (triangularis), depressor labii inferioris (quadratus) and the mentalis muscles are lip depressors and retractors that antagonize the superior perioral muscle groups. They are innervated by the marginal mandibular branch of the facial nerve. The deep mentalis muscle permits chin elevation and depression and protrusion of the lower lip. The bellies of the mentalis muscles have variable proximities to each other. A patient with a chin 'dimple' or 'cleft chin' has a larger distance between mentalis muscles. This is a normal anatomic variant.

The platysma muscle runs from the superficial fascia of the chest across the anterior and lateral neck over the mandible to intercalate with the lower lip depressors and retractors. It is innervated by the cervical branch of the facial nerve and is continuous with the superficial fascia or SMAS of the lower face. It provides only a thin protective cover to the anterior facial vascular bundle and mandibular branch of the trigeminal nerve.

VASCULAR ANATOMY

The internal carotid artery supplies the eyelids, upper nose and nasal dorsum, forehead and scalp via sub-branches of its ophthalmic branch. The ophthalmic artery arises behind the eye and branches into the orbital and ocular group. The orbital group includes the supraorbital, dorsal nasal and the anterior ethmoidal artery (Fig. 142.13). The supraorbital artery exits the orbit through the supraorbital foramen alongside the supraorbital nerve and perforates the frontalis muscle to ultimately course in the subcutaneous tissue of the forehead and scalp. The supratrochlear artery exits the medial orbit and courses medial to the supraorbital artery to supply the nasal root and the low midline forehead. This artery serves as the axial blood supply for the midline forehead flap often used to repair nasal defects. The success of this flap depends upon isolation and preservation of the supratrochlear artery. The anterior ethmoidal artery exits the nasal passage at the interface of the nasal bone and nasal cartilage to provide arterial supply to the nasal dorsum. The dorsal nasal artery crosses the midline over the nasal root and anastomoses with the angular artery, which originates from the external carotid artery.

While the internal carotid artery contributes to some areas of the scalp and upper face, the external carotid artery supplies most of the

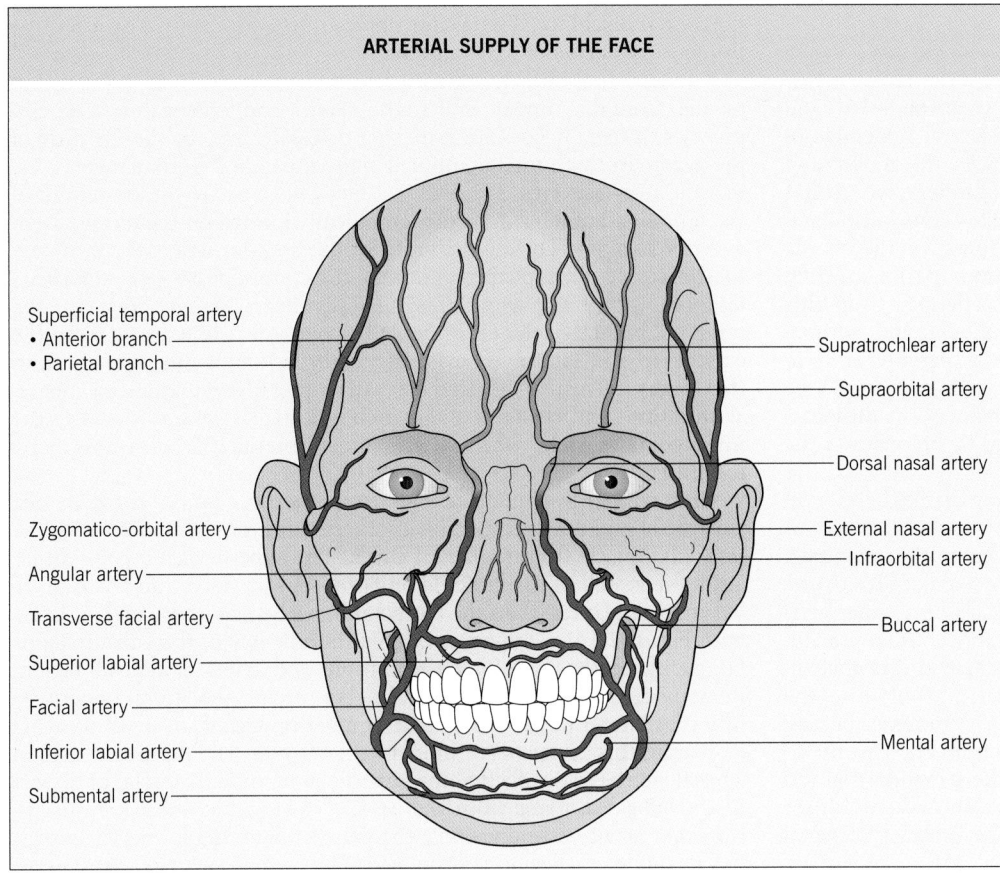

ARTERIAL SUPPLY OF THE FACE

Superficial temporal artery
• Anterior branch
• Parietal branch

Zygomatico-orbital artery

Angular artery

Transverse facial artery

Superior labial artery

Facial artery

Inferior labial artery

Submental artery

Supratrochlear artery

Supraorbital artery

Dorsal nasal artery

External nasal artery

Infraorbital artery

Buccal artery

Mental artery

Fig. 142.13 Arterial supply of the face. Light pink designates arteries derived from the internal carotid artery; dark pink, from the external carotid artery.

face. The facial artery branches off from the external carotid artery and courses deep to the mandible up through or behind the submandibular salivary gland. It passes over the mandibular ridge onto the face anterior to the masseter muscle, where it can be palpated. Its tortuous course maintains a diagonal and superior direction passing alongside the nose and terminating at the medial canthus. The platysma and risorius muscles protect the facial artery near the mandible. As the vessel traverses up the face, it becomes covered by the zygomaticus muscles of the midface and the orbicularis oculi as it nears the medial canthus.

The facial artery gives rise to the inferior and superior labial arteries that course horizontally below and above the lips, respectively. These arteries are found deep to the lip mucosa, but can course more superficially into the submucosa of the lip in elderly patients. After forming the superior labial branch, it becomes known as the angular artery. At its endpoint near the medial canthus tendon, the angular (or facial) artery anastomoses with the dorsal nasal branch of the ophthalmic artery. Since the ophthalmic artery is a branch of the internal carotid system, this anastomosis joins the internal and external carotid arterial systems. During most of their course, the facial artery and vein are covered by the superficial muscles of facial expression. The facial artery also anastomoses with branches of the internal maxillary (the infra-orbital branch) and superficial temporal (transverse facial) arterial tree. This allows excellent blood supply to the facial skin even if distal arterial branches are cut or tied during surgery. The high density of arterial supply to the head and neck accounts for its excellent healing potential and viability of local flaps and grafts.

The lateral face, scalp and forehead are primarily supplied by the superficial temporal artery and its branches. This artery arises in the superficial lobe of the parotid gland as the terminal branch of the external carotid artery. It courses superficially to the main facial nerve trunks, then gives off the transverse facial artery before exiting the parotid gland superficially. The latter transverse artery runs parallel to and 2 cm below the zygomatic arch[4]. The superficial temporal artery exits the parotid and enters the subcutaneous fat in the preauricular crease, where it assumes an ascending vertical course over the zygomatic arch. It can be easily palpated just medial to the upper tragus of the ear. It runs alongside and superficial to the auriculotemporal nerve within, then above the SMAS layer of the temple and lateral forehead. The

most superficial portion of the superficial temporal artery is often visible in aged patients within the subdermal fat above the galea aponeurotica as it courses cephalad above and anterior to the ear. Here it forms the parietal and frontal (anterior) arterial branches that originate just above the uppermost attached portion of the ear. The forehead, eyebrows and lateral scalp receive their arterial supply from these branches of the superficial temporal artery. There are many anastomoses on the scalp between the bilateral superficial temporal arteries. Because of this rich supply chain, the entire scalp tissue remains viable even if one of these arteries is occluded. This rich anastomotic network also explains why scalp surgery can be a very bloody process. Surgical dissection at the level of the galea aponeurotica may serve to avoid transection of the copious subdermal vascular supply.

Most of the arteries of the face run anterior to and parallel with their corresponding veins (see Fig. 142.3). The veins lack valves and therefore permit two-way flow of venous blood. The facial vein connects to the deep facial vein as it drains the cheek. The latter vein parallels the internal maxillary artery and anastomoses with the pterygoid venous plexus medial to the upper mandibular ramus. The facial vein crosses over the submandibular glands, while its corresponding artery passes beneath them. It then drains into the internal jugular vein, which connects with the external jugular vein via the retromandibular vein. The facial vein can communicate with the cavernous sinus of the brain via the ophthalmic vein or the pterygoid plexus. The paranasal area and upper lip are the regions drained by this network. This interface may permit skin or wound infections to gain access to the cavernous sinus of the brain from the draining facial or ophthalmic veins, with potentially devastating consequences.

Arterial blood supply to the face is delivered by a rich subdermal plexus that is fed by larger perforating arteries. Wound healing and flap success depend on maximal blood supply to the area. Axial flaps, such as the midline forehead flap, incorporate a known subcutaneous artery (e.g. the supratrochlear artery) into their design. Random pattern flaps are maintained by the subdermal arterial plexus and do not rely on a single feeder artery to maintain blood flow. The anastomotic vascular network permits facial arteries to be clamped or tied off during surgery without compromising tissue viability. Nearby ipsilateral or contralateral anastomotic arterial branches can often compensate for any loss in local blood supply.

THE FACIAL NERVE

The muscles of facial expression are innervated by the facial nerve, or cranial nerve VII. The facial nerve courses between the SMAS and the deep fascia before its branches penetrate the lateral underside of the facial muscles. There is significant variability in the course and arborization of this nerve from patient to patient. Cranial nerve VII has two major roots, the smaller of which provides sensory innervation and taste sensation to the anterior two-thirds of the tongue via the chorda tympani branch. Sensory innervation to a portion of the external auditory meatus, soft palate, and pharynx is also derived from this small facial nerve root. The submaxillary, submandibular and lacrimal glands contain parasympathetic fibers of the facial nerve that have secretory effects. In addition to the muscles of facial expression (see Table 142.1), the buccinator, stapedius, posterior belly of the digastric, stylohyoid and platysma muscles are all innervated by branches of the facial nerve.

Upon exiting the skull at the stylomastoid foramen near the level of the earlobe, the facial nerve immediately gives off the posterior auricular branch, which provides motor innervation to the occipitalis and posterior auricular muscles (Fig. 142.14). The remainder of the nerve trunk enters the parotid gland and bifurcates into the horizontally oriented temporofacial branch and lower cervicofacial branch. If a line is drawn from the superior border of the tragus to the angle of the mandible, the entrance site of the facial nerve trunk into the parotid gland lies at the midpoint. The temporal, zygomatic, buccal, marginal mandibular, and cervical branches arise from the two major rami of the facial nerve. It courses in between the glandular parotid tissue and becomes more superficial as it follows an upward curvilinear pathway on its way to the ventral surfaces of the muscles of facial expression.

While the facial nerve trunk is well protected in adults at its exit from the skull by the mastoid process, the surgeon must beware when performing procedures in this anatomic region in children. Because the mastoid process is not fully developed until age five, the main facial nerve trunk lies in a superficial subcutaneous plane behind the earlobe and may be damaged in superficial cutaneous procedures. The major facial nerve branches on the cheek are protected only by a small amount of parotid tissue, parotid fascia and subcutaneous fat. If a surgical procedure requires violation of the parotid fascia, meticulous dissection is necessary to avoid major facial nerve damage and subsequent

functional disability. The motor nerves of the face course deeper than the sensory nerves or axial vasculature.

The temporal branch of the facial nerve provides motor innervation to the frontalis, upper orbicularis oculi, and corrugator supercilii muscles. It usually has four rami that originate over the middle third of the zygomatic arch for a combined approximately 2.5 cm 'danger' zone in this area (see Figs 142.5 & 151.5). The most posterior ramus of the temporal branch can be topographically located on the temple 1 cm anterior to a vertical line drawn from the anterior insertion of the ear to the scalp. This posterior ramus runs anterior to the superficial temporal artery and vein. The most significant 'danger zone' for the temporal branch of the facial nerve lies between a line drawn from the earlobe to the lateral edge of the eyebrow and a line drawn from the tragus to just above and lateral to the highest forehead crease. Within this zone, the temporal branch is at highest risk as it crosses the midzygomatic arch, where it lies most superficially over this bony prominence.

The temporal branch of the facial nerve courses between the superficial and deep temporalis fascia, penetrating the underside of the frontalis muscle from its lateral edges. The superficial temporal artery and vein as well as the auriculotemporal sensory nerve run posterior to but more superficial than the temporal nerve branch (compare Fig. 142.3 with Fig. 142.14). This neurovascular bundle lies in the subcutaneous fat overlying the SMAS of the temple and lateral forehead region. Remember that once the temporal nerve reaches the lateral underbelly of its ipsilateral target muscles, it is most protected. In order to avoid damaging this facial nerve branch, the surgeon should either remain superficial to the SMAS (i.e. the superficial temporalis fascia) or dissect in the subgaleal plane from the medial to lateral forehead. Similar to the other facial nerve divisions, the greatest potential for nerve damage lies in the lateral regions of the face. The central face has many nerve arborizations and protective muscles that usually afford a minimal risk for facial motor nerve damage.

Damage to a ramus of the temporal branch of the facial nerve can result in notable cosmetic and functional loss. The temporal branch consists of long, usually singular and often superficially coursing rami that have few arborizations or cross-innervations. These characteristics make nerve damage and permanent sequelae more likely when cutaneous procedures are performed in the forehead and temporal regions. Even though the upper orbicularis oculi and corrugator supercilii muscles are innervated by the temporal branch, minimal functional or cosmetic compromise occurs, due to cross-innervation by other motor nerves. However, only 15% of patients will have any cross-innervation to the frontalis muscle by the more inferior zygomatic branch of the facial nerve. Such arborization permits retention of some functional mobility of the frontalis should the temporal branch be sacrificed. For the other 85% of patients, violation of the temporal nerve results in motor denervation and the inability to raise a now lowered or 'droopy' eyebrow[4]. Flattening of the forehead with diminished visibility of wrinkles and skin tension lines on the ipsilateral side is easily noted. The functional loss of the frontalis muscle significantly hampers a patient's ability to communicate non-verbally via facial expression and may have devastating psychosocial consequences. Over time, the inability to raise one's eyebrow can lead to eyebrow and eyelid ptosis and upper visual field compromise as muscular disuse atrophy progresses. Brow lifts and blepharoplasty may be necessary if the temporal nerve branch is permanently damaged.

The zygomatic branch of the facial nerve provides motor innervation to the lower orbicularis oculi, procerus, mouth elevators and nasal muscles. Its fibers overlie the parotid (Stensen's) duct and course horizontally and upwards after emerging from the parotid gland as the second division of the facial nerve. There is marked variability in the innervation it provides to these muscles; thereby, damage to this nerve branch can have unpredictable outcomes. Generally, injury to the zygomatic branch results in decreased orbicularis oculi function and a diminished ability to close the ipsilateral eyelid tightly. The orbicularis oculi is also innervated in its supraorbital aspect by the temporal branch of the facial nerve. Therefore, complete loss of circumferential periocular motor function is highly unlikely. Other effects may include dysfunction of nasal muscles and lip elevators.

The buccal branch is the third division of the facial nerve, and it courses inferiorly to the zygomatic branch in a downward direction on

THE FACIAL (MOTOR) NERVE

- Superficial temporal artery
- Facial nerve (superior division)
  - Temporal branch
  - Zygomatic branch
  - Temporofacial branch
- Stylomastoid foramen
- Facial nerve (inferior division)
  - Posterior auricular branch
  - Cervicofacial branch
  - Buccal branch
  - Marginal mandibular branch
  - Cervical branch

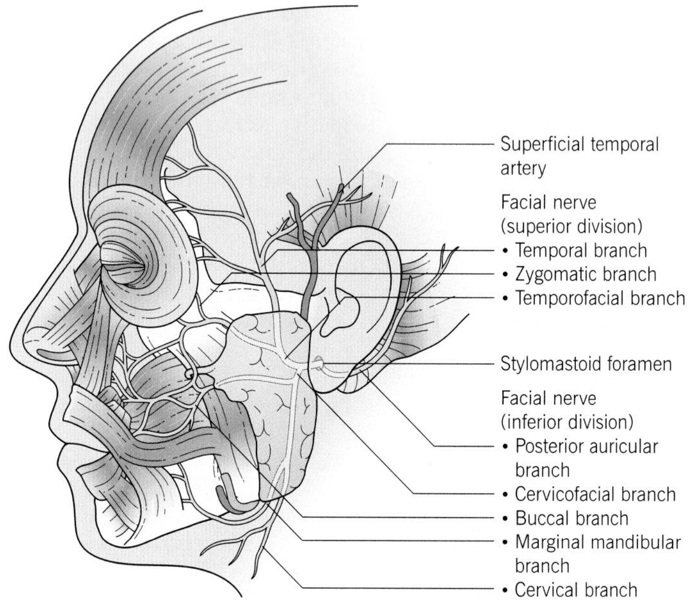

Fig. 142.14 The facial (motor) nerve.

the cheek. It innervates the orbicularis oris muscle, the zygomaticus muscles, the lip elevators, the buccinator muscle and nasal muscles to a variable extent. Damage to this nerve causes buccinator dysfunction that results in accumulation of food between the teeth and the buccal mucosa with chewing. Approximately 80% of patients have anastomoses between the fibers of the zygomatic and buccal branches[13]. Each branch has two points of arborization, with the first occurring 2 cm anterior to the anterior edge of the parotid gland and the second usually occurring under the modiolus 1 cm lateral to the oral commissure at the anterior aspect of the buccal fat pad. Here the nerves may be damaged due to their superficial anatomy, protected only by the thin fascia of the SMAS, an often underdeveloped risorius muscle, and the subcutaneous fat. At the first branching site near the parotid, the zygomatic and buccal nerves lie between the masseter muscle and the posterior side of the buccal fat pad.

Although damage to the zygomatic or buccal branches of the facial nerve may occur during surgical procedures, subsequent motor dysfunction is often temporary and far less debilitating than a similar injury to the temporal nerve. The high degree of anastomoses between the zygomatic and buccal branches minimizes functional damage and promotes nerve recovery after trauma. Partial paralysis of the perioral muscles may occur, causing variable symptomatic defects in facial expression, including a diminished ability or unilateral defect in forming a smile or pucker, lip pursing and lip seal formation. Drooling, food accumulation between the cheeks and gingivae, and muffled speech may occur secondary to buccal or zygomatic nerve damage. Orbicularis oculi defects have already been discussed and include lower eyelid droop, which can lead to chronic conjunctivitis, sicca symptoms, and ectropion. Difficulty wrinkling up the nose and inability to flare the nostrils may also occur with zygomatic or buccal branch trauma. Fortunately, most of these symptoms resolve within 6 months due to the extensive ramification and cross-innervation of these branches of the facial nerve.

The orbicularis oris, mentalis, and lip depressor muscles are innervated by the marginal mandibular branch of the facial nerve. The nerve courses along the angle of the mandible below the parotid gland and continues up over the mandibular body anterior to the facial artery, which can be palpated easily as it courses over the medial mandible. The nerve is very susceptible to damage, due to its superficial location over the bony edge of the jaw (i.e. just inferior and lateral to the lateral oral commissure), where it is covered only by fascia and an often unpredictably thin or poorly developed platysma muscle. This facial nerve branch is often composed of only one ramus. The marginal mandibular nerve 'communicates' with the buccal branch of the facial nerve in only 10% of patients; therefore, damage to the former branch can lead to permanent disfiguring and functional defects in facial expression[4]. Normal symmetric facial expression and function of the mouth depends upon the equal and opposite effects exerted by the lip depressors and elevators in conjunction with the orbicularis oris muscle. Characteristically, a patient with marginal mandibular nerve damage cannot form a symmetric smile. There is inability to pull the ipsilateral lower lip downward and laterally or evert the corresponding vermilion border. The end result is a 'crooked' smile. The defect is appreciated upon smiling, but is not as apparent when the patient is at rest.

The cervical branch of the facial nerve innervates the platysma muscle. This muscle receives nerve fibers from the marginal mandibular nerve as well. Damage incurred to the cervical branch rarely causes functional or cosmetic defects.

SENSORY INNERVATION OF THE HEAD AND NECK

The trigeminal nerve, or cranial nerve V, provides the primary sensory innervation to the face, while the upper cervical nerves (C2, C3) provide sensory supply to the neck, part of the ear, and posterior scalp (Fig. 142.15). The facial, glossopharyngeal and vagus nerves provide a small portion of sensory innervation to the ear. The trigeminal nerve is the largest cranial nerve. It has motor (to the muscles of mastication), sensory and parasympathetic functions, supplying secretory fibers (originating from the facial and glossopharyngeal nerves) to the lacrimal and parotid glands. The sensory branches of the trigeminal nerve course more superficially than the trunk of the facial nerve, and

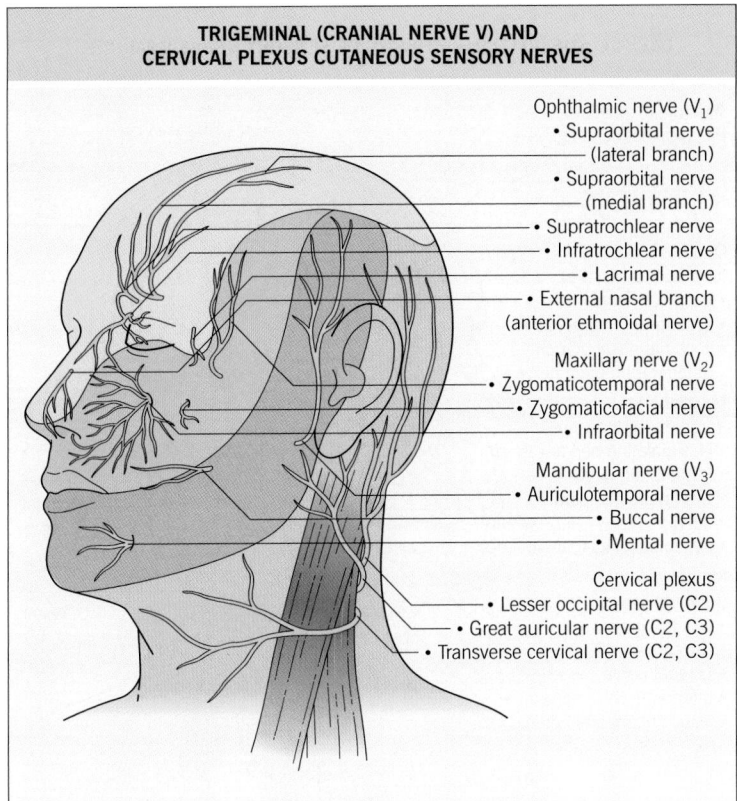

Fig. 142.15 Trigeminal (cranial nerve V) and cervical plexus cutaneous sensory nerves. The concha and external auditory canal are variably innervated by branches of the vagus, glossopharyngeal, and facial nerves.

Labels in figure:
- TRIGEMINAL (CRANIAL NERVE V) AND CERVICAL PLEXUS CUTANEOUS SENSORY NERVES
- Ophthalmic nerve (V$_1$)
  - Supraorbital nerve (lateral branch)
  - Supraorbital nerve (medial branch)
  - Supratrochlear nerve
  - Infratrochlear nerve
  - Lacrimal nerve
  - External nasal branch (anterior ethmoidal nerve)
- Maxillary nerve (V$_2$)
  - Zygomaticotemporal nerve
  - Zygomaticofacial nerve
  - Infraorbital nerve
- Mandibular nerve (V$_3$)
  - Auriculotemporal nerve
  - Buccal nerve
  - Mental nerve
- Cervical plexus
  - Lesser occipital nerve (C2)
  - Great auricular nerve (C2, C3)
  - Transverse cervical nerve (C2, C3)

are thereby readily subject to damage during surgical procedures. Fortunately, most resulting sensory dysfunction is not debilitating or permanent. Transmedian re-innervation after unilateral trigeminal root transection has been demonstrated. This is due to collateral sprouting of sensory nerves from the contralateral trigeminal nerve root[14]. The sensory nerves exist in the superficial plane between the subcutaneous fat and the SMAS and often run together with arteries and veins in neurovascular bundles. Knowledge of the sites where the major branches of sensory nerves emerge from the skull assists the surgeon in performing regional nerve blocks that facilitate facial surgery and improve patient comfort.

The trigeminal nerve is divided into three main branches, called the ophthalmic (V1), maxillary (V2) and mandibular (V3) nerves (see Fig. 142.15). The smallest, uppermost sensory branch is the ophthalmic division, which gives off three branches (nasociliary, frontal and lacrimal nerves) before exiting the orbit (Fig. 142.16). Sensory fibers to the sinuses and upper nasal septal mucosa, as well as secretory parasympathetic fibers (that originate from the facial nerve) to the lacrimal gland are also provided by the ophthalmic branch of the trigeminal nerve. The nasociliary branch gives rise to the infratrochlear nerve and the external branch of the anterior ethmoidal nerve. Sensory innervation to the root of the nose and part of the medial canthus is supplied by the infratrochlear nerve. The nasal dorsum, tip, supratip and columella derive cutaneous innervation from the external nasal branch of the anterior ethmoidal nerve, which emerges between the upper nasal cartilage and nasal bones. Nerve blocks for the nose rely on knowledge of these anatomic relationships among the sensory nerves. The nasociliary branch also supplies the corneal surface via the ciliary nerve. If an episode of zoster (varicella zoster virus) involves the nasal tip, then close ophthalmologic follow-up is warranted due to presumed corneal involvement.

The frontal nerve branch of the ophthalmic division forms the supratrochlear and supraorbital nerves. The exit route (called the supratrochlear ridge) of the supratrochlear nerve lies 1 cm lateral to the midline on the supraorbital ridge. This branch of the frontal nerve provides sensory innervation to the medial upper eyelid, medial forehead, and frontal scalp. The supraorbital foramen (through which emerges the supraorbital neurovascular bundle) lies 2.5 cm lateral to the midline on the supraorbital ridge (see Fig. 142.2). After penetrating

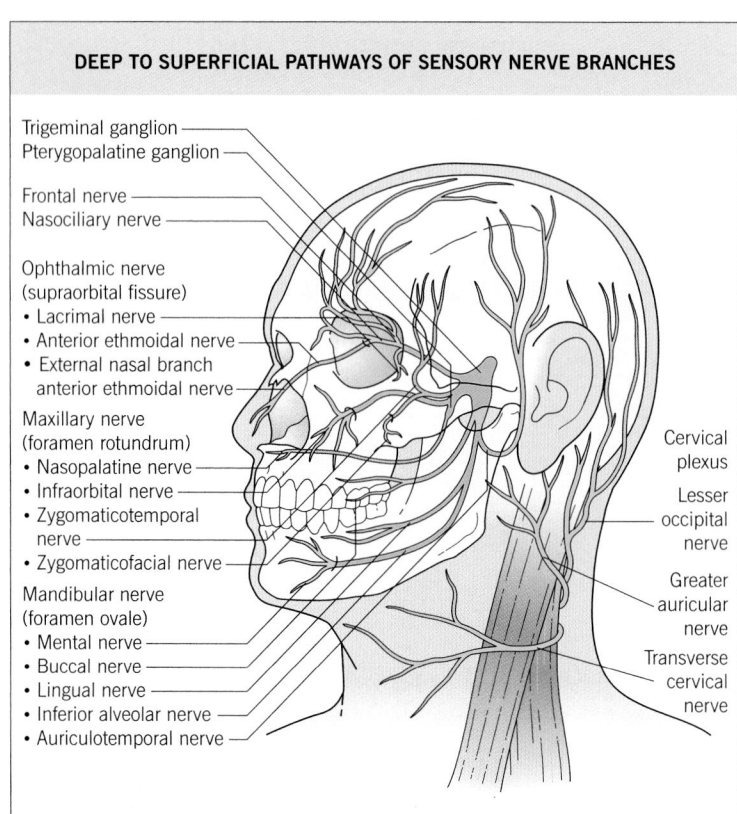

DEEP TO SUPERFICIAL PATHWAYS OF SENSORY NERVE BRANCHES

Trigeminal ganglion
Pterygopalatine ganglion

Frontal nerve
Nasociliary nerve

Ophthalmic nerve
(supraorbital fissure)
• Lacrimal nerve
• Anterior ethmoidal nerve
• External nasal branch
  anterior ethmoidal nerve

Maxillary nerve
(foramen rotundrum)
• Nasopalatine nerve
• Infraorbital nerve
• Zygomaticotemporal
  nerve
• Zygomaticofacial nerve

Mandibular nerve
(foramen ovale)
• Mental nerve
• Buccal nerve
• Lingual nerve
• Inferior alveolar nerve
• Auriculotemporal nerve

Cervical plexus

Lesser occipital nerve

Greater auricular nerve

Transverse cervical nerve

Fig. 142.16 Deep to superficial pathways of sensory nerve branches.

the frontalis muscle to emerge above the frontalis SMAS, the supra-orbital nerve provides cutaneous sensation to the forehead, scalp and upper eyelid. A small lacrimal nerve branch of the ophthalmic division of cranial nerve V innervates the lateral eyelid skin and lies near the upper lateral orbital rim. Frontal nerve blocks, and specifically the supratrochlear and supraorbital block, offer quick and effective anesthesia for surgical procedures of the forehead.

The maxillary branch (V2) of the trigeminal nerve forms the infra-orbital, zygomaticofacial and zygomaticotemporal cutaneous sensory branches (see Fig. 142.15). The infraorbital foramen lies 2.5 cm lateral to midline and 1 cm inferior to the infraorbital rim, in the same vertical line as the supraorbital and mental foramina. The infraorbital neuro-vascular bundle emerges here to provide significant sensory innervation to the medial cheek, upper lip, nasal sidewall and ala, and the lower eyelid. Infraorbital nerve blocks offer simple and effective anesthesia for much of the cheek, lower eyelid and nose. Lateral to the infraorbital foramen, the zygomaticofacial nerve emerges to innervate the skin of the malar eminence. Cutaneous innervation of the temple and supra-temporal scalp region is provided by a third branch of the maxillary division, the zygomaticotemporal nerve. It emerges from the lateral orbital margin at the zygomatic bone. The superior alveolar and palatine nerves are deeper branches of V2 that provide sensory innervation to the upper teeth, palate, nasal mucosa, and gingiva.

The mandibular branch (V3) is the largest division of the trigeminal nerve and the only one to carry both cutaneous sensory and motor fibers. It supplies cutaneous sensory innervation to the face as well as motor innervation to the muscles of mastication. The auriculotemporal, buccal and inferior alveolar nerves represent the three main cutaneous branches of V3. The auriculotemporal nerve emerges from behind the neck of the mandible to course just deep to the superficial temporal artery from the superior margin of the parotid gland in the preauricular sulcus up towards the lateral scalp. It provides sensory innervation to the external ear and auditory canal, temple, temporoparietal scalp, temporomandibular joint and tympanic membrane. It also carries para-sympathetic secretory fibers to the parotid gland.

The buccal nerve supplies sensory innervation to the cheek, buccal mucosa, and gingiva. It runs deep to the parotid over the pterygoid muscle to the upper surface of the buccinator, which it pierces to reach the overlying skin. Because the terminal branches of the buccal nerve are small and numerous, regional buccal nerve block techniques are

not feasible anesthetic options. The inferior alveolar branch of V3 innervates the mandibular teeth as it courses through the mandibular sulcus. Its terminal branch forms the mental nerve, which emerges from the mental foramen in the same topographic line as the supra-orbital and infraorbital neurovascular bundles (i.e. 2.5 cm lateral to the midline). The mental vein, artery and nerve emerge from the mental foramen below the lower second premolar. The lingual nerve supplies sensory innervation to the anterior two-thirds of the tongue, the floor of the mouth, and the lower gingivae. It arises from V3 and courses parallel and superior to the inferior alveolar nerve.

The cervical plexus is a network of arborizing and anastomosing nerve branches of the ventral rami of the four most superior cervical nerves. It emerges from the mid-posterior margin of the sterno-cleidomastoid (SCM) muscle at Erb's point to give off three branches, designated as C2, C3 and C4. C2 and C3 compose the greater auricular nerve, which runs from the posterior edge of the SCM towards the earlobe in the same plane and path as the external jugular vein. It inner-vates the skin of the lateral neck, angle of the jaw, and part of the auricular and postauricular skin.

The lesser occipital nerve (C2) emerges from the same point at the SCM and assumes a course parallel to the SCM upward to innervate the skin of the neck and postauricular scalp. The transverse cervical nerve (C2 and C3) likewise emerges from behind the SCM and arcs anteriorly around and across the SCM in a transverse direction. Its many terminal branches supply the skin of the anterior neck. The supra-clavicular nerve (C3 and C4) emerges from the same point at the SCM posterior margin, then courses inferiorly until it reaches the supra-clavicular region, where it terminates, and provides sensory inner-vation to the anterior chest and shoulder skin (see Fig. 142.4).

Perineural invasion of cutaneous tumors such as basal cell carcinomas, neuropathic melanomas and squamous cell carcinomas may be encountered by the clinician. Patients are often asymptomatic from dermal nerve twig infiltration by tumor cells, with the diagnosis made only by histopathologic tissue examination. Some patients may experience sensory abnormalities and, rarely, motor dysfunction. Most of these scenarios occur in the setting of squamous malignancies (incidence rates range from 3% to 14%), with less than 1% of basal cell carcinomas showing any histologic evidence of perineural spread[13]. Knowledge of the neuroanatomy of the head and neck assists the surgeon in planning adjuvant therapy, such as radiation, for patients with nerve involvement.

LYMPHATIC DRAINAGE OF THE HEAD AND NECK

Squamous cell carcinomas, melanomas, and other cutaneous neoplasms may spread via lymphatics to regional lymph nodes and subsequently metastasize to other organs. It is important for the clinician to have a thorough understanding of the lymphatic drainage of the head and neck in order to appropriately stage and manage patients. Before any surgical endeavor is undertaken for a malignancy in this region, palpation of regional lymph nodes and basins should be performed. Head and neck cancers usually spread to adjacent lymph nodes in a diagonal direction from cephalad to caudad (Fig. 142.17). There is a large degree of variability in drainage pathways, but the anatomic location of individual lymph nodes is more consistent from patient to patient. Cutaneous neoplasms that breach the papillary dermis may spread from small lymph capillaries to progressively larger and deeper lymphatic trunks in the area. Lymph channels often course along the same directional pathway as the head and neck veins. They are more numerous and often more superficial than the corresponding veins and lie predominantly between the super-ficial and deep fascial layers.

Important primary lymphatic drainage patterns of the head and neck region include the following: parotid nodes often collect from the forehead and eyelids (upper lateral face); submandibular nodes from the lower and medial face or from the submental nodes; submental nodes from the central lower lip and chin. Lateral cervical nodes are the common subsequent lymph collection site from these areas. Parotid nodes may be extraglandular or intraglandular. The extraglandular channels are invested within the parotid sheath. Two-thirds of all people will also have one to three pretragal and infra-auricular lymph nodes that are considered part of the parotid node basin[4]. These

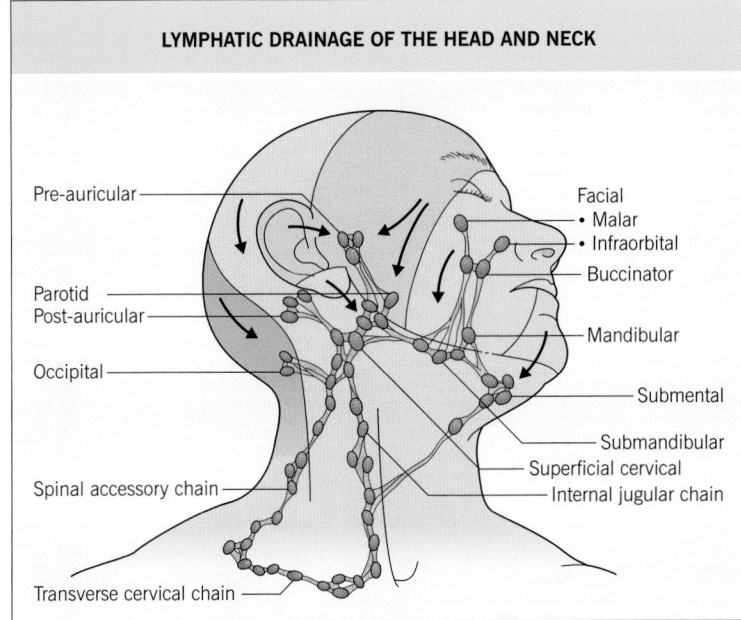

LYMPHATIC DRAINAGE OF THE HEAD AND NECK

Pre-auricular

Parotid
Post-auricular

Occipital

Spinal accessory chain

Transverse cervical chain

Facial
• Malar
• Infraorbital

Buccinator

Mandibular

Submental

Submandibular
Superficial cervical
Internal jugular chain

Fig. 142.17 Lymphatic drainage of the head and neck.

pre-and infra-auricular nodes drain the ear, the lateral lower cheek, the frontolateral scalp and the forehead, as well as the nasal root. Drainage of the parotid unit may then follow the external or internal jugular vein in the jugular lymph node chain; therefore, palpation for nodes from the site of the cutaneous lesion to the supraclavicular and even axillary nodal basins is recommended.

Submandibular nodes should be examined as the patient relaxes the neck muscles and tilts the chin down. This nodal group drains the gingival and mucous membranes, lower eyelids, anterior two-thirds of the tongue, lips, nose and medial cheeks. The submental nodes (up to eight) of the neck lie beneath the platysma and drain the anterior third of the tongue and floor of the mouth, in addition to the lower middle lip, chin and medial lower cheeks. They are best examined by elevating the chin and asking the patient to engage the platysma. Submental nodes frequently drain bilaterally or contralaterally and empty into the submandibular basin or directly into the internal jugular lymphatic chain. Note that up to one-quarter of healthy people have small (less than 1 cm) non-fixed palpable submental nodes[4].

The superficial lateral cervical nodes are adjacent to the infra-auricular parotid nodes and lie near the high external jugular vein. Use the sternocleidomastoid muscle as a landmark to palpate these nodes (up to four) over its cephalad portion. Deeper lateral cervical nodes include the spinal accessory, internal jugular and transverse cervical chains, which form a triangle on the neck. The internal jugular chain is the main lymphatic collection trunk of the head and neck and may contain up to 25 lymph nodes in each patient. The internal jugular chain on the right often drains into the subclavian vein, whereas the left-sided lymphatic chain empties into the thoracic duct. These nodes can be palpated by rolling two fingers over the area of the carotid triangle.

Acute or chronic lymphedema may ensue after transection of larger lymphatic channels or nodes, or even after disruption of smaller channels in areas (e.g. infraorbital) with limited or vulnerable lymphatic drainage. Adequate drainage can be achieved by orienting flaps in the same direction as lymphatic patterns. The surgeon must be mindful of the variability in drainage patterns and sites and the fact that malignancies do not respect the midline. Since cross-communication between lymphatics may result in contralateral drainage, bilateral examination for lymphadenopathy should be undertaken before a neoplasm is excised.

REFERENCES

1. Dzubow LM. Tissue movement – a macrobiomechanical approach. J Dermatol Surg Oncol. 1989;15:389–99.
2. Dzubow LM. Facial Flaps: Biomechanics and Regional Application. Norwalk: Appleton & Lange, 1990.
3. Robinson JK, Sengelmann RD, Hanke CW, Siegel DM. Surgery of the Skin: Procedural Dermatology. St Louis: Mosby, 2005.
4. Salasche SJ, Bernstein G, Senkarik M. Surgical Anatomy of the Skin. Norwalk: Appleton & Lange, 1988.
5. Gosain AK, Yousif NJ, Madiedo G, Larson DL, Matloub HS, Sanger JR. Surgical anatomy of the SMAS: a reinvestigation. Plast Reconstr Surg. 1993;92:1254–65.
6. Burger GC, Menick FJ. Aesthetic reconstruction of the nose. St Louis: Mosby, 1994.
7. Summers BK, Siegle RJ. Facial cutaneous reconstructive surgery: general aesthetic principles. J Am Acad Dermatol. 1993;29:669–81.
8. Zide BM, Jelks GW. Surgical Anatomy of the Orbit. New York: Raven Press, 1985.
9. Stegman SJ, Tromovitch TA, Glogau RG. Cosmetic Dermatologic Surgery, 2nd edn. St Louis: Mosby, 1990.
10. Larrabee WF, Makielski KH. Surgical Anatomy of the Face. New York: Raven Press, 1993.
11. Tromovitch TA, Stegman SJ, Glogau RG. Flaps and Grafts in Dermatologic Surgery. Chicago: Year Book, 1989.
12. Bennett RG. Fundamentals of Cutaneous Surgery. St Louis: Mosby, 1988.
13. Carlson KC, Roenigk RK. Know your anatomy: perineural involvement of basal and squamous cell carcinoma on the face. J Dermatol Surg Oncol. 1990;16:827–33.
14. Robinson PP. Recession of sensory loss from the midline following trigeminal sensory root section: collateral sprouting from the normal side? Brain Res. 1983;259:177–80.

Anesthesia

George J Hruza

143

Key features

- Local anesthetics are classified into two groups – amides and esters, depending upon the linkage in their intermediate chain
- 'Anesthetic allergies' vary from palpitations secondary to epinephrine and vasovagal reactions to urticaria from preservatives or the local anesthetic (especially esters)
- Additives to the local anesthetic include epinephrine, sodium bicarbonate and hyaluronidase
- Nerve blocks are particularly helpful when performing procedures on the face, digits and palmoplantar surfaces

INTRODUCTION

Effective anesthesia is an essential component of dermatologic surgery. Almost all dermatologic surgical procedures can be performed under local anesthesia. Local anesthetics have been in use since the 1880s with the introduction of cocaine, which was extracted from leaves of the South American bush *Erythroxylon coca*[1]. This was followed by procaine in 1904, tetracaine in 1930, and the first amide local anesthetic, lidocaine, was introduced in 1943[1]. The introduction of lidocaine was a major breakthrough because lidocaine is far less likely to cause an allergic reaction than the ester-type anesthetics that preceded it.

Local anesthesia has several advantages over general anesthesia, including reduced morbidity (especially in patients who are poor anesthesia risks), reduced cost, reduced procedure time and faster recovery. The main disadvantages are some limitation on the extent of a procedure and the possibility of greater patient discomfort from the injections. Knowledge of the physiology, dosage, side effects, and proper 'painless' local anesthesia technique are essential for performing dermatologic surgery and to keep patients safe and satisfied.

DISCUSSION

Physiology and Structure

Local anesthetics act by blocking sodium channels in the axon cell membrane from opening. This prevents sodium from entering the nerve cell. The nerve cell is not depolarized and consequently the action potential is blocked. The cationic form of the anesthetic seems to bind to a receptor in the sodium channel[2]. Smaller unmyelinated C-type nerve fibers that conduct pain sensation are blocked more quickly and easily than intermediate fibers that carry sensations of heat and cold. The myelinated A-type fibers that carry pressure sensation and motor fibers are blocked last. Clinically, this is evident when an area seems fully anesthetized for scalpel surgery, but the patient still feels the pressure of the surgeon's fingers at the surgical site.

All local anesthetics consist of three parts (Fig. 143.1):
- a secondary or tertiary amine end
- an aromatic end
- an intermediate connecting chain that contains an ester or amide.

The aromatic portion is hydrophobic and lipophilic. This is essential to allow the anesthetic to diffuse through nerve cell membranes. The amine portion is hydrophilic and is responsible for the anesthetic's water solubility, which is important for preparing, storing and administering the anesthetic[2].

Local anesthetics are weak organic bases, which, to be water soluble and injectable, require the addition of a hydrochloride salt. In aqueous solution, the salt equilibrates between the ionized and non-ionized

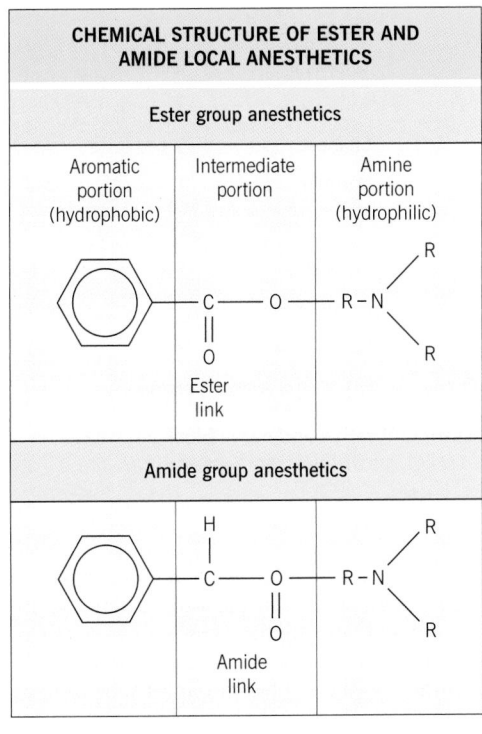

CHEMICAL STRUCTURE OF ESTER AND AMIDE LOCAL ANESTHETICS

Ester group anesthetics

| Aromatic portion (hydrophobic) | Intermediate portion | Amine portion (hydrophilic) |

Ester link

Amide group anesthetics

Amide link

Fig. 143.1 Chemical structure of the ester and amide group local anesthetics. The aromatic (hydrophobic) end is joined to the amine (hydrophilic) end with an ester or amide linkage.

form. The ionized form is water soluble, allowing injection into the tissue. However, it is the non-ionized, lipid-soluble base that diffuses through the tissue to the nerve cell membrane, where the ionized cation is responsible for blocking nerve conduction.

The dissociation constant (pKa) of each anesthetic determines the proportion of the anesthetic base and its cation at a given pH. The pKa of all local anesthetics is higher than physiologic pH. For most local anesthetics at a pH of 7.4, 80% or more is in the cationic ionized form. An anesthetic with a low pKa will have a rapid onset of action. Alkalinization of the anesthetic solution, as is done with the addition of sodium bicarbonate, will speed its onset of action. However, if the pH is raised too much, the anesthetic may precipitate out of solution. Anesthetic sensitivity to pH also helps explain why infected tissue is difficult to effectively anesthetize[3]. The inflammatory response surrounding the infection acidifies the site (reduces the pH), which reduces the proportion of the anesthetic in the non-ionized lipid-soluble form that is needed for anesthetic action at the nerve cell membrane.

Pharmacology

Local anesthetics are classified into two groups, depending on the linkage in the intermediate chain (Table 143.1). Amide anesthetics have an amide linkage and ester anesthetics have an ester linkage. They differ in how they are metabolized and in the risk of sensitization. Ester anesthetics are hydrolyzed by plasma pseudocholinesterase, and the metabolites are excreted by the kidneys. Patients with a deficiency of functional pseudocholinesterase are at an increased risk of ester anesthetic toxicity. The metabolite para-aminobenzoic acid (PABA) is responsible for the allergic reactions seen with ester anesthetics. Amide anesthetics are metabolized by hepatic microsomal enzymes, and the metabolites are excreted by the kidneys. Patients with severe liver disease may be at increased risk of amide anesthetic toxicity.

Local anesthetics differ in the speed of onset, duration of action, and potency, depending on each compound's intrinsic chemical

LOCAL ANESTHETICS FOR INFILTRATIVE AND NERVE BLOCK ANESTHESIA					
Generic name	Trade name®	Onset (min)	Duration plain (h)	Maximum dose plain (mg for 70 kg man)	Maximum dose with epinephrine (mg for 70 kg man)
Amides					
Articaine	Septocaine	2–4	0.5–2	350	500
Bupivacaine hydrochloride	Marcaine	5–8	2–4	175	225
Etidocaine	Duranest	3–5	3–5	300	400
Levobupivacaine hydrochloride	Chirocaine	2–10	2–4	150	Not available
Lidocaine	Xylocaine	Rapid	0.5–2	350	500 (3500 dilute)
Mepivacaine	Carbocaine	3–20	0.5–2	300	500
Prilocaine hydrochloride	Citanest	5–6	0.5–2	400	600
Ropivacaine*	Naropin	1–15	2–6	200	Not available
Esters					
Chloroprocaine hydrochloride	Nesacaine	5–6	0.5–2	800	1000
Procaine	Novocaine	5	1–1.5	500	600
Tetracaine	Pontocaine	7	2–3	100	Not available

Addition of epinephrine has no effect on onset or duration of action of ropivacaine.

Table 143.1 Local anesthetics for infiltrative and nerve block anesthesia. In clinical practice, the duration of anesthesia appears to be less than stated, especially for head and neck areas. Addition of epinephrine prolongs anesthesia by a factor of two.

characteristics (see Table 143.1). A low pKa leads to rapid onset of anesthesia, as most of the anesthetic will be in the ionized active form. Greater lipid solubility is associated with higher anesthetic potency, as the compound penetrates the nerve cell membrane more easily. Duration of action is determined by the strength of anesthetic binding to the sodium channel receptor.

Occasionally, pregnant women need to undergo skin surgery. The local anesthetic of choice in pregnancy is lidocaine. It is classified into pregnancy category B. This means that, in animal studies, no teratogenic effects have been documented. Studies in pregnant women who received lidocaine during the first trimester of pregnancy have shown no increase in anatomic abnormalities in the newborns. However, it is recommended that lidocaine, as with all other pharmacologic agents, be used cautiously during the first 4 months of pregnancy, when maximum organogenesis takes place. Lidocaine crosses the placenta into the fetus. Lidocaine can be safely used in nursing mothers with the realization that some of the anesthetic may be excreted in the mother's milk.

Lidocaine can be safely used in children, but the maximum recommended dosage should be adjusted downward based on the child's weight and age. Parabens, used as preservatives, are bound to albumin. In a jaundiced newborn, they could displace bilirubin from the albumin, worsening the hyperbilirubinemia[4]. For this reason, only paraben-free anesthetics should be used in newborns.

Additions to Local Anesthetics

Epinephrine

All local anesthetics, except for cocaine, relax vascular smooth muscle, which results in vasodilation. This causes increased bleeding at the operative site and reduced duration of anesthetic action as the anesthetic is rapidly removed from the surgical site through the dilated blood vessels. The addition of epinephrine has the beneficial effect of constricting blood vessels. This prolongs the duration of anesthesia 100% to 200% by slowing removal of the anesthetic from the surgical site. Also, there is reduced intraoperative bleeding due to the vasoconstriction. The addition of epinephrine provides more effective anesthesia by decreasing the volume of anesthetic needed. The reduced absorption rate decreases anesthetic toxicity and allows larger doses to be used safely. The vasoconstrictive effect of epinephrine, manifested by skin blanching, takes about 15 minutes to fully develop. While they usually coincide, blanching does not always denote the anesthetized area.

Epinephrine is premixed with local anesthetics at a concentration of 1:100 000 or 1:200 000. However, concentrations as low as 1:1 000 000 achieve effective vasoconstriction, while concentrations greater than 1:100 000 are associated with greater risk of side effects. The concentration used in a given patient should be individualized. Patients who have relative contraindications to epinephrine should receive lower concentrations, while highly vascular areas such as the scalp should receive higher concentrations. The maximum dosage used at a concentration of 1:100 000 is determined by the anesthetic with which the epinephrine is premixed.

Epinephrine is a strong β- and α-agonist and, as such, it must be used cautiously in patients with altered β- and α-receptors. Absolute contraindications to the use of epinephrine include hyperthyroidism and pheochromocytoma. Patients taking β-blockers, monoamine oxidase inhibitors, tricyclic antidepressants, and phenothiazines are more sensitive to epinephrine. Therefore, epinephrine should be used with caution, with the dose and concentration reduced accordingly. Severe hypertension developing after epinephrine-containing anesthetic injection in patients taking β-blockers has been reported[5]. This is probably due to unopposed α-adrenergic activity with its associated vasoconstriction. Fortunately, this reaction seems to be quite rare[6], and mainly occurs when higher doses are used. Patients with severe hypertension or with severe cardiovascular disease (especially coronary artery disease) may have their underlying disease exacerbated if large amounts of epinephrine are administered with the local anesthetic. High doses of epinephrine can induce labor. However, the low doses of epinephrine used in cutaneous surgery can be safely used during pregnancy. Epinephrine use in the periorbital area in patients with narrow angle glaucoma should be avoided, as it may aggravate the patient's glaucoma.

The use of epinephrine on digits has been controversial. Historically, epinephrine was not used on digits for fear of causing vasoconstriction that might result in digital necrosis. More recent studies have not demonstrated any increased risk from epinephrine in digital anesthesia. It appears that most cases of digital necrosis occurred due to vessel compression from too much anesthetic volume being injected (tamponade), constricting circumferential dressings, tourniquets, postoperative hot soaks, infection, use of vasoconstrictive anesthetics such as cocaine, or non-standard mixing of lidocaine with epinephrine[7]. There is no evidence of digital necrosis due solely to commercially available lidocaine with epinephrine[7]. However, epinephrine is clearly contraindicated for digital anesthesia in patients with peripheral vascular disease. I have found that combining lidocaine with dilute epinephrine

DIFFERENTIAL DIAGNOSIS OF LOCAL ANESTHETIC SYSTEMIC REACTIONS

Diagnosis	Pulse rate	Blood pressure	Signs and symptoms	Emergency management
Vasovagal reaction	Low	Low	Excess parasympathetic tone; diaphoresis, hyperventilation, nausea	Trendelenburg, cold compress, reassurance
Epinephrine reaction	High	High	Excess α- and β-adrenergic receptor stimulation; palpitations	Reassurance (usually resolves within minutes), phentolamine, propranolol
Anaphylactic reaction	High	Low	Peripheral vasodilation with reactive tachycardia; stridor, bronchospasm, urticaria, angioedema	Epinephrine 1:1000 0.3 ml sc, antihistamines, fluids, oxygen, airway maintenance
Lidocaine overdose 1–6 µg/ml	Normal	Normal	Circumoral and digital paresthesias, restlessness, drowsiness, euphoria, lightheadedness	Observation
6–9 µg/ml	Normal	Normal	Nausea, vomiting, muscle twitching, tremors, blurred vision, tinnitus, confusion, excitement, psychosis	Diazepam, airway maintenance
9–12 µg/ml	Low	Low	Seizures, cardiopulmonary depression	Respiratory support
>12 µg/ml	None	None	Coma, cardiopulmonary arrest	Cardiopulmonary resuscitation and life support

Table 143.2 **Differential diagnosis of local anesthetic systemic reactions.** In case of systemic reactions during or after local anesthetic injections, hemodynamic signs are helpful in determining the cause of the reaction.

(1:500 000) and small volumes provides safe digital anesthesia. Ring blocks of the digit should be avoided. Fear of the use of epinephrine on the ear or nose is unwarranted, but is still taught to many medical students.

Self-limited systemic side effects of epinephrine include palpitations, anxiety, fear, diaphoresis, headache, tremor, weakness, tachycardia and elevated blood pressure. These signs and symptoms can be seen on occasion even with normal doses used for skin surgery, but they usually resolve within a few minutes (Table 143.2). They are more commonly seen when injecting highly vascular areas, especially the face and scalp. Skin necrosis from vasoconstriction is an extremely rare complication of epinephrine injection and would be an issue only in patients with severe vascular compromise at the injection site.

Serious side effects of epinephrine injection include arrhythmias, ventricular tachycardia, ventricular fibrillation, cardiac arrest and cerebral hemorrhage. None of these should be expected to occur at the doses used for skin surgery. However, it is prudent to limit the total dose injected in patients with severe cardiac disease.

Epinephrine is stable only in an acidic environment. Therefore, when epinephrine is premixed with local anesthetics, the pH is lowered into the 3.5 to 5.5 range with the addition of acidic preservatives such as sodium metabisulfite to stabilize the epinephrine. This acidic solution is not only more painful at the time of injection[8] but it also slows the onset of anesthetic action, as less anesthetic is in the active form. By preparing the mixture fresh daily and using it by the end of the day, the mixture has a higher pH, which is less painful. Adding 0.5 ml epinephrine (1:1000) to 50 ml plain lidocaine will give a final concentration of 1:100 000 epinephrine. Alternatively, the lidocaine with epinephrine can be neutralized with sodium bicarbonate (see below).

Sodium bicarbonate

Injecting the standard lidocaine with epinephrine mixture at a pH of 3.5 to 5.5 is quite painful, with significant stinging due to the acidic pH. The pH can be neutralized with the addition of sodium bicarbonate. Adding one part of 8.4% sodium bicarbonate to ten parts lidocaine with epinephrine will bring the pH into a more physiologic 7 to 8 range. This mixture significantly reduces the pain of anesthetic injection[8,9]. This can be done at the time the syringe is drawn up, immediately before injection. Alternatively, 5 ml bicarbonate can be added to a 50 ml bottle of lidocaine with epinephrine. As the epinephrine activity is lost at a rate of 25% per week in an alkaline or neutral environment, the mixture should be labeled with the date prepared, kept refrigerated, and used within about 1 week.

Hyaluronidase

Hyaluronidase (derived from bovine testicular hyaluronidase) depolymerizes hyaluronic acid, which breaks up the ground substance, allowing anesthetics to diffuse further away from the injection point. In addition, there is less distortion of the injected structures[10]. However, the greater diffusion of anesthetic may decrease its duration of action.

Hyaluronidase is most useful for periorbital surgery and to increase the rate of successful nerve blocks. It is prepared by adding 150 units (one ampule) to 30 ml local anesthetic. Allergic reactions to hyaluronidase are rare, but they can occur. Some surgeons recommend an intradermal skin test before using hyaluronidase. In addition, the preparation contains thimerosal preservative, which can cause contact dermatitis.

Anesthetic Mixtures

In an attempt to take advantage of different anesthetic properties, some surgeons combine two local anesthetics in one syringe. For example, a combination of lidocaine, for its rapid onset of action, with bupivacaine hydrochloride, for its long duration of action, is often used. However, a study looking at such combinations has found that such mixtures do not live up to their promise. The mixture seems to take on the properties of one of the components to the exclusion of the other[11]. Therefore, most surgeons will inject the rapid-onset anesthetic first and the longer-acting anesthetic later, to minimize the pain of injection and maximize the duration of action.

Side Effects

Vasovagal reactions

By far the most common side effect of local anesthetic injection is a vasovagal reaction, in which the vagus nerve discharges due to patient anxiety. This results in an increase in parasympathetic tone (see Table 143.2). Vasovagal reactions are manifested by dizziness, diaphoresis, syncope, bradycardia and hypotension. Placing the patient in the Trendelenburg position will rapidly relieve the patient's symptoms. A cold towel on the forehead can also be helpful. Oxygen, fluids or epinephrine are usually not necessary. To avoid significant vasovagal reactions, all patients should have local anesthetic infiltrated in the recumbent position.

Allergic reactions

The most important side effect of local anesthetics is the development of allergic reactions. The allergy is usually a type I IgE-mediated reaction manifested by urticaria, angioedema, bronchospasm, and, on rare occasions, anaphylaxis with associated hypotension and tachycardia (see Table 143.2). Most true local anesthetic allergies have been reported with ester anesthetics; amide anesthetics are implicated only very rarely. Preservatives added to multidose vials, especially methylparaben and sodium metabisulfite, have frequently been shown to be the cause of 'local anesthetic' allergy[12].

There is some allergy cross-reactivity within the various ester anesthetics and within the amide anesthetics, but there is no cross-reactivity between the ester and amide anesthetic classes. It is PABA (the metabolite of ester anesthetics) that is thought to be responsible for the ester anesthetic allergic reactions. Ester anesthetics can also cause type IV delayed hypersensitivity reactions and cross-react with several contact sensitizers, including PABA, para-amino salicylic acid and para-phenylenediamine.

Patients who present with a history of 'local anesthetic' allergy need to be questioned in detail about the 'allergy' with a review of relevant medical records whenever possible. Often, the 'allergy' is a result of a vasovagal reaction or epinephrine sensitivity. If the reaction seems to represent a true allergic reaction and the offending anesthetic is known (usually an ester), using an anesthetic from the other class (usually an amide) in a preservative-free solution is a reasonable solution. Skin testing, by an allergist, may be warranted if the offending agent is not certain[13]. The testing should include pinprick followed by intradermal tests of an ester anesthetic, an amide anesthetic, methylparaben and sodium metabisulfite. Alternatively, for small procedures, adequate anesthesia can be obtained with intradermal injection of 1% diphen-hydramine solution. Epinephrine may be added to counteract vasodilation caused by diphenhydramine, to enhance the anesthetic effect, and to reduce systemic antihistamine symptoms[14]. Intradermal normal saline with benzyl alcohol preservative will achieve very brief anesthesia through pressure effects on cutaneous nerve endings and the anesthetic properties of the benzyl alcohol preservative. It can be used for very short procedures such as a shave biopsy[15].

Limited allergic reactions can be managed with oral antihistamines and prednisone. However, patients developing bronchospasm, angioedema, or hemodynamic compromise require immediate emergency management including epinephrine, bronchodilators, parenteral antihistamines, corticosteroids, intravenous fluids, and oxygen.

Local side effects

Bruising and edema are frequently seen after local anesthetic infiltration, especially in the periorbital area. Periorbital edema will often develop after surgery on the forehead and frontal scalp. Transient motor nerve paralysis is sometimes seen. This may be delayed for some time after the sensory nerves have become anesthetized, because of the large myelinated nerve fibers involved. The paralysis may persist for several hours after the sensory nerves have returned to normal. Informing the patient when a motor nerve has been affected by the anesthetic will eliminate distressed patient telephone calls later in the day. Prolonged sensory nerve paresthesia may develop if a sensory nerve is injured through intraneural injection. This is most commonly seen after nerve blocks, and it can be minimized by avoiding intraneural injection and by using small gauge needles for injection.

Overdosage

If the local anesthetic dosage administered is kept within the recommended maximums, clinical symptoms of local anesthetic over-dose are unlikely to be encountered. Maximum recommended dosages of lidocaine are 5 mg/kg plain, 7 mg/kg with epinephrine at standard 1–2% concentrations, and 35–50 mg/kg at 0.05–0.1% tumescent lidocaine anesthesia with dilute epinephrine concentrations[16–18].

The symptoms of local anesthetic overdose are directly related to the serum blood level, and include increasing CNS and cardiovascular signs and symptoms (see Table 143.2). CNS symptoms start with circumoral and digital numbness and tingling, followed by lightheaded-ness, tinnitus, visual disturbances, slurred speech, muscle twitching, and, finally, seizures and coma. Cardiovascular symptoms develop at significantly higher doses than early CNS symptoms and include hypotension, arrhythmias, respiratory arrest and cardiac arrest.

Bupivacaine hydrochloride has a greater risk of cardiac toxicity than lidocaine. Prilocaine hydrochloride metabolizes to ortho-toluidine, which is an oxidizing agent capable of converting hemoglobin to methemoglobin. This can become significant with large doses of more than 500 mg.

Topical Anesthetics

Skin

Historically, the only anesthetic used for topical anesthesia of keratinized skin was benzocaine, which is an ester anesthetic. Anesthesia was generally effective only when applied to traumatized skin. Little if any anesthesia was achieved in intact normal skin. Of greater concern was the high rate of allergic contact dermatitis seen with benzocaine. Recently, there have been several topical anesthetics introduced that seem to achieve moderate topical anesthesia of intact skin (Table 143.3).

EMLA cream (AstraZeneca, Wayne, PA) is a eutectic mixture of 2.5% lidocaine and 2.5% prilocaine hydrochloride. It is able to achieve superficial anesthesia, with the degree of anesthesia related to the amount and duration of application before surgery. EMLA is applied as a thick layer under occlusion at least 1 hour before the procedure. It is especially useful for reducing the pain of non-ablative laser procedures and to reduce the pain of local anesthetic or other injections. There are reports of more extensive procedures, such as split-thickness skin graft harvesting, being done with EMLA alone. However, I have found the degree of anesthesia to be too unpredictable to rely on EMLA alone for most surgical procedures. One dermatology group has been able to do CO_2 laser resurfacing solely under EMLA anesthesia. They prepare the skin with vigorous degreasing followed by two applications of EMLA 1 hour apart under occlusion. Additional EMLA is applied to the skin after the first pass with the laser has removed the epidermis.

EMLA appears to be safe, but some caution is advised when using large amounts on skin with a damaged skin barrier and in infants who might be susceptible to methemoglobinemia from too much prilocaine

TOPICAL ANESTHETICS FOR MUCOUS MEMBRANE AND INTACT SKIN ANESTHESIA				
Generic name	Trade name®	Concentration (%)	Type	Primary use
Benzocaine	Americaine otic	20	Ester	Tympanic membrane
Benzocaine	Hurricaine	20	Ester	Mucous membranes
Benzocaine/Tetracaine	Cetacaine	14/2	Ester	Mucous membranes
Benzocaine/lidocaine/tetracaine			Ester/amide	Intact skin
Cocaine		2–10	Ester	Nasal mucosa
Dibucaine (cinchocaine)	Nupercainal	1	Amide	Mucous membranes
Lidocaine	LMX	4–5	Amide	Intact skin
Lidocaine	Topicaine	4	Amide	Intact skin
Lidocaine	Xylocaine	2–5	Amide	Mucous membranes
Lidocaine in acid mantle cream		30–40	Amide	Intact skin
Prilocaine/Lidocaine	EMLA	2.5/2.5	Amide	Intact skin
Proparacaine (proxymetacaine)	Alcaine	0.5	Ester	Conjunctiva
Tetracaine	Pontocaine	0.5	Ester	Conjunctiva
Prilocaine/Lidocaine mix	Betacaine LA	Proprietary	Amide	Intact skin

Table 143.3 Topical anesthetics for mucous membrane and intact skin anesthesia. Anesthetics for topical skin anesthesia require application 0.5–2 hours prior to surgery under occlusion for maximal effect.

hydrochloride absorption. EMLA often blanches the skin after application. Even though this blanching has no effect on treatment efficacy when treating vascular lesions, relatively light-colored lesions may become difficult to identify. I have patients mark out the outline of the vascular lesion before applying EMLA.

Other preparations that have been optimized for epidermal penetration and have been shown to achieve moderate superficial skin anesthesia include Betacaine-LA consisting of a proprietary mixture of lidocaine and prilocaine hydrochloride, LMX (Ferndale Laboratories, Ferndale, MI) containing 4% or 5% lidocaine, Topicaine containing 4% lidocaine, 4% tetracaine gel, 30–40% lidocaine in acid mantle cream, and various other compounded mixtures of lidocaine, benzocaine and tetracaine. In a comparison study, EMLA and LMX were found to achieve superior anesthesia to tetracaine, which was superior to Betacaine-LA, which was superior to control[19]. According to the manufacturers, Betacaine-LA and LMX do not require occlusion to be effective. A comparison of EMLA under occlusion and LMX unoccluded found that LMX achieved equivalent anesthesia to EMLA after less than one-third of application time[20]. None of the topical anesthetics have any significant effectiveness for palmar or plantar surfaces.

Iontophoresis of 1–4% lidocaine with epinephrine can enhance the depth and effectiveness of topical anesthesia. It is practical only for rather small areas, but anesthesia can be achieved within a few minutes with a 1 mA current. The main drawback is the additional equipment and supplies needed.

Topical skin anesthetics are primarily useful for non-invasive laser and intense pulsed light treatments, including laser hair removal, laser acne treatment, tattoo fading, pigmented lesion destruction, vascular lesion photocoagulation and non-ablative photorejuvenation. They are very useful in reducing the pain of needle insertion and some of the pain of injection when injecting local anesthetics, botulinum toxin, or filler materials such as the various hyaluronic acid-based filler materials that, due to their acidity, sting on injection. Anesthesia is too unpredictable to be able to use them even for minor surgical procedures such as skin biopsies, curettage or electrodesiccation.

The various preparations have differing recommended times of application and whether or not occlusion is necessary. However, for maximal effectiveness, the anesthetic should be applied as a thick layer under occlusion to the proposed treatment area for at least 1 hour. Caution should be exercised when large areas are to be anesthetized, especially when using compounded mixtures with high lidocaine concentrations, as several deaths have been reported in patients applying compounded topical anesthetics under occlusion to their entire legs and thighs.

Mucous membranes

Topical anesthetics for mucous membranes are far more effective than skin anesthetics, as the stratum corneum barrier is absent (see Table 143.3). One to two drops of 0.5% tetracaine into each eye achieves complete conjunctival anesthesia after a few seconds of stinging. This allows for insertion of eye shields or painless injection through the conjunctiva. Proparacaine (proxymetacaine) hydrochloride is an equally effective alternative conjunctival anesthetic.

A 2–10% solution of cocaine is the topical anesthetic of choice for intranasal anesthesia because of its excellent vasoconstrictive and hemostatic property. However, onerous record-keeping requirements make it relatively impractical for in-office use. Due to its significant cardiac stimulatory effects, cocaine should be used with caution in patients with significant heart disease.

Oral and anal mucosa can be effectively anesthetized within a couple of minutes with 2–4% lidocaine jelly or viscous lidocaine as well as various benzocaine-containing preparations. Topical intraoral anesthesia is especially helpful in reducing the pain of nerve block injections done through the intraoral route.

Cryoanesthesia

Rapid cooling of the skin surface is used routinely for many non-ablative laser procedures. The anesthesia is achieved with one of the following: a short burst of cryogen onto the skin surface (Dynamic Cooling Device, Candela, Wayland, MA); a cold glass window is placed directly onto the site being treated (contact cooling); an iced gel is placed on the surface being treated (passive cooling); or −5°C

refrigerated air is blown onto the skin surface with a coupling gel in place (Cryo 5, Zimmer Medizin Systems, Irvine, CA). All of these methods cool the skin to reduce pain of laser treatment and to protect the epidermis from laser-induced heat injury.

Cryoanesthesia can also be helpful in skin surgery. Dermabrasion can be done entirely under cryoanesthesia by freezing the skin with a cryogen spray before dermabrading. Unfortunately, the most effective and safe cryogen sprays (Frigiderm, Fluro-Ethyl) contain chlorofluorocarbons that are harmful to the ozone layer, and their manufacture has been discontinued. They are still available in limited quantities at ever-escalating prices. Ethyl chloride spray can, through evaporative cooling, achieve brief anesthesia to reduce the pain of needle insertion. An ice cube or −5°C forced air cooling (Cryo 5) will likewise numb the skin just long enough to reduce the pain of needle insertion. I have found forced air cooling helpful in reducing the pain of palmar and finger injections of botulinum toxin A for hyperhidrosis. However, if the cold air is directed directly onto the needle, the liquid in the needle may freeze momentarily, making it seem that the needle is clogged. Moving the cold air blower away from the needle for 5 to 10 seconds will permit the contents of the needle to thaw out, allowing injection to continue.

Anesthetic Injection Techniques
Local infiltration

The great majority of dermatologic surgical procedures are done under anesthesia achieved with local infiltration. Every attempt should be made to minimize the pain of injecting the anesthetic. There are several maneuvers that can significantly reduce pain of injection[21]. The pain of needle insertion is reduced by reassurance, verbal distraction, and mechanical distraction such as a pinch at the site of injection. Mechanical distraction works based on the gate theory of pain. The pinching will stimulate cutaneous nerves, making them somewhat refractory to the immediately following pinprick sensation from needle insertion. A very useful adjunct taking advantage of the gate theory of pain is the use of vibration at or immediately proximal to the injection site. This is very useful when injecting anesthetic in very anxious or young patients and has made it feasible for us to eliminate the need for nerve block anesthesia when injecting botulinum toxin into the palms and soles in many patients. Care must be taken when applying a vibrator to the injection site, as the needle may move unpredictably across the surface due to the vibration before being inserted into the skin. Small 30-gauge needles that are inserted quickly further reduce pain. Slow, timid needle insertion is felt more by the patient than a quick needle insertion. Topical anesthesia, as noted above, can almost completely eliminate the pain of needle insertion.

The actual injection of the anesthetic causes a significant stinging sensation that is usually far more painful than the needle insertion. Buffering the anesthetic to a physiologic pH and using anesthetic that has been warmed to body temperature will reduce the stinging sensation[8,9,22]. Injecting the anesthetic as slowly as practical will reduce the pain from tissue distention by the anesthetic fluid, and also allows the injection of additional anesthetic to be done through an already numb area. Additional sticks should be through an already numb area, and the injection should start on the side that the sensory innervation is coming from and proceed distally. Using the smallest practical syringe size, usually 1 or 3 ml, will allow for low pressures of injection, which are less painful. Subcutaneous anesthetic injection is less painful than intradermal injection, but the onset of anesthesia is slower and of shorter duration. I usually start by creating a small intradermal wheal, followed by subcutaneous injection, and finish with intradermal injection at the incision line to enhance anesthesia and hemostasis.

Field block anesthesia

Field block anesthesia involves injecting a ring of anesthetic around the proposed surgical site. It is useful for anesthetizing large areas while conserving the amount of anesthetic used. Injecting a ring of anesthesia around a cyst will avoid puncturing the cyst. Ring block anesthesia is practical only in areas where innervation arrives horizontally through the skin, such as is seen on the scalp, rather than vertically from deeper tissues, as is seen on the eyelid. A ring block may achieve anesthesia, but there will be no hemostasis at the incision site. Therefore, the addition of intradermal anesthetic with epinephrine at the proposed incision site is recommended. The most frequent use of ring block anesthesia is on the scalp, nose (for rhinophyma repair), ear pinna, and on the trunk and extremities (where the injection is started as a ring block but often finished with infiltration inside the ring block).

Tumescent anesthesia

Tumescent anesthesia involves the subcutaneous infiltration of large amounts of dilute 0.05–0.1% lidocaine with 1:1 000 000 epinephrine (Table 143.4). It has been used most extensively for liposuction under local anesthesia (see Ch. 156), ambulatory phlebectomy, hair transplantation, and dermabrasion. The anesthetic is infiltrated with the help of any one of several pumps, with the injection carried out through long 18–20-gauge 3.5-inch (8.9-cm) spinal needles or specially designed multiport cannulas. The infiltration is started slowly with small needles and gradually speeded up with spinal needles and finally infiltration cannulas. Infiltration of the deep subcutaneous plane is done first, followed by the superficial fat compartment. The solution is injected until firm tumescence of the tissue has been achieved. Anesthesia and epinephrine- induced hemostasis develop within about 20 minutes and last for several hours, which is significantly longer than the duration of anesthesia achieved with conventional concentrations of lidocaine with epinephrine. In the subcutaneous fat, dilute lidocaine is absorbed at a much slower rate than standard lidocaine concentrations. Doses as high as 35–50 mg/kg lidocaine have been found to be safe when used in tumescent anesthesia[16–18].

Nerve Block Techniques

Nerve blocks are an effective and efficient way to anesthetize large areas using the least amount of anesthetic, minimizing both patient discomfort and distortion of the operative site. When injecting in the region of a nerve, care must be taken not to inject the accompanying blood vessels. Using larger, 25–27-gauge needles allows one to draw back to make sure that the needle is not intravascular. To reduce pain of injection, an intradermal wheal using a 30-gauge needle should be placed first. The aim of nerve block injections is to deposit the anesthetic near, but not into, the nerve, as intraneural injection may cause nerve injury and subsequent dysesthesias. Insertion of the needle into a nerve is usually felt by the patient as a sharp pain radiating along the nerve. If this happens, the needle should be pulled back and repositioned slightly. Intra-foramina injections should also be avoided to minimize the risk of nerve injury. With proper placement, most nerves can be blocked with a 1–2 ml injection. The addition of hyaluronidase will enhance diffusion of the anesthetic and increase the rate of nerve block 'take'.

For most nerve blocks, 1% lidocaine with epinephrine and bicarbonate is used. If prolonged anesthesia is desired, 0.25% bupivacaine hydrochloride with epinephrine can be added. As the sensory nerves are large and myelinated, anesthetic effect may take 10 to 20 minutes to develop[23]. Using 2% lidocaine may increase success of the nerve block. Articaine 4% with or without epinephrine supplied in dental carpules

seems to be especially effective for relatively painless facial nerve blocks, with very small volumes (often less than 0.2 ml/injection site) of anesthetic needed for effective anesthesia. This seems to be due to its more effective diffusion from the site of injection compared to lidocaine. Some surgeons omit epinephrine from the nerve block anesthetic as it is not needed for vasoconstriction at the site of the nerve. I use it as part of my anesthetic mix to prolong the duration of the nerve block. Once a nerve has been effectively blocked, local infiltration of lidocaine with epinephrine along the proposed incision line to achieve local vasoconstriction may be helpful in reducing bleeding.

Facial nerve blocks

The forehead and frontal scalp above the eyebrows are innervated by the supraorbital nerve (Fig. 143.2), which exits the skull through the supraorbital foramen at or immediately above the orbital rim in the midpupillary line (Fig. 143.3). The notch can often be palpated on the patient. The anesthetic is infiltrated through a 0.5-inch (1.3-cm) long needle inserted perpendicularly into the skin immediately superficial to the periosteum at the orbital rim in the midpupillary line (Fig. 143.4). Approximately 1 ml of anesthetic is generally sufficient. The supratrochlear nerve innervates the midforehead, glabella and frontal scalp (see Fig. 143.2). It exits the skull at the upper medial portion of the orbit (see Fig. 143.3). Injecting 1 ml of anesthetic immediately superficial to the periosteum at the superomedial orbital rim at the junction of the glabella and eyebrow will block the supratrochlear nerve (see Fig 143.4). To achieve complete forehead and frontal scalp anesthesia requires extending a line of anesthetic injected in the subcutaneous plane laterally from the supraorbital nerve to the region immediately superior and posterior to the attachment of the ear pinna. This will block the auriculotemporal nerve and greater auricular nerve branches that innervate the forehead, temple and frontal scalp.

The infraorbital nerve exits the skull through the infraorbital foramen (see Fig. 143.3) and innervates the medial cheek, upper lip and nasal ala (see Fig. 143.2). With a 1-inch (2.5-cm) long needle inserted perpendicular to the skin, 2 ml of anesthetic is injected approximately 1 cm inferior to the orbital rim in the midpupillary line, immediately superficial to the maxillary bone periosteum (see Fig. 143.4). A less painful and more reliable alternative is to block the infraorbital nerve through the intraoral approach. The needle is inserted between the first and second premolars (bicuspids), moving cephalad along the periosteum

TUMESCENT ANESTHESIA FORMULA	
Ingredient	Quantity (ml)
Lidocaine 1%	50–100
Epinephrine (1:1000)	1
Sodium bicarbonate 8.4%	10
Hyaluronidase 150 U/ml	6 (optional)
Triamcinolone acetonide 40 mg/ml	0.25 (optional)
Normal saline 0.9%	900–950

Table 143.4 Tumescent anesthesia formula. For tumescent anesthesia, a final concentration of 0.05% to 0.1% lidocaine with 1:1000 000 epinephrine is prepared. Hyaluronidase may be added to enhance diffusion and corticosteroids may be added to reduce inflammation, edema and possibly fibrosis.

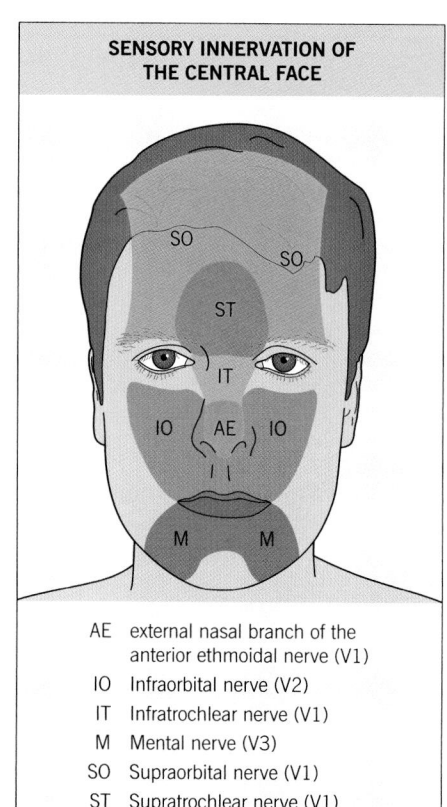

SENSORY INNERVATION OF THE CENTRAL FACE

Fig. 143.2 Sensory innervation of the central face.

AE	external nasal branch of the anterior ethmoidal nerve (V1)
IO	Infraorbital nerve (V2)
IT	Infratrochlear nerve (V1)
M	Mental nerve (V3)
SO	Supraorbital nerve (V1)
ST	Supratrochlear nerve (V1)

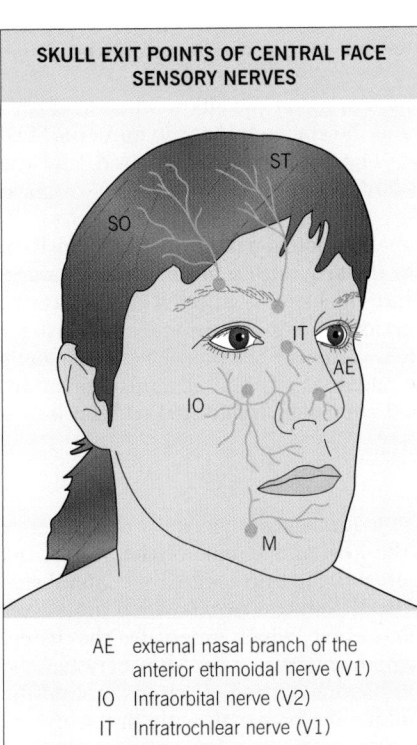

Fig. 143.3 Skull exit points of central face sensory nerves.

SKULL EXIT POINTS OF CENTRAL FACE SENSORY NERVES

AE	external nasal branch of the anterior ethmoidal nerve (V1)
IO	Infraorbital nerve (V2)
IT	Infratrochlear nerve (V1)
M	Mental nerve (V3)
SO	Supraorbital nerve (V1)
ST	Supratrochlear nerve (V1)

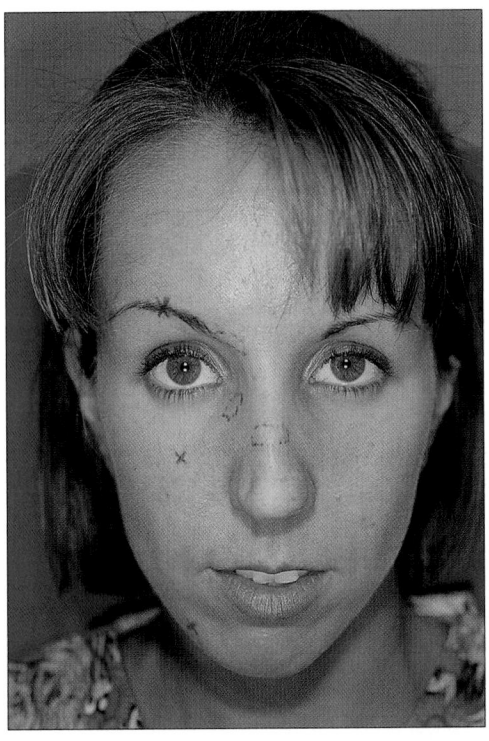

Fig. 143.4 Locations of needle insertions for central face nerve blocks. From superior to inferior, the supraorbital, infraorbital and mental nerves are marked with an 'x' and the supratrochlear, infratrochlear and external nasal nerves are marked with a rectangle.

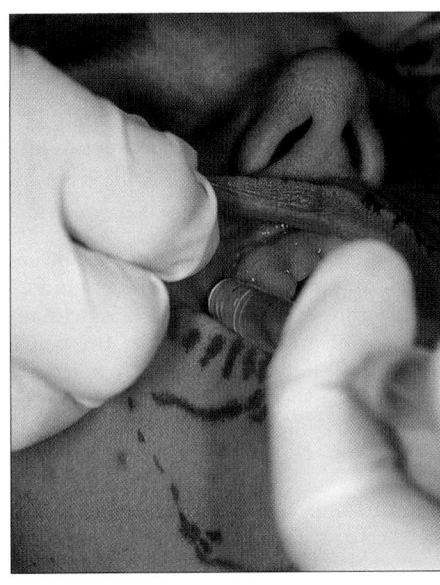

Fig. 143.5 Intraoral route for infraorbital nerve block. The needle is inserted cephalad between the premolar (bicuspid) teeth in the midpupillary line.

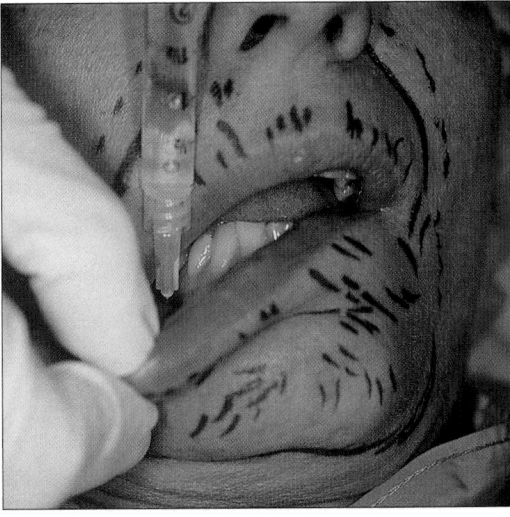

Fig. 143.6 Intraoral route for mental nerve block. The needle is inserted caudally between the premolar (bicuspid) teeth in the midpupillary line.

The lower lip and portions of the chin are innervated by the mental nerve (see Fig. 143.2), which exits the mandible through the mental foramen in the midpupillary line (see Fig. 143.3). A 0.5-inch (1.3-cm) needle is inserted perpendicular to the skin to the level of the periosteum in the midpupillary line, and about halfway cephalad along the mandible, and 1 ml of anesthetic is injected to block the mental nerve (see Fig. 143.4). The intraoral route is less painful and more reliable. The needle is inserted between the first and second premolars (bicuspids) caudally along the periosteum to a halfway point down the mandible (Fig. 143.6).

Digital nerve blocks

Nerve blocks for the fingers and toes are technically very similar. There are two options to anesthetize a digit. The most commonly used technique by dermatologists blocks the sensory nerves coursing laterally along the digit. A 0.5-inch (1.3-cm) needle is inserted perpendicular to the digit near its base in the horizontal plane until the bone is touched. At this point, the needle is withdrawn slightly, positioned dorsally, and anesthetic is injected. Next, the needle is positioned ventrally and additional anesthetic is injected. This process is repeated on the other side of the digit. This block should be done without epinephrine, and small volumes (usually less than 1.5 ml) should be injected to minimize the risk of ischemic injury from mechanical circumferential compression of the blood supply to the digit.

Alternatively, the digit can be blocked at the level of the metacarpal or metatarsal bone. A 1.5-inch (3.8-cm) needle is inserted dorsally between the metacarpal/metatarsal bones, and anesthetic is infiltrated as the needle is advanced ventrally, with most of the anesthetic injected

until bone is reached (Fig. 143.5). The needle is pulled slightly back and the anesthetic is injected. The pain of needle insertion can be lessened by applying a topical anesthetic to the mucosa a couple of minutes prior to injection. The infratrochlear nerve, which innervates the lateral and dorsal nose (see Fig. 143.2), can be blocked by injecting anesthetic superficial to the periosteum at the inferomedial orbital rim at the superior end of the nose–cheek concavity (see Fig. 143.4). The nasal tip receives innervation from the external nasal branch of the anterior ethmoidal nerve (see Fig. 143.2), which emerges at the nasal cartilage and bone junction slightly lateral from the midline (see Fig. 143.3). Perichondrial infiltration of anesthetic at this spot will anesthetize the nasal tip (see Fig. 143.4). To complete nasal anesthesia, a few drops of anesthetic at the base of the columella may be needed as well.

just dorsal to the palmar/plantar skin. This injection will block the metacarpal/ metatarsal nerve, which travels immediately superficial to the flexor retinaculum. The process is repeated on the other side of the metacarpal/ metatarsal bone of the digit being anesthetized. The advantage of this block is that there is less risk of compression injury than can occur with the more commonly performed digital block.

Penile nerve block

The dorsal nerve of the penis is a branch of the pudendal nerve. It divides into major anterior (dorsal) and minor posterior (ventral) branches at the base of the penis. By injecting a ring of anesthesia without epinephrine in the subcutaneous plane around the base of the penis, most of the penis will be anesthetized. The only areas that may require additional anesthetic infiltration will be the periurethral region of the glans and, sometimes, the ventral glans and frenulum.

Hand nerve block

With the popularity of botulinum toxin A for palmar and plantar hyperhidrosis, a method to anesthetize the palmar surface is necessary. Topical anesthetics are ineffective on glabrous skin, and local anesthetic injections are too painful in the palms or soles. Nerve block of the median nerve will anesthetize the palmar surface of the first three and a half fingers plus two-thirds of the palmar surface (Fig. 143.7). Block of the ulnar nerve will anesthetize the rest of the fingers and palm (Fig. 143.7). The median nerve lies in the carpal tunnel, deep to the palmaris longus tendon and between the flexor digitorum superficialis and flexor carpi radialis tendons. By apposing the thumb and fifth finger with the wrist slightly flexed, the palmaris longus tendon will become apparent. A 0.5–1-inch needle is inserted at the first (proximal) wrist crease, immediately medial (ulnar) to the palmaris longus tendon (Fig. 143.8). It is then advanced deep into the carpal tunnel and a few milliliters of anesthetic are injected. A slight 'popping'

or reduction in resistance can be felt as the needle enters the carpal tunnel.

The ulnar nerve is most easily blocked at the elbow where it travels between the olecranon process and the epicondyle of the humerus. The ulnar nerve is the 'funny bone'. The patient's arm is flexed, and the needle is inserted between the bones with several milliliters of anesthetic injected.

An alternative is to have an anesthesiologist perform a Bier block, in which the blood is pushed out of the arm with a compressive bandage, a tourniquet is applied, and dilute lidocaine is injected intravenously. Anesthesia of the hand will develop in 5 to 10 minutes and last for about 1 hour. Once the procedure is complete, the tourniquet is gradually released and the anesthetic is released into the general circulation. Therefore, the dose administered should be monitored to keep it at a safe level.

Foot nerve block

Anesthesia of the plantar surface requires nerve blocks of the posterior tibial nerve, which innervates the heel and middle of the sole of the foot; the sural nerve, which innervates the fifth toe and the lateral side of the sole of the foot; the superficial peroneal nerve, which innervates the skin of the toes; the saphenous nerve, which innervates the instep; and the deep peroneal nerve, which innervates the skin between the first and second toes (Fig. 143.9). Before starting injections around the ankle, the area should be thoroughly prepared with antiseptic to minimize the risk of infection.

The patient is placed in the prone position. The posterior tibial artery is palpated using a Doppler ultrasound probe if needed, and a 1.5-inch (3.8-cm) needle is directed anteriorly and laterally, immediately lateral to the arterial pulse, until the bone is touched. The needle is pulled back slightly, and several milliliters of anesthetic are injected in the groove between the medial malleolus and the Achilles tendon (Fig. 143.10). The sural nerve is blocked by injecting anesthetic in the groove between the lateral malleolus and Achilles tendon in an identical fashion to the tibial nerve injection (see Fig. 143.10).

The patient is placed in the supine position. The saphenous and superficial peroneal nerves are blocked by infiltrating anesthetic subcutaneously from malleolus to malleolus on the dorsal surface of the foot (Fig. 143.11). The deep peroneal nerve is blocked by inserting a 1.5-inch (3.8-cm) needle lateral (toward the middle of the foot) to the extensor hallucis longus tendon down to the bone (see Fig. 143.11). Next, the needle is pulled back slightly, and several milliliters of anesthetic are injected. The tendon is identified by having the patient

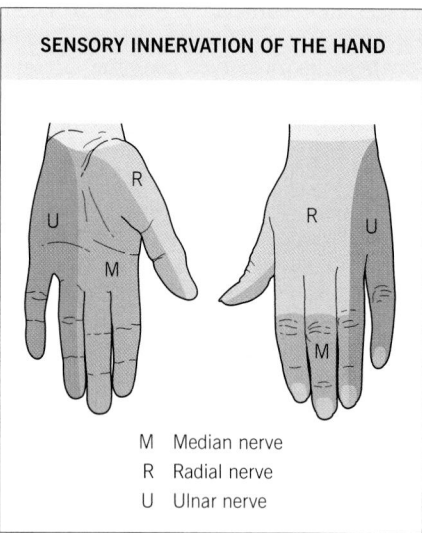

Fig. 143.7 Sensory innervation of the palmar surface and dorsal surface of the right hand.

SENSORY INNERVATION OF THE HAND

M Median nerve
R Radial nerve
U Ulnar nerve

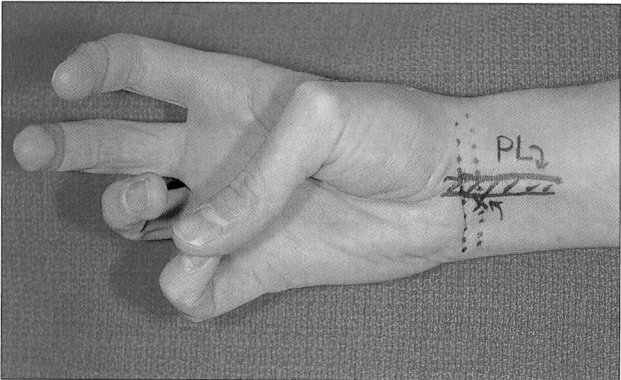

Fig. 143.8 Cutaneous markers for the median nerve location at the wrist. Note thumb and little finger apposition and wrist flexion to visualize the palmaris longus tendon. X, needle entry point; PL, palmaris longus tendon.

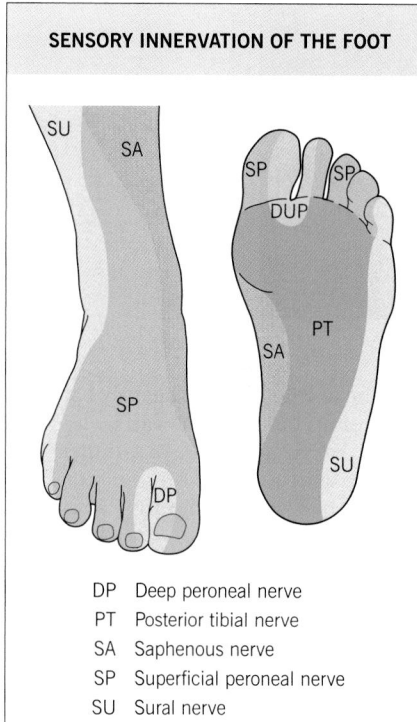

Fig. 143.9 Sensory innervation of the dorsal surface and plantar surface of the right foot.

SENSORY INNERVATION OF THE FOOT

DP Deep peroneal nerve
PT Posterior tibial nerve
SA Saphenous nerve
SP Superficial peroneal nerve
SU Sural nerve

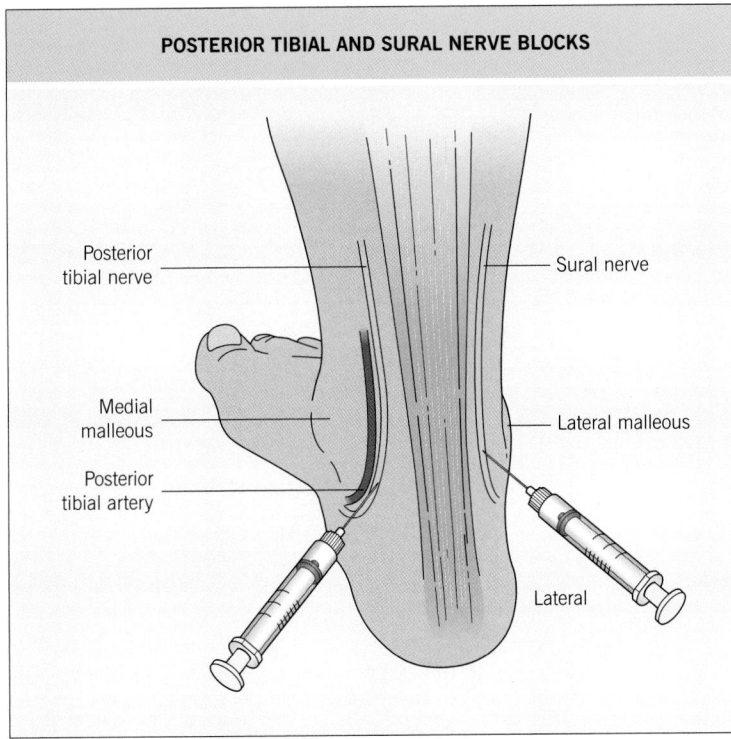

Fig. 143.10 Posterior tibial and sural nerve blocks.

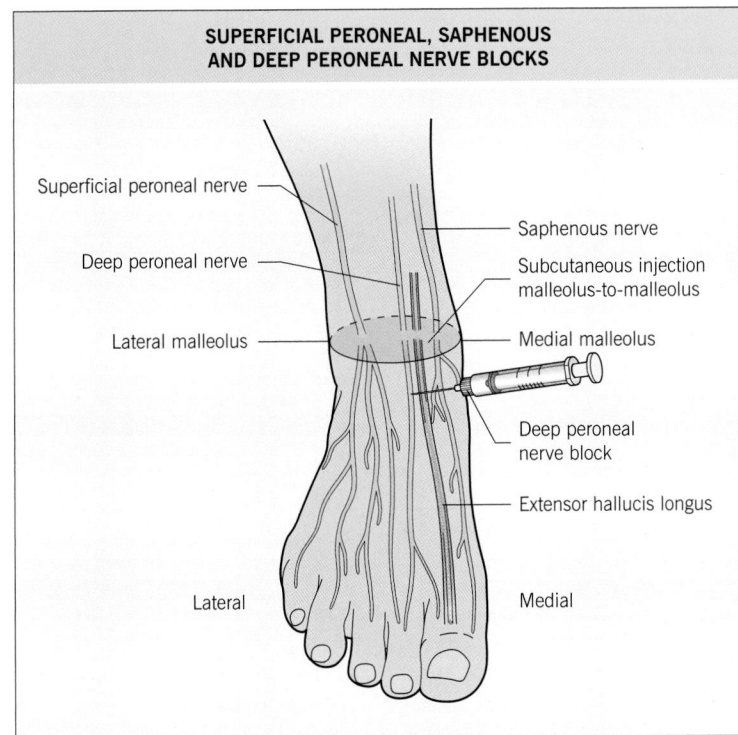

Fig. 143.11 Superficial peroneal, saphenous, and deep peroneal nerve blocks. Great toe dorsiflexion aids in visualizing the extensor hallucis longus tendon.

dorsiflex his or her great toe against resistance. Alternatively, local anesthetic infiltration between the first and second toes may be easier and more expeditious.

Higher Levels of Anesthesia

In anxious patients, or when relatively large areas are to be anesthetized, oral or sublingual anxiolytics such as triazolam (Halcion®) 0.25–0.5 mg or zolpidem tartrate (Ambien®) 5–10 mg will reduce anxiety and may even generate a certain degree of amnesia for the procedure. The addition of a narcotic analgesic such as oxycodone (10 mg)/acetaminophen (650 mg) orally (Percocet®) or meperidine hydrochloride (Demerol®) 50 mg intramuscularly, will act synergistically with the anxiolytics to achieve a greater degree of sedation as well as reducing the pain of local anesthetic infiltration. I find these useful for procedures done under tumescent anesthesia. Of course, patients given any sedating medications should have someone else take them home after the procedure.

Credentialing for higher levels of anesthesia may be regulated by local medical licensure authorities and hospitals, and the physician must be in full compliance with the rules in his or her particular locale. Most of the regulations require procedures done under general anesthesia or with intravenous sedation to be done in an ambulatory surgery center or hospital with a supervising anesthesiologist. Higher levels of anesthesia involving the use of intravenous medications such as midazolam hydrochloride (Versed®) and fentanyl should be done in a monitored environment with appropriate resuscitative equipment readily available. Nitrous oxide administration is a useful form of moderate analgesia, with the degree depending on the concentration administered. At a 20% concentration, the analgesia is equivalent to giving a narcotic analgesic. At an 80% concentration, most patients will become unconscious. The advantage of nitrous oxide is the rapid reversal of anesthetic effect as soon as the gas is turned off. With proper training, nitrous oxide can be safely administered in the office, as it has been done for many years in many dental offices. General inhalation anesthesia or deep intravenous sedation with propofol should generally be performed by anesthesiologists.

REFERENCES

1. Wildsmith JAW, Strichartz GR. Local anaesthetic drugs – an historical perspective. Br J Anaesth. 1984;56:937–9.
2. Hille B. Local anesthetics: hydrophilic and hydrophobic pathways for the drug-receptor reaction. J Gen Physiol. 1977;69:497–515.
3. Bieter RN. Applied pharmacology of local anesthetics. Am J Surg. 1936;34:500–10.
4. Rasmussen LF, Ahlfors CE, Wennberg RP. The effect of paraben preservatives on albumin binding of bilirubin. J Pediatr. 1976;89:475–8.
5. Foster CA, Aston SJ. Propranolol-epinephrine interaction: a potential disaster. Plast Reconstr Surg. 1983;72:74–8.
6. Dzubow LM. The interaction between propranolol and epinephrine as observed in patients undergoing Mohs surgery. J Am Acad Dermatol. 1986;15:71–5.
7. Krunic AL, Wang LC, Soltani K, Weitzul S, Taylor RS. Digital anesthesia with epinephrine: an old myth revisited. J Am Acad Dermatol. 2004;51:755–9.
8. Stewart JH, Chinn SE, Cole GW, Klein JA. Neutralized lidocaine with epinephrine for local anesthesia – II. J Dermatol Surg Oncol. 1990;16:842–5.

9. Stewart JH, Cole GW, Klein JA. Neutralized lidocaine with epinephrine for local anesthesia. J Dermatol Surg Oncol. 1989;15:1081–3.
10. Lewis-Smith PA. Adjunctive use of hyaluronidase in local anaesthesia. Br J Plast Surg. 1986;39:554–8.
11. Galindo A, Witcher T. Mixtures of local anesthetics: bupivacaine-chloroprocaine. Anesth Analg. 1980;59:683–5.
12. Nagel JE, Fuscaldo JT, Fireman P. Paraben allergy. JAMA. 1977;237:1594–5.
13. Glinert RJ, Zachary CB. Local anesthetic allergy. Its recognition and avoidance. J Dermatol Surg Oncol. 1991;17:491–6.
14. Roberts EW, Loveless H. The utilization of diphenhydramine for production of local anesthesia: report of a case. Texas Dent J. 1979;97:13–15.
15. Wiener SG. Injectable sodium chloride as a local anesthetic for skin surgery. Cutis. 1979;23:342–3.
16. Lillis PJ. Liposuction surgery under local anesthesia: limited blood loss and minimal lidocaine absorption. J Dermatol Surg Oncol. 1988;14:1145–8.

17. Klein JA. Tumescent technique for regional anesthesia permits lidocaine doses of 35 mg/kg for liposuction. J Dermatol Surg Oncol. 1990;16:248–63.
18. Klein JA. Improved technique for local anesthesia: improved safety in large volume liposuction. J Plast Reconstr Surg. 1993;92:1085–98.
19. Friedman PM, Fogelman JP, Nouri K, et al. Comparative study of the efficacy of four topical anesthetics. Dermatol Surg. 1999;25:950–4.
20. Altman DA, Gildenberg SR. High-energy pulsed light source hair removal device used to evaluate the onset of action of a new topical anesthetic. Dermatol Surg. 1999;25:816–18.
21. Arndt KA, Burton C, Noe JM. Minimizing the pain of local anesthesia. Plast Reconstr Surg. 1983;72:676–9.
22. Bainbridge LC. Comparison of room temperature and body temperature local anaesthetic solutions. Br J Plast Surg. 1991;44:147–8.
23. Grekin RC, Auletta MJ. Local anesthesia in dermatologic surgery. J Am Acad Dermatol. 1988; 19:599–614.

Wound Closure Materials and Instruments

Glenn Goldman

Key features

- The characteristics ascribed to a suture include:

  - capillarity
  - USP size
  - coefficient of friction
  - plasticity
  - tensile strength
  - physical configurations
  - elasticity
  - memory
  - pliability
  - tissue reactivity

- Sutures used to approximate the dermis and deeper tissue layers are generally absorbable, while surface sutures are usually non-absorbable and require removal

- The most commonly employed needle in dermatologic surgery is a 3/8 circle and triangular in shape, with a size and sharpness that corresponds to the anatomic site

- Needle holders with small smooth jaws accommodate finer needles and those with large serrated jaws grasp larger needles

- The major types of scissors are Gradle, tissue, undermining, suture-cutting, and bandage-cutting

INTRODUCTION

Dermatologic surgeons rely on quality surgical instruments and wound closure materials in order to facilitate excision and repair and to optimize the cosmetic and functional outcome for a given procedure. This chapter will carefully review the wound closure materials and surgical instruments available to the dermatologic surgeon. Helpful hints and model surgical tray setups are included to assist in the preparation for surgery in specific anatomic locations.

DISCUSSION

Sutures

The purpose of a suture is to approximate wound edges and maintain closure until a surgical repair has matured sufficiently to prevent wound dehiscence or a spread scar. Sutures are divided into two categories: (1) absorbable; and (2) non-absorbable. Studies of wound-healing by Levenson et al.[1] have shown that during the first 1–2 weeks postoperatively, the intrinsic tensile strength of the wound is approximately 7–10% of native bursting pressure. At 5 weeks, the intrinsic tensile strength is approximately 60%, and, in general, after 1 month, dehiscence is unlikely with normal activity. During this time period, absorbable buried dermal sutures are utilized to alleviate tension and maintain wound edge approximation. Epidermal, non-absorbable sutures are non-tension bearing, but allow for fine adjustments of the epidermal edges and thus provide an improved cosmetic result.

The ideal suture, were it to exist, would handle easily, hold a secure knot, and have high tensile strength. It would neither cause inflammation nor promote infection, and it would gradually dissolve, thereby obviating suture removal. Because the qualities needed for buried or absorbable sutures are distinct from those needed for surface sutures, each subset balances the best characteristics of the ideal suture with a tolerable set of detriments.

The characteristic attributes ascribed to a suture are defined by the United States Pharmacopeia (USP) as follows:

- **Capillarity** is defined as the ability of a suture to absorb and transfer fluid. Multifilament (braided or twisted) sutures have greater capillarity than monofilament (single-stranded) sutures.

- Two **physical configurations** exist: monofilament and multifilament. Multifilament braided sutures handle and tie more easily[2], but they may increase the risk of infection, due to the potential to harbor organisms between filament strands[3]. Therefore, monofilament suture material such as nylon or polypropylene may be more appropriate for closing contaminated wounds[2,4–7]. Monofilament materials have a low coefficient of friction and slide easily through tissue (see below)[7]. Until recently, monofilament sutures were used primarily for exterior suturing, and most buried sutures were braided. With the introduction of poliglecaprone 25 (Monocryl®), monofilament absorbable suture is now regularly employed for deep sutures.

- The **USP size** of a suture is determined by the diameter of the suture material needed to achieve a given tensile strength, and this is expressed in multiples of zeros; the smaller the cross-sectional diameter of the suture, the more zeros. For example, 7-0 polyglactin 910 (Vicryl®) is a much finer suture than 3-0 Vicryl®. The actual diameter of a given USP size varies depending upon the composition of the suture. For example, 4-0 surgical gut is a larger-diameter suture than 4-0 polypropylene (Prolene®) because polypropylene is innately stronger for a given diameter. In general, the smallest suture that will provide adequate tensile strength for the indicated repair should be utilized.

- **Elasticity** refers to the ability of a suture to regain its original length after being stretched. An elastic suture, such as polybutester (Novafil®), allows for tissue swelling, and then maintains tension on the wound edges after the edema has resolved.

- The **coefficient of friction** determines the ease with which a suture will pull through tissue. A suture with a low friction coefficient, such as polypropylene (Prolene®), slides easily through tissue. For this reason, Prolene® is the material most commonly used for the running subcuticular suture (see Ch. 146). Knot strength is directly proportional to the friction coefficient of the suture material. The more slippery the suture material, the more likely it is that the resulting knot will unravel. Hence, when suturing with Prolene®, it may be useful to place several additional throws for each knot.

- **Memory** is defined as a suture's tendency to retain its natural configuration and is determined by the elasticity and plasticity of the suture material. Memory is a useful property for maintaining closure during the postoperative period, and high-memory sutures such as polypropylene (Prolene®) are widely used for surface approximation. Drawbacks of high-memory sutures are that they do not handle very easily and they have a relatively low knot strength. As with sutures that have a low coefficient of friction, it is helpful to place a few extra throws in order to ensure a secure knot. Suture material with low memory, such as silk, is easy to handle and rarely becomes untied.

- **Plasticity** is the ability of the suture to retain its new length and form as well as tensile strength after it has been stretched. This is an important characteristic for a suture material that is to be used in situations with tissue edema. Sutures with plasticity, such as polypropylene, will stretch to accommodate edema and not cut into tissue[8].

- **Pliability** refers to how easily the suture can be bent. Braided suture materials, such as silk, are the most pliable, and they are capable of readily being tied into a knot. Polyglactin (Vicryl®) is a buried, absorbable braided suture that is easily tied.

- The **tensile strength** of a suture is determined by the force (in pounds) required to snap it. Tensile strength is determined by the composition and diameter of the suture. In general, synthetic materials are stronger than natural materials. A suture that has been knotted has approximately one-third the tensile strength of the same material unknotted[9].

- **Tissue reactivity** is the degree of foreign body inflammatory response evoked by a suture when placed in a wound. In general, natural materials (such as surgical gut and silk) cause much more of an inflammatory response than synthetic materials (such as nylon, polypropylene and polyester)[5,10].

Types of Suture Material

Sutures are characterized as absorbable or non-absorbable, based upon their ability to be enzymatically digested or hydrolyzed. Sutures that lose most of their tensile strength within 60 days of implantation are defined as absorbable. Most absorbable sutures lose their tensile strength long before they are fully absorbed. In general, absorbable sutures are used to close the dermis and deeper subcutaneous layers.

Non-absorbable sutures are resistant to hydrolysis and enzymatic degradation. Non-absorbable sutures such as nylon and polypropylene are usually used as surface sutures, and they are routinely removed 5–10 days postoperatively (earlier on the face and later on the trunk and extremities).

Absorbable Sutures

The most common absorbable sutures are described below and are summarized in Table 144.1[11].

Surgical gut

Surgical gut (catgut), one of the first sutures ever used, is produced from bovine or sheep intestine. It is a natural tan fiber that is packaged wet in alcohol and dries quickly when exposed to air. Plain surgical gut is rarely used today because of its poor tensile strength and high tissue reactivity. When used as a buried suture, plain gut loses its tensile strength in 7 to 10 days, and it is completely digested in 60 to 70 days[12].

Chromic gut is plain gut that has been processed with chromium salts to increase its resistance to enzymatic degradation. The tensile strength of chromic gut typically lasts for 10 to 14 days. Chromic gut is still widely used for surface suturing of mucosal surfaces, where it lasts long enough to maintain wound edge apposition but breaks down reasonably fast.

Fast-absorbing gut is plain gut that has been heated to begin breakdown of the suture prior to use. This suture maintains its tensile strength for 3 to 5 days[13]. Fast-absorbing gut has experienced renewed popularity in the past 5–10 years for suturing skin grafts and for placing surface sutures in wounds that are well approximated by buried sutures. No increase in postoperative wound infections is noted. Fast-absorbing gut is convenient for the surgeon and the patient because suture removal is not necessary[13,14].

Polyglycolic acid

Polyglycolic acid (Dexon®), introduced in 1970, was the first synthetic absorbable suture and represented a vast improvement over surgical gut[15]. It is a braided glycolic acid polymer with easy handling qualities, and it maintains 20% of its tensile strength at 3 weeks. Dexon® produces minimal inflammation, because it is absorbed primarily by hydrolysis, unlike surgical gut, which is degraded by proteolytic enzymes[15,16]. Poloxamer 188-coated and uncoated Dexon® are available. Coated Dexon® is easier to tie, and it passes more easily through tissue than does the non-coated form.

Polyglactin 910

Polyglactin 910 (Vicryl®, Polysorb®), a synthetic, braided copolymer of glycolide and L-lactide, was first introduced in 1974 and supplanted Dexon® as the most popular buried suture in cutaneous surgery[17]. Similar to Dexon®, the absorption of Vicryl® occurs primarily by hydrolysis. The water-repelling properties of lactide delay penetration of water, and thus delay the loss of tensile strength. Polyglactin 910

COMMONLY USED ABSORBABLE SUTURES						
Suture	Configuration	Tensile strength	Ease of handling	Knot security*	Tissue reactivity	Uses
Surgical gut (plain)	Virtually monofilament	Poor at 7–10 days	Fair	Poor	Moderate	Rarely used today in skin
Surgical gut (chromic)	Virtually monofilament	Poor at 21–28 days	Poor	Poor	Less than plain	Skin grafts; surface sutures for mucosae
Surgical gut (fast-absorbing)	Virtually monofilament	50% at 3–5 days	Fair	Poor	Low	Skin grafts, surface sutures
Polyglycolic acid (Dexon®)	Braided†	20% at 21 days	Good	Good	Low	
Polyglactin (Vicryl®, Polysorb®)	Braided†	75% at 14 days; 50% at 21 days	Good	Fair	Low	Subcutaneous closure, vessel ligature
Polydioxanone (PDS II®)	Monofilament	70% at 14 days; 50% at 30 days; 25% at 42 days	Poor	Poor	Low	Subcutaneous closure (high-tension areas)
Glycolide and trimethylene carbonate (Maxon®)	Monofilament	81% at 14 days; 59% at 28 days	Fair	Good	Low	Subcutaneous closure (high-tension areas)
Poliglecaprone 25 (Monocryl®)	Monofilament	50–60% at 7 days	Good	Good	Minimal	When minimal tissue reactivity is essential
Glycomer 631 (Biosyn®)	Monofilament	75% at 14 days; 40% at 21 days	Good	Poor	Minimal	Subcutaneous closure (high-tension areas)

*Directly proportional to the friction coefficient and indirectly proportional to memory.
†Multifilament.

Table 144.1 Commonly used absorbable sutures. Adapted from Garrett AB. Wound closure materials. In: Wheeland R (ed). Cutaneous Surgery. Philadelphia: WB Saunders, 1994:199–205.

(Vicryl®) maintains 75% of its tensile strength at 2 weeks and 50% at 3 weeks. Although stronger than polyglycolic acid, polyglactin 910 absorption is usually complete by 90 days, whereas polyglycolic acid is usually still being absorbed at 120 days[16].

Vicryl® is available either undyed or dyed violet. The violet form may be visible when embedded in the skin, and it should be avoided[18]. A lubricant coating of polyglactin 370 and calcium stearate allows for easier suture passage through tissue. Vicryl® has been immensely popular due to its easy handling characteristics. It holds knots well, does not tear tissue, and has all-round favorable qualities.

Vicryl® is not rapidly absorbed when placed percutaneously, and it can persist as a small nodule in the suture line or extrude as a 'spitting stitch' (which is disturbing to the patient, but is easily snipped out with fine scissors). Burying knots deeply in the dermis and subcutaneous tissue and avoiding wound tension may both help to avoid this reaction. Newer monofilament sutures such as poliglecaprone 25 have supplanted the use of Vicryl® for some indications, but the latter remains a widely used and immensely valuable suture.

Polydioxanone

Polydioxanone (PDS II®) is a monofilament polymer made from the polyester poly (p-dioxanone). Introduced in 1980, the primary advantage of PDS® over polyglycolic acid (Dexon®) and polyglactin 910 (Vicryl®) is prolonged tensile strength[19]. It maintains approximately 70% of its tensile strength at 2 weeks and 50% at 4 weeks. Traces of buried polydioxanone are present in 6-month histologic preparations[7]. PDS® is employed in high-tension areas, such as the proximal extremities and trunk.

Similar to Dexon® and Vicryl®, PDS® has minimal tissue reactivity[19]. As a monofilament suture, it retains packaging memory[7], and it is relatively stiff and difficult to tie[20]. However, polydioxanone demonstrates optimal capacity to glide through tissue[7], and the monofilament configuration allows PDS® to be safely used in contaminated wounds. Nonetheless, due to the difficulty in handling PDS®, it is used relatively less frequently in cutaneous surgery.

Polytrimethylene carbonate

Glycolide and trimethylene carbonate (Maxon®) is a monofilament suture that combines the prolonged tensile strength of PDS® with supple handling and smooth knot formation[20]. Maxon® is much more flexible and manageable than polydioxanone, demonstrating 60% less rigidity[20]. Maxon® maintains 81% of its tensile strength at 2 weeks and 59% at 4 weeks[21], and complete absorption occurs by hydrolysis in approximately 180 days. Despite this prolonged absorption, there is minimal tissue reactivity. Maxon® may be most useful for large surgical procedures on the trunk or extremities that are under substantial tension, and which require prolonged suture-based approximation during healing.

Poliglecaprone 25

Poliglecaprone 25 (Monocryl®) is a newer, relatively expensive, absorbable monofilament suture consisting of a copolymer of glycolide and ε-caprolactone. At 7 days, it maintains approximately 50–60% of its tensile strength, and complete absorption by hydrolysis occurs at around 90 days[7]. Similar to Maxon®, Monocryl® offers supple handling and minimal tissue reactivity. Prolonged support and minimal tissue reactivity led to a lower incidence of hypertrophic scarring in a breast reduction scar model[22]. Furthermore, poliglecaprone 25 demonstrates better knot tying and security than other commonly used absorbable monofilament suture materials[7]. Because Monocryl® apparently leads to less inflammation than Vicryl®, it has supplanted Vicryl® in some applications.

Glycomer 631

Glycomer 631 (Biosyn®) is an absorbable monofilament suture material with physical characteristics similar to poliglecaprone 25 (Monocryl®). Complete absorption of Biosyn® occurs at approximately 6 months, with low tissue reactivity[7]. Because of its relative permanence, Biosyn® has use similar to Maxon® for suturing of large truncal wounds.

Non-absorbable Sutures

The most commonly used non-absorbable sutures are described below and summarized in Table 144.2[11].

Silk

Silk is a braided, natural suture, and it represents the gold standard regarding ease of handling, knot formation and knot stability, by which newer synthetic sutures are measured. Also, braided silk is very soft and pliable, and it is, therefore, commonly used on mucosal surfaces and in intertriginous regions. Despite these advantages, there are major drawbacks to its use in cutaneous surgery. Silk has a low tensile strength, its braided configuration produces a high coefficient of friction, and the high capillarity increases the risk of infection. As an organic, foreign protein (fibroin) made by the silkworm, silk has greater tissue reactivity than any other suture except surgical gut.

Nylon

Nylon (Ethilon®, Dermalon®), a monofilament, polymerized polyamide introduced in 1940, was the first synthetic non-absorbable suture to become commercially available. Nylon quickly became very popular, and because it has high tensile strength and low tissue reactivity and is inexpensive, it is the most commonly used non-absorbable suture in dermatologic surgery[23,24]. The major disadvantages of monofilament nylon are memory and stiffness, which lead to relative knot insecurity[24]. In practice, this can be easily counteracted by firmly setting knots and increasing the number of knot throws. Nylon is available as a braided

COMMONLY USED NON-ABSORBABLE SUTURES						
Suture	Configuration	Tensile strength	Ease of handling	Knot security*	Tissue reactivity	Uses
Silk	Braided†	None in 365 days	Gold standard	Good	Moderate	Mucosal surfaces
Nylon:						
Ethilon®	Monofilament	Decreases 20% per year	Good to fair	Poor	Low	Skin closure
Dermalon®	Monofilament	Good	Good to fair	Poor		
Surgilon®	Braided†	Good	Good	Fair		
Nurolon®	Braided†	Good	Good	Fair		
Polypropylene (Prolene®, Surgilene®, Surgipro®)	Monofilament	Extended	Good to fair	Poor	Minimal	Running subcuticular suture
Polyester (Dacron®, Mersilene®, Ethibond®)	Braided†	Indefinitely	Very good	Good (coating decreases)	Minimal	Mucosal surfaces
Polybutester (Novafil®)	Monofilament	Extended	Good to fair	Poor	Low	

*Directly proportional to the friction coefficient and indirectly proportional to memory.
†Multifilament.

Table 144.2 Commonly used non-absorbable sutures. Adapted from Garrett AB. Wound closure materials. In: Wheeland R (ed). Cutaneous Surgery. Philadelphia: WB Saunders, 1994:199–205.

suture (Surgilon®, Nurolon®) which handles more easily but which is more expensive.

Polypropylene

Polypropylene (Prolene®, Surgilene®, Surgipro®) is a monofilament polymer of propylene[25]. An inert plastic, it has minimal tissue reactivity. The major advantage of this suture is its low coefficient of friction, which allows for a gentle, smooth pull through tissue[25]. This characteristic makes it the suture of choice for the running subcuticular suture. Polypropylene also has high plasticity and stretches with tissue swelling, thus reducing the likelihood of postoperative track marks[8,24]. However, it remains stretched (lack of elasticity), and it may allow wound edge separation once the swelling has subsided[9,24]. The other disadvantages of this suture are its memory (which compromises knot security) and increased cost compared to nylon. Prolene® has become very popular as a surface suture for facial repairs.

Polyester sutures

Polyester sutures (Dacron®, Mersilene®, Ethibond®) are braided, multi-filament sutures with high tensile strength, very good handling, and low tissue reactivity. These sutures last indefinitely in the body. Ethibond® comes coated with polybutilate, which decreases its drag through tissue (decreased friction coefficient). Polyester sutures are of great assistance for approximation of mucosal tissues, particularly the vermilion lip. They combine the soft feel of silk with a lack of tissue reactivity.

Polybutester

Polybutester (Novafil®) is a monofilament suture of polyglycol terephthalate and polybutylene terephthalates. Its major advantages are excellent handling, high elasticity, and low tissue reactivity[26].

Suture Selection

In general, a surgeon should select the smallest suture that will provide adequate strength for a given closure (Table 144.3). For facial repairs, 4-0 or 5-0 polyglactin 910 (Vicryl®) are common absorbable sutures, and 5-0 or 6-0 nylon or polypropylene are typical surface sutures. Poliglecaprone 25 (Monocryl®) is popular as a dermal suture due to its relatively fast absorption and lack of tissue reactivity. Monocryl® is useful in areas where minimal tissue reactivity is essential. 5-0 Prolene® is the suture of choice for the running subcuticular suture.

For larger truncal defects, 3-0 or 4-0 Vicryl® or Monocryl® for buried sutures and 3-0 or 4-0 nylon for epidermal closure are good choices. PDS® is used mainly for dermal and subcutaneous suturing of large truncal defects, because it assures prolonged support; however, this wiry suture is hard to tie and handle. Maxon® can be used when very-long-term wound support is essential. Skin staples offer a quick, strong alternative for epidermal closure of large scalp and truncal defects[27].

Fast-absorbing gut (6-0) is a convenient suture for small full-thickness skin graft closures and for linear repairs that are well approximated with buried sutures. Recent studies have confirmed the safety, convenience and economy of using absorbable sutures (e.g. Vicryl®, surgical gut) for epidermal skin closures in certain clinical situations[14,28].

Octylcyanoacrylate tissue adhesive (Dermabond®) is a practical, but expensive, alternative method of epidermal closure in wounds with minimal to no tension[29,30]. Wound closure tapes offer a non-traumatic alternative to epidermal sutures, and they are useful when applied to healing wounds following suture or staple removal. Additionally, they can be used over a running subcuticular suture at the time of surgery, relieving tension from the wound edges and providing a cosmetic, convenient alternative to a daily dressing change[31]. Maloney and colleagues[32] recently demonstrated that the optimal application of wound closure tapes is in a parallel non-overlapping pattern (perpendicular to wound tension), following complete coating of the skin surface with Mastisol® adhesive (Ferndale Laboratories).

Needles

The ideal needle is sharp and strong, and closely matches the suture diameter. The needle should be strong enough to hold its shape and retain its sharpness, pass after pass. The best needles are made of stainless steel, and the size and shape of the needle should be selected to correspond to the thickness and toughness of the tissue to be sutured.

There are several major brands of suture materials, including: Ethicon, Davis & Geck, Look, US Surgical and DermaGlide. Unfortunately, each suture manufacturer follows different needle nomenclature (Fig. 144.1). Most manufacturers, however, provide needle comparison reference guides. In general, the needle is the most expensive component of the needle/suture unit.

A needle is composed of three parts: the shank, the body and the point (Fig. 144.2)[33]. In dermatologic surgery, most needles have a swaged (eyeless) shank with a hollow proximal end into which the suture is inserted and then crimped. The suture track is determined by the size of the needle shank, not the suture size. The body of the needle can be straight, $\frac{1}{4}$ circle, $\frac{3}{8}$ circle, $\frac{1}{2}$ circle, or $\frac{5}{8}$ circle (Fig. 144.3). The most common shape used in skin surgery is the $\frac{3}{8}$ circle. Flattened needle bodies allow for firm grasping with needle holders to limit 'twisting' during suture placement.

The most common needle-point used in cutaneous surgery is triangular in shape (see Fig. 144.2). Triangular-shaped 'cutting' needles are preferred because they are easier to pass through tissues than are round needles. The conventional cutting needle has a triangular tip and is flat along the outer arc, with a sharp edge on the inside arc of the needle. The reverse cutting tip has a flat edge facing the inside arc of the needle, and a sharp edge facing the outer arc. Reverse cutting

COMMONLY UTILIZED SUTURES BY SITE			
Site	Deep suture	Surface suture	Other suture
Face	4-0 or 5-0 polyglactin or poliglecaprone	5-0 or 6-0 nylon or polypropylene	
Neck and distal extremities	4-0 polyglactin or poliglecaprone	4-0 or 5-0 nylon or polypropylene	
Trunk and proximal extremities	3-0 or 4-0 polyglactin or glycolide and trimethylene carbonate	3-0 or 4-0 nylon or polypropylene	
Mucosa	None	5-0 silk or polyester	
Vascular ligature			4-0 or 5-0 polyglactin

Table 144.3 **Commonly utilized sutures by site.** Note that there is considerable variation, depending upon the preference of the surgeon (bias of author and editors is admitted).

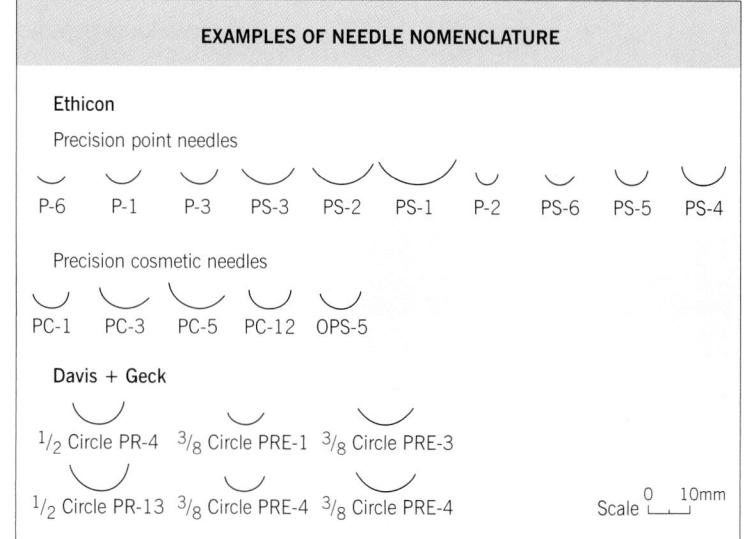

EXAMPLES OF NEEDLE NOMENCLATURE

Ethicon

Precision point needles

P-6   P-1   P-3   PS-3   PS-2   PS-1   P-2   PS-6   PS-5   PS-4

Precision cosmetic needles

PC-1   PC-3   PC-5   PC-12   OPS-5

Davis + Geck

$\frac{1}{2}$ Circle PR-4 $\frac{3}{8}$ Circle PRE-1 $\frac{3}{8}$ Circle PRE-3

$\frac{1}{2}$ Circle PR-13 $\frac{3}{8}$ Circle PRE-4 $\frac{3}{8}$ Circle PRE-4   Scale 0   10mm

Fig. 144.1 **Needle nomenclature by two representative manufacturers.**

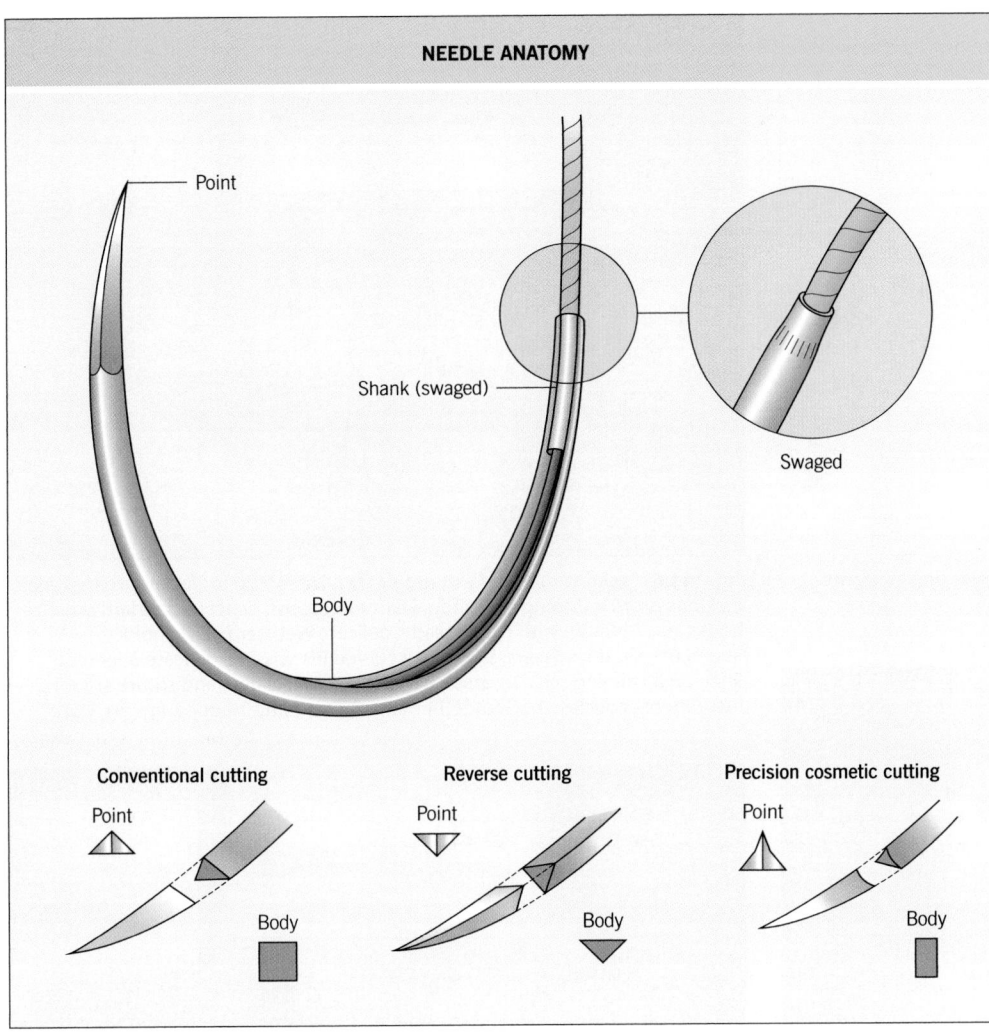

NEEDLE ANATOMY

Fig. 144.2 Needle anatomy. The shank body and point are shown, and specific needle points for different types of cutting.

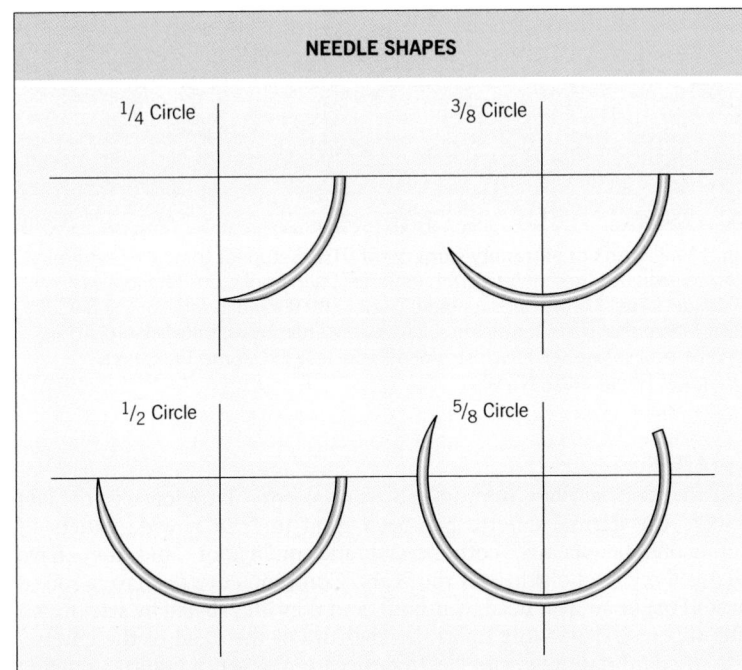

NEEDLE SHAPES

Fig. 144.3 Needle shapes. The most common shape used in skin surgery is the ³/₈ circle.

needles have the advantage of minimizing the risk of tearing through the wound edge during suture placement. The more the needle-point is honed, the sharper the needle is and the greater the cost of the suture unit.

For the majority of wound closures on the face, the Ethicon P ('plastic') and PS ('plastic skin') or an equivalent series are adequate and economical. The PS-3 and P-3 needles are particularly suited to dermatologic surgery. They are hand-honed and reverse cutting. The PC ('precision cosmetic') series represents Ethicon's superior skin surgery needle, and it can be used for fine, delicate work. These are the sharpest, most expensive needles, and they have flattened bodies for better grasping and conventional cutting points. The PC-1 needle is a very fine sharp needle ideal for delicate facial repair.

The FS ('for skin') and equivalent series of needles are not finely honed, and they are less sharp and less expensive. These needles are certainly adequate for skin surgery on the trunk or extremities, although some dermatologic surgeons usually use PS even for these sites.

The number after the series designation denotes the needle size. Most needles are drawn to size on the package (Fig. 144.4). The smallest needle/suture unit that will provide adequate tensile strength for a given repair should be utilized. In areas with thick dermis (e.g. the back), larger needles are much easier to pass through the tissue and do not bend. A PS-2 reverse cutting needle is very useful for this indication.

Instruments

Proper instruments are essential for effective execution of cutaneous surgery. Instruments should be selected to allow the greatest precision and speed for a given procedure. There is a wide variation in the cost and quality of surgical instruments. In general, practices should avoid low-quality, low-cost instruments, for they are poorly finished and, therefore, are more difficult to use and are not durable. With surgical instruments, it is clear that 'you get what you pay for'. A high-quality instrument will more than make up for its cost by performing well day after day in countless procedures. Modern instruments are a blend of surgical stainless steel with carbon alloy, chromium, nickel and tungsten carbide. Tungsten carbide is a very hard alloy that enhances function and durability of blades of scissors and jaws of needle holders. Quality instruments are usually covered by a warranty which will range

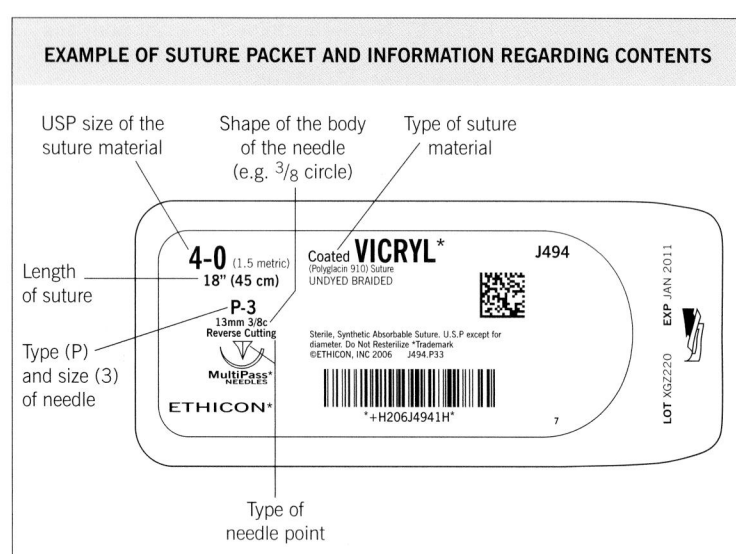

Fig. 144.4 Example of suture packet and information regarding contents.

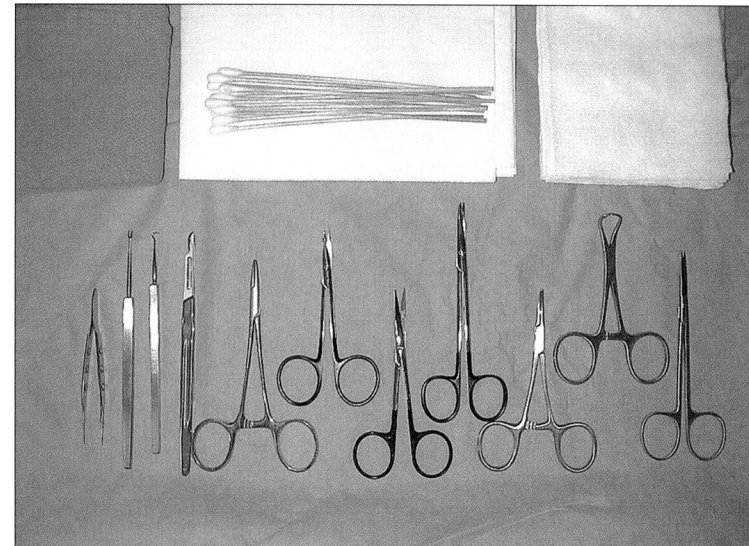

Fig. 144.6 Facial surgery tray or repair tray. Tray setup for facial surgery/repair includes (from left to right) Bishop–Harmon forceps, delicate standard skin hooks, no. 7 handle with no. 15 blade, delicate Webster needle holder, Supercut® Gradle scissors, Supercut® curved iris scissors, delicate Supercut® Shea undermining scissors, small hemostat, towel clamp, and suture scissors. Instruments courtesy of George Tiemann & Company, Hauppauge, NY, USA.

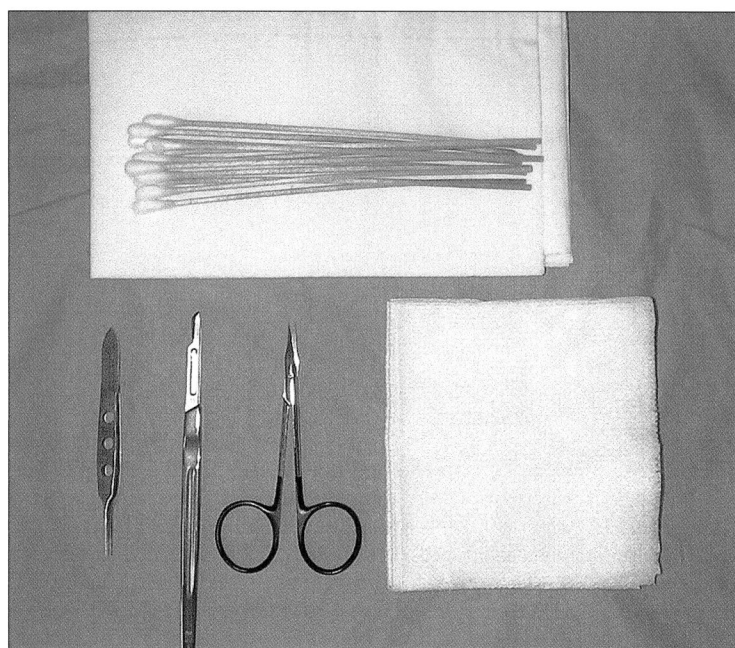

Fig. 144.5 Mohs micrographic surgery tray. Tray setup for basic Mohs micrographic surgery includes (from left to right) Bishop–Harmon forceps, no. 7 handle with no. 15 blade, and Supercut® Gradle scissors. Instruments courtesy of George Tiemann & Company, Hauppauge, NY, USA.

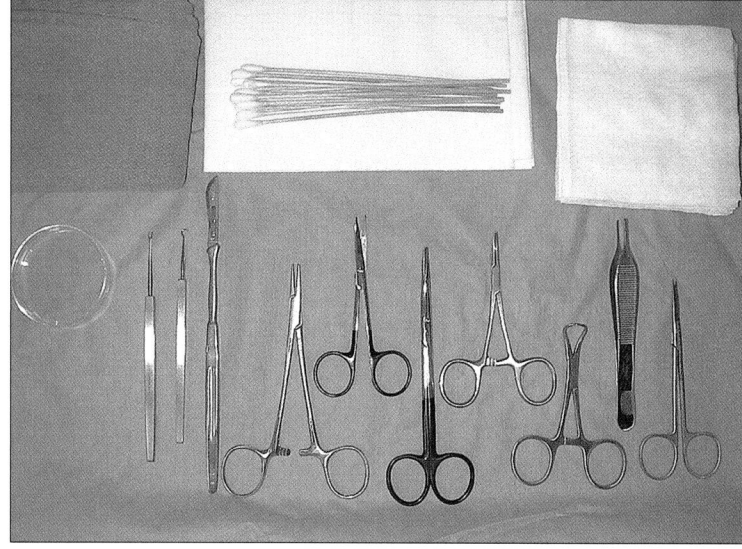

Fig. 144.7 Trunk or extremity surgery tray. Tray setup for truncal or extremity surgery includes (from left to right) Petri dish, skin hooks, no. 7 handle with no. 10 blade, larger Halsey needle holder, Supercut® curved iris scissors, Supercut® baby Metzenbaum undermining scissors, small hemostat, towel clamp, Adson forceps, and suture scissors. Instruments courtesy of George Tiemann & Company, Hauppauge, NY, USA.

from 1 to 5 years, depending on the instrument type and cost. The surgeon should work closely with a reputable dealer to collect a set of instruments that best fulfills his or her special needs. It is important to keep instruments in good condition by caring for them properly and keeping them sharp. A manual of proper instrument care is available from the manufacturer acknowledged in the figures.

Some of the author's instruments of choice for given procedures are listed and shown in Figures 144.5–144.8. Sets of trays for cutaneous surgeries on the face, trunk and extremities are illustrated.

Biopsy blades

Shave biopsies can be performed using a no. 15 blade on a disposable handle. However, an economical alternative that allows great precision is a Gillette® blade. The disadvantage of this blade is that two back-to-back blades must be separated and sterilized by office staff. In addition, the blades may snap and may present a sharp hazard. A similar, more convenient (but more expensive) alternative is the DermaBlade® (Personna Medical), which comes prepackaged and sterilized. The DermaBlade® offers a plastic holder that adds a margin of safety for the operator.

Curettes

The first dermatologic instruments were curettes. Developed in the late 1800s, the dermal curette has been used to treat a wide variety of cutaneous neoplasms, both benign and malignant, and they have changed relatively little over the years. Common curettes have a round head (Fox) or an oval head (Cannon), and they are labeled by size (much like sutures), depending upon the aperture of the head of the curette. For standard curettage and electrodesiccation, a set of curettes ranging from 4.0 or 5.0 down to 1.0 or 2.0 is employed. Curettes must be sharpened periodically. They are used for tumor removal and debulking, and they may allow a surgeon to better define tumor margins prior to excision[34]. Disposable curettes tend to be very sharp and may cut into tissue, and the surgeon must be aware of this drawback.

Scalpels

The choice of scalpel handle and blade is based on the surgical site and personal preference of the surgeon (Fig. 144.9). Available blade handles are flat, round, or long and thin in shape. The flat, standard no. 3

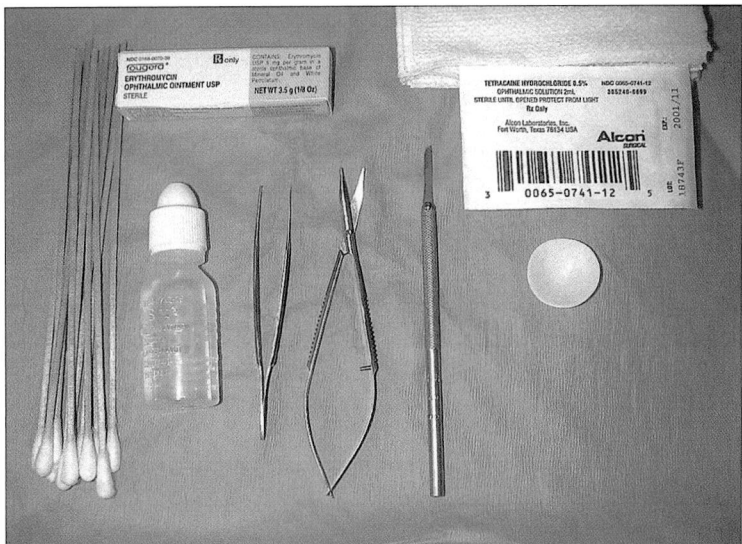

Fig. 144.8 Eyelid tray. Tray setup for eyelid surgery includes (from right to left) topical anesthetic, Teflon® eyeshield, Beaver blade setup, Westcott (or Castroviejo) scissors, Bishop–Harmon forceps, and ophthalmic ointment. Instruments courtesy of George Tiemann & Company, Hauppauge, NY, USA.

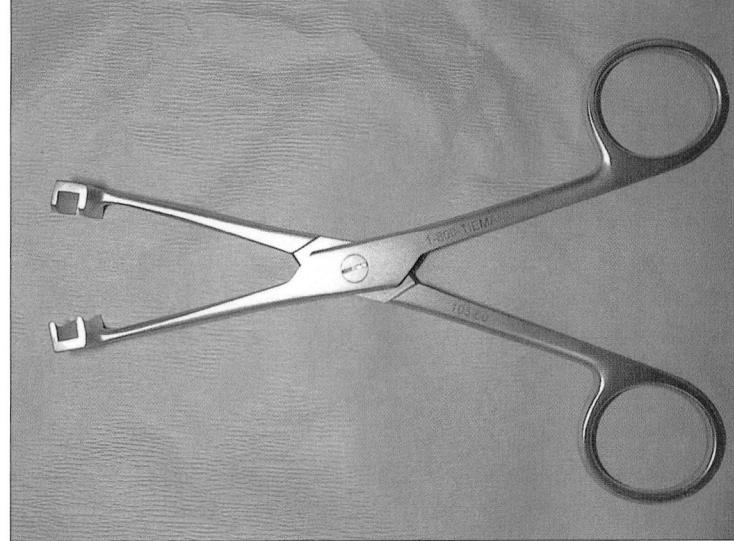

Fig. 144.10 Blade remover. Instrument courtesy of George Tiemann & Company, Hauppauge, NY, USA.

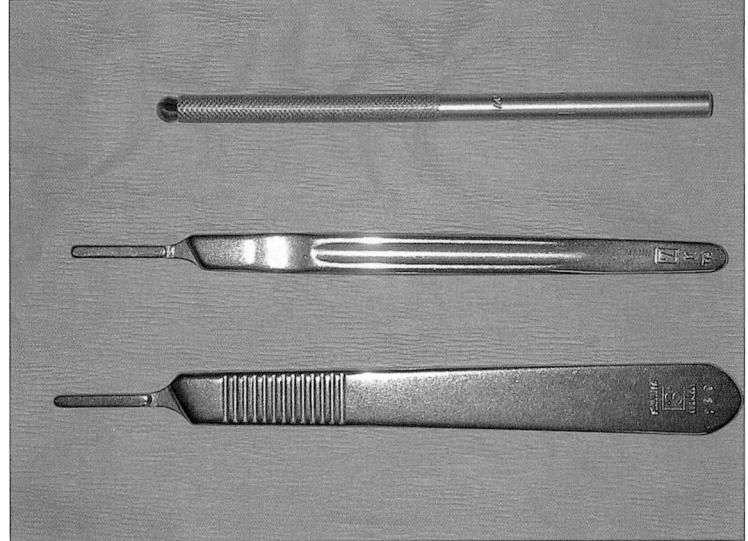

Fig. 144.9 Standard scalpel handles. From top to bottom: Beaver blade handle, no. 7 handle, and no. 3 handle. Instruments courtesy of George Tiemann & Company, Hauppauge, NY, USA.

handle is the most frequently used handle in dermatologic surgery, and it comes with or without an imprinted ruler. This is a durable, inexpensive handle that is adequate for most cutaneous procedures. Many plastic surgeons prefer the rounded, textured no. 7 handle and feel that it gives better control and comfort because the cutting angle of the blade may be changed by rolling the handle with the fingers rather than having to use the wrist to accomplish the same task with a flat no. 3 handle. For small procedures, such as those on the eyelid and/or ear, some surgeons prefer small hexagonal or round knurled blade handles.

The most commonly used blades in dermatologic surgery are no. 15, no. 10 and no. 11. The no. 15 blade is the most popular blade. It is gently curved and is appropriate for the majority of skin surgery. The no. 10 blade is a wide blade, similar in shape to the no. 15 blade, and it is used primarily for larger excisional procedures on sites such as the back. The sharpest area of a curved blade is the belly, not the tip. The no. 11 blade is tapered to a sharp point; it is used for stab incisions in incision and drainage procedures, removal of milia, and for 'through and through' excision. Great care must be exercised with the no. 11 blade, the use of which is associated with a high frequency of operator injury. For small specialty procedures, disposable mini-blades are available for use in conjunction with small hexagonal or round knurled blade holders. Scalpel blades are made of either stainless steel or the

sharper, more expensive carbon steel. Disposable scalpels are available, but they are not weighted and are usually less sharp. For personal protection, blade extractors are available (Fig. 144.10).

Needle holders

Needle holders for facial and hand surgery are small and light with narrow, fine jaws, while larger needle holders with wide sturdy jaws are designed for work on the trunk and proximal extremities. The jaws of needle holders are either smooth or serrated. As a general rule, smaller, smooth jaws can accommodate finer needles and suture materials, and larger, serrated jaws accommodate larger needles and sutures. Serrations prevent 'twisting' of larger needles (e.g. Ethicon PS-2 and FS-2) during suturing. Smooth jaws are less damaging to fine-caliber needles (e.g. Ethicon P-3) and will not tear smaller sutures (6-0), but suture needles may slip if not grasped carefully. There are now some small needle holders that have delicate serrated jaws. These allow for a good grip on fine needles without damaging the needle. Large needles should not be used with fine needle holders as this may lead to damage to the inserts of these delicate instruments, i.e. a fine needle driver used a single time to suture a large wound on the back may never again function properly.

Because of constant metal-to-metal contact, needle holders must be strong and durable. Alloy inserts of tungsten carbide are used to increase the strength and hardness of the jaws and prolong the life of the needle holder. Carbide inserts are more expensive, but they are typically guaranteed for 5 years. Instruments with tungsten carbide have gold finger handles.

Popular models such as the Webster and Halsey needle holders (Fig. 144.11), which have smooth or delicately serrated jaws and tapered tips, are ideal for the small needles and fine suture materials that are commonly used in cutaneous facial surgery. Use of these instruments for procedures on the trunk will lead to their demise. The Crile–Wood needle holder has a gently tapered blunt tip, and it is designed to hold larger needles more appropriate for skin surgery on the trunk or extremities. Baumgartner and Mayo–Hegar holders are durable, strong drivers with serrated jaws, which will stand up to repeated use on the back. The Olsen–Hegar needle holder has suture-cutting scissors behind the jaws and is convenient to use when working alone, although it is very easy to accidentally cut off the needle from the suture when attempting to re-grasp the needle.

Scissors

Surgical scissors are required for cutting skin, undermining the sub-cutis and deeper fascial layers, cutting sutures, and removing wound dressings (Fig. 144.12). Scissors may have long or short handles, and the blades are straight or curved and serrated or smooth. The tips may be sharp or blunt. Scissors used in cutaneous surgery can be either completely stainless steel (most popular, least expensive) or have

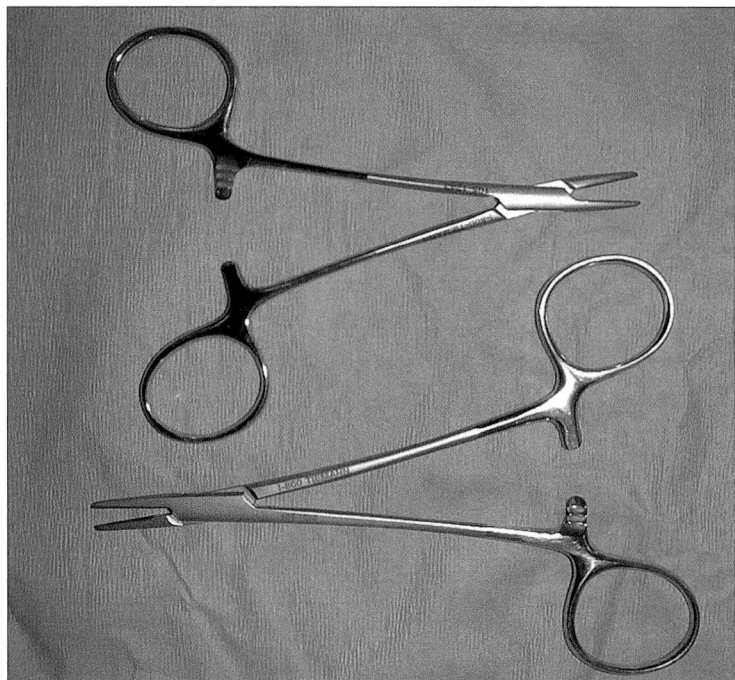

Fig. 144.11 Standard delicate Webster and Halsey needle holders.
Instruments courtesy of George Tiemann & Company, Hauppauge, NY, USA.

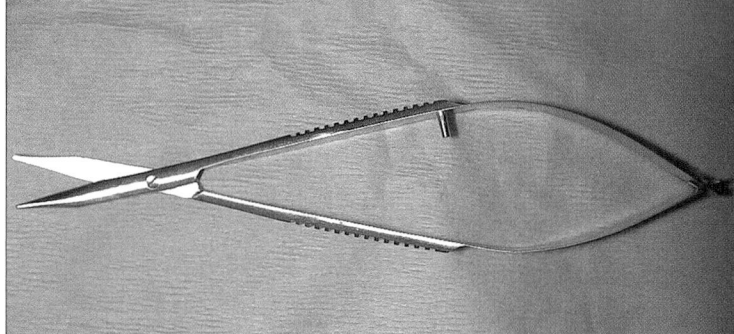

Fig. 144.13 Westcott scissors. Instrument courtesy of George Tiemann & Company, Hauppauge, NY, USA.

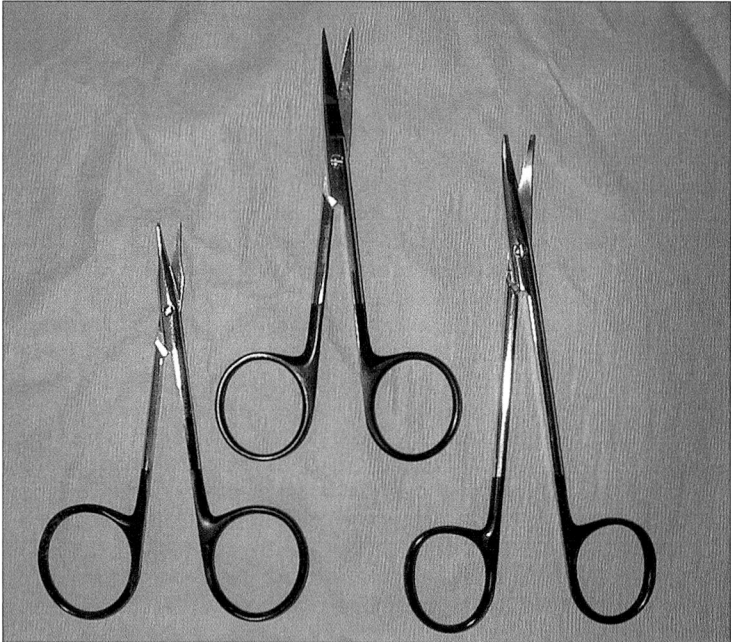

Fig. 144.12 Standard scissors. From left to right: Supercut® Gradle scissors, Supercut® iris scissors, and Supercut® baby Metzenbaum scissors. Instruments courtesy of George Tiemann & Company, Hauppauge, NY, USA.

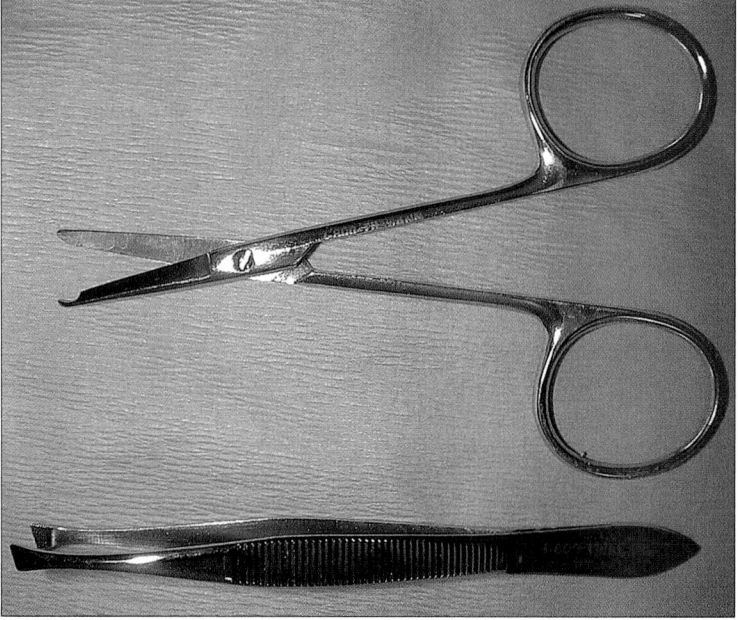

Fig. 144.14 Suture-removal scissors (with groove to grab suture) and forceps. Instruments courtesy of George Tiemann & Company, Hauppauge, NY, USA.

tungsten carbide inserts to strengthen the blades. Tungsten carbide instruments are easily identified by their gold handles.

Gradle scissors are small, delicate, sharp-tipped, and tapered to a very fine point with a gentle curve[35]. Due to their sharpness and precision, Supercut® Gradle scissors are ideal for removing thin stages during Mohs micrographic excision and for removing skin tags. Gradle scissors must be used with care, and they should never be used to cut sutures. With improper use, they are quickly dulled and the tips are easily malpositioned.

Tissue scissors have relatively short handles and sharp tips. They are available in straight or curved models, with or without the serrations that prevent tissue motion during cutting. Of the various models available, the author prefers curved Supercut® iris scissors to cut tissue and for sharp dissection. Supercut® iris scissors have the sharpest edge of the standard tissue scissors available, and they are easily recognized by their black handles. They have a fine bevel angle at the cutting edge,

and they are available with smooth edges or one serrated edge. The 'razor-like' edge of these scissors makes it possible to cut tissue with a smooth, easy cutting motion.

Westcott and Castroviejo scissors are delicate, spring-loaded tissue scissors with very sharp tips (Fig. 144.13). The configuration of their handle and spring-loaded action make them ideal for manipulation in small delicate sites, specifically the eyelid. For this reason, they are popular with oculoplastic surgeons. They should only be used for eyelid surgery or they will quickly dull.

Large, less expensive scissors are sufficient for cutting sutures. Tissue scissors should never be used to cut suture material. Specially designed suture-removal scissors with a half-moon hook on the lower blade are available and the small hooked tip easily grasps the loop and prevents accidental sticks (Fig. 144.14). The O'Brien scissors have a short-angled blade that allows for suture cutting with the very tip of the blade so as to avoid digging into the skin.

Undermining scissors are usually blunt-tipped (for safety) and have longer handles (for comfort). They are available in different sizes to accommodate the various anatomic regions in which skin surgery is performed. Baby Metzenbaum scissors have a high handle-to-blade length ratio (see Fig. 144.12), and, with the resultant small blade arc, they have become the most widely used scissor for sharp or blunt undermining. Larger Metzenbaum scissors are ideal for undermining in fascial planes on the scalp, trunk and extremities. Steven's tenotomy scissors and Supercut® Shea undermining scissors are ideal for more superficial, delicate undermining. The tips of these sutures allow for sharp, less traumatic undermining.

Every skin surgery office needs bandage-cutting scissors. The most popular 5.5-inch Lister scissors have angled blades and large blunt tips that easily slide under a dressing without damaging the underlying skin. The Universal scissor is also a popular choice. The serrated edges and larger rings provide greater cutting power.

Forceps

Proper forceps are essential for delicate, safe handling of tissue and suture needles during skin surgery. The most useful forceps in skin surgery are lightweight and have fine tips. The tips may be either toothed (tissue forceps) or serrated (thumb forceps). Serrated forceps can exert excessive pressure on tissues, resulting in crush injury. Toothed forceps have opposing teeth and allow for gentle handling of tissue. The most popular tissue forceps have 1 × 2 teeth; however, 2 × 3 and multi-toothed patterns are available. Some forceps have both distal teeth for handling of tissue and a more proximal raised platform for firmly grasping suture needles, allowing the surgeon to avoid manual handling of sharp needles.

Forceps are available with delicate (≤0.6 mm), regular (1–1.5 mm) or heavy (≥1.6 mm) tips. Adson forceps are the standard large forceps used for excisional surgery on the trunk and proximal extremities. Both the Bishop–Harmon and Foerster forceps are very lightweight, fine-tipped, and ideal for delicate work on the face and hand, where they are the forceps of choice. Because Bishop–Harmon forceps are easily bent and 'offset', they must be handled with care, and they should not be used for manipulating the thicker skin of the trunk or proximal extremities. 'Bishops' are also very expensive to replace.

Both epilating and jewelers' forceps have a fine, sharp point and are useful for suture removal. Splinter forceps have fine, extra-fine or superfine delicate pointed tips, and they are used in hair transplants, for splinter removal, for removing embedded sutures, and for grasping bleeding vessels prior to cautery or electrodesiccation.

Hemostats

Hemostats are used to grasp bleeding vessels prior to ligation. The most popular hemostat is the Halstead Mosquito model which is available in 3.5-inch and 5-inch lengths, either curved or straight, and either delicate- or regular-tipped.

Skin hooks

Skin hooks enable the surgeon to handle tissue with minimal trauma, and they are particularly useful for elevating flaps and reflecting skin edges during undermining[36]. Many surgeons also use skin hooks to visualize bleeding vessels for hemostasis and for placement of dermal sutures. Since the rise in HIV and hepatitis C viral infections, some surgeons have abandoned the use of the skin hook in exchange for a fine forceps, hoping to decrease the risk of an accidental stick. With caution, however, skin hooks can be valuable when elevating flaps.

Skin hooks are available in single-, double- or multiple-pronged patterns. The multiple-pronged instruments are referred to as skin rakes; they are used mainly for rhytidectomies and larger truncal procedures in which large flaps or margins of tissue are being elevated and/or undermined. Single-pronged hooks are used most frequently in cutaneous surgery for flap elevation and undermining delicate skin. The single shepherd hook – which has a more circular shape – holds tissue better than does the single standard hook, but it does not release as easily.

Special Instruments

For delicate work near the eye, the dermatologic surgeon needs fine instruments that allow for precise cutting and carefully controlled tissue manipulation. The Beaver handle (see Fig. 144.9), which comes in a variety of sizes, can be rolled with one's fingertips, providing greater precision and control. Beaver handles are fitted with specialized smaller, sharper blades. The no. 64 blade has a rounded shape with a blunt tip that one may prefer for work around the eye. The no. 67 blade is smaller but similar in shape to the standard no. 15 blade, and the no. 65 blade is a miniature version of the no. 11 blade for stab incisions. Beaver blades dull more rapidly than do the standard no. 15 blades. (Angled Beaver blades are useful for taking Mohs stages or biopsies in the external ear canal.)

The Castroviejo needle holder, although expensive, is ideal for suturing the delicate skin near the eye or for use by a surgeon with small hands and for whom the rings in the standard needle driver prove cumbersome. This needle holder has spring handles and an optional self-locking device. Castroviejo and Westcott scissors, as discussed earlier, provide precise meticulous control when cutting eyelid skin. Lightweight forceps, such as Bishop–Harmon or Foerster forceps, aid in achieving the delicate handling of tissues necessary in this region. Plastic, Teflon® and metal eye shields are available, and they should be used when the lid margin will be breached and when cautery will be performed near the eye. Metal eye shields conduct heat and reflect laser beams, which may be a disadvantage.

Chalazion clamps are commonly used for immobilizing earlobes, lips and tongues during procedures on these areas. Small chalazion clamps can be particularly valuable on the lip when the labial artery must be transected during a lip wedge procedure.

Nail nippers, splitters and elevators are necessary for nail surgery (see Ch. 149). The double-action nail nipper is extremely strong, and it will cut the thickest nails. Nail splitters have a perpendicular, flat second blade that will not damage the nail bed.

Antiseptics and Sterilization

Several antiseptics are available for preparing the skin prior to cutaneous surgery. The attributes and weaknesses of these preparations are outlined in Table 144.4[37]. Iodophors offer sustained, broad antimicrobial activity, although users must be aware of possible contact dermatitis, as well as skin staining. Chlorhexidine (Hibiclens®) also has sustained, broad antimicrobial activity with the added advantage over iodophors of rapid onset. Use of chlorhexidine around the eye(s) should be avoided due to the risk of keratitis. Alcohol should be allowed to dry sufficiently so as to not ignite or it should not be used at all if electrosurgery is anticipated. A summary of sterilization methods is presented in Table 144.5[38].

Drapes

Table 144.6 outlines the various types of sterile drapes that can be used during cutaneous surgery.

Hemostasis

Most bleeding during cutaneous surgery can be characterized either as superficial or dermal oozing, deep musculature oozing, venular/

ANTISEPTIC AGENTS		
Agent	**Advantages**	**Disadvantages**
Povidone-iodine (Betadine®) Iodoform (triiodomethane)	Broad antimicrobial spectrum, including fungi	Skin irritant; contact dermatitis; residual color; may cross-react with radiopaque iodine and iodides in medications
Chlorhexidine (Hibiclens®)	Broad antimicrobial coverage; no absorption; non-toxic; prolonged suppression of bacterial growth	Irritating to eyes (keratitis) and middle ear (otitis)
Hexachlorophene (pHisoHex®)	Strong effect against Gram-positive cocci	Little effect on Gram-negative organisms or fungi; teratogen; absorbed through skin with potential neurotoxicity in infants
Isopropyl alcohol	Inexpensive; denatures protein, including bacterial cell walls	Weak antimicrobial activity; flammable in the setting of cautery; skin irritant
Hydrogen peroxide		No significant antiseptic properties; cytotoxic to keratinocytes in culture

Table 144.4 Antiseptic agents. Adapted from Leffell DJ, Brown M. Manual of Skin Surgery. New York: Wiley-Liss; 1997:155.

STERILIZATION METHODS		
Method	**Advantages**	**Disadvantages**
Steam autoclave	Most popular in office; easiest; safest	Must use 20–30 min at 2 atm pressure and 121°C; corrosive; may dull sharp instruments
Chemiclave	Lower humidity than steam; less dulling of sharp instruments; instruments are drier	Special chemical needed (mixture of formaldehyde, methyl ethyl ketone, acetone and alcohols)
Dry heat (oven)	Inexpensive; no corrosion or dulling	High temperature, longer time (1 h at 171°C; 6 h at 121°C); cannot use cloth, paper or plastic
Gas sterilization	Good for large volumes (mostly used in hospitals)	Expensive equipment; prolonged times (1 day for paper, 7 days for polyvinyl chloride); toxic and mutagenic gas
Cold sterilization (alcohol, detergent, quaternary ammonium, or more effective glutaraldehyde solutions)	Simple; inexpensive	Irritating to skin; not recommended as only method; not always effective against bacterial spores or hepatitis B virus

Table 144.5 Sterilization methods.

TYPES OF STERILE DRAPES		
Type	**Advantages**	**Disadvantages**
Fenestrated paper and plastic drape	Inexpensive	Less absorbant; central hole often too small for larger cases
Cloth drape pack	Relatively inexpensive; easily customized; can clamp electrocautery cord to drape	Requires laundering
Full-sized operating room boundary package with sterile full-body-length drape	Stricter sterility; large sterile field	Expensive; claustrophobic

Table 144.6 Types of sterile drapes.

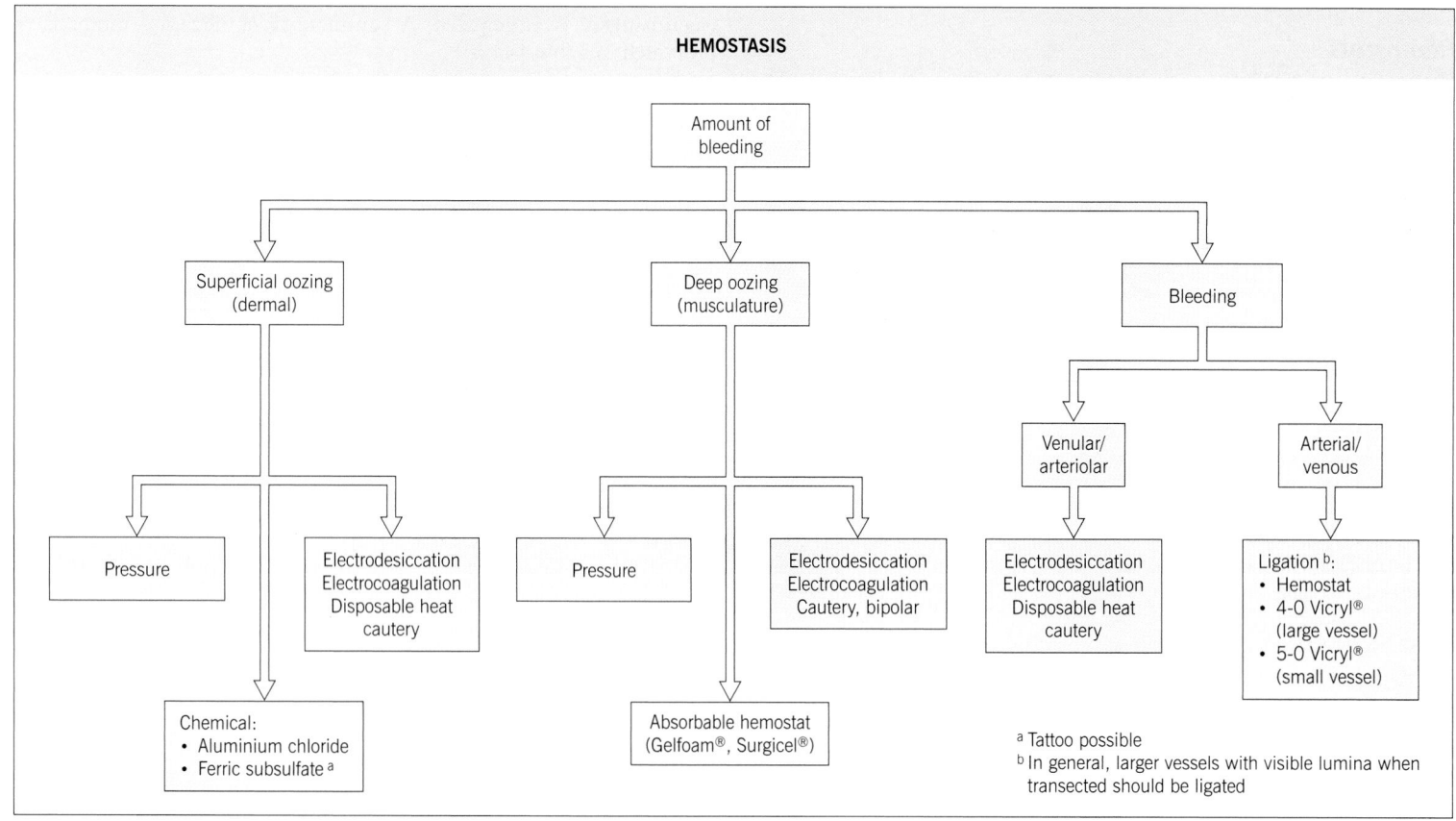

Fig. 144.15 Hemostasis algorithm.

arteriolar bleeding, or venous/arterial bleeding (Fig. 144.15). For 'oozing', mechanical pressure and the use of chemical and absorbable hemostatic agents are usually sufficient. Surface wounds created by shave biopsy are generally best treated with aluminum chloride, which leads to excellent hemostasis of capillary beds without tissue staining. For more vigorous dermal oozing, ferric subsulfate (Monsel's solution) is very effective; however, when combined with blood, ferric subsulfate may lead to a permanent or semipermanent dermal tattoo. In order to avoid this outcome, the wound should be firmly pressed with gauze and then the ferric subsulfate solution should be instantly pressed against the (dry) dermis with a saturated cotton swab. For visible arteriolar and venular bleeding, electrosurgery (electrodesiccation or electrocoagulation) is generally recommended and carries only a minor risk of rebleeding. Heat cautery (e.g. electrocautery) coagulates by transfer of heat to the tissues and is safe to use in patients with older, poorly insulated pacemakers and/or defibrillators. In general, larger vessels with visible lumina when transected should be ligated with 4-0 absorbable suture.

REFERENCES

1. Levenson S, Geever EF, Crowley LV, et al. The healing of rat skin wounds. Ann Surg. 1965;161:293–308.
2. Usher FC, Allen JE, Crosthwait RW, Cogan JE. Polypropylene monofilament: a new biologically inert suture for closing contaminated wounds. JAMA. 1962;179:780–2.
3. Bucknall T. Factors influencing wound complications: a clinical and experimental study. Ann R Coll Surg. 1983;65:71–7.
4. Sharp WV, Belden TA, King PH, et al. Suture resistance to infection. Surgery. 1982;91:61–3.
5. Postlethwait RW, Willigan DA, Ulin AW. Human tissue reaction to sutures. Ann Surg. 1975;181:144–50.
6. Alexander JW, Kaplan JZ, Altemeier WA. Role of suture materials in the development of wound infection. Ann Surg. 1967;165:192–9.
7. Molea G, Schonauer F, Bifulco G, et al. Comparative study on biocompatibility and absorption times of three absorbable monofilament suture materials (Polydioxanone, Poliglecaprone 25, Glycomer 631). Br J Plast Surg. 2000;53:137–41.
8. Holmlund DE. Physical properties of surgical suture materials: stress-strain relationship, stress-relaxation and irreversible elongation. Ann Surg. 1976;184:189–93.
9. Herrmann JB. Tensile strength and knot security of surgical suture materials. Am Surg. 1971;37:209–17.
10. Bennett RG. Selection of wound closure materials. J Am Acad Dermatol. 1988;18:619–37.
11. Garrett AB. Wound closure materials. In: Wheeland R (ed.). Cutaneous Surgery. Philadelphia: WB Saunders, 1994:199–205.
12. Jenkins HP, Hrdina LS, Owen FM, et al. Absorption of surgical gut (catgut). III. Duration in the tissue after loss of tensile strength. Arch Surg. 1942;45:74–102.
13. Webster RC, McCollough EG, Giandello PR, et al. Skin wound approximation with new absorbable suture material. Arch Otolaryngol. 1985;111:517–19.
14. Guyuron B, Vaughan C. A comparison of absorbable and non-absorbable suture materials for skin repair. Plast Reconstr Surg. 1991;89:234–6.
15. Postlethwait R. Polyglycolic acid surgical suture. Arch Surg. 1970;101:489–94.
16. Craig PH, Williams JA, Davis KW, et al. A biologic comparison of polyglactin 910 and polyglycolic acid synthetic absorbable sutures. Surg Gynecol Obstet. 1975;141:1–10.
17. Conn J Jr, Oyasu R, Welsh M, et al. Vicryl (polyglactin 910) synthetic absorbable sutures. Am J Surg. 1974;128:19–23.
18. Aston SJ, Rees TD. Vicryl sutures. Aesthetic Plast Surg. 1977;1:289–93.
19. Lerwick E. Studies on the efficacy and safety of polydioxanone monofilament absorbable suture. Surg Gynecol Obstet. 1983;156:51–5.
20. Rodeheaver GT, Powell TA, Thacker JG, et al. Mechanical performance of monofilament synthetic absorbable sutures. Am J Surg. 1987;154:544–7.
21. Katz AR, Mukherjee DP, Kaganov AL, et al. A new synthetic monofilament absorbable suture made from polytrimethylene carbonate. Surg Gynecol Obstet. 1985;161:213–22.
22. Niessen FB, Spauwen PHM, Kon M. The role of suture material in hypertrophic scar formation: Monocryl vs. Vicryl-rapide. Ann Plast Surg. 1997;39:254–60.
23. Nilsson T. Mechanical properties of Prolene and Ethilon sutures after three weeks in vivo. Scand J Plast Reconstr Surg. 1982;16:11–15.
24. Nilsson T. Mechanical properties of Prolene, Ethilon and surgical steel loops. Scand J Plast Reconstr Surg. 1981;15:111–15.
25. Miller JM, Kimmel LE Jr. Clinical evaluation of monofilament polypropylene suture. Am Surg. 1967;33:666–70.
26. Bang RL, Mustafa MD. Comparative study of skin wound closure with polybutester (Novafil) and polypropylene. J R Coll Surg (Edinb). 1989;34:205–7.
27. Campbell JP, Swanson NA. The use of staples in dermatologic surgery. J Dermatol Surg Oncol. 1982;8:680–90.
28. Fosko SW, Heap D. Surgical pearl: an economical means of skin closure with absorbable suture. J Am Acad Dermatol. 1998;39:248–50.
29. Maw JL, Quinn JV, Wells GA, et al. A prospective comparison of octylcyanoacrylate tissue adhesive and suture for the closure of head and neck incisions. J Otolaryngol. 1997;26:26–30.
30. Quinn J, Wells G, Sutcliffe T, et al. A randomized trial comparing octylcyanoacrylate tissue adhesive and sutures in the management of lacerations. JAMA. 1997;277:1527–30.
31. Taube M, Porter RJ, Lord PH. A combination of subcuticular suture and sterile Micropore tape compared with conventional interrupted sutures for skin closure. A controlled trial. Ann R Coll Surg Engl. 1983;65:164–7.
32. Katz KH, Desciak EB, Maloney ME. The optimal application of surgical adhesive tape strips. Dermatol Surg. 1999;25:686–8.
33. Bernstein G. Needle basics. J Dermatol Surg Oncol. 1985;11:1177–8.
34. Johnson TM, Tromovitch TA, Swanson NA. Combined curettage and excision: a treatment method for primary basal cell carcinoma. J Am Acad Dermatol. 1991;24:613–17.
35. Gibbs RC. A love affair with a gradle scissors. J Dermatol Surg Oncol. 1981;7:771.
36. Boyer JD, Zitelli JA, Brodland DG. Undermining in cutaneous surgery. Dermatol Surg. 2001;27:75–8.
37. Leffell DJ, Brown M. Manual of Skin Surgery. New York: Wiley-Liss, 1997:155.
38. Sebben JE. Sterilization and care of surgical instruments and supplies. J Am Acad Dermatol 1984;11:381–92.

Dressings

Gregg M Menaker and Stephanie L Mehlis

Key features

- Dressings should provide the optimum environment for rapid healing by protecting the wound from further trauma or bacterial invasion

- Dressings that provide a moist environment and prevent eschar formation allow wounds to re-epithelialize and heal faster than if left uncovered

- Semipermeable or occlusive dressings provide a moist environment, retain wound fluid that contains growth factors conducive to healing, and promote a low tissue oxygen tension that stimulates angiogenesis and deposition of collagen

- A traditional layered dressing consists of a non-adherent contact layer, an absorbent contouring layer and a securing layer

- Newer advanced technology dressings include the following types: hydrogels, alginates, foams, films and hydrocolloids

- Recently, tissue-engineered composite skin equivalents have been developed combining living keratinocytes and fibroblasts from human foreskins with bovine collagen

INTRODUCTION

The variety of cutaneous surgical procedures performed by dermatologists, as well as the types of wounds they manage clinically, require dressing materials and techniques that address the specific needs of the injury. In addition to the care of surgical incision sites such as those created by any surgeon, the dermatologist's armamentarium often extends into the care of poorly healing and chronic wounds. The choice of treatment modalities is indeed substantial and ever expanding, giving dermatologists flexibility in wound care strategy.

THE HISTORY OF DRESSINGS

The practice of using dressings dates back thousands of years. The use of fabrics such as linen on wounds continued for at least 4000 years until woven absorbent cotton gauze was introduced in 1871. The Edwin Smith Surgical Papyrus, which is one of the earliest medical treatises (dating back to 1615 BC), describes the use of linen strips and plaster to dress wounds, stating that closed wounds would heal more quickly than open wounds[1]. Ancient documents disclose how lint was used to pack and fill open wounds and how bandages were used to re-approximate wounds in order to facilitate healing. Linen strips were sometimes coated with grease or oil to prevent adherence to wounds or with honey to create a semi-occlusive and adherent dressing[2].

Lister connected the presence of pus with infections. However, this association became linked such that it was held that one is always indicative of the other, which is not always true. It is this link that interfered with the acceptance of occlusive dressings, as well as with progress in the study of their value. Although the work of Pasteur, Koch and Lister in the late 1800s on the cause of bacterial infections began in earnest the investigation of specific therapies for wound management, it was not until the past half-century that the understanding of wound healing completely changed. Until the mid-1900s, it was firmly believed that wounds healed more quickly if they were kept dry and uncovered.

In 1948, Oscar Gilje described a 'moist chamber effect' for healing ulcers[3]. Two years later, Schilling and colleagues published a study in which the treatment of common minor wounds with highly occlusive

or semi-occlusive nylon films was evaluated. They found semi-occlusive dressings to be more effective than open treatment healing. The fact that the semi-occlusive dressing proved to be more effective than the highly occlusive dressing is said to have set back this area of study. In 1962, George Winter conducted what is considered to be the landmark study on moist wound healing, demonstrating a 30% greater benefit of occlusive dressings versus air drying of wounds[4]. Many studies conducted since Winter's work have contributed to the concept of the benefits of moist wound healing by occlusive dressings.

THE FUNCTIONS OF A WOUND DRESSING

A wound dressing is a substitute for native epithelium lost as a result of injury. The process of wound repair occurs in stages (see Ch. 141), each of which may require different dressings. The main function of a dressing is to provide the optimum environment for rapid healing by protecting the wound from further trauma, bacterial invasion or exposure to caustic substances, which is especially important during the early acute, inflammatory stage. The dressing should ideally be able to conform to the wound shape, absorb wound fluid without increasing bacterial proliferation or causing excessive desiccation, provide pressure for hemostasis, and prevent leakage from the bandage. The dressing should also support the wound and surrounding tissues, eliminate pain, promote re-epithelialization during the reparative phase, and be easily applied and removed with minimal injury to the wound. The composition of the dressing is also an important consideration. It should be composed of inert material that does not shed fibers or compounds into the wound that could lead to a foreign body reaction or an irritant or allergic reaction[5]. The 'ideal' dressing that meets all these requirements for every wound type does not yet exist (Table 145.1). However, in the vast array of dressings available, it is quite possible to select or fashion one for achieving one's goal.

MOIST HEALING ENVIRONMENT

A wound dressing's capacity to maintain a moist environment is of prime importance in healing (Fig. 145.1). There are several mechanisms by which moisture assists the reparative process, the most basic of which is the suppression of tissue desiccation and crust formation. A scab or eschar forms as a result of the drying of a wound, particularly of the superficial dermis which itself becomes integrated into the scab. The studies of Winter and Scales illustrated that uncovered, air-dried wounds developed thicker scabs and re-epithelialized at a slower rate. This slower rate has been attributed to the requirement of the regenerating epidermis to migrate deeper below the dry fibrous tissue to a region of moisture where live cells survive. It is only in such an environment that epidermal cells can move toward bridging the defect of the wound; therefore, the thicker the scab, the deeper the migration. This, along with the continuing loss of dermis and collagen and a reduction in adnexal structures, contributes to the depth of the scars and a worse cosmetic outcome[1].

Many endogenous factors that are critical to wound healing (e.g. fibrin degradation products, platelet-derived growth factor) are found in fluid from occluded (or dressed) acute cutaneous wounds and may be more available in a moist environment (see Ch. 141). Another possible value of a moist wound environment may be its ability to confer an electrical gradient between the wound and normal skin. That is, upon injury of skin, an internal battery and a current flow are created until drying of the wound occurs. It is thought that in maintaining moisture, this electrical gradient may promote epidermal cell migration between the wound and surrounding skin[6].

COMPARISON OF THE IDEAL DRESSING VERSUS THE OCCLUSIVE DRESSINGS AND SKIN SUBSTITUTES									
	Characteristics of an ideal dressing								
	Conforms	Absorbs wound fluid	Decreases bacterial proliferation	Provides pressure	Supports surrounding tissue	Eliminates pain	Promotes re-epithelialization	Easily reapplied	Inert material	Does not shed fibers or compounds into the wound
Films					++	+	+		+	+
Foams	+	++		+		+	+	+	+	
Hydrogels	++	+				++	+	+	+	+
Alginates	++	++	+				+	+		
Hydrocolloids	+	++		+		+	+	+		
Epidermal grafts						+	++		+	+
Dermal grafts					+	+	++	+		+
Composite grafts					+	+	++			+

Table 145.1 Comparison of the ideal dressing versus the occlusive dressings and skin substitutes (i.e. ideal dressing versus reality).

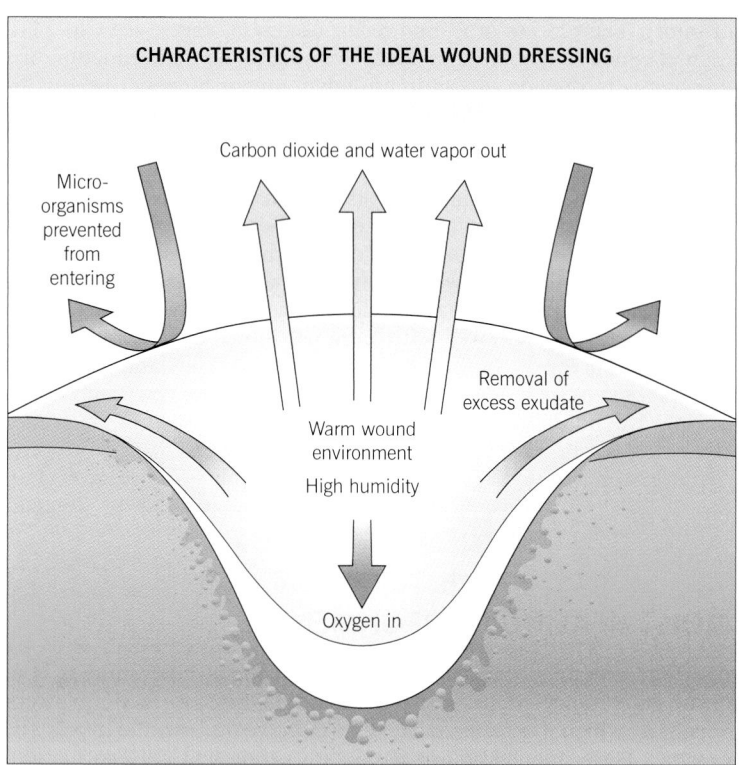

Fig. 145.1 Characteristics of the ideal wound dressing.

THE ROLE OF OXYGEN

For many years, it was believed that oxygen availability was of primary importance in the rate of healing. However, subsequent studies have shown that the oxygen requirement is initially low during the early wound repair stages. After acute injury, wounds experience a temporary but extreme hypoxia due to disruption of blood flow from clotting that prevents exsanguination. This distress is the signal for migration of keratinocytes and fibroblasts as well as the initiation of angiogenesis. Hypoxia has been shown to upregulate proliferation and production of TGF-β by dermal fibroblasts; TGF-β is known to stimulate production of extracellular matrix molecules. Under hypoxic conditions, keratinocytes migrate better along collagen and fibronectin, and low oxygen levels also promote angiogenesis in the acute wound[7]. The use of a semipermeable dressing can provide the appropriate oxygen tension for wound repair to proceed quickly.

In summary, *acute* wounds that heal under occlusion have demonstrated accelerated healing, greater resistance to breaking open, and better cosmetic outcomes than those that heal open to the air. Also, as a result of occlusion, *chronic* wounds are often less painful (particularly upon wound debridement) and they have better formation of granulation tissue.

TRADITIONAL WOUND DRESSINGS

Wound dressings can be categorized either by the composition and structure of the dressing or by the dressing technique and how the dressing is utilized relative to the wound. Traditional or conventional dressings have commonly been made of natural, synthetic or partially synthetic materials[1]. Readily available traditional wound dressings include Band-aids®, Telfa® pads and Exu-dry® dressings. Naturally occurring materials such as cotton, silk, linen or cellulose-based substances have a long history of use and have been produced in various combinations for maximal clinical usefulness. Bleached cotton is processed into balls or fibers which are woven into gauze pads, packing strips, wrapping strips, knitted tubes and compressed felt.

The basic cotton gauze dressing in use today is frequently composed of cotton plus cellulose acetate (added for increased absorbency) and is manufactured with or without various substances incorporated into the fabric. Petrolatum and other ointments such as soft paraffin wax, with or without antibacterials such as povidone-iodine, sulfadiazine, bismuthtribromophenate (Xeroform®), framycetin and chlorhexidine, are examples of impregnated substances; balsam of Peru is found in the tulle gras used predominantly in Western Europe. These medicated dressings are often composites of rayon, nylon or gauze, and are used for malodorous wounds such as chronic ulcers. Activated charcoal cloth (with or without antibacterial silver salt) is also used for exudate absorption plus odor control.

These types of dressings are placed directly against the wound bed and have the advantage of having less chance of adhering to the wound as well as the ability to mold into the depression of deeper wounds for the purpose of filling dead space and providing absorption. The disadvantage of this type of dressing is the potential for maceration of the wound and surrounding skin should the dressing remain in place for an extended period of time. Other pros and cons of traditional dressings are that although relatively inexpensive and readily available, they do require frequent replacement, which is time-consuming for the medical staff and the patient and is potentially costly in healthcare personnel time[8].

The technique used for most conventional dressings is that of the 'layered dressing' and it is either a 'pressure' or 'non-pressure' dressing. A layered dressing is usually constructed in three parts (Fig. 145.2): (1) the contact or interface layer, which is usually a non-adherent, fluid-permeable material that makes direct contact with the wound; (2) the absorbent layer, usually a cotton pad, gauze or other such material, which is placed on top of the contact layer to 'wick in' and retain wound exudate and help the dressing mold to the shape of the wound; and

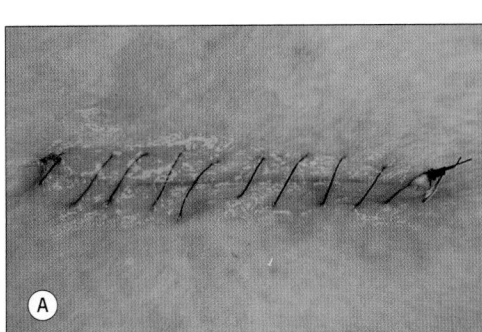
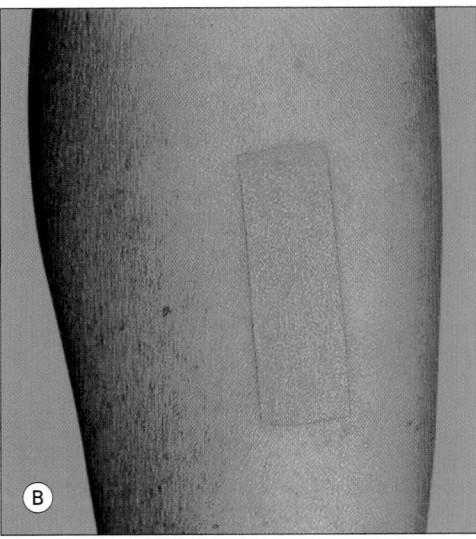
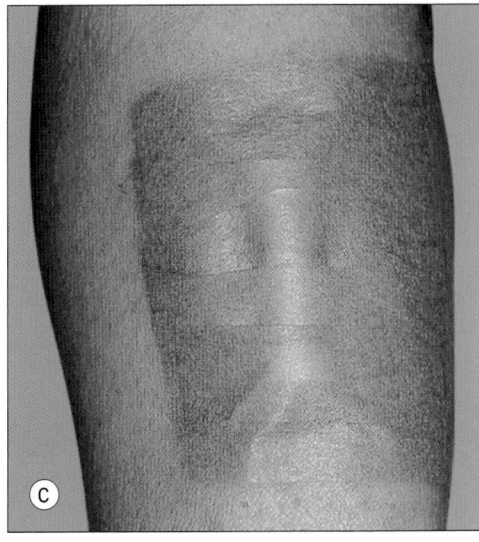

Fig. 145.2 Pressure dressing. A Antibiotic ointment applied over sutures helps to prevent infection and prevents contact layer from adhering directly to the wound. **B** Three layers of paper tape comprise the contact layer. **C** Rolled gauze or a cotton dental roll can be used to: (i) provide pressure for hemostasis; (ii) aid in conforming the dressing to the wound; and (iii) absorb excess exudate. The entire dressing is secured with additional layers of tape.

(3) the outer layer or wrap, often tape or other banding material for retention of the underlying layers. Of note, each layer should be placed in close approximation to the one before it, with no gaps or air pockets, and should increase in size and degree of overlap, from wound bed to outermost layer.

A 'pressure' dressing has more bulk added to the absorbent layer and is arranged so as to create hemostasis at the wound site. Usually applied immediately after surgery and changed to a lighter dressing within 24 hours, the body sites for this type of dressing are most often digits, extremities and the scalp. In addition to limiting bleeding, the pressure dressing also minimizes edema and lends support to the surrounding tissue. It is important to be aware of the amount of pressure exerted upon the wound bed so as not to create localized ischemia, potentially resulting in tissue necrosis[9].

Postsurgical skin wound defects healing by first intention are those that are clean, free of debris and sutured by aseptic technique. Placing sutures postsurgically provides hemostasis, reduces the possibility of wound infection (which may potentiate a delay in healing and chance of dehiscence), and sometimes improves the ultimate cosmetic result. After suture removal, the use of external splinting tape (such as Steri-Strips™) supports the tissues, enabling favorable collagen remodeling that may limit scar formation and hypertrophy.

Second intention healing is often employed following many cutaneous surgical techniques such as punch biopsy, cryosurgery, laser surgery, excision (Fig. 145.3) and curettage. In such cases, moisture at the wound bed is the key to optimal spontaneous healing. A semi-occlusive dressing is the treatment of choice, with the topical application of ointment directly on the wound. Monitoring of the wound as it progresses through stages of healing for signs of infection and prevention of drying of the wound bed until re-epithelialization has

occurred is usually sufficient in the management of this type of surgical wound[10].

TOPICAL ANTIMICROBIAL AGENTS

The usefulness of topical antimicrobial agents for cutaneous wounds is a matter of debate. It is thought by some that a clean wound created with good aseptic technique does not require a topical antimicrobial, as long as the wound is well cared for in the postsurgical period. Also, while it is well known that infection prolongs wound healing, a distinction must be made between bacterial colonization of the wound and true infection that leads to tissue compromise. Lastly, chronic wounds treated with the most commonly used topical antibiotic preparations often require repeated, sometimes painful, dressing changes.

There are, however, more sophisticated methods of providing bacterial control for wounds. For example, nanocrystalline silver comes in a variety of dressing types (e.g. Acticoat™, Actisorb® Silver, Contreet Foam, Contreet Hydrocolloid and Silverlon™) and offers broad-spectrum antibiotic activity against both Gram-positive (including methicillin-resistant *Staphylococcus aureus* [MRSA]) and Gram-negative pathogens[11]. These dressings can release antibacterial levels of silver for 3 to 7 days. Silver ions kill microorganisms by inhibiting bacterial-specific enzymes important in bacterial cell wall synthesis and gene transcription. Despite extensive testing, there has been no documented evidence of either bacterial resistance or cytotoxicity from these dressings[12]. Silver ions also appear to decrease the levels of matrix metalloproteinases that are upregulated in non-healing, chronic wounds. Studies have shown that silver-containing dressings can significantly reduce burn wound-associated sepsis and bacteremia as well as shorten hospitalization time.

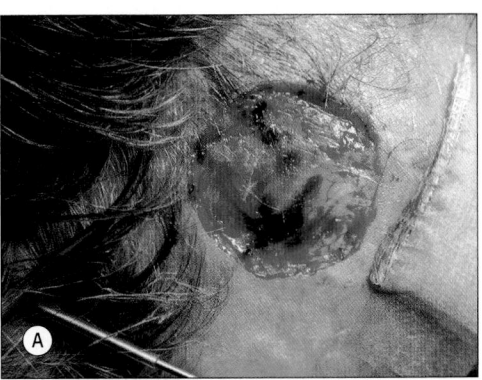
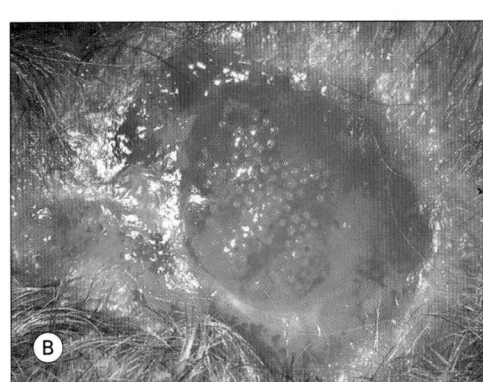
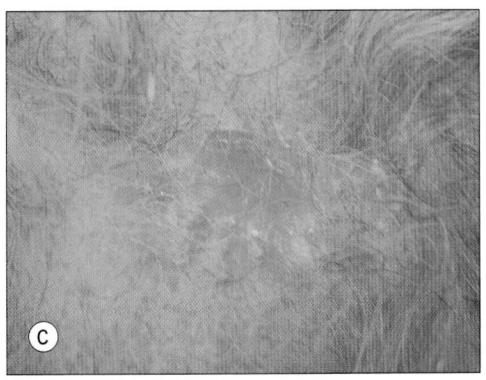

Fig. 145.3 Second intention healing. A Surgical wound immediately following Mohs micrographic surgery; a semi-occlusive dressing will be used. **B** Wound healing by second intention 3 weeks following surgery. Note abundance of pink granulation tissue. **C** Fully re-epithelialized wound 6 weeks following surgery.

OCCLUSIVE DRESSINGS					
Dressing type	Composition	Permeability	Indicated uses	Advantages	Disadvantages
Films	Thin polyurethane sheets	Semipermeable	Intravenous sites Skin tears Split-thickness graft donor sites Laser resurfacing Mohs surgery defects	Translucent Permeable to water vapor Tends to reduce postoperative pain Creates bacterial barrier	Difficult to position properly May adhere to wound as it dries Possible exudate accumulation Non-absorbent
Foams	Bilaminate polyurethane or silicone	Semipermeable	Chronic wounds Dermabrasion Burns Mohs surgery defects Laser resurfacing	Absorbent Permeable to water vapor Conforms to wound shape Thermally insulates Comfortable	Opaque Cannot be used on dry wounds Possible undesirable drying effect on inadequately exudative wounds
Hydrogels	Hydrophilic polymer sheets, gel and impregnated dressings	Semipermeable with outer membrane in place	Ulcers Dermabrasion Laser resurfacing Superficial thermal burns Chemical peels Graft donor sites	Semitransparent Donates fluid to necrotic tissue Soothing, cushioning and cooling effect, reduction of postoperative pain Available in sheets, powdered or pre-mixed amorphous gels Low trauma at dressing changes Reportedly helpful for pruritus	No spontaneous sucking ability Absorption is slow Requires secondary dressing Caution in infected wounds
Alginates	Seaweed-based complex polysaccharide	Semipermeable	Chronic highly exudative wounds Full-thickness burns Surgical wounds Split-thickness graft donor sites Mohs surgery defects	Highly absorbent with spontaneous sucking ability Hemostatic properties Non-adherent Conforms to wound shape Soluble for low trauma dressing changes with normal saline No reports of toxicity Useful in infected wounds	Requires a secondary dressing to prevent desiccation Gel has unpleasant appearance and odor Mild burning sometimes reported upon application
Hydrocolloids	Starch or plastic woven polymer, dextran, polyethylene glycol, water	Semipermeable	Chronic ulcers Burns Trauma wounds Surgery wounds Dermabrasion Bullous disorders Inflammatory disorders (e.g. lichen simplex chronicus)	Capillary action facilitates debris removal Conforms to wound shape Directly adheres to wound site and is easy to use Increased patient comfort Thermal insulation	Risk of maceration of surrounding skin Possible wound trauma with dressing change Gel has unpleasant appearance and odor Opaque Caution in infected wounds

Table 145.2 Occlusive dressings.

Although povidone-iodine, another commonly used antiseptic, can inhibit wound healing, newer formulations – such as cadexomer-iodine polymer, which slowly releases iodine from dextran beads – have not demonstrated toxic effects on keratinocytes. The level of iodine that is slowly released from the beads is sufficiently low as to confer antimicrobial activity, but with little or no cytotoxic effects, while the gel that results from the process works to absorb exudate. Bacteria and cellular debris become trapped in the spaces between the beads and are removed with irrigation at the time of dressing changes. Recommended for exudative wounds such as leg ulcers, a layer of beads is applied to the wound and covered with a pad or other suitable secondary dressing. The frequency of dressing changes is determined by the nature of the wound, perhaps requiring daily changes (if the beads are saturated) to three times per week as the healing progresses[7]. Studies have shown a significant decrease in ulcer size with cadexomer-iodine when compared to hydrocolloid and paraffin gauze dressings[13].

Cadexomer-iodine is also found in multiple types of occlusive dressings (see next section), including hydrocolloids (e.g. Iodosorb®) and hydrogels (e.g. Iodoflex®). Because the iodine is absorbed, caution must be taken when using these dressings in patients with a history of thyroid disease. They should not be used in young children, pregnant and lactating women, or patients with a known or suspected iodine sensitivity, Hashimoto's thyroiditis or a history of Graves disease.

OCCLUSIVE DRESSINGS

Occlusive dressings are a separate category of dressings, commonly divided into five major groups: films, foams, hydrogels, alginates and hydrocolloids (Table 145.2 & Fig. 145.4).

Polymer Films

Polymer films are thin, elastic, transparent sheets of polyurethane or other synthetic semipermeable, self-adhesive polymer dressing (Fig. 145.5). This dressing is gas permeable, allowing for the exchange of oxygen, carbon dioxide and water vapor, but impermeable to larger molecule efflux, due to its pore size. Therefore, proteins and water of wound fluids and bacteria are prevented from moving across the dressing. Its permeability to water vapor allows for the release of insensible water and for sweat from the skin to vaporize. This provides the potential advantage of preventing maceration of the wound and its surrounding skin. The semi-occlusive nature of this dressing allows for passage of oxygen to the wound, which had been considered to be an important feature when these dressings were initially introduced. There has been evidence since then, however, that low pO_2 levels similar to those that actually exist under the dressings facilitate healing.

Uses

Although polymer film dressings may theoretically be used on any uncontaminated wound, they are most commonly used to cover intravenous sites and sites of partial-thickness wounds such as skin tears, superficial decubitus ulcers, split-thickness graft donor sites, burns, laser wounds, dermabrasion, and Mohs surgery defect sites[14]. They are also useful for holding pinch grafts in place for venous ulcer treatment. As the dressing allows for the visual monitoring of the wound, it may be used to hold a graft in place until engraftment. A film dressing can also be used as a 'splint' to hold a thin split-thickness graft stiff as it is being harvested from the donor site. The harvested skin graft is prevented from folding or wrinkling by the attached film as it is sutured into place at the recipient site. An additional piece of film may then be used to secure the graft instead of using sutures[15].

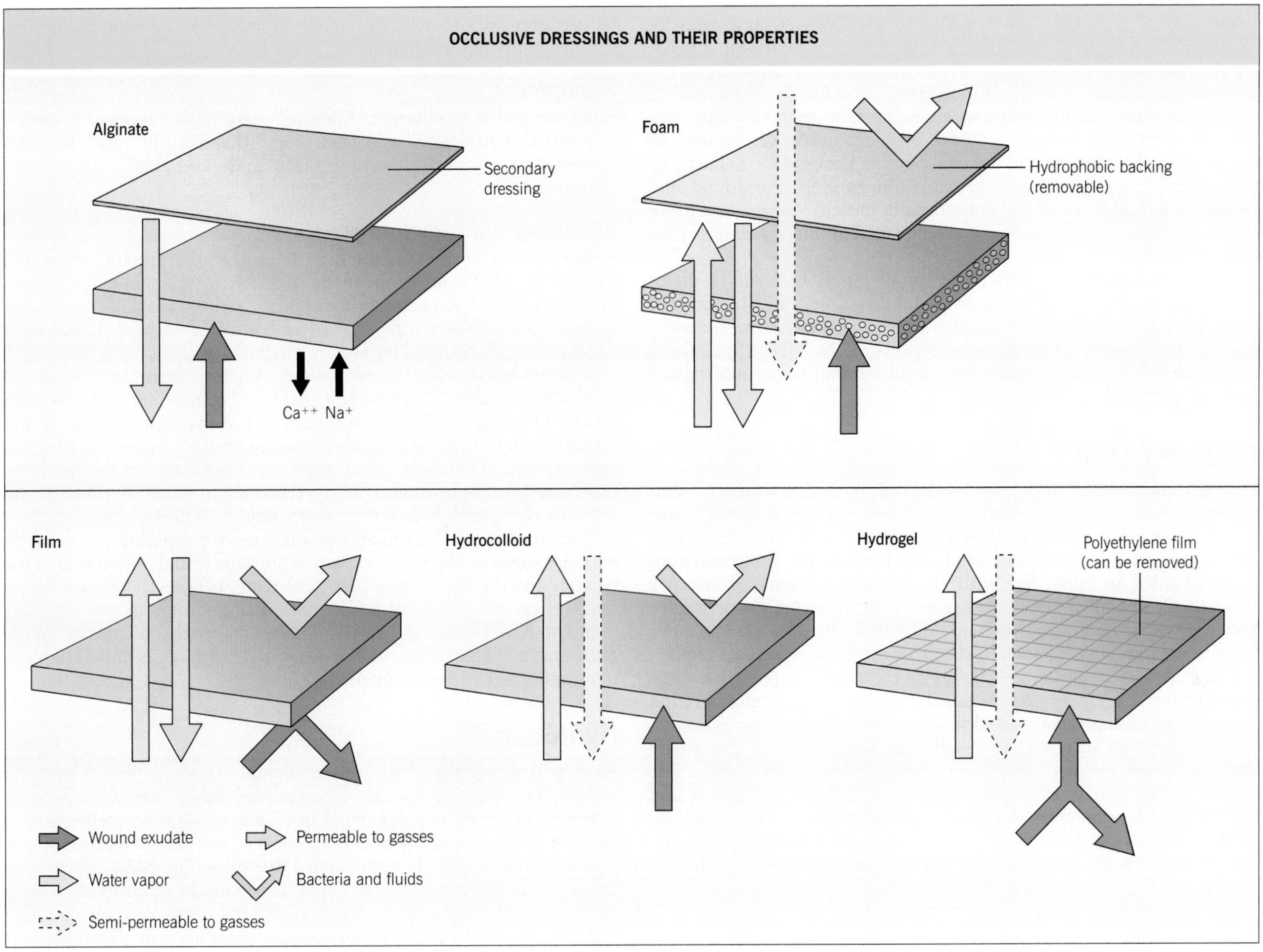

Fig. 145.4 Diagram of occlusive dressings and their properties.

Alginate — Secondary dressing

Ca^{++} Na^+

Foam — Hydrophobic backing (removable)

Film

Hydrocolloid

Hydrogel — Polyethylene film (can be removed)

Wound exudate

Water vapor

Semi-permeable to gasses

Permeable to gasses

Bacteria and fluids

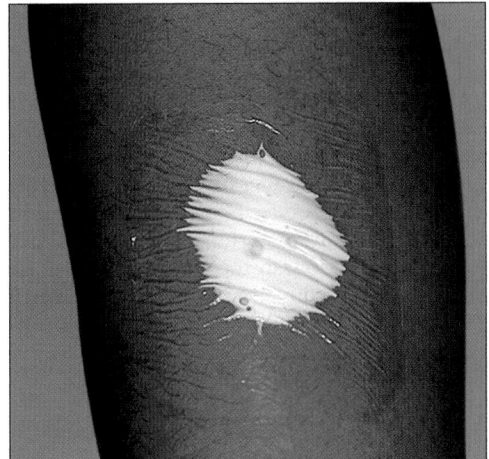

Fig. 145.5 Example of a polymer film used to occlude a topical anesthetic cream.

Examples

Bioclusive™ (Johnson & Johnson); Opsite™ (Smith & Nephew); Polyskin® II (Kendall); ProCyte Transparent Film Dressing (Bard Medical); Silon-TSR® (Bio Med Sciences); and TEGADERM™ (3M).

Advantages/disadvantages

The advantages of this type of dressing are: its translucency, thereby allowing direct visualization of the wound without removal of the dressing; its permeability to water vapor; and its tendency to reduce postoperative pain. It is also thought to enhance re-epithelialization of graft donor sites, with a reported increase in healing rates of 25–45%[16]. One disadvantage of film dressings is that they are difficult to place properly, requiring uniform tension on the film to prevent wrinkling and its adhering to itself. As the film usually only adheres to intact skin, a 1–2 cm application margin is recommended. Films may also adhere to the wound as drying progresses, thereby risking disruption or stripping of the newly formed epithelium, which is not yet tightly bound to the underlying dermal layer. It is possible also to traumatize newly grafted skin tissue during dressing changes. For these reasons, it is advised to allow the film dressing to remain in place until it spontaneously falls off, which can occur after 1–2 weeks.

There are several film dressings, however, that have no adhesive at all or have an adhesive-free zone. Examples of such dressings are Blister Film® (which is composed of polyester rather than polyurethane) and Omniderm®. The dressing with no adhesive maintains contact with the wound via the surface tension created by the fluid layer of the wound. This type of product has been reported to promote wound healing without toxic effects to the underlying tissue[17]. Wrinkling of the film during placement creates a conduit for bacterial penetration and for leakage of wound exudative fluid. It is recommended that the film be placed over the wound with a complete 2–3 cm adhesion margin to prevent this leakage.

Another disadvantage of film dressings is that they are non-absorbent; therefore, wound fluid can accumulate under the dressing layer, especially with highly exudative wounds. This is often the case in the first 7–10 days after the creation of the wound. Exudate accumulation does not adversely affect wound healing; in fact, in a study by Buchan et al.[18] it was shown to have significant bactericidal activity. This aside, fluid could leak out, necessitating frequent changing of the dressing for comfort and appearance sake. The adherent characteristic of film dressings makes frequent changing less desirable, especially for certain types of wounds. A 27- or 30-gauge needle can be used to puncture the film for the purpose of aspirating the exudate, followed by placement of another piece of the same film to reseal the wound site. Another method employs the placement of butterfly tubing as a drain under the film dressing, with the needle inserted into a vacutainer for aspiration.

Numerous studies regarding the proliferation of bacteria under occlusive dressings have documented significant increases in bacterial growth. In such studies, significant increases in bacterial populations, with a shift toward Gram-negative organisms, have been noted and documented[19]. The elevated bacterial counts, however, have not correlated with an increased rate of infection.

Polymer Foams

Polymer foam dressings are semi-occlusive, bilaminate, and polyurethane- or silicone-based. They consist of a hydrophilic foam with a hydrophobic backing, which then prevents leakage, provides a barrier against bacterial penetration, and provides the moist environment afforded by films but with the addition of some absorbency (Fig. 145.6). The inner layer is composed of an absorbent, gas-permeable polyurethane foam mesh, which lies adjacent to the wound. The outer layer is a semipermeable, non-absorbent membrane composed of polyurethane, polyester, silicone or Gore-Tex®, surrounded by a polyoxyethylene glycol foam. This layer protects against outside bacterial contamination to some extent and against the drying out of the underlying layers.

Foam dressings are typically non-adherent, thereby requiring secondary dressing layers to ensure secure placement with a good seal. The quality of the seal is important to prevent leakage, desiccation and problems with adherence. There are, however, some foams available with an adhesive surface, usually surrounding a central absorptive core. Ideally, once a foam dressing has absorbed some amount of exudate, it should be able to retain that fluid, even if exposed to pressure. Some brands are described as having that quality.

Uses

They have been used for: wounds from Mohs surgery, surgical incisions, dermabrasion and burns; chronic wounds such as diabetic ulcers, venous ulcers and pressure ulcers (stages I, II and III); and deep cavity wounds refractory to other methods[20]. They have also gained popularity

for use after laser resurfacing, as they greatly reduce postprocedure discomfort and simplify wound care.

Examples

Adherent and non-adherent: Allevyn™ (Smith & Nephew); Biatain™ (Coloplast); Curafoam™ and Hydrosorb® (Kendall); Flexzan® (Bertek); Lyofoam® (Convatec); Reston™ (3M); and Sof-Foam™ (Johnson & Johnson).

Advantages/disadvantages

Although very absorbent, there is a limit to the amount of wound exudate this type of dressing can absorb. Therefore, it should be changed every 1–3 days. The permeability of foams to both gas and water vapor makes them suitable for mild to moderately exudative wounds, although there are brands designed for heavily exudative wounds.

Silicone-based rubber foams, known as silastic foams, are composed of a silicone mixture to which a stannous octoate catalyst has been added. This type molds and contours to the shape of the wound and therefore can be used for packing cavities or deep ulcers such as pilonidal sinuses. The additional advantages are absorbency, non-adherence, increased comfort for the patient, a tendency to be less expensive, and dressing changes that do not generally require skilled nursing care[21].

The disadvantages of foam dressings are the inability to use them with dry wounds, their opacity, which prevents visual monitoring of the wound, and the need for frequent changing, perhaps as often as every day. Infrequent changing could risk incorporation of the dressing material into the wound itself. There is also the possibility of an undesirable drying effect of the wound if drainage is insufficient to maintain a moist environment.

Hydrogels

As their name implies, hydrogels are composed primarily of water – up to 96%. This dressing type consists of a cross-linked hydrophilic polymer network composed of polyvinyl alcohol, polyacrylamides, polyethylene oxide or polyvinyl pyrrolidone; it is produced as sheets, amorphous gels (pre-mixed or dry), or as impregnated dressings (Fig. 145.7). Hydrogels are semitransparent (allowing visual inspection of the wound), have a high absorptive capacity (between 100% and 200% of their volume), and are able to maintain a moist wound environment. However, this absorptive action is delayed in its onset and increases slowly as it provides for continuous, long-term absorption. Hydrogels are described as semi-adherent or completely non-adherent, depending upon the subtype, and therefore require a secondary dressing to hold them in place[22]. The latter is necessary as hydrogels are poor bacterial barriers and selectively permit Gram-negative organisms to proliferate. For this reason, antibiotic ointment is often applied prior to the application of the dressing[23]. Hydrogels are soothing and actually lower the temperature of cutaneous wounds, a cooling effect that can be augmented by refrigerating the dressing prior to application.

In general, the sheet form of a hydrogel dressing is constructed by sandwiching the hydrophilic polymer between two removable thin sheets of polyethylene film, with some types containing a supportive inner gel mesh. For application to the wound, the film on the contact side is removed, leaving the outer film in place. With this mode of

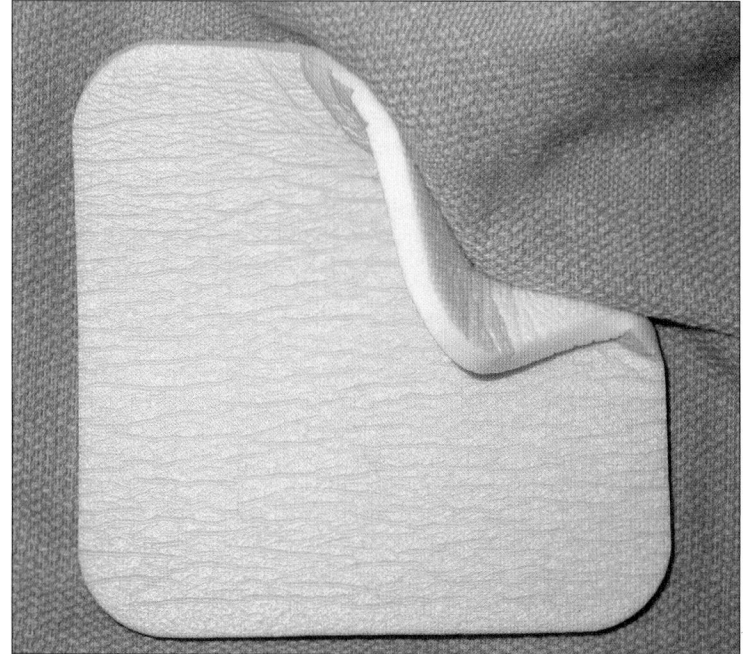

Fig. 145.6 Example of a polymer foam.

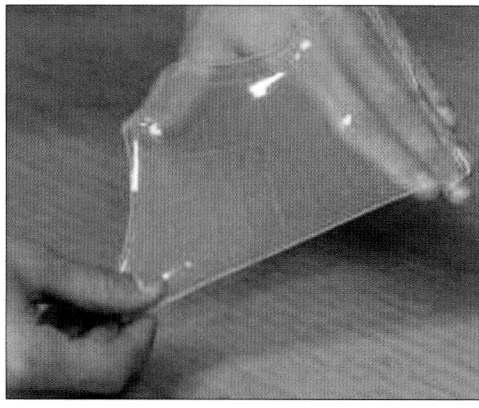

Fig. 145.7 Example of a hydrogel sheet.

application, the dressing is semipermeable to gases (including oxygen) and water vapor. If the outer film is also removed, then the dressing becomes permeable to fluid as well; as a result, exudate can pass to a secondary gauze dressing. The polymer sheets can be removed easily without trauma to the wound bed. The amorphous hydrogel form is a cornstarch-derived polymerized compound that forms a gel upon hydration at the time of use. It is available commercially in a powdered or pre-mixed form, is applied wet to the wound defect, requires a secondary outer dressing and requires water application to the surface for removal.

Uses

Hydrogels are particularly useful with dermabrasion, laser resurfacing, chemical peels, superficial thermal burns, ulcers, surgical wounds such as graft donor sites, and partial-thickness wounds in which an interval of light to moderate exudate production is likely. They are also quite helpful in the prevention of pressure ulcers.

Examples

Hydrogel sheets: CarraDres™ Clear Hydrogel Sheet, CarraSorb™ Freeze Dried Gel (Carrington Labs); Nu-Gel™ (Johnson & Johnson); and Vigilon™ (Bard Medical).

Amorphous gels: Biolex® Wound Gel (Bard); CarraSyn™ Hydrogel (Carrington); GRX Wound Gel (Geritrex Corp.); Intrasite™ Gel (Smith & Nephew); and Tegagel™ Hydrogel Wound Filler (3M Health Care).

Impregnated dressings: DermaGauze™ (DermaRite) and Tegagel™ Wound Filler with gauze (3M Health Care).

Advantages/disadvantages

One significant advantage to hydrogel dressings is a reduction in postoperative pain and inflammation. Another is that hydrogels have been shown to accelerate the rate of wound healing when compared to traditional Telfa® and gauze dressings. For example, Geronemus & Robins[24] found an average 25–45% faster rate of re-epithelialization of split-thickness wounds in pig skin. They reported that 100% of hydrogel-treated wounds were healed by postoperative day 4 compared with 32% of open air control wounds. Hydrogels have also been credited with faster healing rates in studies of dermabrasion and hair transplant donor and recipient sites when compared to standard Telfa® and Adaptic™ dressings[25].

One potential disadvantage is that hydrogels allow bacterial growth at the wound site. However, as with other types of occlusive dressings, studies have not shown an increase in infection rate. The absorptive quality along with the semi- or non-adherent nature of hydrogels often results in more frequent dressing changes than is seen with other occlusive dressings.

Alginates

Alginate dressings are made from a natural, complex polysaccharide derived from various types of algae or kelp (seaweed). An extraction process produces a sodium salt form of alginic acid, and during a second step, sodium ions are exchanged for calcium, zinc and magnesium. The end result is an alginate fiber, and non-woven mats or twists of this fiber are then made into a dressing (Fig 145.8). Upon application of the dressing, a reverse ion exchange occurs between the calcium within the alginate fibers and the sodium from blood or the wound exudate. This results in the formation of a soluble sodium alginate gel that fills and completely covers the wound in a non-adherent manner, providing a moist wound healing environment. The extent and rate of gel formation depends on the amount of wound exudate. Alginate dressing materials have hemostatic properties, believed to be the result of the release of free calcium by the fibers during the ion exchange. This release of calcium augments the clotting cascade, producing the hemostatic advantage.

Alginate gel dressings are highly absorbent, which allows them to remain in place at the wound site for several days at a time, thereby minimizing dressing changes. To secure an alginate dressing, a secondary dressing is required. A dressing change is indicated when the dressing has been in place for several days or when exudate soaks through to the secondary dressing[26]. Removal of the dressing in a dried state can re-injure the wound.

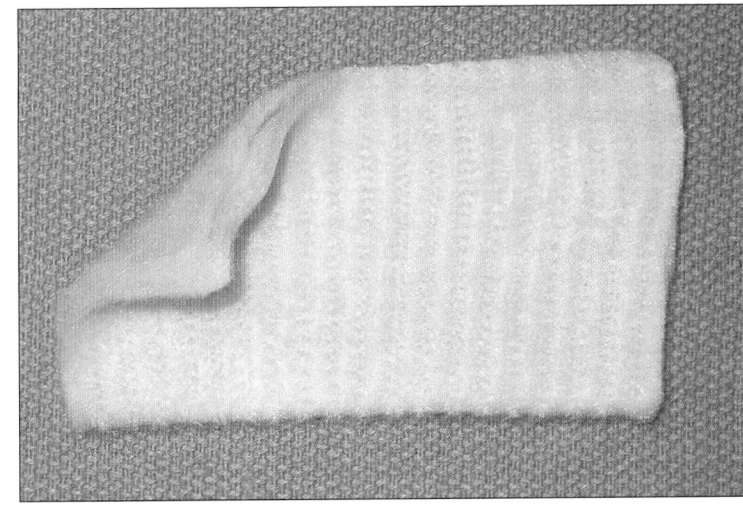

Fig. 145.8 Example of an alginate.

Uses

As alginates are transformed into a gel matrix by wound fluid, they are best employed for highly exudative wounds. Full-thickness burns and surgical wounds, split-thickness graft donor sites, Mohs surgery defects, and refractory decubiti and chronic ulcers may benefit from alginate dressing application. Alginates can reportedly be used on dry wounds as well, but pre-application moistening with saline is necessary and the dressing should be changed on a daily basis to limit desiccation.

Examples

Algiderm® (Bard Medical); AlgiSite™ (Smith & Nephew United); Fibracol® Plus, a collagen–alginate complex dressing (Johnson & Johnson); Kaltostat® (ConvaTec); and Sorbsan® (Bertek).

Advantages/disadvantages

Alginate dressings are soluble and can be removed by saline irrigation, which allows for less painful dressing changes. They have been shown to encourage wound healing and are metabolized by the body, should residual material remain at the wound. Concerns about the potential toxicity of alginates have been met with over 40 years of their use and no commonly reported complications. One disadvantage of alginates is that the gel has a yellow–brown appearance, which can be confused with purulent discharge. Therefore, careful wound monitoring for signs of infection is indicated. Similar to hydrocolloids, alginate gel may have an unpleasant odor associated with its normal use, so patients should be made aware of this feature. Additionally, removal of the secondary outer dressing is necessary to visually inspect the wound and to monitor for desiccation.

Hydrocolloids

Colloid is a Greek term for a two-phase system comprised of a uniform dispersion of one phase of matter (unfilterable small particles) into another phase of matter or matrix. Mutually attractive charges exist between the particles, which contributes to the diffusible properties of colloids. Colloids are characterized by the strength of attraction of the particles to the continuous medium and to the proportion of water within that medium. This property accounts for the absorptive and expansive capacity of colloid gels, which function as a semipermeable membrane. Gel swelling occurs because the particle concentration of the gel is usually higher than that of the surrounding medium, thereby drawing water from the surroundings into the gel.

Since cells and tissues throughout the body are comprised of colloids, it seems reasonable that the creation of an environment similar to that found on cell surfaces would aid in the healing process. Colloid dressings are available in more than one usable form, and they were first used as ostomy products. Chronic ulcers and fissures around ostomy sites were found to heal rapidly when they were bandaged with hydrocolloid products, so these materials were quickly adapted for use as wound dressings.

The most commonly used hydrocolloid dressings (e.g. DuoDERM®) are available as sheets with an inner adhesive layer consisting of a hydrophilic colloid base that is a mixture of pectin, karaya, guar or carboxymethyl cellulose and an adhesive containing polyisobutylene, styrene isoprene or ethylene vinyl acetate (Fig. 145.9). The outer layer is composed of a thin semipermeable material such as polyurethane. A gel is formed in the presence of wound exudate, and as a unit, the dressing is semipermeable to water vapor and gases[27].

Another type of hydrocolloid dressing is a synthetic, non-adherent, high-density plastic woven polymer (e.g. N-Terface®). Fluid is able to flow through this matrix to be absorbed by an overlying dressing without adherence to the new epithelial surface.

Uses

Hydrocolloids are used for the treatment of burns, partial-thickness and dermabrasion wounds, traumatic wounds such as lacerations and abrasions, surgical wounds such as donor graft sites and excisions, chronic ulcers, bullous disorders such as epidermolysis bullosa, and refractory inflammatory diseases such as lichen simplex chronicus and psoriasis.

Examples

Polymer blend: DuoDERM® (Convatec); N-Terface® (Winfield Labs); Tielle™ (Johnson & Johnson); and Sorbex® (Bard Medical).
Cadexomer-iodine beads: Iodosorb® (Smith & Nephew).

Advantages/disadvantages

When in sheet form, these dressings can be cut and conformed to the shape of the wound. They also adhere directly, are waterproof, and therefore do not require a secondary dressing. They also have a cushioning or pressure-relieving effect (especially at bony sites), which increases as the dressing absorbs exudate. The resulting colloidal gel that forms prevents the dressing from adhering to the wound base. Accumulation of the exudate itself in a moist, semipermeable environment becomes a source of phagocytic cells and endogenous enzymes. This feature, along with the gel, results in autolytic debridement that can be washed away with saline irrigation of the wound bed[28].

Due to their semipermeable outer barrier, hydrocolloids have also been shown to stimulate angiogenesis and increase the rate of healing by as much as 40% when compared to open air controls. A comparison of hydrocolloids versus wet-to-dry saline gauze dressings in the treatment of decubiti ulcers found that hydrocolloids do not require as many dressing changes as traditional wound dressings. Although the cost of individual hydrocolloid dressings is greater than gauze dressings and the healing rates were the same, the savings were in the cost of nursing time. In addition, the changes tend to be simple and painless for the patient[29].

One disadvantage of hydrocolloids is that as an occlusive dressing, maceration of the wound's surrounding skin is possible. Leakage of excessive tissue exudate can also occur, resulting in soiling of outer garments and bedding. In addition, there is the possibility of the growth of excessive granulation tissue, the extension of which into a woven matrix (as is found in N-Terface®) could result in trauma to the wound upon attempted removal of the dressing. Similar to alginate dressings, the end product of hydrocolloids is a yellow–brown, thick, foul-smelling gel resembling purulent discharge. As with other occlusive dressings, hydrocolloids are subject to similar bacterial proliferation and colonization within the moist environment underneath the dressing, but have not shown increased rates of infection as a result. Some investigators, in fact, have reported a decrease in the growth of *Pseudomonas*[19].

Composites

The designs of occlusive dressings are constantly changing, with the goal of improved and simplified care for a greater range of wounds. Several new types of composite dressings, which combine two or more types of semi-occlusive dressings into one product, are commercially available. They have three components: (1) a semi- or non-adherent layer that contacts the wound (like a hydrogel, hydrocolloid, foam or alginate); (2) an absorptive layer; and (3) an outer layer (like a film with an adhesive border). This maximizes the efficiency and comfort of the dressing by expanding absorbency as well as lessening the chance of maceration[30]. Other features include the lack of need for secondary retention dressings and better waterproof coverings, which enable the patient to shower or bathe.

DRESSINGS FOR LEG ULCERS

The predominant types of skin ulcers that affect the lower extremity are venous, arterial and neuropathic; less commonly, they are due to inflammation, infection, trauma or malignancy (see Ch. 105). Leg ulcers precipitated by venous disease are by far the most common, causing up to 80% of cases. Moisture retention at the ulcer site is often best accomplished with occlusive dressings. The five major categories of occlusive dressings are simplified in Figure 145.10. Only a few comparative studies of dressings have been conducted, and no particular category has been proven conclusively to enhance rates of healing of acute surgical wounds or chronic ulcers[21,31]. Therefore, the choice of

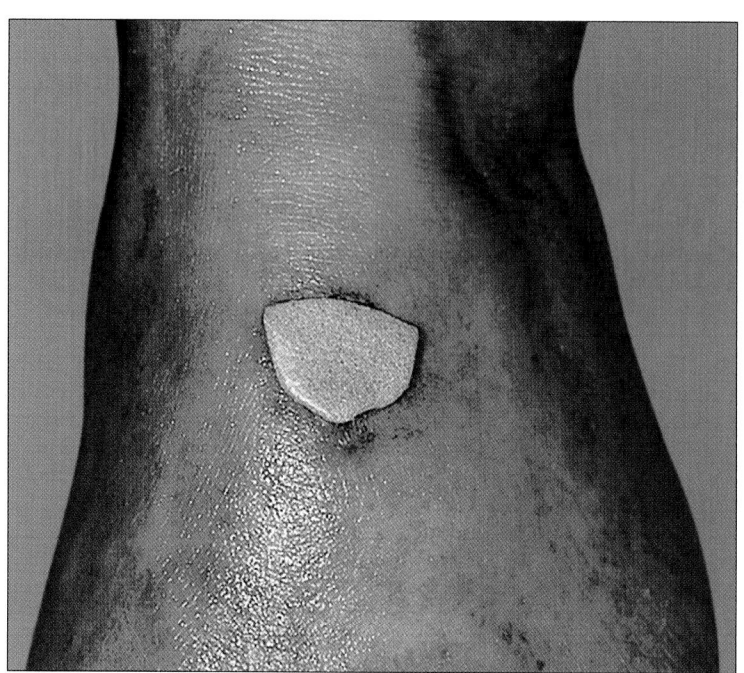

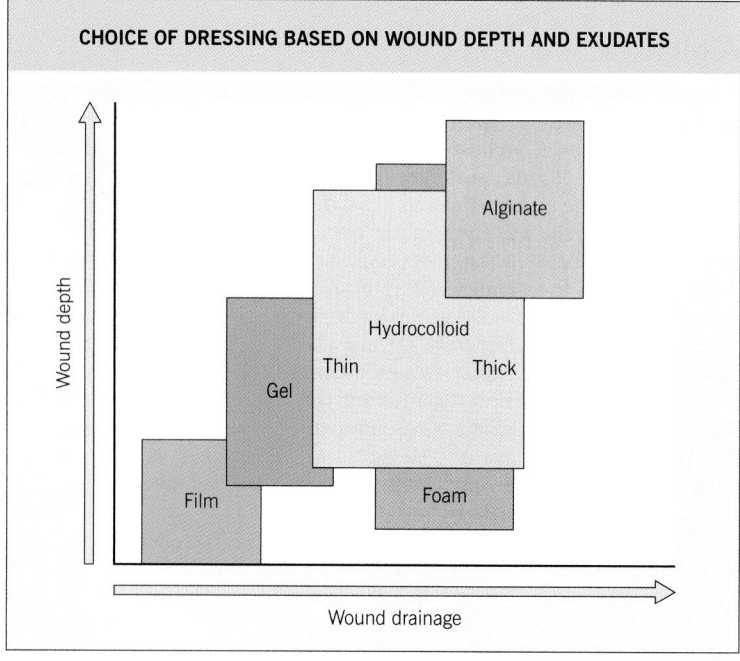

CHOICE OF DRESSING BASED ON WOUND DEPTH AND EXUDATES

Wound depth

Alginate

Hydrocolloid

Thin   Thick

Gel

Film

Foam

Wound drainage

Fig. 145.9 Hydrocolloid wound dressing (DuoDERM®) placed over a healing wound on the foot.

Fig. 145.10 Choice of dressing based on wound depth and exudates.

a moisture-retaining dressing can be left to the preference of the physician and patient.

Compression is considered to be of utmost importance in the care of venous ulcers. It alleviates edema by increasing hydrostatic pressure and decreasing the pressure of surface veins, thereby decreasing macromolecule and fluid extravasation. Compression is also said to promote fibrinolysis and ultimately improve cutaneous blood flow once edema has been mechanically reduced. Studies by Fletcher et al.[32] concluded not only that compression increased healing rates, but that high compression was better than low, and that compression without a moist dressing yielded better results than did a moist dressing without compression.

Types of Compression Dressings

Compression can be accomplished by dressings that range from adhesive, relatively non-absorbent types to those which are moderately compressive and absorbent. Traditionally, compression or 'pressure dressings' are comprised of a non-adherent contact layer, followed by an absorbent layer, and then an outer layer. The efficacy and benefit of the dressing depends upon the role of each of these layers. Although the definitive optimal pressure required to prevent the capillary leakage that occurs with venous hypertension has not been delineated, the general recommendation for leg ulcers is to achieve an ankle pressure of 30–40 mmHg[33].

Compression Stockings

With compression stockings, the patient is afforded some independence in the application of the device, if he or she is physically capable. However, for arthritic and/or elderly patients, application can be difficult. Some stockings are fashioned with silk inner linings or zippers for easier use.

Compression Bandages

The Unna boot has existed for over 100 years. Created for the treatment of venous stasis ulcers and for some use in selected eczematous dermatoses by Paul Gerson Unna during the 1880s, it was originally a cotton bandage impregnated with zinc oxide, gelatin and glycerin paste. It has a history of being the preferred dressing for this type of wound[34]. Applied in a semi-rigid state, it confers (semi-rigid) compression along with the advantages of a moisture-retaining occlusive dressing. It should be applied by a qualified medical professional and changed once a week unless heavy drainage from the wound necessitates more frequent replacement. Correct application of the Unna boot prevents excessive or abnormal pressure to the limb, compromised circulation, skin breakdown, additional ulcer formation or further limb deterioration[35]. In one study, healing time for ulcers treated with Unna boots alone was less than half the time required to heal ulcers treated with only support stockings[36]. Combining compression with occlusive dressings also increased the healing rate of venous ulcers[37].

The use of a flexible compression bandage has the advantage of increased absorbency and compression maintenance as compared to the rigidity of the Unna boot. There is a vast commercially available selection of elasticity gradations and brands. They are categorized as elastic or inelastic, single- or multilayer, long- or short-stretch compression, and cohesive wrap. The greatest difficulty in using elastic compression is determining the proper amount of tension needed to safely and effectively achieve the desired goal. One manufacturer's attempt to help resolve this problem was made by marking the bandage with a drawing that changes as the bandage is stretched to the proper tension during application. However, it is generally thought that multilayered compression bandaging is superior to single-layered techniques.

Multilayer Compression Bandages

The components of this system often are four distinct layers, the first of which is an orthopedic wool layer applied loosely in spiral fashion. It absorbs exudate as well as redistributes pressure around the ankle. The second layer is a crepe bandage, used to smooth the wool layer and to increase absorbency. The third layer is a light elastic compression bandage, followed by the fourth and last layer, which is the outer, elastic, cohesive bandage used to secure all layers in place. The four-layered system can remain in place for up to 1 week and has the advantage of providing absorption as well as evenly distributed pressure throughout the leg. Multilayered compression systems are available commercially in complete kits[38].

Examples

Compression stockings: Jobst: Fast-Fit® Relief, Support Plus, UlcerCare®, and Futuro® (Beiersdorf).

Unna boot: Gelocast® (Beiersdorf-Jobst); Primer Modified Unna Boot (Glenwood, Inc.); Tenderwrap Unna Boot Bandage (Kendall); and UNNA-FLEX® Elastic Unna Boot (Convatec).

Single layer: CircAid, CircAid Thera Boot (CircAid Medical); SurePress® High Compression Bandage (Convatec).

Multilayer: DYNA-FLEX™ Multi-Layer Compression System (Johnson & Johnson Medical); Profore™ (Smith & Nephew).

Cohesive wrap: FLEX-WRAP™ Self Adherent Wrap (Kendall); 3M Coban™ Self Adherent Wrap (3M Health Care).

Types of Paste Dressings

Medicated paste bandages are used underneath graduated compression dressings, but are not designed to confer compression themselves. They are used to treat the chronic dermatitis associated with leg ulcers, by creating an absorptive, protective, contact layer against the wound surface and surrounding skin. These open-weave, cotton bandages are impregnated with zinc paste, calamine or ichthammol, all of which have a soothing action on irritated skin; coal tar, which has an anti-inflammatory effect; or clioquinol, which has deodorizing and anti-bacterial actions (plus some type of preservative). There are also commercially available zinc oxide/preservative-free formulas and combinations of zinc oxide with each of the above components and calamine–clioquinol varieties.

The skin of leg ulcer patients is often easily sensitized to topical medications. Therefore, it becomes important in such patients to perform patch testing prior to bandaging if sensitization is suspected. The bandage can be applied in short strips or in a loose fashion from the base of the toes upward to just below the knee, and may be left in place undisturbed for up to 2 weeks. When used appropriately, this type of dressing can be quite helpful in the management of leg ulcers.

Examples

Calaband®, Ichthaband®, Quinaband®, Steripaste®, Tarband®, Zincaband® (Seton); Viscopaste™ PB7 (Smith & Nephew).

Growth Factors, Heat and Enzymes

It is known that exudate from acute cutaneous wounds contains many endogenous factors that are critical to the wound healing process, including growth factors such as platelet-derived growth factor (PDGF) and epidermal growth factor (EGF). As a result, retaining this fluid over wounds, as is accomplished by the use of occlusive dressings, has been shown to augment wound healing. The potential therapeutic use of exogenous growth factors to enhance healing is reviewed in Chapter 141. The use of infrared energy[39] and radiant heat bandages[40] has been effective in the laboratory as well as in small trials in healing leg ulcers which are refractory to other methods and in ulcers of different etiologies. The value of these therapies could be determined through further study.

Enzyme agents

With the possible exception of ulcers due to pyoderma gangrenosum, the practice of wound debridement is commonly accepted as the standard of care for leg ulcers. Although there is no solid scientific evidence for the benefit of this procedure, it is thought to permit the adequate development of granulation tissue and epithelialization. Debridement can be accomplished by the following mechanisms: surgically; mechanically via irrigation, wet-to-dry dressings or the use of dextranomers; autolytically via compression bandaging and the use of occlusive dressings such as hydrocolloids and alginates; chemically via proteolytic enzymes; and biosurgically via leeches and maggots[41].

As mentioned, a moist wound environment promotes the lytic activity of enzymes that clear residual debris during early wound healing. Topical application of the commercially available enzymatic agents, collagenase, papain and trypsin, can be used to supplement this autolytic activity. Collagenase (Santyl®) is reported to be effective in the removal of devitalized tissue and to contribute to the formation of granulation tissue and ulcer epithelialization, without attacking healthy or new granulation tissue. Papain (e.g. Accuzyme®, Panafil®) is harmless to viable tissue, while functioning as a potent digestive agent to non-viable tissue. Its action, however, requires the presence of an activator such as urea with which it is processed, since papain alone is relatively ineffective; some formulations also contain Chlorophyllin Copper Complex Sodium, which adds to the healing action. Trypsin (e.g. Granulex®, Balsa-Derm®) is processed with balsam of Peru (which is an effective capillary bed stimulant and mild bactericide) and castor oil, which is used to reduce premature epithelial desiccation and cornification, as well as pain.

Fly larvae (order Diptera) have been used for centuries to biosurgically debride chronic ulcers. Today, the most commonly used maggots are those of the green bottle fly *Lucilia sericata*. These maggots only digest necrotic tissue, leaving healthy tissue exposed. This digestion is accomplished though collagenases and trypsin-like enzymes with minimal destruction of normal tissue. They also have antimicrobial effects via secretion of antibacterial compounds (e.g. phenylacetic acid, phenylacetaldehyde) and the ingestion and subsequent killing of Gram-positive (including MRSA) and, to a lesser extent, Gram-negative bacteria. In a small clinical trial, larval therapy was superior to hydrogel therapy with regard to cost-effectiveness and superior wound healing ability[42].

Tissue-Engineered Skin Equivalents

Advances in tissue culture techniques for keratinocytes and fibroblasts, as well as new methods that allow the generation of large quantities of these cells, are rapidly being incorporated into a new group of wound dressings that blur the distinction between wound dressing and tissue-engineered skin (Table 145.3). For chronic ulcers that are resistant to healing, skin equivalents can be used. One advantage is that painful, often slow-to-heal donor sites do not have to be created. These previously unresponsive wounds undergo an 'edge effect', where the skin equivalents promote epithelialization from the edge of the ulcer toward its center, likely due to release of cytokines by the donor cells that stimulate healing[43]. There are three types of skin substitutes: epidermal grafts, dermal replacements, and composite grafts (with both an epidermal and dermal component).

Epidermal grafts

The first epidermal autografts were successfully cultivated in 1975 by Rheinwald and Green. They have been used successfully in a variety of clinical situations, including burns, chronic ulcers, vitiligo and post-surgical wounds. Only one product is currently commercially available in the US: Epicel® (Genzyme Biosurgery). A skin biopsy is first obtained from the patient and then the autologous keratinocytes are co-cultured with irradiated murine fibroblasts that serve as a feeder layer. A sheet of keratinocytes two to eight cells thick forms and is attached to petroleum gauze. The graft must be sutured into place and the gauze backing is removed after 1 week, when the keratinocytes have attached to the wound. Biopsies of skin obtained 6 months to 1 year post grafting show anchoring fibrils and neovascularization. This epidermal autograft is approved for use in partial- and full-thickness burns as well as following removal of congenital melanocytic nevi.

There are several studies demonstrating the efficacy of cultured epidermal autografts. For example, in a review of 30 patients with burns averaging 78% of the body surface area, 69% of the grafts had permanently adhered to the patients[44]. The advantages of this type of graft are the use of autologous keratinocytes and the ability to minimize the amount of tissue harvesting. Epidermal grafts must be placed onto clean wound beds, and the primary disadvantages are the short shelf-life, the expense, and the 3-week interval required for the culture of the keratinocytes.

TISSUE-ENGINEERED SKIN EQUIVALENTS			
Name and description	Use	Advantages	Disadvantages
Epidermal – autologous			
Epicel® – sheet of cultured keratinocytes (derived from a skin biopsy) attached to petrolatum gauze Laserskin® – esterified hyaluronic acid (laser-perforated) and seeded with keratinocytes	Partial- and full-thickness burns Congenital melanocytic nevus excision sites Pyoderma gangrenosum (non-inflammatory; see Ch. 27) Epidermolysis bullosa Chronic ulcers	Capable of self-repair Single application is often sufficient Permanent and cosmetically acceptable Good adherence Covers a large surface area from a small skin biopsy	Very expensive Minimal shelf-life; must be used soon after delivery from manufacturer Needs biopsy of normal skin Available 3 weeks after biopsy Technically difficult to apply Susceptible to infection
Dermal			
Xenogenic (see Table 145.4) Biobrane®, E-Z Derm™ – acellular porcine collagen type I Oasis® – porcine intestinal collagen type 1 and extracellular matrix (Fig. 145.11) Integra™ – bovine tendon collagen and shark chondroitin	Burns Split-thickness donor sites Post-laser resurfacing Chronic ulcers	Translucent Elastic Minimal exudate accumulation Reduces pain of some wounds Long shelf-life Non-human origin avoids human pathogen transmission Immediately available	May adhere to wound strongly enough to damage new epithelium May have higher infection rate Expensive Possible bovine allergy Usually needs multiple applications
Allogenic (see Table 145.4) Alloderm® – cadaveric decellularized dermis Transcyte™ – neonatal foreskin fibroblasts grown on Biobrane (see above) Dermagraft™ – neonatal foreskin fibroblasts grown on a biodegradable mesh	Burns and split-thickness skin graft sites Chronic ulcers Epidermolysis bullosa	Decreased pain Immediate availability Immunologically inert Easy to remove	Theoretical risk of transmission of human pathogens Usually needs multiple applications
Composite – xenogenic & allogenic			
Apligraf®, OrCel® – neonatal foreskin keratinocytes and fibroblasts plus bovine collagen type I; bilayered	Chronic ulcers Wounds resistant to healing Burns Epidermolysis bullosa	Capable of self-repair Single application is often sufficient Immediately available	Very expensive Minimal shelf-life; must be used soon after delivery from manufacturer

Table 145.3 Tissue-engineered skin equivalents.

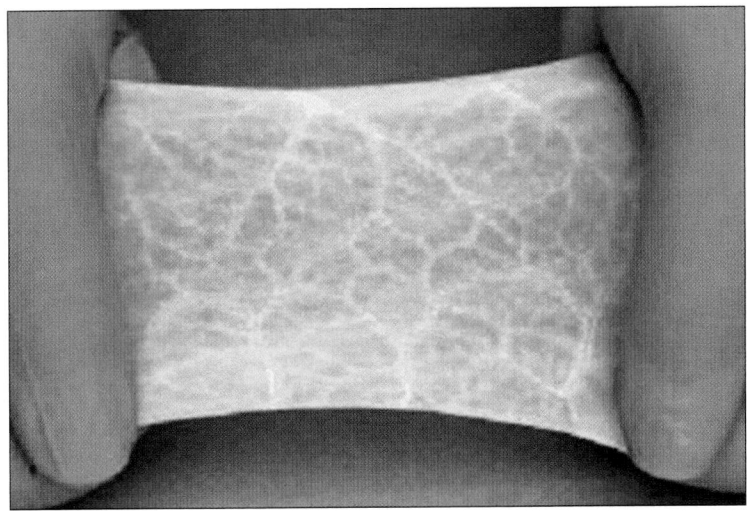

Fig. 145.11 Example of a xenogenic wound matrix derived from porcine small intestine submucosa (Oasis®).

to as 'HYAFF') and is also available without keratinocytes (Hyalofil®) for use as a primary dressing for wounds such as ulcers[46].

Celaderm™ (Celedon Science) is composed of allogenic keratinocytes cultured from neonatal foreskins. It has a much longer shelf-life, but, as an allogenic rather than autologous graft, it is not permanent. The graft is placed on the wound every other week until it heals; pain relief occurs and stimulation of epithelialization is observed. Although clinical trials of both Laserskin® and Celaderm™ are limited, improved healing of diabetic foot ulcers and venous stasis ulcers was noted when compared to saline gauze[47]. They are also used for partial- and full-thickness burns.

Dermal replacements

There are two types of dermal replacements: allogenic and xenogenic (see Table 145.3). Neither of these is permanent: DNA analysis of wounds after the application of non-autologous skin substitutes shows complete disappearance of grafted cells after 2 months[48]. The goal of these dermal grafts is to provide a temporary biologic dressing in order to stimulate the healing process. They are placed over the wound, extending slightly onto normal skin, and then bolstered into place. Secondary dressings must be applied. The major component of dermal replacements is collagen, and occasionally there are additions such as extracellular matrix (including glycosaminoglycans), fibroblasts and basement membrane material.

Xenogenic (Fig 145.11)

Details of the xenogenic dermal replacements are outlined in Table 145.4. The advantages of these products are their ability to affect hemostasis and to provide immediate closure, cosmetically acceptable scars with

There are additional epidermal grafts available outside of the US, such as Laserskin® and Celaderm™. Laserskin® (Fidia Advanced Biopolymers) is another cultured autologous keratinocyte sheet requiring an initial small skin biopsy, but the sheet is attached onto a hyaluronic membrane with laser-drilled microperforations to allow keratinocytes to migrate onto the wound bed[45]. This hyaluronic membrane is a biodegradable biopolymer of esterified hyaluronic acid (referred

DERMAL REPLACEMENT GRAFTS		
	Description	**Comments**
Xenogenic		
Biobrane® (Bertek Pharmaceuticals)	Bilayer dressing: inner nylon mesh fabric coated with porcine type I collagen ('dermis') bonded to a semipermeable silicone film membrane ('epidermis')	Tissue ingrowth into the nylon fabric following binding of collagen to fibrin[49] Two versions: (1) trilaminar nylon (better for clean, partial-thickness burn wounds or donor sites); and (2) monofilament nylon (better for meshed autografts)
E-Z Derm™ (Brennen Medical)	Porcine-derived type I collagen attached to a gauze liner	Gauze liner is discarded upon placement[50]
Oasis® (Healthpoint)	Derived from porcine small intestine submucosa (mucosa and muscle removed) Porcine type I collagen, extracellular matrix (e.g. hyaluronic acid, fibronectin) and growth factors (FGF, TGF-β)	In study of 120 patients with venous leg ulcers, after 12 weeks of treatment, 55% of Oasis® + compression group healed vs 34% in compression alone group; at 6 months, 100% and 70% remained healed, respectively[51] Approved for venous, diabetic and pressure ulcers, and burns
Integra™ (Integra Life Science)	Bilayer dressing: bovine tendon collagen admixed with shark-derived, modified GAGs ('dermis') plus an outer silicone membrane	Debridement required prior to graft placement with sutures or staples Outer silicone cover removed after several weeks; in large wounds, replaced by ultrathin autograft (2-step process) In a controlled trial of matched-pair thermal injuries, as efficacious as other xenografts and synthetic skin substitutes[52] Approved for life-threatening third-degree burns
Allogenic		
Alloderm® (LifeCell)	Human cadaveric skin, chemically treated and purified to remove epidermis, all cellular components and pathogens Cryopreserved (shelf-life of 6 months)	Repopulation of host fibroblasts and endothelial cells seen within 10 days of grafting Treatment of burns and in combination with split-thickness superthin autografts[48]
Transcyte™ (Smith & Nephew)	Biobrane® (see above) plus neonatal foreskin fibroblasts	Approx. 2 weeks for graft take Fibroblasts initially secrete extracellular matrix (including collagen) and growth factors that stimulate granulation tissue and epithelialization but then die In a controlled trial of excised burns, easier to use and similar outcomes when compared to human cadaveric skin Approved for partial- and full-thickness burns
Dermagraft™ (Smith & Nephew) (formerly Transcyte TC™)	Neonatal foreskin fibroblasts are seeded onto a 3-D scaffold of biodegradable polyglactin mesh	Similar time to graft take and similar fibroblast function as Transcyte™ (see above) In 235 patients with diabetic ulcers, improved but not significant difference in healing time compared to conventional therapy Approved for diabetic foot ulcers and epidermolysis bullosa[53]

Table 145.4 Dermal replacement grafts. 3-D, three-dimensional; FGF, fibroblast growth factor; GAGs, glycosaminoglycans; TGF-β, transforming growth factor-β.

second intention healing, safety from potential human pathogen transmission due to their animal origin, and adequate shelf-life, facilitating off-the-shelf access. Biobrane® has significant elasticity, enabling a full range of motion to the covered body part, and has no requirement for dressing changes once it adheres to the wound bed.

The drawbacks are that these dressings need to remain dry and a pressure dressing is often needed to keep the graft in place. They are all ineffective over exposed bone, and because healing time is slower compared to sutured repairs, there is the potential for infection if not cared for adequately. Bovine allergy is also a possibility. Biobrane® may adhere to the wound so tightly that it could damage newly developed epithelium and inhibit wound contraction[54]. Because Integra™ has a complicated application procedure, the FDA requires that all physicians complete a company-sponsored training program.

Allogenic

Details of the allogenic dermal replacements are outlined in Table 145.4. The advantages of these products are their ability to provide immediate closure, cosmetically acceptable scars with second intention healing, and adequate shelf-life, facilitating off-the-shelf access.

Composite grafts

Apligraf® (Organogenesis) is a bilayered human skin equivalent derived from human neonatal foreskins (Fig 145.12). It contains living human keratinocytes within an epidermal layer and a dermal layer equivalent consisting of bovine collagen type I gel seeded with fibroblasts. This composite graft produces its own matrix proteins and growth factors, and if wounded, it can repair itself. Apligraf® has been used to treat both acute and chronic wounds that fail to heal by standard means. Whereas several applications of the material may be required to completely heal chronic wounds, a single application may be sufficient to initiate a satisfactory healing response. Chronic venous ulcers that were randomized to receive compression plus Apligraf® healed in a shorter time period compared to compression alone, especially in the case of larger defects[55]. It is currently approved by the Food and Drug Administration (FDA) for venous and diabetic ulcers, but has also been shown to be useful in epidermolysis bullosa, pyoderma gangrenosum, burns and surgical excisions.

OrCel® (Ortec International) is a similar bilayered skin equivalent. It is composed of neonatal foreskin-derived keratinocytes grown on the non-porous side of a cross-linked bovine collagen I sponge. On the other, porous side of this sponge are human dermal fibroblasts that also produce multiple matrix proteins and growth factors. As with all of the allogenic and xenogenic grafts, this is not a permanent skin replace-

ment, and DNA from the cultured cells is not detectable 2 weeks post grafting. It is FDA-approved for the treatment of full- and partial-thickness donor sites as well as burns[48].

Each of these products is extremely expensive, at approximately US$1000 per graft. However, they have the advantage of mimicking the structure and function of normal human skin. Both products are used in the outpatient setting, and Apligraf® in particular has great safety data based upon its use in over 200 000 patients. Orcel® has the advantage of a 9-month shelf-life because it is cryopreserved, whereas Apligraf® has a shelf-life of only 5 days. Another disadvantage is the potential for disease transmission. Nevertheless, these composite grafts may be justified in certain situations when adequate skin grafts cannot be obtained from the patient.

SPECIAL CONSIDERATIONS

Laser Resurfacing

Laser skin resurfacing has emerged as a useful modality for conditions such as actinic skin damage, acne scarring and rhytides (see Ch. 137). The benefits, safety and reproducibility of this technique have increased its popularity, although it does require a prolonged and often painful recovery period for the patient. The primary goal after laser resurfacing is total and uniform re-epithelialization. In the absence of infection and with the use of occlusive dressings, this is possible within 5–7 days. Delay of re-epithelialization has been attributed to crust formation, to which the wound is most prone during the first 2–3 postoperative days.

Occlusive dressings may be classified as open or closed (Fig. 145.13). An open dressing is defined as the application of an ointment or cream directly to the skin wound without an overlying textile dressing. The choice of this more labor-intensive method requires the commitment of the patient to maintain adequate coverage of the wound by frequent, scheduled ointment reapplication and to be able to tolerate the soiling of bedding and garments during the healing period. However, an open

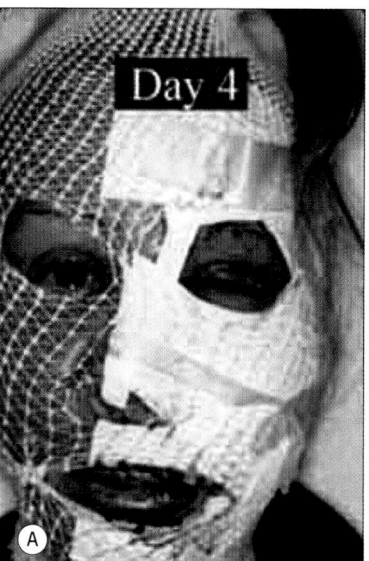
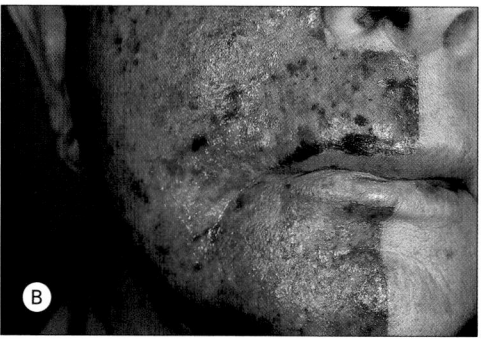

Fig. 145.13 **Occlusive dressings for post-laser resurfacing. A** In this side-by-side comparison, the patient's left face is dressed with a foam dressing. **B** In this side-by-side comparison, the patient's right face is dressed using the open technique.

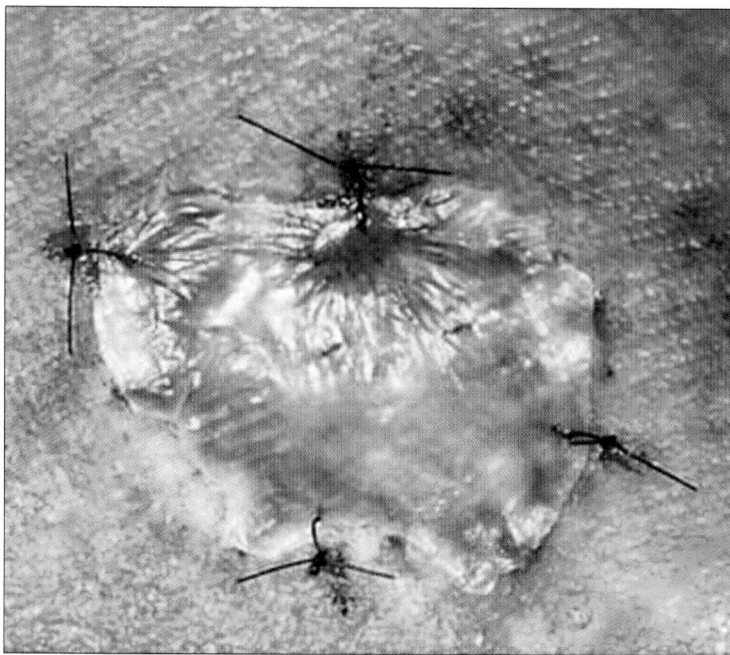

Fig. 145.12 **Example of a composite (xenogenic and allogenic) graft sutured into place (Apligraf®).**

dressing does result in less bacterial colonization than closed dressings, it allows for easy wound monitoring, and it is effective and less expensive than the closed wound care technique. Examples of products used for open dressings are: petrolatum, Aquaphor® (Beiersdorf-Jobst), Complex CU3® ointment (Procyte), and Elta® Crème (Swiss-America Products). Antibiotic ointment applied to facial wounds of less than 48 hours has been reported to significantly increase the rate of contact dermatitis and is therefore not recommended.

Closed dressings are found among any of four main occlusive dressing categories, and all have been produced specifically for post-laser skin resurfacing care. Weinstein et al.[56] examined the most commonly used post-laser resurfacing dressings to compare the clinical advantages and disadvantages of each. Samples from the composite foam (Flexzan®), hydrogel (2nd Skin®), polymer film (Silon-TSR®), and hydrocolloid categories (N-Terface®, Mepitel®) were reviewed.

Among their conclusions were that when compared to open dressing techniques, closed dressings overall resulted in faster re-epithelialization with improved patient comfort. In following their postoperative care protocol, they found that regular wound inspection within the first postoperative week was necessary in order to monitor for signs of infection, healing progress, and patient adherence to care instructions, regardless of the choice of occlusive dressing. The immediate placement of a closed dressing after surgery was followed by return of the patient on postoperative days 1 and 2, at which point the wound was cleaned and the entire dressing was changed. There was no perceptible delay or interference in re-epithelialization by changing the dressing at this point. The replacement dressing remained in place until postoperative day 5, at which time the closed dressing was removed and the patient was converted to open dressing alone[56].

Absorbency without saturation, placement stability, ease of use, patient comfort, and minimal adherence to the newly developing epithelium are the desirable characteristics of a closed dressing for laser resurfacing. Flexzan® is an open cell polyurethane foam with an adhesive coating that is applied in strips and does not need an absorptive secondary dressing. Patients appreciated the light maintenance it required. It is opaque; therefore careful removal with sufficient moistening is necessary for inspection of the wound.

The hydrogel 2nd Skin® was reported to decrease pain and pruritus, but maintaining the dressing in place was challenging. There was a preference for the use of this dressing in areas of prolonged re-epithelialization. Silon-TSR® and N-Terface® are thin, transparent polymer films with slits or mesh to allow passage of exudate into an overlying absorptive secondary dressing. They conformed well to facial contours and did not adhere to new epithelium, but did have the problem of slippage. Mepitel® is a silicone polymer with large pores to allow escape of exudate which is self-adhesive only to dry areas. It had all the benefits of passage of exudate into a secondary dressing without crust formation, stability without slipping from place, and easy removal from the moist wound. It is reported to leave behind an imprint of its mesh pattern on the healing skin, a side effect that fades within a few weeks once conversion to an open dressing has been made[56].

Oxygen mist therapy following CO_2 laser resurfacing has also been explored. In one study, a semipermeable polyurethane foam dressing was applied as the postoperative dressing on one half of the face and oxygen mist therapy was applied on the other half. Mist therapy is comprised of oxygen (93% at 15 l/minute) and a nutrient mist (Aminoplex®) consisting of sterile water, sodium, chloride, potassium, lactate, acetate, glucose, urea, choline, amino acids, and nucleic acid derivatives. The two methods demonstrated comparable healing rates, with no significant differences in the occurrence of erythema, scarring and acne. Patients did, however, express a preference for the oxygen mist therapy over the foam dressing because of a lesser sense of confinement and decreased pain. The additional benefit of oxygen mist therapy was that as an 'open' dressing, it allowed for wound monitoring. Therefore, oxygen mist therapy may be another option to occlusive dressings following laser resurfacing[57].

FUTURE DIRECTIONS

The past 100 years have brought great advances in wound dressing technology. Research into the mechanisms of wound healing has led to our ability to heal wounds in nearly half the time using occlusive dressings. With recent advances in both polymer and tissue-engineering technology, it is likely that the field will continue to change at an even faster pace. Synthetic growth factors will likely speed the healing of all types of wounds, but the cost of these agents will be prohibitive except in the most difficult cases. Bioengineered skin replacements will likely continue to proliferate, and they will eventually become affordable to a larger subset of patients. By the close of the 21st century, it is likely that we will achieve many of the goals of the ideal wound dressing.

REFERENCES

1. Bennett RG. Dressings and miscellaneous surgical materials. In: Fundamentals of Cutaneous Surgery. St Louis: Mosby, 1987:xii, 823.
2. Cho CY, Lo JS. Dressing the part. Dermatol Clin. 1998;16:25–47.
3. Gilje, O. On taping (adhesive tape treatment) of leg ulcers. Acta Derm Venereol. 1948;28:454–67.
4. Winter GD. Formation of the scab and the rate of epithelization of superficial wounds in the skin of the young domestic pig. Nature. 1962;193:293–4.
5. Cunningham BB, Bernstein L, Woodley DT. Wound dressings. In: Roenigk RK, Roenigk HH (eds). Dermatologic Surgery: Principles and Practice, 2nd edn. New York: Marcel Dekker, 1996:131.
6. Eaglstein WH, Davis SC, Mehle AL, Mertz PM. Optimal use of an occlusive dressing to enhance healing. Effect of delayed application and early removal on wound healing. Arch Dermatol. 1988;124:392–5.
7. Li W, Dasgeb B, Phillips T, et al. Wound-healing perspectives. Dermatol Clin. 2005;23:181–92.
8. Matthews DN. Dressing of open wounds and burns with tulle gras. Lancet. 1941;1:43.
9. Ersek RA. Ischemic necrosis and elastic net bandages. Tex Med. 1982;78:47–9.
10. Zitelli JA. Wound healing by first and second intention. In: Roenigk RK, Roenigk HH (eds). Dermatologic Surgery: Principles and Practice, 2nd edn. New York: Marcel Dekker, 1996:101–30.
11. Strohal R, Schelling M, Takacs M, Jurecka W, Gruber U, Offner F. Nanocrystalline silver dressings as an efficient anti-MRSA barrier: a new solution to an increasing problem. J Hosp Infect. 2005;60:226–30.

12. Dunn K, Edwards-Jones V. The role of Acticoat with nanocrystalline silver in the management of burns. Burns. 2004;30(suppl. 1):S1–9.
13. Hansson C. The effects of cadexomer iodine paste in the treatment of venous leg ulcers compared with hydrocolloid dressing and paraffin gauze dressing. Cadexomer Iodine Study Group. Int J Dermatol. 1998;37:390–6.
14. Rubio PA. Use of semiocclusive, transparent film dressings for surgical wound protection: experience in 3637 cases. Int Surg. 1991;76:253–4.
15. Gilmore WA, Wheeland RG. Treatment of ulcers on legs by pinch grafts and a supportive dressing of polyurethane. J Dermatol Surg Oncol. 1982;8:177–83.
16. Hien NT, Prawer SE, Katz HI. Facilitated wound healing using transparent film dressing following Mohs micrographic surgery. Arch Dermatol. 1988;124:903–6.
17. Rosdy M, Clauss LC. Cytotoxicity testing of wound dressings using normal human keratinocytes in culture. J Biomed Mater Res. 1990;24:363–77.
18. Buchan IA, Andrews JK, Land SM. Clinical and laboratory investigation of the composition and properties of human skin wound exudate under semipermeable dressings. Burns. 1980;7:326–34.
19. Gilchrist B, Reed C. The bacteriology of chronic venous ulcers treated with occlusive hydrocolloid dressings. Br J Dermatol. 1989;121:337–44.
20. Viamontes L, Temple D, Wytall D, Walker A. An evaluation of an adhesive hydrocellular foam dressing and a self-adherent soft silicone foam dressing in a nursing home setting. Ostomy Wound Manage. 2003;49:48–52, 54-6, 58.

21. Vermeulen H, Ubbink DT, Goossens A, de Vos R, Legemate DA. Systematic review of dressings and topical agents for surgical wounds healing by secondary intention. Br J Surg. 2005;92:665–72.
22. Eisenbud D, Hunter H, Kessler L, Zulkowski K. Hydrogel wound dressings: where do we stand in 2003? Ostomy Wound Manage. 2003;49:52–7.
23. Mertz PM, Marshall DA, Eaglstein WH. Occlusive wound dressings to prevent bacterial invasion and wound infection. J Am Acad Dermatol. 1985; 12:662–8.
24. Geronemus RG, Robins P. The effect of two new dressings on epidermal wound healing. J Dermatol Surg Oncol. 1982;8:850–2.
25. Mandy SH. A new primary wound dressing made of polyethylene oxide gel. J Dermatol Surg Oncol. 1983;9:153–5.
26. Thomas S. Alginate dressings in surgery and wound management – Part 1. J Wound Care. 2000;9:56–60.
27. Cassidy C, St Peter SD, Lacey S, et al. Biobrane versus Duoderm for the treatment of intermediate thickness burns in children: a prospective, randomized trial. Burns. 2005;31:890–3.
28. Bolton LL, Johnson CL, Van Rijswijk L. Occlusive dressings: therapeutic agents and effects on drug delivery. Clin Dermatol. 1991;9:573–83.
29. Xakellis GC, Chrischilles EA. Hydrocolloid versus saline-gauze dressings in treating pressure ulcers: a cost-effectiveness analysis. Arch Phys Med Rehabil. 1992;73:463–9.
30. Hansbrough JF, Franco ES. Skin replacements. Clin Plast Surg. 1998;25:407–23.

31. Consensus Development Conference on Diabetic Foot Wound Care: 7–8 April 1999, Boston, Massachusetts. American Diabetes Association. Diabetes Care. 1999;22:1354–60.

32. Fletcher A, Cullum N, Sheldon TA. A systematic review of compression treatment for venous leg ulcers. Br Med J. 1997;315:576–80.

33. Stemmer R, Marescaux J, Furderer C. [Compression therapy of the lower extremities particularly with compression stockings]. Hautarzt. 1980;31:355–65.

34. Kikta MJ, Schuler JJ, Meyer JP, et al. A prospective, randomized trial of Unna's boots versus hydroactive dressing in the treatment of venous stasis ulcers. J Vasc Surg. 1988;7:478–83.

35. Callam MJ, Ruckley CV, Dale JJ, Harper DR. Hazards of compression treatment of the leg: an estimate from Scottish surgeons. Br Med J (Clin Res Ed). 1987; 295:1382.

36. Hendricks WM, Swallow RT. Management of stasis leg ulcers with Unna's boots versus elastic support stockings. J Am Acad Dermatol. 1985;12(1 Pt 1):90–8.

37. Cordts PR, Hanrahan LM, Rodriguez AA, Woodson J, LaMorte WW, Menzoian JO. A prospective, randomized trial of Unna's boot versus Duoderm CGF hydroactive dressing plus compression in the management of venous leg ulcers. J Vasc Surg. 1992;15:480–6.

38. Cullum N, Nelson EA, Fletcher AW, Sheldon TA. Compression bandages and stockings for venous leg ulcers. Cochrane Database Syst Rev. 2000;(2):CD000265.

39. Posten W, Wrone DA, Dover JS, Arndt KA, Silapunt S, Alam M. Low-level laser therapy for wound healing: mechanism and efficacy. Dermatol Surg. 2005; 31:334–40.

40. Thomas DR, Diebold MR, Eggemeyer LM. A controlled, randomized, comparative study of a radiant heat bandage on the healing of stage 3-4 pressure ulcers: A pilot study. J Am Med Dir Assoc. 2005;6:46–9.

41. Phillips TJ. Successful methods of treating leg ulcers. The tried and true, plus the novel and new. Postgrad Med. 1999;105:159–61, 165–6, 173–4 passim.

42. Beasley WD, Hirst G. Making a meal of MRSA – the role of biosurgery in hospital-acquired infection. J Hosp Infect. 2004;56:6–9.

43. Kirsner RS, Falanga V, Kerdel FA, Katz MH, Eaglstein WH. Skin grafts as pharmacological agents: pre-wounding of the donor site. Br J Dermatol. 1996;135:292–6.

44. Carsin H, Ainaud P, Le Bever H, et al. Cultured epithelial autografts in extensive burn coverage of severely traumatized patients: a five year single-center experience with 30 patients. Burns. 2000;26:379–87.

45. Lobmann R, Pittasch D, Muhlen I, Lehnert H. Autologous human keratinocytes cultured on membranes composed of benzyl ester of hyaluronic acid for grafting in nonhealing diabetic foot lesions: a pilot study. J Diabetes Complications. 2003; 17:199–204.

46. Campoccia D, Hunt JA, Doherty PJ, et al. Quantitative assessment of the tissue response to films of hyaluronan derivatives. Biomaterials. 1996;17:963–75.

47. Khachemoune A, Bello YM, Phillips TJ. Factors that influence healing in chronic venous ulcers treated with cryopreserved human epidermal cultures. Dermatol Surg. 2002;28:274–80.

48. Bello YM, Falabella AF. Use of skin substitutes in dermatology. Dermatol Clin. 2001;19:555–61.

49. Smith DJ. Use of Biobrane in wound management. J Burn Care Rehabil. 1995;16(3 Pt 1):317–20.

50. Davis DA, Arpey CJ. Porcine heterografts in dermatologic surgery and reconstruction. Dermatol Surg. 2000;26:76–80.

51. Mostow EN, Haraway GD, Dalsing M, Hodde JP, King D; OASIS Venus Ulcer Study Group. Effectiveness of an extracellular matrix graft (OASIS Wound Matrix) in the treatment of chronic leg ulcers: a randomized clinical trial. J Vasc Surg. 2005;41:837–43.

52. Heimbach D, Luterman A, Burke J, et al. Artificial dermis for major burns. A multi-center randomized clinical trial. Ann Surg. 1988;208:313–20.

53. Eisenbud D, Huang NF, Luke S, Silberklang M. Skin substitutes and wound healing: current status and challenges (part 1 of 2). Wounds. 2004;16:2–17.

54. Yang JY, Tsai YC, Noordhoff MS. Clinical comparison of commercially available Biobrane preparations. Burns. 1989;15:197–203.

55. Falanga V, Margolis D, Alvarez O, et al. Rapid healing of venous ulcers and lack of clinical rejection with an allogeneic cultured human skin equivalent. Human Skin Equivalent Investigators Group. Arch Dermatol. 1998;134:293–300.

56. Weinstein C, Ramirez O, Pozner J. Postoperative care following carbon dioxide laser resurfacing. Avoiding pitfalls. Dermatol Surg. 1998;24:51–6.

57. Onouye T, Menaker G, Christian M, Moy R. Occlusive dressing versus oxygen mist therapy following CO_2 laser resurfacing. Dermatol Surg. 2000;26:572–6.

Biopsy Techniques and Basic Excisions

Suzanne Olbricht

INTRODUCTION

The cornerstone of dermatologic diagnosis is the correlation of clinical and histologic findings. A biopsy procedure is required in order to obtain tissue for pathologic examination, and fortunately the skin is more accessible than most other tissues. Nowadays, modern instruments and techniques allow cutaneous biopsies to be performed efficiently with minimal tissue distortion. In some situations, a biopsy procedure is also curative, either coincidentally or intentionally. Knowledge of basic excisional surgical techniques can minimize cosmetic and functional impairment. Performance of a timely skin biopsy may also circumvent the need for more invasive procedures, and even critically ill patients can undergo a skin biopsy with minimal risk.

KEY CONCEPTS

Site Selection

Performance of a biopsy that will yield accurate and relevant histologic information depends upon the selection of an appropriate lesion or site within a lesion (Table 146.1). Biopsying a tumor is often more straightforward: sampling the thickest portion of the tumor and avoiding necrotic tissue. In inflammatory processes, biopsies of two characteristic lesions, one in an early stage and one in a more developed stage, is often most fruitful. For example, in Sweet's syndrome, histologic examination of an erythematous plaque and a papulovesicle should allow one to establish the diagnosis. For blisters, ulcers or necrotic lesions, the biopsy specimen should include normal perilesional skin as well as affected skin so that the pathologist can identify either the plane of separation for a blister or the inflammation, infection or tumor adjacent to the ulceration or necrosis.

The anticipated depth of the lesion to be biopsied must also be considered. In the case of a superficial lesion, e.g. an actinic keratosis versus Bowen's disease, it can be assessed via a more 'superficial' biopsy that extends to the papillary dermis. On the other hand, accurate diagnosis of a subcutaneous nodule, e.g. panniculitis versus polyarteritis nodosa, requires a biopsy that includes subcutaneous tissue. Occasionally, fascia must be obtained, e.g. morphea profunda versus eosinophilic fasciitis. Disorders that primarily affect the collagen and elastic fibers within the dermis may have subtle histologic findings (e.g. atrophoderma of Pasini and Pierini) and longitudinally sectioned wedge biopsies that include both the affected area as well as adjacent normal-appearing skin prove most helpful.

Biopsy Technique Selection

Six major methods are employed to biopsy skin: curettage, snip or scissors biopsy, shave biopsy, punch biopsy, incisional biopsy, and excision *in toto* (Table 146.2). Depending upon the type of lesion and its size, several of these procedures are also curative, especially excision *in toto*. However, these methods do differ with regard to the quality and quantity of skin obtained. Lesional characteristics and operator experience are factors that influence the choice of a particular procedure.

BIOPSY SITE SELECTION	
Lesion/disorder	**Appropriate site**
Tumor	Thickest portion
Blister	Edge of lesion, including perilesional skin
Ulcerated/necrotic lesion	Edge of ulcer or necrosis plus adjacent skin
Generalized polymorphous eruption	Characteristic lesion of recent onset (± more developed lesion)
Small vessel vasculitis	Characteristic lesion of recent onset

Table 146.1 Biopsy site selection.

SELECTION OF TYPE OF BIOPSY TECHNIQUE				
Method	**Indication**	**Type of specimen obtained**	**Anesthetic technique**	**Closure**
Curettage	• Lesions involving the epidermis (e.g. SKs, AKs, verrucae) • Confirm clinical diagnosis of BCC prior to definitive treatment	Epidermal sheet or fragmented	Wheal	Secondary
Scissors biopsy	• Pedunculated lesion	Tissue above connection to the epidermis	None or wheal	Secondary
Shave biopsy	• Lesions involving the epidermis ± superficial dermis • Elevated lesion	Epidermis and papillary dermis; occasionally, reticular dermis (elevated lesions)	Wheal	Secondary
Punch biopsy	• Process (e.g. tumor, inflammation) involves the dermis • Depressed lesion	Epidermis, dermis and sometimes subcutaneous fat	Wheal or deep	Primary; simple suture
Incisional biopsy	• Process (e.g. tumor, inflammation) involves the subcutaneous fat or fascia • Large-sized tumors • Subtle disorders of dermal connective tissue	Epidermis, dermis and subcutaneous fat	Deep	Primary; layered closure
Excision *in toto*	• Biopsy intended to be definitive treatment • Strong clinical suspicion of cutaneous malignancy (e.g. invasive melanoma)	Epidermis, dermis and subcutaneous fat	Deep	Primary; layered closure

Table 146.2 Selection of type of biopsy technique. AKs, actinic keratoses; BCC, basal cell carcinoma; SKs, seborrheic keratoses.

Although *curettage* is frequently used to remove clinically benign epidermal lesions (e.g. verrucae, seborrheic keratoses) as well as actinic keratoses (e.g. in patients with vascular rosacea in whom hypopigmentation from liquid nitrogen application can be problematic), there are situations where histologic confirmation of the presumed diagnosis is desirable. Curettage is also used to confirm the clinical diagnosis of basal cell carcinoma (BCC) just prior to definitive treatment by curettage and electrodesiccation. The specimen obtained can vary from an epidermal sheet to fragments of epidermis and dermis. Its disadvantages as a biopsy specimen include frequent fragmentation of the tissue and difficulty in orientation. *Snip or scissors biopsy* is an efficient technique for assessing pedunculated lesions as well as removing benign growths (e.g. acrochordons, filiform warts).

The *shave biopsy* usually provides a specimen consisting of epidermis, papillary dermis and, sometimes, reticular dermis (particularly in elevated lesions). It is a popular biopsy technique for 'planing' papular, clinically benign lesions (e.g. irritated or unwanted compound and dermal melanocytic nevi, fibrous papules of the nose) where histologic confirmation is desired. Shave biopsy is also a useful procedure for diagnosing superficial carcinomas, e.g. nodular and superficial BCCs, squamous cell carcinoma (SCC) *in situ*, lentigo maligna.

Some authors distinguish a shave biopsy from a saucerization procedure in which the depth of the biopsy specimen is intentionally deeper due to the angulation of the blade (see section on Variations). This latter technique is often used to biopsy melanocytic nevi with atypical features, especially on the trunk, as well as minimally invasive SCCs or keratoacanthomas. Its advantage is that it allows histologic examination of the entire lesion, which increases diagnostic accuracy, especially in the case of larger lesions (as compared to partial punch biopsy).

The *punch biopsy* supplies a cylindrical- to conically shaped specimen consisting of epidermis, dermis and, sometimes, subcutaneous fat. The volume of tissue sampled correlates with the size of the punch biopsy instrument. In general, the diameter of the metal 'barrel' varies from 2 to 6 mm, and the wider the diameter, the greater the likelihood of obtaining subcutaneous fat. However, the thickness of the dermis and the amount of subcutaneous fat required to establish the diagnosis must be kept in mind. Punch biopsies are particularly helpful for examining processes within the dermis, e.g. tumors, inflammation (see Table 146.2). In the case of tumors, sampling a majority of the lesion is desirable, but for large-sized tumors, multiple punch biopsies may be required.

The *incisional* biopsy removes a wedge of tissue from the center or edge of a lesion (see Site selection) and is the best option for obtaining deep subcutaneous fat or fascia for histologic examination. It is also used to sample a significant portion of large-sized tumors. Excision *in toto* removes the entire lesion and includes epidermis, dermis and subcutaneous fat. For these reasons, it is often the biopsy of choice for a presumed invasive cutaneous melanoma[1].

Specimen Handling

Transportation of the biopsy specimen to the laboratory differs according to the processing and type of examination required (Table 146.3). Most specimens are placed in formalin, but, occasionally, special carrier media are necessary, e.g. Michel's medium for direct immunofluorescence. Fresh tissue specimens are sent on saline-moistened gauze and either promptly delivered to the laboratory or packed in ice; the laboratory must be in reasonable proximity and have the capability of processing the tissue immediately.

A protocol must be established within the clinician's practice to ensure that specimens and results are appropriately tracked and assigned to the correct patient. Immediately after the biopsy specimen has been obtained, it should be placed in a container previously labeled with the patient's name and other identifying information. If multiple biopsies are to be performed, prelabeling the containers alphabetically and with the respective sites avoids confusion. The specimen and its accompanying requisition form are then taken to a designated site, where it is first logged into a pathology specimen book and then set aside for delivery to the pathology laboratory.

When the report is received, a notation is made in the pathology book, cross-checking the patient-identifying information. It is also

SPECIMEN HANDLING		
Proposed laboratory test	**Carrier medium**	**Comments**
Routine microscopy	10% neutral buffered formalin	Fixation process begins immediately
Direct immunofluorescence	Michel's medium or fresh*	Depends on laboratory preference or availability
Immunoperoxidase	Formalin, fresh* or Michel's medium	Depends on test to be performed – contact pathologist
Culture for bacteria, mycobacteria or fungi	Fresh* or minced in sterile culture/carrier medium appropriate for organism (usually performed by laboratory)	
Culture for viruses	Viral transport medium (e.g. M4RT)	
Electron microscopy	Glutaraldehyde	

Laboratory must be in close proximity and specimen placed on saline-moistened gauze, but need to avoid bacteriostatic saline solution when culturing for microbes.

Table 146.3 Specimen handling.

useful to have the pathology book identify the plan for the patient and whether the plan has been accomplished. For instance, the book may document that the patient already has an appointment for suture removal. When the suture removal has taken place and the patient has been informed of the results of the biopsy, this information is also logged into the book. Some patients prefer a call regarding any anxiety-provoking biopsy results such as skin cancer, but most patients appreciate a written letter detailing the diagnosis and recommended treatment plan. Regardless, if a biopsy has been performed, it is the physician's responsibility to track the specimen and follow through to notification of the results to the patient and disposition of recommended care.

Patient Preparation

A discussion of the reason(s) to do the biopsy, the site to be biopsied and the technique to be used can be brief and to the point. Informed consent requires a discussion of the major risks, which include bleeding, discomfort, infection and scarring (see Ch. 151). Bleeding can often be controlled by firm pressure at the site of the wound, but may require more aggressive forms of hemostasis. Discomfort is usually minimal, although some sites such as the forehead, fingers and feet may throb.

Infection is unusual. Except when the area to be biopsied is already infected or the site is mucosal, the skin can be prepared by application of antibacterial soaps and the procedure is then considered to be a *clean* procedure. For clean procedures, preoperative prophylactic antibiotics are currently not recommended, even in patients with artificial valves or joints[2–4]. Chapters 150 and 151 review the guidelines for antibiotic prophylaxis as well as regimens for both oral and non-oral sites. Preoperative antibiotics are administered within a 2-hour window before the incision; there is debate as to whether or not a second dose is administered 6 hours later and under which circumstances antibiotics should be continued for 48–72 hours[5].

Most patients are primarily interested in discussing whether or not there will be visible scarring. This is best predicted by the type of biopsy to be performed and the anatomic site. Generally, patients can be reassured that small biopsies may be done without grossly noticeable permanent 'marks'.

Many patients are anxious about the needle sticks required for administration of the local anesthesia and the pain of the procedure. The patient's cooperation is easily obtained in an organized and peaceful environment with a calm and reassuring staff. A well-informed, comfortable patient in a supine position will tolerate the procedure without difficulty.

Site Preparation and Anesthesia

Effective site preparation is most efficient if a standard clinical protocol has been established. Marking the site, cleansing the skin[6], and draping are important procedures prior to the instillation of local anesthesia (Table 146.4). Local anesthesia is adequate for all skin biopsies (see Ch. 143). The agent generally used is lidocaine, either at a 1% or 2% concentration[7]. Epinephrine may be added to the lidocaine in order to reduce bleeding and prolong anesthesia, but it is usually avoided in patients who have a proclivity for cardiac arrhythmias. Use of epinephrine in patients receiving β-adrenergic receptor antagonists ('β-blockers') should be undertaken with care, as a markedly elevated blood pressure may occur because of unopposed α-adrenergic receptor agonist activity[8].

Most adverse reactions to anesthetic agents are vasovagal in nature and can be ameliorated by performing the biopsy on a comfortable patient in a supine position. For patients with true allergic reactions[9], possible agents to use in a controlled environment include paraben-free lidocaine or ester-class anesthetics (e.g. procaine). Injections of saline or diphenhydramine may be somewhat effective in a patient with relative tolerance to pain.

Techniques to decrease the pain associated with instillation of the local anesthesia include slow delivery of the agent through a needle with a small bore (30-gauge) into the compartment containing subcutaneous fat[10] (Fig. 146.1A). Pinching of the site during injection is also often effective. Buffering the lidocaine with sodium bicarbonate[11] and/or applying ice[12] may be helpful. Topical agents that may prove effective in reducing the pain of needle insertion include eutectic mixture of local anesthetics (e.g. EMLA® with lidocaine and prilocaine), tetracaine, liposome-encapsulated tetracaine, and liposome-encapsulated lidocaine[13].

When the local anesthetic agent is instilled in a deep compartment, 5 to 10 minutes is required for anesthesia to develop on the surface of the skin. Gentle massage of the site may assist in spreading the agent subepidermally and achieving good anesthesia. Injection of the agent superficially, creating an edematous wheal, has immediate efficacy but is more painful (Fig. 146.1B). Since a punch or shave biopsy requires very little agent and therefore a very short injection time, superficial instillation is the technique often used. In addition, a wheal is helpful prior to a shave biopsy as the lesion is further elevated from the plane of the surrounding skin. Of note, since epinephrine requires up to 15 minutes to produce maximal vasoconstriction and thereby minimize bleeding[14], lidocaine without epinephrine is sufficient for an immediate biopsy. Regardless of other considerations, it is critical to have the local anesthesia in the compartment that is to be biopsied, i.e. a superficial wheal may be entirely adequate as anesthesia for a shave biopsy but will not suffice for an incisional wedge biopsy that extends into the subcutaneous fat.

Hemostasis

All methods of biopsy require attention to hemostasis of the wound bed. For small-diameter, superficial wounds, compression alone may suffice. However, most wounds require additional treatment. For biopsy sites that are not sutured, styptics such as aluminum chloride hexahydrate (Drysol™, Xerac AC™) and ferric subsulfate (Monsel's solution) are frequently used. Pressure is applied to the edges of the wound so that there is no active bleeding, and the styptic is applied using a cotton-tipped swab along with pressure to the wound bed for approximately 1–2 minutes. Aluminum chloride is generally preferred, as ferric subsulfate may tattoo the wound bed. Another option for hemostasis is to place a small piece of absorbable hemostatic sponge (e.g. Gelfoam®, Instat®) onto the wound bed and then apply a compression bandage[15].

Punch biopsy sites are usually closed primarily and the suturing itself creates sufficient hemostasis. Wounds created during incisional biopsy or excision *in toto* may require electrocoagulation for hemostasis before closure (see Ch. 140). 'Cauterization' of vessels occurs when heat or electricity is delivered to each bleeding point by a metal tip or a monopolar or bipolar electrode attached to an electrosurgical device. First, active bleeding is cleared by pressure with gauze or a cotton-tipped swab and the electric energy or heat is transmitted to the site just as the vessel begins to rebleed. The endpoint is no active bleeding in the wound bed. Bleeding within the dermis in the sides of the wound

SITE PREPARATION PROTOCOL	
Sequential steps	**Comments**
Mark site with surgical pen or ink	Local anesthesia may obscure site, especially when the erythematous color is due to vasodilation or when there is a minimally elevated dermal tumor
Time out for patient and site identification	JCAHO universal protocol for patient safety
Cleanse skin surface	Soap and water, isopropyl alcohol, chlorhexidine scrub or povidone-iodine solution[6]
Drape	Gauze (small biopsies) or sterile cloths
Anesthetize	Local instillation of anesthetic agent

Table 146.4 Site preparation protocol. JCAHO, Joint Commission on Accreditation of Healthcare Organizations.

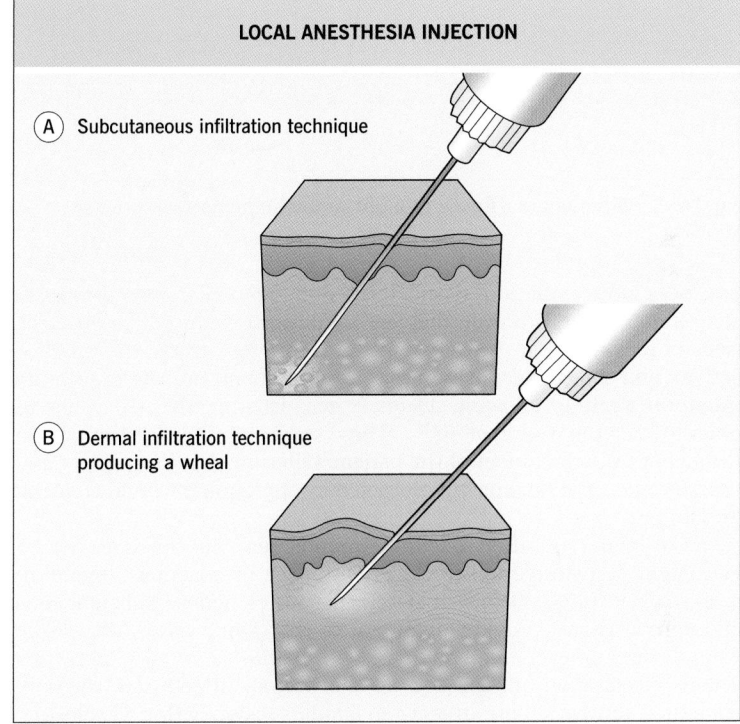

LOCAL ANESTHESIA INJECTION

(A) Subcutaneous infiltration technique

(B) Dermal infiltration technique producing a wheal

Fig. 146.1 Local anesthesia injection. A Deep infiltration. **B** Superficial infiltration.

can be controlled by suturing and does not need cautery. At times, to produce hemostasis, a large actively bleeding vessel may need to be identified, grasped with a hemostat, and tied off with an absorbable suture and a figure-of-eight stitch (Fig. 146.2).

It is important to minimize lateral heat spread (due to tissue resistance to electrical energy) as it may retard normal wound-healing processes and promote necrosis or dehiscence. Use of bipolar forceps or heat cautery is recommended if the patient has a pacemaker or implantable cardioverter-defibrillator (ICD), in order to preclude interference with the device[16].

Wound Closure

Closure of wounds created by a biopsy procedure may occur by either secondary or primary intention healing. Secondary intention healing repairs wounds by the processes of granulation tissue formation, epidermal cell migration, and contraction (see Ch. 141). These processes occur simultaneously, beginning within the first few days after surgery and continuing until the wound has been completely re-epithelialized. For the remainder of the patient's lifetime, maturation of the scar occurs, with gradual improvement in color, texture and contour. Closure of the wound via suturing is regarded as primary intention healing. The same

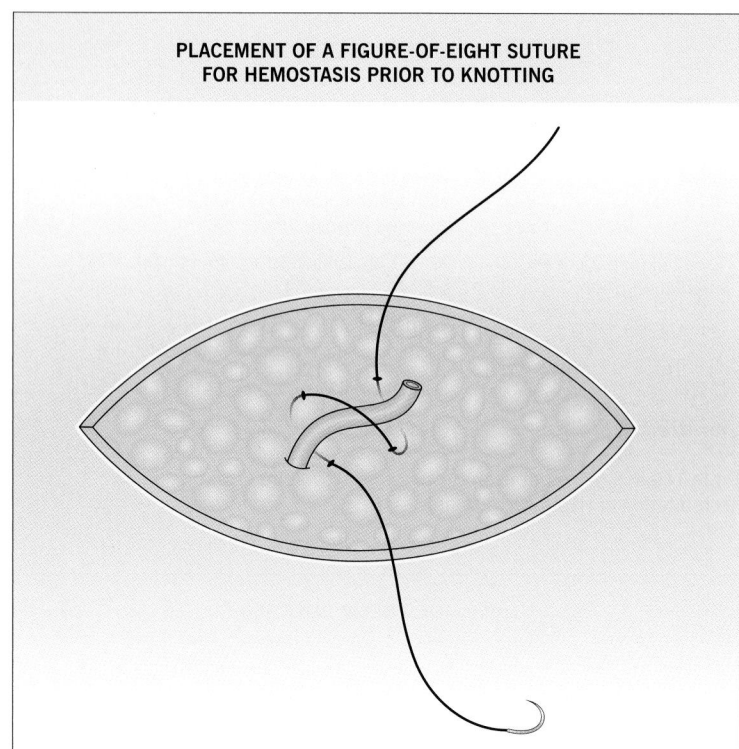

PLACEMENT OF A FIGURE-OF-EIGHT SUTURE FOR HEMOSTASIS PRIOR TO KNOTTING

Fig. 146.2 Placement of a figure-of-eight suture for hemostasis prior to knotting.

processes of granulation tissue formation, epithelial migration and contraction occur; however, they are significantly reduced, because the sides of the wound are already opposed. Processes related to fibroblast activity and collagen deposition play a more important role in primary intention healing, allowing adequate tensile strength to develop in order to keep the wound closed[17]. These scars also undergo maturation throughout the remainder of the patient's lifetime. Both secondary and primary intention healing are promoted by appropriate wound care and dressings.

For primary intention healing, wounds may be closed either by placement of a simple full-thickness suture or by a layered closure. In a layered closure, subepidermal buried sutures oppose subcutaneous and dermal tissue, provide alignment of the wound edges, set up the wound edges for eversion, and assist with hemostasis by occluding any vessels bleeding within the edge of the wound. In addition, the subepidermal sutures supply strength to handle tension within the closure. Although subepidermal sutures are generally absorbable, they remain intact in the tissue for 8 to 12 weeks, the period when the scar is slowly acquiring tensile strength. As a result, they prevent dehiscence and spread of the scar. Epidermal or skin stitches oppose the epidermal edges and complete eversion. They can also correct minor degrees of misalignment in the closure. Satisfying these objectives via conscious placement of stitches improves the function and appearance of the scar[18].

Knotting is the means for stabilizing the placement of the suture, usually produced with an instrument tie (Fig. 146.3). The first throw of the knot is started by pulling the long end of the suture tight with the fingers of the non-dominant hand and looping it around the needle holder once or twice. The needle holder then grasps the short end and pulls it through the loops. The loops are pulled across the wound so that they lie flat. These steps are then repeated to produce the second throw of the knot, but this time with the loop in the opposite direction around the needle holder. When this second loop is pulled across the wound, a square knot is created. Depending on the memory and thickness of the suture material, three to six throws may be required to properly secure the knot. Care is taken to ensure that the knot lies flat without significant tension or tightness[19]. Sometimes, a loose loop is left in the second throw, to allow the suture to adjust to any wound swelling that may develop.

Sutures commonly used for subepidermal placement are composed of synthetic absorbable materials, e.g. braided polyglactin (Vicryl®) and monofilament polydioxanone (PDS®). The *interrupted buried dermal stitch* (Fig. 146.4A) is designed such that the stitch is in the dermis and

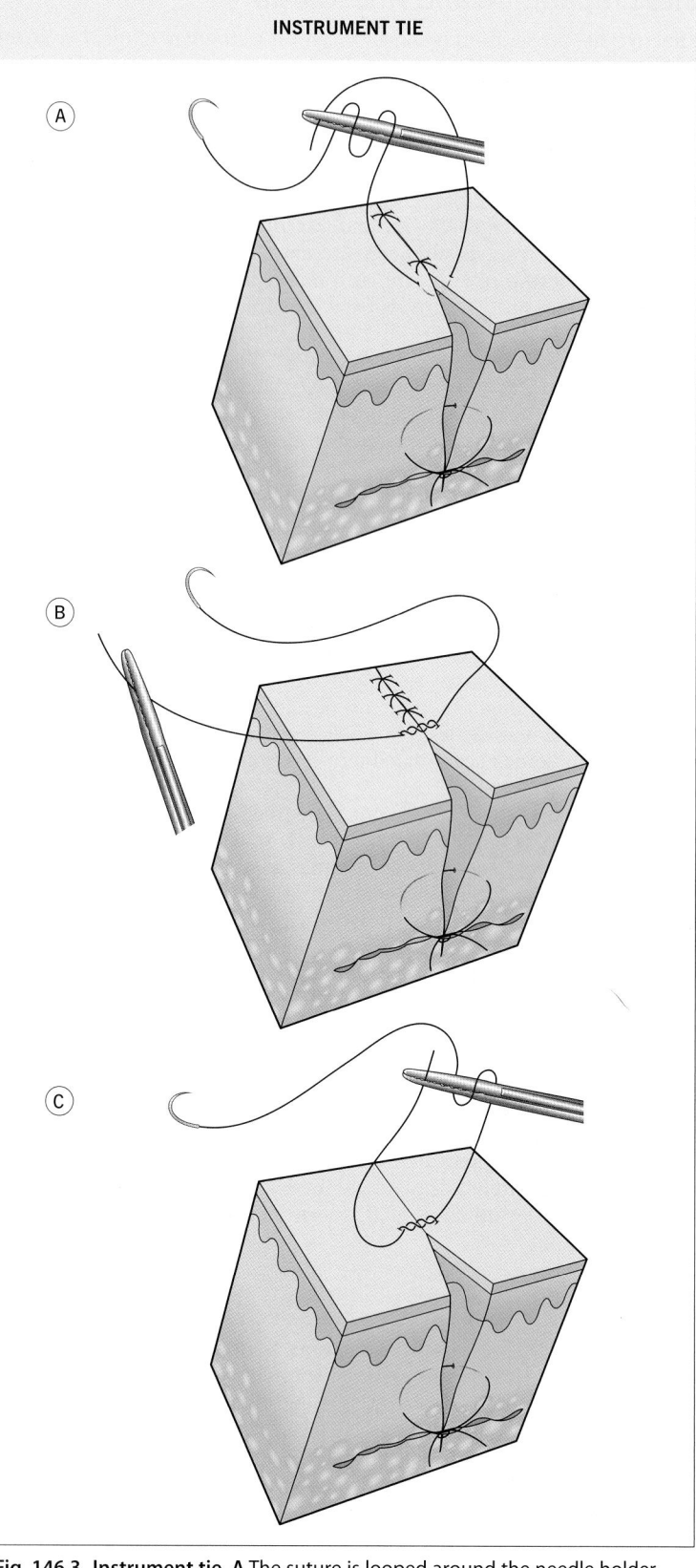

INSTRUMENT TIE

Fig. 146.3 Instrument tie. A The suture is looped around the needle holder, then the needle holder grasps the short end and pulls it through the loops to create a knot. **B** The suture is drawn over the wound so that the knot lies flat across the wound. **C** A loop is made around the needle holder in the opposite direction. The needle holder then grabs the short end and pulls it through so that the knot lies flat on the skin surface.

fat and the knot is inverted (buried). The needle enters the undermined deep surface of the wound and passes up into the dermis. After crossing the wound, it enters the opposite side of the wound at the same level in the dermis and then exits the deep surface. The knot is then tied and the ends of the suture cut. When the suture material is released, the knot settles within the deep portion of the wound, minimizing tissue reaction to the suture and extrusion through the wound. Enough buried

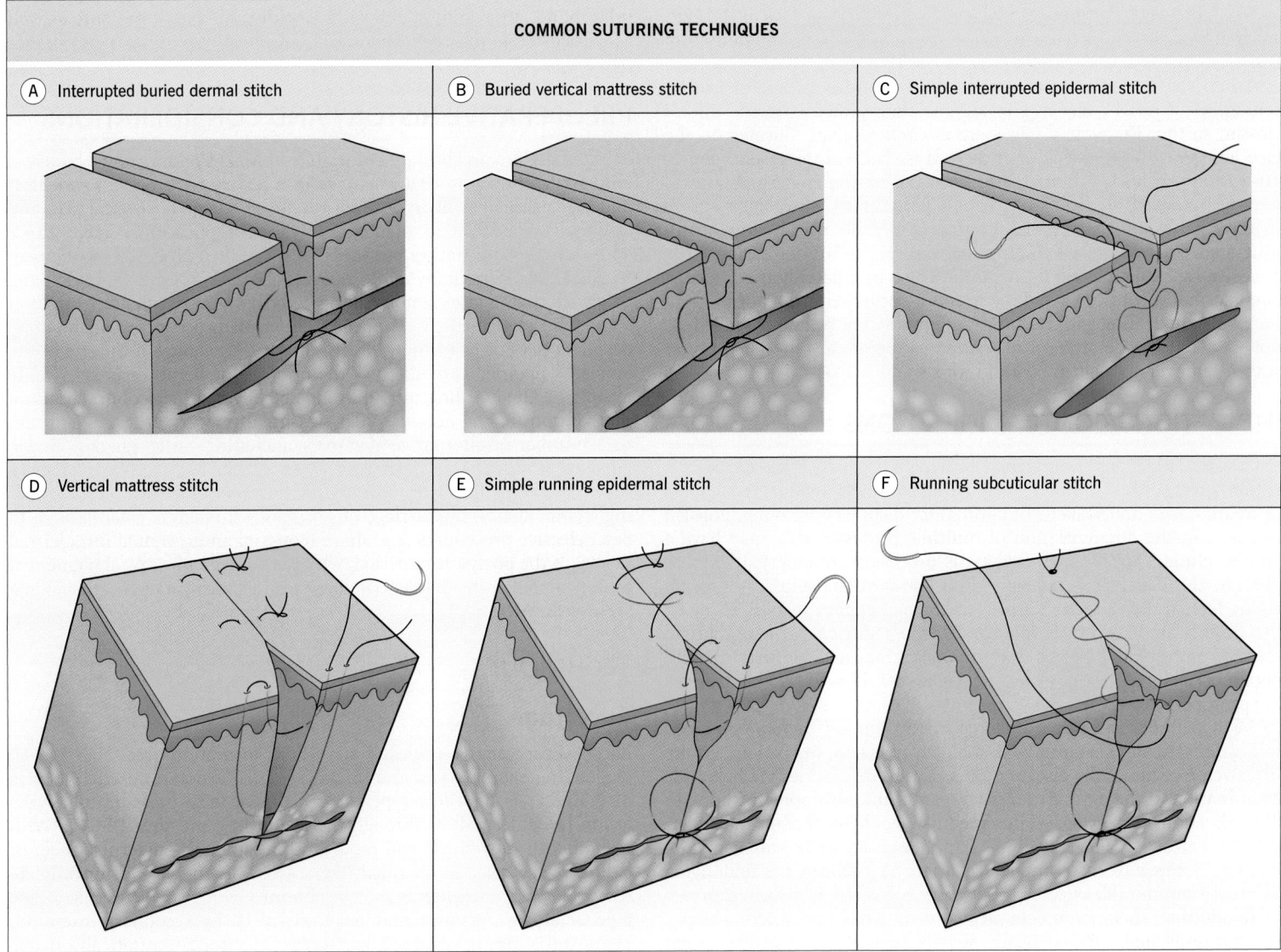

COMMON SUTURING TECHNIQUES

| A Interrupted buried dermal stitch | B Buried vertical mattress stitch | C Simple interrupted epidermal stitch |
| D Vertical mattress stitch | E Simple running epidermal stitch | F Running subcuticular stitch |

Fig. 146.4 Common suturing techniques. A Interrupted buried dermal stitch. **B** Buried vertical mattress stitch. **C** Simple interrupted epidermal stitch. **D** Vertical mattress stitch. **E** Simple running epidermal stitch. **F** Running subcuticular stitch.

dermal stitches are placed such that tension is eliminated and the deep tissues are completely opposed. In order to facilitate eversion, this basic stitch may be modified, creating a *buried vertical mattress stitch*[20]. In this stitch, the suture is nearest to the skin surface (within the superficial dermis) at a point 3–4 mm lateral to the wound edge, and then it exits the wound deeper in the dermis (Fig. 146.4B). A very subtle dimple may be appreciated above the suture where it lies superficially in the dermis.

On occasion, a *running dermal stitch* is used to close the deep component. The stitch is begun similarly to the interrupted buried dermal stitch, but, after tying, only the short end of the suture is cut. The needle then draws the suture through the subcutaneous fat and dermis on one side, passing to the other side, and then continuing along the length of the wound. At each step, the suture is pulled tightly to oppose the edges. At the end of the wound, the knot is achieved by tying the loose end to the last loop. This stitch is only used when there is little tension in the wound, as rupture of the suture material anywhere along the suture line would release the suture for the entire length of the wound, allowing dehiscence or spread of the scar.

Monofilament nylon (Ethilon®) or polypropylene (Prolene®) are commonly used epidermal sutures. The *simple interrupted epidermal stitch* is placed by passing the needle through the epidermis into the superficial dermis in a plane just superior to the buried suture, across the wound, into the dermis on the opposite side and then up through the epidermis (Fig. 146.4C). Eversion is assisted by placing the suture both farther from the wound edge and in a deeper plane (rather than on the surface). Using the curve of the needle to create the path for the suture also facilitates eversion. If there are no buried sutures, the stitch

opposes the edges for the full depth of the wound. The *vertical mattress stitch* (Fig. 146.4D) is sometimes used for wounds where eversion will be difficult and when a single suture opposing the deep and superficial edges is desired. This stitch has four points of entry into the skin. It is started by passing the needle through the epidermis 5–8 mm lateral to the wound edge, exiting from the deep portion of the wound. It re-enters the opposite side of the wound in the same deep position, and exits from the epidermis equidistant from the wound edge as the entry point. The needle is reversed and epidermis is re-entered closer to the wound edge, drawn through upper dermis, crosses the wound, enters the dermis and finally exits close to the wound edge. Once tied, the knot is positioned on one side of the wound, not over the line of closure. Since this suture must be removed within 1–2 weeks, depending upon the site, it is not a good stitch to use as the sole means of closure in a wound with tension. A variant of this stitch, the running combined simple and vertical mattress stitch, also everts well and saves surgical time[21].

In the presence of buried sutures, a *simple running epidermal stitch* may be placed for opposition of the epidermal edges. This running stitch may be passed via the dermis and the epidermis in a fashion similar to the simple interrupted epidermal stitch (Fig. 146.4E). Alternatively, it may be placed in the upper dermis, referred to as a *running subcuticular stitch* (Fig. 146.4F). This stitch is placed with the needle passing in and out of the upper dermis in a plane horizontal to the surface. Two knots are tied, one on each end of the wound, and they are the only visible portion of the suture. Running stitches are frequently used to save time[22]. They do not necessarily prevent track marks, which occur because of tension, inadequate undermining, ineffective buried dermal sutures, and poor placement of the epidermal suture.

Non-absorbable sutures that pass through to the surface of the skin are removed. If they remain in place, they cause tissue inflammation and create a less than optimal functional and cosmetic result. To remove a suture, the thread is severed near the knot with either fine-tipped scissors or a no. 11 blade. The knot is then pulled over the line of closure so that the wound edges are not pulled apart. Sutures on the face are generally removed after 5–7 days, and sutures elsewhere, at 10–14 days. If buried dermal sutures are used, the epidermal sutures may be removed at the earlier times. Sometimes, absorbable suture material is used for superficial closures, especially in the simple running epidermal stitch, precluding the need for suture removal. Sterile adhesive tapes such as Steri-Strips™ are also occasionally used instead of epidermal sutures, to avoid the need for suture removal, but they are ineffective in dealing with tension[23] and producing eversion. They may, however, reduce the amount of scar spreading if they are placed after suture removal and left in position for several weeks[24].

INDICATIONS/CONTRAINDICATIONS

A biopsy is indicated at any time in which the clinical diagnosis of a cutaneous disorder is unclear or must be substantiated before a course of treatment is undertaken. Inflammatory disorders are often biopsied to assist in the differentiation of multiple processes that may have a similar clinical appearance. Infectious processes are biopsied so as to observe the causative organism in tissue sections and/or to obtain tissue for culture. Lesions suspicious for malignancy (e.g. BCC, SCC, melanoma) are biopsied in order to develop a surgical plan appropriate for the tumor type. Biopsies of normal skin may also be performed, to obtain tissue for metabolic or genetic studies[25,26]. Nowadays, skin biopsies are even performed prenatally.

Most patients can safely undergo a skin biopsy; therefore, contraindications are not absolute. A skin biopsy may save the patient a more invasive procedure if the disease process can be determined via histologic examination of the skin. Patients who are immunosuppressed because of medications (e.g. cyclosporine, prednisone, chemotherapy) or underlying diseases (e.g. HIV infection, lymphoma, leukemia) often require biopsies because of the complicated interplay between the underlying disorders and the side effects of therapy (e.g. infections, drug reactions).

In addition, there are no cutaneous or mucosal sites where a biopsy is contraindicated. Diagnostically, it is more useful to biopsy a lesion from the hand or the face that provides accurate information than it is to biopsy a late-stage, non-specific lesion on the arm. Biopsies can be done on the legs of patients with diabetes mellitus and the digits of patients with vascular compromise, although greater attention to postoperative care may be necessary. For patients with coagulation or platelet disorders (due to either underlying diseases or medications), it may be preferable to biopsy a site that can be compressed to produce hemostasis. For example, if an arm or leg were biopsied, postoperative bleeding can be controlled by pressure applied by an elastic circumferential bandage.

In certain anatomic sites, it may be necessary to exercise caution to avoid injuring a vital structure (see Chs 142 & 151). The temporal nerve lies in a superficial location, just beneath thin dermis and subcutaneous fat, midway between the eyebrow and the temporal hairline. The spinal accessory nerve also courses superficially at the posterior edge of the sternocleidomastoid muscle at a point one-third of the distance between the mastoid process and the inferior attachments of the muscle. Severing these nerves leads to motor dysfunction; thus, these sites are best biopsied in a superficial manner. The temporal and thyroid arteries are also relatively superficial. Cutting them leads to temporary difficulty with hemostasis but has no long-term adverse effect.

Some lesions require special consideration before performing a biopsy. A mass that is pulsatile may indicate large arterial vessel involvement, a situation requiring additional clinical evaluation prior to biopsy and special surgical arrangements in case of bleeding. A post-traumatic cephalic mass or cystic midline lesion may need preoperative radiologic examination to determine any possible connection to the intracranial or intraspinal space[27,28]. Biopsy of a lesion on the upper trunk or shoulders of a patient who tends to form keloids must be carefully discussed, weighing the possibility of keloid formation against the utility of the information that will be obtained. Hypertrophic scars, on the

other hand, are common and resolve with time and/or pressure as well as corticosteroid injections, and need not interfere with the performance of a biopsy.

PREOPERATIVE HISTORY AND CONSIDERATIONS

While there are no absolute contraindications to performing a biopsy, a clinician will want to be aware of certain features of a patient's medical and surgical history in order to formulate an adequate surgical plan and to predict the need to manage possible complications. Table 146.5 summarizes information pertinent to the issues previously discussed. In particular, patients who are taking medications or have underlying disorders that lead to abnormalities in coagulation or platelet function should be identified in advance. Almost all procedures can be done despite a patient receiving warfarin, heparin or aspirin if the site of the biopsy is planned carefully and the options for hemostasis are readily available. The bleeding time may also be affected by alcohol ingestion, oral vitamin E, and non-steroidal anti-inflammatory drugs, in addition to a number of alternative therapies, including garlic, gingko, ginger, ginseng, feverfew and green tea[29,30] (see Table 133.3). While biopsies may be done safely during pregnancy[31], the emotional turmoil surrounding a coincidental miscarriage or pregnancy mishap is great enough to defer elective procedures (e.g. shave biopsy of an unwanted intradermal nevus) to the postpartum period, whereas biopsies of atypical pigmented lesions in which the differential diagnosis includes cutaneous melanoma are not deferred.

TECHNIQUES

Curettage

Local anesthesia is achieved by wheal formation (see Fig. 146.1). Depending upon the size and thickness of the lesion, a curette 3–5 mm in diameter is held like a pencil and drawn with pressure under the lesion (if epidermal) or through the lesion (e.g. presumed BCC). With one smooth movement and moderate pressure, an epidermal sheet or ball of tissue may be obtained (Fig. 146.5). In the case of incomplete removal, further fragments may be obtained by repeated curettage. This type of biopsy assumes that healing will be by secondary intention. Hemostasis may be obtained by a styptic, electrodesiccation, absorbable hemostatic sponge, or pressure. The resulting scar is usually minimal in the case of epidermal lesions versus not much of an issue in the case of a BCC, as it is definitive treatment of the latter that produces the final scar.

Snip or Scissors Biopsy

Pedunculated lesions can be biopsied via a snip or scissors biopsy (Fig. 146.6). Local anesthesia is obtained by wheal formation in the upper dermis just under the narrow attachment of the lesion to the skin surface. For tumors with a very narrow neck, this type of biopsy can be done quickly without anesthesia. Scissors, usually fine iris scissors or sharp gradle scissors, are used to separate the lesion from its base at the level of the skin surface. A toothed forceps is often used to

PREOPERATIVE HISTORY
Allergies
Medications, including nutritional supplements and over-the-counter preparations
Past reactions to local anesthesia
Difficulties with hemostasis during previous procedures
Past problems with wound healing, including infection, keloid formation
Pacemaker or implantable cardioverter-defibrillator (ICD)
Disease or past replacement of the cardiac valves
Past orthopedic surgery with joint replacement
Hypertension
Diabetes mellitus
Immunosuppression
Infection or vascular compromise at the biopsy site
Possible pregnancy

Table 146.5 Preoperative history.

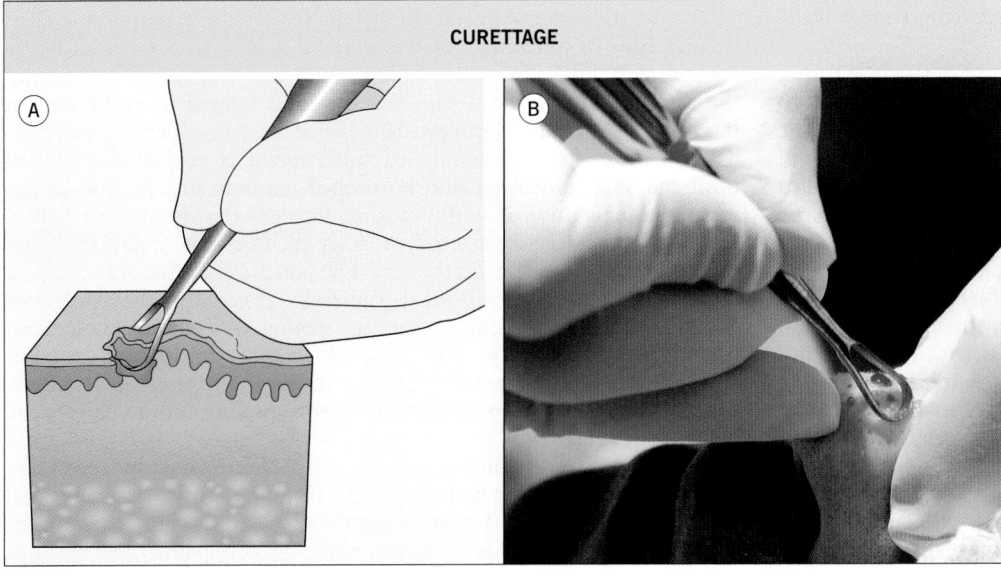

Fig. 146.5 Curettage. A Diagram. **B** Demonstration of technique.

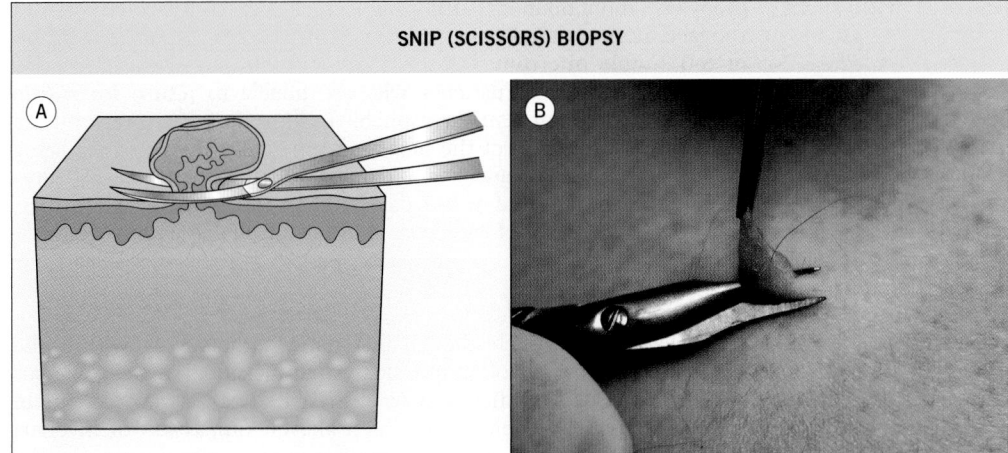

Fig. 146.6 Scissors biopsy. A Diagram. **B** Demonstration of technique.

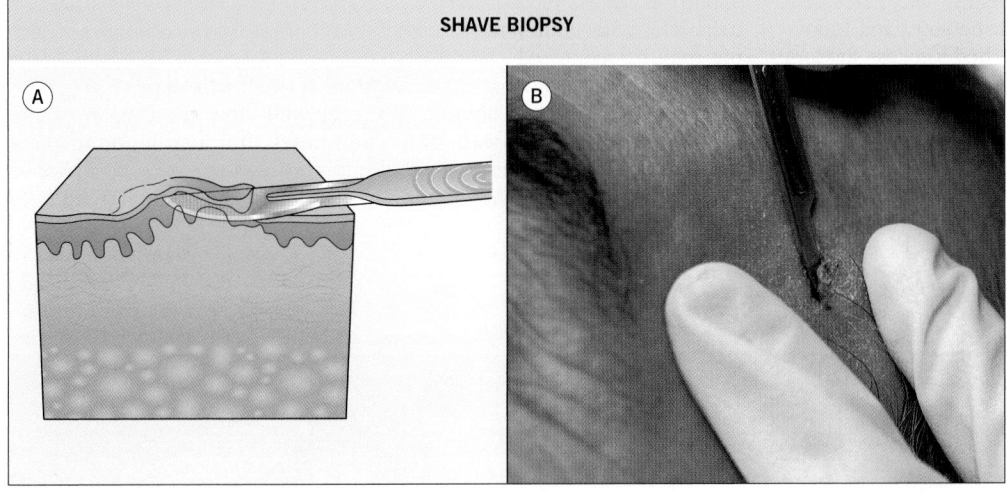

Fig. 146.7 Shave biopsy. A Diagram. **B** Demonstration of technique.

handle the tissue. Healing is by secondary intention, and a styptic, electrodesiccation, absorbable hemostatic sponge, or pressure may be required for hemostasis. Scarring produced by this type of biopsy procedure is a small, often hypopigmented macule and may be very difficult to see.

Shave Biopsy

Shave biopsy is the most commonly used technique for obtaining a skin specimen for histologic examination (Fig. 146.7). If the intention is to remove the entire lesion, then the terms shave excision or tangential excision are used instead of shave biopsy. Obtaining an appropriate specimen is facilitated by the use of the local anesthesia to produce a wheal under the lesion so that it is elevated above the plane of the surrounding skin. A no. 15 blade on a blade handle is used (almost parallel to the skin surface) to cut the specimen from its bed. Alternatively, sometimes only the blade, and not the blade handle, is used. Cutaneous surgeons generally hold the blade or the blade handle like a pencil, to facilitate control of small movements. It is helpful to begin on one edge by holding the blade vertically and incising only through the epidermis. The blade is then turned to a horizontal position and a smooth sawing motion is used to complete the removal of the specimen.

A good specimen may also be obtained by a single-edged razor blade held in a semi-curved shape[32].

The goal is a shallow, saucer-shaped defect and a single piece of unfragmented tissue; edges should be smooth. Forceps may be used to hold the specimen while *in situ* in order to supply traction against the movement of the blade and then to remove the entire specimen and place it in the appropriate container. However, the tissue must be handled gently so that crush artifact does not confuse the microscopic appearance. Toothed, as opposed to smooth or ridged, forceps minimize crushing of the tissue. The specimen should include full-thickness epidermis and superficial dermis. The most common error when first performing shave biopsies is to remove only hyperkeratotic debris or the upper portion of the epidermis. The latter is especially true in areas with thick stratum corneum (e.g. palms, soles). Therefore, the dermatologist needs to appreciate the angulation of the blade that is required in order to obtain the full thickness of the epidermis for histologic examination. Observation of the wound bed and review of the tissue sections will help refine the skills needed to perform this procedure.

Shave biopsy sites heal by secondary intention. As with curettage and snip biopsy, hemostasis is easily obtained with a styptic, electrodesiccation, absorbable hemostatic sponge, and/or pressure. With practice and skill, as well as choosing the appropriate lesion to biopsy in this manner, the resulting mature scar is flat or slightly depressed with slight hypopigmentation.

Punch Biopsy

Punch biopsy is used to sample processes within the dermis (e.g. tumors, inflammation) or the occasional depressed lesion. As discussed above, the volume of tissue obtained varies depending upon the diameter of the metal 'barrel'. For example, the specimen obtained with a 2 mm punch biopsy is very small and may not yield sufficient pathologic findings for an accurate diagnosis. In one study, however, where 2 mm punch biopsy specimens (examined by a dermatopathologist) were compared to excisional specimens, an accurate diagnosis was made in 79 of 84 cases[33]. For most punch biopsies, an instrument with a 3 to 4 mm diameter is adequate. Occasionally, a 6 mm punch biopsy is performed to increase the likelihood of obtaining subcutaneous fat. However, as stated previously, the thickness of the dermis and the amount of subcutaneous fat required to establish the diagnosis must be kept in mind.

Disposable punch biopsy instruments are generally used. Reusable stainless steel instruments are available but must be sterilized following each procedure and sharpened frequently. Toothed forceps, scissors, needle holder and suture material are also required. Local anesthesia is achieved with either superficial or deep instillation of the agent.

An optimal aesthetic result is obtained when the round punch biopsy instrument is used to produce an oval-shaped defect that can be closed without dog-ear formation when sutured into a straight line parallel to the other skin lines in the region. While traction is applied by stretching or spreading the skin in the direction perpendicular to the relaxed skin lines (with the index finger and thumb of one hand), the instrument is pushed into the skin and rotated in one direction (Fig. 146.8). Back-and-forth twisting is not recommended as epidermis may be sheared off. Generally, the instrument is pushed and rotated until the subcutaneous plane is reached, as indicated by loss of the resistance encountered while cutting through the dermis. At times, the punch biopsy is utilized to just incise the skin superficially as when the skin is very thin (e.g. on the ear). The punch biopsy specimen is then removed and forceps are used (peripherally at one superficial edge) to gently extricate the specimen from the wound. Scissors may be needed to detach the base of the specimen, which can then be transferred to the appropriate container. In the case of fibrotic tumors or disorders, pressure may need to be applied to the surrounding skin to elevate the biopsy specimen.

Although a punch biopsy wound can be left to heal by secondary intention after achieving hemostasis, the resulting scar is often depressed and takes several weeks to heal. Usually this wound is closed primarily, and the resulting scar is generally white or hypopigmented and has a linear or cruciate configuration. On the trunk or extremities, one or two simple interrupted epidermal stitches of 4-0 nylon or polypropylene monofilament suture achieve closure and hemostasis. On the face, neck or hands, the resulting scar may be less apparent if 5-0 or 6-0 simple interrupted sutures are utilized. Some physicians use fast-absorbing gut for patients who are unable to return for suture removal. However, it is also reasonable to have the patient return for a face-to-face discussion of the biopsy results, since the biopsy is being done to establish a diagnosis and determine a treatment plan. Sutures on the face are removed at 5–7 days, and on the trunk or extremities, at 10–14 days. A pathology report is usually available within 7 days.

Incisional Biopsy

Large lesions in which the characteristic pathology is within the dermis or subcutis are often biopsied via an incisional or wedge biopsy (Fig. 146.9). The specimen may be entirely lesional or may contain an edge of clinically normal skin, which allows comparison of involved versus uninvolved skin as well as examination for any microscopically apparent early changes at the edge of the lesion. The goal is to obtain a wedge of tissue 3–4 mm wide and as deep as necessary. The tissue should be in one piece for accurate orientation of the specimen during preparation; depending upon the possible diagnoses, longitudinal sectioning may be requested. The length of the wedge varies, but should be long enough to avoid dog-ear formation in the final closure.

Local anesthesia is obtained by deep and slow infiltration of the agent. It is advisable to wait 10 to 15 minutes after instillation to allow for complete anesthesia and to obtain the maximal vasoconstrictive effect of epinephrine. With a no. 15 blade and the blade handle held

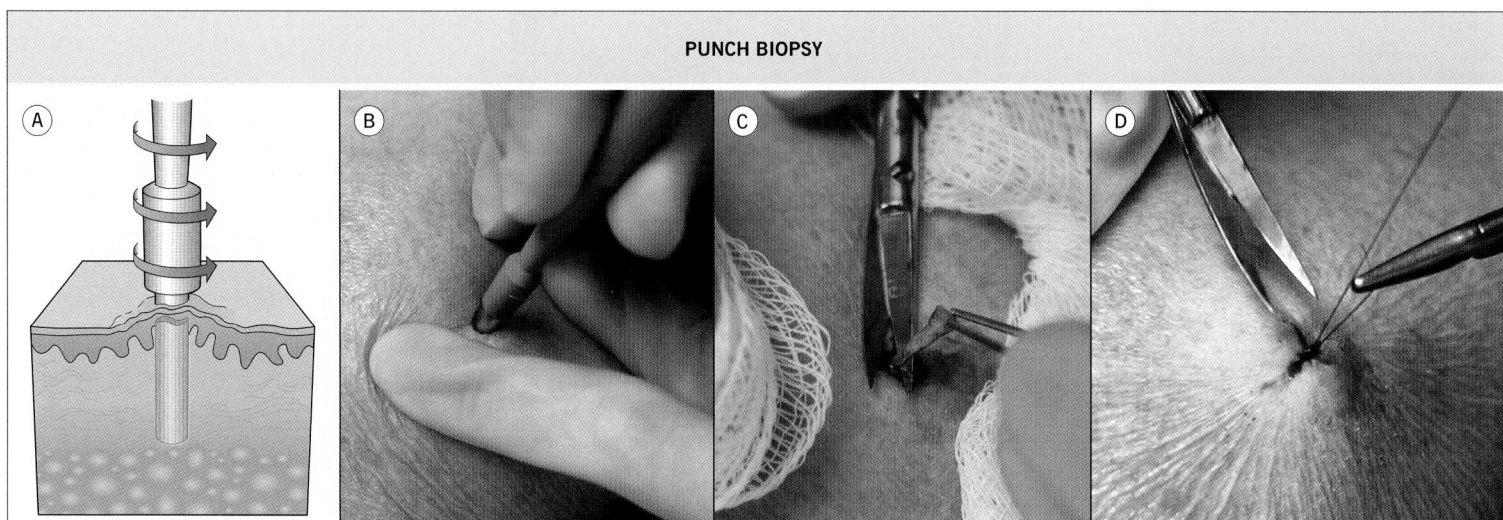

PUNCH BIOPSY

Ⓐ Ⓑ Ⓒ Ⓓ

Fig. 146.8 Punch biopsy. A Diagram. **B** Punch biopsy instrument rotated into the skin. **C** Cutting the base of the specimen. **D** Closure of the biopsy wound with a simple epidermal stitch.

INCISIONAL BIOPSY

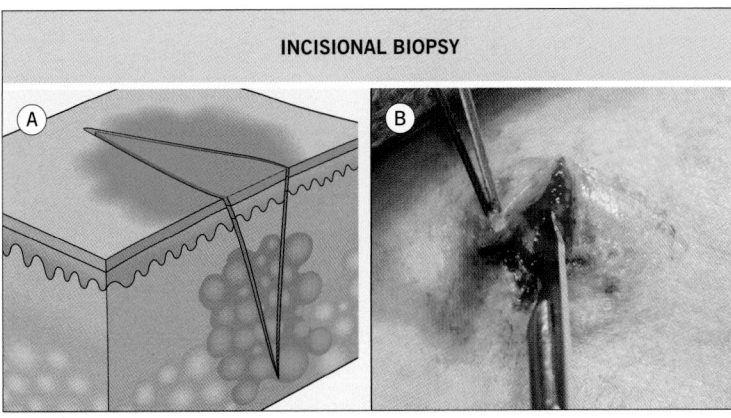

Fig. 146.9 Incisional biopsy. A Diagram. **B** Demonstration of the procedure.

perpendicular to the skin surface, a superficial incision into the epidermis scores one long side of the wedge using a light touch and one long motion, facilitated by traction by the non-dominant hand or an assistant. The second long side is then scored similarly. These lines are then redrawn with the blade held in the same manner but with firm pressure, incising into deep tissue, first one side, then the other. The incision is continued until the desired depth has been reached, usually in one or two more cutting movements. The incision is angled toward the center axis so that deep within the tissue, the two incisions meet and complete the separation of the tissue. A forceps is used to lift the tissue out of the wound. If the tissue is still connected at its base, the blade or tissue scissors may be used to complete the detachment.

Hemostasis is best achieved by point electrocoagulation. Large arterioles may require tying off with absorbable suture. An incisional biopsy wound is generally closed with suturing. In some circumstances, such as a site compromised by necrosis or infection, secondary intention healing may be the best option, even if it is slow and prolonged. Deep interrupted stitches of absorbable suture material, 4-0 or 5-0 in caliber, with the knot inverted are utilized to close the subcutis and the dermis (see Fig. 146.4). The epidermis is then closed with simple interrupted sutures of nylon or polypropylene monofilament. The size of the epidermal suture varies depending upon the site; the face is generally closed with 6-0 suture and other sites by 4-0 or 5-0 suture.

Excisional Biopsy (Excision *in toto*)

Excision represents the workhorse of dermatologic surgery[34]. The procedure is designed to remove entire lesions for histopathologic examination as well as for surgical cure. Lesions such as a clinically typical BCC or an unsightly or troublesome subepidermal lesion presumed to be benign are commonly biopsied (or excised) in this fashion (Table 146.6). Atypical pigmented lesions suspicious for melanoma are excised *in toto* as a biopsy procedure because the degree of atypia and depth of invasion may not be uniform; the excision allows the pathologist to examine the entire lesion and decreases the likelihood of sampling error. In addition, excision is frequently the treatment of choice after the diagnosis of a cutaneous malignancy has been established by a previous biopsy. The excision specimen is again submitted for histologic examination in order to confirm the diagnosis and for comment as to whether the margins of the specimen are clear of pathology. Although the basic concepts discussed above with regard to an incisional biopsy also pertain to this procedure, an excision *in toto* is more complicated because it is intended to be the final definitive procedure. Therefore, margins required for cure, as well as cosmetic and functional challenges with respect to the final scar, must be carefully considered in advance.

Recommended margins for removal of an entire lesion depend on the clinical diagnosis. Most benign lesions can be removed completely by including a 1–2 mm margin of normal-appearing skin around the circumference of the tumor. A clinically well-demarcated, small BCC or SCC is generally, though not always, cured with 4–5 mm margins[36,37]. Atypical nevi are frequently excised with 3–4 mm margins. While 4 mm may not be required for complete removal of the lesion, it may save some patients a second procedure, since it is standard practice to re-excise a nevus with moderate to severe atypia still present at the margins microscopically. The suggested margin for melanoma *in situ* (with the

EXCISION OF COMMON BENIGN CUTANEOUS LESIONS

Lesion	Comments
Epidermoid inclusion cyst	Dissection facilitated by injection of liberal amount of local anesthesia into surrounding tissue; allows surgeon to work in plane between resulting edema and cyst wall[35] Fusiform excision should include any poral opening or scarring attaching the cyst to the surface Fusiform excision may be smaller than the area deformed by the cyst, but enough of the redundant expanded tissue should be excised so that the scar lies flat
Pilar cyst	See epidermoid inclusion cyst; dissection usually easier
Lipoma	The extent can be appreciated by palpation, then marked with surgical marking pen. A linear incision is made in the middle of the skin covering the lipoma. The tumor is more firm and dense than the surrounding normal subcutaneous fat.
Dermatofibroma	Patient needs to be warned that scar may be more noticeable than original lesion, especially on the lower extremities
Melanocytic nevi	See text

Table 146.6 Excision of common benign cutaneous lesions.

possible exception of lentigo maligna, where wider margins may be required) is 5 mm. For invasive melanoma, the recommended margin depends on the Breslow depth, e.g. 1 cm margins for tumors ≤1.0 mm in depth (see Ch. 113). The depth of the defect to be created must also be planned in advance[38]. Primary closure is facilitated when the base of the surgical wound lies within subcutaneous fat. In the case of melanomas, the excision should include full-thickness skin and subcutis, with fascia at the base of the wound.

Although an excision is often referred to as an ellipse, the actual shape is fusiform (Fig. 146.10). The optimal geometry of the wound varies depending on the contour of the site and the elasticity and thickness of the skin[39]. The angle at each end of the excision varies from 30 to 75 degrees[40]. In order to minimize dog-ear formation, each side of the fusiform shape is three to four times as long as it is wide. The central axis becomes the line of closure and dictates where the surface scar will be visible. The mature scar should appear as a thin line, although some spreading may be seen on the upper trunk and shoulders. From a cosmetic standpoint, an optimal scar results when the line of closure is placed within major skin folds, skin lines with minimal tension, wrinkles, or boundaries between distinct cosmetic units[41]. Movement of underlying muscles may distort the line of closure, but this can be predicted in advance and the excision plan adjusted. For hair-bearing areas, the line of closure should follow the normal patterns of hair growth.

The process of excision and repair can be divided into a series of steps (Fig. 146.11). Local anesthesia is best obtained by injection into the subcutaneous tissue. The planned excision, which can be delineated with surgical marking dye *prior* to injection, is ringed by the anesthetic agent, with the needle pointed outward to include the area needed for undermining. After ensuring that anesthesia has developed, the site is

FUSIFORM DESIGN

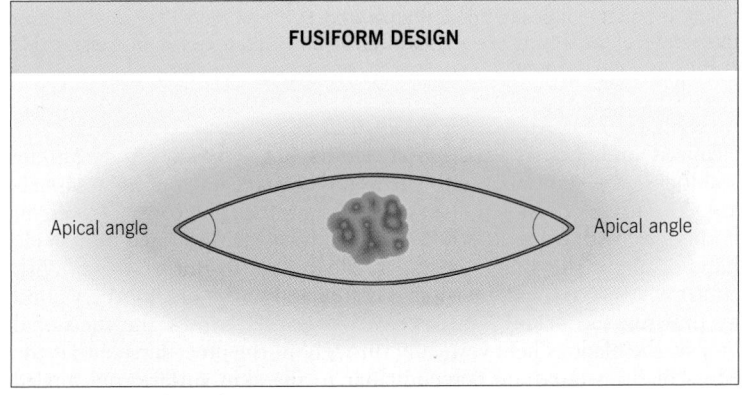

Apical angle   Apical angle

Fig. 146.10 Fusiform design.

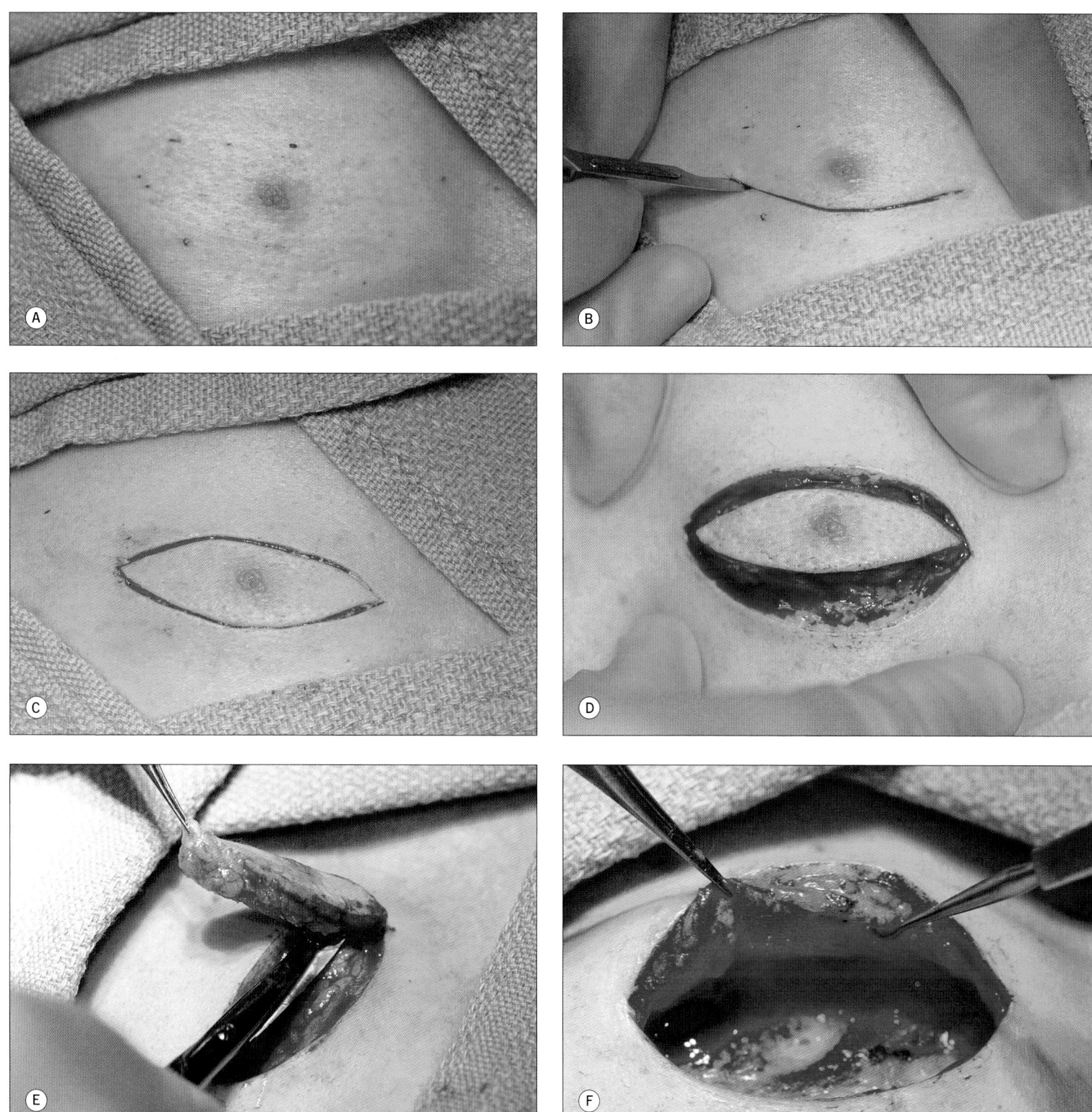

Fig. 146.11 Fusiform excision of an atypical melanocytic nevus. A After the margins are marked, the site is anesthetized, prepared with an antibacterial cleansing agent, and draped with sterile cloths. **B** Stabilizing the site with traction, the epidermis on one side of the fusiform design is scored using a no. 15 blade. **C** The epidermis on the opposite side is then scored. **D** The incision is completed into the appropriate plane in the subcutaneous tissue and the specimen then sits up in the middle of the wound like an island. **E** The base of the specimen is dissected with scissors or a blade. **F** The wound edges are then undermined in the same plane as the base of the wound.

Continued

cleansed and draped with sterile cloths. The excision is begun by stabilizing the site either with the non-dominant hand or by an assistant. As with an incisional biopsy (see above), the epidermis is scored on both sides by drawing lightly with a no. 15 blade (mounted on a blade handle) along the lines chosen to create the fusiform shape. With continued traction, the incision is completed to the base of the wound by drawing the blade with increased pressure. Unlike the incisional biopsy, the blade is held vertically throughout the procedure so that the edges of the wound are perpendicular to the skin surface, not angled inward to create a wedge. Completing the incision in one to two strokes

after scoring minimizes ragged edges. Care is taken at both apical angles to completely incise to the same depth as that reached at the center of the wound. When the fusiform incision is complete, either to the level of the subcutaneous fat or the fascial plane, the specimen sits up from its base like an island. The specimen is then dissected from the base of the wound using scissors or a blade and the specimen is transferred to the appropriate container. The end result of the excision is a fusiform-shaped wound with vertical sides and a flat even base consisting of subcutaneous fat or fascia. Hemostasis is achieved by electrocoagulation.

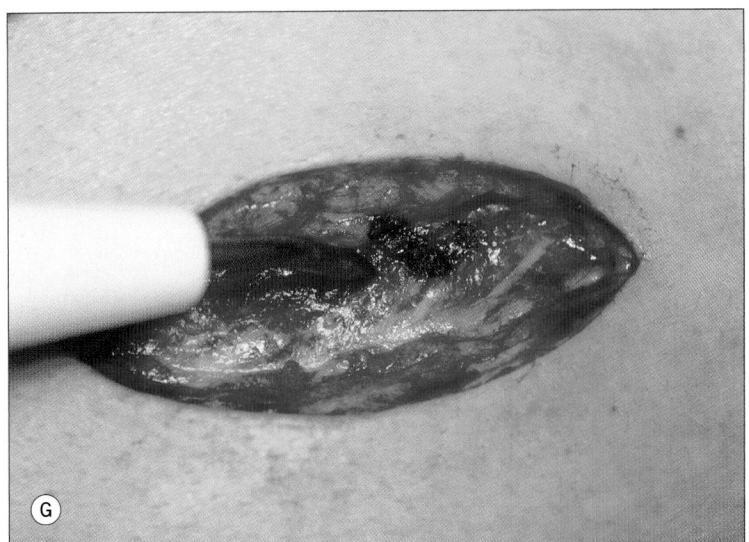

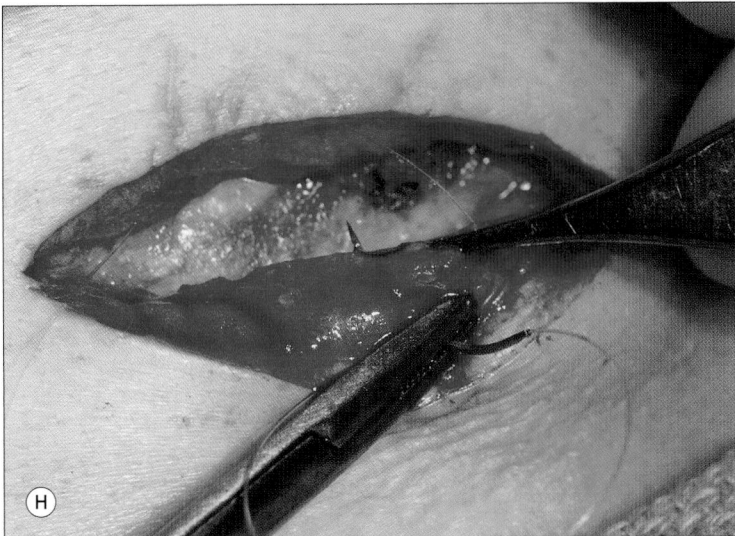

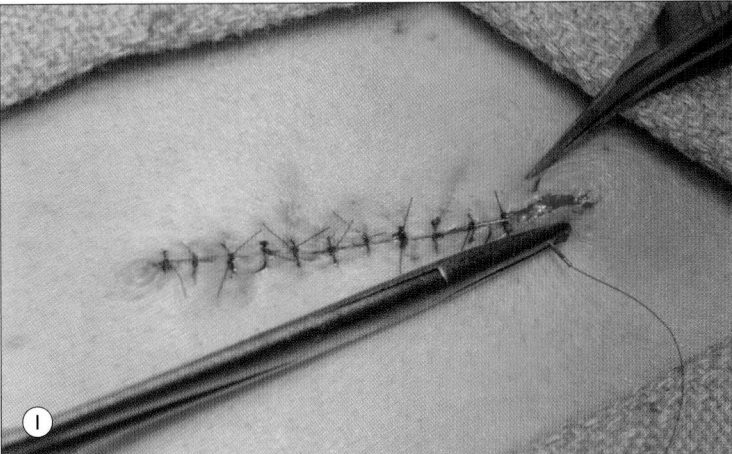

Fig. 146.11, cont'd Fusiform excision of an atypical melanocytic nevus.
G Electrodesiccation or electrocoagulation is used to address small actively bleeding vessels to achieve hemostasis. **H** The subepidermal space is closed with buried stitches. **I** The epidermal edges are opposed by simple interrupted stitches.

The remainder of the procedure deals with the creation of a cosmetically acceptable and functional closure. In order to free tissue for movement into the wound, undermining is performed at the edges of the wound with either scissors or a scalpel. A favorite technique is to use scissors with rounded tips for insertion and then spreading of the tissue to produce blunt dissection in the plane of undermining, a procedure advocated because of the belief that it is less likely to cut

arteries or nerves. Using the same scissors, but with a snipping or cutting motion to sharply dissect, is also safe and more effective in generating a smooth, less ragged unit of skin[42]. Sometimes, the two techniques are combined, with spreading followed by snipping of the intervening tethering strands. Undermining is done in a controlled fashion, and good exposure and visualization is achieved by maintaining adequate hemostasis as the dissection proceeds. Tactile confirmation of the position of the tips of the scissors is also helpful.

In order to fill the defect with skin that matches with regard to thickness, the level of undermining is almost always at the same depth as the base of the wound, i.e. within the subcutaneous fat or at the fascial plane. Rarely, when there are superficially located arteries and nerves to be avoided, the plane of undermining is more superficial than the base of the wound. The use of curved scissors with the tips pointed upwards may facilitate staying in the appropriate plane.

The goals of undermining are to mobilize a unit of skin to move into the defect[43] in order to reduce wound closure tension[44], to allow proper wound edge eversion[45], and to provide a wide area for distribution of redundant tissue over the base of the wound. Undermining around the entire wound to a distance that is at least the diameter of the wound may be required to meet these goals. When little undermining is done, opposed wound edges are pulled inward and redundant tissue bunches up in the wound bed. This redundant tissue has a force and mass that may apply pressure to the healing wound, producing a situation that allows for maturing scars to spread out (Fig. 146.12). During closure, wide undermining disperses the redundant tissue over a large area of wound bed. It may also serve to create a plate-like horizontal scar that distributes the forces of contraction and stabilizes the final result. Undermining must include the apical angles, where it facilitates the rotation that occurs as the two sides of the fusiform shape are brought together. The adequacy of the width of undermining can be tested either by picking up both wound edges with toothed forceps or skin hooks and opposing them or by placing a large temporary suture. The temporary suture may also supply some intraoperative tissue expansion that will facilitate closure. Braided polyester (e.g. Ethibond®) suture is commonly used for this purpose since it is soft and will not cut through tissue. If with these tests, the wound edges cannot be draped easily for closure, undermining can be extended.

Once undermining is adequate and after again ensuring that the wound is dry, subcutaneous and epidermal sutures are placed to complete the closure. As with the incisional biopsy, deep interrupted stitches of absorbable suture material (4-0 or 5-0 in caliber, with the knot inverted) close the subcutis and the dermis. The epidermis is then closed with simple interrupted or running sutures with a smaller caliber. For a fusiform excision *in toto*, the end result of the procedure is a straight or curved line of closure that has the wound edges completely opposed and everted. The line of closure sits above the surrounding skin, sometimes described as having the appearance of the ridge line of a tent or a mountain range. The healing of a tensionless everted wound edge results in a flat, hairline scar.

Dog-ear Repair

Closure of a fusiform excision may create dog-ears, i.e. tissue redundancies that distort the normal contour of the skin at the apical angles[46]. These dog-ears are also referred to as cutaneous cones and may consist of standing cones, lying cones, inverted cones or protruding cones (also called pitcher lip deformities because of their resemblance to the lip of a water pitcher). Inverted cones can be the most difficult to diagnose, as the appearance is that of a subtle dimple rather than a protrusion. Regardless of their subtle nature, these redundancies will distort the final scar unless they are repaired. Dog-ears are also produced by tissue movement during flap closures. Finessing both simple and flap closures demands a knowledgeable and skillful approach to the repair of dog-ears.

Dog-ears primarily result from geometric factors (Fig. 146.13). They may appear in closures of fusiform excisions (with sides of equal length) when the sides are of insufficient length compared to the width of the excision. The resulting apical angles are too wide to rotate in and maintain a flat contour to the skin surface. For this reason, linear closure of a circle, an oval or an ellipse will always create dog-ears. Dog-ears also always form during closure of fusiform shapes that have sides of

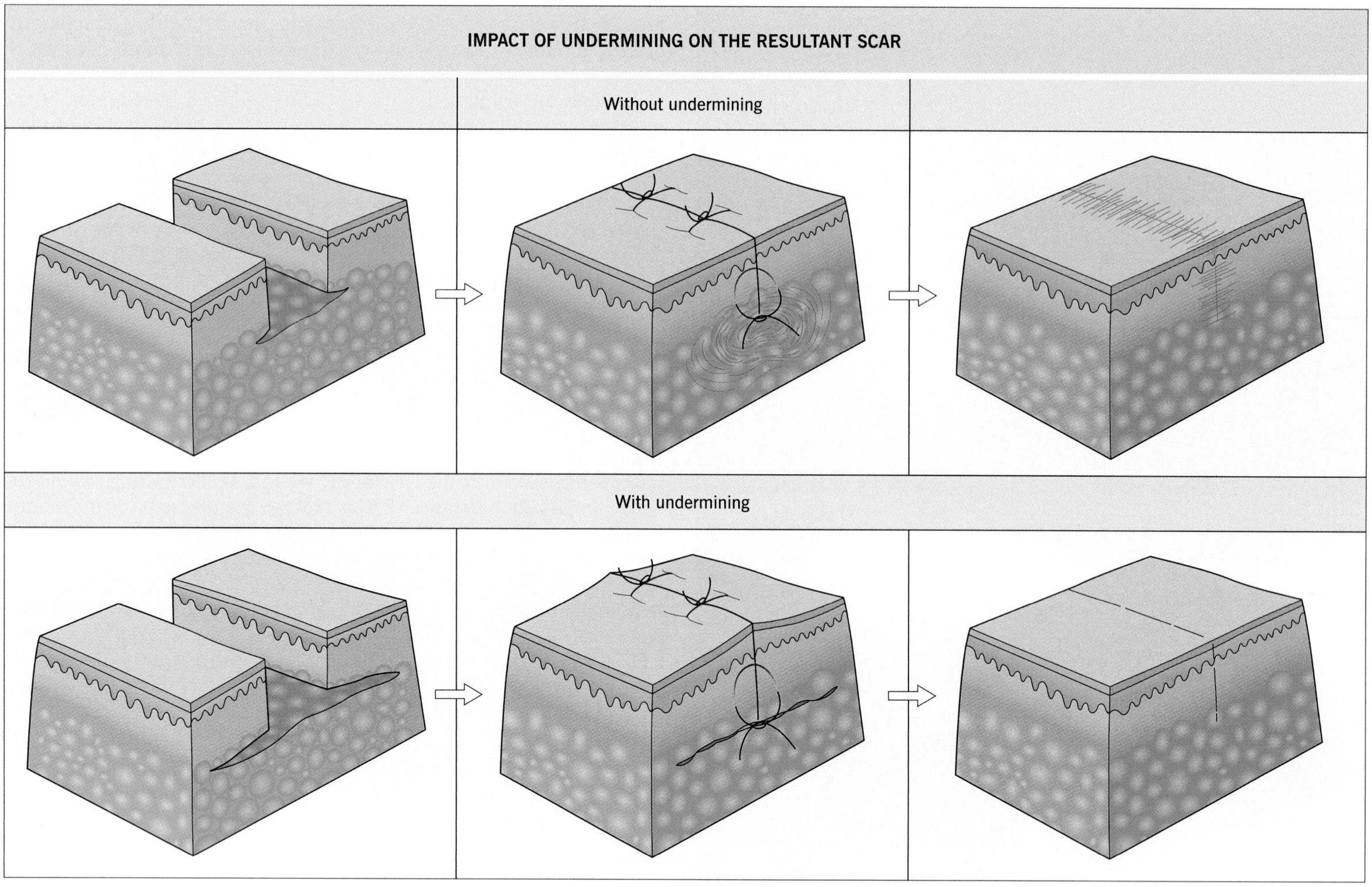

IMPACT OF UNDERMINING ON THE RESULTANT SCAR

Without undermining

With undermining

Fig. 146.12 Impact of undermining on the resultant scar. Without undermining, there is tension on the wound and eversion of the wound edges does not occur. Another consequence is spreading of the scar.

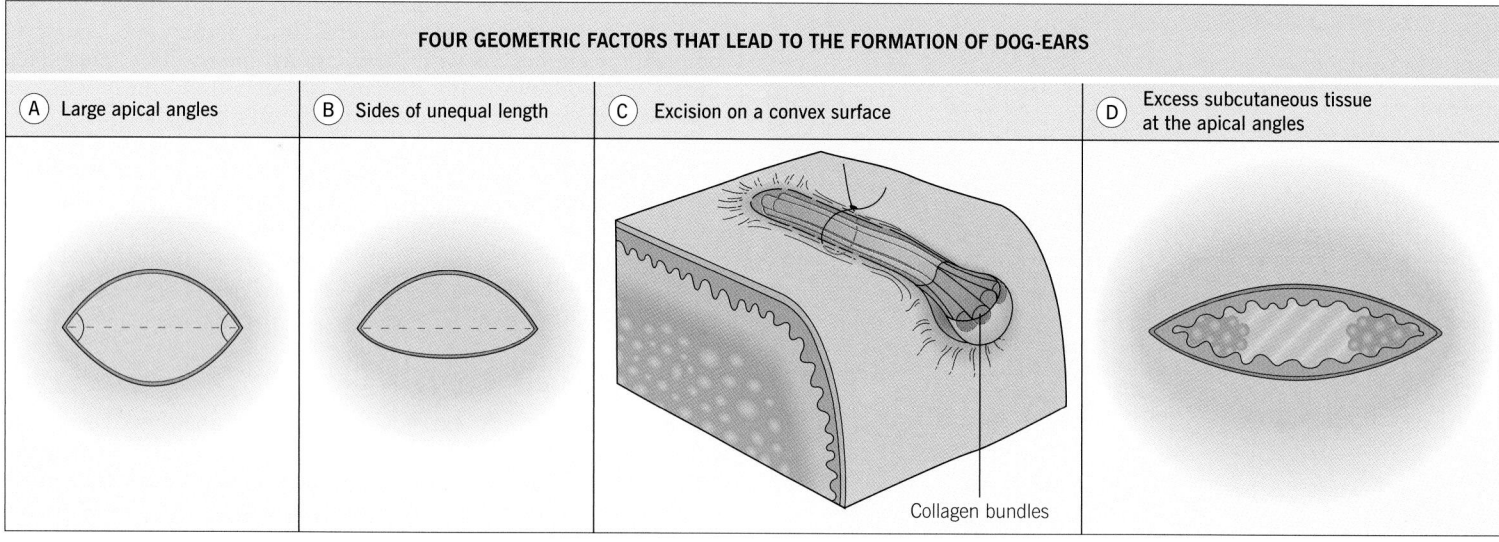

FOUR GEOMETRIC FACTORS THAT LEAD TO THE FORMATION OF DOG-EARS

| (A) Large apical angles | (B) Sides of unequal length | (C) Excision on a convex surface | (D) Excess subcutaneous tissue at the apical angles |

Collagen bundles

Fig. 146.13 Four geometric factors that lead to the formation of dog-ears.

unequal length; redundant tissue becomes apparent on the longer side. Notably, when an excision is performed on a convex surface, dog-ears may occur despite seemingly small apical angles. With suture placement, collagen bundles are pulled together and act as rigid rods that will not lie flat on a curved surface.

In addition to geometric forces, protrusions are produced when there is excessive subcutaneous tissue in the base of the wound at the apices (as compared to the center of the wound). A lack of adequate undermining at the apices will then magnify these protrusions. This process is usually called 'boating' or 'pseudo dog-ear' formation. It is important to distinguish boating from true dog-ear formation because repair of the former requires removal of the excess subcutaneous tissue and appropriate undermining as opposed to the techniques described below.

Many dog-ears are small and can be repaired via a closure that employs the rule of halves (Fig. 146.14). The midpoint of each side is opposed with a suture, bisecting the wound. Each unclosed half is then bisected again and the closure is continued until all tissue has been opposed. For a fusiform shape with unequal sides, repair of dog-ears in this manner produces a curved line of closure. The curvature is directly proportional to the size of the dog-ear such that a small dog-ear produces a slight curvature and a larger dog-ear produces a more pronounced curve. If the wound is in a site such as the forehead, which lacks loose tissue to free

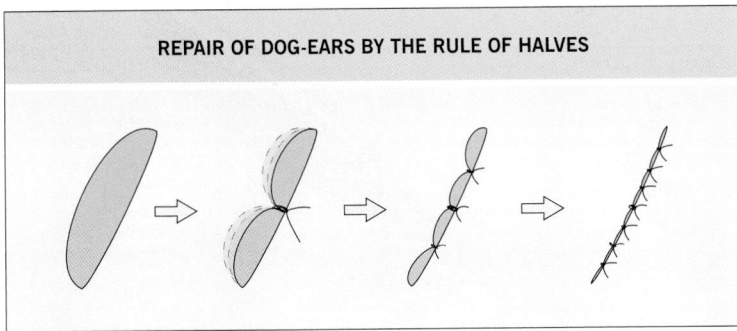

Fig. 146.14 Repair of dog-ears by the rule of halves.

up and mobilize, the line of closure may remain straight; however, there will be noticeable gathering on one side of the line and a depressed contour on the opposite side of the line where the skin thinned as it was stretched to fit.

Simple straight, curvilinear or angled excisions of dog-ears will also restore the desired contour of the site, even though they lengthen the scar (Fig. 146.15). The first step is to close the center portion of the wound with subcutaneous sutures. It is helpful to continue to oppose subcutaneous tissue from the center of the wound outward until the dog-ears become visible. Epidermal sutures may also need to be placed since any gaping at the center of the wound will underestimate the size of the dog-ears. After undermining, one limb of the dog-ear is cut through to

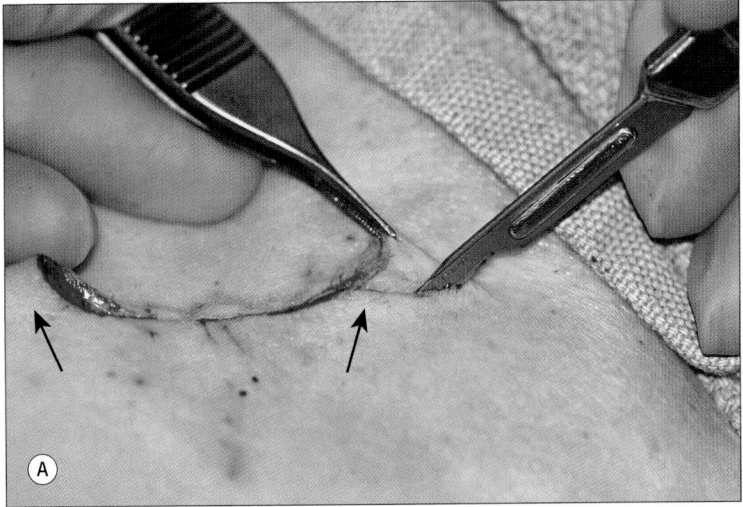

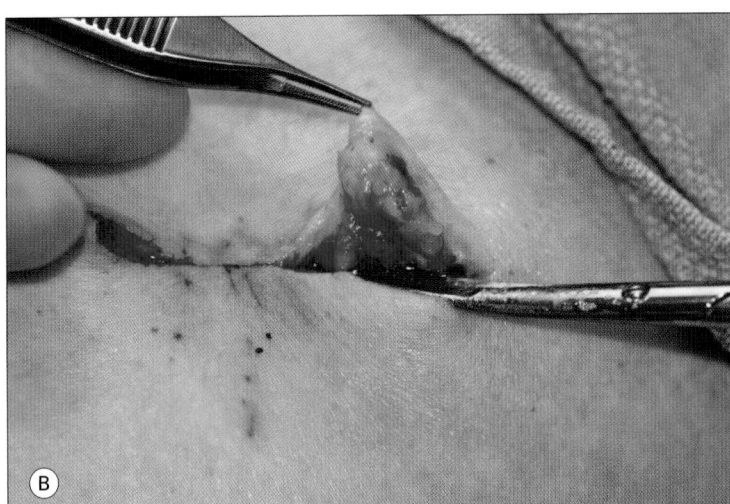

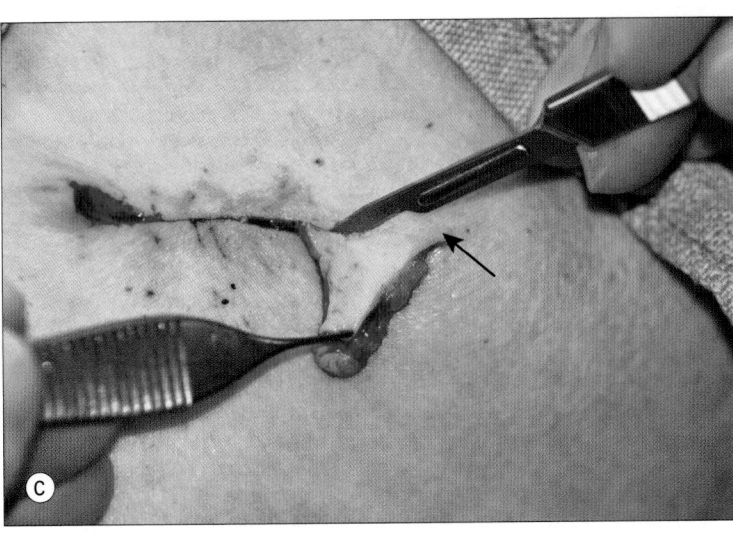

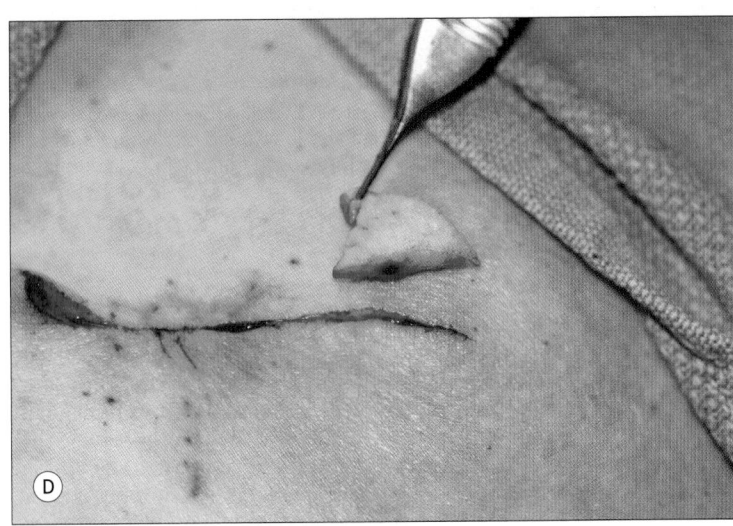

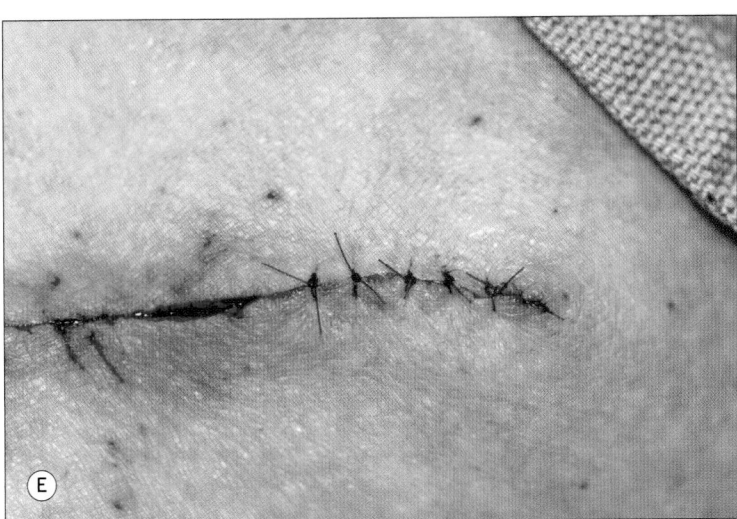

Fig. 146.15 Repair of dog-ears by straight excision. A Dog-ears are protrusions that form at each end during closure of a disc-shaped defect (arrows). The first limb of the dog-ear is incised to the subcutaneous compartment by scissors or a blade. **B** The wound is undermined beneath the entire dog-ear in the same plane as the rest of the defect. **C** The undermined dog-ear is draped over the incision; the arrow indicates the apex which lies flat against the underlying skin surface. Scissors or a blade is used to complete the excision of the second limb of the dog-ear. **D** The redundant tissue removed is in the shape of a triangle, often called a Burow's triangle. **E** Subcutaneous and epidermal sutures are placed to complete the closure.

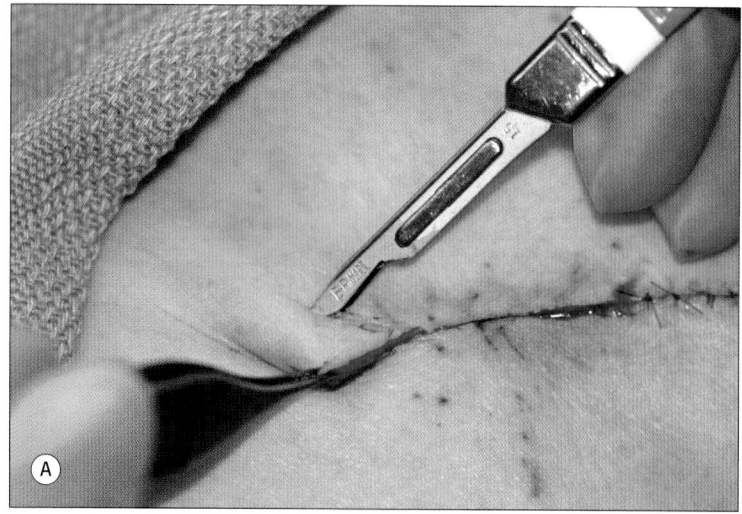
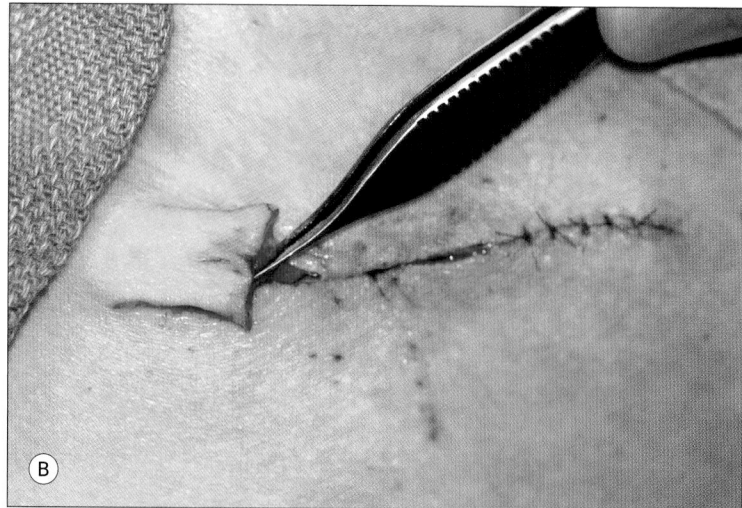
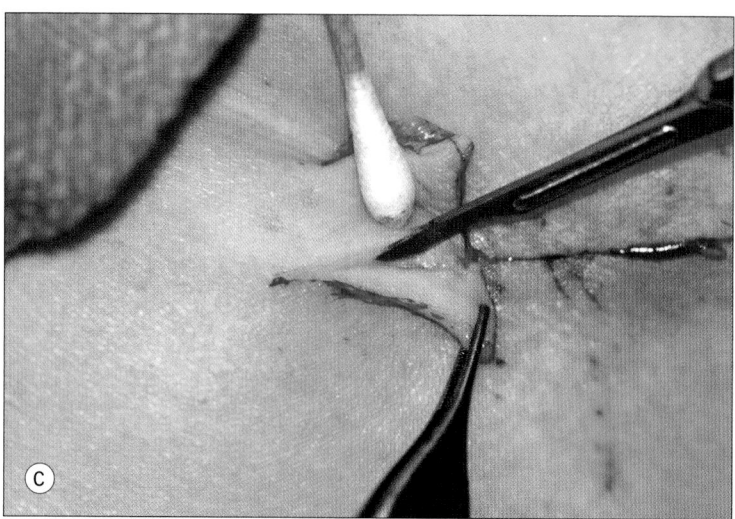
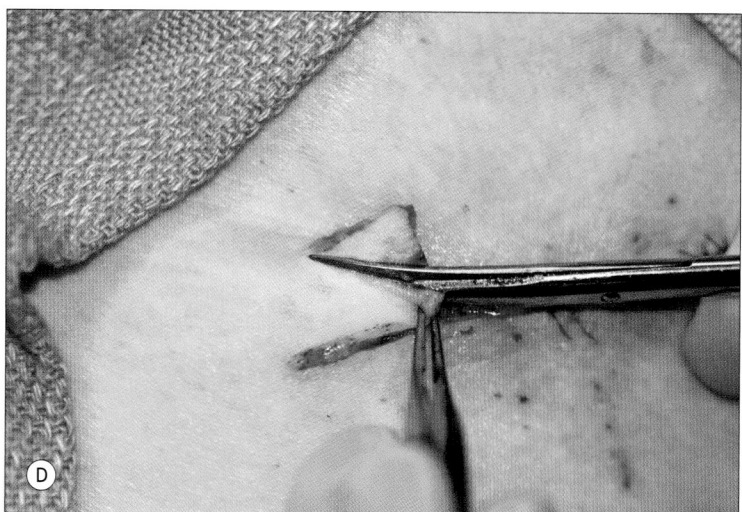

Fig. 146.16 Repair of dog-ears by M-plasty. A Each limb of the dog-ear is cut at a 30–45° angle from the end of the wound to about halfway toward the apex of the redundancy. **B** After both limbs are cut and the wound is fully undermined beneath the dog-ear, the redundant tissue can be draped over the incision. At this point, an M is visible. **C** A Burow's triangle is removed from half of the draped tissue. **D** A second Burow's triangle is excised from the opposite side of the draped tissue.

Continued

the base of the wound along the line that is desired for final closure. Undermining is repeated until the excess tissue can be draped over the cut edge. The new apical angle will lie flat if the limb has been adequately cut and if undermining has been sufficient. The second limb of the dog-ear is then addressed by cutting from the wound to the new apical angle. The excess tissue that is removed will be in the shape of a triangle that is referred to as Burow's triangle[47]. An alternative method, helpful for novices wanting to create a straight closure, is bisection of the dog-ear, laying each half out along the skin surface and then cutting the two triangles of excess tissue. Closure is then completed with subcutaneous and epidermal sutures.

An M-plasty is a dog-ear repair that shortens the total scar length (Fig. 146.16). Depending upon the site, M-plasty scars may also fit within prominent lines and folds more accurately. This procedure is particularly helpful in sites that are not flat. The first step, as above, is to close the center portion of the wound and adequately undermine the apical angle. Both lateral limbs are cut at an obtuse angle from the end of the wound to about halfway toward the apex of the redundancy. The excess tissue is then draped over the cut edge and an M is now apparent. Cutting from the central tip to the two new apical angles removes two pieces of tissue that are also triangular in shape. The area of these two triangles is equal to the area of the single triangle that would have been removed had a simple excision of the dog-ear been performed. If the central tip lies in a good position, then a standard closure is performed. If the tip needs to be advanced to approximate the wound edges and fill the defect, a three-corner stitch is used. Care must be taken with the three-corner stitch, as necrosis of the tip can occur with too much tension[48].

A dog-ear may also be displaced to a distant site. After closure of the central portion of the wound, an incision is made perpendicular to the dog-ear to an appropriate site where there is enough redundant tissue such that it can be removed as a triangle (Fig. 146.17). Undermining is required over a wide area so that tissue can be moved without tension. This procedure is also referred to as a Burow's advancement flap (see Ch. 147). It is commonly used to avoid dog-ear repair in a free margin or in a cosmetically or functionally sensitive area.

Finessing closure of fusiform excisions may require changing the axis of the line of closure so that the scar blends better with the prominent lines and folds of the site. Changing the axis will produce dog-ears that can be repaired by any of these methods.

VARIATIONS/UNUSUAL SITUATIONS

A disc excision (with straight or angled edges) may be performed for either biopsy purposes or for biopsy and definitive treatment. This option is chosen when healing by secondary intention is preferred[49] or when it is desirable to remove the tumor first and then repair the dog-ears during the closure. Secondary intention healing may be advantageous when the risk of adverse reactions with primary closure is high. For example, excisions of even small tumors on the anterior lower leg that are closed primarily can produce wounds with tension and wounds that are more likely than those at other sites to dehisce, become infected or be painful. This is especially true if undermining is inadequate and weight-bearing is not minimized for the first 5–7 postoperative days (including, at times, the use of crutches). Another option for wounds with too much tension in this location is the placement of a skin graft,

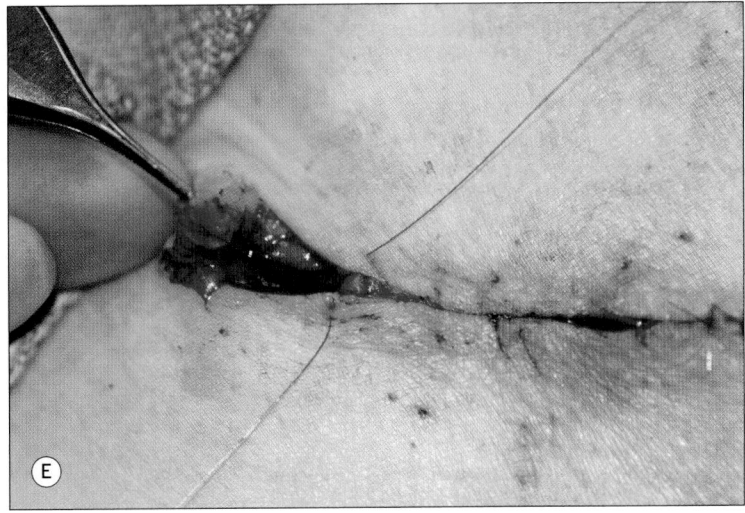

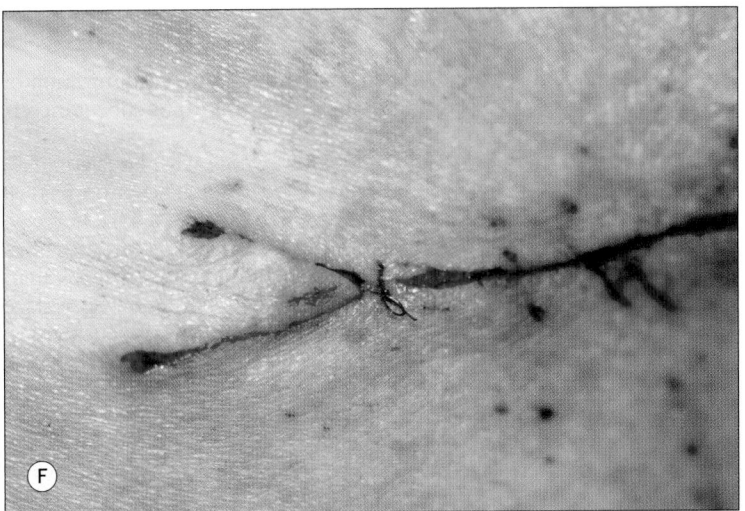

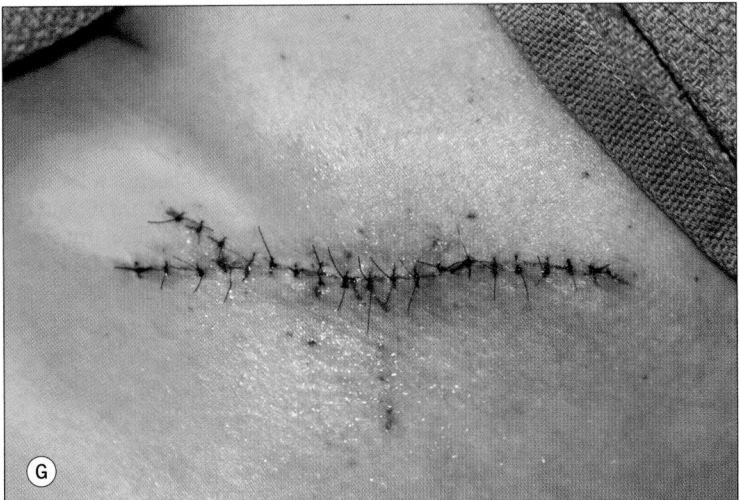

Fig. 146.16, cont'd Repair of dog-ears by M-plasty. E A corner stitch is used to pull the point of the M-plasty into appropriate position. The needle enters the epidermis proximal to the expected position of the point, passes into the dermis, crosses the wound and enters the dermis of the tip. It then passes horizontally through the dermis of the tip, crosses the wound again, enters the opposite dermis and passes to the epidermal surface. **F** The knot of the corner stitch lies across the wound proximal to the position of the point of the M-plasty. **G** The closure can then be completed and the sutured wound lies flat.

but postoperative care requires leg elevation and the absolute avoidance of weight-bearing.

When these wounds heal by secondary intention, postoperative care is less burdensome, as the patient may resume normal activities almost immediately while dressing and bandaging the wound daily. However, compared to a linear excision, re-epithelialization requires a significantly

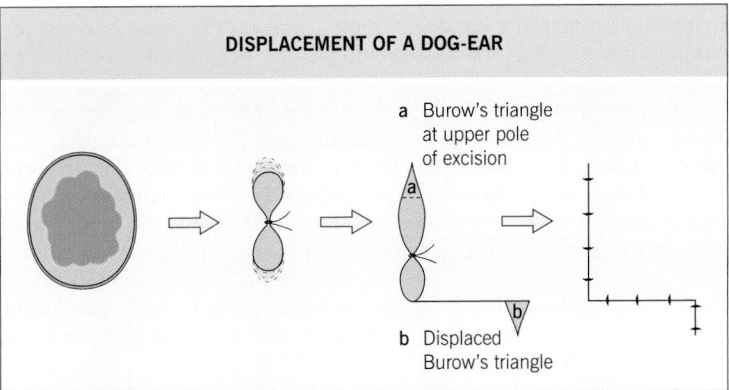

Fig. 146.17 Displacement of a dog-ear.

longer period of time; the latter varies directly with the size of the tumor and can range from 2 weeks to at least 2 months on the distal lower extremities. The patient also needs to consider the resultant scar, i.e. a depressed circular scar versus a graft versus a linear scar.

Removal of melanocytic nevi on the upper trunk and shoulders via disc excision or saucerization (angled edges) results in a smaller, often more cosmetically acceptable scar than does a fusiform excision. Also, the excision of tumors in sites such as the ear may be amenable to disc excision followed by secondary intention healing.

Performing a disc excision and then repairing the dog-ears during the closure allows the surgeon to pay particular attention to the issue of appropriate curative margins without dealing simultaneously with the cosmetic and functional issues of the closure. Once the tumor has been removed and the area widely undermined, the line of closure can be determined, that is, the closure with the least amount of tension that fits into the dominant lines of the site[50,51]. The central portion of the wound is opposed by subcutaneous and epidermal sutures or by a large simple interrupted temporary suture and then the dog-ears are repaired. Since the cosmetic and functional issues are addressed after excision of the tumor and undermining, the resulting scar can be optimized.

POSTOPERATIVE CARE

Wound care and bandaging both play an important role in minimizing the risk of complications and in obtaining optimal cosmetic and functional results. Wound care removes surface debris and promotes re-epithelialization. A good bandage supports and stabilizes the wound in the closed position, wicks away excessive blood or tissue fluid, supplies pressure to the wound for hemostasis, and protects the wound from the dryness and bacterial contamination of the external environment.

A small shallow wound that is supposed to heal by secondary intention is cared for by daily cleansing of the site with mild soap and water, application of an antibiotic ointment or petrolatum, and coverage with an adhesive bandage such as a Band-Aid® (with a central non-adherent area). A newly formulated liquid adhesive bandage has been reported to also be effective, and, in a trial on minor cuts and abrasions, proved easy to use[52]. A large shallow wound that is to close by secondary intention may need a bandage fashioned specifically for that site, usually consisting of layers of antibiotic ointment or petrolatum, Telfa®, gauze or cotton, and tape or other means of adhering the bandage at the site.

A layered bandage is also required for a sutured wound. A liquid adhesive (e.g. Mastisol®) is applied to the skin surface surrounding the sutures. An antibiotic ointment or petrolatum is applied in a thin line onto the wound edge. Sterile tapes such as Steri-Strips™ are placed perpendicular to the line of closure. The final layer is rolled gauze or cotton, which is then taped in place with paper tape or Hy-Tape® ('pink' tape). Elastic dressing (e.g. Coban®) can be used for compression, but should be released and reapplied if it is used circumferentially, so that vascular compromise distally does not occur.

Patients need oral and written instructions regarding the care the wound will require at home. Most simple wounds are cleansed daily with soap and water and redressed until the sutures are removed or the wound has completely re-epithelialized. Patients should understand that they need to remove any crusting or debris from the wound as they cleanse it and they may prefer to use cotton-tipped swabs or gauze.

Instructions regarding bandages should likewise be clear. Leaving the wound open to the air or allowing it to become dry retards re-epithelialization and may compromise the final appearance or the scar[53].

Bandages that minimize the need for wound care are preferred by many patients. In addition, the stability and protection afforded by a bandage that stays in place for a week or more may further optimize the results, especially for wounds closed primarily. These bandages may be constructed in layers as discussed above and should be kept dry to prevent maceration of the covered skin. On the trunk and extremities, a bandage can be made of a polyurethane foam dressing (e.g. Cutinova Hydro®) covered by a water repellent film (e.g. Bioclusive®), precluding the need for any care and allowing ease of movement and a normal regimen for bathing.

Once the sutures have been removed and the wound cleaned, the use of liquid adhesive and sterile tapes for another week or two further stabilizes the wound. Many specialized bandaging systems are available for complicated wounds (see Ch. 145).

COMPLICATIONS

Short-term complications of biopsies and excisions are few in number and generally engender limited morbidity (Table 146.7)[54]. In addition, the smaller the procedure, the fewer the complications, which explains why shave biopsies and snip biopsies are quite safe. Hemorrhage may occur, from the time of the procedure to afterwards when the patient has returned home, and it usually occurs within the first 24 hours. Although many patients take aspirin, warfarin or other agents that affect coagulation or platelet function, hemostasis can be achieved during the procedure, resulting in few adverse bleeding events[55].

Infection occurs rarely, in less than 1% of most procedures[56]. Some patients have difficulty with either irritant or allergic reactions to topical antibiotics[57] or to tapes and bandages. These often pruritic eruptions are managed with a change in the wound care regimen but do not usually require topical corticosteroid creams. Biopsies performed on the lower limbs, limbs affected by lymphedema, intertriginous areas, and ears are most susceptible to infections, but this complication is minimized by appropriate wound care. If an infection develops, oral antibiotics may be required.

Pain is generally minimal. When it occurs 3–5 days after the procedure, infection is the most likely cause, even in the absence of erythema, tenderness and purulence. Very rarely, paresthesias may result and can persist for several months, especially on the forehead. Wounds that are closed primarily may dehisce either because of tension, poor wound healing or infection. These wounds are thereafter managed for secondary intention healing and a delayed reconstruction can be undertaken, if needed, when the attendant inflammation has resolved.

Long-term complications (see Table 146.7) generally consist of functionally or cosmetically adverse scarring[58]. Depressed scars may occur if not enough subcutaneous tissue is brought into the line of closure. Atrophic and widened scars occur in areas where there is intermittent stretching of the scar as it overlies major muscle groups. Careful

---

SHORT-TERM AND LONG-TERM COMPLICATIONS OF BIOPSY PROCEDURES AND EXCISIONS

Short-term complications

- Irritant or allergic reactions to topical antibiotics and/or tapes and bandages
- Hemorrhage
- Poor wound healing; dehiscence of closed wounds
- Pain
- Infection
- Pruritus, paresthesias

Long-term complications

- Atrophic scars (thin, depressed, spread)
- Hypertrophic scars (red, thickened)
- Keloids
- Distortion of normal structures (e.g. ectropion, elevated nasal ala, notching of helix of the ear)
- Hypoesthesia, anesthesia
- Paralysis (e.g. due to injury to facial nerve branches)

Table 146.7 Short-term and long-term complications of biopsy procedures and excisions.

---

surgical technique that includes adequate undermining, minimization of tension at the line of closure and the use of multiple subcutaneous sutures can minimize this complication.

Scars may pursue a prolonged course of healing with erythematous thickening at the line of closure. These hypertrophic scars do resolve with time. To speed their resolution, practitioners often advise massage or inject triamcinolone (10–40 mg/ml) into the scars. Silicone dressings are also recommended, but they are probably no more effective than non-silicone gel dressings[59]. In addition, scars may have a fragile surface (due to reduced dermal–epidermal attachments), pruritus or paresthesias, most of which resolve with time.

A true keloidal scar is one that grows beyond the boundaries of the original surgical injury and appears as a thickened erythematous or hyperpigmented nodule or plaque (see Ch. 98). It occurs in predisposed individuals who may have a history of previous keloid formation. Keloidal scarring is most commonly observed when procedures are performed on the upper trunk and shoulders and may be very difficult to treat.

FUTURE TRENDS

For the foreseeable future, histologic examination of tissue specimens will be the mainstay of dermatologic diagnostic testing. Excisions likewise will be frequently utilized, both to remove a specimen for diagnosis as well as to clear pathologic tissue completely. Future near-term advances will include improved means of anesthesia[60] and improved wound care with the development of agents to speed healing and minimize scarring. It is possible that advances in confocal laser microscopy may visualize *in situ* microscopic tissue architecture and cellular detail, but it is unlikely that this process will replace standard biopsy techniques.

REFERENCES

1. Salopek TG, Slade J, Marghoob AA, et al. Management of cutaneous malignant melanoma by dermatologists of the American Academy of Dermatology. I. Survey of biopsy practices of pigmented lesions suspected as melanoma. J Am Acad Dermatol. 1995;33:441–50.
2. Messingham MJ, Arpey CJ. Update on the use of antibiotics in cutaneous surgery. Dermatol Surg. 2005;31:1068–78.
3. Dajani AS, Taubert KA, Wilson W, et al. Prevention of bacterial endocarditis. Recommendations by the American Heart Association. JAMA. 1997;277:1794–801.
4. Meyer GW, Artis AL. Antibiotic prophylaxis for orthopedic prostheses and GI procedures: report of a survey. Am J Gastroenterol. 1997;92:989–91.
5. Classen DC, Evans RS, Pestotnik SL, et al. The timing of prophylactic administration of antibiotics and the risk of surgical wound infection. N Engl J Med. 1992;326:281–6.
6. Sebben JE. Surgical antiseptics. J Am Acad Dermatol. 1983;9:759–65.

7. Koay J, Orengo I. Application of local anesthetics in dermatology surgery. Dermatol Surg. 2002;28:143–8.
8. Dzubow LM. The interaction between propranolol and epinephrine as observed in patients undergoing Mohs surgery. J Am Acad Dermatol. 1986;15:71–5.
9. Eggleston ST, Lush LW. Understanding allergic reactions to local anesthetics. Ann Pharmacother. 1996;30:851–7.
10. Arndt KA, Burton C, Noe JM. Minimizing the pain of local anesthesia. Plast Reconstr Surg. 1983;72:676–9.
11. Stewart JH, Cole GW, Klein JA. Neutralized lidocaine with epinephrine for local anesthesia. J Dermatol Surg Oncol. 1989;15:1081–3.
12. Kuwahara RT, Skinner RB. EMLA versus ice as a topical anesthetic. Dermatol Surg. 2001;27:495–6.
13. Eidelman A, Weiss JM, Lau J, et al. Topical anesthetics for dermal instrumentation: a systematic review of randomized, controlled trials. Ann Emerg Med. 2005;46:343–51.

14. Lui S, Carpenter RL, Chiu AA, et al. Epinephrine prolongs duration of subcutaneous infiltration of local anesthesia in a dose related manner. Reg Anesth. 1995;20:378–84.
15. Armstrong RB, Nickhols J, Pachance J. Punch biopsy wounds treated with Monsel's solution or a collagen matrix: a comparison of healing. Arch Dermatol. 1988;122:546–9.
16. El-Gamal HM, Dufresne RG, Saddler K. Electrosurgery, pacemakers and ICDs. Dermatol Surg. 2001;27:385–90.
17. Baum CL, Arpey CJ. Normal cutaneous wound healing: clinical correlation with cellular and molecular events. Dermatol Surg. 2005;31:674–86.
18. Perry AW, McShane RH. Fine tuning of the skin edges in the closure of surgical wounds: controlling inversion and eversion with the path of the needle. J Dermatol Surg Oncol. 1981;7:471–6.
19. Annunziata CC, Drake DB, Woods JA, et al. Technical considerations in knot construction. J Emerg Med. 1997;15:351–6.

20. Zitelli JA, Moy RL. Buried vertical mattress suture. J Dermatol Surg Oncol. 1989;15:17–19.
21. Krunic AL, Weitzul S, Taylor RS. Running combined simple and vertical mattress suture: a rapid skin-everting stitch. Dermatol Surg. 2005;31:325–9.
22. Wong NL. Review of continuous sutures in dermatology surgery. J Dermatol Surg Oncol. 1993;19:923–31.
23. Bunker TD. Problems with the use of Op-Site sutureless skin closures in orthopedics procedures. Ann R Coll Surg Engl. 1983;65:260–2.
24. Hodges JM. Management of facial lacerations. South Med J. 1976;69:1413–18.
25. Niyama T, Higuchi I, Sakoda S, et al. Diagnosis of dystrophinopathy by skin biopsy. Muscle Nerve 2002;25:398–401.
26. Prasa A, Kaye EM, Alroy J. Electron microscopic examination of skin biopsy as a cost-effective tool in the diagnosis of lysosomal storage diseases. J Child Neurol. 1996;11:301–8.
27. Kennard CD, Rasmussen JE. Congenital midline nasal masses: diagnosis and management. J Dermatol Surg Oncol. 1990;16:1025–36.
28. Baldwin HE, Berck CM, Lynfield YL. Subcutaneous nodules of the scalp: preoperative management. J Am Acad Dermatol. 1991;25:819–30.
29. Chang LK, Whitaker DC. The impact of herbal medicines on dermatologic surgery. Dermatol Surg. 2001;27:759–63.
30. Heck AM, De Witt BA, Lukes AL. Potential interactions between alternative therapies and warfarin. Am J Health Syst Pharm. 2000;57:1221–7.
31. Richards KA, Stasko T. Dermatology surgery and the pregnant patient. Dermatol Surg. 2002;28:248–56.
32. Harvey DT, Fenske NA. The razor blade biopsy technique. Dermatol Surg. 1995;21:345–7.
33. Todd P, Garioch JJ, Humphreys S, et al. Evaluation of the 2-mm punch biopsy in dermatological diagnosis. Clin Exp Dermatol. 1996;21:11–13.

34. Dunlavey E, Leshin B. The simple excision. Dermatol Clin 1998;16:49–64.
35. Salasche SJ, Giancola JM, Trookman NS. Surgical pearl: hydroexpansion with local anesthesia. J Am Acad Dermatol. 1995;33:510–12.
36. Wolf DJ, Zitelli JA. Surgical margins for basal cell carcinoma. Arch Dermatol. 1987;123:340–4.
37. Brodland DG, Zitelli JA. Surgical margins for excision of primary cutaneous squamous cell carcinoma. J Am Acad Dermatol. 1992;27:241–8.
38. Takenouchi T, Nomoto S, Ito M. Factors influencing the linear depth of invasion of primary basal cell carcinoma. Dermatol Surg. 2001;27:393–6.
39. Chretien-Marquet B, Caillou V, Brasnu DN, et al. Description of cutaneous excision and suture using a mathematical model. Plast Reconstr Surg. 1999;103:145–50.
40. Moody BR, McCarthy JE, Sengelmann RD. The apical angle: a mathematical analysis of the ellipse. Dermatol Surg. 2001;27:61–3.
41. Bernstein G. Lines of elective incision on the skin. In: Lask GP, Moy RL (eds). Principles and Techniques of Cutaneous Surgery. New York: McGraw-Hill, 1996:209–20.
42. Boyer JD, Zitelli JA, Brodland DG. Undermining in cutaneous surgery. Dermatol Surg. 2001;27:75–8.
43. Mackay DR, Saggers GC, Kotwal N, et al. Stretching skin: undermining is more important than intraoperative tissue expansion. Plast Reconstr Surg. 1990;86:722–30.
44. McGuire MF. Studies of the excisional wound: I. Biomechanical effects of undermining and wound orientation on closing tension and work. Plast Reconstr Surg. 1980;66:419–27.
45. Zitelli, JA. Tips for a better ellipse. J Am Acad Dermatol. 1990;22:101–3.
46. Gormley DE. The dog-ear: causes, prevention, and correction. J Dermatol Surg Oncol. 1977;3:194–8.

47. Gormley DE. A brief analysis of the Burow's wedge/triangle principle. J Dermatol Surg Oncol. 1985;11:121–3.
48. Stegman SJ. Suturing techniques for dermatology surgery. J Dermatol Surg Oncol. 1978;4:63–9.
49. Zitelli JA. Wound healing by secondary intention. A cosmetic appraisal. J Am Acad Dermatol. 1983;9:407–15.
50. Davis TS. The circular excision. Ann Plast Surg. 1980;4:21–5.
51. Spicer TE. Techniques of facial lesion excision and closure. J Dermatol Surg Oncol. 1982;8:551–6.
52. Eaglstein WH, Sullivan TP, Giordano PA, et al. A liquid adhesive bandage for the treatment of minor cuts and abrasions. Dermatol Surg. 2002;28:263–7.
53. Eaglstein WH. Moist wound healing with occlusive dressings: a clinical focus. Dermatol Surg. 2001;27:175–81.
54. Salasche SJ. Acute surgical complications: cause, prevention and treatment. J Am Acad Dermatol. 1986;15:1163–85.
55. Otley C, Olbricht SM, Frank EW, et al. Risks of perioperative anticoagulation in dermatologic surgery. Arch Dermatol. 1996;132:161–5.
56. Futoryan T, Grande D. Postoperative wound infection rates in dermatology surgery. Dermatol Surg. 1995;21:509–14.
57. Gette MT, Marks JC, Maloney ME. Frequency of postoperative allergic contact dermatitis to topical antibiotics. Arch Dermatol. 1992;128:365–7.
58. Hayes CM, Whitaker DC. Complications of cutaneous surgery. Adv Dermatol. 1994;9:161–77.
59. De Oliveira GV, Nunes TA, Magna LA, et al. Silicone versus nonsilicone gel dressings: a controlled trial. Dermatol Surg. 2001;27:721–6.
60. Greenbaum SS. Iontophoresis as a tool for anesthesia in dermatologic surgery: an overview. Dermatol Surg. 2001;27:1027–30.

Flaps

David G Brodland and David Pharis

Key features

- A cookbook approach to flap reconstruction is not realistic
- The mnemonic STARTS lists basic reconstruction options: simple side-to-side closures, transposition flaps, advancement flaps, rotation flaps, tissue importation flaps and skin grafts
- The KISS principle (keep it simple, stupid!) indicates that the least complex approach that achieves the desired result is often best
- Extensive undermining, everted wound edges, meticulous hemostasis without excessive electrocoagulation, and technical precision are important in achieving an outstanding result

INTRODUCTION

Cutaneous reconstruction has played an important role in the establishment of dermatologic surgery as a vital discipline within dermatology. An in-depth understanding of reconstructive options, combined with a dermatologist's intimate familiarity with skin, enables optimal aesthetic and functional results. Equally important is an intimate understanding of the tissue dynamics of flaps, why they work, what problems each flap type can address, and their limitations. A cookbook approach to flap reconstruction is not realistic because of the many variables relating to the characteristics of the defect, the donor skin, the patient and the surgeon. It is better to attempt to provide a foundation of basic concepts from which the individual can build his or her skills and, hopefully, his or her unique style in reconstruction. Therefore, this chapter will emphasize the fundamentals of the various types of flaps and their execution. Clinical examples will be used to illustrate these key points.

BACKGROUND

At the patient's side, it is always helpful to have an on-demand recall of the flap options that are available. With experience, this is automatic, but those with less experience may find the mnemonic STARTS helpful (Table 147.1). The basic options for reconstruction include: simple side-to-side closures, transposition flaps, advancement flaps, rotation flaps, tissue importation flaps and skin grafts. It is incumbent upon the surgeon to synthesize the many factors that may affect the choice of the most appropriate flap for a defect. The characteristics of the wound, qualities of the adjacent skin, the functional aspects of the affected anatomic site, the pertinent aesthetic considerations, the anatomic borders in proximity to the defect, and the age and expectations of the patient all contribute to the decision regarding the most appropriate reconstructive approach.

STARTS MNEMONIC
Simple side-to-side closure
Transposition flaps
Advancement flaps
Rotation flaps
Tissue importation flaps
Skin grafts

Table 147.1 STARTS mnemonic.

The most important goal in reconstruction is functional aesthetics. This means that the reconstruction should first and foremost maintain all vital functions and accomplish this with an aesthetic result. It should be remembered that not all aesthetic reconstructions are functional, but all functional reconstructions can be aesthetic.

Fundamentals of Flap Design and Suturing Technique

Technical precision may be the most important variable in achieving an outstanding result. Accomplished reconstructive surgeons with meticulously precise suturing techniques are able to achieve outstanding and nearly imperceptible results, irrespective of the defect presented to them or which flap they use to reconstruct it. On the other hand, surgeons with poor technique may achieve average or poor results using the same flap in similar situations. Suturing techniques are often underemphasized, but will be covered here as an essential component of flap reconstruction.

The first important step is to prepare the wound edges of both the defect and the flap. All incisions should be made at a 90° angle to the skin surface such that the wall of the defect and the skin edge of the flap are square. Secondly, the wound base should be made a uniform depth. Whether reconstructing with an elliptical side-to-side closure or with any of the more intricate flaps, the contour of the wound base will persist and may affect the long-term appearance of the wound. Likewise, the thickness of the flap should be uniform. While the thickness of the flap relative to the depth of the defect merits some consideration, care should be taken when considering the use of a flap with a thick subcutaneous tissue component, since these flaps are much more prone to postoperative edema and 'pincushioning'. Nevertheless, all components of the flap should be fashioned with uniformity in mind.

Widespread undermining of the subcutaneous tissue adjacent to both the defect and the donor site defect is important for creating a broad 'plate-like scar'. This results in the distribution of scar contraction over a greater area and diffuses the effects of contraction such that the latter is not focused on the flap itself or the incision lines of the flap (Fig. 147.1). Undermining should be uniform and complete, including the areas of low tissue tension such as the tips of an ellipse or the pivot points of flaps.

Next, meticulous pinpoint hemostasis with complete visualization of all undermined skin with the help of an assistant is critical. Excessive postoperative bleeding within a sutured wound often results in an inferior outcome. It should be emphasized, however, that extensive tissue injury caused by electrosurgical hemostasis should be avoided as fervently as postoperative bleeding, since this can contribute equally to unwanted results. Suture ties should be used when necessary for larger, high-pressure blood vessels. With a well-prepared wound and flap that are characterized by uniformity in thickness, sharply squared edges, well-loosened tissue margins and excellent hemostasis, the wound is ready for suturing.

There are many ways to suture a wound, and opinions vary as to what method is the most effective. The role of dermal sutures is often debated and some question whether there is a need for these sutures at all. It is our opinion that not only are dermal sutures necessary, they are the most important component in order to consistently achieve outstanding aesthetic results. It is universally agreed that inverted skin edges should be avoided, since they persist as a noticeable, shadow-casting scar. It is preferable instead to try to achieve everted skin edges. Skin edge eversion can be accomplished by either dermal sutures or the external epidermal sutures. Eversion with epidermal sutures can be accomplished by various suturing techniques, e.g. vertical and horizontal mattress suturing, 90° needle insertion technique (see Ch. 146).

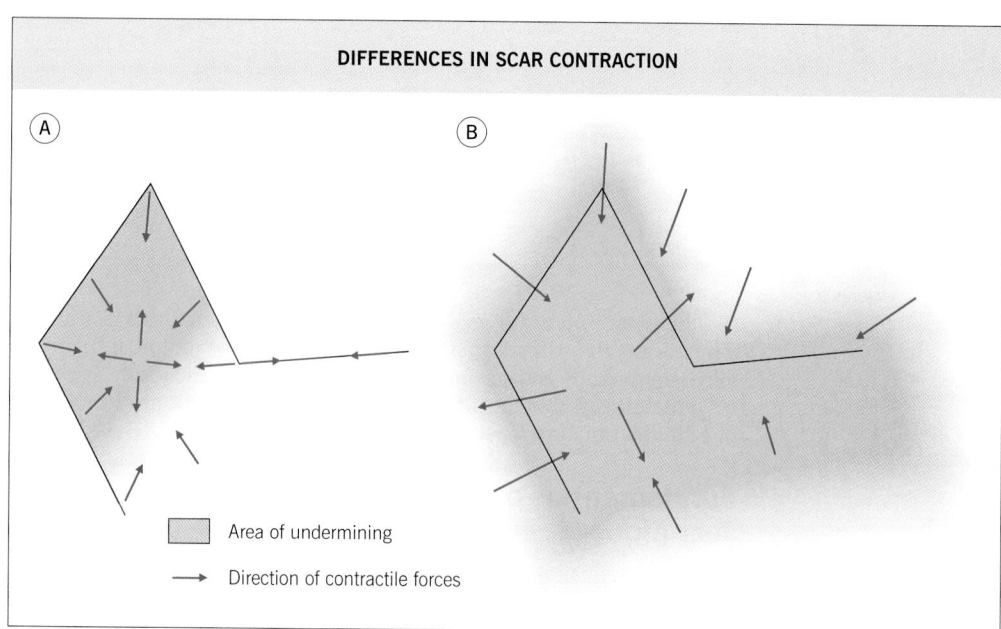

Fig. 147.1 Differences in scar contractions.
Depiction of differences between wounds that are undermined and those that are not undermined prior to suture placement. **A** The contraction forces are focused on the margins of the flap in a wound that was not widely undermined. **B** Broad diffusion of contractile forces that are not concentrated at the flap margins, making 'pincushioning' less likely in the widely undermined flap.

A dermal suturing technique known as the 'buried' or subcutaneous vertical mattress suture is the preferred way of achieving wound edge eversion (see Fig. 146.4B). The reason this is preferred over epidermal eversion sutures is that the buried vertical mattress sutures remain in place, supporting the sutured skin and maintaining eversion for 2 months or longer, depending on the type of suture material used. Conversely, most superficial epidermal sutures either dissolve or are removed within the first week or two following surgery, eliminating the support of eversion and allowing the natural forces of scar contraction to affect the healing incision. The natural course of wound healing is characterized by maximization of scar contraction at 2 months following injury. Therefore, with no suture support to counteract the contractile element in the plane of the incision perpendicular to the skin, it is only natural to expect inversion as the scar shortens in this plane (Fig. 147.2). It is thought that the continued presence of the buried vertical mattress sutures within the dermis helps to maintain the original eversion of the skin edge through the most intense periods of scar contraction. This accounts for an improved cosmetic result at 3, 6 and 12 months compared to wounds without dermal suture support.

Flap Movement Characteristics

It is helpful to broadly characterize flap types according to their mechanism of skin rearrangement. By understanding the dynamics of each flap, it is easier to select one that will provide functionally aesthetic results. Upon consideration of the unique characteristics of the defect, the donor skin, and the functional and aesthetic issues of reconstruction in the context of the mechanisms of flap tissue movement, a rational decision regarding the method of closure can be made.

In a general sense, all flaps have similar components and characteristics that tend to be taken for granted but are very important to understand. These components include the flap body, pedicle or vascular base, primary and secondary defect, and, as an integral part of flap dynamics, the primary and secondary movements (Table 147.2, Fig. 147.3).

Most tissue movement results in some degree of tension. This tension creates vectors of force that tend to return moving skin to its original position. Therefore, the primary movement of a flap creates a primary tension vector, while the secondary movement (during closure

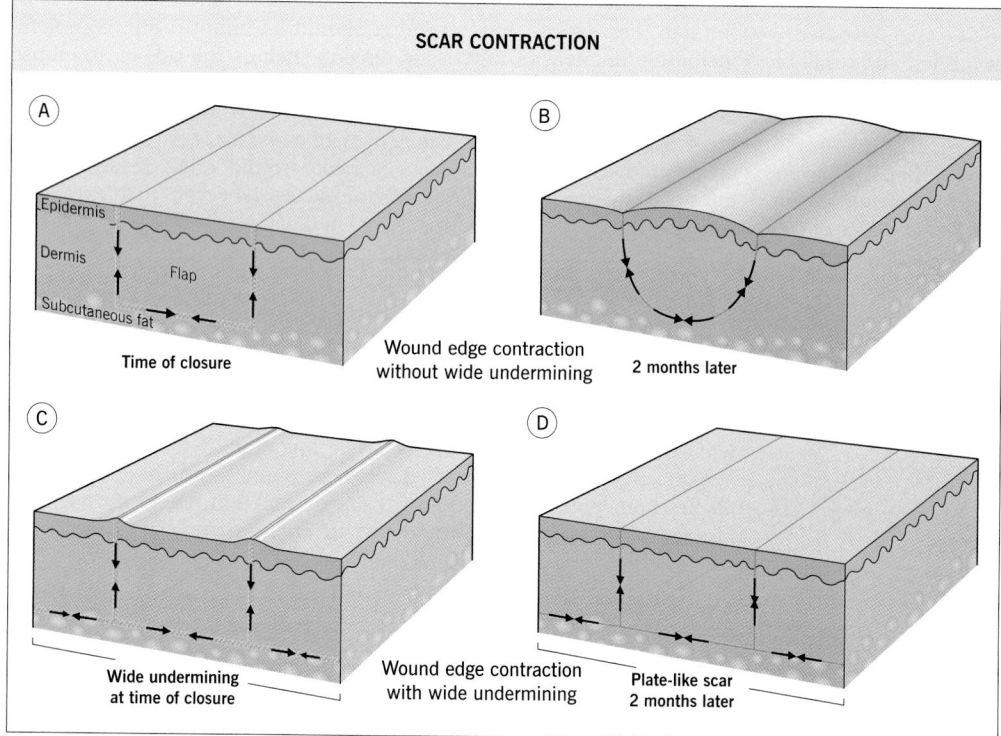

Fig. 147.2 Scar contraction. A Sutured wound without wound edge eversion and without undermining of the surrounding tissue. **B** The results of scar contraction, leading to inversion of the scars and 'pincushioning' of the flap. **C** A wound sutured with eversion and wide undermining. **D** The canceling effect of scar contraction and wound eversion as well as the diffusion of scar contraction in the deep, undermined wound plane.

of the donor site defect) creates a secondary tension vector. Consideration of these forces and the effects of these forces on adjacent tissue and even the blood supply of the flap is the primary factor in selecting one flap over another. The most perfectly executed flap that via tension vectors results in the distortion of a free margin (e.g. a lip or eyelid) is of little value to the patient or the goal of aesthetic restoration. Therefore, the initial and most important skill required for the proper execution of flaps is the ability to anticipate the direction and amount of tension created by particular flaps and to predict what effects this tension will have on adjacent structures. All diagrams in this chapter illustrate the movement of flaps and the anticipated resultant tension vectors.

DEFINITIONS OF FLAP COMPONENTS	
Body	The skin being advanced, transposed, rotated, interpolated or imported into the primary defect
Pedicle	Also known as the vascular base of the flap, it is the conduit of the vascular supply that will remain intact and maintain the vascularization of the body of the flap intraoperatively and for the early postoperative period
Primary defect	The area deficient in skin that will be reconstructed by the movement of the body of the flap
Secondary defect (donor site defect)	The area devoid of skin created by the movement of the body of the flap
Primary flap movement	The movement of the flap body into the defect
Secondary flap movement	The tissue movement necessary to close the void or donor site defect created by the movement of the body of the flap
Primary tension vector	The direction of the force tending to counteract the movement of the body of the flap
Secondary tension vector	The direction of the force created by the closure of the donor site defect

Table 147.2 Definitions of flap components.

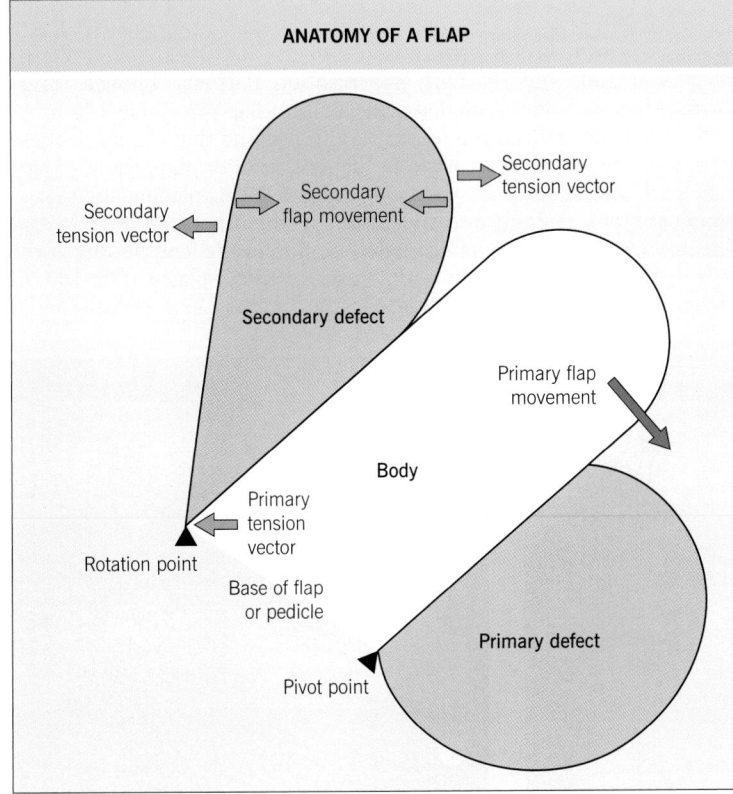

Fig. 147.3 Anatomy of a flap. Definitions of the components of a flap are outlined in Table 147.2.

There are four broad categories of flaps based upon how the tissue is rearranged in order to achieve closure (Table 147.3). The first category of flaps essentially displaces one or both Burow's triangles that would be removed if the wound were closed by a simple side-to-side closure. The second category includes the flaps that reconfigure defects while the third includes flaps that reorient tissue from adjacent pools of laxity into the defect. Finally, there is a category of flaps that enables defect closure by tissue importation.

Burow's triangle displacement flaps

Flaps that displace Burow's triangles to a convenient location distant from the defect include the single tangent advancement flap (Burow's flap), the bilateral single tangent advancement flap (A-to-T flap), the double tangent advancement flap (U-flap), the bilateral double tangent advancement flap (H-flap), and rotation flaps (including the glabellar or Rigor flap, Mustarde flap and the helical advancement flap) (Fig. 147.4). For the most part, these flaps displace Burow's triangles along straight or curved incision(s) tangential to the wound.

The key features of these flaps are: (1) they displace Burow's triangles to a distant site; (2) there is limited reorientation of tissue; and (3) their movement is dependent upon the intrinsic elasticity of the skin. Just as a simple side-to-side closure performed in stiff, inelastic skin would result in a tense closure, so would a Burow's triangle displacement-type flap. When the surrounding skin is elastic and 'loose', the wound edges

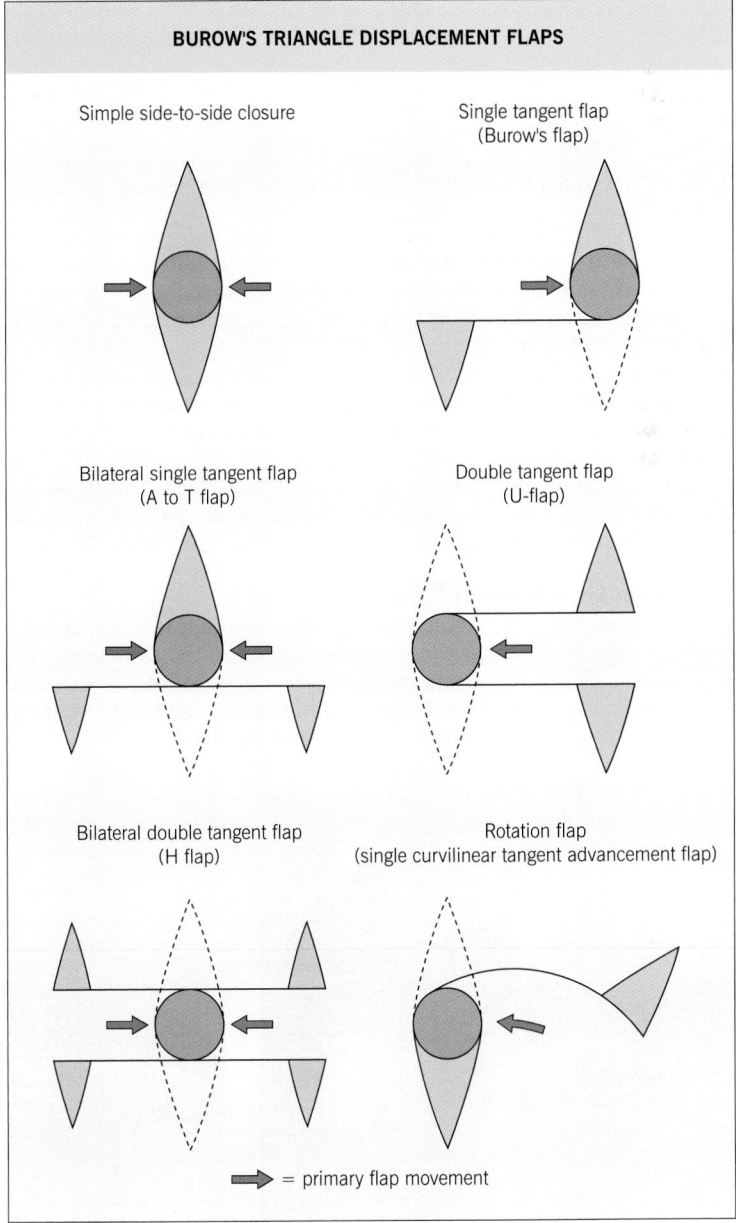

Fig. 147.4 Burow's triangle displacement flaps.

CLASSIFICATION OF FLAPS BASED ON DESIGN CHARACTERISTICS

Flap category	Flap variations	Synonym	Mechanism of tissue movement	Advantages	Disadvantages
Burow's triangle displacement flaps	Single tangent adv flap Bilateral single tangent adv flap Double tangent adv flap Bilateral double tangent adv flap Curvilinear tangent adv flap	Burow's flap A-to-T flap, O-to-T flap U-flap H-flap Rotation flap, Karpandzic flap Mustarde flap	Tissue advancement: dependent upon intrinsic tissue elasticity	• Enables closures adjacent to vital structures through displacement of Burow's triangles • Single tangent flaps have excellent blood supply	• Depends on intrinsic skin laxity of the flap skin • Requires extensive undermining • Double tangent flaps have a more limited blood supply
Defect reconfiguration flaps	Island pedicle flap	Kite flap, Myocutaneous pedicle flap	Tissue advancement: dependent upon intrinsic elasticity of subcutaneous pedicle Tissue movement results in reconfiguration of the defect	• Tissue conservative due to reconfiguration of the defect without removal of Burow's triangle	• Blood supply is limited to the subcutaneous pedicle • Use limited to locations with spongy, elastic subcutaneous tissue
Tissue reorientation flaps	Rhombic transposition flap Bilobed transposition flap Nasolabial transposition flap Nasolabial flap with a twist (Spear's flap)	Limberg flap, Dufourmentel flap, Webster's 30° flap Melolabial fold flap	Reorientation of adjacent tissue laxity	• Effective for tight closures • Directional tissue gain can be achieved in direction of tissue deficit	• Depends on laxity adjacent to the defect • Multidirectional incisions; difficult to place all in RSTL
Tissue importation flaps	Paramedian forehead flap Nasolabial interpolation flap Retroauricular pedicled flap Modified Hughes flap Abbe Cross lip flap	Indian flap Pin back flap	Importation of tissue from a distant site	• Coverage of large wounds • Can provide vascularity for coverage of avascular grafts such as cartilage grafts	• Two-stage flap • Vascular supply limited to narrow pedicle

Table 147.3 Classification of flaps based on design characteristics. adv, advancement; RSTL, relaxed skin tension lines.

can be closed under minimal tension in both a side-to-side closure and with these flaps. Thus, the only advantage that these flaps confer over a side-to-side closure in tight skin is that a larger area of skin is typically undermined, which releases the latter from the tethering effect of the subcutaneous tissue. This allows for a modest decrease in wound closure tension. The most obvious utility of these flaps is in defects where, for functional or aesthetic reasons, it is inconvenient to remove a Burow's triangle immediately adjacent to the defect. An example of this is a defect above or below the eye in which displacement of the Burow's triangle is useful in order to avoid removing a triangle from the eyebrow or eyelid skin (Fig. 147.5).

Defect reconfiguration flaps

The island pedicle advancement flap is unique in that it is an advancement of tissue oriented in a plane perpendicular to the skin and at 90° to the more traditional advancement or rotation flaps. In this case, the tissue redundancy created at the pivot point of the flap is buried in the subcutaneous plane at the advancing edge of the flap.

Tissue reorientation flaps

The tissue reorientation flaps are characterized by the lifting of skin from an adjacent donor site and reorienting it through the transposition of the flap over a peninsula of skin between the donor site and the defect. There is a pivot point at the base of this flap (see Fig. 147.3). The tissue movement depends on the presence of laxity in adjacent tissue. Although intrinsic elasticity of the flap skin may facilitate the ease of execution, without ample laxity in the flap donor site, the transposition can not be performed. Some of the flaps that fall into this category include the rhombic transposition flap, the bilobed transposition flap and the nasolabial transposition flap (see Table 147.3).

To better understand the reorientation of tissue that occurs in these flaps, a review of the most basic tissue reorientation flap, the Z-plasty, is helpful. Z-plasties transpose two angular flaps, placing them in a complementary fashion into the defects of the other flap (Fig. 147.6). This reorientation of tissue ultimately results in the lengthening of the skin in the direction of the middle arm of the Z-plasty (Fig. 147.7). There is a complementary decrease in the length of skin perpendicular

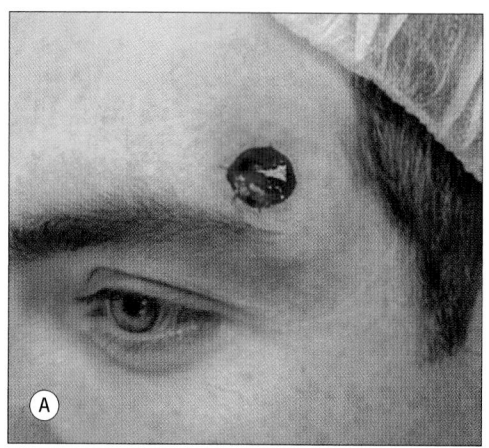
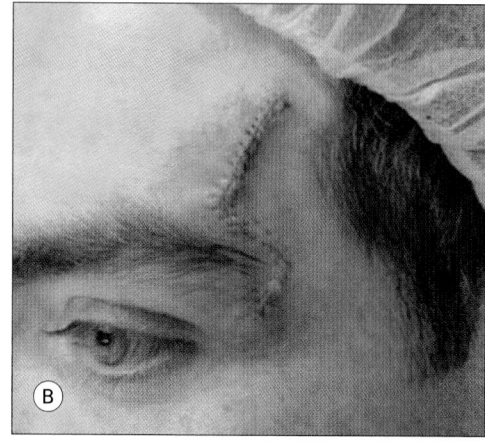
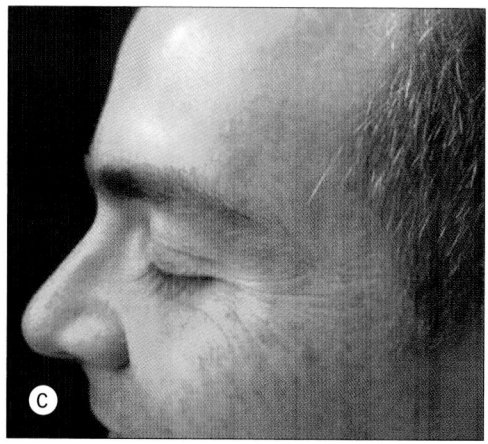

Fig. 147.5 Single tangent advancement flap (Burow's flap). A The wound extends to the brow. **B** Closure with a single tangent advancement flap with the tangent extending lateral to the brow and displacing a Burow's triangle to the temple and lateral orbit. **C** The eyebrow is entirely preserved.

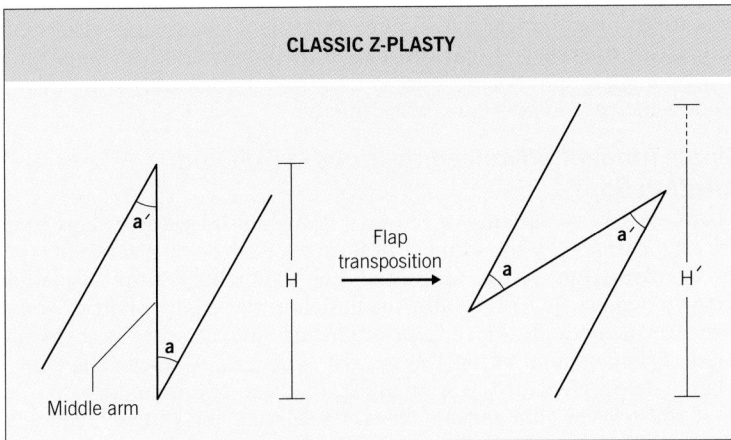

CLASSIC Z-PLASTY

Fig. 147.6 Classic Z-plasty. The directional tissue gain (dotted line) is depicted (H to H') after flap transposition in the direction of the middle arm of the Z-plasty.

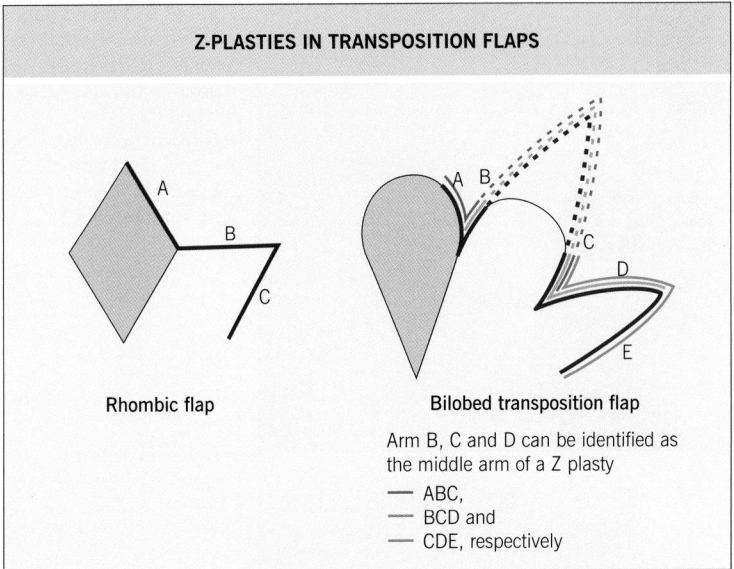

Z-PLASTIES IN TRANSPOSITION FLAPS

Rhombic flap

Bilobed transposition flap

Arm B, C and D can be identified as the middle arm of a Z plasty
— ABC,
— BCD and
— CDE, respectively

Fig. 147.8 Z-plasties in transposition flaps. Z-plasties are highlighted within the designs of both the rhombic and the bilobed transposition flap. Note in the rhombic flap the middle arm of the Z-plasty is line B and is the direction of anticipated tissue lengthening. In the bilobed transposition flap diagram, there is a series of three Z-plasties all contributing to tissue gain in the desired direction of the defect.

to this same arm. The amount of lengthening is proportional to the angles of the flap(s). Put another way, tissue gain in the direction of the middle arm is directly proportional to the width of the base of the flaps. This is effectively the mechanism of tissue reorientation in transposition flaps. Upon careful examination, Z-plasties can be found within the design of transposition flaps (Fig. 147.8). Therefore, just as with Z-plasties, transposition flaps work because the reorientation of the tissue results in lengthening of tissue in the direction of the skin deficit at the expense of the laxity in the donor site.

It is helpful to understand the utility of these principles of reorientation. An example of the utilization of these principles is in the case of a defect on the nasal tip (Fig. 147.9). The skin is typically very tight in this area, making simple side-to-side closure in the vertical direction difficult. Side-to-side closure in the horizontal direction is impractical because of the distortion that would occur to the free margin of the ala. When one looks for donor sites, there is typically a substantial amount of laxity on the mid nasal dorsum and nasal sidewall. A bilobed flap allows utilization of this laxity through tissue reorientation using two lobes. The underlying mechanism of tissue reorientation is a series of Z-plasties inherent in this flap. Since tissue gain in Z-plasties is in the direction of the middle arm of the Z-plasty, a substantial reorientation and lengthening of tissue in the desirable direction for repair of the defect occurs without distortion. In contrast to the Burow's triangle displacement flap, this flap does not rely upon intrinsic elasticity of the flap skin. This is key to avoiding distortion of the alar rim.

Tissue importation flaps

Large defects, or defects in areas where tissue laxity is lacking, may be reconstructed by importing vascularized tissue from a site that is not adjacent to the defect (see Table 147.3). Tissue importation flaps are typically derived from a distant donor site with ample tissue laxity and, most importantly, an excellent blood supply. This blood supply may be based on a particular artery (e.g. paramedian forehead flap based on the supratrochlear artery) or by a rich, random-patterned blood supply (e.g. the retroauricular pedicled flap).

These flaps are typically two-staged flaps requiring a period of vascular ingrowth from the wound bed of the defect. This time period ranges from 2 to 6 weeks, with 3 weeks being the most commonly reported time point for transection of the pedicle. In the head and neck region, defect sites where tissue importation flaps are commonly employed include the nose, the ear, the eyelid and the lip. The appropriate selection and execution of these four broad flap categories are discussed in more detail below.

DESCRIPTION OF TECHNIQUE

Burow's Triangle Displacement Flaps

The group of flaps that comprise the Burow's triangle displacement flaps has the common feature of the displacement of Burow's triangle(s) along an incision made tangential to the defect (see Fig. 147.4). In each case, the basic method of closure is side-to-side advancement of tissue

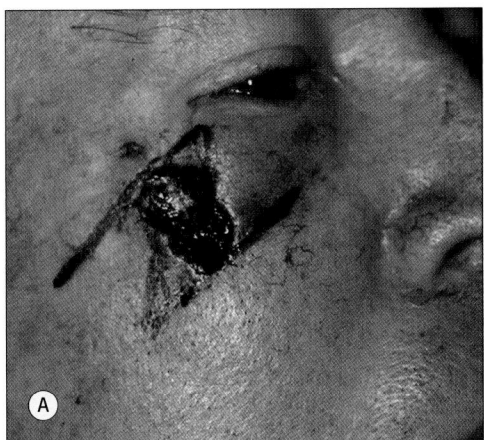 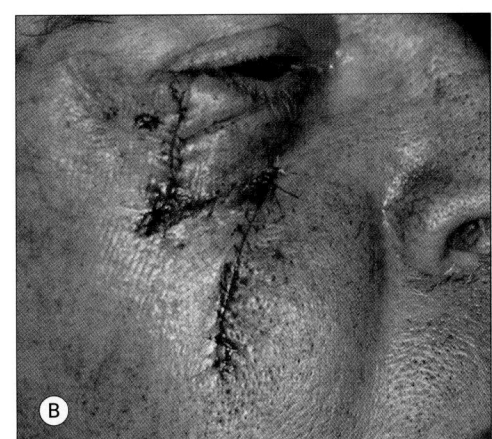 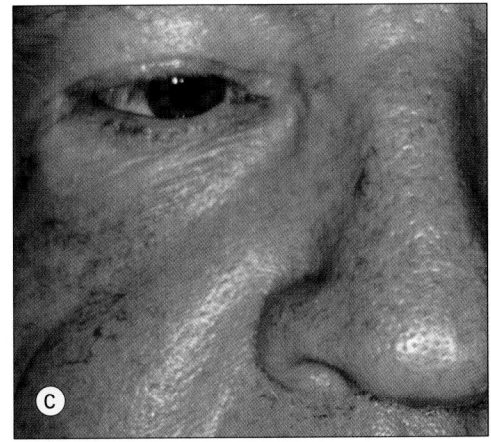

Fig. 147.7 Classic Z-plasty. A Defect close to lid margin. **B** The wound is closed with a Z-plasty closure with the transposition of flaps at the upper medial and lower lateral aspects of the wound. This is done to lengthen tissue in the direction of the palpebral margin in order to prevent ectropion as demonstrated at the 4-month postoperative visit (**C**).

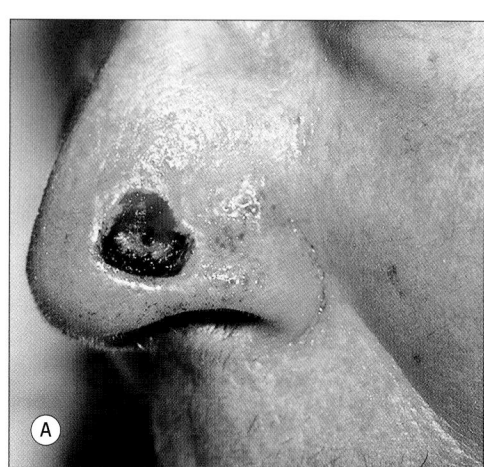

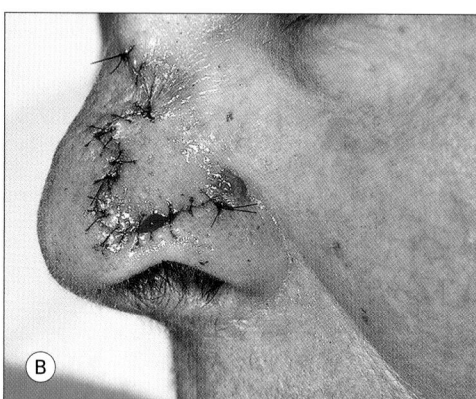

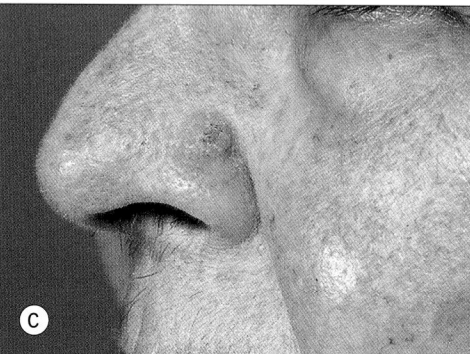

Fig. 147.9 Bilobed flap.
A Defect on the nasal tip adjacent to the free margin of the ala. Bilobed flap reconstruction with minimal distortion of the alar rim (**B**) and long-term result (**C**).

relocation of the triangle(s) to a more convenient location. As discussed earlier, one drawback is that the area of the flap is relatively large and the resulting tissue undermining is increased dramatically with only a modest increase in lax tissue recruitment.

Single tangent advancement flaps (STAF) and rotation flaps

There are several variants of Burow's triangle displacement flaps that are differentiated by the number of Burow's triangle displacements, or the configuration of the tangential line extending to the displaced triangle (see Fig. 147.4). Ideally, the design of these flaps should, when possible, incorporate the concept of placing surgical scars at cosmetic subunit borders and within the relaxed skin tension lines. Therefore, when a defect is located near an arcing junction of a cosmetic subunit or if the relaxed skin tension lines are curved, the Burow's triangle displacement flap, classically known as the rotation flap, may be an excellent option. An example of this would be the cheek rotation flap for a defect on the mid to medial upper cheek (Fig. 147.10). On the other hand, when the cosmetic subunit junctions or relaxed skin tension lines are relatively straight, the single tangent advancement flap, traditionally known as the Burow's advancement flap, may be optimal (Fig. 147.11).

Once the need to displace a Burow's triangle in order to avoid a vital structure is established, the incision lines should be planned in the optimal location. The incision, whether straight or arced, should be made perpendicular to the skin and should extend to the point of preferred displacement of the triangle. The triangle should then be excised to a depth commensurate with the depth of the defect being repaired and the thickness of the flap. The flap should be elevated by dissection in the subcutaneous plane and all other wound edges should be widely undermined at a similar depth. The optimal thickness of a flap will depend upon the location of the flap. Creating a flap that is too thin with dissection at the dermal–subcutaneous junction may compromise the flap's blood supply and may lead to a less natural looking flap. Conversely, if the flap is in a site with very thick subcutaneous tissue and an excessively thick flap is created, flap mobility may be decreased, the flap edges may be more difficult to evert, and the underlying neurovascular structures or facial muscles can be unintentionally damaged. Therefore, the optimal plane of dissection of a flap is normally somewhere between the upper mid subcutaneous tissue and the deep subcutaneous tissue. Flaps involving the movement of hair-bearing skin, cartilage or other special anatomic structures may specifically dictate the thickness of the flap.

Once the flap has been raised and the surrounding skin undermined, the flap is ready to be sutured into place. If the flap is large and heavy and would result in distortion of adjacent structures (e.g. eyelids), it may be necessary to use a flap suspension suture. This is typically achieved by placing a suture in a fixed or rigid structure that underlies the flap. Periosteal placement is often the most effective way of anchoring a suspension suture. The suture is then placed into the flap's undersurface through the subcutaneous tissue, into the deep dermis. Placement within the flap should correspond topographically to its

with the removal of Burow's triangles in the direction perpendicular to the side-to-side tissue movement. The greatest utility of these flaps is in situations where the normal adjacent location of one or both of the Burow's triangles would impinge upon a vital functional or cosmetic structure (see Fig. 147.5). These flaps allow for displacement or

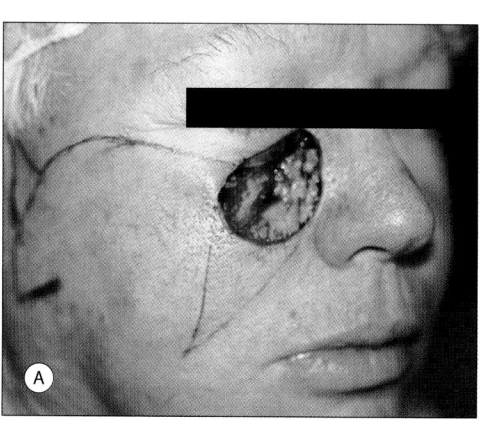

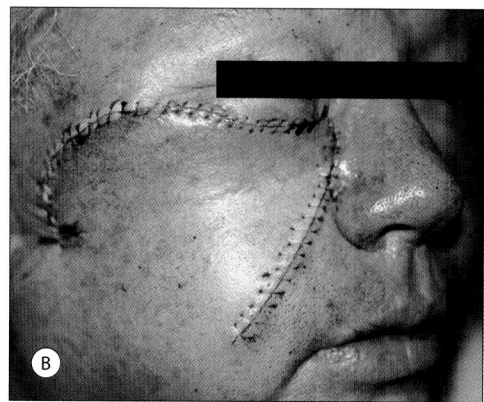

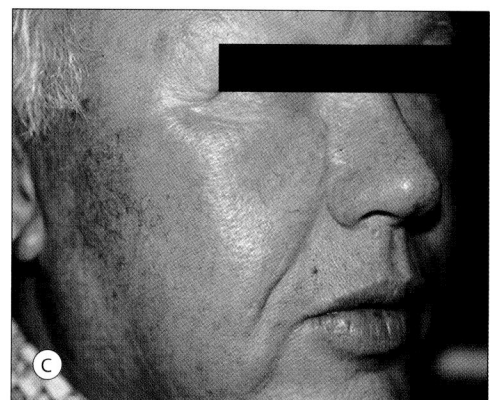

Fig. 147.10 Rotation flap. Large defect (**A**) on the medial cheek and lower eyelid reconstructed with a rotation flap (Mustarde flap) with displacement of the superior Burow's triangle laterally along the curvilinear tangent which follows the relaxed skin tension lines (**B**). **C** Final results with no distortion of the eyelid and incision lines nicely camouflaged along cosmetic subunit borders and relaxed skin tension lines.

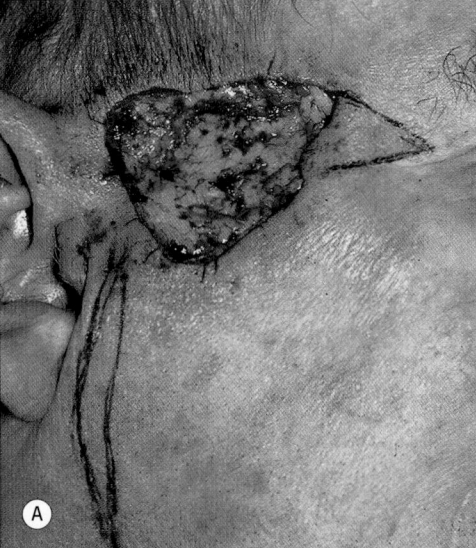

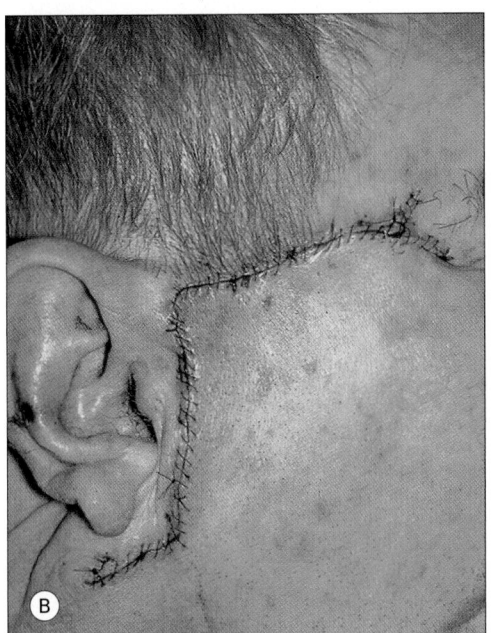

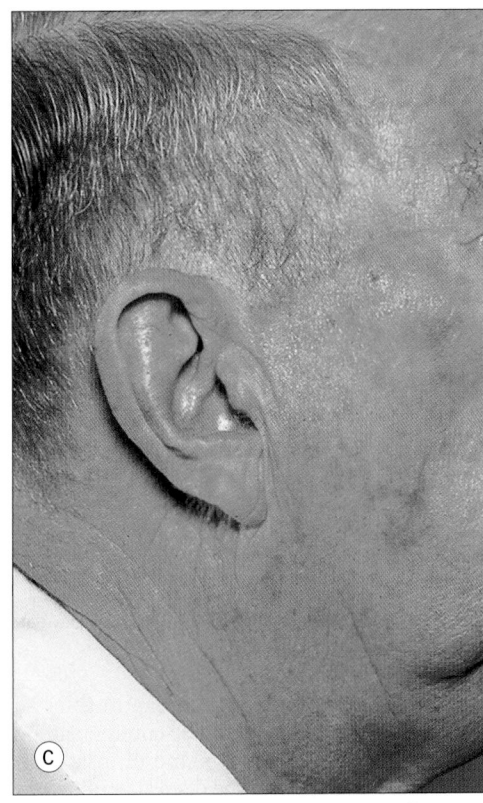

Fig. 147.11 Single tangent advancement flap.
A Large defect situated between the ear and the
eye. **B** A single tangent advancement flap
(Burow's flap) reconstructs the defect by displacing
a Burow's triangle inferiorly to just below the
earlobe. **C** One month after reconstruction.

desired location relative to the periosteal suture. This can be repeated
as necessary, with care to avoid interruption of vascular supply.

The next step of the closure is to suture the skin edges of the two
Burow's triangles, evenly distributing them. The remainder of the
flap can now be completely sutured into the defect in the standard
fashion with even distribution of the wound edges of the flap and
opposing skin.

Double tangent advancement flaps (DTAF)

Double tangent advancement flaps displace both Burow's triangles
along parallel tangents (see Fig. 147.4). Therefore, these flaps are
typically peninsular in configuration with an isolated vascular base at
the distal ends of the tangents. The execution of this flap is very similar
to that of single tangent advancement flaps, except that one must be
mindful of the more limited vascular supply (Fig. 147.12). This isolated

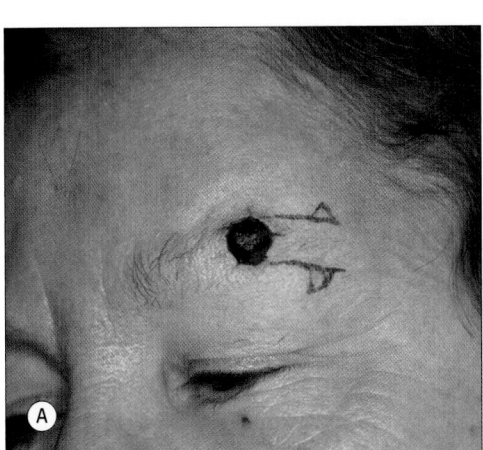

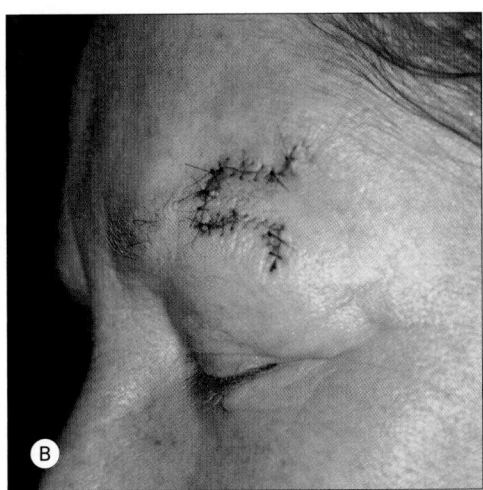

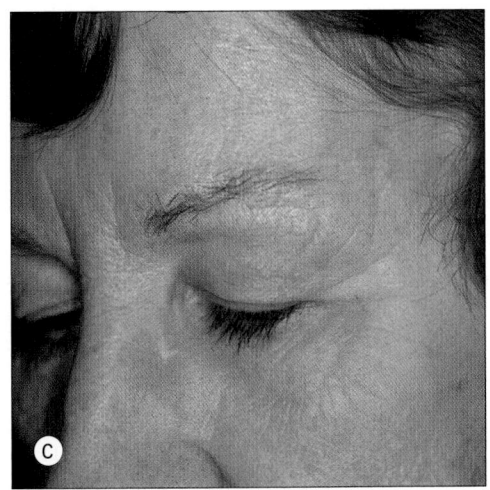

Fig. 147.12 Double tangent advancement flap. This technique was used to reconstruct and preserve the continuity of the eyebrow in this patient.

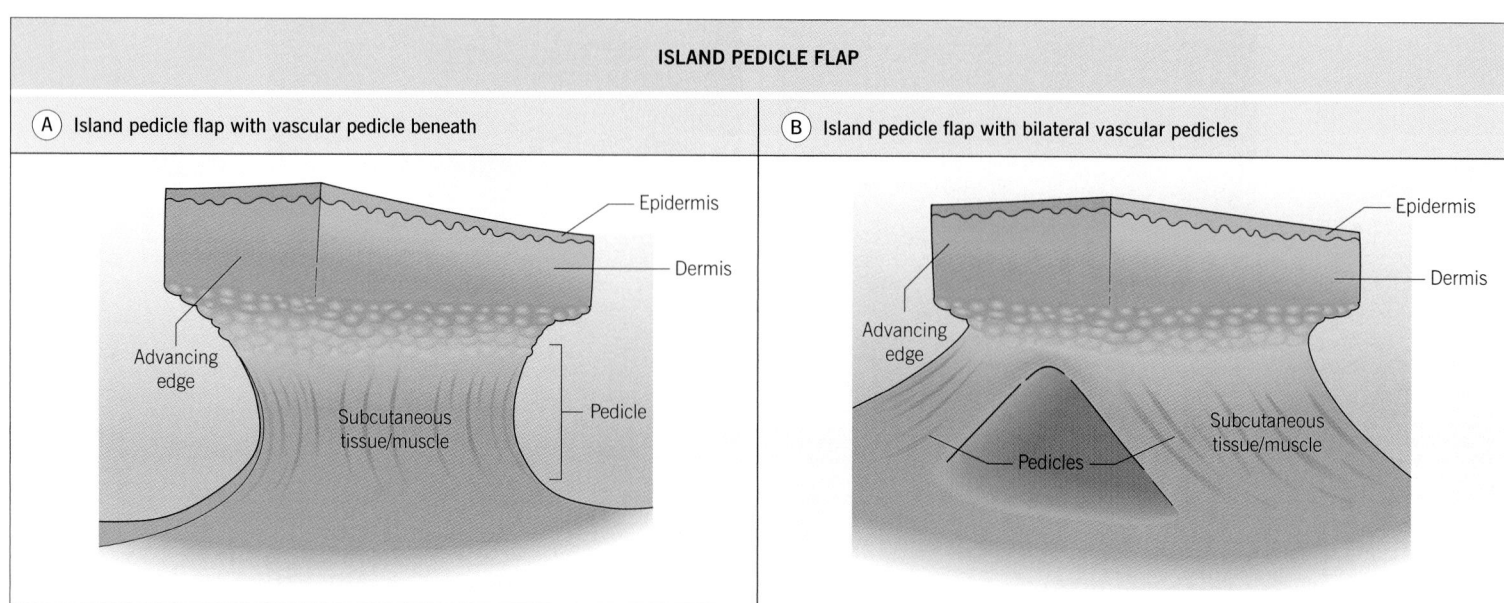

ISLAND PEDICLE FLAP

Ⓐ Island pedicle flap with vascular pedicle beneath

Ⓑ Island pedicle flap with bilateral vascular pedicles

Epidermis

Dermis

Advancing edge

Subcutaneous tissue/muscle

Pedicle

Epidermis

Dermis

Advancing edge

Pedicles

Subcutaneous tissue/muscle

Fig. 147.13 Island pedicle flap. A Vascular pedicle derived immediately beneath the island of skin. **B** Vascular pedicles derived from tissue lateral to the island flap.

vascular supply necessitates limiting the length of the flap to three to four times the width. The thickness of the flap should be commensurate with the thickness of the defect, with the typical plane of dissection between the upper mid subcutaneous tissue and the deep subcutaneous tissue. When suspension sutures are necessary, extreme caution is necessary in order to avoid compromise of the vascular supply to the leading edge of the flap. Again, the first closure points are at the site of the displaced Burow's triangles. Suturing the advancing flap in a standard fashion with even distribution of the flap along the recipient tissue margins completes the execution of this flap.

Defect reconfiguration (island pedicle) flaps

The island pedicle flap is, as previously noted, a unique advancement flap. It is unique in several ways, including the fact that the creation of the island of epidermis and dermis, by definition, eliminates blood supply from the rich vascular plexus within the deep dermis and superficial subcutaneous skin. In effect, the vascular supply is isolated to the subcutaneous tissue. The two variations in pedicle design hinge upon whether the pedicle is created immediately beneath the island or from the subcutaneous tissue lateral to the island (Fig. 147.13). The variant with the pedicle immediately beneath the vascular pedicle is created by dissecting away surrounding superficial subcutaneous tissue and eliminating the tethering effects of the tissue adjacent to the pedicle (Fig. 147.14). The island pedicle flap with laterally based pedicles is created by tunneling immediately beneath the island while carefully maintaining vascularized sheets of subcutaneous tissue, either bilaterally or unilaterally to the side of the island (Fig. 147.15). The authors' preference has been to develop a pedicle immediately under the island because of the more durable and reliable vascular supply. However, there are clearly some anatomic sites where the lateral pedicles provide adequate blood supply and better flap mobility.

In general, it is appropriate to think of the island pedicle flap as an advancement of what would be one of the Burow's triangles in a simple side-to-side closure. It must be located in areas with very elastic and spongy subcutaneous tissue with a rich blood supply. The island pedicle flap is an extremely tissue-efficient flap in which little or no tissue is discarded and yet it often provides outstanding clinical results. The mechanism for tissue conservation involves a reconfiguration of the defect into an angular shape via the use of what would be a Burow's triangle (Fig. 147.16). The original shape of the defect is reconfigured behind the advancing island to a defect of equal area but very angular in shape that can be closed without tissue redundancy, obviating removal of Burow's triangle.

It is useful from the standpoint of flap execution to recognize conceptually that an island pedicle flap (especially those with the pedicle based immediately beneath the island) is essentially a rotation flap turned perpendicular to the surface of the skin (Fig. 147.17). Whereas, in a rotation flap, the vascular source lies parallel with the

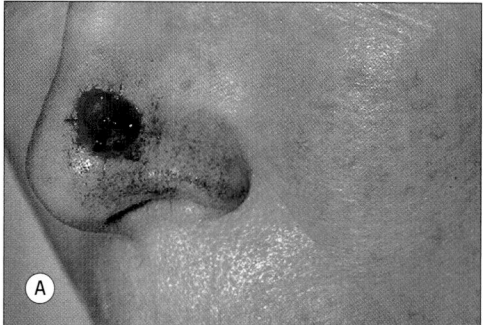

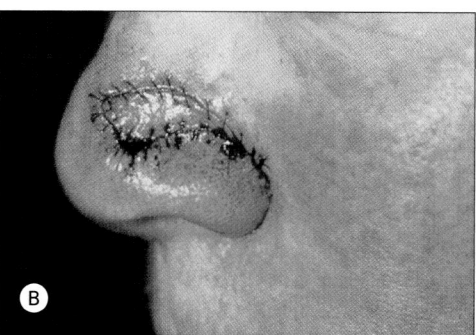

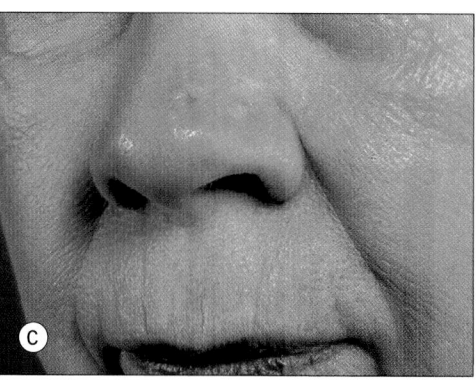

Fig. 147.14 Island pedicle flap. Reconstruction of a nasal defect (**A**) with an island pedicle flap whose pedicle is derived deep to the island along the alar crease (**B**). **C** Cosmetic result at one year.

skin, the analogous vascular supply of the island pedicle flap runs perpendicular to the skin. While the plane of tissue movement in the traditional rotation flap is parallel with the skin, it is perpendicular to the skin in an island pedicle flap. Once this analogy between a rotation flap and an island pedicle flap is understood, it is easy to see that movement of the island pedicle flap is facilitated by the same factors that facilitate movement of a rotation flap. For example, the excision

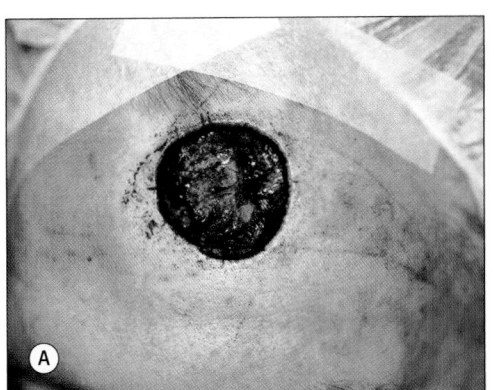

Fig. 147.15 Island pedicle flap. A Large forehead defect. **B** Intraoperatively, an island pedicle flap is derived as a single pedicle based on the rich blood supply of the supratrochlear and supraorbital arteries (inferior to the flap). **C** The defect is now comprised of acute angles which are more easily closed primarily.

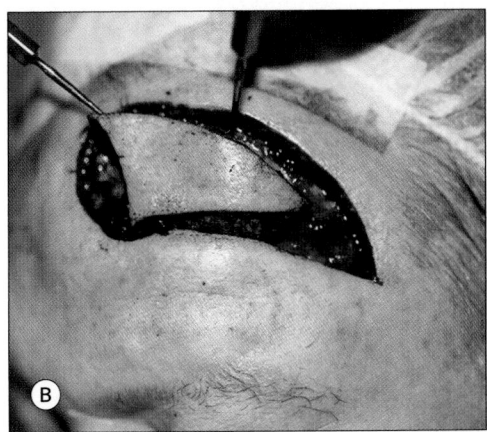

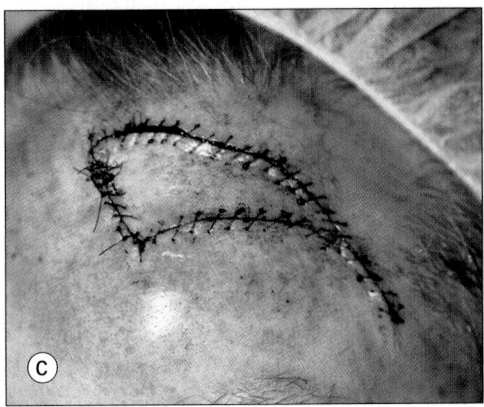

ROTATION FLAP ANALOGY FOR AN ISLAND PEDICLE FLAP

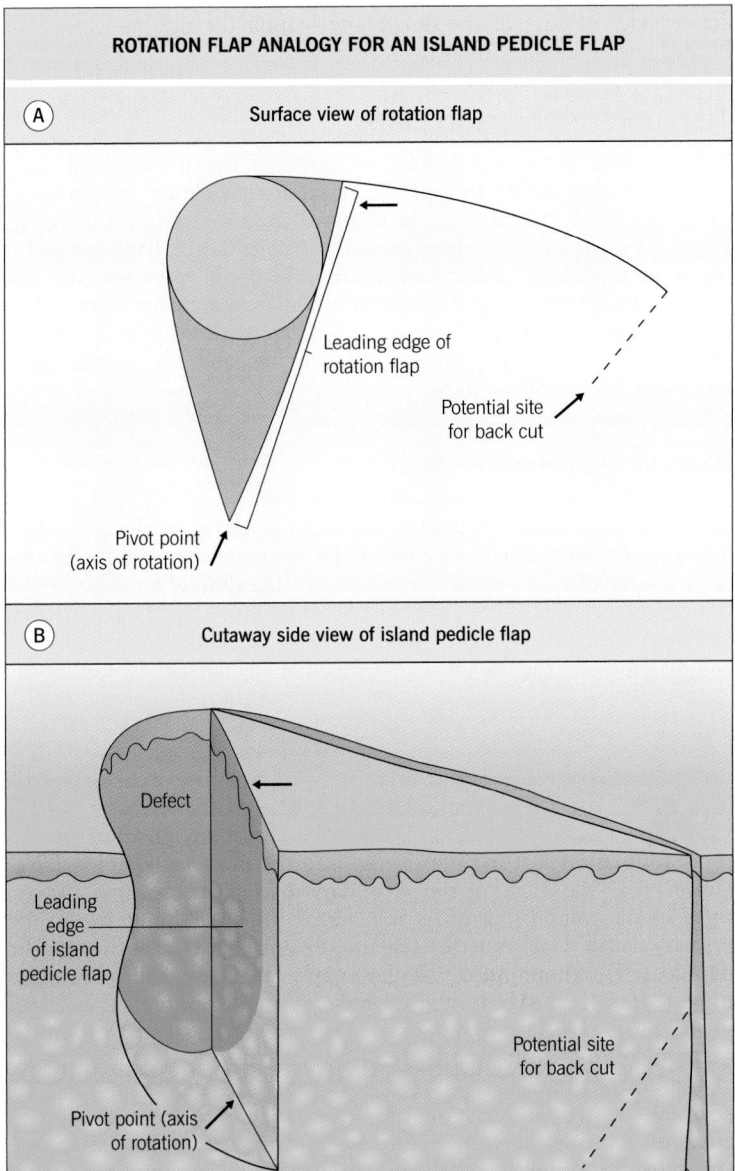

(A) Surface view of rotation flap

Leading edge of rotation flap

Potential site for back cut

Pivot point (axis of rotation)

(B) Cutaway side view of island pedicle flap

Defect

Leading edge of island pedicle flap

Potential site for back cut

Pivot point (axis of rotation)

Fig. 147.17 Rotation flap analogy for an island pedicle flap. A A rotation flap with standard removal of a Burow's triangle adjacent to the defect and the site of a potential back cut which would facilitate flap movement. **B** Side view of a defect and an island pedicle flap. The plane of rotation is perpendicular to the skin surface. The shaded area is where the equivalent of a Burow's triangle has been removed to facilitate flap movement. The dotted line is analogous to the back cut of a rotation flap. Note the similarities between a rotation flap and an island pedicle flap.

ISLAND PEDICLE FLAP

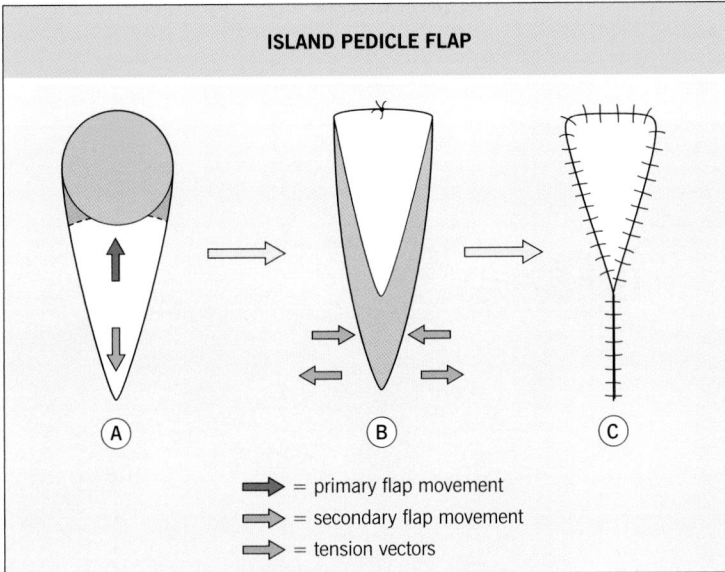

(A) (B) (C)

→ = primary flap movement
⇒ = secondary flap movement
⇒ = tension vectors

Fig. 147.16 Island pedicle flap. Reconfiguration of the defect (shaded area) in **A** to the defect in **B**. The shaded secondary defect in **B** is comprised entirely of acute angles which are easily closed primarily (**C**).

of the Burow's triangle facilitates the rotation and advancement of the rotation flap. Likewise, the advancement of an island pedicle flap is facilitated by the removal of the tissue analogous to the Burow's triangle, i.e. any subcutaneous tissue at the base of the defect (see Fig. 147.17B). Without its removal, the subcutaneous tissue left in the base of the wound serves as a physical impedance to the advancing island pedicle flap.

Another technique for enhancing rotation flap mobility, the back cut, is also applicable to the island pedicle flap. A back cut for a rotation flap releases some of the restraining tension of the flap and is helpful in its mobilization. The equivalent of a back cut can also improve the mobility of an island pedicle flap. This is done by incising the subcutaneous pedicle at the trailing edge of the flap in a direction beveled slightly into the pedicle (see Fig 147.17B).

In order to enable eversion of the skin edges of the island pedicle flap, the island is very slightly undermined at the dermal–subcutaneous junction to facilitate its eversion. Extreme care must be taken to avoid compromise of the vascular supply. The skin surrounding the island pedicle flap is widely undermined in the superficial subcutaneous tissue. Once adequate mobility of the flap is obtained, it is advanced into the defect, with closure of the donor site behind the flap and standard layered closure of all skin edges.

Tissue Reorientation Flaps

Transposition flaps as a whole are some of the most useful flaps because of their ability to tap into adjacent tissue reservoirs in order to repair defects in anatomic locations with minimal inherent laxity. When planned and executed properly, transposition flaps allow for repair of even large defects with minimal or no skin tension and without distortion of important surrounding anatomic structures. The classic transposition flap is the rhombic flap, with other useful transposition flap variants being the bilobed flap and the single-staged nasolabial transposition flap.

Rhombic transposition flap

The classic rhombic flap, originally described by Limberg in 1963, was based on the concept of placing the tension vector of the secondary defect nearly perpendicular to that of the primary defect (Fig. 147.18A). After closure of the donor site, the Limberg flap allowed for repair of the primary defect with essentially no wound edge tension. Dufourmentel added important modifications that made the closure of the donor site easier by placing the secondary defect at an acute angle (60°) to the primary defect. Thus, the flap must pass through a shorter arc in order to be positioned within the primary defect (Fig. 147.18B). Webster modified the rhombic flap further by making the angle of the secondary defect even more acute (30°) to further facilitate closure of the secondary defect (Fig. 147.18C). The smaller flap size of the Webster variant allows the surgeon to position the flap in almost any position relative to the primary defect in order to tap into the most lax skin available. However, as the angle of the secondary defect becomes more acute, more of the wound tension is transferred from the donor site to the primary defect. Care must be taken to ensure that the tension on the flap does not compromise vascular supply and flap viability. Another important concept to bear in mind is that as more tension is transferred to the primary defect, important nearby anatomic structures will be more prone to distortion.

Careful planning is required prior to incising the rhombic transposition flap in order to ensure that the donor site comes from the area adjacent to the defect with the most abundant tissue laxity. This donor site, most commonly, parallels the relaxed skin tension lines. We prefer to remove the Burow's triangle at the pivot point prior to insetting of the flap. This ensures more accurate incision lines and allows more precise suture placement in order to distribute flap tension evenly. The flap and the skin surrounding the defect and the donor site are undermined to ensure all are of the same thickness. Following careful hemostasis, the secondary defect is closed in the standard layered fashion. Next, the flap is inset into the defect, trimmed to fit and then closed in the standard layered fashion.

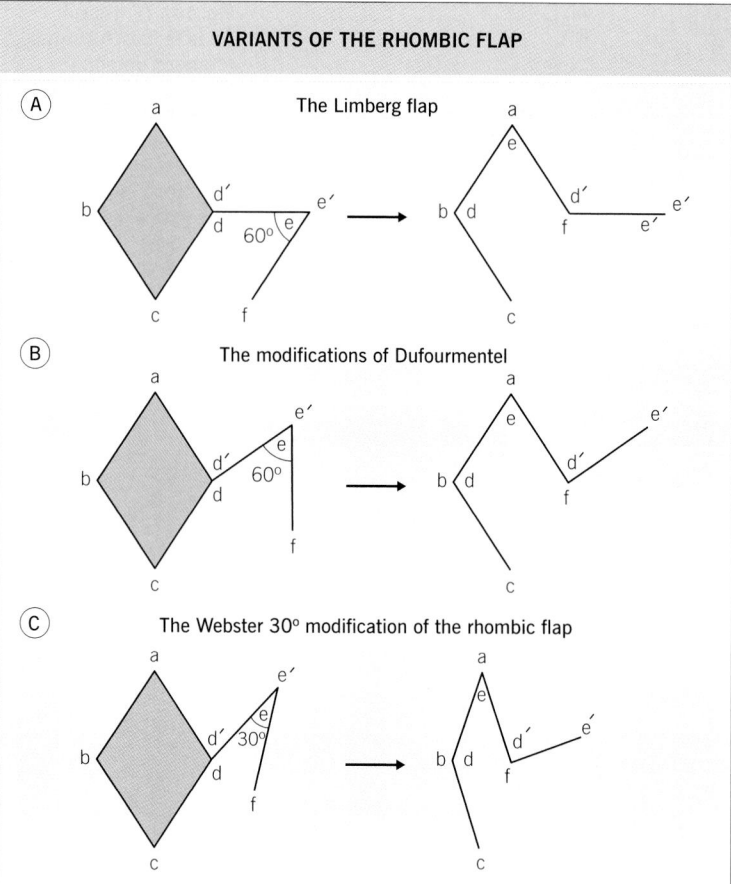

Fig. 147.18 Variants of the rhombic flap. A The Limberg flap is the standard rhombic flap. **B** The modifications of Dufourmentel. **C** The Webster 30° modification of the rhombic flap.

Although extremely versatile, there are specific areas where the rhombic transposition flap provides reliable and reproducible results. The lateral, upper two-thirds of the nose and the lateral forehead are ideally suited for the rhombic flap because of the frequent difficulty in closing defects in these areas primarily (Fig. 147.19). The adjacent tissue laxity available on the nasal sidewall and the lateral cheek provide ample reservoirs of donor tissue. Large defects of the central cheek may occasionally be closed by the rhombic flap when other, more simplistic options are not possible because of the size of the defect. In other anatomic sites on the face, the rhombic flap may be a second or third option for repair, but other options are usually chosen first because of the difficulty in concealing the geometric shape of the incision lines of the rhombic flap.

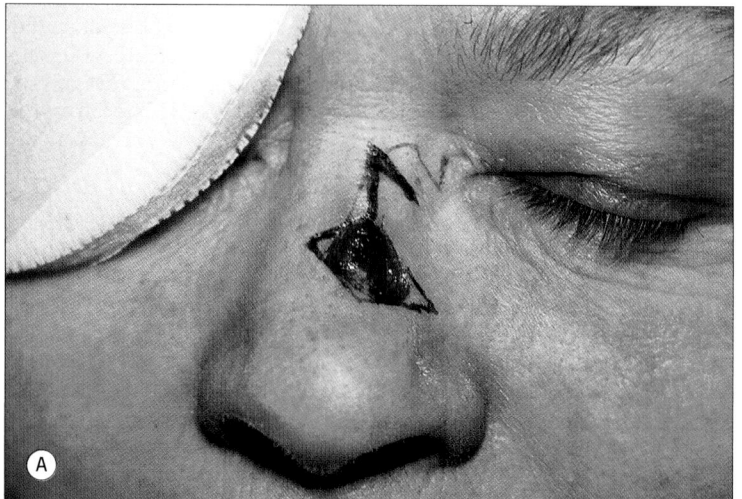

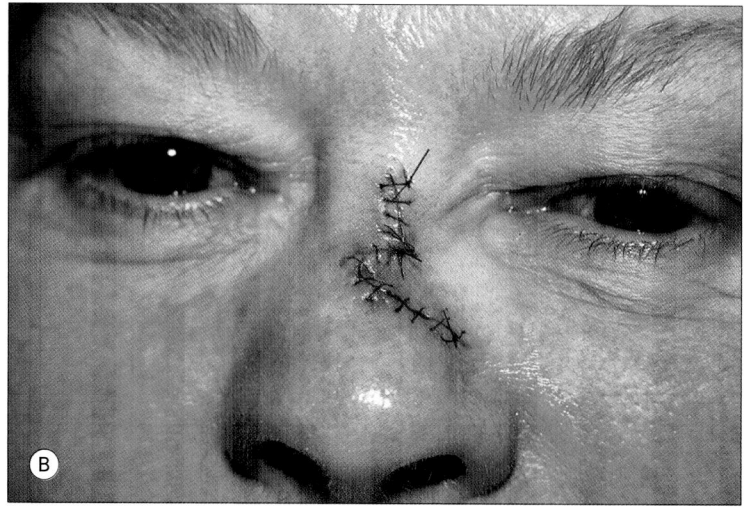

Fig. 147.19 Rhombic transposition flap. Example of a rhombic flap on the upper lateral nose.

Bilobed transposition flap

The bilobed flap is essentially two transposition flaps in series, and it is one of the most useful flaps for repair of defects of the lower one-third of the nose. The bilobed flap was first described by Esser in 1918 and important modifications to the flap were described by Zitelli in 1989. Zitelli modified the classic flap to decrease the pivot angle of the flap from 180° to close to 90–100° (Fig. 147.20). This simple modification helps to minimize two of the most common problems associated with the bilobed flap, the problem of pincushioning of the primary lobe and the tendency for dog-ears to form at the pivot point of the flap.

Careful planning is required for the bilobed flap in order to ensure minimal distortion of surrounding structures. Figure 147.20 depicts a reliable method for planning the incisions of the bilobed flap that may be helpful for those less experienced with implementation of this flap. Drawing with a sterile marker on the patient (prior to incising the flap) ensures that the incision lines are placed in such a way as to maximize both functional and aesthetic results. For nasal defects, the flap should be designed so that the tertiary defect is closed in a fashion that is perpendicular to the line of the alar rim. This ensures that the contra-lateral ala is not lifted during closure of the tertiary defect. We again remove the Burow's triangle when incising the bilobed flap, in order to provide the most accurate placement. Wide undermining of both the donor and recipient sites in a submuscular plane allows for good tissue mobility while providing excellent blood supply. On the side of the flap where the pivot point is located, we carry the plane of undermining to the nasofacial groove in order to facilitate proper placement of the flap, with no distortion of surrounding anatomic structures. Careful hemostasis is followed by closure of the tertiary site in the standard layered fashion followed by careful insetting and suturing of the flap into the primary defect. The secondary flap is then trimmed to match the circular secondary defect and sutured in the standard layered fashion (Fig. 147.21).

Defects of the lower one-third of the nose measuring between 0.5 and 1.5 cm are the ideal size and location for the use of the bilobed flap. Smaller defects can often be closed in a primary fashion and larger defects may need either a skin graft or a two-staged tissue importation flap, depending on other characteristics of both the patient and the defect. Although the bilobed flap is the most common flap chosen for the distal third of the nose, it is rarely used in other anatomic sites because more simplistic options are usually available for those locations.

Nasolabial transposition flap

The single-staged nasolabial (melolabial) flap is a variation of a transposition flap that can be used to reconstruct defects of the nasal sidewall or large alar defects. Traditional designs of the nasolabial flap resulted in significant blunting of the nasofacial groove and frequent flap pincushioning, often requiring one or more postoperative revisions. This is perhaps why this flap has been underutilized in reconstruction of the nose. In 1990, Zitelli described several modifications of the traditional design that helped to minimize the need for surgical revisions. These modifications are outlined below.

The flap should be designed to include the preplanned excision of the Burow's triangle along the lateral nasal sidewall. The donor site should parallel the nasolabial fold and, once incised and elevated, should be widely undermined in a subcutaneous plane across the cheek. The recipient site should be undermined in a submuscular plane on the nose and then the surgeon should transition to the more superficial subcutaneous plane at the nasofacial sulcus. After careful hemostasis has been obtained, a periosteal suture is placed in the undersurface of the flap corresponding to the new location of the nasofacial groove. This is secured to the periosteum of the nasal sidewall and, once tied, recreates this important cosmetic structure while at the same time essentially eliminates any tension on the flap. The periosteal sutures also minimize secondary flap movement that might pull the ala laterally postoperatively. The flap should then be thinned of subcutaneous fat and sutured in place. We frequently utilize tacking sutures on the undersurface of the flap in an attempt to recreate the alar crease and to prevent collapse of the internal nasal valve. The tip of the flap is finally trimmed to match the distal aspect of the defect and sutured in place with minimal tension in order to limit flap ischemia (Fig. 147.22).

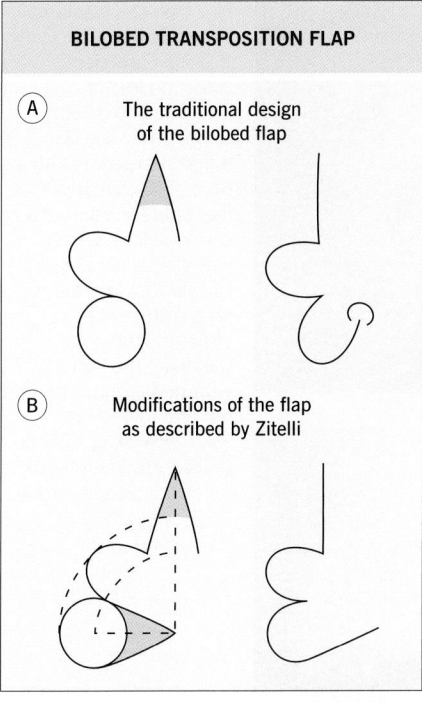

BILOBED TRANSPOSITION FLAP

(A) The traditional design of the bilobed flap

(B) Modifications of the flap as described by Zitelli

Fig. 147.20 Bilobed transposition flap. A The traditional design of the bilobed flap results in tissue protrusion at the pivot point. **B** Modifications of the bilobed flap as described by Zitelli.

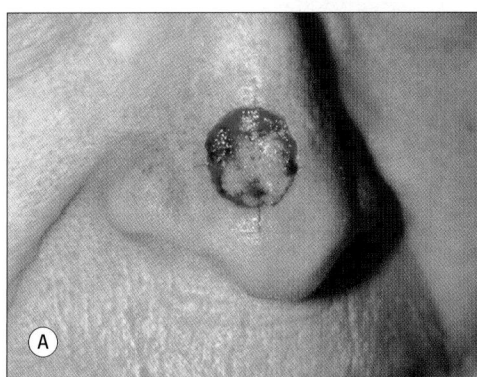
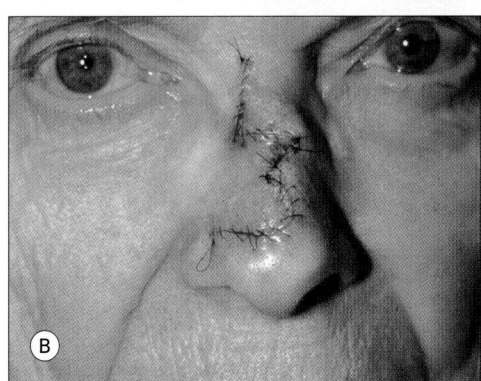
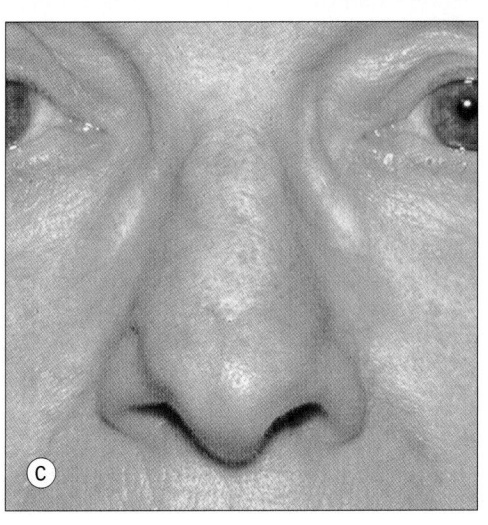

Fig. 147.21 Bilobed flap. A distal nose defect transposition (**A**) reconstructed with a modified bilobed transposition flap (**B**). **C** Cosmetic result at one year postoperatively.

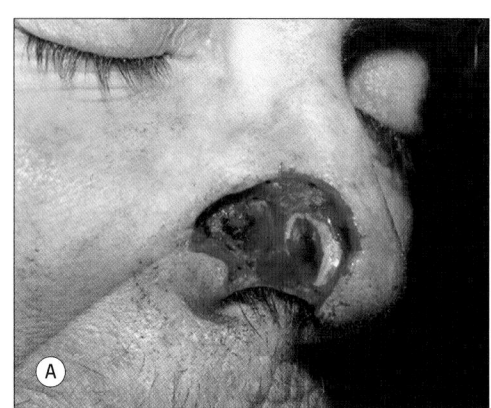

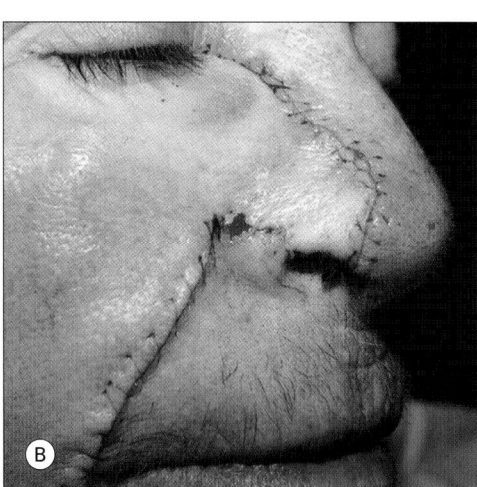

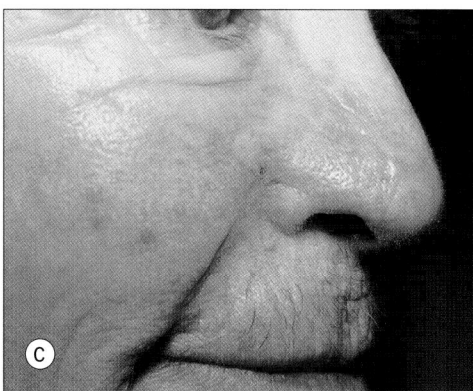

Fig. 147.22 Nasolabial transposition flap.
A Large nasal defect involving loss of cartilage and extending to the intranasal skin. **B** Reconstruction with a nasolabial transposition flap after insertion of a cartilage strut which was placed parallel to the alar rim in order to reconstitute the structural integrity of the nose. The flap is wrapped around the alar rim and folded onto itself, reforming the rim. **C** Cosmetic result at six months postoperatively.

Tissue Importation Flaps

Tissue importation flaps are a loosely associated group of flaps that employ the concept of transferring tissue from a distant reservoir into a defect when other adjacent repair options are unsatisfactory. The flap itself is supported by either: (1) a single vessel as in the paramedian forehead flap (an axial flap); or (2) a rich collection of subcutaneous perforating vessels that enter the flap pedicle through underlying muscle (random pattern flap). Tissue importation flaps are ordinarily two-stage procedures. The first stage includes the initial planning and implementation of the flap. The vascular pedicle is left in place after the first stage of the procedure to ensure adequate blood supply. The second stage involves the separation of the pedicle and the insetting of the proximal flap. Tissue importation flaps are most useful for reconstruction of large defects and are especially valuable when cartilage grafting is required to rebuild normal anatomic substructure and preserve proper function. The most common tissue importation flaps used in dermatologic surgery include the paramedian forehead flap, the nasolabial interpolation flap, the retroauricular flap, and the turnover nasolabial or Spear's flap.

Paramedian forehead flap

The paramedian forehead flap, an axial flap based on the supratrochlear artery, is the most useful flap for reconstruction of subtotal and total

nasal defects. The excellent vascular supply supports both the flap as well as any cartilage grafts that are used to rebuild the cartilage framework of the nose. The paramedian forehead flap also provides the best color and texture match of any of the tissue importation flaps used to reconstruct large defects of the nose and far exceeds the cosmetic results of a skin graft.

An important concept in flap design includes the enlargement of the nasal defect to encompass the entire cosmetic unit when possible. This makes the junction of the flap and the remaining nasal skin less conspicuous and is more likely to result in an excellent cosmetic outcome. If necessary, proper mucosal lining is ensured by using a nasal mucosal flap or split-thickness skin graft. If cartilage support is required, conchal or nasal septal cartilage is used to rebuild the normal subcutaneous cartilage framework. Next, a foil template of the defect is constructed and then transferred to the forehead. Using a length of 4×4 gauze to simulate the length of the pedicle, the surgeon ensures that the flap is long enough to be inset without tension on the tip. The base of the pedicle, fed by the supratrochlear artery, can be located with the use of a Doppler device, but this artery is consistently located 10 mm lateral to the midline of the glabella. When planning the forehead flap, keep in mind that the base of the flap must be thin enough to allow adequate twisting of the base in order to reach the defect. However, too small a pedicle base may risk vascular compromise that would result in disastrous consequences. We find a pedicle width between 8 and 15 mm to be adequate for both flap mobility and vascular supply.

Flap procurement is begun by incising the distal flap (on the upper forehead) in the subcutaneous plane and, as work progresses proximally (toward the inferior forehead), dissecting to a gradually deeper plane. The distal one-third of the flap should be dissected in the superficial subcutaneous plane, the middle one-third in the deep subcutaneous plane, and the proximal one-third (just above the brow) in the submuscular plane. The surgeon must carefully dissect the remaining pedicle above the periosteum, being sure to not sever the supratrochlear artery as it exits the supraorbital foramen. Bilaterally, the forehead is undermined in a subgaleal plane and then closed in a standard layered fashion. The widest part of the forehead defect may not close, but heals well by secondary intention. Finally, the distal end of the flap is thinned to match the thickness of the remaining nasal skin before it is inset.

The second stage of the forehead flap is performed 3 weeks later. The pedicle is severed near both the brow and the edges of both the brow and the pedicle stump are freshened so that an upside-down V is formed by both the pedicle stump and the brow defect. The stump is then trimmed of all fat and inset in a standard layered fashion, being sure to reposition the medial brow to match the contralateral side. After carefully trimming and thinning the proximal edge of the remaining flap, it is inset into the remaining nasal defect (Fig. 147.23).

Nasolabial interpolation flap

The nasolabial (melolabial) interpolation flap, a random pattern pedicle flap, has traditionally been utilized principally for the repair of defects primarily involving the nasal ala. This flap is especially useful for large defects and complex defects involving the alar rim. In certain circumstances, the nasolabial interpolation flap may be utilized for the repair of nasal tip defects when the latter are moderate in size and a paramedian forehead flap is less optimal.

When utilizing the nasolabial interpolation flap for the repair of alar defects, we recommend excising the remainder of the cosmetic unit of the ala in order to ensure a better aesthetic and functional result (Fig. 147.24). After providing any necessary cartilage support, a foil template is made of the contralateral ala and then it is turned over and placed on the ipsilateral nasolabial skin. A length of 4×4 gauze can be utilized to ensure proper flap length prior to outlining the flap on the cheek skin. The flap on the cheek is incised and dissected to a well-vascularized pedicle deep in the subcutis. The cheek and the defect are widely undermined in the superficial subcutaneous plane; the flap is then turned on its pedicle, trimmed, and sutured into place in a standard layered fashion. The donor defect is closed up to the base of the pedicle.

Three weeks later, the patient returns for separation of the pedicle. The surgeon amputates, trims and sutures the flap and the cheek in a standard layered fashion to ensure recreation of the normal complex anatomic features of this aesthetically important area. We find that

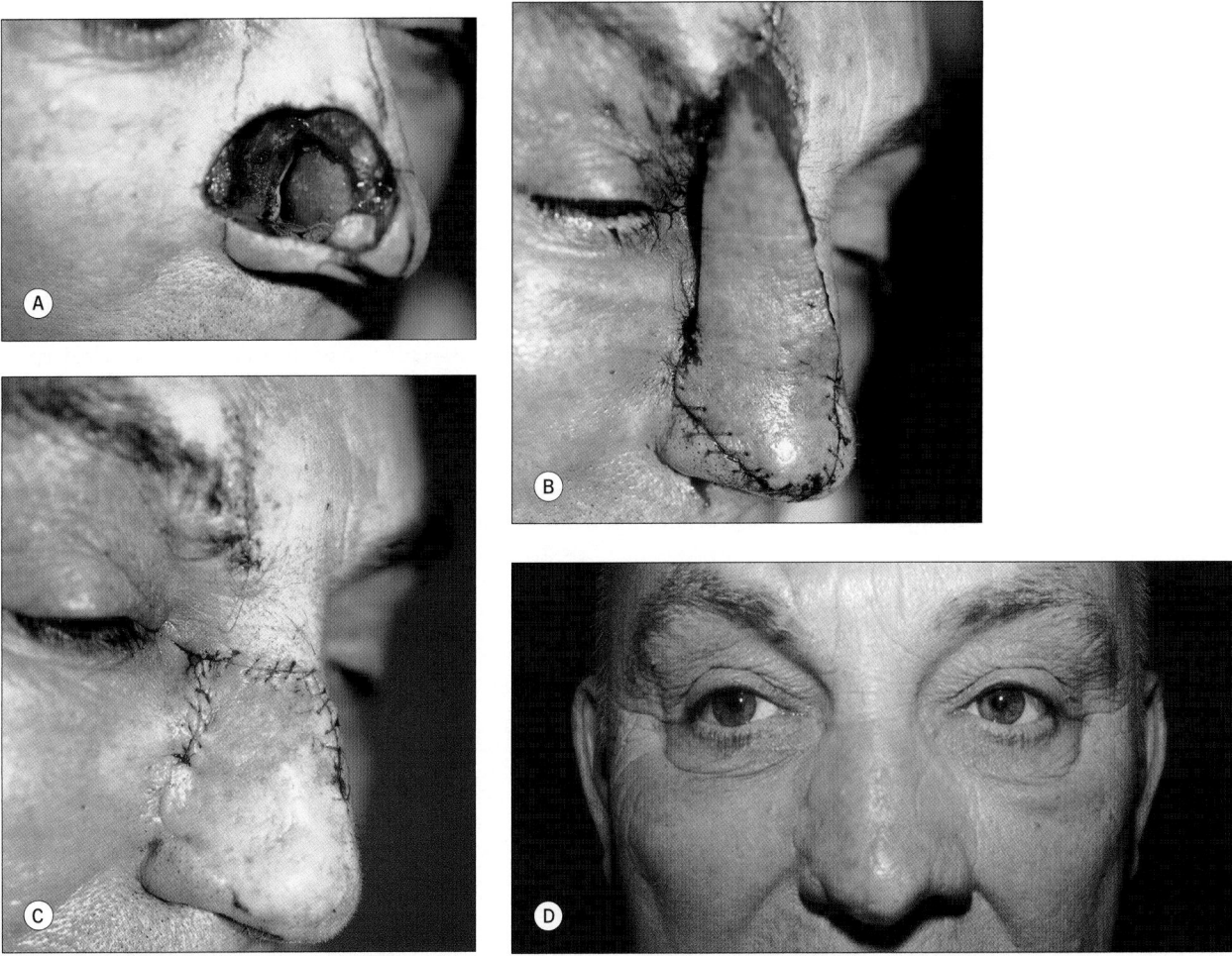

Fig. 147.23 **Paramedian forehead flap. A** Large full-thickness defect of the right half of the distal nose. The mucosal defect was reconstructed with a contralateral septal mucosal pull-through flap. A 15 mm square cartilage graft was harvested from the nasal septum and used to reconstitute the structural integrity of the nasal sidewall. Note that the remainder of the nasal sidewall cosmetic subunit and the right nasal tip subunit will be excised and reconstructed with a forehead flap. **B** Immediately postoperatively. **C** Immediately after takedown of flap 3 weeks later. **D** Early cosmetic results with no revision 2 months postoperatively.

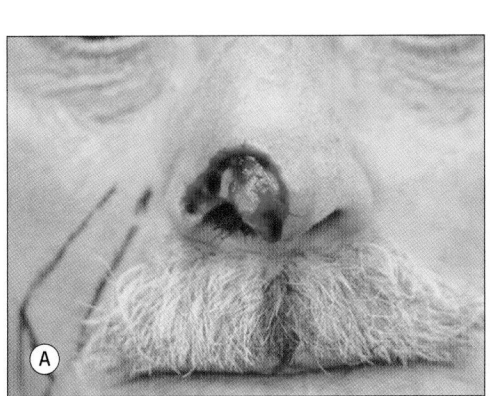

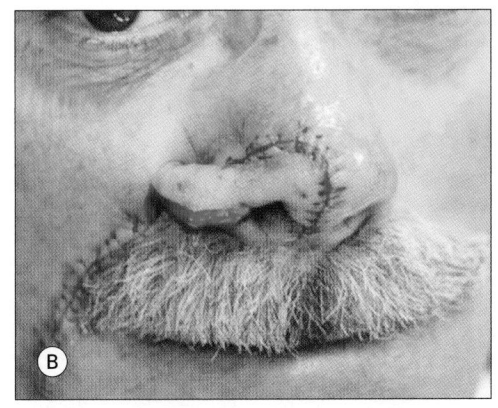

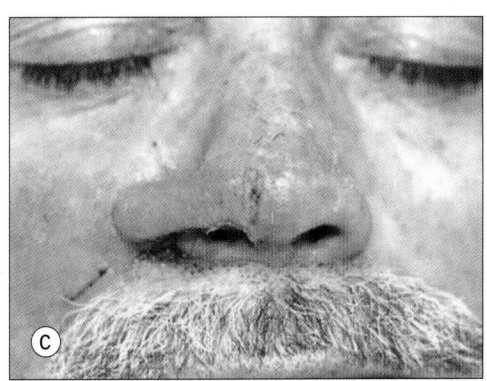

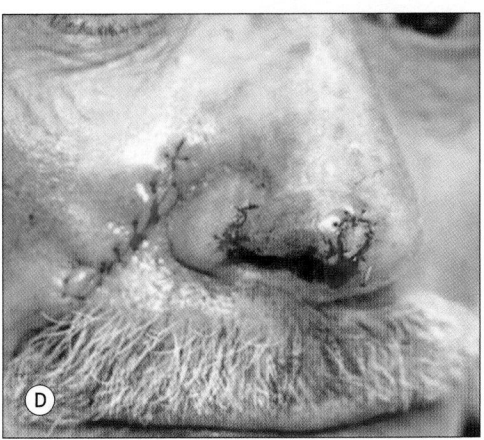

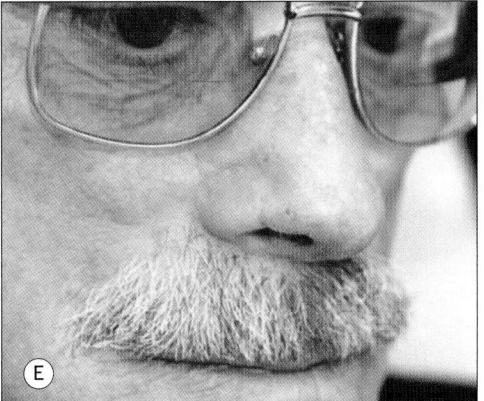

Fig. 147.24 **Nasolabial interpolation flap. A** Large alar defect with severe loss of structural integrity. **B** Nasolabial interpolation flap in place. Cartilage strut from auricle was sutured into wound bed parallel to alar rim to restore structural integrity. **C** Preoperatively (3 weeks after initial reconstruction), small area of flap necrosis in the region of the soft triangle of the nose. **D** Postoperatively, at time of transection of pedicle. Full-thickness skin graft was harvested from the resected pedicle and placed in site of necrosis to prevent notching of the soft triangle. **E** Six months postoperatively.

fusiform excision of the pedicle stump provides for the most aesthetically pleasing repair of the cheek donor site.

Retroauricular flap

The two-staged retroauricular flap is useful for large defects of the helical rim that involve loss of cartilaginous support. The retroauricular flap is a random pattern flap without a single vascular pedicle. Nonetheless, because of the rich blood supply of the scalp skin, this is one of the most well vascularized random pattern tissue importation flaps.

After providing cartilage support (if needed), a foil template of the defect is fashioned and then placed on the skin of the postauricular scalp. The necessary size of the flap is marked and then the flap is incised from the retroauricular sulcus back to the hairline. The flap is dissected in a subcutaneous plane and the tip judiciously thinned to match the thickness of the skin at the defect. The flap is sutured into place in a layered fashion, being sure to minimize tension as the flap curls around the anterior helical rim. We find the use of bolster sutures to be very helpful in recreating the curve of the antihelix. Three weeks later, the pedicle is severed near the scalp and the posterior aspect of the

flap is sutured into place. The donor site can either be closed with a skin graft or left to heal by secondary intention (Fig. 147.25).

Spear's flap

The reverse nasolabial (melolabial) pedicle flap, described by Spear, is useful for reconstruction of full-thickness defects of the ala that involve the attachment point of the lateral ala to the cheek.

The design of the Spear's flap is planned in a manner similar to that of the single-staged nasolabial interpolation flap, with the use of a foil template made from the contralateral ala. This template is placed upside down on the skin of the cheek lateral to the nasolabial fold and the flap is incised to a point just lateral to the edge of the defect. The flap is then dissected to a well-vascularized pedicle deep in the subcutis adjacent to the defect. Next, the flap is twisted on its pedicle and the edge of the mucosal defect adjacent to the nasal tip is sutured to the under-turned skin of the medial edge of the flap; we use a 5.0 chromic gut suture for this portion of the flap. The lateral portion of the under-turned flap is then sutured to the lateral mucosal defect. By folding the flap on itself, the alar rim and the surface of the ala are recreated, and

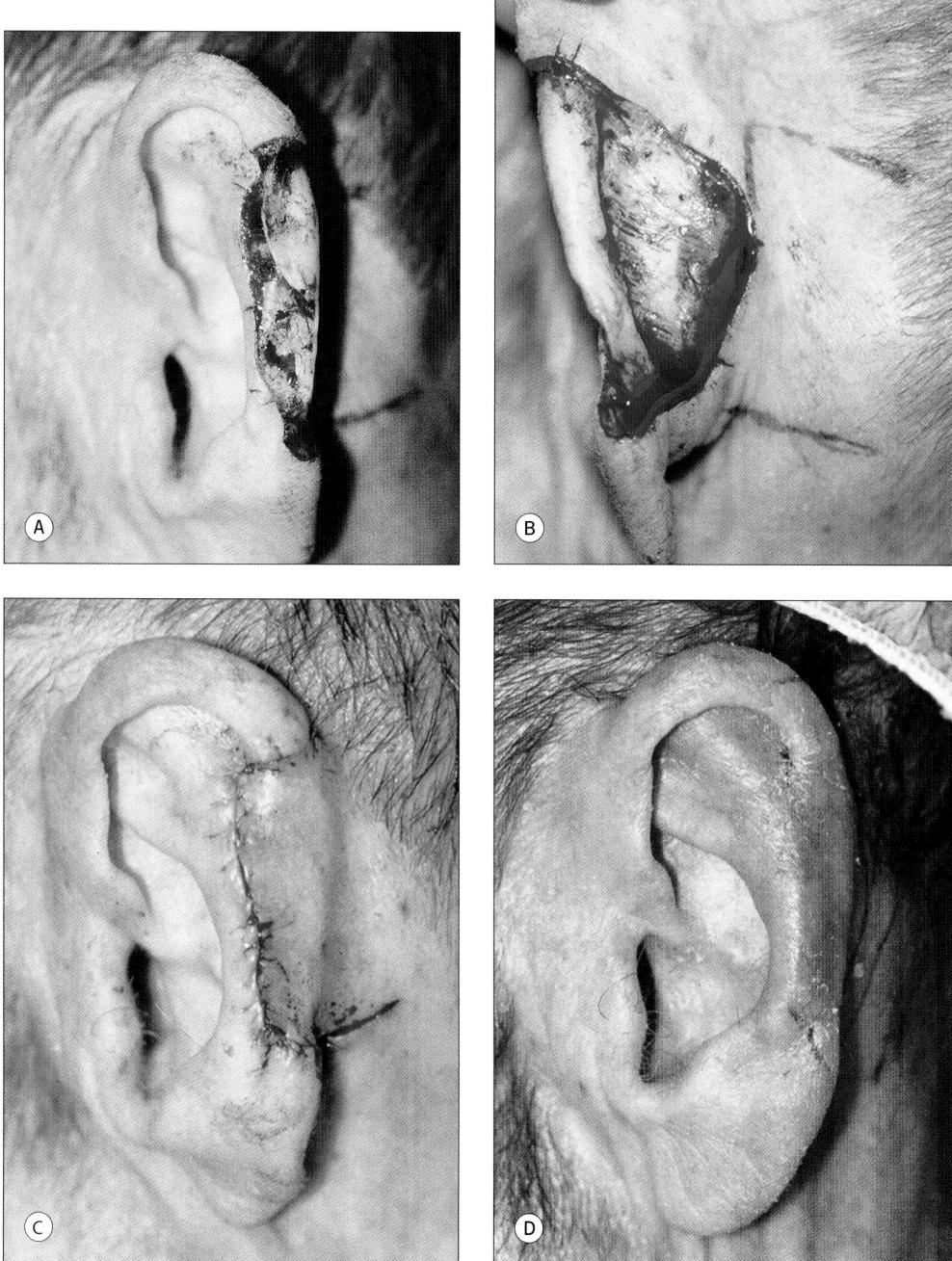

Fig. 147.25 Retroauricular flap. A Large helical rim defect with preservation of much of the auricular cartilage. **B** Posterior ear defect and the planned incisions for the retroauricular flap. **C** Retroauricular flap in place immediately postoperatively. **D** Immediately after takedown.

the tip of the flap is carefully trimmed to match the contralateral ala. The surface of the flap is closed in the standard layered fashion. As with the other nasolabial flaps, the donor site is closed after widely undermining the skin of the cheek. Occasionally, a dog-ear is created superolaterally to the new ala and it needs to be excised and sutured to complete the repair (Fig. 147.26). Usually, a second stage to reposition the new, lateral aspect of the ala is necessary by folding the flap on itself. Typically, the newly formed ala is positioned too far laterally and is shifted up to 1 cm medially to correspond with the position of the contralateral ala.

Table 147.4 summarizes the flaps discussed above and lists the areas of the face where the specific flaps are most useful for providing excellent functional and aesthetic results.

POSTOPERATIVE CARE

Postoperative care after flap surgery varies from practice to practice. Some surgeons have the patient change the bandage once or several times a day, cleansing the wound at each bandage change. Others apply a bandage for a day or two and leave the sutured wounds open to air thereafter. Still others apply a single bandage at the time of the surgery and leave it undisturbed for up to a week. Regardless of how the postoperative care is accomplished, there are common goals to achieve during the postoperative period.

One of these common goals is to prevent postoperative bleeding. The first 48 hours is the time period during which bleeding from the wounds and the formation of hematomas most commonly occur. Efforts to reduce these complications include meticulous intraoperative hemostasis and the application of pressure over the wounds. Pressure can be applied by using taping techniques, pressure wraps or specialized pressure garments. Normally, pressure becomes less important after 24 to 48 hours. In the patient at higher risk for bleeding, it may be necessary to maintain pressure for a more prolonged period of time. In some patients with a very high risk of postoperative bleeding, it may be helpful to use a tie-over bolster dressing directly over the wound to ensure constant firm pressure throughout the postoperative period.

Another common goal in the postoperative care of flaps is to reduce the risk of infection. All forms of infection can complicate the postoperative course and affect the cosmetic and functional results. Prevention of postoperative infections is covered elsewhere (Ch. 151). However, good surgical technique and observance of sterile technique during reconstruction is paramount. One novel approach, particularly well suited for cutaneous reconstructions, is the direct infiltration of the unclosed wound preoperatively with local anesthesia containing antibiotics. The benefit of intralesional nafcillin and clindamycin has been studied and this procedure is used routinely in some practices prior to reconstruction.

An additional important goal in the postoperative care of flap reconstructions is protection of the flap tissue from all environmental

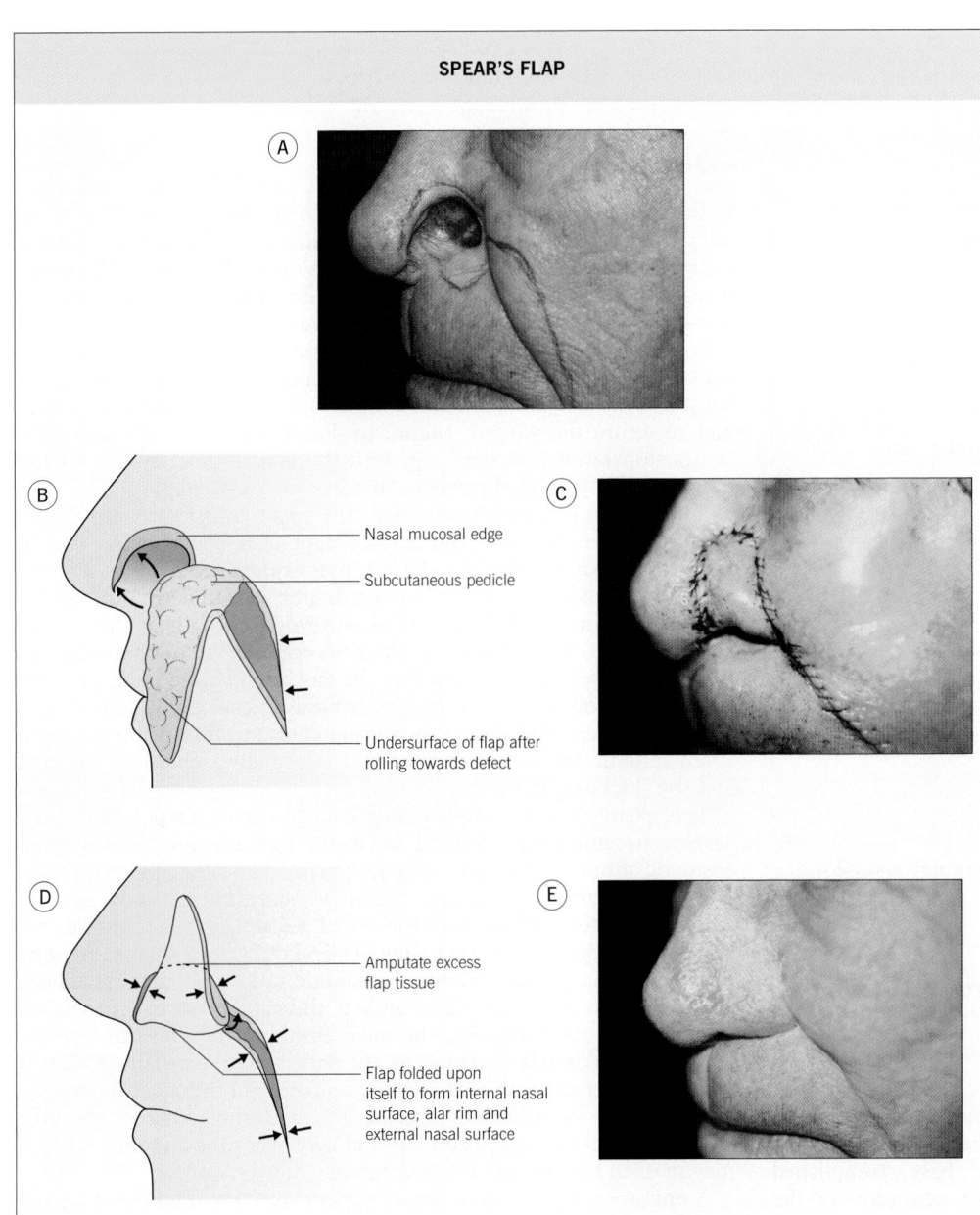

SPEAR'S FLAP

A

B
— Nasal mucosal edge
— Subcutaneous pedicle
— Undersurface of flap after rolling towards defect

C

D
— Amputate excess flap tissue
— Flap folded upon itself to form internal nasal surface, alar rim and external nasal surface

E

Fig. 147.26 Spear's flap. A Nasal defect involving the entire nasal ala and a portion of the nasal sidewall with the plans marked for a nasolabial transposition flap with a twist as described by Spear. **B** Corresponding schematic. **C** Flap in place having been twisted on a subcutaneous pedicle sutured into the mucosal side of the defect and folded upon itself followed by suturing of the cutaneous side of the defect. **D** Corresponding schematic demonstrating placement of the flap and amputation of the distal portion. **E** Early results after second revision.

COMMON LOCATIONS FOR PARTICULAR FLAPS
Burow's triangle displacement flaps
Burow's flap (single tangent advancement flap) and bilateral single tangent advancement flap (A-to-T flap)
– Distal, lateral nasal sidewall – Upper lateral lip – Infranasal upper lip – Eyebrow and suprabrow forehead – Mid helix
Unilateral or bilateral double tangent advancement flaps (U- or H-flap)
– Forehead – Helix – Large defect of upper lip
Rotation flap(s)
– Upper cheek – Medial chin – Nasal dorsum (Rigor flap) – Lower eyelid
Defect reconfiguration flaps
Island pedicle flap
– Upper lateral and mid upper cutaneous lip – Mucosal lip – Lateral chin and lower lip – Distal nasal sidewall – Preauricular cheek – Eyebrow
Tissue reorientation flaps
Rhombic transposition flap
– Nasal sidewall – Temples and lateral forehead – Lateral canthus and lateral lower lid – Lateral chin and lower lip – Superior and anterior helix
Bilobed transposition flap
– Nasal tip and supratip
Nasolabial transposition flap
– Alar defects, especially those involving the lateral portion of the ala – Lateral alar crease and distal nasal sidewall
Tissue importation flaps
Paramedian forehead flap
– Large nasal defects – Moderate-size defect nasal tip – Nasal defects with loss of cartilage and/or nasal lining – Large medial canthus defects
Nasolabial (melolabial) interpolation flap
– Nasal ala and alar rim – Nasal tip – Mid upper lip
Melolabial flap with a twist (Spear's flap)
– Full-thickness alar defects involving the junction of the lateral ala and the cheek/upper lip
Retroauricular flap
– Large defects of the anterior ear or helix – Full-thickness defects requiring cartilage graft reconstruction

Table 147.4 Common locations for particular flaps.

insults, including contamination, physical injury, temperature extremes, excessive movement and stretching of the sutured skin during the early postoperative period, and UV radiation. This is best accomplished by occlusive bandaging techniques and thorough education of the patient.

Presented here are the details of postoperative flap care as routinely implemented in one surgical practice. After the completion of the flap reconstruction, a light bandage is applied over a very thin coat of antibiotic ointment which is placed directly over the incision lines. The light bandage consists of non-stick gauze that is affixed with hypoallergenic paper tape. The tape completely covers the non-stick gauze, resulting in complete occlusion of the sutured skin. A 'bulky' secondary bandage is then applied on top of this thin primary bandage. The bulky bandage consists of rolled or fluffed absorbent gauze, which is affixed again with paper tape, using a technique of taping which applies downward pressure to the bulky gauze. This is accomplished by the placement of one end of the tape on the skin of one side of the wound and stretching it over the top of the bulky gauze and then attaching the other end to the opposite side of the flap under tension. This is repeated numerous times with thin, 1 cm wide strips of tape until the bulky gauze is entirely covered and firmly affixed by the tape. The patient is instructed not to allow the bandage to become wet for 1 week. They are instructed to remove the bulky secondary bandage 24 to 48 hours after the surgery, leaving the thin, primary bandage in place. This bandage is left undisturbed and kept dry for the remainder of the week.

The patient returns to the office in 1 week for bandage removal, suture removal and evaluation of the wound. Any evidence of hematoma, infection or other complications is addressed at that time. The skin is cleansed and another thin bandage with topical antibiotic ointment, non-stick gauze and hypoallergenic paper tape is applied for one more week. The patient is instructed again to keep this bandage dry and to remove it in 1 week (i.e. 2 weeks after the surgery). The patient is encouraged to contact the physician in the postoperative period if there are any problems and to return in 3 months for a final evaluation of the wound healing process. Minor revisions may be made at that time to optimize the aesthetic and functional results.

COMPLICATIONS

In the immediate postoperative period, the potentially serious sequelae are primarily postoperative bleeding and infection. Both adverse events are rare if meticulous surgical technique is used. Nonetheless, failure to recognize either complication and intervene appropriately can lead to disastrous postoperative results. Postoperative bleeding that results in a hematoma requires immediate attention. The most effective intervention is an immediate return to the operating suite to remove the sutures, evacuate the hematoma, locate and ligate the bleeding vessel, and re-suture the wound. Failure to do so likely risks flap necrosis. If a postoperative infection is present, immediate oral antibiotics and drainage of any trapped purulent material are required.

In the mid postoperative period, the most common complication requiring intervention is the development of a hypertrophic scar or trapdoor deformity. This usually becomes evident around 4 to 8 weeks after surgery and occasionally develops despite wide undermining, appropriate flap thinning and meticulous suturing technique at the time of surgery. Often, the patient is advised to aggressively massage the site many times per day. Massage and the tincture of time often promote adequate remodeling of the healing wound. Occasionally, active intervention is necessary. We use a varying concentration of intralesional triamcinolone injections (5–40 mg/ml), depending upon the location and the thickness of the flap.

Late postoperative complications include persistent pincushioning, surface irregularities, blunting or ablation of the junction between cosmetic units, and surface telangiectasias. Persistent pincushioning and minor surface irregularities can be addressed as early as 6 to 12 weeks postoperatively with the use of a scalpel to plane the surface and dermabrasion or dermasanding to blend the planed surface. In order to redefine the junction between cosmetic units that may have been ablated by the placement of a flap (e.g. the alar crease in a nasolabial transposition flap), incising the area, thinning the subcutis and re-suturing the skin edges to recreate the natural fold is usually all that is required. Laser ablation of telangiectasias that not infrequently develop around the incision lines of large nasal flaps can be done at any time. We find that these tend to develop gradually over time and that ablation may need to be repeated at future visits.

Sometimes, regardless of proper patient selection, flap planning and suturing technique, some amount of postoperative refinements may be necessary. These may vary from simple procedures to correct surface irregularities to more complicated interventions requiring further scalpel surgery. The key to a successful outcome from a postoperative intervention is recognizing the circumstances where an intervention would be helpful and then choosing the appropriate intervention. Understanding the normal sequence of healing after a surgical procedure helps the surgeon to decide when and by what means to intervene in this process.

FURTHER READING

Borges AF. The rhombic flap. Plast Reconst Surg. 1981;67:458–66.

Boyer JD, Zitelli JA, Brodland DG. Undermining in cutaneous surgery. Dermatol Surg. 2001;27:65–8.

Brodland DG. Fundamentals of flap and graft wound closure in cutaneous surgery. Cutis. 1994;53:192–200.

Brodland DG. Advancement flaps. In: Roenigk RK, Roenigk HH Jr (eds). Dermatologic Surgery: Principles and Practice, 2nd edn. New York: Marcel Dekker, 1996.

Brodland DG. Complex cutaneous closures. In: Ratz JL (ed.). Textbook of Dermatologic Surgery. Philadelphia: Lippincott-Raven, 1998.

Brodland DG. Paramedian forehead flap reconstruction for nasal defects. Dermatol Surg. 2005;31:1046–52.

Burget GC, Menick FJ. Aesthetic Reconstruction of the Nose. St. Louis: CV Mosby, 1994.

Dzubow LM. Subcutaneous island pedicle flaps. J Dermatol Surg Oncol. 1986;12:591–6.

Dzubow LM. Flap dynamics. J Dermatol Surg Oncol. 1991;17:116–30.

Fazio MJ, Zitelli JA. Principles of reconstruction following excision of nonmelanoma skin cancer. Clin Dermatol. 1995;13:601–16.

Futoryan T, Grande D. Postoperative wound infection rates in dermatologic surgery. Dermatol Surg. 1995;21:509–14.

Griego RD, Zitelli JA. Intra-incisional prophylactic antibiotics for dermatologic surgery. Arch Dermatol. 1998;134:688–92.

Pharis DB, Papadapoulos DJ. Superiorly based nasolabial interpolation flap for repair of nasal tip defects. Dermatol Surg. 2000;26:19–24.

Spear SL, Kroll SS, Romm S. A new twist to the nasolabial flap for reconstruction of lateral alar defects. Plast Reconstr Surg. 1987;79:915–20.

Zitelli JA. The bilobed flap for nasal reconstruction. Arch Dermatol. 1989;125:957–9.

Zitelli JA. Tips for wound closure: pearls for minimizing dog-ears and applications of periosteal sutures. Dermatol Clin. 1989;7:123–8.

Zitelli JA. The nasolabial flap as a single-staged procedure. Arch Dermatol. 1990;126:1445–8.

Zitelli JA. Tips for a better ellipse. J Am Acad Dermatol. 1990;22:101–3.

Zitelli JA, Brodland DG. A regional approach to reconstruction of the upper lip. J Dermatol Surg Oncol. 1991;17:143–8.

Zitelli JA, Fazio MJ. Reconstruction of the nose with local flaps. J Dermatol Surg Oncol. 1991;17:184–9.

Zitelli JA, Moy RL. Buried vertical mattress suture. J Dermatol Surg Oncol. 1989;15:17–19.

Grafts

Désirée Ratner

Key features

- Free skin grafts are pieces of skin that have been severed from their local blood supply and transferred to another location

- Grafts for soft tissue reconstruction can be divided into four types: full-thickness skin grafts, split-thickness skin grafts, composite grafts, and free cartilage grafts

- In dermatologic surgery, grafts are most commonly used to repair defects created after removal of skin cancers; grafts also provide coverage and more rapid healing of leg ulcers

- The clinical situation determines the type of graft to be placed

- A working knowledge of the indications, techniques, donor site considerations, postoperative care, and postoperative complications of all types of skin grafting is essential for optimal soft tissue reconstruction

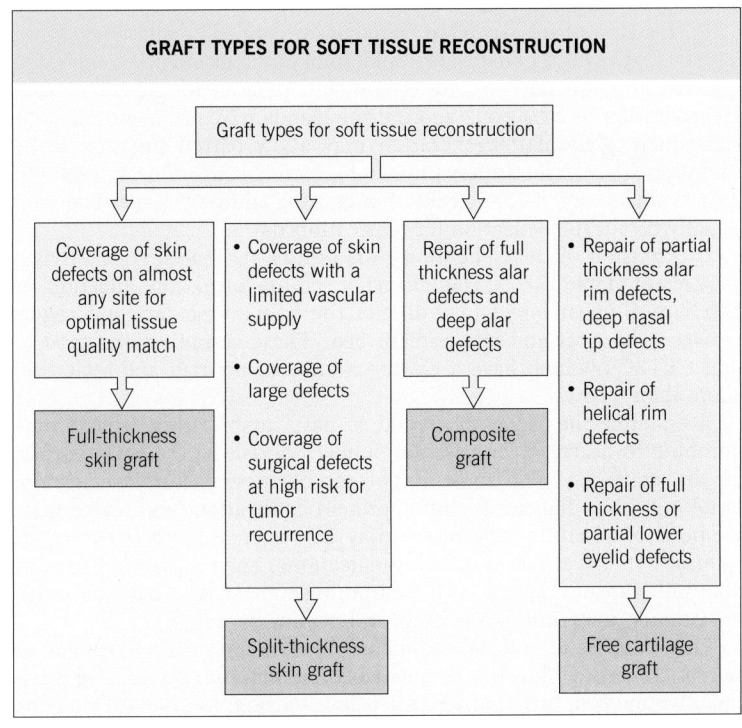

Fig. 148.1 Graft types for soft tissue reconstruction.

INTRODUCTION AND BACKGROUND

Skin grafting procedures originated approximately 2500 to 3000 years ago, when surgeons of the Hindu Tilemaker caste replaced noses amputated as punishment for theft and adultery with skin grafts harvested from the gluteal region[1]. It was not until the 19th century, however, that skin grafting was again introduced as a reconstructive technique. In 1869, Reverdin's account of pinch grafting for leg ulcers was published; in subsequent decades, Ollier and Thiersch's accounts of thin split-thickness skin grafting, and Wolfe and Krause's accounts of full-thickness skin grafting appeared in the literature[2–6]. While these and other 19th century surgeons used skin grafts to address only the most difficult problems of surgical management, skin grafting has since evolved into a reconstructive option that is routinely, and sometimes preferentially, used for the surgical repair of skin defects.

Free skin grafts are pieces of skin that have been severed from their local blood supply and transferred to another location. They can be divided into four types: full-thickness skin grafts (FTSGs), split-thickness skin grafts (STSGs), composite grafts, and free cartilage grafts (Fig. 148.1 & Table 148.1)[7–9a]. FTSGs are composed of the entire epidermis and the full thickness of dermis, including adnexal structures such as hair follicles and sweat glands. STSGs are composed of the full thickness of the epidermis and partial thickness of dermis. These can be subdivided into thin, medium and thick grafts, depending on the amount of dermis included in the graft. Composite grafts are composed of at least two different tissue types, usually skin and

cartilage. Free cartilage grafts consist of cartilage with its overlying perichondrium.

WOUND HEALING CONSIDERATIONS

Wound healing after skin grafting proceeds through a unique series of events[10,11]. The first 24-hour period following placement of the graft is termed the stage of plasmatic imbibition, during which fibrin glue attaches the graft to its recipient bed, allowing it to take up the underlying wound exudate and to become edematous, gaining up to 40% in weight[12]. The graft thereby remains hydrated and obtains a supply of nutrients, which maintains the patency of graft vessels until revascularization begins. The fibrin beneath the graft is subsequently replaced by granulation tissue, which attaches the graft permanently to its bed.

With proper apposition of the graft and its recipient bed, revascularization may proceed. Anastomoses begin to form within 48–72 hours

COMPARISON OF GRAFT TYPES USED IN SOFT TISSUE RECONSTRUCTION								
Graft type	Tissue match	Nutritional requirements	Requirement for recipient bed vascularity	Infection risk	Graft contraction risk	Durability	Sensation	Appendageal functions
FTSG	Good to excellent	High	High	Low	Low	Good to excellent	Good	Excellent
STSG	Poor to fair	Low	Low	Low	High	Fair to good	Fair	Poor
Composite	Good	High	Very high	Moderate	Low	Fair	Fair	Good
Free cartilage	N/A	Moderate	High	Moderate	Migration or deformation possible, with subsequent resorption	Good	N/A	N/A

Table 148.1 Comparison of graft types used in soft tissue reconstruction. FTSG, full-thickness skin graft; STSG, split-thickness skin graft.

of grafting between the recipient bed and pre-existing vessels in the dermis of the graft, a process known as inosculation[13,14]. Vascular proliferation occurs next, with sprouting and budding of vessels in the graft and in the recipient bed[10]. Even relatively avascular tissue may be grafted, as long as the avascular area is small and surrounded by a rich vascular bed. Through a process known as the bridging phenomenon, vascular connections arising from the recipient bed allow blood flow to occur through pre-existing graft vasculature, so that nutrients reach the part of the graft overlying the avascular area. Full circulation is restored to the graft within 4–7 days.

Restoration of the lymphatic circulation parallels restoration of the blood supply over the first week. Epidermal proliferation occurs between the 4th and 8th day post-transplant and persists for several weeks. Degeneration of sebaceous and eccrine glands may occur initially, but subsequent glandular regeneration may allow partial function to be maintained[10]. Graft reinnervation and return of sensory nerve function may begin as early as 2–4 weeks after grafting, although patients do not usually regain full sensation for many months[9,15,16].

If extension of the ischemic period occurs, decreased graft survival may result (Table 148.2). Hematoma or seroma formation, infection, or mechanical shear forces may disrupt the fragile vascular connections between the graft and its recipient bed. These complications tend to affect FTSGs (which have a greater volume to nourish and revitalize) more than STSGs.

Even after the ischemic period is past, many other factors may combine to decrease the vascular supply nourishing the undersurface of the graft[7–9,15]. The most important of these factors is cigarette smoking[17], but diabetes mellitus, protein deprivation, and severe trace element or vitamin deficiencies may also increase the risk of graft failure[7–9,15,18]. Certain systemic medications, such as corticosteroids, chemotherapeutic agents, other immunosuppressive drugs, and anticoagulants, may interfere with wound healing as well.

Other causes of graft failure include: insufficient vascularity due to necrotic debris within the recipient bed, hematoma, seroma, an avascular wound bed, infection, excessive graft tension, mechanical shearing forces, and improper postoperative care (see Table 148.2)[7,9]. The most common infectious agents associated with graft failure include coagulase-positive staphylococci, β-hemolytic streptococci and *Pseudomonas*. Pseudomonal infections are particularly common in auricular grafts. For all of these reasons, a thorough preoperative evaluation, meticulous intraoperative technique, and good postoperative care are essential to maximize graft survival.

FULL-THICKNESS SKIN GRAFTS

Indications/Contraindications

FTSGs are most commonly used to repair facial defects resulting from the removal of skin cancers[7–9,19]. They may be used to repair defects at virtually any site, as long as the recipient bed has a sufficiently rich vascular supply to promote capillary regrowth, as well as fibroblasts to supply collagen for graft adherence. Small avascular areas may be grafted due to the bridging phenomenon. Larger areas of avascular tissue, including patches of exposed bone, cartilage, tendon or nerve devoid of periosteum, perichondrium, peritenon or perineurium, respectively, are unable to support full-thickness grafts. For this reason, FTSGs should not be placed over such avascular tissue.

Under the proper circumstances, FTSGs can provide excellent color, texture and thickness matches for facial defects because they include the full thickness of epidermis and dermis. Wound contraction is minimized since the full thickness of dermis is present, and dermal adnexal structures remain intact[20]. FTSGs may be especially useful for the cosmetically and functionally acceptable repair of defects of the nasal tip, dorsum, ala and lateral sidewall, as well as the lower eyelid and ear (Fig. 148.2)[9].

Preoperative History and Donor Site Considerations

A thorough preoperative evaluation that includes questions regarding bleeding tendencies, alcohol use, use of anticoagulant medications (including aspirin and non-steroidal anti-inflammatory drugs) and a history of hypertension can help reduce the risk of excessive bleeding and clot formation beneath the graft postoperatively[7,8]. Diabetes mellitus, nutritional deficiencies or cigarette smoking may increase the risk of graft failure, and any history of these should be identified preoperatively. As mentioned earlier, immunosuppressive medications may also interfere with wound healing, thereby increasing the risk of graft failure.

Selection of a donor site for full-thickness skin grafting depends upon the color, texture, thickness, and sebaceous qualities of the skin surrounding the defect (Tables 148.3 & 148.4)[7,8,21]. Most FTSGs are taken from the sun-exposed areas above the shoulders whose color, vascular pattern, texture, and distribution and quality of adnexal structures best match the skin surrounding the facial defects. The thinnest grafts are usually harvested from the upper eyelid or the postauricular sulcus. Medium-thickness grafts are often harvested from the preauricular and cervical regions, while thicker grafts may be taken from the supraclavicular or clavicular region or the nasolabial fold[22]. It is important to recognize that donor site thickness, irrespective of site, will vary from one patient to another, and it is therefore important to examine all donor sites carefully to find the best possible tissue match. This approach will ensure the best donor site selection for each individual patient and surgical defect.

A regional approach may at times be used to obtain the best possible match for a given defect. Grafts taken from redundant upper eyelid skin may be used to repair lower eyelid defects, providing a good color and texture match in addition to a well-camouflaged donor site scar. Grafts used for lower eyelid defects should be oversized by 100–200% to allow for contraction and to avoid the possible side effect of ectropion[23]. Due

CAUSES OF GRAFT FAILURE	
Poor graft–bed contact	Hematoma
	Seroma
	Shearing forces due to excessive postoperative activity
	Shearing forces due to inadequate immobilization of graft
Poor recipient bed vascularity	Inadequate vascular bed
	Exposed cartilage, bone, tendon
	Nicotine-induced vasoconstriction
Infection	Coagulase-positive *Staphylococcus*
	Beta-hemolytic *Streptococcus*
	Pseudomonas spp.
Host factors	Diabetes mellitus
	Immunosuppression
	Poor general health
	Nutritional deficiencies
	Systemic conditions with vascular compromise
Technique	Rough handling of tissue
	Excessive devitalized tissue in recipient bed due to cautery
	Increased tension on graft due to inadequate size
	Inadequate hemostasis
	Inadequate trimming of adipose layer
	Placement of upside-down graft (more common with STSG)
	Inadequate anchoring (composite and free cartilage grafts)

Table 148.2 Causes of graft failure. STSG, split-thickness skin graft.

DONOR SITE CONSIDERATIONS FOR FULL-THICKNESS SKIN GRAFTS
• Pattern of sun exposure
• Color
• Vascular pattern
• Texture
• Sebaceous quality
• Skin thickness
• Skin consistency
• Sufficient tissue available for harvesting
• Ability to camouflage donor site scar

Table 148.3 Donor site considerations for full-thickness skin grafts.

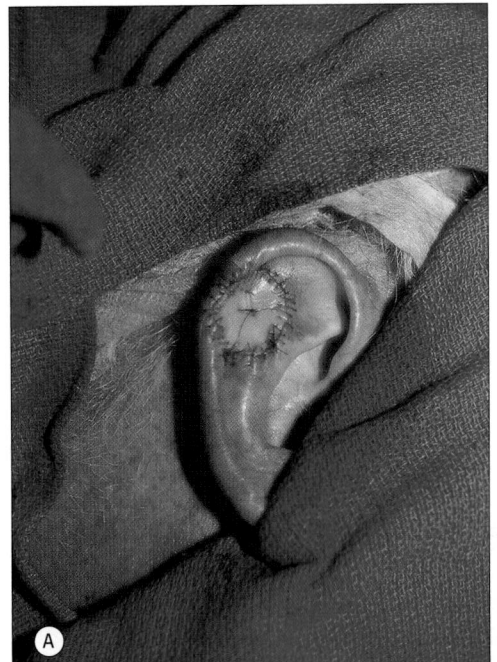

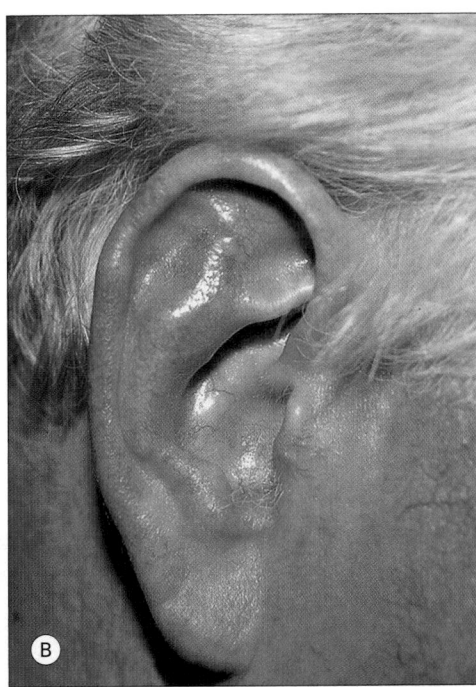

Fig. 148.2 Full-thickness skin graft. A Full-thickness skin graft taken from the preauricular region was used to repair this defect of the right upper anterior ear. **B** Eight-week postoperative result.

SUMMARY OF POSSIBLE FULL-THICKNESS DONOR SITES FOR DEFECTS IN DIFFERENT LOCATIONS	
Defect sites	**Donor sites**
Nasal dorsum, sidewalls, tip	Preauricular region, supraclavicular region or lateral neck (if large)
Nasal tip, ala	Preauricular region, conchal bowl, nasolabial fold
Junction of nasal dorsum/tip	Burow's graft
Ear	Postauricular sulcus, preauricular
Lower eyelid/medial canthus	Upper eyelid, postauricular sulcus
Scalp	Supraclavicular region, lateral neck, inner upper arm
Forehead	Burow's graft, supraclavicular region, lateral neck, inner upper arm (if large)

Table 148.4 Summary of possible full-thickness donor sites for defects in different locations.

to its relatively large size and inconspicuous location, postauricular skin may also be useful as a primary donor site for eyelid defects (including those of the medial canthus), as well as for auricular defects. Because postauricular skin is relatively non-sun-exposed, grafts harvested from this region may not provide a good color or texture match for facial defects in other areas.

Preauricular skin is more versatile, and it can be used to repair most nasal defects, since the thickness and degree of sun exposure of these areas tend to be comparable[24,25]. The donor site scar in this region can be easily camouflaged, as in facelift surgery, to provide a cosmetically desirable result. Even bearded individuals have a 1–2 cm hairless zone in the preauricular region. Care must be taken not to harvest hair-bearing skin in grafts taken from this area, as the dimensions of the preauricular region are relatively small. Accidentally including mature follicular units may produce the undesirable cosmetic result of hair growth within the graft. Hair-bearing skin from the temporoparietal region may be used to repair defects of the eyebrow, where survival of the follicular units after transplantation may help to produce a superior cosmetic result. Skin from the nasolabial fold or from the conchal bowl can sometimes be used to graft small nasal tip defects[26,27]. At times, sufficient laxity of the skin may be present, particularly on the nose or forehead, to allow for partial closure of the defect and use of the adjacent Burow's triangle as a FTSG, providing an excellent tissue match[28–30].

For larger defects requiring full-thickness grafts of sun-damaged skin, such as the forehead and scalp vertex, the supraclavicular region or lateral neck can be used as a donor site[22]. Again, care must be taken not to harvest unwanted hair along with the graft. These donor sites are often more difficult to camouflage, and must be carefully placed, especially in areas that might not always be covered by clothing, such as the lateral neck. Although the color and texture match may not be optimal, areas below the neck with thin, redundant skin, such as the upper inner arms, forearms and inguinal area, can be used.

Description of Technique

Varying techniques for harvesting and placing FTSGs have been described[7–9,23,31]. In order to perform an FTSG, a template of the defect is first made, using any flexible material, such as gauze, Telfa™ or aluminum foil, which can be bent to conform to the defect. After marking the periphery of the recipient site with a marking pen, the template material is pressed against the defect, and the resulting outline of the inked margin serves as a guide to cut a perfect template (Fig. 148.3A,B). The template is applied to the donor site, and inking material applied around it (Fig. 148.3C). The graft should be 3–5% larger in size than the true template to allow for the natural contraction and shrinkage of the graft after its removal from the donor site. Often, just cutting around the outside of the inked margin accounts for this extra 'safety' skin. For eyelid defects, grafts should be oversized significantly, to minimize the risk of ectropion. Marking the donor site prior to local anesthesia prevents incorrect sizing due to tissue stretch from lidocaine infiltration.

After the donor site is marked, local anesthesia may be injected into the donor and recipient sites. Epinephrine may be used without compromising graft survival[32]. If waterproof ink is not available for template marking, the outline of the graft template may be scored on the donor site with a needle. The donor site and recipient beds are then scrubbed with an antibacterial preparation such as chlorhexidine, rinsed with saline, and draped with sterile towels.

The donor site is excised with a scalpel to the level of the subcutaneous fat. The graft is placed in a sterile bowl or Petri dish containing normal saline, where it may remain for up to 1–2 hours. Grafts may be utilized up to 24 hours after harvesting if refrigerated or kept on ice. Before the graft is sutured into place, defatting of the graft should take place (Fig. 148.3D). This is an essential step, since direct contact between the graft and its bed allows for connections between existing vessels as well as new vessel growth and nutritional support from the base of the defect. Adipose tissue adherent to the graft is poorly vascularized and is therefore not a good tissue medium for new vessel growth between the graft and its bed.

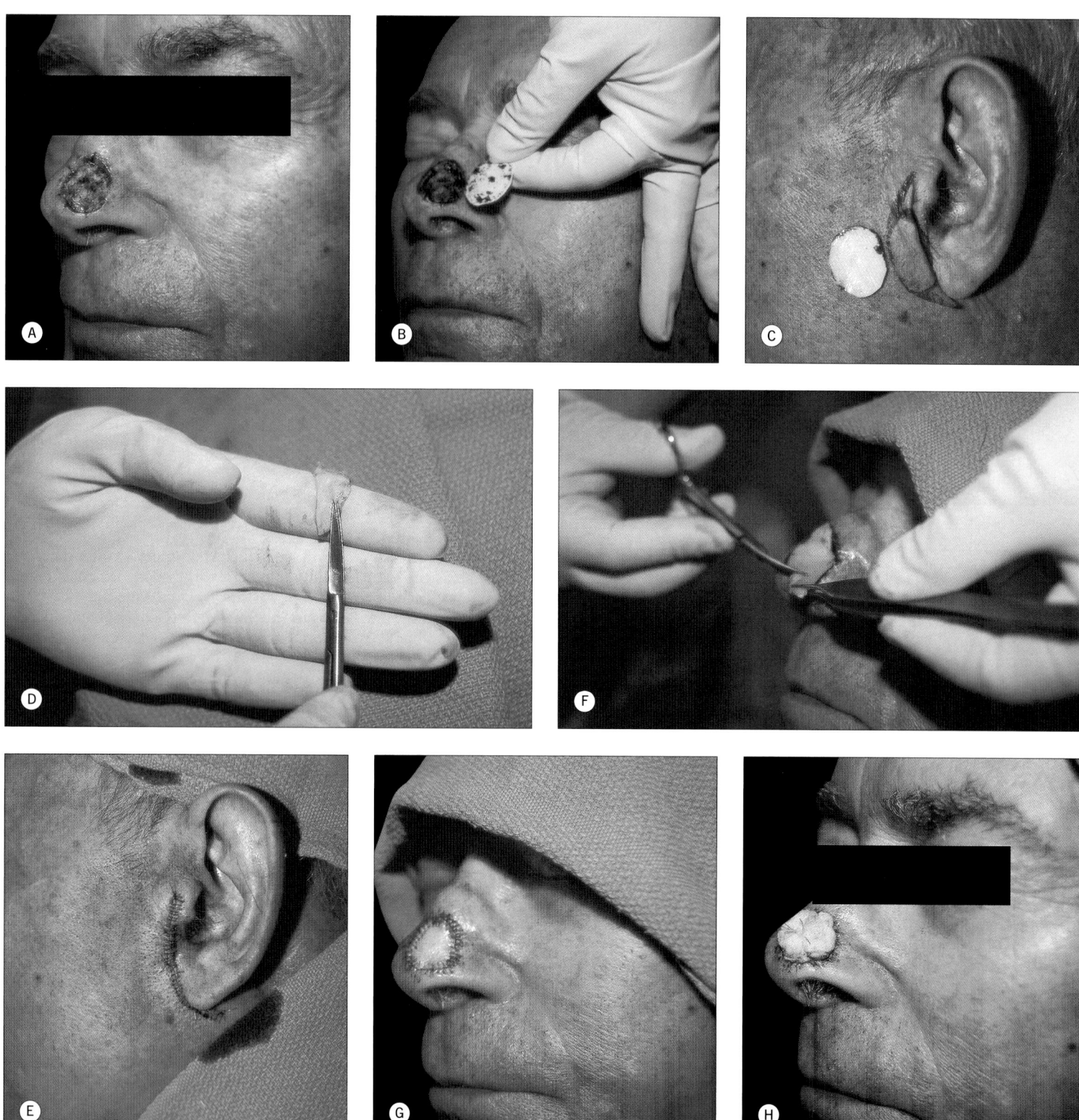

Fig. 148.3 Placement of a full-thickness skin graft. A A 1.7 × 2.0 cm defect of the nasal tip is present after removal of recurrent basal cell carcinoma with Mohs micrographic surgery. A preauricular donor site provides the best match in this case for color, sebaceous quality, degree of photodamage, and thickness. **B** After marking the periphery of the recipient site with a marking pen, the template material is pressed against the defect. The resulting outline of the inked margin serves as a guide to cut a perfect template, seen here adjacent to the nasal defect. **C** The template has been applied to the preauricular donor site, and inking material applied around it. Burow's triangles are outlined on either side of the template to close the site primarily. Marking the donor site prior to local anesthesia prevents incorrect sizing due to tissue stretch from lidocaine infiltration. **D** The graft is carefully defatted with curved iris scissors so that only the white, glistening surface of the dermis remains. **E** Preauricular donor site is closed primarily. **F** Full-thickness skin graft is trimmed with curved iris scissors to ensure a perfect fit. **G** Full-thickness skin graft sewn into place with 6-0 fast-absorbing chromic gut sutures. **H** Xeroform™ bolster sewn into place over full-thickness skin graft with 5-0 polypropylene tie-over sutures.

When defatting is performed, the graft is placed dermal side up on the fingers or in the palm. All fat is trimmed from the underside using sharp scissors. Fat is adequately removed when all of the yellow globular material is gone, and a white glistening surface of dermis remains. If indicated, part of the dermis can also be trimmed to allow for differences in the thickness of the recipient site, although adnexal structures may be removed in the process, potentially altering the cosmetic result. The graft is then placed dermis down in the recipient bed, and rotated and trimmed if necessary, to provide a perfect fit (see Fig. 148.3F). While one surgeon is trimming the graft, another may close the donor site, usually in a linear layered fashion with bilateral removal of dog ears (Fig. 148.3E).

Contouring of donor skin in FTSGs may be challenging, particularly in the reconstruction of defects on the nasal tip, ala, lateral nasal sidewall, helical rim of the ear, and eyelid[33]. Graft contouring often requires multiple trial placements within the graft bed, as well as multiple trimmings, to obtain an optimal aesthetic result (Fig. 148.3F). Removal of cartilage not needed for structural support before grafting may increase the chance of graft survival, particularly for auricular defects, without compromising the aesthetic appearance of the repair[34,35].

Securing the Graft

Perimeter sutures, basting sutures, support dressings, or a combination of any or all of these can be used to anchor the FTSG. Depending upon the size of the graft, four to eight interrupted 5-0 or 6-0 absorbable or non-absorbable sutures may be placed at opposite edges of the graft periphery (e.g. at 3, 6, 9 and 12 o'clock) to tack down its four quadrants. A simple running suture, such as 6-0 fast-absorbing chromic gut suture (Fig. 148.3G), may then be placed around the perimeter of the graft. Great care is taken to achieve perfect epidermal wound approximation. The running suture is placed in almost epicuticular fashion, passing the needle first through the graft and then through the surrounding skin. Placing the suture slightly higher in the dermis on the graft side and slightly deeper in the dermis of the surrounding skin makes suture placement easier, prevents tenting of the edges of the graft, and maximizes graft–recipient bed contact.

The use of tissue adhesives in full-thickness skin grafting has been investigated. In an initial pilot study of 21 patients, it was found that the use of cyanoacrylate tissue adhesive to secure FTSGs to their recipient bed wound edges produced cosmetic results essentially identical to those achieved with suturing[36]. Because these adhesives set virtually instantaneously, the graft must be perfectly trimmed and aligned before application of the adhesive, since fine adjustments in positioning the edge of the graft are not easily made. Tissue adhesives may represent a useful time-saving alternative to suturing for securing the periphery of selected grafts, particularly those in relatively immobile areas such as the temple, forehead and distal nose.

Basting sutures, usually simple interrupted 6-0 fast-absorbing gut sutures, can occasionally be placed to secure the central portion of the graft. They can be useful in securing large grafts to provide extra support against movement, as well as grafts placed on a concave surface where tenting of the graft could possibly occur. All sutures should be snug, but not strangulating, as graft survival can be compromised from sutures that have been tied too tightly.

Immobilization of the graft over its bed can be maximized by the use of pressure dressings. Classically, tie-over bolster dressings have been employed to immobilize grafts, using anchoring stents to ensure direct contact between the graft and its bed[9,37]. These stents may consist of various materials such as Xeroform™ gauze (bismuth tribromophenate-petrolatum-impregnated gauze, Sherwood-Daris & Geck, St Louis, MO), cotton balls, foam rubber, sponges, plastic beads or disks. Although sutures are usually employed to anchor the stent, adhesive wound closure tapes or Steri-strips™ can also be applied to exert an even amount of pressure to the bolster over the graft[38]. Adherence of the dressing to the graft, which tends to pull the graft away from its bed at the time of dressing removal, can be minimized by first applying antibiotic ointment, a non-adherent contact dressing, or Xeroform™ gauze, to the graft site[39]. Pressure or tie-over dressings help to immobilize the newly placed graft during the critical period of revascularization, and they help to prevent hematoma or seroma formation. Some authors postulate that such dressings may not be necessary to secure very small FTSGs[40].

The simplest bolster consists of Xeroform™ gauze alone, which is molded and placed to apply pressure to the graft. One end of each of the peripheral non-absorbable sutures is cut long, to a length of approximately 3–6 cm, and its opposing suture is left uncut. The suture ends can then be tied over the dressing two at a time (i.e. 12 o'clock to 6 o'clock and 3 o'clock to 9 o'clock) to secure the bolster (Fig. 148.3H). A running bolster suture has also been described[41]. A light dressing consisting of Telfa™ and Hypafix® (Hy-Tape Corporation, Yonkers, NY)

may be placed over the graft. The donor site is dressed with a pressure dressing for 24 hours.

Postoperative Care

After the pressure dressings are removed, the patient (or physician) must follow the wound care instructions carefully. One method is to gently clean the donor site and area immediately surrounding the bolster with hydrogen peroxide followed by application of antibiotic or petrolatum ointment (Vaseline®) twice a day. The bolster is not disturbed until dressing removal in 1 week, at which point the bolster and all tie-over sutures are removed. Steri-strips™ may be applied to the donor site as needed after the sutures have been removed.

The ideal graft is light pink in color when the bolster is removed. The color of the graft may range, however, from pink or red to darker blue or purple, depending on the extent of graft revascularization. Patients should be cautioned about these color changes beforehand so that they will not be alarmed if they occur. A bluish tinge may be a sign of ecchymosis rather than graft failure. A black graft signals necrosis and is undesirable. It is possible that the entire epidermal surface may become black and necrotic, and then slough without adversely affecting the dermal portion of the graft, as re-epithelialization can occur from adnexal structures and the epithelial edges, with an acceptable cosmetic result. Therefore, eschars should not be debrided, since they can serve as natural dressings, under which healing will progress. After sutures are removed, gentle cleansing with hydrogen peroxide to remove all crusts is recommended, followed by a thin layer of Vaseline® or antibiotic ointment. Patients should be counseled that the vascular supply of the graft remains fragile for weeks. For this reason, trauma, such as direct shower water to the area, and excessive activity should be avoided for an additional 1 to 2 weeks.

Variations/Unusual Situations

Purse-string suture

The purse-string suture is a subcuticular stitch that is placed around the periphery of a circular or oval surgical defect[42,43]. This type of suture allows partial closure of the defect by advancing skin from the entire periphery of the wound, and may help to cover areas of exposed cartilage or bone at the edge of the wound that could inhibit graft take. The full-thickness graft that is required to cover the remainder of the defect is thereby greatly reduced in size due to an approximately 50% reduction in the area of the defect[42]. Because of the reduced defect size, the skin graft needed to complete the repair may be harvested from traditional preauricular, postauricular or supraclavicular donor sites, which provide the best color, texture and thickness match for most sun-exposed areas. Furthermore, FTSG placement decreases the risk of significant wound contraction, resulting in a better cosmetic and functional result than would be produced by split-thickness skin grafting or second intention healing.

Burow's grafts

Defects of the nasal sidewall and dorsum, and sometimes of the forehead, lateral neck or other areas, may be repaired with Burow's grafts[28]. Because Burow's grafts utilize skin adjacent to the defect, they tend to provide a cosmetically superior match compared to grafts harvested from other locations[29,30,44]. These grafts are harvested from the skin superior to the defect if on the nose, and medial or lateral to the defect if on the forehead. The Burow's triangle is excised (see Ch. 146) and the resulting donor defect is closed primarily, thereby partially decreasing the size of the original defect. The triangle is defatted, trimmed, and sutured into the defect. Operating time is decreased because a separate donor site is not required. Burow's grafts tend to be limited in size. When insufficient laxity is present for partial donor site closure, or if the Burow's triangle does not appear to be sufficiently large to cover the remaining defect, alternative donor sites should be sought.

Deep nasal defects

Deep postsurgical defects on the nose and alar rim may at times pose a challenge for repair. Delaying FTSG placement for 12 to 14 days may increase the likelihood of graft survival over defects of the nasal tip and ala with denuded cartilage[45]. If a depressed defect on the nose is anticipated, but immediate reconstruction is preferred, dermal grafts can be used as a tissue filler prior to FTSG placement[46]. Use of these dermal grafts can effectively fill the defect, with little risk of resorption, and eliminate the need for a more complicated choice of repair. The 'drumhead' graft repair of deep nasal alar defects involves application of an overlying rigid plastic suspension coupled with an undersized graft, thereby preventing graft depression and nasal valve collapse[46a].

Perichondrial cutaneous grafts (PCCGs) are actually composite grafts composed of full-thickness skin and subjacent perichondrium, and may be used as a substitute for FTSGs in the reconstruction of deep nasal tip and alar defects, particularly in defects with exposed cartilage[21,47,48]. These grafts are harvested from the conchal bowl, utilizing the subperichondrial plane as the plane of dissection of the graft. The cartilage is not removed, making this graft more analogous to a FTSG than a cartilage-containing composite graft, which will be discussed in detail later. The advantages of PCCGs over FTSGs include the following: the former grafts are thicker, they have a greater chance of survival under conditions of vascular compromise, and they contract less than FTSGs.

Postoperative Complications

The complications of full-thickness grafting can be divided into short-term problems of graft failure and long-term functional and cosmetic problems[9]. Short-term problems include infection, hematoma, seroma, and shearing forces of the graft over the wound bed. These problems are significant when they occur, but they usually can be avoided. Infection after grafting of facial defects, in particular, is not often encountered, and oral antibiotics are not routinely given postoperatively. Nevertheless, it is important to be gentle while handling tissue intraoperatively, and to minimize devitalized tissue created by electrocautery, to minimize the risk of infection. Prophylactic oral antibiotics that cover *Staphylococcus* and *Streptococcus* species may be helpful in selected patients, especially those with diabetes mellitus, immunosuppression, or a prolonged intraoperative time.

Hematoma and seroma formation can be avoided by meticulous hemostasis intraoperatively, pressure dressings, and postoperative caution[49,50]. After consultation with the patient's internist, cardiologist or primary care physician, patients may be instructed to avoid aspirin for 10 days before surgery, non-steroidal anti-inflammatory drugs for 5 days before surgery, and alcohol for 2 days before and 2 days after surgery. Warfarin can often be discontinued 2 days before surgery and resumed the day after based on the recommendations of the patient's internist or cardiologist. Patients are also advised not to engage in vigorous activity, heavy lifting or bending for at least 1–2 weeks after surgery. The latter measures help to inhibit graft movement and supplement the effectiveness of the bolster in minimizing shearing forces of the graft over its bed.

Long-term complications of FTSGs consist of cosmetic and functional problems. It is imperative to stress to the patient prior to graft placement that FTSGs usually take months to look natural. Good preoperative counseling may help to alleviate the fears concerning the graft's cosmetic appearance during the first weeks after the bolster is removed. Make-up can usually be applied 3–4 weeks after graft placement. It is important to note that FTSGs are often depressed during their first 2–4 weeks. This depression will usually correct itself within 4–6 weeks. Although careful donor site selection will minimize the color, texture and contour deformities that can occur, patient and physician satisfaction with the cosmetic result may not be complete after healing has finished. Delaying skin grafting for 7–14 days if tissue loss is deep, such as on the nasal tip or ala, may allow granulation tissue to fill in the defect such that a better contour may ultimately be achieved[45,51,52]. Spot dermabrasion or laser resurfacing may be performed after 6 weeks to 6 months to correct differences in elevation between the graft and its surrounding skin, as well as to improve color and texture mismatch[53,54]. Resurfacing of the entire cosmetic unit may be helpful in optimizing the cosmetic result. Hyperpigmentation of the graft can be treated with a brief course of topical hydroquinone and/or tretinoin. The use of tretinoin pre- and postoperatively has not been shown to alter the course of healing of FTSGs[55].

Functional complications of FTSGs occur primarily as a result of wound contraction. Grafts contract secondary to the centripetal move-ment of unopposed elastic fibers, and a variable amount of shrinkage can therefore be expected, depending upon the thickness and elasticity of the donor site[7,56]. In one study, it was found that the area of FTSGs contracted by a mean of 38% by 16 weeks after placement, with grafts applied to the periorbital area and nose contracting more than those applied to the scalp and temples[56]. Graft contraction usually increases as the thickness of the graft decreases, and is thought to occur in the fibrous layer under the graft, either in the bed itself or in the layer of scar tissue wedged between the graft and its bed[7]. Complications due to graft contraction are usually minimal in FTSGs. If wound contraction does result in functional or cosmetic abnormalities, secondary revisional surgery may be needed.

Future Directions

For patients with an inadequate vascular bed, full-thickness skin grafting may not be possible, necessitating repair with a less cosmetically elegant STSG. High-density porous polyethylene implants have therefore been designed which permit ingrowth of fibroneovascular tissue without change in the size or shape of the implant[57]. When these prefabricated implants were placed in rabbits, it was found that they developed sufficient vascularity to sustain an FTSG. This technology holds promise for patients with deep nasal and ear defects, in whom an anatomically correct structure could be implanted, after which, time could be allowed for fibrovascular tissue ingrowth, and full-thickness skin grafted later for a superior cosmetic result. In addition, progress is being made on incorporating complex blood vessels into bioengineered skin equivalents.

SPLIT-THICKNESS SKIN GRAFTS

Split-thickness skin grafts (STSGs) consist of epidermis and a portion of the dermis. These grafts vary in thickness from approximately 0.005 to 0.030 inches (0.13–0.78 mm), and are classified as thin (0.005–0.012 inches/0.13–0.31 mm), medium (0.012–0.018 inches/0.31–0.47 mm) or thick (0.018–0.030 inches/0.47–0.78 mm), depending upon the amount of dermis included in the graft (Table 148.5).

Indications/Contraindications

STSGs have less tissue requiring revascularization than FTSGs. They are thus more likely to survive when placed on almost any recipient bed, including those with a limited vascular supply. These grafts may therefore be placed over periosteum, perichondrium, peritenon and perineurium. STSGs are also used to cover large defects, particularly those that cannot be covered by a flap or would heal too slowly by secondary intention, as well as refractory venous leg ulcers[7,11]. STSGs may be useful for covering surgical defects in sites at high risk for tumor recurrence, since deep recurrent tumor is usually visible when growing through split-thickness skin. If the tumor does not recur after 1–2 years, the graft can be removed and a definitive reconstruction performed.

Advantages of STSGs over FTSGs include their improved chance of survival under conditions of vascular compromise, their ease of application, their ability to cover large defects, and their ability to act as a 'window' for recurrence of high-risk lesions. The principal disadvantages of STSGs include their suboptimal cosmetic appearance, the presence of a granulating donor site wound requiring postoperative care, greater graft contraction, and the special equipment required to harvest larger grafts. Furthermore, because of their relative thinness, STSGs may be less durable than FTSGs, necessitating regrafting or partial healing by secondary intention.

CLASSIFICATION OF SPLIT-THICKNESS SKIN GRAFTS	
Thin	0.005–0.012 in/0.13–0.31 mm
Medium	0.012–0.018 in/0.31–0.47 mm
Thick	0.018–0.030 in/0.47–0.78 mm

Table 148.5 Classification of split-thickness skin grafts.

While thicker STSGs tend to be cosmetically superior to thinner STSGs, poor color and texture match with the surrounding skin often occurs after placement of an STSG (Fig. 148.4). STSGs tend to be pale or white in color, hairless, and smooth in texture, with impaired sweating due to the fact that adnexal structures are not removed in their entirety with the graft and do not survive. The contrast between the STSG and its surrounding skin can therefore produce a 'tire-patch' appearance, which is more pronounced than that seen in FTSGs.

Preoperative History and Donor Site Considerations

Cosmesis of the donor site scar should be taken into consideration when selecting a donor site for an STSG. The ease of postoperative donor site care and the type of instrument used to harvest the graft may also help to dictate the donor site. Ideally, STSGs should be harvested from an area from which a broad area of skin can be removed while still concealed beneath clothing. The most common donor sites include the anterior, medial and lateral portions of the upper thigh, the inner and outer aspects of the upper arm, and the inner aspect of the forearm. The anteromedial thigh is most frequently used as the donor site for STSGs, as harvesting and wound care are convenient, and wounds in this location do not interfere with ambulation. Donor site wounds on the buttocks tend to require assisted postoperative care, although their scars are ideally placed from the cosmetic point of view. Power-driven dermatomes and large freehand knives require large flat donor surfaces, which may limit donor sites to the thighs, abdomen and buttocks, while smaller grafts can be harvested freehand or with a Davol-Simon dermatome.

Description of Grafting Techniques

A wide variety of techniques for harvesting and placing STSGs have been described[7,58–60]. The instruments used to harvest STSGs can be classified into freehand and electric dermatomes. Freehand dermatomes include scalpel blades, double-edged razor blades, and knives such as the Weck blade. Although acceptable grafts can be obtained using these freehand devices, considerable technical expertise is required to harvest them.

A standard #15 or #15c blade can be an effective tool for harvesting small STSGs of medium thickness. After a template of the defect is made, the donor site is marked out and anesthetized. The donor site is scored lightly with the blade, after which the graft is harvested by orienting the blade parallel to the skin and gently sweeping the blade just below the level of the epidermis, so that the blade is just visible beneath the skin (Fig. 148.5). It is helpful to have an assistant apply traction to the donor site while the graft is harvested. Several blades may be required to harvest the graft, as the sharpness of the blade diminishes quickly with multiple passes. This technique may be especially useful in harvesting small STSGs of medium thickness for the repair of auricular and postauricular defects.

Power-driven dermatomes became the standard method of harvesting larger STSGs after Brown developed the first such instrument in the 1940s. Until recently, the Brown and Padgett dermatomes were the instruments of choice for harvesting STSGs of various thicknesses and widths, while Davol-Simon dermatomes were used to cut smaller

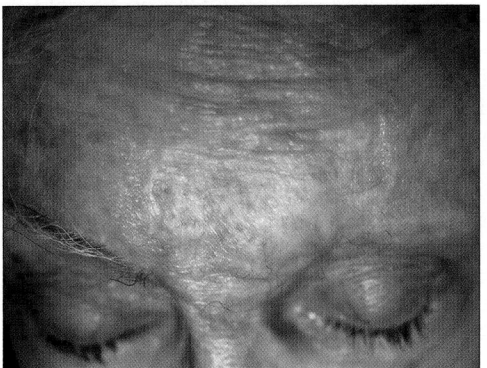

Fig. 148.4 Split-thickness skin graft site on the forehead 1 year after placement. Note hypopigmentation and smooth texture of grafted skin compared with the surrounding normal skin.

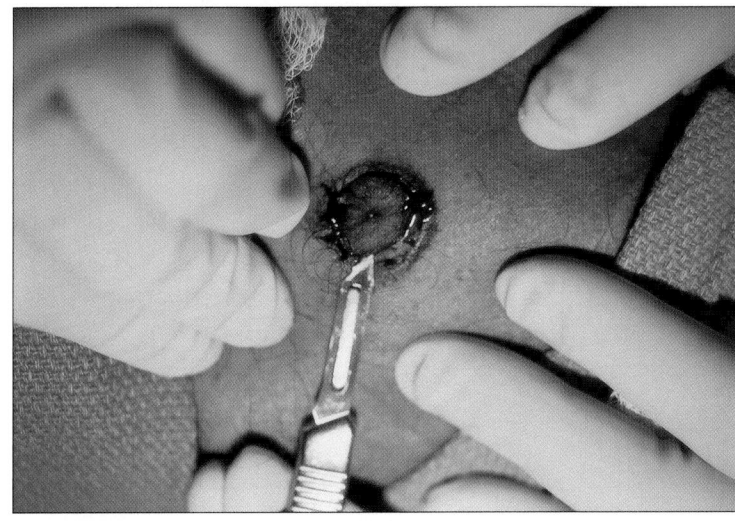

Fig. 148.5 Freehand harvesting of a small split-thickness skin graft from the upper outer arm using a no. 15 scalpel blade. The blade is oriented parallel to the skin, and gently swept just below the level of the epidermis, so that the blade is just visible beneath the graft. An assistant applies traction to the donor site to facilitate harvesting.

STSGs of fixed width and thickness. Although STSGs can be obtained easily and reliably with any of these devices when properly used, the quality of the graft obtained is technique-dependent, and substantial irregularity in graft thickness and width may at times occur. The Zimmer dermatome, a newer dermatome originally powered by compressed water-pumped nitrogen and subsequently modified into an electrically powered version, tends to harvest uniform grafts of predetermined width and thickness such that consistent graft quality tends to be less dependent on the technique of the operator.

After the dermatome is prepared, the donor and recipient sites are anesthetized with lidocaine with or without epinephrine, and the areas are prepped and draped in the usual sterile fashion. If chlorhexidine surgical scrub is used, a saline wash is employed to remove any excess scrub. The donor site is lubricated in advance with sterile mineral oil or another lubricant to ease travel of the dermatome over the skin. The handpiece is held on the donor site at an angle of 30–45°. A throttle control is pressed to start the cut, and the unit is guided forward using light downward pressure to ensure that the cutting edge remains in continuous contact with the donor site. An assistant applies tension by pulling the skin away from the donor area to create a flat, even surface. As the dermatome glides over the donor skin, the graft emerges from the pocket area of the dermatome, and is lifted away from the machine with tissue forceps or hemostats (Fig. 148.6A). Once a sufficiently large graft has been harvested, the dermatome is pulled away from the skin and the graft is placed in sterile saline (Fig. 148.6B).

Securing the Graft

As in the case of FTSGs, STSGs should be secured so that infection, hematoma or seroma formation, and mechanical shearing forces can be prevented. Both the perimeter and the central portion of the graft must be secured for adequate nutritional support and to ensure graft survival. The edges of STSGs need not be as closely approximated to the surrounding wound edge as those of FTSGs, since overlapping skin will slough without affecting the ultimate cosmetic result. After the graft has been placed such that the dermal side is adherent to the recipient bed, the perimeter of the graft may be secured with sutures or staples. Several centrally placed basting sutures may also be helpful in ensuring good apposition of the graft to its bed. Once the graft has been secured and its bolster sewn into place, a non-adhesive dressing or pressure dressing may be applied as an additional precaution. Sutures or staples are removed after 7–10 days.

Donor Site Care

Harvesting STSGs creates a second wound, the donor defect, which often causes more postoperative discomfort than the grafted area itself.

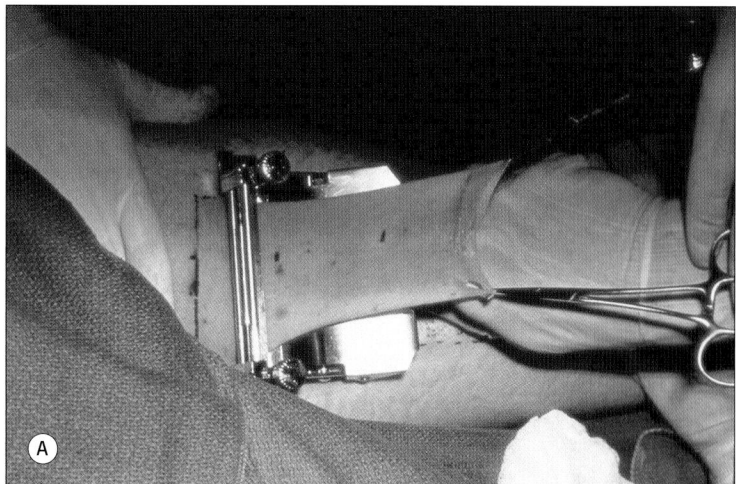

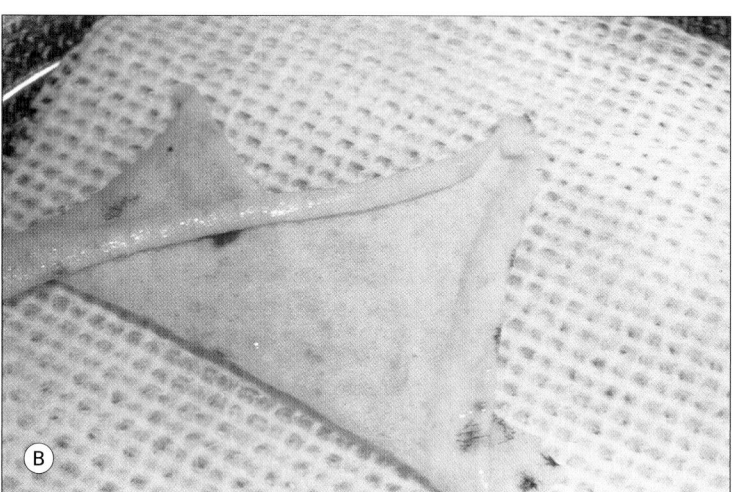

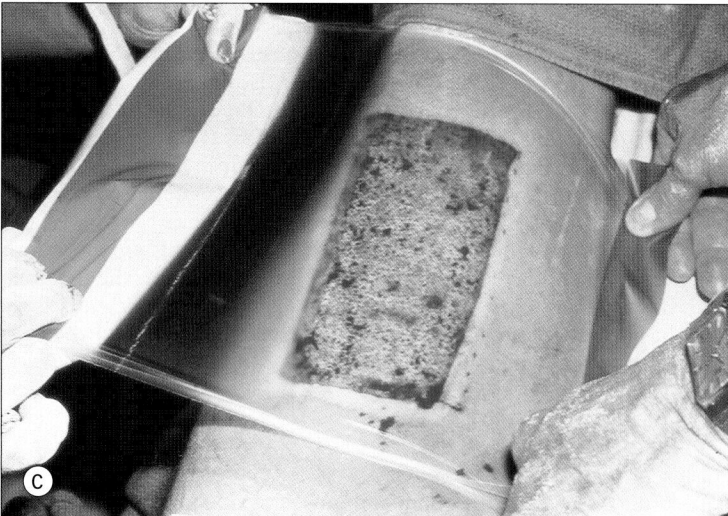

Fig. 148.6 Harvesting of a large split-thickness skin graft with an electric dermatome. A As the Zimmer air dermatome glides over the donor skin, the graft emerges from the pocket area of the dermatome, and is lifted away from the machine with sterile hemostats. **B** Split-thickness skin graft placed on sterile saline-soaked gauze. Note that the edges curl inward toward the dermal surface of the graft. **C** An Opsite® dressing is placed over the donor site on the anterior thigh immediately after harvesting.

This partial-thickness wound heals by secondary intention. While STSG donor sites were once treated with bulky occlusive dressings left in place for 10–14 days, the advent of transparent, vapor-permeable dressings such as Opsite® (Allerderm Laboratories, Petaluma, CA) has made the postoperative period easier in terms of comfort and ease of care (Fig. 148.6C)[61]. These dressings are advantageous in that they allow the serosanguineous drainage that inevitably accumulates at the

donor site to collect, keeping the wound moist and thereby shortening healing time. Because these dressings are transparent, the wound can easily be observed for complications during the healing process. In one review of the literature, these dressings were found to be associated with the fastest healing rates, a low infection rate, the least amount of pain, and minimal cost when compared with other dressings[62].

After the skin around the donor site area is cleaned and dried, a thin coat of an adhesive such as Mastisol® (Ferndale Laboratories, Ferndale, MI) is applied around the wound and allowed to dry. An Opsite® dressing is then placed over the wound. Paper tape is placed around the perimeter of the Opsite®, followed by a gauze dressing and an Ace® wrap (Becton-Dickinson, Rochelle Park, NJ).

Variations/Unusual Situations

Meshing the graft with scalpel slits may be performed to allow for drainage of accumulated blood or serosanguineous material that could otherwise inhibit graft–bed contact. This technique may also be used to expand the surface area of an STSG. A graft meshing machine may be utilized to expand the surface area of the graft by a ratio ranging from 3:1 to 9:1. Meshing can help to provide coverage of a large recipient area with smaller donor grafts. Furthermore, expanded meshed grafts placed experimentally on contaminated recipient beds have been found to exhibit increased take as compared with non-meshed donor skin[63].

Postoperative Care

During the first 24 hours after grafting, a large amount of serosanguineous fluid may accumulate beneath the donor site dressing. Patients need to be forewarned of this so that they do not become alarmed. If this occurs, the fluid can be drained with a needle and syringe, and an Opsite® patch applied. Alternatively, a new Opsite® dressing can be applied. The dressing can then be left in place until healing is complete. Depending on the thickness of the STSG, the donor site should fully re-epithelialize in 7–21 days. The flat scar usually evolves in color from pink to white over a period of months.

Complications

The complications of split-thickness skin grafting can be divided into early complications, which stem from failure of engraftment, and late complications[7,9,19]. Failure of engraftment may result from hematoma or seroma formation, infection, and shearing forces. Late complications can be divided into cosmetic and functional problems.

Color and texture mismatch of STSGs with the surrounding skin is predictable and expected to occur. Grafts often remain erythematous for months to years after placement, but, more importantly, they may exhibit significant hyperpigmentation and hypopigmentation as well. Darker-skinned patients are especially prone to graft hyperpigmentation, despite observance of preventive measures. Patients should minimize graft exposure to the sun without sunscreens for 6 months, and wear sunscreens consistently thereafter to avoid hyperpigmentation. The absence of adnexal structures can predispose to xerosis and a build-up of keratinous debris. The resultant scaling, pruritus and dryness can be minimized with the liberal use of emollients.

Functional considerations are of paramount concern, since STSGs contract more than FTSGs and can create forces powerful enough to produce joint contraction if placed over or near joints[64,65]. Contraction of facial grafts, especially near the nasal ala, the eyelid, the helical rim and the free margins of the vermilion border, may produce significant cosmetic deformities, including retraction of the nasal ala, ectropion, distortion of the helical rim and distortion of the vermilion border, respectively. Hypertrophic scarring of the graft and donor sites may also occur, and can be treated with corticosteroid-impregnated tape or intralesional steroids. Graft fragility and breakdown can occur in areas of trauma, particularly in sites such as the lower leg or in areas with little underlying soft tissue support, such as those directly overlying perichondrium or periosteum. Such complications are not always avoidable, but forewarning patients may reduce the risk of unnecessary trauma to the area. Lastly, bullae can occur within graft sites, presumably related to decreased anchoring properties of the basement membrane zone (see Ch. 34).

Future Directions

In recent years, biosynthetic and tissue-engineered living skin replacements have been the focus of research in skin transplantation. Cultured human keratinocytes have been seeded onto type I collagen membranes to reconstitute the epidermis, enabling transfer of actively proliferating keratinocytes onto partial-thickness wounds[66]. Human epidermal tissues mimicking the biochemical and morphologic properties of human skin have also been established *in vitro* by growing human keratinocytes on a dermal fibroblast-containing collagen gel[67]. Such skin-equivalent cultures may hold promise in reconstituting the epidermis in patients with full-thickness burn wounds and chronic ulcers.

An acellular dermal matrix has been created from normal human skin, which could in the future be used in conjunction with cultured epidermis to graft partial- or full-thickness wounds[68]. An artificial dermis has also been used prior to full-thickness grafting of the skin of the nose[69]. In addition, an acellular allograft dermal matrix has been shown to provide a good bed for STSGs in patients with full- and partial-thickness burns[70]. A tissue-engineered human skin equivalent, a bilayered product containing living human fibroblasts, keratinocytes and bovine collagen, is commercially available for the repair of surgical defects and coverage of lower leg ulcers that would previously have been repaired with STSGs[71]. Dermal–epidermal composites using autologous keratinocytes and human allodermis may in the future be used for grafting full-thickness wounds in patients with burns, leg ulcers or surgical wounds[72].

COMPOSITE GRAFTS

Indications/Contraindications

Composite grafts are modified FTSGs, consisting of two or more tissue layers. In dermatologic surgery, these grafts are usually composed of skin and cartilage, although they may be composed of skin and fat or skin and perichondrium[47,73–75b]. Composite grafts are especially useful for the repair of full-thickness alar rim defects, as well as nasal tip defects with cartilage loss[76,77]. Full-thickness nasal mucosal defects can be repaired using composite grafts to provide mucosal lining and structural support, and a nasolabial or forehead flap can be moved into place thereafter to reconstruct the overlying soft tissue defect[7]. As discussed earlier, conchal bowl composite grafts or PCCGs, consisting of skin and perichondrium, may be used (with or without an underlying cartilage graft) for deeper nasal defects that require skin coverage, especially defects with exposed cartilage[47].

Preoperative History and Considerations

Composite grafts require rapid revascularization for their survival. Early re-establishment of graft circulation occurs via direct vessel anastomoses between the subdermal plexus of the graft and the subdermal plexus of the wound edge. Since composite grafts are dependent upon this bridging phenomenon for their survival, they are of necessity limited in size, with no point being more than 1 cm from a vascular source, as the risk of central necrosis increases significantly at graft diameters greater than 2 cm[78]. Composite grafts for nasal alar and ear reconstruction are possible because of the rich vascular supply of the nose and the ear, and because of the small surface areas generally involved. Composite grafts, like FTSGs, are threatened by excessive shearing forces of the graft over the wound bed, which prevent revascularization from occurring.

During the healing process, composite grafts pass through four stages[79]. After graft placement, the tissue blanches completely. By 6 hours, the graft develops a pale pink color, signifying anastomosis of the vessels of the graft with those of the recipient site. At 12–24 hours, the graft appears dusky blue, reflecting venous congestion, and by 3–7 days, it should be pink, indicating graft survival.

Donor Site Considerations for Composite Grafts

The complexity of the anatomy of the nasal ala makes reconstruction of full-thickness defects involving this area difficult. There may be insufficient skin on the nose to develop adequate local flaps, and

nasolabial flaps, which provide reasonable defect coverage, generate other cosmetic deformities. The loss of alar tissue support also creates a functional deficit, as the alar skin is liable literally to be 'blowing in the breeze' during inspiration and expiration. Composite grafts provide an excellent cosmetic and functional alternative for repair of small full-thickness defects of the alar rim less than 2 cm in diameter[80]. Composite grafts taken from the earlobe have been used successfully for this type of repair, although composite grafts taken from the cartilaginous portion of the ear are more frequently used[74,76,77].

Donor sites for harvesting composite grafts from the ear for alar repair include the crus of the helix, the helical rim and the conchal bowl (see Ch. 142)[76,77,80,81]. Small alar defects involving loss of cartilage can be elegantly repaired using the helical crus as the donor site, while more substantial defects will need to be repaired using the helical rim or conchal bowl, since the crus will not provide sufficient inner lining for the graft. Donor defects involving the crus of the helix can be repaired with minimal scar formation, while wedge excisions are usually necessary to repair helical rim donor sites. The conchal bowl donor site heals by secondary intention.

Advantages of auricular composite grafts in the repair of full-thickness defects of the alar rim relate mainly to the presence of cartilage, which provides structural support and stability, with prevention of alar distortion during inspiration and at rest[77,81]. Disadvantages include a higher risk of graft failure with an increased number of tissue layers, substantial graft size limitations, and limited donor tissue availability. Nevertheless, these grafts, when properly applied, can yield outstanding results.

Composite grafts used for full-thickness nasal mucosal repair are usually obtained from the triangular fossa, scapha, conchal cavum, cymba or helical crus of the ear. The appropriate donor site is that which best matches the contour of the surgical defect. These donor sites are usually allowed to heal by secondary intention, with a good aesthetic outcome.

Description of Technique

Composite grafts used for repair of the nasal ala are performed as follows (Fig. 148.7)[73,77,80,82]. The donor and recipient sites are anesthetized using local anesthesia, and cleaned thoroughly with chlorhexidine. In the event that the alar tissue is scarred and retracted, this area must be vigorously debrided to assure the best possible blood supply for the graft. The defect is then measured and a template made as described previously. The donor site is marked and anesthetized, and the graft is harvested. The tissue is handled very gently and placed in sterile saline until ready for placement.

Due to the fragility of composite grafts, a tongue-in-groove technique is recommended to maximize graft stability and increase graft survival[77,81]. Two cartilaginous wings are marked out and anesthetized on either side of the donor site prior to graft harvesting. After the graft is harvested, the skin overlying these two cartilaginous wings is removed, leaving the cartilage with its overlying perichondrium (Fig. 148.7B). These wings are then inserted into pockets prepared within the alar tissue of both sides of the defect (Fig. 148.7C) such that the graft interlocks with its recipient bed (Fig. 148.7D). Interlocking the graft with its recipient bed may help to minimize shearing forces and to provide a larger surface area for revascularization.

The graft is sutured into place in two layers. The undersurface of the graft, which replaces the inner lining of the nose, can be secured first using a 6-0 absorbable suture. The skin is then closed with a 6-0 non-absorbable suture, taking very small tissue bites so as to minimize vessel strangulation and to maximize the number of potential vessels available for reanastomosis. The needle should pass through the mucosal portion of the graft first, then through the outer epithelial edge of the graft, so that the knots are tied external to the graft, and are not buried between the graft and its recipient bed. The cartilage does not need to be sutured, as it will heal on its own. A Vaseline® gauze or Xeroform™ dressing can then be placed in the nasal vestibule for support, and antibiotic ointment applied to the external suture line. A non-stick dressing is then applied to protect the graft from external injury.

Conchal bowl composite grafts used for reconstruction of deep defects on the nasal ala are harvested in essentially the same way as

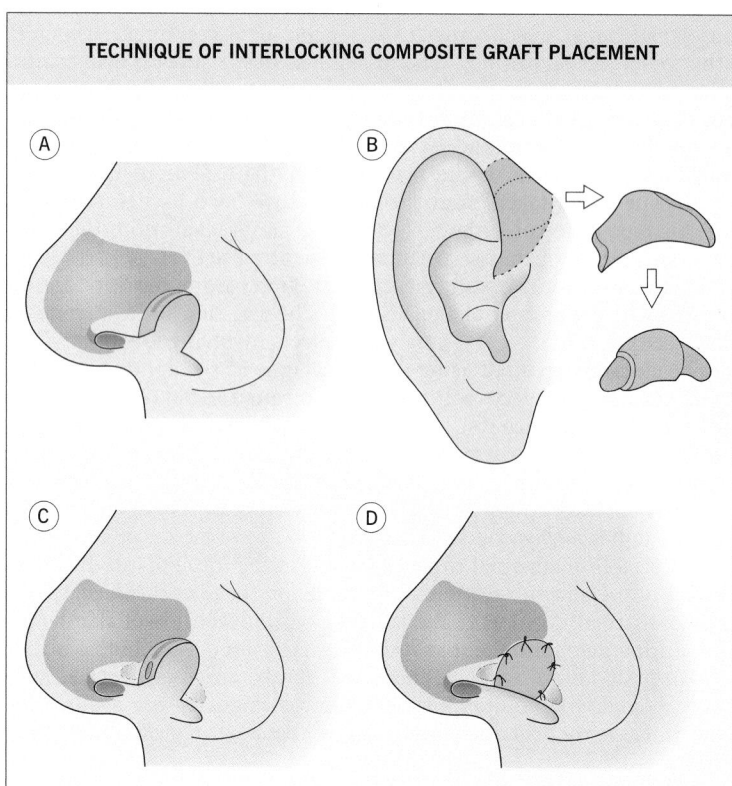

TECHNIQUE OF INTERLOCKING COMPOSITE GRAFT PLACEMENT

Ⓐ Ⓑ

Ⓒ Ⓓ

Fig. 148.7 Technique of interlocking composite graft placement. A A full-thickness nasal alar defect extending through both skin and cartilage requires repair. **B** Donor site at the crus of the helix. An area of skin approximately 5–10% greater in area than the actual defect is marked out, with cartilaginous wings marked out on either side. After the graft is harvested, the skin is removed on both sides to expose the cartilaginous portion of the graft, such that two cartilaginous pegs with their overlying perichondrium frame the lateral aspects of the graft. **C** A pocket is undermined on either side of the recipient site, into which the cartilaginous pegs will be placed. **D** The cartilaginous pegs are inserted into the holes prepared within the alar tissue on either side of the defect. The graft is then sutured into place.

composite grafts taken from the helical crus[81]. Potential advantages of the conchal bowl technique include increased bulk, which may be superior in filling deep partial-thickness defects of the nasal ala, and an excellent cosmetic match for the missing sebaceous skin of the nose.

Donor Site Closure

Helical crus defects can often be closed in a side-to-side fashion. A simple advancement, rotation or transposition flap may also be utilized to take advantage of loose preauricular skin. Helical rim defects are usually closed with an ear wedge resection. Auricular grafts obtained from the triangular fossa, scapha, conchal bowl or cymba heal well by secondary intention. Defects of the conchal bowl may heal more rapidly if a 2 mm punch is used to remove small plugs of conchal cartilage, which allows healing by secondary intention from the soft tissue on the opposite side of the cartilage.

Variations/Unusual Situations

When securing composite grafts of the nasal ala, delayed intranasal knot tying has been recommended by some authors to facilitate wound closure by improving visualization, allowing for gentle manipulation of tissue, and enabling precise placement of sutures in a confined space[83]. When placing the intranasal sutures, the needle of the 6-0 fast-absorbing chromic gut is first passed through the nasal mucosa, and then passed through the corresponding location on the 'mucosal' side of the graft. Sutures are placed at 1–2 mm intervals along the defect and graft, and their free ends are held separately by hemostats to prevent tangling. After all intranasal sutures are placed, the composite graft may be placed into the alar defect and the cartilaginous wings inserted. The most internal intranasal sutures are then tied first, followed by the more accessible, external sutures.

Postoperative Care

Ice packs should be applied to the grafted area as often as possible for up to several days postoperatively. Oral antibiotics are generally advisable because of the high bacterial colonization around the nares and the higher risk of failure with composite grafts. Sutures are removed after 1 week.

Complications

As with other types of grafts, there is a risk of necrosis in the early stages of healing, and contraction, textural changes, atrophy, and contour irregularities thereafter. If the graft survives but the cosmetic result is suboptimal, dermabrasion or laser resurfacing may be performed 6 weeks to 6 months postoperatively to correct textural differences between the graft and the surrounding skin, and to improve the color match between them. Resurfacing of the entire cosmetic unit may provide superior cosmetic results. In the event of composite graft failure, a two-stage revision with placement of a cheek interpolation flap may be performed or, alternatively, a second composite grafting procedure may be undertaken.

Conchal bowl donor sites are at somewhat greater risk of postoperative bleeding than other areas if left to heal by secondary intention. Application of pressure dressings over the front and back of the ear to 'sandwich' the conchal cartilage with placement of hemostatic foam over the donor site itself may decrease this risk.

The ear is also prone to infection with *Pseudomonas*, which resides in the external auditory meatus. Cleaning the ear with a dilute solution of vinegar, applying topical gentamicin ointment, and the use of oral quinolone antibiotics are all helpful prophylactic measures which should be considered after harvesting auricular cartilage. If infection is suspected, oral quinolone antibiotics should be started immediately, and therapy should be guided thereafter by the results of cultures and sensitivities. If the infection does not resolve with appropriate antibiotics, the presence of a fungal infection, most often secondary to *Candida*, should be excluded.

FREE CARTILAGE GRAFTS

Indications/Contraindications

Free cartilage grafts are used most commonly in dermatologic surgery for reconstruction of the nasal ala, tip and sidewall, the ear, and the eyelid[73,75a,80,84–88]. These grafts may be used to restore the architecture of an anatomic site that has undergone significant cartilage loss. Free cartilage grafts are also useful in maintaining the position and contour of free margins against the forces of contraction during wound healing.

Nasal Ala

Partial-thickness alar defects extending into deep soft tissue or approaching the alar rim often lead to collapse of the alar rim, producing a functional as well as a cosmetic deficit. Placement of free cartilage grafts, which consist of cartilage covered by its overlying perichondrium, can be used to avert this potential problem[82,87]. The grafted cartilage provides a rigid but flexible cartilaginous framework that braces the alar rim against collapse during inspiration and expiration. Free cartilage grafts may be used in conjunction with flaps as well as with FTSGs to maintain airway patency and to minimize the risk of alar retraction during wound healing[80,87].

The usefulness of the free cartilage graft lies in its ability to prevent alar retraction. It is possible that long-term survival of the cartilage itself may not ultimately be important, as the mere presence of the rigid framework of the graft in the initial stages of wound healing seems to be sufficient to inhibit alar retraction.

Nasal Sidewall and Tip

Deep defects of the nasal sidewall may at times involve loss of the upper lateral nasal cartilage. Nasal valve obstruction may result, which becomes noticeable with inspiration and resolves on expiration. Delayed nasal valve obstruction can also occur if unresisted scar contracture collapses the remaining cartilaginous structure of the nasal sidewall. Replacement of lost cartilage at the time of reconstruction can avert these potential problems[21,73]. Similarly, loss of cartilage at the distal nasal tip necessitates replacement of structural support for optimal functional and cosmetic results[84–86].

Ear

Auricular defects involving loss of cartilage are generally repaired for cosmetic, rather than functional, reasons. Cartilage grafts may be used as braces along the helical rim to minimize the risk of contracture, and may also be used in the conchal bowl to assist in hearing aid placement[73].

Preoperative History and Donor Site Considerations

Potential donor sites for free cartilage grafts include the conchal bowl, the auricular helix, the antihelix, nasal septum, and ribs[73]. The conchal bowl is most frequently used by dermatologic surgeons, however, as the donor site for free cartilage grafts[82,87,88]. Conchal cartilage is elastic, has a high degree of memory, and has varied contours that can be matched to the desired contour of the ala. Although an anterior approach to the conchal bowl may be used, the posterior approach results in better camouflage of the donor site scar and preservation of the shape of the ear. If the antihelix is used as a donor site, it is recommended that a subtotal resection of the antihelical cartilage be performed, leaving a complete rim of intact cartilage to prevent distortion.

Description of Technique
Nasal ala

The techniques for alar batten cartilage grafting have been well described[73,80,82,87,88]. The alar batten provides a rigid but flexible cartilaginous framework to brace the alar rim against collapse. The length of the cartilage graft is determined by measuring the distance between the lateral border of the defect and the medial border of the defect at the alar rim, and adding to that measurement an extra 4–5 mm. The conchal bowl donor site is incised anteriorly or posteriorly. The skin overlying the cartilage is then undermined with blunt scissor dissection to expose the perichondrial surface of the conchal bowl. The desired length of cartilage is incised with the scalpel (Fig. 148.8A), and a second incision is then made exactly parallel to the first, to create a cartilaginous strip that is 3–6 mm in width, depending upon the desired width of the graft. Alternatively, a larger disk- or oblong-shaped piece may be harvested to match the base of the defect precisely. The cartilage is easily separated from the anterior skin with sharp scissor dissection. The graft is then placed in sterile saline while the donor site is reapproximated with non-absorbable sutures.

The cartilage graft must next be secured into place. If a cartilaginous strip is to be used, the soft tissue of the recipient bed is undermined medially and laterally with a hemostat or blunt-scissor dissection, and the ends of the graft inserted into the undermined pockets such that the graft interlocks with its recipient bed (Fig. 148.8B). The graft is sutured into its recipient bed with one or two 5-0 absorbable sutures for additional security. A disk- or oblong-shaped cartilage graft also requires suturing for secure placement.

After the graft has been anchored, a nasolabial flap or FTSG is sutured into place to complete the closure (Fig. 148.8C–E). A standard tie-over bolster is placed over the FTSG and secured into place with 5-0 non-absorbable sutures. Sutures are removed in 1 week.

Nasal sidewall and tip

The free cartilage grafts used for nasal sidewall and tip reconstruction are harvested in much the same way as free cartilage grafts for nasal alar reconstruction[73]. Nasal sidewall grafts tend to be wider and broader than alar grafts, given the fact that they are bracing a broader surface area against the forces of inspiration. Alternatively, multiple cartilaginous strips can be placed in perpendicular orientation to the lateral nasal sidewall, and secured with absorbable or non-absorbable sutures to brace the side of the nose against collapse. After the cartilaginous

structure is in place, a flap or FTSG may be performed to cover the remaining cutaneous defect.

Nasal tip grafts for distal nasal reconstruction are organized in order to provide both proximal and distal structural support, thus optimizing the aesthetic and functional result[73,84–86]. The proximal grafts consist of bilateral batten grafts secured into place at the sites of the lateral cartilages with 5-0 or 6-0 non-absorbable sutures. On top of these may be sewn a dorsal nasal cartilage graft. A columellar strut of cartilage often provides distal support, on top of which may be sewn an additional tip graft. Alar batten grafts secured to the columellar strut and lateral alar soft tissue provide alar rim support. A paramedian forehead flap or melolabial interpolation flap may be placed thereafter to provide coverage of the cutaneous defect.

Ear

If conchal cartilage is used to repair a large helical defect, the cartilage graft should match the defect as closely as possible in size and shape[73]. Harvesting and placing a narrow strip of cartilage matching the helical defect alone will result in helical rim collapse under the forces of wound contraction. If necessary, a partial wedge closure of the defect may be performed prior to cartilage graft placement to decrease the portion of the defect requiring replacement of structural support. The cartilage graft is secured by sewing it to the intact cartilaginous framework with 6-0 absorbable or non-absorbable sutures. The graft is then generally covered with a pedicled retroauricular advancement flap.

Eyelid

Partial-thickness lower eyelid defects with loss of the tarsal plate, as well as full-thickness lower eyelid defects, may be repaired with cartilage grafts. Stabilization of the eyelid with free cartilage grafts provides structural support, minimizing the risk of ectropion and preventing desiccation of the cornea. The technique of performing free cartilage grafts for the repair of full-thickness and partial-thickness lower eyelid defects is beyond the scope of this chapter, but is well described by Otley & Sherris[73].

Postoperative Care

Regardless of the site of free cartilage grafting, care must be taken postoperatively to minimize movement of the cartilage graft. Routine wound care is performed to the flap or graft overlying the free cartilage graft. Trauma to the area should be minimized.

Complications

Postoperative complications following free cartilage grafting are rare. There is a risk of postoperative infection at the conchal bowl donor site, particularly with Gram-negative bacilli, which reside within the external auditory meatus. Appropriate bacterial and fungal cultures of any tissue exudate should be obtained if infection is suspected. Empiric therapy with quinolone antibiotics should be initiated, and modified as sensitivities dictate. When prophylactic antibiotics and appropriate operative technique are used, the risk of suppurative chondritis is extremely low[89].

Postoperative tenderness, swelling and erythema may herald the occurrence of inflammatory chondritis or perichondritis, which should be treated with cool compresses and non-steroidal anti-inflammatory drugs for several weeks or even months postoperatively.

Later complications may include resorption of the graft, displacement or deformation after placement, and extrusion. Surgical revision may be required if these complications occur. Recipient sites such as the ear are subject to trauma and are therefore at increased risk of graft displacement and resorption. Every effort should therefore be made intraoperatively to utilize grafts of sufficient thickness and stiffness to resist the forces of trauma and wound contracture, and to anchor these grafts so as to maximize their stability.

Future Trends

While autologous cartilage is considered to be the optimal grafting material due to its pliability, accessibility, and ease of harvesting under local anesthesia, the supply of this material may be limited, and

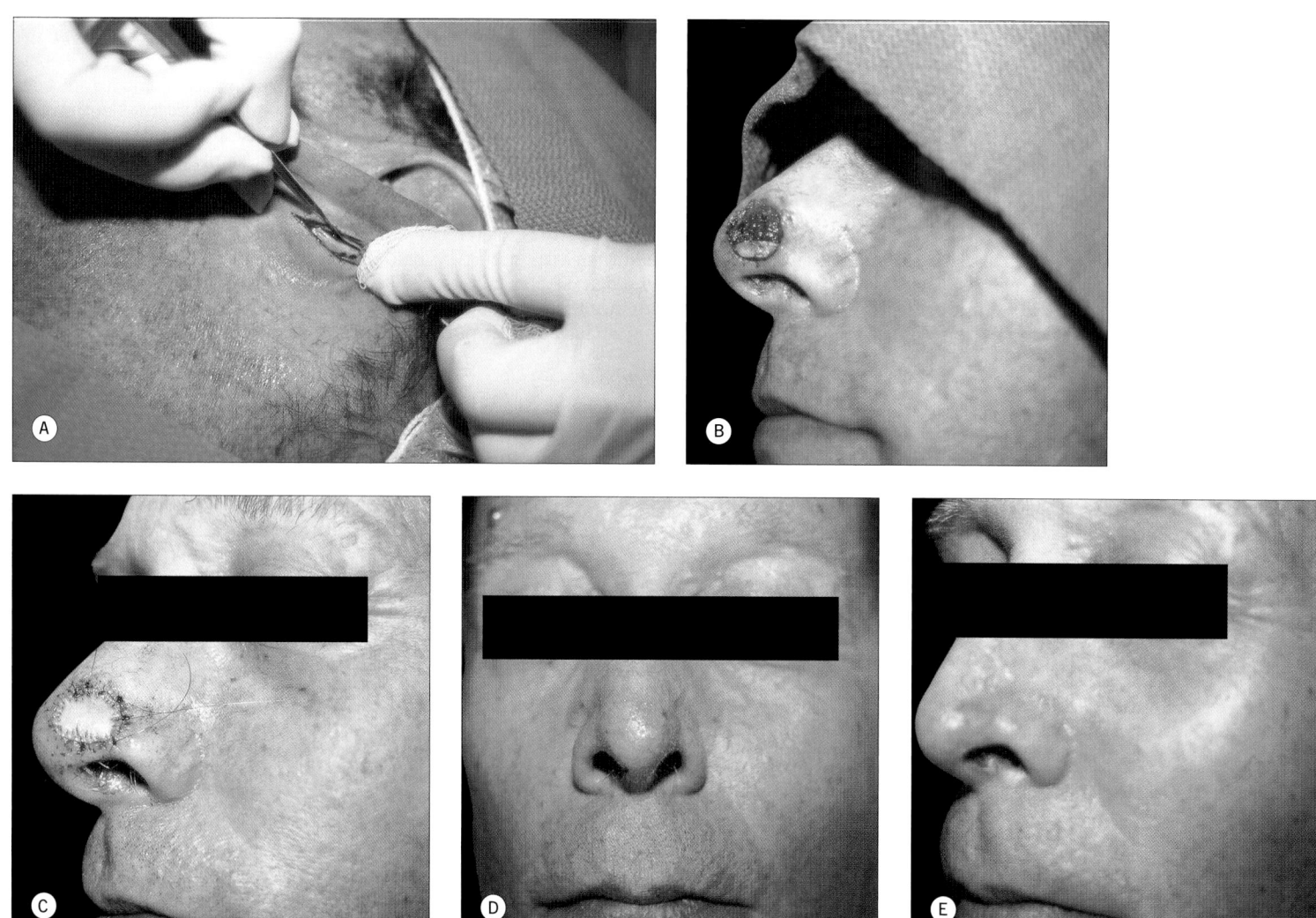

Fig. 148.8 Harvesting and placement of a free cartilage graft. A The posterior conchal bowl donor site has been incised to the level of the perichondrium. The desired length of cartilage was incised with the scalpel, and a second incision made parallel to the first to isolate a cartilaginous strip with its overlying perichondrium. **B** The ends of the cartilaginous strip with its overlying perichondrium have been inserted into pockets undermined on either side of the recipient bed, such that the graft interlocks with its recipient bed on the left nasal ala. The graft is sutured to the underlying dermis with one 5-0 absorbable suture for additional security. **C** A full-thickness skin graft has been sutured into place over the free cartilage graft. **D & E** Eight-week postoperative front and side views of the full-thickness skin graft and underlying free cartilage graft on the left nasal ala. The alar rim remains in perfect alignment.

harvesting may entail additional morbidity for the patient. The use of other implantable materials for nasal reconstruction has been investigated, including porous, high-density polyethylene implants[90]. These polyethylene implants demonstrated the ability to heal by secondary intention and support skin grafts when used to reconstruct auricular cartilage in rabbits[91]. They were also well tolerated as replacements for native cartilage in patients requiring rhinoplasty or nasal reconstruction[92].

Tissue engineering has recently been used to generate autologous cartilage implants to fill defects of the nose or outer ear[93–95]. Chondrocytes can be stimulated with growth factors to increase their proliferative rate and production of extracellular matrix. Such chondrocytes, when implanted on a resorbable synthetic scaffold, can thereby be induced to produce a three-dimensional aggregate of cartilage[90,95,96]. *In vitro* engineering of human cartilage could be the ideal cartilage replacement method, without the risk of infection and with the possibility of reconstructing large defects with different configurations[96]. These and newer implantable materials will, over time, become increasingly

available, and will certainly be of use to dermatologic surgeons who perform nasal reconstruction.

CONCLUSIONS

A working knowledge of the indications, techniques, donor site considerations, and postoperative complications of all types of skin grafting is necessary for soft tissue reconstruction. As the incidence of skin cancer continues to rise, increasing numbers of patients are likely to require reconstructive procedures to repair their defects. Furthermore, split-thickness skin grafting for lower extremity ulcers is an effective, reasonable treatment for patients with refractory leg ulcers. With proper defect assessment, reconstructive planning, and attention to detail preoperatively, intraoperatively and postoperatively, optimal cosmetic and functional results using skin grafting techniques can be achieved. A thorough understanding of skin grafting is invaluable for all physicians performing reconstructive surgery.

REFERENCES

1. Hauben DJ, Baruchin A, Mahler A. On the history of the free skin graft. Ann Plast Surg. 1982;9:242–5.
2. Reverdin J. Greffe épidermique. Bull Soc Imp Chir Paris. 1869;10:493, 511.
3. Ollier L. Sur les greffes cutanées ou autoplastiques. Bull Acad Med Paris. 1872;2:243.
4. Thiersch C. Uber Hautverpflanzung. Zentralbl Chir. 1886;13:17–18.
5. Wolfe J. A new method of performing plastic operations. Br Med J. 1875;2:360–1.
6. Krause F. Ueber die Transplantation grosser ungestielter Hautlappen. Verhandl Deutsch Ges Chir. 1893;22:46.
7. Johnson TM, Ratner D, Nelson BR. Soft tissue reconstruction with skin grafting. J Am Acad Dermatol. 1992;27:151–65.
8. Johnson T, Ratner D. Skin grafts. In: Ratz JL (ed.). Textbook of Dermatologic Surgery. Philadelphia: Lippincott-Raven, 1998:201–21.
9. Ratner D. Skin grafting. From here to there. Dermatol Clin. 1998;16:75–90.
9a. Adams DC, Ramsey ML. Grafts in dermatologic surgery: review and update on full- and split-thickness grafts, free cartilage grafts and composite grafts. Dermatol Surg. 2005;31:1055–67.
10. Smahel J. The healing of skin grafts. Clin Plast Surg. 1977;4:409–24.
11. Kirsner RS, Eaglstein WH, Kerdel FA. Split-thickness skin grafting for lower extremity ulcerations. Dermatol Surg. 1997;23:85–91; quiz 92–3.
12. Converse JM, Uhlschmid GK, Ballantyne DL Jr. "Plasmatic circulation" in skin grafts. The phase of serum imbibition. Plast Reconstr Surg. 1969;43:495–9.
13. Clemmesen T, Ronhovde DA. Restoration of the blood-supply to human skin autografts. Scand J Plast Reconstr Surg. 1968;2:44–6.
14. Converse JM, Smahel J, Ballantyne DL Jr, Harper AD. Inosculation of vessels of skin graft and host bed: a fortuitous encounter. Br J Plast Surg. 1975;28:274–82.
15. Skouge J. Skin Grafting. New York: Churchill Livingstone, 1991.
16. Fitzgerald MJ, Martin F, Paletta FX. Innervation of skin grafts. Surg Gynecol Obstet. 1967;124:808–12.
17. Goldminz D, Bennett RG. Cigarette smoking and flap and full-thickness graft necrosis. Arch Dermatol. 1991;127:1012–15.
18. Harris DR. Healing of the surgical wound. II. Factors influencing repair and regeneration. J Am Acad Dermatol. 1979;1:208–15.
19. Ratner D. Skin grafting. Semin Cutan Med Surg. 2003;22:295–305.
20. Walden JL, Garcia H, Hawkins H, Crouchet JR, Traber L, Gore DC. Both dermal matrix and epidermis contribute to an inhibition of wound contraction. Ann Plast Surg. 2000;45:162–6.
21. Gloster HM Jr. The use of full-thickness skin grafts to repair nonperforating nasal defects. J Am Acad Dermatol. 2000;42:1041–50.
22. Matheson BK, Mellette JR Jr. Surgical pearl: clavicular grafts are "superior" to supraclavicular grafts. J Am Acad Dermatol. 1997;37:991–3.
23. Tromovitch TA, Stegman SJ, Glogau RG. Flaps and Grafts in Dermatologic Surgery. Chicago: Yearbook Medical, 1989:49–54, 65–7.
24. Breach NM. Pre-auricular full-thickness skin grafts. Br J Plast Surg. 1978;31:124–6.
25. Corwin TR, Klein AW, Habal MB. The aesthetics of the preauricular graft in facial reconstruction. Ann Plast Surg. 1982;9:312–15.
26. Beare RL, Bennett JP. The naso-labial full thickness graft. Br J Plast Surg. 1972;25:315–17.
27. Rohrer TE, Dzubow LM. Conchal bowl skin grafting in nasal tip reconstruction: clinical and histologic evaluation. J Am Acad Dermatol. 1995;33:476–81.
28. Zitelli JA. Burow's grafts. J Am Acad Dermatol. 1987;17:271–9.
29. Krishnan R, Hwang L, Orengo I. Dog-ear graft technique. Dermatol Surg. 2001;27:312–14.
30. Kaufman AJ. Adjacent-tissue skin grafts for reconstruction. Dermatol Surg. 2004;30:1349–53.
31. Palkar VM. Full-thickness skin grafting. J Surg Oncol. 2000;73:31.
32. Fazio MJ, Zitelli JA. Full-thickness skin grafts. Clinical observations on the impact of using epinephrine in local anesthesia of the donor site. Arch Dermatol. 1995;131:691–4.
33. Hill TG. Contouring of donor skin in full-thickness skin grafting. J Dermatol Surg Oncol. 1987;13:883–8.
34. Mellette JR Jr, Swinehart JM. Cartilage removal prior to skin grafting in the triangular fossa, antihelix, and concha of the ear. J Dermatol Surg Oncol. 1990;16:1102–5.
35. Larson PO, Ragi G, Mohs FE, Snow SN. Excision of exposed cartilage for management of Mohs surgery defects of the ear. J Dermatol Surg Oncol. 1991;17:749–52.
36. Craven NM, Telfer NR. An open study of tissue adhesive in full-thickness skin grafting. J Am Acad Dermatol. 1999;40:607–11.
37. Hill TG. Enhancing the survival of full-thickness grafts. J Dermatol Surg Oncol. 1984;10:639–42.
38. Orengo I, Lee MW. Surgical pearl: the "unsuture" technique for skin grafts. J Am Acad Dermatol. 1998;38:758–9.
39. Salasche SJ, Winton GB. Clinical evaluation of a nonadhering wound dressing. J Dermatol Surg Oncol. 1986;12:1220–2.
40. Langtry JA, Kirkham P, Martin IC, Fordyce A. Tie-over bolster dressings may not be necessary to secure small full thickness skin grafts. Dermatol Surg. 1998; 24:1350–3.
41. Adams DC, Ramsey ML, Marks VJ. The running bolster suture for full-thickness skin grafts. Dermatol Surg. 2004;30:92–4.
42. Brady JG, Grande DJ, Katz AE. The purse-string suture in facial reconstruction. J Dermatol Surg Oncol. 1992;18:812–16.
43. Harrington AC, Montemarano A, Welch M, Farley M. Variations of the pursestring suture in skin cancer reconstruction. Dermatol Surg. 1999;25:277–81.
44. Silapunt S, Peterson SR, Alam M, Goldberg LH. Clinical appearance of full-thickness skin grafts of the nose. Dermatol Surg. 2005;31:177–83.
45. Robinson JK, Dillig G. The advantages of delayed nasal full-thickness skin grafting after Mohs micrographic surgery. Dermatol Surg. 2002;28:845–51.
46. Meyers S, Rohrer T, Grande D. Use of dermal grafts in reconstructing deep nasal defects and shaping the ala nasi. Dermatol Surg. 2001;27:300–5.
46a. Draper BL, Wentzell JM. The "drumhead" graft repair of deep nasal alar defects. Dermatol Surg. 2007; 33:17–22.
47. Gloster HM Jr, Brodland DG. The use of perichondrial cutaneous grafts to repair defects of the lower third of the nose. Br J Dermatol. 1997;136:43–6.
48. Love CW, Collison DW, Carithers JS, Ceilley RI. Perichondrial cutaneous grafts for reconstruction of skin cancer excision defects. Dermatol Surg. 1995; 21:219–22.
49. Salasche SJ. Acute surgical complications: cause, prevention, and treatment. J Am Acad Dermatol. 1986;15:1163–85.
50. Salasche SJ, Feldman BD. Skin grafting: perioperative technique and management. J Dermatol Surg Oncol. 1987;13:863–9.
51. Ceilley RI, Bumsted RM, Panje WR. Delayed skin grafting. J Dermatol Surg Oncol. 1983;9:288–93.
52. Thibault MJ, Bennett RG. Success of delayed full-thickness skin grafts after Mohs micrographic surgery. J Am Acad Dermatol. 1995;32:1004–9.
53. Robinson JK. Improvement of the appearance of full-thickness skin grafts with dermabrasion. Arch Dermatol. 1987;123:1340–5.
54. Nehal KS, Levine VJ, Ross B, Ashinoff R. Comparison of high-energy pulsed carbon dioxide laser resurfacing and dermabrasion in the revision of surgical scars. Dermatol Surg. 1998;24:647–50.
55. Otley CC, Gayner SM, Ahmed I, Moore E, Roenigk R, Sherris D. Preoperative and postoperative topical tretinoin on high-tension excisional wounds and full-thickness skin grafts in a porcine model: a pilot study. Dermatol Surg. 1999;25:716–21.
56. Stephenson AJ, Griffiths RW, La Hausse-Brown TP. Patterns of contraction in human full thickness skin grafts. Br J Plast Surg. 2000;53:397–402.
57. Can Z, Ercocen AR, Apaydin I, et al. Tissue engineering of high density porous polyethylene implant for three-dimensional reconstruction: an experimental study. Scand J Plast Reconstr Surg Hand Surg. 2000;34:9–14.
58. Skouge JW. Techniques for split-thickness skin grafting. J Dermatol Surg Oncol. 1987;13:841–9.
59. Whitaker DC, Grande DI, Koranda FC, Knabel MR. Rapid application of split-thickness skin grafts. J Dermatol Surg Oncol. 1982;8:499–504.
60. Glogau RG, Stegman SJ, Tromovitch TA. Refinements in split-thickness skin grafting technique. J Dermatol Surg Oncol. 1987;13:853–8.
61. James JH, Watson AC. The use of Opsite, a vapour permeable dressing, on skin graft donor sites. Br J Plast Surg. 1975;28:107–10.
62. Rakel BA, Bermel MA, Abbott LI, et al. Split-thickness skin graft donor site care: a quantitative synthesis of the research. Appl Nurs Res. 1998;11:174–82.
63. Nappi JF, Falcone RE, Ruberg RL. Meshed skin grafts versus sheet skin grafts on a contaminated bed. J Dermatol Surg Oncol. 1984;10:380–1.
64. Rudolph R. The effect of skin graft preparation on wound contraction. Surg Gynecol Obstet. 1976;142:49–56.
65. Rudolph R, Suzuki M, Guber S, Woodward M. Control of contractile fibroblasts by skin grafts. Surg Forum. 1977;28:524–5.
66. Horch RE, Debus M, Wagner G, Stark GB. Cultured human keratinocytes on type I collagen membranes to reconstitute the epidermis. Tissue Eng. 2000; 6:53–67.
67. Margulis A, Zhang W, Garlick JA. In vitro fabrication of engineered human skin. Methods Mol Biol. 2005;289:61–70.
68. Mizuno H, Takeda A, Uchinuma E. Creation of an acellular dermal matrix from frozen skin. Aesthetic Plast Surg. 1999;23:316–22.
69. Suzuki S, Shin-ya K, Kawai K, Nishimura Y. Application of artificial dermis prior to full-thickness skin grafting for resurfacing the nose. Ann Plast Surg. 1999;43:439–42.
70. Wainwright D, Madden M, Luterman A, et al. Clinical evaluation of an acellular allograft dermal matrix in full-thickness burns. J Burn Care Rehabil. 1996;17:124–36.
71. Eaglstein WH, Falanga V. Tissue engineering for skin: an update. J Am Acad Dermatol. 1998;39:1007–10.
72. Chakrabarty KH, Dawson RA, Harris P, et al. Development of autologous human dermal-epidermal composites based on sterilized human allodermis for clinical use. Br J Dermatol. 1999;141:811–23.
73. Otley CC, Sherris DA. Spectrum of cartilage grafting in cutaneous reconstructive surgery. J Am Acad Dermatol. 1998;39:982–92.
74. Haas AF, Glogau RG. A variation of composite grafting for reconstruction of full-thickness nasal alar defects. Arch Dermatol. 1994;130:978–80.
75. Gurunluoglu R, Shafighi M, Gardetto A, Piza-Katzer H. Composite skin grafts for basal cell carcinoma defects of the nose. Aesthetic Plast Surg. 2003;27:286–92.
75a. Adams C, Ratner D. Composite and free cartilage grafting. Dermatol Clin. 2005;23:129–40, vii.
75b. Geyer AS, Pasternack F, Adams C, Ratner D. Use of a skin-fat composite graft to prevent alar notching: an alternative to the delayed postoperative repair. Dermatol Surg. 2005;31:602–7.
76. Field LM. Nasal alar rim reconstruction utilizing the crus of the helix, with several alternatives for donor site closure. J Dermatol Surg Oncol. 1986;12:253–8.
77. Ratner D, Katz A, Grande DJ. An interlocking auricular composite graft. Dermatol Surg. 1995;21:789–92.
78. Ruch MK. Utilization of composite free grafts. J Int Coll Surg. 1958;30:274–5.
79. McLaughlin C. Composite ear grafts and their blood supply. Br J Plast Surg. 1954;7:274–8.
80. Adams C, Ratner D. Composite and free cartilage grafting. Dermatol Clin. 2005;23:129–40, vii.
81. Weisberg NK, Becker DS. Repair of nasal ala defects with conchal bowl composite grafts. Dermatol Surg. 2000;26:1047–51.
82. Otley CC. Alar batten cartilage grafting. Dermatol Surg. 2000;26:969–72.
83. Albertini JG, Ramsey ML. Surgical pearl: delayed intranasal knot tying for composite grafts of the ala. J Am Acad Dermatol. 1998;39:787–8.
84. Burget GC. Aesthetic reconstruction of the tip of the nose. Dermatol Surg. 1995;21:419–29.
85. Burget GC, Menick FJ. Nasal reconstruction: seeking a fourth dimension. Plast Reconstr Surg. 1986;78:145–57.
86. Burget GC, Menick FJ. Nasal support and lining: the marriage of beauty and blood supply. Plast Reconstr Surg. 1989;84:189–202.
87. Ratner D, Skouge JW. Surgical pearl: the use of free cartilage grafts in nasal alar reconstruction. J Am Acad Dermatol. 1997;36:622–4.
88. Byrd DR, Otley CC, Nguyen TH. Alar batten cartilage grafting in nasal reconstruction: functional and cosmetic results. J Am Acad Dermatol. 2000;43:833–6.
89. Kaplan AL, Cook JL. The incidences of chondritis and perichondritis associated with the surgical manipulation

of auricular cartilage. Dermatol Surg. 2004;30:58–62; discussion 62.

90. Sabini P, Sclafani AP, Romo T III, McCormick SA, Cocker R. Modulation of tissue ingrowth into porous high-density polyethylene implants with basic fibroblast growth factor and autologous blood clot. Arch Facial Plast Surg. 2000;2:27–33.

91. Williams JD, Romo T III, Sclafani AP, Cho H. Porous high-density polyethylene implants in auricular reconstruction. Arch Otolaryngol Head Neck Surg. 1997;123:578–83.

92. Romo T III, Sclafani AP, Sabini P. Use of porous high-density polyethylene in revision rhinoplasty and in the platyrrhine nose. Aesthetic Plast Surg. 1998;22:211–21.

93. Vacanti CA, Upton J. Tissue-engineered morphogenesis of cartilage and bone by means of cell transplantation using synthetic biodegradable polymer matrices. Clin Plast Surg. 1994;21:445–62.

94. Vacanti CA, Vacanti JP. Bone and cartilage reconstruction with tissue engineering approaches. Otolaryngol Clin North Am. 1994;27:263–76.

95. Naumann A, Rotter N, Bujia J, Aigner J. Tissue engineering of autologous cartilage transplants for rhinology. Am J Rhinol. 1998;12:59–63.

96. Rotter N, Aigner J, Naumann A, et al. Cartilage reconstruction in head and neck surgery: comparison of resorbable polymer scaffolds for tissue engineering of human septal cartilage. J Biomed Mater Res. 1998;42:347–56.

Nail Surgery

Phoebe Rich

Key features

- A thorough understanding of the anatomy and physiology of the nail unit is crucial to performing successful nail surgery

- The nail matrix forms the nail plate; damage to the nail matrix (including from surgical procedures) can cause permanent nail dystrophy

- There is no subcutaneous tissue in the nail unit, so the dermis of the nail bed sits on the periosteum of the distal digit

- Preoperative evaluation prior to nail surgery is essential and should include a radiograph of the digit when a subungual tumor is suspected

INTRODUCTION

Nail surgery allows the dermatologist to diagnose clinically ambiguous nail lesions or dystrophies, remove nail tumors, and alleviate pain caused by ingrown or traumatized nails. The major goal of nail surgery is to achieve the desired diagnosis or outcome by performing the procedure safely with minimal pain and scarring[1]. Because dermatologists are the physicians who understand and manage nail disorders, they are well suited to perform nail surgery. A solid grasp of the anatomy and physiology of the nail unit is a prerequisite for successful nail surgery. Other necessities for an optimal outcome include a well-prepared patient, adequate anesthesia and hemostasis, and proper technique (Table 149.1).

SURGICAL ANATOMY OF THE NAIL UNIT

As previously emphasized, successful nail surgery requires a comprehensive understanding of the anatomy and physiology of the nail unit. The structures that comprise the nail unit are the nail matrix, the proximal and lateral nail folds, the hyponychium and the nail bed (Fig. 149.1).

The nail matrix is the most vital component of the nail unit, because it is the germinative epithelium from which the nail plate is generated via differentiation of matrix keratinocytes. The distal third of the nail matrix is sometimes visible through the proximal nail plate as the white half-moon-shaped structure called the lunula. Whereas the proximal nail matrix forms the superficial (dorsal) surface of the nail plate, the distal nail matrix forms the inferior (ventral) portion of the nail plate (Fig. 149.2). This observation is key to understanding the clinical presentations of certain pathologic processes and nail tumors and it provides a rationale for basic nail surgical principles and techniques. For example, given that damage to the matrix can cause

permanent nail dystrophy, distal matrix surgery is preferable to proximal matrix surgery, since a defect due to the former would be less obvious on the undersurface of the nail plate[2,3].

The nail bed, sometimes referred to as the sterile matrix, extends from the distal lunula to the hyponychium. Its rich vascular supply

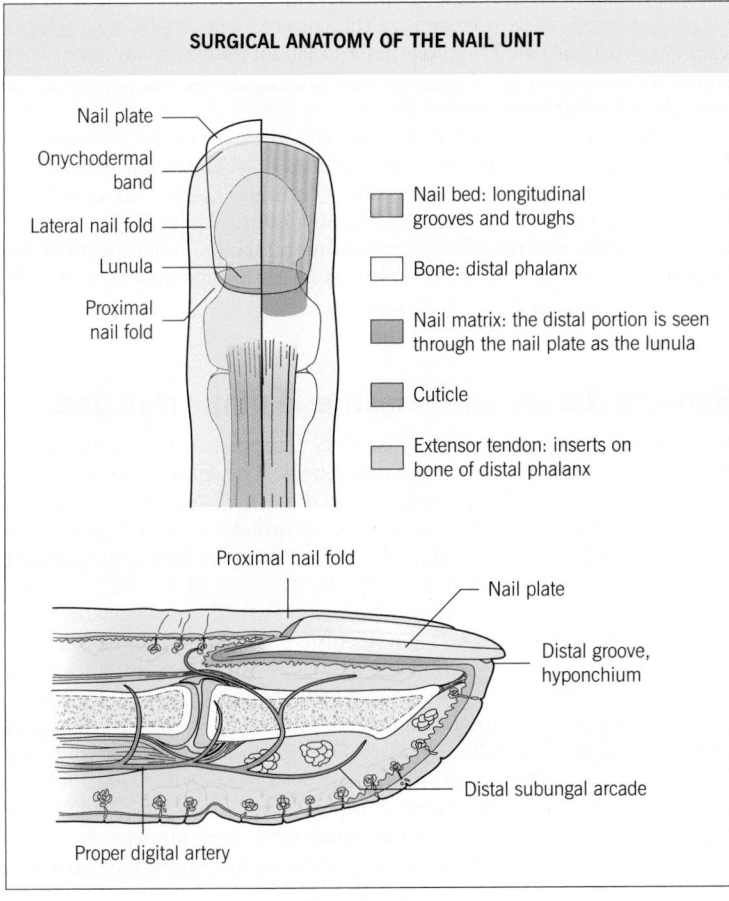

SURGICAL ANATOMY OF THE NAIL UNIT

Nail plate
Onychodermal band
Lateral nail fold
Lunula
Proximal nail fold

Nail bed: longitudinal grooves and troughs

Bone: distal phalanx

Nail matrix: the distal portion is seen through the nail plate as the lunula

Cuticle

Extensor tendon: inserts on bone of distal phalanx

Proximal nail fold
Nail plate
Distal groove, hyponchium
Distal subungal arcade
Proper digital artery

Fig. 149.1 Surgical anatomy of the nail unit.

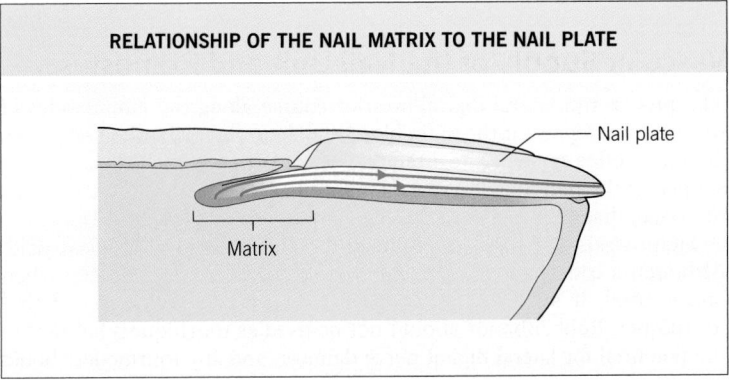

RELATIONSHIP OF THE NAIL MATRIX TO THE NAIL PLATE

Nail plate

Matrix

Fig. 149.2 Relationship of the nail matrix to the nail plate. The proximal part of the nail matrix forms the superficial (dorsal) nail surface; the distal portion of the matrix forms the inferior (ventral) portion of the nail plate. Hence, surgery to the distal matrix is preferable to surgery of the proximal matrix, because, if there is scarring, that associated with the former will be on the undersurface of the nail plate and therefore less obvious.

PREREQUISITES FOR SUCCESSFUL NAIL SURGERY OR NAIL BIOPSY

1. Understanding of nail anatomy and physiology
2. Proper patient selection and preparation
3. Adequate anesthesia
4. Hemostasis
5. A nail condition that has eluded diagnosis by routine clinical inspection, history, diagnostic (radiologic) imaging and/or microbiologic evaluation
6. A dermatopathologist who is familiar with the histopathologic idiosyncrasies of the nail unit

Table 149.1 Prerequisites for successful nail surgery or nail biopsy.

results in the pink color of the nail bed seen through the translucent nail plate. The nail bed is composed of longitudinal ridges and grooves, which explains clinical phenomena such as the longitudinal orientation of splinter hemorrhages. While the bulk of the nail plate is formed by the nail matrix, the nail bed probably contributes a few epithelial cells to the undersurface of the nail plate, which helps to explain the tight adhesion of the nail plate to the nail bed. Surgery of the nail bed rarely leads to a permanent dystrophy of the nail apparatus, but it may result in mild onycholysis. An important feature of the nail bed is that there is no subcutaneous tissue beneath it. The dermis of the nail bed sits directly on the periosteum of the distal digit. The lack of subcutaneous tissue in the nail unit explains why nail surgical specimens extend to the level of the periosteum.

The proximal and lateral nail folds support and protect the nail plate. The end product of the proximal nail fold is the cuticle, which adheres tightly to the proximal nail plate and seals and protects the nail unit from environmental pathogens and irritants. The insertion of the extensor tendon of the digit is approximately 12 mm proximal to the cuticle, and is usually proximal to the surgical field in all but the most extensive nail surgery. The proximal and lateral nail folds are collectively called the paronychium. The perionychium consists of the paronychium plus the hyponychium and nail bed[4].

The hyponychium is located under the free edge of the nail plate. It begins at the most distal part of the nail bed (in the region just proximal to the distal groove) and then becomes contiguous with the volar skin of the digit. Like the cuticle, the hyponychium also functions to seal and protect the nail unit from environmental factors. Disruption of the hyponychium by trauma or disease can result in onycholysis with subsequent bacterial and fungal infections.

Sensory Nerves and Anesthesia of the Nail Unit

For patient acceptance of nail surgery, complete anesthesia and a resultant pain-free procedure are mandatory. The sensory nerves to the nail course along the lateral sides of the digit in close approximation to the digital arteries. Anesthesia can be administered as a digital block and/or a wing block. In a digital block, 2% plain lidocaine (without epinephrine) is injected superficially into the base of the digit on both lateral sides with a 30-gauge needle (Fig. 149.3). To prevent vasospasm and tamponade of the vessels, the volume of local anesthetic should be less than 1.0–1.5 ml on each side of the digit. An adjunctive anesthetic approach is a paronychial or wing block in which plain lidocaine is injected into the proximal and lateral nail folds. A small volume of anesthetic is injected, which blanches the skin of the nail fold and may help somewhat with hemostasis. It is sometimes useful to inject a long-acting anesthetic (e.g. bupivacaine, ropivacaine) around the nail unit at the end of the procedure to provide more prolonged anesthesia, sometimes up to 12 hours. Although the dogma in nail surgery has been to avoid the use of epinephrine in digital blocks, several recent comprehensive reviews describe the safe use of lidocaine with epinephrine in the digits of patients with no history of vascular disease[5].

Vascular Supply of the Nail Unit and Hemostasis

The proper and lateral digital arteries course along the lateral sides of the digit and represent the main blood supply to the nail unit. The proper digital arteries give rise to branches that form the superficial arcade supplying the nail fold and matrix, as well as a second arcade that feeds the bone, distal nail bed, and hyponychial area (see Fig. 149.1).

Hemostasis is necessary to adequately visualize the surgical field. Although a tourniquet is not usually necessary for nail surgery, when one is used, it should be a flat Penrose drain or a Maramed digital tourniquet. Rubber bands should not be used as tourniquets because of the potential for lateral digital nerve damage, and any tourniquet should not be left in place for more than 15 minutes. An assistant applying pressure to the sides of the digit during the procedure usually achieves hemostasis without resorting to a tourniquet. A sterile glove on the patient's hand is sometimes used to impart a sterile field while also providing hemostasis. The tip of the glove finger is removed, and then the remainder is rolled back past the affected nail to the base of the

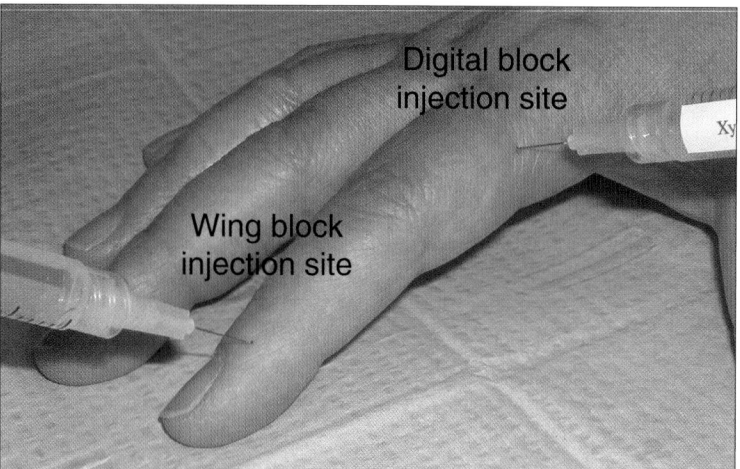

Fig. 149.3 **The location of lidocaine injections for a wing block and a digital block.**

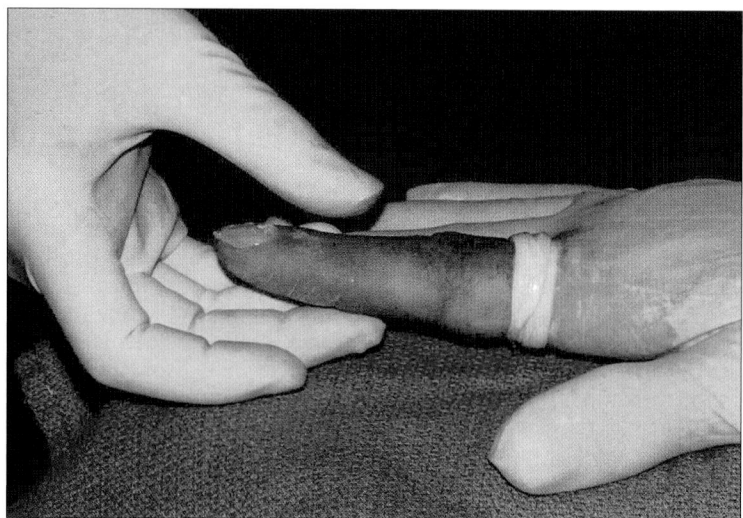

Fig. 149.4 **Sterile glove used as a tourniquet and sterile field.** The tip of the glove finger is removed, then the remainder is rolled back to the base of the finger.

finger to act as a gentle tourniquet and to provide a sterile field for the nail surgery (Fig. 149.4).

PATIENT PREPARATION AND PREOPERATIVE EVALUATION

A well-prepared patient facilitates a successful surgical procedure (see Ch. 151). A complete history and appropriate clinical examination of the nail unit are paramount. The history should include prescribed medications (especially anticoagulants and salicylates) and supplements (see Ch. 133) in addition to a review of systems, with particular attention to the presence or absence of diabetes mellitus, autoimmune connective tissue diseases, peripheral vascular disease, cutaneous conditions with nail manifestations, and prosthetic valves and joints (Table 149.2). Physical examination should include inspection of all 20 nails as well as palpation of peripheral pulses. Appropriate laboratory tests for bacteria, fungi and/or viruses should be obtained when there is a possibility of infection. Radiographic studies to define space-occupying lesions and underlying bony defects are often necessary prior to nail surgery. A full 'procedure, alternatives and risk' (PAR) discussion should include the possibility of permanent nail dystrophy, bleeding, pain and infection. While not mandatory, clinical photographs of the preoperative nail are usually worthwhile. The digit is then washed with surgical soap such as chlorhexidine (e.g. Hibiclens®) or povidone-iodine (e.g. Betadine®) and sterilely draped. A sterile glove on the patient's hand can also provide a sterile field (see Fig. 149.4)[6].

PATIENT EVALUATION PRIOR TO NAIL SURGERY

History

- Medical history
  - Diabetes mellitus
  - Peripheral vascular disease
  - Autoimmune connective tissue disease
  - Raynaud's phenomenon
  - Arthritis
  - Prosthetic joints or heart valves
  - Bleeding diathesis
- Drug history
  - Allergies
  - Use of anticoagulants, salicylates and NSAIDs
  - Use of herbal medicine
- Cutaneous history
  - History of the nail condition (duration, progression, exposures, trauma)
  - Psoriasis, lichen planus or other cutaneous disorders with nail manifestations
  - Previous malignancies
  - Previous fungal, bacterial and/or viral cultures or diagnostic tests
  - Occupation and hobbies

Examination

- All 20 nails, good lighting and magnification
- Mucous membranes, hair and scalp
- Pertinent cutaneous examination
- Peripheral pulses, especially in toenail surgery

Laboratory tests

- Radiography, diagnostic imaging studies (e.g. MRI)
- Mycology, microbiology or virology studies

'Procedure, alternatives and risk' discussion

- Possibility of permanent dystrophy
- Possibility of no diagnosis
- Length of time for nail to regrow
- Bleeding, infection and pain, as with any surgery

Table 149.2 Patient evaluation prior to nail surgery.

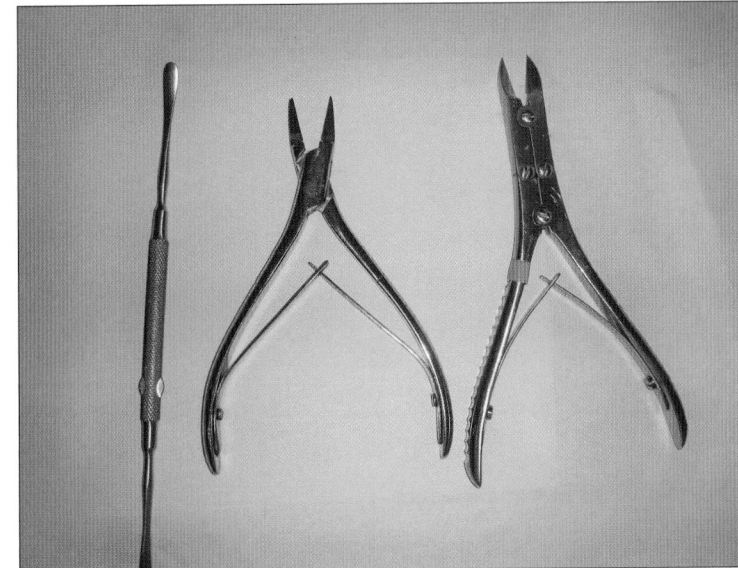

Fig. 149.5 Instruments used in nail surgery. Freer septum elevator, English nail splitter, and double-action nail clipper (left to right).

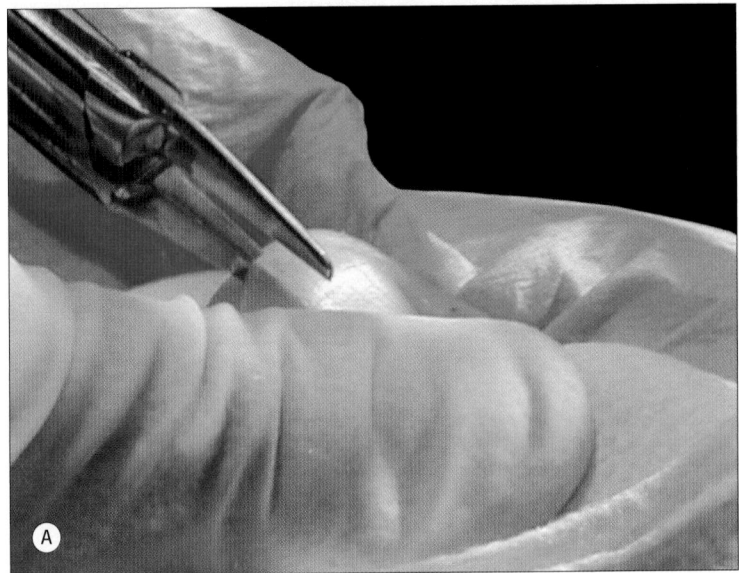

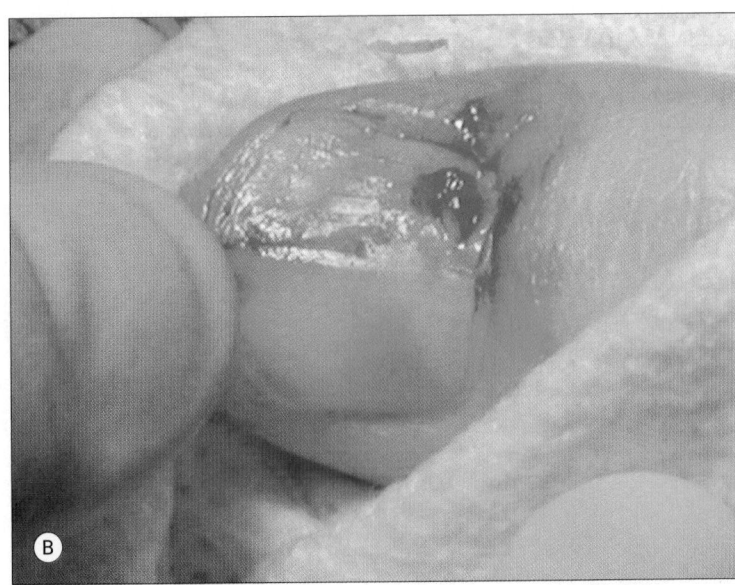

Fig. 149.6 An English nail splitter is used to divide the nail plate prior to partial nail avulsion. A Note the flat, anvil-like blade of the English nail splitter that is inserted under the nail plate. **B** After partial nail avulsion, a glomus tumor is identified prior to excision.

INSTRUMENTS FOR NAIL SURGERY

Most of the instruments used in nail surgery are standard instruments used in cutaneous surgery. However, there are several special instruments that can make nail surgery easier (Fig. 149.5). The Freer septum elevator is an instrument with thin curved blades that facilitates atraumatic nail avulsion. An English nail splitter has a cutting blade opposed to a flat anvil-like surface that facilitates partial longitudinal nail avulsion. A double action nail clipper is an indispensable instrument that easily cuts thickened nail plates.

NAIL AVULSION AND NAIL MATRIX EXPLORATION

Nail avulsion is the most basic procedure in nail surgery and is a prelude to additional surgical procedures that may need to be performed. Avulsion can be partial or total, and it involves removal of the nail by separating the nail plate from its attachments to the nail bed, matrix and nail folds. Avulsion of the nail plate facilitates examination of the nail bed and matrix area for tumors, and thus provides good exposure for subsequent excision or biopsy (Fig. 149.6). Partial longitudinal avulsion is useful in the management of ingrown nails when surgical or chemical (phenol) matricectomy is performed (see below). In an acute bacterial infection of the nail unit, distal and/or lateral partial nail avulsion allows drainage of the subungual purulent material.

As noted previously, nail avulsion is the fundamental procedure in nail surgery. The basic principle is to loosen the nail plate from its attachments to the underlying nail bed, matrix, and proximal and lateral nail folds. There are two approaches to nail avulsion: distal and proximal.

In *distal nail plate avulsion*, after anesthesia, an instrument such as a Freer elevator or dental spatula is inserted under the nail plate in a distal to proximal direction (Fig. 149.7A). As the instrument reaches the area of the matrix where the attachment of the nail plate is looser,

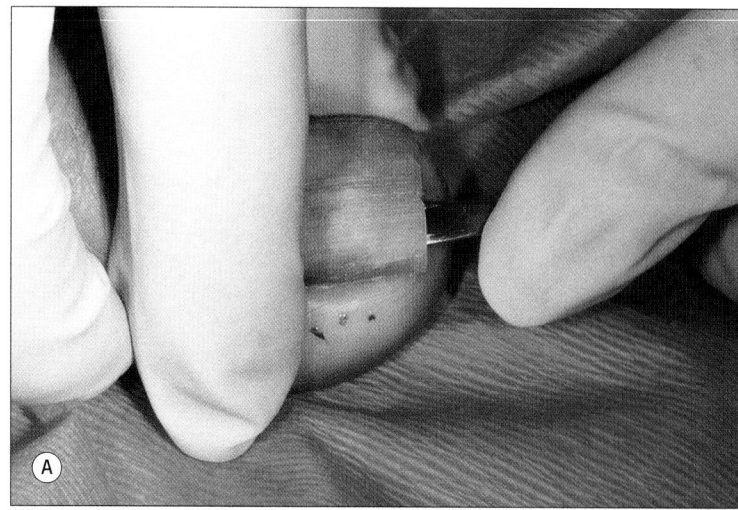

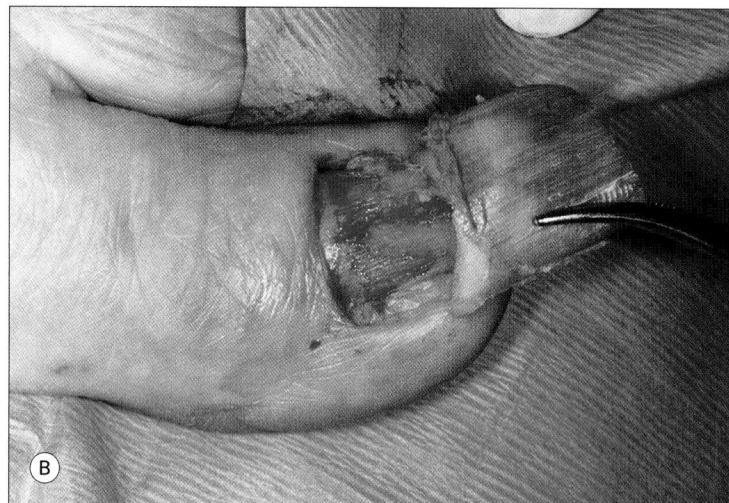

Fig. 149.7 Distal nail plate avulsion. A The Freer septum elevator is inserted under the nail plate (from the hyponychium) in several parallel passes. **B** The loosened nail plate is grabbed with a hemostat and removed.

the decrease in resistance is felt. One must anticipate that change, so that the instrument is not inadvertently jammed into the proximal groove and cul-de-sac with such force as to traumatize that area. It is preferable to insert the instrument from the hyponychium several times rather than to try to slide the instrument back and forth across the nail bed to loosen the nail plate. The attachment of the proximal and lateral nail folds to the nail plate is weak, so those areas are easily separated. Once the attachments to the nail plate are severed, the nail plate can be grasped by a hemostat on one lateral edge and rotated or pulled off the nail bed (Fig. 149.7B).

A *proximal nail plate avulsion* is performed if there is massive distal subungual damage or there is no distal free edge. In a proximal avulsion, the nail plate is loosened from its attachment to the nail matrix by inserting the Freer elevator under the proximal nail at the proximal nail fold (Fig. 149.8A). The nail plate is then removed from that direction, i.e. it is lifted from the proximal end (Fig. 149.8B).

Partial nail plate avulsion is useful when the precise location of the lesion under the nail is known (Fig. 149.9). In some cases it is possible to cut a portion of the overlying nail plate and reflect the partially loosened nail plate to expose the lesion so it can be excised. The nail plate can then be repositioned to cover and protect the wound during the early stages of the healing process. While the piece of replaced nail plate does not reattach and will eventually be shed, it does provide protection and minimizes discomfort for the patient during the immediate postoperative period. The replaced nail plate can be secured with a suture or Steri-Strips™.

The second fundamental nail surgical procedure is *nail matrix exploration*, which allows the clinician to examine the nail matrix and ventral surface of the nail fold for tumors and other pathology. Releasing incisions, about 5 mm in length, are made in the proximal nail fold beginning at the junction of the proximal and lateral nail folds and angling laterally and proximally (Fig. 149.10A). This allows the nail fold to be reflected so that the matrix can be inspected. Skin hooks or sutures (placed through the nail fold and retracted proximally) allow for exposure of the matrix for visual inspection as well as for subsequent biopsy or excision (Fig. 149.10B). At the end of the procedure, the fold is reflected back into place and secured with simple interrupted stitches or Steri-Strips™ (Fig. 149.10C).

NAIL EXCISIONS AND BIOPSIES

The techniques used for nail excision and/or biopsy depend upon the location of the pathology within the nail unit, the type of lesion, and the objective of the procedure. Useful nail surgical techniques are the punch biopsy (with or without prior nail avulsion), the elliptical excision in the nail bed or nail matrix, the lateral longitudinal combined biopsy/excision, and the chemical matricectomy. Surgical procedures should be oriented properly so that the nail unit heals in a manner that minimizes scarring and has the best functional and cosmetic outcome. In the nail bed, an excision is usually oriented in a longitudinal axis, whereas in the matrix the orientation of the excision is horizontal (Fig. 149.11). For biopsies of the nail bed, the size of the surgical specimen is determined by the type of lesion; as a general guideline, excisions of 3 mm or less are preferable and defects should be sutured when possible. Nail punch biopsy, elliptical excision and matricectomy will be discussed separately, based on location within the nail unit.

Surgery of the Proximal Nail Fold

The epidermis of the nail folds is similar to that of other cutaneous sites, with two exceptions: the nail matrix lies beneath the proximal nail fold and should be protected, and the nail fold produces the cuticle

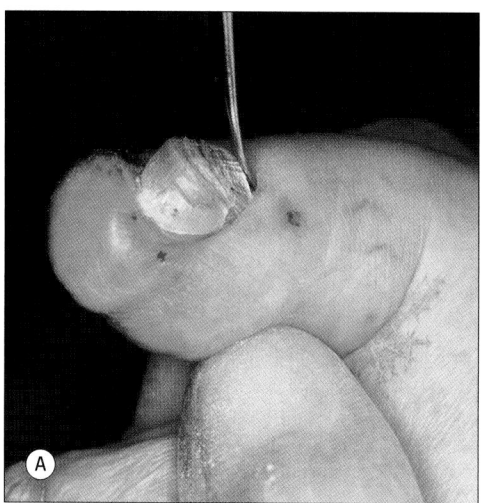

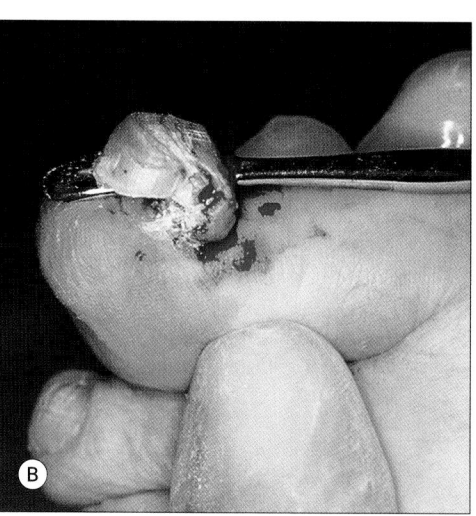

Fig. 149.8 Proximal nail plate avulsion. The Freer elevator is inserted under the proximal portion of the nail plate (**A**) and rotated to lift the thickened nail plate from the nail bed (**B**). Currently, this procedure is being done less frequently than in the past.

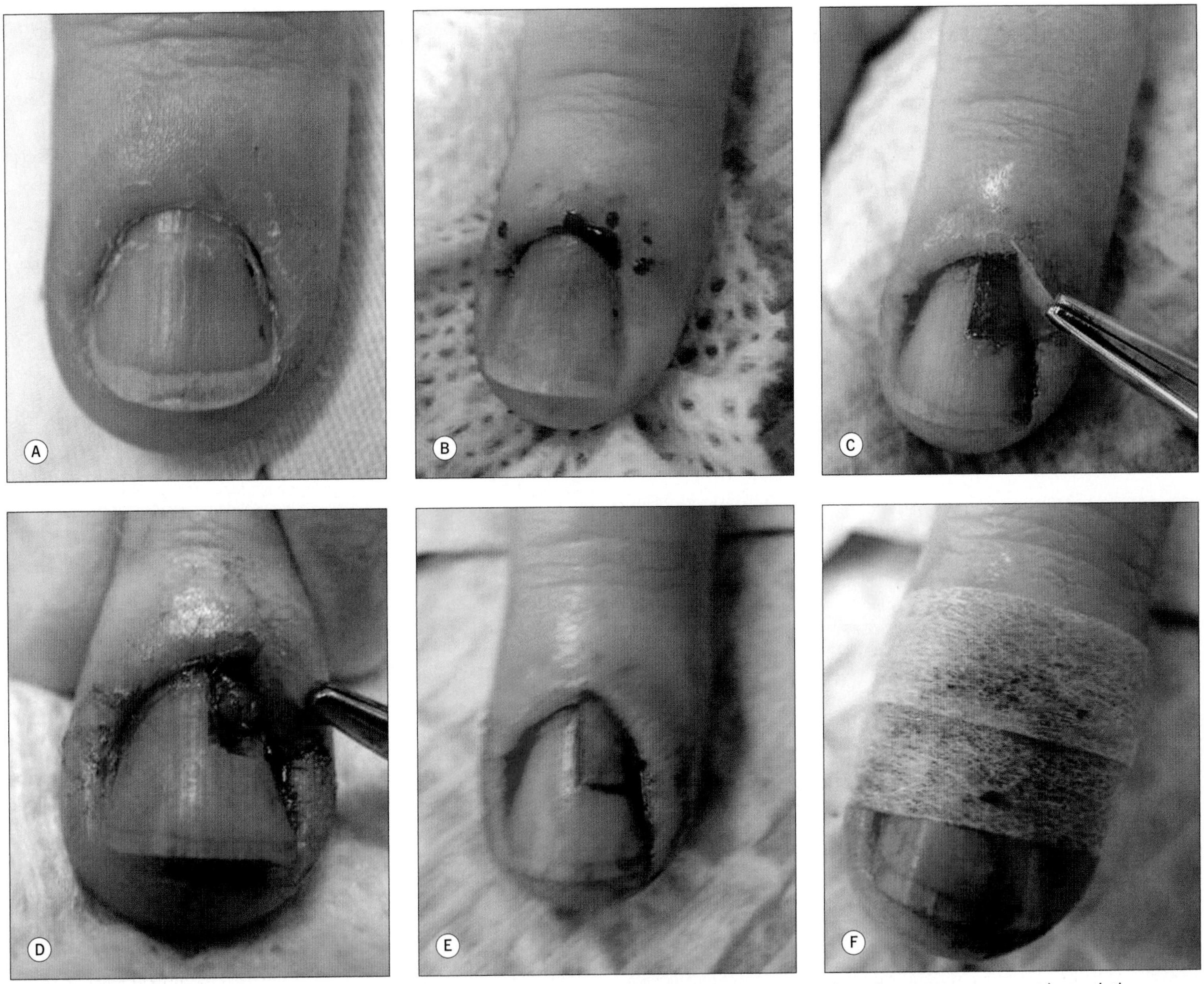

Fig. 149.9 **Focal nail surgery with partial removal and then replacement of loosened nail plate. A** Preoperatively, a glomus tumor is present beneath the proximal nail plate. **B** The nail unit after wing block anesthesia. **C** A cut in the nail plate allows a flap of nail to be reflected (with a hemostat), thereby exposing the subungual area. **D** The glomus tumor is removed, leaving a small defect. The flap of nail is replaced (**E**) and secured with Steri-Strips™ (**F**).

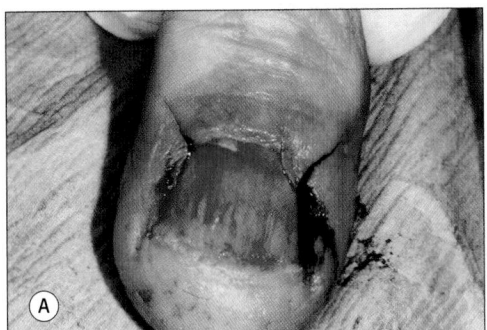
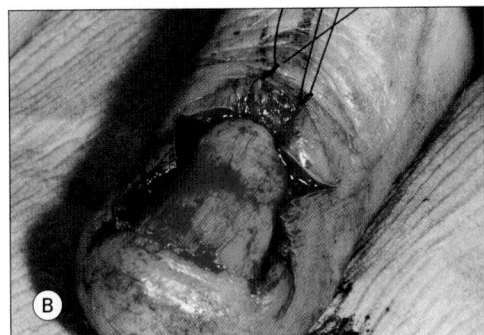
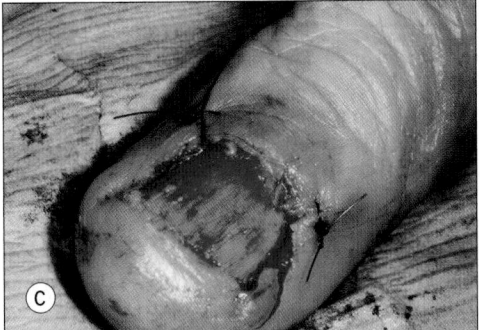

Fig. 149.10 **Nail matrix exploration. A** After nail plate avulsion, releasing incisions in the proximal nail fold (PNF) are made. **B** The PNF is retracted with skin hooks or sutures to allow visualization of the nail matrix. **C** The PNF is replaced and sutured or approximated with Steri-Strips™.

that attaches to the nail plate. A space-occupying lesion in the proximal nail fold, such as a fibroma or myxoid cyst, often presses on the underlying nail matrix and causes a characteristic longitudinal depressed defect in the nail plate immediately distal to its site (see Ch. 70). Lesions of the nail fold can be biopsied via shave, punch or incisional techniques or excised *en bloc*[7]. It is useful to insert a Freer elevator beneath the proximal nail fold in order to shield the matrix from

inadvertent damage from the scalpel (Fig. 149.12). The majority of the time, the nail is not avulsed prior to nail fold surgery. A punch or shave biopsy of the nail fold is performed as for other cutaneous sites. Also, a crescent of nail fold can be removed and allowed to heal by secondary intention; this provides an aesthetically acceptable cosmetic result, just more of the nail plate and lunula is visible. For best results with this latter technique (e.g. when excising a myxoid cyst), it is better to

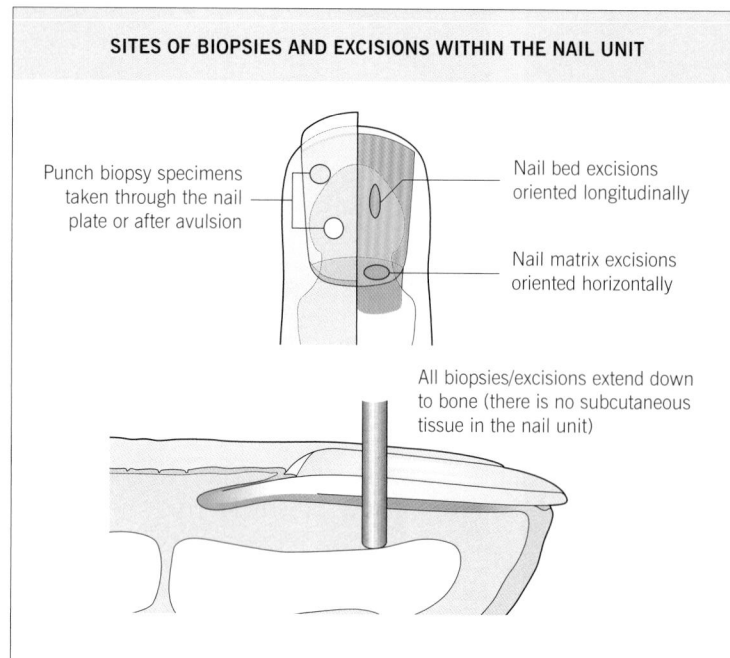

SITES OF BIOPSIES AND EXCISIONS WITHIN THE NAIL UNIT

Punch biopsy specimens taken through the nail plate or after avulsion

Nail bed excisions oriented longitudinally

Nail matrix excisions oriented horizontally

All biopsies/excisions extend down to bone (there is no subcutaneous tissue in the nail unit)

Fig. 149.11 Sites and orientations of biopsies and excisions within the nail unit.

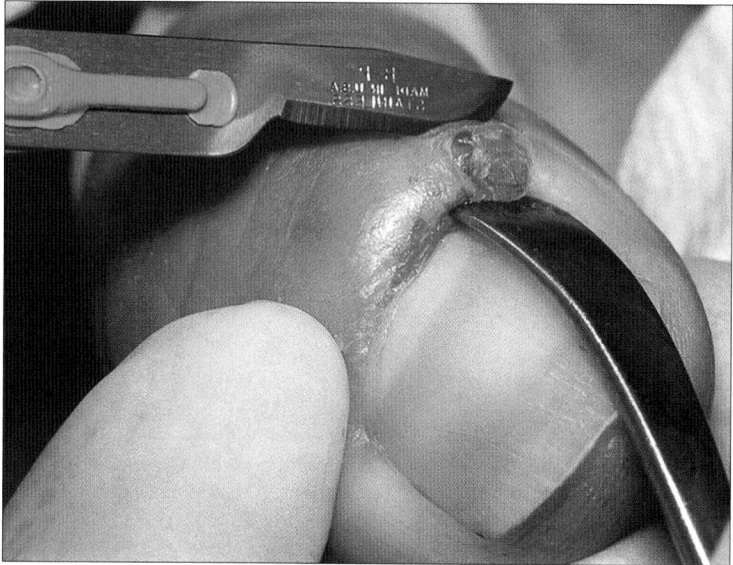

Fig. 149.12 Nail fold biopsy of a space-occupying lesion. A Freer elevator is inserted beneath the proximal nail fold and a crescent of nail fold is removed.

remove the entire width of proximal fold in a symmetric manner to prevent distorted healing.

Biopsy or Surgery of the Nail Bed

In response to pathologic conditions, the nail bed has a limited number of responses, including hyperkeratosis, onycholysis, erosion, dyschromia or a space-occupying mass. The similarity of clinical findings due to dissimilar nail conditions makes nail biopsy a useful diagnostic tool. Nail bed biopsy is a simple and safe technique that facilitates the diagnosis and even treatment of a variety of nail bed disorders (Table 149.3). The nail plate is usually avulsed prior to the nail bed biopsy; however, occasionally the biopsy is performed through the nail plate. When a punch biopsy is performed through the nail plate, a 'double punch' technique is employed, with a trephine of a greater diameter used to make a larger hole in the nail plate, then a trephine with a smaller diameter used to remove the specimen. This facilitates non-traumatic retrieval of the specimen. When an elliptical excision of a nail bed lesion such as a glomus tumor is performed, the nail bed excision is oriented longitudinally (see Fig. 149.11). The area can be undermined

CLINICAL FEATURES OF NAIL BED DISORDERS IN WHICH A BIOPSY MAY FACILITATE DIAGNOSIS AND SUBSEQUENT TREATMENT

Diagnosis	Clinical features
Malignant tumors of the nail bed	
Squamous cell carcinoma, Bowen's disease	Hyperkeratosis, dyschromia, onycholysis, destruction of the nail plate
Keratoacanthoma	Multiple or solitary, nail plate destruction, mass, erosion, granulation tissue, ± pain
Melanoma	Pigmentation of the nail bed, erosion, destruction of the nail plate; 25% are amelanotic
Metastatic carcinomas	Mass, pseudo-clubbing, nail dystrophy, dusky red color, ± pain
Kaposi's sarcoma	Pigmentation, elevation, destruction of the nail plate
Basal cell carcinoma	Rare, variable clinical appearance
Benign tumors of the nail bed	
Pyogenic granuloma	Exuberant friable mass, needs to be distinguished from amelanotic melanoma
Glomus tumor	Spontaneous pain, blue–red mass
Epidermoid cyst	Mass, nail plate deformity
Fibroma	Mass, elevation, distortion of the nail (if presses on matrix, distal groove; if underneath nail plate, elevation of plate)
Exostosis	Mass, elevation of the nail plate, tenderness, secondary infection can occur
Osteochondroma	Enlargement of digit, elevation or destruction of the nail plate
Enchondroma	Mass, alteration of the nail plate, pain
Infectious conditions of the nail bed	
Onychomycosis	Hyperkeratosis, dyschromia, nail dystrophy, onycholysis
Warts	Verrucous mass, sometimes painful, nail plate deformity or destruction, must distinguish from verrucous or squamous cell carcinoma
Subungual scabies	Hyperkeratosis of hyponychium
Inflammatory dermatoses involving the nail bed	
Psoriasis	Onycholysis, hyperkeratosis, splinter hemorrhages, oil drop discoloration
Lichen planus	Violaceous discoloration, atrophy of nail bed; if nail matrix is involved, onychorrhexis, hapalonychia (soft nails), pterygium
Other nail bed conditions	
Hemorrhage, trauma	Red–violet to black discoloration under nail plate; persistent or non-migrating discoloration needs to be distinguished from melanoma

Table 149.3 Clinical features of nail bed disorders in which a biopsy may facilitate diagnosis and subsequent treatment. Adapted from Rich P. Nail biopsy: indications and methods. J Dermatol Surg Oncol. 1992;18:673–82.

at the level of the periosteum and absorbable polyglactin (e.g. Vicryl®) sutures placed to approximate the nail bed wound edges (Fig. 149.13). The nail bed usually heals with minimal scarring, although occasionally there may be onycholysis.

Nail Matrix Biopsy

The nail matrix biopsy has multiple indications, the most important of which is to exclude the diagnosis of subungual melanoma in a patient

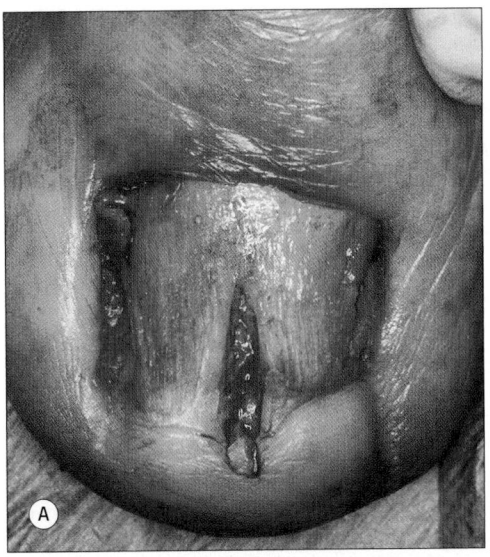

Fig. 149.13 Nail bed excision of a glomus tumor. A Elliptical excision is oriented longitudinally. B Absorbable sutures approximate the wound edges.

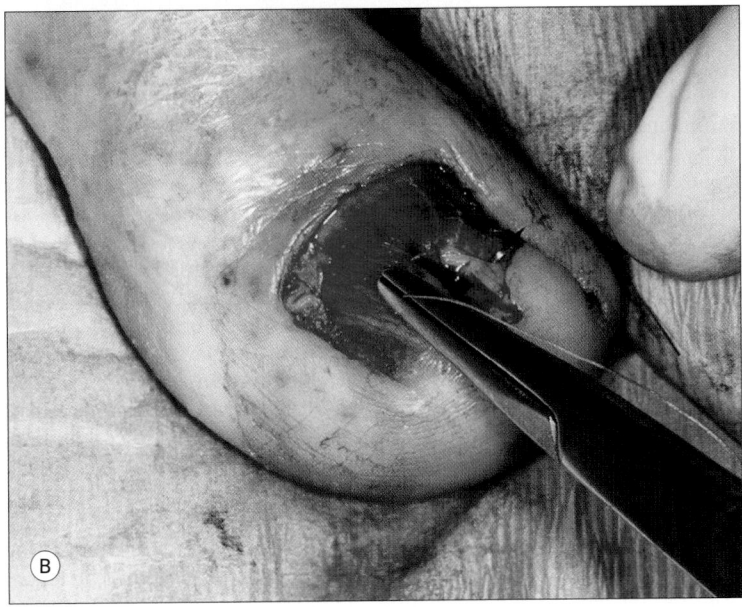

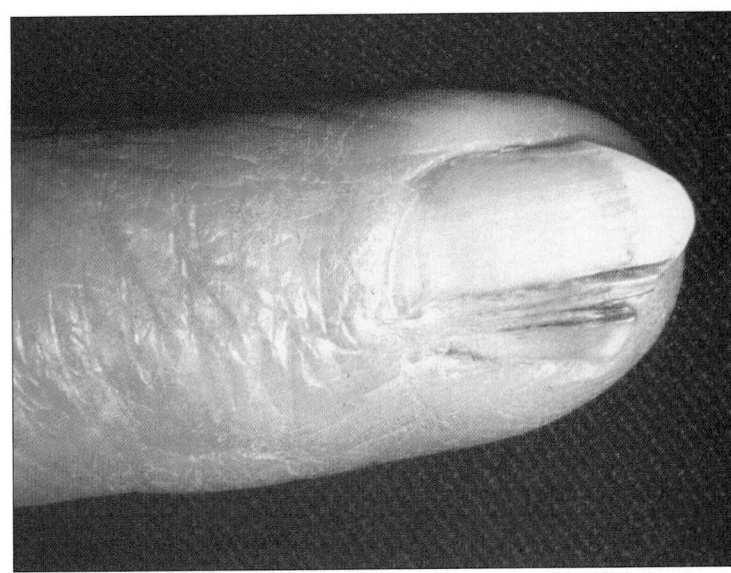

Fig. 149.14 A nail matrix biopsy can result in permanent nail dystrophy. Obtaining the specimen from the distal nail matrix, if possible, and suturing the defect minimize scarring.

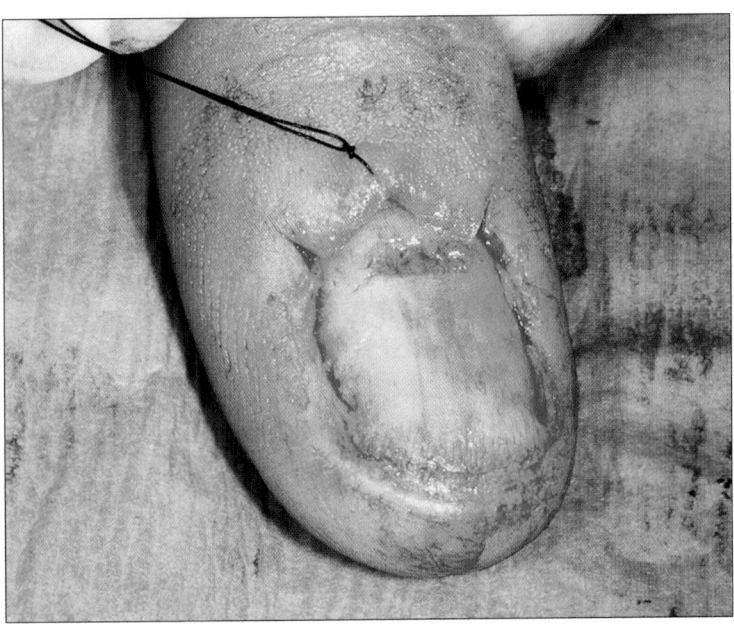

Fig. 149.15 Nail matrix excision in the distal matrix. The excision is oriented in a horizontal axis within the matrix and then sutured.

with abnormal pigmentation of the nail plate (see Ch. 70). A biopsy of a pigmented band (longitudinal melanonychia) must be taken from the nail matrix where the pigment is generated (see below). Of all the locations within the nail unit where a biopsy can be performed, it is the nail matrix that carries the greatest risk in terms of scarring (Fig. 149.14). However, a nail matrix biopsy is a relatively safe and simple procedure when the principles of nail surgery are followed. With regard to nail anatomy and physiology, it is important to remember that the distal matrix forms the inferior (ventral) surface of the nail plate, and the proximal matrix forms its superficial (dorsal) surface (see Fig. 149.2). When there is a choice, the distal matrix is the preferred site for a matrix biopsy because any resultant split or defect will be hidden in the undersurface (ventral aspect) of the nail plate (see Fig. 149.2). Split nails that involve the dorsal surface are unsightly and easily traumatized as they catch on items such as clothing.

Prior to nail matrix biopsy, the nail plate is usually avulsed and the matrix exploration facilitated by releasing incisions that allow the proximal nail fold to be retracted (see Fig. 149.10). The nail plate avulsion can be total or partial. When an elliptical excision is performed in the nail matrix, the preferred orientation is horizontal (Fig. 149.15), and after undermining, absorbable polyglactin (e.g. Vicryl®) interrupted stitches should be used to approximate the wound edges. A punch biopsy 3 mm or smaller in the mid or distal matrix does not need to be sutured.

Nail matrix excision and repair results in a thinner nail plate because the thickness of the nail plate is to a large extent related to the length of the matrix. For the best cosmetic outcome, elliptical excisions within the matrix area should be sutured (see above). As there is no

subcutaneous fat under the nail matrix or bed, biopsies should extend to the periosteum of the underlining distal phalanx, with undermining performed at the periosteal level.

Great care must be exercised when handling the small fragile tissue specimen that is obtained from the nail biopsy. The tissue must be oriented and marked so that it is received by the pathologist in a state that allows for appropriate histologic evaluation. It is best to use surgical markers to identify the biopsy site and to allow the examining pathologist to orient the epidermal surface properly. Cutting down with the scalpel all the way to the periosteum and then undercutting beneath the specimen avoids crush injury[8].

Lateral Longitudinal Nail Biopsy and Excision

A lateral longitudinal nail biopsy is a useful procedure where a length of the lateral nail unit is removed, including the nail matrix, nail folds, nail bed, nail plate and hyponychium. This procedure allows all these parts of the nail unit to be histologically examined simultaneously. It is useful for longitudinal pigmented bands of the lateral one-third of the nail and for inflammatory conditions in which the nail bed, nail matrix, nail plate, nail folds and hyponychium are involved concurrently. In

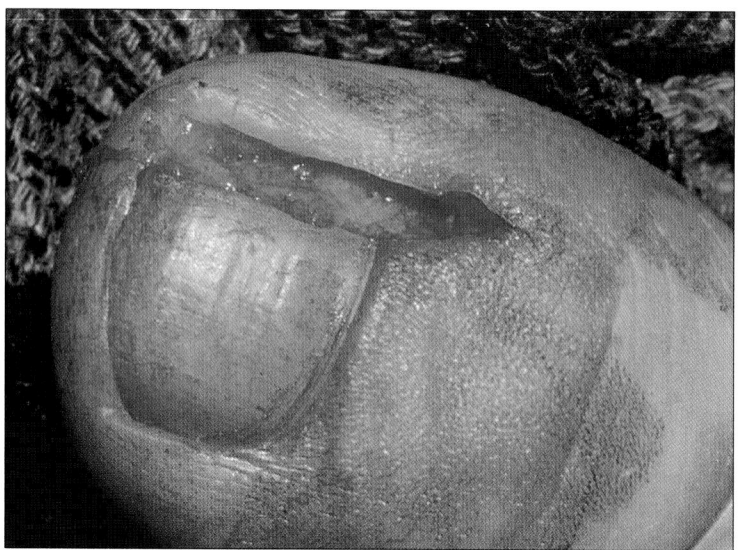

Fig. 149.16 Lateral longitudinal biopsy. The lateral portions of the nail unit are excised *en bloc* including the hyponychium, nail plate, nail bed, nail matrix and proximal nail fold.

NAIL UNIT TUMORS: RADIOGRAPHIC FINDINGS AND SURGICAL TREATMENTS

Tumor	Radiographic findings	Surgical treatment
Subungual exostosis	Radiopaque bone growth that is well circumscribed	Nail plate avulsion followed by surgical removal (can use bone rongeur)[9,10]
Keratoacanthoma	Cup-shaped radiolucent defect (early)	Surgical excision[11]
Enchondroma	Central round radiolucent defect	Surgical excision
Squamous cell carcinoma	Radiolucent defect (late)	Microscopically controlled (Mohs) surgery[12,13]
Glomus tumor	Occasional radiolucent defect	Surgical excision (nail bed – longitudinal axis; nail matrix – horizontal axis)[14]
Myxoid cyst	Osteoarthritis	Cryosurgery, surgical excision (can use Freer elevator to protect matrix)[15]

Table 149.4 Nail unit tumors: radiographic findings and surgical treatments. Adapted from Rich P. Curr Prob Dermatol. 1999;11:161–208.

this technique, the lateral one-third of the nail plate with its surrounding and supporting structures is removed *en bloc*. This is performed by excising through the nail plate and the matrix into the proximal nail fold and then laterally through the lateral nail fold to and including the hyponychium (Fig. 149.16). The scalpel cuts through the nail unit down to the periosteum and the specimen is removed intact by loosening it from the underlying bone. The resultant defect is undermined and sutured or allowed to heal secondarily. The lateral groove heals with a narrower but cosmetically acceptable nail.

DRESSINGS AND POSTOPERATIVE CARE FOLLOWING NAIL SURGERY

Proper dressings can reduce postoperative pain and throbbing and minimize postoperative complications. A layer of antibiotic ointment is applied to the surgical site and covered with a non-stick dressing such as Vaseline™ gauze or Telfa®. A bulky gauze dressing is used for its absorptive and protective functions. Tube gauze such as Xspan® secures the dressing, and tape anchors the dressing to the skin. Given the likelihood of postoperative edema, the dressing should not be too tight and the tape should be non-constrictive. Patients should be instructed to keep the dressing dry. Preoperative non-steroidal anti-inflammatory drugs (NSAIDs) are helpful in controlling mild discomfort and inflammation; narcotic analgesics are sometimes prescribed. Keeping the digit elevated higher than the heart will minimize painful throbbing. Bleeding into the dressing can result in the bandage sticking to the surgical site, in which case discomfort can be minimized by soaking the bandage to loosen it prior to removal.

SPECIAL SITUATIONS IN NAIL SURGERY

Nail Tumors

There are several nail unit tumors that are difficult to diagnosis by clinical appearance alone (e.g. pyogenic granuloma, squamous cell carcinoma) and there are others where a preoperative radiograph points to the correct diagnosis (e.g. osteochondroma). These tumors are discussed in Chapter 70 and their treatment is outlined in Table 149.4.

Management of Malignant Neoplasms of the Nail Unit

Melanoma

Approximately 1–3% of all melanomas in Caucasians and 20% of melanomas in African-Americans occur within the nail unit[16,17]. Due to delays in diagnosis, subungual melanoma has a poor prognosis. In many patients, melanoma of the nail unit is treated as a chronic

paronychia, verruca, onychomycosis or an ingrown nail prior to the biopsy and correct diagnosis being established. A study by Glat et al.[18] reported a delay of nearly 2 years in the diagnosis of 22 subungual melanomas, resulting in 10- and 5-year survival rates of 13% and 30%, respectively[19].

The most reliable way to diagnose ungual melanoma is by histologic examination of the appropriate part of the nail matrix (or, rarely, the nail bed)[20]. Certain clinical features should raise one's suspicion of the possibility of melanoma. These clinical features are outlined in the mnemonic ABCDEF: *a*ge of the patient (older); *b*rown/black and *b*readth greater than 3 mm; *c*hange in the band; *d*igit involved (thumb, great toe); *e*xtension of pigment onto the nail folds (Hutchinson's sign); and *f*amily history of melanoma[21]. Algorithms based on patient age, single or multiple bands, presence of Hutchinson's sign (see below), and ethnic background suggest a logical approach for diagnosis, but the bottom line is that in a Caucasian, a new, unexplained pigmented band in the nail usually should be biopsied, and the biopsy specimen should be taken from the nail matrix at the origin of the pigmented band (Fig. 149.17).

The clinical diagnosis of nail apparatus melanoma is difficult because there are many benign causes of longitudinal melanonychia (melanonychia striata; see Ch. 70). Inactive melanocytes are present in the nail matrix and nail bed of Caucasians. When they are stimulated to proliferate or produce melanin, the pigment is incorporated into the nail plate and appears as a longitudinal brown or black band. Histologically, melanocyte activation is seen much more commonly than nevi; additional causes are listed in Table 70.2.

An additional consideration is that darkly pigmented individuals frequently have benign pigmented bands of the nail. In fact, over 90% of African-Americans have one or more longitudinal pigmented bands by the age of 50 years. Longitudinal melanonychia occurs in over 10–20% of Asians and the incidence is much higher in Hispanics and Middle Eastern populations[17]. Because the precise etiology of longitudinal melanonychia often cannot be ascertained from clinical inspection and history alone, subungual melanoma should always be included in the differential diagnosis and a biopsy of any suspicious lesion is mandatory[20].

The management of longitudinal melanonychia in children presents a particularly challenging problem. Melanomas are rare in children and there is controversy regarding whether all pigmented bands in children need to be biopsied. Several recent reviews have suggested that it may be safe to observe some of these lesions in children[22,23]. In one series of eight children with longitudinal melanonychia who were followed for a period of 5 years, five children had their pigmented bands excised and three were observed. None of the children had melanoma or a change in their bands, and serious disfigurement occurred in two of those who had their bands excised. However, the debate continues regarding biopsy or excision of longitudinal melanonychia in children and hopefully further studies examining the impact of color, width and change will provide guidance.

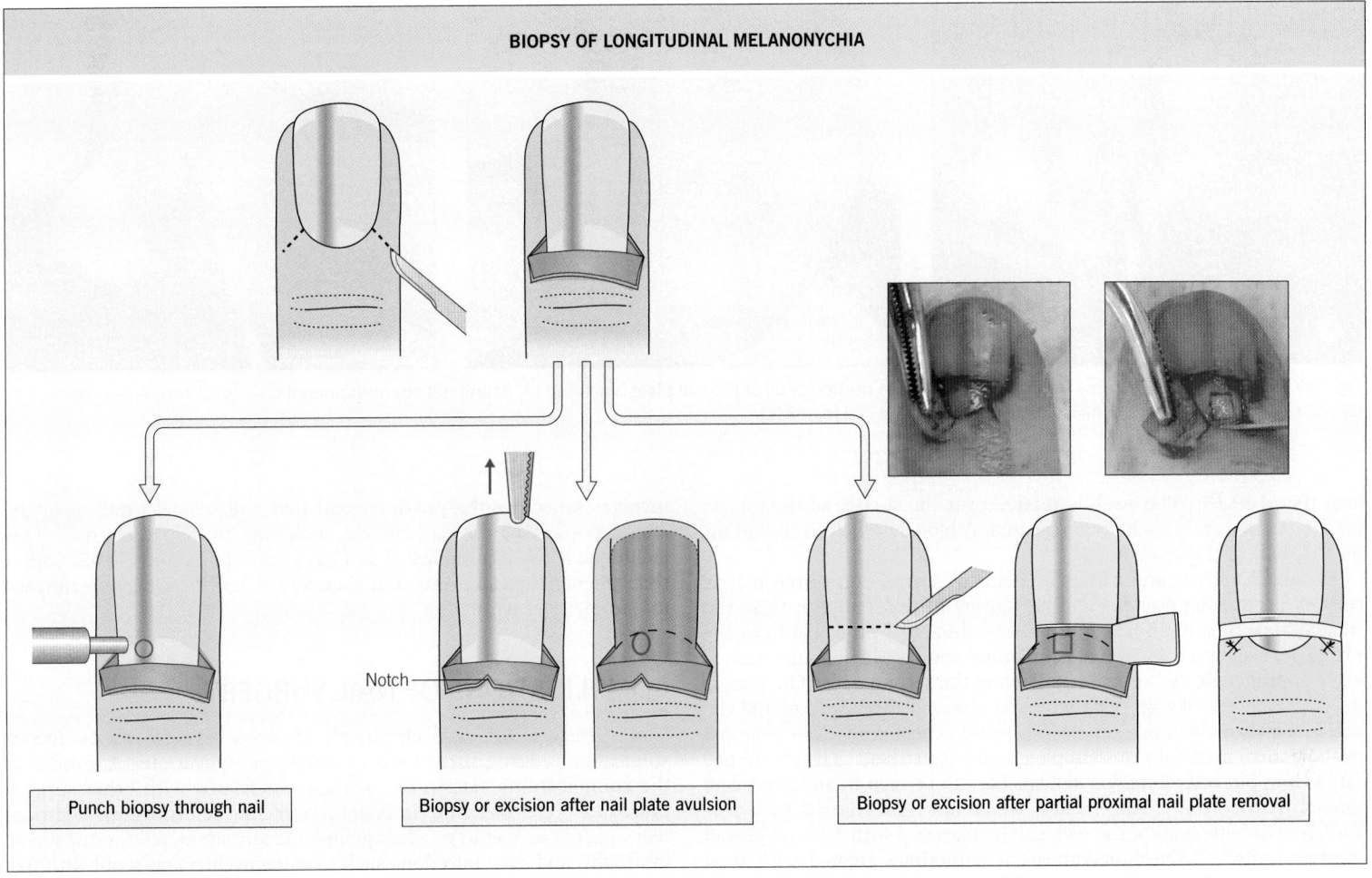

Punch biopsy through nail

Biopsy or excision after nail plate avulsion

Biopsy or excision after partial proximal nail plate removal

Notch

Fig. 149.17 Biopsy of longitudinal melanonychia. Histologic examination of the nail matrix can be achieved via three different surgical approaches.

Much discussion has centered round the presence or absence of Hutchinson's sign, which is the leaching of pigment into the perionychium in association with a melanoma. While at times helpful in confirming the clinical diagnosis of melanoma of the nail unit, it is an inconsistent feature and sometimes not particularly helpful. Melanoma can occur without Hutchinson's sign, and pseudo-Hutchinson's sign can occur in the absence of melanoma. Pseudo-Hutchinson's sign represents the presence or illusion of pigment in the perionychium and can be associated with a variety of disorders (Table 149.5).

Squamous cell carcinoma

Squamous cell carcinoma (SCC) of the nail bed and lateral nail groove is not uncommon. The clinical features of this tumor can be non-specific, such as hyperkeratosis of the lateral groove or slight onycholysis when the nail bed is involved. These carcinomas may have a verrucous appearance and are often treated as verrucae for many years before they are biopsied. However, one should have a high index of suspicion for SCC when recalcitrant verrucous or keratotic lesions are present in the lateral nail groove and fold. In addition, SCC of the nail unit can present as paronychia, persistent onycholysis, a mass, or dystrophy of the nail plate; however, often the clinical features are minimal[24]. Predisposing factors are radiation exposure and infection with human papillomavirus (HPV) types 16 and 18[25]. Mohs surgery is the treatment of choice for SCC of the nail apparatus[12], unless bone involvement requires amputation. Lastly, even though SCC is the most common malignant tumor of the nail unit and there is often a long delay in diagnosis, it rarely metastasizes[26].

Management of Ingrown Toenails

An ingrown toenail occurs when a portion of the nail plate grows into the skin of the lateral nail groove. This sharp nail spicule acts as a foreign body, and secondary infection and formation of granulation tissue often ensue. Heredity, poorly fitting shoes and improper nail grooming can contribute to the development of ingrown toenails. Any associated infection should be treated and conservative measures tried first, e.g. lamb's wool, longer toenails. Surgical management involves partial or total nail plate avulsion followed by chemical or surgical destruction of the lateral portion of the nail matrix.

Phenol matricectomy is used more commonly than surgical matricectomy, because it is easier to perform and causes less post-operative discomfort. The principle of phenol matricectomy is chemical destruction of the portion of the nail matrix associated with the in-growing part of the nail. After anesthetizing the digit, the nail is partially or completely avulsed. Full-strength phenol (88%) is applied to the lateral part of the nail matrix with a small cotton swab fashioned from small wisps of cotton wound around a small wooden stick or toothpick. The swab is dipped into the phenol and the excess is drained off, and it is then carefully inserted under the nail fold in the desired

ETIOLOGIES OF A PSEUDO-HUTCHINSON'S SIGN
Pigment present in paronychium
• Normal variant for skin phototypes IV, V and VI
• Laugier–Hunziker syndrome, Peutz–Jeghers syndrome
• Radiation exposure
• Malnutrition
• Minocycline, zidovudine (AZT)
• Postinflammatory
• Benign melanocytic nevi
• Regressing nevoid melanosis in childhood
• Subungual hematoma
Pigment visible through paronychium
• Neoplasms (benign nevi, squamous cell carcinoma, basal cell carcinoma)
• Subungual hematoma

Table 149.5 Etiologies of a pseudo-Hutchinson's sign. Adapted from Baran R. Hutchinson's sign: a reappraisal. J Am Acad Dermatol. 1996;34:87–90.

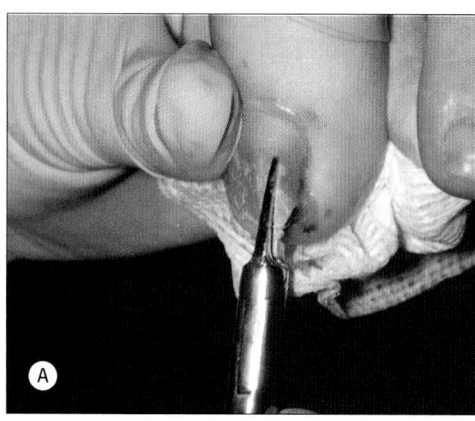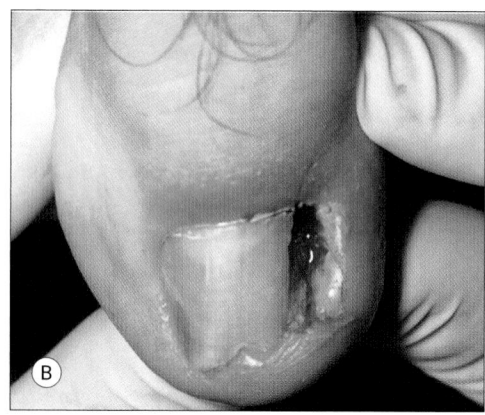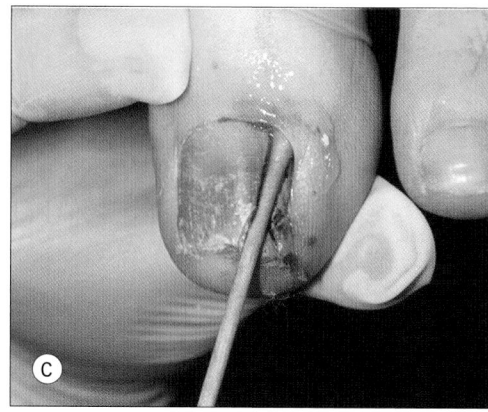

Fig. 149.18 Phenol matricectomy for ingrown toenails. A portion or all of the nail plate is avulsed (**A, B**) and full-strength phenol on a small cotton wisp on a toothpick is inserted under the nail fold and applied to the nail matrix (**C**).

area (Fig. 149.18). The swab is rotated over the surface of the matrix for 30 seconds and this is then repeated. A bloodless field is important for this part of the procedure.

Phenol is caustic and causes a chemical destruction of the matrix cells by denaturing proteins and preventing further nail growth in the treated area. The nail folds and nail bed should be protected from the phenol (can apply a thin layer of petrolatum) and the phenol is neutralized with isopropyl alcohol or saline following the second pass. The digit is dressed with a bulky dressing which is changed the next day and the nail is soaked daily during the healing phase. There is generally minimal postoperative pain with this simple effective treatment. The recurrence rate is low, but occasionally a nail spicule can be seen in an incomplete phenol matricectomy. Pincer nails, which are characterized by hyper-curvature of both sides of the nail, can be managed with bilateral phenol matricectomy[27,28]. Onychogryphosis is sometimes treated with total phenol matricectomy.

Surgical excision of the lateral nail matrix is sometimes performed for the treatment of ingrown toenails and pincer nails. This procedure involves reflecting the proximal nail fold and scalpel excision of the lateral portion of the nail matrix, including the lateral horn[29]. This technique is more complicated and has greater postoperative discomfort than phenol matricectomy and therefore is less frequently performed for simple ingrown nails.

COMPLICATIONS OF NAIL SURGERY

Nail surgery is safe and effective[30]. However, as with all cutaneous surgical procedures, there are occasionally complications. A number of the complications are similar to those associated with other surgical procedures, e.g. bleeding, infection, pain and deformity. In addition, nail surgery can lead to pyogenic granuloma formation, reflex sympathetic dystrophy, and deep infections such as osteomyelitis and septic arthritis. The most characteristic complication of nail surgery is nail plate deformity, which results from nail matrix damage. When care is taken and the principles of nail surgery are strictly followed, complications are rare.

REFERENCES

1. Rich P. Nail biopsy: indications and methods. Dermatol Surg. 2001;27:229–34.
2. Rich P, Scher RK. An Atlas of Diseases of the Nail. New York: Parthenon Publishing Group, 2003.
3. Fleckman P, Allan C. Surgical anatomy of the nail unit. Dermatol Surg. 2001;27;257–60.
4. Haneke E. Surgical anatomy of the nail apparatus. Dermatol Clin. 2006;24:291–6.
5. Denkler K. A comprehensive review of epinephrine in the finger: to do or not to do. Plast Reconstr Surg. 2001;108:114–24.
6. McGinness JL, Parlette HL 3rd. Versatile sterile field for nail surgery using a sterile glove. Dermatol Online J. 2005;11:10.
7. Grover C, Bansal S, Nanda S, Reddy BS, Kumar V. En bloc excision of proximal nail fold for treatment of chronic paronychia. Dermatol Surg. 2006;32:393–8.
8. Scher RK, Daniel CR (eds). Nails: Diagnosis, Therapy, Surgery, 3rd edn. Philadelphia: WB Saunders, 2005.
9. Carrol RE, Chance JT, Inan Y. Subungual exostosis of the hand. J Hand Surg Br. 1992;17:569–74.
10. de Palma L, Gigante A, Specchia N. Subungual exostosis of the foot. Foot Ankle Int. 1996;17:758–63.
11. Baran R, Gottman S. Distal digital keratoacanthoma: a report of 12 cases and review of the literature. Br J Dermatol. 1998;139:512–15.
12. de Berker DA, Dahl MG, Malcolm AJ, Lawrence CM. Micrographic surgery for subungual squamous cell

carcinoma. Br J Plast Surg. 1996;49:414–19.
13. Salasche SJ, Orengo IF. Tumors of the nail unit. J Dermatol Surg Oncol. 1992;18:691–700.
14. Baran R, Dawber RPR, de Berker D, Haneke E, Tosti A (eds). Diseases of the Nails and their Management, 3rd edn. London: Blackwell, 2001.
15. Salasche SJ. Myxoid cysts of the proximal nail fold: a surgical approach. J Dermatol Surg Oncol. 1984;10:35–9.
16. Banfield CC, Redburn JC, Dawber RP. The incidence and prognosis of nail apparatus melanoma: a retrospective study of 105 patients in four English regions. Br J Dermatol. 1998;139:276–9.
17. Baran R, Kechijian P. Longitudinal melanonychia (melanonychia striata): diagnosis and management. J Am Acad Dermatol. 1989;21:1165–75.
18. Glat PM, Spector JA, Roses DF, et al. The management of pigmented lesions of the nail bed. Ann Plast Surg. 1996;37:125–34.
19. Klausner JM, Inbar M, Gutman M, et al. Nail-bed melanoma. J Surg Oncol. 1987;34:208–10.
20. Daniel CR. Longitudinal melanonychia and melanoma: an unusual presentation. Dermatol Surg. 2001; 27:294–5.
21. Levit EK, Kagen MH, Scher RK, et al. The ABC rule for clinical detection of subungual melanoma. J Am Acad Dermatol. 2000;42:269–74.
22. de Berker D. Childhood nail diseases. Dermatol Clin. 2006;24:355–63.

23. Andre J. Pigmented nail disorders. Dermatol Clin. 2006;24:329–49.
24. Hale LR, Dawber RP. Subungual squamous cell presenting with minimal nail changes: a factor in delayed diagnosis? Australas J Dermatol. 1998;39:86–8.
25. Guitart A, Bergfeld WF, Tuthill RJ, et al. Squamous cell carcinoma of the nail bed: a clinicopathological study of 12 cases. Br J Dermatol. 1990;123:215–22.
26. Lumpkin LR III, Rosen T, Tschen JA. Subungual squamous cell carcinoma. J Am Acad Dermatol. 1984;11:735–8.
27. Haneke E. Surgical treatment of ingrowing toenails. Cutis. 1986;37:251–6.
28. Byrne DS, Caldwell D. Phenol cauterization for ingrowing toenails: a review of five years experience. Br J Surg. 1989;76:598–9.
29. Haneke E, Baran R. Nail ablation and matrixectomy. In: Krull EA, Zook EG, Baran R, Haneke E (eds). Nail Surgery: A Text and Atlas. Philadelphia: Lippincott Williams & Wilkins, 2001;83–88.
30. Lecha M, Effendy I, Feuilhade de Chauvin M, et al. Taskforce on onychomycosis education. Treatment options – development of consensus guidelines. J Eur Acad Dermatol Venereol. 2005;19(suppl. 1):25–33.

Mohs Surgery

Clark C Otley and Randall K Roenigk

150

Synonyms: Mohs micrographic surgery, chemosurgery, Mohs chemosurgery (includes fresh tissue technique and fixed tissue technique)

Key features

- 100% micrographic tissue margin examination
- Highest cure rate
- Tissue sparing
- Total tissue control and precise mapping
- Same physician serves as both surgeon and pathologist
- Immediate re-excision of residual cancerous tissue as indicated
- Least complicated reconstruction possible due to tissue sparing

INTRODUCTION

The most common cancer worldwide, non-melanoma skin cancer, causes significant morbidity, occasionally mortality (see Ch. 108), and it consumes substantial healthcare resources. There is a myriad of techniques available for the management of non-melanoma skin cancer, as noted in Table 150.1. Superficial ablative techniques, such as electrodesiccation and curettage or cryotherapy, are employed for minor skin cancers. In general, the superficial ablative therapies are highly cost-effective, and they provide acceptable cure rates with reasonable cosmesis for low-risk, non-melanoma skin cancer. In contrast, deeper non-melanoma skin cancers as well as those with high-risk features are managed with techniques such as radiation therapy (see Ch. 139), excision (see Ch. 146), and Mohs micrographic surgery. Radiation therapy and excisional surgery with frozen or paraffin-embedded ('permanent') section analysis have specific indications in the management of non-melanoma skin cancer, but are not the focus of this chapter. Comprehensive reviews of the management of non-melanoma skin cancer are readily available[1,2].

Mohs surgery is a specialized surgical and pathologic technique used for the removal of high-risk cutaneous neoplasms. The most important innovation associated with Mohs surgery is the method of tissue preparation and devotion to the histologic examination of 100% of the tissue margins. This innovation is accomplished through a variety of technical adaptations, and it forms the basis for the high cure rate and tissue-sparing ability of Mohs surgery. Precise micrographic tissue mapping, complete physical control of the tissue within the dermatologic surgery unit, and the ability of the dermatologic surgeon to function as both the surgeon and the pathologist contribute to unparalleled technical precision.

Mohs surgery offers the highest cure rates for all non-melanoma skin cancers. However, it would be impractical and cost-prohibitive to utilize this highly technical modality for the management of all skin cancers, particularly those that are at low risk for recurrence. Therefore, Mohs surgery is commonly reserved for cancers that are at high risk for recurrence when treated with less rigorous management options.

Mohs surgery is commonly contrasted with routine excision utilizing either delayed paraffin-embedded (permanent) or frozen section margin control. These techniques also offer high cure rates for appropriately selected non-melanoma skin cancer. However, it is important to note the distinct differences between these techniques and Mohs surgery. Conventional histologic sections, whether frozen or permanent, generally examine the peripheral margins of a specimen using a standard 'bread loaf' technique. Thin, cross-sectional slices of representative tissue are taken from the specimen and examined histologically (Fig. 150.1). This offers some opportunity to detect involved margins; however, only a small portion of the total peripheral margin, equivalent to 0.01% of the surface area, is examined by these techniques. In contrast, the unique tissue processing associated with Mohs surgery allows 100% margin control and an optimal cure rate. An additional advantage of Mohs surgery is greater control of the actual tissue specimen due to fewer individuals handling the tissue, as compared with the number involved in performing an excision with frozen sections.

TREATMENT OPTIONS FOR NON-MELANOMA SKIN CANCER

Superficial lesions

- Electrodesiccation and curettage
- Cryotherapy
- Curettage and cryotherapy
- Imiquimod cream
- Photodynamic therapy
- 5-Fluorouracil cream

Deeper/high-risk lesions

- Mohs surgery
- Excision with paraffin-embedded section histology
- Excision with frozen section histology
- Radiation therapy

Table 150.1 Treatment options for non-melanoma skin cancer.

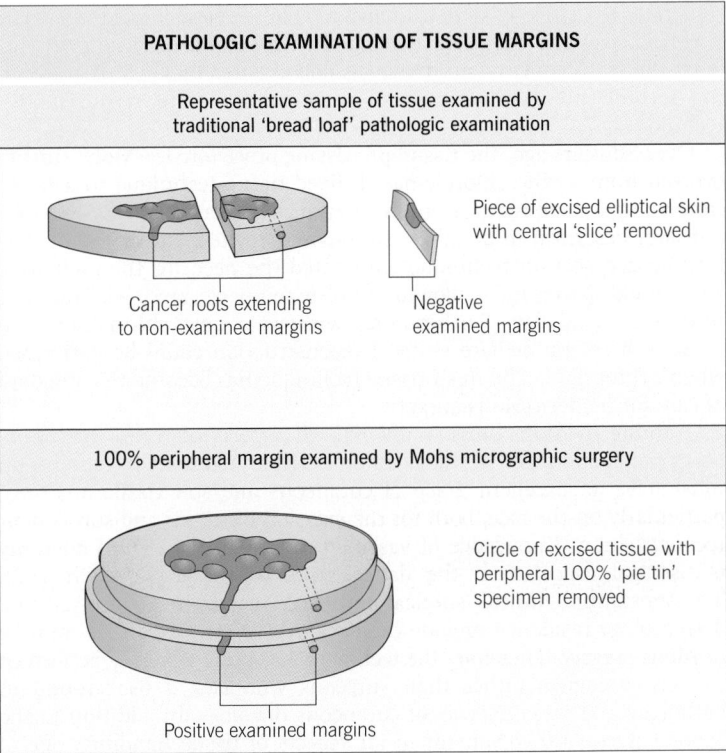

PATHOLOGIC EXAMINATION OF TISSUE MARGINS

Representative sample of tissue examined by traditional 'bread loaf' pathologic examination

Cancer roots extending to non-examined margins

Piece of excised elliptical skin with central 'slice' removed

Negative examined margins

100% peripheral margin examined by Mohs micrographic surgery

Circle of excised tissue with peripheral 100% 'pie tin' specimen removed

Positive examined margins

Fig. 150.1 Pathologic examination of tissue margins. Comparison of traditional 'bread loaf' sections (0.01% of total margin examined) versus Mohs micrographic surgery (100% of total margins examined).

Compared with the results from Rowe and colleagues'[3] large meta-analysis of cure rates with Mohs surgery, cure rates associated with excision plus frozen section pathology have been suboptimal, e.g. a 5% false-negative rate, 6.5% false-positive rate, and 2-year cure rates ranging from 83% to 92% for facial sites[4]. Although a recent randomized trial comparing Mohs surgery with excision for basal cell carcinoma (primary and recurrent) showed lower recurrence rates for Mohs surgery, the differences were not significant[5]. However, there were multiple methodologic shortcomings that impaired the ability of the trial to reveal meaningful differences[5,6]. These shortcomings included referral bias, enrollment bias, randomization bias, crossover bias and rescue bias, as well as inadequate endpoint assessment[6].

HISTORY

Mohs surgery was developed by Dr Frederic E Mohs, whose pioneering work was performed at the University of Wisconsin in the 1930s and first published in 1941[7]. Dr Mohs described his technique as chemosurgery. In his initial experiments, he observed that intralesional injection of 20% zinc chloride solution produced tumor necrosis with preservation of histology. His original clinical technique involved the application of a zinc chloride paste to cancerous tissue 24 hours prior to surgical removal of the tumor. The paste essentially fixed and isolated the tumor *in vivo*. Subsequently, the tumor was excised, sectioned into multiple pieces, and marked with colored dyes for purposes of orientation. A precise and detailed map of the resected tumor was created, including orientation relative to remaining tissue and ink locations. The specimen was flattened with physical pressure so that histologic sections would encompass all lateral and deep margins, and then it was inverted for histologic sectioning. Serial tissue sections were cut on a microtome, arranged on glass slides, and then stained. The precise location of any residual tumor seen on histologic examination was noted on the map. In cases with residual tumor at the margins, zinc chloride paste was applied to cancerous margins for 24 hours, and further tissue resection, processing and analysis were performed until complete tumor clearance was obtained.

With the original fixed tissue technique, the zinc chloride caused tissue necrosis, rendering wounds unacceptable for surgical reconstruction. From this limitation, Dr Mohs' second major innovation emerged: an objective analysis of second intention wound healing. Until that time, surgical dogma held that allowing wounds to heal by second intention (without closure) produced inferior cosmetic results compared to reconstruction, the surgeon's 'first intention'. The acceptable, and, at times, superior, cosmetic outcome associated with second intention healing, particularly on concave surfaces, was documented by Dr Mohs, affording second intention its rightful place among valid reconstructive techniques.

Over 30 years ago, the tissue-processing procedure for Mohs surgery evolved from a zinc chloride-based, fixed tissue technique to a fresh-frozen tissue technique, an innovation initially performed by Dr Mohs but later described in detail by Tromovitch & Stegman in 1974[8]. The fresh-frozen section technique eliminated the need for the escharotic zinc chloride paste, and it allowed complete tumor clearance with multiple resections in 1 day. Furthermore, without a zinc chloride-induced necrotic base, immediate surgical reconstruction could be performed when appropriate. The fresh tissue technique has become the standard of care for modern Mohs surgery.

Training in Mohs surgery involves all aspects of tumor resection, tissue preparation, and histologic interpretation. Additionally, the surgeon must have an excellent grasp of cutaneous and soft tissue anatomy, particularly on the face, both for the excision of tumor and subsequent reconstruction. Knowledge of vascular, muscular and neural anatomy is essential, especially in the 'danger zones' of the face (see Ch. 142). The substantial clinical, surgical and pathologic training received in a dermatology residency provide the background for specialized training in Mohs surgery. Therefore, the technique has been primarily performed by dermatologists rather than surgeons who lack a background in pathology and other aspects of cutaneous oncology. In addition to the Mohs surgeon's involvement in all aspects of tissue handling, one of the unique advantages of Mohs surgical training is the degree of expertise in clinicopathologic correlation, which derives from dual training in both clinical and pathologic tumor assessment. After the

tumor has been excised, the dermatologic surgeon must also have a mastery of soft tissue and cutaneous reconstruction, with an emphasis on both functional and aesthetic restoration. The practice of Mohs surgery has evolved into a major specialty within the field of dermatology. Although utilized throughout the world, Mohs surgery appears to be far more commonly performed in the US than other countries.

INDICATIONS/CONTRAINDICATIONS

The majority of non-melanoma skin cancers are treated with superficial ablative techniques such as electrodesiccation and curettage or cryotherapy. These techniques produce reasonable cure rates and are cost-efficient for the management of most low-risk skin cancers. In contrast, Mohs surgery is ideally suited for skin cancers at high risk of recurrence. The definition of 'high risk' for skin cancer depends on multiple factors, including the characteristics of the tumor (see Ch. 108), the anatomic site, and history of prior treatment.

Generally accepted indications for Mohs surgery are listed in Table 150.2. Because other treatment options outlined in Table 150.1 can also be utilized in some patients, these indications are not considered absolute. However, Mohs surgery is often preferred because of its higher cure rate. A thorough review of indications for Mohs surgery can be found in *Guidelines of Care for Mohs Micrographic Surgery*, issued by the American Academy of Dermatology[9]. Mohs surgery has also been successfully utilized for management of many other types of cutaneous neoplasms, as noted below.

Because of the diligent and complete histologic examination of the surgical margins, Mohs surgery can be utilized to track unpredictable tumor projections, including perineural invasion. These deep and irregular tumor extensions are responsible for the higher recurrence rates with other techniques. We will review the use of Mohs surgery for each of the most commonly managed tumors, which are listed in Table 150.3.

Basal Cell Carcinoma

For primary basal cell carcinoma (BCC), cure rates of 87–95% can be obtained with superficial ablative therapies and excision. Theoretically, the optimal cure rates associated with Mohs surgery could be applied to all BCCs. Practically, however, the majority of BCCs are well managed with superficial ablation techniques and excision. Mohs surgery would be cost-prohibitive if used to manage all BCCs. Therefore, Mohs surgery is usually limited to BCCs that meet the indications listed in Table 150.2.

INDICATIONS FOR MOHS SURGERY FOR NON-MELANOMA SKIN CANCER

Tumor characteristics

- Recurrent
- High-risk* anatomic location (periorbital, perinasal, periauricular, perioral)
- Other anatomic sites where tissue preservation is imperative (fingers, toes, genitals)
- Aggressive histologic subtype:
  – Morpheaform (sclerosing), micronodular, or infiltrating BCC
  – High-grade and deeply penetrating SCC
- Perineural invasion
- Large size (>2 cm diameter)
- Poorly defined clinical borders

Characteristics of background skin

- Prior exposure to ionizing radiation
- Chronic scar (Marjolin's ulcer)
- Site of positive margins on prior excision

Patient characteristics

- Immunocompromised
- Underlying genetic syndrome, e.g. xeroderma pigmentosum, nevoid BCC (Gorlin) syndrome, or Bazex–Dupré–Christol syndrome

High risk for recurrence.

Table 150.2 Indications for Mohs surgery for non-melanoma skin cancer. BCC, basal cell carcinoma; SCC, squamous cell carcinoma.

CUTANEOUS TUMORS MANAGEABLE WITH MOHS SURGERY

- Basal cell carcinoma
- Squamous cell carcinoma
- Keratoacanthoma
- Lentigo maligna
- Other types of melanoma (controversial)
- Dermatofibrosarcoma protuberans
- Atypical fibroxanthoma
- Microcystic adnexal carcinoma
- Other tumors (see text)

Table 150.3 Cutaneous tumors manageable with Mohs surgery.

For high-risk BCCs, Mohs surgery provides superior cure rates. In the meta-analysis by Rowe et al., the 5-year cure rate for *primary* BCC treated with Mohs surgery was 99%, as compared to 90–92% using standard treatments (Table 150.4)[3]. The 5-year cure rate for *recurrent* BCC treated with Mohs surgery was 94.4%, as compared to 80.1% for standard treatments (surgical excision, radiotherapy, cryotherapy, curettage, electrodesiccation)[11]. The basis for the superior cure rates for Mohs surgery is the meticulous examination of all peripheral and deep surgical margins[11a,11b].

Mohs surgery is well suited to treatment of large BCCs (>2 cm), and size has been directly related to recurrence rate. In general, tumors >2 cm have been present for a longer duration and have a greater likelihood of recurring if treated by standard methods. When large lesions are present in cosmetically important areas, the sparing of normal tissue is also a critical advantage of Mohs surgery. Basosquamous carcinoma, a hybrid between basal and squamous cell carcinoma, has a higher risk of recurrence and is well managed with Mohs surgery as well[12].

Squamous Cell Carcinoma

When compared with other treatments, Mohs surgery offers the highest cure rates for patients with high-risk primary or recurrent squamous cell carcinomas (SCCs). The local recurrence rates based upon a retrospective review of Mohs surgery versus non-Mohs surgery modalities for primary SCC are outlined in Table 150.4[10]. There is some inherent bias in these data as the studies quoted in the table did not all use the same patient selection criteria. For example, techniques such as electrodessication and curettage appear to have higher cure rates than excision to adipose, but it is likely that patients who had curettage selected as a definitive treatment had superficial tumors.

As with BCC, Mohs surgery is indicated for management of SCCs with one or more risk factors for recurrence or metastasis, including

large SCCs (>2 cm), recurrent tumors, incompletely excised SCCs, tumors with ill-defined clinical margins, rapid growth or perineural invasion, and tumors arising in chronic scar tissue (see Table 150.2)[12a,12b]. The latter, termed Marjolin's ulcers, can behave aggressively, and a multidisciplinary approach to regional node assessment and reconstruction may be necessary in these cases. Numerous, rapidly arising SCCs may affect immunosuppressed solid-organ transplant recipients, and Mohs surgery is well suited for the management of these neoplasms.

SCC arising in high-risk or anatomically sensitive sites may be managed with Mohs surgery. For example, tumors of the lip have a high propensity for recurrence and metastasis, and cure rates as high as 92% have been obtained with Mohs surgery[13]. Mohs surgery is also well suited for SCCs occurring in anogenital areas and on the digits, where tissue conservation is needed. When compared with conventional methods, Mohs surgery for the treatment of penile SCC offers comparable survival rates. Prior to Mohs surgery, most cases of SCCs involving the nail unit were treated with amputation, electrocoagulation or radiation. Mohs surgery is an excellent choice for treatment of periungual and subungual SCC without osseous involvement – with cure rates up to 96%[14].

Keratoacanthoma

Keratoacanthoma (KA) may be considered a well-differentiated SCC with specific histologic features. KAs classically grow quickly and then spontaneously involute, but there are exceptions and metastasis has been reported. Because KAs may cause significant tissue destruction before involuting, and because definitive differentiation from aggressive SCC can be challenging, most KAs are managed with excisional or Mohs surgery. Mohs surgery may be of particular benefit for large lesions as well as those occurring in anatomically sensitive areas.

Verrucous Carcinoma

Verrucous carcinoma is considered a variant of SCC, and it can be triggered by the human papillomavirus. It occurs most commonly in the oral cavity, on the plantar surface of the foot, or on the penis. Because the tumors are usually localized, Mohs surgery is an excellent treatment option. While considered a low-grade carcinoma, several reports of metastases have been described. Mohs surgery should be considered in the management of verrucous carcinoma, especially for larger lesions.

Melanoma

The role of Mohs surgery in the treatment of melanoma continues to be controversial. This is due, in part, to disagreements regarding the reliability of detecting atypical melanocytes in frozen sections. The use of special stains, such as HMB45, mel-5, melan-A and S100, may increase histologic sensitivity during Mohs surgery for melanocytic lesions[15]. Some dermatologic surgeons advocate the use of formalin-fixed final margins to confirm that the final Mohs surgery margin is negative[16].

Another controversial aspect of Mohs surgery for melanoma involves the advisability of margins that are narrower than published guidelines for a tumor that has a higher capacity to metastasize than BCC and SCC. Although uncontrolled, the extensive experience of Zitelli et al. in the management of melanoma with Mohs surgery provides reassurance that outcomes are equivalent to standard margins[17,18]. While many clinicians do not find significant benefits to Mohs surgery for routine management of melanoma (e.g. most tumors, with the exception of lentigo maligna, are well defined), specific clinical scenarios appear especially appropriate for utilization of Mohs surgery. These include: locally recurrent melanoma; tumors with a large diameter; ill-defined or amelanotic melanoma; and melanoma near critical anatomic structures such as the genitals, digits, eyelids, nose and ears. Of note, many dermatologic surgeons remove a clinically tumor-free margin of at least 5 mm when managing melanoma, a technique termed 'wide Mohs'. Mapped serial sections and the 'square method' are modifications based upon similar histologic principles that attempt to achieve complete margin control with paraffin-embedded pathology only[19,20].

LONG-TERM CURE RATES FOR PRIMARY BCC AND SCC BY TREATMENT MODALITY

Treatment modality	Long-term (5-year) cure rates	
	BCC (%)	SCC (%)
Surgical excision	90	92
Electrodessication & curettage	92	96
Radiation	91	90
Cryotherapy	92	N/A
All non-Mohs modalities	91	92
Mohs surgery	99	97

Table 150.4 Long-term cure rates for primary basal cell carcinoma (BCC) and squamous cell carcinoma (SCC) by treatment modality. Based upon Rowe DE, Carroll RJ, Day CL. Long-term recurrence rates in previously untreated (primary) basal cell carcinoma – implications for patient follow-up. J Dermatol Surg Oncol. 1989;15:315–28 and Rowe DE, Carroll RJ, Day CL Jr. Prognostic factors for local recurrence, metastasis, and survival rates in squamous cell carcinoma of the skin, ear, and lip: implications for treatment modality selection. J Am Acad Dermatol. 1992;26:976–90, with permission from the American Academy of Dermatology, Inc.

Lentigo Maligna

Since lentigo maligna (melanoma *in situ* of sun-damaged skin) may be a clinically ill-defined tumor, it has a high local recurrence rate with standard wide-excisional surgery. Although frozen section histology of lentigo maligna can be challenging, Mohs surgery offers the possibility of complete margin examination and tissue sparing. Lentigo maligna that is at risk of recurrence or in an anatomically sensitive site may be managed with wide Mohs surgery followed by tangential permanent histologic confirmation, with immunostains as needed[15,16]. This dual method employs the advantages of both Mohs surgery and permanent histology, albeit with the disadvantage of delayed closure for complex cases. Some groups also use frozen section immunostains to enhance diagnostic accuracy[15].

Atypical Fibroxanthoma

Atypical fibroxanthoma (AFX) typically presents as an ulcerated nodule within the sun-damaged skin of the head and neck region in an elderly person. Histologically, AFX is composed of spindle cells mixed with bizarre, multinucleated giant cells. It generally grows in a contiguous fashion. Mohs surgery has demonstrated utility in the management of AFX, especially in areas of cosmetic importance[21].

Dermatofibrosarcoma Protuberans

Dermatofibrosarcoma protuberans (DFSP) is an uncommon, slow-growing, locally aggressive soft tissue sarcoma that most often arises on the trunk of young to middle-aged adults. DFSP typically invades beyond clinically visible tumor margins with unpredictable and irregular extensions. Recurrence rates after standard excision range from 11% to 53%. Mohs surgery is ideally suited to track the irregular tumor extensions of DFSP, and offers a cure rate of up to 98.4%[22]. Removal of DFSP with Mohs surgery can be time consuming and can require numerous tissue sections. Some physicians have proposed a modified 'slow Mohs' technique, in which 100% of the tissue margin is examined with tangential permanent histologic sections in tumors with unpredictable margins. This technique has the advantage of higher-quality permanent pathology sections, but the disadvantages of less precise tissue control and potentially incomplete margin examination. Additionally, each tissue resection is delayed by 24–48 hours for tissue processing. CD34 immunostain can be utilized on frozen or permanent sections to aid in tumor mapping.

Microcystic Adnexal Carcinoma

Microcystic adnexal carcinoma (MAC) is an uncommon, locally aggressive tumor that typically involves the face of older adults. Histologically, the cells demonstrate eccrine differentiation and often have an infiltrative growth pattern with frequent perineural invasion. In the literature, the overall recurrence rate for MAC approaches 40%. To date, Mohs surgery appears to offer the highest cure rate while permitting tissue sparing[23]. A study by Chiller et al.[24] demonstrated that defects following Mohs surgery were four times larger than clinical estimates. They concluded that preoperative estimation of margins is generally unreliable, and complete histologic verification of clear margins is advisable. Because MAC appears in elderly patients, and appreciating the propensity for extensive subclinical spread, preoperative scouting biopsies of clinically normal skin at multiple sites around the primary tumor can be helpful in delineating the potential extent of surgery. In cases in which resection of MAC would be considered mutilating in an elderly patient, a strategy of observation can be considered.

Sebaceous Carcinoma

The use of Mohs surgery for management of sebaceous carcinoma has also been debated, primarily due to reports of discontiguous growth. However, discontiguous growth will thwart any method of histologic margin evaluation. The desire for tissue conservation on the eyelid (the most common site of sebaceous carcinoma) makes Mohs surgery a logical approach. The removal of an extra safety margin of tissue for permanent sections may be a reasonable strategy with this type of tumor. The advantages of Mohs surgery for sebaceous cell carcinoma

of the eyelid have been documented in a study showing an 11.1% recurrence rate with Mohs surgery, as compared to 30% with standard excision[25].

Other Tumors and Uses

Mohs surgery has been used to treat a number of other malignant neoplasms, including Merkel cell carcinoma[26], extramammary Paget's disease[27], angiosarcoma, lymphoepithelioma-like carcinoma, mucinous eccrine carcinoma, eccrine porocarcinoma, adenoid cystic carcinoma, papillary eccrine carcinoma, and leiomyosarcoma[28], as well as benign tumors that tend to recur, such as infantile digital fibroma and granular cell tumor. The experience with these rare neoplasms is limited, but the complete margin examination of Mohs surgery may provide enhanced tumor clearance. Mohs surgery has also been used to extirpate difficult-to-treat cutaneous fungal infections.

Contraindications

As mentioned previously, discontiguous tumors can create problems with false-negative margins, but this problem also occurs with all other methods of evaluating surgical margins histologically, and therefore it is not an absolute contraindication (Table 150.5). If a tumor cannot be reliably identified histologically, especially on frozen sections, this can also be a relative contraindication. For example, some examples of lentigo maligna can be difficult to identify as compared to the melanocytic hyperplasia found in adjacent sun-damaged skin uninvolved by malignancy. Also, spindle cell neoplasms can be difficult to distinguish from fibrosis. If patients are unwilling or unable to undergo surgery, including those patients with serious medical problems, then a non-surgical approach such as radiotherapy may be a better option. However, for some patients with serious medical problems, Mohs surgery done under local anesthesia may be safer than more extensive anesthesia and surgery in a hospital operating room facility.

Preoperative History and Considerations

A directed history and physical examination should be performed at the time of consultation (Table 150.6). Indications for antibiotic prophylaxis should be evaluated and then reviewed with the patient's primary physician if necessary (Table 150.7)[29]. Similarly, the management of any implanted cardiac pacemakers and defibrillators should be considered, with cardiology consultation if needed (see Ch. 151). Finally, the management of blood thinners, including warfarin, aspirin and non-steroidal anti-inflammatory drugs (NSAIDs), should be discussed (Table 150.8)[30].

Once the medical evaluation has been completed, the dermatologic surgeon should explain the nature of the tumor and the therapeutic options and obtain informed consent. The risks, benefits and alternatives should be fully explained. The repair options should briefly be described. The patient should be encouraged to continue regular medications and eat a light meal on the morning of surgery, unless conscious sedation is planned. It is recommended that patients bring a friend or spouse with them on the day of surgery.

Patients with extremely large or invasive tumors may require preoperative evaluation with a CT scan, MRI, PET scan or other laboratory testing. A multidisciplinary approach may be useful with these patients. Very complex patients requiring a multidisciplinary approach should be evaluated preoperatively by otorhinolaryngology, oculoplastic, plastic surgery or neurosurgery colleagues as needed. Intraoperatively, the Mohs surgeon can perform tissue resection with margin control, while the repair can be coordinated by the appropriate specialist. The team approach is especially useful in areas such as the periorbital area,

---

CONTRAINDICATIONS TO MOHS SURGERY

- Discontiguous tumor growth
- Tumor undiagnosable on frozen section pathology
- Inability of the patient to tolerate surgery

Table 150.5 Contraindications to Mohs surgery.

PREOPERATIVE CONSIDERATIONS FOR MOHS SURGERY

Medical history

- History of previous skin cancers and treatments
- Cardiac, pulmonary, hepatic and renal disease
- Infectious diseases, including hepatitis and HIV
- Bleeding disorders
- Diabetes mellitus
- Hypertension

History of exposure to

- Ionizing radiation (e.g. acne treatments)
- Ultraviolet light
- Arsenic

Physical examination

- Full skin examination (if not already performed)
- Lymph node examination, if indicated
- Cardiac, pulmonary, and pharyngeal examination (if sedation planned)

Laboratory tests

- Prothrombin time/INR (if patient is on warfarin therapy)
- ECG, chest X-ray, and other radiologic or laboratory studies (if warranted)

Other considerations

- Medications – including warfarin, aspirin, NSAIDs, vitamin E supplementation, herbal remedies (e.g. *Ginkgo biloba*, garlic), other blood thinners. Continue if medically indicated; discontinue if not medically necessary
- Allergies
- Determine if antibiotic prophylaxis is indicated (see Table 150.7)
- Discontinue alcohol 72 hours prior to surgery
- Discontinue tobacco use 1 week prior to surgery if complex repair planned
- Pacemaker/defibrillator management per cardiology
- Explanation of nature of tumor and therapeutic options
- Obtain informed consent and explain the risks, benefits and alternatives of the procedure
- Inform the patient of the estimated duration of surgery
- Review repair options and consider the need for other specialists (e.g. ophthalmology, otolaryngology, neurosurgery or plastic surgery)
- Encourage a light breakfast and routine medications, unless conscious sedation is planned
- Measure and photograph the tumor
- Review pathology report and/or glass slides from skin biopsy

Table 150.6 Preoperative considerations for Mohs surgery.

---

external auditory canal, and in cases involving large, deep tumors such as DFSP.

Mohs surgery is most commonly performed under local anesthesia. Conscious sedation may be an option for managing patients with many tumors who wish to be treated in one session (see Ch. 143).

DESCRIPTION OF TECHNIQUE

Upon arrival, the patient's demographic information is confirmed and a directed medical history and vital signs are recorded. It is wise to review the preoperative biopsy prior to Mohs surgery. For relatively shallow tumors or those at sites favorable for second intention healing, the first Mohs stage ('layer') is planned as a shallow excision. In contrast, for deep tumors or at sites where second intention healing is not a good option, a full-thickness excision to subcutaneous fat is planned for the first Mohs stage.

The sequence of tumor removal is demonstrated in Figure 150.2. The tumor is closely examined with bright illumination, and the clinical margin is marked with ink, such as a gentian violet marker. References to diagrams and photographs are made to ensure correct site identification. Every patient is asked to confirm the tumor location with a mirror. Any prophylactic antibiotic, antianxiety drug or cardiac device management is either administered or performed as indicated during the preoperative period. The planned procedure and possible reconstruction are reviewed and consent is obtained.

The site is then wiped with alcohol, and local anesthetic, usually 1% lidocaine with 1:100 000 epinephrine, is injected to achieve complete

---

GUIDELINES FOR ANTIBIOTIC PROPHYLAXIS FOR THE PREVENTION OF ENDOCARDITIS AND PROSTHESIS INFECTION DURING MOHS SURGERY

Prophylaxis may be given*

High-risk cardiac conditions

- Prosthetic valve
- History of bacterial endocarditis
- Complex cyanotic congenital heart disease[†]
- Surgically constructed systemic–pulmonary shunts or conduits

Moderate-risk cardiac conditions

- Most other cardiac malformations
- Mitral valve prolapse with regurgitation or without regurgitation in men >45 years old
- Any hemodynamically significant valvular dysfunction
- Hypertrophic cardiomyopathy

Other moderate-risk conditions

- Total joint replacement – first 2 years following surgery, previous prosthetic joint infection, or immunocompromised patient
- Shunt/fistula with nearby inflamed/infected tissue

Prophylaxis is not usually given

Negligible-risk cardiac conditions

- History of rheumatic fever without valve dysfunction
- Post coronary artery bypass grafting
- Pacemaker or defibrillator
- Physiologic, functional or innocent murmur
- Mitral valve prolapse without regurgitation (except in men >45 years old)
- Secundum atrial septal defect
- Greater than 6 months status post repair of atrial septal defect, ventricular septal defect, patent ductus arteriosus

Other low-risk conditions

- Dialysis catheters, vascular grafts (without nearby inflamed/infected tissue)[‡]
- Ventriculoperitoneal shunts (without nearby inflamed/infected tissue)
- Orthopedic hardware (e.g. pins, plates, screws), total joint replacement > 2 years previously without complicating factors (see above)
- Penile prostheses
- Breast implants

Antibiotic regimen – single dose given 30–60 minutes before surgery

- Non-oral site:
  Cephalexin 2 g po
  If penicillin allergic: clindamycin 600 mg po, azithromycin 500 mg po, or clarithromycin 500 mg po
- Oral site:
  Amoxicillin 2 g po
  If penicillin allergic: as for non-oral site (see above) or cephalexin 2 g po (if no history of type 1 hypersensitivity reaction)

The American Heart Association recommends endocarditis prophylaxis for procedures involving oral, respiratory, gastrointestinal or genitourinary mucosa in patients with medium- or high-risk cardiac conditions; they do not recommend endocarditis prophylaxis for incision or biopsy of surgically scrubbed non-infected skin, regardless of cardiac risk factors (Dajani AS, Taubert KA, Wilson W, et al. JAMA. 1997;277:1794–801).
[†]*Including single ventricle states, transposition of the great arteries, tetralogy of Fallot.*
[‡]*Risk may be higher in the first 6–12 months after graft placement.*

Table 150.7 Guidelines for antibiotic prophylaxis for the prevention of endocarditis and prosthesis infection during Mohs surgery. Note that indications for non-Mohs excisional surgery may be different (see Ch. 151).

MANAGEMENT OF BLOOD THINNERS DURING MOHS SURGERY

- Warfarin is generally continued, keeping INR in therapeutic range
- Aspirin is usually continued if medically necessary (history of thrombotic event or coronary artery disease)
- Agents not medically necessary (for headache, pain, prevention) discontinued 10–14 days (aspirin) or 3 days (NSAIDs) prior to surgery

Table 150.8 Management of blood thinners during Mohs surgery.

---

local anesthesia. Variations on local anesthesia include diluting the epinephrine to 1:200 000 to decrease the risk of tachycardia or adding bupivacaine to extend the duration of anesthesia (see Ch. 143). Next, the site and ample surrounding tissue is prepared in a sterile manner with chlorhexidine or povidone-iodine, and then draped. The central portion of the tumor is often debulked with a curette prior to Mohs

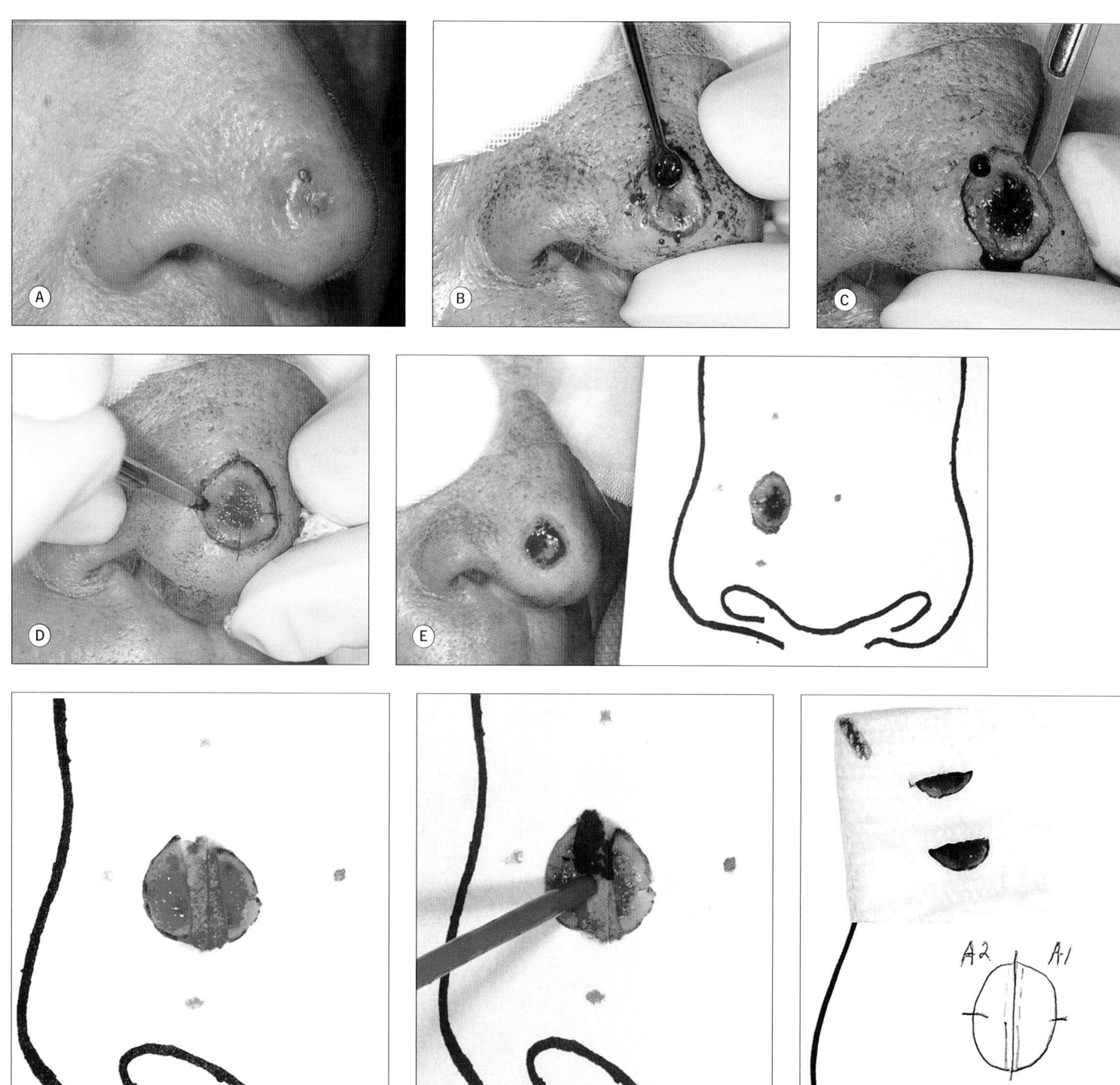

Fig. 150.2 Mohs micrographic surgery technique. A Preoperative appearance of a basal cell carcinoma on the nose. **B** Debulking of the tumor via curettage. **C** Beveled excision (with scalpel at a 45° angle) of all clinically evident tumor plus a small margin of normal-appearing skin. **D** Placement of hash marks at 3, 6, 9 and 12 o'clock positions in adjacent surrounding tissue. **E** Orientation of the excised specimen on an anatomic card. **F** Specimen sectioned into two pieces and flattened. **G** Marking of the cut margins of the specimen with red and blue inks. **H** Matching Mohs map and tissue specimen ready for histologic preparation. A red mark on the gauze denotes the location of the first specimen with the second specimen always placed below. Different systems are used but precision is common to all.

Continued

excision, as a means of further defining subclinical tumor extension. Conservative curettage may also avoid unnecessary removal of unaffected tissue[31]. Sometimes, deeper tumors are debulked by excision with a scalpel prior to the first Mohs excision.

The first micrographic layer includes all clinically evident tumor plus a small margin of normal-appearing tissue. Depending on the histologic subtype and likelihood of subclinical tumor extensions, the margin of normal skin may range from 1 to 10 mm. Narrow margins are also taken in areas where tissue sparing is essential. When confronted by recurrent tumor, the most thorough approach is to resect all tissue involved by the previous treatments, including the primary site and

reconstruction scar. If the recurrence is clearly isolated to one site only, and if complete resection would cause problems, then a localized resection of the clinically recurrent area can be considered with caution.

When excising the Mohs layer, special care should be taken to incise beyond the previously curetted edge. The scalpel is held at a 30–90° angle away from the tumor in order to create a beveled incision. Subsequent incisions are beveled progressively more, so that the incisions under the center of the specimen are horizontal. Before the specimen is completely removed, both the tissue to be removed and the adjacent surrounding tissue are marked with a shallow scalpel cut, or hash

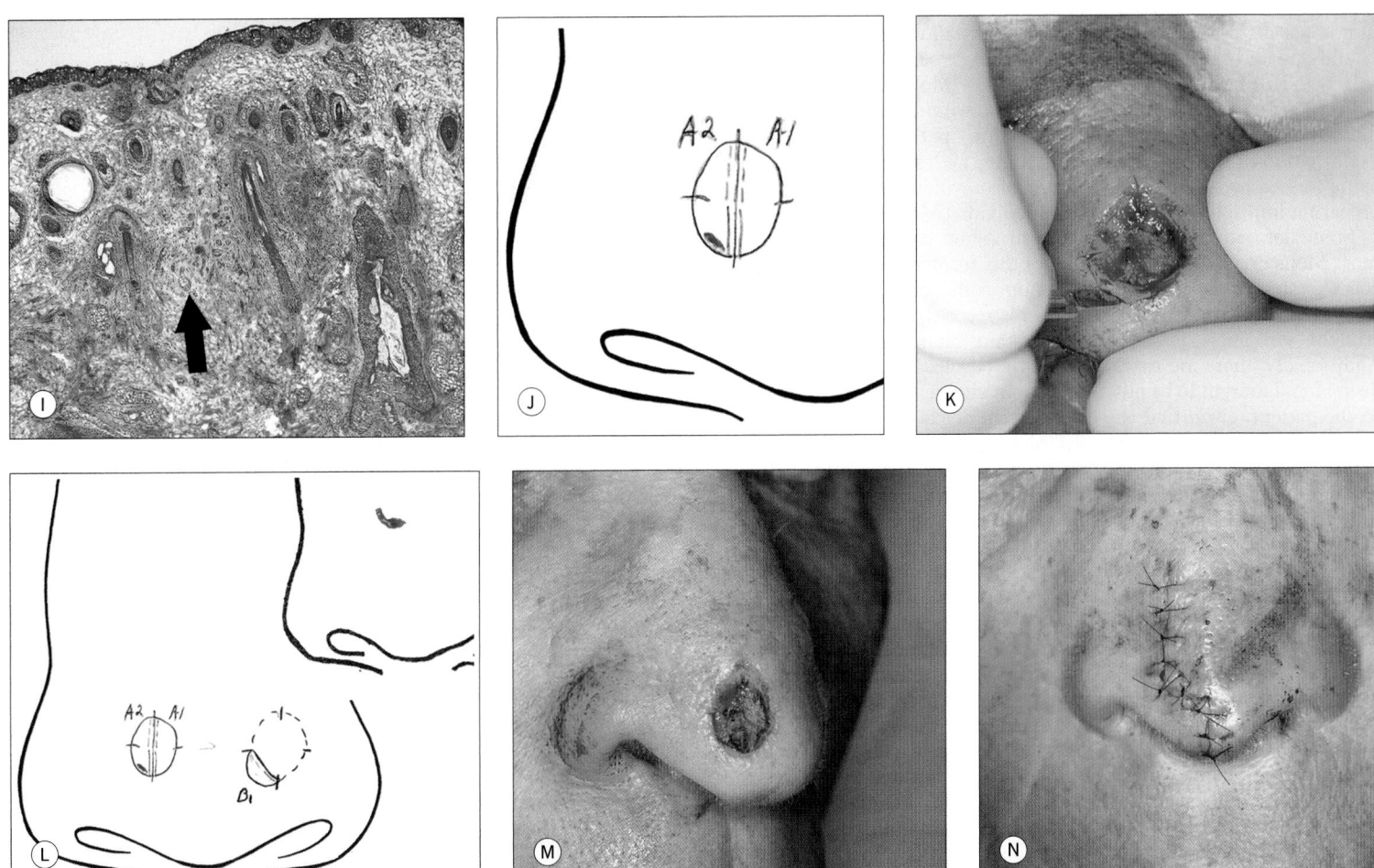

Fig. 150.2, cont'd Mohs micrographic surgery technique. I Histopathologic section with positive tumor denoted by the arrow. **J** Mohs map marked with purple at the site of cancer at the margin. **K** Re-excision of the area of residual basal cell carcinoma. **L** Mohs map from the second layer with corresponding tissue. **M, N** Postoperative tumor-free defect and repair.

mark. Hash marks, sometimes called hatch marks, are commonly placed in the incision margins at 12, 3, 6 and 9 o'clock positions for small specimens, and at locations of planned tissue sectioning for larger specimens. The hash marks are used for orientation of the specimen, both on the patient and histologically. Two hash marks may be useful at the 12 o'clock position in locations with few anatomic landmarks, such as acral and scalp skin, to avoid confusion over orientation.

Once the hash marks are in place, the tissue is removed with either a scalpel or iris scissors. At this point, it is critical that the tissue be placed in the correct orientation as it is lowered onto an anatomic transfer card or marked gauze. We utilize blotter paper cards with outlines of anatomic sites to ensure correct orientation during transfer and processing of tissue. Hemostasis is then obtained using electrofulguration. A sterile pressure dressing is placed on the wound, and the patient may go to a waiting room for 20–45 minutes while the tissue is being processed. Large specimens, such as DFSP or lentigo maligna, may require more than 1 hour to process.

Once the tissue specimen has been excised, a depiction of the surgical defect is drawn on a preprinted anatomic map. The hash marks, which have previously been placed on the tissue, aid in orientation and are marked on the map. The specimen is then cut precisely into sections of sufficient size so that they can fit on a microscope slide and a cryostat chuck. All sectioning is done through hash marks and is recorded on the map. If the specimen is small, it may be submitted as one piece, although commonly two to four pieces are created. Obsessive attention must be paid to maintaining proper orientation of all sections during processing.

After the tissue is sectioned, downward pressure is placed on the edges of the beveled tissue in order to flatten it such that epidermis, dermis and fat all lie parallel against the blotter card in a horizontal plane; as a result, the histologic sections contain the total tissue margin. This is a unique and critical step in Mohs surgery tissue preparation. All cut margins, except the epidermal edges, are marked with two or more colored inks and the colors are noted on the micrographic map. If any epidermal edges curve upward, several partial-thickness relaxing cuts can be placed in the central, tumor-bearing portion of the tissue. The pieces are then numbered on the micrographic map, consecutively placed in a Petri dish with moist gauze, and carried to the laboratory, which is within the operative suite. A mark noting the specific orientation of the specimens in the Petri dish is made on the gauze.

The histotechnician then begins processing by inverting the specimen (deep surface upward), pressing it flat, and then embedding it on a chuck in an embedding medium. Frozen sections are then cut, mounted on slides, and stained with H&E. Most practices utilize a linear automatic stainer for this purpose. Some Mohs surgeons prefer the toluidine blue stain, because it is rapid and the purplish metachromatic stromal staining helps to distinguish BCCs from adnexal structures. High-quality preparation of frozen histologic sections is paramount to the successful practice of Mohs surgery[32]. The sections are then examined histologically by the surgeon, and, if there is residual tumor, the area is marked accordingly on the map. In cases requiring further resection, the surgeon then precisely removes additional tissue only in the area of residual tumor, using the map and hash marks present on the patient for orientation. This process is repeated until all tissue margins are free of tumor. As with the initial layer, the width of the margin removed on subsequent layers can be varied, depending on the aggressiveness of the histology and need for tissue sparing. Once the tumor is completely removed, the final defect is measured and photographed. At this point, repair options can be discussed.

VARIATIONS/UNUSUAL SITUATIONS

The single section method for tissue processing of smaller tumors was described by Randle et al.[33]. The single section method involves a highly beveled specimen processed with relaxing incisions on the superior, tumor-bearing portion of the specimen that allow all peripheral edges to fold outward into a single plane. The single section method is particularly useful for tumors in which a shallow Mohs layer can be taken, with the goal of allowing the resulting wound to heal by second intention. Additionally, the single section method allows unaltered examination of the complete deep margin, with no possibility of areas being missed by tissue subdivision. It also avoids the time involved in preparing multiple sections from a subdivided Mohs layer.

Some dermatologic surgeons perform a non-beveled 90° incision for most Mohs excisions. An advantage of this technique is that the vertical edges created are ideal for reconstruction. Although a traditional beveled edge can be trimmed in preparation for reconstruction, a true, sharp, straight 90° angle is difficult to obtain after resection of tissue. Additionally, there are cases in which a beveled incision may cause a deep lateral margin to be positive without true tissue-sparing advantage to the patient, given that the deep dermal defect will be narrower and potentially tumor-bearing. The 90° Mohs incisions do necessitate more extensive manipulation during tissue preparation, principally by creation of relaxing incisions in the upper portion of the specimen, in order to induce the tissue to flatten into a single plane. Debulking of tumor to adipose prior to the Mohs layer also makes it easier to get the Mohs layer to flatten. With practice, flat specimens are easily and readily obtainable with 90° Mohs incisions, with the advantages mentioned above.

Wide Mohs surgery is a modification of traditional Mohs surgery in which a larger, clinically tumor-free margin is taken either before or after Mohs histologic margin evaluation. This is performed on tumors that have a high propensity for recurrence or metastases, particularly melanoma and cutaneous sarcomas[17]. In utilizing wide Mohs margins, the surgeon is actively deciding to prioritize optimal cure rates over tissue sparing for high-risk tumors. Wide Mohs margins of 5–20 mm can be taken with high-risk tumors, while maintaining the advantages of 100% margin examination, in cases where tissue sparing is a lower priority.

When confronted with frozen pathology that may be challenging, particularly with lentigo maligna and DFSP, some Mohs surgeons elect to complement a complete frozen section Mohs removal of the tumor with a final delayed permanent histologic section. Permanent margin confirmation is utilized in a small minority of Mohs cases in which frozen histology may be less than ideal. This dual frozen–permanent technique utilizes the advantages of each processing method, and permits the addition of immunostains as needed (Fig. 150.3). Obviously, the dual technique comes with the inconvenience of having to delay reconstruction while awaiting permanent section results. The use of microwave fixation for the rapid preparation of permanent sections is being actively explored as a way to optimize final histology, while avoiding the need for delayed reconstruction.

Frozen section immunohistochemistry has been increasingly utilized for high-risk tumors in conjunction with Mohs surgery[15]. With this technique, alternate tissue sections are processed with H&E and rapid immunostains. Commonly used immunostains include cytokeratin stains for SCC, melan-A for melanoma and lentigo maligna, MNF116 for BCC, and CD34 for DFSP. Unfortunately, none of these immunostains are completely sensitive and specific, but they can prove helpful in selected cases.

POSTOPERATIVE CARE

Multiple options exist for management of tissue defects after tumor clearance with Mohs surgery. The management strategy will take into account anatomic location, patient comorbidities, likelihood of surgery in the future, severity of the tumor, and the aesthetic needs of the patient. With experienced guidance from the dermatologic surgeon skilled in cutaneous reconstructive techniques, patients are able to select the best options for their situation.

Allowing surgical defects to heal by second intention may result in excellent cosmetic results in areas that are concave, as demonstrated by the experience of Dr Mohs and others[34]. Second intention healing can also be used for recurrent tumors in which flaps or grafts might hinder surveillance of the treatment site. Second intention healing requires patient commitment in the form of wound care. Patients must be willing to meticulously cleanse the area over a 2- to 8-week healing

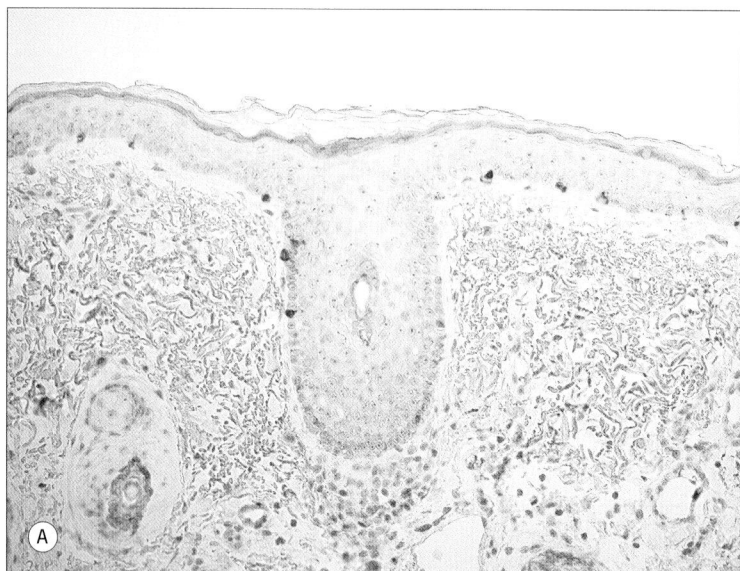

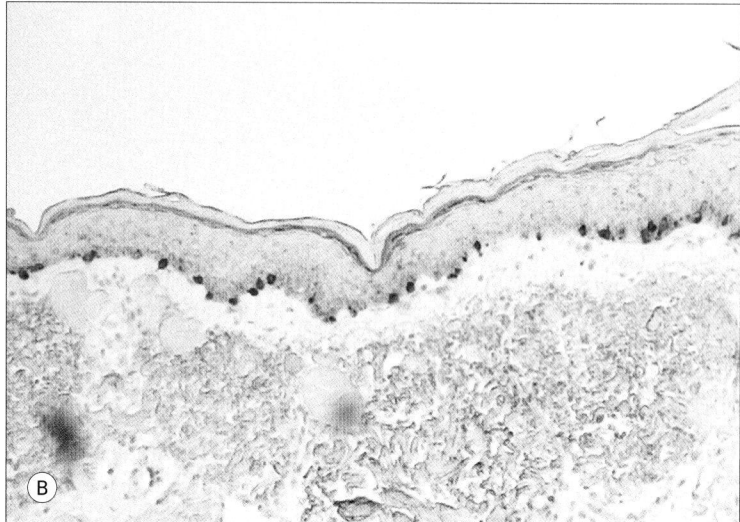

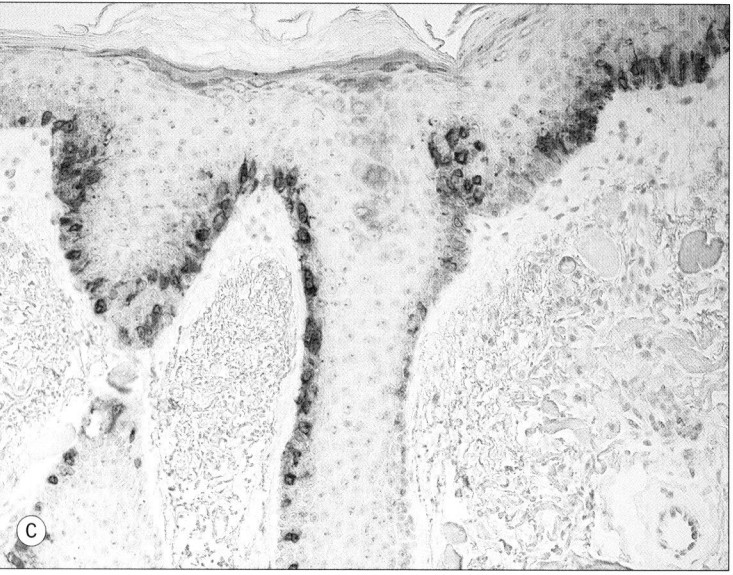

Fig. 150.3 Immunostaining with melan-A. A Normal density of melanocytes. **B** Melanocytic hyperplasia with scattered atypical melanocytes in sun-damaged skin. **C** Lentigo maligna with atypical melanocytic hyperplasia, some pagetoid spread, and adnexal extension.

period. Typically, wound care regimens involve cleansing the wound twice daily with a saline solution or soapy water, applying a layer of ointment (either petroleum jelly or antibiotic ointment), and then covering with a non-adherent dressing. Because of the prolonged time associated with second intention healing, and because wounds on areas other than concavities may heal with unsightly scars, the majority of Mohs surgery defects are closed immediately, either with primary layered closure or with local skin flaps and grafts. Wound care after cutaneous reconstruction is similar to second intention wound care, although limited to 1–2 weeks. A discussion of cutaneous reconstruction can be found in other chapters of this text.

Antibiotics may be given postoperatively for wound infection prophylaxis if surgery is extensive, particularly for procedures involving multiple layers and subsequent reconstruction[29]. Additionally, surgical reconstruction on highly sebaceous noses and other sites with significantly high bacterial colonization may require prophylactic antibiotics. Pain control is assessed on a case-by-case basis. Substantial pain following Mohs surgery is uncommon, and, usually, acetaminophen is sufficient for postoperative discomfort. If warranted, oral narcotic analgesics may be prescribed for patients with low pain thresholds, large tumors, complex reconstruction, or wounds in anatomic locations of high tension.

Ongoing surveillance at least annually for new primary and recurrent cancer is recommended for all patients, given that 50% of patients with non-melanoma skin cancer will experience another skin cancer during the next 5 years. For many patients with susceptible phenotypes, annual surveillance with treatment of precancerous actinic keratoses is advised.

COMPLICATIONS

Fortunately, complications from Mohs surgery are uncommon. Intraoperative considerations include anxiety, pain (with local anesthesia injection), bleeding, nerve damage and allergic reactions. Anxiety should be assessed before surgery begins, and the patient should be directly questioned as to their perceptions of anxiety. If warranted, oral midazolam syrup can be given in the range of 5–15 mg orally for healthy adults. Many patients experience pain when lidocaine is injected into the skin. Using a small-bore needle, pinching the skin, and injecting slowly can minimize the pain. The addition of sodium bicarbonate can buffer the lidocaine mixture and lessen the pain of injection. Hemorrhage is a potential risk during surgery, which can be minimized with meticulous hemostasis and pressure bandaging. Epinephrine included in the local anesthetic may augment hemostasis. To date, there is no evidence that patients taking aspirin or warfarin for serious medical problems experience increased risks of hemorrhage or bleeding complications[30]. The most common site for major arterial transection is the superficial temporal artery, which can result in significant bleeding requiring suture ligation. Smaller bleeding sites are treated with electrocoagulation. Injury to cutaneous sensory nerves occurs during all cutaneous surgery. Transection of significant motor nerves is occasionally necessary for removal of deeply invasive tumors, especially in the temporal region. Whenever possible, the surgeon should inform the patient before surgery of any possible loss of function or sensation. Before beginning surgery, the patient should be thoroughly questioned regarding allergies. Considerations include past reactions to local anesthetics, antibiotics, iodine, latex and tape products. Fortunately, lidocaine allergy is rare, but the surgeon should be prepared for an emergency response if necessary.

After Mohs surgery is completed, potential complications include postoperative bleeding, hematoma/seroma formation, infection, necrosis, dehiscence and scarring (see Ch. 151). Postoperative bleeding is usually easily controlled with a pressure bandage. Hematomas and seromas are an uncommon complication following reconstruction. These complications can be reduced by meticulous hemostasis during surgery, pressure dressings, and proper postoperative wound care by the patient. Infection risk should be assessed before and after surgery. The rate of clinically significant infection after Mohs surgery is very low (0.7%)[35]. Antibiotics should be considered for reconstructed sites on sebaceous noses and for defects requiring multiple Mohs layers for tumor clearance. Antibiotics should also be considered for any debilitated patient when proper wound care is a concern.

Necrosis and scarring are potential risks after any surgery. Necrosis can occur after a wound is closed under tension, or in association with an improperly designed flap with insufficient vascular supply. In the preoperative period, the likelihood and type of postsurgical scar should be assessed and discussed with patients when deciding on reconstructive options. All cutaneous surgery involving removal of tissue into the deep papillary and reticular dermis results in scarring to a degree. Various reconstruction options are available to minimize scarring, and they can be performed immediately after tumor clearance with Mohs surgery. Functional defects resulting from soft tissue removal can be restored with reconstructive techniques as well. Other potential pitfalls associated with suboptimal performance of Mohs surgery may result from lack of attention to detail, incorrect interpretation of histopathology (Fig. 150.4), and lack of appreciation of aggressive tumor characteristics (Table 150.9)[36,37].

FUTURE TRENDS

The history of Mohs surgery is one of continuous innovation and improvement. Given increases in the incidence of skin cancers, the demand for Mohs surgery services will continue to rise. Preoperative tumor definition with confocal scanning laser microscopy is being explored to assist in efficient removal of tumors[38]. Digital technology has been applied to Mohs surgery, enabling telepathology confirmation[39]. Finally, the use of newer immunostains on either frozen or microwave-processed tissue continues to enhance the diagnostic sensitivity and specificity of pathologic examination. These and other innovations promise to bolster the status of Mohs surgery as the gold standard for removal of cutaneous tumors[40,41].

POTENTIAL PITFALLS OF MOHS SURGERY

• Excisional errors
  – Misorientation of tissue
  – Errors in mapping or orientation
• Histology laboratory errors
  – Processing artifacts
  – Incomplete tissue sections
  – Errors in labeling
• Pathology errors
  – Undiagnosed tumor (e.g. inflammation obscuring tumor, perineural invasion)
  – Overdiagnosed tumor (e.g. tangentially sectioned hair follicles)
• Failure to consider discontiguity or the need for adjuvant therapy

Table 150.9 Potential pitfalls of Mohs surgery.

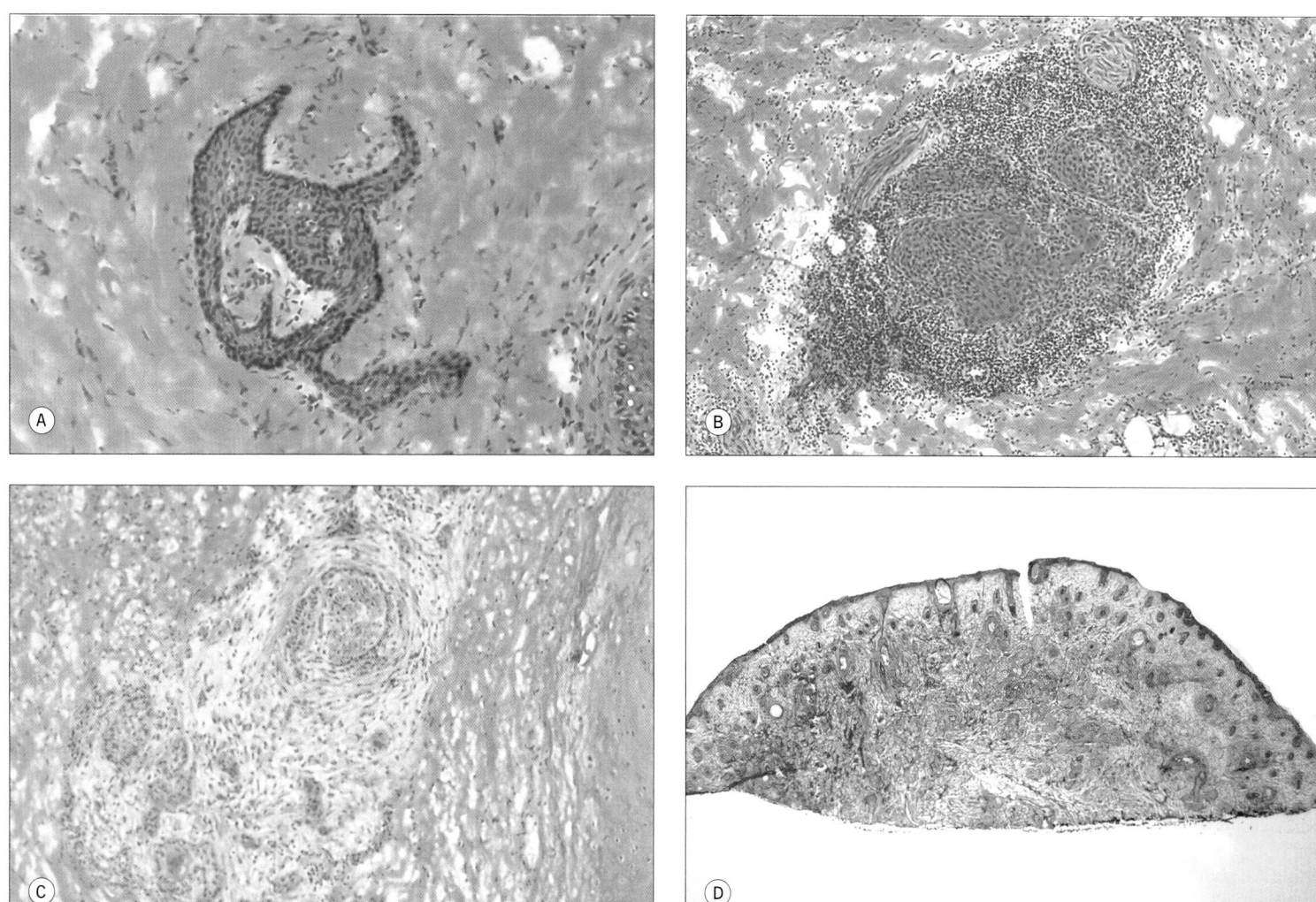

Fig. 150.4 Histologic challenges in Mohs surgery. A Folliculocentric basaloid hyperplasia may mimic basal cell carcinoma; however, the lack of clefting adjacent to the cells, apoptosis or mitotic figures as well as the presence of a fibrous sheath permits distinction. **B** Dense inflammation can obscure tumor cells, as seen here with a squamous cell carcinoma in a patient with chronic lymphocytic leukemia. **C** Careful evaluation is required to identify subtle foci of perineural squamous cell carcinoma. **D** Incomplete histologic margins (e.g. due to a small portion of missing epidermis) can lead to false-negative readings.

REFERENCES

1. Martinez JC, Otley CC. The management of melanoma and non-melanoma skin cancer: a review for the primary care physician. Mayo Clin Proc. 2001;76:1253–65.
2. Thissen MR, Neumann MH, Schouten LJ. A systematic review of treatment modalities for primary basal cell carcinomas. Arch Dermatol. 1999;135:1177–83.
3. Rowe DE, Carroll RJ, Day CL. Long-term recurrence rates in previously untreated (primary) basal cell carcinoma – implications for patient follow-up. J Dermatol Surg Oncol. 1989;15:315–28.
4. Ghauri RR, Gunter AA, Weber RA. Frozen section analysis in the management of skin cancers. Ann Plast Surg. 1999;43:156–60.
5. Smeets NWJ, Krekels GAM, Ostertag JU, et al. Surgical excision vs Mohs micrographic surgery for basal-cell carcinoma of the face: randomized controlled trial. Lancet. 2004;364:1766–72.
6. Otley CC. Mohs' micrographic surgery for basal-cell carcinoma of the face. Lancet. 2005;365:1226–7
7. Mohs FE. Chemosurgery: a microscopically controlled method of cancer excision. Arch Surg. 1941;42:279–95.
8. Tromovitch TA, Stegman SJ. Microscopically controlled excision of skin tumors: chemosurgery (Mohs) fresh tissue technique. Arch Dermatol. 1974;110:231–2.
9. Drake LA, Dinehart SM, Goltz RW, et al. Guidelines of care for Mohs micrographic surgery. J Am Acad Dermatol. 1995;33:271–8.
10. Rowe DE, Carroll RJ, Day CL Jr. Prognostic factors for local recurrence, metastasis, and survival rates in squamous cell carcinoma of the skin, ear, and lip: implications for treatment modality selection. J Am Acad Dermatol. 1992;26:976–90.

11. Rowe DE, Carroll RJ, Day CL. Mohs surgery is the treatment of choice for recurrent (previously treated) basal cell carcinoma. J Dermatol Surg Oncol. 1989;15:424–31.
11a. Leibovitch I, Huilgol SC, Selva D, et al. Basal cell carcinoma treated with Mohs surgery in Australia I. Experience over 10 years. J Am Acad Dermatol. 2005;53:445–51.
11b. Leibovitch I, Huilgol SC, Selva D, et al. Basal cell carcinoma treated with Mohs surgery in Australia II. Outcome at 5-year follow-up. J Am Acad Dermatol. 2005;53:452–7.
12. Leibovitch I, Huilgol SC, Selva D, Richards S, Paver R. Basosquamous carcinoma: treatment with Mohs micrographic surgery. Cancer. 2005;104:170–5.
12a. Leibovitch I, Huilgol SC, Selva D, et al. Cutaneous squamous cell carcinoma treated with Mohs micrographic surgery in Australia I. Experience over 10 years. J Am Acad Dermatol. 2005;53:253–60.
12b. Leibovitch I, Huilgol SC, Selva D, et al. Cutaneous squamous cell carcinoma treated with Mohs micrographic surgery in Australia II. Perineural invasion. J Am Acad Dermatol. 2005;53:261–6.
13. Holmkvist KA, Roenigk RK. Squamous cell carcinoma of the lip treated with Mohs micrographic surgery: outcome at 5 years. J Am Acad Dermatol. 1998; 38:960–6.
14. Zaiac MN, Weiss E. Mohs micrographic surgery of the nail unit and squamous cell carcinoma. Dermatol Surg. 2001;27:246–51.
15. Zalla MJ, Lim KK, DiCaudo DJ, et al. Mohs micrographic excision of melanoma using immunostains. Dermatol Surg. 2000;26:771–84.

16. Cohen LM, McCall MW, Zax RH. Mohs micrographic surgery for lentigo maligna melanoma: a follow-up study. Dermatol Surg. 1998;24:673–7.
17. Zitelli JA, Brown C, Hanusa BH, et al. Mohs micrographic surgery for the treatment of primary cutaneous melanoma. J Am Acad Dermatol. 1997; 37:236–45.
18. Bricca GM, Brodland DG, Ren D, Zitelli JA. Cutaneous head and neck melanoma treated with Mohs micrographic surgery. J Am Acad Dermatol. 2005;52:92–100.
19. Huilgol SC, Selva D, Chen C, et al. Surgical margins for lentigo maligna melanoma: the technique of mapped serial excision. Arch Dermatol. 2004;140:1087–92.
20. Johnson TM, Headington JT, Baker SR, et al. Usefulness of the staged excision for lentigo maligna melanoma: the 'square' procedure. J Am Acad Dermatol. 1997; 37:758–64.
21. Davis JL, Randle HW, Zalla MJ, et al. A comparison of Mohs micrographic surgery with wide excision for the treatment of atypical fibroxanthoma. Dermatol Surg. 1997;23:105–10.
22. Snow SN, Gordon EM, Larson PO, et al. Dermatofibrosarcoma protuberans: a report on 29 patients treated with Mohs micrographic surgery with long-term follow-up and review of the literature. Cancer. 2004;101:28–38.
23. Leibovitch I, Huilgol SC, Selva D, et al. Microcystic adnexal carcinoma: treatment with Mohs micrographic surgery. J Am Acad Dermatol. 2005;52:295–300.
24. Chiller K, Passaro D, Scheuller M, et al. Microcystic adnexal carcinoma: forty-eight cases, their treatment, and their outcome. Arch Dermatol. 2000;136:1355–9.

25. Spencer JM, Nossa R, Tse DT, et al. Sebaceous carcinoma of the eyelid treated with Mohs micrographic surgery. J Am Acad Dermatol. 2001;44:1004–9.

26. O'Connor WJ, Roenigk RK, Brodland DG. Merkel cell carcinoma: comparison of Mohs micrographic surgery and wide excision in eighty-six patients. Dermatol Surg. 1997;23:929–33.

27. O'Connor WJ, Lim KK, Zalla MJ, et al. Comparison of Mohs micrographic surgery and wide excision for extramammary Paget's disease. Dermatol Surg. 2003;29:723–7.

28. Bernstein SC, Roenigk RK. Leiomyosarcoma of the skin: treatment of 34 cases. Dermatol Surg. 1996;22:631–5.

29. Huang CC, Boyce S, Northington M, Desmond R, Soong SJ. Randomized controlled surgical trial of preoperative tumor curettage of basal cell carcinoma in Mohs micrographic surgery. J Am Acad Dermatol. 2004;51:585–91.

30. Maragh SL, Otley CC, Roenigk RK, Phillips PK. Antibiotic prophylaxis in dermatologic surgery: updated guidelines. Dermatol Surg. 2005;31:83–93.

31. Otley CC. Continuation of medically necessary aspirin and warfarin during cutaneous surgery. Mayo Clin Proc. 2003;78:1392–6.

32. Davis DA, Pellowski DM, Hanke CW. Preparation of frozen sections. Dermatol Surg. 2004;30:1479–85.

33. Randle HW, Zitelli J, Brodland DG, et al. Histologic preparation for Mohs micrographic surgery: the single section method. J Dermatol Surg Oncol. 1993;19:522–4.

34. Zitelli JA. Wound healing by first and second intention. In: Roenigk RK, Roenigk HH (eds). Dermatologic Surgery: Principles and Practice, 2nd edn. New York: Marcel Dekker, 1996:101–30.

35. Whitaker DC, Grande DJ, Johnson SS. Wound infection rate in dermatologic surgery. J Dermatol Surg. 1988;14:525–8.

36. Mehrany K, Weenig RH, Pittelkow MR, Roenigk RK, Otley CC. High recurrence rates of squamous cell carcinoma in patients with chronic lymphocytic leukemia. Dermatol Surg. 2005;31:38–42.

37. Mehrany AK, Weenig RH, Pittelkow MR, Roenigk RK, Otley CC. High recurrence rates of basal cell carcinoma after Mohs surgery in patients with chronic lymphocytic leukemia. Arch Dermatol. 2004;140:985–8.

38. Busam KJ, Hester K, Carlos C, et al. Detection of clinically amelanotic malignant melanoma and assessment of its margins by in vivo confocal scanning laser microscopy. Arch Dermatol. 2001;137:923–9.

39. Chandra S, Elliott T, Vinciullo C. Telepathology as an aid in Mohs micrographic surgery. Dermatol Surg. 2004;30:945–7.

40. Phillips PK, Roenigk RK. Statistics. In: Snow SN, Mikhail GR (eds). Mohs Micrographic Surgery, 2nd edn. Madison: University of Wisconsin Press, 2004: 414–20.

41. Gross KG, Steinman HK, Rapini RP. Mohs Surgery: Fundamentals and Techniques. St Louis: Mosby, 1999.

Surgical Complications and Optimizing Outcomes

151

Anna S Clayton and Thomas Stasko

Key features

- A thorough preoperative assessment of the patient is required to increase the chances for a successful outcome for any surgical procedure

- Attention to detail, selection of the simplest procedures that will produce the desired result, and meticulous intraoperative technique will prevent many complications

- Anticipation of avoidable complications and careful management of unavoidable ones optimize the results

- Clear communication between patient and surgeon must begin before the start of the procedure and continue through every stage, including the recovery and healing phases

- Many complications do not manifest until several days to months postoperatively; the patient must be monitored periodically to ensure that all parties are satisfied with the final outcome

INTRODUCTION

The verb 'to complicate' means to make or become intricate and/or difficult. Surgical complications are deviations from the original planned outcome, which usually occur as the result of a series of multiple inter-related events (Fig. 151.1)[1]. Because of the nature of cutaneous surgery, the unexpected can and does happen; however, with careful planning and meticulous attention to technique and detail, many potential complications can be avoided or minimized.

Complications can threaten the patient's life, the ability to heal, and the cosmetic appearance of the scar. Life-threatening emergencies in cutaneous surgery are rare, but the surgeon must be prepared to deal with such problems as cardiac arrhythmias and anaphylaxis. Proper, well-maintained equipment for resuscitation must be readily available. At a minimum, the staff should be trained in Basic Life Support. Physicians in offices where extensive cutaneous surgery is performed should also have training in Advanced Cardiac Life Support. A full discussion of this topic is beyond the scope of this chapter, but it is well covered in other sources[2,3].

The surgeon should conduct a thorough preoperative assessment of the patient, including history and directed physical examination, to identify pre-existing conditions that may affect the patient's ability to heal. Proper informed consent obtained at this time and again just prior to the procedure ensures that the patient is well educated about what to expect. This education may minimize future misunderstandings. An outcome that the patient perceives as unexpected may in reality be an expected outcome for the given procedure. A discussion of the possible risks prior to the procedure may avoid this confusion.

Prevention of an unsatisfactory outcome starts in the planning stage of the procedure, then continues with good intraoperative surgical technique and careful postoperative care. Anticipation of avoidable complications and management of unavoidable ones optimize the results. Throughout the process, it is essential to involve the patient in his or her own care.

DISCUSSION

Preoperative Assessment

A thorough preoperative assessment is an invaluable tool for identifying conditions that could lead to surgical complications. A simple one-page preoperative questionnaire can be completed by the patient – with help from the nurse, technician or physician, as needed – at the time of the initial evaluation. 'Yes' or 'no' answers to specific questions can indicate a need for further evaluation or for a change in operative procedure or plan (Fig. 151.2).

Potential for bleeding

Although some bleeding is an expected part of any surgical procedure, excessive bleeding is a common complication. The discovery of a bleeding disorder prior to surgery allows for an attempt to correct the condition if it is reversible, or postponing or changing plans for surgery if it is not. The bleeding disorder may be due to abnormalities in the *coagulation cascade* (inherited deficiencies in coagulation factors, as in hemophilia) or in the *platelet*, or a combination of the two[4]. Platelet problems can be subdivided into problems with *production* (leukemia, use of myelosuppressive drugs), problems with *survival* (disseminated intravascular coagulation, idiopathic thrombocytopenic purpura), or problems with *function* (drugs, Hermansky–Pudlak syndrome).

If there is no history indicative of a bleeding disorder, and the patient is otherwise well, laboratory testing is usually unnecessary; however, appropriate screening laboratory tests should be checked if there is a suspicion of a hereditary or acquired bleeding disorder. A platelet count as part of the CBC (complete blood count) identifies only a quantitative problem. The bleeding-time test measures platelet function, but it can be difficult to perform and interpret as the results are very much operator-dependent. An *in vitro* bleeding-time assay, the platelet function analyzer 100 (PFA-100), provides an easy method for rapidly assessing platelet function. Unlike the bleeding time, the PFA-100 can be performed on a collected blood specimen. It is useful in detecting platelet defects, most cases of von Willebrand disease, and the effects of aspirin and other antiplatelet agents[6,7]. Additional standard screening tests include a PT (prothrombin time) test, which can determine a defect in the extrinsic clotting pathway and an aPTT (activated partial thromboplastin time) test, which can determine a defect in the intrinsic pathway[8].

A review of medications and nutritional supplements should be a part of the preoperative assessment. Aspirin and aspirin-containing products are well-documented sources of bleeding problems. Platelet aggregation is irreversibly affected when the aspirin acetylates cyclooxygenase. One aspirin affects a platelet throughout its lifespan of 6–10 days. If the patient can safely discontinue aspirin, without a high risk for stroke or myocardial infarction, it should be withheld for 10 days before surgery and then 5–7 days after surgery. Although many recent publications support continuing medically indicated anticoagulant therapy during the perioperative period, several confirm that for patients taking aspirin for primary prevention or pain, the surgeon can safely elect to discontinue that medication[9,10]. Non-steroidal anti-inflammatory drugs, such as ibuprofen and naproxen, affect the same enzyme, though the block is not as severe or irreversible[11]. If possible, the patient should stop these medications 1–4 days prior to surgery, depending on the half-life of the drug.

Fig. 151.1 Interrelated surgical complications.

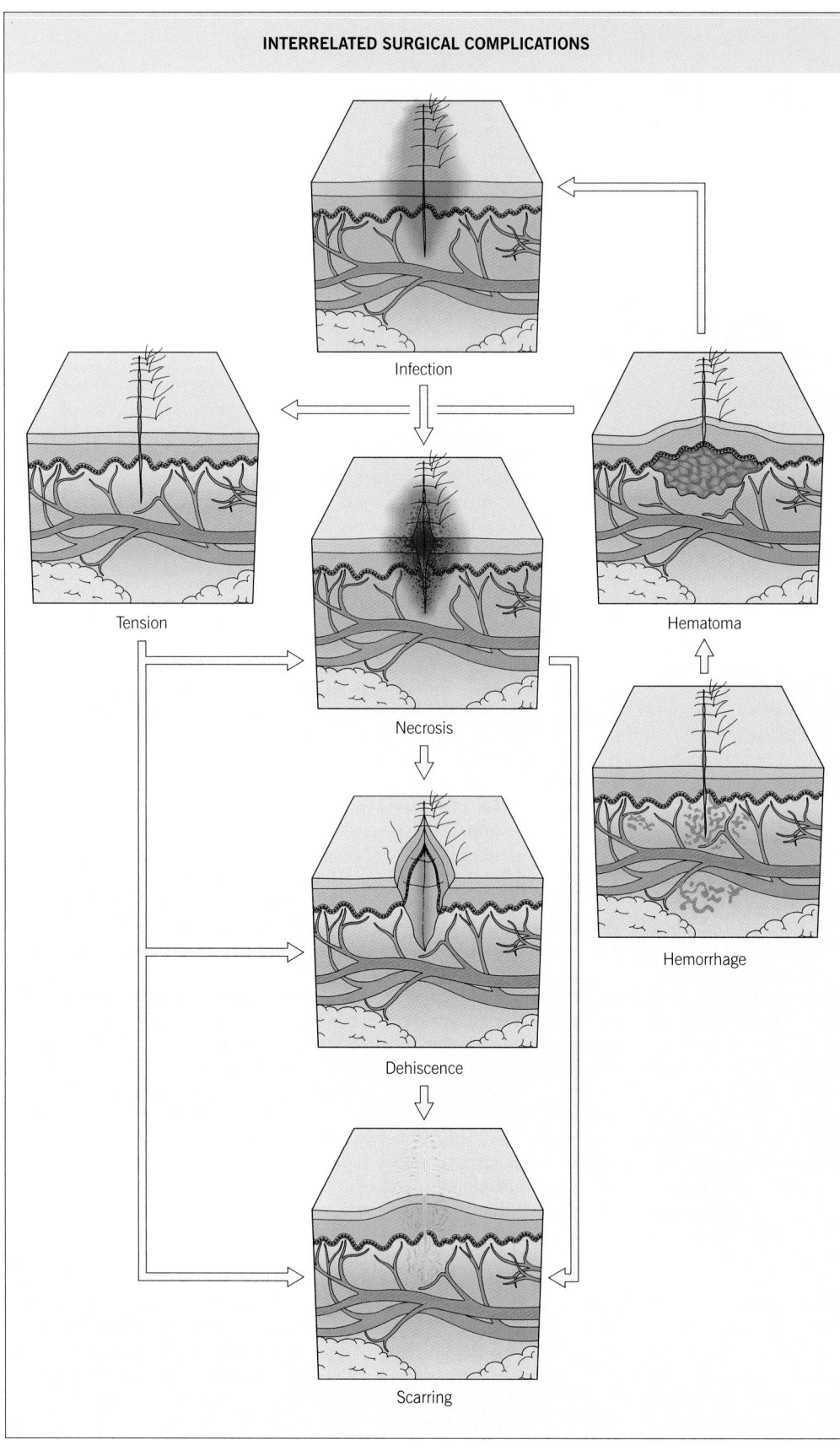

INTERRELATED SURGICAL COMPLICATIONS

Infection

Tension

Hematoma

Necrosis

Hemorrhage

Dehiscence

Scarring

Warfarin is a commonly used anticoagulant. Several studies have been published in the vascular, oral and dermatologic surgery literature that support the viewpoint that surgery can be performed without stopping warfarin as long as the international normalization ratio (INR) equals 2 to 3 or less[12–14]. The surgeon should minimize unnecessary undermining and ensure that intraoperative control of bleeding is meticulous. If, with the help of the physician who is supervising the anticoagulation, the warfarin can be safely held for surgery, it should be discontinued 2–4 days prior to surgery and restarted the evening or morning after surgery. An INR can be checked just before surgery.

Heparin is given parenterally and it acts as an antithrombin factor. When administered intravenously, heparin has a short half-life of approximately 1 hour and can be rapidly reversed by intravenous protamine sulfate. Heparin can be used for patients who need an operative procedure that the surgeon feels should not be attempted in the presence of warfarin, but who cannot go without anticoagulation for prolonged periods of time. The patient is usually hospitalized and heparin is substituted for warfarin. Immediately before the surgery, heparin is discontinued or reversed with protamine sulfate. The heparin is then restarted post procedure, in the controlled inpatient setting[15].

ALGORITHMS GENERATED FROM ANSWERS TO PREOPERATIVE QUESTIONNAIRES

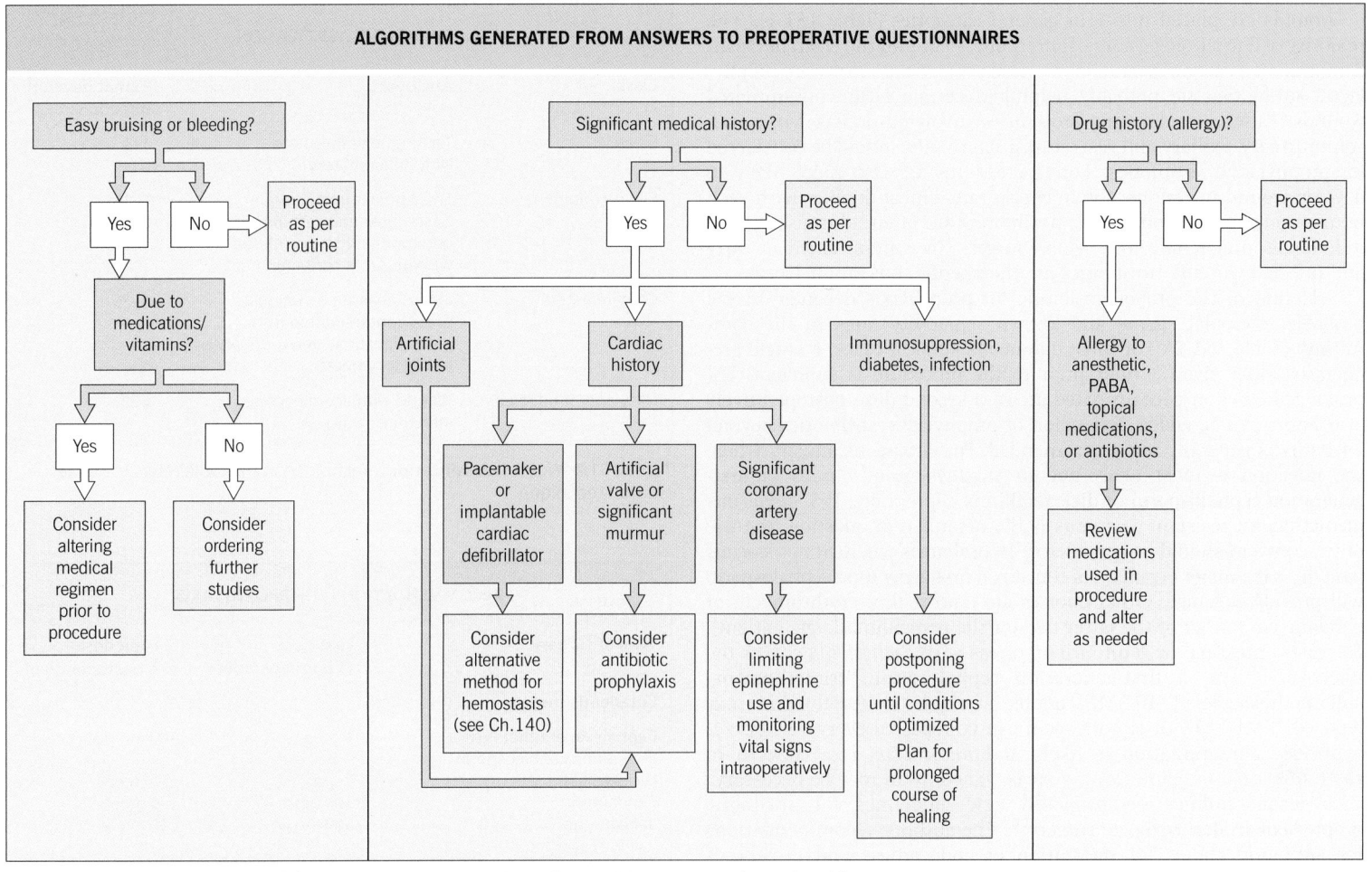

Fig. 151.2 **Algorithms generated from preoperative questionnaires.** PABA, para-aminobenzoic acid.

Studies have shown that vitamin E in doses of 200–400 IU per day reduced platelet adhesion. Patients with abnormal platelets, such as diabetics and renal dialysis patients, treated with vitamin E have decreased platelet aggregation. The effect is synergistic when vitamin E is taken with other antiplatelet agents like aspirin and garlic. Garlic decreases platelet aggregation, and it significantly increases fibrinolytic activity at a dosage of 900 mg per day. Eicosapentaenoic acid (fish oil) decreases platelet aggregation and adhesion and increases bleeding time. Many other dietary supplements such as dong quai, licorice, devil's claw and danshen have the same effect[16]. Patients should be advised to discontinue supplements containing these substances in preparation for a surgical procedure.

Ethanol is a potent vasodilator. It may cause bleeding by inhibiting platelet aggregation and platelet granule release. It may also accentuate the increase in bleeding time caused by aspirin[17]. In addition, alcohol consumption may decrease the patient's attention to optimal wound protection. Patients should be advised to avoid alcohol consumption during the immediate preoperative and postoperative period.

Wound healing

The principles of wound healing are covered in detail in Chapter 141. To forestall complications due to poor wound healing, close attention should be paid to pre-existing medical conditions and medications that may affect wound healing. If the patient is a brittle diabetic, is suffering acutely from congestive heart failure, or has uncontrolled hypertension or a myriad of other severe conditions, it may be best to postpone the procedure until the patient's medical problems are under better control. If the procedure cannot be postponed, the patient should be forewarned that there might be a prolonged postoperative healing phase. In addition, any chronic debilitating illness may predispose patients to developing secondary infections.

Medications such as glucocorticoids may also delay healing and predispose the patient to secondary infections and a prolonged post-operative course. Patients on other immunosuppressives such as cyclosporine may also be prone to infections and prolonged healing.

Cigarette smoking interferes with wound healing. Areas repaired by flaps or grafts are particularly susceptible to poor healing and wound necrosis. If there is refusal to stop smoking completely, the patient should be strongly encouraged to decrease consumption to less than 1 pack per day for 1 week preoperatively and for 3–4 weeks post-operatively, to attempt to maximize wound healing[18].

There is a growing body of literature to support delaying procedures on patients who are on, or have recently completed, isotretinoin therapy, because of poor wound healing and the formation of excessive granulation tissue. In keloid fibroblast cultures, retinoids have been shown to modulate connective tissue metabolism. Most reported problems have been individual case reports involving resurfacing procedures after courses of isotretinoin for acne therapy. It may be prudent to postpone cosmetic procedures in such patients for up to 1 year after the cessation of isotretinoin therapy[19–21].

Reactivation of an HSV infection can dramatically interfere with the postoperative course. Patients with a history of herpes labialis or other facial herpetic infections should receive prophylactic antiviral therapy prior to dermabrasion, laser resurfacing or chemical peels. Antiviral therapy, such as oral acyclovir at a dose of 200 mg five times a day, should start 2–5 days prior to the procedure and continue for 5 days postoperatively or until the skin has re-epithelialized[22]. Similar regimens consisting of oral famciclovir 250 mg three times daily or oral valacyclovir 1 g twice daily can be utilized and are more convenient.

The shoulders, central chest, upper arms and upper back are more prone to hypertrophic scar or spread scar formation during the healing phase. The patient should be counseled about the increased risk of scarring in these areas.

Prophylactic antibiotics

Antibiotic prophylaxis is administered to prevent wound infection, the development of bacterial endocarditis, or infection in implanted prosthetic devices. The risk and consequences of infection must be weighed against the risk and cost of administration of the antibiotic.

Wounds are placed into four general categories (Table 151.1). The majority of dermatologic surgical procedures fall into the clean or clean-contaminated categories and do not need prophylaxis. However, prophylactic antibiotics are probably helpful in certain clean-contaminated wounds. Patients undergoing procedures involving oronasal mucosal, genitourinary, axillary and gastrointestinal tissues should be considered for prophylactic antibiotics. Long procedures are also more likely to develop wound infections: the infection rate almost doubles with each hour of operation. Prophylactic antibiotics are often administered for individuals undergoing long Mohs surgery. In contaminated or dirty and infected wounds, antibiotics are therapeutic, not prophylactic.

Selection of the proper antibiotic for prophylaxis depends on the probable microbial agents and known sensitivity rates in the community (Table 151.2). For most cutaneous surgical cases, a single pre-operative dose given 1 hour prior to the procedure is sufficient. For prolonged cases in contaminated areas, a second dose postoperatively at 6 hours can be added. Extension of prophylactic antibiotics beyond 24 hours is generally not recommended. For cutaneous surgery where the infection is most likely due to *Staphylococcus aureus*, a first-generation cephalosporin or dicloxacillin is appropriate. If *S. epidermis* or methicillin-resistant *S. aureus* is the organism in question, the use of vancomycin should be considered. In oral areas where *Streptococcus viridans* is the major organism of concern, a first-generation cephalosporin will provide coverage. Other choices are amoxicillin, erythromycin or clindamycin (either of the latter two for the penicillin-allergic patient). For gastrointestinal or genitourinary areas with *Escherichia coli* as the likely organism, a first-generation cephalosporin, trimethoprim–sulfamethoxazole (TMP-SMX) double strength or ciprofloxacin may be used. TMP-SMX or ciprofloxacin can be repeated every 12 hours if continued contamination is likely. If *Enterococcus* is a concern in gastrointestinal or genitourinary areas, vancomycin may be necessary.

A recent publication proposed new guidelines for antibiotic prophylaxis in dermatologic surgery[24]. The authors' recommendations for antibiotic choice for prevention of endocarditis and prostheses infections are summarized in Table 151.3. Except for operations lasting 6 hours or longer, they proposed a single oral preoperative dose given 30 to 60 minutes prior to surgery. For surgical site infection prophylaxis, the same antibiotics and dosing were recommended preoperatively, possibly followed by up to 10 days of postoperative antibiotics, depending on the surgeon's estimation of the risk for wound infection.

Antibiotic prophylaxis for endocarditis is generally not required for any patient undergoing non-Mohs surgery for a cutaneous lesion with an intact skin surface. For surgical manipulation of eroded, non-infected skin, prophylaxis should be given to high-risk patients, i.e. those with prosthetic cardiac valves, a history of previous bacterial endocarditis, most congenital cardiac malformations, rheumatic and other acquired valvular dysfunction even after valvular surgery, hypertrophic cardiomyopathy, or mitral valve prolapse with valvular regurgitation.

For surgical manipulation of infected/abscessed skin, or in the presence of distant skin infection, the patients mentioned previously, as well as other high-risk patients (e.g. those with orthopedic prostheses or ventriculoatrial/peritoneal shunts), should receive endocarditis prophylaxis. Unless another organism has been cultured, *S. aureus* should be considered the most likely skin contaminant, and the antibiotic regimen is similar to the coverage for *S. aureus* above. For gastrointestinal/genitourinary (*Enterococcus*) prophylaxis in low-risk patients, amoxicillin may be given (2–3 g orally 1 hour preoperatively ± 1.5 g orally 6 hours postoperatively). For high-risk patients, according to one review article[23], either of the following should be utilized:

- ampicillin plus gentamicin (2 g orally + 1.5 mg/kg intravenously/intramuscularly 1 hour preoperative), then amoxicillin (1.5 g orally 6 hours postoperative) *or*
- vancomycin plus gentamicin (1 g intravenously + 1.5 mg intravenously/intramuscularly 1 hour preoperative); this combination can be repeated in 8 hours and is recommended for patients with newly implanted (<60-day-old) prosthetic valves.

Although the authors of the review cited clearly defined 'high-risk' patients, the population of 'low-risk' patients is not clearly defined.

Consultation with the patient's cardiologist or orthopedic surgeon may be extremely helpful in determining the need for prophylaxis and the regimen to be used.

WOUND CLASSIFICATION		
Class	Attributes	% that develop infections
Clean	Technique immaculate Non-inflammatory	1–4
Clean-contaminated	Small breaks in technique Gastrointestinal, respiratory or genitourinary tracts entered without gross contamination	5–15
Contaminated	Major breaks in technique Gross contamination from gastrointestinal, genitourinary or respiratory tracts	6–25
Dirty and/or infected	Wound with acute bacterial infection ± pus	>25

Table 151.1 Wound classification[1]. Technique in the table refers to sterile surgical technique.

RECOMMENDATIONS FOR PROPHYLAXIS		
Type of surgery	First dose (1 h preoperative)	Second dose (6 h postoperative)
Cutaneous surgery		
Cephalexin or other first-generation cephalosporin	1 g po	500 mg po
Dicloxacillin	1 g po	500 mg po
Clindamycin	300 g po	150 g po
Vancomycin	500 mg iv	250 mg iv
Oral surgery		
Cephalexin or other first-generation cephalosporin	1 g po	500 mg po
Amoxicillin	3 g po	1.5 g po
Erythromycin	1 g po	500 mg po
Clindamycin	300 mg po	150 mg po
Gastrointestinal or genitourinary surgery		
Cephalexin or other first-generation cephalosporin	1 g po	500 mg po
Trimethoprim–sulfamethoxazole, double-strength	1 tablet po	
Ciprofloxacin	500 mg po	
Enterococcus		
Vancomycin	500 mg iv	250 mg iv

Table 151.2 Recommendations for prophylaxis[23].

RECOMMENDATIONS FOR ANTIBIOTIC PROPHYLAXIS IN DERMATOLOGIC SURGERY		
Surgical site	Non-penicillin allergic	Penicillin allergic
Non-oral sites	Cephalexin 2 g po or Dicloxacillin 2 g po	Clindamycin 600 mg po or Clarithromycin 500 mg po or Azithromycin 500 mg po
Oral and nasal mucosal sites	Amoxicillin 2 g po	Clindamycin 600 mg po or Cephalexin 2 g po or Clarithromycin 500 mg po or Azithromycin 500 mg po

Table 151.3 Recommendations for antibiotic prophylaxis in dermatologic surgery[24].

Defibrillators and pacemakers

The electrosurgical instruments often used in cutaneous procedures have the potential to interfere with the function of pacemakers and implantable cardioverter-defibrillators (ICD; see Ch. 140). If the patient's preoperative history reveals the presence of such devices, caution should be exercised to avoid inducing arrhythmias. Alternatives to electrosurgery may be considered. Battery-operated cautery units have been used successfully in dermatologic surgery, and they do not produce high-frequency electromagnetic interference or electrical currents traversing the body. Bipolar instruments concentrate the current across the tips, minimizing the chance of interference with implanted devices. If conventional electrosurgery must be used, the active tip should not be applied to an area within 15 cm of the implanted device whenever possible. Electrocoagulation should also be kept at as low a setting as possible, and it should be delivered in bursts lasting <5 seconds in order to minimize the chance of prolonged inhibition[25].

In consultation with the patient's cardiologist, the ICD can be deactivated for the duration of the procedure. The pacemaker can also be placed in a fixed rate mode, rather than the sensing mode, to minimize the possibility of interference. During the procedure, if conventional electrosurgery is to be used, continuous cardiac monitoring with an ECG or pulse oximeter should be strongly considered. A contingency plan should already be in place to deal with an arrhythmia should it occur. If the device is deactivated or its function altered for the procedure, it is the surgeon's responsibility to ensure that the patient returns to his or her cardiologist within a reasonable time, for readjustment and evaluation post procedure. Electrical equipment should be properly grounded during the procedure. If bipolar forceps or true electrocautery is used instead of electrosurgery, intraoperative monitoring, cardiology consultation and postoperative evaluation may be unnecessary for most stable patients[26].

Allergies

True allergic reactions to local anesthetics may be type I (immediate) or type IV (delayed-type hypersensitivity) (see Ch. 143). Patients who have a type IV sensitivity to one major group of local anesthetics (ester or amide) are usually not allergic to members of the other group. However, patients with a history of para-aminobenzoic acid (PABA) allergy can cross-react with anesthetics in the ester group (e.g. procaine). Type I reactions are more commonly associated with the ester anesthetics and their PABA metabolite. Although the lack of cross-reactivity between ester and amide anesthetics is true for type IV sensitivity, it has not been adequately studied for anaphylaxis. If there is a possibility of a type I amide allergy by history, or if the surgeon is reluctant to substitute an amide in an ester-allergic patient, referral to an allergist for a progressive challenge protocol can be considered to identify a suitable amide anesthetic[27].

Epinephrine (adrenaline) is a vasoconstrictive agent commonly added to local anesthetics because it lessens bleeding and prolongs the duration of anesthesia. Patients will occasionally report a history of an 'allergy' to local anesthetic, describing their symptoms of palpitations, headache, tachycardia, tachypnea or tremor (see Ch. 143). These 'allergic reactions' may be, in truth, reactions to epinephrine given in high dosages or inadvertently injected intravascularly. Since the half-life of epinephrine in serum is short, when these reactions do develop, specific therapy is usually not necessary. In order to avoid them, the lowest dosage and concentration of epinephrine (less than 1:200 000) should be used and injection of significant amounts intravascularly should be avoided using proper infiltration technique[28].

Another very commonly encountered systemic side effect often mistaken by the patient as an allergic reaction is the vasovagal reaction. The patient recalls becoming pale, sweaty and lightheaded, perhaps even fainting. In contrast to a true toxic or allergic reaction, the pulse remains slow and regular and the blood pressure and respiratory rate are normal (see Table 143.2). No loss of bowel or bladder control or prolonged tonic-clonic movement occurs unless the patient has a seizure secondary to brain hypoxia during the vasovagal reaction. Treatment consists of keeping the patient supine or in the Trendelenburg position and giving reassurance until the patient recovers sufficiently to be allowed to gradually sit up and ambulate[29].

Chlorhexidine gluconate is a frequently utilized surgical skin preparation. It is a broad-spectrum antibacterial of the halogenated phenol class. Though it has a very weak sensitizing potential, it has been reported to cause allergic contact dermatitis[30]. Similar reactions have also occurred with the iodophor povidone-iodine (Betadine®)[31]. Both compounds can also be skin irritants, especially when occluded. Care must be taken to ensure that all traces of skin cleanser are removed prior to application of the dressing.

Topical antibiotics can cause allergic contact dermatitis. Neomycin is the most common sensitizer, though bacitracin can also cause sensitization. Co-reactivity against both neomycin and bacitracin is common. Cross-sensitivity between neomycin and gentamicin, kanamycin, streptomycin and tobramycin can also occur. Mupirocin or erythromycin ointment are alternatives if the patient is allergic to both neomycin and bacitracin. As there is no convincing evidence that topical antibiotic ointment prevents infection, plain petrolatum (paraffin) ointment may be the best agent for wound dressing[32].

Informed consent

The lines of communication should be open between the surgeon and the patient before the procedure begins. The physician should make the patient aware of his or her condition, how it affects overall health, if treatment is imperative, and what different treatment options might be available. Pros and cons of surgery as well as alternative therapies should be discussed in a language that the patient can easily understand. To assess how much the patient understands, it helps to ask the patient to describe the procedure in his or her own words. The patient should also be informed about the risks of the procedure and the results to be reasonably expected. Common complications (like bleeding, infection, allergic reactions, scarring) should be addressed and strategies for dealing with them discussed. In turn, the patient must accept responsibility for preoperative preparation and postoperative wound care.

It is the surgeon's responsibility to provide oral and written clear, detailed information delineating the indications for the procedure and describing the procedure, the risks involved, and the postoperative care necessary to ensure the best outcome possible. Should complications arise, as they inevitably will in some cases, the surgeon should be honest with the patient about treatment options and outcome.

Intraoperative Considerations

Contamination

Although good statistics are lacking, the risk of infection in cutaneous surgery is very low. It is certainly less than 5%, and most probably is in the range of 1–2%. The indications for prophylactic antibiotics were discussed previously. Although wound infections usually do not become evident until 4–8 days postoperatively, in most cases the infection truly begins at the time of surgery. The surgical team should prepare the skin and the surgical field, prepare the instruments, and wear the correct protective equipment in order to help reduce the incidence of infection and protect both the patient and caregivers.

The skin cannot be sterilized, but it is possible to remove the majority of the resident flora and pathogenic bacteria by using mechanical cleansing and antiseptic agents. The extent of skin preparation varies with the invasiveness and complexity of the proposed surgical procedure. A 2-second wipe with 70% isopropyl alcohol or a 10-second cleansing with an iodophor swab may be adequate for most shave and superficial biopsies[33]. Chlorhexidine produces rapid bacterial destruction, is effective against a wide range of Gram-positive and Gram-negative bacteria, and binds with the protein of the stratum corneum, providing residual action. These properties make it the most frequently used preoperative preparation for skin surgery. It is, however, irritating to the conjunctiva, and it may be toxic to the cornea or tympanic membrane and middle ear, so caution must be exercised in these areas. Iodophors are another excellent antiseptic; one advantage is that the area that has been prepared is readily apparent because of the brownish-orange color. They are effective against Gram-positive and Gram-negative bacteria and some fungal spores, but they have a slower and shorter duration of action than chlorhexidine. Also, as noted earlier, they can cause skin irritation, and there are patients who may develop an allergic contact dermatitis to this cleanser[34].

The preparation and sterilization of surgical instruments is covered in Chapter 144. Use of the surgical mask may help protect the patient from surgical personnel with active upper respiratory tract infections.

The mask protects the surgical team from contamination by saliva droplets or blood from the patient. It is also essential to protect the eyes from accidental splashes of body fluid. Appropriate surgical attire and glove use is advocated in all surgical situations as part of universal precautions. In cases where sterility is not essential (superficial shave biopsies), non-sterile examination gloves can be used[35].

Bleeding

Intraoperative bleeding can obscure the surgical site. It can be upsetting to both the surgeon and the patient. If it continues after closure, it can cause a hematoma that can lead to infection, increased tension on wound edges, and dehiscence (see Fig. 151.1). A careful history should have helped to identify patients prone to bleeding, and it may have allowed for changes in medical management or medications preoperatively to reduce intraoperative bleeding. When not contraindicated (e.g. procedures on toes or fingers in patients with peripheral vascular disease), use of epinephrine with the anesthetic is helpful (see Ch. 143). Suction can also maintain good visualization in an otherwise bloody field. An assistant can provide traction across the wound surface or pressure at the periphery of the site. Frequent blotting with sponges or cotton-tipped applicators also helps to keep the field clear.

Bleeding should be controlled as soon as is practical; individual small vessels should be isolated and precisely cauterized (to avoid excessive char) or ligated. It may be prudent to ligate visible vessels lying proximal to the wound bed, since they might be nicked or partially cut during the procedure. Large vessels noted in the surgical wound should be tied off or cauterized at both visualized ends as long as the surgeon is sure there is adequate collateral circulation to the area. Bleeding, which may not be apparent at the time of the closure, may develop once the effect of the epinephrine diminishes. The surgeon must ensure that the surgical field is as dry as possible prior to closure. Particular attention should be paid to apices or cut muscle that can steadily ooze.

If, at the beginning of the procedure, bleeding is more than usual, undermining should be kept to a minimum. If appropriate, consideration should be given to a linear closure rather than a more complicated flap or graft. Blood easily accumulates unnoticed in non-visualized 'dead space'. Placement of a drain should be considered for larger flaps or complex multilayered linear closures, to allow egress of small amounts of continued bleeding and to avoid hematoma formation. A simple fenestrated small Penrose drain can suffice (Fig. 151.3). It should be removed 24–48 hours later, once bleeding has lessened and the chance for hematoma formation has diminished.

In open wounds that continue to bleed in spite of adequate attempts at hemostasis, hemostatic materials such as gelatin sponges or powder (Gelfoam®), oxidized cellulose (Oxycel®, Surgicel®), microfibrillar collagen (Avitene®, Collastat®) or topical thrombin can be applied to the wound to provide a matrix to speed coagulation. Caution should be exercised when using oxidized cellulose, because the use of excessive amounts can result in foreign body reactions[36].

Tissue injury

Because of the nature of invasive procedures, some tissue injury is unavoidable. Gentle handling of the wound edges during the procedure can minimize this trauma and allow the viable tissue to heal more rapidly. Skin hooks or single-toothed forceps should be used carefully, without crushing, to grasp tissue, and skin edges should always be handled gently. When using electrocautery to control bleeding, indiscriminate and excessive burning should be avoided. Large areas of charred and necrotic tissue left in the wound increase the risk of inflammation and infection.

Tension

Excessive tension at the closure site can cause tissue necrosis and dehiscence (see Fig. 151.1). Postoperatively, tension can be a source of increased discomfort for the patient once the local anesthesia has dissipated. There is a tendency for the surgeon to tighten surface sutures when wounds gap open. Such action can lead to 'train track' scars. At the time of surgery, the operative site should be thoroughly evaluated and the closure planned to minimize wound tension. Adequate undermining should be accomplished. Buried absorbable sutures should bear the burden of the tension, minimizing the need for

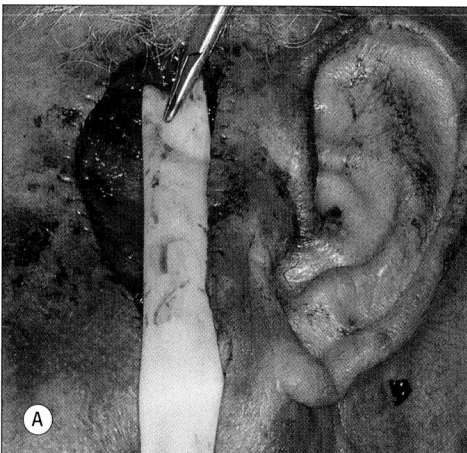

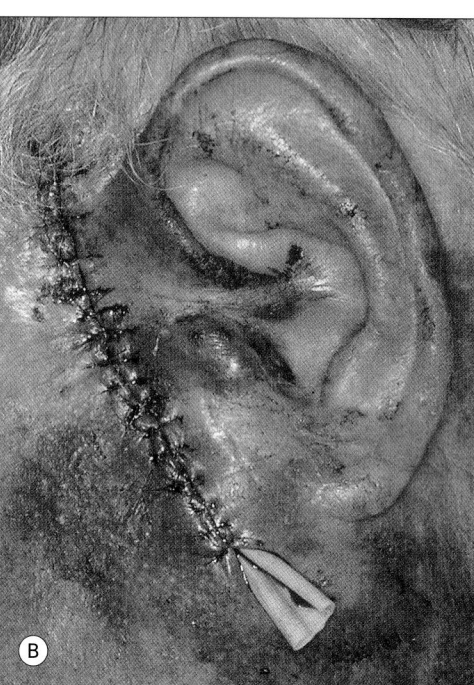

Fig. 151.3 Placement of Penrose drain because of excessive bleeding.

tight surface sutures. The closure should be oriented to take advantage of maximal tissue movement. Instead of a linear closure, using a flap or graft to close the defect can minimize tension in appropriate circumstances. Relaxing incisions can also be performed 2–3 cm from the wound edge, parallel to the incision site, to share tension over a larger area. If the defect cannot be completely closed due to excessive tension, partial closure can be accomplished and the remainder of the wound allowed to heal secondarily. If the site is chosen well, this method yields an excellent cosmetic result. Intraoperative or preoperative tissue expansion may also allow for the safe closure of large defects[37]. If a wound appears too tight at the time of closure, it probably is making complications more likely (Fig. 151.4).

Necrosis

Necrosis is usually the result of a hematoma, an infection, or wound tension compromising the blood flow to the skin edge, resulting in necrotic tissue (see Fig. 151.1). Although pale, poorly perfused tissue at a flap or wound edge may, at times, be a warning of future problems with perfusion, actual necrosis will not become evident until the postoperative time period. The factors leading to necrosis begin preoperatively and continue into the perioperative period. The hazards of smoking have been discussed earlier, but they cannot be overemphasized. Smoking decreases perfusion and increases the risk of necrosis. Patients should be counseled repeatedly to stop, or at the very least decrease, their cigarette consumption.

The blood supply to the skin arises primarily from the subdermal plexus. Extensive superficial undermining may damage this plexus and the segmental arteries supplying it. Hematoma formation may compromise blood flow to and from the area through pressure on this plexus.

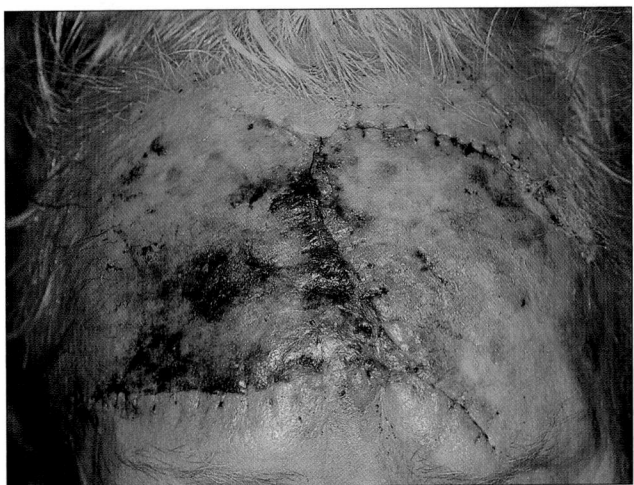

Fig. 151.4 Postoperative appearance of wound closed under tension with resulting necrosis.

Even normal postoperative edema may compromise blood flow. Sutures tied too tightly may also decrease perfusion, leading to necrosis. The use of a loop stitch, leaving space between the first and second loops of the surgeons knot, may allow for tissue expansion from postsurgical edema, decreasing the risk of tissue necrosis[38].

Flap tips may become necrotic because of an inadequate blood supply. If the 3:1 length-to-base ratio is exceeded, circulation to the distal tip may be poor[39]. When correcting redundancies caused by rotation at the base of a flap, the surgeon must ensure that the pedicle is not narrowed. Correction of the redundancy may need to be delayed in order to protect the vascular supply to the flap.

As mentioned earlier, epinephrine is frequently used in combination with the local anesthetic in dermatologic surgery. The vasoconstrictive properties that make it ideal in most locations may be extremely detrimental in areas with limited collateral circulation such as the digits. In such cases, it would be prudent to use smaller amounts of an anesthetic that contains epinephrine, a more dilute epinephrine concentration (e.g. 1:200 000 instead of 1:100 000), or a local anesthetic without epinephrine.

Grafts may become necrotic if an adequate blood supply from the wound bed is not established. In general, full-thickness grafts require more nutrients than split-thickness grafts (see Ch. 148). Areas with a poor or absent vascular supply, such as exposed bone, exposed cartilage or sites of previous therapeutic radiation, often cannot support full-thickness grafts and may not fully support split-thickness grafts. Sites with greater than 1 cm² of exposed bone or cartilage have a greater incidence of graft failure. The graft must also be well apposed to the wound bed. Strict hemostasis is required to prevent blood from accumulating in the space between the graft and the wound. However, excessive electrocoagulation should also be avoided because of the resulting necrotic debris created. Absorbable hemostatic agents may also interfere with the engrafting of the new tissue. The placement of basting sutures and tie-down bolsters may help ensure adequate contact between the graft and the wound bed (see Ch. 148).

Nerve deficits

The preoperative evaluation should include a quick survey of neurologic function in the areas that could be affected by the proposed procedure. During cutaneous surgery, sensory and motor nerves may be injured or cut (see Ch. 142). It is essential to document – and, more importantly, make the patient aware of – pre-existing deficits prior to infiltrating the anesthetic (see Ch. 143). Local anesthesia or nerve blocks can lead to temporary nerve deficits lasting 6–12 hours. Full evaluation of the extent of the injury may have to wait until a day to several weeks after surgery.

Skin surgery will result in the transection of cutaneous nerves. Patients frequently note sensory deficits at the site of primary closures or flaps. Almost all will experience hypoesthesia in skin grafts. Most areas have diverse sensory innervation, and, unless a major nerve is injured, there are very few significant permanent deficits. Sensory nerves often do regenerate, though this process may take months. The

patient should be aware preoperatively that there may be paresthesias in the area as it heals. Occasionally, completely normal sensation never returns. The areas most prone to sensory nerve injury leading to noticeable sensory defects are the digits, the forehead and the scalp.

Injury to motor nerves can be more alarming, since this can result in paralysis of the denervated muscles. The closer to the nerve root that the injury takes place, the more severe the consequence. Thankfully, most of the larger branches of the facial nerve are deep to the muscle fascia and well protected. As a result, injuries to the main trunk of the facial nerve (or its zygomatic and buccal branches) rarely occur in dermatologic surgery, because these nerves lie relatively deep and are somewhat protected. Injuries to these nerves do, however, result in significant sequelae, including inability to close the eyelids, loss of sphincter control around the mouth leading to drooling, and a distorted face.

The area of highest consequence on the cheek lies lateral to a line drawn from the lateral canthus of the eye to the angle of the mouth and medial to where the nerve divides into five major branches near the surface of the parotid gland (Fig. 151.5). Medial to this area, innervation is usually diverse enough to render the results of transection of a single nerve mild. Lateral to this area, the main trunk lies deep within the parotid gland and is relatively well protected by it[40]. Unless the procedure is a deep excision of an infiltrative skin cancer, the majority of cutaneous surgeons are unlikely to cause significant motor nerve injury except in the following important danger areas:

- The *temporal branch of the facial nerve* courses very superficially as it crosses the zygomatic arch, and it is covered only by the superficial temporalis fascia, with very little subcutaneous fat. Paralysis of the frontalis muscle results from transection of the nerve in this location. The ability to elevate the forehead on the affected side is lost (Fig. 151.6A). This loss is often of only cosmetic concern; however, if there is pre-existing brow ptosis, the paralysis may result in a severe ptosis that interferes with vision and requires surgical correction with a brow pexy.
- The *mandibular branch of the facial nerve* is subject to injury as it crosses the mandible, near the facial artery and vein. It is covered at this point only by skin and thin platysma muscle. This nerve innervates the lip depressors, and injury can cause asymmetry visible when the patient smiles or attempts other facial expressions using these muscles. In addition, mouth function may be compromised, resulting in drooling.
- The *spinal accessory nerve* can be damaged as it exits from behind the sternocleidomastoid muscle at Erb's point in the posterior triangle of the neck. Damage leads to winging of the scapula and difficulty abducting the arm, because of paralysis of the trapezius muscle. Pain is a frequent accompaniment of injury to the spinal accessory nerve.

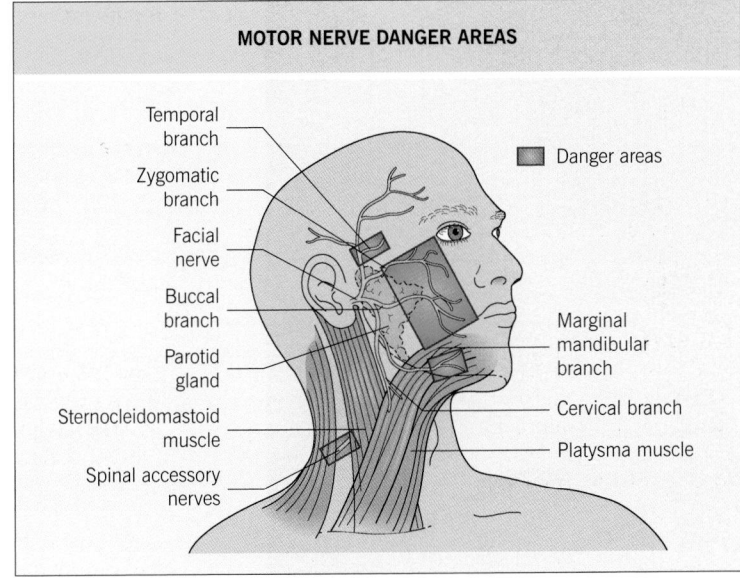

Fig. 151.5 Motor nerve danger areas.

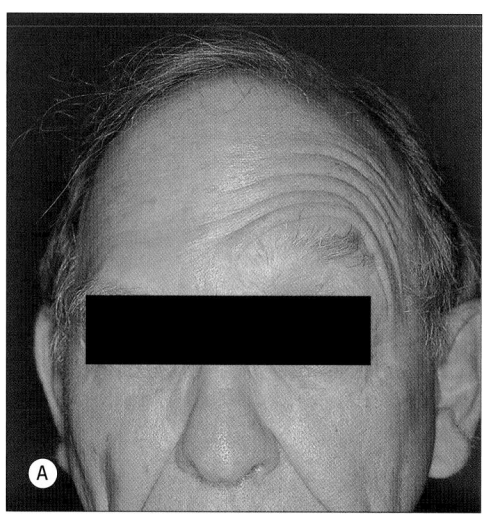

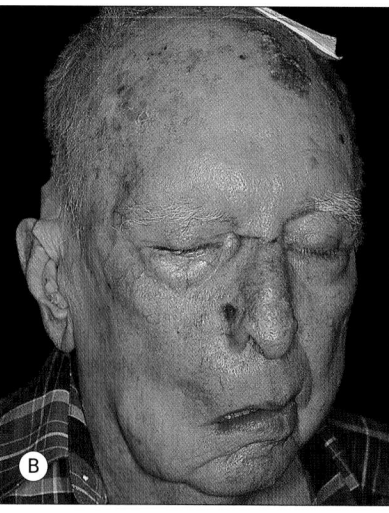

Fig. 151.6 Damage to the facial nerve. A Loss of the ability to elevate the forehead due to transection of the temporal branch. **B** Loss of function of the main branch of the facial nerve. The ability to close the eye has been restored by the placement of a gold weight in the eyelid.

The surgeon must be aware of these danger areas and be on the lookout for these nerves (see Fig. 151.5). Injury is sometimes unavoidable even with the most careful dissection, especially if a neoplasm involves the nerve. Early consultation, even preoperatively, with the appropriate specialties (neurology, neurosurgery, radiation oncology) may allow for optimal management of the problems. Regeneration of motor nerves is possible, but unpredictable. When major motor branches are cut, surgical reapproximation or nerve grafts may be necessary. Muscle stimulation may prevent atrophy while awaiting return of function. At times it may be practical to simply address the functional problems created, such as placing gold weights to allow eye closure (Fig. 151.6B).

Unsatisfactory scarring

Although scars do not acquire their final appearance until months postoperatively, operative techniques can greatly affect the appearance. Spread scars were discussed earlier. Though they may be unavoidable in certain anatomic areas, the surgeon may choose to use longer-lasting absorbable or non-absorbable sutures in the deeper layers of closure, in order to reduce the risk of early spread scars[41].

A trapdoor or pincushion-like appearance may develop in the area of transposition flaps (Fig. 151.7). Wide undermining at the time of repair, and squaring off the corners rather than trimming more circular wound edges, may reduce the incidence of this complication[42]. Removing excess subcutaneous tissue underneath the flap and trimming the flap so that it just covers the defect without any redundancy may also help.

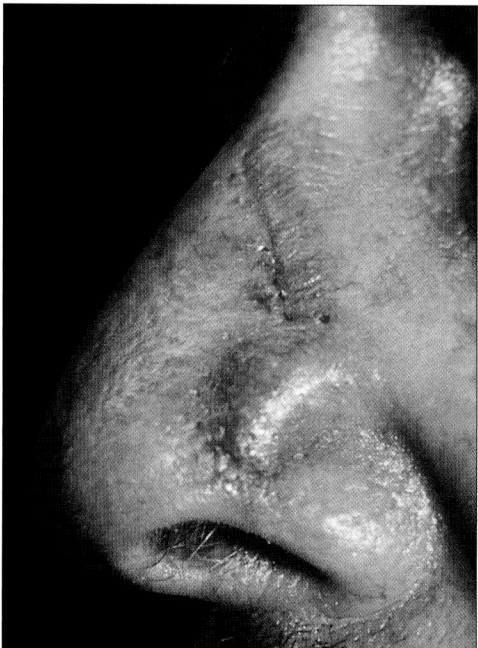

Fig. 151.7 'Trapdoor' or 'pincushion' appearance of a flap reconstruction.

Postoperative Considerations

After the procedure is complete and the patient has left the office, complications may still occur. Before the patient leaves, detailed wound care instructions should be reviewed with the patient and whoever else may be helping to care for the wound site. The surgeon must also ensure that the patient has been provided easy-to-understand, written postoperative wound care instructions. These instructions should include answers to the most commonly asked questions, for example, 'How do I know if it is infected?' 'How much bleeding is too much bleeding?' 'When can I take a shower/bath?' 'When can I play golf/ tennis?' The patient should also have a direct method of contacting the physician or a suitable representative if there are questions or concerns not answered by the handout provided. A little foresight and education can greatly reduce the number of midnight calls or quickly bring to the attention of the physician a complication best addressed earlier rather than later. It is imperative that the contact physician be available and responsive. It is helpful for the physician or designee to call the patient postoperatively to check on his or her progress and answer questions.

Bleeding/hematoma/ecchymosis

Some cases of postoperative bleeding will occur despite exhaustive pre-operative evaluation, preparation, and careful intraoperative hemostasis. Most bleeding occurs within the first 24 hours, with the majority occurring within 6 hours. During this period, clots are still fragile and movement can easily dislodge them. As the epinephrine dissipates, small-vessel bleeding may increase. A pressure dressing applied immediately after the procedure helps to prevent this problem. The patient should be instructed to leave the dressing in place for at least 24 hours. If the surgical procedure was more involved than a superficial shave or punch biopsy, the dressing should consist of multiple layers: ointment, then an initial non-adherent contact layer (e.g. Telfa®, Release®), followed by a bulky absorbent layer consisting of gauze, cotton, sponges or eye pads. An outer layer of tape or stretchable gauze (e.g. Ace Wrap®, Coban®) covers all of these. The bandage should provide pressure but not cause ischemia.

A small amount of bleeding is normal; however, the patient should be told that bleeding which soaks the dressing needs attention. The patient should be instructed to remove the old dressing, as saturated dressings no longer provide any meaningful pressure, and apply firm pressure without release to the site for 15–20 minutes as timed *by the clock*. If pressure stops the bleeding, then the dressing should be reinforced with additional gauze and tape. If bleeding persists, then the patient needs to be evaluated by the surgeon.

The surgeon can once again attempt direct pressure, but, if this fails, the wound should be exposed, and the area reanesthetized and explored. If a single bleeding vessel is identified, then it can be electrocoagulated or ligated. Frequently, a single source is not identified. Bleeding can occur in multiple areas and each must be addressed. A drain may be helpful if a very dry surgical field cannot be achieved. If possible, surgical procedures should be scheduled early in the day to prevent having to bring the patient in during the wee hours of the morning to accomplish this.

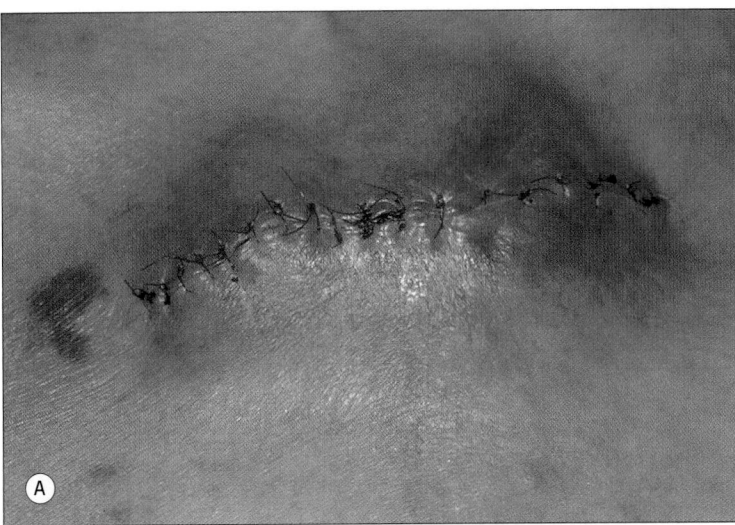

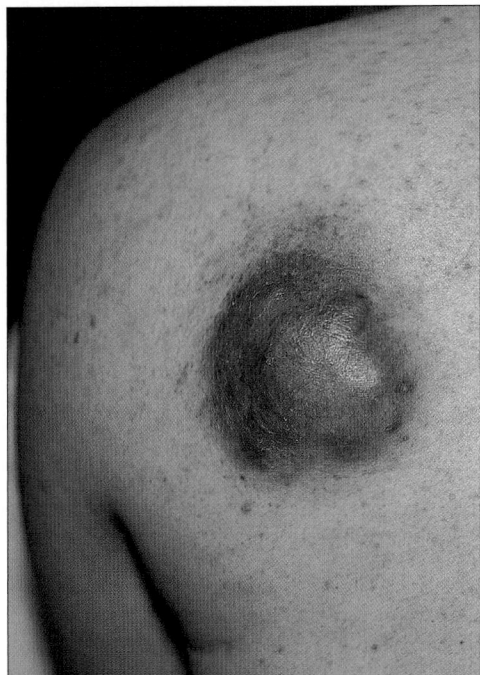

Fig. 151.9 Organized hematoma.

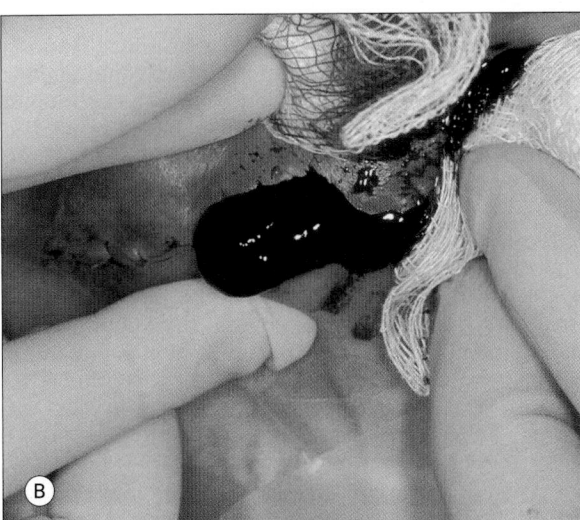

Fig. 151.8 Hematoma. A Postoperative hematoma formation. **B** Evacuation of hematoma.

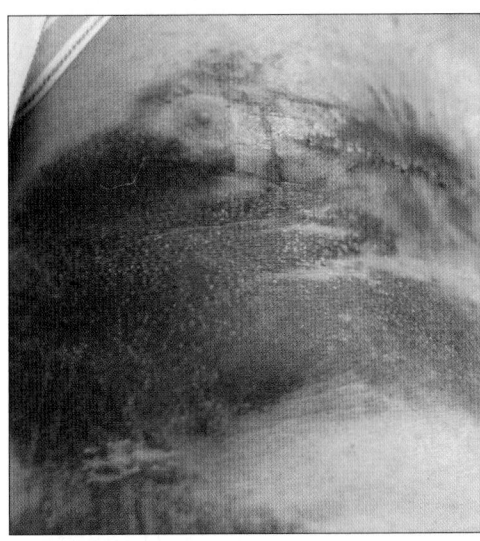

Fig. 151.10 Ecchymosis that has migrated to a dependent area of the lateral trunk.

If blood collects in the open space of a wound instead of seeping out through the wound edge, a hematoma forms. The presenting symptom may be an acute, throbbing pain if the hematoma is a large, expanding one. Smaller hematomas cause more of a pressure sensation. Early, expanding hematomas should be evacuated. Hematomas can lead to dehiscence or necrosis due to pressure, and they may act as a nidus for infection. Hematomas consist of gelatin-like clots that are usually too firm to evacuate without removing sutures (anesthetize the area first!). After evacuation (Fig. 151.8), the site should be irrigated and any residual bleeding controlled. The wound may be re-closed, with particular attention paid to closing any dead space. Placing a drain is often appropriate. Many surgeons advocate empirical antibiotics after hematoma evacuation, because of an increased risk of infection.

If the hematoma goes unnoticed and untreated for several days post surgery, the clot becomes organized (Fig. 151.9). It is then thick, fibrous, and adherent to the surrounding tissue. If large or actively expanding, it should still be evacuated. In most circumstances, the resulting wound should be allowed to heal by secondary intention with possible delayed closure, instead of primary closure.

Small, organized hematomas can be allowed to reabsorb without evacuation. If at around 1–2 weeks postoperatively there is significant liquefaction leading to a fluctuant mass, the fluid can be aspirated with a large bore (16–18-gauge) needle. Warm compresses applied for 30- to 60-minute intervals several times daily can speed resolution[43].

Bromelain, found in the pineapple plant, has been used as a medicinal for ages. One placebo-controlled study found that bromelain decreased the time required for resorption of surgery-associated hematoma. The recommended dose was 500 mg immediately postoperatively and then three to four times a day on an empty stomach until the hematoma resolved. Patients not allergic to pineapple reported no side effects[16].

Ecchymoses occur when there is leakage of a small amount of blood into the interstitial space. A bruised appearance is common following surgical procedures involving areas with loose distensible tissue, such as the periorbital areas or the upper chest in the elderly. It can be alarming to the patient who is not counseled to expect the possibility. The involved area changes in color from deep purple, black and blue, to green, then yellow as the hemoglobin is degraded to bilirubin. The ecchymosis can extend widely, usually migrating to dependent areas (Fig. 151.10). The concern is mainly cosmetic, and temporary, because most resolve with time and leave no sequelae.

Infection

Though most cases of infection begin at the time of surgery, postoperative contamination is possible if good wound care does not occur. Blood-soaked dressings are excellent breeding grounds for bacteria. The patient or caregiver should be instructed to wash their hands carefully prior to changing any dressings or cleaning the wound site. Excessive exposure or manipulation of the wound site during the first 24–48 hours after the procedure should be avoided.

As discussed previously, infection usually does not become evident until 4–8 days after surgery. The patient may note increasing erythema (Fig. 151.11). Instead of dissipating with time, pain and tenderness may increase. Ascending red streaks (lymphangitis), swelling, and a purulent discharge may develop. Systemic symptoms of fever and chills indicate spread of the infection.

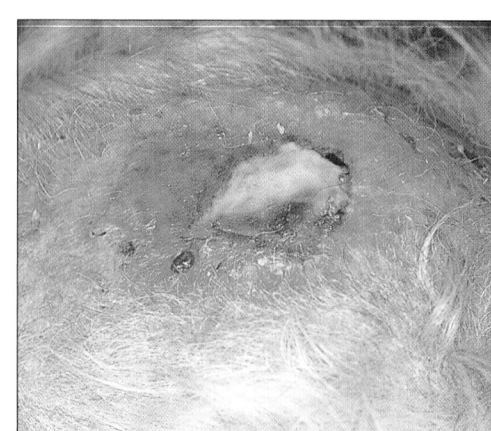

Fig. 151.11 Wound infection and necrosis at full-thickness skin graft site.

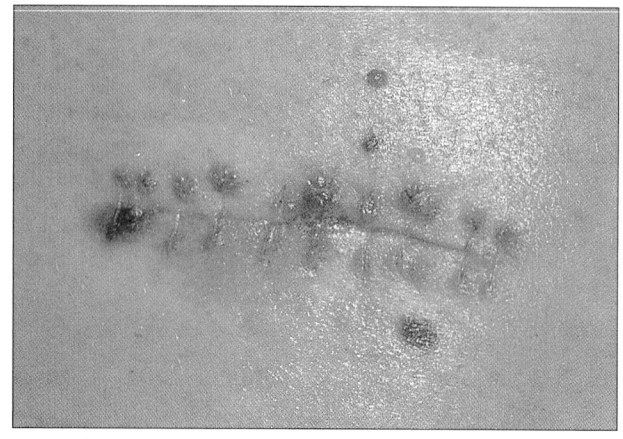

Fig. 151.13 Inflammatory suture reaction.

The area should be placed at rest, elevated, and heat applied. If the infection seems more than just mild, sutures should be removed and the defect left open. If an abscess is present, it should be drained. Deep cavities should be packed lightly with iodoform gauze. Packing needs to be changed daily until drainage stops. Discharge or exudate should be sent for Gram stain and culture. Antibiotics should be initiated based on the most likely causative organism(s) and a Gram stain if available. The choice of antibiotic should be adjusted as necessary once the culture results are available. *S. aureus* is the most frequent culprit in the skin. A first-generation cephalosporin or penicillinase-resistant penicillin would be an appropriate choice. If *Pseudomonas* is suspected, as in postoperative chondritis, a fluoroquinolone would be appropriate. If there is rapid spread, systemic symptoms, or extensive lymphangitis, the patient may need parenteral antibiotics, more aggressive wound care, and possible hospitalization.

Contact dermatitis, or candidal or dermatophyte infections, may mimic bacterial infection. Contact dermatitis due to topical antibiotics frequently presents with pruritus rather than pain and with erythema corresponding to all areas of ointment application rather than being confined to limited portions of the wound (Fig. 151.12). Contact dermatitis from bandage adhesives will usually be strikingly limited to the area of adhesive contact. Inflammatory suture reactions may occur without infection (Fig. 151.13).

Necrosis

The earliest sign of necrosis may be pallor. There may also be cyanosis at the periphery of the flap or graft. Early intervention could include judicious suture removal or replacement to reduce tension, elevation to reduce edema thereby improving blood flow, and gentle heat applied to the area to improve circulation. Treatment with hyperbaric oxygen may be appropriate in the face of early necrosis of a large or vital reconstruction[44].

Once necrosis is established, very minimal cleaning and debridement should be undertaken until the full extent of necrosis is clearly demarcated. More vigorous debridement may extend the process further. An eschar eventually forms and will separate from the wound base as it heals by secondary intention (Fig. 151.14). If infection is present, it should be treated appropriately. Delayed scar revision is an option if the site does not heal with an acceptable appearance.

Dehiscence

Wound edges can separate because of excessive tension, infection and necrosis (see Fig. 151.1). Dehiscence most often occurs at the time of suture removal, though it can certainly happen before or after. Patients are often under the mistaken impression that scar tissue is strong. In reality, tensile strength never exceeds 80% of the strength of uncut skin, and that level is not achieved until months after the procedure. At 2 weeks post surgery, tensile strength is less than 10% of normal (Fig. 151.15)[1]. Patient education must emphasize and re-emphasize this lack of tensile strength. Patients should be told specifically in which activities they may or may not engage (i.e. no lifting more than 'x' pounds, no running, no jogging, no sit-ups, etc.).

If prolonged support is needed, sutures may be removed in stages. Adhesive strips do provide some support after suture removal, but it is not long-lived. Count on no more than 1–2 days at best. If the wound opens at suture removal because of excessive tension or too much activity (Fig. 151.16), the surgeon can consider resuturing if there is no infection, hematoma or necrosis. If dehiscence is due to another underlying complication, such as infection or hematoma, that condition should be treated appropriately.

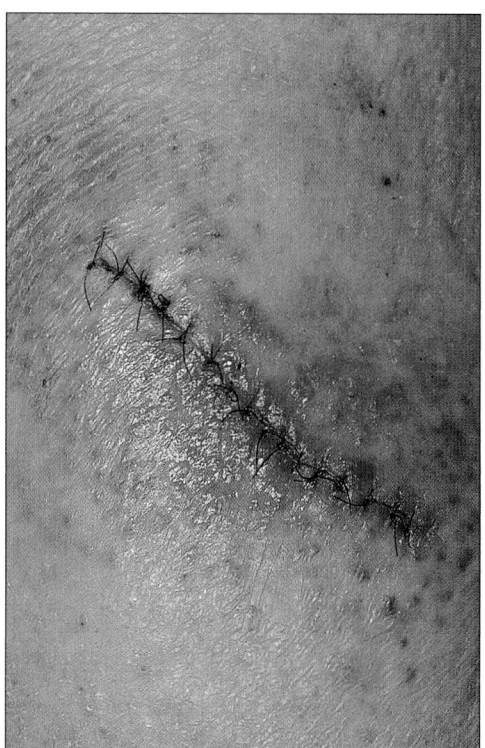

Fig. 151.12 Contact dermatitis to antibiotic ointment.

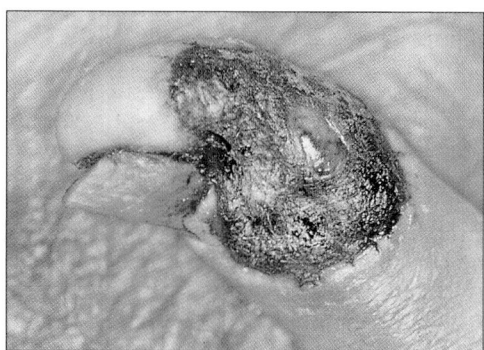

Fig. 151.14 Necrosis of a full-thickness skin graft. Two weeks after placement.

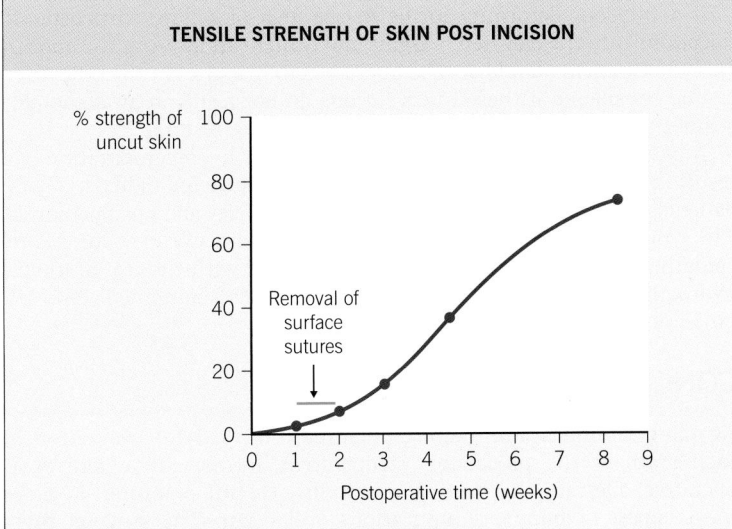

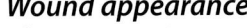

Fig. 151.15 Tensile strength of skin post incision.

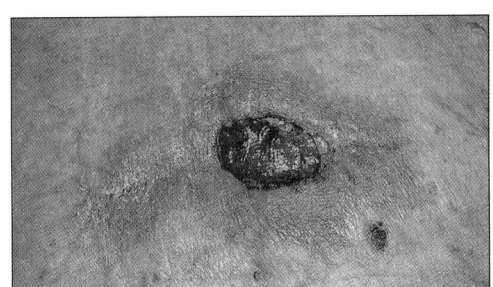

Fig. 151.16 Wound dehiscence after suture removal.

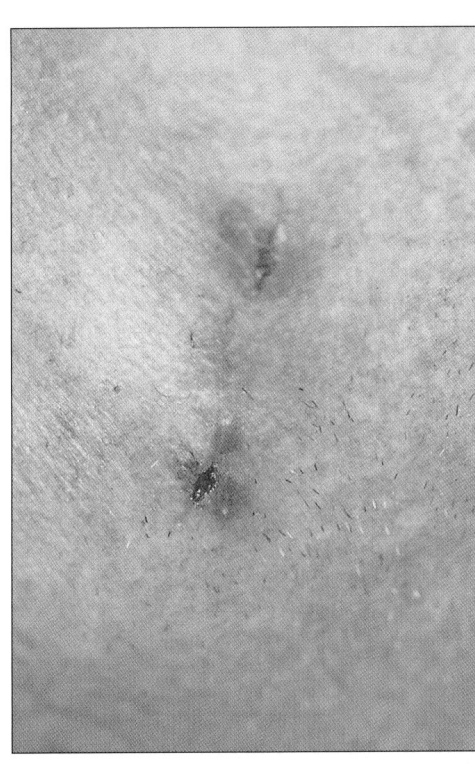

Fig. 151.17 Granulomatous reaction to suture placement.

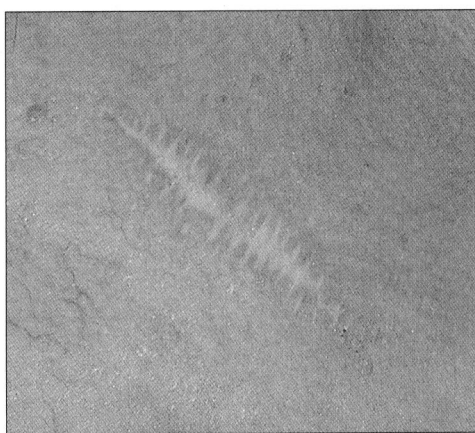

Fig. 151.18 Suture 'tracks' in a spread scar.

Wound appearance

The postoperative wound appearance may be a source of anxiety for both patient and surgeon. Problems may range from the simple (e.g. a spitting subcutaneous suture) to the more complex (e.g. a trapdoor deformity or spread scars). A key to dealing with most of these problems is continued communication between patient and surgeon. The patient who does not feel free to express concern or dissatisfaction in the office may all too readily do so in other places where the surgeon may not hear about it and cannot act to correct what can be corrected.

Buried sutures should be absorbed uneventfully by the body within the period of time specified by the manufacturer. Unfortunately, nature does not always adhere to package inserts. As digestion of the suture takes place, sterile abscesses may form as pustules along the suture track (Fig. 151.17). This event may occur anywhere from 1 to 4 months postoperatively, most commonly at about 6 weeks. The pustules can be opened with a sterile needle and the remaining suture gently removed. Sometimes, the papules are deeper. If the appearance is consistent with a suture reaction, reassure the patient that it is not a recurrence of malignancy, then instruct the patient to gently massage the site. Perform a biopsy if warranted. If the suture is protruding, it can be carefully removed. The ultimate appearance of the scar is usually unaffected by this process.

Suture tracks or railroad tracking is caused by tight sutures left in place too long (Fig. 151.18). The best way to avoid this appearance is planning to minimize wound tension and allow for early suture removal. Proper placement of buried sutures can help relieve wound edge tension.

Some anatomic sites are more prone to the development of keloids and hypertrophic scars (Fig. 151.19), and some individuals may have a genetic predisposition to keloid development. Keloids differ from hypertrophic scars by growing beyond the margins of the original wound (see Ch. 98). Intervention at the early stages of a hypertrophic scar can yield a more acceptable result. High-potency topical corticosteroids or intralesional corticosteroids may decrease the thickness of the scar and the accompanying symptoms of pain and pruritus. However, there is a risk of telangiectasias, atrophy or widening of the scar. Smaller hypertrophic scars may respond to simple massage. Silicone gel sheeting applied to

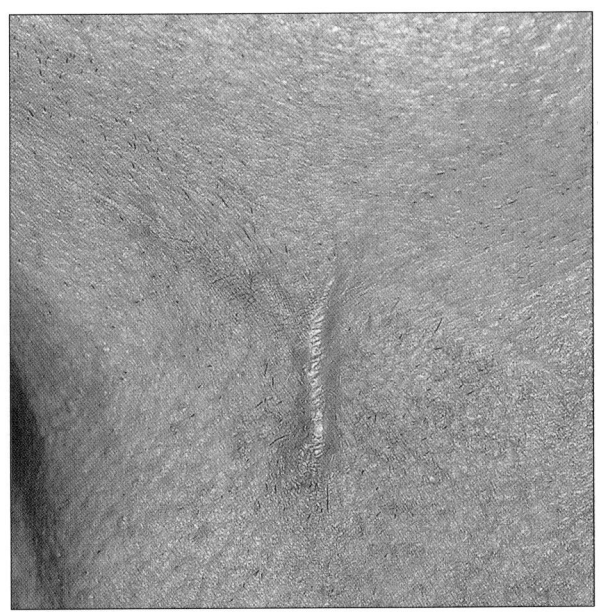

Fig. 151.19 Hypertrophic scar. One month after excisional surgery.

the scars and worn for 12–24 hours per day for at least 2 months has been shown to improve the appearance of hypertrophic scars and keloids[45]. Simple occlusion and hydration may be just as effective without silicone[46]. One study using topical onion extract found that it was ineffective in improving erythema or pruritus of postsurgical scars, while petrolatum-based ointment alone did improve appearance[47].

Scar appearance can also be improved by dermabrasion. When performed during the 4–8-week interval following the initial injury, it superimposes the mechanisms of second intention wound healing on the remodeling phase of the primary scar. This in turn appears to re-establish a normal-appearing epidermis across initial scar boundaries[48]. Lasers such as the pulsed carbon dioxide (CO_2) and the 585-nm pulsed dye laser, or a combination of both, are also used in the treatment of hypertrophic scars and keloids[49,50].

Keloids tend to develop more frequently on the earlobes, neck and trunk. In predisposed individuals, especially those with a personal or family history of keloid formation, even superficial shave biopsies can result in keloid formation. Patients at risk should be counseled about this risk prior to the procedure. There are several treatment modalities used for keloids, with varying degrees of success (see Ch. 98).

Even well-approximated wound edges can produce spread scars. Like hypertrophic scars and keloids, they are more prevalent in certain anatomic areas such as the back, chest and shoulders. Patients who need excisions in these areas should be counseled preoperatively about the possibility that what may initially appear as a thin scar may widen over time. Most of this process occurs within 6 months after the surgery.

If a trapdoor deformity forms in the area of a flap, corticosteroid injections into the elevated margins and center can improve the appearance. The patient should also be instructed to massage the area. Revision can be considered if these interventions do not result in an acceptable cosmetic result. Patience often produces the best results.

Anytime the epidermis is injured, hyper- or hypopigmentation can result. This is more pronounced in dark-skinned individuals. Again, patients should be warned about this possibility pre- and postoperatively. The wound site should be strictly protected from UV exposure. Early epidermal hyperpigmentation can be improved with the use of topical hydroquinones, though this is ineffective unless combined with UV protection.

CONCLUSIONS

Avoiding complications requires planning and careful evaluation at each stage of the procedure: preoperative, intraoperative and postoperative. Despite the best of intentions, careful planning, and the most expert of hands, complications still occur. The surgeon must learn from experience and the experience of others, to improve patient care. Finally, the surgeon must always remember to treat the patient, not just the condition. The patient's expectations and concerns must be addressed, not simply the surgeon's. Like beauty, complications are in the eye of the beholder. The patient who feels abandoned by his or her physician may not be happy with any outcome, no matter how technically perfect.

REFERENCES

1. Stasko T. Complications of cutaneous procedures. In: Roenigk RK, Roenigk HH Jr (eds). Dermatologic Surgery Principles and Practice, 2nd edn. New York: Marcel Dekker,1996;149–75.
2. Fader DJ, Johnson TM. Medical issues and emergencies in the dermatologic office. J Am Acad Dermatol. 1997;36:1–16.
3. Bennett RG. Fundamentals of Cutaneous Surgery. St Louis: Mosby, 1988:553–90.
4. Peterson SR, Joseph AK. Inherited bleeding disorders in dermatologic surgery. Dermatol Surg. 2001;27:885–9.
5. Selva-Nayagam PA, Hill DC. Preoperative assessment of the elderly patient. J Geriatr Dermatol. 1996;4:169–78.
6. Harrison P. Progress in the assessment of platelet function. Br J Haematol. 2000;111:733–44.
7. Vora A, Makris M. An approach to investigation of easy bruising. Arch Dis Child. 2001;84:488–91.
8. Maloney ME. Management of surgical complications and suboptimal results. In: Wheeland RG (ed.). Cutaneous Surgery. Philadelphia: WB Saunders, 1994:921–34.
9. Otley CC. Continuation of medically necessary aspirin and warfarin during cutaneous surgery. Mayo Clin Proc. 2003;78:1392–6.
10. Kovich O, Otley CC. Thrombotic complications related to discontinuation of warfarin and aspirin therapy perioperatively for cutaneous operation. J Am Acad Dermatol. 2003;48:233–7.
11. Salasche SJ. Acute surgical complications: cause, prevention, and treatment. J Am Acad Dermatol. 1986;15:1163–85.
12. Alcalay J, Alkalay R. Controversies in perioperative management of blood thinners in dermatologic surgery: continue or discontinue? Dermatol Surg. 2004;30:1091–4.
13. Caliendo FJ, Halpern VJ, Marini CP, et al. Warfarin anticoagulation in the perioperative period: is it safe? Ann Vasc Surg. 1999;13:11–16.
14. Campbell JH, Alvarado F, Murray RA. Anticoagulation and minor oral surgery: should the anticoagulation regimen be altered? J Oral Maxillofacial Surg. 2000;58:131–5.
15. Bithell TC. Blood coagulation. In: Lee RG (ed.). Wintrobe's Clinical Haematology. Philadelphia: Lea & Febiger, 1993:566–615.
16. Dinehart SM, Henry L. Dietary supplements: altered coagulation and effects on bruising. Dermatol Surg. 2005;31:819–26.
17. Deykin D, Janson P, McMahon L. Ethanol potentiation of aspirin-induced prolongation of the bleeding time. N Engl J Med. 1982;306:852.
18. Smith JB, Fenske NA. Cutaneous manifestations and consequences of smoking. J Am Acad Dermatol. 1996;34:733–4.
19. Rubenstein R, Roenigk HH Jr, Stegman SJ, Hanke CW. Atypical keloids after dermabrasion of patients taking isotretinoin. J Am Acad Dermatol. 1986;15:280–5.
20. Zachariaeae H. Delayed wound healing and keloid formation following argon laser treatment or dermabrasion during isotretinoin treatment. Br J Dermatol. 1988;118:703–6.
21. Bernstein LJ, Geronemus RG. Keloid formation with the 585-nm pulsed dye laser during isotretinoin treatment. Arch Dermatol. 1997;133:111–13.
22. Roenigk RK. Chemical peel with trichloroacetic acid. In: Roenigk RK, Roenigk HH Jr (eds). Dermatologic Surgery Principles and Practice, 2nd edn. New York: Marcel Dekker, 1996:1121–35.
23. Haas AF, Grekin RC. Antibiotic prophylaxis in dermatologic surgery. J Am Acad Dermatol. 1995;32:155–76.
24. Maragh SL, Otley CC, Roenigk RK, Phillips PK. Antibiotic prophylaxis in dermatologic surgery: updated guidelines. Dermatol Surg. 2005;31:83–93.
25. LeVasseur JG, Kennard CD, Finley EM, Muse RK. Dermatologic electrosurgery in patients with implantable cardioverter-defibrillators and pacemakers. Dematol Surg. 1998;24:233–40.
26. El-Gamal HM, Dufresne RG, Saddler KS. Electrosurgery, pacemakers and ICDs: a survey of precautions and complications experienced by cutaneous surgeons. Dermatol Surg. 2001;27:385–90.
27. Skidmore RA, Patterson JD, Tomsick RS. Local anesthetics. Dermatol Surg. 1996;22:511–22.
28. Thomas RM, Amonette RA. Emergencies in skin surgery. In: Roenigk RK, Roenigk HH Jr (eds). Dermatologic Surgery Principles and Practice, 2nd edn. New York: Marcel Dekker,1996:77–89.
29. Vance JW. Anesthesia. In: Roenigk RK, Roenigk HH Jr (eds). Dermatologic Surgery Principles and Practice, 2nd edn. New York: Marcel Dekker,1996:31–9.
30. Ljunggren B, Moller H. Eczematous contact allergy to chlorhexidine. Acta Dermatol. 1972;52:308–10.
31. Marks JG. Allergic contact dermatitis due to povidone-iodine. J Am Acad Dermatol. 1982;6:473.
32. Smack DP, Harrington AC, Dunn C, et al. Infection and allergy incidence in ambulatory surgery patients with white petroleum versus bacitracin ointment. A randomized controlled trial. JAMA. 1996;276:972–7.
33. Takegami KT, Siegle RJ, Ayers LW. Microbiologic counts during outpatient office-based cutaneous surgery. J Am Acad Dermatol. 1990;23:1149.
34. Sebben JE. Surgical preparation, facilities, and monitoring. In: Roenigk RK, Roenigk HH Jr (eds). Dermatologic Surgery Principles and Practice, 2nd edn. New York: Marcel Dekker, 1996:1–24.
35. Haas AF. Antisepsis. In: Robinson JK, Arndt KA, Leboit PE, Wintroub BU (eds). Atlas of Cutaneous Surgery. Philadelphia: WB Saunders, 1996:27–31.
36. Billingsley EM, Maloney ME. Considerations in achieving hemostasis. In: Robinson JK, Arndt KA, Leboit PE, Wintroub BU (eds). Atlas of Cutaneous Surgery. Philadelphia: WB Saunders, 1996:67–73.
37. Greenbaum SS, Greenbaum CH. Intraoperative tissue expansion using a Foley catheter following excision of a basal cell carcinoma. J Dermatol Surg Oncol. 1990;16:45–8.
38. Bernstein G. The loop stitch. J Dermatol Surg Oncol. 1984;10:587.
39. Tromovitch TA, Stegman SJ, Glogau RG. Flaps and Grafts in Dermatologic Surgery. Chicago: Year Book Medical, 1989:1–6.
40. Salasche SJ, Bernstein G, Senkarik M. Surgical Anatomy of the Skin. Norwalk: Appleton & Lange, 1988:100–25.
41. McDonald M, Stasko T. Prevention of unsatisfactory scarring. In: Harahap M (ed.). Surgical Techniques for Cutaneous Scar Revision. New York: Marcel Dekker, 2000:53–80.
42. Kaufman AJ, Kene KL, Moy RL. Role of tissue undermining in the trapdoor effect of transposition flaps. J Dermatol Surg Oncol. 1993;19:128–32.
43. Robinson JK. Management of hematomas. In: Robinson JK, Arndt KA, Leboit PE, Wintroub BU (eds). Atlas of Cutaneous Surgery. Philadelphia: WB Saunders, 1996:73–7.
44. Pellitteri PK, Kennedy TL, Youn BA. The influence of intensive hyperbaric oxygen therapy on skin flap survival in a swine model. Arch Otolaryngol. 1992;118:1050–4.
45. Berman B, Flores F. Comparison of a silicone gel-filled cushion and silicone gel sheeting treatment of hypertrophic or keloid scars. Dermatol Surg. 1999;24:484–6.
46. Ricketts CH, Martin L, Faria DT, et al. Cytokine mRNA changes during the treatment of hypertrophic scans with silicone and nonsilicone gel dressings. Dermatol Surg. 1996;22:955–9.
47. Jackson BA, Shelton AJ. Pilot study evaluating topical onion extract as treatment for post surgical scars. Dermatol Surg. 1999;25:267–90.

48. Harmon CB, Yarborough JM. Scar revision by dermabrasion. In: Roenigk RK, Roenigk HH Jr (eds). Dermatologic Surgery Principles and Practice, 2nd edn. New York: Marcel Dekker,1996:911–21.

49. Alster TS, Lewis AB, Rosenbach A. Laser scar revision: comparison of CO_2 laser vaporization with simultaneous pulsed dye laser treatment. Dermatol Surg. 1998;24:1299–302.

50. Alster TS, Handrick C. Laser treatment of hypertrophic scars, keloids, and striae. Semin Cutan Med Surg. 2000;19:287–92.

Systematic Evaluation of the Aging Face

Richard G Glogau

With advancing years, an aged appearance becomes a presenting complaint. There is a kind of cognitive dissonance when one looks in the mirror, a sense of unhappiness with one's appearance that may reflect:

- competitive job pressures
- divorce and return to dating
- the barrage of advertising media
- wider availability of cosmetic services
- higher discretionary income
- less social stigma surrounding cosmetic rejuvenation procedures
- an explosion of medical and surgical technology.

In Nancy Etcoff's book, *Survival of the Prettiest: The Science of Beauty*, the author states that people tend to respond positively to good-looking people without expectation of reward, and, further, that good-looking people tend to get away with everything from shoplifting to cheating at exams[1]. It is Etcoff's thesis that there are 'hard-wired' responses in human beings that make them respond in predictable ways to beauty in the human face and form. What are the characteristics of beauty in the human face?

THE GENDER DIFFERENCES

While there are exceptions to every rule, the idealized female face tends to exhibit several characteristics that are reproducible from culture to culture and across the ages. In contrast, the attractive masculine face tends to have a very different set of characteristics. These facial features are summarized in Table 152.1.

As the human face ages, one can see a change in all of the anatomic compartments of the face, starting on the outside with the skin and proceeding inwardly to the subcutaneous fat, the underlying musculature, and, finally, even the bony structures. All contribute to the aging appearance in one way or another. By utilizing a systematic approach, an analysis of the aging face can be made that will aid in a rational selection of therapies as well as clarify the points that need to be communicated to patients seeking cosmetic enhancement.

ANATOMIC BASIS FOR AGING APPEARANCE

Too often, patients encounter physicians who have developed a preference for one therapeutic 'hammer', and the patients all become 'nails'. Failure to match a given therapeutic technique to the underlying anatomic basis for the cosmetic problem leads to mediocre results at best and disasters at worst. By knowing the risk:benefit ratio for a given procedure, and communicating this information to the patient, the physician can successfully complete the cosmetic consultation visit.

Among medical professionals there still exists a great deal of confusion, given that, on a regular basis, patients with particular anatomic defects are being matched with the wrong therapeutic procedure. Examples include:

- patients with severe, chronic sun damage having facelifts instead of resurfacing
- patients with jowls and platysmal banding of the neck undergoing liposuction without redraping the superficial musculoaponeurotic system (SMAS) and skin
- patients gaunt with aging lipoatrophy being subjected to laser resurfacing and rhytidectomy, without addressing their subcutaneous volume, producing a skeletonized appearance
- patients with deep glabellar furrows being treated with injectable fillers, but without botulinum toxin to paralyze the intrinsic muscles producing the frown.

In some cases, evolving medical knowledge has made once-standard therapies passé. For example, in the past, blepharoplasty for the lower eyelids routinely included removal of infraorbital fat. Nowadays, the fat is more commonly repositioned medially to fill the 'tear trough' and is not routinely removed, especially in younger patients. Considered in turn, each anatomic compartment lends itself to some therapy, individually or combined with other therapies, to give the desired aesthetic effect.

PHOTOAGING

Cumulative exposure to sunlight remains the largest factor in aging skin, and it is responsible for a large portion of the unwanted aesthetic changes. Clinical signs of cutaneous photoaging include: rhytides, lentigines, keratoses, telangiectasia, loss of translucency, loss of elasticity, and sallow color[2,3].

A simple systematic classification of patient photoaging types (types I through IV) has been developed by the author (Table 152.2 & Fig. 152.1)[4]. The generalizations outlined in Table 152.2, and explained below, apply at different ages and to different degrees in more darkly pigmented skin, partially depending upon the degree of sun exposure. Younger patients, usually in their third or fourth decade, have only the earliest signs of photoaging, primarily a change in homogeneity of color. In general, these individuals have no rhytides at all, even when the face is animated by talking or expression, and they are categorized as type I, 'no wrinkles'.

As the patient ages, cumulative UV damage to the dermal elastic fibers becomes more marked, and the inherent 'snap back' quality of the skin becomes impaired. Wrinkles begin to appear, at first only when the face is in motion, usually as expression lines parallel to the melolabial fold, at the corners of the mouth, in the lateral canthal areas, and over the zygomatic arch and malar eminences. These patients are commonly in their 30's or 40's, and look unlined when their face is at rest. However, as soon as they begin to talk, the lines appear. They are

GENDER DIFFERENCES IN CHARACTERISTICS OF ATTRACTIVE HUMAN FACES	
Idealized female facial features	**Idealized male facial features**
A larger, smooth forehead with a smaller nose	An overhanging, horizontal brow with minimal arch
Eyebrows that have an arch or gull-wing shape	Deeper set eyes that look closer together
Eyes that are set wider apart, creating a bigger look	A somewhat larger nose
Prominent cheekbones	A wider mouth
A heart-shaped taper to the lower face, with a smaller lower:upper face ratio	A squared lower face with a more equal ratio of lower:upper face
Full vermilion lips	A beard or coarser texture to the lower facial skin

Table 152.1 Gender differences in characteristics of attractive human faces. These characteristics are cross-culturally persistent.

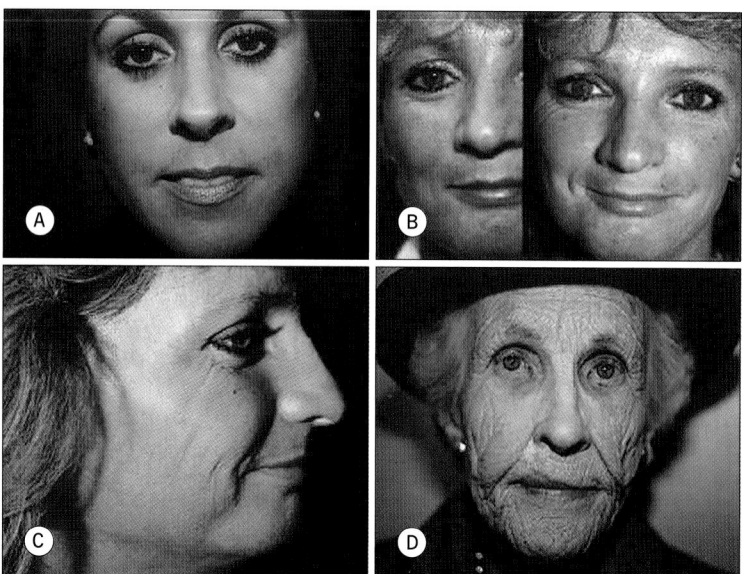

Fig. 152.1 The Glogau wrinkle scale. A Type I ('no wrinkles'): skin is uniform in color. There is an absence of lines even at the corners of the eyes and mouth. **B** Type II ('wrinkles in motion'): when the face is at rest, the patient appears similar to type I. But when the face is animated by expression, there are many parallel lines which appear, first at the corners of the mouth, then parallel to the melolabial folds, then at the corners of the eyes, and finally over the malar cheeks. **C** Type III ('wrinkles at rest'): this patient clearly shows the parallel lines seen with animation in type II, except they are now present with the face at complete rest. **D** Type IV ('only wrinkles'): the perioral skin in particular is likely to demonstrate the total replacement of normal skin with minute, rhomboid and geometric rhytides, clearly seen in this patient. The entire face shows similar rhytides on close inspection.

GLOGAU PHOTOAGING CLASSIFICATION – WRINKLE SCALE
Type I – 'no wrinkles'

• Early photoaging
  – Mild pigmentary changes
  – No keratoses
  – Minimal wrinkles
• Patient age (yrs) – 20's or 30's
• Minimal or no makeup

Type II – 'wrinkles in motion'

• Early to moderate photoaging
  – Early senile lentigines visible
  – Keratoses palpable but not visible
  – Parallel smile lines beginning to appear
• Patient age (yrs) – late 30's or 40's
• Usually wears some foundation

Type III – 'wrinkles at rest'

• Advanced photoaging
  – Obvious dyschromia, telangiectasia
  – Visible keratoses
  – Wrinkles even when not moving facial muscles
• Patient age (yrs) – 50's or older
• Wears heavy foundation

Type IV – 'only wrinkles'

• Severe photoaging
  – Yellow–gray color of skin
  – Prior skin malignancies
  – Wrinkled throughout with no normal skin
• Patient age (yrs) – 60's to 70's
• Can't wear makeup – 'cakes and cracks'

Table 152.2 Glogau photoaging classification – wrinkle scale.

classified as type II, 'wrinkles in motion'. These patients demonstrate the influence the underlying musculature has on the skin, a critical consideration when contemplating the use of botulinum toxin (see Ch. 159).

As the photoaging process advances, damage to the elastic fibers becomes more severe. Eventually, the wrinkles produced by dynamic movement of the face persist, even when the face is at rest. Generally by the sixth or older decade of life, there are visible parallel lines lateral to the eye ('crow's feet'), at the corners of the mouth, and radiating down from the lower eyelids onto the malar cheeks, as well as across the upper lip and lower lip. These patients appear lined, even when their face is at rest, and are classified as type III, 'wrinkles at rest'. The repetitive effect of underlying muscular expression is now permanently 'ironed' into the skin as the passive bystander, i.e. lines are readily visible, even without active muscular contraction.

With continued photoaging, the wrinkles gradually spread to cover the majority of the facial skin, while the dermis becomes totally engorged with accumulations of poorly staining ground substance, giving a thickened, coarse quality to the skin. Usually this occurs by the seventh decade of life, but it happens earlier in the most severely affected individuals. Many of these patients have already had one or more skin cancers. They really have no unlined skin anywhere on their face, and are classified as type IV, 'only wrinkles'.

PIGMENTARY SYSTEM

Patients should also be categorized according to their Fitzpatrick Sun-Reactive Skin Type[5]. This classification scheme (see Table 134.3) is based upon the skin's response to erythema-producing doses of UV light. Patients differ in their reactivity to sunlight, and the skin type serves as a very good indicator of the potential for developing dyschromia following epidermal/papillary dermal injury. The scale also reflects the likelihood of developing postinflammatory hyperpigmentation during the near-term postoperative period, and the potential for permanent leukoderma resulting from destruction of melanocytes.

As part of the evaluation of each patient, the degree of photodamage present and the pigmentary UV response can be assessed and then expressed in a shorthand fashion. A patient who is a Fitzpatrick III, Glogau photoaging III is a very different candidate for resurfacing than is a Fitzpatrick I, Glogau photoaging II person. The risk:benefit ratios are entirely different in these two patients and the presence of lines and wrinkles alone is not necessarily a sufficient indication for resurfacing.

As a general rule, patients with Fitzpatrick skin types I–III will tolerate resurfacing without significant risk of color change. While resurfacing may be undertaken in Fitzpatrick skin types IV–VI, the risk of pigmentary change is certainly high enough such that the patient should be warned there could be color change in the treated skin.

THE LOSS OF SUBCUTANEOUS FAT

A major component of aesthetic disharmony in the aging face is the loss or redistribution of subcutaneous fat. While in some areas (e.g. the submental region), unwanted subcutaneous fat may lend itself to removal via liposuction, in general there is a modern appreciation that removal of fat should be done with caution because of the flattening or hollowing of contours that may occur. Aging produces a profound loss of subcutaneous fat in the forehead, temporal fossae, premalar areas, chin, and perioral area (Fig. 152.2). The older face has a flattened quality to the cheekbones, a sunken appearance to the lips, a bulging of the inferior fat pads of the eye, and, in general, a loss of the fullness and roundness of youth. Experienced plastic surgeons have recognized this, and are moving away from excessive fat removal to fat repositioning or augmentation. Dr Steven Hoefflin has written, 'in the aging face it is not the tightness of the SMAS (platysma aponeurosis) or skin that makes the difference, but the quantity and position of subcutaneous fat'[6].

As an example, the routine removal of the infraorbital fat as a part of blepharoplasty, which often accentuated the deep grooves between the lower eyelid and the cheek, has become outdated. Now surgeons prefer to utilize an arcus marginalis release and mobilize the fat medially and anteriorly to fill in the groove and return a more youthful appearance to the lower eyelids through restoration of lower lid convexity. Similarly, repositioning of the premalar fat has become an important part of routine facelifting, reversing the aged appearance that comes from flattening of the cheekbone contours.

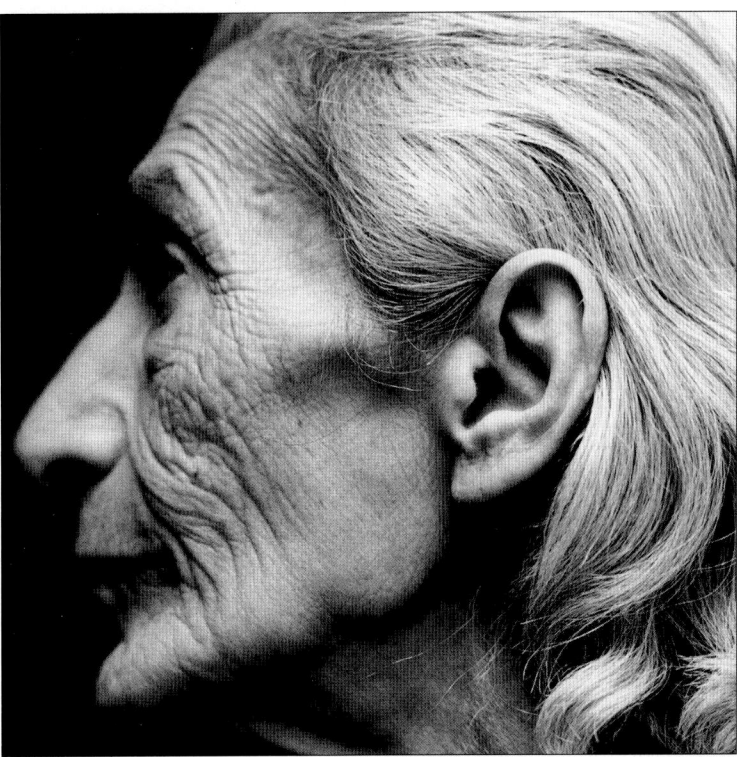

Fig. 152.2 Fat and cartilaginous changes in the aging face. Here we see the ravages of time expressed as loss of almost all the subcutaneous fat, especially of the brow, temple, cheek, chin and perioral area. There is distinct elongation of the cartilaginous structures of the nose leading to a drooping tip as well as a loss of bone (from bony resorption) giving rise to a 'witch's chin' appearance. General sag of the superficial musculoaponeurotic system (SMAS) leads to the overall impression of drooping, sagging skin. From Tan SR, Glogau RG. Filler Esthetics. In: Carruthers J, Carruthers A (eds.): Soft Tissue Augmentation. Philadelphia: Elsevier Saunders, 2005, p. 15.

The ultimate recognition of the importance of the subcutaneous volume of the face comes from the work of surgeons like Fournier, Coleman, Amar and others, who have evolved techniques of fat transfer to restore the volume contours of the aged face. Microlipoinjection in small and larger volumes, placed subcutaneously and intramuscularly, has been used with great success to reshape the aging face. While difficulties remain in the predictability and longevity of fat transfers, the aesthetic effects are often impressive because of the naturalness of the resulting appearance.

The restoration of loss of volume explains the appeal of injectable fillers such as collagen, hyaluronic acid gel, polylactic acid, and micro-droplet silicone (see Ch. 158)[7]. Within the field of aesthetic medicine today, lip augmentation via injectables remains one of the most frequently requested cosmetic procedures. The market is literally over-flowing with new, injectable agents and alloplastic implants.

Analysis of the aging face must include an assessment of the quality and position of the subcutaneous fat. Are the lips thin? Have they lost their shape? Are the cheekbones flattened? Is there wasting in the temporal fossae, above the eyebrows, or in the buccal pads? Resurfacing and/or facelifting will not address these problems, and may actually exacerbate their effects (Fig. 152.3).

CHANGES IN FACIAL MUSCULATURE

Perhaps nothing has driven home the impact of facial musculature on facial aging like the introduction of botulinum toxin for selective chemical denervation of muscles of the face. Paralysis or partial weaken-ing of the glabellar corrugator/procerus complex, the forehead frontalis muscle, and the lateral orbicularis muscles has revolutionized the management of the upper third of the aging face.

Deep glabellar lines, which in the past could only briefly be improved with injectable fillers, now melt away with the placement of botulinum toxin in the corrugator/procerus complex (Fig. 152.4). Crow's feet lines, which routinely reappeared after deep resurfacing, now vanish in a few days. Even the troublesome horizontal lines and creases of the lower eyelid, which persisted after blepharoplasty and/or resurfacing, can now be treated with botulinum toxin. The toxin is both safe and temporary and it has now become a standard therapy in cosmetic surgery[8].

Understanding the psychosocial impact of the position of the eyebrows requires a closer look at the unspoken effects of brow position (Table 152.3). Brow position is closely associated with emotional states, and the medial and lateral portions of the brow function independently in this regard. Surgeons must be conscious of the strong impact that brow shape and position can have on appearance and even the inter-personal relationships that Dr Etcoff has described. That is, people tend to treat you better if you do not have a glabellar scowl, if your eyebrows

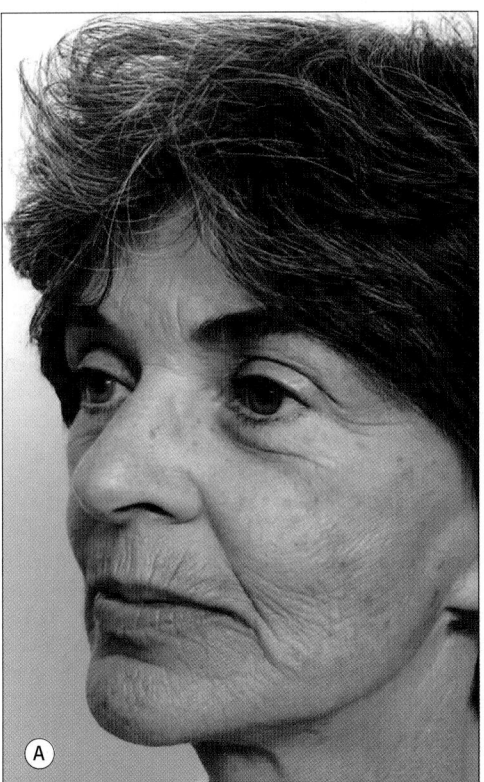

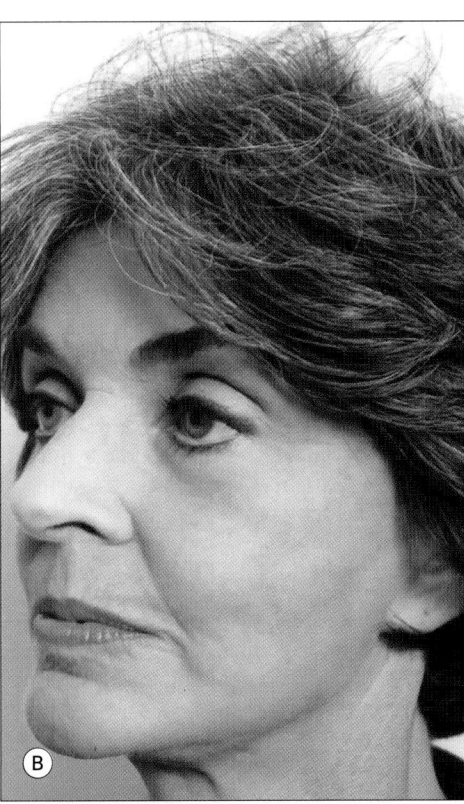

Fig. 152.3 Laser resurfacing. This patient has undergone laser resurfacing to her full face. She looks 'better' but not 'younger', because no attention has been paid to volume changes.

A

B

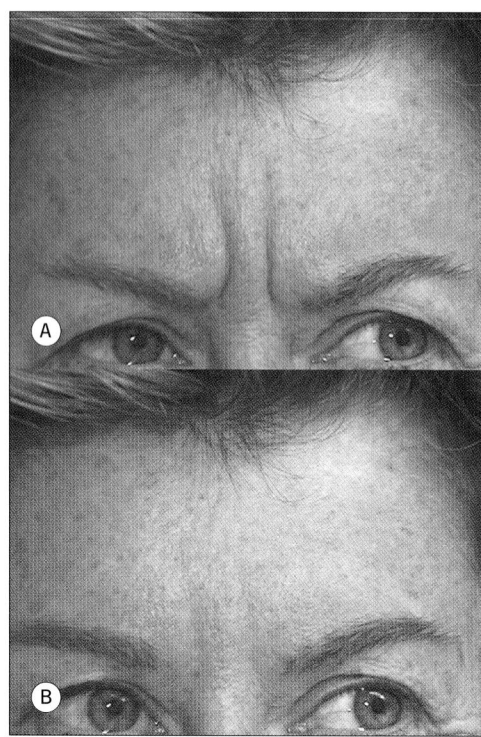

Fig. 152.4 Facial musculature: glabellar frown lines. This patient demonstrates the glabellar muscular complex at maximum frown before (**A**) and after (**B**) treatment with botulinum toxin A.

RELATIONSHIP OF EMOTIONAL STATES WITH BROW POSITIONS			
Medial brow up	Medial brow down	Lateral brow up	Lateral brow down
Expectant	Tired	Surprised	Disapproving
Quizzical	Stern	Elated	Sad
Curious	Angry	Happy	Fatigue
Anticipatory	Unhappy	Approving	Anxious
Friendly	Mystified	Excited	Disappointed
Serene	Puzzled	Alert	Forlorn
Knowing	Worried		Disdainful

Table 152.3 Relationship of emotional states with brow positions.

arch properly (if you are female), and if the relationship between the lateral and medial brow is flattering.

The most striking example of the importance brow position can have on perceived appearance is the development of brow ptosis with age. The most common problem in the patient's own analysis of his or her aging face is the inability to relate the hooding of the upper eyelid skin to malposition of the brows and forehead. How many patients ask for (and receive) upper lid blepharoplasty when the source of their problem is ptosis of the upper brow and forehead?

Overzealous use of botulinum toxin in the upper third of the face routinely produces brow ptosis, a feeling of 'heaviness', and a slightly Neanderthal appearance, because the older forehead does not have the inherent resiliency to maintain any brow position without the support of the underlying frontalis muscle. On the other hand, the surgeon who inappropriately elevates the brow to a position improper for the patient's gender or age also does the patient no favor. The quality of elasticity of the skin and soft tissue must be taken into account before attempting to address the position of the brow, either surgically or with botulinum toxin.

INHERENT LOSS OF ELASTICITY

As the facial soft tissue ages, both the skin and the underlying supporting structures, while sagging under the effects of gravity, lose their inherent resiliency or ability to resist stretching.

In the lower third of the face, a facelift procedure is often essential for a successful aesthetic outcome. Redraping, repositioning, and judicious removal of skin and soft tissue that has lost its elasticity can lead to the restoration of a youthful appearance that cannot be achieved with resurfacing, fillers, fat transfer or botulinum toxin. While, in truth, many of these other techniques when properly applied have made it possible for patients to delay and defray the aging process, virtually no one escapes the effects of gravity and the loss of intrinsic elasticity. The facelift procedure is not in danger of extinction, though it now requires more selective application and execution that is mindful of the other components of aging discussed above.

CHANGES IN UNDERLYING CARTILAGE AND BONE

Due to changes in the underlying cartilage, the aging nose elongates and the tip droops. The aging mouth is affected by bony remodeling of the maxilla, while the chin sharpens and protrudes. The ears appear to lengthen as the lobes droop. The tarsal plate softens and no longer holds the lower lid margin in its proper position or curve. Various surgical procedures address these problems: tip rhinoplasty, tarsal lid tightening, canthoplasty, etc. Newer dental implant procedures and maxillofacial surgery can address intrinsic changes affecting the lower face.

The diagnostic eye of the cosmetic surgeon should not overlook the contribution of the underlying hard structures of the face, particularly when assessing for the presence (or, more commonly, absence) of facial symmetry. Patients often present with requests for the treatment of facial problems without appreciating the contribution of underlying structures to their facial asymmetry. Although subtle, the asymmetry is not due to the soft tissue. As a practical example, no amount of collagen is going to correct an underlying difference in the maxillary structure of the cheekbones.

These pre-existing aspects of facial asymmetry need to be identified so they can be shown to the patient and discussed. Too many patients become dissatisfied with their facelift results and then rail against their surgeons when it is their underlying facial bony structures that are the root cause of the facial asymmetry. Recognizing pre-existing facial asymmetry due to underlying bony or cartilaginous structural differences is an important component of setting realistic patient expectations. One exercise is to have patients carefully examine their earlobes to demonstrate the reality of presurgical asymmetry.

COMBINATION THERAPIES

Optimal improvement in appearance can more often be obtained by combining procedures. At one end of the therapeutic spectrum, topical agents such as tretinoin, α-hydroxy acids, hydroquinone and 5-fluorouracil can inhibit or reverse UV irradiation-associated changes in aging skin. At the other end of the therapeutic spectrum, rhytidectomy, blepharoplasty, brow lift, and suction-assisted lipectomy often provide dramatic results in facial rejuvenation. The choice of specific therapies rests on the ability of the surgeon to look at the face, analyze the anatomic components of the aging appearance, and then prioritize them, matching the risk:benefit ratios of various procedures to each element. Is the predominant problem sun damage, sagging or loss of volume? Often there are overriding constraints, e.g. the 'down time', surgical risk, cost and likelihood of benefit, that all weigh in on the selection of the appropriate therapy. However, underlying all of these choices must be a rational analysis of the various elements that comprise the aging face.

THE NEW PARADIGM

The new paradigm for facial rejuvenation is the four R's: relax, refill, redrape and resurface. By using a systematic anatomic approach to the aging face, the surgeon can quickly and astutely match the individual 'R' to the underlying problem. The more specifically the chosen therapies address the anatomic defects, the better the outcome and the happier the patient.

REFERENCES

1. Etcoff N. Survival of the Prettiest: the Science of Beauty. New York: Doubleday, 1999.
2. Balin A, Pratt L. Physiological consequences of human skin aging. Cutis. 1989;43:431–6.
3. Montagna W, Carlisle K, Kirchner S. Epidermal and Dermal Histological Markers of Photodamaged Human Facial Skin. Shelton: Richardson-Vicks, 1988.
4. Glogau RG. Chemical peeling and aging skin. J Geriatr Dermatol. 1994;2:30–5.
5. Fitzpatrick T. The validity and practicality of sun-reactive skin types I through VI. Arch Dermatol. 1988;124:869–71.
6. Hoefflin SM. The youthful face: tight is not right, repositioning is right. Plast Reconstr Surg. 1998;101:1417.
7. Glogau RG, Tan SR. Filler esthetics. In: Carruthers J, Carruthers A (eds). Soft Tissue Augmentation. In: Dover JS, Alam M (series eds). Procedures in Cosmetic Dermatology. Edinburgh: Elsevier Saunders, 2005:11–18.
8. Glogau RG, Tan SR. Botox esthetics. In: Carruthers J, Carruthers A (eds). Botulinum Toxin. In: Dover JS, Alam M (series eds). Procedures in Cosmetic Dermatology. Edinburgh: Elsevier Saunders, 2005:1–8.

Cosmetics and Cosmeceuticals

Zoe Diana Draelos

Synonyms: ■ Cosmetics ■ Skin care products ■ Cosmeceuticals ■ Bioactive cosmetics ■ Nail products ■ Hair care products ■ Exfoliants ■ Moisturizers ■ Cleansers

Key features

- Colored cosmetics and skin care products have an important role in the prevention of dermatologic disease and the maintenance of skin health

- Hair is a non-living structure that can be beautified through the use of shampoos and conditioners to improve its behavior and appearance

- Nail cosmetics primarily adorn the nails, but improper use can lead to nail disease

- Cosmeceuticals are non-prescription products designed to improve the functioning of the skin, primarily through a reversal of the aging process

- Skin, hair and nail care products have a profound impact on these structures, and they should be part of the knowledge base of the dermatologist

INTRODUCTION

Cosmetics and skin care products are assuming an increasingly important role in dermatology as the sophistication of raw materials and the resulting formulations provide for the development of products that impact the functioning of the skin. It was traditionally thought that the stratum corneum was a non-living, biologically inert layer of skin upon which skin care products and cosmetics impinge. It was also thought that the stratum corneum was a complete barrier unaffected by the application of non-prescription topical agents. An improved understanding of stratum corneum function, primarily obtained through the use of non-invasive bioengineering techniques, has demonstrated that the stratum corneum can be dramatically influenced by non-prescription topical agents, and that these agents can indeed penetrate the stratum corneum and influence skin function.

This new understanding of the biologic importance of the stratum corneum to skin health led to the development of a new category of skin care product, known as the cosmeceutical[1]. A cosmeceutical is a scientifically designed, useful product intended for external application to the human body that has desirable aesthetic characteristics and meets rigid chemical, physical and medical standards[2]. Even though many cosmeceuticals currently exist for use on the skin, hair and nails, there is no regulatory description that acknowledges the current scientific sophistication of these formulations. At present, in the US and Europe, a drug is defined as 'an article intended for the use in the diagnosis, mitigation, treatment or prevention of disease or intended to affect the structure or any function of the body'. Conversely, a cosmetic is defined by the US Federal Food, Drug and Cosmetic Act, written in 1938, as 'articles intended to be rubbed, poured, sprinkled, or sprayed on, introduced into, or otherwise applied to the human body or any part thereof for cleansing, beautifying, promoting attractiveness, or altering the appearance', without affecting structure or function[3].

Cosmeceuticals are now a reality due to the expanding dermatologic knowledge-base, which has rendered obsolete the prior outdated clear distinction between cosmetics and drugs[4]. It is somewhat bewildering to realize that water is a cosmeceutical. Water profoundly influences the structure and function of the viable epidermis. Many substances can function as cosmeceuticals if entry into and through the stratum corneum is facilitated via the use of penetration enhancers, such as propylene glycol, isopropyl myristate, and pyrrolidone derivatives. Propylene glycol profoundly alters the barrier characteristics of the stratum corneum, while isopropyl myristate is capable of penetrating into the lipid bilayer of cell membranes. Pyrrolidone derivatives interact with both keratin and the stratum corneum lipids to drive substances into the skin. These substances are commonly found in cosmetic formulations; however, new understanding of skin physiology allows recognition of their profound effects on the skin, which were previously unknown.

This chapter presents the current dermatologic understanding regarding colored cosmetics, cleansers, moisturizers, cosmeceuticals, and hair and nail care products. It critically evaluates their scientific effect while assessing their aesthetic value. After reading this discourse, the dermatologist should possess a working fund of knowledge regarding these products, which have a tremendous impact on skin, hair and nail health due to their frequency of use.

DISCUSSION

Skin Care Products

The three basic categories of skin care products are cleansers, astringents and moisturizers. Cleansers are designed to remove sebum, desquamating corneocytes, bacteria, fungi and environmental dirt from the face and body, while leaving the intercellular lipid barrier intact. Astringents are actually a subset of cleansers designed to supplement the failure of the cleanser to perform its intended function. Lastly, moisturizers are designed to minimize the barrier damage induced by cleansing. Thus, these three skin care products work together to balance the hygiene needs of the skin with the important task of preserving barrier function. This chapter proceeds by examining the formulation and use of each of these skin care products.

Cleansers

The development of soaps designed to cleanse the skin has been the single most important advance in decreasing disease worldwide. Even though soap is ubiquitous in the developed world, one of the main goals of world health organizations is to introduce the concept of cleansing with soap to areas of the globe where contagious diseases run rampant. In basic chemical terms, soap is a fatty acid salt resulting from a reaction between a fat and an alkali[5]. The soap solubilizes sebum and environmental dirt, such that it can be rinsed away with water. The mechanics of rubbing the soap over the skin with the hand or a bathing implement results in the physical removal of skin scale, bacteria and fungi from the skin surface. In the developed world, where bathing has become a daily ritual, excessive use of soap has resulted in dermatologic conditions, such as xerotic eczema. This has led to the development of cleansers with skin conditioning benefits that are chemically not true soaps, indicated by the nomenclature detergents.

Cleansers, whether formulated as bars or liquids, can be divided into three basic types: soaps, syndets and combars (Table 153.1). True soaps, discussed previously, are composed of long-chain fatty acid alkali salts with a pH of between 9 and 10. This alkaline pH raises the pH of the skin following cleansing, resulting in stratum corneum barrier disruption and the resultant feeling of tightness following bathing. Alkalinization of the skin disrupts the natural acid mantle, which may be significant in dermatitic skin. Recognition of the need to preserve skin pH at 5.4 led to the development of *synthetic detergents*, known as syndets, such as sodium cocoyl isethionate. Syndet cleansers, also known as beauty cleansers, contain less than 10% soap, and are designed

CATEGORIES OF CLEANSING PRODUCTS		
Product type	Composition	Product examples®,™
Bar soap	True soap in bar form; pH 9–10	Ivory Bar Soap (Procter & Gamble) Pure and Natural Bar Soap (Andrew Jergens Corporation)
Syndet bar cleanser	Synthetic detergents (no soap), in bar form; pH 5.5–7	Cetaphil Bar (Galderma) Dove Bar (Unilever) Oil of Olay Bar (Procter & Gamble)
Syndet liquid	Synthetic detergents, in liquid form; pH 5.5–7	Dove Liquid (Unilever) Oil of Olay Foaming Face Wash (Procter & Gamble)
Combar soap	Combination of true soap and synthetic detergent; pH 9–10	Dial (Dial Corporation) Irish Spring (Colgate-Palmolive)
Body wash	Emulsion system applied with a puff, allowing synthetic detergent cleansing combined with enhanced skin moisturization and emolliency	Aveeno Body Wash (Johnson & Johnson) Dove Body Wash (Unilever) Oil of Olay Daily Renewal Body Wash (Procter & Gamble)
Lipid-free cleanser	Cleans without fats; may contain glycerin, cetyl alcohol, stearyl alcohol, sodium lauryl sulfate and, occasionally, propylene glycol	Aquanil (Person & Covey) CeraVe Cleanser (Coria) Cetaphil (Galderma)
Cleansing cream	Waxes and mineral oil with detergent action from borax	Noxema (Noxell Corporation) Pond's Cold Cream
Astringent/ toner	Alcohol-based product that may contain witch hazel, salicylic acid or glycolic acid	Clarifying Lotion 2, 3, 4 (Clinique)
Moisturizing astringent/toner	Glycerin-based humectant moisturizer	Clarifying Lotion 1 (Clinique)
Exfoliant cleanser	Glycolic or salicylic acid-containing cleanser	Oil-free Acne Face Wash (Neutrogena)
Abrasive cleanser	Polyethylene beads or other small particles within the syndet cleanser	Clinique 7th Day Scrub Cream Oil of Olay Age Defying Series Face Wash (Procter & Gamble)

Table 153.1 Categories of cleansing products.

SPECIALTY SOAP FORMULATIONS	
Type of soap	Unique ingredients
Superfatted soap	Increased oil and fat and fat ratio up to 10%
Castile soap	Olive oil used as main fat
Deodorant soap	Antibacterial agents
French milled soap	Additives to reduce alkalinity
Floating soap	Extra air trapped during mixing process
Oatmeal soap	Ground oatmeal added (coarsely ground to produce abrasive soap; finely ground for gentle cleanser)
Acne soap	Sulfur, resorcinol, benzoyl peroxide or salicylic acid added
Facial soap	Smaller bar size, no special ingredients
Bath soap	Larger bar size, no special ingredients
Aloe vera soap	Aloe vera added to soap, no special skin benefit
Vitamin E soap	Vitamin E added, no special skin benefit
Cocoa butter soap	Cocoa butter used as major fat
Nut or fruit oil soap	Nut or fruit oils used as major fat
Transparent soap	Glycerin and sucrose added
Abrasive soap	Pumice, coarse oatmeal, maize meal, ground nut kernels, dried herbs or flowers added
High impact soap	Strong, high concentration fragrance added to scent skin after cleansing
Soap-free soap	Contains synthetic detergents (syndet bar)

Table 153.2 Specialty soap formulations.

are typically noted in direct proportion to the cleansing ability of the cleanser. An attempt to provide cleansing and barrier restoration in the same product has led to the development of body washes. Since body washes are liquids, incorporating both hydrophilic and lipophilic ingredients emulsified into a single phase, it is possible to cleanse and moisturize simultaneously while allowing for rinsing away of the surfactants. Body washes must be used with a puff to induce both water and air into the cleanser emulsion in sufficient quantity to allow cleansing and moisturization to occur. The syndet detergent, primarily ammonium laureth sulfate, solubilizes oil-soluble dirt into the rinse water for removal, while occlusive moisturizing substances (e.g. petrolatum) and emollients (e.g. soybean oil) are left behind to retard transepidermal water loss and improve skin smoothness.

Other cleanser variants for persons with dry, dermatitic skin include lipid-free cleansers and cold creams. These products are excellent at removing cosmetics and low levels of environmental dirt. Lipid-free cleansers are soap-free liquid products applied to dry or moistened skin, rubbed to produce minimal lather, and rinsed or wiped away. They possess low surfactant capabilities, and they can only remove bacteria through mechanical means, yet they are important in persons with barrier disruption[8]. The classic cleanser for dry, dermatitic skin is cold cream, which combines the effect of a lipid solvent, such as wax or mineral oil, with detergent action from borax[9].

Occasionally, a dermatologic need arises for specialty cleansers designed to offer a skin benefit beyond pure removal of sebum and environmental dirt. For example, it may be desirable to induce corneocyte disadhesion in maturing patients requiring an exfoliant cleanser. This can be accomplished through the addition of chemical exfoliants, such as salicylic acid or glycolic acid, to the cleanser formulations discussed previously. Exfoliant cleansers containing benzoyl peroxide or salicylic acid are sometimes used as an adjunct in topical acne treatment. Exfoliation can also be induced mechanically through the incorporation of fine abrasive particles (such as polyethylene beads, aluminum oxide, ground fruit pits, or sodium tetraborate decahydrate granules) in a liquid syndet cleanser to remove skin scale. Lastly, mechanical exfoliation can be encouraged through the use of specially woven face clothes, designed to remove skin scale without inducing epidermal damage.

with a pH of 5.5–7.0 in order to minimize cutaneous alkalinization[6]. The third type of cleanser, known as a combar, is composed of an alkaline soap to which surface active agents with a pH of 9–10 have been added. Combars are milder cleansers than true soaps, but induce more thorough cleansing than syndets. For example, true soap is a good cleansing choice for excessively oily or dirty skin, while a combar is a good cleanser for normal skin with a moderate amount of environmental dirt. Syndets would be the least damaging to the cutaneous barrier in persons with dry skin or any form of dermatitis.

The many brands of cleansers currently on the market fall into one of the three aforementioned groups, yet there must be something unique, for marketing purposes, about each cleanser. The unique aspects of each cleanser are created through the addition of specialty additives (Table 153.2). Common cleanser additives include various fragrances and foaming agents designed to alter the aesthetics of the lather, but the most dermatologically relevant additives are antibacterial agents. The most widely used antibacterial in both bar and liquid cleansers is triclosan[7]. Triclosan works by blocking lipid synthesis in the bacterial cell wall, thus decreasing the skin biofilm bacteria count and reducing odor.

Another important dermatologic need with regard to skin cleansing is minimization of skin barrier dysfunction. Unfortunately, surfactants cannot distinguish between unwanted sebum and oil-soluble dirt and the intercellular lipids. Thus, increases in transepidermal water loss

The development of novel detergents and cleansing specialty additives has created a confusing plethora of consumer products, yet the goal remains the same: to allow adequate skin hygiene without barrier damage. Our next concern is the discussion of moisturizers, designed to replace skin sebum in instances where the stratum corneum barrier has been damaged from overexuberant cleansing.

Moisturizers

The term 'moisturizer' is somewhat misleading to the consumer, who assumes that the cream or lotion actually puts moisture or water back into the skin[10]. Moisturizers do not put water back into the skin externally, nor do they get incorporated into the intracellular lipids. Moisturizers simply attempt to retard transepidermal water loss and create an optimal environment for restoration of the stratum corneum barrier[11]. The optimal water content for the stratum corneum is above 10%, depending on the measurement technique employed, and moisturizers can function to raise the cutaneous water content through occlusion or humectancy with a variety of active agents (Table 153.3)[12].

Occlusive moisturizers prevent evaporative water loss to the environment by placing an oily substance on the skin surface through which water cannot penetrate, thus replenishing the stratum corneum moisture by water movement from the lower viable epidermal and dermal layers[13]. There are many different classes of chemical that can function as occlusive moisturizers[14], for example, hydrocarbon oils and waxes (petrolatum, mineral oil, paraffin, squalene), silicone (cyclomethicone, dimethicone), vegetable oils (castor oil, corn oil, grape seed oil, soybean oil), animal oils (mink oil, emu oil), fatty acids (lanolin acid, stearic acid), fatty alcohol (lanolin alcohol, cetyl alcohol), polyhydric alcohols (propylene glycol), wax esters (lanolin, beeswax, stearyl stearate), vegetable waxes (carnauba wax, candelilla wax), phospholipids (lecithin) and sterols (cholesterol, ceramides).

The most effective occlusive moisturizer is petrolatum, since it reduces transepidermal water loss by 99%[15]. Total occlusion of the stratum corneum is undesirable, since transepidermal water loss is the cellular signal that initiates barrier repair and the resulting synthesis of intercellular lipids[16,17]. Complete cessation of transepidermal water loss results in no barrier repair, allowing water loss to return to its normal pretreatment level once the complete occlusion has been removed[16-18]. Petrolatum allows barrier repair while permeating throughout the interstices of the stratum corneum[19].

Another technique for rehydrating the stratum corneum is the use of humectants. Humectants are substances that attract moisture; they include glycerin, honey, sodium lactate, urea, propylene glycol, sorbitol, pyrrolidone carboxylic acid, gelatin, hyaluronic acid, and some vitamins and proteins[14,20]. The body utilizes hyaluronic acid and other glycosaminoglycans in the dermis as biologic humectants to prevent desiccation of the skin. Humectants can only hydrate the skin from the environment when the ambient humidity exceeds 70%. Consequently, rehydration of the stratum corneum generally occurs by water that is attracted from the deeper epidermal and dermal tissues. Most moisturizers combine both occlusive and humectant moisturizing ingredients, since water drawn by a humectant to a damaged stratum corneum barrier will be lost to the atmosphere unless trapped by an occlusive[21,22]. Humectants also help to improve the smoothness of xerotic skin by inducing corneocyte swelling and minimizing voids between the desquamating corneocytes[23].

In summary, remoisturization of the skin must occur in four steps:
- initiation of barrier repair
- alteration of surface cutaneous moisture partition coefficient
- onset of dermal–epidermal moisture diffusion
- synthesis of intercellular lipids[24].

Moisturizers attempt to increase stratum corneum water content through the principles of occlusion and humectancy.

Astringents

Occasionally, patients use skin care products that either correct the deficiencies of the cleanser or supplement the effects of the moisturizer. These products are known as astringents or toners. They are used after cleansing but before moisturizing, and they are left on the face following use. Astringents are usually liquids wiped over the face with a cotton ball. Originally, astringents were intended to remove soap scum left behind on the face from the use of lye-based soaps and hard water. If left behind, this soap scum could cause irritant contact dermatitis. The original astringents were fragranced isopropyl alcohol or propylene glycol solutions designed to remove oil-soluble residue. The development of synthetic detergents and treated water has made this original intent obsolete, yet astringents remain popular.

Currently, astringents are used to remove the oily residue left behind after cleansing of the face with lipid-free cleansers or cleansing creams, discussed previously. Oily complexion astringents are formulated to remove any remaining sebum from the face following synthetic detergent cleansing or to deliver keratolytics, such as salicylic acid, glycolic acid or witch hazel. Some astringents designed for dry skin contain a humectant liquid moisturizer, such as propylene glycol or glycerin, and skin soothing agents, such as allantoin, guaiazulene or quaternium-19[25]. A complete cosmetic-counter facial treatment routine involves a cleanser followed by an astringent and then a moisturizer. Once the skin has been prepared in this manner, colored cosmetics are applied: the next subject of discussion.

Colored Facial Cosmetics

Colored facial cosmetics are intended to adorn the eyes, lips and cheeks with color for the purposes of creating a fashionable appearance, highlighting certain desirable features, and camouflaging facial flaws. Colored cosmetics are of importance to the dermatologist for their role in maintaining skin health, inducing dermatitis, and camouflaging surgical defects. This section discusses facial foundations, powders, blushes, lipsticks, mascaras and eye shadows.

Facial foundations
Formulation
Facial foundations are the first cosmetic applied to the face following the use of a moisturizer and, therefore, represent the colored facial cosmetic with the greatest impact on the integrity of the skin. Facial foundations are basically pigmented moisturizers worn for 8 hours or longer before removal. Consequently, this class of color cosmetics, more than any other, has an impact on the integrity of the skin. Facial foundations are available for every complexion type and skin color, fulfilling the needs listed in Table 153.4.

There are four basic facial foundation formulations: oil-based, water-based, oil-free, and water-free or anhydrous forms[26]. Oil-based products are designed for dry skin, while water-based products can be adapted for all skin types. Oil-free formulations are used in oily skin foundations, while anhydrous forms are extremely long-wearing and used for camouflage or theatrical purposes.

DIFFERENT TYPES OF MOISTURIZERS		
Moisturizer type	**Composition**	**Product examples®,™**
Oil only	Petrolatum	Vaseline petroleum jelly (Chesebrough Ponds)
Oil-in-water emulsion	Water, petrolatum	Eucerin cream (Biersdorf)
Polymer-based	Water, polyglycerylmethacrylate, petrolatum	Cetaphil cream (Galderma)
Vegetable oil and wax	Castor oil, corn oil, ozokerite, beeswax, paraffin, carnauba wax	Lip moisture (Neutrogena)
Glycerin-rich	Water, glycerin, petrolatum	Norwegian formula hand cream (Neutrogena) Curel lotion (Andrew Jergens)
Dimethicone and ceramides	Water, petrolatum, dimethicone, ceramides	CeraVe (Coria) EpiCeram (Ceragenix)

Table 153.3 Different types of moisturizers. Additional prescription moisturizers are based upon glycyrrhetinic acid and shea butter (Atopiclair®), palmitoylethanolamide (MimyX®), paraffin (Biafine®), and sodium hyaluronate (Hylira™).

FUNCTIONS OF FACIAL FOUNDATION
Add facial color
Blend facial color
Camouflage pigmentation irregularities
Normalize facial skin
Provide sun protection
Act as a treatment product

Table 153.4 Functions of facial foundation.

Oil-based foundations are water-in-oil emulsions containing pigments suspended in oil (e.g. mineral oil) or lanolin alcohol. Vegetable oils (grape seed, coconut, sesame, safflower) and synthetic esters (isopropyl myristate, octyl palmitate, isopropyl palmitate) may also be incorporated. The water evaporates from the foundation following application, leaving the pigment in oil on the face. This creates a moist skin feeling, especially desirable in dry complected patients. Oil-based foundations do not shift color as they mix with sebum, since the color is fully developed in the oily phase of the formulation. These foundations are easy to apply, since the pigment can be spread over the face for up to 5 minutes, prior to setting.

Water-based facial foundations are oil-in-water emulsions containing a small amount of oil, in which the pigment is emulsified, and a relatively large quantity of water. The primary emulsifier is usually a soap, such as triethanolamine, or a non-ionic surfactant. The secondary emulsifier, present in smaller quantity, is usually glyceryl stearate or propylene glycol stearate. These popular foundations are appropriate for minimally dry to normal skin. Since the pigment is already developed in oil, this foundation type is also not subject to color drift. The amount of time the product can be moved over the face, known in the industry as playtime, is shorter than with oil-based foundations. These products are usually packaged in a bottle.

Oil-free facial foundations contain no animal, vegetable or mineral oils. They contain other oily substances, such as dimethicone or cyclomethicone. These foundations are usually designed for oily complected individuals, since they leave the skin with a dry feeling. Silicone is non-comedogenic, non-acnegenic and hypoallergenic, accounting for the tremendous popularity of this type of facial foundation formulation. These products are also usually liquids packaged in a bottle.

Water-free, or anhydrous, foundations are waterproof. Vegetable oil, mineral oil, lanolin alcohol and synthetic esters form the oil phase, which may be mixed with waxes to form a cream. High concentrations of pigment can be incorporated into the formulation, yielding an opaque facial foundation. The coloring agents are based on titanium dioxide with iron oxides, occasionally in combination with ultramarine blue. Titanium dioxide acts both as a facial concealing agent and sunscreen. These products can be dipped from a jar, squeezed from a tube, wiped from a compact, or stroked from a stick. These foundations are well suited for use in people who require facial camouflaging. They can be combined with a high-coverage powder foundation to increase the opacity of the cosmetic.

Application and Cutaneous Effects

Facial foundations must be evenly applied to create the optimal cosmetic appearance and achieve the secondary benefit of sun protection. The iron oxide pigment and other covering agents, for example, titanium dioxide, zinc oxide and kaolin, are physical particulates that block both UVA and UVB radiation (see Ch. 132). A facial foundation without any added chemical sunscreen ingredients, such as cinnamates, para-aminobenzoic acid (PABA) esters or avobenzone, usually has a sun protection factor (SPF) of at least 4. Facial foundations that have greater coverage in order to camouflage underlying pigmentation defects usually possess an SPF of at least 8. The inclusion of additional sunscreen agents to the facial foundation can raise the SPF to 15. Thus, facial foundation is an excellent, cosmetically elegant facial photoprotectant.

An even, cosmetically acceptable application of facial foundation begins with a proper color match to the skin at the jawline and application with the fingertips. A dab of foundation should be placed on the forehead, nose, cheeks and chin, and blended with a light circular motion until it is evenly spread over all the face, including the lips.

Finally, a puff or sponge should be used, stroking in a downward direction, to remove any streaks and to flatten vellus facial hair. Special care should be taken to rub the foundation into the hairline, over the tragus, and beneath the chin. Foundation should also be blended around the eyes, and it may even be applied to the entire upper eyelid if desired. The foundation should be allowed to set or dry until it can no longer be removed with light touch. If additional coverage is desired, a second layer of foundation can be applied.

The most common adverse dermatologic effect related to the use of facial foundation is a condition patients describe as 'breakouts'. Patients typically note small perifollicular papules 48 hours after using a new facial foundation. The appearance is that of acne; however, the 48-hour time course is inconsistent with a diagnosis of acne. This condition may represent a perifollicular irritant contact dermatitis, since facial foundations tend to migrate to the follicular ostia as they mix with eccrine secretions and sebum, which break down the cosmetic film (Fig. 153.1). This observation may explain why facial foundations that have been found on clinical testing to be non-comedogenic and non-acnegenic cause acneiform eruptions in individuals with self-diagnosed sensitive skin. Overall, however, facial foundations are an infrequent cause of dermatologic problems.

Powders

One of the ways of preventing migration of facial foundation, improving its sun protective capabilities, and increasing oil absorption is to apply powder over the foundation. Facial powders contain predominantly talc (hydrated magnesium silicate) and increased amounts of covering pigments. The covering pigments used in face powder are listed in order of increasing opaqueness in Table 153.5. It is generally accepted that the optimum opacity is achieved with a particle size of 0.25 μm.

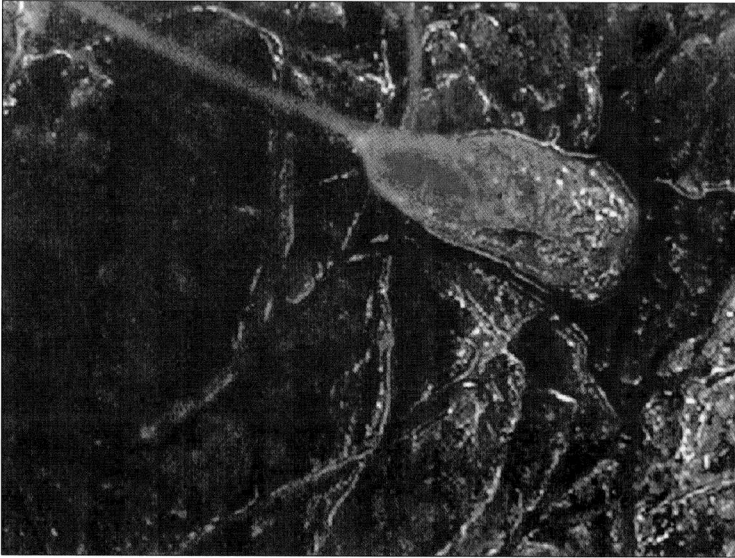

Fig. 153.1 As seen by a 400x video microscope, the iron oxide particles in facial foundation tend to migrate to the follicular ostia as sebum and eccrine secretions mix with the cosmetic film.

COVERING ABILITY OF FACE POWDER INGREDIENTS*
1. Titanium dioxide
2. Kaolin
3. Magnesium carbonate
4. Magnesium stearate
5. Zinc stearate
6. Prepared chalk
7. Zinc oxide
8. Rice starch
9. Precipitated chalk
10. Talc

Table 153.5 Covering ability of face powder ingredients. *Listed in order of increasing opacity.

Facial powders usually also contain magnesium carbonate and/or kaolin (hydrated aluminum silicate) to absorb oil and perspiration. Full-coverage face powders are usually packaged as a cake in a compact and applied to the face with a puff, or loose in a jar and dusted over the face with a brush. Specially pigmented powders are used to redden the cheeks, known as blushes, and to color the eyelids, known as eye shadows.

Facial blushes

Facial blushes are typically powders designed to simulate rosy cheeks, occasionally an unwanted finding in rosacea patients. Blushes have the same basic formulation as face powders, except for the presence of different surface characteristics that can vary from a matte dull finish, to a frosted shine, to a metallic glow, depending on current fashion trends[27]. Some of the rough-edged particles designed to produce light reflection can cause irritation in people with sensitive skin (Fig. 153.2). Powder blush can be used to absorb facial oil, blend the facial erythema of rosacea across the cheeks, and add color to a sallow face by dusting on the central chin, cheeks, nasal tip and forehead.

Eye shadows

Eye shadows are similar to powder blushes in formulation and surface characteristics, except that the color variation is broader, but limited in the US by the Food and Drug Administration (FDA) to the purified natural colors or inorganic pigments listed in Table 153.6[28]. Eye shadow can be used to camouflage misshapen eyes, provide sun protection to the upper eyelid, and minimize the appearance of unwanted periorbital pigmentation. Eye shadows are a common concern to dermatologists, since they may be responsible for eyelid dermatitis. They may contain the same light-reflective particles as blushes and cause pruritus of the eyelids due to irritant contact dermatitis until discontinued (Fig. 153.3).

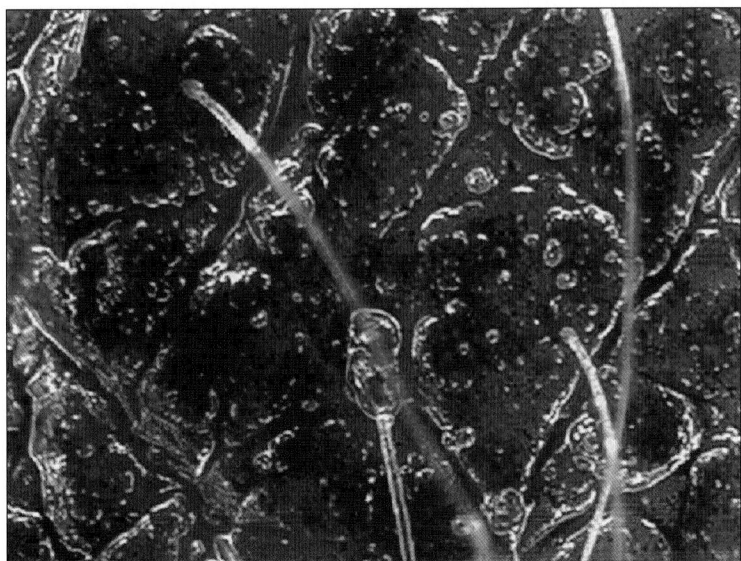

Fig. 153.2 A 400× video microscope captures the appearance of the light-reflective particles and pigment particles following application of a blush to the cheeks.

PIGMENTS ALLOWED BY THE US FDA IN EYE SHADOW COSMETICS
Iron oxides
Titanium dioxide (alone, or combined with mica)
Copper, aluminum and silver powder
Ultramarine blue, violet and pink
Manganese violet
Carmine
Chrome oxide and hydrate
Iron blue
Bismuth oxychloride (alone, or on mica or talc)
Mica

Table 153.6 Pigments allowed by the US Food and Drug Administration (FDA) in eye shadow cosmetics.

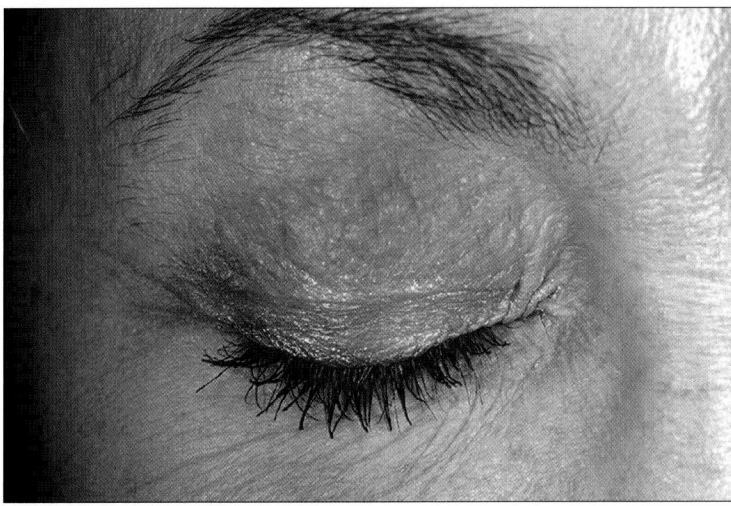

Fig. 153.3 Upper eyelid dermatitis may be exacerbated by the use of heavily pigmented, light-reflective eye shadows.

The North American Contact Dermatitis Group has determined that 12% of cosmetic reactions occur on the eyelid, but only 4% could be linked to eye makeup use[29]. Unfortunately, it can be difficult to determine the etiology of allergic contact eyelid dermatitis with routine patch testing[30], since many substances can be transferred to the eye area by the hands, complicating the dermatologic evaluation[31]. However, eye shadows are a rare cause of eye infections, since the dry powder cake does not support bacterial growth. This is not the case with mascaras.

Mascaras

Mascaras are eyelash cosmetics, as opposed to eye shadows, which are eyelid cosmetics. Mascaras are designed to color, camouflage, elongate and thicken the eyelashes, which are the frame to the eyes. They must be carefully formulated to allow easy and even application without smudging, irritancy or toxicity. Some of the coloring agents employed include iron oxide to produce black, ultramarine blue to create navy, and umber, burnt sienna or synthetic brown oxide to create brown[32].

Most modern mascaras are formulated as liquids then stored in a tube with a multitufted applicator brush. The applicator is inserted into the tube between uses, providing numerous opportunities to inoculate bacteria into the cosmetic. The most dangerous bacterial infection is a *Pseudomonas aeruginosa* corneal infection, which can permanently diminish visual acuity[33,34]. *Staphylococcus epidermidis*, *S. aureus* and fungal organisms may also proliferate in contaminated mascaras[35,36]. Infections are more common if the globe is traumatized with the infected mascara wand. Even though mascaras contain antibacterials, it is still wise to discard all mascara tubes after 3 months and not allow multiple persons to use the same mascara tube[37].

There are several mascara formulations that are less likely to support bacterial and fungal growth (Table 153.7). Mascaras are available as water-based, solvent-based, and a water/solvent hybrid. Water-based mascaras are easily removed with water and less likely to cause eye area irritation, but the presence of water provides welcome media for bacterial growth. Solvent-based mascaras are manufactured without water, must be removed with a special cleanser, and are more irritating; however, they are less likely to support bacterial growth, and they are the formulation of choice for individuals who are carriers of *Staphylococcus* or *Streptococcus* species[38]. The water/solvent hybrid mascaras are an attempt to provide a water-resistant cosmetic with the benefits of both.

Another dermatologic side effect of the use of mascara is conjunctival pigmentation, resulting from the washing of mascara into the conjunctival sac by lacrimal fluid[39]. This colored particulate matter can be observed on the upper margin of the tarsal conjunctiva. Histologically, the pigment is seen within macrophages and extracellularly in association with a variable lymphocytic infiltrate. Electron microscopy suggests that ferritin, carbon and iron oxides are present within the tissues[40]. Unfortunately, there is no treatment for the condition, which is usually asymptomatic.

DIFFERENT TYPES OF MASCARA FORMULATIONS		
Mascara formulation	**Composition**	**Advantages/Disadvantages**
Water-based	Waxes, pigments, resins	Easy to remove with water; runs with tearing; supports bacterial growth
Solvent-based waterproof	Petroleum distillates, pigments, waxes	Must be removed with solvent; waterproof; does not support bacterial growth
Water-resistant water/solvent hybrid	Oil-in-water emulsion, pigments	Removal with water and cleanser; resists running with tearing; less likely to support bacterial growth
Compressed cake	Pigments, talc	Removal with water; runs with tearing; least allergenic; does not support bacterial growth

Table 153.7 Different types of mascara formulations.

Lipsticks

Lipstick is a lip cosmetic designed to frame the teeth. Lipsticks are mixtures of waxes, oils and pigments in various concentrations to yield the characteristics of the final product. For example, a lipstick designed to remain on the lips for a prolonged period of time is composed of high wax, low oil and high pigment concentrations, whereas a product designed for a smooth creamy feel on the lips is composed of low wax and high oil concentrations[41]. The waxes commonly incorporated into lipstick formulations are white beeswax, candelilla wax, carnauba wax, ozokerite wax, lanolin wax, ceresin wax and other synthetic waxes. Usually, lipsticks contain a combination of these waxes carefully selected and blended to achieve the desired melting point. Oils for pigment dispersion are then selected, such as castor oil, white mineral oil, lanolin oil, hydrogenated vegetable oils or oleyl alcohol, to form a film suitable for application to the lips[42,43].

Certain common lipstick ingredients can cause difficulty in the sensitized patient[44]. Castor oil, found in almost all lipsticks due to its excellent ability to dissolve bromo acid dyes, can cause allergic contact dermatitis[45–47]. Even the bromo acid dyes, such as eosin (D & C Red No. 21), found in indelible lipsticks can cause allergic contact dermatitis[48]. Other lipstick ingredients reported to cause allergic contact dermatitis include: ricinoleic acid[49], benzoic acid[50], lithol rubine BCA (Pigment Red 57-1)[51], microcrystalline wax[52], oxybenzone[53], propyl gallate[54] and C18 aliphatic compounds[55].

Facial cosmetics for camouflaging

All of the colored cosmetics previously discussed are used together for facial camouflaging purposes to minimize facial defects while accentuating attractive facial features. Camouflage cosmetics are used by paramedical aestheticians, dermatologists, plastic surgeons, and cosmetic consultants[56]. Their successful use requires a well-formulated, quality product applied with the skill of a stage makeup technician and the artistic abilities of a painter[57]. Facial defects requiring camouflaging are defects of pigmentation, contour, or a combination of both[58].

Pigmentation defects represent abnormalities limited to the color of the skin (in the absence of textural changes), whereas contour defects are defined as areas where the facial skin is hypertrophic or atrophic (with textural changes due to the absence of appendageal structures). Table 153.8 list examples of pigmentary abnormalities frequently encountered by dermatologists that arise from inflammatory disorders, systemic diseases or extrinsic effects (e.g. sun exposure). Pigmentation defects can be camouflaged either by applying an opaque cosmetic that allows none of the abnormal underlying skin tones to be appreciated or by applying foundations of complementary colors. For example, red pigmentation defects can be camouflaged by applying a green foundation, since green is the complementary color to red. The blending of the red skin with the green foundation yields a brown tone, which can be readily covered by a more conventional facial foundation. Furthermore, yellow skin tones can be blended with a complementary-colored purple foundation to also yield brown tones.

CAMOUFLAGE FOR ABNORMALITIES OF FACIAL PIGMENTATION		
Facial color	**Disease process**	**Undercover foundation color**
Red	Psoriasis, lupus, rosacea	Green
Yellow	Solar elastosis, chemotherapy, dialysis	Purple
Brown hyperpigmentation	Melasma, lentigines, nevi	White
Hypopigmentation and depigmentation	Postinflammatory, congenital, vitiligo	Brown

Table 153.8 Camouflage for abnormalities of facial pigmentation.

The camouflaging of facial contour abnormalities is based on the principle that dark colors make protuberances appear to recede while light colors make surface depressions appear more shallow. Creating an even-appearing surface on a scarred face is achieved through artistic shading. Powdered blush-type products are best suited for this purpose. Areas of the face that need to be lightened should be brushed with a light pink or peach pearled blush or buffer. Areas of the face that need to be darkened should be brushed with a deep plum or bronze matte-finish blush or highlighter.

There are special cosmetics manufactured for these camouflaging purposes. A reference list of the websites of the recommended camouflaging cosmetic companies is given in the Appendix.

Hair Care Products

Some of the material discussed above is applicable to hair care products, since shampoos can be likened to skin cleansers, while conditioners are similar to skin moisturizers.

Hair shampoos

Shampoos are simply designed to cleanse the hair; however, this is a complicated task considering that the average woman has 4–8 m^2 of hair surface area to clean[59]. Shampoos are intended to remove sebum, sweat components, desquamated stratum corneum, styling products and environmental dirt from the hair and scalp[60]. They contain detergents, foaming agents, conditioners, thickeners, opacifiers, softeners, sequestering agents, fragrances, preservatives and specialty additives[61]. Synthetic detergents remove sebum and dirt; however, excessive removal of sebum leaves the hair dull, susceptible to static electricity, and difficult to comb, creating the need for hair conditioners[62]. Shampoo detergents can be chemically classified as anionics, cationics, non-ionics, amphoterics and natural surfactants (Table 153.9)[63]. The basic difference between bar soap and shampoo is the addition of a

SHAMPOO DETERGENTS		
Surfactant type	**Chemical class**	**Characteristics**
Anionics	Lauryl sulfates, laureth sulfates, sarcosines, sulfosuccinates	Deep cleansing; may leave hair harsh
Cationics	Long-chain amino esters, ammonio esters	Poor cleansing; poor lather; impart softness and manageability
Non-ionics	Polyoxyethylene fatty alcohols, polyoxyethylene sorbitol esters, alkanolamides	Mildest cleansing; impart manageability
Amphoterics	Betaines, sultaines, imidazolinium derivatives	Non-irritating to eyes; mild cleansing; impart manageability
Natural surfactants	Sarsaparilla, soapwort, soap bark, ivy, agave	Poor cleansing; excellent lather

Table 153.9 Shampoo detergents.

SPECIALTY SHAMPOOS		
Shampoo type	**Function**	**Unique ingredients**
Oily hair	Provide excellent cleansing to remove sebum with minimal conditioning	Strong surfactants such as sodium lauryl sulfate or the sulfosuccinates
Dry hair	Provide mild cleansing and excellent conditioning	Milder surfactants such as sodium laureth sulfate
Conditioning	Contain added conditioners to enhance shine and minimize static electricity	Hydrolyzed proteins designed to penetrate the hair shaft
Baby	Utilize mild detergents that anesthetize the conjunctiva to prevent stinging, burning and irritation	Detergents from the amphoteric group such as the betaines
Medicated	Designed to treat dandruff and seborrheic dermatitis through the use of keratolytics as well as antiproliferative and anti-inflammatory agents	Tar, salicylic acid, sulfur, selenium disulfide, ketoconazole, and zinc pyrithione
Professional	Designed for use following hair dyeing to reduce hair shaft swelling	Cationic acidic shampoos to neutralize residual hair shaft alkalinity following permanent hair dyeing

Table 153.10 Specialty shampoos.

higher concentration of sequestering agents to chelate magnesium and calcium ions, preventing the formation of other salts or insoluble soaps known as soap scum. Without sequestering agents, shampoos would leave the hair dull and contribute to scalp pruritus. There are many different types of shampoo, designed to meet various hair cleansing needs. These are summarized in Table 153.10.

Hair conditioners

The need for hair conditioners arises from the inability of shampoos to remove just enough sebum to leave the hair clean, without removing too much sebum and creating dry, unmanageable, dull hair[64]. Conditioners are also required because permanent waving, permanent dyeing and other chemical hair treatments damage the cuticle, making the hair harsh, brittle and difficult to disentangle (Table 153.11)[65]. Hair conditioners are designed to reverse this hair damage by improving sheen, decreasing brittleness, decreasing porosity, increasing strength, and repairing degradation in hair protein[66,67].

Hair conditioners improve manageability by decreasing static electricity. Following combing or brushing, the hair shafts become negatively charged, causing the hairs to repel one another. Conditioners deposit positively charged ions on the hair shaft, neutralizing the electrical charge. They also improve manageability by reducing hair shaft combing friction by as much as 50%, leading to enhanced disentangling and smoothing the cuticular scale to increase hair shine[68,69]. Maximum hair shine is produced by large-diameter, elliptical hair shafts with a sizable medulla and intact, overlapping cuticular scales[70]. Hair that lacks shine is missing its cuticle, as shown in Figure 153.4.

Special hair conditioner formulations attempt to repair split-ends by temporarily reapproximating the frayed remnants of remaining medulla and cortex. This is accomplished through the use of hydrolyzed animal proteins that can minimally penetrate the hair shaft, enhancing hair tensile strength by 5% until the hair is next shampooed. There are several types of conditioners formulated for a variety of needs (Table 153.12). Leave-in conditioners are specially designed for African-American hair in order to maintain hair water content despite the unavoidable loss that occurs following hair straightening.

Nail Care Products

There are a variety of nail care products, summarized in Table 153.13. The focus of this section is on nail polish and the use of nail sculptures, since these are of most concern to the dermatologist.

Nail polish

Nail polish is a cosmetic designed to temporarily place a pigmented layer over the natural nail plate, and it consists of pigments suspended in a volatile solvent to which film-forming agents have been added[71]. Nitrocellulose is the most commonly employed primary film-forming agent in nail lacquer. It produces a shiny, tough film that adheres well to the nail plate. The film is somewhat oxygen-permeable, thus allowing gas exchange between the atmosphere and the nail plate, which is required to maintain nail strength. It also decreases nail water vapor loss from 1.6 to 0.4 mg/cm^2/h, preventing nail plate dehydration[72].

A resin, such as toluene–sulfonamide–formaldehyde, must be added to the nitrocellulose to decrease hardness, but some individuals are sensitive to this substance, which is found on the standard dermatology patch test tray. This resin has been eliminated in hypoallergenic nail enamels, which instead contain a polyester resin or cellulose acetate butyrate, but allergic contact dermatitis is still possible and the enamel is less durable[73].

A professional nail enamel application requires three layers of polish: a base coat, a pigmented nail enamel, and a top coat. The base coat ensures good adhesion to the nail plate and prevents polish chipping. The second layer is the actual pigmented nail enamel, while the third layer or top coat provides gloss and resistance to chipping.

Problems associated with nail enamels include nail plate discoloration and allergic contact dermatitis. The nail staining is most

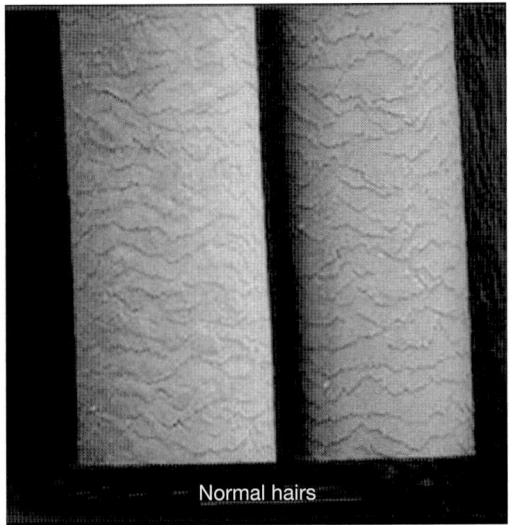
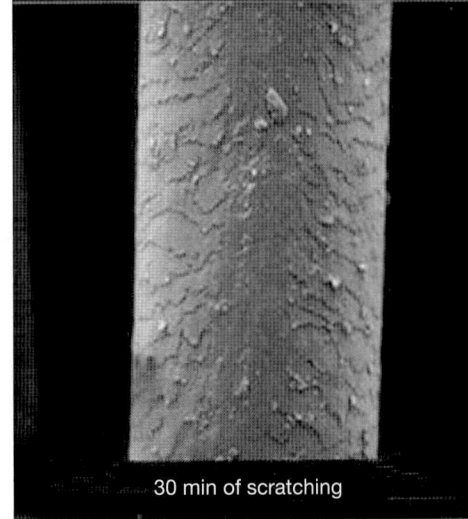
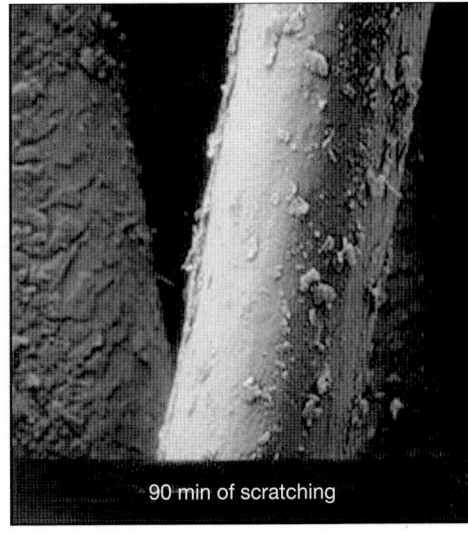

Normal hairs | 30 min of scratching | 90 min of scratching

Fig. 153.4 Electron photomicrographs demonstrating the progressive removal of the hair cuticle as a result of scratching. The most common cause of cuticle removal is scratching and this leads to dull fragile hair.

CHEMICAL HAIR TREATMENTS: COLORING, PERMANENT WAVING AND RELAXING

Treatment	Definition	Chemicals used	Process	Adverse effects
Permanent coloring	Color persists indefinitely (until new growth appears)	• H_2O_2 (referred to as the developer or oxidizing agent) • Ammonia • Dye (e.g. *p*-phenylenediamine, aminophenols)	• H_2O_2 lightens ('lifts') the previous color by oxidizing melanin, and it causes the dye to 'develop' and deposit color • Alkaline pH leads to swelling and disruption of the cuticle, allowing the dye to penetrate into the cortex • To dye dark hair to a light blonde color, the hair must first be bleached (e.g. with a mixture of ammonium persulfate and H_2O_2)	• Dull, brittle hair (especially with permanent color) • Allergic contact dermatitis • Staining of the skin
Demi-permanent coloring	Color lasts 2–3 months (12–24 shampoos)	• Low concentration of H_2O_2 • Non-ammonia alkali (e.g. monoethanolamine) • Dye (e.g. *p*-phenylenediamine, aminophenols)	• Similar to permanent color (but to a lesser degree)	
Semi-permanent coloring	Color lasts 4–6 weeks (6–12 shampoos)	• No H_2O_2 • Mild non-ammonia alkali • Azo dyes, henna, polymerized dyes, aminophenols ± *p*-phenylenediamine	• Small dye particles both coat the cuticle and penetrate into the cortex, or dye polymers coat the cuticle • The hair is not lightened	
Gradual coloring	Color slowly builds up over time	• Metallic dyes (e.g. salts of lead, bismuth or silver)	• Dye particles slowly accumulate in the cuticle, darkening the hair within a limited (brown–black) range	
Temporary coloring	Color is removed with 1–2 shampoos	• Azo and other FD&C dyes	• Dye coats the cuticle of the hair shaft (particles are too large to penetrate the cuticle)	
Permanent waving ('perm')*	Chemical treatments 'permanently' curl hair (until new growth appears)	• Ammonium or sodium thioglycolate (pH 9–10; 'alkaline perm') – *or* – • Glycerol monothioglycolate (pH 6.5–8; 'acid perm'; requires application of heat) – *or* – • Bisulfites or mercaptamine (low/neutral pH, 'thioglycolate-free perms')	• The hair is wrapped around rods and the chemical solution is applied to break disulfide bonds between keratin polypeptide chains • Neutralizing solution is then used to reform the disulfide bridges, and the hair takes the shape of the rod	• Dull, brittle hair (especially with alkaline perms) • Irritant contact dermatitis • Allergic contact dermatitis
Chemical relaxing (lanthionizing)*	Chemical treatments 'permanently' straighten hair (until new growth appears)	• Sodium hydroxide (lye) – *or* – • Guanidine hydroxide (calcium hydroxide cream + guanidine carbonate activator solution; 'no-lye' relaxers) – *or* – • Ammonium thioglycolate ('thio' relaxers)	• Disulfide bonds between keratin polypeptide chains are broken and reformed in a similar manner to permanent waving • Relaxer cream is brushed onto the hair, which is mechanically smoothened section by section; this is followed by use of a neutralizing shampoo	• Dull, brittle hair (breakage may be substantial, especially with sodium hydroxide) • Irritant contact dermatitis/ chemical burns • Allergic contact dermatitis

*Permanent waving or relaxing should be performed before coloring hair, since the former procedures can produce irreversible color loss; to minimize damage to the cuticle, it is best to wait 2–4 weeks before color is applied.

Table 153.11 Chemical hair treatments: coloring, permanent waving and relaxing. FD&C, Federal Food, Drug and Cosmetic Act; H_2O_2, hydrogen peroxide.

HAIR CONDITIONERS

Type	Use	Indication
Instant	Apply following shampoo; rinse	Minimally damaged hair; aids wet combing
Deep	Apply for 20–30 minutes; shampoo; rinse	Chemically damaged hair
Leave-in	Apply to towel-dried hair; style	Prevents hair dryer or hair straightening damage; aids in combing and styling
Rinse	Apply following shampoo; rinse	Aids in disentangling if creamy rinse; removes soap residue if clear rinse

Table 153.12 Hair conditioners.

commonly seen following the use of deep red nail polishes containing D & C Reds No. 6, 7, 34, or 5 Lake[74]. The nail plate will be stained yellow after 7 days of continuous nail polish wear and will fade without treatment in approximately 14 days, once the enamel has been removed (Fig. 153.5)[75]. Allergic contact dermatitis is seen in persons sensitive to toluene–sulfonamide–formaldehyde, who may develop proximal nail-fold erythema and edema, fingertip tenderness and swelling, and/or eyelid dermatitis[76]. The North American Contact Dermatitis Group determined that 4% of positive patch tests were due to toluene-sulfonamide–formaldehyde resin allergy[30]. The latter is sometimes referred to as tosylamide formaldehyde resin.

Nail sculptures

Nail polish is designed to color the nail plate, and it may make the nail somewhat stronger due to the presence of the resin layer, but it cannot elongate fingernails. Since long fingernails are considered attractive

153

NAIL COSMETICS

Nail cosmetic	Main ingredients	Function	Adverse reactions
Nail polish	Nitrocellulose, toluene–sulfonamide–formaldehyde resin*, plasticizers, solvents, colorants	Add color and shine to nail plates	Allergic contact dermatitis to toluene–sulfonamide–formaldehyde resin; nail plate staining
Nail hardener	Formaldehyde, acetates, acrylics or other resins	Increase nail strength and prevent breakage	Allergic contact dermatitis to formaldehyde
Nail enamel remover	Acetone, alcohol, ethyl acetate or butyl acetate	Remove nail polish	Irritant contact dermatitis
Cuticle remover	Sodium or potassium hydroxide	Destroy keratin that forms excess cuticular tissue on nail plate	Irritant contact dermatitis
Nail white	White pigments	Whiten free nail edge	Practically none
Nail bleach	Hydrogen peroxide	Remove nail plate stains	Irritant contact dermatitis
Nail polish drier	Vegetable oils, alcohols or silicone derivatives	Speed drying time of nail polish	Practically none
Nail buffing cream	Pumice, talc or kaolin	Smooth ridges in nails	Practically none
Nail moisturizer	Occlusives, humectants, lactic acid	Increase water content of nails	Practically none

*Also referred to as tosylamide formaldehyde resin.

Table 153.13 Nail cosmetics.

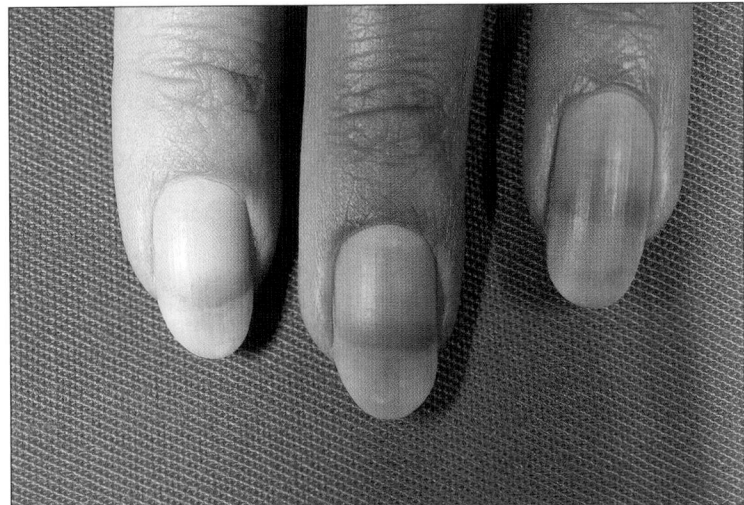

Fig. 153.5 Yellow nail staining due to wearing deeply pigmented red and orange nail polishes. This type of staining is common and reversible.

NAIL SCULPTURE APPLICATION

Nail sculpture application is an involved process requiring approximately 2 hours to sculpt 10 fingernails. The basic process is as follows:
1. All nail polish and oils are removed from the nail.
2. The nail is roughened with a coarse emery board, pumice stone or grinding drill to create an optimal surface for sculpted nail adhesion.
3. An antifungal, antibacterial liquid, such as decolorized iodine, is applied to the entire nail plate to minimize onychomycosis and paronychia.
4. The loose edges of the cuticle are trimmed, removed or pushed back, depending on the operator.
5. A flexible template is fitted beneath the natural nail plate, upon which the elongated sculpted nail will be built. Or, a preformed nail tip is used for this purpose.
6. The acrylic is mixed and applied with a brush to cover the entire natural nail plate and extended onto the template or preformed nail tip to obtain the desired nail length.
7. The final sculpture is sanded to a high shine.
8. Nail polish, jewels, decals, decorative metal strips or airbrushed designs may be added.

Table 153.14 Nail sculpture application.

among some women, this has led to the development of a new industry dedicated to the application of nail prostheses. These nail prostheses, known as nail sculptures, are applied over the natural fingernails and toenails, as described in Table 153.14.

Nail sculptures are formed by mixing liquid ethyl or isobutyl methacrylate monomers with powdered polymethyl methacrylate polymer. The mixture is allowed to polymerize in the presence of a benzoyl peroxide accelerator and a formable acrylic is made, which hardens in 7–9 minutes[77]. Usually, hydroquinone, monomethyl ether of hydroquinone, or pyrogallol is added to slow down polymerization[78].

Many patients are not aware that the finished nail sculptures require more care than natural fingernails. With continued wear of the sculpture, the acrylic loosens from the natural nail, especially around the edges. These loose edges must be clipped and new acrylic applied approximately every 3 weeks to prevent infection and onycholysis[79,80]. However, damage to the natural nail plate is inevitable with the use of nail sculptures (Fig. 153.6). After 2 to 4 months of wear, the natural nail plate becomes yellowed, dry, thin and bendable. This is due to interference with the nail's normal vapor exchange, nail plate trauma during the removal process, and damage to the underlying nail bed[81]. For this reason, it is not advisable to wear sculptured nails for more than 3 months consecutively, allowing 1 month between applications (Fig. 153.7).

Allergic contact dermatitis is an important dermatologic issue, since isobutyl, ethyl and tetrahydrofurfuryl methacrylate are still strong

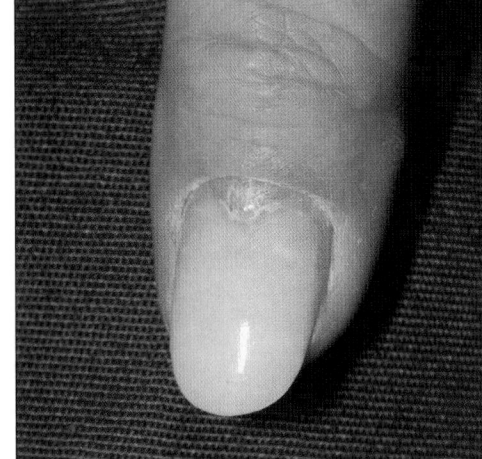

Fig. 153.6 Onychodystrophy of the central nail due to wearing a nail prosthesis. The nail prosthesis grows out with the nail plate and new polymer must be applied to the proximal nailfold. The polymer has damaged the cells of the central nail matrix.

sensitizers[82,83]. However, the polymerized, cured acrylic is not sensitizing, only the liquid monomer[84]. Therefore, a careful operator who avoids skin contact with the uncured acrylic can avoid sensitizing the patient. Patch testing should be performed in suspected sensitized individuals with methyl methacrylate monomer (10% in olive oil) and methacrylate acid esters (1% and 5% in olive oil and petrolatum)[85].

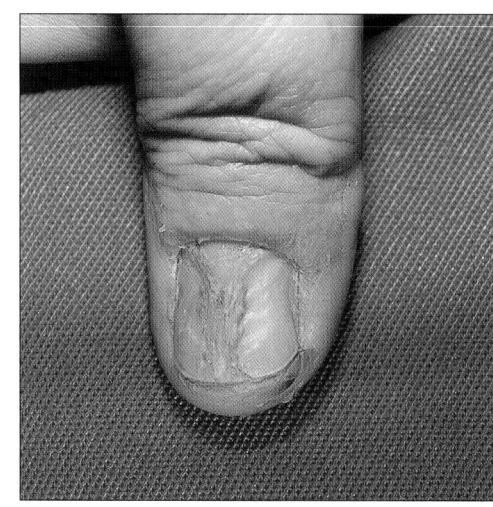

Fig. 153.7 Continuous use of a nail prosthesis can result in dramatic nail plate damage.

DERMATOLOGIC USES OF HYDROXY ACIDS AS TOPICAL PREPARATIONS AND PEELS
Skin conditions
Photodamaged skin
Ichthyosis
Xerotic eczema
Acne
Acne rosacea
Seborrheic keratoses (improves appearance)
Actinic keratoses
Lentigines (improves appearance)
Verrucae
Cutaneous effects
Moisturizing exfoliant
Skin peeling agent
Penetration enhancer
Preventative for corticosteroid-induced skin atrophy

Table 153.15 Dermatologic uses of hydroxy acids as topical preparations and peels.

Current Hydroxy Acid Cosmeceuticals

The discussion so far has focused on products intended to function purely in a cosmetic realm, yet there are cosmeceuticals in the current marketplace known as hydroxy acids. These hydroxy acids address the scaliness and roughness of aged skin that is not due to an inherently lower stratum corneum water content[86]. The roughness associated with mature skin may be due to an abnormal desquamation associated with a possible failure in intercellular communication[87]. This observation has led to the enormous popularity of α- and β-hydroxy acids.

Alpha-hydroxy acids

This group of organic carboxylic acids is distinguished by a substituted hydroxy group covalently bonded to the α-carbon of a carboxylic acid. The linear, aliphatic nature of the α-hydroxy acid (AHA) structure accounts for its water-soluble or hydrophilic properties (Fig. 153.8). The three subcategories of AHA consist of: (1) monocarboxylic acids – glycolic (2-hydroxyethanoic acid), lactic (2-hydroxy-propanoic acid) and mandelic acid (2-hydroxy-2-phenylethanoic acid); (2) dicarboxylic acids – malic (2-hydroxy-1,4-butanedioic acid) and tartaric acid (2,3-dihydroxy-1,4-butanedioic acid); and (3) tricarboxylic acids – citric acid (2-hydroxy-1,2,3-propanetricarboylic acid). The intricacies of the formulation are more important than the nature of the AHA, since the exfoliative effect is similar[88].

AHAs induce immediate epidermal effects through corneocyte disadhesion, which is thought to require disruption of ionic bonding[89,90]. The corneocyte disadhesion occurs initially in the stratum corneum at the level of the stratum granulosum; once the cutaneous barrier has been disrupted, this is followed by dermal penetration[91]. The epidermal effects of AHAs are a thinned stratum corneum with epidermal acanthosis and decreased melanogenesis. The dermal effects of AHAs are delayed and include increased synthesis of glycosaminoglycans, prevention of topical corticosteroid atrophy, and increased dermal thickness, possibly due to enhanced production of collagen via fibroblast proliferation, in a dose-dependent manner[92,93].

Disruption of corneocyte adhesion is ultimately valuable in a large variety of dermatologic conditions (Table 153.15)[94]. For example, AHAs can be incorporated into an acne treatment regimen, given their ability to induce epidermolysis and dislodge comedones; however, AHAs

cannot enter the milieu of the pore[95]. Benefit has also been shown by Briden et al.[96] in the treatment of rosacea with monthly glycolic acid peels. Sloughing of corneocytes and smoothing of seborrheic keratoses, verrucae and calluses can also be achieved[97,98]. Glycolic acid preparations, either formulated as topicals or short-contact peels, appear to be appropriate for both lightly and darkly pigmented skin[99]. Lastly, AHAs have been purported to function as anti-inflammatory agents and antioxidants by alleviating the erythema associated with cutaneous UV exposure[100]. Glycolic acid appears to confer an SPF of 2.4 to the skin[101].

Beta-hydroxy acid

The previously discussed α-hydroxy acids form only one component of the hydroxy acid family, which has been demonstrated to enhance cutaneous functioning. A similar, but chemically different, hydroxy acid is salicylic acid (ortho-hydrobenzoic acid), the only so-called β-hydroxy acid (BHA). Salicylic acid is an organic aromatic carboxylic acid with a hydroxy group in the beta position (Fig. 153.9). This phenolic, hydrophobic, lipophilic compound is a white crystalline powder chemically unrelated to the α-hydroxy acids. Perhaps even labeling it as a hydroxy acid is somewhat of a marketing misnomer.

Salicylic acid is unique among the hydroxy acids, since it can enter the milieu of the sebaceous unit, inducing exfoliation in the oily areas of the face[102]. For this reason, it has been used for years by dermatologists as a comedolytic in over-the-counter (OTC) preparations designed to improve comedonal acne[103,104]. Salicylic acid is approved for the

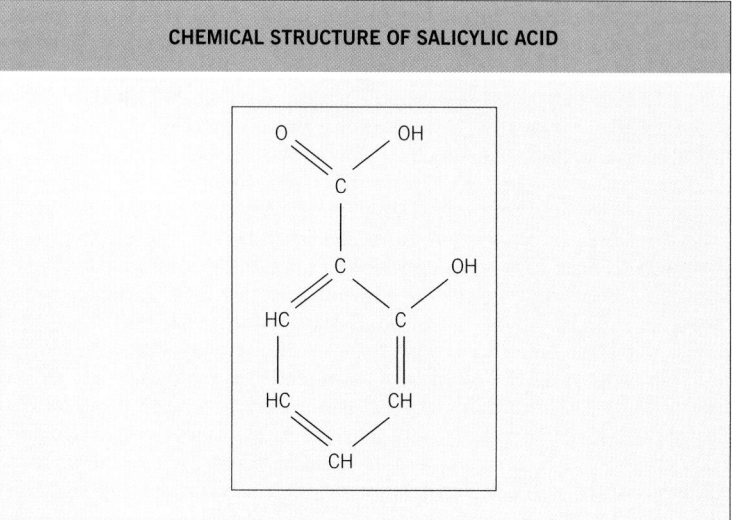

CHEMICAL STRUCTURE OF SALICYLIC ACID

Fig. 153.9 The chemical structure of salicylic acid accounting for its lipophilic properties.

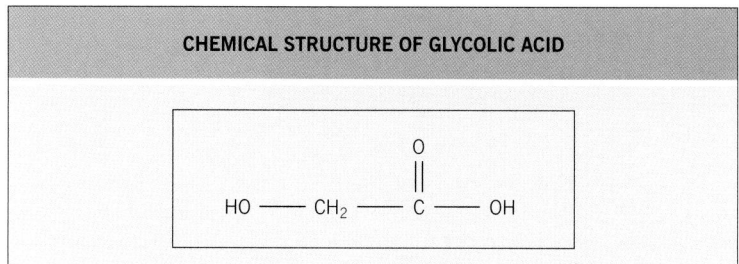

CHEMICAL STRUCTURE OF GLYCOLIC ACID

Fig. 153.8 The chemical structure of glycolic acid accounting for its hydrophilic properties.

treatment of acne as an OTC drug monographed by the FDA at a level of 2% or less. It is also an excellent keratolytic, inducing exfoliation of calluses, corns and warts[105]. Salicylic acid is incorporated into many shampoos designed to remove undesquamated corneocytes from the scalp of patients with seborrheic dermatitis and psoriasis[106].

Salicylic acid is thought to function through solubilization of intercellular cement, thereby reducing corneocyte adhesion. It appears to eliminate the stratum corneum layer by layer from the outermost level downward[107]. This is in contrast to the α-hydroxy acids, which appear to diminish cellular cohesion between the corneocytes at the lowest levels of the stratum corneum. This difference is probably due in part to the water-soluble characteristics of the α-hydroxy acids, which readily penetrate into the stratum corneum, and the oil-soluble characteristics of salicylic acid, which remains on the stratum corneum. Differences in penetration also explain the decreased stinging and burning experienced with topical salicylic acid compared with glycolic acid, since the salicylic acid does not readily penetrate to the dermis.

Topical application of salicylic acid can also take the form of short-contact cutaneous peels. Salicylic acid can be used alone in concentrations of 10–50% or combined with the α-hydroxy acid lactic acid in Jessner's solution. Salicylic acid will remain in solution at concentrations of 20% or less, in 95% ethyl alcohol; however, at concentrations of 30% and above, it precipitates, necessitating shaking of the solution prior to its use. In contrast to glycolic acid peels, salicylic acid is a self-neutralizing peel that ends with the formation of white salicylic acid crystals on the skin[108]. The crystals are easily rinsed from the skin surface with water, but they remain in the follicular ostia, providing a prolonged keratolytic effect. Thus, salicylic acid peels are useful for general exfoliation in patients with photoaging, comedolysis in acne patients, and patients with sensitive skin, such as rosacea patients, where dermal penetration should be minimized.

FUTURE DIRECTIONS

Improved understanding of the physiology of the stratum corneum is leading to new dermatologic developments in the realm of cosmetics and skin care products. This has spurred the growth in cosmeceuticals that promise to improve cutaneous function and enhance appearance. In addition, technology that was originally developed for skin keratin can be directly transferred to hair and nail keratin. Future research will undoubtedly explore methods of preventing cutaneous inflammation, which represents a common thread between dermatologic disease and potential adverse effects of cosmetics.

APPENDIX

Camouflage Cosmetic Manufacturers

Atelier Esthetique, Veil
www.veilcover.com

Ben Nye Company, Inc., Coverette
www.bennyemakeup.com

Cosmetic Specialty Labs
www.aloe-vera.com

Dermablend Corrective Cosmetics
www.dermablend.com

Dermacolor
www.charlesfox.co.uk/Dermacolor/dermacolor.html

Fashion Fair Cosmetics, Cover Tone
www.fashionfair.com

Innoxa Ltd., Keromask Cover Cream
www.beautycafe.com

Il Makiage Cosmetics, Cream Makiage
www.il-makiage.com

Joe Blasco Cosmetics, Dermaceal
www.joeblasco.com

Lydia O'Leary, Covermark
www.covermarkusa.com

REFERENCES

1. Vermeer BJ, Gilchrest BA. Cosmeceuticals. Arch Dermatol. 1996;132:337–40.
2. Epstein H. Factors in formulating cosmeceutical vehicles. Cosmet Toilet. 1997;112:91–9.
3. 21 USC 301–392.
4. Lavrijsen APM, Vermeer BJ. Cosmetics and drugs: is there a need for a third group: cosmeceutics? Br J Dermatol. 1991;124:503–4.
5. Willcox MJ, Crichton WP. The soap market. Cosmet Toilet 1989;104:61–3.
6. Wortzman MS, Scott RA, Wong PS, et al. Soap and detergent bar rinsability. J Soc Cosmet Chem. 1986;37:89–97.
7. Schreiber J. Antiperspirants. In: Barel AO, Paye M, Maibach HI (eds). Handbook of Cosmetic Science and Technology. New York, NY: Marcel Dekker, 2001:689–701.
8. Mills OH, Berger RS, Baker MD. A controlled comparison of skin cleansers in photoaged skin. J Geriatric Dermatol. 1993;1:173–9.
9. Jass HE. Cold creams. In: deNaarre MG (ed.). The Chemistry and Manufacture of Cosmetics, Vol III, 2nd edn. Wheaton, IL: Allured Publishing, 1975:237–49.
10. Baker CG. Moisturization: new methods to support time proven ingredients. Cosmet Toilet. 1987;102:99–102.
11. Goldner R. Moisturizers: a dermatologist's perspective. J Toxicol Cut Ocular Toxicol. 1992;11:193–7.
12. Boisits EK. The evaluation of moisturizing products. Cosmet Toilet. 1986;101:31–9.
13. Wu MS, Yee DJ, Sullivan ME. Effect of a skin moisturizer on the water distribution in human stratum corneum. J Invest Dermatol. 1983;81:446–8.
14. De Groot AC, Weyland JW, Nater JP. Unwanted Effects of Cosmetics and Drugs Used in Dermatology, 3rd edn. Amsterdam: Elsevier, 1994:498–500.
15. Friberg SE, Ma Z. Stratum corneum lipids, petrolatum and white oils. Cosmet Toilet. 1993;107:55–9.

16. Jass HE, Elias PM. The living stratum corneum: implications for cosmetic formulation. Cosmet Toilet. 1991;106:47–53.
17. Holleran W, Feingold K, Man MQ, et al. Regulation of epidermal sphingolipid synthesis by permeability barrier function. J Lipid Res. 1991;32:1151–8.
18. Grubauer G, Feingold KR, Elias PM. Relationship of epidermal lipogenesis to cutaneous barrier function. J Lipid Res. 1987;28:746–52.
19. Ghadially R, Halkier-Sorensen L, Elias PM. Effects of petrolatum on stratum corneum structure and function. J Am Acad Dermatol. 1992;26:387–96.
20. Spencer TS. Dry skin and skin moisturizers. Clin Dermatol. 1988;6:24–8.
21. Rieger MM, Deem DE. Skin moisturizers II. The effects of cosmetic ingredients on human stratum corneum. J Soc Cosmet Chem. 1974;25:253–62.
22. Idson B. Dry skin: moisturizing and emolliency. Cosmet Toilet. 1992;107:69–78.
23. Robbins CR, Fernee KM. Some observations on the swelling of human epidermal membrane. JSCC. 1983;37:21–34.
24. Jackson EM. Moisturizers: What's in them? How do they work? Am J Contact Dermatitis. 1992;3:162–8.
25. Wilkinson JB, Moore RJ. Astringents and skin toners. In: Harry's Cosmeticology, 7th edn. New York: Chemical Publishing, 1982:74–81.
26. Draelos ZK. Cosmetics in Dermatology. Edinburgh: Churchill Livingstone, 1995;1–14.
27. Schlossman ML, Feldman AJ. Fluid foundation and blush make-up. In: deNavarre MG (ed.). The Chemistry and Manufacture of Cosmetics. Wheaton, IL: Allured Publishing, 1988:748–51.
28. Lanzet M. Modern formulations of coloring agents: facial and eye. In: Frost P, Horowitz SN (eds). Principles of Cosmetics for the Dermatologist. St Louis: Mosby, 1982:138–9.
29. Adams RM, Maibach HI. A five-year study of cosmetic reactions. J Am Acad Dermatol. 1985;13:1062–9.

30. Wolf R, Perluk H. Failure of routine patch test results to detect eyelid dermatitis. Cutis. 1992;49:133–4.
31. Nethercott JR, Nield G, Linn Holness D. A review of 79 cases of eyelid dermatitis. J Am Acad Dermatol. 1989;21:223–30.
32. Wilkinson JB, Moore RJ. Coloured make-up preparations. In: Harry's Cosmeticology, 7th edn. New York: Chemical Publishing, 1982:341–7.
33. Wilson LA, Ahearn DG. Pseudomonas-induced corneal ulcer associated with contaminated eye mascaras. Am J Ophthalmol. 1977;84:112–19.
34. MMWR Reports. Pseudomonas aeruginosa corneal infection related to mascara applicator trauma. Arch Dermatol. 1990;126:734.
35. Ahearn DG, Wilson LA. Microflora of the outer eye and eye area cosmetics. Develop Ind Microbiol. 1976;17:23–8.
36. Kuehne JW, Ahearn DG. Incidence and characterization of fungi in eye cosmetics. Develop Ind Microbiol. 1971;12:1973–7.
37. Bhadauria B, Ahearn DG. Loss of effectiveness of preservative systems of mascaras with age. Appl Environ Microbiol. 1980;39:665–7.
38. Ahern DG, Wilson LA, Julian AJ, et al. Microbial growth in eye cosmetics: contamination during use. Develop Ind Microbiol. 1974;15:211–16.
39. Jervey JH. Mascara pigmentation of the conjunctiva. Arch Opthalmol. 1969;81:124–5.
40. Platia EV, Michels RG, Green WR. Eye-cosmetic-induced conjunctival pigmentation. Ann Ophthalmol. 1978;10:501–4.
41. Cunningham J. Color cosmetics. In: Williams DF, Schmitt WH (eds). Chemistry and Technology of the Cosmetics and Toiletries Industry. London: Blackie, 1992:143–9.
42. deNavarre MG. Lipstick. In: deNavarre MG (ed.). The Chemistry and Manufacture of Cosmetics, 2nd edn. Wheaton, IL: Allured Publishing, 1975:778.

43. Boelcke U. Requirements for lipstick colors. J Soc Cosmet Chem. 1961;12:468.

44. Sulzgerger MD, Boodman J, Byrne LA, Mallozzi ED. Acquired specific hypersensitivity to simple chemicals. Cheilitis with special reference to sensitivity to lipsticks. Arch Dermatol. 1938;37:597–615.

45. Sai S. Lipstick dermatitis caused by castor oil. Contact Dermatitis. 1983;9:75.

46. Brandle I, Boujnah-Khouadja A, Foussereau J. Allergy to castor oil. Contact Dermatitis. 1983;9:424–5.

47. Andersen KE, Neilsen R. Lipstick dermatitis related to castor oil. Contact Dermatitis. 1984;11:253–4.

48. Calnan CD. Allergic sensitivity to eosin. Acta Allergol. 1959;13:493–9.

49. Sai S. Lipstick dermatitis caused by ricinoleic acid. Contact Dermatitis. 1983;9:524.

50. Calnan CD. Amyldimethylamino benzoic acid causing lipstick dermatitis. Contact Dermatitis. 1980;6:233.

51. Hayakawa R, Fujimoto Y, Kaniwa M. Allergic pigmented lip dermatitis from lithol rubine BCA. Am J Contact Dermatitis. 1994;5:34–7.

52. Darko E, Osmundsen PE. Allergic contact dermatitis to Lipcare lipstick. Contact Dermatitis. 1984;11:46.

53. Aguirre A, Izu R, Gardeazabal J, et al. Allergic contact cheilitis from a lipstick containing oxybenzone. Contact Dermatitis. 1992;27:267–8.

54. Cronin E. Lipstick dermatitis due to propyl gallate. Contact Dermatitis. 1980;6:213–14.

55. Hayakawa R, Matsunaga K, Suzuki M, et al. Lipstick dermatitis due to C18 aliphatic compounds. Contact Dermatitis. 1987;16:215–19.

56. Rayner V. Clinical Cosmetology: A Medical Approach to Esthetics Procedures. Albany, NY: Milady Publishing, 1993:116–22.

57. Buchman H. Stage Makeup. New York: Watson-Guptill, 1979:15–18.

58. Draelos ZK. Cosmetic camouflaging techniques. Cutis. 1993;52:362–4.

59. Bouillon C. Shampoos and hair conditioners. Clin Dermatol. 1988;6:83–92.

60. Robbins CR. Interaction of shampoo and creme rinse ingredients with human hair. In: Chemical and Physical Behavior of Human Hair, 2nd edn. New York: Springer-Verlag, 1988:122–67.

61. Fox C. An introduction to the formulation of shampoos. Cosmet Toilet. 1988;103:25–58.

62. Zviak C, Vanlerberghe G. Scalp and hair hygiene. In: Zviak C (ed.). The Science of Hair Care. New York: Marcel Dekker, 1986:49–86.

63. Rieger M. Surfactants in shampoos. Cosmet Toilet. 1988;103:59–72.

64. Garcia ML, Epps JA, Yare RS, Hunter LD. Normal cuticle-wear patterns in human hair. J Soc Cosmet Chem. 1978;29:155–75.

65. Corbett JF. Hair conditioning. Cutis. 1979;23:405–13.

66. Zviak C, Bouillon C. Hair treatment and hair care products. In: Zviak C (ed.). The Science of Hair Care. New York: Marcel Dekker, 1986:115–16.

67. Rook A. The clinical importance of 'weathering' in human hair. Br J Dermatol. 1976;95:111–12.

68. Price VH. The role of hair care products. In: Orfanos CE, Montagna W, Stuttgen G (eds). Hair Research. Berlin: Springer-Verlag, 1981:501–6.

69. Robinson VNE. A study of damaged hair. J Soc Cosmet Chem. 1976;27:155–61.

70. Zviak C, Bouillon C. Hair treatment and hair care products. In: Zviak C (ed.). The Science of Hair Care. New York: Marcel Dekker, 1986:134–7.

71. Wing HJ. Nail preparations. In: deNavarre MG (ed.). The Chemistry and Manufacture of Cosmetics. Wheaton, IL: Allured Publishing, 1988:983–1005.

72. Mast R. Nail products. In: Whittam JH (ed.). Cosmetic Safety: A Primer for Cosmetic Scientists. New York: Marcel Dekker, 1987:265–313.

73. Schlossman ML. Nail-enamel resins. Cosmetic Technol. 1979;1:53.

74. Samman PD. Nail disorders caused by external influences. J Soc Cosmet Chem. 1977;28:351.

75. Daniel DR, Osmet LS. Nail pigmentation abnormalities. Cutis. 1980;25:595–607.

76. Scher RK. Cosmetics and ancillary preparations for the care of the nails. J Am Acad Dermatol. 1982;6:523–8.

77. Barnett JM, Scher RK, Taylor SC. Nail cosmetics. Dermatol Clin. 1991;9:9–17.

78. Viola LJ. Fingernail elongators and accessory nail preparations. In: Balsam MS, Sagarin E (eds). Cosmetics, Science and Technology, 2nd edn. New York: Wiley-Interscience, 1972:543–52.

79. Goodwin P. Onycholysis due to acrylic nail applications. J Exp Dermatol. 1976;1:191–2.

80. Lane CW, Kost LB. Sensitivity to artificial nails. Arch Dermatol. 1956;74:671–2.

81. Baden H. Cosmetics and the nail. In: Diseases of the Hair and Nails. Chicago: Yearbook Publishers, 1987:99–102.

82. Marks JG, Bishop ME, Willis WF. Allergic contact dermatitis to sculptured nails. Arch Dermatol. 1979;115:100.

83. Fisher AA. Cross reactions between methyl methacrylate monomer and acrylic monomers presently used in acrylic nail preparations. Contact Dermatitis. 1980;6:345–7.

84. Fisher AA, Franks A, Glick H. Allergic sensitization of the skin and nails to acrylic plastic nails. J Allergy. 1957;28:84.

85. Baran R, Dawber RPR. The nail and cosmetics. In: Samman PD, Fenton DA (eds). The Nails in Disease, 4th edn. Chicago: Yearbook Publishers, 1986:129.

86. Potts RO, Buras EM, Chrisman DA. Changes with age in the moisture content of human skin. J Invest Dermatol. 1984;82:97–100.

87. Wepierre J, Marty JP. Percutaneous absorption and lipids in elderly skin. J Appl Cosmetol. 1988;6:79–92.

88. Stiller MJ, Bartolone J, Stern R, et al. Topical 8% glycolic acid and 8% l-lactic acid creams for the treatment of photodamaged skin. Arch Dermatol. 1996;132:631–6.

89. Dietre CM, Griffin TD, Murphy, GF, et al. Effects of alpha-hydroxy acids on photoaged skin. J Am Acad Dermatol. 1996;34:187–95.

90. Berardesca E, Maibach H. AHA mechanism of action. Cosmet Toilet. 1995;110:30–1.

91. Van Scott EJ, Yu RJ. Hyperkeratinization, corneocyte cohesion and alpha hydroxy acids. J Am Acad Dermatol. 1984;11:867–79.

92. Bernstein EF, Uitto J. Connective tissue alterations in photoaged skin and the effects of alpha hydroxy acids. J Geriatric Dermatol. 1995;3(suppl.):7A–18A.

93. Lavker RM, Kaidbey K, Leyden JJ. Effects of topical ammonium lactate on cutaneous atrophy from a potent topical corticosteroid. J Am Acad Dermatol. 1992;26:535–44.

94. Van Scott EJ, Yu RJ. Alpha hydroxy acids: procedures for use in clinical practice. Cutis. 1989;43:222–8.

95. Van Scott EJ, Yu RJ. Alpha hydroxy acids: therapeutic potentials. Can J Dermatol. 1989;1:108–12.

96. Briden ME, Rendon-Pellerano MI. Treatment of rosacea with glycolic acid. J Geriatric Dermatol. 1996;4(suppl.):17B–21B.

97. Klaus MV. Evaluation of ammonium lactate in the treatment of seborrheic keratoses. J Am Acad Dermatol. 1977;22:199–203.

98. Siskin SB. The effects of ammonium lactate 12% lotion versus no therapy in the treatment of dry skin of the heels. Int J Dermatol. 1993;32:905–7.

99. Kakita LS, Petratos MA. The use of glycolic acid in Asian and darker skin types. J Geriatric Dermatol 1996;4(suppl.):8B–11B.

100. Perricone NV. An alpha hydroxy acid acts as an antioxidant. J Geriatric Dermatol. 1993;1:101–4.

101. Perricone NV, DiNardo JC. Photoprotective and antiinflammatory effects of topical glycolic acid. Dermatol Surg. 1996;22:435–7.

102. Davies M, Marks R. Studies on the effect of salicylic acid on the normal stratum corneum. Br J Dermatol. 1980;103:191–6.

103. DiNardo JC. A comparison of salicylic acid, salicylic acid with glycolic acid and benzoyl peroxide in the treatment of acne. Cosmet Dermatol. 1995;8:12.

104. Kligman A, Kligman AM. Salicylic acid as a peeling agent for the treatment of acne. Cosmet Dermatol. 1997;10:44–7.

105. Huber C, Christopher E. Keratolytic effect of salicylic acid. Arch Dermatol Res. 1977;257:293–7.

106. Draelos ZD. Salicylic acid in the dermatologic armamentarium. Cosmet Dermatol. 1997;10(suppl. 4): 7–8.

107. Roberts DL, Marshall R, Marks R. Detection of the action of salicylic acid on the normal stratum corneum. Br J Dermatol. 1980;103:191–6.

108. Kligman D, Kligman AM. Salicylic acid peels for the treatment of photoaging. Dermatol Surg. 1998;24:325–8.

Chemical and Mechanical Skin Resurfacing

154

Gary D Monheit and Mark A Chastain

Synonyms: ■ Chemical resurfacing: chemical peeling, chemexfoliation ■ Mechanical resurfacing: dermabrasion (includes dermasanding) ■ Cosmeceutical: topical agent possessing pharmacologic and physiologic effects but promoted to a variable degree as a cosmetic ■ Jessner's peel: Combes' peel ■ Baker–Gordon peel: deep phenol peel

---

Key features

- Chemical peeling, dermabrasion and laser ablation are the three main methods of skin resurfacing

- Chemical and mechanical resurfacing procedures have a long history of safety and efficacy in ameliorating various skin conditions

- Resurfacing procedures represent one part of a comprehensive skin care program that should include photoprotective measures and topical medical and/or cosmeceutical agents

- Each resurfacing procedure injures the skin to a specific depth in order to promote the regrowth of new skin with improved surface characteristics

- The degree of clinical improvement, the length of the recovery period, and the risk of complications are all proportionate to the depth of tissue injury

- Selection of suitable patients and proper choice of resurfacing procedure are critical to success

- Prolonged redness, pigmentary or textural irregularities, infection, delayed healing and scarring are potential complications of resurfacing

- Resurfacing procedures are a rewarding part of dermatologic practice, both for the patient and physician

INTRODUCTION

Resurfacing procedures to improve the health and appearance of skin have been utilized by humans for thousands of years. The ancient Egyptians applied various chemicals to the skin and may have even used sandpaper in order to attain a smoother skin surface[1,2]. Resurfacing methods within the practice of dermatology were initially described over 100 years ago, but their role has expanded dramatically over the last several decades. Our society's increasing emphasis on a youthful image and aesthetic appearance has resulted in an explosion in public demand for commercial skin care products, professional assistance from physicians and non-physicians to assure proper medical and cosmeceutical skin therapy, and procedural intervention by physicians.

All ablative resurfacing procedures injure the skin, in a controlled fashion, to a specific depth and thereby promote the growth of new skin with improved surface characteristics. The three fundamental methods used to create the controlled injury are chemical resurfacing (chemical peeling), mechanical resurfacing (motorized dermabrasion or manual dermasanding) and laser resurfacing (see Ch. 137). Chemical resurfacing entails the application of irritating chemical substances, mechanical resurfacing involves skin contact with an abrasive surface, and laser resurfacing is accomplished by irradiating the skin with a

laser beam. In general, skin resurfacing procedures can be classified as superficial, medium-depth or deep, according to their level of injury (Table 154.1). Skin resurfacing is usually performed only on the head and neck, in part because of the critical aesthetic value of this area. Caution must be exercised in treating the neck, due to its propensity for complications; only superficial procedures should be performed on the lower one-third of the neck. Resurfacing of other areas has yielded less predictable and less impressive results and is beyond the scope of this chapter.

In comparison to the other resurfacing modalities available for skin rejuvenation, chemical resurfacing probably has the longest and most well-documented history[1]. Experimentation with various peeling compounds in the late 19th and early 20th centuries led to sporadic reports describing their use in the medical literature. The initial reports were met with skepticism, but further investigation by both dermatologists and plastic surgeons verified their effectiveness in facial skin rejuvenation. Many individuals embraced these procedures as a 'fountain of youth' in the early years, and chemical peeling experienced tremendous growth

---

CLASSIFICATION OF ABLATIVE SKIN RESURFACING METHODS
Superficial – very light
• Low potency formulations of glycolic acid or other α-hydroxy acids
• 10–20% TCA (weight-to-volume formulation)
• Tretinoin
• Salicylic acid
• Microdermabrasion
Superficial – light
• 70% glycolic acid
• Jessner's solution (see Table 154.4)
• 25–30% TCA
• Solid CO_2 slush
• Microdermabrasion
Medium-depth
• 88% phenol (rarely used)
• 35–40% TCA (not recommended)
• Jessner's–35% TCA (the most popular combination)
• 70% glycolic acid–35% TCA
• Solid CO_2–35% TCA (most potent combination)
• Conservative manual dermasanding
• Erbium:YAG laser resurfacing
• Conservative CO_2 laser resurfacing
Deep
• Unoccluded or occluded Baker–Gordon phenol peel (see Table 154.5)
• TCA in concentrations >50%
• Wire-brush or diamond-fraise dermabrasion
• Aggressive manual dermasanding
• Manual dermasanding or motorized dermabrasion after a medium-depth peel
• Aggressive erbium:YAG laser resurfacing
• CO_2 laser resurfacing
• Combination erbium: YAG/CO_2 laser resurfacing

Table 154.1 Classification of ablative skin resurfacing methods. Although this classification represents an oversimplification because the depth of injury actually varies somewhat along a continuum for each different type of resurfacing procedure, it is helpful when discussing the various options with a patient. TCA, trichloroacetic acid.

in popularity. Over the last few decades, chemical peeling has become an important part of our armamentarium in the management of various cosmetic as well as non-cosmetic skin problems.

Since Kromayer's original report of motorized dermabrasion in 1905, there has been considerable growth not only in chemical resurfacing procedures, but also in other forms of mechanical resurfacing. Mechanical resurfacing is most often known as dermabrasion and refers to any procedure that involves surgical planing of the skin using an abrasive surface. The use of dermabrasion was originally limited to the treatment of scars, but its role expanded during the latter half of the 20th century to include a multitude of indications[2]. Recent adaptations of the traditional techniques of dermabrasion have led to the development of a less invasive procedure, known as microdermabrasion[3]. Dermasanding, which is a manual technique for dermabrasion utilizing abrasive paper, has been in use since the early days, but has experienced a recent resurgence in interest[4,5]. Today, mechanical resurfacing procedures remain a popular option for both patients and physicians.

Over the past decade, the practice of skin rejuvenation has been revolutionized by the development of resurfacing lasers. Carbon dioxide (CO_2) laser resurfacing is invaluable in treating cutaneous photoaging because it can consistently deliver impressive results. However, the deep wounds and extensive recovery time seen with CO_2 laser resurfacing (see Table 154.1) have led to the development of less invasive modalities, such as erbium:YAG laser resurfacing, non-ablative laser treatments, and fractional laser ablation. Despite the capabilities of lasers in facial rejuvenation, their use is limited by the considerable monetary cost to either rent the equipment or purchase and maintain it. Furthermore, nearly all the complications associated with chemical peeling and dermabrasion can occur with laser resurfacing. The use of lasers carries additional risks, such as exposure to infectious agents in the plume, fire hazards, and ocular injury by the laser beam. There may also be an increased risk of anesthesia-related problems, as well as higher financial costs of surgery, because of the greater level of sedation often required. The following discussion will focus on chemical peeling and dermabrasion, as laser therapy is covered in Chapter 137.

PREOPERATIVE HISTORY AND CONSIDERATIONS

Indications

The preoperative consultation is important in identifying at-risk patients who are best avoided or who require an extra-cautious approach, as well as in selecting patients who are ideal candidates for intervention. The dermatologist must evaluate the prospective patient and his or her skin condition carefully, to determine if a chemical or mechanical resurfacing procedure is indicated. When resurfacing is deemed appropriate, selection of the proper procedure for each patient is critical to assure that the desired results are achieved in a safe and effective manner. In general, the degree of skin surface irregularities is proportional to the depth of the injury that must be created by resurfacing (see Table 154.1) in order to achieve significant improvement. As listed in Table 154.2, there are six major indications for resurfacing.

Pre-neoplastic or neoplastic skin lesions can certainly be improved with resurfacing procedures. Those originating in the epidermis, such as actinic keratoses or lentigines, are more amenable to treatment than those with a dermal origin. Although some dermatologic conditions may be aggravated by resurfacing, acne and pigmentary dyschromias such as melasma respond favorably to superficial chemical peeling or microdermabrasion. Another indication for chemical and mechanical

skin resurfacing is to blend the effects of other procedures by preventing or eliminating lines of demarcation.

Photoaging is probably the single condition for which skin resurfacing procedures are most often performed. For patients with photoaging and acne scarring, the Glogau system (see Ch. 152) is helpful in deciding upon the most appropriate skin rejuvenation program. It classifies patients into one of four groups based on degree of severity. Patients in category I are often young with minimal photoaging and are best managed with superficial chemical peels or microdermabrasion in conjunction with medical or cosmeceutical therapy. Patients in category II would likely benefit from a medium-depth chemical peel as well as long-term medical therapy to include a retinoid and/or an α-hydroxy acid (AHA). Individuals in category III typically need prolonged medical treatment in conjunction with one of the following: a medium-depth chemical peel (with or without dermasanding), a deep chemical peel, dermabrasion or laser resurfacing. A medium-depth or deep chemical peel, dermabrasion or laser resurfacing as well as adjunctive medical therapy would certainly be indicated in patients with category IV photoaging. However, an invasive surgical operation, such as a rhytidectomy, blepharoplasty or scar revision is often required in addition to resurfacing in order to achieve the desired results.

Contraindications and Patient Selection

When evaluating a patient for chemical or mechanical resurfacing, a careful history and physical examination are important to assess the skin problems which prompted his or her presentation and to identify any factors that may contribute to intraoperative or postoperative difficulties (Table 154.3) The patient should be asked about prior resurfacing procedures, rhytidectomy (facelift) or oral isotretinoin therapy within the last 6 months, as these can increase the risk of complications following medium-depth and deep resurfacing[6,7]. Any history of abnormal scar formation or therapeutic radiation exposure warrants extreme caution when considering a patient for skin resurfacing. Individuals with prior radiation exposure should be examined closely for the presence of intact facial hair in order to ensure that there are enough pilosebaceous units to promote re-epithelialization[8]. Another important element of the patient's history is the presence or absence of a prior herpes simplex infection. Risk factors for HIV infection or viral hepatitis should be identified, and routine laboratory screening is recommended in individuals undergoing dermabrasion with a powered engine. The general health and nutritional status of the patient is also an important consideration, especially for medium-depth and deep resurfacing procedures.

Patients with certain cutaneous disorders, such as rosacea, seborrheic dermatitis, atopic dermatitis, psoriasis or vitiligo, may be

---

MAJOR INDICATIONS FOR CHEMICAL AND MECHANICAL SKIN RESURFACING

- Actinically damaged skin and rhytides
- Scarring
- Pre-neoplastic or neoplastic lesions (e.g. actinic keratoses)
- Underlying skin diseases such as acne
- Pigmentary dyschromias (including tattoos)
- Demarcation lines secondary to other resurfacing procedures

Table 154.2 Major indications for chemical and mechanical skin resurfacing.

CONTRAINDICATIONS TO CHEMICAL AND MECHANICAL SKIN RESURFACING

Absolute

- Poor physician–patient relationship
- Lack of psychologic stability and mental preparedness
- Unrealistic expectations
- Poor general health and nutritional status
- Isotretinoin therapy within the last 6 months*
- Complete absence of intact pilosebaceous units on the face
- Active infection or open wounds (such as herpes simplex, excoriations or open acne cysts)

Relative

- Medium-depth or deep resurfacing procedure within the last 3–12 months*
- Recent facial surgery involving extensive undermining, such as a rhytidectomy*
- History of abnormal scar formation or delayed wound healing
- History of therapeutic radiation exposure
- History of certain skin diseases (such as rosacea, seborrheic dermatitis, atopic dermatitis, psoriasis and vitiligo) or active retinoid dermatitis
- Fitzpatrick skin types IV, V and VI*

*These contraindications apply only to medium-depth and deep resurfacing procedures.

Table 154.3 Contraindications to chemical and mechanical skin resurfacing.

at increased risk for postoperative complications, including disease exacerbation, prolonged erythema, contact dermatitis or even delayed healing. In particular, individuals with rosacea have vasomotor instability and may develop an exaggerated inflammatory response to the resurfacing procedure. Evaluation of the patient's Fitzpatrick skin type (see Ch. 134) is helpful in predicting the chance of postoperative pigmentary dyschromias. Individuals with Fitzpatrick skin types I or II are at low risk for hyperpigmentation or hypopigmentation after medium-depth or deep resurfacing, whereas those with types III through VI are at greater risk for these complications[9].

The patient should understand that chemical and mechanical resurfacing procedures cannot reliably reduce pore size and their ability to improve lax skin and deeper wrinkles and scars is limited, depending on the type of intervention being performed. While dermabrasion may sometimes eliminate telangiectasias, chemical peels cannot accomplish this and can even unmask them by removing the pigmentary irregularities. The patient must fully understand the potential benefits, limitations and risks of the procedure, and an informed consent must be signed. A test spot may be useful in some patients to assess their suitability for resurfacing and may be particularly helpful when there is a great deal of concern about the chances of postoperative pigmentary dyschromias[10]. Although a favorable test spot result does not guarantee a positive outcome following full-face resurfacing, an unfavorable test spot result is useful in identifying high-risk patients. If the dermatologist feels any uncertainty about the patient's suitability or the likelihood of a favorable result, the procedure should not be performed.

Preoperative and Intraoperative Preparations

Another purpose of the preoperative consultation is to ensure that the patient is adequately prepared for the procedure. Almost every patient desiring facial rejuvenation for cutaneous photoaging would benefit from botulinum toxin injections to alleviate dynamic wrinkles (see Ch. 159). These injections appear to enhance the results of deeper resurfacing procedures by immobilizing the muscles implicated in the development of rhytides during the critical time of postoperative collagen remodeling. It is recommended that botulinum toxin injections be administered as an adjunctive therapy preoperatively in patients with photoaging undergoing medium-depth or deep chemical peels, dermabrasion or laser resurfacing.

Due to the significant morbidity associated with herpetic infections in the healing period, patients who undergo medium-depth or deep resurfacing (see Table 154.1) must be treated prophylactically with an antiviral agent, regardless of whether there is a history of herpes simplex infection[11]. These drugs are not routinely given to patients having a superficial chemical peel or microdermabrasion, because the injury is generally not sufficient to activate the virus. However, therapy may be considered in conjunction with superficial resurfacing in patients with a strong personal history of recurrent herpes simplex. Recommended prophylaxis consists of acyclovir 400 mg three times daily or valacyclovir 500 mg twice daily, beginning on the day of the procedure. It is advisable to administer the drug for at least 10 to 14 days[12]. The reason for such a long duration of therapy is that viral replication is possible only in intact epidermal cells, making clinical infection unlikely during the first few days postoperatively. The risk of an eruption increases dramatically with the onset of re-epithelialization and remains high until this process is complete.

It is important that the patient adheres to a strict skin care regimen during the immediate preoperative and postoperative periods in order to achieve optimal results. The authors treat patients with topical tretinoin on a nightly basis prior to the procedure. Because of the tendency for retinoids to cause irritation within 1 to 2 weeks of starting therapy (i.e. retinoid dermatitis), a weaker, more gentle tretinoin formulation should be used in patients with sensitive skin. In patients with active retinoid dermatitis, resurfacing should be delayed, because this condition may lead to a prolongation in postoperative erythema. Decreasing the frequency of therapy or switching to an alternative retinoid will allow the inflammation to subside, so that the procedure can be performed[13].

All-*trans*-retinoic acid, or tretinoin, has been classified as a superficial chemical peeling agent, but it is best considered as an integral component of a complete skin rejuvenation program. With chronic use, this drug has been shown to improve actinically damaged skin both clinically and histologically[14] The use of tretinoin prior to chemical peeling, dermabrasion or laser resurfacing speeds epidermal healing and enhances the effects of the procedure[13,14]. Tretinoin also increases the depth of a chemical peel by decreasing the thickness of the stratum corneum. Its use is restricted, however, during the postoperative healing period until there is complete re-epithelialization and diminished inflammatory erythema.

Hydroquinone blocks the enzyme tyrosinase and can reduce the production of epidermal melanin during the healing phase. Patients with skin type III or higher may benefit from the twice-daily application of a 4% to 8% topical hydroquinone in the preoperative and postoperative (post-healing) periods – even if there is no history of pigmentary abnormalities[9]. It is also necessary to use hydroquinone when peeling for the treatment of pigmentary dyschromias, such as melasma, in patients of any skin type[9]. The use of a Wood's light to localize the pigment to either the epidermis or dermis, or to both locations, may occasionally be helpful in choosing the most appropriate intervention and in predicting a patient's response to therapy.

All patients undergoing any type of skin resurfacing procedure must adhere to strict photoprotective measures during the postoperative period. This issue is critical in patients whose Fitzpatrick skin type is III or higher, in patients with pigmentary disturbances, in patients taking exogenous estrogens, as well as in all patients having medium-depth or deep resurfacing. Specific methods to minimize sun exposure and proper use of sunblocks should be discussed. Patients are also counseled to avoid tobacco use, as smoking in the postoperative period may limit the effectiveness and complications from resurfacing.

The need for intraoperative sedation and analgesia is also discussed with the patient preoperatively, so that plans are made accordingly. Superficial resurfacing procedures usually require only 'talkesthesia', a technique that is extremely helpful in awake patients undergoing a procedure (talking calmly to the patient with encouragement during the procedure). Medium-depth chemical or mechanical resurfacing usually requires a limited degree of perioperative sedation and analgesia, which may include the application of topical amide anesthetics, regional blocks of the supraorbital, infraorbital and mental nerves, as well as oral diazepam, intramuscular meperidine hydrochloride or intramuscular hydroxyzine hydrochloride. Although deep resurfacing procedures can be accomplished entirely with nerve blockade, local injections of lidocaine and mild sedatives, some patients require intravenous or general (endotracheal tube) anesthesia. Application of the tumescent technique (see Ch. 157) to resurfacing has allowed many patients to undergo deep resurfacing procedures without the additional risks of intravenous or general anesthesia[15]. The patient's inherent pain tolerance, level of anxiety, concomitant medical conditions, and willingness to pay the extra costs of heavier sedation are important topics in the preoperative consultation that are used to plan for appropriate anesthesia.

The patient must be given specific instructions to follow on the day of the procedure. Upon awakening, the patient washes his or her face with a gentle cleanser and preferably avoids the application of any cosmetics. Individuals undergoing procedures requiring minimal or no sedation are encouraged to eat a light breakfast, but patients receiving deeper anesthesia should have nothing by mouth except their usual medications. Particularly for the medium-depth and deep resurfacing procedures, the dermatologist should meet with the patient and his or her family preoperatively to re-establish rapport, answer last-minute questions, discuss perioperative and postoperative expectations and instructions, and assure compliance with antimicrobial prophylaxis.

DESCRIPTION OF TECHNIQUES

Chemical Resurfacing Procedures

Although there is currently a wide variety of resurfacing procedures available for facial rejuvenation, chemical peeling remains a popular choice for both patient and physician. In comparison to some of the newer options, chemical peels have a longstanding safety and efficacy record, are performed with ease, are low in cost, and have a relatively quick recovery time. Various acidic and basic compounds are used to produce a controlled skin injury and are classified as superficial, medium-depth and deep peeling agents, according to their level of penetration, destruction and inflammation (see Table 154.1). In general, superficial peels cause epidermal injury and occasionally extend into the papillary dermis, medium-depth peels cause injury through the papillary dermis to the upper reticular dermis, and deep peels cause injury to the mid-reticular dermis.

Prior to the application of peeling solutions, the skin surface must be vigorously cleansed to remove residual oils, debris and excess stratum corneum. The authors use gauze pads containing 0.25% triclosan (an ingredient found in some deodorant soaps), followed by rinsing with water and drying. Because of the defatting and degreasing properties of acetone, gauze pads moistened in an acetone preparation are then used to cleanse the skin even further. Finally, the cleansed skin is palpated immediately prior to peeling, in order to check for the presence of residual oil, and if any is felt, the process is repeated. The importance of cleansing prior to the peeling procedure cannot be over-emphasized. A thorough and evenly distributed cleansing and degreasing of the face assures uniform penetration of the peeling solution and leads to an even result without skipping areas (Fig. 154.1).

The effect of a chemical peel is dependent upon the agent used, its concentration, and the techniques employed before and during its application. Each wounding agent used in peels has unique chemical properties and causes a specific pattern of injury to the skin[15–20]. It is important for the physician using these solutions to be familiar with their cutaneous effects and proper methods of application, to assure correct depth of injury. The marketplace has been flooded with numerous proprietary formulations of these peeling agents, with each product claiming unique advantages. These products are often expensive and have not been shown to be safer or more effective than the conventional solutions. The following discussion on superficial, medium-depth and deep peeling will therefore focus on the specific chemical agents that are actively responsible for producing the various patterns of injury.

Superficial chemical peeling

Superficial chemical peels are indicated in the management of acne and its postinflammatory erythema, mild photoaging (Glogau I and II), epidermal lesions such as lentigines and keratoses, as well as melasma and other pigmentary dyschromias. Multiple peels on a repeated basis are usually necessary to obtain optimal results. The frequency of peels and degree of exposure to the peeling agent may be increased gradually as necessary. Results are enhanced by medical or cosmeceutical therapy, including a retinoid and, if necessary, a bleaching agent. All superficial chemical peels share the advantages of only mild stinging and burning during application as well as minimal time needed for recovery.

Superficial chemical peels are divided into two varieties – very light and light (see Table 154.1). With very light peels, the injury is usually limited to the stratum corneum and only creates exfoliation, but the injury may extend into the stratum granulosum. The agents used for these peels include low-potency formulations of glycolic acid, 10–20% trichloroacetic acid (TCA), Jessner's solution (Table 154.4), tretinoin and salicylic acid[21–23]. Light peels injure the entire epidermis down to the basal layer, stimulating the regeneration of a fresh new epithelium. Agents used for light peels include 70% glycolic acid, 25–35% TCA and solid CO_2 slush[21,22]. During the application of superficial peeling agents, there may be mild stinging followed by a level I frosting, defined as the appearance of erythema and streaky whitening on the surface (Fig. 154.2).

Alpha-hydroxy acids (AHAs) are naturally found in foods and have been used widely in skin rejuvenation programs since the early 1990s. The depth of injury is determined by the specific AHA used, its pH, the concentration of free acid, the volume applied to the skin, and the duration of contact. In low concentrations, AHAs have been shown to decrease the cohesion of corneocytes at the junction of the stratum corneum and the stratum granulosum[24]. Higher concentrations are associated with complete epidermolysis. With chronic use of AHA-containing products on a daily basis, there is an increase in skin thickness, acid mucopolysaccharides, and the density of collagen, as well as an improvement in elastic fiber quality[19]. The most popular of the AHAs, glycolic acid, is available in a variety of over-the-counter preparations and can be purchased by physicians in unbuffered

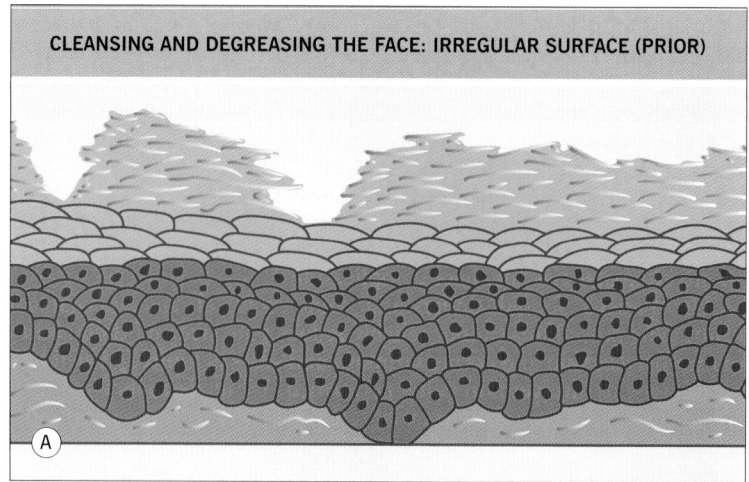

CLEANSING AND DEGREASING THE FACE: IRREGULAR SURFACE (PRIOR)

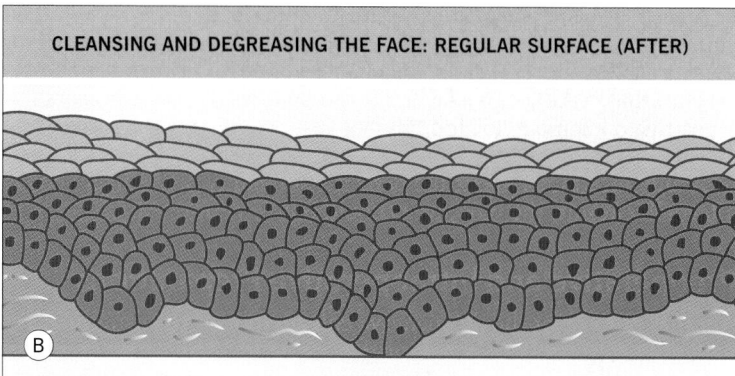

CLEANSING AND DEGREASING THE FACE: REGULAR SURFACE (AFTER)

Fig. 154.1 Cleansing and degreasing the face. A Irregular surface (prior). **B** Clean, regular surface (after).

JESSNER'S SOLUTION (COMBES' FORMULA)	
Resorcinol	14 g
Salicylic acid	14 g
85% lactic acid	14 g
95% ethanol (q.s.ad)	100 ml

Table 154.4 Jessner's solution (Combes' formula). q.s.ad, a sufficient quantity up to.

concentrations as high as 70% for chemical peels. Weekly or biweekly applications of 40–70% unbuffered glycolic acid (with cotton swabs, a sable brush, or 2 in × 2 in gauze pads) have been used most often for acne, mild photoaging, and melasma[25]. The time of application is critical for glycolic acid, as it must be rinsed off with water or neutralized with 5% sodium bicarbonate after 2 to 4 minutes.

Application of 10–20% TCA with either a saturated gauze pad or sable brush produces erythema and a very light frost within 15 to 45 seconds. The depth of penetration of the peeling solution is related to the number of coats applied. Protein precipitation results and leads to exfoliation without vesiculation. Concentrations of TCA up to 30% can also be used alone as a superficial peeling agent, but may create an injury that extends partially into the upper dermis. Jessner's solution is a combination of keratolytic ingredients that has been used for over 100 years in the treatment of inflammatory and comedonal acne as well as hyperkeratotic skin disorders (see Table 154.4). Jessner's solution has intense keratolytic activity, initially causing loss of corneocyte cohesion within the stratum corneum and subsequently creating inter-cellular and intracellular edema within the upper epidermis if application is continued[26]. The mode of application for the Jessner's peel is similar to that of the 10–20% TCA peel. The clinical endpoint of treatment is erythema and blotchy frosting. Salicylic acid, a β-hydroxy acid that is one of the ingredients in Jessner's solution, can also be used alone in superficial chemical peeling[23]. It is a preferred therapy for comedonal acne as it is lipophilic and concentrates in the pilosebaceous apparatus

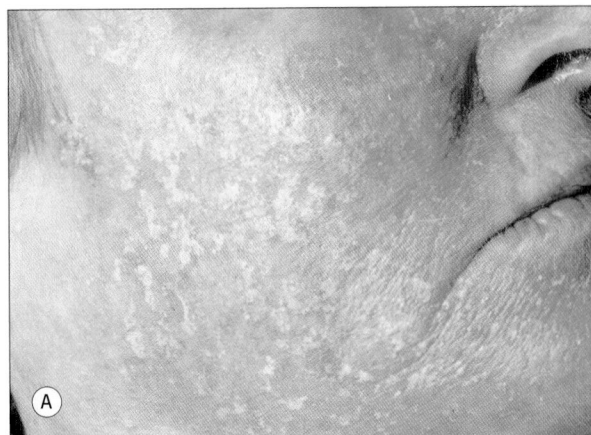

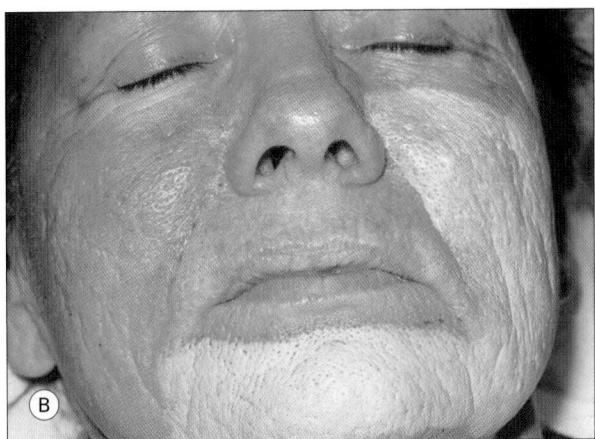

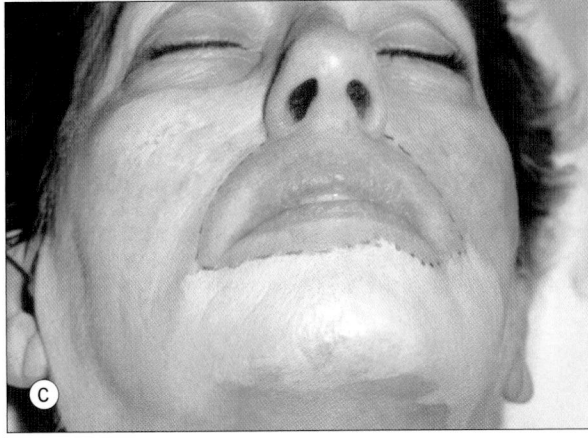

Fig 154.2 **Levels of frosting. A** Level I frosting as found with light chemical peeling: erythema with streaky frosting. **B** Level II frosting: erythema with diffuse white frosting. **C** Level III frosting: solid white enamel frosting.

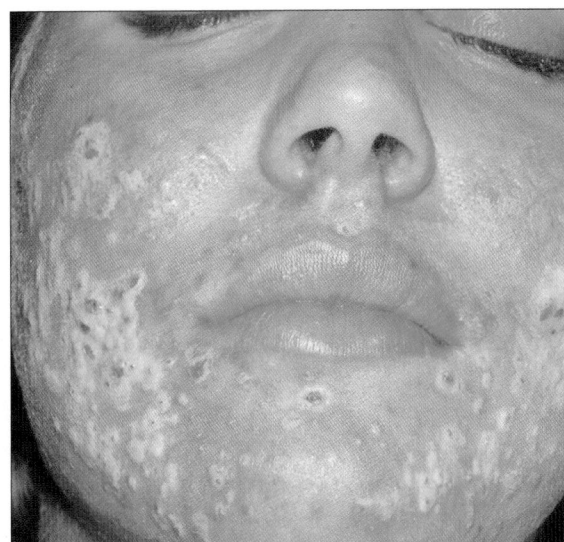

Fig. 154.3 **Salicylic acid peels.** These peels are effective for the treatment of acne, including comedones. Repetitive peels over 6 weeks combined with medical acne treatment will hasten resolution of the condition. Note the perifollicular frosting seen with salicylic acid, a lipophilic chemical.

(Fig. 154.3). It is quite effective as an adjunctive therapy for open and closed comedones and resolving post-acne erythema.

Prior to the initial treatment, the patient must understand that the net effect of repetitive superficial chemical peels never approaches the beneficial effect obtained with a single medium-depth or deep peel. The improvements in cutaneous photoaging following superficial peels are usually subtle because there is little to no effect on the dermis. These peels thus cannot produce an appreciable effect on textural changes such as deep wrinkles and furrows which originate within the dermis. Nevertheless, their ease of use and minimal downtime makes these 'lunchtime' peels rewarding for patients with realistic expectations and are a favorite of busy patients.

Medium-depth chemical peeling

Medium-depth chemical peels consist of controlled damage through the epidermis and papillary dermis, with variable extension to the upper reticular dermis. Both medium-depth and deep chemical peeling produce epidermal necrosis, papillary dermal edema and homogeniza-

tion, and a sparse lymphocytic infiltrate within the first several days[15]. During the next 3 months postoperatively, there is increased collagen production with expansion of the papillary dermis and the development of a mid-dermal band of thick fibers. These changes correlate with continued clinical improvement during this time.

For many years, 40–50% TCA was the prototypical medium-depth peeling agent because of its ability to ameliorate fine wrinkles, actinic changes and 'pre-neoplasias'. TCA as a single agent for medium-depth peeling has fallen out of favor because of the high risk of complications, especially scarring and pigmentary alterations, when used in strengths approaching 50% and higher[27]. Today, most medium-depth chemical peels are performed utilizing 35% TCA in combination with either Jessner's solution, 70% glycolic acid, or solid CO_2 as a 'priming' agent. These combination peels have been found to be as effective as 50% TCA alone, but with fewer risks. The level of penetration is better controlled with these combination peels, thereby preventing the 'hot spots' that can produce dyschromias and scarring seen with higher concentrations of TCA.

Brody and Hailey[28] developed the use of solid CO_2 to freeze the skin prior to the application of 35% TCA. This causes complete epidermal necrosis and significant dermal edema, thereby allowing deeper penetration of the TCA in selected areas. This technique is particularly useful to efface the edges of mild acne scars and to destroy thicker epidermal growths. Monheit[26] then described a combination medium-depth peel in which Jessner's solution is applied, followed by 35% TCA. Similarly, Coleman & Futrell[29] have demonstrated the usefulness of 70% glycolic acid prior to the application of 35% TCA for medium-depth peeling. The Jessner's solution and glycolic acid both appear to effectively weaken the epidermal barrier and allow deeper, more uniform, and more controlled penetration of the 35% TCA.

Current indications for medium-depth chemical peeling include Glogau group II photoaging, epidermal lesions such as actinic keratoses, pigmentary dyschromias and mild acne scarring, as well as blending of the effects of deeper resurfacing procedures. The most popular of the medium-depth peels for facial rejuvenation is the Jessner's–35% TCA peel, with other combination peels being utilized less frequently. This peel has been widely accepted because of its broad range of uses, the large number of individuals in whom it is indicated, its ease of modification according to the situation, and its excellent safety profile.

The Jessner's–35% TCA peel is particularly useful for the improvement of mild to moderate photoaging (Fig. 154.4). It freshens sallow, atrophic skin and softens fine rhytides, with minimal risk of textural or pigmentary complications. Collagen remodeling occurs for as long as 3 to 4 months postoperatively, during which time there is continued improvement in texture and rhytides. Deep furrows, however, are not eliminated with this peel. When used in conjunction with a retinoid, bleaching agent and sunscreens, a single Jessner's–35% TCA peel

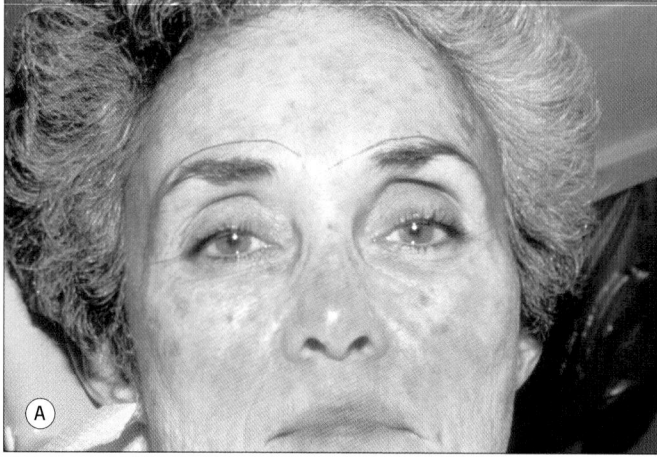

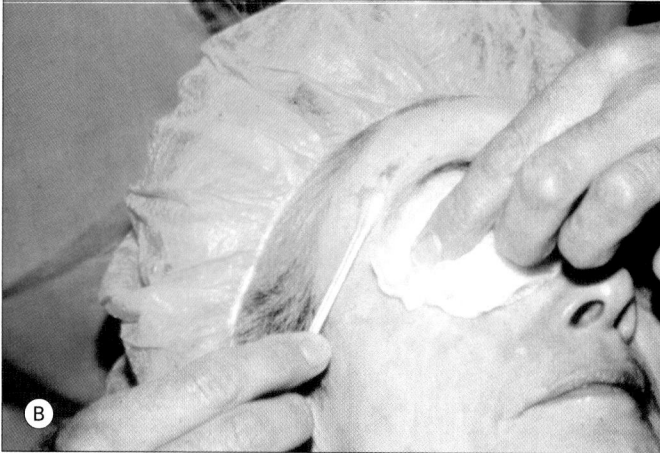

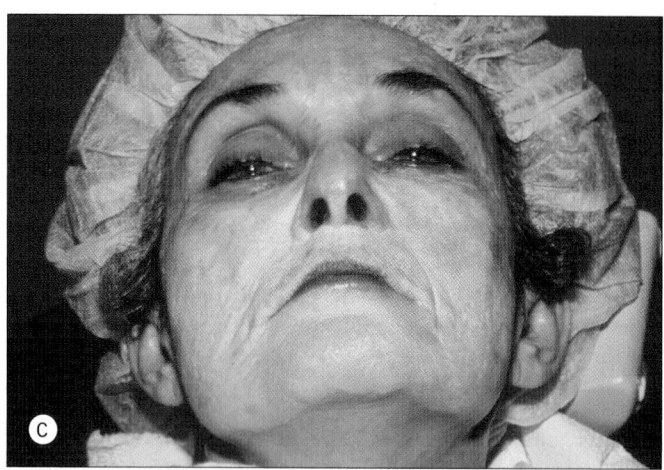

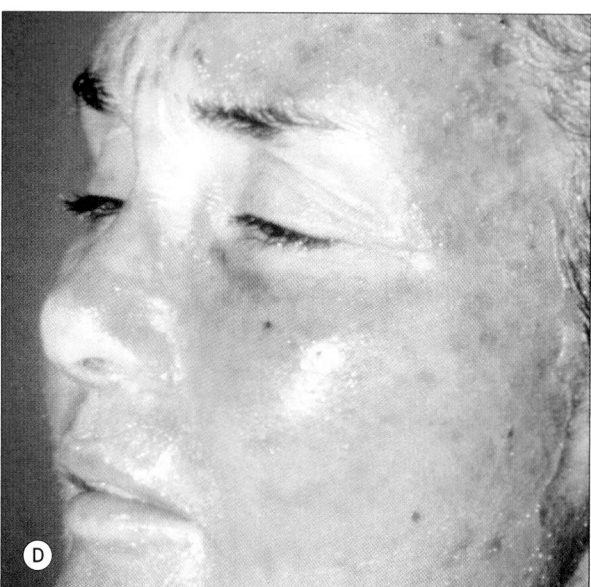

Fig. 154.4 Medium-depth chemical peel used to treat moderate photoaging of the skin. A Preoperative, demonstrating actinic keratoses plus aging textural changes. **B** Application of 35% trichloroacetic acid (TCA) directly after Jessner's solution. **C** White enamel frosting (level III) from 35% TCA. **D** Desquamation and inflammation 4 days after peel. **E** Final results 6 months later.

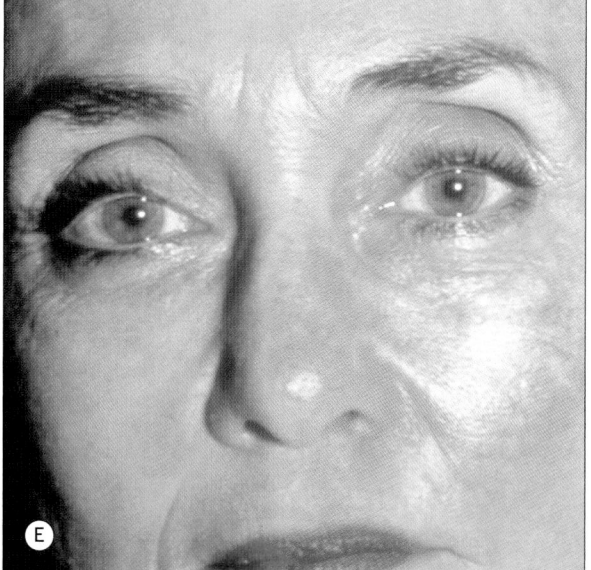

lessens pigmentary dyschromias and lentigines more effectively than repetitive superficial peels (Fig. 154.5). Epidermal growths such as actinic keratoses also respond well to this peel. In fact, the Jessner's–35% TCA peel has been found as effective as topical 5-fluorouracil chemotherapy in removing both grossly visible and clinically undetectable actinic keratoses, but has the added advantages of lower morbidity and greater improvement in associated photoaging[30,31].

Another indication for the Jessner's–35% TCA peel is to blend the effects of other resurfacing procedures with the surrounding skin. Patients who undergo laser resurfacing, deep chemical peeling or dermabrasion to a localized area such as the periorbital or perioral region often develop a sharp line of demarcation between the treated and untreated skin. The treated skin may appear hypopigmented (also

known as pseudohypopigmentation) in comparison to the untreated skin. These irregularities are often conspicuous and are troubling to the patient. A Jessner's–35% TCA peel performed on the adjacent untreated skin helps to blend the treated area into its surroundings. For example, a patient with advanced photoaging in the periorbital region and moderate photoaging on the remaining face may desire CO_2 laser resurfacing only around the eyes. In this patient, medium-depth chemical peeling of the areas not treated with the laser would improve the photoaging in these regions and avoid a line of demarcation[32]. Similarly, a patient having spot dermabrasion to a localized scar would benefit from a Jessner's–35% TCA peel to the remainder of that cosmetic unit or to the rest of the face. It is important to note that when used in combination with other resurfacing procedures such as

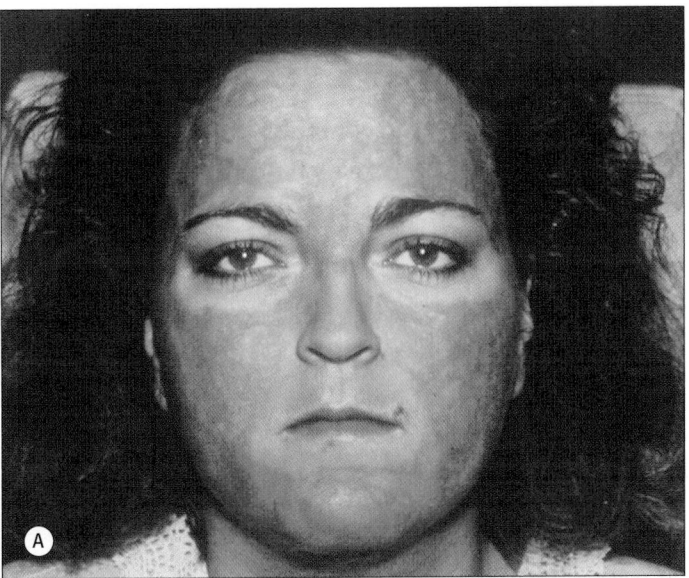

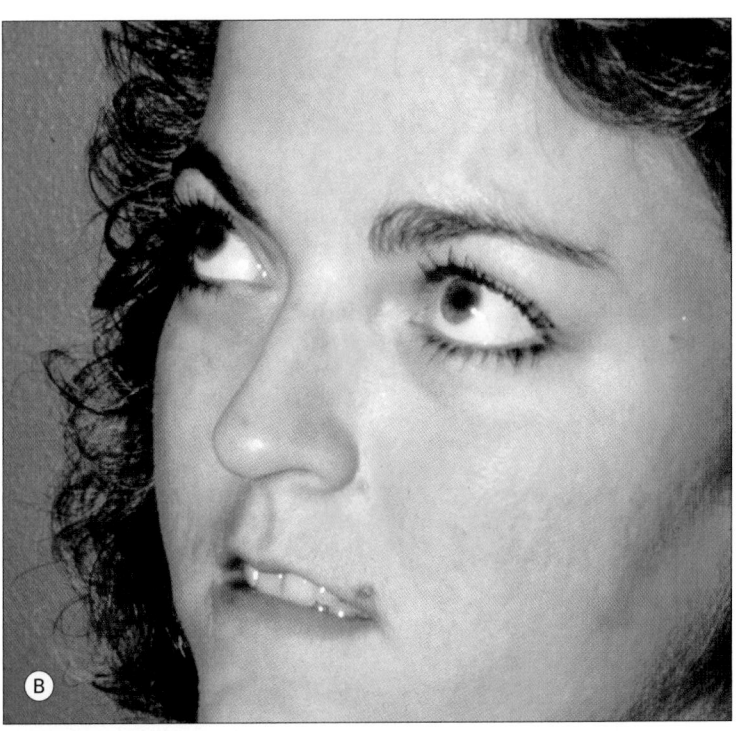

Fig. 154.5 Postinflammatory hyperpigmentation unresponsive to hydroquinone, tretinoin and superficial chemical peeling. Full response to a medium-depth chemical peel and topical agents was observed. **A** Preoperative. **B** Six weeks postoperative.

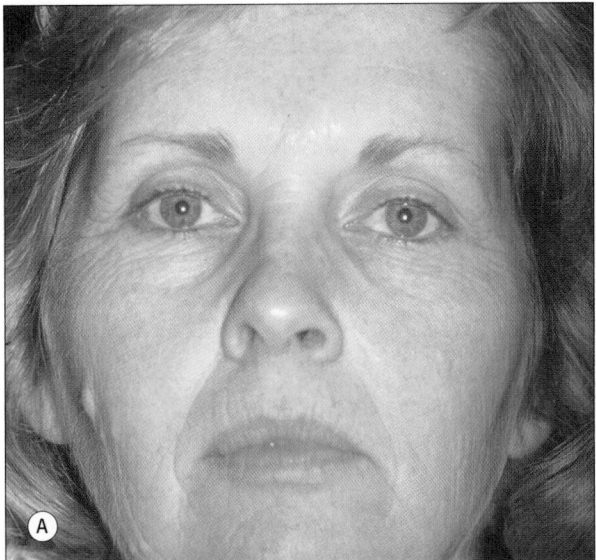

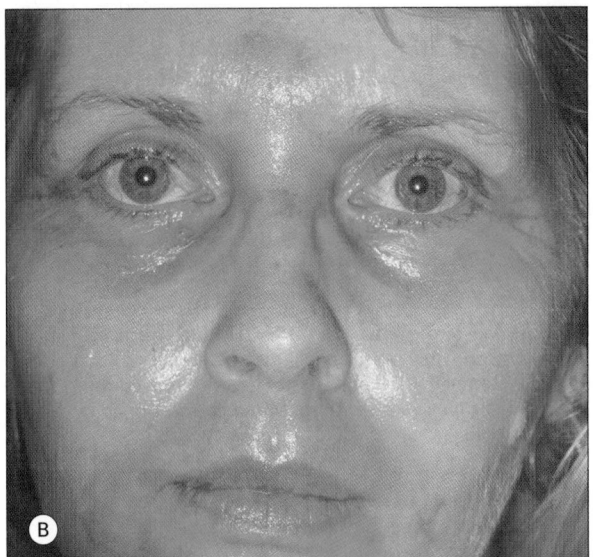

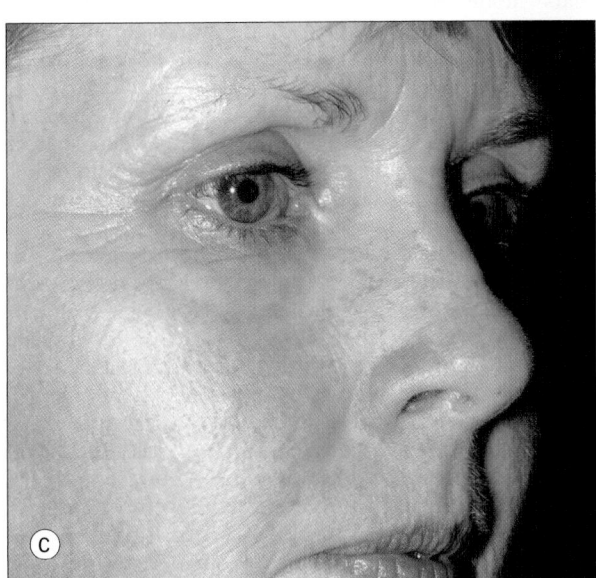

Fig. 154.6 Combination procedure utilizing perioral–periorbital CO$_2$ laser resurfacing with Jessner's + 35% trichloroacetic acid peel to the remainder of the face. The peel will blend the color and texture of the laser treated areas. **A** Preoperative: the eyelids and lips need deeper resurfacing than do the cheeks, which require only medium-depth injury. **B** Four days postoperative: note difference in the rate of healing between laser- and peel-treated areas. **C** One year postoperative.

laser ablation or dermabrasion, the peel should be performed first, in order to avoid accidental application of the peeling agent onto previously abraded areas of skin (Fig. 154.6).

Using either cotton-tipped applicators or gauze pads, a single, even coat of Jessner's solution is applied first to the forehead, then the cheeks, nose and chin, and, lastly, the eyelids. Proper application of Jessner's solution causes minimal discomfort and creates a faint frost within a background of mild erythema (level I; Fig. 154.7A). After waiting 1 to 2 minutes for the Jessner's solution to completely dry, 35% TCA is then applied evenly with one to four cotton-tipped applicators (Fig. 154.7B). The ultimate effectiveness of this peel is directly dependent upon the depth of penetration of the peeling solutions, and this depth is a function of the adequacy of degreasing and the amount

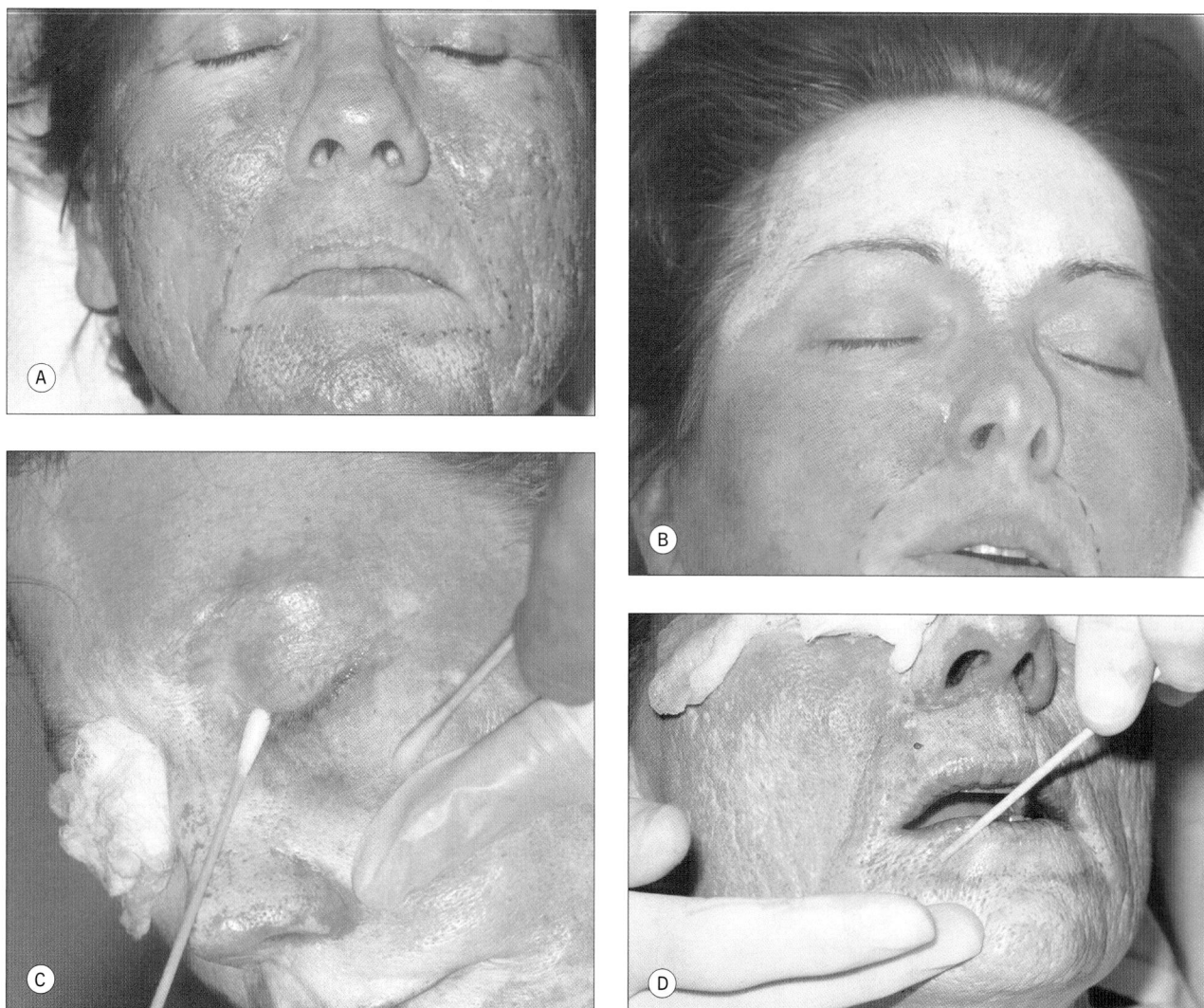

Fig. 154.7 Technical aspects of the Jessner's + 35% trichloroacetic acid (TCA) peel. A Appearance of level I frosting after application of Jessner's solution, erythema with blotchy frosting. **B** 35% TCA applied after Jessner's solution dries with an even application using cotton-tipped applicators, one to four. A level III or white enamel frosting is obtained. **C** Eyelids are treated with one cotton-tipped applicator moistened with 35% TCA. A dry applicator is used to absorb tears during eyelid peeling. **D** Lip rhytides are peeled with saturated cotton-tipped applicators. The wooden shaft is used to rub peel solution further into the lip rhytides.

of both solutions applied. The use of cotton swabs, particularly for the application of TCA, is advantageous because is allows the surgeon to easily vary the amount of solution applied according to the patient's specific needs. The amount of TCA delivered to the skin surface is determined by the number of applicators used, their degree of saturation, the amount of pressure applied to the skin surface, and the duration of their contact with the skin. Four moist cotton-tipped applicators are applied in broad strokes over the forehead and on the medial cheeks. Two mildly soaked cotton-tipped applicators can be used across the lips and chin, and one damp cotton-tipped applicator on the eyelids (Fig. 154.7C).

Anatomic areas of the face are peeled with TCA sequentially from the forehead to temple to cheeks and finally to the lips and eyelids. Careful feathering of the solution into the hairline and around the rim of the jaw and brow conceals the demarcation line between peeled and non-peeled skin. Areas of wrinkled skin are stretched taut with the help of an assistant, to allow even application of the solution into the folds and troughs. This technique is particularly helpful on the skin of the upper and lower lips. For perioral rhytides, TCA is applied with the wooden portion of a cotton-tipped applicator and extended onto the vermilion border (Fig. 154.7D).

Eyelid skin must be treated delicately and carefully to avoid over-application and to prevent exposure of the eyes to TCA solution. The patient should be positioned with the head elevated at 30°. Excess peel solution on the cotton tip should be squeezed out so that the applicator is semi-dry. With the eyes closed, a single applicator is rolled gently from the periorbital skin onto the upper eyelid skin without going beyond the superior aspect of the supratarsal plate. Another semi-dry applicator is

then rolled onto the lower eyelid skin within 2 to 3 mm of the lid margin while the patient is looking superiorly. Excess peel solution should never be left on the lids, because it can roll into the eyes. Any tears should be immediately dried with a cotton-tipped applicator because they may pull the solution into the eye by capillary action (see Fig. 154.7C). Tears can also travel down the cheek and carry TCA onto the neck, resulting in a linear streak.

The white frost from the TCA application appears on the treated area within 30 seconds to 2 minutes. This response is representative of keratocoagulation and indicates that the TCA's physiologic reaction is complete. TCA takes longer to frost than phenol preparations, but a shorter period of time than the superficial peeling agents. The desired endpoint in medium-depth peeling is level II to level III frosting. Level II frosting is defined as a white-coated frosting with a background of erythema (see Fig 154.2B). Level III frosting, which is associated with penetration to the reticular dermis, is a solid white enamel frosting with no background of erythema (see Fig. 154.2C). A deeper level III frosting should be restricted only to areas of thick skin and heavy actinic damage. Most medium-depth chemical peels achieve a level II frosting and this is especially important over the eyelids and areas of sensitive skin. Areas with a greater tendency to form scars, such as the zygomatic arch and the bony prominences of the jawline and chin, should receive no greater than level II frosting.

Before re-treating an area, the surgeon should wait at least 3 to 4 minutes after the application of TCA, to ensure that frosting has reached its peak. Each cosmetic unit is then assessed, and areas of incomplete or uneven frosting are carefully re-treated with a thin application of TCA. Additional applications of TCA increase the depth of penetration as well as the risk of complications, so one should apply more solution only to the underfrosted areas. Thicker keratoses do not frost as well as the surrounding skin, so vigorous rubbing of the lesion may be needed for adequate TCA penetration. If necessary, thicker epidermal lesions may be treated with liquid nitrogen cryotherapy for several seconds prior to the application of TCA. As will be discussed later, mechanical abrasion can also be performed in selected areas at the completion of the Jessner's–35% TCA chemical peel, to enhance the results.

Though there is an immediate burning sensation as the peel solution is applied, the discomfort begins to subside as frosting occurs and resolves fully by the time of discharge. If necessary, a topical amide anesthetic can be applied under occlusion prior to a medium-depth peel, for pain relief[33]. Cool saline compresses offer symptomatic relief at the conclusion of the peel. Unlike the compresses in glycolic acid peels, the saline following a TCA peel simply provides relief and does not 'neutralize' the acid.

TCA Cross

The 'TCA Cross' technique is a new innovative approach to deep ice-pick and fibrotic acne scars. Rather than a peel or method of exfoliation, it is the use of 90% TCA as a full-thickness destructive tool. As applied to an ice-pick scar, it destroys the epidermis and deep dermal tunnel, creating a full-thickness skin wound which will heal with the rejuvenation of new collagen filling the depressed scar. This method offers a new, simpler approach to these full-thickness depressions in which the alternatives are surgical: punch grafts, excision and scar revision. The procedure is performed independently of other resurfacing procedures such as peeling, laser resurfacing or dermabrasion.

After the face is cleansed and degreased with acetone, the ice-pick and depressed fibrotic scars to be treated are outlined with a skin marker and photographed. This serves as a guide for further treatment sessions. The 90% TCA is applied to the interior of the ice-pick scar with a toothpick, being careful not to drip the acid over normal skin. Each of the scars is treated until a brilliant white frosting appears. A topical antibiotic is then placed on each treated site. The procedure is performed with no anesthesia or sedation, as it only produces a brief stinging equivalent to the feeling of cryosurgery.

Healing occurs over the next 2 to 3 weeks, with granulation tissue, fibroplasia and remodeling of new collagen, which will elevate and soften the depressed scars. The procedure is repeated in two to six sessions at 6-week intervals until normal elevation is achieved. Then, a more superficial resurfacing procedure such as medium-depth peeling, laser resurfacing or dermabrasion can be performed to smooth the more superficial scars and blend with other treated areas.

The clinician must warn his patient about potential dyschromia, especially in Fitzpatrick skin types III through VI, as skin destruction of this depth can depigment the areas treated. The multiple procedures may not be able to raise all scars to the surface but will surely give improvement. It does add another simple treatment to our techniques for treating scars and for facial resurfacing.

Deep chemical peeling

Patients in Glogau groups III and IV may require deep chemical peeling, motorized dermabrasion or laser resurfacing to improve their greater degree of skin damage. As discussed to medium-depth peels, deep chemical peeling leads to production of new collagen and ground substance down to a level in proportion to the depth of the peel. Deep chemical peels create an injury through the papillary dermis, into the superficial reticular dermis, and which may extend into the mid-reticular dermis. Deep peeling entails the use of either TCA in concentrations above 50% or a phenol-containing preparation. Because of the risk of scarring and other complications with such potent concentrations of TCA, this agent is not recommended for deep chemical peeling. Therefore, solutions containing phenol remain the agents of choice for deep chemical peels.

The application of pure, undiluted, 88% phenol to the skin causes rapid and complete coagulation of epidermal keratin proteins and is thought to block itself from further penetration. Classified as a medium-depth peeling agent, pure phenol is rarely used for chemical peeling because its limited depth of penetration results in a lesser degree of effectiveness. In contrast, the Baker–Gordon peel utilizes phenol in a

THE BAKER–GORDON FORMULA	
88% liquid phenol, USP	3 ml
Tap water	2 ml
Septisol® liquid soap	8 drops
Croton oil	3 drops

Table 154.5 The Baker–Gordon formula.

formulation that permits deeper penetration into the dermis than is achieved with full-strength phenol[34] (Table 154.5). First described in 1961[35], the Baker–Gordon peel has been used successfully for several decades. The Baker–Gordon formula consists of Septisol® (Vestal Laboratories, St. Louis, MO), croton oil and tap water added to a solution of phenol, reducing its concentration to 50% or 55%. The mixture of ingredients is freshly prepared and must be stirred vigorously prior to application due to its poor miscibility. The liquid soap, Septisol®, is a surfactant that reduces skin tension, allowing a more even penetration. Croton oil is a vesicant epidermolytic agent that enhances phenol absorption. Recent investigations into the effects of this peel using varying concentrations of both phenol and croton oil have suggested that the procedure's efficacy is more related to the amount of croton oil than to that of phenol[34,36]. Modifications of the original Baker–Gordon formula, in order to improve the risk-to-benefit ratio of deep peeling, are currently being investigated[37].

There are two main variations of deep chemical peeling with the Baker–Gordon phenol formula – occluded and unoccluded. Occlusion of the peeling solution with tape is thought to increase its penetration and extend the injury into the mid-reticular dermis. This technique is particularly helpful for deeply lined, 'weather-beaten' faces, but should be utilized only by experienced surgeons because of the higher risk of complications[38]. The unoccluded technique as modified by McCollough involves more cleansing of the skin and the application of more peel solution. This may enhance the efficacy of the solution but without penetration as deeply as in an occluded peel. In the hands of a skilled and knowledgeable surgeon, both methods are safe and reliable in rejuvenating advanced to severe photoaged skin. Deep chemical peeling can significantly improve or even eliminate deep furrows as well as other textural and pigmentary irregularities associated with severe photoaging (Fig. 154.8). A remarkable degree of improvement is the expected result of deep chemical peeling when performed properly on carefully selected patients.

Patients must be made aware of potential complications, including scarring, textural changes such as 'alabaster skin', and pigmentary disturbances (Fig. 154.9). Patients often experience postoperative erythema that can take many months to resolve and may be followed by variable hypopigmentation. Male patients and patients with darker complexions are less favorable candidates for deep chemical peeling, since the hypopigmentation is less easily camouflaged. Because phenol is cardiotoxic and undergoes hepatic and renal elimination, preoperative evaluation includes a complete blood count, liver function tests, blood urea nitrogen, creatinine and electrolyte determinations, and a baseline electrocardiogram. Any patient who has a history of cardiac arrhythmias or who is taking a medication known to precipitate arrhythmias should not undergo a full-face Baker–Gordon phenol peel. Patients with a history of hepatic or renal disease are also poor candidates.

Compared with medium-depth and superficial peeling, the Baker–Gordon phenol peel is a time-consuming procedure and it must only be performed in a properly equipped facility. The required waiting period after the treatment of each cosmetic unit limits the rate of cutaneous absorption, thereby preventing the serum levels of phenol from reaching a dangerous peak during the procedure[39]. Intravenous hydration with a liter of lactated Ringer's solution before the procedure and another liter during the peel also promotes phenol excretion and prevents toxicity. Continuous electrocardiography, pulse oximetry, and blood pressure monitoring are mandatory during the entire perioperative period. Any abnormalities, such as a premature ventricular contraction (PVC) or premature atrial contraction (PAC), necessitate abrupt stoppage of the procedure and careful evaluation for toxicity[40]. Oxygen is supplemented throughout the procedure, as some physicians feel that it has a protective effect against cardiac arrhythmias.

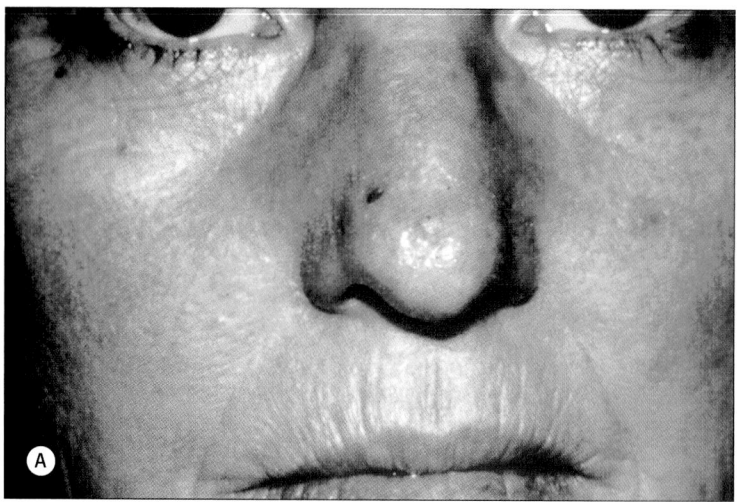

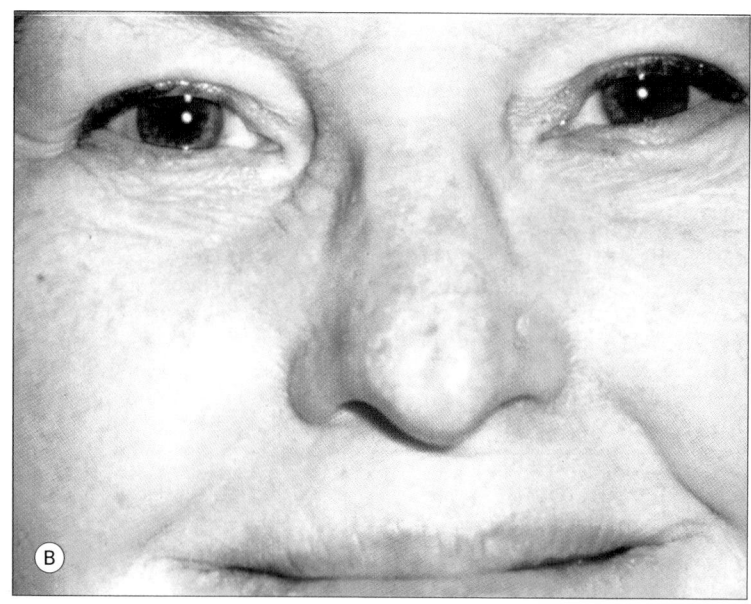

Fig. 154.8 Advanced photoaging in the form of perioral rhytides treated with Baker's phenol peel. A Preoperative, demonstrating perioral rhagades, textural and pigmentary changes, and epidermal lesions. **B** Postoperative: 2 years later. Note the phenol peel maintains correction for many years.

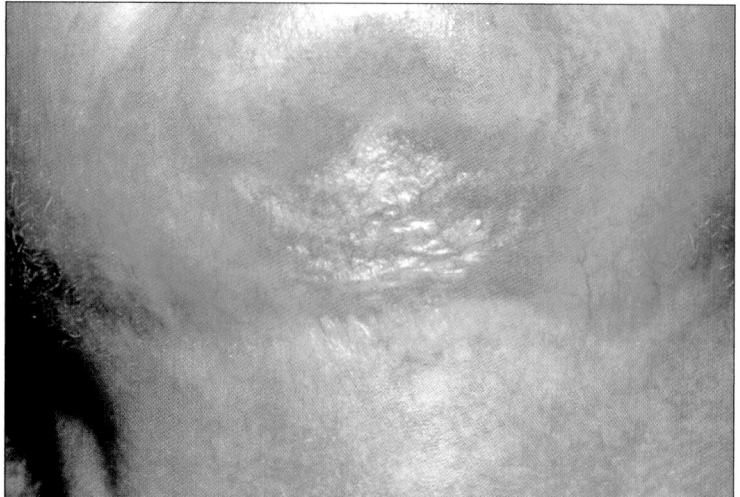

Fig. 154.9 Complications from Baker's phenol peel. There was prolonged non-healing, resulting in hypopigmentation and marbled scarring.

On the morning of the procedure, the patient shaves and cleanses the face and does not eat breakfast or apply cosmetics. Before the administration of anesthesia, the patient is examined while he or she is in a seated position and appropriate landmarks are noted. After thorough cleansing and degreasing of the skin, the chemical agent is applied sequentially to six aesthetic units: forehead, perioral region, right cheek, left cheek, nose and periorbital region. There is a 15-minute time interval between the treatment of each cosmetic area, allowing 60 to 90 minutes for the entire procedure. Cotton-tipped applicators are used with a similar technique as discussed for the medium-depth Jessner's–35% TCA peel. Less solution, though, is used, because frosting occurs very rapidly. Occlusion of the peel can be accomplished with strips of waterproof zinc oxide tape applied to each cosmetic unit just after the phenol is applied and then removed on postoperative day 1 (see below). Care is exercised to extend the peel slightly beyond the mandibular rim to conceal the demarcation between treated and untreated skin.

The last aesthetic unit, the periorbital skin, is treated cautiously and conservatively to avoid overpenetration, which can lead to ectropion or scarring. It is important to remember that diluting a phenol compound with water may increase its penetration, so mineral oil rather than water should be used to flush the eyes if contact occurs. Recent evidence by Hetter indicates that the croton oil may be an important factor in determining depth of penetration of the phenol peel[34]. Using one or two drops rather than the three in the Baker–Gordon formula can limit the risk of phenol complications such as textural effacement or hypopigmentation.

Application of the peeling agent creates an immediate burning sensation which lasts for 15 to 20 seconds, subsides for 20 minutes, and then returns for the next 6 to 8 hours. Ice packs may be applied as necessary for patient comfort. Narcotics are usually prescribed upon discharge for adequate pain control. Systemic corticosteroids are also administered by some surgeons to lessen the inflammatory response. For untaped peels, petrolatum is applied and a biosynthetic dressing can be used for the first 24 hours.

Mechanical Resurfacing Procedures

Over the last five decades, dermabrasion utilizing a rotating abrasive surface attached to a power-driven hand engine has been considered the premier skin resurfacing procedure for facial scars. It has generally been regarded as a deep resurfacing modality based on its depth of injury and its prolonged healing time. The original descriptions of modern dermabrasion involved the use of a wire brush which remains in use today, but there has been a slow trend in favor of more superficial methods of mechanical resurfacing. In 1957, the diamond fraise was introduced and became the preferred instrument for dermabrasion by some surgeons because it is less aggressive and more forgiving than the wire brush[41]. Recently, there has been a resurgence of interest in manual dermasanding which allows for more deliberate and controlled skin planing[4,5]. Microdermabrasion, the mechanical resurfacing procedure developed most recently, is the most conservative of all[3].

Microdermabrasion

Because microdermabrasion removes the stratum corneum and superficial spinous layer, and the injury rarely extends past the basal layer, this modality is considered superficial in depth. Whether it is classified as very light or light in comparison to the other superficial resurfacing procedures depends upon the techniques and aggressiveness of the operator. The microdermabrasion unit's handpiece is a closed system which propels aluminum oxide crystals at the skin at high speeds and simultaneously removes them with suction (Fig. 154.10). These units were developed commercially in the mid-1990s and are currently in widespread use in both physicians' offices and non-medical aesthetic spas. Microdermabrasion may be indicated for acneiform conditions, pigmentary dyschromias, and as a 'lunchtime' procedure for facial rejuvenation in all skin types[42], but it is not generally considered effective at improving the appearance of rhytides[43,44]. Its use in improving the appearance of scars is controversial, but it has been explored with favorable results[3]. Both the patient and physician must understand that the degree of objective improvement with microdermabrasion may be limited. Ideal candidates for microdermabrasion typically desire facial rejuvenation without 'downtime.' Appropriately selected patients have

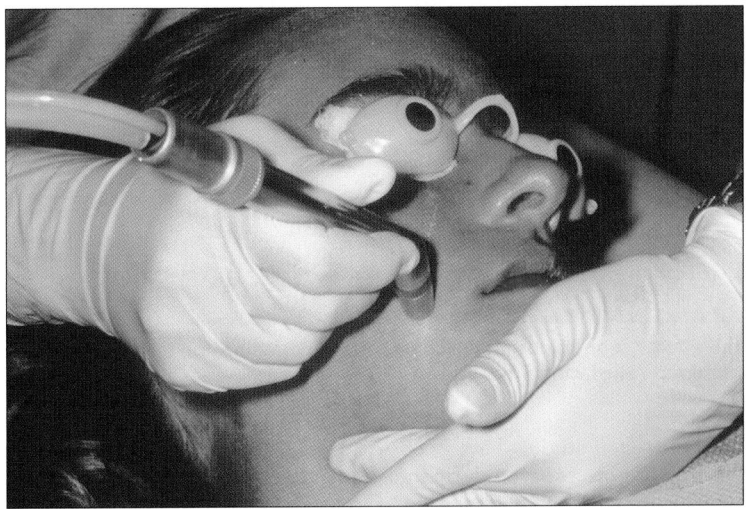

Fig. 154.10 Microdermabrasion. Aluminum oxide crystals are propelled at high speeds within a closed system and removed with suction.

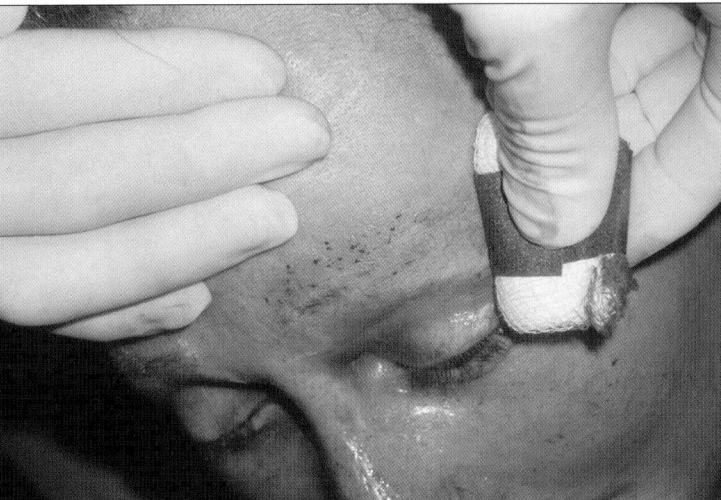

Fig. 154.11 Dermasanding. Manual dermasanding utilizing 320 grit silicon carbide sandpaper to blend CO_2 laser resurfacing into the eyebrow area.

a subjective perception of improvement usually exceeding the objective signs depicted with photographs. Patients often report that their skin has a smoother texture and that cosmetics are easier to apply and blend in with their skin more easily.

Although the role of microdermabrasion in facial rejuvenation grew dramatically after these units were initially developed, the scientific data to justify their use were lacking until more recently. An increase in epidermal and dermal thickness, flattening of the rete pegs, vascular ectasia with perivascular inflammation, papillary dermal hyalinization, and newly deposited collagen and elastic fibers have all been observed[45]. Following microdermabrasion, there also appears to be a significant alteration in epidermal barrier function[46]. Other investigators have observed an elevation of transcription factors, cytokines, and matrix metalloproteinases following microdermabrasion[47].

Manual dermasanding

Manual dermasanding involves abrading the skin by hand using silicon carbide sandpaper or wallscreen commercially available at any hardware store. It is gaining in popularity for skin resurfacing because it has several advantages over power-driven dermabrasion (Table 154.6). Its classification as a wounding agent is entirely dependent upon the type of paper used, the force applied by the surgeon, and the duration of contact with the skin. Although it can be used to produce a wound as deep as with wire-brush dermabrasion or several passes with a pulsed CO_2 laser, manual dermasanding is probably most commonly used as a medium-depth or 'minimally deep' resurfacing modality.

Manual dermasanding can be used to resurface an entire face, but because it is so labor-intensive, it is most often utilized for resurfacing localized regions to minimize the appearance of a scar[48] or to blend or enhance the effects of a medium-depth chemical peel or a combination procedure[49]. It can be used following CO_2 laser resurfacing to feather the transition into hair-bearing areas that are inaccessible to the laser. Manual dermasanding of the eyebrows and hairline and gently abrading the upper neck at the inferior aspect of the laser-irradiated zone are all effective at minimizing lines of demarcation between treated and untreated skin (Fig. 154.11). It can also be useful immediately after laser resurfacing for stubborn rhytides, particularly in the perioral

region. Manual dermasanding can improve the outcome by producing a slightly greater depth of injury in a controlled fashion where further thermal injury would be risky. It will also remove adherent necrotic debris and thermal damage, thus speeding up the healing process. Similarly, a medium-depth chemical peel can be immediately followed by manual dermasanding on the more troublesome areas to enhance the results and also along the borders of the peeled skin to blend the effects.

Our clinical experience suggests that dermasanding after a Jessner's–35% TCA peel may yield impressive postoperative results that approach those seen with either motorized dermabrasion or CO_2 laser resurfacing in patients with cutaneous photoaging. This combination is particularly helpful in patients who may not tolerate the greater degree of sedation often necessary with CO_2 laser resurfacing or who cannot afford the additional fees to cover anesthesia services.

The necessary materials for manual dermasanding include silicon carbide sandpaper or wallscreen. Both may be purchased in a variety of grades: fine grade (#400), medium grade (#220–320) and coarse grade (#180). The sandpaper is easier to use because of its flexibility and is also more easily cut into smaller pieces which can be steam autoclaved. A 4 cm × 8 cm piece of sterilized sandpaper is wrapped around either the barrel of a 3 ml syringe or a rolled-up gauze pad and moistened with saline or a soap-free cleanser for lubrication. A 1% solution of lidocaine with epinephrine may be used if additional anesthesia is necessary. Both back-and-forth and circular motions are used to gradually abrade the skin, layer by layer, until the hills and valleys are softened or adjacent areas are blended to the desired degree. Coarse grades may be used initially for 'debulking', followed by finer grades later in the procedure. The fine grade is used to blend delicate areas of skin such as around the eyelids. At the completion of the procedure, the dark-colored silicon carbide particles remaining on the skin surface should be rinsed off because there is a theoretical risk of their becoming implanted.

Motorized dermabrasion

Although various abrasive materials have long been used for mechanical resurfacing, the development of a power-driven unit to facilitate the procedure was revolutionary. Some of the units most commonly used today are the Bell hand engine (Bell International, Burlingame, CA), the AEV-12 hand engine (Ellis International, Madison, NJ), and the Osada surgical handpiece (Osada, Inc., Los Angeles, CA). A topical refrigerant spray is used to produce anesthesia and to harden the skin as it is abraded (Fig. 154.12). The spray immobilizes the topographic features so that there is no distortion by the pressure of the abrasive instrument. Though concerns over the potential harm to the environment caused by cryogenic sprays have intermittently hampered their commercial availability in recent years, these agents are available for purchase at the time of this writing.

The two abrasive instruments most often employed with these units are the wire brush and the diamond fraise. The wire brush has numer-

ADVANTAGES OF MANUAL DERMASANDING OVER MOTORIZED DERMABRASION
• Greater control over depth of injury, particularly on the lips and orbital rims
• Blending of abraded areas into adjacent unabraded areas accomplished more easily and with better results
• Lower cost and greater simplicity of instrumentation and set-up
• Far less risk of aerosolizing infectious particles
• Possibly lower incidence of postinflammatory hypopigmentation

Table 154.6 Advantages of manual dermasanding over motorized dermabrasion.

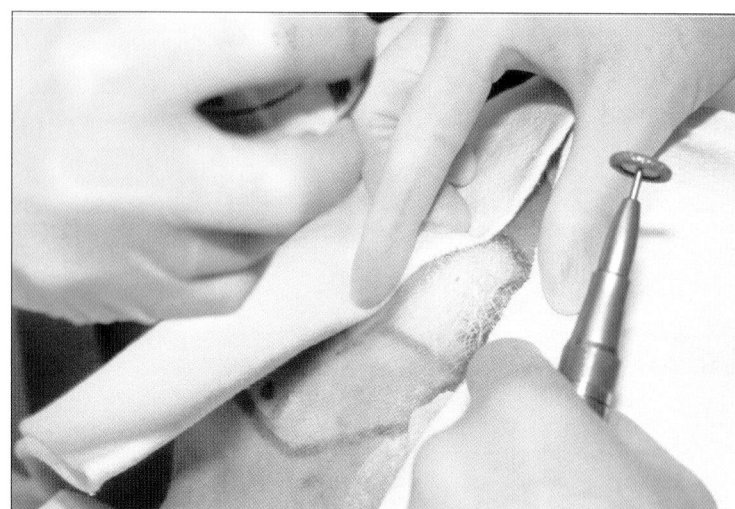

Fig. 154.12 Mechanical dermabrasion. This technique is performed with a diamond fraise over rigid skin cooled with a topical refrigerant spray.

ous small-caliber, stainless-steel wires that project circumferentially from the curved side of a cylindrical hub. A diamond fraise consists of a stainless-steel cylinder to which industrial-grade diamonds are bonded to create the abrasive surface. As compared with wire-brush instruments, diamond fraises are manufactured with a greater variety in shape, width of abrasive surface, wheel diameter, and coarseness of grit. There continues to be considerable controversy about which one of these instruments is superior[41], but surgeons generally agree that the wire brush is more aggressive. The wire brush cuts more quickly and more deeply into the skin with each stroke, thereby posing a greater risk for injury and requiring more skill to operate. Though the diamond fraise is generally safer and more forgiving, it may not yield the degree of improvement possible with the wire brush, especially for more stubborn conditions such as acne scarring.

Because dermabrasion with either instrument is highly technique-dependent and its learning curve is steep, there may be considerable variability in the clinical results obtained by different operators. It is very important for beginner dermabraders to receive hands-on instruction from an experienced operator in order to be adequately trained. The proper techniques for motorized dermabrasion have also been the subject of comprehensive reviews in the literature[41]. Careful evaluation of the depth of injury throughout the procedure is critical to assure sufficient depth for optimal results without penetrating beyond the desired level and risk scarring. Because of the potential for aerosolization of infectious particles during dermabrasion, appropriate precautions are mandatory to protect the operating-room staff.

All of the conditions amenable to treatment with manual dermasanding are also manageable with motorized dermabrasion. Although manual dermasanding is very well suited to combination resurfacing procedures for enhancement and blending, this concept was originally popularized with the use of the motor-driven technique[50]. Motorized dermabrasion may still be preferable to manual dermasanding for full-face resurfacing because less time and energy are expended. It also remains widely utilized for resurfacing localized areas, a procedure known as spot dermabrasion. This procedure, which can also be performed with the manual technique, is most useful for improving the appearance of surgical or traumatic scars[51]. Spot dermabrasion yields the greatest amount of improvement when performed about 6 weeks after the initial injury. A medium-depth peel can be performed on the remainder of the cosmetic unit or on the rest of the face to assure that the adjacent areas are blended.

The resurgence of manual dermasanding and the development of laser technology have led to a decline in the number of motorized dermabrasion procedures. Although all of the major indications for skin resurfacing that were mentioned earlier also apply to dermabrasion, many dermasurgeons continue to use this modality only for selected conditions in which dermabrasion can consistently achieve superior results. A list of these conditions, as compiled by the authors according to their experience, is found in Table 154.7. It should be noted that any such list must be viewed with some degree of hesitation because very

CONDITIONS FOR WHICH MOTORIZED DERMABRASION MAY BE THE PREFERRED RESURFACING MODALITY
• Acne scarring
• Surgical or traumatic scars
• Benign neoplasms (multiple trichoepitheliomas, syringomas, angiofibromas)
• Malignant and pre-malignant neoplasms (skin cancer treatment and prevention in nevoid basal cell carcinoma syndrome and xeroderma pigmentosum, as well as management of extensive carcinoma *in situ*)
• Extensive epidermal lesions such as epidermal nevi
• Decorative or traumatic tattoos unresponsive to the pigmented lesion lasers
• Rhinophyma

Table 154.7 Conditions for which motorized dermabrasion may be the preferred resurfacing modality.

few controlled studies have been performed to evaluate the safety and efficacy of power-driven dermabrasion in comparison with either CO_2 laser resurfacing or manual dermasanding[52–56].

Moderate to severe acne scarring is the most notable of these conditions, for laser resurfacing has yielded variable results and chemical peeling is generally disappointing. Dermabrasion selectively planes off the 'hilltops' that surround the atrophic 'valleys', whereas chemical peeling and laser irradiation may produce an injury of equivalent depth in both areas (Fig. 154.13). Effacing the edges of the atrophic scars can be accomplished with the CO_2 laser or the solid CO_2–35% TCA peel[28], but these methods may be more difficult and their results less predictable as compared with dermabrasion. It is our opinion that conventional motorized dermabrasion remains the gold standard in resurfacing procedures for this condition. The physician, though, must choose the scars most amenable to dermabrasion alone. These include shallow fibrotic scars, hypertrophic scars and undulating, rolling scars. The deeper fibrotic scars, ice-pick scars and scars with significant tissue loss may require a lifting or filling procedure prior to the dermabrasion. In these patients, the results are significantly enhanced with one or more of the following adjunctive procedures 4 to 6 weeks preoperatively: punch or scalpel excision, punch grafting, dermal grafting, fat grafting, TCA Cross, or scar undermining (subcision)[57].

POSTOPERATIVE CARE

Because superficial resurfacing procedures generally do not extend beyond the epidermis, the dermal wound healing mechanisms are not activated. In contrast, medium-depth and deep resurfacing procedures stimulate the following four stages of dermal wound healing (see Ch. 141): (1) inflammation and coagulation; (2) re-epithelialization; (3) fibroplasia and matrix formation; and (4) collagen remodeling.

Because the pronounced edema following medium-depth and deep resurfacing procedures may minimize the appearance of scars, rhytides and other irregularities, the patient's initial perception of his or her improvement may be exaggerated. As swelling subsides postoperatively, patients should be reassured and advised that collagen remodeling continues for several months and leads to further clinical improvement. At some point in the postoperative course, patients often want to know when another resurfacing procedure can be performed if it is necessary. The presence of persistent postoperative erythema may indicate continued collagen remodeling and may serve as a warning that a similar resurfacing procedure performed prematurely could produce scarring. To assure their safety, patients undergoing medium-depth resurfacing should not undergo another medium-depth or deep procedure for the next 3 to 9 months. An individual having a deep resurfacing procedure should avoid another one for at least 12 months postoperatively. Touch-up procedures for the revision of a prior suboptimal outcome are also best avoided during these times, so repeated efforts to counsel and reassure the patient are necessary.

The length of the healing time is generally proportionate to the depth of the resurfacing procedure. Superficial resurfacing procedures cause minimal downtime and necessitate little postoperative care. They usually produce mild erythema and desquamation that lasts from 1 to 4 days depending on the wounding agent and the techniques used. Regular washing with a mild cleanser and the use of routine moisturizers and sunscreens are generally sufficient during the healing period.

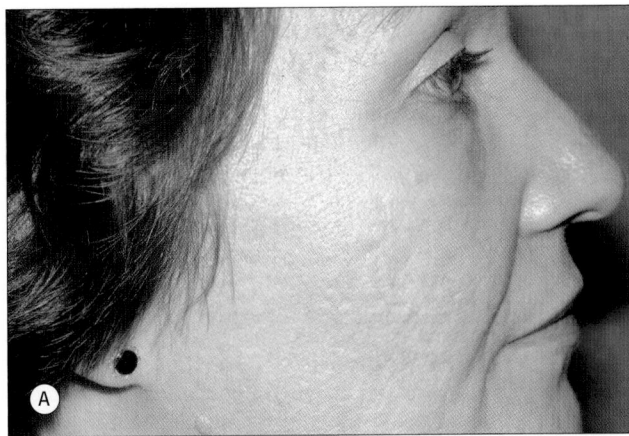

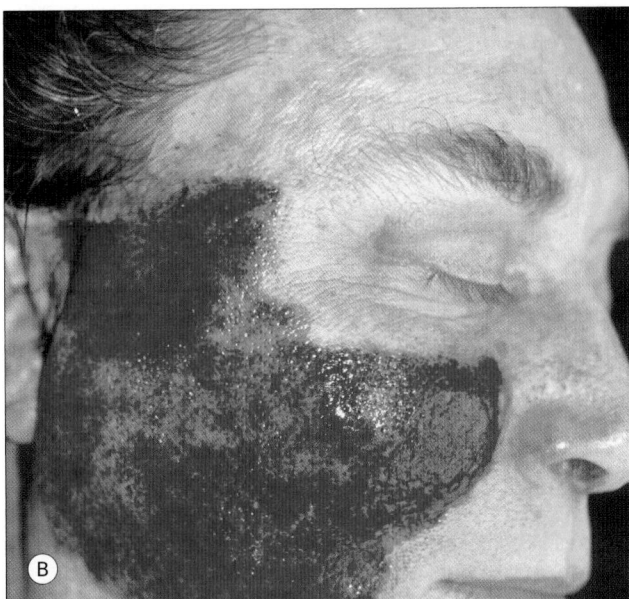

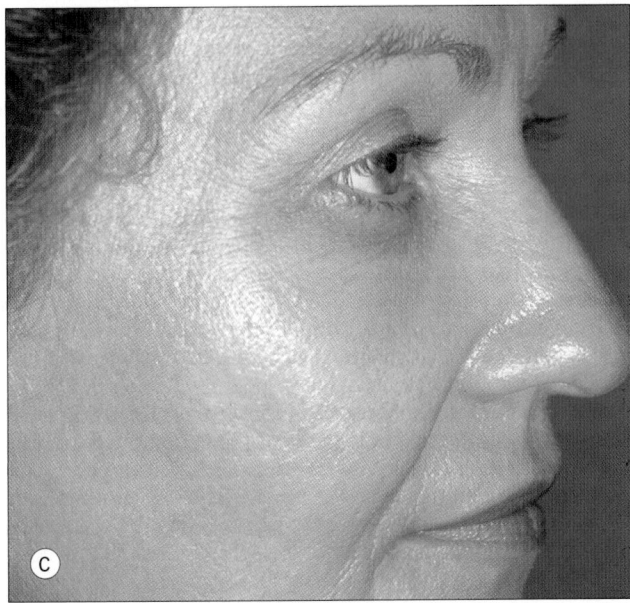

Fig. 154.13 Full-face dermabrasion performed for acne scars. A Preoperative: shallow and atrophic scars most amenable to dermabrasion. **B** Postoperative: dermabrasion prior to biosynthetic dressing. **C** Three months postoperative.

There is a considerably longer healing time and more involved postoperative care is necessary following medium-depth resurfacing procedures. Follow-up visits are scheduled regularly in order to monitor the patient's postoperative course. After a medium-depth chemical peel, occlusive dressings are not necessary because the epidermis, which is not removed intraoperatively, functions as a biologic dressing until peeling occurs. Because areas of medium-depth peeling which

have been enhanced by manual dermasanding do not possess residual epidermis, occlusive dressings may be used on these areas during the first 3 days.

The patient is instructed to soak the areas four times daily with warm compresses and to apply an emollient after each soak and during the intervening periods as necessary. A solution of 0.25% acetic acid (one tablespoon of white vinegar added to one pint of warm water) is preferred for the soaks because the mild acidity is physiologic for healing granulation tissue. It is also a mild debridant and has antibacterial effects, especially against *Pseudomonas* and other Gram-negative organisms. Occlusive emollients, such as petrolatum, Aquaphor® or Eucerin® Creme (both from Beiersdorf AG, Hamburg, Germany), speed the process of re-epithelialization and lessen the tendency for delayed healing[58]. These emollients are also helpful in wound debridement and in the prevention of crust formation and infection.

Following medium-depth resurfacing, edema begins to appear almost immediately and progressively worsens during the first 48 hours. It can even be severe enough to close the eyelids and impair the patient's visual fields. If tolerated, aspirin or other non-steroidal anti-inflammatory drugs (NSAIDs) can be administered preoperatively and during the first 24 hours postoperatively, to alleviate discomfort and reduce swelling. After a medium-depth chemical peel such as the Jessner's–35% TCA peel, there is initially a brawny, dusky erythema which is followed by the formation of a brownish crust that begins to separate from the skin surface between days 4 and 8 postoperatively. The underlying, newly formed epithelium is brightly erythematous but fades to a pink color that resembles a sunburn (see Fig. 154.4D). By postoperative day 7 to 10, re-epithelialization has occurred and the erythema can be camouflaged with cosmetics. Within 2 to 4 weeks after the procedure, the erythema usually resolves fully and retinoids and sunscreens can be restarted as tolerated.

Deep resurfacing procedures, such as the Baker–Gordon phenol peel or dermabrasion, require a follow-up visit the next day, several visits during the first week, and very close monitoring thereafter. At each visit, instructions for wound care are reviewed with the patient and any questions are answered. The immediate postoperative course after deep resurfacing is similar to that following medium-depth procedures, except that edema and erythema may be even more severe and persistent. NSAIDs can provide some relief, but an intramuscular corticosteroid injection is often administered on the day of surgery, even though its effects on wound healing are not completely understood. Pruritus may occur during the healing period following a resurfacing procedure of any depth, but is particularly prevalent after deeper resurfacing. This problem can be alleviated by the use of emollients, ice packs, NSAIDs and antihistamines until the symptom spontaneously resolves. Milia formation, which commonly occurs 3 to 4 weeks after deep chemical peeling or mechanical resurfacing, is easily managed with needle extraction.

Patients undergoing deep mechanical resurfacing with either motorized dermabrasion or manual dermasanding may be managed with an occlusive biosynthetic dressing applied immediately after the procedure. Occlusive tape or a biosynthetic dressing is usually utilized postoperatively in patients undergoing a Baker–Gordon phenol peel. Occlusive tape dressings must be removed on the first postoperative day and this procedure may require analgesia and sedation. For this reason, the authors prefer untaped phenol peels with application of ointment or bio-occlusive dressings. Whenever a biosynthetic dressing is used, it must be removed daily and replaced with a new one for the first 2 or 3 days postoperatively so that the face can be gently debrided with saline soaks and moistened cotton tips. The patient should be instructed to regularly apply an occlusive ointment to areas around the mouth, eyelids and hairline that are not adequately covered by the dressing. Occlusive, biosynthetic dressings have been shown to enhance collagen synthesis and hasten re-epithelialization in superficial wounds. They also minimize the amount of discomfort and obviate the need for repeated soaks by the patient during the first few days after the procedure.

By the third day following deep mechanical or chemical resurfacing, the patient begins open wound care with 0.25% acetic acid soaks four to six times daily and regular applications of an occlusive ointment. By the 7th to the 14th day postoperatively, re-epithelialization is usually complete and the ointment is replaced with a heavy moisturizer, as discussed previously. The marked edema and erythema typically seen after dermabrasion or dermasanding generally resolve after several weeks. The erythema resulting from deep peeling may be more persistent, but is rarely present beyond 2 to 4 months. Strict sun avoidance is critical for 3 to 6 months after dermabrasion or deep chemical peeling. The patient typically restarts sunscreens and retinoid therapy within a couple weeks of re-epithelialization, as tolerated.

COMPLICATIONS

Complications may occur following any method of skin resurfacing involving injury to any depth, but are more common after medium-depth and deep procedures. It is far simpler to prevent the development of a complication than to manage it once it has occurred. Complications may be prevented by proper selection of suitable patients and appropriate resurfacing modalities, precise intraoperative techniques, and proper patient management before and after the procedure (see Table 154.3). The dissatisfied patient represents a complication even when the cosmetic result is favorable. Improper wound care, trauma to the healing area resulting from overzealous debridement, compulsive picking or scratching, and premature use of irritating substances such as depilatories or wax for the removal of hair can each cause the depth of injury to extend beyond the threshold of safety. As discussed in the next section, the development of infection in the postoperative period can also extend the depth of injury and increase the risk of permanent sequelae.

With specific regard to chemical peeling, excessive injury to the skin can result from poor technique during application or problems with the chemical agents utilized. The degree of frosting is monitored closely to assure that the agent has been applied evenly and that the injury extends to the proper depth. Although it does not always correlate completely with the depth of injury, the level of frosting is a very valuable guide for determining the appropriate endpoint of treatment. Injuring the skin too deeply during a chemical peel, as suggested by an excessive degree of frosting, may result not only from overapplication but also from the use of excessively concentrated peeling solutions. The latter error can be caused by the surgeon's choice of an improper peeling agent, such as 50% TCA, or it can be related to unexpected disturbances in a solution's pharmacologic mixture. For Baker–Gordon peels, a new batch should be mixed by the surgeon prior to each procedure in order to be certain that the preparation is made correctly. The other peeling solutions are available in various formulations and strengths for purchase directly from medical supply dealers. Reputable dealers mix and label these solutions properly according to the standard weight-to-volume formula. Storage of peeling solutions in proper containers away from sunlight and immediate replacement of expired solutions are important measures to ensure chemical stability of the agents being used[59]. Immediately prior to peeling, an ample volume of the solution should be poured from the primary storage container into a smaller, secondary cup. The peeling agent is applied directly to the skin surface from this cup and the excess subsequently discarded in order to avoid contamination of the storage container and to avoid the accidental transfer of concentrated crystals from the neck of the storage container to the patient's skin.

Errors during mechanical resurfacing procedures may also lead to an injury of excessive depth and a higher risk of adverse sequelae. This problem can result from poor technique in the handling of the instruments or from failure to recognize the appropriate treatment endpoint. The beginner should first start by conservatively dermasanding small areas to get a comfortable feel for the skin's response to this type of injury. As knowledge and experience is gained, one can then progress on to diamond fraise dermabrasion and later to the use of the wire brush. Observation of experienced surgeons and hands-on training is invaluable. The beginner should always err on the side of conservativism to avoid excessively deep tissue injury that could produce long-term complications, while still yielding favorable results.

Intraoperative exposure of vital structures to the resurfacing agent during chemical peeling or mechanical resurfacing may occur and can have serious adverse consequences. Extreme care must be exercised when dermabrading with a power-driven, rotating instrument, to assure that the dominant hand maintains complete control continuously. During chemical peeling, the moistened applicator should never be passed over the central face, to avoid inadvertent exposure of a vulnerable surface such as the eye to the solution. There should always be appropriate fluids readily available to rinse the area in case such an exposure does occur. In particular, saline is used to dilute TCA, mineral oil is used to dilute Baker–Gordon phenol solutions, and sodium bicarbonate is used to neutralize glycolic acid.

Adverse systemic effects related to a resurfacing procedure are very uncommon but can usually be traced to an identifiable causative factor in the perioperative period. Peeling with phenol solutions has been associated with systemic toxicities, so these procedures must be performed slowly and only on properly selected, healthy patients in an appropriate clinical setting. The use of Jessner's solution poses a theoretical risk of systemic salicylate or resorcinol toxicity, but this is probably not clinically significant when application is limited to the face and neck. Undoubtedly, the most common cause of systemic problems related to resurfacing procedures is an adverse allergic or physiologic reaction to a medication used for anesthesia. It is imperative that the surgeon know all the physiologic effects and the potential adverse consequences of each drug administered systemically, unless there is an attending anesthesiologist who assumes this responsibility. Fortunately, the chemical and mechanical resurfacing procedures utilized most often can be performed with little or no sedation.

It is important to make a distinction between a true complication and an expected side effect of a resurfacing procedure. With medium-depth and deep resurfacing, transient erythema, flushing, increased skin temperature, pruritus, edema, milia formation and mild alterations in mood are typical occurrences, so they should not be classified as true complications. Patient reassurance may be all that is necessary, since these problems usually resolve spontaneously. True complications that may develop within a treated area include infection, delayed wound healing and persistent erythema, scarring, and pigmentary or textural abnormalities[60,61]. Any of these true complications can occur despite proper patient and procedure selection, perfect surgical technique, and appropriate management before and after the operation.

Infection is an uncommon complication that develops in the postoperative period and may be caused by bacterial, viral or fungal organisms. An important preventive measure is the continuous use of soaks for adequate wound debridement. Frequent postoperative visits are helpful to assure early recognition and treatment of any infection so that scarring does not result. An infection may present with delayed wound healing, ulcerations, excessive necrotic material and crusting, purulent drainage, or odor. An acneiform eruption or pustular folliculitis can even be a manifestation of infection and should initially be treated as such. Infection with streptococcal and staphylococcal organisms can occur under biosynthetic membranes or thick, occlusive ointments, so these are best avoided, except in the immediate postoperative period. Other organisms, such as *Escherichia coli* or *Pseudomonas*, may even infect the area if there is improper wound care. *Candida* infections can also occur and are sometimes related to the use of prophylactic antibiotics or occlusive wound care. Clinical suspicion of a wound infection necessitates immediate institution of empiric antimicrobial therapy, laboratory culture for identification of the organism(s), and wound debridement as necessary[62].

Herpes simplex infection can occur during the healing period following medium-depth or deep resurfacing and has the potential for devastating sequelae. An outbreak can even occur in patients on the recommended 10–14-day prophylactic antiviral regimen. The keys to avoiding scar formation are rapid recognition and aggressive therapy started early in the course of infection. The dosage of antiviral drug should be increased to the recommended maximum in cases of active herpetic infection.

Persistent erythema beyond 2 months after a medium-depth procedure may be precipitated by the use of topical or systemic retinoid therapy, contact with various allergens or irritants, an underlying skin condition or genetic susceptibility, or the presence of active infection[60,63]. Persistent erythema may indicate the impending development of scar formation. Especially when indurated, it should be treated promptly and aggressively. Management includes massage therapy, topical, intralesional or even systemic corticosteroids, silicone gel sheeting, and pulsed dye laser therapy. In most cases, scarring can be prevented. Mild scarring may even fade away spontaneously. Ectropion can rarely occur when aggressive resurfacing creates scarring or excessive tightening of periorbital skin in a susceptible patient.

154

Textural abnormalities, skin atrophy and dyspigmentation are additional complications that may occur with medium-depth and deep resurfacing procedures. The return of normal pigmentation in patients whose Fitzpatrick skin type is IV or higher is less predictable, so an extra measure of caution is necessary. Postoperative hyperpigmentation may be prevented and/or treated with a topical retinoid, a 4–8% hydroquinone preparation and strict photoprotection, but hypopigmentation that can follow deeper resurfacing is typically permanent. Another pigmentary problem following deeper resurfacing procedures is a conspicuous demarcation line separating the untreated and treated areas. Although this problem can usually be avoided with adequate planning and proper technique, the approach to its management should focus on lightening the pigment in the adjacent untreated areas.

CONCLUSIONS AND FUTURE TRENDS

The sheer number of patients demanding medical therapy or procedural intervention to rejuvenate their skin mandates that dermatologists be well versed in this area. The field of resurfacing is constantly changing, with the development of new techniques and procedures as well as fluctuations in patient demands and expectations. In all areas of cosmetic surgery, there has been a recent trend in favor of less invasive procedures. Many dermatologists choose to learn and implement only a handful of resurfacing procedures that best fulfill the needs of their practice and meet the demands of their patient population.

REFERENCES

1. Brody HJ, Monheit GD, Resnik SS, Alt TH. A history of chemical peeling. Dermatol Surg. 2000;26:405–9.
2. Lawrence N, Mandy S, Yarborough J, Alt T. History of dermabrasion. Dermatol Surg. 2000;26:95–101.
3. Tsai RY, Wang CN, Chan HL. Aluminum oxide crystal microdermabrasion. A new technique for treating facial scarring. Dermatol Surg. 1995;21:539–42.
4. Harris DR, Noodleman FR. Combining manual dermasanding with low strength trichloroacetic acid to improve actinically injured skin. J Dermatol Surg Oncol. 1994;20:436–42.
5. Chiarello SE. Tumescent dermasanding with cryospraying. A new wrinkle on the treatment of rhytids. Dermatol Surg. 1996;22:601–10.
6. Dingman DL, Hartog J, Siemionow M. Simultaneous deep-plane face lift and trichloroacetic acid peel. Plast Reconstr Surg. 1994;93:86–93; discussion 4–5.
7. Rubenstein R, Roenigk HH, Stegman SJ, Hanke CW. Atypical keloids after dermabrasion of patients taking isotretinoin. J Am Acad Dermatol. 1986;15:280–5.
8. Wolfe SA. Chemical face peeling following therapeutic irradiation. Plast Reconstr Surg. 1982;69:859–62.
9. Monheit GD. Chemical peeling for pigmentary dyschromias. Cosmet Dermatol. 1995;8:10–15.
10. Swinehart JM. Test spots in dermabrasion and chemical peeling. J Dermatol Surg Oncol. 1990;16:557–63.
11. Gilbert S, McBurney E. Use of valacyclovir for herpes simplex virus-1 (HSV-1) prophylaxis after facial resurfacing: a randomized clinical trial of dosing regimens. Dermatol Surg. 2000;26:50–4.
12. Monheit GD. Facial resurfacing may trigger the herpes simplex virus. Cosmet Dermatol. 1995;8:9–16.
13. Monheit GD. Skin preparation: an essential step before chemical peeling or laser resurfacing. Cosmet Dermatol. 1996;9:13–14.
14. Yamamoto O, Bhawan J, Hara M, Gilchrest BA. Keratinocyte degeneration in human facial skin: documentation of new ultrastructural markers for photodamage and their improvement during topical tretinoin therapy. Exp Dermatol. 1995;4:9–19.
15. Goodman G. Dermabrasion using tumescent anesthesia. J Dermatol Surg Oncol. 1994;20:802–7.
16. Stegman SJ. A comparative histologic study of the effects of three peeling agents and dermabrasion on normal and sun-damaged skin. Aesthetic Plast Surg. 1982;6:123–5.
17. Stegman SJ. A study of dermabrasion and chemical peels in an animal model. J Dermatol Surg Oncol. 1980;6:490–7.
18. Nelson BR, Fader DJ, Gillard M, et al. Pilot histologic and ultrastructural study of the effects of medium-depth chemical facial peels on dermal collagen in patients with actinically damaged skin. J Am Acad Dermatol. 1995;32:472–8.
19. Ditre CM, Griffin TD, Murphy GF, et al. Effects of alpha-hydroxy acids on photoaged skin: a pilot clinical, histologic, and ultrastructural study. J Am Acad Dermatol. 1996;34:187–95.
20. Fitzpatrick RE, Tope WD, Goldman MP, Satur NM. Pulsed carbon dioxide laser, trichloroacetic acid, Baker-Gordon phenol, and dermabrasion: a comparative clinical and histologic study of cutaneous resurfacing in a porcine model. Arch Dermatol. 1996;132:469–71.
21. Rubin M. Chemical Peels. Philadelphia: Saunders, 2005.
22. Clark CP. Office-based skin care and superficial peels: the scientific rationale. Plast Reconstr Surg. 1999;104:854–64; discussion 65–6.
23. Kligman D, Kligman AM. Salicylic acid peels for the treatment of photoaging. Dermatol Surg. 1998;24:325–8.
24. Van Scott EJ, Yu RJ. Hyperkeratinization, corneocyte cohesion, and alpha hydroxy acids. J Am Acad Dermatol. 1984;11:867–79.
25. Slavin JW. Considerations in alpha hydroxy acid peels. Clin Plast Surg. 1998;25:45–52.
26. Monheit GD. The Jessner's + TCA peel: a medium depth chemical peel. J Dermatol Surg Oncol. 1989;15:945–50.
27. Brody HJ. Trichloroacetic acid application in chemical peeling, operative techniques. Plast Reconstr Surg. 1995;2:127–8.
28. Brody HJ, Hailey CW. Medium-depth chemical peeling of the skin: a variation of superficial chemosurgery. J Dermatol Surg Oncol. 1986;12:1268–75.
29. Coleman WP, Futrell JM. The glycolic acid trichloroacetic acid peel. J Dermatol Surg Oncol. 1994;20:76–80.
30. Witheiler DD, Lawrence N, Cox SE, et al. Long-term efficacy and safety of Jessner's solution and 35% trichloroacetic acid vs 5% fluorouracil in the treatment of widespread facial actinic keratoses. Dermatol Surg. 1997;23:191–6.
31. Spira M, Freeman R, Arfai P, et al. Clinical comparison of chemical peeling dermabrasion, and 5-fu for senile keratoses. Plast Reconstr Surg. 1970;46:61–6.
32. Monheit GD, Zeitouni NC. Skin resurfacing for photoaging: laser resurfacing versus chemical peeling. Cosmet Dermatol. 1997;10:11–22.
33. Koppel RA, Coleman KM, Coleman WP. The efficacy of EMLA versus ELA-Max for pain relief in medium-depth chemical peeling: a clinical and histopathologic evaluation. Dermatol Surg. 2000;26:61–4.
34. Hetter GP. An examination of the phenol-croton oil peel: Part I. Dissecting the formula. Plast Reconstr Surg. 2000;105:227–39; discussion 49–51.
35. Baker TJ, Gordon HL. The ablation of rhytides by chemical means: a preliminary report. J Fla Med Assoc. 1961;48:451–4.
36. Hetter GP. An examination of the phenol-croton oil peel: Part IV. Face peel results with different concentrations of phenol and croton oil. Plast Reconstr Surg. 2000;105:1061–83; discussion 84–7.
37. Stone PA. The use of modified phenol for chemical face peeling. Clin Plast Surg. 1998;25:21–44.
38. Alt T. Occluded Baker/Gordon chemical peel. Review and update. J Dermatol Surg Oncol. 1989;15:980–93.
39. Wexler MR, Halon DA, Teitelbaum A, et al. The prevention of cardiac arrhythmias produced in an animal model by the topical application of a phenol preparation in common use for face peeling. Plast Reconstr Surg. 1984;73:595–8.
40. Beeson WH. The importance of cardiac monitoring in superficial and deep chemical peeling. J Dermatol Surg Oncol. 1987;13:949–50.
41. Alt TH. Facial dermabrasion: advantages of the diamond fraise technique. J Dermatol Surg Oncol. 1987;13:618–24.
42. Bernard RW, Beran SJ, Rusin L. Microdermabrasion in clinical practice. Clin Plast Surg. 2000;27:571–7.
43. Shim EK, Barnette D, Hughes K, Greenway HT. Microdermabrasion: a clinical and histopathologic study. J Dermatol Surg. 2001;27:524–30.
44. Coimbra M, Rohrich RJ, Chao J, Brown SA. A prospective controlled assessment of microdermabrasion for damaged skin and fine rhytides. Plast Reconstr Surg. 2004;113:1438–43; discussion 1444.
45. Freedman BM, Rueda-Pedraza E, Waddell SP. The epidermal and dermal changes associated with microdermabrasion. J Dermatol Surg. 2001;27:1031–3; discussion 1033–4.
46. Rajan P, Grimes PE. Skin barrier changes induced by aluminum oxide and sodium chloride microdermabrasion. J Dermatol Surg. 2002;28:390–3.
47. Karimipour DJ, Kang S, Johnson TM, et al. Microdermabrasion: a molecular analysis following a single treatment. J Am Acad Dermatol. 2005;52:215–23.
48. Zisser M, Kaplan B, Moy RL. Surgical pearl: manual dermabrasion. J Am Acad Dermatol. 1995;33:105–6.
49. Lusthaus S, Benmeir P, Neuman A, et al. The use of sandpaper in chemical peeling combined with dermabrasion of the face. Ann Plast Surg. 1993;31:281–2.
50. Ayhan S, Baran CN, Yavuzer R, et al. Combined chemical peeling and dermabrasion for deep acne and posttraumatic scars as well as aging face. Plast Reconstr Surg. 1998;102:1238–46.
51. Katz BE, Oca AG. A controlled study of the effectiveness of spot dermabrasion ('scarabrasion') on the appearance of surgical scars. J Am Acad Dermatol. 1991;24:462–6.
52. Nehal KS, Levine VJ, Ross B, Ashinoff R. Comparison of high-energy pulsed carbon dioxide laser resurfacing and dermabrasion in the revision of surgical scars. Dermatol Surg. 1998;24:647–50.
53. Kitzmiller WJ, Visscher M, Page DA, et al. A controlled evaluation of dermabrasion versus CO₂ laser resurfacing for the treatment of perioral wrinkles. Plast Reconstr Surg. 2000;106:1366–72; discussion 73–4.
54. Holmkvist KA, Rogers GS. Treatment of perioral rhytides: a comparison of dermabrasion and superpulsed carbon dioxide laser. Arch Dermatol. 2000;136:725–31.
55. Gin I, Chew J, Rau KA, et al. Treatment of upper lip wrinkles: a comparison of the 950 microsec dwell time carbon dioxide laser to manual tumescent dermabrasion. Dermatol Surg. 1999;25:468–73; discussion 73–4.
56. Chew J, Gin I, Rau KA, et al. Treatment of upper lip wrinkles: a comparison of 950 microsec dwell time carbon dioxide laser with unoccluded Baker's phenol chemical peel. Dermatol Surg. 1999;25:262–6.
57. Goodman GJ. Postacne scarring: a review of its pathophysiology and treatment. Dermatol Surg. 2000;26:857–71.
58. Collawn SS, Boissy RE, Gamboa M, Vasconez LO. Ultrastructural study of the skin after facial chemical peels and the effect of moisturization on wound healing. Plast Reconstr Surg. 1998;101:1374–9; discussion 80.
59. Spinowitz AL, Rumsfield J. Stability-time profile of trichloroacetic acid at various concentrations and storage conditions. J Dermatol Surg Oncol. 1989;15:974–5.
60. Brody HJ. Complications of chemical peeling. J Dermatol Surg Oncol. 1989;15:1010–19.
61. Demas PN, Bridenstine JB. Diagnosis and treatment of postoperative complications after skin resurfacing. J Oral Maxillofac Surg. 1999;57:837–41.
62. Giandoni MB, Grabski WJ. Cutaneous candidiasis as a cause of delayed surgical wound healing. J Am Acad Dermatol. 1994;30:981–4.
63. Maloney BP, Millman B, Monheit G, McCollough EG. The etiology of prolonged erythema after chemical peel. Dermatol Surg. 1998;24:337–41.

Sclerotherapy and Ambulatory Phlebectomy

155

Mitchel P Goldman, Robert A Weiss and Neil S Sadick

Key features

- Superficial telangiectasias, reticular veins and varicose veins of the lower extremities are interconnected and develop after impairment of venous return

- Poor venous return results from venous valvular incompetence or primary muscle pump failure

- A pretreatment physical examination to assess the extent and cause of the problems should be performed with the patient in a standing position

- The physical examination can be supplemented by Doppler or duplex ultrasonography

- Both preoperative and postoperative compression are important in the management of venous insufficiency

- Sclerosing agents should destroy the entire vascular wall, producing permanent fibrosis of the vessel

- The minimal concentration and volume of sclerosing agent should be used to achieve the desired results

- All of the affected portions of the superficial venous system should be treated, starting with the most proximal

- Large veins should be treated before smaller veins, and veins should be treated from proximal to distal

- Currently, the only FDA-approved agents are sodium tetradecyl sulfate and sodium morrhuate; hypertonic saline (11.7–23.4%) and glycerin (72% mixed 2:1 with 1% lidocaine with or without epinephrine) are not approved and represent off-label usage

- The most common local side effects following injection of sclerosing agents are hyperpigmentation, telangiectatic matting, and cutaneous ulcers

- Patients generally require one to three sclerosant injection treatment sessions spaced at 6–8-week intervals

INTRODUCTION

Varicose and telangiectatic leg veins increase in extent and severity with increasing age. The evolution of safe and effective treatment options has made sclerotherapy and ambulatory phlebectomy an increasing part of the dermatologic surgeon's practice. The utilization of improved diagnostic modalities, more efficient sclerosing agents and simplified surgical techniques have made the treatment of venous disease safe, efficient and highly satisfying for both physician and patient. This chapter presents the most recent advances in sclerotherapy and ambulatory phlebectomy as they relate to the management of telangiectasias and intermediate-sized truncal branch (saphenous-related) varicosities.

VENOUS ANATOMY, PHYSIOLOGY AND PATHOPHYSIOLOGY

The peripheral venous system functions both as a reservoir to hold extra blood (e.g. during pregnancy) and as a conduit to return blood from the periphery to the heart and lungs. The correct function of the venous system depends on a complex series of pumps and valves that are individually frail, yet the system as a whole performs well under extremely adverse conditions[1] (Fig. 155.1). Superficial veins carry less than 5% of venous blood, while the deep venous system carries 95% of the blood.

The superficial venous system is a complicated variable network of interconnecting veins, most of which are unnamed[2]. A few larger truncal superficial veins are fairly constant in location. These truncal superficial veins serve as a conduit to pass blood centrally into the deep venous system. The principal named superficial veins are the small saphenous vein (SSV), which runs from the ankle to the knee, and the great saphenous vein (GSV), which runs from the ankle to the groin[3] (Fig. 155.2).

An interconnecting system of perforating veins that pass through the deep fascia connects the superficial veins to the deep veins of the calf or thigh (Figs 155.1 & 155.3). All venous blood eventually is received by the deep venous system on its way back to the right atrium of the heart.

Blood is propelled back to the heart via the pumping action of the foot and calf muscles, which squeeze blood out of the venous segment through one-way valves when muscle contractions increase the pressure within the fascial muscle compartment (Fig. 155.4). Venous pathology can result from primary muscle pump failure due to venous obstruction (thrombotic or non-thrombotic) or from venous valvular incompetence[4].

A genetic predisposition for the development of varicose veins has been observed, and both dominant and recessive patterns of inheritance have been described. Approximately 70% of patients can identify superficial venous disease as a familial trait. Hormonal influences from pregnancy or estrogen and progesterone supplementation are believed to be additional predisposing factors[5].

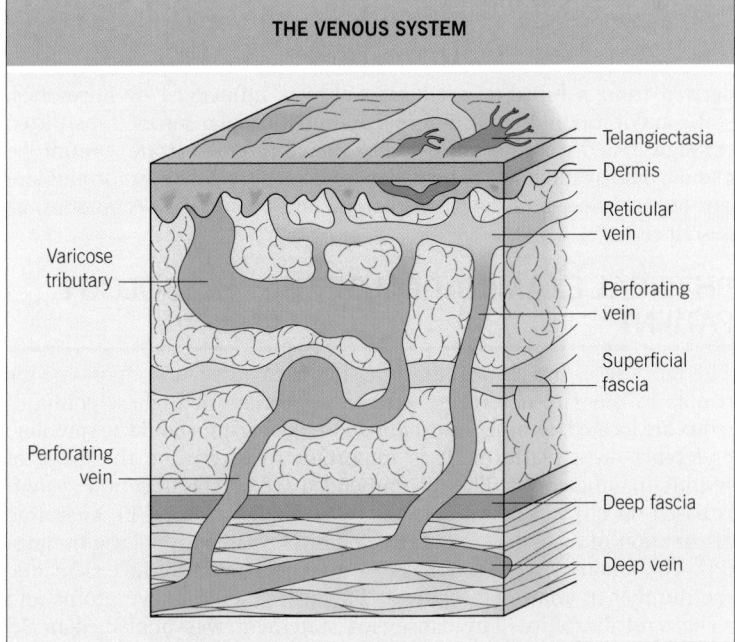

THE VENOUS SYSTEM

Fig. 155.1 **The cutaneous venous system.** The deep venous system drains the superficial venous system, which, in turn, is fed from the skin surface by telangiectasias in the dermis. The latter drain via reticular veins into the larger venous channels located in the reticular dermis and subcutaneous compartments. Redrawn from: Somjen GM, Ziegenbein R, Johnston AH, Royle JP: Anatomical examination of leg telangiectases with duplex scanning. J Dermatol Surg Oncol. 1993;19:940.

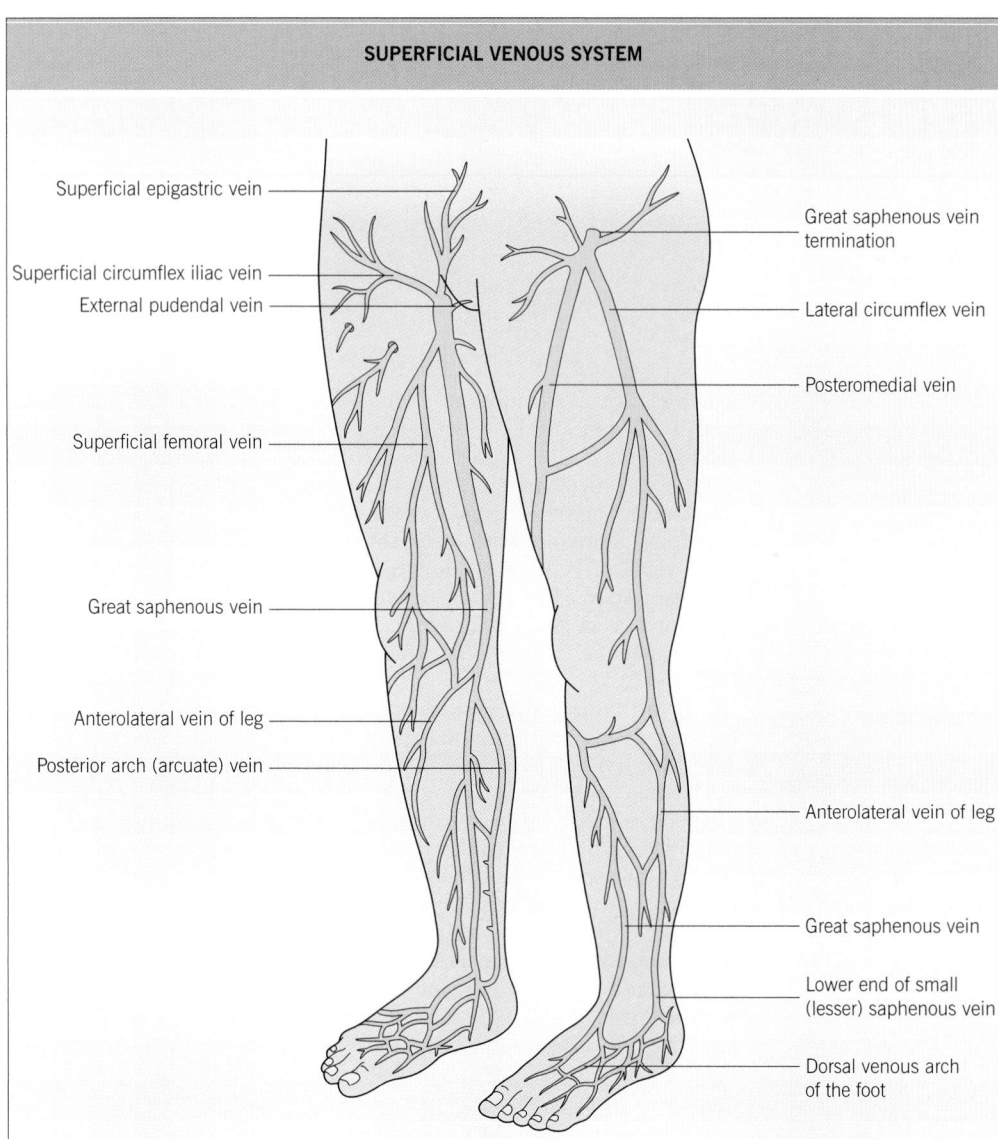

SUPERFICIAL VENOUS SYSTEM

Superficial epigastric vein

Superficial circumflex iliac vein

External pudendal vein

Superficial femoral vein

Great saphenous vein

Anterolateral vein of leg

Posterior arch (arcuate) vein

Great saphenous vein termination

Lateral circumflex vein

Posteromedial vein

Anterolateral vein of leg

Great saphenous vein

Lower end of small (lesser) saphenous vein

Dorsal venous arch of the foot

Fig. 155.2 Superficial venous system. Lateral and medial views of the distribution of the major axial trunks of the superficial venous system, the great and small saphenous veins, and associated tributaries.

In summary, telangiectasias, reticular veins and varicose veins are derived from a hereditary substrate that is influenced by hormones, static gravitational pressures and dynamic muscular forces transmitted through failed venous valves. The hereditary substrate cannot be altered, but the influence of hemodynamic forces and hydrostatic pressure can be modified, both by sclerotherapy and by surgical techniques, as described here.

PHYSICAL EXAMINATION OF THE PHLEBOLOGY PATIENT

The purpose of the clinical examination is to survey the main venous trunks in order to determine where the primary or highest points of reflux are located. During the examination, the patient should be standing, preferably on a platform. It is important to determine the grade of venous insufficiency[6]. The recommended CEAP classification system is based on clinical manifestations (C), etiologic factors (E), anatomic distribution of disease (A), and the underlying pathophysiologic findings (P)[7]. The venous severity scoring (VSS) system is based on three elements: the number of anatomic segments affected, grading of symptoms and signs, and disability. The consensus statement was published in 25 journals and books in eight languages, truly a worldwide distribution.

For the practicing physician, CEAP is an instrument for correct diagnosis, to guide the treatment and to assess to the prognosis. It is important to stress that CEAP is a descriptive classification, while VSS and quality-of-life (QOL) scores are instruments for longitudinal research to assess outcomes. In modern phlebologic practice, the vast majority of patients will have a duplex scan of the venous system of

the leg, which will provide data on E, A and P. In basic CEAP, the single highest descriptor should be used for clinical class, e.g. a patient with varicose veins, swelling and lipodermatosclerosis will be C4b (Table 155.1). To resort to use of the C-classification *only* brings us back to the previous classifications that were based solely on the clinical appearance. Even in basic CEAP, where a duplex scan is performed, classification of E, A and P with multiple descriptors is recommended. For the anatomic classification A in basic CEAP, the simple s, p and d descriptors should be used, e.g. a patient could be classified as C4aS; Ep; As, d; Pr. Use of all components of CEAP should be encouraged. Venous disease is complex, but can be described using this system (see Table 155.1).

A disposable sclerotherapy garment is an excellent means for preserving patient modesty while gaining full access to the entire lower extremity. A two-step examination stool also aids in the clinical assessment. The medial plantar and ankle regions are examined for the presence of specific skin changes, including clusters of telangiectatic veins (referred to as 'corona phlebectasia'), hemosiderin deposition, atrophie blanche, lipodermatosclerosis, and/or active or healed ulceration. These findings suggest a chronic state of venous insufficiency, located in either the saphenous veins or the deep venous systems. The lateral posterior malleolar region is similarly examined. Skin changes in this area most often indicate small saphenous vein insufficiency.

There are three branch veins that are important for evaluating the saphenofemoral junction (SFJ)[8]. Attention is first directed toward the anterior abdominal wall. The presence of varices in this area ('caput medusae') indicates insufficiency of the superficial epigastric vein (see Fig. 155.2); this is always abnormal and should alert the phlebologist

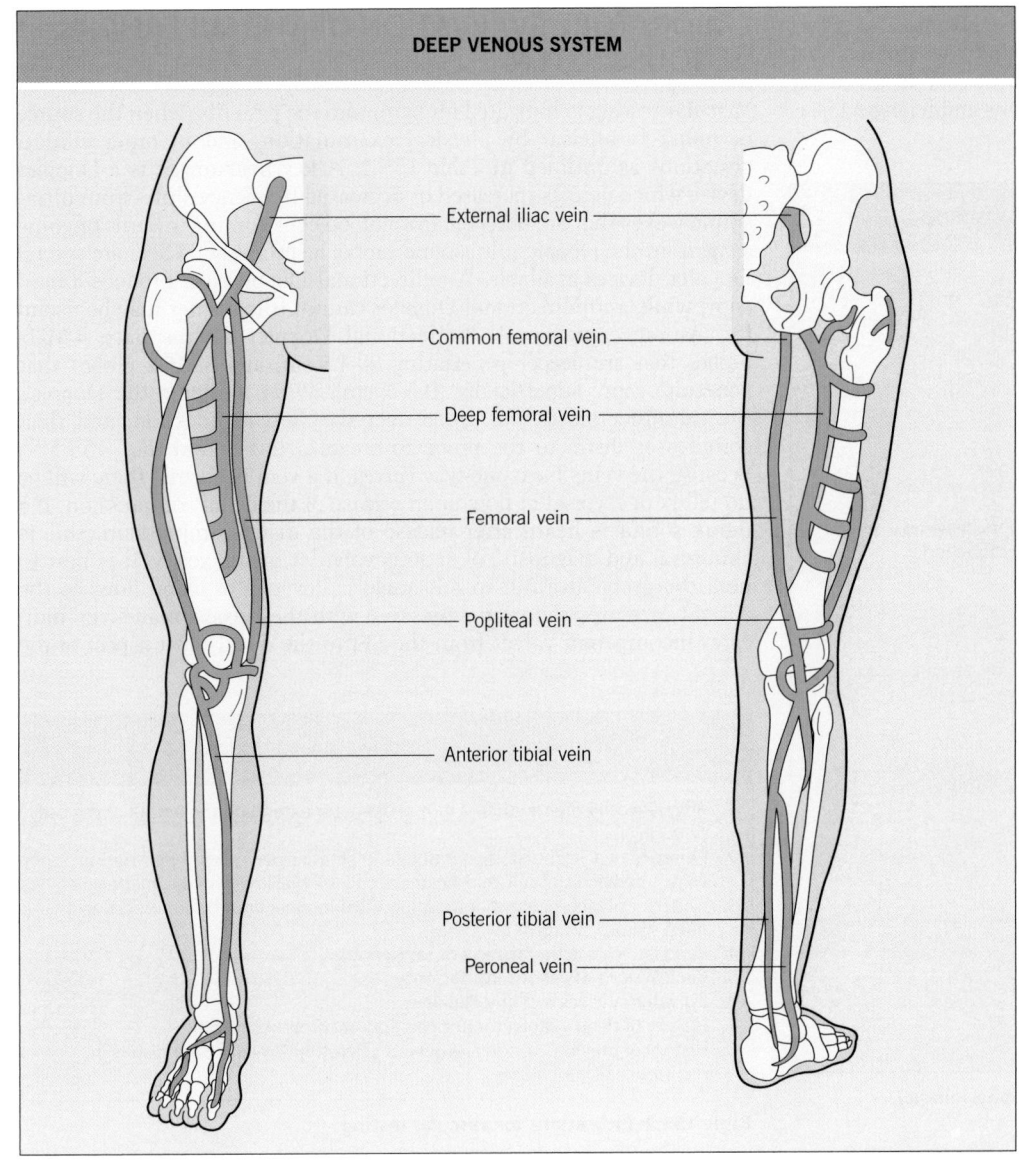

DEEP VENOUS SYSTEM

External iliac vein

Common femoral vein

Deep femoral vein

Femoral vein

Popliteal vein

Anterior tibial vein

Posterior tibial vein

Peroneal vein

Fig. 155.3 Deep venous system. The major drainage vessel below the knee is the popliteal vein, while the femoral vein is the major portal of drainage in the inguinal area of the groin (great saphenous distribution).

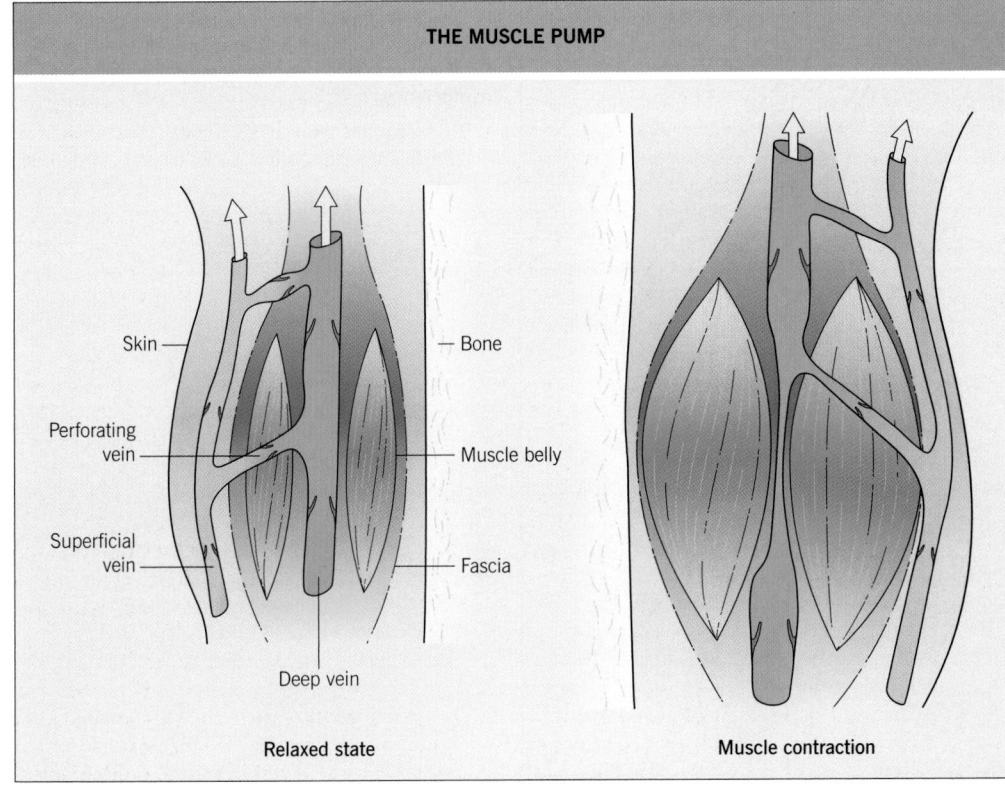

THE MUSCLE PUMP

Skin

Perforating vein

Superficial vein

Bone

Muscle belly

Fascia

Deep vein

Relaxed state

Muscle contraction

Fig. 155.4 The muscle pump, or 'peripheral heart'. This is located primarily in the calves. During muscle contraction, compression of veins transports blood to the heart by means of the deep venous system. Modified from Goldman MP, et al. Sclerotherapy, 4th edition. London: Mosby, 2007.

to underlying deep venous obstruction, usually in the iliofemoral segment (see Fig. 155.3). The posteromedial thigh vein and the anterolateral thigh vein are often also insufficient in patients with GSV insufficiency and usually present as dilated varicose reticular veins and telangiectasias within the involved anatomic zones[7].

CEAP CLASSIFICATION OF CHRONIC VENOUS DISORDERS

Clinical classification

C0: no visible or palpable signs of venous disease
C1: telangiectasias or reticular veins
C2: varicose veins
C3: edema
C4a: hemosiderin pigmentation, eczematous dermatitis
C4b: lipodermatosclerosis, atrophie blanche
C5: healed venous ulcer
C6: active venous ulcer

S: symptoms including aches, pains, tightness, skin irritation, heaviness, muscle cramps, and other complaints attributable to venous dysfunction
A: asymptomatic

Etiologic classification

Ec: congenital
Ep: primary
Es: secondary (post-thrombotic)
En: no venous etiology identified

Anatomic classification

As: superficial veins
Ap: perforator veins
Ad: deep veins
An: no venous location identified

Pathophysiologic classification

Pr: reflux
Po: obstruction
Pr,o: reflux and obstruction
Pn: no venous pathophysiology identified

Table 155.1 CEAP (Clinical, Etiologic, Anatomic, Pathophysiologic) classification of chronic venous disorders.

LABORATORY EVALUATION OF THE SUPERFICIAL VENOUS SYSTEM

Vascular testing is indicated for symptomatic patients, when the source of reflux is unclear by physical examination, and in other clinical situations as outlined in Table 155.2. A key instrument is a Doppler device which detects increased or decreased frequency shifts from ultrasound waves that are reflected from blood cells coming towards or going away from the Doppler ultrasound probe, respectively[9]. There are several Doppler devices available. A bidirectional Doppler can produce a hard copy, while a unidirectional Doppler cannot (the former may be useful for insurance purposes). Bidirectional Doppler devices have 4 MHz probes that are deeper penetrating (4–4.5 cm) and 8 MHz probes that penetrate more superficially (0.5–2 cm). When utilizing the Doppler, the examiner places the probe over the vein in question, and then compresses distal to the probe to create a flux sound (Fig. 155.5)[10]. Because the veins have one-way valves, if a vein is normal there will be no reflux or reversal of flow upon release of the distal compression. If a reflux sound is heard after release of the distal compression, this is abnormal and diagnostic of venous valvular insufficiency. It is best to hold the probe at a 30° to 45° angle[11]. Reversal of blood flow, as the patient increases abdominal pressure with the Valsava maneuver, indicates incompetent valves from the SFJ to the distal-most aspect of the

---

INDICATIONS FOR VASCULAR TESTING

1. Any varicosity greater than 2 mm in diameter extending the length of the calf or thigh
2. Presence of a 'starburst' cluster of telangiectasias over sites of perforating veins (medial distal calf, mid-posterior calf, medial knee, medial midthigh)
3. Evidence of incompetent perforating veins, connecting the superficial and deep venous systems
4. Varicose veins, either truncal or saphenous
5. Clinical signs of venous insufficiency
6. Symptomatic veins of any diameter
7. History of deep venous thrombosis and/or thrombophlebitis
8. History of previous venous surgery or sclerotherapy with poor results or recurrence of varicosities

Table 155.2 Indications for vascular testing.

DOPPLER EXAMINATION OF THE GREAT SAPHENOUS VEIN

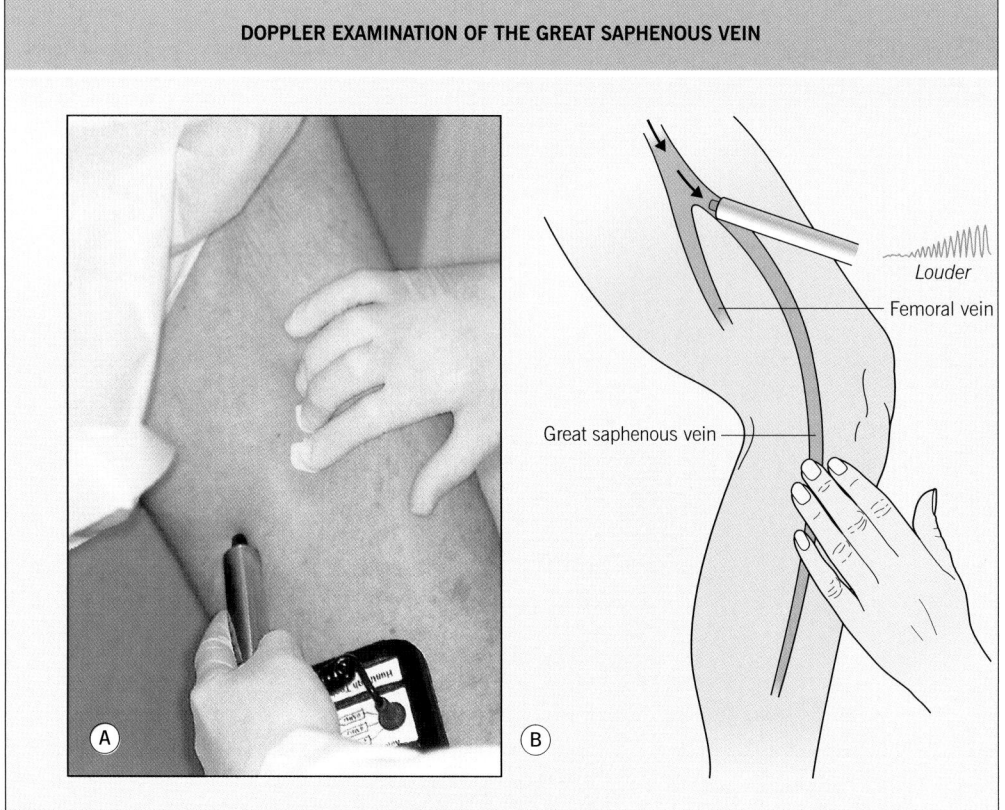

Louder

Femoral vein

Great saphenous vein

(A)   (B)

Fig. 155.5 Doppler examination of the great saphenous vein. A Doppler probe held at a 30° to 45° angle. **B** Doppler examination of the great saphenous vein; a reflux found after the release of distal compression denotes venous valvular insufficiency.

probe. When placed on the medial superior thigh over the GSV a few centimeters distal to the SFJ, reversal of blood flow for >0.5 seconds indicates an incompetent SFJ. These patients require endolumenal radiofrequency or laser closure of the GSV before any treatment is given to the distal varicose, reticular and/or telangiectatic leg veins.

Duplex ultrasonography is a highly accurate, non-invasive technique that can provide both anatomic and physiologic information regarding the venous system[12] (Table 155.3). For this reason, it is rapidly becoming the modality of choice, not only for pretreatment assessment of varicose veins, but also for guidance during newly described endovascular radiofrequency and laser procedures and for performance of follow-up studies. Duplex examination of normal veins involves the use of a ≥7.5 MHz gray-scale, high-resolution β-mode scanner and a 5 MHz Doppler probe. While the β-mode scanner provides real-time anatomic images, the Doppler probe supplies physiologic information in the form of blood flow data. Incorporation of the real-time image allows reproducible positioning of the Doppler probe at a known anatomic site. Using this method, the physician can obtain longitudinal and transverse images of veins and arteries that are up to 8 cm below the skin surface. For deeper assessment, a <7.5 MHz probe may be needed.

COMPRESSION IN SCLEROTHERAPY AND VENOUS DISEASE

Graduated compression has many benefits in patients with venous disease. It reduces the diameter of the veins, thereby increasing flow velocity and decreasing the chance of thrombus formation. Following sclerotherapy (which is essentially a *controlled* thrombophlebitic reaction), compression reduces the diameter of the resulting thrombosis of the treated vein, which minimizes the inflammatory reaction, thereby decreasing the extent and incidence of post-treatment hyperpigmentation, recanalization of the vein and telangiectatic matting. Compression also increases the contact between the sclerosant and the endothelial lining of the vessel wall, potentiating pan-vessel obliteration. There are three main types of graduated compression: graduated elastic compression stockings or bandages, inelastic compression garments or bandages, and pneumatic compression pumps[13]. Compression bandages are not recommended, as they are difficult to apply in a graduated manner and hold their compression for only a few hours after application.

Graduated elastic compression stockings are most commonly employed following sclerotherapy. They come in four classes based upon the pressure generated by the stocking at the ankle level (from 20–30 mmHg [class I] to 50–60 mmHg [class IV]) (see Ch. 105)[14]. Most sclerotherapy patients wear thigh-high or panty-hose stockings. In addition, most manufacturers now offer so-called 'fashion hose' which approximate 18 mmHg pressure and are sheer and associated with greater patient compliance. In a multicenter study performed by Weiss et al.[15], 20 mmHg compression was shown to increase sclerotherapeutic efficacy and diminish post-treatment hyperpigmentation. At least 3 days of compression was necessary to produce this positive effect and 3 weeks of daytime wear was found to be the optimal time required for the maximal effect[15]. We recommend that all patients wear graduated compression stockings for 1 week after the procedure. It is important to wear the stockings 24 hours a day, even while in the shower and sleeping. If one removes the stockings in the shower, the veins dilate. If one removes the stockings at night, the superficial system also dilates. For this reason, it is recommended that all patients wear the thigh-high stockings, which are more hygienic and easier to use than panty-hose that extend higher up to the waist.

SCLEROSING SOLUTIONS

The optimal sclerosing agent is one that induces pan-endothelial destruction or removal[16]. Thrombosis alone will not obliterate vessels because intact endothelium contains tissue plasminogen activator that can dissolve thrombi, leading to recanalization. The ideal sclerosing agent should possess no systemic toxicity and produce local endothelial destruction fully extending to the adventitia with minimal thrombus formation[17]. The resultant vascular destruction induces an inflammatory reaction which leads to fibrosis and eventually obliteration of the vessel.

There are several important points to remember when choosing a particular sclerosing solution and determining the appropriate sclerosant concentration (Table 155.4)[18]:

COMPARISON OF DOPPLER ULTRASOUND AND DUPLEX SCANNING FOR PRESCLEROTHERAPY EVALUATION

	Doppler	Duplex
Portability	Yes	Yes
Easy to use	Yes	Yes
Cost (2007) (approximate in US dollars)	Unidirectional: $750 Bidirectional: $1500	Gray scale: $10 000+ Color: $20 000+
Information obtained	1. Patency, competence of venous valves 2. Detection of deep venous thrombosis in thigh	1. Patency, competence of venous valves 2. Detection of deep venous thrombosis with greater accuracy (thigh > calf) 3. Velocity of reflux 4. Anatomy and anomalies of venous system (number of great saphenous veins) 5. Termination of small saphenous vein 6. Thrombosis versus sclerosis
Reliability	Less reliable because of blind, non-pulsed sound beam	More reliable because of actual visualization of venous anatomy

Table 155.3 Comparison of Doppler ultrasound and duplex scanning for presclerotherapy evaluation.

A GUIDE FOR THE SELECTION OF SCLEROSING SOLUTION CONCENTRATION AND VOLUME BY VESSEL TYPE

Vessel	Solution concentration	Volume (per region)
Telangiectatic matting (after previous treatment)	Glycerin, 72%, diluted 2:1 with 1% lidocaine with epinephrine	0.1–0.2 ml
Telangiectasias (up to 1 mm)	Glycerin, 72%, diluted 2:1 with 1% lidocaine with epinephrine Sodium tetradecyl sulfate, 0.1–0.25% Polidocanol, 0.25–0.5% Hypertonic saline, 11.7% Hypertonic saline, 10% and dextrose, 25% Polyiodide iodide, 0.1%	0.1–0.3 ml
Venulectasias (1–2 mm)	Sodium tetradecyl sulfate, 0.25–0.5% Glycerin, 72% Polidocanol, 0.5–0.75% Hypertonic saline, 11.7–23.4% Hypertonic saline, 10% and dextrose, 25%	0.2–0.5 ml
Reticular veins (2–4 mm subcutaneous blue veins)	Sodium tetradecyl sulfate, 0.1–0.25%, foam Polidocanol, 0.25–0.5%, foam Polyiodide iodide, 0.3–1.0%	0.5 ml (may increase to 1–3 ml if filling of reticular vein is observed by foam)
Non-saphenous varicose veins (3–8 mm)	Sodium tetradecyl sulfate, 0.5–1.0%, foam Polidocanol, 1.0–3.0%, foam Polyiodide iodide, 1.0–2.0%	0.5 ml for liquids 3 ml of foam per injection site in a large-capacity vein
Saphenous varicose trunks (usually >5 mm)	Sodium tetradecyl sulfate, 1.0–3.0%, foam Polidocanol, 3.0–5.0%, foam Polyiodide iodide, 2.0–6.0% (rarely to 12%)	0.5 ml for liquids (low-volume injection critical at high concentrations) 3 ml with foam

Table 155.4 A guide for the selection of sclerosing solution concentration and volume by vessel type. The sclerosing agents are listed in order of preference.

1. If the sclerosant is too weak, insufficient endothelial damage will occur, leading to thrombosis secondary to varicose vessel wall damage. However, there will be no fibrosis and recanalization of the vessel occurs.

2. Too strong a solution may lead to uncontrolled destruction of vascular endothelium and other layers, which may eventuate in hyperpigmentation, neoangiogenesis (telangiectatic matting) and ulceration secondary to sclerosant extravasation.

3. Choose the minimal sclerosant concentration (MSC) that will cause irreversible damage to the cell wall of the abnormal vessel.

Sclerosing agents are classified into three groups based upon the mechanism whereby they cause injury to the endothelium (Table 155.5):

1. Hyperosmotic agents – the osmotic agents include hypertonic saline and hypertonic saline–dextrose. Their primary mechanism of action involves endothelial cell damage through dehydration (Fig. 155.6A).

2. Chemical irritants – the chemical irritants include chromated or non-chromated glycerin and polyiodide iodide. They injure cells by acting as corrosives; their cauterizing effect is thought to be due to the associated heavy metal (Fig. 155.6B).

3. Detergent sclerosants – the detergent sclerosants include sodium tetradecyl sulfate, polidocanol and sodium morrhuate. This group of agents causes vascular injury by altering the surface tension around endothelial cells (Fig. 155.6C).

The only agents that are Food and Drug Administration (FDA)-approved for sclerotherapy in the US are sodium tetradecyl sulfate, sodium morrhuate (fatty acids in cod liver oil) and hypertonic saline[19]; the latter is approved as an abortifacient rather than for treatment of varicose veins. Glycerin is approved as a hyperosmotic agent for the treatment of acute intracerebral edema and acute angle glaucoma. Sclerosing agents lacking FDA approval include polidocanol (Aethoxysklerol®) and polyiodide iodide (Varigloban®). Glycerin, hypertonic saline (11.7–23.4%)

and sodium tetradecyl sulfate (0.25–3%; Sotradecol® or Fibrovein®) remain the sclerosants of choice at this time in the US.

Determining the minimal volume and minimal concentration of the most appropriate sclerosing agent is a key factor in producing effective sclerotherapy results. This concept, termed the minimal sclerosant concentration (MSC), will enable the sclerotherapist to achieve maximal results while minimizing the complication profile[20,21]. A guide to suggested sclerosing agents and initial choices of sclerosant concentrations and volumes for instillation as related to vessel type and diameter is presented in Table 155.4.

It is also important to have a working knowledge of the complication profile of each sclerosing solution (see Table 155.5). The osmotic sclerosants such as hypertonic saline are associated with burning and cramping on injection and an increased incidence of ulcerative necrosis secondary to extravasation.

Sodium tetradecyl sulfate (Sotradecol®) has been associated with a low incidence of allergic reactions, ranging from urticaria to anaphylaxis (<0.01%)[5]. However, with increasing usage, it is now believed that the risk of type I (i.e. immediate hypersensitivity) reactions is extremely minimal. In fact, after over 20 years of use in over 20 000 patients, the authors have never seen an allergic reaction except for one case of urticaria. A similar low incidence of allergic and anaphylactic reactions has been reported with polidocanol (Aethoxysklerol®)[5].

Hyperpigmentation has been reported in 5–30% of patients treated with all sclerosing solutions except glycerin, which has a <1% incidence of pigmentation. However, in the authors' experience, glycerin's true incidence parallels that of other sclerosing agents of similar potency and the incidence of hyperpigmentation is more related to concentration as well as host skin type, vessel type and other vascular fragility factors[22–24].

Creating foaming detergent solutions by mixing them with air (typically in a mixture of 1 ml solution with 4 ml air) has been found to increase

IMPORTANT CHARACTERISTICS OF SCLEROSING SOLUTIONS					
Sclerosing solution (Brand name)	Class	Allergenicity	Risks	FDA approval	Dose limitation
Hypertonic saline [11.7–23.4%]	Hyperosmotic	None	Pain and cramping Necrosis of skin Hyperpigmentation	Yes, as abortifacient [18–30%]	6–10 ml
Hypertonic saline [10%] and dextrose [25%] (Sclerodex®)	Hyperosmotic	Low (due only to added phenethyl alcohol)	Pain (much less than with hypertonic saline alone)	No (sold in Canada)	10 ml of undiluted solution
Sodium tetradecyl sulfate (Sotradecol®, Fibrovein®, Thromboject®)	Detergent	Very rare anaphylaxis	Pain with perivascular injection Necrosis of skin (with higher concentrations) Hyperpigmentation	Yes	10 ml of 3%
Polidocanol (Aethoxysklerol®, Aetoxisclerol®, Sclerovein®)	Detergent	Very rare anaphylaxis	Lowest risk of pain Lowest risk of necrosis Hyperpigmentation (with higher concentrations) Disulfiram-like reaction	No	5 ml of 3% (depends on body weight, see ref. 5)
Sodium morrhuate (Scleromate®)	Detergent	Anaphylaxis, highest risk	Pain Necrosis of skin Hyperpigmentation	Yes	10 ml
Ethanolamine oleate	Detergent	Urticaria, anaphylaxis	Pain Necrosis of skin Hyperpigmentation Viscous, difficult to inject Acute renal failure Hemolytic reactions	Yes (used primarily for esophageal varices)	10 ml
Polyiodide iodide (Varigloban®, Variglobin®, Sclerodine®)	Chemical irritant	Anaphylaxis Iodine hypersensitivity reactions	Pain Necrosis of skin Dark brown color makes intravascular placement more difficult to confirm	No	5 ml of 3%
Glycerin [72%] with chromium potassium alum [8%] (Chromex®, Scleremo®); glycerin [72%]	Chemical irritant	Very rare anaphylaxis (none for glycerin alone)	Pain and cramping Low risk of hyperpigmentation Viscous, difficult to inject Hematuria with injections >10 ml	Yes (for treatment of acute intracerebral edema and acute angle glaucoma)	10 ml

Table 155.5 **Important characteristics of sclerosing solutions.**

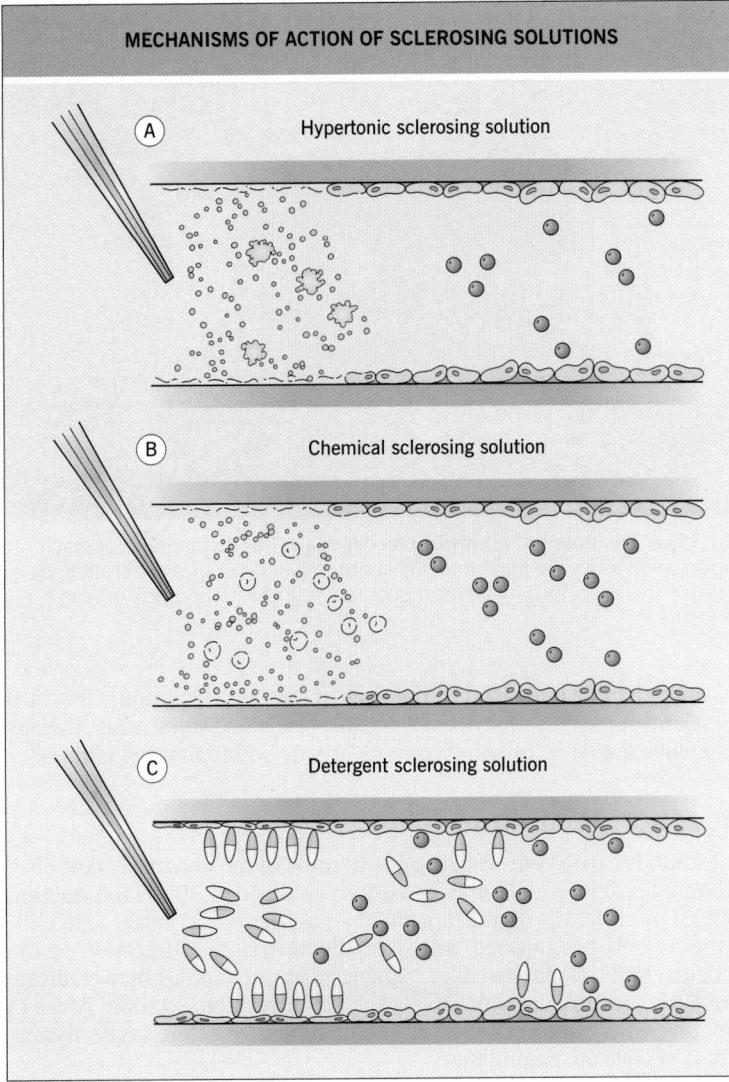

MECHANISMS OF ACTION OF SCLEROSING SOLUTIONS

(A) Hypertonic sclerosing solution

(B) Chemical sclerosing solution

(C) Detergent sclerosing solution

Fig. 155.6 Mechanisms of action of sclerosing solutions. A Hypertonic, which induces endothelial damage via a gradient dehydration effect. **B** Chemical, which injures cells by acting as a corrosive. **C** Detergent, the hydrophobic portion of the detergent molecule attaches to the endothelial cell wall while the hydrophilic portion draws water into the cell, leading to an overhydrated maceration effect. Modified from Goldman MP, et al. Sclerotherapy, 4th edition. London: Mosby, 2007.

the potency of the sclerosing solution twofold while decreasing its adverse effect profile fourfold. Foam displaces blood and remains for an extended time in the target vessel. This makes it more efficient, so that it may be utilized at lower concentrations.

TECHNIQUES FOR TREATING TELANGIECTASIAS AND RETICULAR VEINS

The treatment of telangiectasias and reticular veins is most commonly performed for cosmetic improvement, but up to 50% of these patients also report a variety of symptoms, from dull aching legs to throbbing pain over the telangiectasia[25]. Telangiectasias are best defined as flat, red to blue vessels 0.1–1 mm in diameter (Table 155.6). Venulectasias are bluish vessels, sometimes distended above the skin surface and most often 1–2 mm in diameter. Reticular veins have a cyanotic hue and are visually 2–4 mm in diameter. When a complex of reticular veins is located on the lateral thigh, it is felt to be a vestige of embryonal development and known as the lateral subdermal plexus[26,27].

The treatment of telangiectasias and reticular veins is undertaken only after all sources of reflux have been addressed, as it is important to treat proximal sites of reflux first and to treat larger vessels before smaller veins. Alone or in combination with laser and intense pulsed light technology, sclerotherapy of small-diameter vessels is the most common challenge faced by the dermatologic surgeon who performs sclerotherapy. Preoperative photographic documentation and full informed consent outlining all possible risks and complications as well as treatment expectations should be obtained prior to therapy[28–30].

Materials employed in the treatment of telangiectasias and reticular veins are relatively simple. They may include:

- cotton balls soaked with 70% isopropyl alcohol
- protective gloves
- 3 and 5 cm³ disposable syringes
- 30-gauge disposable ½-inch transparent hub needles
- magnifying lens (2–3×)
- nitroglycerin paste for prolonged blanching
- bronchodilator inhaler in case of bronchospasm
- epinephrine in case of anaphylaxis.

Flow sheets with segmental numerical division of the legs are helpful in documenting areas that are treated at each session. Because successful sclerotherapy that results in pan-luminal endofibrosis can take up to 6 weeks, it is recommended that treatment sessions should not be repeated for at least this interval of time.

There are four techniques that may be employed in the treatment of telangiectatic and reticular veins[30–32]. They include:

	CLASSIFICATION OF VEINS AND CLINICAL APPROACH TO TREATMENT OF VENOUS PATHOLOGY			
Type	**Description**	**Diameter (mm)**	**Color**	**Treatment**
I	Telangiectasias (spider veins)	0.1–1	Usually red	• Microsclerotherapy • Intense pulsed light • Lasers (e.g. pulsed dye)
	Telangiectatic matting		Red network	• Laser (e.g. pulsed dye, 1064 nm Nd:YAG)
II	Venulectasias	1–2	Violaceous	• Sclerotherapy • Laser (e.g. 1064 nm Nd:YAG)
III	Reticular varicosities	2–4	Cyanotic blue to blue–green	• Sclerotherapy • Ambulatory phlebectomy • Laser (e.g. 1064 nm Nd:YAG)
IV	Varicosities (secondary saphenous branch or perforator-related)	3–8	Blue to blue–green	• Ambulatory phlebectomy • Sclerotherapy
V	Saphenous varicosities (truncal or axial varicosities including main saphenous trunks and first-generation branch varicosities)	≥5	Blue to blue–green May be palpable and not visible	• Ambulatory phlebectomy • Radiofrequency obliteration • Sclerotherapy • Endovascular laser obliteration • Surgical ligation/stripping procedures

Table 155.6 Classification of veins and clinical approach to treatment of venous pathology. Nd:YAG, neodymium:yttrium aluminum garnet.

1. Aspiration technique. Aspiration of a small amount of blood into the needle hub may ensure that the dermatologic surgeon has adequately cannulated the vein. The vein may collapse if aspiration is too strong.
2. Puncture-fill technique. This technique relies on the feeling associated with perforating the vein wall. Although it is slightly more precarious for beginners, this technique can be mastered with time.
3. Air bolus technique (Fig. 155.7). Injection of $<0.5 \text{ cm}^3$ of air prior to introduction of sclerosant will displace blood in the vein. Once intravascular access is confirmed, the sclerosant can be safely injected. Air inadvertently introduced into the tissues is not as damaging as the sclerosant might be. Too strong of a push may lead to truncal distention and rupture. The small air bolus technique is ideal for hypertonic saline, as even slight extravasation of solution will cause an epidermal ulceration.
4. Empty vein technique. In an attempt to remove as much blood as possible, the leg is elevated and kneading with gentle pressure is performed before the sclerosant is injected. The persistence of varicose veins after treatment is usually due to recanalization of the intramural thrombus that develops. The empty vein technique may reduce the amount of thrombus. This concept is more important when treating larger veins. Other advantages of this technique are that an empty vein has minimal volume and therefore the endothelium is exposed to a concentration similar to that injected. Also, a smaller volume of sclerosant is necessary to ensure contact with the endothelial surface and lower concentrations of sclerosant may be employed

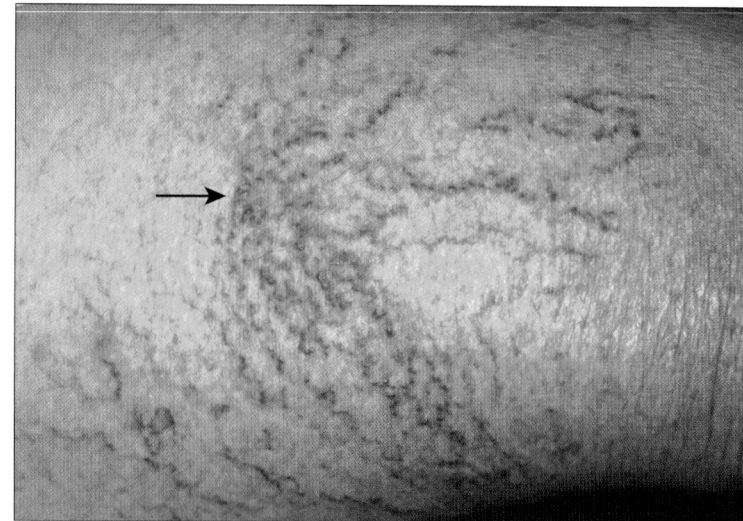

Fig. 155.8 Treatment of arborizing feeder veins. This therapeutic approach (arrow) diminishes the number of injections required in a given sclerotherapy treatment session, thus minimizing potential side effects. Courtesy of Jean L Bolognia MD.

since there is less blood in the vein to dilute the solution[33]. Foamed sclerosing agents, discussed later, displace blood from veins, thereby inducing a de facto empty vein technique with enhanced efficacy.

Injection Technique

Injection is carried out utilizing one or more of the previously described techniques. The needle may be bent at an angle of 30°. Hand traction is used by either the dermasurgeon or an assistant to keep the skin taut. Large vessels are injected before smaller vessels, i.e. injection of the reticular veins feeding smaller telangiectasias or venules may eradicate the latter, minimizing side effects such as hyperpigmentation. Areas of vascular arborization (Fig. 155.8) should be treated before single discrete linear vessels are cannulated[34].

The utilization of alcohol in swabbing the skin prior to injection will increase the index of refraction of light and thus make the vessels more visible at the skin surface. Alternatively, the sclerosing solution itself can be dripped onto the skin just before injection, avoiding the cooling and vasoconstriction resulting from alcohol evaporation. Brisk cannulation of veins causes minimal vascular trauma, less vasoconstriction, and less chance of extravasation of blood. Injection pressure is kept to a minimum by performing the injection slowly in order to prevent

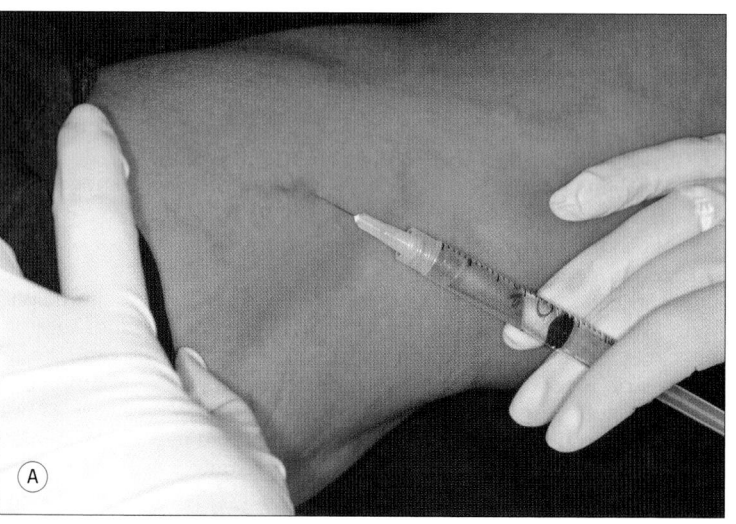

(A)

AIR BOLUS TECHNIQUE

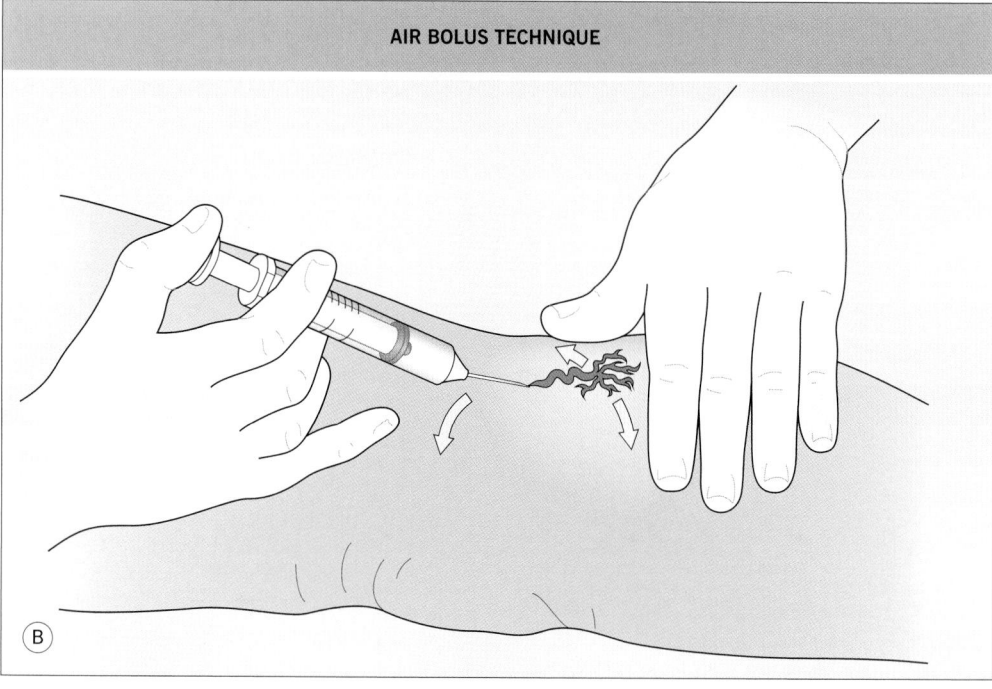

Fig. 155.7 Air bolus technique. A Injection of an air bolus ($<0.5 \text{ cm}^3$) prior to injection of sclerosant can displace blood in the vein and ensure intravascular needle location. Air inadvertently introduced into the tissues is not as damaging as the sclerosant might be. **B** Three point stretching of the skin allows for more accurate canulation of the vessel. B, Redrawn from Goldman MP, et al. Sclerotherapy, 4th edition. London: Mosby, 2007.

(B)

vascular distention, and to allow adequate time for the sclerosing agent to interact with endothelium. A small amount of sclerosant is used at each injection site (0.1–0.4 cm^3) in order to minimize side effects such as telangiectatic matting, postsclerosis pigmentation and ulcerative necrosis due to extravasation. The sclerosing injection is stopped when the solution has filled the targeted veins. Injections are carried out at approximately 3–6 cm intervals until the entire vessel has been treated.

Foamed Detergent Solutions

A detergent solution such as sodium tetradecyl sulfate can be foamed to a thick consistency by rapidly agitating it with air in a ratio of solution to air of 1:4. There are numerous advantages of using foam when treating larger varicosities. For instance, an increased quantity of solution can be injected over longer segments of veins. A foamed sclerosing solution retains more of its potency, as the full concentration of the sclerosant is present on each microbubble residing on the outer micelle. Due to persistence and increased potency, foamed agents reduce the number of treatments and allow treatment of larger vessels. In contrast, for smaller vessels, non-foamable glycerin or hypertonic saline are rapidly diluted but act only within their concentration gradients, thus limiting the extent and intensity of sclerosing action. It is not practical to treat large veins with glycerin or hypertonic saline, as more frequent injections are necessary and the potency is rapidly diminished by concentrations being rapidly diluted by blood within the treated vein.

It may be desirable to have the patient wait for 15–30 minutes following their first treatment session with a sclerosing agent other than hypertonic saline or glycerin, in order to assure that there is no evidence of a type I immediate hypersensitivity reaction[35].

Treatment sessions are carried out at 6–8-week intervals in order to allow enough time for full endosclerosis to occur and for post-treatment inflammation to resolve, and to evaluate the results of the previous treatment session. Most patients will require one to three treatment sessions in order to clear their legs of unwanted telangiectatic and reticular vessels. If a poor response is seen at the end of this treatment schedule, the dermatologic surgeon may:
- increase the concentration of sclerosant
- switch to another sclerosant
- re-examine the patient to find a possible source of reflux previously missed.

Lasers and Intense Pulsed Light Sources for Treatment of Telangiectasias

Laser and intense pulsed light (IPL) therapy of lower extremity vessels may have a synergistic effect when used in combination with sclerotherapy. Although beyond the scope of this chapter, a few words regarding the utilization of lasers (see Ch. 136) and IPL for the treatment of lower extremity telangiectasias is appropriate. Primary indications for laser/IPL treatment of leg veins include ankle telangiectasias, resistance to sclerotherapy, and fine matting postsclerotherapy.

For leg veins, wavelengths of 600–1100 nm have been found to be most useful in delivering sufficient light energy so that the target vessel has its entire diameter thermocoagulated. It has been noted that more superficial red vessels are most efficiently treated by shorter wavelengths of 500–600 nm (green–yellow spectrum), while deeper blue vessels are best targeted by longer wavelengths of infrared light of 755–1100 nm[36]. Longer wavelengths, extended pulse durations and improved cooling technologies have made laser and IPL treatment of small lower extremity veins more consistent, with a lower complication profile than that seen with earlier technologies[37-39].

The longer wavelength 1064 nm Nd:YAG lasers have been shown to be effective in treating reticular veins up to 4 mm in diameter. They also have a distinct advantage in that they may be utilized in treating individuals with more darkly pigmented skin (Fitzpatrick skin types IV–VI)[40,41]. Unfortunately, reticular veins that are 4 mm in diameter are much more painful to treat with a laser than with sclerotherapy. In addition, laser treatment can only 'spot-weld' the vein and will not treat the entire feeding network of veins.

LARGER VARICOSE VEINS

The treatment of large-diameter blood vessels requires greater and more precise attention to details regarding anatomy and points of reflux[42]. Contraindications to treatment of large-diameter veins include pregnancy, lactation, allergy to the sclerosing agent, thrombophilia or a hypercoagulable state, non-ambulation, travel within 48 hours of treatment, and non-compliance[43].

Factors of importance in the treatment of large-diameter veins include:
1. An understanding of the precise anatomy of the varicosity under consideration for treatment.
2. Adherence to a rational treatment plan in which injections begin at the highest point of reflux, with progression to the next highest point in a proximal-to-distal direction.
3. Determination of the most significant reflux point[44,45].

The dermatologic surgeon must determine whether reflux originates in the deep venous system, GSV or SSV, or a perforator (see Figs 155.2 & 155.3). The veins which represent the primary source of reflux must be treated before secondary sources of reflux are treated. Duplex ultrasound guidance (see Table 155.3) is often helpful in the therapeutic approach to larger-diameter vessels, particularly those cases where the anatomy is so intricate that the point of reflux would otherwise be difficult to detect.

Slightly modified techniques and/or positions for large-vein sclerotherapy have been described worldwide (Table 155.6). Three positions for treating large-diameter vessels are: (1) the standing supine elevation direct cannulation (SSDC) technique; (2) the multiple precannulation sites (MPS) technique; and (3) supine cannulation (SC)[5,35,45].

A foamed detergent sclerosing agent is currently recommended. The concentration of foamed agent is determined by the size of the vein to be injected (see Table 155.4). While polyiodide iodide (non-foamed) and foamed polidocanol (Aethoxysklerol®) are widely used outside the US, foamed sodium tetradecyl sulfate is most commonly employed in the US for treatment of large varicosities.

In the standing supine elevation direct cannulation (SDC) position, the patient stands at first, causing the varices to bulge and become more visible (Fig. 155.9)[27]. Injection points are marked at primary sites of reflux into the system and approximately every 3–4 cm along the vein being treated. The patient is then placed in a supine or prone position, the vein is emptied to maximize sclerosant–endothelial contact, and a small volume of sclerosant is injected at each of the marked points along the vein to be treated. A 27–30-gauge needle on a 3 ml syringe is often employed for this technique. The needle is advanced while aspirating into the syringe until aspiration of dark venous blood indicates penetration of the lumen. Concentrated sclerosant (0.5–1.5 ml) is

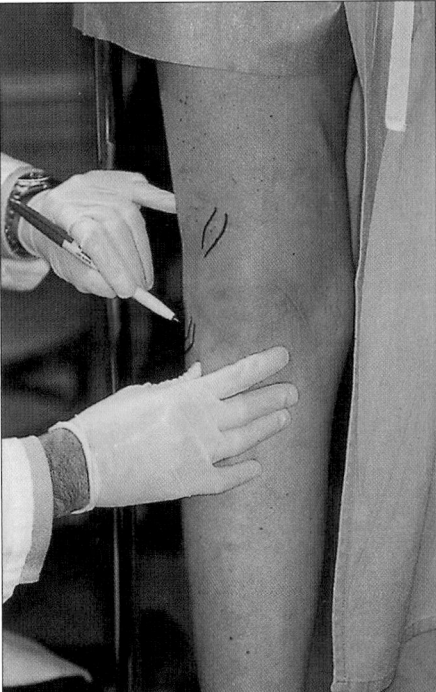

Fig. 155.9 Marking of treatment sites. Prior to large-vein sclerotherapy, marking of treatment sites in a standing position by indelible marker is performed.

injected at each site, followed by massage, again to ensure maximum sclerosant–endothelial contact. The vein appears visually contracted at the end of the treatment. Leg elevation for a minute following the injection of foam allows the larger veins to contract. This may result in further spread and better contact of the sclerosant with the endothelium, improving the results.

In the multiple precannulation sites (MPS) variation, the patient initially stands, in order to induce the varices to bulge and become more visible. Injection points are marked at proximal and distal sites along the distended vein. The veins are subsequently cannulated with a 23-gauge butterfly needle and tubing or a plastic intravenous cannula and extension tubing at *both* proximal and distal sites[46].

The butterfly needles or cannulas must be firmly secured, as the patient then moves to the treatment table and elevates the extremity undergoing treatment. After the intravascular position has been verified, 2–3 ml of sclerosant is infused into the cannula and subsequently into the vein while the surrounding area is observed for swelling or other evidence of extravasation. In the majority of cases, a single proximal and a single distal injection point are sufficient to sclerose a large tortuous vessel[47].

The authors routinely use the supine cannulation position, as it is faster and has less risk of vasovagal responses as compared to the upright position. Just prior to injection, detergent sclerosing solution is foamed by mixing the sclerosing solution with one part solution to four parts air[48]. Larger veins are treated proximal to distal with an appropriate concentration of sclerosing solution. Veins <1 mm diameter are typically treated with 72% glycerin.

Duplex ultrasound (see Table 155.3) may also be a helpful tool in the treatment of large non-junctional varicose veins in selected circumstances. Incomplete endosclerosis presents as a pattern of intravascular thrombosis (multiple echoes), with the vein lumen remaining partially patent. When sclerotherapy has been successful, the vein wall is thickened and non-compressible (non-echogenic)[42,49]. With duplex-guided sclerotherapy, we recommend using only a foamed sclerosing solution. This will decrease the chance for inadvertent arterial injection and allow the sclerotherapist to better visualize the sclerosing solution flowing into the targeted vein. The distribution of sclerosant will be easily visible as a sparkling on duplex ultrasound within the treated veins.

Doppler guidance with a hand-held device may also be an effective tool in large-vein sclerotherapy, particularly when access to duplex ultrasound is not readily available[50]. Doppler ultrasound may pick up points of occult reflux and perforator veins not obvious on physical examination. A change in the position of varicose veins when the patient moves from a standing to a supine position, which may occur in up to 25% of cases, may be assessed by this technique. Finally, it may also serve as a guide to accurate instillation points for sclerosing solutions. Utilizing an 8 MHz probe, the amount of maximal reflux is assessed and the probe is placed approximately 1 cm distal to the injection site with an assistant holding the Doppler probe in place (Fig. 155.10). The injection is then carried out with foamed sclerosing solution, which will make a loud sound 1 cm distal to the point of reflux. Some authorities feel that Doppler is too inferior and should not be used.

POSTSCLEROTHERAPY COMPRESSION

Cotton-roll pads are applied along the entire course of the treated vessels and are held in place by a compression garment. Graduated compression stockings that are class I (20–30 mmHg) or preferably class II (30–40 mmHg) are suggested for all patients following sclerotherapy of telangiectasias and reticular veins[15]. Patients should be instructed to walk 30 minutes after each treatment session, in order to minimize thromboembolic events as well as decrease the diameter of the superficial veins. The optimal duration of compression was shown in a recent study to be a minimum of 3 weeks, although 3 days of compression led to better results than no compression[15]. After large-vein sclerotherapy, we recommend 7 days of uninterrupted compression, during which the patients may bathe or shower by placing a large plastic bag over the compression bandage or stocking or just allow the stocking to get wet and dry it off with a hairdryer. After the first 7 days, the compression pads or cotton rolls are discarded and patients are permitted to remove the stocking, as needed, for bathing and sleeping. Ambulation is begun immediately post-treatment.

COMPLICATIONS

There are three major considerations in anticipating and managing complications of sclerotherapy (Table 155.7). The first is that fastidious technique will minimize the incidence of side effects. Second is an appropriate understanding of maneuvers that may be instituted if something is felt to go wrong. Finally, an appreciation of the management options available for adverse sequelae can minimize the intensity of complications when they occur[51].

Postsclerotherapy Pigmentation

The incidence of postsclerotherapy hyperpigmentation (Fig. 155.11) varies from 4% to 30%[24,48,52,53]. The purple–brown pigmentation has been shown to be due to extravascular deposits of hemosiderin[54]. Hypercoagulability syndromes such as antithrombin III, protein C or protein S deficiencies, use of non-steroidal anti-inflammatory drugs, high total body iron stores, use of minocycline, or the vessel fragility commonly noted in the elderly may predispose to this adverse sequela[55]. Ways to minimize the incidence of post-therapy pigmentation are outlined in Table 155.8. Although various treatment modalities have been tried for this complication, only the utilization of the Q-switched ruby laser has shown any degree of reproducible success[56–58]. Pigmentation usually lasts for 6–12 months. If it persists, the dermatologic surgeon should search for a vessel with persistent reflux into the area or an underlying predisposition.

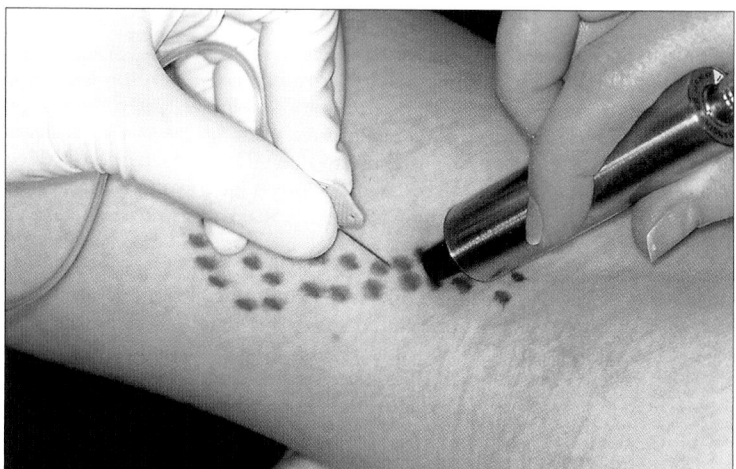

Fig. 155.10 Doppler-guided sclerotherapy. Doppler-guided injection is carried out 1 cm distal to point of reflux as ascertained by Doppler examination.

SCLEROTHERAPY COMPLICATIONS	
Cutaneous complications	**Extracutaneous complications**
Early	**Early**
• Localized urticaria	• Systemic allergic reactions (e.g. anaphylaxis)
• Bruising	• Scotomata (with foam sclerosants)
• Edema	• Vasovagal syncope
• Ischemia/necrosis (e.g. due to arterial injection)	
Delayed	**Delayed**
• Superficial thrombophlebitis	• Deep venous thrombosis/ pulmonary embolus
• Ulceration (secondary to ischemia/necrosis)	• Nerve damage
• Hyperpigmentation	
• Telangiectatic matting (neoangiogenesis)	
• Hypertrichosis	
• Compression-related problems (folliculitis, irritant contact dermatitis)	

Table 155.7 Sclerotherapy complications.

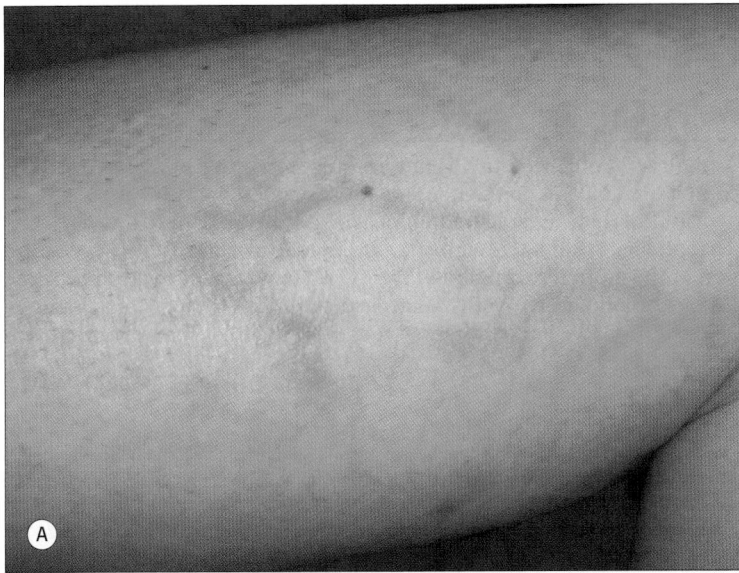

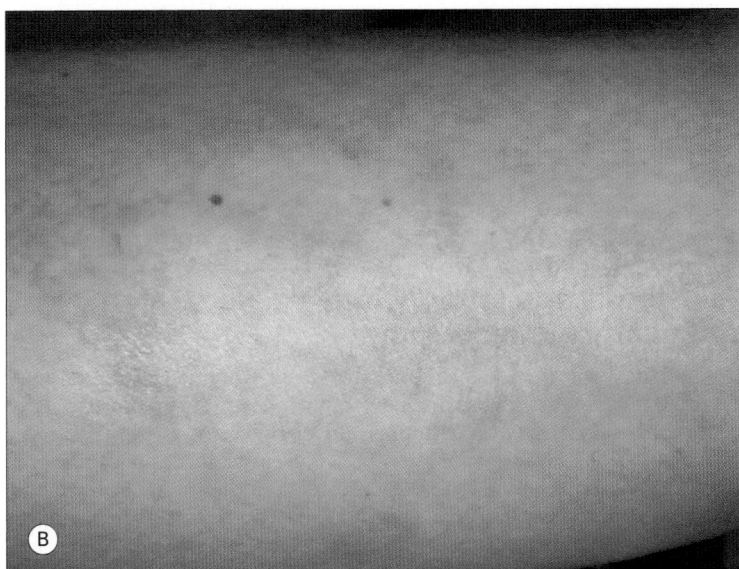

Fig. 155.11 Sclerotherapy-induced hyperpigmentation. A Development of hyperpigmentation along the course of a 3–4 mm diameter reticular vein 3 months after treatment with sodium tetradecyl sulfate 0.5% foam. **B** Six months after treatment with the Q-switched ruby laser at 6 J/cm², 5 mm diameter spot. Note complete resolution of hyperpigmentation.

METHODS TO MINIMIZE POSTSCLEROTHERAPY HYPERPIGMENTATION
Pretreatment planning
• Evaluate for a hypercoagulable state in patients with a history of venous thrombosis (see Table 105.4)
• Avoid treating patients with known defects in iron transport (e.g. hemochromatosis)
• Avoid concomitant use of minocycline, aspirin or NSAIDs
Treatment technique
• Eliminate high-pressure reflux before treating smaller vessels
• Select a sclerosant with the least inflammatory effects
• Use a sclerosant concentration appropriate for the vessel size (see Table 155.4)
• Minimize intravascular pressure by elevating the leg during treatment
• Direct treatment at the deepest site in a telangiectatic cluster
• Minimize risk of vessel rupture (e.g. by slow injection)
• Avoid excessive syringe pressure
Post-treatment care
• Apply compression immediately after treatment
• Remove postsclerotherapy clots as early as possible

Table 155.8 Methods to minimize postsclerotherapy hyperpigmentation. NSAIDs, nonsteroidal anti-inflammatory drugs.

Telangiectatic Matting

Nets of very fine blushes of telangiectasias may occur around sites of previously injected veins or sites of previous surgical interruption, e.g. ligation or ambulatory phlebectomy. They may occur from days to months after treatment and are seen in 5–14% of patients[24,48,59]. Sites of predilection include the thighs, medial malleolus, and medial and lateral calves. Risk factors include obesity, use of estrogen-containing medications, pregnancy and a family history of telangiectatic veins. Excessive postsclerotherapy inflammation may also predispose individuals to this complication, due to inadequate compression or the use of more than the minimal sclerosant concentration (MSC) of sclerosing solution.

Generally, telangiectatic matting resolves within 3–12 months without specific treatment. Persistence should lead the dermatologic surgeon to attempt to locate a source of reflux in the area (usually a feeding reticular vein), although matting may be a sign of underlying saphenous insufficiency. Low injection pressure with the utilization of the MSC is the most effective way to minimize this complication. Additional measures include the use of no more than 1 ml of sclerosant per injection site, limiting the injection blanch to 1–2 cm, encouraging normalization of weight, and discontinuation of oral contraceptives for 1 month prior and 2 months following sclerotherapy. Short-wavelength lasers (595–600 nm) and intense pulsed light sources as well as reinjection of vessels utilizing glycerin solution are the most effective ways of managing this problem[60].

Ulceration

Cutaneous necrosis may occur with any sclerosing agent (although the authors have never seen this with glycerin) and does not necessarily imply physician error. It may be the result of extravasation of a sclerosing agent into the perivascular tissues (especially common with the use of hypertonic saline and non-foamed sodium tetradecyl sulfate >1% in concentration) (Fig. 155.12); injection into a dermal arteriole or an arteriovenous anastomosis; reactive vasospasm of the vessel; or excessive cutaneous pressure created by compression techniques[61]. If hypertonic saline is extravasated outside of the targeted vessel, infiltration of the area with normal saline may dilute the sclerosant. A hemorrhagic bulla may form over the area within 12–24 hours and later progress to an ulcer. If a porcelain-white area appears within the skin immediately postinjection, this indicates arteriole injection or spasm. To reduce the likelihood of ulceration, the physician may rub a small amount of 2% nitroglycerin ointment into the area until a reactive hyperemia is seen. Since most ulcerations are less than 4 mm in diameter, secondary healing usually results in an acceptable scar. Larger

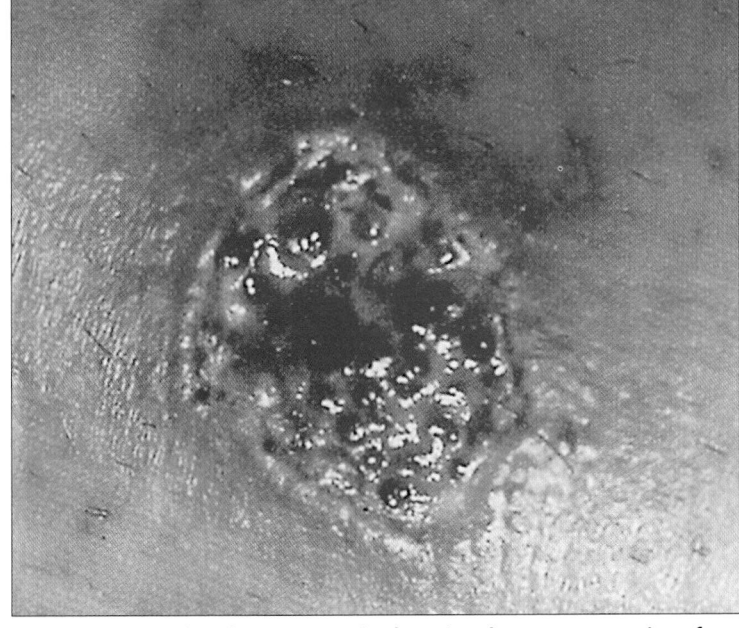

Fig. 155.12 Postsclerotherapy necrotic ulceration due to extravasation of hypertonic saline.

ulcerations may be excised (as early as possible) and closed for faster healing and a smaller scar. Application of topical antibiotic ointments (e.g. mupirocin) and hydrocolloid or hydrophilic dressings may reduce the pain associated with the ulcer and speed the rate of healing[62].

Systemic Allergic Reaction

True allergic reactions following sclerotherapy treatments are extremely rare. Delayed hypersensitivity reactions, which may be urticarial or morbilliform in nature, can occur from 8 to 16 hours after treatment. Type I immediate reactions varying from urticaria to bronchospasm to anaphylaxis eventuating in cardiovascular collapse have been rarely reported. Intrinsically, only hypertonic saline has no potential to act as an allergen. However, the presence of additives such as benzoate or lidocaine may lead to the development of hypersensitivity reactions.

Sodium tetradecyl sulfate has a surprisingly low allergic potential (< 0.01%). The most commonly reported hypersensitivity reactions are morbilliform eruptions developing 30–90 minutes after injection[63]. Polidocanol reactions are similarly rare (<0.01%). Both urticarial and morbilliform reactions have been reported, as well as a rare fatality[63].

Antihistamines and oral corticosteroids (e.g. prednisone 40–60 mg/day for 7–10 days) can be used for the milder reactions, whereas intravenous corticosteroids and subcutaneous epinephrine are often required for more serious reactions.

Arterial Injection

The most feared complication in sclerotherapy is inadvertent injection into an artery. Arterial injection of a sclerosing agent produces a sludge embolus that obstructs small arteries as well as the microcirculation. The most common location for an arterial injection to occur is the popliteal fossa, when attempting to inject the small saphenous vein. After an intra-arterial injection, the patient may or may not note immediate pain. A dusky cyanotic hue and pallor in the distribution of the injected artery usually occurs within a few minutes. Arterial pulsations in the posterior tibial or dorsalis pedis are not usually affected. Sloughing of superficial tissues may result in significant scarring or amputation[64].

Arterial injection is a true sclerotherapy emergency. Immediate intervention has been advocated, but has never been proven to affect outcome. Procaine, 1%, administered via periarterial infiltration, forms a complex with sodium tetradecyl sulfate, rendering it inactive. Cooling of the limb to minimize tissue anoxia, followed by immediate heparinization for 7–10 days and administration of intravenous dextran (10%, 500 mg daily) for 3 days is recommended. Thrombolysis (e.g. 250–750 000 IU streptokinase) and the utilization of long-term vasodilator therapy (e.g. calcium channel blockers) should be considered.

Miscellaneous Complications

Localized urticaria following injection is common and most likely related to mast cell degranulation and cytokine release. No treatment is indicated, although pretreatment with an H_1 antihistamine or immediate application of class I ultra-potent topical corticosteroids may ameliorate the erythema, if bothersome to the patient. Compression-related problems such as ulcers, pressure bullae, contact dermatitis and folliculitis may be minimized by adherence to appropriate compression guidelines[51].

Nerve damage may occur secondary to direct injection of sclerosant or as a result of perivascular inflammation around nerve sheaths. The saphenous and sural veins of the inner leg and foot are high-risk locations and special caution should be taken when injecting these locations. The utilization of non-steroidal anti-inflammatory drugs may shorten the duration of symptoms[65].

Superficial thrombophlebitis may appear 1–3 weeks after injection as a tender erythematous induration over the injected vein. This complication is observed less often if compression is maintained for an adequate period of time following sclerotherapy. When superficial thrombophlebitis occurs, the thrombus should be evacuated and adequate compression, frequent ambulation, and aspirin or a non-steroidal anti-inflammatory drug instituted. The concomitant presence of deep vein thrombosis must be considered[51], and a search for underlying causes

for thrombophlebitis other than the sclerotherapy procedure may be warranted.

AMBULATORY PHLEBECTOMY

Ambulatory phlebectomy is an in-office surgical procedure for the complete removal of diseased venous segments by means of hook avulsion of the targeted vessel, developed in the 1950s by the Swiss dermatologist Robert Mueller[66]. All superficial veins, with the exception of the groin termination of the GSV, may be easily avulsed utilizing this technique. Large veins – in particular, well-demarcated branches of the GSV, SSV or perforators – can be avulsed through microstab incisions[66,67].

Preoperative Considerations

Doppler and duplex ultrasound evaluations are necessary in order to confirm the competence of the saphenofemoral and saphenopopliteal junctions, as well as that of the deep venous system[68]. The varicose veins to be removed are outlined with an indelible pen with the patient in a standing position. Marking of appropriate venous segments is the most important part of this procedure because it allows rapid isolation of desired venous segments to be removed. Because of potential shift of the vein up to 3 to 4 cm when moving from an upright vertical to a transverse horizontal position, the patient is then asked to lie in the operative position and confirmation of venous position by either Doppler or transepidermal illumination (Vein-Lite® or Venoscope®) with separate marking over the veins is performed. This double marking technique has been found to be helpful in determining this positional shift[69,70] (Fig. 155.13).

Anesthesia and Intraoperative Materials for Ambulatory Phlebectomy

Tumescent anesthesia has several advantages when performing ambulatory phlebectomy. These include: rapid anesthesia of an extensive segment of diseased vein; compression of the vein, allowing it to be removed through a 2–3 mm incision; and easier location of the vein owing to the temporary swelling and firmness of the soft tissues pressing the vein against the skin. In addition, tumescent anesthesia reduces blood loss, diminishes bruising, eliminates multiple needle sticks, and produces greater postoperative comfort. Most commonly, a 0.05% concentration of tumescent anesthesia is employed (see Ch. 156)[71,72].

Instrumentation for the ambulatory phlebectomy procedure involves the use of a number of varied hook devices, which come in small, medium and large diameters (sizes 2 to 4) from various manufacturers. The ideal hook should have a comfortable grip to prevent fatigue and a sharp harpoon to catch the adventitia of the vein[66,73] (Fig.155.14).

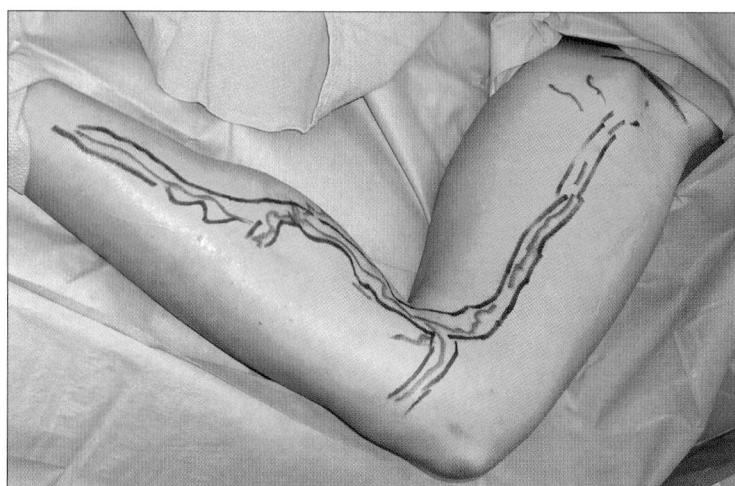

Fig. 155.13 Appearance of the leg after outlining the varicose veins in black ink while the patient is standing and then green ink while the patient is lying down in the operative position with transillumination.

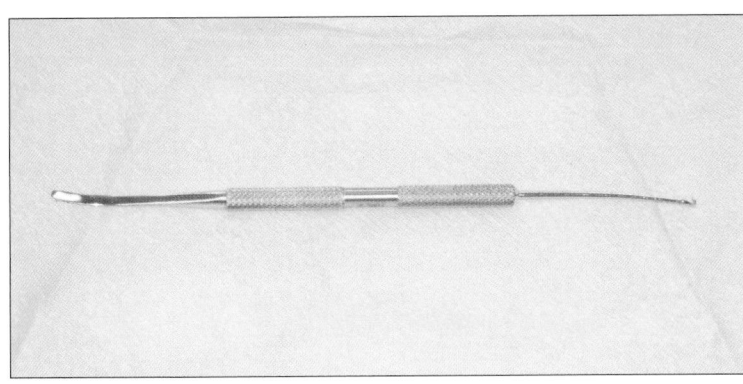

Fig. 155.14 Phlebectomy hook. A classic Mueller type of hook at one end and a Varaday dissector at the other end ('Goldman hook').

intervals along the entire length of the marked vein, until the entire diseased vein has been removed or adequate interruption has been made[74,75].

Special care should be paid to difficult anatomic zones such as the knees, ankles and feet. The 'hooking' should be gentle and slow. Once the vein is hooked, it should come out easily. If it is difficult and if removal of the vein requires a lot of traction, it is possible that a fascial strand structure has been hooked. The hook should be removed, reintroduced, and another attempt should be made. Ambitious 'hooking' in the ankle and foot should be avoided in order to eliminate complications such as swelling, hematomas and nerve damage. Phlebectomy in the pretibial area should also be performed very carefully because many lymphatic vessels are normally located in this area. Aggressive damage to lymphatic vessels can result in a lymphocele. Phlebectomy in the popliteal area should be particularly gentle since the skin of the back of the knee is very soft and microincisions are very easily enlarged by overzealous 'hooking'.

Ambulatory Phlebectomy Technique

Microincisions measuring from 1 to 3 mm in length and parallel to the long axis of the extremity are made with an 18- or 16-gauge hypodermic needle or a no. 11 blade. The microincisions are made vertically and should follow the tension lines. The interval between incisions varies between 3 and 5 cm according to the patient and type of vein being removed. Separation of the vein from the surrounding adventitia may be accomplished utilizing an iris scissor or the spatula component of a phlebectomy hook as developed by Varadey and should follow the tension lines of Langer[70].

The vein is then exteriorized utilizing the phlebectomy hook. The exteriorized vein is then clamped proximally and distally and pushed or pulled, depending on operator preference, from each end until the vein is avulsed (Fig. 155.15). A gentle rotation or rolling motion of the clamp in the same and/or opposite direction pulls and frees the vein from its secondary connective tissue sheath. The process is repeated at 3–5 cm

Postoperative Considerations for Ambulatory Phlebectomy

Postoperatively, the area is cleansed and antibiotic ointment applied to the puncture sites. The leg is then wrapped, first with cotton gauze and then with an elastic compression dressing extending from the dorsum of the foot to the groin. This dressing helps to promote hemostasis in order to reduce swelling of the foot and leg and to speed wound healing. The bandage is removed within 24 hours and then a class II (30–40 mmHg) graduated compression stocking is worn continuously for 1 week and during working hours for a period of 2–4 weeks.

Walking while the patient is still in the office is encouraged, to help mold the pressure wrap and disclose any persistent bleeding. This allows the patient to quickly return to a normal gait, thus generating normal function of the calf muscle pump, minimizing potential thromboembolic complications.

HOOKING AND CLAMPING THE VENOUS SEGMENTS

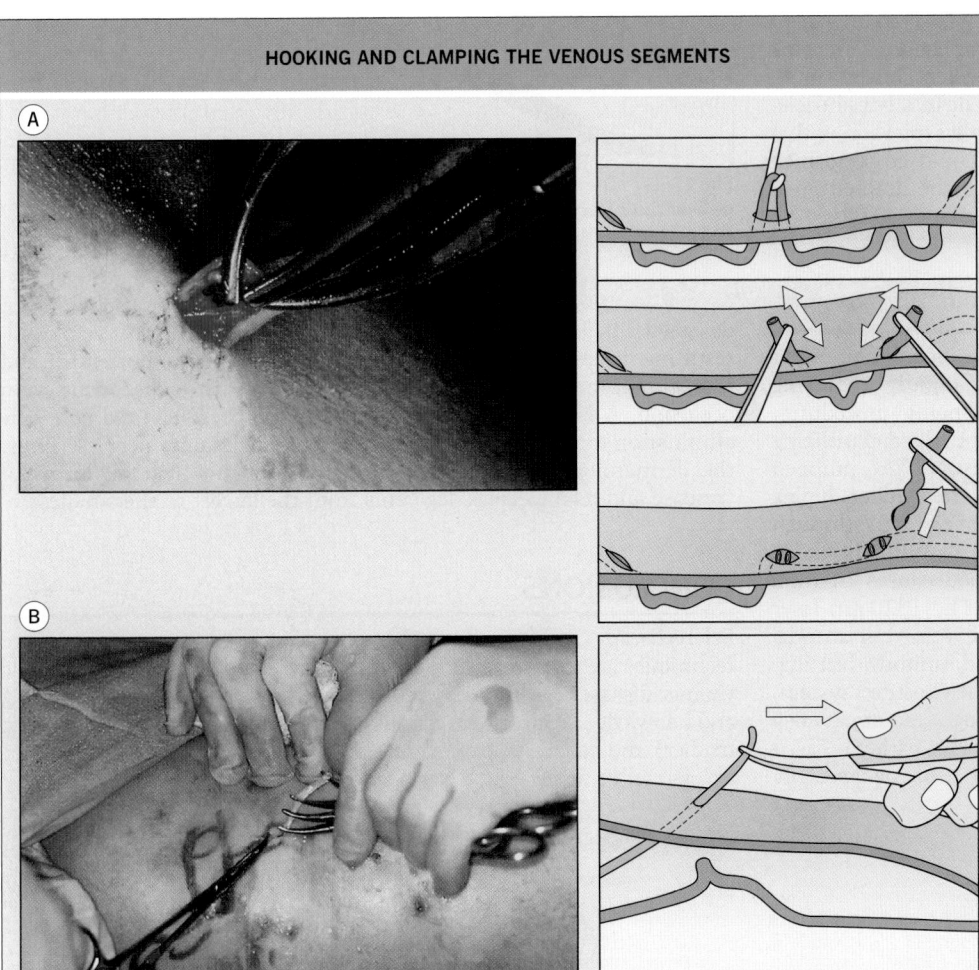

Fig. 155.15 Hooking and clamping venous segments. A After hooking at several sites, the vein is incised and then clamped proximally and distally; it is then pulled and rolled to free it from surrounding connective tissue adventitial attachment. **B** Successive clamping of the hooked vessel with a concomitant pushing or pulling motion allows avulsion of longer venous segments. Redrawn from Ricci S, Georgiev M, Goldman MP: Ambulatory phlebectomy: A practical guide to stab avulsion varicectomy, 2e. London: Taylor & Francis, 2005.

COMPLICATIONS OF AMBULATORY PHLEBECTOMY
Anesthetic complications
Allergic reaction
Vascular complications
Bleeding, seroma Superficial thrombophlebitis Deep venous thrombosis/pulmonary embolus Telangiectatic matting Lymphocele Peristent edema
Neurologic complications
Nerve damage around the ankle Hypesthesia (temporary) Dysesthesia (temporary or permanent) Traumatic neuroma
Cutaneous complications (other than vascular sequelae)
Skin necrosis (blistering, ulceration) related to the procedure or compression bandage Post-operative infection (e.g. cellulitis) Hypo- or hyperpigmentation of the microincision Dimpling Tattooing with marking pen ink Talc granuloma

Table 155.9 Complications of ambulatory phlebectomy.

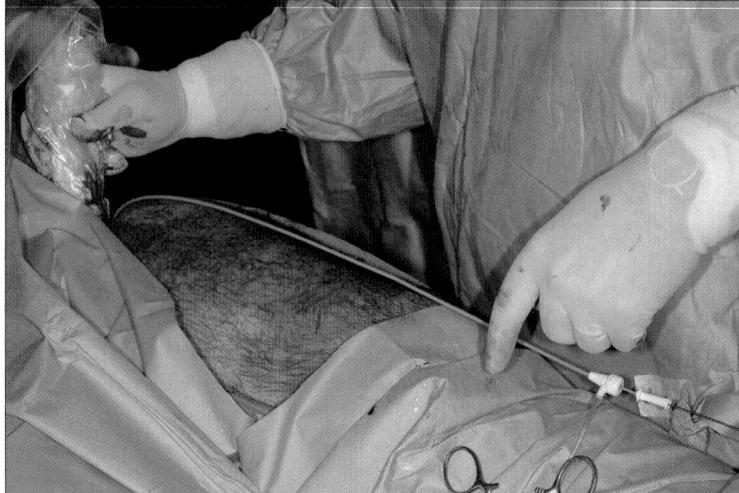

Fig. 155.16 Insertion of the diode laser fiber (815 nm) into the great saphenous vein under duplex guidance.

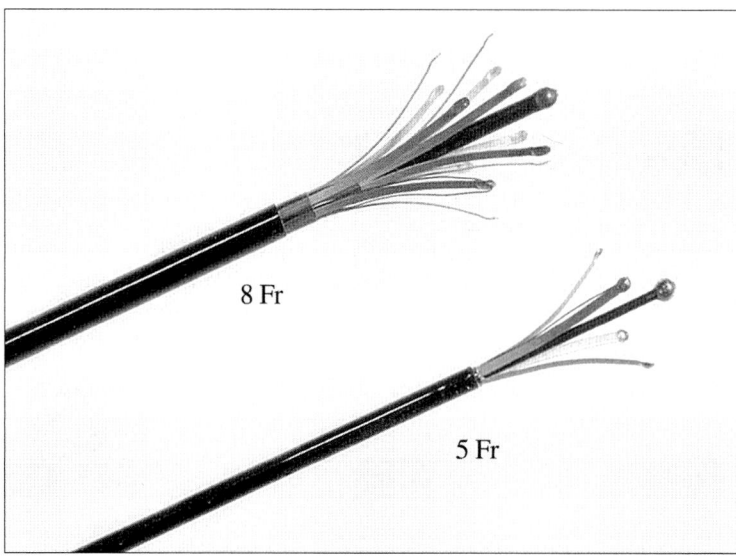

Fig. 155.17 The Closure® system utilizes either the 5-Fr or 8-Fr catheter to deliver radiofrequency energy to the great saphenous vein wall. Courtesy of VNUS Medical Technologies, Sunnyvale, CA, USA.

Complications of Ambulatory Phlebectomy

Ambulatory phlebectomy satisfactorily removes varicosities of different sizes, and results in a series of cosmetic micro-scars that are pleasing to the patient and dermatologic surgeon. The entire procedure can be performed under local anesthesia on an ambulatory basis in all except the most severe and complicated cases[76,77]. Complications may be divided according to the system that has been affected (Table 155.9). The most common complication is the development of a lymphocele. This presents as a firm subcutaneous nodule. Simple aspiration with a 22-gauge needle of yellow–clear lymphatic fluid should be performed every few days, with immediate compression over the drained area. Resolution typically occurs after two to three drainage sessions.

ENDOVASCULAR VEIN CLOSURE

Newly developed endovascular technologies, which incorporate either radiofrequency or laser thermal heating, are rapidly replacing saphenofemoral/saphenopopliteal ligation and stripping procedures. Lasers can be used by placing an optic fiber endoluminally and utilizing various diode lasers (810, 940, 980 nm) or the newest Nd:YAG pumped 1320 nm laser (CTEV®). Typically, the fiber is inserted under duplex guidance into the GSV or through exteriorization of the GSV through a variation of ambulatory phlebectomy (Fig. 155.16). With the diode lasers, the heat energy created by heating of blood causes thermal destruction and contraction of the vein wall[78–82]. The 1320 nm laser operates by targeting water, not blood, so that the vein wall absorbs most of the energy and results in a more controlled, uniform heating. Another system, initially cleared for use in 1999, the Closure® system, occludes veins by utilizing heat generated through radiofrequency energy which is delivered directly to the vein walls. This catheter-based approach delivers radiofrequency energy into the vein via specially designed insulated electrodes (Fig. 155.17) that heat the vein wall, resulting in endothelial denudation, collagen fibril shortening and thickening, and contraction of the vein, with subsequent vein occlusion. A 2-year 90% 'occlusion effect' has been reported, whereby elimination of saphenofemoral incompetence is maintained[83,84]. Thus, the dermatologic surgeon now has the ability to treat all forms of varicose and telangiectatic leg veins from the largest to the smallest.

CONCLUSIONS

Sclerotherapy, ambulatory phlebectomy, and endovenous vein closure techniques are excellent techniques for both cosmetic and symptomatic venous disease[85]. Although they all require some additional training and knowledge of superficial venous anatomy and physiology, remarkable medical and cosmetic improvements in the sensation and appearance of legs can be achieved.

REFERENCES

1. Boisseau MR. Venous valves in the legs: hemodynamic and biological problems and relationship to physiopathology. J Mal Vasc. 1997;22:122–7.
2. Griton P, Vanet P, Cloarec M. Anatomic and functional features of venous valves. J Mal Vasc. 1997;22:97–100.
3. Labropoulos N, Giannoukas AD, Nicolaides AN, et al. The role of venous reflux and calf muscle pump function in nonthrombotic chronic venous insufficiency. Correlation with severity of signs and symptoms. Arch Surg. 1996;131:403–6.
4. Labropoulos N, Delis K, Mansour MA, et al. Prevalence and clinical significance of posterolateral thigh perforator vein incompetence. J Vasc Surg. 1997;26:743–8.
5. Goldman M, Bergan J, Guex J-J. Sclerotherapy. St Louis: Mosby, 2006
6. Butie A. Clinical examination of varicose veins. Dermatol Surg. 1995;21:52–6.
7. Kistner RL, Elkof B, Masuda EM. Diagnosis of chronic venous disease of the lower extremities: the 'CEAP' classification. Mayo Clin Proc. 1996;71:338–45.
8. Furderer CR. Les crosses saphenìennes. anatomie et concepts therapeutiques. Phlebologie. 1986;39:3–14.
9. Weiss RA. Evaluation of the venous system by Doppler ultrasound and photophlethysmography or light reflection rheography before sclerotherapy. Semin Dermatol. 1993;12:78–87.
10. Weiss RA. Vascular studies of the legs for venous or arterial disease. Dermatol Clin. 1994;12:175–90.
11. Weiss RA, Weiss MA. Continuous wave venous Doppler examination for pretreatment diagnosis of varicose and telangiectatic veins. Dermatol Surg. 1995;21:58–62.
12. Thibault PK. Duplex examination. Dermatol Surg. 1995;21:77–82.
13. Veraart JCJM, Neumann, HAM. Interface pressure measurements underneath elastic and non-elastic bandages. Phlebologie. 1996;1(suppl,):56–9.
14. Veraart JCJM, Koster D, Neumann HAM. Compression therapy and the pressure in the deep venous system. Phlebologie. 1996;1(suppl.):68–73.
15. Weiss RA, Sadick NS, Goldman MP, Weiss MA. Post-sclerotherapy compression: controlled comparative study of duration and its effect on clinical outcome. Dermatol Surg.. 1999;25:105–8.
16. Carlin MC, Ratz JL. Treatment of telangiectasia: comparison of sclerosing agents. J Dermatol Surg Oncol. 1987;13:1181–4.
17. Sadick NS. Advances in sclerosing solutions. Cosmet Dermatol. 1996;20:313–16.
18. Sadick NS. Hyperosmolar versus detergent sclerosing agents in sclerotherapy. Effect on distal vessel obliteration. J Dermatol Surg Oncol. 1994;20:313–16.
19. Goldman MP. A comparison of sclerosing agents. Clinical and histologic effects of intravascular sodium morrhuate, ethanolamine oleate, hypertonic saline (11.7%) and sclerodex in the dorsal rabbit ear vein. J Dermatol Surg Oncol. 1991;17:354–62.
20. Sadick NS. Sclerotherapy of varicose and telangiectatic leg veins. Minimal sclerosant concentration of hypertonic saline and its relationship to vessel diameter. J Dermatol Surg Oncol. 1991;20:65–70.
21. Weiss RA, Goldman MP. Advances in sclerotherapy. Dermatol Clin. 1995;13:431–45.
22. Sadick NS. Treatment of varicose and telangiectatic leg veins with hypertonic saline: a comparative study of heparin and saline. J Dermatol Surg Oncol. 1995;16:24–8.
23. Sadick NS, Farber B. A microbiologic study of diluted sclerotherapy solutions. J Dermatol Surg Oncol. 1993;19:450–4.
24. Leach BC, Goldman MP. Comparative trial between sodium tetradecyl sulfate and glycerin in the treatment of telangiectatic leg veins. Dermatol Surg. 2003;29:612–15.
25. Weiss MA, Weiss RA, Goldman MP. Sclerotherapy: how minor varicosities cause leg pain. Contemp Ob Gyn. 1991;36:113–25.
26. Weiss MA, Weiss RA. Sclerotherapy. Curr Opin Dermatol. 1997;4:167–74.
27. Goldman MP, Weiss RA, Bergan JJ. Diagnosis and treatment of varicose veins: a review. J Am Acad Dermatol. 1994;31:393–413.
28. Goldman MP, Bennett RG. Treatment of telangiectasia: a review. J Am Acad Dermatol. 1987;17:167–82.
29. Baccaglini H, Spreafico G, Castro C, Sorrentino P. Consensus conference on sclerotherapy of varicose veins of the lower limbs. Phlebologie. 1997;12:2–16.
30. Guex J-J. Microsclerotherapy. Semin Dermatol. 1993;12:129–34.
31. Duffy DM. Sclerotherapy. Clin Dermatol. 1992; 10:373–80.
32. Bodian EL. Techniques for sclerotherapy for sunburst venous blemishes. J Dermatol Surg Oncol. 1985;11:696–704.
33. Duffy DM. Small vessel sclerotherapy: an overview. Adv Dermatol. 1988;13:221–42.
34. Goldman MP. Advances in sclerotherapy treatment of varicose and telangiectatic leg vein. Am J Cosmet Surg. 1992;9:235–40.
35. Gallagher PL. Varicose veins – primary treatment with sclerotherapy. A personal appraisal. J Dermatol Surg Oncol. 1992;18:39–42.
36. Sadick NS. A dual wavelength approach for laser/intense pulsed light source treatment of lower extremity veins. J Am Acad Dermatol. 2002;46:66–72.
37. Sadick NS. Effective treatment of leg vein telangiectasia with a new 940 nm diode laser (Commentary). Dermatol Surg. 2001;18:141–2.
38. Weiss RA, Sadick NS. Epidermal cooling crystal collar device for improved results and reduced side effects on leg telangiectasias using intense pulsed light. Dermatol Surg. 2000;26:1015–18.
39. Sadick NS, Weiss RA, Goldman MP. Advances in laser surgery for leg veins. Bimodal wavelength approach to lower extremity vessels, new cooling techniques and longer pulse durations. Dermatol Surg. 2002; 28:16–20.
40. Sadick NS, Prieto VG, Shea CR, Nicholson J, McCaffrey T. Clinical and pathophysiologic correlates of 1064-nm Nd:YAG laser treatment of reticular veins and venulectasias. Arch Dermatol. 2001;137:613–17.
41. Sadick NS. Long-term results with a multiple synchronized-pulse 1064 nm Nd:YAG laser treatment of leg venulectasias and reticular veins. Dermatol Surg. 2001;27:365–72.
42. Zummo M, Forrestal M. Sclerotherapy of the long saphenous vein – a prospective Duplex controlled comparative study. Phlebologie. 1995;Suppl. 1:571–3.
43. Baccaglini B, Spreafico G, Costoro C, Sorrentino P. Sclerotherapy of varicose veins of the lower limbs. Consensus paper. Dermatol Surg. 1996;22:883–9.
44. Cornu-Thenard A, de Cottreau H, Weiss RA. Sclerotherapy. Continuous wave Doppler-guided injections. Dermatol Surg. 1995;21:867–70.
45. de Groot WP. Practical phlebology. Sclerotherapy of large veins. J Dermatol Surg Oncol. 1991;17:589–95.
46. Marley WM, Marley NF. Sclerotherapy treatment of varicose veins. Semin Dermatol. 1993;12:98–101.
47. Orbach EJ. Sclerotherapy of varicose veins. Utilization of intravenous air-block technique. Am J Surg. 1944;66:362–6.
48. Barrett JM, Allen B, Ockelford A, Goldman, MD. Microfoam ultrasound guided sclerotherapy of varicose veins in 100 legs. Dermatol Surg. 2004;30:6–12.
49. Raymond-Martimbeau P. Advanced sclerotherapy treatment of varicose veins with duplex ultrasonographic guidance. Semin Dermatol. 1993;12:123–8.
50. Thibault PK, Lewis WA. Recurrent varicose veins. Part 2: Injection of incompetent perforating veins using ultrasound guidance. J Dermatol Surg Oncol. 1992;18:895–900.
51. Leibaschoff G, Brizzio E, Ferreira J, Banf J. Prevention of iatrogenic complications in the treatment of varicosities. Am J Cosmet Surg. 1994;11:51–3.
52. Georgiev M. Postsclerotherapy hyperpigmentations: a one-year follow-up. J Dermatol Surg Oncol. 1990;16:608–10.
53. Georgiev M. Postsclerotherapy hyperpigmentations. Chromated glycerin as a screen for patients at risk (a retrospective study). J Dermatol Surg Oncol. 1993;19:649–52.
54. Thibault P, Wlodarczyk J. Postsclerotherapy hyperpigmentation. The role of serum ferritin levels and the effectiveness of treatment with the copper vapor laser. J Dermatol Surg Oncol. 1992;18:47–52.
55. Goldman MP. Post-sclerotherapy hyperpigmentation: treatment with a flashlamp-excited pulsed dye laser. J Dermatol Surg Oncol. 1992;18:417–22.
56. Goldman MP, Kaplan RP, Duffy DM. Postsclerotherapy hyperpigmentation: a histologic evaluation. J Dermatol Surg Oncol. 1987;13:547–50.
57. Scott C, Seiger E. Postsclerotherapy pigmentation. Is serum ferritin level an accurate indicator? Dermatol Surg. 1997;23:281–3.
58. Tafazzoli A, Rostan E, Goldman MP. Q-switched ruby laser treatment for postsclerotherapy hyperpigmentation. Dermatol Surg. 2000;26:653–6.
59. Goldman MP, Sadick NS, Weiss RA. Cutaneous necrosis, telangiectatic matting, and hyperpigmentation following sclerotherapy. Etiology, prevention and treatment. Dermatol Surg. 1995;21:19–29.
60. Davis LT, Duffy DM. Determination of incidence and risk factors for post-sclerotherapy telangiectatic matting of the lower extremity: a retrospective analysis. J Dermatol Surg Oncol. 1990;16:327–30.
61. Zimmet SE. The prevention of cutaneous necrosis following extravasation of hypertonic saline and sodium tetradecyl sulfate. J Dermatol Surg Oncol. 1993; 19:641–6.
62. Zimmet SE. Hyaluronidase in the prevention of sclerotherapy-induced extravasation necrosis. A dose-response study. Dermatol Surg. 1996;22:73–6.
63. Weiss RA, Weiss MA. Incidence of side effects in the treatment of telangiectasias by compression sclerotherapy: hypertonic saline vs. polidocanol. J Dermatol Surg Oncol. 1990;16:800–4.
64. Biegeleisen K, Neilson RD, O'Shaughnessy A. Inadvertent intra-arterial injection complicating ordinary and ultrasound-guided sclerotherapy. J Dermatol Surg Oncol. 1993;19:953–8.
65. Thibault PK, Wlodarczyk J. Correlation of serum ferritin levels and postsclerotherapy pigmentation. A prospective study. J Dermatol Surg Oncol. 1994 20:684–6.
66. Goldman MP, Geogiev M, Ricci S. Ambulatory Phlebectomy: A Practical Guide for Treating Varicose Veins, 2nd edn. New York: Taylor Francis, 2005.
67. Garde C. Cryosurgery of varicose veins. J Dermatol Surg Oncol. 1994;20:56–8.
68. Georgiev M, Ricci S, Carbone D, Antignani P, Moliterno G. Stab avulsion of the short saphenous vein. Technique and duplex evaluation. J Dermatol Surg Oncol. 1993;19:456–64.
69. Neumann HAM. Ambulatory minisurgical phlebectomy. J Dermatol Surg Oncol. 1992;18:53–4.
70. Weiss RA, Goldman MP. Transillumination mapping prior to ambulatory phlebectomy. Dermatol Surg. 1998;24:447–50.
71. Olivencia JA. Maneuver to facilitate ambulatory phlebectomy. Dermatol Surg. 1996;22:654–5.
72. Smith SR, Goldman MP. Tumescent anesthesia in ambulatory phlebectomy. Dermatol Surg. 1988;24:453–6.
73. Ramelet AA. Muller phlebectomy. A new phlebectomy hook. J Dermatol Surg Oncol. 1991;17:814–16.
74. Sadick NS, Schanzer H. Combined high ligation and stab avulsion for varicose veins in an outpatient setting. Dermatol Surg. 1998;24:475–9.
75. Sadick NS. Multi-focal pull-through endovascular cannulation technique of ambulatory phlebectomy. Dermatol Surg. 2002;28:32–7.
76. Ramelet AA. Complications of ambulatory phlebectomy. Dermatol Surg. 1997;23:947–54.
77. Olivencia JA. Complications of ambulatory phlebectomy. Review of 1000 consecutive cases. Dermatol Surg. 1997;23:51–4.
78. Proebstle TM, Sandhofer MD, Kargl A, et al. Thermal damage of the inner vein wall during endovenous laser treatment: key role of energy absorption by intravascular blood. Dermatol Surg. 2001;28:596–600.
79. Weiss RA. Comparison of endovascular radiofrequency versus 810 nm diode laser occlusion of large veins in an optimal model. Dermatol Surg. 2002;28:56–61.
80. Novarro L, Min RJ, Bone C. Endovenous laser: a new minimally invasive method of treatment for varicose veins: preliminary observations using an 810 nm diode laser. Dermatol Surg. 2001;27:117–22.
81. Goldman MP. Intravascular lasers in the treatment of varicose veins. J Cosmet Dermatol. 2004;3:162–6.
82. Goldman MP, Mauricio M, Rao J. Intravascular 1320nm laser closure of the great saphenous vein: a 6-12 month follow-up study. Dermatol Surg. 2004;30:1380–5.
83. Goldman MP, Amiry S. Closure of the greater saphenous vein with endoluminal radiofrequency thermal heating of the vein wall in combination with ambulatory phlebectomy: 50 patients with more than 6-month follow-up. Dermatol Surg. 2002;28:29–31.
84. Weiss RA, Weiss MA. Controlled radiofrequency endovenous occlusion using a unique radiofrequency catheter under duplex guidance to eliminate saphenous varicose vein reflux: a two-year follow-up. Dermatol Surg. 2002;28:38–42.
85. Alam M, Nguyen T (eds). Treatment of Leg Veins (Procedures in Cosmetic Dermatology). Philadelphia: Saunders, 2006.

Liposuction

William P Coleman III and Timothy Corcoran Flynn

156

Synonyms: ■ Liposculpture ■ Tumescent liposuction ■ Lipoplasty ■ Fat suction

Key features

- Liposuction is indicated for spot reducing areas of localized fat
- Liposuction is ideally suited for healthy patients who are near their ideal body weight
- The tumescent local anesthetic technique is the safest approach to anesthesia for liposuction
- Liposuction consists of avulsion and aspiration of lipocytes through criss-crossing tunnels in the subcutaneous tissue
- Non-cosmetic uses for liposuction include treatment of hyperhidrosis and lipomas as well as breast reduction

INTRODUCTION AND BACKGROUND

Liposuction is an effective method for surgically improving localized areas of excess subcutaneous fat. Modern liposuction is performed using dilute local anesthesia via the tumescent technique, together with small cannulas connected to a vacuum aspirator. Liposuction can be safely performed in an office setting and conservative techniques ensure few complications. Substantial amounts of fat can be aspirated with minimal blood loss and excellent aesthetic results.

The history of modern liposuction traces its roots back to 1975, when Drs Arpad and Giorgio Fischer developed hollow cannulas attached to a suction source which, when placed subcutaneously, were capable of aspirating subcutaneous fat[1]. In Paris, Illouz developed updated equipment for performing liposuction. He also promoted the concept of a 'wet technique' in which saline was injected into the fat before suctioning[2]. Pierre Fournier further refined the techniques of liposuction, teaching many physicians around the world. He also popularized the idea of postoperative compression to help support the suctioned tissue following surgery[3].

American dermatologic surgeons including Lawrence Field, Rhoda Narins, Samuel Stegman and Bruce Chrisman learned the technique early on and advanced the field[4]. Klein developed the tumescent technique in 1985, which allowed liposuction under local anesthesia with minimal blood loss, vastly increasing the safety of the procedure[5–9]. The American Academy of Dermatology and the American Society for Dermatologic Surgery promoted education in liposuction in the Core Surgical Curriculum in Dermatology as early as 1987[10]. Importantly, the American Academy of Dermatology was the first specialty organization to approve and publish guidelines of care for liposuction in 1991 (which have been subsequently updated)[11].

Liposuction is currently among the most common cosmetic procedures performed in the US. A conservative estimate is that there are now from 300 000 to 400 000 procedures performed in the US annually[12].

INDICATIONS AND CONTRAINDICATIONS

Tumescent liposuction is indicated for improving localized adiposities. Certain areas of subcutaneous fat are often not fully responsive to diet and exercise alone[13] and excessive dieting or caloric expenditure as a means of improving body shape can have serious health consequences.

Most liposuction patients complain that the troublesome areas of fat excess 'run in the family'. Furthermore, these areas of excess subcutaneous fat can be resistant to caloric restriction or exercise and tumescent liposuction is a specific solution to correct these localized areas of excess subcutaneous fat. Thus, it is a complement to, not a replacement for, diet and exercise.

Liposuction can be used to treat localized areas of adiposity from the face to the ankles. Common areas improved by liposuction include the abdomen (Fig. 156.1) and inner and outer thighs on women (Fig. 156.2). Other sites include the neck and jowls (Fig. 156.3), male and female breasts, back, flanks (Fig. 156.4), hips (see Fig. 156.2), buttocks, upper arms, knees (Fig. 156.5), calves and ankles. Genetic predisposition determines the location of excess fat storage in each individual.

Non-cosmetic indications for liposuction include aspiration of lipomas[14–17] (Table 156.1). Liposuction is an effective technique for debulking these benign tumors, and, often, large lipomas can be successfully treated, leaving only minimal scars.

Contraindications are few in healthy patients. Individuals seeking liposuction as a surgical weight loss procedure should be discouraged. Liposuction is used to improve the shape of localized areas and is not able to significantly reduce body mass. Patients should be screened carefully for a history of poor wound healing or excessive surgeries in the areas to be improved by liposuction, as well as coagulation or bleeding disorders. Those with evidence of fragility or poor skin elasticity, e.g. Ehlers–Danlos syndrome or cutis laxa, should be identified. Patients must be examined for hernias and hypertrophic or keloidal scarring.

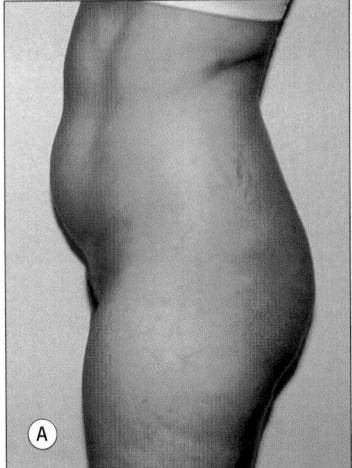 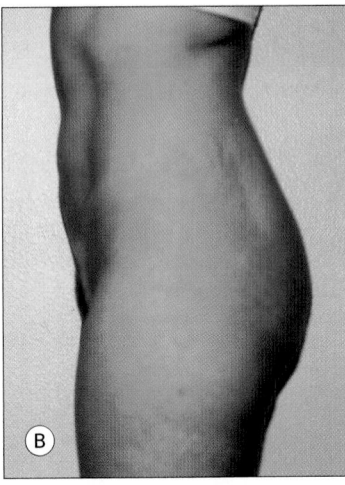

Fig. 156.1 Liposuction of the upper and lower abdomen. A Preoperative. **B** Postoperative, showing improved contours. Courtesy of WP Coleman III MD.

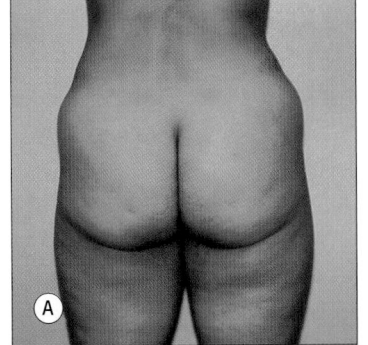 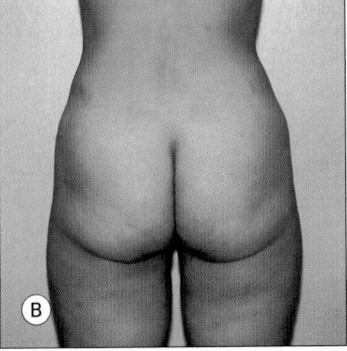

Fig. 156.2 Liposuction of the inner and outer thighs and hips. A Preoperative. **B** Postoperative, showing improved contours. Courtesy of WP Coleman III MD.

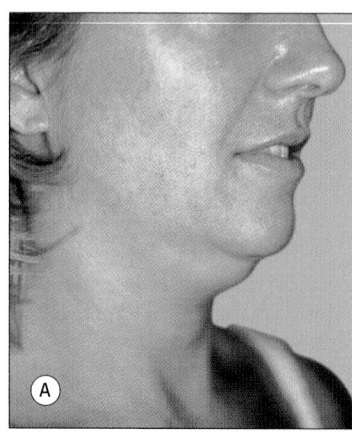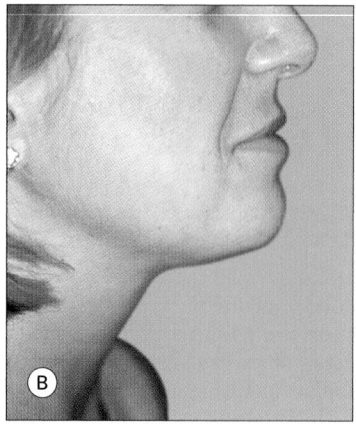

Fig. 156.3 Liposuction of the neck and jowls. A Preoperative. **B** Postoperative, showing improved appearance. Courtesy of WP Coleman III MD.

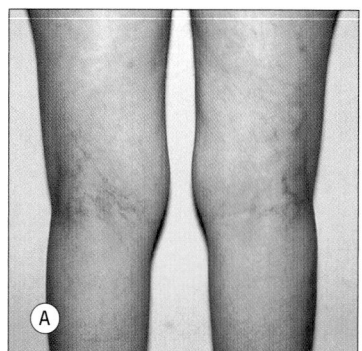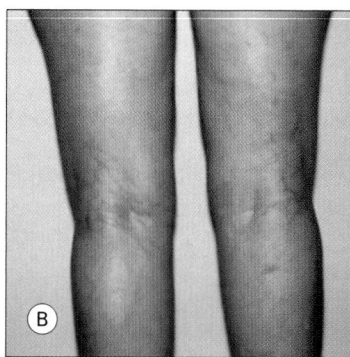

Fig 156.5 Liposuction of the medial knees. A Preoperative. **B** Postoperative, showing more even contours. Courtesy of WP Coleman III MD.

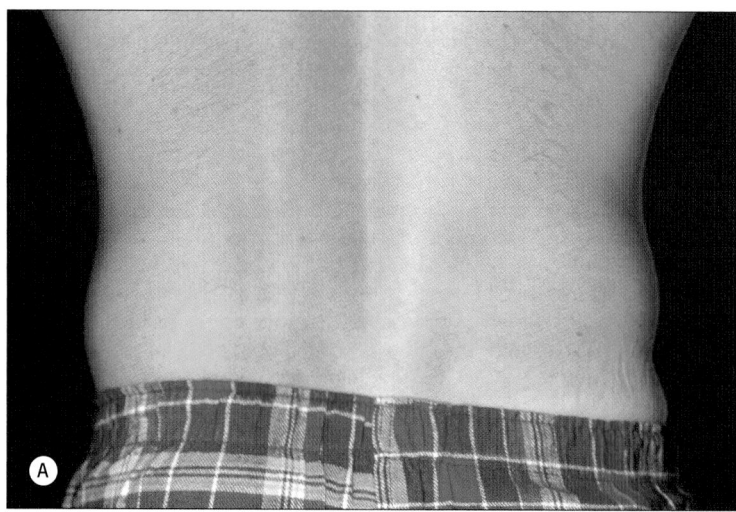

Fig. 156.4 Liposuction of male flanks. A Preoperative. **B** Postoperative, showing the significant improvement. Courtesy of TC Flynn MD.

NON-COSMETIC INDICATIONS FOR LIPOSUCTION
Lipomas
Familial multiple lipomatosis
Adiposis dolorosa (Dercum's disease)
Gynecomastia
Pseudogynecomastia
Insulin-induced lipohypertrophy
HIV/HAART-associated lipodystrophy
Axillary bromhidrosis
Axillary hyperhidrosis (Fig. 156.6)
Undermining flaps
Aspirating hematomas
Lymphedema following axillary lymphadenectomy

Table 156.1 Non-cosmetic indications for liposuction.

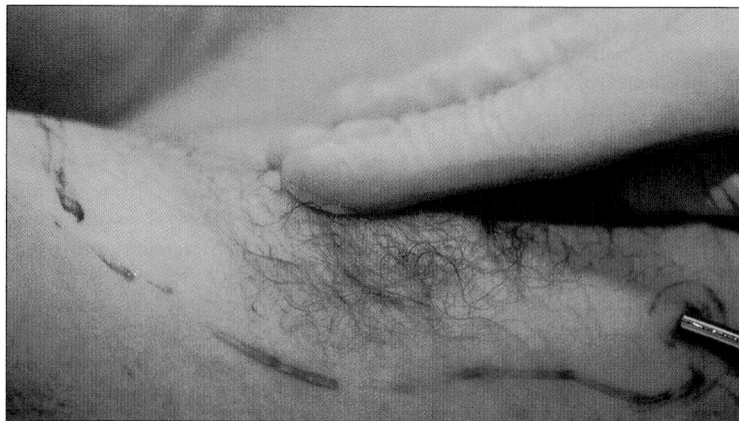

Fig. 156.6 Superficial liposuction of the axilla is performed for improvement of hyperhidrosis. Courtesy of WP Coleman III MD.

Allergy to lidocaine is a relative contraindication for performing tumescent liposuction. Although it is not unusual for patients to give a history of a perceived adverse reaction to epinephrine (adrenaline), liposuction surgeons should be careful when treating individuals who report a previous adverse episode. Patients who are taking pseudoephedrine for upper respiratory tract symptoms, or who may be on herbal supplements which may contain ephedrine-like chemicals, can be predisposed to tachycardias associated with epinephrine. Patients with significant medical problems are usually poor risks for surgery.

PREOPERATIVE HISTORY AND CONSIDERATIONS

Most patients arrive for a liposuction consultation feeling both anxious and conflicted. Many feel guilty that they have not been able to achieve their goals through diet and exercise efforts. Others harbor embarrassment about their bodies. Many are also afraid of surgery and are concerned about pain and convalescence. The liposuction surgeon must keep these issues in mind when meeting with the patient and do everything possible to put him or her at ease.

As with any other medical or surgical consultation, a pertinent review of the past medical history, medications and allergies is essential. The review of systems should be comprehensive enough to exclude any underlying abnormalities which would preclude or modify surgery. Social and psychiatric histories are particularly important since these may reveal details which would make the patient an inappropriate candidate for cosmetic surgery.

The physical examination for liposuction should be performed with patients completely unclothed in the body areas of concern to them. Tight-fitting undergarments can distort fatty bulges and mask contours. The patient should be examined standing up so that the full effects of gravity are apparent. Physical examination consists of both observation and palpation. Grasping the skin and fatty tissues using a 'pinch test' technique will reveal the thickness of areas of adiposity as well as the firmness of underlying fat. The surgeon should look for asymmetries, scars, hernias, musculoskeletal abnormalities, signs of previous liposuction, dimples, skin laxity, and overlying cutaneous lesions. During this examination, it is useful to describe any abnormalities detected to the patient. This will add to the patient's understanding and can show him or her what may or may not be able to be achieved through liposuction. It is important to accurately describe individual body parts in words that the patient will understand, pointing them out to reinforce. Colloquialisms may lead to confusion about which anatomic part is being discussed (Fig. 156.7). Also it is important to remember that the patient has a different vantage point looking down at their areas of adiposity.

The presence of obesity and/or poor muscle tone are two warning signs that the patient may not be an appropriate candidate for liposuction. Many patients arrive at the physician's office with the false idea that liposuction is a substitute for good dietary and exercise habits. In fact, the best candidates are those who have made consistent efforts to control their weight and remain physically active. Some textbooks suggest that patients should be within 10 lb (4.5 kg) of their ideal body weight to be good candidates for liposuction. This is not a hard-and-fast rule since human bodies come in many shapes and sizes. In some situations, it is sensible to perform liposuction on patients who are greater than 10 lb (4.5 kg) over their ideal body weight, in an effort to bring one or two areas of excess fat into harmony with the rest of their bodies. However, in general, the heavier a patient is, the less likely he or she will be happy with the cosmetic results of liposuction. Also, patients who have been unsuccessful in dieting and exercising are unlikely to suddenly change their behavior and maintain their body weight after liposuction. Consequently, they are likely to be disappointed with the results of their procedure. The consultation is an important time to have frank discussions about the limitations of liposuction and the importance of diet and exercise so that patients can develop a realistic attitude about what surgery can accomplish.

A small minority of physicians perform liposuction on obese patients. These large-volume extractions are intrinsically more dangerous, especially when performed on patients who are poor-risk for anesthesia due to their obesity. The notion that atherosclerotic heart disease and diabetes mellitus can be improved with liposuction is still unproven[17].

Some patients are relatively slender except for the abdominal area (Fig. 156.8). Upon physical examination, it is obvious that most of their fat is stored around the viscera. Palpation of the abdominal tissues reveals a firm underlying musculature with very little fat on the pinch test. These patients not only are poor candidates for liposuction but also are at increased risk for cardiovascular disease. This physical finding is most common in men but can be seen in women as well. The surgeon should have a frank discussion with these patients about the implications of the genetic tendency to store fat around the viscera and recommend consultation with an internist and appropriate nutritional experts.

If the physician feels that the patient is an appropriate candidate for liposuction, preliminary discussions may ensue about the suggested areas for surgery. Some patients may have multiple sites of excess localized fat. However, the physician should temper the patient's enthusiasm for extensive surgery when it is inappropriate. In general, operating on over 10% of the body increases liposuction risks. This is analogous to calculating the risks of burns. Guidelines of care published by dermatologic organizations recommend fat extractions of less than 5000 ml[18,19]. This volume should be considered an uppermost

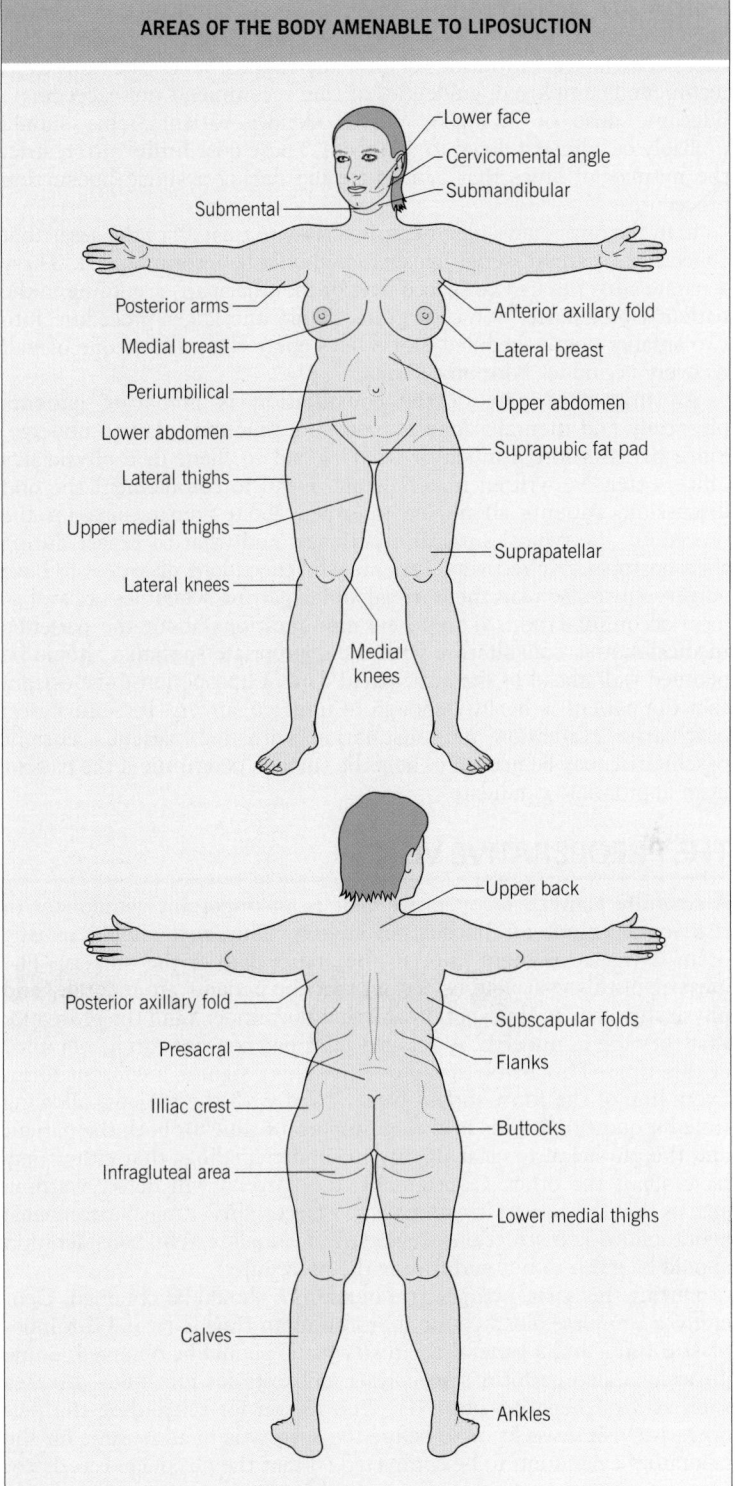

AREAS OF THE BODY AMENABLE TO LIPOSUCTION

Lower face
Cervicomental angle
Submandibular
Submental
Posterior arms
Anterior axillary fold
Medial breast
Lateral breast
Periumbilical
Upper abdomen
Lower abdomen
Suprapubic fat pad
Lateral thighs
Upper medial thighs
Suprapatellar
Lateral knees
Medial knees

Upper back
Posterior axillary fold
Subscapular folds
Presacral
Flanks
Iliac crest
Buttocks
Infragluteal area
Lower medial thighs
Calves
Ankles

Fig 156.7 Areas of the body amenable to liposuction.

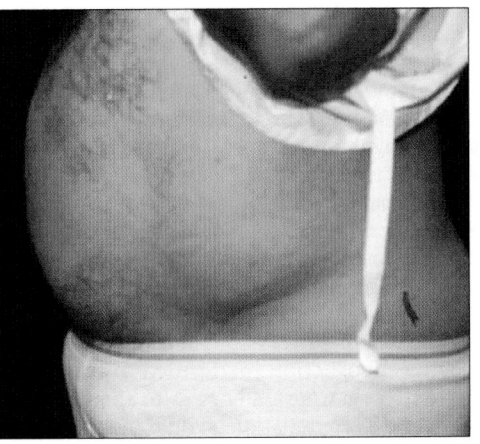

Fig. 156.8 Some patients retain most of their fat intra-abdominally around the viscera. These patients are poor candidates for liposuction and are at increased risk for cardiovascular disease.

limit. Many experienced liposuction surgeons rarely, if ever, remove anywhere near 5000 ml in a single session. Larger extractions also necessitate larger infiltrations of local anesthetics. When the tumescent technique is employed, guidelines of care recommend not exceeding a lidocaine dose of 55 mg/kg[19–21]. In slender patients, this should probably be adjusted down to 45 mg/kg. These dose limits also restrict the number of areas that can be treated during a single liposuction procedure.

If, in the physician's judgment, it is risky to treat all of the areas that concern the patient, serial liposuction should be recommended. These separate surgeries can be spaced days or months apart, according to the patient's preference. Some surgeons divide one larger procedure into two smaller ones scheduled 2 or 3 days apart. This allows one overall recovery period for both procedures.

An important part of the consultation is preparing patients physically and mentally for the procedure that they plan to undergo. Since patients forget much of what is said to them in a physician's office, extensive written materials are useful to complement the oral discussion. Patients should be informed about preparations for the procedure, the typical surgical experience, and what to expect during their postoperative recovery. Patients who travel long distances to have surgery must also plan their arrival and departure schedules, as well as local accommodation. If there are any questions about the patient's medical status, consultation with the appropriate specialist should be planned well ahead of the anticipated date of liposuction to be certain that the patient is healthy enough to undergo surgery. In some cases, psychiatric evaluation or consultation with the patient's current psychiatrist may be needed to help the surgeon determine if the patient is an appropriate candidate.

THE PREOPERATIVE VISIT

A carefully planned preoperative visit is an important component of risk management for liposuction surgery. This visit should usually occur 2 weeks or more prior to the actual date of the surgery. The purpose of this visit is to be certain that the patients are mentally and physically ready for liposuction and that they understand the procedure that they are to undergo. A detailed informed consent can be obtained at this time. This involves more than simply signing a consent form. Every line of the form should be reviewed with the patient, allowing time for questions. This is also an important time for both the patient and the physician to clear up any misunderstandings that either may have about the other. Occasionally, the surgeon will detect warning signals that the patient has unrealistic expectations or may be unreliable about following instructions. In these individuals, careful consideration should be given to not performing the procedure.

During this visit, preoperative bloodwork should be obtained. Generally, a complete blood count, a prothrombin time, a partial thromboplastin time, and a general chemistry panel should be obtained. Some physicians also perform a urinalysis and tests for infectious diseases such as viral hepatitis and HIV. One reason for scheduling the preoperative visit 2 weeks or so before the surgery is to allow time for the laboratory evaluation to be completed so that the physician can detect any abnormalities. Also, occasionally laboratory tests are incorrectly performed and must be repeated.

Detailed pre- and postoperative instructions should be provided to the patient during this visit. Preoperative instructions should include a list of over-the-counter medications that should be avoided. Aspirin, non-steroidal anti-inflammatory drugs (e.g. ibuprofen), vitamin E and alcohol are common anticoagulants that patients should carefully avoid preoperatively. Herbal remedies are also becoming more popular and many of these may have anticoagulant activity (see Table 133.3). It is wise to discontinue all herbal remedies for 2 weeks preoperatively to be certain. Drugs that affect the hepatic cytochrome P-450 system should be discontinued if possible (see later). Patients should also be counseled about proper nutrition. Trying to lose weight rapidly or eating excessively should both be discouraged. Many patients benefit from nutritional counseling on a pre- and postoperative basis.

Patient preparations for the day of surgery should also be reviewed. Individuals who are having liposuction performed under local anesthesia with mild sedation can eat normally prior to their surgery. Those undergoing moderate or deep sedation should not eat after

midnight. Clothing should be loose so that it can fit over postoperative elastic garments. Also, minor fluid leakage or bleeding is possible and may stain clothing, car seats, or bedding following the surgery. Patients should have firm plans for a reliable driver who can take them home after they have fully recovered from anesthesia and are released from care. Patients should stay with an attentive adult for the first postoperative night to be sure that they are doing well and that all their needs are met.

DESCRIPTION OF TECHNIQUES

Tumescent Anesthesia

The technique of using tumescent local anesthesia for liposuction was developed by the dermatologist Dr Jeffrey Klein. In 1987, Klein detailed the infiltration of a dilute solution of lidocaine with epinephrine into fat[5]. The technique allowed for liposuction to be performed totally by local anesthesia as well as for significantly reduced bleeding. The previous common complications of seroma formation and hematomas became uncommon[7]. Bruising was also minimized. The procedure has been proven to be remarkably safe.

Klein demonstrated that dilute concentrations of lidocaine with epinephrine are not absorbed to the same degree as commercially available solutions of lidocaine, even when the total dose is equal. He confirmed that tumescent liposuction performed using only dilute solutions of lidocaine with epinephrine safely allowed dosages of up to 35 mg of lidocaine per kilogram of body weight[6]. This advance allowed larger amounts of fat to be removed with only local anesthesia.

A typical tumescent anesthetic formulation is shown in Table 156.2. Dilute solutions of lidocaine with epinephrine provide safe local anesthesia with excellent vasoconstriction. Sodium bicarbonate is added to adjust the solution to a more physiologic pH closer to the pKa of lidocaine[9]. The combination of dilute solutions of lidocaine with the vasoconstrictive effects of epinephrine ensures minimal systemic absorption of lidocaine[22].

The tumescent technique provides a number of advantages (Table 156.3). There is complete regional anesthesia without the need for nerve blocks. Local anesthesia persists for up to 24 hours after tumescent liposuction, reducing the needs for postoperative analgesia[9]. There is minimal blood loss and the extensive vasoconstriction produced by the dilute epinephrine reduces the volume of whole blood for each liter of pure fat removed by liposuction to less than 12 ml[7,9]. Because there is little blood loss, there is minimal postoperative bruising. Patients can thus return to their normal lives quickly, with a rapid postoperative recovery. Improved aesthetic results are also seen with tumescent liposuction because smaller cannulas can be used, reducing irregularities of the skin[23].

FORMULA FOR TUMESCENT LIPOSUCTION (LIDOCAINE 0.05%, EPINEPHRINE 1:1 000 000)
50 ml 1% plain lidocaine (500 mg)
1 ml 1:1000 epinephrine from ampule (1 mg)
10 ml sodium bicarbonate (of an 8.4% NaHCO₃ solution)
1 liter normal saline (0.9% NaCl solution)

Table 156.2 Formula for tumescent liposuction (lidocaine 0.05%, epinephrine 1:1 000 000).

ADVANTAGES OF TUMESCENT LIPOSUCTION
Complete regional anesthesia without the need for nerve blocks
Local anesthesia persists for up to 24 hours, reducing the need for postoperative analgesia
Minimizes blood loss
Minimal postoperative bruising
Rapid postoperative recovery
Smaller cannulas can be used, reducing irregularities of the skin
Decreased anesthetic risk compared to intravenous or general anesthesia

Table 156.3 Advantages of tumescent liposuction.

An important advantage is the decreased anesthetic risk with tumescent anesthesia for liposuction, compared to intravenous or general anesthesia[12,24–26]. Systemic anesthesia is associated with a significant risk of serious complications[27] and converting liposuction to a local anesthesia procedure increases safety. More recent research has indicated that the maximum safe dosage of lidocaine, when used with the tumescent technique for liposuction, is 55 mg/kg[20,21]. Klein recommends an upper limit of 45 mg/kg for thinner individuals[23].

Fresh tumescent anesthetic solution must be correctly and carefully prepared prior to each procedure by a trained healthcare professional. Personnel must be familiar with the importance of careful records and drug preparation. All individuals who prepare tumescent anesthesia must be familiar with sterile technique. Normal saline should be used as the vehicle for the dilute solutions of lidocaine with epinephrine. Standardization is important in preparing tumescent anesthesia, i.e. by using the same commercial solutions of lidocaine as well as individual 1 ml ampules of 1:1000 epinephrine. This minimizes confusion and limits risk.

The concentrations of lidocaine and epinephrine can be varied depending on the anatomic site. The standard formula of 0.05% lidocaine with 1:1 000 000 epinephrine plus sodium bicarbonate works well for most areas of the body (see Table 156.2). Occasionally, individual 'hot spots' such as the periumbilical area or breast require increased concentrations of lidocaine within the tumescent anesthetic solution.

Proper infiltration of tumescent anesthesia is important. The skin is initially cleansed with an antimicrobial scrub to reduce bacterial contamination. Insertion sites for the infiltration needles are anesthetized with small wheals of 1% lidocaine with epinephrine. While waiting for the intradermal anesthetic to provide cutaneous anesthesia, the prepared tumescent anesthetic bags are suspended from an intravenous pole. Commercially available infiltration tubing is connected to the bag containing the tumescent anesthesia, and the tubing is correctly connected to a peristaltic pump. Air is removed from the infiltration tubing and a blunt-tipped infiltrating cannula or spinal needle is connected to the tubing.

The anesthesia may initially be infiltrated into the subcutaneous fat using 20-gauge spinal needles. More extensive infiltration is then performed using a blunt-tipped side-port 16–18-gauge infiltrating cannula (Fig. 156.9). These small-diameter infiltration cannulas can be passed through slit incisions created in the skin with a no. 15 blade. The peristaltic pump (Fig. 156.10) facilitates infiltration of the anesthetic fluid into subcutaneous fat. The cannula must be repositioned from site to site to ensure an even distribution of the tumescent anesthetic. Moving the needle while infiltrating is associated with increased pain, and consequently, a gentle, slow infiltration technique is preferred. In certain areas where the adipose tissue is more sensitive, infiltration must be done more slowly than in others. Sensitive areas include the inner thighs, breasts, upper abdomen, and periumbilical area.

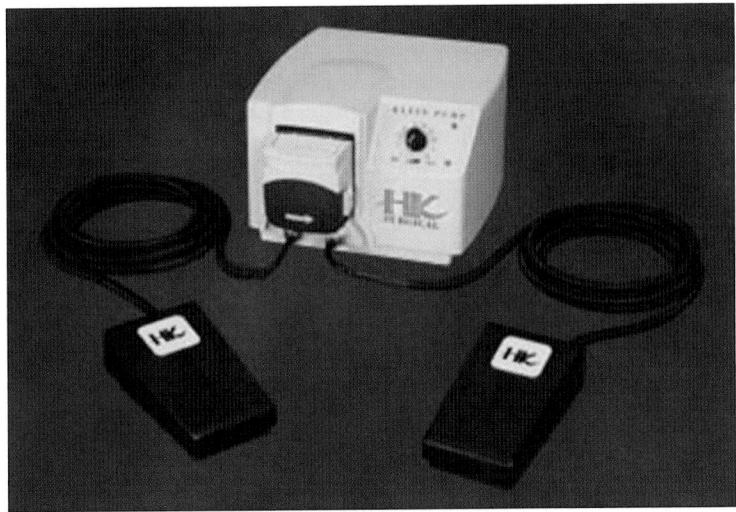

Fig 156.10 Peristaltic pump for infiltration of tumescent anesthetic mixtures. Courtesy of HK Surgical, San Clemente, CA.

Once sufficient tumescent anesthesia has been infiltrated, at least 15 minutes should pass to allow for maximal vasoconstrictive effect of the epinephrine before beginning surgery. An overlying blanching of the skin which is cool to the touch will gradually be noted. The patient is then 'tumesced' and ready for aspiration of adipose tissue.

Drug interactions must be considered when using any form of anesthesia[28]. Caution must be exercised with patients on β-blockers. Although rapid absorption of epinephrine may result in hypertension and bradycardia in these patients, when the epinephrine is absorbed slowly, as in the case of tumescent anesthesia, there is minimal risk[23]. In other words, while tumescent liposuction performed in the setting of β-blockade has not revealed any evidence of hypertension, one must still be cautious in these patients[23]. Patients on propranolol may also experience chest pain following subcutaneous injection of concentrated epinephrine.

Tumescent anesthesia and certain sedatives may have significant interactions[28]. Some sedatives (such as diazepam and flurazepam) can reduce the rate of lidocaine metabolism after liposuction. Because lidocaine is rapidly eliminated by hepatic metabolism and a number of drugs can inhibit lidocaine metabolism, a long list of medications is associated with an increase in lidocaine toxicity[23]. Examples of such drugs are provided in Table 156.4. These medications should be avoided or discontinued prior to liposuction or the total dose of lidocaine should be reduced.

Bupivacaine should not be substituted for lidocaine and is contraindicated for tumescent liposuction[29]. Bupivacaine cardiac toxicity can be subtle and is not preceded by convulsions. Lidocaine usually gives

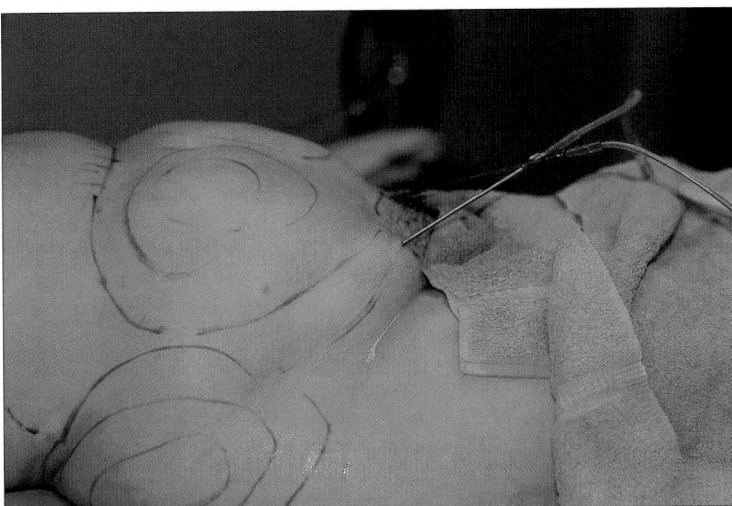

Fig. 156.9 Infiltration of tumescent anesthetic into the previously marked patient. Concentric circles denote areas of increased fat. Sterile towels are positioned to absorb leaking fluids. Courtesy of WP Coleman III MD.

EXAMPLES OF DRUG INTERACTIONS WITH LIDOCAINE	
Drug	**Comments**
Anesthetics • Bupivacaine • Halothane plus nitrous oxide	Lidocaine is displaced from plasma binding proteins by bupivacaine Increase in lidocaine plasma concentration (lowers maximum safe dose)
Amiodarone	Sinus bradycardia, seizures; competes with lidocaine for binding to CYP3A4
Beta-blockers	Decrease in systemic clearance (including hepatic); propranolol and lidocaine both metabolized by CYP2D isoenzymes
Cocaine	Increased risk of seizures and death
Phenytoin	Additive cardiac depressant effects

Table 156.4 Examples of drug interactions with lidocaine. Adapted from Klein JA. Lidocaine Toxicity and Drug Interactions. In: Tumescent Technique. Tumescent Anesthesia and Microannular Liposuction. St. Louis: Mosby, 2000.

warning signs of CNS toxicity long before the onset of dangerous cardiotoxic effects. Furthermore, the cardiotoxicity of bupivacaine is often unresponsive to resuscitation efforts. Prilocaine has been used in Europe for tumescent anesthesia instead of lidocaine[30]. However, rigorous comparative studies have not been performed, and, in the US, prilocaine does not have Food and Drug Administration (FDA) approval to be marketed for local anesthesia for dermatologic surgical procedures. Prilocaine can also produce methemoglobinemia[30]. Ropivacaine is a new long-acting amide local anesthetic that resembles bupivacaine[31,32]. Insufficient data are available at this time to compare dilute tumescent solutions of ropivacaine and dilute solutions of lidocaine in terms of safety and efficacy.

Surgical Technique

Patients are instructed to arrive at the appointed time for surgery freshly bathed and wearing loose clothing. Most patients who are undergoing tumescent liposuction will appreciate pre-sedation with mild oral sedatives such as lorazepam. Consequently, they will need a driver. The staff should coordinate with the driver as to when to return to pick up the patient and to be certain that they will stay with the patient the remainder of the day and night. The mobile phone number for the driver as well as the phone number of the location at which the patient will spend the night should be verified. The driver, who is usually a friend, spouse or parent, should also be instructed in what to expect during the postoperative period and be provided written information on expected care. This attendant should also have phone numbers for reaching the physician and staff for questions or possible emergencies.

The patient is then taken to the preparative area, where he or she changes into a surgical gown. Vital signs are taken, including blood pressure and heart rate. Photographs should then be taken if they have not been done preoperatively. These should include multiple views of the sites of surgery with the areas completely unclothed so as not to distort the areas of adiposity.

Next, the surgeon marks the patient, who is standing to allow for the effects of gravity. Marking can be done according to the custom of the surgeon, but should be devised so that the subsequent distortion by local anesthetic infiltration will not obscure the various thicknesses of the adiposity. One way to mark is to use concentric circles, as in a topographic map (see Fig. 156.9). Pluses or minuses can be drawn on the patient to indicate areas where more or less fat should be removed. Existing dimples and dents should also be outlined for later identification during surgery so that they can be avoided.

The previously marked patient is then placed on the surgical table. If significant sedation is to be employed, intravenous lines and monitoring devices such as pulse oximeters and cardiac monitors can be utilized. Most patients undergoing the tumescent technique, however, require very little ancillary sedation. Those who are still anxious can receive minor additional sedation such as 25 mg of meperidine intramuscularly, a dose which does not impair the protective reflexes.

Once the patient is relaxed, tumescent infiltration can begin (see Fig. 156.9). Slow infiltration is much less painful than rapid infiltration. Physicians who use rapid infiltration techniques typically employ more aggressive forms of systemic anesthesia. Rapid infiltration has increased potential for abdominal perforation. This is compounded by the fact that deeply sedated patients are not awake enough to complain of discomfort associated with muscular penetration. Another disadvantage of moderate and deep sedation is that because of concerns about total anesthesia time, there is usually little or no delay between infiltration of the tumescent fluid and the beginning of the procedure. Significant vasoconstriction from the infiltration of the tumescent fluid does not occur for at least 10 minutes after infiltration. Consequently, it is better to wait for this period of time before beginning suctioning.

INSTRUMENTATION

The basic instruments required for liposuction are suction cannulas, tubing and an aspirator[33]. These are available in various designs (Fig. 156.11). Each surgeon must make individual decisions about instrumentation based on personal style and experience. However, liposuction can be performed using many different types of cannulas

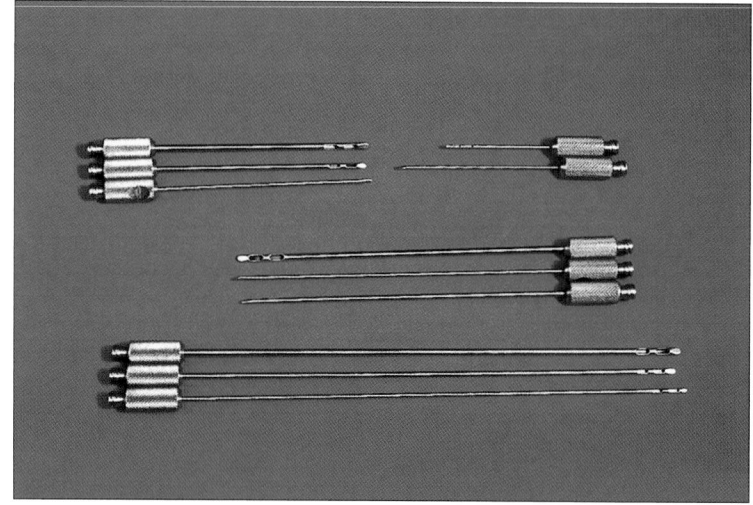

Fig. 156.11 A variety of small-diameter liposuction cannulas. Courtesy of WP Coleman III MD.

and aspirators. The number of holes arranged along the shaft of the cannula is probably unimportant, although two or more holes increase the flow of fat through the instrument. The most important parameter for choosing cannulas is size: the smallest possible cannula should be employed. Smaller-diameter cannulas (3 mm or less) create smaller tunnels through the fat and achieve smoother results. Also smaller-diameter cannulas penetrate the fat more easily and create less tissue trauma. Longer cannulas allow the surgeon to work from fewer skin insertion sites, leaving fewer scars. However, depending on the shape and location of the adiposity, better access often requires multiple incision sites. Shorter cannulas are easier to control as they pass through subcutaneous tissue. The tiny incisions required for insertion of 3 mm cannulas leave nearly invisible scars in most patients, but can be an issue if the patient has a tendency toward keloids or hyperpigmentation.

Ultrasound was introduced into liposuction instruments in the 1990s, but has largely been abandoned by most dermatologic surgeons. External ultrasound involves preoperative use of an ultrasonic probe over the areas to be suctioned, in an attempt to liquefy or loosen the fat. Double-blind studies have found no benefit to this approach[34]. Internal ultrasonic liposuction employs a probe or cannula with an ultrasonic vibration at the tip. These instruments have been shown to liquefy fat prior to suction. Although this makes subsequent liposuction easier, studies have shown increased potential for seromas and burns[35]. Ultrasonic probes also pass through the tissue like a 'hot knife through butter' and do not provide the usual tactile feedback from tissue resistance that manual cannulas do. This makes it difficult for the surgeon to determine in exactly what level of the fat the cannula is located and increases the possibility of intra-abdominal perforation or end hits to the opposing dermis.

The most recent innovation in liposuction technology is powered liposuction. These instruments feature a motorized cannula which moves in a 'to-and-fro' motion, from 800 to 10 000 repetitions per minute (Fig. 156.12). The short motorized strokes vary from 2 to 12 mm, according to the instrument, and allow the surgeon to precisely sculpt small areas of excess fat (Fig. 156.13). Powered liposuction instruments also allow easier penetration of fat, when compared to manual cannulas, but retain the feel of tissue resistance[36]. The key to properly using this technology is to move the cannula slowly and allow the motorized motion to work efficiently. Studies have shown that powered liposuction increases the fat aspirated (per minute) by 30% or more[37]. There have been no significant complications reported when using this approach, although some early users indicated increased problems with seromas. This was probably due to the incidental radial movement of these instruments which enlarges the subcutaneous tissue tunnel. Thus a 4 mm cannula might have the effect of a 5 or 6 mm cannula in the tissue. Therefore, 2 or 3 mm powered liposuction cannulas are preferable and should avoid problems with seromas.

Liposuction is based on the technique of criss-crossing tunnels (from multiple insertion sites) through the subcutaneous tissue. Each area to

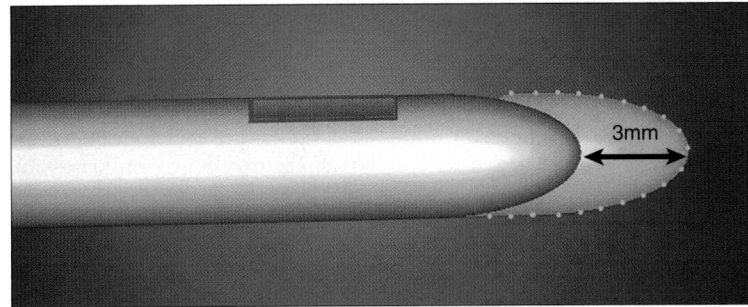

Fig. 156.12 Reciprocating powered cannula. This reciprocating powered cannula has a 3 mm to-and-fro motion. From Coleman WP III, Katz B, Bruck M, et al. The efficacy of powered liposuction. Dermatol Surg. 2001;27:735–8.

POWERED LIPOSUCTION

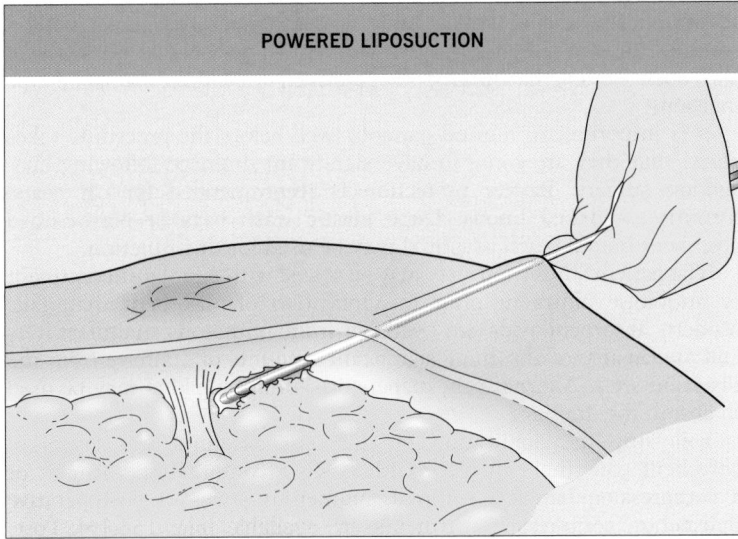

Fig. 156.13 Powered liposuction. Using powered liposuction to more precisely sculpt small areas of fat around the umbilicus.

CONTRACTION OF THE FATTY LAYER

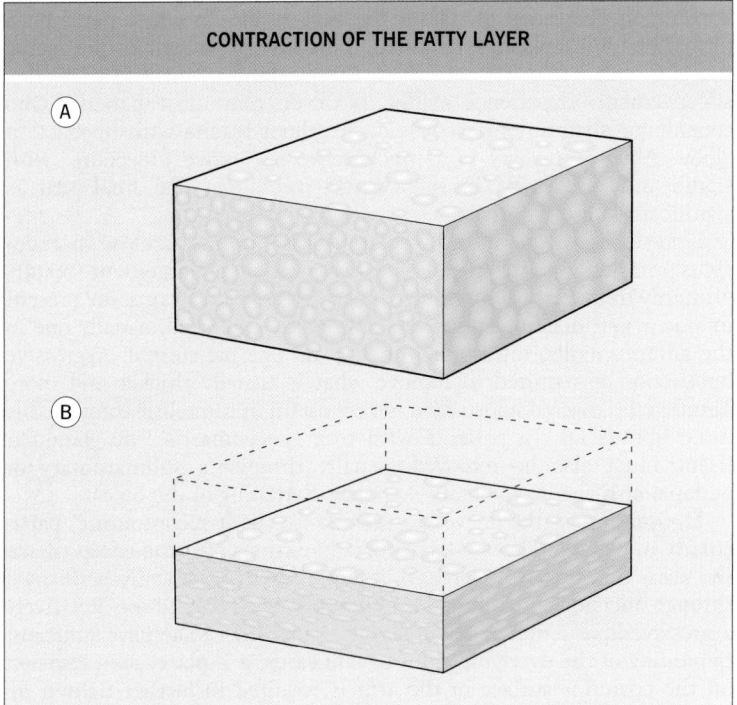

Fig. 156.14 Contraction of the fatty layer. A Immediately after liposuction, the fatty layer resembles a wet sponge. With subsequent subtraction of the fat cells, the thickness of the subcutaneous tissue decreases. **B** Much like a dry sponge, the subcutaneous tissue has compacted.

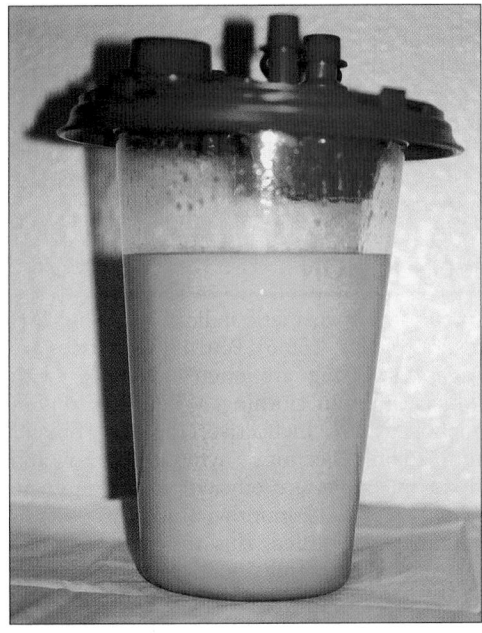

Fig. 156.15 Bloodless liposuction aspirate. Typical, nearly bloodless liposuction aspirate using the tumescent technique. Courtesy of WP Coleman III MD.

be suctioned should be tunneled from at least two different directions, but often three or four are more effective. For instance, in the lower abdomen, suctioning can be performed from pubic, flank and periumbilical incisions. Multiple small tunnels ultimately provide the smoothest contraction of the overlying skin and the most thorough removal of fat. Subsequent contraction of the fatty layer occurs much like a wet sponge becoming dry (Fig. 156.14).

The liposuction aspirate should be yellow or slightly blood tinged (Fig. 156.15). A red aspirate in the suction tubing indicates excessive bleeding and the surgeon should immediately move on to a different tunnel. The surgeon's dominant hand acts as the piston moving the instrument in and out of the tissue, while the non-dominant hand pulls, presses and squeezes the skin to facilitate penetration of the cannula and provides important tactile information about the thickness of the underlying fat. The final surgical endpoint should be a skin thickness in the suctioned areas which is similar to that of the surrounding non-treated skin.

Surgeons may safely aspirate several thousand milliliters of fat during one operative session. The guidelines of care published by the American Academy of Dermatology recommend a maximum fat removal of 4500 ml[19]. However, it is in fact very unusual to extract 4500 ml of fat in a patient who is healthy and near their ideal body weight. Larger fat extractions imply an obese patient. In these cases, consideration should be given to proper dieting and exercise before the procedure. In larger patients, serial liposuction may be performed at different times to avoid exceeding the recommended volume extraction.

VARIATIONS/UNUSUAL SITUATIONS

Guidelines of care published by dermatologic organizations recommend that liposuction be performed as a solo procedure and not combined with other techniques[18,19]. However, there are cases in which liposuction is employed as a fundamental part of a combined surgical

technique. For instance, in facelifting, liposuction of the neck and pre-tunneling of the cheeks are often performed prior to flap dissection and advancement. In patients in whom the neck alone is to be treated, liposuction may be combined with submental resection and platysmal plication with each surgical component contributing to the final result. Cook[38] has also described a technique of laser desiccation of fat over the platysma and subdermally as an added component to improve neck contouring.

In other anatomic sites, skin excision may be combined with liposuction. Where there is a significant abdominal panniculus, a pubic incision may be used to remove excess skin in conjunction with liposuction of the rest of the abdomen. In most patients, however, even with a large panniculus, this is unnecessary because of the significant skin retraction that occurs after liposuction of the lower abdomen. Some surgeons prefer to perform liposuction first and wait at least a year to see whether or not additional excisional surgery or further liposuction is needed to obtain the best result. In some patients, a formal abdominoplasty is required. This involves repair of the rectus muscles and often relocation of the umbilicus with inferior flap advancement. Experience shows, however, that most patients who consult for abdominoplasty achieve excellent results with liposuction alone. Abdominoplasty is a much more aggressive procedure, with significantly increased morbidity and mortality. The final scar is significant and often unattractive as well.

Liposuction is an excellent option for improvement of pseudogynecomastia. In these patients, the breast enlargement results primarily from excess fat rather than the excess glandular tissue present in true gynecomastia. Multiple insertion sites are used, usually one in the anterior axilla, one submammary and one pre-sternal. Aggressive liposuction is required to remove what is usually thicker and more fibrotic fat. Powered liposuction is very useful in tunneling through this more fibrous fat. In patients with true gynecomastia, the glandular tissue must also be removed, usually through a submammary or periareolar incision, to obtain sufficient flattening of the breast.

Liposuction of the arms can provide excellent recontouring, particularly in women. Excessive fatty accumulations over the triceps make the arms unattractively large. Liposuction here is typically performed through incisions in the axilla and superior to the elbow. Relatively aggressive liposuction is usually indicated in order to achieve sufficient tightening of the overlying skin. In rare cases, a Z-plasty skin excision on the posterior surface of the arm is required to further tighten up loose skin.

Recently, thigh-lifting procedures have been reintroduced. These were popular in the 1960s and 1970s before the introduction of liposuction. Large incisions are usually required over the buttocks or inner thighs to lift the thighs. Unfortunately, in many instances, the scars eventually stretch significantly, creating a new deformity. In the inner thigh area, labial ptosis may be produced in some women. Artful liposuction in these areas usually provides excellent results without the need for lifting. Patients with 'cellulite' or a 'cottage cheese' appearance to the skin usually also benefit from targeted muscle training to fill and smooth the overlying skin which has become stretched and distorted from lack of exercise and cycles of weight loss and gain. Currently, there are no creams or surgical procedures which can change cellulite in any significant way.

NON-COSMETIC LIPOSUCTION

Liposuction may also be used for non-cosmetic indications. The chief among these is hyperhidrosis[14] (see Fig. 156.6). Patients with excessive eccrine and apocrine axillary sweating are often miserable, with constantly wet armpits which can ruin clothing. When prescription antiperspirants and iontophoresis are ineffective, the three major options include botulinum toxin injections, sympathectomy and liposuction. Botulinum toxin injections are efficient and require no recovery, but must be repeated every 6–12 months. Since 100 units or more of botulinum A are typically required, this treatment is quite expensive and beyond the reach of many individuals. Sympathectomy is also expensive and has increased morbidity. Liposuction of the axilla is a permanent option preferred by many patients and physicians. For axillary hyperhidrosis, subdermal liposuction is used aggressively to remove as much of the subdermal fat in the axilla as possible. Since many of the eccrine and apocrine sweat glands reside in the upper fat, sweating is diminished postoperatively. The goal is to make the patient a normal sweater, not anhidrotic. A starch iodine test identifies the areas of greatest sweating (see Ch. 40). The axilla is most efficiently approached from inferior and superior insertion sites. The liposuction should be aggressive enough to create some subdermal fibrosis, in an attempt to also eliminate as many dermal eccrine and apocrine structures as possible. Patients are usually comfortable within 24 hours and able to resume normal activities within 2–3 days. Often there is immediate diminished sweating with a rebound 2–3 weeks postoperatively. The final results are often not seen for 6–9 months as fibrosis develops in the subdermal region.

Larger lipomas can also be removed efficiently using liposuction. The goal here is to flatten out the lipoma but not necessarily remove the entire lesion. A portion of it should be submitted for pathologic examination. The advantage of liposuction over standard excisional surgery is that a much smaller scar results. As with any adiposity, the lipoma is tunneled in a criss-cross direction until flat. Subsequent healing and fibrosis usually flattens the remaining lipoma further, resulting in a normal contour. It is difficult to suction smaller lipomas and these are best removed through direct puncture excision. However, lipomas the size of a golf ball or larger are excellent candidates for liposuction.

POSTOPERATIVE CARE

Following the liposuction, the patient enters the postoperative period. Cannula insertion sites are routinely left open rather than being sutured closed. Experience has shown that closing insertion sites with sutures leads to a greater increase in postoperative edema as well as greater bruising. Closing cannula insertion sites allows for less tissue drainage via direct flow out of the subcutaneous space. Klein[23] has advocated the use of small adits: 1–2 mm openings made with a common biopsy punch biopsy instrument. These are more likely to stay open during the initial postoperative period than are 'stab'-type incisions.

It is important to remind patients (well before the procedure takes place) that they are going to have significant drainage following liposuction surgery. Barrier protection is recommended for car seats, furniture, and bed linens. Large plastic trash bags or plastic-lined absorbent drapes (such as Chux) may be used for this function.

The patient's insertion sites may be coated with petrolatum ointment or antibiotic ointment prior to application of absorbent materials. Modern absorbent pads are available from numerous manufacturers and are capable of absorbing significant amounts of drainage from the insertion sites. Alternatively, diapers or sanitary napkins may be used to absorb the drainage.

Following the application of sufficient amounts and layers of absorbent pads (held in place with tape), a compression garment or a compression bandage is fitted. Numerous styles of postoperative liposuction compression garments are available (Fig. 156.16). Postoperative compression minimizes bruising and aids in drainage. An increase in drainage minimizes postoperative edema. It is important to use firm compression immediately following tumescent liposuction[39]. Mild compression is sufficient after 3 or 4 days. Mild compression assists patients in feeling more secure and decreases pain by restricting movement of the treated tissue and by providing a moderate degree of analgesia. Many patients actually enjoy the comfort and feel of a compression garment.

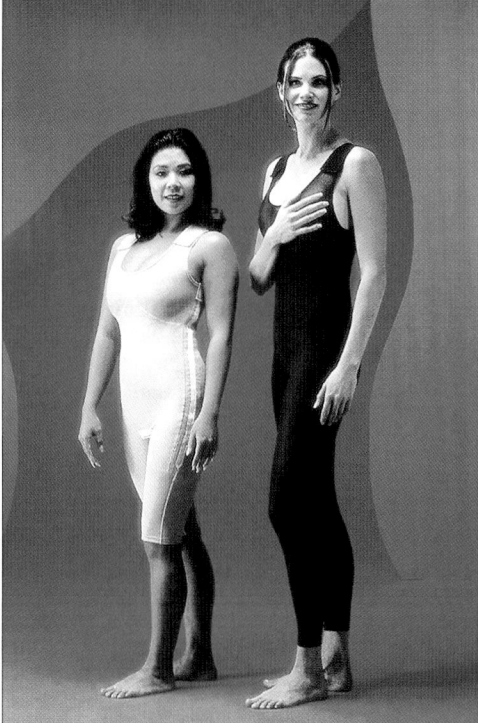

Fig. 156.16 Examples of liposuction compression garments. Courtesy of Miller Medical, Tuscon, AZ.

Infections have occasionally been reported with liposuction and oral antibiotics may provide prophylaxis against more serious infections. Lidocaine is bactericidal[40,41]. This may explain, in part, the relatively few infections seen with tumescent liposuction. Careful local wound care and cleanliness are essential in producing a good liposuction outcome. Our patients continue their preoperative antibiotics for 5 to 7 days following liposuction and are asked to shower daily following their procedure.

Patients are asked to change the absorptive pads and bandages the morning after their liposuction. Most individuals will experience continued drainage for 24–48 hours following liposuction. Patients are advised to take their first shower with the absorbent bandages and the tape in place, as the shower assists in the removal of the tape. Patients then follow the shower by reapplying absorbent pads where needed and their compression garment on top of the pads.

Most patients can return to work and exercise within 48 hours following their liposuction. It is important to ask the patients to ambulate regularly beginning the day following liposuction. This movement encourages further drainage as well as remodeling of the subcutaneous tissue. Movement has the additional benefit of increasing lymphatic drainage through intermittent pumping action of the skeletal muscles. Light exercise may begin 24 hours after surgery. Exercise keeps the patient from losing lean body mass during the postoperative period.

All patients are given a set of written postoperative liposuction instructions including important phone numbers should the patient need to contact the doctor. These postoperative instructions remind the patient that swelling and firmness beneath the skin and a reduced sensation in the skin are common. This will usually resolve over the first 3 to 4 weeks after the surgery. The postoperative instructions also remind patients that the final results are not seen before 6–12 months following the liposuction.

Patients return for their first postoperative appointment 1 day following liposuction. This visit is important to check for problems and reassure the patient. The next visit usually occurs at 1 week. The areas that have been treated are examined and palpated by the liposuction surgeon and the patient's progress is assessed. It is often necessary to remind patients that improvement from liposuction is a gradual process and in the immediate postoperative period they will simply obtain minimal improvement. They can look forward to a gradually improving shape. We have also used this postoperative visit to encourage patients to exercise and maintain an active and healthy lifestyle. We encourage caloric expenditure and emphasize eating a reasonable diet. Many liposuction surgeons recognize that liposuction may be used to 'jump-start' a patient's conversion to a healthy lifestyle and improved dietary pattern. Patients are seen for 3-month and 6-month follow-up visits. If touch-ups are required, it is wise to wait 1 year before proceeding, to be certain that the final results have been achieved.

COMPLICATIONS

Complications of liposuction must be differentiated from common sequelae (Table 156.5). After liposuction, it is common to have prolonged swelling, areas of numbness, bruising, and red incisions. Infections, hematomas and seromas are uncommon complications that require medical attention, but can usually be resolved rapidly[42].

Serious complications of liposuction are closely linked to the type of sedation employed. There have been a number of deaths from liposuction in patients who had moderate or deep sedation[12,24,42]. The authors are not aware of any deaths from liposuction, however, in

COMPLICATIONS OF LIPOSUCTION

Infection (e.g. bacterial, atypical mycobacterial)
Hematomas
Seromas
Skin indentations
Erosions, ulcerations
Thrombophlebitis (non-septic, septic)
Pulmonary embolism
Abdominal perforation

Table 156.5 Complications of liposuction.

patients who underwent the procedure with true tumescent local anesthesia[43].

Thrombophlebitis and pulmonary embolism postoperatively are associated with non-ambulatory patients and prolonged procedures under general anesthesia. This is also true for liposuction. An advantage of the tumescent local anesthetic technique is that patients are ambulatory immediately after surgery, thus minimizing the risks of this potential problem.

Abdominal perforation is one of the leading causes of liposuction deaths[44]. This is exclusively a complication of liposuction under general anesthesia[25]. Deeply sedated patients have decreased muscle tone and are unable to alert the physician to the pain of penetration of the liposuction cannula. Occult abdominal hernias may contribute to this complication.

General anesthesia also increases risks of respiratory failure and cardiac death[27]. Besides the direct effect of the systemic anesthesia, fluid overload may contribute to these problems. Anesthesiologists or anesthetists who are not accustomed to working with patients who have been infiltrated with tumescent anesthetic fluids may inadvertently overhydrate the patient with additional intravenous fluids. A significant amount of the saline infused subcutaneously is absorbed systemically, automatically correcting for surgical fluid losses. No additional intravenous fluids are usually required. Compounding this problem is the recent discovery that intravenous fluid bags are typically overfilled by at least 10%, leading to further errors in calculating fluid replacement in liposuction[45].

The keys to avoiding complications in liposuction lie in proper patient selection, appropriate patient evaluations, monitoring according to the degree of sedation, good surgical technique, avoidance of excessive fat removal or overzealous additional simultaneous procedures, and adequate postoperative care.

FUTURE TRENDS

Liposuction is now a mature procedure and most patients obtain predictable results[46–50]. Technology is constantly providing physicians with new ways to perform liposuction. As of this writing, there are studies underway evaluating the use of external ultrasound to liquefy fat. A 1,064 nm Nd:YAG laser with a 300 μm fiber has been shown to provide minor destruction of fat cells in the neck[51]. Although marketed to physicians as an improvement over older instrumentation, experience to date has been disappointing. It is likely that liposuction will remain one of the most popular cosmetic procedures.

REFERENCES

1. Fischer A, Fischer G. First surgical treatment for molding body's cellulite with three 5 mm incisions. Bull Int Acad Cosmet Surg. 1976;3:35.
2. Illouz YG. Body contouring by lipolysis: a 5-year experience with over 3000 cases. Plast Reconstr Surg. 1983;72:591–7.
3. Fournier PF, Otteni FM. Lipodissection in body sculpturing: the dry procedure. Plast Reconstr Surg. 1983;72:598–609.
4. Field LM. The dermatologist and liposuction – a history. J Dermatol Surg Oncol. 1987;13:1040–1.

5. Klein JA. Tumescent technique for liposuction surgery. Am J Cosmet Surg. 1987;4:263–7.
6. Klein JA. Tumescent technique for regional anesthesia permits lidocaine doses of 35 mg/kg for liposuction. J Dermatol Surg Oncol. 1990;16:248–63.
7. Lillis PJ. Liposuction surgery under local anesthesia: limited blood loss and minimal lidocaine absorption. J Dermatol Surg Oncol. 1988;14:1145–8.
8. Lillis PJ. The tumescent technique for liposuction surgery. Dermatol Clin. 1990;8:439–50.
9. Klein JA. Tumescent technique for local anesthesia

improves safety in large-volume liposuction. Plast Reconstr Surg. 1993;92:1085–98; discussion 99–100.
10. Flynn TC, Coleman WP III, Field LM, Klein JA, Hanke CW. History of liposuction. Dermatol Surg. 2000;26:515–20.
11. Drake LA, Ceilley RI, Cornelison RL, et al. Guidelines of care for liposuction. Committee on Guidelines of Care. J Am Acad Dermatol. 1991;24:489–94.
12. Coleman WP III, Hanke CW, Glogau RG. Does the specialty of the physician affect fatality rates in liposuction? A comparison of specialty specific data. Dermatol Surg. 2000;26:611–15.

13. Flynn TC, Narins RS. Preoperative evaluation of the liposuction patient. Dermatol Clin. 1999;17:729–34.
14. Coleman WP III. Noncosmetic applications of liposuction. J Dermatol Surg Oncol. 1988;14:1085–90.
15. Narins RS. Liposuction surgery for a buffalo hump caused by Cushing's disease. J Am Acad Dermatol. 1989;21:307.
16. Chastain MA, Chastain JB, Coleman WP III. HIV lipodystrophy: review of the syndrome and report of a case treated with liposuction. Dermatol Surg. 2001;27:497–500.
17. Coleman WP III, Letessier S, Hanke CW. Liposuction. In: Coleman WP III, Hanke CW, Alt TH, Asken S (eds). Cosmetic Surgery of the Skin. St Louis: Mosby, 1997:178–205.
18. Lawrence N, Clark RE, Flynn TC, Coleman WP III. American Society for Dermatologic Surgery Guidelines of Care for Liposuction. Dermatol Surg. 2000;26:265–9.
19. Coleman WP III, Glogau RG, Klein JA, et al. Guidelines of care of liposuction. J Am Acad Dermatol. 2001;45:438–47.
20. Ostad A, Kageyama N, Moy RL. Tumescent anesthesia with a lidocaine dose of 55 mg/kg is safe for liposuction. Dermatol Surg.1996;22:921–7.
21. Coleman WP III. Tumescent anesthesia with a lidocaine dose of 55 mg/kg is safe for liposuction (editorial). Dermatol Surg. 1996;22:919.
22. Klein JA. Anesthetic formulation of tumescent solutions. Dermatol Clin. 1999;17:751–9.
23. Klein JA. Tumescent Technique. Tumescent Anesthesia and Microcannular Liposuction. St Louis: Mosby, 2000.
24. Rao RB, Ely SF, Hoffman RS. Deaths related to liposuction. N Engl J Med. 1999;30:1471–5.
25. Coleman WP III, Hanke CW, Lillis P, Bernstein G, Narins R. Does the location of the surgery or the specialty of the physican affect malpractice claims in liposuction? Dermatol Surg. 1999;25:343–7.

26. Hanke CW, Bernstein G, Bullock S. Safety of tumescent liposuction in 15,336 patients. National survey results. Dermatol Surg. 1995;21:459–62.
27. Forrest JB, Rehder K, Cahalan MK, Goldsmith CH. Multicenter study of general anesthesia. III. Predictors of severe perioperative adverse outcomes. Anesthesiology. 1992;76:3–15.
28. Klein JA, Kassarjdian N. Lidocaine toxicity with tumescent liposuction. A case report of probable drug interactions. Dermatol Surg. 1997;23:1169–74.
29. Klein JA. Intravenous fluids and bupivacaine are contraindicated in tumescent liposuction. Plast Reconstr Surg. 1998;102:2516–19.
30. Breuninger H, Wehner-Caroli J. Subcutaneous infusion anesthesia with prilocaine diluted with Ringer's lactate. Hautarzt.1998;49:709–13.
31. Breuninger H, Hobbach PS, Schimek F. Ropivacaine: an important anesthetic agent for slow infusion and other forms of tumescent anesthesia. Dermatol Surg. 1999;25:799–802.
32. Moffitt DL, De Berker DA, Kennedy CT, Shutt LE. Assessment of ropivacaine as a local anesthetic for skin infiltration in skin surgery. Dermatol Surg. 2001;5:437–40.
33. Bernstein G. Instrumentation for liposuction. Dermatol Clin. 1999;17:735–49.
34. Lawrence N, Coleman WP III. Ultrasonic-assisted liposuction. Internal and external. Dermatol Clin. 1999;17:761–71.
35. Lawrence N, Coleman WP III. The biologic basis of ultrasonic liposuction. Dermatol Surg. 1997;23:1197–200.
36. Coleman WP III. Powered liposuction. Dermatol Surg. 2000;26:315–18.
37. Coleman WP III, Katz B, Bruck M, et al. The efficacy of powered liposuction. Dermatol Surg. 2001;27:735–8.
38. Cook W. Laser neck and jowl liposculpture including platysma laser resurfacing, dermal laser resurfacing and

vaporization of subcutaneous fat. Dermatol Surg. 1997;23:1143–8.
39. Klein JA. Post-tumescent liposuction care. Open drainage and bimodal compression. Dermatol Clin. 1999;17:881–9.
40. William BJ, Hanke CW, Bartlett M. Antimicrobial effects of lidocaine, bicarbonate, and epinephrine. J Am Acad Dermatol. 1997;37:662–4.
41. Klein JA. Antibacterial effects of tumescent lidocaine. Plast Reconstr Surg. 1999;104:1934–6.
42. Grazer FM, de Jong RH. Fatal outcomes from liposuction: census survey of cosmetic surgeons. Plast Reconstr Surg. 2000;105:436–46; discussion 447–8.
43. Hanke W, Cox SE, Kuznets N, Coleman WP 3rd. Tumescent liposuction report performance measurement initiative: national survey results. Dermatol Surg. 2004;7:967–77.
44. Talmor M, Hoffman LA, Lieberman M. Intestinal perforation after suction lipoplasty; a case report and review of the literature. Ann Plast Surg. 1997;38:169–72.
45. Coleman WP IV, Flynn TC, Coleman KL. When one liter does not equal 1000 milliliters: implications for the tumescent technique. Dermatol Surg. 2000;26:1024–8.
46. Yoho RA, Romaine JJ, O'Neil D. Review of the liposuction, abdominoplasty, and face-lift mortality and morbidity risk literature. Dermatol Surg. 2005;31:733–43.
47. Shiffman MA, Di Giuseppe A. Liposuction: Principles and Practice. Berlin: Springer-Verlag, 2006.
48. Hanke CW, Sattler G, Sommer B. Textbook of Liposuction. London: Informa Healthcare, 2007.
49. Narins RS. Safe Liposuction and Fat Transfer. London: Informa Healthcare, 2003.
50. Hanke CW, Sattler G. Liposuction (Procedures in Cosmetic Dermatology). St Louis: Saunders, 2005.
51. Kim KH, Geronemus RG. Laser lipolysis using a novel 1,064 nm Nd:YAG laser. Dermatol Surg. 2006;32:241–8.

Hair Restoration

Dow B Stough, Jeffrey M Whitworth and David Julian Seager

157

Key features

- Hair is important in order to frame the face, maintain a youthful appearance, and abet self-esteem
- Realistic expectations are key to patient satisfaction following restoration surgery
- Normal hair grows in follicular unit groupings of one, two, three, or even four hairs
- Modern hair restoration techniques utilize follicular unit grafts
- Donor hair from the occipital area that is not under androgenetic hormonal influence is transplanted to bald areas of the anterior scalp and hairline
- The trend has been to complete hair restoration surgery in fewer high-density sessions; even single transplantation sessions are becoming the norm
- Transplant teams include the physician as well as highly trained counselors and technicians
- Androgenetic hair loss continues throughout life; this may require additional grafting at variable intervals

INTRODUCTION

The field of hair restoration is an exciting and dynamic specialty in contemporary medicine, although the public is largely unaware of results possible with the refined techniques that have evolved over the past 20 years. Advanced technologies enable surgeons to achieve more aesthetically pleasing results than ever before. The specialty of hair restoration includes both medical and surgical modalities. Initially pioneered by dermatologists, the current discipline is a true mixture of all surgical subspecialties as well as physicians from non-surgical specialties. The colorful history of this field is briefly summarized below.

HISTORICAL PERSPECTIVES

The list of individuals who have served as innovators in this field is extensive, with numerous achievements and advancements. We have taken the liberty of arbitrarily separating this brief synopsis into two sections: hair transplantation before follicular unit transplantation and hair transplantation since follicular unit transplantation.

Hair Transplantation Prior to the Follicular Unit

In the early 19th century, J Dieffenbach demonstrated the successful autotransplantation of hair into skin. Subsequent to this, in the 19th and early 20th centuries, sporadic cases and reports of successful transplantation of relatively large grafts, or the use of hair-bearing flaps for restoration of traumatic and other alopecias, were documented in the world literature. The literature credits Okuda in 1939 with demonstrating the successful use of 2- to 4-mm punch grafts for restoration of alopecia of the scalp, eyebrow, mustache and pubic areas. In 1943, Tamura, an often-overlooked author, demonstrated the use of single hair grafts implanted by 'injection' for restoration of the skin overlying the mons pubis in women. Of note, neither Okuda nor Tamura demonstrated the use of hair-bearing autografts for restoration of male pattern baldness (MPB). The successful use of hair-bearing autografts for the correction of MPB was first described in 1959, in a paper authored by Dr Norman Orentreich. Though this was Dr Orentreich's original published report on the subject, his first treatment of a patient with hair-bearing autografts for restoration of MPB was in 1952. It is for his groundbreaking work that Dr Orentreich is duly recognized as the father of hair restoration surgery. From 1959 until the mid 1980s, hair transplantation for the correction of MPB progressed with refinements in the standard punch autograft.

The Follicular Unit

The 1990s represented a period of fierce debate that centered on the use of 'follicular unit grafts' to achieve total hair restoration. The advent of follicular unit transplantation is credited to Dr Bob Limmer in San Antonio, who, in the late 1980s, began using microscopes to create small one- to five-hair grafts that were inserted into needle slits. Dr Limmer removed all excess non-hair-bearing tissue, which allowed for the natural hair groupings to be transplanted into 18-gauge needle sites. While improvements are still being made, most follicular unit transplants performed today are quite similar to Dr Limmer's original technique.

Around 1995, Dr William Rassman documented the natural growth patterns of hair as seen through a hair densitometer. He stated that 'hairs grow in groups, most frequently in pairs, sometimes in groups of three, and more rarely in groups of four and five; understanding this architecture is critical, the incorporation of the patient's growing hair groups is to be exploited in the design of the restoration.' In 1997, Dr Robert Bernstein and Dr Bill Rassman described their technique under the moniker 'follicular unit transplantation', thus contributing the term 'follicular unit' to our nomenclature. Follicular unit 'purists' insist, however, that the term applies only to grafts containing hair in its natural groupings.

In individuals with blonde, red or brown hair, follicular unit grafts are often created utilizing microscopes for tissue dissection (Fig. 157.1); in those with black hair, this is not a necessity. While hair density following transplantation may occasionally be less than optimal, some surgeons feel strongly that the capacity for a (pure) follicular unit

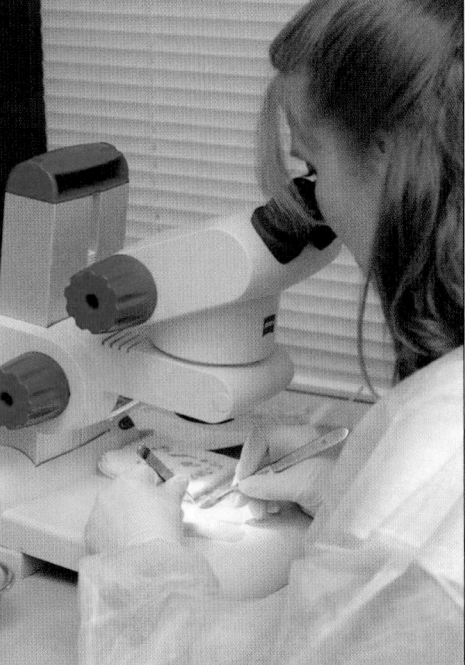

Fig. 157.1 Graft dissection utilizing Zeiss Stemi DV4 microscope.

transplant to produce a natural result, coupled with the demonstrated advantages of stereomicroscopic subsection of donor tissue (related to low hair transection rates), make follicular unit transplantation a superior method of hair restoration. The latest development in the field involves the ability to produce an acceptable single-session result utilizing only follicular unit grafts. Dr David Seager of Canada and others have pioneered this work. This brief history brings us to the present, the era of follicular unit transplantation in which undetectable single-session hair transplantations are becoming the standard of care.

PSYCHOLOGY OF HAIR LOSS

Behavioral scientists have confirmed that an individual's physical features, i.e. face, body frame, size, hair and other physical traits, can shape one's social attitude and attributes which then influence socioeconomic status and occupation. As stated by Dr TF Cash, 'Hair is one of the few body parts we have (that allows) immediate control to express our individual or chosen identity. Rapid hair loss 'matures' the younger man, whereas a full head of hair will result in a more youthful appearance.' Given the latter statement, it is not surprising that studies have demonstrated that androgenetic alopecia is an unwelcome and stressful experience for most men. The desire for hair should not simply be equated with vanity, since hair performs the function of framing the face. The concept of facial framing is paramount to understanding the role of hair restoration surgery. Artists have long recognized that facial features exist in a dimensional relationship with one another. The presence of hair preserves a youthful facial appearance. This effect is achieved by shortening the face so that hair returns the viewer's focus to the center of the face. By restoring hair in a balding individual, the face becomes the central focus and the restored hair paradoxically becomes a 'non-issue'. A permanent framing of the face creates a stable image that becomes familiar and comfortable. This stabilization of one's appearance is one of the chief reasons that hair restoration ranks among the highest in patient satisfaction. This is not to suggest that most men with androgenetic alopecia should seek hair restoration surgery. In fact, it is only recommended for those who are most disturbed by their current appearance and concerned about future loss. Detailed psychological testing is usually not necessary, since men and women who seek medical consultation for androgenetic alopecia obviously are more psychologically distressed with regard to their hair loss than typical patients who suffer from alopecia.

In summary, men and women with androgenetic alopecia often seek alleviation of distressing thoughts and feelings about their appearance. Surgery can lead to a more secure, fulfilling sense of self. The high satisfaction rate among those who undergo hair restoration procedures is testament to the evolution of this specialty.

ANDROGENS

At puberty, boys experience a rise in the circulating levels of testosterone. Testosterone is then metabolized into dihydrotestosterone (DHT) by an enzyme known as 5α-reductase (Fig. 157.2; see Ch. 69). Regional differences in androgen metabolism are present in balding versus non-

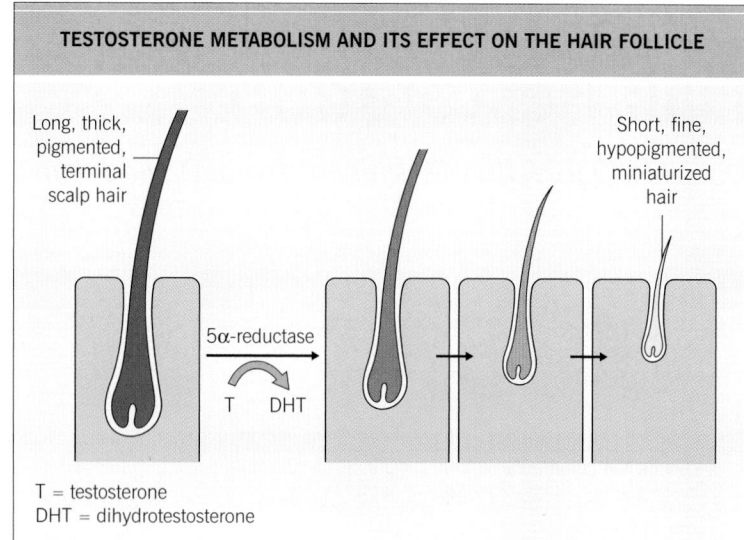

TESTOSTERONE METABOLISM AND ITS EFFECT ON THE HAIR FOLLICLE

Long, thick, pigmented, terminal scalp hair

Short, fine, hypopigmented, miniaturized hair

5α-reductase

T → DHT

T = testosterone
DHT = dihydrotestosterone

Fig. 157.2 Testosterone metabolism and its effect on the hair follicle. Testosterone is metabolized into dihydrotestosterone (DHT) by the enzyme 5α-reductase. This enzyme is found in the hair follicles of the scalp.

balding scalp skin, with 5α-reductase activity higher in areas of balding. Inflammation may play a role in some individuals by stimulating cytokines and growth factors, which retard hair growth.

ANDROGENETIC ALOPECIA

Androgenetic alopecia is multifactorial and has a polygenic form of inheritance. In other words, it can result from an interaction of several genes combined with environmental factors. Miniaturization of terminal anagen hairs to smaller vellus hairs is the hallmark of androgenetic alopecia (see Fig. 157.2). Hair follicles become progressively smaller in size and have decreased periods of hair cycling. This results in small, fine, hypopigmented hairs that are known as vellus hairs. Vellus hairs may be present in large amounts prior to permanent shedding (Fig. 157.3). Most individuals recognize that the progression of alopecia results in a horseshoe-shaped rim of hair around the scalp. Hair in the parietal and occipital regions may thin, but it is unclear whether this hair is affected by the same androgen-mediated processes that typically occur in regions commonly affected by MPB.

CLASSIFICATION OF MALE PATTERN ALOPECIA

Dr O'Tar Norwood developed the Norwood classification system, which has been used for over 20 years and has become the standard classification system for MPB (Fig. 157.4). This classification system recognizes seven grades of baldness, ranging from I to VII. In addition, there are variances of hair loss within these grades, designated as type a variants. The variant baldness has a more diffuse pattern, without the simultaneous development of loss on the vertex (with the exception

Fig. 157.3 Progression of androgenetic alopecia. DHT, dihydrotestosterone.

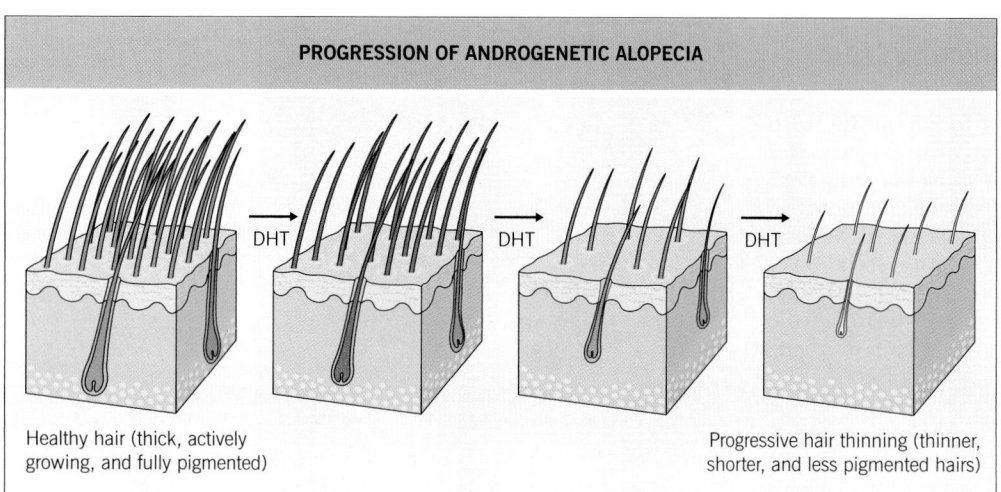

PROGRESSION OF ANDROGENETIC ALOPECIA

DHT → DHT → DHT →

Healthy hair (thick, actively growing, and fully pigmented)

Progressive hair thinning (thinner, shorter, and less pigmented hairs)

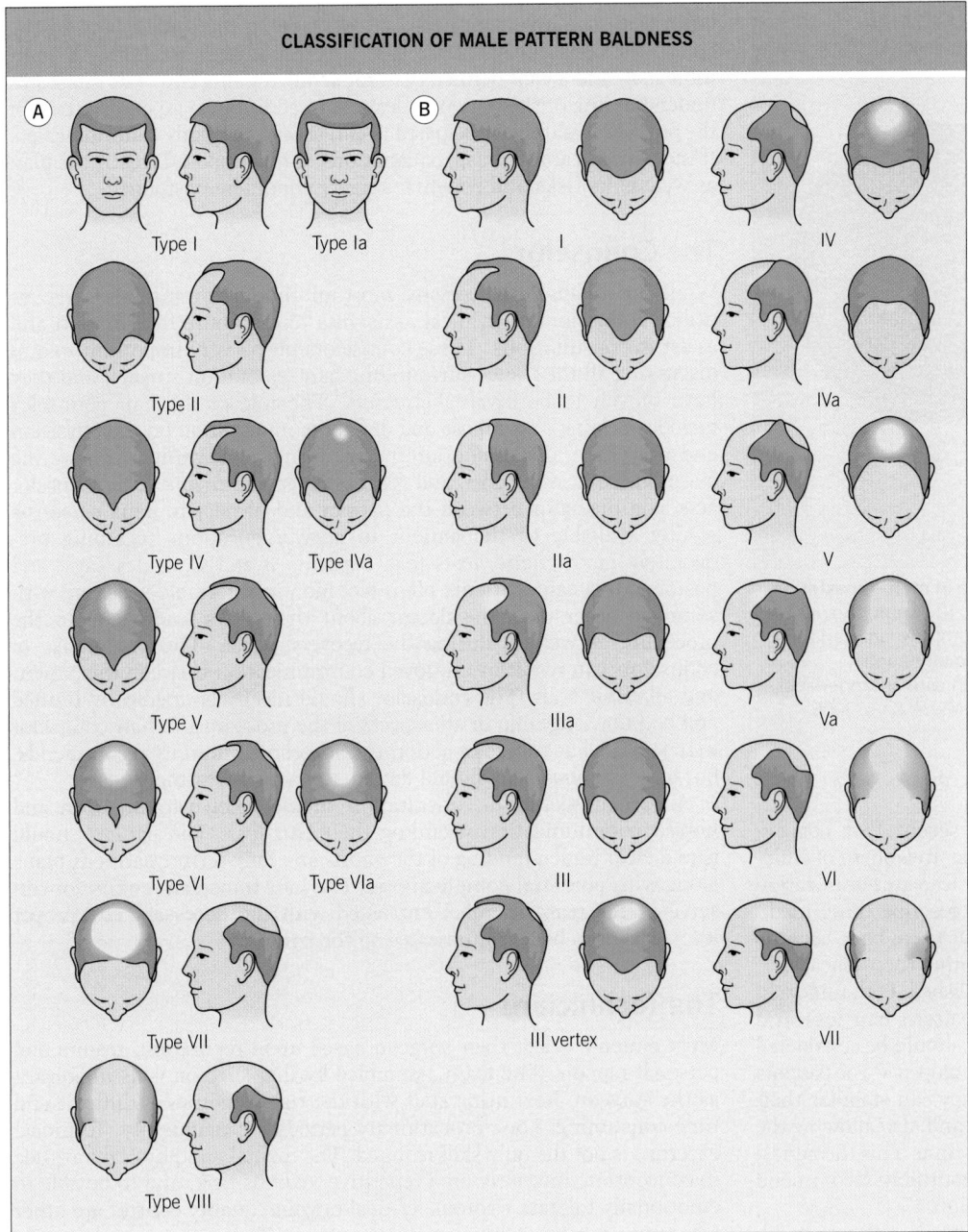

CLASSIFICATION OF MALE PATTERN BALDNESS

A

Type I   Type Ia

Type II

Type IV   Type IVa

Type V

Type VI   Type VIa

Type VII

Type VIII

B

I

II

IIa

IIIa

III

III vertex

IV

IVa

V

Va

VI

VII

Fig. 157.4 Classification of male pattern baldness. **A** Hamilton's classification. **B** Norwood's classification. In the authors' opinion, Norwood's classification is preferred.

of Va). All transplant surgeons routinely recognize patients that fall outside this standard classification regimen. Nevertheless, the Norwood classification system has practical applications for the majority of patients. This system is a time-honored communication tool and should be recognized as such.

MEDICAL TREATMENT

Currently, there are only two medically proven treatments for hair loss: topical minoxidil and oral finasteride. Minoxidil exerts its effects on the cells of the hair follicle, although its precise mechanism of action in androgenetic alopecia is not known. Topical minoxidil is approved by the Food and Drug Administration (FDA) to regrow hair or stop hair loss in both men and women. With continued use of the product, a patient would expect to produce longer, larger-caliber hairs. Common side effects of topical minoxidil include unwanted facial hair growth (especially disconcerting for women) and irritant contact dermatitis; occasionally, allergic contact dermatitis develops secondary to one of the components in the minoxidil solution. Rarely, patients may complain of headache, ankle edema or chest pain.

The only oral medication indicated for the treatment of androgenetic alopecia in men is finasteride (Propecia®; 1 mg/day). Finasteride is a specific inhibitor of Type II 5α-reductase (see Ch. 68), and it leads to a decrease in the conversion of testosterone to DHT in several sites,

including scalp skin (5α-reductase is present in scalp hair follicles). In a controlled trial of oral finasteride (1 mg/day) versus placebo conducted in 305 men with androgenetic alopecia, those who received finasteride had a considerable difference in hair counts after 5 years compared to those who received placebo (Fig. 157.5). This study represented the longest clinical trial performed to date of a hair loss treatment. After 5 years, the men on finasteride had an average of 277 more hairs in a 1-inch diameter circle than those who received placebo. The net benefit of finasteride also increased each year. At the end of the 5-year study, a panel rated 90% of those men treated with finasteride as having no visible hair loss (compared to baseline) versus 25% of the men in the placebo group.

Possible side effects of oral finasteride include changes in sexual function that manifest in men as decreased libido, ejaculatory dysfunction, or erectile dysfunction. It should be noted that overall the incidence of these side effects is less than 2% (only slightly higher than placebo). In one study, all the patients who discontinued finasteride had resolution of this side effect, as did 58% of the men who continued to take the finasteride. Gynecomastia is an infrequent side effect. With regard to the effects of finasteride (1 mg/day) on concentrations of serum prostate-specific antigen (PSA) in men with androgenetic alopecia, a recent randomized controlled trial involving 355 men found a median decrease in serum PSA of 40% (men ages 40–49 years) and 50% (men ages 50–60 years), compared to placebo after 48 weeks. The

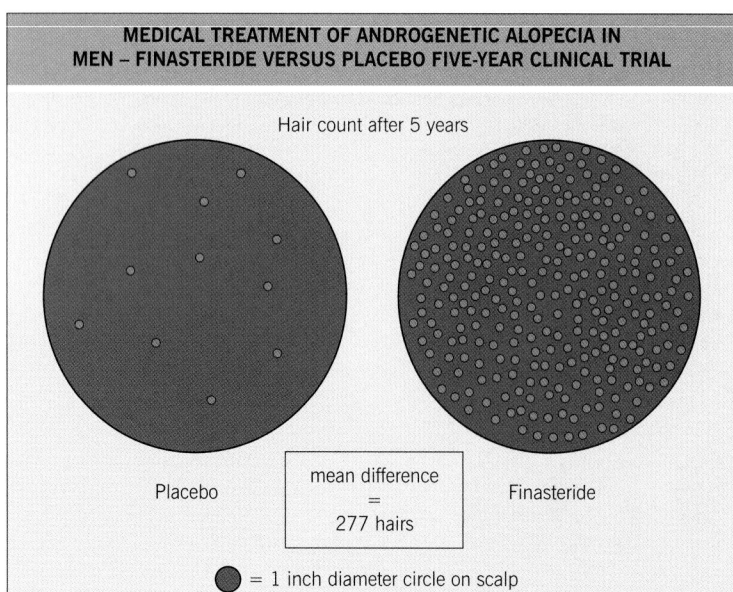

MEDICAL TREATMENT OF ANDROGENETIC ALOPECIA IN MEN – FINASTERIDE VERSUS PLACEBO FIVE-YEAR CLINICAL TRIAL

Hair count after 5 years

Placebo

mean difference
=
277 hairs

Finasteride

● = 1 inch diameter circle on scalp

Fig. 157.5 Medical treatment of androgenetic alopecia in men – finasteride (n = 219) versus placebo (n = 15) five-year clinical trial. The figure shows the mean difference in hair count after 5 years (p<0.001). From: The Finasteride Male Pattern Hair Loss Study Group. Long-term (5-year) multinational experience with finasteride 1 mg in the treatment of men with androgenetic alopecia. Eur J Dermatol. 2002;12:38–49; product insert, Merck & Co, 2006.

recommendation of the authors was to adjust serum PSA concentrations when performing prostate-cancer screening. In women of child-bearing age, finasteride (and spironolactone) can lead to feminization of a male fetus (see Ch. 68). Some physicians prescribe these medications primarily for post-menopausal women, but there have been no prospective randomized controlled trials to determine their efficacy.

The advantages of medical therapy are well established. Both minoxidil and finasteride are likely to slow or halt male pattern hair loss in a given individual. For this reason, medical therapy should be considered in all patients with mild to moderate androgenetic alopecia. For patients who desire hair restoration surgery, medical therapy can stabilize their hair loss, thus necessitating less donor harvesting and also allowing the patient to maintain a more natural appearance over time. This theoretical scenario is why many hair transplant surgeons routinely recommend medical therapy in conjunction with transplantation.

A few individuals will experience impressive regrowth with minoxidil, finasteride, or both. However, a patient must continue to use these medications indefinitely if they desire to maintain the benefit they have obtained. Upon discontinuation of minoxidil or finasteride, one would expect loss of hairs regrown or maintained by these medications.

THE HAIR TRANSPLANT TEAM

Hair transplantation differs from traditional dermatologic surgery in that it involves an entire team of individuals. This team has become a necessity due to the vast amount of preoperative counseling, intensive labor requirements, and division of duties required for the successful completion of a single transplant session. The transplant team consists of the surgeon, the counselor and the technicians. Typically, surgeons will employ two to four technicians per case.

The Surgeon

Individuals considering hair restoration surgery should expect to meet with a physician to discuss surgical and medical options. During the consultation, a plan for hair restoration is sought and received. This process is crucial for both the patient and the physician; an outcome that is satisfactory to both parties hangs in the balance of a successful consultation. This is the time when a patient's preconceived notions and desires, perhaps fraught with emotion, are modified by a physician's knowledge. The doctor will express concerns about patient expectations and gauge what can be feasibly attained. Often the patient and doctor

begin from two divergent perspectives, meet in the middle, and by the end of the consultative phase have a common understanding, a common goal, and a well-defined plan for achieving this end. The surgeon's understanding of the patient's desires, in addition to an explanation of the procedure and the anticipated result, should be clearly communicated. If the patient cannot grasp explanations of the proposed treatment plan as well as its risks and benefits, surgery should be postponed.

The Counselor

While not an absolute necessity, most full-time hair transplant surgeons utilize counselors or medical assistants to distribute information and assist in consultations. These counselors play a very important role in discussing all the issues surrounding hair restoration surgery, and they have proven to be invaluable assets. The role of the hair counselor includes helping to compose and distribute information on the physician and the clinic, discussing alternative forms of treatment, answering questions concerning cost, and scheduling appointments. The counselor acts as a mediator between the patient and physician. This person is readily available to the patient to answer questions regarding pre-operative instructions, tests (e.g. hepatitis B and C viral assays) and postoperative care. Patients often feel more comfortable speaking with someone other than the doctor about their fears leading up to the procedure as well as during the recovery phase. The proper use of counselors can result in improved communication between the patient and all clinic staff. The counselor should ideally be medically trained and be knowledgeable in all aspects of the procedure. A hair counselor may relate what course of action the surgeon commonly recommends, but only the physician should dictate the actual treatment plan.

A patient seeking a consultation should receive frank, open and honest communication regarding their hair loss. The patient should gain a clear understanding of the short- and long-term treatment plans along with potential complications. The hair transplant counselor can serve as the team member entrusted with the necessary and proper information to be communicated to the patient.

The Technicians

Most patients select their surgeon based upon reputation, results and personal rapport. The team assembled by that surgeon is as important as the surgeon. Recruiting staff with the right qualities is difficult and time-consuming. Long probationary periods are mandatory. Technical expertise is not the only skill required. The mental and physical fortitude to concentrate intensely on a repetitive, tedious task, and to be able to emotionally tolerate rigorous, critical ongoing quality control are other rare traits a good technician must possess. Technicians are primarily utilized for two major tasks: cutting and planting. The first task involves tedious sectioning of the donor strip into slivers, followed by further sectioning into follicular units. In this role they are referred to as 'cutters'. Their second task is to create recipient sites and insert follicular unit grafts. Thus, they are termed 'planters'. Additionally, the successful technician must have a personality suitable for working closely and harmoniously without friction for long hours with his or her team-mates. Staff selection and training is the most difficult and expensive component of the entire process.

One must also accept that, even with highly trained and efficient staff, it will take twice as long to place grafts into pre-made recipient sites at a density of 35–40 follicular units/cm² as it does to place the same number of grafts more loosely (i.e. 20–25 follicular units/cm²). Because of the inherently slower planting technique along with the greater number of grafts, the surgery time for sessions utilizing density counts greater than 30 follicular units/cm² can be extremely prolonged. Knowledge of these crucial factors alone will not enable a hair transplant facility to successfully 'dense-pack' grafts. Translation of theory into practice is difficult. Exceptional talent and years of constant tutored training are required before the long learning curve is mastered and staff members become expert at these techniques.

THE CONSULTATION

The consultation process involves communication of a patient's goals as well as what may be reasonably expected of the hair transplant team in achieving these goals. A certain percentage of individuals seeking a consultation for hair restoration surgery must be rejected. These individuals either do not meet the necessary criteria or cannot be satisfied with current technology. It is incumbent upon the physician to identify the patient's spoken and unspoken needs, and to make the expected and attainable results very clear to the patient. The process of consultation is an effort by the physician to communicate his knowledge and apply it to the unique needs of each patient. The following concepts are stressed in the consultation:

- The progressive nature of hair loss. Hair loss will never become static. It is an ongoing process, which will proceed (albeit slowly in some cases) throughout one's lifetime.
- Framing the face. A natural facial framing returns one's familiar appearance and restores the central face as the focus of attention.
- Natural appearance. Baldness is a very natural condition. The treatment of hair loss should also be natural in appearance. Utilizing today's techniques, hair replacement should not look odd or artificial. Hair restoration cannot produce an exact duplicate of nature, but it can give the illusion to onlookers that no surgical intervention has occurred. Therefore, modern hair restoration surgery is natural and undetectable in everyday life.
- Permanent hairline. While the process of hair loss is relentlessly progressive, transplanted hairlines are permanent. The creation of a permanent hairline visually arrests the change in appearance that patients find so distressing. However, hairlines must be acceptable following their initial placement after transplantation and throughout one's lifetime. Lessons of the past have taught us that wide, rounded, youthful hairlines will look odd after the fifth decade of life.

During the consultation, the physician will inquire about the patient's ultimate goal, previous hair transplants or scalp surgeries, and medical history. The question, 'What is your goal?' is the most important question the surgeon can ask. The physician should specifically ask what area of loss is the most disconcerting to the patient. This consideration is of critical significance in the preoperative evaluation, as it is the foundation from which patient expectations can be synchronized with surgical and medical capabilities. Inquiring about a history of previous hair transplants or scalp surgeries, both of which factor into preoperative planning from the standpoint of scalp elasticity, recipient site creation, and donor strip harvesting, is imperative.

Many patients presenting with 3- to 4-mm round punch autografts have an unnatural appearance. This does not automatically equate to a dissatisfied patient. It is imperative that one approaches the subject with caution and does not assume the patient is unhappy with his or her appearance.

A medical history should include questions regarding previous bleeding problems, all medications (prescription, over-the-counter and herbal), and drug allergies. For example, garlic, *Ginkgo biloba*, vitamin E and other supplements have the potential to contribute to intraoperative and postoperative bleeding (e.g. by inhibiting platelet aggregation; see Ch. 133). Evaluation also includes assessing the need for preoperative antibiotics in select cases, such as individuals with prosthetic joints, valvular heart disease or diabetes mellitus (see Ch. 151). The authors do not recommend preoperative antibiotics on a routine basis. A consultation flow sheet specifically designed for hair restoration should be composed (Fig. 157.6).

LIMITATIONS

When hair transplantation is planned, it is important to clearly indicate to patients the limitations of the procedure and what is to be expected. The patient must comprehend the concept of hair loss progressing over time. The rate of hair loss in any given individual is unpredictable, but the success of a particular patient's hair transplant will depend in part on the amount of subsequent hair loss experienced by that person. It is best to avoid quoting the exact number of grafts or procedures required to satisfy an individual. Instead, provide ranges and emphasize that these are estimates only. Be wary of patients who are insistent upon a treatment plan written in stone. An inability to appreciate why an exact total is impossible to predict indicates difficulty in understanding that hair loss is an ongoing process and the fact that successful hair transplantation is dependent upon appreciating this ongoing loss. For example,

a 30-year-old man with isolated bitemporal recession may require only one session of follicular unit grafts. Five years later, he may require further grafting to prevent the unnatural appearance of a separation between his transplanted temporal scalp and receding hair. If he has not understood from the onset that this was likely to occur, he may present for further work with the perception that he is 'repairing' what was inadequately performed in his first transplant session. If, however, he understands that he is likely to need future grafts due to the progressive nature of hair loss, he will rightly view subsequent transplant sessions as an appropriate extension of his earlier procedures. Medical therapy is helpful to prevent ongoing hair loss, but cannot be relied upon as a safety net that will never fail. In addition, there will always be cases where medical therapy is discontinued for various reasons. When predicting how much hair loss an individual will incur, it is safest to assume that all patients will progress to an advanced stage of alopecia, and surgeons should plan any transplant accordingly. Planning for this advancement, patients are assured a transplant that will stand the test of time and remain natural in appearance throughout their lives.

The observation of hair loss subsequent to transplantation is repeatedly noted. Post-transplant telogen effluvium is thought to occur as a result of local tissue trauma. Terminal hairs can be affected, but vellus hairs are the most susceptible to this process. Medical therapy, such as finasteride, may help to modify this loss. Due to the delay of 6 months between the transplant session and the observed result, patients will frequently be forgetful of their initial counseling and their initial appearance. It is our practice to take photographs and to incorporate discussions of the above issues into the consultation and the informed consent.

CANDIDATE SELECTION

Useful criteria for assessing an individual's quality as a candidate for hair transplantation include, but are not limited to, the degree of baldness, caliber of the hair shaft, skin and hair color contrast, donor hair volume, donor hair density, and patient expectations. We routinely refer to 'the big five' when selecting a candidate (Table 157.1).

Donor Hair Density

Patients with a high density of donor hair in the occipital scalp will yield a greater number of follicular units per donor strip. A large donor supply is extremely advantageous. Men require a density count of at least 40 follicular units/cm^2 in their donor area to be considered for transplants. Fortunately, most men presenting for hair transplantation have follicular unit counts greater than 55 hairs/cm^2 in the occipital region. Follicular unit counts vary among different ethnic groups. For example, Caucasians have higher follicular unit counts than Asians. The number of hairs per follicular unit grouping varies (Table 157.2).

Caliber

Hair transplant surgeons generally speak of hair caliber when discussing the size of the hair shaft. Larger width (>80 μm) hair is of higher cosmetic value than fine hair. Patients possessing fine hair (<60 μm) are certain to have a sparse quality to their transplant. These individuals can have 'see through' hair, even with dense packing of more than 25 follicular units/cm^2 in the recipient area. Transplants of fine hair will always cover less surface area than large-caliber hair grafts.

Color Contrast

The skin to hair color contrast is less important with follicular unit grafting than with previous techniques. Individuals with a hair color that closely matches their skin color will have a lower contrast of transplanted hair against the background of scalp skin. These patients obtain optimal short- and long-term results because the follicular unit is less prominent as it exits the scalp. This is the concept behind scalp camouflaging products, which reduce the disparity of hair color to skin color. For this reason, patients with light hair color and fair skin are superior candidates to those possessing dark hair color and fair skin. Both groups can be confidently transplanted provided only one-haired follicular units are utilized in the frontal hairline region.

MEDICAL CONSULTATION FORM FOR HAIR TRANSPLANT PROCEDURE

Date ____/____/____   Time in/out _____/_____

Name_____

Age_____   Skin color _____

Medical history: **Patient goals:**

General health_____   _____

Drug allergies_____   _____

Bleeding tendencies_____   _____

Smoking history_____

Age hair loss began_____   **Treatment plan:**

History of diabetes ☐ , artificial joints ☐ ,   Past scalp reductions_____

   heart valves ☐ , pacemaker ☐ , defibrillator ☐   Previous transplants_____

History of abnormal scarring or keloids ☐   Estimated graft sessions_____

Current medications_____

_____

Family history of hair loss_____   Minoxidil/Finasteride Rx _____

_____

Hair loss treatments used_____   HIV and Hepatitis B and C

_____   blood work explained   ☐

Vitamins/supplements_____   Procedure explained   ☐

_____   Web site explained   ☐

                                               Literature reviewed   ☐

Hair and scalp evaluation:

Grade_____

Current pattern_____   Areas of most concern to patient_____

Anticipated pattern_____   _____

Density_____

Scalp thickness_____

Hair color_____   Areas to be transplanted_____

    Curl_____   _____

    Texture_____   _____

    Vellus_____

    Terminal_____

    Caliber_____

    Problems_____

Comments/Special Instructions

_____

_____

_____

Fig. 157.6 Medical consultation form for hair transplant procedure.

Patient Expectations

The individual's expectations are also an important consideration when assessing a candidate for hair restoration. If a patient approaches the procedure with unrealistic expectations or desires, and these desires cannot be modified through careful consultation and explanations, this person is a poor candidate for hair transplantation. Most unrealistic expectations occur in the realm of density. Individuals with fine hair (<60 mm) cannot expect significant density. Patients who wear hair systems may never be pleased with the comparative density achieved with follicular unit grafting.

Age Considerations

Individuals in good health can be transplanted throughout their lifetime. Men in their late teens and early 20s with the beginnings of frontotemporal recession often desire restoration of their hairline to its original juvenile location. Such cases are problematic. The fear of future baldness is oftentimes the stimulus to seek consultation. Surgery can only provide a 'quick fix' and may result in misplaced hairlines 20 or 30 years later. If a transplant is placed low at an early age, it may eventually appear unnatural. Young men with early hair loss (Norwood I & II) currently maintain enough hair for facial framing and will

FIVE BASIC CRITERIA FOR ASSESSING CANDIDATES FOR HAIR TRANSPLANTATION	
Age	Patients over the age of 25 years are preferable. While patients younger than 25 years of age often seek consultation, there is a hesitancy to operate. The predictive value of future hair loss is much lower for individuals between 15 and 25 years of age. Even with the theoretical safety net of finasteride, physicians should carefully choose candidates under 25 years of age. This subgroup also tends to desire a return to a full head of hair as opposed to a mature pattern of restoration that is routinely performed in older age groups
Hair shaft caliber	The caliber of the hair shaft is crucial. Those with large-caliber hair shafts (greater than 70 μm) obtain much denser coverage than individuals with corn silk quality hair. This can be demonstrated mathematically in that very small volume increases in hair shaft diameter result in exponential increases in surface area coverage
Donor hair	A variety of instruments are available to measure donor hair density. Measuring a 0.25 cm^2 field and multiplying by four is the preferred method. Patients seeking hair transplantation who have >80 follicular units/cm^2 are excellent candidates. Those with donor hair density <40 follicular units/cm^2 are considered poor candidates
Degree of baldness	The degree of baldness is perhaps the most important criterion in candidate selection. Those with complete baldness of the frontal scalp as opposed to baldness limited to the vertex are excellent candidates. When frontal baldness is corrected, this creates the most dramatic positive change in appearance
Hair color	Follicular unit grafting has made hair color less of an issue than when punch grafts were employed. Color contrast between hair and skin can make grafts apparent if not transplanted with great care. Individuals with 'salt-and-pepper' hair, red hair or blonde hair are preferential to those with jet-black hair. Black-haired individuals are not exempt as hair transplant candidates, but should receive only one-hair follicular units in the frontal hairline for the most natural result. Proper technique eliminates most problems with dark-haired candidates

Table 157.1 Five basic criteria for assessing candidates for hair transplantation.

RACIAL VARIATION IN FOLLICULAR UNITS IN THE OCCIPITAL SCALP				
Predominant hair	Caucasians	Asians*	Africans	Chinese
Follicular unit/mm^2	1	1	0.6	0.7
Average density (hairs/mm^2)	2	1.7	1.6	1.4
Predominant hair grouping	Two	Two	Three	Two

*Non-Chinese

Table 157.2 Racial variation in follicular units in the occipital scalp. Reproduced with permission from Tsai RY, Lee SH, Chan HL. The distribution of follicular units in the Chinese scalp: implications for reconstruction of natural-appearing hairlines in Orientals. Dermatol Surg. 2002; 28:500–3.

receive limited aesthetic benefit from surgery. This is also true of patients who are only seeking restoration in areas of thinning. Another consideration when planning a hair restoration procedure is that, due to the progression of MPB, patients can be left with an unnatural zone of baldness between transplanted hair and further recessions. Young individuals who obtain a restoration of their original low-lying hairline will seek corrective surgery later in life as they experience continual progression of androgenetic alopecia.

The Vertex

While some individuals desire full coverage from the vertex to the frontal scalp, this should be discouraged. The vertex is problematic, due to the consumption of an endless supply of donor tissue. There are two primary reasons for this excess, the first being a 360° progression of baldness, and the second, a central gravity pull that always leaves an area of scalp visible. Therefore, the illusion of density is seldom achieved in this area. When density is sufficient, the patient will risk a poor outcome later in life due to peripheral loss of non-transplanted hair. The vertex area does not become 'stable with time'; vertex baldness is a progressive process, and therefore the vertex should be approached with extreme caution. Statistical probability dictates that most individuals will face significant future vertex hair loss that will result in deformity and/or an unpleasant cosmetic outcome.

Female Pattern Alopecia

Women with female pattern alopecia experience hair loss in a different pattern than men (see Ch. 68); thus, the above discussion of the presence or absence of frontal baldness does not typically apply to women. Patterns of female hair loss do bear their own considerations in assessing the patient's qualifications as a candidate for hair restoration.

In female pattern hair loss, the most anterior segment of the frontal hairline is usually maintained. In its mildest form, female pattern alopecia may be noticeable only as a slight expansion of the central part. In its most severe form, it may present as diffuse, severe thinning of hair in all areas of the scalp (diffuse unpatterned alopecia). Women from either end of the clinical spectrum are poor surgical candidates.

Those with mild female pattern alopecia are not suitable surgical candidates since differences in pre-transplanted scalp versus post-transplanted scalp are difficult to appreciate. Those with diffuse unpatterned alopecia are also poor surgical candidates for the obvious reason that the entire scalp is affected; thus, the donor area is of limited value, as it is also susceptible to hair loss. The ideal women for hair transplantation are those with high-density donor hair and extensive hair loss or thinning of the frontal scalp. A frontal thinning pattern of less than 20 hairs/cm^2 is required to proceed with a recommendation for hair transplantation. Patients with greater than 20 hairs/cm^2 will receive only marginal improvement. Of note, in women, especially if there are other signs of possible hyperandrogenemia (e.g. hirsutism) or signs of virilization, hormonal evaluation is recommended, including measurement of circulating levels of free testosterone and DHEA-S.

TECHNICAL ASPECTS

The Natural Hairline

Younger patients always request a lower-than-appropriate hairline. Patients must be reminded that low hairlines placed on a 20-year-old look natural, but the same hairline looks unnatural on a 60-year-old. It is difficult to convince patients that they will eventually regret the placement of a low hairline. There are no surgeons today that can predict or even 'guesstimate' the degree of baldness in a 20-year-old male at age 60. Conservative approaches to hairline design are therefore mandatory. The hairline pattern must look natural for one's lifetime. As a general rule, the vast majority of hairlines will begin in a zone from 7 to 10 cm above the brow region. As physicians, we must provide the patient with what he needs and not necessarily what he desires for the moment. A natural hairline is not a line at all. A natural hairline is an irregular zone of one- and two-hair follicular units. A natural, non-transplanted hairline may appear to begin along a common, well-defined boundary, but upon close inspection will reveal undulations and a striking peninsula-like irregularity to the border (Fig. 157.7). Mimicking this natural irregularity is a challenge for hair restoration surgeons.

One-Session Technology

The goal of current hair transplantation techniques is to produce a one-session result. This goal can be achieved in a significant percentage of patients. In the early 2000s, the 1000- to 2000-graft session became the norm. The ability to produce acceptable density with follicular unit transplantation is largely dependent upon the number of follicular units transplanted per cm^2. Individuals with advanced baldness, i.e. Norwood stage VI or VII, will require placement of transplants into a bald area measuring at least 50 cm^2 in order to achieve facial framing. Surgical

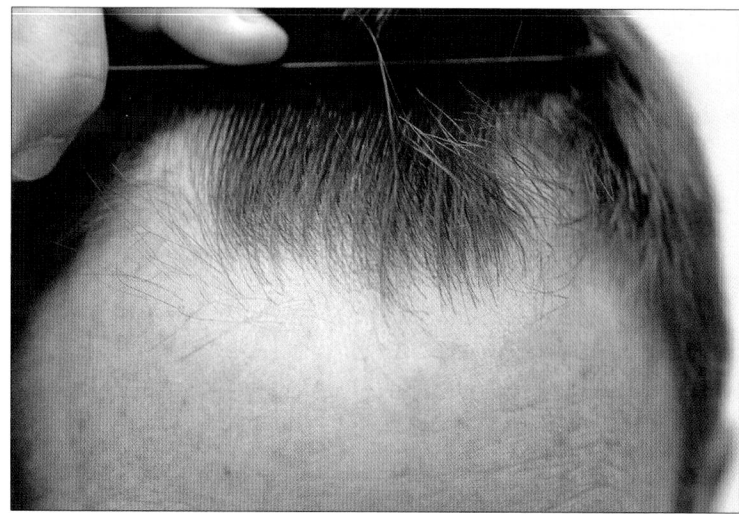

Fig. 157.7 The natural hairline. The photograph shows the natural hairline of a 32-year-old Caucasian man.

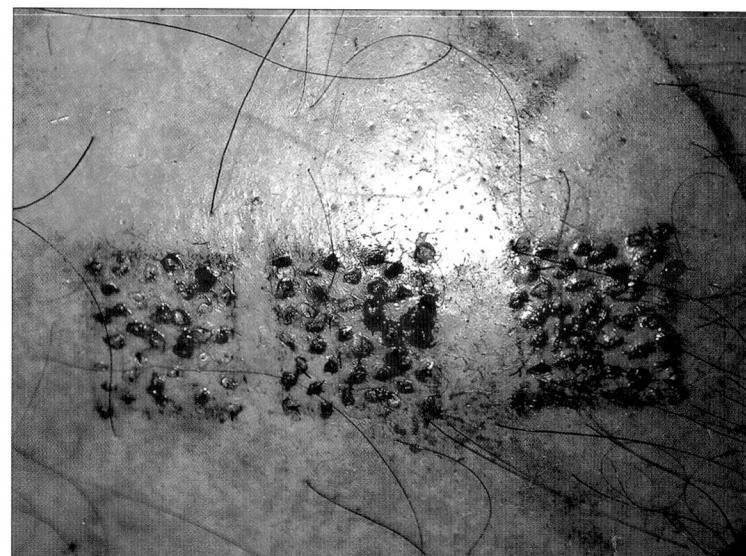

Fig. 157.8 Follicular unit count per cm². The photograph demonstrates the differences between 35, 40 and 45 follicular units/cm² (left to right).

teams previously sought to transplant follicular units into bald recipient zones at densities of 20 units/cm². With these densities, acceptable one-session results can occasionally be achieved, but this is the exception. When follicular unit counts edged to over 30 units/cm² in the early 2000s, one-session results became routine. Experienced transplant teams can expect significant coverage in one to two sessions. This is achieved by producing an average density of 37 follicular units/cm² within a recipient area of about 80 cm². In most patients, an area of 80 cm² covers the frontal third of the scalp. In the average candidate with 75 μm-width hair and baldness involving the frontal half of the scalp, one to two sessions should be adequate for an acceptable result. There are no published norms for single-session follicular unit density, but more than 30 follicular units/cm² has now become the standard most surgeons strive to attain. This goal is not easy to achieve, but is realistic with the use of a 20-gauge needle for recipient site creation. A 1 cm² template drawn onto a bald scalp by a temporary marker will accurately provide a follicular unit count per cm² (Fig. 157.8).

Maximizing Recipient Density

There are sound arguments for maximizing the recipient site density in a single session. One can hypothesize that 'microscarring' forms after each session of hair transplantation. This scarring impairs the vascularity of the area transplanted, reducing the blood supply available to grafts. This hypothesis implies that better growth may be obtained by planting 100 grafts into a given 'virgin' area in one session than by planting 50 grafts into the same-sized area in two separate sessions. Almost all transplant surgeons routinely report superior growth following the first

session of transplants compared to subsequent sessions. This supports the hypothesis that scarring or other effects of previous surgery have a detrimental effect on further sessions. Patient convenience and cost are other legitimate reasons multiple sessions are less appealing than a single session (Fig. 157.9).

Size of Sessions

If the average donor strip width is kept to less than 1.2 cm, then sessions are usually limited to approximately 3000 grafts or less. Donor scalp of average density rarely yields more than an average of 100 follicular units/cm², and removing a strip of tissue greater than 30 cm in length at one time can prove to be problematic. Limited donor area length, increased tension, bleeding, and postoperative pain are some of the problems encountered with a strip extended beyond 30 cm. It is advisable to position the anterior ends of the donor incision posterior to the superficial temporal arteries (see Ch. 142), which in most patients limits the donor strip to a length less than 30 cm.

It generally takes 8 to 12 hours to transplant 3000 grafts in one session, utilizing a staff of five technicians. Sessions of 1500 grafts can be achieved in 5 to 7 hours by a staff of five technicians. These time-frames, however, are illustrative of average cases, and the pace of the procedure is secondary compared to the quality of the work. The number of hairs transferred can be roughly estimated from the number of grafts. For example, individuals with 1000 predominantly two-hair grafts will receive 2000 hairs, while those with an average of 2.5 hairs

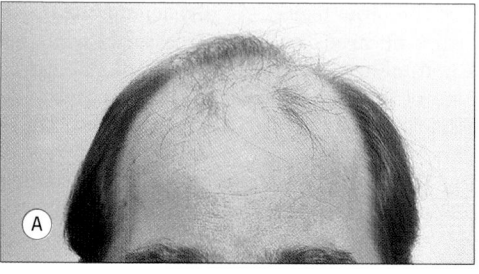
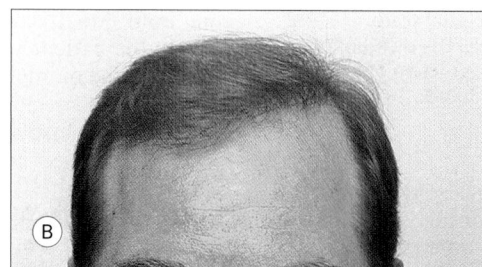
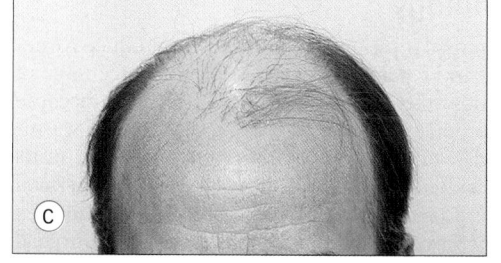
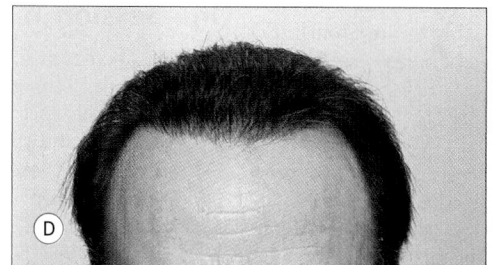

Fig. 157.9 Maximizing recipient density. Before (**A, C**) and after (**B, D**) photographs of patients following a single transplant session.

per follicular unit would receive 5000 hairs in a 2000-graft session. A hair densitometer or any hand-held magnification device enables quick assessment of the number of one-, two-, three- or four-hair follicular units, allowing an estimation of the number of hairs to be transferred prior to donor strip removal.

Donor Strip Harvesting

Most surgeons favor taking a single elliptical donor strip from the occipital scalp that ranges in width from 7 mm to 1.2 cm. This must be determined prior to surgery. In patients with average density, a strip of tissue 20 cm long by 7 mm wide will yield over 1000 follicular units. Likewise, a strip of tissue 11 cm long by 1 cm wide will yield approximately 1000 follicular units. Each case must be individualized based on donor tissue laxity, donor tissue density, and previous scars. The more laxity present, the wider the harvested donor strip can be. Likewise, the greater the donor area density, the shorter the donor strip length required. Previous scars may necessitate a decreased width due to tension.

Prior to surgery, 15 cm³ of 0.5% lidocaine with 1:200 000 epinephrine is administered to the donor area. This is followed by 10 cm³ of 0.2% ropivacaine HCl. Immediately before excising the area, 20 cm³ of saline solution is injected to create dermal turgor. We utilize 3 cm³ syringes to administer this saline. Syringes larger than 3 cm³ cannot achieve firm tumescence of the occipital area, which assists in minimizing follicular unit transection.

The goal of donor strip removal is to minimize transection of hair follicles during this harvesting phase (transection is also avoided during the dissection phase). Using an elliptical incision with a double blade, one scores the surface of the scalp, being careful not to extend beyond 1 mm in depth. The double-bladed knife can be used as a template to insure uniform width of the donor strip. After scoring the epidermis, the removal is completed with a single #10 surgical blade. One donor dissection utilizes four skin hooks exerting tension away from the incision, with the blade being held parallel to the patient's hair follicles. The scalpel blade is then inserted approximately 5 mm into the scalp, enough to reach a depth of 1–2 mm below the terminus of the hair follicles. The strip of tissue is tapered into an elliptical pattern and cut from the base using scissors. Hemostasis is obtained with cautery or, rarely, ligation with sutures. The preferred method of wound closure is with surgical staples (Fig. 157.10).

Graft Dissection

Once the donor tissue is harvested, the strip is immediately placed into a Petri dish containing chilled isotonic saline, where it is kept until dissection. Technicians subsection the elliptical donor tissue into slivers, each approximately 2 mm in width (Fig. 157.11). Considerable skill and experience is required to avoid transection during slivering. Each sliver is further dissected into follicular unit grafts with a surgical razor blade or #10 surgical blade, using backlighting and microscopic magnification. Grafts are observed and separated into those containing one, two, three, or more hairs per follicular unit. The follicular unit grafts are then placed back into chilled isotonic saline (Fig. 157.12). It is imperative these grafts stay cool and moist in order for them to maintain their viability. The benefits of hair in a complete non-transected state are controversial. There is evidence that transected hairs will grow, but these hairs have been found to have a decreased diameter.

Anesthesia

The recipient scalp is anesthetized in preparation for creating the incisions for graft placement. The authors routinely perform a bilateral supraorbital nerve block, which produces anesthesia of the midfrontal portion of the scalp. The nerve blocks are achieved by infiltrating initially with buffered 0.5% lidocaine, followed by 0.2% ropivacaine HCl.

Fifteen to 30 minutes before making the incisions, the area is injected with a saline and epinephrine mixture at a concentration of 1:80 000.

THE RECIPIENT SITE

Success in densely packing follicular units is dependent upon small recipient sites. This necessitates using a rectangular blade varying from

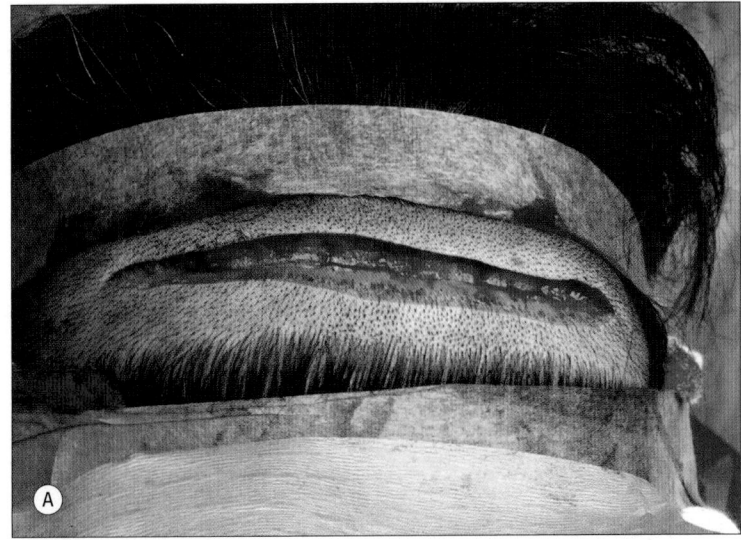

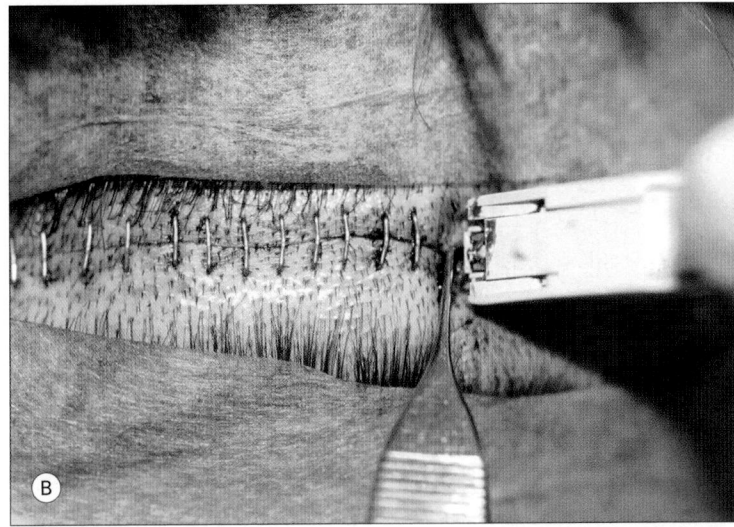

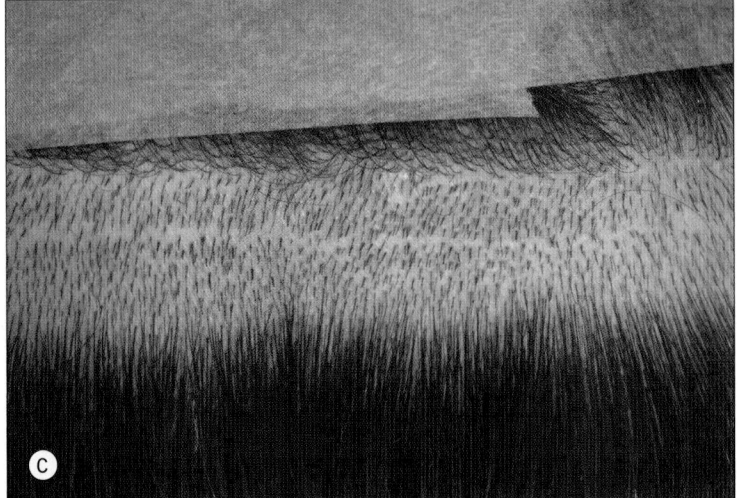

Fig. 157.10 Donor strip harvesting. A The donor strip prior to closure. **B** The donor area closure with staples. **C** A single linear scar 1–2 mm in width is common.

0.7 to 1 mm in size. Alternatively, a 20-gauge needle can be used. Using needles of this small gauge negates any removal of recipient tissue. Some studies have demonstrated that placing over 40 follicular units/cm² results in less than optimal growth. Most of these studies, however, have used 18-gauge needles.

The density of placement varies from case to case due to existing recipient site hair, tissue characteristics, vascularity, and graft size. Angulation is defined as the angle of insertion of the needle into the recipient scalp. A sharp angle of insertion, i.e. less than 20°, is favorable

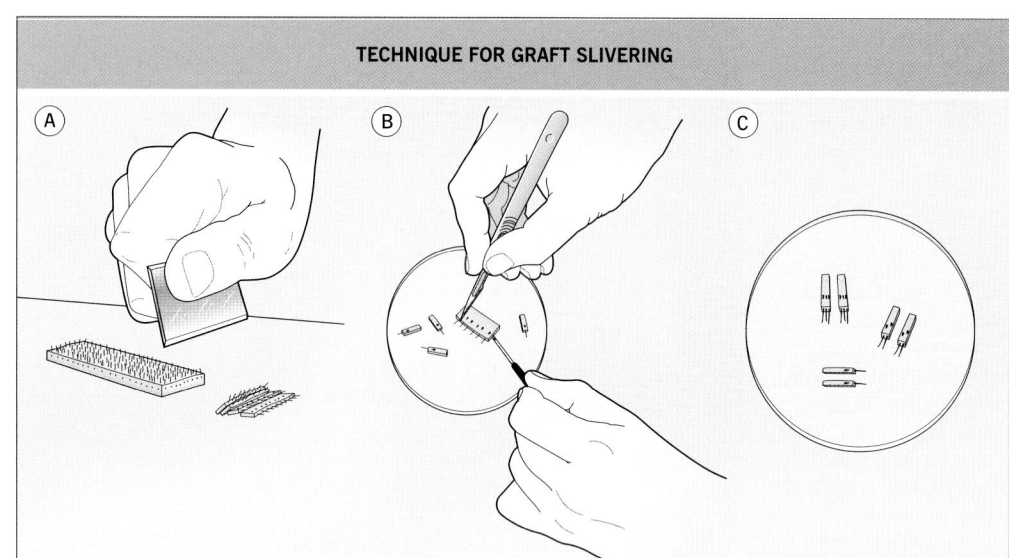

Fig. 157.11 Technique for graft slivering. A Donor slivering producing slivers 2 mm wide by 10 mm long. **B** Slivers being sectioned into follicular units. **C** Follicular unit grafts are placed into dish with saline and separated into one-, two- and three-haired follicular units. **D** A portion of donor strip prior to slivering. **E** Appearance of a sliver. **F** A single follicular unit produced by microscopic dissection of a sliver.

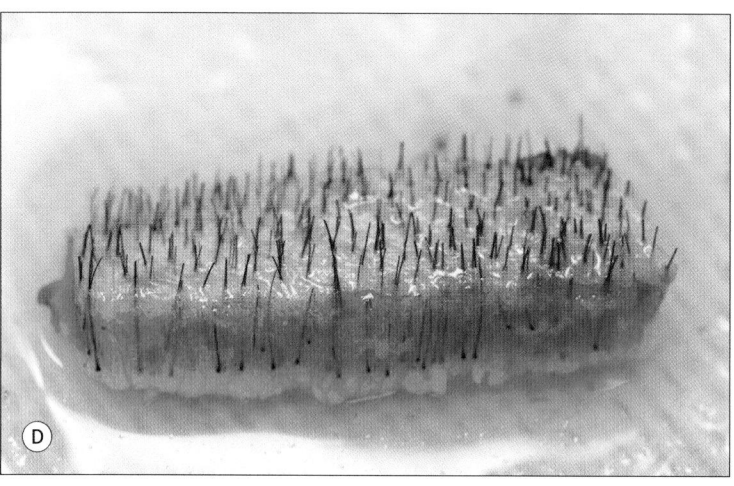

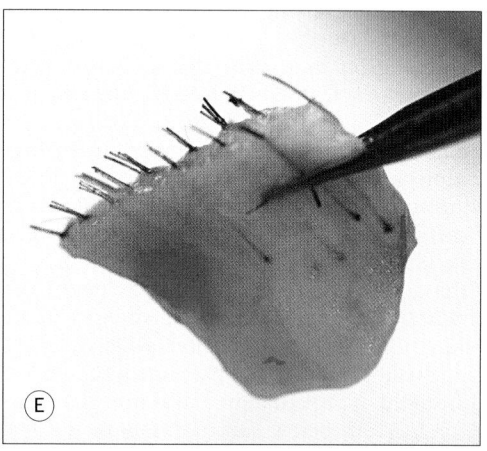

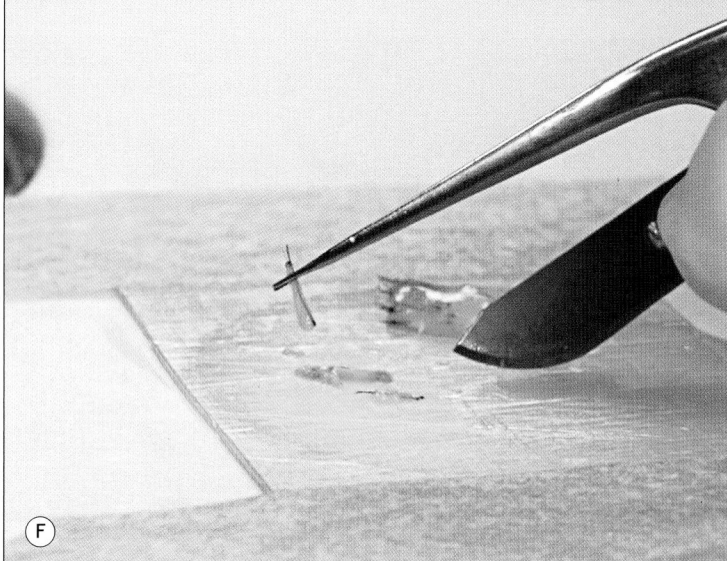

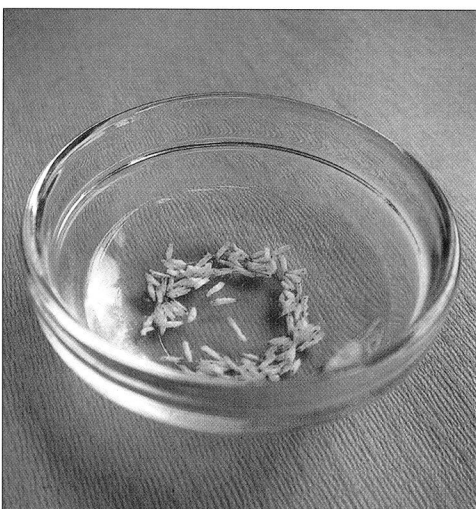

Fig. 157.12 Follicular unit grafts. They are stored in isotonic saline to maintain their viability.

in the anterior hairline. Larger angles (20°–45°) can be used more posteriorly. Dense packing techniques require skillful graft creation and placement, which can only be achieved by experienced technicians. One surgeon inserting all the grafts would be inefficient and offers no benefit to the patient. Thus, a rotating team of well-trained technicians is standard practice.

Insertion Phase

Placing 40 grafts/cm² into 20-gauge-sized sites without excessive trauma to the grafts is achieved by the 'stick and place' method of

planting. The hypodermic needle used to make the recipient site is first used as a dilator; then, as the needle is being withdrawn, it is used to help guide the graft into the minute recipient tunnel. The same technician that makes the site plants the site. Two technicians can work simultaneously in the stick and place method. Each technician works independently of the other in separate areas. In the separated needle stick and graft placement technique, the surgeon has complete control of graft positioning. The surgeon dictates the spacing and angle by recipient site creation. The technicians then insert all the grafts. A modified approach is one in which the physician makes the site and the technician places the grafts, but the technician then simultaneously

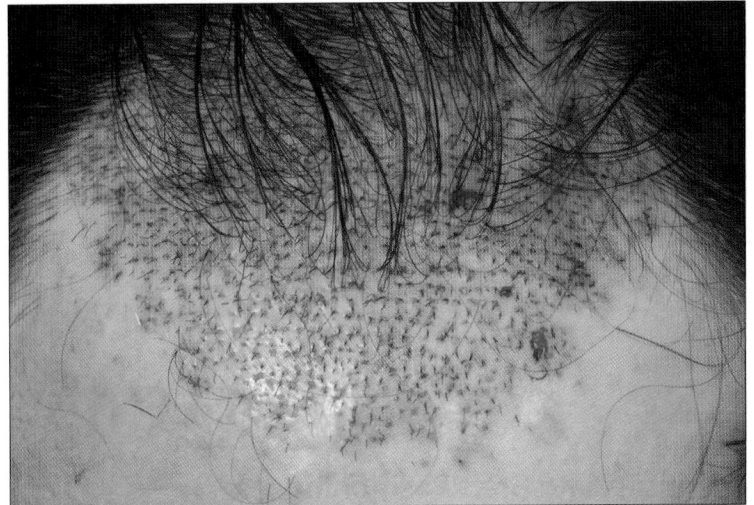

Fig. 157.13 Immediate postoperative photograph demonstrating graft placement and hairline design.

makes additional sites as needed. This is a hybrid of the two methods and can routinely achieve a density of over 30 grafts/cm² in the recipient site (Fig.157.13).

When the angled needle is inserted anterior to existing grafts, compression and popping are minimized. Therefore, planting with a back to front pattern is superior. This results in less displacement, because the graft is pushed against the back wall.

Nuances

The most important factors for successful follicular unit transplantation are: the need for binocular stereoscopic microscopic dissection, skillful atraumatic graft planting, and, above all, the need to keep the grafts completely moist. The latter is by far the most important factor influencing the success of follicular unit transplantation. Partial drying of grafts is the most common reason practitioners are unable to achieve adequate growth from follicular unit transplantation, despite otherwise immaculate technique. The authors advocate total immersion of grafts in saline and believe that drying of grafts even for brief periods (less than 1 minute) is detrimental to survival. Binocular stereoscopic microscopic dissection has become the standard for slivering an intact donor strip. Other methods without magnification can be used, but the transection rates are higher. Growth yield may be affected.

Postoperative

Immediately after hair restoration surgery, the surgeon should supply the patient with instructions on wound care and permissible activities. The patients usually will need approximately 3 days of recovery before the redness and crusting of the scalp resolve. Postoperative explanations are crucial, and compliance is important for the ultimate outcome. Table 157.3 is a summary of the postoperative instructions unique to hair transplantation.

Complications

Possible complications following a procedure include:
- nausea and vomiting caused by medication
- postoperative bleeding (less than 0.5%)
- infection (less than 0.5%)
- excessive swelling (5%)
- temporary headache
- temporary numbness of the scalp
- abnormal scarring around the grafts (less than 1%)
- poor growth of grafts
- fainting (less than 1%)
- folliculitis
- keloid formation
- neuroma
- persistent scalp pain

POSTOPERATIVE INSTRUCTIONS
Following your transplant, relax the rest of the day. Do not get hot. No heavy lifting or strenuous exercise for at least 5 days. Do not lean over to tie shoes or pick up objects from the floor for the first 48 hours. These all could initiate bleeding
Do not drink alcoholic beverages for 2 days following your transplant
Sleep with your head elevated for one or two nights following your procedure
Following your daily shampoo, apply bacitracin–polymyxin ointment* to each graft and the donor area using a Q-tip or clean fingertips
Apply bacitracin–polymyxin ointment* to the grafts for approximately 3 to 4 days and to the donor area every day until your staples are removed
Crusts (scabs) will form over the transplant sites and solidify over the first few days. These crusts will naturally fall off within 2 weeks. Do not pick or scratch at these crusts at any time
Surgical staples in the donor area should be removed by 7 days after the procedure. We will provide you with a staple remover
Wait for at least 2 weeks after the procedure before wearing a hairpiece

If you have a history of itching or redness following application of bacitracin or bacitracin–polymyxin ointment, please let us know.

Table 157.3 Postoperative instructions. Special considerations following hair transplantation surgery.

- telogen effluvium
- arteriovenous fistula formation.

Ergonomics

There are practical difficulties, pertaining to staff, associated with 'megasessions'. In addition to the extra recruitment and training, there is the problem of maintaining staff for the prolonged hours required during large graft sessions. Planting for many hours on a daily basis can and does lead to physical ailments, such as repetitive strain syndrome. To combat this, close attention must be paid to ergonomics. For instance, it is important that planters position their elbows or forearms on a firm, supportive surface while using wrist and finger movements. If the planters have to support the entire weight of their arms throughout their planting, they will often develop muscle fatigue in their neck, shoulders and forearms. The staff should also rotate duties; that is, after a certain interval of planting, they should do some other type of work, such as cutting grafts or administrative work, prior to returning to graft placement. They must have frequent relaxation breaks, and they must do regular stretching exercises at least every hour during their planting and cutting of grafts.

HAIR REPAIR

A critical facet to any modern hair restoration surgery practice lies in addressing problems stemming from previously performed hair restoration surgery. This is a crucial component of the hair restoration industry, given the refinements in surgical technique that have evolved. In earlier days of hair restoration surgery, it was common to see patients managed entirely with the use of large round grafts. At the time, this represented state-of-the-art surgical work; however, this now-antiquated practice has left generations of hair transplant recipients with results that are often more detrimental than helpful to their overall cosmetic appearance. The implications of this practice are far-reaching, having affected the image of the entire field of hair restoration surgery. Terms such as 'plugs', 'cornrows' and 'Barbie-doll' are often used to describe the appearance of hair transplants from the 60s, 70s and 80s. The hair transplant community has suffered and continues to suffer from the public's perception of hair transplantation that was formulated over the course of those decades. Fortunately, follicular unit grafting affords the hair industry an opportunity to undo some of this unnatural, obvious early restoration. Changing the public perception of hair transplantation remains a major goal for the specialty, especially with regard to advances made in hair repair surgery.

Donor Site Repair

Scarring of the donor area is a common complaint of those presenting for hair repair surgery. Older graft harvesting methods consisted of punch harvesting donor hair using trephines of varying diameter. The resulting circular wounds were usually left to granulate, leaving hundreds of white circular scars in the occiput and parietal scalp. This 'shotgun' harvest technique is frequently seen as a source of patient dissatisfaction. When it is encountered in the setting of an individual desiring further grafting, partial redress of the problem can be achieved with a linear strip harvesting technique that removes some of the circular scarring. Removing a linear strip of tissue consisting of two rows of scars flanking a single strip of intact hair allows for maximum removal of scar during strip harvesting. It is important to ensure there is enough tissue laxity to allow for closure of the strip with minimal tension, in order for this to be effective.

Scar Widening

Linear graft harvesting techniques can occasionally result in undesirably wide donor scars. It is important to understand that there is a strong opinion in the hair transplantation literature that revisions of these donor scars are often unsuccessful. Even with flawless surgical technique, buried sutures, extensive undermining and closure under no tension, many experienced and skilled surgeons report widening of the revised scars to the same or an even greater degree than that of the original scar. The use of tissue expansion may improve chances for successful revision, but this option is seldom utilized.

To minimize scarring of the donor area, always inquire regarding a history of keloidal scarring or Ehlers–Danlos syndrome. Both subsets of patients should obviously be approached with caution. Those with the latter tend to develop widened scars regardless of surgical technique. It is the authors' experience that persons with dark hair and fair skin (Fitzpatrick types I and II) may be more susceptible to apparent, broad scars. This statement is based upon observations from clinical experience, but we are unaware of scientific evidence that would provide an adequate explanation. Scar width is directly related to the width of the donor strip. Strip harvesting in individuals with a tendency towards wide scars should be limited to a width of 1 cm or less. This has almost completely alleviated the problem of donor scar widening in the authors' practice.

Recipient Site Repair

True repair work in the recipient area is required when there has been inappropriate positioning of grafts (regardless of size) or use of grafts too large in size (4–5-mm plugs). When individuals with large round grafts present for hair repair, either hair may be removed or, in some cases, follicular unit grafts can be placed in front of and between large grafts. Repair surgery that utilizes only follicular unit transplants should be reserved for those with good skin-to-hair color match and hair positioned in such a way that transplanting around it will not result in further cosmetic detriment. An example of where follicular unit grafting alone would fail to camouflage previously placed large grafts would be their use in trying to conceal an inappropriately low hairline. The majority of the time, a combination of hair removal and retransplantation is necessary to achieve repair in patients in whom grafts of large sizes have resulted in deformity.

As a general rule when dealing with unacceptably large graft sizes, the greater the contrast between hair color and scalp color, the greater the chance that hair will need to be removed to achieve an acceptable restoration. Through hair removal, hair in unnatural clumps or locations is deleted or thinned, thus providing a more natural appearance. Techniques for removal include surgery, laser and electrolysis. Laser hair removal is seldom permanent and should be considered a temporary solution for graft removal. Electrolysis is effective at thinning hair within punch grafts; however, this technique results in scarring and hypopigmentation. Our preferred method involves removal of round grafts using frontal elliptical reductions of the existing punch grafts. This method involves an 'en bloc' removal of all anteriorly situated grafts.

Punch removal is utilized when isolated areas require removal. Resulting wounds are sutured or stapled. Follicular unit grafts are subsequently dissected from the excised round grafts. These 'recycled' grafts are used in front of, behind, and around the remaining round grafts. In this manner, hair is not wasted. Recycled hair from old round grafts can be used to reinforce or create new hairlines, make remaining round grafts less conspicuous, or add density in areas of ensuing alopecia.

Punch Excision

Hair regrowth following the removal of unwanted standard round autografts can be a bothersome problem. Where possible, strip excision of round grafts is preferred over punch excision. Strip excision is more effective, with less incidence of regrowth. If punch excision of round grafts is performed, the use of a punch trephine larger in diameter than the graft to be removed is necessary to prevent regrowth. It is crucial to orient such trephines parallel to the anticipated direction of hair growth.

Inappropriate Graft Positioning

It is important to understand that, regardless of graft size, inappropriately positioned grafts may become problematic. Certainly, examples of this are striking when large round grafts have been used to create a hairline that is too low. However, any-sized grafts used for a crown restoration that has subsequently become isolated due to progression of alopecia will require additional surgery or removal. Even follicular unit transplantation can result in the need for reparative surgery if follicular unit grafts were poorly positioned. In instances of poor graft positioning, repair hinges upon successful removal of malpositioned hair. The same techniques as described previously, with or without recycling of the hair within the follicular units, are used.

Those performing hair restoration surgery should be skilled in the art of hair repair. Persons seeking corrective hair surgery have often endured suboptimal surgery, counseling, or both. Such individuals must always be treated with sensitivity, and each case must be carefully considered prior to embarking on surgical repair. For a successful remedy, each patient must be handled individually.

Scalp Reduction

A scalp reduction is simply an excision of bald scalp. With this technique, hair-bearing skin is brought closer together by removing the center scalp affected by alopecia. There are many different designs employed for the excision of the balding area. Reductions may be performed in conjunction with hair transplantation for the remaining bald scalp; when combined, these two techniques allow for a complete hair restoration. Scalp reductions are seldom employed nowadays, yet a few surgeons remain strong advocates of the procedure.

One problem arising after a scalp reduction is that, with the passage of time, excision scars become noticeable. Usually more than one scalp reduction is necessary to effectively address a person's baldness. This problem may be lessened when individuals are also treated with finasteride. Although scalp reductions are a solution to baldness, their efficacy diminishes over time due to the unpredictable progression of hair loss in any given individual. Resurgence of this technique depends in part upon scarring being adequately concealed and ongoing progression of baldness being arrested by medical therapy.

SUMMARY

One must remember that alopecia progression may impart a desire for further hair restoration procedures. Recessions along the parietal and temporal scalp which result in the isolation of transplanted hair represent one of the most common situations warranting subsequent treatment. Careful planning and appropriate candidate selection will lead to results that withstand the test of time.

Follicular unit hair transplantation surgery, when performed with future hair loss and the patient's own hair characteristics in mind, offers patients an alternative that appears natural. It is important to note that many patients transplanted in the 1990s have results that mimic nature so closely that their spouses and even hairstylists are unaware a hair transplant procedure has been performed. The standard of hair restoration for the 2000s is to achieve this degree of naturalness in a single session (Figs 157.14 & 157.15).

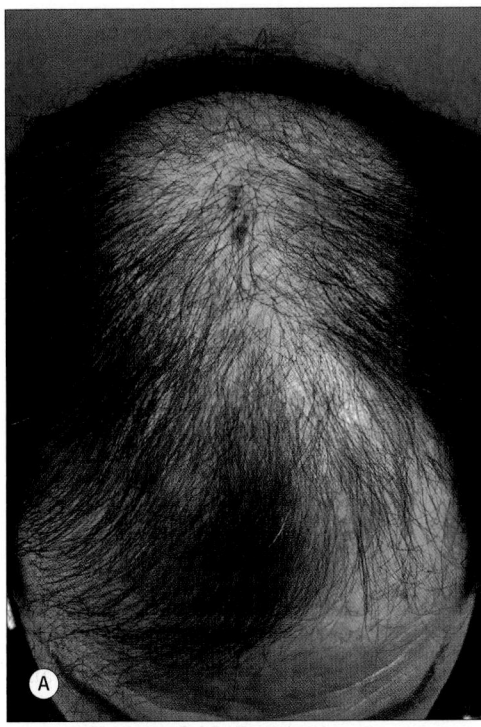

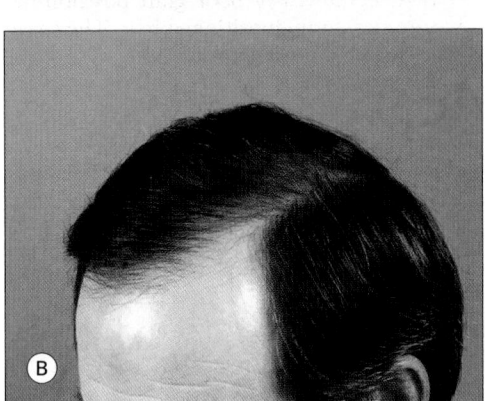

Fig. 157.14 A 40-year-old man with Norwood IV pattern alopecia. The patient underwent a total of 2500 grafts; his vertex was not transplanted. This patient's hairline was started 3 years prior to its completion.

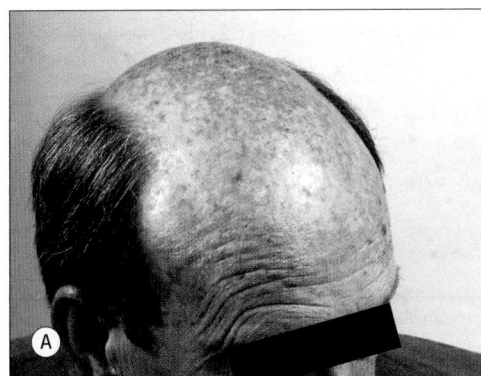

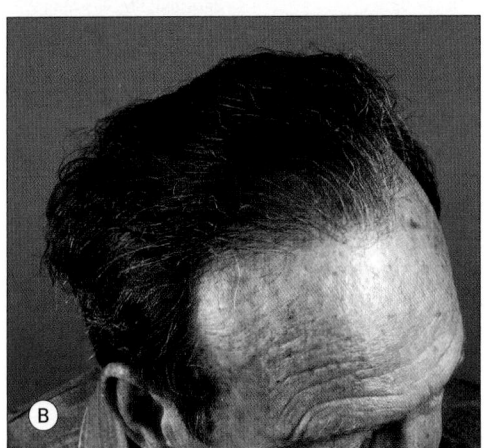

Fig. 157.15 A 62-year-old man with Norwood VI pattern alopecia. The same patient is shown before (**A**) and after (**B**) receiving 3500 grafts. The final hairline was deliberately made irregular with a 2 cm feathering zone.

FURTHER READING

Baden HP. Diseases of the Hair and Nails. London: Year Book Medical, 1987.

Brandy DA. A technique for hair-grafting in between existing follicles in patients with early pattern baldness. Dermatol Surg. 2000;26:801–5.

Camacho FM, Randall VA, Price VH. Hair and Its Disorders – Biology, Pathology and Management. London: Martin Dunitz, 2000.

Cash TF. The psychosocial consequences of androgenetic alopecia: a review of the research literature. Br J Dermatol. 1999;141:398–405.

Cather JC, Lane D, Heaphy MR Jr, et al. Finasteride – an update and review. Dermatol Surg. 1999;64:167–71.

Commo S, Gaillard O, Bernard BA. The human hair follicle contains two distinct k19 positive compartments in the outer root sheath: a unifying hypothesis for stem cell reservoir? Differentiation. 2000;66:157–64.

D'Amico AV, Roehrborn CG. Effect of 1 mg/day finasteride on concentrations of serum prostate-specific antigen in men with androgenetic alopecia; a randomised controlled trial. Lancet Oncol. 2007;8:21–5.

Dawber R, Van Neste D. Hair and Scalp Disorders – Common Presenting Signs, Differential Diagnosis and Treatment. Philadelphia: Martin Dunitz, 1995.

Diani AR, Mulholland MJ, Shull KL, et al. Hair growth effects of oral administration of finasteride, a steroid 5α-reductase inhibitor, alone and in combination with topical minoxidil in the balding stumptail macaque. J Clin Endocrinol Metab. 1992;74:345–50.

Dzubow LM. A redefinition of male pattern baldness and its treatment. Yale University/Glaxo Dermatology Lectureship Series in Dermatology, 1995.

Guess HA, Gormley GJ, Stoner E, et al. The effect of finasteride on prostate specific antigen: review of data. J Urol. 1996;155:3–9.

Headington JT. Telogen effluvium: new concepts and review. Arch Dermatol. 1993;129:356–63.

Kaplan SA, Holtgrewe HL, Bruskewitz R, et al. Comparison of the efficacy and safety of finasteride in older versus younger men with benign prostatic hyperplasia. Urology. 2001;57:1073–7.

Kaufman KD, Olsen EA, Whiting D, et al. Finasteride in the treatment of men with androgenetic alopecia. Finasteride Male Pattern Hair Loss Study Group. J Am Acad Dermatol. 1998;39:578–89.

Limmer BL. Elliptical donor stereoscopically assisted micrografting as an approach to further refinement in hair transplantation. J Dermatol Surg Oncol. 1994;20:789–93.

Ludwig E. Classification of the types of androgenetic alopecia (common baldness) occurring in the female sex. Br J Dermatol. 1977;97:247–54.

Matzkin H, Barak M, Braf Z. Effect of finasteride on free and total serum prostate-specific antigen in men with benign prostatic hyperplasia. Br J Urol. 1996;78:405–8.

Norwood OT. Male pattern baldness: classification and incidence. South Med J. 1975;68:1359–65.

Olsen EA (ed). Disorders of Hair Growth: Diagnosis and Treatment. New York: McGraw-Hill, 1993:257–83.

Orentreich DS. The history of hair restoration surgery. In: Stough DB, Haber B (eds). Hair Replacement: Surgical and Medical. St Louis: Mosby Year Book, 1996:50–62.

Overstreet JW, Fuh VL, Gould J, et al. Chronic treatment with finasteride daily does not affect spermatogenesis or semen production in young men. J Urol. 1999;162:1295–300.

Price VH. Treatment of hair loss. N Engl J Med. 1999;341:964–73.

Price VH, Menefee E. Quantitative estimation of hair growth I. Androgenetic alopecia in women: effect of minoxidil. J Invest Dermatol. 1990;5:683–7.

Price VH, Menefee E, Strauss PC. Changes in hair weight and hair count in men with androgenetic alopecia after application of 5% and 2% topical minoxidil, placebo, or no treatment. J Am Acad Dermatol. 1999;41:717–21.

Price VH, Roberts JL, Hordinsky M, et al. Lack of efficacy of finasteride in postmenopausal women with androgenetic alopecia. J Am Acad Dermatol. 2000;43:768–76.

Rassman WR. Technique – small graft hair transplantation. In: Stough D, Haber R (eds). Hair Replacement: Surgical and Medical. St Louis: Mosby Year Book, 1996.

Roenigk RK, Roenigk HH Jr. Roenigk & Roenigk's Dermatologic Surgery, Principles and Practice, 2nd edn. New York: Marcel Dekker, 1996:1211–12.

Rook A, Dawber R. Diseases of the Hair and Scalp, 2nd edn. Oxford: Blackwell Scientific, 1991.

Staughton RCD. The Color Atlas of Hair and Scalp Disorders. London: RCD Staughton and Wolfe Publishing, 1988.

Stough D, Haber R. Hair Replacement: Surgical and Medical. St Louis: Mosby Year Book, 1996.

Stough D, Whitworth J. Methodology of follicular unit hair transplantation. Hair restoration and laser hair removal. Dermatol Clin. 1999;17:297–306.

Unger WP. Hair Transplantation, 3rd edn. New York: Marcel Dekker, 1995.

Unger WP. The history of hair transplantation. Hair Transplant Forum Int. 2000;10:97–108.

Van Neste D, Fuh V, Sanchez-Pedreno P, et al. Finasteride increases anagen hair in men with androgenetic alopecia. Br J Dermatol. 2000;143:804–10.

Whiting DA. Diagnostic and predictive value of horizontal sections of scalp specimens in male pattern androgenetic alopecia. J Am Acad Dermatol. 1993;29:554.

Whiting DA. Chronic telogen effluvium: increased scalp hair shedding in middle-aged women. J Am Acad Dermatol. 1996;35:899–906.

Whiting DA, Howsden FL. Color Atlas of Differential Diagnosis of Hair Loss. London: Canfield Publishing, 1996.

Whitworth JM, Stough DB, Limmer B, et al. A comparison of graft implantation techniques for hair transplantation. Semin Cutan Med Surg. 1999;18:177-83.

Repair

Avram M. Management of widened donor scars. Hair Transplant Forum Int. 2002;12:116.

Epstein E. Management of widened donor scars. Hair Transplant Forum Int. 2002;12:116.

Kabaker S. Management of widened donor scars. Hair Transplant Forum Int. 2002;12:116.

Leavitt ML. Corrective hair restoration. In: Stough DB, Haber RS (eds). Hair Replacement: Surgical and Medical. St Louis: Mosby Year Book, 1996:306–13.

Mangubat T. Management of widened donor scars. Hair Transplant Forum Int. 2002;12:116.

Puig C. Management of widened donor scars. Hair Transplant Forum Int. 2002;12:116.

Shiell R. Management of widened donor scars. Hair Transplant Forum Int. 2002;12:116.

Swinehart J. Hair repair surgery. Dermatol Surg. 1999;25:523–9.

History

Bernstein RM, Rassman WR. Follicular transplantation: patient evaluation and surgical planning. Dermatol Surg. 1997;23:771–84.

Bernstein RM, Rassman WR. The aesthetics of follicular transplantation. Dermatol Surg. 1997;23:785–99.

Limmer BL. Elliptical donor harvesting. In: Stough DB, Haber RS (eds). Hair Replacement: Surgical and Medical. St Louis: Mosby Year Book, 1996:142–7.

Okuda S. Clinical and experimental studies of transplantation of living hairs. Jpn J Dermatol. 1929;46:135–8.

Orentreich N. Autografts in alopecias and other selected dermatological conditions. Ann NY Acad Sci. 1959;83:463.

Reed W. Rethinking some cornerstones of hair transplantation. Hair Transplant Forum Int. 1999;9:133,138–9.

Tamura H. Pubic hair transplantation. Jpn J Dermatol. 1943;53:76.

Unger WP. Commentary on: Follicular transplantation by Bernstein and Rassman. Dermatol Surg. 1997; 23:801–5.

Unger WP. The history of hair transplantation. Dermatol Surg. 2000;26:181–9.

Soft Tissue Augmentation

158

Seth L Matarasso and Neil S Sadick

Key features

- Filler substances are used to smooth and even out superficial wrinkles and deep folds of the face
- Other indications include atrophic, traumatic, and acne scars; lip augmentation; and loss of subcutaneous fat
- Agents include autologous fat grafts, collagen xenografts from bovine collagen, hyaluronic acid derivatives and synthetic materials
- Selection of an agent depends on the size, depth and location of the defect
- Agents are injected into the dermis or subcutaneous fat by serial puncture or single-entry techniques
- Filler substances can be used as monotherapy or as an adjunct to other rejuvenating injectable techniques or surgical procedures
- Complications are technique-dependent or material-related, and include hypersensitivity reactions, granuloma formation, contour irregularities and vascular occlusion

Interventions for the aging face can be broadly categorized into the four "R's" of facial rejuvenation: Resurfacing (chemical peels, dermabrasion, and ablative and non-ablative lasers); Recontouring (the various facial surgical procedures); Relaxing (chemodenervation with paralytic agents); and Replacement with soft tissue augmentation. Replacement of lost or atrophic subcutaneous tissue with filling agents has recently witnessed a truly remarkable growth. Technology has also kept pace with patient demand for safe and effective dermal fillers and the menu of available agents for soft tissue augmentation has exponentially increased.

Patients often do not adequately appreciate the nature of their defect, and must first be educated about the underlying anatomy of a 'wrinkle'. The distinction must be made between dynamic versus static lines and those changes due to external photodamage as opposed to those secondary to chronology and gravitational pull (Table 158.1). Although these defects often appear in combination, their treatment does require individual assessment. Patients need to be aware of newer, commercially available injectable products. Many of these newer products have different inherent characteristics and indications that may have supplanted traditional agents already familiar to patients.

While the type of defect is clearly important, so, too, are its size, depth and location, as well as the appearance and integrity of the adjacent tissue (Table 158.2). A discussion regarding therapeutic options should include the alternatives of surgery (rhytidectomy, excision punch grafting, etc.), resurfacing (Ch. 137) and chemodenervation agents (botulinum toxin, Ch. 159), as well as no intervention at all. Patients should have an adequate comprehension of the indications and technique, advantages and disadvantages, and inherent risks of each procedure, with an estimation of the financial cost and recuperation time. As with any treatment, the success is largely proportional to the extent of realistic and appropriate goals and expectations set by both the physician and the patient. Patients undergoing elective rhytid effacement with soft tissue augmentation must realize that replacing lost or atrophic subcutaneous tissue is often temporary (Table 158.3). Monotherapy with one agent may not be adequate and multiple agents may be required. All wrinkles are not created equally; they come in many shapes and sizes, and, as such, there is no one filler agent that is suitable for all defects. The choice of an appropriate dermal or subcutaneous implant – whether temporary or permanent or liquid, semi-solid or solid – requires knowledge of the available materials and their characteristics.

CAUSES OF CUTANEOUS DEFECTS

Chronologic aging

- Loss of subcutaneous fat
- Gravity

Photodamage

- Breakdown of collagen and elastin
- Neoplastic changes

Trauma

- Disease
- Inflammation
- Surgery

Table 158.1 Causes of cutaneous defects.

SOFT TISSUE AUGMENTATION: PREINJECTION CONSIDERATIONS

Defect parameters	Patient goals
Medications (anticoagulants)	What defect is of concern to the patient?
History of hypersensitivity reaction	Degree of improvement
History of herpes facialis	Expectations (longevity)
Volume required	Morbidity patient is willing to sustain
Location	Risk/benefit ratio
Alternative/simultaneous treatments	
Medical history	
Pregnancy/lactation	
Autoimmune disease	

Table 158.2 Soft tissue augmentation: preinjection considerations.

SOFT TISSUE AUGMENTATION INDICATIONS

- Non-dynamic rhytides – nasolabial folds, marionette lines
- Distensible scar
  - Acne scar
  - Traumatic/surgical scars
- Perioral – vermillion, oral commissures
- Combination therapy
  - Multiple fillers
  - Paralytic agents (botulinum toxin)

Table 158.3 Soft tissue augmentation indications.

HISTORICAL PERSPECTIVE

The history of soft tissue augmentation dates back to 1893, when Neuber used blocks of autologous fat harvested from the arms for tissue augmentation of depressed facial defects (Table 158.4). In 1899, Gersvny injected paraffin into the scrotum as a testicular prosthesis for a patient with advanced tuberculosis. Brunings first described using the syringe technique to transfer free fat in 1911. Baronders published a review of permanent soft tissue augmentation with liquid silicone in 1953. In 1981, bovine collagen (Zyderm® I) became the first US Food and Drug Administration (FDA)-approved xenogenic agent for soft tissue augmentation, followed by Zyderm® II and Zyplast®. It was not until 20 years later that the FDA rapidly began to approve new fillers for temporary soft tissue augmentation. The CosmoDerm® family

HISTORICAL MILESTONES OF FILLER SUBSTANCES		
Year	Physician	Milestone
1893	Neuberg	First to use autologous fat for tissue augmentation
1899	Gersvny	First to use bioinjectable paraffin to correct cosmetic deformities
1910	Lexor	First to use large-block grafts to treat malar depression associated with chin recession
1911	Brunings	First described transfer of free fat employing the syringe technique
1959	Peer	Reported 50% survival of syringe-aspirated transplanted fat at 1 year
1953	Baronders	Use of liquid silicone in medicine
1976	Fischer	Cellusuctiome extraction of fat
1978	Illouz	Liposuction as fat source
1981		FDA approval of Zyderm I®
1983		FDA approval of Zyderm II®
1985		FDA approval of Zyplast®
1986	Fournier	Microliposuction
2003		FDA approval of CosmoDerm 1® and CosmoPlast®
2003		FDA approval of injectable Restylane®
2005		FDA approval of CosmoDerm 2®

Table 158.4 Historical milestones of filler substances. FDA, Food and Drug Administration.

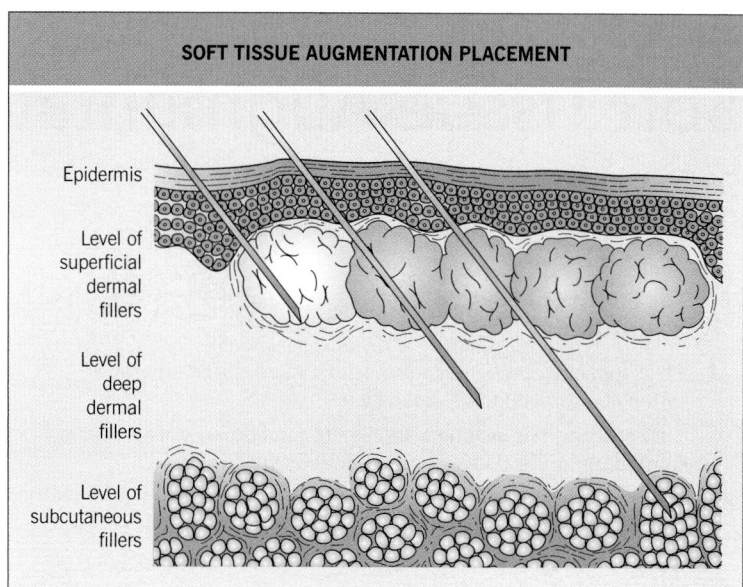

Fig. 158.1 Soft tissue augmentation placement.

(CosmoDerm® 1, CosmoDerm® 2 and CosmoPlast®), of injectable collagens derived from a single human fibroblast source was soon followed by the fast-track release of an entirely new class of agents – the hyaluronans. Restylane®, a non-animal stabilized hyaluronic acid (NASHA), was shortly followed by hyaluronans derived from rooster combs (Hylaform® and then Hylaform Plus®). A survey by the American Society for Aesthetic Plastic Surgery in 2004 revealed that the hyaluronans had become the most popular filling agents. The release, popularity and safety of these new agents prompted further investigation and was shortly followed by the availability of the longer-lasting synthetic products – calcium hydroxylapatite (Radiesse®) and poly-L-lactic acid (Sculptra®) – and a renewed interest in permanent fillers such as silicone oil and polymethylmethacrylate microspheres[1].

FILLER MATERIALS AND GENERAL INJECTION TECHNIQUE

There is an ever-expanding array of materials and devices for soft tissue augmentation (Tables 158.5 & 158.6). They can be divided, based either on site of cutaneous placement into the subcutaneous space or dermis, or on their derivation (autologous, xenograft, allograft, synthetic, or semi-synthetic). Autologous materials (e.g. fat, Isolagen®) are harvested from the patient, and theoretically have no risk of immunologic reaction, but do require an initial harvesting procedure and potentially have a limited donor reservoir. Xenografts are harvested from a different species and are semi-synthetic formulations (e.g. bovine collagen, some hyaluronic acid derivatives). Allograft materials (e.g. Dermalogen®,

Cymetra®, Fascian®) are harvested from human cadaveric tissue. Synthetic substances (e.g. expanded polytetrafluoroethylene, Radiesse®, Sculptra®) often provide longer-lasting results, but may have a greater potential for rejection[2].

To reduce ecchymosis, patients should be instructed to abstain from medications that would inhibit platelet aggregation for at least 10 days prior to injection. Cosmetic makeup and cutaneous debris should be removed. Percutaneous injections can be painful, especially in the central face and perioral areas; surface anesthesia can be achieved by using a topical preparation or ice approximately 15 minutes prior to administration. Some products will require nerve blocks and/or regional anesthesia. To fully appreciate the depth and scope of the defect, patients should be placed in a dependent or seated position, and there should be adequate lighting and, if necessary, magnification. Proper placement of the filler material is crucial (Fig. 158.1). There are two basic injection techniques: serial multiple punctures and single-entry. The former deposits small amounts of filler sequentially, with a small degree of overlap so there are no spaces between the injected material. In the single-entry method, either the full length of the needle is inserted into the proper dermal or subcutaneous plane and the filler is injected in a retrograde manner as the needle is withdrawn, or, conversely, the material can be injected as the needle is advanced (anterograde) creating a blunt dissection within the tissue space.

BOVINE COLLAGEN

Bovine collagen is an injectable with a long safety track record of use in more than a million patients[3]. The three forms (Zyderm® collagen I, Zyderm® collagen II, and Zyplast®) are all derived from a closed US cattle herd that is carefully monitored to prevent transmission of prion-mediated disease (bovine spongiform encephalitis). The products consist primarily of sterile, purified fibrillar suspension and contain 98% type I dermal bovine collagen, with the remainder consisting of type III collagen, suspended in phosphate-buffered physiologic saline containing 0.3% lidocaine[1].

Zyderm® collagen I, the original implant (introduced in 1981), has a concentration of 35 mg/ml, and Zyderm® collagen II (1983) has a concentration of 65 mg/ml. Zyplast®, the third form, received approval in 1985 and is cross-linked by the addition of glutaraldehyde. This characteristic decreases digestion by collagenase and makes it less immunogenic and longer lasting than the 3 months anticipated for the Zyderm® products[4].

All three products are supplied in boxes of preloaded syringes, each containing 0.5–1.5 cm³ of product, and should be kept refrigerated (4°C) to assure homogenicity and fluidity of the fibrils. With each syringe, there is an associated lot number and expiration date that should be

PARTIAL LIST OF CHARACTERISTICS OF THE IDEAL FILLER SUBSTANCE	
Material	Administration
Non-allergenic (minimal risk of hypersensitivity)	Basic instrumentation
FDA-approved	Painless
Non-carcinogenic/non-teratogenic	Outpatient
No migration	(minimal recuperation)
Minimal inflammation	User-friendly
No overt cutaneous change (undetectable)	Large amount available
Reproducible	Easy storage
Durable	
Minimal adverse sequelae (infection, ecchymosis)	
Stable (inert)	
Affordable	

Table 158.5 Partial list of characteristics of the ideal filler substance. FDA, Food and Drug Administration.

		INJECTABLE FILLERS		
Filler	**Material**	**Depth of implantation**	**Duration**	**FDA-approved***
Collagen				
Zyderm® I	Bovine collagen†	Superficial dermis	3–6 mos	✓
Zyderm® II	Bovine collagen†	Mid dermis	3–6 mos	✓
Zyplast®	Bovine collagen cross-linked by glutaraldehyde†	Mid to deep dermis	4–6 mos	✓
Evolence Breeze™	Porcine collagen	Superficial to mid dermis	12+ mos	
Evolence™	Porcine collagen	Mid to deep dermis	12+ mos	
CosmoDerm® 1	Human bioengineered collagen	Superficial dermis	3–6 mos	✓
CosmoDerm® 2	Human bioengineered collagen	Mid dermis	3–6 mos	✓
CosmoPlast®	Human bioengineered collagen cross-linked by glutaraldehyde	Mid to deep dermis	4–6 mos	✓
Hyaluronic acid				
Hylaform Fine Lines®	Hyaluronic acid from rooster combs	Superficial dermis	6–9 mos	
Hylaform®	Hyaluronic acid from rooster combs	Mid dermis	6–9 mos	✓
Hylaform Plus®	Hyaluronic acid from rooster combs	Deep dermis	6–9 mos	✓
Restylane Fine Line®	Hyaluronic acid, non-animal stabilized	Superficial dermis	6–9 mos	
Restylane®	Hyaluronic acid, non-animal stabilized	Mid dermis	6–9 mos	✓
Perlane®	Hyaluronic acid, non-animal stabilized	Deep dermis	6–9 mos	✓
Captique®	Hyaluronic acid, non-animal stabilized	Mid dermis	4–9 mos	✓
Juvéderm Ultra®	Hyaluronic acid, non-animal stabilized	Superficial to mid dermis	6–9 mos	✓
Juvéderm Ultra Plus®	Hyaluronic acid, non-animal stabilized	Mid to deep dermis	6–9 mos	✓
Puragen Plus™	Hyaluronic acid, non-animal stabilized	Mid dermis	6–9 mos	
Other synthetic components				
Laresse™	Carboxymethylcellulose and polyethylene oxide	Mid dermis	4–9 mos	
Sculptra®	Poly-L-lactic acid	Subcutis	1 to 3 y	✓
Radiesse®	Calcium hydroxylapatite microspheres	Subcutis	2 to 5 y	✓
Artefill® (Artecoll®)	Polymethylmethacrylate beads suspended in bovine collagen†	Deep dermis to subcutis	'Permanent'	✓
Silicone	Liquid silicone	Deep dermis	'Permanent'	✓‡
Aquamid™	Polyacrylamide	Subcutis	'Permanent'	

*As of August 2007.
†Requires skin testing prior to injection because of potential hypersensitivity to bovine collagen.
‡Injection for cosmetic purposes represents off-label use.

Table 158.6 Injectable fillers. There are also allograft materials derived from human cadaveric tissue (e.g. Dermalogen®, Cymetra®, and Fascian®) as well as Isolagen® which represents autologous collagen and fibroblasts.

documented for tracking purposes. A 30-gauge, 0.5-inch needle is usually used, but the company also supplies an adjustable depth gauge (ADG) needle to manually adjust the length of the needle.

Prior to initiating therapy, potential allergic response to the products must be excluded. Hypersensitivity to all three formulations can be reduced with double skin testing. The skin test is available in 1.0 cm³ tuberculin syringes that contain 0.3 ml of Zyderm® I, which screens for allergy to all three forms of bovine collagen. Approximately 0.1 cm³ of the contents is injected subcutaneously in an inconspicuous area, such as the volar aspect of the forearm. Localized hypersensitivity is found in 3% of patients and is manifested as swelling, induration, tenderness or erythema that persists or occurs 6 or more hours following implantation. Despite a negative preliminary test, an additional 1–2% of people will subsequently develop an allergic reaction to the products. Therefore, it is generally the standard of practice to perform a second skin test 2 weeks after the initial skin test. This test, using a similar volume, can be injected on the contralateral arm or the periphery of the face (pretragal area, anterior hairline), and should be monitored for 2 additional weeks. A positive reaction occurring with either test is a contraindication and should preclude further therapy with bovine collagen. Conversely, negative double skin testing allows the patient to proceed with treatment 4 weeks after the initial test or 2 weeks after the second test. For patients who have not had collagen injected for a

year or more, a single re-test with a 2-week observation period is suggested, prior to commencing further treatment.

Zyderm® I is implanted into the superficial dermis by introducing the needle at a 20–30° angle to the plane of the skin. Proper placement should be apparent with a flat, yellow blanching of the skin. Because a significant portion of Zyderm® I is water, overcorrection is commonly utilized to maximize the aesthetic result. It is primarily suited to smooth out and fill superficial wrinkles such as perioral and periocular rhytides, and is the most forgiving and versatile of the three collagen preparations. Zyderm® II is more viscous than Zyderm® I; it is suitable for shallow scars and can be used synergistically with botulinum toxin in the glabellar region. When injected too superficially, persistent whiteness can be appreciated.

Zyplast® is injected with the needle at more of an angle (45–90°) to the defect, and is placed deeper in the dermis. If placed properly, it does not cause immediate blanching, but a more subtle and somewhat delayed blanch. Deep nasolabial folds, marionette grooves, and lip augmentation respond best to Zyplast®. Lip enhancement is the most common use of bovine collagen; it is indicated only for the vermilion border, and is not FDA-approved for the mucosa (Fig. 158.2). The different types of collagen may be used simultaneously, particularly when the cosmetic defect has multiple depths or is quite deep. This is well illustrated in the perioral area, where Zyplast® can be injected in a

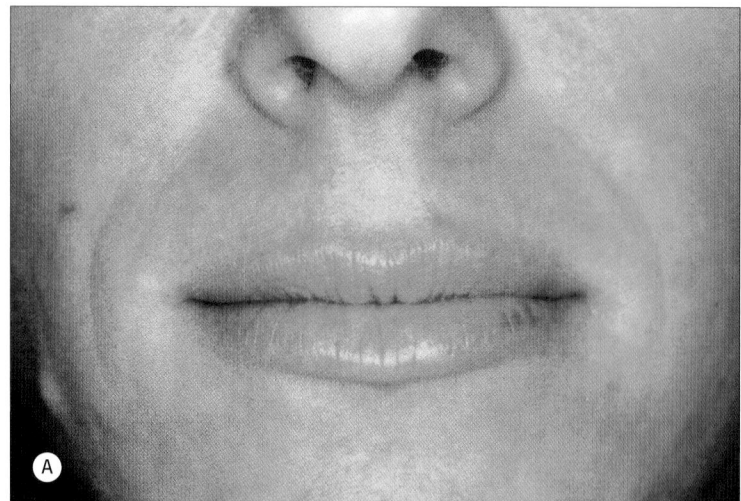

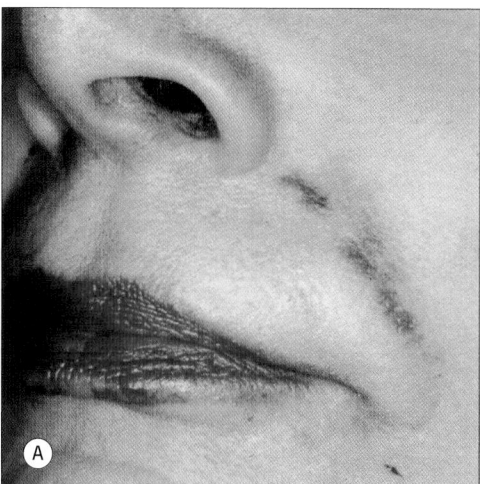

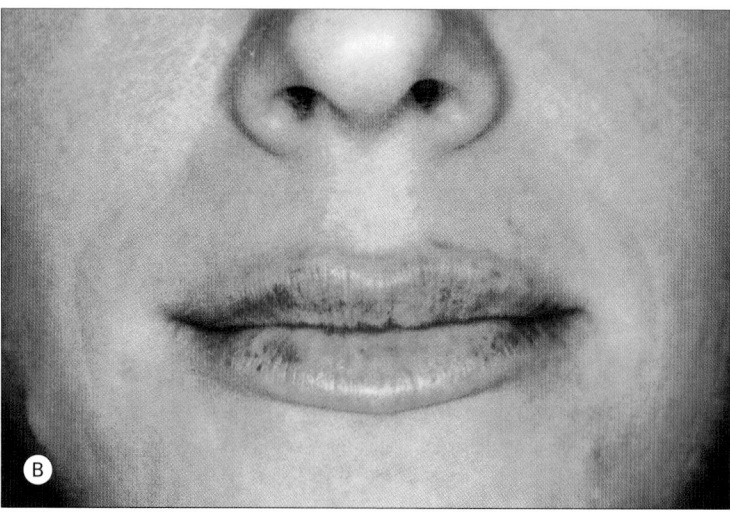

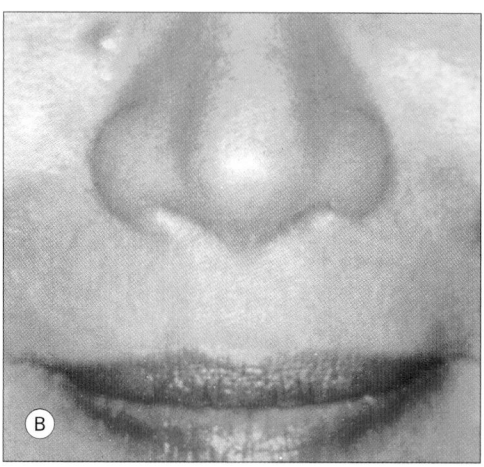

Fig. 158.3 Bovine collagen – adverse reactions. A Excess ecchymosis resulting from injection of Zyplast® with serial puncture technique into the nasolabial folds of a patient on anticoagulation therapy. B Sterile abscesses appeared in the nasolabial folds following injection of Zyplast® (the patient had two prior negative skin tests). Resolution was not complete for 12 months.

Fig. 158.2 Bovine collagen – lip augmentation. Pre- (A) and post-injection (B) of 1 cm³ of Zyplast® into the vermilion of the lips for augmentation.

continuous flow along the vermilion border, and Zyderm® into the radiating vertical lines. Similarly, a deep nasolabial fold can be softened by first injecting Zyplast® into the deep dermis, then layering Zyderm® above it in the superficial papillary dermis.

A common source of frustration for patients receiving collagen injections is the temporary nature of the correction. In general, patients can anticipate 3 to 6 months of improvement, with gradual diminution of results; however, patients can receive additional treatment or maintenance therapy at any time.

The adverse treatment responses to injectable collagen can be divided into non-hypersensitive- and hypersensitive-reaction patterns. Many of the former are technique-dependent, and include injection site ecchymosis (Fig. 158.3A), superficial placement with apparent beading, and deep placement with intravascular occlusion. In fact, Zyplast® is contraindicated in the glabellar area because the deeper placement required can result in vascular injury. Vascular occlusion following dermal placement of collagen presents as an immediate cutaneous blanch associated with pain. Immediate vasodilation with warm compresses and topical nitroglycerin may reduce the vasospasm. Ultimately, if tissue necrosis and slough occur, sustained emotional support and wound care are essential to prompt resolution.

There are two forms of true, classic type IV hypersensitivity to these implants. They develop in about 1% of those patients whose two skin tests are negative and who subsequently receive treatment. Due primarily to Zyderm®, and occurring at approximately 2 weeks after treatment, the more common reaction is manifested by swollen, indurated granulomas at both the treatment and test sites (see Ch. 93). Although they resolve spontaneously and without permanent scarring, they can take up to 1 year to completely dissipate. In addition to reassurance and adequate camouflage makeup, treatment has included

non-steroidal anti-inflammatory drugs and intralesional injections of triamcinolone acetonide. There are reports that oral cyclosporine and topical tacrolimus have expedited resolution of these complications[5,6]. Sterile abscesses are the second form of delayed hypersensitivity that have been associated with bovine collagen. The incidence is low, approximately 1 to 4 in 10 000 treatments, and due in large part to Zyplast®. These reactions are characterized by the sudden onset of pain, usually days to weeks after injection, followed shortly by tense edema and erythema with fluctuant nodules (Fig. 158.3B). The lesions can be treated with drainage, intralesional corticosteroids and oral antibiotics. However, scarring can occur. The circulating antibovine collagen antibodies that occur in these reactions do not cross-react with human collagen, and the FDA has not been convinced of any statistical association between bovine collagen and autoimmune connective tissue disease (Table 158.7).

Koken Atelocollagen® and Resoplast® are non-fibrillar forms of implantable bovine collagen that are not approved for use in the US.

COMPLICATIONS ASSOCIATED WITH USE OF BOVINE COLLAGEN

• Localized hypersensitivity reaction
  – Granulomatous
  – Sterile abscesses
• Intravascular injection
  – Tissue necrosis
  – Vision loss
• Infection
  – Reactivation of herpes simplex
  – Acneiform eruption
• Contour irregularity
  – Superficial placement: beading
• Theoretical unproven risk of autoimmune connective tissue disease

Table 158.7 Complications associated with use of bovine collagen.

POLYMETHYLMETHACRYLATE (PMMA) MICROSPHERES (ARTEFILL®)

Known as Artecoll® outside of the US and designated by the manufacturer as Artefill® for FDA approval, the product contains polymethylmethacrylate (PMMA) microspheres suspended in a solution of 3.5% bovine collagen and 0.3% lidocaine. The collagen serves as a carrier, and, over 1–3 months following injection, it is degraded. The remaining intact, inert, non-biodegradable 30–40 μm PMMA beads, commonly known as Lucite™ or Plexiglas™, are large enough to avoid phagocytosis but small enough to promote permanent augmentation. Once the host's collagen has encapsulated the microspheres, the augmentation has been purported to be permanent. Prepackaged in a 1.0 cm³ syringe, it is injected with a 27-gauge needle. As the collagen vehicle is obtained from a closed herd of cattle, it would be prudent to perform a skin test to reduce the risk of an allergic reaction to the bovine collagen. In an inconspicuous site, a small aliquot (0.05 ml) can be injected at the junction of the dermis and subcutaneous tissue. In addition to hypersensitivity reactions, there is also a risk of delayed granuloma formation.

SYNTHETIC HUMAN COLLAGEN

One of the primary drawbacks to bovine collagen is the risk of hypersensitivity. The CosmoDerm® family of dermal fillers was based on the safety profile following the extensive use of this synthetic human collagen in burns and wounds. Unlike botulinum toxin type A, which is classified as a drug because it 'achieves its primary intended purpose by chemical action or is metabolized by the body', these fillers were classified as devices in the US. Because they were not considered as new products, but simply a change in source material, the FDA approval process was accelerated. All three formulations – CosmoDerm® 1, CosmoDerm® 2, and CosmoPlast® – closely resemble the bovine-sourced products. They have the same consistency, concentration (dispersed in phosphate-buffered saline with 0.3% lidocaine), and injection technique as their Zyderm®/Zyplast® counterparts; the primary distinction is that they are grown from a single human fibroblast cell culture and, unlike other human-derived products, are not cadaveric in nature. They are the result of tissue-engineering technology and have undergone extensive pathology screening for viral and bacterial contamination to avoid the possibility of disease transmission. As these products are non-animal-based, they do not require an initial skin test for hypersensitivity. Therefore, they can be injected on the same day as the initial consultation.

Similar to its bovine analogue Zyderm® I, CosmoDerm® 1 has a concentration of 35 mg/ml and is placed into the superficial papillary dermis with a comparable degree of blanching and overcorrection, and is also primarily indicated for superficial lines and defects. CosmoDerm® 2 has a concentration of 65 mg/ml human-based collagen and has similar indications as Zyderm® II. CosmoPlast®, like Zyplast®, contains 35 mg/ml of human-derived collagen cross-linked with glutaraldehyde, which makes it less immunogenic and increases its durability. It is a deeper implant, to a depth of approximately 2.0 mm, and does not require overcorrection to improve deep folds and wrinkles.

All three CosmoDerm® products are packaged similarly to the three bovine products and are prepackaged as an opaque white material in a box of six preloaded syringes with adhesive labels and 30-gauge, 0.5-inch and adjustable depth gauge (ADG) needles. Upon comparison, the cost of the CosmoDerm® group is slightly higher than that of the Zyderm® group, even though the initial screening process with skin tests is eliminated. The cosmetic result appears to be comparable. Anecdotally, some physicians have noted that human-derived products have better flow characteristics and are easier to inject. A comparison of duration of correction has not yet been scientifically scrutinized[7].

HUMAN-DERIVED CADAVERIC COLLAGEN

In the late 1980s, research began on extracting intact human collagen fibers and acellular dermal matrix from cadavers for human dermal implantation. These products, Dermalogen® and Cymetra®, are available in preloaded syringes and implantable grafts. However, with the introduction and availability of the newer forms of bioengineered human collagen, these products seem to have lost much of their original appeal.

Dermalogen® is the prototype and is an injectable allograft material of human tissue origin composed predominantly of intact collagen and elastin fibers and glycosaminoglycans harvested from the dermal layer of human cadaveric skin. The indications are similar to those for bovine collagen: facial rhytides, atrophic scars, and lip enhancement. Because there is some evidence of neovascularization and host collagen deposition in sites injected with Dermalogen®, early reports suggested that correction may be longer lasting; however, this has yet to be substantiated[8]. Although skin testing was originally recommended, Dermalogen® does not carry the risk of hypersensitivity, and no skin test is currently supplied.

Cymetra® consists primarily of micronized human collagen fibers. It is comparable to other injectable allografts (e.g. Dermalogen®) and is similar in composition and processing. Its acellular nature mitigates skin testing, and to date there have been no reports of hypersensitivity reactions. This feature provides a major advantage for patients with a prior history of bovine collagen hypersensitivity. The indications are the same. One distinction of Cymetra® is that it is in powder form, translating into a prolonged shelf-life. It is rehydrated prior to injection by using 1.0 ml of 1% lidocaine. Once completely saturated, the product changes from a white powder to a cream color with a paste-like consistency.

HUMAN-DERIVED CADAVERIC FASCIA

Fascia lata has long been utilized in surgery, first as suture material and later for repair of hernias and eyelid ptosis and for reconstructive purposes in orthopedic surgery and otolaryngology[9]. Preserved particulate fascia harvested primarily from cadaveric fascia lata became FDA-approved in 1999 (Fascian®) and is registered as a tissue product designed to replace areas of lost fascia or collagen. It is supplied in 3 ml syringes and, as it is in powder form, can be stored at room temperature. Prior to injection, it is hydrated with 1.5 to 3.0 ml of 0.5% lidocaine with 1:100 000 epinephrine or with normal saline and a Luer-to-Luer lock syringe connector is used to emulsify the powder. Syringes containing five different particle sizes (0.1, 0.25, 0.5, 1.0 and 2.0 mm) are available, all with 80 mg of the product. The larger-sized particles give a greater volumetric correction, but are also more likely to clog in the syringe upon injection. Obstructions can be released by aspirating an additional 0.5 ml of saline or replacing the needle. Skin testing is not required[10]. Using a 16- to 18-gauge needle, the reconstituted Fascian® is injected above the superficial subcutaneous fat. Pretunneling (subcision) with the needle prior to injection will create a pocket for the deposition of the Fascian®. Overcorrection is recommended, to anticipate reabsorption of the diluent. Perhaps due to relatively limited use, few adverse reactions have been reported; however, postinjection edema can be significant and should be addressed with cool compresses and, if necessary, systemic corticosteroids.

Unlike other fillers, Fascian® is not marketed as a 'device' in the US, but rather is supplied under the criteria of the Tissue Reference Group (TRG) and comes with no prescribed indications. The grafts are, in theory, applicable to any body defect that would be amenable to other forms of soft tissue augmentation. Fascian® is advantageous not only because of its ease of storage, availability in multiple sizes, and lack of need for skin testing, but also because of the potential for large volumetric correction and applicability to deep subdermal defects. It is, however, limited by the need for preparation and the use of large-bore needles for administration, as well as the lack of controlled studies documenting its longevity.

AUTOLOGOUS FIBROBLASTS AND COLLAGEN

Isolagen® is derived from autologous fibroblasts, rather than bovine or cadaveric or cultured human fibroblasts. It is currently available in the UK and at the time of publication was in phase III clinical trials in the US. Skin obtained from the patient is grown at a separate facility and then injected back into the same donor patient at a later date. A 3 mm punch biopsy is harvested from an inconspicuous area such as the posterior auricular sulcus, and is transported to the manufacturer where it is cultured by a patented process. From the single biopsy, fibroblasts that will produce collagen are stimulated to proliferate into tens of millions of cells. After approximately 6 to 8 weeks, there is a resultant yield of between 1 and 2 cm³ of injectable material containing fibroblasts and native collagen. This can be injected into areas that have traditionally been treated with collagen, such as the perioral area including the nasolabial folds, lips and marionette lines. The injections must be performed within 24 hours of receipt of the material and should be preceded by local anesthesia as the product does not contain lidocaine. It is recommended that the injections be repeated three times at 2-week intervals, which supposedly stimulates the fibroblasts to continue to produce collagen for 6–12 months. The limited yield of product (1–2 cm³), the off-site shipping and processing of the tissue, and the extent to which the fibroblasts continue to produce collagen and effect soft tissue correction are concerns that have limited enthusiasm for this product.

Autologen®, a similar autologous product that was derived from the patient's excess skin following surgery (rhytidectomy, abdominoplasty), is no longer available. Fibrel® was a fibrin foam that required reconstitution with the patient's plasma; soft tissue augmentation was accomplished as clot formation at the site of implantation. It, too, is no longer available.

HYALURONIC ACID DERIVATIVES

The hyaluronic acid derivatives (hyaluronans) have more recently been approved for use in the US. This class of compounds has become the most popular filling agent and has spawned an entire new industry, complete with competing products and brand loyalty. Presently, there are at least three manufacturers, with well over a dozen hyaluronic acid-based injectable agents; all remarkably similar (see Table 158.6). Hyaluronic acid is named for its glossy appearance (the Greek word for glass is *hyalos*). Hyaluronic acid is a glycosaminoglycan or acid mucopolysaccharide that resides in the cutaneous dermal ground substance and fills the extracellular spaces between collagen fibers. It functions as a space-filling and stabilizing molecule. It is a ubiquitous component of connective tissue and is identical in chemical and molecular form in all tissues and mammals and is therefore species non-specific. The hyaluronic acid molecule is a simple chemical structure and is a high-molecular-weight, long-chain polysaccharide of repeating disaccharide units of N-acetylglucosamine and D-glucuronic acid. The intertwining coils are polar in nature and have an enormous ability to attract water (hydrophilic) and impart skin turgor. In connective tissue, hyaluronic acid's main biologic function is to create volume and lubricate extracellular structures by forming a gelatinous matrix in which collagen and elastin fibers are embedded and held together in proper alignment. It also regulates cell movement and function, and is particularly important in development and remodeling of tissues. A direct correlation exists among the amount of hyaluronic acid in dermal tissue, the dermal water content, and the viscoelastic properties of the extracellular matrix. The concentration of naturally occurring hyaluronic acid in the skin decreases with age, resulting in decreased ability to hold water (hydration), which renders the dermis less voluminous and increases its propensity to wrinkle.

A dual mechanism of action accounts for the correction of facial wrinkles: hyaluronic acid integrates into dermal tissue, then attracts and binds water molecules to sustain augmentation. In its natural unmodified state, implanted exogenous hyaluronic acid is rapidly degraded by hyaluronidase and has a half-life of only 12 to 24 hours. It was not until it was determined that the hyaluronic acid molecule required stabilization through chemical cross-linking that its enzymatic breakdown was decreased and its viability and *in situ* residency was increased. Then, it could be used as an acceptable filler.

Its viscoelastic properties, lack of hypersensitivity and migration, and insolubility make it an appropriate agent for soft tissue augmentation. After implantation into tissues, injectable hyaluronic acid is metabolized into carbon dioxide and water and eliminated by the liver[11–13] (Table 158.8).

There are two broad categories of injectable cross-linked hyaluronic acid, each with three distinct formulations. One category (the Hylaform® group) is animal-derived (rooster combs), stabilized hyaluronic acid and the second is non-animal-derived synthetic hyaluronic acid (NASHA).

BENEFITS OF HYALURONIC ACID DERIVATIVES
• Identical in all species and all tissue types
• No skin test required
• Room storage
• Biodegradable
• Long-lasting/stable
• High degree of safety

Table 158.8 Benefits of hyaluronic acid derivatives.

The NASHA group (Restylane®, Captique® and Juvederm®) is generated from bacterial (*Streptococcus*) fermentation. The two categories share many characteristics; they are clear, non-particulate, colorless, thick gels that contain no lidocaine. Without the addition of an anesthetic, they are fairly painful to administer and therefore require some type of topical or regional nerve block anesthesia prior to injection. All are similarly packaged and are available in preloaded single-use syringes that are accompanied by 30-gauge, 0.5-inch needles as well as labels that can be removed and affixed to the patient records. The products do not require skin testing and can be stored at room temperature. Placement should be in the mid to deep dermis to the point of correction but without overcorrecting the defect. These products are more viscous than many other injectables, especially the collagen products, and they have different flow characteristics (rheology), and greater pressure must be applied to the plunger of the syringe. However, they are more malleable and contour irregularities are responsive to manual massage. Augmentation lasts approximately 6–9 months, longer than with most other temporary fillers[14] (Table 158.9). They are approved for 'correction of moderate to severe facial wrinkles and folds, such as the nasolabial folds' but are routinely used for many facial indications inclusive of lip augmentation. Perhaps due to the novelty, durability or malleability of the product, there has been a great deal of interest generated in expanded non-traditional use of the injectable hyaluronic acids. They are used on the face in the supra-brow area to assist in elevating the brow, in the infraocular sulcus, and in the periauricular area to rejuvenate the appearance of the senescent/atrophic ear. Additionally, on the extremities, using hyaluronic acid instead of autologous fat in the dorsum of the hand provides volume and camouflages the vasculature and tendons that appear with increasing age.

Adverse reactions are reportedly less than 2%. One of the major advantages of hyaluronic acid gels over collagen is the decreased incidence of delayed hypersensitivity reactions (see Table 158.9). Since it

COMPARISON OF COLLAGEN AND HYALURONANS		
	Collagen	**Hyaluronans**
Compatibility	Species and tissue specific	Identical in all species and tissues
Duration	3–4 months	4–8 months (longer with subsequent injections)
Origin	Bovine or human	Animal (avian) or bacterial (streptococcal fermentation)
Augmentation	Filler replacement	Water absorption
Pattern of loss	Steady volume loss	Isovolemic degradation
Viscosity	Constant	Dynamic
Anesthesia	0.3% lidocaine	None: requires topical/block
Discomfort	Minimal	Significant
Correction	50–100% overcorrection	No overcorrection
Preinjection skin test	Double skin test	Not required
Allergy prevalence (hypersensitivity)	~3% of population	~0.4% of population
Shipping & storage	Refrigerated	Room temperature

Table 158.9 Comparison of collagen and hyaluronans.

should be nearly impossible to react to pure hyaluronic acid, as it is identical in all species and tissue types, any such reactions are thought to be due to impurities in hyaluronan production: residual avian proteins (Hylaform®) or byproducts of bacterial fermentation (Restylane®)[14a]. Similar to all injectables, other adverse reactions include ecchymosis, acneiform eruptions and reactivation of herpes simplex[15,16]. Injection discomfort and postinjection ache, erythema and edema are expected sequelae.

With most fillers, if the placement is too superficial, a contour irregularity results and resolution occurs only with time. However, with the hyaluronic acids, a 'lump' can often be redistributed into the desired location by physician massage. If is the lump persists, the irregularity can be treated with one of two methods. The easiest is to express the material by simple incision and drainage. With manual pressure, the clear intact hyaluronan is readily extruded. If the administration has been too deep and the localized bump is not readily accessible to drainage, local injection of small amounts of hyaluronidase (Wydase®) can reduce its size. A very unique complication is the appearance of cutaneous blue beading. This, too, is the result of erroneous placement in the superficial dermis and can persist for a significant amount of time. Fortunately, this complication also responds to the intralesional injection of hyaluronidase[16a].

Animal-derived Hyaluronic Acid

The avian-derived form of hyaluronic acid (extracted from rooster combs) is distributed as Hylaform® and there are three concentrations: Hylaform Fine Lines® for superficial lines and wrinkles, Hylaform® for moderate rhytides, and Hylaform Plus® for deep folds. At the time of publication, only the last two agents have received FDA approval. They all have a high molecular weight but low concentration of hyaluronic acid (5.5 mg/ml).

Non-animal-derived Synthetic Hyaluronic Acid

There are currently three major injectable hyaluronic acids produced by streptococcal fermentation (non-animal stabilized hyaluronic acid – NASHA). In the Restylane® family, three forms are available: Restylane Fine Line®, Restylane® and Perlane®; however, only Restylane® and Perlane® are currently FDA-approved and available in the US. Each has a concentration of 20 mg/ml of hyaluronic acid; the difference is the size of the gel particles. Restylane Fine Line® is injected into the upper dermis for superficial lines and contains 500 000 gel particles per milliliter. Restylane®, for mid-dermal applications, has 100 000 gel particles per milliliter. Perlane® (8000 gel particles per milliliter) is for deep dermal augmentation and the more profound facial folds. Post-injection swelling, erythema and bruising are not atypical and may be more prolonged than with other hyaluronic acid fillers (Fig. 158.4).

Captique® is a re-formulation of Hylaform® with 5.5 mg/ml of hyaluronic acid, but, as opposed to being of avian derivation, it is non-animal hyaluronic acid (NASHA). This product has FDA approval for mid-dermal defects. Although it does not have the erythema and reactivity of other NASHA products (Fig. 158.5), its low hyaluronic acid concentration does not sustain long augmentation. However, occasionally adverse reactions can occur (Fig. 158.6).

Juvederm® is similar to Captique® and Restylane® in that it is based on non-animal, cross-linked technology. There are similarly three forms: Juvederm® 18 with a concentration of 18 mg/ml of hyaluronic acid, designed for the superficial dermis; Juvederm® Ultra (24 mg/ml of hyaluronic acid) for deeper mid-dermal defects; and Juvederm® Ultra Plus, which contains 30 mg/ml of hyaluronic acid for correction of the deepest contour irregularities[16]. The two thicker forms, Juvederm® Ultra and Juvederm® Ultra Plus were granted FDA approval in January 2007.

EXPANDED POLYTETRAFLUOROETHYLENE

Expanded polytetrafluoroethylene (ePTFE) is a synthetic solid material that is soft, pliable and clinically inert, with minimal tissue reactivity and high tensile strength. These characteristics have made it useful as a vascular graft in cardiac, urogynecologic, ophthalmologic, and plastic and reconstructive surgery since 1975. It received FDA approval

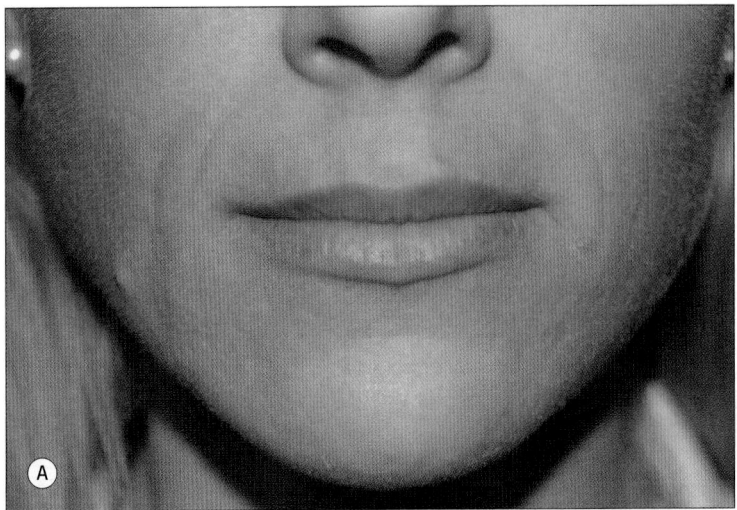

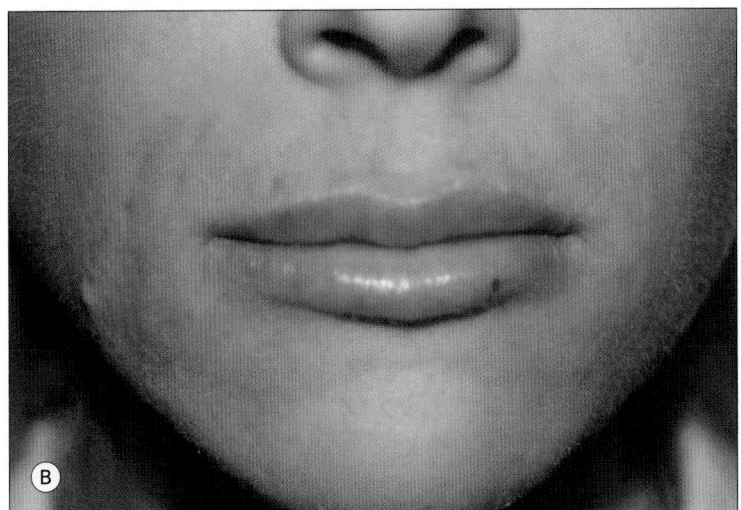

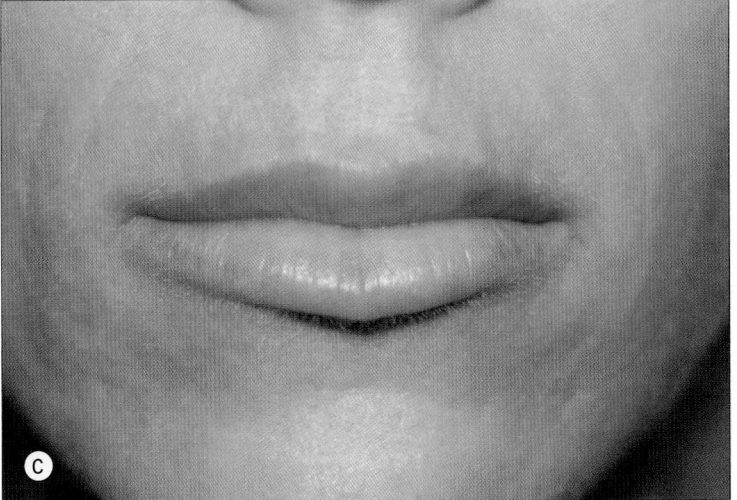

Fig. 158.4 Hyaluronic acid – lip and perioral augmentation. A Prior to injection of Restylane® into the perioral area. **B** Significant edema postoperatively. **C** Three months postinjection with correction maintained.

for soft tissue augmentation in 1993, and currently there are two major products with aesthetic indications. Gore-Tex® Subcutaneous Augmentation Material comes in two forms, single- and multi-stranded, which are both 15 cm in length. In addition, SoftForm® is available as hollow tubes of three lengths (50, 70 and 90 mm) with varying external diameters (2.4, 3.2 and 4.0 mm). They are useful, either as solitary filling agents or in conjunction with other fillers, to address deep nasolabial folds, atrophic lips, and wasting associated with AIDS. Following a combination of nerve blocks and local anesthesia, entry and exit incisions are made and the ePFTE is implanted.

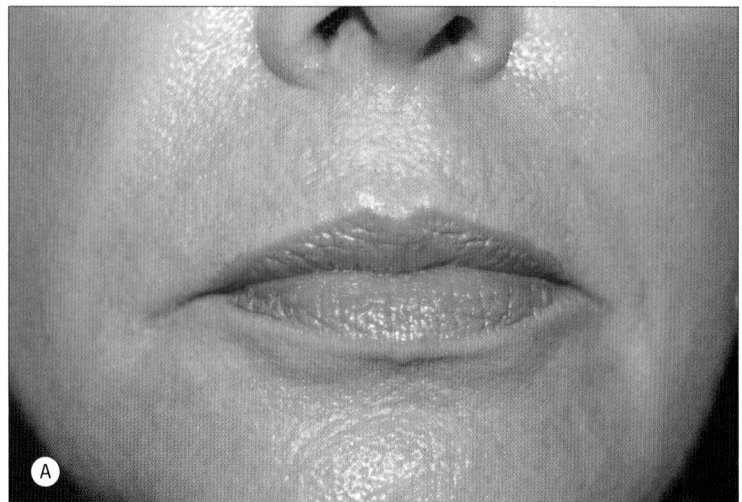

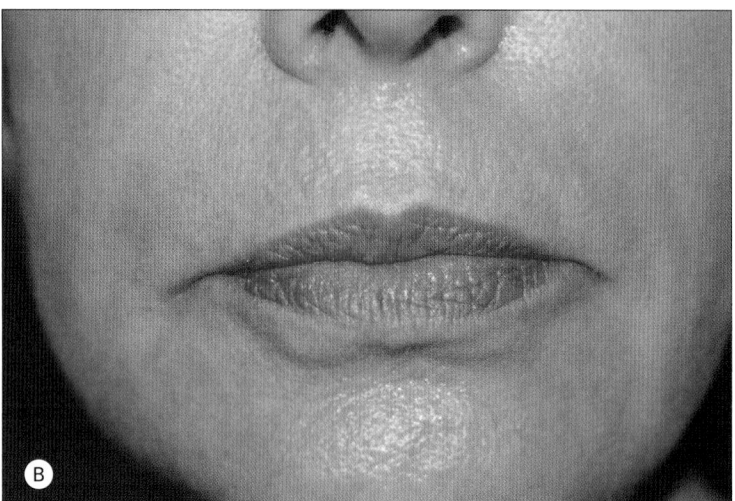

Fig. 158.5 Hyaluronic acid – perioral augmentation. A Before administration of 1 cm³ of Captique®. B Immediate postinjection appearance with minimal erythema.

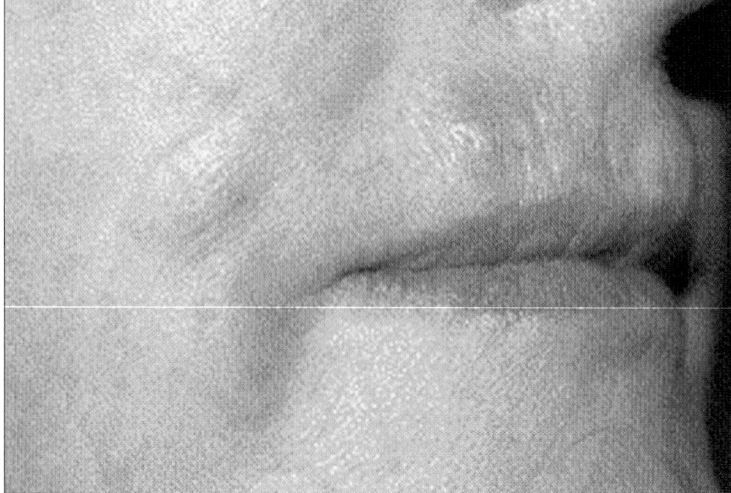

Fig. 158.6 Hyaluronic acid – adverse reactions. Four weeks after placement of 1 cm³ of Captique® into the perioral area, painful, indurated nodules appeared. Cultures did not reveal the presence of any microorganisms. With permission from Matarasso SL, Herwick R. Hypersensitivity reaction to nonanimal stabilized hyaluronic acid. J Am Acad Dermatol. 2006;55:128–31.

A straight Keith needle with a suture (0-silk) attached to the Gore-Tex® implant is used to perpendicularly enter and exit the skin. The Gore-Tex® is pulled through the subcutaneous tissue by pulling the attached suture. There will be some resistance and steady constant pressure will be required. With the implant in place, the sutures are cut

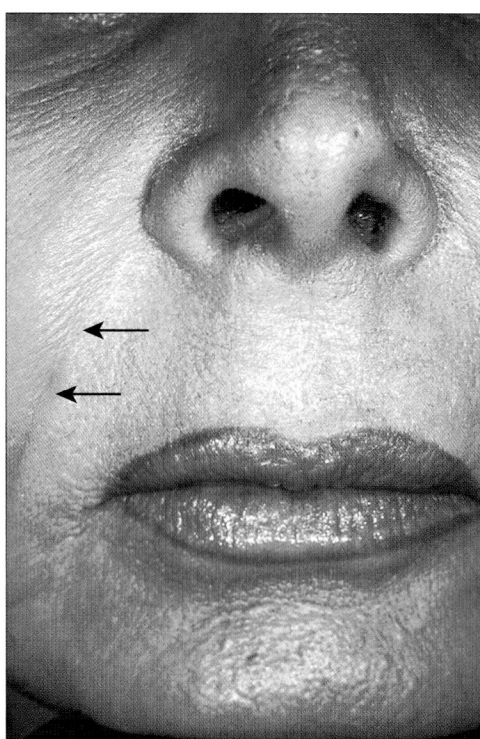

Fig. 158.7 Placement of expanded polytetrafluoroethylene into the nasolabial fold. Superficial placement of SoftForm® is both palpable and visible (arrows).

free and the tips of the implant are buried in the deep dermis. Closure of incision sites may not be necessary. The porosity of the implant leads to fibrous in-growth, improving the degree of augmentation and anchoring the implant via decreased movement[17].

SoftForm® is inserted via a preloaded trochar delivery system. Once the thick delivery apparatus is removed, the implant ends are tapered and buried subdermally; the incision sites will need to be sutured. The hollow-tube configuration of SoftForm® is designed to promote in-growth of fibroblasts with subsequent neocollagenesis. Placement of both ePTFE products is unforgiving and should be directly beneath and parallel to the overlying defect, high in the subcutaneous fat, just underneath the deep reticular dermis[4].

The primary advantage of ePTFE is that it is not degraded and remains intact; it is essentially permanent. However, the disadvantages include: the potential for small incisional scars; the risk of infection, extrusion and migration; and the fact that, even under the best of circumstances, patients can palpate it (Fig. 158.7). In addition, a solid implant placed in a mobile area may intrinsically be counterintuitive and, in fact, may create a new defect. Fortunately, should an adverse event occur, the ePTFE can be removed in a similar fashion to the original insertion. However, the longer the implants remain in place, the more fibrosis there is, and it becomes increasingly difficult to remove them. Compared to other agents, these fillers are technically more difficult to place and have an associated steep learning curve, and their use seems to have significantly decreased[17a].

LIPOTRANSFER

Historically, autologous fat has always been considered one of the safest fillers, with estimations of success as high as 50%. However, two concerns have remained. The original *en bloc* technique required excision of the donor tissue and a resultant second defect; essentially patients traded one defect for another. Furthermore, the non-particulate solid nature of the tissue required implantation, with the potential for incisional scars. The arrival of liposuction in the 1980s solved many of these existing problems. A byproduct of liposuction, the suctioned fat was easily accessible and could be reinjected through small cannulas and needles. Consequently, there has been a renaissance of autologous fat transplantation.

For many, autologous fat is considered to be the optimal filler. The advantages remain the biocompatibility and avoidance of allergy, the relative abundance of graft supply, the ability to address three-dimensional volume correction, and the possibility of permanent correction.

Theoretical disadvantages include the inability to place material into the dermis to address fine lines and wrinkles or small scars, the cumbersome aspects of harvesting the fat and determining the optimal donor site, the inability to predict the percentage of graft survival, and the debate over viability of stored fat. Perhaps the major drawback is that it requires two procedures: harvesting and insertion of the fat[18,19].

Fat may be harvested from any site where there is excess adiposity. Ironically, those patients who most often request this procedure have limited donor subcutaneous supply. Definitive studies have not yet determined if one area is preferable to others; however, areas with easy access, with limited postoperative morbidity, and which appear to be relatively insensitive to dietary fluctuation include the abdomen, medial knee, and upper outer buttock areas[20].

Patients are instructed to abstain from medications that would interfere with blood clotting for 10 days prior to the procedure, and to arrive in comfortable clothes. Written consent is obtained. The donor and recipient sites are photographed and prepared, and the patients are provided with an oral anxiolytic. The subcutaneous space of the donor site is infiltrated with tumescent anesthesia (see Ch. 143)[21]. Through a percutaneous stab incision made with a no. 11 blade, the donor fat can be aspirated using a 12- to 14-gauge single-holed microcannula (1.5–4.0 inches) that has a beveled edge. The needle is mounted on a conventional hypodermic (10–20 ml) Luer-Lok® syringe. Similar to standard liposuction, the non-dominant hand grasps the subcutaneous adipose tissue and, with the dominant hand holding a syringe under negative pressure, the needle/microcannula is placed in the subcutaneous fat. Moving up and down in a vertical motion perpendicular to the skin, a mixture of yellow fat, some anesthetic solution and, as the procedure progresses and the fat store is depleted, some blood will appear in the syringe. The filled syringes are placed upright in a dependent position, allowing gravity to separate the supernatant fat from the infranatant blood and anesthetic fluid, which can be discarded. The relatively pure supernatant fat is injected using a large-bore (16- or 18-gauge) needle. After a small bleb of local anesthesia is introduced, the needle is inserted almost parallel to the skin and is advanced to the farthest point of interest. The plunger is then drawn back to aspirate, to ensure that intravascular placement does not occur. The fat is threaded as the needle is withdrawn; frequently, it dissects along the subcutaneous plane without assistance. Although there is some discomfort associated with the injection, it relates primarily to the sudden stretch and expansion of the subcutaneous space and is generally well tolerated by most patients. Molding is undertaken by firm massage to encourage proper subcutaneous fat distribution and a uniform contour. There remains a great deal of variability in technique. Some physicians prefer multiple passes with an intricate layering of small fat droplets, while others have recently found success with intramuscular placement[22,23]. Sterile pressure dressings are applied to the donor site and ice compresses to both the donor and recipient sites. The patient is instructed in postoperative care, including systemic antibiotics, and pain management without aspirin-containing products. Any remaining fat can be meticulously labeled and frozen. When properly stored, it has been suggested that frozen fat can be utilized for up to 12–18 months[24].

Areas amenable to autologous fat transfer on the aging face include the nasolabial fold, cheeks (Fig. 158.8), infraorbital area, marionette lines, lips, scars from acne, and stable disease processes associated with idiopathic facial subcutaneous atrophy (e.g. linear morphea [including coup de sabre], Parry-Romberg syndrome)[25,26]. The dorsum of the hand often shares all of the signs of aging found in sun-exposed areas, but the advances available for facial rejuvenation often compound the disparity between the aging face and hand. Replacing fat in the back of the hand masks the appearance of protruding tendons and vessels (Figs 158.9 & 158.10). This imparts a more youthful appearance that is compatible with a rejuvenated face. Adipose transfer has also been shown to be effective in treating partial lipodystrophies associated with highly active retroviral therapy (HAART) for patients with HIV infection.

Despite the expanding use of transplanted adipose tissue, the literature has few objective studies documenting persistence of grafted material and rate of resorption[27]. Results seem to depend on repeated injections with smaller amounts over time, rather than single injections of larger amounts, which seem to be subject to lower survival rates and higher volume resorption. Presumably because large volumes cannot be sustained by passive diffusion of the recipient bed, overcorrection is discouraged and the transplanted area should be corrected to 100%. There are still many unanswered questions with regard to

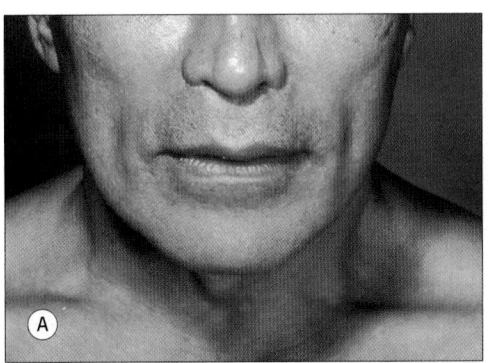
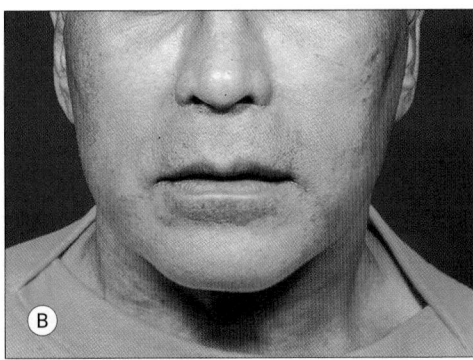

Fig. 158.8 Lipotransfer. Before (**A**) and after (**B**) injection of 10 cm³ of autologous fat into both buccal areas.

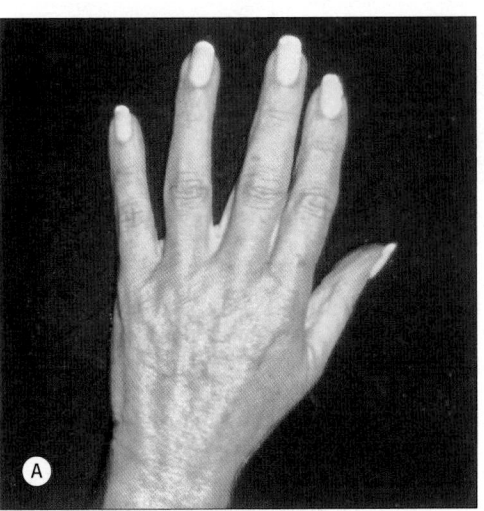
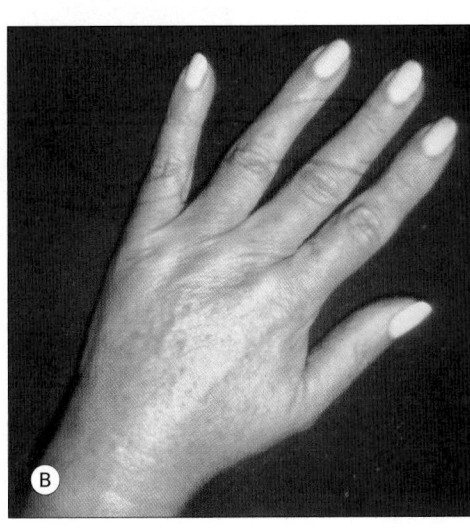

Fig. 158.9 Lipotransfer. Before (**A**) and after (**B**) injection of approximately 10 cm³ of autologous fat into the dorsum of each hand.

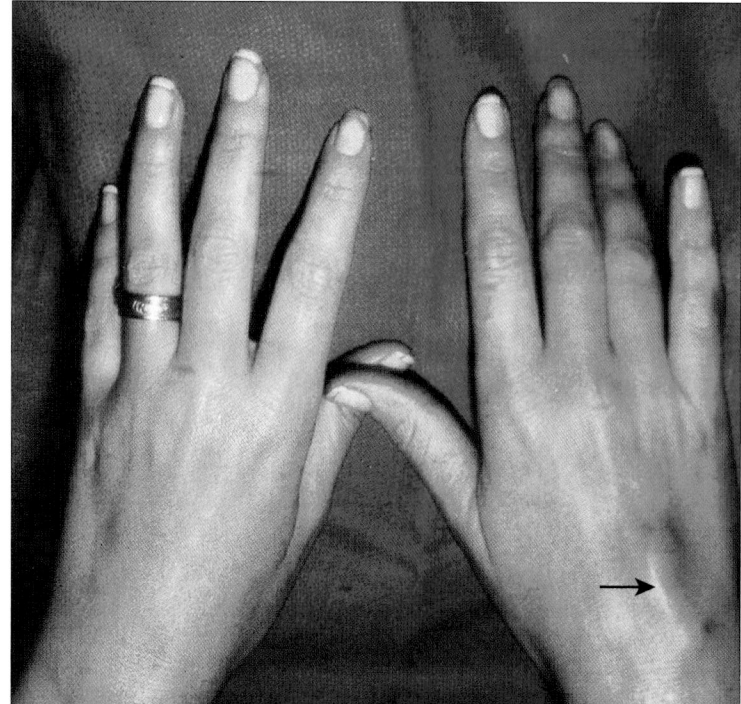

Fig. 158.10 Lipotransfer. Intravascular injection of autologous fat required surgical evacuation (arrow).

lipotransfer technique, viability and persistence of the transplant, and storage[28,29].

CALCIUM HYDROXYLAPATITE

Initially approved for laryngoplasty (vocal cords) and stress-related bladder sphincter incompetence, Radiesse® (previously Radiance FN®) has found a niche in the filler market because its duration is estimated to be up to 1–2 years. It is a milky white suspension comprised of two components: (1) an aqueous gel carrier containing glycerin, sodium carboxymethylcellulose and water; and (2) the matrix particle. Once the carrier dissipates, the matrix, composed of 25–125 µm microspheres of calcium hydroxylapatite, provides the augmentation effect. Calcium hydroxylapatite is a non-allergenic (inert) bioceramic that is identical to the primary mineral constituents found in bone and teeth. This bio-compatible product contains no human, bacterial or animal products and therefore does not pose a risk of hypersensitivity. The material is individually packaged in 1.0 ml syringes. It requires the use of a larger bore needle (25- to 27-gauge). The area to be addressed should be anesthetized with topical or regional anesthesia, and the material is deposited deeply at the dermal–subcutaneous junction.

A unique quality of this product is that it can assume the characteristics of the tissue surrounding it – so, when used for augmentation purposes, it stimulates the fibroblasts to produce collagen. And, when placed into the periosteal space, the material stimulates the production of bone. This product can be used for most facial rhytides and scars and is particularly suitable for patients who have had prior experience with fillers but request a longer duration (Fig. 158.11). Lip augmentation is a contraindication, as there is a greater propensity for mucosal granuloma formation and the constant motion may cause migration of the filler[30,31] (Fig. 158.12). Since the Radiesse® implant is radio-opaque, both the patient and the treating physician should be informed that it may be visible on dental radiographs.

POLY-L-LACTIC ACID

Another dermal filler is polymerized polylactic acid, known as NewFill® or Sculptra®. It was granted FDA approval for the correction of shape and contour deficiencies resulting from facial fat loss associated with HAART for HIV-infected patients[32]. It is powdered lyophilized suture material, i.e. Vicryl® (polyglactin 910). Freeze-dried preparations of polylactic acid are stored at room temperature, and, before injection, each vial must be reconstituted with a total of 5 ml of liquid: 4 ml of

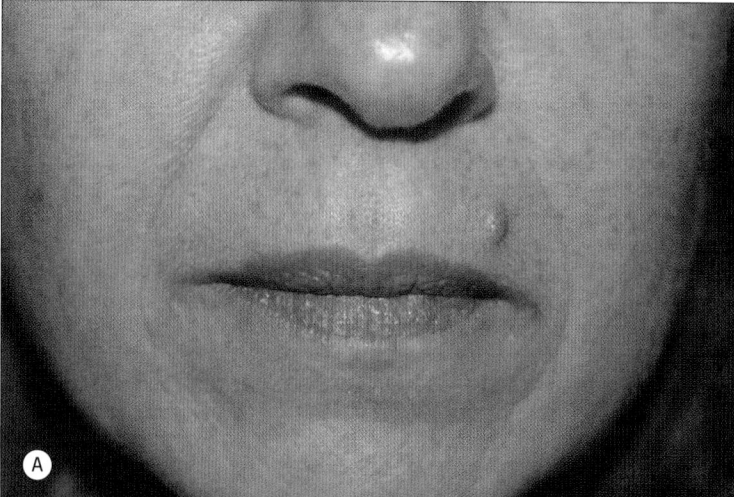

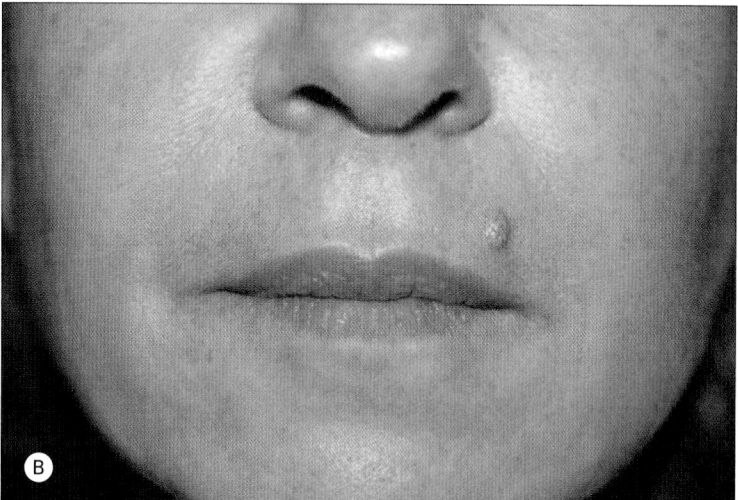

Fig. 158.11 Calcium hydroxylapatite – perioral augmentation. A Prior to injection of 1 cm³ of Radiesse®. **B** Follow-up: softening of nasolabial fold and elevation of lateral oral commissure.

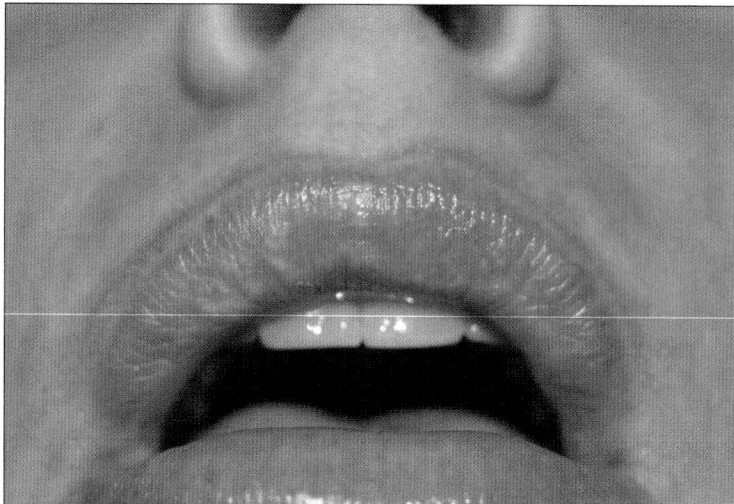

Fig. 158.12 Calcium hydroxylapatite – labial mucosal nodule. Radiesse® was placed too superficially.

sterile water and 1 ml of lidocaine. The result yields a thick suspension of 4.45% polylactic acid. To adequately saturate the powder and obtain a uniform suspension and homogeneous material deposition, it is suggested that the diluent be added approximately 2–4 hours prior to use and that immediately prior to injection the mixture be vigorously agitated. A 26-gauge needle is used to place the product high in the subcutaneous/deep dermal plane without overcorrection. Frequent needle change may be necessary, as the material has a tendency to form clumps. There may be the appearance of some immediate augmentation due to edema, but, to achieve dermal thickness and prolonged neocollagenesis, the recommended protocol is a series of three injections at 3- to 6-week intervals. Persistence of augmentation has varied, but some improvement has been seen at 1.5 to 2 years. There are concerns related to its progenitor suture material; unpredictably, hypersensitivity, granulomas and subcutaneous nodules can arise.

SILICONE

Silicone, polydimethylsiloxane, consists of repeating units of dimethylsiloxane terminated with trimethylsiloxane. Centistoke (cs) refers to the viscosity of silicone oil and is directly related to the chain length of the repeating units. A 1 cs product is equivalent in consistency to water, 350 cs products are oils similar in consistency to mineral oils, and a 1000 cs product is similar in texture to honey. Although useful when injected by an experienced physician, silicone has had a tumultuous history and continues to be controversial. Pure injectable-grade (350 cs) liquid silicone was never approved by the FDA and remains prohibited in the US. However, injectable intraocular silicone (AdatoSil® 5000 centistoke) was approved in 1994 for tamponade to treat complicated retinal detachment. Silikon 1000® was approved for intraocular use in 1997. Under the US FDA Modernization Act, which afforded physicians the right to use medical devices under the same off-label provisions applicable to drugs, physicians could legally use standardized silicone oils for soft tissue augmentation. Since this off-label ruling, there has been an increase in interest and use of silicone for permanent soft tissue augmentation. In 2001, the FDA approved a clinical study of SilSkin®, a highly purified 1000 cs oil, for the treatment of nasolabial folds, marionette lines, and mid-malar depressions. In 2003, the FDA also approved SilSkin® for investigational treatment of HIV-associated lipoatrophy[33,34]. However, prior to administering these products for any purpose, not only is an informed consent required, but physicians must also discuss their use with their medical liability carriers, because they may not cover complications with silicone.

The only form of injectable liquid silicone for soft tissue augmentation is Silikon® 1000. As the placement of the product results in permanent augmentation, there is very little margin for error, and meticulous technique is essential. Many practitioners prefer to use a glass syringe attached to a 30-gauge needle. The silicone is deposited using a microdroplet serial puncture technique, using 0.005–0.01 ml aliquots placed at 2 mm to 5 mm intervals within the dermis without overcorrection. The average treatment should not exceed 0.25–0.75 ml of silicone and the intervals between sessions are usually monthly until the collagen response and cumulative fibroplasia achieve the desired result. As the endpoint of treatment approaches, the volume injected per visit diminishes and the time interval between treatments lengthens. Patients can expect slow and gradual, but permanent, improvement of 30–90%.

Common post-treatment events include erythema, edema and ecchymosis. The incidence of overcorrection with superficial beading, granulomatous and inflammatory reactions, and movement of the product to a distant site (drift) have improved with purer (unadulterated) silicone oil and strict adherence to indications and protocol[35,36].

CONCLUSION

The vast array of available filler products, and those that are on the horizon, are only one means to improve tissue loss associated with aging and trauma. The optimal result may be best achieved by combining fillers of different depth, origin and durability with other aesthetic procedures[30,37]. In short, 'Fillers fill and lifts lift.' The science of soft tissue augmentation is evolving in an exponential manner. Keeping abreast of advances and perfecting a few techniques will be most advantageous for patients; it is not only what is injected, but how it is injected, that determines the degree of success. Finally, regardless of the treatment chosen, it is the combination of clinical judgment, realistic expectations, meticulous preparation, and surgical skill that provides optimal results.

REFERENCES

1. Aschinoff R. Overview: soft tissue augmentation. Clin Plast Surg. 2000;274:479–87.
2. Rohrer TE. Soft tissue filler substances. Curr Probl Dermatol. 2001;13:54–60.
3. Drake L, Dinehart SM, Farmer ER, et al. Guidelines of care for soft tissue augmentation. J Am Acad Dermatol. 1996;34:695–7.
4. Kaminer MS, Krauss MC. Filler substances in the treatment of facial aging. Med Surg Dermatol. 1998;5:215–21.
5. Baumann L, Kerdel F. The treatment of bovine collagen allergy with cyclosporin. Dermatol Surg. 1999;25:247–9.
6. Moody BR, Sengelmann RD. Topical tacrolimus in the treatment of bovine hypersensitivity. Dermatol Surg. 2001;27:789–91.
7. Matarasso SL, Beer K. Injectable collagens. In: Carruthers J, Carruthers A (eds). Soft Tissue Augmentation: Procedures in Cosmetic Dermatology Series. London: Elsevier, 2005:19–31.
8. West TB, Alster TS. Autologous human collagen and dermal fibroblasts for soft tissue augmentation. Dermatol Surg. 1998;24:510–12.
9. Burres S. Preserved particulate fascia lata for injection: a new alternative. Dermatol Surg. 1999;25:790–4.
10. Burres S. Soft tissue augmentation with Fascian. Clin Plast Surg. 2001;28:101–9.
11. Piacquadio S, Jarcho M, Goltz R. Evaluation of Hylan B gel as soft tissue augmentation implant material. J Am Acad Dermatol. 1997;35:544–9.
12. Frank T, Gendler E. Hyaluronic acid for soft tissue augmentation. Clin Plast Surg. 2001;28:121–7.
13. Matarasso SL. Hyaluronic acids: a review and update of available filling agents. Aesthetic Surg J. 2004;24:1–4.
14. Narins RS, Brandt F, Leyden J, et al. A randomized, double blind, multicenter comparison of the efficacy and tolerability of Restylane versus Zyplast for the correction of nasolabial folds. Derrnatol Surg. 2003;29:588–95.
14a. Matarasso SL, Herwick R. Hypersensitivity reaction to injectable non-animal stabilized hyaluronic acid. J Am Acad Dermatol. 2006;55:128–31.

15. Friedman PM, Mafong EA, Kauver AN, Geronemus RG. Safety data of injectable nonanimal stabilized hyaluronic acid gel for soft tissue augmentation. Dermatol Surg. 2002;28:491–4.
16. Lowe NJ, Maxwell A, Lowe P, et al. Hyaluronic acid fillers: adverse reactions and skin testing. J Am Acad Dermatol. 2001;45:930–3.
16a. Brody HJ. The use of hyaluronidase in the treatment of granuomatous hyaluronic acid reactions or unwanted hyaluronic acid misplacement. Dermatol Surg. 2005:31;893–897.
17. Lawrence N. Goretex. In: Narins RS (ed.). Cosmetic Surgery: An Interdisciplinary Approach. New York: Marcel Dekker, 2001:289–311.
17a. Cox SE. Who is still using ePTFE (Gortex/Softform)? Dermatol Surg. 2005;31:163–5.
18. Glogau RG, Matarasso SL, Markey AC. Microlipoinjection: autologous fat grafting. In: Moy R, Lask G (eds). The Principles and Techniques of Cutaneous Surgery. New York: McGraw-Hill, 1996: 437–44.
19. Tzikas TL. Autologous fat grafting for midface rejuvenation. Facial Plast Surg Clin North Am. 2006;14:229–40.
20. Pinski KS, Roenigk HH. Autologous fat transplantation: long-term follow-up. J Dermatol Surg Oncol. 1992;18:179–84.
21. Klein JA. The tumescent technique for liposuction surgery. Am J Cosmet Surg. 1987;4:263–7.
22. Coleman SR. Long-term survival of fat transplants: controlled demonstrations. Aesthetic Plast Surg. 1995;19:421–5.
23. Coleman SR. The techniques of periorbital lipoinfiltration. Oper Tech Plast Reconstr Surg. 1994;1:120–6.
24. Takasu K, Takasu S. Long-term frozen fat for tissue augmentation. J Aesthetic Dermatol Cosmet Surg. 1999;1:173–8.
25. Matarasso A, Matarasso SL. Autologous fat transplantation: a long-term following. Plast Reconstr Surg. 1995;5:988.

26. Chajchir A, Benzaquen I. Liposuction fat grafts in face wrinkles and hemifacial atrophy. Aesthetic Plast Surg. 1986;10:115–17.
27. Carpaneda CA, Ribeiro MT. Percentage of graft viability versus injected volume in adipose autotransplants. Aesthetic Plast Surg. 1994;18:17–19.
28. Sadick NS. Fatty acid analysis of transplanted adipose tissue. Arch Dermatol. 2001;37:723–9.
29. Drake L, Dinehart S, Farmer E, et al. Guidelines of care for soft tissue augmentation with fat transplantation. J Am Acad Dermatol. 1996;34:690–4.
30. Hoffman C, Schuller-Petrovic S, Soyer HP, et al. Adverse reactions after cosmetic lip augmentation with permanent biological inert materials. J Am Acad Dermatol. 1999;40:100–102.
31. Tzikas TL. Evaluation of the Radiance FN soft tissue filler for facial soft tissue augmentation. Arch Facial Plast Surg. 2004;6:234–9.
32. Day JN, Raabe A, Shiner AM, et al Intradermal polylactic acid (NewFill) for treatment of severe HIV-associated facial lipoatrophy. HIV Med. 2002;3:162.
33. Orentreich DS, Orentreich NO. Injectable fluid silicone. In: Roenigk RK, Roenigk HH (eds). Dermatologic Surgery: Principles and Practice. New York: Marcel Dekker, 1989:1349–95.
34. Jones D, Carruthers A, Orentreich D, et al. Highly purified 1000-cst silicone oil for the treatment of human immunodeficiency virus-associated facial lipoatrophy: an open pilot trial. Dermatol Surg. 2004;30:1279–86.
35. Baumann L, Halem M. Lip silicone granulomatous foreign body reaction treated with Aldara (imiquimod 5%). Dermatol Surg. 2003;29:429–32.
36. Duffy DM. The silicone conundrum: A battle of anecdotes. Dermatol Surg. 2002;28:590–4.
37. Miller TA, Klein AW, Lambros VS, Matarasso SL. Soft tissue augmentation. J Aesthetic Surg. 2001;20:309–14.

Botulinum Toxin

159

Alastair Carruthers and Jean Carruthers

Synonyms: ■ Botulinum toxin type A, botulinum A exotoxin, BTX-A, BOTOX®/BOTOX Cosmetic®, Dysport®, Reloxin® ■ Botulinum toxin type B, BTX-B, MYOBLOC®

Key features

- Botulinum toxin (BTX) causes chemodenervation of muscles by blocking acetylcholine release

- Injections of botulinum toxin type A (BTX-A) that weaken or relax muscles can smooth hyperfunctional lines and change the contour of the face and neck

- Adjunctive use of BTX-A with laser resurfacing or soft tissue augmentation is beneficial, particularly in active regions such as the perioral and periocular areas

- The cosmetic effects of BTX-A typically last months and may increase with subsequent injections

- Complications (e.g. eyelid ptosis) are generally caused by diffusion of the toxin to non-targeted muscles and can be avoided by using concentrated doses and careful technique

INTRODUCTION

Botulinum exotoxin (BTX) injections are commonly used to improve facial aesthetics by smoothing hyperdynamic rhytides in the upper face. In recent years, BTX has been used increasingly in the mid- and lower face and neck, in part because of its demonstrated efficacy and safety for indications in the upper face, and in part because of awareness that muscular hyperactivity (in addition to volume depletion) contributes to the aesthetic appearance of the mid- and lower face and neck. Today, BTX therapy is an integral aspect of most cosmetic practices.

PROPERTIES OF BOTULINUM TOXINS

Various strains of the bacterium *Clostridium botulinum* produce, as a group, seven distinct serotypes of BTX that affect neural function: A, B, C1, D, E, F and G[1]. Although all these serotypes produce chemodenervation and atrophy of skeletal muscles by blocking acetylcholine release from motor neurons at the neuromuscular junction (Fig. 159.1), they differ with regard to cellular mechanism of action and clinical profile[2].

BTX type A (BTX-A) was the first toxin developed for clinical use and it is manufactured and distributed by Allergan Inc. under the brand name BOTOX®/BOTOX Cosmetic® and by Ipsen Limited (UK) under

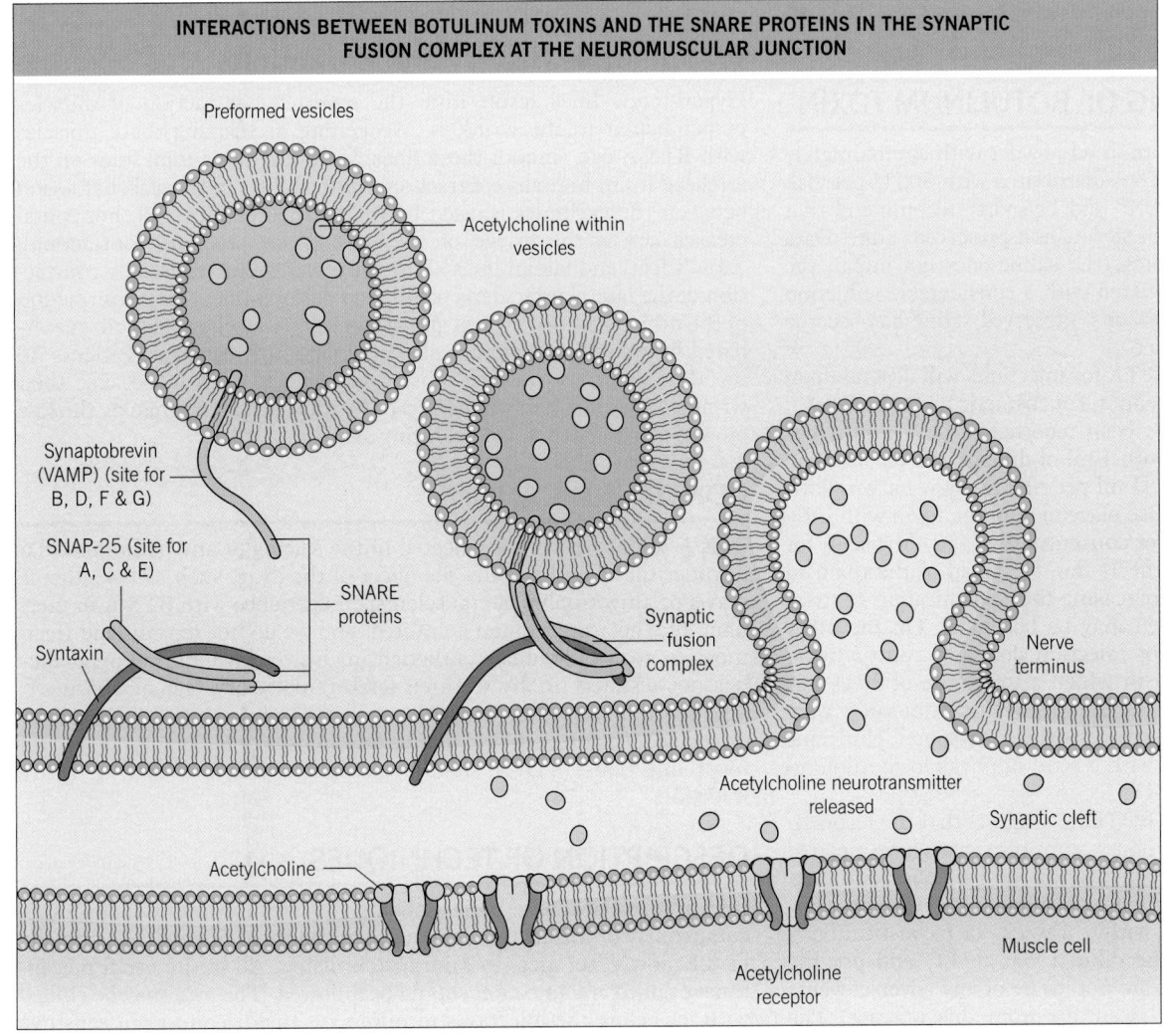

INTERACTIONS BETWEEN BOTULINUM TOXINS AND THE SNARE PROTEINS IN THE SYNAPTIC FUSION COMPLEX AT THE NEUROMUSCULAR JUNCTION

Preformed vesicles

Acetylcholine within vesicles

Synaptobrevin (VAMP) (site for B, D, F & G)

SNAP-25 (site for A, C & E)

SNARE proteins

Syntaxin

Synaptic fusion complex

Nerve terminus

Acetylcholine neurotransmitter released

Synaptic cleft

Acetylcholine

Acetylcholine receptor

Muscle cell

Fig. 159.1 Interactions between botulinum toxins and the SNARE proteins in the synaptic fusion complex at the neuromuscular junction. Botulinum toxins A, C and E catalyze the cleavage of the SNAP-25 protein. Botulinum toxins B, D, F and G catalyze the cleavage of synaptobrevin (or the vesicle-associated membrane protein, VAMP). Adapted from Rohrer TE, Beer K: Background to Botulinum Toxin. In Carruthers A, Carruthers J, editors: Botulinum Toxin, Philadelphia, 2005, Saunders.

the name Dysport® (to be marketed in the US, Canada and Japan as Reloxin® by Medicis in 2008). Other BTX-A preparations on the world market include Linurase® (Prollenium Medical Technologies Inc., Canada), CBTX-A (Lanzhou Biological Products Institute, China), Neuronox® (Medy-Tox Inc., South Korea), and Xeomin® (Merz GmbH, Germany); Mentor Corporation (US) has a preparation (Purtox®) that may be introduced in future years. None of these newer products are licensed for importation into or approved for use in North America at the time of writing. Since all preparations of BTX-A differ in potency and clinical effect, their units are not interchangeable.

Intramuscular injections of BTX-A have become the treatment of choice for a number of disorders characterized by muscular hyper-activity, such as strabismus[3], blepharospasm and hemifacial spasm[4], and cervical dystonia[5]. In addition, the ability of BTX to block acetyl-choline release from autonomic nerve endings innervating glandular tissue or smooth muscle has led to investigation of its use for other indications, including hyperhidrosis[6], migraine[7], tension headaches[8] and myofascial pain[9]. Direct comparisons of BOTOX® and Dysport® for the treatment of hyperhidrosis and cervical dystonia have suggested that Dysport® may be slightly more effective but has a higher incidence of adverse effects[10,11].

The only other commercially available serotype is a formulation of BTX type B (BTX-B; MYOBLOC®, also called Neurobloc® in Europe; marketed by Solstice Neurosciences, Inc.) that was approved in the US by the Food and Drug Administration (FDA) in 2000 for the treatment of cervical dystonia, but has been used off-label to treat facial wrinkles and evaluated in several smaller clinical trials[12–14]. Research indicates that there are key differences in effects between BTX-A and BTX-B for the treatment of facial rhytides: BTX-B has a more rapid onset of action but a shorter duration of effect, diffuses more widely, and is associated with greater pain and other side effects than BTX-A[15,16].

Note: Since most of the information available on the cosmetic uses of BTX, both from published reports and from our personal experience, pertains to the use of BOTOX®/BOTOX Cosmetic®, the following discussion focuses on the cosmetic use of those formulations specifically, and all unit doses given in the description of techniques refer to BOTOX® units, unless otherwise stated.

DILUTION AND HANDLING OF BOTULINUM TOXIN

BOTOX® is distributed as a vacuum-dried powder with approximately 100 U per vial; lyophilized Dysport® is distributed with 500 U per vial. The manufacturers of both BOTOX® and Dysport® recommend that their products be reconstituted with sterile, non-preserved saline. Data suggest that reconstitution with preserved saline does not impair the stability of BTX-A[17,18] and is associated with a considerable reduction of pain on injection[19]. For these reasons, preserved saline has become the reconstitution material of choice.

The optimum concentration of BTX for injections will depend upon the serotype, formulation and procedure. For cosmetic use of BOTOX®, the average volume of diluent has been reported to be 2.5 ml[17], but many users reconstitute the vial with 1 ml of diluent. We recommend using a concentration of 100 U/ml (1 ml per vial) to allow for very-low-volume injections that permit precise placement of the toxin with little spread to non-targeted areas. Lower concentrations may be useful for some indications, but if adverse effects due to spread of the toxin to unintended targets is a problem, increasing the concentration of toxin and decreasing the volume injected may be beneficial. On the other hand, data suggest that volume of injection does not contribute to diffusion; in a dose-dilution study in which a total dose of 30 U was reconstituted in 1, 3, 5 or 10 ml, no differences in efficacy or safety were observed between groups[20]. For the cosmetic use of Dysport®, clinicians recommend diluting a 500 U vial with 2.5 ml of physiologic saline to obtain a concentration of 200 U/ml[21].

Although the package insert for BOTOX® suggests that the reconstituted toxin should be used within 4 hours, some physicians have reported using BTX-A 7 to 10 days after reconstitution with no observed alteration in potency[17], and Hexsel and colleagues found no significant differences in efficacy when injected within 6 weeks of reconstitution[22]. It is common practice to store the diluted vial at 4°C and use the diluted toxin over several days; we are not aware of any adverse events or any significant loss of potency resulting from this practice. The

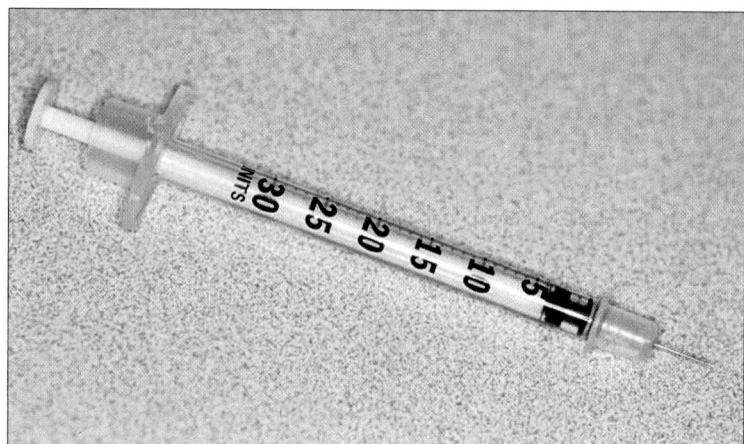

Fig. 159.2 Equipment. A 30-gauge insulin needle has no 'dead volume' and is ideal for injections.

diluted toxin is transferred to a 0.3 ml insulin syringe with a 30-gauge needle that has no 'dead volume' and is ideal for injections (B-D Ultrafine II 0.3 ml syringe, 30-gauge 6 mm needle; Fig. 159.2)[23].

Dosing and Injection Schedules

The effects of BTX-A injections are usually apparent within a day or two and are obvious for 3 or 4 months, although they may last for 6 months or longer. With repeated injections, there is a tendency for later injections to provide aesthetic improvement that lasts longer; it is possible that over the course of treatment, individuals alter their habitual use of muscles that cause expression lines. Long-term remodeling of the dermis and epidermis that helps to sustain the cosmetic effects also occurs in most individuals, because the tissue is no longer subjected to the same forces of muscle contraction.

Preoperative History and Conditions

Hyperkinetic lines result from the repeated contraction of muscles perpendicular to the wrinkles. Weakening or relaxing these muscles with BTX-A can smooth these lines, including horizontal lines on the forehead (from frontalis contraction), vertical lines in the glabellar region between the eyebrows (caused by the corrugator muscles), horizontal creases across the bridge of the nose (from procerus contraction), 'crow's feet' and lateral lines along the lower eyelid (caused by contraction of the lateral orbicularis oculi), and perioral lines (from contraction of the orbicularis oris). Deep grooves or folds elsewhere that are exacerbated by muscle activity are also amenable to treatment. Patients 30 to 50 years of age may be most responsive to BTX-A, because their wrinkles are more likely to be caused by muscle activity than by the loss of skin elasticity that occurs during aging.

CONTRAINDICATIONS

BTX-A therapy is contraindicated in the setting of any neuromuscular disorder that could amplify the effect of the drug, such as myasthenia gravis or amyotrophic lateral sclerosis. Experience with BTX-A in pregnant and lactating women is limited, and we do not recommend treatment in such individuals, although inadvertent use during pregnancy has not resulted in any reported teratogenicity or pregnancy issues[24]. The possibility of drug interactions exists, and patients taking aminoglycoside antibiotics should receive lower doses of BTX-A. As is true for most injections, BTX-A should not be given in any area of active infection.

DESCRIPTION OF TECHNIQUES

Injections for aesthetic indications may be given intramuscularly, subcutaneously or intradermally. We use intradermal injections, especially in the crow's feet area, to minimize bruising. All of the usual precautions prior to any injection should be followed. The area may be chilled with ice before the injections to minimize any discomfort in sensitive individuals. Alternatively, a topical anesthetic can be applied 15 to 30 minutes prior to injection to minimize discomfort, and some physicians report great benefits from vibration analgesia[25].

Electromyographic (EMG) guidance can be used to inject BTX into the most active region of the muscle. Once a thorough understanding of the relevant facial anatomy is attained (Fig. 142.7), injection with an EMG system provides little benefit. However, even experienced clinicians may find EMG guidance to be useful for the occasional difficult-to-treat patient.

Glabellar Frown Lines

Frown lines in the glabellar region are caused by contraction of the corrugator supercilii and orbicularis oculi muscles, which move the brow medially, and the procerus and depressor supercilii, which pull the brow inferiorly. Because the corrugator and procerus are used only to control facial expression, the goal of treatment should be to produce a significant weakening of these muscles. The treatment sites and doses should be individualized because the location, size and use of the frown muscles vary greatly between individuals.

Extensive clinical experience supports the efficacy and safety of BTX-A for the treatment of glabellar rhytides[24,26,27]. We currently use five injection sites when treating glabellar frown lines and vary the dosage depending on the individual brow. Men typically require higher starting doses than women; in dose-ranging studies, a total of 20 to 40 U was significantly more effective than 10 U in women[28], whereas 40 to 80 U were more effective than lower doses in men[29]. We use initial starting doses of approximately 30 and 60 U BTX-A for women and men, respectively, titrating to 50 and 100 U in women and men, respectively, if necessary.

During a typical procedure, the patient is seated with the chin down and head slightly lower than the physician's. We insert the needle just above the superior bony orbital rim, directly above the inner canthus (Fig. 159.3) and inject an appropriate dose – 7 to 10 U in women and 15 to 20 U in men. Regardless of eyebrow position, the injection site is always above the bony supraorbital ridge. We repeat the procedure on the opposite side of the brow to ensure symmetry. Next, we inject 5 to 10 U into the procerus at the midline. In individuals with horizontal brows, we inject an additional 4 to 5 U 1 cm above the bony supraorbital rim in the midpupillary line. Since this injection site is the most likely to cause eyebrow ptosis, it may be omitted if eyebrow ptosis

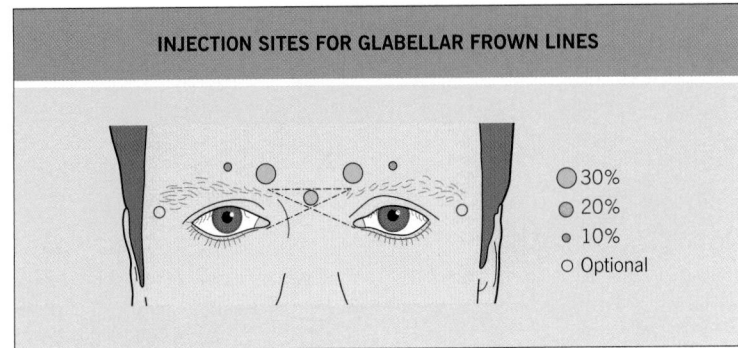

INJECTION SITES FOR GLABELLAR FROWN LINES

○ 30%
○ 20%
○ 10%
○ Optional

Fig. 159.3 Injection sites for glabellar frown lines. The authors currently use five injection sites when treating glabellar frown lines and vary the dosage depending on the individual brow. The injection in the midpupillary line may be omitted if eyebrow ptosis seems likely or possible. Sometimes, an injection is made above the lateral canthus or into the tail of the eyebrow.

appears likely or possible, at the cost of slightly reducing the effectiveness of treating the frown complex. Finally, it is frequently necessary to inject above the lateral canthus or into the tail of the eyebrow, further reducing the ability to frown and improving lateral eyebrow position. The procedure effectively smoothes the glabellar lines at rest and prevents their appearance when the patient attempts to frown for an average of 3 to 4 months (Fig. 159.4).

Crow's Feet

Contraction of the lateral fibers of the orbicularis oculi muscle produces 'crow's feet', lines that radiate from the lateral canthus. Since forceful closure of the eyelids requires orbicularis contraction, the goal of treatment is to produce weakening just in the lateral orbital area, rather than a complete paralysis of the muscle. Because the orbicularis oculi is diffusely innervated, multiple injections are required to weaken broad areas of the muscle.

Reported total doses for the treatment of crow's feet range from 8 to 16 U per side (in women) and 12 to 16 U per side (in men) distributed over multiple injection sites, with 3 to 4 U injected per site[24]. We inject 12 to 15 U of BTX-A per side distributed in equal parts among two to four injection sites (Fig. 159.5). Injections are performed when the patient

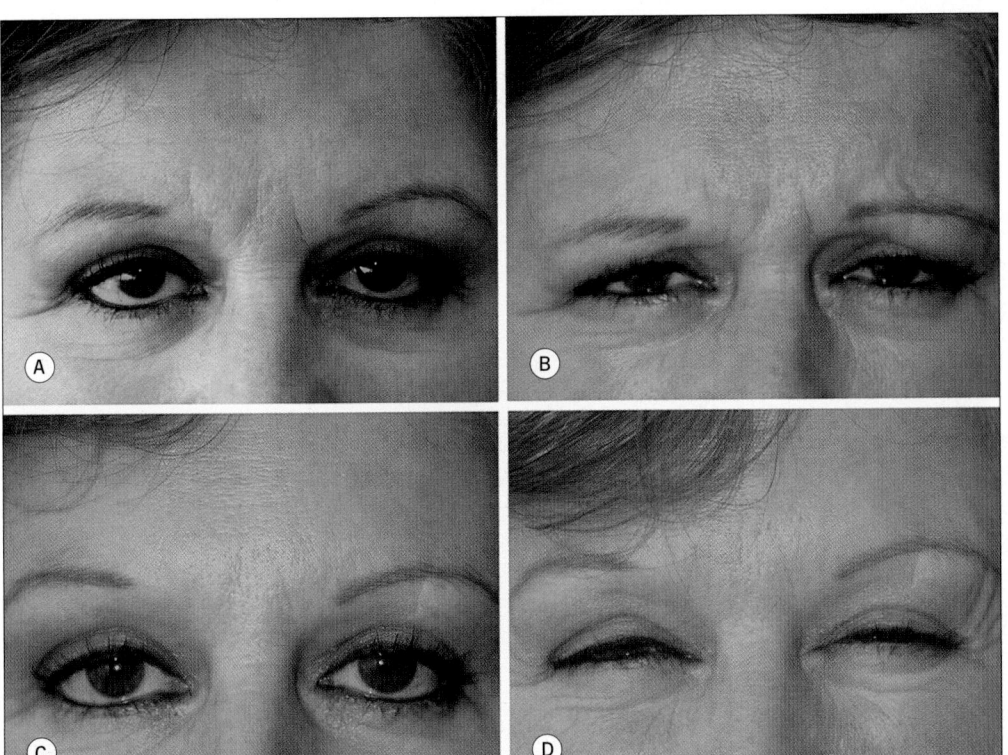

Fig. 159.4 Glabellar lines. In a subject at rest (**A**) and during frowning (**B**). Subject at rest (**C**) and attempting to frown (**D**) 1 week after BTX-A treatment.

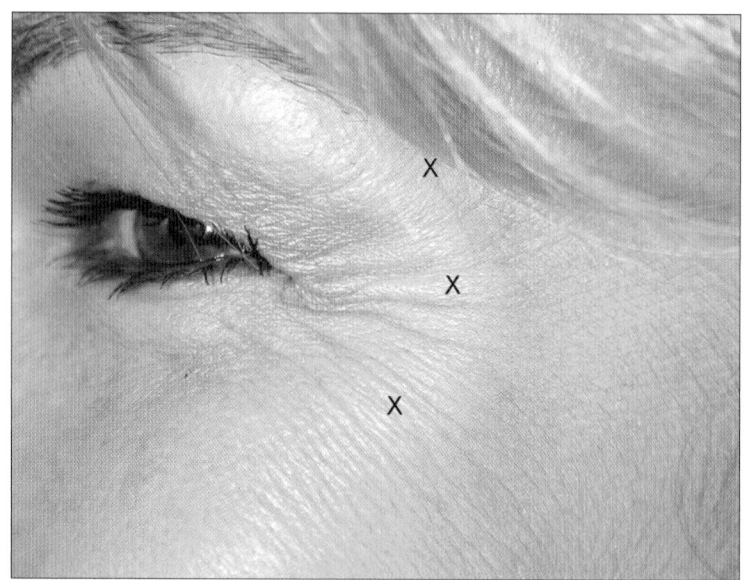

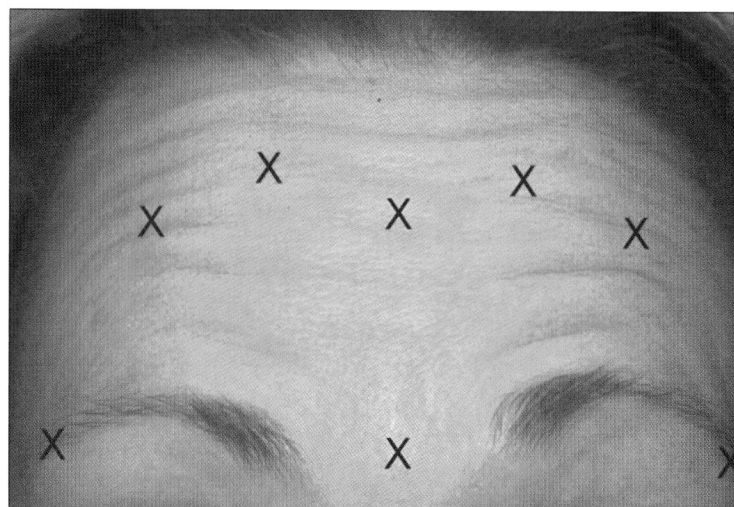

Fig. 159.8 Injection sites for horizontal forehead lines. Injection sites must be kept well above the brow. The lower X's mark the sites of injection of the brow depressors.

Fig. 159.5 Injection sites for crow's feet. The authors inject 12 to 15 U of BTX-A (BOTOX®) per side among two to four injection sites.

is *not* smiling, or the toxin may affect the ipsilateral zygomaticus complex, causing upper lip ptosis. Injections are lateral to the lateral orbital rim, because more medial injections can result in a side effect of temporary lower eyelid droop; at least one case of lateral rectus weakness causing diplopia has been reported following injection in the lateral periocular area. We inject superficially and try to use as few injections as possible to minimize bruising. Care is taken to avoid injecting any superficial veins. Results last approximately 3 months (Fig. 159.6).

Horizontal Forehead Lines

Deep horizontal creases in the forehead are produced by the repeated contraction of the frontalis. This large, vertically oriented muscle is the brow elevator; it inserts superiorly into the galea aponeurotica and inferiorly into the skin of the brow. Unfortunately, weakening the frontalis sufficiently to eliminate hyperkinetic forehead lines can result in undesired brow ptosis or a complete lack of expressiveness. There-

fore, the goal of treatment is to only soften, rather than completely eliminate, forehead lines. Ideally, the individual will still be able to elevate the eyebrows, albeit to a lesser extent, after treatment (Fig. 159.7). We believe that the brow depressors should *always* be treated at the same time as the frontalis, and we use the technique described under 'Brow lift and shaping' below.

A wide range of doses and dilutions have been described for the treatment of horizontal forehead lines, but most reports emphasize that the injection sites should be kept well above the brow to avoid ptosis[24]. In our practice, a total of 10 to 15 U BTX-A is divided among multiple sites distributed horizontally across the mid forehead, 2 to 3 cm above the eyebrows (Fig. 159.8). For individuals with a broad forehead (more than 12 cm between the temporal fusion lines [the slight prominence at the point where the temporalis fascia joins the skull] at the mid-forehead level), we use five injection sites. For individuals with a narrow forehead, we use four injection sites and a slightly lower total dose. Effects typically last from 3 to 6 months.

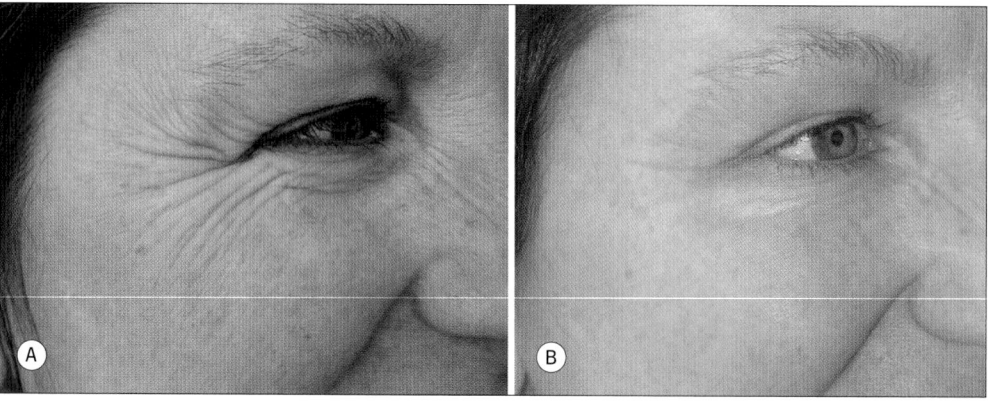

Fig. 159.6 Crow's feet. Subject with crow's feet before (**A**) and 3 weeks after BTX-A treatment (**B**).

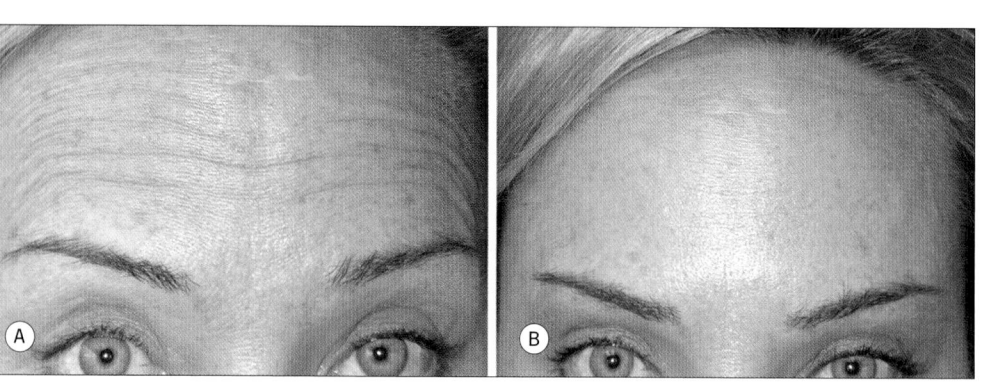

Fig. 159.7 Horizontal forehead lines produced when the subject elevated the brows before (**A**) and 1 month after BTX-A treatment (**B**).

Brow Lift and Shaping

Brow ptosis often occurs during aging, resulting in an angry, scowling expression. The shape and height of the eyebrow are determined by the opposing activity of the frontalis muscle, which elevates the brow, and the brow depressors. The medial brow depressors are the corrugator supercilii, the procerus, and the medial portion of the orbicularis oculi; the lateral depressor is the lateral portion of the orbicularis oculi lateral to the temporal fusion line. Previously, we believed that brow lifts were a result of the inactivation of the brow depressors and published several reports (along with other authors) claiming that treatment of the brow depressors led to brow elevation[30–33]. However, additional analysis of a dosing study showed that central injections of 20 to 40 U of BTX-A into the glabella alone (with the most lateral injection at the mid-pupillary line) led to a dramatic lateral eyebrow elevation, followed by an entire brow lift that peaked at 12 weeks post treatment[34]. Interestingly, too little BTX-A (10 U) led to a brief *fall* in eyebrow position. We now believe that changes in eyebrow position after glabella injection in women is due to diffusion of the BTX-A into the lower frontalis muscle, which causes an improved resting tone in the remainder of the muscle and in eyebrow position.

Hypertrophic Orbicularis Oculi

The pretarsal portion of the orbicularis oculi muscle is involved in the blink reflex. Contraction of the pretarsal orbicularis during smiling tends to decrease the size of the palpebral aperture. Hypertrophy of this muscle can give a 'jelly roll' appearance to the lower eyelid, enough that some individuals may complain that they look overweight. We have found that injection of 2 U of BTX-A into the lower pretarsal orbicularis opens the palpebral aperture both at rest and during smiling (Fig. 159.9)[35,36].

We inject subcutaneously in the midpupillary line, 3 mm below the ciliary margin. The dose is limited to 2 U or occasionally 4 U, because higher doses in this area can result in symptomatic dry eye (keratoconjunctivitis sicca). Lateral orbital injections have a synergistic effect with lower eyelid injections and can be used as a safe way to enhance the lower eyelid effect without using too high a dose in the lower lid orbicularis. This procedure is used only for patients who respond well to a preinjection snap test, in which the lower eyelid is briefly pulled off the globe by downward pressure on the lower eyelid skin, then quickly released, and the speed with which the eyelid snaps back to the globe assessed. Patients who have had previous lower eyelid ablative resurfacing or infralash blepharoplasty without a coexisting canthopexy to support the normal position of the lower eyelid are not good candidates for this procedure.

'Bunny Lines'

Contraction of the upper nasalis muscle causes fanning rhytides ('bunny lines') at the radix root of the nose. BTX-A treatment weakens the upper nasalis effectively and dramatically softens these lines. Bunny lines are typically treated in conjunction with the glabellar complex. We inject 2–4 units of BTX-A into each belly of the upper nasalis as it traverses the lateral bony dorsum of the nose. Usually one injection per side is sufficient (Fig. 159.10). We are careful to inject well above the nasofacial groove to avoid relaxing the levator labii superioris and causing lip ptosis. The area is gently massaged following each injection to facilitate diffusion of the toxin; however, too-vigorous massage or massage in a downward direction could also result in lip ptosis.

Repeated Nasal Flare

Some individuals repeatedly and embarrassingly dilate their nostrils in social situations. The sides of the columella/septum become visible when the nostrils are prominently flared. Contraction of the nasalis muscle accentuates the nasal flare. Injection of 5 to 10 U of BTX-A bilaterally into the lower nasalis fibers covering the lateral nasal ala, at the most active area of muscle contraction, has produced a satisfactory decrease in involuntary nostril flare in some patients for 3 to 4 months.

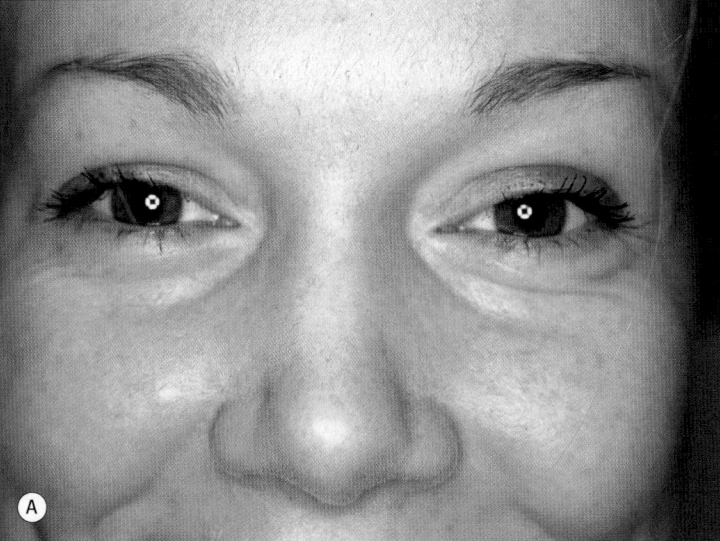
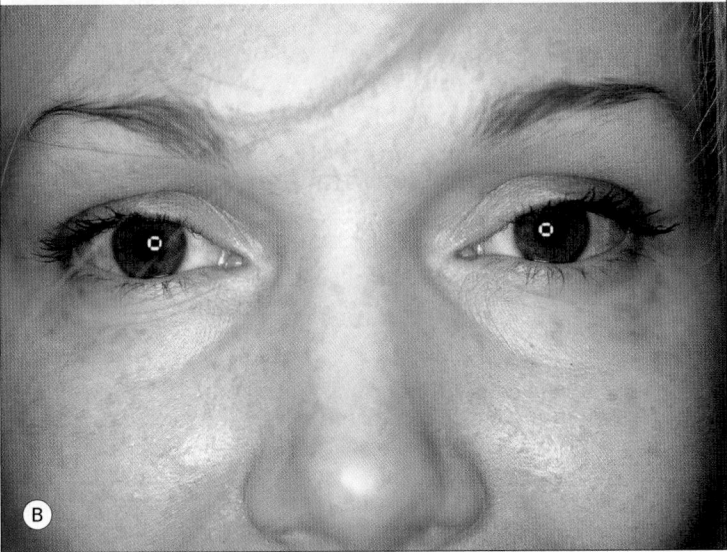

Fig. 159.9 Hypertrophic orbicularis oculi muscle. BTX-A treatment of the lower pretarsal orbicularis opens the palebral aperture. Note the position of the lower eyelids in the subject before (**A**) and after treatment (**B**).

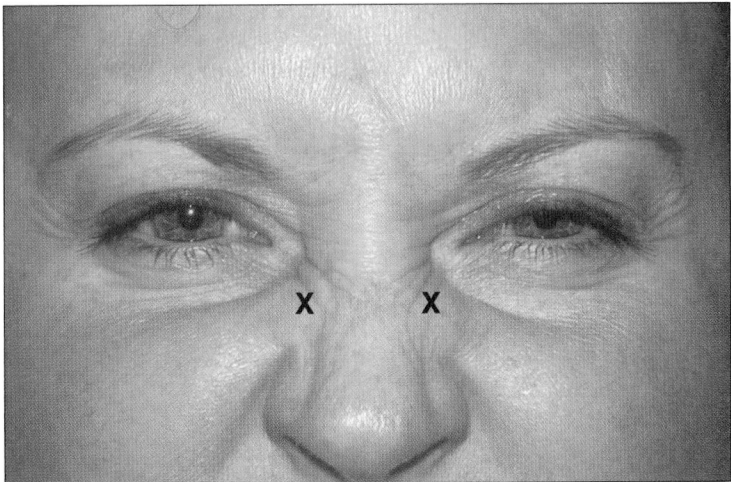

Fig. 159.10 Injection sites for 'bunny lines'. 2–4 units of BTX-A are injected into each belly of the upper nasalis as it traverses the lateral bony dorsum of the nose. Usually one injection per side is sufficient.

Nasolabial Folds in Selected Patients

Nasolabial folds extend from the lateral nasal ala to a point lateral to the external angle of the mouth. Young adults have a shallow indentation, but older individuals who smile excessively or sustain photodamage can develop a permanent, deep crevice. The most common treatments for nasolabial folds have been soft tissue fillers and laser resurfacing. Although muscle contraction contributes to the appearance of the folds, injecting BTX-A directly into the area of the fold is not the treatment of choice, because it is likely to result in an asymmetric smile, flaccid cheek, flattening of the midface, and incomplete or disappointing results. The cutaneous upper lip lengthens vertically, as is often seen during aging. However, for some individuals who have a naturally shorter cutaneous upper lip, very small doses of BTX-A (1 U into each lip elevator complex above the nasofacial groove) can be beneficial for improving nasolabial folds, particularly when the injections are given concurrently with other treatment (fillers or resurfacing).

Because the duration of effect of this procedure is relatively long (~6 months), it is important to be very careful in patient selection and to be clear about the potential results of the procedure.

Nasal Tip Droop

Nasal tip droop is common during aging. Contraction of the depressor septi nasi, a small muscle located at the external base of the nasal septum, pulls the tip of the nose downward. Injection of 2 to 3 U of BTX-A into the depressor septi at the base of the columella slightly elevates the nasal tip. Caution should be taken with individuals who already have a long non-vermilion upper lip, because of an associated risk of lip ptosis.

Vertical Lip Rhytides (Perioral Lines)

During aging, the area of the mouth undergoes characteristic changes: the lateral portions of the lips recede to produce a 'rosebud mouth'; the vertical distance between the columella and the vermilion border of the upper lip increases, and the substance of the vermilion lip rolls inside, producing the thin and disappointed lips characteristic of old age. Dense vertical perioral rhytides are often associated with the lengthening of the cutaneous upper lip during aging. These vertical lines are commonly referred to as 'smokers' lines' but can have other causes, such as heredity, photodamage, or activities such as playing a musical instrument that require pursing of the lips. Radial upper lip wrinkles are exaggerated by the pursestring-like action of the orbicularis oris sphincter muscle of the lip. Multiple fine wrinkles of the upper lip can be effectively treated with fillers such as collagen or hyaluronic acid or with mid-depth or deeper resurfacing. However, deeper wrinkles may be resistant to these treatments.

BTX-A treatment of the lip sphincter is recommended only for deep lines. Small doses that produce localized microparesis of the orbicularis oris can dramatically reduce radial lip lines and improve the appearance of the lips. To maintain competence of the mouth, it is important to be conservative with dosing, and superficial injections are recommended over deep injections. In our practice, we achieve optimal results with doses not exceeding 4 U BTX-A per lip (2 U per lip quadrant). We typically inject 1 U per lip line, which smoothes the lines and also results in a pleasing pseudoeversion of the lip (Fig. 159.11). BTX-A is injected in the area of muscle contraction adjacent to the creases at the vermilion border on either side of the cupid's bow. The corners of the lips are avoided because injection at these sites can cause weakness of the lateral lip elevators resulting in drooping of the lateral lip and drooling, and the midline is avoided to prevent flattening of cupid's bow. Even with conservative dosing, however, BTX-A treatment of perioral lines may result in lip sphincter weakening that subtly affects mouth function. This procedure may not be desirable for musicians who play wind instruments and professional singers or speakers. Some patients have difficulty with lip proprioception after treatment, but eating, drinking and singing are typically not affected.

BTX-A injections for radial lip lines may be particularly useful in combination with perioral laser and electrosurgical resurfacing or in combination with a soft tissue-augmenting agent such as collagen or hyaluronic acid.

Upper Gum Show

When some individuals smile, the upper lip is retracted too far, resulting in excessive exposure of the upper gum. The gum line, upper incisors and canines are fully revealed. The levator labii superioris alaeque nasi muscle retracts the upper lip; chemodenervation of the muscle with BTX-A results in a moderate drop in the upper lip sufficient to cover the upper gum. We inject 1 to 2 U of BTX-A into the levator labii superioris alaeque nasi on each side of the bony nasal prominence. Small concentrated doses are used, often injected with EMG guidance to accurately target the muscle. An undesired side effect of this treatment is the vertical elongation of the cutaneous upper lip. Because this effect is already an undesirable sign of aging, the procedure generally produces unsatisfactory results in patients who are middle-aged and older, and it is usually recommended only for younger patients. For most patients, the best results are obtained when this procedure is used in combination with soft tissue augmentation of the lip margins.

Facial Asymmetry: Functional Muscle Imbalance

Injections of BTX-A can also be used to correct facial asymmetry resulting from facial nerve palsies[37], dystonias[4,38], surgery[39] or trauma[40]. In cases of hemiparesis, BTX-A is used to decrease muscle activity on the unaffected side; for hyperkinesia, the affected muscles are treated.

Normal adult faces usually have some degree of facial asymmetry, but it is generally not noticed unless photographs are examined. Midfacial asymmetry may have bony tissue, soft tissue or innervational/muscular causes. BTX-A treatment can be invaluable for patients with facial asymmetry caused by neuromuscular abnormalities. In hemifacial spasm, repeated clonic and tonic facial movements draw the facial midline over toward the hyperfunctional side. BTX-A treatment of the hyperfunctional zygomaticus, risorius and masseter muscles allows the face to be centered at rest. Hypofunctional asymmetry, such as that seen in Bell's palsy due to unilateral seventh nerve dysfunction, can be relieved by small doses of BTX-A injected into muscles on the normofunctional side[41]. Only 1 to 2 U of BTX-A in the zygomaticus, risorius and orbicularis oris and 5 to 10 U in the masseter are needed to restore facial symmetry.

For patients with asymmetric jaw movement, intraoral injection of 10 to 15 U of BTX-A into the internal pterygoid on the hyperfunctional side can relax the jaw and relieve discomfort. Physicians who are not thoroughly comfortable with facial surface anatomy are well advised to use an EMG guidance system for injections.

Unilateral surgical or traumatic injury of the orbicularis oris or the risorius muscle can cause the mouth to be pulled off center by the unopposed actions of the partner muscles on the uninjured side. Chemodenervation of the risorius immediately lateral to the corner of the mouth on the uninjured side re-centers the mouth when the face is at rest. Similarly, facial asymmetry is evident in individuals with congenital or acquired unilateral weakness of the depressor anguli oris (DAO) muscle who are unable to depress the corner of one side of the mouth. In these cases as well, BTX-A treatment of the partner muscle restores aesthetic balance.

Mouth Frown

The frowning expression created when the lateral corners of the mouth are permanently angled downward can create an impression of dis-

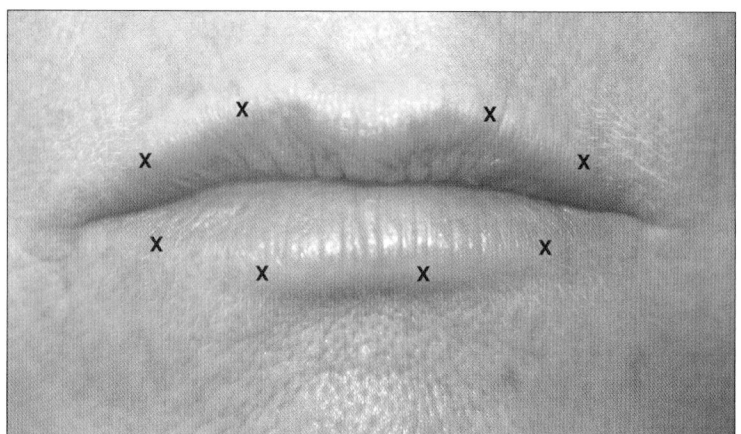

Fig. 159.11 Injection sites for perioral rhytides. The authors typically inject 1 U of BTX-A (BOTOX®) per lip line.

approval and unpleasantness. The DAO muscle pulls down the corner of the mouth in opposition to the zygomaticus major and minor muscles. BTX-A can be used to weaken the DAO and reset muscular balance, allowing the zygomaticus to elevate the corners of the mouth and return them to a horizontal position (Fig. 159.12).

In our practice, we ask patients to frown to aid in the location of the DAO, then inject 2 to 3 U of BTX-A into the posterior aspect of the muscle on each side, close to the mandible as well as 3 U into each insertion of the mentalis for a superior result (Fig. 159.13). The effects of this procedure may be potentiated with repeated treatment.

It is always important to be cautious when injecting toxin close to the mouth. A misplaced injection could result in complications, including a flaccid cheek, incompetent mouth or asymmetric smile. The treatment is not recommended for singers or musicians, or for patients who

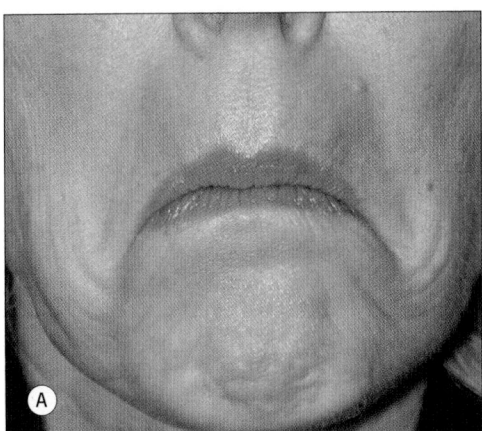

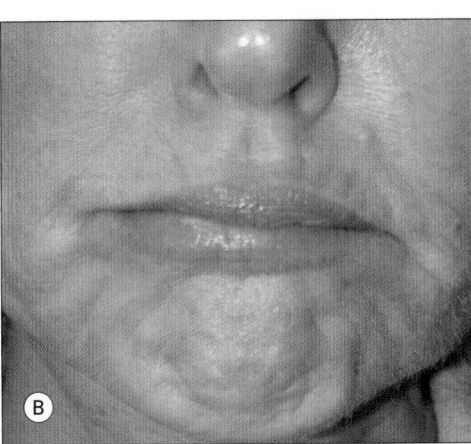

Fig. 159.12 Mouth frown. The subject before (**A**) and after BTX-A treatment (**B**) of the depressor anguli oris muscle.

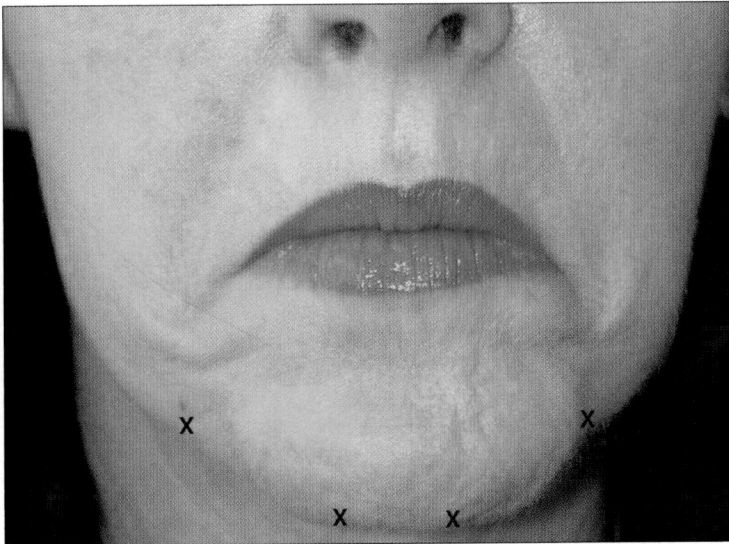

Fig. 159.13 Injection sites for mouth frown. The authors typically inject 2 to 3 U of BTX-A (BOTOX®) into the posterior aspect of the depressor anguli oris muscle and 3 U into each insertion of the mentalis muscle.

use their perioral muscle with intensity. With this procedure, as for others in the perioral area, the most pleasing results may be obtained with BTX-A injections in combination with laser resurfacing.

Melomental Folds (Marionette Lines)

Melomental folds ('drool grooves' or marionette lines) extending from the down-turned corner of the mouth to the lateral mentum involuntarily produce a sad expression and give the appearance of advancing age. Traditionally, soft tissue augmentation has been used; however, the effects are not long lasting, because filling agents do not endure in this highly mobile and expressive region of the face.

Because contraction of the DAO muscle exacerbates the melomental folds, BTX-A treatment is a useful adjunct to soft tissue augmentation. In our practice, we inject 2 to 5 U of BTX-A (depending upon the size of the muscle) into each DAO immediately above the angle of the mandible and 1 cm lateral to the lateral oral commissure. It is crucial that the injection be lateral and low at the junction of the depressor and the superior margin of the mandible, because injection too medial or too high can cause an ipsilateral weakness of the depressor labii inferioris muscle and flattening of the lower lip contour when the mouth attempts to form an 'O', while injection too high can compromise the sphincter function of the orbicularis oris leading to incompetence of the mouth.

Best results in this area are obtained with BTX-A in combination with the soft tissue-augmenting agent most suitable for the individual (see Ch. 158). BTX-A treatment prevents the repeated molding and contortion of the implant, enhancing and extending the duration of the soft tissue augmentation.

Mental Crease

The convexity between the lower lip and the prominence of the chin is called the mental crease. Contraction of the mentalis muscle can produce a deep groove in this region. This area is closely tethered to the bony mentum (chin), and soft tissue augmentation of the mental crease is often unsuccessful because the filling agent visibly beads. BTX-A injections at the level of the crease may also give unsatisfactory results because the orbicularis oris is weakened, sometimes resulting in an incompetent mouth. Fortunately, we have found that injection of the mentalis muscle with 3 to 5 U of BTX-A per mentalis band gives a satisfactory softening of the crease while avoiding complications from weakening of the orbicularis oris. Injections to the mentalis are especially valuable in individuals who have had previous trauma or surgery to this area (Fig. 159.14).

Peau d'Orange (Apple Dumpling) Chin

An 'orange peel' appearance of the chin during aging results from the loss of dermal collagen and subcutaneous fat at the mentum. The appearance worsens when the mentalis and depressor labii inferioris muscles are used together with the orbicularis oris muscle during mastication or speech. *Peau d'orange* chin is frequently seen asymmetrically during and after recovery from unilateral facial paresis (Bell's palsy). Previous treatment options have included soft tissue augmentation to fill in the tissue gaps and ablative and non-ablative laser resurfacing. Depending upon the patient's aesthetic need for chin augmentation, BTX-A and soft tissue augmentation can be used together, or BTX-A can be used alone to improve the appearance of the chin. We inject 5 to 10 U into the mentalis at the most distal point from the orbicularis oris (i.e. the prominence of the chin) in order to avoid complications from orbicularis oris weakening (Fig. 159.15). Following treatment, the chin is massaged to facilitate diffusion of the toxin.

Masseteric Hypertrophy

For facial contouring in patients with masseteric hypertrophy, preliminary investigations have shown that BTX-A may be a simple alternative to surgery, associated with a short recovery period. To and colleagues[42] found that 200 to 300 U of Dysport® led to a 31% reduction in muscle bulk 3 months after treatment, while von Lindern et al.[43] reported a 50% reduction in masseter muscles after treatment with an average of 100 U of Dysport® and Park and colleagues[44] were able to reduce muscle

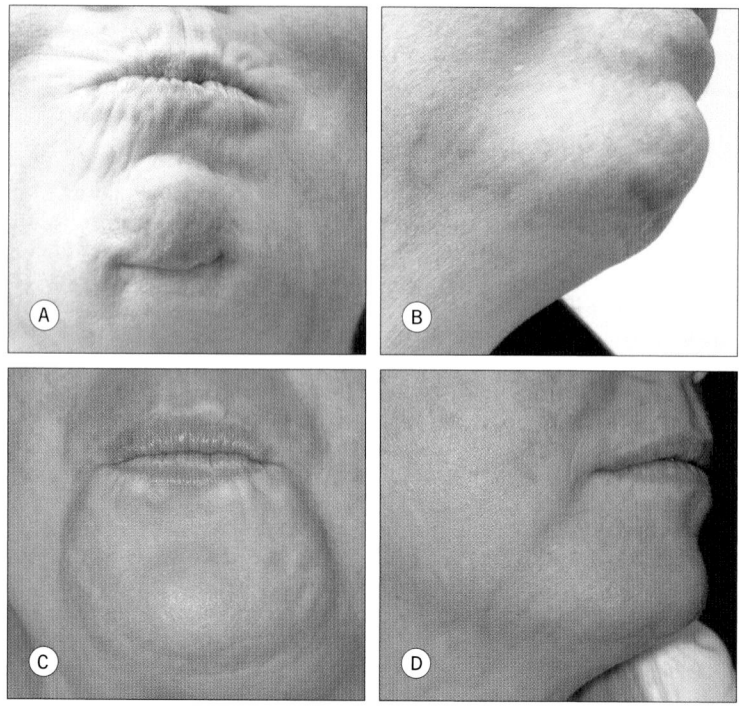

Fig. 159.14 Mental crease. Treatment of traumatically damaged mentalis muscle. Subject puckers before treatment (**A**, **B**). Two weeks after chemodenervation of the mentalis muscle with BTX-A (**C**, **D**).

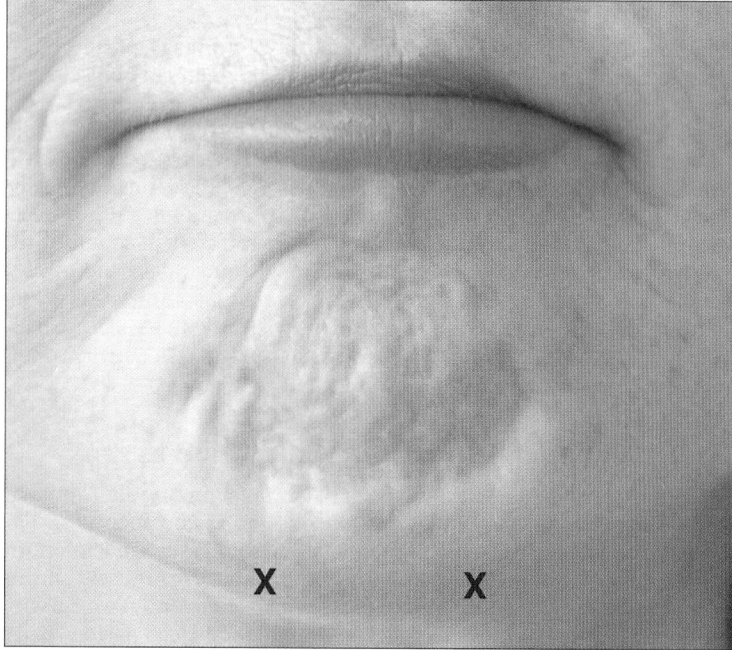

Fig. 159.15 Injection sites for *peau d'orange* chin. The authors inject 5 to 10 U of BTX-A (BOTOX®) into the mentalis muscle at these sites.

thickness by up to 19%. Side effects – mastication difficulty, muscle pain, and verbal difficulty during speech – lasted from 1 to 4 weeks.

Horizontal Neck Lines

Some individuals, especially those with chubbier necks, have two or three horizontal 'necklace' lines of skin indentation caused by the superficial musculoaponeurotic system attachments in the neck. Our treatment approach for softening these lines is to inject small doses of BTX-A at multiple sites along the horizontal lines, generally using no more than a total dose of 10 to 20 U of BTX-A per treatment session. Aliquots of 1 to 2 U are injected into the deep intradermal plane at 2 to 3 cm intervals (Fig. 159.16). The neck is gently massaged following the injections to avoid bruising. The physician is cautioned to use deep dermal rather than subcutaneous injections for two reasons: (1) venous

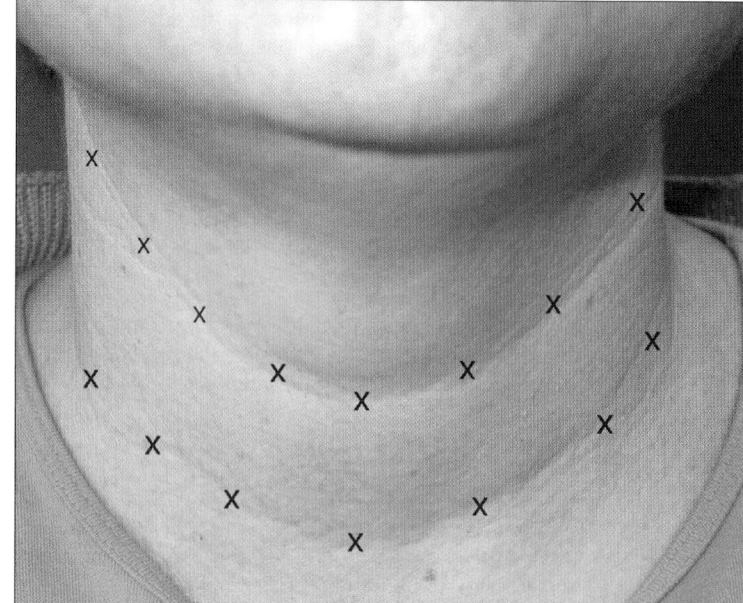

Fig. 159.16 Injection sites for horizontal necklace lines. Aliquots of 1 to 2 U of BTX-A (BOTOX®) are injected into the deep intradermal plane at 2 to 3 cm intervals.

perforators that are deeper in the neck, especially in the lateral neck, can bleed; and (2) the underlying muscles of deglutition are cholinergic and could potentially be affected.

Platysmal Bands

The platysma muscle originates from the superficial fascia of the upper chest and continues superiorly to join the superficial musculoaponeurotic system. The posterior fibers of the platysma blend with the inferior muscles of facial expression, including the depressor anguli oris, mentalis, risorius, and orbicularis oris. Platysmal bands are formed when the anterior fibers of the platysma separate into two discrete vertical bands. The bands often tighten and become more visible when the neck is animated, as when the patient speaks, exercises or plays a musical instrument. The emergence of platysmal bands during aging is often accompanied by other senescent changes, including loss of cervical skin elasticity and accumulation of submental fat. BTX chemodenervation of the anterior part of the platysma muscle can soften the platysmal bands (Fig. 159.17) and produce a gentle anterior neck lift. However, in aging necks with jowl formation and bone resorption, BTX-A treatment of the platysma may emphasize, rather than soften,

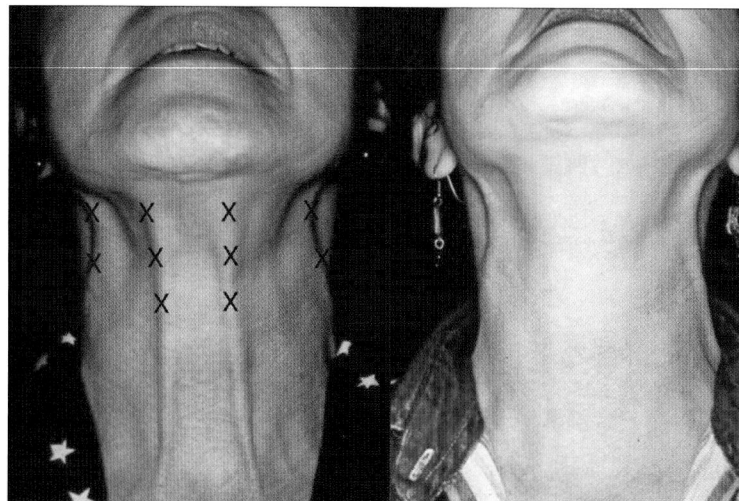

Fig. 159.17 Injection sites for platysmal bands. Before (**A**) and after (**B**) treatment. Each band is injected in three sites at 1 to 1.5 cm intervals with 5 U of BTX-A (BOTOX®) per site. Photographs courtesy of M Carney MD.

the muscle cords. Thus chemodenervation of the platysma is recommended only for patients who have obvious platysmal bands, good cervical skin elasticity and minimal submental fat accumulation.

For many patients, BTX-A may be most useful as an adjunct to traditional facelift surgery; residual muscular banding that becomes apparent in the postoperative period can be simply treated with BTX-A rather than by a second invasive surgical procedure. BTX-A treatment can also be used as a 'rehearsal', so that individuals who are not ready to undergo traditional facelift surgery can experience immediate aesthetic enhancement without a significant period of convalescence. BTX-A treatment might even slow the degenerative changes occurring in the neck and postpone the need for rhytidectomy.

Although some authors have reported injecting up to 250 U of BTX-A per neck with improvement in the appearance of the lower face and neck[45], large doses of BTX-A must be used cautiously in the neck. The platysma is external to the larynx and the muscles of deglutition and neck flexion. Doses from 75 to 100 U of BTX-A can produce weakness in the neck flexors and dysphagia, and we have reported one patient treated with only 60 U in her neck who developed such profound dysphagia that she required a nasogastric tube until she could swallow again[46]. Therefore, we recommend that the physician proceed with caution and inject no more than 30 to 40 U of BTX-A over multiple sites per cervical treatment session.

In the procedure we use, we ask the patient to contract the platysma, then grasp the offending platysmal band and inject BTX-A into three sites at 1.0 to 1.5 cm intervals with 5 U per site (for a total of 15 U/band) (see Fig. 159.17A). A single treatment typically involves injection of two bands with a total dose of 30 U of BTX-A. This dose is safe and effective and has not been associated with any significant adverse events.

Adjunctive Use

BTX-A is beneficial in many patients as an adjunct therapy to enhance or prolong the results of other cosmetic procedures. Prior to surgery, BTX-A treatment to chemodenervate specific muscles can facilitate subsequent manipulation of tissues during the surgery and permit a greater surgical correction or a better concealment of the surgical incision. BTX-A can also be used to reduce tension exerted on a wound or surgical incision by the underlying muscles, thereby promoting better healing with less scar formation.

Although BTX-A can be used alone to create a mild brow lift, an endoscopic brow lift or facelift is often required when brow ptosis is moderate to severe and a greater elevation is desired. Preoperative relaxation of the brow depressors with BTX-A can facilitate a greater brow elevation, and postoperative BTX treatment can help prolong the benefits of surgery by relaxing the muscles that work to re-establish the depressed brow. With upper and lower lid blepharoplasty, BTX-A pretreatment of the crow's feet area relaxes the orbicularis oculi muscle and permits a more accurate estimation of the amount of skin to be resected during surgery, as well as better placement of the incision so that it is concealed within the orbital margin. After lower eyelid ectropion and 'roundeye' repair, dehiscence of the temporal incision can damage the results. Any dehiscence can be prevented with BTX-A treatment to temporarily weaken the lateral fibers of the orbicularis oculi, which pull on the medial side of the incision. BTX-A injections can also be given in combination with all surgeries that correct hyperkinetic lines to delay or prevent the reappearance of wrinkles, and BTX-A treatment is often used adjunctively with traditional rhytidectomy surgery, as described above.

BTX-A in conjunction with ablative resurfacing leads to optimal improvement of dynamic rhytides, with superior and longer-lasting outcomes[47]. Regular postoperative injections, given every 6 to 12 months, prolong the effects of resurfacing[48] and many clinicians now use BTX-A injections as part of their standard laser resurfacing protocol. For example, repeated contraction of the orbicularis oculi can cause deep smile lines. The preferred treatment for smile lines is CO_2 laser resurfacing, which tightens the skin and smoothes the lines. However, we find that prior treatment of the orbicularis oculi muscle with BTX-A enhances the results of laser resurfacing. Indeed, several studies have found that combined BTX-A and laser resurfacing leads to longer-lasting improvements[49–51].

Likewise, combination treatment with BTX-A and intense pulsed light (IPL) therapy may be a synergistic approach to the treatment of facial aging. In one study in which we compared the treatments alone and in combination, we found that patients treated with both therapies experienced a 15% greater global aesthetic improvement (reduction in crow's feet in addition to an improvement in skin tone and texture) compared to IPL alone[52].

BTX-A is also frequently used in combination with soft tissue augmentation, where it prevents the distortion of the filler and prolongs the beneficial effects of tissue augmentation (see above). Preceding the injection of filling agents by approximately 1 week, BTX-A may work on several levels, including reducing the dynamic component of rhytid formation in newly remodeled skin and allowing more permanent eradication of wrinkles[47]. Several studies have documented the synergistic effect of adjunctive BTX-A and fillers, citing a greater aesthetic improvement of longer duration with combination therapy than with fillers alone[53–55].

Hyperhidrosis

BTX-A has been used in the management of hyperhidrosis since early reports of its use to treat Frey's syndrome[56]. Subsequently, a number of authors published reports demonstrating the therapeutic efficacy of BTX-A in patients with hyperhidrosis, both palmoplantar and axillary[6,57–59].

Dramatically effective with minimal side effects, BTX-A was approved for the treatment of axillary hyperhidrosis in Canada and the US in 2001 and 2004, respectively. Typically, 50 to 150 U of BTX-A per axilla are divided among 10 to 20 injection sites (defined by Minor's starch-iodine test, see Ch. 40). Because BTX-A diffuses approximately 1 cm from its injection point, injection sites are located 1.5 to 2 cm apart and approximately 1 cm from the edge of the affected area. The BTX-A is injected intradermally or immediately subdermally. Injections are usually repeated at 6- to 12-month intervals, although, in the experience of the authors, most subjects are far from their preinjection degree of hyperhidrosis when they present for reinjection.

The value of BTX-A in the management of palmoplantar hyperhidrosis, while marked, is not as clear as in axillary hyperhidrosis. This relates to both the need for anesthesia to inject the palmar surface in the majority of individuals as well as the large surface area affected and therefore the high dose of BTX-A required. Local anesthesia is usually accomplished using median and ulnar nerve blocks at the wrist. Typical doses of BTX for the palm are 100 to 200 U distributed among 50 to 100 injection sites, including the distal wrist crease and the thenar and hypothenar eminences.

POSTPROCEDURAL CARE

Manual pressure can be applied to the injection site immediately after withdrawal of the needle to help prevent bruising. Depending upon the site of injection, the physician may massage the area after the injection to spread the toxin, but only if it is possible to do so without spreading the toxin to non-targeted muscles. To minimize undesired toxin diffusion, patients should be directed to remain upright for at least 2 to 4 hours after the procedure and to refrain from rubbing or manipulating the area for 24 hours. Because there is evidence suggesting that BTX-A binds preferentially at actively stimulated muscles, patients are also asked to contract and relax the treated muscles as much as possible for 2 to 3 hours following the injections. Patients should be told to expect some transient redness, swelling or bruising at the injection sites, and patients should be advised that the effects of treatment will probably begin to diminish in 3 or 4 months.

COMPLICATIONS

BTX-A occasionally affects non-targeted muscles or glandular tissue in the areas surrounding the injection, which can result in effects such as eyelid ptosis (Fig. 159.18), lower eyelid laxity, epiphora (excessive tearing), diplopia, brow ptosis, decreased strength of eye closure, dry eye, mouth incompetence, difficulties in speech and the inability to whistle. Use of careful injection technique to target the toxin to the appropriate muscles and the use of concentrated low doses to limit its

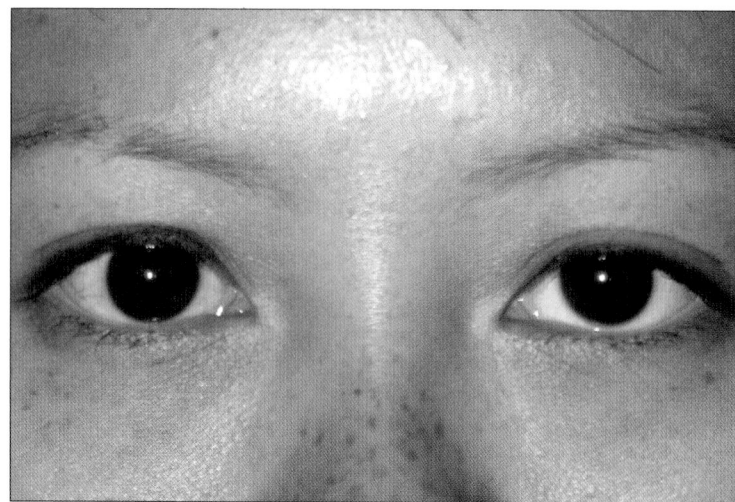

Fig. 159.18 Blepharoptosis. Diffusion of toxin to the levator of the upper eyelid resulted in eyelid ptosis (subject's left eye).

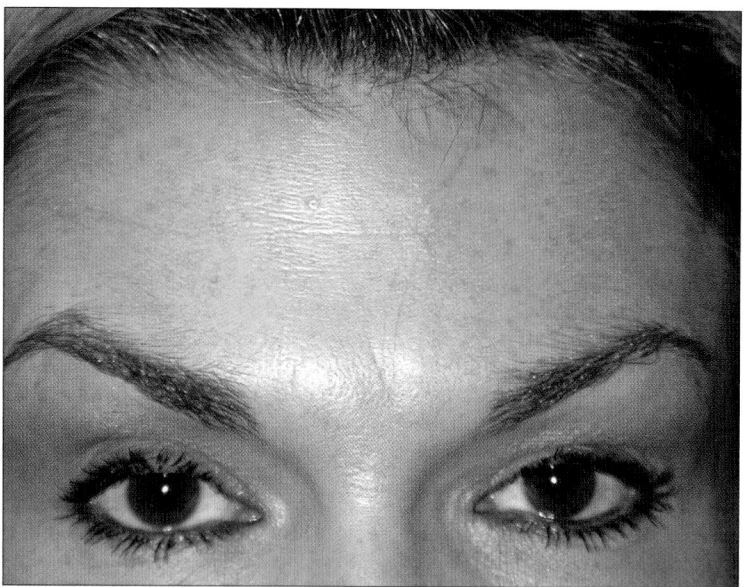

Fig. 159.19 'Cockeyed' brow. A quizzical appearance can occur when the lateral fibers of the frontalis muscle are not injected appropriately, and the untreated lateral fibers of the frontalis muscle pull upward on the brow.

diffusion to non-targeted muscles or glands are recommended to try to prevent the occurrence of these adverse effects[60]. In general, a higher concentration allows for more accurate placement, greater duration of effect, and fewer side effects, since lower concentrations may encourage the spread of toxin. Of note, there is an area of denervation associated with each point of injection of about 1 to 1.5 cm (diameter, 2–3 cm) that is due to toxin spread.

A quizzical or 'cockeyed' appearance can occur in the brow when the lateral fibers of the frontalis muscle have not been injected appropriately and these untreated lateral fibers pull upward on the brow (Fig. 159.19). Brow ptosis may last upwards of 3 months, while upper eyelid ptosis can persist from 2 to 12 weeks. Bruising, diplopia, ectropion, a drooping lateral lower eyelid, and an asymmetric smile (caused by the spread of toxin to the zygomaticus major) are all reported complications of BTX-A injections in the periorbital area. Transient local bruising, ptosis, dry eyes, diplopia, and facial droop can occur with injections into the cheek.

Complications of the lower face involve effects on muscle function and facial expression, usually due to overenthusiastic use of BTX-A in large doses. Injections placed too close to the mouth, injection into the mental fold, and interaction with the orbicularis oris muscle can all result in a flaccid cheek, incompetent mouth or asymmetric smile. Large doses (>100 U) of BTX-A in the platysma have resulted in reports of dysphagia and weakness of the neck flexors.

Although one of the greatest concerns associated with the use of BTX-A is the formation of neutralizing antibodies leading to non-response of subsequent injections, the overall risk is actually low (<5%) when BTX-A is used at recommended doses for neurologic applications. Injecting the lowest effective doses, with the longest feasible intervals between injections, minimizes the potential for immunogenicity. Some believe the total protein concentration to be critical in determining potential immunogenicity; the protein content in current lots of BTX-A is significantly lower than in previous batches and has been shown to be less antigenic than the original product. Clinical experience with BTX-B is currently limited and we await further evidence from the neurologic literature of the risk of resistance. However, although cross-reactive antibodies (to BTX-A and BTX-B) do occur, cross-resistance has not been a problem.

No long-term adverse effects have been reported, and no systemic safety problems have been associated with FDA-approved uses of BTX-A. A recent review of the long-term safety of BTX-A for cosmetic purposes revealed no serious adverse events in over 850 treatment sessions for up to 9 years[61].

FUTURE TRENDS

BTX-A has become the treatment of choice for smoothing hyperkinetic lines in the face and neck, creating a more pleasant and youthful appearance. Alone or in combination with surgery, soft tissue augmentation, or ablative and non-ablative laser resurfacing, BTX-A treatment is both an art and a science, with its use in facial sculpting and enhancing, along with dermatologic correction. Moreover, the number of dermatologic indications for BTX-A is likely to continue to grow. Easy to use, minimally invasive, very well tolerated by patients and extremely safe, injections of BTX-A can be used alone or in combination with other cosmetic procedures and are an integral part of most cosmetic practices.

REFERENCES

1. Jankovic J, Hallett M (eds). Therapy with Botulinum Toxin. New York: Marcel Dekker, 1994.
2. Eleopra R, Tugnoli V, Rossetto O, et al. Different time courses of recovery after poisoning with botulinum neurotoxin serotypes A and E in humans. Neurosci Lett. 1998;256:135–8.
3. Scott AB. Botulinum toxin injection into extraocular muscles as an alternative to strabismus surgery. Ophthalmology. 1980;87:1044–9.
4. Carruthers J, Stubbs HA. Botulinum toxin for benign essential blepharospasm, hemifacial spasm and age-related lower eyelid ectropion. Can J Neurol Sci. 1987;14:42–5.
5. Jankovic J, Schwartz K. Botulinum toxin injections for cervical dystonia. Neurology. 1990;40:277–80.
6. Glogau R. Botulinum A neurotoxin for axillary hyperhidrosis. No sweat Botox. Dermatol Surg. 1998;24:817–19.

7. Silberstein S, Mathew N, Saper J, et al. Botulinum toxin type A as a migraine preventive treatment. Headache. 2000;40:445–50.
8. Blumenfeld A. Botulinum toxin type A as an effective prophylactic treatment in primary headache disorders. Headache. 2003;43:853–60.
9. Porta M. A comparative trial of botulinum toxin type A and methylprednisolone for the treatment of myofascial pain syndrome and pain from chronic muscle spasm. Pain. 2000;85:101–5.
10. Ranoux D, Gury C, Fondarai J, Mas JL, Zuber M. Respective potencies of Botox and Dysport: a double blind, randomised, crossover study in cervical dystonia. J Neurol Neurosurg Psychiatry. 2002;72:459–62.
11. Simonetta Moreau M, Cauhepe C, Magues JP, Senard JM. A double-blind, randomized, comparative study of Dysport vs. Botox in primary palmar hyperhidrosis. Br J Dermatol. 2003;149:1041–5.

12. Ramirez AL, Reeck J, Maas CS. Botulinum toxin type B (Myobloc) in the management of hyperkinetic facial lines. Otolaryngol Head Neck Surg. 2002;126:459–67.
13. Alster TS, Lupton JR. Botulinum toxin type B for dynamic glabellar rhytides refractory to botulinum toxin type A. Dermatol Surg. 2003;29:516–18.
14. Sadick NS. Prospective open-label study of botulinum toxin type B (Myobloc) at doses of 2,400 and 3,000 U for the treatment of glabellar wrinkles. Dermatol Surg. 2003;29:501–7.
15. Lowe N, Lask G, Yamauchi P. Efficacy and safety of botulinum toxins A and B for the reduction of glabellar rhytids in female subjects. Presented at the American Academy of Dermatology 2002 Winter Meeting; 2002 February 22-27; New Orleans, LA.
16. Matarasso SL. Comparison of botulinum toxin types A and B: a bilateral and double-blind randomized

evaluation in the treatment of canthal rhytides. Dermatol Surg. 2003;29:7–13.

17. Klein AW. Dilution and storage of botulinum toxin. Dermatol Surg. 1998;24:1179–80.

18. Huang W, Foster JA, Rogachefsky AS. Pharmacology of botulinum toxin. J Am Acad Dermatol. 2000; 43:249–59.

19. Alam M, Dover JS, Arndt KA. Pain associated with injection of botulinum A exotoxin reconstituted using isotonic sodium chloride with and without preservative: a double-blind, randomized controlled trial. Arch Dermatol. 2002;138:510–14.

20. Carruthers A, Carruthers J. Dose dilution and duration of effect of botulinum toxin type A (BTX-A) for the treatment of glabellar rhytids. Presented at the American Academy of Dermatology 2002 Winter Meeting; 2002 February 22-27; New Orleans, LA.

21. Lowe NJ. Botulinum toxin type A for facial rejuvenation: United States and United Kingdom perspectives. Dermatol Surg. 1998;24:1216–18.

22. Hexsel DM, Trindade de Almeida A, Rutowitsch M, et al. Multicenter, double-blind study of the efficacy of injections with botulinum toxin type A reconstituted up to six consecutive weeks before application. Dermatol Surg. 2003;29:523–9.

23. Flynn TC, Carruthers JA, Carruthers JDA. The use of the Ultra-Fine II short needle 0.3-cc insulin syringe for botulinum toxin injections. J Am Acad Dermatol. 2002;46:931–3.

24. Carruthers J, Fagien S, Matarasso SL; Botox Consensus Group. Consensus recommendations on the use of botulinum toxin type A in facial aesthetics. Plast Reconstr Surg. 2004;114 (suppl.):1S–22S.

25. Smith KC, Comite SL, Balasubramanian S, Carver A, Liu JF. Vibration anesthesia: a noninvasive method of reducing discomfort prior to dermatologic procedures. Dermatol Online J. 2004;10:1.

26. Carruthers JA, Lowe NJ, Menter MA, et al. A multicenter, double-blind, randomized, placebo-controlled study of efficacy and safety of botulinum toxin type A in the treatment of glabellar lines. J Am Acad Dermatol. 2002;46:840–9.

27. Carruthers JD, Lowe NJ, Menter MA, et al. Double-blind, placebo-controlled study of the safety and efficacy of botulinum toxin type A for patients with glabellar lines. Plast Recontr Surg. 2003;112:1089–98.

28. Carruthers A, Carruthers J, Said S. Double-blind, randomized, parallel group, dose-ranging study of botulinum toxin type A in the treatment of glabellar lines. Presented at the European Academy of Dermatology and Venereology Meeting; 2001 October 10; Munich, Germany.

29. Carruthers A, Carruthers J. Botulinum toxin type A for treating glabellar lines in men: a dose ranging study. Presented at the Annual Meeting of the American Academy of Dermatology; 2003 March 21-26; San Francisco, CA.

30. Ahn MS, Catten M, Maas CS. Temporal brow lift using botulinum toxin A. Plast Reconstruct Surg. 2000;105:1129–35.

31. Huang W, Rogachefsky AS, Foster JA. Brow lift with botulinum toxin. Dermatol Surg. 2000;26:55–60.

32. Huilgol SC, Carruthers A, Carruthers JDA. Raising eyebrows with botulinum toxin. Dermatol Surg. 2000;25:373–6.

33. Carruthers A, Carruthers J, Said S. Botulinum toxin type A (BTX-A) in the treatment of glabellar rhytids: an objective analysis of treatment response. Presented at the American Academy of Dermatology 2002 Winter Meeting; 2002 February 22-27; New Orleans, LA.

34. Carruthers A, Carruthers J. Glabella BTX-A injection and eyebrow height: a further photographic analysis. Presented at the Annual Meeting of the American Academy of Dermatology; 2003 March 21-26; San Francisco, CA.

35. Carruthers J, Carruthers A. BOTOX use in the mid and lower face and neck. Semin Cutan Med Surg. 2001;20:85–92.

36. Flynn TC, Carruthers JA, Carruthers JA. Botulinum-A toxin treatment of the lower eyelid improves infraorbital rhytides and widens the eye. Dermatol Surg. 2001;27:703–8.

37. Armstrong MWJ, Mountain RE, Murray JAM. Treatment of facial synkinesis and facial asymmetry with botulinum toxin type A following facial nerve palsy. Clin Otolaryngol Allied Sci. 1996;21:15–20.

38. Blitzer A, Brin MF, Keen MS, Aviv JE. Botulinum toxin for the treatment of hyperfunctional lines of the face. Arch Otolaryngol Head Neck Surg. 1993;119:1018–22.

39. Borodic GE. Botulinum A toxin for (expressionistic) ptosis overcorrection after frontalis sling. Ophthal Plast Reconstr Surg. 1992;8:137–42.

40. Carruthers A, Carruthers J. Clinical indications and injection technique for the cosmetic use of botulinum A exotoxin. Dermatol Surg. 1998;24:1189–94.

41. Carruthers JDA, Carruthers JA. Botulinum A exotoxin in clinical ophthalmology. Can Ophthalmol. 1996;31:389–400.

42. To EW, Ahuja AT, Ho WS, et al. A prospective study of the effect of botulinum toxin A on masseteric muscle hypertrophy with ultrasonographic and electromyographic measurement. Br J Plast Surg. 2001;54:197–200.

43. von Lindern JJ, Niederhagen B, Appel T, Berge S, Reich RH. Type A botulinum toxin for the treatment of hypertrophy of the masseter and temporal muscle: an alternative treatment. Plast Reconstr Surg. 2001;107:327–32.

44. Park MY, Ahn KY, Jung DS. Application of botulinum toxin A for treatment of facial contouring in the lower face. Dermatol Surg. 2003;29:477–83.

45. Matarasso A, Matarasso SL, Brandt FS, Bellman B. Botulinum A exotoxin for the management of platysma bands. Plast Reconstr Surg. 1999;103:645–52.

46. Carruthers J, Carruthers A. Practical cosmetic Botox techniques. J Cutan Med Surg. 1999;3(suppl. 4):S49–S52.

47. Fagien S. Botox for the treatment of dynamic and hyperkinetic facial lines and furrows: Adjunctive use in facial aesthetic surgery. Plast Reconstr Surg. 2003;112;40S–52S.

48. Carruthers J, Carruthers A, Zelichowska A. The power of combined therapies: Botox and ablative facial laser resurfacing. Am J Cosmet Surg. 2000;17:129–31.

49. West TB, Alster TS. Effect of botulinum toxin type A on movement-associated rhytides following CO_2 laser resurfacing. Dermatol Surg. 1999;25:259–61.

50. Zimbler MS, Holds JB, Kokoska MS, et al. Effect of botulinum toxin pretreatment on laser resurfacing results: a prospective, randomized, blinded trial. Arch Facial Plast Surg. 2001;3:165–9.

51. Lowe N, Lask G, Yamauchi P, Moore D, Patnaik R. Botulinum toxin type A (BTX-A) and ablative laser resurfacing (Erbium:YAG): a comparison of efficacy and safety of combination therapy vs. ablative laser resurfacing alone for the treatment of crow's feet. Presented at the American Academy of Dermatology 2002 Summer Meeting; 2002 July 31-August 4; New York, NY.

52. Carruthers J, Carruthers A. The effect of full-face broadband light treatments alone and in combination with bilateral crow's feet botulinum toxin type A chemodenervation. Dermatol Surg. 2004;30:355–66.

53. Carruthers J, Carruthers A, Maberley D. Deep resting glabellar rhytides respond to BTX-A and Hylan B. Dermatol Surg. 2003;29:539–44.

54. Carruthers J, Carruthers A. A prospective, randomized, parallel group study analyzing the effect of BTX-A (Botox) and nonanimal sourced hyaluronic acid (NASHA, Restylane) in combination compared with NASHA (Restylane) alone in severe glabellar rhytides in adult female subjects: treatment of severe glabellar rhytides with a hyaluronic acid derivative compared with the derivative BTX-A. Dermatol Surg. 2003;29:802–9.

55. Patel MP, Talmor M, Nolan WB. Botox and collagen for glabellar furrows: advantages of combination therapy. Ann Plast Surg. 2004;52:442–7.

56. Bushara KO, Jones, JW, Park DM, Schutta HS. Botulinum toxin and sweating [abstr]. Mov Disord. 1995;10:391.

57. Lowe NJ, Yamauchi PS, Lask GP, Patnaik R, Iyer S. Efficacy and safety of botulinum toxin type A in the treatment of palmar hyperhidrosis: a double-blind, randomized, placebo-controlled study. Dermatol Surg. 2002;28:822–7.

58. Lowe PL, Cerdan-Sanz S, Lowe NJ. Botulinum toxin type A in the treatment of bilateral primary axillary hyperhidrosis: efficacy and duration with repeated treatments. Dermatol Surg. 2003;29:545–8.

59. Naumann M, Lowe NJ, Kumar CR, Hamm H. Botulinum toxin type A is a safe and effective treatment for axillary hyperhidrosis over 16 months: a prospective study. Arch Dermatol. 2003;139:731–6.

60. Klein AW. Complications, adverse reactions, and insights with the use of botulinum toxin. Dermatol Surg. 2003;29:549–56.

61. Carruthers A, Carruthers J. Long-term safety of cosmetic botulinum toxin type A: a review. In press 2007.

Index

Page numbers in **bold** refer to major discussions in the text, and usually include aspects such as epidemiology, clinical features, diagnosis, pathology and treatment.
Page numbers in *italics* refer to pages on which tables/figures are to be found.
Entries under 'skin,' and 'cutaneous' have been kept to a minimum; readers are advised to seek more specific index entries.

Index